3RD EDITION

DRUG-INDUCED DISEASES

Prevention, Detection, and Management

JAMES E. TISDALE, PharmD, BCPS, FCCP, FAPhA, FNAP, FAHA

Professor
College of Pharmacy
Purdue University
Indianapolis, Indiana
Adjunct Professor
School of Medicine
Indiana University
Indianapolis, Indiana

DOUGLAS A. MILLER, PharmD

Professor (Emeritus)
College of Pharmacy and Health Sciences
Wayne State University
Detroit, Michigan

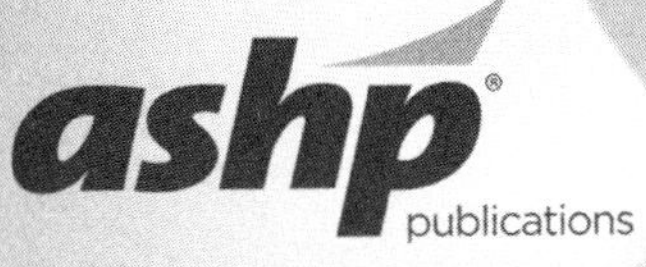

Any correspondence regarding this publication should be sent to the publisher, American Society of Health-System Pharmacists, 4500 East-West Highway, Suite 900, Bethesda, MD 20814, attention: Special Publishing.

Acquisitions Editor: Beth Campbell

Editorial Project Manager, Books and eLearning Courses: Ruth Bloom

Editorial Project Manager, Publications Production Center: Kristin Eckles

Cover and Page Design: David Wade

Library of Congress Cataloging-in-Publication Data

Names: Tisdale, James E., editor. | Miller, Douglas A., editor. | American Society of Health-System Pharmacists, issuing body.

Title: Drug-induced diseases: prevention, detection, and management / James E. Tisdale, Douglas A. Miller.

Other titles: Drug-induced diseases (Tisdale)

Description: Third edition. | Bethesda, Maryland : American Society of Health-System Pharmacists, [2018] | Includes bibliographical references and index.

Identifiers: LCCN 2017061345 | ISBN 9781585285303 (hardback)

Subjects: | MESH: Iatrogenic Disease—prevention & control | Drug-Related Side Effects and Adverse Reactions

Classification: LCC RC90 | NLM QZ 42 | DDC 615.7/042—dc23

LC record available at https://lccn.loc.gov/2017061345

ISBN: 978-1-58528-530-3

10 9 8 7 6 5 4 3 2 1

DEDICATION

When it comes to the future, there are three kinds of people: those who let it happen, those who make it happen, and those who wonder what happened.

—John M. Richardson, Jr.

This book is dedicated to our students, past, present, and future, who we know are well equipped to make it happen.

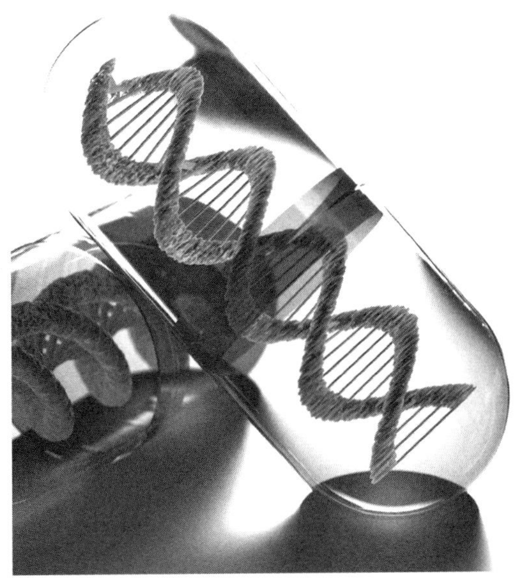

TABLE OF CONTENTS

FOREWORD xi

PREFACE xiii

CONTRIBUTORS xv

REVIEWERS xxi

SECTION I—MAGNITUDE/SIGNIFICANCE OF DRUG-INDUCED DISEASES: IMPACT ON THE HEALTHCARE SYSTEM 1

Chapter 1: Drug Safety and Drug-Induced Diseases: The Regulatory, Legal, and Practice Environments 3
Cynthia Reilly, MS, BS Pharm

Chapter 2: Epidemiology and Public Health Impact of Drug-Induced Diseases 19
John R. Litaker, PhD, MSc, MMedSc, and James P. Wilson, PharmD, PhD, FASHP

Chapter 3: Factors Contributing to Drug-Induced Diseases 31
Tyler Shugg, PharmD, Abdullah Assiri, PharmD, and Brian R. Overholser, PharmD

Chapter 4: Postmarketing Surveillance for Drug-Induced Diseases 47
Tobias Peschel, MD, PhD, MBA, and Hugh H. Tilson, MD, DrPH

Chapter 5: Evaluating Patients for Drug-Induced Diseases 59
Douglas A. Miller, PharmD, and James E. Tisdale, PharmD, BCPS, FCCP, FAPhA, FNAP, FAHA

SECTION II—DRUG-INDUCED DERMATOLOGIC DISEASES 69

Chapter 6: Drug Allergy and Cutaneous Diseases 71
Lynne M. Sylvia, PharmD

Chapter 7: Systemic Lupus Erythematosus-Like Syndrome 123
Karen W. Lee, PharmD, BCPS, and Matthew F. Ambury, PharmD, BCPS

Chapter 8: Photosensitivity 143
Julie M. Koehler, PharmD, FCCP

Chapter 9: Alopecia, Hirsutism, and Hypertrichosis 165
Kristine E. Keplar, PharmD

SECTION III—DRUG-INDUCED NEUROLOGICAL DISEASES 215

Chapter 10: Seizures 217
Timothy E. Welty, PharmD, FCCP, BCPS

Chapter 11: Stroke 229
Denise H. Rhoney, PharmD, FCCP, FCCM, FNCS

TABLE OF CONTENTS

Chapter 12: Movement Disorders 253
Jack J. Chen, PharmD, FASCP, FCCP, BCPS, BCGP; Khashayar Dashtipour, MD, PhD; and David M. Swope, MD

Chapter 13: Peripheral Neuropathy 279
Dennis Parker, Jr., PharmD

Chapter 14: Visual Disturbances 295
Yaman Kaakeh, PharmD, BCPS, BCNSP, CNSC, and Steven R. Abel, PharmD, FASHP

Chapter 15: Delirium 325
Matthew A. Fuller, PharmD, FASHP, BCPP

Chapter 16: Sleep Disorders 347
Lisa L. Forsyth, PharmD, FCCM

Chapter 17: Cognitive Disorders 357
Michele Y. Splinter, PharmD, MS, BCPS, FCCP

SECTION IV—DRUG-INDUCED PSYCHIATRIC DISEASES 373

Chapter 18: Depression 375
Sheila Botts, PharmD, FCCP, BCPP, and Melody Ryan, PharmD, MPH

Chapter 19: Anxiety 399
Julie A. Dopheide, PharmD, BCPP, FASHP, and Seth Gomez, PharmD, BCPP

Chapter 20: Psychosis 415
Jessica L. Gören, PharmD, BCPP

SECTION V—DRUG-INDUCED PULMONARY DISEASES 429

Chapter 21: Interstitial Lung Disease/Pulmonary Fibrosis 431
Jordan R. Covvey, PharmD, PhD, BCPS, and Erin E. Mancl, PharmD, BCPS, BCCCP

Chapter 22: Asthma and Bronchospasm 451
Suzanne G. Bollmeier, PharmD, BCPS, AE-C, and Rebecca L. Stauffer, PharmD, BCPS

SECTION VI—DRUG-INDUCED CARDIOVASCULAR DISEASES 469

Chapter 23: Myocardial Ischemia and Acute Coronary Syndromes 471
Kevin M. Sowinski, PharmD, FCCP

Chapter 24: Heart Failure 501
Yazid N. Al Hamarneh BSc(Pharm), PhD, and Ross T. Tsuyuki, BSc(Pharm), PharmD, MSc, FCSHP, FACC, FCAHS

Chapter 25: Ventricular Arrhythmias 523
James E. Tisdale, PharmD, BCPS, FCCP, FAPhA, FNAP, FAHA

Chapter 26: Supraventricular Arrhythmias 569
James E. Tisdale, PharmD, BCPS, FCCP, FAPhA, FNAP, FAHA

Chapter 27: Hypertension 617
Liza W. Claus, PharmD, BCACP, and Joseph J. Saseen, PharmD, BCPS, BCACP, FCCP, FASHP

Chapter 28: Hypotension 631
Katy E. Trinkley, PharmD, BCACP, and Robert L. Page II, PharmD, MSPH, BCPS (AQ-Cardiology), BCGP, FCCP, FAHA, FASHP, FHFSA

Chapter 29: Valvular and Pericardial Heart Disease 659
Sarah A. Spinler, PharmD, FCCP, FAHA, FASHP, AACC, BCPS (AQ-Cardiology), and Frank E. Silvestry, MD, FACC, FASE

SECTION VII—DRUG-INDUCED ENDOCRINE DISEASES 677

Chapter 30: Glucose and Insulin Dysregulation 679
Devra K. Dang, PharmD, BCPS, CDE, FNAP; Frank Pucino, Jr., PharmD, MPH, FASHP, FCCP; Charles D. Ponte, PharmD, BC-ADM, BCPS, CDE, CPE, FAADE, FAPhA, FASHP, FCCP, FNAP; and Karim Anton Calis, PharmD, MPH, FASHP, FCCP

Chapter 31: Thyroid Diseases 697
Genevieve Lynn Ness, PharmD; Judy T. Chen, PharmD, BCPS, BCACP, CDE, FNAP; Betty J. Dong, PharmD, FASHP, FAPhA, FCCP; Frank Pucino, Jr., PharmD, MPH, FASHP, FCCP; and Karim Anton Calis, PharmD, MPH, FASHP, FCCP

Chapter 32: Hypothalamic, Pituitary, and Adrenal Diseases 729
Andrew Y. Hwang, PharmD, BCPS; Steven M. Smith, PharmD, MPH, BCPS; and John G. Gums, PharmD, FCCP

Chapter 33: Sexual Dysfunction in Males 757
Mary Lee, PharmD, BCPS, FCCP, and Roohollah Sharifi, MD, FACS

Chapter 34: Gynecologic Diseases and Infertility in Women 781
Judith A. Smith, PharmD, BCOP, CPHQ, FCCP, FISOPP

SECTION VIII—DRUG-INDUCED GASTROINTESTINAL DISEASES 807

Chapter 35: Upper Gastrointestinal Ulceration 809
Dianne W. May, PharmD, FCCP, BCPS; Micaela Carroll, PharmD, BCPS; and J. Russell May, PharmD, FASHP

Chapter 36: Diarrhea 821
Sarah A. Nisly, PharmD, BCPS, FCCP, and Alison M. Walton, PharmD, BCPS

Chapter 37: Constipation 835
Sarah A. Nisly, PharmD, BCPS, FCCP, and Carolyn M. Jung, PharmD, BCPS

Chapter 38: Hepatic and Cholestatic Diseases 845
Scott S. Malinowski, PharmD, and Daniel M. Riche, PharmD, FCCP, BCPS, CDE, ASH-CHC, CLS

Chapter 39: Pancreatitis 877
Pramodini B. Kale-Pradhan, PharmD, and Sheila M. Wilhelm, PharmD, FCCP, BCPS

TABLE OF CONTENTS

Chapter 40: Nausea and Vomiting 905

Saeed K. Alzghari, MS, MBA (HOM), PharmD, BCPS; Bonnie A. Labdi, PharmD, BCOP; and Jon D. Herrington, PharmD, BCPS, BCOP

SECTION IX—DRUG-INDUCED DISEASES OF THE KIDNEY AND FLUID & ELECTROLYTE DISORDERS 939

Chapter 41: Acute Kidney Injury 941

Amy Barton Pai, PharmD, BCPS, FASN, FCCP, FNKF, and Nicole M. Wegrzyn, PharmD, BCACP

Chapter 42: Chronic Kidney Disease 965

Mary K. Stamatakis, PharmD

Chapter 43: Syndrome of Inappropriate Antidiuretic Hormone Secretion and Diabetes Insipidus 981

Mark A. Malesker, PharmD, FCCP, FCCM, FASHP, BCPS, and Daniel E. Hilleman, PharmD, FCCP

Chapter 44: Acid–Base Disorders 1001

Lori D. Wazny, BSc(Pharm), PharmD, EPPh; J. Christine Davis, BSc(Pharm), PharmD, ACPR; and Robert E. Ariano, PharmD, BCPS, FCCM

SECTION X—DRUG-INDUCED HEMATOLOGICAL DISORDERS 1023

Chapter 45: Bleeding Disorders 1025

Tiffany Pon, PharmD, BCPS, and Jaekyu Shin, PharmD, MS, BCPS

Chapter 46: Thrombocytopenia 1049

Kellie Jones Weddle, PharmD, BCOP, FCCP, FHOPA, and Patrick J. Kiel, PharmD, BCPS, BCOP

Chapter 47: Thromboembolic Diseases 1063

Candice L. Garwood, PharmD, FCCP, BCPS, BCACP

Chapter 48: Neutropenia and Agranulocytosis 1087

Teresa C. Thakrar, PharmD, BCOP, and Christopher A. Fausel, PharmD, MHA, BCOP

Chapter 49: Anemias 1099

LeAnn B. Norris, PharmD, BCPS, BCOP, and Charles L. Bennett, MD, PhD, MPP

SECTION XI—DRUG-INDUCED BONE, JOINT, AND MUSCLE DISEASES 1117

Chapter 50: Osteoporosis and Osteomalacia 1119

Laura M. Borgelt, PharmD, FCCP, BCPS, and Danielle R. Fixen, PharmD

Chapter 51: Gout and Hyperuricemia 1135

Jasmine D. Gonzalvo, PharmD, BCPS, BC-ADM, CDE, LDE

Chapter 52: Myopathy 1149

Craig Williams, PharmD, FLNA, BCPS

TABLE OF CONTENTS

SECTION XII—MISCELLANEOUS DRUG-INDUCED DISEASES **1163**

Chapter 53: Weight Gain 1165
Amy Heck Sheehan, PharmD

Chapter 54: Temperature Dysregulation 1185
Susan M. Wilson, PharmD, and Ian A. Ross, PharmD

Chapter 55: Ototoxicity 1233
Monica L. Miller, PharmD, MS

Chapter 56: Oral Manifestations of Systemically Administered Drugs 1253
Ashley H. Meredith, PharmD, BCACP, BCPS, CDE

Chapter 57: Neoplastic Diseases 1283
Sandra Cuellar, PharmD, BCOP, and Christina Mactal Haaf, PharmD, BCOP, BCPS

Chapter 58: Teratogenicity 1311
Kylie N. Barnes, PharmD, BCPS

INDEX **1343**

FOREWORD

Much has changed in pharmacotherapy since the publication of the second edition of this text. New drugs have been introduced, and postmarking experience with those previously available has given us a better understanding of associated risks. In addition, patterns of medication use and drug exposure have continued to be affected by the way drugs are promoted, by reclassification of drugs from prescription to nonprescription status, by changes in drug prices, and by product shortages, which, unfortunately, have become commonplace. As a result of an aging population and other factors, more people are using more drugs today than ever before. Nearly half of Americans report having used a prescription medication in the last 30 days, and nearly a quarter used three or more. Perhaps the only things that have stayed about the same are the systems we use for prescribing, dispensing, administering, and monitoring drug therapy, which have not changed appreciably since the mid-1900s. As a consequence, drug-related morbidity and mortality is rampant. Nearly 20 years ago, Ernst and Grizzle[1] estimated that drug-related problems cost Americans more than $177 billion and were responsible for more than 200,000 deaths annually. It is unlikely that those horrifying statistics have improved in the years since.

There are numerous ways we can improve medication use. These include the reassessment of the risks and benefits of direct-to-consumer advertising; possible expansion of the authority of the U.S. Food and Drug Administration to include "nutraceuticals" and dietary supplements; a slower, more controlled launch of newly approved drugs to allow an evaluation of safety and efficacy in population subsets not thoroughly evaluated during clinical trials; more structured, broad-based programs for postmarketing surveillance; and the development of fully integrated and properly aligned systems of prescribing, dispensing, administering, and monitoring drug therapy and for educating consumers about safe and effective medication use.

Change won't be easy (or quick); however, and, until improvements are made, individual practitioners will continue to be their patients' best defense against drug-related morbidity or mortality—a responsibility that requires exceptional vigilance. The third edition of *Drug-Induced Diseases: Prevention, Detection, and Management* will help with that. Editors Tisdale and Miller have assembled a remarkable team of experts to serve as chapter authors and reviewers, and together they have created an essential resource for healthcare practitioners. The text uses a unique disease-oriented approach and organizes critical information in an easily retrievable format. It has been carefully updated using a standardized search strategy to include drugs introduced since the previous edition as well as new information about drugs previously marketed. Tables and figures also have been updated, where appropriate, to enhance readability and the text includes new chapters.

Drug-related morbidity and mortality is rampant. *Drug-Induced Diseases: Prevention, Detection, and Management* is an extraordinary work that continues to be the standard for understanding and preventing drug-induced diseases. It can be a practitioner's most useful tool.

John A. Gans, PharmD
Professor and Dean (Emeritus)
Philadelphia College of Pharmacy
CEO (Emeritus)
American Pharmacists Association

[1]Ernst FR, Grizzle AJ. Drug-related morbidity and mortality: updating the cost-of illness model. *J Am Pharm Assoc.* 2001; 41:192-9.

PREFACE

We are very pleased to present this third edition of *Drug-Induced Diseases: Prevention, Detection, and Management*. The second edition is used throughout the United States and in 20 other countries around the world, and it is gratifying to know that the text is helping fill a previously unmet need for this type of reference.

In the preface to the first edition, readers were reminded of healthcare providers' prime directive, "First, do no harm." Although drug therapy can prolong and improve a patient's quality of life, it is important to remember that drugs are also capable of causing harm by triggering new ailments or exacerbating those that already exist. The potential benefits of drug therapy, therefore, must always be weighed carefully against the potential harm.

Unfortunately, we don't always know all the risks associated with a given drug in advance. Premarketing trials fail to identify serious adverse events in at least 20% of drugs approved by the U.S. Food and Drug Administration (see Chapters 1–5). Despite best efforts to ensure that all drugs are safe and effective, millions of patients each year develop drug-induced diseases—some previously known and some previously unknown. In the second edition's preface, readers were reminded of Heraclitus' admonition, "If you do not expect the unexpected, you will not find it." Whenever drug therapy is employed, healthcare providers must train themselves to be on the lookout for unexpected consequences.

Pharmacists, physicians, nurses, and other healthcare professionals on the front lines of patient care and pharmacotherapy must be knowledgeable about the risk of drug-induced diseases and methods of prevention, detection, and management. Students in the health professions must learn that pharmacotherapy has both benefits and risks. Every time a patient presents with a new disease or an exacerbation of an existing condition, someone needs to ask, "Could this problem be drug-induced?"

The purpose of this book is to provide a comprehensive source of information regarding the prevention, detection, and management of drug-induced diseases for current and future healthcare practitioners. Our hope is that it will also encourage practitioners to weigh the risks and benefits before initiating pharmacotherapy and to always expect the unexpected.

As in the previous editions, we consider drug-induced diseases to be a specific subset of adverse effects caused by drugs—a subset characterized by the severity of symptoms and outcomes. For the purposes of this book, we have defined a drug-induced disease as an unintended effect of a drug that results in mortality or morbidity with symptoms sufficient to prompt a patient to seek medical attention and/or require hospitalization.

The text has been structured to facilitate readers' ability to find specific information related to drug-induced diseases. Section I describes the changing regulatory, legal, and practice landscape as they relate to drug-induced diseases; provides a general overview of the epidemiology and public health impact of these conditions; discusses factors that may contribute to the development of drug-induced diseases; describes the structure and strategy of postmarketing surveillance for their detection and characterization; and provides a general approach to patient evaluation. Sections II through XII are organized around specific diseases in which drugs have been implicated as causative agents or, in some cases, the organ system that is involved.

The disease-related chapters follow a consistent structure: causative agents, epidemiology, mechanisms, clinical presentation and differential diagnosis, risk factors, morbidity and mortality, methods of prevention, management, and information for patients. Each chapter underwent blinded external review by one or more additional content experts.

PREFACE

Numerous changes and, we believe, significant improvements have been incorporated into this edition. Three chapters have been added: Bleeding Disorders, Teratogenicity, and Oral Manifestations of Systemically Administered Drugs. Chapters have been expanded, and information throughout has been carefully updated by the contributors. Chapter authors used a structured and more consistent literature search strategy to ensure relevant information was not inadvertently overlooked.

As in previous editions, each chapter includes a series of standard tables, which are in a consistent format throughout. All of the "Agents Implicated" tables include an indication of the strength of the evidence (Level of Evidence) that links a listed drug to a specific drug-induced disease:

- **Level of evidence A** has been assigned when there is evidence of causality from one or more randomized, controlled clinical trials.
- **Level of evidence B** indicates that there is evidence of causality from nonrandomized clinical trials, prospective observational studies, cohort studies, retrospective studies, case-control studies, meta-analyses, and/or postmarketing surveillance studies.
- **Level of evidence C** has been assigned when evidence of causality is from one or more published case reports or case series.

Undertaking a book such as this is not an easy task, and we gratefully acknowledge the work of the chapter authors and expert external content reviewers. Without their significant contributions, this book could not have been completed. We also want to express our appreciation for the assistance of the ASHP staff. We sincerely hope that this text helps practitioners as they work to continually improve patient outcomes related to drug therapy.

James E. Tisdale
Douglas A. Miller
October 2018

CONTRIBUTORS

Steven R. Abel, PharmD, FASHP
Associate Provost for Engagement
Purdue University
West Lafayette, Indiana

Yazid N. Al Hamarneh, BSc(Pharm), PhD
Associate Director/Scientific Officer
Alberta SPOR Support Unit Consultation and Research Services
EPICORE Centre
Department of Medicine
University of Alberta
Edmonton, Alberta, Canada

Saeed K. Alzghari, MS, MBA (HOM), PharmD, BCPS
Director of Clinical Pharmacy
Gulfstream Diagnostics
Dallas, Texas

Matthew F. Ambury, PharmD, BCPS
Director of Pharmacy
Lemuel Shattuck Hospital
CompleteRx
Boston, Massachusetts

Robert E. Ariano, PharmD, BCPS, FCCM
Clinical Care Pharmacist
Department of Pharmacy
St. Boniface Hospital
Professor
College of Pharmacy
University of Manitoba
Winnipeg, Manitoba, Canada

Abdullah Assiri, PharmD
Purdue University College of Pharmacy
West Lafayette, Indiana
Department of Clinical Pharmacy
King Khalid University
Abha, Saudi Arabia

Kylie N. Barnes, PharmD, BCPS
Clinical Assistant Professor
Department of Pharmacy Practice and Administration
University of Missouri–Kansas City School of Pharmacy
Kansas City, Missouri

Charles L. Bennett, MD, PhD, MPP
Professor and Endowed Chair
Medication Safety and Efficacy
Center of Economic Excellence
South Carolina College of Pharmacy
Columbia, South Carolina

Suzanne G. Bollmeier, PharmD, BCPS, AE-C
Professor, Pharmacy Practice
Division of Ambulatory Care Pharmacy
St. Louis College of Pharmacy
St. Louis, Missouri

Laura M. Borgelt, PharmD, FCCP, BCPS
Associate Dean for Administration and Operations
Professor
Departments of Clinical Pharmacy and Family Medicine
Skaggs School of Pharmacy and Pharmaceutical Sciences
University of Colorado Anschutz Medical Campus
Aurora, Colorado

Sheila Botts, PharmD, FCCP, BCPP
Regional Administrator, Clinical Pharmacy Services
Kaiser Permanente
Aurora, Colorado

Rebecca L. Stauffer, PharmD, BCPS
Assistant Professor
Department of Pharmacy Practice
St. Louis College of Pharmacy
St. Louis, Missouri

Karim Anton Calis, PharmD, MPH, FASHP, FCCP
Director of Clinical Research and Compliance
Eunice Kennedy Shriver National Institute of Child Health and Human Development
National Institutes of Health
Clinical Professor
University of Maryland
Baltimore, Maryland
Clinical Professor
Virginia Commonwealth University
Richmond, Virginia

Micaela Carroll, PharmD, BCPS
Internal Medicine Clinical Pharmacist
UAB Hospital
Birmingham, Alabama

Jack J. Chen, PharmD, FASCP, FCCP, BCPS, BCGP
Professor and Senior Associate Dean for Academic Affairs
Department of Clinical and Administrative Sciences
School of Pharmacy
American University of Health Sciences
Signal Hill, California

CONTRIBUTORS

Judy T. Chen, PharmD, BCPS, BCACP, CDE, FNAP
Clinical Associate Professor
Purdue University College of Pharmacy
Indianapolis, Indiana

Liza W. Claus, PharmD, BCACP
Assistant Professor, Clinical Pharmacy
Skaggs School of Pharmacy and Pharmaceutical Sciences
Assistant Professor, Family Medicine
School of Medicine
University of Colorado Anschutz Medical Campus
Aurora, Colorado

Jordan R. Covvey, PharmD, PhD, BCPS
Assistant Professor of Pharmacy Administration
Division of Pharmaceutical, Administrative, and Social Sciences
Duquesne University School of Pharmacy
Pittsburgh, Pennsylvania

Sandra Cuellar, PharmD, BCOP
Oncology Resident Director/Clinical Pharmacist/Team Leader, Ambulatory Pharmacy Services
Clinical Assistant Professor, Pharmacy Practice
University of Illinois at Chicago College of Pharmacy
Chicago, Illinois

Devra K. Dang, PharmD, BCPS, CDE, FNAP
Associate Clinical Professor of Pharmacy and Medicine
University of Connecticut Schools of Pharmacy and Medicine
Storrs, Connecticut

Khashayar Dashtipour, MD, PhD
Associate Professor
Department of Neurology
Loma Linda University
Loma Linda, California

J. Christine Davis, BSc(Pharm), PharmD, ACPR
Clinical Pharmacist
Manitoba Renal Program
Department of Pharmacy
St. Boniface Hospital
Clinical Assistant Professor
College of Pharmacy
University of Manitoba
Winnipeg, Manitoba, Canada

Betty J. Dong, PharmD, FASHP, FAPhA, FCCP
Professor of Clinical Pharmacy and Family and Community Medicine
Departments of Clinical Pharmacy and Family and Community Medicine
Schools of Pharmacy and Medicine
University of California, San Francisco
San Francisco, California

Julie A. Dopheide, PharmD, BCPP, FASHP
Professor of Clinical Pharmacy, Psychiatry, and the Behavioral Sciences
University of Southern California School of Pharmacy and Keck School of Medicine
Los Angeles, California

Christopher A. Fausel, PharmD, MHA, BCOP
Clinical Manager, Oncology Pharmacy
Indiana University Health
Indianapolis, Indiana

Danielle R. Fixen, PharmD
Assistant Professor
Department of Clinical Pharmacy
Skaggs School of Pharmacy and Pharmaceutical Sciences
University of Colorado Anschutz Medical Campus
Aurora, Colorado

Lisa L. Forsyth, PharmD, FCCM
Beaumont Hospital
Royal Oak, Michigan

Matthew A. Fuller, PharmD, FASHP, BCPP
Clinical Pharmacy Specialist, Psychiatry
Northeast Ohio VA Healthcare System
Louis Stokes Cleveland Department of Veterans Affairs Medical Center
Clinical Professor of Psychiatry and Psychology
Case Western Reserve University School of Medicine
Cleveland, Ohio

Candice L. Garwood, PharmD, FCCP, BCPS, BCACP
Professor (Clinical)
College of Pharmacy and Health Sciences
Wayne State University and Harper University Hospital
Detroit Medical Center
Detroit, Michigan

Seth Gomez, PharmD, BCPP
Senior Pharmacist–Psychiatry
Office of the Medical Director
Alameda County Behavioral Health Care Services
Oakland, California

Jasmine D. Gonzalvo, PharmD, BCPS, BC-ADM, CDE, LDE
Clinical Associate Professor
Purdue University College of Pharmacy
Indianapolis, Indiana

Jessica L. Gören, PharmD, BCPP
Associate Professor
Department of Pharmacy Practice
University of Rhode Island
Kingston, Rhode Island

CONTRIBUTORS

John G. Gums, PharmD, FCCP
Professor of Pharmacy and Medicine
Associate Dean for Clinical and Administrative Affairs
College of Pharmacy
University of Florida
Gainesville, Florida

Christina Mactal Haaf, PharmD, BCOP, BCPS
Clinical Assistant Professor, Clinical Pharmacist
Department of Pharmacy Practice
University of Illinois at Chicago College of Pharmacy
Chicago, Illinois

Jon D. Herrington, PharmD, BCPS, BCOP
Hematology/Oncology Clinical Pharmacy Specialist
Baylor Scott & White Medical Center–Temple
Baylor Scott & White Health
Clinical Professor
Texas A&M University College of Medicine
Temple, Texas
Adjunct Associate Professor
University of Texas College of Pharmacy
Austin, Texas

Daniel E. Hilleman, PharmD, FCCP
Professor of Pharmacy and Medicine
Department of Pharmacy Practice
Creighton University School of Pharmacy and Health Professions
Omaha, Nebraska

Andrew Y. Hwang, PharmD, BCPS
Assistant Professor
Department of Clinical Sciences
Fred Wilson School of Pharmacy
High Point University
High Point, North Carolina

Carolyn M. Jung, PharmD, BCPS
Assistant Professor of Pharmacy Practice
Clinical Pharmacy Specialist
College of Pharmacy & Health Sciences
Butler University/Eskenazi Health
Indianapolis, Indiana

Yaman Kaakeh, PharmD, BCPS, BCNSP, CNSC
Clinical Affiliate Professor of Pharmacy Practice
Purdue University College of Pharmacy
West Lafayette, Indiana

Pramodini B. Kale-Pradhan, PharmD
Professor (Clinical)
College of Pharmacy and Health Sciences
Wayne State University
Detroit, Michigan

Kristine E. Keplar, PharmD
Clinical Pharmacist/Clinical Coordinator
HSHS St. Anthony's Memorial Hospital
Effingham, Illinois

Patrick J. Kiel, PharmD, BCPS, BCOP
Clinical Pharmacy Specialist
Hematology/Oncology–Precision Genomics Program
Indiana University Simon Cancer Center–IU Health
Indianapolis, Indiana

Julie M. Koehler, PharmD, FCCP
Associate Dean for Clinical Education and External Affiliations
Professor of Pharmacy Practice
College of Pharmacy and Health Sciences
Butler University
Indianapolis, Indiana

Bonnie A. Labdi, PharmD, BCOP
Clinical Pharmacy Specialist
Hematology/Oncology
Memorial Hermann Cancer Center–TMC
Houston, Texas
Clinical Assistant Professor
Department of Internal Medicine–Oncology
The University of Texas McGovern Medical School at Houston
Houston, Texas

Karen W. Lee, PharmD, BCPS
Regional Vice President, Clinical
Comprehensive Pharmacy Services
Boston, Massachusetts

Mary Lee, PharmD, BCPS, FCCP
Professor of Pharmacy Practice
Chicago College of Pharmacy
Vice President and Chief Academic Officer
Pharmacy and Optometry Education
Midwestern University
Downers Grove, Illinois

John R. Litaker, PhD, MSc, MMedSc
Managing Director
The Litaker Group
Austin, Texas

Mark A. Malesker, PharmD, FCCP, FCCM, FASHP, BCPS
Professor of Pharmacy Practice and Medicine
Creighton University
Omaha, Nebraska

Scott S. Malinowski, PharmD
Clinical Associate Professor
Department of Pharmacy Practice
University of Mississippi School of Pharmacy
Jackson, Mississippi

CONTRIBUTORS

Erin E. Mancl, PharmD, BCPS, BCCCP
Clinical Pharmacist
Lung Transplant and Advanced Lung Disease
Loyola University Health System
Maywood, Illinois

Dianne W. May, PharmD, FCCP, BCPS
Clinical Professor
Department of Clinical and Administrative Pharmacy
Campus Director for Pharmacy Practice Experiences
Division of Experience Programs
University of Georgia College of Pharmacy
Augusta, Georgia

J. Russell May, PharmD, FASHP
Associate Department Head and Clinical Professor
Department of Clinical and Administrative Pharmacy
University of Georgia College of Pharmacy
Augusta, Georgia

Ashley H. Meredith, PharmD, BCACP, BCPS, CDE
Clinical Associate Professor
Department of Pharmacy Practice
Purdue University
Indianapolis, Indiana

Douglas A. Miller, PharmD
Professor (Emeritus)
College of Pharmacy and Health Sciences
Wayne State University
Detroit, Michigan

Monica L. Miller, PharmD, MS
Clinical Associate Professor
Department of Pharmacy Practice
Purdue University
Indianapolis, Indiana
Internal Medicine Clinical Specialist
Department of Pharmacy Services
Eskenazi Health
Indianapolis, Indiana

Genevieve Lynn Ness, PharmD
Director, Christy Houston Foundation Drug Information Center
Assistant Professor of Pharmaceutical Social and Administrative Sciences
Belmont University College of Pharmacy
Nashville, Tennessee

Sarah A. Nisly, PharmD, BCPS, FCCP
Associate Professor
Wingate University School of Pharmacy
Wingate, North Carolina

LeAnn B. Norris, PharmD, FCCP, BCPS, BCOP
Clinical Associate Professor
South Carolina College of Pharmacy
Columbia, South Carolina

Brian R. Overholser, PharmD
Associate Professor
Department of Pharmacy Practice
Purdue University College of Pharmacy
West Lafayette, Indiana
Division of Clinical Pharmacology
Indiana University School of Medicine
Indianapolis, Indiana

Robert L. Page II, PharmD, MSPH, BCPS (AQ-Cardiology), BCGP, FCCP, FAHA, FASHP, FHFSA
Professor of Clinical Pharmacy
Clinical Specialist, Division of Cardiology
University of Colorado Schools of Pharmacy and Medicine
Aurora, Colorado

Amy Barton Pai, PharmD, BCPS, FASN, FCCP, FNKF
Associate Professor, Clinical Pharmacy
University of Michigan College of Pharmacy
Ann Arbor, Michigan

Dennis Parker, Jr., PharmD
Associate Professor (Clinical)
College of Pharmacy and Health Sciences
Wayne State University and Detroit Receiving Hospital
Detroit Medical Center
Detroit, Michigan

Tobias Peschel, MD, PhD, MBA
Senior Vice President Pharmacovigilance & Epidemiology
Gilead Sciences, Inc.
Foster City, California

Tiffany Pon, PharmD, BCPS
Assistant Professor
Department of Clinical Pharmacy
University of California, San Francisco
San Francisco, California

Charles D. Ponte, PharmD, BC-ADM, BCPS, CDE, CPE, FAADE, FAPhA, FASHP, FCCP, FNAP
Professor of Clinical Pharmacy and Family Medicine
Departments of Clinical Pharmacy and Family Medicine
West Virginia University
Morgantown, West Virginia

Frank Pucino, Jr., PharmD, MPH, FASHP, FCCP
Adjunct Clinical Scientist
Eunice Kennedy Shriver National Institute of Child Health and Human Development
Bethesda, Maryland

CONTRIBUTORS

Cynthia Reilly, MS, BS Pharm
Senior Vice President
Academy of Managed Care Pharmacy
Alexandria, Virginia

Denise H. Rhoney, PharmD, FCCP, FCCM, FNCS
Ron and Nancy McFarlane Distinguished Professor and Chair
Division of Practice Advancement and Clinical Education
UNC Eshelman School of Pharmacy
Chapel Hill, North Carolina

Daniel M. Riche, PharmD, FCCP, BCPS, CDE, ASH-CHC, CLS
Associate Professor
Department of Pharmacy Practice
University of Mississippi School of Pharmacy
Associate Professor
Department of Medicine
University of Mississippi Medical Center
Research Associate Professor
National Center for Natural Products Research
Research Institute of Pharmaceutical Sciences
Jackson, Mississippi

Ian A. Ross, PharmD
Clinical Pharmacist
Intensive Care Unit and Cardiovascular Intensive Care Unit (ICU and CV–ICU)
Ascension Providence Rochester Hospital
Rochester, Michigan

Melody Ryan, PharmD, MPH
Professor
Department of Pharmacy Practice and Science
University of Kentucky College of Pharmacy
Lexington, Kentucky

Joseph J. Saseen, PharmD, BCPS, BCACP, FCCP, FASHP
Professor and Vice Chair, Clinical Pharmacy
Skaggs School of Pharmacy and Pharmaceutical Sciences
Professor, Family Medicine
School of Medicine
University of Colorado Anschutz Medical Campus
Aurora, Colorado

Roohollah Sharifi, MD, FACS
Professor of Surgery and Urology
University of Illinois at Chicago College of Medicine
Section Chief of Urology
Jesse Brown Veterans Administration Medical Center
Chicago, Illinois

Amy Heck Sheehan, PharmD
Associate Professor
Pharmacy Practice
Purdue University College of Pharmacy
West Lafayette, Indiana

Jaekyu Shin, PharmD, MS, BCPS
Associate Professor of Clinical Pharmacy
Department of Clinical Pharmacy
University of California, San Francisco
San Francisco, California

Tyler Shugg, PharmD
Purdue University College of Pharmacy
West Lafayette, Indiana
Division of Clinical Pharmacology
Indiana University School of Medicine
Indianapolis, Indiana

Frank E. Silvestry, MD, FACC, FASE
Associate Professor of Medicine
Perelman School of Medicine
University of Pennsylvania
Philadelphia, Pennsylvania

Judith A. Smith, PharmD, BCOP, CPHQ, FCCP, FISOPP
Associate Professor
Director, WHIM Research Program
McGovern Medical School
University of Texas Health Science Center at Houston
Houston, Texas

Steven M. Smith, PharmD, MPH, BCPS
Assistant Professor of Pharmacy and Medicine
Departments of Pharmacotherapy and Translational Research and Community Health and Family Medicine
Colleges of Pharmacy and Medicine
University of Florida
Gainesville, Florida

Kevin M. Sowinski, PharmD, FCCP
Professor and Associate Head
Department of Pharmacy Practice
Purdue University College of Pharmacy
West Lafayette, Indiana
Adjunct Professor
Division of Clinical Pharmacology
Indiana University School of Medicine
Indianapolis, Indiana

Sarah A. Spinler, PharmD, FCCP, FAHA, FASHP, AACC, BCPS (AQ-Cardiology)
Professor of Clinical Pharmacy
Philadelphia College of Pharmacy
University of the Sciences in Philadelphia
Philadelphia, Pennsylvania

Michele Y. Splinter, PharmD, MS, BCPS, FCCP
Associate Professor
Department of Pharmacy: Clinical and Administrative Sciences
College of Pharmacy
University of Oklahoma Health Sciences Center
Oklahoma City, Oklahoma

CONTRIBUTORS

Mary K. Stamatakis, PharmD
Professor
Department of Clinical Pharmacy
West Virginia University School of Pharmacy
Morgantown, West Virginia

David M. Swope, MD
Senior Faculty
Department of Neurology
Mt. Sinai Hospital
New York, New York

Lynne M. Sylvia, PharmD
Senior Clinical Pharmacy Specialist–Cardiology
Department of Pharmacy
Tufts Medical Center
Boston, Massachusetts

Teresa C. Thakrar, PharmD, BCOP
Clinical Pharmacist, Hematology/Stem Cell Transplant
Indiana University Health
Indianapolis, Indiana

Hugh H. Tilson, MD, DrPH
Adjunct Professor, Epidemiology
Adjunct Assistant Professor, Public Health Leadership Program
University of North Carolina
Chapel Hill, North Carolina

James E. Tisdale, PharmD, BCPS, FCCP, FAPhA, FNAP, FAHA
Professor
College of Pharmacy
Purdue University
Indianapolis, Indiana
Adjunct Professor
School of Medicine
Indiana University
Indianapolis, Indiana

Katy E. Trinkley, PharmD, BCACP
Associate Professor
Department of Clinical Pharmacy
Skaggs School of Pharmacy and Pharmaceutical Sciences
Department of Medicine, School of Medicine
University of Colorado Anschutz Medical Campus
Aurora, Colorado

Ross T. Tsuyuki, BSc(Pharm), PharmD, MSc, FCSHP, FACC, FCAHS
Professor and Chair
Department of Pharmacology
Professor of Medicine (Cardiology)
Department of Medicine
Director, EPICORE Centre
Faculty of Medicine and Dentistry
University of Alberta
Edmonton, Alberta, Canada

Alison M. Walton, PharmD, BCPS
Associate Professor of Pharmacy Practice
College of Pharmacy and Health Sciences
Butler University
Indianapolis, Indiana

Lori D. Wazny, BSc(Pharm), PharmD, EPPh
Extended Practice Pharmacist and Clinical Associate Professor
Manitoba Renal Program
University of Manitoba College of Pharmacy
Winnipeg, Manitoba, Canada

Kellie Jones Weddle, PharmD, BCOP, FCCP, FHOPA
Clinical Professor
Purdue University College of Pharmacy
Indianapolis, Indiana

Nicole M. Wegrzyn, PharmD, BCACP
Clinical Pharmacist, Ambulatory Care
Department of Pharmacy
CareMore Health Clinical Instructor
University of Arizona College of Pharmacy
Tucson, Arizona

Timothy E. Welty, PharmD, FCCP, BCPS
Professor and Chair
Department of Clinical Sciences
College of Pharmacy and Health Sciences
Drake University
Des Moines, Iowa

Sheila M. Wilhelm, PharmD, FCCP, BCPS
Associate Professor (Clinical)
Department of Pharmacy Practice
College of Pharmacy and Health Sciences
Wayne State University
Detroit, Michigan

Craig Williams, PharmD, FLNA, BCPS
Clinical Professor
Oregon State University
Portland, Oregon

James P. Wilson, PharmD, PhD, FASHP
Associate Professor
Division of Health Outcomes and Pharmacy Practice
College of Pharmacy
The University of Texas at Austin
Austin, Texas

Susan M. Wilson, PharmD
Director of Pharmacy
McLaren Flint
Flint, Michigan

REVIEWERS

Jacquelyn L. Bainbridge, BS Pharm, PharmD, FCCP, MSCS
Professor
Department of Clinical Pharmacy, Skaggs School of Pharmacy and Pharmaceutical Sciences
Department of Neurology, School of Medicine
University of Colorado Anschutz Medical Campus
Aurora, Colorado

Gretchen M. Brophy, PharmD, BCPS, FCCP, FCCM, FNCS
Professor of Pharmacotherapy & Outcomes Science and Neurosurgery
Medical College of Virginia Campus
Virginia Commonwealth University
Richmond, Virginia

Susan P. Bruce, PharmD, BCPS
Associate Dean, Pharmacy Education and Interprofessional Studies
Chair and Professor, Pharmacy Practice
Northeast Ohio Medical University
Rootstown, Ohio

Judy Cheng, PharmD, MPH, FCCP, BCPS
Professor of Pharmacy Practice
Interim Chair, Department of Pharmacy Practice
MCPHS University
Boston, Massachusetts

Lily Kung Cheung, PharmD
Associate Professor
Department of Pharmacy Practice
College of Pharmacy and Health Sciences
Texas Southern University
Houston, Texas

Sheryl L. Chow, PharmD, FCCP, FAHA, FHFSA
Associate Professor
Pharmacy Practice and Administration
Western University of Health Sciences
Pomona, California

Kristen Cook, PharmD, BCPS
Clinical Assistant Professor
College of Pharmacy UNMC
Pharmacist
Nebraska Medicine Midtown Clinic
Omaha, Nebraska

John W. Devlin, PharmD, BCCCP, FCCM, FCCP
Professor of Pharmacy
Northeastern University
Boston, Massachusetts

Thomas C. Dowling, PharmD, PhD, FCCP
Assistant Dean
Ferris State University
Grand Rapids, Michigan

Kaelen C. Dunican, PharmD
Professor of Pharmacy Practice
School of Pharmacy–Worcester/Manchester
MCPHS University
Worcester, Massachusetts

Susan C. Fagan, PharmD, BCPS, FCCP
Jowdy Professor and Assistant Dean
University of Georgia College of Pharmacy
Augusta, Georgia

Ema Ferreira, BS Pharm, MSc, PharmD, FCSHP
Full Clinical Professor
Faculty of Pharmacy
University of Montreal/CHU Ste-Justine
Montreal, Quebec, Canada

Lindsay R. Figg, PharmD, BCOP
Clinical Pharmacist, Hematology/Oncology
University of Louisville Hospital
Louisville, Kentucky

Jason C. Gallagher, PharmD, FCCP, FIDSA, BCPS
Clinical Professor
Clinical Pharmacy Specialist, Infectious Diseases
Temple University
Philadelphia, Pennsylvania

Tanna Hassig, PharmD, BCPS
ICU Clinical Lead Pharmacist
Department of Pharmacy
University of Colorado Hospital, Anschutz Medical Campus
Aurora, Colorado

Sheryl J. Herner, PharmD, MHSA, FCCP, BCPS, CPPS
Clinical Pharmacy Chief of Quality and Medication Safety
Kaiser Permanente Colorado
Clinical Associate Professor
University of Colorado Skaggs School of Pharmacy and Pharmaceutical Sciences
Denver, Colorado

REVIEWERS

John B. Hertig, PharmD, MS, CPPS
Associate Director
Center for Medication Safety Advancement
Purdue University College of Pharmacy
West Lafayette, Indiana

Kyle E. Hultgren, PharmD
Director
Center for Medication Safety Advancement
Purdue University College of Pharmacy
West Lafayette, Indiana

Brian K. Irons, PharmD, FCCP, BCACP
Division Head, Ambulatory Care
Professor, Department of Pharmacy Practice
School of Pharmacy
Texas Tech University Health Sciences Center
Lubbock, Texas

Timothy J. Ives, PharmD, MPH, FCCP, CPP
Professor of Pharmacy, Adjunct Professor of Medicine
Eshelman School of Pharmacy
The University of North Carolina at Chapel Hill
Chapel Hill, North Carolina

Melanie S. Joy, PharmD, PhD
Associate Professor
Department of Pharmaceutical Sciences
University of Colorado Anschutz Medical Campus
Skaggs School of Pharmacy and Pharmaceutical Sciences
Aurora, Colorado

Michael P. Kane, PharmD, FCCP, BCPS, BCACP
Professor, Department of Pharmacy Practice
School of Pharmacy and Pharmaceutical Sciences
Albany College of Pharmacy and Health Sciences
Clinical Pharmacy Specialist
Albany Medical Center Division of Community Endocrinology
Albany, New York

Emily Kathol, PharmD, BCOP
Clinical Pharmacist
Nebraska Medicine
Omaha, Nebraska

Adam M. Kaye, PharmD, FASCP, FCPhA
Clinical Professor of Pharmacy
Department of Pharmacy Practice
Thomas J. Long School of Pharmacy and Health Sciences
University of the Pacific
Stockton, California

Michael Kotlyar, PharmD
Associate Professor
Department of Experimental and Clinical Pharmacology
College of Pharmacy
University of Minnesota
Minneapolis, Minnesota

Robert J. Kuhn, PharmD
Professor of Pharmacy Practice and Science
University of Kentucky College of Pharmacy
Lexington, Kentucky

Jeffrey A. Kyle, PharmD, BCPS
Associate Professor of Pharmacy Practice
McWhorter School of Pharmacy
Samford University
Birmingham, Alabama

Rebecca M. Law, PharmD
Associate Professor
School of Pharmacy and Faculty of Medicine
Memorial University of Newfoundland
St. John's, Newfoundland and Labrador, Canada
Visiting Scholar
Department of Dermatology, Faculty of Medicine
University of California, San Francisco
San Francisco, California

Charles Makowski, PharmD, BCPS
Clinical Pharmacy Specialist, Drug Information and Medication Safety
Pharmacy Service Line
Henry Ford Health System
Detroit, Michigan

Janene L. Marshall, PharmD, BCPS
Clinical Associate Professor
Pharmacy Practice
Chicago State University College of Pharmacy
Chicago, Illinois

Joseph E. Mazur, PharmD, BCPS
Clinical Specialist
Medical Intensive Care Unit
Medical University of South Carolina
Charleston, South Carolina

Anna K. Morin, PharmD
Dean
Professor of Pharmacy Practice
School of Pharmacy–Worcester/Manchester
MCPHS University
Worcester, Massachusetts

REVIEWERS

Lynette R. Moser, PharmD
Associate Professor (Clinical), Interim Chair
Department of Pharmacy Practice
College of Pharmacy and Health Sciences
Wayne State University
Detroit, Michigan

Mark A. Munger, PharmD, FCCP, FAHA, FHFSA
Professor, Pharmacotherapy
Adjunct Professor, Internal Medicine
University of Utah
Salt Lake City, Utah

Kimberly Lovin Nealy, PharmD, BCPS, CDE, CPP
Associate Professor of Pharmacy
Levine College of Health Sciences
Wingate University
Wingate, North Carolina

Stefanie C. Nigro, PharmD, BCACP, CDE
Assistant Professor
Department of Pharmacy Practice
MCPHS University
Boston, Massachusetts

Julie H. Oestreich, PharmD, PhD
Assistant Professor
Pharmaceutical Sciences
University of Findlay College of Pharmacy
Findlay, Ohio

Keith M. Olsen, PharmD, FCCP, FCCM
Dean and Professor
College of Pharmacy
University of Arkansas for Medical Sciences
Little Rock, Arkansas

Kari L. Olson, BSc(Pharm), PharmD, FCCP, BCPS (AQ-Cardiology)
Clinical Pharmacy Supervisor
Clinical Pharmacy Cardiac Risk Service
Kaiser Permanente Colorado
Clinical Associate Professor
University of Colorado Skaggs School of Pharmacy and Pharmaceutical Sciences
University of Colorado Anschutz Medical Campus
Aurora, Colorado

Carol A. Ott, PharmD, BCPP
Clinical Professor of Pharmacy Practice
Purdue University College of Pharmacy
West Lafayette, Indiana
Clinical Pharmacy Specialist, Outpatient Psychiatry
Eskenazi Health
Indianapolis, Indiana

Robert B. Parker, PharmD, FCCP
Professor
Department of Clinical Pharmacy
University of Tennessee College of Pharmacy
Memphis, Tennessee

Amy M. Pick, PharmD, BCOP
Professor of Pharmacy Practice
Director of Faculty and Staff Development
School of Pharmacy and Health Professions
Creighton University
Omaha, Nebraska

Theresa R. Prosser, PharmD, FCCP, BCPS, AE-C
Professor of Pharmacy Practice
St. Louis College of Pharmacy
St. Louis, Missouri

Laurajo Ryan, PharmD, MSc, BCPS
Clinical Associate Professor
The University of Texas at Austin College of Pharmacy
Department of Medicine
UT Health San Antonio
San Antonio, Texas

Charles C. Sharkey, MS, MBA, PharmD
Pharmacy Site Manager
Pharmacy Residency Coordinator Postgraduate Year One (PGY 1)
Chairperson Institutional Review Board (IRB)
Pharmacy Service
New York Harbor Healthcare System
Brooklyn, New York

Glen L. Stimmel, PharmD
Associate Dean of Academic Affairs
Professor of Clinical Pharmacy, Psychiatry, and the Behavioral Sciences
School of Pharmacy and Keck School of Medicine
University of Southern California
Los Angeles, California

Steven C. Stoner, PharmD, BCPP
Clinical Professor and Department Chair
Division of Pharmacy Practice and Administration
University of Missouri–Kansas City School of Pharmacy
Kansas City, Missouri

Toby C. Trujillo, PharmD, FCCP, FAHA, BCPS (AQ-Cardiology)
Associate Professor
University of Colorado Skaggs School of Pharmacy and Pharmaceutical Sciences
Aurora, Colorado

REVIEWERS

Elena M. Umland, PharmD
Associate Dean for Academic Affairs
Professor of Pharmacy
Jefferson College of Pharmacy
Thomas Jefferson University
Philadelphia, Pennsylvania

Sara R. Vazquez, PharmD, BCPS, CACP
Clinical Pharmacist
University of Utah Health
Salt Lake City, Utah

Johnathan Voss, PharmD, BCCCP, BCNSP
Clinical Pharmacist–Critical Care
John Peter Smith Hospital
Fort Worth, Texas

Mary L. Wagner, PharmD, MS
Associate Professor
Department of Pharmacy Practice and Administration
Ernest Mario School of Pharmacy
Rutgers, The State University of New Jersey
Piscataway, New Jersey

Barbara S. Wiggins, PharmD
Clinical Pharmacy Specialist–Cardiology
Medical University of South Carolina
Mt. Pleasant, South Carolina

Daniel M. Witt, PharmD, FCCP, BCPS
Professor & Chair
Assistant Dean of Clinical Affairs
Department of Pharmacotherapy
University of Utah College of Pharmacy
Salt Lake City, Utah

Felix K. Yam, PharmD, MAS, BCPS (AQ-Cardiology)
Associate Clinical Professor
Skaggs School of Pharmacy and Pharmaceutical Sciences
University of California–San Diego
La Jolla, California

Mary Ann E. Zagaria, PharmD, MS, BCGP
Clinical Consultant Pharmacist and President
MZ Associates, Inc.
Hallowell, Maine

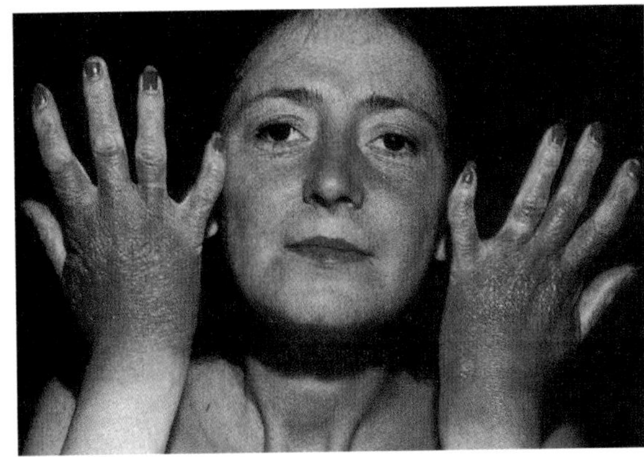

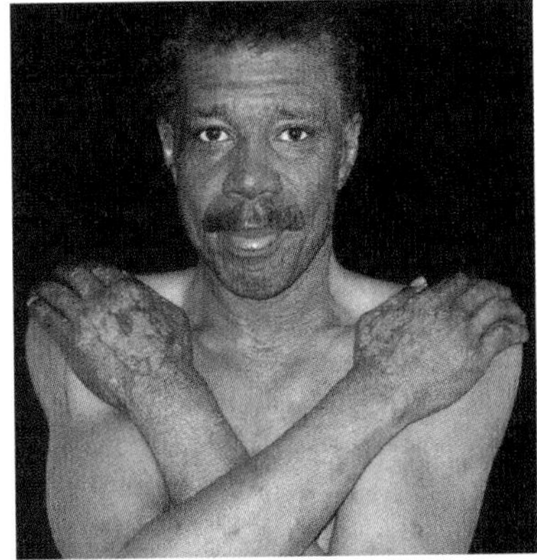

FIGURE 8-3 Drug-Induced Phototoxicity and Photoallergy

The photo on the left depicts a case of drug-induced phototoxicity secondary to demethylchlortetracycline use for treatment of acne. The woman was wearing a hat that protected her face and neck from sunlight exposure, but her hands were exposed to sunlight while holding a railing at a sporting event. The photo on the right depicts a case of drug-induced photoallergy secondary to trimethoprim–sulfamethoxazole use for *Pneumocystis jiroveci* pneumonia prophylaxis. Eczema and hyperpigmentation of the sun-exposed areas are noted. Photos reprinted with permission from Wolff K, Johnson RA, Suurmond D. *Fitzpatrick's Color Atlas and Synopsis of Clinical Dermatology: Common and Serious Diseases*. 5th ed. New York, NY: McGraw-Hill; 2005:226-69.

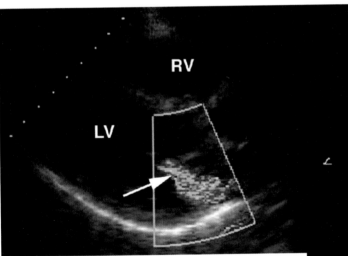

FIGURE 29-2 Transthoracic Echocardiogram with Color Doppler Map from the Parasternal Window in the Long Axis of the Same Patient as in Figure 29-1

Demonstrating a jet of moderate mitral regurgitation (arrow) directed slightly posteriorly, due to mild restriction of the posterior leaflet, as is characteristic of anorexiant-induced valvulopathy. LV = left ventricle, RV = right ventricle.

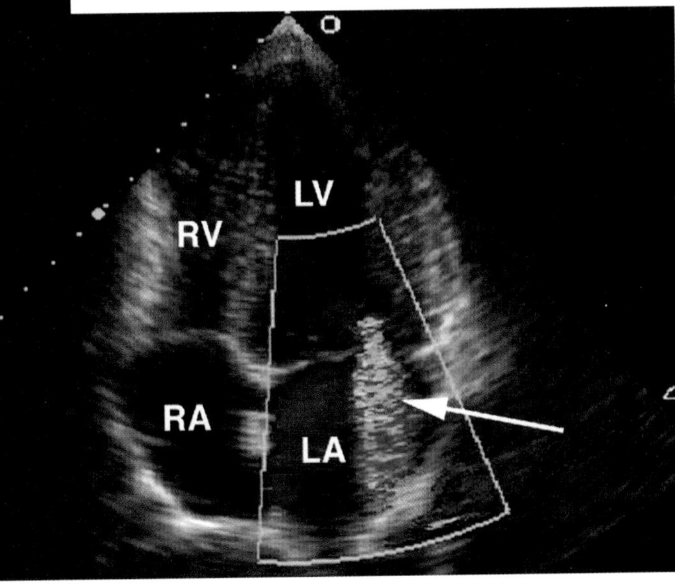

FIGURE 29-3 Apical 4-Chamber View from a Transthoracic Echocardiogram from the Same Patient as in Figures 29-1 and 29-2

Demonstrating a jet of moderate mitral regurgitation (arrow) directed slightly posteriorly and laterally, due to mild restriction of the posterior leaflet, characteristic of anorexiant-induced valvulopathy. LA = left atrium, LV = left ventricle, RA = right atrium, RV = right ventricle.

SECTION I

MAGNITUDE/ SIGNIFICANCE OF DRUG-INDUCED DISEASES: IMPACT ON THE HEALTHCARE SYSTEM

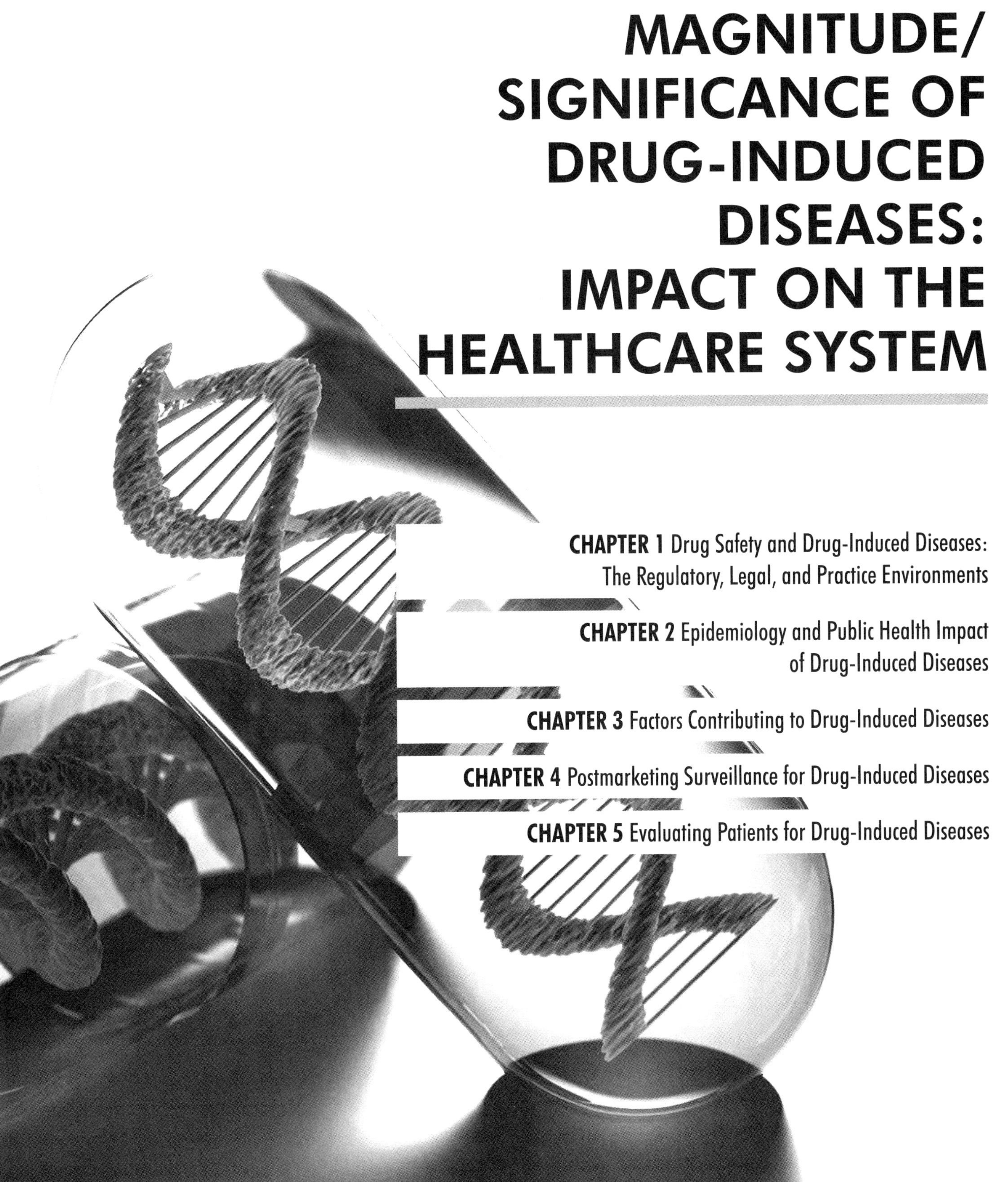

CHAPTER 1 Drug Safety and Drug-Induced Diseases: The Regulatory, Legal, and Practice Environments

CHAPTER 2 Epidemiology and Public Health Impact of Drug-Induced Diseases

CHAPTER 3 Factors Contributing to Drug-Induced Diseases

CHAPTER 4 Postmarketing Surveillance for Drug-Induced Diseases

CHAPTER 5 Evaluating Patients for Drug-Induced Diseases

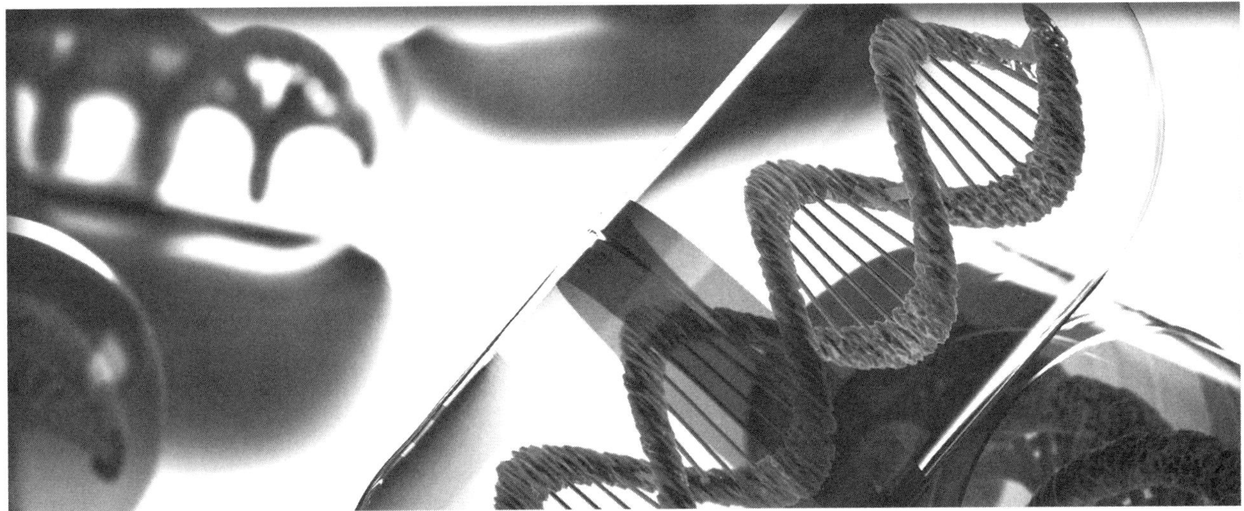

CHAPTER 1

Drug Safety and Drug-Induced Diseases: The Regulatory, Legal, and Practice Environments

Cynthia Reilly

The regulatory, legal, and practice environments in healthcare surrounding drug safety have been the subject of much scrutiny in recent years. In the early 2000s, the highly publicized market withdrawal of widely used drug products, including rofecoxib (Vioxx) and troglitazone (Rezulin) for safety reasons served as a focal point of concerns about the effectiveness of the U.S. drug approval and safety surveillance systems.[1] Eleven new drug and biologic products approved by the U.S. Food and Drug Administration (FDA) between 1996 and 2012 were withdrawn from the U.S. market between the time of approval and 2013.[2] This represents roughly 2% of the 522 products approved during this period. With the exception of drotrecogin alfa (Xigris), which was withdrawn for failing to demonstrate improved outcomes in patients with septic shock, these products were withdrawn for safety reasons that included cardiac and liver effects and opportunistic infections.

Other safety-related regulatory actions (e.g., labeling changes, such as the addition of precautions, contraindications, or black box warnings) are far more common and, although less publicized, have the potential for significant impact on patient safety if these therapies are not properly managed. Among the 522 therapies evaluated in a study encompassing the time period 1996–2012, 180 received a boxed warning either premarket or postmarket.[2] Of these, 105 products received a boxed warning as part of the preapproval review process, and 50 received a boxed warning postapproval based on safety concerns that arose after the products were marketed. Both premarket and postmarket boxed warning information was issued for 25 of the 522 products for which

Note: The author wishes to acknowledge the work of Henri R. Manasse, who co-authored this chapter in a previous edition.

labeling histories were evaluated. Other adverse events associated with medication therapy, such as medication errors, have also heightened awareness among healthcare professionals, policymakers, and other stakeholders concerning all aspects of drug safety.[3] Consumers have also expressed concern, with one survey finding that 71% of respondents had either high or moderate concern about themselves or a family member being harmed by a medication error during hospitalization.[4] As medication experts, pharmacists play a critical role in ensuring drug safety through their activities in selecting and monitoring drug therapy, communicating risk versus benefit to patients to allow for informed decision making, and reporting suspected adverse drug events and drug-induced diseases.

The extent of adverse drug events, which includes but is not limited to drug-induced diseases, is staggering. The FDA's Adverse Event Reporting System (AERS) receives approximately 500,000 reports every year from prescribers, pharmacists, nurses, patients, and others.[5] In total, since its inception in 1969, the system has received roughly 5 million reports. In 2015, the FDA issued 19 public health advisories (i.e., descriptions of safety concern with recommended actions) concerning drug and biologic products.[6] However, it has been reported that 10% or less of the adverse events that occur are reported to this spontaneous reporting system.[7]

Drug-induced disease can result from unanticipated or anticipated drug effects. Disease also can occur from product impurities, as was the case with deaths attributed to the use of contaminated heparin in 2008.[8] Vigilance on the part of regulatory authorities, drug manufacturers, clinicians, and patients is necessary to minimize the potential for harm that is inherent in drug use.

DRUG SAFETY: THE REGULATORY ENVIRONMENT

THE FDA AND REGULATORY EFFORTS TO ENSURE DRUG SAFETY

Until 2007, FDA efforts to provide drug safety had largely focused on premarket strategies. However, as the history of the agency demonstrates (Figure 1–1), much of the FDA's regulatory authority was created in response to harm, or concern for harm, associated with drugs already on the market.[9] The origins of the FDA can be traced back to the late 1860s,

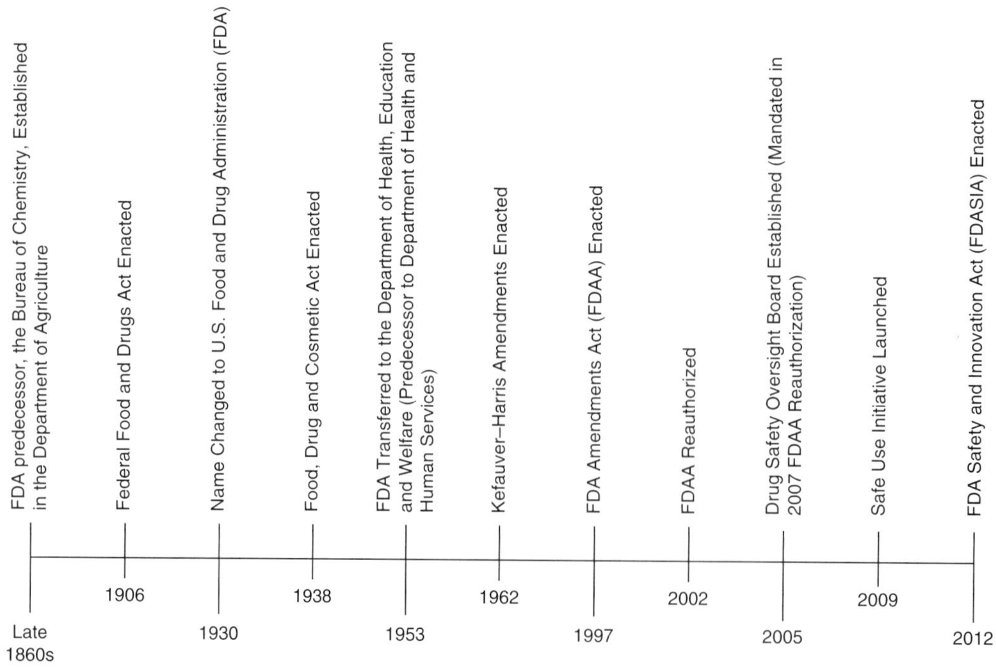

FIGURE 1-1 History of U.S. Food and Drug Administration Drug Safety Activities and Regulations[9]

when its predecessor, the Bureau of Chemistry, was established as part of the Department of Agriculture. Over the years, there were repeated attempts to introduce legislation to address concerns about adulterated drug products from overseas. However, it was not until 1906, when the Federal Food and Drugs Act was passed, that the focus of the agency shifted from scientific to regulatory activities. Although that legislation permitted regulation of drug product labeling, the impetus for the law was not drug safety but rather concerns for *food* safety, which were prompted by Upton Sinclair's *The Jungle*. The novel exposed unsanitary conditions in the meatpacking industry, which at the time were considered the greater threat to public safety.

It wasn't until enactment of the Food, Drug, and Cosmetic Act in 1938 that legislation began to focus on premarket drug safety. Once again, this authority was granted in response to a safety incident in which an antifreeze-like ingredient in the elixir sulfanilamide resulted in more than 100 deaths.[9] In 1962, the Kefauver–Harris Amendments to the 1938 Act introduced a requirement to demonstrate both efficacy and safety prior to drug approval. This was the first legislation that focused on adverse events caused by active ingredients and was spurred by reports of birth defects following the use of thalidomide abroad. Severe malformations, including a flipper-like appearance of limbs caused by very short or absent long bones, resulted in withdrawal of the drug from worldwide markets. A U.S.-based drug manufacturer had applied for, but never received, approval to market the drug in the United States.

Significant efforts to improve drug safety have been addressed within the FDA Amendments Acts (FDAAs) of 1992, 1997, 2002, 2007, and 2012. Most notably, the 2007 reauthorization of the act grants the FDA increased authority to request that manufacturers complete postmarketing safety studies and requires that manufacturers develop and submit risk evaluation and mitigation strategies (REMS) for all drug products for which they seek FDA approval.[10-12] Although patient and prescriber education programs are potential components of REMS programs, more stringent programs, such as patient and provider registries or required laboratory monitoring and reporting, may be included in a more comprehensive restrictive drug distribution system (RDDS). FDAA 2007 also requires that the FDA establish a mechanism to increase and coordinate postmarketing surveillance efforts. The requirement was addressed by the establishment of the Sentinel Initiative in 2008, which is discussed in greater detail in Chapter 4: Postmarketing Surveillance for Drug-Induced Diseases. The 2007 reauthorization also mandated the Drug Safety Oversight Board—an entity that the FDA had already created in 2005 following the market withdrawal of Vioxx—as a mechanism to advise the agency on managing and communicating information about emerging safety issues.[6] The FDA Safety and Innovation Act of 2012 (FDASIA) included a requirement that the FDA create a five-year plan to introduce a structured benefit/risk framework to be used agencywide to assess safety during the new drug approval process.[13] In addition, the agency was directed to use monies collected from user fees to assess the effectiveness of, and make improvements to, the REMS program and evaluate strategies for using data from the Sentinel System to inform regulatory actions. The law also includes a focus on increasing the safety and integrity of the drug supply chain. Although requirements in FDASIA augmented existing work to address drug safety, it also sought to expedite drug development under certain circumstances.[13] Specifically, the law called on the FDA to improve communications with pharmaceutical manufacturers engaged in drug development and to increase staff capacity and expertise to support the review of drugs for rare diseases and the use of biomarkers and pharmacogenomics for drug approval.

THE FDA'S SAFETY-RELATED REGULATORY ACTIONS

The FDA considers and may request a number of regulatory actions when a serious or life-threatening safety concern is identified for a drug. Each action has the potential to decrease or eliminate patient access to drug therapy. Therefore, decisions regarding specific courses of action must carefully balance the effectiveness of the drug, other therapeutic options for the condition being treated, the type of possible harm to patients, and the potential for its occurrence.

Regulatory options following drug approval include clinician and patient warnings, labeling changes, and product withdrawals. To increase transparency as well as consumer and clinician awareness, the Prescription Drug User Fee Act (PDUFA IV, a component of FDAA 2007 that authorizes the FDA to use fees collected from pharmaceutical manufacturers to conduct safety activities) requires the FDA to generate quarterly reports that include information on recently identified potentially serious risks and new safety information generated from the AERS database.[12,15] Introduction of this process and enhanced efforts via the MedWatch program and other FDA drug safety initiatives generate extensive amounts of safety information. Although this is beneficial, concerns have been raised about whether this information effectively reaches or is understood by target audiences, including healthcare professionals and patients.[16,17] Safety information is and always will be an evolving topic, but the FDA and professional associations such as ASHP are collaborating to determine how this information can be made available in ways that are most useful to clinicians and their patients.

In July 2012, the FDA launched the first classwide REMS for opioids after holding a series of stakeholder meetings to discuss options to ensure that the benefits of these drugs continue to outweigh their risks.[18] The effort was in response to an alarming increase in the number of overdose deaths associated with the use of these products. According to the Centers for Disease Control and Prevention (CDC), such deaths have increased more than 300% since 1998, while prescribing rates for these drugs quadrupled between 1999 and 2010.[19] In 2014, deaths from prescription opioids reached an all-time high of roughly 19,000.[20] The REMS, which involved more than 30 products marketed by more than 20 companies, required that manufacturers modify product labeling to include a boxed warning to highlight risks; provide training to prescribers, pharmacists, and other healthcare professionals to ensure proper use; and provide educational materials to patients.[18] The extent of opioid prescribing and the morbidity and mortality associated with their use was highlighted by an advertisement during Super Bowl 50 for a drug to treat a drug-induced disease, opioid-induced constipation.[21] The promotion, which cost an estimated $10 million (based on projected costs of $5 million per 30 seconds for Super Bowl ads), drew criticism from the White House, elected officials, pain and addiction specialists, and the media, among other stakeholders. In February 2015, the FDA announced plans to extend the REMS to include immediate-release opioid products.[22]

When less stringent interventions are unable or deemed unlikely to address safety concerns, RDDS can be used to allow continued availability of drugs that are associated with significant safety concerns but provide a health benefit if used appropriately in specific patient populations. RDDS can include clinician or facility registration, patient registries that are used to track and evaluate response to therapies, and performance-linked access systems. The FDA can request that these programs be established for drugs that are already approved or as a condition for approval. For example, in 1999, the drug thalidomide, which had previously been removed from world markets, was approved in the United States for the treatment of lesions caused by Hansen disease, or leprosy.[23] However, to prevent or reduce the risk of significant drug-induced disease, thalidomide is available only via physicians and pharmacists registered in the System for Thalidomide Education and Prescribing Safety (STEPS) program. The drug cannot be prescribed for women of childbearing age, unless the patient meets certain criteria (e.g., ability to comprehend and follow pregnancy precautions). The physician must also document proof of a negative pregnancy test 24 hours prior to initiation of therapy and on an ongoing basis during therapy. Oral and printed patient education materials are also a significant component of the STEPS program.

Thalidomide is one of dozens of drugs marketed in the United States for which an RDDS is required (Table 1-1).[24] This list is expected to continue to expand based on the FDA's increased authority to require these programs under the PDUFA IV. Although these programs facilitate ongoing availability of drug therapies, they also present challenges to clinicians and patients.[25] RDDS are not currently

Table 1-1 FDA-Approved Drugs with RDDS[24]

Drugs

- α1-proteinase inhibitor
- Alemtuzumab[a]
- Alosetron
  - Avelumab
- Alvimopan
- Ambrisentan
  - Axicabtagene
- Bosentan
- Buprenorphine and buprenorphine/naloxone fixed dose
  - Brodalumab
- Cabozantinib
- Carfilzomib
- Carglumic acid
- Ceritinib
- Cisapride[a]
- Clofazimine[a]
- Clozapine
- Collagenase clostridium histolyticum
- Cysteamine
- Dalfampridine
- Deferasirox
- Deferiprone
  - Deutetrabenazine
- Diphtheria antitoxin (equine)
- Dofetilide
- Droxidopa
- Eculizumab
  - Fentanyl (transmucosal immediate-release and iontophoretic transdermal formulations)
  - Flibanserin
- Gefitinib
- Ibritumomab
- Iloprost
- Isotretinoin
- Lenalidomide
- Lenvatinib
- Lomitapide
- Macitentan
- Mifepristone
- Mipomersen
- Natalizumab
  - Obeticholic acid
- Olanzapine
- Olaparib
- Panobinostat
- Pertuzumab
- Pomalidomide
- Riociguat
- Ruxolitinib
- Sodium oxybate
- Taliglucerase alfa
- Tasimelteon
- Teduglutide
- Tegaserod
- Tetrabenazine
- Thalidomide
- Treprostinil
- Vandetanib
- Vemurafenib
- Vigabatrin

FDA = U.S. Food and Drug Administration, RDDS = restricted drug distribution systems.
[a]Drug is available only through established compassionate-use programs.

standardized, and each drug manufacturer may establish its own management processes, including clinician registration requirements. The variability and complexity of these processes can delay or limit patient access to therapies, especially as patients move between healthcare settings. At the urging of professional organizations and others, the FDA is evaluating strategies to minimize unintended consequences of these programs on continuity of care and patient access to these high-risk drugs.

A significant challenge to the FDA drug approval process is the need to balance safety with more rapid access to innovative and life-saving therapies. Expedited pathways have been developed to meet these objectives.[26] To qualify for these programs—which include fast-track designation, breakthrough therapy designation, accelerated approval, and priority review designation—a drug must meet specific requirements. These include that the drug must (1) address an unmet medical need, (2) provide benefit over available drug treatments, and (3) be used in the treatment of a serious or life-threatening condition. The breakthrough therapy category that was created as part of FDASIA has, as intended, increased the rate of submission and approval of medications with preliminary studies indicating superior efficacy in treating serious conditions compared to existing treatments. From fiscal year (FY) 2012 through FY 2017, the FDA received 500 applications for breakthrough therapies.[27] Of these, 191 applications were granted, 244 were denied, and 65 were withdrawn from consideration. Although this change has been welcomed by many, others have raised concerns that, even though these pathways do not change the standards of quality for evidence required for drug approval, they do alter the extent of evidence that is necessary to demonstrate efficacy and safety.[28]

Often, expedited drug approvals are based on surrogate markers, with requirements for postmarketing safety evaluations to identify adverse events that either did not appear, or could not be fully characterized, during the drug approval process. Historically, the FDA had been criticized for failure to ensure drug manufacturers' timely and adequate compliance with postmarketing requirements. This was, in part, due to the inability to enforce these requirements. With the 2007 reauthorization of FDAA, the agency secured the authority to require studies and impose sanctions if timelines and goals were not met. However, to date, the impact of this change has been limited. An evaluation comparing the status of postmarketing studies between 2007 and 2011 found that the proportion of pending studies (i.e., those not initiated but not yet behind the agreed-upon schedule) decreased from roughly 57% to 44%.[29] However, the proportion of delayed studies (those behind schedule) doubled from 6.8% in 2007 to 13.5% in 2011. When only those studies included under the 2007 FDAA change were considered, 15% of studies were pending and just over 1% were delayed. To a great extent, the lower percentages for FDAA-required studies reflect the fact that these processes had only recently been initiated (i.e., the timelines for these commitments were likely in initial stages and therefore unlikely to be included in the delayed category).

The recent trend toward shorter time frames for drug approval has been criticized as a significant contributor to drug safety problems, but this perception is misleading because it implies a direct cause-and-effect relationship between shortened average time to drug approval and drug withdrawals or other safety issues. Safety concerns can arise throughout a product's life cycle.[30] An example is aprotinin, an antithrombotic agent that was used in cardiac surgery for 14 years before accumulating reports of increased morbidity and mortality resulted in its voluntary withdrawal from the U.S. market in late 2007.[31]

An FDA assessment of the timing of safety-related actions for 444 new molecular entities (NMEs) approved between 1991 and 2006 demonstrated that regulatory actions occur throughout a product's life cycle.[32] Among drugs that the FDA approved during that time period, 78% were associated with at least one safety-related action and 3% were withdrawn from U.S. market. A subanalysis of drugs approved from 1991 through 1995 (i.e., representing drugs that were marketed for a minimum of 13 years) found that 27% of NMEs underwent changes or additions to boxed warnings, warnings, or precautions sections of the FDA-approved labeling. No drugs in this subgroup were removed from the market. For drugs marketed less than 5 years (i.e., those approved from 2003 through 2006), 44% underwent safety-related labeling changes, and there were no market withdrawals. These data demonstrate that safety actions occur on an ongoing basis and that newer drugs are not necessarily more prone to safety issues. Rather, it is likely that new safety signals are generated throughout the life cycle of a drug.

DRUG SAFETY IN THE LEGAL ENVIRONMENT

Drug safety has been the subject of countless court rulings, with most cases focusing on who is responsible for ensuring the safe use of drug products—pharmaceutical manufacturers, prescribers, other healthcare professionals, or a combination of these entities. A summary of cases involving pharmaceutical manufacturers and pharmacies is provided in Table 1-2.

PHARMACEUTICAL MANUFACTURERS

State and federal courts have commonly found pharmaceutical manufacturers to be the primary entity responsible for drug safety. Historically, there has been substantial litigation against pharmaceutical manufacturers alleging that they hid, misrepresented, or otherwise failed to meet the obligation to inform clinicians and patients regarding known or suspected risks associated with a drug's use. In *Feldman v. Lederle Laboratories* (1984), one of the more unusual cases, the New Jersey Supreme Court ruled in favor of plaintiff Feldman, who claimed that the drug manufacturer failed to provide sufficient information and warnings to physicians about the potential for tooth discoloration associated with its tetracycline product, demeclocycline.[33] Ms. Feldman was prescribed and dispensed samples of the drug by her father, a physician and pharmacist, several times when she was an infant and toddler. The company claimed that at the time Ms. Feldman received demeclocycline, information about this adverse effect was not fully known, and therefore not included in the labeling and prescribing information approved by the FDA. However, abnormalities in tooth development and discoloration associated with tetracycline products had been reported previously in published studies of laboratory animals and children with cystic fibrosis who received high doses. A lower court had found the manufacturer not liable because the company had asked the FDA for guidance on whether to include a warning in the labeling of all of its tetracycline products, but the agency advised against including this information

Table 1-2 Examples of Product and Professional Liability Court Rulings[33-40]

Case Name/Parties Involved	Year of Ruling	Type of Case	Outcome
Feldman v. Lederle Laboratories	1984	Product liability	Reversed a lower court decision and found that the drug manufacturer had a responsibility to provide information and warn about potential adverse effects
Jones v. Irvin and K-Mart	1986	Professional liability	Maintained a lower court decision and found that while the pharmacist has a duty to warn, the prescriber's role as learned intermediary is predominant
Brown v. American Home Products Corporation Diet Drugs	2000	Product liability	Approved a class-action settlement after finding that the manufacturer had failed to disclose information about serious adverse effects
Warner Lambert v. Kent	2008	Product liability	Upheld a lower court decision allowing an exemption for patients to sue drug manufacturers for punitive damages, even in the absence of evidence of fraud
Wyeth v. Levine	2009	Product liability	Upheld lower court decisions that awarded damages to a patient after finding that the drug manufacturer failed to provide adequate warning in product labeling about the danger associated with a specific route of administration
Eli Lilly Company v. United States Department of Justice	2009	Product liability and marketing practices	Drug manufacturer pled guilty and agreed to a settlement to redress costs incurred by state and federal public insurers associated with off-label marketing of a drug product that resulted in patient harm
Oleckna v. Daytona Discount Pharmacy	2015	Professional liability	Reversed a lower court decision, and found that a pharmacist's duty extends beyond due and proper care in filling a prescription

in demeclocycline labeling based on a lack of sufficient evidence. However, the state supreme court disagreed with the lower court's decision, noting that the FDA's response did not prevent the manufacturer from providing this information or relieve the company of its responsibility to do so. There are several unusual circumstances in this case, including uncertainty as to whether Ms. Feldman received demeclocycline or another tetracycline. Because samples were used, no prescription or dispensing records were available to confirm the plaintiff's assertion. In addition, most product liability cases include the manufacturer and prescriber as litigants, but in this instance, legal action was directed only toward the drug manufacturer, not the prescriber (the patient's father).

In *Brown v. American Home Products Corporation Diet Drugs*, the federal courts approved a negotiated settlement in the class-action product liability case of fenfluramine–phentermine ("fen-phen") or dexfenfluramine with phenteramine.[34] The class-action lawsuit found that product manufacturers for fenfluramine (marketed as Pondomin by American Home Products, Inc.) and dexfenfluramine (marketed as Redux by Wyeth) possessed extensive information, including published case reports, animal studies, case reports in patients taking drugs with similar effects on serotonin, and unpublished studies conducted by the manufacturer, showing that the drugs could cause damage to heart valves and lead to valvular regurgitation. The court found that despite having this information, the manufacturer continued to market the drug combination until the drugs were withdrawn from the market in 1997, without further investigating these reports or warning prescribers or patients through labeling or other mechanisms. The settlement created a $2.5 billion fund to compensate patients for harm and cover current and future associated healthcare costs based on factors such as length of therapy and extent of harm.

A 2001 U.S. Supreme Court case ruled that patients cannot sue pharmaceutical companies for withholding information during the drug approval process in instances in which the FDA has found no evidence of fraud or failure to disclose information. However, in *Warner Lambert v. Kent*, a split decision by that court upheld a lower court decision allowing an exemption in Michigan law that permitted patients who had received troglitazone to sue the product manufacturers for punitive damages by alleging fraud, even in instances when the FDA did not allege or find evidence of fraud.[35] Similar exemptions exist in seven other states.

A U.S. Supreme Court decision in March 2009 set a precedent that may affect future cases that involve how pharmaceutical manufacturers view and operationalize their duty to warn of significant adverse drug events in product labeling. In *Wyeth v. Levine*, the court upheld a state trial and supreme court decision that awarded damages to a Vermont woman whose arm was amputated because of gangrene that developed following administration of promethazine by intravenous (IV) push.[36] The product's FDA-approved labeling included information on the preferred route of administration (deep intramuscular injection), warnings about the potential for gangrene (especially with intraarterial or subcutaneous administration), and a preference for administration via continuous IV infusion rather than rapid push when the drug is administered via IV. However, the trial court found that the patient's injuries would not have occurred if the product's labeling included adequate warning, including specific information about the danger of IV push administration. The U.S. Supreme Court agreed with the trial court and disagreed with the pharmaceutical manufacturer's argument that it was protected from state law claims because of federal labeling requirements and the FDA's approval of the existing product's label. In general, those requirements allow a manufacturer to change labeling only following FDA approval of the proposed change. However, the court noted that the manufacturer could have strengthened the safety warning through the "Changes Being Affected" regulation, which allows labeling changes that improve safety while the manufacturer is in the process of seeking the FDA's official approval of that change. In issuing its decision, the court emphasized that the pharmaceutical manufacturer, not the FDA, is ultimately responsible for the accuracy and completeness of the product labeling and that the FDA's regulatory authority is intended to be complementary to, not pre-emptive of, a state's role in drug safety. This decision may have a far-reaching impact on other ongoing product liability cases.

In 2009, Eli Lilly, manufacturers of the drug olanzapine (Zyprexa), pled guilty to misdemeanor criminal charges of promoting the drug for off-label use brought by the U.S. Department of Justice.[37] The settlement of $1.415 billion, included a criminal fine of $515 million and up to $800 million to settle civil lawsuits with the federal government and the states to redress costs associated with off-label promotion that resulted in payments from Medicaid and federal programs for unapproved uses, including dementia and psychosis associated with Alzheimer disease in assisted-living nursing home residents. This amount was in addition to state-based consumer protection lawsuits that were resolved in 2008, when Lilly agreed to pay $62 million to 33 states.

PHARMACISTS' AND OTHER CLINICIANS' DUTY TO WARN

According to the National Association of Chain Drug Stores, as of March 2015 there have been approximately 125 state and federal lawsuits involving the pharmacist's duty to warn.[38] The majority of these cases have found that pharmacists are not liable for patient harm resulting from adverse drug events or drug-induced disease. These decisions are generally based on the learned intermediary doctrine, which assigns responsibility for drug selection to the prescriber based on his or her knowledge of the drug and the individual patient. Pharmacists have generally been considered "sellers" of the drug product or service, and the courts have considered dispensing to be an extension of the physicians' order. Several decisions have noted that if pharmacists' liability was permitted, it could undermine the physician–patient relationship by calling prescribers' authority into question.[41] Based on existing case law, it is unclear how the learned intermediary doctrine would be applied to pharmacists who select drug therapy under collaborative practice agreements or with the significant expansion of information that would be available to pharmacists from proposed national or universal electronic health records. In *Jones v. Irvin and K-Mart*, the plaintiff appellate argued that the practice of pharmacy had changed dramatically, that the pharmacist had greater knowledge of the dangers associated with drugs than physicians and, therefore, the pharmacists' duty to warn warranted new consideration. The court found that while this advanced knowledge may be true, the physician's role as learned intermediary is predominant.[39] However, in *Oleckna v. Daytona Discount Pharmacy* in 2015, Florida's 5th circuit court of appeals reversed a lower court ruling that a pharmacist could not be held negligent for a death that occurred after a patient overdosed on a combination of opioids and alprazolam.[40] The plaintiff asserted that the pharmacist allowed the patient to repeatedly receive refills before the supply of drug from previous prescriptions was exhausted. In allowing a civil lawsuit to proceed, the court stated, "We refuse to interpret a pharmacist's duty to use 'due and proper care in filling the prescription' as being satisfied by 'robotic compliance' with the instructions of the prescribing physician." These two cases highlight the fact that courts are beginning to take a more expansive view of the pharmacist's role.

Although the learned intermediary principle has frequently shielded pharmacists and their employers from liability, it negatively affects efforts to establish pharmacists as medication experts and independent practitioners. Most importantly, pharmacists have a professional obligation to ensure safe care, regardless of legal liability. Patient education, including risk communication, is a significant component of the commitment that all pharmacists make through their education, licensure, and subsequent practice.

THE DRUG APPROVAL PROCESS AND OTHER FACTORS THAT AFFECT DRUG-INDUCED DISEASE

The drug approval process is expected to assess the efficacy and, to a certain extent, the safety of new drug products, but it should be noted that several characteristics of that process and the subsequent environment of drug use contribute to drug-induced disease. Patient populations in preapproval clinical trials are, by necessity, narrowly structured and defined. Strict inclusion and exclusion criteria often exclude patients with multiple diseases and advanced disease and patients of a certain sex, age, or race. Even the largest clinical trial conducted across multiple study sites evaluates a drug's use in a number of patients that is small in comparison with that following broader use of the drug postapproval—use that includes individuals with characteristics not studied during the approval process.

Drug-induced disease can also be attributed to conditions of drug use postapproval, which can differ dramatically from established conditions in clinical studies. An evaluation that linked outpatient dispensing and diagnosis information for 160 commonly prescribed drugs found that 21% of drug use was for off-label indications (i.e., did not match indications listed in the FDA-approved labeling).[42] Further, 73% of this off-label use was considered to be based on little or no scientific evidence. Subtle changes in manufacturing processes can also contribute to drug-induced diseases. For example, between 1998 and 2001, there was a dramatic increase in the number of pure red-cell aplasia (PRCA) cases in patients with chronic kidney disease.[43,44] PRCA is a known, but very rare, adverse effect that can occur when antierythropoietin antibodies form in response to erythropoietin treatment. Most events occurred in patients treated with an erythropoietin product supplied by one manufacturer, but cases also occurred in patients treated with a similar product. On further analyses, the dramatic increase in adverse events was attributed to a change in the stabilizers in one manufacturer's product and subsequent storage, handling, and subcutaneous administration of that product. Education regarding proper use of the various formulations resulted in a significant decrease in the number of PRCA cases.

Product contamination has also resulted in significant morbidity and mortality. One example is the case of serious adverse events associated with heparin that occurred from November

2007 through February 2008.[8,45] Adverse events included 62 deaths, with other reports of patients experiencing allergic symptoms or symptomatic hypotension. Voluntary product recalls occurred when a pattern of serious events was determined. The adverse drug events were later linked to the presence of oversulfated chondroitin sulfate in the active pharmaceutical ingredient from an overseas plant that processed heparin from pig intestines. The contaminant was not detected in random sampling of manufacturing plants, in part because it mimics heparin in commonly used tests. FDA-conducted follow-up tests found that the contaminant accounted for 5–20% of the total mass of each sample tested. It was alleged that the contamination with chondroitin was a purposeful act.[46] Plans to increase overseas inspections and to modify current standards for assessing the purity of heparin were also announced. This incident illustrated the importance of oversight and inspection of the complete product development process, including assessment of the raw materials. It also noted that even in a more robust system of inspections, purposeful adulteration may occur at any time by unscrupulous suppliers of raw materials and manufacturers, as well as criminal acts by private citizens, as occurred with acetaminophen adulteration in the early 1980s. Since passage of FDASIA, the FDA has taken substantial steps to improve the safety of an increasing global supply chain, including clarifying the agency's inspection authority and increasing penalties for adulterated and counterfeit drugs.[14]

RECOMMENDATIONS TO IMPROVE DRUG SAFETY

In recent years, a number of public and private entities have assessed drug safety efforts in the United States and made recommendations for improvements. Many of these recommendations, such as development of a national database for enhanced collection and assessment of reports of adverse drug events and drug-induced diseases, were included in PDUFA IV, and their implementation is complete or well underway. The following describes major reports and the current status of their recommendations.

NATIONAL ACADEMY OF MEDICINE

In its landmark 2006 report, *The Future of Drug Safety: Promoting and Protecting the Health of the Public*, the National Academy of Medicine (formerly the Institute of Medicine) issued more than two dozen recommendations to improve drug safety.[47] The report, which focused on postmarketing safety, identified structural and procedural barriers at the FDA that hampered efforts to enhance drug safety. The report stated that preapproval data are inherently limited in their ability to identify infrequent adverse events and that existing approaches for data collection following drug approval are not adequate to address this shortcoming. The report's authors called for increased proactive postmarketing surveillance by the FDA, as well as additional authority for the FDA to control manufacturers' postapproval marketing activities. Many of the academy's recommendations, including strengthened authority to require REMS, were included in PDUFA IV. Strategies to better inform the public, such as establishment of an advisory committee to address communication of risks, have also been implemented. However, the recommendation to prevent potential harm by restricting direct-to-consumer advertising for a period of 2 years following drug approval and requiring that labeling and marketing materials for these products contain a symbol to designate the recent approval status, were controversial and not addressed in the reauthorization of the legislation. Other National Academy of Medicine reports, including *Preventing Medication Errors* (2006) and *Knowing What Works in Health Care: A Roadmap for the Nation* (2008), have also addressed drug safety.[3,48] Although these reports focus on the broader context of avoidable harm from drug therapies and comparative effectiveness, respectively, they include components on drug-induced disease and postmarketing safety surveillance.

GOVERNMENT ACCOUNTABILITY OFFICE

In 2006, the Government Accountability Office (GAO) issued the report, *Drug Safety: Improvement Needed in FDA's Postmarket Decision-Making and Oversight Process*, which evaluated drug safety processes based on an assessment of regulatory actions for four drugs: leflunomide (Arava), cerivastatin (Baycol), valdecoxib (Bextra), and cisapride (Propulsid).[1] Leflunomide remains available in the United States, but the other drugs were withdrawn voluntarily from the U.S. market following several safety assessments by FDA staff and subsequent regulatory actions. A major finding in the GAO report was instances in which divisions within FDA's Center for Drug Evaluation and Research (CDER) made conflicting recommendations. As a result, decisions were either not made or were made counter to the recommendations of another FDA group without a clear process for resolving the disparate views.

The GAO identified a lack of collaboration and communication between what were then the two predominant offices involved in drug safety—the Office of New Drugs (OND), which is responsible for drug approval and for initiating regulatory actions, and the Office of Drug Safety (ODS), which predominantly focused on postmarketing safety. The GAO described the ODS as serving in an advisory capacity to the OND, based on its finding that the ODS had no authority to initiate a regulatory action. The report identified a lack of documented processes for decision-making, including an absence of criteria to determine the appropriate regulatory action when a safety concern is identified.

Since that time, significant progress has been made to address shortcomings identified in the GAO report, including consolidation of safety efforts under the Office of Surveillance and Epidemiology, which is charged with identifying drug safety concerns and recommending actions to improve product safety and protect the public health.[49] In 2007, the CDER launched the Document Archiving, Reporting, and Regulatory Tracking System (DARRTS) system, which facilitates sharing of information about drugs with significant safety concerns across the numerous divisions within the agency.[50] In 2012, the agency also proposed a framework for prioritizing drugs that are tracked in DARRTS. Once identified, FDA staff designate the concern as standard, priority, or emergency based on an assessment of factors that include the size of the population affected and the theoretical frequency of harm. Modulating factors, including the extent and quality of evidence indicating a potential harm and the availability of alternative treatments are also considered. With this work, the FDA has taken substantial steps to address the concerns highlighted in the GAO report that focus on the lack of criteria and processes. However, it should be noted that risk assessment and decisions about drug safety are not an exact science and require careful balancing of the advantages and disadvantages of providing continued availability of a drug, which is based on evidence that, by nature, is constantly evolving.

OFFICE OF THE INSPECTOR GENERAL

In 2013, the Office of the Inspector General (OIG) for the Department of Health and Human Services completed an assessment of the effectiveness of REMS and issued seven recommendations to address shortcomings identified in the agency's processes to monitor these programs.[51] The study, which reviewed drug manufacturers' submission and subsequent FDA assessment of 49 of the 99 REMS that were in place in 2012, found that the FDA determined nearly half of the submissions were incomplete. Further, only seven of the submissions that were reviewed met all goals established by the FDA, according to the agency's own assessment of submitted reports. A common reason for failing to meet established goals was a documented lack of patient or prescriber awareness of potential harm. In other instances, the FDA assessment found that information was lacking to determine if this goal was met either because surveys were not conducted or due to shortcomings in survey design or implementation (e.g., small sample size, patient selection not representative of the target population). The OIG recommendations included developing plans to assess and validate REMS assessments submitted by manufacturers, identify incomplete sponsor submissions and work with sponsors to clarify expectations and ensure timely submissions, and take steps to ensure safety in instances where REMS are not meeting established goals. The OIG also recommended that the agency seek legislative authority to enforce FDA assessment plans. At the time this report was issued, some OIG-recommended improvements were already underway as part of the FDA's REMS Integration Initiative.[52] This initiative, which was introduced in 2011, includes a goal of improving the standardization and assessment of REMS.

FDA

In addition to the activities described above, the FDA has also assessed existing processes and taken numerous steps to enhance drug safety. In late 2007, the FDA's Science Board Subcommittee on Science and Technology published a document entitled, *FDA Science and Mission at Risk: Report of the Subcommittee on Science and Technology*.[53] The report was requested by then Commissioner Andrew von Eschenbach to review the adequacy of the agency's science and technology resources to meet current and future challenges. The report concluded that the agency's resources had diminished, despite an increase in responsibilities that resulted from the speed of scientific discoveries, increased and more complex products, and the increasingly global nature of the pharmaceutical industry. The subcommittee recommended that the existing deficits in scientific research programs; recruitment, development, and retention of expert staff; and information technology must be corrected to meet these challenges.

Among the report's specific recommendations was the need to strengthen and coordinate the science program across the FDA's centers. The need for collaboration was identified with external scientific and research programs, including the Agency for Healthcare Research and Quality's Centers for Education and Research on Therapeutics, the CDC, the National Institutes of Health, and others when the expertise is not available at the FDA. It is anticipated that the Reagan–Udall Foundation, an independent not-for-profit organization mandated by PDUFA IV, will assist in the development of these and other public–private partnerships as part of its charge to assist the FDA in modernizing its activities to address the rapid pace of change in the scientific and regulatory environments.

Other recommendations in the report include broadening staff with the statistical and epidemiologic expertise needed to analyze collected data as well as staff with expertise in risk assessment and its quantitative measurement. A major focus of the report was the need to establish information standards that permit sharing and aggregation of information from public and private postmarketing safety surveillance databases. The report noted that these standards were critical, especially with the establishment of new sciences, including pharmacogenetics, nanotechnology, and cell-based products, for which collection of the necessary extent and types of data will not be supported by current systems.

In terms of funding these improvements, the report stated that appropriation provided by PDUFA IV supplied only a small portion of what was needed. The Science Board called for a 2009 budget to address the identified shortcomings and directed the FDA Commissioner to develop an action plan to implement the report's recommendations. Calls to increase FDA funding are echoed by healthcare professionals, research, and consumer sectors through entities such as the Alliance for a Stronger FDA.[54] The Alliance, whose members include former Secretaries of the Department of Health and Human Services and Commissioners of the FDA, aims to build awareness regarding current deficits in funding and advocate for increased federal appropriations to reduce the FDA's reliance on user fees paid by drug manufacturers.

In 2009, the FDA launched the Safe Use Initiative which functions as a partnership with external public and private stakeholders with the stated goal of reducing preventable harm from medications.[55] This collaborative group identifies specific areas of focus or cases where there is demonstrated harm, and then works with partners to develop and implement interventions to reduce this harm. Since launching, initiative projects have addressed many high-impact issues, such as safety concerns associated with acetaminophen and opioids, as well as the use of atypical antipsychotics in pediatric populations.[56]

Other FDA efforts to enhance drug safety have included improved guidance to industry on premarketing risk assessment, development and use of risk-minimization action plans, and pharmacovigilance and pharmacoepidemiologic assessment.[57-59]

Consumer awareness and education has also been a major focus, including new regulations that require inclusion of MedWatch reporting information on drug packaging and patient information leaflets for prescription and nonprescription drugs and in direct-to-consumer television advertising.[60-62]

IMPROVING DATA COLLECTION AND USE

At the core of efforts to improve drug safety, there is reliance on the extent and quality of information used to inform these decisions. Safety information gained from premarketing as well as postmarketing studies is often described as data that are unreported, underreported, and unpublished. The International Committee of Medical Journal Editors Uniform Requirements for Manuscripts Submitted to Biomedical Journals requirement that researchers register human subjects research on the website www.clincialtrials.gov as a condition of publication and the editor's obligation to publish negative studies represent the combined efforts of regulatory and private entities to address these shortcomings.[63]

Other efforts have focused on developing standards for reporting drug-induced diseases and other adverse drug events. The Consolidated Standards of Reporting Trials (CONSORT), in "Better Reporting of Harms in Randomized Trials: An Extension of the CONSORT Statement," recommends the use of standardized terminology and inclusion of harms information in the publication abstract as mechanisms to assist clinicians, researchers, and patients in the critical appraisal of clinical trial results.[64] Public and private collaborations to improve active surveillance, including data mining in large population-based databases, are described in Chapter 4.

DRUG SAFETY CHALLENGES AND OPPORTUNITIES

As noted in the FDA Science Board report, the rapid rate of new drug development, the evolving role of evidence-based medicine, and advancing science and technology offer ongoing and new challenges to our nation's drug safety system. Novel first-in-class drugs, nanotechnology, cell-based therapies, large-molecule biologics, and biosimilars are among many challenges in assessing and ensuring postmarketing drug safety.

Pharmacogenomics and personalized drug therapy have the potential to improve the prediction and prevention of drug-induced disease from the perspective of both individual patients and entire populations. One of the earliest known genetic variations to result in drug-induced disease is glucose-6-phosphate dehydrogenase deficiency, which results in the destruction of red blood cells when a person is exposed to certain drugs (e.g., antimalarial agents, aspirin, nonsteroidal anti-inflammatory drugs, quinidine, quinine, and sulfonamide antibiotics). More recent discoveries include variations in the organic anion transporter *SLCO1B1*, which are associated with an increased risk of statin-induced myopathy.[65]

Many factors contribute to genetic variation in response to drug therapy. Polymorphisms, which can be affected by the interplay of more than one genetic variation, may lead to differences in drug disposition, including absorption, distribution, and excretion.[66] These differences can lead to decreased or increased pharmacologic effect, with the latter more frequently resulting in toxicity or undesired drug effects. Genetic differences in drug transporters also play a role in response to drug therapies. Examples of drugs, genetic variables, and the proposed associated adverse drug event are described in Table 1-3.[66,67]

Some genetic polymorphisms are more common in certain racial groups; therefore, ethnicity has been used to predict drug response in the absence of more specific genetic information for an individual patient.[68] For example, the relative risk of angioedema or cough associated with the use of angiotensin-converting enzyme (ACE) inhibitors has been estimated at 3 and 2.7 for blacks and East Asians, respectively, as compared with whites. Other studies, including the Gruppo Italiano per lo Studio della Sopravvivenza nell'Infarto Miocardico (GISSI)-1 trial found that intracranial hemorrhage or moderate-to-severe bleeding following thrombolytic therapy was more common in

Table 1-3 Examples of Drug-Induced Diseases Associated with Genetic Variability[66,67]

Drug	Genetic Variation	Adverse Drug Event or Drug-Induced Disease
Abacavir	*HLA*	Hypersensitivity reaction
ACE inhibitors	Bradykinin B_2 receptor	ACE inhibitor-induced cough and angioedema
Carbamazepine	*HLA-B*1502* allele	Stevens–Johnson syndrome, toxic epidermal necrolysis
Cisplatin, carboplatin, and oxaliplatin	Changes in gene expression in the dorsal-root ganglia resulting in apoptosis (*Cdkn1a, Ckap2, Bid3, S100a8, S100a9*), inflammation (*S100a8, S100a9, Cd163, Mmp9*), and nerve growth and regeneration (*Mmp9, Gfap*)	Peripheral neurotoxicity
Digoxin	P glycoprotein *3435TT* genotype	Increased drug accumulation and potential for digoxin toxicity
Mercaptopurine	Thiopurine methyltransferase polymorphism	Hematopoietic toxicity
Oral contraceptives	Variation in prothrombin and factor V	Increased risk of DVT or cerebral vascular thrombosis
Trimethoprim–sulfamethoxazole, clarithromycin, quinidine	*KCNE2* variants in potassium channels	QT interval prolongation, morbidity, and mortality

ACE = angiotensin-converting enzyme, DVT = deep vein thrombosis, HLA = human leukocyte antigen.

black patients.[24,69] Although these and other studies give credence to ethnicity as a determinant of adverse events, shortcomings in the data, including inconsistent definitions and reporting of ethnicity and adverse events, limit its application to clinical practice. Most drug-induced diseases, including ACE-inhibitor–induced cough, have been theorized as a complex interaction of ethnic and other factors such as age, sex, and comorbid disease.[70] When considered in total, these predictive factors can be used to improve drug safety by guiding drug selection and monitoring.

The inclusion of genetic biomarker information and its clinical application in FDA-approved drug labeling is becoming more common. In 2013, the FDA issued guidance to assist manufacturers in applying pharmacogenomics in premarket clinical studies and in labeling decisions.[71] An evaluation of ten drugs previously withdrawn from the market determined that the severe adverse effects that led to this action could all be attributed to genetic variation.[72] The authors concluded that with proper patient selection and monitoring these drugs could have remained on the market. Despite the promise of pharmacogenomics, currently there is no requirement that pharmaceutical manufacturers complete genetic studies. Further, whether these studies are voluntary or required, more research (including practical clinical trials) and better systems for collecting and analyzing these data are needed. Even with improved data, uncertainties will remain regarding the extent to which genetics affects drug response and the interplay of genetics with other variables, including concomitant therapies, diet, and other patient variables. At present, the clinical significance of genetic variation and genetic testing in drug safety and effectiveness are much debated.

As the regulatory and legal environments evolve, clinicians will continue to play a central role in improving drug safety and preventing drug-induced disease. The identification and management of adverse effects, participation in spontaneous reporting efforts, and provision of patient education that addresses both the risk and benefit of therapies are critical and core clinician responsibilities. As illustrated by the example of thalidomide, drugs with significant safety concerns can provide great health benefits when properly managed. Medication-therapy management and other care provided by pharmacists are essential components of the drug safety system.

REFERENCES

1. General Accounting Office. Drug safety: improvement needed in FDA's postmarket decision-making and oversight process. GAO-06-402. http://www.gao.gov/new.items/d06402.pdf (accessed 2018 Jan 4).
2. Cheng CM, Shin J, Guglielmo J. Trends in boxed warnings and withdrawals for novel therapeutic drugs, 1996 through 2012. *JAMA Intern Med.* 2014; 174:1704-5.
3. Institute of Medicine. *Preventing medication errors.* Washington, DC: National Academies Press; 2006.
4. Consumers Union. Consumer reports poll finds high levels of concern about medical harm and support for public ratings on hospital safety. http://safepatientproject.org/press_release/consumer_reports_poll_finds_high_levels_of_concern_about_medical_harm__support_for_public_ratings_on_hospital_safety (accessed 2018 Jan 4).
5. Harpaz R, DuMouchel W, LePendu P et al. Performance of pharmacovigilance signal detection algorithms for the FDA Adverse Event Reporting System. *Clin Pharmacol Ther.* 2013; 93:10.1038/clpt.2013.24.
6. US Food and Drug Administration. Drug Safety Oversight Board. http://www.fda.gov/AboutFDA/CentersOffices/OfficeofMedicalProductsandTobacco/CDER/ucm082129.htm (accessed 2018 Jan 4).
7. Heinrich J. Adverse drug events: substantial problem but magnitude uncertain. Testimony before the Committee on Health, Education, Labor, and Pensions, US Senate. United States General Accounting Office (US GAO). http://www.gao.gov/new.items/he00053t.pdf (accessed 2018 Jan 4).
8. US Food and Drug Administration. FDA media briefing on heparin; April 21, 2008 (transcript). https://wayback.archive-it.org/7993/20170406155133/http://www.fda.gov/bbs/transcripts/2008/heparin_transcript_042108.pdf (accessed 2018 Jan 4).
9. Swann JP. History of the FDA. In: Kurian G, ed. *The historical guide to American government.* New York, NY: Oxford University Press; 1998.
10. 110th Congress. *Food and Drug Administration Amendments Act of 2007, Public law* 110-85. September 27, 2007.
11. US Food and Drug Administration. PDUFA fact sheet. https://wayback.archive-it.org/7993/20171105040618/https://www.fda.gov/ForIndustry/UserFees/PrescriptionDrugUserFee/ucm119175.htm (accessed 2018 Jan 4).
12. US Food and Drug Administration. PDUFA IV five year plan, March 2008. https://www.fda.gov/downloads/ForIndustry/UserFees/PrescriptionDrugUserFee/UCM332680.pdf (accessed 2018 Jan 4).
13. US Food and Drug Administration. PDUFA reauthorization performance goals and procedures fiscal years 2013 through 2017. http://www.fda.gov/downloads/ForIndustry/UserFees/Prescription DrugUserFee/UCM270412.pdf (accessed 2018 Jan 4).
14. US Food and Drug Administration. Regulatory Information. Food and Drug Administration Safety and Innovation Act (FDASIA. https://wayback.archive-it.org/7993/20170404011306/https://www.fda.gov/RegulatoryInformation/LawsEnforcedbyFDA/SignificantAmendmentstotheFDCAct/FDASIA/default.htm (accessed 2018 Jan 4).
15. US Food and Drug Administration. Potential signals of serious risks/new safety information identified from the Adverse Event Reporting System (AERS). http://www.fda.gov/cder/aers/potential_signals/default.htm (accessed 2018 Jan 4).
16. Thompson CA. 'Dear Healthcare Professional' letters may not be effective REMS communication tool. http://www.ajhp.org/content/71/3/177?sso-checked=true (accessed 2018 Jan 4).
17. Levine G. Communication Experts Call on FDA To Improve Message Delivery. *Am J Health-Syst Pharm.* 2008; 65:1791-2.
18. US Food and Drug Administration. Questions and answers: FDA approves a risk evaluation and mitigation strategy (REMS) for extended-release and long-acting (ER/LA) opioid analgesics. http://www.fda.gov/Drugs/DrugSafety/InformationbyDrugClass/ucm309742.htm (accessed 2018 Jan 4).
19. Centers for Disease Control and Prevention. Prescription painkiller overdoses in the US. http://www.cdc.gov/vitalsigns/PainkillerOverdoses/index.html (accessed 2018 Jan 4).
20. Centers for Disease Control and Prevention. Number and age-adjusted rates of drug-poisoning deaths involving opioid analgesics and heroin: United States, 2000–2014. http://www.cdc.gov/nchs/data/health_policy/AADR_drug_poisoning_involving_OA_Heroin_US_2000-2014.pdf (accessed 2018 Jan 4).
21. CNN. Super Bowl drug ad spurs big backlash. http://money.cnn.com/2016/02/11/news/super-bowl-painkiller-constipation-ad/ (accessed 2018 Jan 4).
22. US Food and Drug Administration. FDA announces enhanced warnings for immediate-release opioid pain medications related to risks of misuse, abuse, addiction, overdose and death. https://www.fda.gov/newsevents/newsroom/pressannouncements/ucm491739.htm (accessed 2018 Jan 4).
23. Thalidomide prescribing information. Summit, NJ: Celgene Corporation; 2007.
24. McEvoy GK, ed. *AHFS drug information* 2016. Bethesda, MD: American Society of Health-System Pharmacists; 2016.
25. American Society of Health-System Pharmacists. PDUFA reauthorization: opportunity to improve continuity of care for patients treated with high-risk drugs. https://www.ashp.org/-/media/assets/advocacy-issues/docs/gad-pdufa-reauthorization-improve-continuity-of-care.ashx (accessed 2018 Feb 26).
26. US Food and Drug Administration. Guidance for industry: expedited programs for serious conditions—drugs and biologics. http://www.fda.gov/downloads/drugs/guidancecomplianceregulatoryinformation/guidances/ucm358301.pdf (accessed 2018 Jan 4).
27. US Food and Drug Administration. CDER breakthrough therapy designation requests received by fiscal year. http://www.fda.gov/downloads/Drugs/DevelopmentApprovalProcess/HowDrugsareDevelopedandApproved/DrugandBiologicApprovalReports/INDActivityReports/UCM481540.pdf (accessed 2018 Jan 4).
28. Darrow JJ, Avorn J, Kesselheim AS. New FDA breakthrough-drug category—implications for patients. *N Engl J Med.* 2014; 370: 1252-8.
29. Fain K, Daubresse M, Alexander GC. The Food and Drug Administration Amendments Act and postmarketing commitments. *JAMA.* 2013;310:202-4.
30. Lasser KE, Allen PD, Woolhandler SJ et al. Timing of new black box warnings and withdrawals for prescription medications. *JAMA.* 2002;287:2215-20.
31. FDA News. FDA requests marketing suspension of Trasylol. http://www.fda.gov/bbs/topics/NEWS/2007/NEW01738.html (accessed 2018 Jan 4).
32. US Food and Drug Administration. Maximizing the public health benefit of adverse event collection throughout a product's marketed life cycle. FDA Public Workshop, January 29, 2008.
33. Medical and Public Health Law Site (MPHLS), Louisiana State University. *Feldman v. Lederle Laboratories*, 479 A.2d 374 (N.J. 1984). https://law.justia.com/cases/new-jersey/supreme-court/1984/97-n-j-429-0.html (accessed 2018 Jan 4).
34. MPHLS, Louisiana State University. *Brown v. American Home Products Corporation Diet Drugs*, No. 99-20593 (E.D.Pa. 08/28/2000). http://biotech.law.lsu.edu/cases/Drugs/brown_v_AHPC_brief.htm (accessed 2018 Jan 4).
35. *Warner-Lambert Co. v. Kent.* No 06-1498, 552 US, 2008 WL 552875 (2008).
36. *Wyeth v. Levine.* 555 US 06-1249 (2009).
37. US Department of Justice. Eli Lilly and Company agrees to pay $1.415 billion to resolve allegations of off-label promotion of Zyprexa. https://www.justice.gov/archive/opa/pr/2009/January/09-civ-038.html (accessed 2018 Jan 4).
38. National Association of Chain Drug Stores. Pharmacists' duty to warn: lawsuits claiming that pharmacies must warn consumers about dangers associated with prescription drugs, revised 10/21/08. http://www.nacds.org/pdfs/membership/duty_to_warn.pdf (accessed 2018 Jan 4).

39. *Jones v. Irvin and K-Mart.* 602 F.Supp. 399. (S.D. Ill. 1985).
40. *Oleckna v. Daytona Discount Pharmacy.* 162 So. 3d 178, 181-82 (Fla. 5th DCA 2015).
41. Beck J, Vale A. *Drug and medical device product liability deskbook (litigation series).* New York: Law Journal Press; 2004.
42. Radley DC, Finkelstein SN, Stafford RS. Off-label prescribing among office-based physicians. *Arch Intern Med.* 2006; 166:1021-6.
43. Bennett CL, Luminari S, Nissenson AR et al. Pure red-cell aplasia and epoetin therapy. *N Engl J Med.* 2004; 351:1403-8.
44. Cournoyer D, Toffelmire EB, Wells GA et al. Antierythropoietin antibody-mediated pure red cell aplasia after treatment with recombinant erythropoietin products: recommendations for minimization of risk. *J Am Soc Nephrol.* 2004; 15:2728-34.
45. US Food and Drug Administration. *Information on adverse event reports and heparin.* https://wayback.archive-it.org/7993/20170723181527/https://www.fda.gov/Drugs/DrugSafety/PostmarketDrugSafetyInformationforPatientsandProviders/UCM112669 (accessed 2018 Jan 4).
46. United States House of Representatives Subcommittee on Oversight and Investigations, Committee on Energy and Commerce. Transcript of testimony of Janet Woodcock, Director, Center for Drug Evaluation and Research. http://docs.house.gov/meetings/IF/IF14/20170913/106396/HHRG-115-IF14-Wstate-WoodcockJ-20170913.pdf (accessed 2018 Jan 4).
47. Institute of Medicine. *The future of drug safety: promoting and protecting the health of the public.* Washington, DC: National Academies Press; 2006.
48. Institute of Medicine. *Knowing what works in health care: a roadmap for the nation.* Washington, DC: National Academies Press; 2008:31b.
49. US Food and Drug Administration. Office of Surveillance and Epidemiology (OSE). http://www.fda.gov/AboutFDA/CentersOffices/OfficeofMedicalProductsandTobacco/CDER/ucm106491.htm (accessed 2018 Jan 4).
50. US Food and Drug Administration. Guidance: classifying significant postmarketing drug safety issues. http://www.fda.gov/downloads/Drugs/GuidanceComplianceRegulatoryInformation/Guidances/UCM295211.pdf (accessed 2018 Jan 4).
51. Office of the Inspector General. FDA lacks comprehensive data to determine whether risk evaluation and mitigation strategies improve drug safety. http://oig.hhs.gov/oei/reports/oei-04-11-00510.pdf (accessed 2018 Jan 4).
52. US Food and Drug Administration. REMS integration initiative. http://www.fda.gov/ForIndustry/UserFees/PrescriptionDrugUserFee/ucm350852.htm (accessed 2018 Jan 4).
53. US Food and Drug Administration. FDA science and mission at risk: report of the Subcommittee on Science and Technology. https://www.fda.gov/ohrms/dockets/ac/07/briefing/2007-4329b_02_01_FDA%20Report%20on%20Science%20and%20Technology.pdf (accessed 2018 Jan 4).
54. Alliance for a Stronger FDA. Alliance for a Stronger FDA home page. http://www.strengthenfda.org (accessed 2018 Jul 10).
55. US Food and Drug Administration. FDA's Safe Use Initiative: collaborating to reduce preventable harm from medications. https://www.fda.gov/ohrms/dockets/ac/07/briefing/2007-4329b_02_01_FDA%20Report%20on%20Science%20and%20Technology.pdf (accessed 2018 Jan 4).
56. US Food and Drug Administration. Safe Use Initiative: current projects. http://www.fda.gov/Drugs/DrugSafety/SafeUseInitiative/ucm188762.htm (accessed 2018 Jan 4).
57. US Food and Drug Administration. Guidance for industry: development and use of risk minimization action plans. https://www.fda.gov/ohrms/dockets/ac/05/briefing/2005-4136b1_03_Risk%20Minimization%20Action%20Plans.pdf (accessed 2018 Jan 4).
58. US Food and Drug Administration. Guidance for industry: premarket risk assessment. https://www.fda.gov/downloads/RegulatoryInformation/Guidances/ucm126958.pdf (accessed 2018 Jan 4).
59. US Food and Drug Administration. Guidance for industry: good pharmacovigilance practices and pharmacoepidemiologic assessment. https://www.fda.gov/downloads/Drugs/GuidanceComplianceRegulatoryInformation/Guidances/UCM071696.pdf (accessed 2018 Jan 4).
60. Final rule. Toll-free number for reporting adverse events on labeling for human drug products. *Fed Regist.* 2008;73:63886-63897.
61. Notice: risk communication committee; notice of meeting. *Fed Regist.* 2008;73:22959-22960.
62. Notice: agency information collection activities; proposed collection; comment requested; experimental study: toll-free number for consumer reporting of drug product side effects in direct-to-consumer television advertisements for prescription drugs. *Fed Regist.* 2008;73:72058-62.
63. International Committee of Medical Journal Editors. Uniform requirements for manuscripts submitted to biomedical journals. http://icmje.org/icmje-recommendations.pdf (accessed 2018 Jan 4).
64. Ioannidis JP, Evans SJ, Gøtzsche PC et al. Better reporting of harms in randomized trials: an extension of the CONSORT statement. *Ann Intern Med.* 2004; 141:781-8.
65. Link E, Parish S, Armitage J et al.; SEARCH Collaborative Group. SLCO1B1 variants and statin-induced myopathy—a genomewide study. *N Engl J Med.* 2008; 359:789-99.
66. Evans WE, McLeod HL. Pharmacogenomics—drug disposition, drug targets, and side effects. *N Engl J Med.* 2003; 348:538-49.
67. Alaedini A, Xiang Z, Kim H et al. Up-regulation of apoptosis and regeneration genes in the dorsal root ganglia during cisplatin treatment. *Exp Neurol.* 2008; 210:368-74.
68. McDowell SE, Coleman JJ, Ferner RE. Systematic review and meta-analysis of ethnic differences in risks of adverse reactions to drugs used in cardiovascular medicine. *BMJ.* 2006; 332:1177-81.
69. Bjornsson TD, Wagner JA, Donahue SR et al. A review and assessment of potential sources of ethnic differences in drug responsiveness. *J Clin Pharmacol.* 2003; 43:943-67.
70. Morimoto T, Gandhi TK, Fiskio JM et al. Development and validation of a clinical prediction rule for angiotensin-converting enzyme inhibitor-induced cough. *J Gen Intern Med.* 2004; 19:684-91.
71. US Food and Drug Administration. Clinical pharmacogenomics—premarket evaluation in early-phase clinical studies and recommendations for labeling. https://www.fda.gov/downloads/Drugs/GuidanceComplianceRegulatoryInformation/Guidances/UCM337169.pdf (accessed 2018 Jan 4).
72. Zhang W, Roederer MW, Chen WQ et al. Pharmacogenetics of drugs withdrawn from the market. *Pharmacogenomics.* 2012; 13:223-31.

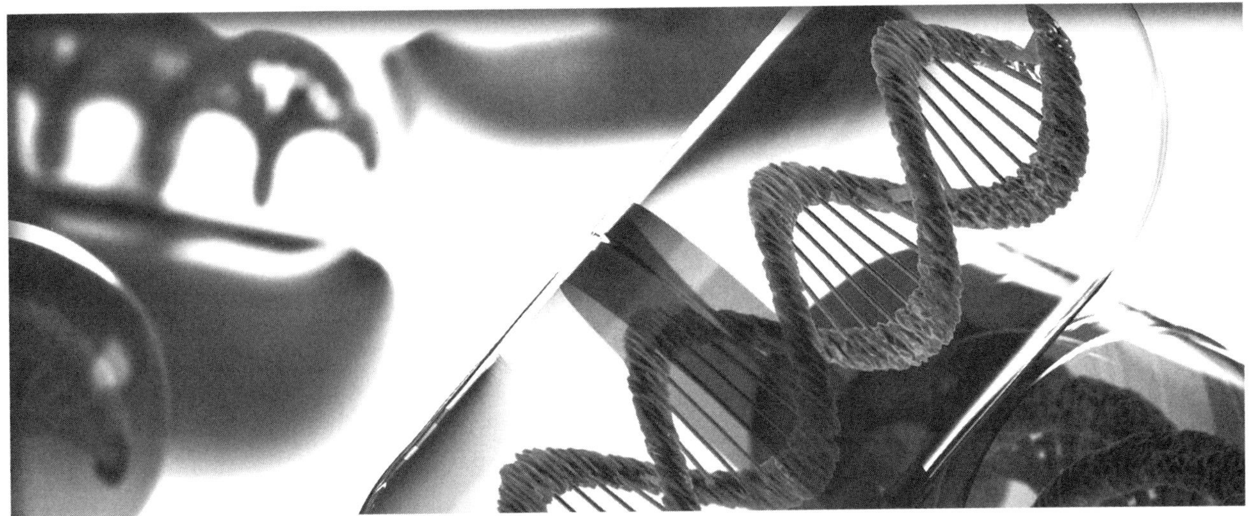

CHAPTER 2

Epidemiology and Public Health Impact of Drug-Induced Diseases

John R. Litaker and James P. Wilson

Medications are an essential component of modern healthcare. Individuals take medications to feel better, overcome illnesses, treat infections, and improve quality of life. Currently, there are thousands of drugs and drug products approved by the U.S. Food and Drug Administration (FDA) available on the American market.[1] Therapeutic benefits associated with prescription and nonprescription medications often imply safety and calculated risks to the general public. However, despite the healing benefits of medications, risks remain that can lead to adverse events and drug-induced diseases. In the seminal report *Preventing Medication Errors* in 2006 the Institute of Medicine acknowledged the seriousness of adverse drug events in hospitals by noting that "[medication] errors are common during all steps of the medication-use process—[from] procuring the drug, prescribing, dispensing, administering, and monitoring the patient's response."[2]

Public assumptions of drug safety may be partially attributable to the FDA's approval and regulatory process. Drugs undergo a rigorous testing and clinical trial process prior to approval to ensure safety and efficacy. Yet some people, including healthcare practitioners, may assume that FDA approval implies absolute safety, despite the fact that there are risks associated with using any medication. Even the FDA recognizes that every approved drug carries some risk and that "for every drug [the] FDA approves, the benefits are balanced against [these] risks."[3] These adverse drug events may be mild or severe depending on the particular product, expected dose, or patient population, and may subsequently manifest as a drug-induced disease.

Medication errors are one cause of drug-induced diseases. In 2000, the Institute of Medicine reported the extent and impact of errors in healthcare in its publication *To Err Is Human*.[4] This report noted that medication errors were "one of the most common types of error" and that substantial numbers of people were affected.[4] Other sources of drug-induced diseases are related to the pharmacologic characteristics of the product itself and do not necessarily involve dispensing or dose errors. Pharmacists and physicians should be keenly aware of the known potential adverse events associated with each drug, because these events are detailed in the product's safety insert. Even well-known products such as aspirin are associated with serious adverse events. Indeed, speculation abounds that aspirin would not meet today's FDA risk-benefit balance because of serious adverse events such as gastrointestinal bleeding.[5]

This chapter focuses on the epidemiology of drug-induced diseases and the impact on both the public's health and the healthcare system. The cost of drug-induced diseases to the healthcare system is also discussed.

OVERVIEW OF EPIDEMIOLOGY

Epidemiology has its historical roots dating back to the philosopher Hippocrates, who, as early as the 4th century B.C., recognized the relationship between disease and environmental, temporal, and geographical factors.[6,7] In more recent times, epidemiology gained considerable attention when John Snow, a physician and epidemiologist, used epidemiologic techniques to identify the source of cholera epidemics in London in the mid-1850s. He mapped the location of each cholera case and noted an association between its geographic location and the company that supplied water to that location. Morbidity and mortality were highest among people who received water from the Southward Company. Further research determined that cholera was spread by contaminated water from this company.

In *A Dictionary of Epidemiology,* John Last defines epidemiology as the "study of the occurrence of disease or other health-related characteristics in human populations,"[8] while Jekel et al.[9] define it as "the study of factors that determine the occurrence and distribution of disease in a population." More specific to drug-induced diseases is the term *pharmacoepidemiology*, which is defined as "the study of the distribution and determinants of drug-related events in populations and the application of this study to efficacious drug treatment."[10] Common to all three definitions is the idea of disease distribution (or diffusion) and disease determinants (or causal factors). Indeed, determining why and how diseases spread from place to place is the essence of epidemiology.

Determining the epidemiology of drug-induced diseases and their impact on the public's health requires a sound methodologic system to establish: (1) the frequency of drug-induced diseases; (2) nonmedical factors contributing to drug-induced diseases; (3) particular medications, doses, and routes of administration associated with drug-induced diseases; (4) the temporal and geographic distribution of drug-induced diseases; and (5) specific patient characteristics associated with drug-induced diseases. Epidemiology and its specific tools are extremely useful and important in understanding drug-induced diseases. Epidemiology provides a scientific and rigorous approach toward answering specific questions and can be used to identify associations, provide strength of evidence, and establish causality. A variety of epidemiologic techniques and research methods are available, including ecologic studies, cohort studies, cross-sectional studies, case–control studies, and randomized, controlled trials. The reader is advised to consult an epidemiology textbook for more detailed explanations of these and other study methods.

LEVELS OF EVIDENCE

Levels of evidence are used to stratify epidemiologic tools according to the strength of influence that these studies may contribute to the decision-making process. The basis for this strength of influence is the study design itself. For example, an experimental-design study will naturally have more influence than a nonexperimental-design study. **Table 2-1** identifies the three levels of evidence, with the associated study type, that are used throughout this book.

However, the reader is cautioned not to rely on the randomized clinical trial as the sole factor in the decision-making process. Each study type has a specific role to play in decision-making, but this role is limited to the type of evidence that the study can provide. In addition, emerging outcomes (whether it is a disease or an adverse drug event) may not readily appear as a problem in its early stages.

Table 2-1 Levels of Evidence for Drug-Induced Diseases Used in This Book

Level of Evidence	Source of Evidence
A	One or more randomized, controlled clinical trial
B	Nonrandomized clinical trials, prospective observational studies, cohort studies, retrospective studies, case–control studies, meta-analyses, and/or postmarketing surveillance studies
C	Evidence from one or more published case reports or case series

In such instances, case reports may be the only source of evidence that such a problem is occurring. A prime example of this is a retrospective review of case reports from the mid-1950s of individuals in Africa, North America, Western Europe, and the Middle East reportedly dying of what was then called a "wasting disease."[11] At the time that the case reports were compiled, blood samples were obtained from the dying individuals and stored. Three decades later, researchers tested these blood samples and found that these individuals were infected with the human immunodeficiency virus.

OVERVIEW OF PUBLIC HEALTH

Public health is concerned with the programs, services, and institutions involved with preventing disease, meeting the health needs of the population, and emphasizing the proper distribution, allocation, and access to health services for all citizens. In England, public health has been defined as "the science and art of preventing disease, prolonging life, and promoting health through organized efforts of society."[12] Public health officials use epidemiology as a tool to help with risk factor analysis, evidence-based policy-setting, and decision analysis.

In addition to epidemiology, biostatistical analyses are used to help public health officials determine the probability and causal relations between drug use and an adverse event. Indeed, biostatistics can help determine at the most basic level whether an occurrence is due to chance alone or to an association with a drug. For example, during the past 10–15 years there has been substantial controversy regarding the administration of the measles, mumps, and rubella (MMR) vaccine in the United Kingdom and the possible link of the vaccination to autism. Biostatistics and epidemiology have been used to determine whether autism is more or less likely to occur in vaccinated children as compared with the general population. The basic premise is that if autism is more likely to develop in vaccinated children (as determined statistically) than in children in the general population, then the association should be further explored to determine whether causality exists. That is, does the vaccine cause autism? Or is there some unaccounted factor that also occurs, but is unrecognized, that causes autism in vaccinated children? Epidemiologic investigations have concluded that there is no evidence linking the MMR vaccination to autism, thus highlighting the importance of epidemiology.[13]

EPIDEMIOLOGY OF DRUG-INDUCED DISEASES

Epidemiology is important in the study of drug-induced diseases. Among other things, epidemiology as applied to pharmaceuticals can be used to investigate the therapeutic effects, risks, and use of drugs in society. Epidemiology is often used to help explain morbidity and mortality questions associated with particular medications. In August 2003, epidemiologists from the U.S. Department of Defense were asked to determine whether there was a causal relationship between the antimalarial drug mefloquine and unexplained domestic killings among recently returned soldiers from Afghanistan.[14] No causal link between mefloquine and the violence was established.

A key obstacle in identifying the cause of drug-induced diseases is recognizing the reaction as a drug-induced disease and distinguishing it from spontaneous (i.e., occurring without taking the drug), yet similar, clinical manifestations that are not drug-related.[15] Another obstacle is determining the numerator (i.e., number of patients with a drug-induced disease) and denominator (i.e., population who took the drug) necessary to calculate the morbidity or mortality rate associated with a particular medication.

In attempting to determine causality of a potential drug-induced disease by a particular agent, it is important to remember that association does not imply causation. Simply put, this means that although a reaction may appear to occur in tandem with a particular drug, it does not necessarily imply that the drug caused the reaction. Indeed, the importance of determining causality was outlined by Professor Sir Austin Bradford Hill, from the London School of Hygiene and Tropical Medicine, in 1965. In particular, Hill stated: "Our observations reveal an association between two variables, perfectly clear-cut and beyond what we would care to attribute to the play of chance. What aspects of that association should we especially consider before deciding that the most likely interpretation of it is causation?"[16] Hill suggested that the following aspects should be considered before causality can be determined, and these are presented with a specific emphasis on drug-induced diseases:

- *Strength of association*—Is there a strong association between a suspected drug-induced disease in people taking the drug versus those not taking the drug? If the association is strong (e.g., a relative risk >3), then one would be more confident that a causal effect exists. An example is the strength of association between pregnant women taking thalidomide and giving birth to a disfigured child. Indeed, this association was so strong that thalidomide was withdrawn from the German market in November 1961 and was not commercially available again until the United States, in July 1998, introduced it to treat erythema nodosum leprosum, but with specific safeguards to prevent it from being used by pregnant women.[17]
- *Consistency*—Does the suspected drug-induced disease occur repeatedly in different persons, at different times, and in different places? Indeed, consistency is a hallmark feature that must occur before causality can even be suggested.
- *Specificity*—Is the suspected drug-induced disease specific to that drug? For example, individuals who take excessive doses of digitalis for heart failure often see "halos." When they stop taking the drug and the plasma digitalis concentrations decrease, the halo effect disappears. Could there be other causes for these patients seeing halos or is it likely only due to digitalis overdose?
- *Temporality*—Does the suspected drug-induced disease manifest before or after drug exposure? To even consider causality, the person must be exposed to the drug before the occurrence of the adverse outcome. If the person is not exposed to the drug before the drug-induced disease occurs, then causality cannot be considered.
- *Biologic gradient*—Does the incidence of the suspected drug-induced disease increase when higher doses of the drug are taken? For example, can we detect increased toxicity with increased doses of a particular drug (e.g., acetaminophen and liver toxicity)?
- *Plausibility*—Is the suspected causation plausible? That is, if a particular adverse event occurs after administration of a particular drug, is it biologically (pharmacologically and physiologically) plausible that the drug caused the event or was it merely coincidental?
- *Coherence*—Does the suspected causation conflict with or support that which is generally known about the disease and its progressive pathology?
- *Experiment*—Is it possible to manipulate the degree of exposure to prevent or enhance the outcome? For example, if a particular drug is suspected of causing a rash in a patient, does the rash disappear after discontinuing the medication, and does subsequent rechallenge cause the rash to reappear? (Note that rechallenge is rarely desirable or ethically appropriate in a clinical setting.)

- *Analogy*—Can the previous experience with a particular medication causing a drug-induced disease be used to enhance our ability to detect or accept a similar outcome with a different drug under similar circumstances? For example, because of the thalidomide debacle of the 1960s, we now know that it is within the realm of possibility that a drug taken during pregnancy can cause birth defects.[17]

In addition to the Hill criteria, Naranjo et al.[18] proposed a method for estimating the probability of adverse reactions. This method uses a probability scale to determine "causality of [adverse drug reactions] in a variety of clinical situations."[19] Although the term *causality* should be replaced with *correlation,* the proposed method is shown to have high between-rater and within-rater reliability on both initial testing and retesting. Clinicians may wish to use this scale as a tool to assess correlation between a medication and an adverse drug event.

CATEGORIZATION OF DRUG-INDUCED ADVERSE EVENTS

Once association between a drug and an adverse event is determined, it is useful to classify the adverse event. Four categories have been suggested to aid in the proper management of any iatrogenic illness[15]:

1. Conscious risk
2. Unexpected complications
3. Inept care
4. Overzealous care

Conscious risk and unexpected complications represent adverse events due to "balanced, informed consideration of benefits and risks."[16] In essence, these two types of drug-induced adverse events are part of the normal risk–benefit consideration inherent when prescribing any drug for any condition to any person. That is, there is always the potential for unintended or unpredictable drug effects on the body. However, both conscious risk and unexpected complications can be mitigated by knowing the risk factors associated with the drug-induced disease, assessing patients for these risk factors, providing optimal doses, and identifying other therapeutic interventions.[16] The latter two categories represent errors of omission and errors of commission, respectively, and represent inappropriate medication use due to a lack of understanding or education about the drug and its impact in the patient for whom it is prescribed.[16]

QUANTIFYING THE IMPACT OF DRUG-INDUCED EVENTS

Determining the quantitative impact of a drug-induced disease to society requires the use of a rigorous and fact-based epidemiologic approach. Several methods for quantifying the impact have been developed, with the simplest being the attributable risk percent measure reported by Cole and MacMahon in 1971.[19] This simple approach relies on the odds ratio (OR) and is expressed as the following:

$$p = (\mathrm{OR} - 1)/\mathrm{OR}$$

where p is the probability that the symptom is the result of taking the drug, and OR is the ratio of the odds of exposure among the cases to the odds of exposure among the controls and is usually accompanied by a 95% confidence interval (CI) to aid in the interpretation of statistical significance.

An example is to determine the quantitative impact of a drug-induced disease of two alternative therapies for the same condition. In 2004, the safety and tolerability of two aerosolized antifungal prophylaxis medications in lung transplant recipients were assessed. Subjects receiving amphotericin B deoxycholate were more likely to have experienced an adverse event than subjects receiving amphotericin B lipid complex (OR 2.16, 95% CI 1.10–4.24, $p = 0.02$).[20] Using the equation above, the quantitative impact of adverse events due to amphotericin B deoxycholate is the following:

$$p = (2.16 - 1)/2.16 = 53.7\%$$

However, additional criteria (e.g., Hill's causality criteria) must also be considered before making a definitive judgment regarding causality.

TRENDS IN REPORTING DRUG-INDUCED EVENTS

The FDA manages the Adverse Event Reporting System (AERS) database, which is a repository of adverse event and medication error reports submitted to the FDA and "serves as a postmarketing safety surveillance program for drug and therapeutic biologic products."[21] Although data and results emanating from AERS should be interpreted with some caution due to limitations inherent in a self-reporting system, the AERS database provides useful information on trends related to the impact of adverse drug events generally and on trends related to new drugs or new drug classes specifically. The nonprofit Institute for Safe Medication Practices monitors and reports on data collected by AERS.

In 2015, the most recent year in which complete data are available, the FDA, through AERS, collected just over 1.16 million reports of adverse drug events.[22] This represents a 32.9% increase from the preceding year. Although the overall increase in number of reports from 2014 to 2015 is substantial, much of this variance can be ascribed to information technology improvements related to how information is reported and regulatory changes that reclassified lower-priority reports into the AERS system.[22] As such, the number of nonserious events increased by 73.2% from 2014 (n = 328,929) to 2015 (n = 569,760) while the number of serious events increased by 9.9% from 2014 (n = 298,979) to 2015 (n = 328,524).[22]

For the domestic serious event category some interesting trends were identified in 2015 data. These include an overall increase in serious adverse drug event reports, a high number of reports for a new class of oral diabetes drugs (the sodium-glucose cotransporter-2 [SGLT2] inhibitors), and the ability to identify drug-associated risks in the post marketing phase of the drug development process.[22] For example, approximately 20% of adults 65 years of age and older are now taking medication to lower their blood glucose concentrations. In the fourth quarter of 2015, over 2 million prescriptions were written for the SGLT2 inhibitors, which promote excretion, rather than reabsorption, of blood glucose and sodium—a nearly sixfold increase from the first quarter of 2014.[22]

The increase in number of prescriptions for a new class of drugs is not in and of itself problematic. Rather the issue is the ability to extrapolate medication safety data to the public at large based on clinical trial data, which are collected from limited and controlled populations. As such, phase IV studies offer postmarketing surveillance to assess "the real world effectiveness of a drug as evaluated in an observational, non-interventional trial in a naturalistic setting which complements the efficacy data that emanates from a pre-marketing randomized controlled trial."[23] In the case of SGLT2 inhibitors, time will ultimately provide evidence on the risk-benefit analysis. However, from current data, there is "evidence [that] multiple safety problems has emerged."[22] From an epidemiology and public health perspective, there is a need to monitor the real impact of new medications in the population. Using the AERS database can support this effort.

PUBLIC HEALTH IMPACT OF DRUG-INDUCED DISEASES

Drug-induced diseases exert a considerable impact on society. They are costly, result in considerable morbidity, and may result in death. Some adverse drug effects are not clinically significant, yet "most [would] agree that any condition that results in hospitalization is significant."[24] In this book, a drug-induced disease is defined as an unintended effect of a drug that may result in mortality or morbidity or cause symptoms sufficient to prompt a patient to seek medical attention and/or require hospitalization. Costs associated with drug-induced diseases have considerable implications for public health policy and planning. For example, costs associated with drug-induced diseases not only divert healthcare resources but also have measurable (e.g., hospitalization) and societal (e.g., lost time from work) costs. From a clinical standpoint, prevention of drug-induced diseases is preferable to treatment after the fact. Fortunately, many drug-induced diseases are preventable. This section explores issues related to the public health implication of drug-induced diseases.

DETERMINING THE INCIDENCE OF DRUG-INDUCED DISEASE

Determining the incidence of drug-induced diseases can be a daunting task, chiefly because it is difficult to determine the associated numerator and denominator. The numerator is defined as the number of new drug-induced disease events occurring during a defined period, while the denominator is defined as the population at risk for the drug-induced disease during the same period. In the general population, the denominator is the number of people exposed to a particular medication and may be identified by using computerized prescription data or medical records. In reality, however, numerous obstacles exist in determining the denominator, because it is difficult to identify the population of interest and to determine how many people in this population have been exposed to the drug. Determining the numerator is also difficult because there is no systematic method of assessing the occurrence of drug-induced diseases in individuals unless the occurrence is serious enough to warrant further medical attention.[24]

Data from hospital admission studies can be used as an appropriate measure of drug-induced disease incidence because (1) medical record data can be used to determine potential association, and perhaps causation, between a particular drug and disease; and (2) drug-induced events precipitating hospitalization are deemed serious enough to be clinically significant and thus would seem to represent a higher burden to society. Indeed, Nelson and Talbert note that "the rate of drug-related admissions is a measure of a subset of the clinically significant related morbidity. Determining this rate could identify some of the cases of drug-related morbidity."[24]

Another obstacle in determining the incidence of drug-induced diseases is that, in many cases, medications are not recognized as the cause of the symptom or disease. Therefore, a particular drug may not be recorded or reported as a potential cause. Clinicians may be slow in recognizing a drug-induced disease because not all adverse events are reported in the literature or necessarily known to the FDA at the time of approval. For rare events (e.g., a drug-induced disease occurring in 1 of every 10,000 people), the likelihood of detection before approval and widespread use is low because the clinical trial process, although rigorous, is not designed to identify all drug-related adverse events. It is often only after a drug reaches the market and is used by a much larger patient population that rare events are identified. Therefore, the importance of postmarketing surveillance activities and signal-detection activities cannot be overstated.

DRUG-RELATED HOSPITAL ADMISSIONS

As noted earlier, drug-induced hospital admissions are a sign of serious clinical events. Sometimes these admissions are avoidable, and other times they are not. For example, a patient with a known allergy to penicillin who is subsequently prescribed this drug and develops anaphylactic shock represents a case of an avoidable hospital admission. On the other hand, a patient may receive a medication that causes a drug–drug, drug–food, or drug–laboratory interaction with subsequent hospitalization that is unavoidable because these interactions were previously undescribed, were previously unknown, or were idiosyncratic in nature.

In a 1993 review, the incidence of drug-related hospital admissions was reported to range from 0.2% to 21.7%, with a median rate of drug-related hospitalizations of 4.9%.[25] The author defined drug-related hospitalizations as adverse events that could cause a side effect, excessive effect, idiosyncratic effect, or hypersensitivity. All of the reviewed studies were conducted in large hospitals, with most located in urban areas. Sample sizes (or total admission numbers) ranged from 41 to 11,891, with a total patient population size of 69,187. Only nine of these studies reported incidence rates above 7%, representing just 6.3% of the patient population assessed (4,420/69,187). The highest reported incidence of 21.7% occurred in a teaching hospital with oncology patients as the predominant population. The primary implicated medications for drug-related admissions in this group were theophylline, cancer chemotherapy agents, and trimethoprim–sulfamethoxazole. In another review, covering the period from 1959 through 1992, 0.3–16.8% (median 5.6%) of all hospital admissions were drug-related.[15]

Determining the rate of drug-induced hospital admissions is dependent on the study population, the ability to extract sufficient medical information, and the study method. Most studies of drug-related admissions rely on a medical record review by a clinical pharmacist. Such a review typically defines a drug-induced admission and establishes criteria for objectively determining whether an admission meets that definition. The definition of *drug-related admission* can include an adverse drug reaction, dose-related therapeutic failures, improperly treated conditions, and drug interactions. Among studies assessing drug-related admissions, wide-ranging results are possible due to variation in prescribing patterns, differences in patient populations, and differences in defining drug-induced illness.

The true extent of drug-related hospital admissions remains a mystery, because it is not possible to make a collective determination of the overall prevalence based on a collection of disparate studies. As Manasse pointed out, although published reports provided useful information about drug misadventuring, these reports were extremely limited "in establishing a national mortality, morbidity, or incidence rate."[26] However, these studies can provide some information about drug-related hospital admissions. For example, reports can inform us about the types of drugs and drug classes frequently implicated in drug-related hospital admissions and potential causes of drug-related problems (e.g., drug–drug interaction, nonadherence, etc.). As an example, in a study published in 2011, researchers in the Netherlands identified the most common reasons for a potentially preventable drug-induced hospital admission as gastrointestinal problems (15%), cardiovascular symptoms (11%), respiratory symptoms (8%), and issues with glycemic control (6%).[27] Reports also can inform us regarding the reason for a medication error. For example, a 2013 report noted drug errors were caused by errors in ordering and prescribing (53%), receiving or administration (13%), monitoring or follow-up (13%), implementing or dispensing (10%), documentation (7%), and others (4%).[28]

Table 2-2 Drug Classes Commonly Associated with Drug-Related Hospital Admissions

- Antidiabetics/hypoglycemics
- Cardiovascular drugs (e.g., ACE inhibitors, diuretics, digoxin)
- Psychotropics
- Gastrointestinal drugs
- NSAIDs
- Anticonvulsants
- Antineoplastics
- Corticosteroids
- Antibiotics

ACE = angiotensin-converting enzyme, NSAID = nonsteroidal anti-inflammatory drug.

Many studies have identified drug types and drug classes frequently implicated in drug-induced hospital admissions. Although the results of these studies vary in terms of drug classes implicated and the number of adverse events associated with each drug class, some general trends are noted. For example, cardiovascular drugs are often implicated in drug-induced hospital admissions. Chiefly among this group are digitalis, diuretics, and angiotensin-converting enzyme inhibitors. See **Table 2-2** for a list of drug classes commonly associated with drug-induced hospital admissions.

COSTS

Costs associated with drug-induced diseases can be quite substantial. Unfortunately, most approaches used to assess the economic impact of a drug-induced disease have methodological limitations that require numerous assumptions, make it difficult to quantify the number and types of medication errors that occur, are often focused on a particular setting, and may lack accurate cost information with which to conduct economic analyses. Additional issues include determining causality and difficulty in properly identifying the numerator and denominator.

Nevertheless, the literature is replete with studies seeking to address the cost burden of drug-induced diseases. A review of the literature from 2010 forward indicates varying assessment methodologies are used with wide ranges in costs purported to be associated with drug-induced diseases. For example, a study in 2011 from The Netherlands reported an average cost for a preventable drug-induced medication-related hospitalization of €5,461[27] while a study in 2015 from Germany reported an average cost for a preventable drug-induced related hospitalization of €2,743.[29]

As with the two studies noted above, findings from articles reporting on the cost burden of drug-induced diseases since the late 1990s are based on a wide range of methodologies, assumptions, and sources of information—all of which are associated with limitations. Samp et al. point out the following:

> Currently published studies on cost of medication errors have many additional limitations. Because of the difficulty in quantifying all types of medication errors, most studies focused on a specific healthcare setting. In addition, many studies examined only errors that were documented in patients' medical records or those errors that resulted in patient harm. Although this information may be more easily available, this type of limited analysis leads to a gross underestimation of the true rate of medication errors and a potential overestimate of medication error costs.[30]

For example, researchers reported on the monetary costs associated with hospitalization due to drug-induced diseases in Australia over an 8-year period from 1988 to 1996.[31] In this study, investigators simply calculated a mean average cost based on average length of stay and average daily cost of hospital care. The report did not include costs of outpatient visits, return visits to a physician's office, pharmacy costs, or additional treatment costs. **Table 2-3** describes items that should be included in a comprehensive health economic assessment.

In 1995, researchers at the Center for Pharmaceutical Economics at the University of Arizona developed a comprehensive cost-of-illness approach associated with drug-related morbidity and mortality based on a probability pathway model.[32] In this model, costs were determined based on specific outcomes associated with treatment. When a patient receives drug therapy, four possible outcomes are possible: (1) optimal therapeutic outcome, in which the patient recovers from the illness; (2) treatment failure; (3) a new medical problem; and (4) a combination of treatment failure and a new medical problem. Therefore, this model went beyond addressing drug-induced diseases, and included drug-related events including treatment failures. It stands to reason that attaining an optimal therapeutic outcome is the desired end result. For patients who do not reach this outcome, additional scenarios are possible: no further treatment, an additional physician visit, additional treatment, an emergency department visit, hospitalization, long-term care admission, or death.

Based on this cost-of-illness model, total estimated morbidity and mortality costs for drug-related diseases were $76.6 billion in 1995.[32] A follow-up study in 2001, using the same cost-of-illness model, reported annual drug-related morbidity and mortality costs (in year 2000 dollars) of $177.4 billion.[33] By comparison, the cost of cardiovascular diseases and stroke were estimated to be $316.6 billion in

Table 2-3 Costs to Consider When Conducting a Health Economic Evaluation

Direct medical costs

- Hospitalization
- Outpatient service (including ancillary services)
- Pharmacy costs
- Diagnostic procedures and tests (e.g., laboratory tests, electrocardiography, chest radiography)
- Surgery
- Extended nursing or home health costs
- Follow-up care (e.g., return visits to the hospital or primary care physician and additional ancillary services such as radiology or laboratory testing)

Direct nonmedical costs

- Transportation to and from the medical provider
- Services (e.g., Meals on Wheels and social assistance)
- Adopting devices and instruments

Indirect costs

- Sick leave
- Reduced productivity
- Early retirement
- Premature death

2011–2012, and the cost for all cancers during this period was estimated at $88.7 billion.[34]

When these figures are analyzed by cost center, hospitalization was the single highest cost driver for drug-related morbidity and mortality, with 1995 expenditures of $47.4 billion and 2000 expenditures of $121.5 billion. In 1995, for example, hospital admissions represented 62% of the total cost. In the 2001 study, hospital admissions accounted for 69% of the total costs. This increase is most likely due to higher costs associated with hospitalizations or medical inflation rather than an increased incidence of drug-related diseases. Costs associated with new medical problems due to a previously prescribed drug therapy are also expensive. Hospitalization costs associated with a new medical problem were estimated to be $5,504 in 1995[32] and $12,797 in 2000.[33]

However, it should be noted that the expenditures presented in this model are estimates. Indeed, hospitalization expenses from the 1995 study assume that 28.2% of all hospitalizations are due to drug-related morbidity and mortality.[32] This figure is high and is at odds with reported estimates of drug-related hospital admissions cited earlier in this chapter.[15,31] As previously discussed, Einarson[25] reported an overall incidence of drug-related hospital admissions ranging from 0.2% to 21.7%, with a median value of 4.9%. Hallis[15] reported an incidence of drug-related hospital admissions ranging from 0.3% to 16.8%, with a median value of 5.8%. Johnson and Bootman[32] acknowledge this discrepancy by noting that estimates (such as by Einarson[25]) focused on hospital admissions due to nonadherence or adverse drug reactions. Johnson and Bootman further note that estimates in their model included "negative therapeutic outcomes owing to all types of drug-related problems" and, as such, the estimated numbers of hospital admissions "would be expected to be greater."[32] Despite this explanation, these numbers appear to be high compared with empirical evidence and should be judged cautiously in this light. From a clinical perspective, the rate of drug-related hospitalizations may be more appropriately in line with the median estimates of 4.9% and 5.6% reported by Einarson[25] and Hallis,[15] respectively, because their studies represent wide reviews of the published literature on the subject.

Table 2-4 Key Components of a Decision Tree Model Used to Assess Potential Outcomes due to Medication Errors[30]

- Is there a medication error?
  - Does this error reach the patient (yes or no)?
- If the error reaches the patient, is the patient harmed (yes or no)?
  - Is the harm permanent or temporary?
- If the patient has permanent harm is this in the form of death, hospitalization, or no hospitalization?
- If the patient has temporary harm does the patient require hospitalization, no hospitalization, or prolonged hospitalization?
- Is life-sustaining intervention required?
- If the error does not reach the patient, is communication needed with the patient regarding the error or can be it be remedied without communication?
  - Is the medication regimen changed (yes or no)?
  - Is medication monitoring required (yes or no)?
  - Is treatment referral required (yes or no)?

In an attempt to provide a more rigorous and comprehensive approach to estimating the cost burden of drug-induced diseases, Samp et al. reported in 2014 on costs associated with medication errors by using a decision-tree model.[30] Such a model allowed for all logical outcomes to be identified along with the unit cost for each outcome. This approach provided a more robust data collection paradigm that could tie a specific medication error end point to the cost of the error and the number of times the error occurred. Components of the Samp et al. decision tree are summarized in **Table 2-4**.[30]

Results from Samp et al.[30] indicated a total of 779 medication errors were observed over a 14-day period with 57.9% (n = 451)* of the errors reaching the patient and 9.3% (n = 42)* of those errors leading to patient harm. The remaining 90.3% (n = 409)* of errors that reached the patient did not lead to patient harm. For those errors that caused harm, 2.5% (n = 1) resulted in permanent harm (in this case death) while 97.5% (n = 41)* resulted in temporary harm.

---

*Samp et al. did not provide individual numbers. Therefore, n is calculated (with appropriate rounding) for each individual subpopulation based on the total number of medication errors (n = 779) and percentages provided by Samp et al.[30]

From an economic perspective, medication errors were deemed to cost on average $88.57.[30] For those medication errors that did not reach the patient the average cost was estimated to be $6.92, while those medication errors that reached the patient the average cost was estimated to be $147.96.[30] Medication errors that did not cause harm were estimated to cost $11.85 while those medication errors that caused harm to the patient were estimated to cost $1,473.40.[30] The authors noted that these values are considerably lower than those in other reported cost estimates, likely because previous studies base cost estimates solely on medication errors resulting in harm, whereas the inclusion of minor medication errors that did not reach the patient or errors that did not cause harm (both of which represent the largest variance of medication errors in this study) were included in the Samp analysis.

Data from published studies indicate a wide margin in terms of the cost burden associated with a drug-induced disease. From a practical perspective, each study adds to the literature and to the discussion of both health outcomes and the economic cost of medication errors. Such information also provides an opportunity for patients, clinicians, and healthcare settings to focus on quality and to develop processes that can reduce medication errors (such as fully implementing meaningful use capabilities for electronic medical records).[35] Caution, however, is in order when reviewing such findings. That is, it is important for the reader to approach these studies with an appreciation of the limitations, assumptions, and methodological issues inherent in the study design.

MORTALITY

Mortality due to drug-induced diseases is a major concern for pharmacists, physicians, and other healthcare providers. Mortality associated with drug-induced diseases presents an emotional and economic burden to society, especially in cases for which the cause is preventable. The mean death rate due to adverse drug reactions was reported to be 5% of all hospitalized patients admitted for a drug-related problem.[26] This is over 16 times higher than the mortality rate of 0.3% for all other hospital admissions.[26] In addition, the cost of hospitalization with resultant mortality is one of the most expensive single pathways identified by Johnson and Bootman as a treatment outcome.[32] In 1995, for example, drug-related mortality due to a new medical problem was associated with a total pathway cost of $5,504.[32] In 2001, drug-related mortality due to a new medical problem that resulted in death was associated with a total pathway cost of $12,797.[33]

Finally, it should be noted that although there are morbidity, mortality, and economic costs associated with drug-induced diseases, there are also significant opportunity costs to public health when medications known to be safe and effective are not used. For example, childhood vaccination rates have declined in some cities throughout the United States because of fears of autism. As such, there has been an increase in the incidence of mumps and measles in some communities. This increase in preventable illnesses not only impacts the individual, but also exerts a concomitant effect on the community population, as herd immunity is reduced and individuals not previously susceptible to the illness may become susceptible.

CONCLUSION

Drug-induced diseases are a continuing concern for patients and healthcare practitioners alike. All drugs have the potential to precipitate an adverse event, which, in its most serious form, can lead to a drug-induced disease. Clinical trials and regulatory approval processes are often very good at identifying the most common types of adverse events and the patients in whom they are likely to occur. However, not all drug-induced diseases can be identified *a priori*, no matter how carefully medications are prescribed or regulated. The interplay of drugs with complex physiologic factors renders drug-induced diseases a consideration as part of the risk-benefit profile associated with the administration of any medication.

Epidemiology is useful in assisting clinicians in identifying potential associative or causal influences on diseases induced by a specific drug.

At the population level, the examples outlined in this chapter demonstrate the potential for epidemiology to not only identify causal inferences (e.g., thalidomide and birth defects), but to also rule out inappropriate causal inferences (e.g., MMR vaccine and autism). At the patient level, causal inferences may be due to the complexity of the patient's condition, physiologic responses, and the specific pharmacodynamic interplay associated with a specific medication. The ability to use tools related to association and causation as described by Hill[16] and Naranjo et al.[18] can be useful in identifying potential causal interactions at the patient level.

REFERENCES

1. US Food and Drug Administration. Approved drug products with therapeutic equivalence evaluations (2016). 36th ed. http://www.accessdata.fda.gov/scripts/cder/ob/ (accessed 2018 Jan 29).
2. Aspden P, Wolcott JA, Bootman L et al., eds. *Preventing medication errors.* Washington, DC: National Academies Press; 2006.
3. US Food and Drug Administration. Frequently asked questions: once the FDA approves a drug, does this mean that the product is perfectly safe? http://www.fda.gov/AboutFDA/CentersOffices/OfficeofMedicalProductsandTobacco/CDER/FAQsaboutCDER/#6 (accessed 2018 Jan 29).
4. Kohn LT, Corrigan JM, Donaldson MS. *To err is human: building a safer health system.* Washington, DC: National Academies Press; 2000.
5. Lowe D. Aspirin: not approvable. *Medical Progress Today.* 2005.
6. Beaglehole R, Bonita R, Kjellström T. *Basic epidemiology.* Geneva: World Health Organization; 1993.
7. Litaker JR, Chou JY, Novak S et al. Implications of SARS: medical geography and surveillance in disease detection. *Ann Pharmacother.* 2003; 37:1841-9.
8. Last JM. *A dictionary of epidemiology.* 3rd ed. New York: Oxford University Press; 1995.
9. Jekel JF, Elmore JG, Katz DL. *Epidemiology, biostatistics, and preventive medicine.* Philadelphia: WB Saunders Company; 1996.
10. Begaud B. *Dictionary of pharmacoepidemiology.* Chichester, England: John Wiley and Sons; 2001.
11. Huminer D, Rosenfield JB, Pitlik SD. AIDS in the pre-AIDS era. *Rev Infect Dis.* 1987; 9:1102-8.
12. Public Health in England. *The Report of the Committee of Inquiry into the Future Development of the Public Health Function.* Cmnd 289. London, England: HMSO; 1988.
13. DeStefano F, Bhasin TK, Thompson WW et al. Age at first measles-mumps-rubella vaccination in children with autism and school-matched control subjects: a population-based study in metropolitan Atlanta. *Pediatrics.* 2004; 113:259-66.
14. News Round-up. US army to investigate side effects of mefloquine. *BMJ.* 2004; 328:660.
15. Hallis J. Drug related hospital admissions in subspecialties of internal medicine. *Dan Med Bull.* 1996; 43:141-55.
16. Hill AB. The environment and disease: association or causation? President's address. *Proc R Soc Med.* 1965; 58:295-300.
17. *FDA Approves Thalidomide for Hansen's Disease Side Effect, Imposes Unprecedented Restrictions on Distribution.* FDA Talk Paper. July 16, 1998.
18. Naranjo CA, Busto U, Sellers EM et al. A method for estimating the probability of adverse drug reactions. *Clin Pharmacol Ther.* 1981; 30:239-45.
19. Cole P, MacMahon B. Attributable risk percent in case control. *Br J Prev Soc Med.* 1971; 25:242-4.
20. Drew RH, Dodds AE, Benjamin DK Jr et al. Comparative safety of amphotericin B limpid complex and amphotericin B deoxycholate as aerosolized antifungal prophylaxis in lung-transplant recipients. *Transplantation.* 2004; 77:232-7.
21. US Food and Drug Administration. Questions and answers on FDA's Adverse Event Reporting System (FAERS). http://www.fda.gov/Drugs/GuidanceComplianceRegulatoryInformation/Surveillance/AdverseDrugEffects/ (accessed 2018 Jan 29).
22. Institute for the Safety of Medicine. Quarter Watch. 2015 annual report (June 29, 2016). https://www.ismp.org/quarterwatch/pdfs/2015Q4.pdf (accessed 2018 Jan 29).
23. Suvarna V. Phase IV of drug development. *Perspect Clin Res.* 2010; 1:57-60.
24. Nelson KM, Talbert RL. Drug-related hospital admissions. *Pharmacotherapy.* 1996; 16:701-7.
25. Einarson TR. Drug-related hospital admissions. *Ann Pharmacother.* 1993; 27:832-40.
26. Manasse HR Jr. Medication use in an imperfect world: drug misadventuring as an issue of public policy, part 1. *Am J Hosp Pharm.* 1989; 46:929-44.
27. Leendertse AJ, Van Den Bemt PMLA, Poolman JB et al. Preventable hospital admissions related to medication (HARM): Cost analysis of the HARM study. *Value in Health.* 2011; 14:34-40.
28. Kuo GM, Touchette DR, Marinac JS. Drug errors and related interventions reported by United States clinical pharmacists: The American College of Clinical Pharmacy Practice-Based Research Network Medication Error Detection, Amelioration and Prevention Study. *Pharmacotherapy* 2013; 33:253-65.
29. Meier F, Maas R, Sonst A. Adverse drug events in patients admitted to an emergency department: An analysis of direct costs. *Pharmacoepidemiol Drug Saf.* 2015; 24:176-86.
30. Samp JC, Touchette, DR, Marinac JS. Economic evaluation of the impact of medication errors reported by US clinical pharmacists. *Pharmacotherapy.* 2014; 34:350-7.
31. Roughead EE, Gilbert AL, Primrose JG et al. Drug-related hospital admissions: a review of Australian studies published 1988–1996. *Med J Aust.* 1998; 168:405-8.
32. Johnson JA, Bootman JL. Drug-related morbidity and mortality. *Arch Intern Med.* 1995; 155:1949-56.
33. Ernst FR, Grizzle AJ. Drug-related morbidity and mortality: updating the cost-of-illness model. *J Am Pharm Assoc.* 2001; 41:192-9.
34. Mozaffarian D, Benjamin EJ, Go AS et al. on behalf of the American Heart Association Statistics Committee and Stroke Statistics Subcommittee. Heart disease and stroke statistics—2016 update: a report from the American Heart Association. *Circulation.* 2016; 133:e38-360.
35. Encinosa WE, Bae J. Will meaningful use electronic medical records reduce hospital costs? *Am J Manag Care.* 2013; 19:eSP19-25.

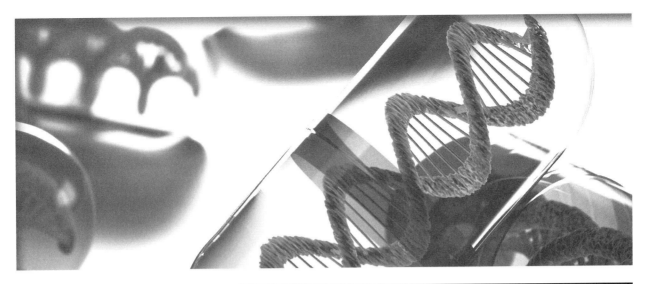

CHAPTER 3

Factors Contributing to Drug-Induced Diseases

Tyler Shugg, Abdullah Assiri, and Brian R. Overholser*

Patients can be predisposed to drug-induced diseases by several modifiable and nonmodifiable factors. Nonmodifiable factors include a patient's age, sex, race, pregnancy status, genetics, and comorbid diseases. These factors should be considered when assessing the risk of a drug-induced disease prior to drug administration. Additionally, efforts should be made to minimize or eliminate modifiable risk factors for drug-induced diseases, including cigarette smoking, alcohol and illicit drug use, drug–drug interactions (DDIs), food–drug interactions, medication adherence, and medication errors. This chapter outlines the most important factors that are known to contribute to drug-induced diseases and provides examples of their clinical consequences.

DEMOGRAPHIC FACTORS

AGE

Advancing age is associated with progressive changes in pharmacokinetic parameters, such as reductions in renal and hepatic clearance and an increased volume of distribution of lipophilic medications.[1] Advancing age can also impact pharmacodynamic responses, such as an exaggerated sensitivity to drugs that affect the central nervous system.[1,2] These physiological changes are associated with a greater risk of drug-induced diseases in elderly patients, prompting the development of special guidance, such as the Beers Criteria from the American Geriatrics Society, to appropriately direct medication therapy in this at-risk population.[3,4]

SEX

Based on data from the U.S. Food and Drug Administration's (FDA's) Adverse Event Reporting System, women experience an increased number of adverse drug events, which tend to be more severe than those reported in men.[5] Although the reasons underlying the greater predisposition for adverse drug events in women remain unclear, potential factors include sex-associated differences in prescribing practices, sex-associated differences in pharmacokinetic

*Tyler Shugg and Abdullah Assiri contributed to this chapter equally.

parameters and pharmacodynamic responses, and the impact of sex hormones on increasing the risk of drug-induced disease.[6-8] As an example, women exhibit a greater risk of the drug-induced arrhythmia torsades de pointes when receiving medications that prolong cardiac repolarization. Torsades de pointes is associated with prolonged QT intervals on the surface electrocardiogram (ECG). The increased risk of this arrhythmia may be mediated by sex hormones, particularly the estrogen to testosterone ratio, which may explain the longer baseline QT intervals in women compared with those in men.[7]

RACE

As technological advances have dramatically improved the understanding of the human genome, pharmacogenetic research has identified genetic factors that influence drug disposition and response. Race, the classification of individuals based on their geographic region of ancestry, is frequently, though somewhat controversially, utilized as an effective marker to predict genotype.[9] Such analyses have identified genetic factors that predispose to drug-induced disease that are more prevalent in specific racial populations.[10] For example, individuals of Han Chinese racial origin have an increased prevalence of the human leukocyte antigen (HLA) variant allele, *HLA-B*1502* (rs3909184G>C and rs2844682G>A), a strong predictor for the development of severe skin reactions, including Stevens–Johnson syndrome (SJS) and toxic epidermal necrolysis (TEN), associated with administration of carbamazepine.[11-13] Therefore, the probability of carrying certain HLA variant alleles can be predicted based on a patient's race. Additionally, there are well-known examples of the impact of race on the risk of drug-induced diseases for which the genetic basis has not been elucidated. For example, the mechanism for the increased risk of angioedema upon administration of angiotensin-converting enzyme (ACE) inhibitors in patients of African origin is not well understood but is largely recognized.[12,14,15]

PREGNANCY

Maternity status greatly impacts the risk of drug-induced disease, particularly in the developing fetus. Exposure to teratogenic drugs during the first trimester can significantly impair organ development, while exposure in later trimesters can have detrimental effects on newborn growth, cognition, and organ function.[16] Accordingly, the FDA requires evaluation of the teratogenic potential of medications during drug development and has released guidance to direct medication use during pregnancy.[17]

Pregnancy is also responsible for physiologic changes that alter maternal pharmacokinetics. Pregnancy is commonly associated with decreases in the rate and extent of drug absorption, increases in the volumes of distribution of several medications, increases in the clearance of renally eliminated drugs, and increases in the activity of drug-metabolizing enzymes, such as cytochrome P450 (CYP) 3A4.[18,19] Although these pharmacokinetic changes greatly impact drug exposure, maternity-associated changes most often result in reduced drug action and do not typically predispose mothers to an increased risk of drug-induced disease.[18]

LIFESTYLE FACTORS

CIGARETTE SMOKING

Cigarette smoking is a risk factor contributing to drug-induced disease by altering pharmacokinetic parameters and pharmacodynamic response.[20] Cigarette smoke contains thousands of compounds, many of which are known to contribute to several types of cancer. Polycyclic aromatic hydrocarbons are among the most studied for their mutagenic effect as well as their potent induction of hepatic CYPs 1A1, 1A2, 2B6, and possibly 2E1.[20,21] Several important widely used drugs, including acetaminophen, diazepam, duloxetine, olanzapine, ondansetron, clozapine, and methadone, are CYP1A2 substrates. Smokers generally require higher doses of these drugs compared to nonsmokers. Thus, abrupt smoking cessation can markedly affect the pharmacokinetics of drugs that are CYP1A2 substrates, leading to potentially serious complications.

Cigarette smoking can also impact the pharmacodynamics of drugs, including diazepam, β-adrenergic receptor blockers (β-blockers), hormonal contraceptives, and opioids.[20,22] For example, the risk of adverse cardiovascular events in female smokers greatly increases with the use of oral contraceptives and is even greater in older compared to younger women.[23] Thus, the use of oral contraceptives by women over the age of 35 years who are heavy smokers is contraindicated due to the heightened potential for drug-induced disease.

ALCOHOL CONSUMPTION

Many drugs can interact with alcohol resulting in serious diseases or even death.[24] Alcohol is primarily metabolized in the liver by alcohol dehydrogenase in addition to CYP enzymes including 2E1, 1A2, and 3A4. Alcohol dehydrogenase converts alcohol to a highly reactive and toxic compound, acetaldehyde, which is metabolized rapidly to form acetate and nicotinamide adenine dinucleotide. Acetaldehyde forms protein adducts by binding to enzymes or microtubules, contributing to tissue damage and liver enlargement.[24,25] Therefore, the hepatic metabolism of many drugs may be affected, leading to reductions in efficacy or increased risk of toxicity. Ethanol is also a CYP2E1 substrate that induces its own metabolism. Thus, ethanol is metabolized by CYP2E1 to a greater extent in chronic alcohol users.[24] More importantly, the administration of the CYP2E1 substrate acetaminophen in chronic consumers of alcohol increases formation of the toxic metabolite *N*-acetyl-p-benzoquinone imine (NAPQI), which enhances the risk of hepatotoxicity.[26,27]

ABUSE SUBSTANCES

Cannabis is one of the most commonly used recreational drugs in the world. Cannabis consists of more than 80 cannabinoids that contribute to its effects.[28] One of these constituents is delta-9-tetrahydrocannabinol, which is used clinically to prevent chemotherapy-related nausea and vomiting and to improve appetite in patients with human immunodeficiency virus (HIV)/acquired immunodeficiency syndrome (AIDS).[29,30] Cannabinoids are highly protein bound, and there is some evidence that they may interact with other highly protein-bound drugs, including warfarin and phenytoin.[31,32] Cannabinoids are also metabolized by CYP2C9 and CYP3A4 and induce CYP1A2 when smoked, similar to cigarettes. Concurrent use of cannabis and CYP1A2 substrates—such as clozapine, olanzapine, haloperidol, and tamoxifen—may necessitate higher doses of these drugs to ensure efficacy.[33] Additionally, patients who are receiving these drugs are at high risk of overdose upon cessation of cannabis because they are likely to be maintained on a higher dose during concomitant cannabis use.

Other widely used illicit drugs include amphetamines and cocaine. Cocaine and amphetamines block the reuptake of monoamines (e.g., dopamine) and inhibit their metabolism. This results in an increased risk of cardiovascular events, hypertensive crisis, and central nervous system adverse events. The risk of these adverse events is enhanced when cocaine or amphetamines are used concurrently with antidepressant drugs, such as selective serotonin reuptake inhibitors and tricyclic antidepressants.[34,35] In addition, amphetamines are metabolized by and inhibit CYP2D6. Concomitant use of drugs that are metabolized by CYP2D6 and amphetamines increases the risk of these drug-induced diseases.[33,35]

COMORBID DISEASES

Comorbid diseases can alter the pharmacokinetics and pharmacodynamics of many drugs and constitute a major cause of drug-induced diseases.[36] Liver and kidney diseases are among the most common disorders that contribute to drug-induced diseases due to decreased drug elimination.

KIDNEY DISEASES

In general, hydrophilic drugs are primarily excreted unchanged through the kidneys.[36] The elimination of these drugs is decreased in patients with kidney diseases due to diminished glomerular filtration and/or tubular secretion. Therefore, patients with kidney disease may be at a higher risk of drug-induced diseases compared to patients with normal kidney function.[37,38] There are several examples of renally eliminated drugs that increase the risk for adverse events, including some β-blockers, nonpotassium-sparing diuretics, insulin, ACE inhibitors, aspirin, warfarin, and clopidogrel.[38]

Kidney diseases may also affect nonrenally excreted drugs by altering absorption, distribution, and clearance. Changes in pharmacokinetics in patients with kidney diseases have been demonstrated for more than 50% of nonrenally excreted drugs approved between 2003 and 2007.[38] The impact of kidney diseases on drug absorption may be a result of gastric pH change, which can alter the bioavailability of certain drugs. Protease inhibitors, immunosuppressants, and erythromycin are examples of drugs with increased bioavailability in patients with chronic kidney diseases.[36,39,40] Proteinuria associated with kidney diseases reduces serum albumin concentrations, which may alter the unbound fractions of highly protein-bound drugs, potentially leading to increased drug effect and toxicity.[41] Hepatic metabolism may also be affected by the marked increase in serum parathyroid hormone concentration that occurs in patients with chronic kidney disease, altering the expression of enzymes involved in phase I and phase II metabolism. Examples of hepatically metabolized drugs for which metabolism is impaired due to kidney disease include midazolam, morphine, and zidovudine.[36]

LIVER DISEASES

The liver is the major organ responsible for drug metabolism. Thus, hepatotoxicity, and in particular liver cirrhosis, can have a substantial impact on drug metabolism and clearance. The extent of impaired drug metabolism is dependent on the severity of injury or disease. Hepatic dysfunction can lead to alterations in absorption, extraction, enterohepatic circulation, and plasma protein binding of hepatically metabolized drugs. There are numerous examples of hepatically metabolized drugs that are associated with an increased risk of drug-induced disease during liver disease, including midazolam, propranolol, morphine, metoprolol, warfarin, and naproxen, among others.[42-45]

OTHER DISEASES

Patients with heart failure, thyroid disease, and electrolyte imbalances are at higher risk of drug-induced diseases due to alterations in the pharmacokinetics or pharmacodynamics of certain drugs. Patients with heart failure with reduced ejection fraction (HFrEF) have decreased cardiac output that results in diminished hepatic blood flow. There is some evidence that a low cardiac output due to HFrEF may result in decreased metabolism of high extraction ratio drugs such as lidocaine.[46] Renal clearance and hepatic blood flow may also be diminished in patients with hypothyroidism. Digoxin and other drugs have been found to provoke exaggerated responses when usual doses are administered to patients with hypothyroidism.[47,48] Additionally, in patients with low serum potassium or magnesium concentrations, there is less competition for digoxin with the Na^+/K^+ ATPase pump, resulting in a higher risk of digoxin-induced arrhythmias.[49]

GENETIC VARIATION

BACKGROUND AND NOMENCLATURE

The overall understanding of the contribution of genetics to drug response has increased in the past decade. Pharmacogenomic studies, including gene candidate and genome-wide scanning approaches, have identified gene variants that increase the risk for drug-related adverse events.[50] The identification of these genetic variants has increased the ability of clinicians to predict drug responses and adverse events that were previously categorized as idiosyncratic adverse drug reactions.[51]

Variability of drug response due to pharmacogenomic factors can be a result of single nucleotide polymorphisms, deletions, insertions, duplications, or any other changes in DNA sequences.[52] Humans are diploid organisms that carry two copies of each gene—one each of maternal and paternal origin—which are referred to as alleles. The variant allele refers to a gene that possesses a genetic mutation while the wild-type allele usually refers to the most common genotype in the population (i.e., nonmutated). The alleles are numbered largely based on the order of discovery with the *1 allele commonly designated as the wild-type. Therefore, a patient that is a carrier of the *1/*1 alleles inherited wild-type alleles for that gene from both their biological mother and father.

By having a copy of the same allele from both sources, this patient would be referred to as being homozygous for the wild-type allele. Conversely, a heterozygous patient has two distinct allele copies of the same gene.

The most common variants that alter drug pharmacokinetics and pharmacodynamics and increase the risk for drug-induced diseases are in genes that encode drug-metabolizing enzymes, drug transporters, drug target receptors, or the human leukocyte antigen.[53,54] As more pharmacogenetic tests are developed and translated to the clinic, there is a need to enhance clinician knowledge in the field. The Pharmacogenomics Knowledgebase and the Pharmacogenomics Research Network have established the Clinical Pharmacogenetics Implementation Consortium (CPIC) guidelines to guide clinicians on the use of available tests to enhance pharmacotherapy efficacy and avoid potential adverse drug events.[55] There are several examples of pharmacogenomic tests that are becoming the standard of care in oncology and with drugs like abacavir, carbamazepine, dapsone, and azathioprine.

DRUG METABOLISM

Drug metabolism pathways can be classified into phase I oxidation/reduction or phase II conjugation reactions.[53,54] A majority of the genes that encode for phase I and II enzymes are polymorphic, and mutations in these genes can result in varying clinical phenotypes. Phenotypic variations can range from ultra-rapid metabolizer (UM), normal or extensive metabolizer (NM or EM, respectively), intermediate metabolizer (IM), and poor metabolizer (PM). EMs are commonly homozygous for the wild-type (i.e., *1) alleles whereas PMs are typically homozygous for decreased function alleles. UMs include carriers of gain-of-function alleles that increase metabolism capacity beyond that of EMs. Therefore, if the patient's genotype is known, their phenotype can be predicted. A final important consideration is the activity of the parent drug versus that of metabolites to facilitate prediction of lack of an appropriate therapeutic response or increased risk of an adverse drug event or drug-induced disease.

The CYP enzymes (e.g., CYP2A6, CYP2B6, CYP2C9, CYP2C19, CYP2D6 and CYP3A4) are predominantly responsible for catalyzing phase I drug metabolism reactions. An example of a polymorphically expressed CYP enzyme is CYP2C9. Substrates for CYP2C9 include phenytoin, glipizide, and S-warfarin (active enantiomer). The phenotype for the drug metabolism capacity of CYP2C9 follows those listed in the preceding paragraph; UM, EM, IM, or PM. The phenotype for CYP2C9 can be predicted based on the patient's genotype (alleles present). Patients that carry decreased function alleles, such as the *CYP2C9*2* or *CYP2C9*3* allele, generally require a smaller starting dose of warfarin than wild-type patients when taking into consideration other genetic and clinical factors that influence warfarin dose determination.[56,57] Furthermore, homozygotes for the *CYP2C9*2* (rs1799853C>T) or *CYP2C9*3* (rs1057910A>C) alleles are at a higher risk of serious bleeding events due to decreased elimination of the active warfarin enantiomer. This example, along with other relevant CYP enzymes and alleles, are summarized in **Table 3-1**.

During phase II metabolism, a small water-soluble chemical entity is conjugated onto the substrate through a covalent bond to enhance renal excretion. Phase II drug metabolism includes glucuronidation, methylation, acetylation, and sulfation conjugation reactions. Most conjugated metabolites are pharmacologically inactive, but there are some examples of active conjugated metabolites such as morphine-6-glucuronide.

Mercaptopurine, a thiopurine drug, is used to treat acute lymphoblastic leukemia or as an immunosuppressant for inflammatory bowel diseases.[58] Mercaptopurine is partially inactivated by an S-methylation reaction via thiopurine S-methyltransferase (TPMT).[54] Several studies have shown that patients with certain genetic variations within the *TPMT* gene (homozygous or heterozygous) have no or low TPMT enzyme activity. Absence of TPMT enzyme activity leads to an increased serum concentration of one of the mercaptopurine active metabolites, 6-thioguanine nucleotide, which may result in severe bone marrow suppression.[59]

Glucuronidation is another important process in Phase II drug metabolism. Irinotecan, a cytotoxic agent, exerts a meaningful uridine 5'-diphospho-glucuronosyltransferase (UGT) effect

Table 3-1 Examples of Genetic Variations Leading to Drug-Induced Diseases

Gene	Example Drug	Alleles of Interest	Response	CPIC Guidelines Recommendation
METABOLIZING ENZYMES				
CYP2C9[117,118]	Warfarin	Presence of at least one allele of *CYP2C*2* or *CYP2C*3*	Increase risk of bleeding	Monitor INR more frequently, and adjust dose accordingly
	Phenytoin	Homozygous variants: presence of two decreased function alleles including **2/*2, *2/*3, or *3/*3*	Increase risk of SJS and TEN	Dose adjustment is recommended
CYP2C19[119]	Clopidogrel	Presence of *CYP2C19*17* allele	Increase risk of bleeding	Dose adjustment is recommended
CYP2D6[120]	Codeine	Ultra-metabolizer: presence of more than 2 functional alleles	Increase risk of death in children and respiratory depression	Consider alternative therapy
Thiopurine methyltransferase[58,59,121]	Azathioprine and mercaptopurine	Homozygote variant leading to low or deficient activity	Myelotoxicity	Consider alternative therapy, or start with very low dose
UGT1A1[122]	Irinotecan	Homozygous of *UGT1A1*28* haplotypes	Myelotoxicity	Dose adjustment is recommended
N-acetyl transferase[123,124]	Isoniazid	n/a	Increase risk of lupus syndrome	n/a
	Hydralazine	n/a	Increase risk of hepatotoxicity	n/a
DRUG TRANSPORTERS				
SLCO1B1[125]	Statins (simvastatin)	Presence of at least one alleles of *SLCO1B1*5 SLCO1B1*15 SLCO1B1*17*	Myopathy Rhabdomyolysis	Consider starting with lower doses or an alternative agent
DRUG TARGETS				
VKORC1[66,117]	Warfarin	Single nucleotide polymorphism: 1639 G>A	Increase risk of bleeding	Monitor INR more frequently, and adjust dose accordingly
G6PD[126]	Rasburicase and dapsone	n/a	Increase risk of hemolytic anemia	Rasburicase is contraindicated when G6PD is deficient
HLA[13,127,128]				
*B*5701*	Abacavir	Presence of at least one *57:01* alleles	Increase risk of hypersensitivity	Not recommended
*B*1502*	Phenytoin	Presence of one or two *57:01* alleles	Increase risk of SJS and TEN	Dose adjustment is recommended
*B*1502 A*3101*	Carbamazepine	Presence of **15:02 or *31:01* alleles	Increase risk of SJS and TEN	Consider alternative therapy
*B*5801*	Allopurinol	Presence of at least one *58:01* alleles	Increase risk of SJS and TEN	Contraindicated

CPIC = Clinical Pharmacogenetics Implementation Consortium, CYP = cytochrome P450, G6PD = glucose-6-phosphate dehydrogenase, HLA = human leukocyte antigen, INR = international normalized ratio, n/a = not applicable (no CPIC recommendation), SJS = Stevens–Johnson syndrome, SLCO1B1 = solute carrier organic anion transporter family 1B1, TEN = toxic epidermal necrolysis, UGT1A1 = uridine diphosphate glucuronosyltransferase 1A1, *VKORC1* = vitamin K-epoxide reductase complex subunit 1.

on drug clearance and drug-related toxicity.[60] The active metabolite of irinotecan is SN-38, the elimination of which is facilitated by glucuronidation through the UGT1A1 enzyme. Patients with Gilbert syndrome are homozygotes for the reduced activity UGT1A1 allele (*UGT1A1*28*, rs34815109) and are predisposed to life threatening myelosuppression. These examples are summarized in Table 3-1.

DRUG TRANSPORT

Drug transporters are expressed in most tissues, including the liver, intestine, kidneys, and the brain.[61,62] They play a role in drug disposition by controlling the uptake and efflux of drugs in cells and by facilitating the movement of drugs between tissues and organs. Drug transporter function can be altered by many factors, including genotype. Organic cation transporter proteins (OCTs) are members of the solute carrier superfamily (SLC) of transporters. OCTs are uptake transporters that are predominantly expressed in the liver and kidney.

Cisplatin is a cancer chemotherapy agent that is widely used to treat solid tumors and is associated with nephrotoxicity and ototoxicity. Patients with minimal expression of both OCT1 and OCT2 or OCT2 alone are less likely to develop cisplatin-induced nephrotoxicity.[63] As an additional example, simvastatin is a widely prescribed medication for the management of dyslipidemias. Patients with polymorphisms in *SLCO1B1* (rs4149056T>C) are predisposed to simvastatin-induced myopathy. Thus, initiating simvastatin therapy with lower doses or considering an alternative agent is recommended in patients with this genotype.[64]

P-glycoprotein (Pgp) is an adenosine triphosphate (ATP)-binding cassette (ABC) transporter that (1) is expressed in the intestine, liver, and kidneys and also at the blood-brain barrier, and (2) protects against foreign substances through efflux from cells. Pgp promotes multidrug resistance by the efflux of pharmacological substrates from cells.[61,62] Pgp limits drug absorption via efflux of its substrates into the intestinal lumen, while in the kidneys and liver it promotes drug excretion into the ultrafiltrate and bile, respectively. Polymorphisms in the *ABCB1* gene have been demonstrated to decrease function and alter plasma drug concentrations by enhancing absorption, decreasing clearance and increasing access to the central nervous system. This may increase the risk of unexpected drug-related adverse events, particularly associated with the Pgp substrate digoxin.[65] The overall clinical relevance of polymorphisms in the *ABCB1* gene needs further delineation but could be an important factor for drug-induced diseases, particularly those associated with digoxin.

DRUG TARGET RECEPTORS

Genetic polymorphisms in drug targets—including enzymes, G-protein coupled receptors, ion channels, and other proteins—contribute to variability in drug efficacy and toxicity. The vitamin K epoxide reductase complex subunit 1 (*VKORC1*) gene encodes for the enzyme that is the primary pharmacological target for warfarin.[66] VKORC1 converts inactive vitamin K epoxide to active vitamin K, which is required for several coagulation factors including VII, IX, and X. An alanine (A) substitution for glycine (G) at position 1639 (1639G>A) in the *VKORC1* gene decreases the promoter activity and expression of VKORC1 protein. Thus, patients with the AA genotype require lower maintenance doses of warfarin and are at higher risk of warfarin-related adverse events, particularly in those patients that also carry reduced function alleles of CYP2C9 (i.e., *2 or *3).[54]

HUMAN LEUKOCYTE ANTIGEN

Several pharmacogenomic studies have demonstrated an important role for the HLA genes in what were previously considered idiosyncratic adverse drug reactions.[50] The major histocompatibility complex region, located on chromosome 6, contains HLA genes class I *(HLA-A, -B and -C)* and class II *(HLA-DR, -DP and -DQ)*, which are important for the function of the human immune system.[67] Several studies have shown various associations between HLA alleles and adverse drug reactions, the most common of which are liver injury and hypersensitivity reactions. The strongest available evidence associating HLA polymorphisms and drug-induced liver injury is with the antimicrobial flucloxacillin, tricyclic antidepressants, diclofenac, amoxicillin-clavulanate, and abacavir.

The most serious adverse drug events that have been associated with HLA polymorphisms are severe skin hypersensitivity reactions.[50] The hypersensitivity response is categorized as early or delayed.[68] The early response is mediated by IgE and the role of genetic polymorphisms in this type of reaction is unclear. The delayed response is T cell-dependent and varies from mild skin rash to very severe hypersensitivity syndrome. The most serious of these reactions affect other organs and tissues resulting in SJS or TEN.[50,68] Carbamazepine is the most commonly prescribed medication that induces SJS/TEN, which is strongly associated with the *HLA-B*1502* allele (rs3909184G>C and rs2844682G>A).[69] Asian populations are at higher risk of carbamazepine-induced SJS/TEN due to a higher allele frequency compared to other populations. The *HLA-A*3101* allele (rs1061235A>T) is associated with SJS/TEN in Caucasian patients, but to a lesser extent. The *HLA-B*1502* allele has not been linked to SJS/TEN in Caucasians due to a low expression frequency. This highlights the importance of the HLA genotype to predict hypersensitivity reactions in Asian populations, which is supported by a "black box" warning in carbamazepine labeling. Other important associations between the HLA genotypes and SJS/TEN, including abacavir, are provided in Table 3-1.[70,71] Pharmacogenetic testing is primarily used in patients of Asian descent to identify individuals at risk of HLA-associated adverse drug reactions prior to initiation of therapy with drugs that are known to induce serious hypersensitivity reactions.

DRUG–DRUG INTERACTIONS

DDIs refer to alterations in the effect of a medication (victim drug) when coadministered with another medication (perpetrator drug).[72] DDIs are the underlying factor in many drug-induced diseases and are attributed to as many as 26% of hospitalizations related to adverse drug reactions.[72-75] Classified by the mechanism that influences the action of the victim drug to increase susceptibility to drug-induced disease, DDIs are broadly divided into pharmacokinetic or pharmacodynamic interactions. Pharmacokinetic-based interactions affect the absorption, distribution, metabolism, or excretion processes, while pharmacodynamic-based interactions alter physiologic systems within the body.

The implications of DDIs on clinical practice are both profound and diverse:

- DDIs can be exploited clinically to achieve synergistic increases in drug efficacy, such as in the use of aminoglycoside and β-lactam antibiotics concomitantly to treat bacterial infections.
- DDIs can result in therapeutic failure, as manifested by the reduced anticonvulsant efficacy of phenytoin during coadministration with rifampin.
- DDIs can result in potentiation of the adverse effects of the victim drug to cause drug-induced disease, such as the development of digoxin-induced nausea, vomiting, anorexia, or arrhythmias when coadministered with amiodarone.

DDIs that result in potentiation of adverse effects constitute an important cause of drug-induced diseases and these interactions will be the focus of this section.

The effective identification and characterization of DDIs are critical to facilitate their prevention and to limit the incidence of drug-induced disease in clinical practice. A complicating factor of DDIs is that they can occur through the simultaneous action of multiple mechanisms. Due to these complexities, DDIs are sometimes difficult to identify and remain an important factor contributing to drug-induced diseases.

PHARMACOKINETIC DRUG–DRUG INTERACTIONS

The many clinical implications of DDIs reflect the vast range of physiologic processes and systems affected. Pharmacokinetic-based DDIs impact drug action by altering drug exposure within the body. Common mechanisms of pharmacokinetic DDIs that cause drug-induced disease, along with clinically relevant examples, are discussed in this section.

Membrane transporters impact the pharmacokinetics of many medications and, therefore, factors that influence transporter activity have implications on both drug efficacy and safety. As indicated in the Genetic Variation section, two important superfamilies of transporters that impact drug disposition include ABCs and SLCs, with members of these two superfamilies contributing to both drug influx and efflux from systemic circulation and/or the drug site of action. Inhibition of drug transport through these mechanisms can increase drug exposure.[76] An important DDI related to drug transporter inhibition involves the novel oral anticoagulant dabigatran when coadministered with a Pgp (member of the ABC superfamily) inhibitor. Serum dabigatran concentrations are elevated when coadministered with verapamil, an inhibitor of Pgp.[77] The decreased Pgp-mediated dabigatran efflux within intestinal epithelial cells increases the risk of major bleeding associated with dabigatran therapy.[78,79] Similarly, the incidence of respiratory depression associated with the antidiarrheal agent loperamide is increased when coadministered with the Pgp inhibitor quinidine.[79] The mechanism involves inhibition of Pgp mediated efflux at the blood-brain barrier. This enhances loperamide access to the central nervous system to precipitate respiratory depression.[80]

Modulations in the activity of drug-metabolizing enzymes are the most common and widely studied mechanism of DDIs. Most frequently, drug-metabolizing enzymes mediate the transformation of a pharmacologically active parent drug into less active or inactive metabolites. Therefore, factors that influence drug metabolism result in changes in exposure of active drug moieties, ultimately resulting in alterations in both the therapeutic and adverse effects of drugs.

The CYP450 enzyme system is primarily responsible for the biotransformation of drugs during phase I metabolism. Clinically relevant DDIs affect the following CYP isoenzymes: CYP1A2, CYP2B6, CYP2C9, CYP2C19, CYP2D6, CYP2E1, and CYP3A4/5.[81-83] Inhibition of CYP enzymes results in increased exposure of parent drugs metabolized by these pathways, increasing both therapeutic activity and the potential for adverse drug effects when the parent drug is the active moiety. Exposure to midazolam is increased during coadministration with the CYP3A inhibitor ketoconazole, resulting in the potentiation and prolongation of midazolam's hypnotic effect.[84] In addition, the induction of CYP enzymes may also precipitate drug-induced diseases. For example, induction of CYP2E1 by isoniazid results in increased metabolism of acetaminophen to its toxic metabolite, NAPQI, resulting in an increased risk for hepatotoxicity.[85-87] There are numerous examples of potential DDIs that precipitate drug-induced diseases. Some of the examples of DDIs involving the inhibition of CYP isoenzymes are displayed in **Table 3-2**.

The kidneys play an important role in the elimination of many drugs. DDIs may potentially influence renal elimination and predispose individuals to drug-induced disease via four distinct mechanisms[88]:

1. Inhibition of tubular secretion, the process by which drugs are moved from the peritubular capillaries to the renal tubular lumen for excretion

Table 3-2 Drug–Drug Interactions Contributing to Drug-Induced Disease Through CYP Inhibition

CYP Enzyme	Victim Drug	Perpetrator Drug	Drug-Induced Disease
CYP1A2[129]	Alosetron	Fluvoxamine	Constipation, gastrointestinal pain, nausea, abdominal distention, ischemic colitis
CYP2B6[130,131]	Efavirenz	Voriconazole	Severe rash, insomnia, vivid dreams, liver failure
CYP2C9[132]	Warfarin	Fluconazole	Increased risk for major bleeding (epistaxis, gastrointestinal bleeding, melena, hematuria)
CYP2C19[133,134]	Diazepam	Isoniazid	Ataxia, somnolence, sedation, respiratory depression
CYP2D6[129,135]	Propranolol	Fluoxetine	Bradyarrhythmia, hypotension, AV block, cardiogenic shock
CYP2E1[136,137]	Theophylline	Disulfiram	Nausea, vomiting, tremor, heart palpitations, tachyarrhythmia, seizures
CYP3A4/5[138-140]	Simvastatin	Clarithromycin	Muscle tenderness, muscle weakness, myalgia, rhabdomyolysis

AV = atrioventricular, CYP = cytochrome P450.

2. Changes in urinary pH that decrease drug excretion
3. Changes in renal blood flow that decrease drug filtration
4. Inhibition of renal drug metabolism

Trimethoprim, when formulated with or without sulfamethoxazole, inhibits OCT2-mediated tubular secretion of the antiparkinsonian drug amantadine, resulting in increased amantadine exposure and the potential for psychiatric symptoms such as delirium, confusion, and combative behavior.[88,89]

PHARMACODYNAMIC DRUG–DRUG INTERACTIONS

The basis for pharmacodynamic DDIs involves alterations of pharmacological targets that accentuate or attenuate a physiological response. Such physiologic alterations are frequently related to the pharmacologic effects of the drug entities but also may occur via off-target effects. Thus, pharmacodynamic DDIs may result in reduced drug efficacy or enhance the risk for drug-induced diseases.

Additive pharmacodynamic effects constitute a very common cause of drug-induced disease. Clinically significant examples of additive pharmacodynamic DDIs include drug-induced hypotension in patients with heart failure as a result of coadministration of multiple agents with hypotensive effects, such as β-blockers, ACE inhibitors, hydralazine, isosorbide dinitrate, and angiotensin receptor blockers. Another example of a pharmacodynamic DDI that can result in a drug-induced disease is the coadministration of multiple drugs known to individually prolong the QT interval on a surface ECG, increasing the risk of torsades de pointes, such as coadministration of the fluoroquinolone levofloxacin, with the antipsychotic agent haloperidol.[90-92]

FOOD–DRUG INTERACTIONS

Food–drug interactions can result in drug-induced diseases. Similar to DDIs, food–drug interactions can occur as a result of the alteration of pharmacokinetic or pharmacodynamic processes due to an interacting component found in the diet. These interactions can contribute to the development of drug-induced disease through a variety of mechanisms, including opposition of a drug's therapeutic activity and potentiation of drug adverse effects and toxicities. Food–drug interactions present a necessary consideration, and their effect on drug action can influence both drug selection and dose determination. Three common and clinically significant examples of food–drug interactions that contribute to drug-induced disease are described below.

Tyramine is a monoamine compound found in aged food and beverage products like cheese and beer, respectively. A potentially life-threatening food–drug interaction occurs when the metabolism of tyramine is inhibited by the class of drugs known as the monoamine oxidase inhibitors (MAOIs), occurring most frequently with older MAOIs such as phenelzine, isocarboxazid, and tranylcypromine. The food–drug interaction dramatically increases tyramine's vasopressive effects and can precipitate severe hypertension, hyperthermia, cardiac arrhythmias, and cerebral hemorrhage.[93]

Caffeine—found in coffee, tea, cola, and chocolate—is involved in a variety of food–drug interactions based on both its pharmacodynamic profile and its similarity in structure and function to certain drugs. Caffeine consumption is contraindicated during use of the structurally similar methylxanthine drug, theophylline. Caffeine increases plasma theophylline concentrations and potentiates its numerous adverse effects. Additionally, caffeine administration has been demonstrated to reduce seizure threshold and may thereby precipitate seizures or diminish the efficacy of anticonvulsant medications.[94-96]

Grapefruit juice is a potent inhibitor of intestinal CYP3A4 metabolism, and it is also implicated in the inhibition of intestinal Pgp efflux transporters and organic anion-transporting polypeptide influx transporters through interactions mediated by furanocoumarin and flavonoid species found in the juice.[97] In fact, trials have demonstrated significant alterations in drug disposition upon coadministration of as little as one 8-ounce glass of grapefruit juice.[98] Food–drug interactions involving grapefruit juice affect a vast number of drugs that rely on the Pgp and CYP3A4 pathways for systemic absorption and metabolism, including antibiotics, antidepressants, antihypertensives, antiarrhythmics, corticosteroids, and medications to manage hypercholesterolemia.[97] For instance, the risk for myopathy and rhabdomyolysis associated with simvastatin may be increased when taken with grapefruit juice.[99]

MEDICATION NONADHERENCE

Medical nonadherence is defined as when patients do not follow provider recommendations about medication therapy with respect to timing, dosage, and frequency. It constitutes a major global healthcare problem and contributes to the incidence of drug-induced disease.[100] The World Health Organization proposes that increasing the effectiveness of adherence interventions may have a greater population-wide health impact than improvements in specific medical treatments.[101] This assertion is supported by recent estimates that as many as 50% of Americans are not adherent to long-term medication therapy, resulting in preventable annual healthcare expenditures of over $100 billion.[102]

The contribution of medication nonadherence to drug-induced disease occurs through a variety of mechanisms. One instance is when a patient nonadherently increases the dose or frequency of drug administration, resulting in enhanced drug exposure. Nonadherence can also contribute to drug-induced disease through indirect mechanisms, such as nonadherent behaviors resulting in decreased medication administration. For example, when a patient omits medication doses, the prescriber may intensify therapy either by increasing the dose or frequency of the medication or through addition of adjunctive medication therapy, thereby predisposing the patient to an increased risk of drug toxicities.[100]

The causes of medication nonadherence are often complex, multifactorial, and highly variable among patients. Six of the most commonly described factors contributing to nonadherence include the following[103]:

1. Lack of patient understanding of the contribution of medication adherence to continued good health
2. Patient perception that the potential risks of medication therapy outweigh the benefits
3. When the complexity of the medication therapy regimen exceeds the patient's mental processing capacity
4. Lack of sufficient patient vigilance
5. When the patient possesses inaccurate, irrational, or conflicting normative beliefs regarding medication therapy
6. Patient disbelief in the therapeutic efficacy of a medication

Addressing the specific cause of patient nonadherence is paramount to effectively improving adherence. Accordingly, strategies to improve medication adherence have focused on combinations of multiple interventions to address the many reasons for nonadherence. For example, patient counseling and provision of health information may improve patient understanding of the benefit and efficacy of medication in promoting health. Interventions such as electronic reminders to take medicine and medication packaging with a calendar feature help increase patient vigilance.[104,105] Despite these multifactorial approaches, strategies to improve adherence have generally demonstrated only modest increases in adherent behavior.[106] As a result, medication nonadherence remains a significant challenge to effective medication therapy and an important factor to consider in relation to drug-induced diseases.

MEDICATION ERRORS

Defined as "any preventable event that may cause or lead to inappropriate medication use or patient harm while the medication is in the control of the healthcare professional, patient, or consumer," *medication errors* constitute a significant cause of drug-induced disease.[107] Medication errors are commonly manifested as administration of the wrong drug, drug overdoses, overlooking of documented patient drug allergies, or failure to detect DDIs—all of which can directly cause adverse drug events.[108] The estimated medication error rate is at 1.6 errors per 1,000 patient days in adult hospitalized patients. This rate is elevated in special patient populations, such as an estimated rate of 13.4 errors per 1,000 patient days in pediatric patients.[109,110]

Medication errors may occur during any step of the medication-use process, including prescribing, transcription, dispensing, administration, and monitoring. A series of studies by the Adverse Drug Event Prevention Study group attributed 28% of discovered adverse drug events to medication errors during a 6-month investigation within two major metropolitan hospitals.[111] The medication errors were most likely to occur during prescribing (56%), administration (34%), transcription (6%), and dispensing (4%).[112] The National Coordinating Council for Medication Error Reporting and Prevention has developed an index for categorizing medication errors based on whether a medication error reaches the patient, whether the error results in patient harm, and the severity of managing the adverse drug event.[113] The index seeks to provide a systematic means to standardize the classification and severity of medication errors to more accurately characterize their burden to medication use.

As medication errors occur over a wide variety of steps in the medication-use process, the reasons that they occur are widely variable. Risk factors that predispose patients to medication errors can be patient-specific (kidney or liver disease, advanced age), prescriber-specific (use of potentially confusing medical abbreviations when prescribing), or factors latent within an institution's system of delivering patient care (poorly structured physical or informational environment, failing to adhere to clinical standards).[114,115] Regardless of medication error etiology, properly identifying the causes is essential in preventing error occurrence.[116] The FDA has instituted efforts to prevent medication errors such as the widely implemented 5 Rights of Medication Administration. The effective use of information technology within the administration of healthcare has been perhaps the greatest advancement in preventing medication errors, as electronic technology has the potential to significantly reduce errors in all steps of the medication-use process.[115] Although the contribution of medication errors to the development of drug-induced disease is well evidenced, strategies for preventing these errors remain a formidable challenge.

SUMMARY

This chapter outlines the most important factors that are known to contribute to drug-induced diseases while demonstrating important clinical consequences. The contribution of age, sex, race, pregnancy status, genetics, comorbid diseases, cigarette smoking, alcohol, illicit drug use, DDIs, food–drug interactions, medication adherence, and medication errors should all be considered to identify the potential for a drug-induced disease.

REFERENCES

1. Bowie MW, Slattum PW. Pharmacodynamics in older adults: a review. *Am J Geriatr Pharmacother.* 2007; 5:263-303.
2. Mangoni AA, Jackson SH. Age-related changes in pharmacokinetics and pharmacodynamics: basic principles and practical applications. *Br J Clin Pharmacol.* 2004; 57:6-14.
3. Routledge PA, O'Mahony MS, Woodhouse KW. Adverse drug reactions in elderly patients. *Br J Clin Pharmacol.* 2004; 57:121-6.
4. American Geriatrics Society. 2015 updated beers criteria for potentially inappropriate medication use in older adults. *J Am Geriatr Soc.* 2015; 63:2227-46.
5. Soldin OP, Chung SH, Mattison DR. Sex differences in drug disposition. *J Biomed Biotechnol.* 2011; 2011:187103.
6. Tran C, Knowles SR, Liu BA et al. Gender differences in adverse drug reactions. *J Clin Pharmacol.* 1998; 38:1003-9.
7. Drici MD, Clement N. Is gender a risk factor for adverse drug reactions? The example of drug-induced long QT syndrome. *Drug Saf.* 2001; 24:575-85.
8. Rademaker M. Do women have more adverse drug reactions? *Am J Clin Dermatol.* 2001; 2:349-51.
9. Bamshad M, Wooding S, Salisbury BA et al. Deconstructing the relationship between genetics and race. *Nat Rev Genet.* 2004; 5:598-609.
10. Coleman JJ, McDowell SE. Ethnicity and adverse drug reactions. *Adv Drug React Bull.* 2005; 234:899-902.
11. Eliasson E. Ethnicity and adverse drug reactions. *BMJ.* 2006; 332:1163-4.
12. Yasuda SU, Zhang L, Huang SM. The role of ethnicity in variability in response to drugs: focus on clinical pharmacology studies. *Clin Pharmacol Ther.* 2008; 84:417-23.
13. Ferrell PB Jr, McLeod HL. Carbamazepine, HLA-B*1502 and risk of Stevens-Johnson syndrome and toxic epidermal necrolysis: US FDA recommendations. *Pharmacogenomics.* 2008; 9:1543-6.
14. Gibbs CR, Lip GY, Beevers DG. Angioedema due to ACE inhibitors: increased risk in patients of African origin. *Br J Clin Pharmacol.* 1999; 48:861-5.
15. Pare G, Kubo M, Byrd JB et al. Genetic variants associated with angiotensin-converting enzyme inhibitor-associated angioedema. *Pharmacogenet Genomics.* 2013; 23:470-8.
16. Gilbert-Barness E. Teratogenic causes of malformations. *Ann Clin Lab Sci.* 2010; 40:99-114.

17. US Food and Drug Administration (FDA), Center for Drug Evaluation and Research. *Reviewer guidance: evaluating the risks of drug exposure in human pregnancies.* Washington DC: FDA; 2005.
18. Costantine MM. Physiologic and pharmacokinetic changes in pregnancy. *Front Pharmacol.* 2014;5:65.
19. Loebstein R, Lalkin A, Koren G. Pharmacokinetic changes during pregnancy and their clinical relevance. *Clin Pharmacokinet.* 1997; 33:328-43.
20. Kroon LA. Drug interactions with smoking. *Am J Health-Syst Pharm.* 2007; 64:1917-21.
21. Washio I, Maeda M, Sugiura C et al. Cigarette smoke extract induces CYP2B6 through constitutive androstane receptor in hepatocytes. *Drug Metab Dispos.* 2011; 3:1-3.
22. Desai HD, Seabolt J, Jann MW. Smoking in patients receiving psychotropic medications: a pharmacokinetic perspective. *CNS drugs.* 2001; 15:469-94.
23. Burkman R, Schlesselman JJ, Zieman M. Safety concerns and health benefits associated with oral contraception. *Am J Obstet Gynecol.* 2004; 190(4 suppl):S5-22.
24. Chan LN, Anderson GD. Pharmacokinetic and pharmacodynamic drug interactions with ethanol (alcohol). *Clin Pharmacokinet.* 2014; 53:1115-36.
25. Zakhari S. Overview: how is alcohol metabolized by the body? *Alcohol Res Health.* 2006; 29:245-54.
26. Schiodt FV, Lee WM, Bondesen S et al. Influence of acute and chronic alcohol intake on the clinical course and outcome in acetaminophen overdose. *Aliment Pharmacol Ther.* 2002; 16:707-15.
27. Hinson JA, Roberts DW, James LP. Mechanisms of acetaminophen-induced liver necrosis. *Handb Exp Pharmacol.* 2010; 196:369-405.
28. Radwan MM, Elsohly MA, Slade D et al. Biologically active cannabinoids from high-potency Cannabis sativa. *J Nat Prod.* 2009; 72:906-11.
29. Jordan K, Sippel C, Schmoll HJ. Guidelines for antiemetic treatment of chemotherapy-induced nausea and vomiting: past, present, and future recommendations. *Oncologist.* 2007; 12:1143-50.
30. Borgelt LM, Franson KL, Nussbaum AM et al. The pharmacologic and clinical effects of medical cannabis. *Pharmacotherapy.* 2013; 33:195-209.
31. Hunt CA, Jones RT. Tolerance and disposition of tetrahydrocannabinol in man. *J Pharmacol Exp Ther.* 1980; 215:35-44.
32. Yamreudeewong W, Wong HK, Brausch LM et al. Probable interaction between warfarin and marijuana smoking. *Ann Pharmacother.* 2009; 43:1347-53.
33. Watanabe K, Yamaori S, Funahashi T et al. Cytochrome P450 enzymes involved in the metabolism of tetrahydrocannabinols and cannabinol by human hepatic microsomes. *Life Sci.* 2007; 80:1415-9.
34. Brownlow HA, Pappachan J. Pathophysiology of cocaine abuse. *Eur J Anaesthesiol.* 2002;19:395-414.
35. Dean A. Pharmacology of psychostimulants. In: Baker A, Lee N, Jenner L, eds. *Models of intervention and care for psychostimulant users.* 2nd ed. Canberra: Australian Government Department of Health and Ageing; 2004:35-50.
36. Naud J, Nolin TD, Leblond FA et al. Current understanding of drug disposition in kidney disease. *J Clin Pharmacol.* 2012; 52:10s-22s.
37. Chapin E, Zhan M, Hsu VD et al. Adverse safety events in chronic kidney disease: the frequency of "multiple hits." *Clin J Am Soc Nephrol.* 2010; 5:95-101.
38. Ginsberg JS, Zhan M, Diamantidis CJ et al. Patient-reported and actionable safety events in CKD. *J Am Soc Nephrol.* 2014; 25:1564-73.
39. Okabe H, Hashimoto Y, Inui KI. Pharmacokinetics and bioavailability of tacrolimus in rats with experimental renal dysfunction. *J Pharm Pharmacol.* 2000; 52:1467-72.
40. Kanfer A, Stamatakis G, Torlotin JC et al. Changes in erythromycin pharmacokinetics induced by renal failure. *Clin Nephrol.* 1987; 27:147-50.
41. Takeuchi A, Masuda S, Saito H et al. Role of kidney-specific organic anion transporters in the urinary excretion of methotrexate. *Kidney Int.* 2001; 60:1058-68.
42. Franz CC, Hildbrand C, Born C et al. Dose adjustment in patients with liver cirrhosis: impact on adverse drug reactions and hospitalizations. *Eur J Clin Pharmaco.* 2013; 69:1565-73.
43. Delco F, Tchambaz L, Schlienger R et al. Dose adjustment in patients with liver disease. *Drug Saf.* 2005; 28:529-45.
44. Verbeeck RK. Pharmacokinetics and dosage adjustment in patients with hepatic dysfunction. *Eur J Clin Pharmaco.* 2008; 64:1147-61.
45. Bergasa NV, Rothman RB, Mukerjee E et al. Up-regulation of central mu-opioid receptors in a model of hepatic encephalopathy: a potential mechanism for increased sensitivity to morphine in liver failure. *Life Sci.* 2002; 70:1701-8.
46. Woosley RL. Pharmacokinetics and pharmacodynamics of antiarrhythmic agents in patients with congestive heart failure. *Am Heart J.* 1987; 114:1280-91.
47. Smith TW. Digitalis. Mechanisms of action and clinical use. *N Engl J Med.* 1988; 318:358-65.
48. Croxson MS, Ibbertson HK. Serum digoxin in patients with thyroid disease. *Br Med J.* 1975; 3:566-8.
49. Raja Rao MP, Panduranga P, Sulaiman K et al. Digoxin toxicity with normal digoxin and serum potassium levels: beware of magnesium, the hidden malefactor. *J Emerg Med.* 2013; 45:e31-4.
50. Daly AK. Pharmacogenomics of adverse drug reactions. *Genome Med.* 2013; 5:5.
51. Uetrecht J, Naisbitt DJ. Idiosyncratic adverse drug reactions: current concepts. *Pharmacol Rev.* 2013; 65:779-808.
52. Ma Q, Lu AY. Pharmacogenetics, pharmacogenomics, and individualized medicine. *Pharmacol Rev.* 2011; 63:437-59.
53. Belle DJ, Singh H. Genetic factors in drug metabolism. *Am Fam Physician.* 2008; 77:1553-60.
54. Sim SC, Kacevska M, Ingelman-Sundberg M. Pharmacogenomics of drug-metabolizing enzymes: a recent update on clinical implications and endogenous effects. *Pharmacogenomics J.* 2013; 13:1-11.
55. Relling MV, Klein TE. CPIC: Clinical Pharmacogenetics Implementation Consortium of the Pharmacogenomics Research Network. *Clin Pharmacol Ther.* 2011; 89:464-7.
56. Aquilante CL, Langaee TY, Lopez LM et al. Influence of coagulation factor, vitamin K epoxide reductase complex subunit 1, and cytochrome P450 2C9 gene polymorphisms on warfarin dose requirements. *Clin Pharmacol Ther.* 2006; 79:291-302.
57. Higashi MK, Veenstra DL, Kondo LM et al. Association between CYP2C9 genetic variants and anticoagulation-related outcomes during warfarin therapy. *JAMA.* 2002; 287:1690-8.
58. Booth RA, Ansari MT, Loit E et al. Assessment of thiopurine S-methyltransferase activity in patients prescribed thiopurines: a systematic review. *Ann of Intern Med.* 2011; 154:814-23, w-295-818.
59. Lennard L, Van Loon JA, Weinshilboum RM. Pharmacogenetics of acute azathioprine toxicity: relationship to thiopurine methyltransferase genetic polymorphism. *Clin Pharmacol Ther.* 1989; 46:149-54.
60. Sim SC, Ingelman-Sundberg M. Pharmacogenomic biomarkers: new tools in current and future drug therapy. *Trends in Pharmaco Sci.* 2011; 32:72-81.
61. DeGorter MK, Xia CQ, Yang JJ et al. Drug transporters in drug efficacy and toxicity. *Annu Rev Pharmacol Toxicol.* 2012; 52:249-73.
62. Schuetz JD, Swaan PW, Tweedie DJ. The role of transporters in toxicity and disease. *Drug Metab Dispos.* 2014; 42:541-5.

63. Filipski KK, Mathijssen RH, Mikkelsen TS et al. Contribution of organic cation transporter 2 (OCT2) to cisplatin-induced nephrotoxicity. *Clin Pharmacol Ther.* 2009; 86:396-402.
64. Ramsey LB, Johnson SG, Caudle KE et al. The clinical pharmacogenetics implementation consortium guideline for SLCO1B1 and simvastatin-induced myopathy: 2014 update. *Clin Pharmacol Ther.* 2014; 96:423-8.
65. Hoffmeyer S, Burk O, von Richter O et al. Functional polymorphisms of the human multidrug-resistance gene: multiple sequence variations and correlation of one allele with P-glycoprotein expression and activity in vivo. *Proc Natl Acad Sci USA.* 2000; 97:3473-8.
66. Rieder MJ, Reiner AP, Gage BF et al. Effect of *VKORC1* haplotypes on transcriptional regulation and warfarin dose. *N Engl J Med.* 2005; 352:2285-93.
67. Stephens C, Lucena MI, Andrade RJ. Genetic variations in drug-induced liver injury (DILI): resolving the puzzle. *Front Genet.* 2012; 3:253.
68. Svensson CK, Cowen EW, Gaspari AA. Cutaneous drug reactions. *Pharmacol Rev.* 2001; 53:357-79.
69. Chung WH, Hung SI, Hong HS et al. Medical genetics: a marker for Stevens-Johnson syndrome. *Nature.* 2004; 428:486.
70. Mallal S, Nolan D, Witt C et al. Association between presence of HLA-B*5701, HLA-DR7, and HLA-DQ3 and hypersensitivity to HIV-1 reverse-transcriptase inhibitor abacavir. *Lancet (London, England).* 2002; 359:727-32.
71. Mallal S, Phillips E, Carosi G et al. HLA-B*5701 screening for hypersensitivity to abacavir. *N Engl J Med.* 2008; 358:568-79.
72. Dechanont S, Maphanta S, Butthum B et al. Hospital admissions/visits associated with drug-drug interactions: a systematic review and meta-analysis. *Pharmacoepidemiol Drug Saf.* 2014; 23:489-97.
73. Prince BS, Goetz CM, Rihn TL et al. Drug-related emergency department visits and hospital admissions. *Am J Hosp Pharm.* 1992; 49:1696-700.
74. McDonnell PJ, Jacobs MR. Hospital admissions resulting from preventable adverse drug reactions. *Ann Pharmacother.* 2002; 36:1331-6.
75. Peyriere H, Cassan S, Floutard E et al. Adverse drug events associated with hospital admission. *Ann Pharmacother.* 2003; 37:5-11.
76. Giacomini KM, Huang SM, Tweedie DJ et al. Membrane transporters in drug development. *Nat Rev Drug Discov.* 2010; 9:215-36.
77. Hartter S, Sennewald R, Nehmiz G et al. Oral bioavailability of dabigatran etexilate (Pradaxa) after co-medication with verapamil in healthy subjects. *Br J Clin Pharmacol.* 2013; 75:1053-62.
78. Kawabata M, Yokoyama Y, Sasano T et al. Bleeding events and activated partial thromboplastin time with dabigatran in clinical practice. *J Cardiol.* 2013; 62:121-6.
79. Finch A, Pillans P. P-glycoprotein and its role in drug-drug interactions. *Australian Prescriber.* 2014; 37:137-9.
80. Sadeque AJ, Wandel C, He H et al. Increased drug delivery to the brain by P-glycoprotein inhibition. *Clin Pharmacol Ther.* 2000; 68:231-7.
81. Zanger UM, Schwab M. Cytochrome P450 enzymes in drug metabolism: regulation of gene expression, enzyme activities, and impact of genetic variation. *Pharmacol Ther.* 2013; 138:103-41.
82. Ogu CC, Maxa JL. Drug interactions due to cytochrome P450. *Proc (Bayl Univ Med Cent).* 2000; 13:421-3.
83. Wang H, Tompkins LM. CYP2B6: new insights into a historically overlooked cytochrome P450 isozyme. *Curr Drug Metab.* 2008; 9:598-610.
84. Olkkola KT, Backman JT, Neuvonen PJ. Midazolam should be avoided in patients receiving the systemic antimycotics ketoconazole or itraconazole. *Clin Pharmacol Ther.* 1994; 55:481-5.
85. Nolan CM, Sandblom RE, Thummel KE et al. Hepatotoxicity associated with acetaminophen usage in patients receiving multiple drug therapy for tuberculosis. *Chest.* 1994; 105:408-11.
86. Moulding TS, Redeker AG, Kanel GC. Acetaminophen, isoniazid, and hepatic toxicity. *Ann Intern Med.* 1991; 114:431.
87. Murphy R, Swartz R, Watkins PB. Severe acetaminophen toxicity in a patient receiving isoniazid. *Ann Intern Med.* 1990; 113:799-800.
88. Bonate PL, Reith K, Weir S. Drug interactions at the renal level. Implications for drug development. *Clin Pharmacokinet.* 1998; 34:375-404.
89. Speeg KV, Leighton JA, Maldonado AL. Toxic delirium in a patient taking amantadine and trimethoprim–sulfamethoxazole. *Am J Med Sci.* 1989; 298:410-2.
90. Sandson NB, Armstrong SC, Cozza KL. An overview of psychotropic drug-drug interactions. *Psychosomatics.* 2005; 46:464-94.
91. Freeman BD, Dixon DJ, Coopersmith CM et al. Pharmacoepidemiology of QT-interval prolonging drug administration in critically ill patients. *Pharmacoepidemiol Drug Saf.* 2008; 17:971-81.
92. Nachimuthu S, Assar MD, Schussler JM. Drug-induced QT interval prolongation: mechanisms and clinical management. *Ther Adv Drug Saf.* 2012; 3:241-53.
93. Rapaport MH. Dietary restrictions and drug interactions with monoamine oxidase inhibitors: the state of the art. *J Clin Psychiatry.* 2007; 68:42-6.
94. Kulkarni C, Joseph T, David J. Influence of adenosine receptor antagonists, aminophylline and caffeine, on seizure protective ability of antiepileptic drugs in rats. *Indian J Exp Biol.* 1991; 29:751-4.
95. Cysneiros RM, Farkas D, Harmatz JS et al. Pharmacokinetic and pharmacodynamic interactions between zolpidem and caffeine. *Clin Pharmacol Ther.* 2007; 82:54-62.
96. Luszczki JJ, Zuchora M, Sawicka KM et al. Acute exposure to caffeine decreases the anticonvulsant action of ethosuximide, but not that of clonazepam, phenobarbital and valproate against pentetrazole-induced seizures in mice. *Pharmacol Rep.* 2006; 58:652-9.
97. Seden K, Dickinson L, Khoo S et al. Grapefruit-drug interactions. *Drugs.* 2010; 70:2373-407.
98. Bressler R. Grapefruit juice and drug interactions. Exploring mechanisms of this interaction and potential toxicity for certain drugs. *Geriatrics.* 2006; 61:12-8.
99. Lilja JJ, Neuvonen M, Neuvonen PJ. Effects of regular consumption of grapefruit juice on the pharmacokinetics of simvastatin. *Br J Clin Pharmacol.* 2004; 58:56-60.
100. Bosworth HB, Granger BB, Mendys P et al. Medication adherence: a call for action. *Am Heart J.* 2011; 162:412-24.
101. World Health Organization. *Adherence to long-term therapies: evidence for action.* Geneva: World Health Organization; 2003.
102. Osterberg L, Blaschke T. Adherence to medication. *N Engl J Med.* 2005; 353:487-97.
103. Marcum ZA, Sevick MA, Handler SM. Medication nonadherence: a diagnosable and treatable medical condition. *JAMA.* 2013; 309:2105-6.
104. Zedler BK, Kakad P, Colilla S et al. Does packaging with a calendar feature improve adherence to self-administered medication for long-term use? A systematic review. *Clin Ther.* 2011; 33:62-73.
105. Haynes RB, Ackloo E, Sahota N et al. Interventions for enhancing medication adherence. *Cochrane Database Syst Rev.* 2008: Cd000011.
106. Bryant J, McDonald VM, Boyes A et al. Improving medication adherence in chronic obstructive pulmonary disease: a systematic review. *Respir Res.* 2013; 14:109.
107. National Coordinating Council for Medication Error Reporting and Prevention. About medication errors. http://www.nccmerp.org/about-medication-errors (accessed 2017 Nov 7).
108. Carmichael JN, Jones WN. Medication therapy and patient care. In: Brown TR, ed. *Handbook of institutional pharmacy practice.* Bethesda, Maryland: American Society of Health-System Pharmacists; 2006.

109. Choi I, Lee SM, Flynn L et al. Incidence and treatment costs attributable to medication errors in hospitalized patients. *Res Social Adm Pharm.* 2016; 12:428-3.

110. McClead RE Jr, Catt C, Davis JT et al. An internal quality improvement collaborative significantly reduces hospital-wide medication error related adverse drug events. *The J Pediatr.* 2014; 165:1222-9.e1221.

111. Leape LL, Bates DW, Cullen DJ et al. Systems analysis of adverse drug events. ADE Prevention Study Group. *JAMA.* 1995; 274:35-43.

112. Bates DW, Cullen DJ, Laird N et al. Incidence of adverse drug events and potential adverse drug events. Implications for prevention. ADE Prevention Study Group. *JAMA.* 1995; 274:29-34.

113. National Coordinating Council for Medication Error Reporting and Prevention. NCC MERP Index for Categorizing Medication Errors. http://www.nccmerp.org/sites/default/files/indexBW2001-06-12.pdf (accessed 2017 Nov 7).

114. Waeschle RM, Bauer M, Schmidt CE. Errors in medicine: Causes, impact and improvement measures to improve patient safety. *Anaesthesist.* 2015; 64:689-704.

115. Wittich CM, Burkle CM, Lanier WL. Medication errors: an overview for clinicians. *Mayo Clin Proc.* 2014; 89:1116-25.

116. Ferner RE. The epidemiology of medication errors: the methodological difficulties. *Br J Clin Pharmacol.* 2009; 67:614-20.

117. Johnson JA, Gong L, Whirl-Carrillo M et al. Clinical Pharmacogenetics Implementation Consortium Guidelines for CYP2C9 and *VKORC1* genotypes and warfarin dosing. *Clin Pharmacol Ther.* 2011; 90:625-9.

118. Caudle KE, Rettie AE, Whirl-Carrillo M et al. Clinical pharmacogenetics implementation consortium guidelines for CYP2C9 and HLA-B genotypes and phenytoin dosing. *Clin Pharmacol Ther.* 2014; 96:542-8.

119. Scott SA, Sangkuhl K, Stein CM et al. Clinical Pharmacogenetics Implementation Consortium guidelines for CYP2C19 genotype and clopidogrel therapy: 2013 update. *Clin Pharmacol Ther.* 2013; 94:317-23.

120. Madadi P, Amstutz U, Rieder M et al. Clinical practice guideline: CYP2D6 genotyping for safe and efficacious codeine therapy. *J Popul Ther Clin Pharmacol.* 2013; 20:e369-96.

121. Relling MV, Gardner EE, Sandborn WJ et al. Clinical pharmacogenetics implementation consortium guidelines for thiopurine methyltransferase genotype and thiopurine dosing: 2013 update. *Clin Pharmacol Ther.* 2013; 93:324-5.

122. Etienne-Grimaldi MC, Boyer JC, Thomas F et al. UGT1A1 genotype and irinotecan therapy: general review and implementation in routine practice. *Fundam Clin Pharmacol.* 2015; 29:219-37.

123. Salazar-Paramo M, Rubin RL, Garcia-De La Torre I. Systemic lupus erythematosus induced by isoniazid. *Ann Rheum Dis.* 1992; 51:1085-7.

124. Stumpf JL. Fatal hepatotoxicity induced by hydralazine or labetalol. *Pharmacotherapy.* 1991; 11:415-8.

125. Wilke RA, Ramsey LB, Johnson SG et al. The clinical pharmacogenomics implementation consortium: CPIC guideline for SLCO1B1 and simvastatin-induced myopathy. *Clin Pharmacol Ther.* 2012; 92:112-7.

126. Relling MV, McDonagh EM, Chang T et al. Clinical Pharmacogenetics Implementation Consortium (CPIC) guidelines for rasburicase therapy in the context of G6PD deficiency genotype. *Clin Pharmacol Ther.* 2014; 96:169-74.

127. Martin MA, Hoffman JM, Freimuth RR et al. Clinical Pharmacogenetics Implementation Consortium Guidelines for HLA-B Genotype and Abacavir Dosing: 2014 update. *Clin Pharmacol Ther.* 2014; 95:499-500.

128. Saito Y, Stamp LK, Caudle KE et al. Clinical Pharmacogenetics Implementation Consortium (CPIC) guidelines for human leukocyte antigen B (HLA-B) genotype and allopurinol dosing: 2015 update. *Clin Pharmacol Ther.* 2016; 99:36-7.

129. Brosen K. Differences in interactions of SSRIs. *Int Clin Psychopharmacol.* 1998; 13:S45-47.

130. Liu P, Foster G, LaBadie RR et al. Pharmacokinetic interaction between voriconazole and efavirenz at steady state in healthy male subjects. *J Clin Pharmacol.* 2008; 48:73-84.

131. Jeong S, Nguyen PD, Desta Z. Comprehensive in vitro analysis of voriconazole inhibition of eight cytochrome P450 (CYP) enzymes: major effect on CYPs 2B6, 2C9, 2C19, and 3A. *Antimicrob Agents Chemother.* 2009; 53:541-51.

132. Black DJ, Kunze KL, Wienkers LC et al. Warfarin–fluconazole. A metabolically based drug interaction: in vivo studies. *Drug Metab Dispos.* 1996; 24:422-8.

133. Ochs HR, Greenblatt DJ, Roberts GM et al. Diazepam interaction with antituberculosis drugs. *Clin Pharmacol Ther.* 1981; 29:671-8.

134. Desta Z, Soukhova NV, Flockhart DA. Inhibition of cytochrome P450 (CYP450) isoforms by isoniazid: potent inhibition of CYP2C19 and CYP3A. *Antimicrob Agents Chemother.* 2001; 45:382-92.

135. Drake WM, Gordon GD. Heart block in a patient on propranolol and fluoxetine. *Lancet (London, England).* 1994; 343(8894):425-6.

136. Loi CM, Day JD, Jue SG et al. Dose-dependent inhibition of theophylline metabolism by disulfiram in recovering alcoholics. *Clin Pharmacol Ther.* 1989; 45:476-86.

137. Upton RA. Pharmacokinetic interactions between theophylline and other medication (Part I). *Clin Pharmacokinet.* 1991; 20:66-80.

138. Lee AJ, Maddix DS. Rhabdomyolysis secondary to a drug interaction between simvastatin and clarithromycin. *Ann Pharmacother.* 2001; 35:26-31.

139. Stirling CM, Isles CG. Rhabdomyolysis due to simvastatin in a transplant patient: Are some statins safer than others? *Nephrol Dial Transplant.* 2001; 16:873-4.

140. Wagner J, Suessmair C, Pfister HW. Rhabdomyolysis caused by co-medication with simvastatin and clarithromycin. *J Neurol.* 2009; 256:1182-3.

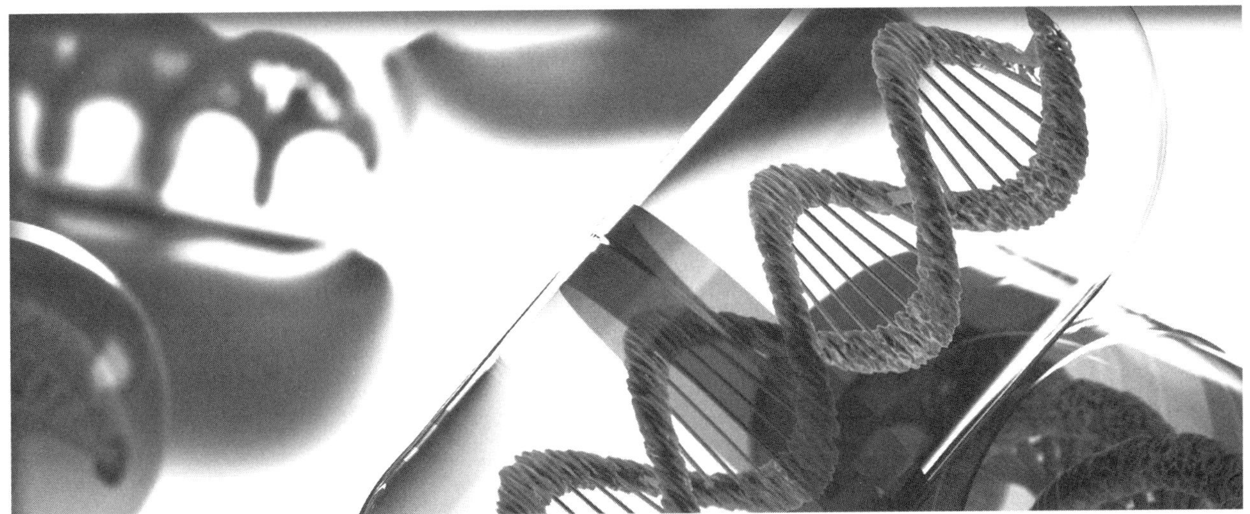

CHAPTER 4

Postmarketing Surveillance for Drug-Induced Diseases

Tobias Peschel and Hugh H. Tilson

The job of ensuring safe therapeutics extends far beyond the drug development, premarketing period. Sustained postmarketing monitoring (surveillance) activities are critically important because premarketing investigation alone cannot define completely the safety profile of a drug. Responsibility for overseeing postmarketing surveillance falls to the U.S. Food and Drug Administration (FDA) in the United States (and comparable divisions of regulatory agencies around the world). However, as in all public health enterprises, the work of postmarketing surveillance is shared by the full spectrum of the healthcare enterprise—from the patient and the individual prescriber, academia and healthcare organizations, to the manufacturer and regulatory agencies. Postmarketing attention to drug-induced diseases encountered in day-to-day practice is the responsibility of every healthcare practitioner and his or her patients. Independent clinical observations and voluntary reporting to manufacturers and regulatory agencies are at the heart of population-level surveillance. However, systems that rely solely on individual observation and voluntary reporting fall short. No individual clinician or patient can be expected to recognize rare drug-associated events and unusual patterns from limited individual experience. Thus, more structured population-based programs of postmarketing surveillance for drug-induced diseases, including structured epidemiological studies, are essential components of our nation's broader public health efforts. The promise of larger and more accessible population-based data for this purpose is great but requires concerted effort to ensure acceptable population-level protections.

RECOGNIZING THE LIMITS OF PREMARKETING DATA

When a drug is approved for marketing under the provisions of the Food, Drug, and Cosmetic Act (FD&C Act), or abroad under similar laws around the world, the product is deemed to meet several official requirements, which often are stated in shorthand as "safe and effective." However, the meaning of that phrase is widely misinterpreted. There is not a broad understanding among the medical community of the burden of proof required to obtain FDA approval to market a drug.

The sponsor of the New Drug Application (NDA) must demonstrate that the product is *efficacious*, usually through well-controlled studies. The approval processes around the world typically require completion of two randomized, blinded, well-controlled clinical trials, with clear separation of efficacy endpoints against placebo when possible or against a rigorous, appropriate standard intervention that is already approved.[1] Thus, the sizes of the preapproval populations under observation are driven by the power of trials to achieve these requirements. Far less clear are the preapproval standards for proof of a new drug's *safety*, distinct from its efficacy. In general, the profile of adverse effects associated with the agent, both self-limiting side effects and serious unexpected and untoward effects induced by the drug, must be such that the threat of these adverse effects is not proven to outweigh the drug's likely benefit. Practicality and necessity often temper the stringency of this requirement in a number of ways. Generally, the number of persons exposed to a new drug before approval for marketing is granted may be as few as 2,000 or 3,000.[1] Indeed, it can be even only a few hundred individuals in the case of orphan drug designation for the treatment of a rare, "orphan" condition. Under these circumstances, the apparent absence of unacceptably frequent or intolerably severe adverse outcomes of treatment can provide only statistical assurance that the likelihood of such drug-induced illnesses, if they exist, is less than about 1/1,000. Moreover, the duration of such preapproval studies is generally only as long as is needed to comply with FDA requirements to meet the prespecified endpoints for efficacy. Thus, the occurrence of an excess of heart attacks following 18 months of therapy could not be detected even in a relatively large preapproval database of studies of 12-month duration. These limitations could be expressed as the *Rule of Too*: to depict population level safety, the preapproval experience alone is too small, too brief, too healthy, and too homogeneous. Absence of data does not prove absence of a problem.

The research environment of the randomized, blinded, well-controlled study further limits what we can know about the new drug's performance in wider clinical use following its approval. Naturally, preapproval studies generally are conducted under tightly controlled circumstances, with carefully designed protocols that exclude patients who appear to present the threat of confusing results. These can include patients affected by concurrent illnesses, taking concomitant medications, and with specific risk factors, or patients belonging to potentially risky population strata, such as the poor, ethnic minorities, children, pregnant women, and the elderly.

In summary, our understanding of the probability (risk) of incurring a drug-induced disease from a newly approved drug is limited by the nature of the system for premarketing study and the approval process.

THE NEED FOR POPULATION-BASED SURVEILLANCE FOLLOWING MARKETING

Systematic approaches to detection, quantification, and education concerning drug-induced disease following marketing have emerged only relatively recently with the advent of clinical trials approximately 50 years ago. Then, as now, the medical community educated itself largely by means of the published word, via clinical and scientific journals. Before randomized, controlled clinical trials were introduced, this "education by publication" typically took the form of anecdotal case histories, describing incidents of illness following drug therapy, where the drug was blamed for the undesired outcome. As part of the reform of the FD&C Act, voluntary reporting of such experiences to the FDA or the manufacturer was introduced as a fledgling surveillance system. The logic for such a system is that the only way to know of potential drug-induced problems that are unlikely to be detected in the preapproval drug development process is to monitor real-world experience after introduction of those products into the marketplace.

The cornerstone of population-based surveillance for medication-induced illness, as with public health monitoring of many emerging problems, is the technique of encouraging all practitioners to participate in a system of spontaneous voluntary reporting. Here the logic is to invite a heightened awareness, particularly regarding new drugs, that adverse outcomes following therapy—particularly those that are otherwise unexpected—may be attributable to the therapy. Therefore, if there is any index of suspicion, any member of the medical team, as well as the patient or his or her family, is encouraged to report, albeit on a voluntary basis.

Clinical detection of any single drug-induced disease or injury in a single patient may be extremely difficult. An immediate anaphylactic reaction to a drug may leave no doubt about its attribution. However, in most cases, drug-induced illness does not manifest itself differently or in dramatic ways from any illness that may be observed in a physician's office or pharmacist's practice. Sudden death, liver or kidney disease, encephalopathy, myocardial infarction, and other events may occur without any likely precipitating event or exposure. Even Stevens-Johnson syndrome, often thought of as a classic drug-induced disease, has as its two most frequent causes—"cause not apparent" and viral infection—with drug-induced problems listed third.[2] Thus, the experiences of the individual clinician alone are inadequate for providing information about population-level issues regarding drug-induced disease, such as prevalence, likely presentation, resolution, and long-term consequences. On one hand, a clinician witnessing one or two dramatic adverse events following the use of a specific drug may consider that drug a "bad actor" when the events may have been a rare coincidence or perhaps not drug-related at all. On the other hand, having never had a problem with the drug may simply be a function of the rarity of the drug-induced illness, the luck of the draw, or a failure to link the kidney disease in a patient or two with the drug or drugs they were taking. There is, in short, no substitute for population-level surveillance to determine the presence or absence of relatively rare problems or an increase in the rates of occurrence of otherwise not-so-rare adverse events over baseline. Thus, as in other public health enterprises, the aggregate experience in a population serves as the most effective sentinel or signaling tool for possible problems.

THE SPONTANEOUS REPORTING SYSTEM IN AMERICA

In this book, we differentiate between adverse drug reactions (ADRs), also referred to as adverse effects or side effects, and drug-induced disease. However, in every sense, the latter are a subset of the former. Thus, our primary system for detecting and tracking drug-induced diseases at the national level is the spontaneous adverse reactions reporting system (SRS), which is the nation's system for tracking all ADRs. Many have criticized the system as a "nonsystem," comprising a loosely administered chain of events in which those in positions to detect ADRs—the patients and the clinicians who work with them—are encouraged, voluntarily and without incentive, to call such incidents to the attention of those who are in a better position to assemble, analyze, and act on the ADRs. Indeed, the activities constituting the SRS are not systematic and are not integrated into the rest of the nation's systems of public health and safety surveillance and intervention/protection. As a result, the protections that this component of the nation's surveillance systems may provide are not guaranteed.

For the system to effectively capture and apply data concerning ADRs, a certain chain of events must transpire. Someone must detect that an adverse event has occurred in association with a drug exposure (an adverse drug event, or ADE) and must suspect that the adverse event might be causally associated with a drug exposure, converting the experience from an ADE to a suspected ADR.[3] This detection and interpretation must then be translated into action—the act of reporting the event, usually to an unseen, remote recipient. This event must be communicated to someone in the system who decides whether to incorporate it with information from other major sources—in the United States, typically either a government agency such as the FDA's MedWatch system, the Vaccine Adverse Event Reporting System, or one or more intermediaries. The primary such intermediary in the United States is the research-based, brand name pharmaceutical company. Pharmaceutical manufacturers receive, process, manage, analyze, and report well over 80% of all ADRs that eventually come to the attention of the FDA.[4] For manufacturers, further ADR reporting spontaneously and voluntarily from the field is mandatory.

In principle, the SRS also could recognize unintended but positive effects such as the unexpected hair growth observed with minoxidil, which led to the development of Rogaine and the sustained penile erection observed as an unexpected side effect of an antihypertensive drug, which eventually became sildenafil (Viagra). Bleeding reported following aspirin use led to eventual understanding of its cardioprotective effects.

THE ACTORS AND THEIR ROLES

It is worthwhile to examine the roles of each of the personal "actors" and the processes involved in the postmarketing surveillance process and explore some of the challenges involved in linking them into an effective system.

THE CLINICIAN

The point of departure for surveillance in the SRS is the reporter—the person, usually a clinician, who recognizes that something untoward, unexpected, and generally unwanted has occurred and suspects that the event is associated with a drug. A patient can introduce this information into the SRS either by reporting it directly to the manufacturer or a regulatory agency via a consumer report or by seeking medical care and calling it to the attention of the provider. Most providers—physicians, nurses, dentists, and pharmacists—claim they have not been trained sufficiently in the detection, management, and reporting of ADRs to function effectively as reporters in this system. Indeed, most indicate they have not reported a single ADR in the past year and they would not know how to report one if necessary.[4] Moreover, most providers state they see very few ADRs in their practice despite the nature and frequency of drug-associated adverse events. Many health profession educators attribute the lack of awareness of ADR prevalence on the failure of health curricula to educate emerging clinicians on the critical balance between a systems-thinking sensibility and the traditional art-and-science approach. More recently, the Association of American Medical Colleges has acknowledged the lack of broad consensus around the competencies required to be taught in professional education for effective participation in the nation's drug safety system. Epidemiology and statistical/probabilistic thinking are important competencies. The result has been a far-reaching comprehensive inventory of such competencies to be incorporated in all training programs.[5]

It also must be noted that very few drug-induced diseases are unique clinical entities. Rather, drugs are partially or broadly responsible for causing or aggravating many common clinical conditions. Identifying drugs as a potential cause requires complex clinical analysis. Furthermore, the drug may have been obtained through another prescriber, self-prescribed from the home medicine cabinet, or combined with an alternate or complementary medicine (prescribed or otherwise) or an unusual or unexpected dietary pattern. The patient may not have adhered to the recommended regimen, resulting in overdosing, underdosing, or (most commonly) episodic dosing, the latter two resulting in the adverse outcome of unexpected or periodic treatment failure. The patient may not recall fully or accurately which medications he or she has taken, or in what quantity, or in the case of illicit drug use, may not wish to disclose it. And, of course, the patient is generally taking medications to treat an underlying or coincident/concomitant illness, the progression of which may be confused with the drug-attributable illness. Clearly, identifying or preventing drug-induced disease requires a partnership between patient, physician, and pharmacist based on full disclosure, open discussions, and awareness of potential risk factors.

The clinician must not merely recognize the illness, but also must go through the process of differential diagnosis and analyses of potential underlying or precipitating factors other than drugs, after which the potential role(s) of drugs in disease need to be considered. This is no easy task, particularly given that the complexities of clinical pharmacology are themselves rapidly evolving. Having made a provisional association between drug and disease, the first concern of the treating provider is to remove and/or counter the offending agent. Simply achieving this goal easily can occupy the whole of a 15-minute patient visit, without the burdensome administrative tasks of reporting to some invisible and remote third party. No economic incentive exists to do so either, as voluntary reporting is expected to be done pro bono. Indeed, reporting an incident likely will generate subsequent questions and requests for more data from the agent receiving the report, creating a potentially significant inconvenience, which could discourage reporting. In the wake of the Institute of Medicine's (IOM; now the National Academy of Medicine) *To Err Is Human* report, we are admonished not to "name, blame, or shame" those who report and attempt to repair errors (in this case in prescribing, warning, or monitoring).[6] Nevertheless, admitting to a decision that caused an adverse outcome could result in a lawsuit or other censure. Widespread physician dread of current tort law and widespread stories of unjustified legal settlements does little to allay this anxiety or encourage reporting. The extent to which these barriers contribute to under-reporting is not known. Based on populations monitored prospectively and objectively, the under-reporting ratio for severe or serious ADRs (actual illnesses induced by medications) is estimated to be tenfold or worse.[7]

THE PATIENT

The patient is the point of departure for the postmarketing surveillance system. Preventing drug-induced disease in the individual patient through awareness of the likely consequences of specific circumstances, such as risk factors and drug interactions, requires a partnership between the physician, pharmacist, and patient and must include full disclosure, open discussion, and awareness of potential risks. In addition, the patient may be a direct reporter of potential drug-induced disease. The SRS receives reports from patients or their advocates every day; up to 20% of reports are from patients/consumers.[8] Although good surveillance practice recommends that patients be referred to a primary caregiver when making a report directly, the Council for International Organizations of Medical Sciences (CIOMS) working group concluded that it is the quality of the report and not the nature of the reporter that is essential.[9] Thus, while in Europe, until recently, consumer reports were generally not included in the SRS, consumer reports have been included for many years in the United States and Canada. The newly emerging European Guidance aligns with these approaches.[10] Thus, patient education regarding potential drug-induced illness and heightened awareness of reporting avenues and action result in a stronger likelihood that the SRS will learn about important drug-induced diseases directly from the patient.

THE MANUFACTURER

In the United States, a much misunderstood and generally underestimated factor in the SRS is the role of the entity marketing the drug (particularly in the early stages of marketing)—the research-based pharmaceutical company. In the regulatory context, these companies also are referred to as sponsors because they sponsor NDAs. The sponsor is responsible, under federal law, for compliance with all applicable federal regulations relating to the safety, efficacy, and purity of its products. These requirements include the conduct of regular ongoing product surveillance.[11] Under these provisions, the sponsor is expected to maintain vigilance regarding the safety of its products, including receipt, management, and further reporting of all ADRs from any source, including the published literature, ongoing clinical trials, and, primarily, the reporters who use, manage, and prescribe their products, as described above. Under the applicable regulations, sponsors are expected to maintain a program that provides an immediate review of any report received from any source, and they can differentiate the serious event from the nonserious.

These tasks and definitions are carefully defined in FDA regulation and the subject of the CIOMS international consensus reports and international management agreements under the International Conferences on Harmonization.

Any report that comes to the company's attention through a spontaneous, voluntary report or product complaint is considered, by definition, potentially attributable to the product(s) involved. If the report also meets the criteria for serious or potentially serious effects and involves one or more events/signs/symptoms that are outside the specific listings in the approved product label (i.e., "unexpected"), such a report must be transmitted to the regulatory authority immediately.[11] This requirement is not limited to the United States as the regulations speak specifically to products sold anywhere in the world. Thus, any report documenting a serious event outside the product label (unexpected, unlabeled, or unlisted, and received by the company, its affiliate, or its agent anywhere the drug is marketed) requires immediate transmittal to FDA. Furthermore, such cases also require sponsors to analyze the completeness of the description carefully and follow up on incomplete data or information needed to ascertain severity and outcome with serious drug-associated illness. Regulatory definitions clearly distinguish between severity (the extent or intensity of the event) and seriousness (the medical impact of the event and its associated outcomes, including the potential for hospitalization or death if not adequately treated). Enough information is needed to help with causality assessments for the individual case and risk factor assessment for evolving case series. This latter requirement results in contacting the reporting practitioner for more information. The CIOMS Working Group has outlined best practices for pharmacovigilance to provide guidance for sponsors in their vital roles in this public health paradigm.[9] These best practices include regular, scheduled, comprehensive reviews of each of their products. The sponsor prepares a summary report for every drug, currently known as a Periodic Safety Update Report, which describes the overall experience over a particular period of time and in the population under surveillance.

The modern scientific research-based pharmaceutical company provides a broad spectrum of services to the healthcare community, including drug information services that constitute a primary interface between the company and healthcare practitioners. A physician, nurse, dentist, or pharmacist may contact the company for information regarding its products and accumulated reported clinical experiences or new information regarding their use. Typically, the purpose of the call is not really to report anything but to learn more about the drug product in question and its use. It is a requirement that the contact be viewed as spontaneous and that information about associated adverse events mentioned by the reporter be considered possible ADRs. In fact, it is not infrequent that during the course of such calls an ADR is revealed. Thus, the better the drug information system, the more calls it receives, and more reports of potential ADRs are generated. This process can introduce significant bias by creating an artifact in the numerator as one attempt to evaluate the relative incidence of ADRs is associated with a particular drug. As communications using web-based social media increase, the reporting criteria for a drug-induced disease will require careful scrutiny and regulatory clarification.

THE REGULATORY AUTHORITY

Ultimately, all ADR reports arrive at the responsible regulatory authority office, either by direct submission (although this is becoming less common) or through the responsible intermediary, the sponsor company. In the U.S. public health model, the role of the government is to ensure conditions in which people can be healthy, a role that requires healthy and active partnerships between government and the private sector, which in this case is the regulated pharmaceutical industry.[12] In recent years, regulatory agencies around the world communicate with each other and share information about drug-induced diseases reported to them. Within the FDA rules, companies notified from abroad are required to handle and report these ADRs as they would domestic reports. The challenge of managing duplicate reporting from multiple sources is always present in the FDA's approach to data management and analysis.

The FDA is the ultimate arbiter of a company's adequacy concerning compliance activities, both on a macro report-by-report level and overall as a partner in public health protection. Each report receives triage in the agency. Serious reports, such as those describing reactions most likely to result in drug-induced disease or injury, receive priority attention, particularly those that also qualify as unexpected. Each sponsor also receives compliance oversight from the agency, including a program of FDA site visits and compliance audits to ensure an intact reporting system with full transparent disclosure from sponsor to agency.

Attribution of a problem being considered for an ADR report requires the clinician to consider the possibility of a causal relationship to a drug, in the context of multiple other possible causal explanations for the same events. Rarely is such a causal relationship unambiguous. Rather, the clinician must apply complex logic, including consideration of the timing of the event, the presence of other possibly causal exposures, the natural history of the underlying disease, and so forth. The SRS operates on the fundamental assumption that a report would not present to the system unless a reporter had some concern or suspicion about a possible causal relationship to the drug. Thus all SRS reports are considered possibly attributable. The evolution of the system, however, brings this assumption into question. More and more, for example, information comes to the attention of the system because of proactive study or detailed information seeking in association with an individual report or engagement with social media. This challenges scientists and practitioners involved in the science of surveillance to differentiate between truly spontaneous and possibly attributable reports and those reports that are elicited.

The pivotal role of the FDA in this public health system has made it particularly vulnerable to public criticism. Recent concerns about unexpected serious drug-induced diseases being undetected for too long (e.g., cardiovascular disease associated with rofecoxib and celecoxib, suicides associated with selective serotonin receptor inhibitors) resulted in the FDA Commissioner's request to the IOM of the National Academies of Science to conduct a thorough ongoing study of the system and the FDA's roles and contributions. In its landmark report, *The Future of Drug Safety*, the IOM calls for sweeping reforms in the way FDA approaches its roles, and specifically defines the critical changes necessary to promote the creation of a new "culture of drug safety."[13] In this new culture, public health efforts at detection of and protection against drug-induced diseases must assume a position equal in importance to those of the review and approval of new drugs.

THE SCIENCE OF SURVEILLANCE

SPONTANEOUS REPORTING

Surveillance is one of the tools of epidemiology, the fundamental science of public health, and the core tool for public health assurances in the pharmaceutical sector. Paradoxically, the surveillance activities in this sector are separated from those at work throughout the rest of the public health landscape. Most public health surveillance activities in the United States are a function of state and local public health agencies. Surveillance information about acute diseases of epidemic potential is consolidated and managed by each of the 50 states and forwarded to the Centers for Disease Control and Prevention (CDC) for aggregation and national reporting through such vehicles as the *Morbidity and Mortality Weekly Report*, and, more recently, the Health Alert Network.

By accident of historic evolution, surveillance for drug safety, and more recently for medication errors, has been handled in the parallel universe of pharmaceutical manufacturers and the FDA. The tools and their applications, however, are remarkably similar to those used in other sectors of public health. Each system designates events of interest. In the case of the CDC, these are reportable suspected cases of infection of epidemic potential, or more recently, conditions of potential for chronic disease epidemics. For the FDA, they are suspected cases of drug-induced disease that could signal potential problems for others taking the drug. Each surveillance system (1) attempts to learn as much about each case as is feasible within the constraints of voluntary reporting; (2) seeks to discern aspects of the case that might give an indication of unusual or unique circumstances (risk factors) to aid in understanding the extent of risk to others; and (3) attempts to develop some estimate of the frequency and evolution of the cases to define the gravity of the public health threat. Thus, a central requirement of both surveillance systems is the participation of well-trained, vigilant public health professionals. These professionals ensure that case reports are analyzed singly and in aggregate by the trained eyes of those who understand the subtleties of epidemiologic signaling systems and can detect patterns and parallels of data gathered from disparate sources.

INDIVIDUAL CASE AND POPULATION-BASED ANALYSIS

The report rate is a key subtlety of the system. Rate calculations require both a numerator (the reported cases) and a denominator (the exposed population). Calculating these elements within a voluntary reporting framework is an intrinsically uncertain process. Whenever surveillance data are accumulated under such voluntary circumstances, inevitably many variations exist in what is reported. When, by whom, to whom, and how reports are submitted become critical elements in surveillance analysis. Put another way, the surveillance numerator, based on voluntary reports, captures a further subset of all such events—those the physician or pharmacist are willing to take the time and trouble to report from among the larger subset of events. Various environmental factors influence reporting and, consequently, may periodically and temporarily change the signaling capacities of the system. A recent journal or newspaper report can cause a cascade of interest and reports from the field, and the passage of time is a well-known cofactor of declining interest in reporting. The emergence of drug information services within industry compounds the challenge and impacts the numerator as described above.

Calculating the denominator—the population exposed to a drug—also is a challenge. Many drugs are "sold" from company to distributor but remain somewhere in the supply pipeline not yet available to patients. Much is prescribed but never dispensed; much is dispensed but never taken. Therefore, efforts to estimate the population exposed requires sophistication and estimates must be used carefully and with many caveats. Thus, the surveillance practitioner must be trained carefully to understand and recognize these factors when attempting to generalize from individual reports to a concern about increased incidence of such reports over a population-expected baseline. The trained professional in the drug-induced disease world refers to reports rates and not incidence when discussing these reports and their trends.

PROACTIVE/SENTINEL SURVEILLANCE

Because of the weaknesses in the existing SRS, many have suggested a more aggressive effort at monitoring populations using methods beyond voluntary reporting, once again turning to the time-honored methods of public health epidemiology. The field specializes in epidemiologic population-based research methods coupled with public health approaches to spontaneous reports, which has been termed *pharmacoepidemiology*.[14,15] Intensive inpatient monitoring, the first major such scheme, was very productive in detecting unexpected increases in the frequencies of otherwise expected diseases in association with drug use, permitting statistical associations to generate signals.[16] However, such systems have proven expensive and limited in numbers of individuals exposed, particularly with new drugs, and have fallen into disuse except as ad hoc studies focused on specific new drugs with an intense effort to discover the degree of exposure nationwide.

LARGE AUTOMATED MULTIPURPOSE POPULATION-BASED SYSTEMS

Contemporary healthcare operates within a continuing revolution in medical informatics, fueled by the advent of large automated databases that support automated medical records, computerized prescribing, and wireless hand-held devices in ambulatory medical practice. As a result, many large components of the healthcare delivery system have automated data describing every drug prescribed, every subsequent major diagnosis associated with a hospitalization (admission and discharge), and, of course, longer term monitoring for late or latent outcomes available to them. These data sets are known as large automated multipurpose population-based systems (LAMPS). LAMPS already have amply demonstrated their value as tools for the pharmacoepidemiologist to use when conducting formal observational studies to test signals from other systems, such as the SRS.

LAMPS, however, have several critical limitations as surveillance tools. The power of a signal generator is tied directly to the size of the exposed population. Thus, a database owned by a single health maintenance organization (HMO), even one reflecting the medical transactions of millions of enrolled individuals, may not include enough exposures to any single drug to detect any but the most commonly associated drug-induced diseases. This includes any new drug in the early phases of marketing and is particularly true in key population subgroups for which a possible increased risk of medication-induced illness may occur.

Public health objectives must be kept clearly in view. Society has the responsibility to monitor for drug-induced diseases that are sufficiently severe to create an unacceptable burden on individuals or that are serious and frequent enough to create a public health burden. For the former, a system to detect the very rare but unacceptably severe reaction is needed. For this, the SRS, with all of its faults, is the only existing tool that can be considered adequate. But for the latter, monitoring and quantitating the occurrence of excess medical adversity risk and documenting excess morbidity, mortality, and cost to society will permit us to accomplish society's public health surveillance tasks. With these objectives clearly in mind, the IOM called for the aggressive development of programs of automated population-based "active surveillance."[13] In response, in the FDA Authorization Act (FDAAA; 2007), Congress mandated the FDA to develop a sentinel surveillance system based in automated population-based data systems with the objective of monitoring a population of 25 million by 2010 and 100 million by 2012.[17] This dramatic vision has spawned major activity across the breadth of the public health system, with emerging LAMPS now recognized and harnessed for drug safety surveillance as well as research. Major health plans, including United Health Care, Wellpoint (Blue Cross/Blue Shield), Aetna, and the collaborative HMO Research Network, among others, have made data available to leading researchers for such explorations.

Academia, in its critical role in the public health system, has organized centers of excellence, such as the Centers for Education and Research on Therapeutics (CERTs) program to assist the FDA in this endeavor.[18] The CERTs convened a think tank to outline the steps forward.[19] Industry, as a key partner in the system, organized and funded (through the Foundation for the National Institutes of Health) an independent effort at testing new methods for cross-system data summary and analysis for prospective (sentinel) development of signals of potential drug-induced diseases (the Pharmaceutical Manufacturers' Association Observational Medical Outcomes Program).[20] In addition, the FDA itself organized and managed a vigorous process for exploring the path to responding to the FDAAA mandate for sentinel surveillance, deemed the *minisentinel*.[21] After 5 years of progressive growth and proofs of concept, the project was adopted in September of 2014 as a standing FDA effort known as the FDA Sentinel Network.[22] The network deploys a distributed data system from 18 organizations including some of the nation's largest health insurers and various disease registries. The FDA and its collaborator, Harvard Medical School, estimate that the system is now capable of monitoring drug exposure for 178 million people, with 48 million currently enrolled/treated, and a growing ability to link drug exposure with validated medical events data, including hospital diagnoses.[22]

In addition to ADRs as a result of the drug, it is also important to monitor potential harm caused by unintentionally administering the incorrect drug (e.g., due to similarities in names or poor legibility of a prescription, or errors along the chain from prescription to patient). This special situation of medication errors demands a third monitoring method. But what system exists to monitor, compile, analyze, and develop proper interventions regarding these errors? Part of the nation's response has been developing institution-based reporting and continuous improvement systems. These are vital because root causes can be locally identified and remedied in institutional systems and practices. They are inadequate, however, in detecting flaws in product presentation or design, name confusion, look-alike packaging, or confusing product information. For these, integration into a more comprehensive national detection system is also required. Therefore, several key leadership organizations have taken decisive action. Notable among these is the MEDMARX system (Quantros, Inc., Milpitas, CA).[23]

THE WAY FORWARD: CAN YOU IMAGINE?

Protecting society against preventable drug-induced diseases and device-associated injury, through early detection of possible problems emerging from therapies, is the primary objective of a public health-oriented drug safety surveillance system. Such protections require, at the population level, an affordable, effective system of monitoring for serious adverse events that occur in the population in excess of what would be expected from disease and natural causes alone. To achieve this objective, progress is needed on three fronts. First, the reporter must be more attuned both to monitoring for possible drug-induced illness and to reporting it effectively. Second, the system needs to be more efficient in retrieving and managing the resulting data and more effective in harnessing it to existing systems of surveillance. Finally, new technologies, made available through the rapid dissemination of automation into medical practice, must be harnessed to the task effectively.

These goals, in turn, require three ambitious sets of activity. First, medical, pharmacy and other health professionals must do a better job of reaching the practitioner with salient messages about drug-induced diseases and with convincing efforts to harness the time and energy of the busy practitioner. We need to do a better job of incorporating these tasks, and the competencies which underlie them, in undergraduate and postgraduate training of our professionals. Continuing education credit for participating in the SRS has been suggested as a promising incentive. But an even more promising strategy is to make the act of reporting one that reaps rewards in terms of useful information to help care for the patient at hand and the other patients under the care of the reporter. Can you imagine a truly easy, user-friendly, and useful system populated by truly public health-oriented satisfied reporters?

Second, public health agencies, notably the CDC and FDA, working with state and local public health surveillance professionals should undertake a thorough and systematic examination of existing methods of population-based surveillance to better align systems and the incentives to strengthen them. Although the SRS may be the most powerful generator of warnings of rare but unacceptable toxicities, better integrated and aligned signal generators are needed for drug-induced diseases that, while possibly less severe, are occurring at greater frequency in the population at large. Certainly these include preventable errors in the use of medications and their avoidable consequences. Can you imagine a truly seamless and integrated system of surveillance for *all* problems of public health importance?

Finally, those working in the field of information technology to support medical practice—such as those involved in developing and promulgating the automated medical record, personal digital assistant, and other hand-held technologies—need to work together to build data systems that are compatible with efficient and accurate conduct of the medical purposes for which they are intended. Equally critical is the development of data standards and refinements needed to provide the public health surveillance system (and, of course, the research enterprise) with the data needed to perform these vital functions in a timely, effective, and affordable way through the game-changing Sentinel Network project. Can you imagine a national surveillance system that does not require therapy team members to report information and to recall where to submit it because the automated system that supports their transactions can do this for them? Can you imagine a system that minimizes the administrative tasks and maximizes patient well-being, perhaps even one that is capable of "finding" problems before they become apparent and enabling us to prevent them from becoming major public health problems? Please imagine these changes as they are vital to a well-functioning integrated, proactive system of postmarketing surveillance. True public health protection requires it.

REFERENCES

1. US Food and Drug Administration. Development and Approval Process (Drugs). www.FDA.gov/Drugs/DevelopmentApprovalProcess (accessed 2017 Nov 8).
2. Strom BL, Carson JL, Halpern AC et al. A population-based study of Stevens-Johnson syndrome—incidence and antecedent drug exposures. *Arch Dermatol.* 1991; 127:831-8.
3. US Food and Drug Administration. An FDA Guide to Drug Safety Terms. https://www.fda.gov/downloads/forconsumers/consumerupdates/ucm107976.pdf (accessed 2017 Dec 13).
4. Ahmad SR. Adverse drug event monitoring at the Food and Drug Administration. *J Gen Int Med.* 2003; 18:57-60.
5. Association of American Medical Colleges. Report X. Contemporary issues in medicine: education in safe and effective prescribing practices: medical school objectives project. https://members.aamc.org/eweb/upload/Contemporary%20Issues%20in%20Med%20Education%20In%20Safe%20and%20Effective%20Report%20X.pdf (accessed 2017 Nov 8).
6. Institute of Medicine. *To err is human. Building a safer health system.* Washington, DC: National Academy Press; 2000.
7. Mittmann N, Knowles SR, Gomez M et al. Evaluation of the extent of under-reporting of serious adverse drug reactions: the case of toxic epidermal necrolysis. *Drug Saf.* 2004; 27:477-87.
8. Strom BL. Risk assessment of drugs, biologics and therapeutic devices. *Pharmacoepidemiol Drug Saf.* 2003; 12:653-62.
9. Council for International Organizations of Medical Sciences (CIOMS). *CIOMS V. Current challenges in pharmacovigilance: pragmatic approaches.* Geneva: CIOMS; 2001.
10. European Medicines Agency. Guidelines on good pharmacovigilance practices (GVP). Module VI—management and reporting of adverse reactions to medicinal products (rev 1). http://www.ema.europa.eu/docs/en_GB/document_library/Scientific_guideline/2014/09/WC500172402.pdf (accessed 2017 Nov 8).
11. US Food and Drug Administration. Guideline for postmarketing reporting of adverse drug experiences. https://www.fda.gov/downloads/drugs/guidancecomplianceregulatoryinformation/guidances/ucm299138.pdf (accessed 2017 Nov 8).
12. Institute of Medicine. The Future of the public's health in the 21st century. Washington DC: The National Academies Press; 2003.
13. Institute of Medicine. The future of drug safety: promoting and protecting the health of the public. Washington, DC: The National Academies Press; 2006.
14. Hartzema A. Pharmacoepidemiology and therapeutic risk management. Cincinnati, OH: Harvey Whitney Books Company; 2008.
15. Strom BL, Kimmel SE. *Textbook of pharmacoepidemiology.* 4th ed. Hoboken, NJ: Wiley; 2007.
16. Boston University School of Public Health. Boston collaborative drug surveillance program. www.bu.edu/bcdsp/ (accessed 2017 Nov 8).
17. US Food and Drug Administration. FDA Authorization Act (FDAAA), Section 905, 2007. https://www.gpo.gov/fdsys/pkg/PLAW-110publ85/pdf/PLAW-110publ85.pdf (accessed 2017 Nov 8).
18. US Department of Health and Human Services. Centers for education and research on therapeutics (CERTs). https://certs.hhs.gov/ (accessed 2017 Nov 8).
19. Behrman RE, Benner JS, Brown JS et al. Developing the sentinel system—a national resource for evidence development. *N Engl J Med.* 2011; 364:498-9.
20. Pharmaceutical Manufacturers' Association. Observational medical outcomes partnership. www.OHDSI.org (accessed 2017 Dec 13).
21. Pasty BM, Breckenridge AM. Mini-sentinel and regulatory science—big data rendered fit and functional. *New Engl J Med.* 2014; 370:2165-7.
22. Findlay S. The FDA's sentinel initiative: health policy brief (June 4, 2015). http://www.healthaffairs.org/healthpolicybriefs/brief.php?brief_id=139 (accessed 2017 Nov 8).
23. Quantros, Inc. MEDMARX. https://www.medmarx.com/ (accessed 2017 Nov 8).

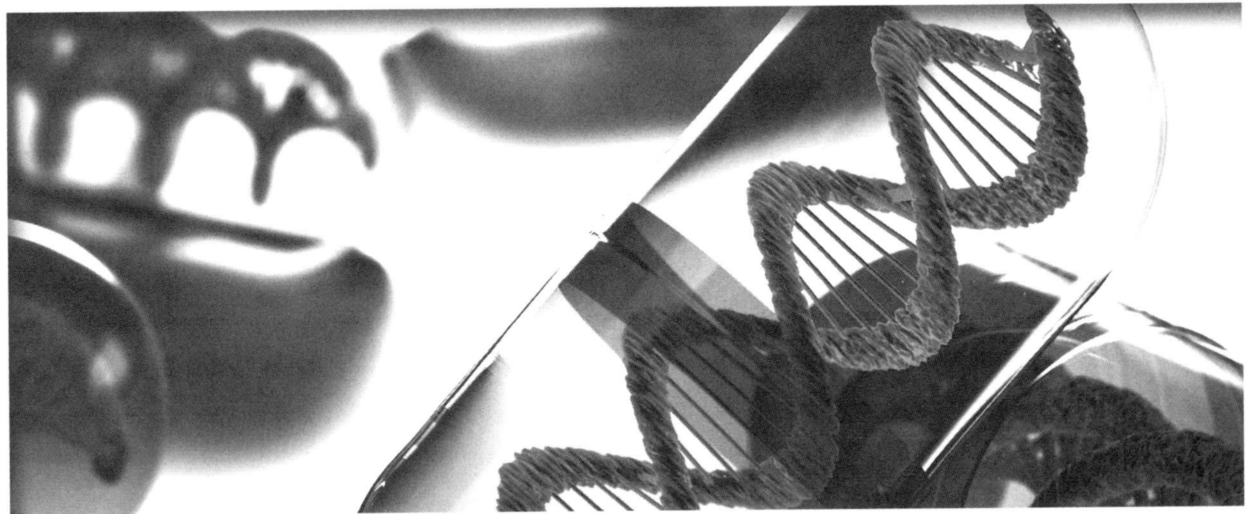

CHAPTER 5

Evaluating Patients for Drug-Induced Diseases

Douglas A. Miller and James E. Tisdale

As discussed in Chapter 2, there are thousands of drugs and drug products available on the market today. Nearly 60% of American adults take at least one prescription drug, and 15% take five or more.[1] In addition, approximately 20% of adults in the United States use natural products (herbs and other botanicals and enzymes).[2] These numbers have increased significantly over the last decade due to a much higher use of most types of medication. Because almost every drug a patient takes has the potential to cause an adverse effect and an associated drug-induced disease, the likelihood is quite high that a healthcare practitioner will encounter patients with one of these drug-related problems.

Unfortunately, clinicians are often slow to recognize adverse drug reactions and their associated drug-induced diseases. Sometimes they are not recognized at all. Patients' symptoms can easily be confused with those of commonly encountered and naturally occurring disease states. Sometimes an adverse drug effect can be mistaken for an exacerbation of a patient's pre-existing condition. As many as 20% of marketed drugs cause serious adverse effects not identified prior to approval and marketing, and serious adverse events have been reported with 33% of drugs following "fast track" approval by the U.S. Food and Drug Administration (FDA).[3] Despite these difficulties, early detection and correction of drug reactions and drug-induced diseases can help reduce morbidity and mortality and is therefore critically important.

Drug reactions can be divided into four general classes[4]:

- *Type A reactions*—These reactions are predictable, common, and relate to the pharmacological action of the drug. These may include reactions associated with drug toxicity or overdose (e.g., acetaminophen-induced hepatic failure), side effects (e.g., sedation with antihistamines), secondary effects (e.g., diarrhea with oral antibiotics), or drug interactions.
- *Type B reactions*—These reactions are unpredictable, uncommon, and usually not related to the pharmacological actions of the drug.

These include allergic reactions as well as those reactions generally described as idiosyncratic (e.g., primaquine-induced hemolytic anemia in a G6PD [glucose-6-phosphate dehydrogenase]-deficient patient). An idiosyncratic reaction is defined as an uncharacteristic, nonimmunological response to a drug that is not related to its pharmacological actions.

- *Type C reactions*—These reactions are associated with long-term drug therapy (e.g., analgesic nephropathy).
- *Type D reactions*—These reactions refer to carcinogenic and teratogenic effects.

About 80% of adverse drug reactions are classified as Type A.[5] Type C and D reactions are delayed in onset and rare compared to Type A and B reactions.

To help ensure that a drug-induced disease is not overlooked in a patient or inappropriately attributed to another cause, clinicians must have a high index of suspicion where drug therapy is concerned. When a patient presents with a new symptom or a symptom that has intensified or changed over time, the clinician must at least entertain the notion that the occurrence might be drug-induced. Every drug a patient is taking or has recently taken should be considered and ruled out as a possible cause. This is easier in some situations and with some drugs and reaction types than others.

PATIENT EVALUATION

Perhaps the most important tool for evaluating a possible drug-induced disease is the medication history. A careful history can yield many clues that will help the clinician rule in or rule out a drug-induced disease. Information that should be collected as part of the medication history is listed in **Table 5-1**. Information may be gathered from many sources including the patient, medication containers, a spouse or caregiver, the patient's medical records, or another healthcare provider such as the patient's primary care physician or pharmacist. The accuracy of the medication history depends not only on the accuracy of the source data but also on the skill and knowledge of the healthcare provider who collects the information and puts it all together. Asking the right questions in the right way can elicit information regarding a patient's medication use that otherwise might be overlooked. **Table 5-2** lists suggestions for obtaining an accurate medication history. Information available to a physician at the time of admission may be inaccurate and could result in an incomplete or inaccurate medication history.[6,7] Due to more extensive knowledge of various drugs and drug products, greater focus on medication therapy issues, and access to more information sources, pharmacists often are able to perform more complete medication histories.[8,9]

Information regarding prescription drugs (including any sample medications, inhalers, creams, ointments, patches, and medications administered in a physician's office, clinic, or infusion center), over-the-counter (OTC; nonprescription) drugs, vitamins, herbals (nutraceuticals, health supplements), and illicit drugs should be collected. Smoking history and alcohol use should also be documented. The name of each medication, its strength, formulation (tablet, capsule, liquid, extended release), dose, route, and frequency should all be recorded. The objective is to determine how a medication has actually been used rather than how it was prescribed. A precise history of when the medication was started and stopped and when the last dose was taken is critical to the investigation of a possible drug-induced disease. In some cases, it is important to know not only about current medications but also about medications that were taken in the past and recently discontinued. Although some patients are very good historians, it is not always advisable to rely solely on the information patients provide. Discussions with a spouse or caregiver or a phone call to the patient's pharmacy to check refill history can sometimes yield additional helpful information.

It is also important to collect a careful history of suspected adverse drug events. What did the patient notice, and when did it start? How did the problem progress? Was there a temporal relationship between the onset of symptoms and the addition or

Table 5-1 Information That Should Be Included in the Medication History

Patient information

- Age (date of birth)
- Sex
- Height
- Weight/BMI
- Race

Current prescription medications being taken or used by the patient

- Name of the medication
- Strength
- Formulation (tablet, capsule, extended release, etc.)
- Dose
- Route
- Frequency
- Reason started
- When started
- Date and time of last dose
- Where medication was procured

Prescription medications taken or used in the last 6 months

- Name of the medication
- Strength
- Formulation (tablet, capsule, extended release, etc.)
- Dose
- Route
- Frequency
- When started and stopped
- Reason discontinued
- Where medication was procured

Current nonprescription (OTC) medications (including vitamins, herbal products, health or dietary supplements, energy enhancers or "nutraceuticals")

- Name of the product
- Strength
- Formulation
- Dose
- Route
- Frequency
- Reason started
- When started
- Date and time of last dose
- Where product was procured

Nonprescription (OTC) medications (including vitamins, herbal products, health or dietary supplements, energy enhancers or "nutraceuticals") taken or used in the past 6 months

- Name of the product
- Strength
- Formulation
- Dose
- Route
- Frequency
- When started and stopped
- Reason for discontinuing use
- Where product was procured

Current and/or past use of tobacco

- Type (cigarettes, pipe, cigar, smokeless tobacco, electronic cigarettes)
- Frequency (e.g., number of packs per day)
- Date started
- Last use

Current and/or past use of alcohol

- Type (liquor, wine, beer)
- Amount and frequency
- Date started
- Last use

Current and/or past use of illicit drugs

- Drug name
- Method of administration (oral, inhaled, smoked, injected)
- Frequency
- Date started
- Last use

Financial issues

- Approximate monthly out-of-pocket medication costs
- Financial burden created by medication purchase

Allergies

- Name of medication or type of food causing allergic reaction
- Type of reaction
- Date of reaction
- Treatment and outcome
- Similar reactions to related drugs or similar foods
- Exposure to common drug allergens (penicillin and sulfa-containing compounds)

Adverse drug reactions

- Name of the medication
- Dosage and frequency
- Reason the medication was being taken
- Nature of the reaction experienced
- How the reaction was treated or managed

BMI = body mass index, OTC = over-the-counter.

Table 5-2 Suggestions for Improving the Accuracy of the Medication History

- Carefully review the patient's medical record and/or other available records before starting the interview to be efficient when questioning and gathering information.
- When possible, set up a special time to do the interview in a private area. The interviewer should not appear rushed and should maintain eye contact and be polite, friendly, and nonjudgmental.
- Use primarily open-ended questions (e.g., "What do you take for back pain?") rather than closed-ended questions (e.g., "Do you take anything for your back pain?") during the interview.
- Be nonjudgmental and make sure to not lead the patient into saying what he or she thinks the interviewer wants to hear. The objective is to find out how medications are actually being used and not how the patient was told to use them.
- Remember to ask patients about medications other than those they take orally (e.g., "Do you use eye drops?"). Patients often forget to mention creams, ointments, patches, eye or ear drops, inhalers, and infusions.
- To help stimulate a patient's memory, ask about medications they take for medical conditions they are known to have (e.g., "What do you take for your glaucoma?").
- Ask patients about medications prescribed by specialists they may see (e.g., "Do you see an allergist? What medications does he or she prescribe for you?").
- Ask patients if their physician recently started, stopped, or made any changes to the medications they are taking.
- Call the patients' community pharmacist to determine an exact medication, dosage strength, directions for use, and adherence (refill history).
- For inquiring about nonprescription medications, additional prompts may include, "What do you take for..."
  - Headache
  - Cold/flu
  - Allergies
  - Sinus
  - Cough
  - Sleeplessness
  - Drowsiness
  - Weight loss/gain
  - Heartburn
  - Stomach upset
  - Gas
  - Constipation
  - Diarrhea
  - Muscle or joint pain
  - Skin problems

discontinuation of any medications and, if so, was the timing of the event similar to that reported previously for a specific drug or drugs for that disease? Has the patient experienced similar reactions in the past? Can the patient provide any insight into what he or she suspects may be causing the problem? Did the patient attempt to self-medicate to treat the problem? If so, what treatment was tried, and was it effective? Do any treatments or activities seem to make the problem better? Does anything seem to make it worse?

A careful physical exam focusing on the organ system(s) involved and the collection of laboratory data can provide objective information helpful in determining whether or not a drug-induced disease is present. Depending on the reaction type and organ system(s) involved, evaluation of kidney function (blood urea nitrogen, serum creatinine, and estimated creatinine clearance), hepatic function (alanine aminotransferase, aspartate aminotransferase, alkaline phosphatase, gamma-glutamyl transferase, total and direct bilirubin, total protein, albumin, international normalized ratio), blood counts, serum drug (and, where appropriate, metabolite) concentrations and/or urinalysis may be helpful and necessary. Special laboratory tests (e.g., antinuclear antibodies, histamine metabolites, complement concentration, patch tests) are available and helpful in some situations. Noninvasive procedures (e.g., electrocardiogram, chest x-ray, computed tomography scan) and even invasive procedures (e.g., kidney or lung biopsy) may be required for some patients. Specific elements of the physical exam and laboratory evaluation important in the differential diagnosis of drug-induced diseases are discussed in Chapters 6–58.

The patient's history and physical exam should be carefully reviewed for the presence of risk factors known to be associated with the suspected drug-induced disease. Race, sex, age, genetic and environmental factors, concomitant drug therapy, comorbidities, immune status, alcohol and tobacco use, and a host of other factors may impact patients' relative risk for developing a drug-induced disease. Specific risk factors for the various drug-induced diseases are included in Chapters 6–58.

DIFFERENTIAL DIAGNOSIS

Once subjective and objective information regarding a suspected drug-induced disease has been collected, the known adverse effect profile of each drug to which the patient has been exposed should be evaluated to determine whether or not there is a likely culprit. Evidence of the ability to cause drug-induced diseases is better for some drugs than others, and, even when evidence is totally lacking, it must be remembered that there was a first report for every adverse drug effect and drug-induced disease recognized today.

Authors of chapters in this text have categorized the strength of evidence that a given drug causes a specific drug-induced disease as Level A, B, or C:

- *Level A*—This level indicates evidence of causation from one or more randomized, controlled clinical trials.
- *Level B*—This level indicates evidence of causation derived from nonrandomized clinical trials, prospective observational studies, cohort studies, case-control studies, meta-analyses and/or postmarketing surveillance studies.
- *Level C*—This level indicates there has been one or more published case reports or case series implicating a given drug as the causative agent of a specific drug-induced disease. Although they may not provide proof of causation, case reports are by far the most common evidence available for most drug-induced diseases and are very important to our understanding of these adverse drug events.

Additional B level evidence should become available as more structured approaches to postmarketing surveillance are implemented (see Chapters 1 and 4).

Perhaps the most challenging aspect of evaluating a patient with a suspected drug-induced disease is assessing causation for the observed signs or symptoms. A conference held in Morges, Switzerland in 1981 was an early attempt to bring organization and structure to causation assessment. Conferees agreed on what became called the 9 *points of consideration* when attempting to determine if a particular drug was the cause of a suspected adverse event.[10]

The considerations included the following:

1. Whether or not the drug was given prior to the event
2. Whether or not the reaction occurred at the site of application
3. Whether or not the interval following exposure to the drug was compatible with the occurrence of the reaction
4. Whether or not the reaction immediately followed drug exposure and had an acute onset
5. Whether or not the patient suffered the same reaction when rechallenged with the suspected drug
6. Whether or not the reaction improved when the drug was discontinued
7. Whether or not multiple drugs were discontinued simultaneously

8. Whether or not the patient had suffered the same reaction to the drug before
9. Whether or not the observed reaction was known to occur with the suspected causative agent

In the years since the Morges conference, a number of approaches to assess causality have been described.[11-18] The World Health Organization–Uppsala Monitoring Center (WHO–UMC) system (**Table 5-3**) allows users to place suspected reactions into one of six categories (from *unlikely* to *certain*) based on identified characteristics.[19] The Naranjo Scale (**Table 5-4**) assigns point values based on a similar set of findings.[20] There are limitations to the use of these methods. To accumulate points for each question with the Naranjo Scale, for example, the dose of the suspected drug would have to be increased or decreased to see if the reaction worsened or improved, the drug would have to be discontinued to see if the reaction subsided and then readministered to see if the reaction reappeared, and the patient would have to receive a placebo to see if it precipitated a similar reaction. These maneuvers are not always practical, possible, or ethical in clinical practice. As a result, few adverse reactions can be classified as *highly probable* or *doubtful*, and most fall somewhere between these extremes (i.e., *possible* or *probable*). Although none of the published causality assessment tools provides precise and reliable quantitative data, they do provide a structured basis for assessment in a standardized and relatively reproducible format and are used widely, particularly by journals assessing case reports submitted for publication.

When it is *possible*, *probable*, or *highly probable* that a medication is causing a drug-induced disease, the clinician must decide whether to continue therapy with that medication or modify the patient's therapeutic regimen. As with all decisions regarding drug therapy, the relative risks and benefits of each course of action must be carefully considered. The substitution of an agent less likely to cause the drug-induced disease may be an option in some cases. When an adverse drug event is known to be dose- or serum concentration-related, reducing the dose of the offending agent or changing the frequency of administration or dosing schedule may be viable options. Although it is not generally a good idea to treat an adverse effect of one drug with a second drug, there are times when this approach is acceptable (e.g., chemotherapy-induced nausea and vomiting). Desensitization is sometimes an option

Table 5-3 The World Health Organization–Uppsala Monitoring Center (WHO–UMC) System for Classification of Suspected Adverse Drug Reactions[19]

WHO–UMC Classification	Characteristics
C1—Certain	Plausible time; not related to underlying condition, concurrent disease, other drugs or chemicals related pharmacologically Positive dechallenge; positive rechallenge
C2—Probable	Reasonable time; unlikely to be related to concurrent disease, other drugs Positive dechallenge; no rechallenge
C3—Possible	Reasonable time; may be due to concurrent disease, other drug No information on dechallenge
C4—Unlikely	Improbable temporal relationship; other confounding factors such as drugs, chemicals, underlying disease
C5—Conditional/ unclassified	Reported as an adverse reaction, but more data are needed for proper assessment
C6—Unassessable/ unclassifiable	Report suggesting an adverse reaction but cannot be judged because of insufficient or contradictory information

Table 5-4 The Naranjo Scale for Estimating the Probability of Adverse Drug Reactions

Question	Points
Are there previous conclusive reports on this reaction? Yes (+1) No (0) Don't know (0)	
Did the adverse event appear after the suspected drug was administered? Yes (+2) No (−1) Don't know (0)	
Did the adverse reaction improve when the drug was discontinued, or a specific antagonist was administered? Yes (+1) No (0) Don't know (0)	
Did the adverse reaction reappear when the drug was readministered? Yes (+2) No (−1) Don't know (0)	
Are there alternative causes (other than the drug) that could on their own have caused the reaction? Yes (−1) No (+2) Don't know (0)	
Did the reaction reappear when a placebo was given? Yes (−1) No (+1) Don't know (0)	
Was the drug detected in the blood (or other fluids) in concentrations known to be toxic? Yes (+1) No (0) Don't know (0)	
Was the reaction more severe when the dose increased, or less severe when dose was decreased? Yes (+1) No (0) Don't know (0)	
Did the patient have a similar reaction to the same or similar drug in any previous exposure? Yes (+1) No (0) Don't know (0)	
Was the adverse event confirmed by any objective evidence? Yes (+1) No (0) Don't know (0)	
Total Points:	
Probability that adverse drug event has occurred: ≥9 highly probable ≥5 probable ≥1 possible 0 doubtful	

Source: Adapted from Naranjo CA, Busto U, Sellers EM et al. A method for estimating the probability of adverse drug reactions. *Clin Pharmacol Ther.* 1981; 30:239-45. Reprinted with permission.

for patients with drug-induced diseases that are immunologically mediated.

Situations in which there is more than one possible culprit drug can create an even greater challenge for clinicians. In some cases, it may be necessary to discontinue all of the possible offending agents and then reinitiate therapy one drug at a time following resolution of the drug-induced disease. In other cases, the WHO–UMC or Naranjo Scale probability rating for each of the possible culprits or the associated level of evidence (e.g., 2 case reports versus 20 case reports versus evidence of causation from one or more randomized, controlled clinical trials) might provide useful clues as to which agent is the most likely offender.

DOCUMENTING AND REPORTING DRUG-INDUCED DISEASES

PATIENT EDUCATION

Patient education and good documentation are critical to the prevention of a recurrent adverse drug event or drug-induced disease in a given patient. The patient needs to know the nature of the reaction that occurred, the generic name and trade names of the causative agent, the generic name and trade names of any other medications that might be expected to cause similar reactions, and whether or not these agents must be avoided entirely or used only with caution. When patients are warned about potential adverse effects of an entire class of drugs (e.g., angiotensin-converting enzyme inhibitors, sulfa-containing compounds, benzodiazepines), they should be given the generic name and trade names of drugs included in that class. All of this information should be reduced to writing, and the patient should receive a copy to keep with important medical records at home and copies to give to each of their other healthcare providers (e.g., physicians, dentists, nurse clinicians, pharmacists). A narrative description of the adverse event should be included in the patient's medical record and, when hospitalization has occurred, in the discharge summary and in any follow-up correspondence with admitting or referring physicians. Depending on the severity and acuity of the reaction, patients should be advised to obtain and wear a medical alert bracelet.

REPORTING DRUG-INDUCED DISEASES

Proper reporting can also be important in efforts to help prevent drug-induced diseases in others who will be exposed to the drug in the future. Some adverse drug effects and their associated drug-induced diseases have been well documented and are well known to healthcare providers. Because they are well known, these adverse events can sometimes be prevented with careful drug use and/or patient monitoring. Unfortunately, some adverse drug effects and drug-induced diseases have not yet been recognized or characterized. These are unexpected and, therefore, not yet preventable. Identifying and characterizing these events, and therefore increasing the likelihood they can be prevented in the future, is the focus of the FDA's voluntary MedWatch program.[21]

The FDA established MedWatch in 1993 as a method to stimulate voluntary reporting of serious adverse events by healthcare professionals and patients. The system collects spontaneous reports of adverse events involving drugs (prescription and OTC), biologics, devices, and special nutritional products including dietary supplements, medical foods, and infant formulas. Adverse reactions associated with vaccines are reported to the FDA through the Vaccine Adverse Event Reporting System, rather than through MedWatch. A spontaneous report is an observation of an adverse event that is made during direct patient care and subsequently reported either directly to the FDA or indirectly to the FDA through the drug's manufacturer. Observations made during clinical trials are not included as part of this spontaneous reporting system. The MedWatch system is also used to collect information regarding product quality problems, reports of suspected counterfeit products, and reports of medication and device use errors that may have been caused by either product name confusion or confusion resulting from packaging and labeling.

The FDA encourages healthcare providers and patients to use MedWatch to submit reports of serious adverse events. For the purpose of this reporting system, an adverse event is defined as any unfavorable and unintended sign, symptom, or disease temporally associated with the use of a medicinal product, whether or not considered related to the product. The FDA defines serious adverse events as those that are fatal, life-threatening, permanently or significantly disabling, those that require or prolong hospitalization, cause a congenital anomaly, or require intervention to prevent permanent impairment or damage. Notwithstanding these definitions, the FDA encourages health professionals to report any adverse event judged clinically significant. The adverse event does not have to be previously unreported or uncommon. Suspicion that a medical product may be related to a serious event is sufficient reason to submit a report and proof of causality is not necessary.

Reports can be filed online (www.fda.gov/Safety/MedWatch), via a toll-free phone line (1-800-FDA-1088), by fax (1-800-FDA-0178) or by prepaid mail. The core elements of the report include the reporter's name, the suspect drug or device, a narrative report of the adverse event or problem, and patient information (identifier, sex, age, and weight). The FDA holds patient identity information in strict confidence. Reporting does not violate provisions of the Health Insurance Portability and Accountability Act, which specifically permits covered entities (such as pharmacists, physicians, or hospitals) to report adverse events and other information related to the quality, effectiveness, and safety of FDA-regulated products both to the manufacturers and directly to the FDA.

Once received by the FDA, reports of adverse events are entered into a postmarketing surveillance database that can be examined for similar reports and used to develop case series. When a report or a series of reports define a previously unrecognized safety issue, the FDA can order a formal epidemiologic evaluation, require labeling changes including boxed warnings, place restrictions on prescribing or dispensing of the drug or, if necessary, order that the product be withdrawn from the market.

Healthcare providers can obtain information generated through the FDA MedWatch program by accessing their website at www.fda.gov/Safety/MedWatch. Information is also disseminated via email to those who subscribe online and through a large number of professional organizations that partner with the FDA for that purpose.

In 2007, the FDA Amendments Act required the agency to develop an active postmarketing risk identification and analysis program for drugs. In response, the FDA embarked on a program to work with public, academic, and private organizations to develop systems to link and analyze drug safety data from multiple sources. The FDA's Sentinel System was launched in February of 2016, and within the first year allowed the agency to access and analyze electronic medication use and safety data from over 193 million patients. The Sentinel System continues to grow and is intended to complement, but not replace, other surveillance tools such as the MedWatch program.

SUMMARY

Morbidity and mortality associated with drug-induced diseases continue to be a major concern for all healthcare practitioners. Drug-induced diseases may also result in substantial healthcare resource utilization and increased costs. Although some drug-induced diseases are identified during clinical trials and the drug approval process, others are not recognized until long after the drug is marketed and available for routine use. Although all drugs have the potential to cause drug-induced diseases, it is easy to overlook them as a possible cause of a patient's illness. All healthcare providers would be well advised to always ask themselves "Could this be drug-induced?" when confronted with a patient experiencing new or worsening symptoms.

REFERENCES

1. Kantor E, Rehm C, Haas JS et al. Trends in prescription drug use among adults in the United States from 1999–2012. *JAMA*. 2015; 314:1818-31.
2. Barnes P, Powell-Griner E, McFann K, Nahin RL. CDC Advance data report #343. Complementary and alternative medicine use among adults: United States, 2002. *Adv Data*. 2004; 343:1-19.
3. Moore, TJ. New drug: caution indicated. *Arch Intern Med*. 2012; 172:1681-2.
4. Rawlins M, Thompson W. Mechanisms of adverse drug reactions. In: Davies D, ed. *Textbook of adverse drug reactions*. New York: Oxford University Press; 1991:18-45.
5. deShazo R, Kemp S. Allergic reactions to drugs and biologic agents. *JAMA*. 1997; 278:1895-906.
6. Gonski PN, Stahters GM, Freiman JS, Smith T. A critical review of admission and discharge medications in the elderly Australian population. *Drugs Aging*. 1993; 3:358-62.
7. Tam VC, Knowles SR, Cornish PL et al. Frequency, type and clinical importance of medication history errors at admission to hospital: a systematic review. *CMAJ*. 2005; 173:510-5.
8. Walchle RD, McKercher PL, Cooper JW. Physician-, nurse-, and pharmacist-conducted patient drug histories. *Contemp Pharm Pract*. 1980; 3:75-8.
9. Reeder TA, Mutnick A. Pharmacist- versus physician-obtained medication histories. *Am J Health-Syst Pharm*. 2008; 65:857-60.
10. Venulet J, Berneker GC, Ciucci AG, eds. *Assessing causes of adverse drug reactions*. London: Academic Press; 1982.
11. Kramer MS, Leventhal JM, Hutchinson TA, Feinstein AR. An algorithm for the operational assessment of adverse drug reactions: background, description, and instructions for use. *JAMA*. 1979; 242:623-32.
12. Karch FE, Lasagna L. Toward the operational identification of adverse drug reactions. *Clin Pharmacol Ther*. 1977; 21:247-54.
13. Koh Y, Li SC. A new algorithm to identify the causality of adverse drug reactions. *Drug Saf*. 2005; 28:1159-61.
14. Berry LL, Segal R, Sherrin TP, Fudge KA. Sensitivity and specificity of three methods of detecting adverse drug reactions. *Am J Hosp Pharm*. 1988; 45:1534-9.
15. Michel DJ, Knodel LC. Comparison of three algorithms used to evaluate adverse drug reactions. *Am J Hosp Pharm*. 1986; 43:1709-14.
16. Benichou C. Criteria of drug-induced liver disorders. Report of an international consensus meeting. *J Hepatol*. 1990; 11:272-6.
17. Maria VA, Victorino RM. Development and validation of a clinical scale for the diagnosis of drug-induced hepatitis. *Hepatology*. 1997; 26:664-9.
18. Fontana RJ, Watkins PB. Drug-Induced Liver Injury Network (DILIN) prospective study; rationale, design, and conduct. *Drug Saf*. 2009; 32:55-68.
19. The Uppsala Monitoring Centre. The Use of the WHO–UMC System for Standardised Case Causality Assessment. https://www.who-umc.org/media/2768/standardised-case-causality-assessment.pdf (accessed 2017 Nov 3).
20. Naranjo CA, Busto U, Sellers EM et al. A method for estimating the probability of adverse drug reactions. *Clin Pharmacol Ther*. 1981; 30:239-45.
21. US Food and Drug Administration. MedWatch: the FDA safety information and adverse event reporting program. http://www.fda.gov/safety/medwatch (accessed 2017 Jun 28).

SECTION II

DRUG-INDUCED DERMATOLOGIC DISEASES

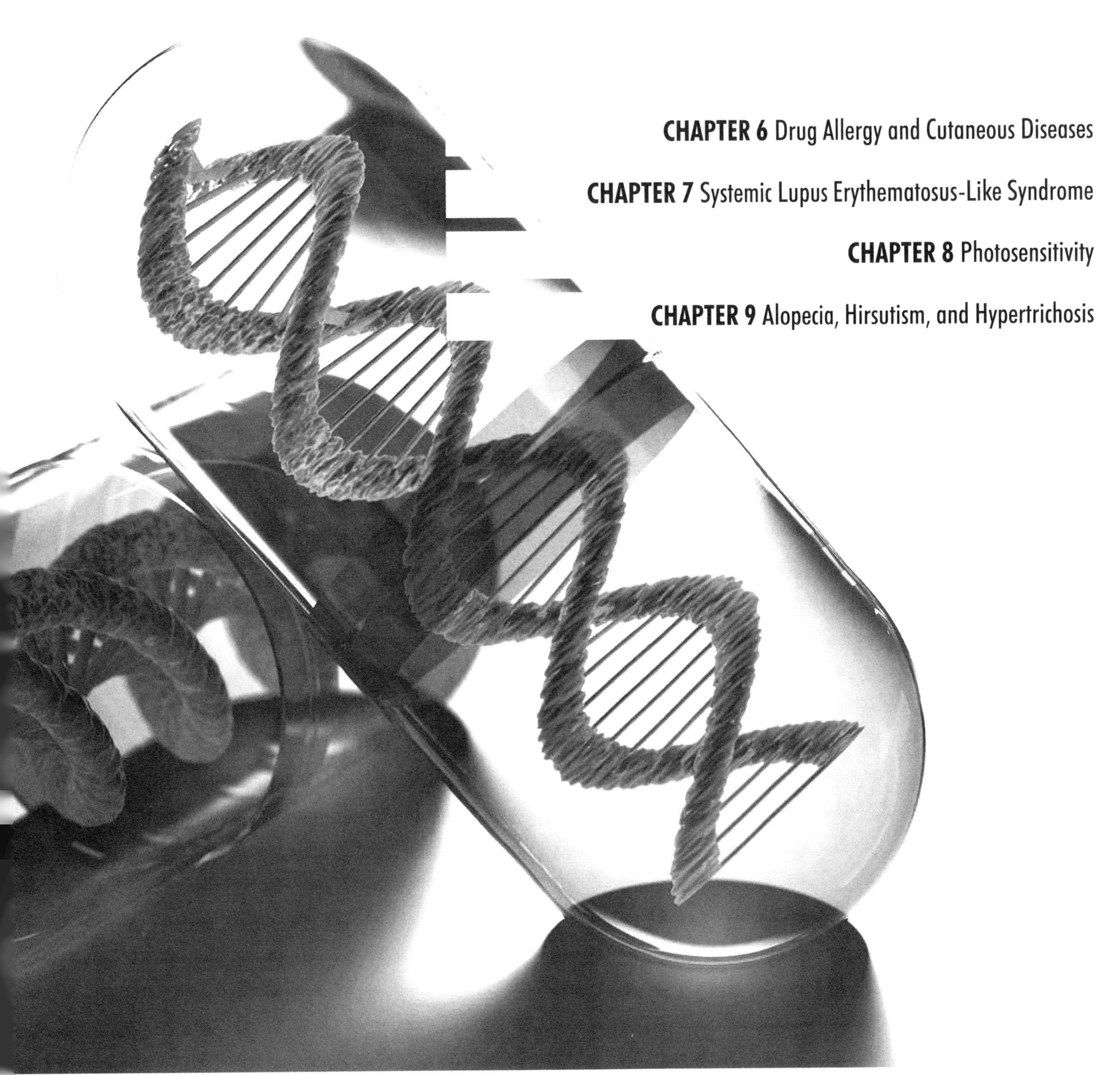

CHAPTER 6 Drug Allergy and Cutaneous Diseases

CHAPTER 7 Systemic Lupus Erythematosus-Like Syndrome

CHAPTER 8 Photosensitivity

CHAPTER 9 Alopecia, Hirsutism, and Hypertrichosis

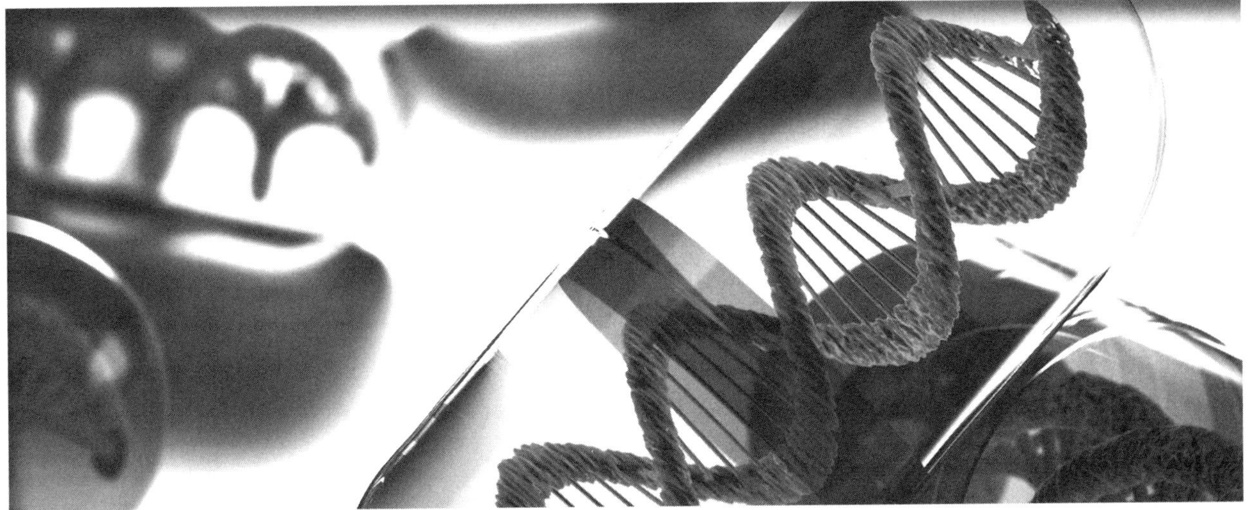

CHAPTER 6

Drug Allergy and Cutaneous Diseases

Lynne M. Sylvia

The terms *drug allergy* and *drug hypersensitivity* are often used synonymously to describe adverse drug reactions mediated by the immune system. According to the International Consensus (ICON) on Drug Allergy, these terms should not be used interchangeably.[1] Drug allergy refers to reactions for which a definite immune mechanism has been proven.[1] The parent drug or its reactive metabolite serves as an antigen, which is subsequently recognized and processed by the immune system, culminating in the production of drug-specific antibodies or sensitized T lymphocytes. The antigen–antibody reaction can target a variety of cells and body tissues, leading to organ-specific or more generalized systemic adverse events. The expert panel on drug allergy recommends that the term *drug hypersensitivity reaction* be used for adverse events that clinically resemble allergy but may or may not be mediated by an immune response.[1] Drug hypersensitivity reactions (DHRs) are more heterogeneous in clinical presentation and underlying mechanism. The implicated drug often has the ability via its chemistry or pharmacology to directly stimulate the release or activation of inflammatory mediators from mast cells, basophils, or other body tissues, causing a reaction that is clinically indistinguishable from drug allergy. The term *drug pseudoallergy*, to describe allergic-like reactions, is no longer recommended. A comparison of the features of drug allergy and DHRs is provided in **Table 6-1**.

Cutaneous eruptions, the most common manifestation of drug-induced disease, can result from both immune- and nonimmune-mediated mechanisms (e.g., pharmacologic effects, idiosyncratic). Therefore, drug-induced skin eruptions and systemic skin diseases are discussed in a separate section of this chapter. Allergic-mediated urticaria, angioedema, and the immune complex diseases associated with dermatologic manifestations (serum sickness-like syndrome, vasculitis) will be discussed in the following section.

DRUG ALLERGY AND DHRs

CAUSATIVE AGENTS

A list of the drugs most frequently implicated in drug allergy is provided in **Table 6-2**.[2,4-139] If a particular drug of concern is not included in this table, it should not be assumed that the drug is

Table 6-1 Differentiating Features of Allergy Versus Drug Hypersensitivity Reactions[1-3]

Characteristic	Allergy	Drug Hypersensitivity Reactions
Clinical presentation	Highly variable; ranging from a localized erythematous rash to life-threatening reactions including anaphylaxis, Stevens–Johnson syndrome, and toxic epidermal necrolysis	Highly variable; ranging from infusion-related reactions such as skin flushing to severe reactions mimicking anaphylaxis
Sensitization period	Required; usually ranging from 5 to 21 days after drug initiation	Not required; reaction can occur within seconds to minutes after administration of first dose
Antibody involvement	Yes; IgE, IgG, IgM, or sensitized T lymphocytes	Not proven; may or may not be mediated by an immune response
Mechanism	Drug can serve as a complete antigen or hapten (parent drug or metabolite) or may bind to T-cell receptor to stimulate immune response	Based on its chemical or pharmacologic properties, drug stimulates release or activation of inflammatory mediators
Risk factors	Highly variable; dependent on drug or patient (host)	Highly variable; dependent on drug or patient (host)
Pretreatment	Not routinely recommended; yield of antibody produced by any given antigenic drug too unpredictable to fully antagonize via pretreatment	Pretreatment regimens are recommended for some drugs; may be recommended to block effects of drug on effector pathways
Treatment	Dependent on signs and symptoms of reaction; includes antihistamines, epinephrine, and corticosteroids	Dependent on signs and symptoms of reaction; may include dose reduction, alteration in rate of infusion, or treatment with antihistamines, epinephrine, or corticosteroids

IgE = immunoglobulin E, IgG = immunoglobulin G, IgM = immunoglobulin M.

Table 6-2 Agents Implicated in Allergic Drug Reactions

Drug	Incidence	Level of Evidence[a]
ANAPHYLAXIS, URTICARIA, ANGIOEDEMA, AND BRONCHOSPASM		
Amphotericin B[4,5]	NK	C
Aprotinin[6]	NK	C
L-asparaginase[7]	NK	C
Aspartame[8,9]	NK	C
Aspirin[10,11]	NK	C
Atracurium[12-14]	NK	C
Azathioprine[15,16]	NK	C
Basiliximab[17]	NK	C
Carboplatin[18]	NK	C
Carboxymethylcellulose[19]	NK	C
Ceftriaxone[20]	NK	C
Cephalosporins[21,22]	0.001–0.1%	C
Cetirizine[23]	NK	C
Cetuximab[24,25]	NK	C
Chlorhexidine[26,27]	NK	C
Chymopapain[28]	NK	C
Cisplatin[7]	NK	C
Clopidogrel[29,30]	NK	C

Table 6-2 Agents Implicated in Allergic Drug Reactions (continued)

Drug	Incidence	Level of Evidence[a]
Clavulanic acid[31]	NK	C
Deferoxamine[32]	NK	C
Diclofenac[10]	NK	C
Etoposide[7]	NK	C
Excipients[8,9,19,33]	NK	C
Fluoroquinolones[34,35]	NK	C
Gentamicin[36]	NK	C
Ibuprofen[10]	NK	C
Infliximab[37]	NK	C
Insulin[38]	NK	C
Iron (intravenous products)[39-41]	NK	C
Isoniazid[42,43]	NK	C
Ketoprofen[44]	NK	C
Lepirudin[45]	NK	C
Leuprorelin[46]	NK	C
Mefenamic acid[10]	NK	C
Mivacurium[14]	NK	C
Omalizumab[47]	0.2%[a]	C
Oxaliplatin[48,49]	NK	C
Paclitaxel[50]	NK	C
Pantoprazole[51]	NK	C
Penicillins[52,53]	0.01–0.05%	B
Phytonadione[54]	NK	C
Polysorbate 80[33]	NK	C
Povidone–iodine[55,56]	NK	C
Prasugrel[57]	NK	C
Protamine[2]	NK	B
Risperidone[58]	NK	C
Rituximab[37]	NK	C
Rocuronium[59]	NK	C
Sodium benzoate[33,60]	NK	C
Streptokinase[61]	NK	C
Sumatriptan[62]	NK	C
Suxamethonium[63]	NK	C
Teniposide[7]	NK	C
Thiopental[12]	NK	C
Ticagrelor[64]	NK	C
Tobramycin[65]	NK	C
Triamcinolone[66]	NK	C
Vancomycin[67]	NK	C
Zidovudine[68]	NK	C

Table 6-2 Agents Implicated in Allergic Drug Reactions (continued)

Drug	Incidence	Level of Evidence[a]
SERUM SICKNESS-LIKE REACTION		
β-lactam antibiotics[69]	NK	C
Bupropion[69-72]	NK	C
Cefaclor[73-75]	NK	B
Ciprofloxacin[76]	NK	C
Fluoxetine[77]	NK	C
Itraconazole[78]	NK	C
Meropenem[79]	NK	C
Minocycline[80-82]	NK	C
Protamine[2]	NK	C
Rituximab[83]	NK	C
Streptokinase[84,85]	NK	C
Sulfites[9,33]	NK	C
Sulfonamides[69]	NK	C
Vaccines[69]	NK	C
VASCULITIS		
Allopurinol[86-88]	NK	C
β-lactam antibiotics[86-88]	NK	C
Celecoxib[89]	NK	C
Cephalosporins[86-88]	NK	C
Colony-stimulating factors[87]	NK	C
Docetaxel[90]	NK	C
Etanercept[87]	NK	C
Fluticasone[91]	NK	C
Fluoroquinolones[87]	NK	C
Hydralazine[87]	NK	C
Infliximab[92]	NK	C
Interferon α-2b[93]	NK	C
Isotretinoin[87]	NK	C
Leukotriene antagonists[94]	NK	C
Methimazole[87]	NK	C
Methotrexate[87]	NK	C
Minocycline[87]	NK	C
Nonsteroidal anti-inflammatory drugs[87]	NK	C
Penicillamine[87]	NK	C
Phenytoin[87]	NK	C
Propylthiouracil[95,96]	NK	C
Rofecoxib[97]	NK	C
Vancomycin[87,98]	NK	C

Table 6-2 Agents Implicated in Allergic Drug Reactions (continued)

Drug	Incidence	Level of Evidence[a]
HYPERSENSITIVITY SYNDROMES		
Abacavir[99,100]	NK	B
Allopurinol[101-103]	NK	C
Carbamazepine[104,105]	NK	B
Dapsone[106-108]	NK	C
Lamotrigine[109]	NK	C
Minocycline[110]	NK	C
Nevirapine[111]	NK	C
Oxcarbazepine[105]	NK	C
Paclitaxel[7]	NK	C
Phenytoin[105]	NK	C
Phenobarbital[105]	NK	C
Valproic acid[112]	NK	C
ALLERGIC-MEDIATED BLOOD DISORDERS		
Cephalosporins[113-115]	NK	C
Heparin[116]	1–5%	B
Histamine H_2-receptor blockers[117-119]	NK	C
Methimazole[120,121]	NK	B
Methyldopa[114]	NK	C
Penicillins[114,115]	NK	C
Piperacillin[122,123]	NK	B
Procainamide[114]	NK	C
Propylthiouracil[120,121]	NK	B
Quinidine[114,115]	NK	C
Quinine[114,115,124]	NK	C
Trimethoprim–sulfamethoxazole[125]	NK	C
Valproic acid[126]	NK	C
Vancomycin[127,128]	NK	C
OTHER		
Cimetidine[129]	NK	C
Clindamycin[130]	NK	C
Corticosteroids[131,132]	NK	C
Diazepam[133]	NK	C
Hetastarch[134]	NK	C
Insulin[38,135]	NK	C
Lidocaine[136]	NK	C
Progesterone[137]	NK	C
Psyllium[138]	NK	C
Vaccines[139]	NK	C

NK = not known.

[a]Definitions for Levels of Evidence: Level A—evidence from one or more randomized, controlled clinical trials; Level B—evidence from nonrandomized clinical trials, prospective observational studies, cohort studies, retrospective studies, case-control studies, meta-analyses and/or postmarketing surveillance studies; and Level C—evidence from one or more published case reports or case series.

incapable of eliciting an immune response. Many drugs are not identified as antigenic until well after approval and use in an extended patient population. To determine a drug's potential to serve as an antigen, three drug-related properties should be considered. First, the molecular weight of a drug can influence its antigenicity. Drugs of molecular weight >4,000 Da, such as erythropoietin, insulin, or other polypeptide hormones, are more capable of serving as complete antigens than are low-molecular-weight drugs (<1,000 Da).[140] Biologic agents (e.g., antisera, antithymocyte globulin, intravenous immunoglobulin) also fit into this category of large polypeptides. Second, drugs containing foreign proteins or large polypeptides of nonhuman origin (e.g., streptokinase, beef or pork insulin, chimeric/murine-derived monoclonal antibodies, L-asparaginase) have the ability to serve as complete antigens.[1,140] However, the most common antigenic drugs (e.g., penicillins, sulfonamides) are of low molecular weight (<1,000 Da) and do not contain a foreign protein. These agents possess a third drug-related property related to conferring antigenic potential, which is the ability of the parent drug or its reactive metabolite to bind covalently to a carrier protein in vivo, thereby forming a complete antigen. The term *hapten* is used to describe a drug (or a metabolite) that must bind to a tissue or cell protein to serve as a complete antigen.[1] Identifying a drug's reactive metabolites and the potential of these metabolites to bind to carrier proteins is not readily achieved in premarketing studies; thus, the allergic potential of many low-molecular-weight drugs is not determined until postmarketing.

Drugs that are commonly associated with DHRs are listed in **Table 6-3**.[141-161] A drug's ability to cause a nonimmune DHR can often be assessed by a review of the drug's chemical and/or pharmacologic properties. Classic examples are anaphylactoid reactions to radiocontrast media, opioid-induced urticaria or generalized pruritus, red man syndrome with vancomycin, and nonsteroidal anti-inflammatory drug (NSAID)-induced asthma or angioedema.

When reviewing Tables 6-2 and 6-3, it should be noted that some drugs are listed as causing both allergy and DHRs. For example, vancomycin-induced red man syndrome is thought to be a nonimmune DHR, whereas vancomycin-associated blood dyscrasias and anaphylaxis are attributed to more rare allergic reactions.[67,127,128] Captopril, ciprofloxacin, and protamine have also been reported to cause both true allergy and nonimmune DHRs. Intravenous immunoglobulin G (IVIG) is most commonly associated with infusion-related reactions such as fever and arthralgias. However, IVIG can also cause an IgE-mediated reaction in patients with selective IgA deficiency.[3] In situations in which a drug can cause both types of reactions, it is often difficult to distinguish between allergy and a nonimmune DHR. Most importantly, the signs, symptoms, and severity of the reaction, rather than its mechanism, should drive clinicians' decision-making.

EPIDEMIOLOGY

Collectively, drug allergy, intolerance, and nonimmune DHRs have been estimated to comprise 25% of all adverse drug events.[2] Drug allergy is considered to be relatively rare, representing 6–10% of all adverse drug reactions.[2,162] In 2002, Hunziker et al.[163] provided an analysis of 12,785 adverse drug reactions of probable or definite association occurring in inpatients between 1974 and 1993. Drug allergy and nonimmune DHRs accounted for 13% of the adverse drug reactions. Differentiation between allergy and nonimmune DHRs as the cause of the adverse event could not be achieved because of the lack of valid skin testing or other in vitro testing methods to determine the presence of drug-specific antibodies.[163]

The epidemiology of anaphylaxis, including drug-induced anaphylaxis, has been re-evaluated by a working group composed of experts in allergy and immunology.[164] The expert panel estimated the frequency of anaphylaxis in 2006 to be 50–2,000 episodes per 100,000 persons, or a lifetime prevalence of 0.05–2%.[164] More recent estimates suggest that the prevalence is increasing, particularly in younger age groups and in patients treated with biologic agents. Neugut et al.[165] reported that the most serious cases of drug-induced anaphylaxis have been associated with the use of penicillin and radiocontrast media. Penicillin is recognized as the most common cause of anaphylaxis and is estimated to account for approximately 75% of fatal

Table 6-3 Agents Implicated in Nonimmune Drug Hypersensitivity Reactions

Drug	Incidence	Level of Evidence[a]
Adrenocorticotropic hormone	NK	C
Angiotensin-converting enzyme inhibitors[2,141-142]	0.1–0.2%	B
Angiotensin receptor blockers[143-146]	0.11%	B
Acetylsalicylic acid (aspirin)[10,11]	NK	C
Ciprofloxacin[147-149]	NK	C
Corticosteroids[150]	NK	C
Cremophor (polyethoxyethylated castor oil)-containing products[7,9]	NK	C
Enoxaparin[151]	NK	C
Infliximab[152-153]	NK	C
Levofloxacin[154]	NK	C
Midazolam[155]	NK	C
Muromonab[156]	NK	C
N-acetylcysteine[157]	NK	C
Nonsteroidal anti-inflammatory drugs[2]	NK	C
Ondansetron[158,159]	NK	C
Opioids[2,160]	NK	C
Paclitaxel[7]	NK	C
Polymyxin B	NK	C
Protamine[2]	0.06–10.7%	B
Radiocontrast media[161]	1.7%	B
Rituximab[37]	NK	C
Sacubitril	NK	C
Somatostatin	NK	C
Urokinase	NK	C
Vaccines[139]	NK	C
Vancomycin	NK	C

NK = not known.

[a]Definitions for Levels of Evidence: Level A—evidence from one or more randomized, controlled clinical trials; Level B—evidence from nonrandomized clinical trials, prospective observational studies, cohort studies, retrospective studies, case-control studies, meta-analyses and/or postmarketing surveillance studies; and Level C—evidence from one or more published case reports or case series.

cases in the United States annually.[2] Nonfatal anaphylaxis attributed to penicillin has been reported in 0.7–10% of the general population, whereas fatal cases occur in 0.002% of the general population.[165] Non-IgE-mediated anaphylaxis (i.e., anaphylactoid reactions) associated with radiocontrast media have occurred in 0.22–1% of patients, particularly in those receiving an agent with high osmolarity.[165]

Angioedema is estimated to occur in 0.1–1.2% of patients treated with angiotensin-converting-enzyme (ACE) inhibitors.[141] However, as many as 25–38% of cases of angioedema presenting to the emergency department (ED) have been attributed to ACE inhibitor therapy.[166,167] In an 8-year retrospective study, 12 of 49 patients (24.5%) presenting to the ED with angioedema reported concomitant therapy with an ACE inhibitor.[166] A second retrospective case-control study revealed an association between ACE inhibitors and angioedema in 15 of 40 patients (38%) presenting to the ED.[167] Compared with a control group of patients without angioedema, patients presenting to the ED with angioedema were 5 times more likely to be taking an ACE inhibitor (OR 5.1, 95% CI 2.03–12.89).[167]

The incidences of allergy and nonimmune DHRs associated with the majority of implicated drugs are unknown. The estimated incidences of allergy and nonimmune DHRs associated with some implicated drugs are presented in Tables 6-2 and 6-3.

MECHANISMS

DRUG ALLERGY

The exact mechanisms by which drugs serve as allergens and elicit immune responses are not well understood. Gaps in our understanding of these mechanisms can be attributed, in part, to the lack of a validated animal model of drug allergy.[168] Another influencing factor is the difficulty in identifying and isolating the antigenic components and metabolites of potential drug allergens. Although much is unknown about the mechanisms by which drugs cause allergy, it is known that a single drug, such as penicillin, can cause a variety of allergic reactions via different mechanisms.[168] At least two theories—the prohapten/hapten concept and the p-i concept—have been described to explain the manner in which drugs stimulate the immune response. Each theory will be discussed separately.

PROHAPTEN/HAPTEN THEORY

In this theory, a number of complex stages appear to be involved in the generation of an immune response to a drug. These stages include the following:

1. Formation of a complete antigen
2. Processing of the complete antigen by antigen-presenting cells
3. Recognition of the antigenic determinant by T lymphocytes
4. Generation of a drug-specific antibody or sensitized T cells
5. Elicitation of a clinical immune response

STAGE 1: FORMATION OF A COMPLETE ANTIGEN

Most drugs that serve as immunogens are low-molecular-weight compounds (<1,000 Da) and are too small to initiate an immune response alone. To be recognized by the immune system, these drugs must bind, usually covalently, to a high-molecular-weight carrier protein, thereby forming a complete antigen. Haptens are drugs that bind to tissue or plasma proteins to form a complete antigen.[1,169] The parent drug rarely has the ability to bind to tissue or cell proteins. For most low-molecular-weight drug immunogens, the hapten is a reactive metabolite of the parent drug, formed via metabolism in the liver, skin keratinocytes, or white blood cells.[168,170] As an example, sulfamethoxazole is well recognized as a highly allergenic compound, but a reactive metabolite, the nitroso-sulfamethoxazole derivative, not the parent compound, serves as the primary hapten.[171] In this regard, the parent drug, sulfamethoxazole, would be considered a prohapten.

STAGE 2: PROCESSING OF THE COMPLETE ANTIGEN BY ANTIGEN-PRESENTING CELLS

Once a hapten–protein conjugate has been formed, it must undergo antigen processing. This crucial stage involves recognition of the complete antigen by antigen-presenting cells (APCs). A number of cells serve as APCs, including macrophages, dendritic cells, cutaneous Langerhans cells, and B lymphocytes.[168-170] With many drug immunogens, the complete antigen is believed to diffuse across the cell membrane of the APC and be internalized into the lysosomes of the APC. Metabolism by proteolytic enzymes in the lysosomes allows for breakdown of the complete antigen to a smaller, hapten–peptide fragment.[172] The last step in this stage of processing is the binding of the hapten–peptide fragment with major histocompatibility complex (MHC) class I or II molecules synthesized by the APC.[1,168,169] Expression of the hapten–MHC complex on the surface of the APC allows recognition by T lymphocytes and further progression of the immune reaction.

STAGE 3: RECOGNITION OF THE ANTIGENIC DETERMINANT BY T LYMPHOCYTES

The manner in which T-helper cells recognize the hapten–MHC complex is not fully understood. It is theorized that three signals must occur for T-helper cells to become activated.[168,170,173,174] The first signal is completed by the interaction of the hapten–MHC complex with an antigen receptor on the surface of the T-helper cell. The second signal is believed to involve an interaction between specific receptors on the APC and the T-helper cell, resulting in the release of cytokines (cell messengers), such as interleukin (IL)-1 or IL-6. If this second signal does not occur, it is believed that the T-helper cells lose their responsiveness to the antigen, and the immune reaction ceases to progress.[168,174] Thus, some patients may process a drug allergen but the immune reaction may be blunted at this stage or at other stages in the process. The third signal involves activation of the CD4+ T lymphocytes with the release of specific cytokines from these activated T lymphocytes. Depending on the cytokines released, the T lymphocytes differentiate into either T-helper type 1 (Th1) or T-helper type 2 (Th2) cells.[173] Differentiation of the T-helper lymphocyte is an important step in the determination of the type of immune reaction to a specific drug allergen. Genetic factors are believed to influence T-helper-cell phenotyping in addition to influencing the type of cytokines released from activated T-helper cells. Dominance of cytokines IL-4 and IL-13 lead to the production of Th2 cells, whereas secretion of IL-2 and interferon β favors the production of Th1 cells.[175]

STAGE 4: GENERATION OF A DRUG-SPECIFIC ANTIBODY OR SENSITIZED T CELLS

Immune responses to a drug can lead to the generation of an antibody (humoral immune response) or sensitized T cells (cellular or delayed immune response). If a patient's response to an allergen is mediated by Th2 cells, a humoral response occurs with IgE, IgG, or IgM as the responding antibody. Th2 cells have the ability to secrete a number of cytokines, primarily IL-4 and IL-13, which stimulate the production of IgE from plasma cells. Th2 cells also secrete IL-5, which activates eosinophils, and IL-3 and IL-10, which are involved in mast cell differentiation.[174] Patients who have a Th1-dominant response to a drug are more likely to generate a cellular immune response with the production of drug-specific sensitized T lymphocytes.[2] At this stage of the immune process, memory cells (either T or B lymphocytes) are also produced to retain memory for the drug allergen. Memory cells allow for a faster onset of an immune reaction upon re-exposure to the antigen.

STAGE 5: ELICITATION OF A CLINICAL IMMUNE RESPONSE

Completion of stages 1 through 4 may not occur until days 5 to 21 of continued drug therapy. This period of sensitization explains the latency in the clinical presentation of the immune reaction. It is also important to consider that some patients may generate an antibody response to a drug allergen, but the event will not progress to a clinical reaction. For example, approximately 40% of patients treated with penicillin for at least 10 days produce drug-specific IgG without manifesting a hypersensitivity response.[2]

The p-i concept: A nonhapten pathway has also been described to explain drug allergy.[1,169,172] Some low-molecular-weight drugs may cause an immune response by "pharmacologically interacting with immune receptors."[1,172] Known as the p-i concept, these drugs do not require binding to a carrier protein or processing by APCs. This theory suggests that drugs bind directly to T-cell receptors in a reversible manner, similar to a ligand binding to a receptor. It is not known whether the drug first binds to the MHC molecule on the APC to signal T-cell activation or whether it directly binds to the T-cell receptor, stimulating the T-cell response. This concept appears most applicable to the initiation of delayed T-cell mediated-reactions, as opposed to humoral reactions.[1,172]

Mechanism-based classification of drug allergy: Since 1968, the Gell and Coombs[176] classification has been used to differentiate allergic drug reactions based on their mechanism and clinical presentation. Using this classification system, allergic reactions are described as types I through IV. It is important to consider that not all allergic drug reactions can be described using this classification. For example, some drug allergies exhibit features of more than one type (e.g., drug rash with eosinophilia and systemic symptoms [DRESS]). In addition, some allergies are mediated by antibodies not included in the classification (e.g., autoantibodies associated with procainamide-induced syndrome resembling systemic lupus erythematosus). The classification system was developed before our understanding of the varied roles of T cells in the immune response. As such, the original classification system has been

Table 6-4 Gell and Coombs Classification of Allergic Drug Reactions[1,2,176,177]

Classification	Timing	Antibody	Targeted Cells	Clinical Presentation
Type I (immediate)	Minutes to 1 hour; usually occurs after the second exposure to the drug; may be delayed for up to 48 hours after exposure	IgE	Mast cells, basophils	Anaphylaxis, isolated urticaria, angioedema, bronchospasm, abdominal cramping, respiratory arrest, cardiovascular collapse, arrhythmias, eosinophilia
Type II (delayed; cytotoxic)	>72 hours and up to weeks after continued initial exposure	IgG or IgM	Blood cells (red cells, platelets, mature neutrophils)	Cytopenias (hemolytic anemia, thrombocytopenia, some neutropenias) Vasculitides (some)
Type III (delayed; immune complex)	>72 hours and up to weeks after continued initial exposure	IgG or IgM	Skin, joint tissue, kidney, liver	Serum sickness-like illness Vasculitides (some) Glomerulonephritis, interstitial nephritis
Type IV (delayed; T-cell mediated)	Variable; >72 hours	Sensitized T lymphocytes	Skin, liver, kidney, lungs	See subtypes below
Type IVa	1–21 days	Th1 cells, interferon γ, monocytes, eosinophils	Skin	Tuberculin reaction, contact dermatitis
Type IVb	1–6 weeks	Th2 cells, interleukin-4, interleukin-5	Skin	Maculopapular rash with eosinophilia
Type IVc	4–28 days	Cytotoxic T cells, perforin, granzyme B, FasL	Skin	Bullous exanthems (SJS, TEN), fixed drug eruptions
Type IVd	>72 hours	T cells and interleukin-8	Skin	Acute generalized exanthematous pustulosis

IgE = immunoglobulin E, IgG = immunoglobulin G, IgM = immunoglobulin M, SJS = Stevens–Johnson syndrome, TEN = toxic epidermal necrolysis, Th = T-helper.

adapted in **Table 6-4** to better represent our current understanding of drug allergy.[1,2,176,177]

It is currently recommended that drug allergies be classified as immediate or nonimmediate based on the onset of the reaction.[1,169] According to the ICON expert panel, immediate reactions are those that culminate in the production of an IgE-mediated response.[1] These reactions typically present as angioedema, bronchospasm, or anaphylaxis and usually occur within 1 hour after first re-exposure to the immunogenic drug. Nonimmediate or delayed drug allergies constitute a broader category of events including maculopapular exanthems, delayed urticaria, immune-mediated blood disorders, and serum sickness reactions. Nonimmediate events are typically mediated by activated T cells and occur at least 1 hour after initial drug exposure and up to weeks or months after initial exposure.[1,169] This classification system, as noted by the expert panel, has limitations because the presence of immune cofactors (e.g., viruses) and the route of drug administration may influence the onset or progression of the immune reaction.[1]

If a patient generates IgE as the responding antibody to a drug allergen, the event is classified as an immediate type I reaction. IgE is commonly referred to as a homocytotropic antibody because of its strong affinity for the Fc receptors on mast cells and basophils.[140] IgE avidly binds to basophils in the blood and mast cells located in the skin and respiratory and gastrointestinal tracts and the connective tissue surrounding the blood vessels.[178] When a patient is re-exposed to the allergenic drug, cross-linking occurs between the hapten–protein complex and IgE bound to the surface of mast cells, basophils, or both. Cross-linking between the drug and two molecules of IgE causes an influx of calcium ions that triggers degranulation of the mast cells and basophils.[178] The end result is the extracellular release of a number of preformed inflammatory mediators such as histamine, heparin, and proteases. Influx of calcium also activates phospholipase A_2 and stimulates the release of arachidonic acids, which can be bio-transformed into a number of secondary mediators, including leukotrienes, prostaglandins, and platelet-activating factor.[164] The cytokine known as tumor necrosis factor α (TNFα) has also been implicated as a mediator. Collectively, these mediators of anaphylaxis can cause increased vascular permeability, a wheal-and-flare reaction, smooth-muscle contraction resulting in bronchospasm, nausea, vomiting, recruitment of inflammatory cells, activation of vagal pathways, decreased coronary blood flow, and delayed atrioventricular conduction.[179,180]

Nonimmediate type II cytotoxic reactions are usually mediated by IgG or IgM. During these reactions, the drug hapten typically binds to a cell-surface protein in the membrane of a blood cell (e.g., red cell, platelet, neutrophil).[113,114] A complexation reaction between the responding antibody (IgG or IgM) and the drug hapten bound to the surface protein leads to destruction of the affected cells (i.e., hemolysis, thrombocytopenia, neutropenia). Cell-bound antibody can also activate complement, a series of 25 plasma proteins that, when activated, assist in cell lysis.[113,114,175] Activated complement proteins possess a variety of properties, including the ability to degranulate mast cells (C3a, C5a), the ability to form a membrane attack complex (C5a and C9a), and the ability to stimulate opsonization to amplify the immune response.[175]

Nonimmediate type III reactions, commonly referred to as immune complex reactions, are usually mediated by IgG. During these events, the drug hapten typically forms a complete antigen by binding covalently with an amino acid component (such as the lysine or cysteine residues) of a plasma protein. The hapten–protein complex then stimulates the production of IgG. Binding between IgG and the circulating complete antigen results in the formation of immune complexes, which often circulate throughout the bloodstream and activate the complement cascade before depositing on targeted cells or tissues.[178] Complement-mediated migration of phagocytes and the release of pyrogens manifests as a fluid phase or serum sickness-like reaction consisting of fever, malaise, and lymphadenopathy. Activation of complement proteins C3a and C5a can also result in degranulation of mast cells with the release of histamine. Eventually, the immune complex may deposit in a variety of tissues, including the walls of blood vessels, glomerular cells, joint tissue, alveoli, and cells in the skin. After deposition on the targeted tissue, the immune complex, with the assistance of complement, mediates cell destruction.

Nonimmediate type IV reactions are subclassified as types IVa through IVd based on the responding T cell, effector mechanism, and clinical manifestations (Table 6-4). On exposure to the antigen, a specific subtype of T cell (e.g., Th1 cell, Th2 cell, cytotoxic T cell) orchestrates an inflammatory response through secretion of specific cytokines (IL-4, IL-5).[1,181] Type IV reactions involve a wide range of clinical events including contact dermatitis from a topically applied medication to more serious dermatologic events such as pustular and bullous exanthems. A complete review of the mechanisms by which drugs cause type IV reactions has been published.[181]

MECHANISMS OF DRUG HYPERSENSITIVITY REACTIONS

DHRs can also be classified as immediate or nonimmediate based on the timing of the event.[1] Drugs cause nonimmune DHRs by a number of mechanisms, including (1) direct stimulation of mast cells resulting in the release of histamine (e.g., opioids, polymyxin, protamine, diamines such as pentamidine, polyethoxylated castor oil), (2) nonimmunologic activation of the complement cascade (e.g., radiocontrast media, protamine), and (3) alteration of the metabolism or production of inflammatory mediators (e.g., ACE inhibitors, aspirin, and NSAIDs).[1,169] The direct stimulatory effects of drugs on mast cells appear to be dose-related and tend to predominate on mast cells in the skin. Ciprofloxacin, vancomycin, and muscle relaxants such as succinylcholine and opiates (e.g., codeine, morphine) have been shown to elicit urticarial reactions in normal skin at concentrations of ≥100 mcg/mL.[182]

The mechanism by which the ACE inhibitors cause angioedema is not completely understood; however, inhibition of the breakdown of bradykinin and substance P may partially explain this adverse event. ACE, a nonspecific dipeptidase enzyme, not only converts angiotensin I to angiotensin II but is also involved in the inactivation of bradykinin, substance P, and neurokinin A.[141] Elevations in plasma concentrations of bradykinin and substance P can lead to inflammation, increased vascular permeability, and vasodilation. Aspirin-induced asthma, also known as aspirin-exacerbated respiratory disease, is believed to result from an imbalance between the production of prostaglandins and leukotrienes from arachidonic acids.[183] Inhibition of cyclooxygenase-1 (COX-1) leads to decreased production of prostaglandin E_2, a modulating prostaglandin in bronchial tissue, and an increased propensity for arachidonic acids to be synthesized via the lipoxy-genase pathway. Increased production of leukotrienes C4, D4, and E4 is associated with smooth-muscle contraction manifesting as bronchospasm, inflammation, and increased mucus production.[183]

CLINICAL PRESENTATION AND DIFFERENTIAL DIAGNOSIS

The signs and symptoms of a number of specific allergic syndromes are provided in **Table 6-5**. The clinical presentation of drug allergy is highly variable and dependent on the responding antibody and the targeted tissues. Allergy may manifest as anaphylaxis; angioedema; urticaria; immune-complex diseases manifesting as a serum sickness-like illness, lupus-like reaction, hypersensitivity vasculitis, or DRESS; and mucocutaneous syndromes such as Stevens–Johnson syndrome (SJS) and toxic epidermal necrolysis (TEN). In addition, allergic drug reactions may be the cause of disorders of the blood, kidney, liver, and pulmonary system. Conditions to consider in the differential diagnoses of these syndromes are listed in **Table 6-6**. The mucocutaneous syndromes and DRESS are discussed in the section Cutaneous Diseases.

Anaphylaxis, the most severe form of an immediate type I reaction, constitutes a medical emergency. The onset of anaphylaxis is usually within minutes to 2 hours after exposure to the causative drug.[184] In rare cases, the onset can be delayed for up to 48 hours after exposure. A consensus panel on allergy has defined anaphylaxis as highly likely when one of the following scenarios is present[184]:

1. Acute onset of a reaction (minutes to several hours) that involves the skin (mucosal tissue) and the respiratory tract and/or a decrease in blood pressure
2. The rapid onset of a reaction after exposure to a likely allergen that involves two organ systems (respiratory tract, skin, decrease in blood pressure, and/or persistent gastrointestinal symptoms)
3. A decrease in blood pressure alone after exposure to a known allergen

An elevated serum tryptase concentration is indicative of the release of stored mediators from mast cells. Concentrations of tryptase, an enzyme that is stored in the secretory granules of the mast cell, become elevated in the serum within 1–2 hours after the onset of anaphylaxis and persist for as long as 6 hours after the event.[164,184] β-tryptase is released only during episodes of mast cell degranulation, whereas concentrations of α-tryptase are elevated in patients with a large mast cell burden (e.g., mastocytosis).[184] Anaphylaxis is most suggestive when the ratio of total (α + β) tryptase to β-tryptase is ≤10.[184] Serum platelet-activating factor may also be a biomarker of anaphylaxis.[185] A late phase of anaphylaxis, characterized by erythema, edema, and excess mucus production with mucus plug formation, occurs 8–12 hours after the initial attack and can last for up to 32 hours.[184] The late-phase reaction is attributed to the effects of leukotrienes, such as leukotriene B4, which stimulate migration of macrophages to the sites of tissue damage.[179,180]

Urticaria with pruritis, a common manifestation of anaphylaxis, can also occur as a sole manifestation of an immediate type I reaction. On subsequent exposure to the causative agent, urticaria may

Table 6-5 Signs and Symptoms Associated with Drug-Induced Allergic Syndromes

Anaphylaxis[2,179,180,184]

- Diffuse urticaria
- Facial flushing
- Angioedema
- Bronchospasm (wheezing, chest tightness, hoarseness)
- Laryngeal edema
- Stridor
- Hypotension
- Cardiac arrhythmias (atrial or ventricular)
- Nausea, vomiting, abdominal cramping, diarrhea
- Lightheadedness, feeling of impending doom
- Eosinophilia
- Elevated tryptase concentrations

Urticaria[285,286]

- Asymmetric, circumscribed erythematous (pink) papular lesions of variable shape ranging from small to geographic in size; lesions have raised borders and areas of central clearing
- Pruritus
- May be associated with angioedema
- May be associated with eosinophilia

Angioedema[184,285,286]

- Asymmetric, nonpitting edema of the face (tongue, lips, eyelids)
- Periorbital edema
- Laryngeal edema
- Tingling of the lips
- Hoarseness, difficulty speaking
- Difficulty swallowing
- Diarrhea, nausea, abdominal pain (if visceral involvement)
- Edema of the extremities, genitalia

Allergic-mediated blood disorders[113,114]

- Hemolytic anemia with positive direct or indirect Coombs test
- Thrombocytopenia, with peripheral count $<100,000\ mm^3$
- Granulocytopenia (agranulocytosis, neutropenia)
- Decreased concentrations of C3, C4
- Evidence of antiplatelet or antineutrophil antibodies

Serum sickness or serum sickness-like reaction[69]

- Fever and malaise
- Skin rash—urticaria, maculopapular rash or mixed presentation of urticarial plaques and maculopapular rash usually starting on the extremities (hands, fingers, toes)
- Arthralgias
- Lymphadenopathy
- Glomerulonephritis
- Elevated erythrocyte sedimentation rate (nonspecific marker)
- Reduced concentrations of C4 and C3; possible elevations in C3a

Vasculitis[86,88,188]

- Skin manifestations—purpura, maculopapular rash, hemorrhagic blisters; skin biopsy revealing leukocytoclastic vasculitis with fibrinoid necrosis and lymphocytic infiltrate
- General—fever, nausea, abdominal pain, polyarthritis, joint swelling
- Kidney—urinalysis revealing proteinuria, granular casts, and red cells; kidney biopsy may reveal deposition of IgG, IgM, or activated complement (C3)
- Pulmonary—hemoptysis, wheezing, pleuritic pain, presence of infiltrate on chest x-ray
- Sore throat, hoarseness
- Synovitis
- Elevated erythrocyte sedimentation rate, presence of antinuclear antibodies or antineutrophilic cytoplasmic autoantibodies

IgG = immunoglobulin G, IgM = immunoglobulin M.

progress to include anaphylaxis. Drug-induced angioedema can also occur as a sole manifestation of allergy, or it can occur with urticaria or as part of an anaphylactic event.[186] Angioedema, also known as giant urticaria or angioneurotic edema, presents as nonpitting edema that extends beyond the epidermis to involve the deep dermis, mucous membranes, and subcutaneous tissues.[186] Angioedema secondary to ACE inhibitors is typically confined to the head and neck, presenting as localized swelling of the face (tongue, lips, and eyelids) with edema of the mucous membranes of the mouth, throat, and nose.[141,142] Rarely, the edematous reaction can extend to the gastrointestinal tract, hands, feet, and genitalia.

The clinical presentation of drug-induced allergic blood disorders is included in Table 6-5. Depending on the causative drug, the patient may present with hemolytic anemia, thrombocytopenia, or granulocytopenia.[113,114] These peripherally mediated blood disorders typically occur within 5–21 days after drug initiation.[113,114] The affected blood cell counts decline rapidly, compared with the

Table 6-6 Conditions to Consider in the Differential Diagnosis of Drug Allergy

Anaphylaxis[179,180,184]

- Asthma
- Carcinoid syndrome
- Cardiogenic shock
- Croup
- Exercise-induced anaphylaxis
- Idiopathic anaphylaxis
- Insect stings or bites
- Latex allergy
- Panic attack
- Septic shock
- Systemic mastocytosis
- Systemic capillary leak syndrome
- Scrombroidosis
- Vasodepressor (vasovagal neurocardiogenic) syncope
- Vocal cord dysfunction syndrome

Angioedema[184,285,286]

- Insect stings or bites
- Food allergy
- Idiopathic or hereditary angioedema
- Hereditary or acquired C1 esterase inhibitor deficiency
- Systemic capillary leak syndrome
- Latex allergy
- Systemic mastocytosis

Urticaria[285,286]

- Cutaneous mastocytosis
- Mastocytosis in association with hematologic disorders (e.g., leukemia)
- Cholinergic urticaria
- Exercise-induced urticaria
- Infection (Epstein–Barr virus; hepatitis A, B, C; gastrointestinal parasites)
- Foods (peanuts, nuts, fish, shellfish, wheat, eggs, milk, soybeans, fruits)
- Food additives (benzoates, sulfites, monosodium glutamate, FD&C [food, drug, and cosmetic] dyes)
- Scrombroidosis
- Occupational exposures (latex, chromates in cement industry, cosmetics, plants)

Serum sickness-like reaction[69]

- Autoimmune disease (rheumatoid arthritis, lupus erythematosus)
- Hepatitis A, B, C
- Hypersensitivity vasculitis
- Infection (aspergillosis, histoplasmosis, coccidioidomycosis, blastomycosis, Epstein–Barr virus, cytomegalovirus)

Hypersensitivity vasculitis[86-88]

- Infection (bacterial endocarditis, hepatitis B or C, occult abscess)
- Rheumatic diseases
- Malignancy (lymphoma, Hodgkin disease, metastatic carcinoma, multiple myeloma)
- Autoimmune disease (rheumatoid arthritis, systemic lupus erythematosus, Wegener granulomatosis)

Hypersensitivity syndrome[188]

- Cutaneous lymphoma

relatively slow decline in the counts observed with bone-marrow-mediated blood disorders. In some patients, drug-specific antibodies (IgM or IgG) and reduced serum concentrations of C3 and C4 can be observed.[113,114]

The immune-complex diseases consist of a group of conditions including serum sickness-like disease (SSLD), hypersensitivity vasculitis, and lupus-like reaction. SSLD is a mild and transient form of the serum sickness that originally occurred with the administration of horse serum in the form of diphtheria antitoxin. The predominant feature of an SSLD is a cutaneous eruption that manifests within 5–21 days after drug initiation.[187] Approximately 90% of patients have either an urticarial reaction due to complement-mediated activation of the mast cells (one third of patients) or a maculopapular rash on the abdomen and extremities with possible extension to the palms and soles (two thirds of patients).[69,187,188] The rash is usually preceded by a prodromal phase consisting of fever and malaise, arthralgias, and lymphadenopathy. In rare instances, the reaction can extend to involve the kidney (i.e., glomerulonephritis). SSLD has been reported in association with a number of drugs, including β-lactam antibiotics, bupropion, cefaclor, ciprofloxacin, minocycline, and sulfonamides.[69-76,80-82] Drug-induced SSLD is often described as a mild condition that is self-limiting after discontinuation of the causative agent. However, in some cases, it progresses to a more serious vasculitis. Any evidence of mucous membrane involvement (i.e., mucocutaneous lesions of the mouth, genitalia, nares) may suggest the development of a more progressive condition, such as SJS.

Drug-induced vasculitides are associated with acute inflammatory and necrotic lesions of the arteries, arterioles, venules, and capillaries. Consistent with other immune-complex diseases, an initial prodromal period is noted within 1-3 weeks after drug initiation and usually consists of fever, arthralgias, and sore throat.[86,188] Cutaneous vasculitis, described as either a purpuric or maculopapular rash of the lower extremities, is the most common presenting manifestation.[87] The purpuric lesions can progress to necrotic ulcerations, and the vasculitic process can extend to include the kidneys, lungs, nasal mucosa, and ears. A number of drugs, such as propylthiouracil, hydralazine, minocycline, phenytoin, and allopurinol, can induce vasculitis through the production of antineutrophil cytoplasmic autoantibodies.[86] Other terms used to describe this condition include leukocytoclastic vasculitis, polyarteritis nodosa, and Churg–Strauss syndrome.

RISK FACTORS

The rarity of drug allergy suggests a reliance on contributory or predisposing factors. Risk factors for drug allergies have been categorized as either drug-related or patient (host)-related. Many extensive reviews have been published describing predisposing factors for both the induction of an immune response to a drug and the elicitation of an allergic drug reaction.[1,182,189,190] However, debate continues as to the influence of these factors on the risk of reactivity. Most risk factors have been identified through small-scale studies and indirect clinical observations. In addition, the majority of the risk assessments have been determined from the study of penicillin. At present, it is not known whether risk factors associated with the penicillins can be extrapolated with confidence to other antigenic drugs. Proposed risk factors for drug allergy are listed in **Table 6-7**. In addition, risk factors associated with specific drugs (e.g., the penicillins, sulfonamides, radiocontrast media) are identified.

The three most commonly described drug-related risk factors for an allergic reaction are increased molecular size (molecular weight ≥4,000 Da), chemical composition consisting of proteins or polypeptides, and the ability of the drug or its reactive metabolite to bind covalently to a carrier protein.[189] The presence of proteins of nonhuman origin (e.g., chimeric monoclonal antibodies containing murine-based components, pork insulin,

Table 6-7 Risk Factors for Allergic and Nonimmune Drug Hypersensitivity Reactions

Allergic reactions

Drug-related factors[182,189,190]

- Chemical properties (molecular weight, polypeptide composition, foreign protein)
- Dose and duration of therapy
- Frequency of treatment courses

Coexisting conditions

- Active infection with Epstein–Barr virus (aminopenicillins)[201]
- Active infection with human immunodeficiency virus (sulfonamides, dapsone, penicillins, ciprofloxacin, phenytoin)[203]
- Cystic fibrosis (β-lactams)[206-208]
- HHV-6 (DRESS)[204,205]

Genetic factors

- HLA B*5701 (abacavir)[193]
- HLA-B*5801 (allopurinol)[335]
- HLA-B*1502 (carbamazepine, phenytoin, fosphenytoin)[355,356]
- HLA-*DRA* (amoxicillin, penicillins)[196]
- CYP2C9*3 (phenytoin)[358]
- HLA-B*13:01 (dapsone)[108]

Patient history

- History of a previous reaction to the specific agent

Pre-existing IgE antibodies against galactose-α-1,3-galactose[24,25]

- Cetuximab

Nonimmune drug hypersensitivity reactions

Drug-related factors[2,3]

- Dose (vancomycin, opiates)
- Infusion rate (vancomycin, paclitaxel)

Patient factors[2,3]

- Female sex (radiocontrast media)[210]
- Atopy (radiocontrast media, aspirin)[211,216]
- Asthma (radiocontrast media, aspirin)[10,11,215]
- Race (angiotensin-converting enzyme inhibitors)[213,214]

Concomitant drug therapy

- β-blockers (radiocontrast media)[21,212]

DRESS = drug rash with eosinophilia and systemic symptoms, HHV-6 = human herpesvirus 6, HLA = human leukocytic antigen.

streptokinase) or the inclusion of antigenic excipients (e.g., FD&C dyes, peanut oil, soybean emulsion, sulfites) also increase the risk of drug reactivity. Other proposed drug-related factors include route of drug administration, dose, and frequency of administration. Sensitization to a drug can occur via any route of administration, and allergic reactions have been reported in association with all routes.[140,182] However, once a patient has been sensitized to a drug, subsequent administration of that drug by the parenteral route has been associated with increased severity of an allergic drug reaction.[190] This observation is largely explained by the higher rate of drug delivery with the parenteral route versus other routes of administration, particularly the oral route.[189] Allergic reactions can occur with any dose of a drug, but sensitization is more likely to be achieved with continuous drug dosing rather than single-dose therapy.[182] Rarely, an allergic reaction may be dose-dependent, as with penicillin-associated hemolytic anemia, which is observed only with continuous intravenous dosing of ≥20 million units daily. More commonly, once a patient has been sensitized to a drug, the severity of the reaction is usually proportional to the dose administered. The frequency of exposure to a given allergic compound has consistently been shown to increase the risk of an immune response, particularly involving IgE. Humoral drug sensitivity is finite, and there is a large degree of interpatient variation in the duration of sensitivity. As such, the shorter the interval between treatment regimens with a sensitizing drug, the more likely the patient will have retained sensitivity and be able to mount an allergic reaction.[2,140,182,189]

Proposed patient-specific risk factors include age, sex, genetic predisposition, and concomitant conditions. Allergic reactions to some drugs have been reported more commonly among patients in specific age groups; however, age has not been consistently identified as a risk factor.[3,191] For example, anaphylaxis associated with penicillin has been reported more commonly in patients between the ages of 20 and 49 years than in children.[192] This finding relates less to the specific age of the patient than to the number of potential exposures to the specific allergenic drug. Within the age of 20–49 years, a greater likelihood exists that a patient has been previously exposed and possibly sensitized to a penicillin, thereby increasing the risk of reactivity on subsequent exposure. Allergic drug reactions do occur in children, particularly in those who receive frequent courses of antibiotics for chronic otitis media, chronic bouts of bronchitis, or infections associated with cystic fibrosis. Therefore, the frequency and number of exposures, rather than age, are more likely to increase risk. For unknown reasons, drug allergy occurs more frequently in female than male patients. Bigby et al.[191] reported a 35% higher incidence of drug-induced allergic cutaneous reactions in women than in men.

Genetic factors may influence a patient's risk of drug allergy. In order for T-helper cells to recognize a drug as an antigen, the drug immunogen must be copresented with MHC class molecules.[169,170,173] In this regard, patients with certain MHC characteristics (or human leukocyte antigens [HLA]) may be at higher risk of reacting to a given antigenic compound as compared with patients without the specific MHC molecules. For example, in patients infected with human immunodeficiency virus (HIV), susceptibility to abacavir-induced hypersensitivity has been found to be associated with the of HLA-B*5701, HLA DR7, and HLA-DQ3.[193,194] HLA-DR4 was present in 19 of 26 patients (73%) with hydralazine-associated lupus-like syndrome, as compared with 4 of 16 hydralazine-treated patients without lupus (25%).[195] Most recently, a single nucleotide polymorphism of HLA-DRA, a MHC Class II gene, was found to be a predictor of skin-test positivity to amoxicillin and other penicillins, but not cephalosporins.[196] A number of HLA alleles have been found to be associated with allergic-mediated severe cutaneous drug reactions (see section Cutaneous Diseases).

In addition to encoding for histocompatibility phenotypes, genetic factors can influence the metabolic deactivation of drugs via phase 1 or phase 2 metabolism. For example, severe reactions to sulfamethoxazole have been noted in patients with hereditary deficiency in *N*-acetyltransferase (slow acetylators).[197] Rieder et al.[198] reported that 19 of 21 patients (90%) with sulfonamide hypersensitivity were slow acetylators, as compared with a 55% frequency of slow acetylators in a race-matched control group (p <0.008). It has also been suggested that patients with a hereditary deficiency in epoxide hydrolase are at higher risk of anticonvulsant hypersensitivity syndrome because of a lesser ability to detoxify the arene oxide metabolite of the aromatic anticonvulsants.[199,200] In addition to encoding for drug metabolic activity, genes also encode for the type of T-cell receptor and costimulatory molecules/cytokines involved in the signaling of allergic reactions.

Although often implicated as a predisposing factor, atopy has not been found to increase the risk of drug allergy.[184,190] Patients who are atopic have high IgE responsiveness to environmental allergens, manifesting as allergic rhinitis, allergic asthma, and atopic dermatitis. Originally, it was theorized that the high IgE responsiveness reported in atopic patients could increase the risk of IgE sensitization to drugs. Studies have shown that a history of atopy does not influence the likelihood of a patient being sensitized to a drug. However, if an atopic patient becomes sensitized to a drug, evidence suggests that the reaction will be more severe than that observed in nonatopic patients.[2,189]

Concomitant viral infections may also predispose a patient to an allergic drug reaction. Pullen et al.[201] reported ampicillin-associated morbilliform rash in 18 of 19 patients (95%) with acute Epstein–Barr virus (EBV) infection. In comparison, a morbilliform skin rash develops in approximately 5% to 10% of the general population exposed to an aminopenicillin (e.g., ampicillin, amoxicillin).[202] Patients infected with other viral pathogens, such as human herpesvirus 6 (HHV-6) and HIV, have also exhibited an increased risk of drug allergy. In HIV-infected patients, 29–65% of those treated with sulfamethoxazole exhibited an allergic or allergic-like reaction, and the risk of reactivity to a number of other drugs (e.g., ciprofloxacin, dapsone, foscarnet, penicillins, phenytoin, rifampin) has also been shown to be increased.[203] HHV-6 has been linked to an increased risk of DRESS.[204,205] The mechanism by which viral infections increase the risk of drug reactivity is not completely understood. Proposed mechanisms include virally mediated alterations in drug metabolism, upregulation of MHC class II molecules on APCs, and increased release of cytokines such as interferon β, which amplify the immune response.[168,173,174]

Cystic fibrosis is a risk factor for allergic reactions to β-lactam antibiotics. At least 20% of patients with cystic fibrosis have an allergic reaction during an antibiotic treatment course, and the risk increases with the number of treatment courses.[206] The most commonly reported allergenic β-lactam antibiotic in these patients was piperacillin in a 1994 study[207]; however, increased rates of reactivity have also been demonstrated with other antipseudomonal penicillins and cephalosporins.[208,209] Evidence suggests that these reactions are not typically mediated by the β-lactam ring, but are more likely to be reactions to the side chains of the agents.[206]

Risk factors for nonimmune DHRs are highly dependent on the specific causative drug. For example, the risk of an anaphylactoid reaction associated with a radiocontrast agent is higher in women, patients with atopy or asthma, and patients receiving nonselective or selective β-adrenergic blocker therapy.[210-212] Risk factors for ACE inhibitor-induced angioedema include black race, a history of idiopathic angioedema secondary to a deficiency in complement-1-esterase inhibitor, and receiving longer-acting agents (i.e., enalapril, lisinopril).[141,213,214] Aspirin intolerance manifesting as aspirin-induced asthma is more commonly observed in patients with history of asthma with or without allergic rhinitis or nasal polys.[10,11,215] Aspirin- or NSAID-induced exacerbations of urticaria or angioedema are more common in atopic patients with history of idiopathic urticaria or angioedema.[216]

The most reliable risk factor for hypersensitivity and most nonimmune DHRs is history of a prior reaction to the drug. For example, patients with a history of an anaphylactoid reaction to a radiocontrast agent have a 16–44% risk of having a reaction on re-exposure particularly to a high-osmolarity agent.[217] For the penicillins, a reliable skin testing method with a high negative predictive value has allowed for more accurate determinations of the risk of reactivity on re-exposure. In a patient with a positive history of an IgE-mediated reaction to a penicillin, a positive skin-prick test revealed a 50–70%

risk of an IgE-mediated reaction on re-exposure.[2,218] In contrast, a negative skin test indicates only a 2–3% risk of an IgE-mediated reaction on re-exposure.[218] Unfortunately, reliable skin-test reagents for other highly allergenic drugs have not been produced, thereby limiting the ability to accurately assess the risk of reactivity to other allergenic drugs.

MORBIDITY AND MORTALITY

In 2002, a task force assembled by the Immunotoxicology Technical Committee, part of the nonprofit Health and Environmental Sciences Institute, provided an estimate of the impact of drug-induced allergic reactions on the healthcare system.[219] On the basis of the assumption that 6–10% of adverse drug reactions are immune-mediated, it was estimated that 137,000–230,000 hospital admissions in 1998 in the United States were attributed to drug-induced allergic reactions. Using cost estimates determined in 1997 for the treatment of adverse drug reactions in hospitalized patients, the task force estimated that the annual cost of hospital-based management of drug allergy is $275 million to $600 million.[219] It was further hypothesized that the total annual cost for management of both inpatient- and outpatient-related drug allergic reactions could approach $1 billion.

PREVENTION

ALLERGIC REACTIONS

Drug-induced allergic reactions have consistently been considered as unpredictable in nature and largely unpreventable. However, continuing advances in pharmacogenomics research may alter the level of preventability of these events. Prospective screening for the presence of the HLA-B*5701 allele has been shown to lower the risk of hypersensitivity to abacavir.[193] In a double-blind, controlled study, 1,956 HIV-infected patients were randomly assigned to undergo either prospective screening for HLA-B*5701 prior to the initiation of abacavir or a standard-of-care approach to abacavir therapy.[193] Prospective screening for HLA-B*5701 with subsequent avoidance of abacavir in identified carriers prevented the occurrence of immunologically confirmed hypersensitivity reactions. Screening was associated with a negative predictive value of 100% and a positive predictive value of 47.9% in this primarily white population.[193] The investigators calculated that only 14 patients would have to be screened to prevent one case of abacavir hypersensitivity. Screening for the HLA-B*5701 allele is currently available. Screening for other HLA alleles is also available for patients considered as high risk for serious cutaneous adverse reactions to allopurinol, carbamazepine, phenytoin, and fosphenytoin (see section Cutaneous Reactions).

Once a patient has had an allergic reaction to a drug, a number of measures can be taken to prevent a subsequent reaction. The most important preventive measure is patient education. In particular, patients should be educated regarding avoidance of the causative drug and any cross-reactive drugs in the future. If a potentially immunogenic medication is deemed necessary, the use of graded challenge and induction of drug tolerance (i.e., desensitization) can often be used to prevent reactions on drug re-exposure.[220,221] A graded challenge procedure, or test dosing, involves the cautious administration of a drug when the risk of a reaction is considered to be low. Graded challenge does not alter the immune or nonimmune response to the drug.[221] Instead, it is used when the risk of an immediate reaction to a drug or related drug on re-exposure is deemed low, no alternative agent is equally effective, and a reliable skin testing method is not available. Classic examples include the slow introduction of furosemide in a patient with history of sulfonamide allergy or the slow introduction of a third-generation cephalosporin in a patient who previously developed a reaction to a first-generation cephalosporin. The starting dose is typically 1/10th–1/100th of the final treatment dose, and doses are increased in two- to fivefold increments every 30 or 60 minutes until the full therapeutic dose is attained.[221,222]

In contrast, temporary induction of drug tolerance, also known as desensitization, is used to modify a patient's response to a drug. Such procedures are intended to alter the immune response and render mast cells less responsive to degranulation.

Table 6-8 Skin Testing for IgE Responsiveness to β-Lactam Antibiotics

Step 1. Epicutaneous (scratch, prick) test with benzylpenicilloyl–polylysine (Pre-Pen) and the minor determinants. Make a nonbleeding scratch of the skin with a lancet. Administer the dose of the reagents (below):

- Pre-Pen, full-strength dilution; 1 drop
- Penicillin G, 10,000 units/mL; 1 drop

Step 2. Evaluate the scratch sites within 10–15 minutes. A positive test result is the presence of itching or an erythematous or wheal reaction at either site of the scratch tests. If the reaction is positive, do not proceed with further testing.

Step 3. If the scratch test is negative, proceed with intradermal testing.

- Pre-Pen, full strength; 0.02 mL intradermally
- Penicillin G, 10,000 units/mL; 0.02 mL intradermally
- Administer a positive control (histamine) and a negative control (saline)

Step 4. Evaluate the sites of intradermal injections within 15–20 minutes. A positive reaction is the presence of itching, erythema or wheal >4 mm, or a wheal reaction >50% the size of the original size of the bleb from the injection of either Pre-Pen or the minor determinants (penicillin G). Assess the site of histamine and saline control. If the histamine control site is not positive, consider interference by antihistaminergic agents.

The term *desensitization* should be used when the underlying mechanism of the drug intolerance is believed to be IgE-mediated (e.g., anaphylaxis due to penicillin).[220] The incremental dosing used in a desensitization protocol allows for downregulation of the immune response and temporary administration of the inciting agent. Reactions most amenable to desensitization are IgE-mediated involving the skin (e.g., angioedema, urticaria), upper and lower respiratory tract (e.g., dyspnea and wheezing), and cardiovascular (e.g., hypotension). Neither graded challenge nor desensitization should be used in patients with history of severe non-IgE-mediated drug allergies manifesting as DRESS, SJS, TEN, exfoliative dermatitis, hemolytic anemia, or hepatitis.

Guidelines for the avoidance of allergic reactions to common drug allergens are provided below.

β-LACTAM ANTIBIOTICS

Whenever possible, a non-β-lactam antibiotic should be used in patients with a history of penicillin allergy. If a β-lactam antibiotic is therapeutically necessary (i.e., treatment of syphilis in a pregnant woman, patient with cystic fibrosis and pneumonia) in a patient with history of IgE-mediated allergy, epicutaneous (prick, scratch) skin testing is the preferred technique for assessing the likelihood of a reaction on re-exposure. The skin-testing procedure is described in **Table 6-8**. Penicillin is rapidly hydrolyzed to a number of reactive metabolites or antigenic determinants. Ninety-five percent of the penicillin molecules that covalently bind to proteins are in the form of benzyl penicilloyl, commonly regarded as the major determinant of penicillin. The parent drug and reactive metabolites found in lesser quantities, such as penilloate and penicilloate, are referred to as minor determinants. Both the major and minor determinants can elicit an IgE-mediated response; thus, both are recommended for use when skin testing for IgE responsiveness. Penicilloyl polylysine (PPL), the major determinant bound to protein, is commercially available as Pre-Pen. The minor determinants are not commercially available in the United States; however, kits containing both the major and minor determinants are available in Europe (Diater Labs, Madrid Spain).[223] In the United States, a dilute concentration of penicillin G (10,000 units/mL) is recommended with PPL for skin testing.[224] Studies have shown a similar reaction rate to oral penicillin in patients with skin-test negativity to PPL plus penicillin G versus those with skin-test negativity to the full set of major and minor determinants.[224,225] When used together for skin testing (i.e., PPL and diluted penicillin G), 97% of patients with a negative skin test have subsequently tolerated a penicillin.[226] Patients with a positive skin test to either determinant and a positive allergy history have a 50–70% risk of reacting with an IgE-mediated response to penicillin on re-exposure.[226] This risk of β-lactam mediated reactivity can also be applied to semisynthetic penicillins and, with lesser certainty, to cephalosporins and carbapenems.[227,228] Little to no risk of a cross-reaction exists between penicillin and aztreonam, a monobactam.[229] A negative penicillin skin test indicates that the risk of an immediate type I reaction to penicillin or another β-lactam is extremely low. These patients are candidates for treatment with full therapeutic doses of a penicillin or a related β-lactam. Of note, skin testing with PPL and the minor determinant(s) does not identify patients who are at risk for unique side-chain mediated reactions to β-lactams (e.g., third-generation cephalosporins, piperacillin).

It is important to keep in mind that skin testing only indicates the potential for an IgE-mediated reaction to penicillin. Skin testing does not quantify the risk of having an IgG-, an IgM- or a cell-mediated reaction. Patients with a history of SJS, exfoliative dermatitis, or TEN associated with a penicillin should not undergo skin testing.

In addition to β-lactam-mediated allergic reactions, side-chain-specific reactions are increasingly reported with a number of penicillins, particularly the aminopenicillins and piperacillin.[230,231] As such, a patient with an allergy to one of these penicillins may not react to other penicillins. Structural similarities and differences between the penicillins are depicted in **Figure 6-1**. In a patient with history of an urticarial or other IgE-mediated reaction to an aminopenicillin or piperacillin, skin testing with Pre-Pen and the minor determinants is the preferred method to rule out β-lactam-mediated allergy. If the skin test result is negative, the patient may be challenged with a penicillin with a structurally different side chain. Dilute concentrations of amoxicillin and piperacillin have also been used to skin test for side-chain-mediated reactions.[232,233] In addition to causing side-chain-mediated allergic reactions, some penicillins have been associated with the development of nonimmunologically mediated drug eruptions. Maculopapular rash with an aminopenicillin (i.e., amoxicillin, ampicillin) may be an idiosyncratic reaction, particularly in a patient with acute EBV infection.[201,230]

The risk of cross-reactivity between penicillins and cephalosporins is low, particularly between penicillin and the second- and third-generation agents. On the basis of laboratory studies, the risk of cross-reactivity between penicillins and the first-generation cephalosporins is less than 10%, and the risk of a cross-reaction between the penicillins and the third-generation cephalosporins is as low as 1%.[2,52] One meta-analysis included nine studies in which the risk of cephalosporin allergy was compared in penicillin-allergic and nonpenicillin-allergic patients. Compared to nonallergic patients, the risk of cross-reactivity in penicillin-allergic patients was highest in association with the first-generation cephalosporins (OR 4.79, 95% CI 3.71–6.17).[234] The first-generation agents included in the analysis (i.e., cephalothin, cephaloridine, cephalexin) had R1 substitutions similar to that of penicillin. The odds ratios for risk of cross-reactivity to the second- and third-generation cephalosporins were not significant at 1.13 (95% CI 0.61–2.12) and 0.45 (95% CI 0.18–1.13), respectively.[234] The lower risk of cross-reactivity between these agents and penicillin may be attributed to structural differences in the R1 substitution on the β-lactam ring. In patients with a history of maculopapular rash associated with a penicillin, the benefits of using a second- or third-generation cephalosporin may substantially outweigh the potential risk of a cross-reaction. In patients with a history of an IgE-mediated reaction and skin-test positivity to penicillin, first-generation cephalosporins should generally be avoided. If deemed medically necessary, a cephalosporin can be administered via a graded challenge, or attempts can be made to desensitize the patient to the cephalosporin.[22]

CARBAPENEMS

Carbapenems contain a β-lactam ring attached to a modified thiazolidine ring with two side chains. The risk of a cross-reaction between a penicillin and a carbapenem appears to be much lower than originally described. In three retrospective studies of patients with a history of penicillin allergy, the rates of cross-reaction to a carbapenem (e.g., imipenem, meropenem) were 9.2%, 9.5%, and 11%.[235-237] Each study was limited by its retrospective design, heavy reliance on self-reported penicillin allergy histories, and the lack of skin testing to confirm IgE reactivity. In prospective studies, both skin testing and carbapenem challenge dosing were used to assess cross-reactive risk.[238-242] In one of these studies, patients

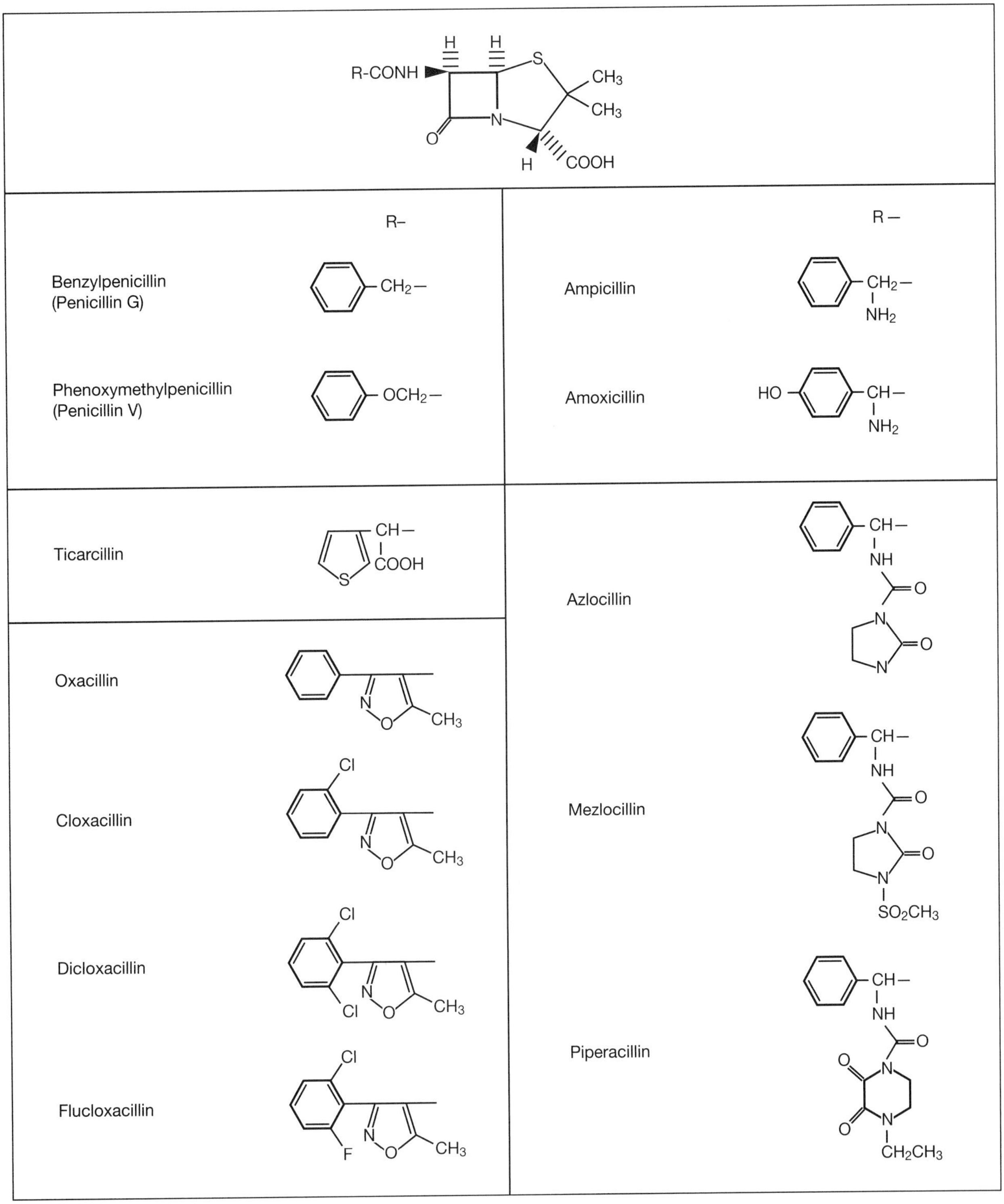

R–	R–
Benzylpenicillin (Penicillin G)	Ampicillin
Phenoxymethylpenicillin (Penicillin V)	Amoxicillin
Ticarcillin	Azlocillin
Oxacillin	Mezlocillin
Cloxacillin	Piperacillin
Dicloxacillin	
Flucloxacillin	

FIGURE 6-1 Similarities and Differences in the Structures of Various Penicillins

Source: Reprinted with permission from Baldo BA. Penicillins and cephalosporins as allergens—structural aspects of recognition and cross-reactions. *Clin Exp Allergy.* 1999; 29:744–9.

with negative results on skin testing for imipenem underwent graded challenge dosing of imipenem to a total dose of 500 mg.[239] None of the 110 patients reacted to imipenem. A low risk of cross-reactivity between meropenem and penicillin was demonstrated in two studies, one involving children ages 3–14 years.[240,241] In both studies, only one patient with skin-test positivity to penicillin had a positive skin test to meropenem. Graded challenge dosing with meropenem was tolerated in 100% of the skin-test-negative patients in both studies.[240,241] Most recently, cross-reactivity between penicillin and ertapenem, meropenem and imipenem was studied in 212 patients with skin-test positivity to a penicillin.[242] None of the 212 patients had skin test positivity to a carbapenem, and 211 successfully completed graded challenge dosing to a full therapeutic dose of each carbapenem.[242] Based on these results, carbapenem use should not be routinely avoided in a patient with history of penicillin allergy. Depending on the allergy history, challenge dosing with the carbapenem may be appropriate. In cases of skin test positivity to penicillin or history of severe penicillin allergy, desensitization may be performed.[243] The risk of cross-reactivity between the carbapenems is also unknown. Imipenem-sensitive patients tolerating meropenem following graded challenge and meropenem desensitization have been reported.[243,244]

CEPHALOSPORINS

A patient with a cephalosporin allergy should be interviewed in depth to obtain information on all antibiotics that have evoked allergic reactions and those that have been administered without adverse incident. Patients with a history of reactivity to one cephalosporin may or may not exhibit reactivity to other cephalosporins or penicillins.[23] Although cephalosporins share the antigenic β-lactam ring of the penicillins, they are more likely to cause allergic reactions mediated by side chains at either the R1 or R2 positions. Structural similarities and differences in the cephalosporins based on R1 and R2 substitutions are depicted in **Figure 6-2**.

In a patient with a history of an urticarial or other IgE-mediated reaction to a cephalosporin, either the antigenic β-lactam ring or an antigenic side chain of the cephalosporin may serve as the antigenic determinant. Skin testing with Pre-Pen and the minor determinant can help to identify the likelihood of a β-lactam allergy. More commonly, allergic reactions to cephalosporins are mediated via the R1 side chain. Examination of the cephalosporin's side chains may aid in the determination of potential cross-reactive agents. For example, cefaclor and cephalexin have identical side chains at the R1 position and cephalothin and cefotaxime have similar side chains at the R2 position.[21] Ceftazidime shares a common side chain with aztreonam.[2,22] Overall, the risk of cross-reactivity between cephalosporin antibiotics is believed to be greater than the risk of cross-reactivity between the cephalosporins and the penicillins.[22] In patients with selective allergy to a cephalosporin, decisions regarding the use of alternative cephalosporins should be based on the severity of the allergic reaction, the availability of equally effective non-β-lactam antibiotics, and the structure-specific feature (i.e., R1 and R2 substitutions) of the cephalosporin.

SULFA DRUGS

In a patient with a documented or reported sulfa allergy, the first step in prevention of a subsequent reaction is accurate and complete history taking. Clarification is needed regarding the specific sulfa drug to which the patient reacted in the past, and whether he or she has taken other sulfa drugs without incident. Sulfa drugs, by definition, possess a sulfamoyl (SO_2NH_2) moiety. Sulfate salts (e.g., morphine sulfate, atropine sulfate), sulfites, and sulfides are not members of the "sulfa" drug class. Sulfa drugs include sulfonamide antibiotics, thiazide diuretics, loop diuretics (e.g., bumetanide, furosemide, torsemide), oral sulfonylurea hypoglycemic agents, carbonic anhydrase inhibitors (e.g., acetazolamide, dorzolamide), celecoxib, metolazone, sumatriptan, and zonisamide.[245] The antiviral agents amprenavir, fosamprenavir, and darunavir are also classified as sulfa drugs. This drug class can be further categorized based on the presence or absence of an aromatic amine group in the N4 position. Sulfonamide antibiotics (e.g., sulfadiazine, sulfamethoxazole, sulfapyridine, amprenavir) have an arylamine at the N4 position, whereas the sulfonamide nonantibiotics (as listed above) do not.[171,245] Presence of

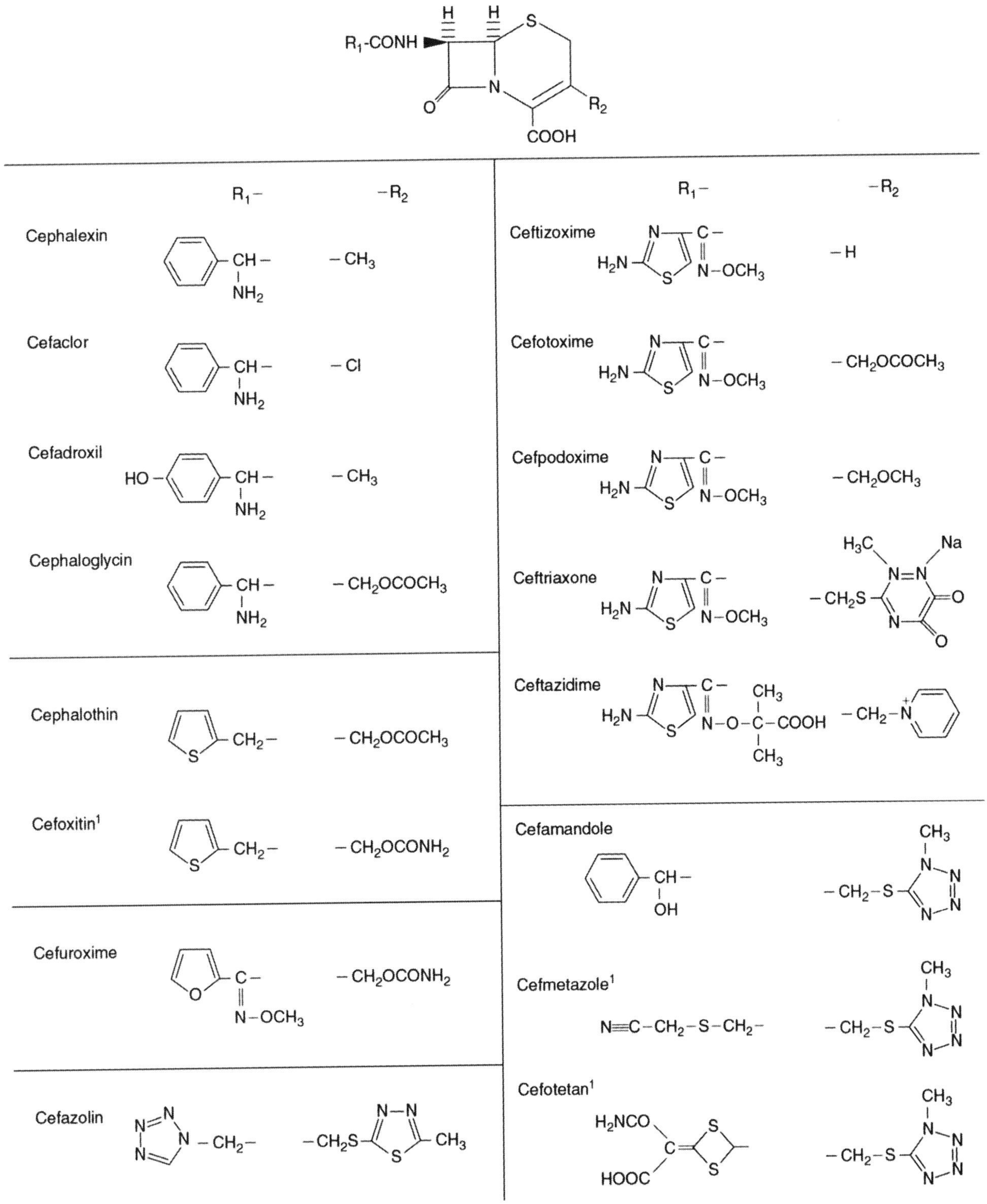

R₁-CONH, H, H, S, N, O, COOH, R₂

	R_1-	$-R_2$
Cephalexin	CH– NH_2	$-CH_3$
Cefaclor	CH– NH_2	–Cl
Cefadroxil	HO– CH– NH_2	$-CH_3$
Cephaloglycin	CH– NH_2	$-CH_2OCOCH_3$
Cephalothin	S CH_2-	$-CH_2OCOCH_3$
Cefoxitin[1]	S CH_2-	$-CH_2OCONH_2$
Cefuroxime	O C– N–OCH_3	$-CH_2OCONH_2$
Cefazolin	N=N N – CH_2- N	$-CH_2S-$ N–N S CH_3

	R_1-	$-R_2$
Ceftizoxime	N C– H_2N- S N–OCH_3	–H
Cefotoxime	N C– H_2N- S N–OCH_3	$-CH_2OCOCH_3$
Cefpodoxime	N C– H_2N- S N–OCH_3	$-CH_2OCH_3$
Ceftriaxone	N C– H_2N- S N–OCH_3	H_3C Na N=N $-CH_2S-$ N O O
Ceftazidime	N C– CH_3 H_2N- S N–O–C–COOH CH_3	$-CH_2-N^+$
Cefamandole	CH– OH	CH_3 N N $-CH_2-S-$ N N
Cefmetazole[1]	N≡C–CH_2–S–CH_2–	CH_3 N N $-CH_2-S-$ N N
Cefotetan[1]	H_2NCO S C= HOOC S	CH_3 N N $-CH_2-S-$ N N

FIGURE 6-2 Similarities and Differences in the Structures of Various Cephalosporins

[1]Cephamycin with an α-methoxy group (–OCH3) at the 7-position.

Source: Reprinted with permission from Baldo BA. Penicillins and cephalosporins as allergens—structural aspects of recognition and cross-reactions. *Clin Exp Allergy.* 1999; 29:744–9.

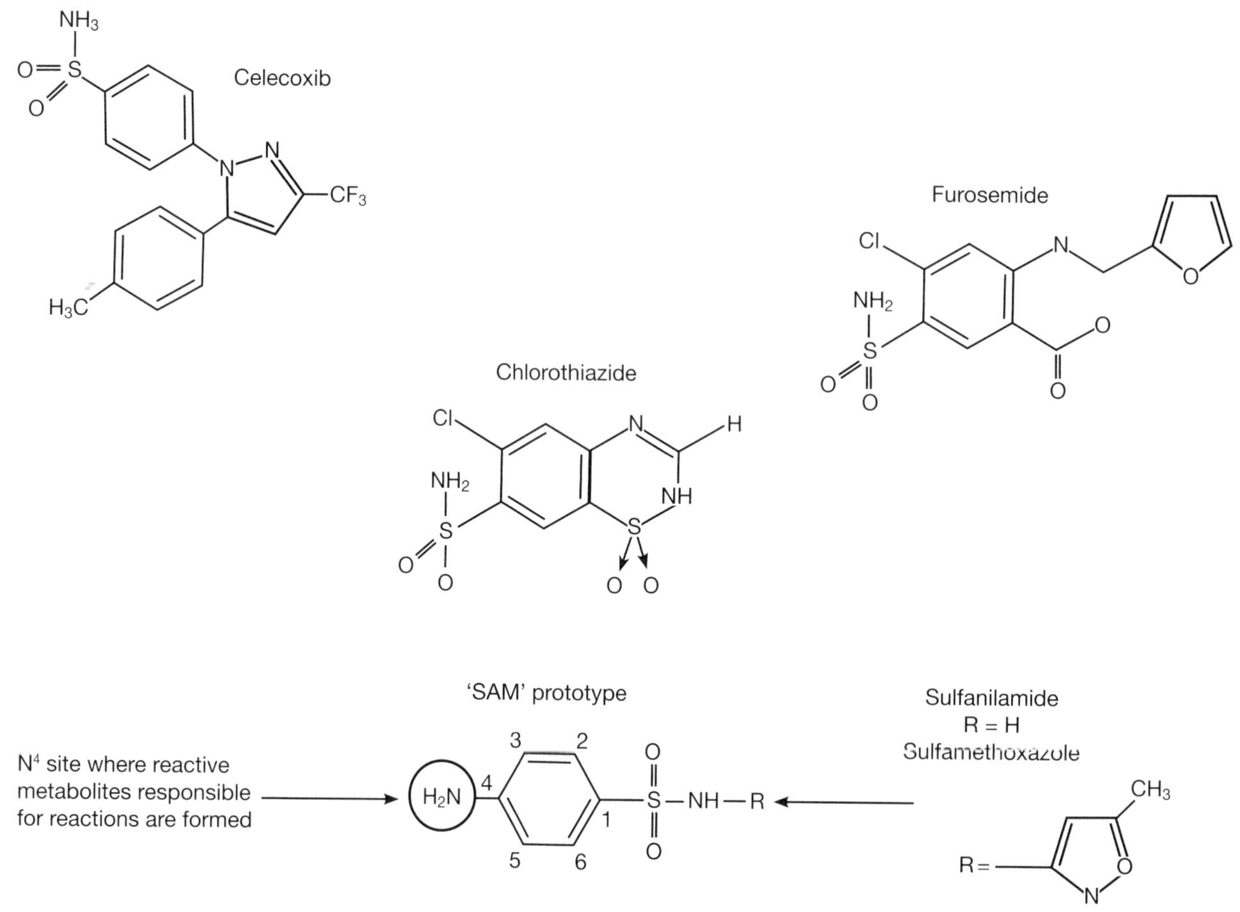

Celecoxib

Furosemide

Chlorothiazide

'SAM' prototype

N^4 site where reactive metabolites responsible for reactions are formed

Sulfanilamide
R = H
Sulfamethoxazole

FIGURE 6-3 Structural Differences Between the Sulfonamide Antibiotics and the Nonantibiotic Sulfonamides

Source: Reprinted with permission from Shapiro LE, Knowles SR, Weber E et al. Safety of celecoxib in individuals allergic to sulfonamide: a pilot study. *Drug Saf.* 2003; 26:187-95.

an arylamine at the N4 position may influence the type of reactivity to a sulfa drug and the potential for the sulfa drug to be reactive.[171,246] Compared with nonantibiotic sulfonamides, the sulfonamide antibiotics are associated with a higher frequency of severe allergic reactions such as SJS. Sulfonamide antibiotics also have an N1 substituent consisting of a 5- to 6-member heterocyclic ring containing >1 nitrogen, which has been linked to the development of IgE-mediated reactions.[171,246] Structural differences between the sulfonamide antibiotics and the nonantibiotic sulfonamides are illustrated in **Figure 6-3**.

Although sulfa drugs are well recognized as allergenic, the risk of reactivity to a specific sulfa drug and the risk of cross-reactivity to other sulfa drugs are not completely known. The lack of a commercially available, reliable reagent for skin testing limits the value of such testing for determination of sulfa allergy. Arndt and Jick, as part of the Boston Collaborative Drug Surveillance program, compared the frequency with which different sulfa drugs caused allergic reactions in a cohort of prospectively monitored inpatients.[247] The risk of reactivity to sulfamethoxazole was the highest at 6% (10 of 169), followed by sulfisoxazole (1.7%, or 8 of 462), chlorothiazide (0.28%, or 2 of 707), hydrochlorothiazide (0%, or 0 of 1,263), and tolbutamide (0%, or 0 of 702).[247] On the basis of this study, sulfamethoxazole is frequently cited as the most reactive of the sulfa class. Strom et al.[248] studied the risk of cross-reactivity between a sulfonamide antibiotic (e.g., sulfamethoxazole) and nonantibiotic sulfonamides (e.g., acetazolamide, loop diuretic, sulfonylurea, thiazide) in a retrospective cohort. Study patients received a nonantibiotic sulfonamide at least 60 days after having experienced an allergic reaction to a sulfonamide antibiotic. The risk of an allergic reaction in these patients within 30 days of receipt of the nonantibiotic sulfonamide was compared with that of a control group of patients without history of sulfa allergy. Of the 969 patients with history of sulfa allergy, 96 (9.9%) had a reaction to the nonantibiotic sulfonamide as compared with 315 (1.6%) of the 19,257 patients without a history of sulfa allergy.[248] Based on the results of this study, the risk of a cross-reaction between the sulfa subclasses is considered low. In fact, patients in this study with a history of sulfonamide antibiotic allergy exhibited a higher risk of subsequent reactivity to a penicillin (14%) than to a nonantibiotic sulfonamide (9.9%). When interpreting the findings of this study, consideration should be given to study design (i.e., retrospective cohort) and the broad definition for drug allergy that included eczematous reactions.

In a patient who is allergic to a specific sulfa drug (e.g., sulfamethoxazole) and requires treatment with another sulfa agent (e.g., a loop diuretic), the severity of the patient's previous allergic reaction is an important factor. Sulfa drugs can cause serious mucocutaneous events such as SJS and TEN, and they can also cause relatively mild maculopapular rash or other isolated skin rash. The severity of the reaction should largely influence the decision as to whether the causative sulfa drug or other sulfa drugs should be administered in the future. Although the structures of the sulfa agents may influence reactivity, cases of suspected cross-reactions between sulfonamide antibiotics and nonantibiotics have been reported.[249,250] If therapy with a sulfa drug is deemed necessary in a patient with history of sulfa allergy, administration of graded challenge doses should be considered. At least two cases have been published describing the successful administration of graded challenge doses of loop diuretics in patients with a history of sulfa allergy.[251,252] Desensitization to hydrochlorothiazide has also been described, starting with 0.025 mg followed by 10-fold incremental dosing every 15 minutes to a final dose of 25 mg.[253]

TETRACYCLINES

The risk of cross-reactivity between the tetracyclines is unknown. Serum sickness-like reactions have been reported in association with tetracycline, doxycycline, and minocycline.[254] Minocycline is considered to be the most antigenic agent in the tetracycline class, based on the number and severity of reported cases (i.e., lupus-like syndrome, serum sickness-like reaction).[82] The antigenicity of minocycline has been attributed to its unique amino acid side chain.[254] Until more is known about the antigenic properties of this drug class, it may be best to avoid the use of all tetracyclines in patients with a history of a severe reaction to any specific tetracycline.

AROMATIC ANTICONVULSANTS

A high degree of cross-reactivity exists between the aromatic anticonvulsants (e.g., carbamazepine, phenobarbital, phenytoin).[255] In vitro lymphocyte testing has revealed cross-reactivity between all three of these anticonvulsants in 40 of 50 patients (80%) with anticonvulsant hypersensitivity syndrome (AHS).[199] Thus, patients with AHS associated with one aromatic anticonvulsant should be advised to avoid the others. Moreover, family members of patients with AHS may be at increased risk of this syndrome.[256] In patients in whom AHS develops, underlying seizure disorders can be safely treated with benzodiazepines, gabapentin, or valproic acid. Oxcarbazepine, the 10-keto derivative of carbamazepine, has exhibited both in vitro and in vivo cross-reactivity with carbamazepine. Some patients with carbamazepine-induced AHS have been subsequently treated with oxcarbazepine without incident, while others have had severe cross-reactions.[257,258] Lamotrigine, a structurally dissimilar anticonvulsant, has also been reported to cause an anticonvulsant hypersensitivity syndrome due to an unknown mechanism.[109] For information on prevention of DRESS and SJS due to anticonvulsants, see section Cutaneous Diseases in this chapter.

BIOLOGICS

The increasing overall prevalence of anaphylaxis is attributed, in part, to the increased use of biologics. This drug class consists of monoclonal antibodies, fusion proteins, and recombinant proteins derived from living sources such as yeast, bacteria, animal cells, or mammalian cells.[259] Examples of biologics include recombinant insulin, erythropoietin, interferon β, human growth hormone, cetuximab, infliximab, omalizumab, adalimumab, ustekinumab, secukinumab, and rituximab. These large proteins can serve as complete antigens. The immunogenicity of these agents is largely related to production methods (e.g., presence of contaminants or stabilizing agents, degree of protein glycosylation, presence of nonhuman protein sequences), and administration (e.g., route of administration, rate of infusion, frequency of use).[259] Some immune reactions to these agents result from the development of neutralizing antibodies that can blunt the biologic agent's ability to exert its intended effect. Neutralizing antibodies occur in up to 60% of patients treated with infliximab, and they have also been shown to develop against natalizumab, interferon β-1b, and interferon β-1a.[259]

Preventive strategies to limit immune-mediated reactions to biologics are highly variable and dependent on the culprit agent. With infliximab, the concomitant administration of prednisone or low-dose methotrexate has been shown to suppress the formation of anti-infliximab neutralizing antibodies.[259,260] Omalizumab, a humanized monoclonal antibody targeted against IgE, is associated with the development of delayed onset anaphylaxis.[261,262] Patients treated with omalizumab are advised to carry an epinephrine auto-injector during and 24 hours after drug administration, and they should be observed for 2 hours after the first three omalizumab injections and for 30 minutes after subsequent injections.[261,262] Cetuximab, a human-murine IgG1 monoclonal antibody, causes anaphylaxis via an oligosaccharide on the Fab portion of the agent's heavy chain.[263] This same oligosaccharide, galactose-α-1,3,-galactose is present in the Lone Star tick and the serum of nonprimate mammals (i.e., certain ingested meats).[25] Up to 20% of cetuximab-treated patients in specific regions of the southern United States developed severe reactions to cetuximab on first exposure, potentially explained by cross-reactions involving pre-existing IgE antibodies against galactose-α-1,3,-galactose.[264] In addition to allergic reactions, biologics may also cause nonimmune DHRs. Depending on the agent, the preventive strategy may include decreasing the rate of drug infusion, pretreatment with antihistamines or corticosteroids, or concomitant administration of corticosteroids. Desensitization protocols have also been described for infliximab, cetuximab, and rituximab.[265,266]

DRUG HYPERSENSITIVITY REACTIONS

Unlike allergic reactions, the administration of pretreatment regimens can prevent many DHRs. Recommended pretreatment regimens for selected agents are provided in **Table 6-9**. In addition, some DHRs are best prevented by avoidance of the causative agent and other pharmacologically similar drugs in the future.

ACE INHIBITORS

Patients with ACE-inhibitor-induced angioedema should be educated to avoid all ACE inhibitors in the future. Re-exposure to the causative agent or to another ACE inhibitor may result in more severe reactions.[267] In addition to women and African Americans, an additional risk factor for ACE-inhibitor-mediated angioedema is concomitant use of the neprilysin inhibitor sacubitril. Inhibition of neprilysin leads to accumulation of bradykinin. To avoid the risk of additive inhibitory effects on bradykinin metabolism, it is recommended that patients undergo a 36-hour washout when switching from ACE inhibitor therapy to combination therapy with sacubitril–valsartan.

Although angiotensin-receptor blockers (ARBs) have no direct effects on the catabolism of bradykinin, angioedema associated with the use of an ARB has been described.[268] In a meta-analysis of 35,000 patients treated with an ARB, the weighted incidence of angioedema was 0.11%.[269] ARBs may cause angioedema by a mechanism independent from that of ACE inhibitors; thus, the term *cross-reactivity* may not directly apply to these events. ARBs are not contraindicated in patients with a history of ACE-inhibitor-induced angioedema, but they should be used with caution after careful weighing of the perceived benefits and risks of therapy. Gavras and Gavras[270] described 10 patients with a history of ACE-inhibitor-induced

Table 6-9 Approaches to Help Prevent Drug Hypersensitivity Reactions

Hypersensitivity reactions (in general)

- With high-risk drugs, monitor for signs and symptoms of allergy during the first 7–30 days of therapy
- Be vigilant in monitoring patients who are frequently exposed to allergenic drugs (e.g., patients with cystic fibrosis, patients with frequent bouts of bronchitis, pneumonia, or otitis media)
- Educate patients about high-risk drugs and the signs of an allergic reaction
- Obtain detailed histories of allergies, with attention to the causative agent(s) and the severity of the reaction(s)
- Educate patients with a documented allergy to avoid the causative drug in the future (depending on the severity of the reaction)
- Educate patients to avoid drugs structurally similar to the causative agent (depending on the severity of the reaction)
- Educate patients to read drug labels, particularly if the patient is reactive to excipients

Immediate reactions to radiocontrast media (high- or low-osmolarity agent)

- Pretreat using prednisone 50 mg orally, administered at 13 hours, 7 hours, and 1 hour before administration of the contrast agent; diphenhydramine 50 mg orally/IV/IM 1 hour before the procedure, and ephedrine 25 mg orally 1 hour before the procedure (avoid ephedrine in patients with unstable angina, hypertension, arrhythmias)[278]
- In an emergency situation, the following pretreatment regimen has been used: hydrocortisone 200 mg IV immediately upon determination of need for the radiocontrast study and every 4 hours until the procedure is completed; diphenhydramine 50 mg IV/IM 1 hour before the procedure[278]

Immediate reaction to paclitaxel

A number of different pretreatment regimens have been used with success:

- Pretreat with dexamethasone 20 mg orally at 12 hours, 6 hours, and 1 hour before paclitaxel infusion; diphenhydramine 50 mg IV 30–60 minutes before the infusion; cimetidine 300 mg IV (or ranitidine 50 mg IV, famotidine 20 mg IV) before the paclitaxel infusion[280]
- Diphenhydramine 50 mg IV, famotidine 20 mg IV and dexamethasone 20 mg IV, each given 30 minutes before the paclitaxel infusion[281]

Vancomycin red man syndrome

- Administer each 1-g vancomycin dose over at least 1 hour; each 1.5-g dose over at least 90 minutes; each 2-g dose over 2 hours
- Pretreat using diphenhydramine 25–50 mg IV, acetaminophen 650 mg orally, hydrocortisone 100 mg IV

IM = intramuscular, IV = intravenous.

angioedema who were subsequently treated with an ARB without incident. In a more comprehensive systematic review of 71 patients with ACE-inhibitor angioedema, the risk of subsequent angioedema associated with an ARB was 9.4% for possible cases and 3.4% for confirmed cases.[146] None of the events was fatal. As a preventive strategy in this setting, consideration should be given to the severity of the event (i.e., diffuse versus localized angioedema) and to prior responsiveness to treatment before switching a patient from therapy with an ACE inhibitor to an ARB.

SALICYLATES

Patients with a history of an allergic or allergic-like reaction to a salicylate present a clinical challenge to the caregiver. Aspirin and NSAIDs can cause both true allergic reactions (e.g., ibuprofen-induced anaphylaxis) and nonimmune DHRs (e.g., exacerbations of asthma, urticaria, angioedema).[271] In this setting, it is crucial to obtain an accurate allergy history. If a patient's history suggests reactivity to a specific NSAID and lack of reactivity to NSAIDs of other chemically dissimilar classes, a true allergic reaction should be suspected.[10] Such patients should be advised to avoid the specific NSAID and any structurally similar agent (e.g., all propionic acid derivatives) because of the risk of cross-reactivity. In patients with asthma who describe an exacerbation after the administration of aspirin or another COX-1 inhibitor, a nonimmune DHR should be suspected.[10] These patients are at risk of severe asthma exacerbations resulting from the pharmacologic effects of aspirin and other potent COX-1 inhibitors on prostaglandin and leukotriene synthesis.[183] Inhibition of COX-1 results in a shifting in the metabolism of arachidonic acids into leukotrienes that cause bronchoconstriction and increased mucus production. Overexpression of leukotrienes may also explain the development of aspirin-induced angioedema and urticaria. Patients with aspirin- or NSAID-induced asthma, urticaria, or angioedema should be advised to avoid all COX-1 inhibitors.[10,183] Studies of short duration involving small numbers of patients with aspirin-induced asthma have shown that the COX-2 inhibitors celecoxib and rofecoxib do not exacerbate asthma.[272-274] In addition, acetaminophen at single doses <1 g, sodium salicylate, choline salicylamide, and magnesium trisalicylate have not been shown to exacerbate asthma because of their lack of effect on the COX-1 enzyme. In patients with aspirin-induced nonimmune DHRs who require aspirin for prevention of cardiovascular disease, both graded challenge and desensitization is recommended.[275] A two-dose challenge of 40.5 mg (one half of an 81-mg tablet) given 90 minutes apart has shown promising results in patients with a history of isolated dermatologic reactions to aspirin.[275] If no reaction occurs after the second dose, cardioprotective therapy with 81 mg of aspirin may commence. In patients with aspirin-induced asthma, desensitization to aspirin has been achieved.[275] Rapid desensitization protocols for patients with cardiovascular disease requiring aspirin have also been described.[275-277]

RADIOCONTRAST MEDIA

Nonimmune DHRs associated with radiocontrast agents may be prevented by the use of pretreatment regimens, as noted in Table 6-9. In addition, administration of a low-osmolarity agent in conjunction with pretreatment has been shown to reduce the risk of reactivity to approximately 1%.[278] Most recently, there is a trend toward skin testing of patients with prior history of reactivity to a radiocontrast agent. Skin testing with a panel of different agents may aid in the identification of an agent of low reactive risk, thereby reducing the risk of reactivity on subsequent exposure.[279]

MANAGEMENT

Recommended treatment regimens for drug allergy vary based on the signs and symptoms of the reaction and the type of allergic syndrome. Reactions mediated by nonimmune mechanisms are treated in a manner similar to those of true allergic reactions, with the choice of therapy based on the patient's signs and symptoms. **Table 6-10** provides a summary of recommended treatments for a variety of allergic syndromes.

In 2015, the Joint Task Force of the American Academy of Allergy, Asthma, and Immunology and the American College of Allergy, Asthma, and Allergy updated the Practice Parameter on the Diagnosis and Management of Anaphylaxis.[184] On the basis of these guidelines, patients with stridor, respiratory distress, wheezing, hypotension, cardiac arrhythmias, shock, or loss of consciousness require immediate treatment. Life-threatening conditions may also develop in patients with nonlife-threatening symptoms on initial presentation (e.g., localized urticaria).[184] Table 6-10 summarizes the Joint Task Force's guidelines for treatment of anaphylaxis. The mainstays of therapy are epinephrine 1 mg/mL dilution administered intramuscularly, oxygen, and aggressive intravenous fluid replacement. In studies of adults and children not experiencing anaphylaxis, epinephrine has been shown to be most efficiently absorbed when administered intramuscularly, rather than subcutaneously.[282] In adults, the preferred intramuscular site of injection is the anterolateral thigh, because of a higher rate of absorption.[283] Consideration should also be given to the addition of a histamine H_1-receptor blocker and histamine H_2-receptor blocker; however, these agents are not rapid-acting and should never be used in place of epinephrine. Patients receiving long-term β-blocker therapy by either oral or topical routes usually require higher doses of epinephrine.[184] In these patients, anaphylaxis is often severe and associated with profound hypotension or bradycardia that are unresponsive to epinephrine. Glucagon may be used in these patients for its inotropic and chronotropic effects that occur independently of α-receptor responsiveness. Corticosteroids have no role in the

Table 6-10 Management of Drug Allergy

Anaphylaxis[179,180,184]

- Discontinue the offending agent
- Establish and maintain airway
- Administer epinephrine 1 mg/mL (adults 0.3–0.5 mg; children 0.01 mg/kg) IM in the lateral aspect of the thigh
- Place patient in a recumbent position
- Oxygen 4–10 L/min through facemask or up to 100% oxygen as needed
- Repeat IM epinephrine every 5–15 minutes for up to 3 injections if the patient is not responding
- Establish IV line for venous access; keep line open with 0.9% saline solution; for hypotension or failure to respond to epinephrine, administer 1–2 L at a rate of 5–10 mL/kg in the first 5–10 minutes; children should receive up to 30 mL/kg in the first hour
- Consider nebulized albuterol 2.5–5 mg in 3 mL saline every 20 minutes for 3 doses; in children, 0.15 mg/kg via nebulizer every 20 minutes for 3 doses
- In cases of refractory bronchospasm or hypotension not responding to epinephrine because a β-adrenergic blocker is complicating management, administer glucagon 1–5 mg (20–30 mcg/kg; maximum 1 mg in children) IV over 5 minutes
- Give epinephrine by continuous IV infusion for patients with inadequate response to IM epinephrine and IV saline; add 1 mg (1 mL of 1 mg/mL) of epinephrine to 1,000 mL of 0.9% saline solution; start infusion at 2 mcg/min and increase up to 10 mcg/min based on blood pressure, heart rate, and cardiac function
- Consider intraosseous access if IV access is unsuccessful in either adults or children
- Consider diphenhydramine 25–50 mg IM/slow IV infusion in adults, then 25–50 mg orally every 4–6 hours; 1 mg/kg (up to 50 mg) in children
- Consider ranitidine 50 mg (adults) or 12.5–50 mg (1 mg/kg) in children, diluted in D5W to a volume of 20 mL administered IV over 5 minutes; given every 6–8 hours
- Consider methylprednisolone 1–2 mg/kg/dose up to 125 mg (or equivalent steroid) to reduce the risk of recurring or protracted anaphylaxis; dose can be repeated every 6 hours as required

Angioedema[184,235,286]

- Discontinue the causative agent
- Establish and maintain airway
- Treatment is based on the extent and severity of the clinical presentation; treatment may include the following:
    - Histamine H_1-receptor antagonist (see Urticaria)
    - Epinephrine (see Anaphylaxis)
    - Corticosteroids (see Anaphylaxis)
    - Nebulized (β_2-agonists (see Anaphylaxis)

Urticaria[285,286]

- Discontinue the causative agent
- Administer epinephrine if the diagnosis of anaphylaxis has not been excluded
- First-line therapy (if tolerated): hydroxyzine hydrochloride 25–150 mg daily at bedtime or in divided doses, diphenhydramine 12.5–50 mg per dose every 4 to 6 hours as needed
- Alternative first-line therapy: nonsedating antihistamines such as cetirizine 10–40 mg daily or in divided doses (adults); loratidine 10–40 mg daily in morning; fexofenadine 180 mg daily or 60 mg twice daily
- Second-line therapy: doxepin 25–100 mg/day (adults); 25–50 mg/day initially up to a maximum of 100 mg/day (adolescents); 1–3 mg/kg/day (children)
- Combinations of antihistamines are also recommended
- Short course of oral corticosteroids if symptoms are severe and not resolving with antihistamines

Serum sickness-like disease[69,188]

- Short course of methylprednisolone
- Corticosteroids (1–2 mg/kg prednisone or equivalent) once daily or administered in 2 divided doses for 5 days (if severe systemic event)

Vasculitis[86-88]

- Discontinue the offending agent
- Histamine H_1-receptor antagonist (diphenhydramine or hydroxyzine) for pruritus
- Corticosteroids (1 mg/kg prednisone or equivalent) in divided doses for 7–14 days or bolus IV therapy with 15 mg/kg/day for 3 days followed by 1 mg/kg/day orally

Hypersensitivity syndrome[188]

- Discontinue the offending agent
- Systemic corticosteroids (>0.5 mg/kg/day prednisone or equivalent)

D5W = 5% dextrose in water, IM = intramuscular, IV = intravenous.

acute treatment of anaphylaxis, except for patients with a history of asthma or idiopathic angioedema; however, these drugs are used adjunctively to prevent the late-phase reaction. Patients treated long term with ACE inhibitors may also require aggressive treatment for hypotension associated with anaphylaxis. In these patients, the release of angiotensin II as a normal compensatory mechanism is blunted. Following treatment and resolution of anaphylaxis, the patient should receive education on the self-administration of epinephrine auto-injectors. Patients at high risk for recurrence of anaphylaxis should be instructed to carry two auto-injectors at all times.[184] Adults should receive the 0.3- or 0.5-mg dose (if available) and children should receive the auto-injector that provides 0.15 mg per dose.[284] The optimal dose for obese patients has not been determined. Concerns in the obese population are optimal weight-based dosing and adequate needle length for intramuscular delivery of epinephrine.[284]

Treatment of immune complex diseases is highly variable and dependent on the patient's presentation. In many cases, discontinuation of therapy with the causative drug is the only treatment required. Supportive therapy may include a mild analgesic/antipyretic, such as acetaminophen, for flu-like symptoms. An oral antihistamine should be considered in patients with pruritus associated with an urticarial, maculopapular, or mixed skin rash. In some patients, a short course of a low-dose oral corticosteroid such as methylprednisolone may be used for treatment of a diffuse erythematous, maculopapular skin rash. High-dose corticosteroids (i.e., prednisone 40–60 mg/day) should be reserved for patients with systemic events involving the kidney or liver, patients with drug hypersensitivity syndromes, or patients with vasculitis.[188] The presence of mucosal involvement (i.e., SJS or TEN) often precludes the use of systemic corticosteroids because of the risk of infectious complications.[188]

INFORMATION FOR PATIENTS

Patients in whom an allergic reaction to a drug develops should be educated as to the name of the specific drug, the terminology used to describe the reaction, and the likelihood of having a similar or more severe reaction upon re-exposure to the drug. If the reaction was severe (e.g., anaphylaxis, SJS), the patient should be advised to wear a medical alert tag or bracelet describing the reaction. In the case of a severe immediate reaction to a drug or chemical, the patient may be prescribed injectable epinephrine in an easily injectable form (e.g., EpiPen or EpiPen Jr.) for use in an emergency situation. Such patients should be advised to have at least two doses of epinephrine in their possession, particularly if they live in a rural area without direct access to emergency care. In addition, these patients must be counseled regarding the appropriate administration technique to ensure rapid absorption (i.e., intramuscularly into the anterolateral thigh).

Patients with a history of allergy to a drug or multiple drugs should be encouraged to ask questions about newly prescribed medications. For example, a patient allergic to a sulfa drug should be advised to question whether any newly prescribed medication is considered a "sulfa medication." Patients with aspirin-induced asthma or reactions to excipients should be encouraged to read the labels of nonprescription medications to identify ingredients of concern. In addition, patients should be educated regarding the avoidance of the causative drug and other cross-reactive drugs in the future.

CUTANEOUS DISEASES

The spectrum of adverse cutaneous reactions ranges from the commonly occurring, often self-limiting erythematous rash to the rare, life-threatening severe cutaneous adverse reactions (SCARs). Approximately 30 different drug-mediated cutaneous reaction patterns have been described.[287] This section will address drug-induced acne, erythematous reactions, fixed drug eruptions, psoriasis, and the SCARs (DRESS, SJS, TEN, warfarin tissue necrosis). The previous section provides discussion of urticaria, angioedema, and skin reactions associated with immune complex diseases. Chapter 8 provides a review of drug-induced photosensitivity.

Standard terms are used to describe the manifestations of skin lesions, including those that are drug-induced. A listing of these terms and their definitions is provided in **Table 6-11**.[287]

CAUSATIVE AGENTS

Identifying the most likely cause of a potential drug-induced cutaneous reaction is complicated by the fact that almost all drugs have been associated with rash as described in the product literature. To streamline the assessment of causality, it is important to consider that antimicrobial agents have been consistently identified as the most frequent

Table 6-11 Glossary of Terms for Skin Lesions[287]

Bullae

- Vesicle filled with serous fluid, >1 cm

Comedone (open)

- Blackhead; dilated hair follicle filled with sebum and bacteria with a blackened mass of skin debris at the surface

Comedone (closed)

- Whitehead; dilated hair follicle filled with sebum and bacteria with an obstructed opening to the skin

Macule

- Circumscribed, nonpalpable, red, flat lesion, <1 cm

Nodule

- Papule that is firm and with depth, 0.5–2 cm

Papule

Solid, palpable, red, elevated lesion, <1 cm

Patch

- Group or cluster of macules

Plaque

- Solid, palpable, elevated solid lesion, 0.5 cm

Pustule

- Vesicle filled with purulent material

Typical target or iris lesion

- Lesion <3 cm in diameter, regular round shape, well-defined border with at least three different zones (two concentric rings around a central area); one ring consists of palpable edema, paler than the central area

Target lesion (flat, atypical)

- Round lesions with only two zones and/or a poorly defined border and nonpalpable, with the exception of a potential central blister

Wheal

- Central blister, irregular, pink in color, superficial area of skin edema

Vesicle

- Circumscribed, elevated lesion filled with serous fluid, 0.5 cm

offenders in cutaneous eruptions, followed in frequency by the NSAIDs.[288,289]

Based largely on reports of single cases, more than 100 drugs have been implicated as causative of SJS or TEN.[288] In a large international case-control study, Roujeau et al.[288] attempted to quantify the association between the use of specific medications and the development of SJS and TEN. Cases (n = 245) were patients admitted to the hospital with a diagnosis of SJS or TEN, and controls (n = 1,147) were patients admitted to the same hospital for an elective procedure or treatment of an acute condition not deemed to be drug related. Of the drugs used for short periods, sulfonamides were the most strongly associated with TEN (crude RR 172, 95% CI 75–396), with trimethoprim–sulfamethoxazole accounting for 69% of these cases.[288] Thiazide diuretics and sulfonylureas were not associated with increased risk. In descending order of frequency, other major drug offenders were chlormezanone (crude RR 62, 95% CI 21–188), cephalosporins (RR 14, 95% CI 3.2–59), quinolones (RR 10, 95% CI 2.6–38), tetracyclines (RR 8.1, 95% CI 1.5–43), and aminopenicillins (RR 6.7, 95% CI 2.5–18).[288] Additionally, acetaminophen was associated with a significant risk (RR 9.3, 95% CI 3.9–22) in all countries other than France. Of the drugs administered for a duration of months to years, carbamazepine, phenobarbital, phenytoin, valproic acid, the oxicam NSAIDs, allopurinol, and corticosteroids were associated with significantly increased risks. The first 2 months of long-term drug administration was identified as the highest-risk period.

In 2007, the results of the Euro-SCAR study offered an update on the risks of SJS/TEN with newly marketed medications.[290] In this international, multicenter case-control study, 379 patients with SCAR and 1,505 controls were enrolled. The results of this study confirmed the high risks previously identified associated with the use of anti-infective sulfonamides, allopurinol, carbamazepine, phenobarbital, phenytoin, and the oxicam NSAIDs.[290] An increased risk of SJS/TEN was also identified with the use of nevirapine (RR >22) and lamotrigine (RR >14), with weaker associations identified with sertraline (RR 11, 95% CI 2.7–46), pantoprazole (RR 18, 95% CI 3.9–85), and tramadol (RR 20, 95% CI 4.4–93).[290] The majority of SCAR cases occurred within 8 weeks of initiation of therapy. Onset of the SCAR within 4–28 days after drug initiation was most suggestive of the drug as the cause.

Medications most commonly associated with the development of skin eruptions are listed in **Table 6-12**.[188,249,250,288,290-334] In addition to

Table 6-12 Agents Implicated in Drug-Induced Cutaneous Diseases

Drug	Incidence	Level of Evidence[a]
ACNE		
Androgenic steroids (methyltestosterone, testosterone, nandrolone)[291]	NK	C
Azathioprine	NK	C
Corticosteroids[292,293]	NK	C
Cyclosporine	NK	C
Danazol	NK	C
EPIDERMAL GROWTH FACTOR RECEPTOR INHIBITORS[294,295]		
Cetuximab	88–90%	B
Erlotinib	75%	B
Gefitinib	25–33%	B
Panitumumab	70–100%	B
Granulocyte colony-stimulating factor[296]	NK	C
Infliximab[297]	NK	C
Iodides[298]	NK	C
Lamotrigine[299]	NK	C
Lithium[300]	NK	C
Tacrolimus[301]	NK	C
FIXED DRUG ERUPTION		
Acetaminophen[302]	NK	C
Allopurinol[302]	NK	C
Barbiturates[298]	NK	C
Carbamazepine[298]	NK	C
Celecoxib[302]	NK	C
Dipyrone[302]	NK	C
Erythromycin[302]	NK	C
Fluconazole	NK	C
Griseofulvin[302]	NK	C
Ibuprofen[302]	NK	C
Metronidazole[302]	NK	C
Paclitaxel[302]	NK	C
Penicillins[302]	NK	C
Phenolphthalein[302]	NK	C
Propofol[303]	NK	C
Pseudoephedrine[302]	NK	C
Quinine[304]	NK	C
Rifampin[302]	NK	C
Sulfamethoxazole[298,302]	NK	C
Tetracyclines[298]	NK	C
Tranexamic acid[305]	NK	C
DRESS		
Allopurinol[188]	NK	C

Table 6-12 Agents Implicated in Drug-Induced Cutaneous Diseases (continued)

Drug	Incidence	Level of Evidence[a]
Azithromycin[306]	NK	C
Captopril[307]	NK	C
Carbamazepine[188]	NK	C
Dapsone[188]	NK	C
Lamotrigine[188]	NK	C
Minocycline[188]	NK	C
NSAIDs[188]	NK	C
Omeprazole[308]	NK	C
Phenytoin[188]	NK	C
Phenobarbital[309]	NK	C
Piperacillin[310]	NK	C
Raltegravir[311]	NK	C
Sulfonamides[188]	NK	B
Teicoplanin[312]	NK	C
Vancomycin[312]	NK	C
PSORIASIS		
ACE inhibitors[313,314]	NK	C
β-blockers[313,314]	NK	B
Chloroquine[313,314]	NK	C
Etanercept[315]	NK	C
Granulocyte colony-stimulating factor	NK	C
Growth hormone[316]	NK	C
Hydroxychloroquine[313,314]	NK	B
Imatinib[313]	NK	C
Infliximab[317]	NK	C
Interferon α and interferon γ[313,314]	NK	C
Lithium[313,314]	NK	B
NSAIDs[313,314]	NK	C
Tetracyclines[313,314]	NK	C
Terbinafine[313,314]	NK	C
Valproate sodium[318]		
STEVENS–JOHNSON SYNDROME/TOXIC EPIDERMAL NECROLYSIS[319]		
Acetaminophen[288, 320,321]	NK	B
Allopurinol[322]	NK	B
Aminopenicillins[188]	NK	B
Celecoxib[249]	NK	C
Cephalosporins[188]	NK	B
Ciprofloxacin[290]	NK	C
Fluconazole[323]	NK	C
Hydralazine[324]	NK	C
Imatinib[325]	NK	C
Imidazole antifungal agents[288,290]	NK	B

Table 6-12 Agents Implicated in Drug-Induced Cutaneous Diseases (continued)

Drug	Incidence	Level of Evidence[a]
Lamotrigine[290]	NK	B
Levofloxacin[326,327]	NK	C
Mesalamine[328]	NK	C
Modafinil[329]	NK	C
Moxifloxacin[330]	NK	C
Nevirapine[290,331]	NK	B
Ofloxacin[332]	NK	C
Pantoprazole[290]	NK	B
Phenobarbital[188]	NK	B
Phenytoin[188]	NK	B
Piroxicam[290]	NK	B
Sertraline[290]	NK	B
Tramadol[290]	NK	C
Trimethoprim–sulfamethoxazole[188,288]	NK	B
Valdecoxib[250]	NK	C
Valproic acid[290]	NK	C
Voriconazole[333]	NK	C
SKIN NECROSIS		
Warfarin[188,298,334]	1 in 10,000[b]	B

ACE = angiotensin-converting enzyme, DRESS = drug rash with eosinophilia and systemic symptoms, HHV-6 = human herpesvirus 6, NK = not known, NSAID = nonsteroidal anti-inflammatory drug.

[a]Definitions for Levels of Evidence: Level A—evidence from one or more randomized, controlled clinical trials; Level B—evidence from nonrandomized clinical trials, prospective observational studies, cohort studies, retrospective studies, case-control studies, meta-analyses and/or postmarketing surveillance studies; and Level C—evidence from one or more published case reports or case series.

[b]Prevalence.

prescription medications, it is important to consider that SCARs have been associated with the use of nonprescription drugs (e.g., acetaminophen, pseudoephedrine) and traditional Chinese herbal medicines.[335]

EPIDEMIOLOGY

Cutaneous and mucocutaneous events are the most commonly reported adverse reactions to medications. Based on the results of the Boston Collaborative Drug Surveillance program conducted in the 1970s and 1980s, it is estimated that a drug-related skin rash develops in 2–3% of all hospitalized patients.[191] In this prospective study of 37,000 hospitalized patients, the majority of the skin reactions were exanthematous (94%), with the remainder urticarial (5%). Approximately 2% of the reactions were fatal.[191] Epidemiologic studies conducted in the 1990s focused on estimating the incidence of SCARs. Compared to exanthematous reactions, SCARs appear to be relatively uncommon. In 1995, Roujeau et al.[188] estimated that serious cutaneous drug events including SJS and TEN occur in 1 of every 1,000 hospitalized patients.

Estimates of the prevalence of drug-induced cutaneous events have been determined from prospective studies of hospitalized patients, outpatients, patients receiving systemic drug therapy, and those exposed to medications via any route of administration.[191,289,336] The estimates have varied based on the type of cutaneous event investigated, the definition used to describe the dermatologic condition, and the population studied. In a 6-month prospective study conducted in 2000–2001, practitioners identified and subsequently a dermatologist assessed all suspected allergic cutaneous reactions that led to hospitalization or occurred during hospitalization.[289] A group of dermatologists and pharmacologists retrospectively evaluated causality. A total of 48 cases were identified, resulting in an estimated prevalence of 3.6 of 1,000 hospitalized patients.[289] The majority of the allergic reactions were exanthematous (56%), and the prevalence was significantly higher in medical (0.5%) versus surgical patients (0.01%).[289] Thirty-four percent of cases were deemed serious on the basis of leading to hospitalization (18%), increasing the duration of hospital stay (14%), or were life-threatening (2%).[289] Compared to other studies reporting an incidence of cutaneous drug reactions of 2% in hospitalized patients, the lower prevalence determined in this study can be attributed to the restricted focus on allergic-mediated skin reactions and on systemic drug exposures.[289]

TEN is estimated to occur in 0.4–1.3 cases per million person-years, while SJS occurs in 1–6 cases per million person-years.[319] The variability in these estimates of incidence can be attributed to differences in the diagnostic criteria for SJS and TEN. The prevalence or incidence of other cutaneous skin disorders is less well described. The incidence of DRESS is highly variable, occurring in 1 of 1,000 to 1 of 10,000 patients exposed to anticonvulsants and sulfonamides, and the mortality rate has been estimated to be approximately 10%.[337] The wide variability in the reported incidence of DRESS can be attributed to the variable presentation of the condition. Fixed drug eruptions occur more frequently, with reported incidences of 2.5–22%.[302] Tissue necrosis has been reported in 1 of 10,000 patients treated with warfarin and in 0.01–0.12% of patients treated with all oral anticoagulants including the coumarin products.[188,334]

MECHANISMS

Cutaneous reactions to drugs can result from both immune and nonimmune mechanisms (i.e., direct pharmacologic effects, nonimmune DHR, idiosyncrasy). Allergy is the underlying mechanism in 50% of the events, including most cases of urticaria, angioedema, serum sickness-like syndrome with maculopapular rash, fixed drug eruptions, vasculitis, and the SCARs, including DRESS, SJS, and TEN. The skin is a target for immunologically mediated reactions because it possesses APCs such as the cutaneous Langerhans cells. The presence of monooxygenases, cytochromes, and transport-associated proteins in the keratinocytes allow for transformation of low-molecular-weight drug haptens into reactive, immunogenic metabolites.[338]

T cells play a major role in the pathophysiology of drug-related cutaneous reactions. An extensive review of the role of the T lymphocyte in the mediation of a variety of drug-induced eruptions has been provided by Naisbett.[339] Based on immunohistologic studies, allergy-mediated maculopapular rashes have been shown to involve the recruitment of CD4 cells and copresentation of the drug hapten with the MHC class II molecule HLA-DR.[339] Maculopapular rashes are also associated with secretion of high levels of IL-5 and eotaxin, two cytokines involved in the recruitment and differentiation of eosinophils. Bullous reactions are more likely to be associated with the recruitment of CD8+ cells and copresentation of the haptenic drug or reactive metabolite with MHC class I molecules.[339] Cell studies of blister fluid from patients who survived TEN also support a dominant role for T lymphocytes, particularly CD8+ cells, in the pathogenesis of this SCAR. In patients with TEN, activation of cytotoxic T lymphocytes ultimately results in dermal-cell apoptosis, which is believed to be triggered via activation of the perforin–granzyme or the Fas-Fas ligand pathways. Stimulation of these pathways triggers activation of caspases, intracellular proteases that cleave a key protein within the cell, leading to keratinocyte apoptosis. In addition to cytotoxic T lymphocytes, other mediators of TEN include monocytes, macrophages, and TNFα. Overexpression of TNFα, interferon α, IL-2, and IL-5 has been reported in skin lesions of patients with SJS and TEN.[337,340]

Mechanisms by which many drugs cause skin eruptions are not known. Pharmacologic effects may be the underlying mechanism by which most drugs cause acneiform eruptions and provocation of psoriasis. Androgenic drugs (e.g., anabolic steroids, danazol, methyltestosterone) aggravate pre-existing acne or cause acneiform eruptions by activating sebaceous-gland hypertrophy and increasing sebum production. The high incidence of acneiform eruptions associated with the use of epidermal growth factor receptor (EGFR) inhibitors may also be explained in part by the known pharmacology of these agents. EGFRs are overexpressed in many solid tumors, explaining the effectiveness of EGFR inhibitors in the treatment of refractory colorectal and lung cancers. EGFRs are also expressed in the basal layer of the epidermis and in the hair follicle.[294,295] Although the mechanism by which EGFR inhibitors cause acne-like rashes is not entirely known, the dose-related incidence may be related to inhibition of EGFR signaling on epidermal epithelium leading to impaired cell growth and differentiation.[294] Provocation of psoriasis by nonselective β-blockers such as propranolol may be explained in part by blockade of epidermal β_2-receptors, resulting in a decrease in intraepidermal cyclic adenosine monophosphate and an increase in epidermal-cell turnover.[313] Cyclooxygenase inhibitors such as indomethacin may induce psoriasis by inhibiting prostaglandin synthesis, thereby shunting the metabolism of arachidonic acids to the lipoxygenase pathway. The resultant increase in leukotriene concentrations may contribute to the exacerbation of psoriasis in patients treated with COX inhibitors.[314] Studies support that leukotriene concentrations are 7–11 times higher in psoriatic lesions as compared with normal skin.[313]

CLINICAL PRESENTATION AND DIFFERENTIAL DIAGNOSIS

The discriminating features of specific drug eruptions are provided in **Table 6-13** and the conditions to consider in the differential diagnoses are provided in **Table 6-14**.

The most common type of drug-induced skin eruption is the exanthematous or maculopapular rash, occurring in 1–5% of first-time users of implicated medications.[342] This red, inflamed cutaneous reaction usually appears as a mixture of discrete macules and papules on the trunk or dependent areas of the body (e.g., lower extremities of an ambulating patient, middle to lower back of a bedridden patient). The lesions typically spread outward in a bilateral, symmetrical pattern to involve the neck, upper and lower extremities, and potentially the face.[298,341,342] The rash is often described as "dot-like" in appearance, or measles (morbilliform)-like, and may or may not be associated with fever and pruritis. The discrete lesions typically coalesce over days into patches with large areas of confluence. The rash usually occurs within 4–14 days after the initiation of therapy with the causative drug or within 1–2 days after drug discontinuation.[341] This reaction is usually self-limited, with resolution in 1–2 weeks after drug discontinuation. Upon re-exposure to the drug, the rash may reappear within hours. In rare instances, a maculopapular rash may be the initial sign of a severe cutaneous event such as SJS. Therefore, all patients who initially present with a maculopapular rash should be assessed for hallmark signs of a more severe, progressive reaction. Lesions in the mucous membranes (e.g., conjunctiva, oral cavity, nares, genitalia) are evident in more than 90% of serious cutaneous events, and extension of the rash to the palms and soles often portends a more protracted course.[188,337]

A commonly encountered clinical challenge is differentiation of a maculopapular rash from an urticarial lesion. Unlike maculopapular lesions, urticarial lesions are typically asymmetrical, pink rather than red, and irregular in shape. These superficial wheals, largely confined to the epidermis, are often described as geographic in shape (i.e., similar in shape to the continent of Africa or Asia). Urticarial lesions are highly pruritic, vary in size from 1 mm to several centimeters in diameter, and typically develop on the chest, face, or neck within minutes to 48 hours after drug exposure.[298] Differentiation of a maculopapular rash from urticaria is important, because the latter often indicates IgE-mediated mast cell degranulation. In a patient with drug-related IgE-mediated urticaria, continuation of the causative drug may lead to a more severe reaction, including angioedema or anaphylaxis. Urticaria may also be caused by foods, insect bites/stings, and environmental factors such as sunlight, cold, and heat.[298]

Fixed drug eruptions (FDEs) are the second most commonly occurring drug-related cutaneous reaction, occurring in 0.5–22% of patients exposed to certain medications.[344] FDEs present as solitary lesions or multiple well-demarcated lesions occurring anywhere on the body, but favoring the

Table 6-13 Signs and Symptoms Associated with Drug-Induced Cutaneous Diseases

Acne[298]
- Papules and pustules on face and upper trunk
- Limited number of comedones to no comedones

Erythematous rash[341,342]
- Symmetrical distribution of macules and papules starting on upper trunk or legs
- Rash may progress to entire body including face
- Pruritus (50%)
- Redness without blistering

DRESS[337,343]
- High fever (38–40°C)
- Diffuse, symmetrical maculopapular rash with pruritus (90%)
- Facial and periorbital edema
- Enlarged lymph nodes at ≥2 sites (cervical and inguinal) in >50% cases
- Involvement of at least one internal organ (hepatitis, pneumonitis, pancreatitis)
- Conjunctivitis
- Eosinophilia
- Atypical lymphocytosis

Fixed drug eruption[287,344]
- Initial burning "stinging" sensation or itching of skin
- Round or oval dusky red to violaceous lesions, 1–20 cm in diameter, favoring the face, lips, hands, feet, perineal area, genitalia
- Lesions recur in the same location(s) upon rechallenge
- Blistering of lesions
- Anorexia and malaise (infrequent)
- High fever (infrequent)
- Hyperpigmentation in the area of the lesion following recovery

Psoriasis
- Red or salmon-pink plaques covered by silvery scales symmetrically distributed on elbows, knees, scalp, and lumbosacral region

SJS/TEN[188,319,337]
- Prodrome of nausea, vomiting, sore throat, cough, arthralgias, myalgias for 2–8 days before rash development
- Widespread erythematous, purpuric rash with flat atypical target lesions
- Burning and painful sensation of the skin
- Fever (10–30% of cases of SJS, 100% of cases of TEN)
- Facial edema
- Mucosal lesions of the mouth, lips, nasal cavity, conjunctivae, genitalia (92–100% of cases of SJS; 85–95% of cases of TEN)
- Epidermal detachment (<10% of body surface area with SJS; >30% of body surface area with TEN)
- Positive Nikolsky sign (TEN)
- Neutropenia (30% of cases of SJS and TEN)
- Lymphopenia (90% of cases of TEN)
- Thrombocytopenia (15% of cases of TEN)
- Prerenal azotemia (TEN)
- Elevated aspartate and alanine aminotransferases (50% of cases of SJS and TEN)
- Hypopigmentation or hyperpigmentation (88% of cases of TEN)
- Keratitis and corneal erosions

Warfarin-induced skin necrosis[188,298,334]
- Poorly demarcated, painful red plaques with soft-tissue edema
- Pain
- Petechial hemorrhages that coalesce into large hemorrhagic bullae with areas of gangrenous tissue
- Lesions usually distributed in areas of fatty tissue (buttocks, breasts, hips)

DRESS = drug rash with eosinophilia and systemic symptoms, SJS = Stevens–Johnson syndrome, TEN = toxic epidermal necrolysis.

face, lips, hands, feet, and genitalia. The lesions are round or oval in shape and range in size from 1–20 cm in diameter.[287,298] The color of the lesions may vary from dusky red, to blue-gray or violaceous. Patients typically describe a burning sensation or itching, or both, associated with the development of lesions. In some patients, the center of the lesion may become bullous and result in denuding of skin. The diagnostic hallmark of FDE is recurrence of the lesion in the same anatomical location after drug rechallenge.[302] Both topical and oral provocation tests have been performed to confirm the diagnosis. However, oral challenge is more likely to lead to the development of generalized bullous lesions.[302] Following resolution of lesions, the affected tissue may remain hyperpigmented for an extended period. As the name implies, the sole cause of FDE is drugs. Therefore, a complete drug history with attention to prescription, nonprescription, and herbal remedies must be obtained to identify the causative agent.

Table 6-14 Conditions to Consider in the Differential Diagnosis of Drug-Induced Cutaneous Disorders

Erythematous rash[298,342]

- Viral exanthema (Epstein–Barr virus, human herpesvirus 6, parvovirus B19)
- Acute graft-versus-host disease
- Bacterial toxin eruption
- Kawasaki disease
- Still disease

Fixed drug eruption[287,302,344]

- Bullous pemphigoid
- Contact dermatitis
- Herpes (simplex) labialis
- Discoid lupus erythematosus
- Insect bite (if a single lesion)
- Phytophotodermatitis

DRESS[188]

- Cutaneous lymphoma
- Psoriasis (aggravation of)[313,314]
- Alcohol consumption
- Physical trauma
- Psychological stress
- Streptococcal infection
- Viral infection

SJS[188,345]

- Postinfectious erythema multiforme (secondary to herpes simplex or mycoplasma infection)
- Kawasaki disease

TEN[188]

- Exfoliative dermatitis
- Staphylococcal scalded-skin syndrome
- Paraneoplastic pemphigus
- Thermal burns

Warfarin-induced skin necrosis[334]

- Disseminated intravascular coagulation
- Purple toe syndrome
- Pyoderma gangrenosum
- Microembolization
- Leukocytoclastic vasculitis
- Necrotizing fasciitis
- Purpura fulminans
- Venous gangrene
- Heparin-induced thrombocytopenia
- Septicemia

DRESS = drug rash with eosinophilia and systemic symptoms, HHV-6 = human herpesvirus-6, SJS = Stevens–Johnson syndrome, TEN = toxic epidermal necrolysis.

Drugs most commonly associated with FDE are listed in Table 6-12.

Acneiform eruptions are an infrequent drug-induced adverse event, accounting for only 1% of all drug-related cutaneous reactions.[298] Unlike acne vulgaris, drug-related acneiform eruptions consist primarily of papules and pustules with limited to no comedones. Similar to those associated with acne vulgaris, these eruptions are typically confined to the face and upper trunk.[298] The classic drug offenders are corticosteroids, adrenocorticotropic hormone, anabolic steroids, combination oral contraceptives, danazol, bromides, iodides, isoniazid, lithium, and azathioprine. Corticosteroids administered orally, parenterally, topically, or by inhalation have been shown to provoke acneiform eruptions or exacerbate underlying conditions of acne.[291,292,293] Steroid-induced acne is common and usually appears within 14 days after initiation of systemic or topical therapy. An acne-like reaction has also been described in association with the use of the EGFR inhibitors (e.g., cetuximab, panitumumab, erlotinib, gefitinib) used in the treatment of colorectal and non-small-cell lung cancer. The acne-like rash is pruritic, with a predominance of pustules and an absence of open or closed comedones.[294,295] The rash is typically mild to moderate in severity, occurs most frequently on the face and V-shaped areas of the chest, back, or both, and appears within 10–14 days after drug therapy initiation. The severity of the rash has been shown to correlate with both increasing drug dose and the antitumor activity of the agent.[295] Some data support a relationship between the occurrence of rash and the increased likelihood of patient survival.[294] In patients with severe rashes, particularly those involving more than 50% of the body surface area, dose modification or interruption of EGFR inhibitor therapy is recommended.[294,295] The rash is typically reversible following discontinuation of therapy.

Psoriasis is a chronic, immunologically mediated skin disease that is characterized by red or salmon-pink plaques covered by silvery or white scales surrounded by normal skin.[313] The plaques are symmetrically distributed on the elbows, knees, scalp, and lumbosacral region. Several clinical phenotypes of psoriasis exist, including pustular, erythrodermic, and nail psoriasis. However, 90% of cases present as plaque psoriasis (psoriasis vulgaris). This chronic condition involves the activation of T lymphocytes with overexpression of a number of cytokines, including TNFα, interferon α, IL-6, IL-2, and IL-8. Drugs can exacerbate pre-existing lesions (e.g., β-blockers, lithium, synthetic antimalarial drugs), provoke the development of new plaques on the normal skin of patients with psoriasis (e.g., β-blockers, lithium), and cause psoriasis in patients with no history or familial predisposition (e.g., growth hormone).[313-315] Most cases of drug-induced psoriasis are clinically indistinguishable from psoriasis from nondrug-induced causes. In some cases, the offending drug can cause a lichenoid pattern of disease or a transformation to the pustular form of psoriasis.[313] The latency period from initiation of therapy with the offending drug to the exacerbation or appearance of psoriatic lesions varies widely. Mean latency periods of 3 weeks, 6 weeks, and 33 weeks have been described for psoriasis induced by the synthetic antimalarial drugs, ACE inhibitors, and lithium, respectively.[313] β-blockers have been associated with a latency period ranging from days to weeks after initiation of therapy. Drugs used to treat psoriasis, including topically applied agents (e.g., coal tar) and systemically administered agents (e.g., etretinate, etanercept, infliximab), can also aggravate the condition. The TNFα-agents infliximab and etanercept have been reported to aggravate psoriasis in patients undergoing treatment for psoriatic arthritis and have provoked psoriasis in patients treated for Crohn disease, ankylosing spondylitis, rheumatoid arthritis, and ulcerative colitis.[315] In patients treated with infliximab or etanercept, new psoriatic lesions developed as soon as after the second injection.[315]

Serious cutaneous adverse reactions include DRESS, SJS, TEN, and warfarin tissue necrosis. DRESS is a distinct clinical syndrome previously described by the more general term, *drug hypersensitivity syndrome*.[99,102,343] DRESS is characterized by the triad of high fever, rash, and internal organ involvement.[188,343] Compared with immune complex diseases such as SSLD, DRESS is associated with a more delayed onset of symptoms, ranging from 3 to 8 weeks after drug initiation, and a more consistent pattern of internal-organ involvement.[99,343] The initial manifestation of DRESS is diffuse, symmetrical maculopapular eruptions on the upper trunk and face. This rash can extend to include the lower extremities and is typically associated with facial and periorbital edema. The edema may lead to gross distortion of the patient's features. Organs affected by this syndrome include the kidney, liver, pancreas, lungs, and hematologic system. A high degree of interpatient variability exists with regard to the targeted organ and the severity of organ involvement. To better define and classify the syndrome, the RegiSCAR scoring system was developed in 2007.[346] Application of this scoring system in 172 cases of suspected DRESS led to the identification of the following features of a probable or definite case: skin rash, hypereosinophilia, lymphadenopathy, and liver involvement.[346]

Both the anticonvulsant hypersensitivity syndrome and the allopurinol hypersensitivity syndrome are classic examples of DRESS. Anticonvulsant hypersensitivity syndrome, associated with the aromatic anticonvulsants (e.g., phenytoin, phenobarbital, carbamazepine), is characterized by the triad of fever (38–40°C), rash (papular, pruritic, often associated with facial or periorbital edema), and lymphadenopathy occurring within 3 months after the initiation of therapy.[255,256] Other diagnostic criteria include hematologic abnormalities (leukocytosis, eosinophilia), myalgias, pharyngitis, and hepatitis or other multisystem involvement (e.g., interstitial nephritis, rhabdomyolysis, pneumonitis).[255,256] Allopurinol hypersensitivity syndrome is associated with a mean (±SD) onset of 47±109 days[102] and also presents with high fever, eosinophilia, and skin rash that may be severe (e.g., SJS or TEN). Kidney failure, hepatomegaly, and abnormalities in liver function tests are also frequently noted. This reaction, attributed to the active metabolite oxypurinol, has been described as a vasculitic immune complex disease.[101,102]

SJS and TEN are related mucocutaneous disorders that are considered by many as drug-induced variants of erythema multiforme. Like erythema multiforme, both SJS and TEN are associated with the widespread development of multiple types of skin lesions, including macules, blisters, purpuric lesions, and the hallmark target iris lesions. The target lesion is discrete, round, <3 cm in diameter, and identified by its central zone of epidermal necrosis surrounded by two concentric rings of edema and erythema.[345] SJS and TEN are progressive bullous disorders that are considered dermatologic emergencies.[288] Unlike erythema multiforme, which is usually self-limiting and related to recurrent herpes simplex viral infections, both SJS and TEN are usually drug-related and extend from diffuse erythematous reactions to include mucous membrane erosion and epidermal detachment. Drugs are the cause of SJS and TEN in 50% and 80% of cases, respectively.[287,347]

Both SJS and TEN typically occur within the first 4 weeks of drug therapy. Before skin lesions become evident, both SJS and TEN are associated with a prodromal syndrome of nausea, vomiting, sore throat, diarrhea, myalgias, and arthralgias. In patients with TEN, high fevers and a burning sensation of the skin are also frequently reported prior to the eruption of skin lesions. Mucous membrane involvement, typically of the mouth and lips, nasal cavity, and conjunctivae, tends to precede the development of skin lesions by 1–3 days.[287,348] The initial lesions are erythematous and appear on the face and upper trunk, after which they rapidly evolve into blisters and target lesions on the face, trunk, and limbs.[348] Full-thickness epidermal detachment occurs within days after the onset of skin lesions. Rather than considered as two distinctly different syndromes, SJS and TEN are often described as a continuous spectrum of a disease, with TEN as the more severe form.[345] The extent of epidermal detachment has been used to distinguish between SJS and TEN. SJS is described by the presence of mucosal erosions with widespread purpuric macules and epidermal detachment of <10% of body surface area, whereas TEN involves widespread purpuric macules and epidermal detachment of >30% of body surface area.[345,349] The term *SJS-TEN overlap* is used to describe cases in which evidence of epidermal detachment is present on 10% to 30% of the body surface area.[345,349] Although regrowth of the epidermis begins within days after the onset of epidermal loss, TEN is sometimes complicated by the development of acute kidney injury, respiratory failure, neutropenia, electrolyte abnormalities, and sepsis. Long-term sequelae of SJS and TEN may include temporary nail loss, permanent visual impairment, cutaneous scarring, and irregular pigmentation. A severity-of-illness scoring system for TEN, known as SCORTEN (SCORe of toxic epidermal necrolysis), has been described and evaluated as a prognostic indicator.[350] With the use of this system, seven independent risk factors, determined within 24 hours of patient presentation with TEN, are used as patient outcome indicators.[350]

Warfarin-induced skin necrosis (WISN) is a severe cutaneous reaction that typically begins within 10 days after initiation of warfarin therapy, with a peak occurrence between days 3 and 6.[298] WISN initially presents with red, poorly demarcated painful plaques usually in areas of high adipose tissue (e.g., breasts, hips, buttocks). The plaques can progress to hemorrhagic blisters and eventually become necrotic, requiring surgical debridement.[188,298] WISN occurs as a result of an imbalance between the concentrations of the endogenous vitamin K-dependent anticoagulant protein C and the vitamin K-dependent clotting factors.[188,298] The half-life of protein C is much shorter (8 hours) compared with those of clotting factors II, IX, and X (24–48 hours). After warfarin initiation, a rapid decline in the concentration of protein C may lead to a hypercoagulable state, resulting in WISN. This theory is supported by the fact that WISN is more likely to occur in patients who receive excessive initial doses of warfarin and have an underlying protein C deficiency. Patients with a deficiency of protein S, the cofactor for protein C activity, may also be at greater risk of WISN. WISN can be fatal if not treated.

RISK FACTORS

Female sex, concomitant viral infection with HIV or EBV, and the presence of autoimmune disease have routinely been identified as risk factors for cutaneous drug eruptions.[191,201,203] In a prospective study of 48 patients with allergic-mediated skin reactions, identified risk factors were HIV (19% of patients), connective-tissue disease (10%), and viral or autoimmune hepatitis (12%).[289] In another prospective cohort study of hospitalized patients with adverse cutaneous drug reactions, those with systemic lupus erythematosus had a relative risk of 4.68 (95% CI 1.79–12.18) and patients with acquired immunodeficiency syndrome had a relative risk of 8.68 (95% CI 2.18–33.19).[351] Studies have also been performed to identify predictors of skin rash associated with specific drugs or drug classes. In the antiepileptic drug class, an increased risk of drug rash was identified in women of reproductive age and in those with history of a rash induced by another antiepileptic medication.[352,353] Other risk factors associated with specific drugs, drug eruptions, or both are provided in **Table 6-15**.

The initial dose, rate of dose titration, and concomitant administration of interacting drugs can be risk factors for cutaneous drug eruptions. Both lamotrigine and nevirapine were identified as strongly associated with SJS/TEN in the EuroSCAR study.[290] In addition to female sex, lack of adherence to the 14-day lead-in period of dosing of nevirapine may increase the risk of SCARs.[290] Factors shown to increase the risk of rash with lamotrigine include age <13 years, history of rash caused by another anticonvulsant agent, exceeding the recommended initial dose or recommended rate of dose escalation, and coadministration with valproic acid.[354] In the EuroSCAR study, daily allopurinol doses >200 mg were associated with a higher risk of SJS/TEN (OR 36, 95% CI 17–76) compared with lower daily doses (OR 3.0, 95% CI 1.1–8.4).[290] In other analyses, both kidney disease and the lack of dose adjustment in patients with impaired kidney function have been identified as risk factors for allopurinol-induced DRESS, SJS, or TEN.[92] Excessive starting doses of warfarin, female sex, and obesity have all been identified as risk factors for WISN.[188,298]

Genetic susceptibility has always been suspected as a risk factor for allergic-mediated cutaneous disorders, and evidence has become available to support this hypothesis. The HLA-B*1502 allele has been strongly linked to the risk of SJS/TEN associated with carbamazepine. In a study of Han Chinese patients, all of whom developed SJS/TEN during carbamazepine therapy, had the HLA-B*1502 allele, whereas only 3% of the patients who tolerated

Table 6-15 Risk Factors for Drug-Induced Cutaneous Diseases

Abacavir

- HHV-6[204,205]
- HLA-B*5701[193]

Allopurinol

- Doses >200 mg per day[322]
- Kidney disease[102,103]
- HLA-B*5801[335]

Amoxicillin and ampicillin

- EBV[201]

Aromatic anticonvulsants (carbamazepine, phenobarbital, phenytoin)

- Previous rash in response to an antiepileptic[353]
- Women of reproductive age[352]
- HLA-B*1502 (carbamazepine, phenytoin, fosphenytoin)[355,356]
- HLA-A*3101 (carbamazepine)[357]
- CYP2C9*3 (phenytoin)[358]

Lamotrigine

- Age <13 years[290]
- Exceeding the recommended initial dose[290]
- Coadministration with valproic acid[290]

Nevirapine

- Female sex[290]
- Lack of adherence to recommendation for 14-day lead-in dosing[290]
- HLA-B*3505[359]

Penicillins

- HIV[203]

Sulfonamides

- HIV[203]

Warfarin

- Female sex[334]
- Hereditary protein C or S deficiency[334]
- Large initial doses[334]
- Obesity[334]

EBV = Epstein–Barr virus, HIV = human immunodeficiency virus, HLA = human leukocyte antigen, HHV-6 = human herpesvirus 6.

carbamazepine had the allele.[355] This allele occurs almost exclusively in patients of Asian and South Asian Indian ancestry. In this same patient population, presence of HLA-B*1502 has been shown to increase the risk of SJS and TEN associated with carbamazepine, phenytoin, and fosphenytoin.[356] In European and North Asian populations, HLA-A*3101 has been related to the development of nonblistering reactions such as DRESS induced by carbamazepine.[357] Most recently, a genetic variant in the CYP2C isozyme, CYP2C9*3, was found in association with phenytoin-induced SCARs.[358] Presence of the HLA-B*5701 allele has been shown to increase the risk of abacavir hypersensitivity,[194] and studies in Han Chinese suggest that the HLA-B*5801 allele may be a genetic marker for allopurinol-induced SJS and TEN.[335] Preliminary evidence also suggests a higher frequency of FDEs in association with the HLA-B22 and HLA-C1 antigens.[302]

MORBIDITY AND MORTALITY

Using four national databases, Stern[336] quantified hospitalizations and visits to office-based physicians and hospital clinics for a primary diagnosis of a skin condition. The U.S. Census estimates for 2000 were used to calculate the rates of hospitalization or office visits for a diagnosis of SJS/TEN, drug eruption, drug allergy, and urticaria/angioedema. Overall, 0.06% of hospital admissions were attributed to a skin condition related to drug use.[336] Approximately 5,000 hospitalizations per year resulted from a diagnosis of erythema multiforme, SJS, or TEN, 35% of which were attributed to drug use.[336] The rates of hospitalization for a primary diagnosis of SJS/TEN and drug eruptions were calculated as 16 and 21 admissions per million person-years, respectively. During the 6 years of study (1995–2000), there were 650,000 office visits with a primary diagnosis of erythema multiforme, SJS, or TEN and 1 million visits with a primary diagnosis of drug eruption.[336] Urticaria, angioedema, and anaphylaxis were the most frequent diagnoses associated with outpatient visits, accounting for 3 times as many visits as SJS/TEN, drug rash, and drug allergy combined.[336] When the data were annualized, more than 500,000 office visits per year were attributed to drug eruptions and drug allergies including a dermatologic component.

Although rare in occurrence relative to other dermatologic conditions, SJS and TEN are associated with substantial morbidity, with the potential for lasting disabilities and complications (e.g., corneal ulcers, corneal neovascularization, skin grafts, coagulopathies, hepatitis, glomerulonephritis) in 30–45% of patients.[319] Moreover, estimates of mortality associated with SJS and TEN range from 1% to 5% and 10% to 70%, respectively.[319] In at least one study, the death rate associated with SJS and TEN was found to positively correlate with age and was 10 times higher in patients >65 years of age.[336] In cases of SJS and TEN, the most common causes of death are sepsis, pulmonary embolism, gastrointestinal bleeding, and hypovolemia.

PREVENTION

Advances in genetic testing allow for prospective screening for the HLA-B*1502 and the HLA-B*5701 alleles, biomarkers of an increased risk of severe hypersensitivity reactions to carbamazepine and abacavir, respectively. Screening for the presence of these and other biomarkers may ultimately lead to the prevention of allergy-mediated severe cutaneous reactions. Genetic tests for HLA-B*1502 and HLA-B*5701 are currently available.

Other preventive measures include the avoidance of drugs with a propensity to cause cutaneous diseases in high-risk populations (**Table 6-16**), adherence to recommended dosing guidelines specifically for dosing titration, and avoidance of drug–drug interactions. Patients who have experienced a SCAR associated with a specific drug should be counseled to avoid the use of that drug and any structurally related drug for the rest of their lives. When initiating therapy with a medication known to present a high risk of a severe cutaneous reaction, counseling should be provided regarding the initial warning signs and symptoms (i.e., burning sensation of skin, mucous membrane involvement).

Table 6-16 Approaches to Help Prevent Drug-Induced Cutaneous Diseases

Drug	Condition	Prevention
Abacavir	DRESS	Test for HLA-B*5701[194]
Allopurinol	DRESS/SJS/TEN	Adjust dose in patients with kidney disease[102] Avoid concomitant therapy with thiazide diuretics[103]
Aromatic anticonvulsants (carbamazepine, phenytoin, phenobarbital)	SJS, TEN	Avoid use in patients with history of severe rash caused by another aromatic anticonvulsant
Carbamazepine	SJS, TEN	Test for HLA-B*1502[355]
Lamotrigine	SJS/TEN	Adhere to recommended dose and dose-escalation recommendations[354] Avoid concomitant therapy with valproic acid[354]
Nevirapine	SJS/TEN	Adhere to 14-day lead-in dosing recommendation
Warfarin	WISN	Avoid loading or large initial doses In patients with protein C or S deficiency or previous history of WISN, overlap therapy with heparin for at least 5 days and initiate warfarin at low doses[334]

DRESS = drug rash with eosinophilia and systemic symptoms, SJS = Stevens–Johnson syndrome, TEN = toxic epidermal necrolysis, WISN = warfarin-induced skin necrosis.

MANAGEMENT

Table 6-17 provides recommended treatment methods for the drug eruptions presented in this section. Of note, maculopapular rashes are generally self-limited and usually do not require treatment. If associated with pruritus, oral antihistamines are advised. Topical corticosteroid creams such as 1% hydrocortisone may be used in patients with nondiffuse limited areas of involvement. In patients with a diffuse maculopapular rash and evidence of systemic symptoms (e.g., arthralgias, muscle pain or weakness), an oral, self-tapering, low-dose steroid regimen (e.g., methylprednisolone) may be appropriate. The recommended treatment of drug-induced urticaria and angioedema is provided in Table 6-10.

Drug-induced psoriasis is usually resistant to treatment and requires discontinuation of the offending agent (e.g., β-blockers, lithium, synthetic antimalarial drug). However, in one case series, 50% of the patients in whom psoriasis associated with either infliximab or etanercept developed were able to continue therapy and their lesions responded favorably to treatment with topical corticosteroids.[315]

Treatment of SJS and TEN is focused on supportive therapy (nutritional support, pain management, fluid replacement) and the prevention of complications such as acute kidney injury and sepsis. Depending on the extent of blistering and epidermal detachment, patients may require treatment in an intensive care or burn unit. Recommended treatment methods for SJS and TEN are provided in Table 6-17. In particular, the topical administration of silver sulfadiazine should be avoided because of the high risk of SJS and TEN associated with sulfonamides and the potential for cross-reactivity with sulfadiazine.[287] The use of systemic corticosteroids remains controversial.[345] To date, there are no large randomized, controlled studies to support the concept that systemic corticosteroids either reduce the time to recovery or prevent the development of complications. In a systematic review, a significant impact on mortality (OR 0.4, 95% CI 0.2–0.9) was demonstrated with corticosteroid use in only 1 of 6 retrospective cohort studies.[361] IVIG has emerged as a potential treatment of SJS and TEN in children and adults.[362-366] IVIG is postulated to inhibit dermal-cell apoptosis triggered via the Fas-Fas ligand pathway.[348] When administered early in the course of the disease, IVIG has shown promising effects on wound healing, progression of disease, and mortality.[362-365] Both low dose (0.2–0.5 g/kg) and high dose (2–3 g/kg) IVIG regimens have been described. Most studies support the use of a

Table 6-17 Management of Drug-Induced Cutaneous Diseases

Disease	Recommended Treatment
Acne[291-298]	May or may not require discontinuation of the offending agent Topical benzoyl peroxide or retinoids
Erythematous reaction[341,342]	Discontinue offending agent Histamine H_1-antagonist (diphenhydramine 25–50 mg orally every 6 hours as needed for itching) Methylprednisolone (6-day self-tapering oral regimen starting with 24 mg on day 1) (if diffuse rash)
FDE[344]	Discontinue offending agent Sunscreen for 6 months to 1 year if areas of hyperpigmentation
DRESS[188,343,360]	Discontinue the offending agent Topical corticosteroids may be of some benefit but most cases are resistant to standard therapies
Psoriasis[270]	Discontinue offending agent Topical corticosteroids may be of some benefit but most cases are resistant to standard therapies
SJS and TEN[188,345,347,349]	IV fluid replacement (saline or lactated Ringer's solution) Nutritional support (enteral or parenteral routes) Pain control (systemic opiate therapy) Eye care—antibiotic eye drops, lubricants Oral hygiene: hydrogen peroxide gargle; anesthetics (viscous lidocaine or benzocaine); antiseptic mouthwash Topical antiseptics (0.5% silver nitrate or 0.05% chlorhexidine) Wound care with biologic dressings (porcine xenografts), synthetic dressings, or silicone dressings Surgical debridement of blisters and necrotic tissue Consider IVIG (1–2 g/kg) or cyclosporine (3–5 mg/kg/day for 7 days)
WISN[188,334]	Discontinue warfarin Vitamin K or fresh-frozen plasma to restore protein C or S Initiate heparin to prevent further thrombosis Protein C concentrate if patient has known protein C deficiency Skin grafting and/or surgical debridement

FDE = fixed drug eruption, DRESS = drug rash with eosinophilia and systemic symptoms, IV = intravenous, IVIG = intravenous immunoglobulin, SJS = Stevens–Johnson syndrome, TEN = toxic epidermal necrolysis, WISN = warfarin-induced skin necrosis.

mean total dose of not less than 2 g/kg.[366] Cyclosporine (3–5 mg/kg/day for 7 days) was shown to offer a greater mortality benefit compared to IVIG (1 g/kg for 3 days) in a single-center retrospective study of 64 patients.[367] Similar to corticosteroids, the optimal doses of IVIG and cyclosporine, times of initiation, and durations of therapy are yet to be determined.

INFORMATION FOR PATIENTS

Patients in whom a drug-induced adverse cutaneous event develops should be educated as to the name of the specific offending drug, the terminology used to describe the rash, and the likelihood of the occurrence of a similar or more severe reaction following re-exposure to the drug. If the reaction was allergic-mediated, the patient should be instructed to question all newly prescribed medications regarding similarity to the offending agent in chemical structure or chemical class. If the cutaneous event was severe, the patient should be advised to wear a medical alert bracelet. Patients with underlying skin conditions such as acne or psoriasis should be instructed to question whether any newly prescribed medication may aggravate the condition.

REFERENCES

1. Demoly P, Adkinson NF, Brockow K et al. International consensus on drug allergy. *Allergy.* 2014; 69:420-37.
2. Bernstein I, Gruchalla R, Lee R et al. Disease management of drug hypersensitivity: a practice parameter. Joint Task Force on Practice Parameters, the American Academy of Allergy, Asthma and Immunology and the Joint Council of Allergy, Asthma and Immunology. *Ann Allergy Asthma Immunol.* 1999; 83:665-700.

3. Chowdhury BA, Lieberman PL. Drug allergens, haptens and anaphylatoxins. In: Lockey RF, Bukantz SC, eds. *Allergens and Allergen Immunotherapy.* 2nd ed. New York, NY: Marcel Dekker; 1999.
4. Vaidya SJ, Seydel C, Patel SR et al. Anaphylactic reaction to liposomal amphotericin B. *Ann Pharmacother.* 2002; 36:1480-81.
5. Ringden O, Andstrom E, Remberger M et al. Allergic reactions and other rare side effects of liposomal amphotericin. *Lancet.* 1994; 344:1156-7.
6. Ceriana P, Maurelli M, Locatelli A et al. Anaphylactic reaction to aprotinin. *J Cardiothorac Vasc Anesth.* 1995; 9:477-8.
7. Shepard GM. Hypersensitivity reactions to chemotherapeutic drugs. *Clin Rev Allergy Immunol.* 2003; 24:253-62.
8. Kulczycki A. Aspartame induced urticaria. *Ann Intern Med.* 1986; 104:207-8.
9. Barbaud A. Place of excipients in drug-related allergy. *Clin Rev Allergy Immunol.* 1995; 13:253-63.
10. Berkes EA. Anaphylactic and anaphylactoid reactions to aspirin and other NSAIDs. *Clin Rev Allergy Immunol.* 2003; 24:137-47.
11. Woessner KM. Aspirin desensitization for cardiovascular disease. *Curr Opin Allergy Clin Immunol* 2015; 15:314-22.
12. Mertes PM, Laxenaire MC, Alia R. Anaphylactic and anaphylactoid reactions occurring during anesthesia in France in 1999-2000. *Anesthesiology.* 2003; 99:536-45.
13. Harle DG, Baldo BA. Atracurium and anaphylaxis. *MedJ Aust.* 1986; 144:220.
14. Thomas AN, Cain S. Cross-sensitivity between atracurium and mivacurium. *Anaesthesia.* 1995; 50:185.
15. Hinrichs R, Schneider LA, Ozdemir C et al. Azathioprine hypersensitivity in a patient with peripheral demyelinating polyneuropathy. *Br J Dermatol.* 2003; 148:1076-7.
16. Sinico RA, Sabadini E, Borlandelli S et al. Azathioprine hypersensitivity: report of two cases and review of the literature. *J Nephrol.* 2003; 16:272-6.
17. Barros VR, Rocha V, Garcia VD et al. Anaphylactic shock after retreatment with basiliximab. *Transplant Proc.* 2003; 35:579.
18. Bruchim I, Goldberg A, Fishman A et al. Carboplatin hypersensitivity: evaluation and successful desensitization protocol. *Immunotherapy* 2014; 6:905-12.
19. Patterson DL, Yunginger JW, Dunn WF et al. Anaphylaxis induced by the carboxymethylcellulose component of injectable triamcinolone acetonide suspension (Kenalog). *Ann Allergy Asthma Immunol.* 1995; 74:163-6.
20. Atanaskovic-Markovic M, Gavrovic-Jankulovic M et al. Type 1 hypersensitivity to ceftriaxone and cross-reactivity with cefazolin and ampicillin. *Allergy.* 2003; 58:537-8.
21. Romano A, Torres MJ, Namour F et al. Immediate hypersensitivity to cephalosporins. *Allergy.* 2002; 57(suppl 72):52-7.
22. Kelkar PS, Li JTC. Cephalosporin allergy. *N Engl J Med.* 2001; 345:804-9.
23. Telia R, Gaig P, Bartra J et al. Urticaria to cetirizine. *J Investig Allergol Clin Immunol.* 2002; 12:136-7.
24. Chung CH, Mirahhur B, Chan E et al. Cetuximab-induced anaphylaxis and IgE specific for galactose-alpha-1,3-galactose. *New Engl J Med.* 2008; 358:1109-17.
25. Berg EA, Platts-Mills TAE, Commins SP. Drug allergens and food—the cetuximab and galactose-alpha-1,3-galactose story. *Ann Allergy Asthma Immunol.* 2014; 112:97-101.
26. Nakonechna A, Dore P, Dixon T et al. Immediate hypersensitivity to chlorhexidine is increasingly recognized in the United Kingdom. *Allergol Immunopathol.* 2014; 42:44-9.
27. Lim KS, Kam PCA. Chlorhexidine—pharmacology and clinical applications. *Anaesth Intensive Care.* 2008; 36: 502-12.
28. Hall BB, McCulloch JA. Anaphylactic reactions following the intradiscal injection of chymopapain under local anesthesia. *J Bone Joint Surg Am.* 1983; 65:1215-19.
29. Campbell KL, Cohn JR, Fischman DL et al. Management of clopidogrel hypersensitivity without drug interruption. *Am J Cardiol.* 2011; 107:812-16.
30. Felix-Getzik E, Sylvia LM. Prasugrel use in a patient allergic to clopidogrel: effect of a drug shortage on drug selection of dual antiplatelet therapy. *Am J Health-Syst Pharm.* 2013; 70:511-13.
31. Fernandez-Rivas M, Perez CC, Cuevas M et al. Selective allergic reactions to clavulanic acid. *J Allergy Clin Immunol.* 1995; 95:748-50.
32. Patriarca G, Schiavino D, Nucera E et al. Successful desensitization of a child with desferrioxamine hypersensitivity. *J Investig Allergol Clin Immunol.* 1995; 5:294-5.
33. Barbaud A. Place of excipients in systemic drug allergy. *Immunol Allergy Clin N Am.* 2014; 34:671-9.
34. Campi P, Pichler WJ. Quinolone hypersensitivity. *Curr Opin Allergy Clin Immunol.* 2003; 3:255-60.
35. Solensky R, Khan DA. Evaluation of antibiotic allergy: the role of skin tests and drug challenges. *Curr Allergy Asthma Rep.* 2014; 14:459.
36. Schulze S, Wollina U. Gentamicin-induced anaphylaxis. *Allergy.* 2003; 58:88-9.
37. Vultaggio A, Castells MC. Hypersensitivity to biologic agents. *Immunol Allergy Clin N Am.* 2014;34:615-32.
38. Jacquier J, Chik CL, Senior PA. A practical, clinical approach to the assessment and management of suspected insulin allergy. *Diabet Med.* 2013; 30:977-85.
39. Walters BA, VanWyck DB. Benchmarking iron dextran sensitivity: reactions requiring resuscitative medication in incident and prevanet patients. *Nephrol Dial Transplant.* 2005; 20:1438-42.
40. Rampton D, Folkersen J, Fishbane S et al. Hypersensitivity reactions to intravenous iron: guidance for risk minimization and management. *Haematologica.* 2014; 99:11.
41. Bircher AJ, Auerbach M. Hypersensitivity from intravenous iron products. *Immunol Allergy Clin N Am* 2014; 24:707-23.
42. Patel AM, McKeon J. Avoidance and management of adverse reactions to antituberculosis drugs. *Drug Saf.* 1995; 12:1-25.
43. Crook MJ. Isoniazid-induced anaphylaxis. *J Clin Pharmacol.* 2003; 43:545-6.
44. De Pasquale T, Buonomo A, Illuminati I et al. IgE mediated anaphylaxis to ketoprofen: a case report. *J Invest Allergol Clin Immunol.* 2015; 25:79-80.
45. Grienacher A, Lubenow N, Eichler P. Anaphylactic and anaphylactoid associated with lepirudin in patients with heparin-induced thrombocytopenia. *Circulation.* 2003; 108:2062-5.
46. Taylor JD. Anaphylactic reaction to LHRH analogue, leuprorelin. *Med J Aust.* 1994; 161:455.
47. Cox L, Platts-Mills TAE, Finegold I et al. American Academy of Allergy, Asthma and Immunology/American College of Allergy, Asthma and Immunology Joint Task Force Report on omalizumab-associated anaphylaxis. *J Allergy Clin Immunol.* 2007; 120: 1373-7.
48. Saif MW. Hypersensitivity reactions associated with oxaliplatin. *Expert Opin Drug Saf.* 2006; 5:687–94.
49. Toki MI, Saif MW, Syrigos KN. Hypersensitivity reactions associated with oxaliplatin and their clinical management. *Expert Opin Drug Saf.* 2014; 13:1545-54.
50. Van Herpen CM, Van Hoesel QG, Punt CJ. Paclitaxel-induced severe hypersensitivity reaction occurring as a late toxicity. *Ann Oncol.* 1995; 6:852.
51. Fardet L, Izzedine H, Ciroldi M et al. Pantoprazole-induced recurrent anaphylactic shock. *Am J Gastroenterol.* 2002; 97:2933.
52. Salkind AR, Cuddy PG, Foxworth JW. Is this patient allergic to penicillin? An evidence-based analysis of the likelihood of penicillin allergy. *JAMA.* 2001; 285:2498-505.
53. Macy E. Penicillin and beta-lactam allergy: epidemiology and diagnosis. *Curr Allergy Asthma Rep.* 2014; 14:476-7.
54. Riegert-Johnson DL, Volcheck GW. The incidence of anaphylaxis following intravenous phytonadione: a 5-year retrospective review. *Ann Allergy Clin Immunol.* 2002; 89:400-6.
55. Waran KD, Munsick RA. Anaphylaxis from povidone-iodine. *Lancet.* 1995; 345:1506.

56. Shroff AP, Jones JK. Reactions to povidone iodine preparation. *JAMA*. 1980; 243:230-1.
57. Mutnick JLM. Desensitization to prasugrel: cardiology's increased need for allergy consultation. *Ann Allergy Asthma Immunol*. 2012; 108:124-5.
58. Cooney C, Nagy A. Angioedema associated with risperidone. *BMJ*. 1995; 311:1204.
59. Russell WJ, Lee C, Milne D. Is allergy to rocuronium a high probability cross-reaction with suxamethonium? *Anaesth Intensive Care*. 2003; 31:333.
60. Michils A, Vandermoten G, Duchateau J et al. Anaphylaxis with sodium benzoate. *Lancet*. 1991; 337:1424-5.
61. Dykewicz MS, McGrath KG, Davison R et al. Identification of patients at risk for anaphylaxis due to streptokinase. *Arch Intern Med*. 1986; 146:305-7.
62. Dachs R, Vitillo J. Angioedema associated with sumatriptan administration. *Am J Med*. 1995; 99:684-5.
63. Harrison GG. Suxamethonium, anaphylaxis and cardiovascular collapse. *S Afr Med J*. 1986; 69:86-7.
64. Quinn KL, Connelly KA. First report of hypersensitivity to ticagrelor. *Canadian J Cardiol*. 2014; 30:957.e3-4.
65. Schretlen-Doherty JS, Troutman WG. Tobramycin-induced hypersensitivity reaction. *Ann Pharmacother*. 1995; 29:704-6.
66. Gonzalo FE, Montagut LB, Vecina ST. Anaphylactic shock caused by triamcinolone acetonide. *Ann Pharmacother*. 1994; 28:1310.
67. Anne S, Middleton E, Reisman RE. Vancomycin anaphylaxis and successful desensitization. *Ann Allergy*. 1994; 73:402-4.
68. Wassef M, Keiser P. Hypersensitivity of zidovudine: report of a case of anaphylaxis and review of the literature. *Clin Infect Dis*. 1995; 20:1387-9.
69. Erffmeyer JE. Serum sickness. *Ann Allergy*. 1986; 56:105-9.
70. Wooltorton E. Bupropion: reports of deaths, seizures and serum sickness. *Can Med Assoc J*. 2002; 166:68.
71. McCollom RA, Elbe DH, Ritchie AH. Bupropion-induced serum sickness-like reaction. *Ann Pharmacother*. 2000; 34:471-3.
72. Yolles JC, Armenta WA, Alao AO. Serum sickness induced by bupropion. *Ann Pharmacother*. 1999; 33:931-3.
73. Kearns GL, Wheeler JG, Childress SH et al. Serum sickness like reactions to cefaclor: role of hepatic metabolism and individual susceptibility. *J Pediatr*. 1994; 125: 805-11.
74. McCullough H. Cefaclor serum sickness. *JAMA*. 1996; 275:1152-3.
75. Kelsey DK. Cefaclor and serum-sickness like reaction. *JAMA*. 1996; 276:950-1.
76. Slama TG. Serum sickness like illness associated with ciprofloxacin. *Antimicrob Agents Chemother*. 1990; 34: 904-5.
77. Shapiro LE, Knowles SR, Shear NH. Fluoxetine-induced serum sickness like reaction. *Ann Pharmacother*. 1997; 31:927.
78. Park H, Knowles S, Shear NH. Serum sickness like reaction to itraconazole. *Ann Pharmacother*. 1998; 32:1249.
79. Ralph ED, John M, Rieder MJ et al. Serum sickness-like reaction possibly associated with meropenem use. *Clin Infect Dis*. 2003; 36:E149-51.
80. Puyana J, Urena V, Quirce S et al. Serum sickness-like syndrome associated with minocycline therapy. *Allergy*. 1990; 45:313-15.
81. Harel L, Amir J, Livni E et al. Serum sickness-like reaction associated with minocycline therapy in adolescents. *Ann Pharmacother*. 1996; 30:481-3.
82. Knowles SR, Shapiro L, Shear NH. Serious adverse reactions induced by minocycline: report of 13 patients and review of the literature. *Arch Dermatol*. 1996; 132:934-9.
83. Herishanu Y. Rituximab-induced serum sickness. *Am J Hematol*. 2002; 70:329.
84. Creamer JD, McGrath JA, Webb-Peploe M et al. Serum-sickness like illness following streptokinase therapy: a case report. *Clin Exp Dermatol*. 1995; 20:468-70.
85. Schweitzer DH, van der Wall EE, Bosker HA et al. Serum-sickness like illness as a complication after streptokinase therapy for acute myocardial infarction. *Cardiology*. 1991; 78:68-71.
86. Merkel PA. Drug-induced vasculitis. *Rheum Dis Clin North Am*. 2001; 27:849-62.
87. Ten Holder SM, Joy MS, Falk RJ. Cutaneous and systemic manifestations of drug-induced vasculitis. *Ann Pharmacother*. 2002; 36:130-47.
88. Calabrese LH, Duna GR Drug-induced vasculitis. *Curr Opin Rheumatol*. 1996; 8:34-40.
89. Jordan KM, Edwards CJ, Arden NK. Allergic vasculitis associated with celecoxib. *Rheumatology*. 2002; 41:1453-5.
90. Leonard GD, Zujewski JA. Docetaxel-related skin, nail and vascular toxicity. *Ann Pharmacother*. 2003; 37:148.
91. English J, Greer KE, McCrone SA et al. Fluticasone-associated cutaneous allergic granulomatous vasculitis. *J Drugs Dermatol*. 2003; 2:326-9.
92. Mcllwain L, Cater JD, Bin-Sagheer S et al. Hypersensitivity vasculitis with leukocytoclastic vasculitis secondary to infliximab. *J Clin Gastroenterol*. 2003; 36:411-3.
93. Pinto JM, Marques MS, Correia TE. Lichen planus and leukocytoclastic vasculitis induced by interferon alpha-2b in a subject with HCV-related chronic active hepatitis. *J Eur Acad Dermatol Venereol*. 2003; 17:193-5.
94. Choi IS, Koh YI, Joo JY et al. Churg-Strauss syndrome may be induced by leukotriene modifiers in severe asthma. *Ann Allergy Asthma Immunol*. 2003; 91:98.
95. Nakamori Y, Tominaga T, Inoue Y et al. Propylthiouracil (PTU) induced vasculitis associated with antineutrophil antibody against myeloperoxidase (MPO-ANCA). *Intern Med*. 2003; 42:529-33.
96. Kitahara T, Hiromura K, Maezawa A et al. Case of propylthiouracil-induced vasculitis associated with antineutrophil cytoplasmic antibody (ANCA): review of literature. *Clin Nephrol*. 1997; 47:336-40.
97. Lillicrap MS, Merry P. Cutaneous vasculitis associated with rofecoxib. *Rheumatology*. 2003; 42:1267-8.
98. Felix-Getzik E, Sylvia LM. Vancomycin-induced leukocytoclastic vasculitis. *Pharmacother*. 2009; 29:846-51.
99. Sullivan JR, Shear NH. The drug hypersensitivity syndrome: what is the pathogenesis? *Arch Dermatol*. 2001; 137:357-64.
100. Clay PG. The abacavir hypersensitivity reaction: a review. *Clin Ther*. 2002; 24:1502-14.
101. Anderson BE, Adams DR. Allopurinol hypersensitivity syndrome. *J Drugs Dermatol*. 2002; 1:60-2.
102. Arellano R, Sacristan JA. Allopurinol hypersensitivity syndrome: a review. *Ann Pharmacother*. 1993; 27:337-43.
103. Kumar A, Edward N, White MI et al. Lesson of the week: allopurinol, erythema multiforme and renal insufficiency. *BM J*. 1996; 312:173-4.
104. Vittorio CC, Muglia JJ. Anticonvulsant hypersensitivity syndrome. *Arch Intern Med*. 1995; 155:2285-90.
105. Ye YM, Thog BYH, Park HS. Hypersensitivity to antiepileptic drugs. *Immunol Allergy Clin N Amer*. 2014; 34:633-43.
106. Kinehara Y, Kijima T, Inoue K et al. Dapsone hypersensitivity syndrome-related lung injury without eosinophilia in the bronchoalveolar lavage fluid. *Intern Med*. 2015; 54:827-31.
107. Urosevic-Maiwald M, Keri K, Harr T et al. Dapsone-induced erythema multiforme with neutropenia in a patient with linear IgA dermatosis: case report and review of the literature. *International J Dermatol*. 2013; 52:1369-71.
108. Zhang FR, Irwanto A, Fu XA et al. HLA-B*13:01 and the dapsone hypersensitivity syndrome. *New Engl J Med*. 2013; 369:1620-8.
109. Schlienger RG, Knolwes SR, Shear NH. Lamotrigine-associated anticonvulsant hypersensitivity syndrome. *Neurology*. 1998; 51:1172-5.
110. Kanno K, Sakai H, Yamada Y et al. Drug-induced hypersensitivity syndrome due to minocycline complicated by severe myocarditis. *J Dermatol*. 2014; 41:160-2.
111. Bourezane Y, Salard D, Hoen B et al. DRESS (drug rash with eosinophilic and systemic symptoms) syndrome associated with nevirapine therapy. *Clin Infect Dis*. 1998; 27:1321-2.

112. Arevalo-Lorido JC, Carretero-Gomez J, Bureo-Dacal JC et al. Antiepileptic drug hypersensitivity syndrome in a patient treated with valproate. *Br J Clin Pharmacol.* 2003; 55:415-6.
113. McDonnell PJ. Drug-induced blood dyscrasias. *Pharm Times.* 2001; April:73-83.
114. Patton WN, Duffull SB. Idiosyncratic drug-induced haematological abnormalities. *Drug Saf.* 1994; 11:445-62.
115. Aster RH. Drug-induced immune thrombocytopenia, an overview of pathogenesis. *Semin Hematol.* 1999; 36:2-6.
116. Greinacher A. Heparin-induced thrombocytopenia *N Engl J Med.* 2015; 373:252-61.
117. Gafter U, Zevin D, Komlos L et al. Thrombocytopenia associated with hypersensitivity to ranitidine, possible cross-reactivity with cimetidine. *Am J Gastroenterol.* 1989; 84:560-62.
118. Shalev O, Seror D. Cimetidine and ranitidine may not cross-react to cause thrombocytopenia. *J Intern Med.* 1991; 230:87-8.
119. Gentilini BR, Curtis BR, Aster RH. An antibody from a patient with ranitidine-induced thrombocytopenia recognizes a site on glycoprotein IX that is a favored site for drug-induced antibodies. *Blood.* 1998; 92:2359-65.
120. Cooper DS, Goldminz D, Levin AA et al. Agranulocytosis associated with antithyroid drugs: effects of patient age and drug dose. *Ann Intern Med.* 1983; 98:26-9.
121. Wing SS, Fantus IG. Adverse immunologic effects of antithyroid drugs. *CMAJ.* 1987; 136:121-5.
122. Perez-Vasquez A, Pastor JM, Riancho JA. Immune thrombocytopenia caused by piperacillin/tazobactam. *Clin Infect Dis.* 1998; 27:650-1.
123. Reichardt P, Handrick W, Linke A et al. Leukocytopenia, thrombocytopenia and fever related to piperacillin/tazobactam treatment: a retrospective analysis of 38 children with cystic fibrosis. *Infection.* 1999; 27:355-6.
124. Kojouri K, Vesely SK, George JN. Quinine-associated thrombotic thrombocytopenia purpura-hemolytic uremic syndrome: frequency, clinical features and long term outcomes. *Ann Intern Med.* 2001; 135:1047-51.
125. Yamreudeewong W, Fosnocht BJ, Weixelman JM. Severe thrombocytopenia possibly associated with trimethoprim/sulfamethoxazole therapy. *Ann Pharmacother.* 2002; 36:78-82.
126. Conley EL, Coley KC, Pollaock BG et al. Prevalence and risk ol thrombocytopenia with valproic acid: experience at a psychiatric teaching hospital. *Pharmacotherapy.* 2001; 21:1325-30.
127. Schwartz MD. Vancomycin-induced neutropenia in a patient positive for an antineutrophil antibody. *Pharmacotherapy.* 2002; 22:783-8.
128. Von Drygalski A, Curtis BR, Bougie DW et al. Vancomycin-induced immune thrombocytopenia. *N Engl I Med.* 2007; 356:904-10.
129. Whalen JP. Hypersensitivity to cimetidine. *J Clin Pharmacol.* 1985; 25:610.
130. Vidal C, Iglesias A, Saez A et al. Hypersensitivity to clindamycin. *DICP.* 1991; 25:317.
131. Butani L. Corticosteroid-induced hypersensitivity reactions. *Ann Allergy Asthma Immunol.* 2002; 89:439-45.
132. Young PC, Montemarano AD, James WD. Contact hypersensitivity to topical corticosteroids. *Am Fam Physician.* 1995; 52:779-82.
133. Asero R. Hypersensitivity to diazepam. *Allergy.* 2002; 57:1209.
134. Kreimeier U, Christ F, Kraft D et al. Anaphylaxis due to hydroxyethy-starch-reactive antibodies. *Lancet.* 1995; 346:49-50.
135. Takuma H, Kawagishi T, Kyogoku I et al. A case of primary and generalized allergy to human insulin with no history of any prior insulin exposure. *Diabetes Res Clin Pract.* 1995; 30:69-73.
136. Mackley CL, Marks JG, Anderson BE. Delayed type hypersensitivity reaction to lidocaine. *Arch Dermatol.* 203; 139:343-6.
137. Phy JL, Weiss WT, Weiler CR et al. Hypersensitivity to progesterone-in-oil after in vitro fertilization and embryo transfer. *Fertil Steril.* 2003; 80:1272-5.
138. Freeman GL. Psyllium hypersensitivity. *Ann Allergy.* 1994; 73:490-2.
139. Ponvert C, Scheinmann P. Vaccine allergy and pseudo-allergy. *Eur I Dermatol.* 2003; 13:10-15.
140. De Week AL. Pharmacologic and immunochemical mechanisms of drug hypersensitivity. *Immunol Allergy Clin North Am.* 1991; 11:461-74.
141. Campo P, Fernandez TD, Canto G et al. Angioedema induced by angiotensin-converting enzyme inhibitors. *Curr Opin Allergy Clin Immunol.* 2013; 13:337-44.
142. Pavletic AJ. Late angioedema in patients with angiotensin-converting enzyme inhibitors. *Lancet.* 2002; 360:493-4.
143. Lo KS. Angioedema with candesartan. *Pharmacotherapy.* 2002; 22:1176-9.
144. Borazan A, Ustun H, Yilmaz A. Angioedema induced by angiotensin II blocker telmisartan. *Allergy.* 2003; 58:454.
145. Irons BK, Kumar A. Valsartan-induced angioedema. *Ann Pharmacother.* 2003; 37:1024-7.
146. Haymore BR, Yoon J, Mikita CP et al. Risk of angioedema with angiotensin receptor blockers in patients with prior angioedema associated with angiotensin-converting enzyme inhibitors: a meta-analysis. *Ann Allergy Asthma Immunol.* 2008; 101:495-9.
147. Assouad M, Willcourt RJ. Anaphylactoid reaction to ciprofloxacin. *Ann Intern Med.* 1995; 122:396-7.
148. Ho DY, Song JC, Wang CC. Anaphylactoid reaction to ciprofloxacin. *Ann Pharmacother.* 2003; 37:1018-23.
149. Davis H, McGoodwin E, Reed TG. Anaphylactoid reactions reported after treatment with ciprofloxacin. *Ann Intern Med.* 1989; 111:1041-3.
150. Ventura MT, Muratore L, Calogiuri GF et al. Allergic and pseudoallergic reactions induced by glucocorticoids: a review. *Curr Pharm Des.* 2003; 9:1956-64.
151. MacLauglin EJ, Fitzpatrick KT, Sbar E et al. Anaphylactoid reaction to enoxaparin in a patient with deep venous thrombosis. *Pharmacotherapy.* 2002; 2:1511-5.
152. Cheifetz A, Smerdley M, Martin S et al. The incidence and management of infusion reactions to infliximab: a large center experience. *Am J Gastroenterol.* 2003; 98:1315-24.
153. Lobel EZ, Korelitz BI, Warman JI. Red man syndrome and infliximab. *J Clin Gastroenterol.* 2003; 36:186.
154. Smythe MA, Cappelletty DM. Anaphylactoid reaction to levofloxacin. *Pharmacotherapy.* 2000; 20:1520-3.
155. Fujita Y, Ishikawa H, Yokota K. Anaphylactoid reaction to midazolam. *Anesth Analg.* 1994; 79:811-2.
156. Berkowitz RJ, Possidente CJ, McPherson BR et al. Anaphylactoid reaction to muromonab-CD3 in a pediatric renal transplant recipient. *Pharmacotherapy.* 2000; 20:100-4.
157. Appelboam AV, Dargan PI, Knighton J. Fatal anaphylactoid reaction to *N*-acetylcysteine: caution in patients with asthma. *Emerg Med J.* 2002; 19:594-5.
158. Kossey JL, Kwok KK. Anaphylactoid reactions associated with ondansetron. *Ann Pharmacother.* 1994; 28:1029-30.
159. Ross AK, Ferrero-Conover D. Anaphylactoid reaction due to the administration of ondansetron in a pediatric neurosurgical patient. *Anesth Analg.* 1998; 87:779-80.
160. Lee AF, Gawkrodger DJ, Thomas WE. Generalized pruritus with opioids. *Lancet.* 1994; 344:1031.
161. Brockow K, Sanchez-Borges M. Hypersensitivity to contrast media and dyes. *Immunol Allergy Clin N Am.* 2014; 34:547-64.
162. Borda I, Slone D, Jick H. Assessment of adverse reactions within a drug surveillance program. *JAMA.* 1968; 205:645-7.
163. Hunziker T, Bruppacher R, Kuenzi UP et al. Classification of ADRs: a proposal for harmonization and differentiation based on experience with the Comprehensive Hospital Drug Monitoring Bern/St. Gallen, 1974-1993. *Pharmacoepidemiol Drug Saf.* 2002; 11:159-63.
164. Lieberman P, Camargo CA, Bohlke K et al. Epidemiology of anaphylaxis: findings of the American College of Allergy, Asthma and Immunology Epidemiology of Anaphylaxis Working Group. *Ann Allergy Asthma Immunol.* 2006; 97:596-602.

165. Neugut A, Ghatak A, Miller R. Anaphylaxis in the United States: an investigation into its epidemiology. *Arch Intern Med.* 2001; 161:15-21.
166. Pigman EC, Scott JL. Angioedema in the emergency department: the impact of angiotensin-converting enzyme inhibitors. *Am J Emerg Med.* 1993; 11:350-4.
167. Gabb GM, Ryan P, Wing LM et al. Epidemiologic study of angioedema and ACE inhibitors. *Aust N Z J Med.* 1996; 26:777-82.
168. Gruchalla RS. Drug metabolism, danger signals and drug-induced hypersensitivity. *J Allergy Clin Immunol.* 2001; 108:475-88.
169. Wheatley LM, Plaut M, Schwaninger JM et al. Report from the National Institute of Allergy and Infectious Diseases workshop on drug allergy. *J Allergy Clin Immunol.* 2015; 136:262-71.
170. Naisbett DJ, Pirmohamed M, Park BK. Immunopharmacology of hypersensitivity reactions to drugs. *Curr Allergy Asthma Rep.* 2003; 3:22-9.
171. Knowles S, Shapiro L, Shear NH. Should celecoxib be contraindicated in patients who are allergic to sulfonamides? Revisiting the meaning of sulfa allergy. *Drug Saf.* 2001; 24:239-47.
172. Adam J, Pichler WJ, Yerly D. Delayed drug hypersensitivity: models of T-cell stimulation. *Br J Clin Pharmacol.* 2011; 71:701-7.
173. Ju C, Uetrecht JP. Mechanism of idiosyncratic drug reactions: reactive metabolites formation, protein binding and the regulation of the immune system. *Curr Drug Metab.* 2002; 3:367-77.
174. Pirmohamed M, Naisbett DJ, Gordon F et al. The danger hypothesis: potential role in idiosyncratic drug reactions. *Toxicology.* 2002; 181-182:55-63.
175. Parkin J, Cohen B. An overview of the immune system. *Lancet.* 2001; 357:1777-89.
176. Coombs PR, Gell PG. Classification of allergic reactions responsible for clinical hypersensitivity and disease. In: Gell RR, ed. *Clinical Aspects of Immunology.* Oxford, England: Oxford University Press; 1968:575-96.
177. Demoly P, Hillaire-Buys D. Classification and epidemiology of hypersensitivity drug reactions. *Immunol Allergy Clin North Am.* 2004; 24:345–56.
178. Roitt I, Brostoff J, Male D. Hypersensitivity: types 1-4. In: *Immunology.* 2nd ed. London, England: Gower Medical Publishing; 1985:19.1-22.9.
179. Kemp SF, Lockey RF. Anaphylaxis: a review of causes and mechanisms. *J Allergy Clin Immunol.* 2002; 110:341-8.
180. Tang AW. A practical guide to anaphylaxis. *Am Fam Physician.* 2003; 68:1325-32;1339-40.
181. Pichler WJ. Delayed drug hypersensitivity reactions. *Ann Intern Med.* 2003; 139:683-93.
182. DeShazo RD, Kemp SF. Allergic reactions to drugs and biologic agents. *JAMA* 1997; 278:1895-906.
183. Stevenson DD, Zuraw BL. Pathogenesis of aspirin-exacerbated respiratory disease. *Clin Rev Allergy Immunol.* 2003; 24:169-87.
184. Lieberman P, Nicklas RA, Randolph C et al. Anaphylaxis—a practice parameter update 2015. *Ann Allergy Asthma Immunol.* 2015; 115:341-84.
185. Vadas P, Gold M, Perelman B et al. Platelet-activating factor, PAF acetylhydrolase, and severe anaphylaxis. *N Engl J Med.* 2008; 358:28-35.
186. Agostoni A, Cicardi M. Drug-induced angioedema without urticaria. *Drug Saf.* 2001; 24:599-606.
187. Levenson DE, Arndt K, Stern RS. Cutaneous manifestations of adverse drug reactions. *Immunol Allergy Clin North Am.* 1991; 11:493-516.
188. Roujeau JC, Stern RS. Severe cutaneous reactions to drugs. *N Engl J Med.* 1994; 331:1272-85.
189. Adkinson NF. Risk factors for drug allergy. *J Allergy Clin Immunol.* 1984; 74:567-72.
190. VanArsdel PP. Classification and risk factors for drug allergy. *Immunol Allergy Clin North Am.* 1991; 11:475-91.
191. Bigby M, Jick S, Jick H et al. Drug-induced cutaneous reactions: a report from the Boston Collaborative Drug Surveillance Program on 15,438 consecutive inpatients, 1975-1982. *JAMA.* 1986; 256:3358-63.
192. Idsoe O, Guthe T, Wilcox RR et al. Nature and extent of penicillin side chain with particular reference to fatalities from anaphylaxis. *Bull World Health Organ.* 1968; 38:159-88.
193. Mallal S, Nolan D, Witt C et al. Association between presence of HLA-B 5701, HLA-DR7 and HLA-DQ3 and hypersensitivity to HIV-1 reverse transcriptase inhibitor abacavir. *Lancet.* 2002; 359:727-32.
194. Mallal S, Phillis E, Carosi G et al. HLA-B*5701 screening for hypersensitivity to abacavir. *N Engl J Med.* 2008; 358:568-79.
195. Batchelor JR, Welsh KI, Tinoco RM et al. Hydralazine-induced systemic lupus erythematosus: influence of HLA-DR and sex on susceptibility. *Lancet.* 1980; 1:1107-9.
196. Gueant JL, Romano A, Cornejo-Garcia JA et al. HLA-DRA variants predict penicillin allergy in genome-wide fine-mapping genotyping. *J Allergy Clin Immunol.* 2015; 135:253-9.
197. Shear NH, Spielberg SP, Grant DM et al. Differences in metabolism of sulfonamides predisposing to idiosyncratic toxicity. *Ann Intern Med.* 1986; 105:179-84.
198. Rieder MJ, Shear NH, Kanee A et al. Prominence of slow acetylator phenotype among patients with sulfonamide hypersensitivity reactions. *Clin Pharmacol Ther.* 1991; 49:13-7.
199. Shear NH, Spielberg SP, Cannon M et al. Anticonvulsant hypersensitivity syndrome: in vitro risk assessment. *J Clin Invest.* 1988; 82:1826-32.
200. Pirmohamed M, Graham A, Roberts P et al. Carbamazepine hypersensitivity: assessment of clinical and in vitro chemical cross-sensitivity with phenytoin and oxcarbazepine. *Br J Clin Pharmacol.* 1991; 32:741-9.
201. Pullen H, Wright N, Murdoch J. Hypersensitivity reactions to antibacterial drugs in infectious mononucleosis. *Lancet.* 1967; 1:1176-8.
202. Shepherd GM. Allergy to beta-lactam antibiotics. *Immunol Allergy Clin N Am* 1991; 11:611-31.
203. Carr A, Cooper DA, Penny R. Allergic manifestations of human immunodeficiency virus (HIV) infection. *J Clin Immunol.* 1991; 11:55-64.
204. Descamps V, Valance A, Edkinger C et al. Association of human herpes virus 6 infection with drug reaction with eosinophilia and systemic symptoms. *Arch Dermatol.* 2001; 137:301-4.
205. Descamps V, Collot S, Mahe E et al. Active human herpes virus 6 infection in a patient with drug rash with eosinophilia and systemic symptoms. *J Invest Dermatol.* 2003; 121:215-6.
206. Ramesh S. Antibiotic hypersensitivity in patients with CF. *Clin Rev Allergy Immunol.* 2002: 23:123-41.
207. Pleasants RA, Walker TR, Samuelson WM. Allergic reactions to parenteral beta-lactam antibiotics in patients with cystic fibrosis. *Chest.* 1994; 106:1124-8.
208. Wills R, Henry RL, Francis JL. Antibiotic hypersensitivity reactions in cystic fibrosis. *J Paediatr Child Health.* 1998; 34:325-9.
209. Koch C, Hjelt K, Pederson SS et al. Retrospective clinical study of hypersensitivity reactions to aztreonam and six other beta-lactam antibiotics in cystic fibrosis patients receiving multiple treatment courses. *Rev Infect Dis.* 1991; 13(suppl 7):S608-11.
210. Lang DM, Alpern MB, Visintainer PF et al. Gender risk for anaphylactoid reaction to radiographic contrast media. *J Allergy Clin Immunol.* 1995; 95:813-7.
211. Lang DM, Alpern MB, Visintainer PF et al. Increased risk for anaphylactoid reaction from contrast media in patients on beta-adrenergic blockers or with asthma. *Ann Intern Med.* 1991; 115:270-6.
212. Toogood JH. Risk of anaphylaxis in patients receiving beta-blocker drugs. *J Allergy Clin Immunol.* 1988; 81:1-5.
213. Brown NJ, Ray WA, Snowden M et al. Black Americans have an increased rate of angiotensin converting enzyme inhibitor-associated angioedema. *Clin Pharmacol Ther.* 1996; 60:8-13.

214. Brown NJ, Nadeau JH. Does race predispose to angiotensin-associated angioneurotic edema? *Ann Intern Med.* 1993; 119:1224.

215. Settipane GA, Chafee FH, Klein DE. Aspirin intolerance. *J Allergy Clin Immunol.* 1974; 53:200-4.

216. Sanchez-Borges M, Capriles-Hulett A, Caballero-Fonseca F. NSAID-induced urticaria and angioedema: a reappraisal of its clinical management. *Am J Clin Dermatol.* 2002; 3:599-607.

217. Lieberman P. Anaphylactoid reactions to radiocontrast material. *Immunol Allergy Clin North Am.* 1992; 12:649-70.

218. Green GR, Rosenblum AH, Sweet LC. Evaluation of penicillin hypersensitivity: value of clinical history and skin testing with penicilloyl-polylysine and penicillin G. *I Allergy Clin Immunol.* 1977; 60:339-45.

219. Health and Environmental Sciences Institute Task Force. Task Force Report: future research needs for the prevention and management of immune-mediated drug hypersensitivity reactions. *J Allergy Clin Immunol.* 2002: 109:S461-78.

220. Solensky R, Khan DA, Bernstein IL et al. Drug allergy: an updated practice parameter. *Ann Allergy Asthma Immunol.* 2010; 105:259–73.

221. Solensky R. Drug desensitization. *Immunol Allergy Clin North Am.* 2004; 24:425–43.

222. Yates AB. Management of patients with history of allergy to beta-lactam antibiotics. *Am J Med.* 2008; 121:572–6.

223. Liu A, Fanning L, Chong H et al. Desensitization regimens for drug allergy: state of the art in the 21st century. *Clin Exp Allergy* 2011; 41:1679–89.

224. Macy E. Penicillin and beta-lactam allergy: epidemiology and diagnosis. *Curr Allergy Asthma Rep.* 2014; 14:476-7.

225. Khan DA, Solensky R. Drug allergy. *J Allergy Clin Immunol.* 2010; 125(suppl):S126–37.

226. Green GR, Rosenblum AH, Sweet LC. Evaluation of penicillin hypersensitivity: value of clinical history and skin testing with penicilloyl-polylysine and penicillin G. *I Allergy Clin Immunol.* 1977; 60:339-45.

227. Saxon A, Beall GN, Rohr AS et al. Immediate hypersensitivity reactions to beta-lactam antibiotics. *Ann Intern Med.* 1987; 107:204-15.

228. Solensky R. Hypersensitivity reactions to beta-lactam antibiotics. *Clin Rev Allergy Immunol.* 2003; 24:201-19.

229. Saxon A, Hassner A, Swabb EA et al. Lack of cross-reactivity between aztreonam, a monobactam antibiotic, and penicillin in penicillin-allergic subjects. *J Infect Dis.* 1984; 149:16-22.

230. Romano A, Quaratino D, Papa G et al. Aminopenicillin allergy. *Arch Dis Child.* 1997; 76:513-7.

231. Romano A, DiFonso M, Viola M et al. Selective hypersensitivity to piperacillin. *Allergy.* 2000; 55:787.

232. Bousquet PJ, Co-Minh HB, Amoux B, Daures JP, Demoly P. Importance of mixture of minor determinants and benzylpenicilloyl polylysine skin testing in the diagnosis of beta-lactam allergy. *J Allerg Clin Immunol.* 2005; 115:1314–6.

233. Blanca M, Mayorga C, Torres MJ et al. Side chain specific reactions to beta-lactams: 14 years later. *Clin Exp Allergy.* 2002; 32:192–7.

234. Pichichero ME, Casey JR. Sale use of selected cephalosporins in penicillin-allergic patients: a meta-analysis. *Otolaryngol Head Neck Surg.* 2007; 136:340-7.

235. Sodhi M, Axtell SS, Callahan J et al. Is it sale to use carbapenems in patients with history of allergy to penicillin? *J Antimicrob Chemother.* 2004; 54:1155-7.

236. McConnell SA, Penzak SR, Warmack TS et al. Incidence of imipenem hypersensitivity reactions in febrile neutropenic bone marrow transplant patients with a history of penicillin allergy. *Clin Infect Dis.* 2000; 31:1512-4.

237. Prescott WA, DePestel DD, Ellis JJ et al. Incidence of carbapenem-associated allergic-type reactions among patients with versus patients without a reported penicillin allergy. *Clin Infect Dis.* 2004; 38:1102-7.

238. Saxon A, Adelman DC, Patel A et al. Imipenem cross-reactivity with penicillin in humans. *J Allergy Clin Immunol.* 1988; 82:213-7.

239. Romano A, Viola M, Gueant-Rodriguez RM et al. Imipenem in patients with immediate hypersensitivity to penicillins. *N Engl J Med.* 2006; 354:2835-7.

240. Romano A, Viola M, Gueant-Rodriguez RM et al. Brief communication: tolerability of meropenem in patients with IgE-mediated hypersensitivity to penicillins. *Ann Intern Med.* 2007; 146:266-9.

241. Atanaskovic-Markovic M, Gaeta F, Medjo B et al. Tolerability of meropenem in children with IgE-mediated hypersensitivity to penicillins. *Allergy.* 2008; 63:237-40.

242. Gaeta F, Valluzzi RL, Alonzi C et al. Tolerability of aztreonam and carbapenems in patients with IgE-mediated hypersensitivity to penicillins. *J Allergy Clin Immunol.* 2015; 135:972-6.

243. Wilson DL, Owens RC, Zuckerman JB. Successful meropenem desensitization in a patient with cystic flbrosis. *Ann Pharmacother.* 2003; 37:1424-8.

244. Baer SL, Wall GC, Skoglund KJ et al. Lack of cross-reactivity to meropenem in a patient with an allergy to imipenem. *J Allergy Clin Immunol.* 2004: 113:173-5.

245. Wulf NR, Matuszewski KA. Sulfonamide cross-reactivity: is there evidence to support broad cross-allergenicity? *Am J Health-Syst Pharm.* 2013; 70:1483-94.

246. Brackett CC, Singh H, Block JH. Likelihood and mechanisms of cross-allergenicity between sulfonamide antibiotics and other drugs containing a sulfonamide functional group. *Pharmacother.* 2004; 24:856-70.

247. Arndt KA, Jick H. Rates of cutaneous reactions to drugs: a report of the Boston Collaborative Drug Surveillance Program. *JAMA.* 1976; 235:918-22.

248. Strom BL, Schinnar R, Apter AJ et al. Absence of cross-reactivity between sulfonamide antibiotics and sulfonamide nonantibiotics. *N Engl J Med.* 2003; 349:1628-35.

249. Ernst EJ, Egge JA. Celecoxib-induced erythema multiforme with glyburide cross-reactivity. *Pharmacotherapy.* 2002; 22:637-40.

250. Glasser DL, Burrouughs SH. Valdecoxib-induced toxic epidermal necrolysis in a patient allergic to sulla drugs. *Pharmacotherapy.* 2003 ;23:551-3.

251. Wall GC, Bigner D, Craig S. Ethacrynic acid and the sulla-sensitive patient. *Arch Intern Med.* 2003; 163:116-7.

252. Earl G, Davenport J, Narula J. Furosemide challenge in patients with heart failure and adverse reactions to sulla-containing diuretics. *Ann Intern Med.* 2003; 138:358-9.

253. Li J, Fernando SL. Successful rapid desensitization to hydrochlorothiazide. *Ann Allergy Asthma and Immunol.* 2013; 110:307-8.

254. Shapiro LE, Knowles SR, Shear NH. Comparative safety of tetracycline, minocycline and doxycycline. *Arch Dermatol.* 1997; 133:1224-30.

255. Ye YM, Thong, BYH, Park HS. Hypersensitivity to antiepileptic drugs. *Immunol Allergy Clin N Am.* 2014; 34:633-43.

256. Bohan KH, Mansuri TF, Wilson NM. Anticonvulsant hypersensitivity syndrome: implications for pharmaceutical care. *Pharmacotherapy.* 2007; 27:1425-39.

257. Zakrzewska JM, Ivanyi L. In vitro lymphocyte proliferation by carbamazepine, carbamazepine-10,11-epoxide and oxcarbazepine in the diagnosis ol drug-induced hypersensitivity. *J Allergy Clin Immunol.* 1988; 82:110-5.

258. Beran RG. Cross-reactive skin eruption with both carbamazepine and oxcarbazepine. *Epilepsia.* 1993; 34:163-5.

259. Purcell RT, Lockey RF. Immunologic responses to therapeutic biologic agents. *J Investig Allergol Clin Immunol.* 2008; 18:335-42.

260. Kapetanovic MC, Larsson L, Truedsson L et al. Predictors of infusion reactions during infliximab treatment in patients with arthritis. *Arthritis Res Ther.* 2006; 8:R131.

261. Limb SL, Starke PR, Lee CE et al. Delayed onset and protracted progression of anaphylaxis after omalizumab administration in patients with asthma. *J Allergy Clin Immunol.* 2007; 120:1378-81.
262. Cox L, Platts-Mills TAE, Finegold T et al. American Academy of Allergy, Asthma and Immunology/American College of Allergy, Asthma and Immunology Joint Task Force Report on omalizumab-associated anaphylaxis. *J Allergy Clin Immunol.* 2007; 120:1373–7.
263. Vultaggio A, Castells MC. Hypersensitivity to biologic agents. *Immunol Allergy Clin N Am.* 2014; 34: 615-32.
264. ONeil BH, Allen R, Spigel DR et al. High incidence of cetuximab-related infusion reactions in Tennessee and North Carolina and the association with atopic history. *J Clin Oncol.* 2007; 25:3644-8.
265. Liu A, Fanning L, Chong H et al. Desensitization regimens for drug allergy: state of the art in the 21st century. *Clin Exp Allergy.* 2011; 41:1679–89.
266. Jareth MR, Kwan M, Kannarkat M et al. A desensitization protocol for the mAb cetuximab. *J Allergy Clin Immunol.* 2009; 123:260-2.
267. Brown NJ, Snowden M, Griffin MR. Recurrent ACEI-associated angioedema. *JAMA.* 1997; 278:232-3.
268. Warner KK, Visconti JA, Tschampel MM. Angiotensin II receptor blockers in patients with ACE inhibitor-induced angioedema. *Ann Pharmacother.* 2000; 34:526-8.
269. Makani H, Messerli FH, Romero J et al. Meta-analysis of randomized trials of angioedema associated with the use of drugs that target the renin-angiotensin-aldosterone system. *Arch Intern Med.* 2012; 172:1582-9.
270. Gavras I, Gavras H. Are patients who develop angioedema with ACE inhibitors at risk of the same problem with ATI receptor blockers? *Arch Intern Med.* 2003; 163:240.
271. Kang LW, Kidon MI, Chin CW et al. Severe anaphylactic reaction to ibuprofen in a child with recurrent urticaria. *Pediatrics.* 2007; 120:e742-4.
272. Martin-Garcia C, Hinojosa M, Berges P et al. Safety of a cyclo-oxygenase-2 inhibitor in patients with aspirin-sensitive asthma. *Chest.* 2002; 121:1812-7.
273. Gyllfors P, Bochenek G, Overholt J et al. Biochemical and clinical evidence that aspirin-intolerant asthmatic subjects tolerate the cyclo-oxygenase-2 selective analgesic drug, celecoxib. *Allergy Clin Immunol.* 2003; 111:1116-21.
274. West PM, Fernandez C. Safety of COX-2 inhibitors in asthma patients with aspirin hypersensitivity. *Ann Pharmacother.* 2003; 37:1497-1501.
275. Woessner KM. Aspirin desensitization for cardiovascular disease. *Curr Opin Allergy Clin Immunol.* 2015; 15:314-22.
276. Stevenson DD. Aspirin desensitization in patients with AERD. *Clin Rev Allergy Immunol.* 2003; 24:159-67.
277. Page NA, Schroeder WS. Rapid desensitization for patients with cardiovascular disease and aspirin hypersensitivity in an era of dual antiplatelet therapy. *Ann Pharmacother.* 2007; 41:61-7.
278. Greenberger PA, Patterson R. The prevention of immediate generalized reactions to radiocontrast media in high-risk patients. *J Allergy Clin Immunol.* 1991; 87:867-72.
279. Brockow K, Sanchez-Borges M. Hypersensitivity to contrast media and dyes. *Immunol Allergy Clin N Am.* 2014; 34:547-64.
280. Kintzel PE. Prophylaxis for paclitaxel hypersensitivity reactions. *Ann Pharmacother.* 2001; 35:1114-7.
281. Markham M, Kennedy A, Webster K et al. An effective and more convenient drug regimen for prophylaxis against paclitaxel-associated hypersensitivity reactions. *J Cancer Res Clin Oncol.* 1999; 125:427-9.
282. Sicherer SH. Advances in anaphylaxis and hypersensitivity reactions to foods, drugs and insect venom. *J Allergy Clin Immunol.* 2003; 111:S829-34.
283. Simons FE, Gu X, Simons KJ. Epinephrine absorption in adults: intramuscular versus subcutaneous injections. *J Allergy Clin Immunol.* 2001; 108:871-3.
284. Song TT, Lieberman P. Epinephrine in anaphylaxis: doubt no more. *Curr Opin Allergy Clin Immunol.* 2015; 15:323-8.
285. Bernstein JA, Lang DM, Khan DA. The diagnosis and management of acute and chronic urticaria: 2014 update. *J Allergy Clin Immunol.* 2014; 133:1270-7.
286. Joint Task Force on Practice Parameters. The diagnosis and management of urticaria: a practice parameter Part II. Chronic urticaria/angioedema. *Ann Allergy Asthma Immunol.* 2000; 85:521-44.
287. McKenna JK, Lieferman KM. Dermatologic drug reactions. *Immunol Allergy Clin North Am.* 2004; 24:399-423.
288. Roujeau JC, Kelly JP, Naldi L et al. Medication use and the risk of Stevens-Johnson syndrome or toxic epidermal necrolysis. *N Engl J Med.* 1995; 333:1600-7.
289. Fiszenson-Albala F, Auzerie V, Mahe E et al. A 6-month prospective survey of cutaneous drug reactions in a hospital setting. *Br J Dermatol.* 2003; 149:1018-22.
290. Mockenhaupt M, Viboud C, Dunant A et al. Stevens-Johnson syndrome and toxic epidermal necrolysis: assessment of medication risks with emphasis on recently marketed drugs. The EuroSCAR-study. *J Invest Dermatol.* 2008; 128:35-44.
291. Hurwitz RM. Steroid acne. *J Am Acad Dermatol.* 1989; 21:1179-81.
292. Monk B, Cunliffe WJ, Layton AM et al. Acne induced by inhaled corticosteroids. *Clin Exp Dermatol.* 1993; 18:148-50.
293. Fung MA. A prospective study of acute onset steroid acne associated with administration of intravenous corticosteroids. *Dermatology.* 2000; 200:43-4.
294. Agero ALC, Dusza SW, Benvenuto-Andrade C et al. Dermatologic side effects associated with the epidermal growth factor receptor inhibitors. *J Am Acad Dermatol.* 2006; 55:657-70.
295. Segaert S, Van Cutsen E. Clinical signs, pathophysiology and management of skin toxicity during therapy with epidermal growth factor receptor inhibitors. *Ann Oncol.* 2005; 16:1425-33.
296. Lee PK, Dover JS. Recurrent exacerbation of acne by granulocyte colony-stimulating factor administration. *J Am Acad Dermatol.* 1996; 34(5 Pt. 1):855-6.
297. Bassi E, Poli F, Charachon A et al. Infliximab-induced acne: report of 2 cases. *Br J Dermatol.* 2007; 156:402-3.
298. Valeyrie-Allanore L, Sassolas B, Roujeau JC. Drug-induced skin, nail and hair disorders. *Drug Saf.* 2007; 30:1011-30.
299. Nielson JN, Licht RW, Fogh K. Two cases of acneiform eruption associated with lamotrigine. *J Clin Psychiatry.* 2004; 65:1720-2.
300. Oztas P, Aksakal AB, Oztas MO. Severe acne with lithium. *Ann Pharmacother.* 2001; 35:961-92.
301. Bakos L, Bakos RM. Focal acne during topical tacrolimus therapy for vitiligo. *Arch Dermatol.* 2007; 143:1223-4.
302. Sehgal VN, Srivastava G. Fixed drug eruption (FDE): changing scenario of incriminating drugs. *Int J Dermatol.* 2006; 45:897-908.
303. Allchurch LG, Crilly H. Fixed drug eruption to propofol. *Anaesth Intensive Care.* 2014; 42:777-81.
304. Genest G, Thomson DM. Fixed drug eruption to quinine: a case report and review of the literature. *J Allergy Clin Immunol Pract.* 2014; 2:469-70.
305. Kaku Y, Ito T, Kudo K et al. Generalized fixed drug eruption induced by tranexamic acid. *European J Dermatol.* 2014; 24:408-9.
306. Sriatanaviriyakul N, Nguyen LP, Henerson MC et al. Drug reaction with eosinophilia and systemic symptoms (DRESS) syndrome associated with azithromycin presenting like septic shock: a case report. *J Med Case Rep.* 2014; 8:332.
307. Goodfield MJ, Milard LG. Severe cutaneous reactions to captopril. *BMJ.* 1985; 290:111.
308. Bourneau-Marin D, Leclech C, Jamet, A et al. Omeprazole-induced drug reaction with eosinophilia and systemic symptoms (DRESS). *Eur J Dermatol.* 2014; 24:413-5.
309. Chaabane A, Fadhel N, Chadli Z et al. Phenobarbital-induced DRESS: a lichenoid picture. *Iran J Allergy Asthma Immunol.* 2014; 13:435-5.

310. Cabanas R, Calderon O, Ramirez E et al. Piperacillin-induced DRESS: distinguishing features observed in a clinical and allergy study of 8 patients. *J Investig Allergol Clin Immunol.* 2014; 24:425-30.
311. Ripamonti D, Benatti SV, DiFilippo E et al. Drug reaction with eosinophilia and systemic symptoms associated with raltegravir use: case report and review of the literature. *AIDS.* 2014; 28:1077-9.
312. Tamagawa-Mineoka R, Katoh N, Nara T et al. DRESS syndrome caused by teicoplanin and vancomycin associated with reactivation of HHV-6. *Int J Dermatol.* 2007; 46:654-5.
313. Tsankov N, Kazandjieva J, Drenovska K. Drugs in exacerbation and provocation of psoriasis. *Clin Dermatol.* 1998; 16:333-51.
314. Dika E, Varotti C, Bardazzi F et al. Drug-induced psoriasis: an evidence-based overview and the introduction of a psoriatic drug eruption probability score. *Cutan Ocul Toxicol.* 2006; 25:1-11.
315. Cohen JD, Bournerias I, Buffard V et al. Psoriasis induced by tumor necrosis factor-alpha antagonist therapy: a case series. *J Rheumatol.* 2007; 34:380-5.
316. Pirgon O, Atabek ME, Sert A. Psoriasis following growth hormone therapy in a child. *Ann Pharmacother.* 2007; 41:157-60.
317. Verea MM, DelPozo J, Yebra-Pimental MT et al. Psoriasiform eruption induced by infliximab. *Ann Pharmacother.* 2004; 38:54-7.
318. Kwan Z, Che Ismail RB, Wong SM et al. Sodium valproate-aggravated psoriasiform eruption. *International J Dermatol.* 2014; 53:e477-9.
319. Letko E, Papialiodis DN, Papaliodis GN et al. Stevens-Johnson syndrome and toxic epidermal necrolysis: a review of the literature. *Ann Allergy Clin Immunol.* 2005; 94:419-36.
320. Biswal S, Sahoo SS. Paracetamol induced Stevens-Johnson syndrome-toxic epidermal necrolysis overlap syndrome. *Int J Dermatol.* 2014; 53:1042-4.
321. FDA Drug Safety Communication: FDA warns of rare but serious skin reactions with the pain reliever/fever reducer acetaminophen. http://www.fda.gov/downloads/Drugs/DrugSafety/UCM363052.pdf (accessed 2017 Dec 19).
322. Halevy S, Ghiskain PD, Mockenhaupt M et al. Allopurinol is the most common cause of Stevens-Johnson syndrome and toxic epidermal necrolysis in Europe and Israel. *J Am Acad Dermatol.* 2008; 58:25-32.
323. Islam S, Singer M, Kulhanjian JA. Toxic epidermal necrolysis in a neonate receiving fluconazole. *J Perinatal.* 2014; 34:792-4.
324. Chan JC, Yap DY, Yeung CK. Hydralazine-induced toxic epidermal necrolysis in a patient on continuous ambulatory peritoneal dialysis. *J Clin Pharm Ther.* 2014; 39:322-4.
325. Bois E, Holle LM, Farooq U. Late onset imatinib-induced Stevens Johnson syndrome. *J Oncology Pharmacy Practice* 2014; 20:476-8.
326. Digwood-Lettieri S, Reilly KJ, Haith LR et al. Levofloxacin-induced TEN in an elderly patient. *Pharmacotherapy* 2002; 22:789-93.
327. Islam AF, Rahman MS. Levofloxacin-induced fatal toxic epidermal necrolysis. *Ann Pharmacother* 2005; 39:1136-7.
328. Fukuraga K, Ohda Y, Inoue T et al. TEN associated with mesalamine in a patient with ulcerative colitis. *Inflamm Bowel Dis.* 2007; 13:1055-6.
329. FDA Medwatch Safety Alert. Provigil (modafinil tablets). http://www.fda.gov/Safety/MedWatch/SafetyInformation/SafetyAlertsforHumanMedicalProducts/ucm152701.htm (accessed 2017 Dec 19).
330. Howard-Thompson A, Cartmell B, Suda KJ. Toxic epidermal necrolysis reaction associated with moxifloxacin. *Int J Antimicrob Agents.* 2014; 44:178-9.
331. Jao J, Sturdevant M, del Rio Martin J et al. Nevirapine-induced Stevens Johnson syndrome and fulminant hepatic failure requiring liver transplantation. *Am J Transplant.* 2010; 10:1713-6.
332. Parmar NV, Kuruvila S, Ganguly S et al. Ofloxacin eyedrops-induced toxic epidermal necrolysis treated with intravenous immunoglobulin. *Int J Dermatol.* 2014; 53:e547-8.
333. Huang DB, Wu JJ, Lahart CJ. TEN as a complication of treatment with voriconazole. *South Med J.* 2004; 97:1116-7.
334. Gelwix TJ, Beeson MS. Warfarin-induced skin necrosis. *Am J Emerg Med.* 1998; 16:541-3.
335. Chia FL, Leong KP. Severe cutaneous adverse reactions to drugs. *Curr Opin Allergy Clin Immunol.* 2007; 7:304-9.
336. Stern RS. Utilization of hospital and outpatient care for adverse cutaneous reactions to medications. *Pharmacoepidemiol Drug Saf.* 2005; 14:677-84.
337. Wolf R, Orion E, Marcos B et al. Life-threatening acute adverse cutaneous reactions. *Clin Dermatol.* 2005; 23:171-81.
338. Merk HF, Baron JM, Neis MM et al. Skin: major target organ of allergic reactions to small molecular weight compounds. *Toxicol Appl Pharmacol.* 2007; 224:313-7.
339. Naisbett DJ. Drug hypersensitivity reactions in skin: understanding mechanisms and the development of diagnostic and predictive tests. *Toxicology.* 2004; 194:179-96.
340. Roberts RJ, Sylvia LM. Drug-induced integumentary disease In: Papadopoulos J, Cooper B, Kane-Gill S et al, eds. *Drug-induced complications in the critically ill patient: A guide for recognition and treatment.* Mt Prospect, IL: Society of Critical Care Medicine; 2012:223-42.
341. Yawalkar N. Drug-induced exanthems. *Toxicology.* 2005; 209:131-4.
342. Stern RS. Exanthematous drug eruptions. *New Engl J Med.* 2012; 366:2492-501.
343. Kardaun SH, Sidoroff A, Valeyrie-Allanore L et al. Variability in the clinical pattern of cutaneous side-effects of drugs with systemic symptoms: does a DRESS syndrome really exist? *Br J Dermatol.* 2007; 156:575-612.
344. Flowers H, Brodell R, Brents M et al. Fixed drug eruptions: presentation, diagnosis and management. *South Med J.* 2014; 107:724-7.
345. Prendiville J. Stevens-Johnson syndrome and toxic epidermal necrolysis. *Adv Dermatol.* 2002; 18:151-73.
346. Caroub P, Musette P, Descamps V et al. The DRESS syndrome: a literature review. *Am J Med.* 2011; 124:588-97.
347. Volcheck GW. Clinical evaluation and management of drug hypersensitivity. *Immunol Allergy Clin North Am.* 2004; 24:357-71.
348. Pereira FA, Mudgil AV, Rosmarin DM. Toxic epidermal necrolysis. *J Am Acad Dermatol.* 2007; 56:181-200.
349. Bastuji-Garin S, Rzany B, Stern RS et al. Clinical classification of cases of TEN, SJS and erythema multiforme. *Arch Dermatol.* 1993; 129:92-6.
350. Bastuji-Garin S, Fouchard N, Bertucci M et al. SCORTEN: a severity of illness score for TEN. *J Invest Dermatol.* 2000; 115:149-53.
351. Hermandez-Salazar A, Rosales SPL, Rangel-Frausto S et al. Epidemiology of adverse cutaneous drug reactions: a prospective study in hospitalized patients. *Arch Med Res.* 2006; 37:899-902.
352. Arif H, Buchsbaum R, Weintraub D et al. Comparison and predictors of rash associated with 15 antiepilepticdrugs. *Neurology.* 2007; 68:1701-9.
353. Alvestad S, Lydersen S, Brodtkorb E. Rash from antiepileptic drugs: influence by gender, age and learning disability. *Epilepsia.* 2007; 48:1360-5.
354. Hirsch LJ, Weintraub DB, Buchsbaum R et al. Predictors of lamotrigine-associated rash. *Epilepsia.* 2006; 47:318-22.
355. Chung WH, Hung SI, Hong HS et al. A marker for Stevens Johnson syndrome. *Nature.* 2004; 428:486.
356. Man CBL, Kwan P, Baum L et al. Association between HLA-B*1502 and antiepileptic drug-induced cutaneous reactions in Han Chinese. *Epilepsia.* 2007; 48:1015-8.

357. Ozeki T, Mushiroda T, Yowang A et al. Genome-wide association study identified HLA-B*3101 allele as a genetic risk factor for carbamazepine-induced cutaneous adverse drug reactions in Japanese population. *Hum Mol Genet.* 2011; 20:1034-41.

358. Chung WH, Chang WC, Lee YS et al. Genetic variants associated with phenytoin-related severe cutaneous adverse reactions. *JAMA.* 2014; 312:525-34.

359. Chantarangsu S, Mushiroda T, Mahasirimongkol S et al. HLA-B*3505 allele is a strong predictor for nevirapine-induced skin adverse drug reactions in HIV infected Thai patients. *Pharmacogenet Genomics.* 2009; 19:139-46

360. Funck-Brentano E, Duong TA, Bouvresse S et al. Therapeutic management of DRESS: a retrospective study of 38 cases. *J Am Acad Dermatol.* 2015; 72:246-52.

361. Law EH, Leung M. Corticosteroids in Stevens-Johnson syndrome/toxic epidermal necrolysis: current evidence and implications for future research. *Ann Pharmacol.* 2015; 49:335-42.

362. Metry DW, Jung P, Levy ML. Use of intravenous immunoglobulin in children with SJS and TEN: seven cases and review of the literature. *Pediatrics.* 2003; 112:1430-6.

363. Ruetter A, Luger TA. Efficacy and safety of IV immunoglobulin for immune-mediated skin disease. *Am J Clin Dermatol.* 2004; 5:153-60.

364. Bachot N, Roujeau JC. Intravenous immunoglobulins in the treatment of severe drug eruptions. *Curr Opin Allergy Clin Immunol.* 2003; 3:269-74.

365. Stella M, Clemente A, Bollero D et al. Toxic epidermal necrolysis (TEN) and Stevens-Johnson syndrome (SJS): experience with high-dose intravenous immunoglobulins and topical conservative approach: a retrospective analysis. *Burns.* 2007; 33:452-9.

366. French LE, Trent JT, Kerdel FA. Use of intravenous immunoglobulin in toxic epidermal necrolysis and Stevens-Johnson syndrome: our current understanding. *Int Immunopharmacol.* 2006; 6:543-9.

367. Kirchof MG, Miliszewski MA, Sikora S et al. Retrospective review of Stevens-Johnson syndrome/toxic epidermal necrolysis treatment comparing intravenous immunoglobulin with cyclosporine. *J Am Acad Dermatol.* 2014; 71:941-7.

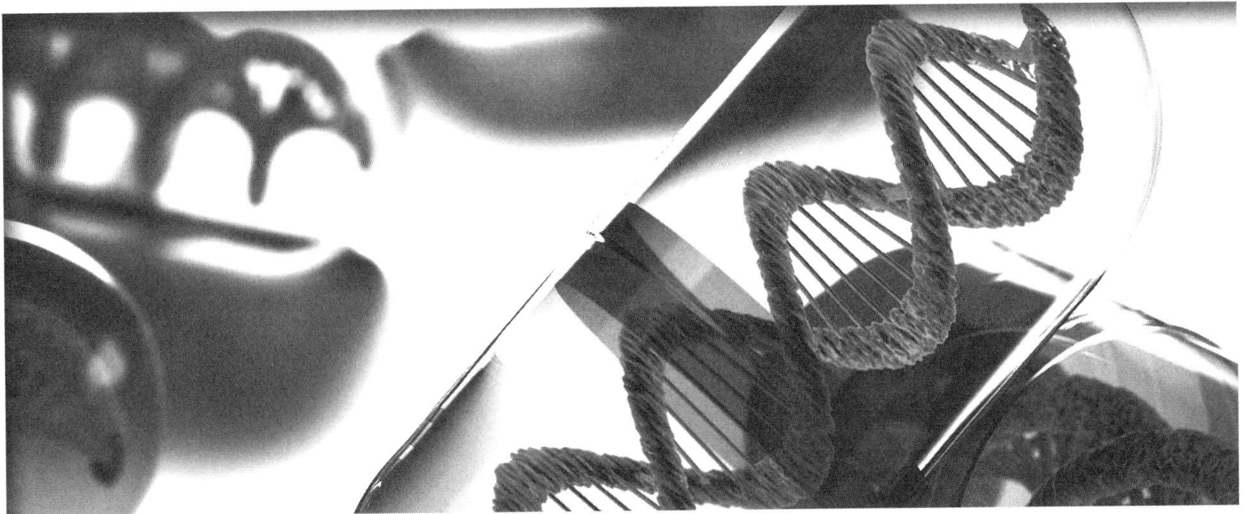

CHAPTER 7

Systemic Lupus Erythematosus-Like Syndrome

Karen W. Lee and Matthew F. Ambury

Idiopathic systemic lupus erythematosus (SLE) is an autoimmune disease of unclear etiology and pathogenesis. Clinical and laboratory findings characterizing SLE involve various organs of the body including the musculoskeletal system, skin, kidneys, and the central nervous system.[1-4] Certain drugs have been reported to cause signs and symptoms that closely mimic the presentation of SLE, and this drug-induced syndrome is often referred to as drug-induced lupus, drug-related lupus, drug-induced lupus-like syndrome, drug-induced lupus erythematosus, lupus erythematosus medicamentosus, and drug/medication-induced SLE.[1,5] For the purpose of this chapter, this syndrome will be referred to as *drug-induced lupus*.

CAUSATIVE AGENTS

Drugs that have been reported to cause drug-induced lupus are listed in **Table 7-1**.[6-202] Since sulfadiazine was first reported to cause drug-induced lupus in 1945, over 90 medications have been associated with the disease.[199,203] Although drug-induced lupus has been reported as an adverse effect in clinical trials, most of the literature is in the form of case reports.

EPIDEMIOLOGY

Approximately 5–10% of cases of SLE are drug-induced.[6,204] Using more recently published data on national prevalence of SLE, approximately 16,000–32,000 people in the Unites States are afflicted by drug-induced lupus, with some estimates as high as 50,000.[6,204,205] The estimated annual incidence of drug-induced lupus ranges from 3.2 to 9.4 cases per 100,000 persons, depending on patient-specific risk factors.[204,205] The true incidence of drug-induced lupus may in fact be much higher, as some patients may experience mild symptoms that remain unrecognized and undiagnosed.

The incidence of drug-induced lupus associated with specific agents is presented in Table 7-1.[6-202] Because the literature associating many medications

Table 7-1 Agents Implicated in Drug-Induced Lupus

Drug	Incidence	Level of Evidence[a]
MOST COMMON		
Chlorpromazine[6-20]	1%	C
Hydralazine[6,14-28]	2–21%	C
Isoniazid[6,16,18-20,29-32]	NK	C
Methyldopa[16,33-35]	NK	C
Minocycline[16,36-51]	0.05%	B
Procainamide[6,14,20,52-62]	15–35%	C
Quinidine[16,20,63-68]	NK	C
ANTICONVULSANTS		
Carbamazepine[16,69-73]	1%	C
Ethosuximide[6,16,69,74-76]	NK	C
Lamotrigine[77-79]	NK	C
Mephenytoin[75]	NK	C
Phenytoin[16,18,69,75]	NK	C
Primidone[6,16,69]	NK	C
Trimethadione[16,67,74,75]	NK	C
Troxidone[6]	NK	C
Valproate[80,81]	NK	C
Zonisamide[82]	NK	C
ANTITHYROID DRUGS		
Methimazole[6,83-85]	NK	C
Methylthiouracil[6,83]	NK	C
Propythiouracil[6,16,35,83,86,87]	NK	C
Thiamazole[83]	NK	C
CARDIOVASCULAR DRUGS		
Acebutolol[6,16,88-90]	NK	C
Amiodarone[91,92]	NK	C
Atenolol[6,16,93]	NK	C
Calcium-channel blockers (diltiazem, nifedipine, verapamil)[94,95]	NK	C
Captopril[6,16,96,97]	NK	C
Chlorthalidone[16,93]	NK	C
Clonidine[6,16,98]	NK	C
Disopyramide[16,93]	NK	C
Enalapril[16,99]	NK	C
Gemfibrozil[100,101]	NK	C
Guanoxan[6]	NK	C
HMG-CoA reductase inhibitors (atorvastatin, fluvastatin, lovastatin, pravastatin, simvastatin)[6,16,100-105]	NK	C
Hydrochlorothiazide[16,106-108]	NK	C
Labetalol[6,16,109]	NK	C

Table 7-1 Agents Implicated in Drug-Induced Lupus (continued)

Drug	Incidence	Level of Evidence[a]
Lisinopril[99]	NK	C
Metoprolol[82]	NK	C
Minoxidil[6,16,93]	NK	C
Oxprenolol[82]	NK	C
Pindolol[16,110]	NK	C
Practolol[6,111]	NK	C
Prazosin[6,16,112]	NK	C
Propafenone[16,93]	NK	C
Propranolol[113]	NK	C
Reserpine[14]	NK	C
Spironolactone[114]	NK	C
Ticlopidine[115]	NK	C
Timolol (ophthalmic)[16,93]	NK	C
Triamterene[101]	NK	C
ANTIBACTERIAL/ANTIFUNGAL AGENTS		
Cefepime[82]	NK	C
Cefuroxime[116]	NK	C
Ciprofloxacin[117]	NK	C
Doxycycline[38]	NK	C
Griseofulvin[6,118,119]	NK	C
Nafcillin[120]	NK	C
Nitrofurantoin[6,16,121,122]	NK	C
Para-aminosalicylic acid[6,83]	NK	C
Penicillin[6,123]	NK	C
Rifabutin[124]	NK	C
Streptomycin[125]	NK	C
Sulfasalazine[16,35,126,127]	NK	C
Sulfonamides[14,20,123,128]	NK	C
Terbinafine[129-131]	NK	C
Tetracycline[38,132]	NK	C
Trimethoprim–sulfamethoxazole[133]	NK	C
CENTRAL NERVOUS SYSTEM AGENTS		
Chlorprothixene[6,10,16,134]	NK	C
Clobazam[135]	NK	C
Clozapine[136,137]	NK	C
Donepezil[138]	NK	C
Lithium[6,16,139,140]	NK	C
Perphenazine[114]	NK	C
Phenelzine[6,16,93]	NK	C
Sertraline[141]	NK	C

Table 7-1 Agents Implicated in Drug-Induced Lupus (continued)

Drug	Incidence	Level of Evidence[a]
OTHER		
Adalimumab[28,142-145]	NK	C
Allopurinol[14]	NK	C
Aminoglutethimide[6,93]	NK	C
Anastrozole[146]	NK	C
Bevacizumab[147]	NK	C
Bupropion[148]	NK	C
Capecitabine[147,149]	NK	C
Certolizumab[82]	NK	C
Cimetidine[114]	NK	C
Cyclophosphamide[149]	NK	C
Dabigatran[150]	NK	C
Danazol[151]	NK	C
Denosumab[151]	NK	C
Diclofenac[82]	NK	C
Docetaxel[152]	NK	C
Doxorubicin[149,153]	NK	C
D-Penicillamine[6,18,35,154-160]	0.4–2%	C
Estrogens[161]	NK	C
Etanercept[28,162-167]	NK	B
Fluorouracil[149]	NK	C
Flutamide[168]	NK	C
Gemcitabine[149]	NK	C
Gold salts[6,83]	NK	C
Hepatitis B vaccine[169]	NK	C
Hydrazine[63,64]	NK	C
Hydroxyurea[170]	NK	C
Ibuprofen[82]	NK	C
Infliximab[28,162,163,166,171-176]	0.22%	C
Interferon α[6,16,177-179]	NK	C
Interferon β[180,181]	NK	C
Interleukin-2[182,183]	NK	C
Leuprolide acetate[184]	NK	C
Levodopa[6,16]	NK	C
Mesalamine[185]	NK	C
Methysergide[6]	NK	C
Naproxen[146]	NK	C
Oral contraceptives[6,14,186-194]	NK	C
Phenylbutazone[6,16,195,196]	NK	C
Piroxicam[146]	NK	C
Promethazine[114]	NK	C
Proton pump inhibitors (esomeprazole, lansoprazole, omeprazole, pantoprazole)[196-198]	NK	C

Table 7-1 Agents Implicated in Drug-Induced Lupus (continued)

Drug	Incidence	Level of Evidence[a]
Ranitidine[146]	NK	C
Sulfadiazine[199]	NK	C
Tamoxifen[149]	NK	C
Taxanes[149,152,200,201]	NK	C
Tiotropium[146]	NK	C
Tocainide[83,202]	NK	C
Zafirlukast[82]	NK	C

HMG-CoA = 3-hydroxy-3-methylglutaryl-coenzyme A, NK = not known.

[a]Definitions for Levels of Evidence: Level A—evidence from one or more randomized, controlled clinical trials; Level B—evidence from nonrandomized clinical trials, prospective observational studies, cohort studies, retrospective studies, case-control studies, meta-analyses and/or postmarketing surveillance studies; and Level C—evidence from one or more published case reports or case series.

with drug-induced lupus is primarily in the form of case reports, the incidence associated with specific medications is largely unknown or assumed to be less than 1%.[93] It is challenging to determine the incidence of drug-induced lupus associated with newer agents. However, drugs such as procainamide and hydralazine have been strongly associated with drug-induced lupus, and the incidence of drug-induced lupus associated with these agents is more easily estimated. Growing evidence supports a strong association between drug-induced lupus and other medications, such as chlorpromazine, isoniazid, methyldopa, quinidine, and minocycline.[83,206]

MECHANISMS

Possible mechanisms of drug-induced lupus are summarized in **Table 7-2.**[50,51,83,90,207-217] Mechanisms of drug-induced lupus involve alterations in immunologic pathways or drug metabolism. Although precise mechanisms are unknown, several hypotheses have been proposed, including one or often a combination of the following mechanisms for a given lupus-inducing agent: molecular mimicry, nucleic acid alterations, immunoregulatory alterations, interference in the complement pathway, and predisposing genetic factors. Molecular mimicry involves the interaction between an implicated medication and a nucleic acid. Drugs or drug metabolites with structures that are similar to the structure of a particular nucleic acid may stimulate the production of autoantibodies to that nucleic acid, the drug, or its metabolite. This hypothesis has been supported by several studies showing structural similarities between hydralazine and the nucleic acid adenosine.[17,218]

The nucleic acid alteration hypothesis suggests that the offending drug or its metabolite may somehow alter the immune process, increasing the immunogenicity of nuclear antigens. Alternatively, the drug or metabolite may couple with an antigen to form a hapten, triggering the formation of autoantibodies. The drug or its metabolites may also damage deoxyribonucleic acid (DNA), which may also result in the formation of autoantibodies.[17,83,219] For drugs that undergo hepatic acetylation, acetylator phenotype may affect response to this damage. Fast acetylators require less DNA repair, suggesting that less damage to DNA occurs in patients with this phenotype.[17,83,219]

Defective methylation of DNA in T cells has been suggested in the pathogenesis of idiopathic SLE and may also contribute to the development of drug-induced lupus. Hypomethylation of DNA in T cells alters T-cell gene expression and function.[51] Both procainamide and hydralazine inhibit DNA methylation, which may be an important component of the development of drug-induced lupus associated with these drugs.

The immunoregulatory alteration hypothesis suggests that drug or drug metabolites may alter

Table 7-2 Mechanisms of Drug-Induced Lupus[a]

Drug	Hypothesized Mechanism(s)
MOST COMMON	
Chlorpromazine[83]	Direct cytotoxicity due to formation of reactive metabolite(s)
Hydralazine[17,83,207-210]	Interaction between hydralazine and nucleic acid adenosine leading to an increase in immunogenicity of nuclear antigens and/or formation of autoantibodies; inhibition of covalent binding reactions between C3 and C4 leading to prohibited clearing of immune complexes; slow acetylation and/or presence of certain HLA alleles; inhibition of DNA methylation; direct cytotoxicity due to formation of reactive metabolite(s)
Isoniazid[83,207,209]	Inhibition of covalent binding reactions between C3 and C4 leading to prohibited clearing of immune complexes; slow acetylation; direct cytotoxicity due to formation of reactive metabolite(s)
Methyldopa	NK
Minocycline[50,211]	Genetic predisposition due to presence of certain HLA alleles; incomplete inhibition of apoptosis pathways resulting in autoimmunity
Procainamide[51,83,209,210,212-216]	Alters function of immunoregulatory cells, including the interference of T-cell maturation, via direct cytotoxicity due to formation of the procainamide-hydroxylamine reactive metabolite; inhibition of covalent binding reactions between C3 and C4 leading to prohibited clearing of immune complexes; slow acetylation; inhibition of DNA methylation
Quinidine[83]	Direct cytotoxicity due to formation of reactive metabolite(s)
OTHERS	
Acebutolol[90]	Direct cytotoxicity due to formation of reactive metabolite(s)
Etanercept[217]	Inhibition of cytotoxic T lymphocyte induction causing down regulation in control of B-cell hyperactivity
Infliximab[217]	Inhibition of cytotoxic T lymphocyte induction causing down regulation in control of B-cell hyperactivity
Propythiouracil[83]	Direct cytotoxicity due to formation of reactive metabolite(s)
Sulfonamides[210]	Slow acetylation

DNA = deoxyribonucleic acid, HLA = human leukocyte antigen, HMG = 3-hydroxy-3-methyl-glutaryl-coenzyme, NK = not known.
[a]For drugs listed in Table 7-1 that are not listed in this table, the mechanism of drug-induced lupus is unknown.

the function of immunoregulatory cells via direct cytotoxicity. Studies examining this hypothesis have produced inconsistent results.[220] Procainamide alters the function of T lymphocytes in vitro, enhancing or suppressing the proliferative response in a concentration-dependent fashion; high concentrations of procainamide suppress lymphocyte response, whereas low concentrations enhance this response.[213] Macrophages and mononuclear cells may also be involved in immunoregulation. It is proposed that during drug metabolism, these cells may release a variety of oxygen free radicals, which may be directly cytotoxic to lymphocytes. This cytotoxicity may lead to the loss of T suppressor cells, stimulation of B cells, and increased antibody production.[17,221] Drugs or drug metabolites may bind to the major histocompatibility antigens on monocytes, rendering them immunogenic.[17,222] The drug or the metabolite may also bind to histone antibodies, stimulating the production of antihistone antibodies.[17,217] Antitumor necrosis factor α (anti-TNF α) may promote humoral autoimmunity by selectively downregulating the induction of cytotoxic T lymphocyte response, a mechanism normally involved in controlling B-cell hyperactivity, which may induce lupus in some patients.[164,217]

Another immunoregulatory alteration hypothesis involves the interference of T-cell maturation in the thymus by a reactive metabolite of procainamide, procainamide-hydroxylamine. These immature T cells are then exported to the periphery and are reactive to chromatin. The T cells assist autoreactive B cells that are already in the periphery to stimulate an autoantibody response.[212,214]

It is well established that hereditary deficiencies in complements 1, 2, and 4 (C1, C2, and C4) predispose patients to idiopathic lupus and other autoimmune diseases.[17] One of the roles of the complement system is to scavenge immune complexes, promoting their clearance from the body.[223] Drug-induced lupus may occur as a result of interference in the complement pathway. Some drugs or drug metabolites may inhibit C3 activation, preventing complement from clearing immune complexes and possibly stimulating autoimmune processes. Isoniazid, hydralazine, and the hydroxylamine metabolite of procainamide have been shown to inhibit covalent binding reactions between C3 and C4.[17,209]

It has been proposed that genetic factors may play a role in the development of drug-induced lupus. The term *lupus diathesis* refers to a predisposition to idiopathic lupus. Patients with lupus diathesis are those with a personal or family history of arthritis, myalgia, drug reaction, pleuritic pain, epilepsy, or leukopenia.[207,224] In patients with lupus diathesis, certain drugs may cause the clinical expression of the disease; in contrast, medications known to cause drug-induced lupus may be used in patients with idiopathic SLE without exacerbating disease.[207,224] Other genetic factors may be important in the development of drug-induced lupus. The incidence of lupus induced by hydralazine and, to a lesser extent, procainamide is higher in slow acetylators.[210,213] This is most likely due to metabolism of hydralazine or procainamide resulting in the formation of an active metabolite. Other genetic factors have also been associated with the development of drug-induced lupus, including the presence of certain human leukocyte antigen (HLA) alleles. HLA-DR4 is found in 73% of patients with hydralazine-induced lupus, which is higher than the rate in patients with SLE (25%).[208] The HLA-DR2 and HLA-DQB1 alleles have also been found in patients with minocycline-induced lupus.[211] The presence of null alleles for the fourth component of complement (C4) has been associated with drug-included lupus.[51,225] Another hypothesis suggests that minocycline-induced lupus may occur as a result of incomplete inhibition of apoptosis pathways, leading to autoimmunity.[50]

CLINICAL PRESENTATION AND DIFFERENTIAL DIAGNOSIS

Signs and symptoms associated with drug-induced lupus are listed in **Table 7-3**. Signs and symptoms of drug-induced lupus typically present within 3 weeks to 2 years after initiation of therapy with the suspected agent.[5,19,51] Patients typically present with prodromal symptoms of arthralgia and arthritis before progression to a lupus-like syndrome, potentially affecting numerous organs.[19] Arthralgia is present in up to 90% of patients with drug-induced lupus.[206,226] Patients typically present with only one or two symptoms. Initial presentation usually involves articular symptoms characterized by polyarticular and symmetric joint

Table 7-3 Signs and Symptoms Associated with Drug-Induced Lupus

- Anemia (serum hemoglobin <11.5 g/dL)
- Anti-dsDNA
- Antihistone antibodies
- Antinuclear antibodies
- Anti-Sm antibodies
- Anti-ssDNA
- Arthralgia
- Arthritis
- Drug-specific skin manifestations (e.g., butterfly rash, purpura, erythema nodosum, and erythematous papules)
- Elevated erythrocyte sedimentation rate
- Fever
- Hepatosplenomegaly
- Hypergammaglobulinemia
- Leukopenia (white cell count <4,000/mm^3)
- Lupus erythematosus cells
- Malaise
- Mild kidney involvement (e.g., glomerulonephritis)
- Myalgia
- Pericarditis
- Pleural effusion
- Pleuritis
- Positive Coombs test
- Pulmonary infiltrate
- Weight loss

DNA = deoxyribonucleic acid, dsDNA = double-stranded DNA, Sm = Smith nuclear antigen, ssDNA = single-stranded DNA.

involvement.[20,227] Constitutional symptoms associated with drug-induced lupus include fever, malaise, musculoskeletal symptoms (i.e., myalgia, arthralgia, arthritis), serositis (i.e., pleurisy, pericarditis, pleural effusion, pulmonary infiltrate), hepatomegaly, splenomegaly, and skin manifestations, including the signature "butterfly rash" associated with SLE.[5,17,19,20,35,227] Weight loss has also been reported in association with drug-induced lupus.[20,21,52] Autoimmune hepatitis has been reported with an incidence of 32–54% in patients with minocycline-induced lupus.[1,40,41] Pulmonary involvement with pleuropericarditis and pulmonary infiltrates is most commonly reported with lupus induced by procainamide.[16,19,52,59,60,228] Cutaneous involvement is generally less frequent in drug-induced lupus, although certain skin manifestations are actually more common as compared with idiopathic SLE, including purpura, erythema nodosum, and erythematous papules. Cutaneous manifestations occur in up to 39% of patients with quinidine- and hydralazine-induced lupus but are rarely associated with minocycline- or procainamide-induced lupus.[1,83,229] Certain drugs may induce characteristic skin manifestations unique to the medication.[5,230]

Serologic evidence in patients with drug-induced lupus typically includes a positive antinuclear antibody (ANA) test, lupus erythematosus cells, antihistone antibodies, and the absence of antibodies to DNA.[1,20,126,227,231] It is important to note that some drugs cause a positive ANA test without evidence of clinical disease.[35,231,232] Likewise, patients taking either quinidine or minocycline and exhibiting rheumatologic symptoms of lupus may not present with a positive ANA test.[16] Depending on the drug, antibody formation may be directed toward individual histones (i.e., H1, H2A, H2B, H3, H4) and/or histone complexes (i.e., H2A-2B, H3-4).[20,233,234] The antibodies present as either immunoglobulin G or immunoglobulin M.[17,19,20] Binding to single-stranded DNA has been reported in a few cases, but binding to double-stranded DNA has not been reported.[17,222] Antiphospholipid antibodies have been reported predominantly in cases of lupus induced by chlorpromazine but also in association with lupus induced by other drugs, such as hydralazine, procainamide, quinidine, valproic acid, amoxicillin, propranolol, and streptomycin.[20,235,236] Antibodies against Smith nuclear antigen (anti-Sm) are not commonly present in patients with drug-induced lupus.[2,19,20,231,237]

Elevations in the erythrocyte sedimentation rate (ESR) are very common, indicative of an inflammatory process.[1,16,17,19,51,227,231] Serum complement concentrations are generally normal; however, several reports of transient lowering of serum complement concentrations (i.e., C3 and C4) have been published.[16,17,19,20,227,231,238,239] Anemia, leukopenia, thrombocytopenia, and hypergammaglobulinemia are less common and are usually mild.[16,17,19,20,227] A positive Coombs test has been reported in cases of lupus induced by methyldopa, procainamide, and hydralazine.[19,20,52,240-244] Circulating lupus anticoagulants, due to binding of autoantibodies to phospholipids and proteins associated with the cell membrane, have been reported in patients taking chlorpromazine; however, the association of these lupus anticoagulants with the diagnosis and prognosis of drug-induced lupus is unclear.[231,245]

Drug-induced lupus is less likely than idiopathic SLE to involve the central nervous system or the kidneys.[5,17,20,123,126,231] Nonetheless, neuropathy has been reported in patients diagnosed with lupus induced by procainamide or hydralazine, and mild and reversible kidney involvement, particularly glomerulonephritis, has been noted in cases of drug-induced lupus caused by D-penicillamine, hydralazine, griseofulvin, procainamide, propylthiouracil, quinidine, and anticonvulsants.[5,14,17,19,20,126,227,231,246-253] The signs and symptoms of idiopathic SLE and drug-induced lupus are compared and contrasted in **Table 7-4**.[1,2,17,19,51,52,93,206,227,230,232,247,254-259] No specific diagnostic criteria for drug-induced lupus exist.[1,17,35] However, several investigators have identified cases of drug-induced lupus based on four patient criteria: (1) adequate exposure (dose and duration) of a drug suspected of inducing lupus, (2) temporal association of clinical manifestation upon drug ingestion with no history of idiopathic SLE prior to drug administration, (3) positive ANA test with at least one clinical symptom of SLE, and (4) remission of clinical symptoms and gradual decline in

Table 7-4 Comparison of Signs and Symptoms Associated with Drug-Induced Lupus Versus Idiopathic SLE

Manifestations	Idiopathic SLE	All Drug-Induced Lupus	Procainamide-Induced Lupus	Hydralazine-Induced Lupus
	% of patients experiencing sign/symptom			
Alopecia	42	Unusual	0	0
Anemia (hemoglobin <11.5 g/dL)	57	0–46	9–21	30–35
Anti-dsDNA	25–80	5	Rare	Rare
Antihistone antibodies	20–60	70–95	90–95	90–95
Antinuclear antibodies	95	95	100	100
Anti-Sm antibodies	40–50	5	10–20	10–20
Anti-ssDNA	50–90	30–48	70–80	70–80
Arthralgia	92–95	75	74–95	84–95
Arthritis	86–95	75	18	50
CNS involvement	25–70	0	0–2	0
Complement concentrations	Reduced	Normal/reduced	NK	NK
Discoid lesions	23	Unusual	0	0
Erythrocyte sedimentation rate	Elevated	Elevated (80)	Elevated	Elevated
Fever	75–85	25–50	45	14–50
Hepatosplenomegaly	9–46	25	20–41	3–75
Hypergammaglobulinemia	NK	10–50	NK	NK
Kidney involvement	38–75	5	0–5	0–20
Leukopenia (white cell count <4,000/mm^3)	43–50	2–33	2–32	26
Lupus erythematosus cells	Up to 70	90	NK	NK
Malaise	75	25–50	NK	NK
Mucosal ulcers	42	Unusual	0	0
Myalgia	48	NK	20–50	2–34
Pericarditis	18–50	50	14–18	0–2
Pleural effusion	16–33	NK	33	10
Pleuritis	42–60	NK	52	14–25
Positive Coombs test	18–25	0–33	33	0–5
Pulmonary infiltrate	0–10	NK	5–20	3–25
Skin manifestations	50–75	0–10	5–18	2–39
Thrombocytopenia	NK	Unusual	NK	NK

CNS = central nervous system, DNA = deoxyribonucleic acid, dsDNA = double-stranded DNA, NK = not known, SLE = systemic lupus erythematosus, Sm = Smith nuclear antigen, ssDNA = single-stranded DNA.

serum ANA concentrations following drug discontinuation.[5,14,16,17,19,226,231] At least one clinical symptom of SLE must be present for diagnosis because many patients can convert from ANA-negative to ANA-positive with no clinical signs or symptoms of lupus.[17] Recurrence of lupus symptoms after a rechallenge with the implicated drug strengthens the probability that the syndrome is drug-induced, although rechallenge is seldom performed.[1,39]

To confirm a case of drug-induced lupus, one must recognize key differences between the clinical and laboratory findings characteristic of idiopathic SLE and those of drug-induced lupus. Although the presentation of SLE and drug-induced lupus appear similar on initial assessment, the underlying characteristics of each condition are not the same. The two conditions differ in terms of known risk factors, affected organs, serologic features, and severity. The diagnosis of SLE is based on the presence of four clinical or laboratory findings in a variety of organs according to guidelines compiled by the American College of Rheumatology.[2] However, no specific diagnostic criteria have been adopted for drug-induced lupus.

Idiopathic SLE presents in a younger population, ranging from 15 to 40 years of age, with an average age at presentation of 29 years. Idiopathic SLE is reported more commonly in females.[5,17,258] Unlike drug-induced lupus, idiopathic SLE often presents with antibodies to double-stranded DNA, and is less likely to be associated with antibodies to antihistones.[1] Antihistone antibodies are present in 25% of SLE cases, whereas 90% of drug-induced lupus cases present with antihistone antibodies.[5,20,227] Anemia, leukopenia, and thrombocytopenia are more common and usually more severe in patients with idiopathic SLE as compared with drug-induced lupus.[227] Other symptoms, such as butterfly rash, alopecia, discoid lesions, and mucosal ulcers are more common in idiopathic SLE.[5,231]

Because drug-induced lupus-like syndrome is characterized by a multisystem presentation, a broad spectrum of illnesses must be ruled out during a differential diagnosis. Viral or bacterial conditions must be ruled out because of the common presentation of fever and malaise. Because patients with lupus induced by certain drugs (e.g., procainamide) may present with pleuropulmonary involvement, other pulmonary diseases (e.g., pneumonia, pulmonary embolus) must be ruled out.[17] Refer to **Table 7-5** for conditions to consider in the differential diagnosis of drug-induced lupus.

Table 7-5 Conditions to Consider in the Differential Diagnosis of Drug-Induced Lupus

- Antiphospholipid antibody syndrome
- Connective-tissue diseases
- Fibromyalgia
- Idiopathic systemic lupus erythematosus
- Pleuropulmonary conditions (pneumonia, pulmonary embolus)
- Rheumatoid arthritis
- Scleroderma
- Systemic sclerosis
- Vasculitis (Wegener granulomatosis)
- Viral/bacteriologic conditions

Other chemical agents and environmental toxins may contribute to lupus-like syndrome and must be ruled out. Such factors include exposure to hydrazines (e.g., mushrooms, tobacco, tobacco smoke), aromatic amines (e.g., hair-coloring solutions), eosin (ingredient in cosmetics), tartrazine (i.e., food colorant), insecticide, and heavy metals (e.g., mercury, cadmium).[5,17,131]

Two other forms of drug-induced lupus include drug-induced subacute cutaneous lupus erythematosus (SCLE) and drug-induced chronic cutaneous lupus erythematosus (CCLE). Drugs including terbinafine, hydrochlorothiazide, acebutolol, bupropion, interferons α and β, immunosuppressive or cancer chemotherapy agents, certain angiotensin-converting enzyme inhibitors, 3-hydroxy-3-methylglutaryl coenzyme A reductase inhibitors (statins), and calcium-channel blockers have been associated with drug-induced SCLE.[89,129,154,260-263] This condition appears to be more common in females than in males, and anti-Sjögren syndrome A/B (also known as anti-Ro/La), antihistone, and ANA have been detected. Fluorouracil agents have been associated with drug-induced CCLE. Limited information regarding these types of drug-induced lupus exists.[226]

Investigation of the patient's medication profile is an important step in diagnosing potential drug-induced lupus. Because the published literature documenting drug-induced lupus is limited to case reports and does not often include medications that have recently entered the market, an understanding of the characteristics that influence the likelihood of a drug to cause lupus is critical. The biochemical structure of a drug may influence the potential for drug-induced lupus.[5,220,227] A common structural feature shared by many drugs associated with lupus is the presence of a nitrogen or sulfur heteroatom in a functional group such as the aromatic amine, hydrazine, sulfhydryl, or thionosulfur. Many of the drugs that have been implicated in drug-induced lupus produce chemically reactive metabolites; these drugs include aromatic amines (e.g., procainamide, dapsone, sulfadiazine, aminosalicylic acid, aminoglutethimide, sulfasalazine, practolol, acebutolol), hydrazines (e.g., hydralazine, isoniazid, phenelzine, hydrazine), or drugs containing a sulfhydryl or thiono group (e.g., propylthiouracil, methimazole, penicillamine, and captopril). Drugs characterized as hydantoin anticonvulsants (e.g., phenytoin, mephenytoin, ethosuximide, trimethadione) may also cause drug-induced lupus because of their similar reactive metabolites. The association between the production of reactive metabolites based on the biochemical structure of a drug and its potential to induce lupus is merely hypothesized. Lithium is associated with lupus but undergoes no metabolism at all.

RISK FACTORS

Risk factors for drug-induced lupus are listed in **Table 7-6** and are often specific to the causative agent. Patient characteristics that influence drug metabolism have been associated with drug-induced lupus.[19] In the past, investigators identified lupus diathesis as a risk factor for drug-induced lupus. However, this has not been proven.

Many reported cases of drug-induced lupus are in older patients (mean age = 62 years).[5,17,35,227] This may be because patients who take these drugs, typically prescribed for cardiac and other diseases, tend to be older.[17,27,35,253] However, cases of anticonvulsant-induced lupus have been reported most commonly in children.[19,20,75,262,264]

According to case reports published in the United States, white patients are six times more likely to be affected by drug-induced lupus as compared with black individuals.[6,20,21,35,265] The ratio of occurrence of idiopathic SLE in blacks versus whites is 2.7:1. However, this ratio is 0.3:1 for procainamide-induced lupus and 0.2:1 for hydralazine-induced lupus.[17]

Idiopathic SLE occurs more commonly in females, with a reported female-to-male ratio of 9:1.[20] Conversely, drug-induced lupus tends to affect both sexes equally, although females may still be at a slightly increased risk; female-to-male ratios range from 1:1 to 1.6:1.[1,17,20,256-258,262,266] An exception is patients with minocycline-induced lupus, with which women are 14 times more likely than men to be affected.[1] It has been hypothesized that women may often have a higher risk of minocycline-induced lupus because of the estrogen-related increase of calcineurin activity causing enhanced T-cell activation.[267]

Many cases of drug-induced lupus occur after prolonged administration of the causative agent for 1 month or longer.[83] Drugs such as antiepileptics, antiarrhythmics (procainamide), and other medications (e.g., hydralazine, isoniazid, chlorpromazine) cause lupus in a dose-dependent manner.[5,17,19,35] This dose relationship may correlate to the accumulation of unacetylated drug in the body.[17,19] Hydralazine doses >200 mg/day or cumulative doses of more than 100 g have been associated with lupus-like syndrome.[20,265,268]

Certain drugs undergo acetylation to be inactivated. Patients who are slow acetylators often are at a higher risk of adverse effects from these drugs because of the potential for accumulation of the active drug. For instance, sulfasalazine is metabolized into sulfapyridine and 5-aminosalicylic acid; the sulfapyridine component is typically acetylated in the liver by the enzyme *N*-acetyltransferase 2 (NAT2). Individuals with a mutation on the *NAT2* gene have impaired enzyme function ("slow acetylators") and present with higher concentrations of the active sulfapyridine component rather than its inactivated form.[126,269] Slow acetylators of procainamide experience lupus-like symptoms four times more rapidly than fast acetylators, and positive ANA tests develop at lower cumulative drug doses in slow acetylators than in fast acetylators.[227,270] Other drugs that are acetylated in the liver through NAT2 include hydralazine, isoniazid, and sulfonamides.[5,17,20,210,227]

Table 7-6 Risk Factors for Drug-Induced Lupus

- Certain HLA allele expression (HLA-DR2, HLA-DR4, HLA-DQB1)
- Duration of drug use (3 weeks to 2 years)
- Female sex
- High single dose or high cumulative dose of drug
- Older age (mean age, 62 years)
- Presence of null alleles for fourth component of complement (C4)
- Slow acetylator phenotype
- White race

HLA = human leukocyte antigen.

The severity of hydralazine-induced lupus is greatly influenced by acetylator phenotype. One study reported that 60% of slow acetylators taking <400 mg of hydralazine had a positive ANA test, whereas 0% of fast acetylators taking the same dose of hydralazine showed positive serum ANA titers.[269] On the other hand, although the incidence of procainamide-induced lupus is higher in slow acetylators, the severity of procainamide-induced lupus is influenced minimally by acetylator type.[207,269] Because both fast and slow acetylators may experience procainamide-induced lupus, it has been hypothesized that a reactive, nonacetylated metabolite of procainamide may be responsible for the syndrome.[270] The influence of the acetylator phenotype is supported by the evidence that no cases of drug-induced lupus associated with the administration of the acetylated form of procainamide, *N*-acetylprocainamide, have been reported.[17,19] Acetylator phenotype is not necessarily a risk factor for lupus induced by all drugs reported to induce this disease; this risk factor is exclusive to certain drugs (Table 7-2). It is also important to note that acetylator status does not influence idiopathic SLE.[271]

Various HLA types, especially HLA-DR2 and DR4, are associated with SLE.[20] However, only HLA-DR4, which is associated with slow acetylation, has been shown to be strongly associated with hydralazine-induced lupus.[5] For example, in one study, 73% of patients with hydralazine-induced lupus had HLA-DR4.[208] The presence of a null allele for C4 is also a risk factor for drug-induced lupus.[51,225]

MORBIDITY AND MORTALITY

Drug-induced lupus usually resolves within weeks to months after discontinuation of the offending drug, although the ANA test may remain positive for months to years.[5,20] It is fatal only in extremely rare circumstances, usually as a result of kidney failure.[5] The psychosocial impact of a drug-induced lupus diagnosis is not as severe as that of idiopathic SLE due to the relatively shorter duration and better prognosis associated with drug-induced lupus. Healthcare utilization is short-term for drug-induced lupus but, with either condition, emotional support, symptomatic treatment, and intentional patient involvement to gather information for an accurate assessment are vital to a timely diagnosis and appropriate treatment.[272]

PREVENTION

Monitoring parameters for prevention and detection of drug-induced lupus are presented in **Table 7-7**. Drug-induced lupus is an idiosyncratic drug reaction that may not be explained by the known pharmacologic actions of the specific drug. To prevent drug-induced lupus, drugs known to cause the lupus-like syndrome should be avoided. However, avoidance of certain drugs may not be an option in many medical circumstances. The lupus-inducing potential of only a select number of drugs has been substantiated with results from prospective studies. The potential for other drugs to cause lupus is supported only by spontaneous, and often single, case reports. As a routine screening process, baseline serum ANA titers should be determined when initiating a medication documented to induce lupus.[35] Periodic ANA testing should be initiated based on clinical judgment, remembering that serum ANA titers alone are not diagnostic of drug-induced lupus. A common recommendation is to obtain a complete blood count, ANA titer, and ESR every 3 months in a patient receiving a drug with the potential to cause lupus.[20] Periodic assessment of constitutional signs and symptoms associated with the syndrome helps guide the clinical decision to continue or discontinue therapy with the implicated drug.

There are no data to support cross-sensitivity between medications implicated in drug-induced lupus; therefore, it is not possible to say with certainty

Table 7-7 Approaches to Help Prevent Drug-Induced Lupus

Monitor the following at baseline and every 3 months during therapy:

- Serum antinuclear antibody titers
- Complete blood count
- Erythrocyte sedimentation rate
- Signs and symptoms of drug-induced lupus

that patients experiencing drug-induced lupus while taking one medication will develop the same reaction to another potential lupus-causing drug. However, careful clinical decision making is necessary when considering treatment with these medications. Patients should be followed carefully and appropriate baseline testing should be performed to ensure patient safety during the course of treatment.

MANAGEMENT

Strategies for managing drug-induced lupus are presented in **Table 7-8**. Symptoms of drug-induced lupus do not subside with continued administration of the offending agent, although they are reversible on discontinuation of therapy.[19,227,231] Therefore, discontinuation of the offending drug is required. Clinical and laboratory findings associated with drug-induced lupus typically disappear within weeks. Rarely, clinical and laboratory findings may take years to resolve after the termination of therapy with the lupus-inducing drug.[5,19,20,126,262] Although symptoms often resolve quickly, serum ANA titers may fall gradually over several months to 2 years.[5,35,51] Clinical symptoms of lupus do not develop in most asymptomatic patients with positive ANA titers, and discontinuation of therapy is not required in these cases.[8,51]

Patients often improve dramatically without treatment. Patients experiencing musculoskeletal and mild constitutional symptoms (e.g., pyrexia, arthralgia, myalgia) may be treated with anti-inflammatory agents such as aspirin and nonsteroidal anti-inflammatory drugs if there are no contraindications to their use.[17,19,20,227,231,273] However, patients presenting with more severe symptoms (e.g., pleurisy, pericarditis, kidney involvement, neuropsychiatric) require treatment with empirical, short-term low-dose systemic corticosteroids (e.g., prednisone 0.5–1.0 mg/kg/day) tapered over 1 week to several months, which may require an additional immunosuppressant and/antihypertensive therapy, if refractory.[5,16,17,19,20,227,256,257,262,273-275] Patients presenting with drug-induced lupus-associated skin manifestations have been treated with antimalarial agents (i.e., chloroquine–hydroxychloroquine).[5,231,273,275] Several case reports describe rechallenge of the offending agent; lupus symptoms promptly reappeared on reinitiation of the drug.[39,227]

INFORMATION FOR PATIENTS

When patients are initiated on a drug that is strongly associated with drug-induced lupus, the healthcare professional should counsel the patient regarding the fact that symptoms of arthralgia or arthritis may occur at any time during the therapy—up to and including 2 years after the first dose. Regardless of whether or not the patient has

Table 7-8 Management of Drug-Induced Lupus

Sign/Symptom	Management
Positive antinuclear antibody only	Continue drug if asymptomatic
Any lupus-like symptoms	Discontinue drug immediately
Persistent constitutional symptoms and/or musculoskeletal symptoms	Discontinue drug immediately; treat symptoms with aspirin or nonsteroidal anti-inflammatory drugs
Cardiovascular (e.g., pleurisy, pericarditis), kidney involvement (e.g., increasing proteinuria/creatinine, active urinary sediment), neuropsychiatric symptoms	Discontinue drug immediately Initiate low-dose corticosteroids (e.g., prednisone 0.5–1.0 mg/kg daily) tapered over 1 week to several months; combine with another immunosuppressant (e.g., azathioprine, mycophenolate mofetil, cyclophosphamide, methotrexate) for refractory cases requiring long-term steroid use Initiate or change/escalate antihypertensive therapy if at least two blood pressure readings over 3 months include systolic blood pressure readings >130 mm Hg or diastolic blood pressure readings >80 mm Hg
Skin and joint manifestations, and constitutional symptoms including fever, malaise, and fatigue	Initiate hydroxychloroquine at 200 mg twice daily and continue indefinitely

an arthritis-related medical condition before the initiation of the drug, symptoms of fever, malaise, and skin manifestations of unknown origin should be reported promptly. The patient should also be counseled regarding other specific symptoms associated with the implicated drugs (e.g., pulmonary symptoms with procainamide, symptoms of hepatotoxicity with minocycline) and educated on sun avoidance. The healthcare professional must educate the patient regarding the importance of reporting symptoms because of (1) the progression of the syndrome if ignored, and (2) the reversibility of the syndrome on cessation of therapy with implicated drug.

REFERENCES

1. Schlienger RG, Bircher AJ, Meier CR. Minocycline-induced lupus. *Dermatology.* 2000;200:223-31.
2. American College of Rheumatology; Ad Hoc Committee on Systemic Lupus Erythematosus Guidelines. Guidelines for referral and management of systemic lupus erythematosus in adults. *Arthritis Rheum.* 1999; 42:1785-96.
3. Resman-Targoff BH. Systemic lupus erythematosus. In: DiPiro JT, Talbert RL, Yee GC et al., eds. *Pharmacotherapy: a pathophysiologic approach.* 9th ed. New York: McGraw-Hill; 2014.
4. Hahn B. Systemic lupus erythematosus. In: Kasper D, Fauci A, Hauser S et al., eds. *Harrison's principles of internal medicine.* 19th ed. New York: McGraw-Hill; 2015.
5. Pramatarov KD. Drug-induced lupus erythematosus. *Clin Dermatol.* 1998; 16:367-77.
6. Yung RL, Richardson BC. Drug-induced lupus. *Rheum Dis Clin North Am.* 1994; 20:61-86.
7. Alarcon-Segovia D, Fishbein E, Cetina JA et al. Antigenic specificity of chlorpromazine induced antinuclear antibodies. *Clin Exp Immunol.* 1973; 15:543.
8. Dubois EL, Tallman E, Wonka RA. Chlorpromazine-induced systemic lupus erythematosus. *JAMA.* 1972; 221:595-6.
9. Berglund S, Gottfries CG, Gottfries I et al. Chlorpromazine-induced antinuclear factors. *Ada Med Scand.* 1970; 187:67-74.
10. Fabius AJM, Faulhofer WK. Systemic lupus erythematosus induced by psychotropic drugs. *Ada Rheum Scand.* 1971; 17:137-47.
11. Goldman LS, Hudson JI, Weddington WW. Lupus-like illness associated with chlorpromazine. *Am J Psychiatry.* 1980; 137:1613-4.
12. Pavlidakey GP, Hashimoto K, Heller GL et al. Chlorpromazine-induced lupus-like disease: case report and review of the literature. *Am J Acad Dermatol.* 1985; 13:109-15.
13. Steen VD, Ramse-Goldman R. Phenothiazine-induced systemic lupus erythematosus with superior vena cava syndrome: case report and review of the literature. *Arthritis Rheum.* 1988; 31:923-6.
14. Lee SL, Chase PH. Drug-induced systemic lupus erythematosus—a critical review. *Semin Arthritis Rheum.* 1975; 5:83-103.
15. Benton JW, Tynes B, Register HB. Systemic lupus erythematosus occurring during anticonvulsant drug therapy. *JAMA.* 1962; 180:115.
16. Rubin RL. Etiology and mechanisms of drug-induced lupus. *Curr Opin Rheumatol.* 1999; 11:357-63.
17. Hess EV, Mongey AB. Drug-related lupus. *Bull Rheum Dis.* 1991; 40:1-8.
18. Harpey JP. Lupus-like syndromes induced by drugs. *Ann Allergy.* 1974; 33:256-61.
19. Weinstein A. Drug-induced systemic lupus erythematosus. *Prog Clin Immunol.* 1980;4 :1-21.
20. Price EJ, Venables PJ. Drug-induced lupus. *Drug Saf.* 1995; 12:283-90.
21. Cameron HA, Ramsay LE. The lupus syndrome induced by hydralazine—a common complication with low dose treatment. *BMJ.* 1984;289:410-2.
22. Sturman SG, Kumararatne D, Beevers DG. Fatal hydralazine induced systemic lupus erythematosus. *Lancet.* 1988; 2:1304.
23. Dustan HP, Taylor RD, Corcoran AC et al. Rheumatic and febrile syndrome during prolonged hydralazine therapy. *JAMA.* 1954; 154:23-9.
24. Perry HM Jr, Schroeder HA. Syndrome simulating collagen disease caused by hydralazine (Apresoline). *JAMA.* 1954; 154:670-3.
25. Condemi JJ, Moore-Jones D, Vaughan JH et al. Antinuclear antibodies following hydralazine toxicity. *N Engl J Med.* 1967; 276:486-91.
26. Carey RM, Coleman M, Feder A. Pericardial tamponade: a major presenting manifestation of hydralazine-induced lupus syndrome. *Am J Med.* 1973; 54:84-7.
27. Finks SW, Finks AL, Self TH. Hydralazine-induced lupus: maintaining vigilance with increased use in patients with heart failure. *South Med J.* 2006; 99:18-22.
28. Quaresma MV, Brando de Oliveira F, Dias MFRG et al. Anti-TNF-alpha and hydralazine drug-induced lupus. *An Bras Dermatol.* 2015; 90:S125-9.
29. Cannat A, Seligmann M. Possible induction of antinuclear antibodies by isoniazid. *Lancet.* 1966; 1:185.
30. Rothfield NF, Bierer WG, Garfield JW. Isoniazid induction of antinuclear antibodies: a prospective study. *Ann Intern Med.* 1978; 88:650-2.
31. Masel MA. A lupus-like reaction to anti-tuberculosis drugs. *Med J Aust.* 1967; 2:738-40.
32. Hothersall TE, Mowat AG, Duthie JJR et al. Drug-induced lupus syndrome: a case report implicating isoniazid. *Scott Med J.* 1968; 13:245-7.
33. Harrington TM, Davis DE. Systemic lupus-like syndrome induced by methyldopa therapy. *Chest.* 1981; 79:696-7.
34. Dupont A, Six R. Lupus-like syndrome induced by methyldopa. *BMJ.* 1982; 285:693-4.
35. Skaer TL. Medication-induced systemic lupus erythematosus. *Clin Ther.* 1992; 14:496-506.
36. Quilty B, McHugh N. Lupus-like syndrome associated with the use of minocycline. *Br J Rheumatol.* 1995; 33:1197-8.
37. Farver DK. Minocycline-induced lupus. *Ann Pharmacother.* 1997; 31:1160-3.
38. Shapiro LE, Knowles SR, Shear NH. Comparative safety of tetracycline, minocycline, and doxycycline. *Arch Dermatol.* 1997; 133:1224-30.
39. Lawson TM, Amos N, Bulgen D et al. Minocycline-induced lupus: clinical features and response to rechallenge. *Br Soc Rheumatol.* 2001; 40:329-35.
40. Gough A, Chapman S, Wagstaff K et al. Minocycline induced autoimmune hepatitis and systemic lupus-erythematosus-like syndrome. *BMJ.* 1996; 312:169-73.
41. Knights SE, Leandro MJ, Khamashta MA et al. Minocycline-related lupus arthritis. *Clin Exp Rheumatol.* 1998; 16:587-90.
42. Matsuura T, Shimizu Y, Fijimoto H et al. Minocycline-related lupus. *Lancet.* 1992; 340:1553.
43. Allston LL. Lupus-like syndrome from minocycline. *Schoch Lett.* 1984; 34:29.
44. Byrne PA, Williams BD, Pritchard MH. Minocycline-related lupus. *Br J Rheumatol.* 1994;33:674-6.
45. Unoue CN, Konda Y, Suwabe N et al. Minocycline-related lupus in childhood. *Eur J Pediatr.* l994; 153:540.

46. Gordon PM, White MI, Herriot R et al. Minocycline-associated lupus erythematosus. *Br J Dermatol.* 1955; 132:120-1.
47. Goldstein Ph, Deviere J, Cremer M. Acute hepatitis and drug-related lupus by minocycline treatment. *Am J Gastroenterol.* 1997; 92:143-6.
48. Benjamin RW, Calkoglu AS. Hyperthyroidism and lupuslike syndrome in an adolescent treated with minocycline for acne vulgaris. *Pediatr Dermatol.* 2007; 24:246-9.
49. Geddes R. Minocycline-induced lupus in adolescents: clinical implications for physical therapists. *J Orthop Sports Phys Ther.* 2007; 37:65-71.
50. Van Steensel MAM. Why minocycline can cause systemic lupus—a hypothesis and suggestions for therapeutic interventions based on it. *Med Hypotheses.* 2004; 63:31-4.
51. Borchers AT, Keen CL, Gershwin ME. Drug-induced lupus. *Ann NY Acad Sci.* 2007; 1108:166-82.
52. Blomgren SE, Condemi JJ, Vaughan JH. Procainamide-induced lupus erythematosus-clinical laboratory observations. *Am J Med.* 1972; 52:338-48.
53. Muna W, Osterman FA, Stevens MB et al. Procainamide-induced lupus. *Johns Hopkins Med J.* 1976 ;138:289-95.
54. Ladd AT. Procainamide-induced lupus erythematosus. *N Engl J Med.* 1962; 267:1357-8.
55. Ghose MK. Pericardial tamponade: a presenting manifestation of procainamide induced lupus erythematosus. *Am J Med.* 1975; 58:581-5.
56. Hope PR, Bates LA. The frequency of procainamide-induced systemic lupus erythematosus. *Med J Aust.* 1972; 2:298-303.
57. Jackson C, Phillips PE. Procainamide-induced lupus with vasculitis. *Clin Exp Rheumatol.* 1986; 4:290-2.
58. Fakhro AM, Ritchie RF, Lown B. Lupus-like syndrome induced by procainamide. *Am J Cardiol.* 1967; 20:367-73.
59. Byrd RB, Schanzer B. Pulmonary sequelae in procainamide induced lupus-like syndrome. *Dis Chest.* 1969; 55:170-2.
60. Anderson RJ, Genton E. Procainamide-induced pericardial effusion. *Am Heart J.* 1972; 83;798-800.
61. Dubois EL. Procainamide induction of a systemic lupus erythematosus-like syndrome. *Medicine (Baltimore).* 1969; 48:217-28.
62. Anastassiades TP, Milliken JA. Lupus-like syndrome, with persistent immunological abnormalities related to procainamide therapy. *Can Med Assoc J.* 1972; 107:312-5.
63. West SG, McMahon M, Portanora JP Quinidine-induced lupus erythematosus. *Ann Intern Med.* 1984; 100:840-2.
64. Kendall MJ, Hawkins CF. Quinidine-induced systemic lupus erythematosus. *Postgrad Med J.* 1970; 46:729-31.
65. Anderson FP, Wanerfa GR. Drug-induced systemic lupus erythematosus due to quinidine. *Conn Med.* 1972; 36:84-5.
66. Yudis M, Meehan JJ. Quinidine-induced lupus nephritis. *JAMA.* 1976; 253:2000.
67. McCormack GD, Barth WF. Quinidine-induced lupus syndrome. *Semin Arthritis Rheum.* 1985; 15:73-9.
68. Cohen MG, Kevat S, Prowse MV, Ahern MI. Two distinct quinidine-induced rheumatic syndromes. *Ann Intern Med.* 1988; 108:369-71.
69. Drory VE, Korczyn AD. Hypersensitivity vasculitis and systemic lupus erythematosus induced by anticonvulsants. *Clin Neuropharmacol.* 1993; 16:19-29.
70. Schmidt S, Welcker M, Schattenkirchner M. Carbamazepine-induced systemic lupus erythematosus. *Br J Psychiatry.* 1991; 161:560-1.
71. Kanno T, Miyata M, Kazuta Y et al. Carbamazepine-induced systemic lupus erythematosus-like disease. *Intern Med.* 1992; 31:1303-5.
72. Amerio P, Inocente C, Feliciani C et al. Drug-induced cutaneous lupus erythematosus after 5 years of treatment with carbamazepine. *Eur J Dermatol.* 2006; 16:281-3.
73. Molina-Ruiz AM, Lasanta B, Barcia A et al. Drug induced systemic lupus erythematosus in a child after 3 years of treatment with carbamazepine. *Austalas J Dermatol.* 2017; 58:e20-2.
74. Singsen BH, Fishman L, Hanson V. Antinuclear antibodies and lupus-like syndromes in children receiving anticonvulsants. *Pediatrics.* 1976; 57:529-34.
75. Beernink DH, Miller JJ III. Anticonvulsant induced antinuclear antibodies in lupus-like disease in children. *J Pediatrics.* 1973; 82:113-7.
76. Ansell BM. Drug-induced systemic lupus erythematosus in a 9 year old boy. *Lupus.* 1993; 2:193-4.
77. Sarzi-Puttini P, Panni B, Cazzola M et al. Lamotrigine-induced lupus. *Lupus.* 2000; 9:555-7.
78. Chang RS, Cole AJ. Lamotrigine-induced lupus-like syndrome: a case report and literature review. *Am J Ther.* 2014; 21:e85-7.
79. Cabanillas M, Suarez-Amor O, Ramirez-Santos A et al Lamotrigine induced subacute cutaneous lupus erythematosus. *Dermatol Online J.* 2012; 18:12.
80. Bleck TP, Smith MC. Possible induction of systemic lupus erythematosus by valproate. *Epilepsia.* 1990; 31:343-5.
81. Park-Matsumoto YC, Tazawa T. Valproate induced lupuslike syndrome. *J Neurol Sci.* 1996; 143:185-6.
82. Araújo-Fernández S, Ahijón-Lana M, Isenberg DA. Drug-induced lupus: Including anti-tumour necrosis factor and interferon induced. *Lupus.* 2014; 23:545-53.
83. Sarzi-Puttini P, Atzeni F, Capsoni F et al. Drug-induced lupus erythematosus. *Autoimmunity.* 2005; 38:507-18.
84. Mei X, Li Y, Qui P et al. Anti-thyroid drug-induced lupus. A case report and review of the literature. *Arch Endocrinol Metab.* 2015; 60:290-3.
85. Seo JY, Byun HJ, Cho KH et al. Methimazole-induced bullous systemic lupus erythematosus: a case report. *J Korean Med Sci.* 2012; 27:818-21.
86. Aloush V, Litinsky I, Caspi D et al. Propylthiouracil-induced autoimmune syndromes: two distinct clinical presentations with different course and management. *Semin Arthritis Rheum.* 2006; 36:4-9.
87. Tetikkurt C, Yuruyen M, Tetikkurt S et al. Propylthiouracil-induced lupus-like or vaculitis syndrome. *Multidiscip Respir Med.* 2012; 7:14.
88. Record NB. Acebutolol-induced pleuropulmonary lupus syndrome. *Ann Intern Med.* 1981; 95:326-7.
89. Fenniche S, Dhaoui A, Ammar FB et al. Acebutolol-induced subacute cutaneous lupus erythematosus. *Skin Pharmacol Physiol.* 2005; 18:230-3.
90. Muta K, Kukami T, Nakajima M. A proposed mechanism for the effects of acebutolol: CES2 and CYP2C19-mediated metabolism and antinuclear antibody production. *Biochem Pharmacol.* 2015; 98:659-70.
91. Sheikhzadeh A, Schafer U, Schnabet A. Drug-induced lupus erythematosus by amiodarone. *Arch Intern Med.* 2002; 162:834-6.
92. Yachoui R, Saad W. Amiodarone-induced lupus-like syndrome. *Am J Ther.* 2015; 22:e20-1.
93. Rubin RL. Drug-induced lupus. *Toxicology.* 2005; 209:135-47.
94. Crawson AN, Magro CM. Subacute cutaneous lupus erythematous arising in the setting of calcium-channel blockers therapy. *Hum Pathol.* 1997; 28:67-71.
95. Kwong HL, Teo RY. An uncommon cutaneous reaction for a common drug. Diagnosis: drug-induced subacute lupus erythematosus (DI-SCLE). *Ann Acad Med Singapore.* 2014; 43:433-4.
96. Sieber C, Grimm E, Follath F. Captopril and systemic lupus erythematosus syndrome. *Br Med J.* 1990; 301:669.
97. Pelayo M, Vargas V, Gonzales A et al. Drug-induced lupus-like reaction with captopril. *Ann Pharmacother.* 1993; 27:1541-2.
98. Heilmann G, Hien P. Clonidine therapy as cause of lupus erythematosus. *Dtsh Med Wochenschr.* 1994; 119:858-9.

99. Leak D. Absence of cross-reaction between lisinopril and enalapril in drug-induced lupus. *Ann Pharmacother.* 1997; 31:1406-7.
100. Goldman JA, Fishman AM, Lee JE, Johnson RJ. The role of cholesterol lowering agents in drug-induced rhabdomyolysis and polymyositis. *Arthritis Rheum.* 1989; 32:358-9.
101. Fusella J, Strosberg JM. Polymyositis exacerbated by gemfibrozil. *J Rheumatol.* 1990; 17:572-3.
102. Ahmed S. Lovastatin induced lupus erythematosus. *Arch Intern Med.* 1991; 151:1667-8.
103. Sridhar MK, Abdulla A. Fatal lupus-like syndrome and ARDS induced by fluvastatin. *Lancet.* 1998; 352:114.
104. Moulis G, Bene J, Sommet A et al. Statin-induced lupus: a case/non-case study in a nationawide pharmacovigilance database. *Lupus.* 2012; 21:885-9.
105. De Jong HJ, Tervaert JW, Saldi SR et al. Association between statin use and lupus-like syndrome using spontaneous reports. *Semin Arthritis Rheum.* 2011; 41:373-81.
106. Darken M, McBurney E. Subacute cutaneous-like drug eruption due to combination diuretic hydrochlorothiazide and triamterene. *J Am Acad Dennatol.* 1988; 18:38-42.
107. Goodrich A, Kohn S. Hydrochlorothiazide-induced lupus erythematosus: a new variant? *J Am Acad Dermatol.* 1993; 28:1001-2.
108. Brown CW, Deng JS. Thiazide diuretics induce lupus-like adverse reaction. *J Clin Toxicol.* 1995; 33:729-33.
109. Brown RC, Cooke J, Losowsky MS. SLE syndrome, probably induced by labetalol. *Postgrad Med J.* 1981; 57:189-90.
110. Bensaid J, Aldigier JC, Gaulde N. SLE syndrome induced by pindolol. *Br Med J.* 1979; 1:1603-4.
111. Raferty EB, Denman AM. Systemic lupus erythematosus induced by practolol. *Br Med J.* 1973; 2:452.
112. Marshall AJ, McGraw ME, Barritt DW. Positive antinuclear factor tests with prazosin. *Br Med J.* 1979; 1:165-6.
113. Harrison T, Siscats J, Wood WH. Propranolol-induced lupus syndrome. *Postgrad Med J.* 1976;58:241-4.
114. Chang C, Gershwin ME. Drug-induced lupus erythematosus: incidence, management and prevention. *Drug Saf.* 2011; 34:357-74.
115. Speira RF, Berman RS, Werner AJ et al. Ticlopidine-induced lupus. *Arch Intern Med.* 2002; 162:2240-3.
116. Uz E, Bavbek N, Turgut FH et al. Cefuroxime-induced lupus. *J Natl Med Assoc.* 2007; 99:1066-7.
117. Mysler E, Paget SA, Kimberly R. Ciprofloxacin reactions mimicking lupus flares. *Arthritis Rheum.* 1994; 37:1112-3.
118. Alexander S. Lupus erythematosus in two patients after griseofulvin treatment of Trichophyton rubrum infection. *Br J Dermatol.* 1962; 74:72-4.
119. Bonilla-Felix M, Verani R, Vanasse LG et al. Nephrotic syndrome related to systemic lupus erythematosus after griseofulvin therapy. *Pediatr Nephrol.* 1995; 9:478-9.
120. Blazes DL, Martin GJ. Drug-induced lupus erythematosus secondary to nafcillin: the first reported case. *Rheumatol Int.* 2004; 24:242-3.
121. Black O, Lundgren R, Wiman L. Nitrofurantoin-induced pulmonary fibrosis and lupus syndrome. *Lancet.* 1974; 1:930.
122. Selroos O, Edgren J. Lupus-like syndrome associated with pulmonary reaction to nitrofurantoin: report of three cases. *Ada Med Scand.* 1975; 197:125-9.
123. Gold S. Role of sulphonamides and penicillin in the pathogenesis of systemic lupus erythematosus. *Lancet.* 1951; 1:268-72.
124. Anyimadu H, Saadia N, Mannheimer S. Drug-induced lupus associated with rifabutin: a literature review. *J Int Assoc Provid AIDS Care.* 2013; 12:166-8.
125. Popkhristov P, Kapnilov S. Streptomycin producing and aggravating lupus erythematosus. *Vestn Dermatol Venereol.* 1960; 34:10-5.
126. Gunnarsson I, Kanerud L, Pettersson E et al. Predisposing factors in sulphasalazine-induced systemic lupus erythematosus. *Br J Rheumatol.* 1997; 36:1089-94.
127. Rafferty P, Yound A, Haeney M. Sulfasalazine-induced cerebral lupus erythematosus. *Postgrad Med J.* 1982; 58:98-9.
128. Cohen P, Gardner BH. Sulfonamide reactions in systemic lupus erythematosus. *JAMA.* 1966; 197:163-5.
129. Callen JP, Hughes AP, Kulp-Shorten C. Subacute cutaneous lupus erythematosus induced or exacerbated by terbinaflne: a report of 5 cases. *Arch Dermatol.* 2001; 137:1196-8.
130. Mancano MA. Patient with terbinafine-induced subactute cutaneous lupus erythematosus. *Hosp Pharm.* 2015; 50:13-7.
131. Farhi D, Viguier M, Cosnes A et al. Terbinafine-induced subacute cutaneous lupus erythematosus. *Dermatology.* 2006; 212:59-65.
132. Domz CA, McNamara DH, Holzapfel HF. Tetracycline provocation in LE. *Ann Intern Med.* 1959; 50:1217-726.
133. Jose A, Cramer AK, Davar K, Guiterrez G. A case of drug-induced lupus erythematosus secondary to trimethoprim/sulfamethoxazole presenting with pleural effusions and pericardial tamponade. *Lupus.* 2017; 26:316-9.
134. Hald A. Case of lupus erythematosus caused by chlorprothixene (Truxal). *Ugeskr Laeger.* 1964; 126:1112-4.
135. Caramaschi P, Biasi D, Carletto A et al. Clobazam-induced lupus erythematosus. *Clin Rheumatol.* 1995; 14:116.
136. Wickert WA, Campbell NR, Martin L. Acute severe adverse clozapine reaction resembling systemic lupus erythematosus. *Postgrad Med J.* 1994; 70:940-1.
137. Rami AF, Barkan D, Mevorach D et al. Clozapine-induced systemic lupus erythematosus. *Ann Pharmacother.* 2006; 40:983-5.
138. Manzo C, Putignano S. Drug-induced lupus erythematosus associated with donepezil: a case report. *Age Ageing.* 2015; 44:1062-3.
139. Presley AP, Kahn A, Williamson N. Antinuclear antibodies in patients on lithium carbonate. *Br Med J.* 1976; 2:280-1.
140. Johnstone EC, Whaley K. Antinuclear antibodies in psychiatric illness: their relationship to diagnosis and treatment. *Br Med J.* 1975; 2:724-5.
141. Hussain HM, Zakaria M. Drug-induced lupus secondary to sertraline. *Aust N Z J Psychiatry.* 2008; 42:1074-5.
142. Spillane AP. Drug-induced lupus erythematosus in a patient treated with adalumimab. *J Am Acad Dermatol.* 2007; 56:S114-6.
143. Amarante CF, Acedo LM, Rabay FM et al. Drug-induced lupus with leukocytoclastic vasculitis: a rare expression associated with adalimumab. *An Bras Dermatol.* 2015; 90:121-4.
144. West ES, Nanda K, Ofodile O et al. Adalimumab-induced cutaneous lupus erythematosus in a 16-year-old girl with juvenile idiopathic arthritis. *Pediatr Dermatol.* 2015; 32:e140-4.
145. Kelly D, O'Connell O, Henry M. Adalimumab-induced lupus serositis. *BMJ Case Rep.* 2015 Mar 4; 2015.
146. Lowe GC, Henderson CL, Grau RH et al. A systematic review of drug-induced subacute cutaneous lupus erythematosus. *Br J Dermatol.* 2011; 164:465-72.
147. Ozaslan E, Eroglu E, Gok K et al. Drug induced lupus erythematous due to capecitabine and bevacizumab treatment presenting with prolonged thrombocytopenia. *Rom J Intern Med.* 2015; 53:282-5.
148. Vasoo S. Drug-induced lupus: an update. *Lupus.* 2006; 15:757-61.
149. Wiznia LE, Subtil A, Choi JN. Subacute cutaneous lupus erythematosus induced by chemotherapy: Gemcitabine as a causative agent. *JAMA Dermatol.* 2013; 149:1071-5.
150. Stöllberger C, Krutisch G, Finsterer J et al. Dabigatran-induced lupus temporaily preventing blood group determination. *Blood Coagul Fibrinolysis.* 2014; 25:625-7.
151. Michalopoulos G, Vrakas S, Makris K et al. Systemic lupus erythematosus in Crohn's disease: drug-induced or idiopathic? *Ann Gastroenterol: Hellenic Society of Gastroenterology.* 2015; 28:408-9.
152. Wong NY, Parsons LM, Trotter MJ et al. Drug-induced subacute cutaneous lupus erythematosus associated with docetaxel chemotherapy: a case report. *BMC Res Notes.* 2014; 7:785.
153. Chen JK, Chen TS, Lim P et al. Drug-induced subacute cutaneous lupus erythematosus associated with doxorubicin. *J Am Acad Dermatol.* 2012; 67:e273-5.

154. Chalmers A, Thompson D, Stein HE et al. Systemic lupus erythematosus during penicillamine therapy for rheumatoid arthritis. *Ann Intern Med.* 1982; 97:659-63.
155. Tsankov N, Lazarova A, Vasileva S et al. Lupus erythematosus-like eruption due to D-penicillamine in progressive systemic sclerosis. *Int J Dermatol.* 1990; 29:571-4.
156. Walshe J. Penicillamine and the SLE syndrome. *J Rheumatol.* 1981; 8:155-60.
157. Enzenauer RJ, West SG, Rubin RL. D-Penicillamine-induced lupus erythematosus. *Arthritis Rheum.* 1990; 33;13S2-3.
158. Chin GL, Kong NCT, Lee BC, Rose IM. Penicillamine induced lupus-like syndrome in a patient with classical rheumatoid arthritis. *J Rheumatol.* 1991; 18:947-8.
159. Oliver I, Liberman UA, DeVries A. Lupus-like syndrome induced by penicillamine in cystinuria. *JAMA.* 1972; 22:588.
160. Harkcom TM, Conn DL, Holley KE. D-Penicillamine and lupus erythematosus-like syndrome. *Ann Intern Med.* 1978; 89:1012.
161. Carroll DG, Cavanagh LE. Drug-induced lupus associated with synthetic conjugated estrogens. *Ann Pharmacother.* 2002; 41:702-6.
162. Cairns AP, Duncan MKJ, Hinder AE et al. New onset of systemic lupus erythematosus in a patient receiving etanercept for rheumatoid arthritis. *Ann Rheum Dis.* 2002; 61:1031-2.
163. Debandt M, Vittecoq O, Descamps V et al. Anti-TNF alpha systemic lupus syndrome. *Clin Rheumatol.* 2003; 22:56-61.
164. DeBandt MD, Sibilia J, Le Loet X et al. Systemic lupus erythematosus induced by anti-tumour necrosis factor alpha therapy: a French national survey. *Arthritis Res Ther.* 2005; 7:R545-51.
165. Haraoui B, Keystone E. Musculoskeletal manifestations and autoimmune diseases related to new biologic agents. *Curr Opin Rheumatol.* 2006; 18:96-100.
166. Cush JJ. Unusual toxicities with TNF inhibition: heart failure and drug-induced lupus. *Clin Exp Rheumatol.* 2004; 22:S141-7.
167. Feldman M, Maini RN. Anti-TNF therapy of rheumatoid arthritis: what have we learned? *Annu Rev Immunol.* 2001; 19:163-96.
168. Reid MB, Glode LM. Flutamide induced lupus. *J Urol.* 1998; 159:2098.
169. Agmon-Levin N, Zafrir Y, Paz Z et al. Ten cases of systemic lupus erythematosus related to hepatitis B vaccine. *Lupus.* 2009; 18:1192-7.
170. Layton AM, Cotterill JA, Tomlisson LW. Hydroxyurea-induced lupus erythematosus. *Br J Dermatol.* 1994; 130:687-8.
171. Favalli EG, Sinigaglia L, Vaenna M, Arnoldi C. Drug-induced lupus following treatment with infliximab in rheumatoid arthritis. *Lupus.* 2002; 11:753-5.
172. Benucci M, Li Gobbi F, Fossi F et al. Drug-induced lupus alter treatment with infliximab in rheumatoid arthritis. *J Clin Rheumatol.* 2005; ll:47-9.
173. Moulis G, Sommet A, Lapeyre-Mestre M et al. Is the risk of tumour necrosis factor inhibitor-induced lupus or lupus-like syndrome the same with monoclonal antibodies and soluble receptor? A case/non-case study in a nationwide pharmacovigilance database. *Rheumatology (Oxford).* 2014; 53:1864-71.
174. Thiebault H, Boyard-Lasselin P, Guignant C et al. Paradoxical articular manifestations in patients with inflammatory bowel diseases treated with infliximab. *Eur J Gastrenterol Hepatol.* 2016; 28:876-81.
175. Lupu A, Tieranu C, Constantineescu CL et al. TNF-alpha inhibitor induced lupus-like symdrome (TAILS) in a patient with IBD. *Curr Health Sci J.* 2014; 40:285-8.
176. Dang LJ, Lubel JS, Gunatheesan S et al. Drug-induced lupus and autoimmune hepatitis secondary to infliximab for psoriasis. *Australas J Dermatol.* 2014; 55:75-9.
177. Ronnblom LE, Aim GV, Oberg KE. Possible induction of systemic lupus erythematosus by interferon-alpha in a patient with a malignant carcinoid tumour. *J Intern Med.* 1990; 227:207-10.
178. Wandl UB, Nagel-Hiemke M, May D et al. Lupus-like autoimmune disease induced by interferon therapy for myeloproliferative disorders. *Clin Immunol Immunopathol.* 1992; 65:70-4.
179. Reyes HA, Cativo EH, Sy AM. Drug-induced subacute cutaneous lupus erythematosus in a patient receiving therapy for chronic hepatitis. *C Am J Ther.* 2016; 23:e1965-7.
180. Sladkova V, Mares J, Lubenova B et al. Drug-induced systemic lupus erythematosus in interferon beta-1b therapy. *Neuro Endocrinol Lett.* 2011; 32:4-6.
181. Buchanan S, Rosemergy I, Healy P. Drug-induced subacute cutaneous lupus erythematosus due to treatment with interferon beta-1a. *N Z Med J.* 2013; 126:98-101.
182. Gonzalo JA, Cuende E, Alés-Martínez JE et al. Interleukin-2: a possible trigger ol autoimmunity. *Int Arch Allergy Immunol.* 1992; 97:251-7.
183. Kroemer G, Andreu JL, Gonzalo JA et al. Interleukin-2, autotolerance, and autoimmunity. *Adv Immunol.* 1991; 150:147-235.
184. Crayton H, Bohlmann T, Suflt R et al. Drug-induced polymyositis secondary to leuprolide acetate (Lupron) therapy for prostate carcinoma. *Clin Exp Rheumatol.* 1991; 9:525-8.
185. Dent MT, Ganapathy S, Holdsworth CD et al. Mesalamine induced-lupus like syndrome. *Br Med J.* 1992; 305:159.
186. Schleicher E. LE cells after oral contraceptives. *Lancet.* 1968; 1:821-2.
187. Bole GG, Friedlander MM, Smith CK. Rheumatic symptoms and serological abnormalities induced by oral contraceptives. *Lancet.* 1969; 1:323-6.
188. Spiera H, Plotz CM. Rheumatic symptoms and oral contraceptives. *Lancet.* 1969; 1:571-2.
189. Elias PM. Erythema nodosum and serological systemic lupus erythematosus: simultaneous occurrence in a patient using oral contraceptives. *Arch Dermatol.* 1973; 108:716-8.
190. Chapel TA, Burns RE. Oral contraceptives and exacerbation of lupus erythematosus. *Am J Obstet Gynecol.* 1971; 110:366-9.
191. Travers RL, Hughes GRV. Oral contraceptive therapy and systemic lupus erythematosus. *J Rheumatol.* 1978; 5:448-51.
192. Pimstone B. Systemic lupus erythematosus exacerbated by oral contraceptives. *S Afr J Obstet Gynecol.* 1966; 4:62-3.
193. Dubois EL, Strain L, Ehn M et al. LE cells after oral contraceptives. *Lancet.* 1968; 2:679.
194. Garovich M, Agudelo C, Pisko E. Oral contraceptives and systemic lupus erythematosus. *Arthritis Rheum.* 1980; 23:1396-8.
195. Farid N, Anderson J. SLE-like reaction to phenylbutazone therapy. *Lancet.* 1971; 1:1022-3.
196. Grayson MF, Martin VM, Markham RL. Antinative DNA antibodies as a reaction to pyrazole drugs. *Ann Rheum Dis.* 1975; 34:373-5.
197. Sandholdt LH, Laurinaviciene R, Bygum A. Proton pump inhibitor-induced subacute cutaneous lupus erythematosus. *Br J Dermatol.* 2014; 170:342-51.
198. Aggarwal N. Drug-induced subacute lupus erythematosus associated with proton pump inhibitors. *Drugs—Real World Outcomes.* 2016; 3:145-54.
199. Hoffman BJ. Sensitivity to sulfadiazine resembling acute disseminated lupus erythematosus. *Arch Dermatol Syphilol.* 1945; 51:190-2.
200. Marchetti MA, Noland MM, Dillon PM et al. Taxane associated subacute cutaneous lupus erythematosus. *Dermatol Online J.* 2013; 19:19259.
201. Lamond NW, Younis T, Purdy K et al. Drug-induced subacute cutaneous lupus erythematosus associated with nab-paclitaxel therapy. *Curr Oncol.* 2013; 20:e484-7.
202. Gelfand MS, Yunus F, White FL. Bone marrow granulomas, fever, pancytopenia and lupus-like syndrome due to tocainide. *South Med J.* 1994; 87:839-41.
203. Araujo-Fernandez S, Ahijon-Lana M, Isenberg DA. Drug-induced lupus: Including anti-tumor necrosis factor and interferon induced. *Lupus.* 2014; 23:545-53.
204. Kauffman CL, Amin CO, Fredeking AE. Drug-induced lupus erythematosus—epidemiology. Elston DM, ed. *Medscape.* https://emedicine.medscape.com/article/1065086-overview#a6 (accessed 2018 Jan 2).

205. Helmick CG, Felson DT, Lawrence RC et al. Estimates of the prevalence of arthritis and other rheumatic conditions in the United States: Part I. *Arthritis Rheum.* 2008; 58:15-25.
206. Atzeni F, Marrazza MG, Sarzi-Puttini P et al. Drug-induced lupus erythematosus. *Reumatismo.* 2003; 55:147-54.
207. Uetrecht JP, Woosley RL. Acetylators phenotype and SLE. *Clin Pharmacokinet.* 1981; 6:118-34.
208. Batchelor JR, Welsh KI, Tinoco RM et al. Hydralazine-induced systemic lupus erythematosus: Influence of HLA-DR and sex on susceptibility. *Lancet.* 1980; 24:1107-9.
209. Sim E, Gill EW. Drugs that induce systemic lupus erythematosus inhibit complement component C4. *Lancet.* 1984; 2:422-4.
210. Uetrecht JP. Mechanism of drug-induced lupus. *Chem Res Toxicol.* 1988; 1:133-43.
211. Dunphy J, Oliver M, Rands AL et al. Antineutrophil cytoplasmic antibodies and HLA class II alleles in minocycline-induced lupus-like syndrome. *Br J Dermatol.* 2000; 142:461-7.
212. Kretz-Rommel A, Rubin RL. Early cellular events in systemic autoimmunity driven by chromatin-reactive cells. *Cell Immunol.* 2001; 208:125-36.
213. Bluestein HG, Redelman D, Zvaifler NJ. Procainamide lymphocyte reactions: a possible explanation for drug-induced autoimmunity. *Arthritis Rheum.* 1981; 24:1019-23.
214. Kretz-Rommel A, Rubin RL. Disruption of positive selection of thymocytes causes autoimmunity. *Nat Med.* 2000; 6:298-305.
215. Datta SK. Positive selection for autoimmunity. *Nat Med.* 2000; 6:259-61.
216. Kretz-Rommel A, Rubin RL. Persistence of autoreactive T cell drive is required to elicit anti-chromatin antibodies in a murine model of drug-induced lupus. *J Immunol.* 1999; 162:813-20.
217. Via CS, Shustov A, Rus V et al. In vivo neutralization of TNF-alpha promotes humoral autoimmunity by preventing the induction of CTL. *J Immunol.* 2001; 167:6821-6.
218. Cameron DJ, Erlanger BF. Nucleic acid-reactive antibodies of restricted heterogenicity. *Immun Chem.* 1976; 13:265-9.
219. Eldredge NT, Robertson WVB, Miller JJ III. The interaction of lupus-inducing drugs with deoxyribonucleic acid. *Clin Immunol Immunopathol.* 1974; 3:263-71.
220. Hughes GRV, Pynes RI, Gharavi A et al. The heterogenicity of serologic findings and predisposing host factors in drug-induced lupus erythematosus. *Arthritis Rheum.* 1987; 25:1070-3.
221. Allan IM, Lunec J, Salmon M et al. Selective lymphocyte killing by lack of reactive oxygen species (ROS). *Agents Actions.* 1986; 19:351-2.
222. Holers VM, Kotzin BL. Human peripheral blood monocytes display surface antigens recognized by monoclonal antinuclear antibodies. *J Clin Invest.* 1985; 76:991-8.
223. Walport MJ. Complement: second of two parts. *N Engl J Med.* 2001; 344:1140-4.
224. Alarcon-Segovia D, Worthington JW, Ward JW et al. Lupus diathesis and the hydralazine syndrome. *N Engl J Med.* 1965; 272:462-6.
225. Speirs C, Chapel H, Fielder AL et al. Complement system protein C4 and susceptibility to hydralazine-induced systemic lupus erythematosus. *Lancet.* 1989; 1:922-4.
226. Antanov D, Kazandjieva J, Etugov D et al. Drug-induced lupus erythematosus. *Clin Dermatol.* 2004;22:157-166.
227. McDonald E, Marino C. Procainamide-induced lupus in elderly. *Hosp Pract (Off Ed).* 1993; 28:95-8.
228. Auerbach RC, Snyder NE, Bragg DG. The chest roentgenographic manifestations of pronestyl-induced lupus erythematosus. *Radiology.* 1973; 109:287-90.
229. Alloway JA, Salata MP. Quinidine-induced rheumatic syndromes. *Semin Arthritis Rheum.* 1995; 24:315-22.
230. Peterson LL. Hydralazine-induced systemic lupus erythematosus presenting as pyoderma gangrenosum-like ulcers. *J Am Acad Dermatol.* 1984; 10:379-84.
231. Solinger AM. Drug related lupus-clinical and etiologic considerations. *Rheum Dis Clin North Am.* 1988; 14:187-202.
232. Uetrecht J. Drug metabolism by leukocytes and its role in drug-induced lupus and other idiosyncratic drug reactions. *Crit Rev Toxicol.* 1990; 3:137-66.
233. Burlingame RW, Rubin RL. Drug-induced anti-histone antibodies display two patterns of reactivity with substructures of chromatin. *J Clin Invest.* 1991; 88:680-90.
234. Portanova JP, Arndt RE, Tan EM et al. Anti-histone antibodies in idiopathic and drug-induced lupus recognize distinct intrahistone regions. *J Immunol.* 1987; 138:446-51.
235. McNeil HP, Chesterman CN, Krilis SA. Immunology and clinical importance of antiphospholipid antibodies. *Adv Immunol.* 1991; 49:193-280.
236. Derksen RHWM, Kater L. Lupus anticoagulant: revival of an old phenomenon. *Clin Exp Rheumatol.* 1985; 3:349-57.
237. Rubin RL. Complement-fixing properties of antinuclear antibodies distinguish drug-induced lupus from systemic lupus erythematosus. *Lupus.* 2004; 13:249-56.
238. Weinstein A, Bordwell B, Rothfield N. Antinative DNA antibodies and serum C3 levels-candidates for the ARA preliminary criteria for the classification of systemic lupus erythematosus. *Arthritis Rheum.* 1978; 21:602.
239. Utsinger PD, Zvaifler NJ, Bluestein RM. Hypocomplementemia in procainamide-associated systemic lupus erythematosus. *Ann Intern Med.* 1976; 84:293.
240. Sherman JD, Love DE, Harrington JF. Anemia, positive lupus and rheumatoid factors with methyldopa. a report of 3 cases. *Arch Intern Med.* 1967; 120:321-6.
241. Breckenridge A, Dollery CT, Worlledge SM et al. Positive direct Coombs tests and antinuclear factor in patients treated with methyldopa. *Lancet.* 1967; 2:1265-7.
242. Perry HM Jr. Chaplin H Jr, Carmody S et al. Immunological findings in patients receiving methyldopa—a prospective study. *J Lab Clin Med.* 1971; 78:905-17.
243. Hahn BH, Charpe GC, Irvin WS et al. Immune responses to hydralazine and nuclear antigens in hydralazine-induced lupus erythematosus. *Ann Intern Med.* 1972; 76:365-74.
244. Weinstein J. Hypocomplementemia in hydralazine-associated lupus erythematosus. *Clin Res.* 1976; 24:306A.
245. Zarrabi MH, Zucker S, Miller F et al. Immunologic and coagulation disorders in chlorpromazine-treated patients. *Ann Intern Med.* 91; 1979:194-9.
246. Alarcon-Segovia D, Wakim KG, Worthington JW et al. Clinical and experimental studies on the hydralazine syndrome and its relationship to systemic lupus erythematosus. *Medicine (Baltimore).* 1967; 46:1-33.
247. Shaenk Z, Mendel JR, Rossio JL et al. Polyradiculoneuropathy accompanying procainamide-induced lupus erythematosus and evidence for drug-induced enhanced sensitization to peripheral nerve myelin. *Ann Neurol.* 1977; 1:378-84.
248. Dammin GJ, Nora JR, Reardan JB. Hydralazine reaction: case with LE cells antemortem and postmortem, and pulmonary, renal, splenic, and muscular lesions of disseminated lupus erythematosus. *J Lab Clin Med.* 1955; 46:806.
249. Bendersky G, Ramirez C. Hydralazine positioning. *JAMA.* 1960; 173:1789-94.
250. Whittingham S, Mackay IR. Systemic lupus erythematosus induced by procainamide. *Aust Ann Med.* 1970; 19:358-61.
251. Whittle TS, Ainsworth SK. Procainamide-induced systemic lupus erythematosus-renal involvement with deposition of immune complexes. *Arch Pathol Lab Med.* 1976; 100:469-74.
252. Rallison ML, Carlisle JW, Lee RE Jr et al. Lupus erythematosus and the Stevens-Johnson syndrome: occurrence as reactions to anticonvulsant medication. *Am J Dis Child.* 1961; 101:725-38.
253. Stokes MB Foster K, Markowitz GS et al. Development of glomerulonephritis during anti-TNF alpha therapy for rheumatoid arthritis. *Nephrol Dial Transplant.* 2005; 20:1400-6.

254. Hess EV. Introduction to drug-induced lupus. *Arthritis Rheum.* 1981; 24:6-9.
255. Harmon CE, Portanova JP. Drug-induced lupus-clinical and serological studies. *Clin Rheum Dis.* 1982; 8:121-35.
256. Hess EV, Mongrey AB. Drug-induced lupus: the same or different from idiopathic disease? In: Lahita RG, ed. *Systemic Lupus Erythematosus.* New York: Churchill-Livingstone; 1992: 893-904.
257. Rich MW. Drug-induced lupus. *Postgrad Med.* 1996; 100:299-308.
258. Stratton MA. Drug-induced systemic lupus erythematosus. *Clin Pharm.* 1985; 4:657-63.
259. Kale SA. Drug-induced lupus erythematosus-differentiating it from the real thing. *Postgrad Med.* 1985; 77:231-5.
260. Noel B. Lupus erythematosus and other autoimmune diseases related to statin therapy: a systematic review. *J Eur Acad Dennatol Venereol.* 2007; 21:17-24.
261. Srivastava M, Rencic A, Diglio G et al. Drug-induced, Ro/SSA-positive cutaneous lupus erythematosus. *Arch Dermatol.* 2003; 139:45-9.
262. Ansell BM. Drug-induced systemic lupus erythematosus in childhood. *Lupus.* 1993; 2:139-40.
263. Callen JP. Drug-induced subacute cutaneous lupus erythematosus. *Lupus.* 2010; 19:1107-11.
264. Jacobs JC. Drug-induced lupus. In: *Pediatric Rheumatology for the Practitioner.* New York: Springer-Verlag; 1982:365-7.
265. Mansilla-Tinoco R, Harland SJ, Ran PJ. Hydralazine, antinuclear antibodies and the lupus syndrome. *Br Med J.* 1982; 284:936-9.
266. Krohn K, Bennett R. Drug-induced autoimmune disorders. *Immunol Allergy Clin North Am.* 1998; 18:897-911.
267. Rider V, Abdou NI. Gender differences in autoimmunity: molecular basis for estrogen effects in systemic lupus erythematosus. *Int Immunopharmacol.* 2001; 1:1009-24.
268. Hildreth EA, Biro CE, McCreary TA. Persistence of the "hydralazine syndrome"—a follow-up study of eleven cases. *JAMA.* 1960; 173:657-60.
269. Perry HM Jr, Tan EM, Carmody S et al. Relationship of acetyl transferase activity to antinuclear antibodies and toxic symptoms in hypertensive patients treated with hydralazine. *J Lab Clin Med.* 1970; 76:114-25.
270. Woosley RL, Drayer DE, Reidenberg MM et al. Effect of acetylator phenotype on the rate at which procainamide induces antinuclear antibodies and the lupus syndrome. *N Engl J Med.* 1978; 298:1157-9.
271. Morris RJ, Freed CR, Kohler PF. Drug acetylation phenotype unrelated to development of spontaneous systemic lupus erythematosus. *Arthritis Rheum.* 1978; 21;192-5.
272. National Institutes of Health (NIH); National Institute of Arthritis and Musculoskeletal and Skin Diseases. *Lupus: A patient care guide for nurses and other health professionals.* 3rd ed. Bethesda, MD: NIH; 2006.
273. Bertsias G, Ioannidis JP, Boletis J et al. EULAR recommendations for the management of systemic lupus erythematosus. Report of a Task Force of the EULAR Standing Committee for International Clinical Studies Including Therapeutics. *Ann Rheum Dis.* 2008; 67:195-205.
274. Mosca M, Tani C, Aringer M et al. European League Against Rheumatism recommendations for monitoring patients with systemic lupus erythematosus in clinical practice and in observational studies. *Ann Rheum Dis.* 2010; 69:1269-74.
275. Yazdany J, Panopalis P, Gillis JZ et al. A quality indicator set for systemic lupus erythematosus. *Arthritis Rheum.* 2009; 61:370-7.

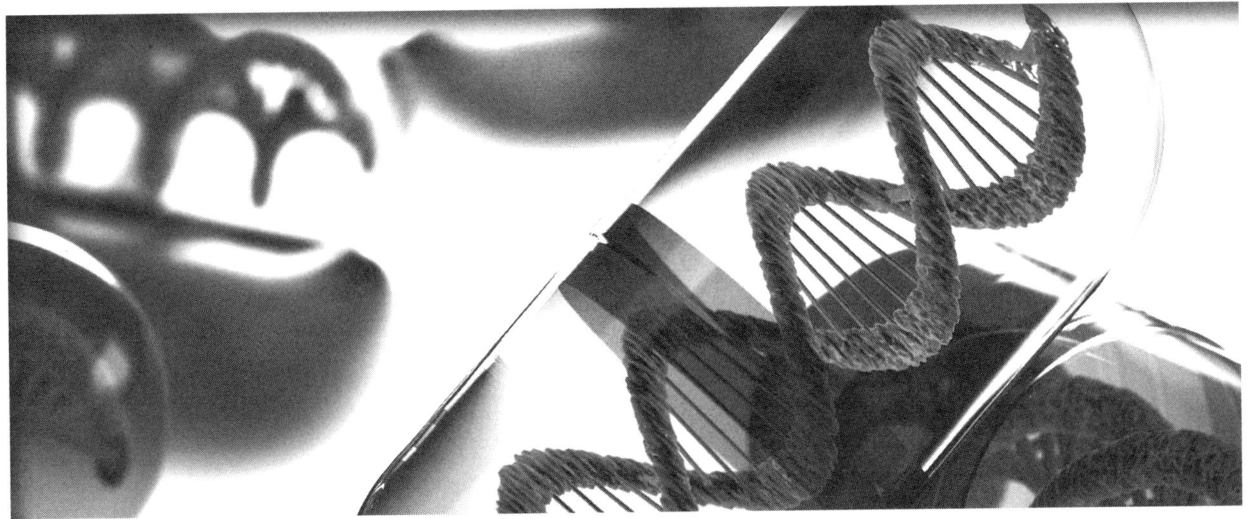

CHAPTER 8

Photosensitivity

Julie M. Koehler

Drug-induced photosensitivity is a term used to describe an undesirable pharmacologic reaction to ultraviolet radiation (UVR), which is categorized as either ultraviolet A (UVA) or ultraviolet B (UVB).[1-3] Although UVB radiation causes erythema, UVA radiation is largely responsible for tanning, photoaging, and drug-induced photosensitivity.[4] Drug-induced photosensitivity reactions are quite common today as a result of an increased number of photosensitizing chemicals found in many drug products.[1] Drug-induced photosensitivity reactions are typically classified as either phototoxic or photoallergic.

CAUSATIVE AGENTS

Several drugs and drug classes, including both systemic drugs and topically applied compounds, have been implicated in causing clinically significant photosensitivity reactions (**Table 8-1**).[5-368] Drug classes that have been reported to cause phototoxic reactions include, but are not limited to, nonsteroidal anti-inflammatory drugs (NSAIDs), tetracyclines, sulfonamides, fluoroquinolones, phenothiazines, and diuretics.[2-371] Drug classes that may cause photoallergic reactions include, but are not limited to, tetracyclines, sulfonamides, diuretics, phenothiazines, and antihistamines.[369-371] Furthermore, many of the drugs within these classes have been linked to the development of both types of photosensitivity (i.e., phototoxic and photoallergic) reactions.

EPIDEMIOLOGY

Although there are many case reports describing drug-induced photosensitivity reactions, it is challenging to estimate the true incidence of such reactions, given the difficulty in distinguishing between sunburn and a mild drug-induced photosensitivity reaction and the resultant potential for bias or inaccuracy in reporting. This is further confounded by patients' ability to control the occurrence of photosensitivity reactions by taking protective action against sunlight exposure.[370] Although the exact incidence of drug-induced photosensitivity in the general population has not been defined, results from a retrospective review from a skin-treatment referral center in Singapore indicated that 11.3% of all cases of photodermatoses were the result of

Table 8-1 Agents Implicated in Drug-Induced Photosensitivity[5-368]

Drug	Incidence	Level of Evidence[a]
Acebutolol[5]	NK	C
Acetazolamide[6]	NK	C
Alectinib[7]	9.9%	A
Alfalfa[8]	NK	C
Alitretinoin[9]	NK	C
Alprazolam[10,11]	NK	C
Amantadine[12]	NK	C
Aminolevulinic acid[13,14]	NK	C
Amiodarone[15-22]	3–10%	B
Amitriptyline[23,24]	NK	C
Amlodipine[25,26]	NK	C
Anagrelide[27]	NK	B
Aripiprazole[3,28]	0.1–1%	A
Atovaquone–proguanil[29]	NK	C
Azathioprine[30]	NK	B
Benazepril[31]	<1%	A
Benzocaine[32]	NK	C
Bergamot oil[33]	NK	B
Bexarotene[34]	NK	C
Bicalutamide[35]	NK	C
Bishop's weed[36]	NK	C
Bitter orange[37]	NK	B
Calcipotriene[38]	NK	C
Canagliflozin[38]	0.2%	A
Captopril[39]	NK	C
Carbamazepine[40]	NK	C
Carvedilol[41]	0.1–1%	A
Cefazolin[42]	NK	C
Ceftazidime[43]	NK	C
Celecoxib[44]	NK	C
Cetirizine[3]	<2%	A
Chlordiazepoxide[45,46]	NK	C
Chlorella[47]	NK	C
Chloroquine[48]	NK	C
Chlorothiazide[49-51]	NK	C
Chlorpromazine[52-55]	NK	C
Chlorpropamide[56]	NK	C
Chlorthalidone[57]	NK	C
Chrysanthemum[58-63]	NK	B
Ciprofloxacin[3,64-67]	<1%	A
Clioquinol[68]	NK	C
Clofazimine[69]	<1%	B

Table 8-1 Agents Implicated in Drug-Induced Photosensitivity[5-368] (continued)

Drug	Incidence	Level of Evidence[a]
Clomipramine[70]	NK	C
Clopidogrel[71]	NK	C
Clozapine[72]	NK	C
Coal tar[73-75]	NK	B
Cobimetinib[76]	47%	A
Crizotinib[77]	NK	C
Cyclobenzaprine[78]	<1%	A
Cyproheptadine[79]	NK	C
Dacarbazine[3,80]	<0.1%	B
Dantrolene[81]	NK	C
Dapsone[82,83]	NK	C
Demeclocycline[84]	NK	C
Desipramine[85]	NK	C
Desoximetasone[86]	NK	C
Desvenlafaxine[87]	<2%	A
Dibucaine[88,89]	NK	C
Dichlorphenamide[90]	NK	C
Diclofenac[3,91,92]	3%[b]	B
Diflunisal[93,94]	NK	C
Diltiazem[3,95-97]	<2%	B
Diphenhydramine[98-100]	NK	C
Doxepin[101]	NK	B
Doxycycline[102-105]	NK	C
Dronedarone[106]	<1%	A
Efavirenz[107,108]	NK	C
Enalapril[3,109,110]	0.5–1%	B
Enoxacin[111]	NK	B
Epirubicin[112]	NK	C
Estrogen–progestin[113-116]	NK	C
Ethionamide[117]	NK	C
Felodipine[118]	NK	C
Fenofibrate[119,120]	NK	C
Flucytosine[121]	NK	C
Fluorouracil[122,123]	NK	C
Fluoxetine[124]	NK	C
Fluphenazine[125]	NK	C
Flutamide[126-131]	NK	C
Fluvastatin[132]	NK	C
Fosinopril[3]	0.2–1%	B
Furosemide[132-135]	NK	C
Ganciclovir[136]	<1%	A
Gemifloxacin[137]	NK	B

Table 8-1 Agents Implicated in Drug-Induced Photosensitivity[5-368] (continued)

Drug	Incidence	Level of Evidence[a]
Glimepiride[3]	NK	C
Glipizide[138]	NK	B
Glyburide[139,140]	NK	C
Gotu kola[141]	NK	C
Griseofulvin[142-145]	NK	C
Haloperidol[146]	NK	C
Hexachlorophene[147]	NK	C
Hydrochlorothiazide[47,148-152]	NK	B
Hydrocortisone[153]	NK	C
Hydroxocobalamin[154]	NK	B
Hydroxyurea[155]	NK	C
Ibuprofen[156,157]	5.3%	B
Imatinib[158-160]	0.1–1%	B
Imipramine[161]	NK	C
Indapamide[162]	NK	C
Isotretinoin[163-166]	NK	C
Itraconazole[167]	NK	C
Ketoconazole[168]	NK	C
Ketoprofen[3,169-177]	<1%	B
Leflunomide[178]	NK	C
Lemon oil[32]	NK	B
Levofloxacin[179]	<0.1%	A
Lime oil[34]	NK	B
Lisinopril[3]	NK	C
Lomefloxacin[180-182]	NK	A
Loratadine[183]	NK	C
Losartan[184]	<1%	A
Lovastatin[3]	NK	C
Maprotiline[3,185]	0.1–1%	B
Mequinol–tretinoin[186,187]	NK	C
Methazolamide[3]	NK	C
Methotrexate[188-197]	3–10%	B
Methoxsalen[198]	NK	C
Methyclothiazide[199]	NK	B
Methyldopa[200]	NK	C
Methylene blue[201,202]	NK	C
Minocycline[3,105,203,204]	NK	C
Mirtazapine[205]	0.1–1%	A
Mitomycin C[206]	NK	C
Moexipril[207]	<1%	B
Moxifloxacin[208,209]	<0.1%	A
Nabumetone[3,210]	<1%	A

Table 8-1 Agents Implicated in Drug-Induced Photosensitivity[5-368] (continued)

Drug	Incidence	Level of Evidence[a]
Nalidixic acid[211-221]	NK	B
Naproxen[222-226]	<1%	B
Nifedipine[3,227,228]	<1%	A
Norfloxacin[229]	NK	C
Nortriptyline[230]	NK	B
Ofloxacin[3,231,232]	<1%	A
Olanzapine[3,233]	0.1–1%	A
Oxaprozin[234]	<1%	A
Paclitaxel[235,236]	NK	C
Panitumumab[237]	NK	B
Pantoprazole[238,239]	NK	C
Paroxetine[3,240]	0.1–1%	A
Peginterferon α-2b[241]	<1%	A
Pentostatin[3,242]	<3%	A
Pirfenidone[243]	9%	A
Phenelzine[244]	NK	C
Piroxicam[3,245-250]	<1%	B
Porfimer[3,251-258]	~20%[c]	A
Promethazine[219,259]	NK	C
Protriptyline[260]	NK	C
Pyrazinamide[3,119,261-262]	<0.1%	B
Pyridoxine[15,263-267]	NK	C
Pyrimethamine[268]	NK	C
Quinethazone[51]	NK	C
Quinidine[269-276]	NK	C
Quinine[277-282]	NK	C
Ramipril[283]	<1%	A
Ranitidine[284,285]	NK	C
Risperidone[286]	<1%	A
Ritonavir[287]	<2%	A
Saquinavir[288,289]	<2%	A
Selegiline[290]	NK	C
Sertraline[3,291]	0.1–1%	A
Simeprevir[292]	5–7%	A
Shitake mushroom[293]	NK	C
Simvastatin[294,295]	NK	C
Sotalol[296]	<0.1%	B
Sparfloxacin[297-302]	2–7.9%	A
Spironolactone[303]	NK	C
St. John's wort[304-316]	NK	B
Sulfadiazine[317]	NK	B
Sulfamethoxazole–trimethoprim[318]	NK	B

Table 8-1 Agents Implicated in Drug-Induced Photosensitivity[5-368] (continued)

Drug	Incidence	Level of Evidence[a]
Sulfisoxazole[319,320]	NK	C
Sulindac[3]	<1%	A
Tacrolimus[3,321,322]	NK	A
Tazarotene[323]	1%[d]	A
Terbinafine[324]	NK	B
Tetracycline[325-328]	NK	C
Thioridazine[3,329,330]	<0.1%	B
Tigecycline[331]	NK	B
Tolazamide[332]	NK	B
Tolbutamide[333]	NK	C
Torsemide[334]	NK	C
Trandolapril[335]	NK	C
Trazodone[336]	<1%	A
Triamterene[337,338]	NK	C
Trimethoprim[339]	NK	C
Trimipramine[340]	NK	C
Tretinoin[341,342]	NK	B
Valacyclovir[343]	NK	B
Valproic acid[344]	NK	C
Valsartan[345]	NK	C
Vandetanib[346,347]	13%	A
Vemurafenib[348-351]	33–49%	A
Venlafaxine[3,352]	0.1–1%	A
Verteporfin[3,353-356]	1–10%	A
Vinblastine[357]	NK	C
Voriconazole[358-367]	7%	A
Zaleplon[368]	<1%	A
Zolpidem[3]	<0.1%	A

NK = not known.
[a]Definitions for Levels of Evidence: Level A—evidence from one or more randomized, controlled clinical trials; Level B—evidence from nonrandomized clinical trials, prospective observational studies, cohort studies, retrospective studies, case-control studies, meta-analyses and/or postmarketing surveillance studies; and Level C—evidence from one or more published case reports or case series.
[b]Incidence reported is for topical gel only.
[c]Incidence varies according to type of cancer being treated.
[d]Incidence reported is for topical foam only.

drug-induced photosensitivity.[372] A more recent review by Dawe et al. reports an incidence of drug-induced photosensitivity ranging between 2% and 15% in patients who were referred to tertiary photodermatology centers.[373] In general, drug-induced phototoxic reactions occur more commonly than photoallergic reactions, and phototoxic reactions may occur in almost any person who receives a sufficiently high dose of the offending agent coupled with enough exposure to UVR.[374,375] The occurrence of drug-induced phototoxicity reactions are, therefore, dependent on the concentration (or amount) of the sensitizing agent (drug) and the amount of light exposure. The recorded incidence, where known, of photosensitivity associated with the administration of specific drugs is included in Table 8-1.[5-368]

MECHANISMS

Photosensitivity reactions can be classified according to the underlying mechanism or pathogenesis of the reaction. Specifically, photosensitivity reactions are the result of either phototoxicity or photoallergy. Phototoxic reactions represent the most common form, and photoallergic reactions are generally uncommon.

Phototoxic reactions are a type of nonimmunologic reaction. During phototoxic reactions, the drug, after ingestion or topical application, is believed to potentiate solar energy by acting as a chromophore (i.e., a chemical group that absorbs light at a specific frequency and imparts color to a molecule), causing absorption of ultraviolet (UV) light and yielding damage to skin tissues, including molecular and cellular damage as well as potential generation of reactive oxygen species.[1] In contrast to photoallergic reactions, drug-induced phototoxic reactions typically occur on first exposure to the drug and are often dose-related.[1,2,369,375] **Figure 8-1** illustrates the underlying mechanism of drug-induced phototoxic reactions.[4,369,371,374]

Unlike phototoxic reactions, drug-induced photoallergic reactions are the result of an immunologic response. The proposed mechanism of photoallergic reactions is that of a type IV cell-mediated hypersensitivity response (i.e., a delayed reaction, mediated by T cells rather than by antibodies, as opposed to a type I reaction, which involves IgE-mediated histamine release from mast cells and basophils; a type II reaction, which involves IgG or IgM antibodies bound to cell surface antigens; or a type III reaction, which involves deposition of circulating antigen-antibody immune complexes).[1,369,374] Specifically, it is postulated that when UV light reacts with either the drug or the drug's metabolites in the skin, a structural change in the drug occurs such that it behaves as a hapten (i.e., a small, separable part of an antigen that reacts with an antibody and is only capable of antibody production when combined with a carrier protein), which then combines with proteins in the skin (a tissue antigen) to form a hapten-protein complex (complete antigen).[1,374] On subsequent exposure to the drug, a hypersensitivity (photoallergic) response is elicited. Once the patient is "sensitized" to the drug, subsequently only minimal amounts of drug exposure are required to produce a photoallergic reaction.[1] In general, photoallergic reactions occurring in sensitized patients are not dose-dependent.[2] Because photoallergic reactions involve the immune system, there is typically a delay between the time of drug exposure and the onset of the skin eruption.[1] **Figure 8-2** illustrates the underlying mechanisms of drug-induced photoallergic reactions.[371,374]

Although the general underlying mechanisms of drug-induced photoallergy and phototoxicity are well-described in the literature, information

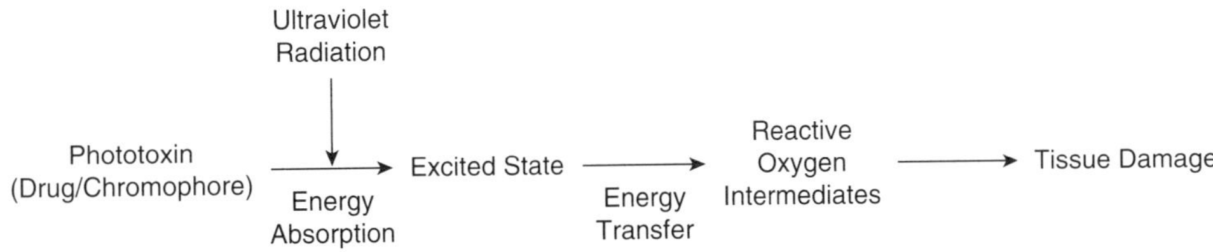

FIGURE 8-1 Mechanism of Drug-Induced Phototoxicity[371]

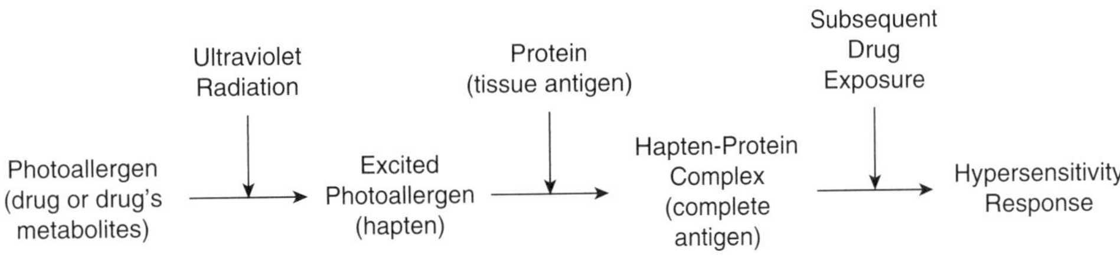

FIGURE 8-2 Mechanism of Drug-Induced Photoallergy[371]

regarding the exact mechanisms of photosensitivity associated with specific drug classes and individual agents are not as well understood. **Table 8-2** summarizes possible underlying mechanisms of drug-induced photosensitivity reactions for selected agents.

DIURETICS AND PHENOTHIAZINES

Diuretics such as hydrochlorothiazide, chlorthalidone, and furosemide and phenothiazines such as chlorpromazine and promethazine contain chlorine substituents within their chemical structures. It has been postulated that UV light exposure causes dissociation of the chlorine substituents, which is believed to lead to free radical formation, producing a photosensitivity reaction.[370] Complement, proteases, and histamine may also play a role in phenothiazine-induced phototoxicity, however, suggesting a nonoxidative mechanism.[371]

NSAIDs

Many NSAIDs have been reported to cause photosensitivity reactions. Within the NSAID class, drugs such as ketoprofen, naproxen, and nabumetone, which contain a 2-aryl propionic acid group, are thought to be the most photoactive.[370,371,375] It is believed that a decarboxylation reaction occurs on exposure to UV light, resulting in free radical formation and a subsequent photosensitivity reaction. NSAIDs lacking the 2-aryl propionic acid group, such as ibuprofen, have also been reported to cause photosensitivity, however, via a less well-understood mechanism.[370,375]

ANTIBACTERIALS

Many antibacterial agents are known to elicit a high degree of photosensitivity. Tetracyclines, fluoroquinolones, and sulfonamides are among the classes that are most commonly implicated.[370,373,375] Within the tetracycline class in particular, oxidative reactions involving free radical formation are believed to play a role.[371] Polymorphonuclear cells and complement have also been identified as potential inflammatory mediators involved in the mechanism of tetracycline-induced photosensitivity.[371]

PSORALENS

Psoralen derivatives, such as methoxsalen, represent a unique class of drugs in that their inherent photosensitizing mechanism is used therapeutically in combination with controlled UV light exposure to produce a melanogenic effect for the treatment of disorders such as idiopathic vitiligo.[371] Thus, the photosensitizing potential of such agents is a known and, for the most part, intended effect. Methoxsalen, when activated by UVA light, becomes highly erythemogenic and melanogenic. Although the precise mechanism by which these agents induce phototoxic reactions is not completely known, it is believed that psoralen-induced phototoxicity involves nonoxygen-dependent pathways and may be linked most closely to the alteration of deoxyribonucleic acid (DNA) synthesis and direct induction of an inflammatory skin reaction to enhance melanin formation.[371]

Table 8-2 Mechanisms of Drug-Induced Photosensitivity

Drug Classes	Mechanism(s)
Diuretics	Dissociation of chlorine substituent on ultraviolet light exposure, causing free radical formation[370]
Nonsteroidal anti-inflammatory drugs	Decarboxylation reaction on ultraviolet light exposure, causing free radical formation[370,371,375]
Phenothiazines	Dissociation of chlorine substituent on ultraviolet light exposure, causing free radical formation[370] Complement, proteases and histamine may also play a role[371]
Photosensitizing agents	Free radical formation on ultraviolet light exposure
Psoralens	Possible alteration of DNA synthesis and direct inflammatory effect, leading to increased melanin production and an erythemogenic effect[371]
Tetracyclines	Oxidative reaction on ultraviolet light exposure, causing free radical formation Polymorphonuclear cells and complement may also serve as inflammatory mediators[371]

DNA = deoxyribonucleic acid.

PHOTOSENSITIZING AGENTS

Porfimer (indicated for palliative treatment in esophageal cancer, for endobronchial non-small cell lung cancer, and for high-grade Barrett esophageal dysplasia) and verteporfin (used for neovascularization associated with age-related macular degeneration, pathologic myopia, or presumed ocular histoplasmosis) represent drugs that are used therapeutically because of their known photosensitizing properties. Both of these agents are used in photodynamic therapy for which UV light exposure is required for pharmacologic activation. On exposure to UV light, these photosensitizers become activated in the presence of oxygen, and free radicals are generated, enhancing the potential for phototoxicity.[371]

CLINICAL PRESENTATION AND DIFFERENTIAL DIAGNOSIS

Classic signs and symptoms associated with drug-induced photosensitivity are listed in **Table 8-3**.[369] Symptoms of drug-induced photosensitivity reactions are very similar to those of a sunburn. Typical photosensitivity reactions may result in the development of erythema, edema, and papules, and in severe cases, may also progress to the development of plaque-like urticarial lesions and possible vesicle formation.[1,369] When differentiating between photosensitivity and other types of skin eruptions, clinicians should note that photosensitivity eruptions classically manifest on areas of the skin that are most routinely exposed to sunlight (e.g., nose, cheeks, tops of the ears, neck, forearms, backs of the hands).[1,369] In general, sharp lines of demarcation between sunlight-exposed and uninvolved skin are noted.[369] In some cases, however, skin eruptions can appear on areas of the skin that receive little to no sun exposure and may be generalized over the entire body. In general, while differentiation between drug-induced photosensitivity and other adverse skin reactions to sunlight may be somewhat challenging (**Table 8-4**), differentiation between cases of drug-induced phototoxicity and photoallergy can also be difficult, given that many drugs have been implicated in causing both types of reactions.[2,371] Differences between the characteristics of phototoxic and photoallergic reactions are highlighted in **Table 8-5**.[2,371] Examples of the clinical appearance of drug-induced phototoxic and photoallergic reactions are presented in **Figure 8-3**.

Cases of drug-induced phototoxic reactions are associated with a much more rapid onset (e.g., within 30 minutes to several hours after exposure to UV light) than those of drug-induced photoallergy.[2] In general, phototoxic reactions are less severe than photoallergic reactions and resemble an exaggerated sunburn.[2] Phototoxic reactions are associated with erythema and pain, and occasionally may progress to blistering and vesicle

Table 8-3 Signs and Symptoms Associated with Drug-Induced Photosensitivity[369]

- Edema
- Erythema
- Erythroderma
- Hyperpigmentation
- Pain
- Papules
- Petechiae
- Pruritus
- Scaly patches
- Scarring
- Swelling
- Vesicles
- Wheals

Table 8-4 Conditions to Consider in the Differential Diagnosis of Drug-Induced Photosensitivity[369]

- Actinic prurigo
- Allergic contact dermatitis
- Epidermolysis bullosa
- Epidermolysis bullosa acquisita
- Erythropoietic protoporphyria
- Hydroa vacciniforme
- Irritant contact dermatitis
- Lichen planus
- Plant-induced photosensitivity reaction (phytophotodermatitis)
- Polymorphic light eruption
- Solar urticaria
- Sunburn
- Systemic lupus erythematosus (subacute cutaneous lupus erythematosus)

Table 8-5 Differentiating Characteristics of Phototoxicity and Photoallergy[2,371]

Characteristic	Phototoxicity	Photoallergy
Frequency of occurrence	Common	Uncommon
Mechanism	Nonimmune-mediated	Immune-mediated
Onset after exposure to drug and sunlight	Immediate (minutes to hours); may occur after single exposure to drug	May be delayed (hours to days); usually occurs after more than one exposure to drug
Distribution	Usually confined to exposed skin	May affect both exposed and unexposed skin
Potential for pigmentary changes	High	Low
Dose-dependency	Yes	No
Potential for cross reactivity	No	Yes
Potential for persistent light reaction	No	Yes

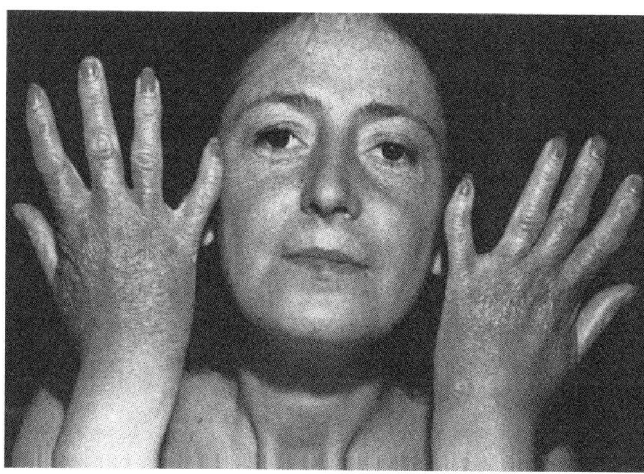

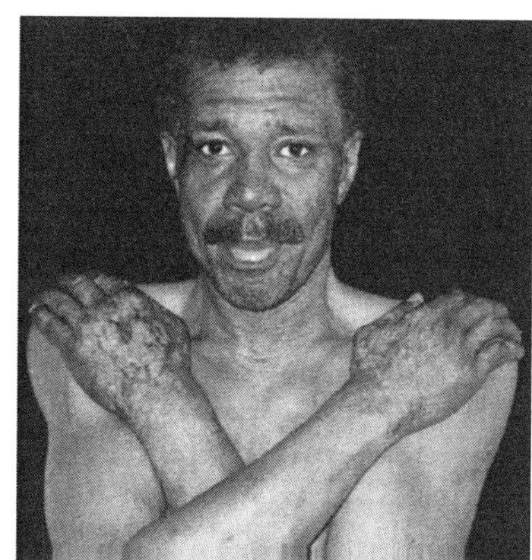

FIGURE 8-3 Drug-Induced Phototoxicity and Photoallergy

The photo on the left depicts a case of drug-induced phototoxicity secondary to demethylchlortetracycline use for treatment of acne. The woman was wearing a hat that protected her face and neck from sunlight exposure, but her hands were exposed to sunlight while holding a railing at a sporting event. The photo on the right depicts a case of drug-induced photoallergy secondary to trimethoprim–sulfamethoxazole use for *Pneumocystis jiroveci* pneumonia prophylaxis. Eczema and hyperpigmentation of the sun-exposed areas are noted. Photos reprinted with permission from Wolff K, Johnson RA, Suurmond D. *Fitzpatrick's Color Atlas and Synopsis of Clinical Dermatology: Common and Serious Diseases*. 5th ed. New York, NY: McGraw-Hill; 2005:226-69. (See color section.)

formation.[369] Within several days of the onset of the reaction, the damaged skin may begin to desquamate (i.e., peel off in scales).[369]

In some cases, epidermal thickening, elastosis, telangiectasia, and pigmentary changes (hyperpigmentation or hypopigmentation) may occur in association with phototoxic reactions.[1] Pigmentary changes occur commonly (4–9%) as a manifestation of photosensitivity in patients receiving long-term, high-dose amiodarone therapy.[371,376-381] Specifically, a blue-gray discoloration commonly develops on areas of the skin that are subjected to unprotected light exposure because of the deposition of amiodarone and its metabolites within the dermis.[371,378,379,381]

The skin damage that occurs in phototoxic reactions is typically confined to areas of exposed skin only. However, occasionally the nails may also be affected. This phototoxic effect is a well-known phenomenon known as photo-onycholysis (i.e., separation of the nail from the distal nailbed in conjunction with sun exposure and simultaneous drug use).[2,4,369] Histologically, dermal edema (swelling of the skin), dyskeratosis (aberrant development of the epidermis with abnormal keratinization), and keratinocytic necrosis (injury to keratinocytes, the predominant cell in the epidermis) may be observed.[4,369]

Cases of drug-induced photoallergic reactions are typically associated with an onset ranging from 24 to 48 hours to up to 14 days after initial exposure to the sun. The initial eruption is usually described as a papulovesicular, intensely pruritic, eczematous dermatitis.[369] In some cases, the rash may involve lichenoid, urticarial, bullous, or purpuric lesions. Histopathologic findings in cases of drug-induced photoallergy are typically similar to those found in cases of contact dermatitis.[1] In general, photoallergic reactions involve only areas directly exposed to the sun, but in severe cases, these reactions may also affect areas that are normally protected from UV light. It is important to note that after discontinuation of therapy with the offending agent, the clinical effects of drug-induced photoallergy may persist for some time. Over time, the eruptions may even become hyperpigmented or hypopigmented.[371]

If the diagnosis of a drug-induced photoreaction remains uncertain after obtaining a thorough history and conducting a full skin exam, photopatch testing may be useful and may further aid in the identification of the offending agent. During photopatch testing, template test sites are exposed to increasing doses of UVA while the patient is taking the suspected drug.[382] In patients with a phototoxicity or photoallergy secondary to a drug, the UVA minimal erythema dose (MED, or the minimum UVA dose that produces a clearly marginated erythema in the irradiated site 24 hours after a single exposure) is significantly lower than the MED for a normal individual of the same skin type. Once the drug is excreted and eliminated from the skin, repeat UVA photopatch testing yields an increase in the MED result.[382]

RISK FACTORS

Several risk factors may increase a person's susceptibility to drug-induced photosensitivity reactions (**Table 8-6**).[2,369,371,374] For any patient who is taking a known photosensitizing agent, use of sunscreens and protective clothing is warranted to minimize the risk of a photosensitivity reaction. It should be noted, however, that occasionally sunscreens themselves can act as photosensitizing agents. Sunscreens containing para-aminobenzoic acid (PABA) contain a sulfa moiety, which may aggravate photodermatitis in sensitized individuals. Although PABA-based sunscreens became widely available in the 1970s, the use of PABA as an ingredient in sunscreens today is much less common, and the majority of commercially available products are promoted as "PABA-free." Padimate O (also known as octyl dimethyl-PABA) is a PABA ester that is chemically similar to PABA but is not as irritating and today can be found in some sunscreen products, including lip balms. In general, sunscreens containing PABA or PABA esters should be avoided in susceptible individuals.[369,371,375]

Table 8-6 Risk Factors for Drug-Induced Photosensitivity Reactions[2,369,371,374]

- Drug–drug interactions
- High drug dose (phototoxic reactions only)
- Immunocompromised state
- Lack of protection against sunlight exposure
- Light skin (types I and II)/fair complexion
- Use of sunscreen products containing PABA or PABA esters (e.g., padimate O)

PABA = para-aminobenzoic acid.

In cases of phototoxicity, the dose of the photosensitizing agent itself may be a risk factor. For example, dose-related increases in the incidence of light eruptions have been reported in association with doxycycline.[383] Reduction of the dose of the offending agent during phototoxic reactions has been shown to yield symptom and reaction resolution in some cases, supporting the theory that dose can be an important risk factor.[384,385]

In cases of photoallergy, the patient's immune status may be an important risk factor. For example, human immunodeficiency virus (HIV) photodermatitis is estimated to occur in approximately 5% of HIV-positive patients with CD4 T lymphocyte counts of 50 cells/μL or lower, with the risk for development increasing as CD4 T lymphocyte counts decline.[2,386-389]

Drug–drug interactions involving photosensitizing agents may play a role in photosensitivity.

Concomitant administration of photosensitizing agents such as porfimer, verteporfin, or psoralens (e.g., methoxsalen) and other agents reported to cause photosensitivity reactions (Table 8-1), such as tetracyclines, phenothiazines, diuretics, sulfonamides, NSAIDs, and others may produce additive photosensitizing effects, thereby increasing the potential for a photosensitivity reaction. In cases of amiodarone-induced photosensitivity, coadministration of pyridoxine has been demonstrated to worsen the photosensitivity reaction, possibly because of a metabolic effect resulting in damage to the skin's structural integrity.[15,381] More specifically, amiodarone is believed to induce phototoxic damage when, following the absorption of a photon, an excited (triplet) state is created, and the excited molecules then interact with a biological target to form a radical species. This species is then susceptible to interaction with molecular oxygen, leading to peroxidation.[263,390] Although the mechanism is not fully understood, pyridoxine enhancement of amiodarone phototoxicity has been demonstrated in vitro through induction of photosensitizing enzyme processes by pyridoxal phosphate, a catalytically active form of vitamin B6.[263,390] Evidence of this has also been suggested in one small randomized, double-blind, placebo-controlled trial.[15] Thami et al. reported a reactivation of photodermatitis caused by the concomitant administration of haloperidol and methotrexate in a patient with psoriasis.[391] Although both drugs have been reported to cause photosensitivity reactions, a possible drug interaction, in which haloperidol likely interfered with tryptophan metabolism, was suggested to play a role in the development of the adverse reaction.[391] With respect to phototoxicity, for which the dose of the drug may be an important factor, any drug interaction that may cause a significant increase in the plasma concentration of the photosensitizing drug may contribute to the development of photosensitivity reactions.

MORBIDITY AND MORTALITY

In general, drug-induced photosensitivity reactions rarely involve significant morbidity or mortality (although voriconazole-induced photosensitivity has been linked to squamous cell carcinoma).[359,392-396] Most reactions are reversible after discontinuation of the offending agent.[2] In some cases, complete resolution of a drug-induced photosensitivity reaction may require weeks to months. In 5–10% of patients who experience photoallergy, however, a chronic condition known as persistent light reaction (PLR) may develop; this is also occasionally described as chronic actinic dermatitis.[397] In such patients, the photosensitivity reaction persists after drug discontinuation, and relapse of the reaction occurs on minimal exposure to UV light in the absence of the offending agent. Although PLR may occur in patients sensitized to systemic photosensitizing agents, it is believed to occur more commonly in patients sensitized to topical photosensitizers.[2]

PREVENTION

Some methods for preventing drug-induced photosensitivity reactions are listed in **Table 8-7**.[369,375] In the case of both photoallergic and phototoxic reactions, the best means of prevention includes both the avoidance of sunlight and the use of broad-spectrum sunscreens that block both UVA and UVB sunlight.[369,375,398-400] Because of their potential to cause or aggravate photodermatitis, sunscreen products containing PABA or PABA esters should specifically be avoided. For patients who are receiving photodynamic therapy with agents such as porfimer and verteporfin, it is important to note that opaque sunscreens such as zinc oxide should

Table 8-7 Approaches to Help Prevent Drug-Induced Photosensitivity[369,400]

- Avoid sunlight
- Use broad-spectrum sunscreens that block both ultraviolet A and B sunlight (minimum sun protection factor of 30[a])
- Avoid sunscreens containing PABA
- Use protective clothing (e.g., wide-brimmed hats, sunglasses, and long-sleeved shirts)
- Use dietary supplements containing antioxidants[b]

PABA = para-aminobenzoic acid.
[a]Although the U.S. Food and Drug Administration recommends a minimum sun protection factor of 15, the American Academy of Dermatology currently recommends a minimum of 30.
[b]Further study is needed to confirm the efficacy of this method.

be used, as nonopaque sunscreens are ineffective for prevention of the photosensitivity induced by these agents.[256,354] Further, it should be noted that sunscreen protection may not always be sufficient to prevent drug-induced photosensitivity reactions. Therefore, the use of protective clothing may also be necessary to prevent adverse reactions to light exposure.

Based on the underlying mechanism of photosensitivity reactions, it has also been suggested that dietary supplementation with antioxidants may help prevent adverse cutaneous photoreactions.[370,398] However, further study is needed to validate this method of prevention.

MANAGEMENT

The appropriate treatment of drug-induced photosensitivity reactions depends to some degree on the type of reaction (i.e., photoallergic or phototoxic). Treatment of patients with phototoxic reactions is similar to that of patients with routine sunburn. Discontinuation of the offending drug often accelerates resolution. In some cases of phototoxicity, reducing the dose of the offending agent (rather than drug discontinuation) may result in resolution of the reaction.[69,371,375,398] In cases of amiodarone-induced photosensitivity in which blue-gray discoloration of the skin has occurred, dose reduction has resulted in gradual disappearance of the pigmentary changes.[380] Systemic corticosteroids are not effective for the management of drug-induced phototoxicity.[1,398,399] Similarly, topical antihistamines have also been shown to be ineffective.[1]

For patients experiencing a photoallergic reaction, both antihistamines and corticosteroids may be prescribed to assist with symptom relief. Oral prednisone in doses of 1 mg/kg/day administered as a short burst (e.g., 3–10 days) or tapered over the course of 3 weeks has been shown to be highly effective in symptomatic patients suffering from photoallergy.[1,369] Topical corticosteroids (e.g., betamethasone valerate 0.1% cream) or NSAIDs (e.g., indomethacin 25 mg three times daily or ibuprofen 400 mg four times daily) may help to reduce pain and inflammation.[369] The use of NSAIDs or corticosteroids should be avoided, however, in cases where such medications have been identified as the potential causative agent of the photoreaction (refer to Table 8-1 for specific NSAIDs and corticosteroids that have been reported to cause photosensitivity). In photoallergic reactions, discontinuation of the offending drug is almost always necessary.[2,371,375] For both types of photosensitivity reactions, the use of ice packs or cold water compresses may occasionally provide symptomatic relief.[369] Treatment options that may be employed in the management of photosensitivity reactions are listed in **Table 8-8**.[1,2,369,399]

Table 8-8 Treatment Options for Drug-Induced Photosensitivity[1,2,369,371,398-400]

- Discontinuation of the offending drug
- Reduction in dose of the offending drug[a]
- Nonsteroidal anti-inflammatory drugs
- Topical corticosteroids[b]
- Antihistamines[b]
- Systemic corticosteroids[b]
- Ice packs or cold water compresses

[a]May be effective only in certain cases of phototoxicity. Photoallergy reactions require discontinuation of the offending agent.
[b]Only shown to be effective in cases of photoallergy.

INFORMATION FOR PATIENTS

Patients for whom medications that have been reported to cause photosensitivity reactions are prescribed should be informed of the potential for this adverse effect prior to the initiation of therapy. During the course of therapy with the potentially photosensitizing agent, patients should be encouraged to avoid excessive exposure to sunlight, particularly from the hours of 10:00 a.m. to 4:00 p.m. and especially in the absence of protection against UV light. The patient should wear protective clothing (e.g., wide-brimmed hats, sunglasses, long-sleeved shirts) and use broad-spectrum sunscreens with a minimum sun protection factor of 30 (especially for patients with light, fair, pale, or albino skin tones; for patients with olive, brown, or black skin tones, a minimum sun protection factor of 15 may be sufficient) throughout the duration of therapy.[369,400]

Zinc oxide and titanium dioxide provide a physical barrier that reflects and scatters the full spectrum of UVR; therefore, sunscreens containing these agents may provide the best protection against sunlight exposure. Although the majority of commercially available sunscreens today are marketed as "PABA-free," consumers should be aware of sunscreens containing PABA or PABA esters, such as padimate O, and such products should generally be avoided in sensitized patients because of the potential to aggravate or worsen photodermatitis.[371,369]

REFERENCES

1. Law R, Law DTS. Dermatologic drug reactions and common skin conditions. In: DiPiro JT, Talbert RL, Yee GC et al., eds. *Pharmacotherapy: a pathophysiologic approach.* 8th ed. New York: McGraw-Hill; 2011:1661-72.
2. Vasssileva SG, Mateev G, Parish LC. Antimicrobial photosensitive reactions. *Arch Intern Med.* 1998; 158:1993-2000.
3. Dufner KS, Buss LA, Kizito J. Drug-induced photosensitivity. *Hosp Pharm.* 2006; 41:196-206.
4. Choi D, Kannan S, Lim HW. Evaluation of patients with photodermatoses. *Dermatol Clin.* 2014; 32:267-75.
5. Maugars Y, Prost A. Photosensitivity and acebutolol. *Rheumatology.* 1988; 40:53-8.
6. Acetazolamide [package insert]. Bedford, OH: Bedford Laboratories; 2002.
7. Alecensa [package insert]. South San Francisco, CA: Genentech USA; 2015.
8. Brown R. Potential interactions of herbal medicines with antipsychotics, antidepressants and hypnotics. *Eur J Herbal Med.* 1997; 3:25-8.
9. Panretin [package insert]. San Diego, CA: Ligand Pharmaceuticals; 1999.
10. Kanwar AJ, Gupta R, Das Mehta S et al. Photosensitivity due to alprazolam. *Dermatologica.* 1990; 181:75.
11. Watanabe Y, Kawada A, Ohnishi Y et al. Photosensitivity due to alprazolam with positive oral photochallenge test after 17 days administration. *J Am Acad Dermatol.* 1999; 40:832-3.
12. Van den Berg WH, van Ketel WG. Photosensitization by amantadine (Symmetrel). *Contact Dermatitis.* 1983; 9:165.
13. Yokoyama S, Nakano H, Nishizawa A et al. A case of photocontact urticaria induced by photodynamic therapy with topical 5-aminolevulinic acid. *J Dermatol.* 2005; 132:996-9.
14. Gupta AK, Ryder JE. Photodynamic therapy and topical aminolevulinic acid: An overview. *Am J Clin Dermatol.* 2003; 4:699-708.
15. Mulrow JP, Mulrow CD, McKenna WJ. Pyridoxine and amiodarone-induced photosensitivity. *Ann Intern Med.* 1985; 103:68-9.
16. Marcus FI, Fontaine GH, Frank R et al. Clinical pharmacology and therapeutic applications of the antiarrhythmic agent, amiodarone. *Am Heart J.* 1981; 101:480-93.
17. Roupe G, Larko O, Olsson SB. Amiodarone photoreactions. *Ada Derm Venereol.* 1987; 67:76-9.
18. Walter JF, Bradner H, Curtis GP. Amiodarone photosensitivity. *Arch Dermatol.* 1984; 120:1591-4.
19. Waitzer S, Butany J, From L et al. Cutaneous ultrastructural changes and photosensitivity associated with amiodarone therapy. *J Am Acad Dermatol.* 1987; 16:779-87.
20. Ammoury A, Michaud S, Paul C et al. Photodistribution of blue-gray hyperpigmentation after amiodarone treatment: molecular characterization of amiodarone in the skin. *Arch Dermatol.* 2008; 144:92-6.
21. Shah N, Warnakulasuriya S. Amiodarone-induced peri-oral photosensitivity. *J Oral Pathol Med.* 2004; 33:56-8.
22. Yones SS, O'Donoghue NB, Palmer RA et al. Persistent severe amiodarone-induced photosensitivity. *Clin Exp Dermatol.* 2005; 30:500-2.
23. Taniguchi S, Hamada T. Photosensitivity and thrombocytopenia due to amitriptyline. *Am J Hematol.* 1996; 53:49-50.
24. Elavil [package insert]. West Point, PA: Merck and Co; 1999.
25. Collins P, Ferguson J. Photodistributed nifedipine-induced facial telangiectasia. *Br J Dermatol.* 1993; 129:630-3.
26. Erbagci Z. Amlodipine associated hyperpigmentation. *Saudi Med J.* 2004; 25:103-5.
27. Agrylin [package insert]. Wayne, PA: Shire US; 2015.
28. Gregorion S, Karagiorga T, Stratigos A et al. Photoonycholysis caused by olanzapine and aripiprazole. *J Clin Psychopharmacol.* 2008; 28:219-20.
29. Malarone [package insert]. Research Triangle Park, NC: GlaxoSmithKline; 2007.
30. Perrett CM, Walker SL, O'Donovan P et al. Azathioprine treatment photosensitizes human skin to ultraviolet A radiation. *Br J Dermatol.* 2008; 159:198-204.
31. Lotensin [package insert]. Sufferin, NY: Novartis Pharmaceuticals; 2007.
32. Kaidbey KH, Allen H. Photocontact allergy to benzocaine. *Arch Dermatol.* 1981; 117:77-9.
33. Naganuma M, Hirose S, Nakayama Y et al. A study of the phototoxicity of lemon oil. *Arch Dermatol Res.* 1985; 278:31-6.
34. Targretin [package insert]. San Diego, CA: Ligand Pharmaceuticals; 2001.
35. Lee K, Oda Y, Sakaguchi M et al. Drug-induced photosensitivity to bicalutamide—case report and review of the literature. *Phtodermatol Photoimmunol Photomed.* 2016; 32:161-4.
36. Ossenkoppele PM, van der Sluis WG, van Vloten WA. Phototoxic dermatitis following the use of Ammi majus fruit for vitiligo. *Ned Tijdschr Geneeskd.* 1991; 135:478-80.
37. McKenna KE, Stern RS. Photosensitivity associated with combined UV-B and calcipotriene therapy. *Arch Dermatol.* 1995; 131:1305-7.
38. Invokamet [package insert]. Titusville, NJ: Janssen Pharmaceuticals; 2014.
39. O'Neil MB, Balfe JW, Geary DF. Captopril related hyperpigmentation (letter). *Br Med L.* 1987; 295:333.
40. Tegretol [package insert]. East Hanover, NJ: Novartis Pharmaceuticals; 2007.
41. Coreg CR [package insert]. Research Triangle Park, NC: GlaxoSmithKline; 2007.
42. Garza LA, Yoo EK, Junkins-Hopkins JM et al. Photo recall effect in association with cefazolin. *Cutis.* 2004; 73:79-80, 85.
43. Vinks SATMM, Heijerman HGM, De Jonge P et al. Photosensitivity due to ambulatory intravenous ceftazidime in cystic fibrosis patient. *Lancet.* 1993; 341:1221-2.
44. Yazici AC, Baz K, Ikizoglu G et al. Celecoxib-induced photoallergic drug eruption. *Int J Dermatol.* 2004; 43:459-61.
45. Luton EF, Finchum RN. Photosensitivity reaction to chlordiazepoxide. *Arch Dermatol.* 1965; 91:362.
46. Blair III HM. Fixed drug eruption from chlordiazepoxide. *Arch Dermatol.* 1974; 109:914.
47. Jitsukawa K, Suizu R, Hidano A. Chlorella photosensitization: new phytophotodermatosis. *Int J Dermatol.* 1984; 23:263-8.
48. Martin-Garcia RF, del R Camacho N, Sanchez JL. Chloroquine-induced, vitiligo-like depigmentation. *J Am Acad Dermatol.* 2003; 48:981-3.

49. Addo HA, Ferguson J, Frain-Bell W. Thiazide-induced photosensitivity: a study of 33 subjects. *Br J Dermatol.* 1987; 116:749-60.
50. Harber LC, Lashinsky AM, Baer RL et al. Skin manifestations of photosensitivity due to chlorothiazide and hydrochlorothiazide. *J Invest Dermatol.* 1959; 33:83-4.
51. Miller RC, Beltrani VC. Quinethazone photosensitivity dermatitis. *Arch Dermatol.* 1966; 93:346.
52. Epstein TH. Photoallergy. *Arch Dermatol.* 1972;106:741.
53. Coleman WP. Unusual cutaneous manifestations of drug hypersensitivity. *Med Clin North Am.* 1967; 51:1073.
54. Epstein S. Chlorpromazine photosensitivity phototoxic and photoallergic reactions. *Arch Dermatol.* 1968; 98:354.
55. Thorazine [package insert]. Philadelphia, PA: SmithKline Beecham Pharmaceuticals; 2002.
56. Diabinese [package insert]. New York, NY: Pfizer; 2001.
57. Thalitone [package insert]. Bristol, TN: Monarch Pharmaceuticals; 2003.
58. Kuno Y, Kawabe Y, Sakakibara S. Allergic contact dermatitis associated with photosensitivity, from alantolactone in a chrysanthemum farmer. *Contact Dermatitis.* 1999; 40:224-5.
59. Paulsen E, Sogaard J, Andersen KE. Occupational dermatitis in Danish gardeners and greenhouse workers (III): compositae-related symptoms. *Contact Dermatitis.* 1998; 38:140-6.
60. dejong NW, Vermeulen AM, van Wijik RG et al. Occupational allergy caused by flowers. *Allergy.* 1998; 53:204-9.
61. Yu XY. A prospective clinical study on reversion of 200 precancerous patients with hua-sheng-ping. *Zhongguo Zhong Xi Yi fie He Za Zhi.* 1993; 13:147-9.
62. Camplimi P, Sertoli A, Fabbri P et al. Alantolactone sensitivity in chrysanthemum contact dermatitis. *Contact Dermatitis.* 1978; 4:93-102.
63. Bleumink E, Mitchell JC, Geismann TA et al. Contact hypersensitivity to sesquiterpene lactones in Chrysanthemum dermatitis. *Contact Dermatitis.* 1976; 2:81-8.
64. Cipro [package insert]. Kenilworth, NJ: Schering-Plough; 2008.
65. Ferguson J, Dawe R. Phototoxicity in quinolones: comparison of ciprofloxacin and grepafloxacin. *J Antimicrob Chemother.* 1997; 40:93-8.
66. Urbina F, Barrios M, Sudy E. Photolocalized purpura during ciprofloxacin therapy. *Photodermatol Photoimmunol Photomed.* 2006; 22:111-2.
67. Tolland J, Elborn S, McKenna K. Ciprofloxacin-induced phototoxicity in patients with cystic fibrosis. *J Am Acad Dermatol.* 2005; 52:158.
68. Rivara G, Barile M, Guarrera M. Photosensitivity in a patient with contact allergic dermatitis from clioquinol. *Photodermatol Photoimmunol Photomed.* 1991; 8:225-6.
69. Lamprene [package insert]. East Hanover, NJ: Novartis Pharmaceuticals; 1999.
70. Ljunggren B, Bojs G. A case of photosensitivity and contact allergy to systemic tricyclic drugs, with unusual features. *Contact Dermatitis.* 1991; 24:259-65.
71. Dogra S, Kanwar AJ. Clopidogrel bisulphate-induced photosensitive lichenoid eruption: first report. *Br J Dermatol.* 2003; 148:609-10.
72. Clozaril [package insert]. East Hanover, NJ: Novartis Pharmaceuticals; 2002.
73. Diette KM, Gange RW, Stern RS et al. Coal tar phototoxicity: kinetics and exposure parameters. *J Invest Dermatol.* 1983; 81:347-50.
74. Kaidbey KK, Kligman AM. Clinical and histological study of coal tar phototoxicity in humans. *Arch Dermatol.* 1977; 113:592-5.
75. Pathak MA, Joshi PC. The nature and molecular basis of cutaneous photosensitivity reactions to psoralens and coal tar. *J Invest Dermatol.* 1983; 80:66-74.
76. Cotellic [package insert]. South San Francisco, CA: Genentech USA; 2015.
77. Oser MG, Janne PA. A severe photosensitivity dermatitis caused by crizotinib. *J Thorac Oncol.* 2014; 9:e51-3.
78. Amrix [package insert]. North Wales, PA: Teva Pharmaceuticals USA; 2013.
79. Cyproheptadine [package insert]. Madison, MS: Cypress Pharmaceuticals; 2005.
80. Truedler R, Georgieva J, Geilen CC et al. Dacarbazine but not temozolomide induces phototoxic dermatitis in patients with malignant melanoma. *J Am Acad Dermatol.* 2004; 50:783-5.
81. Dantrium [package insert]. Cincinnati, OH: Procter and Gamble Pharmaceuticals; 1999.
82. Vandersteen PR, Jordon RE. Dermatitis herpetiformis with discoid lupus erythematosus: occurrence of sulfone-induced discoid lupus erythematosus. *Arch Dermatol.* 1974; 110:95-8.
83. De D, Dogra S, Kaur I. Dapsone induced acute photosensitivity dermatitis: a case report and review of the literature. *Lepr Rev.* 2007; 78:401-4.
84. Frost P, Weinstein GD, Gomez EC. Methacycline and demeclocycline in relation to sunlight. *JAMA.* 1971; 216:326.
85. Narurkar V, Smoller BR, Hu CH et al. Desipramine-induced blue-gray photosensitive pigmentation. *Arch Dermatol.* 1993; 129:474-6.
86. Stierstorfer MB, Baughman RD. Photosensitivity to desoximetasone emollient ream (letter). *Arch Dermatol.* 1988; 124:1870-1.
87. Khedezla [package insert]. Spring Valley, NY: Par Pharmaceutical Companies; 2013.
88. Urrutia I, Jauregui I, Gamboa P et al. Photocontact dermatitis from cinchocaine (dibucaine). *Contact Dermatitis.* 1998; 39:139-40.
89. Horio T. Photosensitivity reaction to dibucaine: case report and experimental induction. *Arch Dermatol.* 1979; 115:986-7.
90. Daranide [package insert]. West Point, PA: Merck and Co; 1996.
91. Montoro J, Rodríguez M, Díaz M et al. Photoallergic contact dermatitis due to diclofenac. *Contact Dermatitis.* 2003; 48:115.
92. Al-Kathiri L, Al-Asmaili A. Diclofenac-induced photoonycholysis. *Oman Med J.* 2016; 31:65-8.
93. Street ML, Winkelmann RK. Lichenoid photoreactive epidermal necrosis with diflunisal. *J Am Acad Dermatol.* 1989; 20:850-1.
94. Roetzheim RG, Hero Id AH, Van Durme DJ. Nonpigmenting fixed drug eruption caused by diflunisal. *J Am Acad Dermatol.* 1991; 24:1021-2.
95. Boyer M, Katta R, Markus R. Diltiazem-induced photo distributed hyperpigmentation. *Dermatol Online J.* 2003; 9:10.
96. Kubo Y, Fukumoto D, Ishigami T et al. Diltiazem-associated photodistributed hyperpigmentation: report of two Japanese cases and published work review. *J Dermatol.* 2010; 37:807-11.
97. Desai N, Alexis AF, DeLeo VA. Facial hyperpigmentation caused by diltiazem hydrochloride. *Cutis.* 2010; 86:82-4.
98. Horio T. Allergic and photoallergic dermatitis from diphenhydramine. *Arch Dermatol.* 1976; 112:1124.
99. Emmett E. Diphenhydramine photoallergy. *Arch Dermatol.* 1974; 110:249.
100. Yamada S, Tanaka M, Kawahara Y et al. Photoallergic contact dermatitis due to diphenhydramine hydrochloride. *Contact Dermatitis.* 1998; 38:282.
101. Sinequan [package insert]. New York, NY: Pfizer; 2007.
102. Carroll LA, Laumann AE. Doxycycline-induced photo-onycholysis. *J Drugs Dermatol.* 2003; 2:662-3.
103. Lim DS, Triscott J. O'Brien's actinic granuloma in association with prolonged doxycycline phototoxicity. *Australas J Dermatol.* 2003; 44:67-70.
104. Lim DS, Murphy GM. High-level ultraviolet A photoprotection is needed to prevent doxycycline phototoxicity: lessons learned in East Timor. *Br J Dermatol.* 2003; 149:213-4.
105. Frost P, Weinstein GD, Gomez EC. Phototoxic potential of minocycline and doxycycline. *Arch Dermatol.* 1972; 105:681-3.

106. Multaq [package insert]. Bridgewater, NJ: Sanofi-Aventis US; 2009.
107. Treudler R, Husak R, Raisova M et al. Efavirenz-induced photoallergic dermatitis in HIV. *AIDS.* 2001; 15:1085-6.
108. Yoshimoto E, Konishi M, Takahashi K et al. The first case of efavirenz-induced photosensitivity in a Japanese patient with HIV infection. *Intern Med.* 2004; 43:630-1.
109. Roten SV, Mainetti C, Donath R et al. Enalapril-induced lichen planus-like eruption. *J Am Acad Derm.* 1995; 32:293-5.
110. Kanwar AJ, Dhar S, Ghosh S. Photosensitive lichenoid eruption due to enalapril. *Dermatology.* 1993; 187:80.
111. Petri H, Tronnier H. Efficacy of enoxacin in the treatment of bacterial infections of the skin with regards to photosensitization. *Infection.* 1986;14:S213-6.
112. Ellence [package insert]. Kalamazoo, MI: Pharmacia and Upjohn Company; 2003.
113. Erickson LR, Peterka ES. Sunlight sensitivity from oral contraceptives. *JAMA.* 1968; 203:980-1.
114. Jelinek JE. Cutaneous side effects of oral contraceptives. *Arch Dermatol.* 1970; 101:181.
115. Morison WL. Solar urticaria due to progesterone compounds in oral contraceptives. *Photodermatol Photoimmunol Photomed.* 2003; 19:155-6.
116. Cooper SM, George S. Photosensitivity reaction associated with use of the combined oral contraceptive. *Br J Dermatol.* 2001; 144:641-2.
117. Holdiness MR. Adverse cutaneous reactions to antituberculosis drugs. *Int J Dermatol.* 1985; 24:280-5.
118. Silvestre JF, Albares MP, Carnero L et al. Photodistributed felodipine-induced facial telangiectasia (letter). *J Am Acad Dermatol.* 2001; 45:323-4.
119. Gardeazabal J, Gonzalez M, Izu R et al. Phenofibrate-induced lichenoid photodermatitis. *Photodermatol Photoimmunol Photomed.* 1993; 9:156-8.
120. Leenutaphong V, Manuskiatti W. Fenofibrate-induced photosensitivity. *J Am Acad Dermatol.* 1997; 35:775-7.
121. Anchobon [package insert]. Nutley, NJ: Roche Pharmaceuticals; 1999.
122. Moyer DB. Continued treatment with fluorouracil for colon cancer despite severe phototoxic dermatitis. *J Allergy Clin Immunol.* 1996; 97:341.
123. Adrucil [package insert]. Irvine, CA: Sicor Pharmaceuticals; 2003.
124. Gaufberg E, Ellison JM. Photosensitivity reaction to fluoxetine. *J Clin Psychiatry.* 1995; 56:486.
125. Prolixin [package insert]. Princeton, NJ: Apothecon; 1998.
126. Tsien C, Souhami L. Flutamide photosensitivity. *J Urol.* 1999; 162:494.
127. Euflex [package insert]. Kenilworth, NJ: Schering; 1986.
128. Fujimoto M, Kikuchi K, Imakado S et al. Photosensitive dermatitis induced by flutamide (letter). *Br J Dermatol.* 1996; 135:489-504.
129. Moraillon I, Jeanmougin M, Manciet JR et al. Photoallergic reaction induced by flutamide. *Photodermatol Photoimmunol Photomed.* 1991; 8:264-5.
130. Vilaplana J, Romaguera C, Azon A et al. Flutamide photosensitivity-residual vitiliginous lesions. *Contact Dermatitis.* 1998; 38:68-70.
131. Kaur C, Thami GP. Flutamide-induced photosensitivity: is it a forme fruste of lupus? *Br J Dermatol.* 2003; 148:593-611.
132. Thual N, Penven K, Chevallier JM et al. Fluvastatin-induced dermatomyositis. *Ann Dermatol Venereol.* 2005; 132:996-9.
133. Burry JN, Lawrence JR. Phototoxic blisters from high frusemide dosage. *Br J Dermatol.* 1976; 94:495-9.
134. Koch CA, Mazzaferri EL, Larry JA et al. Bullous pemphigoid after treatment with furosemide. *Cutis.* 1996; 58:340-4.
135. Panayiotou BN, Prasad MVR, Zaman MN. Frusemide-induced bullous pemphigoid. *Br J Clin Pract.* 1997; 51:49-50.
136. Cytovene [package insert]. Nutley, NJ: Roche Laboratories; 2000.
137. Factive [package insert]. Cary, NC: Cornerstone Pharmaceuticals; 2011.
138. Glucotrol [package insert]. New York, NY: Roerig; 2009.
139. Micronase/Glynase [package insert]. Kalamazoo, MI: Pharmacia and Upjohn Company; 1997.
140. Fox GN, Harrell CC, Mehregan DR. Extensive lichenoid drug eruption due to glyburide: A case report and review of the literature. *Cutis.* 2005; 76:41-5.
141. Aguirre A, Gardeazabal J, Izu R et al. Allergic contact dermatitis due to plant extracts in a multisensitized patient. *Contact Dermatitis.* 1993; 28:186-7.
142. Guillaume JC, Roujeau JC, Revuz J et al. The culprit drugs in 87 cases of toxic epidermal necrolysis (Lyell's syndrome). *Arch Dermatol.* 1987; 123:1166-70.
143. Kawabe Y, Mizuno N, Miwa N et al. Photosensitivity induced by griseofulvin. *Photodermatol Photoimmunol Photomed.* 1988; 5:272-4.
144. Kojima T, Hasegawa T, Ishida H et al. Griseofulvin-induced photodermatitis: report of six cases. *J Dermatol.* 1988; 15:76-82.
145. Matsuo I, Inukai N, Fujita H et al. Possible involvement of oxidation of lipids in inducing griseofulvin photosensitivity. *Photodermatol Photoimmunol Photomed.* 1990; 7:213-7.
146. Haldol [package insert]. Raritan, NJ: Ortho-McNeil Pharmaceuticals; 2007.
147. pHisoHex [package insert]. New York, NY: Sanofi-Synthelabo; 2003.
148. Diffey BL, Langtry J. Phototoxic potential of thiazide diuretics in normal subjects. *Arch Dermatol.* 1989; 125:1355-8.
149. Gomez-Bernal S, Alvarez-Perez A, Rodriguez-Pazos L et al. Photosensitivity due to thiazides. *Actas Dermosifiliogr.* 2014; 105:359-66.
150. Reed BR, Huff JC, Jones SK et al. Subacute cutaneous lupus erythematosus associated with hydrochlorothiazide therapy. *Ann Intern Med.* 1985; 103:49-51.
151. Johnston GA. Thiazide-induced lichenoid photosensitivity. *Clin Exp Dermatol.* 2002; 27:670-2.
152. Robinson HN, Morison WL, Hood AF. Thiazide diuretic therapy and chronic photosensitivity. *Arch Dermatol.* 1985; 121;522-4.
153. Rietschel RL. Photocontact dermatitis to hydrocortisone. *Contact Dermatitis.* 1978; 4:334-7.
154. Cyanokit [package insert]. Napa, CA: Dey LP; 2006.
155. León-Mateos A, Zulaica A, Caeiro JL et al. Photo-induced granulomatous eruption by hydroxyurea. *J Eur Acad Dermatol Venereol.* 2007; 21:1428-9.
156. Bergner T, Przybilla B. Photosensitization caused by ibuprofen. *J Am Acad Dermatol.* 1992; 26:114-6.
157. *Micromedex(r) Healthcare Series* [intranet database]. Version 5.1. Greenwood Village, CO: Thomson Healthcare.
158. Gleevec [package insert]. East Hanover, NJ: Novartis; 2005.
159. Valeyrie L, Bastuji-Garin S, Revuz J et al. Adverse cutaneous reactions to imatinib (STI571) in Philadelphia chromosome-positive leukemias: a prospective study of 54 patients. *J Am Acad Dermatol.* 2003; 48:201-6.
160. Brazzelli V, Muzio F, Manna G et al. Photoinduced dermatitis and oral lichenoid reaction in a chronic myeloid leukemia patient treated with imatinib mesylate. *Photodermatol Photoimmunol Photomed.* 2012; 28:2-5.
161. Hashimoto K, Joselow SA, Tye MJ. Imipramine hyperpigmentation: a slate-gray discoloration caused by long-term imipramine administration. *J Am Acad Dermatol.* 1991; 25:357-61.
162. Rutherford T, Sinclair R. Photo-onycholysis due to indapamide. *Australas J Dermatol.* 2007; 48:35-6.
163. Wong RC, Gilbert M, Woo TY et al. Photosensitivity and isotretinoin therapy (letter). *J Am Acad Dermatol.* 1985; 14:1095-6.

164. Diffey BL, Spiro JG. Photosensitivity studies and isotretinoin therapy (letter). *J Am Acad Dermatol.* 1985; 12:119-20.
165. McCormack LS, Turner MLC. Photosensitivity and isotretinoin therapy (letter). *J Am Acad Dermatol.* 1983; 9:273-4.
166. Accutane [package insert]. Nutley, NJ: Roche Laboratories; 2003.
167. Alvarez-Fernandez JG, Castano-Suarez E, Cornejo-Navarro P et al. Photosensitivity induced by oral itraconazole. *J Eur Acad Dermatol Venereol.* 2000; 14:501-3.
168. Mohamed KN. Severe photodermatitis during ketoconazole therapy. *Clin Exp Dermatol.* 1988; 13:54.
169. Pigatto PD, Legori A, Bigardi AS et al. Gruppo Italiano Ricerca Dermatiti da Contatto ed Ambientali Italian multicenter study of allergic contact photodermatitis: epidemiological aspects. *Am J Contact Dermatitis.* 1996; 7:158-63.
170. Orudis [package insert]. Philadelphia, PA. Wyeth-Ayerst Laboratories; 1997.
171. Devleeschouwer V, Roelandts R, Garmyn M et al. Allergic and photoallergic contact dermatitis from ketoprofen: results of (photo) patch testing and follow-up of 42 patients. *Contact Dermatitis.* 2008; 58:159-6.
172. Bagheri H, Lhiaubet V, Montastruc JL et al. Photosensitivity to ketoprofen: Mechanisms and pharmacoepidemiological data. *Drug Saf.* 2000; 22:339-49.
173. Albes B, Marguery MC, Schwarze HP et al. Prolonged photosensitivity following contact photoallergy to ketoprofen. *Dermatology.* 2000; 201:171-4.
174. Alomar A. Ketoprofen photodermatitis. *Contact Dermatitis.* 1985; 12:112-3.
175. Catrani S, Calista D, Arcangeli F et al. Photo-allergic dermatitis to topical ketoprofen: a study of five cases. *G Ital Dermatol Venereol.* 1992; 127:167-8.
176. Cusano F, Rafenelli A, Bacchilega R et al. Photo-contact dermatitis from ketoprofen. *Contact Dermatitis.* 1987; 17:108-9.
177. Tosti A, Gaddoni G, Valeri F et al. Contact allergy to ketoprofen: report of 7 cases. *Contact Dermatitis.* 1990; 23:112-3.
178. Rivarola de Gutierrez E, Abaca H. Photodistributed lichenoid drug eruption with rhabdomyolysis occurring during leflunomide therapy. *Dermatology.* 2004; 208:232-3.
179. Levaquin [package insert]. Raritan, NJ: Ortho-McNeil Pharmaceuticals; 2007.
180. Kimura M, Kawada A. Photosensitivity induced by lomefloxacin with cross-photosensitivity to ciprofloxacin and fleroxacin. *Contact Dermatitis.* 1998; 38:180.
181. Kurumaji Y, Shono M. Scarified photopatch testing in lomefloxacin photosensitivity. *Contact Dermatitis.* 1992; 26:5-10.
182. Hunt TL, Adams MA. Pharmacokinetics and safety of lomefloxacin following multiple doses. *Diagn Microbiol Infect Dis.* 1989; 12:181-7.
183. Claritin [package insert]. Kenilworth, NJ: Schering; 2000.
184. Cozaar [package insert]. Whitehouse Station, NJ: Merck and Company; 2002.
185. Koch P, Bahmer FA. Photoallergic dermatitis caused by the herbicide phenmedipham. *Derm Beruf Umwelt.* 1989; 37:203-5.
186. Kligman AM. Topical retinoic acid (tretinoin) for photoaging: conceptions and misperceptions. *Cutis.* 1996; 57:142-4.
187. Solage [package insert]. Buffalo, NY: Westwood-Squibb Pharmaceuticals; 1999.
188. Methotrexate [package insert]. Florence, KY: Xanodyne Pharmacal; 2003.
189. Roenigk HH, Fowler-Bergfled W, Curtis GH. Methotrexate for psoriasis in weekly oral doses. *Arch Dermatol.* 1969; 99:86-93.
190. Moller H. Cytostatic drugs and inflammation. *Lancet.* 1970; 2:427.
191. Moller H. Reactivation of acute inflammation by methotrexate. *J Invest Dermatol.* 1969; 52:437-41.
192. Vogler WR, Huguley CM, Kerr W. Toxicity and antitumor effects of divided doses of methotrexate. *Arch Intern Med.* 1965; 115:285-93.
193. Corder MP, Stone WH. Failure of leucovorin rescue to prevent reactivation of a solar burn after high dose methotrexate. *Cancer.* 1976; 37:1660-2.
194. Dunagin WG, Millikan LE. Drug eruptions. *Med Clin North Am.* 1980; 64:983-1003.
195. Kaplan AP. Drug-induced skin disease. *J Allergy Clin Immunol.* 1984; 74:573-9.
196. LeVine MJ. Erythema resulting from suberythemogenic doses of ultraviolet radiation and methotrexate. *Arch Dermatol.* 1981; 117:656-8.
197. Korossy KS, Hood AF. Methotrexate reactivation of sunburn reaction. *Arch Dermatol.* 1981; 117:310-1.
198. Vella Briffa D, Warin AP. Photo-onycholysis caused by photochemotherapy. *BML* 1977; 2:1150.
199. Methyclothiazide [package insert]. Morgantown, WV: Mylan Pharmaceuticals; 2012.
200. Vaillant L, Le Marchand D, Grognard C et al. Photosensitivity to methyldopa. *Arch Dermatol.* 1988; 124:326-7.
201. George M. Methylene blue-induced hyperbilirubinemia and phototoxicity in a neonate. *Clin Pediatr.* 2000; 39:659.
202. Porat R, Gilbert S, Magilner D. Methylene blue-induced phototoxicity: an unrecognized complication. *Pediatrics.* 1996; 97:717-21.
203. Kestel JL. Photo-onycholysis from minocycline: side effects of minocycline therapy. *Cutis.* 1981; 28:53.
204. Allen JC. Minocycline. *Ann Intern Med.* 1976; 85:482-7.
205. Remeron [package insert]. West Orange, NJ: Organon; 2002.
206. Fuller B, Lind M, Bonomi P. Mitomycin C extravasation exacerbated by sunlight. *Ann Intern Med.* 1981; 94:542.
207. Univasc [package insert]. Milwaukee, WI: Schwarz Pharma; 1998.
208. Barman-Balfour JA, Wiseman LR. Moxifloxacin. *Drugs.* 1999; 57:363-73.
209. Avelox [package insert]. West Haven, CT: Bayer Health Care; 2008.
210. Krischer J, Scolari F, Kondo-Oestreicher M et al. Pseudoporphyria induced by nabumetone. *J Am Acad Dermatol.* 1999; 40:492-3.
211. Boisvert A, Barbeau G. Nalidixic acid-induced photodermatitis after minimal sun exposure. *Drug lntell Clin Pharm.* 1981; 15:126-7.
212. Burry JN. Persistent phototoxicity due to nalidixic acid. *Arch Dermatol.* 1974; 109:263.
213. Bisland D, Douglas WS. Sunbed pseudoporphyria induced by nalidixic acid (letter). *Br J Dermatol.* 1990; 123:547.
214. Mathew TH. Nalidixic acid. *Med J Aust.* 1966; 2:243.
215. Ramsay CA, Obreshkova E. Photosensitivity from nalidixic acid. *Br J Dermatol.* 1974; 91:523.
216. Ramsay CA. Photosensitivity from nalidixic acid. *Proc R Soc Med.* 1973; 66:747.
217. Susskind W. Suspected reactions to nalidixic acid. *BMJ.* 1965; 1:316.
218. Brauner GJ. Bullous photoreaction to nalidixic acid. *Am J Med.* 1975; 58:576.
219. Rosen K, Swanbeck G. Phototoxic reactions from some common drugs provoked by a high-intensity UVA lamp. *Ada Derm Venereol.* 1982; 62:246-8.
220. Wainwright NJ, Collins P, Ferguson J. Photosensitivity associated with antibacterial agents. *Drug Saf.* 1993; 9:437-40.
221. NegGram [package insert]. New York, NY: Sanofi-Winthrop Pharmaceuticals; 1997.
222. Naprosyn [package insert]. Nutley NJ: Roche Laboratories; 2006.
223. Levy ML, Barron KS, Eichenfield A et al. Naproxen-induced pseudoporphyria: a distinctive photodermatitis. *J Pediatr.* 1990; 117:660-4.

224. Rivers JK, Barnetson RS. Naproxen-induced bullous photodermatitis. *Med J Aust.* 1989; 151:167-8.

225. Suarez SM, Cohen PR, DeLeo VA. Bullous photosensitivity to naproxen: "pseudoporphyria." *Arthritis Rheum.* 1990; 33:903-8.

226. Habbema L, Bruynzeel DR. Fixed drug eruption due to naproxen. *Dermatologica.* 1987; 174:184-5.

227. Collins P, Ferguson J. Photodistributed nifedipine-induced lacial telangiectasia. *Br J Dermatol.* 1993; 129:630-3.

228. Tsele E, Chu AC. Nifedipine and telangiectasias. *Lancet.* 1992; 339:365-6.

229. Noroxin [package insert]. West Point, PA: Merck and Co; 2001.

230. Pamelor [package insert]. Ontario, Canada: Patheon; 2007.

231. Baran R, Brun P. Photoonycholysis induced by the fluoroquinolones pefioxacine and ofioxacine: report on 2 cases. *Dermatologica.* 1986; 173:185-8.

232. Scheile RT, Cramer WR, Decker EL. Photosensitizing potential ol ofioxacin. *Int J Dermatol.* 1993; 32:413-6.

233. Gregorion S, Karagiorga T, Stratigos A et al. Photoonycholysis caused by olanzapine and aripiprazole. *J Clin Psychopharmacol.* 2008; 28:219-20.

234. Daypro [package insert]. Chicago, IL: GD Searle and Co; 1999.

235. Cohen AD, Mermershtain W, Gellen DB et al. Cutaneous photosensitivity induced by paclitaxel and trastuzumab therapy associated with aberrations in the biosynthesis olporphyrins. *J Dermatol Treat.* 2005; 15:19-21.

236. Cohen PR. Photodistributed erythema multiforme: Paclitaxel-related, photosensitive conditions in patients with cancer. *J Drugs Dermatol.* 2009; 8:61-4.

237. Vectibix [package insert]. Thousand Oaks, CA: Amgen; 2008.

238. Ricciardi L, Fedele R, Mazzeo L et al. Adverse reactions to pantoprazole. *Scand J Gastroenterol.* 2003; 38:800.

239. Correia O, Lomba VH, Azevedo R et al. Possible phototoxicity with subsequent progression to discoid lupus following pantoprazole administration. *Clin Exp Dermatol.* 2001; 26:455-6.

240. Vilaplana J, Botey E, Lecha M et al. Photosensitivity induced by paroxetine. *Contact Dermatitis.* 2002; 47:118-9.

241. PegIntron [package insert]. Whitehouse Station, NJ: Schering; 2011.

242. Nipent [package insert]. San Ramon, CA: SuperGen; 1999.

243. Esbriet [package insert]. Brisbane, CA: Intermune; 2014.

244. Case JD, Yusk JW, Callen JP. Photosensitive reaction to phenelzine: a case report. *Photodermatol.* 1988; 5:101-2.

245. de Castro JLC, Freitas JP, Menezes F et al. Sensitivity to thimerosal and photosensitivity to piroxicam. *Contact Dermatitis.* 1991; 24:187-92.

246. Figueiredo A, Ribeiro CAF, Goncalo S et al. Piroxicam-induced photosensitivity. *Contact Dermatitis.* 1987; 17:73-9.

247. Goncalo M, Figueiredo A, Tavares P et al. Photosensitivity to piroxicam: absence of cross-reaction with tenoxicam. *Contact Dermatitis.* 1992; 27:287-90.

248. Kurumaji Y. Ampiroxicam-induced photosensitivity. *Contact Dermatitis.* 1996; 34:298-9.

249. McKerrow KJ, Greig DE. Piroxicam-induced photosensitive dermatitis. *J Am Acad Dermatol.* 1986; 15:1237-41.

250. Toyohara A, Chen K-R, Miyakawa S-I et al. Ampiroxicam-induced photosensitivity. *Contact Dermatitis.* 1996; 35:101-2.

251. Furuse K, Fukuoka M, Kato H et al. A prospective phase II study on photodynamic therapy with photofrin II for centrally located early stage lung cancer. *J Clin Oncol.* 1993;11:1852-1857.

252. Kato H, Horai T, Furuse K et al. Photodynamic therapy for cancers: A clinical trial of porfimer sodium in Japan. *Jpn J Cancer Res.* 1993; 84:1209-14.

253. Moriwaki SI, Misawa J, Yoshinari Y et al. Analysis of photosensitivity in Japanese cancer-bearing patients receiving photodynamic therapy with porfimer sodium (Photofrin). *Photodermatol Photoimmunol Photomed.* 2001; 17:241-3.

254. Lam S, Palcic B, McLean D et al. Detection of early lung cancer using low dose photofrin II. *Chest.* 1990; 97:333-7.

255. Nseyo UO, Dougherty TJ, Sullivan L. Photodynamic therapy in the management of resistant lower urinary tract carcinoma. *Cancer.* 1987; 60:3113-9.

256. Photofrin [package insert]. Carolina, Puerto Rico: Wyeth-Ayerst; 2003.

257. Van Hillegersberg R, Kort WJ, Wilson JHP. Current status of photodynamic therapy in oncology. *Drugs.* 1994; 48:510-27.

258. Wilson BD, Mang TS, Stoll H et al. Photodynamic therapy for the treatment of basal cell carcinoma. *Arch Dermatol.* 1992; 128:1597-601.

259. Phenergan [package insert]. Philadelphia, PA: Wyeth Pharmaceuticals; 2004.

260. Vivactil [package insert]. East Hanover, NJ: Odyssey Pharmaceuticals; 2004.

261. Pyrazinamide [package insert]. Pearl River, NY: Lederle Laboratories; 1997.

262. Choonhakarn C, Janma J. Pyrazinamide-induced lichenoid photodermatitis (letter). *J Am Acad Dermatol.* 1999; 40:645-6.

263. Guerciolini R, Del Favero A, Cannistraro S. Amiodarone-induced photosensitivity and pyridoxine (letter). *Lancet.* 1984; 1:962.

264. Kawada A, Kashima A, Shiraishi H et al. Pyridoxine-induced photosensitivity and hypophosphatasia. *Dermatology.* 2000; 201:356-60.

265. Morimoto K, Kawada A, Hiruma M et al. Photosensitivity Irom pyridoxine hydrochloride (vitamin B6). *J Am Acad Dermatol.* 1996; 35:304-5.

266. Baer RL. Cutaneous skin changes probably due to pyridoxine abuse (letter). *J Am Acad Dermatol.* 1984; 10:527-8.

267. Murata Y, Kumano K, Ueda T et al. Photosensitive dermatitis caused by pyridoxine hydrochloride. *J Am Acad Dermatol.* 1998; 39:314-7.

268. Ortel B, Sivayathorn A, Hönigsmann H. An unusual combination ol phototoxicity and Stevens-Johnson syndrome due to antimalarial therapy. *Dermatologica.* 1989; 178:39-42.

269. Bruce S, Wolf JE. Quinidine-induced photosensitive livedo reticularis-like eruption. *J Am Acad Dermatol.* 1985; 12:332-6.

270. Berger TG, Sesody ST. Quinidine-induced lichenoid photodermatitis. *Cutis.* 1982; 29:595-600.

271. Armstrong RB, Leach EE, Whitman G et al. Quinidine photosensitivity. *Arch Dermatol.* 1985; 121:525-8.

272. Bogoch ER, Ross JB. Photosensitive dermatitis probably due to quinidine. *Arch Dermatol.* 1976; 112:559-60.

273. De Groot WP, Wuite J. Livedo racemosa-like photosensitivity reaction during quinidine Durettes medication. *Dermatologica.* 1974; 48:371-6.

274. Gammer S, Gross PR. Photoallergy induced by quinidine. *Cutis.* 1976; 17:72-4.

275. Lang Jr PG. Quinidine-induced photodermatitis confirmed by photopatch testing. *J Am Acad Dermatol.* 1983; 9:124-8.

276. Sun DK, Reiner D, Frishman W et al. Adverse dermatologic reactions from antiarrhythmic drug therapy. *J Clin Pharmacol.* 1994; 34:953-66.

277. Dawson TAJ. Side effect of quinine for nocturnal cramps (letter). *BMJ.* 1995; 310:738.

278. Wagner GH, Diffey BL, Ive FA. 'I'll have mine with a twist of lemon': quinine photosensitivity from excessive intake of tonic water (letter). *Br J Dermatol.* 1994; 131:734-5.

279. Ferguson J, Addo HA, Johnson BE et al. Quinine induced photosensitivity: clinical and experimental studies. *Br J Dermatol.* 1987; 117:631-40.

280. Ljunggren B, Hindsen M, Isaksson M. Systemic quinine photosensitivity with photoepicutaneous cross-reactivity to quinidine. *Contact Dermatitis.* 1992; 26:1-4.

281. Ljunggren B, Sjovall P. Systemic quinine photosensitivity. *Arch Dermatol.* 1986; 122:909-11.

282. Okun MM, Henner M, Paulson C. A quinine-induced drug reaction of photosensitive distribution with histological features mimicking mycosis fungoides. *Clin Exp Dermatol.* 1994; 19:246-8.

283. Wagner SN, Welke F, Goos M. Occupational UVA-induced allergic photodermatitis in a welder due to hydrochlorothiazide and ramipril. *Contact Dermatitis.* 2000; 43:245-6.
284. Todd P, Norris P, Hawk JLM et al. Ranitidine-induced photosensitivity. *Clin Exp Derm.* 1995; 20:146-8.
285. Kondo S, Kagaya M, Yamada Y et al. UVB photosensitivity due to ranitidine. *Dermatology.* 2000; 201:71-3.
286. Risperdal [package insert]. Titusville, NJ: Janssen Pharmaceuticals; 2007.
287. Norvir [package insert]. North Chicago, IL: Abbott Laboratories; 2001.
288. Winter AJ, Pywell JM, Ilchyshyn JM et al. Photosensitivity due to saquinavir. *Genitourin Med.* 1997; 73:323.
289. Invirase [package insert]. Nutley NJ: Roche Laboratories; 2001.
290. Selegiline [package insert]. Spring Valley, NY: Par Pharmaceuticals; 2003.
291. Zoloft [package insert]. New York, NY: Pfizer; 2008.
292. Olysio [package insert]. Titusville, NJ: Janssen Therapeutics; 2013.
293. Hanada K, Hashimoto I. Flagellate mushroom (Shiitake) dermatitis and photosensitivity. *Dermatol.* 1998; 197:255-7.
294. Granados MTR, de la Torre C, Cruces MJ et al. Chronic actinic dermatitis due to simvastatin. *Contact Dermatitis.* 1998; 38:294-5.
295. Holme SA, Pearse AD, Anstey AV. Chronic actinic dermatitis secondary to simvastatin. *Photodermatol Photoimmunol Photomed.* 2002; 18:313-4.
296. Betapace [package insert]. Wayne, NJ: Berlex Laboratories; 2001.
297. Dawe RS, Ibbotson SH, Sanderson JB et al. A randomized controlled trial (volunteer study) of sitafloxacin, enoxacin, levofloxacin, and sparfloxacin phototoxicity. *Br J Dermatol.* 2003; 149:1232-41.
298. Hamanaka H, Mizutani H, Shimizu M. Sparfloxacin-induced photosensitivity and the occurrence of a lichenoid tissue reaction after prolonged exposure. *J Am Acad Dermatol.* 1998; 38:945-9.
299. Rubinstein E. Safety profile of sparfloxacin in the treatment of respiratory tract infection. *J Antimicrob Chemother.* 1996; 37:145-60.
300. Lipsky BA, Unowsky J, Zhang H et al. Treating acute bacterial exacerbations of chronic bronchitis in patients unresponsive to previous therapy: sparfloxacin versus clarithromycin. *Clin Ther.* 1999; 21:954-65.
301. Mahajan VK, Sharma NL. Photo-onycholysis due to sparfloxacin. *Australas J Dermatol.* 2005; 46:104-5.
302. Zagam [package insert]. Collegeville, PA: Rhone-Poulenc Rorer Pharmaceuticals; 1998.
303. Anon. Spironolactone: first report of photosensitivity: case report. *Reactions Weekly.* 2003; 937:14.
304. Duran N, Song P-S. Hypericin and its photodynamic action. *Photochem Photobiol.* 1986; 43:677-80.
305. Jacobson JM, Feinman L, Liebes L et al. Pharmacokinetics, safety, and antiviral effects of hypericin, a derivative of St. John's Wort plant, in patients with chronic hepatitis C virus infection. *Antimicrob Agents Chemother.* 2001; 45:517-24.
306. Kerb R, Brockmoller J, Staffeldt B et al. Single-dose and steady-state pharmacokinetics of hypericin and pseudohypericin. *Antimicrob Agents Chemother.* 1996; 40:2087-93.
307. Brockmoller J, Reum T, Bauer S et al. Hypericin and pseudohypericin: pharmacokinetics and effects on photosensitivity in humans. *Pharmacopsychiatry.* 1997; 30:94-101.
308. Pace N, MacKinney G. Hypericin, the photodynamic pigment from St. John's Wort. *J Am Chem Soc.* 1941; 63:2570-4.
309. Roots T. Evaluation of photosensitization of the skin and multiple dose intake of Hypericum extract. Second International Congress on Phytomedicine. Munich, Germany; 1996.
310. Schempp CM, Muller K, Windhofer B et al. Single-dose and steady-state administration of hypericum perforatum extract (St. John's Wort) does not influence skin sensitivity to UV radiation, visible light, and solar-stimulated radiation. *Arch Dermatol.* 2001; 137:512-3.
311. Schempp CM, Ludtke R, Winghofer B et al. Effect of topical application of hypericum perforatum extract (St. John's Wort) on skin sensitivity to solar stimulated radiation. *Photodermatol Photoimmunol Photomed.* 2000; 16:125-8.
312. Southwell IA, Campbell MH. Hypericin content variation in Hypericum perforatum in Australia. *Phytochemistry.* 1991; 30:475-8.
313. Siegers CP, Biel S, Wilhelm KP. Phototoxicity caused by hypericum. *Dtsch Z Nervenheilkd.* 1993; 12:320-2.
314. Gulick RM, McAuliffe V, Holden-Wiltse J et al. Phase I studies of hypericin, the active compound in St. John's Wort, as an antiretroviral agent in HIV-infected adults: AIDS Clinical Trials Group Protocols 150 and 258. *Ann Intern Med.* 1999; 130:510-4.
315. Golsch S, Vocks E, Rakoski J et al. Reversible increase in photosensitivity to UV-B caused by St. John's Wort extract. *Hautarzt.* 1997; 48:249-52.
316. Brockmoller J, Reum T, Bauer S et al. Hypericin and pseudohypericin: pharmacokinetics and effects on photosensitivity in humans. *Pharmacopsychiatry.* 1997; 30:94-101.
317. Sulfadiazine [package insert]. Princeton, NJ: Sandoz; 2008.
318. Sulfamethoxazole–trimethoprim [package insert]. Philadelphia, PA: AR Scientific; 2010.
319. Flach A. Photosensitivity to sulfisoxazole ointment. *Arch Ophthalmol.* 1981; 99:609-10.
320. Gantrisin [package insert]. Nutley, NJ: Roche Laboratories; 1995.
321. De D, Kanwar AJ. Tacrolimus-induced hyperpigmentation in a patch of vitiligo. *Skinmed.* 2008; 7:93-4.
322. Prograf [package insert]. Deerfield, IL: Fujisawa USA; 2001.
323. Fabior [package insert]. Research Triangle Park, NC: Stiefel Laboratories; 2012.
324. Lamisil [package insert]. East Hanover, NJ: Novartis Pharmaceuticals; 2013.
325. Epstein JH, Seibert JS. Porphyria-like cutaneous changes induced by tetracycline hydrochloride photosensitization. *Arch Dermatol.* 1976; 112:661-6.
326. Bethell HJN. Photo-onycholysis caused by demethylchlortetracycline. *Br Med J.* 1977; 2:96.
327. Ory EM. The tetracyclines. *Med Clin North Am.* 1970; 54:1173.
328. Hawk JLM. Skin changes resembling hepatic cutaneous porphyria induced by oxytetracycline photosensitization. *Clin Exp Dermatol.* 1980; 5:321-5.
329. Kardaun SH, Scheffer E, Vermeer BJ. Drug-induced pseudolymphomatous skin reactions. *Br J Dermatol.* 1988; 118:545-52.
330. Llambrich A, Lecha M. Photoinduced lichenoid reaction by thioridazine. *Photodermatol Photoimmunol Photomed.* 2004; 20:108-9.
331. Tygacil [package insert]. Philadelphia, PA: Wyeth Pharmaceuticals; 2013.
332. Tolazamide [package insert]. Morgantown, WV: Mylan Pharmaceuticals; 2009.
333. Kar PK, Das Gupta SK, Das KD. Tolbutamide photosensitivity. *J Indian Med Assoc.* 1984; 82:289-91.
334. Byrd DR, Ahmed I. Photosensitive lichenoid reaction to torsemide—a loop diuretic. *Mayo Clin Proc.* 1997; 72:930-1.
335. Varik [package insert]. Wiesbaden, Germany: Albert-Roussel-Pharma GmbH: 1997.
336. Oleptro [package insert]. Dublin, Ireland: Labopharm Europe Limited; 2010.
337. Fernández de Corres L, Bernaola G, Fernández E et al. Photodermatitis from triamterene. *Contact Dermatitis.* 1987; 17:114-5.
338. Dyrenium [package insert]. Pittsburgh, PA: SmithKline Beecham Pharmaceuticals; 1998.
339. Chandler MJ. Recurrence of phototoxic skin eruption due to trimethoprim. *J Infect Dis.* 1986: 153:1001.
340. Surmontil [package insert]. Pomma, NY: Duramed Pharmaceuticals; 2007.

341. Avita [package insert]. Morgantown, WV: Mylan Pharmaceuticals; 2011.
342. Retin-A Micro [package insert]. Los Angeles, CA: Ortho Dermatologics; 2010.
343. Valtrex [package insert]. Research Triangle Park, NC: GlaxoSmith-Kline; 2007.
344. Depakote [package insert]. Chicago, IL: Abbott Laboratories; 1998.
345. Frye CB, Petticrew TJ. Angioedema and photosensitive rash induced by valsartan. *Pharmacotherapy.* 1998; 18:866-8.
346. Kong HH, Fine HA, Stern JB, Tuner ML. Cutaneous pigmentation after photosensitivity induced by vandetanib therapy. *Arch Dermatol.* 2009; 145:925.
347. Caprelsa [package insert]. Wilmington, DE: Astra Zeneca Pharmaceuticals LP; 2011.
348. Zelboraf [package insert]. Nutley, NJ: Hoffmann-LaRoche; 2011.
349. Gelot P, Dutartre H, Khammari A et al. Vemurafenib: An unusual UVA-induced photosensitivity. *Exp Dermatol.* 2013; 22:297-8.
350. Boussemart L, Routier, Mateus C et al. Prospective study of cutaneous side-effects associated with the BRAF inhibitor vemurafenib: a study of 42 patients. *Ann Oncol.* 2013; 24:1691-7.
351. Lacouture ME, Duvic M, Hauschild A et al. Analysis of dermatologic events in vemurafenib-treated patients with melanoma. *Oncologist.* 2013; 18:314-22.
352. Vaccaro M, Borgia F, Barbuzza O et al. Photodistributed eruptive telangiectasia: an uncommon adverse drug reaction to venlafaxine. *Br J Dermatol.* 2007; 157:822-4.
353. Lui H, Anderson RR. Photodynamic therapy in dermatology: recent developments. *Dermatol Clin.* 1993; 11:1-13.
354. Lui H. Photodynamic therapy in dermatology with porfimer sodium and benzoporphyrin derivative: an update. *Semin Oncol.* 1994; 21:11-4.
355. Levy JG. Photosensitizers in photodynamic therapy. *Semin Oncol.* 1994; 21:4-10.
356. Visudyne [package insert]. Duluth, GA: Novartis Ophthalmics; 2001.
357. Velban [package insert]. Indianapolis, IN: Eli Lilly and Company; 1997.
358. Tolland JP, McKeown PP, Corbett JR. Voriconazole-induced pseudoporphyria. *Photodermatol Photoimmunol Photomed.* 2007; 23:29-31.
359. McCarthy KL, Playford EG, Looke DF et al. Severe photosensitivity causing multifocal squamous cell carcinoma secondary to prolonged voriconazole therapy. *Clin Infect Dis.* 2007; 44:e55-6.
360. Racette AJ, Roenigk HH Jr, Hansen R et al. Photoaging and phototoxicity from long-term voriconazole treatment in a 15-year-old girl. *J Am Acad Dermatol.* 2005; 52:581-5.
361. Rubenstein M, Levy ML, Metry D. Voriconazole-induced retinoid-like photosensitivity in children. *Pediatr Dermatol.* 2004; 21:675-8.
362. Patel AR, Turner ML, Baird K et al. Voriconazole-induced phototoxicity masquerading as chronic graft-versus-host disease of the skin in allogeneic hematopoietic cell transplant recipients. *Biol Blood Marrow Transplant.* 2009; 15:370-6.
363. Willis ZI, Boyd AS, Di Pentima MC. Phototoxicity, pseudoporphyria, and photo-onycholysis due to voriconazole in a pediatric patient with leukemia and invasive aspergillosis. *J Pediatric Infect Dis Soc.* 2015; 4:e22-4.
364. Vohringer S, Schrum J, Ott H, Hoger PH. Severe phototoxicity with long-term voriconazole treatment. *J Dtsch Dermatol Ges.* 2011; 9:274-6.
365. Hansford JR, Cole C, Blyth CC, Gottardo NG. Idiosyncratic nature of voriconazole photosensitivity in children undergoing cancer therapy. *J Antimicrob Chemother.* 2012; 67:1807-9.
366. Haylett AK, Felton S, Denning DW, Rhodes LE. Voriconazole-induced photosensitivity: Photobiological assessment of a case series of 12 patients. *Br J Dermatol.* 2013; 168:179-85.
367. VFEND [package insert]. New York, NY: Pfizer; 2002.
368. Sonata [package insert]. Philadelphia, PA: Wyeth Laboratories; 2007.
369. Wolff K, Johnson RA, Saavedra AP. Photosensitivity, photo-induced disorders, and disorders by ionizing radiation. In: *Fitzpatrick's color atlas and synopsis of clinical dermatology.* 7th ed. New York: McGraw-Hill; 2013:191-225.
370. Moore DE. Drug-induced cutaneous photosensitivity: incidence, mechanism, prevention and management. *Drug Saf.* 2002; 25:345-72.
371. Gould JW, Mercurio MG, Elmets CA. Cutaneous photosensitivity diseases induced by exogenous agents. *J Am Acad Dermatol.* 1995; 33:551-76.
372. Khoo SW, Tay YK, Tham SN. Photodermatoses in a Singapore skin referral centre. *Clin Exp Dermatol.* 1996; 21:263-8.
373. Dawe RS, Ibbotson SH. Drug-induced photosensitivity. *Dermatol Clin.* 2014; 32:363-8.
374. Allen JE. Drug-induced photosensitivity. *Clin Pharm.* 1993; 12:580-7.
375. Drucker AM, Rosen CF. Drug-induced photosensitivity: Culprit drugs, management, and prevention. *Drug Saf.* 2011; 34:821-37.
376. Heger JJ, Prystowsky EN, Zipes DP. Relationships between amiodarone dosage, drug concentrations, and adverse side effects. *Am Heart J.* 1983; 106:931-5.
377. Jafari-Fesharaki M, Scheinman MM. Adverse effects of amiodarone. *Pacing Clin Electrophysiol.* 1998; 21:108-20.
378. Kounis NG, Frangides C, Papadaki PJ et al. Dose-dependent appearance and disappearance of amiodarone-induced skin pigmentation. *Clin Cardiol.* 1996; 19:592-4.
379. Matheis H. Amiodarone pigmentation. *Dermatologica.* 1972; 145:304-18.
380. Cordarone [package insert]. Philadelphia, PA: Wyeth-Ayerst Laboratories; 1998.
381. Jaworski K, Walecka I, Rudnicka L et al. Cutaneous adverse reactions of amiodarone. *Med Sci Monit.* 2014; 20:2369-72.
382. Heckman CJ, Chandler R, Kloss JD et al. Minimal erythema dose (MED) testing. *J Vis Exp.* 2013; 75: e50175.
383. Layton AM, Cunliffe WJ. Phototoxic eruptions due to doxycycline-a dose-related phenomenon. *Clin Exp Dermatol.* 1993; 18:425-7.
384. Wainwright NJ, Collins P, Ferguson J. Photosensitivity associated with antibacterial agents. *Drug Saf.* 1993;9:437-40.
385. Johnson BE, Ferguson J. Drug and chemical photosensitivity. *Semin Dermatol.* 1990; 9:39-46.
386. Toback AC, Longley J, Cardullo AC et al. Severe chronic photosensitivity in association with acquired immunodeficiency syndrome. *J Am Acad Dermatol.* 1986; 15:1056-7.
387. Bilu D, Mamelak AJ, Nguyen RHN et al. Clinical and epidemiologic characterization of photosensitivity in HIV-positive individuals. *Photodermatol Photoimmunol Photomed.* 2004; 20:175-83.
388. Rodwell GEL, Berger TG. Pruritis and cutaneous inflammatory conditions of HIV disease. *Clinics in Dermatology.* 2000; 18:479-84.
389. Vin-Christian K, Epstein JH, Maurer TA et al. Photosensitivity in HIV-infected individuals. *J Dermatol.* 2000; 27:361-9.
390. Cozzani I, Jori G. Photo-oxidation of L-glutamate decarboxylase from Escherichia coli, sensitized by the co-enzyme pyridoxal phosphate and proflavin. *Biochim Biophys Acta.* 1980; 623:84-8.
391. Thami GP, Kaur S, Kanwar AJ. Delayed reactivation of haloperidol induced photosensitive dermatitis by methotrexate. *Postgrad Med J.* 2002; 78:116-7.
392. Cowen EW, Nguyen JC, Miller DD et al. Chronic phototoxicity and aggressive squamous cell carcinoma of the skin in children and adults during treatment with voriconazole. *J Am Acad Dermatol.* 2010; 62:31.
393. Ibrahim SF, Singer JP, Arron ST. Catastrophic squamous cell carcinoma in lung transplant patients treated with voriconazole. *Dermatol Surg.* 2010; 36:1752-5.

394. Singer JP, Boker A, Metchnikoff C et al. High cumulative dose exposure to voriconazole is associated with cutaneous squamous cell carcinoma in lung transplant recipients. *J Heart Lung Transplant.* 2012; 31:694-9.

395. Epaulard O, Villier C, Ravaud P et al. A multistep voriconazole-related phototoxic pathway may lead to skin carcinoma: results from a French nationwide study. *Clin Infect Dis.* 2013; 57:e182-8.

396. Williams K, Manish M, Chin-Hong P et al. Voriconazole-associated cutaneous malignancy: a literature review on photocarcinogenesis in organ transplant recipients. *Clin Infect Dis.* 2014; 58:997-1002.

397. Paek Sy, Lim HW. Chronic actinic dermatitis. *Dermatol Clin.* 2014; 32:355-61.

398. Gozali MV, Shou B, Luo D. Update on treatment of photodermatosis. *Dermatol Online J.* 2016; 22:2.

399. Knowles SR, Shear NH. Cutaneous drug reactions with systemic features. In: Wolverton SE, ed. *Comprehensive dermatologic drug therapy.* 3rd ed. China; Elsevier Saunders; 2013:747-56.

400. Diaz JH, Nesbitt LT. Sun exposure behavior and protection: Recommendations for travelers. *J Trav Med.* 2013; 20:108-18.

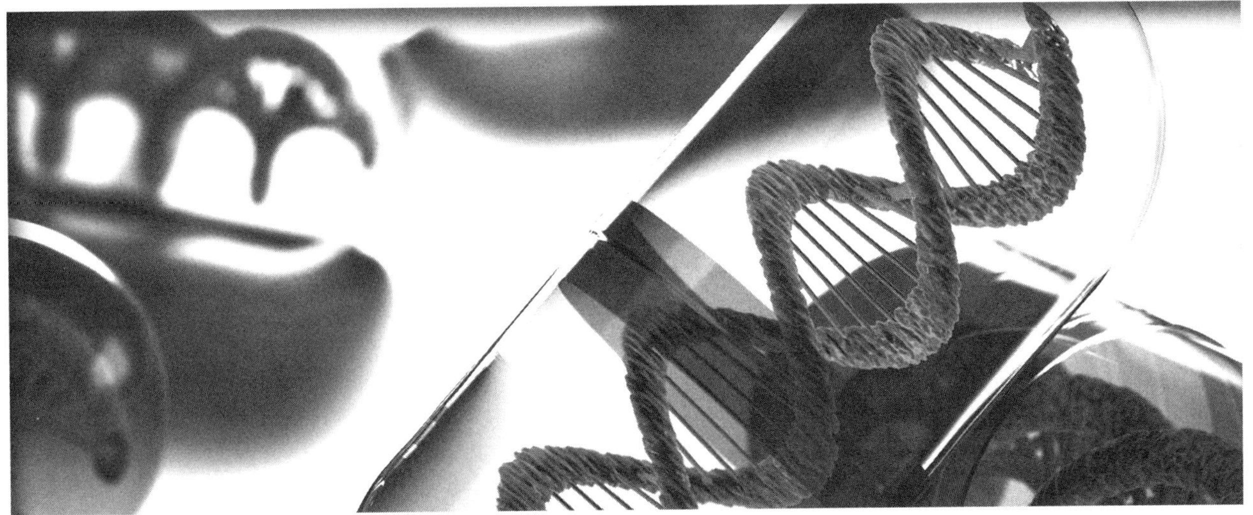

CHAPTER 9

Alopecia, Hirsutism, and Hypertrichosis

Kristine E. Keplar

ALOPECIA

Alopecia is hair loss due to a disturbance of the hair growth cycle and may be manifested as complete or partial hair loss. Although the scalp is most often involved, the disorder can affect all hair-bearing areas of the body.[1-3] Most cases are caused by androgenetic alopecia, also known as male pattern baldness, secondary to hormonal and genetic factors. A relatively small percentage of alopecia cases are drug-induced.[4] Although drug-induced alopecia is not an extremely common event, it is quite distressing to the patient and, therefore, important to recognize.[5]

The three phases of hair growth are anagen, catagen, and telogen (**Figure 9-1**).[6-8] The anagen, or growth, phase is the most active phase of the growth cycle and lasts from several months to years. During this phase, the hair follicle produces hair continuously. Intense mitotic activity occurs, and follicles are highly susceptible to noxious events.[6] The catagen cycle, or transition period, lasts only 1–2 weeks. During this phase, the inferior portion of the hair follicle significantly thins. The third and final phase of hair growth is the telogen, or resting, phase. This phase usually lasts 2–4 months, after which the follicle re-enters the anagen phase. At any given time, 80–90% of the follicles of the typical scalp are in the anagen phase, and 10–15% of follicles are in the telogen phase. Hair is shed during the telogen phase; telogen follicles usually shed between 30 and 100 hairs daily.[6,8,9] Follicles in the telogen and catagen phases, unlike those in the anagen phase, typically are not sensitive to noxious agents, such as cancer chemotherapy drugs, because of their inconsistent mitotic and metabolic activity.[6]

Androgenetic alopecia, or male pattern baldness, is hair thinning that occurs in an M-shaped pattern, during which hair loss occurs on the crown and temple areas of the head but spares the back and sides of the head. It is termed *androgenetic alopecia* because it generally follows the distribution of androgen-sensitive hair follicles. Androgenetic hair loss is often familial and is thought to involve a physiologic process incited in genetically predisposed hair follicles under the influences of androgens. Drugs with androgenic activity can also induce this type of hair loss.[10-13]

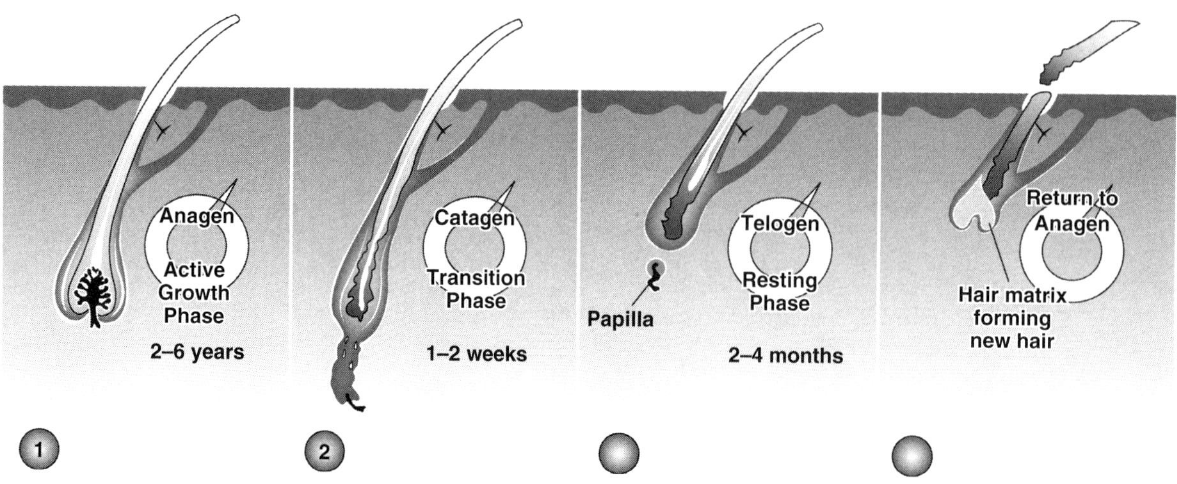

FIGURE 9-1 Diagram of the Hair Growth Cycle

During the normal hair cycle, the active growth phase (anagen) can last from 2 to 6 years. This is followed by a short transition phase (catagen), which lasts 1–2 weeks, and then by a resting phase (telogen), lasting 2–4 months. The hair is then shed, the anagen phase begins again, and a new hair is developed.[6-9]

Alopecia areata, an autoimmune inflammatory disease, is another type of alopecia that includes patchy hair loss, complete loss of scalp hair, or complete loss of scalp and body hair. Alopecia areata has been postulated to have an autoimmune pathogenesis involving inflammatory cytokines, including tumor necrosis factor alpha (TNFα). Alopecia areata is very rare, and only a few drugs have been associated with it. At this time, the precise pathogenesis of drug-induced alopecia areata has not been elucidated, but it is thought to involve the person's own immune system, which attacks healthy hair follicles by mistake.[13-17]

CAUSATIVE AGENTS

The primary medications that may induce alopecia are anticoagulants, androgenetic agents, hormone therapy, psychotropic drugs, thyroid medications, antiretroviral drugs, and cancer chemotherapy agents.[3,6,11,18] Drugs known to induce alopecia are listed in **Table 9-1**.[18-169]

ANTICOAGULANTS

Heparin and heparinoid drugs primarily affect scalp hairs. Hair loss usually occurs approximately 3 months after the initiation of treatment. In one report, the onset of hair loss varied from 1 week to 3 months after the last dose of heparin.[170] Although unfractionated heparin has been the primary anticoagulant linked to drug-induced alopecia, low-molecular-weight heparins, warfarin, and direct-acting oral anticoagulants have also been implicated as causative agents.[4,10,11,28,171-173] Warfarin typically induces mild, diffuse alopecia with an onset between 3 and 20 weeks after the initiation of therapy. Most cases of hair loss secondary to warfarin or heparinoid drugs go unnoticed by the patient. Only 20% of those who experience hair loss associated with these drugs exhibit clinically evident alopecia. Scalp hair is the primary target, but eyebrows, axillary, and pubic hair also may be affected. Total alopecia is extremely rare.[19,28]

RETINOL/RETINOIDS

Vitamin A, or retinol, is often prescribed for the treatment of hair disorders. However, alopecia of the telogen effluvium type can occur in association with ingestion of vitamin A in doses >50,000 international units daily (whether dietary, such as cod liver oil, or pharmaceutical) over a period of several months.[18] Other retinoids such as acitretin, etretinate, and isotretinoin also cause hair loss.[26] Alopecia associated with these agents usually occurs after 3–8 weeks of therapy. Alopecia may occur after exposure to lower doses, but the onset is longer than

Table 9-1 Agents Implicated in Drug-Induced Alopecia[18-169]

Drug	Incidence	Level of Evidence[a]
AMPHETAMINES/CNS STIMULANTS		
Amphetamine aspartate[18-20,b]	<1%	C
Benzphetamine[18-20,b]	NK	C
Dextroamphetamine[18-20,b]	NK	C
Dexmethylphenidate[18-20,b]	NK	C
Diethylpropion[18-21,b]	NK	C
Lisdexamfetamine[18-20,b]	NK	C
Methamphetamine[18-20,b]	NK	C
Methylphenidate[18-21,b]	NK	C
ANABOLIC STEROIDS/ANDROGENS		
Fluoxymesterone[6,13,20,22,23]	NK[c]	C
Danazol[6,13,20,22,23]	NK[c]	C
Dihydroepiandrosterone (DHEA)[6,13,20,22,23]	NK[c]	C
Methyltestosterone[6,13,20,22,23]	NK[c]	C
Nandrolone[6,13,20,22,23]	NK[c]	C
Oxandrolone[6,13,20,22,23]	NK[c]	C
Oxymetholone[6,13,20,22,23]	NK[c]	C
Progesterone[6,13,20,22-24]	NK[c]	A
Stanozolol[6,13,20,22,23]	NK[c]	C
Testolactone[6,13,20,22,23,25]	Up to 66%	A
Testosterone[6,13,20,22,23]	NK[c]	C
ANGIOTENSIN-CONVERTING ENZYME INHIBITORS		
Benazepril[26]	<1%	C
Captopril[26]	1–5%	C
Enalopril[26]	NK	C
Lisinopril[26]	NK	C
Quinapril[26]	NK	C
Ramipril[11]	NK	C
ANTIARRHYTHMICS		
Amiodarone[27]	1–4%	C
ANTICOAGULANTS		
Apixaban[28]	NK	C
Dabigatran[28]	NK	C
Dalteparin[28]	NK[d]	C
Enoxaparin[28]	NK[d]	C
Heparin[23,28]	0–50%	C
Nadroparin[16]	NK[d]	C
Rivaroxaban[28]	NK	C
Warfarin[11,28-31]	>5%	C

Table 9-1 Agents Implicated in Drug-Induced Alopecia[18-169] (continued)

Drug	Incidence	Level of Evidence[a]
ANTICONVULSANTS		
Carbamazepine[9,32,33]	0.01–6%	C
Ezogabine[21]	<2%	C
Felbamate[26]	NK	C
Gabapentin[26,34]	0.1–1%	A
Lamotrigine[10]	1–5%	C
Levetiracetam[35]	NK	C
Oxcarbazepine[21]	1–10%	C
Phenobarbitol[33]	1.2%	C
Pregabalin[36]	0.1–1%	C
Primidone[33]	1.5%	A
Tiagabine[26]	>1%	C
Topiramate[21,37,38,e]	1–5%	C
Valproic acid[9,26,32,39-42,f]	2.6–13% 24–28% with higher doses[10,42]	A A
ANTIFUNGALS		
Fluconazole[43,g]	NK	C
Isavuconazonium[21,g]	<5%	C
Voriconazole[43,g]	82%	C
ANTIVIRALS		
Acyclovir[11,26]	1–5%	C
Atazanavir[26,44]	NK	C
Didanosine[26,45]	NK	C
Indinavir[26,h]	NK	C
Lamivudine[21,26]	<1%	C
Saquinavir[26]	NK	C
Valacyclovir[26,46]	NK	C
Zalcitabine[26]	<1%	C
Zidovudine[26]	NK	C
β-BLOCKERS		
Acebutolol[26]	NK	C
Atenolol[26]	NK	C
Betaxolol[26]	<2%	C
Carvedilol[26,47]	≤1%	B
Metoprolol[26]	NK	C
Nadolol[26]	NK	C
Propranolol[26,48]	NK	C
Timolol[11,26]	>5%	C
CALCIUM-CHANNEL BLOCKERS		
Nifedipine[11]	1–5%	C
Verapamil[11]	<1%	C

Table 9-1 Agents Implicated in Drug-Induced Alopecia[18-169] (continued)

Drug	Incidence	Level of Evidence[a]
CANCER CHEMOTHERAPY AGENTS		
Ado-trastuzumab emtansine[49]	1–13%	B
Afatinib[49]	9–15%	B
Alemtuzumab[49]	1–30%	B
Altretamine[50,51]	<1%	A
Amsacrine[18,21]	>10%	C
Anastrozole[21]	1–13%	C
Axitinib[21,49]	4–13%	B
Bevacizumab[49]	3–27%	B
Bleomycin[11,52,h]	50%	C
Bortezomib[49]	1–11%	B
Brentuximab[21,49]	10–19%	B
Busulfan[11,18,53]	>10%	C
Cabazitaxel[21,54]	10%	C
Cabozantinib[21,49,i]	12–22%	B
Carboplatin[11,21]	3–17%	A
Cetuximab[48,54]	2–30%	B
Cisplatin[11,55-57]	>10%	A
Cyclophosphamide[11,55-57]	40–60%	C
Dabrafenib[21,49]	11–32%	B
Dactinomycin[58,i]	>30%	C
Dasatinib[49,59]	1≤19%	A
Daunorubicin[11,60]	>10%	C
Docetaxel[60-63,k]	38%	A
Doxifluridine[64]	9–10%	C
Doxorubicin[11,21,55-57,60,65,66,i]	16–100%	A
Edatrexate[67]	Up to 35%	C
Efaproxiral[68]	28%	C
Epirubicin[18,69]	25–100%	C
Eribulin[70]	33%	B
Erlotinib[49,71,72]	5–14%	B
Estramustine[73]	1%	A
Etoposide[52,55-57,74,75,i]	44%	B
Everolimus[21,49]	1–13%	B
Exemestanel[6,76,77]	2–15%	A
Fluorouracil[11]	>10%	C
Gefitinib[78,79]	10–11%	A
Gemcitabine[80-83]	10–61%	A
Idarubicin[84]	1–10%	C
Ifosfamide[21,74]	75–100%	C
Imatinib[21,49]	1–11%	B

Table 9-1 Agents Implicated in Drug-Induced Alopecia[18-169] (continued)

Drug	Incidence	Level of Evidence[a]
Ipilimumab[49]	1–18%	B
Irinotecan (conventional)[18,21,85,86]	46–72%	C
Irinotecan (liposomal)[21]	14%	C
Ixabepilone[21,87,88]	43–92%	A
Lapatinib[21,89]	13%	C
Lenalidomide[21]	≥1%	C
Lenvatinib[21]	12%	C
Letrozole[21,90]	3–5%	C
Lobaplatin[91]	26–33%	C
Methotrexate[8,18,21,74,92-95,l]	≥10%	A
Mitomycin[21,96]	4%	B
Mitoxantrone[18,97]	0.4–11%	B
Nilotinib[21,49,98]	12–20%	B
Omacetaxine[21]	15%	C
Oxaliplatin[21]	3%	C
Paclitaxel[18,21,65,99-101,m]	87–92%	A
Palbociclib[21]	22%	C
Panitumumab[54]	4–9%	C
Pazopanib[21,49,j]	8–17%	B
Pemetrexed[102]	6–11%	A
Pertuzumab[21]	52–65%	C
Pirarubicin[103-105]	12–94%	C
Regorafenib[21,49]	8–47%	B
Sonidegib[21]	53%	C
Sorafenib[21,106-109]	14–38%	A
Sunitinib[109-111,j]	5–14%	A
Tacrolimus[21]	<15%	C
Tamoxifen[21,112,113]	<1–5%	A
Temozolomide[114,115]	9%	C
Temsirolimus[49]	1–26%	B
Teniposide[21,74,116]	9%	A
Thiotepa[18,72]	NK[d]	C
Tipiracil[21]	7%	C
Topotecan[18,65,117-122]	49–77% 10% (oral)	A
Trametinib[49]	6–26%	B
Trastuzumab[123]	NK	C
Trifluridine[21]	7%	C
Vandetanib[21]	8%	C
Vemurafenib[21,47]	9–48%	C
Vinblastine[11,18]	>10%	C
Vincristine[11,18,52]	20–70%	C

Table 9-1 Agents Implicated in Drug-Induced Alopecia[18-169] (continued)

Drug	Incidence	Level of Evidence[a]
Vindesine[18,124,125]	6–92%	B
Vinorelbine[18,82,124-128]	1–15%	A
Vismodegib[21,49]	50.6–63.1%	C
CHOLESTEROL-LOWERING AGENTS		
Atorvastatin[129]	<2%	C
Cholestyramine[129]	NK	C
Clofibrate[129]	NK	C
Lovastatin[11]	1–5%	C
Pravastatin[11]	<1%	C
COLONY-STIMULATING FACTORS		
Eltrombopag[21]	2–10%	C
Filgrastim[21]	≥5%	C
Pegfilgrastim[21]	<1%	C
CONTRACEPTIVES (oral/intrauterine)		
All agents with high progesterone content which include products containing a first- and second-generation progestin[11,15,127-132]	NK[c]	B
CORTICOSTEROIDS		
Budesonide[21]	<5%	C
Dexamethasone[21]	NK	C
Hydrocortisone[21]	NK	C
Methylprednisolone[21]	NK	C
Triamcinolone[21]	NK	C
DOPAMINE AGONISTS		
Bromocriptine[18,133]	<1%	C
Cabergoline[18,133]	<1%	C
Dopamine[18,133]	<1%	C
Levodopa[18,133]	<1%	C
Pergolide[18,133]	<1%	C
Ropinirole[18,133]	<1%	C
GONADOTROPIN-RELEASING HORMONE-RELEASING AGONISTS		
Goserelin[18,21]	1–10%	C
GOUT MEDICATIONS		
Allopurinol[18,19,21]	NK	C
Colchicine[19,21,133,134]	1–10%	C
Febuxostat[21]	<1%	C
HISTAMINE$_2$-RECEPTOR ANTAGONISTS		
Cimetidine[26,135]	NK	C
HEAVY METALS/TOXINS		
Arsenic, bismuth, lead, mercury, thallium[136-138,n]	NK	C

Table 9-1 Agents Implicated in Drug-Induced Alopecia[18-169] (continued)

Drug	Incidence	Level of Evidence[a]
IMMUNOSUPPRESSANTS		
Azathioprine[11]	<1%	C
Belatacept[21]	<10%	C
Cyclosporine[11]	1–5%	C
Gold[11,138]	1–5%	C
Leflunomide[18,139]	9–17%	A
Methotrexate[8,18,21,74,92,94,140]	0.5–10%	A
Mycophenolate[21]	3–20%	C
Sulfasalazine[21,26,141]	6%	A
Tacrolimus[18,142]	28%	C
INTERFERONS[6,26,143]		
Interferon alfa-N3[6,26,143]	2–30%	A
Interferon alfacon-1[6,26,143]	2–30%	A
Interferon alfa-2a, recombinant[6,26,143]	2–30%	A
Interferon alfa-2b[6,26,143]	2–30%	A
Peginterferon alfa-2a and alfa-2b[6,26,143]	14–44%	A
MULTIPLE SCLEROSIS AGENTS		
Alemtuzumab[21]	3%	C
Fingolimod[21]	1–10%	C
Teriflunomide[21]	10–13%	C
NSAIDs		
Diclofenac[21]	<1%	C
Etodolac[21]	<1%	C
Ibuprofen[21]	<1%	C
Indomethacin[21]	<1%	C
Ketoprofen[21]	<1%	C
Ketorolac[21]	<1%	C
Meloxicam[21]	<2%	C
Nabumetone[21]	<1%	C
Naproxen[11]	<1%	C
Oxaprozin[21]	<1%	C
Piroxicam[21]	<1%	C
Sulindac[21]	<1%	C
OPIOIDS		
Fentanyl[21]	1–10%	C
PSYCHOTROPIC DRUGS[9,11,32]		
Amitriptyline[9,11,21,32]	NK	C
Amoxapine[9,11,21,32]	NK	C
Aripiprazole[9,11,21,32,144]	<1%	A
Bupropion[9,11,32,145]	<0.1%	C
Buspirone[9,10,11,32]	1–5%	C
Citalopam[9,11,32,146]	<1%	B
Clomipramine[6,9,21,32]	NK	C

Table 9-1 Agents Implicated in Drug-Induced Alopecia[18-169] (continued)

Drug	Incidence	Level of Evidence[a]
Clonazepam[9]	NK[d]	C
Desipramine[9,11,21,32]	NK	C
Doxepin[9,11,21,32]	NK	C
Escitalopam[9,11,21,32,147]	<1%	C
Fluoxetine[9,11,21,32]	NK	C
Fluvoxamine[9,11,21,32,148]	<1%	B
Haloperidol[9,10,11,21,32,133]	<1%	C
Imipramine[9,11,21,32,149]	0.01%	C
Lithium[3,9,11,18,33,133,150-152,o]	12–20%	A
Nortriptyline[9,11,21,32]	NK	C
Olanzapine[9,11,21,32,153]	0.1–1%	A
Paroxetine[9,11,21,32,154]	<1%	B
Protriptyline[21]	NK	C
Quetiapine[9,155]	NK	C
Risperidone[9,21,32,149]	NK	C
Sertraline[9,11,21,32,156]	<1%	B
St John's Wort (Hypericum perforatum)[9,11,21,32,157]	NK	C
Tranylcypromine[32,158]	NK	C
Trazodone[9,11,21,32]	<1%	C
Trimipramine[9,11,21,32]	NK	C
Venlafaxine[9,11,32, 159]	NK	C
Ziprasidone[9,11,32,160]	0.1–1%	B
RETINOIDS		
Acitretin[6,18,19,161]	20–30%	C
Etretinate[6,18,19,161]	20–30%	C
Isotretinoin[6,18,19,161]	20–30%	C
Retinoic acid[6,18,19,161]	20–30%	C
THYROID MEDICATIONS		
Carbimazole[11,162,163]	3.5–10%	C
Levothyroxine[11,21,162,163]	NK[p]	C
Liothyronine[11,21,162,163]	NK[p]	C
Methimazole[11,21,162,163]	NK[p]	C
Propylthiouracil[11,21,162,163]	NK[p]	C
TUMOR NECROSIS FACTOR INHIBITORS		
Adalimumab[9,11,21,32,164]	<1%	C
Certolizumab pegol[9,11,21,32]	<5%	C
Etanercept[165]	NK	C
Golimumab[166]	NK	C
Infliximab[164,167]	NK	C
MISCELLANEOUS DRUGS		
Aminoglutethimide[24]	NK	C
Boceprevir[121]	22–27%	C

Table 9-1 Agents Implicated in Drug-Induced Alopecia[18-169] (continued)

Drug	Incidence	Level of Evidence[a]
Cetirizine[11]	1–5%	C
Clonidine[21]	1–10%	C
Diazoxide[21]	NK	C
Ethionamide[21]	NK	C
Exenatide[21]	<1%	C
Gentamicin[168]	NK	C
Imiquimod[61]	1%	C
Isoniazid[169]	NK	C
Nitrofurantoin[21]	NK	C
Naltrexone[21]	<1%	C
Onabotulinumtoxin A[21]	<1%	C
Pasireotide[21]	2–18%	C
Vasopressin[11,14]	>10%	C
Vitamin A[18,21]	NK	C

CNS = central nervous system, NK = not known; NSAIDs= nonsteroidal anti-inflammatory drugs.
[a]Definitions for Levels of Evidence: Level A—evidence from one or more randomized, controlled clinical trials; Level B—evidence from nonrandomized clinical trials, prospective observational studies, cohort studies, retrospective studies, case-control studies, meta-analyses and/or postmarketing surveillance studies; and Level C—evidence from one or more published case reports or case series.
[b]Weight loss may play a role in amphetamine-induced hair loss.
[c]Although the incidence is not known, it is believed to occur commonly.
[d]Although the incidence is not known, it is believed to occur rarely.
[e]Abnormal hair texture has been observed in association with topiramate.
[f]"Perming" effects may be observed in association with valproic acid.[39]
[g]Incidence only reported when antifungal agents were administered for months at high doses.
[h]Combinations of indinavir plus ritonavir may be associated with severe hair loss.[18] Thoracic, axillary, pubic, thigh, and leg hair loss are also frequently adverse effects of indinavir.
[i]Bleomycin, dactinomycin, doxorubicin, and etoposide may cause delayed alopecia.[11,21,52,55-58]
[j]Hair color changes have been reported such as depigmentation[21,49]; incidence of hair color changes associated with cabozantinib was reported as 34%[49]; (incidence of hair discoloration from pazopanib was noted to be 23–39%[21-49]; incidence of hair discoloration from sunitinib was noted to be 20–29%).[109]
[k]Hair loss associated with docetaxel, is sudden in onset (usually during the third week after the first 1-hour infusion) and complete in many patients, including loss of axillary and pubic hair, eyelashes, and eyebrows.[60,61]
[l]Methotrexate causes dose-related alopecia.[8,21,74,92-94]
[m]Paclitaxel has been reported to cause loss of all body hair.[14,99-101]
[n]Degree and incidence of alopecia depends on dose and time of exposure.[136,137]
[o]Changes in hair texture, such as loss of curl or wave, often may occur at high hair lithium concentrations.[150]
[p]All thyroid replacement agents implicated, since hyperthyroidism and hypothyroidism are associated with hair loss.[11,21,162,163]

8 weeks. Alopecia is diffuse and involves not only the scalp but also eyelashes, eyebrows, pubic and axillary hair.[19] Lightening of hair color and hair kinking can also occur in association with retinoids.[18]

IMMUNOSUPPRESSANTS

Medications used for rheumatoid arthritis, notably disease-modifying antirheumatic drugs (DMARDs), have been associated with mild, reversible alopecia.[11,26,138] Gold therapy may cause exfoliative dermatitis leading to alopecia. There is a case report of scarring alopecia following gold therapy.[138] Methotrexate-induced alopecia is thought to be dose-dependent.[74,92] Other DMARDs that may cause alopecia include leflunomide and sulfasalazine. Cyclosporine, tacrolimus, and mycophenolate, which are often used following organ transplantation, have also been associated with hair loss.[18,142]

DOPAMINE AGONISTS

Dopamine agonists implicated in alopecia include bromocriptine, levodopa, pergolide, pramipexole, and ropinirole. Alopecia caused by these agents is considered to be a rare adverse effect.[18,174]

INTERFERONS

No correlation has been established between interferon dose and the onset or severity of hair loss. In some patients, alopecia resolves despite continued treatment.[6] Transient localized alopecia has been noted at the injection site in patients treated with interferon alfa. There are also reports of hair shape and hair color changes associated with interferon use.[18]

THYROID MEDICATIONS

Antithyroid medications, including iodine, propylthiouracil, carbimazole, and methimazole can cause iatrogenic hypothyroidism leading to alopecia. Papadopoulos and Harden reported that carbimazole, an agent similar in structure to methimazole, induced alopecia in a small percentage of patients.[162] However, hair regrowth occurred in all cases after carbimazole therapy was discontinued.[162] This reversible type of hair loss is telogen effluvium and is associated with dry scalp and dry and brittle hair.[4,6] In a few case reports, carbimazole-induced alopecia occurred in euthyroid patients.[163] Sometimes the hair loss terminates despite continuation of therapy with carbimazole and methimazole.[19] Thyroid replacement medications can also cause drug-induced alopecia.[175]

ANTIEPILEPTICS

Several antiepileptic drugs have been associated with alopecia.[19] Of these, valproic acid is associated with the highest incidence of hair loss, reported between 2.6% and 12%. Alopecia occurs within 3 months after initiating therapy and is believed to be of the telogen effluvium type. The hair loss is usually transient and may terminate even if the medication is continued.[19] Valproic acid can also affect hair by causing a "perming" effect or "diffuse curliness of the hair." One report stated that this curliness occurred while taking valproic acid for approximately 1 year. The curliness persisted for approximately 30 months of therapy and subsided within approximately 6 months after discontinuation of the therapy.[39] Carbamazepine may also cause hair loss.[6,9,32,33] Other antiepileptic medications that have been associated with hair loss have all been implicated via case reports. In one case, alopecia developed after 2 months of topiramate therapy in a 15-year-old female. Hair loss resolved after discontinuation of therapy and recurred upon reinitiation of topiramate treatment.[37]

PSYCHOTROPICS

Psychotropic drug-induced alopecia tends to manifest with transient mild to moderate hair loss and is reversible upon discontinuation of therapy.[3] In some cases, improvement has occurred spontaneously despite continuation of lithium therapy. Lithium has been associated with dry and limp hair as well as texture changes. There have been some rare reports of loss of body hair associated with lithium use. This effect reversed upon discontinuation of therapy.[32] Lithium-induced hair loss may be a result of lithium-induced hypothyroidism; resolution of the hypothyroid state may reverse the hair loss.[150] Antidepressant agents such as the tricyclic antidepressants, selective serotonin reuptake inhibitors, new-generation antidepressants and the antianxiety agent buspirone have all been implicated in causing alopecia, although this occurs rarely.[32] Atypical and typical antipsychotic agents have also been reported to induce hair loss, which usually occurs several months after the initiation of therapy and is characterized as nonscarring, diffuse alopecia with generalized or localized hair loss commonly affecting the scalp. The alopecia is reversible, usually within 2–5 months after discontinuation of therapy.[176]

HORMONES/ANDROGENS

Two types of oral contraceptive-induced hair loss have been identified. In the first type, hair loss occurs about 3 months after discontinuation of therapy with oral contraceptives. This type of alopecia is similar to postpartum hair loss, in which increased telogen loss is a consequence of the higher percentage of anagen hair maintained during pregnancy. Although hair shedding can appear dramatic, it usually is not noticeable.[6,173]

The androgenic effects of progestin are responsible for the second type of oral contraceptive-induced alopecia. In these cases, modifying therapy to an oral contraceptive with a lower dose of progestin often results in resolution of the alopecia. The incidence of this type of drug-induced alopecia is decreasing because of the lower progestin content of new formulations of oral contraceptives.[18,173,177,178]

Any medication containing androgens or anabolic steroids can produce or aggravate alopecia in women.[11,26,179] For instance, androgenetic alopecia occurs in a small percentage of women receiving hormone-replacement therapy.[18] Methyltestosterone and progestin derivatives such as medroxyprogesterone and norethindrone may, in rare instances, aggravate scalp alopecia. Estrogen also has been associated with increased hair shedding.[177] A review of hormone-replacement therapy with esterified estrogen 0.65–1.25 mg and methyltestosterone 1.25–2.5 mg in 2,556 patients over 13 years verified the occurrence of drug-induced alopecia associated with both hormone replacement combinations.[131] Anabolic steroids such as testosterone and nandrolone may also cause androgen-induced hair loss.[26,163] Antiestrogens and aromatase inhibitors such as tamoxifen and letrozole and gonadotropin-releasing hormone agonists may also be associated with androgenetic alopecia.[18]

TUMOR NECROSIS FACTOR–BLOCKING AGENTS

Several case studies have implicated anti-TNFα agents (also known as biologic agents) with alopecia. This only occurs in certain individuals who are genetically susceptible. This drug-induced alopecia may present months to years after starting a biologic agent.[164,167]

CANCER CHEMOTHERAPY

Cancer chemotherapy-induced alopecia occurs commonly.[6,11,55,175] The agents that are most commonly implicated include bleomycin, cisplatin, cyclophosphamide, daunorubicin, doxorubicin, fluorouracil, methotrexate, and vincristine.[6,11,55,175]

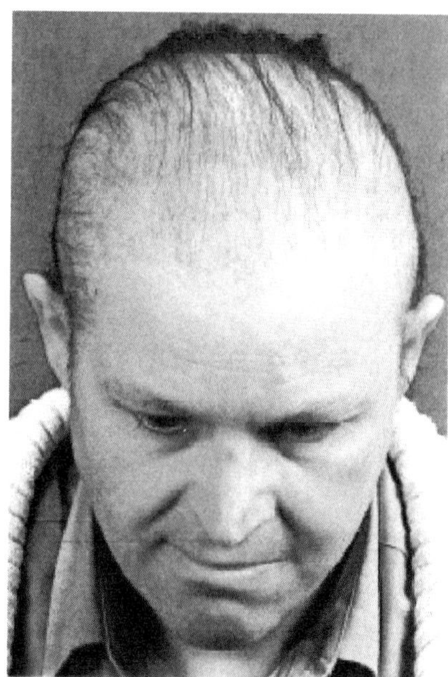

FIGURE 9-2 Diffuse Alopecia Caused by 5-Fluorouracil[19]

Source: Reprinted with permission from Bork K, ed. *Cutaneous side effects of drugs*. Philadelphia: Saunders; Copyright ©1988:249-58.

Figure 9-2 depicts a patient with alopecia induced by fluorouracil.[19] Although chemotherapy-induced alopecia is classified as anagen effluvium, it may present with different clinical patterns and be caused by different mechanisms. Evidence shows that the hair follicle may react to the same insult capable of stopping mitosis with shedding patterns consistent with both anagen effluvium and telogen effluvium. When mitotic activity of the hair cycle is arrested, several factors influence hair shedding. Consequently, hair may fall out very quickly or gradually. The onset of anagen effluvium hair loss is typically days to weeks; however, because chemotherapy can induce telogen effluvium, hair loss can start within months. Although hair loss begins in days to weeks, it might not be prominent until 1–2 months.[18,180,181] The onset and degree of hair loss is highly variable depending on the specific medication, dose, pharmacokinetic variables such as half-life and duration of therapy. Combination therapy increases the risk and severity of alopecia.[182] Hair may appear patchy or patterned and typically falls out spontaneously or with brushing or combing.[4,129,138] Chemotherapy-induced alopecia may also involve the beard, eye brows, eye lashes, axillary, and pubic hairs if the chemotherapy is given at high doses for a sufficiently long period of time and with repeated exposures.[180] The majority of male patients with cancer chemotherapy-induced alopecia report that the frequency of shaving is reduced to one to three times a week.[129]

Scarring alopecia has been noted in association with gefitinib and erlotinib, two tyrosine kinase inhibitors used for treatment of tumors that test positive for the human epidermal growth factor receptor (HER). This alopecia shows chronic folliculitis and perifolliculitis with lymphocytes, plasma cells, and some neutrophils and eosinophils; the upper follicle revealed perifollicular fibrosis, all of which are suggestive of drug-induced scarring alopecia. In the case of the erlotinib, improvement in the scalp occurred after discontinuing erlotinib therapy for 3 weeks. Reintroduction of erlotinib therapy caused a recurrence of the scalp lesions.[72,79] Treatment with lapatinib and trastuzumab, two other agents used for HER-positive tumors, has been reported to cause tufted hair folliculitis, a type of scarring alopecia.[89,123,164,167,183]

Permanent alopecia may occur after conditioning regimens used commonly in hematopoietic stem-cell transplantation and in association with certain cancer chemotherapy agents administered in high doses (e.g., carboplatin).[53,184,185] Combination antineoplastic therapy can also lead to permanent alopecia. Examples include cyclophosphamide, thiotepa, and carboplatin combination therapy, as well as cyclophosphamide administered with busulfan.[184,185]

POISONING AND NONMETAL ELEMENTS

Poisoning with arsenic, bismuth, copper, lead, mercury, or thallium can result in pronounced hair loss, which occurs relatively quickly after exposure.[4,6,136] Hair loss associated with thallium, gold, arsenic, and bismuth usually begins 2–4 weeks after exposure.[13,137] Thallium can affect not only the scalp but also the eyelashes, eyebrows (lateral aspects), arms, and legs. Total epilation may occur approximately 1 month after the initiation of therapy.[4,6] Severe hair shedding usually occurs only in association with the cytotoxic agents. Noncytotoxic drug-induced hair loss rarely results in total hair loss, and is normally reversible upon discontinuation of the offending drug.[18]

ANTIFUNGAL AGENTS

Prior to 2012, antifungals had not been widely associated with alopecia; however, in September 2012, a multistate outbreak of mold-induced meningitis required the use of high-dose and long-term therapy with antifungal agents. Voriconazole was one of the two antifungal drugs used in this outbreak. After several months of therapy, many patients complained of alopecia as well as nail changes including brittle nails, split nails, thinning nails and, in some cases, complete loss of nails. Prior to this, the only antifungal agents that had been associated with alopecia were fluconazole and voriconazole from one case report in one child.[43] In a cross-sectional survey of patients taking a high dose of voriconazole (6 mg/kg every 12 hours) for at least 1 month, 82% reported alopecia. Hair loss occurred on the scalp in 96% of cases, eyebrows and eye lashes in 38%, and arms and legs in 42%. Extensive hair loss requiring a wig or hat was reported in 15% of patients. After discontinuing therapy with voriconazole, 82% of those with alopecia reported that the hair loss had stopped, and 69% indicated that hair regrowth had begun.[43]

EPIDEMIOLOGY

Drug-induced alopecia is not uncommon, although the exact incidence is not known. The incidence of alopecia associated with specific drugs, where known, is presented in Table 9-1.[18-169] Alopecia associated with cancer chemotherapy and cytotoxic drugs, whether noticed or unnoticed, occurs in nearly 100% of patients who do not undergo hair loss prophylaxis. The prevalence and severity depend on the drug as well as on individual predisposition. Hair loss can occur in association with some drugs when administered in usual doses, while alopecia associated with other drugs is unpredictable and occurs only occasionally.[6,11,18,55] Heparin and heparinoid drugs can lead to telogen effluvium, with an incidence that varies from 0% to >50%.[170] Vitamin A (retinol)-induced alopecia has been reported in approximately 20–30% of patients.[6,19]

The incidence of DMARD-induced alopecia ranges from 1% to 10%.[13,138-141,170] Alopecia caused by dopamine agonists occurs rarely and is more common in females.[18,174] Nearly 20–30% of patients receiving interferon experience alopecia of the telogen effluvium type.[6] The incidence of alopecia induced by carbimazole ranges from 3.5% to 10%.[162] The overall incidence of hair loss provoked by antiepileptic medications is 0.01–12%, with valproic acid therapy associated with the highest incidence (2.6–12%).[19,37,41] Alopecia induced by carbamazepine has been reported to be a very rare adverse event in some case reports, while others estimate the incidence to be as high as 6%.[6,9,32,33] The incidence of lithium-induced hair loss is 12–17%.[3] Hormone-replacement therapy with esterified estrogen 0.625–1.25 mg and methyltestosterone 1.25–2.5 mg induces alopecia with a reported incidence of 8.8%.[131] Cytostatic agents have been reported to cause total scalp hair loss in roughly 10% of patients. Hair loss was reversed after therapy was discontinued.[4,19,129,186]

MECHANISMS

Mechanisms of drug-induced alopecia are listed in **Table 9-2**.[5,6,43,72,79,166,176,180,187,188] Drugs that induce alopecia can be classified according to their effects on the phases of the hair growth cycle.[1,67] There are two patterns of drug-induced alopecia: anagen effluvium and telogen effluvium.[5,186]

During anagen effluvium, drugs may partially or completely suppress mitosis and cause metabolic impairment of hair growth. This leads to failure to form a hair shaft or the formation of a thinned, weakened hair shaft.[5,186] Eighty-five percent of hair follicles on the scalp are in the anagen phase. Therefore, this is a major target for drugs that cause anagen effluvium alopecia. Hair loss also can be manifested in axillary, pubic, and other body regions. Cytotoxic agents such as cancer chemotherapy drugs and toxic plasma concentrations of certain metals cause drug-induced alopecia by affecting follicles during the anagen phase of hair growth. Because the duration of the anagen phase is the primary determinant of hair length, the maximum length of the new anagen hair is shorter than that of the hair it is replacing. Eventually, the anagen phase is shortened to the point at which the hair cannot reach the skin surface. At this point, the only visible part of the hair cycle on the skin is the pore, as the hair follicle can no longer be seen.[8] In patients with anagen alopecia, hair loss is almost always reversible when therapy with the offending agent is terminated. However, hair grows at a rate of only about 1 cm per month, so several months are required for complete reversal of the hair loss.[6] The medications most commonly associated with anagen effluvium are cancer chemotherapy agents.[5]

The majority of drug-induced hair loss is primarily considered telogen effluvium hair loss, because the majority of drugs that induce hair loss disrupt the telogen effluvium growth phase. In telogen effluvium, drugs provoke hair loss by causing premature termination of the anagen, or growing, phase of the hair cycle, resulting in an increased number of shed hairs. This type of hair loss often can be identified by the presence of a clubbed root on shed hair. Hair loss is typically diffuse rather than patchy, and patients often are asymptomatic. Telogen effluvium is primarily noted on the scalp; however, it sometimes may be detected in other locations.[1,5,6,9] Telogen hair loss often occurs secondary to events such as severe illness, nutritional deficiencies (protein, vitamins, and minerals), childbirth, fever, and hemorrhage. It can be caused by drugs including warfarin, heparin, low-molecular-weight heparins, lithium, certain β-blockers (metoprolol, nadolol, propranolol), and α- and λ-interferon. A few cytotoxic agents also may cause telogen effluvium by shifting the hair follicles into a premature resting cycle.[187,189]

Alopecia areata has been postulated to have an autoimmune pathogenesis involving inflammatory cytokines, including TNFα. Drugs have typically not been associated with alopecia areata, but there are several case reports of biologic agents inducing this type of hair loss.[166,167,190] It has been proposed that anti-TNFα agents lead to the development of other autoimmune diseases, in which the body's immune system is inappropriately activated by the anti-TNFα agents, which then attacks hair follicles.[166,167,191,192] The mechanism is unknown but

Table 9-2 Mechanisms of Drug-Induced Alopecia[5,6,43,72,79,166,176,180,187,188]

Drug	Mechanism
Amphetamines	Telogen effluvium
Anabolic steroids/androgens	Androgenetic alopecia
Anesthetics	Telogen effluvium
Angiotensin-converting enzyme inhibitors	Telogen effluvium
Antiarrhythmics	Telogen effluvium
Anticoagulants	Telogen effluvium
Anticonvulsants	Telogen effluvium
Antifungals	Telogen effluvium
Antivirals	Telogen effluvium
β-blockers	Telogen effluvium
Calcium-channel blockers	Telogen effluvium
Cancer chemotherapy agents	Anagen effluvium
Erlotinib	Plus scarring alopecia
Gefitinib	Plus scarring alopecia
Lapatinib	Plus scarring alopecia
Trastuzumab	Plus scarring alopecia
Cholesterol-lowering agents	Telogen effluvium
Colony-stimulating factor	Telogen effluvium
Contraceptives (oral/intrauterine)	Androgenetic alopecia
Corticosteroids	Telogen effluvium
Dopamine agonists	Telogen effluvium
Gonadotropin-releasing hormone-releasing agonists	Androgenetic alopecia
Gout medications	Telogen effluvium
Histamine$_2$-receptor antagonists	Telogen effluvium
Heavy metals/toxins	Anagen effluvium
Immunosuppressants	Telogen effluvium/alopecia areata
Interferons	Telogen effluvium
Multiple sclerosis agents	Unknown
NSAIDs	Telogen effluvium
Psychiatric medications	Telogen effluvium
Retinoids	Telogen effluvium
Thyroid medications	Telogen effluvium
Tumor necrosis factor–blocking agents	Psoriatic alopecia or alopecia areata
MISCELLANEOUS AGENTS	
Aminoglutethimide	Telogen effluvium
Boceprevir	Telogen effluvium
Cetirizine	Telogen effluvium
Clonidine	Telogen effluvium
Diazoxide	Telogen effluvium
Ethionamide	Telogen effluvium
Exenatide	Telogen effluvium
Gentamicin	Telogen effluvium

Table 9-2 Mechanisms of Drug-Induced Alopecia[5,6,43,72,79,166,176,180,187,188] (continued)

Drug	Mechanism
Imiquimod	Telogen effluvium
Isoniazid	Telogen effluvium
Nitrofurantoin	Telogen effluvium
Naltrexone	Telogen effluvium
Onabotulinumtoxin A	Telogen effluvium
Pasireotide	Telogen effluvium
Vasopressin	Telogen effluvium

NSAID = nonsteroidal anti-inflammatory drug.

a proposed hypothesis is that the alopecia is caused when an alternative signaling pathway leads other autoimmune diseases to develop such as psoriatic alopecia or alopecia areata.[164,167]

Drugs also may induce hair loss by increasing androgen activity. Hair loss occurring by this mechanism is termed *androgenic alopecia* or *androgenetic alopecia*, also known as male pattern baldness. Women with androgenetic alopecia have lower scalp follicle concentrations of 5α-reductase (which converts testosterone to dihydrotestosterone), lower scalp follicle concentrations of the gene encoding aromase CYP19A1 (which converts testosterone to estrogen), and greater density of androgen receptors. However, these patients do not have higher plasma concentrations of androgens and tend to have normal fertility, menses, and endocrine function.[193-195] Drugs implicated in androgenetic alopecia include danazol, metyrapone, progestins, estrogen receptor antagonists, and anabolic steroids.[5,13,58] In many cases, hair loss is not reversible upon discontinuation of therapy with the offending agent.[5]

CLINICAL PRESENTATION AND DIFFERENTIAL DIAGNOSIS

Signs and symptoms associated with drug-induced alopecia are listed in **Table 9-3**.[1,4-6,12,13,58,175,193,196-198] Features of different types of drug-induced alopecia are compared in **Table 9-4**.[4-6,11-13,18,58,167,173,193,197,198] To determine the type of drug-induced alopecia, patients should be evaluated for the presence of shedding or fragile hair (or both), slowed rate of hair growth, inability to regenerate new hair, and any related local or systemic disorders. In addition to a visual inspection, specific diagnostic procedures such as the hair-pull test, hair plucks, microscopic examination of hair and scalp, as well as cultures and biopsies may be used.[1] The hair-pull test is one of the easiest tests used to evaluate alopecia. Patients are advised not to shampoo the hair for 24 hours prior to the test.[193] The clinician grasps approximately 60 hairs using the thumb and index and middle fingers. The hairs are gently but firmly pulled. The test is considered positive for active shedding when more than six hairs are pulled free.

When a definitive diagnosis is needed or if the routine testing is inconclusive, a scalp biopsy can be performed. The scalp biopsy provides histologic features, the number of anagen and telogen hairs, and the number of terminal and vellus hairs per area, which provides a more definitive analysis of the hair loss. A scalp biopsy leaves a small scar on the patient's scalp, as it is an invasive procedure. Patients may refuse the biopsy because of the scar if the hair loss is potentially irreversible. A scalp biopsy is usually not necessary for routine diagnosis of hair loss.[12] The biopsy is usually reserved for alopecia that lacks identifiable triggers, chronic hair loss, miniaturized hair shafts, or failure to exclude alopecia areata.[200]

Patients with drug-induced anagen alopecia present with hair that is thin and fragile, and shed hairs are narrow, broken, and have no roots.[5] Because

Table 9-3 Signs and Symptoms Associated with Drug-Induced Alopecia[1,4-6,12,13,58,175,193,196-198]

Anagen effluvium alopecia

- Acute severe hair shedding with an onset of days to weeks after the initiation of therapy
- Hair loss from other sites is less common
- May cause loss of hair from entire scalp, eyebrows, and eyelashes; often >200 hairs are shed daily
- Photograph/visualization of scalp reveals diffuse thinning, which may progress to loss of entire scalp hair
- Positive hair-pull test
- Trichogram/TrichoScan reveals weakening and thinning of hair shaft, hair shaft breaks easily at the base with minimal trauma, and/or dystrophic hair (toxically damaged hair)

Telogen effluvium alopecia

- Hair loss is usually diffuse and mild; many times, it is not noticeable at all
- Hair loss occurs usually within 2–4 months after the initiation of therapy
- Increased hair shedding can vary from day to day (often ~100–150 hairs per day)
- Occasional loss of pubic or body hairs can occur
- Photograph/visualization of scalp reveals diffuse thinning; may progress to entire scalp hair loss
- Positive hair-pull test
- Scalp biopsy shows absence of inflammation with increased telogen count
- Shed hair has clubbed roots
- Trichogram/TrichoScan often reveals that scalp and hair shafts appear normal

Androgenetic alopecia

- Hair loss is nonscarring
- Hair-pull test reveals high telogen count
- Photograph and/or visualization of scalp reveals diffuse thinning, specific areas of hair loss, progression of hair loss in androgenetic pattern
- Scalp biopsy (possible histologic features) reveals fraction of terminal hair is decreased, nonspecific focal perivascular basophilic degeneration of the lower third of the connective-tissue sheaths of otherwise normal anagen follicles, perifollicular lymphocyte infiltrate at the level of the sebaceous duct, and/or fibrotic streamers present
- Trichogram/TrichoScan reveals shorter, finer, and often lighter-colored hair shafts

Female androgenetic alopecia

- Diffuse thinning typically occurs at vertex but can spread to the crown
- For the most part, the frontal hair line is preserved

Male androgenetic alopecia

- Hair loss begins at the frontal hairline and causes a receding hairline and possibly thins the hair at the crown, then can spread
- Hair loss is nonscarring
- Preservation of the follicular ostia is observed

Alopecia areata

- Biopsy reveals peri- and intrafollicular inflammatory infiltrate of the hair follicle (around anagen stage)
- Often hair loss is in patches but can involve total scalp hair loss and rarely total body hair loss
- Positive hair-pull test
- Short hairs that taper near the scalp are found near margin of the alopecia ("exclamation point" hairs)

the hair is weakened, it is susceptible to fracture with minimal trauma.[5,201] Microscopic examination of hair from patients with cancer chemotherapy-induced alopecia reveals fragmentation, trichorrhexis, decreased diameter, and depigmentation of the hair shaft. The hair breaks off nearly as quickly as it issues from the hair follicle.[187,197] Anagen effluvium alopecia usually develops within days to weeks after the initiation of therapy with the causative agent, and the hair shedding is acute but may not be prominent until 1–2 months.[180] Hair may appear patchy or patterned, and typically falls out spontaneously or with brushing or combing.[4,18,129] Often, the hair loss is very severe, especially when

Table 9-4 Comparison of Features of Drug-Induced Alopecia[4-6,11-13,18,58,167,173,193,197,198]

Feature	Anagen Effluvium	Telogen Effluvium	Androgenetic Alopecia	Alopecia Areata
Onset of hair loss	Days to weeks	Becomes evident within 2–4 months	2–4 months (gradual with progression)	1 month to years
Description of hair loss	Extensive or severe hair loss can occur Sometimes complete hair loss can occur, especially with certain cancer chemotherapy agents	Usually mild and diffuse, often not noticed at all	First appears as telogen effluvium then proceeds to androgenetic alopecia if drug therapy is continued In males, primarily bitemporal recession of the hairline; in women, a diffuse thinning over the scalp with more noticeable thinning in the frontal and parietal areas with preservation of the anterior hairline	Typically starts with a patch of hair loss, then can progress to multiple patches of hair loss In rare events, total scalp hair loss and total body hair loss can occur
Evaluation of the hair follicle	Weakening and thinning of hair shaft; breaks easily at the base with minimal trauma	Scalp and hair shafts often appear normal Shed hair has clubbed roots	Shorter, finer, and often lighter-colored hair shafts often present	Bald areas are usually circular or oval shaped and smooth to touch Short hairs that taper near the scalp are found near margin of the alopecia ("exclamation point" hairs)
Results if therapy with causative drug is discontinued	Usually resolves; however, if long-term exposure to drug, may result in a scarring alopecia (which does not resolve with discontinuation of therapy)	Nearly always resolves with discontinuation of therapy or lower doses of the causative drug	In many cases, it is not reversible upon discontinuing the causative agent	Usually resolves completely with discontinuation of agent in conjunction with treatment In cases of alopecia totalis or alopecia universalis, may see treatment failure or not have complete resolution of the alopecia

two or more alopecia-provoking drugs are administered.[182] Anagen effluvium alopecia may produce loss of most of the scalp hair, eyelashes, and eyebrows. This type of alopecia occurs almost exclusively in association with cytotoxic drugs such as cancer chemotherapy agents. Normally, hair regrowth occurs rapidly if therapy with the causative agent is discontinued and minimal damage to the hair follicles occurred.[18,19,129,175,180,182]

Patients with drug-induced telogen alopecia typically present with mild, diffuse hair loss. Shed hair typically has clubbed roots and the hair comes out by the roots. Miniaturized hairs are generally not found.[1,5,6,8,202] Alopecia in patients with telogen effluvium is usually subclinical and rarely involves more than 50% of the hairs.[6,186,202,203] Although presentation depends on the percentage of hair follicles involved, hair loss in patients with drug-induced telogen alopecia often does not become evident until 2–4 months after the initiation of therapy with the offending drug.[197] As the hair loss is mild and often occurs long after therapy with the offending agent has been initiated, this condition can be easily overlooked. Hair loss is generally diffuse rather than patchy, and patients often are asymptomatic. Telogen effluvium is noted primarily on the scalp; however, it sometimes may be detected in other locations.[1,5,6,9] Examination of shed hair reveals the presence of a clubbed root. If on microscopic exam a white bulb is found on the shaft of extracted hair, the test is considered positive for telogen effluvium.[10] Progressive miniaturization of the hair follicles is noted. If the offending drug is continued, with each successive growth cycle, hair follicles become smaller and produce shorter, finer hairs that cover the scalp poorly.[170] In telogen effluvium, the hair root is not damaged so hair will, in most cases, spontaneously regrow once therapy with the offending drug is discontinued.[6,186,203] Severe shedding is uncommon and occurs exclusively in association with interferons, anti-retroviral drugs, heparin and heparinoids, and, on occasion, cancer chemotherapy agents.[18] Hair regrowth normally occurs within 2–6 months after discontinuing therapy with the causative agent.[11,18,26,175]

Drug-induced androgenetic alopecia may be suspected in patients taking an androgenic drug and in whom hair loss is mediated by the presence of androgen dihydrotestosterone in hair and/or plasma, the hair loss is male-pattern type (no effects on nonscalp hair), the shedding is usually not severe, and the hair comes out by the roots.[11,18,26,175,193,196] Miniaturization of hairs with various lengths and diameters is a classic sign of androgenetic alopecia. With successive anagen cycles, the hair follicles become smaller, manifesting as finer, shorter hair; over time, nonpigmented vellus hairs replace pigmented terminal hairs. In women, androgenetic alopecia often manifests as a diffuse thinning but more concentrated thinning over the top of the scalp with preservation of the anterior hairline, or as complete baldness and loss of all hair except the occipital and temporal fringes.[1,5,58,196] Evaluation of plasma testosterone concentrations is of value in these patients; testing for drug-induced alopecia is expected to yield normal or low concentrations in the absence of other features consistent with androgen excess (e.g., hirsutism, acne, or irregular menses).[5,11,179,193,198] Biopsy of the scalp in women with androgenetic alopecia shows increased aromatase activity compared to that in men with androgenetic alopecia.[177]

Alopecia aerata presents often with bald areas that are usually oval or circular, well-defined, and a smooth patch or patches. The affected area can range from just patches on the scalp to total scalp hair loss (alopecia totalis) and in rare cases to total body hair loss (alopecia universalis). Inflammation is present but usually deep in the skin and is revealed via a scalp biopsy. The hair-pull test reveals pencil point and telogen shafts. In some instances, there is mild itching, tingling, tenderness or a burning sensation in the affected area.[191,192,197] Reports of drug-induced alopecia areata reveal hair loss after several months of therapy which usually progresses if the causative agent is not discontinued. After terminating therapy with the offending medication, hair loss with treatment usually returns but very slowly, often months later.[166,167] Trichotillomania, a result of a psychiatric disorder such as obsessive-compulsive disorder, psychosis, anxiety disorder, is another cause of alopecia and involves a compulsion to pull out one's hair. The hair loss involves patchy hair loss with incomplete thinning and stubble present. Another cause of alopecia is traction alopecia where the hair is pulled back tightly repeatedly or for long periods of time. It usually presents a frontal and/or temporal hair loss.[10] Conditions to consider in the differential diagnosis of drug-induced alopecia are listed in **Table 9-5**.[4,10]

RISK FACTORS

Risk factors for drug-induced alopecia are listed in **Table 9-6**.[11,161,173,175] Route of administration has been shown to influence the risk of alopecia associated with some drugs. Cancer chemotherapy agents administered intravenously may cause complete alopecia within a short time, whereas oral therapy tends to be associated with a lower risk of alopecia, regardless of the total dose administered. Drug combinations, higher doses, and longer duration of drug therapy as well as drug interactions that lead to increased plasma concentrations can contribute to the risk of alopecia.[187] For example, lithium-induced changes in hair texture, such as a loss of a natural wave or curl, are more likely to occur in patients with significantly higher hair lithium concentrations than in those who do not experience hair changes.[150] The risk of anticoagulant-induced hair loss is not related to age but appears

Table 9-5 Conditions to Consider in the Differential Diagnosis of Drug-Induced Alopecia[4,10]

Alopecia areata, scarring alopecia, telogen effluvium
- Systemic/chronic illness (e.g., autoimmune disorder, cancer)

Alopecia areata, telogen effluvium
- Hypothyroidism

Androgenetic alopecia (women)
- Hirsutism (combined hirsutism/alopecia in polycystic ovary disease)
- Amenorrhea
- Infertility

Scarring alopecia, telogen effluvium, tinea capitis
- Infection (systemic or local)

Telogen effluvium
- Physical stress (e.g., surgery, pregnancy, malnutrition)
- Life-threatening psychological stress

Telogen effluvium; anagen effluvium
- Serious illness within previous 3–4 months

Traction alopecia
- Tight braids
- "Pulled-back" hairstyle

Trichotillomania
- If taking psychoactive medication, also consider telogen effluvium, as both types of alopecia could be occurring simultaneously
- Psychiatric disorder (e.g., psychosis, anxiety, obsessive-compulsive disorder)

Table 9-6 Risk Factors for Drug-Induced Alopecia[11,161,173,175]

Risk factors related to drug administration:
- Combination therapy
- Drug interactions leading to higher drug concentrations
- Higher doses
- Intravenous route of administration
- Longer duration of exposure

Disease states:
- Autoimmune disease
- Endocrine abnormalities
- Hyperandrogenic disorders
- Hypothyroidism or hyperthyroidism
- Illness/fevers/infection
- Increased blood loss
- Inflammatory diseases (i.e., seborrheic dermatitis, psoriasis)
- Iron deficiency anemia
- Parturition
- Polycystic ovary syndrome
- Poor nutritional status/crash diets (low serum iron or ferritin concentrations or deficiency of protein, zinc, selenium)

Family history of androgenetic alopecia

Recent surgery

Stress

to be dose-related and seems to be more frequent in women than men.[6,19] Alopecia caused by dopamine agonists is also more common in women.[18,174] Vitamin A (retinol)-induced alopecia occurs more frequently in women receiving higher doses. Vitamin E, taken concurrently with vitamin A, may potentiate vitamin A toxicity.[6,19] Patients with pre-existing thyroid disease, polycystic ovary disease, inflammatory diseases such as seborrheic dermatitis, psoriasis, malnutrition, or certain metabolic disorders such as liver disorders and chronic kidney disease are at risk for alopecia.[1,204] Concomitant systemic and chronic illness such as autoimmune disorders and cancer may also increase the risk. Stress, crash dieting, nutritional deficiencies (protein, vitamins, and minerals), iron deficiency infection, fever, and childbirth are other factors that can lead to telogen effluvium.[4,10,177,189] Women with androgenetic alopecia who take a progestin with high androgenic activity for oral contraception or hormone-replacement therapy are at increased risk for further hair loss. Testosterone and related substances such as dehydroepiandrosterone (DHEA) should be avoided in women with androgenetic alopecia because of the increased risk for worsening the condition.[196]

Postoperative alopecia is the temporary or permanent loss of hair that occurs following prolonged immobilization during general anesthesia and intubation.[199] Localized pressure-induced ischemia is the likely cause. Patients at highest risk for permanent hair loss include those undergoing cardiac or gynecologic surgical procedures for which the combined intraoperative and postoperative intubation time exceeds 24 hours.

MORBIDITY AND MORTALITY

Although drug-induced hair loss is usually reversible, it can be quite traumatic for both men and women.[79] In one study, cancer chemotherapy-induced alopecia ranked third on patients' lists of distressing symptoms, behind nausea and vomiting.[205] Patients sometimes refuse cancer chemotherapy for fear of hair loss.[74] It is important that clinicians appreciate their patients' views regarding the social impact of hair loss, even in cases in which patients experience only hair thinning. Understanding patients' feelings regarding hair loss and openly discussing the matter may reduce the risk that they will abruptly discontinue medications and suffer potentially serious health consequences as a result.[32]

PREVENTION

Avoiding therapy with medications that may cause alopecia is the best method of prevention, but in many cases this is not feasible. In situations in which drug-induced alopecia may occur, continuation of therapy may be necessary, particularly with cancer chemotherapy agents, anticoagulants, or psychiatric medications. In such cases, clinicians should use the lowest possible dose of the potentially causative agents and avoid, when possible, the use of multiple drugs with the potential to cause hair loss. In addition, the duration of exposure should be limited to the extent possible, and the oral, rather than intravenous, route should be used whenever possible.[178,187] Delivery of anthracyclines via liposomes significantly reduces the risk of hair loss compared with other routes of administration.[52] Avoiding drug interactions that lead to increased plasma concentrations of alopecia-inducing drugs is also important, especially if the alopecia is dose-dependent. Approaches to help prevent drug-induced alopecia are presented in **Table 9-7**.[6,10,11,52,177,178,187,206-209]

Other preventive measures include ensuring proper nutritional status and management of stress. Stress and anxiety are often present in patients who are taking psychotropic medications and are also symptoms of malnutrition. Stress, anxiety, and malnutrition are each well-documented causes of hair loss. Therefore, patients taking drugs known to cause alopecia may experience hair loss due to the medication, stress, anxiety, or any combination of these factors. Consequently, helping the patient cope and gain better control of his or her disease state may reduce stress and anxiety and may decrease the risk or severity (or both) of hair loss induced by psychotropic medications.[11,26]

Table 9-7 Approaches to Help Prevent Drug-Induced Alopecia[6,10,52,177,178,187,206-209]

- Avoid drug interactions that could increase plasma concentrations of potentially causative agents associated with dose-dependent alopecia
- Avoid drugs with potential to induce alopecia where possible
- Avoid, when possible, the use of multiple drugs with the potential to cause hair loss
- Check plasma iron and ferritin concentrations and thyroid function at first sign of hair loss
- For patients undergoing cancer chemotherapy, consider scalp cooling or hypothermia
- Identify and manage comorbid diseases and conditions that can cause or exacerbate hair loss, such as infections, fevers, malnutrition, polycystic ovary syndrome, hyperinsulinemia, inflammatory diseases, and autoimmune diseases
- Identify any family history of androgenetic alopecia, hirsutism, amenorrhea, or infertility prior to initiation of therapy with medications known to cause hair loss; this may allow the clinician to identify and correct potential risk factors for alopecia
- Limit duration of exposure to potentially causative agents
- Maintain proper nutritional status
- Manage stress
- Monitor kidney and/or liver function in patients taking renally eliminated or hepatically metabolized drugs known to cause dose-dependent alopecia
- Recognize patients at high risk for alopecia or existing alopecia to avoid alopecia-inducing medication if possible or consider prophylactic therapy such as minoxidil
- Use liposomal delivery of the anthracyclines to significantly lower risk of hair loss
- Use the lowest possible dose of potentially causative agents
- Use the oral route rather than the intravenous route whenever possible
- Warn patients with breast cancer or lymphoproliferative disorders of the potential for interference with drug delivery if using scalp cooling; scalp cooling should be avoided in patients with hepatic dysfunction

Diseases or conditions that can cause or exacerbate hair loss, such as infections, fever, malnutrition, polycystic ovary disease, hyperinsulinemia, inflammatory diseases, and autoimmune disorders should be identified and managed appropriately and ameliorated, if possible. Prior to the initiation of therapy with drugs known to cause alopecia, assessment of plasma iron and ferritin concentrations and thyroid function, identifying any family history of androgenetic alopecia, and detection of conditions associated with androgen excess, such as hirsutism, amenorrhea, or infertility may allow the clinician to identify and correct potential risk factors.[10,11,177] Methotrexate-induced alopecia may be prevented with folic acid supplementation.[74,92] There are a few reports that valproic acid-induced hair loss may be prevented with zinc and selenium supplementation, dose reduction, or both.[32,40,41,210] In general, maintaining patients' euthyroid status will aid in preventing antithyroid-induced alopecia.[210] The risk of postoperative alopecia may be reduced with frequent intraoperative and postoperative head repositioning.[199]

Patients with a family history of androgenetic alopecia are at high risk for androgenetic-induced alopecia associated with certain oral contraceptives. In these patients, selection of an oral contraceptive with little to no androgenic effects, such as norgestimate or ethynodiol diacetate, may reduce the risk of alopecia.[161,196] Prophylactic therapy with topical minoxidil can be prescribed when a patient with a family history of androgenetic alopecia requires long-term therapy with a medication known to induce androgenetic alopecia. Minoxidil is not effective for prevention of cancer chemotherapy-induced alopecia, but it will help reduce the severity and duration of the alopecia.[211,212]

Scalp cooling and hypothermia are of questionable efficacy for the prevention of cancer chemotherapy-induced alopecia, but it can possibly help the degree of chemotherapy-induced alopecia. Scalp cooling involves applying a cooling turban around the scalp with a tourniquet pressure ranging from 30 to 50 mm Hg above systolic blood pressure 10 minutes prior to drug administration, followed by removal 30 minutes after drug administration application. Hypothermia involves cooling the scalp to at least 24°C for 5 minutes before, during, and 20 minutes after the infusion of cancer chemotherapy.[6,52] Some investigators have raised concerns that, in some cases, these methods may be detrimental because of a possible reduction of delivery of chemotherapy drugs to intended areas, or when chemotherapy is being used for generalized hematogenic metastases or there is a high likelihood of metastasis to the scalp, such as in patients with breast cancer or lymphoproliferative disorders.[52,206] Liver dysfunction may also impair the potential efficacy of these preventive measures, as it inhibits the metabolism of some chemotherapy agents, thereby allowing drug concentrations to persist beyond the protective time frame of induced scalp hypothermia.[207,208,209]

A scalp cooling device, DigniCap, has been approved by the U.S. Food and Drug Administration (FDA) in the United States with the indication of decreasing the risk of chemotherapy-induced alopecia among women battling breast cancer. In a trial of more than 100 women with breast cancer, only 34% of those who used the cap lost over half their hair, compared to 100% in the control group. No serious adverse events were noted. The tight-fitting silicone cap has a coolant that circulates throughout the cap with a temperature that never goes below 32°F (0°C). The DigniCap is an important device as some women have opted out of chemotherapy due to the alopecia and with the prevention of hair loss in these patients may be a significant benefit to their quality of life. The FDA concluded from the studies that the risk of a decrease in chemotherapy delivery to an isolated grouping of the breast cancer cells in the scalp via the use of the cold cap is extremely rare.[213]

MANAGEMENT

DRUG THERAPY

Retinoid-induced alopecia is quickly reversible when the dose is decreased or vitamin A supplementation is discontinued. Hair regrowth occurs in approximately 2–3 months.[6,19] Dopamine-induced alopecia is reversible following discontinuation of therapy.[18,133] Chemotherapy-induced alopecia almost always resolves after discontinuation of therapy, and hair regrowth tends to occur rapidly. However, the texture and color of regrown hair may be different.[18] In rare cases associated with exposure to cancer chemotherapy over a long period, atrophy of the hair bulb may occur. However, most believe that this atrophy is always reversible after discontinuation of therapy with the causative agent.[19,129] In the case of lapatinib-induced alopecia, after a dose reduction, there was improvement.[89,123]

For patients with drug-induced telogen alopecia, hair growth returns when the causative agent is discontinued or the dose is decreased. Usually, additional treatment is not necessary.[18,186,202,209] When discontinuation of therapy or dose adjustment is not possible, a trial with topical minoxidil is recommended (**Table 9-8**).[1,6,8,10,11,13,52,173,193,203,206-209,211,213-221]

Use of minoxidil for the prevention and treatment of chemotherapy-induced alopecia does not prevent the onset of hair loss but has shortened the duration or reduced the severity of the hair loss.[212,222] In one study, minoxidil shortened the period of hair loss to regrowth from 137 to 50 days.[222]

Minoxidil can be used for the management of any type of drug-induced hair loss. The American Academy of Dermatology guidelines recommend minoxidil as first-line treatment for androgenetic alopecia in men or women.[223] Minoxidil is the only topical agent with proven efficacy for androgenetic

Table 9-8 Treatment Options for Drug-Induced Alopecia[1,6,8,10,11,13,52,173,193,203,206-209,211,213,215-221]

Treatment	Dose and Administration	Comments
TOPICAL TREATMENT		
Minoxidil	2% solution (men and women), apply twice daily 5% solution (men only), apply twice daily 5% foam (men only), apply twice daily	Solution: A dropper or extended-spray applicator must be used to apply the solution directly to the scalp Foam: Place a capful in hand and apply foam directly to the scalp; monitor for hypertrichosis and skin irritation; wait 4 hours before washing or swimming; after applying, do not allow scalp to become wet from the rain; should not be used in pregnant or nursing women
Anthralin cream (alopecia areata only)	0.1%, 0.25%, 0.5%, and 1% creams Apply once daily; start with 5-minute duration of therapy at a time and work up to as long as 1 hour After each application period, the scalp should be rinsed thoroughly with cool-to-lukewarm water and then cleansed with shampoo	New hair growth becomes apparent in 2–3 months Adverse effects include erythema, pruritus, scaling folliculitis, pyoderma, and regional lymphadenopathy Withholding treatment for a few days results in rapid resolution of adverse effects; treatment then can be restarted, but anthralin should be left on for shorter periods Staining of clothes and skin can occur
Topical steroids (alopecia areata only)	Twice daily application of an intermediate-potency corticosteroid solution or lotion to the entire scalp Commonly used agents: Fluocinolone acetonide cream 0.2% and betamethasone dipropionate cream 0.05%	Typically not as effective as intradermal steroid treatment Primarily used in combination therapy and not monotherapy Commonly used with corticosteroid injections, anthralin, or minoxidil Treatment duration is a minimum of 3 months before hair regrowth can be expected; maintenance therapy is often necessary

Table 9-8 Treatment Options for Drug-Induced Alopecia[1,6,8,10,11,13,52,173,193,203,206-209,211,213,215-221] (continued)

Treatment	Dose and Administration	Comments
INTRALESIONAL INJECTIONS		
Corticosteroids: triamcinolone acetonide (alopecia areata only)	Strength range: 2.5–10 mg/mL, but the 5-mg/mL concentration is the most often used; inject intralesionally in multiple sites 1 cm apart; inject 0.1 mL into each site; a maximum volume of 3 mL on the scalp in one visit is recommended Use 0.5-inch long, 30-gauge needle	Hair grown usually apparent in 4 weeks Treatment every 4–6 weeks as needed Adverse effects: local skin atrophy and telangiectasia, which can be minimized by specifically injecting into mid-dermis rather than into the more superficial epidermis or the subdermal fat Topical anesthetic may be applied 30–60 minutes before the treatment to alleviate injection pain
ORAL TREATMENT		
5α-reductase inhibitors	Finasteride: 1 mg orally once daily (male and female) Dutasteride: 0.5 mg orally once daily (male and female)	Benefits not evident for 4 months or longer May be combined with minoxidil For women: rule out pregnancy before use; if child-bearing age, use contraception
Corticosteroids: prednisone (alopecia areata only)	For extensive or rapidly spreading alopecia areata in adults >60 kg: 40 mg prednisone daily × 7 days; then taper slowly by 5 mg every few days × 6 weeks For less extensive alopecia areata: 20 mg prednisone daily or every other day followed by slow tapering in increments of 1 mg when hair loss is stable	Seldom used due to adverse effects Reserved for use with progressive alopecia areata Used in combination with topical or injected corticosteroid therapy as well as with topical minoxidil therapy
Cyproterone (for use in women only; not available in the United States)	50 mg orally daily OR 50–100 mg for 10 days/month if premenopausal	Rule out pregnancy before use; use contraception, if applicable May be used with minoxidil Monitor for dyslipidemias, weight gain, depression
Flutamide (for use in women only)	250–500 mg orally daily (doses of 250–375 mg may be less hepatotoxic)	Reserved for refractory disease due to potential for hepatotoxicity
Oral contraceptives (for use in women only)	Ethinyl estradiol + drospirenone Ethinyl estradiol + norgestimate Ethinyl estradiol + ethynodiol diacetate 1 tablet orally at bedtime (low-androgenic-activity progestin)	Efficacy studies are lacking Often combined with spironolactone
Spironolactone (for use in women only)	100–300 mg orally daily (often need ≥200 mg/day)	Rule out pregnancy before use; use contraception, if applicable May be used with minoxidil Monitor serum potassium concentrations, blood pressure, dizziness

Table 9-8 Treatment Options for Drug-Induced Alopecia[1,6,8,10,11,13,52,173,193,203,206-209,211,213,215-221] (continued)

Treatment	Dose and Administration	Comments
PRIOR TO CANCER CHEMOTHERAPY		
Scalp cooling	Involves applying a cooling turban around the scalp with tourniquet pressure ranging from 30 to 50 mm Hg above systolic blood pressure 10 minutes prior to drug administration and then removed 30 minutes after drug administration	These methods may be detrimental because of a possible reduction of distribution of chemotherapy to intended areas or when chemotherapy is being used for generalized hematogenic metastases or if there is a high likelihood of metastasis to the scalp such as in breast cancer or lymphoproliferative disorders
DigniCap (approved only for females with breast cancer)	The silicone cooling cap is fitted onto the head 30 minutes prior to chemotherapy; the cap is worn throughout the chemotherapy infusion and continued after therapy depending on the chemotherapy drug and dose; this postinfusion cooling time usually lasts 30–150 minutes; once postinfusion cooling is complete, the cap will be kept on the head for 15 minutes as the cap warms up to diminish any discomfort	FDA concluded minimal risk of reduced chemotherapy to intended areas when treating breast cancer The most common adverse effects of the cooling system include cold-induced headaches, chills, neck and shoulder discomfort, and pain associated with wearing the cooling cap for the required period of time DigniCap is not recommended for use in patients with hematological malignancies
Hypothermia therapy	Cool the scalp to at least 24°C for 5 minutes before, during, and 20 minutes after the infusion of chemotherapy	
AFTER CHEMOTHERAPY, IF SCARRING OCCURS		
	Topical steroids (Clobetasol topical solution) Acitretin 25 mg orally once daily Isotretinoin 15 mg orally twice daily	Skin dryness; erythema
COSMETIC OPTIONS		
Hairpiece, wig, hairstyling		Often used by patients faced with temporary or permanent alopecia
SURGICAL OPTIONS		
Hair transplantation	Cylindrical grafts Elliptical grafts Minigrafts and micrografts	Can be expensive For more extensive balding, more than one method is necessary
Scalp reduction Transposition flap Soft-tissue expansion		
MISCELLANEOUS OPTION		
Low-level laser therapy (LLLT)	655 nm wavelength Focus light for several minutes to each infected area	Relatively inexpensive No adverse effects; can be combined with other methods

FDA = U.S. Food and Drug Administration.

alopecia and is the only drug that is FDA-approved for hair loss for both men and women. The drug works by affecting the hair cycle, causing premature termination of the telogen phase, and may also prolong the anagen phase.[215] A 2% strength is available for both men and women and a 5% strength is approved only for men.[11,12] For women who do not respond to the 2% strength, the 5% strength can be used, as it has been shown to provide greater patient satisfaction in one study.[11] However, the incidence of hypertrichosis and scalp contact dermatitis were higher in association with the 5% strength as compared with the 2% strength.[11] Minoxidil solution or minoxidil foam should be applied twice daily to a dry scalp. If the solution is used, a dropper or extended-spray applicator must be used to apply the solution directly to the scalp.[173,196] A capful of the foam product should be applied directly to the scalp with the hands. Patients should be told that at least 4–6 months of treatment is necessary before the effects of minoxidil become evident, and maximum effects may not occur for approximately 1 year.[12,173] Adverse effects of tachycardia and hypotension are very rare (0.001%).[12]

Minoxidil treatment may be required indefinitely, unless therapy with the alopecia-inducing drug is discontinued. However, if minoxidil treatment is discontinued, some if not all of the regained hairs are shed within 3 months.[12,202] Minoxidil has been reported to cause scalp irritation, although the incidence is lower in association with the new foam product. In addition, the foam product contains much less propylene glycol, which is thought to be the cause of the contact dermatitis.[163]

Oral medications are also available for androgen-induced alopecia. However, these drugs have not been studied for the management of drug-induced alopecia. Finasteride and dutasteride exert their effects by inhibiting 5α-reductase type 2, which results in a decrease in plasma dihydrotesterone (DHT) concentrations. Finasteride reduces plasma prostate-specific antigen (PSA) concentrations and, thereby, could impair early detection of prostate cancer. Monitoring PSA concentrations prior to treatment and annually is recommended taking into account its effect when interpreting the results.[221] Finasteride has been on the market for years and has been widely used for the management of androgenetic alopecia in men, whereas dutasteride is relatively new for the treatment of androgenetic alopecia. Dutasteride 2.5 mg daily was found to be superior to finasteride 5 mg daily in increasing scalp hair growth in men.[221] The difference may be that finasteride inhibits only one isoenzyme of 5α-reductase, resulting in a 70% reduction of serum DHT concentrations, while dutasteride inhibits both type 1 and type 2 isoenzymes, reducing serum DHT concentrations by 94–95%.[224] Adverse sexual effects of finasteride and dutasteride such as erectile dysfunction, low libido, and infertility are uncommon and resolve spontaneously in most patients even without discontinuing therapy.[225]

Despite initial failures of finasteride for treatment of women with androgenetic alopecia, more recent data have demonstrated clinical efficacy. One case found that dutasteride 0.5 mg orally once daily provided clinical improvement, accompanied by an increase in mean hair diameter, reduction in variability of hair diameter, and normalization of trichogram results in a 46-year-old female.[224] Both finasteride and dutasteride are well tolerated by women.[224] Dutasteride may have the potential for efficacy in the management of androgenetic alopecia in women as well as men if large, long-term studies demonstrate efficacy.

Recently, topical formulations of finasteride and dutasteride (with and without topical minoxidil) have been used in men and women. Initial reports are promising; however, the necessary research to ensure efficacy and safety is lacking.[221]

For women, other oral antiandrogens that can be used to treat androgen-induced alopecia include spironolactone, cyproterone acetate (which is not available in the United States), and flutamide. However, flutamide is associated with hepatic toxicity and is rarely used.[10,11] Spironolactone, an aldosterone antagonist with antiandrogenic effects, is commonly used in women with androgenetic alopecia at doses of 100–300 mg daily.[13] In patients taking spironolactone, periodic serum potassium concentrations should be determined, as the drug can cause hyperkalemia. In an unblinded trial of 80 women taking spironolactone 200 mg daily or cyproterone acetate

50 mg daily (or 100 mg for 10 days/month in women who were premenopausal), 85% of women in both groups experienced no worsening of female pattern hair loss. If oral antiandrogens such as finasteride or spironolactone are prescribed to females of reproductive age, pregnancy should be excluded prior to use and oral contraceptive therapy or other methods of contraception should be prescribed concomitantly, as these agents are known teratogens.[11,13] Oral antiandrogens have been used alone or in combination with topical minoxidil in men and women.[10,12,226] Some trials in men have shown superior efficacy when minoxidil is combined with finasteride.[12]

Newer oral contraceptives with antiandrogenic effects such as ethinyl estradiol in combination with drospirenone, norgestimate, or ethynodiol are potential treatments for female alopecia.[227] Some premenopausal women taking antiandrogens are using these newer low-dose progesterone oral contraceptives to prevent pregnancy (because antiandrogens are teratogenic) while benefiting from their antiandrogenic effects. Unfortunately, topical and oral antiandrogens such as progestins and estrogens for the treatment of alopecia have not been studied in large trials, and the safety and efficacy of these agents are unknown. These drugs are not used in men because of the potential for sexual adverse effects.[26,161]

There are no supportive data for using oral estrogens, spironolactone, cyproterone acetate, or flutamide to treat or prevent drug-induced androgenetic alopecia in males; however, a case report involving a male-to-female transsexual person with severe male androgenetic alopecia reported flutamide to be effective in partial reversal of hair loss.[221]

The treatment of alopecia areata centers on anti-inflammatory and immunosuppressive therapy. These treatments commonly include corticosteroid injections, corticosteroid topical products, minoxidil, and anthralin. The choice of one agent over another depends on the extent of condition (localized versus extensive), and the patient's personal preference. If more than 50% of the scalp is involved, topical minoxidil plus either anthralin or topical steroid is typically used. Oral corticosteroids are also used at higher dose for 7 days followed by a taper over at least 6 weeks. Unfortunately, patients with alopecia totalis or alopecia universalis usually respond less well to treatment, and therapeutic failure occurs in most of these patients with any mode of management. If the hair loss involves less than 50% of the scalp, intralesional corticosteroid injections are usually prescribed first. Topical minoxidil, topical corticosteroid or oral prednisone can also be administered with the intralesional corticosteroid treatment or as monotherapy.[193,218,228]

Other less popular therapies with mixed reviews include psoralen and ultraviolet A phototherapy, topical immunotherapy, topical retinoids, bexarotene, sulfasalazine, methotrexate, and cyclosporine.[193,218,228] Psoralen and ultraviolet A phototherapy involve controlled exposure of the affected skin to ultraviolet light. The rate of response to this therapy is highly unpredictable (ranging from 15% to more than 70%). If treatment is successful, there is a relapse rate of 26%. Diphenylcyclopropenone is the drug of choice for topical immunotherapy, but it is associated with adverse effects of including cervical lymphadenopathy, a severe eczematous reaction, urticaria, and postinflammatory pigment changes. Topical retinoids such as topical tretinoin lack data from large, double-blind, placebo-controlled studies. In one study of topical retinoids, efficacy was only 55% compared to 70% with topical steroids. In a study of bexarotene gel, only 26% of patients experienced hair regrowth in at least 50% of treated sites. Sulfasalazine, methotrexate, and cyclosporine are all oral immunomodulatory and immunosuppressive drugs with potentially harmful adverse effects and require blood monitoring for white cell counts, serum creatinine and blood urea nitrogen, hematologic toxicity (methotrexate and sulfasalazine), hepatotoxicity (methotrexate and cyclosporine), and serum drug, lipid, potassium, and magnesium concentrations (cyclosporine).[218,228]

An experimental treatment option for various types of alopecia is platelet-rich plasma (PRP), which involves subcutaneous cap injections of autologous plasma with >1,000,000 platelets. PRP contains high concentrations of growth factors to potentially stimulate hair regrowth. PRP can be used in combination with other treatments, is inexpensive, and lacks significant adverse effects; however, thus far, its efficacy remains controversial.[221,229,230]

NONDRUG THERAPY

Cosmetic treatments are also available for addressing all types of drug-induced alopecia and are applicable to both men and women. Common cosmetic treatment options for temporary or permanent drug-induced alopecia include wigs, hair pieces, hair extensions, and hair weaves. There are also dyes available that can be sprayed or applied to the scalp that aid in camouflaging balding areas. Special hairstyling techniques also can be of benefit. These cosmetic measures often can produce satisfactory results.[10]

Surgical procedures are rarely needed for patients with drug-induced alopecia, but they are an option for patients with alopecia that is either permanent or severe or in situations in which therapy with the offending drug cannot be discontinued.[12,173] Hair transplantation or surgical hair restoration is popular with males with androgenetic alopecia. Robotic systems for harvesting hair follicles have been introduced that have improved this procedure. However, the efficacy of these systems has been disappointing for both sexes, due to a wide variation in results associated with different patient characteristics, surgical techniques, and skill levels of surgeons and teams. Another limitation is that these systems cannot arrest the progression of alopecia, which is a problem if the offending drug is continued.[191,221] Other surgical interventions include scalp reduction, transposition flap, and soft-tissue expansion procedures. Table 9-8 provides a list of the various treatment options for drug-induced alopecia.[1,6,8,10,11,13,52,173,193,203,206-209,211,213,215-221]

Low-level laser therapy is one of the newest nondrug treatments for alopecia. It has been studied for therapy of androgenetic alopecia but can be applied to alopecia areata and cancer chemotherapy-induced alopecia. Low-level laser therapy involves the use of low levels of red or near-infrared light, known as photobiomodulation or low-level laser therapy (LLLT), which is believed to work by inducing proliferative activity in the hair follicles resulting in terminalization of vellus hair follicles. There is some debate as to the optimal wavelength, but 655 nm is the wavelength used in clinical studies. LLLT is easy to use and resembles a hairbrush that one places on the head for a few minutes in the affected area while it emits the light therapy. LLLT is relatively inexpensive, can be used in both men and women, is associated with no known adverse effects, and can be easily obtained without a prescription. LLLT can be used both as monotherapy and in combination therapy, such as with topical minoxidil.[191,231]

INFORMATION FOR PATIENTS

Patients experiencing hair loss, whether permanent or temporary, should be informed that it is safe for them to style, blow dry, and tease the hair and use hair spray, hair color, and permanents. This helps patients deal with the cosmetic effects of alopecia.[193,196] Patients with alopecia often decrease the frequency of shampooing because they associate it with increased hair shedding. Patients should be educated regarding the hair growth cycle and should understand the cumulative nature of hair loss. With once-weekly shampooing, patients may experience 7 days' cumulative hair loss at one time, while daily shampooing allows a more realistic assessment of the actual daily hair loss and improves scalp health.[173,177]

If significant alopecia occurs, head coverings, wigs, and hairpieces should be encouraged, and patients should be assured that these cosmetic devices will not interfere with hair regrowth. Use of these cosmetic aids may improve patients' morale.[5] Patients also may benefit from use of a wide-toothed comb or soft-bristled brush and should be instructed to comb hair gently and to avoid excessive brushing, especially if undergoing cancer chemotherapy. Baby shampoo or a protein-enriched shampoo may be optimal in patients with alopecia, and use of a satin pillowcase will minimize friction. If alopecia is excessive, short hairstyles tend to disguise hair thinning, but enough length should be left to possibly allow for arrangement of hair to cover areas of baldness. If hair loss becomes pronounced, some patients prefer to shave the head, which may promote regrowth once the treatment is stopped. If a wig is worn, care should be taken to ensure that the lining is comfortable and not irritating. Applying baby oil, mineral oil, or ointment containing petrolatum and lanolin with some mineral oil and cod liver oil (which contain vitamins A and D) and massaging the scalp may reduce itching and keep the skin soft. Avoiding sun exposure helps protect the scalp.[74]

Patients should be educated regarding the risk of alopecia when a potentially causative agent is prescribed. Although patients find hair loss to be disturbing, alopecia is often tolerable, provided that wigs are available and advance warning regarding hair loss is provided.[74] Patients should also be informed that hair regrowth following chemotherapy may involve new hair that is coarse and has a color change. Hair also may be thinner than it was prior to therapy.[74,187] Patients should be counseled regarding proper nutrition, such as dietary protein intake, and should avoid fad or crash dieting while receiving medications with the potential to induce alopecia.[177]

Patients using topical minoxidil should be warned of its primary adverse effect, which is hypertrichosis or excessive hair growth. Hypertrichosis primarily occurs above the eyebrows, in the malar region, and on the lateral cheek area. Occasionally, hair growth is also noted above the lip and on the chin.[193] Some rare hair growth on the limbs has been noted in association with the 5% solution. Local adverse effects from irritation and contact dermatitis also have been reported with continued use.[202] Switching to the foam product may help minimize the risk of these adverse effects. Patients should be told that an increase in scalp hair shedding may occur during the first months of therapy as the follicles cycle from the telogen to the anagen phase. Patients should be informed that 4–6 months may be required before the effects of minoxidil become evident, and up to 1 year may be required for maximum effects.[12] Patients should be warned that if minoxidil treatment is discontinued and the alopecia-inducing agent is still present, hair loss will resume.[12,13,175] After each use of the topical solution, the hands should be washed to avoid applying solution on other parts of the body. Topical minoxidil should remain on the scalp for at least 4 hours before showering or shampooing.[12] When appropriate, it is important to assure patients that once the drug causing alopecia is discontinued, the alopecia tends to resolve.

Patients taking 5α-reductase inhibitor therapy may experience decreased libido or impotence rarely during therapy that resolves spontaneously in most patients even without discontinuing therapy.[225] To prevent pregnancy in a partner of child-bearing age, men should use barrier contraceptives (even though the risk is negligible) and women of child-bearing age should be told to use contraception, because these medications can lead to fetal abnormalities.[12,13,221] Women who are prescribed antiandrogenetic medications should be warned, if applicable, not to become pregnant as these medications are teratogenic.[11] Effects on libido and changes in menstrual patterns may occur. Because kidney function could be compromised, patients with severe heart failure should be instructed to have their serum potassium concentrations and kidney function measured at 3 days and 1 week after initiating therapy with spironolactone and with every increase in dose, then every 2–4 weeks for 3 months, then every 3 months for a year, then every 6 months thereafter. If serum creatinine is >4 mg/dL or serum potassium is >5 mEq/L, interrupt or discontinue therapy. Spironolactone should be avoided in patients with kidney disease or conditions associated with hyperkalemia.[21]

HIRSUTISM AND HYPERTRICHOSIS

Both hirsutism and hypertrichosis are patterns of excessive hair growth that may be highly distressing to patients. Hirsutism occurs only in women and involves excessive growth of hair with masculine characteristics or "male-like" pattern of hair growth on the body and face, usually as a result of excessive androgenic stimulation. The effects of androgens on the hair follicles differ based on the body site. Androgen excess can lead to suppression of growth of scalp hair as excess androgens cause androgen-sensitive hair follicles to shorten during the anagen phase, resulting in miniaturization of the scalp hair, less scalp coverage, and alopecia. Conversely, androgen excess can cause hair growth in women in a pattern consistent with androgen-sensitive areas such as the face, axilla, pubis, chest, buttocks, lower back, abdomen, inner thighs, and shoulders. This is primarily due to increased sensitivity of the pilosebaceous units to androgens. Androgen excess can also cause acne and menstrual irregularities.[216,232-234]

In contrast, hypertrichosis is excessive hair growth that is independent of androgen influence. Hypertrichosis describes hair growth on any part of the body that is in excess of the amount that is usually present in persons of the same race, sex, and age. The hair growth is manifested by the uniform and superfluous growth of vellus (nonterminal) hair over the body, particularly in nonsexual areas. Unlike hirsutism, hypertrichosis can occur in both men and women. Drug-induced hirsutism can be induced by androgenic drugs, while drug-induced hypertrichosis usually is not associated with androgen production.[1,6,161,235,236]

CAUSATIVE AGENTS

HIRSUTISM

Drug-induced hirsutism is caused by androgenic agents such as danazol, testosterone, adrenocorticotropic hormones, and glucocorticoids (**Table 9-9**).[6,18,19,23,25,177,198,201,203,217,235-242] Hirsutism has been reported in 0.1% of women taking oral contraceptives. Hair growth has been reported on the face and is most likely caused by the progestin component. It may take some time for the hair growth to resolve following discontinuation. Hormone-replacement therapies containing moderate-to-high amounts of progestin are more likely to induce hirsutism.[177,235]

Valproic acid was shown in one prospective longitudinal trial in Indian women to increase serum testosterone concentrations and lead to polycystic ovary syndrome (POS). The incidence of hirsutism associated with valproic acid was 20%.[217,241] It is debatable as to whether phenytoin, high dose glucocorticoids, and acetazolamide induce hirsutism versus hypertrichosis; these drugs are reported in the literature to cause hirsutism or hypertrichosis via an unknown mechanism.[6,18,19,201,217,236,239,240] Cyclosporine and minoxidil are often listed in the nondermatological literature as causes of hirsutism (technically drug-induced hypertrichosis as this hair growth is independent of androgen influence).[217,242]

HYPERTRICHOSIS

Drugs associated with hypertrichosis are listed in **Table 9-10**.[6,18,19,21,201,217,235,238,243-269] The primary drugs known to cause hypertrichosis are cyclosporine, phenytoin, and oral and topical minoxidil. Other agents reported to induce hypertrichosis include diazoxide, erythropoietin, penicillamine, and psoralens.[18,235] Ophthalmic prostaglandin analogs have been well documented to cause hypertrichosis.[261] Drug-induced hyperprolactinemia can induce unwanted hair growth.[270]

Cyclosporine-induced hypertrichosis usually occurs within the first 3 months of therapy, generally peaks at about 6 months and is dose dependent.[260] Patients taking cyclosporine for prevention of rejection following organ transplantation at doses as high as 6 mg/kg/day are at higher risk (30–60%) for hypertrichosis versus only a 3% risk when taking lower doses (<5 mg/kg/day) for dermatological diseases.[6,201,271,272] Children and adolescents are at higher risk of developing moderate-to-severe hypertrichosis associated with cyclosporine than adults. Children experience excessive hair growth on the scalp, arms, legs, upper lip, parotid area of the face, eyebrows, ear lobes, nose, and back of neck. In addition, adults experience increase in body hair. The condition is reversible upon discontinuation of therapy, but it may take months for complete resolution.[260]

Long-term phenytoin therapy has been well documented as a cause of hypertrichosis (**Figure 9-3**), which typically occurs approximately 2–3 months after the initiation of therapy.[19] The limbs and sometimes the face and trunk are the most commonly affected areas. Hypertrichosis is reversible upon discontinuation of the drug. Dose reduction, when possible, may attenuate abnormal hair growth.[246]

Both oral and topical minoxidil cause hypertrichosis that primarily affects the malar areas, forehead, and sides of the face. Facial hypertrichosis is believed to be due to a systemic effect or via the transfer of the drug from the hands.[13] Hypertrichosis may disappear after approximately 1 year, even

Table 9-9 Agents Implicated in Drug-Induced Hirsutism[6,18,19,24,25,177,198,201,203,217,235-242]

Drug	Incidence	Level of Evidence[a]
Acetazolamide[236,c]	NK	C
Betamethasone[6,19,c]	NK	C
Carbamazepine[18,201,237]	NK	C
Cortisone[6,19,c]	1–10%	C
Corticotropin (adrenocorticotropic hormone)[6,18,19,201,238]	NK	C
Danazol[6,18,201,239]	NK	A
Dehydroepiandrosterone (DHEA)[216,240,217]	NK	C
Dexamethasone[6,19,c]	NK	C
Fludrocortisone[6,19,c]	NK	C
Fluoxymesterone[18,177,201,203,235]	NK[b]	C
Hydrocortisone[6,19,c]	NK	C
Methylprednisolone[6,19,c]	NK	C
Methyltestosterone[18,177,201,203,235]	NK	C
Metoclopramide[198]	NK	C
Metyrapone[201]	NK	C
Nandrolone[6,18,201]	NK	C
Oral contraceptives/hormones with androgenic activity[18,177,201,217,235]	NK[b]	C
Oxandrolone[18,177,201,203,235]	NK	C
Oxymetholone[6,18,201]	NK	C
Phenytoin[19]	NK	C
Prednisolone[6,19,c]	NK	C
Progesterone[6,19,24,201]	NK	C
Stanozolol[6,18,201]	NK	C
Testolactone[18,25,177,201,203,235]	NK	C
Testosterone[18,177,201,203,235]	NK	C
Triamcinolone[6,19,c]	NK	C
Valproic acid[217,241]	NK	C

NK = not known.

[a]Definitions for Levels of Evidence: Level A—evidence from one or more randomized, controlled clinical trials; Level B—evidence from nonrandomized clinical trials, prospective observational studies, cohort studies, retrospective studies, case-control studies, meta-analyses and/or postmarketing surveillance studies; and Level C—evidence from one or more published case reports or case series.

[b]Believed to be common in susceptible women.

[c]It is debated as to whether acetazolamide, glucocorticoids, and phenytoin cause hirsutism versus hypertrichosis.

if the medication is continued, and usually resolves in 1–6 months if minoxidil application is discontinued.[193] Diazoxide can also lead to hypertrichosis that is often observed within a few weeks of initiating therapy and is more severe on the face and limbs. Diazoxide-induced hypertrichosis is reversible, but resolution can take as long as 2 years.[6,241] Erythropoietin, when used in patients with chronic kidney disease, can induce hypertrichosis. Erythropoietin-induced hypertrichosis is reversible upon discontinuation of therapy.[6]

Vaccines have been reported to cause hypertrichosis. This may be due to a rare hypersensitivity reaction to aluminum-containing antigen solutions and the aluminum hydroxide in the vaccines. Affected areas often develop nodules with hyperpigmentation, hypopigmentation, hypertrichosis, and lichenification.[273]

Table 9-10 Agents Implicated in Drug-Induced Hypertrichosis[6,18,19,21,201,217,235,238,243-269]

Drug	Incidence	Level of Evidence[a]
ANTIHYPERTENSIVES		
β-blockers[18,201]	NK	C
Diltiazem[6,18]	NK	C
Minoxidil[243,244]	80% (oral)[245,246] 22–46% (topical)[247]	A
Nifedipine[18,201]	NK	C
Verapamil[6,18,201]	NK	C
ANTICONVULSANTS		
Phenytoin[6,18,248,249,250, 251,252,253]	8.5–12%	A
ANTIVIRAL AGENTS		
Acyclovir[254]	NK	C
Zidovudine[6,18,201,238]	NK	C
CHELATING AGENT		
Penicillamine[6,18,19,235]	NK	C
CANCER CHEMOTHERAPY AGENTS		
Cetuximab[21,255,256]	1–10%	C
Erlotinib[257] (eyelash trichomegaly; hypertrichosis)	1–10%	C
Everolimus[21]	1–10%	C
Sorafenib[258]	NK	C
Tacrolimus[21]	<15%	C
CORTICOSTEROIDS[259,b]		
Budesonide[18,201,217,235,238]	NK	C
Betamethasone[18,201,217,235]	NK	C
Cortisone[18,201,217,235]	NK	C
Dexamethasone[18,201,217,235]	NK	C
Fludrocortisone[18,201,217,235]	NK	C
Hydrocortisone[18,201,217,235]	NK	C
Methylprednisolone[18,201,217,235]	NK	C
Prednisone[18,201,217,235]	NK	C
Prednisolone[18,201,217,235]	NK	C
Triamcinolone[18,201,217,235]	NK	C
ERYTHROPOIESIS-STIMULATING AGENTS		
Erythropoietin[6,18]	NK	C
IMMUNOSUPPRESSANTS		
Cyclosporine[6,201,260]	30–60% with organ transplantation doses such as 6 mg/kg/day 3% with doses <5 mg/kg/day	A A
INTERFERONS[c]		
Interferon alfa-N3[235]	NK	C
Interferon alfacon-1[235]	NK	C
Interferon alfa-2a, recombinant[235]	NK	C

Table 9-10 Agents Implicated in Drug-Induced Hypertrichosis[6,18,19,21,201,217,235,238,243-269] (continued)

Drug	Incidence	Level of Evidence[a]
Interferon alfa-2b[235]	NK	C
Peginterferon alfa-2a and alfa-2b[235]	NK	C
NONSTEROIDAL ANTI-INFLAMMATORY DRUGS		
Benoxaprofen[6,18]	NK	C
OPHTHALMIC AGENTS WITH PROSTAGLANDIN ANALOGS[c]		
Latanoprost[18,235,261,262]	Up to 77%	C
Bimatoprost[18, 235,261,262]	Up to 77%	C
Travoprost[18,235,261,262]	Up to 77%	C
PRENATAL EXPOSURE		
Alcohol abuse[249]	NK	C
Hydantoin[249]	NK	C
Minoxidil[249]	NK	C
PSYCHIATRIC DRUGS		
Aripiprazole[21]	<1%	C
Citalopram[263]	NK	C
Phenothiazines[6,18,201]	NK	C
Trazodone[21]	<1%	C
RETINOIDS		
Tretinoin (retinoic acid)[6,18,201]	NK	C
VACCINES		
Bacillus Calmette-Guerin (BCV) vaccination[264]	NK	C
Diphtheria-pertussis-tetanus[265,266]	NK	C
Measles[265,267]	NK	C
Smallpox[265,268]	NK	C
MISCELLANEOUS DRUGS		
Diazoxide[18,19,269]	>1%	C
Polidocanol[21]	NK	C
Psoralens[6,18,238]	NK	C
Streptomycin[6,18,238]	NK	C

NK = not known.
[a]Definitions for Levels of Evidence: Level A—evidence from one or more randomized, controlled clinical trials; Level B—evidence from nonrandomized clinical trials, prospective observational studies, cohort studies, retrospective studies, case-control studies, meta-analyses and/or postmarketing surveillance studies; and Level C—evidence from one or more published case reports or case series.
[b]Hypertrichosis reported in children using inhaled corticosteroids.
[c]Eyelash trichomegaly.

Ophthalmic agents used to treat glaucoma that contain prostaglandin F analogs such as latanoprost, bimatoprost, and travoprost can induce trichomegaly of the eyelashes and can also darken the eyelashes. In one case report, latanoprost promoted the regrowth of eyelashes in a patient suffering eyelash loss due to alopecia.[261]

EPIDEMIOLOGY

The overall incidences of drug-induced hirsutism and hypertrichosis are unknown. The incidences of hirsutism and hypertrichosis associated with specific drugs, where known, are presented in Table 9-9 and Table 9-10.[6,18,19,21,23,25,177,198,201,203,217,235-269]

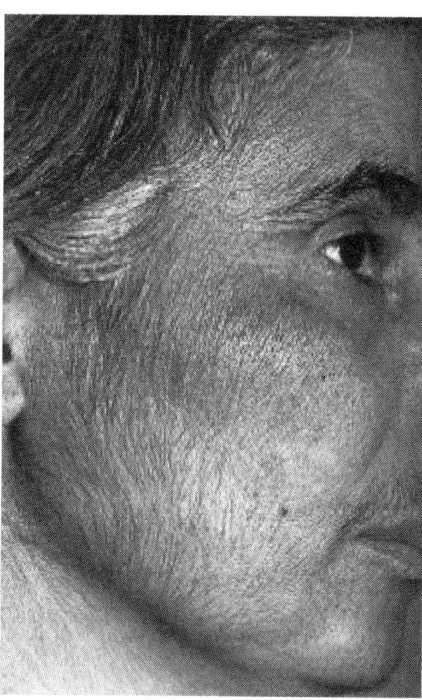

FIGURE 9-3 Hypertrichosis Caused by Phenytoin[19]

Source: Reproduced with permission from Bork K, ed. *Cutaneous side effects of drugs*. Philadelphia, PA: Saunders; Copyright©1988:249-58.

Although neither drug-induced disease is considered to occur commonly, these are well-recognized complications associated with drugs such as anabolic steroids, cyclosporine, and minoxidil.[241] When minoxidil is taken orally for at least 1 month, over 80% of patients experience reversible hypertrichosis.[6] Topical minoxidil has been reported to cause hypertrichosis in 3–5% of women using the 2% solution and in more than 5% of those using the 5% solution.[245,247] Erythropoietin has been reported to cause hypertrichosis in 13% of patients with chronic kidney disease. With the lower cyclosporine doses used in the treatment of dermatologic diseases, the risk of hypertrichosis declines to approximately 3%.[6] The incidence of drug-induced hypertrichosis associated with diazoxide in children treated for idiopathic hypoglycemia is nearly 100%. Two investigators reported incidences of hypertrichosis of 2% and 6% in children receiving phenytoin. Another study found that 35% of children experienced hair growth; however, this report included cases in which only moderate hypertrichosis occurred.[274] Hirsutism is known to affect 5–15% of women, but drugs are not a frequent cause.[216] Drug-induced hypertrichosis appears to be less common than hirsutism except in the treatment of organ transplantation with cyclosporine therapy, during which drug-induced hirsutism is manifested in 30–60% of patients.

MECHANISMS

HIRSUTISM

Terminal hair (coarse, longer, pigmented hair) is found primarily on the scalp and eyebrows. Vellus hair is the short fine, unpigmented hair found in all other areas. As androgen concentrations increase during puberty, the vellus hair of androgen-sensitive follicles is converted to terminal hair. Exposure to exogenous androgens such as testosterone can also cause vellus hair to be converted to terminal hair resulting in drug-induced hirsutism (**Table 9-11**).[18,19,177,201,216,217,235-239,242,275-277] Nondrug-related hirsutism is commonly associated with hormonal abnormalities associated with POS. Hirsutism involving virilization, especially in women over 25 years of age, is commonly associated with an androgen-producing tumor. Drug-induced androgenic stimulation of hair follicles is a less common cause of hirsutism.[33,58,278-281] Hyperinsulinemia can also lead to hirsutism via inhibition of aromatase, the enzyme that converts testosterone to estrogen. Valproic acid can cause hirsutism by provoking hyperinsulinemia.[278]

HYPERTRICHOSIS

Although mechanisms of hypertrichosis are not well understood, it is, by definition, not associated with androgen excess or exposure to androgenic agents. The disorder is not common and describes an increase in nonsexual hair. Hypertrichosis may be congenital (e.g., Hurler syndrome, fetal alcohol syndrome, or trisomy 18 syndrome), or associated with anorexia nervosa, malnutrition, hypothyroidism, porphyria, epidermolysis bullosa, dermatomyositis, or following skin trauma. It also can be caused by drugs that stimulate hair growth.[241,270,274] Hair growth induced by erythropoietin may be caused by a decrease in plasma cortisol concentrations. At higher serum concentrations, cortisol has

Table 9-11 Mechanisms of Drug-Induced Hirsutism and Hypertrichosis[18,19,177,201,216,217,235-239,242,275-277]

HIRSUTISM DRUGS	Mechanism
Acetazolamide[236]	Androgenic activity
Androgens/anabolic steroids[18,177,216,217,235,239,275,276]	Androgenic activity
Carbamazepine[18,201,237]	Androgenic activity
Contraceptives/hormones with androgenic activity[18,177,216,217,235,239,275,276]	Androgenic activity
Corticosteroids[18,201,217,235]	Androgenic activity
Corticotropin (adrenocorticotropic hormone)[18,19,238]	Androgenic activity
Metoclopramide[216]	Androgenic activity
Phenytoin[19]	Androgenic activity
Valproic acid[216,217,242,277]	Androgenic activity
HYPERTRICHOSIS DRUGS	
All offending agents	Stimulates hair growth[a]

[a]Mechanism is unknown.

been shown to inhibit follicular activity. Many antipsychotic agents are known to cause hyperprolactinemia, which can indirectly cause hypertrichosis. The mechanism of cyclosporine-induced hypertrichosis is unknown and appears to be independent of androgens as the hair grows in nonandrogen dependent sites and no other androgen effects are present like virilization. Pre- and postcyclosporine treatment studies showed no significant difference in testosterone, DHEA, and hydroxyprogesterone concentrations. Cyclosporine may exert its effect on skin structures as it is highly lipophilic and accumulates in the skin.[241] The proposed mechanism of diazoxide-induced hypertrichosis involves altered cutaneous blood flow leading to changes in hair growth.[241]

Several underlying pathologic conditions are associated with acquired generalized hypertrichosis, such as human immunodeficiency virus-infection (HIV) and acquired immunodeficiency syndrome (AIDS). Patients with HIV or AIDS can experience eyelash trichomegaly or a generalized form of hypertrichosis. The pathogenesis remains unknown but may be multifactorial, associated with malnutrition, metabolic changes, and immunologic dysregulation, such as elevated serum interferon concentrations. In addition, drugs such as interferon and zidovudine may contribute to hypertrichosis.[235]

Hypertrichosis can appear after a head injury or other cerebral disturbances. Hypertrichosis was originally attributed to phenytoin therapy administered following head injury, but hypertrichosis has also occurred in patients with head injury who have not received phenytoin. Malnutrition and anorexia nervosa may, in rare instances, lead to hypertrichosis. Excessive hair growth of the limbs and trunks has been recorded in children with celiac disease as well as in young women on low-carbohydrate diets.[282] These acquired conditions as well as conditions such as juvenile hypothyroidism and malignancy are rare causes of hypertrichosis, and the mechanism is not fully understood.

CLINICAL PRESENTATION AND DIFFERENTIAL DIAGNOSIS

HIRSUTISM

Signs and symptoms associated with drug-induced hirsutism and hypertrichosis are listed in **Table 9-12**.[216,217,235] Women with drug-induced hirsutism present with excessive hair growth in a somewhat masculine pattern, such as the appearance of coarse facial hair in the upper lip or chin area. The chest, lower abdomen, back, and limbs also may be affected.[283] Patients with hirsutism often present with other dermatologic symptoms of virilization, such as acne, androgenetic alopecia,

Table 9-12 Signs and Symptoms Associated with Drug-Induced Hirsutism and Hypertrichosis[216,217,235]

Hirsutism

- The development of larger, curlier, and darker hair in a male pattern; examples of sexual hair: mustache, beard, inner thighs, chest, back, buttocks area, and/or abdomen found on women
- Ferriman–Gallwey score[a]: score of 8 or higher

May be associated with

- Elevated serum testosterone concentration; the normal upper limit for total plasma testosterone concentrations in women is 70–90 ng/dL
- Insulin resistance
- A total plasma testosterone concentration that is normal or marginally elevated (within approximately 20 ng/dL of the upper limits of normal) in the absence of other features of concern (polycystic ovary syndrome, risk of neoplasm, risk of endocrinopathy, thyroid dysfunction, metabolic syndrome) probably indicates idiopathic hirsutism or idiopathic hyperandrogenism
- Pelvic ultrasonogram: polycystic ovaries or neoplasm
- Menstrual irregularities
- Metabolic syndrome (central obesity, hypertension, glucose abnormalities, and dyslipidemias)

Hypertrichosis

- Hair growth is distributed in a generalized, nonsexual pattern on men or women; the hair involved may be vellus, lanugo, or terminal hair
- Hair growth normally involves face, limbs (front and back), eyelashes, elbows, pinnae auris, elbows, anterior or posterior neck, lumbosacral region or trunk
- Ferriman–Gallwey scale[a]: score of <8
- No elevation in free testosterone concentrations following start of hypertrichosis-inducing agent
- No laboratory test evaluation required

[a]See Figure 9-4 for the Ferriman–Gallwey scoring system for hirsutism.[216,217]

and seborrhea oleosa.[6] A physical examination typically facilitates differentiation between hirsutism and hypertrichosis. The Ferriman–Gallwey scoring system for hirsutism (**Figure 9-4**), which evaluates hair growth in nine body areas, can be helpful.[216,217,284] The nine body areas that are androgen-sensitive are graded from 0 (no terminal hair) to 4 (frankly virile) to obtain a total score. A normal score is less than 8.[216,217,274,284] A careful medication history should be obtained, and patients should be questioned regarding the onset and progression of hair growth, family history of similar disorders, exposure to skin irritants, menstrual and reproductive history, presence of hair loss, acne, and any changes in extremity or head size, facial contour, or weight.[33,216,217,274]

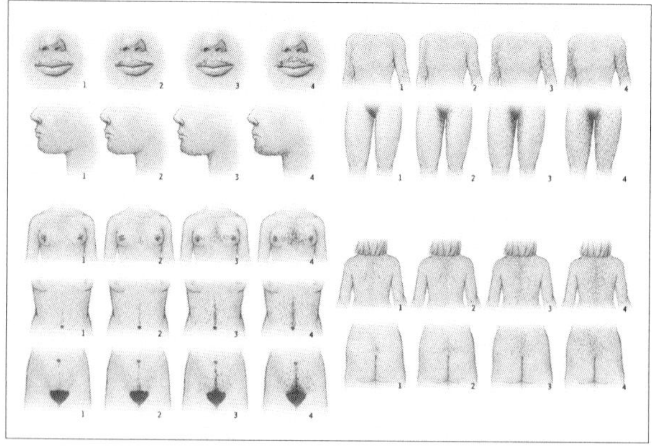

FIGURE 9-4 The Ferriman–Gallwey Scoring System for Hirsutism[216,217]

Source: Rosenfield RL. Hirsutism. *N Engl J Med.* 2005; 353:2578-88. Copyright© Massachusetts Medical Society. Reprinted with permission from Massachusetts Medical Society.

During evaluation of hirsutism, it is important to rule out nondrug causes such as POS, ovarian tumor, adrenal tumor, hyperprolactinemia, congenital adrenal hyperplasia, Cushing syndrome, diabetes, and thyroid disease.[33,216,217,274,285] In particular, in women with epilepsy who present with hirsutism, POS should be excluded. POS is characterized by hyperinsulinemia due to insulin resistance, which promotes androgen production. Women with epilepsy have a higher incidence of POS and higher plasma androgen concentrations,

Table 9-13 Conditions to Consider in the Differential Diagnosis of Drug-Induced Hirsutism and Hypertrichosis[177,241,285,286]

- Adrenal tumor
- Congenital adrenal hyperplasia
- Cushing syndrome
- Diabetes
- Familial
- Hyperprolactinemia
- Idiopathic
- Insulin resistance
- Ovarian tumor
- Polycystic ovary syndrome
- Thyroid disease

which medications may further exacerbate. Laboratory evaluations for patients with hirsutism should include measurement of serum total and unbound testosterone, DHEA, DHEA sulfate (DHEA-S), follicle-stimulating hormone, luteinizing hormone, and prolactin concentrations. An ovarian tumor is considered when the total serum testosterone concentration is >200 ng/dL in the presence of a mildly elevated DHEA-S concentration.[177] For drug-induced hirsutism, the history of hair growth is very important in determining whether androgenic drugs have been used because most androgenic drugs are not detected by testosterone assays except for valproic acid, which increases plasma testosterone concentrations.[217] Drug-induced hirsutism should be suspected in female patients with hair growth exhibiting masculine characteristics who have been exposed to drugs known to have androgenic effects. Conditions to consider in the differential diagnosis of drug-induced hirsutism and hypertrichosis are listed in **Table 9-13.**[177,241,285,286] In addition, specific diagnostic tests that can be used to differentiate drug-induced hirsutism from other causes of hirsutism are listed in **Table 9-14.**[270,274]

HYPERTRICHOSIS

In patients with hypertrichosis, the excessive hair growth involves terminal and/or vellus hair and a

Table 9-14 Clinical and Diagnostic Evaluation of Hirsutism[245,248,270-274]

Diagnosis	Abnormal Laboratory Values		Other Tests
Drugs/familial/idiopathic	Laboratory values are within normal limits		
Congenital adrenal hyperplasia	Cortisol	Low to normal	ACTH stimulation test can be helpful for diagnosis
	DHEA-S	High to normal	
	Testosterone	High to normal	
	17-α-hydroxyprogesterone	High	
Polycystic ovary syndrome	Follicle-stimulating hormone	Low to normal	Insulin, glucose, and lipid concentrations
	Luteinizing hormone prolactin	Normal to high	
	Testosterone	Normal to high	
Tumors • Adrenal tumor • Ovarian • Pituitary	Cortisol	High	Imaging[a]
	DHEA-S	Normal to high	
	Testosterone	High	Imaging[a]
	Testosterone	High	Imaging[a]
	Prolactin	High	

ACTH = adrenocorticotropic hormone, DHEA-S = dehydroepiandrosterone sulfate.

[a]Plasma prolactin concentrations may be high if drug-induced (e.g., risperidone) hyperprolactinemia is present. May need venous catheterization to help identify a tumor when imaging is negative in the face of strong clinical suspicion.

nonmale pattern of hair growth is noted on areas of the body where the hair is normally short. Hypertrichosis may be generalized or circumscribed and is independent of hormone stimulation.[6] Examples of hypertrichosis in a male patient include hair in the forehead area or coarser, prominent hair on one area of the shoulder or forearm.[283] Drug-induced hypertrichosis should be suspected in male or female patients who exhibit abnormal growth of nonsexual hair (nonandrogen-dependent hair) and who are taking potentially causative drugs that are not associated with increased androgenic activity.[217,240,241] Drug-induced hypertrichosis usually becomes apparent within a few weeks to a few months following initiation of therapy.[6,19,235,287] Diazoxide induces hair growth within a few weeks after initiation of treatment.[6] Phenytoin-induced hypertrichosis may not appear until after 2–3 months of therapy.[287] Topical minoxidil induces hair growth after approximately 4 months of therapy, whereas systemic minoxidil causes hypertrichosis within a few weeks of treatment initiation.[6,235] Hypertrichosis induced by cyclosporine may become evident within the first month of therapy, but symptoms generally worsen over the first 6 months of therapy before remaining constant.[241] After the offending drug is stopped, hypertrichosis resolves within several months to 1 year depending on the hair cycling characteristics of the affected site (i.e., if face is involved, resolution generally occurs within 3 months; resolution of hypertrichosis involving the arms requires approximately 1 year).[235]

RISK FACTORS

Women who are already at risk for hirsutism from other causes, such as menopause, pregnancy, excessive ovarian androgen production, family history of hirsutism, and those of Mediterranean origin may be at greater risk of hirsutism or experience more pronounced hirsutism when exposed to medications with androgenic effects.[276,282,283,285] Risk factors for drug-induced hirsutism are summarized in **Table 9-15**.[177,216,235,270,283,286]

Table 9-15 Risk Factors for Drug-Induced Hirsutism[177,216,235,270,283,286]

- Female sex
- Drug administration
  - Higher doses
  - Intravenous route
  - Longer duration of exposure
- Combination of two or more drugs that can cause hair growth
- Cushing syndrome, hyperprolactinemia, acromegaly, thyroid dysfunction, and tumors
- Drug interactions that lead to increased serum concentrations of drug that cause hirsutism
- Endocrine abnormalities, such as insulin resistance
- Female patients already at risk for hirsutism
- Genetic predisposition
- Hormonal abnormalities, such as menstrual irregularity, endometrial cancer, polycystic ovary syndrome, infertility
- Metabolic abnormalities, such as metabolic syndrome often involving central obesity, hypertension, glucose abnormalities, and dyslipidemia

Drug dose and duration of therapy can be risk factors for drug-induced hirsutism and hypertrichosis, as some drugs induce hair growth only at higher doses and following long-term exposure. For instance, the risk of hypertrichosis associated with cyclosporine is lower in patients taking smaller doses for the management of dermatologic diseases compared with patients taking higher doses for other indications.[6] The addition of tretinoin solution to topical minoxidil therapy leads to increased absorption of minoxidil and an associated increased risk of hypertrichosis.[288] Children and adolescents appear to be at greater risk for cyclosporine–induced hypertrichosis than adults.[241]

In prepubertal children, hypertrichosis is typically not associated with an underlying endocrine disorder but is commonly an adverse effect of drug administration.[289] Concomitant administration of two or more drugs known to cause abnormal hair growth increases the risk, as do drug interactions that lead to increased serum concentration of a hirsutism-provoking drug. Increased serum concentrations of drugs that induce hypertrichosis usually increase the risk; however, psoralen-induced hypertrichosis appears not to be dose-related.[241,274] **Table 9-16** summarizes risk factors for drug-induced hypertrichosis.[18,235,241,283]

Table 9-16 Risk Factors for Drug-Induced Hypertrichosis[6,235,241,283]

- Drug administration
  - Higher doses
  - Intravenous route
  - Longer duration of exposure
- Combination of two or more drugs that can cause hair growth
- Drug interactions that lead to increased serum concentrations of drug that cause hypertrichosis
- Acquired immunodeficiency syndrome
- Anorexia nervosa
- Familial trait or congenital
- Head injuries and other cerebral disturbances
- Hepatic porphyria caused by chemical exposure such as hexachlorobenzene
- Juvenile dermatomyositis
- Juvenile hypothyroidism
- Malignancy
- Malnutrition

Table 9-17 Approaches to Help Prevent Drug-Induced Hirsutism and Hypertrichosis[18,235,241,274,283]

- Avoid drugs with potential to induce hirsutism or hypertrichosis when possible
- Use the lowest possible dose of the potentially causative agent
- Avoid, when possible, the use of multiple drugs with the potential to cause hirsutism or hypertrichosis
- Limit the duration of exposure
- Use the oral route rather than the intravenous route whenever possible
- Avoid drug interactions that could increase serum concentrations of drugs with the potential to cause dose-dependent hirsutism or hypertrichosis; adjust appropriately doses of renally-eliminated or hepatically-metabolized drugs with the potential to cause hirsutism or hypertrichosis in patients with kidney or liver disease, respectively
- Identify any family history of androgenetic alopecia, hirsutism, amenorrhea, or infertility prior to initiating therapy with medications known to cause hirsutism or hypertrichosis to allow the clinician to identify and correct potential risk factors

MORBIDITY AND MORTALITY

Drug-induced hirsutism and hypertrichosis, while often unpleasant, are not associated with increased morbidity or mortality.

PREVENTION

Drug-induced hair growth is best prevented by avoiding the use of agents known to cause hirsutism or hypertrichosis, especially in patients with pre-existing risk factors. Patients should not be exposed to two or more drugs with a known potential to cause abnormal hair growth unless absolutely necessary. Lower doses and shorter periods of exposure to potentially causative drugs are also advised.[6] Using a contraceptive medication with a lower progestin content may be of benefit in reducing the risk of hirsuitism.[19] The potential for minoxidil-associated hypertrichosis is increased if the topical solution is accidentally transferred to the face from the hands or from residual minoxidil on pillows, bed sheets, and garments. Topical minoxidil also may be distributed via local intravascularization, but this is not normally preventable.[193,283,287] Avoiding drug interactions that lead to increased serum concentrations of drugs that cause hirsutism or hypertrichosis is also important, especially if the hirsutism or hypertrichosis is dose-dependent. **Table 9-17** provides some approaches to help prevent drug-induced hirsutism and hypertrichosis.[18,235,241,274,283]

MANAGEMENT

HIRSUTISM

Medications for managing hirsutism include those that inhibit androgen action at the hair follicles and suppress androgen production. Response to these medications is very slow, and desired effects may not be evident for 6 months or more; consequently, hair removal techniques may also be warranted. Clinical management of drug-induced hirsutism includes discontinuing the causative agent, if possible, administering topical pharmacological treatment, using cosmetic procedures for hair removal, using light sources and lasers for hair removal, and administering oral systemic drug therapy (oral contraceptives, antiandrogens, 5α-reductase inhibitors).[235]

A detailed list of the topical and nonpharmacologic procedures for the treatment of both hirsutism and hypertrichosis is provided in **Table 9-18**.[216,235,244,290] Systemic agents used for the treatment of hirsutism are listed in **Table 9-19**.[161,186,211,216]

If the offending medication can be discontinued, then no treatment is needed if the excess hair growth is mild. Discontinuation of therapy with some drugs (e.g., cortisol) usually leads to resolution of hirsutism.[29] However, drug-induced hirsutism is not always reversible, and resolution, when it does occur, may require longer than 6 months after discontinuation of therapy. In this case, if the hair growth is moderate to severe, or if the patient cannot tolerate even mild hirsutism, short-term use of cosmetic procedures, topical

Table 9-18 Cosmetic Measures for Management of Hypertrichosis and Hirsutism[216,235,244,290]

Cosmetic Measure	Information
Bleaching	Commercial products contain persulfate to boost peroxide bleach but can lead to anaphylaxis Home product: 40 mL hydrogen peroxide + 7 mL 20% ammonia Apply to hair and leave on hair until the color is removed (average time is 5–10 minutes) Duration of effect: Up to 4 weeks Disadvantages: Does not work well for dark-skinned patients; skin irritation
Chemical depilatories	Chemicals that damage the hair leading to breakage at the skin's surface Thioglycolates are commonly used in concentrations of 2–4% and act within 5–15 minutes Duration of effect: ~1 week Disadvantage: Potent skin irritant; not for use in children unless for small localized sites to avoid toxicity from systemic thioglycolate absorption Adverse effects: Skin irritation, allergic contact dermatitis, and, with inadvertent eye contact, corneal alkali burns
Electrosurgical epilation	Three types of electrolysis: Galvanic electrolysis; thermolysis electrolysis; blend method of electrolysis (considered the most effective) Considered a permanent mode of hair removal Target: Localized coarse hair Duration of effect: Hair regrows in 20–40% of the follicles treated Disadvantage: Expensive, painful, requires multiple treatment sessions and is time-consuming Adverse effects: Hyperpigmentation or hypopigmentation, perifollicular inflammation, punctate scarring
Light source and laser treatments	Several effective systems available: Ruby laser, alexandrite laser, diode laser, neodymium:yttrium-aluminum-garnet (Nd:YAG) laser, and intense pulsed-light sources (590–1,200 nm) Longer pulse durations and longer wavelength lasers such as the Nd:YAG laser should be used on dark skin to lessen risk of scarring or dyspigmentation; these lasers are less efficacious but involve less risk to skin; pulsed diode lasers are generally more reliable and less expensive than other laser sources for hair removal; Q-switch YAG lasers are optimal for darker skinned patients; however, they are ineffective for permanent hair removal Duration of effect: Permanent hair removal often occurs primarily in patients with dark hair after multiple treatments, although hyperpigmentation is a risk Patients with blonde, red, or white hair may not have permanent hair removal, but the regrowing hairs are thinner and more lightly pigmented Disadvantages: Cost and rare adverse reaction of thermal damage-related cutaneous side effects (blistering, crusting, scabbing, pigmentary alteration, scarring); if occurs, this usually requires treatment with topical corticosteroid or topic antibiotic Adverse effects: Pain/discomfort (icing treated areas postprocedure is helpful); immediate perifollicular edema and mild erythema, which lasts ~minutes to hours following treatment
Plucking	Appropriate for targeting only small areas, as it is painful, slow, and tedious Duration of effect: Up to 2 weeks Adverse effects: Hyperpigmentation; folliculitis, distorted hair follicles, scarring Risk of metaplastic ossification

Table 9-18 Cosmetic Measures for Management of Hypertrichosis and Hirsutism[216,235,244,290] (continued)

Cosmetic Measure	Information
Shaving	Does not affect the rate or width of regrowth; it will, however, result in stubble that grows out without the softer and finer unshaven hair tip Duration of effect: 24 hours Disadvantages: Requires daily shaving; skin irritation
Topical hair growth retardant (cell-cycle inhibitor)	Eflornithine hydrochloride, 13.9%; topical cream applied twice daily; slows excessive hair growth but does not remove excessive hair; noticeable results take about 6–8 weeks; patients must also use hair removal methods Clinical trials have shown efficacy for facial hirsutism improvement Target: Facial areas of unwanted hair growth Contraindications: Pregnancy, breastfeeding Disadvantages: Expensive; hair grows back after discontinuation; must use hair-removal techniques Adverse effects: Burning, stinging, acne, rash may occur at application site
Trimming	Does not accelerate hair regrowth Good option for young children with either local or generalized hypertrichosis Duration of effect: ~24 hours or longer Disadvantage: Hypertrichosis may still be noticeable
Waxing	Cold, warm, or hot wax is applied to the area of unwanted hairs; then the wax is stripped off, thus epilating the embedded hairs Target: Any vellus hairs in all areas of the body Duration of effect: 2–6 weeks Disadvantage: Poor results when attempting removal of short hair Adverse effects: Pain, skin irritation, folliculitis

pharmacologic treatment for hair removal, or both may be desirable.

If the causative agent cannot be discontinued, a variety of treatment options exist. Nonsystemic drug treatment is appropriate for mild hirsutism. For patients with moderate-to-severe hirsutism or those with mild hirsutism who desire more aggressive treatment, systemic therapy should be considered along with nonpharmacologic and topical treatments. Weight loss in overweight women can decrease serum concentrations of androgens and lessen hirsutism.[270]

Measures include bleaching, wax stripping, shaving, plucking (tweezing), using hair-removal creams (depilatories), and electrolysis. The FDA has approved electrolysis as an option for permanent hair removal, because it has been associated with a 30% reduction in the number of hair follicles. Laser therapy is a newer development, and several types are available, including the ruby, alexandrite, pulsed diode, and Q-switched yttrium-aluminum-garnet (YAG) lasers. Pulsed-diode lasers are often more reliable and less expensive than other laser sources for hair removal. Q-switched YAG lasers work best for darker-skinned patients with dark hair. Unfortunately, laser therapy is not always effective for long-term hair removal. After a single laser treatment, hair growth is delayed for 2–6 months, and hair removal is permanent in some patients after multiple treatments. The cost of these approaches is sometimes an issue, because most patients require repeated treatments.[216,270,280]

Oral contraceptives containing lower amounts of androgenic progestins (e.g., norgestimate desogestrel, ethynodiol diacetate, gestodene, and norethindrone acetate) are preferable for the management of mild to moderate hirsutism. This treatment should reduce the need for shaving by 50% and can usually arrest the progression of hirsutism but will not reverse it.[216] Women with clinically significant hirsutism may require therapy with an androgen-inhibiting agent either as monotherapy or in addition to oral contraceptive treatment.[216,219,222,227] The addition of the oral contraceptive ensures menstrual cycling and minimizes the risk of pregnancy, as antiandrogens and α_2-reductase inhibitors are teratogenic.[216] It has been

Table 9-19 Common Medications Used for Treatment of Hirsutism[21,161,186,211,216,217]

Type of Therapy	Agent	Dose	Contraindications/ Precautions	Major Adverse Effects
Androgen inhibition	Spironolactone	50–100 mg orally twice daily (300 mg daily for pronounced hirsutism or for obese patients)	Lack of contraception, kidney disease, liver failure	Teratogenic; irregular menstrual bleeding unless oral contraceptive administered; decreased libido; nausea; hyperkalemia; hypotension; liver dysfunction
	Cyproterone (not available in the United States)	Induction: 50–100 mg orally at bedtime, days 5–15 of the menstrual cycle Maintenance: 5 mg orally at bedtime, days 5–15	Lack of contraception	Teratogenic; irregular menstrual bleeding unless estrogen administered cyclically; decreased libido; nausea
	Flutamide	125–250 mg orally twice daily	Lack of contraception; liver disease	Teratogenic; reserved for severe hirsutism because of hepatotoxicity
Androgen suppression	Ethinyl estradiol + drospirenone OR ethinyl estradiol + norgestimate OR ethinyl estradiol + ethynodiol diacetate (all low androgenic activity)	1 tablet orally at bedtime (higher estrogen doses may be necessary in heavier women for menstrual regularity)	Breast cancer, smoking, history of thrombosis, cardiovascular disease, uncontrolled hypertension	Irregular vaginal bleeding, venous thrombosis, bloating
5α-reductase inhibitors	Finasteride	1–5 mg orally daily	Lack of contraception	Teratogenic; minimal adverse effects in females
	Dutasteride	0.5–2.5 mg orally daily	Lack of contraception	Teratogenic; limited data on dutasteride use in hirsutism; minimal adverse effects in females
Other hormones	Glucocorticoids	Example: prednisone 5–7.5 mg orally at bedtime	Uncontrolled diabetes; obesity	Changes typical of Cushing syndrome; adrenal atrophy
	Gonadotropin-releasing agonists	Leuprolide acetate, depot suspension 7.5 mg monthly intramuscularly, with 25–50 mcg transdermal estradiol	Osteoporosis	Osteoporosis without estrogen-progestin replacement

reported that combined therapy with an oral contraceptive and an androgen-receptor inhibitor may produce clinical improvement in up to 75% of women with hirsutism.[270]

Antiandrogenic drugs include spironolactone, flutamine, and cyproterone. Spironolactone and flutamine are the most widely used and are equally effective. Spironolactone is an aldosterone antagonist and appears to be the safest androgen-receptor inhibitor. Flutamide may cause hepatotoxicity, and liver function should be monitored in patients receiving this agent. Cyproterone is not available in the United States. Therapy with spironolactone or cyproterone often provides significant attenuation of hirsutism within 6 months and maximum benefit within 9–12 months.[216]

Other hormonal therapies include finasteride, a 5α-reductase inhibitor that has been shown to be effective for the treatment of hirsutism. However, finasteride is teratogenic, causing feminization in male infants exposed to finasteride during the first trimester; therefore, while not contraindicated in women of childbearing potential, finasteride is recommended only for women who are postmenopausal with no chance of becoming pregnant. If used in premenopausal women, measures must be implemented to prevent pregnancy. Finasteride is usually reserved for severe or refractory cases of hirsutism. Once initiated, treatment should be continued for at least 2 years for maximum benefit.[270,279] Combination therapy with finasteride and spironolactone demonstrated additive reduction in hirsutism scores.[286,291]

Dutasteride, also a 5α-reductase inhibitor, has not been extensively studied for the management of hirsutism. Other hormonal therapies include glucocorticoids and gonadotropin-releasing hormone agonists. The efficacy of glucocorticoids for drug-induced hirsutism is unknown. Gonadotropin-releasing hormone agonists are considered alternatives to oral contraceptives.[216]

Treatment with eflornithine, a topical hair growth inhibitor, has been shown to reduce rates of hair growth. Eflornithine therapy results in the reduction of the frequency of use of other methods of hair removal. Eflornithine is indicated for facial hirsutism and is marketed as an 11.5% topical cream that is applied twice daily. The cream is effective for slowing excessive hair growth but not for removing excess hair. The cream must remain on the skin for at least 4 hours. Unfortunately, if therapy is discontinued, hair growth will likely return.[177,235,282]

HYPERTRICHOSIS

Although drug-induced hypertrichosis nearly always resolves after discontinuation of therapy with the causative agent, reversal of hair growth takes time. During that period, cosmetic methods for hair removal are suggested and are effective (Table 9-18).[235,274,280] Consequently, the management of drug-induced hypertrichosis includes discontinuation of therapy with the offending agent, if possible, as well as nonsystemic approaches including cosmetic procedures for removal of excess hair; hair removal using light sources and lasers; and topical pharmacologic treatment.[235] Systemic therapy with agents such as antiandrogens or oral contraceptives should not be used. Treatment with eflornithine may be effective for hypertrichosis. See Table 9-19 for details on eflornithine.[161,186,211,216]

Cosmetic measures for the treatment of hirsutism include bleaching, wax stripping, shaving, plucking (tweezing), using hair-removal creams (depilatories), electrolysis and laser therapy. A discussion of these measures is provided in Table 9-18.[216,235,244,290]

INFORMATION FOR PATIENTS

Patients should have realistic expectations regarding the time frame for resolution of drug-induced hirsutism and hypertrichosis, and must understand that it may take a long time for these conditions to resolve even after therapy with the causative agent is discontinued. When certain medications are used to treat hirsutism, hormonal suppression for several months or longer may be necessary before reduction of hair growth becomes evident.[216,217,282] When oral drug therapy is used to manage hirsutism, patients should be instructed that treatment must continue during therapy with the causative agent. For patients with drug-induced hypertrichosis, when the offending drug is discontinued, resolution of excess hair growth may require several months to 1 year, depending on the hair-cycling characteristics of the site of hypertrichosis. For example, it takes an average of 3 months for hypertrichosis resolution if the excess hair growth is on the face but an average of 1 year if the excessive hair growth is on the arms.[235]

Patients with drug-induced hirsutism or hypertrichosis should be counseled regarding the potential benefit of cosmetic measures, and these can be encouraged even if oral therapy is prescribed. Patients should be informed of the cosmetic options available, their adverse effects, duration, effectiveness, and cost. Inform patients that although shaving can lead to a stubble-like hair, it does not worsen hirsutism. Depilating agents, though effective, can cause chronic skin irritation and may even worsen hair growth if used excessively or indiscriminately. Waxing or plucking in androgenized skin may lead to folliculitis and trauma to the hair shaft, and does not kill the hair follicles. Methods that can permanently destroy the hair follicle, such as electrolysis and laser, often work well, but require time to be effective. These methods may also be costly and usually require repeated treatments.[216,217,280]

REFERENCES

1. Bergfeld WF. Hair disorders. In: Moschella SL, Hurley HJ, eds. *Dermatology.* Vol 1. Philadelphia: Saunders; 1992:1541-60.
2. Levantine A, Almeyda J. Drug induced alopecia. *Br J Dermatol.* 1973; 89:549-53.
3. Warnock JK. Psychotropic medication and drug-related alopecia. *Psychosomatics.* 991; 32:149-52.
4. Nielsen TA, Reichel M. Alopecia: diagnosis and management. *Am Fam Physician.* 1995; 51:1513-22.
5. Maguire HC Jr. Drug-induced alopecia. *Am Fam Physician.* 1979; 19:178-9.
6. Tosti A, Misciali C, Piraccini BM et al. Drug-induced hair loss and hair growth: incidence, management, and avoidance. *Drug Saf.* 1994; 10:310-7.
7. Ramos PM, Miot HA. Female pattern hair loss: a clinical and pathophysiological review. *An Bras Dermatol.* 2015; 90:529-43.
8. Ellis JA, Sinclair R, Harrap SB. Androgenetic alopecia: pathogenesis and potential for therapy. *Expert Rev Mol Med.* 2002; 4:1-11.
9. Mercke Y, Sheng H, Khan T et al. Hair loss in psychopharmacology. *Ann of Clin Psych.* 2000; 12:35-42.
10. Springer K, Brown M, Stulbuerg DL. Common hair loss disorders. *Am Fam Physician.* 2003; 68:93-102.
11. Shapiro J. Hair loss in women. *N Engl J Med.* 2007; 357:1620-30.
12. Otberg N, Finner AM, Shapiro J. Androgenic alopecia. *Endocrinol Metab Clin North Am.* 2007; 36:379-98.
13. O'Mara NB. Treatment of androgenic alopecia in women. *Pharmacist's Letter.* 2003; 19:1-3.
14. Beccastrini E, Squatrito D, Emmilabel G et al. Alopecia areata universalis during off-label treatment with Infliximab in a patientwith Behcet disease. *Dermatol Online J.* 2010; 16:15.
15. Mulinari-Brenner F, Bergfeld WF. Hair loss: an overview. *Dermatol Nursing.* 2001; 13:269-72.
16. Lazzarini R, Capareli GC, Buense R et al. Alopecia universalis during treatment with leflunomide and adalimumab-case report. *An Bras Dermatol.* 2014; 89:320-2.
17. Lindsey SF, Tosti A. Hair loss induced by tumor necrose factor alpha inhibitors. *J Clin Investigat Dermatol.* 2013; 1:1-6.
18. Tosti A, Pazzaglia M. Drug reactions affecting hair: diagnosis. *Dermatol Clin.* 2007; 25:223-31.
19. Bork K, ed. *Cutaneous side effects of drugs.* Philadelphia: Saunders; 1988:249-58.
20. Hall J, ed. *Sauer's manual of skin diseases.* 8th ed. Philadelphia: Lippincott Williams and Wilkins; 2000.
21. Lexicomp. Home page. https://online.lexi.com/lco/action/home (accessed 2017 Nov 15).
22. Hosea SW, Santaella ML, Brown EJ et al. Long-term therapy of hereditary angioedema with danazol. *Ann Intern Med.* 1980; 93:809-12.
23. Wiebke A. Androgen therapy in women. *Eur J Endocrinol.* 2006; 154:1-11.
24. Progesterone [package insert]. Corona, California: Watson Laboratories; 2005.
25. Teslac [package insert]. Princeton, New Jersey: Bristol-Myers Squibb; 2004.
26. Allen J. Drug-induced hair loss. *Pharmacist's Letter.* 1999; 17:1-3.
27. Jafari-Fesharaki M, Scheinman MM. Adverse effects of amiodarone. *PACE.* 1998; 21:108-20.
28. Watra MM, Patel JP, Arya R. Traditional anticoagulants and hair loss: a role for direct oral anticoagulants. *Drugs-Real World Outcomes.* 2016; 3:1.
29. Rook A. Endocrine influences on hair growth. *BMJ.* 1965; 1:609-14.
30. Spencer LV, Callen JP. Hair loss in systemic disease. *Dermatol Clin.* 1987; 5:565-70.
31. Criscitiello M, Levine H. Thromboembolism and prosthetic heart valves. *Hosp Pract.* 1992:69-96.
32. Gautam M. Alopecia due to psychotropic medications. *Ann Pharmacother.* 1999; 33:631-7.
33. Herranz JL, Armijo JA, Arteaga R. Clinical side effects of phenobarbital, primidone, phenytoin, carbamazepine, and valproate during monotherapy in children. *Epilepsia.* 1988; 29:794-804.
34. Neurontin [package insert]. New York: Pfizer; 2007.
35. Keppra [package insert]. Smyrna, GA: UCB Group; 2008.
36. Lyrica [package insert]. New York: Pfizer; 2007.
37. Chuang YC, Chang WN, Chen IL et al. Topiramate-induced hair loss: case report. *Dermatol Psychosom.* 2002; 3:183-4.
38. Topiramate [package insert]. Princeton, NJ: Zydus Pharmaceuticals; 2009.
39. Gupta AK. "Perming" effects associated with chronic valproate therapy. *Br J Clin Pract.* 1988; 42:75-7.
40. Pinder Rm, Brogden RN, Speight TM et al. Sodium valproate: a review of its pharmacological properties and therapeutic efficacy in epilepsy. *Drugs.* 1977; 13:81-123.
41. Rimmer EM, Richens A. An update on sodium valproate. *Pharmacotherapy.* 1985; 5:171-84.
42. Depakote [package insert]. North Chicago, IL: Abbott Laboratories; 2006.
43. Malani AN, Kerr L, Obear J et al. Alopecia and nail changes associated with voriconazole therapy. *CID.* 2014; 59:e61-5.
44. Reyataz [package insert]. Princeton, New Jersey: Bristol-Myers Squibb; 2009.
45. Videx [package insert]. Princeton, New Jersey: Bristol-Myers Squibb Company; 2007.
46. Valtrex [package insert]. Greenville, NC: GlaxoSmithKline; 2007.
47. Coreg [package insert]. Research Triangle Park, North Carolina: GlaxoSmithKline; 2008.
48. England JRF, England GOF. Alopecia and propranolol therapy. *Aust Fam Physician.* 1982; 11:225-6.
49. Belum VR, Marulanda K, Ensslin C et al. Alopecia in patients treated with molecularly targeted anticancer therapies. *Ann Oncol.* 2015; 26:2496-502.
50. Hansen LA, Hughes TE. Altretamine. *DICP.* 1991; 25:146-52.
51. Hexalen [package insert]. Bloomington, Minnesota: MGI Pharma; 2003.
52. Wyatt AJ, Leonard GD, Sachs DL. Cutaneous reactions to chemotherapy and their management. *Am J Clin Dermatol.* 2006; 7:45-63.
53. Tosti A, Piraccini BM, Vincenzi C et al. Permanent alopecia after busulfan chemotherapy. *Br J Dermatol.* 2005 ;152:1056-8.
54. Lynch TJ Jr, Kim ES, Eaby B et al. Epidermal growth factor receptor inhibitor-associated cutaneous toxicities: an evolving paradigm in clinical management. *Oncologist.* 2007; 12:610-21.
55. Botchkarev VA. Molecular mechanisms of chemotherapy-induced hair loss. *JID Symposium Proceedings.* 2003; 8:72-5.
56. Hubbard SM. Chemotherapy-induced alopecia. *Clin Oncol.* 1985; 387-457.

57. Hussein AM. Chemotherapy-induced alopecia. New developments. *Southern Med J.* 1993; 489-96.
58. Lee A, Thomson J. Drug-induced skin reactions. In: Lee A. *Adverse drug reactions.* London: Pharmaceutical Press; 2002:19-43.
59. Sprycel [package insert]. Princeton, New Jersey: Bristol-Myers Squibb Company; 2008.
60. Elis A, Blickstein D, Manor Y et al. Association between alopecia and response to chemotherapy in patients with Hodgkin lymphoma. *Ther Drug Monit.* 2005; 27:287-9.
61. Francis PA, Rigas JR, Kris MG et al. Phase II trial of docetaxel in patients with stage II and IV non-small cell lung cancer. *J Clin Oncol.* 1994; 12:1232-7.
62. Extra JM, Rousseau F, Bruno R et al. Phase I and pharmacokinetic study of taxotere (RP56976; NSC 628503) given as a short intravenous infusion. *Cancer Res.* 1993; 53:1037-42.
63. Taxotere [package insert]. Bridgewater, NJ: Sanofi-Aventis; 2008.
64. Bajetta E, Colleoni M, Rosso R et al. Prospective randomised trial comparing fluorouracil versus doxifluridine for the treatment of advanced colorectal cancer. *Eur J. Cancer.* 1993; 29A:1658-63.
65. Forbes C, Shirran L, Bagnall AM. A rapid and systematic review of the clinical effectiveness and cost-effectiveness of topotecan for ovarian cancer. *Health Technol Assess.* 2001; 5:1-110.
66. Katsumata N, Fujiwara Y, Kamura T. Phase II clinical trial of pegylated liposomal doxorubicin (JNS2002) in Japanese patients with mullerian carcinoma (epithelial ovarian carcinoma, primary carcinoma of fallopian tube, peritoneal carcinoma) having a therapeutic history of platinum-based chemotherapy: a phase II study of the Japanese gynecologic oncology group. *Jpn J Clin Oncol.* 2008; 38:777-85.
67. Vandenberg TA, Pritchard KI, Eisenhauer EA et al. Phase II study of weekly edatrexate as first-line chemotherapy for metastatic breast cancer: a National Cancer Institute of Canada Clinical Trials Group study. *J Clin Oncol.* 1993; 1241-4.
68. Shaw E, Scott C, Suh J et al. RSR13 plus cranial radiation therapy in patients with brain metastases: comparison with the radiation therapy oncology group recursive partitioning analysis brain metastases database. *J Clin Oncol.* 2003; 21:2364-71.
69. Cersosimo RJ, Hong WK. Epirubicin: a review of pharmacology, clinical activity, and adverse effects of an adriamycin analogue. *J Clin Oncol.* 1986; 4:425-39.
70. Tan AR, Rubin EH, Walton DC et al. Phase 1 study of eribulin mesylate administered once every 21 days in patients with advanced solid tumors. *Clin Cancer Res.* 2009; 15:4213-9.
71. Tarceva [package insert]. Melville, New York: OSI Pharmaceuticals; 2008.
72. Hepper DM, Wu P, Anadkat MJ. Scarring alopecia associated with the epidermal growth factor receptor inhibitor erlotinib. [Letter to Editor]. *J Am Acad Dermatol.* 2011; 64:996-8.
73. Emcyt [package insert]. New York: Pharmacia and Upjohn Company; 2007.
74. Batchelor D. Hair and cancer chemotherapy: consequences and nursing care—a literature review. *Eur J Cancer Care.* 2001; 10:147-63.
75. Etopophos [package insert]. Princeton, New Jersey: Bristol-Myers Squibb Company; 2005.
76. Aromasin [package insert]. Kalamazoo, Michigan: Pharmacia and Upjohn Company; 2003.
77. Aromasin [package insert]. New York: Pharmacia and Upjohn Company; 2008.
78. Ray-Coquard I, Cesne AL, Whelan JS et al. A phase II study of Gefitinib for patients with advanced HER-1 expresing synovial sarcoma refractory to doxorubicin-containing regimens. *Oncologist.* 2008; 13:467-73.
79. Donovan JC, Ghazarian DM, Shaw JC. Scarring alopecia associated with the use of epidermal growth factor inhibitor getitinib. *Arch Dermatol.* 2008; 144:1524-5.
80. Gemzar [package insert]. Indianapolis, IN: Eli Lilly and Company; 2007.
81. Tonato M, Mosconi AM, Martin C. Safety profile of gemcitabine. *Anticancer Drugs.* 1995; 6:27-32.
82. Clegg A, Scott DA, Sidhu M et al. A rapid and systematic review of the clinical effectiveness and cost-effectiveness of paclitaxel, docetaxel, gemcitabine, and vinorelbine in non-cell lung cancer. *Health Technol Assess.* 2001; 5:1-195.
83. Akaza H, Naito S, Usami M et al. Efficacy and safety of gemcitabine monotherapy in patients with transitional cell carcinoma after cisplatin-containing therapy: a Japanese experience. *Jpn J Clin Oncol.* 2007; 37:201-6.
84. Idarubicin [package insert]. New York: Pharmacia and Upjohn; 2006.
85. Shimada Y, Yoshino M, Wakui A et al. Phase II study of CPT-11, a new camptothecin derivative, in metastatic colorectal cancer. *J Clin Oncol.* 1993; 11:909-13.
86. Raymond E, Fabbro M, Boige V et al. Multicentre phase II study and pharmacokinetic analysis of irinotecan in chemotherpy-naïve pateints with glioblastoma. *Ann Oncol.* 2003; 14:603-14.
87. Conlin AK, Vahdat L. Dermatological toxicity of ixabepilone. *Anticancer Res.* 2006; 26:2279-80.
88. Goodin S. Ixabepilone: a novel microtubule-stabilizing agent for the treatment of metastatic breast cancer. *Am J Health-Syst Pharm.* 2008; 65:2017-26.
89. Ena P, Fadda GM, Ena L et al. Tufted hair folliculitis in a woman treated with lapatinib for breast cancer. *Clin Exp Dermatol.* 2008; 33:776-94.
90. Simpson D, Curran MP, Perry CM. Letrozole: a review of its use in postmenopausal women with breast CA. *Drugs.* 2004; 64:1213-30.
91. Fiebig HH, Henss H, von Pawell et al. Phase II clinical trial of lobaplatin (D-19466) in pretreated patients with small-cell lung cancer. *Onkologie.* 1996; 19:328-32.
92. Nyfors A. Benefits and adverse drug experiences during long-term methotrexate treatment of 248 psoriatics. *Dan Med Bull.* 1978; 25:208-11.
93. Methotrexate for Injection [package insert]. Paramus, New Jersey: Mayne Pharma (USA); 2005.
94. Methotrexate [package insert]. Liberty Corner, New Jersey: Intas Pharmaceteuticals; 2007.
95. Hande KR, Oldham RK, Fer MF et al. Randomized study of high-dose versus low-dose methotrexate in the treatment of extensive small cell lung cancer. *Am J Med.* 1982; 73:413-9.
96. Mitamycin [package insert]. Princeton, New Jersey: Bristol-Myers Squibb Company; 2000.
97. Smith IE. Mitoxantrone (novantrone): a review of experimental and early clinical studies. *Cancer Treat Rev.* 1983; 10:103-15.
98. Kantarijian H, Giles F, Wunderle L et al. Nilotinib in imatinib-resistant CML and Philadelphia chromosome-positive ALL. *N Engl J Med.* 2006; 354:2542-51.
99. Park YH, Ryoo B, Choi S et al. A phase II study of paclitaxel plus cisplatin chemotherapy in an unfavourable group of patients with cancer of unknown primary site. *Jpn J Clin Oncol.* 2004; 34:681-5.
100. Rowinsky EK, Cazenave LA, Donehower RC. Taxol: a novel investigational antimicrobule agent. *J Natl Cancer Inst.* 1990; 82:1247-59.
101. Taxol [package insert]. Princeton, NJ: Bristol-Myers Squibb; 2007.
102. Alimta [package insert]. Indianapolis, IN: Eli Lilly and Company; 2008.
103. Samonigg H, Kaskparek AK, Stoger H et al. 4'-O-tetrahydropyranyl-docorubicin in advanced breast cancer. A phase II study. *Cancer Chemother Pharmacol.* 1990; 26:293-6.
104. Scheithauer W, Samonigg H, Depisch D et al. Pirarubicin (4'-O-tetrahydropyranyl-adriamycin) for the treatment of advanced breast cancer. *Invest New Drugs.* 1990; 8:207-10.
105. Spielmann M, Kerbrat P, Delozier T et al. Pirarubicin in advanced breast cancer: a French cooperative phase II study. *Eur J Cancer.* 1990; 26:821-3.

106. McKeage K, Wagstaff AJ. Sorafenib in advanced renal cancer. *Drugs.* 2007; 67:475-83.

107. Llovet JM, Ricci S, Mazzaferro V et al. Sorafenib in advanced hepatocellular carcinoma. *N Engl J Med.* 2008; 359:378-90.

108. Eisen T, Ahmad T, Flaherty KT et al. Sorafenib in advanced melanoma: a phase II randomised discontinuation trial analysis. *Br J Cancer.* 2006; 95:581-6.

109. Lee WJ, Lee JL, Chang SE et al. Cutaneous adverse effects in patients treated with the multitargeted kinase inhibitors sorafenib and sunitinib. *Br J Dermatol.* 2009; 1045-51.

110. Faivre S, Delbaldo C, Vera K et al. Safety, pharmacokinetic, and antitumor activity of SU11248, a novel oral multitarget tyrosine kinase inhibitor, in patients with cancer. *J Clin Oncol.* 2006; 24:25-35.

111. Sutent [package insert]. New York: Pfizer Labs; 2008.

112. Fisher B, Costantino JP, Wickerham DL et al. Tamoxifen for Prevention of Breast Cancer: Current Status of the National Surgical Adjuvant Breast and Bowel Project P-1 Study. *J Natl Cancer Inst.* 2005; 97:1652-62.

113. Ayoub J, Audet-Lapointe P, Methot Y et al. Efficacy of sequential cyclical hormonal therapy in endometrial cancer and its correlation with steroid receptor status. *Gynecol Oncol.* 1988; 31:327-37.

114. Trudeau ME, Crump M, Charpentier D et al. Temozolomide in metastatic breast cancer (MBC): a phase II trial of the National Cancer Institute of Canada—clinical trials group (NCIC-CTG). *Ann Oncol.* 2006; 17:952-6.

115. Bleehen NM, Newlands ES, Lee SM et al. Cancer research campaign phase II trial of temozolomide in metastatic melanoma. *J Clin Oncol.* 1995; 13:910-3.

116. Vumon [package insert]. Princeton, New Jersey: Bristol-Myers Squibb Company; 2009.

117. van Warmerdam LJC, Verweij J, Schellens JHM et al. Pharmacokinetics and pharmacodynamics of topotecan administered daily for 5 days every 3 weeks. *Cancer Chemother Pharmacol.* 1995; 35:237-45.

118. Perez-Soler R, Fossella FV, Glisson BS et al. Phase II study of topotecan in patients with advanced non-small-cell lung cancer previously untreated with chemotherapy. *J Clin Oncol.* 1996; 14:503-13.

119. Creemers GJ, Wanders J, Gamucci T et al. Topotecan in colorectal cancer: a phase II study of the EORTC early clinical trials group. *Ann Oncol.* 1995; 6:844-6.

120. Treat J, Huang cH, Lane SR. Topotecan in the treatment of relapsed small cell lung cancer patients with poor performance status. *Oncologist.* 2004; 9:173-81.

121. Hycamptin for Injection [package insert]. Research Triangle, North Carolina: GlaxoSmithKline; 2007.

122. Hycamptin capsules [package insert]. Research Triangle, North Carolina: GlaxoSmithKline; 2007.

123. Rosman HS, Anadkat MJ. Tufted hair follicutis in a woman treated with trastuzumab. *Target Oncol.* 2010; 5:295-6.

124. Cersosimo RJ, Bromer R, Licciardello JTW et al. Pharmacology, clinical efficacy and adverse effects of vindesine sulfate, a new vinca alkaloid. *Pharmcotherapy.* 1983; 3:259-74.

125. Smith IE, Hedley DW, Powles TJ et al. Vindesine: a phase II study in the treatment of breast carcinoma, malignant melanoma, and other tumors. *Cancer Treat Rep.* 1978; 62:1427-33.

126. Marty M, Extra JM, Dieras V et al. A review of the antitumour activity of vinorelbine in breast cancer. *Drugs.* 1992; 44:29-35.

127. Depierre A, Lemarie E, Dabouis G et al. A phase II study of navelbine (vinorelbine) in the treatment of non-small-cell lung cancer. *Am J Clin Oncol.* 1991; 14:115-9.

128. Canobbio L, Boccardo F, Pastorino G et al. Phase-II study of navelbine in advanced breast cancer. *Semin Oncol.* 1989; 16:33-6.

129. Merk HF. Drugs affecting hair growth. In: Merk HF, ed. *Hair and hair disease.* Heidelberg, Germany: Springer-Verlag; 1990:601-9.

130. Jones EE. Androgenic effects of oral contraceptives; implications for patient compliance. *Am J Med.* 1995; 98:116S-9S.

131. Phillips ER, Ryan S, Ferrari R et al. Estratest and Estratest HS (esterified estrogens and methyltestosterone) therapy: a summary of safety surveillance data, January 1989 to August 2002. *Clin Ther.* 2003; 25:3027-43.

132. Cerel-Suhl SL, Yeager BF. Update on oral contraceptive pills. *Am Fam Physician.* 1999; 60:2073-84.

133. Mira H, Kondo T. Hair loss induced by dopamine agonist: case report and review of the literature. *Parkinsonism Relat Disord.* 2003; 10:51-5.

134. Atas B, Caksen H, Tuncer O et al. Four children with colchicine poisoning. *Hum Exp Toxicol.* 2004; 23:353-6.

135. Tullio CJ, Roberts MA. Cimetidine-induced alopecia. *Clin Pharm.* 1985; 4:145.

136. Pierard GE. Toxic effects of metals from the environment on hair growth and structure. *J Cutan Pathol.* 1979; 6:237-42.

137. Moore D, House I, Dixon A. Thallium poisoning. Diagnosis may be elusive but alopecia is the clue. *BMJ.* 1993; 306:1527-9.

138. Burrows NP, Grant JW, Crisp AJ et al. Scarring alopecia following gold therapy. *Acta Derm Venereol.* 1994; 74:486.

139. Arava [package insert]. Bridgewater, NJ: Sanofi-Aventis; 2007.

140. Roenigk HH, Fowler-Bergfeld W, Curtis GH. Methotrexate for psoriasis in weekly oral doses. *Arch Dermatol.* 1969; 99:86-93.

141. Kremer JM. Rational use of new and existing disease-modifying agents in rheumatoid arthritis. *Ann Intern Med.* 2001; 134:695-706.

142. Tricot L, Lebbe C, Pillebout E et al. Tacrolimus-induced alopecia in female kidney-pancreas transplant patients. *Transplantation.* 2005; 1546-9.

143. Shepherd J, Jones J, Takeda A et al. Adefovir dipivoxil and pegylated interferon alfa-2a for the treatment of chronic hepatitis B: a systematic review and economic evaluation. *Health Technol Assess.* 2006; 20:iii-iv, xi-xiv, 1-188.

144. Abilify [package insert]. Princeton, New Jersey: Bristol-Myers Squibb Company; 2008.

145. Bupropion [package insert]. Sellersville,PA: Teva Pharmaceuticals; 2007.

146. Celexa [package insert]. St. Louis, Missouri: Forest Pharmaceuticals; 2009.

147. Lexapro [package insert]. St. Louis, Missouri: Forest Pharmaceuticals, Inc; 2009.

148. Luvox CR [package insert]. Palo Alto, California: Jazz Pharmaceutics; 2008.

149. Rebora A. Changes in growth and distribution of hair associated with psychotropic drug use. Incidence and mechanisms. *CNS Drugs.* 1997; 8:323-34.

150. McCreadie RG, Farmer JG. Lithium and hair texture. *Acta Psychiatr Scand.* 1985; 72:387-8.

151. Chan HH, Wing Y, Su R et al. A control study of the cutaneous side effects of chronic lithium therapy. *J Affect Disord.* 2000; 57:107-13.

152. Sarantidis D, Waters B. A review and controlled study of cutaneous conditions associated with lithium carbonate. *Br J Psychiatry.* 1983; 143:42-50.

153. Zyprexa [package insert]. Indianapolis, IN: Eli Lilly and Company; 2005.

154. Paxil CR [package insert]. Research Triangle Park, North Carolina: GlaxoSmithKline; 2009.

155. McLean RM, Harrison-Woolrych M. Alopecia associated with quetiapine. *Int Clin Psychopharmacol.* 2007; 22:117-9.

156. Sertraline [package insert]. New York: Pfizer; 2009.

157. Parker V, Wong AHC, Boon HS et al. Adverse reactions to St John's Wort. *Can J Psychiatry.* 2001; 46:77-9.

158. Lesse S. Tranylcypromine (Parnate)—a study of 1000 patients with severe agitated depressions. *Am J Psychother.* 1979; 32:220-42.

159. Pitchot W, Ansseau M. Venlafaxine-induced hair loss. *Am J Psychiatry*. 2001; 158:1159-60.
160. Geodon [package insert]. New York: Pfizer; 2008.
161. Goodman NF. AACE Hyperandrogenism Guidelines: American association of clinical endocrinologists medical guidelines for clinical practice for the diagnosis and treatment of hyperandrogenic disorders. *Endocrine Practice*. 2001; 7:121-34.
162. Papadopoulos S, Harden RM. Hair loss in patients treated with carbimazole. *BMJ*. 1966; 17:1502-3.
163. Dinh QQ, Sinclair R. Female pattern hair loss: current treatment concepts. *Clin Interv Aging*. 2007; 2:189-99.
164. Ferran M, Calvet J, Almirall M et al. Alopecia areata as another immune-mediated disease developed in patients treated with tumor necrosis factor-α blocker agents. Report of five cases and review of the literature. *J Eur Acad Dermatol Venereol*. 2011; 25:479-84.
165. Garcovich S, Manco S, Zampetti A et al. Onset of lichen planopilaris during treatment with etanercept. *Br J Dermatol*. 2008; 158:1161-3.
166. Huynh C, Reguiai Z, Lambrecht L et al. First two cases of alopecia areata during golimumab therapy. *Joint Bone Spine*. 2016; 83:367-8.
167. Ribeiro LBP, Rego JCG, Duque-Estrada B et al. Alopecia secondary to anti-tumor necrosis factor-alpha therapy. *An Bras Dermatol*. 2015; 90:232-5.
168. Hajime Y, Ichiro M. Loss of hair related to gentamicin treatment. *JAMA*. 1970; 211:123.
169. Gupta KB, Kumar V, Vishukarma S, Shandily R. Isoniazid-induced alopecia. *Lung India*. 2011; 28:60-1.
170. Klingman AM. Pathologic dynamics of human hair loss. *Arch Dermatol*. 1961; 83:175-97.
171. Wang YY, Po HL. Enoxaparin-induced alopecia in patients with cerebral venous thrombosis. *J Clin Pharm Ther*. 2006; 31:513-7.
172. Aspner R, Horl WH, Sunder-Plassmann G. Dalteparin-induced alopecia in hemodialysis patients: reversal by regional citrate anticoagulation. *Blood*. 2001; 97:2914-5.
173. Burke KE. Hair loss. What causes it and what can be done about it. *Postgrad Med*. 1989; 85:52-8, 67-73, 77.
174. Tabamo RE, DiRocco A. Alopecia induced by dopamine agonists. *Neurology*. 2002; 58:829-30.
175. Shapiro J, Wiseman M, Lui H. Practical management of hair loss. *Can Fam Physician*. 2000; 46:1469-77.
176. Warnock JK, Morris DW. Adverse cutaneous reactions to antipsychotics. *Am J Clin Dermatol*. 2002; 3:629-36.
177. Hordinsky M, Sawaya M, Roberts JL. Hair loss and hirsutism in the elderly. *Clin Geriatr Med*. 2002; 18:121-33.
178. Cormia FE. Alopecia from oral contraceptives. *JAMA*. 1967; 201:141-3.
179. Zouboulis CC, Degitz K. Androgen action on human skin—from basic research to clinical significance. *Exp Dermatol*. 2004; 13:5-10.
180. Trueb RM. Chemotherapy-induced alopecia. *Curr Opin Support Palliat Care*. 2010; 4:281-4.
181. Blankenship ML. Drugs and alopecia. *Aust J Derm*. 1983; 24:100-4.
182. Pillans PI, Woods DF. Drug-associated alopecia. *Int J Derm*.1995; 34:149-58.
183. Shapiro J, ed. Hair disorders: current concepts in pathophysiology, diagnosis and management. In: *An issue of dermatologic clinics*. 1st ed. Oxford, UK: Elsevier Health Sciences; 2012.
184. Machado M, Moreb JS, Khan SA. Six cases of permanent alopecia after various conditioning regimens commonly used in hematopoietic stem cell transplantation. *Bone Marrow Transplant*. 2007; 40;979-82.
185. Tran D, Sinclair RD, Schwarer AP et al. Permanent alopecia following chemotherapy and bone marrow transplantation. *Australas J Dermatol*. 2000; 41:106-8.
186. Smith AG. Skin disorders. In: Davies DM, Ferner RE, DeGlanville H, eds. *Davies's textbook of adverse drug reactions*. 5th ed. London: Lippincott-Raven Publishers; 1998:566-84.
187. Pai GS, Vimala AM, Dinesh M. Occurrence and severity of alopecia in patients on combination chemotherapy. *Indian J Cancer*. 2000; 37:95-104.
188. Johns Hopkins Medicine. Immunosuppressive medications. http://www.hopkinslupus.org/lupus-treatment/lupus-medications/immunosuppressive-medications/ (accessed 2017 Nov 15).
189. Mulinari-Brenner F, Bergfeld WF. Hair loss: diagnosis and management. *Clev Clin J Med*. 2003; 70:705-12.
190. Bene J, Moulis G, Auffret M et al. Alopecia induced by tumour necrosis factor-alpha antagonists: description of 52 cases and disproportionality analysis in a nationwide pharmacovigilance database. *Rheumatology*. 2014; 53:1465-9.
191. Santos Z, Avci P, Hamblin MR. Drug discover for alopecia: gone today, hair tomorrow. *Expert Opin*. 2015; 101-17.
192. Vidal CI. Overview of alopecia: a dermatopathologist's perspective. *Mo Med*. 2015; 112:308-12.
193. Thiedke CC. Alopecia in women. *Am Fam Physician*. 2003; 67:1007-14, 1017-18.
194. Drake LA, Dinehart SM, Farmer ER et al. Guidelines of care for androgenetic alopecia. *J Am Dermatol*. 1996; 35:465-9.
195. Levy LL, Emer JJ. Female pattern alopecia: current perspectives. *Int J Womens Health*. 2013; 5:541-56.
196. Price VH. Treatment of hair loss. *N Engl J Med*. 1999; 341:964-73.
197. Rebora A. Telogen effluvium: an etiopathogenetic theory. *Int J Dermatol*. 1993; 32:339-40.
198. Barth JH. Rational investigations in the diagnosis and management of women with androgenic alopecia. *Clin Dermatol*. 2001; 10:147-63.
199. Boyer JD, Vidmar DA. Postoperative alopecia: a case report and literature review. *Cutis*. 1994; 54: 321-22.
200. Harrison S, Bergfeld W. Diffuse hair loss: Its triggers and management. *Cleve Clin J Med*. 2009; 76:361-7.
201. Piraccini BM, Iorizzo M, Rech G et al. Drug-induced hair disorders. *Curr Drug Saf*. 2006; 1:301-5.
202. Sommer M, Wilson C. Therapeutic approaches to the management of common baldness. *Int J Clin Pract*. 1999; 53:381-5.
203. Barth JH, Dawber PR. Drug-induced hair loss. *BMJ*. 1989; 298:675.
204. Grover C, Khurana A. Telogen effluvium. *Indian J Dermatol Venereol Leprol*. 2013; 79:591-603.
205. Coates A, Abraham S, Kaye SB et al. On the receiving end—patient perception of the side-effects of cancer chemotherapy. *Eur J of Cancer*. 1983; 19:203-8.
206. Grevelman EG, Breed WP. Prevention of chemotherapy-induced hair loss by scalp cooling. *Ann Oncol*. 2005; 16:352-9.
207. Dorr, VJ. A practitioner's guide to cancer-related alopecia. *Sermin Oncol*. 1998; 25:562- 70.
208. Vendelbo Johansen, LV. Scalp hypothermia in the prevention of chemotherapy-induced alopecia. *Acta Radiol Oncol*. 1985; 24:113-6.
209. Lotfi-Jam K, Carey M, Jefford M et al. Nonpharmacologic strategies for managing common chemotherapy adverse effects: a systematic review. *J Clin Oncol*. 2008; 26:5618-29.
210. Weigand DA. Alopecias. Diagnostic and pathogenetic considerations. *Nebr State Med J*. 1969; 54:26-37.
211. Bandaranayake I, Mirmirani P. Hair loss remedies—separating fact from fiction. *Cutis*. 2004;73:107-14.
212. Wang J, Lu Z, Au JL. Protection against chemotherapy-induced alopecia. *Pharm Res*. 2006; 23:2505-14.
213. ClinicalTrials.gov. Efficacy and safety of Dignicap System for preventing chemotherapy-induced alopecia. https://clinicaltrials.gov/ct2/show/NCT01831024 (accessed 2017 Dec 14).
214. Shapiro J, Otberg N. *Hair loss and restoration*. 2nd ed. Boca Raton, FL: CRC Press/Taylor and Francis Group; 2015.

215. Messenger AG, Rundegren J. Minoxidil: mechanisms of action on hair growth. *Br J Dermatol.* 204; 150:186-94.
216. Bona G, Bozzola M, Buzi F et al. Hirsutism. *Minerva Pediatr.* 2007: 59:289-98.
217. Rosenfield RL. Hirsutism. *N Engl J Med.* 2005; 353:2578-88.
218. Alsantali A. Alopecia areata: a new treatment plan. *Clin Cosmet Investig Dermatol.* 2011; 4:107-15.
219. Gutzmer R, Werfel T, Mao R et al. Successful treatment with oral isotretinoin of acneiform skin lesions associated with cetuximab therapy. *Br J Dermatol.* 2005; 153:849-51.
220. Pomerantz RG, Chirinos RE, Falo LD, Geskin LJ. Acitretin for treatment of EGFR inhibitor-induced cutaneous toxic effects. *Arch Dermatol.* 2008; 144:949-50.
221. Varothai S, Bergfeld WF. Androgenetic alopecia: an evidence-based treatment update. *Am J Clin Dermatol.* 2014; 15:217-30.
222. Duvic M, Lemak NA, Valero V et al. A randomized trial of minoxidil in chemotherapy-induced alopecia. *J Am Acad Dermatol.* 1996; 35:74-8.
223. Drake LA, Dinehart SM, Farmer ER et al. Guidelines for care for androgenetic alopecia. *J Am Acad Dermatol.* 1996; 35:465-9.
224. Olszewaska M, Rudnicka L. Case reports: effective treatment of female androgenic alopecia with dutasteride. *J Drugs Dermatol.* 2005; 4:637-40.
225. Yim E, Nole KL, Tosti A. 5α-reducatse inhibitors in androgenetic alopecia. *Curr Opin Endocrinol Diabetes Obes.* 2014; 21:493-8.
226. Hoedemaker C, van Egmond S, Sinclair R. Treatment of female pattern hair loss with a combination of spironolactone and minoxidil. *Australas J Dermatol.* 2007; 48:43-5.
227. Millikan L. Hirsutism, postpartum telogen effluvium, and male pattern alopecia. *J Cosmet Dermatol.* 2005; 5:81-6.
228. Majid I, Keen A. Management of alopecia areata: an update. *BJMP.* 2012; 5:a530.
229. Singhal P, Agarwal S, Dhot PS, Sayal SK. Efficacy of platelet-rich plasma in treatment of androgenic alopecia. *Asian J Transfus Sci.* 2015; 9:159-62.
230. Khatu SS, More YE, Gokhale NR et al. Platelet-rich plasma in androgenic alopecia: myth or an effective tool. *J Cutan Aesthet Surg.* 2014; 7:107-10.
231. Tin SS, Wiwanitkit V. Low-level laser therapy for androgenic alopecia. *Int J Trichology.* 2014; 6:189.
232. Townsend KA, Marlowe. Relative safety and efficacy of finasteride for treatment of hirsutism. *Ann Pharmacother.* 2004; 38:1070-3.
233. Goodman NF, Cogin RH, Futterweit W et al.; American Association of Clinical Endocrinologists, American College of Endocrinology, and Androgen Excess and PCOS Society Disease State Clinical Review. Guide to the Best Practices in the Evaluation and Treatment of Polycystic Ovary Syndrome—part 1. *Endocr Pract.* 2015; 21:1291-300.
234. Goolsby JM. AACE Hyperandrogenism guidelines. *J Am Acad Nurse Pract.* 2001; 13:492-4.
235. Trueb RM. Causes and management of hypertrichosis. *Am J Clin Dermatol.* 2002; 3:617-27.
236. Weiss IS. Hirsutism after chronic administration of acetazolamide. *Am J Ophthal.* 1974; 78:327.
237. Luef G, Abraham I, Haslinger M et al. Polycystic ovaries, obesity and insulin resistance in women with epilepsy. A comparative study of carbamazepine and valproic acid in 105 women. *J Neurol.* 2002; 249:835-41.
238. Valeyri-Allanore L, Sassolas B, Roujeau J. Drug-induced skin, nail and hair disorders. *Drug Saf.* 2007; 30:1011-30.
239. Barbieri RL, Evans S, Kistner RW. Danazol in the treatment of endometriosis: analysis of 100 cases with a 4-year follow-up. *Fertil Steril.* 1982; 37:737-46.
240. Sachdeva S. Hirsutism: evaluation and treatment. *Indian J Dermatol.* 2010; 55:3-7.
241. Miwa LJ, Shaefer MS, Stratta R et al. Drug-induced hypertrichosis: case report and review of the literature. *DICP.* 1990; 24:365-8.
242. Harper JI, Kendra JR. Dermatological aspects of the use of cyclosporine A for prophylaxis of graft-versus-host disease. *Br J Derm.* 1984; 110:469-74.
243. González M, Landa N, Gardeazabal J et al. Generalized hypertrichosis after treatment with topical minoxidil. *Clin Exp Dermatol.* 1994; 19:157-8.
244. Dawber RP, Rundegren J. Hypertrichosis in females applying minoxidil topical solution and in normal controls. *J Eur Acad Dermatol Venereol.* 2003; 17:271-5.
245. Novak E, Franz TJ. Topically applied minoxidil in baldness. *Int J Dermatol.* 1985; 24:82-7.
246. Kosman ME. Evaluation of a new antihypertensive agent Minoxidil. *JAMA.* 1980; 244:73-5.
247. Lucky AW, Piacquadio DJ. A randomized, placebo-controlled trial of 5% and 2% topical minoxidil solutions in the treatment of female pattern hair loss. *J Am Acad Dermatol.* 2004; 50:541-53.
248. Sparberg M. Diagnostically confusing complications of diphenylhydantoin therapy: A review. *Ann Intern Med.* 1963; 59:914-30.
249. Baumeister FAM, Schwarz HP, Stengel-Rutkowski S. Childhood hypertrichosis: diagnosis and management. *Arch Dis Child.* 1995; 72:457-9.
250. Herberg KP. Effects of diphenylhydantoin in 41 epileptics institutionalized since childhood. *South Med J.* 1977; 70:19-24.
251. Livingston S, Peterson D, Boks LL. Hypertrichosis occurring in association with Dilantin therapy. *J Pediatr.* 1955; 47:351-2.
252. Scheinfeld N. Phenytoin in cutaneous medicine: its uses, mechanisms, and side effects. *Dermatol Online J.* 2003; 9:6.
253. Guerreiro MM, Vigonius U, Pohlmann H et al. A double-blind controlled clinicaltrial of oxcarbazepine versus phenytoin in children and adolescents with epilepsy. *Epilepsy Res.* 1997; 27:205-13.
254. Acyclovir [package insert]. Schaumburg, IL: APP Pharmaceuticals; 2008.
255. Cohen PR, Escudier SM, Kurzrock R. Cetuximab-associated elongation of the eyelashes: case report and review of eyelash trichomegaly secondary to epidermal growth factor receptor inhibitors. *Am J Clin Dermatol.* 2011; 12:63-7.
256. Kerob D, Dupuy A, Reygagne P et al. Facial hypertrichosis induced by cetuximab, an anti-EGRF monoclonal antibody. *Arch Dermatol.* 2006; 142:1656-7.
257. Lane K, Goldstein SM. Erlotinib-associated trichomegaly. *Ophthal Plast Reconstr Surg.* 2007; 23:65-6.
258. Ahmad T, Eisen T. Kinase inhibition with BAY 43-9006 in renal cell carcinoma. *Clin Cancer Res.* 2004; 10:6388s-92s.
259. de Vries TW, de Langen-Wouterse JJ, de Jong-Van den Berg LT et al. Hypertrichosis as a side effect of inhaled steroids in children. *Pediatr Pulmonol.* 2007; 42:370-3.
260. Wysocki GP, Daley TD. Hypertrichosis in patients receiving cyclosporine therapy. *Clin Exp Dermatol.* 1987; 12:191-6.
261. Mansberger SL, Cioffi GA.Eyelast formation secondary to latanoprost treatment in a patient with alopecia. *Arch Ophthalmol.* 2000; 118:718-19.
262. Demitsu T, Manabe M, Harima N. Hypertrichosis induced by latanoprost. *J Am Acad Dermatol.* 2001; 44:721-3.
263. Bode D, Seehusen DA, Baird D. Hirsutism in women. *Am Fam Physician.* 2012; 85:373-80.
264. Oztas P, Catal F. Dilmen U. Localized hypertrichosis following BCG vaccination: case report. *Nigerian J Paediatrics.* 2003; 30:93.
265. Cox NH, Moss C, Forsyth A. Cutaneous reactions to aluminum in vaccines: an avoidable problem. *Lancet.* 1988; 2:43.
266. Pembroke A, Marten RH. Unusual cutaneous reactions following diphtheria and tetanus immunization. *Clin Exp Dermatol.* 1979; 43:345-8.
267. Ozkan H, Dündar NO, Ozkan S. Hypertrichosis following measles immunization. *Pediatric Dermatol.* 2001; 18:457-8.
268. Kumar LR, Goyal BG. Pigmented hairy scar following smallpox vaccination. *Indian J Pediatr.*1968; 35:283-4.

269. Koblenzer PJ, Baker L. Hypertrichosis lanuginose associated with diazoxide therapy in prepubertal children: a clinicopathologic study. *Ann N Y Acad Sci.* 1968; 11;150:373-82.

270. Hunter MH, Carek PJ. Evaluation and treatment of women with hirsutism. *Am Fam Physician.* 2003; 67:2565-72.

271. Lutz G. Effects of cyclosporine A on hair. *Skin Pharmacol.* 1994; 7:101-4.

272. Tejani A, Butt KMH. Cyclosporine experience in renal transplantation in children. *Mt Sinai J Med.* 1987; 54:467-74.

273. Garcia-Patos V, Pujol RM, Alomar A. Persistent subcutaneous nodules in patients hyposensitized with aluminum-containing allergen extracts. *Arch Dermatol.* 1995; 131:1421-4.

274. Azziz R. The evaluation and management of hirsutism. *Obstet Gynecol.* 2003; 101:995-1007.

275. Ginsburg J, White M. Hirsutism and virilisation. *Br Med J.* 1980; 280:369-71.

276. Sakiyama R. Approach to patients with hirsutism. *West J Med.* 1996; 165:386-91.

277. Prabhakar S. Sahota P, Kharbanda PS. Sodium valproate, hyperandrogenism and altered ovarian function in Indian women with epilepsy: a prospective study. *Epilepsia.* 2007; 48:1371-7.

278. Hendrick V. Women and mental illness: how gender affects presentation and treatment. *Drug Benefit Trends.* 2007; 19:359-72.

279. O'Driscoll JB, Mamtora H, Higginson J. A prospective study of the prevalence of clear-cut endocrine disorders and polycystic ovaries in 350 patients presenting with hirsutism or androgenic alopecia. *Clin Endocrinol.* 1994; 41:231-42.

280. Speroff L, Shaw JC. Hirsutism and hyperandrogenism in women. In: Noble J, ed. *Textbook of primary care medicine.* 2nd ed. St. Louis, MO: Mosby-Year Book; 1996:824-1826.

281. Harman MS, Blackman MR. Common problem in reproductive endocrinology. In: Parker RL, Burton JR, Zieve PD, eds. *Principles of ambulatory medicine.* 5th ed. Philadelphia: Lippincott, Williams and Wilkins; 1999:1168-97.

282. Dawber RPR. Guidance for the management of hirsutism. *Curr Med Res Opin.* 2005; 21:1227-34.

283. Powell J, Stone E, Dawber RPR. Hirsutism and hypertrichosis. In: Powell J, Stone, E, Dawber RRR, eds. *An atlas of hair and scalp diseases.* New York: The Parthenon Publishing Group; 1999:37-42.

284. Ehrmann DA, Barnes RB, Rosenfield RL. Hyperandrogenism, hirsutism, and the polycystic ovary syndrome. In: DeGroot LJ, Jameson JL, eds. *Endocrinology.* 5th ed. Philadelphia: Elsevier Saunders; 2006.

285. Kologlu S, Baskal N, Kologlu LB et al. Hirsutism due to the treatment with l-thyroxine in patients with thyroid pathology. *Endocrinologie.* 1988; 26:179-85.

286. Falsetti P, Gambera A, Andrico S et al. Acne and hirsutism in polycystic ovary syndrome: clinical, endocrine-metabolic and ultrasonographic differences. *Gynecol Endocrinol.* 2002; 16:275-84.

287. Wendelin DS, Pope DN, Mallory SB. Hypertrichosis. *J Am Acad Dermatol.* 2003; 161-79.

288. Bolduc C, Shapiro J. Management of androgenic alopecia. *Am J Clin Dermatol.* 2000; 1:151-8.

289. Vashi RA, Mancini AJ, Paller AS. Primary generalized and localized hypertrichosis in children. *Arch Dermatol.* 2001; 137:877-84.

290. Battle EF Jr, Hobbs LM. Laser-assisted hair removal for darker skin types. *Dermatol Ther.* 2004; 17:177-83.

291. Kelestimur F, Everest H, Unluhizarci K et al. A comparison between spironolactone and spironolactone plus finasteride in the treatment of hirsutism. *Eur J Endocrinol.* 2004; 150:351-4.

SECTION III

DRUG-INDUCED NEUROLOGICAL DISEASES

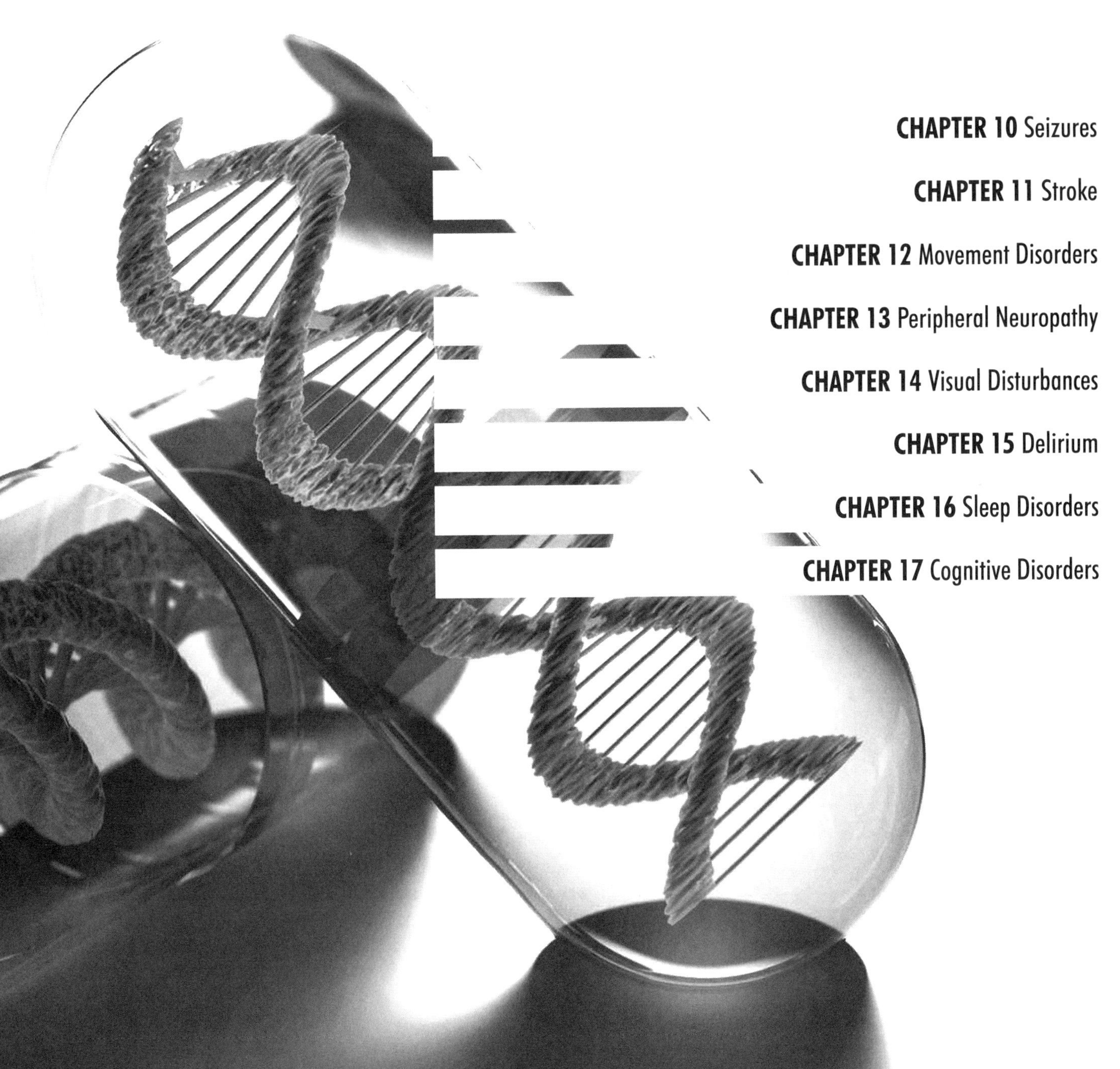

CHAPTER 10 Seizures

CHAPTER 11 Stroke

CHAPTER 12 Movement Disorders

CHAPTER 13 Peripheral Neuropathy

CHAPTER 14 Visual Disturbances

CHAPTER 15 Delirium

CHAPTER 16 Sleep Disorders

CHAPTER 17 Cognitive Disorders

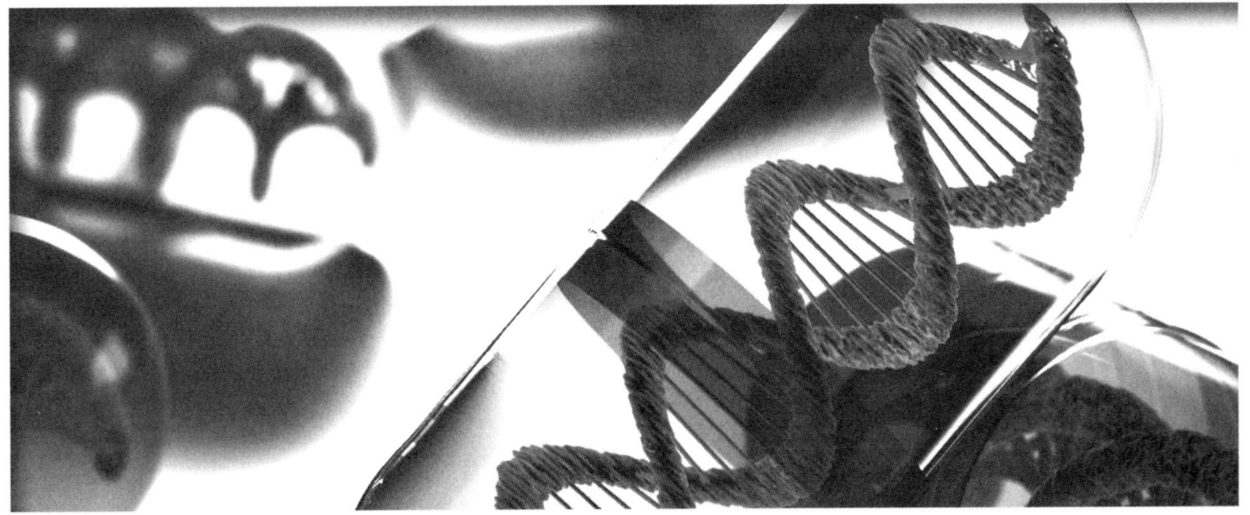

CHAPTER 10

Seizures

Timothy E. Welty

Seizures, including those induced by drugs, are serious neurologic events; without prompt and proper recognition, diagnosis, and treatment, seizures can result in permanent neurologic deficits. Drug-induced seizures can present as a single limited seizure event, convulsive status epilepticus, or nonconvulsive status epilepticus. It is important to rapidly recognize drug-induced seizures and to provide immediate, effective treatment.

CAUSATIVE AGENTS

Numerous drugs have been identified as possible causes of seizures. Because drug-induced seizures are relatively rare events, it is difficult to determine incidence and causality for many drugs. Most reports of drugs causing seizures are based on individual cases, epidemiologic studies, and very few prospective studies.[1] A list of drugs associated with seizures is presented in **Table 10-1**.[1-37]

Drugs can induce seizures in a number of clinical situations. The scenario that most people recognize is the setting of an intentional or unintentional overdose. Seizures can also occur as an adverse effect of a drug even when administered at therapeutic doses. These events are not predictable and may occur even in patients with no history of or risk factors for seizures. Abrupt discontinuation of therapy with some drugs can also result in a seizure. Many illicit drugs are associated with this type of seizure. In addition, ethanol, baclofen, antiepileptic drugs, and benzodiazepines may be associated with withdrawal seizures. Caution must be exercised when using an antagonist to one of these drugs because of the potential for precipitating a seizure.

EPIDEMIOLOGY

First-time seizures from all causes occur with an incidence of 70–100 per 100,000 individuals annually.[38] Of these, 23–61 per 100,000 are single events in patients in whom epilepsy does not develop. The mortality rate associated with a first unprovoked seizure is 1–4%. Limited data indicate that seizures as a toxic complication of drugs comprise approximately 6% of new onset seizures, and nearly 9% of cases with status epilepticus are related to drug toxicity.[39,40] The incidence of pediatric cases of drug-induced seizures was reported as 4.7% in

Table 10-1 Agents Implicated in Drug-Induced Seizures[1-37]

Drug	Incidence	Level of Evidence[a]
ANTIARRYTHMICS		
Lidocaine[1]	20–25%	A
Mexiletine[2]	NK	B
ANALGESICS		
Hydromorphone[3]	NK	C
Meperidine[4,5]	2.1%	B
Morphine[5]	NK	B
Naloxone[5]	NK	B
Nefopam[5]	NK	B
Tramadol[6,7]	13–50%	B
ANESTHETICS		
Propofol[8,9]	23–40%	B
Sevoflurane[10-12]	50–100%	A
ANTIBIOTICS		
Carbapenems[13]	0.9%[b] 2–3%[c]	B
Cephalosporins[14]	NK	B
Fluoroquinolones[3]	NK	B
Penicillins[14]	NK	B
ANTIDEPRESSANTS		
Bupropion[15,16]	0.5–4%	A
Tricyclic/tetracyclic antidepressants[16,17]	0.25–2%	A
ANTIEPILEPTIC DRUGS		
Benzodiazepines[3]	NK	B
Carbamazepine[18-20]	NK	A
Felbamate[21]	NK	B
Oxcarbazepine[12,18]	NK	C
Phenobarbital[3]	NK	B
Phenytoin[3]	NK	B
Topiramate[3]	NK	B
ANTIMALARIAL DRUGS		
Hydroxychloroquine[23]	NK	B
ANTINEOPLASTIC DRUGS		
5-fluorouracil[24,25]	NK	C
Busulfan[27]	1.8–40%	B
Chlorambucil[24]	NK	B
Interferon α[3,26]	0.16%	B
Methotrexate[24]	NK	B
ANTIPSYCHOTIC DRUGS		
Phenothiazines[28-30]	2.1%	A
Clozapine[31,32]	1–4%	B
Haloperidol[3,32]	NK	B
ASTHMA DRUGS		
Theophylline–aminophylline[3]	NK	B

Table 10-1 Agents Implicated in Drug-Induced Seizures[1-37] (continued)

Drug	Incidence	Level of Evidence[a]
CONTRAST MEDIA		
Iodinated and noniodinated[3]	0.2–0.5% 15%[d]	B
HERBAL COMPOUNDS		
Ephedra (Ma huang)[33]	NK	B
Eucalyptus[34,35]	NK	C
Gingko[34,35]	NK	C
Ginseng[34,35]	NK	C
Pennyroyal[34]	NK	C
Sage[34]	NK	C
Shankhapusphi (Ayurveda)[34]	NK	C
Star anise[34]	NK	C
Star fruit[34]	NK	C
IMMUNOSUPPRESSANTS		
Cyclosporine[3]	0.5–3.9%	B
STIMULANT DRUGS FOR ADHD		
Atomoxetine[36,37]	NK	C
Methylphenidate[37]	NK	C

ADHD = attention deficit/hyperactivity disorder, NK = not known.
[a]Definitions for Levels of Evidence: Level A—evidence from one or more randomized, controlled clinical trials; Level B—evidence from nonrandomized clinical trials, prospective observational studies, cohort studies, retrospective studies, case-control studies, meta-analyses and/or postmarketing surveillance studies; and Level C—evidence from one or more published case reports or case series.
[b]Used alone.
[c]Used in combination with other antibiotics.
[d]In patients with brain metastases.

an analysis of data from the Toxicology Investigators Consortium Case Registry.[41]

The precise incidences of seizures induced by specific drugs are unclear. One of the first reported studies on drug-induced seizures by the Boston Collaborative Drug Surveillance Program found a rate of 0.08% in 32,812 patients.[42] Another review of emergency cases of status epilepticus showed that ethanol ingestion and drug overdose were responsible for 13% and <5%, respectively, of these cases.[43] Twenty-five percent of the seizures related to a drug overdose were fatal. A review of 1993 data from the California Poison Control System showed that cyclic antidepressants, stimulants, antihistamines, theophylline, and isoniazid were the most common causes of drug-induced seizures.[44] A follow-up to this study 10 years later showed that the most common causes of drug-induced seizures were bupropion, diphenhydramine, cyclic antidepressants, tramadol, amphetamines, isoniazid, and venlafaxine.[45] Of patients included in this series, 68% had a single seizure, 27% had more than one seizure, and 3.6% experienced status epilepticus. In a study of drug-induced seizures among children, the most common causative agents were antidepressants and anticholinergics/antihistamines.[41] In this study, sympathomimetics were the most common causative drugs in children younger than 2 years old. However, these data are derived only from calls to poison centers or admissions to an emergency department and do not account for drug-induced seizures that occur outside these settings. Most likely, the incidence of drug-induced seizures is greater than is reflected in these reports. Even so, drug-induced seizures are relatively rare events that typically occur as a single, isolated seizure.

ANALGESICS

Tramadol is associated with drug-induced seizures. In a review of 190 cases of tramadol toxicity reported to a poison control center, 13.7% of patients experienced a seizure.[6] A similar study reported that 55% of patients with tramadol intoxication experienced a seizure.[7] Ninety percent of these seizures were single events, and 84% occurred within 24 hours of ingesting a toxic dose. Chronic use of tramadol predisposed these patients to a seizure. Most cases are associated with toxic doses or prolonged chronic use, but seizures are possible at therapeutic doses, especially in patients with underlying epilepsy.[7]

ANESTHETICS

Although propofol is used in the treatment of refractory status epilepticus, it is also associated with drug-induced seizures. Several case series have suggested that 24–40% of patients receiving propofol experience seizures or epileptiform electroencephalogram (EEG) activity during induction, emergence, and recovery from anesthesia.[8,9]

Sevoflurane is associated with a high incidence of drug-induced seizures. Studies of EEG activity during the induction of anesthesia have shown epileptiform activity in 50–60% of children and adults, and this increases to nearly 100% of patients when combined with hyperventilation and hypocapnia.[10,11] Additional study of EEGs in patients receiving sevoflurane has demonstrated a dose-dependent relationship in the EEG change.[12] At a 1.5 minimum alveolar concentration, epileptiform EEG discharges were present in 100% of patients.

ANTIBIOTICS

Carbapenems have been reported to cause seizures. Approximately 0.9% of patients taking imipenem as monotherapy experience a seizure.[13] The incidence of seizures in patients taking imipenem in combination with other antibiotics is 2–3%. In one study, 28% of $n = 21$ children treated with imipenem for bacterial meningitis experienced a seizure.[46] In contrast, meropenem caused no seizures in a study of adult patients with bacterial meningitis.[47] In another study, 12% of children receiving therapy with meropenem experienced a seizure.[48]

Cephalosporins are associated with neurotoxicity, with 10% of individuals with neurotoxicity experiencing convulsive seizures and another 10% having EEG-confirmed nonconvulsive status epilepticus.[49] About 50% of these cases were related to inappropriate dose adjustment in kidney disease. Penicillins have also been associated with seizures, typically in association with inappropriate dosing in patients with acute kidney injury or chronic kidney disease.[14]

There are several case reports of seizures associated with isoniazid, especially in children.[50] Reports of seizures with other antibiotics include quinolones and macrolides.[51] However, it is difficult to determine if the seizure resulted from the antibiotic or complications of an infectious process.

ANTICHOLINERGICS

In a study of drug-induced seizures in adults, nearly 10% of the cases were associated with ingestion of an anticholinergic agent.[44] A study in pediatric patients showed that 22% of children with drug-induced seizures had ingested an anticholinergic agent or antihistamine.[41] Diphenhydramine, chlorpheniramine, and doxylamine were the most common anticholinergic agents associated with drug-induced seizures in children.

ANTIDEPRESSANTS

Overdoses with tricyclic antidepressants are responsible for over 40% of seizures encountered in the emergency department.[17,52] Most of these seizures are generalized tonic-clonic seizures, but partial seizures may occur in individuals with a history of epilepsy.[42,45]

Other antidepressant agents can cause seizures in the setting of an overdose. Approximately 2% of patients with an overdose of a selective serotonin reuptake inhibitor experience a seizure.[53] Overdose of bupropion is also associated with a high incidence of seizures.[15]

Antidepressant drugs may also cause seizures at therapeutic doses. The incidence varies from approximately 0.1% with lower doses of imipramine to over 2% with higher doses of bupropion.[30] The risk of seizures appears lowest with trazadone, fluoxetine, and fluvoxamine. In contrast, the risk of seizures is highest in association with maprotiline, amoxapine, and bupropion, and these drugs should be avoided in patients with epilepsy. The risk of antidepressant-associated seizures is dose-dependent; for example, the incidence of seizures associated with bupropion at doses above 450 mg/day is 2–4%, while at lower doses the incidence is 0.5–1%.

ANTIEPILEPTIC DRUGS

Paradoxically, antiepileptic drugs have been associated with drug-induced seizures.[19-22] It is unclear if the seizures were due to an actual adverse event associated with the antiepileptic drug, a result of pre-existing seizures, due to an overdose of the antiepileptic drug, or breakthrough seizures following discontinuation of the antiepileptic drug.

ANTIFIBRINOLYTIC DRUGS

Although antifibrinolytic drugs are considered to be safe, seizures have been reported with their use.[54] Unlike aprotinin, tranexamic acid and EACA (ε-aminocaproic acid) are associated with seizures.[54] Most reports of seizures are in patients who are in the early postoperative period following cardiac surgery.[55,56] The incidence of seizures associated with tranexamic acid in retrospective studies is reported to be 0.5–1% with standard doses but increases to 6.4–7.3% with higher doses (>100 mg/kg). In a prospective study, the incidence of tranexamic acid-induced seizures was 3%. Seizures associated with tranexamic acid also have been reported in patients with kidney disease, other surgeries, and hemoptysis.

ANTIPSYCHOTICS

Among older antipsychotic agents, chlorpromazine is associated with the greatest risk of seizures, with an incidence of 2.1%.[28] At chlorpromazine doses <200 mg/day, 200–900 mg/day and >900 mg/day, the incidence of seizures is 0.3%, 0.7%, and 9%, respectively.[29] Concomitant treatment with other psychoactive agents increases the risk of chlorpromazine-induced seizures. Other older antipsychotic agents, such as trifluoperazine and thiothixene, are associated with a much lower risk of seizures than chlorpromazine.

Of the newer atypical antipsychotic agents, clozapine is associated with the greatest risk of seizures. The cumulative risk of seizures associated with clozapine over nearly 4 years of treatment has been estimated to be 10%.[31] At clozapine doses <300 mg/day, the incidence of seizures is approximately 1%, which increases to 4% at doses >600 mg/day.[32]

ANTINEOPLASTIC AGENTS

Approximately 13% of patients with cancer experience a seizure, and seizures account for 5% of neurologic complications.[57] Children with cancer are especially susceptible to seizures, which occur with a much higher incidence than in adults.[58] The causes of seizures among patients with cancer vary greatly and include primary brain tumors, brain metastases, metabolic derangements, and medications.[22] Drug-induced seizures are more common during intensive cancer chemotherapy that involves prolonged hospitalization, in patients with liver or kidney disease, and with high doses of antineoplastic agents, such as those recommended in protocols for bone marrow transplantation.

HERBAL MEDICINES AND TRADITIONAL CHINESE MEDICINE

Several herbal medicines and ingredients have been connected with drug-induced seizures. Actual incidences in humans are unknown due to poor mechanisms for detecting, reporting, and tracking adverse effects associated with these products.[59,60] Administration of typical doses of some of these substances has resulted in a seizure incidence of nearly 100% in animal models. Herbal products associated with seizures include nux vomica (strychnine), *Illicium henryi*, betel nut, *Morus alba* L. (mulberry), ephedra, eucalyptus, *Gingko biloba*, pennyroyal, sage, shankhapushpi, star anise, and star fruit.

STIMULANT DRUGS FOR ATTENTION DEFICIT/ HYPERACTIVITY DISORDER

Drugs such as methylphenidate and atomoxetine have been implicated as a cause of seizures in cases of overdose and abuse.[61,62] Early reports of seizures associated with drugs for attention deficit/hyperactivity disorder (ADHD) in children were complicated by the fact that this population is at increased risk for seizures. Two studies indicate that these drugs do not increase the risk of seizures in children with ADHD.[61,62] In one of these studies, children with epileptiform discharges on EEG were studied separately from those with normal EEG recordings.[61,62] Stimulant medications did not increase the risk of seizures in children with normal EEGs. A greater risk of seizures was reported in children with epileptiform discharges, but this could not be attributed to stimulant use. These data indicate that stimulant medications may be safely used in children with ADHD with little added risk of seizures.

MECHANISMS

Seizures are acute neurologic events resulting from hypersynchronous and hyperactive discharges of neurons. The precise mechanisms that result in this type of neuronal activity are poorly understood, in part because there are multiple causes of hypersynchronous activity. Proposed mechanisms of action of antiepileptic drugs involve excitatory neurotransmitters, ion channels (sodium, potassium, and calcium), and inhibitory neurotransmitters, providing limited understanding of the pathophysiology of seizures. However, other mechanisms are likely involved in the genesis of seizures due to toxicity and overdoses of medications.

Although specific mechanisms are not fully understood, there is some limited insight regarding potential mechanisms of seizures induced by some drugs. Proposed mechanisms by which specific drugs induce seizures are summarized in **Table 10-2.**[3,7,63-76] Meperidine is a well-documented causative agent in drug-induced seizures, most likely as a result of accumulation of the active metabolite normeperidine. The mechanism of seizures induced by penicillin and carbapenems is believed to be inhibition of the inhibitory neurotransmitter gamma-aminobutyric acid (GABA). Seizures caused by theophylline overdose in children, adults, and the elderly may occur as a result of saturation of hepatic metabolism of the drug, resulting in progressive theophylline accumulation. Premature infants may be somewhat protected from theophylline-induced seizures because of the different metabolic pathways for theophylline in immature hepatic enzyme systems.[64]

Table 10-2 Mechanisms of Drug-Induced Seizures

Drug	Mechanism
5-fluorouracil[65]	Genetic polymorphism of dihydropyrimidine dehydrogenase leading to accumulation
Bupropion[66]	Increased noradrenergic activity
Carbapenems[49]	GABA antagonist; NMDA agonist
Cisplatin[67]	Hypomagnesemia, hypokalemia, hyponatremia
Clozapine[3]	Anticholinergic activity and reduced affinity for striatal dopaminergic receptors
Cyclosporine[68]	Direct neurotoxin
Fluoroquinolones[69]	Displacement of GABA from receptors
Tramadol[7]	Increased neuronal excitability
Interferon α[70]	Increased neuronal excitability
Isoniazid[71,72]	Disruption of pyridoxine metabolism
Maprotiline[73]	Increased noradrenergic activity
Meperidine[3]	Accumulation of metabolite, normeperidine, with CNS excitation activity
Methotrexate[74]	Mineralizing microangiopathy of cerebral vasculature
Penicillins[3]	GABA antagonist
Phenothiazines[75]	Dopamine antagonist activity
Theophylline[64]	Disruption of pyridoxine metabolism
Tricyclic antidepressants[76]	Increased noradrenergic activity

CNS = central nervous system, GABA = gamma-aminobutyric acid, NMDA = *N*-methyl-D-aspartic acid.

CLINICAL PRESENTATION AND DIFFERENTIAL DIAGNOSIS

A major problem with drug-induced seizures is accurate detection and diagnosis. The clinical presentation of seizures may be variable, ranging from decreased levels of consciousness to a major generalized tonic-clonic event (**Table 10-3**). Symptoms of a seizure can be extremely subtle, and unless caregivers are aware of the various presentations of seizures, these symptoms can be overlooked or misdiagnosed. In addition, seizures are usually brief

Table 10-3 Signs and Symptoms Associated with Drug-Induced Seizures

- "Blacking out" spells, lapses in memory
- Sudden, unexplained alteration in consciousness
- Daydreaming
- Falling
- Shaking or convulsions of all limbs
- Jerks, shoulder shrugs
- Sudden episodes of various stereotypical sensations or automatic, uncontrolled movements

and unpredictable events, complicating detection and diagnosis. Caregivers of individuals who are at increased risk for drug-induced seizures and who are receiving medications known to cause seizures should be trained regarding the typical symptoms of a seizure, including alteration of consciousness and uncontrolled muscle movement of part or all of the body.

Seizures generally last for seconds to a couple of minutes, but drug-induced seizures can develop into status epilepticus, which requires immediate medical intervention. Patients with status epilepticus may not experience convulsions, but may present only with decreased levels of consciousness. When a patient experiences unexplained alterations in consciousness, seizures should be considered as a possible diagnosis.

Although the clinical presentation of a seizure is the primary method of detection, a definitive diagnosis is only possible with an EEG. Many other disorders are associated with clinical presentations that are similar to those of seizures (**Table 10-4**). The EEG should demonstrate abnormal neuronal activity that is consistent with a seizure. An EEG is preferably performed during a seizure to ensure that the abnormal activity is recorded, but the brief duration of most seizures makes this difficult to accomplish. Between seizures, the EEG can be completely normal, and is not helpful in determining whether the patient had a seizure. However, an abnormal EEG between seizures is indicative of an ongoing propensity for further seizures. The EEG should be performed by a skilled EEG technician and interpreted by a neurologist. It is particularly important to distinguish drug-induced seizures from seizures caused by neurological injuries or lesions, such as in patients with cancer, who

Table 10-4 Conditions to Consider in the Differential Diagnosis of Drug-Induced Seizures

- Seizures due to other causes
- Anxiety or panic attack
- Cardiac arrhythmia
- Complicated migraine headache
- Hypoglycemia
- Psychogenic events
- Stroke
- Syncope
- Tics
- Transient ischemic attack

may have brain metastases. Seizures that occur due to antineoplastic drug therapy may not be ongoing, and can often be treated or prevented by dose adjustments of chemotherapy agents. Criteria have been developed to assist in determining whether seizures are drug-induced or due to a different cause, and include development of encephalopathy and seizures soon after administration of a cancer chemotherapy agent, exclusion of metabolic and structural causes, and exclusion of seizures due to other drugs.[23,77]

Beyond seizures associated with antineoplastic therapy, it is important to determine the risk for ongoing seizures, which would result in a diagnosis of epilepsy. Most drug-induced seizures are single events associated with the presence of the toxic agent. When therapy with the offending drug is discontinued, further seizures do not recur. However, if the patient experiences additional seizures after discontinuation of the causative drug with sufficient time for the drug to be eliminated, it is likely that epilepsy has developed and maintenance treatment should be initiated with an antiepileptic drug.

RISK FACTORS

Precise risk factors for drug-induced seizures have not been clearly identified. Possible risk factors for drug-induced seizures are listed in **Table 10-5**. Drugs known to cause seizures at therapeutic doses should be used with caution in patients with a history of epilepsy or seizures, or in patients with preexisting neurological disorders involving the central nervous system. However, a history of epilepsy

Table 10-5 Risk Factors for Drug-Induced Seizures

- History of epilepsy or seizures
- Cancer
- Compromised blood–brain barrier
- Pre-existing neurological disorders
- Concomitant use of central nervous system stimulant drugs
- Impaired metabolism of hepatically metabolized drugs in patients with liver disease
- Impaired elimination of renally eliminated drugs in patients with kidney disease

is not an absolute contraindication to therapy with drugs that may be associated with seizures, and treatment decisions should be made on an individual basis. Patients with compromised kidney or liver function are at risk for the accumulation of renally eliminated or hepatically metabolized drugs. For example, the risk of meperidine-induced seizures is increased sevenfold in patients with kidney disease.[3] In other patients, disorders or infections that compromise the blood–brain barrier may allow excessive penetration of a drug into the central nervous system and result in seizures. Finally, drugs known to cause metabolic disruptions such as hyponatremia or hypoglycemia could produce seizures, and serum sodium and/or glucose concentrations should be monitored carefully when using these drugs. Antiepileptic drugs can cause seizures when a drug is improperly chosen for management of a seizure or epilepsy syndrome. Juvenile myoclonic epilepsy is an example of an epilepsy syndrome that can be exacerbated by the use of the incorrect antiepileptic drug. Carbamazepine and oxcarbazepine have been shown to increase the risk of myoclonic and absence seizures in patients with juvenile myoclonic epilepsy.[18,19,22] Accurate diagnosis of seizure and proper selection of an antiepileptic drug therapy are essential to prevent worsening of seizures in this patient population. In addition, discontinuation of antiepileptic drugs can precipitate seizures, especially in patients with epilepsy. This typically occurs in association with abrupt discontinuation of an antiepileptic drug, but seizures can occur even during controlled withdrawal of therapy.[20,22] Withdrawal seizures have been reported in association with discontinuation of therapy with carbamazepine, oxcarbazepine, phenobarbital, phenytoin, felbamate, and benzodiazepines. Seizures resulting from the discontinuation of antiepileptic drugs can be severe and result in status epilepticus.

Seizures associated with antiepileptic drugs are most likely to occur with doses resulting in supratherapeutic serum concentrations. For example, serum phenytoin concentrations >30 mcg/mL have been associated with seizures.[78] Topiramate has also been reported to cause seizures at supratherapeutic doses.[79] In addition, drug-induced metabolic disturbances such as hyponatremia induced by carbamazepine or oxcarbazepine result in seizures.

Seizures associated with fluoroquinolones are relatively uncommon, and often occur in patients with a prior diagnosis of epilepsy, neurotrauma, or anoxia.[80] Some evidence exists that concomitant use of nonsteroidal anti-inflammatory agents increases the risk of fluoroquinolone-induced seizures. There appears to be a relationship between the chemical structure of the fluoroquinolone and the propensity to cause seizures. Compounds that contain the 7-piperazine or 7-pyrrolidine moieties (e.g., ciprofloxacin, enoxacin, norfloxacin, tosufloxacin, clinafloxacin) have an increased potential to cause seizures.[81] The majority of reported cases of carbapenem-induced seizures have occurred in patients with kidney disease or a compromised blood–brain barrier, allowing greater penetration of the drug into the brain.

Theophylline-induced seizures can occur at any dose. Older children, adults, and the elderly are particularly vulnerable to seizures associated with theophylline, especially in overdose. In one case series, seizures related to theophylline developed in 6% of elderly patients.[82]

MORBIDITY AND MORTALITY

Drug-induced seizures are typically single events of short duration that are associated with a low risk of morbidity or mortality. However, during these events, an individual may experience an injury, such as lacerations or broken bones from falling, or may injure others if the seizure occurs while driving a motor vehicle or operating equipment or machinery. It is unlikely that typical drug-induced seizures result in repeated seizures, as may occur in patients with epilepsy.

Status epilepticus occurs rarely as a result of drug-induced seizures, but is associated with increased morbidity and mortality. Uncontrolled, prolonged seizures can result in permanent neurologic damage and increase the risk of ongoing seizures. Additionally, uncontrolled status epilepticus can result in death.

PREVENTION

As the mechanisms and causes of drug-induced seizures are diverse, it is difficult to describe specific plans for prevention (**Table 10-6**). Caution should be exercised when using medications known to cause seizures in patients with a history of epilepsy or seizures. Efforts should be made to ensure proper dose adjustments of drugs in patients with kidney or liver disease. Increased monitoring of metabolic function parameters may be helpful in preventing seizures due to drug effects on serum chemistry and homeostasis. Premedication and combination anesthesia may reduce the risk of seizures associated with sevoflurane. To minimize the risk of seizures, pretreatment with benzodiazepines and/or narcotics and concomitant use of nitrous oxide have been suggested.[83] In addition, hypocapnia should be avoided and a maximum of 1.5 minimum alveolar concentration of sevoflurane should be used during anesthesia to prevent sevoflurane-induced seizures.

To reduce the risk of withdrawal seizures, therapy with antiepileptic drugs should be withdrawn over 1–2 months, unless potentially life-threatening adverse effects are occurring, in which case more rapid discontinuation of therapy is warranted. Care should be taken to ensure proper doses and laboratory monitoring of antiepileptic drug therapy, including serum antiepileptic drug concentrations, serum electrolyte concentrations, and kidney and liver function tests.

Appropriate dose adjustment of penicillins and carbapenems in patients with kidney disease or a compromised blood–brain barrier is the best method of preventing seizures associated with these agents. These drugs and fluoroquinolone antibiotics should be used with caution in patients with a history of seizures. Similarly, other drugs, such as hydroxychloroquine and antipsychotic agents should be used with caution in patients with a history of epilepsy.[84,85] Some have suggested initiating therapy with an antiepileptic drug in patients in whom therapy with clozapine is initiated in an attempt to prevent seizures.[28]

Many of the reported cases of seizures associated with ephedra or ma huang occurred in patients without a history of epilepsy, and often occurred with the coadministration of other stimulant drugs, like phenylpropanolamine or caffeine.[34] Clearly, other stimulant drugs should not be administered in combination with ephedra.

Table 10-6 Approaches to Help Prevent Drug-Induced Seizures

- Appropriate dose adjustment of potentially seizure-inducing drugs in patients with liver or kidney disease
- Appropriate monitoring of laboratory values (e.g., serum electrolytes, kidney function, liver function, serum glucose concentrations)
- Avoid concomitant use of drugs that are central nervous system stimulants
- Avoid abrupt discontinuation of therapy with drugs with central nervous system activity

MANAGEMENT

Because drug-induced seizures can occur through a variety of mechanisms, treatment strategies should be approached carefully and should be individualized. The first step is to immediately discontinue the causative agent, or in the case of withdrawal seizures, to reinitiate therapy with the discontinued medication. If the risk of a second acute seizure appears to be low, then pharmacologic interventions to treat seizures are probably not necessary. However, if the risk of another acute seizure is high, then seizures should be treated aggressively. The focus of treatment is prevention of additional acute seizures.

Some drugs induce seizures by altering metabolism leading to disorders such as hypoglycemia or hyponatremia. In these cases, the underlying metabolic abnormality should be identified and corrected before the initiation of therapy with drugs commonly used to treat seizures. Antiepileptic drugs are associated with numerous adverse drug reactions, and indiscriminate use should be avoided.

Management of drug-induced seizures is dependent on the causative agent. However, a general treatment approach to seizures can be used.[86] The key to treatment and prevention of additional seizures is rapid identification of the causative agent and rapid implementation of an appropriate treatment plan. When the likelihood of repeated acute seizures is low, more time is available to discontinue the offending agent or take alternative actions.

The acute treatment of seizures typically involves provision of supportive care followed by drug therapy to control the seizures. Usually a benzodiazepine such as lorazepam, diazepam, or midazolam is administered to provide rapid control of seizures. Most patients respond to these measures. If seizures are not controlled or recur, administration of a benzodiazepine can be repeated or therapy with an antiepileptic drug can be initiated. New evidence suggests that phenytoin should be avoided when treating drug-induced seizures.[86] In the very rare situations in which patients do not respond to additional doses of a benzodiazepine, other agents such as short-acting barbiturates, general anesthetics, exceptionally high doses of a benzodiazepine, or other antiepileptic drugs may be used.

Benzodiazepines are usually effective in treating and preventing carbapenem-induced seizures, because benzodiazepines enhance GABA activity.[87] For patients with seizures induced by tricyclic antidepressants, benzodiazepines are the preferred drugs for treatment.[17] In this situation, phenytoin should be avoided, because of its lack of efficacy and the possibility of enhancing the arrhythmogenic effects of tricyclics. Benzodiazepines are recommended for the management of seizures induced by antimalarial drugs.[88] However, benzodiazepines may not be as effective for the management of theophylline-induced seizures.[89] Theophylline may antagonize the effects of benzodiazepines, rendering them less effective. Therefore, barbiturates are the preferred agents for treating theophylline-induced seizures. Loading doses of phenobarbital or pentobarbital, 5–15 mg/kg, should be administered, with additional loading doses given until seizures terminate.[90] Patients should be intubated and mechanically ventilated prior to initiation of intravenous doses of barbiturates because of the respiratory and cardiovascular adverse effects of these agents.

If it is determined that seizures are induced by an antineoplastic agent, the general recommendation is not to treat the seizures, when possible, but to adjust the cancer chemotherapy doses and regimen.[22] Care should also be taken to address underlying metabolic changes associated with antineoplastic drugs that can result in seizures. However, if there are other potential causes of the seizures, especially central nervous system tumors, ongoing use of antiepileptic therapy is indicated.

INFORMATION FOR PATIENTS

As drug-induced seizures are rare events and are usually very short in duration, education of all patients regarding the seizure risk when receiving potentially seizure-inducing drugs may not be productive. Individuals who are at increased risk for seizures should be advised regarding signs and symptoms. Caregivers should be instructed concerning first aid for seizures. If a seizure occurs, caregivers should protect the patient from self-injury or injuring others by laying the person on his or her side, placing a pillow under the head, making sure the airway remains clear, and helping the individual become reoriented once the seizure subsides. In addition, timing the duration of the seizure with a clock is important, and emergency medical care should be called if a seizure lasts longer than 5 minutes or when a seizure occurs in an individual without a history of seizures. Forcing objects into the patient's mouth or restraining the patient should never be attempted. In addition to instruction on managing seizures, individuals with a history of epilepsy should be advised to avoid medications that may cause seizures, particularly nonprescription drugs and herbal products, and to avoid abrupt discontinuation of antiepileptic agents.

REFERENCES

1. Fuzier R, Lapeyre-Mestre M, Samili K et al. Adverse drug reactions to local anaesthetics. *Drug Saf.* 2009; 32:345-56.
2. Borowicz KK, Banach M. Antiarrhythmic drugs and epilepsy. *Pharmacol Rep.* 2014; 66:545-51.
3. Ruffmann C, Boglium G, Beghi E. Epileptogenic drugs: a systematic review. *Exp Rev Neurother.* 2006; 6:575-89.
4. Nadvi S, Sarnaik S, Ravindranath Y. Low frequency of meperidine-associated seizures in sickly cell disease. *Clin Pediatr.* 1999; 38:459-62.
5. Kaiko RF, Foley KM, Gabrinski PY et al. Central nervous system excitatory effects of meperidine in cancer patients. *Ann Neurol.* 1983; 13:180-5.
6. Marquardt KA, Alsop JA, Albertson TE. Tramadol exposures reported to statewide poison control system. *Ann Pharmacother.* 2005; 39:1039-44.
7. Jovanovic-Cupic V, Martinovic Z, Nesic N. Seizures associated with intoxication and abuse of tramadol. *Clin Toxicol.* 2006; 44:143-6.
8. Walder B, Tramèr MR, Seeck M. Seizure-like phenomena and propofol. *Neurology.* 2002; 58:1327-32.
9. San-Juan D, Chiappa KH, Cole AJ. Propofol and the electroencephalogram. *Clin Neurophysiol.* 2010; 121:998-1006.
10. Yli-Hankala A, Vakkuri A, Särkelä M et al. Epileptiform electroencephalogram during mask induction of anesthesia with sevoflurane. *Anesthesiology.* 1999; 91:1596-603.
11. Vakkuri A, Yli-Hankala A, Särkelä M et al. Sevoflurane mask induction of anaesthesia is associated with epileptiform EEG in children. *Acta Anaesthesiol Scand.* 2001; 45:805-11.
12. Jääskeläinen SK, Kaisti K, Suni L et al. Sevoflurane is epileptogenic in healthy subjects at surgical levels of anesthesia. *Neurology.* 2003; 61:1073-8.
13. Calandra G, Lydick E, Carrigan J et al. Factors predisposing to seizures in seriously ill infected patients receiving antibiotics: experience with imipenem/cilastatin. *Am J Med.* 1988; 84:91-110.
14. Misra UK, Kalita J, Chandra S et al. Association of antibiotics with status epilepticus. *Neurol Sci.* 2013; 34:327-31.
15. Pesola GR, Avasarala J. Bupropion seizure proportion among new-onset generalized seizures and drug related seizures presenting to an emergency department. *J Emerg Med.* 2002; 22:235-9.
16. Pisani F, Spina E, Oteri G. Antidepressant drugs and seizure susceptibility: from in vitro data to clinical practice. *Epilepsia.* 1999; 40:S48-56.
17. Citak A, Soysal DD, Uçsel R et al. Seizures associated with poisoning in children: tricyclic antidepressant intoxication. *Pediatr Int.* 2006; 48:582-5.
18. Chaves J, Sander JW. Seizure aggravation in idiopathic generalized epilepsies. *Epilepsia.* 2005; 46:133-9.
19. Liporace JD, Sperling MR, Dichter MA. Absence seizures and carbamazepine in adults. *Epilepsia.* 1994; 35:1026-8.
20. DeToledo JC, Ramsay RE, Lowe MR et al. Increased seizures after discontinuing carbamazepine: results from the gabapentin monotherapy trial. *Ther Drug Monit.* 2000; 22:753-6.
21. Welty TE, Privitera M, Shukla R. Increased seizure frequency associated with felbamate withdrawal in adults. *Arch Neurol.* 1998; 55:641-5.
22. Gelisse P, Genton P, Kuate C et al. Worsening of seizures by oxcarbazepine in juvenile idiopathic generalized epilepsies. *Epilepsia.* 2004; 45:1282-6.
23. Taylor WRJ, White NJ. Antimalarial drug toxicity. *Drug Saf.* 2004; 27:25-61.
24. Singh G, Rees JH, Sander JW. Seizures and epilepsy in oncological practice: causes, course, mechanisms and treatment. *J Neurol Neurosurg Psychiatry.* 2007; 78:342-9.
25. Yeh KH, Cheng AL. High-dose 5-fluorouracil infusional therapy is associated with hyperammonaemia, lactic acidosis and encephalopathy. *Br J Cancer.* 1997; 75:464-5.
26. Furqaan AM, Jacobson IL, Herrera B et al. Seizures during pegylated interferon and ribavirin therapy for chronic hepatitis C: observations from the WIN-R trial. *J Clin Gastroenterol.* 2011; 45:286-92.
27. Eberly AL, Anderson GD, Bubalo JS et al. Optimal prevention of seizures induced by high-dose busullan. *Pharmacotherapy.* 2008; 28:1502-10.
28. Hedges D, Jeppson K, Whitehead P. Antipsychotic medication and seizures: a review. *Drugs Today.* 2003; 39:551-7.
29. Logothetis J. Spontaneous epileptic seizures and electroencephalographic changes in the course of phenothiazine therapy. *Neurology.* 1967; 17:869-77.
30. Pisani F, Oteri G, Costa C et al. Effects of psychotropic drugs on seizure threshold. *Drug Saf.* 2002; 25:91-110.
31. Devinsky O, Honigleld G, Patin J. Clozapine-related seizures. *Neurology.* 1991; 41:369-71.
32. Stimmel GL, Dopheide JA. Psychotropic drug-induced reductions in seizure threshold: incidence and consequences. *CNS Drugs.* 1996; 5:37-50.
33. Haller CA, Benowitz NL. Adverse cardiovascular and central nervous system events associated with dietary supplements containing ephedra alkaloids. *N Engl J Med.* 2000; 343:1833-8.
34. Spinella M. Herbal medicines and epilepsy: the potential for benefit and adverse effects. *Epilepsy Behav.* 2001; 2:524-32.
35. Samuels N, Finkelstein Y, Singer SR et al. Herbal medicine and epilepsy: proconvulsive effects and interactions with antiepileptic drugs. *Epilepsia.* 2008; 49:373-80.
36. Kashani J, Ruha AM. Isolated atomoxetine overdose resulting in seizure. *J Emerg Med.* 2007; 32:175-8.
37. Klein-Schwartz W. Abuse and toxicity of methylphenidate. *Curr Opin Pediatr.* 2002; 14:219-23.
38. Hauser WA, Beghi E. First seizure definitions and worldwide incidence and mortality. *Epilepsia.* 2008; 49:8-12.
39. Lowenstein DH, Alldredge BK. Status epilepticus at an urban public hospital in the 1980s. *Neurology.* 1993; 43:483-8.
40. Pesola GR, Avasarala J. Bupropion seizure propogation among new-onset generalized seizures and drug related seizures presenting to an emergency department. *J Emerg Med.* 2002; 22:235-9.
41. Finkelstein Y, Hutson JR, Freedman SB et al. Drug-induced seizures in children and adolescents presenting for emergency care: Current and emerging trends. *Clin Toxicol.* 2013; 51:761-6.
42. Boston Collaborative Drug Surveillance Program. Drug-induced convulsions. *Lancet.* 1972; 2:677-9.
43. DeLorenzo RJ, Hauser WA, Towne A et al. A prospective, population-based epidemiologic study of status epilepticus in Richmond, Virginia. *Neurology.* 1996; 46:1029-35.
44. Olson KR, Kearney TE, Dyer JE et al. Seizures associated with poisoning and drug overdose. *Am J Emerg Med.* 1994; 12:392-5.
45. Thundiyil JG, Kearney TE, Olson KR. Evolving epidemiology of drug-induced seizures reported to a poison control center system. *J Med Toxicol.* 2007; 3:15-19.
46. Wong VK, Wright HT Jr, Ross LA et al. Imipenem/cilastatin treatment of bacterial meningitis in children. *Pediatr Infect Dis J.* 1991; 10:122-5.
47. Schmutzhard E, Williams KJ, Vukmirovits G et al. A randomised comparison of meropenem with cefotaxime or ceftriaxone for the treatment of bacterial meningitis in adults. Meropenem Meningitis Study Group. *Antimicrob Chemother.* 1995; 36:85-97.
48. Odio CM, Puig JR, Feris JM et al.; Meropenem Meningitis Study Group. Prospective, randomized, investigator-blinded study of the efficacy and safety of meropenem vs. cefotaxime therapy in bacterial meningitis in children. *Pediatr Infect Dis J.* 1999; 18:581-90.

49. Misra UK, Kalita, J, Chandra S et al. Association of antibiotics with status epilepticus. *Neurol Sci.* 2013; 34:327-31.
50. Minns AB, Ghafouri N, Clark RF. Isoniazid-induced status epileptics in a pediatric patient after inadequate pyridoxine therapy. *Pediatri Emerg Care.* 2010; 26:380-81.
51. Douros A, Grabowski K, Stahlmann R. Safety issues and drug-drug interactions with commonly used quinolones. *Expert Opin Drug Metabol Toxicol.* 2015; 11:25-39.
52. Ellison DW, Pentel PR. Clinical features and consequences of seizures due to cyclic antidepressant overdose. *Am J Emerg Med.* 1989; 7:5-10.
53. Isbister GK, Bowe SJ, Dawson A et al. Relative toxicity of selective serotonin reuptake inhibitors (SSRIs) in overdose. *J Toxicol Clin Toxicol.* 2004; 42:277-85.
54. Ortmann E, Besser MW, Klein AA. Antifibrinolytic agents in current anaesthetic practice. *Br J Anaesth.* 2013; 111:549-63.
55. Sharma V, Katznelson R, Jerath A et al. The association between tranexamic acid and convulsive seizures after cardiac surgery: a multivariate analysis. *Amaestjesoa.* 2014; 69:124-30.
56. Lecker I, Wang DS, Whissell PD et al. Tranexamic acid-associated seizures: causes and treatment. *Annal Neurol.* 2016; 79:18-26.
57. Clouston PD, DeAngelis LM, Posner JB. The spectrum of neurological disease in patients with systemic cancer. *Ann Neurol.* 1992; 31:26S-273.
58. DiMario FJ Jr, Packer RJ. Acute mental status changes in children with systemic cancer. *Pediatrics.* 1990; S5:353-60.
59. Wu M, Fang M, Hu Y et al. Four types of traditional Chinese medicine inducing epileptic seizures. *Seizure.* 2012; 21:311-5.
60. Chan K, Zhang H, Lin ZX. An overview on adverse drug reactions to traditional Chinese medicines. *Br J Clin Pharmacol.* 2014; 80:834-3.
61. Hemmer SA, Pasternak JF, Zecker SG et al. Stimulant therapy and seizure risk in children with ADHD. *Pediatr Neurol.* 2001; 24:99-102.
62. Wernicke JF, Holdridge KC, Jin L et al. Seizure risk in patients with attention-deficit-hyperactivity disorder treated with atomoxetine. *Dev Med Child Neurol.* 2007; 49:498-502.
63. De Sarro G, Ammendola D, Nava F et al. Effects of some excitatory amino acid antagonists on imipenem-induced seizures in DBA/2 mice. *Brain Res.* 1995; 671:131-40.
64. Lowry JA, Jarrett RV, Wasserman et al. Theophylline toxicokinetics in premature newborns. *Arch Pediatr Adolesc Med.* 2001; 155:934-9.
65. van Kuilenburg AB. Dihydropyrimidine dehydrogenase and the efficacy and toxicity of 5-fluorouracil. *Eur J Cancer.* 2004; 40:939-50.
66. Ascher JA, Cole JO, Colin JN et al. Bupropion: a review of its mechanism of antidepressant activity. *J Clin Psychiatry.* 1995; 56:395-401.
67. Lyass O, Lossos A, Hubert A et al. Cisplatin-induced nonconvulsive encephalopathy. *Anticancer Drugs.* 1998; 9:100-4.
68. Erer B, Polchi P, Lucarelli G et al. CsA-associated neurotoxicity and ineffective prophylaxis with clonazepam in patients transplanted for thalassemia major: analysis of risk factors. *Bone Marrow Transplant.* 1996; 18:157-62.
69. Mehlhorn AJ, Brown DA. Safety concerns with fluoroquinolones. *Ann Pharmacother.* 2007; 41:1859-66.
70. Calvet MC, Gresser I. Interferon enhances the excitability of cultured neurons. *Nature.* 1979; 278:558-60.
71. Wood JD, Peesker SJ. The effect on GABA metabolism in brain of isonicotinic acid hydrazide and pyridoxine as a junction of time after administration. *J Neurochem.* 1972; 19:1527-37.
72. Bonner AB, Peterson SL, Weir MR. Seizures induced by theophylline and isoniazid in mice. *Vet Hum Toxicol.* 1999; 41:175-7.
73. Baumann PA, Maitre L. Neurobiochemical aspects of maprotiline (Ludiomil) action. *J Int Med Res.* 1979; 7:391-400.
74. Price RA, Birdwell DA. The central nervous system in childhood leukaemia. III. Mineralizing microangiopathy and dystrophic calcification. *Cancer.* 1978; 42:717-28.
75. Itil TM, Soldatos C. Epileptogenic side effects of psychotropic drugs: practical recommendations. *JAMA.* 1980; 244:1460-3.
76. Ebert U. Basic mechanisms of psychotropic drugs. *Epilepsia.* 2002; 43:2-7.
77. Pirzada NA, Ali II, Dafer RM. Fluorouracil-induced neurotoxicity. *Ann Pharmacother.* 2000; 34:35-8.
78. Stilman N, Masdeu JC. Incidence of seizures with phenytoin toxicity. *Neurology.* 1995; 35:1769-72.
79. Anand JS, Chodorowski Z, Wisniewski M. Seizures induced by topiramate overdose (letter). *Clin Toxicol (Phila).* 2007; 45:197.
80. Owens RC Jr, Ambrose PG. Antimicrobial safety: locus on fluoroquinolones. *Clin Infect Dis.* 2005; 41:S144-57.
81. Owens RC Jr, Ambrose PG. Clinical use of the fluoroquinolones. *Med Clin North Am.* 2000; 84:1447-69.
82. Sessler CN. Theophylline toxicity: clinical features of 116 consecutive cases. *Am J Med.* 1990; 88:567-76.
83. Constant I, Seeman R. Inhalational anesthetics in pediatric anesthesia. *Curr Opin Anaesthesiol.* 2005; 18:277-81.
84. Fish DR, Espir ML. Convulsions associated with prophylactic antimalarial drugs: implications for people with epilepsy. *BML.* 1988; 297:526-7.
85. Koch-Stoecker S. Antipsychotic drugs and epilepsy: indications and treatment guidelines. *Epilepsia.* 2002; 43:19-24.
86. Chen HY, Albertson TE, Olson KR. Treatment of drug-induced seizures. *Brit J Clin Pharmacol.* 2016; 81:412-9.
87. Koppel BS, Hauser WA, Politis C et al. Seizures in the critically ill: the role of imipenem. *Epilepsia.* 2001; 42:1590-3.
88. Marquardt K, Albertson TE. Treatment of hydroxychloroquine overdose. *Am J Emerg Med.* 2001; 19:420-4.
89. Yoshikawa H. First-line therapy for theophylline-associated seizures. *Ada Neurol Scand.* 2007; 186:57-61.
90. Willmore LJ. Epilepsy emergencies: the first seizure and status epilepticus. *Neurology.* 1998; 51:S34-8.

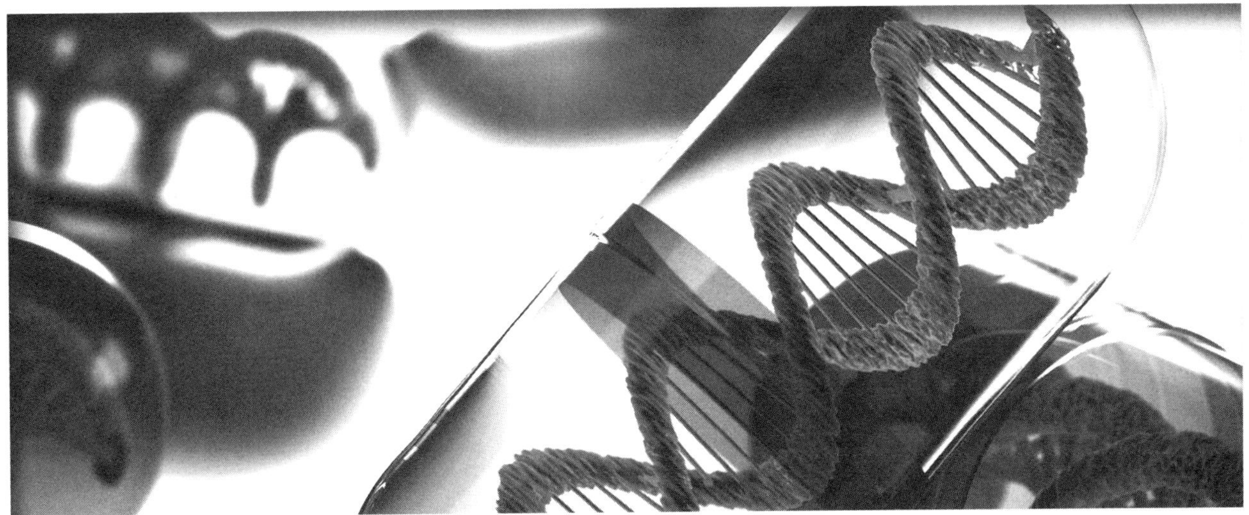

CHAPTER 11

Stroke

Denise H. Rhoney

Stroke, the fifth leading cause of death in the United States, refers to a sudden onset of focal neurologic deficit.[1,2] There are two main types of stroke: ischemic and hemorrhagic. Drugs should always be considered as a possible etiology of either type of stroke. A secondary cause of drug-induced stroke could be associated with medications that induce other diseases discussed elsewhere in this text that are also risk factors for stroke, such as hypertension, hyperlidemia, or atrial fibrillation.

ISCHEMIC STROKE

CAUSATIVE AGENTS

Drugs that have been reported to cause ischemic stroke are listed in **Table 11-1**.[3-53] Many of the agents listed in the table have been associated with both ischemic and hemorrhagic stroke. For many medications, the potential association with drug-induced stroke is controversial.

There is substantial controversy as to whether oral contraceptives are a cause of stroke. Many studies have attempted to assess the possible relationship between oral contraceptives and stroke, but the results are contradictory. Higher-dose formulations have been shown to increase the risk of stroke in specific subgroups of patients: smokers; those with hypertension; age >35 years; prior history of stroke; those with hyperlipidemia; and those with a history of migraine headaches. Although the potential increased risk of stroke appears to be diminished with lower-dose formulations of oral contraceptives, meta-analyses have reported conflicting results.[54,55] Therefore, oral contraceptives should be used with caution in women at risk for stroke.[56-58] The rate of ischemic stroke among users of the norelgestromin/ethinyl estradiol (Ortho EVRA) contraceptive patch is 13.6/100,000 woman–years, which is similar to the stroke rate in users of norgestimate-containing oral contraceptives (11.3/1000,000 woman–years).[59]

Data from postmenopausal women receiving hormone replacement therapy with estrogen provide some additional information regarding the risk of stroke in patients receiving oral contraceptives. In the Women's Health Initiative, a randomized trial of 16,500 generally healthy postmenopausal women, the combination of estrogen and progestin increased the relative risk of ischemic stroke by 44%.[60] Although patients in this trial were relatively healthy, they were substantially older than typical patients

Table 11-1 Agents Implicated in Drug-Induced Ischemic Stroke

Agent	Incidence	Level of Evidence[a]
Alcohol abuse (≥5 drinks daily)[3,4]	RR 1.69, 95% CI 1.34–2.15	B
Amphetamines[5-7]	NK	C
Cisplatin[8-15]	0.137%	B
Cocaine[6,16-23]	NK	B
Ecstasy[6,24]	NK	C
Haloperidol[25]	6.43 per 1,000 person-years	B
Heroin[4,6,26]	NK	C
Hormone replacement in postmenopausal women[27]	RR 1.31, 95% CI 1.02–1.68	A
Intranasal phenoxazoline or oxymetazoline[28]	NK	C
Intravenous immunoglobulin[29]	NK	C
Isometheptene mucate[30]	NK	C
Marijuana[4,31]	NK	C
Methylphenidate[6]	NK	C
Nicotine[4,32,33]	25% RR 1.8, 95% CI 1.3–3.6	A
Nonsteroidal anti-inflammatory agents[34-36]	NK	B
Olanzapine[37-39,b]	NK	C
Oral contraceptives (women age 25–44 years >50 mcg estradiol)[40,41]	0.9–10/100,000 RR 2.8, 95% CI 1.2–4.4	B
Prothrombin complex concentrate[42-44]	1.9%	A
Recombinant factor VIIa[45]	NK[b]	B
Risperidone[25,37,38,c]	2.88 per 1,000 person-years	B
Selective serotonin reuptake inhibitors[46-50,d]	OR 1.48, 95% CI 1.08–2.02	B
Serotonin–norepinephrine reuptake inhibitors[48,d]	NK	B
Sumatriptan[3,51]	NK	C
Tamoxifen[52,53]	RR 1.49, 95% CI 1.16–1.90	B

CI = confidence interval, NK = not known, OR = odds ratio, RR = relative risk.
[a]Definitions for Levels of Evidence: Level A—evidence from one or more randomized, controlled clinical trials; Level B—evidence from nonrandomized clinical trials, prospective observational studies, cohort studies, retrospective studies, case-control studies, meta-analyses and/or postmarketing surveillance studies; and Level C—evidence from one or more published case reports or case series.
[b]Primarily reported in patients with dementia; total of 39 cases reported.
[c]A total of 151 thromboembolic events reported with rFVIIa in Food and Drug Administration Adverse Event Reporting System.
[d]Primarily reported with high doses.

receiving therapy with oral contraceptives; therefore, it may not be appropriate to draw inferences from these results regarding the risk of stroke associated with oral contraceptive therapy in younger patients.

In December 2004, the U.S. Food and Drug Administration (FDA) issued a health advisory concerning the use of nonsteroidal anti-inflammatory agents (NSAIDs) and cyclooxygenase (COX)-2 selective drugs.[36] There is evidence that these agents increase the risk for myocardial infarction and stroke when used for extended periods of time or in high-risk settings (such as immediately after cardiac surgery).[34] In 2004 and 2005, respectively, rofecoxib and valdecoxib were withdrawn from the U.S. market. A National Institutes of Health (NIH) clinical trial with celecoxib was suspended due to increased cardiovascular events, but the drug was not removed from the market. However, the FDA recommends the use of other agents or the lowest effective dose and required the addition of a "black box" warning to the labeling. Additionally, the NIH halted an Alzheimer disease trial that showed an increase in the risk of cardiovascular events in patients receiving naproxen but not celecoxib.[35] Recently the extended follow-up data from the Adenomatous Polyp PRevention On Vioxx study found an increased risk of ischemic stroke associated with rofecoxib compared to placebo and reported that 7 of the 18 ischemic strokes occurred after rofecoxib therapy had been discontinued.[34] This finding raises concern regarding the risk of stroke in patients who have a previous exposure to rofecoxib. The FDA-issued public health advisory is as follows[36]:

1. Physicians prescribing COX-2 selective agents should consider this emerging information when weighing the benefits against risks for individual patients. Patients who are at a high risk of gastrointestinal bleeding, have a history of intolerance to nonselective NSAIDs, or are not doing well on nonselective NSAIDs may be appropriate candidates for COX-2 selective agents.
2. Individual patient risk for cardiovascular events and other risks commonly associated with NSAIDs should be taken into account for each prescribing situation.
3. Consumers are advised that all nonprescription pain medications, including NSAIDs, should be used in strict accordance with the label directions. If an NSAID is needed for longer than 10 days, a physician should be consulted.

The American Heart Association (AHA) has recommended a stepped-care approach for the management of musculoskeletal symptoms in patients with risk factors or known cardiovascular disease.[35,61]

EPIDEMIOLOGY

The most common type of nondrug-induced stroke is ischemic, which accounts for 85% of all cases. Of ischemic strokes, 65% are atherothrombotic with the remainder cardioembolic in origin. The overall incidence of drug-induced stroke is unknown, but generally considered to be low. In young adults (<50 years of age) drug-related etiologies can be identified in 15–38% of ischemic strokes.[6,62] Illicit drug use, particularly cocaine, is commonly implicated in younger patients who lack other known vascular risk factors. Since the emergence of the more potent alkaloidal cocaine ("crack"), there has been a significant increase in the number of case reports of cocaine-associated stroke.[63] The incidence of all drug-induced strokes may be on the rise.[6] The incidence of stroke associated with specific agents is presented in Table 11-1.

Table 11-2 Mechanisms of Drug-Induced Ischemic Stroke

Drug	Mechanism(s)
Intravenous drugs of abuse (e.g., heroin) Cocaine Methylphenidate (from injection of oral product) Tamoxifen	Cerebral embolism
Cocaine Amphetamines Methylphenidate Sumatriptan SSRI SNRI	Vasoconstriction/vasospasm
Amphetamines Cocaine Alcohol Caffeine Cigarette smoking	Acute hypertension
Heroin Cocaine Amphetamines	Vasculitis
Cocaine Cigarette smoking Nonsteroidal anti-inflammatory agents Cisplatin	Induces direct vascular damage and subsequently promotes platelet aggregation and vasoconstriction
Olanzapine Risperidone	Orthostatic hypotension

SSRI = selective serotonin reuptake inhibitor, SNRI = serotonin norepinephrine reuptake inhibitor.

MECHANISMS

There are many proposed mechanisms for drug-induced strokes. Mechanisms by which drugs result in stroke may be multifactorial and are discussed below and presented in **Table 11-2**.

EMBOLIC MECHANISMS

Embolism can produce a stroke when a clot, plaque, platelet aggregate, or foreign body breaks off into the circulation and obstructs a cerebral artery. Intravenous drugs of abuse (i.e., heroin) can be associated with cerebral infarction due to embolic vessel occlusion, infective endocarditis, or hemorrhage due to rupture of a septic (mycotic) aneurysm. Stroke is a complication in about 20% of patients with infective endocarditis. Cocaine and other drugs may cause heart disease, which results in release of emboli to the brain. Foreign body emboli, primarily from talc fillers, have been reported after injection of agents intended for oral administration (i.e., methylphenidate).[64] Foreign substances injected into the systemic circulation may embed in the lung, resulting in granulomatous reactions that ultimately provide a path for this foreign material to reach the brain. Tamoxifen may be associated with a paradoxical embolism and subsequent cerebral venous thrombosis.[53]

VASOCONSTRICTION/VASOSPASM

Systemic vasoconstriction can lead to hypertension and intracerebral hemorrhage (ICH), whereas cerebral vasoconstriction can lead to infarction. Vasoconstriction may be transient or prolonged. Vasospasm with subsequent cerebral infarction may occur in association with cocaine, amphetamines, phenylpropanolamine, ephedrine, and methylphenidate.[65] Cocaine temporarily causes vasoconstriction, thus reducing blood supply to various brain regions. Cocaine may potentiate the effects of serotonin by blocking its reuptake, resulting in vasoconstriction.[66] In addition, cocaine exerts direct effects on calcium channels leading to release of intracellular calcium in cerebral vascular smooth muscle cells.[63] Other possible mechanisms of cocaine-induced vasospasm are via endothelin-1 release and reuptake of dopamine at presynaptic nerve terminals. There appears to be a cumulative effect of cocaine exposure and the risk of stroke.[63] The use of selective serotonin reuptake inhibitors and serotonin-norepinephrine reuptake inhibitors can cause vasoconstrictive stroke (Call–Fleming syndrome) or vasospasm.[46,47] Underlying atherosclerosis may augment this vasoconstriction. Sumatriptan binds to a particular subpopulation of 5-hydroxytryptamine (5-HT_1) receptors in the pia and dural vessels, leading to vasconstriction.[67] Subcutaneous administration of sumatriptan has been shown to result in vasoconstriction of the middle cerebral and internal carotid arteries within 30 minutes.[68] There have been case reports of stroke associated with triptan use; however, patients with migraine are also at increased risk of stroke.[69]

ACUTE HYPERTENSION

The primary mechanism of hypertension-associated drug-induced stroke is drug effects on neurotransmitters. Many drugs increase catecholamine release from central noradrenergic nerve terminals (i.e., amphetamines, ephedra, nonprescription sympathomimetics), block reuptake of catecholamines into adrenergic nerve terminals (i.e., cocaine), or increase plasma catecholamine concentrations (i.e., ethanol, cocaine). Hypertension related to drug use may disrupt cerebral autoregulation, promote reperfusion of brain tissue, or damage cerebral arterioles leading to hemorrhage. Cigarette smoking acutely elevates blood pressure and reduces cerebral blood flow.[70-72] Alcohol acutely and chronically increases blood pressure related to increased adrenergic activity and increased plasma concentrations of cortisol, renin, aldosterone, and vasopressin.[73-75]

VASCULITIS

Inflammation of small-, medium-, and large-size intracranial arteries and subsequent development of arteritis is a reported mechanism of stroke induced by drugs such as heroin, amphetamines, cocaine, ephedra, and pseudoephedrine.[76] These agents are associated with an inflammatory vasculopathy and vessel wall necrosis.[77]

CLOTTING DERANGEMENTS

Platelets play an important role in the development of thrombosis. With endothelial damage, vessel collagen can be exposed to blood, and acts as a triggering mechanism for platelet activation, resulting in release of adenosine diphosphate from the platelets, causing platelets to aggregate. Thromboxane A_2 is produced, which also promotes platelet aggregation and vasoconstriction. Cocaine may stimulate platelet aggregation and inhibit prostacyclin.[78] Cigarette smoking aggravates atherosclerosis and increases arterial wall stiffness, ultimately increasing the likelihood of plaque formation. Smoking increases platelet reactivity and inhibits prostacyclin formation.[79] Alcohol consumption may elevate blood pressure and interfere with platelet function; chronic use may result in coagulation abnormalities due to liver impairment. Nonsteroidal anti-inflammatory agents act primarily via inhibition of COX, which consists of 2 major isoenzymes (COX-1 and COX-2). Experimental evidence suggests that inhibition of COX-2 results in a shift in the prothrombotic/antithorombotic balance toward thrombosis. The differential biological effects of these agents are a result of the degree of selectivity for COX-2 versus COX-1.[35] Cisplatin induces direct endovascular damage and also indirect damage via free radical-induced lipid peroxidation. An increase in plasma concentrations of von Willebrand factor has been reported during cisplatin chemotherapy regimens and is evidence of direct endovascular damage leading to platelet aggregation and vasoconstriction.[80] In addition, cisplatin may reduce activity of the anticoagulant protein C.[13]

ORTHOSTATIC HYPOTENSION

A potential mechanism for stroke associated with atypical antipsychotic agents is orthostatic hypotension leading to "watershed" strokes. Hyperprolactinemia induced by these drugs may also result in promotion of platelet aggregation.[81]

CLINICAL PRESENTATION AND DIFFERENTIAL DIAGNOSIS

Clinically, it is difficult to distinguish drug-induced stroke from nondrug-induced etiologies. The diagnosis of drug-induced stroke is often made by exclusion of other causes, or through serum or urine drug testing. The typical patient experiencing a stroke presents with an abrupt onset of neurologic deficits, which can include hemiparesis, speech disturbance, hemisensory loss, monocular or visual field loss, and/or ataxia. The clinical presentation of both ischemic stroke and ICH is dependent on the anatomical location of the infarction. It is not possible to distinguish an ischemic stroke from ICH based on clinical examination alone, although several characteristics are more indicative of ICH, including headache, impaired level of consciousness, nausea and vomiting, and extreme elevations of blood pressure. Subarachnoid hemorrhage must be suspected in a patient who experiences a sudden new severe headache. Drug-induced stroke can occur at any time during therapy with a potentially causative agent. Common signs and symptoms of drug-induced ischemic stroke are presented in **Table 11-3**.

Table 11-3 Signs and Symptoms Associated with Drug-Induced Ischemic Stroke

Signs	Symptoms
Anterior cerebral artery occlusion	Contralateral hemiparesis Confusion Gait apraxia
Middle cerebral artery blockage	Contralateral hemiparesis Dysarthria Hemianesthesia Contralateral homonymous hemianopia Aphasia Apraxia Sensory neglect
Posterior cerebral artery blockage	Contralateral homonymous hemianopia Unilateral cortical blindness Memory loss Unilateral 3rd cranial nerve palsy
Ophthalmic artery blockage	Monocular loss of vision
Vertebrobasilar system blockage	Unilateral or bilateral cranial nerve deficits (e.g. nystagmus, vertigo, dysphagia, dysarthria, diplopia, blindness) Ataxia Impaired consciousness Coma

Drug-induced stroke must be distinguished from stroke due to other etiologies. Conditions to consider in the differential diagnosis of drug-induced stroke are presented in **Table 11-4**. It is difficult to distinguish between drug-induced and nondrug-induced causes of stroke unless symptoms are temporally related to the ingestion of substances of abuse or agents with surrogate monitoring parameters (i.e., drug screen) that can quantitatively be assessed.

Table 11-4 Conditions to Consider in the Differential Diagnosis of Drug-Induced Ischemic Stroke

- Brain tumor
- Cerebral abscess
- Cerebral hemorrhage
- Cranial trauma
- Encephalitis
- Malingering/somatization
- Meningitis
- Metabolic encephalopathy (hypoglycemia, diabetic keto-acidosis, hyperosmolar coma, hepatic encephalopathy, renal failure, hypercapnia, sepsis)
- Migraine headache
- Peripheral neuropathy
- Postcardiac arrest ischemia
- Psychiatric symptoms
- Seizure disorder (with postictal paralysis)
- Syncope

Diagnosis of stroke consists of a thorough evaluation of patient history, clinical examination, laboratory evaluation, and imaging studies, including computerized tomography (CT) scan, cerebral angiography, and magnetic resonance imaging (MRI). Laboratory studies should consist of serum electrolyte and glucose concentrations, complete blood count, coagulation parameters, and drug screen evaluation. A CT scan is essential to differentiate between ischemic and hemorrhagic stroke.

RISK FACTORS

Risk factors for drug-induced stroke are presented in **Table 11-5**. An underlying history of hypertension is one of the most common risk factors. In addition, any patient with other risk factors for stroke is at a higher risk for drug-induced stroke. The Framingham study identified five factors that placed the general population at increased risk of ischemic stroke: elevated systolic blood pressure, elevated serum cholesterol concentration, glucose intolerance, cigarette smoking, and left ventricular hypertrophy by electrocardiogram.[82] Risk factors for ischemic stroke have been outlined in recent guidelines from the American Stroke Association/AHA.[83]

Table 11-5 Risk Factors for Drug-Induced Ischemic Stroke[83]

- Concurrent caffeine use
- Concurrent tobacco use
- Dementia
- Diabetes
- Elderly
- Exposure to drugs of abuse
- High doses of potentially causative agents
- History of vascular events
- Hypertension
- Migraine headaches with aura
- Physical inactivity
- Polydrug use
- Pregnancy
- Previous stroke

MORBIDITY AND MORTALITY

Stroke is one of the most devastating diseases, yet one of the most preventable. The overall direct and indirect economic impact of stroke is approximately $40.9 billion annually.[84] Stroke is the fifth leading cause of death in the United States and a leading cause of disability in hospitalized patients.[1,2] Long-term sequelae of a stroke, whether induced by drugs or other etiologies, include: memory loss, depression, behavioral changes, emotional lability, difficulty performing activities of daily living, communication problems, paralysis, and neglect on the side of the body corresponding to the location of the stroke.

PREVENTION

The most effective means of prevention of drug-induced stroke is avoidance of agents known to be associated with stroke, especially in high-risk patients. Strategies for prevention of drug-induced stroke are listed in **Table 11-6**.[83] Drug-induced stroke may also be prevented by minimizing other risk factors for ischemic stroke (e.g., hypertension, hyperlipidemia, smoking, diabetes). However, the mainstay of prevention is patient education and identification of risk factors, particularly in those patients that are at high risk.

Table 11-6 Approaches to Help Prevent Drug-Induced Ischemic Stroke[83]

Drug	Condition	Prevention
Alcohol	Moderation	Men should consume no more than 2 drinks/day and nonpregnant women should consume no more than 1 drink/day Control hypertension
All drugs	General risk factor reduction	Control of hypertension Glucose control Cholesterol-lowering therapy Weight management Atrial fibrillation management Sleep apnea management Physical activity Discontinue drugs known to be associated with stroke in patients at high risk
Cigarette smoking	Smoking cessation	Encourage patient and family to stop smoking Provide counseling, nicotine replacement and formal programs
Drug abuse	Cessation	Rehabilitation program
Hormone replacement therapy	Avoid use for primary prevention of stroke	If used for other indications the patient should be informed of vascular risks
NSAID	Musculoskeletal pain	Refer to scientific statement for stepped care approach recommendations[50]
Oral contraceptive use	Avoid in those at high risk	Inform patients about stroke risk and encourage alternative forms of birth control among women who smoke cigarettes, have migraines (especially with older age or smoking), are >35 years of age, or have had prior thromboembolic events
SSRI/SNRI	Possibly dose-related	Use lowest effective dose for all indications

NSAID = nonsteroidal anti-inflammatory drug, SNRI = serotonin norepinephrine reuptake inhibitor, SSRI = selective serotonin reuptake inhibitor.

MANAGEMENT

The management of any stroke patient includes many phases: prevention of stroke or other vascular disease; supportive and medical management during the acute phase; measures to mitigate the ongoing pathologic process; and rehabilitation. In addition, discontinuation of the offending agent (if identified) is essential.

Approaches to treatment of drug-induced acute ischemic stroke are similar to those of stroke due to other etiologies (please refer to treatment guidelines published for the acute management of ischemic stroke).[85] Hospital admission is indicated for any patient presenting with an acute stroke. Neurologic progression and cardiac sequelae are common in the early stages of a stroke. Preventing and recognizing secondary complications such as aspiration pneumonia and pulmonary embolism are essential. The only proven specific treatment for acute ischemic stroke at present is the thrombolytic agent recombinant tissue plasminogen activator (rt-PA). In appropriately selected patients, rt-PA significantly increases the likelihood of a good neurologic recovery.[86,87] To be eligible for rt-PA therapy, patients should have a well-described time of symptom onset within 4.5 hours of initiation of rt-PA treatment. Every effort should be made to shorten any delays in the initiation of treatment, because earlier treatment is associated with increased outcome benefits. The dose of rt-PA for stroke is 0.9 mg/kg intravenously over 1 hour, 10% as an initial bolus. The maximum total dose is 90 mg. During the first 24 hours after treatment, therapy with antithrombotic agents such as heparin and aspirin should be withheld, blood pressure should be strictly maintained at

<180/105 mm Hg, and close neurologic and cardiac monitoring should be performed in an intensive care unit or stroke unit.[85]

The new guidelines also include recommendations for endovascular interventions including mechanical thrombectomy and intra-arterial thrombolysis.[85] If a patient meets criteria for undergoing endovascular therapy, this should be considered in addition to receiving rt-PA, and the patient should be transferred to a comprehensive stroke center. The guidelines recommend that patients should undergo endovascular therapy with a stent retriever if they meet the following criteria: prestroke modified Rankin score of 0 to 1; acute ischemic stroke with receipt of intravenous rt-PA within 4.5 hours of symptom onset; causative occlusion of the internal carotid artery or proximal (M1) middle cerebral artery; age 18 years or older; NIH Stroke Scale (NIHSS) score of 6 or greater; Alberta Stroke Program Early CT score of 6 or greater; and treatment that can be initiated (groin puncture) within 6 hours of symptom onset.[85] Other recommendations suggest that intra-arterial rt-PA could be administered in carefully selected patients who have contraindications to the use of intravenous rt-PA and that endovascular approaches may be reasonable in patients who do not meet the criteria listed above.[85]

Fever (temperature >38°C) and glucose disorders should be treated aggressively in patients with acute stroke because both conditions exacerbate cerebral ischemia and may worsen neurologic outcome.[88] A twofold increase in short-term mortality has been reported in patients with hyperthermia within the first 24 hours of hospitalization with acute stroke.[88] Persistent in-hospital hyperglycemia during the first 24 hours is associated with worse outcomes when compared to normoglycemia; therefore, hyperglycemia treatment to achieve a target blood glucose range of 140–180 mg/dL is recommended. Additionally, hypoglycemia (blood glucose <60 mg/dL) should be treated.[85]

Arterial blood pressure is a dynamic parameter that may fluctuate substantially and is associated with clinical consequences. Studies have found a U-shaped relationship between admission blood pressure and favorable clinical outcomes, with optimal systolic and diastolic blood pressure ranges of 121–200 mm Hg and 81–110 mm Hg, respectively.[89] In-hospital elevations in blood pressure immediately following acute stroke have shown an inverse relationship to outcome; that is, increased blood pressure is associated with worse outcomes.[90,91] The appropriateness of treating acute hypertension in patients who do not qualify for reperfusion therapies is challenging. In fact, lowering blood pressure excessively may exacerbate cerebral ischemia in patients experiencing stroke. In many patients, blood pressure spontaneously decreases during the first 24 hours following a stroke. The most recent guidelines recommend, for patients not receiving reperfusion therapies, withholding of antihypertensive therapy unless the systolic pressure is >220 mm Hg or the diastolic pressure is >120 mm Hg. If antihypertensive therapy is initiated in patients who exceed these thresholds, then it is reasonable to lower blood pressure by 15% from baseline during the first 24 hours.[85]

If antihypertensive therapy is needed in the acute stage of drug-induced stroke, intravenous agents should be used, particularly those for which doses can be easily titrated. Labetalol may be administered initially as intravenous boluses of 10–20 mg until the desired blood pressure is achieved. Labetalol should be avoided in patients with contraindications to β-blockers. Nicardipine therapy may be initiated as a continuous intravenous infusion of 5 mg/hr, and the infusion rate can be adjusted to achieve the desired blood pressure. Other agents may also be useful depending on the clinical situation.[85]

After the acute phase of a drug-induced stroke, risk factor management is essential.[92] The appropriate specific preventive agent may be aspirin, clopidogrel, combination aspirin/extended-release dipyridamole, or an oral anticoagulant. Of these, aspirin is the most frequently prescribed for thrombotic causes of stroke. There is a lack of consensus regarding the optimal dose for stroke prevention. Doses of 50–325 mg have been shown to be effective. For patients with cardioembolic sources of stroke including atrial fibrillation, oral anticoagulation is recommended. For those with nonvalvular atrial fibrillation the guidelines currently recommend warfarin, apixaban, dabigatran, or rivaroxaban as reasonable options. Dose selection of these newer target-specific oral anticoagulants should be performed with careful attention to kidney function and drug interactions. Warfarin is indicated for patients with atrial fibrillation associated with valvular disease. The standard target range for the international normalized ratio (INR) is 2–3, however, patients with mechanical prosthetic valves may require a higher INR (2.5–3.5), but this places them at increased risk for ICH. In addition, any other risk factor that may be present (e.g., hyperlipidemia, hypertension, diabetes) should be managed aggressively. Please refer to secondary prevention guidelines for specific recommendations.[92]

INFORMATION FOR PATIENTS

Risk factor assessment is essential for prevention of drug-induced stroke. Because patients do not obtain many of the drugs known to cause stroke at pharmacies, it is extremely important that patients at risk are counseled to consult healthcare professionals before purchasing nonprescription drugs. For example, patients with hypertension should be advised that cough and cold medicines or herbal products might contain sympathomimetic drugs that could place them at increased risk for drug-induced stroke. Patients should be instructed to inform their healthcare professionals of all medications that they are taking, to facilitate a full evaluation of potential agents that may be associated with drug-induced stroke. Because medications that may induce stroke include a large number of recreational drugs of abuse, appropriate counseling regarding risks associated with these agents should be performed and referral to rehabilitation programs should be considered. In addition, all patients should be counseled regarding the signs and symptoms of and risk factors for drug-induced ischemic stroke and should be instructed to seek medical attention at the onset of symptoms.

INTRACEREBRAL HEMORRHAGE

CAUSATIVE AGENTS

ICH describes bleeding into the brain parenchyma with possible extension into the ventricular system or subarachnoid space. This chapter will focus on ICH, although studies provide information for hemorrhagic stroke, which includes ICH and subarachnoid hemorrhage; therefore, the term *hemorrhagic stroke* will be used when applicable. Drugs that have been reported to cause hemorrhagic stroke are listed in **Table 11-7**.[4,6,16,20,26,47,50,86,87,93-162] Many of the agents that are associated with ICH are used as therapeutic agents for other disease states. Symptomatic ICH is one of the most feared complications associated with the use of rt-PA for ischemic stroke and occurs in approximately 6% of treated patients. It is estimated that for every 100 patients treated with rt-PA, one will experience severe disability or death associated with symptomatic ICH.[163] Most patients who experience this devastating complication have more severe baseline infarcts.[163-165] Other risk factors for symptomatic ICH associated with rt-PA will be discussed later in the chapter (i.e., Table 11-11).

Vitamin K antagonists (warfarin) have been the standard of care for the treatment of thromboembolic diseases for many years. Target-specific oral anticoagulants (dabigatran, rivaroxaban, apixaban, edoxaban) have been developed and found to be at least noninferior to warfarin (target INR 2–3). The rate of major bleeding among long-term users of warfarin is 1.5–5.2% per year with a mortality rate from major bleeding that exceeds 13%.[166,167] Intracranial bleeding is the most feared complication and accounts for 8.7% of the major bleeding episodes with a 46–55% mortality rate.[168,169] A recent meta-analysis compared the risk of bleeding associated with target specific oral anticoagulants with that of warfarin in patients with atrial fibrillation and venous thromboembolism.[170] The results indicate that the use of target-specific oral anticoagulants is associated with significant reductions in the risk of major bleeding (RR 0.72,

Table 11-7 Agents Implicated in Drug-Induced Intracerebral Hemorrhage

Agent	Incidence	Level of Evidence[a]
Abciximab[93,94]	5.5%	B
Amphetamines[95-97]	NK	C
Apixaban[98]	0.33%/yr	A
Aspirin[99,100]	12/10,000	A
Aspirin + clopidogrel[101]	0.4%/yr	A
Cocaine[4,6,16,20,102-104]	NK	B
Dabigatran[105,106]	150 mg = 0.31%/yr 110 mg = 0.23%/yr	A
Edoxaban[107]	0.26%/yr	A
Ephedra-containing products (32 mg/day)[108-111,b]	NK	B
Glycoprotein IIb/IIIa inhibitors[111-114] With heparin Without heparin	0.12% 0.07%	B
Heparin[115-117]	0.3%	A
Heavy alcohol use (>60 g/day or >3 drinks/day)[4,118-122]	NK	B
Herbal energy drinks (adaptogenic blend *Eleutherococcus senticosus, Schisandra, Panax* species)[123]	NK	C
Heroin[6,26]	NK	C
Intra-arterial thrombolytics for management of stroke[124-126]	6.8–15%	A
Low-molecular weight heparins[127-130]	NK	A
Nicotine[131-133]	Two- to fourfold increased risk	A
Phenylpropanolamine[134-138] Dietary supplements Cough and cold preparations	NK NK	B
Pseudoephedrine[139]	NK	C
Rivaroxaban[140]	0.67%/yr	A
rt-PA for management of ischemic stroke[86,87,141,142]	1.9–10.6%	A
SSRI[47,50,143-146]	0.01%/yr OR 1.32, 95% CI 1.02–1.71	B
High-dose statin[147-153]	NK	B
Thrombolytic therapy for management of acute myocardial infarction[154-156]	0.46–1.9%	A
Warfarin[116,117,157-162]	0.3-1%/yr	A

CI = confidence interval, NK = not known, OR = odds ratio, rt-PA = recombinant tissue plasminogen activator, SSRI = selective serotonin reuptake inhibitor.

[a]Definitions for Levels of Evidence: Level A—evidence from one or more randomized, controlled clinical trials; Level B—evidence from nonrandomized clinical trials, prospective observational studies, cohort studies, retrospective studies, case-control studies, meta-analyses and/or postmarketing surveillance studies; and Level C—evidence from one or more published case reports or case series.

[b]Including the herbal source ma huang.

95% CI 0.62–0.85, NNT 156), fatal bleeding (RR 0.53, 95% CI 0.43–0.64, NNT 454), intracranial bleeding (RR 0.43, 95% CI 0.37–0.50, NNT 185), clinically relevant bleeding (RR 0.78, 95% CI 0.68–0.90, NNT 99), and total bleeding (RR 0.76, 95% CI 0.71–0.82, NNT 18). Data from the clinical trials also suggest that the rates of major bleeding associated with these newer agents are 2–3% per year, and rates of hemorrhagic stroke are 0.1–0.5% per year.[106,171-175]

Alcohol abuse remains an important risk factor for ICH with the risk related to the quantity consumed. Individuals who consume 41–120 g (~5 fluid ounces) daily have a 4.6 times higher risk of ICH compared to nondrinkers, and those who consume

121 g or greater daily are at 11.3 times higher risk.[176] Other drugs of abuse have also been implicated in ICH. Cocaine and other sympathomimetics have been implicated in both ischemic stroke and ICH.[77]

Both epidemiological and clinical trials have suggested that very low cholesterol concentrations achieved with high-dose statin therapy are associated with ICH.[147-153] It has been suggested that adequate cholesterol concentrations are necessary to maintain the integrity of the small vessels to prevent rupture.[177] In the Heart Protection Study, there was a trend toward a higher risk of ICH after treatment with simvastatin compared to placebo in patients who had a previous history of stroke or transient ischemic attack (TIA).[178] In the only study to evaluate high-dose statin therapy in primarily ischemic stroke patients (Stroke Prevention by Aggressive Reduction in Cholesterol Levels), patients randomized to atorvastatin had a higher rate of ICH compared to those in the placebo group (HR 1.66, 95% CI 1.08–2.55).[147-152] However, the overall net vascular benefit associated with statins in this trial outweighed the risk of ICH, so it is reasonable to conclude that the majority of ischemic stroke patients receive benefit from statin therapy. A meta-analysis of 31 randomized controlled trials that included 91,588 statin-treated patients found no significant association between statin use and ICH.[179] There are also data from a small study to suggest that continuing statin therapy after ICH is associated with early neurological improvement and reduced 6-month mortality.[180] Currently there is insufficient evidence to provide definitive recommendations regarding the use of statins in ICH patients.[181]

Many drugs theoretically may increase the risk of hemorrhagic stroke, although, for some, such an association has not been reported. Direct thrombin inhibitors such as hirudin or bivalirudin have not been shown to increase the risk of hemorrhagic stroke in clinical trials, and the risk of bleeding associated with these drugs is lower than that associated with heparin.[182] However, clinicians should be aware of the possibility of intracranial hemorrhage associated with these agents, especially when used in combination with other antiplatelet drugs such as the glycoprotein IIb/IIIa receptor antagonists. Intracranial bleeding events have been reported in association with glycoprotein IIb/IIIa receptor antagonists, especially when used in combination with heparin, and are associated with increased mortality.[114] The Abciximab in Emergency Treatment of Stroke Trial, which was terminated prematurely, was designed to evaluate the impact of abciximab on outcome following ischemic stroke. Compared to placebo, abciximab was associated with an increased rate of symptomatic or fatal ICH without improved efficacy.[93] Conflicting information has been reported regarding the risk of bleeding complications associated with the use of enoxaparin for prevention of venous thromboembolism in patients undergoing neurosurgery, but concern has been expressed regarding the use of low molecular weight heparins in this population.[127-129] There was also concern regarding the risk of ICH associated with the use of nonaspirin nonsteroidal anti-inflammatory agents (NANSAIDs). However, a recently published multicenter case-control study did not find an increased risk of ICH associated with NANSAIDs.[183]

Selective serotonin reuptake inhibitors (SSRIs) are used commonly to treat poststroke depression and for facilitating functional recovery after stroke. Observational studies suggest that SSRIs are associated with several adverse effects in older people (age >65 years) including increased risk for ICH (adjusted risk ratio 1.42, 95% CI 1.23–1.64).[146] These data suggest that SSRIs may cause one additional ICH per 10,000 persons (0.01%) treated for 1 year. Recently a cross-sectional epidemiological study of 4,945 patients who received antidepressants found that 5.5% developed cerebral microbleeds, but there was no significant causal relationship between exposure to SSRIs and ICH.[184] For the general population and patients with previous hemorrhagic or ischemic stroke who warrant treatment with an SSRI, there remain insufficient reliable data to make recommendations about any risk of ICH associated with an SSRI, with or without concurrent antiplatelet or anticoagulant therapy.[185]

EPIDEMIOLOGY

Approximately 37,000–52,000 people per year suffer from ICH (approximately 8–13% of all strokes) in the United States.[186] Although ICH only accounts for a small proportion of all strokes, it is associated with the highest mortality rate. Drug-related etiologies can be identified in 14–27% of patients

Table 11-8 Mechanisms of Drug-Induced Intracerebral Hemorrhage

Drug	Mechanism(s)
Alcohol abuse Amphetamines Cocaine Ephedra Nicotine Phenylpropanolamine Pseudoephedrine	Acute hypertension
Aspirin Glycoprotein IIb/IIIa inhibitors Heparin High-dose statin Low-molecular weight heparin SSRI Thrombolytics Warfarin	Bleeding diathesis

SSRI = selective serotonin reuptake inhibitor.

with ICH.[6,62] The incidence of drug-induced hemorrhagic stroke may be increasing.[6] Anticoagulant therapy is implicated in roughly 10% of all cases of ICH. The incidence of hemorrhagic stroke associated with specific drugs is presented in Table 11-7.

MECHANISMS

There are many proposed mechanisms for drug-induced hemorrhagic strokes. Mechanisms by which drugs result in ICH may be multifactorial and are discussed below and presented in **Table 11-8**.

ACUTE HYPERTENSION

Acute hypertension is an often under-recognized mechanism, particularly for drug-induced ICH. The primary mechanism behind drug-associated hypertension is related to the effect of drugs on neurotransmitters. Many drugs increase catecholamine release from central noradrenergic nerve terminals (i.e., amphetamines, ephedra, nonprescription sympathomimetics), inhibit reuptake of catecholamines into adrenergic nerve terminals (i.e., cocaine), or increase plasma catecholamine concentrations (i.e., ethanol, cocaine). Hypertension related to drug use may disrupt cerebral autoregulation, promote reperfusion of injured brain tissue, or damage cerebral arterioles, which may eventually rupture.

Ephedra products increase sympathomimetic activity, leading to acute hypertension. In combination with caffeine, ephedrine 20 mg increases systolic blood pressure by 14 mm Hg.[187] Caffeine acts by competitively antagonizing adenosine receptors, thus inhibiting adenosine-mediated dilatation, resulting in vasoconstriction. Caffeine also augments the release of catecholamines, enhancing the effects of ephedra.[188,189] Cigarette smoking acutely elevates blood pressure and reduces cerebral blood flow.[70,71,122] Alcohol acutely and chronically increases blood pressure related to increased adrenergic activity and increased plasma concentrations of cortisol, renin, aldosterone, and vasopressin.[73-75]

BLEEDING DIATHESIS

The mechanism by which anticoagulants increase the incidence of ICH is unclear. Anticoagulants may cause spontaneous subclinical hemorrhages that eventually become clinically significant. Drugs that cause thrombocytopenia (platelets $<50{,}000 \times 10^3/\mu L$), such as heparin, may increase the risk for drug-induced ICH. Drugs that cause severe hepatic failure or hepatitis may cause clotting derangements and a subsequent risk of ICH. Cocaine and heroin may also induce an illness identical to autoimmune thrombocytopenic purpura that places patients at higher risk of stroke. SSRIs may increase the risk of ICH through their antiplatelet effects.[190] Serotonin in platelets is essential for maintenance of hemostatic functioning and SSRIs deplete platelet serotonin storage leading to attenuation of platelet activity.[191] The antiplatelet effects of SSRIs are considered to be dose-dependent.[143,145]

CLINICAL PRESENTATION AND DIFFERENTIAL DIAGNOSIS

It is not possible to distinguish an ischemic stroke from hemorrhagic stroke due to ICH based on clinical examination alone, although several characteristics are more indicative of ICH: headache, impaired level of consciousness, nausea and vomiting, and extreme elevations of blood pressure. Drug-induced hemorrhagic stroke can occur at any time during therapy with a potentially causative agent. Common clinical features of drug-induced ICH are presented in **Table 11-9.**

Table 11-9 Signs and Symptoms Associated with Drug-Induced Intracerebral Hemorrhage

Signs	Symptoms
Brainstem hemorrhage	Altered consciousness Ataxia Coma Difficulty breathing Diplopia Disconjugate gaze Dysmetria Nystagmus
Increased intracranial pressure	Loss of consciousness Nausea/vomiting Sudden headache
Lobar hemorrhage	Aphasia Contralateral sensory-motor deficits Gaze deviation Hemianopia Hemispatial and/or sensory neglect Seizure

Table 11-10 Conditions to Consider in the Differential Diagnosis of Drug-Induced Intracerebral Hemorrhage

- Arterial dissection of the carotid or vertebral artery
- Arteriovenous malformation
- Central nervous system infection/brain abscess
- Cerebral aneurysm
- Encephalitis
- Hemorrhagic conversion of ischemic infarct
- Hypertensive encephalopathy
- Intracranial tumors
- Ischemic stroke
- Metabolic encephalopathy
- Seizure
- Trauma

Drug-induced hemorrhagic stroke must be distinguished from hemorrhagic stroke due to other etiologies. Conditions to consider in the differential diagnosis of drug-induced ICH are presented in **Table 11-10**. It is difficult to distinguish between drug-induced and nondrug-induced causes of hemorrhagic stroke unless symptoms are temporally related to the ingestion of substances of abuse, quantification drug concentration (i.e., illicit drug screen), or agents with surrogate monitoring parameters (i.e., warfarin or heparin) that can be assessed quantitatively.

Diagnosis of stroke consists of a thorough evaluation of patient history, clinical examination, laboratory evaluation, and imaging studies, including CT scan, cerebral angiography, and MRI. Laboratory studies should consist of serum electrolyte and glucose concentrations, complete blood count, coagulation parameters, and drug screen evaluation. A CT scan is essential to differentiate between ischemic and hemorrhagic stroke.

RISK FACTORS

Risk factors for drug-induced ICH are presented in **Table 11-11**. Thrombolysis has become a mainstay of therapy for both acute myocardial infarction and acute ischemic stroke. Although this therapy improves morbidity and mortality in these patients, there is an inherent risk of ICH. Risk factors for ICH associated with thrombolytic therapy following acute myocardial infarction include advanced age, female, African-American, systolic blood pressure ≥160 mm Hg, diastolic blood pressure ≥100 mm Hg, previous stroke, rt-PA dose >1.5 mg/kg, and low body weight (≤50 kg).[192] Risk of thrombolysis-related ICH in patients with acute ischemic stroke include NIH Stroke Scale score >20 (severe stroke), advanced age, thrombocytopenia, early infarct signs on pretreatment CT scan, increased time to treatment, history of heart failure, elevated serum glucose (>200 mg/dL), low plasminogen activator inhibitor concentration, history of diabetes mellitus and cardiac disease, increasing stroke severity, use of antiplatelet agents other than aspirin, elevated pretreatment mean blood pressure, and lower platelet counts.[165,193] In addition, use of rt-PA in patients that do not meet the inclusion criteria and/or meet exclusion criteria detailed in the National Institutes of Neurological Diseases Study—especially administration of rt-PA to patients that present >4.5 hours from the onset of symptoms—increases the risk of ICH in patients with acute ischemic stroke.[194,195] The GRASPS (Glucose Race Age Sex Pressure Stroke Severity) clinical risk score is a validated scoring system for predicting risk of symptomatic ICH after receiving rt-PA.[196] This score includes six predictor variables: glucose at presentation, race (Asian), age, sex (male), systolic blood pressure at presentation, and severity

Table 11-11 Risk Factors for Drug-Induced Intracerebral Hemorrhage

General risk factors

- Age >65 years
- History of hypertension
- Amyloid angiopathy
- Cigarette smoking
- Sedentary lifestyle
- Coagulation disturbances
- Thrombocytopenia

Aspirin-induced intracerebral hemorrhage[99]

- History of stroke
- Hypertension
- Age >75 years
- Race (black population)
- Dose ≥650 mg/day
- Amyloid accumulation
- Epistaxis
- Concurrent use with anticoagulants
- Neoplasm
- Vascular malformations or aneurysms

Oral anticoagulant-induced intracerebral hemorrhage[200]

- Advanced age (>85 years)
- Previous cerebral ischemic event
- Cerebral amyloid angiopathy
- Addition of antiplatelet agents
- Intensity of anticoagulation
- Duration of therapy
- History of bleeding
- Drug interactions
- Time in therapeutic range
- Kidney disease

Intra-arterial thrombolytic-induced intracerebral hemorrhage[209]

- National Institutes of Health Stroke Scale >20
- Longer time to recanalization
- Lower platelet count
- Hyperglycemia

Intravenous thrombolytic-induced intracerebral hemorrhage[193,208]

- Severity of neurologic deficit at time of presentation (measured by National Institutes of Health Stroke Scale >20)
- Thrombolytic dose used for ischemic stroke (>0.9 mg/kg or 90 mg)
- Early signs of infarction with brain edema or mass effect on imaging studies
- Age >80 years
- Hypertension
- Timing of revascularization therapy (i.e., longer stroke onset-to-treatment times)
- Hyperglycemia (glucose >200 mg/dL) or history of diabetes
- Coadministration of antithrombotic agents
- History of heart failure
- Thrombocytopenia

Heparin-induced intracerebral hemorrhage

- Hypertension
- Use of bolus dosing
- Thrombocytopenia
- Size of stroke

Low molecular weight heparin and glycoprotein IIb/IIIa inhibitor-induced intracerebral hemorrhage

- Age >75 years
- Kidney disease
- Thrombocytopenia

Selective serotonin reuptake inhibitor-induced intracerebral hemorrhage[47]

- Heavy alcohol use
- Cigarette smoking
- Vulnerability to bleeding diathesis

High-dose statin-induced intracerebral hemorrhage[147,149]

- Age >65 years
- Stage 2 hypertension
- Middle-aged men
- Previous ischemic stroke or transient ischemic attack

of stroke at presentation (NIHSS). The score calculator can be accessed at the following site: http://www.strokeassociation.org/STROKEORG/General/Get-With-The-Guidelines-Stroke-sICH-Calculator_UCM_453748_SubHomePage.jsp.

The FDA banned phenylpropanolamine, which was marketed in combination with caffeine as a weight-loss aid, after numerous adverse cardiovascular and central nervous system events.[137] Used in combination, these drugs have an additive effect on blood pressure.[197] Women between the ages of 18 and 49 years who use phenylpropanolamine as an appetite suppressant are 17 times more likely to experience an ICH compared with women of that age group that do not take this medication.[138] The risks associated with cough and cold preparations are less clear. The risks in men taking phenylpropanolamine are also unclear because the case-control study included too few men from which to draw conclusions.[137] The association between sympathomimetic drugs and ICH appears to be dose-related and additive when used in combination with other agents with similar activity. Patients receiving phenylpropanolamine in cough and cold products were three times more likely to develop ICH than those patients not receiving these products.[137,198] Herbal preparations that contain ephedra or ma huang also increase the risk of ICH in a dose-related fashion. The risk of ICH is fourfold greater in patients receiving ephedra doses >32 mg/day than those receiving no ma huang or lower doses.[108,109,199] This is an important issue with respect to counseling of patients regarding nonprescription drug products or the use of herbal supplements/energy drinks that may have sympathomimetic effects.

Anticoagulant therapy is used commonly to treat many thromboembolic disorders, particularly in the elderly population. Patients with an INR >3 or an activated partial thromboplastin time (aPTT) >80–90 seconds are at increased risk of ICH associated with warfarin and heparin, respectively. Factors that increase the risk of anticoagulant-related ICH include advanced age, level of anticoagulation, prior stroke, and hypertenson.[117,159,200] The risk for ICH with warfarin therapy is particularly high at age ≥85 years. INR <2 is not associated a with lower risk of ICH compared with INR between 2 and 3, but the risk is increased with INR >3.5, which should be avoided.[117,157,200] Therefore, for prevention of recurrent ischemic stroke, warfarin therapy should be focused on maintaining INR between 2 and 3.[117] The risk of anticoagulant-related bleeding is highest during the first month of therapy.[201] The HAS-BLED score has been validated to assess the bleeding risk in atrial fibrillation patients and assigns one point for the presence of each of the following: hypertension (uncontrolled systolic blood pressure >160 mm Hg), abnormal renal and/or liver function, previous stroke, bleeding history or predisposition, labile INR, elderly (age >65 years), and concomitant drugs (antiplatelets or nonsteroidal anti-inflammatory drugs) and/or alcohol excess. The HAS-BLED scores range from 0 to 9 with scores ≥3 indicating the highest risk of bleeding.[167] There is an increased rate of cerebral bleeding associated with intermittent intravenous heparin therapy compared with that associated with continuous intravenous infusion. Subcutaneous heparin is associated with bleeding rates similar to those due to continuous intravenous infusion.[115,117] Increased bleeding incidences have been reported in patients in whom aPTT is prolonged to more than twice the upper limit of the therapeutic range in at least 50% of the tested samples. For every 10-second increase in aPTT, major bleeding complications are increased by 7%.[117]

Patients with acute kidney injury or chronic kidney disease (serum creatinine >2 mg/dL) are at greater risk of bleeding associated with low molecular heparins or glycoprotein IIb/IIIa receptor antagonists than patients with normal kidney function.[202,203] Many of these agents are excreted renally and may accumulate in patients with kidney disease. Dose adjustments may be necessary; however, there currently are no published data regarding the optimal dosing regimen in patients with kidney disease. Patients ≥75 years of age have a higher rate of ICH after treatment with glycoprotein IIb/IIIa receptor antagonists.[113]

The use of aspirin for both primary and secondary prevention of vascular events including ischemic stroke has been associated with increased risk of ICH (RR 1.35).[99] Because significant benefit is achieved with the use of aspirin, evaluation of possible risk factors for ICH may assist in judging if the risk exceeds the benefit. Risk factors for aspirin-induced ICH include age (older than 75 years), race (black), hypertension, amyloid accumulation, history of epistaxis, high dose (>650 mg/day), bleeding disorders, and neoplasm.[99]

Use of combinations of agents such as antiplatelet drugs, anticoagulants, or thrombolytics may provide additive beneficial effects in patients with heart disease or stroke or TIAs, but these combinations also increase the risk of ICH. Concomitant use of aspirin with warfarin or heparin and glycoprotein IIb/IIIa antagonists is associated with an increased incidence of bleeding.[117] The use of combinations of oral antiplatelet agents for secondary prevention of stroke or acute coronary syndromes has become a common practice, based on the results of clinical

Table 11-12 Approaches to Help Prevent Drug-Induced Intracerebral Hemorrhage

Drug	Condition	Prevention
Alcohol	Moderation	Men should consume no more than 2 drinks/day and nonpregnant women should consume no more than 1 drink/day Control hypertension
All drugs	General risk factor modification	Control of hypertension (blood pressure <130/80 mm Hg) Discontinue drugs known to be associated with stroke in patients at high risk
Cigarette smoking	Smoking cessation	Encourage patient and family to stop smoking Provide counseling, nicotine replacement and formal programs
Substance abuse	Cessation	Rehabilitation program
Target specific oral anticoagulants		Control of hypertension Combination of aspirin and clopidogrel may accentuate ICH risk Evaluate for potential drug interactions
Thrombolytic therapy	Assess risk benefit and monitor patients closely	Follow recommended inclusion/exclusion selection criteria outlined in acute ischemic stroke guidelines[85]
Warfarin[102]	Assess risk benefit and monitor patients closely	Maintain INR <3 Control of hypertension Caution in elderly patients who are at highest risk Avoid combinations of warfarin with antiplatelet agents Evaluate for potential drug interactions

ICH = intracerebral hemorrhage, INR = international normalized ratio.

trials showing additive benefit when combining therapy with extended-release dipyridamole or clopidogrel with aspirin. However, a study that evaluated the combination of aspirin and clopidogrel for prevention of recurrent stroke or TIA reported an absolute 1.3% increase in the risk of life-threatening bleeding. This combination therapy was not associated with a reduction in vascular events, so the risks of the combination therapy appeared to outweigh the benefits.[204] There are newer ongoing trials that are assessing the safety of short-term use of dual antiplatelet drugs following minor stroke or TIA that will identify the risk-benefit ratio.

MORBIDITY AND MORTALITY

ICH accounts for only a small percentage of all stroke cases but is associated with the highest incidence of mortality (in-hospital mortality of ~34%). Therefore, the mortality rates associated with drug-induced ICH may be high.

PREVENTION

The most effective means of prevention of drug-induced stroke is avoidance of agents known to be associated with ICH, especially in high-risk patients. Strategies for prevention of drug-induced hemorrhagic stroke are listed in **Table 11-12.** Patients receiving anticoagulant therapy should be closely monitored for intensity of anticoagulation, kidney function, and the possibility of drug interactions. Careful selection of ischemic stroke patients as candidates to receive intravenous rt-PA is also important. However, the mainstay of prevention is patient education and identification of risk factors, particularly in those patients that are at high risk.[181]

MANAGEMENT

The management of any ICH patient has many phases: prevention of ICH, supportive and medical management during the acute phase, measures to mitigate the ongoing pathologic process, and rehabilitation. In addition, discontinuation of the offending agent (if identified) is essential.

All patients with acute drug-induced ICH should be hospitalized, and most require care in an intensive care unit. Guidelines for the management of patients with ICH have been published previously.[181] Patients with ICH often present with severe acute hypertension. There is no consensus regarding the ideal target range for blood pressure control. The decision regarding the appropriate target lower blood pressure is a balance between minimizing hematoma volume and preventing ischemic changes. There is an ongoing study to assess the efficacy of early (within 4.5 hours of symptom onset) intensive blood pressure lowering (systolic blood pressure <140 mm Hg) for improving outcome after ICH. Until completion of this study, guidelines suggest that, in patients presenting with systolic blood pressure between 150 and 220 mm Hg and without contraindication to acute intervention, lowering blood pressure to a systolic pressure of 140 mm Hg is safe. For those presenting with systolic blood pressure above 220 mm Hg, blood pressure should be reduced aggressively via continuous intravenous infusion of antihypertensive agents.[181] Surgical evacuation of the hematoma may be necessary in some patients. General medical management and supportive care are indicated for all patients to prevent complications (i.e., intracranial hypertension, hyperthermia, hyperglycemia).[181]

If ICH occurs in the setting of thrombolytic, anticoagulant, or antiplatelet therapy, immediate cessation of therapy with the causative agent is indicated, with rapid reversal of the impaired clotting profile. Patients with ICH who are receiving unfractionated heparin or low-molecular weight heparin should receive protamine sulfate (1 mg/100 units of heparin or 1 mg of enoxaparin). The dose of protamine should be adjusted according to the time elapsed from last heparin dose. For example, if heparin was discontinued within the previous 30–60 minutes, the protamine dose is 0.5–0.75 mg/100 units of heparin; if the heparin infusion was discontinued within the previous 60–120 minutes, the protamine dose is 0.375–0.5 mg/100 units of heparin; if the heparin infusion was discontinued more than 120 minutes ago, the protamine dose is 0.25–0.375 mg/100 units of heparin. Protamine sulfate should be administered intravenously over 10 minutes in doses not to exceed 50 mg because of the potential risk of severe systemic hypotension.[181] Patients with bleeding caused by platelet dysfunction should receive platelet transfusions (6 units) and/or a single dose of desmopressin (0.3 mcg/kg). For ICH related to thrombolytic therapy, the currently recommended management is platelet infusion (6–8 units) and cryoprecipitate that contains factor VIII.[181]

Patients who are receiving warfarin with INR elevation and experiencing ICH should undergo INR reversal immediately. The treatment options include fresh frozen plasma (FFP), prothrombin-complex concentrates (PCCs), activated PCC FEIBA (factor VIII inhibitor bypassing activity), vitamin K, and recombinant activated factor VIIa (rFVIIa).[205] Therapy should never be withheld to check coagulation profiles because normalization of the INR with some of these approaches may require several hours. Administration of PCCs normalizes the INR more rapidly than FFP, and PCCs can be given in smaller volumes, thus decreasing the risk of heart failure exacerbation associated with FFP. Therefore, PCCs may be preferred over FFP.[181] Recombinant activated factor VIIa does not replace all clotting factors and, although the INR may be lowered, clotting may not be restored in vivo; therefore rFVIIa is not recommended for warfarin reversal in patients with ICH.[181] Administration of intravenous vitamin K alone is insufficient for warfarin reversal during the first hours, but should be part of all acute warfarin reversal strategies at a dose of 5–10 mg.

Idarucizumab is currently the only antidote available for reversing the effects of the target-specific oral anticoagulants (specifically dabigatran). However, other antidotes, including andexanet alfa and aripazine, have been developed and have shown promise in early clinical trials evaluating their efficacy and safety for reversal of factor Xa inhibitors.[206] The newer target-specific oral anticoagulants are different from warfarin in that they have relatively short half-lives of 5–15 hours in patients with normal kidney function. Evaluation of prothrombin time with selected agents (apixaban, rivaroxaban, edoxaban) and thrombin time (dabigatran) may be helpful for individualization of care. Until the newer antidotes are available, potential reversal strategies for apixaban, rivaroxaban, and edoxaban include using FEIBA, PCCs, or rFVIIa.[207] Fresh frozen plasma and vitamin K are not useful for reversal of the target-specific oral anticoagulants. Activated charcoal can be used if the most recent dose of these drugs was taken within 2 hours. Hemodialysis is also another option for management of ICH associated with dabigatran, but less so for the other agents because they are more highly protein bound.[181] For a more complete review of reversing the effects of antithrombotic agents, please refer to the guidelines from the Neurocritical Care Society published in 2016.[210]

A difficult decision after anticoagulation-induced ICH is deciding whether to reinitiate anticoagulant therapy. There are no strict guidelines on the length of time to withhold anticoagulation therapy following ICH. Avoidance of oral anticoagulation for at least 4 weeks in patients without mechanical heart valves might decrease the risk of ICH recurrence. The guidelines also recommend avoidance of long-term anticoagulation with warfarin in patients with nonvalvular atrial fibrillation after warfarin-associated spontaneous lobar ICH because of the high risk of recurrence.[181] The safety of the target-specific oral anticoagulants in patients with atrial fibrillation and past ICH is unknown.

INFORMATION FOR PATIENTS

Risk factor assessment of patients and drug profile review for potential drug interactions is essential for prevention of drug-induced ICH. Because patients do not obtain many of the drugs that are known to cause ICH at pharmacies, it is extremely important that patients at risk are counseled to consult their healthcare professionals before purchasing non-prescription drug or herbal products. For example, patients with hypertension should be advised that cough and cold products or herbal products, including energy drinks may contain sympathomimetic agents that could place them at increased risk for drug-induced hemorrhagic stroke. Prevention of head injury is very important, especially when patients are taking anticoagulants or antiplatelets that might cause intracranial bleeding if they hit their head. It is important that patients realize they can still have a healthy active lifestyle, but just be cautious of activities (e.g., skiing, hockey, soccer) that might place them at high risk for falling or hitting their head. Patients receiving combinations of agents that are known to cause hemorrhagic stroke (such as anticoagulants and aspirin) should be informed regarding the increased risk. Patients should be instructed to inform their healthcare professionals of all medications that they are taking, to facilitate a full evaluation of potential agents that may be associated with drug-induced hemorrhagic stroke. It is important for patients to closely adhere to the regimens prescribed including scheduled laboratory monitoring to minimize the risk associated with the use of some of these agents.

REFERENCES

1. Go AS, Mozaffarian D, Roger VL et al. Heart disease and stroke statistics—2014 update: a report from the American Heart Association. *Circulation.* 2014; 129:e28-292.
2. Heron M. Deaths: leading causes for 2007. *Natl Vital Stat Rep.* 2011; 59:1-95.
3. Reynolds K, Lewis B, Nolen JD et al. Alcohol consumption and risk of stroke: a meta-analysis. *JAMA.* 2003; 289:579-88.
4. Kaplan EH, Gottesman RF, Llinas RH et al. The association between specific substances of abuse and subcortical intracerebral hemorrhage versus ischemic lacunar infarction. *Front Neurol.* 2014; 5:174.
5. Bostwick DG. Amphetamine induced cerebral vasculitis. *Hum Pathol.* 1981; 12:1031-3.
6. Kaku DA, Lowenstein DH. Emergence of recreational drug abuse as a major risk factor for stroke in young adults. *Ann Int Med.* 1990; 113:821-7.
7. De Silva DA, Wong MC, Lee MP et al. Amphetamine-associated ischemic stroke: clinical presentation and proposed pathogenesis. *J Stroke Cerebrovasc Dis.* 2007; 16:185-6.
8. Azak A, Oksuzoglu B, Deren T et al. Cerebrovascular accident during cisplatin-based combination chemotherapy of testicular germ cell tumor: an unusual case report. *Anticancer Drugs.* 2008; 19:97-8.
9. Dietrich J, Marienhagen J, Schalke B et al. Vascular neurotoxicity following chemotherapy with cisplatin, ifosfamide, and etoposide. *Ann Pharmacother.* 2004;3 8:242-6.
10. El Amrani M, Heinzlef O, Debroucker T et al. Brain infarction following 5-fluorouracil and cisplatin therapy. *Neurology.* 1998; 51:899-901.
11. Gerl A, Clemm C, Wilmanns W. Acute cerebrovascular event after cisplatin-based chemotherapy for testicular cancer. *Lancet.* 1991; 338:385-6.
12. Li SH, Chen WH, Tang Y et al. Incidence of ischemic stroke post-chemotherapy: a retrospective review of 10,963 patients. *Clin Neurol Neurosur.* 2006; 108:150-6.
13. Russmann S, Winkler A, Lovblad KO et al. Lethal ischemic stroke after cisplatin-based chemotherapy for testicular carcinoma and cannabis inhalation. *Eur Neurol.* 2002; 48:178-80.
14. Serrano-Castro PJ, Guardado-Santervas P, Olivares-Romero J. Ischemic stroke following cisplatin and 5-fluorouracil therapy: a transcranial Doppler study. *Eur Neurol.* 2000; 44:63-4.
15. Meattini I, Scotti V, Pescini F et al. Ischemic stroke during cisplatin-based chemotherapy for testicular germ cell tumor: case report and review of the literature. *J Chemother.* 2010; 22:134-6.
16. Cregler LL, Mark H. Medical complications of cocaine abuse. *New Engl J Med.* 1986; 315:1495-500.
17. Daras M, Tuchman AJ, Marks S. Central nervous system infarction related to cocaine abuse. *Stroke.* 1991; 22:1320-5.
18. Fredericks RK, Lefkowitz DS, Challa VR et al. Cerebral vasculitis associated with cocaine abuse. *Stroke.* 1991; 22:1437-9.
19. Klonoff DC, Andrews BT, Obana WG. Stroke associated with cocaine use. *Arch Neurol.* 1989; 46:989-93.
20. Levine SR, Washington JM, Jefferson MF et al. "Crack" cocaine-associated stroke. *Neurology.* 1987; 37:1849-53.
21. Levine SR, Welch KM. Cocaine and stroke. *Stroke.* 1988; 19:779-83.
22. Siniscalchi A, Bonci A, Mercuri NB et al. Cocaine dependence and stroke: pathogenesis and management. *Curr Neurovasc Res.* 2015; 12:163-72.

23. Sordo L, Indave BI, Barrio G et al. Cocaine use and risk of stroke: a systematic review. *Drug Alcohol Depend.* 2014; 142:1-13.
24. Reneman L, Habraken JB, Majoie CB et al. MDMA ("Ecstasy") and its association with cerebrovascular accidents: preliminary findings. *AJNR.* 2000; 21:1001-7.
25. Shin JY, Choi NK, Lee J et al. Risk of ischemic stroke associated with the use of antipsychotic drugs in elderly patients: a retrospective cohort study in Korea. *PloS one.* 2015; 10:e0119931.
26. Brust JC, Richter RW. Stroke associated with addiction to heroin. *J Neurol Neurosurg Psychiatry.* 1976; 39:194-9.
27. Viscoli CM, Brass LM, Kernan WN et al. A clinical trial of estrogen-replacement therapy after ischemic stroke. *New Engl J Med.* 2001; 345:1243-9.
28. Magargal LE, Sanborn GE, Donoso LA et al. Branch retinal artery occlusion after excessive use of nasal spray. *Ann Ophthalmol.* 1985; 17:500-1.
29. Caress JB, Cartwright MS, Donofrio PD et al. The clinical features of 16 cases of stroke associated with administration of IVIg. *Neurology.* 2003; 60:1822-4.
30. Meschia JF, Malkoff MD, Biller J. Reversible segmental cerebral arterial vasospasm and cerebral infarction: possible association with excessive use of sumatriptan and Midrin. *Arch Neurol.*1998; 55:712-4.
31. Zachariah SB. Stroke after heavy marijuana smoking. *Stroke.* 1991; 22:406-9.
32. Wolf PA, D'Agostino RB, Kannel WB et al. Cigarette smoking as a risk factor for stroke. The Framingham Study. *JAMA.* 1988; 259:1025-9.
33. Shah RS, Cole JW. Smoking and stroke: the more you smoke the more you stroke. *Expert Rev Cardiovasc Ther.* 2010; 8:917-32.
34. Afilalo J, Coussa-Charley MJ, Eisenberg MJ. Long-term risk of ischemic stroke associated with rofecoxib. *Cardiovasc Drugs Ther.* 2007; 21:117-20.
35. Antman EM, Bennett JS, Daugherty A et al. Use of nonsteroidal antiinflammatory drugs: an update for clinicians: a scientific statement from the American Heart Association. *Circulation.* 2007; 115:1634-42.
36. Bennett JS, Daugherty A, Herrington D et al. The use of nonsteroidal anti-inflammatory drugs (NSAIDs): a science advisory from the American Heart Association. *Circulation.* 2005; 111:1713-6.
37. Wooltorton E. Risperidone (Risperdal): increased rate of cerebrovascular events in dementia trials. *CMAJ.* 2002; 167:1269-70.
38. Pasternak B, Svanstrom H, Ranthe MF et al. Atypical antipsychotics olanzapine, quetiapine, and risperidone and risk of acute major cardiovascular events in young and middle-aged adults: a nationwide register-based cohort study in Denmark. *CNS Drugs.* 2014; 28:963-73.
39. Shin JY, Choi NK, Jung SY et al. Risk of ischemic stroke with the use of risperidone, quetiapine and olanzapine in elderly patients: a population-based, case-crossover study. *J Psychopharmacol.* 2013; 27:638-44.
40. Hannaford PC, Croft PR, Kay CR. Oral contraception and stroke. Evidence from the Royal College of General Practitioners' Oral Contraception Study. *Stroke.* 1994; 25:935-42.
41. Roach RE, Helmerhorst FM, Lijfering WM et al. Combined oral contraceptives: the risk of myocardial infarction and ischemic stroke. *Cochrane Database Syst Rev.* 2015; 8:CD011054.
42. Milling TJ Jr, Refaai MA, Goldstein JN et al. Thromboembolic events after vitamin k antagonist reversal with 4-factor prothrombin complex concentrate: exploratory analyses of two randomized, plasma-controlled studies. *Ann Emerg Med.* 2016; 67:96-105.
43. Majeed A, Eelde A, Agren A et al. Thromboembolic safety and efficacy of prothrombin complex concentrates in the emergency reversal of warfarin coagulopathy. *Thromb rRes.* 2012; 129:146-51.
44. Zareh M, Davis A, Henderson S. Reversal of warfarin-induced hemorrhage in the emergency department. *West J Emerg Med.* 2011; 12:386-92.
45. O'Connell KA, Wood JJ, Wise RP et al. Thromboembolic adverse events after use of recombinant human coagulation factor VIIa. *JAMA.* 2006; 295:293-8.
46. Noskin O, Jafarimojarrad E, Libman RB et al. Diffuse cerebral vasoconstriction (Call-Fleming syndrome) and stroke associated with antidepressants. *Neurology.* 2006; 67:159-60.
47. Ramasubbu R. SSRI treatment-associated stroke: causality assessment in two cases. *Ann Pharmacother.* 2004; 38:1197-201.
48. Ramasubbu R. Cerebrovascular effects of selective serotonin reuptake inhibitors: a systematic review. *J Clin Psychiatry.* 2004; 65:1642-53.
49. Trifiro G, Dieleman J, Sen EF et al. Risk of ischemic stroke associated with antidepressant drug use in elderly persons. *J Clin Psychopharmacol.* 2010; 30:252-8.
50. Shin D, Oh YH, Eom CS et al. Use of selective serotonin reuptake inhibitors and risk of stroke: a systematic review and meta-analysis. *J Neurol.* 2014; 261:686-95.
51. Hall GC, Brown MM, Mo J et al Triptans in migraine: the risks of stroke, cardiovascular disease, and death in practice. *Neurology.* 2004 ;62:563-8.
52. Braithwaite RS, Chlebowski RT, Lau J et al. Meta-analysis of vascular and neoplastic events associated with tamoxifen. *J Gen Intern Med.* 2003; 18:937-47.
53. Bushnell CD, Goldstein LB. Risk of ischemic stroke with tamoxifen treatment for breast cancer: a meta-analysis. *Neurology.* 2004; 63:1230-3.
54. Chan WS, Ray J, Wai EK et al. Risk of stroke in women exposed to low-dose oral contraceptives: a critical evaluation of the evidence. *Arch Int Med.* 2004; 164:741-7.
55. Gillum LA, Mamidipudi SK, Johnston SC. Ischemic stroke risk with oral contraceptives: A meta-analysis. *JAMA.* 2000; 284:72-8.
56. Goldstein LB, Adams R, Alberts MJ et al. Primary prevention of ischemic stroke: a guideline from the American Heart Association/American Stroke Association Stroke Council. *Stroke.* 2006; 37:1583-633.
57. Lidegaard O. Oral contraception and risk of a cerebral thromboembolic attack: results of a case-control study. *BMJ (Clinical research ed.)* 1993; 306:956-63.
58. Lidegaard O. Oral contraceptives, pregnancy and the risk of cerebral thromboembolism: the influence of diabetes, hypertension, migraine and previous thrombotic disease. *BJOG.* 1995; 102:153-9.
59. Jick SS, Jick H. The contraceptive patch in relation to ischemic stroke and acute myocardial infarction. *Pharmacotherapy.* 2007; 27:218-20.
60. Wassertheil-Smoller S, Hendrix SL, Limacher M et al. Effect of estrogen plus progestin on stroke in postmenopausal women: the Women's Health Initiative: a randomized trial. *JAMA.* 2003; 289:2673-84.
61. Patrono C, Baigent C. Nonsteroidal anti-inflammatory drugs and the heart. *Circulation.* 2014; 129:907-16.
62. Sloan MA, Kittner SJ, Rigamonti D et al. Occurrence of stroke associated with use/abuse of drugs. *Neurology.* 1991; 41:1358-64.
63. Treadwell SD, Robinson TG. Cocaine use and stroke. *Postgrad Med J.* 2007; 83:389-94.
64. Chillar RK, Jackson AL. Reversible hemiplegia after presumed intracarotid injection of Ritalin. *New Engl J Med.* 1981; 304:1305.
65. Kaufman MJ, Levin JM, Ross MH et al. Cocaine-induced cerebral vasoconstriction detected in humans with magnetic resonance angiography. *JAMA.* 1998; 279:376-80.
66. Friedman E, Gershon S, Rotrosen J. Effects of acute cocaine treatment on the turnover of 5-hydroxytryptamine in the rat brain *Br J Pharmacol.* 1975; 54:61-4.
67. Luman W, Gray RS. Adverse reactions associated with sumatriptan. *Lancet.* 1993; 341:1091-2.
68. Tfelt-Hansen P, Ferrari MD, Olesen J. Association between sumatriptan and stroke. *Lancet.* 1993; 342:303.

69. O'Quinn S, Davis RL, Gutterman DL et al. Prospective large-scale study of the tolerability of subcutaneous sumatriptan injection for acute treatment of migraine. *Cephalalgia.* 1999; 19:223-31; discussion 200.
70. Kool MJ, Hoeks AP, Struijker Boudier HA et al. Short- and long-term effects of smoking on arterial wall properties in habitual smokers. *J Am Coll Cardiol.* 1993; 22:1881-6.
71. Kubota K, Yamaguchi T, Abe Y et al. Effects of smoking on regional cerebral blood flow in neurologically normal subjects. *Stroke.* 1983; 14:720-4.
72. Rogers RL, Meyer JS, Shaw TG et al. Cigarette smoking decreases cerebral blood flow suggesting increased risk for stroke. *JAMA.* 1983; 250:2796-800.
73. Beevers DG. Alcohol and hypertension. *Lancet.* 1977; 2:114-5.
74. Brackett DJ, Gauvin DV, Lerner MR et al. Dose- and time-dependent cardiovascular responses induced by ethanol. *J Pharmacol Exp Ther.* 1994; 268:78-84.
75. Lip GY, Beevers DG. Alcohol, hypertension, coronary disease and stroke. *Clin Exp Pharmacol Physiol.* 1995; 22:189-94.
76. Konzen JP, Levine SR, Garcia JH. Vasospasm and thrombus formation as possible mechanisms of stroke related to alkaloidal cocaine. *Stroke.* 1995; 26:1114-8.
77. O'Connor AD, Rusyniak DE, Bruno A. Cerebrovascular and cardiovascular complications of alcohol and sympathomimetic drug abuse. *Med Clin North Am* 2005; 89:1343-58.
78. Togna G, Tempesta E, Togna AR et al. Platelet responsiveness and biosynthesis of thromboxane and prostacyclin in response to in vitro cocaine treatment. *Haemostasis.* 1985; 15:100-7.
79. Renaud S, Blache D, Dumont E et al. Platelet function after cigarette smoking in relation to nicotine and carbon monoxide. *Clin Pharmacol Ther.* 1984; 36:389-95.
80. Doll DC, Ringenberg QS, Yarbro JW. Vascular toxicity associated with antineoplastic agents. *J Clin Oncol.* 1986; 4:1405-17.
81. Smith DA, Beier MT. Association between risperidone treatment and cerebrovascular adverse events: examining the evidence and postulating hypotheses for an underlying mechanism. *J Am Med Dir Assoc.* 2004; 5:129-32.
82. Wolf PA, D'Agostino RB, Belanger AJ et al. Probability of stroke: a risk profile from the Framingham Study. *Stroke.* 1991; 22:312-8.
83. Meschia JF, Bushnell C, Boden-Albala B et al. Guidelines for the primary prevention of stroke: a statement for healthcare professionals from the American Heart Association/American Stroke Association. *Stroke.* 2014; 45:3754-832.
84. Taylor TN, Davis PH, Torner JC et al. Lifetime cost of stroke in the United States. *Stroke.* 1996; 27:1459-66.
85. Powers WJ, Rabinstein AA, Ackerson T et al.; American Heart Association Stroke Council. 2018 guidelines for the early management of patients with acute ischemic stroke: a guideline for healthcare professionals from the American Heart Association/American Stroke Association. *Stroke.* 2018; 49:e46-110.
86. The National Institute of Neurological Disorders and Stroke rt-PA Stroke Study Group. Tissue plasminogen activator for acute ischemic stroke. *New Engl J Med.* 1995; 333:1581-7.
87. Hacke W, Kaste M, Bluhmki E et al. Thrombolysis with alteplase 3 to 4.5 hours after acute ischemic stroke. *New Engl J Med.* 2008; 359:1317-29.
88. Prasad K, Krishnan PR. Fever is associated with doubling of odds of short-term mortality in ischemic stroke: an updated meta-analysis. *Acta Neurol Scand.* 2010; 122:404-8.
89. Vemmos KN, Tsivgoulis G, Spengos K et al. U-shaped relationship between mortality and admission blood pressure in patients with acute stroke. *J Int Med.* 2004; 255:257-65.
90. Rodriguez-Garcia JL, Botia E, de La Sierra A et al. Significance of elevated blood pressure and its management on the short-term outcome of patients with acute ischemic stroke. *Am J Hypertens.* 2005; 18:379-84.
91. Yong M, Kaste M. Association of characteristics of blood pressure profiles and stroke outcomes in the ECASS-II trial. *Stroke.* 2008; 39:366-72.
92. Kernan WN, Ovbiagele B, Black HR et al. Guidelines for the prevention of stroke in patients with stroke and transient ischemic attack: a guideline for healthcare professionals from the American Heart Association/American Stroke Association. *Stroke.* 2014; 45:2160-236.
93. Adams HP Jr, Effron MB, Torner J et al. Emergency administration of abciximab for treatment of patients with acute ischemic stroke: results of an international phase III trial: Abciximab in Emergency Treatment of Stroke Trial (AbESTT-II). *Stroke.* 2008; 39:87-99.
94. Walsh RD, Barrett KM, Aguilar MI et al. Intracranial hemorrhage following neuroendovascular procedures with abciximab is associated with high mortality: a multicenter series. *Neurocritical Care.* 2011; 15:85-95.
95. Goodman SJ, Becker DP. Intracranial hemorrhage associated with amphetamine abuse. *JAMA.* 1970; 212:480.
96. Nakagawa K, Vento MA, Ing MM et al. Racial disparities in methamphetamine-associated intracerebral hemorrhage. *Neurology.* 2015; 84:995-1001.
97. McEvoy AW, Kitchen ND, Thomas DG. Intracerebral haemorrhage and drug abuse in young adults. *Br J Neurosurg.* 2000; 14:449-54.
98. Granger CB, Alexander JH, McMurray JJ et al. Apixaban versus warfarin in patients with atrial fibrillation. *New Engl J Med.* 2011; 365:981-92.
99. Gorelick PB, Weisman SM. Risk of hemorrhagic stroke with aspirin use: an update. *Stroke.* 2005; 36:1801-7.
100. He J, Whelton PK, Vu B et al Aspirin and risk of hemorrhagic stroke: a meta-analysis of randomized controlled trials. *JAMA.* 1998; 280:1930-5.
101. Hart RG, Tonarelli SB, Pearce LA. Avoiding central nervous system bleeding during antithrombotic therapy: recent data and ideas. *Stroke.* 2005; 36:1588-93.
102. Green RM, Kelly KM, Gabrielsen T et al. Multiple intracerebral hemorrhages after smoking "crack" cocaine. *Stroke.* 1990; 21:957-62.
103. Nolte KB, Brass LM, Fletterick CF. Intracranial hemorrhage associated with cocaine abuse: a prospective autopsy study. *Neurology.* 1996; 46:1291-6.
104. Martin-Schild S, Albright KC, Hallevi H et al. Intracerebral hemorrhage in cocaine users. *Stroke.* 2010; 41:680-4.
105. Connolly SJ, Ezekowitz MD, Yusuf S et al. Dabigatran versus warfarin in patients with atrial fibrillation. *New Engl J Med.* 2009; 361:1139-51.
106. Hart RG, Diener HC, Yang S et al. Intracranial hemorrhage in atrial fibrillation patients during anticoagulation with warfarin or dabigatran: the RE-LY trial. *Stroke.* 2012; 43:1511-7.
107. Giugliano RP, Ruff CT, Braunwald E et al. Edoxaban versus warfarin in patients with atrial fibrillation. *New Engl J Med.* 2013; 369:2093-104.
108. Bruno A, Nolte KB, Chapin J. Stroke associated with ephedrine use. *Neurology.* 1993; 43:1313-6.
109. Haller CA, Benowitz NL. Adverse cardiovascular and central nervous system events associated with dietary supplements containing ephedra alkaloids. *New Engl J Med.* 2000; 343:1833-8.
110. Morgenstern LB, Viscoli CM, Kernan WN et al. Use of Ephedra-containing products and risk for hemorrhagic stroke. *Neurology.* 2003; 60:132-5.
111. Samenuk D, Link MS, Homoud MK et al. Adverse cardiovascular events temporally associated with ma huang, an herbal source of ephedrine. *Mayo Clin Proc.* 2002; 77:12-6.
112. Ali A, Hashem M, Rosman HS et al. Glycoprotein IIb/IIIa receptor antagonists and risk of bleeding: a single-center experience in 1020 patients. *J Clin Pharmacol.* 2004; 44:1328-32.

113. Iakovou I, Dangas G, Mintz GS et al. Comparison of frequency of hemorrhagic stroke in patients <75 years versus > or =75 years of age among patients receiving glycoprotein IIb/IIIa inhibitors during percutaneous coronary interventions. *Am J Cardiol.* 2004; 93:346-9.
114. Qureshi AI, Hussain MS, Nasar A et al. Intracranial hemorrhages associated with intravenous platelet glycoprotein IIB/IIIA receptor inhibitors in the United States. *Cardiovasc Drugs Ther.* 2005; 19:371-3.
115. The International Stroke Trial (IST): a randomised trial of aspirin, subcutaneous heparin, both, or neither among 19435 patients with acute ischaemic stroke. International Stroke Trial Collaborative Group. *Lancet.* 1997; 349:1569-81.
116. Kase CS, Robinson RK, Stein RW et al. Anticoagulant-related intracerebral hemorrhage. *Neurology.* 1985; 35:943-8.
117. Levine MN, Raskob G, Beyth RJ et al. Hemorrhagic complications of anticoagulant treatment: the Seventh ACCP Conference on Antithrombotic and Thrombolytic Therapy. *Chest.* 2004; 126:287S-310S.
118. Beghi E, Boglium G, Cosso P et al. Stroke and alcohol intake in a hospital population—a case-control study. *Stroke.* 1995; 26:1691-696.
119. Ben-Shlomo Y, Markowe H, Shipley M et al. Stroke risk from alcohol consumption using different control groups. *Stroke.* 1992; 23:1093-8.
120. Donahue RP, Abbott RD, Reed DM et al. Alcohol and hemorrhagic stroke—The Honolulu Heart Program. *JAMA.* 1986; 255:2311-4.
121. Monforte R, Estruch R, Graus F et al. High ethanol consumption as risk factor for intracerebral hemorrhage in young and middle-aged people. *Stroke.* 1990; 21:1529-32.
122. Rodgers H, Aitken PD, French JM et al. Alcohol and stroke. A case-control study of drinking habits past and present. *Stroke.* 1993; 24:1473-7.
123. Worrall BB, Phillips CD, Henderson KK. Herbal energy drinks, phenylpropanoid compounds, and cerebral vasculopathy. *Neurology.* 2005; 65:1137-8.
124. del Zoppo GJ, Higashida RT, Furlan AJ et al. PROACT: a phase II randomized trial of recombinant pro-urokinase by direct arterial delivery in acute middle cerebral artery stroke. *Stroke.* 1998; 29:4-11.
125. Kase CS, Furlan AJ, Wechsler LR et al. Cerebral hemorrhage after intra-arterial thrombolysis for ischemic stroke: the PROACT II trial. *Neurology.* 2001; 57:1603-10.
126. Singer OC, Berkefeld J, Lorenz MW et al. Risk of symptomatic intracerebral hemorrhage in patients treated with intra-arterial thrombolysis. *Cerebrovasc Dis.* 2009; 27:368-74.
127. Agnelli G, Piovella F, Buoncristiani P et al. Enoxaparin plus compression stockings compared with compression stockings alone in the prevention of venous thromboembolism after elective neurosurgery. *New Engl J Med.* 1998; 339:80-5.
128. Geerts WH, Jay RM, Code KI et al. A comparison of low-dose heparin with low-molecular-weight heparin as prophylaxis against venous thromboembolism after major trauma. *New Engl J Med.* 1996; 335:701-7.
129. Nurmohamed MT, van Riel AM, Henkens CM et al. Low molecular weight heparin and compression stockings in the prevention of venous thromboembolism in neurosurgery. *J Thromb Haemost.* 1996; 75:233-8.
130. The Publications Committee for the Trial of ORG 10172 in Acute Stroke Treatment (TOAST) Investigators. Low molecular weight heparinoid, ORG 10172 (danaparoid), and outcome after acute ischemic stroke: a randomized controlled trial. *JAMA.* 1998; 279:1265-72.
131. Kurth T, Kase CS, Berger K et al. Smoking and risk of hemorrhagic stroke in women. *Stroke.* 2003; 34:2792-5.
132. Bonita R, Scragg R, Stewart A et al. Cigarette smoking and risk of premature stroke in men and women. *BMJ (Clinical research ed.)* 1986; 293:6-8.
133. Colditz GA, Bonita R, Stampfer MJ et al. Cigarette smoking and risk of stroke in middle-aged women. *New Engl J Med.* 1988; 318:937-41.
134. Cantu C, Arauz A, Murillo-Bonilla LM et al. Stroke associated with sympathomimetics contained in over-the-counter cough and cold drugs. *Stroke.* 2003; 34:1667-72.
135. Fallis RJ, Fisher M. Cerebral vasculitis and hemorrhage associated with phenylpropanolamine. *Neurology.* 1985; 35:405-7.
136. Forman HP, Levin S, Stewart B et al. Cerebral vasculitis and hemorrhage in an adolescent taking diet pills containing phenylpropanolamine: case report and review of literature. *Pediatrics.* 1989; 83:737-41.
137. Kernan WN, Viscoli CM, Brass LMet al. Phenylpropanolamine and the risk of hemorrhagic stroke. *New Engl J Med.* 2000; 343:1826-32.
138. Yoon BW, Bae HJ, Hong KS et al. Phenylpropanolamine contained in cold remedies and risk of hemorrhagic stroke. *Neurology.* 2007; 68:146-9.
139. Montalban J, Ibanez L, Rodriguez C et al Cerebral infarction after excessive use of nasal decongestants. *J Neurol Neurosurg Psychiatry.* 1989; 52:541-3.
140. Hankey GJ, Stevens SR, Piccini JP et al. Intracranial hemorrhage among patients with atrial fibrillation anticoagulated with warfarin or rivaroxaban: the rivaroxaban once daily, oral, direct factor Xa inhibition compared with vitamin K antagonism for prevention of stroke and embolism trial in atrial fibrillation. *Stroke.* 2014; 4:1304-12.
141. Rao NM, Levine SR, Gornbein JA et al. Defining clinically relevant cerebral hemorrhage after thrombolytic therapy for stroke: analysis of the National Institute of Neurological Disorders and Stroke tissue-type plasminogen activator trials. *Stroke.* 2014; 45:2728-33.
142. Wahlgren N, Ahmed N, Davalos A et al. Thrombolysis with alteplase for acute ischaemic stroke in the Safe Implementation of Thrombolysis in Stroke-Monitoring Study (SITS-MOST): an observational study. *Lancet.* 2007; 369:275-82.
143. Bak S, Tsiropoulos I, Kjaersgaard JO et al. Selective serotonin reuptake inhibitors and the risk of stroke: a population-based case-control study. *Stroke.* 2002; 33:1465-73.
144. de Abajo FJ. Effects of selective serotonin reuptake inhibitors on platelet function: mechanisms, clinical outcomes and implications for use in elderly patients. *Drugs & Aging.* 2011; 28:345-67.
145. de Abajo FJ, Jick H, Derby L et al. Intracranial haemorrhage and use of selective serotonin reuptake inhibitors. *Br J Clin Pharmacol.* 2000; 50:43-7.
146. Hackam DG, Mrkobrada M. Selective serotonin reuptake inhibitors and brain hemorrhage: a meta-analysis. *Neurology.* 2012; 79:1862-5.
147. Amarenco P, Bogousslavsky J, Callahan A III et al. High-dose atorvastatin after stroke or transient ischemic attack. *New Engl J Med.* 2006; 355:549-59.
148. Ariesen MJ, Claus SP, Rinkel GJ et al. Risk factors for intracerebral hemorrhage in the general population: a systematic review. *Stroke.* 2003; 34:2060-5.
149. Iso H, Jacobs Dr Jr, Wentworth D et al. Serum cholesterol levels and six-year mortality from stroke in 350,977 men screened for the multiple risk factor intervention trial. *New Engl J Med.* 1989; 320:904-10.
150. Sturgeon JD, Folsom AR, Longstreth WT Jr et al. Risk factors for intracerebral hemorrhage in a pooled prospective study. *Stroke.* 2007; 38:2718-25.
151. Thrift A, McNeil J, Donnan G. Reduced frequency of high cholesterol levels among patients with intracerebral haemorrhage. *J Clin Neurosci.* 2002; 9:376-80.
152. Goldstein LB, Amarenco P, Szarek M et al. Hemorrhagic stroke in the Stroke Prevention by Aggressive Reduction in Cholesterol Levels study. *Neurology.* 2008; 70:2364-70.

153. Hackam DG, Austin PC, Huang A et al. Statins and intracerebral hemorrhage: a retrospective cohort study. *Arch Neurol.* 2012; 69:39-45.
154. Gebel JM, Sila CA, Sloan MA et al. Thrombolysis-related intracranial hemorrhage: a radiographic analysis of 244 cases from the GUSTO-1 trial with clinical correlation. *Stroke.* 1998; 29:563-9.
155. Gurwitz JH, Gore JM, Goldberg RJ et al. Risk for intracranial hemorrhage after tissue plasminogen activator treatment for acute myocardial infarction. *Ann Int Med.* 1998; 129:597-604.
156. Kase CS, Pessin MS, Zivin JA et al. Intracranial hemorrhage after coronary thrombolysis with tissue plasminogen activator. *Am J Med.* 1992; 92:384-90.
157. Fang MC, Chang Y, Hylek EM et al. Advanced age, anticoagulation intensity, and risk for intracranial hemorrhage among patients taking warfarin for atrial fibrillation. *Ann Int Med.* 2004; 141:745-52.
158. Gorter JW. Major bleeding during anticoagulation after cerebral ischemia: patterns and risk factors. *Neurology.* 1999; 53:1319-27.
159. Hart RG, Boop BS, Anderson DC. Oral anticoagulants and intracranial hemorrhage. Facts and hypotheses. *Stroke.* 1995; 26:1471-7.
160. Hylek EM, Evans-Molina C, Shea C et al. Major hemorrhage and tolerability of warfarin in the first year of therapy among elderly patients with atrial fibrillation. *Circulation.* 2007; 115:2689-96.
161. Steiner T, Rosand J, Diringer M. Intracerebral hemorrhage associated with oral anticoagulant therapy: current practices and unresolved questions. *Stroke.* 2006; 37:256-62.
162. Fang MC, Go AS, Hylek EM et al. Age and the risk of warfarin-associated hemorrhage: the anticoagulation and risk factors in atrial fibrillation study. *J Am Geriatr Soc.* 2006; 54:1231-6.
163. Saver JL. Hemorrhage after thrombolytic therapy for stroke: the clinically relevant number needed to harm. *Stroke.* 2007; 38:2279-83.
164. Lansberg MG, Albers GW, Wijman CA. Symptomatic intracerebral hemorrhage following thrombolytic therapy for acute ischemic stroke: a review of the risk factors. *Cerebrovasc Dis.* 2007; 24:1-10.
165. Lansberg MG, Thijs VN, Bammer R et al. Risk factors of symptomatic intracerebral hemorrhage after tPA therapy for acute stroke. *Stroke.* 2007; 38:2275-8.
166. Gage BF, Yan Y, Milligan PE et al. Clinical classification schemes for predicting hemorrhage: results from the National Registry of Atrial Fibrillation (NRAF). *Am Heart J.* 2006; 151:713-9.
167. Pisters R, Lane DA, Nieuwlaat R et al. A novel user-friendly score (HAS-BLED) to assess 1-year risk of major bleeding in patients with atrial fibrillation: the Euro Heart Survey. *Chest.* 2010; 138:1093-100.
168. Fang MC, Go AS, Chang Y et al. Death and disability from warfarin-associated intracranial and extracranial hemorrhages. *Am J Med.* 2007; 120:700-5.
169. Linkins LA, Choi PT, Douketis JD. Clinical impact of bleeding in patients taking oral anticoagulant therapy for venous thromboembolism: a meta-analysis. *Ann Int Med.* 2003; 139:893-900.
170. Chai-Adisaksopha C, Crowther M, Isayama T et al. The impact of bleeding complications in patients receiving target-specific oral anticoagulants: a systematic review and meta-analysis. *Blood.* 2014; 124:2450-8.
171. Ruff CT, Giugliano RP, Braunwald E et al. Comparison of the efficacy and safety of new oral anticoagulants with warfarin in patients with atrial fibrillation: a meta-analysis of randomised trials. *Lancet.* 2014; 383:955-62.
172. Hylek EM, Held C, Alexander JH et al. Major bleeding in patients with atrial fibrillation receiving apixaban or warfarin: the ARISTOTLE Trial (apixaban for reduction in stroke and other thromboembolic events in atrial fibrillation): predictors, characteristics, and clinical outcomes. *J Am Coll Cardiol.* 2014; 63:2141-7.
173. Piccini JP, Garg J, Patel MR et al. Management of major bleeding events in patients treated with rivaroxaban vs. warfarin: results from the ROCKET AF trial. *Eur Heart J.* 2014; 35:1873-80.
174. Hankey GJ, Patel MR, Stevens SR et al. Rivaroxaban compared with warfarin in patients with atrial fibrillation and previous stroke or transient ischaemic attack: a subgroup analysis of ROCKET AF. *Lancet Neurol.* 2012; 11:315-22.
175. Connolly SJ, Eikelboom J, Joyner C et al. Apixaban in patients with atrial fibrillation. *New Engl J Med.* 2011; 364:806-17.
176. Juvela S, Hillbom M, Palomaki H. Risk factors for spontaneous intracerebral hemorrhage. *Stroke.* 1995; 26:1558-64.
177. Ooneda G, Yoshida Y, Suzuki K et al. Smooth muscle cells in the development of plasmatic arterionecrosis, arteriosclerosis, and arterial contraction. *Blood Vessels.* 1978; 15:148-56.
178. Third Report of the National Cholesterol Education Program (NCEP) Expert Panel on Detection, Evaluation, and Treatment of High Blood Cholesterol in Adults (Adult Treatment Panel III) final report. *Circulation.* 2002; 106:3143-21.
179. McKinney JS, Kostis WJ. Statin therapy and the risk of intracerebral hemorrhage: a meta-analysis of 31 randomized controlled trials. *Stroke.* 2012; 43:2149-56.
180. Tapia-Perez JH, Rupa R, Zilke R et al. Continued statin therapy could improve the outcome after spontaneous intracerebral hemorrhage. *Neurosurg Rev.* 2013; 36:279-87; discussion 287.
181. Hemphill JC, 3rd, Greenberg SM, Anderson CS et al. Guidelines for the management of spontaneous intracerebral hemorrhage: a guideline for healthcare professionals from the American Heart Association/American Stroke Association. *Stroke.* 2015; 46:2032-60.
182. Weitz JI, Buller HR. Direct thrombin inhibitors in acute coronary syndromes: present and future. *Circulation.* 2002; 105:1004-11.
183. Choi NK, Park BJ, Jeong SW et al. Nonaspirin nonsteroidal anti-inflammatory drugs and hemorrhagic stroke risk: the acute brain bleeding analysis study. *Stroke.* 2008; 39:845-9.
184. Aarts N, Akoudad S, Noordam R et al. Inhibition of serotonin reuptake by antidepressants and cerebral microbleeds in the general population. *Stroke.* 2014; 45:1951-7.
185. Lopponen P, Tetri S, Juvela S et al. Association between warfarin combined with serotonin-modulating antidepressants and increased case fatality in primary intracerebral hemorrhage: a population-based study. *J Neurosurg.* 2014; 120:1358-63.
186. Qureshi AI, Tuhrim S, Broderick JP et al. Spontaneous intracerebral hemorrhage. *New Engl J Med.* 2001; 344:1450-60.
187. Haller CA, Jacob P III, Benowitz NL. Pharmacology of ephedra alkaloids and caffeine after single-dose dietary supplement use. *Clin Pharmacol Ther.* 2002; 71:421-32.
188. Benowitz NL. Clinical pharmacology of caffeine. *Ann Rev Med.* 1990; 41:277-88.
189. Robertson D, Frolich JC, Carr RK et al. Effects of caffeine on plasma renin activity, catecholamines and blood pressure. *New Engl J Med.* 1978; 298:181-6.
190. Skop BP, Brown TM. Potential vascular and bleeding complications of treatment with selective serotonin reuptake inhibitors. *Psychosomatics.* 1996; 37:12-6.
191. De Clerck F. The role of serotonin in thrombogenesis. *Clin Physiol Biochem.* 1990; 8:40-9.
192. Huynh T, Cox JL, Massel D et al. Predictors of intracranial hemorrhage with fibrinolytic therapy in unselected community patients: a report from the FASTRAK II project. *Am J Heart.* 2004; 148:86-91.
193. Khatri P, Wechsler LR, Broderick JP. Intracranial hemorrhage associated with revascularization therapies. *Stroke.* 2007; 38:431-40.
194. Katzan IL, Furlan AJ, Lloyd LE et al. Use of tissue-type plasminogen activator for acute ischemic stroke: the Cleveland area experience. *JAMA.* 2000; 283:1151-8.
195. Tanne D, Bates VE, Verro P et al. Initial clinical experience with IV tissue plasminogen activator for acute ischemic stroke: a multicenter survey. The t-PA Stroke Survey Group. *Neurology.* 1999; 53:424-7.

196. Sung SF, Chen SC, Lin HJ et al. Comparison of risk-scoring systems in predicting symptomatic intracerebral hemorrhage after intravenous thrombolysis. *Stroke.* 2013; 44:1561-6.

197. Brown NJ, Ryder D, Branch RA. A pharmacodynamic interaction between caffeine and phenylpropanolamine. *Clin Pharmacol Ther.* 1991; 50:363-71.

198. Loizou LA, Hamilton JG, Tsementzis SA. Intracranial haemorrhage in association with pseudoephedrine overdose. *J Neurol Neurosurg Psychiatryy.* 1982; 45:471-2.

199. Wooten MR, Khangure MS, Murphy MJ. Intracerebral hemorrhage and vasculitis related to ephedrine abuse. *Ann Neurol.* 1983; 13:337-40.

200. Hughes M, Lip GY. Risk factors for anticoagulation-related bleeding complications in patients with atrial fibrillation: a systematic review. *QJM.* 2007; 100:599-607.

201. Torn M, Algra A, Rosendaal FR. Oral anticoagulation for cerebral ischemia of arterial origin: high initial bleeding risk. *Neurology.* 2001; 57:1993-9.

202. Farooq V, Hegarty J, Chandrasekar T et al. Serious adverse incidents with the usage of low molecular weight heparins in patients with chronic kidney disease. *Am J Kidney Dis.* 2004; 43:531-7.

203. Fernandez JS, Sadaniantz BT, Sadaniantz A. Review of antithrombotic agents used for acute coronary syndromes in renal patients. *Am J Kidney Dis.* 2003; 42:446-55.

204. Diener HC, Bogousslavsky J, Brass LM et al. Aspirin and clopidogrel compared with clopidogrel alone after recent ischaemic stroke or transient ischaemic attack in high-risk patients (MATCH): randomised, double-blind, placebo-controlled trial. *Lancet.* 2004; 364:331-7.

205. Holbrook A, Schulman S, Witt DM et al. Evidence-based management of anticoagulant therapy: antithrombotic therapy and prevention of thrombosis, 9th ed: American College of Chest Physicians Evidence-Based Clinical Practice Guidelines. *Chest.* 2012; 141:e152S-184S.

206. Mo Y, Yam FK. Recent advances in the development of specific antidotes for target-specific oral anticoagulants. *Pharmacother.* 2015; 35:198-207.

207. Kaatz S, Crowther M. Reversal of target-specific oral anticoagulants. *J Thromb Thrombolysis.* 2013; 36:195-202.

208. Mazya M, Egido JA, Ford GA et al. Predicting the risk of symptomatic intracerebral hemorrhage in ischemic stroke treated with intravenous alteplase: safe implementation of treatments in stroke (SITS) symptomatic intracerebral hemorrhage risk score. *Stroke.* 2012; 43:1524-31.

209. Kidwell CS, Saver JL, Carneado J et al. Predictors of hemorrhagic transformation in patients receiving intra-arterial thrombolysis. *Stroke.* 2002; 33:717-24.

210. Frontera JA, Lewin JJ 3rd, Rabinstein AA et al. Guidelines for reversal of antithrombotics in intracranial hemorrhage: a statement for healthcare professionals from the Neurocritical Care Society and Society of Critical Care Medicine. *Neurocrit Care.* 2016; 24:6-46.

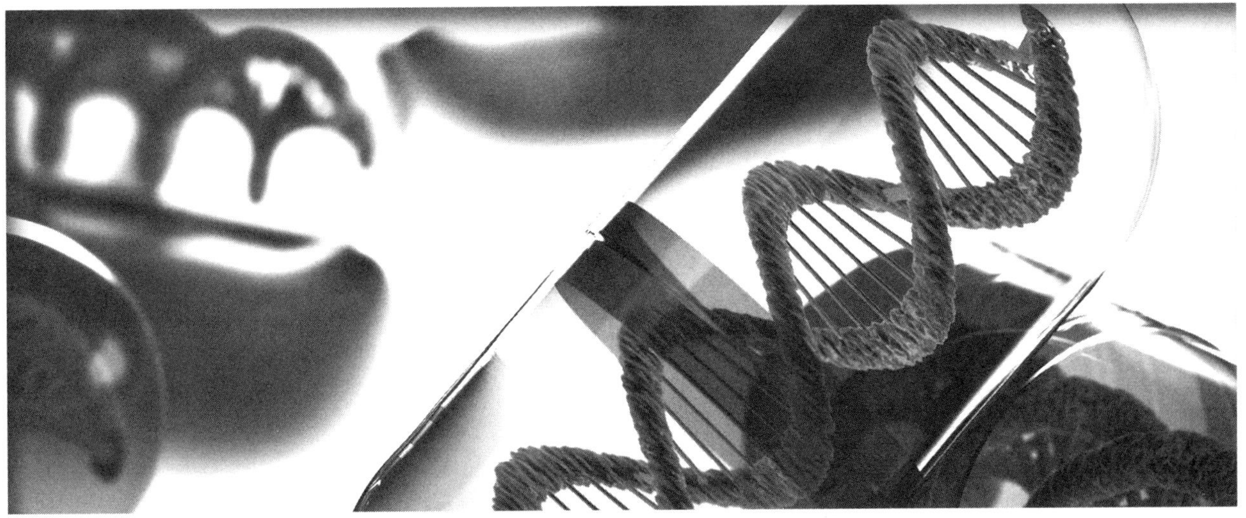

CHAPTER 12

Movement Disorders

Jack J. Chen, Khashayar Dashtipour, and David M. Swope

In the United States and across the globe, drug-induced movement disorders (DIMDs) are a significant iatrogenic burden among selected patient populations, such as those receiving psychotropic agents for psychiatric disorders or antiemetic drugs (e.g., droperidol, metoclopramide, prochlorperazine) for gastrointestinal disorders.[1] DIMDs refer to a variety of distinct, treatment-emergent, involuntary movements, including akathisia, tardive dyskinesia (TDk), dystonia, and parkinsonism, which may interfere with medication adherence, performance of motor tasks, and psychosocial interactions. In patients with psychiatric disorders, DIMDs are a significant source of distress and discomfort resulting in medication nonadherence or refusal, subsequent relapse and rehospitalization, and increased use of healthcare resources.[2] In one study, patients with schizophrenia or schizoaffective disorder in whom antipsychotic-induced DIMD developed were 40 times more likely to discontinue maintenance medication therapy.[3] DIMDs are under-recognized iatrogenic conditions. In one study, resident physicians failed to detect or recognize more than 50% of cases of TDk and drug-induced parkinsonism.[4]

DIMDs can be described as acute or tardive. Acute DIMDs (e.g., acute akathisia, acute dystonia) occur within hours to days after exposure. Tardive (i.e., delayed onset) DIMDs (e.g., tardive akathisia, TDk, tardive dystonia) occur months to years after drug exposure. Patients with DIMDs commonly present with two or more coexistent movement disorders.[5,6] Examples of DIMD combinations include TDk with parkinsonism, TDk with tardive dystonia, and TDk with akathisia.

Soon after the introduction of conventional antipsychotics in the 1950s, it became obvious that these agents were a cause of iatrogenic movement disorders. These DIMDs were termed *extrapyramidal symptoms* (EPS) or *side effects*, which implies the involvement of extrapyramidal regions (i.e., basal ganglia and thalamus) as opposed to the corticospinal pyramidal motor system. Subsequently, as induction of EPS became viewed as a typical and expected correlate to antipsychotic efficacy, the term *neuroleptic* ("seize the nerves") was coined.[7] The introduction of clozapine, an antipsychotic nearly devoid of EPS, in the late 1980s demonstrated that development of EPS was not a requisite for antipsychotic efficacy, and thus the newer antipsychotics are referred to as atypical. It is important to note that EPS is not synonymous with DIMDs. The former refers collectively to drug-induced dystonia, parkinsonism, and TDk. Drug-induced akathisia is considered a DIMD but not an EPS.

It has been clearly established that atypical antipsychotics are associated with a significantly lower risk of DIMDs compared with that associated with conventional neuroleptics (with or without concurrent antimuscarinic prophylaxis).[8-13] However, among the category of atypical antipsychotics, differences in risk of EPS exist. Clozapine and pimavanserin are associated with the lowest risk of EPS. Lurasidone, olanzapine, paliperidone, risperidone, and ziprasidone are associated with higher risks of dose-dependent EPS.

Movement disorders are also associated with other psychotropic drugs, such as lithium, selective serotonin reuptake inhibitors (SSRIs), psychostimulants, and tricyclic antidepressants (TCAs). Tremor commonly occurs in association with lithium treatment, which also occasionally causes chorea.[14] Treatment with SSRIs may cause akathisia and tremor, but rarely induces dyskinesia, dystonia, or parkinsonism.[15,16] Psychostimulants (e.g., amphetamine, methylphenidate, pemoline) have occasionally been reported to produce a variety of movement disorders such as dyskinesias, dystonia, stereotypic behavior, and tics.[17] The most common movement disorders associated with TCAs are akathisia, myoclonus, and tremor.[18,19] Antiepileptic agents rarely induce movement disorders, with the exception of valproate, which is frequently associated with tremor and, to a lesser extent, parkinsonism. Carbamazepine, ethosuximide, felbamate, gabapentin, phenobarbital, and phenytoin have rarely been associated with dyskinesia or dystonic reactions.[20] For many years, chorea has been recognized as a complication of estrogen- and progesterone-containing products (e.g., oral contraceptives).[21] Antiemetics that block central dopamine receptors (i.e., droperidol, metoclopramide, prochlorperazine) are also commonly implicated in the various DIMDs.[22-25]

Drug-induced tremor, although not uncommon, will not be discussed in this chapter, and readers are referred elsewhere for further reading.[26] Readers are also referred elsewhere for discussions on drug-induced myoclonus (abrupt, brief, and sudden "shock-like" involuntary movements), levodopa-induced dyskinesias, neuroleptic malignant syndrome, restless legs syndrome, and motor tics.[27-32] The primary topics that will be covered in this chapter are drug-induced akathisias, TDk, dystonias, and parkinsonism.

AKATHISIA (ACUTE AND TARDIVE)

The term *akathisia* is derived from Greek ("not sitting still"), and was initially used at the turn of the 20th century to describe the restlessness and pacing observed in patients diagnosed with hysteria and neuroses. Akathisia is now used extensively to describe the restlessness and pacing behavior induced by neuroleptics and other drugs. Akathisia induced by psychotropic agents can be a distressing adverse effect, resulting in poor treatment adherence and, consequently, an increased risk of relapse or exacerbation of the underlying psychiatric disorder.

CAUSATIVE AGENTS

Agents implicated in drug-induced akathisia are listed in **Table 12-1**.[24,25,33-44] Conventional neuroleptics and antidopaminergic antiemetics are the most commonly implicated drugs in acute and tardive akathisia. Several atypical antipsychotics also induce akathisia, albeit with lower incidences as compared with conventional neuroleptics. The SSRIs and the serotonin–norepinephrine reuptake inhibitor mirtazapine are also commonly implicated in acute akathisia, but rarely in tardive akathisia.

EPIDEMIOLOGY

Acute akathisia occurs in 20–30% of patients taking conventional neuroleptics but has been reported in up to 76% of patients.[34-36] The incidence of tardive akathisia is approximately 30%.[36]

The atypical antipsychotics (e.g., aripiprazole, clozapine, iloperidone, olanzapine, paliperidone, quetiapine, risperidone, ziprasidone) also induce akathisia, although the risk is lower than

Table 12-1 Agents Implicated in Drug-Induced Akathisia

Drug	Incidence	Level of Evidence[a]
ANTIEMETICS/GASTRIC MOTILITY AGENTS		
Droperidol[24]	20–30%	B
Metoclopramide[24,25]	20–30%	B
Prochlorperazine[24]	20–30%	B
Promethazine[33]	20–30%	B
ANTIEPILEPTICS		
Carbamazepine[41]	NK	C
PSYCHOTROPICS		
Amoxapine[42]	NK	C
Atypical antipsychotics[37-39,b]	5–15%	A
Conventional neuroleptics[34-37,c]	20–30%	A
Lithium[43]	NK	C
Selective serotonin-reuptake inhibitors[40,d]	5%	B
Tricyclic antidepressants[44,e]	5%	C

NK = not known.
[a]Definitions for Levels of Evidence: Level A—evidence from one or more randomized, controlled clinical trials; Level B—evidence from nonrandomized clinical trials, prospective observational studies, cohort studies, retrospective studies, case-control studies, meta-analyses and/or postmarketing surveillance studies; and Level C—evidence from one or more published case reports or case series.
[b]Amisulpride, aripiprazole, asenapine, brexpiprazole, cariprazine, clozapine, iloperidone, lurasidone, olanzapine, paliperidone, quetiapine, risperidone, sertindole, ziprasidone.
[c]Chlorpromazine, fluphenazine, haloperidol, mesoridazine, molindone, perphenazine, promazine, thioridazine, thiothixene, trifluoperazine, triflupromazine.
[d]Citalopram, escitalopram, fluoxetine, fluvoxamine, paroxetine, sertraline.
[e]Amitriptyline, clomipramine, desipramine, doxepin, imipramine, nortriptyline.

that associated with conventional neuroleptics. In one study, the prevalence of akathisia associated with clozapine, risperidone, and conventional neuroleptics was 7.3%, 13%, and 23.8%, respectively.[37] However, at daily doses >6 mg, the frequency of risperidone-induced akathisia increases significantly. The incidence of akathisia in iloperidone-treated patients is low and similar to that of placebo.[38,39]

Akathisia is also induced by SSRIs and TCAs. Although the incidence of SSRI- and TCA-induced akathisia has not been studied systematically, it appears to occur in at least 5% of patients treated with SSRIs, with higher rates associated with stimulating SSRIs (e.g., fluoxetine, paroxetine).[40] Treatment-emergent anxiety, agitation, and restlessness are commonly reported in association with antidepressants (especially within the first 2 weeks of initiating treatment), and it is possible that a subset of these patients are experiencing akathisia.

Akathisia also frequently occurs in association with antidopaminergic antiemetics. In one study, acute, transient akathisia occurred in 71.4%, 25%, 35.3%, and 11.1% of patients treated with droperidol, metoclopramide, prochlorperazine, and placebo, respectively.[24] Rapid intravenous infusion of metoclopramide is associated with a higher incidence of akathisia compared with slow infusion.[25]

MECHANISMS

The pathophysiologic mechanism of drug-induced acute akathisia is not well understood, but involves altered dopaminergic and serotonergic activity (**Table 12-2**). This theory is supported by the observation that akathisia is a well-recognized effect of centrally-acting dopamine-receptor–blocking agents (DRBAs). The dopaminergic pathway of the mesolimbic tract appears to be affected, and the stronger the antidopaminergic effect of a drug, the higher the

Table 12-2 Mechanisms of Drug-Induced Akathisia

Drug	Mechanism
Amoxapine Atypical antipsychotics[a] Conventional neuroleptics[b] Droperidol Metoclopramide Prochlorperazine Promethazine	Postsynaptic blockade of dopamine type 2 receptors in the mesocortical pathway
Selective serotonin reuptake inhibitors[c] Tricyclic antidepressants[d]	Stimulation of 5-hydroxytryptophan (serotonin) type 2 receptors in the ventral tegmental area, resulting in hypofunction of the dopaminergic mesocortical pathway
Carbamazepine Lithium	Unknown

[a]Amisulpride, aripiprazole, asenapine, brexpiprazole, cariprazine, clozapine, iloperidone, lurasidone, olanzapine, paliperidone, quetiapine, risperidone, sertindole, ziprasidone.
[b]Chlorpromazine, fluphenazine, haloperidol, mesoridazine, molindone, perphenazine, promazine, thioridazine, thiothixene, trifluoperazine, triflupromazine.
[c]Citalopram, escitalopram, fluoxetine, fluvoxamine, paroxetine, sertraline.
[d]Amitriptyline, clomipramine, desipramine, doxepin, imipramine, nortriptyline.

incidence of akathisia.[45] Serotonergic and noradrenergic input in the ventral tegmental area exerts an inhibitory effect on mesocortical dopamine transmission. This is supported by the observation that akathisia may be caused by serotonergic agents such as SSRIs, and the positive therapeutic response to antiserotonergic therapies such as 5-hydroxytryptophan (serotonin) type 2 (5-HT_2) receptor blockers (e.g., cyproheptadine) and the noradrenergic β-receptor blocker propranolol (which also possesses antiserotonergic activity). In addition, the atypical antipsychotics, which also block 5-HT_2 receptors, are associated with lower rates of akathisia compared to those of conventional neuroleptics. Iron deficiency has been implicated as a component of the pathophysiologic mechanism for akathisia, but the data are inconsistent.[46] The mechanism underlying the tardive form of akathisia is less well understood, but is probably distinct from that of acute akathisia.

CLINICAL PRESENTATION AND DIFFERENTIAL DIAGNOSIS

According to the *Diagnostic and Statistical Manual of Mental Disorders,* 5th Edition (*DSM-V*), medication-induced akathisia is comprised of both a subjective and an objective component.[47] The core features are subjective symptoms of restlessness (commonly referable to the legs) and at least one of the following objective findings: fidgety movements or leg swinging while seated, marching on the spot while standing, rocking from one foot to another, pacing to relieve subjective restlessness, or an inability to sit or stand still for several minutes (**Table 12-3**). Subjective dysphoria is a major component of neuroleptic-induced akathisia and includes apprehension, an inner sense of restlessness (often in the legs), anxiety, and the urge to move. Significant mental distress is experienced if the patient is asked to not move or is restrained from moving. Unlike most movement disorders, which are involuntary, the movements associated with akathisia (e.g., fidgeting, leg or body shifting, toe tapping, walking) are voluntary, and occur in response to the subjective feeling of restlessness or discomfort. As with other movement disorders, anxiety or stress exacerbates pre-existing akathisia.

Symptoms of acute akathisia may occur within an hour (as with intravenously administered antidopaminergic antiemetics) to within several weeks of initiating or increasing the dose of the offending drug, and may also develop after neuroleptic therapy cessation or dose reduction (i.e., withdrawal akathisia). Occasionally, the discontinuation of

Table 12-3 Signs and Symptoms Associated with Drug-Induced Movement Disorders

Akathisia

- Subjective feeling of restlessness and need to move
- Objective symptoms of pacing, walking in place, foot or toe tapping, rocking while seated
- Distress if restrained or unable to move
- Symptoms may improve during sleep or in a supine position

Tardive dyskinesia

- Abnormal involuntary choreoathetoid movements affecting the orofacial region, tongue, upper and lower extremities, and trunk
- Symptoms are not painful but may result in embarrassment in social settings and difficulty with chewing, speaking, and swallowing
- Lip smacking, chewing movements, and tongue protrusion are common

Dystonia

- Sustained involuntary muscle contractions or spasms resulting in abnormal postures or twisting and repetitive movements
- Affected body parts include the neck, upper and lower extremities, jaw, larynx, and trunk
- Symptoms associated with distress, pain, and disability
- Difficulty with walking, breathing, head turning, speech, and swallowing

Parkinsonism

- Tremor, rigidity, slowness of movement affecting bilateral upper and lower extremities, and truncal regions
- Masked facies, micrographia, slow shuffling gait, and stooped posture

therapy with a concurrent antiakathisia agent (e.g., propranolol) may unmask akathisia. Although the temporal criteria for tardive akathisia are debatable, the onset of symptoms after 3 months of stable drug therapy is considered tardive.

Drug-induced akathisia may be mistaken for anxiety, psychotic agitation, drug withdrawal symptoms, or restless legs syndrome (**Table 12-4**). Acute drug-induced akathisia should be suspected if symptoms develop soon after the initiation of therapy with potentially causative drugs and in the absence of other conditions associated with restlessness. In contrast to restless legs syndrome, patients with akathisia may report improvement when lying down or sleeping, absence of lower extremity paresthesias, absence of diurnal pattern, and absence of periodic leg movements in sleep.

Table 12-4 Conditions to Consider in the Differential Diagnosis of Drug-Induced Movement Disorders

Akathisia

- Alcohol or drug withdrawal
- Anxiety disorder
- Psychic agitation
- Restless legs syndrome

Tardive dyskinesia

- Edentulism
- Huntington disease
- Hyperthyroidism
- Levodopa-induced dyskinesia
- Neuroacanthocytosis (choreoacanthocytosis)
- Sydenham chorea
- Wilson disease

Dystonia

- Arthritis
- Atlantoaxial rotary subluxation
- Catatonia
- Conversion reaction
- Dopa-responsive dystonia
- Huntington disease
- Idiopathic dystonia
- Inherited dystonias
- Neuroleptic malignant syndrome
- Orthopedic disorder
- Tetanus
- Wilson disease

Parkinsonism

- Essential tremor
- Hypothyroidism
- Parkinson disease (nondrug-induced)
- Severe depression
- Wilson disease

Tardive akathisia may be suspected in the absence of other conditions associated with restlessness. The symptoms of tardive akathisia are similar to those of acute akathisia, except that patients with tardive akathisia tend to report less distressing subjective symptoms and are able to suppress movements or remain still for longer periods. The Barnes Akathisia Rating Scale (BARS) may be used for akathisia detection and assessment.[48] The BARS

Table 12-5 Risk Factors for Drug-Induced Akathisia

- Advanced age
- Cognitive impairment
- Female sex
- High dose neuroleptic therapy
- High potency neuroleptic therapy
- History of akathisia
- Intellectual disability
- Iron deficiency
- Mood disorder
- Presence of negative symptoms of schizophrenia
- Rapid neuroleptic dose escalation

is a clinician-rated assessment tool, composed of four items used to assess the presence and severity of drug-induced akathisia. The BARS rates both objective items (e.g., observed restlessness) and subjective items (e.g., patients' awareness of restlessness and related distress), in addition to a global clinical assessment of akathisia.

RISK FACTORS

Risk factors for drug-induced akathisia are not well described, but include older age, concurrent mood disorder (e.g., anxiety, bipolar disorder, depression), cognitive impairment, female sex, history of akathisia, intellectual disability, iron deficiency, presence of negative symptoms of schizophrenia, use of high-dose neuroleptics, rapid neuroleptic dose escalation, and use of high-potency neuroleptics (**Table 12-5**).[36,37,49]

MORBIDITY AND MORTALITY

When left untreated, the symptoms of acute drug-induced akathisia may gradually subside or may fluctuate over time. In some patients, acute akathisia may become chronic and persist for months or years. Acute akathisia has been associated with promoting aggression, suicidal behavior, and treatment nonadherence in patients with schizophrenia.[50-52] Worsening of anxiety and aggressive behavior may result in an increase in neuroleptic dose, which in turn may exacerbate the underlying akathisia. Although tardive akathisia may slowly remit upon drug discontinuation, it often persists.

Table 12-6 Approaches to Help Prevent Drug-Induced Akathisia

Amoxapine, atypical antipsychotics, conventional neuroleptics, lithium, metoclopramide

- Use lowest effective dose
- Use standardized dose titration to avoid excessive dose escalation
- Correct underlying iron deficiency
- If high risk for akathisia (e.g., prior history of akathisia) exists, concurrent administration of an antimuscarinic agent or β-blocker is recommended

Droperidol, prochlorperazine, promethazine, selective serotonin reuptake inhibitors, tricyclic antidepressants

- Use lowest effective dose

Carbamazepine

- None known

PREVENTION

Approaches to help prevent drug-induced akathisia are summarized in **Table 12-6**. As with most drug-induced diseases, prevention is very important. Primary prevention aided by knowledge and recognition of risk factors is a key factor for minimizing the burden of akathisia. The necessity of short- or long-term use of potentially causative agents should be carefully evaluated. If indicated, the lowest effective dose should be used, and patients should undergo regular evaluations for emergence of akathisia. Standardized titration of doses of antipsychotic agents to avoid excessive dose escalation and the use of atypical antipsychotics are successful means of prevention. Although iron deficiency has been associated with acute and tardive akathisia, routine iron supplementation as a preventive or treatment intervention is not supported by available evidence.[53] In patients at high risk of akathisia (e.g., history of akathisia), concurrent administration of an antimuscarinic agent or β-blocker is reasonable.

MANAGEMENT

Early detection is a key factor in the probability of eventual remission of drug-induced akathisia. If treatment with an implicated agent has been

Table 12-7 Management of Drug-Induced Akathisia

- Discontinue or reduce dose of causative agent
- If due to neuroleptic, switch to an atypical antipsychotic
- Consider trial of antimuscarinic agent or nonselective β-blocker (i.e. propranolol)
- Miscellaneous other agents may be effective (amantadine, benzodiazepine, clonidine, cyproheptadine, mianserin, mirtazapine)

extended for 3 months or longer, the patient should be examined periodically to determine the presence of subjective and objective features of akathisia. When akathisia is detected, several management approaches can be initiated (**Table 12-7**).

For patients with acute akathisia, the causative agent should be discontinued, if possible. For neuroleptic-treated patients, a switch to an atypical antipsychotic or alternative agent should be considered. In patients in whom causative agents have been discontinued, the akathisia may promptly resolve, only to be replaced with increased agitation and anxiety. Care should be taken to differentiate these symptoms from those of persistent akathisia. Administration of a lipophilic β-blocker, such as propranolol, is effective and well-tolerated.[54] β_2-receptor inhibition appears to be crucial for efficacy, as β_1-receptor selective agents are less effective.[55] However, a trial of a cardioselective, β_1-receptor blocker is reasonable if β_2-blockade is undesirable. The hydrophilic β-blockers (e.g., atenolol, nadolol) do not appear to be effective. β-blockers should be avoided in patients with a history of cardiac conduction blocks, orthostatic hypotension, or reactive airway disease. Administration of antimuscarinic agents (e.g., benztropine, diphenhydramine), benzodiazepines, or antiserotonergic agents (cyproheptadine) is also effective and may be preferable if sedation is desired.[54,56-58] However, these agents should be used with caution in elderly patients with cognitive impairment. Less commonly used agents include amantadine, amitriptyline, clonidine, mianserin, mirtazapine, and mild opioids (e.g., codeine or propoxyphene).[59-64]

Treatment of drug-induced tardive akathisia is difficult, as no drug therapy consistently provides benefit. If possible, therapy with the suspected agent should be discontinued, or modification of therapy from a conventional neuroleptic to an atypical antipsychotic should be performed. Antimuscarinic agents and β-blockers may be considered. However, compared with their use in patients with acute akathisia, improvement is less likely to occur.

INFORMATION FOR PATIENTS

Before initiating therapy with antipsychotic agents, clinicians should inform patients regarding the purpose of antipsychotic treatment and the potential risk of movement disorders, such as akathisia, and to document that this counseling has been performed. Informed consent is recommended by some clinicians, and should be updated yearly or when there is a change in antipsychotic therapy. The patient's family members or caregivers can play a role in monitoring and reporting any abnormal movements. Patients and caregivers should be educated regarding the symptoms of akathisia and the importance of timely reporting, because early detection reduces the risk of irreversible abnormal movements.

TARDIVE DYSKINESIA

TDk (also referred to as tardive stereotypy) presents as delayed-onset movements manifesting as repetitive, coordinated, seemingly purposeful movements affecting the orofacial area (e.g., lips, tongue, mouth). TDk does not present as parkinsonism-based resting tremor. Many patients with TDk develop a combination of movement disorders, and the presence of multiple movement disorders should alert the clinician to the possibility of DIMDs.

CAUSATIVE AGENTS

TDk is a persistent DIMD that develops after at least 1 month of treatment with DRBAs. Agents implicated in TDk are listed in **Table 12-8**.[9-13,23,65] The term *tardive dyskinesias* emphasizes the delayed or tardive onset of choreoathetoid, stereotypic movements.

Table 12-8 Agents Implicated in Drug-Induced Tardive Dyskinesia

Drug	Incidence	Level of Evidence[a]
ANTIEMETICS/GASTRIC MOTILITY AGENTS		
Metoclopramide[23]	12–40%	B
Prochlorperazine[23]	NK	C
PSYCHOTROPICS		
Amoxapine[65]	NK	C
Atypical antipsychotics[9-11,13,b]	5–15%	A
Conventional neuroleptics[12,13,c]	20–30%	A

NK = not known.

[a]Definitions for Levels of Evidence: Level A—evidence from one or more randomized, controlled clinical trials; Level B—evidence from nonrandomized clinical trials, prospective observational studies, cohort studies, retrospective studies, case-control studies, meta-analyses and/or postmarketing surveillance studies; and Level C—evidence from one or more published case reports or case series.

[b]Amisulpride, aripiprazole, asenapine, brexpiprazole, cariprazine, iloperidone, lurasidone, olanzapine, paliperidone, quetiapine, risperidone, sertindole, ziprasidone.

[c]Chlorpromazine, fluphenazine, haloperidol, mesoridazine, molindone, perphenazine, promazine, thioridazine, thiothixene, trifluoperazine, triflupromazine.

EPIDEMIOLOGY

Since the initial reports in the late 1950s and early 1960s, TDk has become one of the most recognized DIMDs.[66-68] In the early 1970s, product labeling for all antipsychotic drugs was revised to include information regarding TDk. Although symptoms may initially be mild, many patients develop progressively severe TDk, resulting in meaningful disability. In a study of antipsychotic-naive patients with first-episode schizophrenia, the incidence of persistent TDk increased with longer duration of treatment.[69] The cumulative incidence of TDk was 4.8% after 1 year, 7.2% after 2 years, and 15.6% after 4 years. Increasing antipsychotic drug dose was associated with a modestly increased risk of TDk, with each 100-mg chlorpromazine equivalent unit increase associated with a 5% increase in the risk of TDk. In the Hillside Hospital TDk study, young patients (mean age 29 years) were followed prospectively for several years.[70] The incidence of TDk associated with neuroleptic treatment was 5.3% per year, similar to that in other prospective studies.[12] The authors concluded that, at the end of 5 years, approximately one in four patients treated with neuroleptics were at risk for TDk. It is important to note that peculiar, choreiform orofacial movements were observed in patients with schizophrenia before the advent of conventional neuroleptic therapy and that dyskinesias may be an intrinsic motor feature of schizophrenia.[71] Although spontaneous dyskinesias occur, the data provide strong evidence demonstrating an increased incidence of TDk associated with neuroleptic drug exposure.

The overall incidence of TDk associated with neuroleptic drug therapy ranges from 0.5 to 70%.[72,73] This range reflects differences in diagnostic criteria, duration of follow-up, sampled population, and study design. Overall, TDk develops in approximately 20–30% of patients treated with conventional neuroleptics.[72,73] On the basis of studies in young patients, estimates of incidence suggest that TDk develops in about 5% of patients per year of neuroleptic exposure.[74] The highest incidence and prevalence of TDk appears to occur in the geropsychiatric population. In a study of elderly psychiatric patients who had never previously received neuroleptic agents, 35.4% developed TDk during neuroleptic treatment.[75] In a prospective study of previously neuroleptic-naive patients 55 years of age or older, the cumulative incidence of TDk was 25%, 34%, and 53% after 1, 2, and 3 years, respectively, of antipsychotic therapy.[76] In another study of middle-aged and elderly patients, the cumulative incidence of neuroleptic-induced TDk was 26%, 52%, and 60% after 1, 2, and 3 years, respectively.[77]

Neuroleptic-induced TDk is a class effect among the conventional neuroleptics. Although debatable, the risk appears to be similar for all agents within the class regardless of formulation (e.g., oral or depot injection). However, the risk of TDk is lower in association with atypical antipsychotics, regardless of prior neuroleptic exposure.[9-13] In one review of 11 long-term studies that were published between 1999 and 2002 (n >2,700 patients), the atypical antipsychotics (olanzapine, quetiapine, risperidone, ziprasidone) were associated with a mean annual incidence of new-onset TDk of 0.8% in adults, compared with 5.4% of those treated with haloperidol.[9] Despite the fact that most patients had been exposed to conventional neuroleptics prior to treatment with an atypical antipsychotic, the incidence of TDk was lower compared to that in haloperidol-treated patients. In this study, the risk of TDk associated with atypical antipsychotics was one-fifth that of conventional neuroleptics. A subsequent systematic review of 12 newer long-term studies published between 2004 and 2006 (n >30,000 patients) confirmed that atypical antipsychotics are associated with a significantly lower incidence of TDk as compared with conventional neuroleptics.[10]

Long-term use of antidopaminergic antiemetics or gastric-motility agents is also associated with a significant risk of TDk. In one study of 434 patients diagnosed with TDk in a movement disorders clinic, the causative agent was metoclopramide in 39.4% of patients, followed by prochlorperazine and promethazine in 11.8% and 9.4% of patients, respectively.[23] In 2009, the U.S. Food and Drug Administration issued a mandate that metoclopramide product labeling regarding TDk must be strengthened to a black box warning.

MECHANISMS

The pathophysiologic basis of drug-induced TDk remains speculative. Results from a study utilizing population pharmacokinetic analysis and D_2 receptor occupancy modeling suggests that higher trough D_2 receptor occupancy (i.e., high trough D_2 receptor blockade) is associated with greater risk of developing TDk.[78] Chronic D_2 receptor blockade results in various neurochemical sequelae including striatal dopaminergic hypersensitivity, cholinergic deficiency within the basal ganglia, dysfunction of striatonigral gamma-aminobutyric acid (GABA)-mediated neurons, maladaptive *N*-methyl-D-aspartate (NMDA)-mediated synaptic plasticity, glutamate-induced excitotoxicity, and oxidative stress.[79-84] Support for some of these hypotheses is derived from observations that antimuscarinic agents worsen TDk, whereas agents with GABAergic, antiglutamatergic, and antioxidant activity suppress TDk. Other mechanistic factors may include attenuation of nitric oxide–mediated neuromodulation in the striatum, genetic polymorphisms of dopamine, NMDA and serotonin receptor genes, and neuroleptic-induced neuronal apoptosis.[85-91] Ex vivo data from animal models of TDk suggest that presynaptic areas such as the substantia nigra are involved.[92] The most popular mechanistic hypothesis for TDk involves long-term blockade of striatal dopamine D_2 receptors resulting in receptor upregulation and hypersensitization. A postmortem study in neuroleptic-treated patients with schizophrenia was unable to detect significant differences in striatal dopamine D_1 or D_2 receptors between patients with and those without TDk.[93] However, an in vivo study using radioligand positron-emission tomography demonstrated that patients with the highest degree of dopamine D_2 receptor upregulation had severe TDk.[94] Within the striatum, GABA and glutamate are the major neurotransmitters that modulate the motor circuit. Evidence suggests that GABA deficiency enhances dyskinesia, and excess glutamate is implicated in neuronal toxicity. Given that several hypotheses are plausible, the pathophysiology of TDk most likely involves multiple mechanisms and events. A unifying hypothesis can be proposed: use of DRBAs results in increased dopamine turnover followed by excess free radical production and subsequent damage to striatal GABAergic fibers and reduced inhibitory activity on motor circuits. Concurrently, long-term blockade of dopamine receptors results in excessive glutamate activity and resultant excitotoxicity. Likewise, long-term dopamine receptor blockade results in receptor supersensitivity and persistent changes within the basal ganglia motor circuit.

CLINICAL PRESENTATION AND DIFFERENTIAL DIAGNOSIS

Symptoms of drug-induced TDk are characterized by a combination of involuntary choreiform (rapid, jerky, nonrepetitive), athetoid (slow, sinuous, writhing), and stereotypic (rhythmic, repetitive) movements (Table 12-3). Regions of the mouth and face (i.e., oral, buccal, lingual, masticatory) are most commonly affected, followed by upper and lower limbs. Choreiform movements commonly affect the proximal muscles, whereas athetoid movements affect the distal muscles. Frequently, TDk occurs in the presence of other movement disorders such as akathisia, dystonia, or parkinsonism. The onset of drug-induced TDk is insidious, and symptoms are initially mild and often unnoticeable to patients. The vast majority of TDk cases are associated with antipsychotic treatment. Patients receiving long-term metoclopramide or phenothiazine antiemetic treatment are also at risk for TDk. Rarely, TDk may occur in association with other agents, such as antiepileptics, lithium, oral contraceptives, and SSRIs. If the offending drug is not discontinued, remission of TDk is rare. Occasionally, TDk may also occur after discontinuation of long-term DRBA treatment. This is reported most commonly in children, but in one study 34% of adult patients—with no prior evidence of TDk in whom neuroleptic therapy was withdrawn—developed emergent dyskinesia within 3 weeks.[74,95] In general, withdrawal dyskinesia improves within 3 months. Also, latent TDk may be "unmasked" during a reduction in neuroleptic dose and during a switch to an atypical antipsychotic.

When assessing a patient presenting with TDk symptoms, the clinician should keep in mind that orofacial dyskinesias can be a feature of several other conditions, including Huntington disease, hyperthyroidism, levodopa-induced dyskinesias, neuroacanthocytosis (choreoacanthocytosis), Sydenham chorea, and Wilson disease (Table 12-4). In addition, orofacial dyskinetic-like movements may be observed in edentulous individuals as well as patients with schizophrenia who are DRBA-naive.[96,97] In one large study of over 2,000 subjects, spontaneous dyskinesia was reported in 1.3% of healthy elderly individuals, 4.8% of medical geriatric inpatients, and up to 2% of neuroleptic-naive psychiatric patients.[74]

The diagnosis of drug-induced TDk is straightforward in most cases. For assessment purposes, the Abnormal Involuntary Movement Scale (AIMS) developed by the National Institute of Mental Health is commonly used, particularly in the psychiatric field.[98] The AIMS rates dyskinetic movements in seven body regions and includes assessments for global severity, functional impairment, and self-awareness of symptoms. Orofacial features include involuntary blinking, chewing and lower jaw movements, grimacing, lip puckering and smacking, tongue protrusion and twisting, and facial tic-like movements. Many patients also experience concurrent choreoathetoid or stereotypic movements of the feet, hands, limbs, trunk, head, and neck. Movements of the fingers may appear as though the patient is playing an invisible guitar or piano. Occasionally, patients exhibit pelvic rocking or "copulatory dyskinesia" and grunting or moaning due to respiratory and pharyngeal dyskinesia.[99] Factors associated with exacerbation of TDk symptoms include administration of antimuscarinics or sympathomimetic stimulants and emotional extremes. Symptoms of TDk can be suppressed for brief periods. Distraction during voluntary movements of unaffected body parts (e.g., finger-tapping test) or during performance of mental tasks (e.g., arithmetic) unmasks latent dyskinesia in other body parts. As with most dyskinesias, symptoms subside during sleep and, in mild cases, patients may be unaware of the movements.

Rabbit syndrome is a rare and peculiar EPS that involves a slow, rhythmic, vertical-only tremor of the perioral region that resembles the chewing motions of a rabbit. Rabbit syndrome is very specific to the buccal region only and differs from orofacial TDk in that tongue involvement is absent. Rabbit syndrome is associated predominantly with neuroleptics, with an incidence ranging from 2.3 to 4.4%.[100] Some clinicians consider rabbit syndrome to be a form of drug-induced parkinsonism.

RISK FACTORS

In general, if patients do not develop TDk during the initial 5 years of neuroleptic treatment, the risk of TDk developing during later years of therapy is reduced. Risk factors for the development of TDk include older age, mood disorder symptomatology, alcoholism or substance-use disorder, concomitant anticholinergic use, conventional (as opposed to atypical) neuroleptic use, daily drug dose, diabetes mellitus, duration of treatment, previous electroconvulsive treatment, female sex, history of EPS, intermittent (as opposed to continuous) neuroleptic treatment, iron deficiency, intellectual disability, and organic brain disorder (**Table 12-9**).[69,76,101-114] Older age is also a well-established risk factor. The risk of TDk is at least five times greater in elderly patients compared to that in young individuals.[115] Not only is TDk more common in the elderly, but TDk also tends to be more severe and irreversible in this age group. If multiple risk factors are present, an additive effect on risk potential is observed. For example, elderly women are very susceptible to TDk. Interestingly, diabetes has been associated as a risk factor for TDk in patients with schizophrenia.[108,109] Diabetic patients treated with metoclopramide are also at increased risk of TDk, compared with metoclopramide-treated nondiabetic patients.[116] However, although some atypical antipsychotics may induce glucose intolerance and diabetes mellitus, the overall risk of TDk remains low compared with that of conventional neuroleptics. The presence of a mood disorder has also been implicated as a risk factor for TDk, although supportive data are equivocal.[117,118]

Table 12-9 Risk Factors for Drug-Induced Tardive Dyskinesia

- Advanced age
- Alcoholism or substance abuse disorder
- Anticholinergic use
- Daily neuroleptic dose
- Diabetes mellitus
- Duration of neuroleptic treatment
- Female sex
- History of electroconvulsive therapy
- History of extrapyramidal symptoms
- Intermittent neuroleptic treatment
- Intellectual disability
- Iron deficiency
- Mood disorder
- Organic brain disorder

MORBIDITY AND MORTALITY

Once TDk develops, remission rates are low if therapy with the antipsychotic drug is continued. In one study, only 11% of patients improved over the course of 5 years with continued therapy.[119] If treatment is discontinued upon early detection, remission rates are favorable, especially in the younger population, but complete remission may require several months to years. However, discontinuation of antipsychotic therapy for the purpose of treating TDk is associated with risks, primarily psychotic decompensation. Mild cases of TDk are often associated with social impairment such as employment difficulties, social isolation, and stigma. Anxiety and stress further exacerbate symptoms. In more severe cases, functional impairment occurs. Patients experience difficulties with chewing, speaking, and swallowing. Orofacial dyskinesias may also result in dental problems, denture displacement, and damage to the soft tissues within the oral cavity. Gait abnormality associated with lower-extremity dyskinesia may result in falls and injury.

PREVENTION

Approaches to help prevent drug-induced TDk are summarized in **Table 12-10**. Primary prevention aided by knowledge and recognition of risk factors is key to minimizing the burden of TDk. The necessity for long-term therapy with DRBAs such as conventional neuroleptics, metoclopramide, and antidopaminergic antiemetics should be carefully evaluated. Standardized dose titration to avoid excessive dose escalation and the use of atypical antipsychotics, rather than conventional antipsychotics, are successful means of prevention. Other strategies include use of lowest effective DRBA dose and eliminating unnecessary, prolonged drug therapy. Although the use of intermittent antipsychotic treatment (or drug holidays), compared with continuous treatment, may seem like a logical strategy for reducing TDk

Table 12-10 Approaches to Help Prevent Drug-Induced Tardive Dyskinesia

Amoxapine, metoclopramide, prochlorperazine

- Carefully evaluate the necessity for long-term administration
- Avoid unnecessary, prolonged drug therapy

Atypical antipsychotics

- Carefully evaluate the necessity for long-term administration
- Use standardized dose titration to avoid excessive dose escalation
- Use lowest effective dose

Conventional neuroleptics

- Carefully evaluate the necessity for long-term administration
- Use standardized dose titration to avoid excessive dose escalation
- Use lowest effective dose
- Consider use of atypical antipsychotic agent

risk, it is actually associated with an increased risk of TDk and higher rates of psychosis relapse and rehospitalization.[111,120] The American Psychiatric Association has published specific indications for short- and long-term antipsychotic drug treatment.[121]

MANAGEMENT

Early detection of drug-induced TDk is imperative, as remission rates are inversely correlated with duration and severity of TDk. For patients with dyskinesias induced by non-DRBAs (e.g., antiepileptics, lithium, oral contraceptives, SSRIs), abnormal movements generally reverse or improve within weeks after discontinuation of the offending drug. For neuroleptic-induced TDk, the movements may improve (generally within weeks) in up to 50% of patients after discontinuation of the causative agent. Thus, routine assessment for TDk (approximately every 3–6 months) is recommended. The most consistent predictor of improvement after discontinuation of neuroleptic therapy is younger age, with an inverse correlation between rates of remission and age.[122] Remission is less likely in patients with severe TDk and the elderly.

Evidence-based guidelines are available for the treatment of tardive syndromes (TDS), including TDk.[123,124] The American Academy of Neurology (AAN) guidelines address the following questions:

1. Is withdrawal of the dopamine receptor blocker an effective treatment for TDS?
2. Does switching from typical to atypical dopamine-blocking agents reduce TDS symptoms?
3. What is the efficacy of drugs in treating TDS?
4. Do patients with TDS benefit from chemodenervation with botulinum toxin?
5. Do patients with TDS benefit from surgical therapy?

The guidelines state that data are insufficient to support or refute discontinuation of therapy with the causative agent as treatment; however, from a clinical context, if TDk is present, it is recommended that the clinician discontinue therapy with the antipsychotic (applies only to patients who can tolerate this). Occasionally, discontinuation of an antipsychotic results in emergence or worsening of dyskinesia (i.e., withdrawal dyskinesia); however, withdrawal dyskinesias are generally self-limiting within 3 months.

The AAN guidelines note that short-term withdrawal may worsen TDk. In clinical practice, switching from a typical antipsychotic to an atypical antipsychotic often results in improvement, and is considered an appropriate approach if maintenance antipsychotic treatment is indicated. However, from an evidence-based perspective, the AAN panel found that data were insufficient to support or refute replacing a typical antipsychotic with an atypical agent to reduce TDk symptoms. The AAN panel reviewed studies involving several drugs for the treatment of TDk and found high levels of evidence to establish deutetrabenazine and valbenazine as effective treatments for TDk. Thus, if pharmacologic intervention is required, deutetrabenazine or valbenazine are recommended as first-line agents. Only moderate evidence is available to support the use of clonazepam and ginkgo biloba and weak evidence to support the use of amantadine and tetrabenazine. The AAN panel found

Table 12-11 Management of Drug-Induced Tardive Dyskinesia

- Discontinue or reduce dose of causative agent
- Discontinue concurrent antimuscarinic agents
- If due to neuroleptic, switch to an atypical antipsychotic
- Consider deutetrabenazine or valbenazine as first-line pharmacologic interventions
- Consider deep brain stimulation (globus pallidus) for medically refractory and severe cases
- Miscellaneous agents (amantadine, baclofen, botulinum toxin, branched-chain amino acids, clonazepam, donepezil, gabapentin, ginkgo biloba, levetiracetam, melatonin, ondansetron, pregabalin, thiamine, verapamil, vitamin B_6, vitamin E) may be considered if other interventions ineffective or not tolerated

insufficient evidence to support or refute the use of acetazolamide, α-methyldopa, aripiprazole, botulinum toxin type A, buspirone, bromocriptine, baclofen, clozapine, fluperlapine, flupenthixol, haloperidol, levetiracetam, melatonin, nifedipine, olanzapine, quetiapine, reserpine, selegiline, sertindole, sulpiride, thiamine, thiopropazate, vitamin B_6, vitamin E, yi-gan san, ziprasidone, and electroconvulsive therapy.

Management approaches for drug-induced TDk are summarized in **Table 12-11**. Of note, because anxiety often exacerbates signs and symptoms of TDk, concomitant anxiety should be treated appropriately. Treatment of rabbit syndrome involves reduction of the neuroleptic dose as much as possible and therapy with an antimuscarinic agent may be attempted. This contrasts with orofacial TDk, for which addition of an antimuscarinic agent tends to exacerbate the movements.

INFORMATION FOR PATIENTS

Before initiating therapy with antipsychotics, clinicians should inform patients about the purpose of antipsychotic treatment and the potential risk of TDk and document that this counseling has been performed.[125] Some clinicians believe that such discussion concerning the risk of TDk should occur after the patient's acute psychiatric condition is stabilized, and at the time that treatment for longer than 3 months is considered.[126] Informed consent is recommended and should be updated yearly or when there is a change in antipsychotic medication.[127] The benefits and need for long-term treatment with antipsychotics should be discussed, and patients should be informed that long-term treatment can result in TDk, especially with the conventional neuroleptics. Patients should understand that movement disorders may also occur in association with the atypical antipsychotics, but are much less common and that early detection of any antipsychotic movement disorder is important and reduces the risk of irreversible abnormal movements. The patient's family members or caregivers can play a role in monitoring and reporting any abnormal movements.

DYSTONIA (ACUTE AND TARDIVE)

Drug-induced acute dystonia (DIAD) occurs shortly after the introduction of a dopamine-receptor blocking agent (e.g., antipsychotic agent) and occasionally after a dose increase or switch to a more potent antipsychotic agent, particularly an injectable high-potency antipsychotic drug. Dystonic reactions are variable in anatomical location and severity and are occasionally painful. The usual manifestations are orofacial dystonia, back arching, and neck extension (retrocollis). The term *tardive dystonia* is used to describe late-onset dystonia. Tardive dystonia is often indistinguishable from idiopathic torsion dystonia. However, patients with tardive dystonia may also have concomitant orobuccolingual dyskinesia.

CAUSATIVE AGENTS

Agents implicated in drug-induced dystonia are listed in **Table 12-12**.[11,13,37,128-136]

EPIDEMIOLOGY

The reported incidence of DIAD varies widely, from 2% to 94% of patients treated with conventional neuroleptics.[128-130] This variance may be attributed to the study method, the study setting (e.g., inpatient or outpatient), and the characteristics of the study population, including age, concurrent use of antimuscarinic agents, and type of neuroleptic agent.

Table 12-12 Agents Implicated in Drug-Induced Dystonia

Drug	Incidence	Level of Evidence[a]
ANTIEMETICS/GASTRIC MOTILITY AGENTS		
Metoclopramide[132]	1–5%	B
Prochlorperazine[131]	1–5%	B
PSYCHOTROPICS		
Atypical antipsychotics[11,13,37,b]	1–5%	A
Conventional neuroleptics[13,37,128-130,133-136,c]	1–50%	A

[a]Definitions for Levels of Evidence: Level A—evidence from one or more randomized, controlled clinical trials; Level B—evidence from nonrandomized clinical trials, prospective observational studies, cohort studies, retrospective studies, case-control studies, meta-analyses and/or postmarketing surveillance studies; and Level C—evidence from one or more published case reports or case series.
[b]Amisulpride, aripiprazole, asenapine, brexpiprazole, cariprazine, iloperidone, lurasidone, olanzapine, paliperidone, quetiapine, risperidone, sertindole, ziprasidone.
[c]Chlorpromazine, fluphenazine, haloperidol, mesoridazine, molindone, perphenazine, promazine, thioridazine, thiothixene, trifluoperazine, triflupromazine.

Other DRBAs (e.g., metoclopramide, prochlorperazine) are also associated with DIAD.[131,132] A prospective study of neuroleptic-treated psychiatric patients reported a prevalence of acute dystonia of 8.5% in those not receiving concurrent therapy with antimuscarinic agents.[137] The prevalence of acute dystonia was lower (2.8%) in patients concurrently taking an antimuscarinic drug. In the same study, DIAD was more commonly associated with butyrophenone antipsychotics (e.g., haloperidol) compared with phenothiazine antipsychotics (e.g., chlorpromazine). In an analysis of pooled data from nine studies, the overall incidence of antipsychotic-induced acute dystonia in patients not receiving antimuscarinic prophylaxis was 14.8%.[133] However, in patients receiving high-potency neuroleptics (e.g., haloperidol), the incidence was 51.2%. One retrospective study of 159 patients found the incidence of neuroleptic-induced dystonia to be 15.7%, while another retrospective study reported an incidence of 31% in young patients.[134,135] A prospective, 14-day study reported an incidence of acute dystonia of 33% associated with haloperidol treatment in young inpatients with psychosis not receiving concurrent therapy with antimuscarinic agents.[136]

Tardive dystonia is distinct from TDk, although the two often coexist. Tardive dystonia, originally known as dystonia tarda, is defined as an involuntary movement predominated by dystonia and associated with the use of a DRBA.[138,139] Tardive dystonia occurs in approximately 2–4% of patients treated with conventional neuroleptics.[140,141] However, the true incidence may be much greater. In one study of inpatient veterans receiving long-term neuroleptic treatment, the prevalence of tardive dystonia was 21.6%.[142]

MECHANISMS

Mechanisms of acute and tardive dystonias are unclear. Dopaminergic hypofunction within the basal ganglia with subsequent overactivity of the cholinergic system has been proposed, and this hypothesis is supported by the antidystonia activity of antimuscarinic agents. A contrasting hypothesis implicates striatal dopaminergic hyperactivity. In addition, other neurotransmitter systems such as GABA and serotonin may contribute.

CLINICAL PRESENTATION AND DIFFERENTIAL DIAGNOSIS

In most cases, the first signs and symptoms of DIAD generally appear within 48 hours of the initiation of drug therapy and, in virtually all cases, signs and symptoms appear within 5 days. Signs and symptoms of DIAD can also occur after an increase in the dose of the DRBA or a reduction in the dose of a concomitant antimuscarinic agent. The risk of DIAD appears to be greater in younger patients and in those receiving DRBAs via the parenteral route. Symptoms include sustained muscular contractions or spasms that result in abnormal fixed postures or positions of the jaw, neck, shoulders, trunk, and extremities (Table 12-3). The severity of symptoms and anatomical distribution varies, but the classic clinical presentation is characterized by the three Os: oculogyric crisis (conjugate deviation of the eyes upward or laterally), opisthotonos or extensor axial dystonia (involuntary posturing in which the head, neck, and spine are arched backward), and oromandibular dystonia (forceful contractions of the jaw causing difficulty in opening or closing the mouth). Blepharospasm (involuntary eyelid closure), trismus (jaw-closing dystonia), laryngeal spasm, tongue protrusion, and respiratory stridor may also be present. Symptoms are usually painful and can interfere with walking, breathing, speaking, swallowing, and vision. In severe cases (e.g., laryngeal spasm), DIAD may be life-threatening. Rhabdomyolysis due to sustained muscle contraction may also occur. Acute dystonia is not only painful and frightening to the patient but the bizarre posturing may be mistaken for hysterical conversion by observers. If acute dystonia occurs in the presence of fever, generalized rigidity, altered level of consciousness, and autonomic instability, a diagnosis of neuroleptic malignant syndrome should be considered (Table 12-4). Dystonia may also resemble catatonia because of the underlying psychiatric disorder. However, in contrast to catatonic patients, those in whom dystonia develops report anxiety and discomfort and seek treatment. Because of the discomfort associated with DIAD, patients are at higher risk for medication nonadherence.

Tardive dystonia develops after months to years during treatment with a DRBA or within 3 months after discontinuation of therapy, and often coexists with TDk. Remission of tardive dystonia is uncommon. DRBAs are most commonly implicated in tardive dystonia. SSRIs have been rarely implicated.[16] In general, the diagnosis of tardive dystonia can be made based on the presence of persistent dystonia (for longer than 1 month), a documented history of DRBA use, and the absence of a general medical or neurologic condition that may account for dystonia (e.g., *DYTI* gene mutations and genetic forms of dystonia, focal lesions of the basal ganglia, stiff person syndrome). In contrast to DIAD, symptoms of tardive dystonia develop insidiously over weeks to months. Symptoms may or may not be painful and can be isolated to one body part (e.g., jaw, cervical area) or may spread to contiguous body parts (segmental dystonia) or even generalize to multiple body parts. Patients often report that anxiety and stress exacerbate symptoms transiently, resulting in daily variations of symptomatology. The clinical presentation of tardive dystonia resembles that of an idiopathic focal, segmental, or generalized dystonia. Cervical tardive dystonia resembles that of idiopathic cervical dystonia. In patients with cervical dystonia, the neck muscles contract involuntarily and sustained contractions cause abnormal head and neck posturing (**Figure 12-1**), whereas periodic muscular spasms cause jerky head movements that may resemble head tremors. The abnormal posturing may vary from mild to severe, pain may or may not be present, and a dystonic head tremor may be present. The concurrent presence of oromandibular dystonia with blepharospasm resembles Meige syndrome. Blepharospasm affects both eyelids and should not be mistaken for hemifacial spasm, which is a peripheral nerve disorder that is generally unilateral and involves twitching or myoclonic spasms affecting the eyelids, cheeks, and mouth regions. Tardive oromandibular dystonia is associated with persistent difficulty in opening or closing the mouth and affects chewing, speech,

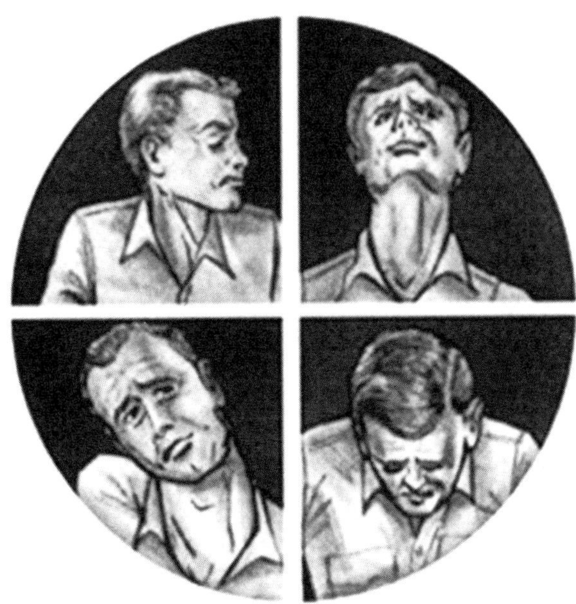

FIGURE 12-1 Cervical Dystonia

Upper left: rotational; upper right: retrocollis; lower right: anterocollis; lower left: laterocollis.

and swallowing. Bruxism may also accompany jaw-closing dystonia.

Pisa syndrome is a form of axial dystonia that is most commonly associated with neuroleptic treatment and is characterized by sustained truncal lateroflexion.[143] Drug-induced Pisa syndrome is more common in elderly patients, females, those receiving combination antipsychotics, or patients who have organic brain pathology (e.g., dementia).[144] The onset of Pisa syndrome may be acute or tardive. Treatment consists of administering antimuscarinic agents and discontinuing or reducing daily doses of the causative agent. As with tardive dystonia, Pisa syndrome responds more favorably to antimuscarinic treatment than TDk. However, unlike tardive dystonia, symptoms of Pisa syndrome generally abate after discontinuation of therapy with the causative agent. Thus, Pisa syndrome may be considered an atypical subtype of tardive dystonia. Rarely, patients with tardive dystonia may experience *status dystonicus*, a life-threatening condition associated with severe dystonic spasms resulting in rhabdomyolysis, myoglobinuria, and acute kidney injury.

In addition to idiopathic dystonia, other conditions, such as atlantoaxial rotary subluxation, conversion reaction, dopa-responsive dystonia, inherited dystonias (e.g., *DYT1*), Huntington disease, and Wilson disease must be ruled out (Table 12-4). Other conditions that cause a twisted neck, such as orthopedic or congenital problems of the neck, ophthalmologic conditions resulting in head tilt to compensate for double vision, stiff neck, arthritis, or wry neck should also be considered.

RISK FACTORS

Risk factors for the development of acute dystonia include young age (<35 years),[135] previous electroconvulsive therapy, male sex, intellectual disability, and use of high-potency neuroleptics (**Table 12-13**). As with other DIMDs, the presence of multiple risk factors confers an additive effective on risk; for example, young men are very susceptible to dystonic reactions.[137] An inverse relationship exists between the incidence of DIAD and age. In contrast to TDk, dystonia is uncommon in older patients. In one retrospective study, antipsychotic-induced acute dystonia was 15 times more common in patients under 35 years of age compared with patients older than 35 years (31% versus 2%, respectively).[135] The highest risk population is young male patients receiving high-potency neuroleptics.[145]

Table 12-13 Risk Factors for Drug-Induced Dystonia

- High-potency neuroleptics
- History of electroconvulsive therapy
- Intellectual disability
- Male sex
- Mood disorder
- Young age (<35 years)

Patients with mood disorders may be at greater risk of DIAD. In a study of 181 male patients with mania or schizophrenia treated with conventional neuroleptics, a significantly higher proportion of the manic patients (26.1%) developed acute dystonia compared to those with schizophrenia (5.9%).[146] However, subsequent studies have failed to find a significant difference in the prevalence of DIAD between manic and schizophrenic patients. In a prospective study of 31 patients, neuroleptic-induced dystonia occurred in 62.5% of patients with mania and 66.7% of those with schizophrenia.[147] In another prospective study of 83 male patients, neuroleptic-induced acute dystonia was reported in 24% of patients with mania and 15% of patients with schizophrenia.[148] Manic patients received higher peak doses of neuroleptics during the risk period for dystonia, and analysis revealed that peak neuroleptic dose and younger age were strongly related to the occurrence of dystonia.

Risk factors for tardive dystonia overlap with some of the risk factors for DIAD and include young age, male sex, and the presence of TDk. Children are considered high risk for drug-induced tardive dystonia. Duration of therapy is not consistently correlated with the risk of drug-induced tardive dystonia, which may develop after a relatively short duration of therapy or after years of treatment. In some cases, drug-induced tardive dystonia may develop following a dose increase despite a long stable period of treatment.[16]

MORBIDITY AND MORTALITY

Although drug-induced dystonia generally does not affect mortality, except in rare cases of laryngeal spasm or status dystonicus, patients are at higher risk for medication nonadherence or refusal because of the discomfort that accompanies a dystonic reaction. In moderate-to-severe cases of tardive dystonia, task-specific impairment can occur, the likelihood of which depends on the affected body part. For example, blepharospasm may impair driving abilities, anterocollis or retrocollis can interfere with maintaining an appropriate line of vision that is required for walking and other sight-directed activities, and jaw-closing dystonia can damage dentition.

PREVENTION

Approaches to help prevent drug-induced dystonia are summarized in **Table 12-14**. Primary prevention aided by knowledge and recognition of risk factors is key to minimizing the burden of drug-induced dystonia. The necessity of short- or long-term use of potentially causative DRBAs such as conventional neuroleptics, metoclopramide, and antidopaminergic antiemetics should be evaluated carefully. If indicated, the lowest effective dose should be administered, and patients should undergo regular evaluation for the emergence of dystonic posturing. Standardized dose titration to avoid excessive dose escalation and the use of atypical antipsychotics are successful means of prevention.

Several studies comparing the incidence of neuroleptic-induced acute dystonia report that administration of concurrent antimuscarinic agents (e.g., benztropine, diphenhydramine, trihexyphenidyl) reduces the overall rate of dystonia by at least twofold.[133,136,137] In patients treated with high-potency neuroleptics (e.g., haloperidol), the risk reduction is even greater (5- to 11-fold).[133,149] Because the greatest risk of neuroleptic-induced acute dystonia occurs within the first week of drug treatment, short-term administration of an oral antimuscarinic agent should be considered, especially in young patients receiving high-potency antipsychotics.[145,150,151]

Table 12-14 Approaches to Help Prevent Drug-Induced Dystonia

Amoxapine, metoclopramide, prochlorperazine

- Carefully evaluate the necessity for short- or long-term therapy
- Use standardized dose titration to avoid excessive dose escalation
- Administer lowest effective dose

Atypical antipsychotics

- Carefully evaluate the necessity for short- or long-term therapy
- Use standardized dose titration to avoid excessive dose escalation
- Administer lowest effective dose
- Short-term administration of oral antimuscarinic agent (e.g., benztropine, diphenhydramine, trihexyphenidyl) may be considered for young patients receiving high-dose olanzapine, paliperidone, or risperidone

Conventional neuroleptics

- Carefully evaluate the necessity of short- or long-term therapy
- Use standardized dose titration to avoid excessive dose escalation
- Administer lowest effective dose
- Consider use of atypical antipsychotic agent
- Short-term administration of oral antimuscarinic agent (e.g., benztropine, diphenhydramine, trihexyphenidyl) may be considered, especially in young patients receiving high-potency neuroleptics

The efficacy of antimuscarinic prophylaxis appears to be inversely related to age.[133] Because of reduced prophylactic efficacy and undesirable antimuscarinic adverse reactions (e.g., cognitive impairment, sedation), the use of antimuscarinic agents in elderly patients for the primary prevention of DIAD is disfavored. Although antimuscarinic agents reduce the severity of EPS, these drugs are also associated with adverse effects, such as blurred vision, cognitive impairment, constipation, dry mouth, sexual dysfunction, and urinary retention. Currently, the practice of primary prophylaxis of drug-induced dystonia with antimuscarinic agents is controversial, but appears to be reasonable in patients at high risk for dystonia (e.g., young men receiving conventional neuroleptics).

Table 12-15 Management of Drug-Induced Dystonia

Acute dystonia

- Discontinue causative agent
- Administer antimuscarinic agent

Tardive dystonia

- Discontinue or reduce dose of causative agent
- If due to neuroleptic, switch to an atypical antipsychotic
- A trial of an antimuscarinic agent may be used
- Consider tetrabenazine
- Consider botulinum toxin for focal dystonias
- A trial of muscle relaxant (e.g., baclofen) may be used
- Miscellaneous agents (amantadine, clonidine, levetiracetam, pregabalin) may be used
- Consider deep brain stimulation (globus pallidus) or pallidotomy

MANAGEMENT

Management approaches for drug-induced dystonia are summarized in **Table 12-15**. Acute dystonia can be relieved effectively with a short course of therapy with a potent antimuscarinic agent (e.g., benztropine, diphenhydramine) administered orally, intramuscularly, or intravenously. If drug-induced dystonia is life-threatening (e.g., stridor due to laryngospasm), intravenous administration of antimuscarinic drugs is warranted and supportive measures such as tracheostomy may be required. Benzodiazepines may be administered to relieve anxiety in conjunction with antimuscarinic therapy.

Symptoms of tardive dystonia also may be improved with antimuscarinic therapy. In addition, atypical antipsychotics (e.g., clozapine, quetiapine), benzodiazepines, muscle relaxants (e.g., baclofen), and dopamine-depleting drugs such as tetrabenazine are also effective. Less commonly used drugs include amantadine, β-blockers, benzodiazepines, clonidine, dantrolene, levodopa, and antiepileptics such as levetiracetam, pregabalin, tiagabine, and zonisamide.

For patients with symptoms of focal dystonia (e.g., cervical, mandibular), local injections of botulinum toxin are highly effective and are preferred because of a low incidence of systemic adverse effects. In refractory and severe cases, intrathecal baclofen and deep brain stimulation of the globus pallidus or ablative pallidotomy should be considered.[152,153]

INFORMATION FOR PATIENTS

Before initiating therapy with DRBAs, clinicians should inform patients regarding the purpose of treatment and the potential risk of dystonia and document that this counseling has been performed. If long-term treatment with a DRBA is anticipated, informed consent is recommended and should be updated yearly. Patients should also understand that early detection of any DRBA-induced movement disorder is important and reduces the risk of irreversible abnormal movements. The patient's family members or caregivers can play a role in monitoring and reporting any abnormal movements.

PARKINSONISM

CAUSATIVE AGENTS

After idiopathic Parkinson disease, drug-induced parkinsonism (DIP) is considered the second most common form. DIP is associated with up to 15% of all cases of parkinsonism worldwide. In one study of elderly patients, 51% of newly referred cases of parkinsonism were believed to be caused by drugs.[154] Agents implicated in drug-induced parkinsonism are listed in **Table 12-16**.[6,37,155-165] The DRBAs are the most commonly implicated agents, and are responsible for 70–80% of DIP cases worldwide. Valproate is a common cause of DIP.[159] Valproate-induced parkinsonism is often characterized by concurrent cognitive and hearing impairment and is underreported because of its insidious onset. The SSRIs are rarely associated with DIP, although SSRI-induced tremor is common.

EPIDEMIOLOGY

In patients treated with conventional neuroleptics, the prevalence of DIP ranges from 20% to 66%.[6,155,156] The prevalence of parkinsonism associated with atypical antipsychotics is much lower. In one study, the prevalence of parkinsonian rigidity associated with clozapine, risperidone, and

Table 12-16 Agents Implicated in Drug-Induced Parkinsonism

Drug	Incidence	Level of Evidence[a]
ANTIEMETICS/GASTRIC MOTILITY AGENTS		
Metoclopramide[157]	1–5%	B
Prochlorperazine[158]	1–5%	B
ANTIEPILEPTICS		
Valproate[159]	5%	B
CARDIOVASCULAR DRUGS		
Methyldopa[159]	NK	C
Reserpine[161]	NK	C
PSYCHOTROPICS		
Amoxapine[162]	NK	C
Atypical antipsychotics[37,b]	5–20%	A
Conventional neuroleptics[6,155,156,c]	20–60%	A
VESTIBULAR SEDATIVES		
Cinnarizine[163,d]	30%	B
Flunarizine[163,d]	30%	B
MISCELLANEOUS		
Tetrabenazine[164,165]	15%	A

NK = not known.
[a]Definitions for Levels of Evidence: Level A—evidence from one or more randomized, controlled clinical trials; Level B—evidence from nonrandomized clinical trials, prospective observational studies, cohort studies, retrospective studies, case-control studies, meta-analyses and/or postmarketing surveillance studies; and Level C—evidence from one or more published case reports or case series.
[b]Amisulpride, aripiprazole, asenapine, brexpiprazole, cariprazine, iloperidone, lurasidone, olanzapine, paliperidone, quetiapine, risperidone, sertindole, ziprasidone.
[c]Chlorpromazine, fluphenazine, haloperidol, mesoridazine, molindone, perphenazine, promazine, thioridazine, thiothixene, trifluoperazine, triflupromazine.
[d]Not marketed in the United States.

conventional neuroleptics was 4.9%, 17.4%, and 35.7%, respectively.[37]

MECHANISMS

The mechanism of DRBA-induced parkinsonism involves occupancy and blockade of striatal dopamine receptors (**Table 12-17**).[166-169] Relative to the conventional neuroleptics, the affinity of atypical antipsychotic agents for striatal dopaminergic receptors is lower, which helps to explain the dose-dependent incidence of parkinsonism induced by conventional neuroleptics and some of the atypical antipsychotics, such as olanzapine, paliperidone, and risperidone. However, receptor affinity and dissociation also play a role, and rapid dissociation from dopamine D_2 receptors (i.e., "fast-off-D_2") plays a role in mitigating EPS risk.[170,171] According to the fast-off-D_2 model,

Table 12-17 Mechanisms of Drug-Induced Parkinsonism

Drug	Mechanism
Amoxapine Atypical antipsychotics[a] Cinnarizine Conventional neuroleptics[b] Flunarizine Metoclopramide Prochlorperazine	Blockade of striatal dopamine-2 receptors
Methyldopa Reserpine Tetrabenazine	Neuronal dopamine depletion
Valproate	Unknown

[a]Amisulpride, aripiprazole, asenapine, brexpiprazole, cariprazine, iloperidone, lurasidone, olanzapine, paliperidone, quetiapine, risperidone, sertindole, ziprasidone.
[b]Chlorpromazine, fluphenazine, haloperidol, mesoridazine, molindone, perphenazine, promazine, thioridazine, thiothixene, trifluoperazine, triflupromazine.

atypical antipsychotics bind loosely to dopamine D_2 receptors, resulting in a short duration of binding, which is sufficient to produce antipsychotic activity without inducing EPS. Conventional neuroleptics bind tightly to dopamine D_2 receptors and thus produce antipsychotic activity, but with an increased risk of inducing EPS. Furthermore, among the atypical antipsychotics, fast-off-D_2 occurs more readily with low-potency agents compared with high-potency agents. For example, EPS is rarely associated with clozapine (an agent that requires higher doses for efficacy) compared with risperidone (an agent that requires lower doses). In addition, the atypical antipsychotics also block 5-HT_{2A} receptors that project to the presynaptic aspect of nigrostriatal dopamine neurons. Because activation of 5-HT_{2A} receptors inhibits dopamine release, blockade of these 5-HT_{2A} receptors enhances dopamine release sufficiently to mitigate the risk of EPS.

In addition to the DRBAs (e.g., antipsychotics, metoclopramide), drugs that deplete presynaptic dopamine (e.g., reserpine, tetrabenazine) or act as dopamine "false transmitters" (e.g., α-methyldopa) can also induce parkinsonism.

CLINICAL PRESENTATION AND DIFFERENTIAL DIAGNOSIS

In general, the clinical features of DIP are indistinguishable from those of idiopathic parkinsonism and include at least two of the following: tremor (rest or postural), rigidity, and bradykinesia (Table 12-3). In the absence of an accurate drug history, DIP can be easily mistaken for idiopathic Parkinson disease. Recognition of DIP may be difficult, as symptoms such as diminished facial expression, reduced energy and motivation, and bradykinesia can mimic negative symptoms of schizophrenia as well as psychomotor retardation associated with depressive disorders (Table 12-4). Tremor is often the most visible feature of DIP, but the presence of tremor in the absence of bradykinesia or rigidity is not parkinsonism. Symptoms of bradykinesia and rigidity often result in masked facies, shuffling gait, slowness of movement, and difficulty with daily tasks (e.g., walking, dressing, eating, grooming, writing). Some investigators define classic DIP as characterized by symmetrical distribution of symptoms, the additional presence of a chin or jaw tremor, and greater postural instability (balance problems and falling) upon initial presentation.[172,173] Single-photon emission computed tomography using a dopamine transporter ligand (e.g., ^{123}I-ioflupane) can be used to differentiate DIP from idiopathic Parkinson disease; results of this test should be normal in patients with DIP. In the majority of cases, DIP develops within 3 months of initiating therapy with the causative agent or, in some cases, after a dose increase, and is reversible upon drug discontinuation. Occasionally, the onset may be acute. Generally, DIP remits (over a period of several months) following discontinuation of therapy. However, some patients may have persistent DIP. The Simpson-Angus Scale is a 10-item rating scale that has been used widely for assessment of DIP in both clinical practice and research settings.[174] The scale consists of one item measuring gait (hypokinesia), six items measuring rigidity, and three items measuring glabella tap, tremor, and salivation, respectively.

RISK FACTORS

Risk factors for the development of DRBA-induced parkinsonism include vulnerability to EPS (e.g., older age, dementia, or pre-existing parkinsonism), female sex, and use of central DRBAs (e.g., metoclopramide, phenothiazine, and butyrophenone antipsychotics) (**Table 12-18**). Patients with acquired immunodeficiency syndrome (AIDS) appear to be very susceptible to DIP. In one study, the likelihood of EPS was 2.4 times higher among patients with AIDS as compared with patients with psychiatric disorders who did not have AIDS.[175]

Table 12-18 Risk Factors for Drug-Induced Parkinsonism

- Acquired immunodeficiency syndrome
- Advanced age
- Dementia
- Female sex
- Underlying Parkinson disease

Table 12-19 Approaches to Help Prevent Drug-Induced Parkinsonism

Amoxapine, atypical antipsychotics, cinnarizine, flunarizine, metoclopramide, prochlorperazine, tetrabenazine

- Carefully evaluate the necessity for long-term therapy
- Use standardized dose titration to avoid excessive dose escalation
- Administer the lowest effective dose

Conventional neuroleptics

- Carefully evaluate the necessity for long-term therapy
- Use standardized dose titration to avoid excessive dose escalation
- Administer the lowest effective dose
- Consider use of atypical antipsychotics
- Initiation of therapy with antimuscarinic agent for primary prevention is controversial, especially for the elderly

Methyldopa, reserpine, valproate

- No known means of prevention

MORBIDITY AND MORTALITY

Discontinuation of therapy with the offending agent often results in some improvement of parkinsonian features within 2 weeks. However, complete improvement is often not achieved for months or up to a year. In a subset of patients, features of parkinsonism remain indefinitely, despite discontinuation of therapy with the offending agent. Of the motor features, tremor typically confers the smallest degree of impairment of activities of daily living, as compared with bradykinesia.

PREVENTION

Approaches to help prevent drug-induced parkinsonism are summarized in **Table 12-19**. Primary prevention aided by knowledge and recognition of risk factors is key to minimizing the burden of DIP. The necessity for long-term use of potentially causative DRBAs such as conventional neuroleptics, metoclopramide, and antidopaminergic antiemetics should be carefully evaluated. If indicated, the lowest effective dose should be used and patients should undergo regular evaluation for emergence of symptoms of parkinsonism. Standardized dose titration to avoid excessive dose escalation and the use of atypical antipsychotics are successful means of prevention. In practice, some clinicians routinely use antimuscarinic agents for primary prophylaxis of DIP, but this approach is controversial, especially for elderly patients.

Table 12-20 Management of Drug-Induced Parkinsonism

- Discontinue or reduce dose of causative agent
- If due to neuroleptic, switch to an atypical antipsychotic
- Consider a trial of antimuscarinic, amantadine, dopamine agonist, or levodopa

MANAGEMENT

Strategies for the management of DIP include discontinuation of therapy with the causative agent, reducing the dose of the offending drug, changing therapy from a conventional neuroleptic to an atypical antipsychotic agent, and the use of antiparkinsonism drugs such as amantadine, antimuscarinics, carbidopa–levodopa, and dopamine agonists (**Table 12-20**). For symptom management, dopamine agonists and carbidopa–levodopa are effective, but a severe neuroleptic-induced parkinsonian tremor may be resistant. Alternatively, antimuscarinic agents can be used and are better tolerated in younger patients. Amantadine is another alternative and is better tolerated than anticholinergic drugs in the elderly.

INFORMATION FOR PATIENTS

Before initiating therapy with DRBAs, clinicians should inform patients regarding purpose of treatment and the potential risk of DIP and document that this counseling has been performed. If long-term treatment with a DRBA is anticipated, informed consent is recommended and should be updated yearly. Patients should also understand that early detection of any DRBA-induced movement disorder is important and reduces the risk of irreversible abnormal movements. The patient's family members or caregivers can play a role in monitoring and reporting any abnormal movements.

REFERENCES

1. Burkhard PR. Acute and subacute drug-induced movement disorders. *Parkinsonism Relat Disord* 2014; 20(suppl 1):S108-12.
2. Perkins DO. Predictors of noncompliance in patients with schizophrenia. *J Clin Psychiatry.* 2002; 63:1121-8.
3. Robinson DG, Woerner MG, Alvir JM et al. Predictors of medication discontinuation by patients with first-episode schizophrenia and schizoaffective disorder. *Schizophr Res.* 2002; 57:209-19.
4. Hansen TE, Brown WL, Weigel RM et al. Underrecognition of tardive dyskinesia and drug-induced parkinsonism by psychiatric residents. *Gen Hosp Psychiatry.* 1992; 14:340-4.
5. van Harten PN, Matroos GE, Hoek HW et al. The prevalence of tardive dystonia, tardive dyskinesia, parkinsonism and akathisia: The Curacao Extrapyramidal Syndromes Study: I. *Schizophr Res.* 1996; 19:195-203.
6. Muscettola G, Barbato G, Pampallona S et al. Extrapyramidal syndromes in neuroleptic-treated patients: prevalence, risk factors, and association with tardive dyskinesia. *J Clin Psychopharmacol.* 1999; 19:203-8.
7. Delay J, Deniker P. Neuroleptic effects of chlorpromazine in therapeutics of neuropsychiatry. *J Clin Exp Psychopathol.* 1955; 16:104-12.
8. Weiden PJ. Discontinuing and switching antipsychotic medications: understanding the CATIE Schizophrenia trial. *J Clin Psychiatry.* 2007; 68(suppl 1):12-9.
9. Correll CU, Leucht S, Kane JM. Lower risk for tardive dyskinesia associated with second-generation antipsychotics: a systematic review of 1-year studies. *Am J Psychiatry.* 2004; 161:414-25.
10. Correll C, Schenk EM. Tardive dyskinesia and new antipsychotics. *Curr Opin Psychiatry.* 2008; 21:151-6.
11. Caroff SN, Mann SC, Campbell EC et al. Movement disorders associated with atypical antipsychotic drugs. *J Clin Psychiatry.* 2002; 63(suppl 4):12-9.
12. Kane JM. Extrapyramidal side effects are unacceptable. *Eur Neuropsychopharmacol.* 2001; 11(suppl 4):S397-403.
13. Solmi M, Murru A, Pacchiarotti I et al. Safety, tolerability, and risks associated with first- and second-generation antipsychotics: a state-of-the-art clinical review. *Ther Clin Risk Manag.* 2017; 13:757-7.
14. Gelenberg AJ, Jefferson JW. Lithium tremor. *J Clin Psychiatry.* 1995; 56:283-7.
15. Gerber PE, Lynd LD. Selective serotonin-reuptake inhibitor-induced movement disorders. *Ann Pharmacother.* 1998; 32:692-8.
16. Zesiewicz TA, Sullivan KL. Drug-induced hyperkinetic movement disorders by nonneuroleptic agents. *Handb Clin Neurol.* 2011; 100:347-63.
17. Weiner WJ, Sanchez-Ramos J. Movement disorders and dopaminomimetic stimulant drugs. In: Lang AE, Weiner WJ, eds. *Drug-Induced Movement Disorders.* Mount Kisco, NY: Futura Publishing; 1992:315-37.
18. Raethjen J, Lemke MR, Lindemann M et al. Amitriptyline enhances the central component of physiological tremor. *J Neurol Neurosurg Psychiatry.* 2001; 70:78-82.
19. Vandel P, Bonin B, Leveque E et al. Tricyclic antidepressant-induced extrapyramidal side effects. *Eur Neuropsychopharmacol.* 1997; 7:207-12.
20. Chadwick D, Reynolds EH, Marsden CD. Anticonvulsant induced dyskinesias: a comparison with dyskinesias induced by neuroleptics. *J Neurol Neurosurg Psychiatry.* 1976; 39:1210-8.
21. Vela L, Sfakianakis GN, Heros D et al. Chorea and contraceptives: case report with pet study and review of the literature. *Mov Disord.* 2004; 19:349-52.
22. Miller LG, Jankovic J. Metoclopramide-induced movement disorders: clinical findings with a review of the literature. *Arch Intern Med.* 1989; 149:2486-92.
23. Kenney C, Hunter C, Davidson A et al J. Metoclopramide, an increasingly recognized cause of tardive dyskinesia. *J Clin Pharmacol.* 2008; 48:379-84.
24. Braude D, Soliz T, Crandall C et al. Antiemetics in the ED: a randomized controlled trial comparing 3 common agents. *Am J Emerg Med.* 2006; 24:177-82.
25. Parlak I, Atilla R, Cicek M et al. Rate of metoclopramide infusion affects the severity and incidence of akathisia. *Emerg Med J.* 2005; 22:621-4.
26. Morgan JC, Sethi KD. Drug-induced tremors. *Lancet Neurol.* 2005; 4:866-76.
27. Jimenez-Jimenez FJ, Puertas I, de Toledo-Heras M. Drug induced myoclonus: frequency, mechanisms and management. *CNS Drugs.* 2004; 18:93-104.
28. Susman VL. Clinical management of neuroleptic malignant syndrome. *Psychiatr Q.* 2001; 72:325-36.
29. Satija P, Ondo WG. Restless legs syndrome: pathophysiology, diagnosis and treatment. CNS. *Drugs.* 2008; 22:497-518.
30. Jankovic J. Differential diagnosis and etiology of tics. *Adv Neurol.* 2001; 85:15-29.
31. Vijayakumar D, Jankovic J. Drug-induced dyskinesia, part 1: treatment of levodopa-induced dyskinesia. *Drugs.* 2016; 76: 759-77.
32. Fabbrini G, Brotchie JM, Grandas F et al. Levodopa induced dyskinesias. *Mov Disord.* 2007; 22:1379-89.
33. Gattera JA, Charles BG, Williams GM et al. A retrospective study of risk factors of akathisia in terminally ill patients. *J Pain Symptom Manage.* 1994; 9:454-61.
34. McCreadie RG, Todd N, Livingston M et al. A double blind comparative study of remoxipride and thioridazine in the acute phase of schizophrenia. *Acta Psychiatr Scand.* 1988; 78:49-56.
35. Van Putten T, May PR, Marder SR. Akathisia with haloperidol and thiothixene. *Arch Gen Psychiatry.* 1984; 41:1036-9.
36. Sachdev P. The epidemiology of drug-induced akathisia: part II. Chronic, tardive, and withdrawal akathisias. *Schizophr Bull.* 1995; 21:451-61.
37. Miller CH, Mohr F, Umbricht D et al. The prevalence of acute extrapyramidal signs and symptoms in patients treated with clozapine, risperidone, and conventional antipsychotics. *J Clin Psychiatry.* 1998; 59:69-75.
38. Weiden PJ, Cutler AJ, Polymeropoulos MH et al. Safety profile of iloperidone: a pooled analysis of 6-week acute phase pivotal trials. *J Clin Psychopharmacol.* 2008; 28(2 suppl 1):S12-19.
39. Kane JM, Lauriello J, Laska E et al. Long-term efficacy and safety of iloperidone: results from 3 clinical trials for the treatment of schizophrenia. *J Clin Psychopharmacol.* 2008; 28(2 sppl 1):S29-35.
40. Baldassano CF, Truman CJ, Nierenberg A et al. Akathisia: a review and case report following paroxetine treatment. *Compr Psychiatry.* 1996; 37:122-4.
41. Milne IK. Akathisia associated with carbamazepine therapy. *N Z Med J.* 1992; 105:182.
42. Hullett FJ, Levy AB. Amoxapine-induced akathisia. *Am J Psychiatry.* 1983; 140:820.
43. Patterson JF. Lithium-induced akathisia. *J Clin Psychopharmacol.* 1988; 8:445.
44. Gill HS, DeVane CL, Risch SC. Extrapyramidal symptoms associated with cyclic antidepressant treatment: a review of the literature and consolidating hypotheses. *J Clin Psychopharmacol.* 1997; 17:377-89.
45. Stahl SM, Lonnen AJ. The mechanism of drug-induced akathsia. *CNS Spectr.* 2011; 16:7-10.
46. Sachdev P, Loneragan C. Acute drug-induced akathisia is not associated with low serum iron status. *Psychopharmacology (Berl).* 1991; 103:138-139.
47. American Psychiatric Association. *Diagnostic and statistical manual of mental disorders.* 5th ed. Washington, DC: American Psychiatric Association; 2013.

48. Barnes TR. The Barnes Akathisia Rating Scale—revisited. *J Psychopharmacol.* 2003; 17:365-70.
49. Kuloglu M, Atmaca M, Ustundag B et al. Serum iron levels in schizophrenic patients with or without akathisia. *Eur Neuropsychopharmacol.* 2003; 13:67-71.
50. Leong GB, Silva JA. Neuroleptic-induced akathisia and violence: a review. *J Forensic Sci.* 2003; 48:187-9.
51. Hansen L. A critical review of akathisia and its possible association with suicidal behaviour. *Hum Psychopharmacol.* 2001; 16:495-505.
52. Duncan EJ, Adler LA, Stephanides M et al. Akathisia and exacerbation of psychopathology: a preliminary report. *Clin Neuropharmacol.* 2000; 23:169-73.
53. Gold R, Lenox RH. Is there a rationale for iron supplementation in the treatment of akathisia? A review of the evidence. *J Clin Psychiatry.* 1995; 56:476-83.
54. Fischel T, Hermesh H, Aizenberg D et al. Cyproheptadine versus propranolol for the treatment of acute neuroleptic induced akathisia: a comparative double-blind study. *J Clin Psychopharmacol.* 2001; 21:612-5.
55. Zubenko GS, Lipinski JF, Cohen BM et al. Comparison of metoprolol and propranolol in the treatment of akathisia. *Psychiatry Res.* 1984; 11:143-9.
56. Vinson DR. Diphenhydramine in the treatment of akathisia induced by prochlorperazine. *J Emerg Med.* 2004; 26:265-70.
57. Lima AR, Weiser KV, Bacaltchuk J et al. Anticholinergics for neuroleptic-induced acute akathisia (Cochrane Review). In: *The Cochrane Library, Issue 2.* Chichester, UK: John Wiley and Sons; 2004.
58. Lima AR, Soares-Weiser K, Bacaltchuk J et al. Benzodiazepines for neuroleptic-induced acute akathisia (Cochrane Review). In: *The Cochrane Library, Issue 2.* Chichester, UK: John Wiley and Sons; 2004.
59. Zubenko GS, Barreira P, Lipinski JF Jr. Development of tolerance to the therapeutic effect of amantadine on akathisia. *J Clin Psychopharmacol.* 1984; 4:218-20.
60. Danel T, Servant D, Goudemand M. Amitriptyline in the treatment of neuroleptic-induced akathisia. *Biol Psychiatry.* 1988;23:186-188.
61. Zubenko GS, Cohen BM, Lipinski JF Jr et al. Use of clonidine in treating neuroleptic-induced akathisia. *Psychiatry Res.* 1984;13:253-259.
62. Poyurovsky M, Weizman A. Serotonergic agents in the treatment of acute neuroleptic-induced akathisia: open label study of buspirone and mianserin. *Int Clin Psychopharmacol.* 1997; 12:263-8.
63. Hieber R, Dellenbaugh T, Nelson LA. Role of mirtazapine in the treatment of antipsychotic-induced akathisia. *Ann Pharmacother.* 2008; 42:841-6.
64. Walters A, Hening W, Chokroverty S et al. Opioid responsiveness in patients with neuroleptic-induced akathisia. *Mov Disord.* 1986; 1:119-27.
65. Tao GK, Harada DT, Kootsikas ME et al. Amoxapine induced tardive dyskinesia. *Drug Intell Clin Pharm.* 1985; 19(7-8):548-9.
66. Sigwald J, Bouttier D, Courvoisier S. Neurological complications of neuroleptic medication. *Rev Neurol (Paris).* 1959; 100:553-95.
67. Kruse W. Persistent muscular restlessness after phenothiazine treatment: report of 3 cases. *Am J Psychiatry.* 1960; 117:152-3.
68. Druckman R, Seelinger D, Thulin B. Chronic involuntary movements induced by phenothiazines. *J Nerv Ment Dis.* 1962; 135:69-76.
69. Chakos MH, Alvir JM, Woerner MG et al. Incidence and correlates of tardive dyskinesia in first episode of schizophrenia. *Arch Gen Psychiatry.* 1996; 53:313-9.
70. Kane JM. Tardive dyskinesia: epidemiological and clinical presentation. In: Bloom FE, Kupfer DJ, eds. *Psychopharmacology: the fourth generation progress.* 4th ed. New York; Raven Press; 1995:1485-95.
71. Kraepelin EP, Barclay RM, trans., Robertson GM, ed. *Dementia praecox and paraphrenia.* Edinburgh, Scotland: E and S Livingstone; 1919.
72. Kane JM, Smith JM. Tardive dyskinesia: prevalence and risk factors, 1959 to 1979. *Arch Gen Psychiatry.* 1982; 39:473-81.
73. Yassa R, Jeste DV. Gender differences in tardive dyskinesia: a critical review of the literature. *Schizophr Bull.* 1992; 18:701-15.
74. Woerner MG, Kane JM, Lieberman JA et al. The prevalence of tardive dyskinesia. *J Clin Psychopharmacol.* 1991; 11:34-42.
75. Yassa R, Nastase C, Dupont D, Thibeau M. Tardive dyskinesia in elderly psychiatric patients: a 5-year study. *Am J Psychiatry.* 1992; 149:1206-11.
76. Woerner MG, Alvir JM, Saltz BL et al. Prospective study of tardive dyskinesia in the elderly: rates and risk factors. *Am J Psychiatry.* 1998; 155:1521-8.
77. Jeste DV, Caligiuri MP, Paulsen JS et al. Risk of tardive dyskinesia in older patients: a prospective longitudinal study of 266 outpatients. *Arch Gen Psychiatry.* 1995; 52:756-65.
78. Yoshida K, Bies RR, Suzuki T et al. Tardive dyskinesia in relation to estimated dopamine D2 receptor occupancy in patients with schizophrenia: analysis of the CATIE data. *Schizophr Res.* 2014; 153:184-8.
79. Aquino CC, Lang AE. Tardive dyskinesia syndromes: current concepts. *Parkinsonism Relat Disord.* 2014; 20(suppl 1):S113-7.
80. Kelley JJ, Roberts RC. Effects of haloperidol on cholinergic striatal interneurons: relationship to oral dyskinesias. *J Neural Transm.* 2004; 111:1075-91.
81. Vijayakumar D, Jankovic J. Drug-induced dyskinesia, part 2: treatment of tardive dyskinesia. *Drugs.* 2016; 76:779-87.
82. Teo JT, Edwards MJ, Bhatia K. Tardive dyskinesia is caused by maladaptive synaptic plasticity: a hypothesis. *Mov Disord.* 2012; 27:1205-15.
83. Andreassen OA, Jorgensen HA. Neurotoxicity associated with neuroleptic-induced oral dyskinesias in rats: implications for tardive dyskinesia? *Prog Neurobiol.* 2000; 61:525-41.
84. Zhang XY, Zhou DF, Cao LY et al. Blood superoxide dismutase level in schizophrenic patients with tardive dyskinesia: association with dyskinetic movements. *Schizophr Res.* 2003; 62:245-50.
85. Nel A, Harvey BH. Haloperidol-induced dyskinesia is associated with striatal NO synthase suppression: reversal with olanzapine. *Behav Pharmacol.* 2003; 14:251-5.
86. Malhotra AK, Murphy GM Jr, Kennedy JL. Pharmacogenetics of psychotropic drug response. *Am J Psychiatry.* 2004; 161:780-96.
87. Segman RH, Goltser T, Heresco-Levy U et al. Association of dopaminergic and serotonergic genes with tardive dyskinesia in patients with chronic schizophrenia. *Pharmacogenomics J.* 2003; 3:277-83.
88. Ohmori O, Shinkai T, Hori H et al. A perspective on molecular genetic studies of tardive dyskinesia: one clue for individualized antipsychotic drug therapy. *Prog Neuropsychopharmacol Biol Psychiatry.* 2003; 27:581-6.
89. Lohmann PL, Bagli M, Krauss H et al. CYP2D6 polymorphism and tardive dyskinesia in schizophrenic patients. *Pharmacopsychiatry.* 2003; 36:73-8.
90. Crowley JJ, Kim Y, Szatkiewicz JP et al. Genome-wide association mapping of loci for antipsychotic-induced extrapyramidal symptoms in mice. *Mamm Genome.* 2012; 23:322-35.
91. Galili R, Mosberg, Gil-Ad I et al. Haloperidol-induced neurotoxicity: possible implications for tardive dyskinesia. *J Neural Transm.* 2000; 107:479-90.
92. Andreassen OA, Ferrante RJ, Aamo TO et al. Oral dyskinesias and histopathological alterations in substantia nigra after long-term haloperidol treatment of old rats. *Neuroscience.* 2003; 122:717-25.
93. Crow TJ, Cross AJ, Johnstone EC et al. Abnormal involuntary movements in schizophrenia: are they related to the disease process or its treatment? Are they associated with changes in dopamine receptors? *J Clin Psychopharmacol.* 1982; 2:336-40.

94. Silvestri S, Seeman MV, Negrete JC et al. Increased dopamine D2 receptor binding after long-term treatment with antipsychotics in humans: a clinical PET study. *Psychopharmacology.* 2000; 152:174-80.
95. Rodnitzky RL. Drug-induced movement disorders in children and adolescents. *Expert Opin Drug Saf.* 2005; 4:91-102.
96. McCreadie RG, Padmavati R, Thara R et al. Spontaneous dyskinesia and parkinsonism in never-medicated, chronically ill patients with schizophrenia: 18-month follow-up. *Br J Psychiatry.* 2002; 181:135-7.
97. Fenton WS. Prevalence of spontaneous dyskinesia in schizophrenia. *J Clin Psychiatry.* 2000; 61(suppl 4):10-4.
98. Guy W. Abnormal Involuntary Movements Scale (AIMS). *ECDEU assessment manual for psychopharmacology.* Washington, DC: United States Government Printing Office; 1976:534-7.
99. Kruk J, Sachdev P, Singh S. Neuroleptic-induced respiratory dyskinesia. *J Neuropsychiatry Clin Neurosci.* 1995; 7:223-9.
100. Schwartz M, Hocherman S. Antipsychotic-induced rabbit syndrome: epidemiology, management and pathophysiology. *CNS Drugs.* 2004; 18:213-20.
101. Smith JM, Baldessarini RJ. Changes in prevalence, severity, and recovery in tardive dyskinesia with age. *Arch Gen Psychiatry.* 1980; 37:1368-73.
102. Miller DD, McEvoy JP, Davis SM et al. Clinical correlates of tardive dyskinesia in schizophrenia: baseline data from the CATIE schizophrenia trial. *Schizophr Res.* 2005; 80:33-43.
103. Davis KL, Berger PA, Hollister LE. Tardive dyskinesia and depressive illness. *Psychopharmacol Commun.* 1976; 2:125-30.
104. Kane JM. Tardive dyskinesia in affective disorders. *J Clin Psychiatry.* 1999; 60(suppl 5):43-7.
105. Dixon L, Weiden PJ, Haas G et al. Increased tardive dyskinesia in alcohol-abusing schizophrenic patients. *Compr Psychiatry.* 1992; 33:121-2.
106. Lieberman JA, Stroup TS, McEvoy JP et al. Effectiveness of antipsychotic drugs in patients with chronic schizophrenia. *N Engl J Med.* 2005; 353:1209-23.
107. Oosthuizen PP, Emsley RA, Maritz JS et al. Incidence of tardive dyskinesia in first-episode psychosis patients treated with low-dose haloperidol. *J Clin Psychiatry.* 2003; 4:1075-80.
108. Caligiuri MP, Jeste DV. Association of diabetes with dyskinesia in older psychosis patients. *Psychopharmacology (Berl).* 2004; 2004;176:281-6.
109. Woerner MG, Saltz BL, Kane JM et al. Diabetes and development of tardive dyskinesia. *Am J Psychiatry.* 1993; 150:966-8.
110. Sachdev P. Early extrapyramidal side-effects as risk factors for later tardive dyskinesia: a prospective study. *Aust N Z J Psychiatry.* 2004; 38:445-9.
111. van Harten PN, Hoek HW, Matroos GE et al. Intermittent neuroleptic treatment and risk for tardive dyskinesia: Curacao Extrapyramidal Syndromes Study III. *Am J Psychiatry.* 1998; 155:565-7.
112. Wirshing DA, Bartzokis G, Pierre JM et al. Tardive dyskinesia and serum iron indices. *Biol Psychiatry.* 1998; 44:493-8.
113. Sachdev P. Drug-induced movement disorders in institutionalised adults with mental retardation: clinical characteristics and risk factors. *Aust N Z J Psychiatry.* 1992; 26:242-8.
114. Pourcher E, Cohen H, Cohen D et al. Organic brain dysfunction and cognitive deficits in young schizophrenic patients with tardive dyskinesia. *Brain Cogn.* 1993; 23:81-7.
115. Jeste DV. Tardive dyskinesia rates with atypical antipsychotics in older adults. *J Clin Psychiatry.* 2004; 65(suppl 9):21-4.
116. Ganzini L, Casey DE, Hoffman WF et al. The prevalence of metoclopramide-induced tardive dyskinesia and acute extrapyramidal movement disorders. *Arch Intern Med.* 1993; 153:1469-75.
117. Keck PE Jr, McElroy SL, Strakowski SM et al. Antipsychotics in the treatment of mood disorders and risk of tardive dyskinesia. *J Clin Psychiatry.* 2000; 61(suppl 4):33-8.
118. Schulze TG, Muller DJ, Krauss H et al. Affective symptomatology in schizophrenia: a risk factor for tardive dyskinesia? *Eur Psychiatry.* 2001; 16:71-4.
119. Bergen JA, Eyland EA, Campbell JA et al. The course of tardive dyskinesia in patients on long-term neuroleptics. *Br J Psychiatry.* 1989; 154:523-8.
120. Goldman MB, Luchins DJ. Intermittent neuroleptic therapy and tardive dyskinesia: a literature review. *Hosp Community Psychiatry.* 1984; 35:1215-9.
121. Task Force of the American Psychiatric Association. *Tardive dyskinesia.* Washington, DC: American Psychiatry Association Press; 1992.
122. Glazer WM, Morgenstern H, Schooler N et al. Predictors of improvement in tardive dyskinesia following discontinuation of neuroleptic medication. *Br J Psychiatry.* 1990; 157:585-92.
123. Bhidayasiri R, Jitkritsadakul O, Friedman JH, Fahn S. Updating the recommendations for treatment of tardive syndromes: a systematic review of new evidence and practical treatment algorithm. *J Neurol Sci.* 2018 Feb 5. pii: S0022-510X(18)30068-6.
124. Bhidayasiri R, Fahn S, Weiner WJ et al. Evidence-based guideline: treatment of tardive syndromes: report of the Guideline Development Subcommittee of the American Academy of Neurology. *Neurology.* 2013; 81:463-9.
125. Schachter DC, Kleinman I. Psychiatrists' attitudes about and informed consent practices for antipsychotics and tardive dyskinesia. *Psychiatr Serv.* 2004; 55:714-7.
126. Ayd FJ. Ethical and legal dilemmas posed by tardive dyskinesia. *Int Drug Ther Newsl.* 1977; 12:29-36.
127. Gupta S, Frank B, Madhusoodanan S. Tardive dyskinesia: legal issues and consent. *Psychiatr Ann.* 2002; 32:245-48.
128. Ayd FJ Jr. A survey of drug-induced extrapyramidal reactions. *JAMA.* 1961; 175:1054-60.
129. Chiles JA. Extrapyramidal reactions in adolescents treated with high-potency antipsychotics. *Am J Psychiatry.* 1978; 135:239-40.
130. Ayers JL, Dawson KP. Acute dystonic reactions in childhood to drugs. *N Z Med J.* 1980; 92:464-5.
131. Olsen JC, Keng JA, Clark JA. Frequency of adverse reactions to prochlorperazine in the ED. *Am J Emerg Med.* 2000; 18:609-11.
132. Bateman DN, Darling WM, Boys R et al. Extrapyramidal reactions to metoclopramide and prochlorperazine. *Q J Med.* 1989; 71:307-11.
133. Arana GW, Goff DC, Baldessarini RJ et al. Efficacy of anticholinergic prophylaxis for neuroleptic-induced acute dystonia. *Am J Psychiatry.* 1988; 145:993-6.
134. Ballerini M, Bellini S, Niccolai C et al. Neuroleptic induced dystonia: incidence and risk factors. *Eur Psychiatry.* 2002; 17:366-8.
135. Addonizio G, Alexopoulos GS. Drug-induced dystonia in young and elderly patients. *Am J Psychiatry.* 1988; 145:869-71.
136. Goff DC, Arana GW, Greenblatt DJ et al. The effect of benztropine on haloperidol-induced dystonia, clinical efficacy and pharmacokinetics: a prospective, double blind trial. *J Clin Psychopharmacol.* 1991; 11:106-12.
137. Spina E, Sturiale V, Valvo S et al. Prevalence of acute dystonic reactions associated with neuroleptic treatment with and without anticholinergic prophylaxis. *Int Clin Psychopharmacol.* 1993; 8:21-4.
138. Keegan DL, Rajput AH. Drug induced dystonia tarda: treatment with L-dopa. *Dis Nerv Syst.* 1973; 34:167-9.
139. Burke RE, Fahn S, Jankovic J et al. Tardive dystonia: late onset and persistent dystonia caused by antipsychotic drugs. *Neurology.* 1982; 32:1335-46.
140. Yassa R, Nair V, Dimitry R. Prevalence of tardive dystonia. *Acta Psychiatr Scand.* 1986; 73:629-33.
141. Raja M. Tardive dystonia. Prevalence, risk factors, and comparison with tardive dyskinesia in a population of 200 acute psychiatric inpatients. *Eur Arch Psychiatry Clin Neurosci.* 1995; 245:145-51.

142. Sethi KD, Hess DC, Harp RJ. Prevalence of dystonia in veterans on chronic antipsychotic therapy. *Mov Disord.* 1990; 5:319-21.
143. Suzuki T, Matsuzaka H. Drug-induced Pisa syndrome (pleurothotonus): epidemiology and management. *CNS Drugs.* 2002; 16:165-74.
144. Stubner S, Padberg F, Grohmann R et al. Pisa syndrome (pleurothotonus): report of a multicenter drug safety surveillance project. *J Clin Psychiatry.* 2000; 61:569-74.
145. Boyer WF, Bakalar NH, Lake CR. Anticholinergic prophylaxis of acute haloperidol-induced acute dystonic reactions. *J Clin Psychopharmacol.* 1987; 7:164-6.
146. Nasrallah HA, Churchill CM, Hamdan-Allan GA. Higher frequency of neuroleptic-induced dystonia in mania than in schizophrenia. *Am J Psychiatry.* 1988; 145:1455-6.
147. Remington GJ, Voineskos G, Pollock B et al. Prevalence of neuroleptic-induced dystonia in mania and schizophrenia. *Am J Psychiatry.* 1990; 147:1231-3.
148. Khanna R, Das A, Damodaran SS. Prospective study of neuroleptic-induced dystonia in mania and schizophrenia. *Am J Psychiatry.* 1992; 149:511-3.
149. Stern TA, Anderson WH. Benztropine prophylaxis of dystonic reactions. *Psychopharmacology (Berl).* 1979; 61:261-2.
150. Winslow RS, Stillner V, Coons DJ et al. Prevention of acute dystonic reactions in patients beginning high potency neuroleptics. *Am J Psychiatry.* 1986; 143:706-10.
151. Sramek JJ, Simpson GM, Morrison RL et al. Anticholinergic agents for prophylaxis of neuroleptic induced dystonic reactions: a prospective study. *J Clin Psychiatry.* 1986; 7:305-9.
152. Dressler D, Oeljeschlager RO, Ruther E. Severe tardive dystonia: treatment with continuous intrathecal baclofen administration. *Mov Disord.* 1997; 12:585-7.
153. Kupsch A, Kuehn A, Klaffke S et al. Deep brain stimulation in dystonia. *J Neurol.* 2003; 250(suppl 1):I47-52.
154. Stephen PJ, Williamson J. Drug-induced parkinsonism in the elderly. *Lancet.* 1984;2:1082-3.
155. Janno S, Holi M, Tuisku K et al. Prevalence of neuroleptic-induced movement disorders in chronic schizophrenia inpatients. *Am J Psychiatry.* 2004; 161:160-3.
156. Halliday J, Farrington S, Macdonald S et al. Nithsdale Schizophrenia Surveys 23: movement disorders: 20-year review. *Br J Psychiatry.* 2002; 181:422-7.
157. Yamamoto M, Ujike H, Ogawa N. Metoclopramide induced parkinsonism. *Clin Neuropharmacol.* 1987; 10:287-9.
158. Bateman DN, Rawlins MD, Simpson JM. Extrapyramidal reactions to prochlorperazine and haloperidol in the United Kingdom. *Q J Med.* 1986; 59:549-6.
159. Jamora D, Lim SH, Pan A et al. Valproate-induced Parkinsonism in epilepsy patients. *Mov Disord.* 2007; 22:130-3.
160. Nouzeilles M, Garcıa M, Rabinowicz A et al. Prospective evaluation of parkinsonism and tremor in patients treated with valproate. *Parkinsonism Relat Disord.* 1999; 5:67-8.
161. Llau ME, Nguyen L, Senard JM et al. Drug-induced parkinsonian syndromes: a 10-year experience at a regional center of pharmaco-vigilance. *Rev Neurol (Paris).* 1994; 50:757-62.
162. Hunt-Fugate AK, Zander J, Lesar TS. Adverse reactions due to dopamine blockade by amoxapine: a case report and review of the literature. *Pharmacotherapy.* 1984; 4:35-39.
163. Teive HA, Troiano AR, Germiniani FM et al. Flunarizine and cinnarizine-induced parkinsonism: a historical and clinical analysis. *Parkinsonism Relat Disord.* 2004; 10:243-5.
164. Kenney C, Hunter C, Jankovic J. Long-term tolerability of tetrabenazine in the treatment of hyperkinetic movement disorders. *Mov Disord.* 2007; 22:193-7.
165. Jankovic J. Treatment of hyperkinetic movement disorders with tetrabenazine: a double-blind crossover study. *Ann Neurol.* 1982; 11:41-7.
166. Tauscher J, Kufferle B, Asenbaum S et al. Striatal dopamine-2 receptor occupancy as measured with 123Iodobenzamide and SPECT predicted the occurrence of EPS in patients treated with atypical antipsychotics and haloperidol. *Psychopharmacology (Berl).* 2002; 162:42-9.
167. Kapur S, Zipursky R, Jones C et al. Relationship between dopamine D(2) occupancy, clinical response, and side effects: a double-blind PET study of first-episode schizophrenia. *Am J Psychiatry.* 2000; 157:514-20.
168. Broich K, Grunwald F, Kasper S et al. D2-dopamine receptor occupancy measured by IBZM-SPECT in relation to extrapyramidal side effects. *Pharmacopsychiatry.* 1998; 31:159-62.
169. Seeman P. Atypical antipsychotics: mechanism of action. *Can J Psychiatry.* 2002; 47:27-38.
170. Kapur S, Seeman P. Does fast dissociation from the dopamine d(2) receptor explain the action of atypical antipsychotics? A new hypothesis. *Am J Psychiatry.* 2001; 158:360-9.
171. Kapur S, Seeman P. Antipsychotic agents differ in how fast they come off the dopamine D2 receptors: implications for atypical antipsychotic action. *J Psychiatry Neurosci.* 2000; 25:161-6.
172. Alvarez MV, Evidente VG. Understanding drug-induced parkinsonism: separating pearls from oysters. *Neurology.* 2008; 70:e32-4.
173. Diaz-Corrales FJ, Sanz-Viedma S, Escobar-Delgado T. Clinical features and ^{123}I-FP-CIT SPECT imaging in the differentiation between drug-induced parkinsonism and Parkinson's disease. *Mov Disord.* 2008; 23(suppl 1):S59.
174. Simpson GM, Angus JWS. A rating scale for extrapyramidal side effects. *Acta Psychiatr Scand.* 1970; (suppl 212):11-9.
175. Hriso E, Kuhn T, Masdeu JC et al. Extrapyramidal symptoms due to dopamine-blocking agents in patients with AIDS encephalopathy. *Am J Psychiatry.* 1991; 148:1558-61.

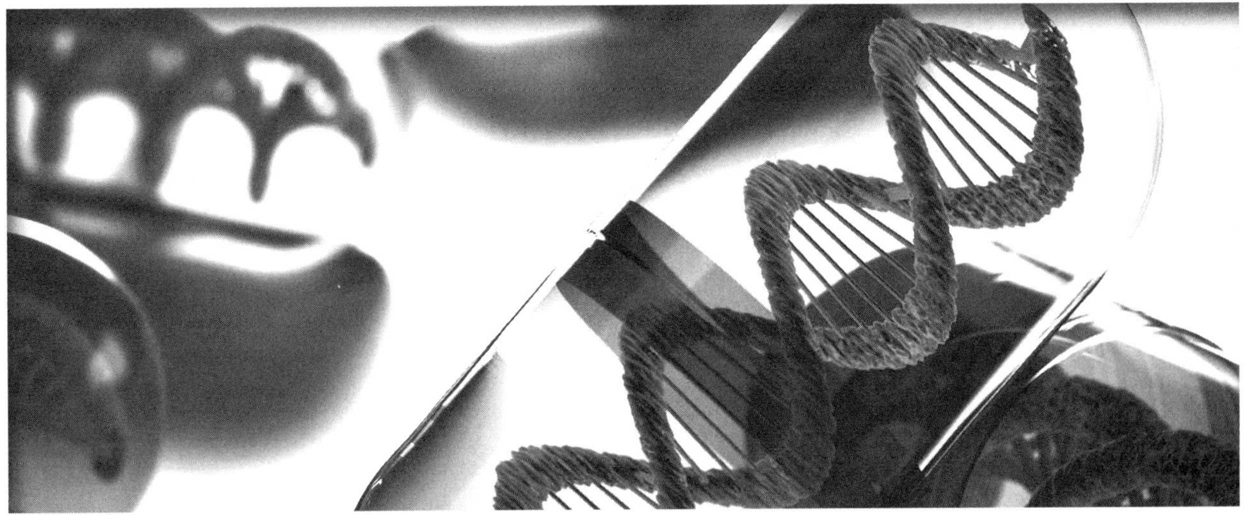

CHAPTER 13

Peripheral Neuropathy

Dennis Parker, Jr.

Peripheral neuropathy is defined as a dysfunction or lesion in the peripheral nervous system that is usually characterized by pain, abnormal sensory symptoms, or both.[1] Although this syndrome is most commonly a complication of chronic illnesses such as diabetes mellitus, alcoholism, or human immunodeficiency virus (HIV) infection, it may also be drug-induced.

CAUSATIVE AGENTS

Many drugs have been associated with peripheral neuropathy. The most common agents that have been implicated include antineoplastic and antiretroviral drugs. Drugs known to cause peripheral neuropathy are listed in **Table 13-1**.[2-93]

EPIDEMIOLOGY

The precise incidence of drug-induced peripheral neuropathy is unknown. Despite few epidemiologic data, it seems likely that the overall incidence of drug-induced peripheral neuropathy is low, and varies depending on the specific medication, its duration of use and dose, and patient-specific factors.[94] The risk of peripheral neuropathy is notably high in association with certain drug classes. Cancer chemotherapy agents (platinum derivatives, taxanes, vinca alkaloids) and antiretroviral drugs (nucleoside reverse-transcriptase inhibitors) are commonly associated with peripheral neuropathy. The incidence of peripheral neuropathy has been reported to be as high as 85–100% in patients receiving higher doses of cisplatin or oxaliplatin and 30–80% in patients with HIV who receive zalcitabine.[25,34,95-97] Most other associations of peripheral neuropathy with drugs are limited to case reports or small case series. Some population-based cohort studies examining the risk of peripheral neuropathy associated with lipid-lowering agents such as statins have been published. One group conducted a study in 166 patients and reported a 4- to 14-fold increased risk of idiopathic polyneuropathy in those on long-term (median 2.8 years) therapy with statins.[55] A subsequent analysis of four cohort trials estimated the incidence of neuropathy associated with statin use to be low (12 per 100,000 person-years).[98] More recent data suggest a clear association between long-term statin exposure and risk of peripheral neuropathy.

Table 13-1 Agents Implicated in Drug-Induced Peripheral Neuropathy

Drug	Incidence	Level of Evidence[a]
ANTI-INFECTIVES		
Chloramphenicol[2,3]	NK	C
Chloroquine[4,5]	NK	C
Ciprofloxacin[6]	NK	C
Dapsone[7,8]	NK	C
Didanosine[9,10]	Up to 23%	B
Ethambutol[11,12]	NK	C
Isoniazid[13-15]	NK	C
Lamivudine[16]	NK	C
Levofloxacin[6]	NK	C
Linezolid[17]	NK	C
Lomefloxacin[6]	NK	C
Mefloquine[18]	NK	C
Metronidazole[19-21]	NK	C
Nitrofurantoin[22]	NK	C
Ofloxacin[6]	NK	C
Podophyllin[23]	NK	C
Stavudine[24]	6–31%	A
Trovafloxacin[6]	NK	C
Zalcitabine[25-27]	>30%	A
ANTINEOPLASTICS		
Fluorouracil[28]	1%	C
Bortezomib[29]	30–47%	A
Capecitabine[30]	NK	C
Carboplatin[31-33]	15–85%	A
Chlorambucil[31]	NK	C
Cisplatin[31,34,35]	15–85%	A
Cytarabine[36]	NK	C
Docetaxel[37,38]	50%	A
Etoposide[39]	NK	C
Ifosfamide[40]	NK	C
Oxaliplatin[41-43]	85%	A
Paclitaxel[44-46]	50%	A
Procarbazine[47]	10–20%	C
Suramin[48]	NK	C
Thalidomide[49,50,51]	50%	A
Vincristine[46,52]	50%	A
CARDIOVASCULAR DRUGS		
Amiodarone[53,54]	NK	C
Atorvastatin[55]	NK	C
Clofibrate[56]	NK	C
Disopyramide[57]	NK	C

Table 13-1 Agents Implicated in Drug-Induced Peripheral Neuropathy (continued)

Drug	Incidence	Level of Evidence[a]
Enalapril[58,59]	NK	C
Hydralazine[60,61]	NK	C
Indomethacin[62]	NK	C
Pravastatin[55]	NK	C
Propafenone[63]	NK	C
Rosuvastatin[55]	NK	C
Simvastatin[55]	NK	C
MISCELLANEOUS		
Acetazolamide[64,65]	NK	C
Alcohol[66]	NK	C
Allopurinol[67]	NK	C
Colchicine[68]	NK	C
Cyclosporine[69,70]	NK	C
Disulfiram[71-74]	NK	C
Gold salts[75-77]	NK	C
Interferons alfa 2a and 2b[78-80]	NK	C
Infliximab[81]	NK	C
Leflunomide[82,83]	3–10%	B
Lithium[84]	NK	C
Nitrous oxide[85]	NK	C
Penicillamine[86]	NK	C
Phenelzine[87,88]	NK	C
Phenytoin[89,90]	NK	C
Pyridoxine[91]	NK	C
Sulfasalazine[92]	NK	C
Tacrolimus[93]	NK	C

NK = not known.

[a]Definitions for Levels of Evidence: Level A—evidence from one or more randomized, controlled clinical trials; Level B—evidence from nonrandomized clinical trials, prospective observational studies, cohort studies, retrospective studies, case-control studies, meta-analyses and/or postmarketing surveillance studies; and Level C—evidence from one or more published case reports or case series.

MECHANISMS

Peripheral neuropathy is associated with damage to the peripheral nervous system, namely the dorsal-root ganglia and dorsal roots. The cell bodies of sensory neurons lie in the dorsal-root ganglia, which give rise to the dorsal roots (axons). It is postulated that drugs may affect the peripheral nervous system selectively because these anatomical structures have a somewhat porous blood–nerve barrier, thus allowing access of harmful toxins.[94,99] Others have pointed out that increased access to sensory neurons alone could not explain susceptibility, as autonomic neurons lack a blood–brain barrier and autonomic dysfunction is commonly absent in patients with drug-induced peripheral neuropathy.[44]

Although mechanisms by which drugs induce peripheral neuropathy have not been fully elucidated, the general pathogenesis of drug-induced peripheral neuropathy primarily involves axonal or cell-body degeneration, demyelination, or both. Axonal degeneration is often associated with the "dying back" phenomenon, in which the most distal portion of the axon degenerates and the myelin sheath begins to break down more proximally toward the cell body.[100]

Table 13-2 Mechanisms of Drug-Induced Peripheral Neuropathy

Drug	Mechanism
Nucleoside reverse-transcriptase inhibitors	Depletion of mitochondrial DNA in neurons
Taxanes and vinca alkaloids	Disruption of neuronal axonal transport
Platinum compounds	Cross-linkage of DNA strands to impair cell division; demyelination and axonal swelling in dorsal-root ganglia
Oxaliplatin (acute)	Interaction with ion channels in dorsal root to enhance Na^{++} transmission; chelation of Ca^{++} ions. Overall shift to more negative membrane potential
Thalidomide Bortezomib	Down regulation of the production of tumor necrosis factor α and inhibition of nuclear factor-κβ leading to reduced nerve growth factor–mediated neuron survival
Isoniazid	Inhibition of phosphorylation of pyridoxine, which leads to neuronal cellular dysfunction
Linezolid	May disrupt neuronal mitochondrial protein synthesis
Statins	Inhibition of HMG-CoA reductase leading to reduced cholesterol synthesis, which is necessary for maintenance of cell-membrane integrity in neurons

DNA = deoxyribonucleic acid, HMG-CoA = 3-hydroxy-3-methyl-glutaryl-coenzyme A.

For some drugs with well-established associations with peripheral neuropathy, several cellular pathways have been identified using in vitro methods and animal models (**Table 13-2**).[101-104] In some cases individual agents are associated with multiple neurotoxic mechanisms.[104] The therapeutic mechanism of action of some drugs is also associated with detrimental consequences to sensory neurons. Nucleoside reverse-transcriptase inhibitors cause peripheral neuropathy by depleting mitochondrial deoxyribonucleic acid (DNA) in neurons. These agents exert a therapeutic effect on HIV reverse-transcriptase DNA but are also substrates for gamma DNA polymerase, which is responsible for replication of neuronal mitochondrial DNA.[105] Vinca alkaloids destroy cancer cells by binding with tubulin to prevent microtubular formation, which disrupts mitosis. Axonal transport is dependent on microtubular function. Dysfunction of axoplasmic transport has been demonstrated in animal models.[35,106,107] Other important mechanisms for chemotherapy associated neuropathy have been identified, including the release of proinflammatory mediators, enhanced oxidative stress, disruption of voltage-gated ion channels, and neuronal apoptosis.[108] Other drugs may affect important mediators of metabolic function. Isoniazid inhibits phosphorylation of pyridoxine, which causes neuronal cellular dysfunction.[109] Paradoxically, pyridoxine overdose is also associated with peripheral neuropathy.[110]

CLINICAL PRESENTATION AND DIFFERENTIAL DIAGNOSIS

A wide spectrum of clinical features can be observed in patients with drug-induced peripheral neuropathy (**Table 13-3**). Symptoms are most often sensory or sensorimotor in nature, and patients present in a similar fashion to those afflicted with peripheral neuropathy due to other causes. The clinical syndrome may be dependent on many factors. Drugs that affect large myelinated axons (e.g., paclitaxel) cause disturbances of proprioception, vibration, and light touch. Others, such as cisplatin, are more selective for small fibers and may cause pain or abnormal temperature sensation.[25,34] Patients with sensorimotor neuropathy present with sensory as well as motor symptoms such as weakness or muscle cramps. The onset and severity of these symptoms vary. Most commonly, neurotoxicity is a dose-related phenomenon that occurs after prolonged, cumulative exposure to the offending agent (weeks to months). In some instances, however,

Table 13-3 Signs and Symptoms Associated with Drug-Induced Peripheral Neuropathy[a]

- Orthostatic hypotension (autonomic neuropathy)
- Reduced sensation (vibration, pinprick)
- Reduced (abnormal) reflexes in affected area
- Reduced nerve action potential amplitude (nerve conduction studies)
- Paresthesias
- Burning sensations
- Shock-like sensations
- Decreased sensations or numbness
- Shooting or stabbing pain
- Radiating pain
- Ataxia

[a]Symptoms are typically distal and symmetrical in nature.

acute symptoms may appear after a single exposure to the drug (e.g., oxaliplatin, paclitaxel).[34] Oxaliplatin induces a unique form of acute neuropathy in a majority of patients, who experience paresthesias in the extremities. Rarely, pharyngolaryngeal dysesthesia may occur, which is manifested as unusual sensations in the mouth or throat and difficulty in swallowing or breathing.[33] Symptoms may begin during the infusion of the drug or shortly thereafter. This syndrome usually resolves spontaneously within days of onset but can recur with subsequent infusions.

Neurotoxic antiretroviral drugs may provoke a syndrome known as "coasting," in which symptoms begin to occur some time after the drug has been discontinued.[111,112] Symptoms may actually worsen for a period of 1–2 months after the offending agent is discontinued. Some drugs known to cause peripheral neuropathy also cause autonomic or optic neuropathies or purely motor abnormalities.

Identifying the cause of peripheral neuropathy can be challenging. Even with extensive investigation, the exact cause is often elusive. In a small study, nearly 50% of cases of sensory neuropathy were categorized as idiopathic.[99] It follows, therefore, that distinguishing drug-induced peripheral neuropathy from nondrug causes can be a daunting task. Drug-induced peripheral neuropathy is often a diagnosis of exclusion, because numerous causes of peripheral neuropathy exist, many of which present in a fashion similar to those that are drug-related. A careful medical history and physical examination are important for diagnosis, and additional tests may be required to establish the most likely cause.

It is important that clinicians inquire specifically about the frequency, quality, and duration of symptoms of peripheral neuropathy. Knowledge of the onset and duration of symptoms is particularly helpful in discerning the etiology of neuropathy, because drug-induced peripheral neuropathy usually presents as a subacute process over several weeks to months. The patient's medical history should be assessed for trauma, infectious diseases (especially HIV), conditions such as diabetes mellitus, kidney or liver disease, cancer, and family history of neuropathy. The patient should also be evaluated for alcohol abuse and for exposure to other potentially neurotoxic chemicals or medications.

On physical examination, drug-induced peripheral neuropathy is usually distal, symmetrical, and sensorimotor in nature. The neurologic exam may reveal a reduced sensation on pinprick as well as reduced vibratory sense bilaterally in the extremities.[113] The reduction in sensation may result in subsequent formation of ulcers. In some cases, hyperesthesia or allodynia may be present. Weakness or clumsiness may be observed in patients with motor involvement secondary to neuropathy. Deep tendon reflexes may be absent or reduced in affected areas.

Grading scales for neuropathy—particularly chemotherapy-induced peripheral neuropathy (CIPN)—are widely used by clinicians to assess the scope and severity of drug-induced peripheral neuropathy as a component of patient monitoring and during clinical trials. The most widely used scales are the National Cancer Institute of Canada Common Toxicity, Eastern Cooperative Oncology Group, and World Health Organization grading scales. These scales generally classify patients from 0 (no symptoms) to up to 4 or 5 (severe, disabling symptoms). Although these tools are helpful, a substantial amount of variability exists between examiners using these scales because of the subjective nature of some classification schemes. More in-depth descriptions of these scales are published elsewhere.[114-116]

Nerve-conduction studies (NCS) and electromyography (EMG) are the primary tools used in electrodiagnostic studies. These tests are usually performed in concert to identify disorders occurring in the nerves, muscle, or both. EMG is used to study the electrical activity of muscles, whereas NCS assess motor and sensory function of the nerves. EMG and NCS are performed by generating a small electrical current via a stimulator placed on the skin along a nerve. Electrical activity is recorded—using either surface electrodes (i.e., NCS) or needle electrodes inserted into muscles (i.e., EMG)—and is visualized as waveforms on a monitor. The amplitude of the waveform estimates the amount of electrically active tissue. Conduction velocity is a measurement of how quickly neurons are propagating impulses. Both amplitude and conduction velocity data generated during NCS can aid in the determination of the level of peripheral nerve disease (i.e., demyelination versus axonal degeneration). In general, axonal destruction produces a reduction in amplitude. This represents the most common consequence of neuropathy induced by medications. In contrast, demyelination is associated with a reduction in conduction velocity, which may occur in patients who receive amiodarone. Although electrophysiologic testing may be useful in identifying the presence of peripheral neuropathy in some patients, many investigators have found a poor correlation between performance on NCS and clinical symptoms of the disease.[117,118] Furthermore, it has yet to be shown that NCS are useful in predicting the future development of peripheral neuropathy in patients receiving potentially neurotoxic drugs. Mileshkin et al.[118] studied the utility of serial NCS in 75 patients receiving thalidomide for relapsed or refractory multiple myeloma in an effort to identify those at risk for developing peripheral neuropathy. Electrophysiologic monitoring was found to be no better than clinical assessment for identifying patients at risk for thalidomide-induced peripheral neuropathy. Therefore, the utility of the routine use of NCS to identify patients at risk for peripheral neuropathy remains unclear.

Conditions to consider in the differential diagnosis of drug-induced peripheral neuropathy are listed in **Table 13-4**. A wide variety of systemic diseases, particularly diabetes mellitus, kidney disease, and thyroid disease may play a role in producing neuropathy. Therefore, complete blood count, fasting blood glucose, blood urea nitrogen and creatinine, and thyroid-stimulating hormone concentrations should be evaluated. Serum vitamin B_{12} concentrations can also be easily obtained and should be included in the patient evaluation. A serum concentration of 100 pg/mL or less with symptoms is usually indicative of vitamin B_{12} deficiency. Malignancy has also been associated with peripheral neuropathy, which is a common presenting feature in patients with small-cell lung cancer.[99] In these patients, symptoms of sensory neuropathy often occur rather abruptly, a presentation that differs from the more common subacute presentation of drug-induced peripheral neuropathy. Therefore, a routine cancer evaluation including chest radiography and measurement of anti-Hu antibodies should be performed in any patient presenting with acute symptoms of neuropathy. Cerebrospinal fluid evaluation may be useful in screening patients for immune-related causes such as Guillain-Barré syndrome and chronic inflammatory demyelinating polyradiculoneuropathy, as elevated plasma protein concentrations may be found in patients with these illnesses. Nerve biopsy, which involves removing and examining nerve tissue, is generally

Table 13-4 Conditions to Consider in the Differential Diagnosis of Drug-Induced Peripheral Neuropathy

- Immune-related disorders
  - Guillain-Barré syndrome
  - Sjögren syndrome
  - Chronic inflammatory demyelinating polyradiculoneuropathy
- Infectious diseases
  - Human immunodeficiency virus
  - Herpes simplex
- Metabolic/systemic diseases
  - Nutritional deficiency
  - Diabetic neuropathy
  - Hypothyroidism
- Traumatic injury
- Hereditary sensory neuropathies
- Idiopathic sensory neuropathy
- Paraneoplastic neuropathy

poorly tolerated and can cause complications of neuropathy. Therefore, this technique is reserved for patients for whom the diagnosis of neuropathy cannot be determined by other means.[99,100,119]

RISK FACTORS

Risk factors for the development of drug-induced peripheral neuropathy are listed in **Table 13-5**. For the most part, cumulative drug exposure increases the risk of peripheral neuropathy, and repeated exposure to an agent that has caused peripheral neuropathy further increases the risk. However, evidence indicates that some patients can be safely rechallenged with cisplatin.[120] For many anticancer drugs, the risk of neurotoxicity appears to be related to both the amount of drug administered in each individual dose and the cumulative dose. Postma et al.[121] studied the effect of dose-dependent neurotoxicity in 227 patients with cancer receiving paclitaxel in doses ranging from 135 to 300 mg/m^2 every 3 weeks. The incidence of neuropathy was higher in patients who had received both a higher cumulative dose and a higher dose per cycle. Similar effects have been noted in patients receiving high doses of oxaliplatin, cisplatin, and vincristine. Therefore, it appears that both total drug exposure and dose intensity can influence the risk of chemotherapy-induced neuropathy.[122,123]

Concomitant administration of neurotoxic HIV medications may result in a substantial increase in the risk of peripheral neuropathy.[124] In addition, HIV infection itself is associated with peripheral neuropathy, and the incidence is higher in patients with a high viral load or low CD4 count.[125] Genetic factors appear to play a role in the development of drug-induced peripheral neuropathy in many patients. The risk of peripheral neuropathy associated with isoniazid and hydralazine may be higher in patients with reduced activity of hepatic *N*-acetyltransferase (i.e., "slow acetylators"). Roughly 50% of Caucasians and African-Americans are slow acetylators. Acetylation status may also be of importance with respect to thalidomide-induced peripheral neuropathy.[117] One study in patients with HIV receiving combination antiretroviral therapy found that genetic polymorphisms in iron-transport genes were associated with a higher risk of sensory neuropathy.[125] Several genetic polymorphisms are postulated to modulate the risk of chemotherapy-induced neuropathy with drugs such as bortezomib, vincristine, and platinum derivatives. However, clinical findings are inconsistent and thus the benefit of pharmacogenomic testing in individual patients remains to be determined.[126-128]

Table 13-5 Risk Factors for Drug-Induced Peripheral Neuropathy

- Prolonged duration of therapy with potentially causative agents
- High drug doses
- Human immunodeficiency virus
- Diabetes mellitus
- Hypothyroidism
- Pre-existing neuropathy
- Concomitant administration of multiple agents known to cause neuropathy
- Possible genetic predisposition
- Impaired hepatic or renal drug metabolism/elimination
- Rapid infusion of some antitumor agents

Diabetes mellitus, alcohol abuse, and nutritional deficiencies all pose a significant risk for the development of peripheral neuropathy. Patients with severe hepatic disease are at an increased risk of neuropathy. In many cases, thiamine deficiency secondary to alcohol abuse has been implicated as a potential mechanism of nerve damage, although some data suggest that toxicity occurs in the absence of chronic alcoholism. Patients with chronic kidney disease are also at risk of vitamin deficiencies. Furthermore, uremia can expose patients with end-stage kidney disease to a variety of toxic substances (phenols, myoinositol) that have been associated with neurotoxicity. Therefore, caution must be used when prescribing potentially neurotoxic medications to these patients who are at a higher risk for drug-induced peripheral neuropathy.[129-133]

MORBIDITY AND MORTALITY

Drug-induced peripheral neuropathy can produce symptoms ranging from mild, annoying paresthesias to painful sensations that can exert a significant impact on the quality of life. Some drugs can induce autonomic neuropathy, which can lead to troublesome symptoms including orthostatic hypotension, severe constipation, and impotence.[134] Rarely, anti-tumor necrosis factor-α therapy has been associated with symptoms similar to multifocal motor neuropathy, which is characterized by severe muscle weakness.[135] Fortunately, the majority of patients with drug-induced neuropathy demonstrate at least partial improvement in symptoms following discontinuation of the offending agent, and many patients experience complete recovery.[35] The coasting phenomenon may occur, however, in some patients after the drug is discontinued. The time to improvement in symptoms after discontinuing some agents may take as long as several months to years. Resolution is dependent on underlying mechanisms and the duration and extent of neuronal damage. Recovery from axonal damage may be prolonged, whereas recovery from a demyelinating process may be more rapid.[119]

PREVENTION

The most effective means for preventing drug-induced peripheral neuropathy is avoidance of use of drugs known to cause the disease in patients with known risk factors (**Table 13-6**). Clinicians should be cognizant of the neurotoxic potential of medications so that patients can be screened for risk factors before initiation of therapy. Medications with a potential to cause peripheral neuropathy should be administered at the smallest effective dose for the shortest possible duration, and doses should be adjusted appropriately in patients with kidney or liver disease.[119] Drugs that can potentially induce vitamin B deficiency, such as isoniazid, should be coadministered with pyridoxine 25–50 mg/day.

Although CIPN is predictable and well established, pharmacologic measures to prevent this complication have generally been disappointing. Although no drugs are currently recommended for the prevention or treatment of CIPN, several strategies have been used to attempt to reduce the risk of this complication (**Table 13-7**).[136] Many agents (amifostine, vitamin E, glutathione, adrenocorticotropic hormone, acetyl-L-carnitine) have been found to be initially effective in mitigating pain in animal models or small trials. Unfortunately, all of these compounds were later found ineffective in large randomized studies.[114,137-143] A recent trial evaluating acetyl-L-carnitine for the prevention of neuropathy in bortezomib-treated patients with multiple myeloma found that the intervention was not only ineffective, but acetyl-L-carnitine may have attenuated the effectiveness of the chemotherapy regimen against myeloma cells.[143]

Acute neuropathy associated with oxaliplatin occurs commonly. Symptoms may be triggered by exposure to cold, and consequently patients should be instructed to avoid extremes in temperatures and cold beverages. Long-term exposure can also cause cumulative toxicity similar to that associated with other platinum compounds. It is postulated that neurotoxicity after oxaliplatin exposure is the result of hyperexcitability due an interaction with ion channels (channelopathy) that results in a relative increase of sodium current. This is likely a result of calcium ion chelation by oxaliplatin or its oxalate metabolite.[104] Some data suggest that prophylactic administration of the sodium-channel blocker carbamazepine or oxcarbazepine may prevent acute oxaliplatin neurotoxicity. Results of unblinded trials showed that neuropathy was less severe in patients receiving oxaliplatin therapy who also received

Table 13-6 Approaches to Help Prevent Drug-Induced Peripheral Neuropathy

- Limit/monitor for potential predisposing risk factors
  - Use lowest dose possible to achieve desired effect
  - Monitor blood urea nitrogen and serum creatinine concentration in patients taking renally eliminated drugs; adjust dose appropriately if kidney disease occurs
  - Monitor liver function in patients taking hepatically eliminated agents; adjust dose if hepatic impairment occurs
- Monitor for signs/symptoms of peripheral neuropathy
- Educate patients about potential symptoms of neuropathy
- Routine clinical neurologic assessment
- Electrophysiologic testing may be useful (NCS, EMG)
- Drugs
  - Routine pyridoxine therapy in patients receiving drugs that may induce vitamin B_{12} deficiency (e.g., isoniazid)

EMG = electromyography, NCS = nerve conduction studies.

Table 13-7 Experimental Pharmacological Approaches to Prevent Drug-Induced Peripheral Neuropathy

Drug	Clinical Condition	Proposed Mechanism
Acetyl-L-carnitine[157,171-173]	CIPN and antiretroviral-induced PN	• Antioxidant effects, and stimulates mitochondrial DNA synthesis • Facilitates expression of nerve-growth factor
Amifostine[30,173-175]	CIPN	• Free radical scavenger
Calcium and magnesium salts[30,148,173-175]	CIPN	• Combats chelation of calcium and magnesium, thus preventing neuronal voltage-gated sodium channelopathy
Carbamazepine/ oxcarbazepine[144,145,176]	CIPN	• Sodium-channel blockade to combat oxaliplatin-induced channelopathy
Erythropoeitin[114]	CIPN	• Erythropoietin receptor activation in neurons stimulates an antiapoptotic effect
Glutamine[105,114,141,142,177]	CIPN	• May upregulate or downregulate nerve growth factor, thus converting glutamine to the excitatory neurotransmitter glutamate
Vitamin E[173,174,177]	CIPN	• Reduction of oxidative stress induced by chemotherapy
Cannabinoids[178]	CIPN	• Activation of cannabinoid and/or 5-HT_{1A} receptors to modulate pain

5-HT = 5-hydroxytryptamine, CIPN = chemotherapy-induced peripheral neuropathy, DNA = deoxyribonucleic acid, PN = peripheral neuropathy.

carbamazepine or oxcarbazepine.[144,145] Conversely, in another study, prophylactic carbamazepine administration failed to confer a significant benefit on electrophysiologic studies or symptomatic relief.[146] Much attention has been devoted to the use of calcium and magnesium to prevent chelation and reduce oxaliplatin-induced excitation, based on theoretical beneficial effects. Many clinicians advocated the use of prophylactic infusions of calcium and magnesium salts, particularly after the publication of a retrospective study of 161 patients with colorectal cancer, which reported that calcium and magnesium administration was effective for reducing the incidence and severity of oxaliplatin-induced neuropathy.[147] These results led to widespread routine use of calcium and magnesium infusions for neuroprotection. A subsequent prospective trial was halted early at an interim analysis, because it was determined that patients who were treated with calcium and magnesium infusions responded less well to chemotherapy. It was later determined that this conclusion was erroneous, as an independent radiologist reviewed computed tomography CT scan data from the trial and determined that there was no negative effect on chemotherapy response in calcium- and magnesium-treated patients.[30,148] A more recent double-blind study confirmed the lack of efficacy of calcium and magnesium infusions for prevention of oxaliplatin-induced neuropathy in patients with colon cancer.[149]

A small placebo-controlled trial found that venlafaxine was effective for prevention of CIPN associated with oxaliplatin. Patients were randomized to venlafaxine or matching placebo to start 1 hour prior to the first oxaliplatin dose (50 mg of immediate-release venlafaxine). Treatment was continued with extended-released venlafaxine (37.5 mg twice daily) on days 2–11. Patients treated with venlafaxine experienced significantly lower rates of CIPN than those in the placebo group.[150]

MANAGEMENT

Unfortunately, pharmacologic measures to reliably treat drug-induced peripheral neuropathy have not been identified. The severity of symptoms of peripheral neuropathy can vary widely. Thus, although neuropathy may occur commonly in association with many drugs, it is often a predictable and tolerable occurrence, such that discontinuation of the causative drug is unnecessary. However, if symptoms are severe, initial treatment of drug-induced peripheral neuropathy should include discontinuation, or at least a reduction in the dose, of the offending agent. After discontinuation of therapy, pharmacologic measures to treat neuropathic pain should be used if symptoms are persistent. In cases such as cancer or HIV treatment, in which drug discontinuation is not possible, other approaches may be helpful. Strategies widely used for patients with peripheral neuropathy induced by antineoplastic regimens include reduction in dose intensity, extending drug-free intervals, and prolonging infusion times.[96,122,151] Another beneficial strategy is an alteration of the administration route. The most prominent example of this strategy involves the use of bortezomib for the treatment of multiple myeloma. In a pivotal phase III trial, subcutaneous administration was found to be as effective as intravenous administration, but was associated with a lower incidence of neuropathy.[152]

Discontinuation of therapy with antiretroviral agents may result in loss of HIV virologic control, and dose reduction is generally undesirable. Similarly, antituberculosis regimens including isoniazid and ethambutol can cause drug-induced peripheral neuropathy, but clinicians may resist modifying the dosage regimen because of concerns regarding the potential for the development of multidrug resistant tuberculosis (MDR-TB). Shin et al.[153] reviewed the management of peripheral neuropathy in patients undergoing treatment for MDR-TB. Antituberculosis medications were not discontinued in any of the 10 patients with presumed drug-induced peripheral neuropathy. The addition of amitriptyline therapy resulted in a favorable response in most patients. Therefore, medications to treat drug-induced peripheral neuropathy can be effective in reducing the frequency or severity of symptoms even if current neurotoxic medications are continued.

Unfortunately, although there are several medications that have shown promise in unblinded studies of drug-induced peripheral neuropathy or in anecdotal reports, evidence from randomized trials demonstrating efficacy is sparse. Duloxetine demonstrates efficacy for reducing pain in CIPN. In a randomized, double-blind study, taxane- or oxaliplatin-treated patients who received duloxetine experienced a greater reduction in pain than those receiving placebo.[154]

A triple agent topical gel containing baclofen, amitriptyline, and ketamine (BAK) has been used to treat peripheral neuropathic pain syndromes. This drug combination has the advantage of blending multiple mechanisms of action that could theoretically work synergistically. A placebo-controlled study of BAK in patients with CIPN reported a trend toward improvement of symptoms of neuropathic pain with minimal adverse effects.[155]

Acetyl-L-carnitine may be a promising agent for managing chemotherapy and antiretroviral toxic neuropathy. Two small unblinded studies in patients experiencing CIPN found acetyl-L-carnitine to be effective for reducing pain scores for up to 1 year, and therapy appeared to be well tolerated.[114,156] One placebo-controlled trial in patients with HIV and antiretroviral-induced neuropathy found a reduction in pain scores in patients treated acutely with intramuscular acetyl-L-carnitine compared to those treated with placebo, as well as improvements in symptoms during follow-up therapy with oral acetyl-L-carnitine.[157] Larger studies are necessary to confirm the results of these preliminary data.

Nerve growth factor (NGF)-1 therapy has been associated with encouraging results in patients with HIV-related neuropathy. Results of a double-blind study and the long-term (48-week) follow-up study showed a reduction in pain symptoms associated with subcutaneous NGF-1, although pain severity was not consistently reduced.[158-161] Unfortunately, the results of phase III studies with this agent in patients with diabetic neuropathy were negative, which limited further large-scale studies.[124] It must be reiterated that results from clinical studies regarding treatment of drug-induced peripheral neuropathy are often confounded by the fact that the disease state itself (HIV, cancer) often plays a role in causing neuropathy.

Other measures to treat pain or other neurologic manifestations are limited to symptomatic treatments used in other types of neuropathic pain, such as diabetic neuropathy or postherpetic neuralgia. Simple analgesics such as nonsteroidal anti-inflammatory drugs or acetaminophen often are associated with limited efficacy but are safe and inexpensive. Other drugs that are generally more effective for neuropathic pain tend to be either more costly or carry the burden of undesirable toxicities or drug interactions.

Tricyclic antidepressants have been used for several years and have been found to be effective in some clinical trials in patients with painful neuropathy. The results of two placebo-controlled trials, however, demonstrated only nonsignificant trends toward efficacy.[162,163]

Gabapentin has been shown to be effective in randomized clinical trials in patients with diabetic neuropathy and postherpetic neuralgia and is associated with few serious adverse effects or drug interactions.[164,165] Small studies have noted that gabapentin may be effective for the management of both HIV and cancer-related pain. An unblinded trial in 20 patients with cancer and neuropathy revealed that gabapentin not only reduced pain scores but also reduced the need for rescue pain medication.[166] In a small study in patients with HIV and sensory neuropathy, both pain and sleep scores improved in gabapentin-treated patients compared with those receiving placebo.[167] The incidence of gabapentin-induced somnolence was high in this particular cohort (80%), but otherwise this agent was generally well tolerated. In contrast, however, a phase III trial of gabapentin in 115 patients with CIPN proved disappointing. After 6 weeks of therapy with either gabapentin or matching placebo, the severity of pain scores was not improved in the treatment group.[168]

Lamotrigine, which has also been studied for the treatment of neuropathic pain syndromes, has demonstrated some benefit for the treatment of peripheral neuropathy in patients with HIV. In a double-blind, randomized trial, Simpson et al.[169] studied the effects of lamotrigine versus placebo in patients with HIV who were afflicted with peripheral neuropathy. Patients were stratified according to whether or not they were receiving neurotoxic antiretroviral agents. Pain scores were significantly improved in lamotrigine-treated patients who were currently receiving neurotoxic HIV medications. Other antiepileptic drugs, such as carbamazepine, topiramate, valproic acid, and pregabalin can be used if other treatments fail. Some of these antiepileptic medications, including topiramate and valproic acid, inhibit the metabolism of drugs that are substrates for the cytochrome P-450 system. Venlafaxine may also be effective for the treatment of drug-induced peripheral neuropathy. Topical preparations such as capsaicin and lidocaine are associated with a low incidence of systemic adverse effects and have been shown to be effective in treating neuropathic pain. Results with these agents, unfortunately, have been generally disappointing in patients with HIV-associated neuropathy, and thus their use should be restricted to adjunctive therapy if other options are ineffective.[158,170] Opioid analgesics and tramadol are also options in patients experiencing inadequate relief or intolerable neuropathy associated with other agents.

INFORMATION FOR PATIENTS

Patients for whom potentially neurotoxic drugs are prescribed should be instructed regarding the signs and symptoms of drug-induced peripheral neuropathy. Patients should understand that for many drugs, symptoms might not appear until late in therapy or even after therapy has been completed or discontinued. Patients should be instructed to consult their pharmacist or physician as soon as they begin to experience abnormal sensations or pain occurring in the extremities so that peripheral neuropathy can be identified sufficiently early to permit intervention. Finally, patients should make their pharmacist and physician aware of all medications they are taking to prevent the occurrence of drug interactions that may predispose them to drug-induced peripheral neuropathy.

REFERENCES

1. Schneider BP, Hershman DL. Symptoms: chemotherapy-induced peripheral neuropathy. *Adv Exp Med Biol.* 2015; 862:77-87.
2. Holt D, Harvey D, Hurley R. Chloramphenicol toxicity. *Adverse Drug React Toxicol Rev.* 1993; 12:83-95.
3. Joy RJ, Scalettar R, Sodee DB. Optic and peripheral neuritis. Probable effect of prolonged chloramphenicol therapy. *JAMA.* 1960; 173:1731-4.
4. Estes ML, Ewing-Wilson D, Chou SM et al. Chloroquine neuromyotoxicity. Clinical and pathologic perspective. *Am J Med.* 1987; 82:447-55.
5. Wasay M, Wolfe GI, Herrold JM et al. Chloroquine myopathy and neuropathy with elevated CSF protein. *Neurology.* 1998; 51:1226-7.
6. Cohen JS. Peripheral neuropathy associated with fluoroquinolones. *Ann Pharmacother.* 2001; 35:1540-7.

7. Gutmann L, Martin JD, Welton W. Dapsone motor neuropathy—an axonal disease. *Neurology.* 1976; 26:514-6.
8. Koller WC, Gehlmann LK, Malkinson FD et al. Dapsone-induced peripheral neuropathy. *Arch Neurol.* 1977; 34:644-6.
9. Cooley TP, Kunches LM, Saunders CA et al. Once-daily administration of 2′,3′-dideoxyinosine (ddI) in patients with the acquired immunodeficiency syndrome or AIDS-related complex. Results of a Phase I trial. *N Engl J Med.* 1990; 322:1340-5.
10. Kieburtz KD, Seidlin M, Lambert JS et al. Extended follow-up of peripheral neuropathy in patients with AIDS and AIDS-related complex treated with dideoxyinosine. *J Acquir Immune Defic Syndr.* 1992; 5:60-4.
11. Forester D. Toxic effects of ethambutol. *Chest.* 1980; 78:496-7.
12. Nair VS, LeBrun M, Kass I. Peripheral neuropathy associated with ethambutol. *Chest.* 1980; 77:98-100.
13. Ochoa J. Isoniazid neuropathy in man: quantitative electron microscope study. *Brain.* 1970; 93:831-50.
14. Evans DA, Manley KA, Mc KV. Genetic control of isoniazid metabolism in man. *Br Med J.* 1960; 2:485-91.
15. Hughes HB, Biehl JP, Jones AP et al. Metabolism of isoniazid in man as related to the occurrence of peripheral neuritis. *Am Rev Tuberc.* 1954; 70:266-73.
16. Cupler EJ, Dalakas MC. Exacerbation of peripheral neuropathy by lamivudine. *Lancet.* 1995; 345:460-1.
17. Bressler AM, Zimmer SM, Gilmore JL et al. Peripheral neuropathy associated with prolonged use of linezolid. *Lancet Infect Dis.* 2004; 4:528-31.
18. Watt-Smith S, Mehta K, Scully C. Mefloquine-induced trigeminal sensory neuropathy. *Oral Surg Oral Med Oral Pathol Oral Radiol Endod.* 2001; 92:163-5.
19. Boyce EG, Cookson ET, Bond WS. Persistent metronidazole-induced peripheral neuropathy. *DICP.* 1990; 24:19-21.
20. Bradley WG, Karlsson IJ, Rassol CG. Metronidazole neuropathy. *Br Med J.* 1977; 2:610-1.
21. Coxon A, Pallis CA. Metronidazole neuropathy. *J Neurol Neurosurg Psychiatry.* 1976; 39:403-5.
22. Jacknowitz AI, Le Frock JL, Prince RA. Nitrofurantoin polyneuropathy: report of two cases. *Am J Hosp Pharm.* 1977; 34:759-62.
23. Filley CM, Graff-Richard NR, Lacy JR et al. Neurologic manifestations of podophyllin toxicity. *Neurology.* 1982; 32:308-11.
24. Browne MJ, Mayer KH, Chafee SB et al. 2′,3′-didehydro-3′-deoxy thymidine (d4T) in patients with AIDS or AIDS-related complex: a phase I trial. *J Infect Dis.* 1993;167:21-9.
25. Berger AR, Arezzo JC, Schaumburg HH et al. 2′,3′-dideoxycytidine (ddC) toxic neuropathy: a study of 52 patients. *Neurology.* 1993; 43:358-62.
26. Dubinsky RM, Dalakas M, Yarchoan R et al. Follow-up of neuropathy from 2′,3′-dideoxycytidine. *Lancet.* 1988; 1:832.
27. Dubinsky RM, Yarchoan R, Dalakas M et al. Reversible axonal neuropathy from the treatment of AIDS and related disorders with 2′,3′-dideoxycytidine (ddC). *Muscle Nerve.* 1989; 12:856-60.
28. Saif MW, Wilson RH, Harold N et al. Peripheral neuropathy associated with weekly oral 5-fluorouracil, leucovorin and eniluracil. *Anticancer Drugs.* 2001; 12:525-31.
29. Cata JP, Weng HR, Burton AW et al. Quantitative sensory findings in patients with bortezomib-induced pain. *J Pain.* 2007; 8:296-306.
30. Kannarkat G, Lasher EE, Schiff D. Neurologic complications of chemotherapy agents. *Curr Opin Neurol.* 2007; 20:719-25.
31. Argov Z, Mastaglia FL. Drug-induced peripheral neuropathies. *Br Med J.* 1979; 1:663-6.
32. Cavaletti G, Bogliun G, Zincone A et al. Neuro- and ototoxicity of high-dose carboplatin treatment in poor prognosis ovarian cancer patients. *Anticancer Res.* 1998; 18:3797-802.
33. Gent P, Massey K. An overview of chemotherapy-induced peripheral sensory neuropathy, focusing on oxaliplatin. *Int J Palliat Nurs.* 2001; 7:354-9.
34. Quasthoff S, Hartung HP. Chemotherapy-induced peripheral neuropathy. *J Neurol.* 2002; 249:9-17.
35. Windebank AJ. Drug-induced neuropathies. *Baillieres Clin Neurol.* 1995; 4:529-73.
36. Russell JA, Powles RL. Letter: neuropathy due to cytosine arabinoside. *Br Med J.* 1974; 4:652-3.
37. Hilkens PH, Verweij J, Stoter G et al. Peripheral neurotoxicity induced by docetaxel. *Neurology.* 1996; 46:104-8.
38. New PZ, Jackson CE, Rinaldi D et al. Peripheral neuropathy secondary to docetaxel (Taxotere). *Neurology.* 1996; 46:108-11.
39. Imrie KR, Couture F, Turner CC et al. Peripheral neuropathy following high-dose etoposide and autologous bone marrow transplantation. *Bone Marrow Transplant.* 1994; 13:77-9.
40. Patel SR, Vadhan-Raj S, Papadopolous N et al. High-dose ifosfamide in bone and soft tissue sarcomas: results of phase II and pilot studies—dose-response and schedule dependence. *J Clin Oncol.* 1997; 15:2378-84.
41. de Gramont A, Figer A, Seymour M et al. Leucovorin and fluorouracil with or without oxaliplatin as first-line treatment in advanced colorectal cancer. *J Clin Oncol.* 2000; 18:2938-47.
42. Giacchetti S, Perpoint B, Zidani R et al. Phase III multicenter randomized trial of oxaliplatin added to chronomodulated fluorouracil-leucovorin as first-line treatment of metastatic colorectal cancer. *J Clin Oncol.* 2000; 18:136-47.
43. Raymond E, Chaney SG, Taamma A et al. Oxaliplatin: a review of preclinical and clinical studies. *Ann Oncol.* 1998; 9:1053-71.
44. Windebank AJ. Chemotherapeutic neuropathy. *Curr Opin Neurol.* 1999; 12:565-71.
45. Bastuji-Garin S, Ochonisky S, Bouche P et al. Incidence and risk factors for thalidomide neuropathy: a prospective study of 135 dermatologic patients. *J Invest Dermatol.* 2002; 119:1020-6.
46. Casey EB, Jellife AM, Le Quesne PM et al. Vincristine neuropathy. Clinical and electrophysiological observations. *Brain.* 1973; 96:69-86.
47. Spivack SD. Drugs 5 years later: procarbazine. *Ann Intern Med.* 1974; 81:795-800.
48. La Rocca RV, Meer J, Gilliatt RW et al. Suramin-induced polyneuropathy. *Neurology.* 1990; 40:954-60.
49. Chaudhry V, Cornblath DR, Corse A et al. Thalidomide-induced neuropathy. *Neurology.* 2002; 59:1872-5.
50. Fullerton PM, Kremer M. Neuropathy after intake of thalidomide (distaval). *Br Med J.* 1961; 2:855-8.
51. Grover JK, Uppal G, Raina V. The adverse effects of thalidomide in relapsed and refractory patients of multiple myeloma. *Ann Oncol.* 2002; 13:1636-40.
52. DeAngelis LM, Gnecco C, Taylor L et al. Evolution of neuropathy and myopathy during intensive vincristine/corticosteroid chemotherapy for non-Hodgkin's lymphoma. *Cancer.* 1991; 67:2241-6.
53. Jacobs JM, Costa-Jussa FR. The pathology of amiodarone neurotoxicity. II. Peripheral neuropathy in man. *Brain.* 1985; 108(pt 3):753-69.
54. Meier C, Kauer B, Muller U et al. Neuromyopathy during chronic amiodarone treatment. A case report. *J Neurol.* 1979; 220:231-9.
55. Gaist D, Garcia Rodriguez LA et al. Are users of lipid-lowering drugs at increased risk of peripheral neuropathy? *Eur J Clin Pharmacol.* 2001; 56:931-3.
56. Gabriel R, Pearce JM. Clofibrate-induced myopathy and neuropathy. *Lancet.* 1976; 2:906.
57. Dawkins KD, Gibson J. Peripheral neuropathy with disopyramide. *Lancet.* 1978; 1:329.
58. Hormigo A, Alves M. Peripheral neuropathy in a patient receiving enalapril. *BMJ.* 1992; 305:1332.
59. Ahmad S. Enalapril and peripheral neuropathy. *J Am Geriatr Soc.* 1995; 43:1182.
60. Raskin NH, Fishman RA. Pyridoxine-deficiency neuropathy due to hydralazine. *N Engl J Med.* 1965; 273:1182-5.

61. Tsujimoto G, Horai Y, Ishizaki T et al. Hydralazine-induced peripheral neuropathy seen in a Japanese slow acetylator patient. *Br J Clin Pharmacol.* 1981; 11:622-5.
62. Eade OE, Acheson ED, Cuthbert MF, Hawkes CH. Peripheral neuropathy and indomethacin. *Br Med J.* 1975; 2:66-7.
63. Galasso PJ, Stanton MS, Vogel H. Propafenone-induced peripheral neuropathy. *Mayo Clin Proc.* 1995; 70:469-72.
64. Vahedi K, Taupin P, Djomby R et al. Efficacy and tolerability of acetazolamide in migraine prophylaxis: a randomised placebo-controlled trial. *J Neurol.* 2002; 249:206-11.
65. Zasorin NL, Baloh RW, Myers LB. Acetazolamide-responsive episodic ataxia syndrome. *Neurology.* 1983; 33:1212-4.
66. Koike H, Sobue G. Alcoholic neuropathy. *Curr Opin Neurol.* 2006; 19:481-6.
67. Azulay JP, Blin O, Valentin P et al. Regression of allopurinol-induced peripheral neuropathy after drug withdrawal. *Eur Neurol.* 1993; 33:193-4.
68. Kuncl RW, Duncan G, Watson D et al. Colchicine myopathy and neuropathy. *N Engl J Med.* 1987; 316:1562-8.
69. Palmer BF, Toto RD. Severe neurologic toxicity induced by cyclosporine A in three renal transplant patients. *Am J Kidney Dis.* 1991;18:116-21.
70. Yoshiyama Y, Nakajima M, Kuwabara S et al. Demyelinating brachial neuropathy complicating syngeneic graft-versus-host disease. *Neurology.* 1997; 48:287-8.
71. Bergouignan FX, Vital C, Henry P et al Disulfiram neuropathy. *J Neurol.* 1988; 235:382-3.
72. Gardner-Thorpe C, Benjamin S. Peripheral neuropathy after disulfiram administration. *J Neurol Neurosurg Psychiatry.* 1971; 34:253-9.
73. Moddel G, Bilbao JM, Payne D et al. Disulfiram neuropathy. *Arch Neurol.* 1978; 35:658-60.
74. Mokri B, Ohnishi A, Dyck PJ. Disulfiram neuropathy. *Neurology.* 1981; 31:730-5.
75. Fam AG, Gordon DA, Sarkozi J et al. Neurologic complications associated with gold therapy for rheumatoid arthritis. *J Rheumatol.* 1984; 11:700-6.
76. Koh WH, Boey ML. Polyneuropathy following intra-muscular sodium aurothiomalate for rheumatoid arthritis—a case report. *Ann Acad Med Singapore.* 1992; 21:821-2.
77. Schlumpf U, Meyer M, Ulrich J et al. Neurologic complications induced by gold treatment. *Arthritis Rheum.* 1983; 26:825-31.
78. Emir S, Kutluk T, Chan KW et al. Peripheral neuropathy during alpha-interferon therapy in a child with Hodgkin's disease. *Pediatr Hematol Oncol.* 1999; 16:557-60.
79. Zuber M, Gause A. Peripheral neuropathy during interferon-alpha therapy in patients with cryoglobulinemia and hepatitis virus infection. *J Rheumatol.* 1997; 24:2488-9.
80. Tambini R, Quattrini A, Fracassetti O et al. Axonal neuropathy in a patient receiving interferon-alpha therapy for chronic hepatitis C. *J Rheumatol.* 1997; 24:1656-7.
81. Tektonidou MG, Serelis J, Skopouli FN. Peripheral neuropathy in two patients with rheumatoid arthritis receiving infliximab treatment. *Clin Rheumatol.* 2007; 26:258-60.
82. Richards BL, Spies J, McGill N et al. Effect of leflunomide on the peripheral nerves in rheumatoid arthritis. *Intern Med J.* 2007; 37:101-7.
83. Martin K, Bentaberry F, Dumoulin C et al. Peripheral neuropathy associated with leflunomide: is there a risk patient profile? *Pharmacoepidemiol Drug Saf.* 2007; 16:74-8.
84. Pamphlett RS, Mackenzie RA. Severe peripheral neuropathy due to lithium intoxication. *J Neurol Neurosurg Psychiatry.* 1982; 45:656.
85. Kreul JF. Neuropathy and nitrous oxide exposure. *JAMA.* 1981; 245:1411.
86. Pool KD, Feit H, Kirkpatrick J. Penicillamine-induced neuropathy in rheumatoid arthritis. *Ann Intern Med.* 1981; 95:457-8.
87. Goodheart RS, Dunne JW, Edis RH. Phenelzine associated peripheral neuropathy–clinical and electrophysiologic findings. *Aust N Z J Med.* 1991; 21:339-40.
88. Heller CA, Friedman PA. Pyridoxine deficiency and peripheral neuropathy associated with long-term phenelzine therapy. *Am J Med.* 1983; 75:887-8.
89. Lovelace RE, Horwitz SJ. Peripheral neuropathy in long-term diphenylhydantoin therapy. *Arch Neurol.* 1968;18:69-77.
90. Birket-Smith E, Krogh E. Motor nerve conduction velocity during diphenylhydantoin intoxication. *Acta Neurol Scand.* 1971; 47:265-71.
91. Dalton K, Dalton MJ. Characteristics of pyridoxine overdose neuropathy syndrome. *Acta Neurol Scand.* 1987; 76:8-11.
92. Price TR. Sensorimotor neuropathy with sulphasalazine. *Postgrad Med J.* 1985; 61:147-8.
93. Wilson JR, Conwit RA, Eidelman BH et al. Sensorimotor neuropathy resembling CIDP in patients receiving FK506. *Muscle Nerve.* 1994; 17:528-32.
94. Weimer LH. Medication-induced peripheral neuropathy. *Curr Neurol Neurosci Rep.* 2003; 3:86-92.
95. Dalakas MC, Semino-Mora C, Leon-Monzon M. Mitochondrial alterations with mitochondrial DNA depletion in the nerves of AIDS patients with peripheral neuropathy induced by 2′3′-dideoxycytidine (ddC). *Lab Invest.* 2001; 81:1537-44.
96. Extra JM, Marty M, Brienza S et al. Pharmacokinetics and safety profile of oxaliplatin. *Semin Oncol.* 1998; 25:13-22.
97. Fischl MA, Olson RM, Follansbee SE et al. Zalcitabine compared with zidovudine in patients with advanced HIV-1 infection who received previous zidovudine therapy. *Ann Intern Med.* 1993; 118:762-9.
98. Gaist D, Jeppesen U, Andersen M et al. Statins and risk of polyneuropathy: a case-control study. *Neurology.* 2002; 58:1333-7.
99. Mitsumoto H, Wilbourn AJ. Causes and diagnosis of sensory neuropathies: a review. *J Clin Neurophysiol.* 1994; 11:553-67.
100. Poncelet AN. An algorithm for the evaluation of peripheral neuropathy. *Am Fam Physician.* 1998; 57:755-64.
101. Badros A, Goloubeva O, Dalal JS et al. Neurotoxicity of bortezomib therapy in multiple myeloma: a single-center experience and review of the literature. *Cancer.* 2007; 110:1042-9.
102. Chong PH, Boskovich A, Stevkovic N et al. Statin-associated peripheral neuropathy: review of the literature. *Pharmacotherapy.* 2004; 24:1194-203.
103. Mileshkin L, Prince HM. The troublesome toxicity of peripheral neuropathy with thalidomide. *Leuk Lymphoma.* 2006; 47:2276-9.
104. Pasetto LM, D'Andrea MR, Rossi E et al Oxaliplatin-related neurotoxicity: how and why? *Crit Rev Oncol Hematol.* 2006; 59:159-68.
105. Carozzi VA, Canta A, Chiorazzi A. Chemotherapy-induced peripheral neuropathy: What do we know about mechanisms? *Neurosci Lett.* 2015; 596:90-107.
106. Shiraishi S, Le Quesne PM, Gajree T. The effect of vincristine on nerve regeneration in the rat. An electrophysiological study. *J Neurol Sci.* 1985; 71:9-17.
107. Cho ES, Lowndes HE, Goldstein BD. Neurotoxicology of vincristine in the cat. Morphological study. *Arch Toxicol.* 1983; 52:83-90.
108. Diezi M, Buclin T, Kuntzer T. Toxic and drug-induced peripheral neuropathies: updates on causes, mechanisms and management. *Curr Opin Neurol.* 2013; 26:481-8.
109. Siskind MS, Thienemann D, Kirlin L. Isoniazid-induced neurotoxicity in chronic dialysis patients: report of three cases and a review of the literature. *Nephron.* 1993; 64:303-6.
110. Schaumburg H, Kaplan J, Windebank A et al. Sensory neuropathy from pyridoxine abuse. A new megavitamin syndrome. *N Engl J Med.* 1983; 309:445-8.
111. Berger AR, Schaumburg HH, Schroeder C et al. Dose response, coasting, and differential fiber vulnerability in human toxic neuropathy: a prospective study of pyridoxine neurotoxicity. *Neurology.* 1992; 42:1367-70.

112. Jongen JL, Broijl A, Sonneveld P. Chemotherapy-induced peripheral neuropathies in hematological malignancies. *J Neurooncol.* 2015; 121:229-37.

113. Smith EM, Bridges CM, Kanzawa G et al. Cancer treatment-related neuropathic pain syndromes–epidemiology and treatment: an update. *Curr Pain Headache Rep.* 2014; 18:459.

114. Bhagra A, Rao RD. Chemotherapy-induced neuropathy. *Curr Oncol Rep.* 2007; 9:290-9.

115. Hausheer FH, Schilsky RL, Bain S et al. Diagnosis, management, and evaluation of chemotherapy-induced peripheral neuropathy. *Semin Oncol.* 2006; 33:15-49.

116. Saad M, Tafani C, Psimaras D et al. Chemotherapy-induced peripheral neuropathy in the adult. *Curr Opin Oncol.* 2014; 26:634-41.

117. Hess CW, Hunziker T, Kupfer A et al. Thalidomide-induced peripheral neuropathy. A prospective clinical, neurophysiological and pharmacogenetic evaluation. *J Neurol.* 1986; 233:83-9.

118. Mileshkin L, Stark R, Day B et al. Development of neuropathy in patients with myeloma treated with thalidomide: patterns of occurrence and the role of electrophysiologic monitoring. *J Clin Oncol.* 2006; 24:4507-14.

119. Olesen LL, Jensen TS. Prevention and management of drug-induced peripheral neuropathy. *Drug Saf.* 1991; 6:302-14.

120. van den Bent MJ, van Putten WL, Hilkens PH et al. Retreatment with dose-dense weekly cisplatin after previous cisplatin chemotherapy is not complicated by significant neuro-toxicity. *Eur J Cancer.* 2002; 38:387-91.

121. Postma TJ, Vermorken JB, Liefting AJ et al. Paclitaxel-induced neuropathy. *Ann Oncol.* 1995; 6:489-94.

122. Verstappen CC, Heimans JJ, Hoekman K et al. Neurotoxic complications of chemotherapy in patients with cancer: clinical signs and optimal management. *Drugs.* 2003; 63:1549-63.

123. Grisold W, Cavaletti G, Windebank AJ. Peripheral neuropathies from chemotherapeutics and targeted agents: diagnosis, treatment, and prevention. *Neuro Oncol.* 2012; 14(suppl 4):45-54.

124. Simpson DM. Selected peripheral neuropathies associated with human immunodeficiency virus infection and antiretroviral therapy. *J Neurovirol.* 2002; 8 (suppl 2):33-41.

125. Kallianpur AR, Jia P, Ellis RJ et al. Genetic variation in iron metabolism is associated with neuropathic pain and pain severity in HIV-infected patients on antiretroviral therapy. *PLoS One.* 2014; 9:e103123.

126. Miltenburg NC, Boogerd W. Chemotherapy-induced neuropathy: a comprehensive survey. *Cancer Treat Rev.* 2014; 40:872-82.

127. Broyl A, Corthals SL, Jongen JL et al. Mechanisms of peripheral neuropathy associated with bortezomib and vincristine in patients with newly diagnosed multiple myeloma: a prospective analysis of data from the HOVON-65/GMMG-HD4 trial. *Lancet Oncol.* 2010; 11:1057-65.

128. Cavaletti G, Alberti P, Marmiroli P. Chemotherapy-induced peripheral neurotoxicity in the era of pharmacogenomics. *Lancet Oncol.* 2011; 12:1151-61.

129. Kharbanda PS, Prabhakar S, Chawla YK et al. Peripheral neuropathy in liver cirrhosis. *J Gastroenterol Hepatol.* 2003; 18:922-6

130. Perretti A, Gentile S, Balbi P et al. Peripheral neuropathy in liver cirrhosis. A clinical and electrophysiological study. *Ital J Gastroenterol.* 1995; 27:349-54.

131. Tegnér R, Lindholm B. Uremic polyneuropathy: different effects of hemodialysis and continuous ambulatory peritoneal dialysis. *Acta Med Scand.* 1985; 218:409-16.

132. Fraser CL, Arieff AI. Nervous system complications in uremia. *Ann Intern Med.* 1988; 15:143-53

133. Krishnan AV, Kiernan MC. Uremic neuropathy: clinical features and new pathophysiological insights *Muscle Nerve.* 2007; 35:273-90.

134. Balayssac D, Ferrier J, Descoeur J et al. Chemotherapy-induced peripheral neuropathies: from clinical relevance to preclinical evidence. *Expert Opin Drug Saf.* 2011; 10:407-17.

135. Fernandez-Menendez S, Gonzalez Nafria N, Redondo-Robles L et al. Multifocal-motor-neuropathy-like disease associated with Infliximab treatment in a patient with Crohn's disease. *J Neurol Sci.* 2015; 349:246-8.

136. Hershman DL, Lacchetti C, Dworkin RH et al. Prevention and management of chemotherapy-induced peripheral neuropathy in survivors of adult cancers: American Society of Clinical Oncology clinical practice guideline. *J Clin Oncol.* 2014; 32:1941-67.

137. van der Hoop RG, Vecht CJ, van der Burg ME et al. Prevention of cisplatin neurotoxicity with an ACTH(4-9) analogue in patients with ovarian cancer. *N Engl J Med.* 1990; 322:89-94.

138. Koeppen S, Verstappen CC, Korte R et al. Lack of neuroprotection by an ACTH (4-9) analogue. A randomized trial in patients treated with vincristine for Hodgkin's or non-Hodgkin's lymphoma. *J Cancer Res Clin Oncol.* 2004; 130:153-60.

139. Roberts JA, Jenison EL, Kim K et al. A randomized, multicenter, double-blind, placebo-controlled, dose-finding study of ORG 2766 in the prevention or delay of cisplatin-induced neuropathies in women with ovarian cancer. *Gynecol Oncol.* 1997; 67:172-7.

140. Cascinu S, Catalano V, Cordella L et al. Neuroprotective effect of reduced glutathione on oxaliplatin-based chemotherapy in advanced colorectal cancer: a randomized, double-blind, placebo-controlled trial. *J Clin Oncol.* 2002; 20:3478-83.

141. Vahdat LT, Thomas ES, Roche HH et al. Ixabepilone-associated peripheral neuropathy: data from across the phase II and III clinical trials. *Support Care Cancer.* 2012; 20:2661-8.

142. Wang WS, Lin JK, Lin TC et al. Oral glutamine is effective for preventing oxaliplatin-induced neuropathy in colorectal cancer patients. *Oncologist.* 2007; 12:312-9.

143. Callander N, Markovina S, Eickhoff J et al. Acetyl-L-carnitine (ALCAR) for the prevention of chemotherapy-induced peripheral neuropathy in patients with relapsed or refractory multiple myeloma treated with bortezomib, doxorubicin and low-dose dexamethasone: a study from the Wisconsin Oncology Network. *Cancer Chemother Pharmacol.* 2014; 74:875-82.

144. Eckel F, Schmelz R, Adelsberger H et al. Prevention of oxaliplatin-induced neuropathy by carbamazepine. A pilot study. *Dtsch Med Wochenschr.* 2002; 127:78-82.

145. Argyriou AA, Chroni E, Polychronopoulos P et al. Efficacy of oxcarbazepine for prophylaxis against cumulative oxaliplatin-induced neuropathy. *Neurology.* 2006; 67:2253-5.

146. Wilson RH, Lehky T, Thomas RR et al. Acute oxaliplatin-induced peripheral nerve hyperexcitability. *J Clin Oncol.* 2002; 20:1767-74.

147. Gamelin L, Boisdron-Celle M, Delva R et al. Prevention of oxaliplatin-related neurotoxicity by calcium and magnesium infusions: a retrospective study of 161 patients receiving oxaliplatin combined with 5-fluorouracil and leucovorin for advanced colorectal cancer. *Clin Cancer Res.* 2004; 10:4055-61.

148. Hochster HS, Grothey A, Childs BH. Use of calcium and magnesium salts to reduce oxaliplatin-related neurotoxicity. *J Clin Oncol.* 2007; 25:4028-9.

149. Loprinzi CL, Qin R, Dakhil SR et al. Phase III randomized, placebo-controlled, double-blind study of intravenous calcium and magnesium to prevent oxaliplatin-induced sensory neurotoxicity (N08CB/Alliance). *J Clin Oncol.* 2014; 32:997-1005.

150. Durand JP, Deplanque G, Montheil V et al. Efficacy of venlafaxine for the prevention and relief of oxaliplatin-induced acute neurotoxicity: results of EFFOX, a randomized, double-blind, placebo-controlled phase III trial. *Ann Oncol.* 2012; 23:200-5.

151. Markman M. Managing taxane toxicities. *Support Care Cancer.* 2003; 11:144-7.

152. Moreau P, Pylypenko H, Grosicki S et al. Subcutaneous versus intravenous administration of bortezomib in patients with relapsed multiple myeloma: a randomised, phase 3, non-inferiority study. *Lancet Oncol.* 2011; 12:431-40.

153. Shin SS, Hyson AM, Castaneda C et al. Peripheral neuropathy associated with treatment for multidrug-resistant tuberculosis. *Int J Tuberc Lung Dis.* 2003; 7:347-53.

154. Smith EM, Pang H, Cirrincione C et al. Effect of duloxetine on pain, function, and quality of life among patients with chemotherapy-induced painful peripheral neuropathy: a randomized clinical trial. *JAMA.* 2013; 309:1359-67.
155. Barton DL, Wos EJ, Qin R et al. A double-blind, placebo-controlled trial of a topical treatment for chemotherapy-induced peripheral neuropathy: NCCTG trial N06CA. *Support Care Cancer.* 2011; 19:833-41.
156. Maestri A, De Pasquale Ceratti A et al. A pilot study on the effect of acetyl-L-carnitine in paclitaxel- and cisplatin-induced peripheral neuropathy. *Tumori.* 2005; 91:135-8.
157. Youle M, Osio M. A double-blind, parallel-group, placebo-controlled, multicentre study of acetyl L-carnitine in the symptomatic treatment of antiretroviral toxic neuropathy in patients with HIV-1 infection. *HIV Med.* 2007; 8:241-50.
158. Estanislao L, Carter K, McArthur J et al. A randomized controlled trial of 5% lidocaine gel for HIV-associated distal symmetric polyneuropathy. *J Acquir Immune Defic Syndr.* 2004; 37:1584-6.
159. McArthur JC, Yiannoutsos C, Simpson DM et al. A phase II trial of nerve growth factor for sensory neuropathy associated with HIV infection. AIDS Clinical Trials Group Team 291. *Neurology.* 2000; 54:1080-8.
160. Pace A, Savarese A, Picardo M et al. Neuroprotective effect of vitamin E supplementation in patients treated with cisplatin chemotherapy. *J Clin Oncol.* 2003; 21:927-31.
161. Schifitto G, Yiannoutsos C, Simpson DM et al. Long-term treatment with recombinant nerve growth factor for HIV-associated sensory neuropathy. *Neurology.* 2001; 57:1313-6.
162. Kieburtz K, Simpson D, Yiannoutsos C et al. A randomized trial of amitriptyline and mexiletine for painful neuropathy in HIV infection. AIDS Clinical Trial Group 242 Protocol Team. *Neurology.* 1998; 51:1682-8.
163. Shlay JC, Chaloner K, Max MB et al. Acupuncture and amitriptyline for pain due to HIV-related peripheral neuropathy: a randomized controlled trial. Terry Beirn Community Programs for Clinical Research on AIDS. *JAMA.* 1998; 280:1590-5.
164. Backonja M, Beydoun A, Edwards KR et al. Gabapentin for the symptomatic treatment of painful neuropathy in patients with diabetes mellitus: a randomized controlled trial. *JAMA.* 1998; 280:1831-6.
165. Rowbotham M, Harden N, Stacey B et al. Gabapentin for the treatment of postherpetic neuralgia: a randomized controlled trial. *JAMA.* 1998; 280:1837-42.
166. Lossignol DA, Plehiers B, Body JJ. Gabapentin (Neurontin) and cancer pain: a pilot study. *Rev Med Brux.* 2004; 25:429-35.
167. Hahn K, Arendt G, Braun JS et al. A placebo-controlled trial of gabapentin for painful HIV-associated sensory neuropathies. *J Neurol.* 2004; 251:1260-6.
168. Rao RD, Michalak JC, Sloan JA et al. Efficacy of gabapentin in the management of chemotherapy-induced peripheral neuropathy: a phase 3 randomized, double-blind, placebo-controlled, crossover trial (N00C3). *Cancer.* 2007; 110:2110-8.
169. Simpson DM, McArthur JC, Olney R et al. Lamotrigine for HIV-associated painful sensory neuropathies: a placebo-controlled trial. *Neurology.* 2003; 60:1508-14.
170. Bianchi G, Vitali G, Caraceni A et al. Symptomatic and neurophysiological responses of paclitaxel- or cisplatin-induced neuropathy to oral acetyl-L-carnitine. *Eur J Cancer.* 2005; 41:1746-50.
171. Flatters SJ, Xiao WH, Bennett GJ. Acetyl-L-carnitine prevents and reduces paclitaxel-induced painful peripheral neuropathy. *Neurosci Lett.* 2006; 397:219-23.
172. Stillman M, Cata JP. Management of chemotherapy-induced peripheral neuropathy. *Curr Pain Headache Rep.* 2006; 10:279-87.
173. Albers J, Chaudhry V, Cavaletti G et al. Interventions for preventing neuropathy caused by cisplatin and related compounds. *Cochrane Database Syst Rev.* 2007:CD005228.
174. Openshaw H, Beamon K, Synold TW et al. Neurophysiological study of peripheral neuropathy after high-dose Paclitaxel: lack of neuroprotective effect of amifostine. *Clin Cancer Res.* 2004; 10:461-7.
175. von Delius S, Eckel F, Wagenpfeil S et al. Carbamazepine for prevention of oxaliplatin-related neurotoxicity in patients with advanced colorectal cancer: final results of a randomised, controlled, multicenter phase II study. *Invest New Drugs.* 2007; 25:173-80.
176. Stubblefield MD, Vahdat LT, Balmaceda CM et al. Glutamine as a neuroprotective agent in high-dose paclitaxel-induced peripheral neuropathy: a clinical and electrophysiologic study. *Clin Oncol (R Coll Radiol).* 2005; 17:271-6.
177. Argyriou AA, Chroni E, Koutras A et al. Vitamin E for prophylaxis against chemotherapy-induced neuropathy: a randomized controlled trial. *Neurology.* 2005; 64:26-31.
178. Ward SJ, McAllister SD, Kawamura R et al. Cannabidiol inhibits paclitaxel-induced neuropathic pain through 5-HT(1A) receptors without diminishing nervous system function or chemotherapy efficacy. *Br J Pharmacol.* 2014; 171:636-45.

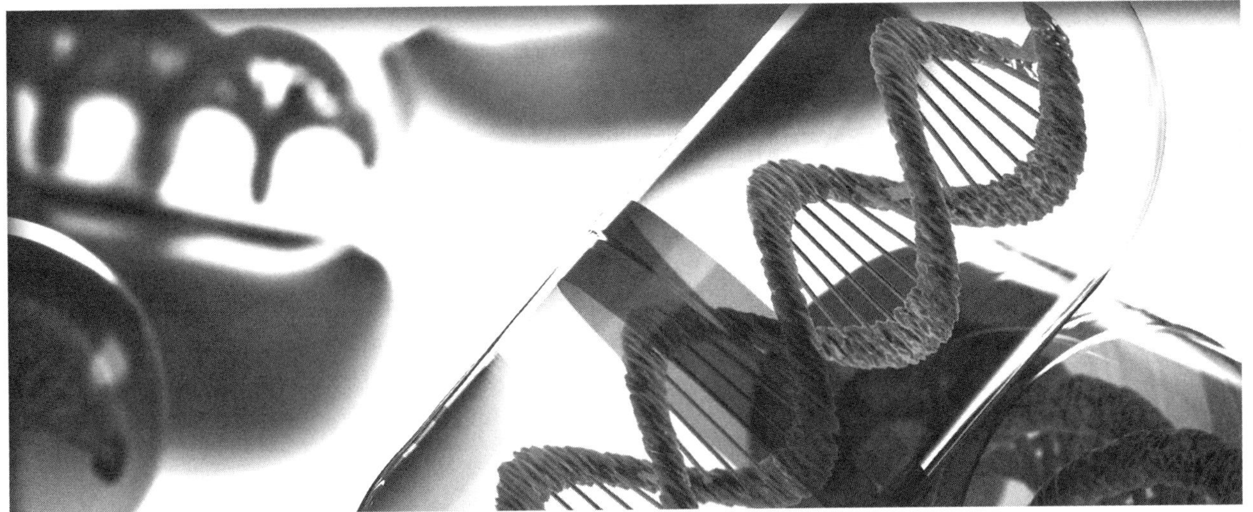

CHAPTER 14

Visual Disturbances

Yaman Kaakeh and Steven R. Abel

Over 20 classes of drugs have been associated with the development of visual disturbances and ocular toxicities. The reported ocular effects range from benign and transient to very severe. Healthcare practitioners should be aware of these drug-induced visual disturbances in order to assess the cause of specific and sometimes serious ocular problems associated with medications.

CAUSATIVE AGENTS

Drugs and herbal supplements that have been reported to cause or exacerbate visual disturbances are listed in **Table 14-1.**[1-204] A wide array of medications can cause visual disturbances through various mechanisms. These ocular problems can occur despite administration at the recommended daily dose.

Many drug classes, such as antihistamines, antipsychotics, and tricyclic antidepressants possess anticholinergic properties that are known to induce visual disturbances. Some medications with strong anticholinergic effects may cause mydriasis, the basis of photophobia that may occur in patients using these agents. Often, these visual disturbances are associated with overdose (e.g., diphenhydramine) or topical or accidental introduction into the eye (e.g., scopolamine patch). Anticholinergics may also precipitate angle-closure glaucoma and aggravate open-angle glaucoma. Cycloplegia occurs to a lesser extent.[1-3,29]

Amiodarone, a widely used antiarrhythmic drug, is known to cause bilateral corneal deposits, especially when used for long durations at higher doses. Only minimal deposits develop in patients taking 100–200 mg daily. However, at doses exceeding 400 mg daily, corneal deposits develop in nearly 100% of patients. The majority of patients are unaffected by these deposits; only 4–9% of users report visual disturbances. Anterior subcapsular lens opacities and halo vision have been associated with amiodarone therapy, although to a lesser extent. One serious complication is optic neuropathy, which is relatively rare but can gradually progress to blindness. Because of its long half-life, amiodarone-induced optic neuropathy may progress even after discontinuation of therapy.[1,2,6,13,23-36]

The antimalarial agents chloroquine and hydroxychloroquine are known to cause ocular disturbances, although the former to a lesser extent.[1,2]

Table 14-1 Agents Implicated in Drug-Induced Visual Disturbances

Drug	Effect(s)	Incidence	Level of Evidence[a]
Acetazolamide[1-4,b]	Angle-closure glaucoma	NK	C
	Myopia	NK	B
Adalimumab[5]	Cataracts	<5%	A
Albuterol[1,4,c]	Mydriasis	NK	C
Alendronate[6-14]	Blurred vision	NK	B
	Conjunctivitis	NK	B
	Ocular pain	NK	B
	Scleritis	NK	B
	Uveitis	NK	B
Alfuzosin[6]	Amblyopia	NK	B
	Blurred vision	NK	B
	Floppy iris syndrome	NK	B
Allopurinol[1,15-19]	Cataracts	NK	B
Amantadine[1,4,20-22,d]	Corneal edema	0.1–1%[e]	A
	Corneal lesions	0.1–1%[e]	A
	Decreased vision	0.1–1%[e]	A
	Keratitis	NK	B
	Mydriasis	NK	B
	Oculogyric crises	NK	B
	Optic nerve palsy	0.1–1%	A
	Photosensitivity	0.1–1%	A
	Visual hallucinations	NK	B
Amiodarone[1,2,6,13,23-36,f]	Blurred vision	NK	B
	Corneal deposits	69–100%	A
	Halo vision	1.4–40%[e]	B
	Lens opacities	22–60%	A
	Optic neuropathy	1.3–1.8%	A
	Photophobia	NK	B
Amphetamine[1,2,4,g]	Decreased vision	NK	B
	Disturbed color vision	NK	B
	Mydriasis	NK	B
	Visual hallucinations	NK	B
Anidulafungin[37]	Blurred vision	<2%	A
	Ocular pain	<2%	A
Aripiprazole[38-40]	Chorioretinopathy	NK	C
	Myopia	NK	C
Anticholinergics[1-3,29,h]	Cycloplegia	NK	B
	Decreased accommodation	NK	B
	Decreased vision	NK	B
	Mydriasis	NK	B
	Photophobia	NK	B

Table 14-1 Agents Implicated in Drug-Induced Visual Disturbances (continued)

Drug	Effect(s)	Incidence	Level of Evidence[a]
Aspirin[1,3,29,41]	Aggravation of sicca	NK	C
	Blurred vision	NK	C
	Intraocular hemorrhage	NK	C
	Myopia (transient)	NK	C
	Periorbital edema	NK	C
	Superficial punctate keratitis	NK	C
Atorvastatin[3,42-44]	Amblyopia	<2%	A
	Dry eyes	<2%	A
	Eye hemorrhage	<2%	A
	Glaucoma	<2%	A
	Ophthalmoplegia	NK	C
	Ptosis	NK	C
Barbiturates[1,2,i]	Disturbed horizontal ocular movement	NK	B
	Miosis	NK	B
	Mydriasis	NK	B
	Ptosis	NK	B
Benzonatate[45]	Blindness	NK	C
Bevacizumab[46]	Excessive lacrimation	>10%	A
Bishop's weed (*Ammi visnaga*)[47,48]	Phototoxicity	NK	C
Bitter orange (*Citrus aurantium*)[47,48]	Phototoxicity	NK	C
Black mustard (*Brassica nigra*)[47-49]	Eye irritation	NK	C
Botulinum toxin[50,51]	Bilateral inferior oblique palsies	NK	C
	Blindness	NK	C
	Diplopia	NK	C
Bromocriptine[35,52]	Blurred vision	NK	C
	Myopia	NK	C
Bupivacaine[53]	Cortical blindness	NK	C
Burning bush (*Dictamnus albus*)[47,48]	Phototoxicity	NK	C
Busulfan[1,32,54-56,j]	Cataracts	12–47%	B
Calcium-channel blockers[1,2,k]	Blurred vision	NK	B
	Transient blindness	NK	B
Canthaxanthine[6,13,47,48,57]	Crystalline retinopathy	NK	C
	Retinal deposits[e]	NK	C
Carbamazepine[1,35,41,58-60,l]	Blurred vision	Up to 5%[e]	B
	Conjunctivitis	NK	C
	Diplopia	Up to 17%[e]	B

Table 14-1 Agents Implicated in Drug-Induced Visual Disturbances (continued)

Drug	Effect(s)	Incidence	Level of Evidence[a]
	Lens opacities	NK	C
	Oculogyric crises	NK	C
	Retinopathy	NK	C
Carmustine[1-3,35,41,61,62,m]	Arterial narrowing	NK	C
	Blurred vision	NK	C
	Conjunctivitis	NK	C
	Intraretinal hemorrhage	NK	C
	Neuroretinitis	NK	B
	Ocular pain	NK	C
	Retinal infarction	NK	C
Celecoxib[13,14,63-69]	Blurred vision	0.1–1.9%	A
	Chromatopsia	NK	C
	Conjunctivitis	0.1–1.9%	A
	Glaucoma	0.1–1.9%	A
	Ocular pain	0.1–1.9%	A
Celery (*Apium graveolens*)[47,48]	Phototoxicity	NK	C
Cetirizine[9,36,70,71]	Blindness	<2%	A
	Blurred vision	NK	C
	Keratoconjunctivitis sicca	NK	C
	Oculogyric crises	NK	C
	Pupillary changes	NK	C
	Xerophthalmia	<2%	A
Chamomile (*Matricaria chamomilla*)[6,13,47-49]	Allergic conjunctivitis	NK	C
Chaulmoogra (*Hydrocarpus*)[47,48]	Visual disturbances	NK	C
Chloramphenicol[1,3,29,n]	Optic neuritis	NK	B
	Retrobulbar neuritis	NK	B
Chlorella[47,48]	Photosensitivity	NK	C
Chloroquine[6,13,29,32,35,72-76,o]	Blurred vision	NK[e]	A
	Corneal deposits	Up to 95%[e]	A
	Maculopathy	<1%[e]	A
	Nyctalopia	NK	C
	Oculogyric crises	NK	C
	Retinopathy	<1%[e]	A
Chlorpheniramine[1-3,p]	Blurred vision	1%	B
	Decreased lacrimation	NK	B
	Mydriasis	NK	B
Chlorpromazine[1,3,29,32,35,77,q]	Cataracts/lens deposits	NK	B
	Conjunctival pigmentation	Up to 46%	B
	Corneal deposits	Up to 95%	B
	Epithelial keratopathy	NK	C

Table 14-1 Agents Implicated in Drug-Induced Visual Disturbances (continued)

Drug	Effect(s)	Incidence	Level of Evidence[a]
	Eyelid pigmentation	NK	B
	Pupillary changes	NK	B
	Retinal pigment deposits	NK	C
Cimetidine[1,2,4]	Decreased vision	NK	B
	Mydriasis	NK	B
	Photophobia	NK	B
	Visual hallucinations	NK	B
Ciprofloxacin[78]	Blurred vision	<1%	A
	Decreased vision	<1%	A
	Diplopia	<1%	A
	Disturbed color vision	<1%	A
	Ocular pain	<1%	A
Clomiphene[1-3,79,r]	Blurred vision	1.5–10%[e]	A
	Mydriasis	5–10%[e]	B
	Optic neuropathy	NK	B
	Visual field changes	5–10%[e]	B
	Visual sensations	5–10%[e]	B
Clonidine[1,2,s]	Dry, itchy eyes	NK	B
	Miosis	NK	B
Contrayerva (*Dorstenia contrayerva*)[47,48]	Phototoxicity	NK	C
Corticosteroids[1,2,26,29,32,35,56,80,t]	Cataracts	10–40%[e]	A
	Decreased vision	NK	B
	Exophthalmos	NK	C
	Increased IOP	30%[e]	A
	Mydriasis	NK	B
	Myopia	NK	B
	Optic neuropathy	NK	C
	Papilledema	NK	B
	Pseudotumor cerebri	NK	B
Crizotinib[81]	Blindness	NK	C
	Optic neuropathy	NK	C
Cyclophosphamide[1,2,41,56,u]	Blepharoconjunctivitis	NK	B
	Blurred vision	Up to 17%	B
	Keratoconjunctivitis sicca	Up to 50%	B
	Optic neuropathy	NK	C
	Pinpoint pupils	NK	B
Cyclosporine[3,35,82,83]	Conjunctivitis	<2%	A
	Cortical blindness	NK	B
	Optic disk edema	2.5%	A
Cypress spurge (*Euphorbia cyparissias*)[47-49]	Conjunctivitis	NK	C
	Corneal defects	NK	C
	Eyelid swelling	NK	C

Table 14-1 Agents Implicated in Drug-Induced Visual Disturbances (continued)

Drug	Effect(s)	Incidence	Level of Evidence[a]
Cytarabine[3,48,84,85,v]	Blurred vision	NK	B
	Corneal toxicity	Up to 80%	A
	Keratoconjunctivitis	Up to 100%	A
	Ocular burning	NK	B
	Photophobia	NK	B
Dapsone[86]	Vision loss	NK	C
Datura (*D. stramonium*, *D. wrightii*)[6,13,47,48]	Mydriasis	NK	C
Deferoxamine[87-89]	Blurred vision	<2%	B
	Maculopathy	NK	C
	RPE changes	<2%	B
Dextroamphetamine[1,2,4,g]	Decreased vision	NK	B
	Mydriasis	NK	B
	Visual hallucinations	NK	B
Diazepam[1,4,31,59,90]	Blurred vision	NK	B
	Conjunctivitis	NK	B
	Diplopia	NK	B
	Nystagmus	NK	B
Diazoxide[1,2,w]	Epiphora	Up to 20%	B
Diclofenac[29,63,91]	Abnormal vision	Up to 2%	B
	Corneal infiltrates	NK	C
	Photosensitivity	NK	C
Digitalis[1-3,29,35,92,x]	Blurred vision	16–20%[e]	B
	Decreased visual acuity	16–20%[e]	B
	Disturbed color vision	16–20%[e]	B
	Halo vision	16–20%[e]	B
	Retrobulbar neuritis	NK	C
Dimethyl sulfoxide[47,48]	Ocular burning	NK	C
Docetaxel[3,4,32,93,94]	Conjunctivitis	1.1–5.1%	A
	Epiphora	Up to 10%	A
	Open-angle glaucoma	NK	C
Doxazosin[6,95]	Amblyopia	NK	B
	Blurred vision	<1%	B
	Floppy iris syndrome	<1%	B
Doxorubicin[1,2,56,y]	Blurred vision	NK	B
	Conjunctivitis	NK	B
	Epiphora	Up to 25%	B
Duloxetine[96]	Blurred vision	3%	A
Echineacea purpurea[6,13,47,48]	Conjunctivitis	NK	C
Erlotinib[97-99]	Trichomegaly	NK	C
Ethambutol[1,2,5,12,25,28,31,34,100,z]	Retrobulbar neuritis	1–50%[e]	B

Table 14-1 Agents Implicated in Drug-Induced Visual Disturbances (continued)

Drug	Effect(s)	Incidence	Level of Evidence[a]
Ethanol[1,3]	Decreased accommodation	NK	B
	Diplopia	NK	B
	Disturbed color vision	NK	B
	Mydriasis	NK	B
	Nystagmus	NK	B
Etidronate[6-9,13,14]	Blurred vision	NK	B
	Conjunctivitis	NK	B
Etodolac[61,101]	Blurred vision	1–3%	A
	Conjunctivitis	NK	C
Fingolimod[102-105]	Macular edema	0.5–1.5%	A
Fluorouracil[1,2,35,56,aa]	Cicatricial ectropion	NK	C
	Conjunctivitis	NK	C
	Corneal erosions	NK	C
	Epiphora	NK	C
	Optic nerve atrophy	NK	C
	Periorbital edema	NK	C
	Photophobia	NK	C
Fluoxetine[1,3,4,106,107,bb]	Abnormal vision	2%	A
	Conjunctivitis	0.1–1%	A
	Dry eyes	0.1–1%	A
	Eye tics	NK	C
	Mydriasis	0.1–1%	A
	Photophobia	0.1–1%	A
Fluvoxamine[4]	Amblyopia	3%	A
	Mydriasis	NK	C
Furosemide[1]	Blurred vision	NK	B
	Xanthopsia	NK	B
Gabapentin[1,108]	Amblyopia	2.7–4.2%	A
	Diplopia	1.2–5.9%	A
	Nystagmus	1–8.3%	A
	Visual hallucinations	0.1–1%	A
Gemcitabine[109]	Retinopathy	NK	C
Gentamicin[1,2,cc]	Pseudotumor cerebri	NK	B
Ginkgo biloba[6,13,47,48]	Spontaneous hyphema	NK	C
	Retinal hemorrhage	NK	C
	Retrobulbar hemorrhage	NK	C
Goa powder (*Andira araroba*)[47-49]	Conjunctivitis	NK	C
Gold[1,3,29,35,dd]	Corneal/conjunctival deposits	Up to 80%	A
	Lenticular deposits	36–55%	A
	Ophthalmoplegia	NK	C

Table 14-1 Agents Implicated in Drug-Induced Visual Disturbances (continued)

Drug	Effect(s)	Incidence	Level of Evidence[a]
Guanethidine[1,2,ee]	Blurred vision	Up to 17%	A
	Conjunctivitis	NK	B
	Miosis	NK	B
	Ptosis	NK	B
Haronga (*Haronga madagascariensis*)[47,48]	Phototoxicity	NK	C
Henbane (*Hyoscyamus niger*)[47,48]	Impaired accommodation	NK	C
	Mydriasis	NK	C
Heparin[35]	Subconjunctival hemorrhage	NK	C
Herb paris (*Paris quadrifolia*)[47,48]	Miosis	NK	C
Hogweed (*Heracleum sphondylium*)[47,48]	Phototoxicity	NK	C
Horse chestnut (*Aesculus hippocastanum*)[47,48]	Visual disturbances	NK	C
Huperzine A[47,48]	Blurred vision	NK	C
Hyaluronic acid[110-112]	Diplopia	NK	C
Hydrochlorothiazide[1,4,29,41,b]	Angle-closure glaucoma	NK	B
	Decreased lacrimation	NK	B
	Myopia	NK	B
	Photosensitivity	NK	C
5-hydroxytryptophan[47,48]	Blurred vision	NK	C
	Mydriasis	NK	C
Hydroxychloroquine[1-3,6,13,29,32,35,36,72-74,113,ff]	Blurred vision	NK	B
	Corneal deposits	Up to 100%[e]	A
	Diplopia	NK	C
	Maculopathy	<1%[e]	A
	Retinopathy	<1%[e]	A
	Visual-field defects	NK	B
Hyoscine patches[114]	Photophobia	Up to 60%	B
Ibandronate[14,48,115]	Conjunctivitis	NK	B
	Scleritis	NK	C
	Uveitis	NK	C
Ibuprofen[3,29,35,63,116-120,gg]	Amblyopia	<1%	C
	Blurred vision	<1%	C
	Decreased vision	<1%	C
	Diplopia	NK	C
	Disturbed color vision	<1%	C
	Scotomata	<1%	C
	Uveitis	NK	C
	Visual field defects	<1%	C
	Vortex keratopathy	NK	C

Table 14-1 Agents Implicated in Drug-Induced Visual Disturbances (continued)

Drug	Effect(s)	Incidence	Level of Evidence[a]
Imatinib[36,49,121-124]	Blurred vision	1–10%	A
	Conjunctivitis	1–10%	A
	Dry eyes	0.1–1%	A
	Epiphora	7–18%	A
	Glaucoma	<0.1%	A
	Macular edema	<0.1%	A
	Periorbital edema	Up to 74%	A
	Vitreous hemorrhage	<0.1%	A
Indomethacin[3,29,35,63,hh]	Blurred vision	NK	C
	Corneal deposits	NK	C
	RPE changes	NK	C
	Retinopathy	NK	C
	Retinopathy of prematurity	NK	C
Interferon[1,3,26,56]	Conjunctivitis	NK	B
	Decreased vision	NK	B
	Disk edema	NK	C
	Retinopathy	Up to 57%	B
Interleukin-2[1,2,125,ii]	Diplopia	NK	C
	Palinopsia	NK	C
	Visual field defects	NK	C
Isoniazid[1,13,jj]	Optic neuritis	NK	B
Isotretinoin[3,9,13,14,29,36,48,126-132]	Blepharoconjunctivitis	20–43%	B
	Blurred vision	16–27%	B
	Cataracts	NK	C
	Corneal deposits	5–7%	B
	Decreased vision	5.9%	B
	Dry eyes	14–33%	B
	Impaired dark adaptation	8%	B
	Intracranial hypertension	10%	B
	Myopia	NK	C
	Optic neuritis	1.9%	C
	Photophobia	5%	B
	Subconjunctival hemorrhage	1.4%	C
	Superficial punctate keratitis	Up to 22%	B
Kava kava (*Piper methysticum*)[47,48]	Impaired accommodation	NK	C
Ketorolac[133]	Abnormal vision	<1%	A
	Blurred vision	<1%	A
Lamotrigine[1,14,59,134,135]	Blurred vision	11–25%	A
	Conjunctivitis	NK	B
	Diplopia	24–49%	A
	Nystagmus	<5%	B

Table 14-1 Agents Implicated in Drug-Induced Visual Disturbances (continued)

Drug	Effect(s)	Incidence	Level of Evidence[a]
Licorice[6,13,47,48]	Decreased vision	NK	C
	Visual disturbances	NK	C
Lily of the valley (*Convallaria majalis*)[47,48]	Disturbed color perception	NK	C
Linezolid[32,136,137,kk]	Blindness	NK	C
	Optic neuropathy	NK	C
Lithium[1-3,41]	Blurred vision	NK	B
	Decreased accommodation	Up to 10%	B
	Exophthalmos	11%	B
	Nystagmus	NK	B
	Ocular teratogenesis	NK	B
	Oculogyric crises	NK	C
	Papilledema	NK	C
	Photophobia	NK	C
Lorazepam[1]	Blurred vision	NK	B
	Conjunctivitis	NK	B
	Diplopia	NK	B
	Nystagmus	NK	B
Lovage (*Levisticum officinale*)[47,48]	Phototoxicity	NK	C
Lovastatin[3,34,138,139]	Blurred vision	1%	A
Mandrake (*Mandragora officinarum*)[47,48]	Mydriasis	NK	C
Marijuana[3,6]	Blurred vision	NK	C
	Dry eyes	NK	C
	Mydriasis	NK	C
	Photophobia	NK	C
	Nystagmus (with overdose)	NK	C
Masterwort (*Peucedanum ostruthium*)[47,48]	Phototoxicity	NK	C
Mechlorethamine[2,3,56]	Necrotizing uveitis	25%	B
Metformin[140]	Vision loss	NK	C
Methamphetamine[1,2,4,g]	Decreased vision	NK	B
	Mydriasis	NK	B
	Visual hallucinations	NK	B
Methanol[141-146]	Blindness	NK	B
	Blurred vision	NK	B
	Optic neuropathy	NK	B
	Optic nerve atrophy	NK	C
Methotrexate[1,3,29,56]	Blurred vision	NK	B
	Conjunctivitis	10–19%	B
	Periorbital edema	20–49%	B
	Optic neuropathy	NK	B

Table 14-1 Agents Implicated in Drug-Induced Visual Disturbances (continued)

Drug	Effect(s)	Incidence	Level of Evidence[a]
Metronidazole[35,41]	Myopia	NK	C
	Oculogyric crises	NK	C
	Optic neuritis	NK	C
	Photophobia	NK	C
	Visual field defects	NK	C
Midazolam[1,3]	Blurred vision	<1%	B
	Conjunctivitis	NK	B
	Decreased accommodation	<1%	B
	Diplopia	<1%	B
	Miosis	<1%	B
	Nystagmus	<1%	B
Mountain laurel (*Kalmia latifolia*)[47,48]	Temporary loss of vision	NK	C
Nalidixic acid[1,2,ll]	Papilledema	NK	B
	Vision loss	NK	B
	Visual sensations	NK	B
Naproxen[1,3]	Cataracts	NK	C
	Corneal opacities	<1%	B
	Decreased vision	<5%	B
	Optic disk edema	<1%	B
	Optic neuritis	<1%	B
	Optic papillitis	<1%	B
Narcotics[1,2,mm]	Decreased accommodation	NK	B
	Diplopia	NK	B
	Epiphora	NK	B
	Irregular pupils	NK	B
	Miosis	NK	B
Niacin[6,13,47,48,147]	Blurred vision	25%	B
	Dryness	20%	B
	Eyelid edema	10%	B
	Cystoid macular edema	NK	B
Ocriplasmin[148-155]	Vision loss	NK	B
	Retinal dysfunction	NK	B
Oral contraceptives[1,3,26,35,nn]	Disturbed color vision	NK	B
	Optic neuritis	NK	B
	Pseudotumor cerebri	NK	B
	Retrobulbar neuritis	NK	B
Paclitaxel[1,3,4,32]	Decreased vision	20%[e]	B
	Open-angle glaucoma	NK	C
	Scintillating scotoma	43%[e]	B
	Vision loss	NK	C
Pamidronate[3,6-9,13,14,156,157]	Blurred vision	NK	B
	Conjunctivitis	<1%	B

Table 14-1 Agents Implicated in Drug-Induced Visual Disturbances (continued)

Drug	Effect(s)	Incidence	Level of Evidence[a]
	Episcleritis	<1%	B
	Nerve palsy	NK	C
	Ocular pain	NK	B
	Photophobia	NK	B
	Ptosis	NK	C
	Retrobulbar neuritis	NK	C
	Scleritis	<1%	B
	Uveitis (anterior)	NK	B
	Xanthopsia	NK	C
Paroxetine[3,4,158]	Anisocoria	<0.1%	A
	Blurred vision	2–5%	A
	Conjunctivitis	0.1–1%	A
	Mydriasis	0.1–1%	A
	Optic neuritis	NK	B
Parsnip (*Pastinaca sativa*)[47,48]	Photosensitivity	NK	C
Phenmetrazine[1,2,4,oo]	Cataracts	NK	C
	Decreased vision	NK	B
	Mydriasis	NK	B
	Retinal venous thrombosis	NK	B
	Visual hallucinations	NK	B
Phenylbutazone[1,2,pp]	Conjunctivitis	NK	B
	Decreased vision	NK	B
	Optic neuritis	NK	C
	Retinal hemorrhage	NK	B
Phenytoin[29,35]	Cataracts	NK[e]	B
	Diplopia	NK	B
	Disturbed color vision	NK	B
	Nystagmus	NK	B
	Ophthalmoplegia	NK	C
Pimpinella (*Pimpinella major*)[47,48]	Photosensitivity	NK	C
Pregabalin[159]	Abnormal vision	Up to 5%[e]	A
	Blurred vision	1–12%[e]	A
	Diplopia	Up to 12%[e]	A
Propofol[3,35,160,qq]	External ophthalmoplegia	NK	C
	Conjunctival chemosis	NK	C
Propolis[47,48]	Conjunctivitis	NK	C
Psyllium (*Plantago ovata, P. afra*)[47-49]	Allergic conjunctivitis	NK	C
Pyrethrum (*Chrysanthemum cinerarifolium*)[47,49]	Irritative conjunctivitis	NK	C
	Keratitis	NK	C
Quetiapine[6,rr]	Cataracts	<0.1%	C

Table 14-1 Agents Implicated in Drug-Induced Visual Disturbances (continued)

Drug	Effect(s)	Incidence	Level of Evidence[a]
Ranitidine[1,2,4]	Diminished vision	NK	B
	Disturbed color vision	NK	C
	Mydriasis	NK	B
	Photophobia	NK	B
	Visual hallucinations	NK	B
Reserpine[1,2,ss]	Conjunctivitis	NK	B
	Miosis	NK	B
Risedronate[6-9,13,14]	Blurred vision	NK	B
	Conjunctivitis	NK	B
	Ocular pain	NK	B
	Scleritis	NK	B
	Uveitis	NK	B
Risperidone[161]	Abnormal vision	1–7%	A
	Conjunctivitis	<1%	A
Rosiglitazone[162]	Macular edema	NK	C
Rue (*Ruta graveolens*)[47,48]	Photosensitivity	NK	C
Scopolia[47,48]	Impaired accommodation	NK	C
Sertraline[163]	Diplopia	NK	C
Sildenafil[3,6,13,32,36,164-170,tt]	Blurred vision	3–50%[e]	A
	Disturbed color vision	3–50%[e]	A
	Increased brightness	3–50%[e]	A
	NAION	NK	B
	Other ocular effects in clinical trials[uu]	<2%	A
	Ocular effects in postmarketing phase[vv]	NK	B
Solifenacin[171]	Blurred vision	3.8–4.8%[e]	A
	Dry eyes	0.3–1.6%[e]	A
Spironolactone[1]	Decreased vision	NK	B
	Myopia	NK	B
St. John's wort (*Hypericum perforatum*)[47,48]	Photosensitivity	NK	C
Streptokinase[172]	Blindness	NK	C
Strophanthus (*Strophanthus kombe*)[47,48]	Disturbed color perception	NK	C
Sulfamethoxazole–trimethoprim[2,4,41,173]	Angle-closure glaucoma	NK	B
	Myopia	NK	B
	Uveitis	NK	B
Sulfonamides[1,4,14,35,41,173-175,ww]	Decreased vision	NK	B
	Myopia	NK	B
	Optic neuritis	NK	B
	Photosensitivity	NK	B
	Uveitis	NK	C

Table 14-1 Agents Implicated in Drug-Induced Visual Disturbances (continued)

Drug	Effect(s)	Incidence	Level of Evidence[a]
Tacrolimus[176]	Maculopathy	NK	C
Tadalafil[3,6,13,169,177,178,e]	Blurred vision	<2%	A
	Conjunctivitis	<2%	A
	Disturbed color vision	<0.1%	A
	Eyelid edema	<2%	A
	Increased lacrimation	<2%	A
	NAION	NK	B
	Ocular pain	<2%	A
	Retinal artery occlusion	NK	B
	Retinal vein thrombosis	NK	B
	Visual field defect	NK	B
Tamoxifen[1,3,6,13,29,32,35,179-181,xx]	Cataracts	8%	A
	Corneal opacities	1–11%	B
	Disturbed color vision	NK	B
	Optic neuritis	<2%	B
	Retinopathy	1–6.3%	B
Tamsulosin[1,182]	Amblyopia	NK	B
	Blurred vision	Up to 2%	A
	Floppy iris syndrome	NK	B
Terazosin[6,183]	Amblyopia	Up to 1.3%	A
	Blurred vision	Up to 1.6%	A
	Floppy iris syndrome	<1%	B
Testosterone[184]	Chorioretinopathy	NK	B
Tetracyclines[1,3,35,41,yy]	Conjunctival deposits	NK	B
	Diplopia	NK	B
	Disturbed color vision	NK	B
	Myopia	NK	B
	Papilledema	NK	B
	Pseudotumor cerebri	NK	B
	Scleral discoloration	NK	B
Thioridazine[1,29,32,35,185,186,e,zz]	Oculogyric crises	NK	C
	Retinopathy	NK[e]	B
Tiagabine[3,13]	Amblyopia	4–9%[e]	A
	Disturbed color vision	50%	B
Tiludronate[8,187]	Cataracts	3%	A
	Conjunctivitis	3%	A
	Glaucoma	3%	A
	Scotoma	NK	C
Tiotropium[188,189]	Blurred vision	>1%	B
	Cataracts	1–3%	A
Tolu balsam (*Myroxylon balsamum*)[47,48]	Phototoxicity	NK	C

Table 14-1 Agents Implicated in Drug-Induced Visual Disturbances (continued)

Drug	Effect(s)	Incidence	Level of Evidence[a]
Topiramate[4,6,9,13,36,190,191]	Abnormal/blurred vision	Up to 13%	A
	Conjunctivitis	1–2%	A
	Diplopia	Up to 14%[e]	A
	Eye pain	At least 1%	A
	Glaucoma	NK	B
	Myopia	NK	A
	Nystagmus	Up to 15%	A
Tranexamic acid[192]	Blindness	NK	C
	Disturbed color vision	NK	C
	Retinopathy	NK	C
Trastuzumab[193]	Macular ischemia	NK	C
	Vision loss	NK	C
Tricyclic antidepressants[1,2,4,35,aaa]	Cycloplegia	NK	B
	Decreased vision	NK	B
	Mydriasis	NK	B
Trimethadione[1,2,bbb]	Diplopia	NK	B
	Photophobia	NK	B
	Visual glare	NK	B
Valerian (*Valeriana officinalis*)[47,48]	Mydriasis	NK	C
Valproic acid[194]	Visual field defect	NK	C
Vardenafil[3,6,13,169,195,196,e]	Blurred vision	<2%	A
	Chromatopsia	<2%	A
	Conjunctivitis	<2%	A
	Dim vision	<2%	A
	Disturbed color vision	<2%	A
	Glaucoma	<2%	A
	NAION	NK	B
	Ocular pain	<2%	A
	Photophobia	<2%	A
	Reduced visual acuity	NK	B
	Retinal vein occlusion	NK	B
Venlafaxine[3,4,197,198]	Blurred vision	4–6%	A
	Glaucoma	NK	B
	Mydriasis	>1%	A
Vigabatrin[1,3,13,199,200]	Diplopia	2%	B
	Visual field constriction	0.1–52%	B
Vinca alkaloids[1,2,3,35,57,ccc]	Blindness	NK	C
	Diplopia	Up to 32%[e]	B
	Extraocular muscle paresis	Up to 50%[e]	B
	Optic neuropathy	NK	B
	Ptosis	32–78%[e]	B

Table 14-1 Agents Implicated in Drug-Induced Visual Disturbances (continued)

Drug	Effect(s)	Incidence	Level of Evidence[a]
Voriconazole[3,201,202,ddd]	Abnormal vision	21–33%	A
	Blurred vision	21–33%	A
	Disturbed color vision	21–33%	A
	Photophobia	21–33%	A
	Visual hallucinations	16.7%	B
Wafer ash (*Ptelea rifoliate*)[47,48]	Phototoxicity	NK	C
Warfarin[1-4,26]	Angle-closure glaucoma	NK	C
	Decreased vision	NK	C
	Ocular hemorrhage	5–11%	B
	Ocular teratogenic effect	NK	B
Wormseed (*Artemisia cina*)[47,48]	Visual disturbances	NK	C
Yellow jasmine (*Gelsemium sempervirens*)[47,48]	Abnormal eye movements	NK	C
	Diplopia	NK	C
	Heavy eyelids	NK	C
Zoledronic acid[3,6,7,14,36,203]	Blurred vision	NK	B
	Conjunctivitis	NK	B
	Eye irritation	NK	B
	Mydriasis	NK	C
	Scleritis	NK	B
	Uveitis	NK	B
Zonisamide[204]	Angle-closure glaucoma	NK	C

IOP = intraocular pressure, NAION = nonarteritic anterior ischemic optic neuropathy, NK = not known, RPE = retinal pigment epithelium.

[a]Definitions for Levels of Evidence: Level A—evidence from one or more randomized, controlled clinical trials; Level B—evidence from nonrandomized clinical trials, prospective observational studies, cohort studies, retrospective studies, case-control studies, meta-analyses and/or postmarketing surveillance studies; and Level C—evidence from one or more published case reports or case series.

[b]Acute myopia may last 24–48 hours. Probably caused by an increase in anteroposterior diameter of the lens, which may be reversible even if drug use is continued.

[c]Only 30 reported cases of mydriasis; 1 case of bilateral narrow-angle glaucoma precipitated by use of albuterol.

[d]Diffuse, white punctate subepithelial corneal opacities have been reported, occasionally associated with superficial punctate keratitis. Onset has been 1–2 weeks after initiation of therapy with doses of 200–400 mg/day. Resolves with drug discontinuation.

[e]Dose-dependent ocular effect.

[f]Corneal deposits are dose- and duration-related; resembles chloroquine keratopathy. Deposits are bilateral, reversible, and unassociated with visual symptoms. Patients taking 100–200 mg/day have only minimal deposits. Deposits occur in ~100% patients receiving 400 mg/day. In addition, anterior subcapsular lens opacities have been reported. Rarely, such opacities may progress, increasing in density and in the diffuse distribution of the deposits. Because of amiodarone's photosensitizing properties, it is thought that light exposure may result in lens changes.

[g]Ocular effects reported with high doses; can induce or exacerbate narrow-angle glaucoma.

[h]Systemic and transdermal anticholinergic agents may cause mydriasis and, less frequently, cycloplegia. Mydriasis may precipitate angle-closure glaucoma. Photophobia is related to the mydriasis. Accommodation is decreased for near objects.

[i]Most significant ocular adverse effects occur in long-term users or in toxic states. Pupillary responses are variable; miosis occurs most frequently, except in toxicity, when mydriasis predominates. Nystagmus and weakness in extraocular muscles may be seen. Chronic abusers exhibit a characteristic ptosis.

[j]Reported with high doses.

[k]Primarily blurred vision; transient blindness at peak concentrations has been observed in several patients.

[l]Ocular adverse effects when dose >1–2 g/day; disappears when dose decreased.

[m]These ocular effects are not well established. Evidence of delayed bilateral ocular toxicity in 2 of 50 patients treated with high-dose intravenous carmustine (800 mg/m^2). Symptoms of ocular toxicity became evident 4 weeks after intravenous treatment. Evidence of delayed ocular toxicity (mean onset, 6 weeks) ipsilateral to the site of infusion developed in 7 of 10 patients treated with intraarterial carotid doses of carmustine to a cumulative minimum of 450 mg/m^2 in two treatments.

[n]Optic neuritis occurs more frequently than retrobulbar neuritis. Rare unless a total dose of 100 g and duration >6 weeks are exceeded. Vision usually improves after drug discontinuation.

Table 14-1 Agents Implicated in Drug-Induced Visual Disturbances (continued)

[o]Patients using ordinary doses may have white-yellow corneal deposits in as little as 3 weeks; little effect on visual function. Serious retinopathy when total dose >100g; usually develops after 1–3 years, but can occur in 6 months. Visual loss may progress from peripheral to central and be associated with changes in color vision. Blurred vision is rare and usually associated with high doses (500–700 mg/day). Macular changes may progress even after the drug is discontinued.
[p]Blurred vision occurs rarely (~1% of patients taking 12–14 mg/day). Decreased lacrimation may lead to contact lens intolerance or aggravate keratoconjunctivitis sicca. Mydriasis is rare, but may precipitate angle-closure glaucoma.
[q]Deposits rare when total dose <500 g. Visible after a total dose of 1 kg in most cases; incidence may increase to 90% after ≥2.5 kg. Usually, deposits do not affect vision. The cornea and conjunctiva may be affected after the lens shows pigment changes. Minimal retinal pigment deposits; further documentation is necessary.
[r]Ocular adverse effects occur in 5–10% of patients. Blurred vision is the most common effect, although visual sensations such as flashing lights, distortion of images, and various colored lights (primarily silver) may occur.
[s]Dry eyes are rare; reversible upon discontinuation of therapy. Miosis may occur in overdose.
[t]Posterior subcapsular cataracts have been associated with systemic administration. Risk is increased in patients who have received >15 mg/day of prednisone or its equivalent for >1 year. Bilateral posterior subcapsular cataracts associated with nasal or inhalation of beclomethasone diproprionate have been reported rarely. Most patients have received therapy for >5 years, often at higher-than-recommended doses. About 40% of patients also were receiving systemic corticosteroids. An elevation in IOP is more common with topical corticosteroids than with systemic therapy, but this is of little consequence in patients without pre-existing glaucoma. Patients with glaucoma should be monitored routinely if receiving systemic corticosteroids. Papilledema is primarily associated with long-term therapy, and the incidence appears to be greater in children than in adults. Intracranial hypertension or pseudotumor cerebri associated with systemic corticosteroids has been well-documented.
[u]Blurred vision is common; onset within 24 hours of receiving high-dose intravenous cyclophosphamide; resolves within 1 hour to 2 weeks. Conjunctivitis is a well-established adverse effect of therapy. Miosis occurs secondary to parasympathomimetic effects. In addition, cyclophosphamide has been reported to potentiate cataract formation when used in combination with corticosteroids. However, more information is needed before a causal relationship can be confirmed.
[v]Corneal toxicity and conjunctivitis have been reported with high-dose (3 g/m^2) therapy.
[w]Increased lacrimation may continue after drug is discontinued.
[x]A glare phenomenon and a snowy appearance in objects have been associated primarily with digitalis intoxication. In a small number of cases, reversible reduction in visual acuity has been noted. Also associated with changes in the visual fields.
[y]Effects may last for several days after discontinuation of treatment.
[z]At doses of 15 mg/kg/day, virtually devoid of ocular adverse effects. Such effects are rare at doses of 25 mg/kg/day for a duration of a few months. Patients treated for prolonged periods should undergo routine visual examinations including visual fields. Most effects are reversible after therapy is discontinued.
[aa]Ocular effects are reversible and seldom interfere with continued therapy.
[bb]Administration of 20–40 mg/day has been associated with paroxysmal contractions of the muscles around the lateral aspect of the eye. This effect occurred 3–4 weeks after initiation of fluoxetine therapy and resolved within 2 weeks following discontinuation.
[cc]Rare, but has been well documented with secondary papilledema and visual loss.
[dd]Deposition in the conjunctiva and superficial cornea more common than in the lens or deep cornea. Incidence in cornea of 40–80% in total doses of ≥1.5 g. Lens deposits observed in 36–55% of patients on long-term therapy (>3 years; lowest cumulative dose, 2.5 g). Visual acuity is unaffected and deposits resolve 3–12 months after discontinuation of therapy.
[ee]Sporadically documented. One study reported a 17% incidence of blurred vision in patients taking 70 mg/day.
[ff]See chloroquine comments (n). Incidence of corneal deposits up to 100% after 4 or more years of therapy. At <4 years incidence is ~1–28%, much lower than that associated with chloroquine.
[gg]Rare; blurred vision has been reported in patients taking from four 200-mg tablets/week to six tablets/day. Changes in color vision have rarely been reported.
[hh]Rare; changes in color vision have rarely been reported.
[ii]Visual complications have occurred during the first or second treatment cycle, usually within 5–6 days after initiation of therapy. Ocular symptoms included diplopia, binocular negative scotomata (isolated areas of varying size and shape in which vision is absent or depressed. These are not perceived ordinarily but may be apparent upon completion of a visual-field examination), and palinopsia (abnormal recurring visual imagery). In most cases, treatment was continued for the entire planned duration of therapy. Symptoms resolved after discontinuation of therapy.
[jj]Prevalence not well defined, but appears to be significantly less common than peripheral neuritis. Evaluation is difficult because most patients are malnourished, chronic alcoholics, or receiving multiple medications. Pre-existing eye disease does not appear to be a predisposing factor.
[kk]Only 12 reported cases of optic neuropathy associated with extended use (>28 days). Duration of therapy ranged from 5–11 months before development of optic neuropathy.
[ll]Visual sensations are most common. Main feature: a brightly colored appearance of objects, occurring soon after the drug is taken. Although quinolone antibiotics are nalidixic acid derivatives, they have rarely been associated with these ocular side effects. Visual loss appears to be temporary; lasting between 30 minutes and 72 hours. Papilledema can also occur, secondary to increased intracranial pressure, primarily in infants and young children. This is reversible upon discontinuation.
[mm]Miosis often with morphine in normal doses; slight with other agents. The effect is secondary to central nervous system action on the pupilloconstrictor center. Other effects are associated with narcotic withdrawal.
[nn]Optic neuritis is quite rare. In patients with retinal vascular abnormalities, use of oral contraceptives may not be prudent. Numerous other possible ocular adverse effects are associated with these agents, and further documentation is required.
[oo]Ocular effects reported with high doses; can induce or exacerbate narrow-angle glaucoma. There have only been a few case reports linking phenmetrazine with cataracts; further documentation is needed.

Table 14-1 Agents Implicated in Drug-Induced Visual Disturbances (continued)

[pp]Diminished vision is the most common ocular adverse effect; may be caused by increased lens hydration. Conjunctivitis is less prevalent and may be associated with development of Stevens–Johnson syndrome or an allergic reaction.
[qq]In 6 of 50 patients undergoing ear, nose, and throat procedures using standardized anesthesia with propofol, there was inability to open the eyes either spontaneously or in response to verbal commands. This effect lasted between 3 and 20 minutes after the end of anesthetic administration. Complete loss of ocular motility occurred in two patients. This was a transient, myasthenia-like weakness.
[rr]There have been 34 cases of cataracts reported with use of quetiapine. At this time, the association remains classified as "unlikely," because cataract development in these patients may have been due to other causes such as age-related lens changes. A causal relationship has not been established.
[ss]Conjunctivitis is common and secondary to dilation of conjunctival blood vessels. Miosis can result, although the symptoms are generally mild and can last up to 1 week after a single dose.
[tt]Color vision alterations are mild to moderate. Blurred vision does not impair visual acuity. Visual alterations usually subside within 4 hours after the dose.
[uu]Ocular effects of sildenafil identified in premarketing clinical trials occurring in <2% of patients: cataracts, conjunctivitis, dry eyes, eye hemorrhage, mydriasis, ocular pain, and photophobia.
[vv]Ocular effects of sildenafil identified in postmarketing phase (incidence not known): decreased vision, diplopia, increased intraocular pressure, ocular burning, ocular redness, ocular swelling/pressure, retinal vascular disease, vitreous detachment/traction.
[ww]Myopia is the most common ocular effect (acute and reversible). Optic neuritis can occur even in association with low doses, although it is usually reversible with complete recovery of vision.
[xx]Generally occur in patients taking higher-than-normal doses for 12–18 months.
[yy]Myopia appears to be acute, transient, and rare. Papilledema is also rare; more prevalent in children and adolescents.
[zz]Pigmentary retinopathy is primarily associated with maximal daily doses or average doses >1000 mg. Daily doses up to 600 mg are relatively safe; the risk associated with daily doses of 600–800 mg is uncertain, but rarely suspected. If doses >800 mg/day are used, periodic ophthalmoscopic examinations may uncover problems before visual acuity is compromised.
[aaa]Mydriasis is the most common ocular adverse effect. Cycloplegia is rare. Precipitation of angle-closure glaucoma has been reported.
[bbb]A prolonged glare or dazzle occurs when eyes are exposed to light. The glare is reversible, occurs at the retinal level, and is more common in adolescents and adults; rare in young children.
[ccc]Onset of extraocular muscle paresis/paralysis may be seen as early as 2 weeks. Dose-related. Most recover fully when therapy is discontinued.
[ddd]Transient; onset within 30 minutes and usually persist for 30 minutes. Most common in first week of therapy, resolving with continued drug administration. May be dose-related.

Like amiodarone, these drugs can cause corneal deposits in nearly all patients, even at therapeutic doses. The majority of adverse ocular effects associated with these drugs are dose- and time-dependent. Maculopathy and retinopathy are rare and most commonly associated with long-term, high-dose therapy. Maculopathy is very serious, and is reversible only if diagnosed in its early phase. Macular changes may progress even after therapy is discontinued. Serious retinal toxicity associated with chloroquine can develop with cumulative doses exceeding 100 g. Retinopathy may develop after 1–3 years, but case reports have described onset in as little as 6 months. In contrast, the total daily dose, rather than the cumulative dose, appears to be more important with hydroxychloroquine. The risk of retinopathy is much lower when the daily dose is 6.5 mg/kg or less for up to 10 years. Blurred vision is rare and usually associated with high doses (500–700 mg/day). Cases of nyctalopia (night blindness) and oculogyric crisis have been reported in association with chloroquine.[2]

Ocular adverse effects associated with the antiepileptic medications are not uncommon. Blurred vision, diplopia, and nystagmus are well-documented adverse effects of carbamazepine and phenytoin.[135] Downbeat nystagmus has been described as a consequence of lamotrigine therapy in two patients. In both cases, plasma lamotrigine concentrations were supratherapeutic, and the nystagmus was reversible upon correction of plasma concentrations.[134] There have also been numerous case reports linking topiramate with acute secondary bilateral angle-closure glaucoma.[190]

The bisphosphonate drugs have been linked to a number of ocular inflammatory adverse effects, including nonspecific conjunctivitis and anterior uveitis. They are currently the only drugs reported to cause scleritis.[7,8,156] Although this is a rare occurrence, scleritis is a serious condition associated with ocular pain and may lead to vision loss.[7] Selective phosphodiesterase-5 inhibitors, such as sildenafil, tadalafil, and vardenafil are commonly associated with transient visual disturbances, namely changes in color perception, blurred vision, and photophobia. These effects are largely dose-dependent. Sildenafil appears to carry the greatest dose-dependency, with impaired color perception observed at the standard 50-mg dose (3%), and increasing in incidence to 11% and 40–50% in association with the 100-mg and 200-mg doses, respectively. There are also reports of nonarteritic anterior ischemic optic neuropathy (NAION) in patients using selective phosphodiesterase-5 inhibitors. However, a causal relationship cannot yet be confirmed, as other risk factors may have been involved.[6,164,166,168]

Other drug classes associated with ocular adverse effects include analgesics, anticoagulants, antidepressants, anti-infectives, antihyperlipidemics, antineoplastic agents, barbiturates, benzodiazepines, β-adrenergic blockers, calcium-channel blockers, corticosteroids, hypouricemics, immune modulators, and oral contraceptives.[1,2] Numerous visual disturbances have also been reported in association with the use of herbal and nutritional supplements.[3,6,13,47-49,57]

EPIDEMIOLOGY

The exact incidence of drug-induced visual disturbances is not known. Numerous factors including the specific medication, frequency of administration, cumulative dose, genetic factors, and route of administration may influence the occurrence of drug-induced visual disturbances. For example, 5% of patients undergoing therapy with topical corticosteroids experience an increase in intraocular pressure of 16 mm Hg or greater, while 30% experiences an increase of 6–15 mm Hg following 4 weeks or more of treatment.[205,206] Further assessment documented that primary open-angle glaucoma developed in 13% of high corticosteroid responders (defined as >15 mm Hg increase) and ocular hypertension occurred in 63.8%. Open-angle glaucoma developed in no low responders (<5 mm Hg increase) and ocular hypertension occurred in only 2.4%.[207]

Corneal opacities occur in 70–100% of patients receiving amiodarone, while optic neuropathy develops in approximately 2%. The anticonvulsant lamotrigine causes diplopia and blurred vision with incidences of 22% and 15%, respectively.[1] Agents used for erectile dysfunction (sildenafil, vardenafil, tadalafil) are associated with dose-dependent changes in color vision, blurred vision, increased light perception, and visualization of flashing lights in 3–50% of patients.[1] High-dose cytarabine has been associated with blurred vision and keratitis in 100% of treated patients. Decreased visual acuity, diplopia, and color vision defects have been reported with nonsteroidal anti-inflammatory drugs (NSAIDs) even in patients taking small doses infrequently.[1] The known incidences of visual disturbances associated with specific drugs are provided in Table 14-1.

MECHANISMS

The pathogenesis of drug-induced visual disturbances appears to be multifactorial. Cumulative or daily dose, duration of therapy, properties of specific medications, and site of drug action all appear to play a role. Although we are knowledgeable about mechanisms of visual disturbances associated with some drugs, mechanisms have yet to be described for the majority of medications. Known mechanisms can be divided into direct and indirect drug effects on the ocular structures (**Table 14-2**).

The blood–aqueous barrier and posterior blood–retinal barrier serve to naturally defend the intraocular structures of the eye from exogenous compounds or toxins. However, some compounds may penetrate the tight junctional areas between retinal pigment epithelium (RPE) cells and within the retinal capillary endothelium. Over time, this can lead to a number of ocular problems, such as epithelial keratopathy or pigmentary deposition. Medications may also interact directly with RPE cells, resulting in retinotoxicity. For example, the antimalarial drugs chloroquine and hydroxychloroquine exhibit high affinity for melanin in RPE and may induce photoreceptor degradation, leading to the development of a "bulls-eye" maculopathy.[34,208]

Amphiphilic compounds, such as amiodarone, accumulate in lysosomes and cannot be eliminated effectively. This leads to the accumulation of the drug in intracytoplasmic lamellar bodies in the eye. The resulting complex with cellular phospholipids on the epithelium cannot be metabolized

Table 14-2 Mechanisms of Drug-Induced Visual Disturbances

Effect	Mechanisms
Angle-closure glaucoma	Associated with mydriasis, which causes closure of the anterior chamber angle, preventing elimination of aqueous humor from the eye; may also result from swelling of the lens or other ocular tissues
Blepharoconjunctivitis	Drug concentrating in the tears causing irritation and subsequent inflammation of the eyelids and conjunctiva
Blurred vision	Direct ocular effects (see: Dry eyes, keratoconjunctivitis sicca, mydriasis) or indirect effects in nonocular areas (central nervous system depression, cranial-nerve damage, hypertension, etc.)
Cataracts/lens opacities	Medications may precipitate as fine granules, typically in the superficial cortex of the lens and in the anterior capsule
Color vision disturbances	Impairment of retinal-cell function through direct effect of medications on the ocular tissues; may occur at therapeutic plasma drug concentrations
Conjunctival pigmentation	Direct deposition of medication in cysts within conjunctival epithelium
Corneal deposits	Accumulation of the drug in the intracytoplasmic lamellar bodies in the eye; these bodies form complexes with cellular phospholipids that cannot be metabolized by lysosomal phospholipids, and corneal deposits result; may be time- or concentration-dependent, or both
Diplopia	See: Dry eyes, keratoconjunctivitis sicca, mydriasis
Dry eyes	Secretion of medication by lacrimal gland, leading to local eye irritation; medications may also indirectly lead to inadequate tear production and subsequent irritation
Epiphora	Excessive lacrimation due to local irritation of the eye or obstruction of tear ducts, thus preventing the drainage of tears
Exophthalmos	Unknown
Extraocular muscle paresis	Cranial-nerve palsy, which may lead to dysfunction in one or more extraocular muscles
Floppy iris syndrome	$\alpha 1$-adrenergic blocking effect (alfuzosin, terazosin, etc.) may also selectively block receptors in the iris dilator muscle, leading to atrophy of the iris dilator smooth muscle
Halo vision	Unknown
Intraocular pressure increases	See: Angle-closure glaucoma
Keratoconjunctivitis sicca	Secretion of medication by lacrimal gland, leading to local eye irritation; medications may also lead indirectly to inadequate tear production and subsequent irritation
Mydriasis	Sympathetic stimulation may cause contraction of the radial muscle, and subsequent dilation of the iris; mydriasis may precipitate or exacerbate angle-closure glaucoma
Necrotizing uveitis	Medications may cause uveitis through direct toxicity or indirect mechanisms, including stimulation of the immune system to develop antidrug antibodies; drug combining with melanin and inducing uveitis by reducing the pigment's free radical scavenger properties; antibiotics stimulating the immune system by liberating antigens from dead microorganisms
Nonarteritic anterior ischemic optic neuropathy (NAION)	Caused by reduced blood flow to the optic nerve; the most common ocular adverse effect found in nearly all patients treated with long-term amiodarone is reversible keratopathy, known as vortex keratopathy; this neuropathy is typically bilateral and symmetric; NAION, nonarteric ischemic optic neuropathy, rarely occurs simultaneously in both eyes; its symptoms often resolve in weeks; the onset is more insidious, and the degree of visual loss is less
Nystagmus	Cerebellovestibular dysfunction; dose-related, potentially irreversible cerebellar deficits
Optic neuropathy	Decrease in axoplasmic flow may lead to vascular occlusion, resulting in optic disk edema that progresses to optic neuropathy; compromised axonal transport in optic nerve that leads to optic neuropathy; may be time or concentration-dependent, or both

Table 14-2 Mechanisms of Drug-Induced Visual Disturbances (continued)

Effect	Mechanisms
Periorbital edema	Allergic reaction; with imatinib, it is presumed that inhibition of platelet-derived growth factor in dermal dendrocytes of the periorbital skin may result in a decrease in interstitial fluid pressure, which may lead to localized edema
Ptosis	Cranial nerve palsy, which may lead to dysfunction in one or both upper eyelid elevator muscles
Retrobulbar neuritis	Drug chelates retinal-cell copper, which acts as a cofactor for mitochondrial functioning in the optic nerve; consequentially, axonal transport in the optic nerve may be compromised and progress to optic neuropathy
Superficial punctate keratitis	Unknown

by lysosomal phospholipids, and corneal deposits occur. These deposits are dose- and duration-related and resemble chloroquine-induced keratopathy.[33,34,208] Amiodarone also causes optic neuropathy, although the mechanism is less clear. It is thought that a vascular occlusion from a decrease in axoplasmic flow may be involved. This may result in optic disk edema that progresses to optic neuropathy.[31,33] Amiodarone-induced optic neuropathy is sometimes difficult to distinguish from NAION because patients may already have underlying vascular disease.[6]

The mechanism of ethambutol-induced optic neuropathy remains incompletely understood. It is postulated that ethambutol chelates retinal-cell copper, which acts as a cofactor for mitochondrial functioning in the optic nerve. As a result, axonal transport in the optic nerve may be compromised, leading to optic neuropathy. These effects appear to be dose- and time-dependent.[13]

An increase in intraocular pressure, caused by certain medications such as corticosteroids, can exacerbate open-angle glaucoma. Mydriatics and mydriatic/cycloplegics could exacerbate angle-closure glaucoma, because this is an anatomical event. Secretion of medications through the lacrimal gland can lead to blurred vision, eye and contact-lens discomfort, dry eye symptoms, and conjunctivitis.

Drug-induced ocular effects are time-dependent, suggesting that tissue accumulation likely plays a role in the pathophysiology.[33] Visual disturbances can also result from the indirect actions of certain medications on nonocular structures. Blurred vision is a common adverse effect of anticholinergic medications and benzodiazepines. Phenytoin may cause cerebellar degeneration and eventually lead to irreversible cerebellar deficits. Vision changes may be an indication of toxic plasma drug concentrations.[1] Drugs that lead to hypertension, metabolic abnormalities, sedation, or dehydration may also lead to visual problems. Nystagmus induced by carbamazepine and phenytoin may be due to cerebellovestibular dysfunction.[58]

CLINICAL PRESENTATION AND DIFFERENTIAL DIAGNOSIS

Signs and symptoms of drug-induced visual disturbances are listed in **Table 14-3**. The onset of signs and symptoms is largely time-dependent, meaning that they are more likely to occur later in therapy. In some cases, drug-induced visual disturbances may mimic the signs and symptoms of other diseases, requiring clinicians to carefully evaluate each contributing factor that might result in their patients' visual disturbances. Various methods of diagnosis are used to identify drug-induced eye disease. These are similar to diagnostic tests and methods used with eye disease that is not drug-induced. Principles such as onset of symptoms in relationship to the initiation of drug therapy are key. The time frame for certain adverse ocular effects of drugs is known, and should stimulate certain diagnostic tests. One example is the increase in intraocular pressure that may be associated with the administration of topical corticosteroids. The maximum intraocular pressure increase occurs within

Table 14-3 Signs and Symptoms Associated with Drug-Induced Visual Disturbances[209]

- Blepharitis
- Blindness
- Blurred vision
- Cataracts
- Color vision alterations
- Conjunctivitis
- Decreased vision (miosis, mydriasis)
- Diplopia
- Glaucoma
- Halos around lights
- Hallucinations
- Hazy vision
- Increased intraocular pressure
- Keratopathy
- Night blindness
- Optic neuropathy
- Photophobia
- Pseudotumor cerebri
- Scleritis
- Tunnel vision
- Vertigo
- Visual field constriction

Table 14-4 Conditions to Consider in the Differential Diagnosis of Drug-Induced Visual Disturbances[31,34,209]

- Stroke
- Concussion
- Dehydration
- Encephalopathy
- Exposure to environmental toxins
- Drug intoxication
- Glaucoma
- Head trauma
- Hypertension
- Intracranial lesions/infarction
- Macular degeneration
- Migraine
- Metabolic disorders (i.e., diabetes, Wilson disease)
- Neoplasm
- Psychiatric disease
- Retinal disease/detachment
- Seizures
- Vitreous detachment

4 weeks, so it makes sense that intraocular pressure should be measured once or twice during that time period. **Table 14-4** lists conditions that should be considered in the differential diagnosis of drug-induced visual disturbances.

Hypersensitivity reactions including dermatitis are most likely to affect the eyelids. Quinolones may cause hyperpigmentation of the eyelids, while 5-fluorouracil is associated with blepharitis and conjunctivitis involvement.[32] Keratoconjunctival disorders present mainly as conjunctival hyperemia (red eye) with or without superficial corneal involvement.[31] Medications that are structurally related to sulfonamides may induce swelling of the ciliary body leading to the development of angle-closure glaucoma.[32]

Agents that dilate the pupil (adrenergics, anticholinergics) may cause blurred vision or precipitate angle-closure glaucoma in patients with narrow anterior chamber angles. Angle-closure glaucoma is a medical emergency. Symptoms include swelling of the eye, clouding of the cornea, and severe pain. Corticosteroids can increase intraocular pressure (IOP) in genetically predisposed patients, resulting in ocular hypertension of open-angle glaucoma.[205,206] Although corticosteroid-induced increases in IOP are associated most frequently with topical ophthalmic preparations, systemic corticosteroids may cause a similar response, although with a lesser magnitude.[210]

Docetaxel and paclitaxel have also been associated with the development of open-angle glaucoma.[32] Unlike angle-closure glaucoma, ocular hypertension and open-angle glaucoma are silent diseases that are frequently symptom-free until there has been significant damage to the optic nerve, resulting in a reduction of the visual field. Patients may describe a loss of central or peripheral vision.

Corticosteroids, allopurinol, phenothiazines, and busulfan have been reported to cause cataracts.[31] Symptoms of cataracts include a reduction in visual clarity and a reduced ability to see in low light or darkness. Many drugs administered systemically reach the retina via the systemic circulation. Phenothiazines may bind to melanin, causing a severe phototoxic retinopathy.[32] Amiodarone appears to cause a bilateral optic neuropathy that is similar to

NAION, a condition also associated with the use of cGMP (cyclic guanosine monophosphate)–specific phosphodiesterase-5 inhibitors for erectile dysfunction.[32] Amiodarone has also been associated with lens deposits and keratopathy due to corneal alterations related to a drug-induced lipid storage disorder.[211] Symptoms of keratopathy include glare and photophobia.

RISK FACTORS

In some instances, the risk of visual disturbances associated with medications is influenced by genetic factors. An example of this is the propensity for topical corticosteroids to cause increases in intraocular pressure. Myocilin is a protein, encoded by the *MYOC* gene, which is linked to the most common form of glaucoma (open angle). Overexpression of myocilin due to corticosteroid administration augments the pressure response.[212] Studies suggest that heterozygotes are at medium risk, while homozygotes are at higher risk.[213] Unfortunately, there is no reliable genomic test to assess individuals prior to treatment to determine the likelihood for exaggerated and potentially adverse response to these medications.

In other cases, the risk for visual disturbances is increased with the daily drug dose, the cumulative drug dose, or both, as well as the use of combinations of medications associated with the development of visual disturbances. Underlying disease states may predispose patients taking certain medications to visual disturbances. The risk of corticosteroid-induced ocular hypertension is greater in patients with high myopia, diabetes mellitus, or connective-tissue disease (particularly rheumatoid arthritis).[210] The best approach to minimize the risk of drug-induced visual disturbances involves accurate diagnosis, including all underlying disease states and pre-existing drug therapy (prescription and nonprescription drugs and natural remedies), past therapeutic response to medications, including adverse events, and careful patient monitoring based on the benefit-to-risk ratio of medications administered. Practitioners must also recognize that some ocular disorders will occur regardless of careful prescribing or monitoring practices. For example, while age-related cataracts are slowly progressive, the potential for their development exists in everyone, depending upon longevity. Ocular symptoms often occur at plasma concentrations within the therapeutic range. The effects may be more marked at higher plasma concentrations.[214] **Table 14-5** lists other risk factors associated with drug-induced visual disturbances.

Table 14-5 Risk Factors for Drug-Induced Visual Disturbances

- Anatomic predisposition (e.g., narrow anterior chamber angles)
- Concomitant use of multiple drugs, including herbal therapies, that may cause visual disturbances (see Table 14-1)
- Cumulative dose (e.g., chloroquine, >100 g)
- Daily dose (e.g., hydroxychloroquine 500–700 mg/day)
- Genetics (e.g., myocilin and topical ophthalmic corticosteroids)
- Underlying disease states/conditions (see Table 14-4)

MORBIDITY AND MORTALITY

In general, the ocular side effects of drugs should have minimal overall adverse impact on the healthcare system in terms of hospitalizations or length of stay, and pose a relatively small risk of mortality. Most adverse events are managed through consultation within the office setting. Certain adverse events such as acute angle-closure glaucoma could result in emergency department visits. Conceivably, drug-induced loss of vision could result in a situation associated with bodily harm or death (i.e., personal or motor vehicle accident).

Left untreated, acute emergencies such as drug-induced angle-closure glaucoma could result in the permanent loss of sight in one or both eyes. Any acute or chronic reduction in visual acuity, as well as clinically significant reactions such as conjunctivitis could be associated with diminished quality of life.

PREVENTION

Some topically administered ocular medications are associated with systemic toxicities that can include visual disturbances. Topical atropine has been associated with blood pressure changes that affect vision. The use of punctal occlusion minimizes systemic absorption of the topically administered medication and therefore reduces, but does not eliminate, the associated risk. Punctal occlusion involves the application of pressure to the inner canthus with the index finger following topical administration of ophthalmic medication. Ideally, pressure should be applied for approximately 2 minutes. However, use of this technique, even for shorter periods, reduces the potential for systemic absorption of the topically administered medication.

The development of visual disturbances associated with systemic medications is frequently related to the average daily dose administered, the duration of treatment, and the cumulative dose. Prescribers are encouraged to consider the potential for visual disturbances associated with prescribed medications and to appropriately monitor patients. Healthcare providers may consider avoiding certain drugs, such as phosphodiesterase-5 inhibitors, in patients already at high risk for certain ocular diseases, such as NAION. Although there are only case reports linking these agents to NAION, these patients may already have compromised optic nerves due to vascular disease. It is postulated that these medications can lead to further neural function damage.

In some situations, visual disturbances occur in association with medications that may be monitored via the assessment of plasma concentrations (e.g., phenytoin). In such cases, therapeutic drug monitoring is suggested as appropriate based on clinical management of the patient and the potential for or suspicion of visual disturbances associated with the medication.

Routine ophthalmic examinations should be completed in all individuals. The usual frequency for examinations in patients without risk is every 2 years for individuals 18–60 years of age, and yearly thereafter. Patients with risk factors, including medications that may be associated with visual disturbances, should be seen more frequently (at least annually). In addition, patients should be educated regarding the necessity for follow-up visits if they receive medications that might be associated with the development of visual disturbances. Prescribers should carefully consider any underlying conditions that might make a patient more susceptible to visual disturbances associated with medications. Product information is another valuable tool in enabling individuals to assess the potential for a medication to induce visual disturbances. Approaches to help prevent drug-induced visual disturbances are outlined in **Table 14-6**.

Table 14-6 Approaches to Help Prevent Drug-Induced Visual Disturbances

- Be aware of the potential for visual disturbances
- Discontinue therapy prior to reaching total cumulative dose associated with visual disturbances
- Use punctal occlusion for topical ophthalmic medications with the potential for systemic adverse effects
- Restrict daily dose to minimize risk of visual disturbances
- Routine ophthalmic examinations

MANAGEMENT

Relatively little information exists regarding the effective management of drug-induced visual disturbances and ocular toxicities. The decision to discontinue, change, or even continue therapy with the offending agent is dependent on multiple factors (risk versus benefit, availability of alternative agents, severity of disease). The key to appropriate management is early identification.

Nonprescription or prescription medications (decongestants, artificial tears, NSAIDs) may be used to manage mild visual disturbances such as blurred vision or conjunctivitis. Discontinuation of the offending agent is usually necessary to ameliorate drug-induced visual disturbances. This is especially true for more serious ocular problems, such as retinopathy or maculopathy. Discontinuation of bisphosphonates is necessary for resolution of scleritis. Visual effects associated with cyclooxygenase-2 inhibitors typically resolve within 72 hours of drug discontinuation. Ocular adverse effects induced by phenytoin often resolve with discontinuation of therapy or dose reduction, although in some cases nystagmus may persist for 20 months or longer.[1] Intraocular pressure elevation, such as that caused by corticosteroids, is an indication to taper therapy. Left uncontrolled, significant increases in intraocular pressure could result in blindness. The antimalarial medications chloroquine and hydroxychloroquine may produce retinopathy and maculopathy. These effects are usually irreversible unless identified in the very early stage. Progression may occur and management may be limited to interventional pharmacology or surgical intervention.

In situations in which discontinuation of therapy is not always feasible (i.e., amiodarone), reducing the dose may help attenuate some of the visual disturbances. This is especially true for obese patients, who may be receiving above-normal doses of certain medications, such as gentamicin.

INFORMATION FOR PATIENTS

Appropriate patient education is the key to preventing and reducing the impact of drug-induced visual disturbances. The use of punctal occlusion when administering topical ophthalmic medications reduces the potential incidence of systemic side effects. The risks and benefits of a particular therapy should be thoroughly conveyed to the patient. Routine ophthalmic examinations are central to eye health assessment, and patients should have follow-up examinations at the recommended frequency. Patients should be advised to disclose all prescription, nonprescription, and herbal medications to their healthcare provider. Any rapid or sudden changes in visual acuity should also be reported.

REFERENCES

1. Fraunfelder FT, Fraunfelder FW. *Drug-induced ocular side effects.* 5th ed. Woburn, MA: Butterworth-Heinemann; 2001.
2. Grant WM, Schuman JS, eds. *Toxicology of the eye.* 4th ed. Springfield, IL: Charles C Thomas Publishing; 1993.
3. Micromedex Healthcare Series. http://www.micromedexsolutions.com/micromedex2/librarian/ (accessed 2018 Jan 31).
4. Tripathi RC, Tripathi BJ, Haggerty C. Drug-induced glaucomas: mechanism and management. *Drug Saf.* 2003; 26:749-67.
5. Humira [package insert]. North Chicago, IL: AbbVie; 2015.
6. Fraunfelder FT, Fraunfelder FW. Drug-related adverse effects of clinical importance to the ophthalmologist. www.eyedrugregistry.com (accessed 2018 Jan 31).
7. Fraunfelder FW. Ocular side effects associated with bisphosphonates. *Drugs Today (Barc)* 2003; 39:829-35.
8. Fraunfelder FW, Fraunfelder FT. Bisphosphonates and ocular inflammation. *N Engl J Med.* 2003; 348:1187-8.
9. Fraunfelder FW, Fraunfelder FT. Adverse ocular drug reactions recently identified by the National Registry of Drug-Induced Ocular Side Effects. *Ophthalmology.* 2004; 111:1275-9.
10. Coleman CI, Perkerson KA, Lewis A. Alendronateinduced auditory hallucinations and visual disturbances. *Pharmacotherapy.* 2004; 24:799-802.
11. Malik AR, Campbell SH, Toma NMG. Bilateral acute anterior uveitis after alendronate. *Br J Ophthalmol.* 2002; 86:1443.
12. Mbekani JN, Slamovits TL, Schwartz BH et al. Ocular inflammation associated with alendronate therapy. *Arch Ophthalmol.* 1999; 117:837-8.
13. Santaella RM, Fraunfelder FW. Ocular adverse effects associated with systemic medications. *Drugs.* 2007; 67:75-93.
14. Fraunfelder FW. Drug-induced ocular inflammatory disorders. *Drugs Today (Barc).* 2007; 43:117-23.
15. Fraunfelder FT, Hanna C, Dreis MW et al. Cataracts associated with allopurinol therapy. *Am J Ophthalmol.* 1982; 94:137-40.
16. Jick H, Brandt DE. Allopurinol and cataracts. *Am J Ophthalmol.* 1984; 98:355-8.
17. Lerman S, Megaw JM, Gardner K. Allopurinol therapy and cataractogenesis in humans. *Am J Ophthalmol.* 1982; 94:141-6.
18. Rudy MA, Zigman S, Schenk E. Lack of photosensitization of ocular tissues by allopurinol. *Arch Ophthalmol.* 1981; 99:2030-3.
19. Clair WK, Chylack LT, Cook EF et al. Allopurinol use and the risk of cataract formation. *Br J Ophthalmol.* 1989; 73:173-6.
20. Fraunfelder FT, Meyer SM. Amantadine and corneal deposits. *Am J Ophthalmol.* 1990; 110:96-7.
21. Nogaki H. Superficial punctate keratitis and corneal abrasion due to amantadine hydrochloride. *J Neurol.* 1993; 240:388-9.
22. Symmetrel [package insert]. Chadds Ford, PA: Endo Pharmaceuticals; 2007.
23. Dolan BJ, Flach AJ, Peterson JS. Amiodarone keratopathy and lens opacities. *J Am Optom Assoc.* 1985; 56:468-70.
24. Domingues MF, Barros H, Falcao-Reis FM. Amiodarone and optic neuropathy. *Acta Ophthalmol Scand.* 2004; 82:277-82
25. Flach AJ, Dolan BJ. Amiodarone-induced lens opacities: an 8-year follow-up study. *Arch Ophthalmol.* 1990; 108:1668-9
26. Hampson JP, Harvey JN. A systematic review of druginduced ocular reactions in diabetes. *Br J Ophthalmol.* 2000; 84:144-9.
27. Ikaheimo K, Kettunen R, Mantyjarvi M. Visual functions and adverse ocular effects in patients with amiodarone medication. *Acta Ophthalmol Scand.* 2002; 80:59-63.
28. Ingram DV, Jaggarao NS, Chamberlain DA. Ocular changes resulting from therapy with amiodarone. *Br J Ophthalmol.* 1982; 66:676-9.
29. Jaanus SD. Ocular side effects of selected systemic drugs. *Optom Clin.* 1992; 2:73-96.
30. Kaplan LJ, Cappaert WE. Amiodarone keratopathy: correlation to dosage and duration. *Arch Ophthalmol.* 1982; 100:601-2.
31. Koneru PB, Lien EJ, Koda RT. Oculotoxicities of systemically administered drugs. *J Ocul Pharmacol* 1986; 2:385-404.
32. Li J, Tripathi RC, Tripathi BJ. Drug-induced ocular disorders. *Drug Saf.* 2008; 31:127-41.
33. Mantyjarvi M, Tuppurainen K, Ikaheimo K. Ocular side effects of amiodarone. *Surv Ophthalmol.* 1998; 42:360-6.
34. Moorthy RS, Valluri S. Ocular toxicity associated with systemic drug therapy. *Curr Opin Ophthalmol.* 1999; 10:438-46.
35. Rennie IG. Clinically important ocular reactions to systemic drug therapy. *Drug Saf.* 1993; 9:196-211.
36. Fraunfelder FW. Ocular adverse drug reactions and the National Registry of Drug-Induced Ocular Side Effects. *Insight.* 2004; 29:7-11.
37. Eraxis [package insert]. New York: Pfizer Inc; 2007.
38. Faure C, Audo I, Zeitz C et al. Aripiprazole-induced chorioretinopathy: multimodal imaging and electrophysiological features. *Doc Ophthalmol.* 2015; 131:35-41
39. Nair AG, Nair AG, George RJ et al. Aripiprazole induced transient myopia: a case report and review of literature. *Cutan Ocul Toxicol.* 2012; 31:74-6.
40. Karadağ H, Acar M, Özdel K. Aripiprazole induced acute transient bilateral myopia: a case report. *Balkan Med J.* 2015; 32:230-2.
41. Abdollahi M, Shafiee A, Bathaiee FS et al. Drug-induced toxic reactions in the eye: an overview. *J Infus Nurs.* 2004; 27:386-98.

42. Negvesky GJ, Kolsky MP, Laureno R et al. Reversible atorvastatin-associated external ophthalmoplegia, antiacetylcholine receptor antibodies, and ataxia. *Arch Ophthalmol.* 2000; 118:427-8.
43. Ertas FS, Ertas NM, Atmaca Y et al. Unrecognized side effect of statin treatment: unilateral blepharoptosis. *Ophthal Plast Reconstr Surg.* 2006; 22:222-4.
44. Lipitor [package insert]. New York: Pfizer Inc; 2007.
45. Cohen V, Jellinek SP, Stansfield L et al. Cardiac arrest with residual blindness after overdose of Tessalon (benzonatate) perles. *J Emerg Med.* 2011; 41:166-71.
46. Avastin [package insert]. South San Francisco: Genentech; 2015.
47. Fraunfelder FW. Ocular side effects associated with dietary supplements and herbal medicines. *Drugs Today (Barc).* 2005; 41:537-45.
48. Fraunfelder FW. Ocular side effects from herbal medicines and nutritional supplements. *Am J Ophthalmol.* 2004; 138:639-47.
49. Fraunfelder FW. Corneal toxicity from topical ocular and systemic medications. *Cornea.* 2006; 25:1133-8.
50. Dubois V, Vickers S. Bilateral inferior oblique palsies following botulinum toxin injections to the frontalis muscle. *J Plast Reconstr Aesthet Surg.* 2006; 59:1122.
51. Kim YJ, Choi KS. Bilateral blindness after filler injection. *Plast Reconstr Surg.* 2013; 131: 298e-299e.
52. Manor RS, Dickerman Z, Llaron Z. Myopia during bromocriptine treatment. *Lancet.* 1981; 1:102.
53. Visser WA, Kolling JB, Groen GJ et al. Persistant corticol blindness after a thoracic epidural test dose of bupivacaine. *Anesthesiology.* 2010; 112:493-5.
54. Kaida T, Ogawa T, Amemiya T. Cataract induced by shortterm administration of large doses of busulfan: a case report. *Ophthalmologica.* 1999; 213:397-9.
55. Socie G, Clift RA, Blaise D et al. Busulfan plus cyclophosphamide compared with total-body irradiation plus cyclophosphamide before marrow transplantation for myeloid leukemia: long-term follow-up of 4 randomized studies. *Blood.* 2001; 98:3569-74.
56. Imperia PS, Lazarus HM, Lass JH. Ocular complications of systemic cancer chemotherapy. *Surv Ophthalmol.* 1989; 34:209-30.
57. Espaillat A, Aiello LP, Arrigg PG et al. Canthaxanthine retinopathy. *Arch Ophthalmol.* 1999; 117:412-3.
58. Remler BF, Leigh RJ, Osorio I et al. The characteristics and mechanisms of visual disturbances associated with anticonvulsant therapy. *Neurology.* 1990; 40:791-6.
59. Verrotti A, Manco R, Matricardi S et al. Antiepileptic drugs and visual function. *Pediatr Neurol.* 2007; 36:353-60.
60. Livingston S, Pauli LL, Berman W. Carbamazepine (Tegretol) in epilepsy: nine year follow-up study with special emphasis on untoward reactions. *Dis Nerv Syst.* 1974; 35:103-7.
61. Shingleton BJ. Ocular toxicity associated with high-dose carmustine. *Arch Ophthalmol.* 1982; 100:1766-72.
62. BiCNU [package insert]. Princeton, NJ: Bristol-Myers Squibb Company; 2007.
63. Coulter DM, Clark DWJ, Savage RL. Celecoxib, rofecoxib, and acute temporary visual impairment. *BMJ.* 2003; 327:1214-5.
64. Coulter DM, Clark DW. Disturbance of vision by COX-2 inhibitors. *Expert Opin Drug Saf.* 2004; 3:607-14.
65. Fraunfelder FT, Fraunfelder FW. Drug-related adverse effects of clinical importance to the ophthalmologist. www.eyedrugregistry.com (accessed 2018 Jan 31).
66. Fraunfelder FW, Solomon J, Mehelas TJ. Ocular adverse effects associated with cyclooxygenase-2 inhibitors. *Arch Ophthalmol.* 2006; 124:277-9.
67. Gehrs KM. Visual disturbance associated with celecoxib—a comment. *Pharmacotherapy.* 2001; 21:1014.
68. Lund BC, Neiman RF. Visual disturbance associated with celecoxib. *Pharmacotherapy.* 2001; 21:114-5.
69. Celebrex [package insert]. New York: Pfizer Inc; 2008.
70. Fraunfelder FT, Fraunfelder FW. Drug-related adverse effects of clinical importance to the ophthalmologist (accessed 2018 Jan 31).
71. Zyrtec [package insert]. New York: Pfizer Inc; 2006.
72. Easterbrook M. Is corneal deposition of antimalarial any indication of retinal toxicity? *Can J Ophthalmol.* 1990; 25:249-51.
73. Easterbrook M. Long-term course of antimalarial maculopathy after cessation of treatment. *Can J Ophthalmol.* 1992; 27:237-9.
74. Easterbrook M. Detection and prevention of maculopathy associated with antimalarial agents. *Int Ophthalmol Clin.* 1999; 39:49-57.
75. Marmor MF, Carr RE, Easterbrook M et al. Recommendations on screening for chloroquine and hydroxychloroquine retinopathy: a report by the American Academy of Ophthalmology. *Ophthalmology.* 2002; 109:1377-82.
76. Rynes RI. Ophthalmologic considerations in using antimalarials in the United States. *Lupus.* 1996;5(suppl 1):S73-74.
77. Chlorpromazine hydrochloride tablets, USP [package insert]. Minneapolis: Upsher-Smith Laboratories Inc; 2003.
78. Cipro [package insert]. West Haven, CT: Bayer Pharmaceuticals Corp; 2007.
79. Clomid [package insert]. Bridgewater, NJ: Sanofi-Aventis US, LLC; 2006.
80. Fraunfelder FT, Meyer SM. Posterior subcapsular cataracts associated with nasal or inhalation corticosteroids. *Am J Ophthalmol.* 1990; 109:489-90.
81. Chun SG, Iyengar P, Gerber DE et al. Optic neuropathy and blindness associated with crizotinib for non–small-cell lung cancer with EML4-ALK translocation. *J Clin Oncol.* 2015; 33:e25-6
82. Avery R, Jabs DA, Wingard JR et al. Optic disc edema after bone marrow transplantation: possible role of cyclosporine toxicity. *Ophthalmology.* 1991; 98:1294-301
83. Sandimmune [package insert]. East Hanover, NJ: Novartis Pharmaceuticals Corp; 2007.
84. Hopen G, Mondino BJ, Johnson BL et al. Corneal toxicity with systemic cytarabine. *Am J Ophthalmol.* 1981; 91:500-4.
85. Lass JH, Lazarus HM, Reed MD. Topical corticosteroid therapy for corneal toxicity from systemically administered cytarabine. *Am J Ophthalmol.* 1982; 94:617-21.
86. Hanuschk D, Kozyreff A, Tafzi N et al. Acute visual loss following dapsone-induced methemoglobinemia and hemolysis. *Clin Toxicol.* 2016; 53:489-92.
87. Baath JS, Lam WC, Kirby M, Chun A. Deferoxamine-related ocular toxicity: incidence and outcome in a pediatric population. *Retina.* 2008; 28:894-9.
88. Lu M, Hansen RM, Cunningham MJ et al. Effects of Desferoxamine on Retinal and Visual Function. *Arch Ophthalmol.* 2007; 125:1581-2.
89. Gelamn R, Kiss S, Tsang SH. Multimodal imaging in case of deferoxamine-induced maculopathy. *Retin Cases Brief Rep.* 2014; 8:306-9.
90. Lutz EG. Allergic conjunctivitis due to diazepam. *Am J Psychiatry.* 1975; 132:548.
91. Tabbara KF. Peripheral corneal infiltrates following oral diclofenac administration. *Arch Ophthalmol.* 2000; 118:1451.
92. Butler VP Jr, Odel JG, Rath E et al. Digitalis-induced visual disturbances with therapeutic serum digitalis concentrations. *Ann Intern Med.* 1995; 123:676-80.
93. Stemmler HJ, Gutschow K, Sommer H et al. Weekly docetaxel (Taxotere) in patients with metastatic breast cancer. *Ann Oncol.* 2001;12:1393-8.
94. Taxotere [package insert]. Bridgewater, NJ: Sanofi-Aventis US, LLC; 2007.
95. Cardura XL [package insert]. New York: Pfizer Inc; 2006.
96. Cymbalta [package insert]. Indianapolis: Eli Lilly and Company; 2007.
97. Goel V, Raina S, Chandragouda D et al. Trichomegaly of eyelashes after treatment with erlotinib in carcinoma pancreas. *Int J Trichology.* 2014; 6:23-4.

98. Celik T, Kosker M. Ocular side effects and trichomegaly of eyelashes induced by erlotinib: a case report and review of the literature. *Cont Lens Anterior Eye*. 2015; 38:59-60.
99. Carser JE, Summers YJ. Trichomegaly of the eyelashes after treatment with erlotinib in non-small cell lung cancer. *J Thorac Oncol.* 2006; 1:1040-1.
100. Fraunfelder FW, Sadun AA, Wood T. Update on ethambutol optic neuropathy. *Expert Opin Drug Saf.* 2006; 5:615-8.
101. Lodine [package insert]. Philadelphia: Wyeth Pharmaceuticals Inc; 2005.
102. Gilenya [package insert]. East Hanover, NJ: Novartis Pharmaceuticals Corporation; 2015.
103. Jain N, Bhatti MT. Fingolimod-associated macular edema: incidence, detection, and management. *Neurology.* 2012; 78:672-80.
104. Gaskin JC, Coote M. Postoperative cystoid macular oedema in a patient on fingolimod. *BMJ Case Rep.* 2015; May 12:2015.
105. Zarbin MA, Jampol LM, Jager RD et al. Ophthalmic evaluations in clinical studies of fingolimod (FTY720) in multiple sclerosis. *Ophthalmology.* 2013; 120:1432-9.
106. Cunningham M, Cunningham K, Lydiard RB. Eye tics and subjective hearing impairment during fluoxetine therapy. *Am J Psychiatry.* 1990; 147:947-8.
107. Prozac [package insert]. Indianapolis: Eli Lilly and Company; 2007.
108. Neurontin [package insert]. New York: Pfizer Inc; 2007.
109. Sheyman A, Wald K, Pahk P et al. Gemcitabine associated retinopathy and nephropathy. *Retin Cases Brief Rep.* 2014; 8: 107-9.
110. Kashkouli MB, Heirati A, Pakdel F et al. Diplopia after hyaluronic acid gel injection for correction of facial tear trough deformity. *Orbit.* 2012; 31:330-1.
111. He MS, Sheu MM, Huang ZL et al. Sudden bilateral vision loss and brain infarction following cosmetic hyaluronic acid injection. *JAMA Ophthamology.* 2013; 131:1234-5.
112. Kim EG, Eom TK, Kang SJ. Severe visual loss and cerebral infarction after injection of hyaluronic acid gel. *J Craniofac Surg.* 2014; 25:684-6.
113. Plaquenil [package insert]. Bridgewater, NJ: SanofiAventis US LLC; 2006.
114. Saeed M, Henderson G, Dutton GN. Hyoscine skin patches for drooling dilate pupils and impair accommodation: spectacle correction for photophobia and blurred vision may be warranted. *Dev Med Child Neurol.* 2007; 49:426-8.
115. Boniva [package insert] Nutley, NJ: Roche Laboratories Inc; 2006.
116. Jain S. Ibuprofen-induced thrombocytopenia. *Br J Clin Pract.* 1994; 48:51.
117. Levy NS. Ibuprofen and visual function. *Arch Ophthalmol.* 1976; 94:86.
118. Nicastro NJ. Visual disturbances associated with over-thecounter ibuprofen in three patients. *Ann Ophthalmol.* 1989; 29:447-50.
119. Tullio CJ. Ibuprofen-induced visual disturbance. *Am J Hosp Pharm.* 1981; 38:1362.
120. Palungwachira P, Palungwachira P, Ogawa H. Localized periorbital edema induced by ibuprofen. *J Dermatol.* 2005; 32:969-71.
121. Fraunfelder FW, Solomon J, Druker BJ et al. Ocular sideeffects associated with imatinib mesylate (Gleevec). *J Ocul Pharmacol Ther.* 2003; 19:371-5.
122. Kusumi E, Arakawa A, Kami M et al. Visual disturbance due to retinal edema as a complication if imatinib. *Leukemia.* 2004; 18:1138-9.
123. Gleevec [package insert]. East Hanover, NJ: Novartis Pharmaceuticals Corp; 2007.
124. Demetri G, von Mehren M, Blanke CD et al. Efficacy and safety of imatinib mesylate in advanced gastrointestinal stromal tumors. *N Engl J Med.* 2002; 347:472-80.
125. Friedman DI, Hu EH, Sadun AA. Neuro-ophthalmic complications of interleukin 2 therapy. *Arch Ophthalmol.* 1991; 109:1679-80.
126. Fraunfelder FT, LaBraico JM, Meyer SM. Adverse ocular reactions possibly associated with isotretinoin. *Am J Ophthalmol.* 1985; 100:534-7.
127. Fraunfelder FW, Fraunfelder FT, Corbett JJ. Isotretinoinassociated intracranial hypertension. *Ophthalmology.* 2004; 111:1248-50.
128. Fraunfelder FW, Fraunfelder FT, Edwards R. Ocular side effects possibly associated with isotretinoin usage. *Am J Ophthalmol.* 2001; 132:299-305.
129. Caffery BE, Josephson JE. Ocular side effects of isotretinoin therapy. *J Am Optom Assoc.* 1988; 9:221-4.
130. Ellies P, Dighiero P, Legeais JM et al. Persistent corneal opacity after oral isotretinoin therapy for acne. *Cornea.* 2006; 19:238-9.
131. Blackman HJ, Peck GL, Olsen TG et al. Blepharoconjunctivitis: a side effect of 13-cis-retinoic acid therapy for dermatologic diseases. *Ophthalmology.* 1979; 86:753-9.
132. Milson J, Jones DH, King K et al. Ophthalmological effects of 13-cis-retinoic acid therapy for acute acne vulgaris. *Br J Dermatol.* 1982; 107:491.
133. Toradol [package insert]. Nutley, NK: Roche Laboratories Inc; 2007.
134. Alkawi A, Kattah JC, Wyman K. Downbeat nystagmus as a result of lamotrigine toxicity. *Epilepsy Res.* 2005; 63:85-8.
135. Hilton EJ, Hosking SL, Betts T. The effect of antiepileptic drugs on visual performance. *Seizure.* 2004; 13:113-28.
136. Azamfirei L, Copotoiu SM, Branzaniuc K et al. Complete blindness after optic neuropathy induced by short-term linezolid treatment in a patient suffering from muscle dystrophy. *Pharmacoepidemiol Drug Saf.* 2007; 16:402-4.
137. Joshi L, Taylor SR, Large O et al. A case of optic neuropathy after short-term linezolid use in a patient with acute lymphocytic leukemia. *Clin Infect Dis.* 2009; 48:e73-4.
138. Schlienger RG, Haefeli WE, Jick H et al. Risk of cataract in patients treated with statins. *Arch Intern Med.* 2001; 161:2021-6.
139. Mevacor [package insert]. Whitehouse Station, NJ: Merck and Company Inc; 2007.
140. Kreshak AA, Clark RF. Transient vision loss in a patient with metformin-associated lactic acidosis. *Am J Emerg Med.* 2010; 28:1059.
141. Paasma R, Hovda KE, Jacobsen D. Methanol poisoning and long term sequelae—a six year follow-up after a large methanol outbreak. *BMC Clin Pharmacol* 2009; 9:1-5.
142. Lu JJ, Kalimullah EA, Bryant SM. Unilateral blindness following acute methanol poisoning. *J Med Toxicol.* 2010; 6:459-60.
143. Sanaei-Zadeh H, Zamani N, Shadnia S. Outcomes of visual disturbances after methanol poisoning. *Clin Toxicol.* 2011; 49:102-7.
144. Koehrer P, Creuzot-Garcher C, Bron AM. Methanol poisoning: two case studies of blindness in Indonesia. *Int Ophthalmol.* 2011; 31:517-24.
145. Sonkar SK, Soni D, Soni DK et al. Drowsy man with breathlessness and blurred vision. methanol toxicity. *Ann Emerg Med.* 2012; 59:255-64.
146. Gee P, Martin E. Toxic cocktail: methanol poisoning in a tourist in Indonesia. *Emerg Med Australas.* 2012; 24:451-3.
147. Fraunfelder FW, Fraunfelder FT, Illingworth DR. Adverse ocular effects associated with niacin therapy. *Br J Ophthalmol.* 1995; 79:54-6.
148. Fahim AT, Khan NW, Johnson MW. Acute panretinal structural and functional abnormalities after intravitreous ocriplasmin injection. *JAMA Ophthalmol.* 2014; 132:484-6.
149. Tibbetts MD, Reichel E, Witkin AJ. Vision Loss After Intravitreal ocriplasmin: correlation of spectral-domain optical coherence tomography and electroretinography. *JAMA Ophthalmol.* 2014; 132:487-90.

150. Kim JE. Safety and complications of ocriplasmin: ocriplasmin, ocriplasmin; oh, how safe art thou? *JAMA Ophthalmol.* 2014; 132:379-80.
151. Thanos A, Hernandez-Siman J, Marra KV, Arroya JG. Reversible vision loss and outer retinal abnormalities after intravitreal ocriplasmin injection. *Retin Cases Brief Repl.* 2014; 8:330-2.
152. Tibbetts MD, Reichel E, Witkin AJ. understanding the adverse effects of ocriplasmin—reply. *JAMA Ophthalmol.* 2015; 133:229-30.
153. Johnson MW, Fahim AT. Understanding the adverse effects of ocriplasmin—reply. *JAMA Ophthalmol.* 2015; 133:230.
154. Beebe DC. Understanding the adverse effects of ocriplasmin. *JAMA Ophthalmol.* 2015; 133:229.
155. Reiss B, Smithen L, Mansour S. Transient vision loss after ocriplasmin injection. *Retina.* 2015; 35:1107-10.
156. Fraunfelder FW, Fraunfelder FT, Jensvold B. Scleritis and other ocular side effects associated with pamidronate disodium. *Am J Ophthalmol.* 2003; 135:219-22.
157. Macarol V, Fraunfelder FT. Pamidronate disodium and possible ocular adverse drug reactions. *Am J Ophthalmol.* 1994; 118:220-24.
158. Paxil CR [package insert]. Research Triangle Park, NC: GlaxoSmithKline; 2008.
159. Lyrica [package insert]. New York: Pfizer Inc; 2007.
160. Marsch SC, Schaefer HG. Problems with eye opening after propofol anesthesia. *Anesth Analg.* 1990; 70:127-8.
161. Risperdal [package insert]. Titusville, NH: Janssen LP; 2008.
162. Colucciello M. Vision loss due to macular edema induced by rosiglitazone treatment of diabetes mellitus. *Arch Ophthamol.* 2005; 123:1273-5.
163. Alao A, Lewokwicz C. Seeing double: sertraline and diplopia: a case report. *Int J Psychiatry Med.* 2015; 49;107-10.
164. Pomeranz HD, Smith KH, Hart WM Jr et al. Sildenafil associated nonarteritic anterior ischemic optic neuropathy. *Ophthalmology.* 2002; 109:584-7.
165. Egan RA, Fraunfelder FW. Viagra and anterior ischemic optic neuropathy. *Arch Ophthalmol.* 2005; 123:709-10.
166. Viagra [package insert]. New York: Pfizer Inc; 2007.
167. Laties AM, Fraunfelder FT. Ocular safety of Viagra (sildenafil citrate). *Trans Am Ophthalmol Soc.* 1999; 97:115-25.
168. Fraunfelder FW, Pomeranz HD, Egan RA. Nonarteritic anterior ischemic optic neuropathy and sildenafil. *Arch Ophthalmol.* 2006;124:733-4.
169. Fraunfelder FW. Visual side effects associated with erectile dysfunction agents. *Am J Ophthalmol.* 2005;723-4.
170. Fraunfelder FW, Shults T. Non-arteritic anterior ischemic optic neuropathy, erectile dysfunction agents, and amiodarone: is there a relationship? *J Neuro-Ophthalmol.* 2006; 26:1-3.
171. Vesicare [package insert]. Research Triangle Park, NC: GlaxoSmithKline; 2008.
172. Peyman, M and Subrayan V. Irreversible blindness following intravenous streptokinase. *JAMA Ophthalmology.* 2013; 131:1368-9.
173. Bovino BA, Marcus DF. The mechanism of transient myopia induced by sulfonamide therapy. *Am J Ophthalmol.* 1982; 84:99-102.
174. Flach AJ. Photosensitivity to sulfisoxazole ointment. *Arch Ophthalmol.* 1981; 99:609-10.
175. Flach AJ. Photosensitivity to topically applied sulfisoxazole ointment: evidence for a phototoxic reaction. *Arch Ophthalmol.* 1982; 100:1286-7.
176. Koh T, Baek SH, Han JI et al. Maculopathy associated with tacrolimus (FK 506). *Korean J Ophthalmol.* 2011; 25:69-71.
177. Escaravage GK Jr, Wright JD Jr, Givre SJ. Tadalafil associated with anterior ischemic optic neuropathy. *Arch Ophthalmol.* 2005; 123:399-400.
178. Cialis [package insert]. Indianapolis: Eli Lilly and Company; 2008.
179. Heier JS, Dragoo RA, Enzenauer RW et al. Screening for ocular toxicity in asymptomatic patients treated with tamoxifen. *Am J Ophthalmol.* 1994; 117:772-5.
180. Pavlidis NA, Petris C, Briassoulis E et al. Clear evidence that long-term, low-dose tamoxifen treatment can induce ocular toxicity: a prospective study of 63 patients. *Cancer.* 1992; 69:2961-4.
181. Noureddin BN, Seoud M, Bashshur Z et al. Ocular toxicity in low-dose tamoxifen: a prospective study. *Eye.* 1999; 13(pt 6):729-33.
182. Flomax [package insert]. Norman, OK: Astellas Pharma Inc; 2007.
183. Hytrin [package insert]. North Chicago, IL: Abbott Laboratories; 1999.
184. Nudleman E, Witmer MT, Kiss S et al. Central serous chorioretinopathy in patients receiving exogenous testosterone therapy. *Retina.* 2014; 34:2128-32.
185. Hadden PW, Tay-Kearney ML, Barry CJ et al. Thioridazine retinopathy. *Clin Experiment Ophthalmol.* 2003; 31:533-44.
186. Marmor MF. Is thioridazine retinopathy progressive? Relationship of pigmentary changes to visual function. *Br J Ophthalmol.* 1990; 74:739-42.
187. Skelid [package insert]. Bridgewater, NJ: Sanofi-Aventis US LLC; 2006.
188. Spiriva [package insert]. Ridgefield, CT: Boehringer Ingelheim Pharmaceuticals Inc; 2014.
189. Oba Y, Zaza T, Thameem DM. Safety, tolerability, and risk benefit analysis of tiotropium in COPD. *Int J Chron Obstruct Pulmon Dis.* 2008; 3:575-84.
190. Fraunfelder FW, Fraunfelder FT, Keates EU. Topiramateassociated acute, bilateral, secondary angle-closure glaucoma. *Ophthalmology.* 2004; 111:109-11.
191. Topamax [package insert]. Titusville, NH: Janssen LP; 2007.
192. Cravens GT, Brown MJ, Brown DR et al. Antifibrinolytic therapy use to mitigate blood loss during staged complex major spine surgery: postoperative visual color changes after tranexamic acid administration. *Anesthesiology.* 2006; 105:1274-6.
193. Saleh M, Bourcier T, Noel G et al. Bilateral macular ischemia and severe visual loss following trastuzumab therapy. *Acta Oncologica* 2011; 50:477-8.
194. Tilz C, Wang-Tils Y, Junemann A. Visual field defect during therapy with valproic-acid. *Eur J Neurol.* 2007; 14:929-32.
195. Levitra [package insert]. West Haven, CT: Bayer Healthcare; 2007.
196. Porst H, Rosen R, Padma-Nathan H et al. The efficacy and tolerability of vardenafil, a new, oral, selective phosphodiesterase type 5 inhibitor, in patients with erectile dysfunction: the first at-home clinical trial. *Int J Impot Res.* 2001; 13:192-9.
197. Effexor [package insert]. Philadelphia: Wyeth Pharmaceuticals Inc; 2008.
198. Ng B, Sanbrook GM, Malouf AJ et al. Venlafaxine and bilateral acute angle closure glaucoma. *Med J Aust.* 2002; 176:241.
199. Daneshvar H, Racette L, Coupland SG et al. Symptomatic and asymptomatic visual loss in patients taking vigabatrin. *Ophthalmology.* 1999; 106:1792-8.
200. Wilton LV, Stephens MDB, Mann RD. Visual field defect associated with vigabatrin: observational cohort study. *BMJ.* 1999; 319:1165.
201. Coleman D. [Letter]. New York: Pfizer Global Pharmaceuticals; 2008.
202. Zonios DI, Gea-Banacloche J, Childs R et al. Hallucinations during voriconazole therapy. *Clin Infect Dis.* 2008; 47:e7-10.
203. Zometa [package insert]. East Hanover, NJ: Novartis Pharmaceuticals Corp; 2007.
204. Weiler DL. Zonisamide-induced angle closure and myopic shift. *Optom Vis Sci.* 2015; 92:e4651.
205. Armalay MF. Statistical attributes of the steroid hypertensive response in the clinically normal eye. *Invest Ophthalmol.* 1965; 4:187.
206. Becker B, Ballin N. Glaucoma and corticosteroid provocative testing. *Arch Ophthalmol.* 1965; 74:621.

207. Lewis JM, Priddy T, Judd J et al. Intraocular pressure response to dexamethasone as a predictor for the development of primary open-angle glaucoma. *Am J Ophthalmol.* 1988; 106:607-12.

208. Hollander DA, Aldave AJ. Drug-induced corneal complications. *Curr Opin Ophthalmol.* 2004; 15:541-8.

209. Fraunfelder FW. Ocular and systemic side effects of drugs. In: Riordan-Eva P, Whitcher JP, eds. *Vaughan and Asbury's general ophthalmology*. New York: The McGraw Hill Companies; 2008.

210. Tripathi RC, Parapuram SK, Tripathi BJ et al. Corticosteroids and glaucoma risk. *Drugs Aging.* 1999; 15:439-50.

211. D'Amico DJ, Kenyon KR, Ruskin JN. Amiodarone keratopathy: drug-induced lipid storage disease. *Arch Ophthalmol.* 1981; 99:257-61.

212. Wentz-Hunter K, Xiang S, Kazushiro O et al. Overexpression of myocilin in cultured human trabecular meshwork cells. *Exp Cell Res.* 2004; 297:39-48.

213. Kersey JP, Broadway DC. Corticosteroid-induced glaucoma: a review of the literature. *Eye.* 2006; 20:407-16.

214. Plaa GL. Acute toxicity of antiepileptic drugs. *Epilepsia.* 1975; 16:183-91.

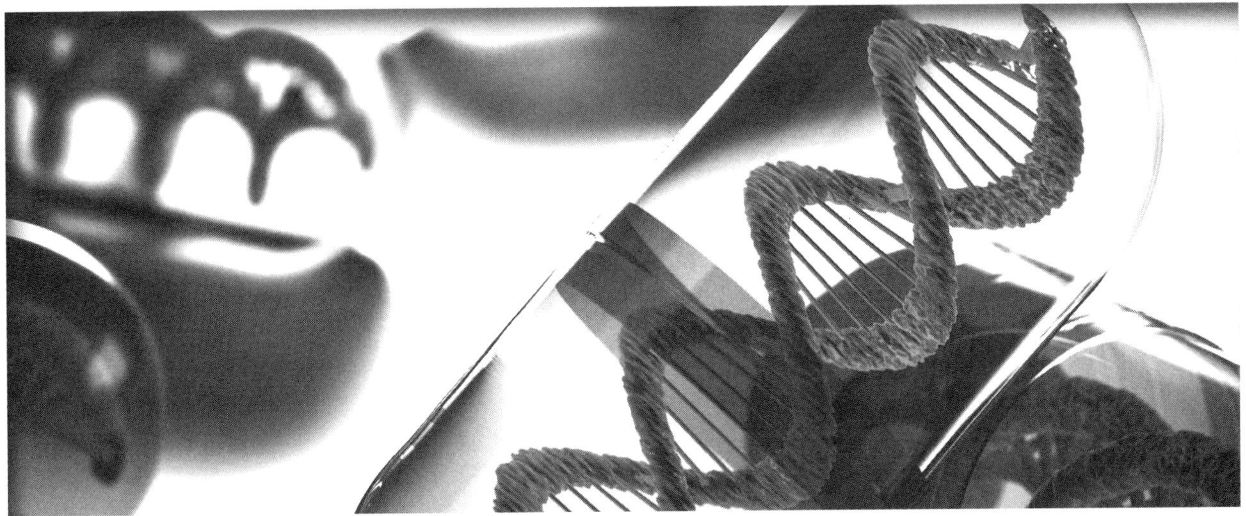

CHAPTER 15

Delirium

Matthew A. Fuller

Delirium is a common and sometimes fatal disorder characterized by disturbance of consciousness and change in cognition that develops over a short period of time.[1] Delirium may have numerous etiologies, including drugs.

CAUSATIVE AGENTS

Drug-induced delirium may be caused by a wide array of drugs; however, there are a few agents that are consistently associated with the development of the disorder.[2-6] These include high-risk drugs that possess anticholinergic properties, such as low potency antipsychotics, tricyclic antidepressants, older antihistamines, sedative hypnotics, corticosteroids, and narcotics (**Table 15-1**).[7-100]

Other drugs vary in their propensity to cause delirium. For instance, exposure to opioids has been shown to increase the risk of delirium in patients with cancer; however, effectively treating pain with opioids in postoperative patients may actually reduce the risk of developing delirium.[17,101,102] The incidence of postoperative delirium approaches 50%.

In a meta-analysis, the association between psychoactive medications and the development of delirium in hospitalized patients was assessed.[103] This meta-analysis reviewed 28 studies that included several classes of psychoactive medications such as antiparkinsons, anticonvulsants, anticholinergics, antiemetics, antidepressants, antipsychotics, benzodiazepines, corticosteroids, histamine-type H_2 antagonists, nonsteroidal anti-inflammatory drugs, and opioid analgesics. Only psychoactive medications (grouped together) were found to be associated with the development of delirium. No individual medication was significantly associated with delirium.

EPIDEMIOLOGY

Delirium is very common and has been reported in 14–24% of patients at hospital admission, up to 56% of hospitalized patients, as many as 60%

Table 15-1 Agents Implicated in Drug-Induced Delirium

Drug	Incidence	Level of Evidence[a]
ANTIPSYCHOTICS		
Clozapine[7]	10.1%	B
Fluphenazine[13]	NK	C
Haloperidol[12]	NK	C
Loxapine[16]	NK	C
Olanzapine[11,96]	1.4%	B
Perphenazine[14]	NK	C
Quetiapine[9]	NK	C
Risperidone[10]	NK	C
Thioridazine[15]	NK	C
Ziprasidone[8]	NK	C
OPIOIDS[27]		
Fentanyl[18,19]	NK	B
Meperidine[19,95]	RR 2.4, 95% CI 1.3–4.4	B
Morphine[17,19]	NK	B
CORTICOSTEROIDS		
Prednisone[20,21,27,97]	13%	C
ANTIARRHYTHMICS		
Amiodarone[25]	NK	C
Lidocaine[23]	NK	C
Quinidine[26]	NK	C
Tocainide[24]	NK	C
DIGOXIN[26,27]	NK	B
ALCOHOL WITHDRAWAL[22]	NK	B
ANTIASTHMATICS		
Theophylline	NK	C
ANTICONVULSANTS		
Phenytoin[28]	NK	C
Acetazolamide[29]	NK	C
Lamotrigine[30]	NK	C
Pregabalin[31]	NK	C
Tiagabine[32]	NK	C
Valproic acid[33,57]	4.1/100 person-years	B
ANTIDEPRESSANTS		
Tricyclics		
Protriptyline[34]	NK	C
Desipramine[35,36]	NK	B
Clomipramine[37]	NK	C
Amitriptyline[14,38]	NK	C
Imipramine[39]	NK	C
Doxepin[40]	NK	C
Selective Serotonin Reuptake Inhibitors		
Fluoxetine[34,41]	NK	C

Table 15-1 Agents Implicated in Drug-Induced Delirium (continued)

Drug	Incidence	Level of Evidence[a]
Paroxetine[42]	NK	C
Sertraline[12]	NK	C
Miscellaneous		
Bupropion[43]	NK	C
Venlafaxine[44]	NK	C
Mirtazapine[45]	NK	C
Monoamine Oxidase Inhibitors		
Phenelzine[47]	NK	C
Tranylcypromine[46]	NK	C
DOPAMINERGIC AGENTS		
Amantadine[48]	NK	C
Levodopa[49]	NK	C
Bromocriptine[50]	NK	C
BENZODIAZEPINES[95]	OR 3, 95% CI 1.3–6.8	B
Lorazepam[51]	NK	C
Diazepam[52]	NK	C
Clonazepam[53]	NK	C
Alprazolam[54]	NK	C
Triazolam[55]	NK	C
Clorazepate[56]	NK	C
LITHIUM[16,57]	2.8/100 person-years	B
NSAIDs		
Diclofenac[58]	NK	C
Ibuprofen[59]	NK	C
Ketoprofen[60]	NK	C
Sulindac[61]	NK	C
Indomethacin[62]	NK	C
Salicylic acid[63]	NK	C
COX-II INHIBITORS		
Celecoxib[64]	NK	C
ACE INHIBITORS[65]		
Enalapril	NK	C
Captopril	NK	C
MISCELLANEOUS ANTIHYPERTENSIVES[65]		
Reserpine	NK	C
Clonidine	NK	C
Methyldopa	NK	C
CALCIUM CHANNEL BLOCKERS		
Nifedipine[67]	NK	C
Verapamil[66]	NK	C
BETA BLOCKERS		
Atenolol[69]	NK	C
Metoprolol[70]	NK	C

Table 15-1 Agents Implicated in Drug-Induced Delirium (continued)

Drug	Incidence	Level of Evidence[a]
Propranolol[13,68]	NK	C
ANTIMICROBIALS		
Aminoglycosides		
Tobramycin[71]	NK	C
Macrolides		
Azithromycin[72]	NK	C
Clarithromycin[73]	NK	C
Cephalosporins		
Cephalexin[74]	NK	C
Cephalothin[75]	NK	C
Cefazolin[76]	NK	C
Penicillins		
Piperacillin–tazobactam[77]	NK	C
Fluoroquinolones[98]		
Ciprofloxacin[78]	NK	C
Gatifloxacin[79]	NK	C
Ofloxacin[80]	NK	C
Levofloxacin[81]	NK	C
Miscellaneous		
Chloramphenicol[82]	NK	C
Trimethoprim–sulfamethoxazole[83]	NK	C
Linezolid[84]	NK	C
Ertapenem[99]	3.3–5.1%	C
HISTAMINE-H_2 ANTAGONISTS		
Cimetidine[85]	NK	C
Ranitidine[86]	NK	C
Nizatidine[87]	NK	C
Famotidine[88]	NK	C
ANTICHOLINERGICS[89,100]		
Atropine[90]	NK	C
Benztropine[12,13,91]	NK	C
Diphenhydramine[84,94]	OR 2.3, 95% CI 1.4–3.6	B
Scopolamine[92]	NK	C
Tolterodine[93]	NK	C

ACE = angiotensin-converting enzyme, CI = confidence interval, COX = cyclo-oxygenase, NK = not known, NSAID = nonsteroidal anti-inflammatory drug, OR = odds ratio, RR = relative risk.

[a]Definitions for Levels of Evidence: Level A—evidence from one or more randomized, controlled clinical trials; Level B—evidence from nonrandomized clinical trials, prospective observational studies, cohort studies, retrospective studies, case-control studies, meta-analyses and/or postmarketing surveillance studies; and Level C—evidence from one or more published case reports or case series.

of individuals in nursing homes, and up to 88% of those in palliative care.[104-106] Most patients have multiple etiologies rather than a single cause of delirium, especially if they are burdened with medical problems or are elderly.

Although the majority of cases are believed to be multifactorial, medications, particularly when patients are taking multiple drugs (polypharmacy), have been cited as the single cause of delirium in 12–39% of cases.[4] Aside from drug causes, other frequently identified etiologies of delirium include sensory and environmental issues (poor vision and hearing), infection, and fluid and electrolyte disturbances.[107]

MECHANISMS

There is a paucity of data describing mechanisms of drug-induced delirium. Some mechanisms have been determined through electrophysiological and biochemical studies and brain scans (**Table 15-2**).[108] The presence of anatomical lesions may lead to development of delirium; symptoms are related to the location of the lesion.

Acetylcholine has been implicated as the major neurotransmitter involved in the development of delirium. Despite various locations of lesions or other neurochemical changes, acetylcholine appears to be the final common pathway involved.[109] This is consistent with the acetylcholine hypothesis of cognitive impairment in neurocognitive disorders such as those due to Alzheimer disease. Elderly patients develop an age-related decrease in acetylcholine reserve, making them more vulnerable to acute changes in plasma acetylcholine concentrations. Further support for this theory is the relationship between the administration of anticholinergic drugs and cognitive deficits, particularly a reduction in the ability to focus or maintain attention and short-term memory deficits. Tune and Egeli[109] studied 88 patients meeting criteria for delirium (n = 47) or dementia (n = 41) and found that those with delirium were taking a significantly larger number of anticholinergic medications than those with dementia. It is unlikely that acetylcholine is the sole neurotransmitter involved in the development of delirium, given its interaction with dopamine transmission.[110] Dopamine exerts an inhibitory effect on the release of acetylcholine.

Table 15-2 Mechanisms of Drug-Induced Delirium

Drug(s)	Mechanism
Amitriptyline Atropine Benztropine Clomipramine Clozapine Desipramine Doxepin Imipramine Olanzapine Protriptyline Quetiapine Scopolamine Thioridazine Tolterodine	Decreased acetylcholine function
Amantadine Levodopa Bromocriptine	Excess dopamine function
Prednisone	Excess glucocorticoid activity
Alprazolam Clonazepam Clorazepate Diazepam Lorazepam Triazolam	Decreased GABA concentration
Fluoxetine Paroxetine Sertraline	Serotonin dysfunction

GABA = gamma-aminobutyric acid.

Glucocorticoid excess also has been implicated in the development of delirium.[111] Preclinical and clinical data support the hypothesis that increases in plasma glucocorticoid concentrations associated with various disorders, including depression, dementia, and Cushing syndrome, lead to cognitive impairment. Even modest increases in plasma glucocorticoid concentrations over a period of 5–6 years have led to reduced hippocampus-dependent memory and hippocampus volumes. There also may be a diminishment in the hypothalamic-pituitary-adrenal axis negative feedback loop in response to elevated plasma glucocorticoid concentrations as well as an increased sensitivity to adrenocorticotrophic hormone stimulation.

Other possible neurotransmitters involved in the pathogenesis of delirium include gamma-aminobutyric acid (GABA), glutamate, β-endorphins, and serotonin.[112] Cerebrospinal fluid sampling in elderly patients with delirium revealed diminished somatostatin-like and β-endorphin-like immunoreactivity. Therefore, although acetylcholine most commonly has been implicated in the development of delirium, the complete pathogenesis remains unknown but is likely multifactorial. A detailed review of the neuropathogenesis of delirium has been published.[113]

CLINICAL PRESENTATION AND DIFFERENTIAL DIAGNOSIS

The Diagnostic and Statistical Manual of Mental Disorders, Fifth Edition (DSM-5), characterizes delirium as a disturbance in attention, awareness, and cognition that develops over a brief period of time.[1] Symptoms of drug-induced delirium do not differ from those associated with delirium from other causes (**Table 15-3**).[1,2,5] There may be a prodromal syndrome of anxiety, changes in sleep patterns, disorientation, irritability, and restlessness 1–3 days prior to the full onset of delirium. Following the prodromal syndrome, patients develop disturbances of consciousness, cognition, psychomotor function, and, in some cases, sleep patterns. These disturbances develop over a short period of time (hours to days), and the symptoms fluctuate throughout the course of the day, making recognition of the disorder difficult.[5,104] Patients may be easily distracted and have a decreased awareness of their environment. Cognitive deficits such as disorientation to place and time, dysarthria, and loss of recent memory are common. Some patients develop perceptual disturbances such as delusions, illusions, or hallucinations. Psychomotor activity may present as hyperactive, hypoactive, or mixed types. Hyperactivity is characterized by agitation, restlessness, and emotional lability. Hypoactivity is characterized by withdrawal, flat affect, lethargy, and diminished responsiveness. Hypoactivity occurs more frequently than hyperactivity, and is unrecognized in as many as 66–84% of hospitalized patients.[114] In a study of patients in an intensive care unit (ICU), 1.6%, 43.5%, and 54.1% of patients were diagnosed with hyperactive, hypoactive, and mixed delirium, respectively.[114] Patients with mixed psychomotor symptoms fluctuate between hypoactive and hyperactive symptoms throughout the day. The sleep-wake cycle is often disrupted, and patients may experience insomnia, daytime drowsiness, or a complete reversal of the sleep cycle. Emotional disturbances such as anxiety, depression, fear, anger, irritability, aggression, or euphoria occur commonly.

Table 15-3 Signs and Symptoms Associated with Drug-Induced Delirium

- Autonomic activation (dilated pupils, dry mouth, flushing, sweating, tachycardia)
- Coma
- Decreased ability to sustain or focus attention
- Disorientation to time or place
- Dysarthria
- Dysgraphia
- Dysnomia
- Easily distracted
- Electroencephalogram abnormalities (generalized theta or delta slow-wave activity)
- Emotional disturbances (anger, anxiety, fear, euphoria, apathy, depression)
- Emotional lability
- Hallucinations
- Hyperactivity (picking at things, trying to get out of bed)
- Illusions
- Memory deficit (recent memory)
- Misinterpretations/misperceptions
- Neurologic abnormalities (unsteady gait and tremor)
- Rambling, pressured, or incoherent speech
- Restlessness
- Sleep disturbances
- Sluggishness or lethargy
- Stupor

The incidence of delirium is very high in certain populations, including older postoperative patients (15–53%), those in an ICU (70–87%) or nursing home (60%), and patients at the end of life (up to 83%).[104] Geriatric, oncologic, pediatric, and psychiatric patients are also at significant risk for developing delirium.[103,108]

Any evaluation of a patient for drug-induced delirium must include a careful and thorough medication history. One must assess patients' use of herbal products, complementary medicines, nonprescription medications, and drugs of abuse, as they have been implicated in provoking delirium. Furthermore, a social history that includes alcohol or illicit drug use should alert the clinician to the potential for delirium, which may occur in association with drug or alcohol withdrawal.[2,115] In the majority of cases, a multitude of etiologies exists, including drugs, and all possibilities must be considered.

The diagnosis of drug-induced delirium is purely clinical, as there are no laboratory tests that can definitively diagnose the disorder. Along with the medical history and clinical observation, the use of rating scales may assist in confirming the diagnosis. In just a few minutes, clinicians can complete a simple screening tool for delirium, the confusion assessment method (CAM), which has been adapted to other settings, such as the ICU (CAM-ICU).[116,117] The mini-mental state examination (MMSE) may also be used to screen patients for delirium. Other scales, such as the delirium rating scale (DRS) and the memorial delirium assessment scale (MDAS), are used to monitor symptoms over time.[118,119] Differentiating delirium from other disorders may be difficult as symptoms may overlap considerably. Delirium is frequently underdiagnosed. Studies report that delirium occurring in patients on general medical units is not diagnosed in 32–67% of cases.[120] It may also be difficult to distinguish drug-induced delirium from that occurring as a result of other etiologies. Conditions to consider in the differential diagnosis of drug-induced delirium are listed in **Table 15-4**.

Patients with drug-induced delirium usually develop symptoms during intoxication, over an extended period of time with continuous drug use, or during drug or alcohol withdrawal. Delirium during acute intoxication presents within minutes to hours after ingestion of the substance (e.g., cocaine, hallucinogens).[121] The potential for delirium is increased if additional agents with anticholinergic activity also are ingested. A drug-induced delirium also may develop secondary to the accumulation of a drug or its metabolite over an extended period of time (e.g., barbiturates, alcohol) or as a result of a combination of a suspect medication and a pre-existing medical condition.[1,122] Withdrawal delirium may last a few hours to several weeks, depending on the half-life of the causative agent. This type of delirium results from lower tissue and body fluid concentrations than those to which the body has become accustomed.

Table 15-4 Conditions to Consider in the Differential Diagnosis of Drug-Induced Delirium

- Dehydration
- Delirium not caused by drugs
- Dementia
- Depression
- Drug/alcohol use or withdrawal
- Fever
- Heart failure
- Hepatic insufficiency
- Hypercalcemia
- Hypo-, hypernatremia
- Hypoglycemia
- Hypoxia
- Infection
- Intoxication
- Kidney disease
- Mania
- Metabolic disturbances
- Shock
- Uremia

Withdrawal delirium may also be precipitated by a drug interaction, lowering the dose of a medication, or increased drug clearance such as that which may occur during dialysis or due to changes in kidney or liver function.[123]

Although most underlying causes of delirium often can be easily ruled out, dementia is often confused with delirium.[1,5,122] Memory impairment is common to both delirium and dementia; however, delirium is associated with impairment in consciousness during which patients are not alert or oriented to time or place. In addition, symptoms that develop rapidly and fluctuate throughout the day are more consistent with delirium than dementia. Differentiation between the two disorders is important and may require a more complete history from family or caregivers (**Table 15-5**).[124]

RISK FACTORS

Specific risk factors for delirium have been identified (**Table 15-6**). It is unknown if the risk factors for drug-induced delirium are different from those for delirium secondary to other causes.

Table 15-5 Clinical Features That Distinguish Delirium and Dementia[124]

Clinical Feature	Delirium	Dementia
Onset	Sudden	Insidious
Course	Fluctuating	Stable
Attention	Disordered	Normal
Cognition	Disordered	Impaired
Consciousness	Reduced	Clear
Delusions	Fleeting	Usually absent
Hallucinations	Usually visual	Usually absent
Involuntary movements	Asterixis or course tremor	Usually absent
Orientation	Usually impaired	Often impaired
Physical illness or drug toxicity	Present	Often present
Psychomotor activity	Altered	Normal
Speech	Often incoherent	Word finding difficulty and perseveration

Table 15-6 Risk Factors for Drug-Induced Delirium

- Acid–base imbalance
- Advanced age
- Anemia
- Cardiac arrhythmias
- Concomitant alcohol use
- Concomitant use of multiple drugs that may cause delirium
- Heart failure
- Dementia
- Depression
- Fever
- Fluid/electrolyte abnormality
- Head trauma
- Hepatic insufficiency
- Hypoalbuminemia
- Hypoglycemia
- Hypoxia
- Impaired physical function
- Infection
- Kidney disease
- Myocardial infarction
- Neoplasm
- Pain
- Parkinson disease
- Poor nutrition
- Respiratory failure
- Seizure disorder
- Sensory deprivation
- Severe illness
- Shock
- Sleep deprivation

A decrease in the metabolism or elimination of psychoactive drugs is a risk factor for drug-induced delirium. In some patients, diminished metabolism may be linked to drug interactions, heart failure, hepatic insufficiency, and/or kidney disease. The anticholinergic effects of psychoactive compounds may contribute to delirium via increased neuronal excitability and rate of neuronal adenosine triphosphate consumption, release of dopamine and glutamate, and stimulation of the sympathetic nervous system. Postoperative pain is also a risk factor for delirium (moderate pain: OR 2.2, 95% CI 1.2–4; severe pain: OR 3.7, 95% CI 1.5–9).[102]

A number of medical conditions are recognized as potential risk factors for the development of delirium and may also increase the risk of drug-induced delirium. Diagnoses of dementia or cognitive impairment have been identified as risk factors for delirium.[5,125] Disorders that affect neuronal functioning may cause delirium, including cerebral infarction, seizures, head trauma, vascular disease, Parkinson disease, and dementia.[2,5,125] Various metabolic abnormalities may contribute to the development of delirium, including electrolyte disturbances, kidney disease, hepatic insufficiency, edema from heart failure, thiamine deficiency, and acid-base imbalance.[2,121] Conditions that lead to changes in the delivery of oxygen or nutrients to the central nervous system also may predispose patients to delirium, such as myocardial infarction, cardiac arrhythmias, heart failure, respiratory failure, chronic obstructive pulmonary disease, anemia, hypoxia, or shock. Recently, alcohol abuse, hypertension, and higher APACHE (Acute Physiology and Chronic Health Evaluation) II scores have been identified as risk factors for delirium.[126]

Infection and fever also increase the risk of delirium. Hyperthermia causes a central release of norepinephrine, glutamate, and dopamine, which may predispose the patient to delirium.[121] Patients with human immune deficiency virus (HIV) infection may develop delirium caused by viral infection of neuronal tissue, opportunistic infection of the central nervous system, or metabolic encephalopathy.[127,128] Antibiotics, antivirals, or antifungal agents may be involved in drug interactions contributing to delirium.

Cancer increases the risk of delirium possibly due to associated liver or kidney disease, prerenal azotemia, hyperosmolality, dehydration, medications (e.g., opioids), hypoxia, disseminated intravascular coagulation, recent surgery, metastasis to the brain or other areas of the central nervous system, and infection.[129,130] In addition, patients undergoing treatment for cancer are often undergoing therapy with complex medication regimens associated with drug interactions that increase the potential for delirium.

The increased risk of delirium in postoperative patients appears to be linked to common occurrences such as infection, hypoxia, myocardial ischemia, metabolic derangement, decreased mobility, and exposure to anticholinergic drugs.[123,131] The increased risk in this population does not correlate with the number of previous surgeries, the duration of the surgical procedure, the type of anesthesia used, or the surgical technique employed.

Conditions of deprivation, including both sleep and sensory deprivation (hearing loss, visual impairment, and immobility), such as that which occurs in an ICU, have been found to be risk factors for delirium.[132] An interventional study of patients with deprivation-associated delirium found that nonpharmacologic interventions such as providing a relaxing night-time environment, hearing aids, glasses or magnifying glasses, large print materials, other forms of communication, and exercise may lower the incidence of delirium.[133] Benzodiazepine use may also be a risk factor for the development of delirium in adult ICU patients.[117]

Advanced age is considered to be a risk factor for delirium, because elderly patients are more likely to have multiple predisposing risk factors.[1,3,110,121-123,132,134] Physiologic changes in the elderly may alter drug transport across the blood-brain barrier making them more vulnerable to central nervous system effects. The presence of at least one copy of the apolipoprotein e4 allele on chromosome 19 increased the risk of postoperative delirium in elderly patients (OR 3.64, 95% CI 1.51–8.77).[133] The National Institute for Health and Care Excellence (NICE) reported that the greatest risk for delirium was associated with chronic cognitive decline or dementia (OR 6.30, 95% CI 2.89–3.74) and aortic aneurysm surgery (OR 8.3, 95% CI 3.6–19.4).[135] In addition, there may be age-related changes in metabolism or elimination that lead to drug accumulation in the elderly.[115] As patients age, the number of concomitant medical conditions and medications generally increases. These factors, along with the potential for increased sensitivity to some psychoactive medications, may contribute to the increased incidence of drug-induced delirium in this age group.

MORBIDITY AND MORTALITY

Few data are available regarding morbidity and mortality specifically associated with drug-induced delirium. However, delirium in general is associated with higher rates of long-term care placement and increased mortality rates.[132] Medical complications such as immobility, skin breakdown, falls, and aspiration pneumonia occur more commonly in patients with delirium.[5,136] These additional medical problems lead to prolonged duration of hospitalization, an increased rate of functional decline necessitating institutionalization, and increased mortality.[5,132,137-142] Drug-induced delirium is an unfortunate event that leads to increased healthcare costs that are almost completely avoidable.[132]

In the months to years after a delirium episode, patients are at risk for delayed recovery and poor functional status.[114,143] Of 126 patients who were diagnosed with delirium in one study, 64% reported the same number of delirium symptoms 1 week later, and 12% had a larger number of symptoms.[143] Patients with persistent delirium had lower activities of daily living scores than those who did not develop delirium. Another study of 77 elderly patients on medical, surgical, and geriatric hospital units indicated that frailty (OR 2, 95% CI 1.2–3.5) and poor recognition of delirium (OR 18.2, 95% CI 2.2–153.2) were associated with an increased risk of poor outcome including functional decline or death.[144]

Other serious outcomes of delirium include persistent or worsening cognitive function and an increased risk of developing dementia.[114] Rockwood and colleagues examined the risk of dementia and death over a 3-year period in previously hospitalized patients over the age of 65 years.[138] After adjusting for age, sex, and comorbid illnesses, there was an increased risk of dementia after an episode of delirium (OR 5.97, 95% CI 1.83–19.54). Delirium was also associated with an increased risk of death (OR 1.71, 95% CI 1.02–1.87). Kelly and colleagues reported that 18% of elderly nursing home residents who were hospitalized for acute medical illness and developed delirium died during their inpatient stay.[142] Of those who were discharged, an additional 18.4% died within 1 month, and another 13.3% died within 3 months. The cumulative mortality in this study was 46.6% at 3 months after hospital discharge.

In a prospective cohort study of 243 patients with delirium and 118 controls, delirium was associated with a twofold increase in mortality during a 12-month period following hospitalization (HR 2.11, 95% CI 1.18–3.77).[145] The 1-year mortality rate associated with delirium is 40–63%.[108,145] It is likely that similar outcomes could be expected in patients with drug-induced delirium.

Delirium was associated with an increased risk of in-hospital mortality (OR 1.49, 95% CI 1.08–2.08) in 11,079 patients hospitalized in a referral coronary care unit. In addition, the 1-year mortality among patients with delirium who survived to be discharged from the coronary care unit was also increased (HR 1.46, 95% CI 1.12–1.87).[146]

Delirium has been reported to be responsible for 49% of all hospital days for elderly patients and accounts for an estimated $38–152 billion in annual healthcare expenditures.[110,147] Daily costs were 2.5 times higher in delirium survivors compared to those who did not develop delirium ($461 ± $570 versus $166 ± $570, p <0.001). Prolonged hospital stays account for a portion of these costs, but expenses are compounded by the need for rehabilitation, long-term care, and home healthcare.[132,147]

PREVENTION

There are few studies regarding primary prevention of drug-induced delirium.[132,148] However, methods of prevention of delirium in general may also be effective for prevention of drug-induced delirium (**Table 15-7**). A prospective, controlled trial was conducted in which standardized protocols were implemented for managing specific risk factors for delirium, such as cognitive impairment, sleep deprivation, immobility, visual and hearing impairments, and dehydration in a group of hospitalized patients.[132] Risk factor management in the treatment group reduced the incidence of delirium compared to that in the control (usual care) group (9.9% versus 15%, p = 0.02). Risk factor management was also associated with significantly fewer days of delirium and a smaller number of delirium episodes. Those in the risk factor management group that were most adherent to the prevention protocol carried a significantly lower risk of delirium (adjusted OR 0.69, 95% CI 0.56–0.87).[149] These techniques for the prevention of delirium may also be applied to those at risk for the development of drug-induced delirium.

Table 15-7 Approaches to Help Prevent Drug-Induced Delirium

- Avoid anticholinergic, sedative/hypnotic, and opioid medications in the elderly
- Obtain a careful medication history and perform periodic reviews of all drug therapy
- Perform a brief mental status exam on acutely ill patients at admission to assist in the detection of drug-induced delirium
- Avoid medications known to cause drug-induced delirium

Antipsychotic agents have been used to prevent delirium in postoperative patients. Some studies found a decreased incidence of delirium associated with prophylactic antipsychotic administration while others did not.[150-156] Given the conflicting evidence, the use of prophylactic antipsychotic therapy to prevent delirium cannot be recommended.[157] The prophylactic use of acetylcholinesterase inhibitors has also been studied in postoperative delirium patients, but this practice was found to be ineffective in preventing delirium and cannot be recommended.[158-161]

Melatonin has been evaluated for the prevention of postoperative delirium.[162-164] Hanania and Kitain reported the first successful use of melatonin in a nondemented patient with a history of postsurgical delirium.[162] Sultan evaluated the incidence of delirium in a randomized controlled trial in 222 patients receiving hip arthroplasty. Melatonin 5 mg was administered at bedtime on the night before surgery, and another 5 mg was given 90 minutes prior to surgery. Melatonin prophylaxis was associated with a lower risk of delirium (10%) compared to that in the control group (33%).[163] Al-Aama and colleagues evaluated the use of low-dose melatonin in a randomized, double-blind, placebo-controlled trial of 145 patients. Patients received melatonin 0.5 mg or placebo at bedtime for 14 days or until discharge. Patients receiving melatonin had a lower risk of delirium (12% versus 31%, $p = 0.014$).[164]

Ramelteon, a synthetic analog of melatonin and a melatonin (MT)1 and MT2 receptor agonist, has also been evaluated for the prevention of delirium.[165] Hatta and colleagues conducted a multicenter trial in 67 elderly hospitalized patients who were randomized to receive ramelteon 8 mg or placebo at bedtime for 7 days. Ramelteon was associated with a lower risk of delirium (3%) compared to placebo (32%).[165]

Nursing staff on an orthopedic unit were educated regarding the appropriate use of pharmacological and nonpharmacological interventions to prevent and treat delirium.[166] Suggestions regarding medication use included avoiding or minimizing the use of routine anticholinergics to prevent/treat nausea, prescribing morphine in the lowest doses for the shortest possible duration after surgery, and using antipsychotic agents for management of psychotic symptoms of delirium. Medication use was evaluated in the 6 months prior to and after the education session. There was a significant decrease in the use of anticholinergic medications, but the use of opioids and antipsychotics did not change significantly. Data regarding the rates of delirium were incomplete. Effective treatment of pain with opioids led to a reduced risk of development of delirium (OR 0.4, 95% CI 0.2–0.7).[102]

A large randomized controlled trial of a computerized system to identify medications that may contribute to delirium risk and trigger a pharmacist review of patients' medication regimen reported a decrease in delirium incidence (12-month HR 0.42, 95% CI 0.34–0.51) but no significant reduction in falls, hospital admission rate, or mortality.[167]

Because delirium is likely the result of multiple issues, including drugs, management of non-drug risk factors is important for the prevention of drug-induced delirium. Wherever possible, anticholinergic, hypnotic/sedative, and opioid medications should be avoided in elderly patients.[6] A careful medication history should be obtained from patients at risk and periodic reviews of all drug therapy should be performed. All elderly patients who present with an acute illness should be screened for the presence of drug-induced delirium.

MANAGEMENT

Principles of management of drug-induced delirium are presented in **Table 15-8**. Management of drug-induced delirium requires that clinicians recognize the presence of delirium and consider that it may be caused by drugs.[5,6] This can be extremely difficult, particularly in intubated patients in the ICU or those with underlying dementia.[168,169] The most critical step in the diagnosis is a careful medication history. Clinicians must carefully consider any new medications, including nonprescription and herbal and complementary medicines that the patient is taking, and the time to onset of signs and symptoms. Other steps in diagnosis include a physical examination and a toxicology screen, which may help in identifying the drug(s) involved. Determination of serum concentrations

Table 15-8 Management of Drug-Induced Delirium

- Identify the causative agent
    - Medication history
    - Physical examination
    - Plasma concentrations
    - Toxicology screen
- Discontinue or reduce the dose of the causative agent; substitute with another drug that does not cause delirium if possible
- Identify and eliminate any other contributors of the drug-induced delirium
- Use a specific antidote (e.g. flumazenil, naloxone) if available
- Use nonpharmacological methods
    - Provide support and orientation
    - Provide an unambiguous environment
    - Maintain competency
- Use drug therapy
    - Atypical antipsychotics
    - Benzodiazepines
    - Haloperidol
    - Melatonin agonists

of suspected drugs may be helpful; however, some agents may cause drug-induced delirium even at therapeutic concentrations.[2,5] When a particular medication is determined to be the causative agent, therapy should be discontinued or the dose should be reduced whenever possible.[121] A drug that is less likely to cause delirium should be substituted if possible.[2]

Management of drug-induced delirium should include supporting and maintaining basic vital functions, including adequate oxygenation, hydration, nutrition, and body temperature. Specific pharmacological and/or physiological precipitants should be identified and discontinued/reversed whenever possible. After treatment is initiated, careful monitoring for signs and symptoms of recovery as well as for treatment-associated adverse effects is important. Any medications used in the treatment of drug-induced delirium should be tapered to discontinuation as soon as possible after recovery to minimize risk of further complications.[121] Care should be taken to prevent dehydration, falls, decubitus ulcers, and aspiration during management of these patients.[101]

Management of drug-induced delirium can include both pharmacological and nonpharmacological treatments.[6] Basic nonpharmacological interventions should always be initiated first because of the ease with which they can be implemented and their proven efficacy.[149] Nonpharmacological approaches to managing delirium include ensuring that patients have their eyeglasses, hearing aids, and dentures, arranging all treatments to be completed during the daytime to permit the maximum amount of sleep at night, reducing nighttime noise, placing familiar objects from home in the room, ensuring clear and concise communications, and encouraging patients to participate in their care and perform their own activities of daily living. The use of physical restraints should be avoided unless patients are likely to harm themselves or others, as deaths have been reported in association with their use.[2,5,170] Constant staff observation in a specialized delirium unit or observation by a sitter or family member is preferable to physical restraint.[169] Often, discontinuation of the causative agent alone is not sufficient, and drug therapy must be used to control symptoms of agitation and psychosis after nonpharmacological measures have been implemented.[6,171]

Psychotropic agents, typical and atypical antipsychotics, and benzodiazepines are the most frequently prescribed classes of medication for the management of delirium. Guidelines from the American Psychiatric Association and NICE recommend psychotropic agents as adjunctive therapy.[2,135] However, these drugs have also been linked to the development of delirium.[103] There are no medications that are approved by the U.S. Food and Drug Administration for the management of drug-induced delirium. Psychotropic agents should be considered after nonpharmacological measures have been implemented, suspected offending drug(s) have been discontinued, and when control of severe agitation is required for the patient's safety or for the safety of others.

Various medications have been utilized for the management of patients with nondrug-induced delirium. However, there is a paucity of evidence supporting the use of medications for the management of drug-induced delirium except where specific antidotes are available (such as naloxone). It seems reasonable, therefore, to discuss literature pertaining to nondrug-induced delirium in this section.

Benzodiazepines may be considered for the treatment of drug-induced delirium, particularly in hyperactive or agitated patients.[172] However, there is little evidence to support the use of benzodiazepines as monotherapy. One study comparing haloperidol, chlorpromazine, and lorazepam in patients with acquired immune deficiency syndrome and delirium reported that lorazepam was less effective than either antipsychotic drug.[168] It is appropriate to initiate benzodiazepine therapy in cases of delirium associated with alcohol or sedative withdrawal or in combination with an antipsychotic agent such as haloperidol when a patient cannot tolerate increases in antipsychotic doses.

Lorazepam is the most commonly used benzodiazepine in patients with delirium because of its rapid onset of action, short half-life, and availability in various dosage forms.[171] This drug is relatively safe for use in patients with hepatic dysfunction, as it has no active metabolites.[172] Lorazepam can be administered orally, intramuscularly (IM), or intravenously (IV) in doses ranging from 0.5 to 2 mg.[169] The dose can be repeated or doubled every 30–60 minutes, depending on the degree of agitation and sedation. Diazepam is recommended as an alternative to physostigmine in patients with anticholinergic toxicity because of its longer duration of action and more favorable adverse effect profile.[6] Haloperidol and phenothiazines should be avoided in this situation.

When benzodiazepines are administered parenterally, they may cause respiratory depression and arrhythmias, and therefore cardiopulmonary function must be monitored.[171] There is also the potential for the occurrence of a paradoxical reaction, in which the patient becomes more agitated with continued benzodiazepine administration. Paradoxical reactions tend to occur more often in the elderly, in those with liver dysfunction, and in patients with low plasma albumin concentrations. Caution should be exercised when using benzodiazepines as they may worsen delirium and cause excessive sedation in some patients.[173]

In a small case series, melatonin 2 mg was administered to two postoperative patients for 3–4 nights. One patient received melatonin for the prevention of delirium and the other for treatment of delirium. In both cases, melatonin effectively reduced the severity of delirium symptoms or prevented delirium. No adverse events were reported.[161] Ramelteon has also been reported to be effective for management of a case of hypoactive delirium.[174]

Haloperidol is the most widely used antipsychotic medication for the symptomatic management of delirium, despite few prospective studies of its effectiveness for agitation and hallucinations in this setting. Haloperidol offers several advantages over the low-potency antipsychotics, including a relative absence of anticholinergic activity, alpha adrenergic blockade, and sedation.[6,172] In nonelderly patients, oral haloperidol doses of 2 mg may be administered for mild agitation, 5 mg for moderate agitation, and 10 mg for severe agitation.[175] In elderly patients, recommended oral haloperidol doses are 0.5 mg for mild agitation, 1 mg for moderate agitation, and 2 mg for severe agitation.[176] Response may occur within 30–60 minutes. The dose may be repeated every 30–60 minutes until the patient is sedated or calm. In some cases, the dose may be doubled until the agitation is controlled. Haloperidol therapy can be continued on a tapering schedule for 3–5 days.[175] The goal is to use the lowest possible haloperidol dose for the shortest possible duration.

In cases in which agitation is severe, the patient is at serious risk of self-injury or is unable or unwilling to take medications orally, haloperidol may be administered IM or IV.[171] Doses vary greatly, from as low as 0.25 mg IM or as high as 10 mg in a single IV dose. A continuous IV infusion of haloperidol may be administered at rates ranging from 2–10 mg/hr.[177] IV administration of haloperidol has been shown to produce a lower incidence of extrapyramidal adverse effects, presumably due to lower concentrations of the pyridinium metabolite; however, IV haloperidol is associated with a risk of prolongation of the corrected QT (QTc) interval and, in some cases, torsades de pointes.[171,178] The maximum daily IV dose should be limited to <35 mg.[179]

Patients receiving treatment with IV haloperidol should undergo a baseline electrocardiogram for determination of the heart rate–corrected QT (QTc) interval. Prolongation of the QTc interval to >0.45 seconds or more than 25% above baseline is cause for concern, and the relative risks and benefits of continued therapy must be carefully considered.

The use of high-dose haloperidol for the treatment of delirium is not without controversy. Dopamine D_2 receptor blockade in the mesolimbic region is believed to be the primary mechanism of action; a threshold of 60% of D_2 receptor blockade is necessary for antipsychotic effects. Some argue that very high doses of haloperidol are unlikely to be more effective than lower doses, because 53–85% of D_2 receptors are occupied by haloperidol at doses of 2–20 mg/day.[180] Therefore, large doses should offer no additional benefit, with the potential for a higher incidence of adverse effects. In fact, there are numerous reports of extrapyramidal symptoms (EPS) including pseudoparkinsonism, acute or tardive dystonia, dyskinesias, and akathisia associated with high-dose IV haloperidol or withdrawal from haloperidol therapy.[181,182] Worsening symptoms may be the result of EPS, especially akathisia, which often goes unrecognized and is sometimes inappropriately managed by increasing haloperidol doses.

Some clinicians prefer to use droperidol in the critical care setting, as it is a more potent, rapid-acting antipsychotic that is more sedating than haloperidol and may be associated with a lower incidence of extrapyramidal effects.[183] Bolus IV injections of droperidol have been associated with hypotension, tachycardia, and torsades de pointes.[183] Baseline QTc interval assessment and cardiac monitoring are necessary when administering high doses of droperidol as prolongation of the QTc interval and torsades de pointes can occur. This drug should be reserved for use only in the ICU setting, where patients are closely monitored and resuscitation equipment is immediately available.

A psychiatric consultation service's experience with the use of thiothixene for treatment of delirium was reviewed in a case series. Hospital records were reviewed over a 32-month period to assess response and adverse effects. Resolution or improvement of delirium was documented in 78% of patients and tolerability was documented in 82% of patients.[184]

Newer antipsychotic agents including aripiprazole, olanzapine, quetiapine, risperidone, and ziprasidone have been reported to be effective for the management of delirium. The use of aripiprazole for the management of delirium was reported in a small case series of two patients.[185] One patient's MMSE score improved from 5 to 28, while his DRS score decreased from 28 to 6. The second patient's MMSE score improved from 7 to 27 while her DRS score decreased from 18 to 6. In another series, 12 of 14 patients with delirium treated with aripiprazole demonstrated a greater than 50% reduction in the DRS score, while 13 showed improvement on the Clinical Global Impressions (CGI) scale scores.[186] There was a low incidence of adverse effects. Aripiprazole (mean daily dose 18.3 mg) was also evaluated in 21 hospitalized patients with cancer to determine response based on delirium subtypes. Patients with hypoactive delirium had a 100% resolution rate compared to 58% in patients with hyperactive delirium. No clinically significant side effects were noted.[187] Patients who received aripiprazole for the treatment of delirium (n = 21) were compared to 21 case-matched patients treated with haloperidol. The overall delirium resolution rates were similar in the two groups. In patients with hypoactive delirium, the resolution rates were 100% in the aripiprazole group and 78% in patients receiving haloperidol. For patients with hyperactive delirium, the resolution rates in the aripiprazole and haloperidol groups were 58% and 75%, respectively.[188]

Olanzapine has been reported to be effective for delirium in several clinical trials. One study enrolled medically ill patients (mean age = 46 years).[189] The mean maximum dose of olanzapine was 8.8 mg/day and the mean time to response was 3.8 days. In another study, patients with cancer (mean age = 61 years) were enrolled.[190] The mean maximum dose was only 6.3 mg/day. Approximately 76% of patients responded within 4–7 days; however, patients ≥70 years of age had a lower response rate of 42%. Sipahimalani and Masand conducted a retrospective medical record review of 22 mixed medical-surgical patients.[191] Five of 11 patients treated with olanzapine (mean dose 8.2 mg daily) showed a significant improvement in their DRS score compared to 6 of 11 patients treated with haloperidol. In a prospective, randomized, single-blind study, the efficacy of therapy with olanzapine (n = 28) was compared with that of haloperidol (n = 45) in a mixed group of critically ill medical-surgical patients.[192] Delirium index scores improved similarly in both groups, and the need for rescue therapy did not differ between groups. Six patients receiving haloperidol experienced mild EPS compared with none in the olanzapine group. Elsayem and colleagues conducted a prospective unblinded study to evaluate the effectiveness of subcutaneous olanzapine for the management of hyperactive or mixed delirium in 24 patients with advanced cancer. Patients received olanzapine 5 mg or 10 mg subcutaneously every 8 hours for 3 days. Efficacy was observed in 9 of 24 (37.5%) of patients. No injection site reactions were reported, but adverse effects (hypotension, agitation, diabetes insipidus, and seizures) were observed in four patients.[193]

Several case reports indicate that quetiapine may be a reasonable option for management of delirium.[194-196] Sasaki et al. reported the effect of quetiapine therapy in 12 patients with delirium of multiple etiologies.[197] Patients were treated for an average of 4.8 days ± 3.5 days with a flexible dose of quetiapine (mean maximum dose was 63.5 mg/day). Delirium rating scale scores improved significantly, and no patient experienced significant adverse events. In a retrospective review of the medical records of 22 mixed medical-surgical patients, quetiapine (median dose = 211 mg daily) was as effective as haloperidol in improving DRS score by more than 50% from baseline.[198] One patient receiving quetiapine experienced mild-to-moderate sedation and two patients receiving haloperidol developed EPS. In another study, the efficacy of therapy with quetiapine at doses of 25–100 mg daily for 7 days was assessed in 22 patients with delirium.[199] The DRS and CGI scores on days 2–7 were significantly lower than those on day 0. Two patients (9.1%) developed mild tremor. Tahir and colleagues conducted a randomized, double-blind, placebo-controlled trial evaluating the effectiveness of quetiapine in 42 patients with delirium. The primary outcome measure was the DRS Revised 98 (DRS-R-98). No differences at individual time points (day 3 and day 10) were statistically significant.[200] Devlin and colleagues conducted a multicenter, prospective, randomized, double-blind, placebo-controlled study to evaluate the efficacy of quetiapine 50 mg every 12 hours for management of delirium in 36 critically ill patients. Patients who received quetiapine spent less time in delirium compared to those in the placebo group (36 hours versus 120 hours, p = 0.006) and less time agitated (6 hours versus 36 hours, p = 0.02). Mortality and length of ICU stay were similar between the groups.[201] Quetiapine was compared to haloperidol in a prospective, double-blind, randomized controlled trial of 52 medically ill patients with delirium. Patients were randomized to receive quetiapine 25–100 mg/day (n = 24) or haloperidol 0.5–2 mg/day (n = 28). The mean change in DRS-R-98 score for quetiapine (−22.9) was not significantly different from that in patients receiving haloperidol (−21.7; p = 0.59).[202]

Risperidone at mean doses of 0.75–1.7 mg daily has been reported to be effective for the management of delirium.[203,204] In an unblinded study, 64 medically ill hospitalized patients with delirium received oral risperidone in daily doses of 1.85–2.97 mg (mean daily dose 2.6 mg ± 3.3 mg).[205] Risperidone was effective in 58 of 64 patients and significantly improved all symptoms measured by DRS, Positive and Negative Syndrome Scale, MMSE, and CGI during a period of 7 days. The comparative efficacy of risperidone and haloperidol for treatment of delirium was assessed in a prospective, randomized, double-blind study of acutely ill inpatients.[206] The MDAS improved significantly in both groups at 7 days; there was no significant difference in efficacy between the groups. In another study, the relationship between response and genetic polymorphisms in the dopamine transporter was studied in 42 patients treated with either haloperidol or risperidone for management of delirium.[207] There was no difference in efficacy between the groups, indicating that dopamine transporter polymorphisms did not significantly influence the effects of the antipsychotics. In a randomized, double-blind study of 126 patients undergoing cardiac surgery with cardiopulmonary bypass, patients were randomly assigned to receive risperidone 1 mg or placebo sublingually.[153] The incidence of postoperative delirium was significantly lower in the risperidone group. Miyaji et al. compared the adverse effects of risperidone with those of haloperidol in a retrospective study of 266 Japanese inpatients treated for delirium; the incidence of adverse effects was significantly lower in risperidone-treated patients.[208] Kim and colleagues conducted a randomized, comparative clinical trial of risperidone and olanzapine in 32 patients with delirium. The mean initial dose and the mean last dose in the risperidone group were 0.6 mg and 0.9 mg, respectively, and 1.8 mg and 2.4 mg, respectively, in the olanzapine group. The primary outcome measure was the DRS-R-98. There was no significant difference in response rate (≥50% reduction from baseline in the DRS-R-98 score) between the risperidone and olanzapine groups (64.7%, 73.3%; $p = 0.71$).[209] Kishi and colleagues evaluated the use of risperidone (mean dose 1.4 mg/day) in 29 patients with cancer and delirium. DRS-R-98 scores improved in 23 of 29 (79%) patients, showed no change in 4 of 29 (14%), and worsened in 2 of 29 (7%). The response rate (defined as a 25% reduction in DRS-R-98 score) was achieved in 14 of 29 (48%) of risperidone-treated patients.[210]

Ziprasidone has also been used for the treatment of delirium.[211,212] This drug is associated with a low risk of sedation and EPS. In a case report in which ziprasidone was administered for delirium, the drug was effective; however, the patient exhibited QTc interval prolongation requiring drug discontinuation.[211] Girard and colleagues conducted a multicenter, randomized, double-blind, placebo-controlled trial in 101 mechanically ventilated ICU patients. Patients were randomized to receive haloperidol, ziprasidone, or placebo every 6 hours for up to 14 days. The primary outcome was the number of days patients were alive without delirium or coma. Patients in the haloperidol group spent a similar number of days alive without delirium or coma (median interquartile range 14 days) as the patients in the ziprasidone (15) and placebo groups (12.5; $p = 0.66$).[213]

Overall, haloperidol and atypical antipsychotics appear to be equally efficacious for the treatment of delirium in acutely ill hospitalized patients.[214-219] However, this statement must be tempered by the fact that large randomized placebo-controlled trials supporting the efficacy of these agents for the treatment of delirium are lacking. In addition, all antipsychotic agents include a boxed warning in their labeling regarding an increased risk of mortality in elderly patients treated for dementia-related psychosis. Clinicians should weigh the benefits and risks associated with antipsychotic drug therapy prior to prescribing these agents for the management of drug-induced delirium.[220] Further studies are required to determine the role of antipsychotics in the management of delirium.

Pharmacological strategies for management of drug-induced delirium should be implemented after nonpharmacological measures have been attempted, suspected offending drug(s) have been discontinued, when control of severe agitation is required for the patient's safety or for the safety of others, and when psychosis is present.

INFORMATION FOR PATIENTS

Patients taking medications implicated in causing delirium and their caregivers should be instructed to be vigilant for early signs and symptoms of the disorder. In addition, they should be taught about available nonpharmacological treatment approaches and instructed to implement these measures should the patient develop signs or symptoms.[6] Early recognition and intervention may prevent or ameliorate this disabling condition.

REFERENCES

1. American Psychiatric Association. *Diagnostic and statistical manual of mental disorders*. 5th ed. Washington, DC: American Psychiatric Association; 2013.
2. American Psychiatric Association. Practice guideline for the treatment of patients with delirium. *Am J Psychiatry*. 1999; 156:1-20.
3. Karlsson I. Drugs that induce delirium. *Dement Geriatr Cogn Disord*. 1999;10:412-5.
4. Alagiakrishnan K, Wiens CA. An approach to drug induced delirium in the elderly. *Postgrad Med J*. 2004; 80:388-93.
5. Francis J. Drug-induced delirium: diagnosis and treatment. *CNS Drugs*. 1996; 5:103-14.
6. Carter GL, Dawson AH, Lopert R. Drug-induced delirium. *Drug Safety*. 1996; 15:291-301.

7. Centorrino F, Albert MJ, Drago-Ferrante G et al. Delirium during clozapine treatment: incidence and associated risk factors. *Pharmacopsychiatry.* 2003; 36:156-60.
8. House M. Overdose of ziprasidone. *Am J Psychiatry.* 2002; 159:1061-2.
9. Balit CR, Isbister GK, Hackett LP et al. Quetiapine poisoning: a case series. *Ann Emerg Med.* 2003; 42:751-8.
10. Morikawa M, Kishimoto T. Probable dementia with Lewy bodies and risperidone-induced delirium. *Can J Psychiatry.* 2002; 47:976.
11. Morgan M, Hackett LP, Isbister GK. Olanzapine overdose: a series of analytically confirmed cases. *Int Clin Psychopharmacol.* 2007; 22:183-6.
12. Byerly MJ, Christensen RC, Evans OL. Delirium associated with a combination of sertraline, haloperidol, and benztropine. *Am J Psychiatry.* 1996; 153:965-6.
13. Lima BR, Vanneman D. Propranolol, benztropine, fluphenazine decanoate, and delirium. *Am J Psychiatry.* 1983; 140:659-60.
14. Rawson RA, Lipscomb WR, Rozynko J. Acute delirium in amitriptyline-perphenazine therapy of alcoholism. *Clin Toxicol.* 1971;4 :5-10.
15. Spring GK. Delirium associated with lithium and thioridazine. *Am J Psychiatry.* 1983; 140:1257-8.
16. Fuller MA, Sajatovic M. Neurotoxicity resulting from a combination of lithium and loxapine. *J Clin Psychiatry.* 1989; 50:187
17. Gaudreau JD, Gagnon P, Roy MA et al. Opioid medications and longitudinal risk of delirium in hospitalized cancer patients. *Cancer.* 2007;109: 2365-73.
18. Okon TR, George ML. Fentanyl-induced neurotoxicity and paradoxic pain. *J Pain Symptom Manage.* 2008; 35:327-33.
19. Fong HK, Sands LP, Leung JM. The role of postoperative analgesia in delirium and cognitive decline in elderly patients: a systematic review. *Anesth Analg.* 2006; 102:1255-66.
20. Lewis DA, Smith RE. Steroid-induced psychiatric syndromes. A report of 14 cases and a review of the literature. *J Affect Disord.* 1983; 5:319-32.
21. Stoudemire A, Anfinson T, Edwards J. Corticosteroid-induced delirium and dependency. *Gen Hosp Psychiatry.* 1996; 18:196-202.
22. McKeon A, Frye MA, Delanty N. The alcohol withdrawal syndrome. *J Neurol Neurosurg Psychiatry.* 2008; 79:854-62.
23. Saravay SM, Marke J, Steinberg MD et al. "Doom anxiety" and delirium in lidocaine toxicity. *Am J Psychiatry.* 1987; 144:159-63.
24. Bikadoroff S. Mental changes associated with tocainide, a new antiarrhythmic. *Can J Psychiatry.* 1987; 32:219-21
25. Athwal H, Murphy G Jr, Chun S. Amiodarone-induced delirium. *Am J Geriatr Psychiatry.* 2003; 11:696-7.
26. Eisenman DP, McKegney FP. Delirium at therapeutic serum concentrations of digoxin and quinidine. *Psychosomatics.* 1994; 35:91-3
27. Wang PS, Schneeweiss S, Glynn RJ et al. Use of the case-crossover design to study prolonged drug exposures and insidious outcomes. *Ann Epidemiol.* 2004; 14:296-303.
28. Khan AY, Kalimuddin MN, Gorman JM. Neuropsychiatric manifestations of phenytoin toxicity in an elderly patient. *J Psychiatr Pract.* 2007; 13:49-54.
29. Rowe TO. Acetazolamide delirium. *Am J Psychiatry.* 1977; 134:587-8.
30. Selek S, Savas HA. Psychosis, delirium, or manic switch due to lamotrigine? *Epilepsy Behav.* 2007; 11:476.
31. Oaklander AL, Buchbinder BR. Pregabalin-withdrawal encephalopathy and splenial edema: a link to high-altitude illness? *Ann Neurol.* 2005; 58:309-12.
32. Forbes RA, Kalra H, Hackett LP et al. Deliberate self-poisoning with tiagabine: an unusual toxidrome. *Emerg Med Australas.* 2007; 19:556-8.
33. Chae BJ, Kang BJ. A case of delirium and subsequent pancytopenia associated with the oral loading of valproic acid. *J Clin Psychiatry.* 2005; 66:801-2.
34. Paul KL, Bhatara VS. Anticholinergic delirium possibly associated with protriptyline and fluoxetine. *Ann Pharmacother.* 1997; 31:1260-1.
35. Nelson JC, Jatlow PI, Bock J et al. Major adverse reactions during desipramine treatment: relationship to plasma drug concentrations, concomitant antipsychotic treatment, and patient characteristics. *Arch Gen Psychiatry.* 1982; 39:1055-61.
36. Kutcher SP, Shulman KI. Despiramine-induced delirium at subtherapeutic concentrations: a case report. *Can J Psychiatry.* 1985; 30;368-89.
37. Ueda N, Yoshimura R, Eto S et al. Delirious episodes induced by intravenous administration of clomipramine associated with an acute increase in its plasma concentrations. *Psychiatry and Clin Neurosci.* 2000; 54:669-72.
38. Gomolin IH, Melmed CA. Prolonged delirium without anticholinergic signs following amitriptyline overdose. *Can Med Assoc J.* 1983; 129:1203-4.
39. Kramer M. Delirium as a complication of imipramine therapy in the aged. *Am J Psychiatry.* 1963: 120:502-3.
40. Santos AB, Mccurdy L. Delirium after abrupt withdrawal from doxepin: case report. *Am J Psychiatry* 1980; 137:239-40.
41. Leionen E, Koponen H, Lepola U. Delirium during fluoxetine treatment. A case report. *Ann Clin Psychiatry.* 1993; 5:255-7.
42. Wakeno M, Okugawa G, Takekita Y et al. Delirium associated with paroxetine in an elderly depressive patient: a case report. *Pharmacopsychiatry.* 2007; 40:199-200.
43. Liberzon I, Dequardo JR, Silk KR. Bupropion and delirium. *Am J Psychiatry.* 1990; 147:1689-90.
44. Howe C, Ravasia S. Venlafaxine-induced delirium. *Can J Psychiatry.* 2003;48:129.
45. Bailer U, Fischer P, Kufferle B et al. Occurrence of mirtazapine-induced delirium in organic brain disorder. *Int Clin Psychopharmacol.* 2000; 15:239-43.
46. Blansjaar BA, Egberts TC. Delrium in a patient treated with disulfiram and tranylcypromine. *Am J Psychiatry.* 1995; 152:296.
47. Alvine G, Black DW, Tsuang D. Case of delirium secondary to phenelzine/L-tryptophan combination. *J Clin Psychiatry.* 1990; 51:311.
48. Postma JU, Van Tilburg W. Visual hallucinations an delirium during treatment with amantadine (Symmetrel). *J Am Geriatr Soc.* 1975; 23:212-5.
49. Nymeyer L, Grossberg GT. Delirium in a 75 year old woman receiving ECT and levodopa. *Convuls Ther.* 1997; 13:114-6.
50. Serby M, Angrist B, Lieberman A. Mental disturbances during bromocriptine and lergotrile treatment of Parkinson's disease. *Am J Psychiatry.* 1978; 135:1227-9.
51. Olshaker JS, Flanigan J. Flumazenil reversal of lorazepam-induced acute delirium. *J Emerg Med.* 2003; 24:181-3.
52. Madan R, Muralidhar V, Kalia PK et al. Diazepam induced delirium. *Indian J Ophthalmol.* 1989; 37:35-6.
53. Fish DE, Neff R, Benedek D. Clonazepam induced delirium in Bosnia. *Mil Med.* 1997; 162:iii.
54. Zalsman G, Hermesh H, Munitz H. Alprazolam withdrawal delirium: a case report. *Clin Neuropharmacol.* 1998; 21:201-2.
55. Goodchild JH, Donaldson M. Hallucinations and delirium in the dental office following triazolam administration. *Anesth Prog.* 2005; 52:17-20.
56. Allgulander C, Borg S. Case report: a delirious abstinence syndrome associated with clorazepate (Tranxilen). *Br J Addict Alcohol Other Drugs.* 1978; 73:175-7.
57. Shulman KI, Sykora K, Gill S et al. Incidence of delirium in older adults newly prescribed lithium or valproate: a population-based cohort study. *J Clin Psychiatry.* 2005; 66:424-7.
58. Okumura A, Fukumoto Y, Hayakawa F et al. Antipyretics and delirious behavior during febrile illness. *Pediatr Int.* 2006; 48:40-3.
59. Hooten WM, Pearlson G. Delirium caused by tacrine and ibuprofen interaction. *Am J Psychiatry.* 1996; 153:842.

60. Tavcar R, Dervnovsek MZ, Brosch S. Ketoprofen intoxication delirium. *J Clin Psychopharmacol.* 1999; 19:95-6.
61. Thornoton TL. Delirium associated with sulindac. *JAMA.* 1980; 243:1630-1.
62. Morrison RL, Katz IR. Drug-related cognitive impairment: Current progress and recurrent problems. *Am Rev Gerontol Geriatr.* 1989; 9:233-79.
63. Bailey RB, Jones SR. Chronic salicylate intoxication: a common cause of morbidity in the elderly. *J Am Geriatri Soc.* 1989; 37:556-1.
64. Macknight C, Rojas-Fernandez CH. Celecoxib and rofecoxib-induced delirium. *J Neuropsychiatry Clin Neurosci.* 2001; 3:305-6.
65. Gray SL, Lai KV, Larson EB. Drug-induced cognition disorders in the elderly: incidence, prevention and management. *Drug Saf.* 1999; 21:101-22.
66. Jacobsen FM, Sack DA, James SP. Delirium induced by verapamil. *Am J Psychiatry.* 1987; 144:248.
67. Myrhed M, Wiholm BE. Nifedipine-a survey of adverse effects *Acta Pharmacol Toxicol (Copenh).* 1986; 58:133-6.
68. Kogoj A. Suspected propranolol-induced delirium. *Can J Psychiatry.* 2004; 49:645.
69. Arber N. Delirium induced by atenolol. *BMJ.* 1988; 297:1048.
70. Fisher AA, Davis M, Jeffery I. Acute delirium induced by metoprolol. *Cardiovasc Drugs Ther.* 2002; 16:161-5.
71. McCartney CF, Hatley LH, Kessler JM. Possible tobramycin delirium. *JAMA.* 1982; 247:1319.
72. Cone LA, Padilla L, Potts BE. Delirium in the elderly resulting from azithromycin therapy. *Surg Neurol.* 2003; 59:509-11.
73. Mermelstein HT. Clarithromycin-induced delirium in a general hospital. *Psychosomatics.* 1998; 39:540-2.
74. Penttila J, Pasila K, Tiisala A et al. Delirium in an adolescent patient during treatment with cephalexin. *J Adolesc Health.* 2006; 39:782-3.
75. Tollefson G. Neuropsychiatric sequelae and cephalothin. *J Clin Psychiatry.* 1984; 45:96.
76. Herd AM, Ross CA, Bhattacharya SK. Acute confusional state with postoperative intravenous cefazolin. *BMJ.* 1989; 299:393-4.
77. Tong MK, Siu YP, Yung CY et al. Piperacillin/tazobactam-induced acute delirium in a peritoneal dialysis patient. *Nephrol Dial Transplant.* 2004; 19:1341.
78. Altes J, Gasco J, de Antonio J et al. Ciprofloxacin and delirium. *Ann Intern Med.* 1989; 110:170-1.
79. Satyanarayana S, Campbell B. Gatifloxacin-induced delirium and psychosis in a n elderly demented woman. *J Am Geriatr Soc.* 2006; 54:871.
80. Fennig S, Mauas L. Ofloxacin-induced delirum. *J Clin Psychiatry.* 1992; 53:137-8.
81. Hakko E, Mete B, Ozaras R et al. Levofloxacin-induced delirium. *Clin Neurol Neurosurg.* 2005; 107:158-9.
82. Levine PH, Regelson W, Holland JF. Chloramphenicol-associated encephalopathy. *Clin Pharmacol Ther.* 1970; 11:194-9.
83. Salkind AR. Acute delirium induced by intravenous trimethoprim-sulfamethoxazole therapy in a patient with the acquired immunodeficiency syndrome. *Hum Exp Toxicol.* 2000; 19:149-51.
84. Serio RN. Acute delirium associated with combined diphenhydramine and linezolid use. *Ann Pharmacother.* 2004; 38:62-5.
85. Jenike MA, Levy JC. Physostigmine reversal of cimetidine-induced delirium and agitation. *J Clin Psychopharmacol.* 1983; 3:43-4.
86. Eisendrath SJ, Ostroff JW. Ranitidine-associated delirium. *Psychosomatics.* 1990; 31:98-100.
87. Galynker II, Tendler DS. Nizatidine-induced delirium in a nonagenarian. *J Clin Psychiatry.* 1997; 58:327.
88. Catalano G, Catalan MC, Alberts VA. Famotidine-associated delirium. A series of six cases. *Psychosomatics.* 1996; 37:349-55.
89. Golinger RC, Peet L, Tune LE. Association of elevated plasma anticholinergic activity with delirium in surgical patient. *Am J Psychiatry.* 1987; 144:1218-20.
90. Hammon K, DeMartino BK. Postoperative delirium secondary to atropine premedication. *Anesth Prog.* 1985; 32:107-8.
91. Roth A, Akyol S, Nelson JC. Delirium associated with the combination of a neuroleptic, an SSRI, and benztropine. *J Clin Psychiatry.* 1994; 55:492-5.
92. Smiler BG, Bartholomew EG, Sivak BJ et al. Physostigmine reversal of scopolamine delirium in obstetric patients. *Am J Obstet Gynecol.* 1973; 1169:326-9.
93. Edwards KR, O'Connor JT. Risk of delirium with concomitant use of tolterodine and acetylcholinesterase inhibitors. *J Am Geriatr Soc.* 2002; 50:1165-6.
94. Agostini JV, Leo-Summers LS, Inouye SK. Cognitive and other adverse effects of diphenhydramine use in hospitalized older patients. *Arch Int Med.* 2001; 161:2091-7.
95. Marcantonio ER, Juarez G, Goldman L et al. The relationship of postoperative delirium with psychoactive medications. *JAMA.* 1994; 272:1518-22.
96. Luedecke D, Schottle D, Karow A et al. Post-injection delirium/sedation syndrome in patients treated with olanzapine pamoate: mechanism, incidence, and management. *CNS Drugs.* 2015; 29:41-6.
97. Kenna HA, Poon AW, Paula de los Angeles C et al. Psychiatric complícations of treatment with corticosteroids : review with case report. *Psychiatry Clin Neurosci.* 2011; 65:549-60.
98. Tome AM, Filipe A. Quinolones review of psychiatric and neurologic adverse reactions. *Drug Saf.* 2011; 34:465-88.
99. Apodaca K, Baker J, Bin-Bilal H et al. Ertapenem-induced delirium : a case report and literature review. *Psychosomatics.* 2015; 56:561-6.
100. Fox C, Smith T, Maidment I et al. Effect of medications with anti-cholinergic properties on cognitive function, delirium, physical function and mortality : a systematic review. *Age Ageing.* 2014; 43:604-15.
101. Gaudreau JD, Gagnon P, Harel F, Roy MA et al. Psychoactive medications and risk of delirium in hospitalized cancer patients. *J Clin Oncol.* 2005; 23:6712-8.
102. Vaurio LE, Sands LP, Wang Y et al. Postoperative delirium: the importance of pain and pain management. *Anesth Anal.* 2006; 102:1267-73.
103. Gaudreau JD, Gagnon P, Roy MA et al. Association between psychoactive medications and delirium in hospitalized patients: a critical review. *Psychosomatics.* 2005; 46:302-16.
104. Inouye SK. Delirium in older persons. *N Engl J Med.* 2006; 3545:1157-65.
105. Boorsma M, Joling KJ, Frijters DH et al. The prevalence, incidence and risk factors for delirium in Dutch nursing homes and residential care homes. *Int J Geriatr Psychiatry.* 2012; 27:709-15.
106. Grassi L, Caraceni A, Mitchell AJ et al. Management of delirium in palliative care: a review. *Curr Psychiatry Rep.* 2015; 13.
107. Brauer C, Morrison S, Silberzweig SB et al. The cause of delirium in patients with hip fracture. *Arch Intern Med.* 2000; 160:1856-60.
108. Cole MG. Delirium in elderly patients. *Am J Geriatr Psychiatry.* 2004; 21:7-21.
109. Tune LE, Egeli S. Acetylcholine and delirium. *Dement Geriatr Cogn Disord.* 1999; 10:342-4.
110. Trzepacz PT. Update on the neuropathogenesis of delirium. *Dement Geriatr Cogn Disord.* 1999; 10:330-4.
111. Olsson T. Activity in the hypothatlic-pituitary-adrenal axis and delirium. *Dement Geriatr Cogn Disord.* 1999; 10:345-9.
112. Koponen HJ. Neurochemistry and delirium. *Dement Geriatr Cogn Disord.* 1999; 10:339-41.
113. Maldonado J. Neuropathogenesis of delirium: review of current etiologic theories and common pathways. *Am J Geriatr Psychiatry.* 2013; 21:1190-222.
114. Pun BT, Ely EW. The importance of diagnosing and managing ICU delirium. *Chest.* 2007; 132:624-36.

115. Irwin P, Murray S, Bilnski A et al. Alcohol withdrawal as an underrated cause of agitated delirium and terminal restlessness in patients with advanced malignancy. *J Pain Symptom Manage.* 2005; 29:104-8.
116. Inouye SK, van Dyck CH, Alessi CA et al. Clarifying confusion: the confusion assessment method. A new method for the detection of delirium *Ann Intern Med.* 1990; 113:941-8.
117. Jacobi J, Fraser GL, Coursin DB. Clinical practice guidelines for the sustained use of sedatives and analgesics in the critically ill adult. *Crit Care Med.* 2002; 30:119-41.
118. Trzepacz PT, Baker R, Greenhouse J. A symptoms rating scale for delirium. *Psychiatr Res.*1988; 23:89-97.
119. Breitbart W, Rosenfeld B, Roth A. The Memorial Delirium Assessment Scale. *J Pain Symptom Manage.* 1997; 13:128-37.
120. Mittal D, Majithia D, Kennedy R et al. Differences in characteristics and outcome of delirium as based on referral patterns. *Psychosomatics.* 2006; 47:367-75.
121. Brown TM. Drug-induced delirium. *Sem Clin Neuropsychiatry.* 2000; 5:113-24.
122. Johnson J. Identifying and recognizing delirium. *Dement Geriatr Cogn Disord.* 1999; 10:353-8.
123. Elie M, Cole MG, Rimeau FJ et al. Delirium risk factors in elderly hospitalized patients. *J Gen Intern Med.* 1998; 13:204-12.
124. Lipowski ZJ. Delirium in the elderly patient. *N Engl J Med.* 1989; 320:578-82.
125. Inouye SK. Predisposing and precipitating factors for delirium in hospitalized older patients. *Dement Geriatr Cogn Disord.* 1999; 10:393-400.
126. Ouimet S, Kavanagh BP, Gottfried SB et al. Incidence, risk factors and consequences of ICU delirium. *Intensive Care Med.* 2007; 33:66-73.
127. Alciati A, Fusi A, D'Arminio Monforte A et al. New-onset delusions and hallucinations in patients infected with HIV. *J Psychiatry Neurosci.* 2001; 26:229-34.
128. Rausch DM, Stover ES. Neuroscience research in AIDS. *Prog Neuropsychopharmacol Biol Psychiatry.* 2001; 25:231-57.
129. Morita T, Tei Y, Tsunoda J et al. Underlying pathologies and their associations with clinical features in terminal delirium of cancer patients. *J Pain Symptom Manag.* 2001; 22:997-1006.
130. Tuma R, DeAngelis LM. Altered mental status in patients with cancer. *Arch Neurol.* 2000; 57:1727-31.
131. Winawer N. Postoperative delirium. *Med Clin North Am.* 2001; 85:1229-39.
132. Inouye SK, Bogardus ST Jr, Charpentier PA et al. A multicomponent intervention to prevent delirium in hospitalized older patients. *N Engl J Med.* 1999; 340:669-76.
133. Leung JM, Sands LP, Wang Y et al. Apolipoprotein E e4 allele increases the risk of early postoperative delirium in older patients undergoing noncardiac surgery. *Anesthesiology.* 2007; 107:406-11.
134. The American Geriatrics Society Expert Panel on postoperative delirium in older adults. Postoperative delirium in older adults: best practice statement from the American Geriatrics Society. *J Am Coll Surg.* 2015; 220:136-48.
135. NICE. Delirium: diagnosis, prevention and management of delirium. *Clin Gudel.* 2010; 103:512-39.
136. Kallin K, Jensen J, Olsson LL et al. Why the elderly fall in residential care facilities, and suggested remedies. *J Fam Practice.* 2004; 53:41-52.
137. O'Keeffe S, Lavan J. The prognostic significance of delirium in older hospital patients. *J Am Geriatr Soc.* 1997; 45:174-8.
138. Rockwood K, Cosway S, Carver D et al. The risk of dementia and death after delirium. *Age Ageing.* 1999; 28:551-6.
139. Uldall KK, Ryan R, Berghuis JP et al. Association between delirium and death in AIDS patients. *AIDS Patient Care STDS.* 2000; 14:95-100.
140. Marcantonio E, Ta T, Duthie E et al. Delirium severity and psychomotor types: their relationship with outcomes after hip fracture repair. *J Am Geriatr Soc.* 2002; 50:850-7.
141. Curyto KJ, Johnson J, TenHave T et al. Survival of hospitalized elderly patients with delirium: a prospective study. *Am J Geriatr Psychiatry.* 2001; 9:141-7.
142. Kelly KG, Zisselman M, Cutillo-Schmitter T et al. Severity and course of delirium in medically hospitalized nursing facility residents. *Am J Geriatr Psychiatry.* 2001; 9:72-7.
143. Marcantonio ER, Simon SE, Bergmann MA et al. Delirium symptoms in post-acute care: prevalent, persistent, and associated with poor functional recovery. *J Am Geriatr Soc.* 2003; 51:4-9
144. Andrew MK, Freter SH, Rockwood K. *BMC Geriatrics.* 2005; 5:5.
145. McCusker J, Cole M, Abrahamowicz M et al. Delirium predicts 12-month mortality. *Arch Intern Med.* 2002; 162:457-63.
146. Naksuk N, Thongprayoon C, Park JY et al. Clinical impact of delirium and antipsychotic therapy: 10-year experience from a referral coronary care unit. *Eur Heart J Acute Cardiovasc Care.* 2015; 6:1-9.
147. Leslie DL, Marcantonio ER, Zhang Y et al. One year health care costs associated with delirium in the elderly population. *Arch Intern Med.* 2008; 168:27-32.
148. Inouye S, Bogardus S, Williams C et al. The role of adherence on the effectiveness of nonpharmacologic interventions: Evidence from the delirium prevention trial. *Arch Intern Med.* 2003; 63:958-64.
149. Flaherty JH, Tariq SH, Raghavan S et al. A model for managing delirious older inpatients. *J Am Geriatr Soc.* 2003; 51:1031-5.
150. Larsen KA, Kelly SE, Stern TA et al. Administration of olanzapine to prevent postoperative delirium in elderly joint-replacement patients: a randomized, controlled trial. *Psychosomatics.* 2010; 51:409-18.
151. van den Boogaard M, Schoonhoven L, van Achterberg T et al. Haloperidol prophylaxis in critically ill patients with a high risk of delirium. *Crit Care.* 2013; 17:R9.
152. Wang W, Li HI, Wang DX et al. Haloperidol prophylaxis decreases delirium incidence in elderly patients after noncardiac surgery: a randomized controlled trial. *Crit Care Med.* 2012; 40:731-9.
153. Prakanrattana U, Prapaitrakool S. Efficacy of risperidone for prevention of postoperative delirium in cardiac surgery. *Anaesth Intensive Care.* 2007; 35:714-9.
154. Kalisvaart KJ, de Jonghe JFM, Bogaards MJ et al. Haloperidol prophylaxis for elderly hip surgery patients at risk for delirium: a randomized placebo controlled study. *J Am Geriatr Soc.* 2005; 53:1658-66.
155. Page VJ, Ely EW, Gates S et al. Effect of intravenous haloperidol on the duration of delirium and coma in critically ill patients (Hope-ICU): a randomized, double-blind, placebo-controlled trial. *Lancet Respir Med.* 2013; 1:515-23.
156. Vochteloo AJ, Moerman S, van der Burg BL et al. Delirium risk screening and haloperidol prophylaxis program in hip fracture patients is a helpful tool in identifying high-risk patients, but does not reduce the incidence of delirium. *BMC Geriatr.* 2010; 11:39.
157. Inouye SK, Westendorp RGJ, Saczynski JS. Delirium in elderly people. *Lancet.* 2014; 383:911-22.
158. Sampson EL, Raven PR, Ndhlova PN et al. A randomized, double-blind, placebo-controlled trial of donepezil hydrochloride (Aricept) for reducing the incidence of postoperative delirium after elective total hip replacement. *In J Geriatr Psychiatry.* 2007; 22:243-349.
159. Marcantonio ER, Palihnich K, Appleton P et al. Pilot randomized trial of donepezil hydrochloride for delirium after hip fracture. *J Am Geriatr Soc.* 2011; 59:S282-8.
160. Gamberini M, Bolliger D, Lurati Buse GA et al. Rivastigmine for the prevention of postoperative delirium in elderly patients undergoing elective cardiac surgery-a randomized controlled trial. *Crit Care Med.* 2009; 37:1762-768.
161. Liptzin B, Laki A, Garb JL et al. Donepezil in the prevention and treatment of post-surgical delirium. *Am J Geriatr Psychiatry.* 2005; 13:1100-6.

162. Hanania M, Kitain E. Melatonin for treatment and prevention of postoperative delirium. *Anesth Analg.* 2002; 94:338-9.

163. Sultan SS. Assessment of role of perioperative melatonin in prevention and treatment of postoperative delirium after hip arthroplasty under spinal anesthesia in the elderly. *Saudi J Anesth.* 2010; 4:169-73.

164. Al-Aama T, Brymer C, Gutmanis I et al. Melatonin decreases delirium in elderly patients: a randomized, placebo-controlled trial. *Int J Geriatr Psychiatry.* 2011; 26:687-94.

165. Hatta K, Kishi Y, Wada K et al. Preventive effects of ramelteon on delirium: a randomized placebo-controlled trial. *JAMA Psychiatry.* 2014; 71:397-403.

166. Hunter KF, Cyr D. The effect of delirium education on use of target prn medications in older orthopaedic patients. *Age Ageing.* 2007; 36:98-101.

167. Lapane KI, Hughes CM, Daiello LA et al. Effect of a pharmacist-led multicomponent intervention focusing on the medication monitoring phase to prevent potential adverse drug events in nursing homes. *J Am Geriatr Soc.* 2011; 59:1238-45.

168. Brietbart W, Marotta R, Platt M et al. A double-blind trial of haloperidol, chlorpromazine, and lorazepam in the treatment of delirium in hospitalized AIDS patients. *Am J Psychiatry.* 1996; 153:231-7.

169. Jacobson SA. Delirium in the elderly. *Psychiatr Clin North Am.* 1997; 20:91-110.

170. Gleason OC. Delirium. *Am Fam Physician.* 2003; 67:1027-34.

171. Jacobson S, Schreibman B. Behavioral and pharmacologic treatment of delirium. *Am Fam Physician.*1997; 56:2005-12.

172. Adams F. Emergency intravenous sedation of the delirious, medically ill patient. *J Clin Psychiatry.* 1988; 49:22-7.

173. Samuels S, Evers M. Pragmatic guidance for managing a common, confounding, and sometimes lethal condition. *Geriatrics.* 2002; 57:33-8.

174. Miura S, Furuya M, Yasuda H et al. Novel therapy with ramelteon for hypoactive delirium. A case report. *J Clin Psychopharmacol.* 2015; 35:1-2.

175. Yudofsky SC, Hales RE, eds. *The American Psychiatric Press textbook of neuropsychiatry.* Washington, DC: American Psychiatric Press; 1992.

176. Jacobson SA, Leuchter AF. Delirium. In: Reichman WE, Katz PR, eds. *Psychiatric care in the nursing home.* New York: Oxford University Press; 1996:57-66.

177. Seneff MG, Mathews RA. Use of haloperidol infusions to control delirium in critically ill adults. *Ann Pharmacother.* 1995; 29:690-4.

178. Rollema H, Skolnik M, D'Engelbronner J et al. MPP(+)-like neurotoxicity of a pyridinium metabolite derived from haloperidol: in vivo microdialysis and in vitro mitochondrial studies. *J Pharmacol Exp Ther.* 1994; 268:380-7.

179. Sharma ND, Rosman HS, Padhi ID et al. Torsades de Pointes associated with intravenous haloperidol in critically ill patients. *Am J Cardiol.* 1998; 81:238-40.

180. Tauscher J, Tauscher-Wisniewski S, Kasper S. Treatment of patients with delirium (letter). *Am J Psychiatry.* 2000; 157:1711.

181. Riker RR, Fraser GL, Richen P. Movement disorders associated with withdrawal from high-dose intravenous haloperidol therapy in delirious ICU patients. *Chest.* 1997; 111:1778-81.

182. Blitzstein SM, Brandt GT. Extrapyramidal symptoms from intravenous haloperidol in the treatment of delirium. *Am J Psychiatry.* 1997; 154:1474-5.

183. Frye MA, Coudreaut MF, Hakeman SM et al. Continuous droperidol infusion for management of agitated delirium in an intensive care unit. *Psychosomatics.* 1995; 36:301-5.

184. Leung JG, Dare FY, Flowers LM et al. Thiothixene in the management of delirium: a case series. *Psychosomatics* 2015; 56:542-64.

185. Alao AO, Moskowitz L. Aripiprazole and delirium. *Ann Clin Psychiatry.* 2006; 18:267-9.

186. Straker DA, Shapiro PA, Muskin PR. Aripiprazole in the treatment of delirium. *Psychosomatics.* 2006; 47:385-91.

187. Boettger S, Breitbart W. An open trial of aripiprazole for the treatment of delirium in hospitalized cancer patients. *Palliat Support Care.* 2011; 9:351-7.

188. Boettger S, Friedlander M, Breitbart W et al. Aripiprazole and haloperidol in the treatment of delirium. *Aust N Z J Psychiatry.* 2011; 45:477-82.

189. Kim K, Pae C, Chae J et al. An open pilot trial of olanzapine for delirium in the Korean population. *Psych Clin Neurosci.* 2001; 55:515-9.

190. Breitbart W, Tremblay A, Gibson C. An open trial of olanzapine for the treatment of delirium in hospitalized cancer patients. *Psychosomatics.* 2002; 43:175-82.

191. Sipahimalani A, Masand PS. Olanzapine in the treatment of delirium. *Psychosomatics.* 1998; 39:422-30.

192. Skrobik YK, Bergeron N, Dumont M et al. Olanzapine vs haloperidol: treating delirium in a critical care setting. *Intensive Care Med.* 2004; 30:444-9.

193. Elsayem A, Bush SH, Munsell MF et al. Subcutaneous olanzapine for hyperactive or mixed delirium in patients with advanced caner: a preliminary study. *J Pain Symptom Manage.* 2010; 40:774-82.

194. Al-Samarrai S, Dunn J, Newmark T et al. Quetiapine for treatment-resistant delirium. *Psychosomatics.* 2003; 44:350-1.

195. Torres R, Mittal D, Kennedy R. Use of quetiapine in delirium. *Psychosomatics.* 2001; 42:347-8.

196. Kim K, Bader G, Kotlyar V et al. Treatment of delirium in older adults with quetiapine. *J Geriatr Psychiatry Neurol.* 2003; 16:29-31.

197. Sasaki Y, Matsuyama T, Inoue S et al. A prospective, open-label, flexible-dose study of quetiapine in the treatment of delirium. *J Clin Psychiatry.* 2003; 64:1316-21.

198. Schwartz TL, Masand PS. Treatment of delirium with quetiapine. *Prim Care Companion J Clin Psychiatry.* 2000; 2:10-12.

199. Maneeton B, Maneeton N, Srisurapanont M. An open-label study of quetiapine for delirium. *J Med Assoc Thai.* 2007; 90:2158-63.

200. Tahir TA, Eeles E, Karapareddy V et al. A randomized controlled trial of quetiapine versus placebo in the treatment of delirium. *J Psychosom Res.* 2010; 69:485-90.

201. Devlin JW, Roberts RJ, Fong JJ et al. Efficacy and safety of quetiapine in critically ill patients with delirium: a prospective, multicenter, randomized, double-blind, placebo-controlled pilot study. *Crit Care Med.* 2010; 38:419-27.

202. Maneeton B, Maneeton N, Srisurapanont M et al. Quetiapine versus haloperidol in the treatment of delirium: a double-blind, randomized, controlled trial. *Drug Des Devel Ther.* 2013; 7:657-67.

203. Horikawa N, Yamazaki T, Miyamoto K et al. Treatment for delirium with risperidone: results of a prospective open trial with 10 patients. *Gen Hosp Psychiatry.* 2003; 25:289-92.

204. Mittal D, Jimerson NA, Neely EP et al. Risperidone in the treatment of delirium: results from a prospective open-label trial. *J Clin Psychiatry.* 2004; 65:662-7.

205. Parellada E, Baeza I, de Pablo J et al. Risperidone in the treatment of patients with delirium. *J Clin Psychiatry.* 2004; 65:348-53.

206. Han CS, Kim YK. A double-blind trial of risperidone and haloperidol for the treatment of delirium. *Psychosomatics.* 2004; 45:297-301.

207. Kim JY, Jung IK, Han C et al. Antipsychotics and dopamine transporter gene polymorphisms in delirium patients. *Psychiatry Clin Neurosci.* 2005; 59:183-8.

208. Miyaji S, Yamamoto K, Hoshino S et al. Comparison of the risk of adverse events between risperidone and haloperidol in delirium patients. *Psychiatry Clin Neurosci.* 2007; 61:275-82.

209. Kim SW, Yoo JA, Lee SY et al. Risperidone versus olanzapine for the treatment of delirium. *Hum Psychopharmacol Clin Exp.* 2010; 25:298-302.

210. Kishi Y, Kato M, Okuyama T et al. Treatment of delirium with risperidone in cancer patients. *Psychiatry Clin Neurosci.* 2012; 66:411-7.
211. Leso L, Schwartz T. Ziprasidone treatment of delirium. *Psychosomatics.* 2002; 43:61-2.
212. Young CC, Lujan E. Intravenous ziprasidone for treatment of delirium in the intensive care unit. *Anesthesiology.* 2004; 101:794-5.
213. Girard TD, Pandharipande PP, Carson SS et al. Feasibility, efficacy, and safety of antipsychotics for ICU delirium: the MIND randomized, placebo-controlled trial. *Crit Care Med.* 2010; 38:428-37.
214. Rea RS, Battistone S, Fong JJ et al. Atypical antipsychotics versus haloperidol for treatment of delirium in acutely ill patients. *Pharmacotherapy.* 2007; 27:588-94.
215. Ozbolt LB, Paniagua MA, Kaiser RM. Atypical antipsychotics for the treatment of delirious elders. *J Am Med Dir Assoc.* 2008; 9:18-28.
216. Khan BA, Zawahiri M, Campbell NL et al. Delirium in hospitalized patients: implications of current evidence on clinical practice and future avenues for research—a systematic evidence review. *J Hosp Med.* 2012; 7:580-9.
217. Yoon HJ, Park KM, Choi WJ et al. Efficacy and safety of haloperidol versus atypical antipsychotic medications in the treatment of delirium. *BMC Psychiatry.* 2013; 13:240.
218. Grover S, Kumar V, Chakrabarti S. Comparative efficacy study of haloperidol, olanzapine and risperidone in delirium. *J Psychosom Res.* 2011; 71:277-81.
219. Wang HR, Woo YS, Bahk WM. Atypical antipsychotics in the treatment of delirium. *Psychiatry Clin Neurosci.* 2013; 67:323-31.
220. MedWatch, the FDA safety information and adverse event reporting system. Antipsychotics, conventional and atypical. http://www.fda.gov/medwatch/safety/2008/safety08.htm#Antipsychotics. (accessed 2017 Dec 12).

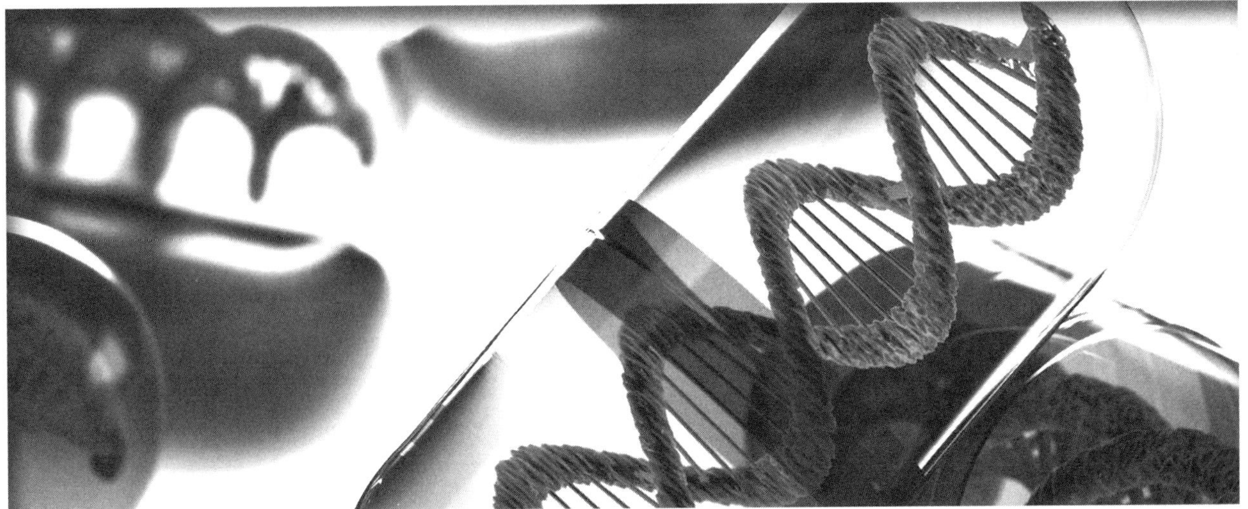

CHAPTER 16

Sleep Disorders

Lisa L. Forsyth

Sleep is essential, comprising approximately one third of life.[1] Drug-induced sleep disorders, such as insomnia, may be reported as difficulty falling asleep, not feeling rested despite adequate time to sleep, and/or daytime sleepiness. Although sleep disturbances may be caused by a variety of medical or psychiatric conditions, drugs always must be carefully considered as a potential cause of these symptoms.

CAUSATIVE AGENTS

Drugs that affect the central nervous system may cause altered patterns of sleep and wakefulness. These effects may be present immediately upon initiation of therapy or following withdrawal of therapy. In addition, drugs may exacerbate primary sleep disorders. Drugs that are reported to cause sleep disorders are listed in **Table 16-1**.[2-60]

EPIDEMIOLOGY

Insomnia is reported in approximately one third of adults in the United States and is considered to be a serious problem in about 50% of those afflicted.[61-63] The overall incidence of drug-induced sleep disturbances in the general population is not known, but individual agents are associated with incidences ranging from 1% to 55% (Table 16-1).[64]

MECHANISMS

Humans, along with most mammals, undergo two phases of sleep: rapid eye movement (REM) and nonrapid eye movement sleep (NREM).[65] NREM sleep is subdivided into stages 1 through 4. A full cycle of NREM and REM sleep requires approximately 90 minutes; and this cycle is repeated approximately four to six times throughout the night. Researchers do not yet fully understand all the functions of REM and NREM sleep and their relationship to the symptoms of sleep disturbance. Elderly individuals experience alterations in sleep patterns manifested typically as decreases in REM, stages 3 and 4 of NREM, and total sleep time. These changes have been found to correspond to added awakenings and total time spent awake at night.[66-68]

Several neurotransmitters are responsible for the sleep cycle.[69] The neurochemistry responsible

Table 16-1 Agents Implicated in Drug-Induced Sleep Disorders

Drug	Incidence	Level of Evidence[a]
α_2 AGONISTS[5,6]	30–75%	B
Clonidine	Sedation, nightmares	
Methyldopa	Insomnia, sedation, nightmares	
ANTICONVULSANTS[7-12]		
Carbamazepine	NK	C
Felbamate	8.6%	B
Lamotrigine	NK	C
Phenytoin	NK	C
ANTIPARKINSONIAN AGENTS[13-19]		
Amantadine	14%	B
Entacapone	30%	B
Levodopa–carbidopa	75%	B
Pergolide, bromocriptine	42%	B
Selegiline	10–32%	B
Trihexyphenidyl, benztropine	NK	C
β-BLOCKERS[5,20-22] (lipophilic: propranolol, timolol)	2–4.3%	B
β-BLOCKERS WITH α-BLOCKING ACTIVITY[23,24]		B
Carvedilol	3–11%	
Labetalol	1–4%	
MAO INHIBITORS[40]		
Phenelzine, tranylcypromine	NK, daytime sleepiness	B
SNRIs		
Desvenlafaxine[41]	6–15%	B
Duloxetine[42,43]	12.6%	B
Venlafaxine[25,44-47]	Insomnia 8% Sedation 13–31%	B
SSRIs		
Citalopram[48]	NK	C
Escitalopram[43]	4.9%	B
Fluoxetine[25,48-51]	Insomnia 5–19% Daytime sedation 5–18%	B
Fluvoxamine[25,49,52]	Insomnia 10–15% Daytime sedation 14–26%	B
Paroxetine[25,49,51,53,54]	Insomnia 8–14% Daytime sedation 2–21%	B
Sertraline[25,48]	Insomnia 7–16% Daytime sedation 7–13%	B
STATINS		
Atorvastatin[56]	3%	C
Lovastatin[57,58]	0.5–1%	C

Table 16-1 Agents Implicated in Drug-Induced Sleep Disorders (continued)

Drug	Incidence	Level of Evidence[a]
MISCELLANEOUS		
Alcohol[2]	NK	C
Bupropion[25,26]	5–19%	B
(Naltrexone–bupropion)	9.2%	C
Corticosteroids[27-38]	12–70%	B
Locaserin[39]	3.5%	C
Stimulants[30,59,60] (e.g., caffeine, cocaine, methylphenidate, theophylline)	46–55%	B

MAO = monoamine oxidase, NK = not known, SNRI = serotonin-norepinephrine reuptake inhibitor, SSRI = selective serotonin reuptake inhibitor.
[a]Definitions for Levels of Evidence: Level A—evidence from one or more randomized, controlled clinical trials; Level B—evidence from nonrandomized clinical trials, prospective observational studies, cohort studies, retrospective studies, case-control studies, meta-analyses and/or postmarketing surveillance studies; and Level C—evidence from one or more published case reports or case series.

for sleepiness and wakefulness has not been fully elucidated, and it is unknown whether one or more neurotransmitters is responsible for sleeping or awakening.[70] A primary function of norepinephrine-containing neurons is to regulate the sleep pattern. Wakefulness is believed to be mediated by norepinephrine, dopamine, acetylcholine, and serotonin.[71] Hypocretin (orexin) is a neuropeptide secreted by the hypothalamus and believed to promote sleep.[69] Melatonin is secreted by the pineal gland in conjunction with dark-light cycles and may promote sleep.

There are three primary mechanisms of drug-induced sleep disturbances (**Table 16-2**).[72-75] First, the desired effects of a drug may affect the neurotransmitters or receptor sites responsible for sleepiness. Second, the sedative effects of drugs used to treat insomnia may carry over into the daytime hours. Third, withdrawal of therapy may produce a sleep disturbance.

CLINICAL PRESENTATION AND DIFFERENTIAL DIAGNOSIS

Patients suffering from sleep disturbance often report an inability to fall asleep, to maintain sleep, or both, or of not feeling rested after having time to sleep.[72-75] Often these complaints are followed by daytime sleepiness and an inability to concentrate. The common signs and symptoms of sleep disorders are listed in **Table 16-3**. A number of medical and psychiatric conditions (**Table 16-4**) are known to affect sleep, and these must be considered when evaluating a patient for a possible drug-induced sleep disorder.[73,74] Polysomnography (PSG) is an assessment of electrophysiologic parameters during sleep and includes an electroencephalogram, electrooculogram, and electromyelogram.[74] Other measures of sleep include sleep latency (time to fall asleep), REM latency (time to first REM sleep), number of awakenings, and the number of stage shifts during sleep.[65,74]

The effects of drugs on sleep are often identified and characterized based on subjective data, PSG measures, objective evidence of sleepiness and alertness from a Multiple Sleep Latency Test (MSLT), wrist actigraphy, and/or by objective performance data.[65,69] The MSLT measures the time to fall asleep in order to evaluate excessive daytime sleepiness. Wrist actigraphy determines the sleep time by measuring wrist movements. Evidence of sleep disturbance on the PSG does not always correlate with patients' subjective complaints.[72-74] Bupropion and venlafaxine have been reported to induce insomnia in as little as 4 days and up to 4 weeks, respectively, following initiation of therapy.[64,75] The time of onset of insomnia associated with the other agents listed in Table 16-1 is highly variable.

Patient assessment should begin with a medication history and physical examination. Further

Table 16-2 Mechanisms of Drug-Induced Sleep Disorders

Drug	Mechanism (neurotransmitter/PSG data)
Alcohol[2-4]	Mechanism unknown, occurs upon withdrawal ↑W, ↓TST
α_2 agonists[5,6]	α_2 receptor agonism No PSG studies available
Antiparkinson agents[13-19]	Effect on various neurotransmitters specific to each drug ↑W, ↓TST
β-blockers[5,20-22]	β-adrenergic inhibitor, lipophilic agents ↑W, ↓TST, ↑S1, ↓REM
β-blockers with α-blocking activity[23,24]	β- and α-antagonism No PSG studies available
Bupropion[25,26]	DA uptake inhibition Minimal PSG data
Corticosteroids[27-38]	Mechanism unknown ↑W, ↑S2, ↓REM
MAO inhibitors[40]	Inhibits MAO enzyme that degrades NE, 5-HT, DA ↓REM, ↑W, ↓TST
SNRIs[25,41-47]	5-HT, NE uptake inhibition, weak affects on DA uptake; ↑W, ↓TST
SSRIs[25,43,48-54]	5-HT uptake inhibition In general ↑W, ↓TST
Statins[56-58]	Mechanism unknown Minimal PSG data, ↑W observed
Stimulants[30,59,60]	Release of various neurotransmitters ↑W, ↓TST

5-HT = 5-hydroxytryptamine (serotonin), DA = dopamine agonists, MAO = monoamine oxidase, NE = norepinephrine, PSG = polysomnography, REM = rapid eye movement, SNRI = serotonin-norepinephrine reuptake inhibitor, SSRI = selective serotonin reuptake inhibitor, S1 = stage 1 sleep, S2 = stage 2 sleep, TST = total sleep time, W = wakefulness.

Table 16-3 Signs and Symptoms Associated with Drug-Induced Sleep-Disorders[72,74]

- Inability to fall asleep
- Inability to maintain sleep
- Not feeling rested following adequate sleep duration
- Excessive daytime sleepiness
- Poor cognitive performance
- Lack of concentration

psychiatric assessment should be undertaken if indicated. When a drug-induced sleep disorder is suspected, patients should be questioned regarding the use of medications known to affect neurotransmitters, the frequency and timing of drug administration, and any history of recent discontinuation of medication.[72] The utility of sleep studies in the diagnosis and characterization of drug-induced sleep disturbance has not been determined.

RISK FACTORS

Specific risk factors for drug-induced sleep disorders have not been definitively elucidated. Older age (beginning in middle-aged adults) and female sex are known risk factors for insomnia, but it is not known if they also are risk factors for drug-induced sleep disorders.[64] Most studies that have attempted to evaluate drug effects on sleep have been conducted in healthy individuals, primarily men, who

Table 16-4 Conditions to Consider in the Differential Diagnosis of Drug-Induced Sleep Disorders[73,74]

Medical

Neurologic

- Delirium
- Epilepsy
- Parkinson disease

Respiratory

- Asthma
- Obstructive sleep apnea

Cardiovascular

- Arrhythmias
- Heart failure

Gastrointestinal

- Gastroesophageal reflux
- Peptic ulcer disease

Endocrine

- Diabetes mellitus
- Hyperthyroidism

Chronic pain

Pregnancy

Psychiatric

Mood Disorders

- Depression
- Mania

Anxiety Disorders

- Generalized anxiety disorder
- Obsessive-compulsive disorder
- Panic

Situational

- Work or financial
- Interpersonal conflict
- Major life events
- Jet lag
- Shift work

Table 16-5 Risk Factors for Drug-Induced Sleep Disorders[64,74]

- Female sex
- Older age
- Concomitant therapy with ≥2 agents with central nervous system effects
- Drug interaction

may respond differently than patients with disease.[64] In addition, the treatment population may already have sleep disturbances or impaired daytime performance prior to the initiation of drug therapy. Both age and drug dose contribute to the frequency of sleep disturbances associated with β-blockers.[64] Potential risk factors for drug-induced sleep disorders are listed in **Table 16-5**.

In addition to directly causing sleep disturbances, drugs may exacerbate symptoms and increase the risk of primary sleep disorders. One example is obstructive sleep apnea, which is characterized by loud snoring and gasping or apneic episodes during sleep. Patients with sleep apnea typically experience excessive daytime sleepiness and poor performance. A patient's apneic episodes may worsen in association with the use of sedative/hypnotic agents, and daytime symptoms may become more severe.[64,72] In addition, the menopausal symptom of "hot flashes" during nighttime hours has been reported as a cause of insomnia following the discontinuation of hormone-replacement therapy.

MORBIDITY AND MORTALITY

Sleep disorders may impair quality of life beyond excessive daytime sleepiness. It has been reported that those who suffer insomnia receive fewer career promotions, demonstrate poor productivity, and have a higher rate of absenteeism.[74,75] In addition to poor performance during the daytime hours at work, there is an increased risk of motor vehicle accidents reported in individuals experiencing insomnia. Nearly 70 million Americans suffer from a sleep disorder, which may have negative consequences on their overall health and well-being.[76] The total cost of insomnia in 2011 was estimated at nearly $63 billion.[75] It is difficult to quantify the financial burden of insomnia because patients often have other comorbidities that contribute to the expenses.[76] Healthcare costs are up to 60% higher in patients with insomnia.[77]

Obstructive sleep apnea has been associated with hypertension, the primary mechanism of which is sympathetic hyperactivity.[78] In addition, sleep deprivation experienced for one night has been linked to hypertension in the ambulatory care setting.[79,80]

Decreased sleep duration may impair glucose tolerance and insulin sensitivity.[81-84] Insulin resistance, like hypertension, may be linked to the increased sympathetic outflow associated with reduced sleep duration. One investigation that spanned 10 years suggested that sleep duration of 5 hours or less may be a significant risk factor for the development of diabetes.[81] Currently, there are no data regarding the incidence of morbidity or mortality directly associated with drug-induced sleep disorders.

PREVENTION

Prevention of drug-induced sleep disorders requires a better understanding of the basic functions and different stages of sleep. Basic and clinical research is necessary to allow clinicians to anticipate possible sleep disturbances based on the pharmacological properties of specific drugs. Nonpharmacological measures to improve sleep hygiene (**Table 16-6**) are useful and have been shown to improve sleep patterns in 70–80% of patients.[85]

Table 16-6 Approaches to Help Prevent Drug-Induced Sleep Disorders[65,85]

Sleep hygiene

- Establish a regular bedtime and wake up time including weekends
- Sleep only as much as necessary
- Go to bed only when sleepy, using the bed only for sleep and intimacy
- Avoid long periods of wakefulness while in bed
- Avoid trying to force sleep; after 30 minutes, leave the bed to do something relaxing (watch television, listen to music, or read)
- Avoid daytime naps
- Do not take your worries to bed
- Exercise regularly (three to four times weekly); however, exercising near bedtime may cause arousal
- Create comfortable sleeping environment (steady temperature, lack of light source)
- Reduce or discontinue the use of alcohol, caffeine, or nicotine
- Avoid hunger or fullness at bedtime
- Avoid drinking large amounts of liquids in the evening to prevent trips to the restroom at night
- Engage in a relaxing or enjoyable activity before bedtime

Pharmacologic approach

- Discontinue agents with potential to cause drug-induced sleep disturbances when possible
- If unable to discontinue potentially causative agents:
  - Change time of administration to earlier in the day
  - Reduce dose to decrease symptoms (e.g., selegiline)

MANAGEMENT

As sleep disturbances may affect all aspects of an individual's life, all symptoms should be investigated carefully. Management of drug-induced sleep disorders requires a thorough understanding of the pharmacology, especially the neurotransmitter activity, of each of the patient's medications. It also is important to consider drug combinations with possible additive central nervous system effects and drug interactions that may potentiate drug effects by altering pharmacokinetics or pharmacodynamics. The first step in management involves discontinuation of agents with potential to cause drug-induced sleep disorders (Table 16-1 and 16-6). The time frame for resolution of symptoms following drug discontinuation is a function of the agent's half-life.

In some cases, such as in patients with seizure disorders, discontinuation of the potentially causative agent is not possible and alternative measures are required. Changing the time of drug administration to earlier in the day may help reduce symptoms for some patients. With some drugs (e.g., selegiline) symptoms are reported most often in association with higher doses, and dose reduction may be helpful.

It is reasonable to employ drug therapy for insomnia when all other measures to resolve a drug-induced sleep disorder have failed. For insomnia requiring short-term treatment, there is no difference in efficacy between benzodiazepines, antidepressants, or sedative-hypnotic agents.[74,85,86] Patients with difficulty falling asleep or with excessive daytime sleepiness may benefit from therapy with a short-acting benzodiazepine such as triazolam or a hypnotic agent such as zolpidem, zaleplon, or eszopiclone.[56,84-87] Patients who are unable to maintain sleep or have trouble awakening may benefit from therapy with an intermediate-acting benzodiazepine such as estazolam or temazepam. The long-acting benzodiazepines (flurazepam and quazepam) may be helpful when there is daytime anxiety in addition to sleep disturbance. There is no rationale, however, for the concomitant use of two benzodiazepines for the treatment of insomnia and anxiety. In all cases, the lowest effective dose should be administered for the shortest possible period of time. Tolerance can develop in as little as 2 weeks with continuous use of some benzodiazepines.[75] One strategy used to help prevent tolerance involves the administration of benzodiazepines for only 3–4 days per week rather than daily.

Two medications recently approved by the U.S. Food and Drug Administration may be effective for treating insomnia: suvorexant and ramelteon. Suvorexant, an orexin antagonist, increases total sleep time by reducing time to sleep onset and awakening after falling asleep.[87] Ramelteon, a melatonin-receptor agonist, modestly improved time to sleep onset but had no effect on total sleep time.[88] There are currently no published data regarding the efficacy of these agents for managing drug-induced sleep disorders.

When long-term treatment of insomnia is required, antidepressants are among potential options.[86] Trazodone may be effective at doses of 50–100 mg for insomnia associated with fluoxetine and bupropion.[89] An advantage of trazodone is its lack of anticholinergic activity. Doxepin has also shown promise in treating antidepressant-induced insomnia and maintains normal nocturnal melatonin secretion.[86] Several other agents, such as antipsychotics (mirtazapine) and melatonin, have been used for the long-term treatment of insomnia but supporting data are limited, and these agents are associated with adverse effects.

Most patients initially seek a nonprescription remedy for the treatment of sleep symptoms. Unfortunately, there are limited data regarding the efficacy of nonprescription drugs.[90] Of the many options available, melatonin is the only agent that has undergone extensive evaluation of its circadian effects and hypnotic properties. Limited and contradictory evidence is available for the efficacy of histamine H_1-receptor antagonists and valerian. Other alternative agents for which some supportive data exist include passionflower, chamomile, St. John's Wort, kava, wild lettuce, patrinia root, and vitamins and supplements (calcium, vitamin A, nicotinamide, magnesium, and vitamin B_{12}).[90] Potential harm of these agents should be considered as the products are not standardized, which discourages healthcare providers from recommending them for routine treatment.[65]

When a treatment is initiated for a sleep disorder, the lowest effective dose should be prescribed. Ideally, these agents should be used for the shortest period of time possible, but this may not be feasible for those patients requiring a longer duration of therapy. Patients under treatment for drug-induced sleep disorders should be routinely monitored to assess the effectiveness of drug therapy and to ensure the resolution of symptoms.

INFORMATION FOR PATIENTS

Patients who are prescribed medications that are known to cause sleep disorders should be instructed to contact their healthcare provider if they experience difficulty falling asleep, do not feel rested after having adequate time to sleep, or are excessively tired during the day. Sleep hygiene education should be provided to patients to identify opportunities to improve sleep disturbances. Patients should be advised to consult with their physician or pharmacist before beginning treatment with any nonprescription medication to avoid interactions that could precipitate sleep disturbances. Finally, patients should be warned not to change the dose or administration times of prescribed medications without consultation with their physician or pharmacist.

REFERENCES

1. Kirkwood CK. Management of insomnia. *J Am Pharm Assoc.* 1999; 39:688-96.
2. Gillin JC, Smith TL, Irwin M et al. EEG sleep studies in "pure" primary alcoholism during subacute withdrawal: Relations to normal controls, age and other clinical variables. *Biol Psychiatry* 1990; 27:477-88.
3. Landolt HP, Roth C, Dijk DJ, Borbély AA. Late-afternoon ethanol intake affects nocturnal sleep and the sleep EEG in middle-aged men. *J Clin Psychopharmacol.* 1996; 6:428-36.
4. Vitiello MV. Sleep, alcohol and alcohol abuse. *Addict Biol.* 1997; 2:151-8.
5. Paykel ES, Fleminger R, Watson JP. Psychiatric side effects of antihypertensive drugs other than reserpine. *J Clin Psycopharmacol.* 1982; 2:14-39.
6. Kostis JB, Rosen RC, Holzer BC et al. CNS side effects of centrally-active antihypertensive agents: a prospective, placebo-controlled study of sleep, mood state, and cognitive and sexual function in hypertensive males. *Psychopharmacology.* 1990; 102:163-70.

7. Roder-Wanner UU, Noachtar S, Wolf P. Response of polygraphic sleep to phenytoin treatment for epilepsy: a longitudinal study of immediate, short- and long-term effects. *Acta Neurol Scand.* 1987; 76:157.
8. Wolf P, Roder-Wanner U-U, Brede M. Influence of therapeutic phenobarbital and phenytoin medication on the polygraphic sleep of patients with epilepsy. *Epilepsia.* 1984; 25:467.
9. Foldvary N, Perry M, Lee J et al. The effect of lamotrigine on sleep in patients with epilepsy. *Epilepsia.* 2001; 42:1569-73.
10. US Food and Drug Administration. Carbamazepine (Carbatrol) package insert. http://pi.shirecontent.com/PI/PDFs/Carbatrol_USA_ENG.pdf (accessed 2017 Dec 14).
11. US Food and Drug Administration. Felbamate (Felbatol) package insert. http://www.accessdata.fda.gov/drugsatfda_docs/label/2009/020189s022lbl.pdf (accessed 2017 Dec 14).
12. Sammaritano M, Sherwin A. Effect of anticonvulsants on sleep. *Neurology.* 2000; 54:S16-24.
13. Navsieda PA, Glantz R, Weber S et al. Psychiatric complications of levodopa therapy of Parkinson's disease. *Adv Neurol.* 1984; 40:271-7.
14. Navsieda PA, Weiner WJ, Kaplan LR et al. Sleep disruption in the course of chronic levodopa therapy:an early feature of the levodopa psychosis. *Clin Neuropharmacol.* 1982; 5:183-4.
15. Chrisp P, Mammen GJ, Sorkin EM. Selegiline. A Review of its pharmacology, symptomatic benefits and protective potential in Parkinson's disease. *Drugs Aging.* 1991; 1:228-48.
16. Jeanty P, van der Kerchove M, Lowental A et al. Pergolide therapy in Parkinson's disease. *J Neurol.* 1984; 231:148-52.
17. Vardi J, Glaubman H, Rabey J et al. EEG sleep patterns in parkinsonian patients treated with bromocryptine and L-dopa: a comparative study. *J Neural Transm.* 1979; 45:307-16.
18. Schwab RS, Poskanzer DC, England AC et al. Amantadine in Parkinson's disease: review of more than two years' experience. *JAMA.* 1972; 222:792-5.
19. Larsen JP, Worm-Peterson J, Siden A et al. The tolerability and efficacy of entacapone over 3 years in patients with Parkinson's disease. *Eur J Neur.* 2003; 10:137-46.
20. Rosen, RC, Kostis JB. Biobehavioral sequellae associated with adrenergic-inhibiting antihypertensive agents: a critical review. *Health Psychol.* 1985; 4:579-604.
21. McAinsh J, Cruickshank JM. Beta-blockers and central nervous system side effects. *Pharmacology.* 1990; 46:163-97.
22. Gleiter CH, Deckert J. Adverse CNS-effects of beta-adrenoceptor blockers. *Pharmacopsychiatry.* 1996; 29:201-11.
23. Pearce CJ, Wallin JD. Labetalol and other agents that block both alpha- and beta-adrenergic receptors. *Cleve Clin J Med.* 1994; 61:59-69.
24. Dunn CJ, Lea AP, Wagstaff AJ. Carvedilol: a reappraisal of its pharmacological properties and therapeutic use in cardiovascular disorders. *Drugs.* 1997; 54:161-85.
25. Preskorn SH. Comparison of the tolerability of bupropion, fluoxetine, imipramine, nefazodone, paroxetine, sertraline, and venlafaxine. *J Clin Psychiatry.* 1995; 56(suppl 6):12-21.
26. US Food and Drug Administration. Naltrexone-bupropion (Contrave) package insert. http://general.takedapharm.com/content/file.aspx?filetypecode=CONTRAVEPI&cacheRandomizer=7516104b-c0aa-4933-a1cd-d15c644e8ee0 (accessed 2017 Dec 14).
27. Chrousos GA, Kattah JC, Beck RW et al.; the Optic Neuritis Study Group. Side effects of glucocorticoid treatment: experience of the optic neuritis treatment trial. *JAMA.* 1993; 269:2110-2.
28. Drigan R, Spirito A, Gleber RD. Behavioral effects of corticosteroids in children with acute lymphoblastic leukemia. *Med Pediatric Oncol.* 1992; 20:13-21.
29. Harris JC, Carel CA, Rosenberg LA et al. Intermittent high dose corticosteroid treatment in childhood cancer: behavioral and emotional consequences. *J Am Acad Child Adolesc Psychiatry.* 1988; 27:720-5.
30. Bailey WC, Richards JM, Manzella BA et al. Characteristics and correlates of asthma in a university clinic population. *Chest.* 1990; 98:821-8.
31. Gillin JC, Jacobs LS, Fram DH et al. Acute effect of a glucocorticoid on normal human sleep. *Nature.* 1972; 237:398-9.
32. Born J, Zwick A, Roth G et al. Differential effects of hydrocortisone, fluocortolone, and aldosterone on nocturnal sleep in humans. *Acta Endocrinol.* 1987; 116:129-37.
33. Fehm HL, Benkowitsch R, Kern W et al. Influences of corticosteroids, dexamethasone and hydrocortisone on sleep in humans. *Neuropsychobiology.* 1986; 16:198-204.
34. Rosenthal L, Folkerts M, Helmus T et al. Administration of dexamethasone and its effects on sleep and daytime alertness. *Sleep Res.* 1995; 24:58.
35. Janson C, Gislason T, Boman G et al. Sleep disturbances in patients with asthma. *Respir Med.* 1990; 84:37-42.
36. Wolkowitz OM, Rubinow D, Doran AR et al. Prednisone effects on neurochemistry and behavior: preliminary findings. *Arch Gen Psychiatry.* 1990; 47:963-8.
37. Lozada F, Silverman S, Migliorati C. Adverse side effects associated with prednisone in the treatment of patients with oral inflammatory ulcerative diseases. *J Am Dent Assoc* 1984; 109:269-70.
38. Kenna H, Poon A, de los Angeles C, Koran L. Psychiatric complications of treatment with corticosteroids: review with case report. *Psychiatry Clin Neurosci.* 2011; 65:549-60.
39. US Food and Drug Administration. Locaserin package insert. http://www.accessdata.fda.gov/drugsatfda_docs/label/2012/022529lbl.pdf (accessed 2017 Dec 14).
40. Remick RA, Froese C, Keller FD. Common side effects associated with monoamine oxidase inhibitors. *Prog Neuropsychopharmacol Biol Psychiatry.* 1989; 13:497-504.
41. US Food and Drug Administration. Desvenlafaxine (Pristiq) package insert. http://www.accessdata.fda.gov/drugsatfda_docs/label/2012/021992s030lbl.pdf (2017 Dec 14).
42. Wade A, Gembert K, Florea I. A comparative study of the efficacy of acute and continuation treatment with escitalopram versus duloxetine in patients with major depressive disorder. *Curr Med Res Opin.* 2007; 23:1605-14.
43. Wohlreich NM, Mallinckrodt CH, Watkin JG et al. Immediate switching of antidepressant therapy: results from a clinical trial of duloxetine. *Ann Clin Psychiatry.* 2005; 17:259-68.
44. Cunningham LA, Borison RL, Carman JS et al. A comparison of venlafaxine, trazodone, and placebo in major depression. *J Clin Psychopharmacol.* 1994; 14:99-106.
45. Augustin BF, Cold JA, Jann MW. Venlafaxine and nefazodone, two pharmacologically distinct antidepressants. *Pharmacotherapy.* 1997; 17:511-530.
46. Nelson JC. Safety and tolerability of the new antidepressants. *J Clin Psychiatry.* 1997; 58(suppl 6):26-31.
47. Salin-Pascual RJ, Galicia-Polo L, Drucker-Colin R. Sleep changes after 4 consecutive days of venlafaxine administration in normal volunteers. *J Clin Psychiatry.* 1997; 58:348-350.
48. Bech P, Ciadella P. Citalopram in depression: meta-analysis of intended and unintended effects. *Int Clin Psychopharmacol.* 1992; 6(suppl 5):45-54.
49. Grimsley SR, Jann MW. Paroxetine, sertraline, and fluvoxamine: new selective serotonin reuptake inhibitors. *Clin Pharm.* 1992; 11:930-57.
50. Dorsey CM, Lukas SE, Cunningham SL. Fluoxetine-induced sleep disturbance in depressed patients. *Neuropsychopharmacology.* 1996; 14:437-42.
51. Saletu B, Frey R, Krupka M et al. Sleep laboratory studies on the single-dose effects of serotonin reuptake inhibitors paroxetine and fluoxetine on human sleep and awakening qualities. *Sleep.* 1991; 14:439-447.

52. Kupfer DJ, Perel JM, Pollock BF et al. Fluvoxamine versus desipramine: comparative polysomnographic effects. *Biol Psychiatry*. 1991; 29:23-40
53. Oswald I, Adam K. Effects of paroxetine on human sleep. *Br J Clin Pharmacol*. 1986; 22:97-9.
54. Richels K, Schwizer E. Clinical overview of serotonin re-uptake inhibitors. *J Clin Psychiatry*. 1990; 51(suppl B):9-12.
55. Sharpley SL, Williamson DJ, Attenburrow MEJ et al. The effects of paroxetine and nefazodone on sleep: a placebo controlled trial. *Psychopharmacology (Berl)*. 1996; 126:50-4.
56. US Food and Drug Administration. Atorvastatin (Lipitor) package insert. http://www.accessdata.fda.gov/drugsatfda_docs/label/2009/020702s056lbl.pdf (accessed 2017 Dec 14).
57. Tobert JA, Shear CL, Chremos AN et al. Clinical experience with lovastatin. *Am J Cardiol*. 1990; 65:23-6.
58. Rosenson RS, Goranson NL. Lovastatin-associated sleep and mood disturbances. *Am J Med*. 1993; 95:548-9.
59. Kaplan J, Fredrickson PA, Renaux SA et al. Theophylline effect on sleep in normal subjects. *Chest*. 1993; 103:193-5.
60. Janson C, Gislason T, Almqvist M et al. Theophylline disturbs sleep mainly in caffeine-sensitive persons. *Pulm Pharmacol*. 1989; 2:125-9.
61. Kupfer DJ, Reynolds CF. Management of insomnia. *N Engl J Med*. 1997; 336:341-6.
62. National Sleep Foundation. 2014 sleep in America poll: sleep in the modern family. https://sleepfoundation.org/sites/default/files/2014-NSF-Sleep-in-America-poll-summary-of-findings—FINAL-Updated-3-26-14-.pdf (accessed 2017 Dec 14).
63. Farney RJ, Walker JM. Office management of common sleep-wake disorders. *Med Clin North Am*. 1995; 79:391-414.
64. Schweitzer PK, Randazzo AC. Drugs that disturb sleep and wakefulness. In: Kryger MH, Roth T, Dement WC, eds. *Principles and practice of sleep medicine*. 6th ed. Philadelphia: Elsevier; 2017.
65. Duong M, Passarella S. Diagnosis and treatment of insomnia. *Am J Health-Syst Pharm*. 2008; 65:927-34.
66. Neylan TC, Reynolds CF, Kupfer DJ. Sleep disorders. In: Hales RE, Yudofsky SC, Talbott JT, eds. *American Psychiatric Press textbook of psychiatry*. 2nd ed. Arlington, VA: American Psychiatric Press; 1994:844.
67. Ancoli-Isreal S. Insomnia in the elderly: A review for the primary care practitioner. *Sleep*. 2000; 23:S23-30.
68. Espiritiu JRD. Aging-related sleep changes. *Clin Geriatr Med*. 2008; 24:1-14.
69. Stevens S, Hening WA. Sleep and wakefulness. In: Goetz CG, ed. *Textbook of clinical neurology*. 3rd ed. Philadelphia: Elsevier; 2007.
70. Roehrs T, Carskadon MA, Dement WC et al. Daytime sleepiness and alertness. In: Kryger MH, Roth T, Dement WC, eds. *Principles and practice of sleep medicine*. 6th ed. Philadelphia: Elsevier; 2017.
71. Krystal AD. Antidepressant and antipsychotic drugs. *Sleep Med Clin*. 2010; 5:571-89.
72. Rajput V, Bromley SM. Chronic insomnia: a practical review. *Am Fam Physician*. 1999; 60:1431-42.
73. Novak M, Shapiro CM. Drug-induced sleep disturbances. *Drug Safety*. 1997;16:133-49.
74. Schutte-Rodin S, Broch L, Buysse D et al. Clinical guideline for the evaluation and management of chronic insomnia in adults. *J Clin Sleep Med*. 2008; 4:487-504.
75. Buysse DJ. Insomnia. *JAMA*. 2013; 309:706-16.
76. American academy of sleep medicine. Insomnia costing US workforce $63.2 billion a year in lost productivity, study shows. http://www.aasmnet.org/articles.aspx?id=2521 (accessed 2017 Dec 14).
77. Fullerton DS. The economic impact of insomnia in managed care: a clearer picture emerges. *Am J Manag Care*. 2006; 12:S246-52.
78. Narkiewicz K, Pesek CA, Kato M et al. Baroreflex control of sympathetic nerve activity and heart rate in obstructive sleep apnea. *Hypertension*. 1998; 32:1039-43.
79. Lusardi P, Mugellini A, Preti P et al. Effects of a restricted sleep regimen on ambulatory blood pressure monitoring in normotensive subjects. *Am J Hyperten*. 1996; 9:503-5.
80. Zhong X, Hilton HJ, Gates GJ et al. Increased sympathetic and decreased parasympathetic cardiovascular modulation in normal humans with acute sleep deprivation. *J App Physiol*. 2005; 98;2024-32.
81. Gangwisch JE, Heymsfield SB, Boden-Albala B et al. Sleep duration as a risk factor for diabetes incidence in a large US sample. *Sleep*. 2007; 30:1667-73.
82. VanHelder T, Symons JD, Radomski MW. Effects of sleep deprivation and exercise on glucose tolerace. *Aviat Space Environ Med*. 1993; 6:487-92.
83. Spiegel K, Leproult R, Van Cauter E. Impact of sleep debt on metabolic and endocrine function. *Lancet*. 1999; 354:1435-39.
84. Mander B, Colecchia E, Spiegel K et al. Short sleep: a risk factor for insulin resistance and obesity. *Diabetes*. 2001; 50(suppl 2):A45.
85. Morin AK, Jarvis CI, Lynch AM. Therapeutic options for sleep-maintenance and sleep-onset insomnia. *Pharmacotherapy*. 2007; 27:89-110.
86. Wiegand MH. Antidepressants for the treatment of insomnia: a suitable approach? *Drugs*. 2008; 68:2411-7.
87. Winkelman JW. Insomnia disorder. *N Engl J Med*. 2015; 373:1437-44.
88. Mayer G, Wang-Weigand S, Roth-Schechter B et al. Efficacy and safety of 6-month nightly ramelteon administration in adults with chronic primary insomnia. *Sleep*. 2009; 32:351-60.
89. Nierenberg AA, Adler LA, Peselow E et al. Trazodone for antidepressant-associated insomnia. *Am J Psychiatry*. 1994; 151:1069-72.
90. Meoli AL, Rosen C, Kristo D et al. Oral nonprescription treatment for insomnia: An evaluation of products with limited evidence. *J Clin Sleep Med*. 2005; 1:173-87.

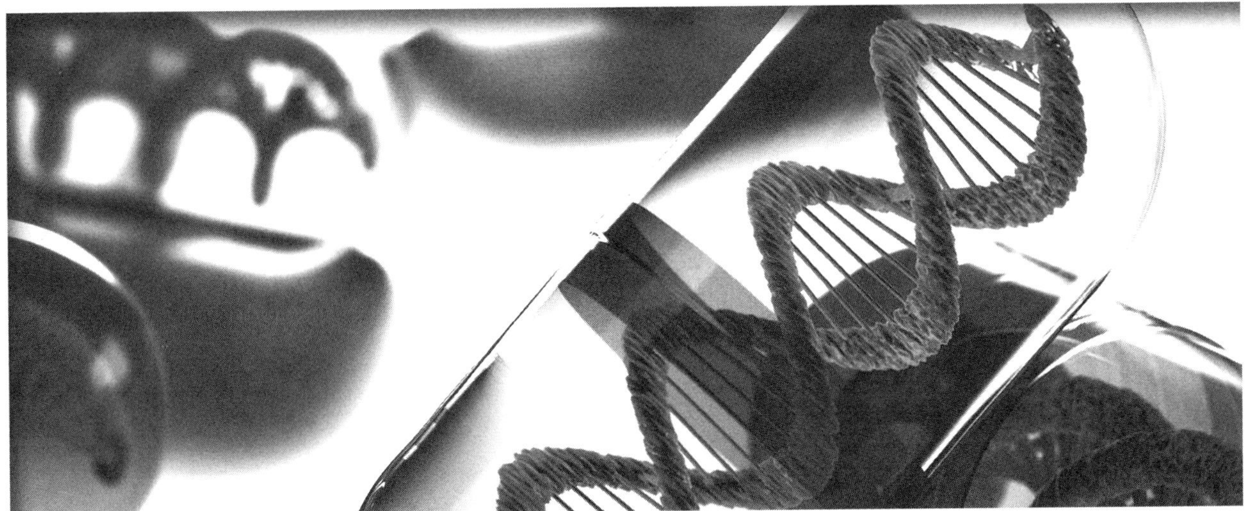

CHAPTER 17

Cognitive Disorders

Michele Y. Splinter

Cognitive function is a multidimensional concept for higher-order mental functions and processes.[1,2] Cognitive domains described in the *Diagnostic and Statistical Manual of Mental Disorders, 5th edition* (*DSM-5*), are perceptual-motor function, language, executive function, learning and memory, complex attention, and social cognition.[3] The *DSM-5* divides the neurocognitive disorders into three syndromes: delirium, mild cognitive disorders, and major cognitive disorders (dementia). Delirium is a disturbance in attention and awareness developing over a short period and is a consequence of another medical condition, substance intoxication or withdrawal, exposure to a toxin, or due to multiple etiologies, and is most often reversible after the insult is removed. Mild and major neurocognitive disorders represent a cognitive decline in performance in one or more cognitive domains and can be due to a number of etiologies including Alzheimer disease, vascular disease, frontotemporal lobar degeneration, and substance or medication use. The ability to live an independent life or not differentiates mild from major neurocognitive disorders.

CAUSATIVE AGENTS

Drugs that have been implicated as causes of cognitive disorders are listed in **Table 17-1**.[4-33] Effects associated with some medications, such as sedation from opiates, are experienced acutely. Cognitive effects of other medications are subtle and are often recognized only with long-term use. An example is slowing of cognitive processing speed in children leading to attention and memory deficits associated with phenobarbital.[34,35]

EPIDEMIOLOGY

It is difficult to determine the relative frequency of drug-induced cognitive disorders because of the diversity of drugs capable of causing cognitive impairment and the divergent demographic characteristics of study populations.[8] In one study, 22% of 229 consecutive hospitalized patients over 70 years of age experienced delirium.[35] Drug toxicity was identified as the most definitive cause of delirium and was the third most probable contributor, after infection and fluid and electrolyte imbalance.

Table 17-1 Agents Implicated in Drug-Induced Cognitive Disorders

Drug Class/Medication	Incidence	Level of Evidence[a]
Androgen-deprivation therapy[4]	NK	B
Anticholinergics[5,6]	18–20%[b]	A
Antiarrhythmics (amiodarone, digoxin, lidocaine)[7,8]	NK	C
Antibiotics[8,9]	NK	C
Antifungals[8,9]	NK	C
Antiretrovirals[8,9]	NK	C
Anticonvulsants	NK	B
Phenobarbital[10]	NK	B
Topiramate[11,12]	35%[c] 7–71%[d]	A
Valproic acid[13]	22%[e]	B
Antineoplastic agents[14,15]	4–75%[f]	A
Cyclophosphamide, thiotepa, carboplatin[1,7]	25%[g]	A
Antipsychotics[16,17]	NK	B
Antiparkinson agents[7,8,18]	NK	C
Benzodiazepines (chronic)[19]	22.2%	B
Glucocorticosteroids[8]	NK	C
Histamine-2-receptor antagonists[20]	0.2% (outpatient) 1.6–1.9% (inpatient)	B
Interferon alfa[21-24]	30–77%	B
Lithium[25,26]	NK	B
Non-nucleoside reverse transcriptase inhibitors[27,28]	18.9–23%	B
Nonsteroidal anti-inflammatory drugs[29-31]	NK	B
Opioids[32]	20–70%[h]	B
Selective serotonin reuptake inhibitors[33]	0.5%	B

NK = not known.
[a]Definitions for Levels of Evidence: Level A—evidence from one or more randomized, controlled clinical trials; Level B—evidence from nonrandomized clinical trials, prospective observational studies, cohort studies, retrospective studies, case-control studies, meta-analyses and/or postmarketing surveillance studies; and Level C—evidence from one or more published case reports or case series.
[b]Elderly.
[c]Healthy volunteers.
[d]Obese children—memory (71%), psychomotor speed (36%), language (29%), attention (29%), visual–spatial perception (14%), and intelligence (7%).
[e]Children of epileptic mothers who took valproate scoring ≤69 on verbal intelligence quotient (IQ).
[f]Varies depending on medication, regimen, population, stage of cancer, domain measured, time of measurement.
[g]High-risk patients with breast cancer receiving high-dose chemotherapy (cyclophosphamide, thiotepa, and carboplatin after receiving standard-dose chemotherapy).
[h]Varies depending on population (healthy, patient with cancer, or patient with nonmalignant pain—and whether tolerant to medication).

In another prospective study, 7% of 1,500 hospital neurologic consultations were for delirium, 17% of which were attributed to drugs.[37]

In an outpatient study of 308 patients older than 60 years of age with pre-existing global cognitive impairment, 35 (11.4%) experienced adverse drug reactions contributing to cognitive dysfunction.[38] Upon follow-up 1 year after enrollment, medications were determined to be the sole cause of cognitive changes in 10 of these patients, and in the others, cognitive function improved after discontinuation of the offending agent.

Commonly used instruments that can be administered within 10 minutes to screen for decline in cognition include the Mini-Mental State Exam and the Montreal Cognitive Assessment (MoCA).[39,40]

Table 17-2 Mechanisms of Drug-Induced Cognitive Disorders

Drug	Mechanisms
Anesthetics[43]	Neuronal apoptosis from activation of caspase and amyloid-β aggregation; tau phosphorylation; alteration of central cholinergic transmission through nicotinic and muscarinic receptors; upregulation of NMDA receptors causing excitotoxicity and apoptosis from calcium influx
Anticholinergics[44,45]	Age-related loss of acetylcholine and cholinergic cell bodies in nucleus basalis of Meynert; accumulation of amyloid-beta peptides in the cortex, hippocampus, and amygdala
Anticonvulsants[34,46,47]	Reduction of neuronal excitability; decrease in the expression of neurotrophins and β-estradiol causing dose-dependent apoptotic neurodegeneration in fetal brains
Antineoplastic agents[48-51]	Leukoencephalopathy, direct cytotoxic effects, cytokine-induced inflammatory response, chemotherapy-induced anemia and menopause; genetic risk factors (low-efficiency efflux pumps, deficits in DNA repair mechanisms), shortened telomere length, and decreased neurotransmitter activity and functional connectivity
Antipsychotics[52]	Decreased cholinergic enzyme choline acetyltransferase; decreased nicotinic and muscarinic acetylcholine receptors due to antagonist activity at dopaminergic-D_2 receptors; decreased nerve growth factor and brain-derived growth factor
Barbiturates[53,54]	Enhancement of GABA, decreased calcium uptake by neuronal membranes depressing excitability; reduction in number of fetal neurons and the length and branching frequency of dendrites
Benzodiazepines[53]	Enhancement of GABA activity
Glucocorticosteroids[55,56]	Hippocampal cell loss
Histamine-2-receptor antagonists[57]	Blockade of histamine-2 receptors in the cerebral cortex and corpus striatum
Interferon alfa[58]	Inhibition of dopaminergic activity
Nonsteroidal anti-inflammatory drugs[30]	Hypersensitivity response types 1 and 3 (aseptic meningitis) Inhibition of lipid beta-oxidation and mitochondrial disarrangement (Reye syndrome)
Opioids[32,59]	Inhibition of the cholinergic system; modulation of behavior of microglia and immune cells that mediate inflammation; apoptosis of microglia and neurons
Selective serotonin reuptake inhibitors[60,61]	Hyponatremia secondary to inappropriate antidiuretic hormone secretion
Tricyclic antidepressants[53]	Anticholinergic and antihistaminic effects

DNA = deoxyribonucleic acid, GABA = gamma-aminobutyric acid, NMDA = *N*-methyl-D-aspartate.

Reported incidences of cognitive disorders depend on the cognitive domain investigated and the measurement instrument used.[41] For example, more than 80 instruments have been employed to assess the different domains of cognitive function in patients with cancer. Several challenges to using cognitive assessments in cancer research have been identified, including the fact that baseline data may not reflect function before the cancer diagnosis, moderating variables (education, race, age, sex) may affect comparisons between groups or established norms, tests may be subject to practice and learning effects, and a valid comparison group is difficult to identify because cancer treatment is specific to diagnosis, stage, and biological factors characteristic of the specific malignancy.[1]

MECHANISMS

Several neuronal processes in the brain are associated with states of awareness.[42] Specific mechanisms of cognitive disorders associated with several classes of medications are summarized in **Table 17-2**.[30,34,43-61]

It has been proposed that neural pathways mediated by acetylcholine regulate conscious awareness and its intensity. Anticholinergic agents are used as antiemetics, antiparkinson agents, and antispasmodics, and have been associated with cognitive impairment.[7,18,62-64] In addition, drugs in many other classes possess anticholinergic properties, including tricyclic antidepressants, antipsychotics, antihistamines, and antiarrhythmics.[7,44] Memory loss in patients with Alzheimer disease or Parkinson disease with prominent dementia has been associated with a significant decline of cortical cholinergic innervation due to cell loss in the nucleus basalis.[65] High-frequency oscillations that unite information related to different aspects of a perceived object from widely distributed cortical neurons appear to emanate from the thalamus.[42] The action of acetylcholine in the cortex and thalamus and the interactions between the neurotransmitters acetylcholine, gamma-aminobutyric acid (GABA), and glutamate appear to be central to the maintenance of conscious awareness. Alzheimer disease is associated with amyloid plaque and formation of neurofibrillary tangles.[66] In a histological study from brains of patients over 70 years of age with Parkinson disease, anticholinergic use for greater than 2 years increased amyloid plaque and neurofibrillary tangle densities by twofold.[66] Authors hypothesized that there was acceleration of β amyloidosis and plaque formation in aging brains in these subjects induced by the antimuscarinic drugs. Rebound insomnia and anxiety have been reported in association with benzodiazepine and barbiturate withdrawal, and hallucinations and delirium have been associated with barbiturate withdrawal.[53] Down-regulation of high-affinity GABA receptors occurs during benzodiazepine and barbiturate therapy, and the withdrawal syndrome probably reflects a state of GABA underactivity in conjunction with a surge in output of excitatory neurotransmitters normally inhibited by GABA. There also appears to be a noradrenergic mechanism contributing to consciousness, as α_2-receptor antagonists and variations in norepinephrine concentrations alter anesthetic dose requirements.[42] In addition, α_2-receptor agonists increase the depth of anesthesia.

Anticonvulsant medications diminish neuronal irritability and therefore may inhibit neuronal excitability and impair cognitive function.[34,46] High serum concentrations of valproate have been shown to affect both function and morphology of the brain, possibly due to interference with pituitary adrenal function, hyperammonemia, or changes in blood–brain barrier permeability.[67] Histologic examination of brains of rats aged 3–30 days who had received phenytoin, phenobarbital, valproate, vigabatrin, diazepam, or clonazepam revealed apoptotic neurodegeneration.[47,54] Anticonvulsants not found to cause apoptosis include carbamazepine, lamotrigine, levetiracetam and topiramate.[68] In addition, anticonvulsants have been implicated in impairing developing brains by diminishing neurogenesis and synaptogenesis.[68]

The hippocampus, which is critical for the formation of new memories, possesses the highest concentration of corticosteroid-binding sites in the brain.[69] Glucocorticoids inhibit glucose transport into cells by 25–30%, thereby accelerating the usual decline in adenosine triphosphate concentrations after ischemia or hypoglycemia.[55] This lessens the cell's ability to inhibit neuronal insults, leading to neuronal death. In several studies involving children with acute lymphoblastic leukemia, those treated with dexamethasone performed less well on cognitive testing than children treated with prednisone.[70,71] It has been hypothesized that dexamethasone may be more neurotoxic than prednisone because of a lesser degree of plasma protein binding and due to the presence of a fluoride atom in its chemical structure.[70] Altered brain membrane lipid content and synaptic transmission in hippocampal neurons have been associated with fluoride anions.[70]

Acute changes in mental status can occur in association with selective serotonin reuptake inhibitors (SSRIs) as a result of hyponatremia due to the syndrome of inappropriate antidiuretic hormone (ADH) secretion.[33,60,61] Increased concentrations of ADH result in the inability of renal tubules to excrete diluted urine, decreasing serum osmolality and serum sodium, resulting in neurological changes that may include lethargy, confusion, seizures, coma, and death.[61] This syndrome may also be caused by other medications, including carbamazepine, oxcarbazepine, tricyclic antidepressants, monoamine oxidase inhibitors, and neuroleptics.[61] These classes of medications may facilitate the secretion of ADH or increase renal responsiveness to ADH.[61]

A substantial decline in cognitive function has been reported in studies of patients with some malignancies, particularly breast cancer.[1] It has been hypothesized that two distinct pathways are involved: psychological and social factors associated with the diagnosis of cancer and a physiologic effect of cancer treatment, particularly with medications that cross the blood–brain barrier. These effects include decreased functional connectivity, dysregulation of proinflammatory cytokine concentrations, and direct cytotoxic effects to the visual system.[48,49,72] Nonsteroidal anti-inflammatory drugs are believed to cause aseptic meningitis through hypersensitivity responses.[30] Only a small number of nonsteroidal anti-inflammatory drugs (diclofenac, ibuprofen, ketoprofen, naproxen, sulindac, and tolmetin) have been associated with aseptic meningitis, which may be attributable to degree of lipophilicity and penetration of the blood–brain barrier.[31] Reye syndrome has been associated with aspirin use in children less than 18 years of age.[30] The mechanism is thought to be inhibition of lipid beta-oxidation and mitochondrial disarrangement, leading to urea genesis and ketogenesis and ultimately hyperammonemia, hypoglycemia, elevated serum lactate, free fatty acids and dicarboxylic acid release.[30] The cyclooxygenase-2 inhibitors rofecoxib and valdecoxib have been associated with increased incidences of stroke and myocardial infarction by inhibiting prostacyclin, producing a prothrombotic state.

CLINICAL PRESENTATION AND DIFFERENTIAL DIAGNOSIS

The clinical presentation of patients with drug-induced cognitive disorders is diverse and may involve acute or chronic changes in states of wakefulness, attention, or memory.[73] Anticholinergic drugs have been associated with memory impairment, confusion, hallucinations, sedation, and dysphoria.[18] The most common cognitive effects associated with anticonvulsants are psychomotor slowing, reduced vigilance, and impairment in memory and mood.[35] In contrast, many patients receiving corticosteroids exhibit mood elevation, and some may experience euphoria, insomnia, restlessness, and increased motor activity.[74] Others become anxious, depressed, or present with psychotic symptoms. Common central nervous system adverse signs and symptoms caused by medications are listed in **Table 17-3**.[1,7,18,25,27,28,35,50,69,74-76]

Table 17-3 Signs and Symptoms Associated with Drug-Induced Cognitive Disorders[1,7,18,25,27,28,35,50,69,74-76]

- Sedation/drowsiness
- Insomnia
- Decreased attention
- Impaired concentration
- Memory disorders
- Confusion
- Myoclonus
- Hallucinations
- Delirium
- Seizure disorders
- Impaired performance on assessment instruments (e.g., Wechsler Adult Intelligence Scale, Digit Span/Digit Symbol, CogHealth, Hopkins Verbal Learning Test) to assess executive function, attention, concentration, intelligence, memory and recall, psychomotor ability, processing verbal ability, vigilance, and visuospatial and visuomotor ability
- Seizure activity on electroencephalogram
- Magnetic resonance imaging changes (e.g., cerebral atrophy, diffuse white matter hyperintensities, ventricular enlargement, cortical calcifications)

Central nervous system effects of benzodiazepines include sedation, hypnosis, decreased anxiety, muscle relaxation, anterograde amnesia, and anticonvulsant activity.[75] As the dose is increased, sedation progresses to hypnosis and then stupor. There have been reports of delirium in hospitalized patients receiving benzodiazepines, more often associated with long-acting agents and higher doses of all benzodiazepines.[7] Long-term use of benzodiazepines in the elderly has been associated with a higher risk for cognitive decline than with episodic, recurrent, or no use of benzodiazepines.[19] Benzodiazepines may also cause paradoxical effects or disinhibition reactions.[75] Euphoria, hallucinations, sleep-walking, sleep-talking, hypomanic behavior, hostility, and rage have been reported with use of various benzodiazepines. These reactions are rare and may be dose-related.

Cases of reversible pseudoatrophy of the brain and mental deterioration have been reported in association with valproate in children.[67] In these reports, the serum valproate concentration was near or above 100 mg/L, magnetic resonance imaging documented pseudoatrophy, and there was a loss of 18–26 intelligence quotient (IQ) points as tested on the Wechsler Intelligence Scale for Children III. The scores with this test are normative IQs with a mean of 100 and a standard deviation of 15.[77] Some of these reports also mentioned the simultaneous presence of other adverse effects of valproate, such as tremor, weight gain, alopecia, ataxia, and nystagmus.[76]

Differentiating between cognitive dysfunction that is drug-induced with that due to a nondrug-induced disease process can be complex. This is especially true in patients with disorders such as epilepsy, Parkinson disease, and human immunodeficiency virus (HIV).[18,78,79] The "five foes" of mental competence in patients with epilepsy have been described as heredity, brain damage, seizures, anticonvulsant medications, and psychosocial issues.[78] Some studies found earlier seizure onset, higher lifetime number of seizures, and having multiple seizure types contributed to lower IQ scores in pediatric patients with epilepsy. Neuropsychiatric problems of Parkinson disease, such as hallucinations, memory loss, confusion, and major neurocognitive disorder can be aggravated by antiparkinson medications.[18] Cognitive and motor impairment occurs in 20% of patients with advanced HIV.[79] Robertson and colleagues conducted a prospective study of HIV-positive patients enrolled in randomized antiretroviral trials and found that a history of immunosuppression (nadir CD4 cell count <200 cells/mm^3) was associated with an increase in neurocognitive impairment.[79] Of 458 patients who were classified as having mild impairment at baseline, 389 had a minimum of one follow-up visit with 172 (44%) improving while receiving highly active antiretroviral therapy.

The differential diagnosis of a patient with altered mental status can be extensive.[7,76,80] Because patients may not be able to provide an accurate history, interviews of family members or care providers may be essential to determine the patient's baseline mental status.[9] It is important to determine the timeline of development of the cognitive dysfunction, which may be described as either acute or insidious. The rate of drug absorption and penetration into the brain determines the speed of onset of acutely occurring drug-induced events.[53] A careful history of current prescription and nonprescription medication use, as well as the use of herbal supplements or other remedies is essential and should include information regarding any recent alterations in drug, dose, or adherence.[7]

The most common causes of cognitive disorders are mild and major neurocognitive disorders due to Alzheimer disease, vascular disorders, Parkinson disease, and substance/medication intoxication.[80] Other degenerative disorders that cause dementia include dementia with Lewy bodies, frontotemporal dementia, and multiple sclerosis.[80] Major neurocognitive disorders associated with chronic alcoholism may be linked to the associated malnutrition and deficiency of the B vitamins or to withdrawal syndromes. Thiamine (vitamin B_1) deficiency can lead to Wernicke encephalopathy, which in turn can progress to irreversible Korsakoff psychosis and death. Vitamin B_{12} deficiency, in addition to damaging peripheral nerves and causing sensory loss, can damage cerebral myelinated fibers, thereby inducing dementia. Another insidious cause of memory loss is chronic metal intoxication, such as that associated with lead, mercury, and aluminum poisoning.

Acute and chronic infections can also impair cognition.[80] Chronic diseases such as tuberculosis, cryptococcosis, advanced stages of HIV infection, and neurosyphilis must be considered. Prion illnesses such as Creutzfeldt–Jakob disease and bovine spongiform encephalopathy are rare. Elderly patients may experience delirium in association with acute infections such as urinary tract infections and pneumonia.[76]

Acute changes in mental status can serve as an alert for an underlying life-threatening medical problem.[73] Metabolic and endocrine disorders, including dehydration, hyperammonemia, hypercalcemia, hyponatremia, hypothyroidism, kidney disease, liver failure, and hypoxemia should be considered in the differential diagnosis.[80-82] Withdrawal from certain agents, including alcohol, barbiturates, benzodiazepines, and tricyclic antidepressants can also cause cognitive disturbances.[53,73]

Table 17-4 Conditions to Consider in the Differential Diagnosis of Cognitive Disorders[73,80,81]

Neoplastic disease

- Primary brain tumor
- Metastatic brain tumor

Central nervous system disorders

- Extradural hemorrhage
- Chronic subdural hematoma
- Vascular dementia
- Postanoxia
- Normal-pressure hydrocephalus
- Stroke

Metabolic disorders

- Dehydration
- Hyperammonemia
- Hypercalcemia
- Hyperglycemia/hypoglycemia
- Hypoadrenalism
- Hyponatremia
- Hypothyroidism/hyperthyroidism
- Kidney disease
- Liver failure
- Hypoxemia

Infections

- Central nervous system infection (meningitis, encephalitis, brain abscess)
- Human immunodeficiency virus
- Neurosyphilis
- Prion diseases (Creutzfeldt–Jakob disease)
- Acute infection/sepsis

Vitamin deficiencies

- Thiamine (B_1) (Wernicke encephalopathy)
- B_{12} (pernicious anemia)
- Nicotinic acid (pellagra)

Toxic disorders

- Intoxication with drugs of abuse/alcohol and/or prescription medications
- Heavy metal intoxication
- Dialysis dementia (aluminum)
- Organic toxins

Psychiatric disorders

- Conversion disorder
- Depression
- Schizophrenia

Recurrent nonconvulsive seizures

Degenerative disorders

- Alzheimer disease
- Dementia with Lewy bodies
- Frontotemporal dementia
- Parkinson disease
- Multiple sclerosis

Psychiatric diseases must also be considered in the differential diagnosis. Some patients with severe depression express confusion and inability to perform routine tasks.[80] Patients with schizophrenia or with a conversion disorder (mental disorders presenting as physical illnesses but lacking a physiologic basis) may experience cognitive dysfunction. In patients with conversion disorders, psychometric testing does not confirm memory loss. Schizophrenia is usually associated with delusions and hallucinations and initially with an intact memory, but unexplained progressive dementia develops in some patients late in life.

Table 17-4 provides a list of conditions to consider in the differential diagnosis of drug-induced cognitive disorders.[73,80,81] Diagnostic tests that can be performed to confirm or assist in the diagnosis are listed in **Table 17-5**.[75,76,80-82]

Table 17-5 Tests for Evaluation of Patients with Cognitive Dysfunction[75,76,80-82]

- Thyroid function
- Vitamin B_{12}
- Complete blood count
- Electrolytes
- Computed tomography/magnetic resonance imaging
- Venereal Disease Research Laboratory (VDRL)
- Human immunodeficiency virus
- Chest x-ray
- Lumbar puncture
- Kidney function
- Liver function
- Serum ammonia concentration
- Urine toxin screen
- Urine heavy metals
- Psychometric testing
- Electroencephalogram

RISK FACTORS

Certain predisposing or precipitating factors may increase the risk of drug-induced cognitive dysfunction (**Table 17-6**).[7,34,63,73,81,83,84] Predisposing characteristics include age, cerebral damage, chronic illness, functional impairment, genetics, polypharmacy, and underlying cognitive impairment.[7,34,81] Precipitating factors include acute illness, infection, metabolic disturbances, dehydration, acute urinary retention, malnutrition, environmental and psychosocial factors, surgery, drug interactions, and dose–response relationships.[7,34,64,73,83,84] Confounding factors, such as those experienced with cancer treatment, may include dose intensity, duration of treatment, concomitant medications, radiation therapy, and other chemotherapy toxicities, including anemia, vascular injury and neurotoxicity.[1]

In one study, altered mental status was present in 40% of patients older than 70 years of age who presented to the emergency department.[73] There are a number of pharmacokinetic changes in the elderly that place them at higher risk of cognitive dysfunction. In elderly patients there is a lesser degree of gastric acid secretion, reduced gastrointestinal blood flow, and a diminished rate of gastric emptying, translating to reduced ionization and solubility of certain drugs and a delay in drug absorption.[85] As a person ages, there is a decrease in lean body mass and an increase in body fat. These changes affect the distribution and volume of distribution of lipophilic and hydrophilic drugs. Binding to serum albumin and α_1-acid glycoprotein is a determinant of drug distribution and the fraction of drug available for activity. Albumin primarily binds with acidic and some basic drugs; albumin concentrations decrease with increasing age. Conversely, α_1-acid glycoprotein binds to basic and neutral drugs; there is either no change or an increase in the α_1-acid glycoprotein concentration with advancing age. In addition, serum drug concentrations may be increased in patients with infection, trauma, myocardial infarction, and chronic disease. Hepatic metabolic activity—especially phase 1 reactions, including oxidation, reduction, and hydrolysis—is diminished in the elderly.[86] Benzodiazepines that are only metabolized by conjugation (lorazepam, oxazepam, and temazepam) are preferred in the elderly to benzodiazepines that also undergo phase 1 reactions to prevent accumulation.[8] Glomerular filtration rate, creatinine clearance, and tubular secretion and absorption all decline in elderly patients. Older patients may also be more sensitive to the effects of some medications because of pharmacodynamic changes.[7,85,86] There may be reduced cholinergic transmission and decreases in receptor numbers and sensitivity.[7,86] Exposure to at least three possible anticholinergic agents for a minimum of 90 days in adults ≥65 years of age was associated with an odds ratio (OR) for a diagnosis of mild cognitive impairment of 2.73 (95% CI 1.27–5.87) compared to those having no anticholinergic exposure.[87] Older age, smoking and excessive perspiration are risk factors for cognitive dysfunction associated with

Table 17-6 Risk Factors for Drug-Induced Cognitive Disorders[7,34,63,73,81,83,84]

Predisposing characteristics

- Elderly
- Children
- Genetic predisposition
- Underlying cognitive impairment
- Chronic illness (e.g., alcoholism, HIV)
- Cerebral damage
- Functional impairment
- Polypharmacy

Precipitating factors

- Acute illness
- Acute infections/sepsis (brain abscess, encephalitis, meningitis, pneumonia, urinary tract infection)
- Metabolic disturbances (hyperammonemia, hypercalcemia, hyperglycemia or hypoglycemia, hyponatremia, hypothyroidism)
- Hypoxemia
- Dehydration
- Acute urinary retention
- Malnutrition
- Environmental (heavy metal intoxication, organic toxins, aluminum toxicity associated with dialysis)
- Psychosocial factors (drug abuse, depression)
- Surgery
- Drug interactions leading to elevated serum concentrations of causative agents and/or additive pharmacodynamic effects
- Elevated serum concentrations of causative agents

HIV = human immunodeficiency virus.

the syndrome of drug-induced inappropriate antidiuretic hormone secretion.[61]

Younger age has also been implicated as a risk factor for specific drug-induced alterations of cognitive function. In a 16-week double-blind, placebo-controlled, randomized add-on study in 86 children with partial seizures, topiramate was associated with difficulty with attention and concentration (12% versus 2%) and forgetfulness and impaired memory (7% versus 0%).[88] Phenobarbital has been shown to slow cognitive processing speed compared with carbamazepine and valproate in children.[10,34] Detriments to attention and memory caused by anticonvulsant medications may impact long-term neurodevelopment in children.[35] Phenobarbital use in 217 children 8–36 months of age resulted in an IQ that was 8.4 points lower on the Standfort-Binet Intelligence Scale, Form L-M compared to that in controls (95% CI −13.3 to −3.5, $p = 0.0057$) after 2 years of treatment.[89] Six months later after a taper and discontinuation, the IQ was lower by 5.2 points in the phenobarbital group (95% CI −10.5 to −0.04, $p = 0.052$).[89] Children ($n = 139$) were retested after completing at least first grade and after 86% had discontinued therapy for 3 or more years.[90] There was no significant difference in IQ points at that time for the phenobarbital group (102.2 versus 105.7 for placebo, $p = 0.09$) but a significantly lower score on the Wide Range Achievement Test reading achievement standard score (87.6 versus 95.6, $p = 0.007$).

Genetic polymorphisms (deoxyribonucleic acid sequence variation) are responsible for inherited differences in drug metabolism and disposition and the resulting effects.[91] In addition, polymorphism in genes encoding drug transporters and targets cause modifications in drug response. Genetic variability affects sensitivity to opioid analgesia and may determine a predisposition to adverse effects.[81] In studies of the addition of topiramate or valproate to carbamazepine therapy, a subgroup of patients who are particularly sensitive to the adverse cognitive effects of topiramate was identified.[92,93] Galimberti and colleagues identified a mutation in the *MT-ATP8* (mitochondrially-encoded adenosine triphosphate synthase 8) gene of a child who developed reversible mental deterioration with brain pseudoatrophy while undergoing valproate therapy.[94] In patients who received androgen-deprivation therapy for prostate cancer, there were 15 single nucleotide polymorphisms (SNPs) associated with impaired cognitive performance (from a total of 384 SNPs) as measured with the International Cognition and Cancer Task Force recommended criteria.[4] Patients with the wild type (GG) of one variant (rs1047726 in G protein subunit B3, GNB3) had higher odds of impaired cognitive performance at 12 months compared to those with one or more A alleles (OR 14, 95% CI 2.97–66.09).[4] Womack and Heilman described the case of a 46-year-old woman in whom memory loss and abnormal memory test results developed, but improved upon discontinuation of tolterodine therapy.[63] The authors suggested that she might be one of the 7% of the population lacking the cytochrome P-450 2D6 enzyme responsible for converting tolterodine to the active 5-hydroxymethyl metabolite. In poor metabolizers, the more lipophilic parent compound predominates and crosses the blood–brain barrier more easily than the metabolite, which is more hydrophilic. Cattie and colleagues found patients with hepatitis C virus genotype 1 had significantly greater neurocognitive decline than patients with other genotypes when treated with pegylated interferon and ribavirin.[24]

Cognitive adverse effects of many medications occur more commonly in association with higher serum concentrations and with polypharmacy.[35,84] Therapeutic serum concentration ranges have been identified for many narrow therapeutic index medications, including phenytoin (10–20 mg/L), carbamazepine (4–12 mg/L), phenobarbital (10–40 mg/L), valproic acid (50–100 mg/L), lithium (0.5–1.2 mEq/L), digoxin (0.5–2 ng/mL), theophylline (5–15 mg/L), lidocaine (1–5 mg/L), and combined amitriptyline + nortriptyline (120–250 ng/mL).[84] Many patients experience cognitive adverse events when the upper limit of the therapeutic range is exceeded. Doses must be individualized for efficacy and to prevent toxicity. Some patients may not tolerate the medication at a lower serum concentration, while others may tolerate much higher concentrations. Additive effects are often observed when sedative or hypnotic medications are taken concurrently.[75] Tolerance may develop to some effects of medications, but other effects may linger. With benzodiazepines, patients report subjectively that drowsiness subsides after a few days, but tolerance to the impairment of some measures of psychomotor performance, such as visual tracking, does not occur.

Adverse central nervous system reactions have been attributed to histamine-2-receptor blockers.[20,57,95] Slugg and colleagues determined that ranitidine-induced adverse central nervous system reactions are more likely to occur in patients with estimated creatinine clearances <50 mL/min than in those with estimated creatinine clearances >50 mL/min.[95] Patients with creatinine clearances <50 mL/min had higher peak plasma concentrations, higher average plasma concentrations, and larger areas under the plasma concentration: time curve than patients who did not have kidney disease.

Postoperative confusion occurs commonly, with a reported incidence between 5% and 45% in the elderly.[96] Common causes include opioids, benzodiazepines, and anticholinergics.[34,96] Short-term and long-term postoperative cognitive dysfunction has been evaluated in both elderly and middle-aged patients.[97,98] Postoperative cognitive dysfunction was present in 25.8% and 9.9% of 1,218 patients ≥60 years of age at 1 week and 3 months after surgery, respectively, as compared with 3.4% and 2.8% in nonsurgical control subjects from the United Kingdom ($p < 0.0001$ and $p = 0.0037$).[97] Risk factors were increasing age, duration of anesthesia, minimal education, a second procedure, postoperative infections, and respiratory complications. In a study investigating patients 40–60 years of age who underwent surgery, cognitive dysfunction was reported in 19.2% at 1 week postoperatively, as compared with 4% of nonsurgical control subjects ($p < 0.001$).[98] The major risk factors for cognitive dysfunction at 7 days were supplementary epidural analgesia and reported avoidance of alcohol consumption.

MORBIDITY AND MORTALITY

There are few published data regarding the influence of drug-induced cognitive impairment on morbidity or mortality. However, one prospective study of hospitalized elderly patients demonstrated that the presence of delirium prolonged the duration of hospitalization from 7.2 days to 12.1 days, and increased the mortality rate from 1% to 8%.[36]

Table 17-7 Approaches to Help Prevent Drug-Induced Cognitive Disorders[35,38,76,99-102]

- Adjust dose for patients with kidney and/or liver disease where applicable
- Limit total dose where possible
- Limit total number of medications
- Use adjunctive medications
- Use around-the-clock regimen
- Perform routine plasma concentration monitoring of medications with defined ranges for efficacy and toxicity
- Upon initiation of medications, use a slow titration to target range
- Use alternative medications with less association for cognitive adverse events
- Use consensus guidelines for safe medication use in specific populations

PREVENTION

A number of strategies have reduced the likelihood of occurrence of drug-induced cognitive disorders including adjusting drug doses in patients with liver or kidney disease, limiting the total dose of medications with known dose–toxicity relationships, monitoring plasma concentrations, slowly titrating the dose, using alternative agents with a lower risk of inducing cognitive dysfunction, limiting the total number of medications, and using consensus criteria. **Table 17-7** provides a summary of measures that can be taken to reduce the risk of drug-induced cognitive disorders.[35,38,76,99-102]

Adjusting drug doses and/or dosing intervals in patients with liver or kidney disease is not only important when initiating therapy, but it is also critical in patients with severe illness in which organ function may decline suddenly and precipitously. Histamine-2-receptor blockers are an example of a class of medications for which careful dose adjustment is necessary.[95] Other medications should be avoided altogether in patients with liver or kidney disease. Meperidine, for example, has a neurotoxic active metabolite, normeperidine, that accumulates after repeated doses in patients with kidney disease.[99]

Another risk reduction strategy is to limit the total dose of a potentially offending agent for which a known dose–toxicity relationship exists.[81] In patients requiring pain management with opioids, for example, the addition of a nonopioid coanalgesic or an adjuvant analgesic and around-the-clock administration can decrease the total required opioid dose.[81,99] Proper management of pain is important, as was demonstrated in a study of postoperative patients 50–80 years of age, which found that pain, not analgesic intake, predicted a decline in mental status during the first 5 days after surgery.[100] Other pain management approaches to consider include the use of a therapy targeting the cause of pain (antitumor therapies such as radiotherapy, chemotherapy, and surgery) or use of a regional anesthetic or neuroablative intervention.[81]

Medications such as anticonvulsants and lithium require routine plasma concentration monitoring to maintain concentrations within specified ranges.[84] Even though plasma topiramate concentrations are not tested routinely, in a study of correlates of topiramate-induced cognitive impairment, the largest causal relationship was plasma concentrations, which varied by 55-fold among 158 healthy volunteers.[103] The authors performed a genome-wide association study (GWAS), including a focused analysis near genes considered candidates for influencing topiramate cognitive response. No significant association was found among the healthy volunteers or with a comparison of a GWAS of cognitive adverse effects in patients with epilepsy taking topiramate. For some medications, minor adverse effects often appear as the plasma concentrations rise before major cognitive toxicities are experienced.[84] To an astute clinician, these minor adverse effects serve as a warning that more serious cognitive impairment may be imminent. For example, gastrointestinal distress may be an early symptom of valproic acid toxicity, while fatigue may be an early indicator of impending toxicity associated with phenytoin or topiramate. Patients become tolerant to some of the adverse cognitive effects of some medications when doses are slowly titrated upward. This is the case with topiramate, for which therapy should be initiated at a low dose and titrated to the target dose over a period of 1–2 months.[92]

Another strategy for the prevention of cognitive disturbances involves the use of medications with lower risk. In a single site retrospective study of 2860 adult outpatients with epilepsy, topiramate (18.5%, 95% CI 1.78–7.49%) and phenytoin (11%, 95% CI 1.08–3.77%) were most likely to be associated with intolerable cognitive adverse effects.[104] Gabapentin, pregabalin, and carbamazepine were the least likely of the antiepileptic medications to cause these adverse effects. Residual daytime sedation has been associated with the use of benzodiazepines and the benzodiazepine-receptor agonist zoldipem.[35,101]

The potential for drug interactions and additive pharmacodynamic effects should be considered as new medications are added to a patient's treatment regimen. The odds for experiencing adverse drug reactions, adjusted for age and duration of symptoms, were shown to increase as the number of drugs used increased in an elderly population.[38] Compared to patients taking zero or one prescription medication, the odds ratio for adverse drug reactions was 2.7 (95% CI 0.9–7.8) in those taking two or three medications, 9.3 (95% CI 3.3–26.6) for those taking four or five medications and 13.7 (95% CI 3.6–51.9) for those taking six or more medications.[38] In a prospective study of 72 children with epilepsy, in which siblings of 45 of the children served as controls, investigators reported that 11% of children with a persistent decrease in IQ score had a significantly higher incidence of toxic plasma drug concentrations, took a larger number of medications simultaneously, had seizures that were more difficult to control, had a higher total number of seizures, and began to have seizures at a younger age.[78]

A tool used to minimize impact of polypharmacy is the Anticholinergic Cognitive Burden (ACB) list, which scores the anticholinergic activity of medications as mild (ACB score 1) or severe (ABC score 2 or 3).[87] Drugs with mild anticholinergic effects have serum anticholinergic activity or in vitro affinity to muscarinic receptors but no known clinically relevant negative cognitive effects. Drugs assigned higher scores have established and clinically relevant cognitive anticholinergic effects.

Federal regulations have been enacted to protect the elderly, a population that is at increased risk for the development of adverse events due to medications. The Omnibus Budget Reconciliation Act of 1987 contained the Federal Nursing Home Reform Bill, which gave the right of long-term care residents to be free from unnecessary physical and chemical restraints.[105] Reportable quality measures, such as the Minimum Data Set for nursing home residents, improve quality for residents by providing regular organized assessments of each resident's physical and mental status.[106] The Beers criteria, first published in 1997 and updated in 2003 and 2012, provide a consensus statement of medications that are potentially inappropriate in older adults in general and in older adults with common medical conditions.[102,107,108] The Beers criteria were accepted by the Centers for Medicare and Medicaid Services for nursing home regulation in 1999.[107] The 2012 update used a comprehensive and systematic review to divide 53 medications or classes of medications into three categories: (1) potentially inappropriate medications and classes to avoid in older adults, (2) potentially inappropriate medications and classes to avoid in older adults with certain diseases and syndromes that the listed drugs can exacerbate, and (3) medications to be used with caution in older adults.[108]

Prognostic molecular testing, as in the case of patients with breast cancer, can assist with identifying patients that might not benefit from prolonged cancer chemotherapy or those at low risk for recurrence, thus preventing overtreatment and limiting adverse events for those populations.[109]

MANAGEMENT

A summary of management strategies for drug induced cognitive disorders is provided in **Table 17-8**.[20,25,81,110,111] Treatment of drug-induced cognitive disorders may include discontinuation of the offending agent with or without adjuvant medications, dose reduction, substitution of a sustained-release formulation, symptomatic management, cognitive rehabilitation, and/or complementary therapies. In some instances, such as in patients with epilepsy or bipolar disease, it may be necessary to initiate treatment with another medication before therapy with the offending agent can be discontinued.[25,35] Use of a sustained-release formulation that may ameliorate toxicity associated with peak plasma concentrations has been recommended for patients with lithium-induced cognitive impairment.[25]

Table 17-8 Management of Drug-Induced Cognitive Disorders[20,25,81,110,111]

- Distinguish between medication effects and symptoms caused by comorbid conditions
- Discontinue the offending agent and use alternative medications
- Reduce the dose of the offending agent
- Where available, use a sustained-release formulation to prevent peak serum concentrations associated with adverse events
- Provide symptomatic treatment
- Treat comorbidities
- Provide cognitive rehabilitation and training
- Complementary therapies
- Provide supportive measures

Discontinuation of some medications such as benzodiazepines and SSRIs may cause a withdrawal reaction.[110,112] Withdrawal symptoms peak from 24 to 72 hours after discontinuation of short- to intermediate-acting agents.[113] These reactions occur more often in patients receiving higher daily doses, with agents having shorter half-lives, those undergoing a longer duration of daily drug therapy, and in association with more rapid rates of tapering.[110] Other predictors of poor outcome following discontinuation of benzodiazepines include a diagnosis of panic disorder, higher levels of anxiety or depression before tapering, higher levels of personality psychopathology (e.g., neuroticism, dependency), and concomitant alcohol and/or substance dependence or abuse. Tapering of therapy has been recommended for patients receiving daily diazepam doses of >10 mg or its equivalent (2 mg lorazepam, 1 mg alprazolam) after patients' anxiety or panic symptoms have been reduced. One recommended schedule is to taper by 25% per week until 1–2 mg equivalents of alprazolam is achieved, then decrease by 25% of the remaining dose every week.[113] Therapy with carbamazepine 200–800 mg/day, imipramine 25 mg/day, valproate 500–2,500 mg/day, and trazodone 100–500 mg/day has been shown to improve benzodiazepine tapering success rates, but has not been shown to diminish withdrawal severity.[114-116] The Physician Withdrawal Checklist (PWC-20) for benzodiazepines and the Discontinuation Emergent Signs and Symptoms (DESS) checklist for SSRIs are helpful tools to differentiate between discontinuation symptoms of rebound/withdrawal and return of anxiety/depression.[112,117] Psychostimulant agents antagonize opioid-induced sedation and cognitive impairment in postsurgical patients and in those with chronic cancer.[81] However, these agents can also cause cognitive adverse effects, including hallucinations, delirium, and psychosis, as well as noncognitive adverse events such as decreased appetite and tachycardia. A short-acting benzodiazepine such as lorazepam is often administered for severe agitation, and antipsychotic drugs such as haloperidol are often administered for the treatment of patients with delirium. Several studies have shown that opioid rotation, also referred to as opioid switching or opioid substitution, can minimize delirium or agitated confusion. Dose conversion tables should be used cautiously as guidelines. Because of incomplete cross-tolerance to opioids in tolerant patients, it has been recommended to decrease the dose of the new opioid by 30–50%. Cherny and colleagues published detailed instructions regarding the manner in which to perform opioid rotation.[81] Liothyronine 25–50 mcg daily was found to improve cognitive functioning in patients receiving lithium, even in the absence of hypothyroidism.[25]

The pharmacokinetic properties of a medication most often determine the duration of adverse cognitive effects.[53] The duration may be affected by redistribution from the brain into other tissues, as occurs with highly lipid-soluble drugs such as diazepam. With other central nervous system depressants, drug metabolism and elimination determine the duration of effect of the parent drug and any active or toxic metabolites. These factors may be influenced by age, disease, genetics, and concomitant medications.

It is important to also screen and treat possible underlying causes of cognitive dysfunction such as metabolic disturbances and infections as well as comorbidities such as anxiety, depression, fatigue and insomnia, which may be associated with drug-induced cognitive dysfunction such as that associated with cancer chemotherapy.[73,111]

Nonpharmacologic interventions have also been shown to be of benefit. Cognitive rehabilitation approaches may significantly improve patient functioning.[118] One approach is for caregivers and family members to orient confused patients to person, place, and time.[99] Supportive measures include convenient arrangement of the home or work environment, use of notes, and avoidance of distractions.[14] Cognitive training (memory and speed process training) and physical activity interventions (bicycling with speed feedback and modified hatha yoga) improved cognitive function in patients with breast cancer.[119] Other complementary/integrative medicine therapies include acupuncture, hypnosis, massage therapy, meditation, relaxation and biofeedback.[111]

INFORMATION FOR PATIENTS

Patients and/or their caregivers should be informed that the prescribed medication has been known to cause cognitive dysfunction, and they should be informed of associated signs and symptoms. Patients should be warned regarding the potential hazards of driving or using machinery and should be aware that alcohol could have additive effects when used concurrently. Patients and their caregivers should be instructed that healthcare providers should be contacted if the prescribed therapy causes intolerable cognitive effects so that appropriate changes in therapy can be implemented.

REFERENCES

1. Hess LM, Insel KC. Chemotherapy-related change in cognitive function: a conceptual model. *Oncol Nurs Forum*. 2007; 34:981-94.
2. Bender CM, Paraska KK, Sereika SM et al. Cognitive function and reproductive hormones in adjuvant therapy for breast cancer: a critical review. *J Pain Symptom Manage*. 2001; 21:407-24.
3. American Psychiatric Association. *Diagnostic and statistical manual of mental disorders*. 5th ed. Arlington, VA: American Psychiatric Association; 2013.
4. Gonzalez BD, Jim HSL, Booth-Jones M et al. Course and predictors of cognitive function in patients with prostate cancer receiving androgen-deprivation therapy: a controlled comparison. *J Clin Oncol*. 2015; 33:2021-7.

5. Lechevallier-Michel N, Molimard M, Dartigues JF et al. Drugs with anticholinergic properties and cognitive performance in the elderly: results from the PAQUID Study. *Br J Clin Pharmacol.* 2004; 59:143-51.
6. Fox C, Smith T, Maidment I et al. Effect of medications with anticholinergic properties on cognitive function, delirium, physical function and mortality: a systematic review. *Age Ageing.* 2014; 43:604-15.
7. Gray SL, Lai KV, Larson EB. Drug-induced cognition disorders in the elderly: incidence, prevention and management. *Drug Saf.* 1999; 21:101-22.
8. Bowen JD, Larson EB. Drug-induced cognitive impairment. Defining the problem and finding solutions. *Drugs Aging.* 1993; 3:349-57.
9. Medwatch. Dear Healthcare Professional Letter and Tamiflu Prescribing Information. http://www.fda.gov/medwatch/safety/2008/safety08.htm#Tamiflu (accessed 2017 Dec 18).
10. Calandre EP, Dominguez-Granados R, Gomez-Rubio M et al. Cognitive effects of long-term treatment with phenobarbital and valproic acid in school children. *Acta Neurol Scand.* 1990; 81:504-6.
11. Meador KJ, Loring DW, Vahle VJ et al. Cognitive and behavioral effects of lamotrigine and topiramate in healthy volunteers. *Neurology.* 2005; 64:2108-14.
12. Aarsen FK, van den Akker ELT, Drop SLS et al. Effect of topiramate on cognition in obese children. *Neurology.* 2006; 67:1307-8.
13. Adab N, Kini U, Vinten J et al. The longer term outcome of children born to mothers with epilepsy. *J Neurol Neurosurg Psychiatry.* 2004; 75:1575-83.
14. Raffa RB, Duong PV, Finney J et al. Is 'chemofog'/'chemo-brain' caused by cancer chemotherapy? *J Clin Pharm Ther.* 2006; 31:129-38.
15. Schagen SB, Muller MJ, Boogerd W et al. Change in cognitive function after chemotherapy: a prospective longitudinal study in breast cancer patients. *J Natl Cancer Inst.* 2006; 98:1742-5.
16. McShane R, Keene J, Gedling K et al. Do neuroleptic drugs hasten cognitive decline in dementia? Prospective study with necropsy follow up. *BMJ.* 1997; 314:266-70.
17. Schneider LS, Dagerman K, Insel PS. Efficacy and adverse effects of atypical antipsychotics for dementia: metaanalysis of randomized, placebo-controlled trials. *Am J Geriatr Psychiatry.* 2006; 14:191-210.
18. Olanow CW, Watts RL, Koller WC. An algorithm (decision tree) for the management of Parkinson's disease (2001): treatment guidelines. *Neurology.* 2001; 56(suppl 5):S1-88.
19. Paterniti S, Dufouil C, Alpérovitch A. Long-term benzodiazepine use and cognitive decline in the elderly: the epidemiology of vascular aging study. *J Clin Psychopharmacol.* 2002; 22:285-93.
20. Cantú TG, Korek JS. Central nervous system reactions to histamine-2 receptor blockers. *Ann Intern Med.* 1991; 114:1027-34.
21. Kraus MR, Schäfer A, Wissmann S et al. Neurocognitive changes in patients with hepatitis C receiving interferon alfa-2b and ribavirin. *Clin Pharmacol Ther.* 2005; 77:90-100.
22. Reichenberg A, Gorman JM, Dieterich DT. Interferon-induced depression and cognitive impairment in hepatitis C virus patients: a 72 week prospective study. *AIDS.* 2005; 19(suppl 3):S174-8.
23. Scheibel, RS, Valentine AD, O'Brien S et al. Cognitive dysfunction and depression during treatment with interferon-alpha and chemotherapy. *J Neuropsychiatry Clin Neurosci.* 2004; 16:185-91.
24. Cattie JE, Letendre SL, Woods SP et al. Persistent neurocognitive decline in a clinic sample of hepatitis C virus-infected persons receiving interferon and ribavirin treatment. *J Neurovirol.* 2014; 20:561-70.
25. Honig A, Arts BM, Ponds RW et al. Lithium induced cognitive side-effects in bipolar disorder: a qualitative analysis and implications for daily practice. *Int Clin Psychopharmacol.* 1999; 14:167-71.
26. Balanzá-Martinez V, Selva G, Martínez-Arán A et al. Neurocognition in bipolar disorders-A closer look at comorbidities and medications. *Eur J Pharmacol.* 2010; 626:87-96.
27. Lochet P, Peyrière H, Lotthé A et al. Long-term assessment of neuropsychiatric adverse reactions associated with efavirenz. *HIV Med.* 2003; 4:62-6.
28. Wise ME, Mistry K, Reid S. Drug points: neuropsychiatric complications of nevirapine treatment. *BMJ.* 2002; 324:879.
29. Saag KG, Rubenstein LM, Chrischilles EA et al. Nonsteroidal antiinflammatory drugs and cognitive decline in the elderly. *J Rheumatol.* 1995; 22:2142-7.
30. Auriel E, Regev K, Korczn AD. Nonsteroidal anti-inflammatory drugs exposure and the central nervous system. *Handb Clin Neurol.* 2014; 119:577-84.
31. Morgan A, Clark D. CNS adverse effects of nonsteroidal antiinflammatory drugs. *CNS Drugs.* 198; 9:281-90.
32. Vella Brincat J, Macleod AD. Adverse effects of opioids on the central nervous systems of palliative care patients. *J Pain Palliat Care Pharmacother.* 2007; 21:15-25.
33. Wilkinson TJ, Begg EJ, Winter AC et al. Incidence and risk factors for hyponatraemia following treatment with fluoxetine or paroxetine in elderly people. *Br J Clin Pharmacol.* 1999; 47:211-7.
34. Meador KJ. Cognitive side effects of medications. *Neurol Clin North Am.* 1998; 16:141-55.
35. Loring DW, Meador KJ. Cognitive and behavioral effects of epilepsy treatment. *Epilepsia.* 2001; 42(suppl 8):24-32.
36. Francis J, Martin D, Kapoor WN. A prospective study of delirium in hospitalized elderly. *JAMA.* 1990; 263:1097-101.
37. Moses H 3rd, Kaden I. Neurologic consultations in a general hospital. Spectrum of iatrogenic disease. *Am J Med.* 1986; 81:955-8.
38. Larson EB, Kukull WA, Buchner D et al. Adverse drug reactions associated with global cognitive impairment in elderly persons. *Ann Intern Med.* 1987; 107:160-73.
39. Folstein MF, Folstein SE, McHugh PR. "Mini-Mental-State" A practical method for grading the cognitive state of patients for the clinician. *J Psychiatr Res.* 1975; 12:189-98.
40. Nasreddine ZS, Phillips NA, Bédirian V et al. The Montreal Cognitive Assessment, MoCA: a brief screening tool for mild cognitive impairment. *J Am Geriatr Soc.* 2005; 53:695-9.
41. Nail LM. Cognitive changes in cancer survivors. Cancer and cancer treatment often cause cognitive deficits, but no guidelines exist for screening or treatment. *Am J Nurs.* 2006; 106(suppl 3):48-54.
42. Beattie C. History and principles of anesthesiology. In: Hardman JG, Limbird LE, Gilman AG, eds. *Goodman & Gilman's the pharmacological basis of therapeutics.* 10th ed. New York: McGraw-Hill; 2001.
43. Hussain M, Berger M, Eckenhoff RG et al. General anesthetic and the risk of dementia in elderly patients: current insights. *Clin Interv Aging.* 2014; 9:1619-28.
44. Donnellan CA, Fook L, McDonald P et al. Lesson of the week: oxybutynin and cognitive dysfunction. *BMJ.* 1997; 315:1363-4.
45. Caccamo A, Oddo S, Billings L et al. M1 receptors play a central role in modulating AD-like pathology in transgenic mice. *Neuron.* 2006; 49:671-82.
46. Meador KJ. Cognitive outcomes and predictive factors in epilepsy. *Neurology.* 2002; 58(suppl 5):S21-6.
47. Bittigau P, Sifringer M, Ikonomidou C. Antiepileptic drugs and apoptosis in the developing brain. *Ann NY Acad Sci.* 2003; 993:103-14.
48. Dumas JA, Makarewicz J, Schaubhut GJ et al. Chemotherapy altered brain functional connectivity in women with breast cancer: a pilot study. *Brain Imaging Behav.* 2013; 7:524-32.
49. Raffa RB, Tallarida RJ. Effects on the visual system might contribute to some of the cognitive deficits of cancer chemotherapy-induced 'chemo'fog'. *J Clin Pharm Ther.* 2010; 35:249-55.
50. Jansen C, Miaskowski C, Dodd M et al. Potential mechanisms for chemotherapy-induced impairments in cognitive function. *Oncol Nurs Forum.* 2005; 32:1151-61.
51. Ahles TA, Saykin AJ. Candidate mechanisms for chemotherapy-induced cognitive changes. *Nat Rev Cancer.* 2007; 7:192-201.

52. Terry AV, Mahadik SP. Time-dependent cognitive deficits associated with first and second generation antipsychotics: cholinergic dysregulation as a potential mechanism. *J Pharmacol Exp Ther.* 2007; 320:961-8.
53. Ashton CH, Teoh R, Davies DM. Drug-induced stupor and coma: some physical signs and their pharmacological basis. *Adverse Drug React Acute Poisoning Rev.* 1989; 8:1-59.
54. Ransom BR, Elmore JG. Effects of antiepileptic drugs on the developing central nervous system. *Adv Neurol.* 1991; 55:225-37.
55. Bijlsma JW, Boers M, Saag KG et al. Glucocorticoids in the treatment of early and late RA. *Ann Rheum Dis.* 2003; 62:1033-7.
56. Wolkowitz OM, Reus VI, Canick J et al. Glucocorticoid medication, memory and steroid psychosis in medical illness. *Ann NY Acad Sci.* 1997; 823:81-96.
57. Odeh M, Oliven A. Central nervous system reactions associated with famotidine: report of five cases. *J Clin Gastroenterol.* 1998; 27:253-4.
58. Capuron L, Ravaud A, Dantzer R. Timing and specificity of the cognitive changes induced by interleukin-2 and interferon-α treatments in cancer patients. *Psychosom Med.* 2001; 63:376-86.
59. Dublin S, Walker RL, Gray SL et al. Prescription opioids and risk of dementia or cognitive decline: A prospective cohort study. *J Am Geriatr Soc.* 2015; 63:1519-26.
60. McSwan KL, Gontkovsky ST, Splinter MY. Acute changes in mental status secondary to selective serotonin reuptake inhibitor-induced hyponatremia. *Rehabil Psychol.* 2003; 48:202-6.
61. Spigset O, Hedenmalm K. Hyponatraemia and the syndrome of inappropriate antidiuretic hormone secretion (SIADH) induced by psychotropic drugs. *Drug Saf.* 1995; 12:209-25.
62. Mesulam M. Cholinergic neurons, pathways, diseases. In: Adelman G, ed. *Encyclopedia of neuroscience.* Boston, MA: Birkhäuser; 1987.
63. Womack KB, Heilman KM. Tolterodine and memory: dry but forgetful. *Arch Neurol.* 2003; 60:771-3.
64. Miller CA. Medications that may cause cognitive impairment in older adults. *Geriatr Nurs.* 1995; 16:47.
65. Tune LE. Serum anticholinergic activity levels and delirium in the elderly. *Semin Clin Neuropsychiatry.* 2000; 5:149-53.
66. Perry EK, Kilford L, Lees AJ et al. Increased Alzheimer pathology in Parkinson's disease related to antimuscarinic drugs. *Ann Neurol.* 2003; 54:235-8.
67. Guerrini R, Belmonte A, Canapicchi R et al. Reversible pseudo-atrophy of the brain and mental deterioration associated with valproate treatment. *Epilepsia.* 1998; 39:27-32.
68. Inoyama K, Meador KJ. Cognitive outcomes of prenatal antiepileptic drug exposure. *Epilepsy Res.* 2015; 114:89-97.
69. Loring DW, Meador KJ. Corticosteroids and cognitive function in humans: methodological considerations. *J Pediatr Hematol Oncol.* 2000; 22:193-6.
70. Waber DP, Carpentieri SC, Klar N et al. Cognitive sequelae in children treated for acute lymphoblastic leukemia with dexamethasone or prednisone. *J Pediatr Hematol Oncol.* 2000; 22:206-13.
71. Kingma A, Van Dommelen RI, Mooyaart EL et al. No major cognitive impairment in young children with acute lymphoblastic leukemia using chemotherapy only: a prospective longitudinal study. *J Pediatr Hematol Oncol.* 2002; 24:106-14.
72. Ng T, Chan M, Khor CC et al. The genetic variants underlying breast cancer treatment-induced chronic and late toxicities: a systematic review. *Cancer Treat Rev.* 2014;4 0:1190-214.
73. American College of Emergency Physicians. Clinical policy for the initial approach to patients presenting with altered mental status. *Ann Emerg Med.* 1999; 33:251-81.
74. Schimmer BP, Funder JW. Adrenocorticotropic hormone, adrenal steroids, and the adrenal cortex. In: Brunton LL, Hilal-Dandan R, Knollmann B, eds. *Goodman & Gilman's: the pharmacological basis of therapeutics.* 13th ed. http://accesspharmacy.mhmedical.com/content.aspx?bookid=2189§ionid=172482605 (accessed 2018 Feb 1).
75. Mihic S, Mayfield J, Harris R. Hypnotics and sedatives. In: Brunton LL, Hilal-Dandan R, Knollmann BC, eds. *Goodman & Gilman's: the pharmacological basis of therapeutics.* 13th ed. http://accesspharmacy.mhmedical.com/content.aspx?bookid=2189§ionid=169518968 (accessed 2018 Feb 1).
76. Zuccala G, Cocchi A, Gambassi G et al. Postsurgical complications in older patients: the role of pharmacological intervention. *Drugs Aging.* 1994; 5:419-30.
77. Wechsler D. *The Wechsler intelligence scale for children.* 3rd ed. San Antonio, TX: The Psychological Corporation; 1991.
78. Bourgeois BF. Antiepileptic drugs, learning, and behavior in childhood epilepsy. *Epilepsia.* 1998; 39:913-21.
79. Robertson KR, Smurzynski M, Parsons TD et al. The prevalence and incidence of neurocognitive impairment in the HAART era. *AIDS.* 2007; 21:1915-21.
80. Bird TD. Memory loss and dementia. In: Braunwald E, Fauci AS, Kasper DL et al., eds. *Harrison's principles of internal medicine.* 15th ed. New York: McGraw-Hill; 2001.
81. Cherny N, Ripamonti C, Pereira J et al. Strategies to manage the adverse effects of oral morphine: an evidence-based report. *J Clin Oncol.* 2001; 19:2542-54.
82. Farkas J, Farkas P, Hyde D. Liver and gastroenterology tests. In: Lee M, ed. *Basic skills in interpreting laboratory data.* 6th ed. Bethesda, MD: ASHP; 2017.
83. Boggs JG. Elderly patients with systemic disease. *Epilepsia.* 2001; 42:18-23.
84. MacKichan JJ. Interpretation of serum drug concentrations. In: Lee M, ed. *Basic skills in interpreting laboratory data.* 6th ed. Bethesda, MD: ASHP; 2017.
85. Bourdet SV, Gidal BE, Alldredge BK. Pharmacologic management of epilepsy in the elderly. *J Am Pharm Assoc.* 2001; 41:421-36.
86. Arryoyo S, Kramer G. Treating epilepsy in the elderly. *Drug Saf.* 2001; 24:991-1015.
87. Cai X, Campbell N, Khan B et al. Long-term anticholinergic use and the aging brain. *Alzheimer Dement.* 2013; 9:377-85.
88. Elterman RD, Glauser TA, Wyllie E et al. A double-blind, randomized trial of topiramate as adjunctive therapy for partial-onset seizures in children. Topiramate YP Study Group. *Neurology.* 1999; 52:1338-44.
89. Farwell JR, Lee YJ, Hirtz DG et al. Phenobarbital for febrile seizures: effects on intelligence and on seizure recurrence. *N Engl J Med.* 1990; 322:364-9.
90. Sulzbacher S, Farwell JR, Temkin N et al. Late cognitive effects of early treatment with phenobarbital. *Clin Pediatrics.* 1999; 38:387-94.
91. Evans WE, Relling MV. Moving towards individualized medicine with pharmacogenomics. *Nature.* 2004; 429:464-8.
92. Aldenkamp AP, Baker G, Mulder OG et al. A multicenter, randomized clinical study to evaluate the effect on cognitive function of topiramate compared with valproate as add-on therapy to carbamazepine in patients with partial-onset seizures. *Epilepsia.* 2000; 1:1167-78.
93. Meador KJ, Loring DW, Hulihan JF et al. Differential cognitive and behavioral effects of topiramate and valproate. *Neurology.* 2003; 60:1483-8.
94. Galimberti CA, Diegoli M, Sartori I et al. Brain pseudoatrophy and mental regression on valproate and a mitochondrial DNA mutation. *Neurology.* 2006; 67:1715-7.
95. Slugg PH, Haug MT III, Pippenger CE. Ranitidine pharmacokinetics and adverse central nervous system reactions. *Arch Intern Med.* 1992; 152:2325-9.
96. Herrick IA, Ganapathy S, Komar W et al. Postoperative cognitive impairment in the elderly: choice of patient controlled analgesia opioid. *Anaesthesia.* 1996; 51:356-60.
97. Moller JT, Cluitmans P, Rasmussen LS et al. for the ISPOCD investigators. Long-term postoperative cognitive dysfunction in the elderly: ISPOCD1 study. *Lancet.* 1998; 351:857-61.

98. Johnson T, Monk T, Rasmussen LS et al.; the ISPOCD2 investigators. Postoperative cognitive dysfunction in middle-aged patients. *Anesthesiology*. 2002; 96:1351-7.
99. Pasero CL, McCaffery M. Reluctance to order opioids in elders. *Am J Nurs*. 1997; 97:20-3.
100. Duggleby W, Lander J. Cognitive status and postoperative pain: older adults. *J Pain Symptom Manage*. 1994; 9:19-27.
101. Farkas RH, Unger EF, Temple R. Zoldipem and driving impairment—identifying persons at risk. *N Engl J Med*. 2013; 369:689-91.
102. Fick DM, Cooper JW, Wade WE et al. Updating the Beers criteria for potentially inappropriate medication use in older adults: results of a US consensus panel of experts. *Arch Intern Med*. 2003; 163:2716-24.
103. Cirulli ET, Urban TJ, Marino SE et al. Genetic and environmental correlates of topiramate-induced cognitive impairment. *Epilepsia*. 2012; 53:e5-38.
104. Javed A, Choeh B, Detyniecki K et al. Rates and predictors of patient-reported cognitive side effects of antiepileptic drugs: An extended follow-up. *Seizure*. 2015; 29:34-40.
105. Federal Regulations: 42 CFR 483.25. http://www.access.gpo.gov/nara/cfr/waisidx_02/42cfr483_02.html (accessed 2017 Dec 18).
106. Department of Health and Human Services. Collecting and updating nursing home data. http://www.medicare.gov/NHCompare/Static/Related/DataCollection.asp?des=NAV. (accessed 2017 Dec 18).
107. Beers MH. Explicit criteria for determining potentially inappropriate medication use by the elderly. An update. *Arch Intern Med*. 1997; 157:1531-6.
108. American Geriatrics Society; 2012 Beers Criteria Update Expert Panel. American Geriatrics Society updated Beers criteria for potentially inappropriate medication use in older adults. *J Am Geriatr Soc*. 2012; 60:616-31.
109. Zwart W, Terra H, Linn SC et al. Cognitive effects of endocrine therapy for breast cancer: keep calm and carry on? *Nat Rev Clin Oncol*. 2015; 12:597-606.
110. Rickels K, DeMartinis N, Rynn M et al. Pharmacologic strategies for discontinuing benzodiazepine treatment. *J Clin Psychopharmacol*. 1999; 19(suppl 2):12S-16S.
111. Avisar A, River Y, Schiff E et al. Chemotherapy-related cognitive impairment: does integrating complementary medicine have something to add? Review of the literature. *Breast Cancer Res Treat*. 2012; 136:1-7.
112. Rosenbaum JF, Fava M, Hoog SL et al. Selective serotonin receptor inhibitor discontinuatioin syndrome: a randomized clinical trial. *Biol Psychiatr*. 1998; 44:77-87.
113. Bailey L, Ward M, Musa M. Clinical pharmacokinetics of benzodiazipines. *J Clin Pharmacol*. 1994; 34:804-11.
114. Schweizer E, Rickels K, Case WG, Greenblatt DJ. Carbamazepine treatment in patients discontinuing long-term benzodiazepine therapy. Effects on withdrawal severity and taper outcome. *Arch Gen Psychiatry*. 1991; 48:448-52.
115. Rynn M, Garcia-Espana F, Greenblatt DJ et al. Imipramine and buspirone in patients with panic disorder who are discontinuing long-term benzodiazepine therapy. *J Clin Psychopharmacol*. 2003; 23:505-8.
116. Rickels K, Schweizer E, Garcia-España F et al. Trazodone and valproate in patients discontinuing long-term benzodiazepine therapy: effects of withdrawal symptoms and taper outcome. *Psychopharmacology (Berl)*. 1999; 141:1-5.
117. Rickels K, Garcia-Espana F, Mandos LA et al. Physician withdrawal checklist (PWC-20). *J Clin Psychopharm*. 2008; 28:447-51.
118. Ahles TA, Saykin AJ, Furstenberg CT et al. Neuropsychologic impact of standard-dose systemic chemotherapy in long-term survivors of breast cancer and lymphoma. *J Clin Oncol*. 2002; 20:485-93.
119. Chan RJ, McCarthy AL, Devenish J et al. Systematic review of pharmacologic and non-pharmacologic interventions to manage cognitive alterations after chemotherapy for breast cancer. *Eur J Cancer*. 2015; 51:437-50.

SECTION IV

DRUG-INDUCED PSYCHIATRIC DISEASES

CHAPTER 18 Depression

CHAPTER 19 Anxiety

CHAPTER 20 Psychosis

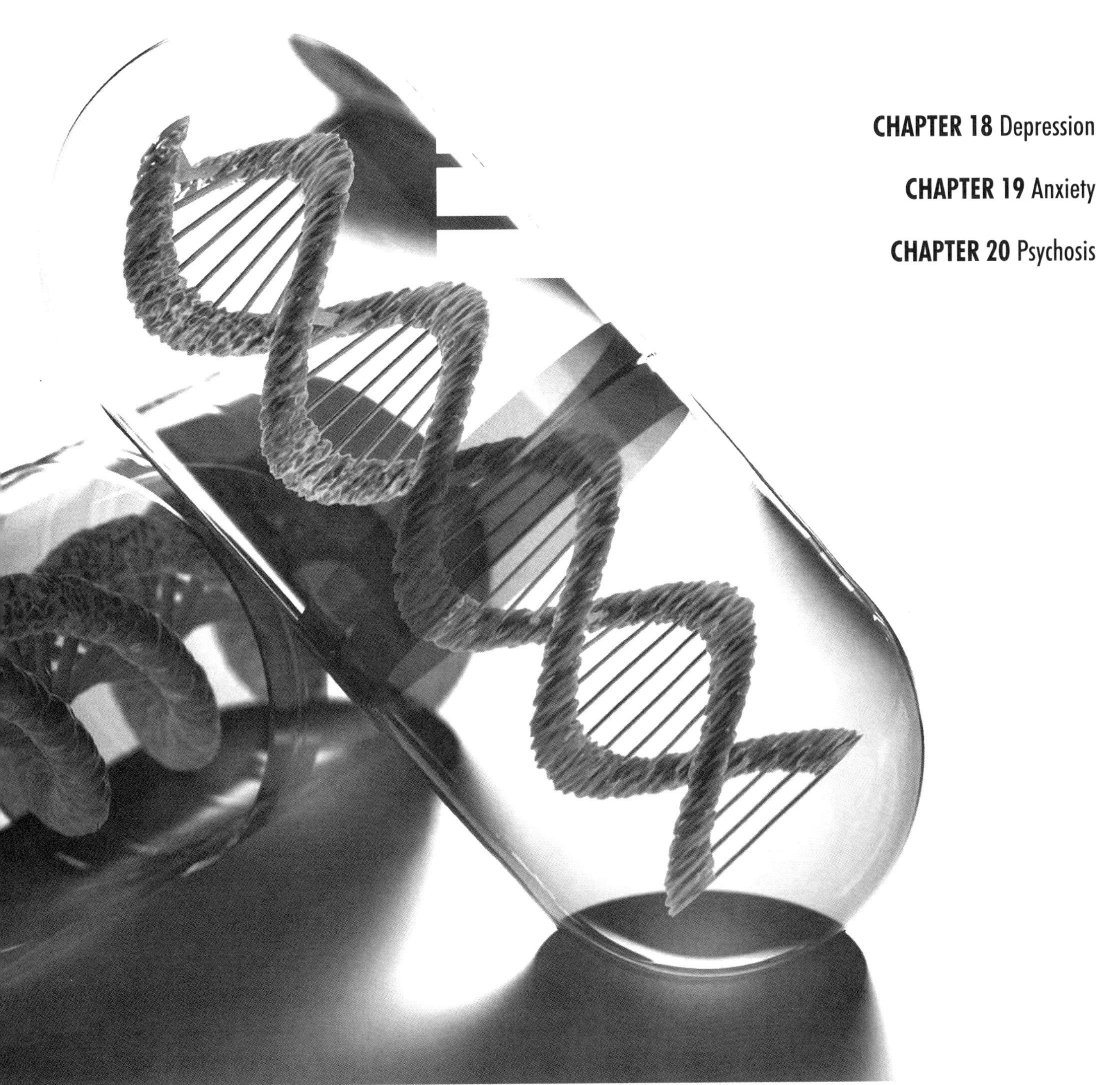

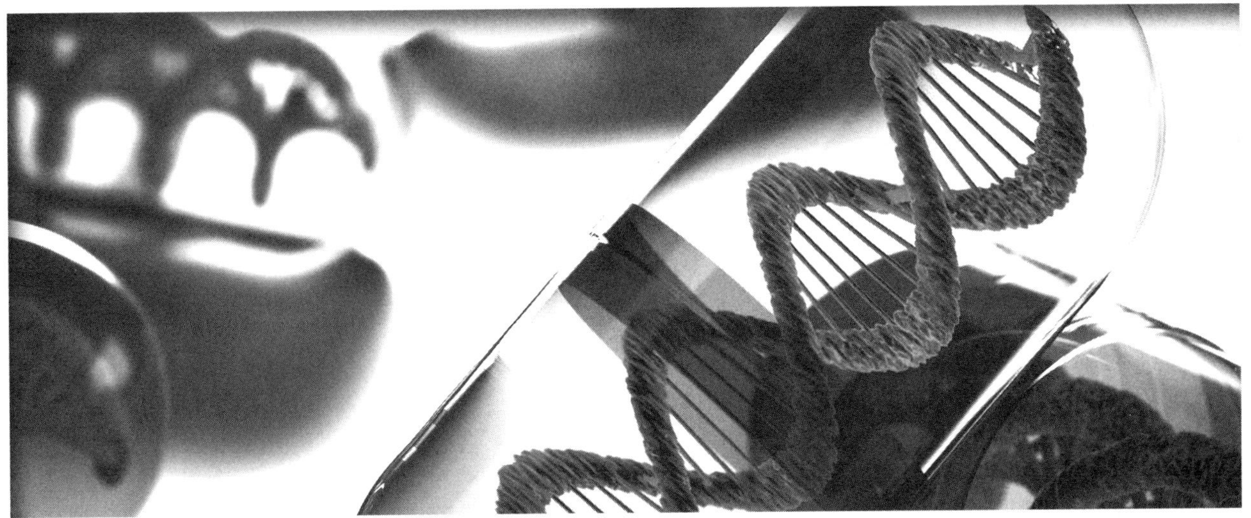

CHAPTER 18

Depression

Sheila Botts and Melody Ryan

Depression is one of the most common psychiatric illnesses. Depression may interfere significantly with a patient's daily functioning and quality of life. Untreated depression is associated with substantial morbidity and increases the risk of suicide and death. The lifetime risk of suicide among patients with depression is 2.2–15%.[1,2] Depression is a biologic illness with an unknown cause. Drug-induced depression is similar in presentation to idiopathic depression and carries similar risks of morbidity and mortality. Although the overall prevalence is unknown, drug-induced depression poses a significant challenge for practitioners, as it may undermine the effectiveness of much-needed treatment. Treatment-emergent suicidality (e.g., suicidal ideation and behavior) has been characterized independently, even though it often occurs with mood changes and poses significant risks to the patient.

CAUSATIVE AGENTS

Depression has been associated with many drugs, including anti-infectives, cardiovascular agents, central nervous system (CNS) drugs, dermatologic agents, hormonal treatments, and immunologic and cancer chemotherapy drugs. The *Diagnostic and Statistical Manual of Mental Disorders, 5th Edition* (*DSM-5*), defines *medication-induced depression* as a "prominent and persistent disturbance of mood that occurs during use of a medication causally related to depression, or within 1 month of intoxication or withdrawal of therapy with a medication."[1] Symptoms must be severe enough to result in clinically significant distress in social, occupational, or other areas of functioning. The clinical features of medication-induced depression may be similar to those of a major depressive disorder (MDD) but do not have to meet full diagnostic criteria. In the evaluative literature, depression may be characterized as a specific symptom (i.e., depressed mood), a cluster of depressive symptoms, or as a diagnostic entity (e.g., MDD) although the latter is less common. For the purposes of this chapter, depression is defined as the presence of any one of these three characterizations and which is severe enough to cause a disruption in daily function. Suicide and suicidality are often associated with depression. Suicidality associated with antidepressants, antipsychotics, and anticonvulsants is defined as suicidal thoughts or behaviors or suicide.

Table 18-1 Agents Implicated in Drug-Induced Depression

Drug	Reported Incidence[a]	Level of Evidence[b]
ANTI-INFECTIVE AGENTS[3-15]		
Cycloserine	NK	C
Ethionamide	NK	C
Fluoroquinolones	NK	C
Mefloquine	NK	C
ANTIVIRAL AGENTS[16-22]		
Efavirenz[29]	1.6–2%	A
CARDIOVASCULAR DRUGS[23-36]		
β-blockers	NK	C
Clonidine	1.5%	C
Digitalis	NK	B
Guanethidine	1.5%	C
Methyldopa	3.6%	B
Reserpine	7%	B
CENTRAL NERVOUS SYSTEM AGENTS[36-89]		
Anticonvulsants[36-73]		
Levetiracetam	4%	A
Phenobarbital	40%	B
Primidone	70%	B
Phenytoin	NK	C
Tiagabine	3%	A
Topiramate	5–10%	A
Vigabatrin	12.1%	A
ANTIDEPRESSANTS[74,c]		
SSRIs, SNRIs, TCAs	1–4%	A
Aripiprazole	NK	C
Quetiapine	NK	C
Lurasidone	NK	C
ANTIMIGRAINE[75]		
Triptans	23%	B
MISCELLANEOUS[76-89]		
Sodium oxybate	10%	B
Tetrabenazine	15%	B
Varenicline	1–3%	A[d]
HORMONAL AGENTS[90-114]		
Corticosteroids	1.3–18%	B
Oral contraceptives	NK	B
GnRH agonists	26–54%	B
Tamoxifen	1–20%	A[d]
Aromatase inhibitors	5–13%	A
Finasteride	NK	B

Table 18-1 Agents Implicated in Drug-Induced Depression (continued)

Drug	Reported Incidence[a]	Level of Evidence[b]
IMMUNOLOGIC AND CANCER CHEMOTHERAPY AGENTS[115-146]		
INFα	13–33%	A
INFβ	0–33%	A
Interleukin-2	NK	C
TNFα inhibitors	NK	C
Vincristine	NK	C
RETINOIC ACID DERIVATIVES[145-165]		
Isotretinion[3-21]	1–5.5%	B

GnRH = gonadotropin-releasing hormone, INF = interferon, NK = not known; SNRI = serotonin-norepinephrine reuptake inhibitor, SSRI = selective serotonin reuptake inhibitor, TCA = tricyclic antidepressant; TNF = tumor necrosis factor.

[a]Incidence reported in the treated population.

[b]Definitions for Levels of Evidence: Level A—evidence from one or more randomized, controlled clinical trials; Level B—evidence from nonrandomized clinical trials, prospective observational studies, cohort studies, retrospective studies, case-control studies, meta-analyses and/or postmarketing surveillance studies; and Level C—evidence from one or more published case reports or case series.

[c]Refers to risk of suicidal ideation when used as antidepressant.

[d]Randomized studies do not support an increased risk of depression.

All drugs associated with inducing depression for which evaluative support is available in the literature are reviewed in this chapter.[3-182] The literature supporting an association of drugs with depression is largely comprised of case reports, postmarketing surveillance, and retrospective observational studies, making the case for causality difficult. There are few prospective, controlled trials with objective assessments of depressive symptoms or diagnostic criteria. When available, these data are discussed for each agent. A list of drugs associated with depression and the estimated incidence for each are presented in **Table 18-1**.[3-165]

EPIDEMIOLOGY

The estimated lifetime prevalence of depression in the general population is approximately 17%.[183] Depression occurs at a much higher rate in patients with chronic illnesses such as diabetes and cardiovascular disease.[184] Although many drugs have been associated with depression, few have been adequately studied to identify the degree of risk that they impart above and beyond that normally present in the population of patients with disease.

ANTI-INFECTIVE AGENTS

Adverse psychiatric effects have been reported in association with most antibiotics, but are still considered relatively rare events.[3] Depression has been reported in patients taking fluoroquinolones, the antitubercular agents cycloserine and ethionamide, and the antimalarial agent mefloquine.[3-15] These data, however, are limited to case reports, and the overall prevalence is unknown.

ANTIVIRAL AGENTS

Both non-nucleoside reverse transcriptase inhibitors (NNRTIs) and protease inhibitors have been associated with depression. The NNRTI efavirenz appears to confer the greatest risk. In over 1,000 patients treated with efavirenz in clinical trials for an average of 1.6 years, severe depression was reported with an incidence of 1.6%, and suicidal ideation occurred in 0.6% of patients.[16] The risk of depression and suicidal ideation increased to 2% in patients with a history of psychiatric disorders. In contrast, several prospective trials have not shown an increased risk of depression associated with efavirenz treatment. A 48-week randomized, controlled trial of patients receiving a protease inhibitor–containing regimen or efavirenz-containing once-daily regimen failed to find a difference in the risk of depression during maintenance treatment.[17] An additional prospective trial compared neuropsychiatric effects of an efavirenz-containing antiviral regimen with those in patients on therapy that did not contain efavirenz.[18] The proportion of efavirenz-treated patients who reached the threshold Center for Epidemiologic Studies—Depression (CES-D) score for clinical depression declined over the course of the study from 34.1% at baseline to 22.3% at week 184. Finally, a large cohort study of patients newly diagnosed with human immunodeficiency virus (HIV) also did not find an increased incidence of depression in those taking efavirenz-containing regimens.[19] In summary, it is difficult to assess the true incidence of efavirenz-associated depression, because depression has been associated with other agents with which efavirenz is almost always prescribed in combination. Other NNRTIs (nevirapine, abacavir), and protease inhibitors (indinavir) have also been noted in clinical case reports to cause depression.[18-22]

CARDIOVASCULAR AGENTS

Antihypertensive agents, including angiotensin-converting enzyme inhibitors, β-blockers, calcium channel blockers, antiadrenergic agents (e.g., reserpine, methyldopa, guanethidine, and clonidine), and thiazide diuretics have been implicated in causing depression in case reports. With the exception of antiadrenergic agents, β-blockers and digoxin, little empirical evidence exists to support this association. Reserpine, methyldopa, and guanethidine increase patients' risk of depression, but these agents are no longer commonly used.[23-27] Case report data support the association between clonidine and depression. However, larger evaluative studies suggest that the incidence of depression in patients taking clonidine is similar to that in the general population.[28] The risk of depression associated with β-blocker therapy remains somewhat controversial. In addition to case reports, two epidemiologic studies support an association with depression, but this link was not confirmed in two prospective studies.[29-32] It has been suggested that depressive disorders rarely develop in patients treated with β-blockers, but that these patients experience typical β-blocker adverse effects, which leads to misdiagnosis of depression. Studies that have incorporated diagnostic criteria for depressive disorders have failed to identify an association between β-blockers and depression.[33,34] Digoxin has been associated with depression in case reports and two small prospective studies.[34-36] In a community sample, Palinkas reported that elderly women taking digoxin had higher rates of significant depressive symptoms than women not taking digoxin (10.5% versus 6.5%), although this difference was not statistically significant.[35] In a second study of 335 patients postmyocardial infarction, digoxin exposure was associated with an increased risk of depression at the 3- to 4-month follow-up visit.[36]

CENTRAL NERVOUS SYSTEM AGENTS

Several CNS-acting drugs have been associated with depression, including antiepileptic drugs (AEDs), benzodiazepines, physostigmine, and 5-hydroxytryptamine $(5\text{-HT})_1$ agonists (triptans). Most AEDs have been reported to cause depression. Conversely, many AEDs may be used to stabilize patients with mood disorders. Sodium valproate, carbamazepine, and lamotrigine have U.S. Food and Drug Administration (FDA)-approved indications for bipolar disorder. In addition, several AEDs including phenytoin and carbamazepine have demonstrated effectiveness in the management of unipolar depression.[37,38] It is important to note that, because of ethical considerations, very few of the AED trials are placebo-controlled. Because of the various CNS activities of the AEDs used as comparators, it is difficult to judge the exact prevalence of depression caused by these agents. Also, the rate of depression in patients with epilepsy is very high (32–48%) and the lifetime prevalence of suicide and suicide attempts is 5–14% in this population.[39] Therefore, this increase in the incidence of mood disorders can be only partially attributed to the AEDs. All of the AEDs, particularly at higher doses, are associated with lethargy, fatigue, drowsiness, and asthenia, which may mimic depression. All AEDs have FDA-mandated warnings regarding suicidality.[40] This requirement stems from data from 199 placebo-controlled trials of 11 AEDs (carbamazepine, felbamate, gabapentin, lamotrigine, levetiracetam, oxcarbazepine, pregabalin, tiagabine, topiramate, valproate, zonisamide).[40] The investigators reported suicidal ideation or behavior in 0.43% of patients taking AEDs compared with 0.22% of those taking placebo. The relative risk of suicidal behavior or ideation in patients taking AEDs for epilepsy was 3.53 (95% CI 1.28–12.1), compared with 1.51 (95% CI 0.95–2.45) for those taking AEDs for psychiatric reasons and 1.87 (95% CI 0.81–4.76) for those taking AEDs for other reasons.[40] No specific AED appears to confer greater risk, and no demographic group appears to be at higher risk. In the wake of this study and subsequent warning, several other investigations have been conducted to attempt to provide clarity regarding the risks of suicidal ideation, behavior, and depression.

A large cohort study of 8,211 patients found no excess risk of suicidal ideation associated with AED use.[41] However, a nested case-controlled study of 44,300 patients ever given AEDs found increased odds (OR 3.08, 95% CI 1.22–7.77) of self-harm or suicidal behavior with a group of newer AEDs associated with depression (levetiracetam, vigabatrin, topiramate, tiagabine) compared with patients not currently taking AEDs.[42] The odds of suicidal behavior or self-harm were not higher in patients taking other AEDs, conventional agents, barbiturates, and newer AEDs with low association with depression compared to those in patients not currently prescribed AEDs. A retrospective database analysis of 2.15 million military veterans over the age of 65 years reported that taking AEDs was associated with an increased hazard of suicidal behavior (HR 4.10, 95% CI 3.85–6.63).[43] Gabapentin, lamotrigine, levetiracetam, phenytoin, topiramate, and valproic acid were all significantly associated with suicidal behavior in this study. Another study of 449,269 veterans older than 65 years of age who were prescribed AEDs did not find an increased risk of suicidal behaviors associated with AED use; however, there was a trend toward an increase in suicidal behavior in patients who were taking levetiracetam or lamotrigine (OR 10.2, 95% CI 1.1–97).[44] A consensus statement of the World Psychiatric Association section of pharmacopsychiatry declined to identify suicidal behavior as a class effect.[45] An expert consensus statement from the International League Against Epilepsy stated that depression was associated with barbiturates, tiagabine, topiramate, vigabatrin, and zonisamide.[46] This panel further stated that withholding AED therapy to prevent depression and suicidality can also be harmful, even resulting in patient death.

Of the AEDs, the barbiturates are most strongly associated with depression in both adult and pediatric populations.[47,50] In one cross-sectional sample of adult patients in Mexico City, primidone use was strongly associated with depression, with an odds ratio of 4.089 (95% CI 2.094–7.985). In this sample, 70% of the patients treated with primidone were depressed.[50] In another study, phenobarbital was associated with an incidence of depression of 40%.[49] Data relating phenytoin use to depression are much less convincing. There are case reports of two patients with epilepsy with supratherapeutic serum phenytoin concentrations (22.7 mcg/mL and 25.5 mcg/mL) who had depressive symptoms. When the phenytoin dose was decreased or the medication was discontinued, the symptoms resolved.[51] A prospective study of 277 patients in whom tiagabine or placebo was added to baseline AED therapy found depression in 3% of those treated with tiagabine.[52] Topiramate treatment has been associated with new-onset depression in 5–10% of patients.[53] Pooled data analysis of perampanel trials found one case of suicidal ideation; 2.4% of patients taking 12 mg/day reporting depression, compared to 1.6% of patients given placebo (no statistical analysis performed).[54] Depression was reported in 4% of levetiracetam-treated patients compared to 2% treated with placebo.[55] Levetiracetam has been implicated as a cause of depression in a prospective study, a retrospective case series, and an additional case report.[56-58] In a prospective study of 71 treatment-refractory epilepsy patients administered levetiracetam, there was no mean change in the Beck's Depression Inventory (BDI) score from baseline to week 24.[59] However, five patients discontinued treatment due to psychiatric symptoms, of whom four had suicidal ideation. Vigabatrin-associated depression occurred in 12.1% of patients treated in double-blind, placebo-controlled clinical trials (p <0.001).[60] In a small, prospective study (n = 23) of patients with previous psychiatric diagnoses who were prescribed zonisamide, one patient developed major depressive disorder.[61] Pregabalin has also been associated with depression in case reports.[62,63] Two cases of depression activation in patients with bipolar disorder have been reported in association with rufinamide.[64]

Depression often is cited as an adverse effect of benzodiazepines, both during therapy and after discontinuation.[65] However, the literature supporting incident depression in patients taking benzodiazepines is not robust, and depression is reported infrequently in controlled clinical trials. Case reports and observational studies have identified an increased risk of depression in patients taking benzodiazepines.[66-69] These reports, however, do not control for confounding variables, such as history of depression, presence of comorbid depression, or concomitant medications, and are therefore difficult to interpret. One large cohort study of 8,211 patients found a relationship between benzodiazepine use and depressive symptoms and suicidality.[41] However, when results were adjusted for comorbid psychiatric conditions, including depression and anxiety, there was no association between benzodiazepine use and suicidal ideation. A prospective trajectory study conducted in 2,590 patients found increasing depression associated with baseline benzodiazepine use.[70] In an historical cohort of 58,967 people, an association between benzodiazepine use and severe anxiety, depression, and poor sleep outcomes was found.[71] In another study, the CES-D 10 was administered to 1,331 people age ≥65 years, of whom 288 (21.6%) had type 2 diabetes mellitus.[72] The investigators found an increased odds of depression in those using benzodiazepines or nonbenzodiazepine hypnotics compared to nonusers (OR 1.66, 95% CI 1.10–2.51). Depression and anxiety are highly comorbid syndromes, and the emergence of depression during benzodiazepine therapy may occur from a relapse or as a coincidental finding. Moreover, alprazolam administered in higher doses has been shown to have an antidepressant effect.[73]

Antidepressant medications are associated with an increased risk of suicidality in patients younger than 25 years of age.[74] Pooled analyses of 24 short-term placebo-controlled antidepressant trials in over 4,400 children and adolescents with MDD, obsessive–compulsive disorder, or other psychiatric disorders revealed that these drugs increase the risk of suicidality, although no suicides were reported. Antidepressant use in patients younger than 18 years of age resulted in an additional 14 cases of suicidality per 1,000 patients treated. A pooled analysis of 295 short-term placebo-controlled studies of antidepressants in over 77,000 adults aged 18–24 years with MDD or other psychiatric disorders showed an additional five cases of suicidality per 1,000 patients treated. There was no increased risk in adults aged 25–64 years, and there was a reduced risk in adults 65 years and older (six fewer cases per 1,000 patients). All antidepressant medications, including antipsychotics with an FDA indication for MDD or bipolar depression (e.g., aripiprazole and quetiapine, lurasidone), have a boxed warning for suicidality in the product information. Suicidality is an inherent risk in patients with major depression and should be considered when balancing the potential risks and benefits of antidepressant therapy in all age groups.

Only a single published epidemiologic study exists to implicate the antimigraine agents, triptans, as causative agents for depression. A cohort analysis of the West Midlands General Practice Research Database in the United Kingdom (UK) examined the incidence of depression in migraineurs receiving any oral triptan, sumatriptan, or the more lipophilic agents in this class (naratriptan or zolmitriptan).[75] A larger proportion of the 1,062 patients (23.2%) receiving any oral triptan were diagnosed with depression, as compared with 16.8% of 18,033 patients not receiving an oral triptan (p <0.001). No difference in the number of patients diagnosed with depression after their first prescription was found between those receiving sumatriptan (4.2%) and those receiving naratriptan or zolmitriptan (3.9%, $p = 0.87$).

Physostigmine was associated with immediate depressive symptoms in nine normal volunteers administered high intravenous doses.[76] Whether the results of this study apply to patients with myasthenia gravis who take oral physostigmine is unknown. Sodium oxybate has been associated with depression, suicidal ideation, and suicide in controlled and uncontrolled clinical trials for sleep disorders as well as in postmarketing case reports.[77-79] In a 12-month open-label study, depression was reported in 10% of patients.[79] Tetrabenazine is associated with new onset or worsening depression in up to 15% of patients treated for chorea or other movement disorders.[80]

In placebo-controlled trials of 4,400 patients, varenicline was associated with a higher risk of depression than placebo.[81] However, patients with a history of psychiatric disorders were excluded from these trials. A postmarketing analysis of the FDA Adverse Event Reporting System found increased odds of suicidal/self-injurious behavior or depression associated with varenicline treatment compared to nicotine replacement therapy (OR 8.4, 95% CI 6.8–10.4).[81] Although smoking cessation may be associated with nicotine withdrawal symptoms including depression and agitation, there appears to be an increased risk of these symptoms associated with varenicline, because some of these cases occurred while patients were still smoking.[81,82] Several large cohort trials have been conducted to help clarify risks associated with varenicline. A large cross-sectional database study of 12,159 patients who were prescribed varenicline was performed, in which questionnaires were sent to participants' primary care physicians to ascertain adverse effects.[83] There were 103 reports of depression occurring during treatment (1%); there was no control group in this study. A retrospective cohort study of 35,800 individuals in the Department of Defense database did not reveal an increased incidence of depression associated with varenicline compared to nicotine replacement therapy.[84] An additional cohort study in the UK also did not find evidence of increased self-harm, suicidal ideation, or initiation of antidepressant therapy in patients taking varenicline.[85] A New Zealand cohort study of 3,415 patients prescribed varenicline reported new or worsening depression in 2.98%.[86] In another large retrospective cohort of 164,766 patients the hazards of new depression actually decreased in association with varenicline.[87] Two prospective, randomized, placebo-controlled studies of varenicline have been performed. In 525 smokers with a past or current history of depression, the incidence of depression associated with varenicline was similar to that of placebo.[88] A much larger study (n = 8144) was conducted in patients with and without pre-existing psychiatric conditions. Patients were assigned to receive therapy with a nicotine patch, varenicline, or bupropion. There was a larger incidence of psychiatric adverse effects in the psychiatric cohort than the nonpsychiatric cohort (5.8% versus 2.1%, p <0.001) but no difference between the treatment groups, either overall or within the cohorts.[89] It appears that the incidence of depression with varenicline is low; however, the FDA requires warnings about depression in the product information for this drug.

HORMONAL AGENTS

The prevalence of drug-induced depression associated with hormonal agents ranges from 1% to 54%. Agents that affect sex-steroid hormone production appear to be associated with significant risks for inducing depression. Gonadotropin-releasing hormone (GnRH) agonists induce a profoundly hypoestrogenic state and are associated with significant depressive symptoms in approximately 50% of patients.[90-95] Tamoxifen, an antiestrogenic agent, does not appear to confer the same risk. Depression as an adverse effect of tamoxifen was not supported by early placebo-controlled trials in patients with breast cancer.[96] However, several published reports suggest that depression may occur in up to 15–20% of tamoxifen-treated patients with breast cancer and that it is often overlooked or erroneously attributed to the illness.[97-99] These reports do not control for confounding factors, such as the effects of the illness, diagnosis, or adverse effects of chemotherapy, and may overestimate the incidence of tamoxifen-induced depression. The Breast Cancer Prevention (P-1) Study of the National Surgical Adjuvant Breast and Bowel Project provided additional controlled data regarding the association between tamoxifen and depression.[100] The P-1 study was a multicenter randomized, double-blind, placebo-controlled chemoprevention trial in which 11,064 women were assigned to receive tamoxifen or placebo for 5 years. The frequency of depression, as assessed by the CES-D, was similar in both groups during the first 36 months of the trial. The presence of risk factors at baseline including history of depression, current or previous treatment with an antidepressant, or extended periods of dysphoric mood (≥12 months) was associated with significant depressive symptoms regardless of treatment arm.[101]

Aromatase inhibitors (anastrozole, letrozole, exemestane) have been commonly associated with depression in clinical trials for treatment of breast cancer.[102] In a retrospective cohort study from the National Health Insurance Research Database in Taiwan, 35,586 breast cancer survivors receiving adjuvant therapy were observed for up to 6 years to determine the incidence of new onset depression.[103] Overall, 3.67% of the population were diagnosed with depression. Both tamoxifen (adjusted HR 1.45, 95% CI 1.11–1.91) and aromatase inhibitors (HR 1.36, 95% CI 1.19–1.55) were identified as independent risk factors for developing a depressive disorder.

Although depression is the most commonly cited reason for discontinuing therapy with oral contraceptives (OCs), the literature does not provide overwhelming evidence of significant OC-induced depression.[104] The Royal College of General Practitioners' Oral Contraception Study reported that depression occurred at a rate of 70 per 1,000 person-years in women taking OCs. This is similar to the expected rate of affective disorders in females in the U.S.-based Epidemiologic Catchment Area studies.[185] Moreover, the rate of depression in women receiving low-dose estrogen (≤35 mcg) was similar to that observed in the control group, suggesting that commonly used low-dose preparations do not carry an increased risk of depression. More recent evaluations have focused on affective changes rather than on identifying a depressive syndrome or disorder. A review of 13 controlled, prospective studies evaluated affective changes during OC treatment and concluded that women taking OCs experience less variability in affect across the menstrual cycle and less negative affect during the time of menstruation.[105]

Finasteride, a competitive inhibitor of 5 α-reductase that inhibits peripheral conversion of testosterone to dihydrotestosterone, is associated with treatment-emergent depression, although the prevalence is unknown. In a prospective study of 128 men initiated on finasteride for androgenic alopecia, depressive symptoms as measured by the BDI were noted during the first 2 months of treatment. However, this change was clinically insignificant, and no patient reported more than mild symptoms.[106] A case-control study demonstrated that 61 men who formerly used finasteride and experienced persistent sexual adverse effects had higher rates of depression and suicidal thoughts than a control group receiving no treatment for male pattern baldness. Depression, measured with the BDI-II, was present in 75% of former finasteride users versus 10% of controls and suicidal thoughts were present in 44% versus 3%.[107] The rate of depression may have been increased in relation with the presence of sexual side effects.

Drugs that affect the hypothalamic-pituitary-adrenal (HPA) axis are associated with depression. Corticosteroids have been associated with significant psychiatric adverse effects, including depression, mania, and psychosis.[108] The occurrence of severe depression in patients taking corticosteroids is supported by case reports.[109,110] Data from case series, observational studies, and controlled trials also support an association with depression. However, many of these reports fail to quantify the prevalence of significant depressive symptoms.[108,111,112] The largest observational study, the Boston Collaborative Drug Surveillance Program, found that severe psychiatric symptoms, including depression, were relatively uncommon (1.3%) in patients without a psychiatric history who were taking low doses of corticosteroids (<40 mg/day prednisone equivalents).[113] However, the incidence increased to 18% in patients taking >80 mg/day prednisone equivalents. A cross-sectional study in patients with chronic obstructive pulmonary disease reported significantly higher self-reported depression scores in the corticosteroid-using group compared with patients who were not taking corticosteroids.[111] Furthermore, in a short-term prospective cohort study of medical inpatients, corticosteroid exposure was associated with a threefold increased risk of incident depressive symptoms.[114]

IMMUNOLOGIC AGENTS

Several medications used in immunotherapy and cancer chemotherapy, including interferon alfa (INFα), interferon beta (INFβ), tumor necrosis factor alpha (TNFα) inhibitors, and interleukin (IL)-2, are associated with depression. In addition, the immunosuppressant agent mycophenolate was reported to cause depression in a patient using the drug for myasthenia gravis.[115] Multiple INFαs are available: recombinant INFα-2a; recombinant

INFα-2b; INFα-n3, a mixture of at least 15 different INF subtypes produced from human leukocytes; peginterferon alfa-2a, a combination of recombinant INFα-2a and an inert 40kD polyethylene glycol polymer; peginterferon alfa-2b, a combination of recombinant INFα-2b and an inert 12-kD polyethylene glycol polymer; and INF alfacon-1 (consensus INF), a recombinant synthetic product. Depression has been reported in association with each type of INFα.[116-124] Several trials investigating the relationship between depression and the various INFαs have been conducted, with treatment-emergent depression reported in 16–96% of patients.[116-145] Although none of these trials were placebo-controlled, many used standardized instruments to assess depression. One study examined the effect of INFα over time and found decreased numbers of patients with depression after 6 months of therapy (8–33%) as compared with 1 month (79–96%, $p = 0.03$).[118]

Two INFβs are available in the United States for treatment of multiple sclerosis: INFβ-1a (intramuscular or subcutaneous injection) and INFβ-1b for subcutaneous administration. Peginterferon beta-1a is also available. The data regarding INFβ-precipitated depression are less clear than those for depression induced by INFα. Two controlled trials suggest an increased risk of depression associated with INFβ-1a, with incidences ranging from 20% to 33%.[125,126] Two other studies of INFβ-1a, have not revealed an increased incidence of depression compared with that associated with placebo.[127,128] Only one trial compared two commercially available formulations of INFβ-1a. The Evidence for Interferon Dose-Effect: European-North American Comparative Efficacy study assigned 677 patients receiving either INFβ-1a 44 mcg subcutaneously three times weekly or INFβ-1a 30 mcg intramuscularly weekly for 24 weeks.[129] No difference in the incidence of depression between the two treatment groups was reported (17% versus 18%, respectively).

A long-term seminal trial of INFβ-1b demonstrated higher rates of depression associated with the clinically used 8 million international units dose compared with those associated with placebo at each yearly timepoint.[130] Two trials have been conducted with the objective of assessing rates of depression associated with INFβ-1b. One study reported depression in a mean (±SD) 13 ± 4% of patients, although no formal testing for depression was performed.[131] Another small study found a decreasing rate of reported depression over the 1-year study period, from 21.4% of patients at baseline to 6.3% of patients at 12 months.[132] Only one study comparing two INFβ products examined depressive symptoms. The Independent Comparison of Interferon trial noted depression in 18 of 88 (22%) of patients administered INFβ-1a 30 mcg intramuscularly weekly and in 18 of 94 (19%) who received INFβ-1b 8 mcg subcutaneously every other day ($p = 0.68$).[133] A prospective cohort of 182 patients initiated on any INFβ treatment was administered the Hamilton Rating Scale for Depression and the BDI at baseline and after a mean treatment duration of 65.6 months. There was no increase in the number of patients demonstrating depression over this time.[134] A Canadian database analysis of antidepressant prescription claims for patients with multiple sclerosis failed to detect a significant difference in the percentage of patients receiving antidepressant prescriptions between those treated with INF and those who received glatiramer acetate. However, the proportion of patients in all cohorts receiving antidepressant medications was high (40%).[135] An Internet-based survey of 2,457 patients with multiple sclerosis collected self-reported information and administered the Patient Health Questionnaire depression module short version to participants.[136] Compared to those who were on no therapy, the risk of depression was higher in patients taking INFβ (OR 1.47, 95% CI 1.07–2.02).

TNFα inhibitors have been reported to cause depression. Case reports of worsening depression and suicidal behavior in patients taking adalimumab, etanercept, infliximab, and ustekinumab have been published.[137-140] In one very small study of 16 patients with ankylosing spondylitis, the number of patients with depression as measured by the Hospital Anxiety and Depression Scale (HADS) and the BDI decreased with ongoing treatment.[141] Similarly, in a study of 92 patients with Crohn disease, infliximab therapy was associated with a decreased incidence of depression as measured by the HADS.[142]

IL-2 has been reported to cause depression. In two studies of patients with metastatic carcinoma, those administered IL-2 were significantly more likely to have depression than those not receiving IL-2 therapy.[143,144] The association between other cancer chemotherapy agents and depression is more tenuous. One trial examined two regimens for the treatment of small-cell lung carcinoma in 77 patients.[145] Regimen 1 consisted of methotrexate, doxorubicin, lomustine, and cyclophosphamide. Regimen 2 comprised cyclophosphamide, doxorubicin, vincristine, and lomustine. Patients were tested with the Profile of Mood States rating scale at baseline and after completion of therapy. Increased depression ratings following therapy were reported in 30% (not statistically significant compared with baseline) of those receiving regimen 1 and 48% (p = 0.03 compared with baseline) of those receiving regimen 2. The authors speculated that the increased depression rating scores in patients who received regimen 2 may be attributable to vincristine. A case report also implicates vincristine as a cause of depression.[146] A patient treated for acute myoblastic leukemia who received vincristine 10 mg instead of 1 mg experienced severe depression with uncontrollable crying. The symptoms dissipated over a 3-week period following the overdose.

RETINOIC ACID DERIVATIVES

Several literature sources suggest a possible association between isotretinoin and depression. There have been a relatively large number of reports of isotretinoin and serious depression submitted to the FDA, documenting a temporal relationship between isotretinoin use and onset or worsening of depression.[147] In addition, cases of positive dechallenge with discontinuation of isotretinoin therapy and initiation of psychiatric treatment and positive rechallenge have been reported.[148-150] These reports have led to several types of trials examining the potential link between isotretinoin use and depression; however, no randomized, controlled studies have been performed. Conflicting reports from retrospective studies found either a relative risk of 2.68 (95% CI 1.10–6.48) for depression associated with isotretinoin use or no increased risk of depression or suicide.[151,152] Several prospective studies have assessed patients prescribed isotretinoin using various depression scales. These trials enrolled between 33 and 126 patients. Although some studies reported significant worsening in depression scores over time with isotretinoin, others saw no change in depression, and others demonstrated statistically significant improvements in mood.[153-160] Four prospective, controlled studies have been performed comparing isotretinoin to other treatments. In the first prospective, case-controlled study, 100 patients treated with isotretinoin were compared to 100 patients treated with topical acne cream or oral antibiotics.[161] This study used two depression scales and collected information on the severity of acne, social support, stress, and family history as potential confounders. Depression developed in two patients treated with isotretinoin, but the difference between the two groups was not statistically significant.[161] A second prospective, controlled study administered isotretinoin 1 mg/kg/day or vitamin C to 46 patients.[162] There was no difference between the groups in scores on the BDI. The third prospective, controlled study compared 75 patients administered isotretinoin to those treated with topical antibiotics or retinoids.[163] The HADS and BDI were administered at baseline, month two, and month four following initiation of therapy. Improvement in mood occurred over time. The fourth prospective, controlled study included 190 patients in three arms: one group treated with isotretinoin, one group administered antibiotics with or without a topical cream, and the third group included individuals of similar age who did not have acne.[164] Compared with baseline, there was no difference in CES-D scores after 6 months of treatment. It should be noted that prospective trials have been underpowered to detect changes in depression risk if the true incidence is low. Despite the lack of consensus in the literature, the product labeling for isotretinoin contains a warning about depression and other neuropsychiatric effects. Therefore, many healthcare providers prescribe isotretinoin with caution and consider depression a substantial risk associated with this drug.[165]

Several other drugs not discussed above have been implicated in causing depression in postmarketing case reports, but a causal association has not been established. These include 3-hydroxy-3-methylglutaryl coenzyme A reductase inhibitors (statins), histamine$_2$ receptor blockers, amiodarone, nonsteroidal anti-inflammatory drugs, metoclopramide, ondansetron, psychostimulants, and monteleukast.[166-182]

MECHANISMS

Drug-induced depression occurs through several mechanisms, including direct alteration of bioamine function, disturbance of HPA axis function, dramatic hormonal changes, and elevation of cytokine production (**Table 18-2**).

The antihypertensive agents reserpine, guanethidine, and methyldopa all induce depression likely by depleting CNS bioamine activity.[185] Guanethidine and reserpine deplete norepinephrine at the synapse. Methyldopa is transformed into α-methyl norepinephrine, which is less active than norepinephrine and replaces it at the sympathetic nerve endings, thus acting as a false neurotransmitter. Tetrabenazine, a monoamine depleter used for hyperkinetic movement disorders, depletes central norepinephrine, dopamine and serotonin.[80] Notably, the norepinephrine depletion caused by reserpine generated one of the early theories of the pathogenesis of depression (e.g., the monoamine hypothesis).[186,187] Clonidine also reduces central norepinephrine output via stimulation of α_2-adrenergic receptors.[188]

The mechanism of digoxin-induced depression is unknown, although alteration of CNS norepinephrine synthesis is suspected. In animal models, digitalis has been shown to inhibit CNS synthesis of norepinephrine and to decrease norepinephrine uptake by CNS tissue, with an apparent overall activation of CNS noradrenergic function. Altered activity of CNS dopaminergic and serotonergic systems also has been demonstrated, particularly in association with high digitalis doses.[36] Similarly, the mechanism of isotretinoin-induced depression is not clear, but animal studies suggest alterations in the dopaminergic, serotonin, and possibly norepinephrine systems.[154,189]

GnRH agonists induce a hypogonadal state, resulting in a significant reduction in both estrogen and androgen production. Significant fluctuation in serum estrogen concentrations and low estrogenic states have been associated with substantial mood symptoms in patients with premenstrual dysphoric disorder and during menopause. The significant decline in estrogen production associated with GnRH agonist therapy is believed to be the cause of depressive symptoms in these patients. Estrogen may affect mood in several ways, such as by increasing the availability of neurotransmitters, including serotonin, through enhancement of the degradation of monoamine oxidase.[190] Estrogen modulates

Table 18-2 Mechanisms of Drug-Induced Depression

Drug	Mechanism
Clonidine	Reduces norepinephrine output via α_2-adrenergic receptor agonism
Cortisone	Elevates plasma cortisol concentrations
Digitalis	Inhibits central nervous system synthesis of norepinephrine
Efavirenz	Increases proinflammatory cytokines IL-1β and TNFα[a]
Guanethidine	Depletes neuronal norepinephrine
INFα	Increases interleukin-6 production
Isotretinoin	Alters dopaminergic, serotonin, and possibly norepinephrine systems
Leuprolide	Reduces both estrogen and androgen production
Methyldopa	Partial agonism of norepinephrine receptor
Phenobarbital	Reduces plasma unbound tryptophan, which influences serotonin
Reserpine	Depletes neuronal norepinephrine, serotonin, and dopamine
Tamoxifen	Reduces estrogen function via antagonism of estrogen receptors
Tetrabenazine	Depletes neuronal norepinephrine, serotonin, and dopamine
Tiagabine	GABA modulation
Topiramate	GABA modulation
Vincristine	Prevents the conversion of dopamine to norepinephrine
Varenicline	$\alpha_4\beta_2$-nicotinic receptor agonist, indirectly modulates dopamine

GABA = gamma-aminobutyric acid, IL = interleukin, INF = interferon, TNF = tumor necrosis factor.
[a]Animal data.

serotonin in other ways, including regulation of tryptophan, a serotonin precursor, and increasing the number of serotonin transport sites.[191] Tamoxifen, an estradiol receptor antagonist, also may produce depressive symptoms caused by a decline in estrogen function. However, raloxifene, a selective estradiol receptor antagonist without CNS activity, does not appear to induce depression.[192]

A number of mechanisms have been proposed regarding the mood effects of OCs. Estrogen may induce pyridoxine deficiency resulting in a decrease in serotonin and gamma-aminobutyric acid (GABA) concentrations in the CNS.[193] Other possible mechanisms include estrogen- and progesterone-mediated augmentation of GABA's inhibition and suppression of glutamate, and progesterone-mediated increase in monoamine oxidase activity.[194]

Corticosteroids are believed to induce mood symptoms by elevating plasma cortisol concentrations. Patients with Cushing syndrome have been reported to have high rates of depressive symptoms.[195] Moreover, abnormalities of the HPA axis due to hypercortisolemia are found in patients with MDD.[196] However, corticosteroids are as likely to induce mania as depression, suggesting a complex interaction.[109]

The mechanism of AED-induced depression likely involves GABA, an inhibitory neurotransmitter, alterations in serotonin activity, or a combination of these effects. Some evidence suggests that antidepressant agents enhance activity at GABA-B receptors and decrease activity at GABA-A receptors.[197] Therefore, agents that primarily act at the GABA-A receptors (phenobarbital, tiagabine, or topiramate) or that indiscriminately increase the amount of GABA available to both receptors (tiagabine) may be associated with greater potential for inducing depression. Both phenobarbital and phenytoin reduce unbound plasma tryptophan concentrations, which influences serotonin turnover.[198] In addition, the enzyme-inducing AEDs can cause a folate deficiency. Decreases in plasma folate concentrations may reduce methylation reactions involving neurotransmitters and monoamines, which may be implicated in depression induction.[199]

Mechanisms of depression caused by the immunologic agents have not been elucidated completely. Most work in this area has been conducted with INFα, and several mechanisms have been proposed that may be applicable to INFβ and IL-2. INFα induces the production of proinflammatory cytokines, such as IL-6, which may lead to depression.[119] An increase in the Montgomery–Asberg Depression Rating Scale (MADRS) scores was significantly and positively correlated with increases in serum IL-6 concentrations.[118] INFα increases serotonin transporter messenger ribonucleic acid and uptake activity, reduces serotonin concentrations in brain or serum, and induces the catabolism of tryptophan.[119] The net effect of these alterations in the serotonin system is to decrease the amount of serotonin at the active receptor sites and potentiate depression. INFα administration is also associated with HPA activation, which has been associated with depression and with increases in serum IL-6 concentrations.[119,200,201] Thus, it is unclear mechanistically why anti-TNF monoclonal antibodies might cause depression.[141] In fact, infliximab has been studied to relieve treatment-resistant depression,[202] particularly in patients with elevated baseline inflammatory biomarkers.[203] Depletion of tryptophan, the amino acid precursor to serotonin, caused by INFα administration has also been hypothesized.[204] Polymorphisms of the allele coding for the 5-HT_{1A} receptor have also been implicated in the development of INFα-induced depression.[204,205] Efavirenz has been shown in rat models to increase concentrations of proinflammatory cytokines IL-1β and TNFα, which may be linked to depression.[206]

Vinca alkaloids inhibit the transport of dopamine hydroxylase, thereby preventing the conversion of dopamine to norepinephrine,[146] possibly resulting in depression. The mechanism of varenicline-induced depression is unknown, but the partial α_4-β_2-nicotinic receptor agonist indirectly modulates dopamine,[207] which may in turn modulate mood.

CLINICAL PRESENTATION AND DIFFERENTIAL DIAGNOSIS

The key feature of diagnosis is the temporal association between the development of depressive symptoms and the use of a causative drug. The disturbance

Table 18-3 Signs and Symptoms Associated with Drug-Induced Depression

- Depressed mood
- Diminished interest or pleasure in most activities
- Sleep changes (insomnia or hypersomnia)
- Appetite increase or decrease
- Hopelessness/helplessness
- Suicidal ideation
- Fatigue
- Diminished ability to concentrate
- Psychomotor agitation or retardation

of mood or presence of depression should be severe enough to result in impairment of daily function. In addition, the clinician must rule out the possibility of pre-existing depression and the influence of the disease state being treated, particularly psychological stressors.

Symptoms associated with drug-induced depression (**Table 18-3**) are similar to those observed in patients with MDD, with few exceptions. More severe symptoms including suicidal ideation and psychosis have been reported in association with INFα, corticosteroids, and varenicline.[82,109,113,120] With most agents, the onset of depression generally occurs during the first weeks of treatment. The median onset of symptoms in FDA-reported cases of isotretinoin-associated depression during the first course of therapy was 30 days, and the median recovery time was 4.5 days.[150] During the rechallenge course, the time to onset of symptoms was shorter.[208] In patients treated with GnRH agonists, the onset of depressive symptoms is consistent with the time to reach a hypogonadal state.[90,91] When the hypogonadal state is of short duration, as with in vitro fertilization treatment, depressive symptoms are transient and less severe.[95] During sustained treatment for endometriosis, depressive symptoms appear to be persistent and generally more severe, sometimes resulting in the need for discontinuation of treatment.[92,96,209] Drug-induced suicidality is temporally associated with initiation of treatment and represents a marked change in thoughts and behavior from baseline.[74] Suicidality associated with anticonvulsants and antidepressants occurs early in treatment, and must be distinguished from the underlying mood disorder for which they were prescribed.

Table 18-4 Conditions to Consider in the Differential Diagnosis of Drug-Induced Depression

- Substance-use disorder
- Pre-existing mood disorder
- General medical conditions
    - Endocrine (e.g., diabetes, hypothyroidism)
    - Infections, human immunodeficiency virus
    - Anemia, folate deficiency
    - Collagen disorders (e.g., systemic lupus erythematosus, scleroderma, rheumatoid arthritis)
- Neurologic disorders (e.g., epilepsy, multiple sclerosis, Parkinson disease)
- Cardiovascular and respiratory disease
- Malignant disease

Conditions and diseases associated with depression must be ruled out to arrive at a diagnosis of drug-induced depression (**Table 18-4**). The incidence of depression in patients with epilepsy ranges from 4% to 62%, depending on the method of diagnosis and the population studied.[210,214] One study found that patients with hypertension were three times more likely to have depression than normotensive patients.[212] Many chronic health conditions for which immunologic agents are used have been associated with high rates of depression. The prevalence of depression in patients with chronic hepatitis C is 11–30%, while the prevalence of depression in patients with cancer is 28%.[213,214] Multiple sclerosis is also associated with a 15–30% point prevalence of depression and a lifetime depression incidence of 40–60%.[215] Fatigue, a symptom common to all of the disease states in this category, often can be confused with depression. Alternatively, depression may be underdiagnosed because of the expectation that patients will present with fatigue. Other conditions that may cause misdiagnosis of depression include hyperthyroidism or hypothyroidism and unrealistic expectations, leading to discouragement and frustration.[216]

RISK FACTORS

Female sex, family history of mood disorder, childhood abuse, anxiety disorders, sleep disorders, and neurologic disorders are known risk factors for MDD.[1] It is unclear, however, whether these factors also increase the risk of drug-induced depression.

Table 18-5 Risk Factors for Drug-Induced Depression

Risk factors common to all drugs

- History of major depressive disorder or prior depression episode
- History of drug-induced depression
- Psychosocial stressors (e.g., financial, relationship, or job stress)

Risk factors associated with specific drugs

- Corticosteroids
  - Dose (>80 mg/day prednisone equivalents)
- Efavirenz
  - Plasma concentrations >2.74 mcg/mL during long-term treatment
- Topiramate
  - Dose (higher starting dose of 50 mg/day, titration of 50 mg/day every 2 weeks)
  - Temporal-lobe epilepsy with hippocampal sclerosis
  - Presence of cognitive adverse effects
  - Family history of epilepsy
  - History of febrile seizures
- INFα
  - Homozygous for the HTR1A-1019G allele
  - Increased immune activation (e.g., increased soluble IL-2 receptor, IL-6, and IL-10 serum concentrations) prior to treatment for hepatitis C
- Oral contraceptives
  - History of premenstrual depression or pregnancy-related depression
  - History of dysmenorrhea
  - Family history of depression while taking oral contraceptives
  - Predisposition to vitamin B_6 deficiency
  - High degree of psychological distress prior to oral contraceptive use
  - Age <20 years experience negative affect more often
  - High estrogen/progesterone content

HTR1A = 5-hydroxytryptamine receptor 1A, IL = interleukin, INF = interferon.

Much of the literature regarding drug-induced depression arises from case reports, database evaluations, and observational studies, which are not designed to identify risk factors. Factors that appear to increase the risk of drug-induced depression are listed in **Table 18-5**.

A history of depression or another psychiatric disorder is the most consistently identified risk factor for depression associated with most of the causative drugs. In addition, the presence of psychological stressors has been noted to increase the risk. Although increased stress may be expected in patients with serious medical illnesses, it is unclear whether increased stress increases the risk of depression associated with drugs such as immunologic or cancer chemotherapy agents. Patients with a history of drug-induced depression are likely to be at greater risk upon repeated exposures.[28]

Dose may be an important risk factor for depression associated with some drugs. Depression is more likely to occur when higher doses of corticosteroids are used (>80 mg/day prednisone equivalents).[114] It is unclear whether multiple courses of corticosteroids increase the risk of depression. However, patients with a history of corticosteroid-induced depression should be monitored closely. Likewise, OCs with higher estrogen content are more commonly associated with depression. Some open-label data suggest that the risk of neuropsychiatric adverse effects associated with long-term treatment (>6 months) with efavirenz were more than five times greater in patients with plasma efavirenz concentrations >2.74 mcg/mL.[217] One case of levetiracetam-induced depression was likely dose-associated.[218] A small study that compared low- and high-dose INFα also showed increased rates of depression with the higher dose.[120]

A prospective, cross-sectional study determined a gene association with depression induced by isotretinoin. The T allele at the *rs9303285* gene encoding the retinoic acid receptor alpha was linked to an approximately 40% risk of isotretinoin-associated depression.[154]

Several factors have been associated with an increased risk of treatment of emergent depression or negative affect in patients taking OCs (Table 18-5). Whereas the overall risk for depression caused by these drugs is considered low, patients presenting with any of these factors should be considered at greater risk. The risk may vary with the type of OC used. Monophasic OCs exert greater mood-stabilizing effects than triphasic products. In addition, patients with premenstrual mood symptoms may have an increased risk of negative mood effects with OCs containing low amounts of progesterone or a low progesterone-to-estrogen ratio. Women without premenstrual mood symptoms appear to have increased risk with a higher progesterone content.[108]

A retrospective study of patients with temporal lobe epilepsy who were initiated on topiramate therapy revealed that those with hippocampal sclerosis in association with temporal-lobe epilepsy were significantly more likely to develop depression than those without hippocampal sclerosis. Patients without hippocampal sclerosis who had cognitive adverse effects such as psychomotor slowing or word-finding difficulties associated with topiramate were also more likely to be diagnosed with depression.[219] A case series of patients initiated on topiramate therapy found that a higher starting dose (50 mg daily) and a faster titration schedule (increase of 50 mg/day every 2 weeks) as well as the presence of cognitive adverse effects caused by topiramate increased the odds of any psychiatric adverse event, including depression. Other related factors were family or personal history of psychiatric conditions, family history of epilepsy, and a history of febrile convulsions.[53] One small study of women with epilepsy found that the odds of development of postpartum depression was increased with multiparity (OR 12.5, 95% CI 1.9–82.7) and AED polytherapy (OR 9.3, 95% CI 1.5–58).[220] However, no specific AED was implicated. One retrospective study of topiramate demonstrated a five-fold increased risk of depression in patients who initiated treatment with rapid titration.[221]

Risk factors for depression associated with INFα treatment include younger age, poor baseline sleep, hepatitis C, and an increase in vegetative symptoms of depression on the Zung depression rating scale after 4 weeks of treatment.[222-225] A polymorphism (C1019G) on the allele coding for the 5-HT_{1A} receptor (HTR1A) has also been implicated in the development of INFα-induced depression.[205,226] Patients who were homozygous for the HTR1A-1019G allele had an approximate threefold increased risk of depression induced by INFα.[227] The HTR1A receptor is the major auto-receptor on the serotonergic raphe neurons. Alterations in this receptor can lead to decreased secretion of serotonin. This polymorphism is relatively common, with approximately 48% of people having at least one C1019G allele. This finding may help explain the very common occurrence of depression in patients treated with INFα.[205] One small study of 16 patients undergoing treatment with various INFα regimens for hepatitis C found that patients with higher levels of immune activation as demonstrated by increased soluble IL-2 receptor, IL-6, and IL-10 serum concentrations prior to treatment were more likely to have major depressive disorder as measured by *DMS-IV* criteria and the MADRS score.[228] A small study of 50 patients with hepatitis C found that the hepatitis C virus genotype 1 was associated with a 2.1 greater odds of developing INFα-associated depression.[229] Conversely, a separate cohort study of 278 patients with hepatitis C determined that hepatitis C virus genotype 2 was associated with a higher risk of developing depression with INFα treatment (OR 2.27, 95% CI 1.07–4.78).[222]

The risk for suicidality associated with antidepressants is inversely related to age, with patients <18 years at greatest risk, and adults 18–24 years at greater risk than older adults (25–64 years).[74] Antidepressant selection, dose, or indication do not significantly change the risk of suicidality within the stratified age groups. Conversely, patients receiving an AED for epilepsy are at greater risk for suicidality than patients with psychiatric disorders (OR 3.53, 95% CI 1.28–12.1).[74]

MORBIDITY AND MORTALITY

Drug-induced depression can be associated with significant morbidity and mortality. Many drugs associated with depressive symptoms are used to treat chronic medical disorders or are components of lifesaving or life-prolonging therapeutic regimens. Patients experiencing significant depressive symptoms as a result of their treatment may be less likely to adhere to therapy and may be less optimistic about potential treatment benefits. Furthermore, the development of severe depressive symptoms may necessitate the discontinuation of life-prolonging treatments.

The presence of depression or severe depressive symptoms may increase the risk of suicide or suicidal ideation. Although the prevalence of suicide risk in patients with drug-induced depression is unknown, up to 15% of patients with severe MDD die as a result of suicide.[1] Moreover, patients with MDD have decreased physical, social, and role functioning as well as increased pain and physical illness.[230] The risk of suicidality associated with antidepressant treatment must be balanced with the much greater risk of suicidality with untreated depression.

PREVENTION

There is very little information available regarding preventive strategies for drug-induced depression. However, some interventions may prove useful (**Table 18-6**). Identifying patients with risk factors (e.g., history of depressive episodes) and implementing a prospective screening and monitoring plan seems prudent, but will not prevent drug-induced depression. Careful monitoring and early detection may, however, minimize the negative sequelae associated with depression. Treating psychosocial stressors with interventions such as counseling and education may also prove beneficial, but this strategy has not been systematically evaluated. One study has examined the role of social support on the development of depression in 127 patients with melanoma who were treated with INFα. Those with more social support had smaller increases in BDI scores during one year of therapy.[231]

Pretreatment or prophylaxis for depressive symptoms may be useful in some cases. Sabet-Sharghi reported the successful pretreatment (with lithium and protriptyline) of an individual with a history of corticosteroid-induced depression.[232] In a retrospective review of patients receiving leuprolide for treatment of endometriosis, concomitant therapy with sertraline minimized the emergence of depressive symptoms.[209] Convincing evidence exists regarding the benefits of pretreatment for depression in patients with melanoma receiving INFα. Musselman et al.[233] randomly assigned 40 patients with melanoma to receive pretreatment with paroxetine (n = 20) or placebo (n = 20) 2 weeks prior to and throughout the 12-week INFα regimen. The risk of developing depression was lower in the paroxetine group (11% versus 35%, RR 0.24, 95% CI 0.08–0.93) and pretreated patients were less likely to discontinue INFα because of depressive symptoms (5% versus 35%, RR 0.14, 95% CI 0.05–0.85). Three meta-analyses of patients with hepatitis C found that prophylactic administration of selective serotonin reuptake inhibitors during INFα treatment reduced the incidence of depression compared to placebo.[234-236] Amantadine, a medication with both antiviral and dopaminergic effects, was studied in 14 patients who were treated with peginterferon alfa-2a and ribavirin for hepatitis C. Compared with the control group, amantadine-treated patients were significantly less likely to develop depression by week 24 of treatment.[237] One small placebo-controlled study in patients receiving efavirenz therapy found that HDRS and BDI scores improved in patients who received cyproheptadine 8 mg/day for 1 week followed by 12 mg/day for 3 weeks.[238]

Table 18-6 Approaches to Help Prevent Drug-Induced Depression

Assess patient for history of depressive episodes or history of drug-induced depression at baseline. *If yes*:

- Consider individual risk–benefit of drug therapy
- Encourage healthy lifestyle behaviors and supportive therapy
- Pretreat with selective serotonin reuptake inhibitor if undergoing therapy with interferon- or gonadotropin-releasing hormone agonist
- Select alternative drug within therapeutic category, if possible

MANAGEMENT

Appropriate management (**Table 18-7**) of drug-induced depression begins with prompt recognition of the emergence of depressive symptoms. In some cases, symptoms may be transient or mild, as in patients receiving GnRH agonist therapy as part of in vitro fertilization treatment.[95] For many patients, education and support may be the only intervention needed. Psychological interventions or psychotherapy are beneficial for patients with mild-to-moderate symptoms of MDD, but the benefit of psychotherapy in patients with drug-induced depression is unclear. For more severe or persistent depressive symptoms, therapy with the offending agent will likely have to be discontinued or antidepressant treatment may need to be initiated, and in some cases, both strategies are required. Children, adolescents, and young adults (18–24 years) receiving antidepressants for depression or other psychiatric disorders should be monitored frequently (weekly to biweekly) during the first few weeks for treatment-emergent suicidality or worsening of depression. The emergence of suicidal ideation or psychotic symptoms should always be considered

Table 18-7 Management of Drug-Induced Depression

- Discontinue the offending agent, if possible
- Substitute medication within therapeutic class
- Counseling or supportive therapy for mild depressive symptoms
- Initiate antidepressant therapy for persistent or moderate-to-severe depressive symptoms

serious, and these patients should receive immediate intervention, including hospitalization.

There are insufficient data to recommend specific doses of antidepressant therapy for the treatment of drug-induced depression, although in most reports doses similar to those used in patients with idiopathic depression have been administered. Duration of therapy should be based on patient response and clinical judgment. In cases in which it would be best for a patient to continue to receive therapy with the causative agent, clinicians should consider factors such as severity of presentation, current mood, and level of psychological stress before deciding to discontinue drug therapy.

Although not always possible, in some cases substituting another medication in the same drug or therapeutic class but with a lower risk of causing depression may represent the best management strategy. For example, patients experiencing β-blocker-induced depression may benefit from receiving a hydrophilic β-blocker or an antihypertensive drug from a different class (e.g., ACE inhibitor or diuretic).[239] Similarly, patients experiencing OC-induced depression may benefit from an OC with a lower estrogen content or different estrogen:progesterone ratio. Patients with varenicline-induced neuropsychiatric side effects should be considered for nicotine replacement or bupropion for smoking cessation. One prospective, observational study substituted nevirapine for efavirenz in 116 patients with neuropsychiatric disturbances. Patients had resultant improvement on the HADS without loss of viral suppression.[240]

No specific treatments have been proposed for depression associated with the immunologic agents. Discontinuation of therapy is sometimes considered, but remission of depression does not always occur simultaneously with the discontinuation of interferon.[213] For patients with hepatitis C, selective serotonin reuptake inhibitors may be the best choice for management, as they are well tolerated by patients with liver disease, whereas tricyclic antidepressants with significant anticholinergic effects may increase the cognitive dysfunction that occurs in these patients.[211] Gleason et al.[241] conducted a study using citalopram to treat depression in patients with hepatitis C. Of the 15 patients participating in the trial, four had previously taken INFα and four were currently receiving INFα therapy. Citalopram 10–40 mg/day was administered to all patients with a resultant improvement in mood. In another study, of 13 patients undergoing therapy with INFα who experienced depression, 85% were responsive to treatment with citalopram.[242] Similar results were achieved with citalopram in another study.[227] Bupropion therapy resulted in remission or improvement in nine of ten patients with INFα-associated depression in an open-label study.[243] The authors postulated that the response may be due to anti-inflammatory effects of bupropion.[244] There are case reports of patients with INFα-induced depression who were responsive to treatment with methylphenidate or venlafaxine.[245,246]

Selection of specific INFα therapy based on patients' depressive symptoms has been proposed. For patients with suicidal tendencies, INFα-n3 is preferred, while INFα-2a is suggested for patients experiencing depersonalization. Patients with paranoia may experience fewer symptoms with INFα-2a or INFα-2b, while those patients exhibiting obsessive or compulsive symptoms may improve during treatment with INFα-n1.[193] However, these recommendations are based on relatively small numbers of patients and the symptoms expressed by those individuals require evaluation in a prospective study. Sertraline has proven effective for the management of depressive symptoms associated with GnRH agonists.[90,91,216] Lithium, selective serotonin reuptake inhibitors, and electroconvulsive therapy have been used to manage corticosteroid-induced depression.[109]

There is inherent difficulty in recommending antidepressant therapy for patients with epilepsy because of the epileptogenic potential of most antidepressant drugs. Bupropion may exert proconvulsant properties in persons without epilepsy, particularly in doses >450 mg/day.[247] Tricyclic antidepressants, particularly amoxapine, clomipramine, maprotiline, and mianserin, also may have epileptogenic potential.[199] Although selective serotonin-reuptake inhibitors are generally preferred in patients with epilepsy, they have been associated with seizures in case reports. This may be due, in part, to an increased incidence of hyponatremia.[248]

INFORMATION FOR PATIENTS

Patients should be informed regarding the possibility of the emergence of depressive symptoms when prescribed a drug associated with depression. They should be instructed to report any symptoms of depressed mood or extreme irritability, anxiety, anhedonia, difficulty sleeping, fatigue, feelings of hopelessness or helplessness, change in appetite or weight, or thoughts of death. Patients with a history of depression may be at greater risk for experiencing drug-induced depression. Patients should be encouraged to inform their provider of any history or treatment of any psychiatric disorder.

The FDA requires pharmacists to distribute medication guides to patients receiving medications with specific warnings of suicidality or other severe neuropsychiatric side effects. Medication guides are intended to inform patients about a known serious side effect of a drug. These guides are available at https://www.fda.gov/drugs/drugsafety/ucm085729.htm.

REFERENCES

1. American Psychiatric Association. *Diagnostic and statistical manual of mental disorders.* 5th ed. Washington, DC: American Psychiatric Association; 2013.
2. Friedman, RA, Leon AC. Expanding the black box—depression, antidepressants, and the risk of suicide *N Engl J Med.* 2007; 356:2343-6
3. Sternbach H, State R. Antibiotics: neuropsychiatric effects and psychotropic interactions. *Harv Rev Psychiatry.* 1997; 5:214-26.
4. Christ W. Central nervous system toxicity of quinolones: human and animal findings. *J Antimicrob Chemother.* 1990; 26(suppl B):219-25.
5. Feinberg SS. Fluoroquinolone-induced depression. *Am J Psychiatry.* 1995; 152:954-5.
6. Labay-Kamara U, Manning S, McMahon T. Fluoroquinolone – induced suicidal ideation and suicidality. *Psychosomatics.* 2012; 53:97-8.
7. LaSalvia EA, Domek GJ, Gitlin DF. Fluoroquinolone-induced suicidal ideation. *Gen Hosp Psychiatry.* 2010; 32:108-10.
8. Ahmed AIA, van der Heijden FMMA, van den Berkmortel H, Kramers K. A man who wanted to commit suicide by hanging himself: an adverse effect of ciprofloxacin. *Gen Hosp Psychiatry.* 2011; 33:82.e5-7.
9. Mitchell RS, Lester W. Clinical experience with cycloserine in the treatment of tuberculosis. *Scand J Respir Dis Suppl.* 1970; 71:94-108.
10. Weinstein HJ, Hallett WY, Sarauw AS. The absorption and toxicity of ethionamide. *Am Rev Respir Dis.*1962; 86:576-8.
11. Dietz A, Frolich L. Mefloquine-induced paranoid psychosis and subsequent major depression in a 25-year-old student. *Pharmacopsychiatry.* 2002; 35:200-2.
12. Whitworth AB, Aichhorn W. First-time diagnosis of severe depression: induced by mefloquine? *J Clin Psychopharm.* 2005; 25:399-400.
13. Meier CR, Wilcock K, Jick SS. The risk of severe depression, psychosis, or panic attacks with prophylactic antimalarials. *Drug Saf.* 2004; 27:203-13.
14. Petersen E, Ronne T, Ronn A et al. Reported side effects to chloroquine, chloroquine plus proguanil, and mefloquine as chemoprophylaxis against malaria in Danish travelers. *J Travel Med.* 2000; 7:79-84.
15. van Reimsdijk MM, Sturkenboom MC, Ditters JM et al. Atovaquone plus chloroguanide versus mefloquine for malaria prophylaxis: a focus on neuropsychiatric adverse events. *Clin Pharm Therap.* 2002; 72:294-301.
16. Sustiva product information. Princeton, NJ: Bristol-Myers Squibb Company; 2009.
17. Journot V, Chene G, De Castro N et al. Use of efavirenz is not associated with a higher risk of depressive disorders: a substudy of the randomized clinical trial ALIZE-ANRS 099. *Clin Infect Dis.* 2006; 42:1790-9.
18. Clifford DB, Evans S, Yang Y et al. Long-term impact of efavirenz on neuropsychological performance and symptoms in HIV-infected individuals (ACTG 5097s). *HIV Clin Trials.* 2009; 10:343-55.
19. Gutierrez F, Garcia L, Padilla S et al. Risk of clinically significant depression in HIV-infected patients: effect of antiretroviral drugs. *HIV Med.* 2014; 15:213-23.
20. Colebunders R, Hilbrands R, De Roo A et al. Neuropsychiatric reaction induced by abacavir. *Am J Med.* 2002; 113:616.
21. Wise MEJ, Mistry K, Reid S. Neuropsychiatric complications of nevirapine treatment. *BMJ.* 2002; 324:879.
22. Harry TC, Matthews M, Salvary I. Indinavir use: associated reversible hair loss and mood disturbance. *Int J STD AIDS.* 2000; 11:474-6.
23. Dollery CT, Emslie-Smith D, Milne MD. Guanethidine in the treatment of hypertension. *Lancet.* 1960; 3:381-7.
24. Seedat YK, Pillay VKG. Further experience with guanethidine: a clinical assessment of 103 patients. *S Afr Med J.* 1966; 1:140-2.
25. Stocks AE, Robertson A. The long-term therapy of severe hypertension with guanethidine. *Am Heart J.* 1967; 73:569-70.
26. Evanson JM, Seers HTN. Comparison of bretylium tosylate with guanethidine in the treatment of severe hypertension. *Lancet.* 1960; 3:387-9.
27. Goodwin FK, Ebert MH, Bunney WE. Mental effects of reserpine in man: a review. In: Shader RI, ed. *Psychiatric complications of medical drugs.* New York: Raven Press; 1972:73-101.

28. Raftos J, Bauer GE, Lewis RG et al. Clonidine in the treatment of severe hypertension. *Med J Aust.* 1973; 1:786-93.
29. Stoudemire A, Brown JT, Harris RT et al. Propranolol and depression: a reevaluation based on a pilot clinical trial. *Psychiatr Med.* 1984; 2:211-8.
30. Griffin SJ, Freidman MJ. Depressive symptoms in propranolol users. *J Clin Psychiatry.* 1986; 47:453-7.
31. Avorn J, Everett DE, Weiss S. Increased antidepressant use in patients prescribed beta-blockers. *JAMA.* 1986; 255:357-60.
32. Thiessen BQ, Wallace SM, Blackburn JL et al. Increased prescribing of antidepressants subsequent to beta-blocker therapy. *Arch Intern Med.* 1990; 150:2286-90.
33. Patten SB, Love EJ. Drug-induced depression. *Psychother Psychosom.* 1997; 66:63-73.
34. Schleifer SJ, Slater WR, Macari-Hinson NM et al. Digitalis and beta-blocking agents: effects on depression following myocardial infarction. *Psychiatric Med.* 1984; 2:211-8.
35. Palinkas LA, Wingard DL, Barrett-Connor E. Chronic illness and depressive symptoms in the elderly: a population based study. *J Clin Epidemiol.* 1990; 43:1131-41.
36. Schleifer SJ, Slater WR, Macari-Hinson MM et al. Digitalis and beta-blocking agents: effects on depression following myocardial infarction. *Am Heart J.* 1991; 121:1397-402.
37. Nemets B, Bersudsky Y, Belmaker RH. Controlled double-blind trial of phenytoin vs. fluoxetine in major depressive disorder. *J Clin Psychiatry.* 2005; 66:586-90.
38. Zhang ZJ, Tan QR, Tong Y et al. The effectiveness of carbamazepine in unipolar depression: a double-blind, randomized, placebo-controlled study. *J Affect Disord.* 2008; 109:91-7.
39. Jones JE, Hermann BP, Barry JJ et al. Rates and risk factors for suicide, suicidal ideation, and suicide attempts in chronic epilepsy. *Epilepsy Behav.* 2003; 4:S31-38.
40. US Food and Drug Administration. Antiepileptic drugs and suicidality. http://www.fda.gov/ohrms/dockets/ac/08/briefing/2008-4372b1-01-FDA.PDF (accessed 2017 Dec 19).
41. Rissanen I, Jaaskelainen E, Isohanni M et al. Use of antiepileptic or benzodiazepine medication and suicidal ideation—the Northern Finland Birth Cohort 1966. *Epilepsy Behav.* 2015; 46:198-204.
42. Andersohn F, Schade R, Willich SN, Garbe E. Use of antiepileptic drugs in epilepsy and the risk of self-harm or suicidal behavior. *Neurology.* 2011; 75:335-40.
43. Pugh MJV, Copeland LA, Zeber JE et al. Antiepileptic drug monotherapy exposure and suicide-related behavior in older veterans. *J Aging Ger Soc.* 2012; 60:2042-7.
44. VanCott AC, Cramer JA, Copeland LA et al. Suicide-related behaviors in older patients with new anti-epileptic drug use: data from the VA hospital system. *BMC Medicine.* 2010; 8:4.
45. Fountoulakis KN, Gonda X, Baghai TC et al. Report of the WPA section of pharmacopsychiatry on the relationship of antiepileptic drugs with suicidality in epilepsy. *Int J Psychiatry Clin Pract.* 2015; 19:158-67.
46. Mula M, Kanner AM, Schmitz B, Schater S. Antiepileptic drugs and suicidality: an expert consensus statement from the Taskforce on Therapeutic Strategies of the ILAE Commission on Neuropsychobiology. *Epilepsia.* 2013; 54:199-203.
47. Dodrill CB. Behavioral effects of antiepileptic drugs. In: Smith D, Treiman D, Trimble M, eds. *Advances in neurology.* New York: Raven Press; 1991:213-24.
48. Robertson MM, Trimble MR, Townsend HRA. Phenomenology of depression in epilepsy. *Epilepsia.* 1987; 28:364-72.
49. Brent DA, Crumrine PK, Varna RR et al. Phenobarbital treatment and major depressive disorder in children with epilepsy. *Pediatrics.* 1987; 80:909-17.
50. Lopez-Gomez M, Ramirez-Bermudez J, Campillo C et al. Primidone is associated with interictal depression in patients with epilepsy. *Epilepsy Behav.* 2005;6:413-6.
51. Garrison SJ, Henson HK. Dilantin toxicity and vegetative depression: a report of two cases. *Arch Phys Med Rehabil.* 1990; 71:422-3.
52. Dodrill CB, Arnett JL, Deaton R et al. Tiagabine versus phenytoin and carbamazepine as add-on therapies: effects on abilities, adjustment, and mood. *Epilepsy Res.* 2000; 42:123-32.
53. Mula M, Trimble MR, Lhatoo SD et al. Topiramate and psychiatric adverse events in patients with epilepsy. *Epilepsia.* 2003; 44:659-63.
54. Rugg-Gunn F. Adverse and safety profile of perampanel: a review of pooled data. *Epilepsia.* 2014; 55(suppl 1):13-5.
55. Keppra [package insert]. Smyrna, GA: UCB; 2008.
56. Hagemann A, May TW, Nieder E et al. Quality of life, anxiety, and depression in adult patients after add-on of levetiracetam and conversion to levetiracetam monotherapy. *Epilep Res.* 2013; 104:140-50.
57. Mula M, Trimble MR, Yuen A et al. Psychiatric adverse events during levetiracetam therapy. *Neurology.* 2003; 61:704-6.
58. Wier LM, Tavares SB, Tyrka AR et al. Levetiracetam-induced depression in a healthy adult. *J Clin Psychiatry.* 2006; 67:1159-60.
59. Lee JJ, Song HS, Hwang YH et al. Psychiatric symptoms and quality of life in patients with drug-refractory epilepsy receiving adjunctive levetiracetam therapy. *J Clin Neurol.* 2011; 7:128-36.
60. Levinson DF, Devinsky O. Psychiatric adverse events during vigabatrin therapy. *Neurology.* 1999; 53:1503-11.
61. Cavanna AE, Seri S. Psychiatric adverse effects of zonisamide in patients with epilepsy and mental disorder comorbidities. *Epilepsy Behav.* 2013; 29:281-4.
62. Hall T, Shah S, Ng B et al. Changes in mood, depression, and suicidal ideation after commencing pregabalin for neuropathic pain. *Austral Fam Physician.* 2014; 43:705-8.
63. Kustermann A, Mobius C, Oberstein T et al. Depression and attempted suicide under pregabalin therapy. *Ann Gen Psychiatry.* 2014; 3:37.
64. Kaufman KR, Struck PJ. Activation of suicidal ideation with adjunctive rufinamide in bipolar disorder. *Epilepsy Behav.* 2011; 20:396-9.
65. Janicak P, Davis JM, Preskorn SH et al. *Principles and practice of psychopharmacotherapy.* 3rd ed. Baltimore: Wilkins and Wilkins; 1997.
66. Lydiard RB, Laraia MT, Ballenger JC et al. Emergence of depressive symptoms in patients receiving alprazolam for panic disorder. *Am J Psychiatry.* 1987; 144:664-5.
67. Nagy LM, Krystal JH, Woods SW et al. Clinical and medication outcome after short-term alprazolam and behavioral group treatment in panic disorder: 2.5 year naturalistic follow-up study. *Arch Gen Psychiatry.* 1989; 46:993-9.
68. Hall RCW, Joffe JR. Aberrant response to diazepam: a new syndrome. *Am J Psychiatry.* 1972; 129:114-8.
69. Hall RCW, Zisook S. Paradoxical reactions to benodiazepines. *Br J Clin Pharmacol.* 1981; 11:99s-104s.
70. Montagnier D, Dartigues J, Rouillon F et al. Ageing and trajectories of depressive symptoms in community-dwelling men and women. *Int J Geriat Psychiatry.* 2014; 29:720-9.
71. Nordfjaern T. A population-based cohort study of anxiety, depression, sleep and alcohol outcomes among benzodiazepine and z-hypnotic users. *Addictive Behav.* 2012; 37:1151-7.
72. Tsai M, Huang C, Lai Y et al. The effect of benzodiazepine and non-benzodiazepine prescriptions for diabetes mellitus type 2 in elderly Taiwanese with depressive symptoms. *Psychogeriatrics* 2016; 16:93-101.
73. Borison RL, Sinha D, Albrecht JW et al. Double-blind comparison of 3- and 6-mg fixed doses of alprazolam vs. placebo in outpatients with major depressive disorder. *Psychopharmacol Bull.* 1989; 25:186-9.
74. Hamad T. Relationship between psychotropic drugs and pediatric suicidality: review and evaluation of clinical data. http://www.fda.gov/ohrms/dockets/ac/04/briefing/2004-4065b1-10-TAB08-Hammads-Review.pdf (accessed 2017 Dec 19).

75. Millson D, Mrischer M, Croft P et al. Are triptans with enhanced lipophilicity used for the acute treatment of migraine associated with an increased consulting rate for depressive illness? *Cephalalgia.* 2000; 20:732-7.
76. Risch SC, Cohen RM, Janowsky DS. Physostigmine induction of depressive symptomatology in normal human subjects. *Psychiatry Res.* 1981; 4:89-94.
77. XYREM oral solution, sodium oxybate oral solution product information. Palo Alto, CA: Jazz Pharmaceuticals; 2014.
78. Rossetti AO, Heinzer RC, Tafti M, Buclin T. Rapid occurrence of depression following addition of sodium oxybate to modafinil. *Sleep Med.* 2010; 11 497-501.
79. Xyrem Study Group. A 12-month, open-label, multicenter extension trial of orally administered sodium oxybate for the treatment of narcolepsy. *Sleep.* 2003; 26:31-5.
80. Kenney C, Hunter C, Mejia N, Jankovic J. Is history of depression a contraindication to treatment with tetrabenazine? *Clin Neuropharmacol.* 2006; 29:259-64.
81. Moore TJ, Furberg CD, Glenmullen J et al. Suicidal behavior and depression in smoking cessation treatments. *PLoS One.* 2011;6:e27016.
82. Kuehn BM. FDA warns of adverse events linked to smoking cessation drug and antiepileptics. *JAMA.* 2008; 299:1121-2.
83. Buggy Y, Cornelius V, Fogg C et al. Neuropsychiatric adverse effects with varenicline: a modified prescription-event monitoring study in general practice in England. *Drug Saf.* 2013; 36:521-31.
84. Gibbons RD, Mann JJ. Varenicline, smoking cessation, and neuropsychiatric adverse effects. *Am J Psychiatry,* 2013; 170:1460-7.
85. Gunnel D, Irvine D, Wise L et al. Varenicline and suicidal behaviour: a cohort study based on data from the General Practice Research Database. *Br J Med.* 2009; 339:b3805.
86. Harrison-Woolrych M, Ashton J. Psychiatric adverse events associated with varenicline: an intensive postmarketing prospective cohort study in New Zealand. *Drug Saf.* 2011; 34:763-72.
87. Kotz D, Viechtbauer W, Simpson C et al. Cardiovascular and neuropsychiatric risks of varenicline: a retrospective cohort study. *Lancet Respir Med.* 2015; 3:761-8.
88. Anthenelli RM, Morris C, Ramey TS et al. Effects of varenicline on smoking cessation in adults with stably treated current or past major depression. *Ann Intern Med.* 2013; 159:390-400.
89. Anthenelli RM, Benowitz NL, West R et al. Neuropsychiatric safety and efficacy of vareniclinie, bupropion, and nicotine patch in smokers with and without psychiatric disorders (EAGLES): a double-blind, randomised, placebo-controlled clinical trial. *Lancet.* 2016; 387:2507-20.
90. Warnock JK, Bundren JC. Anxiety and mood disorders associated with gonadotropin-releasing hormone agonist therapy. *Psychopharmacol Bull.* 1997; 33:311-6.
91. Warnock JK, Bundren JC, Morris DW. Depressive mood symptoms associated with ovarian suppression. *Fertil Steril.* 2000; 74:984-6.
92. Lupron Depot 3.75 product information. Lake Forest, IL: TAP Pharmaceuticals; 1995.
93. Zoladex 3.6 mg product information. London: Zeneca Pharmaceuticals; 1995.
94. Toren P, Dor J, Mester R et al. Depression in women treated with a gonadotropin-releasing hormone agonist. *Biol Psychol.* 1996; 39:378-82.
95. Steingold KA, Cedars M, Lu JK. Treatment of endometriosis with a long-acting gonadotropin-releasing hormone agonist. *Obstet Gynecol.* 1987; 69:403-11.
96. Early Breast Cancer Trialists' Collaborative Group. Systemic treatment of early breast cancer by hormonal, cytotoxic, or immune therapy: 133 randomised trials involving 31,000 recurrences and 24,000 deaths among 75,000 women. *Lancet.* 1992; 339:71-85.
97. Cathcart CK, Jones SE, Pumroy CS et al. Clinical recognition and management of depression in node negative breast cancer patients treated with tamoxifen. *Breast Cancer Res Treat.* 1993; 27:277-81.
98. Shariff S, Cumming CE, Lees A et al. Mood disorder in women with early breast cancer taking tamoxifen, an estradiol receptor antagonist: an expected or unexpected effect? *Ann N Y Acad Sci.* 1995; 761:365-68.
99. Anelli TF, Anelli A, Tran KN et al. Tamoxifen administration is associated with a high rate of treatment-limiting symptoms in male breast cancer patients. *Cancer.* 1994; 74:74-77.
100. Day R, Ganz PA, Costantino JP et al. Health-related quality of life and tamoxifen in breast cancer prevention: a report from the National Surgical Adjuvant Breast and Bowel Project P-1 Study. *J Clin Oncol.* 1999; 17:2659-69.
101. Day R, Ganz PA, Constantino JP. Tamoxifen and depression: more evidence from the national surgical adjuvant breast and bowel project's breast cancer prevention (P-1) randomized study. *J Natl Cancer Inst.* 2001; 93:1615-23.
102. ARIMIDEX oral tablets, anastrozole oral tablets product information. Wilmington, DE: AstraZeneca Pharmaceuticals; 2013.
103. Chang CH, Chen SJ, Liu CY Adjuvant treatments of breast cancer increase the risk of depressive disorders: a population-based study. *J Affect Disord.* 2015; 182:44-9.
104. Kay CR. The Royal College of General Practitioners' Oral Contraception Study: some recent observations. *Clin Obstet Gynecol.* 1984; 11:759-86.
105. Oinonen KA, Mazmanian D. To what extent do oral contraceptives influence mood and affect? *J Affect Disord.* 2002; 70:229-40.
106. Rahimi-Ardabili B, Pourandarjani R, Habibollahi P, Mualeki A. Finasteride induced depression: a prospective study. *BMC Clin Pharmacol.* 2006; 6:7
107. Irwig MS. Depressive symptoms and suicidal thoughts among former users of finasteride with persistent sexual side effects. *J Clin Psychiatry.* 2012; 73:1220-3.
108. Brown ES, Suppes T. Mood symptoms during corticosteroid therapy: a review. *Harv Rev Psvchiatry.* 1998; 5:239-46.
109. Grigg JR. Prednisone mood disorder with associated catatonia. *J Geriatr Psychiatry Neurol.* 1989; 2:41-4.
110. Sutor B, Wells LA, Rummans TA. Steroid-induced depressive psychosis responsive to electroconvulsive therapy. *Convuls Ther.* 1996; 12:104-7.
111. Gift AG, Wood RM, Cahill CA. Depression, somatization, and steroid use in chronic obstructive pulmonary disease. *Int J Nurs Stud.* 1989; 26:281-6.
112. Patten SB, Williams JV, Love EJ. Self-reported depressive symptoms following treatment with corticosteroids and sedative hypnotics. *Int J Psychiatry Med.* 1996;26:15-24.
113. Boston Collaborative Drug Surveillance Program. Acute adverse reactions to prednisone in relation to dosage. *Clin Pharmacol Ther.* 1972; 13:694-8.
114. Patten SB, Williams JV, Love EJ. Self-reported depressive symptoms in association with medication exposures among medical inpatients: a cross-sectional study. *Can J Psychiatry.* 1995; 40:264-69.
115. Draper HM. Depressive disorder associated with mycophenolate mofetil. *Pharmacotherapy.* 2008; 28:136-9.
116. Schaefer M, Schmidt F, Folwaczny C et al. Adherence and mental side effects during hepatitis C treatment with interferon alfa and ribavirin in psychiatric risk groups. *Hepatology.* 2003; 34:443-51.
117. Bonaccorso S, Puzella A, Marino V et al. Immunotherapy with interferon-alpha in patients affected by chronic hepatitis C induces an intercorrelated stimulation of the cytokine network and an increase in depressive and anxiety symptoms. *Psychiatry Res.* 2001; 105:45-55.
118. Maes M, Bonaccorso S, Marino V et al. Treatment with interferon-alpha (IFN alpha) of hepatitis C patients induces lower serum dipeptidyl peptidase IV activity, which is related to IFN alpha-induced depressive and anxiety symptoms and immune activation. *Mol Psychiatry.* 2001; 6:475-80.
119. Malaguarnera M, Laurino A, di Fazio I et al. Neuropsychiatric effects and type of IFN-alpha in chronic hepatitis C. *J Interferon Cytokine Res.* 2001; 21:273-8.

120. Fried MW, Shiffman ML, Reddy KR et al. Peginterferon alfa-2a plus ribavirin for chronic hepatitis C virus infection. *N Engl J Med.* 2002; 347:975-82.
121. Zigante F, Bastie A, Buffet C et al. Incidence of interferon alfa-induced depression inpatients with chronic hepatitis C. *Hepatology.* 2002; 35:978-9.
122. Sjogren MH, Sjogren R, Lyons MF et al. Antiviral response of HCV genotype 1 to consensus interferon and ribavirin versus pegylated interferon and ribavirin. *Dig Dis Sci.* 2007; 52:1540-7.
123. Quarantini LC, Bressan RA, Galvao A et al. Incidence of psychiatric side effects during pegylated interferon-α retreatement in nonresponder hepatitis C virus-infected patients. *Liver Int.* 2007; 27:1098-1102.
124. Lotrich FE, Rabinovitz M, Gironda P et al. Depression following pegylated interferon-alpha: characteristics and vulnerability. *J Psychosomatic Res.* 2007; 63:131-5.
125. Galetta SL. The controlled high risk Avonex multiple sclerosis trial (CHAMPS Study). *J Neuroophthalmol.* 2001; 21:292-5.
126. PRISMS Study Group and the University of British Columbia MS/MRI Analysis Group. PRISMS-4: long-term efficacy of interferon-beta-1a in relapsing MS. *Neurology.* 2001;56:1628-36.
127. Patten SB, Metz LM. Interferon beta1a and depression in secondary progressive MS: data from the SPECTRIMS trial. *Neurology.* 2002;59:744-746.
128. The Once Weekly Interferon for MS Study Group (OWIMS). Evidence of interferon beta-1a dose response in relapsing-remitting MS: the OWIMS Study. *Neurology.* 1999; 53:679-86.
129. Panitch H, Goodin DS, Francis G. Randomized, comparative study of interferon beta-1a treatment regimens in MS: The EVIDENCE Trial. *Neurology.* 2002; 59:1496-506.
130. The IFNB Multiple Sclerosis Study Group and The University of British Columbia MS/MRI Analysis Group. Interferon beta-1b in the treatment of multiple sclerosis: final outcome of the randomized controlled trial. *Neurology.* 1995; 45:1277-85.
131. Neilley KL, Goodin DS, Goodkin DE et al. Side effect profile of interferon beta-1b in MS: results of an open label trial. *Neurology.* 1996; 46:552-4.
132. Feinstein A, O'Connor P, Feinstein K. Multiple sclerosis, interferon beta-1b and depression: a prospective investigation. *J Neurol.* 2002; 249:815-20.
133. Durelli L, Verdun E, Barbero P et al. Every-other-day interferon beta-1b versus once-weekly interferon beta-1a for multiple sclerosis: results of a 2-year prospective randomized multicentre study (INCOMIN). *Lancet.* 2002; 359:1453-60.
134. Porcel J, Rio J, Sanchez-Betancourt A et al. Long-term emotional state of multiple sclerosis patients treated with interferon beta. *Mult Scler.* 2006; 12:802-7.
135. Patten SB, Williams JV, Metz LM. Anti-depressant use in association with interferon and glatiramer acetate treatment in multiple sclerosis. *Mult Scler.* 2008; 14:406-11.
136. Taylor KL, Hadgkiss EJ, Jelinek GA et al. Lifestyle factors, demographics, and medications associated with depression risk in an international sample of people with multiple sclerosis. *BMC Psychiatry.* 2014; 14:327.
137. Davis JC, van der Heijde D, Braun J et al. Recombinant human tumor necrosis factor (etanercept) for treating ankylosing spondylitis: a randomised controlled trial. *Arthritis Rheum.* 2003; 48:3230-6.
138. Ellard R, Ahmed A, Shah R, Bewley A. Suicide and depression in a patient with psoriasis receiving adalimumab: the role of the dermatologist. *Clin Exper Derm.* 2014; 39:62-7.
139. Roblin X, Oltean P, Heluwaert F, Bonaz B. Panic attack with suicide: an exceptional adverse effect of infliximab. *Dig Dis Sci.* 2006; 51:1056.
140. Eshuis EJ, Magnin KMMY, Stokkers PCF et al. Suicide attempt in ulcerative colitis patient after 4 months of infliximab therapy—a case report. *J Crohn's Colitis.* 2010; 4:591-3.
141. Ertinli I, Ozer S, Kiraz S et al. Infliximab, a TNF-α antagonist treatment in patients with ankylosing spondylitis: the impact of depression, anxiety, and quality of life level. *Rheumatol Int.* 2012; 32:323-30.
142. Iglesais M, Barreiro de Acosta M, Vazquez I et al. Psychological impact of Crohn's disease on patients in remission: anxiety and depression risks. *Rev Esp Enfirm Dig.* 2009; 101:249-57.
143. Capuron L, Ravaud A, Dantzer R. Early depressive symptoms in cancer patients receiving interleukin 2 and/or interferon alfa-2b therapy. *J Clin Oncol.* 2000; 18:2143-51.
144. Capuron L, Ravaud A, Gualde N et al. Association between immune activation and early depressive symptoms in cancer patients treated with interleukin-2-based therapy. *Psychoneuroendocrinology.* 2001; 26:797-808.
145. Silberfarb PM, Holland JCB, Anbar D et al. Psychological response of patients receiving two drug regimens for lung carcinoma. *Am J Psychiatry.* 1983; 140:110-11.
146. Yoffe G, Rice L, Alfrey CP et al. Case report: depressive reaction to vincristine overdose. *Clin Lab Haematol.* 1986; 8:80-1.
147. Hazen PG, Carney JF, Walker AE et al. Depression: a side effect of 13-cis retinoic acid therapy. *J Am Acad Dermatol.* 1983; 9:278-9.
148. Scheinman PL, Peck GL, Rubinow DR et al. Acute depression from isotretinoin. *J Am Acad Dermatol.* 1990; 22:1112-4.
149. Hanson N, Leachman S. Safety issues in isotretinoin therapy. *Semin Cutan Med Surg.* 2001;20:166-83.
150. Wysowski DK, Pitts M, Beitz J. An analysis of reports of depression and suicide in patients treated with isotretinoin. *J Am Acad Dermatol.* 2001; 45:515-9.
151. Azoulay L, Blais L, Koren G et al. Isotretinoin and the risk of depression in patients with acne vulgaris: a case-crossover study. *J Clin Psychiatry.* 2008; 69:e1-e7.
152. Jick SS, Kremers HM, Vasilakis-Scaramozza C. Isotretinoin use and risk of depression, psychotic symptoms, suicide, and attempted suicide. *Arch Dermatol.* 2000; 136:1231-6.
153. Fakour Y, Ameri H, Ehsani AH et al. The effect of isotretinoin (Roaccutane) therapy on depression and quality of life of patients with severe acne. *Iran J Psychiatry.* 2014; 9:237-40.
154. Alzoubi KH, Kahbour OF, Hassan RE et al. The effect of genetic polymorphisms at the RARA gene on the adverse effects profile of isotretinoin-treated acne patients. *Internat J Clin Pharmacol Therapeutics.* 2013; 51:631-40.
155. Ergun T, Seckin D, Ozaydin N et al. Isotretinoin has no negative effect on attention, executive function and mood. *J Eur Acad Dermatol Venereology.* 2012; 26:431-9.
156. Nevoralova Z, Dvorakova D. Mood changes, depression, and suicide risk during isotretinoin treatment: a prospective study. *Int J Dermatol.* 2013; 52:163-8.
157. Kellett SC, Gawkrodger DJ. A prospective study of the responsiveness of depression and suicidal ideation in acne patients to different phases of during isotretinoin therapy. *Eur J Dermatol.* 2005; 15:484-88.
158. Marron SE, Tomas-Aragones L, Boira S. Anxiety, depression, quality of life, and patient satisfaction in acne patients treated with oral isotretinoin. *Acta Derm Venereol.* 2013; 93:701-6.
159. Yesilova Y, Bez Y, Ari M et al. Effects of isotretinoin on obsessive compulsive symptoms, depression, and anxiety in patients with acne vulgaris. *J Derm Treat.* 2012; 23:268-71.
160. Rehn LMH, Meririnne E, Hook-Nikanne J et al. Depressive symptoms and suicidal ideation during isotretinoin treatment: a 12-week follow-up study of male Finnish military conscripts. *J Eur Acad Dermatol Venereology.* 2009; 23:1294-7.
161. Cohen J, Adams S, Patten S. No association found between patients receiving isotretinoin for acne and the development of depression in a Canadian prospective cohort. *Can J Clin Pharmacol.* 2007; 14:e227-33.
162. Simic D, Situm M, Letica E et al. Psychological impact of isotretinoin therapy in patients with moderate and severe acne. *Coll Antropol.* 2009; 33(suppl 2):15-9.

163. Kaymak Y, Taner E, Taner Y. Comparison of depression, anxiety, and quality of life in acne vulgaris patients who were treated with either isotretinoin or topical agents. *Int J Dermatol.* 2009; 48:41-6.
164. McGrath EJ, Lovell CR, Gillison F et al. A prospective trial of the effects of isotretinoin on quality of life and depressive symptoms. *Brit J Dermatol.* 2010; 163:1323-9.
165. Rowe C, Spelman L, Ozimeski M et al. Isotretinoin and mental health in adolescents: Australian consensus. *Australasian J Dermatol.* 2014; 55:162-7.
166. Lechleitner M, Hoppichler F, Konwalinka G et al. Depressive symptoms in hypercholesterolemic patients treated with pravastatin. *Lancet.* 1992; 340:910.
167. Duits N, Bos FM. Depressive symptoms and cholesterol-lowering drugs. *Lancet.* 1993; 341:114.
168. Billings RF, Tang SW, Rakoff VM. Depression associated with cimetidine. *Can J Psychiatry.* 1981; 26:260-1.
169. Crowder MK, Pate JK. A case-report of cimetidine-induced depressive syndrome. *Am J Psychiatry.* 1980; 137:1451.
170. Billings RF, Stein MB. Depression associated with ranitidine. *Am J Psychiatry.* 1986; 143:915-6.
171. Stocky A. Ranitidine and depression. *Aust N Z J Psychiatry.* 1991; 25:415-8.
172. Blechman WJ, Schmid FR, April PA et al. Ibuprofen or aspirin in rheumatoid arthritis therapy. *JAMA.* 1975; 233:336-69.
173. Cochrane GM. A double-blind comparison of naproxen with indomethacin in osteoarthritis. *Scand J Rheumatol.* 1973; 2:89-93.
174. Adams CD. Metoclopromide and depression. *Ann Intern Med.* 1985; 103:960.
175. Feder R. Metoclopromide and depression. *J Clin Psychiatry.* 1987; 48:38.
176. Oren DA. Dysphoria after treatment with ondansetron. *Am J Psychiatry.* 1995; 152:1101.
177. Ambrose A, Salib E. Amiodarone-induced depression. *Brit J Psychiatry.* 1999; 174:366-7.
178. Farmer P, Unis AS, Hsu G. Pemoline, depressive symptoms and escape from dexamethasone suppression. *J Clin Psychopharmacol.* 1983; 3:331-2.
179. Rosenfeld AA. Depression and psychotic regression following prolonged methylphenidate use and withdrawal: case report. *Am J Psychiatry.* 1979; 136:226-8.
180. Twerski B. Sympathomimetic-induced depression. *Am J Psychiatry.* 1987; 144:252.
181. Grassi L, Biancosino B, Pavanati M et al. Depression or hypoactive delirium? A report of ciprofloxacin-induced mental disorder in a patient with chronic obstructive pulmonary disease. *Psychother Psychosom.* 2001; 70:58-9.
182. US Food and Drug Administration; Center for Drug Evaluation and Research. Early communication about an ongoing safety review of montelukast (Singulair). https://www.fda.gov/Drugs/DrugSafety/PostmarketDrugSafetyInformationforPatientsandProviders/DrugSafetyInformationforHeathcareProfessionals/ucm070618.htm (accessed 2017 Dec 19).
183. Blazer DG, Kessler RC, McGonagle KA et al. The prevalence and distribution of major depression in a national community sample: the national comorbidity study. *Am J Psychiatry.* 1994; 151:979-86.
184. Robins LN, Wing J, Wittchen HU et al. One-month prevalence of mental disorders in the United States: based on 5 epidemiologic catchment area sites. *Arch Gen Psych.* 1988; 45:1069-77.
185. Keller S, Frishman WH. Neuropsychiatric effects of cardiovascular drug therapy. *Cardiol Rev.* 2003; 11:73-93.
186. Schildkraut JJ. Neuropharmacology and the affective disorders. *N Engl J Med.* 1969; 281:302.
187. Maas JW. Biogenic amines and depression. *Arch Gen Psychiatry.* 1975; 32:1357.
188. Beers MH, Passman CJ. Antihypertensive medications and depression. *Drugs.* 1990; 40:792-9.
189. Bremner JD, McCaffery P. The neurobiology of retinoic acid in affective disorders. *Prog Neuropsychopharmacol Biol Psychiatry.* 2008; 32:315-31.
190. Sherwin BB. Hormones, mood, and cognitive functioning in postmenopausal women. *Obstet Gynecol.* 1996; 87(suppl 2):20-26S.
191. Sherwin BB, Suranyi-Cadotte BE. Up-regulatory effect of estrogen on 3H-imipramine binding sites in surgically menoDausal women. *Biol Psychol.* 1990: 28:339-48.
192. Jarkova NB, Martenyi F, Masanauskaite D et al. Mood effect of raloxifene in postmenopausal women. *Maturitas.* 2002; 42:71-5.
193. Adams PW, Rose DP, Folkard J et al. Effect of pyridoxine hydrochloride (vitamin B6) upon depression associated with oral contraception. *Lancet.* 1973; 1;897-904.
194. Smith S, Waterhouse BD, Chapin JK et al. Progesterone alters GABA and glutamate responsiveness: a possible mechanism for its anxiolytic action. *Brain Res.* 1987; 400:353-9.
195. Haskett RF. Diagnostic categorization of psychiatric disturbance in Cushing's syndrome. *Am J Psychiatry.* 1985; 142:911-6.
196. Gerner RH, Wilkins JN. CSF cortisol in patients with depression, mania, or anorexia nervosa and in normal subjects. *Am J Psychiatry.* 1983; 140:92-4.
197. Fernandez-Teruel A, Escorihuela RM, Boix F et al. Imipramine and desipramine decreased the GABA-stimulated chloride uptake, and antiGABAergic agents enhance their action in the forced swimming test in rats. *Neuropsychobiology.* 1990; 23:147-52.
198. Prat JA, Jenner P, Johnson Al et al. Anticonvulsant drugs alter plasma tryptophan concentrations in epileptic patients: implications for antiepileptic action and mental function. *J Neurol Neurosurg Psychiatry.* 1984; 27:1131-3.
199. Lambert MV, Robertson MM. Depression in epilepsy: etiology, phenomenology, and treatment. *Epilepsia.* 1999; 40(suppl 10):S21-47.
200. Shimizu H, Ohtani K, Sato N et al. Increases in serum interleukin-6, plasma ACTH and serum cortisol levels after systemic interferon-alpha administration. *J Endocrinol.* 1995; 42:551-6.
201. Maes M, Wauters A, Verkerk R et al. Lower L-tryptophan availability in depression: a marker of a more generalized disorder in protein metabolism. *Neuropsychopharmacology* 1996; 15:243-51.
202. Mehta D, Raison C, Woolwine BJ et al. Transcriptional signals related to glucose and lipid metabolism predict treatment response to the tumor necrosis factor antagonist infliximab in patients with treatment-resistant depression. *Brain Behav Immun.* 2013; 31:205-15.
203. Raison CL, Rutherford RE, Woolwine BJ et al. A randomized controlled trial of the tumor necrosis factor-alpha antagonist infliximab in treatment resistant depression: role of baseline inflammatory biomarkers. *JAMA Psychiatry.* 2013; 70:31-41.
204. Kraus MR, Al-Taie O, Schafer A et al. Serotonin-1A receptor gene HTR1A variation predicts interferon-induced depression in chronic hepatitis C. *Gastroenterol.* 2007; 132:1279-86.
205. Galvao-de Almedia A, Quarantini LC, Tartaglioni A et al. Serononin-1A receptor CC genotype is associated with persistent depression related to interferon-alpha in hepatitis C patients. *Gen Hosp Psychiatry.* 2014; 36:255-60.
206. O'Mahony SM, Myint AM, Steinbusch H et al. Efavirenz induces depressive-like behaviour, increased stress response, and changes in the immune response in rats. *Neuroimmunomodulation.* 2005; 12:293-8.
207. Hays JT, Ebbert JO, Sood A. Efficacy and safety of varenicline for smoking cessation. *Am J Med.* 2008; 121(4 suppl 1):S32-42.
208. O'Donnell J. Overview of existing research and information linking isotretinoin, depression, psychosis and suicide. *Am J Ther.* 2003; 10:148-59.
209. Warnock JK, Bundren JC, Morris DW. Sertraline in the treatment of depression associated with gonadotropin-releasing hormone agonist therapy. *Biol Psych.* 1998; 43:464-5.
210. Jacoby A, Baker GA, Steen N et al. The clinical course of epilepsy and its psychosocial correlates: findings from a UK community study. *Epilepsia.* 1996; 37:148-61.
211. Victoroff JI, Benson DF, Engel J et al. Interictal depression in patients with medically intractable complex partial seizures: electroencephalography and cerebral metabolic correlates [abstract]. *Ann Neurol.* 1990; 28:221.

212. Rabkin JE, Charles E, Kass F. Hypertension and DSM-III depression in psychiatric outpatients. *Am J Psychiatry.* 1983; 140:1072-4.
213. Zdilar D, Franco-Bronson K, Buchler N et al. Hepatitis C, interferon alfa, and depression. *Hepatology.* 2000; 31:1207-11.
214. Hosaka T, Aoki T. Depression among cancer patients. *Psychiatry Clin Neurosci.* 1996; 50:309-12.
215. Sadovnick AD, Remick RA, Allen J et al. Depression and multiple sclerosis. *Neurology.* 1996; 46:628-32.
216. Patten SB. Psychopharmacology for the clinician psychopharmacologie pratique. *J Psychiatry Neurosci.* 2001; 26:66.
217. Gutiérrez F, Navarro A, Padilla S et al. Prediction of neuropsychiatric adverse events associated with long-term efavirenz therapy, using plasma drug level monitoring. *Clin Infect Dis.* 2005; 41:1648-53.
218. Kaufman KR, Bisen V, Zimmerman A et al. Apparent dose-dependent levetiracetam-induced de novo major depression with suicidal behavior. *Epil Behav Case Reports.* 2013; 1:110-2.
219. Mula M, Trimble MR, Sander JWAS. The role of hippocampal sclerosis in topiramate-related depression and cognitive deficits in people with epilepsy. *Epilepsia.* 2003; 44:1573-7.
220. Galanti M, Newport DJ, Pennell PB et al. Post-partum depression in women with epilepsy: influence of antiepileptic drugs in a prospective study. *Epilepsy Behav.* 2009; 16:426-30.
221. Mula M, Hesdorffer DC, Trimble M, Sander JW. The role of titration schedule of topiramate for the development of depression in patients with epilepsy. *Epilepsia.* 2009; 50:1072-6.
222. Whale R, Fiahlo R, Rolt M et al. Psychomotor retardation and vulnerability to interferon alpha induced major depressive disorder: prospective study of a chronic hepatitis C cohort. *J Psychosomatic Res.* 2015; 79:640-5.
223. Marron MM, Anderson SJ, Garrity J et al. Association of baseline sleep quality with trajectories of depressive symptoms in patients undergoing interferon treatment. *Psychosomatic Med.* 2015; 77:911-20.
224. Marcellin P, Lau GK, Zeuzem S et al. Comparing the safety, tolerability and quality of life in patients with chronic hepatitis B vs chronic hepatitis C treated with peginterferon alpha-2a. *Liver Int.* 2008; 28:477-85.
225. Robaeys G, DeBie J, Wichers MC et al. Early prediction of major depression in chronic hepatitis C patients during peg-interferon a-2b treatment by assessment of vegetative-depressive symptoms after four weeks. *World J Gastroenterol.* 2007; 13:5736-40.
226. Cozzolongo R, Porcelli P, Cariola F et al. Serotonin gene polymorphisms and lifetime mood disorders in predicting interferon-induced depression in chronic hepatitis C. *J Affective Disord.* 2015; 183:90-7.
227. Kraus MR, Schafer A, Schottker K et al. Therapy of interferon-induced depression in chronic hepatitis C with citalopram: a randomized, double-blind, placebo-controlled study. *Gut.* 2008; 57:531-6.
228. Wichers MC, Kenis G, Leue C et al. Baseline immune activation as a risk factor for the onset of depression during interferon-alpha treatment. *Biol Psychiatry.* 2006; 60:77-9.
229. Cunha ECM, Behrensdorf MF, Bavaresco V et al. Genotype 1 of hepatitis C virus increases the risk of major depression: a 12-week prospective study. *Gen Hosp Psychiatry.* 2015; 37:283-7.
230. Wells KB, Stewart A, Hays RD et al. The functioning and well-being of depressed patients: results from the Medical Outcomes Study. *JAMA.* 1989; 262:914-9.
231. Kovacs P, Panczel G, Balatoni T et al. Social support decreases depressogenic effect of low-dose interferon alpha treatment in melanoma patients. *J Psychosom Res.* 2015; 78:579-84.
232. Sabet-Sharghi F, Hutzler JC. Prophylaxis of steroid induced psychiatric syndromes. *Psychosomatics.* 1990; 31:113-4.
233. Musselman DL, Lawson DH, Gumnick JF et al. Paroxetine for the prevention of depression induced by high-dose interferon alfa. *N Engl J Med.* 2001; 344:961-6.
234. Ehret M, Sobierja DM. Prevention of interferon-alpha-associated depression with antidepressant medications in patients with hepatitis C virus: a systematic review and meta-analysis. *Int J Clin Pract.* 2014; 68:255-61.
235. Hou X, Xu J, Wang J, Yu Y. Can antidepressants prevent pegylated interferon-α/ribavirin-associated depression in patients with chronic hepatitis C: meta-analysis of randomized, double-blind, placebo-controlled trials? *PLOS One.* 2013; 8:e76799.
236. Udina M, Higdalgo D, Navines R et al. Prophylactic antidepressant treatment of interferon-induced depression in chronic hepatitis C: a systematic review and meta-analysis. *J Clin Psychiatry.* 2014; 75:10.
237. Quarantini LC, Miranda-Scippa A, Schinoni MI et al. Effect of amantadine on depressive symptoms in chronic hepatitis C patients treated with pegylated interferon: a randomized, controlled pilot study. *Clin Neuropharmacol.* 2006; 29:138-43.
238. Dabaghzadeh F, Ghaeli P, Kahalili H et al. Cyproheptadine for prevention of neuropsychiatric adverse effects of efavirenz: a randomized clinical trial. *AIDS Patient Care STDs.* 2013; 27:146-54.
239. Yudofsky SC. Beta-blockers and depression: the clinician's dilemma. *JAMA.* 1992; 267:1826-7.
240. Pedrol E, Llibre JM, Tasias M et al. Outcome of neuropsychiatric symptoms related to an antiretroviral drug following its substitution by nivirapine: the RELAX study. *HIV Med.* 2015; 16:628-34.
241. Gleason OC, Yates WR, Isbell MD et al. An open-label trial of citalopram for major depression in patients with hepatitis C. *J Clin Psychiatry.* 2002; 63:194-8.
242. Hauser P, Khosla J, Aurora H et al. A prospective study of the incidence and open-label treatment of interferon-induced major depressive disorder in patients with hepatitis C. *Mol Psychiatry.* 2002; 7:942-7.
243. Chen W, Lai H, Su W et al. Bupropion for interferon-alpha-induced depression in patients with hepatitis C viral infection: an open-label study. *Psychiatry Investig.* 2015; 12:142-5.
244. Brustolium D, Ribiero-dos-Santos R, Kast RE et al. A new chapter opens in anti-inflammatory treatments: the antidepressant bupropion lowers production of tumor necrosis factor-alpha and interferon-gamma in mice. *Int Immunopharmacol.* 2006; 6:903-7.
245. Camacho A, Ng B. Methylphenidate for alpha-interferon induced depression. *J Psychopharm.* 2006; 20:687-9.
246. Malek-Ahmadi P, Prabhu F. Venlafaxine for treatment of interferon alfa-induced depression. *Ann Pharmacother.* 2006; 40:2075.
247. Davidson J. Seizures and bupropion: a review. *J Clin Psychiatry.* 1989; 50:256-61.
248. De Picker L, Van Den Eede F, Dumont G et al. Antidepressants and the risk of hyponatremia: a class-by-class review of literature. *Psychosomatics.* 2014; 55:536-47.

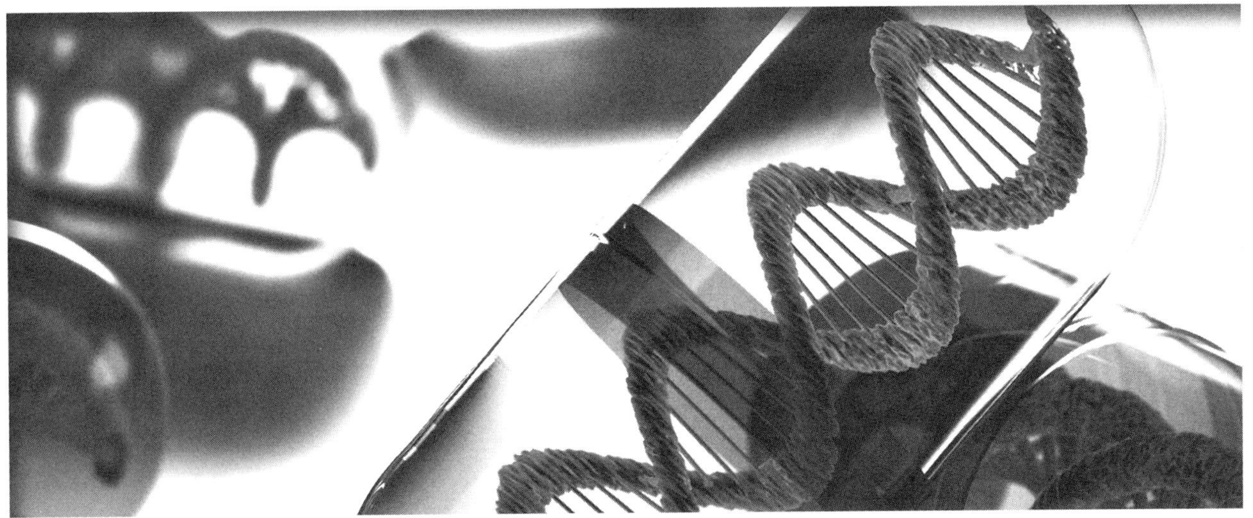

CHAPTER 19

Anxiety

Julie A. Dopheide and Seth Gomez

Each individual, no matter how healthy, has experienced symptoms of anxiety at some point in his or her life. Anxiety can be adaptive and help individuals to prepare and enhance their performance; it also drives one to be more cautious in potentially dangerous circumstances. For example, occasional low-level anxiety can motivate an individual to prepare for an examination, professional presentation, or help one avoid walking alone in a high crime area. In contrast, when persistent anxiety above an individual's tolerability threshold causes undue distress, discomfort, and impairs functioning, it is considered maladaptive and therefore a disorder. If left untreated, anxiety may lead to other conditions, such as depression or alcohol abuse.[1-4] The *Diagnostic and Statistical Manual of Mental Disorders, Fifth Edition* (*DSM-5*), includes a diagnosis of substance or medication-induced anxiety, a clear indication that medications are an increasingly well-recognized contributor to signs and symptoms of anxiety.[1] A patient presenting with anxiety symptoms should be carefully assessed to determine whether a primary anxiety disorder is present, whether the symptoms are situational, or whether the symptoms are secondary to a drug. A combination of these factors is also possible.[1,4]

CAUSATIVE AGENTS

Drugs that may induce anxiety are listed in **Table 19-1**.[4-80] Drugs from a variety of classes have been implicated as causes of anxiety. These include central nervous system (CNS) agents, cardiovascular drugs, anti-infectives, hormonal products, cancer chemotherapy agents, nonprescription medications and herbal supplements, and illicit drugs, among others. The *DSM-5* diagnostic criteria for substance/medication-induced anxiety involves predominant panic attacks or symptoms of anxiety developing soon after substance intoxication or withdrawal, or after exposure to a medication. To meet the criteria, the symptoms should cause clinically significant distress or impairment in social, occupational, or other important areas of functioning.[1] Individuals who develop anxiety after taking drugs listed in this chapter experience a wide range of symptoms and symptom severity. Individual agents that cause specific symptoms of anxiety are

Table 19-1 Agents Implicated in Drug-Induced Anxiety[a]

Drug	Incidence	Level of Evidence[b]
Amphetamines[4-8,c]	10–50%	A
Anabolic steroids[7,9,73]	10–50%	B
Antipsychotics[10,11]	10–30%	B
Aripiprazole[10,12]	10–20%	B
Armodafinil[50-53,c]	1–10%	A
Atomoxetine[7,56,57]	NK	B
Abacavir[62]	NK	C
Baclofen[7,d]	NK	C
Barbiturates[7,d]	NK	B
Benzodiazepines[6,7,13,14,d]	10–50%	A
β-agonists[64]	NK	B
β-blockers[7,15,16,d]	10–40%	B
Bitter orange (synephrine)[38]	NK	B
Brexpiprazole[76]	2–4%	B
Bupropion[4,7,c]	10–20%	B
Caffeine[4,7,17,18,c,d]	10–30%	A
Cannabis[1,19,d]	30–70%	B
Cariprazine[77]	10–20%	B
Carisoprodol[63,d]	NK	C
Clomiphene[49]	NK	B
Cocaine[1,4]	10–50%	A
Cycloserine[20]	30–60%	B
Dopamine agonists[7,21]	10–30%	B
Dopamine antagonists[7,10,21,d]	10–30%	B
Dronabinol[7]	NK	C
Efavirenz[7,60,61,c]	NK	B
Ephedrine[7,22]	NK	A
Estrogen[23-25,72,e]	NK	A
Flumazenil[7,20,c]	NK	A
Fluoroquinolones[7,26]	NK	C
Gabapentin[27,d]	NK	B
Glucocorticoids[71]	NK	B
Gonadotropin-releasing hormone agonists[28]	NK	B
Guarana[7,22]	NK	B
Ifosfamide[7]	NK	C
Levodopa[7,58,59,d]	40–90%	B
Lidocaine[7]	NK	C
Montelukast[65,c]	NK	C
Mefloquine[29,30,c]	NK	C
Methylphenidate, dexmethylphenidate[4-8,31]	10–30%	A
Metoclopramide[7,d]	NK	C
Modafinil[8,32]	5–20%	A
Nicotine[4,7,33,d,f]	NK	A

Table 19-1 Agents Implicated in Drug-Induced Anxiety[a] (continued)

Drug	Incidence	Level of Evidence[b]
Nonsteroidal anti-inflammatory drugs[7,34,c]	NK	C
Opioids[20,23,54,d]	30–70%	B
Phencyclidine[1,4]	10–50%	A
Pregabalin[7,55,d]	NK	C
Progesterone[24,78]	10–30%	B
Pseudoephedrine[4,7,35]	NK	A
Raltegravir[80]	NK	C
Selective serotonin reuptake inhibitors[4,7,36,37,c,d]	10–40%	A
Serotonin norepinephrine reuptake inhibitors[7,c,d]	NK	C
Statins[79]	NK	C
Theophylline[7,41,c]	20–50%	A
Thyroid hormone supplementation[4,74,75,c]	10–50%	B
Topiramate[66-69,c]	NK	C
Valerian[42,43,d]	NK	B
Varenicline[44,45,70]	NK	A
Vinblastine[46,47,c]	NK	C
Yohimbine[4,7,48,c]	NK	B
Ziprasidone[10,11]	10–20%	B

NK = not known.

[a]For all drugs listed, anxiety may occur during both treatment and withdrawal unless otherwise specified.

[b]Definitions for Levels of Evidence: Level A—evidence from one or more randomized, controlled clinical trials; Level B—evidence from nonrandomized clinical trials, prospective observational studies, cohort studies, retrospective studies, case-control studies, meta-analyses and/or postmarketing surveillance studies; and Level C—evidence from one or more published case reports or case series.

[c]Anxiety only occurs during treatment (not during withdrawal).

[d]Anxiety only occurs during withdrawal (not during treatment).

[e]Anxiety may occur during fluctuations in plasma concentrations.

[f]Includes cigarettes and nicotine replacement therapies (gum, lozenge, inhalers, patches).

presented when a description of the type of drug-induced anxiety is available.

CNS-ACTIVE AGENTS

Anxiety is associated with intoxication and withdrawal from drugs of abuse such as cocaine, methamphetamine, and phencyclidine.[4,7] Anxiety is also a well-known effect of stimulating substances such as caffeine, nasal decongestants (e.g., pseudoephedrine), and amphetamines.[1,17,18,35] Stimulant medications including dextroamphetamine, amphetamine, methylphenidate, and dexmethylphenidate have been associated with new-onset or worsening anxiety in susceptible individuals.[4-8] Anxiety is uncommon when these agents are used at recommended doses for attention deficit/hyperactivity disorder (ADHD). In fact, some studies report improvements in anxiety symptoms when patients with ADHD are treated with methylphenidate (children) and mixed amphetamine salts (adults).[31,82] The use of atomoxetine, a nonstimulant medication for ADHD, may prompt early discontinuation due to anxiety symptoms. Atomoxetine-associated anxiety may be particularly problematic in individuals with developmental disabilities or epilepsy.[56,57]

Selective serotonin reuptake inhibitors (SSRIs), serotonin norepinephrine reuptake inhibitors (SNRIs), and some tricyclic antidepressants (TCAs) are effective treatments for anxiety and depressive disorders when used at recommended doses for longer than 4 weeks. It is also important to recognize that new-onset or worsening anxiety is possible during the initiation of treatment, during a dose increase, or after abrupt discontinuation of therapy with these agents.[36]

Anxiety is also common when CNS depressant agents such as barbiturates, benzodiazepines, and opioids are discontinued abruptly after long-term use.[4,13,23,54] Benzodiazepines relieve anxiety via potentiation of γ-aminobutyric acid (GABA), an inhibitory neurotransmitter.[4,23] After 2–4 weeks of treatment with benzodiazepines, receptor dependence develops and significant withdrawal symptoms can occur when a dose is missed or when therapy is discontinued.[4,13,14] Anxiety associated with benzodiazepine withdrawal is frequently described as worse than the pretreatment anxiety for which therapy was initiated. Abrupt discontinuation of high-dose benzodiazepines produces the most severe withdrawal-associated anxiety. Abrupt discontinuation of benzodiazepines with shorter half-lives and no significant active metabolite (e.g., alprazolam) is particularly anxiety-provoking.[13,14]

Carisoprodol, a muscle relaxant, is increasingly recognized for its abuse potential and is now considered a controlled substance (C-IV) in the United States. As more individuals misuse and abuse carisoprodol, the number who experience withdrawal and associated anxiety will also likely increase.[63] Valerian is an herbal product that modulates GABA in the CNS and is used for anxiety and insomnia.[42,75] Symptoms of worsening anxiety and insomnia have been reported after abrupt discontinuation of valerian, suggesting that dependence occurs over time, an effect similar to that associated with benzodiazepines.[42,43]

Certain anticonvulsants may also precipitate drug-induced anxiety symptoms. Gabapentin and pregabalin employ similar mechanisms of action and both are associated with anxiety upon withdrawal of therapy.[7,27,55] Topiramate-induced anxiety can also be problematic at low doses (<100 mg/day) leading to discontinuation or requiring additional treatment in 2–5.5% of migraneurs.[66] Three case reports of topiramate-induced new onset panic attacks occuring 3–6 weeks after intiation have also been described.[67-69]

Varenicline is a selective $\alpha_4\beta_2$-nicotinic acetylcholine partial receptor agonist that is indicated for smoking cessation. During a controlled clinical trial in 250 Asian patients taking varenicline, 5.6% developed anxiety compared with 2.4% in the placebo group.[44] Case reports of insomnia, anxiety, depression, and psychosis associated with varenicline therapy for smoking cessation prompted the U.S. Food and Drug Administration (FDA) to issue a public health advisory in January 2008.[45] More detailed evaluations of the neuropsychiatric effects of varenicline have since been conducted that show the risk of varenicline-associated anxiety may be confined to individuals with pre-existing psychiatric disorders.[70,83] In individuals without pre-existing psychiatric disorders, there was a nonsignificant trend toward increased anxiety associated with varenicline.[70] Available evidence indicates that any person taking varenicline is at risk for treatment emergent anxiety, but this is more likely to occur in individuals with pre-existing psychiatric disorders.

STEROIDS AND HORMONES

Steroids and several hormones have been associated with mood swings, including anxiety. Anxiety is a well-known adverse effect associated with the use of glucocorticoids and anabolic steroids, including nandrolone, oxymetholone, stanozolol, and oxandrolone.[7,9,71] Anxiety provoked by these steroidal agents is less common than rage, aggression, and irritability, but panic attacks and worsening anxiety have all been described.[7,9,71] The steroidal hormones estrogen, progesterone, and testosterone, are associated with anxiety, particularly during fluctuating plasma concentrations that occur in association with certain medical conditions or age-related decline (e.g., hypogonadism, reproductive-age transitions), and from exogenous hormone supplementation or withdrawal.[23,24,72] The severity of anxiety induced by hormone changes is related to sex, individual susceptibility, and the degree of fluctuation in plasma concentrations. For example, estrogen replacement and withdrawal have been linked to worsening anxiety, insomnia, and panic attacks in susceptible women.[7,23,72] A wide range in severity of anxiety symptoms associated with estrogen concentration changes have been reported in premenstrual, postpartum, and perimenopausal women; plasma estrogen concentrations decline before stabilizing at menopausal concentrations.[84,85] Similarly, low concentrations of testosterone in women with age-related decline in androgens and men with hypogonadism may induce anxiety or depression; testosterone replacement in these individuals may improve anxiety symptoms.[86] Furthermore, new onset anxiety occurs in 8.9% of older males treated with the gonadotropin-releasing hormone (GnRH) agonists leuprolide and goserelin for treatment of prostate cancer, emphasizing the role of low testosterone concentrations in the emergence of anxiety symptoms.[28] Dependence and abuse of testosterone and testosterone analogues for recreational use and performance enhancement is also associated with greater self-report of anxiety and anxiety disorders.[9,73] Therefore, anxiety symptoms may occur during times when plasma testosterone concentrations are in excess or deficient and may occur in both women and men.[39,81,87,88] Danazol is an androgen that may be used for the treatment of endometriosis and fibrocystic breast disease. The risk of danazol-induced anxiety and irritability is similar to that associated with leuprolide and goserelin.[7]

Clomiphene is a selective estrogen receptor modulator used to induce ovulation in the treatment of infertility. In a self-reported survey using the State-Trait Anxiety Inventory, 25.9% (n = 162) of patients reported anxiety as an adverse effect of clomiphene, while other possible symptoms of anxiety including forgetfulness and difficulty concentrating occurred in approximately 19% of patients.[49] In the same study, human menopausal gonadotropin use was associated with even higher rates of anxiety; however, anxiety rates were also correlated with the number of years spent trying to conceive. This suggests that the duration of infertility is also anxiety-provoking.[49]

Thyroid hormone supplementation does not routinely lead to anxiety. However, excessive doses may result in emotional symptoms, such as feeling "on edge" or jittery, as well as physical symptoms, including sweating or tachycardia.[4] One study of 40 women with subclinical hypothyroidism describes significantly elevated anxiety scores in 8 of 20 women treated with thyroxine 50–100 mcg/day, as compared with only 1 of 14 women treated with placebo.[74] Thyroid supplements containing triiodothyronine, thyroxine, desiccated thyroid, or tiratricol can cause tachycardia and general anxiety symptoms as well.[75]

ANTI-INFECTIVE AGENTS

Anti-infective agents have been associated with neuropsychiatric adverse effects including anxiety, although the frequency is difficult to predict because of multiple possible mechanisms and confounding variables.[7,26,89] Fluoroquinolones are the class of antibiotic agents associated with the highest incidence of adverse CNS effects, including anxiety and insomnia.[7,26] Efavirenz is the most well-known antiretroviral agent to cause neuropsychiatric effects including anxiety.[60,61] One case report of abacavir-induced anxiety in a pediatric male and postmarketing reports of worsening anxiety associated with raltegravir in patients with pre-existing psychiatric disorders have been documented.[62,80] Although other neuropsychiatric effects may occur, it is uncommon for antiretroviral medications other than efavirenz to induce anxiety.[61]

Antimalarial agents, especially mefloquine, may cause adverse neuropsychiatric effects including depression and anxiety, in children and adults.[29,30,90] In one published case a 10-year-old child experienced feelings of impending doom, panic, a spider phobia, separation anxiety, and multiple physical symptoms of anxiety (hyperventilation, restlessness, insomnia) after taking mefloquine for 2 weeks during a trip to Africa. Symptoms slowly resolved over 1–3 months after the drug was discontinued.[29,30]

OTHER AGENTS

Cancer chemotherapy regimens can provoke a variety of neuropsychiatric effects such as emotional lability associated with ifosfamide, anxiety symptoms induced by vinblastine, or hallucinations and confusion attributed to chlorambucil or cytarabine, respectively. However, intolerable anxiety symptoms are not commonly reported with these agents.[7,46,47]

Angiotensin-converting enzyme inhibitors, β-blockers, statins, and nonsteroidal anti-inflammatory agents (NSAIDs) may cause anxiety.[7,16,34] Among the NSAIDs, indomethacin is associated with the largest number of case reports of treatment-associated anxiety and other psychiatric symptoms.[34] Physical symptoms of anxiety including tremors and tachycardia are a known adverse effect of bronchodilator agents such as albuterol and theophylline. The leukotriene receptor antagonist montelukast, an optional adjunctive treatment for asthma, has been increasingly recognized as an inducer of CNS adverse effects including anxiety, particularly in children, adolescents, and young adults. The increase in reporting is likely related to increased awareness due to a 2008 FDA alert highlighting the behavioral and mood changes associated with montelukast.[65,91] Though montelukast-induced anxiety is possible, the combined effects of concurrent use of inhaled corticosteroids, oral corticosteroids, or β-agonists should also be considered.[65] Irritability attributed to montelukast has also been reported in an adult female with human immunodeficiency virus concurrently taking efavirenz, suggesting a possible interaction between these drugs.[92] Due to the lack of systematic reports and routine assessment for neuropsychiatric adverse effects, it is impossible to determine an incidence of anxiety associated with most of the aforementioned agents.

Table 19-2 12-Month Prevalence of *DSM-5* Anxiety Disorders in the General Population[1]

Anxiety Disorder	Prevalence (%)
Substance or medication-induced anxiety disorder	0.002[a]
Generalized anxiety disorder	2.9
Separation anxiety disorder	0.9–1.9
Social anxiety disorder	7
Agoraphobia	1.7
Panic disorder	2–3
Panic attacks (isolated)	11.2
Post-traumatic stress disorder[b]	3.5
Obsessive–compulsive disorder[b]	1.2

DSM-V = Diagnostic and Statistical Manual of Mental Disorders, Fifth Edition.

[a]*DSM-5* states the prevalence is likely higher in clinical populations relative to that reported in epidemiological studies.

[b]*DSM-5* has reclassified post-traumatic stress disorder and obsessive-compulsive disorder into trauma and stress related disorders and obsessive-compulsive and related disorders, respectively.

EPIDEMIOLOGY

Estimates of the relative likelihood of anxiety induced by specific drugs based on available evidence are provided in Table 19-1. The 12-month prevalence of primary anxiety disorders in the general population is provided in **Table 19-2.**[1]

MECHANISMS

For most agents, mechanisms of drug-induced anxiety are poorly or incompletely understood. Possible or probable mechanisms of drug-induced anxiety, where known, are presented in **Table 19-3.**[3-7,18,20,23,35,93] One of the best-understood mechanisms for drug-induced anxiety involves increasing noradrenergic outflow from the locus coeruleus of the CNS. Stimulants, yohimbine, and withdrawal from benzodiazepines or opioids all appear to increase noradrenergic outflow from the CNS.[6,7,23,93,94] Pseudoephedrine, ephedrine, and bitter orange (synephrine) produce dose-related symptoms of anxiety via α_1-adrenergic stimulation that increases nervousness centrally, causing vasoconstriction and a "jittery" or restless feeling. Anxiety associated with withdrawal from carisoprodol is believed to be due to declining concentrations of one of its metabolites, meprobamate, a compound that may activate $GABA_A$ receptors in a manner similar to that of benzodiazepines.[63] Topiramate inhibits the enzyme carbonic anhydrase leading to elevations in central concentrations of CO_2, which is thought to provoke panic symptoms.[67-69] Gabaminergic mechanisms are likely involved when anxiety occurs during abrupt discontinuation of therapy with gabapentin or pregabalin; however, mechanisms of anxiety associated with these anticonvulsants require further study.[27,55]

Caffeine and guarana (an herbal form of caffeine derived from the plant *Paullinia cupana*) exert anxiogenic effects through antagonism of adenosine receptors and the phosphodiesterase enzyme, resulting in excessive neurotransmitter activity.[17,18,23] Anxiety associated with nicotine withdrawal is believed to occur because of a lack of stimulation of dopaminergic reward centers in the brain upon abrupt discontinuation.[6,23] Although overuse of inhalers containing β-agonists such as albuterol can also provoke anxiety symptoms,

Table 19-3 Mechanisms of Drug-Induced Anxiety

Drug	Mechanism
Amphetamines, methylphenidate, stimulants, bupropion, ziprasidone[3-7,35,93,97]	Inhibition of norepinephrine and dopamine reuptake in the presynaptic neuron and stimulation of dopamine receptors
Benzodiazepine withdrawal[4,13,20,23]	Decreased GABA activity and increased noradrenergic outflow from the CNS associated with benzodiazepine withdrawal
Caffeine, guarana, theophylline[4,17,18,20,22,23]	Antagonism of adenosine receptors and phosphodiesterase inhibition
Carisoprodol withdrawal[63]	Decreased GABA activity due to declining concentrations of the metabolite meprobamate
Dopamine agonists and antagonists[20,23,97]	Fluctuating dopaminergic tone in the CNS
Gonadotropin-releasing hormone analogues[28]	Suppresses secretion of gonadotropins LH and FSH from the pituitary gland which leads to decreased production of estrogen or testosterone
Steroidal hormones[23,78,87,a] Estrogen Progesterone	Dysregulation of neurotransmitters in the CNS Estrogen concentration decline causes 5-HT dysregulation Progesterone metabolism modulates GABA
Opioid withdrawal[20,23,54,94]	Decreased opioid receptor activity and increased noradrenergic outflow from CNS
Selective serotonin reuptake inhibitors, serotonin norepinephrine reuptake inhibitors, tricyclic antidepressants[4,20,23]	Neurotransmitter reuptake inhibition (serotonin, norepinephrine, dopamine)
Topiramate[61-69]	Possibly through inhibition of carbonic anhydrase leading to an increase in central CO_2

5-HT = 5-hydroxytryptamine, GABA = gamma-aminobutyric acid, CNS = central nervous system, CO_2 = carbon dioxide, LH = luteinizing hormone, FSH = follicle-stimulating hormone.
[a]Anxiety may occur during fluctuations in plasma concentrations.

tremors and anxiety are common in individuals taking these drugs even at normal doses. The likely mechanism is direct stimulation of postsynaptic β-adrenergic receptors causing palpitations, tremors, and the general feeling of anxiety.

Withdrawal from levodopa therapy may trigger a plethora of nonmotor symptoms including anxiety in people with Parkinson disease. Off periods, including early mornings, appear to be associated with higher rates and greater severity of anxiety symptoms due to the decline of dopamine concentrations in the brain.[58,59,95] Interestingly, use of dopaminergic agonists, such as rotigotine and pramipexole, may be associated with fewer nonmotor symptoms compared to levodopa formulations due to their longer duration of action.[58,59,96] However their impact on reducing anxiety symptoms has not been determined. Withdrawal of therapy with dopaminergic agonists or administration of dopaminergic antagonists can cause significant functional-impairing anxiety in individuals with dopaminergic deficits caused by Parkinson disease.[7,96]

Antipsychotics and antidepressants may induce akathisia on initiation and during dose titration. Antagonism of dopamine receptors in the nigrostriatal tract associated with first-generation antipsychotics such as haloperidol, or second-generation antipsychotic agents including risperidone, ziprasidone, aripiprazole, brexpiprazole, and cariprazine can lead to extrapyramidal effects including akathisia, which is a subjective feeling of inner restlessness. Akathisia is frequently accompanied by, or described as, an intolerable feeling of anxiety.[10,12,76,77] Furthermore, aripiprazole, brexpiprazole, and cariprazine act to some degree as partial dopamine agonists at dopamine receptors leading to behavioral activation and anxiety in some individuals. In general, antipsychotic agents that block dopamine receptors but exert no significant anticholinergic blockade are more likely to cause anxiety or akathisia. Additionally, ziprasidone inhibits the reuptake of norepinephrine and serotonin to a degree similar to that of the TCA imipramine, which may initially exacerbate anxiety symptoms in susceptible individuals.[97] Neurotransmitter reuptake inhibition with SSRIs, SNRIs, and TCAs can precipitate anxiety due to acute changes in neurotransmitter activity that occur during intiation of therapy or a dose increase, and can also occur during abrupt discontinuation of therapy leading to withdrawal symptoms.[36,37]

Anxiety caused by fluctuating plasma concentrations of hormones has been well described, although the mechanism of anxiogenesis is poorly understood. Estrogen exerts multiple complex effects on neurotrophins, cortisol, and neurotransmitter systems.[24] One theory linking estrogen dysregulation to anxiety involves estrogen's role in effective serotonin use. When plasma estrogen concentrations decline significantly, the associated serotonin dysregulation causes anxiety.[23] Progesterone deficiency and supplementation has been linked with anxiety and irritability in women.[23,24] One potential mechanism involves progesterone's neuroactive steroid metabolites (e.g., 5-tetrahydroprogesterone, allopregnanolone), which are allosteric modulators of $GABA_A$, causing anxiolytic effects in some and anxiogenic effects in others, depending on an individual's genetic susceptibility to anxiety and progesterone metabolite formation.[78,87] In addition, progesterone possesses some antiestrogen activity that can precipitate anxiety in some individuals.[23] GnRH agonists are synthetic derivatives of the native decapeptide produced by the hypothalamus, and may cause anxiety via reversible suppression of the synthesis and release of luteinizing and follicle-stimulating hormones which ultimately leads to reduced synthesis of sex hormones (e.g., testosterone).[28] Similarly, GnRH antagonists can be expected to induce anxiety by suppressing gonadotropin hormone release.

CLINICAL PRESENTATION AND DIFFERENTIAL DIAGNOSIS

Signs and symptoms associated with drug-induced anxiety are listed in **Table 19-4**. An individual with significant anxiety experiences a combination of physical, emotional, and cognitive symptoms that may challenge his or her ability to interact with others, think clearly, or participate in the activities of daily living. Table 19-4 differentiates physical, emotional, and cognitive symptoms of anxiety that may be further rated as mild, moderate, or severe, depending on the impact of these symptoms on the individual's ability to function.

Table 19-4 Signs and Symptoms Associated with Drug-Induced Anxiety[1-4,8-16]

Emotional

- Fear of "going crazy"
- Fear of losing control
- Feeling "on edge"
- Feeling jittery
- Feeling of impending doom
- Feelings of inferiority
- Irritability
- Sadness
- Tearfulness

Cognitive

- Blanking out
- Difficulty concentrating
- Extreme worries
- Intrusive thoughts
- Irritability
- Obsessive thoughts
- Rapid or racing thoughts

Physical

- Chest pain
- Choking sensation
- Diarrhea
- Difficulty speaking
- Exaggerated startle response
- Exhaustion
- Fatigue
- Fidgeting
- Flushing
- Hypervigilance
- Insomnia
- Nausea, vomiting
- Palpitations
- Poor eye contact
- Restlessness
- Shaky voice
- Tearfulness
- Tremulousness

Patient assessment should begin by documenting the patient's experience of anxiety subjectively and objectively. Both clinician-rated (e.g., Hamilton Anxiety Rating Scale) and self-rated standardized anxiety scales (e.g., Beck Anxiety Inventory) are useful to establish objective measures of anxiety and to monitor persistence or remittance of symptoms over time.[4,98] However, these tools are unable to link the symptoms to the cause (e.g., drug-induced anxiety). The clinician's interview is crucial to investigate whether symptoms are likely drug-induced by establishing the time course of the onset of anxiety in relation to initiation or discontinuation of drug therapy.

An individual's sensitivity to experiencing caffeine-induced anxiety can vary greatly, but emotional, cognitive, and physical symptoms are all possible. During acute consumption, symptoms of anxiety generally manifest within 15–30 minutes after ingesting between 200 and 500 mg of caffeine or 3–5 cups of brewed coffee or may occur as caffeine withdrawal 1–2 days after abrupt discontinuation.[1,17,18] The onset of anxiety symptoms associated with benzodiazepine withdrawal is related to the half-life of the specific agent. For short- to intermediate-acting agents such as alprazolam or lorazepam, withdrawal symptoms can occur within 6–24 hours of abrupt cessation, whereas withdrawal symptoms can occur within 2–3 days of discontinuing benzodiazepines with longer half-lives, such as clonazepam or diazepam.[13,14] Withdrawal syndromes associated with carisoprodol include symptoms of anxiety, tremors, restlessness, and irritability, among other somatic and neuropsychiatric effects such as headache and insomnia.[63] Restlessness, irritability, tremor, and sweating combined with elevated blood pressure have been reported during pregabalin withdrawal.[7,55] Similar anxiety symptoms accompanied by diaphoresis and palpitations are reported with gabapentin therapy.[27]

It can be difficult to distinguish drug-induced anxiety from other possible causes of anxiety in many patients. Conditions to consider in the differential diagnosis of drug-induced anxiety are listed in **Table 19-5**.[1,4,10,15-17,31,96] A thorough physical examination and medication and substance abuse history are necessary for a comprehensive assessment. Associated symptoms that are more indicative of substance-induced anxiety versus a primary anxiety disorder include new-onset panic attacks after the age of 45 years, vertigo or loss of balance, loss of bladder or bowel control, and slurred speech or amnesia. Also, drug-induced anxiety typically does not meet the duration criteria for a primary anxiety disorder. For example, to meet the criteria for generalized anxiety disorder, anxiety symptoms must cause functional impairment for 6 months.[1,4] In individuals with cancer, distinguishing drug-induced anxiety is particularly difficult because of high levels of situational anxiety related to the diagnosis and the need to endure treatment over months to years.[46]

Table 19-6 outlines a systematic approach to patient assessment and lists key questions useful in assessing drug-induced anxiety and differentiating

Table 19-5 Conditions to Consider in the Differential Diagnosis of Drug-Induced Anxiety[1,4,10,15-17,31,96]

- Addison disease
- Akathisia
- Asthma
- Attention-deficit hyperactivity disorder
- Cardiomyopathies
- Chronic obstructive pulmonary disease
- Chronic pain
- Cushing syndrome
- Delirium
- Dementia
- Electrolyte abnormalities
- Fibromyalgia
- Hypertension
- Hyperthyroidism or Graves disease
- Hypoglycemia
- Irritable bowel syndrome
- Mitral valve prolapse
- Multiple sclerosis
- Parkinson disease
- Perimenopause
- Pheochromocytoma
- Premenstrual dysphoric disorder
- Premenstrual syndrome
- Seizure disorder or epilepsy
- Systemic lupus erythematosus
- Traumatic brain injury

Table 19-6 Clinical Assessment and Differential Diagnosis of Drug-Induced Anxiety[4,88]

Diagnostic interview

1. Record emotional, cognitive and physical symptoms of anxiety.
2. Rate each symptom as mild, moderate or severe using standardized anxiety rating scales (e.g., HAM-A, GAD-7)
3. Document functional impairment from anxiety
4. Conduct medication and substance abuse history

Key questions

"Yes" responses increase likelihood of drug-induced anxiety

1. Does individual have current psychiatric illness?
2. Does individual have a chronic medical illness?
3. Is situational anxiety considered unlikely?
4. Did the onset of anxiety happen within 1 week of the initiation of a substance or an ↑ or ↓ in dose of a substance?

Physical assessment

1. Physical examination
2. Record vital signs
3. Obtain toxicology screen
4. Obtain appropriate laboratory and diagnostic tests (e.g., TFTs if hyperthyroidism, ECG if cardiac symptoms reported)

ECG = electrocardiogram, HAM-A = Hamilton Anxiety Rating Scale, GAD-7 = generalized anxiety disorder 7-item scale, TFT = thyroid-function test.

Table 19-7 Risk Factors for Drug-Induced Anxiety[1-4,13,14,24,37,88,93,108,109]

- Primary anxiety disorder(s)
- Presence of any chronic psychiatric illness (e.g., bipolar disorder, major depression, schizoaffective disorder, schizophrenia)
- Presence of chronic medical condition(s)
- Use of more than one drug(s)/substance(s) known to provoke anxiety
- Currently withdrawing from sedative–hypnotic medication
- Currently withdrawing from alcohol or another substance of abuse
- Elevated plasma concentrations of potentially anxiety-provoking agents
- *ADORA2A2* gene polymorphisms in panic disorder, caffeine and amphetamine users

it from a primary anxiety disorder.[4,97] Laboratory or other diagnostic tests are useful to determine whether there is an underlying medical cause or associated medical problem such as hyperthyroidism or mitral-valve prolapse and to identify substances potentially involved via urine toxicology tests.

RISK FACTORS

Risk factors for drug-induced anxiety are listed in **Table 19-7**.[1-4,13,14,24,39,96,97] Clinical studies show that individuals with an existing anxiety disorder or elevated levels of anxiety, particularly panic disorder (PD) or post-traumatic stress disorder (PTSD), are especially sensitive to worsening panic attacks, hypervigilance, and exacerbated anxiety when taking even low doses of drugs known to cause anxiety.[23,38,43,99,100] For example, a controlled trial of the anxiogenic effects of the dopaminergic agonist bromocriptine and the dopaminergic antagonist sulpiride found that stimulation of dopaminergic function may cause anxiety in high-anxiety individuals at baseline and may exert anxiolytic effects in low-anxiety and otherwise healthy individuals.[21] Furthermore, individuals with primary anxiety disorders including social anxiety disorder (SAD), generalized anxiety disorder (GAD), and obsessive–compulsive disorder (OCD) are more susceptible to worsening anxiety associated with well-known anxiogenic substances such as caffeine or stimulants. Patients with a history of PD are more likely to experience panic attacks after use of glucocorticoids, especially in younger adults between the ages of 18 and 30 years.[71] Other psychiatric illnesses, including schizophrenia, schizoaffective disorder, bipolar disorder, and ADHD are associated with higher rates of anxiety and anxiety disorders compared with the nonaffected population. For this reason, drug-induced anxiety is also more common in these patients.[1,2,4] Parkinson disease can be considered a risk factor given the high rates of anxiety in this population and particularly during the off-period where anxiety is significantly more severe.[96]

Multiple genes encoding for proteins or enzymes have been identified that confer risk of developing an anxiety disorder.[99] For example, in PD, polymorphisms in genes encoding monoamine oxidase-A (MAO-A) in females, cholecystokinin receptors, several serotonin receptor subtypes (e.g., 5-HT_{1A}), and tryptophan hydroxylase 2 are possible risk factors.[100-103] Serotonin gene polymorphisms (5-HTTLPR), particularly the SS genotype, are probable risk factors for developing PTSD in non-hispanic black veterans and following exposure to combat or genocide trauma.[104-105] The SS genotype may also confer risk of developing social anxiety symptoms.[106]

Despite the growing evidence of candidate genes involved in the psychopathogenesis of anxiety disorders, PTSD, and OCD, the influence of genetic polymorphisms and their phenotypes on exacerbation or development of anxiety symptoms upon exposure to anxiogenic drugs is not well defined. Single nucleotide polymorphisms, rs5751876 (1976 C/T) and rs35320474 (2952 C/Tins), within the ADORA2A genotype may confer risk of anxiety in light caffeine users (<300 mg of caffeine per week).[107] The genetic polymorphism 1976T/T-2592 Tins/Tins may also be a factor that contributes to the heightened anxiety observed after 10–20 mg of amphetamine administration in individuals who are light smokers (<10 cigarettes per week) and moderate caffeine consumers (1–2 cups per day).[107-109] The A2A polymorphism may also be a shared genetic trait in individuals with PD, which could explain the increased sensitivity to caffeine in this population.[18,107]

Risk and intensity of anxiety during nicotine withdrawal is a function of the amount of daily nicotine use and individual sensitivity to withdrawal discomfort. However, nicotine-dependent individuals with a comorbid primary anxiety or mood or substance use disorders are more likely to experience a greater number of withdrawal symptoms and have higher risk of relapse upon cessation attempts.[110,111] Thus, nicotine withdrawal anxiety can occur after abrupt cessation of cigarette smoking but also after abrupt discontinuation of nicotine replacement therapies such as gum, inhalers, lozenges, or, less often, nicotine patches.[33] Combining smoking cessation products to increase chances of sustained abstinence, such as with varenicline and bupropion, also increases the risk of secondary anxiety compared to that associated with varenicline monotherapy.[112]

Individuals who misuse or abuse stimulants or those with narcolepsy taking high doses are the most likely to experience intolerable anxiety symptoms.[5-7] Modafinil and its R-enantiomer, armodafinil, are nonstimulant compounds that are anxiogenic. Although higher doses (e.g., modafinil doses >400 mg) pose a greater risk, individual sensitivity should be considered as anxiogenic effects can occur with lower doses.[32,50] Modafinil 200 mg and armodafinil 150 mg appear to cause anxiety symptoms at comparable rates when used for shift-work sleep disorder.[50] In addition, severe anxiety, restlessness, and palpitations with armodafinil doses of 150 mg or more have required discontinuation in clinical trials when used for a variety of sleep disorders, schizophrenia, and bipolar depression.[51-53]

Drug-induced anxiety is more pronounced at higher drug doses. For example, it is uncommon for patients to experience anxiety associated with pseudoephedrine at doses as low as 30 mg. However, the 120-mg sustained-release dose is associated with a greater risk of anxiety.[35] Anxiety associated with ephedrine, bitter orange (*Cypraea aurantium*, synephrine), caffeine, guarana, yohimbine, and steroids is also dose-related.[7,13,22,33,38,71] In addition, drug-induced anxiety is more likely in patients with impaired hepatic or renal function who are taking potentially causative agents for which the liver or kidney, respectively, contribute substantially to drug clearance.

MORBIDITY AND MORTALITY

There is no direct connection between drug-induced anxiety and increased mortality. However, there is increasing evidence linking anxiety to negative health consequences including heart disease, impaired disease recovery, and increased propensity for poor health habits such as cigarette smoking and abuse of alcohol and other substances.[2,3,113-116] Anxiety disorders may cause altered hypothalamic-pituitary axis responses secondary to imbalances of cortisol and anti-inflammatory and proinflammatory cytokines.[117] For example, tumor necrosis factor-α has been found in higher concentrations in individuals with GAD and PTSD.[117] Imbalances of cortisol have also been associated with PTSD, GAD, and OCD. However, it is unclear if cortisol imbalances contribute to PD, SAD, or to drug-induced anxiety. The impact of these associations on morbidity remain to be elucidated. Although elevatations in pro-inflammatory cytokines are recognized as risk factors for cardiovascular morbidity, the impact of drug-induced anxiety on risk of cardiovascular morbidity or death is unknown.

PREVENTION

Approaches to prevention of drug-induced anxiety are listed in **Table 19-8.** Preventing drug-induced anxiety starts with patient assessment to determine whether risk factors are present. If one or more risk factors exist, the clinician should carefully weigh the risk versus the benefits of initiating therapy with a drug known to cause anxiety. Alternative treatments with a lower risk for inducing anxiety should be considered. If the drug in question represents the most appropriate treatment option, initiation of therapy should be gradual, with careful dose titration and monitoring to detect the emergence of anxiety and determine the need for treatment with psychotherapeutic or pharmacologic interventions. If discontinuation of antidepressant therapy is necessary, the dose should be reduced gradually over 2–6 weeks to prevent serotonin withdrawal syndrome (symptoms include worsening anxiety or insomnia).[4,37] If discontinuation of therapy with agents known to cause anxiety upon drug withdrawal is necessary (e.g., benzodiazepine, barbituates), tapering the dose gradually over weeks to months can minimize the risk of anxiety.[4,13] Doses of drugs known to cause anxiety that predominantly undergo renal or hepatic clearance should be reduced appropriately in patients with kidney or liver disease, respectively.

Table 19-8 Approaches to Help Prevent Drug-Induced Anxiety[1-4]

- Assess patient for an underlying anxiety disorder or history of drug-induced anxiety to determine the risk of drug-induced anxiety
- Counsel patient regarding the risk of anxiety when initiating or discontinuing therapy with a potentially causative drug
- Initiate therapy with potentially anxiety-provoking medications slowly, with gradual dose titration. For example, initial doses of selective serotonin reuptake inhibitors can be reduced by half
- Minimize use of multiple medications with a risk for inducing anxiety

MANAGEMENT

Management of drug-induced anxiety is largely supportive and typically involves lowering doses or discontinuation of the causative agent. For example, anxiety symptoms associated with steroid supplementation or hormone replacement typically resolve within 2–4 weeks of cessation of therapy.[24,72] Supportive treatment may include reassurance, instruction on relaxation techniques, and avoidance of other substances known to cause anxiety. Antidepressant-induced anxiety is usually transient during initiation or abrupt discontinuation of therapy. Slower dose titration during initiation of therapy and gradual dose tapering during discontinuation can minimize or alleviate anxiety symptoms and is critical in patients with a history of antidepressant-induced anxiety. Effective management of antipsychotic-induced anxiety involves a dose reduction, substituting therapy with an antipsychotic agent with lower dopaminergic antagonist activity and more histamine antagonism, or treating the anxiety with a β-adrenergic blocker or benzodiazepine when the former is not appropriate.[10,11]

In cases in which therapy with the anxiety-provoking agent cannot be discontinued (e.g., in patients who are undergoing cancer chemotherapy), temporary management with a benzodiazepine can be considered. Lorazepam 0.5–1 mg administered two or three times daily offers the advantage of rapid onset (30–45 minutes), intermediate duration of effect (~6–8 hours), and no active metabolites that can accumulate. Clonazepam 0.25–0.5 mg administered once or twice daily can be considered if less frequent administration is desired, but the onset of effect may be longer (1–2 hours) and the drug can accumulate over time because of a long half-life of 20–50 hours. The duration of supportive therapy varies based on the necessary duration of treatment with the causative agent.[4] Withdrawing therapy slowly and over a longer period of time (over months instead of weeks) may attenuate anxiety related to abrupt benzodiazepine discontinuation. Alternatively, therapy with an agent that increases GABA activity, such as valproic acid, can be initiated to diminish withdrawal symptoms and associated anxiety.[13]

Caffeine-induced anxiety and withdrawal symptoms abate with time (typically 3–7 days) and may be managed with mild analgesics to treat headache symptoms.[6,17,22] There is evidence that exercise attenuates caffeine-induced state anxiety in nonsmoking males.[118] Nicotine supplementation with gradual tapering can lessen anxiety associated with nicotine withdrawal.[23]

The management of anxiety induced by thyroid supplementation includes reducing the dose or discontinuing the thyroid supplement and providing patient counseling and reassurance as necessary.[74] A clinician with expertise in hormone regulation should be consulted when patients present with anxiety related to hormonal imbalance. Management strategies include hormonal supplementation or discontinuation, treatment with antianxiety medication (e.g., SSRIs), or both.

INFORMATION FOR PATIENTS

Individuals prescribed medications known to cause anxiety during treatment or withdrawal and those who elect to take nonprescription drugs known to cause anxiety should be warned of the risks. Patient education regarding the risk of withdrawal symptoms after discontinuation of a CNS-active agent is essential. Individualized discontinuation regimens should be developed based on patient tolerance. For example, decreasing the dose of a benzodiazepine by 25% per week is well tolerated by some patients, but others may require more gradual tapering over weeks or even months.[4,13] Patients who have difficulty withdrawing from benzodiazepine therapy because of excessive anxiety should be offered the option of therapy with anticonvulsant drugs, as these agents have been used effectively to prevent anxiety and other benzodiazepine withdrawal symptoms such as insomnia and tremulousness.[13,14]

When drug-induced anxiety occurs, the caregiver should reassure the patient that drug-induced anxiety is usually of short duration (days to weeks) and will improve after a dose decrease or discontinuation of the causative agent along with supportive treatment. Patients at risk for anxiety should be counseled regarding the type of anxiety symptoms that may occur in association with the drug (e.g., panic attacks, jitteriness, fearful thoughts), the typical time of onset of symptoms, and available interventions should anxiety occur.

REFERENCES

1. American Psychiatric Association. *Diagnostic and statistical manual of mental disorders.* 5th ed. Arlington, VA: American Psychiatric Association; 2013.
2. Kessler RC, Chiu WT, Demler O et al. Prevalence, severity and comorbidity of *DSM-IV* disorders in the National Comorbidity Survey Replication. *Arch Gen Psychiatry.* 2005; 62:617-27.
3. Goodwin RD, Stayner DA, Chinman MJ et al. The relationship between anxiety and substance use disorders among individuals with severe affective disorders. *Compr Psychiatry.* 2002; 43:245-52.
4. Guthrie SK, Bostwick JR. Anxiety disorders. In: Alldredge BK, Corelli RL, Ernst ME et al, eds. *Koda-Kimble & Young's applied therapeutics: the clinical use of drugs.* 10th ed. Philadelphia: Lippincott Williams and Wilkins; 2013.
5. O'Malley MB, Gleeson SK, Weir ID. Wake-promoting medications. In: Kryger MH, Roth T, Dement WC, eds. *Principles and practice of sleep medicine.* 5th ed. St. Louis, MO: WB Saunders; 2011.
6. Roehrs T, Roth T. Medication and substance abuse. In: Kryger MH, Roth T, Dement WC, eds. *Principles and practice of sleep medicine.* 5th ed. St. Louis: WB Saunders; 2011.
7. Drugs that cause psychiatric symptoms. *Med Lett Drugs Ther.* 2008; 50:1301-2.
8. Mitler MM, Hayduk R. Benefits and risks of pharmacotherapy for narcolepsy. *Drug Saf.* 2002; 25:791-809.
9. Piacentino D, Kotzalidis GD, Del Casale A et al. Anabolic-androgenic steroid use and psychopathology in athletes: a systematic review. *Curr Neuropharmacol.* 2015; 13:101-21.
10. Bratti IM, Kane JM, Marder SR. Chronic restlessness with antipsychotics. *Am J Psychiatry.* 2007; 164:1648-54.
11. Geodon package insert. New York: Pfizer Incorporated; August 2015.
12. Lea JW, Stoner SC, Lafollette J. Agitation associated with aripiprazole initiation. *Pharmacotherapy.* 2007; 27:1339-42.
13. Rickels K, DeMartinis N, Rynn M et al. Pharmacologic strategies for discontinuing benzodiazepine treatment. *J Clin Psychopharmacol.* 1999; 19(suppl 2):12-6.
14. Salzman C. Benzodiazepine dependency: summary of the APA task force on benzodiazepines. *Psychopharmacol Bull.* 1990; 26:61.
15. Keller S, Frishman WH, Epstein J. Neuropsychiatric manifestations of cardiovascular therapy. *Heart Dis.* 1999; 1:241-54.
16. Davies S, Jackson PR, Ramsey LE et al. Drug intolerance due to nonspecific adverse effects related to psychiatric morbidity in hypertensive patients. *Arch Intern Med.* 2003; 163:592-600.
17. Lara DR. Caffeine, mental health, and psychiatric disorders. *J Alzheimers Dis.* 2010; 20:S239-248.
18. Vilarim MM, Araujo DMR, Nardi AE. Caffeine challenge test and panic disorder: a systematic literature review. *Expert Rev Neurother.* 2011; 11:1185-95.

19. Lee D, Schroeder JR, Karschner EL et al. Cannabis withdrawal in chronic, frequent cannabis smokers during sustained abstinence within a closed residential environment. *Am J Addict.* 2014; 23:234-42.
20. Brunton LL, Chabner BA, Knollmann BC. *Goodman & Gilman's: the pharmacological basis of therapeutics.*12th ed. McGraw-Hill; 2011.
21. Mizuki Y, Suetsugi M, Ushijima I et al. Differential effects of dopaminergic drugs on anxiety and arousal in healthy volunteers with high and low anxiety. *Prog Neuropsychopharmacol Biol Psychiatry.* 1997; 21:573-90.
22. Haller CA, Jacob P, Benowitz NL. Pharmacology of ephedra and caffeine after single-dose dietary supplement use. *Clin Pharmacol Ther.* 2002; 71:421-32.
23. Stahl SM. *Essential psychopharmacology.* 4th ed. Cambridge University Press: New York; 2013.
24. Seeman MV. Psychopathology in women and men: focus on female hormones. *Am J Psychiatry.* 1997; 154:164-1647.
25. Sivin J. Risks, benefits, advantages and disadvantages of levonorgestrel-releasing contraceptive implants. *Drug Saf.* 2003; 26:303-35.
26. Kahn JB. Latest industry information on the safety profile of levofloxacin in the US. *Chemotherapy.* 2001; 47(suppl 3):32-37, 44-48.
27. Norton JW. Gabapentin withdrawal syndrome. *Clin Neuropharmacol.* 2001; 24:245-6.
28. DiBlasio CJ, Hammett J, Malcolm JB et al. Prevalence and predictive factors for the development of de novo psychiatric illness in patients receiving androgen deprivation therapy for prostate cancer. *Can J Urol.* 2008; 15:4249-56.
29. van Riemsdijk MM, van der Klauw MM, van Heest JA et al. Neuropsychiatric effects of antimalarials. *Eur J Clin Pharmacol.* 1997; 52:1-6.
30. Clattenburg RN, Donnelly CL. Case study: neuropsychiatric symptoms associated with the antimalarial agent mefloquine. *J Am Acad Child Adolesc Psychiatry.* 1997; 36:1606-8.
31. Gurkan K, Bilgic A, Turkoglu S et al. Depression, anxiety and obsessive-compulsive symptoms and quality of life in children with attention-deficit hyperactivity disorder (ADHD) during three-month methylphenidate treatment. *J Psychopharmacol.* 2010; 24:1810-18.
32. Wong YN, Simcoe D, Hartman LN et al. A double-blind, placebo-controlled, ascending-dose evaluation of the pharmacokinetics and tolerability of modafinil tablets in healthy male volunteers. *J Clin Pharmacol.* 1999; 39:30-40.
33. Haustein KO, Haffner S, Woodcock BG. A review of the pharmacological and psychopharmacological aspects of smoking and smoking cessation in psychiatric patients. *Int J Clin Pharmacol Ther.* 2002; 40:404-18.
34. Onder G, Pellicciotti F, Gambassi G et al. NSAID-related psychiatric adverse events: who is at risk? *Drugs.* 2004; 64:2619-27.
35. Wellington K, Jarvis B. Cetirizine/pseudoephedrine. *Drugs.* 2001; 61:2231-40.
36. Goethe JW, Wooley SB, Cardoni AA et al. Selective serotonin reuptake inhibitor discontinuation: side effects and other factors that influence medication adherence: *J Clin Psychopharmacology.* 2007; 27:451-8.
37. Fava GA, Gatti A, Belaise C et al. Withdrawal symptoms after selective serotonin reuptake inhibitor discontinuation: a systematic review. *Psychother Psychosom.* 2015; 84:72-81.
38. Nykamp DL, Fackih MN, Compton AL. Possible association of acute lateral-wall myocardial infarction and bitter orange supplement. *Ann Pharmacother.* 2004; 38:812-6.
39. Cooper MA, Ritchie EC. Testosterone replacement therapy for anxiety. *Am J Psychiatry.* 2000; 157:1884.
40. Okun MS, McDonald WM, DeLong MR. Refractory nonmotor symptoms in male patients with Parkinson Disease due to testosterone deficiency: a common unrecognized comorbidity. *Arch Neurol.* 2002; 59:807-11.
41. Bender B, Milgrom H. Theophylline-induced behavior change in children: an objective evaluation of parents' perceptions. *JAMA.* 1992; 267:2621-4.
42. Plushner SL. Valerian: valeriana officinalis. *Am J Health-Syst Pharm.* 2000; 57:328-35.
43. Garges HP, Varia I, Doraiswamy PM. Cardiac complications and delirium associated with valerian root withdrawal. *JAMA.* 1998; 280:1566-7.
44. Tsai ST, Cho HJ, Cheng HS et al. A randomized controlled trial of varenicline, a selective α_4, β_2 nicotinic acetylcholine receptor partial agonist, as a new therapy for smoking cessation in Asian smokers. *Clin Ther.* 2007; 29:1027-39.
45. US Food and Drug Administration. Varenicline Public Health Advisory. https://www.fda.gov/Drugs/DrugSafety/PostmarketDrugSafetyInformationforPatientsandProviders/ucm051136.htm (accessed 2017 Dec 20).
46. Nystedt M, Berglund G, Bolund C et al. Side effects of adjuvant endocrine treatment in premenopausal breast cancer patients: a prospective randomized study. *J Clin Oncol.* 2003; 21:1836-44.
47. Beisecker A, Cook MR, Ashworth J et al. Side effects of adjuvant chemotherapy: perceptions of node-negative breast cancer patients. *Psychooncology.* 1997; 6:85-93.
48. Stine SM, Southwick SM, Petrakis IL et al. Yohimbine-Induced Withdrawal and Anxiety Symptoms in Opioid-Dependent Patients. *Biol Psychiatry.* 2002; 51:642-51.
49. Choi SH, Shapiro H, Robinson GF et al. Psychological side-effects of clomiphene citrate and human menopausal gonadotrophin. *J Psychosom Obstet Gynaecol.* 2005; 26:93-100.
50. Tembe DV, Dhavele A, Desai H et al. Armodafinil versus modafinil in patients with excessive sleepiness associated with shift work sleep disorder: a randomized double blind multicentric clinical trial. *Neurol Res Int.* 2011; 2:1.
51. Black JE, Hull SG, Tiller J et al. The long-term tolerability and efficacy of armodafinil in patients with excessive sleepiness associated with treated obstructive sleep apnea, shift work disorder, or narcolepsy: an open-label extension study. *J Clin Sleep Med.* 2010; 6:458-66.
52. Calabrese JR, Frye MA, Yang R et al. Efficacy and safety of adjunctive armodafinil in adults with major depressive episodes associated with bipolar I disorder: A randomized, double blind placebo-controlled multicenter trial. *J Clin Psychiatry.* 2014; 75:1054-61.
53. Kane JM, D'Souza DC, Patkar AA et al. Armodafinil ascar adjunctive therapy in adults with cognitive deficits associated with schizophrenia: a 4-week, double-blind, placebo-controlled study. *J Clin Psychiatry.* 2010; 71:1475-81.
54. Amato L, Davoli M, Minozzi S et al. Methadone at tapered doses for the management opioid withdrawal. *Cochrane Database Syst Rev.* 2013; 2:CD003409.
55. Grosshans M, Mutschler J, Hermann D et al. Pregabalin abuse, dependence, and withdrawal: a case report. *Am J Psychiatry.* 2010; 167:869-86.
56. Torres A, Whitney J, Rao S et al. Tolerability of atomoxetine for treatment of pediatric attention-deficit/hyperactivity disorder in the context of epilepsy. *Epilepsy Behav.* 2011; 20:95-102.
57. Aman MG, Smith T, Arnold LE et al. A review of atomoxetine effects in young people with developmental disabilities. *Res Dev Disabil.* 2014; 35:1412-24.
58. Rizos A, Martinez-Martin P, Odin P et al. Characterizing motor and non-motor aspects of early-morning off periods in Parkinson's disease: an international multicenter study. *Parkinsonism Relat Disord.* 2014; 20:1231-5.
59. Witjas T, Kaphan E, Azulay JP et al. Nonmotor fluctuations in Parkinson's disease: frequent and disabling. *Neurology.* 2002; 59:408-13.
60. Abers MS, Shandera WX, Kass JS. Neurological and psychiatric adverse effects of antiretroviral drugs. *CNS Drugs.* 2014; 28:131-45.

61. Ford N, Shubber Z, Pozniak A et al. Comparative safety and neuropsychiatric adverse events associated with efavirenz use in first-line antiretroviral therapy: a systematic review and meta-analysis of randomized trials. *J Acquir Immune Defic Syndr.* 2015; 69:422-9.
62. Soler Palacin P, Aramburo A, Moraga FA. Neuropsychiatric reaction induced by abacavir in a pediatric human immunodeficiency virus-infected patient. *Pediatr Infect Dis J.* 2006; 25:382.
63. Reeves RR, Burke RS. Carisoprodol: abuse potential and withdrawal syndrome. *Drug Alcohol Depend.* 2012; 123(1-3):29-34.
64. Horikawa YT, Udaka TY, Crow JK et al. Anxiety associated with asthma exacerbations and overuse of medication: the role of cultural competency. *J Dev Behav Pediatr.* 2014; 35:154-7.
65. Calapai G, Casciaro M, Miroddi et al. Montelukast-induced adverse drug reactions: a review of case reports in the literature. *Pharmacology.* 2014; 94:60-70.
66. Lainez MJ, Freitag FG, Ascher S et al. Time coure of adverse events most commonly associated with topiramate for migraine prevention. *Eur J Neurol.* 2007; 14:900-6.
67. Goldberg JF. Panic attacks associated with the use of topiramate. *J Clin Psychopharmacol.* 2001; 21:461-2.
68. Damsa C, Warczyk S, Cailhol L et al. Panic attacks associated with topiramate. *J Clin Psychiatry.* 2006; 67:326-7.
69. Christensen RC, Garces LK. New-onset panic attacks associated with topiramate. *Psychiatry (Edgemont).* 2006; 3:10-18.
70. Molero Y, Lichtenstein P, Zetterqvist J. Varenicline and risk of psychiatric conditions, suicidal behaviour, criminal offending, and transport accidents and offences: population based cohort study. *BMJ.* 2015; 350:h2388.
71. Fardet L, Petersen I, Nazareth I. Suicidal behavior and severe neuropsychiatric disorders following glucocorticoid therapy in primary care. *Am J Psychiatry.* 2012; 169:491-7.
72. Kunte H, Harms L, Plag J et al. Acute onset of panic attacks after transdermal estrogen replacement. *Gen Hosp Psychiatry.* 2014; 36:e7.
73. Ip EJ, Lu DH, Barrnett MJ et al. Psychological and physical impact of anabolic-androgenic steroid dependence. *Pharmacotherapy.* 2012; 32:910-9.
74. Kong WM, Sheikh MH, Lumb PJ et al. A 6-month randomized trial of thyroxine treatment in women with mild subclinical hypothyroidism. *Am J Med.* 2002; 112:348-54.
75. Natural Medicines. Therapeutic Research Center (2016). https://naturalmedicines-therapeuticsresearch.com (accessed 2018 Jan 30).
76. Rexulti package insert. Rockville, MD: Otsuka America Pharmaceutical; July 2015.
77. Vraylar package insert. Parisppany, NJ: Actavis Pharma; September 2015.
78. Lovick TA. Estrous cycle and stress: influence of progesterone on the female brain. *Braz J Med Biol Res.* 2012; 45:314-20.
79. Tuccori M, Montagnani S, Mantarro S. Neuropsychiatric adverse events associated with statins. *CNS Drugs.* 2014; 28:249-72.
80. Isentress package insert. Whitehouse Station, NJ: Merck and Co; February 2015.
81. Davis S. Testosterone deficiency in women. *J Reprod Med.* 2001; 46(3 suppl):291-6.
82. Gabriel A. The mixed amphetamine salt extended release (Adderal XR, Max-XR) as an adjunctive to SSRIS or SNRIS in the treatment of adult ADHD patients with comorbid partially responsive generalized anxiety: an open-label study. *Atten Defic Hyperact Disord.* 2010; 2:87-92.
83. Thomas K, Martin RM, Knipe DW et al. Risk of neuropsychiatric adverse events associated with varenicline: systematic review and meta-analysis. *BMJ.* 2015; 350:h1109.
84. Siegel AM, Mathews SB. Diagnosis and treatment of anxiety in the aging woman. *Curr Psychiatry Rep.* 2015; 17:93.
85. Rapkin AJ, Mikacich JA, Moatakef-Imani B et al. The clinical nature and formal diagnosis of premenstrual, postpartum, and perimenopausal affective disorders. *Curr Psychiatry Rep.* 2002; 4:419-28.
86. McHenry J, Carrier N, Hull E et al. Sex difference in anxiety and depression: Role of testosterone. *Front Neuroendocrinol.* 2014; 35:42-57.
87. Strohle A, Romeo E, di Michele F et al. Induced panic attacks shift gamma-aminobutyric acid type A receptor modulatory neuroactive steroid composition in patients with panic disorder: preliminary results. *Arch Gen Psych.* 2003; 60:161-8.
88. Wells KB, Golding JM, Burnam MA. Chronic medical conditions in a sample of the general population with anxiety, affective, and substance use disorders. *Am J Psychiatry.* 1989; 146:1440-6.
89. Sternbach H, State R. Antibiotics: neuropsychiatric effects and psychotropic interactions. *Harv Rev Psychiatry.* 1997; 5:214-26.
90. Tran TM, Browning J, Dell ML. Psychosis and paranoid delusions after a therapeutic dose of mefloquine: a case report. *Malar J.* 2006; 5-74:1-5.
91. Perona A, Garcia-Saiz M, Alvarez S. Psychiatric disorders and montelukast in children: a disproportionality analysis of the VigiBase. *Drug Saf.* 2016; 39:69-78.
92. Ibarra-Barrueta O, Palacio-Zabalza I, Mora-Attorasagasti O et al. Effect of concomitant use of montelukast and efavirenz on neuropsychiatric adverse events. *Ann Pharmacother.* 2014; 48:145-8.
93. Sullivan GM, Coplan JD, Kent JM et al. The noradrenergic system in pathological anxiety: a focus on panic with relevance to generalized anxiety and phobias. *Biol Psychiatry.* 2000; 46:1205.
94. Kosten TR, George TP. The neurobiology of opioid dependence: implications for treatment. *Sci Pract Perspect.* 2002; 1:13-20.
95. Storch A, Schneider CB, Wolz M et al. Nonmotor fluctuations in parkinson disease: severity and correlation with motor complications. *Neurology.* 2013; 80:800-9.
96. Walsh K, Bennett G. Parkinson's disease and anxiety. *Postgrad Med.* 2001; 77:89-93.
97. Möller HJ. Antipsychotic and antidepressant effects of second generation antipsychotics: two different pharmacological mechanisms? *Eur Arch Psychiatry Clin Neurosci.* 2005; 255:190-201.
98. Marques L, Chosak A, Simon NM et al. Rating scales for anxiety disorders. In: Baer L, Blais MA, ed. *Handbook of clinical rating scales and assessment in psychiatry and mental health.* New York: Humana Press; 2010:37-72.
99. Domschke K, Maron E. Genetic factors in anxiety disorders. In: Baldwin DS, Leonard BE, eds. *Anxiety disorders mod trends pharmacopsychiatry.* Basel, Switzerland: S. Karger; 2013:24-46.
100. Reif A, Domschke K, Klauke B et al. Meta-analysis argues for a female specific role of MAOA-uVNTR in panic disorder in four European populations. *Am J Med Genet B Neuropsychiatr Genet.* 2012; 159B:786-93.
101. Maron E, Toru I, Tasa G et al. Association testing of panic disorder candidate genes using CCK-4 challenge in healthy volunteers. *Neurosci Lett.* 2008; 446:88-92.
102. Wilson J, Markle D, Fitches A. Cholecystokinin system genes: associations with panic and other psychiatric disorders. *J Affect Disord.* 2012; 136:902-8.
103. Blaya C, Salum GA, Moorjani P et al. Panic disorder and serotonergic genes (SLC6A4, HTR1A and HTR2A): Association and interaction with childhood trauma and parenting. *Neurosci Lett.* 2010; 485:11-15.
104. Liu Y, Garrett ME, Dennis MF et al. An examination of the association between 5-HTTLPR, combat exposure, and PTSD diagnosis among US veterans. *PLoS One.* 2015; 10:e0119998.
105. Gressier F, Calati R, Balestri M et al. The 5-HTTLPR polymorphism and posttraumatic stress disorder: a meta-analysis. *J Trauma Stress.* 2013; 26:645-53.
106. Miu AC, Vulturar R, Chis A et al. Reappraisal as a mediator in the link between 5-HTTLPR and social anxiety symptoms. *Emotion.* 2013; 13:1012-22.
107. Yang A, Palmer AA, de Wit H. Genetics of caffeine consumption and responses to caffeine. *Psychopharmacology.* 2010; 211:245-57.
108. Alsene K, Deckert J, Sand P, de Wit H. Association between A2a receptor gene polymorphisms and caffeine-induced anxiety. *Neuropsychopharmacology.* 2003; 28:1694-702.

109. Hohoff C, McDonald JM, Baune BT et al. Inter-individual variation in anxiety response to amphetamine: possible role for adenosine A2A receptor gene variants. *Am J Med Genet B Neruopsychiatr Genet.* 2005; 139B:42-4.

110. Weinberger A, Desai RA, McKee SA. Nicotine withdrawal in US smokers with current mood, anxiety, alcohol use and substance use disorders. *Drug Alcohol Depend.* 2010;108:7-12.

111. Piper ME, Cook JW, Schlam TR et al. Anxiety diagnoses in smokers seeking cessation treatment: relations with tobacco dependence, withdrawal, outcome and response to treatment. *Addiction.* 2010; 106:418-27.

112. Ebbert J, Hatsukami DK, Croghan IT et al. Combination varenicline and bupropion SR for tobacco-dependence treatment in cigarette smokers: a randomized trial. *JAMA.* 2014; 311:155-63.

113. Anisman H, Merali Z. Cytokines, stress and depressive illness: brain-immune interactions. *Ann Med.* 2003; 35:2-11.

114. Kiecolt-Glaser JK, McGuire L, Robles TF et al. Emotions, morbidity and mortality: new perspectives from psychoneuroimmunology. *Ann Rev Psychol.* 2002; 53:83-107.

115. Huffman JF, Smith FA, Blais MA et al. Anxiety, independent of depressive symptoms, is associated with in-hospital cardiac complications after acute myocardial infarction. *J Psychosom Res.* 2008; 65:557-63.

116. Moser DK, McKinley S, Riegel B et al. Relationship of persistent symptoms of anxiety to morbidity and mortality outcomes in patients with coronary heart disease. *Psychosom Med.* 2011; 73:803-9.

117. Furtado M, Katzman MA. Neuroinflammatory pathways in anxiety, posttraumatic stress, and obsessive compulsive disorders. *Psychiatry Res.* 2015; 229:37-48.

118. Motl RW, Dishman RK. Effects of acute exercise on the soleus H-reflex and self-reported anxiety after caffeine ingestion. *Physiol Behav.* 2004; 80:577-85.

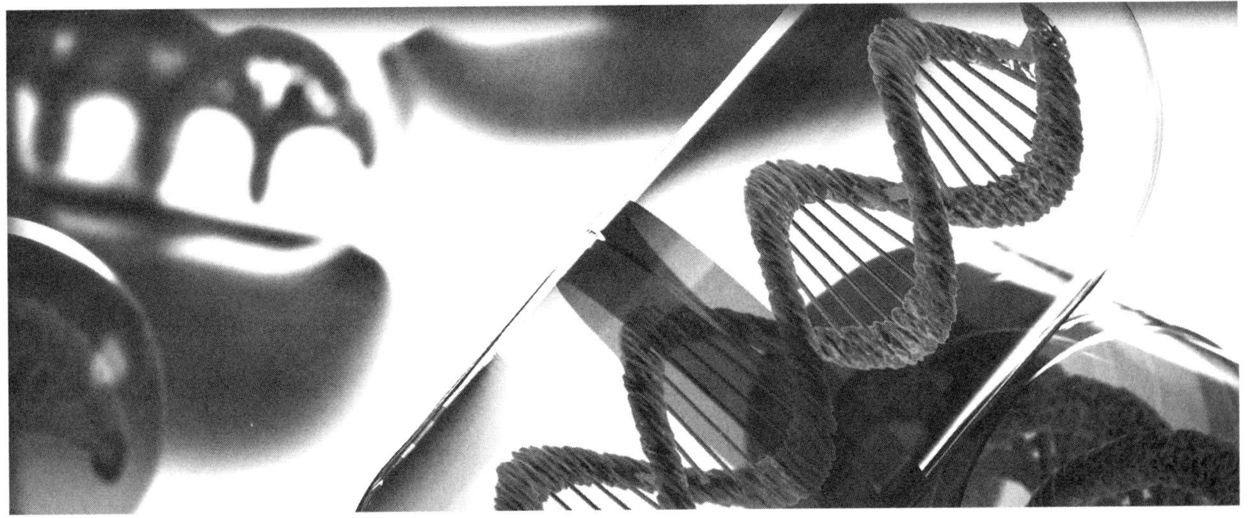

CHAPTER 20

Psychosis

Jessica L. Gören

The term *psychosis* was first introduced in the 19th century to describe the manner in which mental illness, manifested as aberrant behavior, related to both psychological and physical well-being. Psychosis is currently defined as an impairment of reality testing due to gross distortion or disorganization of reality.[1-5] Patients with psychosis experience gross inaccuracy of perception, even with evidence to the contrary. Visual, auditory, tactile, and olfactory hallucinations, delusions or fixed false beliefs, and illusions (distortion in perception) often characterize the impaired reality testing associated with psychosis. The associated physical symptoms can include agitation, anxiety, aggression, pacing, unusual behaviors such as talking to someone not visible to others, and withdrawal from society. Although psychosis is a relatively common medical disorder, it is not a specific diagnosis but rather a feature of many disease states.[1-8]

CAUSATIVE AGENTS

Many medications are associated with drug-induced psychosis (**Table 20-1**) and withdrawal psychosis (**Table 20-2**).[9-124] Agents more commonly implicated include amphetamines, anticholinergics, corticosteroids, anabolic steroids, dopaminergic agents, ma huang (ephedrine), and tacrolimus.[2,3,5-8] The pharmacological diversity of these drugs clearly indicates that no single mechanism of action can be fully responsible for drug-induced psychosis. In fact, the mechanisms seem to be as complex and poorly understood as those associated with idiopathic psychosis.

The causes of drug-induced psychosis extend beyond U.S. Food and Drug Administration (FDA)-approved medications to include herbal and nutritional supplements used by many. Several illicit drugs such as lysergic acid diethylamide (LSD), psilocybin, and phencyclidine (PCP) induce psychotic states similar in presentation to psychosis induced by legal medications.[42,125-127] Increasingly, newer synthetic drugs of abuse such as synthetic cathinones (e.g., bath salts) and synthetic cannabinoids (e.g., K2, spice) have been associated with psychosis.[128,129] For all of these agents, drug-induced psychosis may occur at normal doses, excessive doses (intoxication) or, occasionally, as a component of a withdrawal phenomenon. Chronic exposure can also lead to drug-induced psychosis, particularly with synthetic cathinones and cannabinoids.[128,129]

Table 20-1 Agents Implicated in Drug-Induced Psychosis

Drug	Incidence	Level of Evidence[a]
Albuterol[9-11]	NK	C
Amantadine[12,13]	1–10%	C
Amphetamines[14-16]	0.25%[b]	A
Anabolic steroids[17]	12%	B
Angiotensin-converting enzyme inhibitors[18-20]	NK	C
Anticholinergics[21-29]	7%	A
Bupropion[30-32]	NK	C
Caffeine[33,34]	NK	C
Carbamazepine[35-37]	NK	C
Celecoxib[38]	NK	C
Chloroquine[39]	NK	C
Ciprofloxacin[40,41]	NK	C
Cocaine[42]	NK	C
Corticosteroids[43-47]	1%	B[d]
Cyclobenzaprine[48,49]	<1%	C
Cycloserine[50,51]	15%	B
Dapsone[52]	NK	C
Dextromethorphan[53,54]	NK	C
Digoxin[20,55]	NK	C
Diphenhydramine[26,29]	NK	C
Disulfuram[56,57]	NK	C[d]
Dopamine agonists[58-63]	>1%	C
Doxazosin[20]	NK	C
Dronabinol[64,65]	3–10%	C
Efavirenz[66]	1%	C
Ephedrine[67-69]	NK	C
Guanfacine[70,71]	NK	C
Ganciclovir[72]	<1%	C
Histamine$_2$ blockers[73-76]	NK	C
HMG CoA reductase inhibitors[77,78]	NK	C
Ifosfamide[79]	<12%	B
Indomethacin[80,81]	<1%	C
Isoniazide[50]	<1%	C
Lacosamide[82,83]	NK	C
Lidocaine[84]	NK	C
Ketamine[85]	12%	B
Levetiracetam[86,87]	1% adult 2% pediatric	A
Levodopa–carbidopa[58,88]	NK	A
Levothyroxine[89]	NK	C
Mefloquine[90,91]	NK	C
Meperidine[92,93]	NK	C
Methylphenidate[16,94]	0.25%[b]	A

Table 20-1 Agents Implicated in Drug-Induced Psychosis (continued)

Drug	Incidence	Level of Evidence[a]
Metoprolol[95,96]	NK	C
Modafinil[97]	NK	C
Monoamine oxidase inhibitors[98-100,c]	NK	C
Nitrous oxide[101,102]	NK	C
Pseudoephedrine[59,103,104]	NK	C
Quinidine[105,106]	<1%	C
Sibutramine[107-109]	NK	C
Tacrolimus[110,111]	<15%	C
Tiagabine[112]	0.8%	B
Trimethoprim–sulfamethoxazole[113,114]	NK	C
Vigabatrin[115,116]	NK	C
Zolpidem[117,118]	1–10%	C
Zonisamide[115,119]	2%	A

HMG CoA = 3-hydroxy-3-methylglutaryl-coenzyme A, NK = not known.
[a]Definitions for Levels of Evidence: Level A—evidence from one or more randomized, controlled clinical trials; Level B—evidence from nonrandomized clinical trials, prospective observational studies, cohort studies, retrospective studies, case-control studies, meta-analyses and/or postmarketing surveillance studies; and Level C—evidence from one or more published case reports or case series.
[b]Therapeutic doses of prescription amphetamines and methylphenidate.
[c]Varies by agent.
[d]Most commonly in association with mania.

Table 20-2 Drugs Implicated in Withdrawal Psychosis

Drug	Incidence	Level of Evidence[a]
Alcohol[120]	5%	B
Benzodiazepines[121,122]	NK	B
Opiates–opioids[123,124]	NK	C

NK = not known.
[a]Definitions for Levels of Evidence: Level A—evidence from one or more randomized, controlled clinical trials; Level B—evidence from nonrandomized clinical trials, prospective observational studies, cohort studies, retrospective studies, case-control studies, meta-analyses and/or postmarketing surveillance studies; and Level C—evidence from one or more published case reports or case series.

EPIDEMIOLOGY

In the 19th century, Jacques-Joseph Moreau de Tours was the first psychiatrist to describe drug-induced psychosis.[2] Despite such a long period of awareness of the problem, the incidence of drug-induced psychosis is still unknown. Limited data exist regarding the incidence of drug-induced psychosis associated with specific medications or conditions. In addition, drug-induced psychosis often occurs more commonly in patients with certain diseases and when drugs are abused chronically or in high doses. The incidence of psychosis in methamphetamine users was reported to be 11 times greater than that of the general population, with 23% of users reporting at least one psychotic symptom in the past year.[130] In an FDA meta-analysis, therapeutic doses of stimulants caused psychosis in one in 400 children.[14] Up to 21% of patients with Parkinson disease receiving a dopamine agonist experience psychotic symptoms, while fewer than 1% of patients with bipolar disorder exhibit similar symptoms.[58] Predisposing factors such as very young or older age groups, psychiatric and neurologic illnesses, and polypharmacy are known to increase the incidence of drug-induced psychosis.

MECHANISMS

Psychosis is not a single disorder, but rather a symptom induced by multiple mechanisms. **Table 20-3** lists some drugs and their mechanism for inducing psychosis. The precise pathophysiology of idiopathic psychosis is not well understood and even less is known about drug-induced psychosis.

Table 20-3 Mechanisms of Drug-Induced Psychosis[2,3,5-8,125-127,131-137]

Drug(s)	Mechanism(s)
Amantadine Apomorphine Bromocriptine Levodopa Pramipexole Ropinirole Rotigotine	Increased dopamine concentrations in CNS
Albuterol Disulfiram Dronabinol Ephedrine Ketamine Nitrous oxide	Increased norepinephrine concentrations
Amphetamine Bupropion Cyclobenzaprine Monoamine oxidase inhibitors Methylphenidate Pseudoephedrine Sibutramine	Increased dopamine concentrations in CNS Increased norepinephrine concentrations in CNS
Dextromethorphan Ketamine Phencyclidine	Glutamate NMDA receptor antagonist
Anabolic steroids	Down regulation of serotonin 1B receptor density in the hippocampus and globus pallidus Up regulation of serotonin 2 receptor density in the nucleus accumbens
Anticholinergics	Decreased cholinergic function
Anticonvulsants Zolpidem	Enhanced GABAergic effects
Chloroquine Fluoroquinolones	NMDA agonist GABA antagonist
Cycloserine	NMDA partial agonist
HMG CoA reductase inhibitors	Decreased brain cell membrane cholesterol leading to decreased serotonin receptors and altered serotonergic functioning

CNS = central nervous system, GABA = gamma-aminobutyric acid, HMG CoA = 3-hydroxy-3-methylglutaryl-coenzyme A, NMDA = *N*-methyl-D-aspartate.

Overlap in clinical presentation of idiopathic psychosis and psychosis caused by both legal and illicit drugs suggests similar mechanisms. Understanding of drug-induced psychosis, therefore, may be enhanced by a discussion of the pathophysiology of idiopathic psychosis and the psychosis associated with illicit drug use.

Psychosis is often associated with alterations of dopamine concentrations in various regions of the brain.[2,6] Increased dopaminergic function in the mesolimbic pathway is associated with hallucinations, delusions, and paranoia.[2,5-8] Increased release of dopamine and/or decreased metabolism or uptake of dopamine can cause psychotic symptoms. This is supported by the observation that administration of mesolimbic dopamine antagonists leads to clinical improvement of psychotic symptoms.[6] Although a hyperdopaminergic state is an important mechanism of both idiopathic and iatrogenic psychotic states, studies indicate it is only one mechanism involved in the provocation of psychotic symptoms.[2,5-8]

Other neurotransmitters may indirectly alter synaptic concentrations of dopamine leading to psychosis. Glutamate, serotonin, norepinephrine, and acetylcholine are believed to exert secondary affects on dopamine neurotransmission and to play a role in psychosis.[2,5-8]

Altered serotonin [5-hydroxytryptamine (5-HT)] receptor functioning is also associated with psychosis. Patients with schizophrenia have abnormal 5-HT receptor functioning, and many antipsychotic agents exert significant effects on serotonergic functioning.[6,131-136] LSD, an agent known to induce hallucinations, is structurally related to serotonin. LSD and psilocybin induce psychosis through stimulation of the 5-HT_{2A} receptor.[126,127]

Glutamate is the major excitatory neurotransmitter in the brain.[5-7] Antagonism of the glutamate *N*-methyl-D-aspartate (NMDA) receptor by PCP and ketamine induces states that may be the best model of idiopathic psychosis.[137,138] Biologic changes associated with hypoglutamatergic function in schizophrenia include decreased glutamate in the cerebrospinal fluid, altered NMDA receptor densities, and decreased glutamate release.[139-141]

It has been hypothesized that altered intracellular signal transduction may be involved in psychosis.[142,143] Gene induction associated with antipsychotics leads to increased expression of the oncogene c-fos or its protein product, which may alter expression of other genes, the products of which are involved directly in psychosis. Another mechanism posited to play a role in psychosis is episodic dysfunction of myelin sheaths disrupting subcortical and cortical processes, which may lead to positive psychotic symptoms and cognitive dysfunction.[142,143]

Alteration of dopamine and serotonin are consistently associated with psychosis. However, the biologic mechanism of psychosis is complex, involves multiple pathways, and has not been fully elucidated. Therefore, the ability to predict drugs that are less likely to induce psychosis based on pharmacological activity is limited at this time.

CLINICAL PRESENTATION AND DIFFERENTIAL DIAGNOSIS

Many symptoms in patients with drug-induced psychosis are similar to those of patients with idiopathic psychoses such as schizophrenia, which is defined by a triad of symptoms: positive, negative, and cognitive.[2-4,8,144] Positive symptoms include delusions, hallucinations, and disorganized speech and behavior.[2-8] Negative symptoms include flat affect, avolition, and social isolation.[2-8] Cognitive symptoms can be diverse but often present as difficulties with concentration and memory.[7,8] Positive symptoms are more typically associated with drug-induced psychosis than negative symptoms (**Table 20-4**).

There is no individual test that is diagnostic for drug-induced psychosis. Diagnosis depends on identification of a temporal relationship between the ingestion of the potentially causative substance and the onset of psychotic symptoms, clinical presentation, medical history and a thorough medication history.[4,8,144] Patients who are acutely psychotic may or may not be able to provide an accurate history. Consultation with family, friends, and other healthcare providers is useful in understanding any pre-existing mental health issues and recent changes in behavior or medical treatment.

A thorough medication history is crucial to the differential diagnosis of drug-induced psychosis. A clear understanding of a patient's baseline psychiatric state and the medications used to treat the disorder may help clinicians distinguish between an underlying disorder that is worsening and a drug-induced psychosis.[2-8,144] **Table 20-5** lists conditions that should be ruled out prior to the diagnosis of drug-induced psychosis.

Table 20-4 Symptoms Associated with Drug-Induced Psychosis[2-8,144]

Symptom	Examples
Auditory hallucinations	Hearing voices
Visual hallucinations	Seeing thing that are not there
Tactile hallucinations	Feeling bugs crawling on skin
Paranoia	Feelings of persecution
Thought removal/insertion/ broadcasting	Feeling that thoughts are being withdrawn, inserted or broadcasted
Thought blocking	Sudden derailment of speech
Ideas of reference	Feeling that there are hidden messages or special meaning in things unrelated to oneself
Grandiosity	Feeling overly self important
Disorganized speech/ behavior	Tangential Illogical Perseveration
Anxiety	Pacing, excessive worry
Agitation	State of extreme anxiety
Delusions	Fixed false beliefs

Table 20-5 Conditions to Consider in the Differential Diagnosis of Drug-Induced Psychosis[2-8,144]

- Infection (including HIV)
- Metabolic abnormalities
- Liver disease
- Hyperthyroidism
- Substance abuse
- Seizure disorder
- Parkinson disease
- Huntington disease
- Tumor/lesions
- Stroke
- Autoimmune disorders
- Alzheimer disease

HIV = human immunodeficiency virus.

Table 20-6 Duration of Detection of Drugs in Urine[145]

Drug	Duration of Detection
Alcohol	12 hours
Amphetamine	Up to 2 days
Opioids	Up to 4 days
Benzodiazepines	1 day to weeks[a]
Barbiturates	1 day to 3 weeks
Cocaine metabolites	2–4 days
Marijuana	1 day to weeks[a]

[a]Depends on quantity and frequency of use.

The medication history should include use of prescription, nonprescription, and illicit drugs and should document any herbal or nutritional supplements being taken. Although drug-induced psychosis is often associated with recent changes in medication therapy (hours to days), the onset may occur much later in treatment with some agents, such as corticosteroids.[43-47] Also, recent discontinuation of medications should be documented, because drug withdrawal can be accompanied by psychotic symptoms.[120-124] Additionally, recent changes in nonpsychotomimetic medications can play a role in drug-induced psychosis. For example, a nonpsychotomimetic drug could antagonize the psychotomimetic effects of another agent or induce its metabolism.[2,6,8] When questions exist about the veracity of a patient's response to queries regarding substance abuse, urine and blood toxicology screening should be performed. **Table 20-6** lists common drugs of abuse and duration of detection in the urine following the last dose.[145]

The psychotomimetic effects of many medications are dose-related.[8,29,31,34,49,52,56,57,89,144] However, interpatient variability exists in the dose at which a medication can cause psychotic symptoms. The recent initiation of therapy with a new psychotomimetic medication or a dose increase in current therapy should always be considered as possible causes when a patient experiences a new onset of psychotic symptoms.

Laboratory monitoring can be helpful to rule out alternate causes of psychosis.[2,3,5,7,8,144] **Table 20-7** provides a list of laboratory tests useful in the differential diagnosis of psychosis. In many cases, the decision to perform laboratory monitoring is based on history and clinical presentation.

Table 20-7 Tests to Aid in the Differential Diagnosis of Drug-Induced Psychosis[3,5,7,8,144]

Standard laboratory monitoring

- Complete blood cell count with differential
- Electrolytes
- Liver function
- Thyroid function
- Toxicology screen

Monitoring if clinically indicated by patient history

- HIV
- Antinuclear antibodies
- Sedimentation rate
- EEG
- Head CT/MRI

CT = computed tomography, EEG = electroencephalogram, HIV = human immunodeficiency virus, MRI = magnetic resonance imaging.

Diagnosis of drug-induced psychosis is a diagnosis of exclusion.[2,3,5,7,8,144] The integral components of diagnosis are accurate medication, medical, psychiatric, and physical histories, physical examination, and laboratory monitoring.[2,3,5,7,8,144] In many instances, a thorough history is sufficient to diagnose drug-induced psychosis.

The *Diagnostic and Statistical Manual of Mental Disorders, 5th Edition,* includes several diagnoses that encompass drug-induced psychosis (termed *substance/medication induced*), including substance/medication-induced psychosis and substance/medication-induced bipolar and related disorders. A key criterion of substance-induced psychosis is absence of delirium.[4] Delirium is differentiated from psychosis by its fluctuating course, disturbances of consciousness, and changes in cognitive processes such as memory.[4] Although these problems may occur in drug-induced psychosis, they are more often indicative of delirium. Research demonstrates that the clinical diagnosis of drug-induced psychosis remains accurate in greater than 70% of cases at 24 months, indicating standard interview, history gathering, and routine laboratory monitoring are sufficient for an accurate diagnosis in most cases.[146]

Prominent hallucinations or delusions are typically present in patients with drug-induced psychosis.[2,3,8,144] Often hallucinations are visual, tactile, and gustatory, whereas auditory hallucinations predominate in idiopathic psychotic disorders.[2,3,8,144] Patients who have insight into psychiatric symptoms that are drug-induced do not meet the criteria for a substance/medication-induced psychosis and should be diagnosed as substance intoxication or withdrawal with perceptual disturbances.[4] However, patient insight is a controversial diagnostic exclusion, as many patients who have insight into their symptoms nonetheless require treatment for psychotic symptoms.[144]

Onset of illness must be assessed to accurately diagnose drug-induced psychosis. Idiopathic psychotic disorders tend to occur during specific periods in life and have a slow progressive and degenerative course.[2,3,5-8,144] Abrupt onset or atypical presentations such as a late age of onset may indicate drug-induced psychosis, which is usually associated with recent medication changes and occurs within hours to days of the change.[2,3,5-8,144] In some rare cases the onset may be more protracted, as is the case with corticosteroid-associated psychosis, which may occur as late as 3 months after medication changes.[43-47]

Duration of symptoms may also help clarify the diagnosis. When symptoms do not remit within 4 weeks after discontinuation of the potentially causative agent, other causes of psychosis must be considered.[4,8,144] Protracted psychosis is not common when the disorder is drug-induced.

Physical symptoms may differ between drug-induced psychosis, intoxication, and idiopathic psychotic states. Typically, drug-induced psychosis is not associated with gross physical abnormalities.[4,8,144] Slurred speech or ataxia are more commonly associated with intoxication and delirium rather than idiopathic or drug-induced psychosis.[2,3,5-7,8,144] Intoxication, drug withdrawal, or delirium are often associated with physical characteristics such as changes in pupil size, tachycardia, sweating, pain and cramping, altered gastrointestinal motility, and drug cravings that are often not present in patients with drug-induced psychosis.[4,5,7,8,144]

Some drugs are associated with a pattern of signs and symptoms that may help identify them as causative agents. Stimulant-induced psychosis is often associated with mydriasis, tachycardia, arrhythmias, and brisk reflexes.[2,3,5-8,14-16] Benzodiazepine withdrawal is associated with tremors, fever, and seizures.[2,3,5-8,121,122,144] Mydriasis, tachycardia, urinary retention, and constipation accompany anticholinergic-induced psychosis.[2,3,5-8,24,144] Although anticholinergic-induced psychosis occurs more commonly in association with oral or parenteral administration, it has also been reported with transdermal use.[27]

RISK FACTORS

Specific risk factors for drug-induced psychosis are listed in **Table 20-8**. Older age, underlying bipolar or psychotic disorder, compromised kidney or liver function, polypharmacy, concomitant use of multiple psychoactive drugs, and metabolic abnormalities (e.g., electrolyte abnormalities) all increase the risk of drug-induced psychosis. Post-traumatic head injury can cause organic psychosis as well as predispose a patient to drug-induced psychosis.[144,147,148] As the number of risk factors increases, so does the likelihood of drug-induced psychosis.

Patient populations in need of special attention are the elderly, infants and children, and patients

Table 20-8 Risk Factors for Drug-Induced Psychosis[2,3,5-8,144,147-149]

- Age >40 years
- Infants and children
- Altered liver or kidney function
- Substance abuse
- Concomitant medications
  - Increased burden of medications with additive effects such as anticholinergic agents
  - Drug interactions (including withdrawal of medications)
- Underlying disease states
  - Systemic lupus erythematosus
  - Parkinson disease
  - Psychiatric illnesses
  - HIV
- Head injury

HIV = human immunodeficiency virus.

with concomitant illnesses. Weight- and age-based dosing are important to decrease risk of drug-induced psychosis for the elderly and children. Prescribing information for individual drugs provides recommendations for dose adjustments for patients with concomitant illnesses such as liver and kidney disease.

In people of any age, concurrent administration of multiple drugs may affect both pharmacokinetic and pharmacodynamic properties of drugs.[5,7,149-153] Increased anticholinergic burden from multiple medications or taking more than nine medications daily substantially increases the risk of drug-induced psychosis.[2,5,7]

Drug interactions that enhance the pharmacological effects and/or increase serum concentrations of potentially causative agents increase the risk of drug-induced psychosis. Pharmacodynamic interactions occur when two medications with similar pharmacological effects have additive or synergistic effects. For example, stimulants and bupropion both increase dopamine and norepinephrine concentrations in the brain. The addition of a stimulant to bupropion treatment could lead to psychotic symptoms that were not present with bupropion monotherapy.

Another potential pharmacodynamic interaction could result from the combination of two drugs that antagonize one other.[154] For example, when a dopamine antagonist is used to treat psychosis, addition of a dopamine agonist can result in the return of psychotic symptoms. Although one would not expect a particularly robust change in dopaminergic antagonism, other pharmacological effects such as anticholinergic transmission could be enhanced leading to increased side effects.

Medications commonly associated with pharmacokinetic drug interactions include antibiotics (ketoconazole, erythromycin), psychotropics (fluvoxamine, fluoxetine, nefazodone), and others (cimetidine, quinidine, protease inhibitors).[149,150,152] Addition of a cytochrome P-450 inhibitor may lead to diminished metabolism of a drug, increased plasma concentrations, and potential for adverse effects.[152,153] Alternately, discontinuation of an agent that was inducing the metabolism of a drug could lead to decreased drug metabolism, increased plasma concentrations, and increased adverse effects, including psychosis.[150] Some agents vulnerable to drug interactions and resulting drug-induced psychosis include stimulants, steroids, opiates/opioids, anticholinergics, antibiotics, β-blockers, angiotensin converting enzyme inhibitors, dopaminergic agents, and antiepileptic medications.[2,3,5,20,149,150,152]

Diligent assessment of medication profiles can help clinicians identify and prevent or treat drug-induced psychosis attributable to drug interactions. Familiarity with those drugs commonly implicated in such drug interactions can help avoid adverse consequences.

MORBIDITY AND MORTALITY

Drug-induced psychosis often requires medical attention to protect the safety of the patient or those around them, although harm due directly to the psychotic state is not typical. Death is rarely directly related to psychosis.[2,3] Death associated with a drug that is causing psychosis is most often the result of a severe intoxication (as may occur with stimulants) or drug withdrawal (as may occur with benzodiazepines).[2-5,121,122]

There is limited information available on the utilization of emergency departments and hospitalizations associated with drug-induced psychosis. One study estimated that 1% of all emergency department visits were related to psychosis.[155] However, the authors did not differentiate between idiopathic and drug-induced psychosis.

Psychosis impairs judgment and insight, which can cause a person to make poor decisions and/or engage in risky behaviors resulting in poor outcomes such as motor vehicle accidents, suicide, or assault.[2,3,8,144] During a psychotic state, patients may misinterpret surrounding events or participate in illegal activities that could lead to incarceration.[2,3,8,144]

PREVENTION

Drug-induced psychosis may be prevented by minimizing risk factors (**Table 20-9**). A thorough history of past and current psychiatric and medical illnesses

Table 20-9 Approaches to Help Prevent Drug-Induced Psychosis

- Utilize lowest dose possible
- Minimize number of concomitant potentially causative medications
- Limit medications with anticholinergic properties
- Adjust doses for elderly
- Avoid use of multiple psychotomimetic medications
- Complete a thorough medication history including nonprescription medications, herbals, alcohol, and illicit drugs

should be completed. Awareness of all prescription and nonprescription medications and herbal and nutritional supplements is essential to accurately assess risk. Direct inquiry regarding the use of herbal and nutritional supplements is necessary because patients often do not volunteer this information spontaneously.[156,157] Nonpejorative inquiry into illicit drug use and alcohol consumption is important.

Using the lowest effective doses, age- and weight-appropriate dose selection, avoidance of polypharmacy, and awareness of drug interactions can reduce the risk of drug-induced psychosis. Additionally, in populations with impaired liver or kidney function, aggressive monitoring may help prevent drug-induced psychosis.

No specific monitoring parameters exist for drug-induced psychosis. However, educating the patients, their families, and caregivers regarding the signs and symptoms of drug-induced psychosis may facilitate early identification and treatment.

MANAGEMENT

Drug-induced psychosis is generally self-limiting following discontinuation of therapy with the offending agent. Resolution of symptoms occurs quickly (hours to days) in most patients.[5,7,8,144] Knowledge of the causative medication's half-life provides guidance regarding the likely time frame for symptom resolution. Treatment should include discontinuation of the offending agent, except when it is determined to be medically necessary and no alternate treatments exist. In those situations, decreasing the dose to below psychotomimetic levels and/or treatment of the psychosis with antipsychotic medications may be appropriate. In some cases, the offending agent may be temporarily discontinued and then reinitiated at a lower dose after resolution of psychosis. The dose may then be carefully increased as appropriate for the clinical situation.

Some patients may be detained against their will for observation and medicated if the risk of harm to themselves or others is deemed unacceptable in a court of law. Some states allow for administration of medication without a court order in emergent situations. Duration of confinement is based on presentation and state law, and therefore treatment options differ from state to state.

Keeping the patient in a safe environment is an important component of treatment during acute psychosis. A safe environment is typically one in which the patient can be observed in a contained location if necessary. Several hours in an emergency department is often sufficient for resolution of symptoms. Drug treatment is rarely necessary following discontinuation of the offending agent.

Medical management is needed if the patient is clearly dangerous to her- or himself or others. In an acute psychotic state, dangerous behaviors may include suicidal or homicidal ideation, violence, extreme paranoia, or unpredictable behaviors. Patients who may hurt themselves or others or may put themselves in dangerous situations typically require acute hospitalization. The goal of acute treatment is to calm the patient and maintain safety. Short-term use of antipsychotics or benzodiazepines may be warranted, provided they are used only during the period of psychosis. Long-term use of these medications places patients at unnecessary risk for complications such as tardive dyskinesia or weight gain and associated metabolic abnormalities. Oral drug administration is preferred; however, in some cases, parenteral administration may be required. Hydration to decrease the risk of delirium is also necessary. Indications of the need for medical management include an inability to maintain a patient's safe behaviors with nondrug measures such as a calm environment, close observation, containment in a limited area or room, or supportive contact with medical professionals, family, or friends.

The choice of medication should be based on efficacy, patient acceptability, and adverse effect profile. The anxiolytic and sedative effects of benzodiazepines render them useful for the treatment of acute agitation and anxiety. Should a patient be disinhibited or become disinhibited with benzodiazepine use, antipsychotics are the drugs of choice. An anticholinergic agent is often administered concomitantly with any antipsychotic agent likely to cause acute extrapyramidal reactions. In patients who are overtly hostile, violent, or aggressive, a combination of benzodiazepines and antipsychotics may be useful.

In cases where withdrawal from a medication is the cause of the psychosis, supportive care is the treatment of choice. Monitoring of subjective complaints and vital signs is useful for identification of patients experiencing withdrawal syndromes. If the discontinuation syndrome places the patient at risk of death or injury, therapy with medication may be reinstituted and the dose then slowly tapered downward for the patient's safety. In the case of benzodiazepines, conversion to a longer-acting agent before downward titration may improve the tolerability of medication discontinuation.[158] However, this is controversial and tapering the original drug can be appropriate treatment.

In instances where discontinuing the offending agent is undesirable (i.e., anti-Parkinsonian agents, corticosteroids), lowering the dose may be sufficient to resolve psychotic symptoms. In cases where drug-induced psychosis is unavoidable to successfully treat the underlying illness, long-term antipsychotic therapy is warranted. In patients with Parkinson disease and drug-induced psychosis, low doses of quetiapine or clozapine are treatments of choice to avoid exacerbation of the underlying movement disorder. Due to adverse effects and associated monitoring procedures required during clozapine therapy, quetiapine is typically viewed as preferred management.[159,160]

In patients with a history of drug-induced psychosis, a rechallenge of the drug may be clinically appropriate. Ideal candidates are patients for whom drug-induced psychosis was the result of high drug doses or concomitant use of multiple psychomimetic medications. Patients who experience psychotic symptoms at low drug doses should not typically be rechallenged. If rechallenge is considered, discussion of the potential risks and benefits of therapy with the patient is important. The drug should be reintroduced at a low dose and with careful monitoring for early signs of psychosis (mild paranoia, agitation, irritability, behavioral changes). Dose increases should be performed over extended time intervals and in smaller increments than usual. In any case, the dose of the agent that is reintroduced should be maintained below previous psychotomimetic doses.

Antidotes are available for several drugs known to cause psychosis (**Table 20-10**). These antidotes are usually necessary only in cases of overdose.[5,154,161-163] Discontinuation of the causative medication and supportive care are often sufficient.[8,144] In cases where an antidote is used, close monitoring to avoid induction of a withdrawal psychosis is necessary.[158,163,164] Specific withdrawal psychosis protocols are limited but are outlined in **Table 20-11**.

Table 20-10 Specific Antidotes for Drug-Induced Psychosis[154,158,161-163]

Anticholinergics

- Physostigmine 0.5–2 mg IM/IV/sub-Q to start, repeating every 20 minutes until response or adverse drug reaction

Opioids

- Naloxone 0.1–0.2 mg IV every 2–3 minutes and repeat every 20–60 minutes

Benzodiazepines

- Flumazenil 0.01 mg/kg over 15 seconds (max 0.2 mg); repeat with 0.005–0.01 mg/kg as needed; do not exceed 3 mg

IM = intramuscular, IV = intravenous, sub-Q = subcutaneous.

Table 20-11 Drug Withdrawal Treatment Protocols[158,164]

Substance	Treatment
Alcohol/benzodiazepine	Chlordiazepoxide 25–50 mg orally every 2 hours as needed for signs/symptoms of withdrawal Supportive care
Opiates/opioids	Methadone 10–20 mg orally every 12 hours; taper over 5–10 days Supportive care

INFORMATION FOR PATIENTS

Patients and their caregivers should be alerted to the potential risks and signs of psychosis whenever psychotomimetic drugs are prescribed. The extent of counseling should be dependent on several factors, including the number of risk factors present, number and severity of comorbidities, polypharmacy, and the dose and number of psychotomimetic medications to be used. Patients and/or caregivers should be instructed to contact their clinician if paranoia, agitation or hallucinations occur.

Patients should be instructed not to take nonprescription medications without first consulting a clinician. Some nonprescription agents associated with psychotomimetic properties include pseudoephedrine, ma huang (ephedra), diphenhydramine, dextromethorphan, and caffeine.[26,29,33,34,53,54,67-69,103] The combination of pseudoephedrine and dextromethorphan in particular increases the risk of psychosis.[103] In addition, patients should be instructed to avoid excessive consumption of caffeinated products.[34,144] Education concerning foods and beverages that are high in caffeine may be necessary depending on the medical sophistication of the patient.

Drug-induced psychosis is often a preventable iatrogenic disease. Careful inquiry about all medications being taken, including nonprescription drugs, complimentary therapies and illicit substances should be completed before making recommendations for nonprescription or prescription drugs. Careful attention should be paid to the combination of agents with high propensity for drug interactions.

Although the outcome of drug-induced psychosis is often favorable, it is important to adequately assess all patients for their risk. Appropriate drug doses, disease and drug monitoring, and minimization of risk factors can improve patient outcomes. Individualization of patient assessments is important because multiple risk factors may substantially increase the risk.

REFERENCES

1. Dirck JH, ed. *Stedman's concise medical dictionary for the health professions.* 7th ed. Philadelphia: Wolters Kluwer, Lippincott Williams and Wilkins; 2012.
2. Sadock BJ, Sadock VA, Ruiz P, eds. *Kaplan and Sadock's comprehensive textbook of psychiatry.* 9th ed. Philadelphia: Lippincott Williams and Wilkins; 2009.
3. Ebert MH, Loosen PT, Nurcombe B, eds. *Current diagnosis and treatment in psychiatry.* 2nd ed. New York: Lange Medical Books/McGraw-Hill; 2008.
4. American Psychiatric Association. *The diagnostic and statistical manual of mental disorders: DSM-5.* Washington, DC: American Psychiatric Association; 2013.
5. Kasper DL, Fauci AS, Hauser SL et al. *Harrison's principles of internal medicine.* 19th ed. New York: McGraw Hill; 2015.
6. Stahl SM. *Essential psychopharmacology.* Cambridge, UK: Cambridge University Press; 2013.
7. Schatzberg AF, Nemeroff CB. *Essentials of clinical psychopharmacology.* 3rd ed. Arlington, VA: American Psychiatry Press; 2013.
8. Sciolla A. Iatrogenic psychosis. *Semin Clin Neuropsychiatry.* 1998; 3:61-9.
9. Ray I, Evans CJ. Paranoid psychosis with ventolin (salbutamol tablets b.p.) *Can Psychiatr Assoc J.* 1978; 23:427.
10. Martin W, Unutzer J, Szuba MP. Exacerbation of psychosis with inhaled albuterol. *J Clin Psychopharmacol.* 1995; 15:446-7.
11. Gluckman L. Letter: Ventolin induced psychosis. *N Z Med J.* 1974; 80:411.
12. Snoey ER, Bessen HA. Acute psychosis after amantadine overdose. *Ann Emerg Med.* 1990; 19:668-70.
13. Borison RL. Amantadine-induced psychosis in a geriatric patient with renal disease. *Am J Psychiatry* 1979; 136:111-2.
14. US Food and Drug Administration. Medwatch Safety Alert—adderall. July 2006. http://www.fda.gov/medwatch/safety/2006/Jul_PIs/Adderall_PI.pdf (accessed 2018 Jan 3).
15. Surles LK, May HJ, Garry JP. Adderall-induced psychosis in an adolescent. *J Am Board Fam Pract.* 2002; 15:498-500.
16. Ross RG. Psychotic and manic like symptoms during stimulant treatment of ADHD. *Am J Psychiatry.* 2006; 163:1149-52.
17. Pope HG, Katz DL. Affective and psychotic reactions associated with anabolic steroid use. *Am J Psychiatry.* 1988; 145:487-90.
18. Tarlow MM, Sakaris A, Scoyni R, Wolf-Klein G. Quinapril-associated acute psychosis in an older woman. *J Am Geriatr Soc.* 2000; 48:1533.
19. Ahmad S. Enalapril-induced acute psychosis. *DICP.* 1991; 25:558-9.
20. Keller S, Frishman WH, Epstein J. Neuropsychiatric manifestations of cardiovascular drug therapy. *Heart Dis.* 1999; 1:241-54.
21. Kuhn JA, Savage GJ. Belladonna alkaloid psychosis: a study of scopolamine hydrobromide vs. methscoplolamine bromide. *Del Med J.* 1974; 46:239-42.
22. Cancelli I, Valentinis L, Merlino G et al. Drugs with anticholinergic properties as a risk factor for pscyhosis in patients affected by Alzheimer's disease. *Clin Pharmacol Ther.* 2008; 84:63-8.
23. Milgrom H, Bender B. Adverse effects of medications for rhinitis. *Ann Allergy Asthma Immunol.* 1997; 78:439-44.
24. Hall RC, Feinsilver DL, Holt RE. Anticholinergic psychosis: differential diagnosis and management. *Psychosomatics.* 1982; 22:581-3.
25. Gopel C, Laufer C, Marcus A. Three cases of angel's trumpet tea-induced psychosis in adolescent substance abusers. *Nord J Psychiatry.* 2002; 56:49-52.
26. Jones J, Dougherty J, Cannon L. Diphenhydramine-induced toxic psychosis. *Am J Emerg Med.* 1986; 4:369-71.
27. Ziskind AA. Transdermal scopolamine-induced psychosis. *Postgrad Med.* 1988; 84:73-6.

28. Hamdan-Allen G, Nixon M. Anticholinergic psychosis in children: a case report. *Hosp Comm Psychiatry.* 1991; 42:191-2.
29. Radovanovic D, Meier PJ, Gruiguis M et al. Dose-dependent toxicity of diphenhydramine overdose. *Hum Exp Toxicol.* 2000; 19:489-95.
30. Golden RN, James SP, Sherer MA et al. Psychosis associated with bupropion treatment. *Am J Psychiatry.* 1985; 142:1459-62.
31. Goren JL, Levin GM. Mania with bupropion: a dose related phenomenon? *Ann Pharmacother.* 2000; 34:619-21.
32. Kumar S, Kodela S, Detweiler JG et al. Bupropion-inudced psychosis: folklore or a fact? A systematic review of the literature. *Gen Hosp Psychiatry.* 2011; 33:612-7.
33. Shaul PW, Farrell MK, Maloney MJ. Caffeine toxicity as a cause of acute psychosis in anorexia nervosa. *J Pediatr.* 1984; 105:493-5.
34. Kruger A. Chronic psychiatric patients' use of caffeine: pharmacological effects and mechanisms. *Psychol Rep.* 1996; 78:915-23.
35. Pleek RR, Birmaher B, Gavrilescu A et al. Mania and neuropsychiatric excitation following carbamazepine. *J Am Aced Child Adolsec Psychiatry.* 1988; 27:500-2.
36. Cavanna AE, Ali F, Rickards HE, McCorry D. Behavioral and cognitive effects of anti-epileptic drugs. *Discov Med.* 2010; 9:138-44.
37. Drake ME, Peruzzi WT. Manic state with carbamazepine therapy of seizures. *J Natl Med Assoc.* 1986; 78:1105-7.
38. Lantz MS, Giambanco V. Acute onset of auditory hallucinations after initiation of celocoxib therapy. *Am J Psychiatry.* 2000; 157:1022-3.
39. Good MI, Shader RI. Lethality and behavioral side effects of chloroquine. *J Clin Psychopharmacol.* 1982; 2:40-7.
40. Cipro [package insert]. West Haven, CT: Bayer; 2009.
41. Tome AM, Filipe A. Quinolones: a review of psychiatric and neurologic adverse-reactions. *Drug Saf.* 2011; 34:465-88.
42. Rosse RB, Collins JP Jr, Fay-McCarthy M et al. Phenomenologic comparison of the idiopathic psychosis of schizophrenia and drug-induce cocaine and phencyclidine psychosis: a retrospective study. *Clin Neuropharmacol.* 1994; 17:359-69.
43. Brown ES, Khan DA, Nejtek VA. The psychiatric side effects of corticosteroids. *Ann Allergy Asthma Immunol.* 1999; 83:495-503.
44. Wolkowitz OM, Reus VI, Canick J et al. Glucocorticoid medication, memory and steroid psychosis in medical illness. *Ann N Y Acad Sci.* 1997; 14:81-96.
45. Patten SB, Neutel CI. Corticosteroid-induced adverse psychiatric effects. *Drug Saf.* 2000; 22:111-22.
46. Gable M, Depry D. Sustained corticosteroid-induced mania and psychosis despite cessation: a case study and brief literature review. *Int J Psychiatry Med.* 2015; 50:398-404.
47. Warrington TP, Bostwick JM. Psychiatric adverse events of corticosteroids. *Mayo Clin Proc.* 2006; 81:1361-7.
48. Douglas MA, Levine DP. Hallucinations in an elderly patient taking recommended doses of cyclobenzaprine. *Arch Int Med.* 2000; 160:1373.
49. Linden CH, Mitchiner JC, Lindzon RD. Cyclobenzaprine overdosage. *J Toxicol Clin Toxicol.* 1983; 20:281-8.
50. Singh R, Gothi D, Joshi J. Multi-resistant tuberculosis: Role of previous treatment with second line therapy on treatment outcomes. *Lung India.* 2007; 24:54-7.
51. Sharma B, Honda R, Nagpol K et al. Cycloserine induced psychosis in a young female with drug resistant tuberculosis. *Gen Hosp Psychiatry.* 2014; 36:451.
52. Krishna Murthy K, Raji Babu KK. Toxic psychosis after accidental ingestion of dapsone: review and case report. *Lepr India.* 1980; 52:443-5.
53. Price LH, Lebel J. Dextromethorphan-induced psychosis. *Am J Psychiatry.* 2000; 157:304.
54. Miller SC. Dextromethorphan psychosis, dependence and physical withdrawal. *Addict Biol.* 2005; 10:325-7.
55. Carney MW, Rapp S, Pearce K. Digoxin toxicity presenting with psychosis in a patient with chronic phobic anxiety. *Clin Neuropharmacol.* 1985; 8:193-5.
56. Li MY, Shen YC. Manic episode with psychosis following a lower than recommended dosage regimen of disulfiram. *Prog Neuropsychopharmacol Biol Psychiatry.* 2008; 32:311-2.
57. Ceylan ME, Turkcan A, Mutlu E, Onal O. Manic episode with psychotic symptoms associated with high dose of disulfiram: case report. *J Clin Psychopharmacol.* 2007; 27:224-5.
58. Young BK, Camiciolo R, Ganzini L. Neuropsychiatric adverse effects of antiparkisonian drugs. Characteristics, evaluation and treatment. *Drugs Aging.* 1997; 10:367.
59. Reeves RR, Pinkofsky HB. Postpartum psychosis induced by bromocriptine and pseudoephedrine. *J Fam Pract.* 1997; 45:164-6.
60. Stoner SC, Dahmen MM, Makos M et al. An exploratory retrospective evaluation of ropinirole-associated psychotic symptoms in an outpatient population treated for restless legs syndrome or Parkinson's disease. *Ann Pharmacother.* 2009; 43:1426-32.
61. Bilal L, Ching D. Cabergoline-induced psychosis in a paiant with undiagnosed depression. *J Neuropsychiatry Clin Neurosci.* 2012; 24:E54.
62. Burback L. Management of a microprolactinoma with Aripiprazole in a woman with cabergoline-induced mania. *Endocrinol Diabetes Metab Case Rep.* 2015; 2015:150100.
63. Aiken CB. Pramipexole in psychiatry: a systematic review of the literature. *J Clin Psych.* 2007; 68:1230-6.
64. Nottage JF, Stone J, Murray RM et al. Delta-9 tetrahydrocannabinol, neural oscillations above 20 Hz and induced psychosis. *Psychopharmacol.* 2015; 232:519-28.
65. Linszen D, van Amelsvoort T. Cannibis and psychosis: an update on course and biological plausible mechanism. *Curr Opin Psychiatry.* 2007; 20:116-20.
66. Welch KJ, Morse A. Association between efavirenz and selected psychiatric and neurologic conditions. *J Infec Dis.* 2002; 185:268-9.
67. Boerth JM, Caley CF. Possible case of mania associated with mahuang. *Pharmacotherapy.* 2003; 23:380-3.
68. Tormey WP, Bruzzi A. Acute psychosis due to the interaction of legal compounds—ephedra alkaloid in "vigueur fit" tablets, caffeine in "red bull" and alcohol. *Med Sci Law.* 2001; 41:331-6.
69. Maglione M, Mioyyo K, Iguchi M et al. Psychiatric effects of ephedra use: an analysis of the Food and Drug Administration reports of adverse effects. *Am J Psychiatry.* 2005; 162:189-91.
70. Mancano M. *Garcinia cambogia*-induced acute hepatitis; varenicline-induced parkinsonism; resistant hypocalcemia after zoledronic acid administration; zonisamide-induced acute kidney injury; psychosis associated with guanfacine. *Hosp Pharm.* 2015; 50:564-8.
71. Kim RK, Chayer R. Psychosis associated with guanfacine. *J Clin Psychopharmacol.* 2015; 35:213.
72. Southworth MR, Dunlap SH. Psychotic symptoms and confusion associated with intravenous granciclovir in a heart transplant patient. *Pharmacother.* 2000; 20:479-83.
73. Catalano G, Catalano MC, Alberts VA. Famotidine associated delirium:a series of six cases. *Psychosomatics.* 1996; 37:349-55.
74. Rodgers PT, Brengel GR. Famotidine associated mental status changes. *Pharmacotherapy.* 1998;18:404-7.
75. Papp KA, Curtis RM. Cimetidine induced psychosis in a 14-year-old girl. *Can Med Assoc J.* 1984; 131:1081-4.
76. Price W, Coli L, Brandsletter RD, Gotz VP. Ranitidine associated hallucinations. *Eur J Clin Pharmacol.* 1985; 29:375-6.
77. Tatley M, Savage R. Psychiatric adverse reactions with statins, fibrates, and ezetimibe. *Drug Saf.* 2007; 30:195-201.
78. Lilly SM, Mortensen EM, Frei CR et al. Comparison of the risk of psychological and cognitive disorders between persistent and nonpersistent statin use. *Am J Cardiol.* 2014; 114:1035-9.
79. Ifosfamide [prescribing information]. Schaumburg, IL: Abraxis Pharmaceutical Products; June 2006.
80. Tharumaratnam D, Bashford S, Khan SA. Indomethacin induced psychosis. *Postgrad Med J* 2000; 76:736-7.
81. Indocin [prescribing information]. Whitehouse Station, NJ: Merck and Company; March 2007.

82. Pinkasov A, Lam T, Hayes D et al. Lacosamide induced psychosis: case report, review of differential diagnosis and relevant pharmacokinetics. *Clin Neuropharmacol.* 2015; 38:198-200.
83. Chatzefanidis D, Karvouni E, Kyritisis AP et al. First case of lacosamide-induced psychosis. *Clin Neuropharmacol.* 2013; 36:27-8.
84. Turner WM. Lidocaine and psychotic reactions. *Arch Intern Med.* 1982; 97:149-50.
85. Wan LB, Levitch CF, Perez AM et al. Ketamine safety and tolerability in clinical trials for treatment-resistant depression. *J Clin Psychiatry.* 2015; 76:247-52.
86. Keppra XR [package insert]. Smyma, GA: UCN Inc; 2015.
87. Goldberg-Stern H, Feldman L, Eidlitz-Markus T et al. Levetiracetam in children, adolscents and young adults with intractable epilepsy: efficacy tolerability and effect on electroencephalogram-a pilot study. *Eur J Paediatr Neurol.* 2013; 17:248-53.
88. Normann C, Hesslinger B, Frauenknecht S et al. Psychosis during chronic levodopa therapy triggered by the new antidepressant drug mirtazepine. *Pharmacopsychiatry.* 1997; 30:263-5.
89. Brownlie BEW, Rae AM, Walshe JWB et al. Psychosis associated with thyrotoxicosis—'thyrotoxic psychosis.' A report of 18 cases with statistical analysis of incidence. *EurJ Endocrinol.* 2000; 142:438-44.
90. van Riemsdijk MM, Ditters JM, Sturkenboom MC et al. Neuropsychiatric events during prophylactic use of mefloquine before traveling. *Eur J Clin Pharmacol.* 2002; 58:441-5.
91. Sowunmi A, Adio RA, Oduola AM et al. Acute psychosis after mefloquine. Report of six cases. *Trop Geogr Med.* 1995; 47:179-80.
92. MacVicar AA. Psychiatric symptoms due to meperidine intoxication (letter). *Can Med Assoc J* 1974; 110:1237.
93. Fogarty T, Murray GB. Psychiatric presentation of meperidine toxicity. *J Clin Psychopharmacol.* 1987; 7:116-7.
94. Kraemer M, Uekermann J, Wiltfang J, Kis B. Methylphenidate-induced psychosis in adult attention deficit/hyperactivity disorder: report of 3 new cases and review of the literature. *Clin Neuropharmacol.* 2010; 33:204-6.
95. Zhao Y, Xu W, Qui L, Yang W. Metoprolol-induced psychosis in a young patient. *Gen Hosp Psychiatry.* 2013; 35:102,e1-2.
96. Rietveld L, van der Hoek T, van Beek MHCT, Schellekens AFA. Familial liability for metoprolol-induced psychosis. *Gen Hosp Psychiatry.* 2015; 37:620.e5-e6.
97. Davies M, Wilton L, Shakir S. Safety profile of modafanil across a range of prescribed indications, including off-label use, in a primary care setting in England: results of a modified prescription-event monitoring. *Drug Saf.* 2013; 36:237-46.
98. Hollan S, Vecsei L, Magyar K. Adverse effects of dopamine potentiation by long-term treatment with selegeline. *Movt Disorders.* 2004; 19:107-9.
99. Sheehy LM, Maxmen JS. Phenelzine-induced psychosis. *Am J Psychaitry.* 1978; 135:1422-3.
100. Aizenberg D, Schwartz B, Zemishlany Z. Delusional parasitosis associated with phenelzine. *Br J Psychiatry.* 1991; 159:716-7.
101. Wong SL, Harrison R, Mattman A et al. Nitrous oxide (N2O)-induced acute psychosis. *Can J Neurol Sci.* 2014; 41:672-4.
102. Sethi NK, Mullin P, Torgovnick J, Capasso G. Nitrous oxide "whippit" abuse presenting with cyanacobalamin responsive psychosis. *J Med Toxicol.* 2006; 2:71-4.
103. Soutullo CA, Cottingham EM, Keck Paul Jr. Psychosis associated with pseudoephedrine and dextromethorphan. *J Am Acad Child Adolesc Psychiatry.* 1999; 38:1471-2.
104. Alevios B. Dependence and chronic psychosis with D-nor-pseudoephedrine. *Eur Psychiatry.* 2003; 18:423-5.
105. Johnson AG, Day RO, Seldon WA. A functional psychosis precipitated by quinidine. *Med J Aust.* 1990; 153:47-9.
106. Deleu D, Schmedding E. Acute psychosis as an idiosyncratic reaction to quinidine: report of 2 cases. *Br Med J (Clin Res Ed).* 1987; 294:1001-2.
107. Lee J, Teoh T, Lee TS. Catatonia and psychosis associated with sibutramine: a case report and pathophysiologic correlation. *J Psychosom Res.* 2008; 64:107-9.
108. Litvan L, Alcoverro-Fortuny O. Sibutramine and psychosis. *J Clin Psychopharmacol.* 2007; 27:727-7.
109. Shah KA, Abraham MA, Espinosa JB. A case of psychosis assocaitied with Pai You Gua slimming capsules containing sibutramine. *J Clin Psych.* 2015; 76:e893-4.
110. Chegounchi M, Hanna MG, Neild GH. Progressive neurologic disease induced by tacrolimus in a renal transplant recipient: case presentation. *BMC Nephrol.* 2006; 31:7.
111. Emiroglu R, Ayvaz I, Moray G et al. Tacrolimus-related neurologic and renal complications in liver transplant: A single-center experience. *Transplant Proc.* 2006; 38:619-21.
112. Seckellares JC, Krauss G, Summerville KW, Deaton R. Occurance of psychosis in patients with epilepsy randomized to tiagabine or placebo treatment. *Epilepsia.* 2003; 43:394-8.
113. Gregor JC, Zilli CA, Gotlib IH. Acute psychosis associated with oral trimethoprim-sulfamethoxazole therapy. *Can J Psychiatry.* 1993; 38:56-8.
114. Mattappalil A, Mergenhagen KA. Neurotoxicity with antimicrobials in the elderly: a review. *Clin Ther.* 2014; 36:1489-511.
115. Besag FM. Behavioral effects of newer antiepileptic drugs: an update. *Expert Opin Drug Saf.* 2004; 3:1-8.
116. Sander JW, Hart YM, Trimble MR, Shorvan SD. Vigabatrin and psychosis. *J Neurol Neurosurg Psychiatry.* 1991; 54:435-9.
117. Markowitz JS, Brewerton TD. Zolpidem-induced psychosis. *Ann Clin Psychiatry.* 1996; 8:89.
118. Eslami-Shahrbabaki M, Barfeh B, Nasirian M. Persistent psychosis after abuse of high dose zolpidem. *Addict Health.* 2014; 6:159-62.
119. Abdoh M, Mersfelder TL, Melgar TA. Psychosis induced by zonisamide: a case report and review of the literature. *Am J Ther.* 2014; 21:e15-6.
120. Turner RC, Lichstein PR, Peden JG Jr et al. Alcohol withdrawal syndromes: a review of pathophysiology, clinical presentation, and treatment. *J Gen Intern Med.* 1989; 4:432-4.
121. Petursson H. The benzodiazepine withdrawal syndrome. *Addiction.* 1994; 89:1455-9.
122. Preskorn SH, Denner LJ. Benzodiazepine and withdrawal psychosis. Report of three cases. *JAMA.* 1977; 3:36-8.
123. Levinson I, Galynker II, Rosenthal RN. Methadone withdrawal psychosis. *J Clin Psychiatry.* 1995; 56:73-6.
124. Shreeram SS, McDonald T, Dennison S. Psychosis after ultra rapid opiate detoxification. *Am J Psychiatry.* 2001; 158:970.
125. Murray RM, Paparelli A, Morrison PD et al. What can we learn about schizophrenia from studying the human model, drug-induced psychosis? *Am J Med Genet B Naeuropsychiatr Genet.* 2013; 162B:661-70.
126. Vollenweider FX, Hell D. Psilocybin induces schizophrenia-like psychosis in humans via a serotonin-2 agonist action. *Neuroreport.* 1998; 9:3897-902.
127. Marek GJ, Aghajanian GK. Indoleamine and the phenethylamine hallucinogens: mechanism of psychotomimetic action. *Drug Alcohol Depend.* 1998; 51:189-98.
128. Nelson ME, Bryant SM, Aks SE. Emerging drugs of abuse. *Emerg Med Clin North Am.* 2014; 31:1-28.
129. Baumann MH, Solis E Jr, Watterson L et al. Bath salts, spice and related designer drugs: The science behind the headlines. *J Neurosci.* 2014; 34:15150-8.
130. McKetin R, McLaren J, Lubman Di, Hides L. The prevalence of psychotic disorders among methamphetamine users. *Addiction.* 2006; 101:1473-8.
131. Arora RC, Meltzer HY. Serotonin 2 (5-HT) receptor binding in the prefrontal cortex of schizophrenic patients. *J Neural Transm.* 1991; 85:19-29.

132. Gurevich EV, Joyce JN. Alteration in the cortical serotonergic system in schizophrenia: a postmortem study. *Biol Psychiatry.* 1997; 42:529-45.
133. Joyce JN, Shane A, Lexow N et al. Serotonin uptake sites and serotonin receptors are altered in the limbic system of schizophrenics. *Neuropsychopharmacology.* 1993; 8:315-36.
134. Laruelle M, Abi-Dargham A, Casanova F et al. Selective abnormalities of prefrontal serotonergic receptors in schizophrenia. *Arch Gen Psychaitry.* 1993; 50:810-8.
135. Schott K, Schaefer JE, Richartz E et al. Autoantibodies to serotonin in serum of patients with psychiatric disorders. *Psychiatry Res.* 2003; 121:51-7.
136. Juckel G, Gallinat J, Riedel M et al. Serotonergic dysfunction in schizophrenia assessed by the loudness dependence measure of primary auditory cortex evoked activity. *Schizophr Res.* 2003; 64:115-24.
137. Anis NA, Berry SC, Burton NR, Lodge D. The dissociative anesthetics, ketamine and phencyclidine selectively reduce excitation of central mammalian neurons by *N*-methyl-D-aspartate. *Br J Pharmacol.* 1983; 79:565-75.
138. de Bartolemeis A, Sarappa C, Buonaguro EF et al. Different effects of the NMDA receptor antagonists ketamine, MK-801, and memantine on postsynaptic density transcripts and their topography: role of Homer signaling, and implications for novel antipsychotic and pro-cognitive targets in psychosis. *Prog Neuropsychopharmacol Biol Psychiatry* 2013; 46:1-12.
139. Di Maria E, Gulli R, Begni S et al. Variations in the NMDA receptor subunit 2B gene (GRIN2B) and schizophrenia: a case-control study. *Am J Med Genet.* 2004; 128B:27-9.
140. Breese GR, Knapp DJ, Moy SS. Integrative role for serotonergic and glutamatergic receptor mechanisms in the action of NMDA antagonists: potential relationships to antipsychotic drug actions on NMDA antagonist responsiveness. *Neurosci Biobehav Rev.* 2002; 26:441-55.
141. Woo TU, Walsh JP, Benes FM. Density of glutamic acid decarboxylase 67 messenger RNA-containing neurons that express the *N*-methyl-D-aspartate receptor subunit NR2A in the anterior cingulate cortex in schizophrenia and bipolar disorder. *Arch Gen Psychiatry.* 2004; 61:649-57.
142. Anwyl R. Metabotropic glutamate receptors. Electrophysiological properties and role in plasticity. *Brain Res Brain Res Rev.* 1999; 29:83-120.
143. Garver DL. Evolution of antipsychotic intervention in the schizophrenic psychosis. *Curr Drug Targets* 2006; 7:1207-15.
144. Mathais S, Lubman DI, Hides L. Substance-induced psychosis: a diagnostic conundrum. *J Clin Psych.* 2008; e1-10.
145. Moeller KE, Lee KC, Kissack JC. Urine drug screening: a practical guide for clinicians. *Mayo Clin Proc.* 2008; 83:66-76.
146. Salvatore P, Baldessarini RJ, Tohen M et al. McLean-Harvard international first-episode project: two-year stability of ICD-10 diagnoses in 500 first-episode psychotic disorder patients. *J Clin Psychiatry.* 2011; 72:189-93.
147. Arciniegas DB, Topkoff J, Silver JM. Neuropsychiatric aspects of traumatic brain injury. *Curr Treat Options Neurol.* 2000; 2:169-86.
148. Hurley RA, Taber KH. Emotional disturbances following traumatic brain injury. *Curr Treat Options Neurol.* 2002; 4:59-75.
149. Sternbach H, State R. Antibiotics: neuropsychiatric effects and psychotropic interactions. *Harv Rev Psychiatry.* 1997; 5:214-26.
150. Chien JY, Mohutsky MA, Wrighton SA. Physiological approaches to the prediction of drug-drug interactions in study populations. *Curr Drug Metab.* 2003; 4:347-56.
151. Gandhi M, Aweeka F, Greenblatt RM, Blaschke TE. Sex differences in pharmacokinetics and pharmacodynamics. *Annu Rev Pharmacol Toxicol.* 2004; 44:499-523.
152. Ingelman-Sundberg M. Pharmacogenomics of the cytochrome P450 and its application in drug therapy: the past, present and future. *Trends Pharmacol Sci.* 2004: 25:193-200.
153. Ley RH, Hachad H, Yao C, Ragueneau-Majlessi I. Relationship between extent of inhibition and inhibitor dose: literature evaluation based on the metabolism and transport drug interaction database. *Curr Drug Metab.* 2003; 4:371-80.
154. Cowen JP. Toxic psychosis with antihistamines reversed by physostigmine. *Postgrad Med J.* 1979; 55:556-57.
155. Hazlett SB, McCarthy ML, Londner MS, Onyike CU. Epidemiology of adult psychiatric visits to US emergency departments. *Acad Emerg Med.* 2004; 11:193-5.
156. Kaufman DW, Kelly JP, Rosenberg L et al. Recent patterns of medication use in the ambulatory adult population of the United States: the Slone survey. *JAMA.* 2002; 287:337-44.
157. Eisenberg DM, Davis RB, Ettner SL et al. Trends in alternative medicine use in the United States, 1990–1997: results of a follow-up national survey. *JAMA.* 1998; 280:1569-75.
158. Rickels K, DeMartinis N, Rynn M, Mandos L. Pharmacologic strategies for discontinuing benzodiazepine treatment. *J Clin Psychopharmacol.* 1999; 19(suppl 2):12S-16S.
159. Klein C, Gordon J, Pollak L et al. Clozapine in Parkinson's disease psychosis: 5-year follow-up review. *Clin Neuropharmacol.* 2003; 26:8-11.
160. Parkinson's Study Group. Low-dose clozapine for the treatment of drug-induced psychosis in Parkinson's disease. *New Eng J Med.* 1999; 340:757-63.
161. Kelly AM, Kerr D, Dietze P et al. Randomised trial of intranasal versus intramuscular naloxone in prehospital treatment for suspected opioid overdose. *Med J Aust.* 2005; 182:24-7.
162. Teoh R, Page AV, Hardern R. Physostigmine as treatment for severe CNS anticholinergic toxicity. *Emerg Med J.* 2001; 18:412.
163. Weinbroum AA, Flaishon R, Sorkine P et al. A risk benefit assessment of flumazenil in the management of benzodiazepine overdose. *Drug Saf.* 1997; 17:181-96.
164. Amato L, Davoli M, Ferri M, Ali R. Methadone at tapered doses for the management of opioid withdrawal. *Cochrane Database Syst Rev.* 2003;CD003409.

SECTION V

DRUG-INDUCED PULMONARY DISEASES

CHAPTER 21 Interstitial Lung Disease/Pulmonary Fibrosis

CHAPTER 22 Asthma and Bronchospasm

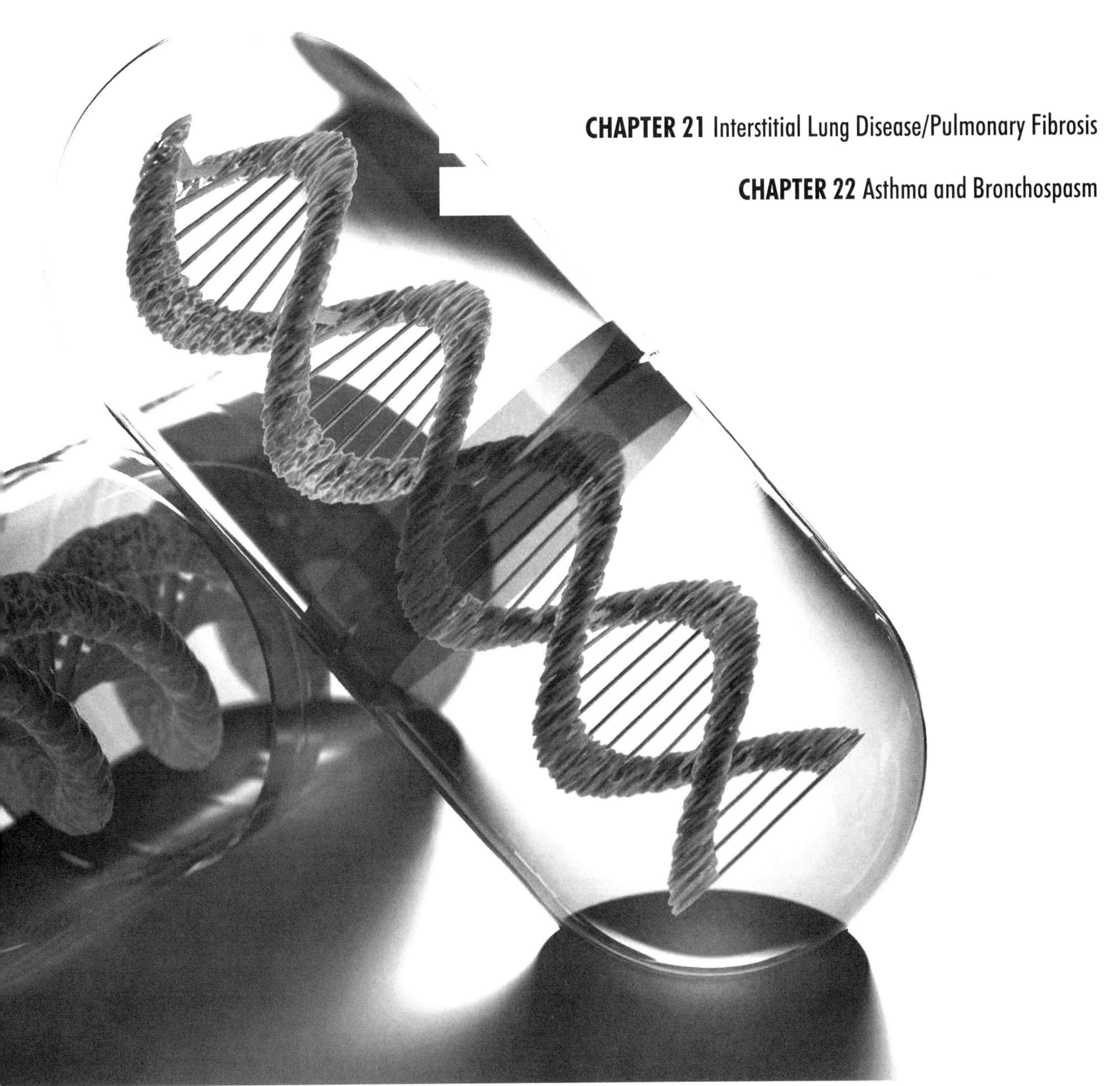

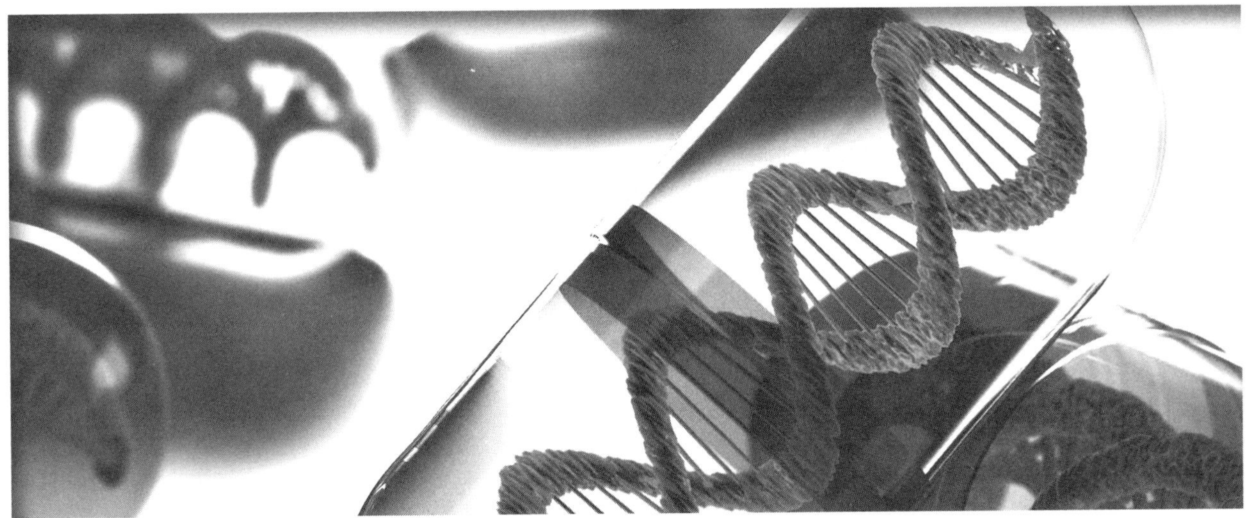

CHAPTER 21

Interstitial Lung Disease/ Pulmonary Fibrosis

Jordan R. Covvey and Erin E. Mancl

Interstitial lung disease (ILD) is a collection of more than 300 related lung disorders with diverse pathophysiology that result in progressive thickening/scarring of the tissue surrounding the alveolar sacs. ILD is broadly split into those disorders with known etiology (approximately 35% of cases), and those of idiopathic origin (65%).[1] Drug-induced ILD falls within the former category as an identifiable cause, alongside environmental exposures, autoimmune diseases, cancer, and certain infections. ILD can exist both acutely and/or subacutely as pneumonitis, or may progress over time to chronic pulmonary fibrosis, which is generally irreversible. Although they are separate entities by classification, drug-induced ILD demonstrates some clinical overlap with the most common form of idiopathic ILD, idiopathic pulmonary fibrosis (IPF). In 2014, the U.S. Food and Drug Administration (FDA) approved the first two therapies specifically indicated for the treatment of IPF, ushering in a hopeful era for the treatment for ILD. This chapter will discuss pertinent aspects of drug-induced ILD, with additional discussion of IPF where appropriate.

CAUSATIVE AGENTS

A wide array of drugs have been identified as causing pulmonary toxicity of several types, such as edema, hemorrhaging, pleural disorders, and vasculopathies. For quick reference, an updated online database of drug-induced and iatrogenic causes of pulmonary toxicity can be found at http://www.pneumotox.com, which currently includes over 1,100 identified agents and 23,000 references.[2] Drugs can be searched by name and are listed by the pattern of drug-induced pulmonary toxicity reported in the literature (covering 20 types and hundreds of subclassifications) as well as notation of how many cases have been reported (<10, 10–50, 50–100, 100–200 or >200 cases). Therapies identified as potential causes of drug-induced ILD populate a large list and encompass a number of different mechanisms and chemical structures (**Table 21-1**).[3-298] The most common therapeutic category associated with drug-induced ILD is cytotoxic (chemotherapeutic) agents, including bleomycin, busulfan, and cyclophosphamide, among others. Because many cancer

Table 21-1 Agents Implicated in Drug-Induced Interstitial Lung Disease/Pulmonary Fibrosis

Drug	Incidence	Level of Evidence[a]
Amiodarone[3-19]	1–15%	A
Anagrelide[20-22]	NK	C
Antiandrogens[23]		
Bicalutamide[24-28]	NK	C
Flutamide[29-30]	NK	C
Nilutamide[31-33]	NK	C
Aurothiopropanosulfonate (gold salt)[34-36]	NK	C
Azacitidine[37-40]	NK	C
Bepridil[41-44]	3.6%	B
Bleomycin[45-53]	3–40%	A
Bromocriptine[54-61]	1–5.7%	B
Busulfan[62-77]	3–29%	B
Chlorambucil[78-86]	NK	C
Cyclophosphamide[87-97]	1%	B
EGFR inhibitors		
Cetuximab[98-102]	1–1.7%	A
Erlotinib[103-107]	0.4–1%	B
Gefitinib[107-109]	0.3–4%	A
Panitumumab[110-112]	1–1.3%	A
Vandetanib[113]	NK	C
Gemcitabine[114-121]	0.6–7.6%	B
HMG-CoA reductase inhibitors[122-124]	NK	C
Hydroxyurea[125-127]	NK	C
Interferon[128-131]	NK	B
Lenalidomide[132-134]	NK	B
Melphalan[135-140]	NK	C
Methotrexate[141-158]	1–7%	A
Methysergide[159-164]	NK	C
Mitomycin C[165-172]	5–17.6%	B
mTOR inhibitors		
Everolimus[173-175]	13.5%–23%	A
Temsirolimus[176-179]	2–29%	A
Mycophenolate mofetil[180-182]	NK	C
Nitrofurantoin[183-211]	0.02%	B
Nitrosoureas		
Carmustine (BCNU)[212-228]	10–30%	B
Lomustine (CCNU)[229-234]	NK	C
Oxaliplatin[235,236]	NK	C
Pemetrexed[237,238]	NK	C
Penicillamine[239-245]	3%	B
Procarbazine[246-248]	NK	C
Rituximab[249-251]	3.7–10%	B
Sirolimus[252-254]	5–16.7%	B
Sulfasalazine[255-263]	NK	C

Table 21-1 Agents Implicated in Drug-Induced Interstitial Lung Disease/Pulmonary Fibrosis (continued)

Drug	Incidence	Level of Evidence[a]
Taxanes		
Docetaxel[264-266]	1–5.3%	A
Paclitaxel[267,268]	0–6%	B
TK inhibitors		
Imatinib[269-278]	NK	C
Sorafenib[279-281]	NK	C
Sunitinib[282-284]	NK	C
TNFα inhibitors[155,285-287]		
Adalimumab[288-291]	NK	B
Etanercept[292-296]	NK	B
Infliximab[297,298]	NK	B

BCNU = bis-chloroethylnitrosourea, CCNU = 1-(2-chloroethyl)-3-cyclohexyl-1-nitrosourea, EGFR = epidermal growth factor receptor, HMG-CoA = 3-hydroxy-3-methylglutaryl-coenzyme A, mTOR = mammalian target of rapamycin, NK = not known, TK = tyrosine kinase, TNFα = tumor necrosis factor alpha.

[a]Definitions for Levels of Evidence: Level A—evidence from one or more randomized, controlled clinical trials; Level B—evidence from nonrandomized clinical trials, prospective observational studies, cohort studies, retrospective studies, case-control studies, meta-analyses and/or postmarketing surveillance studies; and Level C—evidence from one or more published case reports or case series.

chemotherapy regimens utilize combination therapies, in some cases, pinpointing the causative agent is difficult. For instance, both FOLFOX (folinic acid, fluorouracil, and oxaliplatin) and FOLFIRI (folinic acid, fluorouracil, and irinotecan) regimens for colorectal cancer have been associated with drug-induced ILD, but the precise pharmacological cause in these cases is unclear.[299] Beyond cancer chemotherapy drugs, causative agents include many others, including cardiovascular drugs, anti-inflammatory agents, antimicrobials, biologics, and miscellaneous therapies.[300] Notably, several newer molecularly targeted class-wide effects of interest pertaining to drug-induced ILD have emerged recently, including tumor necrosis factor alpha (TNFα) inhibitors and epidermal growth factor receptor (EGFR) inhibitors. There are limited data associating nonprescription drugs and herbal supplements with drug-induced ILD. However, there are reports linking illicit drugs such as cocaine and heroin with ILD, but the association is somewhat tenuous, and therefore, they are not included in this chapter.[2]

EPIDEMIOLOGY

Estimates of the incidence and prevalence of drug-induced ILD are limited due to the rare nature of the disease and the fact that the diagnosis is one of exclusion. Identification of a single therapeutic agent as a definitive cause is difficult in concert with other confounding factors, such as comorbid disease states and therapies, which may compound risk such as immunosuppressive agents and/or radiation therapy. For instance, in one systematic review of ILD among patients with rheumatoid arthritis, over 40% of patients had disease-related ILD prior to exacerbation that was subsequently attributed to TNFα therapy.[155] Therefore, the actual incidence of drug-induced ILD may be greatly underestimated. An important registry of patients with ILD established in New Mexico estimated the incidence and prevalence of drug/radiation-induced ILD to be 1.1–1.8 per 100,000 annually and 1.2–2.2 per 100,000, respectively.[301] ILD associated with drugs or radiation accounted for 2–3% of ILD cases overall, which is the most commonly cited estimate for drug-induced ILD.[301] A more recent epidemiological study using the United Kingdom (UK)-based General Practice Research Database identified an incidence of drug and radiation-induced ILD of 4.1 per 1,000,000 person-years (95% CI 3.4–4.9) from 1997–2008, with only 17% of included cases resulting from drug therapy (the remainder from radiation).[302] IPF is one of the most common forms of ILD.[303] The prevalence of IPF in the United States has been estimated from 4 to 27.9 per 100,000 to as high as 42.7 to 63 per 100,000, depending on the specificity of case definitions.[304] Similarly, incidence estimates were reported at 6.8–8.8 per 100,000 using narrow diagnostic criteria and 16.3–17.4 per 100,000 with broader criteria.[304] Despite these more defined estimates, there is a call for an international registry of patients with IPF, a movement that could also greatly enhance epidemiological estimates of drug-induced ILD.[305] Benefits associated with such a registry could include identification of key comorbidities, characterization of natural disease course, and provision of evidence to support advances in care.[305]

The incidence of ILD associated with specific drugs (Table 21-1) varies widely. Because ILD includes both pneumonitis and fibrosis, estimates can be inconsistent as pneumonitis is encountered more commonly. As mentioned previously, combined use of many of the implicated agents also renders incidence estimates variable. Lastly, most estimates of drug-induced ILD are obtained from case reports and observational studies, which can make identification of the true incidence difficult. For instance, the incidence of pulmonary toxicity associated with bleomycin in one study was estimated at 6.8%; however, this effect was highly dose dependent, with higher doses conferring a hazard ratio (HR) of 4.3 (95% CI 2.2–8.2) compared to lower doses.[306] Carmustine-induced lung injury follows a similar pattern and also appears more common in females due to differences in pharmacokinetics.[212] The incidence of ILD among patients treated with gefitinib has been estimated to be as high as 8% among Japanese patients in clinical trials but significantly lower (<1%) in other parts of the world, possibly as a result of differences in genetic susceptibility.[307]

MECHANISMS

The precise mechanism of drug-induced ILD is not well elucidated, although existing data have produced some theories regarding the pathophysiology. In IPF, it was originally hypothesized that fibrosis was the result of longstanding intra-alveolar inflammation and subsequent induction of fibrogenesis.[308] However, current research supports the concept that fibrosis may actually result from injury to alveolar epithelial cells and an induced state of abnormal wound healing.[308] Under this theory, microinjuries to the epithelium promote formation of a wound clot, increase secretion of growth factors, and increase proliferation of fibroblasts to the site of injury. Neovascularization develops, extracellular matrix is deposited, and alveolar epithelial cell death occurs, resulting in fibrosis.[308]

In drug-induced ILD, mechanisms may vary according to therapeutic class of the inciting agent (**Table 21-2**), as well as the patient's inherent genetic susceptibility.[121,124,133,236,309-314] It should be noted that the majority of proposed mechanisms of drug-induced ILD are theories at best, with limited evidence for confirmation. However, despite the fact that drugs may differ with respect to the events induced prior to lung insult, it is conceivable that drugs induce ILD via the same pathophysiological pathway as IPF, resulting in the similar appearance of fibrotic lesions from a radiological and histopathological perspective. The pathophysiology underlying drug-induced pneumonitis and fibrosis generally progresses over weeks to months, although the onset may be more rapid (days to weeks) for drugs with a hypersensitivity-type component associated with the induced pulmonary injury.[315]

CLINICAL PRESENTATION AND DIFFERENTIAL DIAGNOSIS

The reduced lung compliance that is characteristic of pulmonary fibrosis is similar to that which occurs in other restrictive lung diseases. Therefore, the diagnosis of drug-induced ILD requires a thorough clinical history and exclusion of other known causes of ILD. The signs and symptoms of drug-induced ILD are listed in **Table 21-3**. Nearly all patients present with dyspnea, and some also experience a nonproductive cough.[316] The onset varies from days to weeks or even years, and is usually correlated with the duration of therapy with the causative agent. For instance, short-term use of an offending medication is more likely to present with acute onset ILD, whereas chronic therapy is likely to be associated with gradual development of symptoms, which the patient may or may not immediately

Table 21-2 Mechanisms of Drug-Induced Interstitial Lung Disease/Pulmonary Fibrosis

Drug	Mechanism(s)
Nitrofurantoin	Generation of free oxygen radicals[309]
Methotrexate	Hypersensitivity reaction[310,311] Generation of free oxygen radicals[309]
Bleomycin	Activation of immune cells and inflammatory cascade Generation of free oxygen radicals[312] Deficiency of hydrolase activity[313]
Paclitaxel, docetaxel	Delayed hypersensitivity reaction[314]
EGFR inhibitors	Impairment of alveolar repair mechanisms[309]
Oxaliplatin	Depletion of glutathione[236]
Gemcitabine	Systemic release of cytokines causing endothelial dysfunction[309] Radiosensitizer[121]
Amiodarone	Induction of phospholipidosis[312] Disruption of lysosomal membranes through protein C activation and release of toxic oxygen radicals[309]
Lenalidomide	Prostaglandin inhibition and fibroblast proliferation[133]
HMG-CoA reductase inhibitors	Induction of phospholipidosis[124]

EGFR = epidermal growth factor receptor, HMG-CoA = 3-hydroxy-3-methylglutaryl-coenzyme A.

Table 21-3 Signs and Symptoms Associated with Drug-Induced Interstitial Lung Disease/Pulmonary Fibrosis

Signs/Symptoms

- Dyspnea (at rest and/or exertional)
- Nonproductive cough
- Crackles in lung bases
- Rash
- Wheezing
- Fatigue
- Digital clubbing
- Cyanosis
- Pulmonary hypertension
  - Peripheral edema
  - Right ventricular enlargement or failure
- Chest radiograph
  - Diffuse ground glass opacity
- HRCT
  - Diffuse opacity
  - Honeycombing
- PFTs
  - Reduced TLC or FVC
  - Reduced DL_{CO} >15% from baseline
- Laboratory tests
  - Leukocytosis
  - Eosinophilia
  - Elevated ESR

DL_{CO} = diffusion capacity of the lungs for carbon monoxide, ESR = erythrocyte sedimentation rate, FVC = forced vital capacity, HRCT = high resolution computed tomography, PFT = pulmonary function test, TLC = total lung capacity.

recognize. With acute forms of drug-induced ILD, pneumonitis usually presents with acute shortness of breath, often with rash, wheezing, and peripheral eosinophilia. For more chronic ILD, progressive dyspnea and reduced exercise tolerance are commonly encountered. On physical examination, digital clubbing is present in 25–50% of patients, and end expiratory crackles are detected on auscultation in more than 80% of cases of IPF.[317] After progression to fibrosis, cyanosis and signs of pulmonary hypertension such as right ventricular dysfunction or peripheral edema may also be present.

Pulmonary function tests (PFTs), widely obtained through the use of spirometry (which can be performed in office-based settings), should be completed during the diagnostic evaluation and monitoring for drug-induced ILD. Key measures include forced vital capacity (FVC; the amount of air forcefully exhaled after a full inspiration) and forced expiratory volume in one second (FEV_1; the amount of air expired in the first second of the FVC test). PFTs progress from normal to a restrictive pattern (reduced total lung capacity [TLC] and FVC) with the addition of reduced carbon monoxide diffusing capacity (DL_{CO}).[318] A reduced DL_{CO} by more than 15% from baseline indicates a pathologic disturbance of alveolar-capillary interface and resultant disruption of gas exchange, and should prompt further assessment. In practice, patients presenting with advanced ILD are often too deconditioned to perform PFTs, and arterial oxygen saturation is determined instead. Hypoxia at rest and with exertion is observed commonly.

Chest imaging should be obtained to diagnose drug-induced ILD. A chest radiograph may be useful to exclude edema or infection and is performed commonly, but it is neither sensitive nor specific for the diagnosis of drug-induced ILD.[318] In fully developed fibrosis, a chest radiograph reveals diffuse "ground glass" opacity and reduced lung volumes.[300] High resolution computed tomography (HRCT) is now a standard test in patients with suspected ILD. HRCT is 90% accurate in diagnosis of IPF and, when coupled with clinical findings and history, 60–80% accurate in diagnosis of drug-induced ILD.[317,318] The histopathological criteria for IPF are those of usual interstitial pneumonia, characterized by a honeycombing pattern from the subpleural cystic airspaces formed.

Bronchoscopy may be performed to obtain bronchoalveolar lavage samples with which to exclude infection and malignancy. Cell differentials with a lymphocytic, neutrophilic, or eosinophilic pattern can be useful for diagnosis when combined with clinical and radiographic data.[300] Transbronchial biopsies are not usually performed, as these tissue samples are too small to allow histological classification of ILD other than sarcoidosis. An open lung biopsy is definitive in the diagnosis of drug-induced ILD; however, it is not often a practical approach in patients with advanced ILD as the procedure can be associated with respiratory compromise, acute exacerbations, pulmonary hypertension, and increased mortality.

In general, laboratory data are not helpful in establishing the diagnosis of drug-induced ILD. Patients may have an elevated white blood cell count with increased eosinophils; however, absence of eosinophilia does not exclude the diagnosis.[318] Amiodarone-induced pulmonary toxicity is often associated with an elevated erythrocyte sedimentation rate; however, this does not contribute meaningfully to the diagnosis.[319] Testing for antinuclear antibodies, anticytoplasmic antibodies, and antiglomerular basal membrane autoantibodies is essential if there is concern regarding the potential for diffuse alveolar hemorrhage, as these antibodies differentiate autoimmune versus nonautoimmune causes.[319]

Because drug-induced ILD is a diagnosis of exclusion, there are several considerations in the differential diagnosis (**Table 21-4**), which may only be distinguished by a positive history of exposure to a causative agent. The symptoms, physical findings, laboratory information, and imaging studies are similar in nearly all types of ILD including connective tissue disease with pulmonary fibrosis, IPF, and certain pneumonias such as those induced by viruses or *Pneumocystis jiroveci*.[31] It should be noted that patients with drug-induced ILD often have pre-existing conditions that increase their risk of lung injury (**Table 21-5**). One proposed set of criteria for the diagnosis of carmustine-induced ILD, which may be applicable to other types of drug-induced ILD, are (1) typical symptoms of nonproductive cough and dyspnea with or without fever; (2) decrease of DL_{CO} capacity by >10% as compared with baseline; and (3) no clinical evidence of active pulmonary infection.[320]

Table 21-4 Conditions to Consider in the Differential Diagnosis of Drug-Induced Interstitial Lung Disease/Pulmonary Fibrosis

Conditions

- Acute respiratory distress syndrome
- Aspiration pneumonitis
- Bronchiolitis obliterans organizing pneumonia (nondrug-induced)
- Connective tissue disease–related pulmonary fibrosis
- Heart failure
- Hyperthyroidism
- Hypoxemia
- Idiopathic pneumonia syndrome after bone marrow transplantation
- Idiopathic pulmonary fibrosis
- Miliary tuberculosis
- *Pneumocystis jiroveci* pneumonia
- Radiation pneumonitis
- Systemic lupus erythematosus
- Viral infection
- Wegener granulomatosis

Table 21-5 Risk Factors for Drug-Induced Interstitial Lung Disease/Pulmonary Fibrosis

Risk factors

- Age (young or old)
- Concomitant use of other cytotoxic drugs
- Dose
    - Amiodarone >400 mg daily
    - Carmustine >1,400 mg/m^2 cumulative
    - Bleomycin >360 units cumulative
- Drug interactions (increased drug concentration or concomitant use of drugs that compound risk)
- Environmental factors (e.g. asbestos, cigarette smoke)
- Genetic factors
- Oxygen therapy (high concentration, e.g., 60% or more FiO_2)
- Radiation therapy (mantle, thoracic, total body)
- Underlying obstructive or restrictive lung disease

FiO_2 = fraction of inspired oxygen.

RISK FACTORS

In general, the likelihood of developing pulmonary toxicity from drugs is unpredictable. Although several risk factors have been identified (Table 21-5), none are consistent for all drugs or patient populations. Patients at risk of developing drug-induced ILD include those with cancer or inflammatory conditions receiving chemotherapy or concurrent therapy with multiple toxic agents. Dose-related toxic effects have been identified in the development of drug-induced ILD for several drugs. Risk factors for lung toxicity associated with amiodarone are a combination of daily dose (>400 mg daily) and duration of therapy (cumulative dose).[319] The risk for pulmonary toxicity is greatest at cumulative doses above 1,400 mg/m^2 for carmustine and above 360 units for bleomycin.[46,216] However, ILD has also been reported at low doses of these drugs, and therefore a strong association between dose and pulmonary toxicity does not always exist. In general, extremes of age can be associated with an increased risk of lung toxicity, depending on the drug. The incidence of bleomycin-induced pulmonary fibrosis increases in patients older than 70 years of age, possibly as a result of diminished antioxidant defenses and impaired drug clearance.[45,306] Conversely, an inverse relationship between age and carmustine-induced pulmonary toxicity has been suggested, with patients under 7 years of age at greatest risk.[214,216]

Environmental factors, such as exposure to asbestos and cigarette smoke, can increase the risk of pulmonary toxicity. It is unknown whether a history of pulmonary adverse effects associated with a specific drug or related compounds increases the risk for future lung toxicity. Certain genetic and other factors may be important in the development of drug-induced ILD. Acute and organizing diffuse alveolar damage associated with bortezomib was first reported in Japan and then in African-American patients, and higher rates of gefitinib-induced ILD have been noted for Japanese patients compared to other populations.[307,321,322] Genetic polymorphisms may explain some differences in drug toxicity across populations, but intrinsic and disease-related sensitivity to ILD in general may cloud the picture. For instance, Japanese patients with rheumatoid arthritis and the HLA-A*31:01 allele may be at higher risk of methotrexate-induced ILD, while HLA-B40, B54, and DR4 antigen sites have been related more generally to increased susceptibility for ILD in the setting of rheumatoid arthritis (for which methotrexate is a commonly used therapy).[323] Concomitant therapies and conditions that may influence the cytochrome P-450 system or detoxification pathways or alter pharmacokinetics of the offending agent may also increase risk of toxicity.[324] Concomitant therapy with radiation or high fractions of inspired oxygen (e.g., >60%) are associated with an increased risk of drug-induced ILD.[324] Radiation therapy can injure lung deoxyribonucleic acid (DNA) and proteins associated with lung tissue repair, which can exert a synergistic effect with drug-induced pulmonary toxicity. The risk associated with oxygen is similar, as higher concentrations of oxygen generate reactive metabolites, leading to further oxidative stress. Underlying disease is known to play a role, primarily in the presence of pre-existing pulmonary disease.[324] However, this association is controversial. The risk of bleomycin-induced pulmonary fibrosis may be increased in patients with kidney disease due to impaired drug clearance. A glomerular filtration rate of <80 mL/min was found to be an independent risk factor for development of bleomycin-induced pulmonary toxicity.[306]

MORBIDITY AND MORTALITY

The morbidity associated with drug-induced ILD from personal, societal, or financial perspectives has not been described; however, it is likely substantial due to the potential impact of pulmonary symptomology (dyspnea, persistent cough, etc.) on the ability to work and conduct activities of daily living. Some data describing healthcare utilization specific to IPF are available. In one case-control analysis, patients with IPF incurred all-cause hospitalizations (0.5/person/year), hospital days (3.1 days/person/year), and outpatient visits (28 visits/person/year) at approximately twice the rate of controls, with an extrapolated incremental IPF-associated cost estimated at over $1 billion/year.[325]

Mortality figures for ILD are imprecise for a number of reasons, including comorbidities in patients that may render the cause of death unclear (lung cancer, cerebrovascular disease, pneumonias) or the lack of a classification system for the various forms of ILD.[301] Pulmonary fibrosis (both idiopathic and otherwise), as the progressive endpoint of ILD, has generated some global figures. Using data from the National Center for Health Statistics, median survival for patients with pulmonary fibrosis was estimated to be 3–5 years, with an average age- and sex-adjusted mortality rate of 50.8 per 1,000,000.[326] Mortality was higher among men, although deaths in women increased at a faster rate (41.3%) over the 1992–2003 study period compared to men (28.4%).[326] In the UK-based study of drug- and radiation-induced ILD, the risk of death was found to be 7 times greater (HR 7.13, 95% CI 3.40–14.93) among those with ILD compared to population-matched controls.[302]

Because of the heterogeneity of conditions under the ILD umbrella, a multidimensional index—the modified gender, age, and physiology (GAP) model—has been created to predict mortality in patients with ILD.[327,328] First established specifically for IPF and then generalized to other ILD, the model assigns points based on gender, age, and physiology including FVC % predicted and DL_{CO} % predicted as well as subtype of ILD.[328] Scores can then be correlated to 1-, 2- and 3-year predicted mortality rates.[328] For instance, a nonelderly woman with IPF and preserved lung function could expect a 1-year mortality rate of 3.1%, compared to 18.2% in an elderly man with the same condition but with pulmonary function at 50% of predicted.[328] This tool may help clinicians better evaluate patients with ILD; however, it should be noted that this index is not specific to drug-induced forms of ILD and may only be applicable broadly.

Mortality rates for ILD induced by specific drugs are of greater pertinence. Mortality due to pneumonitis associated with bleomycin has been estimated at approximately 10 to 20%.[329] Among a case series literature review of 123 patients with methotrexate-induced pneumonitis, the respiratory-related fatality rate was 13%.[142] Mortality due to amiodarone-induced pneumonitis has been estimated at 10%, although it may be 2–3 times higher in those requiring hospital admission.[14] A recent review of seven classes of targeted therapies for non-small-cell lung cancer (EGFR inhibitors, anaplastic lymphoma kinase inhibitors, angiogenesis inhibitors, tyrosine kinase [TK] inhibitors, human epidermal growth factor receptor 2 [HER2] inhibitors, anti-CD20 antibodies, and mammalian target of rapamycin inhibitors) reported a wide range of mortality rates.[330] For instance, among reports of ILD induced by gefitinib, erlotinib, and sorafenib, mortality rates were estimated at >30%, while ILD-related deaths among patients receiving rituximab, temsirolimus, and everolimus were significantly less common.[330]

PREVENTION

Prevention of drug-induced ILD should focus on avoidance of potentially causative agents in patients who are at risk and careful selection for use in other populations. Other general strategies are summarized in **Table 21-6**. In general, the lowest effective dose of a drug should be utilized so as to avoid excessive exposure and additional associated risk of drug-induced ILD. Beyond careful dose selection, there remains minimal evidence supporting strategies for prevention or risk reduction.

Table 21-6 Approaches to Help Prevent Drug-Induced Interstitial Lung Disease/ Pulmonary Fibrosis

Prevention and early detection

- Use lowest dose for shortest duration possible for desired effect
- Avoid combinations of drugs known to increase risk
- Frequent follow-up to monitor for symptoms of dyspnea and nonproductive cough
- PFTs and DL_{CO} at baseline and every 2 weeks to every 2–4 months for high-risk drugs
- Consider chest radiograph every 3–6 months for high-risk drugs
- Consider HRCT every 6 months for high-risk drugs
- Inhaled corticosteroids (fluticasone 880 mcg every 12 hours) for prophylaxis of carmustine-induced pulmonary toxicity

DL_{CO} = diffusion capacity of the lungs for carbon monoxide, HRCT = high resolution computed tomography, PFT = pulmonary function test.

All recommended strategies focus on frequent screening to maximize the likelihood of early diagnosis. In patients at risk for drug-induced ILD, pretreatment and routine on-treatment PFTs should be determined because a change may be indicative of toxicity development; however, reductions in TLC and FVC may not become evident until after disease is established. The measurement of DL_{CO} should be considered for patients taking drugs associated with a high incidence of pulmonary fibrosis (Table 21-1), although little is known about whether this reduces the incidence or simply aids in more prompt diagnosis.[331] In addition, the significance of asymptomatic reductions in DL_{CO} is unknown. Monitoring frequency is largely left to the discretion of health-care providers and tends to be both patient-specific and drug-dependent, with usual frequency of every 2 weeks to every 2–4 months.[332] The positive predictive value of serial DL_{CO} monitoring with spirometry for amiodarone-induced pulmonary toxicity is 21%.[333] Despite this low value, it is recommended to consider chest radiography, PFTs, and DL_{CO} monitoring prior to initiation of therapy and every 3–6 months in patients taking maintenance amiodarone therapy.[319] Monitoring of DL_{CO} and PFTs is probably less likely to detect early disease for patients taking drugs with lower rates of pulmonary fibrosis. As discussed previously, HRCT is a more sensitive test for diagnosis of drug-induced ILD, but there is no evidence supporting HRCT in the routine monitoring for drug-induced pneumonitis.[9]

Limited options exist for pharmacologic prevention of drug-induced ILD. Inhaled corticosteroids have been studied for prophylaxis of carmustine-associated lung toxicity in patients with breast cancer.[334] Inhaled fluticasone 880 mcg every 12 hours preserved pulmonary function and decreased the incidence of pulmonary toxicity in patients with breast cancer treated with a conditioning regimen of cyclophosphamide, cisplatin, and carmustine for autologous stem cell transplantation.[335] Some prevention strategies for drug-induced ILD with other medications show early promise. Inhibition of HER2 with recombinant monoclonal antibodies may reduce the risk of bleomycin-induced pulmonary toxicity.[336] In addition, thalidomide reduced the incidence of bleomycin-induced pulmonary toxicity in a mouse model, possibly due to its known inhibitory effect on interleukin-6–dependent cell growth.[337] Finally, two therapies in development, JNJ7777120 plus naproxen and NCX 466, which target a dual mechanism with a cyclooxygenase inhibitor and nitric oxide donor, both reduced incidence of bleomycin-induced pulmonary fibrosis.[338,339] However, further research in prevention strategies for ILD associated with all causative medications continues to be warranted.

MANAGEMENT

The goals of drug-induced ILD management include early detection, discontinuation of the causative agent, and, in some cases, initiating corticosteroid therapy. Monitoring for signs and symptoms of drug-induced pulmonary fibrosis is essential, in view of the fact that, in most documented cases, a positive clinical response has been reported within the first 7–10 days after discontinuing the causative agent and initiating therapy with corticosteroids. In some cases, positive response may occur even sooner. Acute episodes of drug-induced ILD such as pneumonitis may resolve within 48 hours after discontinuation of the causative agent. However, pulmonary fibrosis may take longer to resolve, if improvement occurs at all. The primary goal of any treatment option is to inhibit the inflammatory response and prevent deposition and progression of fibrotic tissue. Extrapolating guidelines for management of IPF, a favorable response is depicted by a decrease in symptoms, reduction in parenchymal abnormalities on HRCT, and two or more of the following: (1) >10% increase in TLC or FVC, (2) >15% improvement in DL_{CO}, or (3) improvement or normalization of oxygen saturation (>4% increase) or partial pressure of oxygen (>4 mm Hg from previous measurement) achieved during a formal cardiopulmonary exercise test.[317] If improvement does not occur, however, referral to a lung transplantation center is an important consideration, given that some patients with IPF or drug-induced ILD benefit from a lung transplant.[317]

Historically, corticosteroid therapy is regarded as the standard treatment for drug-induced ILD, although compelling evidence supporting this practice is lacking for most forms of ILD. Of note, standard doses of corticosteroid therapy have not been established, and the risk of adverse drug reactions such as immune system compromise, hypertension, hyperglycemia, fluid retention, and bone density alterations must be considered prior to initiation of therapy.

More data exist regarding treatment options for IPF than for drug-induced ILD. The American Thoracic Society (ATS) guidelines for IPF do not recommend the use of corticosteroid monotherapy or corticosteroids in combination with cyclophosphamide (a historic and empirically used therapy for IPF), due to the lack of evidence supporting any survival benefit.[317] Guidance also recommends against use of several other therapies including colchicine, imatinib, acetylcysteine alone or in combination with corticosteroids and azathioprine, or endothelin receptor antagonists.[317] The ATS guidelines, however, recommend the use of nintedanib or pirfenidone, two novel therapies approved for use in IPF in 2014.[317] Treatment with nintedanib, a TK inhibitor, has been associated with an increased likelihood of preserving lung function and fewer acute exacerbations in patients with mild-to-moderate IPF.[340,341] Pirfenidone is an oral antifibrotic medication associated with a reduction in mortality, FVC decline, and improved symptoms in patients with IPF.[342,343] It should be emphasized that these agents are currently only FDA-approved for use in IPF, and therefore other types of ILD (drug-induced or otherwise) are unapproved indications.

Treatment recommendations exist for ILD induced by specific drugs, including carmustine, bleomycin, and amiodarone. An algorithm to help guide treatment is provided in **Figure 21-1**. For management of carmustine-induced ILD, a clinical scoring system has been developed to determine the necessity for adjunctive corticosteroids during carmustine therapy for breast cancer.[334] Patients with a score ≥6 were initiated on prednisone therapy (60 mg twice daily for 10 days, followed by 30 mg daily for 1 week, then 20 mg daily for 1 week, with a gradual taper of 5 mg weekly until discontinuation), while patients with a score <6 were monitored weekly.[334] The prednisone regimen produced clinical improvement within 72 hours of initiation with no patients progressing to chronic pulmonary fibrosis or death.[334] Therefore, corticosteroids may inhibit development of carmustine-induced chronic pulmonary fibrosis when initiated upon early signs of acute toxicity.

For management of bleomycin-induced ILD, drug discontinuation and corticosteroid therapy are recommended. No specific doses have been studied, but prednisone 0.75–1 mg/kg daily for an initial 4–6 weeks (followed by a careful and gradual taper) to assess clinical response is a reasonable option. Drugs that have been investigated in animals include thalidomide, curcumin, aerosolized heparin, aerosolized urokinase, and oral acetylcysteine.[336,344-346] Pirfenidone therapy was initiated in two patients who experienced severe bleomycin pulmonary toxicity; however, both patients died.[347] Prospective trials are needed to better establish any potential benefit of drug therapy for treatment of bleomycin-induced ILD.

Some limited evidence supports the use of corticosteroids for the management of amiodarone-induced pulmonary toxicity. Amiodarone-induced lung injury can be particularly difficult to manage because some patients require continued treatment for refractory arrhythmia management, even in the presence

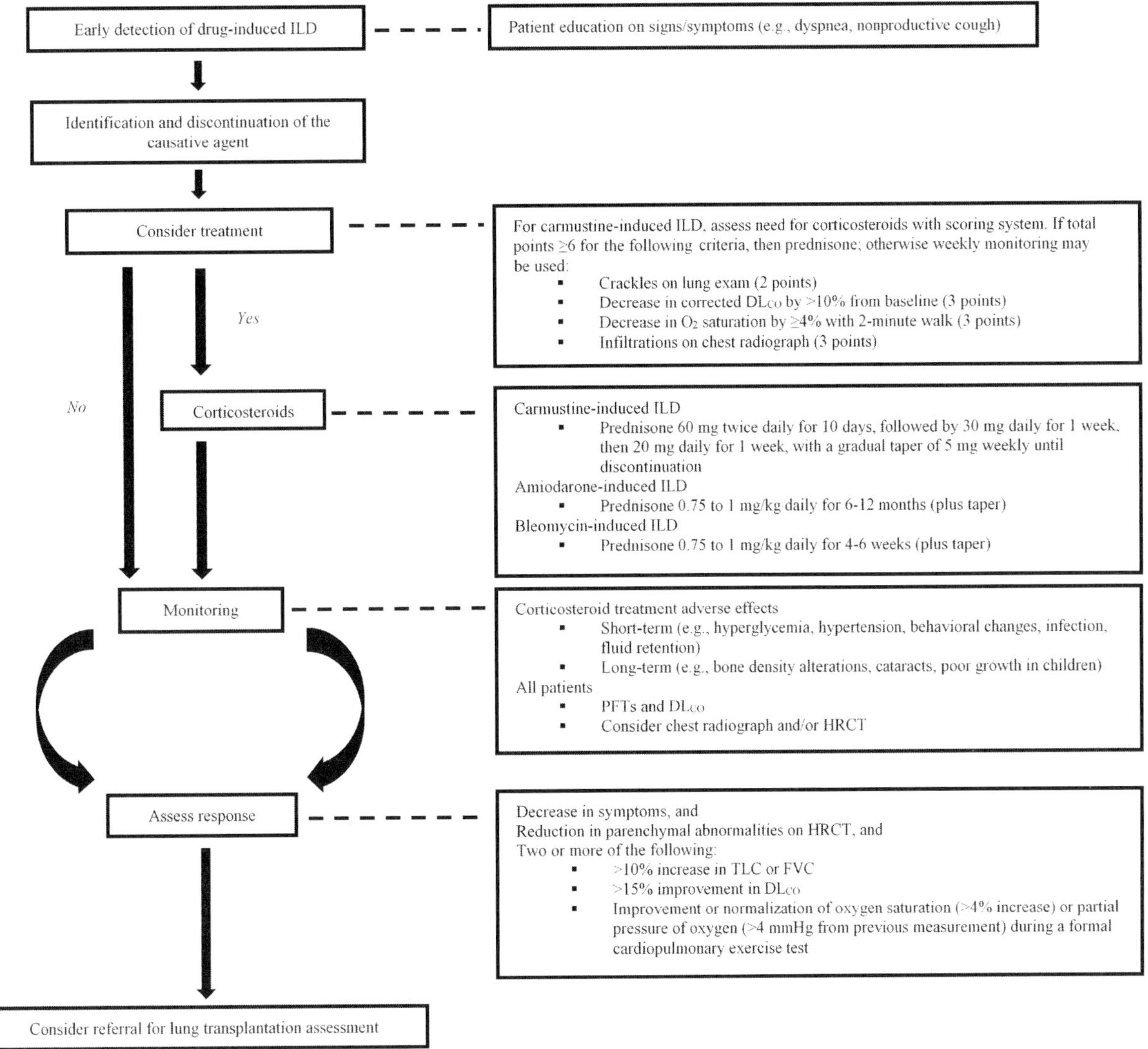

FIGURE 21-1 Treatment Algorithm for Selected Agents in Drug-Induced Interstitial Lung Disease/Pulmonary Fibrosis

DL_{CO} = diffusion capacity of the lungs for carbon monoxide, FVC = forced vital capacity, HRCT = high resolution computed tomography, ILD = interstitial lung disease, PFTs = pulmonary function tests, TLC = total lung capacity.

of pulmonary fibrosis. Prednisone (0.75–1 mg/kg daily) is often administered until clinical and radiographic improvement occurs, with tapering of therapy recommended. The total corticosteroid treatment duration for amiodarone-induced lung toxicity should be approximately 6–12 months, due to the long half-life of amiodarone and the risk of recurrence. Early discontinuation of corticosteroid therapy has resulted in recurrence of amiodarone-induced pulmonary fibrosis.[319]

INFORMATION FOR PATIENTS

Healthcare providers must guide patients in their understanding of the risk of drug-induced ILD. Patients should be reminded of the balance of risks and benefits of the associated therapies. Patients should understand the risk factors associated with drug-induced ILD, as well as the common symptoms of shortness of breath and nonproductive cough.[348] It should be emphasized to notify the prescriber immediately of any of these symptoms in order to detect early signs of pulmonary toxicity. All patients should be counseled to cease tobacco use prior to starting therapy with any medication associated with drug-induced ILD. Finally, in the event that drug-induced ILD occurs, providers should ensure patient understanding of the disease. All relevant medical specialties should weigh in on the decision regarding optimal therapies for the disease upon cessation of the offending agent. If patients receive corticosteroids, counseling regarding adverse effects and referrals for dietitian and exercise programs to manage these effects should be emphasized. Communication about drug-induced ILD between patients and their providers is critical for effective management due to the risk of rapid progression and high mortality rates associated with the disease.

REFERENCES

1. European Respiratory Society. Interstitial lung diseases. In: *European lung white book.* http://www.erswhitebook.org/chapters/interstitial-lung-diseases/ (accessed 2018 Jan 3).
2. Pneumotox online. http://www.pneumotox.com (accessed 2018 Jan 3).
3. Sunderji R, Kanji Z, Gin K. Pulmonary effects of low dose amiodarone: a review of the risks and recommendations for surveillance. *Can J Cardiol.* 2000; 16:1435-40.
4. Parambil JG, Myers JL, Aubry MC et al. Causes and prognosis of diffuse alveolar damage diagnosed on surgical lung biopsy. *Chest.* 2007; 132:50-7.
5. Kanji Z, Sunderji R, Gin K. Amiodarone-induced pulmonary toxicity. *Pharmacotherapy.* 1999; 19:1463-6.
6. Donaldson L, Grant IS, Naysmith MR et al. Acute amiodarone-induced lung toxicity. *Intensive Care Med.* 1998; 24:626-30.
7. Jafari-Fesharaki M, Scheinman MM. Adverse effects of amiodarone. *PACE.* 1998; 21(1 pt 1):108-20.
8. Nicolet-Chatelain G, Prevost MC, Escamilla R et al. Amiodarone-induced pulmonary toxicity: immunoallergologic tests and bronchoalveolar lavage phospholipid content. *Chest.* 1991; 99:363-9.
9. Jessurun GA, Boermsa WG, Crijns HJ. Amiodarone induced pulmonary toxicity: predisposing factors, clinical symptoms and treatment. *Drug Saf.* 1998; 18:339-44.
10. Bedrossian CW, Warren CJ, Ohar J et al. Amiodarone pulmonary toxicity: cytopathology, ultrastructure, and immunocytochemistry. *Ann Diagn Pathol.* 1997; 1:47-56.
11. Vorperian VR, Havighurst TC, Miller S et al. Adverse effects of low dose amiodarone: a meta-analysis. *J Am Coll Cardiol.* 1997; 30:791-8.
12. Tisdale JE, Follin SL, Ordelova A et al. Risk factors for the development of specific non-cardiovascular adverse effects associated with amiodarone. *J Clin Pharmacol.* 1995; 35:351-6.
13. Weinberg BA, Miles WM, Klein LS et al. Five-year follow up of 589 patients treated with amiodarone. *Am Heart J.* 1993; 125:109-20.
14. Papiris SA, Triantafillidou C, Kolilekas L et al. Amiodarone: review of pulmonary effects and toxicity. *Drug Saf.* 2010; 3:539-58.
15. Singh SN, Fletcher RD, Fisher SG et al. Amiodarone in patients with congestive heart failure and asymptomatic ventricular arrhythmia. *N Engl J Med.* 1995; 333:77-82.
16. Range FT, Hilker E, Breithardt G et al. Amiodarone-induced pulmonary toxicity – a fatal care report and literature review. *Cardiovasc Drugs Ther.* 2013; 27:247-54.
17. Jackevicius CA, Tom A, Essebag V et al. Population-level incidence and risk factors for pulmonary toxicity associated with amiodarone. *Am J Cardiol.* 2011; 108:705-10.
18. Ernawati DK, Stafford L, Hughes JC. Amiodarone-induced pulmonary toxicity. *Br J Clin Pharmacol.* 2008; 66:81-7.
19. Ott MC, Khoor A, Leventhal JP et al. Pulmonary toxicity in patients receiving low-dose amiodarone. *Chest.* 2003; 123:646-51.
20. Raghavan M, Mazer MA, Brink DJ. Severe hypersensitivity pneumonitis associated with anagrelide. *Ann Pharmacother.* 2003; 37:1228-31.
21. Tirgan AM, Lunbin A, Sherman BW. Anagrelide associated pulmonary interstitial fibrosis. *Blood.* 1992; 80(suppl 1):455a.
22. Spencer EM, Lawrence DS. 'Double hit' from streptococcal pneumonia and hypersensitivity pneumonitis associated with anagrelide. *Clin Lab Haematol.* 2006; 28:63-5.
23. Bennett CL, Raisch DW, Sartor O. Pneumonitis associated with nonsteroidal antiandrogens: presumptive evidence of a class effect. *Ann Intern Med.* 2002; 137:625.
24. Masago T, Watanabe T, Nemoto R et al. Interstitial pneumonitis induced by bicalutamide given for prostate cancer. *Int J Clin Oncol.* 2011; 16:763-5.
25. Shioi K, Sakai N, Yoshida M et al. Successful recovery from interstitial pneumonitis, induced by bicalutamide and leuprorelin acetate given as treatment for prostate cancer. *Hinyokika Kiyo.* 2005; 51:211-4.
26. Shioi K, Yoshida M, Sakai N. Interstitial pneumonitis induced by bicalutamide and leuprorelin acetate for prostate cancer. *Int J Urol.* 2003; 10:625-6.
27. McCaffrey JA, Scher HI. Interstitial pneumonitis following bicalutamide treatment for prostate cancer. *J Urol.* 1998; 160:131.
28. Wong PW, Macris N, DiFabrizio L et al. Eosinophilic lung disease induced by bicalutamide: a case report and review of the medical literature. *Chest.* 1998; 113:548-50.
29. Azuma T, Kurimoto S, Mikami K et al. Interstitial pneumonitis related to leuprorelin acetate and flutamide. *J Urol.* 1999; 161:221.
30. Nomura M, Sato H, Fujimoto N et al. Interstitial pneumonitis related to flutamide monotherapy for prostate cancer. *Int J Urol.* 2004; 11:798-800.
31. Wieder JA, Soloway MS. Interstitial pneumonitis associated with neoadjuvant leuprolide and nilutamide for prostate cancer. *J Urol.* 1998; 159:2099.
32. Gomez JL, Dupont A, Cusan L et al. Simultaneous liver and lung toxicity related to the nonsteroidal antiandrogen nilutamide (Anandron): a case report. *Am J Med.* 1992; 92:563-6.
33. Akoun GM, Liote HA, Liote F et al. Provocation test coupled with bronchoalveolar lavage in diagnosis of drug (nilutamide)-induced hypersensitivity pneumonitis. *Chest.* 1990; 97:495-8.
34. Schwartzman KJ, Bowie DM, Yeadon C et al. Constrictive bronchiolitis obliterans following gold therapy for psoriatic arthritis. *Eur Respir J.* 1995; 8:2191-3.
35. Ettensohn DB, Roberts NJ, Condemi JJ. Bronchoalveolar lavage in gold lung. *Chest.* 1984; 85:569-70.
36. Sinha A, Silverstone EJ, O'Sullivan MM. Gold-induced pneumonitis: computed tomography findings in a patient with rheumatoid arthritis. *Rheumatology.* 2001; 40:712-4.
37. Hueser CN, Patel AJ. Azacitidine-associated hyperthermia and interstitial pneumonitis in a patient with myelodysplastic syndrome. *Pharmacotherapy.* 2007; 27:1759-62.

38. Adams CD, Szumita PM, Baroletti SA et al. Azacitidine induced interstitial and alveolar fibrosis in a patient with myelodysplastic syndrome. *Pharmacotherapy.* 2005; 25:765-8.
39. Kuroda J, Shimura Y, Mizutani S et al. Azacitadine-associated acute interstitial pneumonitis. *Intern Med.* 2014; 53:1165-9.
40. Sekhri A, Palaniswamy C, Kurmayagari K et al. Interstitial lung disease associated with azacitidine use: a case report. *Am J Ther.* 2012; 19:e98-100.
41. Gaku S, Naoshi K, Teruhiko A. A case of bepridil induced interstitial pneumonitis. *Heart.* 2003; 89:1415.
42. Yamasaki K, Yatera K, Noguchi S et al. Incidence and outcomes of bepridil-induced interstitial pneumonia. *Resp Med.* 2013; 107:2088-91.
43. Suzuki T, Hanaoka M, Yokoyama T et al. Graduate progression of interstitial pneumonia induced by bepridil. *Intern Med.* 2009; 48):2033-5.
44. Watanbe M, Takata Y, Fukasawa S et al. Two patients with bepridil-induced interstitial pneumonia. *Circ J.* 2009; 73:1352-5.
45. Saxman SB, Nichols CR, Einhorn LH. Pulmonary toxicity in patients with advanced-stage germ cell tumors receiving bleomycin with and without granulocyte colony stimulating factor. *Chest.* 1997; 111:657-60.
46. Jules-Elysee K, White D. Bleomycin-induced pulmonary toxicity. *Clin Chest Med.* 1990; 11:1-20.
47. Ngan HYS, Liang RHS, Lam WK et al. Pulmonary toxicity in patients with non-Hodgkin's lymphoma treated with bleomycin-containing combination chemotherapy. *Cancer Chemother Pharmacol.* 1993; 32:407-9.
48. Comis RL. Bleomycin pulmonary toxicity: current status and future directions. *Semin Oncol.* 1992; 19(2 suppl 5):64-70.
49. Wolkowicz J, Sturgeon J, Rawji M et al. Bleomycin induced pulmonary function abnormalities. *Chest.* 1992; 101:97-101.
50. Goldiner PL, Carlol GC, Cvitkovic E et al. Factors influencing post-operative morbidity and mortality in patients treated with bleomycin. *BMJ.* 1978; 1:1664-7.
51. Tryka AF, Skornik WA, Godleski JJ et al. Potentiation of bleomycin-induced lung injury by exposure to 70% oxygen. *Am Rev Respir Dis.* 1982; 126:1074-9.
52. Douglas MJ, Coppin CM. Bleomycin and subsequent anesthesia: a retrospective study at Vancouver General Hospital. *Can Anaesth Soc J.* 1980; 27:449-52.
53. Haas CD, Coltman CA, Gottlieb JA et al. Phase II evaluation of bleomycin: a Southwest Oncology Group Study. *Cancer.* 1976; 38:8-12.
54. Rinne UK, Krupp P, LeWitt PA et al. Pleuropulmonary changes during long-term bromocriptine treatment for Parkinson's disease. *Lancet.* 1981; 1:44-5.
55. Brunt ER, Boeree MJ. Low dose bromocriptine-induced pleural effusion and pleuropulmonary fibrosis. *Eur J Neurol.* 1995; 2:127-32.
56. Hillerdal G, Lee J, Blomkvist A et al. Pleural disease during treatment with bromocriptine in patients previously exposed to asbestos. *Eur Respir J.* 1997; 10:2711-5.
57. Kinnunen E, Viljanen A. Pleuropulmonary involvement during bromocriptine treatment. *Chest.* 1988; 94:1034-6.
58. Comet R, Domingo C, Such JJ et al. Pleuropulmonary disease as a side-effect of treatment with bromocriptine. *Respir Med.* 1998; 92:1172-4.
59. Ward CD. Pleuropulmonary and retroperitoneal fibrosis associated with bromocriptine treatment. *Lancet.* 1987; 50:1706-7.
60. Wiggins J, Skinner C. Bromocriptine-induced pleuropulmonary fibrosis. *Thorax.* 1986; 41:328-330.
61. Pfitzenmeyer P, Foucher P, Dennewald G et al. Pleuropulmonary changes induced by ergoline drugs. *Eur Respir J.* 1996; 9:1013-9.
62. Ringdin O, Remberger M, Ruutu T et al. Increased risk of chronic graft-versus-host disease, obstructive bronchiolitis, and alopecia with busulfan versus total body irradiation: long-term results of a randomized trial in allogeneic marrow recipients with leukemia. *Blood.* 1999; 93:2196-201.
63. Hartsell WF, Czyzewski EA, Ghalie R et al. Pulmonary complications of bone marrow transplantation: a comparison of total body irradiation and cyclophosphamide to busulfan and cyclophosphamide. *Int J Radiat Oncol Biol Phys.* 1995; 32:69-73.
64. Morgan M, Dodds A, Atkinson K et al. The toxicity of busulphan and cyclophosphamide as the preparative regimen for bone marrow transplantation. *Br J Haematol.* 1991; 77:529-34.
65. Oakhill A, Green I, Knowlson GT et al. Busulphan lung in childhood. *J Clin Pathol.* 1981; 34:495-500.
66. Manning DM, Strimlan CV, Turbiner EH. Early detection of busulfan lung: report of a case. *Clin Nucl Med.* 1980; 5:412-4.
67. Hankins DG, Sanders S, Mac Donald FM et al. Pulmonary toxicity recurring after a six week course of busulfan therapy and after subsequent therapy with uracil mustard. *Chest.* 1978; 73:415-6.
68. Miyashita T, Ojima A, Tuji T et al. Varied pulmonary lesions with intra-alveolar large lamellar bodies in an autopsy case with busulfan therapy. *Acta Pathol Jpn.* 1977; 27:239-49.
69. Pearl M. Busulfan lung. *Am J Dis Child.* 1977; 131:650-2.
70. Soble AR, Perry H. Fatal radiation pneumonia following subclinical busulfan injury. *Am J Roentgenol.* 1977; 128:1518.
71. Stott H, Stephens R, Fox W et al. An investigation of the chest radiographs in a controlled trial of busulfan, cyclophosphamide and a placebo after resection for carcinoma of the lung. *Thorax.* 1976; 31:265-70.
72. Vernof H, Miller HJ, Vye MV. Busulfan toxicity. *Ill Med J.* 1975; 147:357-60.
73. Podoll LN, Winkler SS. Busulphan lung: report of two cases and review of the literature. *Am J Roentgenol Radium Ther Nucl Med.* 1974; 120:151-6.
74. Bredeson C, LeRademacher J, Kato K et al. Prospective cohort study comparing intravenous busulfan to total body irradiation in hematopoietic cell transplantation. *Blood.* 2013; 122:3871-8.
75. Copelan EA, Hamilton BK, Avalos B et al. Better leukemia-free and overall survival in AML in first remission following cyclophosphamide in combinationwith busulfan compared with TBI. *Blood.* 2013; 122:3863-70.
76. Uhlving HH, Bang CL, Christensen IJ et al. Lung function after allogeneic hematopoietic stem cell transplantation in children: a longitudinal study in a population-based cohort. *Biol Blood Marrow Transplant.* 2013; 19:1348-54.
77. Kalaycio M, Pohlman B, Kuczkowski E et al. High-dose busulfan and the risk of pulmonary mortality after autologous stem cell transplant. *Clin Transplant.* 2006; 20:783-7.
78. Crestani B, Jaccard A, Israel-Biet D et al. Chlorambucil associated pneumonitis. *Chest.* 1994; 105:634-6.
79. Mohr M, Kingreen D, Ruhl H et al. Interstitial lung disease: an underdiagnosed side-effect of chlorambucil? *Ann Hematol.* 1993; 67:704-6.
80. Giles FJ, Smith MP, Goldstone AH. Chlorambucil lung toxicity. *Acta Haematol.* 1990; 83:156-8.
81. Lane SD, Besa EC, Justh G et al. Fatal interstitial pneumonitis following high-dose intermittent chlorambucil therapy for chronic lymphocytic leukemia. *Cancer.* 1981; 47:32-6.
82. Godard P, Marty JP, Michel FB. Interstitial pneumonia and chlorambucil. *Chest.* 1979; 76:471-3.
83. Cole SR, Myers TJ, Kiatsky AU. Pulmonary disease with chlorambucil therapy. *Cancer.* 1978; 41:455-9.
84. Shafqat H, Olszewski AJ. Chlorambucil-induced acute interstitial pneumonitis. *Case Rep Hematol.* 2014; 2014:575417.

85. Kalambokis G, Stefanou D, Arkoumani E et al. Bronchiolitis obliterans organizing pneumonia following chlorambucil treatment for chronic lymphocytic leukemia. *Eur J Haematol.* 2004; 73:139-42.
86. Khong HT, McCarthy J. Chlorambucil-induced pulmonary disease: a case report and review of the literature. *Ann Hematol.* 1998; 77:85-7.
87. Twohig KJ, Matthay RA. Pulmonary effects of cytotoxic agents other than bleomycin. *Clin Chest Med.* 1990; 11:31-54.
88. Segura A, Yuste A, Cercos A et al. Pulmonary fibrosis induced by cyclophosphamide. *Ann Pharmacother.* 2001; 35:894-7.
89. Schaap N, Raymakers R, Schattenberg A et al. Massive pleural effusion attributed to high-dose cyclophosphamide during conditioning for BMT. *Bone Marrow Transplant.* 1996; 18:247-8.
90. Usui Y, Aida H, Kimula Y et al. A case of cyclophosphamide-induced interstitial pneumonitis diagnosed by bronchoalveolar lavage. *Respiration.* 1992; 59:125-8.
91. Tsukamoto NT, Matsukuma K, Matsuyama T et al. Cyclophosphamide-induced interstitial pneumonitis in a patient with ovarian carcinoma. *Gynecol Oncol.* 1984; 17:41-51.
92. Abdel Karim FW, Ayash RE, Allam C et al. Pulmonary fibrosis after prolonged treatment with low-dose cyclophosphamide. *Oncology.* 1983; 40:174-6.
93. Burke DA, Stoddart JC, Ward MK et al. Fatal pulmonary fibrosis occurring during treatment with cyclophosphamide. *Br Med J (Clin Res Ed).* 1982; 285:696.
94. Ge Y, Peng Q, Zhang S et al. Cyclophosphamide treatment for idiopathic inflammatory myopathies and related interstitial lung disease: a systematic review. *Clin Rheumatol.* 2015; 34:99-105.
95. Ochoa R, Bejarano PA, Glück S et al. Pneumonitis and pulmonary fibrosis in a patient receiving adjuvant docetaxel and cyclophosphamide for stage 3 breast cancer: a case report and literature review. *J Med Case Rep.* 2012; 6:413.
96. Hamada K, Nagai S, Kitaichi M et al. Cyclophosphamide-induced late-onset lung disease. *Intern Med.* 2003; 42:82.
97. Malik SW, Myers JL, DeRemee RA, Specks U. Lung toxicity associated with cyclophosphamide use. Two distinct patterns. *Am J Respir Crit Care Med.* 1996; 154(6 pt 1):1851.
98. Hoag JB, Azizi A, Doherty TJ et al. Association of cetuximab with adverse pulmonary events in cancer patients: a comprehensive review. *J Exp Clin Cancer Res.* 2009; 28:113.
99. Satoh T, Gemma A, Kudoh S et al. Incidence and clinical features of drug-induced lung injury in patients with advanced colorectal cancer receiving cetuximab: results of a prospective multicenter registry. *Jpn J Clin Oncol.* 2014; 44:1032-9.
100. Shablak A, Conn A. A case of fatal cetuximab-induced interstitial lung disease during the first weeks of treatment. *Targ Oncol.* 2014; 9:177-80.
101. Achermann Y, Frauenfelder T, Obrist S et al. A rare but severe pulmonary side effect of cetuximab in two patients. *BMJ Case Rep.* 2012; 2012.
102. De Vos FY, Driessen CM, Jaspers HC et al. Cetuximab-induced pneumonitis in head and neck cancer patient. *Oral Oncol.* 2012; 48:e17-8.
103. Bugés C, Carcereny E, Moran T et al. Interstitial lung disease arising from erlotinib treatment in a Caucasian patient. *Clin Lung Cancer.* 2015; 16:e1-3.
104. ter Heine R, van den Bosch RT, Schaefer-Prokop CM et al. Fatal interstitial lung disease associated with high erlotinib and metabolite levels. A case report and a review of the literature. *Lung Cancer.* 2012; 75:391-7.
105. Ren S, Li Y, Li W et al. Fatal asymmetric interstitial lung disease after erlotinib for lung cancer. *Respiration.* 2012; 84:431-5.
106. Spigel DR, Lin M, O'Neill V et al. Final survival and safety results from a multicenter, open-label, phase 3b trial of erlotinib in patients with advanced nonsmall cell lung cancer. *Cancer.* 2008; 112:2749-55.
107. Hotta K, Kiura K, Takigawa N et al. Comparison of the incidence and pattern of interstitial lung disease during erlotinib and gefitinib treatment in Japanese patients with non-small cell lung cancer: the Okayama Lung Cancer Study Group experience. *J Thorac Oncol.* 2010; 5:179-84.
108. Cohen MH, Williams GA, Sridhara R et al. United States Food and Drug Administration Drug Approval summary: Gefitinib (ZD1839; Iressa) tablets. *Clin Cancer Res.* 2004; 10:1212-8.
109. Kudoh S, Kato H, Nishiwaki Y et al. Interstitial lung disease in Japanese patients with lung cancer: a cohort and nested case-control study. *Am J Respir Crit Care Med.* 2008; 177:1348-57.
110. Giusti RM, Shastri K, Pilaro AM et al. US Food and Drug Administration approval: panitumumab for epidermal growth factor receptor-expressing metastatic colorectal carcinoma with progression following fluoropyrimidine-, oxaliplatin-, and irinotecan-containing chemotherapy regimens. *Clin Cancer Res.* 2008; 14:1296-302.
111. Osawa M, Kudoh S, Sakai F et al. Clinical features and risk factors of panitumumab-induced interstitial lung disease: a postmarketing all-case surveillance study. *Int J Clin Oncol.* 2015; 20:1063-71.
112. Yamada T, Moriwaki T, Matsuda K et al. Panitumumab-induced interstitial lung disease in a case of metastatic colorectal cancer. *Onkologie.* 2013; 36:209-12.
113. Ernesto S, Arpin D, Nesme P et al. Diffuse interstitial lung disease linked to vandetanib. *Clin Lung Cancer.* 2012; 13:236-8.
114. Takada M, Negoro S I, Kudo S et al. Activity of gemcitabine in non-small-cell lung cancer: results of the Japan gemcitabine group (A) phase II study. *Cancer Chemother Pharmacol.* 1998; 41:217-22.
115. Linskens RK, Golding R P, van Groeningen C J et al. Severe acute lung injury induced by gemcitabine. *Neth J Med.* 2000; 56:232-5.
116. Maruchella A, Fiorenzano G, Merizzi A et al. Diffuse alveolar damage in a patient treated with gemcitabine. *Eur Respir J.* 1998; 11:504-6.
117. Vander Els NJ, Miller V. Successful treatment of gemcitabine toxicity with a brief course of oral corticosteroid therapy. *Chest.* 1998; 114:1779-81.
118. Pavlakis N, Bell DR, Millward MJ et al. Fatal pulmonary toxicity resulting from treatment with gemcitabine. *Cancer.* 1997; 80:286-91.
119. Belknap SM, Kuzel TM, Yarnold PR. Clinical features and correlates of gemcitabine-associated lung injury: findings from the RADAR project. *Cancer.* 2006; 106:2051-7.
120. Ioka T, Katayama K, Tanaka S et al. Safety and effectiveness of gemcitabine in 855 patients with pancreatic cancer under Japanese clinical practice based on post-marketing surveillance in Japan. *Jpn J Clin Oncol.* 2013; 43:139-45.
121. Umemura S, Yamane H, Suwaki T et al. Interstitial lung disease associated with gemcitabine treatment in patients with non-small-cell lung cancer and pancreatic cancer. *J Cancer Res Clin Oncol.* 2011; 137:1469-75.
122. Xu JF, Washko GR, Nakahira K et al. Statins and pulmonary fibrosis: the potential role of NLRP3 inflammasome activation. *Am J Respir Crit Care Med.* 2012; 185:547-56.
123. Fernández AB, Karas RH, Alsheikh-Ali AA et al. Statins and interstitial lung disease: a systematic review of the literature and of Food and Drug Administration adverse event reports. *Chest.* 2008; 134:824-30.
124. Huang LK, Tsai MJ, Tsai HC et al. Statin-induced lung injury: diagnostic clue and outcome. *Postgrad Med J.* 2013; 89:14-9.
125. Blanc PL, Joasson JM, Jammoud H et al. Acute interstitial pneumonia with fever after administration of hydroxyurea. *Presse Med.* 2000; 29:242-5.
126. Quintas-Cardama A, Perez-Encinas M, Gonzalez S et al. Hydroxyurea-induced acute interstitial pneumonitis in a patient with essential thrombocythemia. *Ann Hematol.* 1999; 78:187-8.
127. Internullo M, Giannelli V, Sardo L et al. Hydroxyurea-induced interstitial pneumonitis: case report and review of the literature. *Eur Rev Med Pharmacol Sci.* 2014; 18:190-3.

128. Salvenburg S, Heijdra YF, Drenth JPH. Pneumonitis as a consequence of (peg)interferon-ribavirin combination therapy for hepatitis C: a review of the literature. *Dig Dis Sci.* 2010; 55:579-85.
129. Arase Y, Suzuki F, Suzuki Y et al. Hepatitis C virus enhances incidence of idiopathic pulmonary fibrosis. *World J Gastroenterol.* 2008; 14:5880-6.
130. Foster GR, Zeuzem S, Pianko S et al. Decline in pulmonary function during chronic hepatitis C virus therapy with modified interferon alfa and ribavirin. *J Viral Hepat.* 2013; 20:e115-23.
131. Elhelaly S, Elgazzar AM, Ragab M et al. Pulmonary hazards of chronic hepatitis C infection treatment with pegylated interferon and ribavirin vs. untreated patients. *Egyptian J Chest Dis Tuberculosis.* 2013; 62:325-9.
132. Chen Y, Kiatsimkul P, Nugent K et al. Lenalidomide-induced interstitial lung disease. *Pharmacotherapy.* 2010; 30:325.
133. Supariwala AA, Grosu H, Jean RE. Severe lenalidomide-induced interstitial pneumonitis requiring mechanical ventilation: case report and review of literature. *Clin Pulm Med.* 2012; 19:113-8.
134. Rajkumar SV, Hayman SR, Lacy MQ et al. Combination therapy with lenalidomide plus dexamethasone (Rev/Dex) for newly diagnosed myeloma. *Blood.* 2005; 106:4050-3.
135. Akasheh MS, Freytes CO, Vesole DH. Melphalan-associated pulmonary toxicity following high-dose therapy with autologous hematopoietic stem cell transplantation. *Bone Marrow Transplant.* 2000; 26:1107-9.
136. Mufti GJ, Hamblin TJ, Gordon J. Melphalan-induced pulmonary fibrosis in osteosclerotic myeloma. *Acta Haematol.* 1983; 69:140-1.
137. Goucher G, Rowland V, Hawkins J. Melphalan-induced pulmonary interstitial fibrosis. *Chest.* 1980; 77:805-6.
138. Major PP, Laurin S, Bettez P. Pulmonary fibrosis following therapy with melphalan: report of two cases. *Can Med Assoc J.* 1980; 123:197-202.
139. Codling BW, Chakera TMH. Pulmonary fibrosis following therapy with melphalan for multiple myeloma. *J Clin Pathol.* 1972; 25:668-73.
140. Buxhofer-Ausch V, Ruckser R, Kier P et al. A rare case of interstitial pneumonitis after tandem high-dose melphalan conditioning and autologous stem cell transplantation in multiple myeloma. *Eur J Haematol.* 2004; 73:143-6.
141. Carroll GJ, Thomas R, Pathouros CC et al. Incidence, prevalence and possible risk factors for pneumonitis in patients with rheumatoid arthritis receiving methotrexate. *J Rheumatol.* 1994; 21:51-4.
142. Imokawa S, Colby TV, Leslie KO et al. Methotrexate pneumonitis: review of the literature and histopathological findings in nine patients. *Eur Respir J.* 2000; 15:373-81.
143. Aaron SD, Dales RE, Pham B. Management of steroid-dependent asthma with methotrexate: a meta-analysis of randomized clinical trials. *Respir Med.* 1998; 92:1059-65.
144. Kremer JM. Experience with methotrexate-associated pneumonitis in northeastern England. *Arthritis Rheum.* 1998; 41:1327-8.
145. Weinblatt ME. Long-term prospective study of methotrexate in the treatment of rheumatoid arthritis: 84-months update. *Arthritis Rheum.* 1992; 35:129-37.
146. Hanrahan PS, Scrivens GA, Russell AS. Prospective long-term follow-up of methotrexate therapy in rheumatoid arthritis: toxicity, efficacy and radiological progression. *Br J Rheumatol.* 1989; 28:147-53.
147. Weinblatt ME, Maier AL, Fraser PA et al. Long-term prospective study of methotrexate in the treatment of rheumatoid arthritis: conclusion after 132 months of therapy. *J Rheumatol.* 1998; 25:238-42.
148. Buchbinder R. Methotrexate therapy in rheumatoid arthritis: a life table review of 587 patients treated in community practice. *J Rheumatol.* 1993; 20:639-44.
149. Furst DE, Erikson N, Clute L et al. Adverse experience with methotrexate during 176 weeks of a longterm prospective trial in patients with rheumatoid arthritis. *J Rheumatol.* 1990; 17:1628-35.
150. Salaffi F, Manganelli P, Carotti M et al. Methotrexate-induced pneumonitis in patients with rheumatoid arthritis and psoriatic arthritis: report of five cases and review of the literature. *Clin Rheumatol.* 1997; 16:296-304.
151. Whitcomb ME, Schwartz MI, Tormey DC. Methotrexate pneumonitis: case report and review of the literature. *Thorax.* 1972; 27:636-9.
152. Filip DJ, Logue GL, Harle TS et al. Pulmonary and hepatic complications of methotrexate therapy for psoriasis. *JAMA.* 1971; 216:881-2.
153. Robertson JH. Pneumonia and methotrexate. *BMJ.* 1970; 2:156.
154. Schwartz IR, Kajani MK. Methotrexate therapy and pulmonary disease. *JAMA.* 1969; 210:1924.
155. Roubille C, Haraoui B. Interstitial lung diseases induced or exacerbated by DMARDS and biologic agents in rheumatoid arthritis: a systematic literature review. *Sem Arthritis Rheum.* 2014; 43:613-26.
156. Conway R, Low C, Coughlan RJ et al. Methotrexate and lung disease in rheumatoid arthritis: a meta-analysis of randomized controlled trials. *Arthritis Rheumatol.* 2014; 66:803-12.
157. Hozumi H, Nakamura Y, Johkoh T et al. Acute exacerbation in rheumatoid arthritis-associated interstitial lung disease: a retrospective case control study. *BMJ Open.* 2013; 3:e003132.
158. Shidara K, Hoshi D, Inoue E et al. Incidence of and risk factors for interstitial pneumonia in patients with rheumatoid arthritis in a large Japanese observational cohort, IORRA. *Mod Rheumatol.* 2010; 20:280-6.
159. Claes I, Slabbynck H, Bedert L et al. A 47-year-old man with non-productive cough and right-sided chest pain. *Eur Respir J.* 1997; 10:2171-3.
160. Hindle W, Posner E, Sweetnam MT et al. Pleural effusion and fibrosis during treatment with methysergide. *BMJ.* 1970; 1:605-6.
161. Kok-Jensen A, Lindeneg O. Pleurisy and fibrosis of the pleura during methysergide treatment for hemicranias. *Scand J Resp Dis.* 1970; 51:218-22.
162. Graham RG. Cardiac and pulmonary fibrosis during methysergide therapy for headache. *Am J Med Sci.* 1967; 254:1-12.
163. Schrijvers D, Catimel G, Highley M et al. KW-2149-induced pulmonary toxicity is not prevented with corticosteroids: a phase I and pharmacokinetic study. *Anti-Cancer Drugs.* 1999; 10:633-9.
164. Graham JR, Suby HI, LeCompte PR et al. Fibrotic disorders associated with methysergide therapy for headache. *N Engl J Med.* 1966; 274:359-68.
165. Castro M, Veeder MH, Mailliard JA et al. A prospective study of pulmonary function in patients receiving mitomycin. *Chest.* 1996; 109:939-44.
166. Linette DC, McGee KH, McFarland JA. Mitomycin induced pulmonary toxicity: case report and review of the literature. *Ann Pharmacother.* 1992; 26:481-4.
167. Verweij J, van der Burg MEL, Pinedo HM. Mitomycin C-induced hemolytic uremic syndrome: six case reports and review of the literature on renal, pulmonary and cardiac side effects of the drug. *Radiother Oncol.* 1987; 8:33-41.
168. Boven E, Pinedo HM. Mitomycin C: interstitial pneumonitis and haemolytic-uraemic syndrome. *Neth J Med.* 1983; 26:153-6.
169. Gunstream SR, Seidenfeld JJ, Sobonys RE et al. Mitomycin-associated lung disease. *Cancer Treat Rep.* 1983; 67:301-4.
170. Saif MW, Dai T. Mitomycin-induced interstitial pneumonitis in a patient with BRCA2 associated metastatic pancreatic carcinoma. *JOP.* 2010; 11:277-9.
171. Wada H, Nakano Y, Yamada H et al. Intravesical mitomycin-C-induced interstitial pneumonia. *Respiration.* 2010; 80:256-9.
172. González-Moreno S, Lambert LA, Mansfield PF. Interstitial pneumonitis: an exceptional toxicity of hyperthermic intraperitoneal mitomycin C. *Eur J Surg Oncol.* 2008; 34:482-4.
173. White DA, Camus P, Endo M et al. Noninfectious pneumonitis after everolimus therapy for advanced renal cell carcinoma. *Am J Respir Crit Care Med.* 2010; 182:396-403.

174. Ellard SL, Clemons M, Gelmon KA et al. Randomized phase II study comparing two schedules of everolimus in patients with recurrent/metastatic breastcancer: NCIC Clinical Trials Group IND.163. *J Clin Oncol.* 2009; 27:4536-41.
175. Motzer RJ, Escudier B, Oudard S et al. Efficacy of everolimus in advanced renal cell carcinoma: a double-blind, randomised, placebo-controlled phase III trial. *Lancet.* 2008; 372:449-56.
176. Atkinson BJ, Cauley DH, Ng C et al. Mammalian target of rapamycin (mTOR) inhibitor-associated non-infectious pneumonitis in patients with renal cell cancer: predictors, management, and outcomes. *BJU Int.* 2014; 113:376-82.
177. Maroto JP, Hudes G, Dutcher JP et al. Drug-related pneumonitis in patients with advanced renal cell carcinoma treated with temsirolimus. *J Clin Oncol.* 2011; 29:1750-6.
178. Hudes G, Carducci M, Tomczak P et al. Temsirolimus, interferon alfa, or both for advanced renal-cell carcinoma. *N Engl J Med.* 2007; 356:2271-81.
179. Bellmunt J, Szczylik C, Feingold J et al. Temsirolimus safety profile and management of toxic effects in patients with advanced renal cell carcinoma and poor prognostic features. *Ann Oncol.* 2008; 19:1387-92.
180. Morrissey P, Gohh R, Madras P et al. Pulmonary fibrosis secondary to administration of mycophenolate mofetil. *Transplantation.* 1998; 65:1414.
181. Gross DC, Sasaki TM, Buick MK et al. Acute respiratory failure and pulmonary fibrosis secondary to administration of mycophenolate mofetil. *Transplantation.* 1997; 64:1607-9.
182. Reynolds BC, Paton JY, Howatson AG et al. Reversible chronic pulmonary fibrosis associated with MMF in a pediatric patient: a case report. *Pediatr Transplant.* 2008; 12:228-31.
183. Jick SS, Jick H, Walker AM et al. Hospitalizations for pulmonary reactions following nitrofurantoin use. *Chest.* 1989; 96:512-5.
184. Holmberg L, Boman G. Pulmonary reactions to nitrofurantoin: 447 cases reported to the Swedish Adverse Drug Reaction Committee 1966–1976. *Eur J Respir Dis.* 1981; 62:180-9.
185. Koch-Weser J, Sidel VW, Dexter M et al. Adverse reactions to sulfisoxazole, sulfamethoxazole, and nitrofurantoin: manifestations and specific reaction rates during 2,118 courses of therapy. *Arch Intern Med.* 1971; 128:399-404.
186. Rosenow EC 3rd, DeRemee RA, Dines DE. Chronic nitrofurantoin pulmonary reaction: report of five cases. *N Engl J Med.* 1968; 279:1258-62.
187. Cameron RJ, Kolbe J, Wilsher ML et al. Bronchiolitis obliterans organising pneumonia associated with the use of nitrofurantoin. *Thorax.* 2000; 55:249-351.
188. Boggess KA, Benedetti TJ, Raghu G. Nitrofurantoin-induced pulmonary toxicity during pregnancy: a report of a case and review of the literature. *Obstet Gynecol Surv.* 1996; 51:367-70.
189. Chudnovsky CR, Otten EJ. Acute pulmonary toxicity to nitrofurantion. *J Emerg Med.* 1989; 7:15-9.
190. Bucknall CE, Adamson MR, Banham SW. Non-fatal pulmonary haemorrhage associated with nitrofurantoin. *Thorax.* 1987; 42:475-6.
191. Willcox PA, Maze SS, Sandler M et al. Pulmonary fibrosis following long-term nitrofurantoin therapy. *S Afr Med J.* 1982; 61:714-7.
192. Hainer BL, White AA. Nitrofurantoin pulmonary toxicity. *J Fam Pract.* 1981; 13:817-23.
193. Simonian SJ, Kroeker EJ, Boyd DP. Chronic interstitial pneumonitis with fibrosis after long-term therapy with nitrofurantoin. *Ann Thorac Surg.* 1977; 24:284-88.
194. Bone RC, Wolfe J, Sobonya RE et al. Desquamative interstitial pneumonia following chronic nitrofurantoin therapy. *Chest.* 1976; 69(2 suppl):296-7.
195. Kursch ED, Mostyn EM, Persky L et al. Nitrofurantoin pulmonary complications. *J Urol.* 1975; 113:392-5.
196. Pearsall HR, Ewalt J, Tsoi MS et al. Nitrofurantoin lung sensitivity: report of a case with prolonged nitrofurantoin lymphocyte sensitivity and interaction of nitrofurantoin-stimulated lymphocytes with alveolar cells. *J Lab Clin Med.* 1974; 83:728-37.
197. Pinerua RF, Hartnett BJS. Acute pulmonary reaction to nitrofurantoin. *Thorax.* 1974; 29:599-602.
198. Selroos O, Edgren J. Lupus-like syndrome associated with pulmonary reaction to nitrofurantoin: report of three cases. *Acta Med Scand.* 1975; 197:125-9.
199. Strandberg I, Wengle B, Fagrell B. Chronic interstitial pneumonitis with fibrosis during long-term treatment with nitrofurantoin. *Acta Med Scand.* 1974; 196:483487.
200. Larsson S, Cronberg S, Denneberg T et al. Pulmonary reaction to nitrofurantoin. *Scand J Respir Dis.* 1973; 54:103-10.
201. Stein JJ, Martin DC. Nitrofurantoin pulmonary hypersensitivity reaction. *J Urol.* 1973; 110:577-8.
202. Ruikka I, Vaissalo T, Saarimaa H. Progressive pulmonary fibrosis during nitrofurantoin therapy: a case history with autopsy report. *Scand J Respir Dis.* 1971; 52:162-6.
203. Brander L, Selroos O. Pulmonary reaction to nitrofurantoin. *Acta Med Scand.* 1969; 185:215-20.
204. Hailey FJ, Glascock HWJ, Hewitt WF. Pleuropneumonic reactions to nitrofurantoin. *N Engl J Med.* 1969; 281:10871090.
205. Harrow BR. Pulmonary reaction to nitrofurantoin. *N Engl J Med.* 1969; 280:389.
206. Howard EJ. Pulmonary reaction to nitrofurantoin. *N Engl J Med.* 1969; 280:389.
207. Strauss WG, Griffin LM. Nitrofurantoin pneumonia. *JAMA.* 1967; 199:175-6.
208. Dawson RB Jr. Pulmonary reactions to nitrofurantoin. *N Engl J Med.* 1966; 274:522.
209. Robinson B. Pleuropulmonary reaction to nitrofurantoin. *JAMA.* 1964; 189:239-40.
210. Israel HL, Diamond P. Recurrent pulmonary infiltration and pleural effusion due to nitrofurantoin sensitivity. *N Engl J Med.* 1962; 266:1024-6.
211. Goemaere NN, Grijm K, van Hal PT et al. Nitrofurantoin-induced pulmonary fibrosis: a case report. *J Med Case Rep.* 2008; 2:169.
212. Schmitz N, Diehl V. Carmustine and the lungs. *Lancet.* 1997; 349:1712-3.
213. Jones RB, Matthes S, Shpall EJ et al. Acute lung injury following treatment with high-dose cyclophosphamide, cisplatin, and carmustine: pharmacodynamic evaluation of carmustine. *J Natl Cancer Inst.* 1993; 85:640-7.
214. O'Driscoll BR, Hasleton PS, Taylor PM et al. Active lung fibrosis up to 17 years after chemotherapy with carmustine (BCNU) in childhood. *N Engl J Med.* 1990; 32:378-82.
215. Smith AC. The pulmonary toxicity of nitrosoureas. *Pharmacol Ther.* 1989; 41:443-60.
216. Aronin PA, Mahaley MS, Rudnick SA et al. Prediction of BCNU pulmonary toxicity in patients with malignant gliomas. *N Eng J Med.* 1980; 303:183-8.
217. Selker RG, Jacobs SA, Moore PB et al. 1,3-Bis(2chloroethyl)-1-nitrosourea (BCNU)-induced pulmonary fibrosis. *Neurosurgery.* 1980; 7:560-5.
218. Parish JM, Muhm JR, Leslie KO. Upper lobe pulmonary fibrosis associated with high-dose chemotherapy containing BCNU for bone marrow transplantation. *Mayo Clinic Proc.* 2003; 78:630-4.
219. Thomas PS, Agrawal S, Gore M et al. Recall lung pneumonitis due to carmustine after radiotherapy. *Thorax.* 1995; 50:1116-8.
220. Lena H, Desrues B, Le Coz A et al. Severe diffuse interstitial pneumonitis induced by carmustine (BCNU). *Chest.* 1994; 105:1602-3.
221. Melato M, Tuveri G. Pulmonary fibrosis following low dose 1 3-bis (2-chloro-ethyl)-1-nitrosourea (BCNU) therapy. *Cancer.* 1980; 45:1311-4.
222. Richter JE, Hastedt R, Dalton JF et al. Pulmonary toxicity of bischloronitrosourea: report of a case with transient response to corticosteroid therapy. *Cancer.* 1979; 43:1607-12.
223. Weiss RB, Shah S, Shane SR. Pulmonary toxicity from carmustine (BCNU): a case report. *Med Pediatr Oncol.* 1979; 6:255-9.

224. Lohani E, O'Driscoll R, Woodcock AA. 25-year study of lung fibrosis following carmustine therapy for brain tumor in childhood. *Chest*. 2004; 126:1007.

225. Reithmeier T, Graf E, Piroth T et al. BCNU for recurrent glioblastoma multiforme: efficacy, toxicity, and prognostic factors. *BMC Cancer*. 2010; 10:30.

226. Lane AA, Armand P, Feng Y et al. Risk factors for development of pneumonitis after high-dose chemotherapy with cyclophosphamide, BCNU and etoposide followed by autologous stem cell transplant. *Leuk Lymphoma*. 2012; 53:1130-6.

227. Reardon DA, Quinn JA, Rich JN et al. Phase 2 trial of BCNU plus irinotecan in adults with malignant glioma. *Neuro Oncol*. 2004; 6:134-44.

228. Alessandrino EP, Bernasconi P, Colombo A et al. Pulmonary toxicity following carmustine-based preparative regimens and autologous peripheral blood progenitor cell transplantation in hematological malignancies. *Bone Marrow Transplant*. 2000; 25:309-13.

229. Stone MD, Richardson MG. Pulmonary toxicity of lomustine. *Cancer Treat Rep*. 1987; 71:786-7.

230. Tucci E, Verdiani P, Di Carlo S et al. Lomustine (CCNU)-induced pulmonary fibrosis. *Tumori*. 1986; 72:95-8.

231. Cordonnier C, Vernant JP, Mital P et al. Pulmonary fibrosis subsequent to high doses of CCNU for chronic leukemia. *Cancer*. 1983; 51:1814-8.

232. Dent RG. Fatal pulmonary toxic effects of lomustine. *Thorax*. 1982; 37:627-9.

233. Vats T, Trueworthy RC, Langston CM. Pulmonary fibrosis associated with lomustine (CCNU): a case report. *Cancer Treat Rep*. 1982; 66:1181-2.

234. Stuart MJ, Chao NS, Horning SJ et al. Efficacy and toxicity of a CCNU-containing high-dose chemotherapy regimen followed by autologous hematopoietic cell transplantation in relapsed or refractory Hodgkin's disease. *Biol Blood Marrow Transplant*. 2001; 7:552-60.

235. Watkins J, Slade JH, Phan A et al. Fatal diffuse alveolar damage associated with oxaliplatin administration. *Clin Colorectal Cancer*. 2011; 10:198-202.

236. Prochilo T, Abeni C, Bertocchi P et al. Oxaliplatin-induced lung toxicity. Case report and review of the literature. *Curr Drug Saf*. 2012; 7:179-82.

237. Hochstrasser A, Benz G, Joerger M et al. Interstitial pneumonitis after treatment with pemetrexed: a rare event? *Chemotherapy*. 2012; 58:84-8.

238. Kim KH, Song SY, Lim KH et al. Interstitial pneumonitis after treatment with pemetrexed for non-small cell lung cancer. *Cancer Res Treat*. 2013; 45:74-7.

239. Wolfe F, Schurle DR, Lin JJ et al. Upper and lower airway disease in penicillamine treated patients with rheumatoid arthritis. *J Rheumatol*. 1983; 10:406-10.

240. Yamakado S, Yoshida Y, Yamada T et al. Pulmonary infiltration and eosinophilia associated with sulfasalazine therapy for ulcerative colitis: a case report and review of the literature. *Intern Med*. 1992; 31:108-13.

241. Kumar A, Bhat A, Gupta DK et al. D-penicillamine induced acute hypersensitivity pneumonitis and cholestatic hepatitis in a patient with rheumatoid arthritis. *Clin Exp Rheumatol*. 1985; 3:337-9.

242. Lahdensuo A, Mattila J, Vilppula A. Bronchiolitis in rheumatoid arthritis. *Chest*. 1984; 85:705-8.

243. Scott DL, Bradby GVH, Aitman TJ et al. Relationship of gold and penicillamine therapy to diffuse interstitial lung disease. *Ann Rheum Dis*. 1981; 40:136-41.

244. Davies D, Lloyd Jones JK. Pulmonary eosinophilia caused by penicillamine. *Thorax*. 1980; 35:957-8.

245. Seo JY, Kim SY, Choi WC. Education and imaging. Hepatobiliary and pancreatic: hypersensitivity pneumonitis induced by penicillamine. *J Gastroenterol Hepatol*. 2009; 24:700.

246. Lewis LD. Procarbazine associated alveolitis. *Thorax*. 1984; 39:206-7.

247. Mahmood T, Mudad R. Pulmonary toxicity secondary to procarbazine. *Am J Clin Oncol*. 2002; 25:187-88.

248. Garbes ID, Henderson ES, Gomez GA et al. Procarbazine-induced interstitial pneumonitis with a normal chest x-ray: a case report. *Med Pediatr Oncol*. 1986; 14:238-41.

249. Liote H, Liote F, Seroussi B et al. Rituximab-induced lung disease: a systematic review. *Eur Respir J*. 2010; 35:691-7.

250. Zayen A, Rais H, Rifi H et al. Rituximab-induced interstitial lung disease: case report and literature review. *Pharmacology*. 2011; 87:318-20.

251. Hadjinicolaou AV, Nisar MK, Parfrey H et al. Non-infectious pulmonary toxicity of rituximab: a systematic review. *Rheumatology*. 2012; 51:653-62.

252. Morelon E, Stern M, Kreis H. Interstitial pneumonitis associated with sirolimus therapy in renal-transplant recipients. *N Engl J Med*. 2000; 343:225-6.

253. Lopez P, Kohler S, Dimri S. Interstitial lung disease associated with mTOR inhibitors in solid organ transplant recipients: results from a large phase III clinical trial program of everolimus and review of the literature. *J Transplant*. 2014; 2014:305931.

254. Weiner SM, Sellin L, Vonend O et al. Pneumonitis associated with sirolimus: clinical characteristics, risk factors and outcome—a single-centre experience and review of the literature. *Nephrol Dial Transplant*. 2007; 22:3631-7.

255. Manchanda S, Rees PJ. A case of severe lung disease caused by sulphasalazine. *Int J Clin Pract*. 1999; 53:233-5.

256. Peters FP, Engels LG, Moers AM. Pneumonitis induced by sulphasalazine. *Postgrad Med J*. 1997; 73:99-100.

257. Salerno SM, Ormseth EJ, Roth BJ et al. Sulfasalazine pulmonary toxicity in ulcerative colitis mimicking clinical features of Wegener's granulomatosis. *Chest*. 1996; 110:556-9.

258. Hamadeh M, Atkinson J, Smith LJ. Sulfasalazine-induced pulmonary disease. *Chest*. 1992; 101:1033-7.

259. Yamakado S, Yoshida Y, Yamada T et al. Pulmonary infiltration and eosinophilia associated with sulfasalazine therapy for ulcerative colitis: a case report and review of the literature. *Intern Med*. 1992; 31:108-13.

260. Parry SD, Barbatzas C, Peel ET et al. Sulphasalazine and lung toxicity. *Eur Resp J*. 2002; 19:756-64.

261. Uittenbogaart SB, Klemt-Kropp M. Mesalazine and sulphasalazine for Crohn's disease: few indications, severe adverse reactions. *Ned Tijdschr Geneeskd*. 2011; 155:A3842.

262. Karmakar GC, Wong CA, Horwood F et al. Sulphasalazine lung toxicity: report of two cases. *N Z Med J*. 2010; 123:86-7.

263. Haroon M, Harney S. A case of severe pulmonary infiltration with eosinophilia (PIE) syndrome induced by sulphasalazine. *Int J Rheum Dis*. 2012; 15:e150-2.

264. Kim ES, Hirsh V, Mok T et al. Gefitinib versus docetaxel in previously treated non-small-cell lung cancer (INTEREST): a randomised phase III trial. *Lancet*. 2008; 372:1809-18.

265. Maruyama R, Nishiwaki Y, Tamura T et al. Phase III study, V-15-32, of Gefitinib versus docetaxel in previously treated Japanese patients with non-small-cell lung cancer. *J Clin Oncol*. 2008; 26:4244-52.

266. Kawaguchi T, Ando M, Asami K et al. Randomized phase III trial of Erlotinib versus docetaxel as second- or third-line therapy in patients with advanced non-small-cell lung cancer: docetaxel and Erlotinib Lung Cancer Trial (DELTA). *J Clin Oncol*. 2014; 32:1902-8.

267. Yasuda K, Igishi T, Kawasaki Y et al. Phase II trial of weekly paclitaxel in previously untreated advanced non-small-cell lung cancer. *Oncology*. 2003; 65:224-8.

268. Bielopolski D, Evron E, Moreh-Rahav O et al. Paclitaxel-induced pneumonitis in patients with breast cancer: case series and review of the literature. *J Chemother*. 2015; 15:1973947815Y0000000029.

269. Lin JT, Yeh KT, Fang HY et al. Fulminant, but reversible interstitial pneumonitis associated with imatinib mesylate. *Leuk Lymphoma.* 2006; 47:1693-5.

270. Yamasawa H, Sugiyama Y, Bando M et al. Drug-induced pneumonitis associated with imatinib mesylate in a patient with idiopathic pulmonary fibrosis. *Respiration.* 2008; 75:350-4.

271. Rajda J, Phatak PD. Reversible drug-induced interstitial pneumonitis following imatinib mesylate therapy. *Am J Hematol.* 2005; 79:80-1.

272. Yokoyama T, Miyazawa K, Kurakawa E et al. Interstitial pneumonia induced by imatinib mesylate: pathologic study demonstrates alveolar destruction and fibrosis with eosinophilic infiltration. *Leukemia.* 2004; 18:645-6.

273. Ma CX, Hobday TJ, Jett JR. Imatinib mesylate-induced interstitial pneumonitis. *Mayo Clinic Proc.* 2003; 78:15781579.

274. Bergeron A, Bergot E, Vilela G et al. Hypersensitivity pneumonitis related to imatinib mesylate. *J Clin Oncology.* 2002; 20:4271-2.

275. Ohnishi K, Sakai F, Kudoh S, Ohno R. Twenty-seven cases of drug-induced interstitial lung disease associated with imatinib mesylate. *Leukemia.* 2006; 20:1162-4.

276. Go SW, Kim BK, Lee SH et al. Successful rechallenge with imatinib in a patient with chronic myeloid leukemia who previously experienced imatinib mesylate induced pneumonitis. *Tuberc Respir Dis.* 2013; 75:256-9.

277. Dao K, Védy D, Lopez J et al. Imatinib-induced dose-dependent interstitial lung disease successfully switched to nilotinib: a case report with concentration exposure data. *Int J Hematol.* 2013; 97:299-300.

278. Nakashima S, Kakugawa T, Motomura H et al. Development of Imatinib mesylate-induced interstitial lung disease 2?weeks after discontinuation of the treatment: a case report. *Multidiscip Respir Med.* 2012; 7:48.

279. Myung HJ, Jeong SH, Kim JW et al. Sorafenib-induced interstitial pneumonitis in a patient with hepatocellular carcinoma: a case report. *Gut Liver.* 2010; 4:543-6.

280. Takeda H, Nishikawa H, Iguchi E et al. Sorafenib-induced acute interstitial pneumonia in patients with advanced hepatocellular carcinoma: report of three cases. *Clin J Gastroenterol.* 2012; 5:407-12.

281. Ide S, Soda H, Hakariya T et al. Interstitial pneumonia probably associated with sorafenib treatment: An alert of an adverse event. *Lung Cancer.* 2010; 67:248-50.

282. Boyle HJ, Chatté G, Rivoire M et al. Lung toxicity in a patient treated with sunitinib. *Eur Respir J.* 2012; 40:1300-3.

283. Yuasa T, Kitsukawa S, Sukegawa G et al. Early onset recall pneumonitis during targeted therapy with sunitinib. *BMC Cancer.* 2013; 13:3.

284. Ivanyi P, Fuehner T, Adam M et al. Interstitial lung disease during targeted therapy in metastatic renal cell carcinoma: a case series from three centres. *Med Oncol.* 2014; 31:147.

285. Nakashita T, Ando K, Kaneko N et al. Potential risk of TNF inhibitors on the progression of interstitial lung disease in patients with rheumatoidarthritis. *BMJ Open.* 2014; 4:e005615.

286. Ramos-Casals M, Perez-Alvarez R, Perez-de-Lis M et al. Pulmonary disorders induced by monoclonal antibodies in patients with rheumatologic autoimmune diseases. *Am J Med.* 2011; 124:386-94.

287. Perez-Alvarez R, Perez-de-Lis M, Diaz-Lagares C et al. Interstitial lung disease induced or exacerbated by TNF-targeted therapies: analysis of 122 cases. *Semin Arthritis Rheum.* 2011; 41:256-64.

288. Allanore Y, Devos-Francois G, Caramella C et al. Fatal exacerbation of fibrosing alveolitis associated with systemic sclerosis in a patient treated with adalimumab. *Ann Rheum Dis.* 2006; 65:834-5.

289. Schoe A, van der Laan-Baalbergen N E, Huizinga TWJ et al. Pulmonary fibrosis in a patient with rheumatoid arthritis treated with adalimumab. *Arthritis Rheum.* 2006; 5:157-9.

290. Reid JD, Bressler B, English J. A case of adalimumab-induced pneumonitis in a 45-year-old man with Crohn's disease. *Can Respir J.* 2011; 18:262-4.

291. Casanova MJ, Chaparro M, Valenzuela C et al. Adalimumab-induced interstitial pneumonia in a patient with Crohn's disease. *World J Gastroenterol.* 2015; 21:2260-2.

292. Yousem SA, Dacic S. Pulmonary lymphohistiocytic reactions temporally related to etanercept therapy. *Mod Pathol.* 2005; 18:651-5.

293. Phillips K, Weinblatt M. Granulomatous lung disease occurring during etanercept treatment. *Arthritis Rheum.* 2005; 53:618-20.

294. Peno-Green L, Lluberas G, Kingsley T et al. Lung injury linked to etanercept therapy. *Chest.* 2002; 122:1858-60.

295. Horai Y, Miyamura T, Shimada K et al. Etanercept for the treatment of patients with rheumatoid arthritis and concurrent interstitial lung disease. *J Clin Pharm Ther.* 2012; 37:117-21.

296. Koike T, Harigai M, Inokuma S et al. Postmarketing surveillance of safety and effectiveness of etanercept in Japanese patients with rheumatoid arthritis. *Mod Rheumatol.* 2011; 21:343-51.

297. Ostor AJ, Chilvers ER, Somerville MF et al. Pulmonary complications of infliximab therapy in patients with rheumatoid arthritis. *J Rheum.* 2006; 33:622-8.

298. Sen S, Peltz C, Jordan K et al. Infliximab-induced nonspecific interstitial pneumonia. *Am J Med Sci.* 2012; 344:75-8.

299. Shimura T, Fuse N, Yoshino T et al. Clinical features of interstitial lung disease induced by standard chemotherapy (FOLFOX or FOLFIRI) for colorectal cancer. *Ann Oncol.* 2010; 21:2005-2010.

300. Schwaiblmair M, Behr W, Haeckel T et al. Drug induced interstitial lung disease. *Open Respir Med J.* 2012; 6:63-74.

301. Coultas DB, Zumwalt RE, Black WC et al. The epidemiology of interstitial lung diseases. *Am J Respir Crit Care Med.* 1994; 150:967-72.

302. Amar RK, Jick SS, Rosenberg D et al. Drug-/radiation-induced interstitial lung disease in the United Kingdom general population: incidence, all-cause mortality and characteristics at diagnosis. *Respirology.* 2012; 17:861-8.

303. Ley B, Collard HR. Epidemiology of idiopathic pulmonary fibrosis. *Clin Epidemiol.* 2013; 5:483-92.

304. Nalysnyk L, Cid-Ruzafa J, Rotella P et al. Incidence and prevalence of idiopathic pulmonary fibrosis: review of the literature. *Eur Respir Rev.* 2012; 21:355-61.

305. Wilson JW, du Bois RM, King TE Jr. Challenges in pulmonary fibrosis: 8—the need for an international registry for idiopathic pulmonary fibrosis. *Thorax.* 2008; 63:285-7.

306. O'Sullivan JM, Huddart RA, Norman AR et al. Predicting the risk of bleomycin lung toxicity in patients with germ-cell tumours. *Ann Oncol.* 2003; 14:91-6.

307. Min JH, Lee HY, Lim H et al. Drug-induced interstitial lung disease in tyrosine kinase inhibitor therapy for non-small cell lung cancer: a review on current insight. *Cancer Chemother Pharmacol.* 2011; 68:1099-1109.

308. Selman M, King TE, Pardo A et al. Idiopathic pulmonary fibrosis: prevailing and evolving hypotheses about its pathogenesis and implications for therapy. *Ann Intern Med.* 2001; 134:136-51.

309. Matsuno O. Drug-induced interstitial lung disease: mechanisms and best diagnostic approaches. *Respir Res.* 2012; 13:39.

310. Cooper JA Jr, White DA, Matthay RA. Drug-induced pulmonary disease. Part 1: Cytotoxic drugs. *Am Rev Respir Dis.* 1986; 133:321.

311. Lynch JP 3rd, McCune WJ. Immunosuppressive and cytotoxic pharmacotherapy for pulmonary disorders. *Am J Respir Crit Care Med.* 1997; 155:395.

312. Cooper JA Jr, Zitnik RJ, Matthay RA. Mechanisms of drug-induced pulmonary disease. *Annu Rev Med.* 1988; 39:395-404.

313. Lazo JS, Merrill WW, Pham ET et al. Bleomycin hydrolase activity in pulmonary cells. *J Pharmacol Exp Ther.* 1984; 231:583.

314. Wang GS, Yang KY, Perng RP. Life-threatening hypersensitivity pneumonitis induced by docetaxel (taxotere). *Br J Cancer.* 2001; 85:1247.

315. Fagan NL, Foral PA, Malesker MA et al. Therapeutic update on drug-induced pulmonary disorders. *US Pharm.* 2011; 36:HS3-8.

316. Daba MH, El-Tahir KE, Al-Arifi MN et al. Drug-induced pulmonary fibrosis. *Saudi Med J.* 2004; 25:700-6.

317. Raghu G, Collard HR, Egan JJ et al. An official ATS/ERS/JRS/ALAT statement: idiopathic pulmonary fibrosis: evidence-based guidelines for diagnosis and management. *Am J Respir Crit Care Med.* 2011; 183:788-824.

318. Wallis A, Spinks K. The diagnosis and management of interstitial lung diseases. *BMJ.* 2015; 350:h2072.

319. Camus P, Martin WJ II, Rosenow EC III. Amiodarone pulmonary toxicity. *Clin Chest Med.* 2004; 25:65-75.

320. Cao TM, Negrin RS, Stockerl-Goldstein KE et al. Pulmonary toxicity syndrome in breast cancer patients undergoing BCNU-containing high-dose chemotherapy and autologous hematopoietic cell transplantation. *Biol Blood Marrow Transplant.* 2000; 6:387-94.

321. Miyakoshi S, Kami M, Yuji K et al. Severe pulmonary complications in Japanese patients after bortezomib treatment for refractory multiple myeloma. *Blood.* 2006; 107:3492-4.

322. Ohri A, Arena F. Severe pulmonary complications in African-American patient after bortezomib therapy. *Am J Ther.* 2006; 13:553-5.

323. Iqbal K, Kelly C. Treatment of rheumatoid arthritis-associated interstitial lung disease: a perspective review. *Ther Adv Musculoskelet Dis.* 2015; 7:247-67.

324. Camus P, Fanton A, Bonniaud P et al. Interstitial lung disease induced by drugs and radiation. *Respiration.* 2004; 71:301-26.

325. Collard HR, Ward AJ, Lanes S et al. Burden of illness in idiopathic pulmonary fibrosis. *J Med Econ.* 2012; 15:829-35.

326. Olson AL, Swigris JJ, Lezotte DC et al. Mortality from pulmonary fibrosis increased in the United States from 1992 to 2003. *Am J Respir Crit Care Med.* 2007; 176:277-84.

327. Ley B, Ryerson CJ, Vittinghoff E et al. A multidimensional index and staging system for idiopathic pulmonary fibrosis. *Ann Intern Med.* 2012; 156:684-91.

328. Ryerson CJ, Vittinghoff E, Ley B et al. Predicting survival across chronic interstitial lung disease: the ILD-GAP model. *Chest.* 2014; 145:723-8.

329. Simpson AB, Paul J, Graham J et al. Fatal bleomycin pulmonary toxicity in the west of Scotland 1991-95: a review of patients with germ cell tumours. *Br J Cancer.* 1998; 78: 1061-6.

330. Chen Y, Luo Y. Interstitial lung disease induced by targeted therapy for non-small cell lung cancer: a review of diagnosis, workup, and management. *J Palliat Care Med.* 2015; 5:1-5.

331. Chetta A, Marangio E, Olivieri D. Pulmonary function testing in interstitial lung diseases. *Respiration.* 2004; 71:209-13.

332. Limper AH, Rosenow EC. Drug-induced interstitial lung disease. *Curr Opin Pulm Med.* 1996; 2:396-404.

333. Gleadhill IC, Wise RA, Schonfeld SA et al. Serial lung function testing in patients treated with amiodarone: a prospective study. *Am J Med.* 1989; 86:4-10.

334. Chap L, Shpiner R, Levine M et al. Pulmonary toxicity of high-dose chemotherapy for breast cancer: a noninvasive approach to diagnosis and treatment. *Bone Marrow Transplant.* 1997; 20:1063-7.

335. McGaughey DS, Nikcevich DA, Long GD et al. Inhaled steroids as prophylaxis for delayed pulmonary toxicity syndrome in breast cancer patients undergoing high-dose chemotherapy and autologous stem cell transplantation. *Biol Blood Marrow Transplant.* 2001; 7:272-8.

336. Faress JA, Nethery DE, FO Kern E et al. Bleomycin-induced pulmonary fibrosis is attenuated by a monoclonal antibody targeting HER2. *J Appl Physiol.* 2007; 103:2077-83.

337. Tabata C, Tabata R, Kadokawa Y et al. Thalidomide prevents bleomycin-induced fibrosis in mice. *J Immunol.* 2007; 179:708-14.

338. Rosa AC, Pini A, Lucarini L et al. Prevention of bleomycin-induced lung inflammation and fibrosis in mice by naproxen and JNJ7777120 treatment. *J Pharmacol Exp Ther.* 2014; 351:308-16.

339. Pini A, Viappiano S, Bolla M, Masini E, Bani D. Prevention of bleomycin-induced fibrosis in mice by a novel approach of parallel inhibition of cyclooxygenase and nitric-oxide donation using NCX 466, a prototype cyclooxygenase inhibitor and nitric-oxide donor. *J Pharmacol Exp Ther.* 2012; 341:493-9.

340. Richeldi L, Costabel U, Selman M et al. Efficacy of a tyrosine kinase inhibitor in idiopathic pulmonary fibrosis. *N Engl J Med.* 2011; 365:1079-87.

341. Richeldi L, du Bois RM, Raghu G et al. Efficacy and safety of nintedanib in idiopathic pulmonary fibrosis. *N Engl J Med.* 2014; 370:2071-82.

342. Noble PW, Albera C, Bradford WZ et al. Pirfenidone in patients with idiopathic pulmonary fibrosis (CAPACITY): two randomised trials. *Lancet.* 2011; 377:1760-9.

343. King TE Jr, Bradford WZ, Castro-Bernardini S et al. A phase 3 trial of pirfenidone in patients with idiopathic pulmonary fibrosis. *N Engl J Med.* 2014; 370:2083-92.

344. Günther A, Lübke N, Ermert M et al. Prevention of bleomycin-induced lung fibrosis by aerosolization of heparin or urokinase in rabbits. *Am J Respir Crit Care Med.* 2003; 168:1358-65.

345. Punithavathi D, Venkatesan N, Babu M. Curcumin inhibition of amiodarone-induced pulmonary fibrosis in rats. *Br J Pharmcol.* 2003; 139:1342-50.

346. Mata M, Ruis A, Cerda M et al. Oral *N*-acetylcysteine reduces bleomycin-induced lung damage and mucin Muc5ac expression in rats. *Eur Respir J.* 2003; 22:900-5.

347. Bendstrup E, Hyldgaard C, Agerbaek M et al. No effect of pirfenidone treatment in fulminant bleomycin-induced pneumonitis. *Respir Med Case Rep.* 2014; 12:47-9.

348. Michaelson JE, Aguayo SM, Roman J. Idiopathic pulmonary fibrosis: a practical approach for diagnosis and management. *Chest.* 2000; 118:788-94.

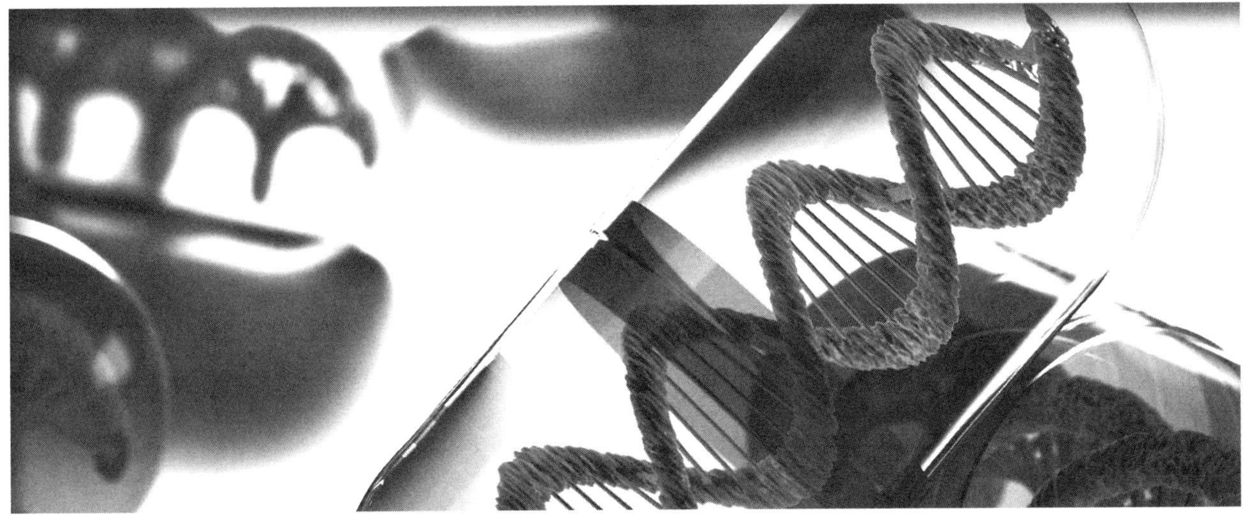

CHAPTER 22

Asthma and Bronchospasm

Suzanne G. Bollmeier and Rebecca L. Stauffer

Asthma is a common disease affecting approximately 1–18% of the population in different countries worldwide[1] and is characterized by airway inflammation, bronchial hyperresponsiveness, and airway obstruction that is usually reversible spontaneously or with treatment. Airway obstruction causes most of the clinical signs and symptoms of asthma, which include shortness of breath and bronchospasm, cough, mucus secretion, and bronchial hyperresponsiveness. Acute asthma exacerbations, or deterioration in status, can be triggered by several factors, including airborne pollens, dust, animal dander, and chemicals, as well as medications.[2] Among known asthma triggers, medications are perhaps the least common.[3] Drugs can lead to bronchospasm by a variety of mechanisms, and drug-induced bronchospasm may present as an isolated event or as a symptom of immunologic (anaphylaxis) or nonimmunologic (anaphylactoid) reactions.[4] Although drug-induced bronchospasm occurs primarily in patients with pre-existing asthma, it may also occur in patients with other forms of airway hyperresponsiveness or drug allergies.[5]

CAUSATIVE AGENTS

Drugs that have been reported to cause bronchospasm or worsen asthma symptoms are listed in **Table 22-1**.[6-103] Most evidence comes from case reports, but for some medications, stronger evidence exists. Although bronchospasm occurs rarely in association with most of the listed causative agents, aspirin, nonsteroidal anti-inflammatory agents (NSAIDs), β-adrenergic receptor antagonists (β-blockers), radiocontrast dyes, sulfites, and angiotensin-converting enzyme (ACE) inhibitors can cause bronchospasm more frequently.[3]

EPIDEMIOLOGY

The prevalence of asthma is increasing, especially among children, in many areas of the world, including Africa, Latin America, Eastern Europe, Asia, and the United States.[104] For example, in the United States, the prevalence of asthma increased by 14.8% in less than 10 years (2001–2010).[105] The overall incidence of drug-induced bronchospasm is unknown.

Table 22-1 Agents Implicated in Drug-Induced Asthma and Bronchospasm

Drug	Incidence	Level of Evidence[a]
Acetaminophen[6-8]	0–32%	A
N-acetylcysteine[9]	NK	B
α-agonists[10]	NK	C
Amiodarone[11,12]	NK	C
Angiotensin-converting enzyme inhibitors[13-16]	0–44% (cough) NK (bronchospasm)	A
Aspirin[17-19]	4–44%	A
Benzalkonium chloride[20,21]	NK	A
β-blockers[22,23]	NK	A
Betahistine[24]	NK	C
Bromelin[25]	NK	C
Carbamazepine[26]	NK	C
Carboprost[27]	NK	C
Cisapride[28]	NK	C
Cocaine[29,30]	NK	C
Colistin[31]	NK	A
Cromolyn[32]	NK	C
Cyclophosphamide[33]	NK	C
D-tubocurarine[34-36]	NK	C
D-penicillamine[37,38]	NK	C
Desensitization extracts[39]	NK	C
Dipyridamole[40]	NK	B
Estrogen[41,42]	NK	B
Ethanol[43]	NK	B
Ethylenediaminetetraacetic acid[44-46]	NK	A
Etidronate[47]	NK	C
Gallamine[48]	NK	C
Glucosamine and chondroitin[49]	NK	C
Heroin[50,51]	NK	B
Hydrocortisone sodium succinate[52,53]	2%	A
Interferon alfa[54]	NK	C
Interleukin-2[55,56]	NK	A
Iodinated radiocontrast media[57]	0.22–1%	B
Isotretinoin[58,59]	NK	C
Losartan[60,61]	NK	C
Menthol[62]	NK	C
Meperidine[63]	NK	C
Methimazole[64]	NK	C
Methotrexate[65,66]	NK	C
Methyldopa[67]	NK	C
Methylprednisolone[68,69]	NK	C
Mivacurium[70]	NK	C
Neostigmine[71]	NK	C

Table 22-1 Agents Implicated in Drug-Induced Asthma and Bronchospasm (continued)

Drug	Incidence	Level of Evidence[a]
Nonsteroidal anti-inflammatory drugs (COX-1)[72-75]	4–44%	A
Oxytocin[76]	NK	C
Pancuronium bromide[77]	NK	C
Pentazocine[78]	NK	C
Pentamidine[79-81]	NK	A
Propafenone[82]	NK	A
Propofol[83]	NK	C
Propylthiouracil[84]	NK	C
Psyllium[85,86]	5–12%	B
Pyrethrin[87,88]	NK	C
Sodium benzoate[89]	NK	C
Sodium salicylate[90]	NK	C
Sulfites[91,92]	5–11%	A
Tamoxifen[93]	NK	C
Tartrazine[94,95]	0–2.4%	B
Tetramethrin[96]	NK	C
Tobramycin[97-99]	NK	A
Venlafaxine[100]	NK	C
Verapamil[101]	NK	C
Yohimbine[102]	NK	C
Zanamivir[103]	NK	C

COX = cyclooxygenase, NK = not known.
[a]Definitions for Levels of Evidence: Level A—evidence from one or more randomized, controlled clinical trials; Level B—evidence from nonrandomized clinical trials, prospective observational studies, cohort studies, retrospective studies, case-control studies, meta-analyses and/or postmarketing surveillance studies; and Level C—evidence from one or more published case reports or case series.

Aspirin can exacerbate symptoms in patients with diagnosed asthma. A recent meta-analysis found the prevalence to be 7% in typical adult patients with asthma, and as high as 14% in those with severe asthma at baseline.[17] Aspirin-induced bronchospasm in patients without a prior diagnosis of asthma is rare, with a prevalence of <1%.[18,19] Due to similar mechanisms, patients with aspirin-exacerbated respiratory disease (AERD) also experience symptoms of asthma or bronchospasm associated with NSAIDs that inhibit cyclooxygenase-1 (COX-1). NSAID-associated hypersensitivity occurs in approximately 26% of patients with asthma.[72] Drugs that are poor inhibitors of COX-1 (acetaminophen and nonacetyl salicylates such as salsalate) and highly selective COX-2 inhibitors (celecoxib) are generally safe to use in this patient population.[73] However, there are case reports of COX-2 inhibitors, such as celecoxib, inducing asthma attacks.[74,75] Meloxicam is a partially selective inhibitor of COX-2 but may be tolerated in aspirin-intolerant patients.[106]

The prevalence of acetaminophen-induced bronchospasm in aspirin-sensitive patients with asthma is 0–6% with single doses ≤650 mg,[8] and most patients can tolerate single acetaminophen doses ≤500 mg.[107] A case-control study evaluating the cross-reactivity of acetaminophen in aspirin-intolerant patients reported bronchospasm in 24% and 32% after an oral challenge with acetaminophen 1,000 mg or 1,500 mg, respectively. No patient with aspirin-tolerant asthma developed acetaminophen-associated bronchospasm.[8] Furthermore, case-control studies have found that increasing frequency of acetaminophen use is associated with asthma in adults.[6,7]

Guidelines recommend against the routine use of β-blockers in patients with asthma, and some experts consider them contraindicated.[2,108] However, due to their beneficial effects on cardiac morbidity and mortality following events such as a myocardial infarction and in patients with heart failure with reduced ejection fraction (HFrEF), β-blockers are often prescribed to patients even with respiratory diseases including asthma. It is estimated that 2.2% of patients with asthma are prescribed β-blockers every year.[23] The prevalence of bronchospasm associated with nonselective β-blockers is unknown, but it has been estimated that 50–100% of patients with asthma exhibit symptoms of bronchospasm after a single dose of a nonselective β-blocker.[3,22] In addition to problems caused by oral or intravenous administration of these drugs, fatal asthma has also been reported in association with ophthalmic administration of timolol.[109,110] Cardioselective β-blockers decrease the risk of, but do not eliminate, β-blocker–induced bronchospasm.[23] Decreased forced expiratory volume in 1 second (FEV_1) and symptoms of bronchospasm have been demonstrated in asthmatic patients receiving cardioselective β-blockers.[23] However, two meta-analyses evaluating the safety of cardioselective β-blockers in patients with reactive airway disease concluded that these agents do not produce clinically significant adverse respiratory effects in this population.[23,111] Also, cardioselective β-blockers were found to be well tolerated in trials that included patients with cardiovascular diseases, including hypertension, angina, and heart failure.[111]

ACE inhibitor-induced cough appears to be a class effect.[13] The prevalence of ACE inhibitor-induced cough in the general population is approximately 5–35%.[13] Interestingly, nonsmoking patients are thought to be at higher risk.[14] Cigarette smoking is believed to negatively impact the cough reflex; therefore, nonsmokers may be more likely to respond to a normal cough reflex exacerbated by an ACE inhibitor. The prevalence of ACE inhibitor-induced cough and bronchospasm in patients with reactive airway disease appears to be similar to that in the general population.[15] Although the incidence of cough and bronchospasm associated with angiotensin receptor blockers (ARBs) is low, and they are often used in patients with ACE inhibitor-induced cough, cases of bronchospasm and cough have been reported in patients taking losartan.[60]

Paradoxical bronchospasm is an unexpected bronchoconstriction associated with inhaled bronchodilators.[112] Although rare, paradoxical bronchospasm associated with bronchodilators delivered by metered-dose inhaler or nebulization has been reported.[46,113-116] This underrecognized reaction may occur in up to 1% of salbutamol inhalations.[112] The cause is unknown, but it is postulated that propellants, preservatives, or the osmolality or pH of the inhalant may play a role.[117] Bronchospasm occurs in up to 6.9% of asthmatic patients following inhalation from a placebo metered-dose inhaler containing only inert ingredients.[118] The incidence of bronchospasm decreases from 4% to 1.55% when active drug is added.[119] Inactive ingredients in metered-dose inhalers implicated include chlorofluorocarbons, sorbitan trioleate, oleic acid, and soya lecithin.[119] Some reports have also implicated newer metered-dose inhalers containing hydrofluoroalkane delivery systems as a cause of paradoxical bronchospasm as many of these inhalers contain similar inert ingredients.[113,114,120,121]

Similarly, preservatives like benzalkonium chloride and medication additives including sulfites, sodium benzoate, and ethylenediamine tetraacetic acid (EDTA) can cause asthma symptoms.[21,89,115] Sulfites are no longer used in inhaled asthma drugs. However, sulfites are still used in injectable forms of isoproterenol and epinephrine. Sulfite-induced bronchospasm rarely occurs in patients without airway hyperresponsiveness.[119] The prevalence of sulfite sensitivity in patients with asthma is 5–11% and increases with age in children with severe asthma.[119,122,123]

Benzalkonium chloride is a common preservative used as a bacteriostatic agent used in nebulizer solutions.[115] EDTA is a stabilizing agent that is also found in some nebulizer preparations. Both compounds have been implicated as a potential cause of paradoxical bronchoconstriction induced by nebulized medications.[115,119,124] Benzalkonium chloride may stimulate histamine release from mast cells, resulting in cumulative dose-related bronchoconstriction.[115,119] EDTA is added to some pharmaceutical preparations as a chelating agent to prevent solution discoloration.[124] Although EDTA has been shown to cause bronchoconstriction when large doses are inhaled, clinically important bronchospasm did not occur when concentrations similar to those found in commercial products were used.[45,115,125]

MECHANISMS

Several mechanisms are associated with drug-induced asthma or bronchospasm. Most reports of bronchospasm are isolated cases, and the mechanism is unknown. Mechanisms of bronchospasm associated with individual drugs, when known, are listed in **Table 22-2.**[8,9,23,126-131]

Bronchospasm can be provoked by direct irritation of the airway from *N*-acetylcysteine or bisulfites, IgE-mediated reactions in anaphylaxis, precipitation of IgG antibodies that may occur in association with methyldopa, mast-cell degranulation, or as a result of an intended or unintended pharmacologic effect in patients taking aspirin or β-blockers.[132] Aspirin-exacerbated respiratory disease is characterized by airway inflammation and hyperresponsiveness associated with drugs that inhibit COX-1 such as aspirin and NSAIDs.[127] This nonallergic hypersensitivity is characterized by an association between aspirin intolerance, asthma, nasal polyps, and chronic rhinosinusitis, referred to as the aspirin tetrad.[127] The mechanism of AERD is not completely understood. It is unlikely that the response to aspirin is caused by an IgE-dependent mechanism but is more likely due to inhibition of COX-1 and prostaglandin synthesis. This leads to activation of inflammatory mast cells, eosinophils, and the subsequent release of leukotrienes and other mediators within the nasal mucosa.[72] Currently proposed mechanisms of AERD are presented in **Figure 22-1.**[133]

Aspirin-exacerbated respiratory disease is characterized by increased production of cysteinyl leukotrienes (CysLTs; leukotrienes C_4, D_4, and E_4) and eosinophilic infiltration.[72,134] Cys-LTs are metabolic products of phospholipid metabolism. Once phospholipid is liberated from the nuclear membrane, it is converted by phospholipase A_2 to arachidonic acid, which is then biotransformed into thromboxanes, prostaglandins, and 5-hydroperoxyeicosatetraenoic acid (5-HETE), which is ultimately biotransformed to leukotriene E_4 (LTE_4).[134,135] Cys-LTs are believed to be the primary mediators of AERD, as biosynthesis of Cys-LTs appears to be upregulated in AERD.[72] Cys-LTs are potent inflammatory mediators causing eosinophil chemotaxis, microvascular permeability, mucous-gland secretion, and bronchoconstriction.[136] Compared with eosinophils from aspirin-tolerant asthmatics, circulating blood eosinophils from patients with AERD carry larger amounts of leukotriene C_4 (LTC_4) synthase, the rate-limiting enzyme for Cys-LT production. Patients with AERD have a larger quantity of eosinophils in bronchial tissue compared to patients with aspirin-tolerant asthma, and Cys-LT concentrations in bronchial lavage fluids correlate with the degree of eosinophilic infiltration of bronchial tissue in patients with AERD.[137] In addition, LTC_4 synthase is overexpressed in the bronchial mucosa of patients with AERD.[137,138]

It is postulated that COX inhibition by aspirin and NSAIDs drives arachidonic acid through the leukotriene metabolic pathway.[139] COX exists

Table 22-2 Mechanisms of Drug-Induced Asthma and Bronchospasm

Drug	Mechanism
Acetaminophen[8]	Not clearly understood; weak inhibition of cyclooxygenase
N-acetylcysteine[9]	Airway irritation
Angiotensin-converting enzyme inhibitors[126]	Not clearly understood; may be related to increased concentrations of bradykinin and substance P with related alterations in prostaglandin homeostasis
Aspirin[127]	Inhibition of COX forces the metabolism of arachidonic acid through the lipoxygenase pathway, resulting in increased concentrations of leukotrienes (see Figure 22-1)
Benzalkonium chloride[128]	Anaphylactoid mast-cell degranulation and stimulation of cholinergic and noncholinergic nerves in the airways
β-blockers[23]	β_2-receptor blockade, leading to bronchoconstriction
Nonsteroidal anti-inflammatory drugs (COX-1 inhibitors)[129]	Inhibition of COX forces the metabolism of arachidonic acid through the lipoxygenase pathway, resulting in increased concentrations of leukotrienes (see Figure 22-1)
Sulfites[130,131]	Sulfur dioxide is liberated during nebulization; inhalation can lead to increased concentrations of proinflammatory mediators such as interleukin-6 and tumor necrosis factor α

COX = cyclooxygenase.

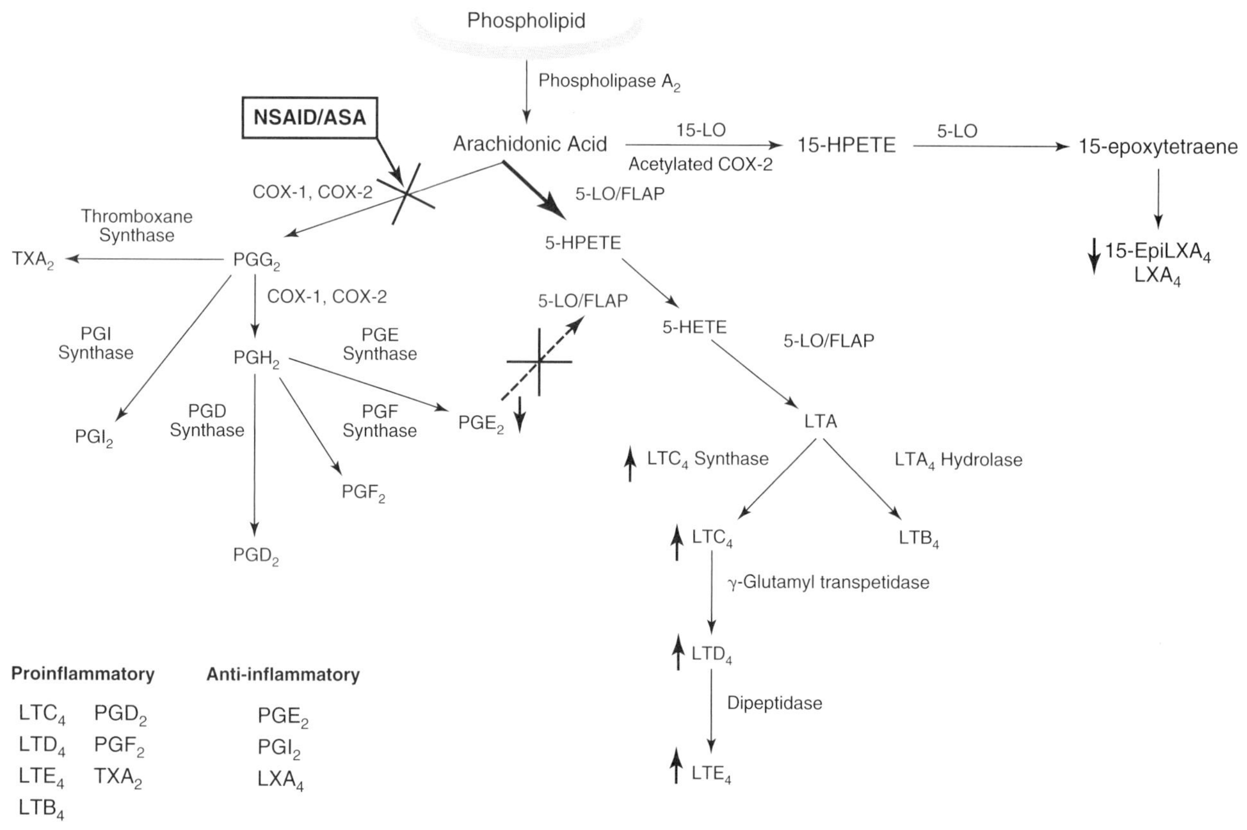

FIGURE 22-1 Mechanisms of Aspirin-Exacerbated Respiratory Disease

Aspirin/NSAID inhibition of cyclooxygenase (COX-1, COX-2) pathways forces the metabolism of arachidonic acid through the lipoxygenase pathway. Decreased prostaglandin E_2 production and increased leukotriene synthase activity results in increased production of the proinflammatory cysteinyl leukotrienes. Production of lipoxin and lipoxin epimers also appears to be decreased. ASA = acetylsalicylic acid (aspirin), COX = cyclooxygenase, 15-EpiLXA$_4$ = 15-epilipoxin A$_4$, HETE = hydroxyeicosatetraenoic acid, HPETE = hydroperoxyeicosatetraenoic acid, LT = leukotriene, LXA$_4$ = lipoxin A$_4$, LO = lipoxygenase, FLAP = 5-lipoxygenase activating protein, NSAID = nonsteroidal anti-inflammatory drug, PG = prostaglandin, TXA$_2$ = thromboxane A$_2$.

in several isoforms, with COX-1 expressed constitutively in most tissues and COX-2 induced by inflammatory mediators.[140] COX enzymes metabolize arachidonic acid to the proinflammatory mediators prostaglandins D$_2$ (PGD$_2$) and F$_2$α (PGF$_2$α), and the anti-inflammatory mediator prostaglandin E$_2$ (PGE$_2$).[141] Exposure to aspirin and most NSAIDs results in decreased production of COX metabolic products such as PGE$_2$, which normally inhibits 5-lipooxygenase (5-LO) and 5-LO activating protein (FLAP). The "braking effects" of PGE$_2$ are greatly minimized, leaving 5-LO unopposed. This leads to oversynthesis of leukotrienes, a reduction in mast-cell stabilization, and the release of histamine and tryptase.[140]

Both β$_1$ and β$_2$-adrenergic receptors are present in the heart and the lungs, but β$_1$-receptors are found primarily in the heart and β$_2$-receptors are mainly found in bronchial smooth muscle.[3] β-blockers competitively inhibit stimulation of β-adrenergic receptors, resulting in unopposed parasympathetic tone, which can result in bronchoconstriction.[3,23,142] Stimulation of β$_2$-receptors (as with β$_2$-receptor agonists) results in relaxation of bronchial smooth muscle, while blocking these receptors results in airway constriction.[22] It is important to consider all routes of administration of β-receptor active agents. Up to 80% of the volume of topically administered β-blocker eyedrops drains into the nasolacrimal duct and is absorbed via the nasal mucosa.[110] Nonselective β-receptor inhibition substantially shifts the dose–response curve of inhaled β$_2$-adrenergic agonists (β$_2$-agonists), limiting their effectiveness in reversing bronchospasm caused by nonselective β-blockers. Cardioselective β-blockers preferentially bind to β_1-adrenergic receptors, but this selectivity is attenuated at higher doses. Bronchospasm caused by cardioselective β-blockers may be easier to reverse with inhaled β_2-agonists.[143]

The mechanism of ACE-inhibitor–induced cough has not been clearly elucidated, although increased concentrations of proinflammatory substances like bradykinin, substance P, prostaglandins, and thromboxane are likely involved.[13] ACE converts angiotensin I to angiotensin II and is also responsible for metabolism of bradykinin, substance P, and neurokinin A.[3] ACE-inhibitor–induced cough may result from the accumulation of these substances in the lungs. Bradykinin and substance P activate mast cells, releasing proinflammatory mediators. In addition, bradykinin is a vasodilator and increases vascular permeability. Inhaled bradykinin causes bronchospasm, possibly through increases in the production of thromboxane A_2, prostacyclin I_2 (PGI_2), and PGE_2, which can activate rapidly acting receptors of the afferent neuronal pathway, stimulating the cough reflex. The accumulation of substance P may also play a role in ACE-inhibitor–induced cough, as it serves as a neurotransmitter for the afferent neurons, in particular sensory C fibers, and can cause bronchoconstriction.[144] A genetic predisposition for ACE-inhibitor–induced cough may exist.[126]

Several different mechanisms may cause paradoxical bronchospasm, including turbulent airflow due to inappropriate inhaler use, the deep inspiratory maneuver used for drug inhalation, IgE-mediated reactions to product excipients (e.g., soy lecithin), excipients in metered-dose inhalers (e.g., oleic acid), and hyperosmolar or acidic nebulizer solutions.[46]

CLINICAL PRESENTATION AND DIFFERENTIAL DIAGNOSIS

The signs and symptoms of drug-induced bronchospasm can be nonspecific and may be difficult to differentiate from other causes of bronchospasm, such as asthma and chronic obstructive pulmonary disease (COPD) (**Table 22-3**).[145,146] Conditions that should be considered in the differential diagnosis of drug-induced asthma or bronchospasm are listed in **Table 22-4**.[12,147] Recent drug exposure and the presence of other risk factors (**Table 22-5**) are usually required for the diagnosis.[3,14,16,129,148] When in doubt, specialists in clinics with the ability to treat anaphylactic reactions should challenge the patient with the suspected causative agent in a controlled environment.

Table 22-3 Signs and Symptoms Associated with Drug-Induced Asthma and Bronchospasm

Drug-induced asthma and bronchospasm[145]

- Tachypnea
- Tachycardia
- Wheezing
- Diaphoresis
- Cyanosis
- Dyspnea
- Cough
- Shortness of breath
- Chest tightness
- Anxiety
- Agitation

ACE-inhibitor–induced cough[146]

- Tickling sensation in the back of the throat
- Dry, hacking, irritating nonproductive, paroxysmal cough
- Hoarseness

ACE = angiotensin-converting enzyme.

Aspirin-exacerbated respiratory disease is an acquired condition that may develop as adult-onset asthma or be superimposed on pre-existing asthma. The typical presentation is that of the classic aspirin tetrad of rhinitis, nasal polyps, asthma, and aspirin intolerance. Typically, symptoms of chronic rhinitis present in the late teen years to middle age and often follow a viral infection.[127] Rhinitis usually worsens, becomes refractory to treatment, and progresses to chronic hyperplastic eosinophilic sinusitis with nasal polyposis.[72] Asthma may develop 1–5 years after the development of rhinitis with polyposis.[127] The development of aspirin or NSAID sensitivity can occur at any point during the disease. Most patients with AERD are not clinically distinguishable from aspirin-tolerant patients with asthma until challenged with aspirin/NSAIDs. Patients may have an acute asthma attack with symptoms of rhinorrhea and conjunctival infection within minutes

Table 22-4 Conditions to Consider in the Differential Diagnosis of Drug-Induced Asthma and Bronchospasm

Drug-induced asthma and bronchospasm[12]

- Pre-existing chronic asthma
- Pre-existing chronic obstructive pulmonary disease
- Allergic rhinitis and sinusitis
- Upper respiratory tract infection
- Foreign body in the trachea or bronchus
- Vocal cord dysfunction
- Vascular rings or laryngeal webs
- Laryngotracheomalacia, tracheal stenosis, bronchostenosis
- Laryngeal edema
- Viral bronchitis or obliterative bronchiolitis
- Cystic fibrosis
- Bronchopulmonary dysplasia
- Aspiration
- Gastroesophageal reflux
- Heart failure
- Pulmonary embolism
- Tumor causing mechanical obstruction
- Acute bronchitis
- Pulmonary infiltration with eosinophilia

ACE-inhibitor–induced cough[147]

- Upper respiratory tract infection
- Allergic rhinitis and sinusitis
- Asthma
- Chronic obstructive airway disease
- Gastroesophageal reflux
- Laryngitis
- Heart failure
- Mitral stenosis
- Pneumonia
- Pulmonary emboli
- Acute bronchitis
- Smoker's cough
- Tuberculosis
- Lung carcinoma

Table 22-5 Risk Factors for Drug-Induced Asthma and Bronchospasm

Aspirin-induced asthma[129]

- Pre-existing asthma
- Nasal polyps
- Age (30s or 40s)
- Female sex

β-blockers[3]

- Pre-existing airway hyperreactivity

ACE-inhibitor–induced cough[14,16,148]

- Female sex
- African-American or Asian race
- Elderly
- Heart failure
- Genetic polymorphism (bradykinin metabolism gene *XPNPEP₂* and bradykinin receptor gene *BDKRB₂*)

ACE = angiotensin-converting enzyme.

to 3 hours of ingestion of aspirin or NSAIDs.[138] A small number of patients present with nonrespiratory symptoms such as urticaria or angioedema after aspirin ingestion.[72] Often, reactions are severe and can be life-threatening.

Diagnosis of AERD begins with a detailed medical history. However, the history may not be helpful because the patient may have taken aspirin or NSAIDs successfully in the past, without bronchospasm or other adverse respiratory effects. Aspirin or NSAID-induced asthma should be suspected when symptoms of persistent and intractable rhinorrhea and nasal congestion occur after ingestion of aspirin or NSAIDs in patients with current nasal polyps or loss of smell and mucosal hypertrophy on CT scan. Patients with AERD tend to have more severe asthma symptoms with an increased risk of severe exacerbations. There is no in vitro test available for the diagnosis of AERD; the definitive diagnosis is made using aspirin provocation tests, during which aspirin may be administered by the oral, inhaled, nasal, or intravenous route (of these, only oral administration is available in the United States). Patients should be challenged when asthma is in remission with an FEV_1 >70% of the predicted value, and the provocation test should be carried out by specialists in clinics with immediate access to emergency equipment and ability to treat anaphylactic reactions. Discontinuation of asthma controller medications is not recommended, as it may lead to severe reactions.[72]

In an oral provocation test, the patient receives placebo capsules the day prior to the challenge to allow for estimation of bronchial stability. On day 2, patients receive 10–30 mg of aspirin, and the dose is doubled every 1.5–3 hours until a positive reaction (nasal congestion, rhinorrhea, or at least a

20% decrease in FEV_1) occurs. If the final aspirin dose is 312 mg (equivalent to 500-mg cumulative dose) and well tolerated, the patient is considered aspirin tolerant.[72] A nasal provocation test involves the administration of lysine-aspirin 8 mg into each nostril (total dose, 16 mg) with rhinomanometry performed every 10 minutes for 2–3 hours.[149] A positive test is defined as a decrease in nasal flow of >40% compared with baseline in at least one nostril that is sustained for at least two rhinomanometry measurements and is accompanied by clinical symptoms persisting for ≥30 minutes.[150,151] During oral inhaled provocation tests, an inhalation of normal saline is administered, and if FEV_1 does not decrease by >10%, increasing oral inhaled doses of lysine aspirin are given every 30 minutes to a maximum cumulative dose of 182 mg. Spirometry is performed at 10, 20, and 30 minutes after each dose. A decrease in FEV_1 of >20% from baseline or the occurrence of substantial extrabronchial symptoms is considered positive for aspirin-induced asthma. Bronchial provocation with lysine-aspirin is as sensitive as, but less specific than, oral provocation testing.[152] The oral route is generally recommended over both intranasal and inhaled routes for the provocation test. Patients with significant nasal obstruction or turbulent nasal flow should not be administered intranasal aspirin. Similarly, those with chronic rhinosinusitis without asthma or those with a history of only upper airway symptoms after NSAID ingestion cannot undergo the inhaled challenge.[72]

Bronchospasm due to β-blockade cannot be distinguished clinically from an acute asthma attack. Drug-induced bronchospasm should be suspected in any asthmatic patient who wheezes while taking a β-blocker. A single dose of a cardioselective β-blocker can result in a significant decrease in FEV_1, whereas chronic β-blocker administration may not cause a significant reduction in FEV_1.[153]

ACE-inhibitor–induced cough is typically characterized as dry, irritating, and nonproductive with a persistent tickling sensation in the back of the throat.[146,154] The cough may present within hours of the first dose, or it may be delayed up to 12 months after the initiation of therapy. ACE-inhibitor–induced cough may cause hoarseness, vomiting, and stress incontinence, and the cough may worsen in the supine position or at night.[147,155] Although the cough may resolve within a week after the discontinuation of ACE-inhibitor therapy, it may linger for 1–3 months in some individuals.[147,154] The differential diagnosis of ACE-inhibitor–induced cough includes asthma, chronic smoking, COPD, postnasal drip, heart failure, upper-respiratory-tract infection, and gastroesophageal reflux.[147,155,156] Diagnosis of ACE-inhibitor–induced cough requires discontinuation of therapy and monitoring of the cough. Diagnosis is confirmed by resolution of the cough within 1–4 weeks after discontinuation, although, as mentioned above, in a subgroup of patients the cough may last up to 3 months.[154]

Patients with paradoxical responses to inhaled drugs demonstrate a lower-than-expected response to the drug or worsening of their pulmonary symptoms. The response is usually rapid and may occur within minutes of inhaling the agent.[157] Patients with known severe asthma have often reported severe wheezing, chest tightness, and dyspnea after ingesting sulfite-containing foods. Reactions to sulfites rarely occur in patients without reactive airway disease. The diagnosis of sulfite sensitivity is made by taking a detailed history and may be confirmed by rechallenge.[119]

RISK FACTORS

Risk factors for drug-induced asthma and bronchospasm are listed in Table 22-5. The principal risk factor for drug-induced bronchospasm is pre-existing asthma. However, smoking, pre-existing airway disease, older age, and respiratory infection may also increase the risk for drug-induced bronchospasm.[4]

Aspirin-exacerbated respiratory disease occurs primarily in adults and generally does not manifest until the 30s or 40s.[129] The frequency of AERD increases with age, and the incidence is fourfold higher in patients 40 years of age or older compared with those younger than 20 years.[2] The risk of AERD also increases with a patient's asthma severity; the prevalence is doubled in patients with severe persistent asthma.[17] Women are affected 2–2.5 times more often than men.[18,158,159] In a study of 500 aspirin-intolerant asthmatic patients from

10 European countries, the prevalence of AERD was 2.3 times greater in women than in men. In women, the onset of symptoms occurred earlier in life, and the disease was more progressive and severe.[158] A study of 300 patients in the United States found the prevalence of AERD to be only 1.3 times greater in women than in men, and the severity of the disease was similar in both sexes.[160] There appears to be no ethnic or familial distribution of AERD, with only 6% of patients in the European study and 1% in the U.S. study having a family history of AERD.[158,160] Patients with nasal polyps or chronic rhinosinusitis had a 9.69% prevalence and 8.7% prevalence, respectively.[17]

ACE-inhibitor–induced cough occurs more often in female patients, in those of Chinese origin, and in nonsmokers.[126,154,161,162] ACE-inhibitor–induced cough is not dose-related and can occur in patients taking initial starting doses.[147] Patients with chronic lung diseases such as COPD or asthma do not appear to be at a greater risk for cough associated with ACE inhibitors.[163] Patients with heart failure that are treated with an ACE inhibitor have a higher incidence of cough than those treated with ACE inhibitors for hypertension.[154] There is speculation regarding the potential for a genetic predisposition to ACE-inhibitor–induced cough. Some evidence implicates polymorphisms in the bradykinin metabolism gene (*XPNPEP*$_2$) and bradykinin receptor genes (*BDKRB*$_2$).[148]

MORBIDITY AND MORTALITY

Any drug reaction that causes acute bronchospasm or exacerbates asthma has the potential to negatively impact patient morbidity and mortality. In patients with AERD, who tend to have more severe asthma, aspirin therapy may be associated with aggressive airway remodeling and, in some, decreased diffusion capacity. A study evaluating factors associated with the development of severe asthma found that 9.44% of patients had experienced aspirin intolerance; of those, 30.67% had severe asthma. Aspirin was a significant risk factor for the development of severe asthma (OR 5.44, 95% CI 2.47–8.41).[164] Another study evaluating 3,307 adult patients with severe or difficult-to-treat asthma demonstrated that the mean percent predicted postbronchodilator FEV_1 was significantly decreased in those who were aspirin-intolerant (75.3%) as compared with those who were aspirin-tolerant (79.9%), and patients with aspirin-intolerant asthma were more likely to have severe asthma based on physician assessment (66% versus 49%).[165] A greater percentage of aspirin-intolerant subjects had a history of intubation (20% versus 11%), and over a 3-month period had more unscheduled office visits (54% versus 44%), emergency department visits (18% versus 13%), and requirement for burst doses of steroids (56% versus 46%).[165] A survey of 500 patients with AERD in 10 European countries found that inhaled and oral corticosteroids were required in 80% and 50% of patients, respectively. The average corticosteroid dose was equivalent to prednisone 8 mg daily.[158] NSAID exposure has also been shown to be a risk factor for rapid-onset fatal or near-fatal asthma.[166]

The responses to a survey administered to 200 patients with AERD indicated that it can also influence quality of life. When asked how badly AERD affected their lives, with a score of one representing mild and score of nine representing severe, most respondents ranked their quality of life with a score of seven. The two categories that diminished quality of life most severely were decreased sense of smell (89%) and chronic nasal symptoms (87%).[167]

The risk of increased morbidity and mortality due to β-blocker-induced bronchospasm is unknown, but fatalities due to bronchospasm caused by these agents have occurred. Single-dose exposure to selective β-blockers can cause a mean decrease in FEV_1 of 7.46% with no change in symptoms.[153] In a meta-analysis of randomized controlled trials evaluating acute nonselective β-blocker exposure in patients with asthma, there was a mean change in FEV_1 of −10.2% and symptoms affecting one in 13 patients. In patients with asthma exposed to acute selective β-blocker therapy, there was a mean change in FEV_1 of −6.9% and symptoms affecting 1 in 33 patients. This meta-analysis also showed an attenuation of concomitant β_2-agonist response of −10.2% in patients exposed to acute selective β-blocker therapy and −20% in patients exposed to acute nonselective β-blocker therapy.[23] Although bronchoconstriction may occur after a single dose of a β-blocker, some researchers suggest that β-blockers may have a beneficial effect for patients with asthma. In one small study, including patients with mild asthma, the nonselective β-blocker nadolol exerted a dose-dependent and significant attenuation in airway hyperresponsiveness from baseline in 80% of the patients.[168]

The largest impact of the persistent cough associated with ACE inhibitors is the potential for patient self-discontinuation of therapy. Discontinuation rates as high as 50% have been reported.[147] The chronic, bothersome cough may also decrease quality of life and potentially increase the use of healthcare resources to determine cough etiology.[147] Patients may also seek nonprescription or prescription medication to relieve the cough.[169]

The morbidity and mortality associated with paradoxical bronchospasm is unknown. However, an ineffective or worsening response from a bronchodilator during an active asthma attack could lead to significant morbidity.

PREVENTION

The primary strategy for preventing drug-induced asthma or bronchospasm is avoidance of causative agents (**Table 22-6**). Alternative analgesic treatments for patients with AERD include acetaminophen, salsalate, meloxicam, and celecoxib.[138] Cases of successful use of COX-2 inhibitors have been reported.[170] However, there have also been reports of COX-2 inhibitors inducing bronchospasm.[171,172] Eight combined studies (n = 206) demonstrated that COX-2–selective NSAIDs may be used safely in patients with AERD.[173] Aspirin-induced asthma is not a risk factor for mortality if aspirin and NSAID avoidance is ensured.[174]

The frequency of cross-sensitivity between aspirin and acetaminophen is uncertain, but is likely between 0 and 6%. Studies show that patients with AERD can usually tolerate single acetaminophen doses of up to 650 mg safely. Single doses of 1,000 mg, however, induce bronchospasm in up to 20% of patients. These reactions associated with acetaminophen tend to be less severe than those associated with aspirin.[73] Aspirin desensitization is a possible alternative if avoidance of aspirin, aspirin-containing products, or NSAIDs is not possible in patients with AERD. Aspirin desensitization, a process involving repeated exposure to aspirin in increasing doses to eliminate adverse effects related to its use, allows patients to take aspirin or cross-reacting NSAIDs. Desensitization and daily aspirin use can significantly improve patient symptoms and quality of life, decrease nasal polyps, and reduce the need for oral corticosteroids and sinus surgery. Desensitization also has been shown to improve nasal and asthma symptom scores in patients with AERD. Contraindications to desensitization include pregnancy, unstable asthma, gastric ulcers, and bleeding disorders. Numerous aspirin desensitization protocols exist. One such protocol desensitizes patients over several days. Patients should have a baseline FEV_1 ≥60% predicted (at least 1.5 L). Therapy with a leukotriene modifier should be initiated if one is not currently taken, and patients should continue therapy with oral or inhaled corticosteroids and long-acting bronchodilators. Antihistamines and short-acting β-agonists should be held prior to the challenge. The protocol starts with administration of aspirin 20–40 mg every 3 hours. If a reaction occurs, it is treated before continuing. This initial provocation dose is then repeated. The effects of aspirin desensitization last indefinitely, but long-term therapy is necessary to

Table 22-6 Approaches to Help Prevent Drug-Induced Asthma and Bronchospasm

Drug	Condition	Prevention
Aspirin	Asthma	Avoidance of aspirin Aspirin desensitization Acetaminophen, salsalate, meloxicam, or celecoxib may be used instead of aspirin
β-blockers	Bronchospasm	Use cardioselective β-blockers at lowest possible dose
ACE inhibitors	Cough	Avoidance of ACE inhibitors Use angiotensin receptor blocker or antihypertensive agent from a different class

ACE = angiotensin-converting enzyme.

maintain desensitization. Maintenance treatment with aspirin should be at least 325 mg and ideally twice daily to ensure adequate anti-inflammatory activity in the respiratory tract. For patients who need primary cardiovascular prophylaxis with aspirin, 81-mg doses may maintain the desensitized state.[175]

Because of the mortality benefits demonstrated with β-blockers, their use may be necessary in patients with HFrEF and/or a history of myocardial infarction.[143] Nonselective β-blockers are contraindicated in patients with asthma. However, one meta-analysis concluded that β_1-selective β-blockers should not be avoided in patients who may benefit from their use.[153] Reports of bronchospasm with low doses and β_2-receptor blockade associated with high doses of cardioselective β-blockers have been documented. Therefore, the chosen cardioselective β-blocker should have a short half-life and be initiated at the lowest possible dose, and upward dose titration should occur slowly.[143] Although cardioselective β-blockers are associated with a lower incidence of respiratory adverse effects than nonselective β-blockers, both types should be avoided in patients with severe asthma. Patients requiring therapy with a topical ophthalmic β-blocker to decrease intraocular pressure should also be prescribed a cardioselective agent such as betaxolol.[143]

MANAGEMENT

Based on one of the proposed mechanisms of AERD, both cys-LT_1 receptor antagonists (zafirlukast and montelukast) and 5-lipoxygenase inhibitors (zileuton) should play a role in the management of AERD.[173,176] A study involving 46 patients evaluated the impact of long-term montelukast therapy in protecting against AERD in aspirin-intolerant patients. Patients with mild or moderate asthma received montelukast 10 mg daily for 12 weeks. The decline in FEV_1 following aspirin challenge decreased from 28.6% ± 1.9% to 10.2% ± 1.7% ($p = 0.0001$). Patients were were considered poor responders if they demonstrated >15% decline in FEV_1 after aspirin challenge. Poor responders ($n = 14$, 30%) had a higher incidence of rhinosinusitis, history of aspirin hypersensitivity, and larger decline in FEV_1 following aspirin challenge before treatment compared with good responders (37.6% ± 3.8% versus 24.7% ± 1.8%; $p = 0.005$).[177]

Numerous smaller studies have evaluated the impact of zileuton in patients with AERD. In one study, $n = 7$ patients demonstrated a mean maximal decrease in FEV_1 of 2.9% while taking with zileuton compared with 4.9% during placebo after an aspirin challenge. However, only two patients in the study experienced complete inhibition of aspirin-induced respiratory adverse effects.[178] Another small study ($n = 6$) evaluated the effect of zileuton and placebo before and during an aspirin challenge. The mean aspirin dose provoking a respiratory reaction was 57 mg (30–100 mg) during initial challenge and increased to 122 mg (45–325 mg) in patients taking zileuton 600 mg four times daily. No participants could tolerate typical aspirin doses, and the authors concluded that the dose of zileuton was inadequate in preventing aspirin-induced respiratory reactions.[179] A study of similar design ($n = 8$) demonstrated much different results with zileuton, showing decreased urinary LTE_4 excretion and a FEV_1 decrease of 4.4% associated with zileuton, compared with 18.6% during placebo.[180] Differences between the studies may be due to differences in zileuton doses. One study used escalating doses of zileuton, whereas the other used a previously determined threshold dose. Differences between the studies may also be related to differences in the patients' disease severity.[181] Patients taking a 5-lipoxygenase inhibitor or a Cys-LT_1 receptor antagonist should continue to exercise caution with aspirin, NSAIDs, and other cross-reacting agents, because bronchospasm may occur.[173]

Omalizumab was shown to facilitate aspirin desensitization in a case report. A patient who had been previously unresponsive to aspirin desensitization received 16 weeks of omalizumab therapy (four doses), after which she underwent 10 days of aspirin desensitization, resulting in aspirin tolerance. Two years later the patient was still able to tolerate aspirin 600 mg daily, did not require asthma control treatment, did not have urticaria, and denied nasal polyp recurrences.[182] The biologic agent mepolizumab, which targets eosinophils, may also have potential for the management of AERD.

A survey of patients with a diagnosis of AERD reported that 88% of patients had been treated with a leukotriene-modifier agent, 24% underwent a trial of zileuton therapy, and 8% had been treated with omalizumab. The greatest benefit was associated with leukotriene receptor antagonists, with 50% of patients remaining on chronic leukotriene receptor antagonist therapy for AERD.[167]

Ipratropium is the preferred treatment for β-blocker–induced bronchospasm.[2] Oxitropium, an antimuscarinic, has also been shown to prevent acute propranolol-induced bronchoconstriction.[183] In addition, evidence has shown that tiotropium may prevent propranolol-induced bronchoconstriction after acute dosing during up-titration to 80 mg. There was no significant difference observed in methacholine or histamine airway hyperresponsiveness for patients receiving propranolol or placebo and no adverse impact on asthma control. Albuterol may be used to treat β-blocker–induced bronchospasm, but acute effects may be attenuated. In one study, after methacholine challenge, patients received albuterol and ipratropium. There was a significant decrease in area under the curve for patients treated with propranolol versus placebo; however, after 20 minutes the difference was no longer significant.[184]

Once ACE-inhibitor–induced cough is suspected, the drug should be discontinued to determine whether the cough is ACE-inhibitor–induced.[147] The cough usually resolves within 1–4 weeks but may take up to 3 months in some individuals.[147,154] A rechallenege may be performed with the same or a different agent to determine if cough recurs. In some patients the cough may abate with long-term therapy or subside spontaneously.[147] Alternatives to ACE inhibitor therapy include ARBs or antihypertensive agents from different drug classes. ARBs are effective for the management of hypertension or heart failure but do not directly inhibit ACE activity or inhibit bradykinin metabolism. Randomized, controlled studies of ARBs have demonstrated a lower incidence of cough in patients with a history of ACE-inhibitor–induced cough.[185,186] In one meta-analysis of studies conducted in patients with intolerance to ACE inhibitors, the incidence of cough associated with ARBs was 24%, compared with 67% associated with ACE inhibitors.[187] If a patient with ACE-inhibitor–induced cough must remain on ACE inhibitor therapy, there are limited drug therapy options to manage cough. Drug therapy, including inhaled cromolyn, theophylline, sulindac, indomethacin, amlodipine, nifedipine, ferrous sulfate, and picotamide (not available in the United States) has been reported to exert some beneficial effects on ACE-inhibitor–induced cough in small, randomized, double-blind, placebo-controlled trials. Small, unblinded, uncontrolled studies have provided limited evidence supporting the use of baclofen, ozagrel, and aspirin (500 mg/day) for management of ACE-inhibitor–induced cough. After discontinuation of the ACE inhibitor and resolution of the cough, a repeat trial of an ACE inhibitor may be attempted in patients with a compelling reason to use an ACE inhibitor and who are unable to take an ARB.[154] Some evidence suggests that ACE-inhibitor–induced cough occurs less frequency with concomitant calcium channel blocker or diuretic therapy compared to that associated with ACE inhibitor monotherapy. There was also a lower frequency of cough when the ACE inhibitor was taken at bedtime.[188]

INFORMATION FOR PATIENTS

Patients with AERD should be instructed to avoid potent COX-1 inhibitors such as aspirin, ibuprofen, ketoprofen, and others. Weak peripheral inhibitors of COX-1 and COX-2 (e.g., acetaminophen, salsalate) may be used, but patients should be informed that there is a chance of exacerbation of asthma with these drugs and to immediately discontinue therapy if this is suspected.[1,3,172,173] Aspirin or NSAID allergy must be documented in all medical records, including at the patient's pharmacy. Patients should be instructed to consult their pharmacist to select nonprescription products with no cross-reactivity with aspirin. Because cross-reactivity is dose-related for some medications, patients should be advised to take only doses recommended by a healthcare provider.

Patients with a respiratory condition such as asthma or COPD should inform providers of their condition. If a patient is prescribed a β-blocker, the patient should be instructed not to take more than the prescribed dose. It is necessary for patients taking β-blockers to inform healthcare providers about their use and be warned that they may exacerbate respiratory conditions.

If patients experience cough due to ACE inhibitors, they should be instructed to contact their healthcare provider and not to treat the cough with nonprescription products. ACE-inhibitor–induced cough is treated with antitussive therapy in approximately 15% of all cases.[189] In one study, treatment with prescription antitussive therapy was twice as likely in patients taking ACE inhibitors compared to patients who did not receive ACE inhibitor therapy. This study did not assess the use of nonprescription antitussives, which would likely increase the risk of misdiagnosis and mistreatment of ACE-inhibitor–induced cough.[169] Patients using ACE inhibitors who experience a chronic cough should be referred to their medical provider to determine the etiology.

REFERENCES

1. The Gobal Strategy for Asthma Management and Prevention. Global Initiative for Asthma (GINA) 2016. http://ginasthma.org/wp-content/uploads/2016/04/wms-GINA-2016-main-report-final.pdf (accessed 2018 Jan 26).
2. National Heart, Lung, and Blood Institute, National Asthma Education and Prevention Program. Expert Panel Report 3: Guidelines for the diagnosis and management of asthma. http://www.nhlbi.nih.gov/health-pro/guidelines/current/asthma-guidelines/full-report (accessed 2018 Jan 26).
3. Covar RA, Macomber BA, Szefler SJ. Medications as asthma triggers. *Immunol Allergy Clin North Am.* 2005; 25:169-90.
4. Babu KS, Marshall BG. Drug-induced airway diseases. *Clin Chest Med.* 2004; 25:113-22.
5. Takafuji S, Nakagawa T. Drug-induced pulmonary disorders. *Intern Med.* 2004; 43:169-70.
6. Shaheen SO, Sterne JA, Songhurst CE et al. Frequent paracetamol use and asthma in adults. *Thorax.* 2000; 55:266-70.
7. Barr RG, Wentowski CC, Curhan GC et al. Prospective study of acetaminophen use and newly diagnosed asthma among women. *Am J Respir Crit Care Med.* 2004; 169:836-41.
8. Settipane RA, Schrank PJ, Simon RA et al. Prevalence of cross-sensitivity with acetaminophen in aspirin-sensitive asthmatic subjects. *J Allergy Clin Immunol.* 1995; 96:480-5.
9. Sandilands EA, Bateman DN. Adverse reactions associated with acetylcysteine. *Clin Toxicol (Phila).* 2009; 47:81-8.
10. Marcelle R. Alpha-adrenergic bronchoconstriction in man. *Arch Physiol Biochem.* 1996; 104:851-4.
11. Imamura H, Kinoshita O, Maruyama K et al. Two cases of bronchial asthma after treatment with amiodarone. *Pacing Clin Electrophysiol.* 2001; 24:1563-5.
12. Yavuzgil O, Goksel T, Gurgun C et al. New-onset bronchial asthma induced by low-dose amiodarone. *Ann Pharmacother.* 2005; 39:385-6.
13. Bezalel S, Mahlab-Guri K, Asher I et al. Angiotensin-converting enzyme inhibitor-induced angioedema. *Am J Med.* 2015; 128:120-5.
14. McEwan JR, Fuller RW. Angiotensin converting enzyme inhibitors and cough. *J Cardiovasc Pharmacol.* 1989; 13(suppl 3):S67-9.
15. Barnes PJ, Woolcock AJ. Difficult asthma. *Eur Respir J.* 1998; 12:1209-18.
16. Morimoto T, Gandhi TK, Fiskio JM et al. Development and validation of a clinical prediction rule for angiotensin-converting enzyme inhibitor-induced cough. *J Gen Intern Med.* 2004; 19:684-91.
17. Rajan JP, Wineinger NE, Stevenson DD, White AA. Prevalence of aspirin-exacerbated respiratory disease among asthmatic patients: A meta-analysis of the literature. *J Allergy Clin Immunol.* 2015; 135:676-81.e671.
18. Schiavino D, Nucera E, Milani A et al. The aspirin disease. *Thorax.* 2000; 55(suppl 2):S66-9.
19. Hedman J, Kaprio J, Poussa T et al. Prevalence of asthma, aspirin intolerance, nasal polyposis and chronic obstructive pulmonary disease in a population-based study. *Int J Epidemiol.* 1999; 28:717-22.
20. Menendez R, Lowe RS, Kersey J. Benzalkonium chloride and bronchoconstriction. *J Allergy Clin Immunol.* 1989; 84:272-4.
21. Fabiano V, Mameli C, Zuccotti GV. Paediatric pharmacology: remember the excipients. *Pharmacol Res.* 2011; 63:362-5.
22. Craig TJ. Drugs to be used with caution in patients with asthma. *Am Fam Physician.* 1996; 54:947-53, 957-48.
23. Morales DR, Jackson C, Lipworth BJ et al. Adverse respiratory effect of acute beta-blocker exposure in asthma: a systematic review and meta-analysis of randomized controlled trials. *Chest.* 2014; 145:779-86.
24. Jimenez I, Anton E, Picans I et al. Betahistine-induced bronchospasm. *Allergy.* 1996; 51:185-8.
25. Galleguillos F, Rodriguez JC. Asthma caused by bromelin inhalation. *Clin Allergy.* 1978; 8:21-4.
26. Lee T, Cochrane GM, Amlot P. Pulmonary eosinophilia and asthma associated with carbamazepine. *Br Med J (Clin Res Ed).* 1981; 282:440.
27. Harber CR, Levy DM, Chidambaram S et al. Life-threatening bronchospasm after intramuscular carboprost for postpartum haemorrhage. *Bjog.* 2007; 114:366-8.
28. Pillans P. Bronchospasm associated with cisapride. *BMJ.* 1995; 311:1472.
29. Caponnetto P, Auditore R, Russo C et al. "Dangerous relationships": asthma and substance abuse. *J Addict Dis.* 2013; 32:158-67.
30. Osborn HH, Tang M, Bradley K et al. New-onset bronchospasm or recrudescence of asthma associated with cocaine abuse. *Acad Emerg Med.* 1997; 4:689-92.
31. Alothman GA, Ho B, Alsaadi MM et al. Bronchial constriction and inhaled colistin in cystic fibrosis. *Chest.* 2005; 127:522-9.
32. Katayama H, Yokoyama A, Fujino S et al. Near-death asthmatic reaction induced by disodium cromoglycate. *Intern Med.* 1996; 35:976-8.
33. Thong BY, Leong KP, Thumboo J et al. Cyclophosphamide type I hypersensitivity in systemic lupus erythematosus. *Lupus.* 2002; 11:127-9.
34. Farmer BC, Sivarajan M. An anaphylactoid response to a small dose of d-tubocurarine. *Anesthesiology.* 1979; 51:358-9.
35. Yeung ML, Ng LY, Koo AW. Severe bronchospasm in an asthmatic patient following alcuronium and D-tubocurarine. *Anaesth Intensive Care.* 1979; 7:62-4.
36. Takki S, Tammisto T. Severe bronchospasm and circulatory collapse following the administration of d-tubocurarine. *Ann Clin Res.* 1971; 3:112-5.
37. Camus P. [The respiratory complications of D-Penicillamine therapy (author's transl)]. *Rev Fr Mal Respir.* 1982; 10:7-20.
38. Tanphaichitr K. D-penicillamine-induced bronchial spasm. *South Med J.* 1980; 73:788-90.

39. Boisseau N, Bouregba M, Vivinus M et al. Acute severe asthma after immunotherapy with Friedmann's vaccine. *Intensive Care Med.* 2000; 26:481.
40. Hillis GS, al-Mohammad A, Jennings KP. Respiratory arrest during dipyridamole stress testing. *Postgrad Med J.* 1997; 73:301-2.
41. Bonnelykke K, Raaschou-Nielsen O, Tjonneland A et al. Postmenopausal hormone therapy and asthma-related hospital admission. *J Allergy Clin Immunol.* 2015; 135:813-6.e815.
42. Barr RG, Wentowski CC, Grodstein F et al. Prospective study of postmenopausal hormone use and newly diagnosed asthma and chronic obstructive pulmonary disease. *Arch Intern Med.* 2004; 164:379-86.
43. Tachibana K, Sasaki S, Nakamura T et al. Bronchospasm induced by ethanol injection for a craniofacial venous malformation. *A A Case Rep.* 2014; 2:149-51.
44. Laborde-Casterot H, Villa AF, Rosenberg N et al. Occupational rhinitis and asthma due to EDTA-containing detergents or disinfectants. *Am J Ind Med.* 2012; 55:677-82.
45. Beasley CR, Rafferty P, Holgate ST. Bronchoconstrictor properties of preservatives in ipratropium bromide (Atrovent) nebuliser solution. *Br Med J (Clin Res Ed).* 1987; 294:1197-8.
46. Spooner LM, Olin JL. Paradoxical bronchoconstriction with albuterol administered by metered-dose inhaler and nebulizer solution. *Ann Pharmacother.* 2005; 39:1924-7.
47. Rolla G, Bucca C, Brussino L. Bisphosphonate-induced bronchoconstriction in aspirin-sensitive asthma. *Lancet.* 1994; 343:426-7.
48. Okazaki K, Saito T, Wakisaka K et al. Bronchospasm possible due to gallamine. A case report. *Tokushima J Exp Med.* 1969; 16:9-14.
49. Tallia AF, Cardone DA. Asthma exacerbation associated with glucosamine-chondroitin supplement. *J Am Board Fam Pract.* 2002; 15:481-4.
50. Doshi V, Shenoy S, Ganesh A et al. Profile of acute asthma exacerbation in drug users. *Am J Ther.* 2014.
51. Elia D, Marinou A, Chetta A. Life-threatening asthma after heroin inhalation. A case report and a review of the literature. *Acta Biomed.* 2010; 81:63-7.
52. Holz W, Ludwig A, Forst H. [Anaphylactic shock following intravenous hydrocortisone succinate administration]. *Anaesthesist.* 2002; 51:187-90.
53. Currie GP, Paterson E, Keenan F et al. An unexpected response to intravenous hydrocortisone succinate in an asthmatic patient. *Br J Clin Pharmacol.* 2005; 60:342.
54. Bini EJ, Weinshel EH. Severe exacerbation of asthma: a new side effect of interferon-alpha in patients with asthma and chronic hepatitis C. *Mayo Clin Proc.* 1999; 74:367-70.
55. Barutca S, Meydan N, Barlak A. Prevention of interleukin-2-induced severe bronchospasm with salbutamol. *J Aerosol Med.* 2003; 16:183-4.
56. Loppow D, Huland E, Heinzer H et al. Interleukin-2 inhalation therapy temporarily induces asthma-like airway inflammation. *Eur J Med Res.* 2007; 12:556-62.
57. Pradubpongsa P, Dhana N, Jongjarearnprasert K et al. Adverse reactions to iodinated contrast media: prevalence, risk factors and outcome—the results of a 3-year period. *Asian Pac J Allergy Immunol.* 2013; 31:299-306.
58. Kapur N, Hughes JR, Rustin MH. Exacerbation of asthma by isotretinoin. *Br J Dermatol.* 2000; 142:388-9.
59. Sabroe RA, Staughton RC, Bunker CB. Bronchospasm induced by isotretinoin. *BMJ.* 1996; 312:886.
60. Dicpinigaitis PV, Thomas SA, Sherman MB et al. Losartan-induced bronchospasm. *J Allergy Clin Immunol.* 1996; 98(Pt 1):1128-30.
61. Conigliaro RL, Gleason PP. Losartan-induced cough after lisinopril therapy. *Am J Health-Syst Pharm.* 2000; 57:996-7.
62. Marlowe KF. Urticaria and asthma exacerbation after ingestion of menthol-containing lozenges. *Am J Health-Syst Pharm.* 2003; 60:1657-9.
63. Elloway R, Sherman S, Maas L et al. Meperidine-associated bronchospasm. *Gastrointest Endosc.* 1992; 38:93.
64. Shtessel M, Toh J, Gavrilova T. Anaphylaxis as a delayed reaction of methimazole therapy. *Ann Allergy Asthma Immunol.* 2015; 115:245-7.
65. Shulimzon TR, Shiner RJ. A risk-benefit assessment of methotrexate in corticosteroid-dependent asthma. *Drug Saf.* 1996; 15:283-90.
66. Jones G, Mierins E, Karsh J. Methotrexate-induced asthma. *Am Rev Respir Dis.* 1991; 143:179-81.
67. Harries MG, Taylor AN, Wooden J et al. Bronchial asthma due to alpha-methyldopa. *Br Med J.* 1979; 1:1461.
68. Schonwald S. Methylprednisolone anaphylaxis. *Am J Emerg Med.* 1999; 17:583-5.
69. Fernandez S, Reano M, Vives R et al. 6-Methylprednisolone-induced bronchospasm. *Allergy.* 1997; 52:780-2.
70. Burburan SM, Xisto DG, Rocco PR. Anaesthetic management in asthma. *Minerva Anestesiol.* 2007; 73:357-65.
71. Hazizaj A, Hatija A. Bronchospasm caused by neostigmine. *Eur J Anaesthesiol.* 2006; 23:85-6.
72. Makowska J, Lewandowska-Polak A, Kowalski ML. Hypersensitivity to aspirin and other NSAIDs: diagnostic approach in patients with chronic rhinosinusitis. *Curr Allergy Asthma Rep.* 2015; 15:47.
73. Simon RA. Treatment of patients with respiratory reactions to aspirin and nonsteroidal anti-inflammatory drugs. *Curr Allergy Asthma Rep.* 2004; 4:139-43.
74. Baldassarre S, Schandene L, Choufani G et al. Asthma attacks induced by low doses of celecoxib, aspirin, and acetaminophen. *J Allergy Clin Immunol.* 2006; 117:215-7.
75. Passero M, Chowdhry S. Cyclooxygenase-2 inhibitors in aspirin-sensitive asthma. *Chest.* 2003; 123:2155-6; author reply 2156.
76. Cabestrero D, Perez-Paredes C, Fernandez-Cid R et al. Bronchospasm and laryngeal stridor as an adverse effect of oxytocin treatment. *Crit Care.* 2003; 7:392.
77. Heath ML. Bronchospasm in an asthmatic patient following pancuronium. *Anaesthesia.* 1973; 28:437-40.
78. Delaney JC. Pentazocine-induced bronchospasm. *Lancet.* 1972; 2:338.
79. Katzman M, Meade W, Iglar K et al. High incidence of bronchospasm with regular administration of aerosolized pentamidine. *Chest.* 1992; 101:79-81.
80. Gearhart MO, Bhutani MS. Intravenous pentamidine-induced bronchospasm. *Chest.* 1992; 102:1891-2.
81. Acute pulmonary effects of aerosolized pentamidine. A randomized controlled study. Toronto Aerosolized Pentamidine Study (TAPS) Group. *Chest.* 1990; 98:907-10.
82. Hill MR, Gotz VP, Harman E et al. Evaluation of the asthmogenicity of propafenone, a new antiarrhythmic drug. Comparison of spirometry with methacholine challenge. *Chest.* 1986; 90:698-702.
83. You BC, Jang AS, Han JS et al. A case of propofol-induced oropharyngeal angioedema and bronchospasm. *Allergy Asthma Immunol Res.* 2012; 4:46-8.
84. Nguyen LT, Luong KV. Propylthiouracil-induced asthma. *Allergy.* 2004; 59:889-90.
85. Vaswani SK, Hamilton RG, Valentine MD et al. Psyllium laxative-induced anaphylaxis, asthma, and rhinitis. *Allergy.* 1996; 51:266-8.
86. Cartier A, Malo JL, Dolovich J. Occupational asthma in nurses handling psyllium. *Clin Allergy.* 1987; 17:1-6.
87. Wagner SL. Fatal asthma in a child after use of an animal shampoo containing pyrethrin. *West J Med.* 2000; 173:86-7.
88. Proudfoot AT. Poisoning due to pyrethrins. *Toxicol Rev.* 2005; 24:107-13.
89. Michils A, Vandermoten G, Duchateau J et al. Anaphylaxis with sodium benzoate. *Lancet.* 1991; 337:1424-5.
90. Park HS, Lim YS, Suh JE et al. Sodium salicylate sensitivity in an asthmatic patient with aspirin sensitivity. *J Korean Med Sci.* 1991; 6:113-7.

91. Steiner M, Scaife A, Semple S et al. Sodium metabisulphite induced airways disease in the fishing and fish-processing industry. *Occup Med (Lond).* 2008; 58:545-50.
92. Marenco Arellano V, Reano-Martos M, Rodriguez-Cabreros M et al. Sulfite sensitivity in a patient with allergic asthma. *Allergol Immunopathol (Madr).* 2011; 39:306-7.
93. Smith RP, Dewar JA, Winter JH. Tamoxifen-induced asthma. *Lancet.* 1993; 341:772.
94. MacCara ME. Tartrazine: a potentially hazardous dye in Canadian drugs. *Can Med Assoc J.* 1982; 126:910-4.
95. Beausoleil JL, Fiedler J, Spergel JM. Food Intolerance and childhood asthma: what is the link? *Paediatr Drugs.* 2007; 9:157-63.
96. Vandenplas O, Delwiche JP, Auverdin J et al. Asthma to tetramethrin. *Allergy.* 2000; 55:417-8.
97. Ting JY. Ocular tobramycin-induced bronchospasm in an adult without asthma or atopy. *Can J Ophthalmol.* 2007; 42:883-4.
98. Nikolaizik WH, Trociewicz K, Ratjen F. Bronchial reactions to the inhalation of high-dose tobramycin in cystic fibrosis. *Eur Respir J.* 2002; 20:122-6.
99. Santos RP, Awa E, Anbar RD. Inhaled tobramycin solution-associated recurrent eosinophilia and severe persistent bronchospasm in a patient with cystic fibrosis: a case report. *BMC Pediatr.* 2007; 7:11.
100. Melien O, Skaali T, Myhr K et al. Venlafaxine and asthma. *Nord J Psychiatry.* 2005; 59:538-40.
101. Ben-Noun L. Acute asthma associated with sustained-release verapamil. *Ann Pharmacother.* 1997; 31:593-5.
102. Landis E, Shore E. Yohimbine-induced bronchospasm. *Chest.* 1989; 96:1424.
103. Williamson JC, Pegram PS. Respiratory distress associated with zanamivir. *N Engl J Med.* 2000; 342:661-2.
104. From the Global Strategy for Asthma Management and Prevention. Global Initiative for Asthma (GINA) 2015. http://ginasthma.org/wp-content/uploads/2016/01/GINA_Report_2015_Aug11-1.pdf (accessed 2018 Feb 16).
105. Centers for Disease Control and Prevention. Survey reveals growing national impact of asthma; 2012. http://www.cdc.gov/media/releases/2012/p0515_asthma_impact.html (accessed 2018 Jan 26).
106. Borges MD, Capriles-Hulett A, Caballero-Fonseca F et al. Tolerability to new COX-2 inhibitors in NSAID-sensitive patients with cutaneous reactions. *Ann Allergy Asthma Immunol.* 2001; 87:201-4.
107. Stevenson DD, Szczeklik A. Clinical and pathologic perspectives on aspirin sensitivity and asthma. *J Allergy Clin Immunol.* 2006; 118:773-86; quiz 787-8.
108. Barnett MJ, Milavetz G, Kaboli PJ. beta-Blocker therapy in veterans with asthma or chronic obstructive pulmonary disease. *Pharmacotherapy.* 2005; 25:1550-9.
109. Odeh M, Oliven A, Bassan H. Timolol eyedrop-induced fatal bronchospasm in an asthmatic patient. *J Fam Pract.* 1991; 32:97-8.
110. Dunn TL, Gerber MJ, Shen AS et al. The effect of topical ophthalmic instillation of timolol and betaxolol on lung function in asthmatic subjects. *Am Rev Respir Dis.* 1986; 133:264-8.
111. Salpeter SR Ormiston TM, Salpeter EE. Cardioselective beta-blockers for chronic obstructive pulmonary disease (Review). http://onlinelibrary.wiley.com/doi/10.1002/14651858.CD003566.pub2/abstract (accessed 2018 Jan 26).
112. Zhong G, Shen NY, Sammut J. Nebulised salbutamol challenge confirming life-threatening paradoxical bronchospasm. *Emerg Med Australas.* 2014; 26:202-3.
113. Raghunathan K, Nagajothi N. Paradoxical bronchospasm: a potentially life threatening adverse effect of albuterol. *South Med J.* 2006; 99:288-9.
114. Broski SE, Amundson DE. Paradoxical response to levalbuterol. *J Am Osteopath Assoc.* 2008; 108:211-3.
115. Asmus MJ, Sherman J, Hendeles L. Bronchoconstrictor additives in bronchodilator solutions. *J Allergy Clin Immunol.* 1999; 104(Pt 2):S53-60.
116. Trautlein J, Allegra J, Field J et al. Paradoxic bronchospasm after inhalation of isoptroterenol. *Chest.* 1976; 70:711-4.
117. Bonniaud P, Favrolt N, Collet E et al. Salbutamol, terbutaline and pirbuterol allergy in an asthmatic patient. *Allergy.* 2007; 62:1219-20.
118. Yarbrough J, Mansfield LE, Ting S. Metered dose inhaler induced bronchospasm in asthmatic patients. *Ann Allergy.* 1985; 55:25-7.
119. American Academy of Pediatrics Committee on Drugs. "Inactive" ingredients in pharmaceutical products: update (subject review). *Pediatrics.* 1997; 99:268-78.
120. Perrio MJ, Wilton LV, Shakir SA. A modified prescription-event monitoring study to assess the introduction of Seretide Evohaler in England: an example of studying risk monitoring in pharmacovigilance. *Drug Saf.* 2007; 30:681-95.
121. Hendeles L, Colice GL, Meyer RJ. Withdrawal of albuterol inhalers containing chlorofluorocarbon propellants. *N Engl J Med.* 2007; 356:1344-51.
122. Mathison DA, Stevenson DD, Simon RA. Precipitating factors in asthma. Aspirin, sulfites, and other drugs and chemicals. *Chest.* 1985; 87(suppl 1):50s-54s.
123. Yang WH, Purchase EC. Adverse reactions to sulfites. *CMAJ.* 1985; 133:865-7, 880.
124. Beasley R, Fishwick D, Miles JF et al. Preservatives in nebulizer solutions: risks without benefit. *Pharmacotherapy.* 1998; 18:130-9.
125. Asmus MJ, Barros MD, Liang J et al. Pulmonary function response to EDTA, an additive in nebulized bronchodilators. *J Allergy Clin Immunol.* 2001; 107:68-72.
126. Israili ZH, Hall WD. Cough and angioneurotic edema associated with angiotensin-converting enzyme inhibitor therapy. A review of the literature and pathophysiology. *Ann Intern Med.* 1992; 117:234-42.
127. Chang JE, White A, Simon RA et al. Aspirin-exacerbated respiratory disease: burden of disease. *Allergy Asthma Proc.* 2012; 33:117-21.
128. Beasley R, Rafferty P, Holgate ST. Adverse reactions to the non-drug constituents of nebuliser solutions. *Br J Clin Pharmacol.* 1988; 25:283-7.
129. Kowalski ML, Makowska JS, Blanca M et al. Hypersensitivity to nonsteroidal anti-inflammatory drugs (NSAIDs)—classification, diagnosis and management: review of the EAACI/ENDA(#) and GA2LEN/HANNA*. *Allergy.* 2011; 66:818-29.
130. Koepke JW, Christopher KL, Chai H et al. Dose-dependent bronchospasm from sulfites in isoetharine. *JAMA.* 1984; 251:2982-3.
131. Wang XB, Du JB, Cui H. Sulfur dioxide, a double-faced molecule in mammals. *Life Sci.* 2014; 98:63-7.
132. Hengameh H, Raissy MH, Marshik P. Drug induced pulmonary diseases. In: Joseph T. DiPiro, Robert L. Talbert, Gary C. Yee, eds. *Pharmacotherapy: a phathophysiologic approach.* 6th ed. New York: McGraw Hill; 2005:577-90.
133. Hamad AM, Sutcliffe AM, Knox AJ. Aspirin-induced asthma: clinical aspects, pathogenesis and management. *Drugs* 2004; 64:2417-32.
134. Kim SH, Park HS. Pathogenesis of nonsteroidal antiinflammatory drug-induced asthma. *Curr Opin Allergy Clin Immunol.* 2006; 6:17-22.
135. Sanak M, Pierzchalska M, Bazan-Socha S et al. Enhanced expression of the leukotriene C(4) synthase due to overactive transcription of an allelic variant associated with aspirin-intolerant asthma. *Am J Respir Cell Mol Biol.* 2000; 23:290-6.
136. Namazy JA, Simon RA. Sensitivity to nonsteroidal anti-inflammatory drugs. *Ann Allergy Asthma Immunol.* 2002; 89:542-50.
137. Cowburn AS, Sladek K, Soja J et al. Overexpression of leukotriene C4 synthase in bronchial biopsies from patients with aspirin-intolerant asthma. *J Clin Invest.* 1998; 101:834-46.
138. Szczeklik A, Stevenson DD. Aspirin-induced asthma: advances in pathogenesis, diagnosis, and management. *J Allergy Clin Immunol.* 2003; 111:913-21; quiz 922.

139. Babu KS, Salvi SS. Aspirin and asthma. *Chest.* 2000; 118:1470-6.
140. Stevenson DD. Aspirin sensitivity and desensitization for asthma and sinusitis. *Curr Allergy Asthma Rep.* 2009; 9:155-63.
141. Obase Y, Matsuse H, Shimoda T et al. Pathogenesis and management of aspirin-intolerant asthma. *Treat Respir Med.* 2005; 4:325-36.
142. Self T, Soberman JE, Bubla JM et al. Cardioselective beta-blockers in patients with asthma and concomitant heart failure or history of myocardial infarction: when do benefits outweigh risks? *J Asthma.* 2003; 40:839-45.
143. Tafreshi MJ, Weinacker AB. Beta-adrenergic-blocking agents in bronchospastic diseases: a therapeutic dilemma. *Pharmacotherapy.* 1999; 19:974-8.
144. Fuller RW, Dixon CM, Cuss FM et al. Bradykinin-induced bronchoconstriction in humans. Mode of action. *Am Rev Respir Dis.* 1987; 135:176-80.
145. Leader WG. Asthma. In: Chisholm-Burns MA, Wells BG, Schwinghammer TL, eds. *Pharmacotherapy: principles and practice.* New York: McGraw Hill; 2006:209-30.
146. Sica DA, Brath L. Angiotensin-converting enzyme inhibition-emerging pulmonary issues relating to cough. *Congest Heart Fail.* 2006; 12:223-6.
147. Luque CA, Vazquez Ortiz M. Treatment of ACE inhibitor-induced cough. *Pharmacotherapy.* 1999; 19:804-10.
148. Mas S, Gasso P, Alvarez S et al. Pharmacogenetic predictors of angiotensin-converting enzyme inhibitor-induced cough: the role of *ACEI, ABO,* and *BDKRB2* genes. *Pharmacogenet Genomics.* 2011; 21: 531-8.
149. Nizankowska-Mogilnicka E, Bochenek G, Mastalerz L et al. EAACI/GA2LEN guideline: aspirin provocation tests for diagnosis of aspirin hypersensitivity. *Allergy.* 2007; 62:1111-8.
150. Bochenek G, Niz Ankowska E, Szczeklik A. Testing for aspirin hypersensitivity. *Allergy.* 2002; 57:562-5.
151. Milewski M, Mastalerz L, Nizankowska E et al. Nasal provocation test with lysine-aspirin for diagnosis of aspirin-sensitive asthma. *J Allergy Clin Immunol.* 1998; 101:581-6.
152. Nizankowska E, Bestynska-Krypel A, Cmiel A et al. Oral and bronchial provocation tests with aspirin for diagnosis of aspirin-induced asthma. *Eur Respir J.* 2000; 15:863-9.
153. Salpeter S, Ormiston T, Salpeter E. Cardioselective beta-blockers for reversible airway disease. *Cochrane Database Syst Rev.* 2002:Cd002992.
154. Dicpinigaitis PV. Angiotensin-converting enzyme inhibitor-induced cough: ACCP evidence-based clinical practice guidelines. *Chest.* 2006; 129(suppl 1):169s-73s.
155. Pylypchuk GB. ACE inhibitor- versus angiotensin II blocker-induced cough and angioedema. *Ann Pharmacother.* 1998; 32:1060-6.
156. Morice AH, Fontana GA, Sovijarvi AR et al. The diagnosis and management of chronic cough. *Eur Respiratory J.* 2004; 24:481-92.
157. Nichol GM, Nix A, Chung KF et al. Characterisation of bronchoconstrictor responses to sodium metabisulphite aerosol in atopic subjects with and without asthma. *Thorax.* 1989; 44:1009-14.
158. Szczeklik A, Nizankowska E, Duplaga M. Natural history of aspirin-induced asthma. AIANE Investigators. European Network on Aspirin-Induced Asthma. *Eur Respir J.* 2000; 16:432-6.
159. Szczeklik A, Nizankowska E. Clinical features and diagnosis of aspirin induced asthma. *Thorax.* 2000; 55(suppl 2):S42-44.
160. Berges-Gimeno MP, Simon RA, Stevenson DD. The natural history and clinical characteristics of aspirin-exacerbated respiratory disease. *Ann Allergy Asthma Immunol.* 2002; 89:474-s8.
161. Os I, Bratland B, Dahlof B et al. Female sex as an important determinant of lisinopril-induced cough. *Lancet.* 1992; 339:372.
162. Os I, Bratland B, Dahlof B et al. Female preponderance for lisinopril-induced cough in hypertension. *Am J Hypertens.* 1994; 7:1012-5.
163. Packard KA, Wurdeman RL, Arouni AJ. ACE inhibitor-induced bronchial reactivity in patients with respiratory dysfunction. *Ann Pharmacother.* 2002; 36:1058-67.
164. Kupczyk M, Kuprys I, Gorski P et al. Aspirin intolerance and allergy to house dust mites: important factors associated with development of severe asthma. *Ann Allergy Asthma Immunol.* 2004; 92:453-8.
165. Mascia K, Haselkorn T, Deniz YM. Aspirin sensitivity and severity of asthma: evidence for irreversible airway obstruction in patients with severe or difficult-to-treat asthma. *J Allergy Clin Immunol.* 2005; 116:970-5.
166. Plaza V, Serrano J, Picado C et al. Frequency and clinical characteristics of rapid-onset fatal and near-fatal asthma. *Eur Respir J.* 2002; 19:846-52.
167. Ta V, White AA. Survey-defined patient experiences with aspirin-exacerbated respiratory eisease. *J Allergy Clin Immunol Pract.* 2015; 3:711-8.
168. Hanania NA, Singh S, El-Wali R et al. The safety and effects of the beta-blocker, nadolol, in mild asthma: an open-label pilot study. *Pulm Pharmacol Ther.* 2008; 21:134-41.
169. Vegter S, de Boer P, van Dijk KW et al. The effects of antitussive treatment of ACE inhibitor-induced cough on therapy compliance: a prescription sequence symmetry analysis. *Drug Saf.* 2013; 36:435-9.
170. Marks F, Harrell K, Fischer R. Successful use of cyclooxygenase-2 inhibitor in a patient with aspirin-induced asthma. *South Med J.* 2001; 94:256-7.
171. Looney Y, O'Shea A, O'Dwyer R. Severe bronchospasm after parenteral parecoxib: cyclooxygenase-2 inhibitors: not the answer yet. *Anesthesiology.* 2005; 102:473-5.
172. Umemoto J, Tsurikisawa N, Nogi S et al. Selective cyclooxygenase-2 inhibitor cross-reactivity in aspirin-exacerbated respiratory disease. *Allergy Asthma Proc.* 2011; 32:259-61.
173. Knowles SR, Drucker AM, Weber EA et al. Management options for patients with aspirin and nonsteroidal antiinflammatory drug sensitivity. *Ann Pharmacother.* 2007; 41:1191-200.
174. Matsuse H, Shimoda T, Matsuo N et al. Aspirin-induced asthma as a risk factor for asthma mortality. *J Asthma.* 1997; 34:413-7.
175. Lee RU, Stevenson DD. Aspirin-exacerbated respiratory disease: evaluation and management. *Allergy Asthma Immunol Res.* 2011; 3:3-10.
176. Steinke J, Wilson J. Aspirin-exacerbated respiratory disease: pathophysiological insights and clinical advances. *J Asthma Allergy.* 2016; 9:45-53.
177. Park JS, Jang AS, Park SW et al. Protection of leukotriene receptor antagonist against aspirin-induced bronchospasm in asthmatics. *Allergy Asthma Immunol Res.* 2010; 2:48-54.
178. Nasser SM, Bell GS, Foster S et al. Effect of the 5-lipoxygenase inhibitor ZD2138 on aspirin-induced asthma. *Thorax.* 1994; 49:749-56.
179. Pauls JD, Simon RA, Daffern PJ et al. Lack of effect of the 5-lipoxygenase inhibitor zileuton in blocking oral aspirin challenges in aspirin-sensitive asthmatics. *Ann Allergy Asthma Immunol.* 2000; 85:40-5.
180. Israel E, Fischer AR, Rosenberg MA et al. The pivotal role of 5-lipoxygenase products in the reaction of aspirin-sensitive asthmatics to aspirin. *Am Rev Respir Dis.* 1993; 148(Pt 6 1):1447-51.
181. Volkman JA, Pontikes PJ. Leukotriene modifiers to prevent aspirin-provoked respiratory reactions in asthmatics. *Ann Pharmacother.* 2002; 36:1457-61.
182. Guillen D, Bobolea I, Calderon O et al. Aspirin desensitization achieved after omalizumab treatment in a patient with aspirin-exacerbated urticaria and respiratory disease. *J Investig Allergol Clin Immunol.* 2015; 25:133-5.
183. Ind PW, Dixon CM, Fuller RW et al. Anticholinergic blockade of beta-blocker-induced bronchoconstriction. *Am Rev Respir Dis.* 1989; 139:1390-4.

184. Short PM, Williamson PA, Anderson WJ et al. Randomized placebo-controlled trial to evaluate chronic dosing effects of propranolol in asthma. *Am J Respir Crit Care Med.* 2013; 187:1308-14.

185. Lacourciere Y, Brunner H, Irwin R et al. Effects of modulators of the renin-angiotensin-aldosterone system on cough. Losartan Cough Study Group. *J Hypertens.* 1994; 12:1387-93.

186. Paster RZ, Snavely DB, Sweet AR et al. Use of losartan in the treatment of hypertensive patients with a history of cough induced by angiotensin-converting enzyme inhibitors. *Clin Ther.* 1998; 20:978-89.

187. Caldeira D, David C, Sampaio C. Tolerability of angiotensin-receptor blockers in patients with intolerance to angiotensin-converting enzyme inhibitors: a systematic review and meta-analysis. *Am J Cardiovasc Drugs.* 2012; 12:263-77.

188. Sato A, Fukuda S. A prospective study of frequency and characteristics of cough during ACE inhibitor treatment. *Clin Exp Hypertens.* 2015; 37:563-8.

189. Vegter S, de Jong-van den Berg LT. Misdiagnosis and mistreatment of a common side-effect—angiotensin-converting enzyme inhibitor-induced cough. *Br J Clin Pharmacol.* 2010; 69:200-3.

SECTION VI

DRUG-INDUCED CARDIOVASCULAR DISEASES

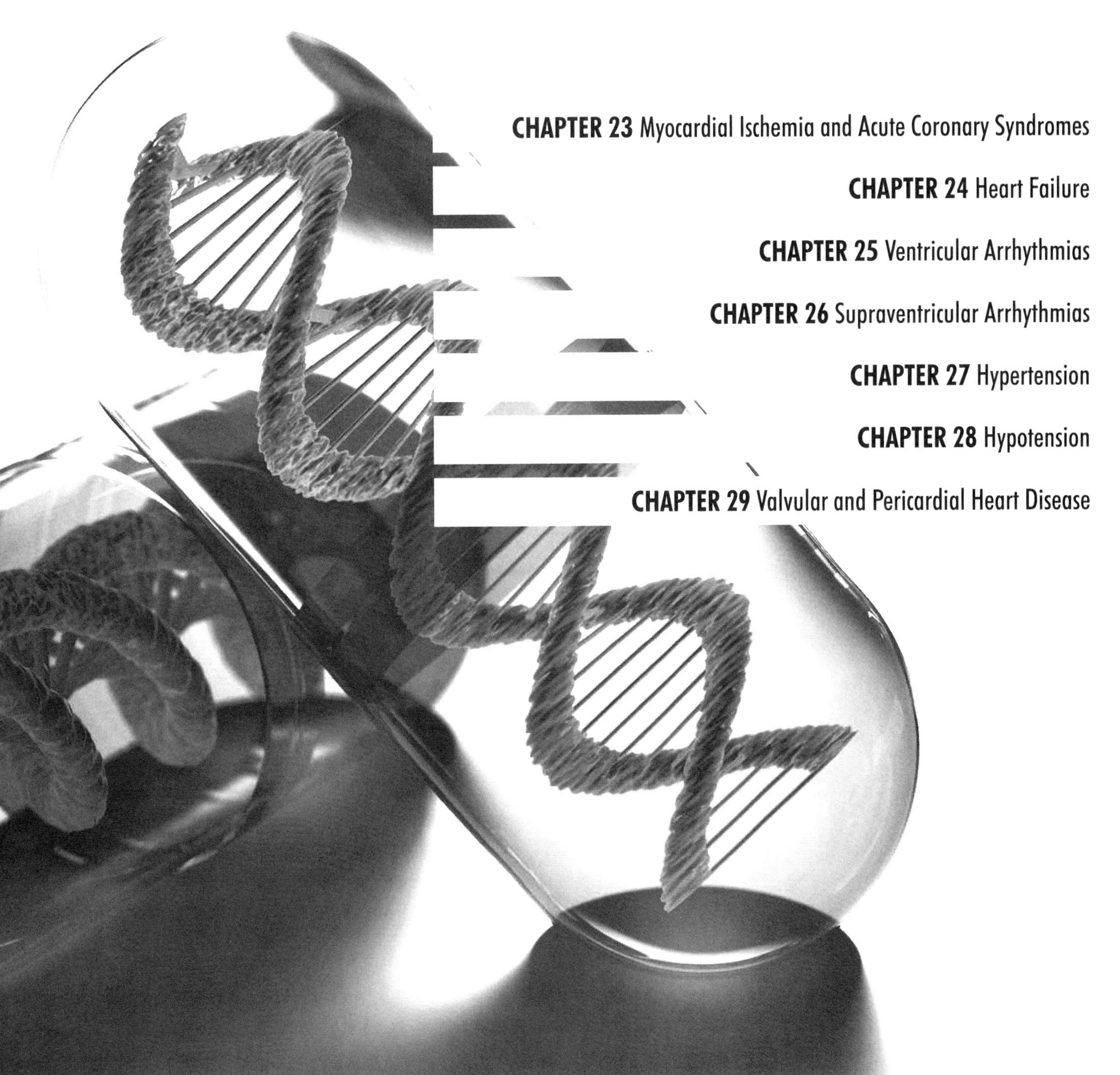

CHAPTER 23 Myocardial Ischemia and Acute Coronary Syndromes

CHAPTER 24 Heart Failure

CHAPTER 25 Ventricular Arrhythmias

CHAPTER 26 Supraventricular Arrhythmias

CHAPTER 27 Hypertension

CHAPTER 28 Hypotension

CHAPTER 29 Valvular and Pericardial Heart Disease

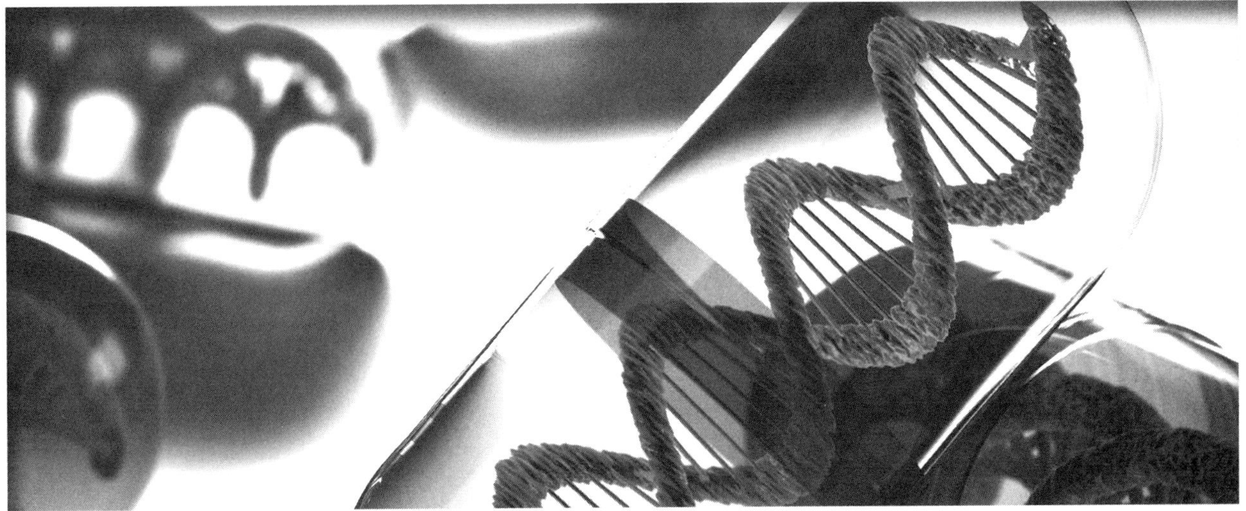

CHAPTER 23

Myocardial Ischemia and Acute Coronary Syndromes

Kevin M. Sowinski

Myocardial ischemia occurs as a result of increased myocardial demand, decreased myocardial oxygen supply, or both, and most commonly occurs in patients with atherosclerotic coronary artery disease. This chapter discusses the specific mechanisms by which drug therapy may cause increased myocardial oxygen demand or decreased supply.

Angina pectoris is a clinical syndrome of chest discomfort caused by reversible myocardial ischemia that produces disturbances in myocardial function but no myocardial necrosis. Myocardial ischemia can also occur without any symptoms of angina and is typically referred to as silent myocardial ischemia. Acute myocardial infarction (MI) is a clinical syndrome associated with the development of a prolonged occlusion of a coronary artery leading to decreased oxygen supply, myocardial ischemia, and irreversible damage to myocardial tissue. MI in patients with coronary artery disease is usually associated with a coronary artery thrombosis superimposed on a ruptured atherosclerotic plaque. The specific mechanisms by which drugs may facilitate or cause MIs will be discussed.

An acute coronary syndrome is associated with three clinical manifestations: ST-segment elevation MI, non-ST-segment elevation MI, and unstable angina.[1,2] For the purposes of this chapter, it is difficult to separate the acute coronary syndromes because, for the most part, the individual case data in the literature do not provide sufficient detail. Therefore, in most cases, the specific acute coronary syndromes will not be discussed separately. Furthermore, based on the available literature, it is difficult to distinguish drugs based on whether they cause myocardial ischemia or infarction.

CAUSATIVE AGENTS

Drugs reported to cause angina pectoris, myocardial ischemia, an acute coronary syndrome, or all three are listed in **Table 23-1**.[3-462] Drug-induced myocardial ischemia or acute coronary syndrome

Table 23-1 Agents Implicated in Drug-Induced Myocardial Ischemia and/or Acute Coronary Syndromes

Therapeutic Area (drug class, drugs)	Incidence/Index of Risk	Level of Evidence[a]
Drug Discontinuation[3-16]	NK	C
Argatroban, aspirin, β-blockers, clonidine, clopidogrel, heparin, nitroglycerin		
Analgesics[7,17-28]		
NSAIDs	Highly variable, dependent on drug and drug dose	A, B, C
Selective COX-2 inhibitors (rofecoxib, celecoxib, valdecoxib)	Celecoxib: RR 1.86, 95% CI 1.33–2.54	
Nonselective NSAIDs (diclofenac, ibuprofen)	Ibuprofen: RR 1.51, 95% CI 0.96–2.37 Diclofenac: RR 1.63, 95% CI 1.12–2.37	
Opioids (methadone, dihydrocodeine, morphine)	NK	C
Others (ketamine, gold sodium thiomalate, nefopam, penicillamine)	NK	C
Anesthetics[29-32]	NK	C
Benzocaine, enflurane, isoflurane, mepivacaine, sevoflurane, propofol		
Anticancer/Cancer-Associated Agents[33-112]	NK	C
5-fluorouracil, bleomycin, capecitabine, carboplatin, carmustine, cisplatin, cyclophosphamide, epirubicin, etoposide, gemcitabine, hydroxyurea, floxuridine, flutamide, L-asparaginase, lapatinib, ixabepilone, methotrexate, paclitaxel, sorafenib, vinblastine, vincristine, vinorelbine		
Antidepressants[17,113-123]	NK	C
Selective serotonin reuptake inhibitors (fluvoxamine, fluoxetine, sertraline, venlafaxine)		
Tricyclic antidepressants		
Others (bupropion, doxepin, maprotiline, trazodone, phenelzine)		
Anti-HIV[124-131]		
Abacavir, didanosine	Abacavir: RR 1.89, 95% CI 1.47–2.45	B
	Didanosine: RR 1.49, 95% CI 1.14–1.95	B
Protease inhibitors	Protease inhibitors: RR 1.16, 95% CI 1.10–1.23	B
Anti-Infectives[17,132-139]	NK	C
Amoxicillin, amphotericin, azithromycin, cinoxacin, clarithromycin, co-trimoxazole, fluconazole, ketoconazole, mefloquine, mesalamine, metronidazole, nitrofurantoin, norfloxacin, penicillin G, roxithromycin		
Antipsychotics[17,120,140,141]	NK	C
Clozapine		
Antimigraine[17,142-176]	NK	C
Dihydroergotamine, ergonovine, ergotamine, methylergonovine, methylergometrine, methysergide, sumatriptan, zolmitriptan		
Blood Modifiers[17,177-181]	NK	C
Coagulation factor VIIA, darbepoetin, erythropoietin, factor VIII inhibitor/prothrombin complex concentrates, tranexamic acid		
Cardiovascular Drugs		
Calcium-channel blockers[17,182-207] (diltiazem, lacidipine, felodipine, isradipine, nifedipine, nisoldipine, verapamil)	NK	C
ACE inhibitors[17,208,209] (captopril, enalapril, lisinopril, perindopril)	NK	C
β-adrenergic blockers[17,198,201,210-213] (ophthalmic and systemic)	NK	C
Stress testing agents/β-adrenergic receptor agonists[214-237] (adenosine, arbutamine, atropine, dipyridamole, dopexamine, dobutamine, milrinone)	NK	C
Other cardiovascular drugs[17,238-244] (alfuzosin, diazoxide, disopyramide, diuretics, encainide, fenoldopam, hydralazine, levosimendan, minoxidil, nitroprusside, prazosin, propafenone, sublingual isosorbide dinitrate)	NK	C

Table 23-1 Agents Implicated in Drug-Induced Myocardial Ischemia and/or Acute Coronary Syndromes (continued)

Therapeutic Area (drug class, drugs)	Incidence/Index of Risk	Level of Evidence[a]
Hormones/Hormone Modifying Agents[17,139,245-289]		
Female sex hormones (oral contraceptives, estrogens)	0- to 5-fold increase in risk (the risk is highly variable, dose and drug specific)	A, B, C
Other hormones (desmopressin, leuprolide, megestrol acetate, oxytocin, oral corticosteroids, prostaglandin F_2 [dinoprost], prostaglandin E_2 [sulprostone], tamoxifen, testosterone, thyroid hormone, vasopressin)	NK	C
Illicit Drugs[17,26,142,290-359]		
Amphetamines (methamphetamine, dextroamphetamine, 3,4-methylene-dioxymethamphetamine, dexfenfluramine)	NK	C
Cocaine	MI: 0.7–6% Chest pain: 39.4%	A, B, C
Others (anabolic steroids, butane inhalation, glue sniffing, LSD, marijuana, heroin, cannabinoids, toluene inhalation)	NK	C
Immune Modulators[360-364] Interferon (alpha-2b), interleukins (alpha-2 and alpha-4), IVIG, smallpox vaccine, rituximab	NK	C
Sympathomimetics[17,116,316,328,365-395] Albuterol, ephedra, ephedrine, epinephrine, formoterol, isoproterenol, methylphenidate, pseudoephedrine, phenylephrine, phenylpropanolamine, salbutamol, salmeterol, sibutramine, terbutaline	NK	C
Other[36,124-126,139,142,350,396-462] Acetylcholine, allopurinol, azaribine, betamethasone, beclomethasone, bromocriptine, caffeine, capsaicin, cetirizine, cimetidine, cisapride, domperidone, dolasetron, ethanol, iloprost, ioversol, metoclopramide, lithium, nicotine, ondansetron, rosiglitazone, sildenafil, terfenadine, theophylline, tegaserod, varenicline	NK Rosiglitazone: OR 1.43, 95% CI 1.03–1.98	C B

ACE = angiotensin-converting enzyme, CI = confidence interval, COX = cyclooxygenase, HIV = human immunodeficiency virus, IVIG = intravenous immunoglobulin, LSD = lysergic acid diethylamide, MI = myocardial infarction, NSAID = nonsteroidal anti-inflammatory drug, NK = not known, OR = odds ratio, RR = relative risk.
[a]Definitions for Levels of Evidence: Level A—evidence from one or more randomized, controlled clinical trials; Level B—evidence from nonrandomized clinical trials, prospective observational studies, cohort studies, retrospective studies, case-control studies, meta-analyses and/or postmarketing surveillance studies; and Level C—evidence from one or more published case reports or case series.

can occur in association with short-term drug administration or during long-term therapy. Because of the temporal nature of case reporting of these drug-induced diseases, in most cases the chapter will review drugs that cause myocardial ischemia or infarction acutely. In some cases, larger and longer-term clinical trials or epidemiologic evidence support a relationship between the development of myocardial ischemia or infarction and long-term administration of a drug. Chronic use of drugs such as cocaine, oral contraceptives, nicotine, rosiglitazone, protease inhibitors, selective cyclooxygenase-2 (COX-2) inhibitors and nonselective nonsteroidal anti-inflammatory drugs (NSAIDs), and others may facilitate or increase the risk of atherosclerotic coronary artery disease and associated myocardial ischemia and infarction. This phenomenon may be thought of as analogous to other factors that increase the risk of coronary artery disease (such as hypertension, diabetes mellitus, obesity, and others). This subject area has received considerable attention from the media, patients, and regulatory agencies because of studies suggesting an increased risk of cardiovascular disease associated with selective COX-2 inhibitors and nonselective NSAIDs.[7,18-22,27,463] Finally, drugs may cause myocardial ischemia or acute coronary syndrome if therapy is abruptly discontinued.

Data regarding drugs that may cause myocardial ischemia or infarction were summarized in a paper describing 20 years of reports (1975–1994) to a Netherlands national center for adverse drug reporting.[17] During this period, 19,141 adverse drug reactions were reported, of which 220 described likely cases of drug-induced chest pain or MI. The article describes 183 cases for which sufficient data were provided to evaluate the cases and adjudicate the findings. Data obtained from spontaneous reporting systems such as that in this article or from reports to the U.S. Food and Drug Administration (FDA) must be interpreted cautiously, as they typically suffer from both underreporting and/or selective reporting. Of particular note in this article is the absence of several classes of drugs or drug classes that are well known to cause myocardial ischemia or infarction, specifically cocaine and cytotoxic drugs. In addition, the underlying diseases of those patients for which adverse drug reactions were reported are not described.

Two recent papers have attempted to determine those at risk for drug-induced acute coronary syndromes and/or myocardial ischemia using two different methods. The first study used computer-based modeling to make predictions regarding protein targets that may be associated with the development of drug-induced MI.[464] The second utilized electronic health record databases in three countries—Denmark, Italy, and the Netherlands—to identify potential drugs that may cause drug-induced MI. The approach in this paper was to first detect potential drug-induced MI and then to identify whether the identified potential offending agent had been reported to cause this in the past. Based on available data, the authors then addressed the biological plausibility.[139] Initially, 163 drugs were identified as being associated with increased risk of MI. After eliminating drugs due to bias and lack of biological plausibility, only nine "prime suspects" were identified: azithromycin, erythromycin, roxithromycin, metoclopramide, cisapride, domperidone, betamethasone, fluconazole, and megestrol acetate (Table 23-1).

EPIDEMIOLOGY

The incidence of drug-induced myocardial ischemia and acute coronary syndromes in the general population is unknown and, with the exception of a small number of drugs, nearly impossible to determine. Nonetheless, drug-induced acute coronary syndrome and myocardial ischemia are not trivial. Both chest pain and MI were among the most common adverse events with serious outcomes reported to the FDA's voluntary reporting system between 1969 and 2002.[465] Although these reporting systems are flawed for the reasons discussed previously, they nevertheless suggest that drug-induced myocardial ischemia and acute coronary syndromes are a common and important problem. Due to the nature of these reports, the underlying conditions of the patients cannot be determined.

With the exception of certain groups (e.g., cocaine users, patients with chronic coronary artery disease, or those at high risk for coronary events) the incidence of drug-induced acute coronary syndromes and myocardial ischemia is likely low. However, several drugs/drug classes, including cocaine, oral contraceptives/hormone-replacement therapy, cytotoxic agents, ergot alkaloids, and triptans, may cause myocardial ischemia or acute coronary syndromes in individuals who do not have clinically evident cardiovascular disease.[323] To put into perspective the difficulty of determining the incidence of drug-induced myocardial ischemia and acute coronary syndromes, it is helpful to review the epidemiology of myocardial ischemia and acute coronary syndromes associated with cocaine and oral contraceptives, the drugs for which the most data are available. The risk of cocaine-induced MI is estimated to be 24–31 times greater than the baseline risk during the first hour after cocaine exposure.[319,320,324] The reported lifetime risk of acute MI in chronic cocaine users is six to seven times greater than that in nonusers. In view of the fact that 25 million Americans have used cocaine at least once in their lifetime, cocaine-induced myocardial ischemia/infarction has the potential to be a major public health problem. In 2011, 505,224 emergency department visits were cocaine-related.[466] Estimates suggest that as many as 40% of these emergency department visits included patients with chest discomfort. In patients whose urine is tested, cocaine or cocaine metabolites are detectable in 14–25% and 7% of those presenting to the emergency department with nontraumatic chest pain in urban and suburban hospitals, respectively. Although these data do not provide the actual incidence of chest pain or acute coronary syndrome associated with cocaine, they do provide some alarming information regarding the epidemiology and potential impact of this drug-induced disease.[319,320,322,324] The actual incidence of cocaine-induced MI among patients who present to the emergency department with cocaine-induced chest pain is highly variable, but ranges between 0.7% and 6%.[467-472]

Soon after oral contraceptives became available in the early 1960s, the first case report of MI associated with these drugs was published.[473] Since then, controversy regarding the potential for myocardial ischemia/infarction induced by oral contraceptives and other female hormones has lingered. Because exogenous female hormones (i.e., oral contraceptives and hormone-replacement therapy) are used by millions of women worldwide, the importance of the potential for myocardial ischemia or acute coronary syndromes associated with these agents is clear. Usually, oral contraceptives are taken by otherwise healthy young women with a low background risk of coronary artery disease and resulting myocardial ischemia or acute coronary syndromes. Numerous studies have been conducted to determine the risk of an acute coronary syndrome or other coronary event associated with oral contraceptive drugs, but the risk remains poorly defined. Depending on the study, type and dose of oral contraceptive used, and population studied, the degree of increased risk of myocardial ischemia/infarction associated with oral contraceptives varies widely, from no increased risk to a fivefold higher risk.[286,473] The hazard increases in women who smoke, have hypertension, diabetes, dyslipidemia, or are over the age of 35 years.[286,473] The effect of hormone-replacement therapy on the risk of coronary events is more strongly established. Numerous studies have called into question the safety of hormone-replacement therapy for reducing the risk of primary or secondary coronary events.[474,475] In January 2003, the FDA approved new labeling for all estrogen and estrogen/progesterone products, highlighting "the increased risk for heart disease, heart attacks" and that "these products are not approved for heart disease prevention."[476]

Selective COX-2 inhibitors were introduced into the U.S. market in the late 1990s, with the potential to revolutionize the manner in which pain and inflammatory disorders were managed. However, several randomized active and placebo-controlled trials, observational studies, and meta-analyses have raised concerns that the selective COX-2 inhibitors and nonselective NSAIDs may increase the risk of MI.[7,18,463] Prospective well-designed studies comparing the effects of COX-2 inhibitors to those of other NSAIDs are not available, although until recently it was thought that nonselective NSAIDs did not increase cardiovascular risk. These trials have limitations, but it seems clear that there is an increase in risk associated with both selective and nonselective NSAIDs and that the risk is variable within each group of agents. The data suggest that the cardiovascular risk is highest with rofecoxib, followed by celecoxib and diclofenac, followed by naproxen and ibuprofen. Whether this is due to decreasing COX-2 selectivity from rofecoxib to ibuprofen is a topic of considerable debate.[22]

Two of the selective COX-2 inhibitors, rofecoxib and valdecoxib, were withdrawn voluntarily from the worldwide market in 2004 and 2005, respectively. "Black box" warnings for the remaining selective COX-2 inhibitor, celecoxib, and all other NSAIDs except aspirin were added to package inserts in 2006, stating: "NSAIDs may cause an increased risk of serious cardiovascular thrombotic events, MI, and stroke, which can be fatal. This risk may increase with duration of use. Patients with cardiovascular disease or risk factors for cardiovascular disease may be at greater risk." At the very least, these warnings should cause healthcare professionals to question the routine use of these agents in patients with cardiovascular disease. In 2013, the European Medicines Agency (EMA) further warned that diclofenac is associated with the same risk as the COX-2 selective inhibitors.[477] This warning was rendered in part due to the publication of a meta-analysis suggesting that COX-2 inhibitors and diclofenac increased vascular risk significantly, whereas ibuprofen and naproxen did not.[478] Subsequent papers suggest that this risk is increased regardless of the amount of time that has passed following an MI. Finally, a recent Danish registry study suggests that in post-MI patients receiving antithrombotic therapy, the risk of MI is independent of the type or duration of NSAID therapy.[479] In 2015, the EMA further warned that high-dose ibuprofen (>2,400 mg/day) was associated with a small increase in cardiovascular risk.[480] A scientific statement from the American Heart Association (AHA) with recommendations for the clinical use of these agents as well as numerous reviews and editorials expressing caution regarding the use of these drugs in patients with cardiovascular disease have been published.[478,479,481-484] Further research is needed in this area, but in the interim, cautious use of all NSAIDs is necessary, and the drugs should be used only in patients who understand the risk.

Two thiazolidinedione drugs, rosiglitazone and pioglitazone, are available for use in the United States for treating type 2 diabetes mellitus. Numerous meta-analyses and observational studies have reported an association between rosiglitazone and an increased risk of MI.[485] A randomized controlled trial designed to further investigate this association was not helpful in answering the important question due to design limitations. As a result of the increased risk of MI suggested by these studies, the FDA issued new prescribing information regarding the potential risk of rosiglitazone-associated myocardial ischemia, particularly in patients taking concomitant nitrate therapy, and instituted a highly restrictive prescribing program in 2010.[485,486] In 2011, the EMA went further and suspended the sale of rosiglitazone. The concerns have led to a scientific statement from the AHA/American College of Cardiology Foundation (ACCF) with recommendations for the clinical use of these agents.[485] Restrictions to the use of rosiglitazone were eased in 2013 based on an FDA advisory panel's recommendations. The FDA's action has met with conflicting opinions regarding the safety and appropriate use of rosiglitazone.[486] The majority of published studies do not suggest an increased risk of ischemic events associated with pioglitazone, and no black box warning is mandated for that drug.

The association between testosterone therapy and the risk of cardiovascular outcomes has been the focus of study recently, fueled by the marked increase in the use of testosterone therapy in men with low serum testosterone concentrations.[487-489] In response to several studies in which an association of increased cardiovascular risk was observed, the FDA issued warnings regarding the use of these products and concluded that despite conflicting and inconclusive evidence, there is the possibility that the testosterone increases cardiovascular risk. These studies were followed by intense media coverage and comment. The FDA mandated the addition of warnings regarding the possibility for increased risk of MI and stroke in patients taking these agents. The Endocrine Society issued a statement suggesting that, until randomized trials are available, patients should be aware of the potential increase in risk, and prescribers should use these agents in accordance with established treatment guidelines.[490] To date there are no large, long-term, randomized, placebo-controlled trials to provide definitive conclusions regarding testosterone therapy and cardiovascular risk. However, numerous smaller studies and a large meta-analysis argue that there is no increase in cardiovascular risk.[491] A published comprehensive literature review that assessed the available evidence concluded that there is no convincing relationship between testosterone therapy (for the treatment of low testosterone concentrations) and enhanced cardiovascular risk.[491]

MECHANISMS

Mechanisms of drug-induced myocardial ischemia and/or acute coronary syndromes are listed in **Table 23-2**.

DRUG-INDUCED MYOCARDIAL ISCHEMIA

Myocardial ischemia results from an imbalance in coronary blood flow, myocardial oxygen supply, and the metabolic needs of the myocardium (myocardial oxygen demand). Myocardial ischemia occurs when myocardial oxygen demand exceeds myocardial oxygen supply. The three major determinants of myocardial oxygen demand are heart rate, contractility, and left ventricular systolic wall tension.[492] Heart rate is the easiest of these factors to assess clinically; an increase in heart rate leads

Table 23-2 Mechanisms of Drug-Induced Myocardial Ischemia and/or Acute Coronary Syndrome

Drug-Induced Disease and Mechanism	Examples (This is a partial list of examples only; for most drugs the mechanism of increased risk is not known.)
Drug-Induced Myocardial Ischemia	
Increased myocardial oxygen demand	
Increased heart rate	**Directly:** Cocaine, adrenergic β-agonists, sympathomimetics, abrupt discontinuation of β-blockers **Indirectly:** Potent vasodilators (nifedipine, minoxidil, hydralazine)
Increased myocardial contractility	**Directly:** Cocaine, adrenergic β-agonists, sympathomimetics, abrupt discontinuation of β-blockers **Indirectly:** Potent vasodilators (nifedipine, minoxidil, hydralazine, etc.)
Increased left-ventricular systolic wall tension (increased preload or increased afterload)	**Increased Preload:** NSAIDs **Increased Afterload:** Drugs that increase blood pressure (cocaine, phenylephrine, amphetamines, etc.)
Decreased myocardial oxygen supply (temporary, nontotal occlusion)	
○ Increased coronary vascular resistance (vasospasm, thrombosis)	Cocaine, phenylephrine, amphetamines, anti-migraine agents (ergot alkaloids, triptans)
○ Decreased coronary diastolic perfusion pressure	Enalapril, nifedipine, minoxidil, hydralazine, nitroprusside, adenosine, dipyridamole
Decreased oxygen carrying capacity	
Drug-Induced Acute Coronary Syndrome	
Acute coronary syndrome associated with acute drug therapy	
Coronary artery thrombosis, superimposed on a damaged atherosclerotic plaque	Cocaine, oral contraceptives, estrogens, COX-2 inhibitors, NSAIDs
Coronary artery vasospasm (with or without a superimposed coronary artery thrombosis)	Cocaine, antimigraine agents (ergot alkaloids, triptans)
Acute coronary syndrome associated with chronic drug therapy (drugs that increase cardiovascular risk)	Cocaine, estrogens, COX-2 inhibitors, NSAIDs, anti-HIV agents/protease inhibitors, oral contraceptives, rosiglitazone

COX = cyclooxygenase, HIV = human immunodeficiency virus, NSAID = nonsteroidal anti-inflammatory drug.

to increased myocardial oxygen demand. Myocardial contractility is reflected by the rate of rise in the intraventricular pressure during isovolumetric contraction and is influenced by a number of variables, including the autonomic nervous system, heart rate, blood calcium concentration, and body temperature. The third determinant, systolic wall tension, is directly related to ventricular systolic pressure and ventricular wall radius and is inversely related to wall thickness. Preload and afterload are important determinants of these components. Reducing systolic blood pressure reduces afterload, which ultimately decreases myocardial oxygen demand. A drug may cause myocardial ischemia simply by modifying any one of these factors. For example, drugs that increase heart rate, either directly (e.g., cocaine, β-adrenergic receptor agonists, abrupt discontinuation of β-blockers) or indirectly by reflex mechanisms (e.g., potent vasodilators such as nifedipine, minoxidil, and hydralazine) may induce myocardial ischemia. Similarly, drugs that increase systolic blood pressure (e.g., cocaine, phenylephrine) may also induce myocardial ischemia. Clinicians should be aware of drugs that modify any of these factors, as they may cause myocardial ischemia.

Myocardial oxygen supply is determined by coronary blood flow and the oxygen-carrying capacity of blood.[492] The most important of these determinants clinically is coronary blood flow. Normally, the arteriolar resistance vessels are the most important regulators of coronary blood flow, whereas large epicardial vessels are low-resistance vessels. Complex factors that determine coronary blood flow include duration of diastole and coronary vascular resistance. Coronary vascular resistance is determined by metabolic control, autoregulation, extravascular compressive forces, and humoral and neural factors. Drug therapy may reduce myocardial oxygen supply by influencing any of these determinants. Agents that cause thrombosis or vasospasm of large coronary epicardial vessels may reduce myocardial oxygen supply. However, drugs that cause microvascular changes should also be considered. Unfortunately, these changes are more difficult to assess clinically. Finally, oxygen-carrying capacity can be affected by conditions such as anemia.

There are several examples of drugs that may precipitate ischemia by decreasing myocardial oxygen supply. Cocaine causes myocardial ischemia not only via increases in heart rate and blood pressure but also via coronary vasoconstriction, which is mediated by cocaine-induced blockade of norepinephrine reuptake, leading to increased plasma norepinephrine concentrations and enhanced α_1-adrenoceptor-mediated vasoconstriction.[319,323,327,329] Some data also suggest that cocaine increases plasma concentrations of endothelin-1, a powerful vasoconstrictor that contributes to coronary vasospasm.[323] Each of these mechanisms contributes to cocaine-induced coronary artery vasospasm. The ergot alkaloids and associated derivatives are widely known to cause coronary vasoconstriction, the mechanism of which is simply an extension of the drug's therapeutic effect, cerebral vasoconstriction. Triptans, which are also used for the treatment of migraines, are contraindicated in patients with coronary artery disease. Like ergot alkaloids, the purported mechanism of increased myocardial ischemia associated with triptans is coronary artery vasoconstriction or vasospasm or both; in the case of triptans, this is mediated by agonism of 5-hydroxytriptophan receptors.

Drugs may reduce myocardial oxygen supply through aggressive reduction of blood pressure via arterial vasodilation, leading to reductions in diastolic perfusion pressure and coronary blood flow. Patients with existing coronary atherosclerosis are particularly at risk for drug-induced myocardial ischemia via this mechanism. Any drug that reduces blood pressure, especially potent vasodilators, may cause myocardial ischemia or an acute coronary syndrome. An observational study suggested that the short-acting dihydropyridine calcium-channel blocker nifedipine may increase the risk of ischemic events and MI in patients with coronary artery disease, likely through this mechanism.[186,204] This study was highly controversial and led to debate for many years. Although the debate was contentious in many ways, there was general agreement that short-acting dihydropyridine calcium-channel blocking agents such as the immediate-release formulations of nifedipine or nicardipine should be avoided in patients with coronary artery disease.[187] Whether or not these restrictions should be applied to all calcium-channel blockers remains a topic of debate. Another drug believed to increase the risk of acute MI by reducing coronary perfusion pressure is enalapril. In a landmark clinical trial, the Cooperative North Scandinavian Enalapril Survival Study-II, early intravenous administration of enalaprilat followed by oral enalapril therapy was not associated with a reduction in the incidence of mortality.[493] One postulated mechanism for this lack of benefit was early drug-induced hypotension resulting in reduced coronary perfusion pressure. Reduction in coronary perfusion pressures during the acute phase of an MI may lead to larger areas of subendocardial tissue damage. An additional example of this phenomenon is the concomitant use of phosphodiesterase-5 inhibitors, such as sildenafil, with nitrates, the combination of which may cause marked hypotension leading to reduced myocardial oxygen supply and consequent myocardial ischemia or infarction.[494] The combined use of these drug classes is discouraged by the manufacturers, national organizations, and government regulators.

An alternative to exercise stress testing as a means to functionally evaluate the clinical and cardiovascular responses is pharmacologic stress testing. These tests provide some prognostic and diagnostic information about the underlying coronary artery disease. Two types of drugs are used: coronary artery vasodilators (adenosine and dipyridamole) and agents that increase cardiac work (dobutamine and arbutamine). Unlike agents that increase cardiac work, adenosine and dipyridamole do not cause ischemia by increasing myocardial oxygen demand. Rather, these coronary artery vasodilators may cause myocardial ischemia by preferentially dilating normal coronary arteries versus diseased vessels. This "steals" blood flow away from diseased segments (frequently referred to as coronary steal). These drugs are used in a controlled setting and frequently cause myocardial ischemia, but MI induced by these drugs is uncommon.

DRUG-INDUCED ACUTE CORONARY SYNDROMES

The mechanism by which a drug can induce an acute coronary syndrome may be thought of in two different, yet complementary, pathways, related to the temporal nature of the event. First, acute drug therapy may cause an acute coronary syndrome. Second, drugs may increase the risk of an acute coronary syndrome with continued, long-term exposure, as a result of the drug increasing the underlying degree of cardiovascular risk. Certain drugs may increase both the acute and chronic risk. The following discussion addresses each of these situations.

ACUTE CORONARY SYNDROME ASSOCIATED WITH SHORT-TERM DRUG THERAPY

Classically, the pathogenesis of an acute coronary syndrome is an occlusion of an epicardial coronary artery caused by a coronary artery thrombosis superimposed on a ruptured atherosclerotic plaque.[495] Less commonly, an acute coronary syndrome may occur despite an absence of clinically significant coronary atherosclerosis and is caused by coronary artery vasospasm with or without a superimposed coronary artery thrombosis.[495] Even though this mechanism is believed to be less common, in one study, 31 prescription, nonprescription, and illicit drugs and approximately 100 cases were associated with drug-induced acute coronary syndrome caused by coronary artery spasm in teenagers and young adults.[142] The acute induction of a drug-induced acute coronary syndrome may occur in association with either of the above-described situations. In either case, for drug-induced MI to occur, coronary blood flow must be occluded for a sufficient amount of time to result in necrosis of myocardial tissue. Thus, a drug-induced acute coronary syndrome could result from drug-induced coronary vasospasm (e.g., cocaine) or drug-induced coronary artery thrombosis (e.g., estrogens, cocaine, COX-2 inhibitors). For example, in theory, selective COX-2 inhibitors, which do not inhibit COX-1 and therefore do not decrease plasma concentrations of platelet-derived thromboxane, may exert different influences on the occurrence of cardiovascular events than other nonselective NSAIDs such as aspirin or naproxen. Inhibition of COX-2 is believed to suppress the endothelial production of prostacyclin, while leaving the production of thromboxane A2, mediated by COX-1, relatively unaffected. This may lead to vasoconstriction, platelet aggregation, thrombosis, and ultimately an acute coronary syndrome.[20,22]

ACUTE CORONARY SYNDROME ASSOCIATED WITH LONG-TERM DRUG THERAPY/INCREASED CARDIOVASCULAR RISK

Drugs may also increase the risk of development of coronary artery disease by accelerating the natural course of pathogenesis of atherosclerosis. The following have been identified as modifiable risk factors by the AHA: cigarette smoking, elevated plasma low-density lipoprotein cholesterol concentrations, reduced plasma high-density lipoprotein cholesterol concentrations, hypertension, obesity, and diabetes.[496,497] Thus, any drug that alters these risk factors in a negative way has the potential to increase the risk of a coronary event. Examples of drugs that have been shown to accelerate the development of coronary atherosclerosis include protease inhibitors (via induction of dyslipidemia) and cocaine. Postmortem studies of cocaine abusers have shown that cocaine accelerates the development of atherosclerosis by causing structural changes in the endothelial membrane, resulting in increased permeability to low-density lipoproteins.

In addition, cocaine has been shown to enhance white-cell migration and increase the expression of adhesion molecules in the endothelium.[323] Other examples of drug-associated acceleration of coronary atherosclerosis include oral contraceptives, COX-2 inhibitors, and rosiglitazone. Finally, there is evidence that statins may increase the risk for development of type 2 diabetes, although there is no evidence that this translates into an increase in the risk of MI.[498,499]

DRUG DISCONTINUATION

Several drugs are known to cause myocardial ischemia or acute coronary syndromes when therapy is abruptly discontinued, in most cases in patients who have underlying coronary artery disease (Table 23-1). There are several mechanisms by which this may occur. For example, abrupt discontinuation of β-blockers may lead to increased myocardial oxygen demand secondary to β-adrenoceptor upregulation and hypersensitivity to catecholamine stimulation. Following the short-term treatment of an acute coronary syndrome, discontinuation of heparin and aspirin leads to an increase in adverse cardiovascular events.[14] These events seem to "cluster" early (~10 hours) after discontinuation and have been attributed to rethrombosis in coronary arteries. Maintenance of aspirin therapy has been proposed as a means of reducing the risk of this phenomenon. Additional data have suggested that discontinuation of clopidogrel therapy may result in an increased risk of death or recurrent acute coronary syndrome.[6] In that study, the incidence of death and recurrent MI was higher during the first 90 days following clopidogrel discontinuation in patients with acute coronary syndromes who were treated medically or with intervention. The theoretical mechanism of this increased risk is platelet activation and increased thrombotic risk immediately upon discontinuation of therapy.[500] This has led to considerable research regarding the appropriate duration of dual antiplatelet therapy.[6] Some suggest that the risk of MI upon discontinuation of antiplatelet therapy is only increased in the presence of elevated thrombotic risk. Decisions regarding discontinuation of dual antiplatelet therapy are challenging, particularly in those individuals who require surgery and those with elevated thrombotic risk.[500] Finally, there is some evidence, although conflicting, that abrupt discontinuation of statins may increase the risk of cardiovascular events.[16] Further research in this area is required.

In summary, there are numerous mechanisms by which drugs may cause myocardial ischemia or acute coronary syndromes. Cocaine is an example of a drug that may cause this disease by multiple mechanisms, including increased myocardial oxygen demand (increased heart rate, contractility, blood pressure, and development of left ventricular hypertrophy), decreased myocardial oxygen supply (platelet aggregation and thrombus formation, coronary artery vasoconstriction), and enhanced development of coronary artery disease (premature atherosclerosis).

CLINICAL PRESENTATION AND DIFFERENTIAL DIAGNOSIS

DRUG-INDUCED MYOCARDIAL ISCHEMIA

The clinical presentation of a patient with drug-induced myocardial ischemia is similar to that of any patient with angina or ischemia associated with atherosclerotic coronary artery disease. The most apparent difference is that drug-induced myocardial ischemia may occur in individuals who do not have, or who are not at risk for, coronary artery disease. For example, it is unusual for a young individual to present with symptoms consistent with myocardial ischemia. Pharmacists and other healthcare professionals must be aware of drugs, both licit and illicit, that may precipitate angina or an acute coronary syndrome and evaluate the causality in appropriate patients.

Typical signs and symptoms associated with angina pectoris are summarized in **Table 23-3**. Briefly, angina typically presents as substernal, retrosternal, or transsternal discomfort that radiates, usually, to the neck and left arm. The discomfort is usually characterized by a dull sensation, rather

Table 23-3 Clinical Presentation and Signs and Symptoms of Chest Pain Associated with Myocardial Ischemia

Quality

- Sensation of pressure or heavy weight on the chest
- Burning sensation in chest
- Chest tightness
- Shortness of breath with feeling of constriction about the larynx or upper trachea
- Visceral pain quality (deep, heavy, squeezing, aching)
- Gradual increase in intensity followed by gradual fading away

Location

- Over the sternum or very near the sternum
- Anywhere between epigastrum and pharynx
- Occasionally limited to left shoulder and left arm; rarely limited to right arm
- Limited to lower jaw
- Lower cervical or upper thoracic spine
- Left interscapular or suprascapular area

Precipitating factors

- Relationship to exercise
- Effort that involves use of arms above the head
- Weather factors (cold, warm and humid); walking against wind
- Large meal
- Emotional factors involved with exercise, fright, and/or anger
- Coitus
- Drugs

Nitroglycerin relief

- Relief of pain

Radiation

- Left arm and shoulder
- Jaw
- Right arm (occasionally)

Duration

- 0.5–30 minutes

than a sharp or stabbing pain, and patients may describe it as a strangling or constricting sensation. Patients often use the following words to describe the discomfort: pressure, heaviness, fullness, squeezing, burning, aching, gas, vise-like, or anxiety. Anginal discomfort usually has a gradual onset and lasts only a few minutes if the precipitating factor is removed. In addition, relief is usually afforded by rest, sublingual nitroglycerin, or both. Longer durations of angina may imply severe myocardial ischemia, coronary vasospasm, unstable angina, or impending or ongoing MI.

DRUG-INDUCED ACUTE CORONARY SYNDROME

In most situations, the clinical presentation of a patient with drug-induced acute coronary syndrome is similar to that of any patient with nondrug-induced acute coronary syndrome. However, there are several exceptions to this generalization. Like myocardial ischemia, acute coronary syndromes are relatively unusual in young populations (<50 years of age). Approximately 25% of all acute MIs in individuals 18–45 years of age have been associated with frequent cocaine use.[329] The typical patient who presents with cocaine-induced acute coronary syndromes is a relatively young man who smokes cigarettes but does not have any other obvious cardiovascular risk factors. Thus, in younger patients without any obvious risk for acute coronary syndromes, the use of cocaine or other drugs that are known to be associated with drug-induced acute coronary syndromes should be considered. However, clinicians must contemplate the possibility of cocaine use in any patient who presents with an acute coronary syndrome. Because cocaine accelerates cardiovascular risk, it is certainly possible that its use is associated with acute coronary syndromes in older patients. Current recommendations suggest that urine screening for cocaine metabolites should be employed only in patients who are unable to communicate or when other sources of a reliable patient history are unavailable.[324]

As with cocaine, acute coronary syndromes associated with oral contraceptives usually occur in younger patients. The typical woman who presents with an acute coronary syndrome secondary to oral contraceptive therapy is usually over the age of 35 years and smokes cigarettes. The risk increases with age and appears to be higher in those with other cardiovascular risk factors, such as diabetes, hypertension, and dyslipidemia.[286]

Acute coronary syndromes classically present as prolonged chest discomfort described as oppressive pain, choking, squeezing, or burning that may radiate to the neck, throat, jaw, shoulders, or both arms. The discomfort associated with an acute coronary syndrome is generally similar in quality and location to anginal pain, except that the duration is longer (>30 minutes), it occurs at rest, and is not relieved by sublingual nitroglycerin or rest. Patients may present with other symptoms, such as nausea, vomiting, diaphoresis, shortness of breath, weakness, lightheadedness, or a sense of impending doom. Not all patients present with classic symptoms; some present with atypical signs or symptoms, are asymptomatic, or are unable to provide a history. The physical examination is not necessarily helpful in establishing the diagnosis of an acute coronary syndrome. However, the findings are important as a guide to immediate management and as a baseline for future comparison. Signs or symptoms of left or right ventricular dysfunction may be detected. Patients may present with bradycardia or tachycardia, low-grade fever, elevated respiratory rate, and leukocytosis. Most of these findings are nonspecific and do not confirm the diagnosis of an acute coronary syndrome.[425] The presentation of a drug-induced acute coronary syndrome is likely similar to that of other causes of acute coronary syndromes, although data are not available, except for that associated with cocaine. Patients with cocaine-induced acute coronary syndromes experience pressure-like chest discomfort, anxiety, palpitations, dizziness, and nausea. Dyspnea and diaphoresis occur in 60% and 40% of patients, respectively. However, it has been suggested that fewer than 50% of patients actually experience chest pain with cocaine-associated acute coronary syndromes, making the diagnosis more difficult.[324]

The classification and diagnosis of an acute coronary syndrome is based on three important features: chest pain, electrocardiographic changes, and serum biomarker (troponin) concentrations.[1,2,501] The diagnostic features of an acute MI are provided in **Table 23-4**. The classification and diagnosis of drug-induced acute coronary syndromes is generally performed in the same manner as with those that are nondrug-induced. Interested readers are directed to these guidelines for more in-depth discussion of the classification and diagnosis of an acute coronary syndrome.[1,2,501] These diagnostic features are likely to help differentiate drug-induced myocardial ischemia from drug-induced acute coronary syndromes. Conditions to consider in the differential diagnosis of drug-induced acute coronary syndromes are presented in **Table 23-5**.

RISK FACTORS

Specific risk factors for drug-induced myocardial ischemia or acute coronary syndromes are likely to be similar to those for nondrug-induced myocardial ischemia or acute coronary syndromes (**Table 23-6**). Although it may be difficult to predict which specific risk factors are necessary for increasing the risk of this disease associated with many of the causative agents, certain risk factors are well known to increase the risk of myocardial ischemia or acute coronary syndromes associated with cocaine, oral contraceptives, and estrogen-replacement therapy. Most patients with cocaine-related chest pain or acute coronary syndromes are younger than 50 years of age, nonwhite, male tobacco smokers with no history of coronary atherosclerosis. In fact, nearly 50% of patients with cocaine-related chest pain or MI do not have evidence of coronary atherosclerosis.[323,502] Tobacco smoking also increases the risk of a coronary event while taking oral contraceptives or hormone-replacement therapy.[473] This increase in the risk of a coronary event associated with smoking is consistent with the increased risk associated with smoking in patients with coronary artery disease or in those at high risk for a coronary event.

MORBIDITY AND MORTALITY

Patients with a history of coronary artery disease and ischemic heart disease who experience drug-induced chest pain and angina often attribute symptoms to those associated with their underlying disease process and may not seek additional medical care. However, depending on the severity of the drug-induced myocardial ischemia, these individuals may suffer recurrent disease exacerbations

Table 23-4 Definition of Myocardial Infarction Based on the ESC/ACCF/AHA/WHF[501] Guidelines

Third Universal Definition of Myocardial Infarction

The term *myocardial infarction* should be used when there is evidence of myocardial necrosis in a clinical setting consistent with myocardial ischemia.

Under these conditions any one of the following criteria meets the diagnosis for myocardial infarction:

1. Detection of rise and/or fall of cardiac biomarkers [cTn] with at least one value above the 99th percentile of the URL together with at least one of the following:
   - Symptoms of ischemia
   - New/presumed new significant ST-T wave changes or new LBBB on the ECG
   - Development of pathological Q waves on the ECG
   - Imaging evidence of new loss of viable myocardium or new regional wall motion abnormality
   - Identification of an intracoronary thrombus
2. Cardiac death with symptoms suggestive of myocardial ischaemia and presumed new ischaemic ECG changes or new LBBB, but death occurred before cardiac biomarkers were obtained, or before cardiac biomarker values would be increased.
3. PCI-related MI is arbitrarily defined by elevation of cTn values (>5 × 99th percentile URL) in patients with normal baseline values or a rise of cTn values >20% if the baseline values are elevated and are stable or falling. In addition, either (a) symptoms suggestive of myocardial ischemia or (b) new ischemic ECG changes or (c) angiographic findings consistent with a procedural complication or (d) imaging demonstration of new loss of viable myocardium or new regional wall motion abnormality are required.
4. Stent thrombosis associated with MI when detected by coronary angiography or autopsy in the setting of myocardial ischaemia and with a rise and/or fall of cardiac biomarker values with at least one value above the 99th percentile URL.
5. Coronary artery bypass grafting-related MI is arbitrarily defined by elevation of cardiac biomarker values (>10 × 99th percentile URL) in patients with normal baseline cTn values (≤99th percentile URL). In addition, either (a) new pathological Q waves or new LBBB, or (b) angiographic documented new graft or new native coronary artery occlusion, or (c) imaging evidence of new loss of viable myocardium or new regional wall motion abnormality.

ACCF = American College of Cardiology Foundation, AHA = American Heart Association, cTn = cardiac troponin, ECG = electrocardiogram, ESC = European Society of Cardiology, LBBB = left bundle branch block, MI = myocardial infarction, PCI = percutaneous coronary intervention, URL = upper reference limit, WHF = World Heart Foundation.

Table 23-5 Conditions to Consider in the Differential Diagnosis of Drug-Induced Myocardial Ischemia and/or Acute Coronary Syndrome

All drugs

- Nondrug-induced acute coronary syndrome and myocardial ischemia

Cocaine-induced acute coronary syndrome/ myocardial ischemia

- Aortic dissection
- Pulmonary hypertension
- Acute pulmonary syndrome ("crack lung")

requiring additional care or alterations in drug regimens. It is likely that this situation occurs very commonly, but the cause is attributed to disease-induced ischemia rather than to drug-induced myocardial ischemia.

Table 23-6 Risk Factors for Drug-Induced Myocardial Ischemia and/or Acute Coronary Syndrome

All drug-induced acute coronary syndrome/ myocardial ischemia

- Pre-existing coronary artery disease

Cocaine-induced acute coronary syndrome/ myocardial ischemia

- Smoking/tobacco use
- Ethanol use

Oral contraceptive-induced acute coronary syndrome

- Age >35 years
- High-dose estrogen
- Smoking/tobacco use
- Hypertension
- Diabetes
- Dyslipidemia

On the other hand, most patients in whom persistent chest pain develops with no history of coronary artery disease and those in whom a drug-induced acute coronary syndrome occurs seek medical attention, whether or not they have underlying coronary artery disease. Many of these patients require hospitalization and urgent treatment. Drug-induced acute coronary syndromes, like those that are nondrug-induced, may increase the risk of sudden death or death related to associated complications, including the development of left ventricular dysfunction, ventricular arrhythmias, or both.

There are considerable data describing the mortality associated with nondrug-induced acute coronary syndromes, and the statistics are alarming. Annual mortality rates for patients who experience a coronary event or MI are 37% and 16%, respectively.[429] Unfortunately, data regarding mortality associated with drug-induced chest pain and acute coronary syndromes are sparse, with the exception of those related to cocaine-induced coronary syndromes. The risk of mortality and recurrent MI associated with cocaine-induced chest pain is low (1-year risk approximately 2% and 1%, respectively).[503] With continued cocaine use, the risk of recurrent chest pain is very high. In patients who suffer a cocaine-induced MI, the risk of complications is substantially higher. In a study of patients with cocaine-induced MI, the risk of cardiac complications, most commonly heart failure and arrhythmias, was 38%.[321] The majority of complications occurred within the first 12 hours of hospitalization. Interestingly, no patients died during the hospitalization period. In another series, the risk of death associated with continued cocaine use was approximately 5%.[504]

PREVENTION

Approaches to help prevent drug-induced myocardial ischemia or acute coronary syndromes are listed in **Table 23-7**. Because patients with underlying coronary artery disease and those at high risk for the development of coronary artery disease are also likely to be at higher risk for the development of drug-induced myocardial ischemia or infarction, it is prudent to avoid drugs that may cause myocardial ischemia or infarction (Table 23-1) in this population unless treatment is absolutely necessary. If a potentially causative agent must be used, extra caution and monitoring should be used with these agents in patients at high risk for a coronary event (i.e., those with multiple risk factors, such as smoking, dyslipidemia, hypertension, diabetes mellitus, or others). In addition, the use of illicit drugs known to cause myocardial ischemia or infarction should be discouraged both in individuals and as a public health strategy. In patients with a history of coronary artery disease, particular attention to increased frequency of angina symptoms and/or use of sublingual nitroglycerin is warranted. More aggressive monitoring of chronic antianginal medications may be necessary.

Table 23-7 Approaches to Help Prevent Drug-Induced Myocardial Ischemia/Infarction

- Instruct patients who have a history of coronary artery disease to avoid, if possible, drugs that may cause myocardial ischemia or infarction.
- For patients who have underlying coronary artery disease and a previous history of anginal symptoms, self-care of angina symptoms should be the same as if the pain was associated with exertion or some other precipitant of an ischemic event.
- Individuals who do not have a history of coronary artery disease, acute coronary syndrome, or myocardial ischemia should be made aware that specific drugs that they are taking may, in unusual circumstances, precipitate a coronary event, and patients should be counseled regarding the symptoms that could result.
- Women >35 years of age should be assessed for cardiovascular risk (hypertension, smoking, diabetes, nephropathy and other vascular diseases) prior to initiation of oral contraceptives.
- Avoidance of drug toxicities through public health initiatives that warn about the dangers of illicit drug use.

There are no strong recommendations for considering drugs to be absolutely contraindicated in patients with known coronary artery disease for the avoidance of drug-induced myocardial ischemia and MI, with a few exceptions. The use of phosphodiesterase-5 inhibitors in patients receiving long-term nitrate therapy for exertional angina (i.e., patients with chronic coronary artery disease and angina) has been strongly discouraged by the AHA.[401] This strong statement is necessary because of the increased risk of coronary events and death when sildenafil is used in combination with short- or long-term nitrate therapy. Ergot alkaloids should also be avoided in patients with underlying coronary artery disease. In response to the clinical data suggesting an increase in cardiovascular events, NSAIDs have come under intense scrutiny. The next section discusses the use of NSAIDs in patients with cardiovascular disease.

In patients without a history of coronary artery disease, strategies for avoidance of drug-induced myocardial ischemia or infarction may be less clear. The approach in these patients should be increased awareness of drugs that have been associated with drug-induced myocardial ischemia or infarction. Unfortunately, no routine monitoring or prevention strategies can prevent drug-induced myocardial ischemia or infarction in all individuals. Recommendations for avoidance of use in specific conditions are available for only a few drugs. Regarding use of oral contraceptives, the Centers for Disease Control and Prevention (CDC) uses the following four classifications as a means for determining the risk–benefit ratio: **1** = A condition for which there is no restriction for the use of the contraceptive method; **2** = A condition for which the advantages of using the method generally outweigh the theoretical or proven risks; **3** = a condition for which the theoretical or proven risks usually outweigh the advantages of using the method; or **4** = a condition that represents an unacceptable health risk if the contraceptive method is used.[505] With respect to cardiovascular disease, the CDC indicates a rating of 3 or 4 for the following conditions: hypertension, multiple risk factors for atherosclerotic cardiovascular disease, vascular disease, current and history of ischemic heart disease and smoker with age >35 years. Dyslipidemia is rated as a 2 or 3 depending on the patient situation.[505]

MANAGEMENT

With the exception of the management of cocaine-induced chest pain and MI, there are very few specific data regarding the appropriate therapy for patients with drug-induced myocardial ischemia or acute coronary syndromes. Because the risk of the development of either disease in an otherwise normal population is very low, the consensus guidelines for the treatment of stable angina, unstable angina, or acute MI provide limited guidance about drug-induced diseases. More recent focused updates and scientific statements[1,2,324] have addressed cocaine-induced disease. However, limited information is available regarding other drugs known to cause myocardial ischemia or acute coronary syndromes.

With that introduction, it is most appropriate to consider treatment of three general groups: (1) patients with a history of chronic coronary artery disease who experience drug-induced ischemia; (2) patients with no history of coronary artery disease who experience drug-induced ischemia; and (3) patients with drug-induced acute coronary syndromes. In all three cases, it should be obvious that illicit drugs that are the cause of any of these drug-induced or drug-exacerbated diseases should be discontinued immediately and permanently.

DRUG-INDUCED MYOCARDIAL ISCHEMIA IN PATIENTS WITH CORONARY ARTERY DISEASE

Standard therapy for nondrug-induced myocardial ischemia secondary to coronary artery disease typically includes short-term management, long-term (prophylactic) therapy, and risk-factor modification.[506] Acute therapy typically involves the administration of sublingual nitrates when an anginal attack occurs or just before exertion in an effort to prevent or treat myocardial ischemia. In addition, most patients also require long-term prophylactic therapy with a β-blocker, calcium-channel blocker, a long-acting nitrate, or all three. The treatment of drug-induced myocardial ischemia is no different from that of classic nondrug-induced ischemia. Unless patients have been warned that a particular drug they are taking has the propensity to increase the risk of myocardial ischemia and subsequent angina, most patients will not associate an increase in the incidence of chest pain with specific drug therapy. Patients should be made aware that specific drugs they are taking might cause angina and potentially exacerbate their disease. When possible, the most effective treatment is to discontinue therapy with the offending agent. In some cases, this is not possible, and maximization of the patient's medical therapy for the underlying myocardial ischemia is necessary.

DRUG-INDUCED MYOCARDIAL ISCHEMIA IN PATIENTS WITH NO HISTORY OF CORONARY ARTERY DISEASE

In most cases, the most effective and logical therapy is to treat the anginal episode with standard therapy as necessary and immediately discontinue therapy with the offending agent. Inasmuch as there is no apparent underlying disease (i.e., no atherosclerotic coronary artery disease), discontinuation of the offending drug removes the sole cause of the symptoms.[506] In certain situations, discontinuation of a culprit agent is impractical or even life threatening. For example, withholding therapy with a cancer chemotherapy agent may not be possible, because it may be the only effective treatment. In these cases, although no specific data are available to support this on all occasions, use of short-term or prophylactic therapies, such as sublingual nitrates, may be necessary to minimize the ischemia. In most other cases, however, discontinuation of the offending agent is the most effective treatment approach. Finally, as discussed in the section above, it is prudent to treat these individuals with therapies that reduce the risk factors.

DRUG-INDUCED ACUTE CORONARY SYNDROMES

The therapies for acute coronary syndromes are outlined in consensus guidelines and reviews and are summarized in **Table 23-8.**[1,2,324] The consensus guidelines outlined in the table illustrate standard treatment of acute coronary syndromes (ST-segment elevation [STSE] acute coronary syndromes and non-ST-segment elevation [NSTSE] acute coronary syndromes) and management of cocaine-induced acute coronary syndromes from two distinct guidelines. Management of methamphetamine-induced acute coronary syndromes is also described as analogous to treatment of cocaine-induced acute coronary syndromes. The only drug-induced acute coronary syndromes for which therapeutic guidance exists are those caused by cocaine and methamphetamine; a specific section is devoted to treatment of these.

The management of conventional (nondrug-induced) acute coronary syndromes typically includes antiplatelet agents, unfractionated heparin or low-molecular-weight heparin, nitrates, β-blockers, anxiolytic drugs, and analgesics. In patients with STSE acute coronary syndromes, the addition of revascularization therapy with percutaneous coronary intervention (PCI) or thrombolytic therapy is generally indicated, and glycoprotein IIb/IIIa receptor antagonists are used in selected patients. In patients with NSTSE acute coronary syndromes, thrombolytic agents are not indicated, but PCI and glycoprotein IIb/IIIa receptor antagonists may be used. In general, therapy for a drug-induced acute coronary syndrome is the same as that for a nondrug-induced acute coronary syndrome. The therapies are similar primarily because there are few data to suggest that they should be different. Following in-hospital care, patients with evidence of drug-induced MI or atherosclerosis should be treated in a manner similar to that of patients with a nondrug-induced acute coronary syndrome. Aggressive cardiovascular risk-factor reduction with smoking cessation therapy and control of hypertension, diabetes, and dyslipidemia is necessary. Treatment with traditional secondary prevention therapies, including aspirin, clopidogrel, β-blockers, statins, and angiotensin-converting enzyme inhibitors should also be administered in these patients.

TREATMENT OF COCAINE-INDUCED ACUTE CORONARY SYNDROMES

As illustrated in Table 23-8, treatment guidelines for cocaine-induced acute coronary syndromes have been published. In addition, new sections regarding cocaine have been added to consensus guidelines for the management of acute coronary syndromes.[1,2,324] Mechanisms of cocaine-induced acute coronary syndrome are multifactorial (increased myocardial oxygen demand, decreased myocardial oxygen supply due to vasoconstriction, and thrombus formation), but, unlike nondrug-induced acute coronary syndromes, a major component of cocaine's effect is secondary to coronary vasoconstriction (in

Table 23-8 Therapy of Acute Coronary Syndromes

STEMI ACCF/AHA 2013 Guidelines[2]	NSTEMI/UA-ACCF/AHA 2014 Guidelines[1]		Cocaine-Associated Chest Pain and MI-AHA Scientific Statement[324]
	Overall Guidelines	Cocaine–Methamphetamine-Specific Guidelines	
Oxygen	Oxygen		Oxygen
Oral antiplatelet agents Aspirin $P2Y_{12}$ inhibitors	Oral antiplatelet agents Aspirin $P2Y_{12}$ inhibitors		Oral antiplatelet agents Aspirin $P2Y_{12}$ inhibitors
Benzodiazepine anxiolytics	Benzodiazepine anxiolytics	Benzodiazepines alone or in combination with nitroglycerin are reasonable for management of hypertension and tachycardia with signs of acute cocaine or methamphetamine intoxication	Benzodiazepine anxiolytics
Analgesics (morphine)	Analgesics (morphine)		Not discussed
Intravenous nitroglycerin	Intravenous nitroglycerin		Intravenous nitroglycerin (nitroprusside or phentolamine may be considered for persistent hypertension)
β-blockers	β-blockers	β-blockers should not be administered to patients with a recent history of cocaine or methamphetamine use who demonstrate signs of acute intoxication due to the risk of potentiating coronary spasm	β-blocker use should be avoided in the acute phase Labetalol does not offer any advantage; carvedilol has not been studied
Reperfusion Thrombolytics Primary PCI	Reperfusion Primary PCI	Not discussed	If ST-segment elevation present, PCI is preferred over thrombolytic therapy If NSTSE, evaluate with cardiac catheterization
Unfractionated heparin, enoxaparin, fondaparinux, bivalirudin	Unfractionated heparin, enoxaparin, fondaparinux, bivalirudin		Unfractionated heparin, enoxaparin, direct thrombin inhibitors
IV GP IIb/IIIa receptor antagonists	IV GP IIb/IIIa receptor antagonists		IV GP IIb/IIIa receptor antagonists
CCBs only when patients are unresponsive to NTG and β-blockers	CCBs only when patients are unresponsive to NTG and β-blockers		CCBs may be considered for patients who do not respond to benzodiazepines and nitroglycerin

ACCF = American College of Cardiology Foundation, AHA = American Heart Association, CCB = calcium-channel blocker, GP = glycoprotein, MI = myocardial infarction, NSTSE = non-ST-segment elevation, NSTEMI = non-ST-segment elevation myocardial infarction, NTG = nitroglycerin, PCI = percutaneous coronary intervention, STEMI = ST segment elevation myocardial infarction, WHO = World Health Organization, UA = unstable angina.

contrast to that of a classic acute coronary syndrome). Therefore, treatment approaches target the vasoconstrictive component as well as the classic therapeutic targets. In addition, cocaine toxicity affects other organ systems, particularly the central nervous system, increasing the risk of seizures, hyperthermia, and subarachnoid hemorrhage. These factors must be considered when treating cocaine-induced acute coronary syndromes. The AHA's recommendations for treatment of cocaine-induced chest pain are provided in Table 23-8 and are based on risk profile. All patients should be evaluated in a chest pain unit and receive aspirin and benzodiazepines initially. If pain is not responsive, nitroglycerin, nitroprusside (for persistent hypertension not controlled with nitroglycerin) or phentolamine (alternative) are recommended. Please note that the two guidelines differ slightly in their approach.

Considerable controversy exists regarding whether β-blockers, thrombolytic therapy, and calcium-channel blockers should be used for the management of cocaine-induced acute coronary syndromes. In theory, β-blockers have the potential to exacerbate coronary artery and systemic vasoconstriction. As described above, cocaine inhibits peripheral norepinephrine reuptake, leading to increased plasma norepinephrine concentrations and enhanced α_1-adrenoceptor-mediated vasoconstriction. When administered to patients who have ingested cocaine, β-blockers, especially nonselective agents, may further enhance coronary vasoconstriction through enhancement of unopposed α_1-adrenoceptor agonism, potentially further increasing blood pressure and heart rate and possibly increasing the risk of seizures and mortality.[319] Available data suggest that labetalol (a β-adrenergic and α_1-receptor inhibitor) may convey benefit in patients with cocaine-induced acute coronary syndromes, but labetalol administration has also been associated with increased seizure activity and mortality in animal models and little effect on coronary vasoconstriction in humans. Carvedilol, which is also a β-adrenergic and α_1-receptor inhibitor, may theoretically benefit patients with cocaine-induced acute coronary syndromes as well, although data supporting carvedilol use in this situation are not available. Several treatment guidelines[1,2,324] and expert reviews suggest that β-blockers of any kind should not be administered during the acute phase of an acute coronary syndrome. However, these recommendations have been questioned. Results of a retrospective study indicated that β-blockers are associated with a substantially lower risk of cocaine-induced MI.[507] The authors of this study suggested that warnings against β-blocker use may apply only to patients with acute cocaine intoxication. The AHA guidelines published in 2014 share these recommendations, whereas the cocaine-specific guidelines published in 2008 recommended against acute β-blocker administration. Further research since the publication of the 2008 guidelines suggests no difference in outcomes between the β-blocker cohort and patients not receiving a β-blocker.[508] However, it is difficult to determine if the patients in that study were acutely intoxicated. Both guidelines specifically recommend against the use of β-blockers in patients acutely intoxicated with cocaine.

Thrombolytic administration to individuals with cocaine-induced acute coronary syndrome is also very controversial. There have been several reports of intracranial hemorrhage or death secondary to thrombolytic use in this population.[317,509,510] Therefore, patients should receive benzodiazepines, aspirin, and nitrates followed by calcium-channel blockers or phentolamine.[317] Therapy with thrombolytics should be reserved for patients who are clearly having an ST-segment elevation MI who cannot undergo revascularization with PCI. These issues related to cocaine-induced acute coronary syndromes suggest that the standard treatment of drug-induced acute coronary syndromes is less than clear and is sometimes dependent on the specific drug causing the acute coronary syndrome.

The use of calcium-channel blockers for the treatment of cocaine-induced chest pain and acute coronary syndromes is also controversial. In theory, calcium-channel blockers should reverse the vasoconstriction frequently associated with cocaine ingestion. In cardiac catheterization studies, verapamil has been shown to reverse cocaine-associated vasospasm. However, results of animal studies regarding the effects of calcium-channel blockers on survival, seizure frequency, and arrhythmias associated with cocaine-induced ischemia have been variable. Current recommendations suggest that the short-acting dihydropyridine calcium-channel blockers should never be administered in patients with cocaine-induced acute coronary syndromes. This recommendation is consistent with that of standard treatment of chronic and acute coronary syndromes. Verapamil or diltiazem should not be used in the presence of left ventricular systolic dysfunction. Therapy with calcium-channel blockers should be reserved for patients with cocaine-induced acute coronary syndromes who do not respond to therapy with nitroglycerin and benzodiazepines.[324]

Finally, after hospitalization, outpatient treatment of patients with evidence of cocaine-induced MI or atherosclerosis should be similar to that used for patients with a nondrug-induced acute coronary syndrome. Aggressive cardiovascular risk-factor reduction with smoking cessation therapy and control of blood pressure, diabetes, and plasma lipid concentrations is necessary. Traditional secondary prevention therapies including aspirin, clopidogrel, statins, and angiotensin-converting enzyme inhibitors should be administered in these patients. Therapy with β-blockers should be used if required based on risk and in consideration of the potential for continued cocaine use.

Finally, while there are limited options for drug treatment programs to reduce cocaine use, there are numerous options for psychosocial intervention. The combination of group and intensive individual counseling has promise for the treatment of cocaine dependence.

ALTERNATIVES TO THE USE OF NSAIDs

Current guidelines recommend against the routine use of nonselective NSAIDs and selective COX-2 NSAIDs in patients with acute coronary syndromes.[2,511] Although these recommendations are focused on the treatment of acute coronary syndromes, they should likely be applied to all patients with cardiovascular disease. During the acute period, narcotic analgesics such as morphine should be administered for pain management. Following discharge from the hospital and during the postinfarction period, the AHA recommends a stepped-care approach for managing musculoskeletal pain.[481] These recommendations strongly advise clinicians to closely evaluate symptoms and to use nonpharmacologic approaches initially. If these techniques are ineffective for pain control, first-line agents may include acetaminophen, aspirin, tramadol, short-term narcotic analgesics or nonacetylated salicylates. The next tier of therapy involves a progression from non-COX-2 selective NSAIDs (e.g., naproxen, ibuprofen) to NSAIDs with some selectivity (e.g., diclofenac, celecoxib) to COX-2 selective NSAIDs (e.g., rofecoxib, etoricoxib). The recommendations also suggest that once the second tier of agents is chosen, the lowest dose of NSAID should be used, and additional therapy should include aspirin 81 mg daily and a proton pump inhibitor.[481] These recommendations have been met with some disagreement, as they are based primarily on cardiovascular risk, rather than the need for pain management.

INFORMATION FOR PATIENTS

Information for patients regarding prevention of these drug-induced conditions is provided in Table 23-7. Patients who are taking drugs that may cause myocardial ischemia or acute coronary syndromes should be instructed that the specific drug may, in some cases, cause chest pain. For patients who have underlying coronary artery disease and a history of anginal symptoms, self-care of angina symptoms should be the same as if the pain was associated with exertion or some other precipitant of an ischemic event. Individuals who do not have a history of coronary artery disease, acute coronary syndrome, or myocardial ischemia should be made aware that specific drugs that they are taking may, in unusual circumstances, precipitate a coronary event, and patients should be counseled regarding the symptoms that could result. Patients should be instructed to consult their pharmacist or physician or go to an emergency department if chest pain, palpitations, light-headedness, dizziness, or shortness of breath occur. Finally, and most unfortunately, many cases of drug-induced ischemia and infarction are associated with illicit-drug use (e.g., cocaine, amphetamines). The best method to avoid these toxicities is through public health initiatives that warn about the dangers of illicit-drug use. Finally, referral of these patients to drug rehabilitation programs is essential for appropriate treatment.

REFERENCES

1. Amsterdam EA, Wenger NK, Brindis RG et al. 2014 AHA/ACC guideline for the management of patients with non-ST-elevation acute coronary syndromes: a report of the American College of Cardiology/American Heart Association Task Force on Practice Guidelines. *Circulation*. 2014; 130:e344-426.
2. O'Gara PT, Kushner FG, Ascheim DD et al. 2013 ACCF/AHA guideline for the management of ST-elevation myocardial infarction: a report of the American College of Cardiology Foundation/American Heart Association Task Force on Practice Guidelines. *Circulation*. 2013; 127:e362-425.
3. Ben-David A. Cardiac arrest in an explosives factory worker due to withdrawal from nitroglycerin exposure. *Am J Ind Med.* 1989; 15:719-22.
4. Berge KH, Lanier WL. Myocardial infarction accompanying acute clonidine withdrawal in a patient without a history of ischemic coronary artery disease. *Anesth Analg.* 1991; 72:259-61.
5. Frye CB, Vance MA. Hypertensive crisis and myocardial infarction following massive clonidine overdose. *Ann Pharmacother.* 2000; 34:611-5.
6. Ho PM, Peterson ED, Wang L et al. Incidence of death and acute myocardial infarction associated with stopping clopidogrel after acute coronary syndrome. *JAMA*. 2008; 299:532-9.
7. Howard PA, Delafontaine P. Nonsteroidal anti-Inflammatory drugs and cardiovascular risk. *J Am Coll Cardiol.* 2004; 43:519-25.
8. Legrand V, Deliege M, Henrard L et al. Patients with myocardial infarction and normal coronary arteriogram. *Chest.* 1982; 82:678-85.
9. Mullins ME, Horowitz BZ, Linden DH et al. Life-threatening interaction of mibefradil and beta-blockers with dihydropyridine calcium channel blockers. *JAMA*. 1998; 280:157-8.
10. Pepine CJ, Lopez LM, Bell DM et al. Effects of intermittent transdermal nitroglycerin on occurrence of ischemia after patch removal: results of the second transdermal intermittent dosing evaluation study (TIDES-II). *J Am Coll Cardiol.* 1997; 30:955-61.
11. Przybojewski JZ, Heyns MH. Acute myocardial infarction due to coronary vasospasm secondary to industrial nitroglycerin withdrawal. A case report. *S Afr Med J.* 1983; 64:101-4.
12. Psaty BM, Koepsell TD, Wagner EH et al. The relative risk of incident coronary heart disease associated with recently stopping the use of beta-blockers. *JAMA*. 1990; 263:1653-7.
13. Reeves WC, Cook L, Wood MA, Whitesell L. Coronary artery spasm after abrupt withdrawal of nitroglycerin in rabbits. *Am J Cardiol.* 1985; 55:1066-9.
14. Theroux P, Waters D, Lam J et al. Reactivation of unstable angina after the discontinuation of heparin. *N Engl J Med.* 1992; 327:141-5.
15. Frishman WH. Beta-adrenergic blocker withdrawal. *Am J Cardiol.* 1987; 59:26F-32F.
16. McGowan MP. There is no evidence for an increase in acute coronary syndromes after short-term abrupt discontinuation of statins in stable cardiac patients. *Circulation.* 2004; 110:2333-5.
17. Ottervanger JP, Wilson JH, Stricker BH. Drug-induced chest pain and myocardial infarction. Reports to a national centre and review of the literature. *Eur J Clin Pharmacol.* 1997; 53:105-10.
18. Gislason GH, Jacobsen S, Rasmussen JN et al. Risk of death or reinfarction associated with the use of selective cyclooxygenase-2 inhibitors and nonselective nonsteroidal antiinflammatory drugs after acute myocardial infarction. *Circulation*. 2006; 113:2906-13.
19. Joshi GP, Gertler R, Fricker R. Cardiovascular thromboembolic adverse effects associated with cyclooxygenase-2 selective inhibitors and nonselective antiinflammatory drugs. *Anesth Analg.* 2007; 105:1793-804.
20. Martinez-Gonzalez J, Badimon L. Mechanisms underlying the cardiovascular effects of COX-inhibition: benefits and risks. *Curr Pharm Des.* 2007; 13:2215-27.
21. Mukherjee D, Nissen SE, Topol EJ. Risk of cardiovascular events associated with selective COX-2 inhibitors. *JAMA*. 2001; 286:954-9.
22. Warner TD, Mitchell JA. COX-2 selectivity alone does not define the cardiovascular risks associated with non-steroidal anti-inflammatory drugs. *Lancet.* 2008; 371:270-3.
23. Ward J, Standage C. Angina pain precipitated by a continuous subcutaneous infusion of ketamine. *J Pain Symptom Manage.* 2003; 25:6-7.
24. Gottlieb NL, Brown HE Jr. Acute myocardial infarction following gold sodium thiomalate induced vasomotor (nitritoid) reaction. *Arthritis Rheum.* 1977; 20:1026-30.
25. Backmund M, Meyer K, Zwehl W et al. Myocardial Infarction associated with methadone and/or dihydrocodeine. *Eur Addict Res.* 2001; 7:37-9.
26. Ioseliani DG, Semitko SP, Gromov DG et al. [Development of transmural myocardial infarction in young persons with intact coronary arteries during methadone use for the treatment of heroine addiction]. *Kardiologiia.* 2004; 44:107-12.
27. Solomon DH, Schneeweiss S, Glynn RJ et al. Relationship between selective cyclooxygenase-2 inhibitors and acute myocardial infarction in older adults. *Circulation.* 2004; 109:2068-73.
28. Akgullu C, Eryilmaz U, Gungor H et al. Myocardial infarction secondary to morphine-induced Kounis syndrome. *Herz.* 2014; 39:874-6.
29. Slogoff S, Keats AS. Isoflurane and outcome after coronary artery surgery. *Anesth Analg.* 1991; 72:842-3.
30. Inoue K, Reichelt W, el-Banayosy A et al. Does isoflurane lead to a higher incidence of myocardial infarction and perioperative death than enflurane in coronary artery surgery? A clinical study of 1178 patients. *Anesth Analg.* 1990; 71:469-74.
31. Merin RG, Lowenstein E, Gelman S. Is anesthesia beneficial for the ischemic heart? III. *Anesthesiology.* 1986; 64:137-40.
32. Pearson AC, Labovitz AJ, Kern MJ. Accelerated hypertension complicated by myocardial infarction after use of a local anesthetic/vasoconstrictor preparation. *Am Heart J.* 1987; 114:662-3.
33. Anderson NR, Lokich JJ, Moore C. The syndrome of 5-fluorouracil cardiotoxicity: an elusive cardiopathy. *Cancer.* 1993; 72:2287-8.
34. Arbuck SG, Strauss H, Rowinsky E et al. A reassessment of cardiac toxicity associated with Taxol. *J Natl Cancer Inst Monogr.* 1993: 117-30.
35. Bachmeyer C, Joly H, Jorest R. Early myocardial infarction during chemotherapy for testicular cancer. *Tumori.* 2000; 86:428-30.
36. Bosek V, Hu P, Robinson LA. Acute myocardial ischemia after administration of ondansetron hydrochloride. *Anesthesiology.* 2000; 92:885-7.
37. Chasen MR, Ebrahim IO. Carboplatin hypersensitivity presenting as coronary vasospasm—a case report. *Cancer Chemother Pharmacol.* 2002; 50:429-31.
38. Cheng JW, Behar L. Calcium channel blockers: association with myocardial infarction, mortality, and cancer. *Clin Ther.* 1997; 19:1255-68; discussion 3-4.
39. Clark JI, Kancharla K, Qamar R et al. Pilot study of sequential vinorelbine and cisplatin followed by docetaxel for selected IIIB and stage IV non-small cell lung cancer. *Lung Cancer.* 2001; 34:271-7.
40. Dow E, Schulman H, Agura E. Cyclophosphamide cardiac injury mimicking acute myocardial infarction. *Bone Marrow Transplant.* 1993; 12:169-72.
41. Fonte CE, Cardello F. Chest pain in a cancer patient on chemotherapy. *Hosp Pract* (Off Ed). 1991; 26:145-6.
42. Gerl A. Vascular toxicity associated with chemotherapy for testicular cancer. *Anticancer Drugs.* 1994; 5:607-14.
43. Icli F, Karaoguz H, Dincol D et al. Severe vascular toxicity associated with cisplatin-based chemotherapy. *Cancer.* 1993; 72:587-93.

44. Kanj SS, Sharara AI, Shpall EJ et al. Myocardial ischemia associated with high-dose carmustine infusion. *Cancer.* 1991; 68:1910-2.

45. Keefe DL, Roistacher N, Pierri MK. Clinical cardiotoxicity of 5-fluorouracil. *J Clin Pharmacol.* 1993; 33:1060-70.

46. Kragel AH, Travis WD, Steis RG et al. Myocarditis or acute myocardial infarction associated with interleukin-2 therapy for cancer. *Cancer.* 1990; 66:1513-6.

47. Kuzel T, Esparaz B, Green D, Kies M. Thrombogenicity of intravenous 5-fluorouracil alone or in combination with cisplatin. *Cancer.* 1990; 65:885-9.

48. Laufman LR, Jones JJ, Morrice B et al. Case report of a lethal cardiac toxic effect following high-dose cyclophosphamide. *J Natl Cancer Inst.* 1995; 87:539-40.

49. Mancuso L, Marchi S, Canonico A. Dynamic left ventricular outflow obstruction and myocardial infarction following doxorubicin administration in a woman affected by unsuspected hypertrophic cardiomyopathy. *Cancer Treat Rep.* 1985; 69:241-4.

50. Mandel EM, Lewinski U, Djaldetti M. Vincristine-induced myocardial infarction. *Cancer.* 1975; 36:1979-82.

51. Mermershtain W, Dudnik J, Gusakova I, Ariad S. Acute myocardial infarction in a young man receiving chemotherapy for testicular cancer: case report. *J Chemother.* 2001; 13:658-60.

52. Nora R, Abrams JS, Tait NS et al. Myocardial toxic effects during recombinant interleukin-2 therapy. *J Natl Cancer Inst.* 1989; 81:59-63.

53. Punt KC, Jansen RL, De Mulder PH et al. Repetitive weekly cycles of 4-day continuous infusion of recombinant interleukin-2: a phase I study. *J Immunother.* 1992; 12:277-84.

54. Roth BJ, Yeap BY, Wilding G et al. Taxol in advanced, hormone-refractory carcinoma of the prostate. A phase II trial of the Eastern Cooperative Oncology Group. *Cancer.* 1993; 72:2457-60.

55. Samuels BL, Vogelzang NJ, Kennedy BJ. Severe vascular toxicity associated with vinblastine, bleomycin, and cisplatin chemotherapy. *Cancer Chemother Pharmacol.* 1987; 19:253-6.

56. Schecter JP, Jones SE, Jackson RA. Myocardial infarction in a 27-year-old woman: possible complication of treatment with VP-16-213 (NSC-141540), mediastinal irradiation, or both. *Cancer Chemother Rep.* 1975; 59:887-8.

57. Schmeller N. [A 79-year-old man with metastatic prostate cancer, treated with Zoladex, flutamide, calcitonin and Ostac, suffers from frequent troublesome sweating with palpitation and angina pectoris, especially at night. Is there a therapy?]. *Internist (Berl).* 1992; 33:284.

58. Schober C, Papageorgiou E, Harstrick A et al. Cardiotoxicity of 5-fluorouracil in combination with folinic acid in patients with gastrointestinal cancer. *Cancer.* 1993; 72:2242-7.

59. Subar M, Muggia FM. Apparent myocardial ischemia associated with vinblastine administration. *Cancer Treat Rep.* 1986; 70:690-1.

60. Vos AH, Splinter TA, van der Heul C. Arterial occlusive events during chemotherapy for germ cell cancer. *Neth J Med.* 2001; 59:295-9.

61. Yano S, Shimada K. Vasospastic angina after chemotherapy by with carboplatin and etoposide in a patient with lung cancer. *Jpn Circ J.* 1996; 60:185-8.

62. Zabernigg A, Gattringer C. Myocardial infarction associated with vinorelbine (Navelbine). *Eur J Cancer.* 1996; 32A:1618-9.

63. Airey CL, Dodwell DJ, Joffe JK, Jones WG. Etoposide-related myocardial infarction. *Clin Oncol (R Coll Radiol).* 1995; 7:135.

64. Akhtar SS, Wani BA, Bano ZA et al. 5-fluorouracil-induced severe but reversible cardiogenic shock: a case report. *Tumori.* 1996; 82:505-7.

65. Aydiner A, Bugra Z, Topuz E, Meric M. Acute myocardial infarction in man treated with epirubicin for non-Hodgkin lymphoma. *Am J Clin Oncol.* 1995; 18:444-8.

66. Bergeron A, Raffy O, Vannetzel JM. Myocardial ischemia and infarction associated with vinorelbine. *J Clin Oncol.* 1995; 13:531-2.

67. Doll DC, List AF, Greco FA et al. Acute vascular ischemic events after cisplatin-based combination chemotherapy for germ-cell tumors of the testis. *Ann Intern Med.* 1986; 105:48-51.

68. Doll DC, Yarbro JW. Vascular toxicity associated with antineoplastic agents. *Semin Oncol.* 1992; 19:580-96.

69. Dumontet C, Morschhauser F, Solal-Celigny P et al. Gemcitabine as a single agent in the treatment of relapsed or refractory low-grade non-Hodgkin's lymphoma. *Br J Haematol.* 2001; 113:772-8.

70. Ensley JF, Patel B, Kloner R et al. The clinical syndrome of 5-fluorouracil cardiotoxicity. *Invest New Drugs.* 1989; 7:101-9.

71. Erol MK, Acikel M, Senocak H. Non-Q-Wave acute anterior myocardial infarction associated with 5-fluorouracil and cisplatin chemotherapy. *South Med J.* 2003; 96:99.

72. Farooqi IS, Aronson JK. Latrogenic chest pain: a case of 5-fluorouracil cardiotoxicity. *QJM.* 1996; 89:953-5.

73. Federman DG, Henry G. Chemotherapy-induced myocardial necrosis in a patient with chronic lymphocytic leukemia. *Respir Med.* 1997; 91:565-7.

74. Fragasso G, Pastore MR, Vicari A et al. Myocardial infarction in a patient with acute lymphoblastic leukemia during L-asparaginase therapy. *Am J Hematol.* 1995; 48:136-7.

75. Frickhofen N, Beck FJ, Jung B et al. Capecitabine can induce acute coronary syndrome similar to 5-fluorouracil. *Ann Oncol.* 2002; 13:797-801.

76. Gryn J, Gordon R, Bapat A et al. Pentostatin increases the acute toxicity of high dose cyclophosphamide. *Bone Marrow Transplant.* 1993; 12:217-20.

77. Harris AL, Wong C. Myocardial ischaemia, radiotherapy, and vinblastine. *Lancet.* 1981; 1:787.

78. Hekmat E. Fatal myocardial infarction potentially induced by paclitaxel. *Ann Pharmacother.* 1996; 30:1110-2.

79. House KW, Simon SR, Pugh RP. Chemotherapy-induced myocardial infarction in a young man with Hodgkin's disease. *Clin Cardiol.* 1992; 15:122-5.

80. Jameson M, Thompson P, Hastie B. 5 Fluorouracil cardiotoxicity. *N Z Med J.* 1995; 108:21.

81. King M, Fernando I. Vascular toxicity associated with cisplatin. *Clin Oncol (R Coll Radiol).* 2003; 15:36-7.

82. Kleiman NS, Lehane DE, Geyer CE Jr et al. Prinzmetal's angina during 5-fluorouracil chemotherapy. *Am J Med.* 1987; 82:566-8.

83. Labianca R, Beretta G, Clerici M et al. Cardiac toxicity of 5-fluorouracil: a study on 1083 patients. *Tumori.* 1982; 68:505-10.

84. Labianca R, Luporini G. 5-fluorouracil cardiotoxicity: the risk of rechallenge. *Ann Oncol.* 1991; 2:383.

85. Laher S, Karp SJ. Acute myocardial infarction following paclitaxel administration for ovarian carcinoma. *Clin Oncol (R Coll Radiol).* 1997; 9:124-6.

86. Law H. Chemotherapy-induced myocardial infarction. *Eur Heart J.* 1996; 17:966-7.

87. Lejonc JL, Vernant JP, Macquin J, Castaigne A. Myocardial infarction following vinblastine treatment. *Lancet.* 1980; 2:692.

88. Leone B, Rabinovich M, Ferrari CR et al. Cardiotoxicity as a result of 5-fluorouracil therapy. *Tumori.* 1985; 71:55-7.

89. McKendall GR, Shurman A, Anamur M, Most AS. Toxic cardiogenic shock associated with infusion of 5-fluorouracil. *Am Heart J.* 1989; 118:184-6.

90. Monk MR, Sanchez JD, Phelps CD, Miller DM. Myocardial ischemia with fluorouracil and floxuridine therapy. *Clin Pharm.* 1987; 6:659-61.

91. Nguyen-Ho P, Kleiman NS, Verani MS. Acute myocardial infarction and cardiac arrest in a patient receiving paclitaxel. *Can J Cardiol.* 2003; 19:300-2.

92. Rowinsky EK, McGuire WP, Guarnieri T et al. Cardiac disturbances during the administration of taxol. *J Clin Oncol.* 1991; 9:1704-12.
93. Schnetzler B, Popova N, Collao Lamb C, Sappino AP. Coronary spasm induced by capecitabine. *Ann Oncol.* 2001; 12:723-4.
94. Schwarzer S, Eber B, Greinix H, Lind P. Non-Q-wave myocardial infarction associated with bleomycin and etoposide chemotherapy. *Eur Heart J.* 1991; 12:748-50.
95. Shanmugasundaram S, Bharathithasan R, Elangovan S. 5-fluorouracil-Induced cardiotoxicity. *Indian Heart J.* 2002; 54:86-7.
96. Singer M. Cardiotoxicity and capecitabine: a case report. *Clin J Oncol Nurs.* 2003; 7:72-5.
97. Somers G, Abramov M, Witter M, Naets JP. Letter: Myocardial infarction: a complication of vincristine treatment? *Lancet.* 1976; 02:690.
98. Villani F, Guindani A, Pagnoni A. 5-fluorouracil cardiotoxicity. *Tumori.* 1979; 65:487-95.
99. Wang WS, Hsieh RK, Chiou TJ et al. Toxic cardiogenic shock in a patient receiving weekly 24-h infusion of high-dose 5-fluorouracil and leucovorin. *Jpn J Clin Oncol.* 1998; 28:551-4.
100. Weinstein P, Greenwald ES, Grossman J. Unusual cardiac reaction to chemotherapy following mediastinal irradiation in a patient with Hodgkin's disease. *Am J Med.* 1976; 60:152-6.
101. Weng MC, Wang WB, Chao TY. Cardiotoxicity related to 5-fluorouracil chemotherapy: a report of two cases. *Zhonghua Yi Xue Za Zhi (Taipei).* 1995; 55:266-9.
102. Ambrosy AP, Kunz PL, Fisher GA, Witteles RM. Capecitabine-induced chest pain relieved by diltiazem. *Am J Cardiol.* 2012; 110:1623-6.
103. Basselin C, Fontanges T, Descotes J et al. 5-fluorouracil-induced Tako-Tsubo-like syndrome. *Pharmacotherapy.* 2011; 31:226.
104. Conti E, Romiti A, Musumeci MB et al. Arterial thrombotic events and acute coronary syndromes with cancer drugs: are growth factors the missed link?: what both cardiologist and oncologist should know about novel angiogenesis inhibitors. *Int J Cardiol.* 2013; 167:2421-9.
105. Kalsch H, Wieneke H, Erbel R. Acute myocardial infarction in a patient with chronic myelocytic leukemia during chemotherapy with hydroxyurea. *Herz.* 2010; 35:420-2.
106. Manojlovic N, Babic D, Stojanovic S et al. Capecitabine cardiotoxicity—case reports and literature review. *Hepato-gastroenterology.* 2008; 55:1249-56.
107. Paiva CE, Paiva BS, Garita R et al. Acute coronary syndrome associated with continuous 5-fluorouracil infusion in a patient with metastatic colorectal cancer—a case report with a discussion on this clinical dilemma. *J Gastrointest Cancer.* 2009; 40:133-7.
108. Scott PA, Ferchow L, Hobson A, Curzen NP. Coronary spasm induced by capecitabine mimicks ST elevation myocardial infarction. *Emerg Med J.* 2008; 25:699-700.
109. Shah K, Gupta S, Ghosh J et al. Acute non-ST elevation myocardial infarction following paclitaxel administration for ovarian carcinoma: a case report and review of literature. *J Cancer Res Ther.* 2012; 8:442-4.
110. Stewart T, Pavlakis N, Ward M. Cardiotoxicity with 5-fluorouracil and capecitabine: more than just vasospastic angina. *Intern Med J.* 2010; 40:303-7.
111. Tsiamis E, Synetos A, Stefanadis C. Capecitabine may induce coronary artery vasospasm. *Hellenic J Cardiol.* 2012; 53:320-3.
112. Arima Y, Oshima S, Noda K et al. Sorafenib-induced acute myocardial infarction due to coronary artery spasm. *J Cardiol.* 2009; 54:512-5.
113. Jefferson JW. A review of the cardiovascular effects and toxicity of tricyclic antidepressants. *Psychosom Med.* 1975; 37:160-79.
114. Rodstein M, Oei LS. Cardiovascular side effects of long-term therapy with tricyclic antidepressants in the aged. *J Am Geriatr Soc.* 1979; 27:231-4.
115. Patterson RN, Herity NA. Acute myocardial infarction following bupropion (Zyban). *QJM.* 2002; 95:58-9.
116. Pederson KJ, Kuntz DH, Garbe GJ. Acute myocardial ischemia associated with ingestion of bupropion and pseudoephedrine in a 21-year-old man. *Can J Cardiol.* 2001; 17:599-601.
117. Reznik I, Rosen Y, Rosen B. An acute ischaemic event associated with the use of venlafaxine: a case report and proposed pathophysiological mechanisms. *J Psychopharmacol.* 1999; 13:193-5.
118. Sunderji R, Press N, Amin H, Gin K. Unstable angina associated with sertraline. *Can J Cardiol.* 1997; 13:849-51.
119. Chamsi-Pasha H, Barnes PC. Myocardial infarction: a complication of amitriptyline overdose. *Postgrad Med J.* 1988; 64:968-70.
120. Chong SA, Mythily, Mahendran R. Cardiac effects of psychotropic drugs. *Ann Acad Med Singapore.* 2001; 30:625-31.
121. Cohen HW, Gibson G, Alderman MH. Excess risk of myocardial infarction in patients treated with antidepressant medications: association with use of tricyclic agents. *Am J Med.* 2000; 108:2-8.
122. DeFeudis FV. Are vascular mechanisms involved in antidepressant action? *Gen Pharmacol.* 1985; 16:553-6.
123. Ngo AS, Ho RY, Olson KR. Phenelzine-induced myocardial injury: a case report. *J Med Toxicol.* 2010; 6:431-4.
124. Flynn TE, Bricker LA. Myocardial infarction in HIV-infected men receiving protease inhibitors. *Ann Intern Med.* 1999; 131:548.
125. Friis-Moller N, Reiss P, Sabin CA et al. Class of antiretroviral drugs and the risk of myocardial infarction. *N Engl J Med.* 2007; 356:1723-35.
126. Gallet B, Pulik M, Genet P et al. Vascular complications associated with use of HIV protease inhibitors. *Lancet.* 1998; 351:1958-9.
127. Holmberg SD, Moorman AC, Williamson JM et al. Protease inhibitors and cardiovascular outcomes in patients with HIV-1. *Lancet.* 2002; 360:1747-8.
128. Jutte A, Schwenk A, Franzen C et al. Increasing morbidity from myocardial infarction during HIV protease inhibitor treatment? *AIDS.* 1999; 13:1796-7.
129. Muise A, Arbess G. The risk of myocardial infarction in HIV-infected patients receiving HAART: a case report. *Int J STD AIDS.* 2001; 12:612-3.
130. Stein JH. Cardiovascular risks of antiretroviral therapy. *N Engl J Med.* 2007; 356:1773-5.
131. Vittecoq D, Escaut L, Monsuez JJ. Vascular complications associated with use of HIV protease inhibitors. *Lancet.* 1998; 351:1959.
132. Lopez-Abad R, Rodriguez F, Garcia-Abujeta JL et al. Myocardial ischemia due to severe amoxicillin allergy. *J Investig Allergol Clin Immunol.* 2004; 14:162-4.
133. Bilgin M, Akyel A, Dogan M et al. Acute coronary syndrome secondary to clarithromycin: the first case and review of the literature. *Turk Kardiyol Dern Ars.* 2014; 42:461-3.
134. Schembri S, Williamson PA, Short PM et al. Cardiovascular events after clarithromycin use in lower respiratory tract infections: analysis of two prospective cohort studies. *BMJ.* (Clinical research ed). 2013; 346:f1235.
135. Bezgin T, Gecmen C, Ozkan B et al. Kounis syndrome secondary to simultaneous oral amoxicillin and parenteral ampicillin use in a young man. *Cardiovasc J Afr.* 2013; 24:e10-2.
136. Biteker M, Duran NE, Biteker FS et al. Kounis syndrome secondary to amoxicillin/clavulanic acid use in a child. *Int J Cardiol.* 2009; 136:e3-5.
137. Tok D, Ozcan F, Senturk B, Golbasi Z. [A case of acute coronary syndrome following the use of parenteral penicillin: Kounis syndrome]. *Turk Kardiyol Dern Ars.* 2012; 40:615-9.
138. Viana-Tejedor A, Espinosa MA, Cuesta J et al. Kounis syndrome secondary to amoxicillin use in an asthmatic patient. *Int J Cardiol.* 2011; 150:e113-5.
139. Coloma PM, Schuemie MJ, Trifiro G et al. Drug-induced acute myocardial infarction: identifying 'prime suspects' from electronic healthcare records-based surveillance system. *PLoS One.* 2013; 8:e72148.
140. Ketch J, Herd A, Ludwig L. ST segment elevations without myocardial infarction in a patient on clozapine. *Am J Emerg Med.* 1996; 14:111-2.

141. Wooltorton E. Antipsychotic clozapine (Clozaril): myocarditis and cardiovascular toxicity. *CMAJ.* 2002; 166:1185-6.
142. El Menyar AA. Drug-induced myocardial infarction secondary to coronary artery spasm in teenagers and young adults. *J Postgrad Med.* 2006; 52:51-6.
143. Kurth T. Migraine and ischaemic vascular events. *Cephalalgia.* 2007; 27:965-75.
144. Peterlin BL, Tietjen G, Meng S et al. Post-traumatic stress disorder in episodic and chronic migraine. *Headache.* 2008; 48:517-22.
145. Schoenen J, Delree P, Moonen G. Acute myocardial infarction in a young female migraineur: sumatriptan suspected, but found not guilty. *Cephalalgia.* 1994; 14:305.
146. Abbrescia VD, Pearlstein L, Kotler M. Sumatriptan-associated myocardial infarction: report of case with attention to potential risk factors. *J Am Osteopath Assoc.* 1997; 97:162-4.
147. Cheng TO. Irreversible coronary occlusion and ergonovine. *Circulation.* 1982; 65:640.
148. Chester AH, O'Neil GS, Yacoub MH. Sumatriptan and ischaemic heart disease. *Lancet.* 1993; 341:1419-20.
149. Fujiwara Y, Yamanaka O, Nakamura T et al. Acute myocardial infarction induced by ergonovine administration for artificially induced abortion. *Jpn Heart J.* 1993; 34:803-8.
150. Hillis WS, Macintyre PD. Sumatriptan and chest pain. *Lancet.* 1993; 342:683.
151. Hudgson P, Foster JB, Walton JN. Methysergide and coronary artery disease. *Am Heart J.* 1967; 74:854-5.
152. Klein LS, Simpson RJ Jr, Stern R et al. Myocardial infarction following administration of sublingual ergotamine. *Chest.* 1982; 82:375-6.
153. Liao JK, Cockrill BA, Yurchak PM. Acute myocardial infarction after ergonovine administration for uterine bleeding. *Am J Cardiol.* 1991; 68:823-4.
154. Liston H, Bennett L, Usher B Jr, Nappi J. The association of the combination of sumatriptan and methysergide in myocardial infarction in a premenopausal woman. *Arch Intern Med.* 1999; 159:511-3.
155. Lloyd DK, Simmons V. Adverse reactions associated with sumatriptan. *Lancet.* 1993; 341:1092.
156. Main ML, Ramaswamy K, Andrews TC. Cardiac arrest and myocardial infarction immediately after sumatriptan injection. *Ann Intern Med.* 1998; 128:874.
157. Meyler WJ. Side effects of ergotamine. *Cephalalgia.* 1996; 16:5-10.
158. O'Connor P, Gladstone P. Oral sumatriptan-associated transmural myocardial infarction. *Neurology.* 1995; 45:2274-6.
159. Ottervanger JP, Paalman HJ, Boxma GL, Stricker BH. Transmural myocardial infarction with sumatriptan. *Lancet.* 1993; 341:861-2.
160. Ottervanger JP, van Witsen TB, Valkenburg HA et al. Adverse reactions attributed to sumatriptan. A postmarketing study in general practice. *Eur J Clin Pharmacol.* 1994; 47:305-9.
161. Roithinger FX, Punzengruber C, Gremmel F et al. Myocardial infarction after chronic ergotamine abuse. *Eur Heart J.* 1993; 14:1579-81.
162. Taylor GJ, Cohen B. Ergonovine-induced coronary artery spasm and myocardial infarction after normal delivery. *Obstet Gynecol.* 1985; 66:821-2.
163. Tsui BC, Stewart B, Fitzmaurice A, Williams R. Cardiac arrest and myocardial infarction induced by postpartum intravenous ergonovine administration. *Anesthesiology.* 2001; 94:363-4.
164. Wolf NM, Meister SG. Irreversible coronary occlusion and ergonovine. *Circulation.* 1982; 66:252.
165. Yasue H, Omote S, Takizawa A, Nagao M. Acute myocardial infarction induced by ergotamine tartrate: possible role of coronary arterial spasm. *Angiology.* 1981; 32:414-8.
166. Mousa HA, McKinley CA, Thong J. Acute postpartum myocardial infarction after ergometrine administration in a woman with familial hypercholesterolaemia. *BJOG.* 2000; 107:939-40.
167. Nall KS, Feldman B. Postpartum myocardial infarction induced by methergine. *Am J Emerg Med.* 1998; 16:502-4.
168. Sutaria N, O'Toole L, Northridge D. Postpartum acute MI following routine ergometrine administration treated successfully by primary PTCA. *Heart.* 2000; 83:97-8.
169. Yaegashi N, Miura M, Okamura K. Acute myocardial infarction associated with postpartum ergot alkaloid administration. *Int J Gynaecol Obstet.* 1999; 64:67-8.
170. Bateman BT, Huybrechts KF, Hernandez-Diaz S et al. Methylergonovine maleate and the risk of myocardial ischemia and infarction. *Am. J. Obstet. Gynecol.* 2013; 209:459.e1-.e13.
171. de Labriolle A, Genee O, Heggs LM, Fauchier L. Acute myocardial infarction following oral methyl-ergometrine intake. *Cardiovasc Toxicol.* 2009; 9:46-8.
172. Kocaoglu I, Gokaslan S, Karagoz A et al. Zolmitriptan-induced acute myocardial infarction. *Cardiol J.* 2012; 19:76-8.
173. Acikel S, Dogan M, Sari M et al. Prinzmetal-variant angina in a patient using zolmitriptan and citalopram. *Am J Emerg Med.* 2010; 28:257.e3-6.
174. Schenkat DH, Schulz LT, Johnson BD. Dihydroergotamine-induced vasospastic angina in a patient taking a calcium channel blocker. *Ann Pharmacother.* 2011; 45:e41.
175. Smith M, Golwala H, Lozano P. Zolmitriptan induced acute coronary syndrome: a unique case. *Am J Ther.* 2011; 18:e153-6.
176. Stillman MJ, Tepper S, Tepper DE, Cho L. QT prolongation, Torsade de Pointes, myocardial ischemia from coronary vasospasm, and headache medications. Part 1: review of serotonergic cardiac adverse events with a triptan case. *Headache.* 2013; 53:208-16.
177. Ehrlich HJ, Henzl MJ, Gomperts ED. Safety of factor VIII inhibitor bypass activity (FEIBA): 10-year compilation of thrombotic adverse events. *Haemophilia.* 2002; 8:83-90.
178. Karayalcin G, Goldberg B, Cherrick I et al. Acute myocardial infarction complicating prothrombin complex concentrate therapy in an 8-year-old boy with hemophilia A and factor VIII inhibitor. *Am J Pediatr Hematol Oncol.* 1993; 15:416-9.
179. Mekontso-Dessap A, Collet JP, Lebrun-Vignes B et al. Acute myocardial infarction after oral tranexamic acid treatment initiation. *Int J Cardiol.* 2002; 83:267-8.
180. Ruel MA, Wang F, Bourke ME et al. Is tranexamic acid safe in patients undergoing coronary endarterectomy? *Ann Thorac Surg.* 2001; 71:1508-11.
181. Sullivan DW, Purdy LJ, Billingham M, Glader BE. Fatal myocardial infarction following therapy with prothrombin complex concentrates in a young man with hemophilia A. *Pediatrics.* 1984; 74:279-81.
182. Early treatment of unstable angina in the coronary care unit: a randomised, double blind, placebo controlled comparison of recurrent ischaemia in patients treated with nifedipine or metoprolol or both. Report of The Holland Interuniversity Nifedipine/Metoprolol Trial (HINT) Research Group. *Br Heart J.* 1986; 56:400-13.
183. Leavitt AD, Zweifler AJ. Nifedipine, hypotension, and myocardial injury. *Ann Intern Med.*1988; 108:305-6.
184. Estacio RO, Jeffers BW, Hiatt WR et al. The effect of nisoldipine as compared with enalapril on cardiovascular outcomes in patients with non-insulin-dependent diabetes and hypertension. *N Engl J Med.* 1998; 338:645-52.
185. Flicker MR, Quigley MA, Caldwell EG. Diltiazem withdrawal syndrome: an opposing viewpoint. *Am J Med.* 1987; 82:1273-5.
186. Furberg CD, Psaty BM, Meyer JV. Nifedipine. Dose-related increase in mortality in patients with coronary heart disease. *Circulation.* 1995; 92:1326-31.
187. Kloner RA. Nifedipine in ischemic heart disease. *Circulation.* 1995; 92:1074-8.
188. Myrhed M, Wiholm BE. Nifedipine—a survey of adverse effects. Four years' reporting in Sweden. *Acta Pharmacol Toxicol (Copenh).* 1986; 58(suppl 2):133-6.
189. Oei SG, Oei SK, Brolmann HA. Myocardial infarction during nifedipine therapy for preterm labor. *N Engl J Med.* 1999; 340:154.

190. O'Mailia JJ, Sander GE, Giles TD. Nifedipine-associated myocardial ischemia or infarction in the treatment of hypertensive urgencies. *Ann Intern Med.* 1987; 107:185-6.
191. Sia ST, MacDonald PS, Triester B et al. Aggravation of myocardial ischaemia by nifedipine. *Med J Aust.* 1985; 142:48-50.
192. Staffurth JS, Emery P. Adverse interaction between nifedipine and beta-blockade. *Br Med J (Clin Res Ed).* 1981; 282:225.
193. Sundstedt CD, Ruegg PC, Keller A, Waite R. A multicenter evaluation of the safety, tolerability, and efficacy of isradipine in the treatment of essential hypertension. *Am J Med.* 1989; 86:98-102.
194. Amorim S, Dias P, Rocha G et al. Poisoning with calcium channel blockers—a case report and review of the literature. *Rev Port Cardiol.* 2001; 20:1249-57.
195. Cohen JD. 1995: the year of the calcium antagonist controversy. *Curr Opin Nephrol Hypertens.* 1996; 5:214-8.
196. Dougall HT, McLay J. A comparative review of the adverse effects of calcium antagonists. *Drug Saf.* 1996; 15:91-106.
197. Endersby CA, Brown EG, Perelman MS. Safety profile of lacidipine: a review of clinical data. *J Cardiovasc Pharmacol.* 1991; 17(suppl 4):S45-7.
198. Henry M, Kay MM, Viccellio P. Cardiogenic shock associated with calcium-channel and beta blockers: reversal with intravenous calcium chloride. *Am J Emerg Med.* 1985; 3:334-6.
199. Jackson G. Calcium antagonists: when the content does not justify the headline. *Br J Clin Pract.* 1995; 49:283-4.
200. Kloner RA, Vetrovec GW, Materson BJ, Levenstein M. Safety of long-acting dihydropyridine calcium channel blockers in hypertensive patients. *Am J Cardiol.* 1998; 81:163-9.
201. Lee DW, Cohan B. Refractory cardiogenic shock and complete heart block after verapamil SR and metoprolol treatment. A case report. *Angiology.* 1995; 46:517-9.
202. Leor J, Battler A. Calcium channel blocker debate: true lies? *Cardiovasc Drugs Ther.* 1996; 10:413-5.
203. Mackay JA, Sever PS. Calcium channel blockers in the dock: innocent or guilty? *J Hum Hypertens.* 1996; 10:277-80.
204. Mancia G, van Zwieten PA. How safe are calcium antagonists in hypertension and coronary heart disease? *J Hypertens.* 1996; 14:13-7.
205. Massie BM. The safety of calcium-channel blockers. *Clin Cardiol.* 1998; 21:II12-7.
206. Messerli FH. Safety of calcium antagonists: dissecting the evidence. *Am J Cardiol.* 1996; 78:19-23.
207. Opie LH. Calcium channel blockers for hypertension: dissecting the evidence for adverse effects. *Am J Hypertens.* 1997; 10:565-77.
208. Baker KM, Johns DW, Ayers CR, Carey RM. Ischemic cardiovascular complications concurrent with administration of captopril. A clinical note. *Hypertension.* 1980; 2:73-4.
209. Davis JB. Chest pain after captopril. *Br Med J (Clin Res Ed).* 1988; 296:214.
210. Canning BS, Green AT, Mulcahy R. Coronary heart disease in the puerperium. A case report. *J Obstet Gynaecol Br Commonw.* 1969; 76:1018-20.
211. Drakos SG, Anastasiou-Nana MI, Nanas JN. Exacerbation of variant angina by metoprolol resulting in syncope due to transient atrioventricular block. *Int J Cardiol.* 2002; 82:83-5.
212. Nanas JN, Sutton RB, Alazraki N, Tsagaris TJ. Acute myocardial infarction in post infarct patient possibly through beta blocker-induced coronary artery spasm. *Am Heart J.* 1987; 113:388-91.
213. Pantridge JF. Letter: Infarction in patients treated with propranolol. *JAMA.* 1974; 230:1126.
214. Beller GA. Dipyridamole thallium 201 imaging. How safe is it? *Circulation.* 1990; 81:1425-7.
215. Biddle P, Lanspa TJ, Mohiuddin SM et al. Myocardial infarction after dipyridamole-assisted thallium-201 imaging. *DICP.* 1989; 23:665-7.
216. Blumenthal MS, McCauley CS. Cardiac arrest during dipyridamole imaging. *Chest.* 1988; 93:1103-4.
217. Brady WJ, Perron AD. Administration of atropine in the setting of acute myocardial infarction: potentiation of the ischemic process? *Am J Emerg Med.* 2001; 19:81-3.
218. Druz RS. Dobutamine stress testing revisited. *J Am Coll Cardiol.* 2002; 39:1708-9.
219. Jahangiri M, Holdright DR. Myocardial infarction secondary to dipyridamole overdose. *Arch Emerg Med.* 1992; 9:62-4.
220. Jamison M, Widerhorn J, Weber L et al. Central and renal hemodynamic effects of a new agonist at peripheral dopamine- and beta-2 adrenoreceptors (dopexamine) in patients with heart failure. *Am Heart J.* 1989; 117:607-14.
221. Lee DS, Yeo JS, Chung JK et al. Transient prolonged stunning induced by dipyridamole and shown on 1- and 24-hour post-stress 99mTc-MIBI gated SPECT. *J Nucl Med.* 2000; 41:27-35.
222. Lette J, Tatum JL, Fraser S et al. Safety of dipyridamole testing in 73,806 patients: the Multicenter Dipyridamole Safety Study. *J Nucl Cardiol.* 1995; 2:3-17.
223. Lewis WR, Arena FJ, Galloway MT, Bommer WJ. Acute myocardial infarction associated with dobutamine stress echocardiography. *J Am Soc Echocardiogr.* 1997; 10:576-8.
224. Marwick TH, Hollman J. Acute myocardial infarction associated with intravenous dipyridamole for rubidium-82 PET imaging. *Clin Cardiol.* 1990; 13:230-1.
225. Nedeljkovic MA, Ostojic M, Beleslin B et al. Dipyridamole-atropine-induced myocardial infarction in a patient with patent epicardial coronary arteries. *Herz.* 2001; 26:485-8.
226. Pressman GS. Acute infarction of a previously stented coronary artery precipitated by dobutamine stress echocardiography. *J Am Soc Echocardiogr.* 2000; 13:150-1.
227. Ranhosky A. Dipyridamole-induced myocardial ischemia. *JAMA.* 1987; 258:203-4.
228. Ranhosky A, Kempthorne-Rawson J. The safety of intravenous dipyridamole thallium myocardial perfusion imaging. Intravenous Dipyridamole Thallium Imaging Study Group. *Circulation.* 1990; 81:1205-9.
229. Sanchis J, Munoz J, Chorro FJ et al. Stunned myocardium after thrombolytic treatment. Identification by dobutamine echocardiography and role of the residual stenosis in the infarction artery. *Int J Cardiol.* 1996; 53:5-13.
230. Svendsen P, Wilson J. Adverse reactions during urography and modification by atropine. *Acta Radiol Diagn (Stockh).* 1971; 11:427-33.
231. Takeuchi M, Sonoda S, Hanada H et al. Acute myocardial infarction in a patient during dobutamine stress echocardiography. *Cathet Cardiovasc Diagn.* 1997; 41:404-6.
232. Dakik HA, Alam S. Myocardial stunning induced and detected by adenosine stress perfusion imaging. *J Nucl Cardiol.* 2001; 8:711-2.
233. Dennis CA, Pool PE, Perrins EJ et al. Stress testing with closed-loop arbutamine as an alternative to exercise. The International Arbutamine Study Group. *J Am Coll Cardiol.* 1995; 26:1151-8.
234. Kiat H, Iskandrian AS, Villegas BJ et al. Arbutamine stress thallium-201 single-photon emission computed tomography using a computerized closed-loop delivery system. Multicenter trial for evaluation of safety and diagnostic accuracy. The International Arbutamine Study Group. *J Am Coll Cardiol.* 1995; 26:1159-67.
235. Polad JE, Wilson LM. Myocardial infarction during adenosine stress test. *Heart.* 2002; 87:E2.
236. Santiago JF, Heiba SI, Jana S et al. Transient ischemic stunning of the myocardium in stress thallium-201 gated SPET myocardial perfusion imaging: segmental analysis of myocardial perfusion, wall motion and wall thickening changes. *Eur J Nucl Med Mol Imaging.* 2002; 29:979-83.
237. Matsumoto N, Nagao K, Hirayama A, Kasama S. Adenosine-induced coronary vasospasm following drug-eluting stent implantation. *BMJ Case Reports.* 2014 Feb 11; 2014.
238. Friedman E, Mandel M, Katznelson D, Sack J. Pheochromocytoma and hydralazine-induced myocardial ischaemia in a 14-year-old boy. *Eur J Pediatr.* 1986; 145:318-20.

239. Satoh H, Morikaw S, Fujiwara C et al. A case of acute myocardial infarction associated with topical use of minoxidil (RiUP) for treatment of baldness. *Jpn Heart J.* 2000; 41:519-23.
240. Scardi S, Zingone B, Pandullo C. Myocardial infarction following sublingual administration of isosorbide dinitrate. *Int J Cardiol.* 1990; 26:378-9.
241. [No authors listed.] Diazoxide therapy: use and risks. *Ann Intern Med.* 1976; 85:529-31.
242. Barron JT, Billhardt RA. Angina pectoris with encainide in dilated cardiomyopathy. *Am Heart J.* 1989; 117:701-2.
243. Falko JM. Hazards in antihypertension therapy. *Ann Intern Med.* 1977; 86:111-2.
244. Barilla F, Giordano F, Jacomelli I et al. ST-segment elevation during levosimendan infusion. *J Cardiovasc Med.* 2012; 13:454-6.
245. Burkman RT. Cardiovascular issues with oral contraceptives: evidenced-based medicine. *Int J Fertil Womens Med.* 2000; 45:166-74.
246. Burkman RT. Oral contraceptives: current status. *Clin Obstet Gynecol.* 2001; 44:62-72.
247. Chasan-Taber L, Stampfer M. Oral contraceptives and myocardial infarction—the search for the smoking gun. *N Engl J Med.* 2001; 345:1841-2.
248. Hannaford P. Health consequences of combined oral contraceptives. *Br Med Bull.* 2000; 56:749-60.
249. Hannaford P. Competing interests and controversy about third generation oral contraceptives. Science is not a dispassionate activity. *BMJ (Clinical research ed).* 2000; 320:382.
250. Hannaford P. Cardiovascular events associated with different combined oral contraceptives: a review of current data. *Drug Saf.* 2000; 22:361-71.
251. Hannaford P. Oral contraceptives and the risk of myocardial infarction. *N Engl J Med.* 2002; 346:1826-9.
252. Hoey J. Oral contraceptives and myocardial infarction. *CMAJ.* 2002; 166:931.
253. Kahlenborn C. Oral contraceptives and the risk of myocardial infarction. *N Engl J Med.* 2002; 346:1826-9.
254. La Vecchia C, Franceschi S. Third generation oral contraceptives and vascular risks. *Eur J Public Health.* 2002; 12:81-2.
255. Landau E, Lessing JB, Weintraub M, Michowitz M. Acute myocardial infarction in a young woman taking oral contraceptives. A case report. *J Reprod Med.* 1986; 31:1008-10.
256. Li SF. Oral contraceptives and the risk of myocardial infarction. *N Engl J Med.* 2002; 346:1826-9.
257. Mann JI, Inman WH. Oral contraceptives and death from myocardial infarction. *Br Med J.* 1975; 2:245-8.
258. McCoy MJ. Angina and myocardial infarction with use of leuprolide acetate. *Am J Obstet Gynecol.* 1994; 171:275-6.
259. Merki-Feld GS, Rosselli M, Dubey RK et al. Long-term effects of combined oral contraceptives on markers of endothelial function and lipids in healthy premenopausal women. *Contraception.* 2002; 65:231-6.
260. Pierce EJ. Angina pectoris and myocardial infarction with the use of leuprolide acetate. *Am J Obstet Gynecol.* 1995; 172:1323.
261. Roy S. Effects of smoking on prostacyclin formation and platelet aggregation in users of oral contraceptives. *Am J Obstet Gynecol.* 1999; 180:S364-8.
262. Shapiro S. Oral contraceptives and the risk of myocardial infarction. *N Engl J Med.* 2002; 346:1826-9.
263. Shulman LP. Oral contraceptives. Risks. *Obstet Gynecol Clin North Am.* 2000; 27:695-704, v-vi.
264. SoRelle R. Myocardial infarction and oral contraceptives. *Circulation.* 2002; 105:E9063.
265. Spitzer WO, Faith JM, MacRae KD. Myocardial infarction and third generation oral contraceptives: aggregation of recent studies. *Hum Reprod.* 2002; 17:2307-14.
266. Tanis BC. Oral contraceptives and the risk of myocardial infarction. *Eur Heart J.* 2003; 24:377-80.
267. Tanis BC, van den Bosch MA, Kemmeren JM et al. Oral contraceptives and the risk of myocardial infarction. *N Engl J Med.* 2001; 345:1787-93.
268. Vandenbroucke JP. Oral contraceptives and the risk of myocardial infarction. *N Engl J Med.* 2002; 346:1826-9.
269. Shigematsu S, Niwa H, Saikawa T. Vasospastic angina induced by prostaglandin F2 alpha. *Br Heart J.* 1993; 69:364-5.
270. Bergeron GA, Goldsmith R, Schiller NB. Myocardial infarction, severe reversible ischemia, and shock following excess thyroid administration in a woman with normal coronary arteries. *Arch Intern Med.* 1988; 148:1450-3.
271. Bond L, Bevan D. Myocardial infarction in a patient with hemophilia treated with DDAVP. *N Engl J Med.* 1988; 318:121.
272. Feenstra J, Borst F, Huige MC et al. [Acute myocardial infarct following sulprostone administration]. *Ned Tijdschr Geneeskd.*1998; 142:192-5.
273. Godsland IF, Winkler U, Lidegaard O, Crook D. Occlusive vascular diseases in oral contraceptive users. Epidemiology, pathology and mechanisms. *Drugs.* 2000; 60:721-869.
274. Grant EC. Hormones for coronary disease. *Lancet.* 2003; 361:612.
275. Hiasa Y, Ishida T, Aihara T et al. Acute myocardial infarction due to coronary spasm associated with L-thyroxine therapy. *Clin Cardiol.* 1989; 12:161-3.
276. Lauer M, Berentelg J. [Severe cardiovascular complications relating to Gemeprost therapy]. *Zentralbl Gynakol.* 2000; 122:324-7.
277. Lindhardt TB, Walker LR, Colov NS, Hansen PS. [Vasospastic angina pectoris following abortion induced by prostaglandin analogue]. *Ugeskr Laeger.* 2000; 162:6536-7.
278. Locker GJ, Kotzmann H, Frey B et al. Factitious hyperthyroidism causing acute myocardial infarction. *Thyroid.* 1995; 5:465-7.
279. Mannucci PM. How I treat patients with von Willebrand disease. *Blood.* 2001; 97:1915-9.
280. Mannucci PM, Carlsson S, Harris AS. Desmopressin, surgery and thrombosis. *Thromb Haemost.* 1994; 71:154-5.
281. McLeod BC. Myocardial infarction in a blood donor after administration of desmopressin. *Lancet.* 1990; 336:1137-8.
282. Nakagawa T, Yasuno M, Tanahashi H et al. A case of acute myocardial infarction. Intracoronary thrombosis in two major coronary arteries due to hormone therapy. *Angiology.* 1994; 45:333-8.
283. Orti G, Mira Y, Vaya A. Acute myocardial infarction associated with Yasmin oral contraceptive. *Clin Appl Thromb Hemost.* 2007; 13:336-7.
284. Paulus D, Saint-Remy A, Jeanjean M. Oral contraception and cardiovascular risk factors during adolescence. *Contraception.* 2000; 62:113-6.
285. Rosenberg L, Palmer JR, Rao RS, Shapiro S. Low-dose oral contraceptive use and the risk of myocardial infarction. *Arch Intern Med.* 2001; 161:1065-70.
286. Lidegaard O, Lokkegaard E, Jensen A et al. Thrombotic stroke and myocardial infarction with hormonal contraception. *N Engl J Med.* 2012; 366:2257-66.
287. Vivo RP, Krim SR. ST elevation myocardial infarction in a teenager: case report and review of the literature. *Southern Med J.* 2009; 102:523-6.
288. Einecke D. [Testosterone supplementation: good feeling in the pants, pain in the chest]. *MMW Fortschritte der Medizin.* 2014; 156:22.
289. Shah SN, Tran HA, Assal A et al. In-stent thrombosis following DDAVP administration: case report and review of the literature. *Blood Coagul. Fibrinolysis.* 2014; 25:81-3.
290. Lindsay AC, Foale RA, Warren O, Henry JA. Cannabis as a precipitant of cardiovascular emergencies. *Int J Cardiol.* 2005; 104:230-2.
291. Bashour TT. Acute myocardial infarction resulting from amphetamine abuse: a spasm-thrombus interplay? *Am Heart J.* 1994; 128:1237-9.
292. Carson P, Oldroyd K, Phadke K. Myocardial infarction due to amphetamine. *Br Med J (Clin Res Ed).* 1987; 294:1525-6.

293. Costa GM, Pizzi C, Bresciani B et al. Acute myocardial infarction caused by amphetamines: a case report and review of the literature. *Ital Heart J.* 2001; 2:478-80.
294. Diercks DB, Kirk JD, Turnipseed SD, Amsterdam EA. Evaluation of patients with methamphetamine- and cocaine-related chest pain in a chest pain observation unit. *Crit Pathw Cardiol.* 2007; 6:161-4.
295. Farnsworth TL, Brugger CH, Malters P. Myocardial infarction after intranasal methamphetamine. *Am J Health-Syst Pharm.* 1997; 54:586-7.
296. Furst SR, Fallon SP, Reznik GN, Shah PK. Myocardial infarction after inhalation of methamphetamine. *N Engl J Med.* 1990; 323:1147-8.
297. Hong R, Matsuyama E, Nur K. Cardiomyopathy associated with the smoking of crystal methamphetamine. *JAMA.* 1991; 265:1152-4.
298. Huang CN, Wu DJ, Chen KS. Acute myocardial infarction caused by transnasal inhalation of amphetamine. *Jpn Heart J.* 1993; 34:815-8.
299. Hung MJ, Kuo LT, Cherng WJ. Amphetamine-related acute myocardial infarction due to coronary artery spasm. *Int J Clin Pract.* 2003; 57:62-4.
300. Packe GE, Garton MJ, Jennings K. Acute myocardial infarction caused by intravenous amphetamine abuse. *Br Heart J.* 1990; 64:23-4.
301. Ragland AS, Ismail Y, Arsura EL. Myocardial infarction after amphetamine use. *Am Heart J.* 1993; 125:247-9.
302. Waksman J, Taylor RN Jr, Bodor GS et al. Acute myocardial infarction associated with amphetamine use. *Mayo Clin Proc.* 2001; 76:323-6.
303. Qasim A, Townend J, Davies MK. Ecstasy induced acute myocardial infarction. *Heart.* 2001; 85:E10.
304. Bowman S. Anabolic steroids and infarction. *BMJ (Clinical research ed).* 1990; 300:750.
305. Fisher M, Appleby M, Rittoo D, Cotter L. Myocardial infarction with extensive intracoronary thrombus induced by anabolic steroids. *Br J Clin Pract.* 1996; 50:222-3.
306. Goldstein DR, Dobbs T, Krull B, Plumb VJ. Clenbuterol and anabolic steroids: a previously unreported cause of myocardial infarction with normal coronary arteriograms. *Southern Med J.* 1998; 91:780-4.
307. Kennedy C. Myocardial infarction in association with misuse of anabolic steroids. *Ulster Med J.* 1993; 62:174-6.
308. Kennedy MC, Corrigan AB, Pilbeam ST. Myocardial infarction and cerebral haemorrhage in a young body builder taking anabolic steroids. *Aust N Z J Med.* 1993; 23:713.
309. Lorimer DA, Hart LL. Cardiac dysfunction in athletes receiving anabolic steroids. *DICP.* 1990; 24:1060-1.
310. McNutt RA, Ferenchick GS, Kirlin PC, Hamlin NJ. Acute myocardial infarction in a 22-year-old world class weight lifter using anabolic steroids. *Am J Cardiol.* 1988; 62:164.
311. Melchert RB, Welder AA. Cardiovascular effects of androgenic-anabolic steroids. *Med Sci Sports Exerc.* 1995; 27:1252-62.
312. Toyama M, Watanabe S, Kobayashi T et al. Two cases of acute myocardial infarction associated with aplastic anemia during treatment with anabolic steroids. *Jpn Heart J.* 1994; 35:369-73.
313. Varriale P, Mirzai-tehrane M, Sedighi A. Acute myocardial infarction associated with anabolic steroids in a young HIV-infected patient. *Pharmacotherapy.* 1999; 19:881-4.
314. Azarisman SM, Magdi YA, Noorfaizan S, Oteh M. Myocardial infarction induced by appetite suppressants in Malaysia. *N Engl J Med.* 2007; 357:1873-4.
315. El-Menyar AA, El-Tawil M, Al Suwaidi J. A teenager with angiographically normal epicardial coronary arteries and acute myocardial infarction after butane inhalation. *Eur J Emerg Med.* 2005; 12:137-41.
316. Ashchi M, Wiedemann HP, James KB. Cardiac complication from use of cocaine and phenylephrine in nasal septoplasty. *Arch Otolaryngol Head Neck Surg.* 1995; 121:681-4.
317. Bush HS. Cocaine-associated myocardial infarction. A word of caution about thrombolytic therapy. *Chest.* 1988; 94:878.
318. Coleman DL, Ross TF, Naughton JL. Myocardial ischemia and infarction related to recreational cocaine use. *West J Med.* 1982; 136:444-6.
319. Hollander JE. The management of cocaine-associated myocardial ischemia. *N Engl J Med.* 1995; 333:1267-72.
320. Hollander JE, Hoffman RS. Cocaine-induced myocardial infarction: an analysis and review of the literature. *J Emerg Med.* 1992; 10:169-77.
321. Hollander JE, Hoffman RS, Burstein JL, Shih RD, Thode HC Jr. Cocaine-associated myocardial infarction. Mortality and complications. Cocaine-Associated Myocardial Infarction Study Group. *Arch Intern Med.* 1995; 155:1081-6.
322. Kloner RA, Rezkalla SH. Cocaine and the heart. *N Engl J Med.* 2003; 348:487-8.
323. Lange RA, Hillis LD. Cardiovascular complications of cocaine use. *N Engl J Med.* 2001; 345:351-8.
324. McCord J, Jneid H, Hollander JE et al. Management of cocaine-associated chest pain and myocardial infarction: a scientific statement from the American Heart Association Acute Cardiac Care Committee of the Council on Clinical Cardiology. *Circulation.* 2008; 117:1897-907.
325. McKee SA, Applegate RJ, Hoyle JR et al. Cocaine use is associated with an increased risk of stent thrombosis after percutaneous coronary intervention. *Am Heart J.* 2007; 154:159-64.
326. Minor RL Jr, Scott BD, Brown DD, Winniford MD. Cocaine-induced myocardial infarction in patients with normal coronary arteries. *Ann Intern Med.* 1991; 115:797-806.
327. Mittleman MA, Mintzer D, Maclure M et al. Triggering of myocardial infarction by cocaine. *Circulation.* 1999;99:2737-41.
328. Noorily SH, Noorily AD. Cocaine and phenylephrine. *Arch Otolaryngol Head Neck Surg.* 1996; 122:207-8.
329. Vasica G, Tennant CC. Cocaine use and cardiovascular complications. *Med J Aust.* 2002; 177:260-2.
330. Wang T, Hadidi F, Triana F, Bargout M. Myocardial infarction associated with the use of cocaine. *Am J Med Sci.* 1988; 295:569-71.
331. Welder AA, Melchert RB. Cardiotoxic effects of cocaine and anabolic-androgenic steroids in the athlete. *J Pharmacol Toxicol Methods.* 1993; 29:61-8.
332. Charles R, Holt S, Kirkham N. Myocardial infarction and marijuana. *Clin Toxicol.* 1979; 14:433-8.
333. Coutselinis A, Michalodimitrakis M. Myocardial infarction and marijuana. *Clin Toxicol.* 1981; 18:389-90.
334. Mittleman MA, Lewis RA, Maclure M et al. Triggering myocardial infarction by marijuana. *Circulation.* 2001; 103:2805-9.
335. Pearl W, Choi YS. Marijuana as a cause of myocardial infarction. *Int J Cardiol.* 1992; 34:353.
336. Sidney S. Cardiovascular consequences of marijuana use. *J Clin Pharmacol.* 2002; 42:64S-70S.
337. Bilkoo P, Thomas J, Riddle CD, Kagaoan G. Clenbuterol toxicity: an emerging epidemic. A case report and review. *Conn Med.* 2007; 71:89-91.
338. Halford S, Simpson H. Towards evidence based emergency medicine: best BETs from the Manchester Royal Infirmary. Diamorphine or morphine for ischaemic cardiac chest pain. *Emerg Med J.* 2003; 20:263-4.
339. Melandri R, De Tommaso I, Zele I et al. [Myocardial involvement in rhabdomyolysis caused by acute heroin intoxication]. *Recenti Prog Med.* 1991; 82:324-7.
340. Yu SL, Liu CP, Lo YK, Lin SL. Acute myocardial infarction after heroin injections. *Jpn Heart J.* 2004; 45:1021-8.
341. Carder JR, Fuerst RS. Myocardial infarction after toluene inhalation. *Pediatr Emerg Care.* 1997; 13:117-9.
342. Hussain TF, Heidenreich PA, Benowitz N. Recurrent non-Q-wave myocardial infarction associated with toluene abuse. *Am Heart J.* 1996; 131:615-6.

343. Appleby M, Fisher M, Martin M. Myocardial infarction, hyperkalaemia and ventricular tachycardia in a young male body-builder. *Int J Cardiol.* 1994; 44:171-4.
344. Choi YS, Pearl WR. Cardiovascular effects of adolescent drug abuse. *J Adolesc Health Care.* 1989; 10:332-7.
345. Crook D. Testosterone, androgens and the risk of myocardial infarction. *Br J Clin Pract.* 1996; 50:180-1.
346. Ferenchick GS, Adelman S. Myocardial infarction associated with anabolic steroid use in a previously healthy 37-year-old weight lifter. *Am Heart J.* 1992; 124:507-8.
347. Fineschi V, Baroldi G, Monciotti F et al. Anabolic steroid abuse and cardiac sudden death: a pathologic study. *Arch Pathol Lab Med* 2001; 125:253-5.
348. Gotway MB, Marder SR, Hanks DK et al. Thoracic complications of illicit drug use: an organ system approach. *Radiographics.* 2002; 22 Spec No:S119-35.
349. Hourigan LA, Rainbird AJ, Dooris M. Intracoronary stenting for acute myocardial infarction (AMI) in a 24-year-old man using anabolic androgenic steroids. *Aust N Z J Med.* 1998; 28:838-9.
350. McLeod AL, McKenna CJ, Northridge DB. Myocardial infarction following the combined recreational use of Viagra and cannabis. *Clin Cardiol.* 2002; 25:133-4.
351. Mewis C, Spyridopoulos I, Kuhlkamp V, Seipel L. Manifestation of severe coronary heart disease after anabolic drug abuse. *Clin Cardiol.* 1996; 19:153-5.
352. Casier I, Vanduynhoven P, Haine S et al. Is recent cannabis use associated with acute coronary syndromes? An illustrative case series. *Acta Cardiologica.* 2014; 69:131-6.
353. Hawley LA, Auten JD, Matteucci MJ et al. Cardiac complications of adult methamphetamine exposures. *J Emerg Med.* 2013; 45:821-7.
354. Hoggett K, McCoubrie D, Fatovich DM. Ecstasy-induced acute coronary syndrome: something to rave about. *Emerg Med Australas.* 2012; 24:339-42.
355. Mir A, Obafemi A, Young A, Kane C. Myocardial infarction associated with use of the synthetic cannabinoid K2. *Pediatrics.* 2011; 128:e1622-7.
356. Okunoye GO, Dutton P. Acute myocardial infarction in pregnancy following unlicensed use of methylenedioxymethamphetamine ('Ecstasy'). *Scott Med J.* 2013; 58:e4-6.
357. Safaa AM, Markham R, Jayasinghe R. Marijuana-induced recurrent acute coronary syndrome with normal coronary angiograms. *Drug Alcohol Rev.* 2012; 31:91-4.
358. Sharma J, de Castro C, Chatterjee P, Pinto R. Acute myocardial infarction induced by concurrent use of adderall and alcohol in an adolescent. *Pediatr Emerg Care.* 2013; 29:84-8.
359. Armitage JD, Montero C, Benner A et al. Acute coronary syndromes complicating the first infusion of rituximab. *Clin Lymphoma Myeloma.* 2008; 8:253-5.
360. Cooper MR, Fefer A, Thompson J et al. Interferon alfa-2b/melphalan/prednisone in previously untreated patients with multiple myeloma: a phase I-II trial. *Invest New Drugs.* 1987; (suppl 5): S41-6.
361. Fisman DN, Smilovitch M. Intravenous immunoglobulin, blood viscosity and myocardial infarction. *Can J Cardiol.* 1997; 13:775-7.
362. Laghi Pasini F, Di Perri T, van der Plas K et al. Myocardial injury after interleukin-2 therapy. *Lancet.* 1989; 1:674.
363. Lengfelder E, Berger U, Hehlmann R. Interferon alpha in the treatment of polycythemia vera. *Ann Hematol.* 2000; 79:103-9.
364. Macedo G, Ribeiro T. Interferon plus ribavirin: a cautionary note. *Am J Gastroenterol.* 1999; 94:3087-8.
365. Cardiovascular effects of epinephrine in hypertensive dental patients. *Evid Rep Technol Assess (Summ).* 2002: 1-3.
366. Butte MJ, Nguyen BX, Hutchison TJ et al. Pediatric myocardial infarction after racemic epinephrine administration. *Pediatrics.* 1999; 104:e9.
367. Chelliah YR, Manninen PH. Hazards of epinephrine in transsphenoidal pituitary surgery. *J Neurosurg Anesthesiol.* 2002; 14:43-6.
368. Cockings JG, Brown M. Ephedrine abuse causing acute myocardial infarction. *Med J Aust.* 1997; 167:199-200.
369. Derreza H, Fine MD, Sadaniantz A. Acute myocardial infarction after use of pseudoephedrine for sinus congestion. *J Am Board Fam Pract.* 1997; 10:436-8.
370. Ferry DR, Henry RL, Kern MJ. Epinephrine-induced myocardial infarction in a patient with angiographically normal coronary arteries. *Am Heart J.* 1986; 111:1193-5.
371. Gavras H, Kremer D, Brown JJ et al. Angiotensin- and norepinephrine-induced myocardial lesions: experimental and clinical studies in rabbits and man. *Am Heart J.* 1975; 89:321-32.
372. Kurland G, Williams J, Lewiston NJ. Fatal myocardial toxicity during continuous infusion intravenous isoproterenol therapy of asthma. *J Allergy Clin Immunol.* 1979; 63:407-11.
373. Matson JR, Loughlin GM, Strunk RC. Myocardial ischemia complicating the use of isoproterenol in asthmatic children. *J Pediatr.* 1978; 92:776-8.
374. Nissen SE. ADHD drugs and cardiovascular risk. *N Engl J Med.* 2006; 354:1445-8.
375. Rezkalla SH, Mesa J, Sharma P, Kloner RA. Myocardial infarction temporally related to ephedra—a possible role for the coronary microcirculation. *WMJ.* 2002; 101:64-6.
376. Samenuk D, Link MS, Homoud MK et al. Adverse cardiovascular events temporally associated with ma huang, an herbal source of ephedrine. *Mayo Clin Proc.* 2002; 77:12-6.
377. Traub SJ, Hoyek W, Hoffman RS. Dietary supplements containing ephedra alkaloids. *N Engl J Med.* 2001; 344:1096-7.
378. Turk MP. Ephedrine's deadly edge. *US News World Rep.* 1997; 123:79-80.
379. Wahl A, Eberli FR, Thomson DA, Luginbuhl M. Coronary artery spasm and non-Q-wave myocardial infarction following intravenous ephedrine in two healthy women under spinal anaesthesia. *Br J Anaesth.* 2002; 89:519-23.
380. Wiener I, Tilkian AG, Palazzolo M. Coronary artery spasm and myocardial infarction in a patient with normal coronary arteries: temporal relationship to pseudoephedrine ingestion. *Cathet Cardiovasc Diagn.* 1990; 20:51-3.
381. Fraunfelder FT, Scafidi AF. Possible adverse effects from topical ocular 10% phenylephrine. *Am J Ophthalmol.* 1978; 85:447-53.
382. Hecker RB, Hays JV, Champ JD, Rubal BJ. Myocardial ischemia and stunning induced by topical intranasal phenylephrine pledgets. *Mil Med.* 1997; 162:832-5.
383. Lai YK. Adverse effect of intraoperative phenylephrine 10%: case report. *Br J Ophthalmol.* 1989; 73:468-9.
384. Leo PJ, Hollander JE, Shih RD, Marcus SM. Phenylpropanolamine and associated myocardial injury. *Ann Emerg Med.* 1996; 28:359-62.
385. Modica PA, Tempelhoff R, Rich KM, Grubb RL Jr. Computerized electroencephalographic monitoring and selective shunting: influence on intraoperative administration of phenylephrine and myocardial infarction after general anesthesia for carotid endarterectomy. *Neurosurgery.* 1992; 30:842-6.
386. Oosterbaan R, Burns MJ. Myocardial infarction associated with phenylpropanolamine. *J Emerg Med.* 2000; 18:55-9.
387. Haft JI. Cardiovascular injury induced by sympathetic catecholamines. *Prog Cardiovasc Dis.* 1974; 17:73-86.
388. Santo M, Sidi Y, Pinkhas Y. Acute myocardial infarction following intravenous salbutamol. *S Afr Med J.* 1980; 58:394.
389. Shovlin CL, Tam FW. Salbutamol nebuliser and precipitation of critical cardiac ischaemia. *Lancet.* 1990; 336:1258.
390. Szczeklik A, Nizankowski R, Mruk J. Myocardial infarction in status asthmaticus. *Lancet.* 1977; 1:658-9.
391. Cunnington C, McDonald JE, Singh RK. Epinephrine-induced myocardial infarction in severe anaphylaxis: is nonselective betablockade a contributory factor? *Am J Emerg Med.* 2013; 31:759.e1-2.

392. Hay E, Shklovski V, Blaer Y, Shlakhover V, Katz A. Intravenous methylphenidate: an unusual way to provoke ST-elevation myocardial infarction. *Am J Emerg Med.* 2015; 33:313.e1-3.
393. Izgi C, Cevik C, Nugent K. Severe myocardial ischemia after concentrated epinephrine use for the treatment of anaphylaxis: Kounis syndrome or epinephrine effect? *Heart Lung.* 2010; 39:160-3.
394. Gomez-Barrado JJ, Turegano S, Garciperez de Vargas FJ, Porras Y. Acute coronary syndrome in a young woman treated with sibutramine. *Rev Esp Cardiol.* 2010; 63:243.
395. Yim KM, Ng HW, Chan CK et al. Sibutramine-induced acute myocardial infarction in a young lady. *Clin Toxicol.* 2008; 46:877-9.
396. Arole A, Kroll HR, Brown M. Coronary vasospasm leading to an acute myocardial infarction after the administration of dolasetron. *J Clin Anesth.* 2005; 17:72-4.
397. Bugiardini R, Galvani M, Ferrini D et al. Effects of iloprost, a stable prostacyclin analog, on exercise capacity and platelet aggregation in stable angina pectoris. *Am J Cardiol.* 1986; 58:453-9.
398. Lewis PS, Boyd CM, Hubert NE, Steele MC. Ethanol-induced therapeutic myocardial infarction to treat hypertrophic obstructive cardiomyopathy. *Crit Care Nurse.* 2001; 21:20-2, 6-8, 30-4.
399. Moreyra AE, Kostis JB, Passannante AJ, Kuo PT. Acute myocardial infarction in patients with normal coronary arteries after acute ethanol intoxication. *Clin Cardiol.* 1982; 5:425-30.
400. Rubin JM, de la Tassa CM, Arias JC. Cisapride can make Prinzmetal angina worse. *Int J Cardiol.* 1998; 65:315-6.
401. Cheitlin MD, Hutter AM Jr, Brindis RG et al. ACC/AHA expert consensus document. Use of sildenafil (Viagra) in patients with cardiovascular disease. American College of Cardiology/American Heart Association. *J Am Coll Cardiol.* 1999; 33:273-82.
402. Dacosta A, Guy JM, Tardy B et al. Myocardial infarction and nicotine patch: a contributing or causative factor? *Eur Heart J.* 1993; 14:1709-11.
403. Dunn N. Cardiovascular events in users of sildenafil. Paper does not provide any reassurance. *BMJ (Clinical research ed).* 2001; 323:50-1.
404. Eid JF. Sildenafil citrate: current clinical experience. *Int J Impot Res.* 2000; 12(suppl 4):S62-6.
405. Feenstra J, van Drie-Pierik RJ, Lacle CF, Stricker BH. Acute myocardial infarction associated with sildenafil. *Lancet.* 1998; 352:957-8.
406. Arnaot MR. Treating heart disease. Nicotine patches may not be safe. *BMJ (Clinical research ed).* 1995; 310:663-4.
407. Arora RR, Timoney M, Melilli L. Acute myocardial infarction after the use of sildenafil. *N Engl J Med.* 1999; 341:700.
408. Ballard HS, Bottino G, Bottino J. Ondansetron and chest pain. *Lancet.* 1992; 340:1107.
409. Curatolo PW, Robertson D. The health consequences of caffeine. *Ann Intern Med.* 1983; 98:641-53.
410. Dutt S, Wong F, Spurway JH. Fatal myocardial infarction associated with bromocriptine for postpartum lactation suppression. *Aust N Z J Obstet Gynaecol.* 1998; 38:116-7.
411. Eickman FM. Recurrent myocardial infarction in a postpartum patient receiving bromocriptine. *Clin Cardiol.* 1992; 15:781-3.
412. Endoh Y, Shibata N, Takeichi K, Shinya W. Coronary thrombosis induced by intracoronary acetylcholine injection in a patient with normal coronary myocardial infarction. *Intern Med.* 1995; 34:171-5.
413. Forman J, Aizer A, Young CR. Myocardial infarction resulting from caffeine overdose in an anorectic woman. *Ann Emerg Med.* 1997; 29:178-80.
414. Hopp L, Haider B, Iffy L. Myocardial infarction postpartum in patients taking bromocriptine for the prevention of breast engorgement. *Int J Cardiol.* 1996; 57:227-32.
415. Hopp L, Weisse AB, Iffy L. Acute myocardial infarction in a healthy mother using bromocriptine for milk suppression. *Can J Cardiol.* 1996; 12:415-8.
416. Iffy L, TenHove W, Frisoli G. Acute myocardial infarction in the puerperium in patients receiving bromocriptine. *Am J Obstet Gynecol.* 1986; 155:371-2.
417. James JE, Stirling KP. Caffeine: a survey of some of the known and suspected deleterious effects of habitual use. *Br J Addict.* 1983; 78:251-8.
418. Keefer RA, Roenigk HH Jr, Hawk WA. Azaribine therapy for psoriasis. Evaluation of potential effects on the liver and other organ systems. *Arch Dermatol.* 1975; 111:853-6.
419. Kirigaya H, Aizawa T, Ogasawara K et al. Incidence of acetylcholine-induced spasm of coronary arteries subjected to balloon angioplasty. *Jpn Circ J.* 1993; 57:883-90.
420. Larrazet F, Spaulding C, Lobreau HJ et al. Possible bromocriptine-induced myocardial infarction. *Ann Intern Med.* 1993; 118:199-200.
421. Maeda N, Hiraoka H, Nakamura T et al. Acetylcholine-induced coronary microvascular vasospasm in a patient with angina pectoris and normal coronary angiogram—a case report. *Angiology.* 1997; 48:995-9.
422. Sekiya M, Okayama H, Suzuki M et al. Acetylcholine-induced myocardial ischemia without epicardial coronary artery spasm: a possible vasospasm of small coronary arteries—a case report. *Angiology.* 1993; 44:811-5.
423. Sueda S, Saeki H, Otani T et al. Major complications during spasm provocation tests with an intracoronary injection of acetylcholine. *Am J Cardiol.* 2000; 85:391-4, A10.
424. Gowda RM, Khan IA, Vasavada BC, Sacchi TJ. Alcohol-triggered acute myocardial infarction. *Am J Ther.* 2003; 10:71-2.
425. Regan TJ, Ettinger PO. How does alcohol affect the heart? *Med Times.* 1978; 106:29-35.
426. Regan TJ, Ettinger PO, Lyons MM et al. Ethyl alcohol as a cardiac risk factor. *Curr Probl Cardiol.* 1977; 2:1-35.
427. Starc R, Brucan A, Bunc M. Acute myocardial infarction induced by alcohol ingestion in an asymptomatic individual. *Eur J Emerg Med.* 1999; 6:403-6.
428. Guigui N, Luyt CE, Vincent F. Coronary spasm after injection of ondansetron: case report and review of the literature. *Int J Cardiol.* 2008; 123:341-2.
429. Hall MC, Ahmad S. Interaction between sildenafil and HIV-1 combination therapy. *Lancet.* 1999; 353:2071-2.
430. Kimmel SE, Berlin JA, Miles C et al. Risk of acute first myocardial infarction and use of nicotine patches in a general population. *J Am Coll Cardiol.* 2001; 37:1297-302.
431. Kloner RA. Cardiovascular risk and sildenafil. *Am J Cardiol.* 2000; 86:57F-61F.
432. Lee TS, Hou X. Nicotine is hazardous to your heart. *Chest.* 1996; 109:584-5.
433. Lopez-Lazaro L, Garcia-Arenillas M, Portoles-Perez A et al. Acute myocardial infarction associated with sildenafil. *Lancet.* 1998; 352:1936-7.
434. Mathew TP, Herity NA. Acute myocardial infarction soon after nicotine replacement therapy. *QJM.* 2001; 94:503-4.
435. Morrison H. Sildenafil (Viagra): cardiac risks. *CMAJ.* 2000; 163:86-7, 90-1.
436. Muniz AE, Holstege CP. Acute myocardial infarction associated wiht Sildenafil (Viagra) ingestion. *Am J Emerg Med.* 2000; 18:353-5.
437. Ottervanger JP, Festen JM, de Vries AG, Stricker BH. Acute myocardial infarction while using the nicotine patch. *Chest.* 1995; 107:1765-6.
438. Porter A, Mager A, Birnbaum Y et al. Acute myocardial infarction following sildenafil citrate (Viagra) intake in a nitrate-free patient. *Clin Cardiol.* 1999; 22:762-3.
439. Drazen JM, Morrissey S, Curfman GD. Rosiglitazone—continued uncertainty about safety. *N Engl J Med.* 2007; 357:63-4.
440. Home PD, Pocock SJ, Beck-Nielsen H et al. Rosiglitazone evaluated for cardiovascular outcomes—an interim analysis. *N Engl J Med.* 2007; 357:28-38.

441. Klatsky AL, Friedman GD, Armstrong MA. Coffee use prior to myocardial infarction restudied: heavier intake may increase the risk. *Am J Epidemiol.* 1990; 132:479-88.

442. Nathan DM. Rosiglitazone and cardiotoxicity—weighing the evidence. *N Engl J Med.* 2007; 357:64-6.

443. Nissen SE. Perspective: effect of rosiglitazone on cardiovascular outcomes. *Curr Cardiol Rep.* 2007; 9:343-4.

444. Nissen SE, Wolski K. Effect of rosiglitazone on the risk of myocardial infarction and death from cardiovascular causes. *N Engl J Med.* 2007; 356:2457-71.

445. Panagiotakos DB, Rallidis LS, Pitsavos C et al. Cigarette smoking and myocardial infarction in young men and women: a case-control study. *Int J Cardiol.* 2007; 116:371-5.

446. Psaty BM, Furberg CD. The record on rosiglitazone and the risk of myocardial infarction. *N Engl J Med.* 2007; 357:67-9.

447. Psaty BM, Furberg CD. Rosiglitazone and cardiovascular risk. *N Engl J Med.* 2007; 356:2522-4.

448. Rosenberg L, Slone D, Shapiro S et al. Case-control studies on the acute effects of coffee upon the risk of myocardial infarction: problems in the selection of a hospital control series. *Am J Epidemiol.* 1981; 113:646-52.

449. Rosenberg L, Slone D, Shapiro S et al. Coffee drinking and myocardial infarction in young women. *Am J Epidemiol.* 1980; 111:675-81.

450. Rosenberg L, Werler MM, Kaufman DW, Shapiro S. Coffee drinking and myocardial infarction in young women: an update. *Am J Epidemiol.* 1987; 126:147-9.

451. Singh S, Loke YK, Furberg CD. Long-term risk of cardiovascular events with rosiglitazone: a meta-analysis. *JAMA.* 2007; 298:1189-95.

452. Smith IK. Trouble brewing. A steaming cup is a great comfort, but consider the effects of unfiltered coffee on the heart. *Time.* 2000; 155:80.

453. Zieske AW, McMahan CA, McGill HC Jr et al. Smoking is associated with advanced coronary atherosclerosis in youth. *Atherosclerosis.* 2005; 180:87-92.

454. Benowitz NL. Cigarette smoking and cardiovascular disease: pathophysiology and implications for treatment. *Prog Cardiovasc Dis.* 2003; 46:91-111.

455. Furlong FW. Possible psychiatric significance of excessive coffee consumption. *Can Psychiatr Assoc J.* 1975; 20:577-83.

456. Heyden S, Tyroler HA, Cassel JC et al. Coffee consumption and mortality in a community study—Evans Co., Ga. *Z Ernahrungswiss.* 1976; 15:143-50.

457. Megalla S, Shaqra H, Bhalodkar NC. Non-ST-segment elevation myocardial infarction in the setting of sexual intercourse following the use of cocaine and sildenafil. *Rev Cardiovasc Med.* 2011; 12:e113-7.

458. Wang CC, Chen WL, Kao TW et al. Incidence of cardiovascular events in which 2 thiazolidinediones are used as add-on treatments for type 2 diabetes mellitus in a Taiwanese population. *Clin Ther.* 2011; 33:1904-13.

459. Akcay AB, Ozcan T, Seyis S, Acele A. Coronary vasospasm and acute myocardial infarction induced by a topical capsaicin patch. *Turk Kardiyol Dern Ars.* 2009; 37:497-500.

460. Harrison-Woolrych M, Maggo S, Tan M et al. Cardiovascular events in patients taking varenicline: a case series from intensive postmarketing surveillance in New Zealand. *Drug Saf.* 2012; 35:33-43.

461. Ware JH, Vetrovec GW, Miller AB et al. Cardiovascular safety of varenicline: patient-level meta-analysis of randomized, blinded, placebo-controlled trials. *Am J Ther.* 2013; 20:235-46.

462. Puhr J, Hack J, Early J et al. Lithium overdose with electrocardiogram changes suggesting ischemia. *J Med Toxicol.* 2008; 4:170-2.

463. McGettigan P, Henry D. Cardiovascular risk and inhibition of cyclooxygenase: a systematic review of the observational studies of selective and nonselective inhibitors of cyclooxygenase 2. *JAMA.* 2006; 296:1633-44.

464. Ivanov SM, Lagunin AA, Pogodin PV et al. Identification of drug-induced myocardial infarction-related protein targets through the prediction of drug-target interactions and analysis of biological processes. *Chem Res Toxicol.* 2014; 27:1263-81.

465. Wysowski DK, Swartz L. Adverse drug event surveillance and drug withdrawals in the United States, 1969-2002: the importance of reporting suspected reactions. *Arch Intern Med.* 2005; 165:1363-9.

466. Stankowski RV, Kloner RA, Rezkalla SH. Cardiovascular consequences of cocaine use. *Trends Cardiovasc Med.* 2015; 25:517-26.

467. Feldman JA, Fish SS, Beshansky JR et al. Acute cardiac ischemia in patients with cocaine-associated complaints: results of a multicenter trial. *Ann Emerg Med.* 2000; 36:469-76.

468. Hollander JE, Hoffman RS, Gennis P et al. Prospective multicenter evaluation of cocaine-associated chest pain. Cocaine Associated Chest Pain (COCHPA) Study Group. *Acad Emerg Med.* 1994; 1:330-9.

469. Kontos MC, Schmidt KL, Nicholson CS et al. Myocardial perfusion imaging with technetium-99m sestamibi in patients with cocaine-associated chest pain. *Ann Emerg Med.* 1999; 33:639-45.

470. Weber JE, Chudnofsky CR, Boczar M et al. Cocaine-associated chest pain: how common is myocardial infarction? *Acad Emerg Med.* 2000; 7:873-7.

471. Finkel JB, Marhefka GD. Rethinking cocaine-associated chest pain and acute coronary syndromes. *Mayo Clin Proc.* 2011; 86:1198-207.

472. Maraj S, Figueredo VM, Lynn Morris D. Cocaine and the heart. *Clin Cardiol.* 2010; 33:264-9.

473. Rosendaal FR, Helmerhorst FM, Vandenbroucke JP. Female hormones and thrombosis. *Arterioscler Thromb Vasc Biol.* 2002; 22:201-10.

474. Hulley S, Grady D, Bush T et al. Randomized trial of estrogen plus progestin for secondary prevention of coronary heart disease in postmenopausal women. Heart and Estrogen/progestin Replacement Study (HERS) Research Group. *JAMA.* 1998; 280:605-13.

475. Writing Group for the Women's Health Initiative Investigators. Risks and Benefits of Estrogen Plus Progestin in Healthy Postmenopausal Women: Principal Results From the Women's Health Initiative Randomized Controlled Trial. *JAMA.* 2002; 288:321-33.

476. FDA News. 2003. http://www.fda.gov/bbs/topics/NEWS/2003/NEW00863.html.

477. Arlett P, Sarac SB, Thomson A et al. The European Medicines Agency's use of prioritised independent research for best evidence in regulatory action on diclofenac. *Pharmacoepidemiol Drug Saf.* 2014; 23:431-4.

478. Coxib, traditional NTC, Bhala N et al. Vascular and upper gastrointestinal effects of non-steroidal anti-inflammatory drugs: meta-analyses of individual participant data from randomised trials. *Lancet.* 2013; 382:769-79.

479. Schjerning Olsen AM, Gislason GH, McGettigan P et al. Association of NSAID use with risk of bleeding and cardiovascular events in patients receiving antithrombotic therapy after myocardial infarction. *JAMA.* 2015; 313:805-14.

480. PRAC recommends updating advice on use of high-dose ibuprofen. European Medicines Agency, 4/13/2015. http://www.ema.europa.eu/ema/index.jsp?curl=pages/news_and_events/news/2015/04/news_detail_002306.jsp&mid=WC0b01ac058004d5c1 (accessed 2018 Feb 9).

481. Antman EM, Bennett JS, Daugherty A et al. Use of nonsteroidal antiinflammatory drugs: an update for clinicians: a scientific statement from the American Heart Association. *Circulation.* 2007; 115:1634-42.

482. Griffin MR. High-dose non-steroidal anti-inflammatories: painful choices. *Lancet.* 2013; 382:746-8.

483. McGettigan P, Henry D. Cardiovascular risk with non-steroidal anti-inflammatory drugs: systematic review of population-based controlled observational studies. *PLoS Med.* 2011; 8:e1001098.

484. Olsen AM, Fosbol EL, Lindhardsen J et al. Long-term cardiovascular risk of nonsteroidal anti-inflammatory drug use according to time passed after first-time myocardial infarction: a nationwide cohort study. *Circulation*. 2012; 126:1955-63.

485. Kaul S, Bolger AF, Herrington D et al. Thiazolidinedione drugs and cardiovascular risks: a science advisory from the American Heart Association and American College of Cardiology Foundation. *Circulation*. 2010; 121:1868-77.

486. Mitka M. Panel recommends easing restrictions on rosiglitazone despite concerns about cardiovascular safety. *JAMA*. 2013; 310:246-7.

487. Vigen R, O'Donnell CI, Baron AE et al. Association of testosterone therapy with mortality, myocardial infarction, and stroke in men with low testosterone levels. *JAMA*. 2013; 310:1829-36.

488. Finkle WD, Greenland S, Ridgeway GK et al. Increased risk of non-fatal myocardial infarction following testosterone therapy prescription in men. *PLoS One*. 2014; 9:e85805.

489. Basaria S, Coviello AD, Travison TG et al. Adverse events associated with testosterone administration. *N Engl J Med*. 2010; 363:109-22.

490. Bhasin S, Cunningham GR, Hayes FJ et al. Testosterone therapy in men with androgen deficiency syndromes: an Endocrine Society clinical practice guideline. *J Clin Endocrinol Metab*. 2010; 95:2536-59.

491. Morgentaler A, Miner MM, Caliber M et al. Testosterone therapy and cardiovascular risk: advances and controversies. *Mayo Clin Proc*. 2015; 90:224-51.

492. Ardehali A, Ports TA. Myocardial oxygen supply and demand. *Chest*. 1990; 98:699-705.

493. Swedberg K, Held P, Kjekshus J et al. Effects of the early administration of enalapril on mortality in patients with acute myocardial infarction. Results of the Cooperative New Scandinavian Enalapril Survival Study II (CONSENSUS II). *N Engl J Med*. 1992; 327:678-84.

494. Scanlon PJ, Faxon DP, Audet AM et al. ACC/AHA guidelines for coronary angiography: executive summary and recommendations. A report of the American College of Cardiology/American Heart Association Task Force on Practice Guidelines (Committee on Coronary Angiography) developed in collaboration with the Society for Cardiac Angiography and Interventions. *Circulation*. 1999; 99:2345-57.

495. Boersma E, Mercado N, Poldermans D et al. Acute myocardial infarction. *Lancet*. 2003; 361:847-58.

496. Mosca L, Banka CL, Benjamin EJ et al. Evidence-based guidelines for cardiovascular disease prevention in women: 2007 update. *Circulation*. 2007; 115:1481-501.

497. Goff DC, Lloyd-Jones DM, Bennett G et al. 2013 ACC/AHA Guideline on the Assessment of Cardiovascular Risk: A Report of the American College of Cardiology/American Heart Association Task Force on Practice Guidelines. *Circulation*. 2014; 129:S49-S73.

498. Shah RV, Goldfine AB. Statins and risk of new-onset diabetes mellitus. *Circulation*. 2012; 126:e282-4.

499. Cederberg H, Stancakova A, Yaluri N et al. Increased risk of diabetes with statin treatment is associated with impaired insulin sensitivity and insulin secretion: a 6 year follow-up study of the METSIM cohort. *Diabetologia*. 2015; 58:1109-17.

500. Ford I. Coming safely to a stop: a review of platelet activity after cessation of antiplatelet drugs. *Ther Adv Drug Saf*. 2015; 6:141-50.

501. Thygesen K, Alpert JS, White HD et al. Universal definition of myocardial infarction. *Circulation*. 2007; 116:2634-53.

502. Gupta N, Washam JB, Mountantonakis SE et al. Characteristics, management, and outcomes of cocaine-positive patients with acute coronary syndrome (from the National Cardiovascular Data Registry). *Am J Cardiol*. 2014; 113:749-56.

503. Hollander JE, Todd KH, Green G et al. Chest pain associated with cocaine: an assessment of prevalence in suburban and urban emergency departments. *Ann Emerg Med*. 1995; 26:671-6.

504. Hollander JE, Hoffman RS, Gennis P et al. Cocaine-associated chest pain: one-year follow-up. *Acad Emerg Med*. 1995; 2:179-84.

505. Centers for Disease Control and Prevention. U S. Medical Eligibility Criteria for Contraceptive Use, 2016. *MMWR Recomm Rep*. 2016; 65:1-104.

506. Fihn SD, Blankenship JC, Alexander KP et al. 2014 ACC/AHA/AATS/PCNA/SCAI/STS Focused Update of the Guideline for the Diagnosis and Management of Patients With Stable Ischemic Heart Disease: A Report of the American College of Cardiology/American Heart Association Task Force on Practice Guidelines, and the American Association for Thoracic Surgery, Preventive Cardiovascular Nurses Association, Society for Cardiovascular Angiography and Interventions, and Society of Thoracic Surgeons. *Circulation*. 2014; 130:1749-67.

507. Dattilo PB, Hailpern SM, Fearon K et al. Beta-blockers are associated with reduced risk of myocardial infarction after cocaine use. *Ann Emerg Med*. 2008; 51:117-25.

508. Fanari Z, Kennedy KK, Lim MJ et al. Comparison of in-hospital outcomes for beta-blocker use versus non-beta blocker use in patients presenting with cocaine-associated chest pain. *Am J Cardiol*. 2014; 113:1802-6.

509. LoVecchio F, Nelson L. Intraventricular bleeding after the use of thrombolytics in a cocaine user. *Am J Emerg Med*. 1996; 14:663-4.

510. Hollander JE, Wilson LD, Leo PJ, Shih RD. Complications from the use of thrombolytic agents in patients with cocaine associated chest pain. *J Emerg Med*. 1996; 14:731-6.

511. Amsterdam EA, Wenger NK, Brindis RG et al. 2014 AHA/ACC Guideline for the Management of Patients with Non-ST-Elevation Acute Coronary Syndromes: a report of the American College of Cardiology/American Heart Association Task Force on Practice Guidelines. *J Am Coll Cardiol*. 2014; 64:e139-228.

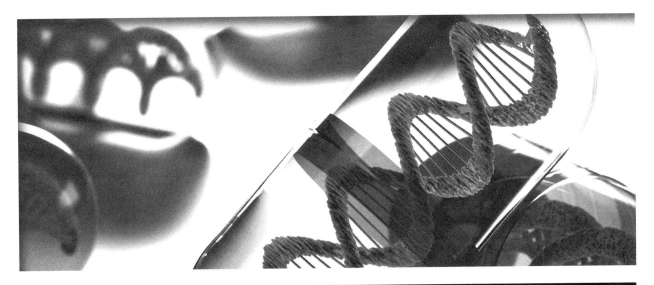

CHAPTER 24

Heart Failure

Yazid N. Al Hamarneh and Ross T. Tsuyuki

Heart failure is a major cause of morbidity and mortality in Western society.[1-4] It is one of the most common reasons for hospitalization, with over 5 million hospitalizations per year in the United States and 106,000 per year in Canada.[4,5] The duration of stay for patients hospitalized with heart failure is long, averaging about 13 days, and in-hospital mortality is high, between 3.2 and 15%.[4,6]

Coronary artery disease is by far the most common cause of heart failure in the United States, accounting for approximately two thirds of cases.[7] Other causes include hypertension, myocarditis, and cardiac toxins, including drugs, which can cause or exacerbate a stable pattern of heart failure.[7,8] Drug-induced heart failure in patients without pre-existing left ventricular dysfunction is quite rare, and drug-induced exacerbation of symptoms of heart failure occurs more frequently in those with established heart failure.[9] This chapter will focus on drug-induced heart failure, primarily heart failure with reduced ejection fraction (HFrEF), including causative agents, epidemiology, mechanism of action, and clinical presentation.

CAUSATIVE AGENTS

Left ventricular ejection fraction (LVEF), also simply referred to as ejection fraction (EF), is used as the primary term to define heart failure.[10] Based on LVEF, heart failure can be divided into heart failure with reduced ejection fraction (HFrEF) if EF is <40% or heart failure with preserved ejection fraction (HFpEF) if the EF is >50%.[10,11]

The agents implicated in drug-induced heart failure are listed in **Table 24-1**.[12-109] Causality is often difficult to ascertain because of the multiplicity of factors that can exacerbate heart failure symptoms. Most calcium-channel blockers (except felodipine and amlodipine), antihyperglycemic agents (dipeptidyl peptidase 4 [DPP-4] inhibitors and thiazolidinediones ["glitazones": rosiglitazone and pioglitazone]), antiarrhythmic agents, anthracyclines (doxorubicin), biologics (bevacizumab, infliximab, lapatinib, trastuzumab), nonsteroidal anti-inflammatory agents (NSAIDs), selective cyclooxygenase-2 (COX-2) inhibitors, and adrenergic β-receptor antagonists (β-blockers) have all been implicated in drug-induced heart failure.

Table 24-1 Agents Implicated in Drug-Induced Heart Failure

Drug	Incidence	Level of Evidence[a]
α_1-antagonists		
Doxazosin[12]	RR 2.04, 95% CI 1.79–2.32	A
Amantadine[13]	NK	C
Aminocaproic acid[14]	NK	C
Amphotericin B[15,16]	NK	C
Anagrelide[17]	2.4%	B
Anthracyclines[18,19]		
Doxorubicin[20-22,24]	0–16%	A
Epirubicin[24]	20%	A
Digoxin immune antibody fragments[25]	NK	C
Antiarrhythmic agents[25,26]	5–10%[24]	A
Disopyramide[29]	16%	A
Dronedarone[30]	3.2%	A
Encainide[28]	2.6%	A
Flecainide[27]	(NYHA class III HF) 13.5%	A
Lidocaine[26]	9%	A
Lorcainide[28]	0.7%	A
Mexiletine[28]	0.9%	A
Moricizine[28]	2.4%	A
Propafenone[28]	4.7%	A
Tocainide[28]	1.6%	A
β-blockers[31]	2%	B
Propranolol[32]	1–5.4%	B
Biologic agents		
Bevacizumab[137]	RR 4.74, 95% CI 1.66–11.18	A
Infliximab[138]	RR 2.84, 95% CI 1.01–7.97	A
Trastuzumab[98]	14% vs 10% (control) Monotherapy: 3–7%[99,100,102,103] NYHA class III or IV: 0–3.9%[101] LVEF decrease >10%: 3–34%[101]	A
Blue cohosh[33]	NK	C
Bromocriptine[34]	NK	C
Buflomedil[185]	NK	C
Cabergoline[35-37]	NK	C
Calcium-channel blockers		A
Diltiazem[38]	20.5%	A
Nifedipine[39]	24–26%	A
Verapamil[40]	NK	C
Carbamazepine[110]	NK	C
Clozapine[41-44]	NK	C
Corticosteroids[45]	Adjusted OR 2.7, 95% CI 2.5–2.9[2]	B
Prednisolone[46]	Dose <7.5 mg/day: RR 1.5, 95% CI 1.3–1.8 Dose ≥7.5 mg/day: RR 3.7, 95% CI 2.7–5.1	B
Cyclophosphamide[47,48]	NK	C

Table 24-1 Agents Implicated in Drug-Induced Heart Failure (continued)

Drug	Incidence	Level of Evidence[a]
Cytarabine[49]	NK	C
Dapsone[50]	NK	C
DPP-4 inhibitors		
Saxagliptin[122]	HR 1.27, 95% CI 1.07–1.51	A
Dutasteride[186]	NK	A
Etanercept[187,188]	NK	B
Fluorouracil[52]	NK	C
Foscarnet[53]	NK	C
Glitazones[54-58]	RR 1.72, 95% CI 1.21–2.42[62]	
Rosiglitazone[59-61]	OR 2.1, 95% CI 1.08–4.08 vs. placebo[63]	A
Pioglitazone[65,66]	HR 1.8, 95% CI 1.4–2.2[64]	A
	0.1–14.1%	
	HR 2.15–7.03	
	RR 2.09, 95% CI 1.52–2.88	
	11%[65]	
	HR 1.41, 95% CI 1.14–1.76[66]	
Hydralazine[34]	NK	C
Ifosfamide[18,67]	NK	C
Imatinib[189]	NK	B
Interferon α[70-72]	NK	C
Itraconazole[73]	NK	C
Licorice[74]	NK	C
Mannitol[75]	NK	C
Megestrol[76]	NK	C
Minoxidil[77]	NK	C
Mitoxantrone[78]	1.5%	C
NSAIDs[79-86]	RR 1.8–9.9, 95% CI 1.4–2.4	B
COX-2 inhibitors		
Celecoxib[87-89]	0.4–1.9%	A
Rofecoxib[85-89]	0–1.9%	A
	RR 1.4, 95% CI 1.17–1.80	
Paclitaxel[90,91]	NK	C
Parkinson disease agents[190]	NK	B
Cabergoline[190]		
Pergolide[190]		
Pramipexole[190]		
Ropinirole[190]		
PEG lavage solution[92]	NK	C
Penicillins[93,94]	NK	C
Ampicillin[94]	NK	C
Pergolide[95,96]	NK	C
Pregabalin[97]	NK	C
Sodium-containing antacids[34]	NK	C

Table 24-1 Agents Implicated in Drug-Induced Heart Failure (continued)

Drug	Incidence	Level of Evidence[a]
Sunitinib[191]	NK	B
Tricyclic antidepressants[104-107]	NK	C
Imipramine	NK	C
Amitriptyline	NK	C
Protriptyline	NK	C
Nortriptyline	NK	C
Clomipramine	NK	C
Venlafaxine[108]	NK	C
Zidovudine[109]	NK	C

CI = confidence interval, COX = cyclooxygenase, DPP = dipeptidyl peptidase, HF = heart failure, HR = hazard ratio, LVEF = left ventricular ejection fraction, NK = not known, NSAID = nonsteroidal anti-inflammatory drug, NYHA = New York Heart Association, OR = odds ratio, PEG = polyethylene glycol, RR = relative risk.

[a]Definitions for Levels of Evidence: Level A—evidence from one or more randomized, controlled clinical trials; Level B—evidence from nonrandomized clinical trials, prospective observational studies, cohort studies, retrospective studies, case-control studies, meta-analyses and/or postmarketing surveillance studies; and Level C—evidence from one or more published case reports or case series.

Isolated case reports have identified other agents as possible causes of drug-induced heart failure (see Table 24-1 for details). Because causality related to these agents is much less certain, these will not be discussed in detail in this chapter. The reader is referred to a comprehensive review by Amabile and Spencer[110] that outlines medications to avoid in patients with heart failure and review papers by Feenstra et al.,[9] Slordal and Spigset,[111] and Maxwell and Jenkins[112] for further discussion of heart failure associated with these agents.

Although drug-induced heart failure in patients without pre-existing left ventricular dysfunction is relatively rare, drug-induced exacerbations of symptoms in those with pre-existing left ventricular dysfunction is more common. Drug-induced causes, expressed as a proportion of all heart-failure exacerbations, are shown in **Table 24-2**. In a prospective study of factors associated with acute exacerbation of heart failure, Tsuyuki et al.[113] reported on 323 episodes of worsening HFrEF in 180 patients during the 43 weeks of the Randomized Evaluation of Strategies for Left Ventricular Dysfunction (RESOLVD) pilot study. Although the most commonly identified precipitant of exacerbations of acute HFrEF was excessive salt intake (22%), antiarrhythmic agents, study medications (which were metoprolol and candesartan and/or enalapril administered in a blinded fashion), and calcium-channel blockers were all implicated. Interestingly, however, medications were not thought to be the primary cause of any of these exacerbations; rather, nonadherence to salt restrictions, followed by other noncardiac causes (such as upper respiratory tract infections), were the most common causes of excerbations.[113]

Table 24-2 Proportion of Heart Failure Exacerbations That Are Drug-Induced[a]

Study	Precipitating Agent(s)	Incidence
Tsuyuki et al.[113,b]	Antiarrhythmic agents	15%
	"Study medications" (β-blockers or placebo)	15%
	Calcium channel blockers	13%
	Nonstudy open-label β-blockers	9%
	NSAIDs	5%
Rich et al.[114]	Fluids (excessive intravascular volume expansion)	5.5%
	β-blockers	0.25%
	Verapamil	0.25%
Garcia Robles et al.[31]	β-blockers	2%

NSAID = nonsteroidal anti-inflammatory drug.

[a]Does not include underuse of drugs (i.e., discontinuation of therapy with diuretics).

[b]Categories not mutually exclusive.

In a review of 401 patients over the age of 70 years hospitalized with HFrEF or HFpEF (average LVEF was 52% in iatrogenic heart failure group and 44% in the noniatrogenic group), Rich et al.[114] determined that iatrogenic causes were present in 28 patients (7%). The most common cause was excessive intravascular volume expansion (22 patients) followed by administration of blood products (3 patients) or verapamil (1 patient).[114] In a review of 100 hospitalizations of patients over 65 years of age with HFrEF, Garcia Robles et al. identified two cases (2%) caused by β-blockers.[31] Other studies revealed acute angina, respiratory infection, uncontrolled hypertension, arrhythmias, and poor adherence to medication therapy as common precipitants of exacerbations of HFrEF and HFpEF.[113-117]

EPIDEMIOLOGY

The incidence of drug-induced heart failure (HFrEF, HFpEF, heart failure with unreported EF) is outlined in Table 24-1. The precise incidence of drug-induced heart failure is difficult to determine because it is often challenging to differentiate drug-induced heart failure from the many other precipitants of this syndrome.[113]

CALCIUM-CHANNEL BLOCKERS

In a post hoc analysis of the Multicentre Diltiazem Postinfarction Trial (MDPIT), Goldstein et al.[38] reported new or worsened HFrEF in 12% and 20.5% of 623 patients receiving placebo or diltiazem, respectively ($p = 0.004$). There was no difference in the incidence of new or worsened heart failure (in patients with LVEF > 0.40) at baseline, highlighting the significant hazard of diltiazem use in patients with left ventricular dysfunction after myocardial infarction.[38] In a randomized, double-blind crossover study of 8 weeks of treatment with isosorbide dinitrate alone, isosorbide dinitrate in combination with nifedipine, or nifedipine alone in 28 patients with mild-to-moderate HFrEF, there were higher incidences of hospitalization due to worsening heart failure in the isosorbide dinitrate plus nifedipine (26%) and nifedipine alone (24%) groups compared to that in the isosorbide dinitrate alone group (0%).[39]

In the second Prospective Randomized Amlodipine Survival Evaluation (PRAISE-2) study, 1,654 patients with HFrEF were randomized to receive amlodipine or placebo. The hazard ratio for death was 1.09 (95% CI 0.92–1.29), indicating no survival benefit (or adverse effect on survival) associated with amlodipine. Many have interpreted these results to mean that amlodipine can be used in patients with HFrEF who need it for reasons other than heart failure (e.g., hypertension or angina not controlled by other agents).[118] Similar recommendations have been made regarding felodipine based on the results of the third Vasodilators in Heart Failure Trial (V-HeFT III), in which patients with HFrEF were randomized to receive felodipine or placebo; there were no differences between the groups in mortality or hospitalization rates.[119]

ANTIHYPERGLYCEMIC AGENTS

GLITAZONES

The glitazone drugs are a well-known cause of fluid retention.[54,55,57,58] Tang et al.[55] reviewed the records of 111 consecutive patients with HFrEF and diabetes who were prescribed a glitazone agent and reported that the incidence of fluid retention was 17%. Of those who fulfilled the criteria for fluid retention, 26% were hospitalized to manage the condition and 11% had pulmonary edema. There was no difference in the baseline New York Heart Association (NYHA) functional heart failure class between patients who developed fluid retention and those who did not. In the randomized A Diabetes Outcome Progression Trial (ADOPT), a higher incidence of heart failure was reported in the rosiglitazone group compared to that in the glyburide group (HR 2.2, 95% CI 1.01–4.79, $p = 0.05$) though not compared to that in the metformin group (HR 1.22, 95% CI 0.66–2.26, $p = 0.52$).[120] A higher incidence of pulmonary edema and use of loop diuretics was also reported in the rosiglitazone group (14.1%) compared to that associated with glyburide (8.5%; $p < 0.001$) or metformin (7.2%; $p < 0.001$).[120]

More recently, several clinical trials and meta-analyses have investigated the impact of glitazone therapy on cardiovascular outcomes, including the incidence of heart failure. In the Diabetes Reduction Assessment with Ramipril and Rosiglitazone Medication (DREAM) study, 5,269 adults with impaired fasting glucose or impaired glucose tolerance or both and no previous cardiovascular disease were randomly assigned to receive rosiglitazone or placebo.[60] A higher proportion of patients in the rosiglitazone group developed heart failure than in the placebo group (0.5% versus 0.1%, respectively, $p = 0.01$). In the Rosiglitazone Evaluated for Cardiac Outcomes and Regulation of Glycemia (RECORD) study, 4,447 patients with inadequate glycemic control were randomly assigned to receive add-on rosiglitazone therapy or metformin plus sulfonylurea (control group). In an interim analysis, the hazard ratio for the development of heart failure associated with rosiglitazone was 2.15 (95% CI 1.30–3.57).[61] Pioglitazone has also been associated with an increased rate of heart failure. In the Prospective Pioglitazone Clinical Trial In Macrovascular Events (PROactive) study, 5,238 patients with type 2 diabetes and evidence of macrovascular disease were randomly assigned to receive pioglitazone or placebo. Pioglitazone was associated with a higher incidence of heart failure (11% versus 8%; $p < 0.0001$).[65] Several meta-analyses have also documented an increased incidence of heart failure (new cases and worsening symptoms) in patients receiving glitazones (Table 24-1).[59,62,63,66]

Notably, although both rosiglitazone and pioglitazone have been associated with an increased incidence of heart failure (new cases and worsening symptoms), to date only rosiglitazone has been shown to be associated with an increased risk of myocardial infarction (OR 1.43, 95% CI 1.03–1.98).[121] Neither rosiglitazone nor pioglitazone has been shown to increase the risk of cardiovascular mortality.[59,62,66] A joint consensus statement by the American Heart Association and the American Diabetes Association recommended cautious use of lower doses of glitazones in patients with NYHA functional class I–II symptoms and avoidance of these agents in those with NYHA class III–IV symptoms.[56] It is best to avoid glitazones in patients with heart failure, in view of the fact that there are many oral antihyperglycemic agents that can be used in this population.

DIPEPTIDYL PEPTIDASE (DPP)-4 INHIBITORS

In light of the latest evidence, the focus of many diabetes trials has shifted toward cardiovascular safety outcomes (rather than an expectation of reducing cardiovascular risk). Scirica et al.[122] conducted a multicenter, randomized, double-blind, placebo-controlled trial to assess the cardiovascular safety and efficacy of saxagliptin in patients with type 2 diabetes who had a history of established cardiovascular disease or multiple risk factors for vascular disease. There was no significant difference between the saxagliptin and placebo groups in the primary endpoint (composite of cardiovascular death, nonfatal myocardial infarction, or nonfatal ischemic stroke) (HR 1, 95% CI 0.89–1.12, $p = 0.99$) nor in the major secondary endpoints (composite of cardiovascular death, nonfatal myocardial infarction, nonfatal ischemic stroke, hospitalization for unstable angina, coronary revascularization, or heart failure (HR 1.02, 95% CI 0.94–1.11, $p = 0.66$). However, saxagliptin increased the risk of hospitalization for heart failure (HR 1.27, 95% CI 1.07–1.51, $p = 0.007$). White et al.[123] conducted a multicenter, randomized, double-blind noninferiority trial of the effects of alogliptin on major cardiovascular events in patients with type 2 diabetes who had an acute coronary syndrome within 15–90 days before randomization. Alogliptin did not increase the risk of hospitalization for heart failure (HR 1.19, 95% CI 0.89–1.59, $p = 0.24$). Green et al.[124] employed a similar design to assess the cardiovascular safety of sitagliptin versus placebo in patients with type 2 diabetes who had established cardiovascular disease. Sitagliptin did not increase the risk of cardiovascular death, nonfatal myocardial infarction, nonfatal stroke, or hospitalization for unstable angina (HR 0.98, 95% CI 0.8–1.08, $p = 0.65$) or the risk of hospitalization for heart failure (HR 1, 95% CI 0.83–1.20, $p = 0.98$). Weir et al.[125] assessed the effects of sitagliptin on patients with type 2 diabetes and heart failure in a population-based retrospective cohort study. When compared to metformin or a sulfonylurea, sitagliptin did not increase the risk of all-cause mortality and hospitalization (adjusted OR 0.84, 95% CI 0.69–1.03, $p = 0.10$). However patients who received sitagliptin were at higher risk of hospital admission due to heart failure (adjusted OR 1.84, 95% CI 1.16–2.92, $p = 0.01$).

ANTIARRHYTHMIC AGENTS

Ravid et al.[28] reviewed the incidence of drug-induced heart failure in 407 patients during 1,133 serial electrophysiologic drug tests with encainide, moricizine, lorcainide, mexiletine, propafenone, or tocainide. Using a strict definition of HFrEF, they reported an overall incidence of drug-induced heart failure of 1.8%. The incidence increased to 3.8% in patients with a history of heart failure. In this study, lorcainide (not available in the United States) was associated with the lowest incidence of heart failure (0.7%), while propafenone was associated with the highest incidence (4.7%). In a randomized, controlled trial investigating the impact of antiarrhythmic therapy postmyocardial infarction, Greene et al.[27] reported no significant difference in the proportion of patients who developed heart failure symptoms or diagnoses requiring hospitalization in patients receiving imipramine (which at the time was studied for possible antiarrhythmic effects), encainide, flecainide, or moricizine (26%) compared with those receiving placebo (18%).[27] Pfisterer estimated that the incidence of drug-induced heart failure associated with older antiarrhythmic agents (excluding ibutilide and dofetilide) is about 5% overall and approximately 10% in those with a history of heart failure.[29] Disopyramide has well-known negative inotropic effects, and flecainide has also been reported to worsen heart failure.[126,127]

Amiodarone, ibutilide, and dofetilide appear to exert minimal negative inotropic effects, and amiodarone and dofetilide are neutral with respect to survival in patients with heart failure.[1] Therefore, amiodarone and dofetilide are recommended for prevention of recurrent atrial fibrillation in patients with HFrEF.[1,2] In contrast, the Antiarrhythmic Trial with Dronedarone in Moderate to Severe CHF Evaluating Morbidity Decrease (ANDROMEDA) trial found that dronedarone, an antiarrhythmic drug with properties similar to those of amiodarone, was associated with increased early mortality related to the worsening of heart failure symptoms in patients who were hospitalized with symptomatic severe HFrEF.[30] During a median follow-up of 2 months, 8.1% of patients receiving dronedarone died, compared with 3.8% receiving placebo (HR 2.13, 95% CI 1.07–4.25, $p = 0.03$), and this excess mortality was predominantly related to worsening of heart failure (3.2% versus 0.6%; p value not reported). An increase in mortality associated with dronedarone was not observed in another trial in which patients with decompensated NYHA class IV HFrEF were excluded (no difference in all-cause mortality, and a reduction in death from cardiovascular causes—dronedarone, 2.7%, versus placebo, 3.9%; HR 0.71, 95% CI 0.51–0.98).[128] It is recommended that dronedarone should be avoided in patients with HFrEF.[129] Overall, heart failure is a known risk factor for proarrhythmic effects and most antiarrhythmic agents worsen heart failure symptoms. Risk versus benefit evaluation is extremely important in this patient population. Amiodarone and dofetilide appear to be the antiarrythmic agents that are least likely to induce or exacerbate heart failure.[130]

ANTHRACYCLINES

The incidence of drug-induced HFrEF is best characterized for the cancer chemotherapy agent doxorubicin. Von Hoff et al.[20] reviewed eight National Cancer Institute trials involving over 3,900 patients and reported an overall incidence of doxorubicin-induced heart failure of 2.2%. However, a retrospective analysis of three clinical trials, which included 630 patients receiving doxorubicin, reported a higher overall incidence of doxorubicin-related HFrEF of 5.1%.[21] In a systematic review of 30 studies, the frequency of anthracycline-induced heart failure in children was reported to be 0–16%.[22] In a cohort of 830 children treated with a mean cumulative anthracycline dose of 288 mg/m^2 during a mean follow-up of 8.5 years, the incidence of anthracycline-induced heart failure was 2.5%.[23] Although anthracyclines can be lifesaving in patients with cancer, the known cardiotoxicity of these agents requires close monitoring with respect to dose and cardiac function.

BIOLOGIC AGENTS

TRASTUZUMAB

Although trastuzumab has clearly been associated with cardiac dysfunction, determination of the incidence is complicated by the coadministration of other cardiotoxic medications such as anthracyclines and cyclophosphamide. In the first large Phase III trial of trastuzumab in patients with metastatic breast cancer that overexpressed human epidermal growth factor receptor 2 (HER2), patients were assigned randomly to standard cancer chemotherapy plus trastuzumab (doxorubicin, epirubicin, or cyclophosphamide for those who had not previously received adjuvant anthracycline therapy or paclitaxel for those who had received previous adjuvant anthracycline therapy) or standard chemotherapy alone. Cardiac dysfunction (based on NYHA criteria) occurred in 27% of the patients receiving an anthracycline, cyclophosphamide, and trastuzumab; in 8% in those who received only an anthracycline and cyclophosphamide; in 13% in those receiving trastuzumab plus paclitaxel; and in 1% of patients receiving paclitaxel alone.[98] In addition, five major trials investigating trastuzumab as adjuvant therapy for patients with HER2 positive breast cancer reported an incidence of severe heart failure (NYHA class III or IV) of 0–3.9% in trastuzumab-treated patients compared with 0–1.3% in control groups.[101,131-135] In these studies, 3–34% of trastuzumab-treated patients experienced >10% reduction in LVEF, compared with 2–17% of patients in control groups (*p* value not reported).[101] In addition, trastuzumab has been used as a single agent in several trials in which the incidence of cardiac dysfunction associated with the drug has been 3–7%.[102] Finally, in a retrospective review of 173 women with metastatic breast cancer who received trastuzumab for at least 1 year at a single institution, 10.9% experienced symptomatic heart failure or had a LVEF between 20% and 40%.[136]

BEVACIZUMAB

Choueiri et al.[137] conducted a meta-analysis of randomized controlled trials of bevacizumab in patients with metastatic breast cancer to evaluate the incidence and the risk of heart failure. They reported that patients who received bevacizumab were at a much higher risk of developing heart failure compared to those who did not receive the drug (RR 4.74, 95% CI 1.84–12.19, $p = 0.001$). No significant difference in the relative risk of heart failure was found between the two approved doses of bevacizumab (2.5 mg/kg and 5 mg/kg, $p = 0.81$).

INFLIXIMAB

Chung et al.[138] conducted a randomized controlled trial to assess the influence of infliximab on clinical outcomes in patients who have moderate-to-severe HFrEF. Patients in this trial were randomized to receive placebo, infliximab 5 mg/kg or infliximab 10 mg/kg (to a maximum of 1 g) immediately after randomization and at 2 and 6 weeks after randomization and were followed for 28 weeks. Patients who received infliximab 10 mg/kg were more likely to have worsened clinical status (NYHA and global assessment) at 14 and 28 weeks compared to patients in the other two groups (placebo and infliximab 5 mg/kg). Those patients were also more likely to die or be hospitalized for HFrEF when compared to the placebo group (HR 2.84, 95% CI 1.01–7.97, $p = 0.043$) and were also more likely to be hospitalized for HFrEF or any other reason when compared to those who received infliximab 5 mg/kg. Of note, reduction in LVEF has been reported in association with lapatinib.[139]

NSAIDs

In a study of more than 10,000 patients over 55 years of age, the adjusted relative risk of hospitalization for heart failure was 1.8 (95% CI 1.4–2.4) in patients receiving diuretics and NSAIDs compared to those taking diuretics only.[79] Bleumink et al.[80] reviewed five studies (including the aforementioned trial) and reported an approximate twofold increase in the relative risk/odds ratio for development of heart failure in patients taking NSAIDs (range between 1.8 [95% CI 1.4–2.4] to 2.2 [95% CI 1–3.4]). Zhao et al.[89] reviewed employers' drug insurance databases to evaluate the cost of heart failure in patients with stable hypertension (and without a history of coronary artery disease or heart failure) who started new treatment with anti-inflammatory medications between January 1999 and September 2000. They reported 102 new outpatient visits for heart failure (based on diagnosis codes and international classification of diseases code) among 20,838 new recipients of prescriptions for traditional NSAIDs (adjusted rate per 1,000 patient-days, 0.124 [95% CI 0.91–1.41, $p = 0.28$]).[89]

COX-2 INHIBITORS

Although the COX-2 inhibitors were originally believed to be free of renal and hemodynamic effects, this has ultimately not proven to be the case. In a randomized, double-blind trial in 1,092 patients ≥65 years of age with hypertension and osteoarthritis, Whelton et al.[87] reported that 0.4% of the patients in the celecoxib group and 0.6% of those in the rofecoxib group developed new onset or worsening of heart failure.[87] In the aforementioned review of patients with stable hypertension in an administrative database, Zhao et al.[89] reported 377 new outpatient visits for heart failure among 19,663 users of celecoxib (adjusted rate per 1,000 patient-days, 0.11) and 228 among 12,218 users of rofecoxib (adjusted rate per 1,000 patient-days, 0.139 [95% CI 1.06–1.48, $p = 0.007$]). In a population-based cohort study in elderly patients, there was an increased risk of hospital admission in patients taking rofecoxib (adjusted rate ratio 1.8, 95% CI 1.4–2.4) and nonselective NSAIDs (adjusted rate ratio 1.4, 95% CI 1–1.9) when compared to those taking celecoxib.[85]

β-BLOCKERS

Although it has been known for some time that β-blockers can precipitate heart failure in susceptible individuals, use of these drugs is now standard care in the management of heart failure, based on morbidity and mortality benefits demonstrated in numerous randomized trials.[1,2,140-142] In 1974, Greenblatt and Koch-Weser[32] reported an incidence of HFrEF of 1% in 319 consecutive hospitalized patients who were prescribed propranolol. These investigators also reviewed 23 studies of 797 outpatients receiving propranolol and reported an incidence of HFrEF of 5.4%. These early results should be balanced against the now incontrovertible evidence supporting the benefit of β-blockers on mortality and morbidity in patients with HFrEF.[1,2,140-142] Indeed, in systematic reviews and clinical trials, the use of β-blockers has been shown consistently to reduce the incidence of mortality in HFrEF by 34% and hospitalizations by 40–50% as compared with placebo.[140,142] In a systematic review of 13 randomized trials of β-blockers, HFrEF was reported as an adverse event in 16.7% of patients receiving β-blockers, compared with 25.1% in those receiving placebo.[140] In an overview of randomized, controlled trials of patients with heart failure comparing β-blockers to placebo, Ko et al.[143] reported that although β-blocker therapy was associated with significant increases in the risk of bradycardia, hypotension, and dizziness, it was also associated with reductions in the incidence of all-cause mortality, hospitalizations for HFrEF, worsening symptoms of HFrEF, and proportion of patients who discontinued therapy with their medications.

MECHANISMS

Mechanisms by which many drugs can induce heart failure can be categorized as those reducing myocardial contractility (calcium-channel blockers, antiarrhythmic agents, anthracyclines, β-blockers), increasing preload (glitazones, NSAIDs, COX-2 inhibitors, corticosteroids), and those increasing afterload (sympathomimetic agents, NSAIDs, and COX-2 inhibitors [via mismatch of vasodilatory and vasoconstrictive prostaglandins]). Mechanisms of drug-induced heart failure are listed in **Table 24-3**. There are several drugs for which the mechanism is unknown, including alogliptin, amantadine, aminocaproic acid, amphotericin B, ampicillin, digoxin immune antibody fragments, bromocriptine, clozapine, cytarabine, dapsone, doxazosin, etanercept, foscarnet, hydralazine, ifosfamide, infliximab, mannitol, pregabalin, saxagliptin, venlafaxine, and zidovudine.

CALCIUM-CHANNEL BLOCKERS

The common mechanism of heart failure associated with the heterogeneous group of calcium-channel blockers is antagonism of L-type calcium channels. All calcium-channel blockers are negative inotropes to varying degrees, but their net effect on cardiac output and symptoms of heart failure depends on other hemodynamic effects in association with the patient's underlying cardiac dysfunction.[144] Verapamil and diltiazem exert strong negative inotropic effects and should be avoided in all patients with HFrEF.[145] Nifedipine

Table 24-3 Mechanisms of Drug-Induced Heart Failure

Drug	Mechanism
Doxorubicin, epirubicin, mitoxantrone	Believed to be related to reduced myocardial contractility Potential mechanisms: Formation of a toxic metabolite Generation of oxygen free radicals Interference with β-adrenergic stimulation of the heart Disturbances in intracellular calcium transport Reduced adenosine diphosphate-stimulated respiration Release of excessive vasoactive compounds such as histamine and catecholamines
Amitriptyline, carbamazepine, clomipramine, diltiazem, disopyramide, encainide, moricizine, flecainide, fluorouracil, imipramine, itraconazole, lidocaine, lorcainide, mexiletine, nifedipine, nortriptyline, propranolol, propafenone, protriptyline, tocainide, verapamil	Reduced myocardial contractility (i.e., negative inotropic effect)
Cabergoline, pergolide	Valvular fibrosis
Aspirin (non-low-dose), celecoxib, diclofenac, diflunisal, etodolac, fenoprofen, flurbiprofen, ibuprofen, indomethacin, ketoprofen, licorice, mefenamic acid, megestrol, meloxicam, minoxidil, nabumetone, naproxen, PEG lavage solution, pioglitazone, piroxicam, prednisolone, rofecoxib, rosiglitazone, sodium-containing antacids, sulindac, tenoxicam, tiaprofenic acid	Increased preload (i.e., fluid retention)
Cyclophosphamide	Endothelial damage, toxic metabolite
Interferon α	Impairment of myocyte metabolism Increased oxygen demand
Blue cohosh, imatinib, anagrelide	Cardiac toxicity
Paclitaxel	Potential exacerbation of anthracycline-induced cardiotoxicity
Sunitinib	Can cause cardiac myocyte apoptosis and mitochondrial injury
Parkinson disease agents	Mechanism unknown, but heart failure may be caused by cardiac valve fibrosis
Etanercept	Blocking the effect of TNFα combined with the other cardiovascular risks of rheumatoid arthritis may cause heart failure

PEG = polyethylene glycol, TNF = tumor necrosis factor.

demonstrates strong negative inotropic effects in vivo and also causes neurohormonal activation via the renin–angiotensin–aldosterone system.[146] Indeed, nifedipine has been associated with serious exacerbations of HFrEF requiring hospitalization and should be avoided in all patients with left ventricular dysfunction.[39] Second-generation dihydropyridine calcium-channel blockers appear to be more vascular-selective, with a lower potential for worsening heart failure.[118,119] In fact, felodipine and amlodipine have both been evaluated as potential therapeutic agents for heart failure. Neither agent was associated with beneficial effects with respect to patient outcomes. However, neither drug provoked an excess of HFrEF exacerbations compared with placebo, suggesting that these agents may be used safely for other purposes (e.g., hypertension, ischemia) in patients with HFrEF, although other alternatives are available such as long-acting nitrates, β-blockers, and ivabradine.

ANTIHYPERGLYCEMIC AGENTS

GLITAZONES

Although the glitazones appear to have predominantly favorable hemodynamic effects in patients with heart failure, their use has been associated with fluid retention and heart failure.[54-58] Glitazones increase plasma volume by 6–7%.[55] The mechanism of fluid retention is not known, but may be related to increased endothelial-cell permeability or effects on renal hemodynamics.[54] Fluid retention associated with glitazones appears to be refractory to treatment with loop diuretics but is reversible upon discontinuation of therapy.[54,57] However, more recent reports and mechanistic studies suggest that diuretics active in the distal collecting duct (i.e., hydrochlorothiazide and spironolactone) may be effective for reducing the degree of fluid retention associated with glitazones.[147,148]

DPP-4 INHIBITORS

Mechanisms by which DPP-4 inhibitors (saxagliptin and alogliptin) cause an increase in hospitalizations for heart failure is unknown.[149] The results of the currently running large trials (such as the CArdiovascular and Renal Microvascular outcomes study with LINAgliptin in patients with type 2 diabetes mellitus at high vascular risk [CARMELINA] study) will help address questions regarding increasing hospitalization due to heart failure associated with this class of agents.[150]

ANTIARRHYTHMIC AGENTS

Many antiarrhythmic drugs reduce myocardial contractility; the net clinical effects reflect the balance of other hemodynamic effects.[29,151] Disopyramide, flecainide, propafenone, and nondihyropyridine calcium-channel blockers appear to have the strongest negative inotropic effects, whereas amiodarone, ibutilide, and dofetilide appear to have negligible adverse negative inotropic effects.[27,28,151] The ANDROMEDA investigators postulated that dronedarone may directly or indirectly worsen heart failure especially in those with pre-existing poor systolic function, but the mechanism remains unknown.[30]

ANTHRACYCLINES

Although the mechanisms of anthracycline-induced heart failure have not been entirely elucidated, oxidative damage may play a role.[152] Formation of a toxic metabolite, generation of oxygen-free radicals, interference with myocardial β-adrenergic stimulation, disturbances in intracellular calcium transport, reduced adenosine diphosphate–stimulated respiration, or release of excessive vasoactive compounds such as histamine and catecholamines have all been suggested as possible mechanisms.[152,153] Although anthracycline-induced heart failure is generally considered irreversible, case reports of complete recovery after doxorubicin-induced cardiac dysfunction have been published.[9,152,154] The risk of doxorubicin-induced cardiac dysfunction is largely dose-dependent, yet cardiotoxicity can occur with low doses in high-risk individuals.[155]

BIOLOGIC AGENTS

Mechanisms by which biologic agents induce cardiovascular toxicity are not well understood. However, the mechanism of therapeutic effect may play an important role. Mechanisms of heart failure induced by specific biologic agents are described below.

TRASTUZUMAB

The mechanism of trastuzumab-induced HFrEF is unknown but is different from that induced by the anthracyclines.[101] Trastuzumab cardiotoxicity is associated with decreased contractility rather than myocyte death.[156] This is supported by myocardial biopsies obtained from patients with trastuzumab-induced cardiac dysfunction, which do not show typical ultrastructural changes (vacuolization or myocyte dropout) on electron microscopy.[157] Data from in vivo and in vitro studies suggest that the mechanism of trastuzumab-induced heart failure may be partially related to direct HER2 blockade and may be associated with disruption of the epidermal growth factor signaling system that is present within the heart.[101,158] Trastuzumab-induced cardiac dysfunction does not appear to be related to cumulative trastuzumab dose and is largely reversible (although the reduction in LVEF persisted in certain patients after discontinuing therapy with trastuzumab), and rechallenge is generally well tolerated.[101,159]

BEVACIZUMAB

Bevacizumab inhibits vascular endothelial growth factor (VEGF) receptors, which may lead to reduction in LVEF and HFrEF via inhibition of angiogenisis and myocardial tissue growth in the heart.[137]

INFLIXIMAB

Infliximab binds with high affinity to the soluble and transmembrane forms of tumor necrosis factor α (TNFα), inhibiting binding of TNFα to its receptor.[150] Blocking the effect of TNFα, combined with other cardiovascular risk factors (such as diabetes, hypertension, and history of cardiovascular events) in patients with rheumatoid arthritis can cause HFrEF or HFpEF.[112]

NSAIDs AND COX-2 INHIBITORS

NSAIDs are a chemically diverse group of compounds associated with a common mechanism of action, which is inhibition of the COX enzyme. In patients with heart failure, kidney homeostasis is maintained mostly by renal prostaglandin E_2 (PGE_2). Inhibition of COX by NSAIDs disrupts kidney homeostasis and leads to sodium and water retention and exacerbation of symptoms of heart failure.[80,160] These drugs have also been reported to antagonize the actions of angiotensin-converting enzyme (ACE) inhibitors and diuretics.[160] There appears to be little clinically important difference between these agents in terms of their potential to exacerbate symptoms of heart failure.[160,161] The mechanism of sodium and fluid retention associated with COX-2 inhibitors is similar to that of NSAIDs.[89,161]

β-BLOCKERS

β-blockers reduce myocardial contractility through competitive antagonism of β1-receptors. β-blockers may initially exacerbate heart failure, especially if initiated at a high dose or with rapid dose increases. However, during chronic therapy, carvedilol, metoprolol, and bisoprolol have been shown to improve LVEF and to reduce the incidence of HFrEF hospitalization and mortality.[140,142] Several mechanisms have been postulated to explain the beneficial effect of β-blockers in heart failure, including reduction in long-term exposure to catecholamines; restoration of myocardial inotropic and chronotropic responsiveness; reduction in circulating plasma concentrations of vasoconstrictors such as norepinephrine, renin, and endothelin reduction in myocardial gene production of inflammatory cytokines; attenuation of left ventricular remodeling; and reduction in the frequency of ventricular premature beats and incidence of sudden cardiac death.[162]

CLINICAL PRESENTATION AND DIFFERENTIAL DIAGNOSIS

The clinical presentation of patients with drug-induced heart failure is not different from that from other causes. Symptoms may occur gradually following initiation of a culprit drug. Signs and symptoms associated with drug-induced heart failure are presented in **Table 24-4**.

The differential diagnosis of drug-induced versus other causes of heart failure or exacerbation of heart failure symptoms may be difficult to distinguish from other common precipitants, such as sodium and fluid excess, ischemia, poor adherence to medical therapy, uncontrolled hypertension, arrhythmias (especially atrial fibrillation), systemic infections, impairment in kidney function, anemia, thyrotoxicosis, ethanol ingestion, pulmonary embolism, and respiratory insufficiency (**Table 24-5**).[31,112-117] In general, a temporal sequence of administration of a new potentially offending agent (or dose increase) with increasing symptoms of heart failure heightens the suspicion of a drug-induced cause.

For most drugs that induce heart failure, worsening symptoms of heart failure begin shortly (within days) after initiation of therapy with the drug or increasing the dose. For those drugs causing fluid retention, plasma volume expansion may take several days to manifest in symptoms of dyspnea.

Table 24-4 Signs and Symptoms Associated with Drug-Induced Heart Failure

- Abdominal pain
- Ascites
- Bloating
- Cough
- Diminishing cognitive function (especially in older patients)
- Dyspnea
- Fatigue
- Gallop rhythm
- Hemoptysis
- Hepatojugular reflux
- Hepatomegaly
- Jugular venous distention
- Nausea
- Nocturia
- Orthopnea
- Paroxysmal nocturnal dyspnea
- Peripheral edema
- Pleural effusion
- Pulmonary edema
- Rales
- Third heart sound (S3)
- Weakness

Table 24-5 Conditions to Consider in the Differential Diagnosis of Drug-Induced Heart Failure

- Anemia
- Arrhythmias (especially atrial fibrillation)
- Hypertensive emergency
- Impairment in kidney function
- Myocardial ischemia/infarction
- New onset heart failure (nondrug-induced)
- Pulmonary embolism
- Respiratory insufficiency
- Sodium and fluid excess
- Systemic infections
- Thyrotoxicosis
- Uncontrolled hypertension
- Valve disease

RISK FACTORS

Risk factors for drug-induced heart failure are presented in **Table 24-6**. The most important risk factor for the development of drug-induced heart failure is pre-existing symptomatic or asymptomatic left ventricular dysfunction.[9] In general, older patients are more susceptible to drug-induced diseases; whether this factor applies to drug-induced heart failure is not known.

ANTIHYPERGLYCEMIC AGENTS

GLITAZONES

In their review of 111 consecutive patients with diabetes and systolic heart failure treated with a glitazone, Tang et al.[55] noted upon univariate analyses that females and insulin users were at increased risk of fluid retention. Interestingly, these authors found no association between baseline severity of heart failure and the occurrence of fluid retention. Risk factors for glitazone-induced heart failure, including those described by the American Heart Association/American Diabetes Association consensus statement, are presented in Table 24-6.[56]

DPP-4 INHIBITORS

To be eligible to take part in the published cardiovascular safety trials of DPP-4 inhibitors, patients had to be at high risk for cardiovascular events, including acute coronary syndrome, clinical events associated with atherosclerosis (age 40 years or over) and dyslipidemia, or hypertension or smoking combined with age 55 years or older (males) or 60 years or older (females).[122-124] Pre-existing heart failure was the predominant risk factor for the development of heart failure associated with DPP4-inhibitors.[122-124]

ANTIARRHYTHMIC AGENTS

As with most other heart failure–inducing agents, the predominant risk factor for the development of antiarrhythmic-induced HFrEF is pre-existing left ventricular dysfunction.[29] Unfortunately, patients with HFrEF are also at high risk for sudden cardiac death. Risk versus benefit evaluation is extremely important in this patient population as many antiarrhythmic agents worsen heart failure symptoms. Amiodarone, dofetilide, and ibutilide are the antiarrythmic agents that are associated with minimal effects on myocardial contractility.[130]

Table 24-6 Risk Factors for Drug-Induced Heart Failure

Antiarrhythmic agents

- Pre-existing heart failure

DPP-4 inhibitors

- Pre-existing heart failure

Glitazones

- Pre-existing left ventricular dysfunction
- History of myocardial infarction
- History of symptomatic coronary artery disease
- Hypertension
- Left ventricular hypertrophy
- Significant aortic or mitral valve disease
- Advanced age (>70 years)
- Long-standing diabetes (>10 years)
- Pre-existing edema
- Current treatment with loop diuretics
- Development of edema or weight gain
- Insulin coadministration
- Chronic kidney disease

Anthracyclines

- Cumulative doxorubicin dose (≥550 mg/m^2)
- Three-week schedule of administration
- Older age
- Concomitant cardiac irradiation
- Concomitant use of cyclophosphamide, amsacrine, fluorouracil, dactinomycin, mithramycin, mitomycin, or vincristine
- Children:
  - Higher cumulative dose
  - Cardiac irradiation
  - Age at treatment (<4 years)
  - Maximal dose within 1 week (>45 mg/m^2)
  - Time since treatment (within 1 week of treatment)
  - Use of daunorubicin (as opposed to doxorubicin)
  - Amsacrine
  - Black race
  - Female sex
  - Trisomy 21

Biologic agents

- Older age
- Higher body-mass index
- Antihypertensive therapy
- Lower pretrastuzumab left ventricular ejection fraction
- Concurrent anthracycline use
- Cumulative anthracycline dose
- Concurrent taxanes and capecitabine
- Pre-existing rheumatoid arthritis
- History of coronary heart disease

DPP = dipeptidyl peptidase.

ANTHRACYCLINES

Risk factors for anthracycline-induced HFrEF have been well-described (Table 24-6).[20,22,152,153] Von Hoff et al.[20] reported an increasing risk of heart failure associated with increasing cumulative doses of doxorubicin. The schedule of administration also appears to influence the risk of doxorubicin-induced heart failure; weekly doses were associated with a significantly lower incidence of HFrEF as compared with larger doses on a 3-week schedule (single dose repeated every 3 weeks or three consecutive daily doses repeated every 3 weeks).[20] There is a general increase in the risk of development of doxorubicin-induced heart failure with increasing age. However, the incidence of doxorubicin-induced heart failure is higher in children (younger than 15 years of age) than in adults. All three of these risk factors (total dose, schedule of administration, and age) remained as independent predictors of the development of heart failure after multivariate analysis.[20] The use of other antitumor therapies such as cardiac irradiation and specific antineoplastic agents may also increase the risk.[152] Risk factors for drug-induced heart failure in children receiving anthracycline therapy are also presented in Table 24-6. Kremer et al.[22] determined that the multivariate risk factors were a maximal dose >45 mg/m^2 within 1 week and the use of daunorubicin.

BIOLOGIC AGENTS

Risk factors for heart failure induced by biologic agents include older age, higher body-mass index, antihypertensive therapy, lower pretrastuzumab LVEF, concurrent anthracycline therapy, concomitant therapy with taxanes and capecitabine, cumulative anthracycline dose, rheumatoid arthritis, and history of coronary heart disease.[98,112,131,132,137,163,164]

MORBIDITY AND MORTALITY

Mortality associated with heart failure is very high, with an annual mortality incidence of 5–10% in patients with mild disease and up to 30–40% in those with more advanced disease.[3] The incidence of in-hospital mortality associated with heart failure is 3.5–15%.[4,6] Moreover, about 20–50% of patients discharged alive from the hospital with heart failure are readmitted within the subsequent 6–12 months.[4,165]

Specific data regarding the incidence of morbidity and mortality associated with drug-induced heart failure are scarce. Doxorubicin-induced heart failure is associated with a mortality rate between 30 and 60%.[20,153] Clearly, there is a need for more epidemiologic data to address the prognosis associated with drug-induced heart failure.

PREVENTION

Obviously, the best preventive measure is to avoid the offending agents (**Table 24-7**). Although this is not always possible, particular caution should be exercised in patients with pre-existing left ventricular dysfunction.

Because of the high incidence of drug-induced heart failure, diltiazem, verapamil, disopyramide, flecainide, and propafenone should be considered contraindicated in patients with heart failure or asymptomatic left ventricular dysfunction (LVEF <0.40). As mentioned previously, felodipine and amlodipine are safer alternatives in patients with heart failure, as compared with nondihydropyridine calcium-channel blockers or nifedipine. In general, patients with diabetes and heart failure should be treated in a similar manner to those without heart failure, with the exception that diabetes-related comorbidities may influence drug doses and monitoring of therapy. Alternatives to glitazones for blood-glucose control include insulin secretagogues (e.g., sulfonylureas, meglitinides), metformin (in those with an estimated glomerular filtration rate >30 mL/min), α-glucosidase inhibitors, incretin agents, and insulin.[166,167] To date, DPP-4 inhibitors are the most studied class of diabetes medications.[168] Overall, these agents do not increase the risk of cardiovascular death, stroke, or myocardial infarction, but their association with the risk of heart failure remains uncertain.[126,168] More well-powered studies are required to determine this relationship.[168] The Empagliflozin Cardiovascular Outcome Event Trial in Type 2 Diabetes Mellitus Patients (EMPA-REG Outcomes) study investigators compared the effect of empagliflozin and placebo on cardiovascular morbidity and mortality in adults with type 2 diabetes and established cardiovascular disease.[169] They reported lower rates of death from cardiovascular causes, nonfatal myocardial infarction, or nonfatal stroke in the empagliflozin group when compared to placebo (HR 0.86, 95% CI 0.74–0.99, p <0.001). They also reported less hospitalization for heart failure in the empagliflozin group (HR 0.65, 95% CI 0.50–0.85, p = 0.002).[169]

Table 24-7 Approaches to Help Prevent Drug-Induced Heart Failure

- Avoid potentially causative agents
- Prevent anthracycline-induced cardiomyopathy with coenzyme Q10, carnitine, pretreatment with antihistamines, cromolyn sodium, probucol, or dexrazoxane (when the cumulative dose of doxorubicin reaches 300 mg/m^2)
- Prevent β-blocker–induced heart failure by starting at low doses with slow careful titration of doses over 6–8 weeks

A number of agents have been suggested for reducing the incidence of anthracycline-induced cardiomyopathy including coenzyme Q10, carnitine, pretreatment with antihistamines, antiadrenergics, cromolyn sodium, probucol, dexrazoxane, *N*-acetylcysteine, vitamin E, amifostine, carvedilol, ACE inhibitors, vitamin A, vitamin C, selenium and glutathione.[152,170,171] Dexrazoxane (60–900 mg/m^2 with 60 mg/m^2 of doxorubicin or 500 mg/m^2 with 50 mg/m^2 of doxorubicin) is indicated for reduction of the incidence and severity of cardiomyopathy associated with doxorubicin in women with breast cancer who received a cumulative dose of 300 mg/m^2 and who would benefit from further doxorubicin administration.[152] Dexrazoxane is not indicated for use during the initiation of therapy with doxorubicin. Other potential strategies to limit anthracycline toxicity include limiting the cumulative dose of anthracycline, replacing bolus administration with slow infusion, and using liposomal anthracyclines in place of traditional formulations.

Depending on the indication, several alternatives to NSAIDs or COX-2 inhibitors exist. For example, for the treatment of osteoarthritis in the presence of heart failure, nonpharmacologic (e.g., physical therapy), traditional pharmacologic (e.g., acetaminophen, intraarticular steroid injections), and nontraditional pharmacologic (e.g., glucosamine) therapies may be preferable. It has been reported that if administered in low doses for a short period of time, nonprescription NSAIDs may be associated with much lower risk of adverse events and drug–drug interactions.[172,173] In patients initiated on β-blockers for heart failure, starting therapy at low doses with slow and careful titration over 6–8 weeks or more will help to minimize the likelihood of an exacerbation of HFrEF.[1,2,142]

Excessive alcohol consumption is associated with cardiomyopathy.[174] The mechanism of this change is not well understood but reduced myocardial contractility has been suggested as one of the main causes.[175] Individuals who consume excessive amounts of alcohol were at higher risk for developing heart failure when compared to those who do not drink alcohol.[176] It has been reported that low-to-moderate alcohol consumption is associated with reduced risk of heart failure, but due to the lack of a high-level evidence, more studies are required to understand this relationship.[177]

MANAGEMENT

The management of drug-induced new-onset heart failure and acute exacerbations of heart failure symptoms includes aggressive diuresis and general supportive care.[1,178] Following discontinuation of therapy with the offending agent, management of drug-induced heart failure exacerbations is the same as the usual management of heart failure. Generally, recovery of the myocardium is related to the elimination half-life of the offending agent (the exception is doxorubicin, with an average onset of recovery of 30 days after the last dose).[20] Reduction or abstinence from alcohol consumption was associated with improvement in cardiac function in patients with alcoholic cardiomyopathy.[179] After the acute event, clinicians should be vigilant in ensuring that all patients with heart failure are receiving all efficacious therapies (and at target doses), including ACE inhibitors or angiotensin receptor blockers, neprilysin inhibitors, β-blockers, and, in selected patients, spironolactone or digoxin or both.[1,2] Traditional NSAID and COX-2 inhibitor–induced heart failure is a particularly vexing clinical problem, as many patients with heart failure have osteoarthritis and gout, which negatively impact quality of life, and these patients could otherwise benefit from these therapies. In these situations, alternative nonpharmacologic and pharmacologic therapies (e.g., acetaminophen) may be preferable. Rechallenge with drugs that have induced or exacerbated heart failure is generally not recommended.

The high prevalence of heart failure and the clinical fragility of such patients suggest that pharmacists' close monitoring can have a great impact. In a systematic review of 12 randomized trials that included 2,060 patients, the addition of a pharmacist to the heart failure team resulted in a 31% reduction in heart failure hospitalizations.[180] Pharmacists can identify patients at risk for drug-induced heart failure, identify drug-induced causes of exacerbations of symptoms of heart failure, guide treatment choices to avoid agents that could exacerbate heart failure, institute appropriate preventive measures when necessary, counsel patients with heart failure on the use of nonprescription medications, and ensure that patients are receiving all proven efficacious therapies for heart failure (ACE inhibitors, neprilysin inhibitors, β-blockers, spironolactone, digoxin) at target doses.

INFORMATION FOR PATIENTS

When the use of a potentially offending agent is unavoidable in patients with HFrEF, patients should be alerted to the signs and symptoms of heart failure. Early detection and treatment of drug-induced heart failure may prevent hospitalization or death. Healthcare personnel should be alerted if the patient develops any of the following: shortness of breath, loss of appetite, rapid weight gain, swelling in lower limbs, abdominal swelling and/or pain, frequent dry hacking cough, increased fatigue with less effort, or difficulty falling asleep.[181,182] This is particularly important in light of studies that have shown that even in patients with long-standing heart failure, knowledge of signs and symptoms is very poor.[183,184] All patients with heart failure should be alerted to the dangers of nonprescription therapies such as NSAIDs, licorice-containing herbal remedies, and sympathomimetics such as those in cough and cold preparations. Patients with heart failure should consult their physician or pharmacist prior to initiating therapy with any new medications, including nonprescription and herbal remedies. Education of patients and their families and friends is very important to improve patients' recognition of early warning symptoms and signs, ensure early intervention before acute heart failure deterioration, and avoidance of exacerbations of drug-induced heart failure. In addition, patients should weigh themselves daily to track changes in body weight that might be indicative of fluid retention (>1 kg/day). In certain situations, patients may be taught how to adjust their diuretic dose based on these changes in body weight and symptoms.

REFERENCES

1. Yancy CW, Jessup M, Bozkurt B et al. 2016 ACC/AHA/HFSA Focused Update on New Pharmacological Therapy for Heart Failure: An Update of the 2013 ACCF/AHA Guideline for the Management of Heart Failure. A Report of the American College of Cardiology/American Heart Association Task Force on Clinical Practice Guidelines and the Heart Failure Society of America. *J Am Coll Cardiol.* 2016; 68:1476-88.
2. McKelvie RS, Moe GW, Ezekowitz JA et al. The 2012 Canadian Cariovascular Society heart failure management guideline update: focus on acute and chronic heart failure. *Can J Cardiol.* 2013; 29:168-81.
3. Massie BM, Shah NB. Evolving trends in the epidemiologic factors of heart failure: rationale for preventive strategies and comprehensive disease management. *Am Heart J.* 1997; 133:703-12.
4. Tsuyuki RT, Shibata MC, Nilsson C et al. Contemporary burden of illness of congestive heart failure in Canada. *Can J Cardiol.* 2003; 19:436-8.
5. DeFrances C, Cullen K, Kozak L. National Hospital Discharge Survey: 2005 annual summary with detailed diagnosis and procedure data. National Centre for Health Statistics. *Vital Health Stat.* 2007; 13.
6. Fonarow GC, Heywood JT, Heidenreich PA et al. Temporal trends in clinical characteristics, treatments, and outcomes for heart failure hospitalizations, 2002 to 2004: findings from Acute Decompensated Heart Failure National Registry (ADHERE). *Am Heart J.* 2007; 153:1021-8.
7. Baliga RR, Haas GJ. *Management of heart failure.* 2nd ed. London, England: Springer-Verlag; 2015.
8. American Heart Association. *Causes and risks for heart failure.* http://www.heart.org/HEARTORG/Conditions/HeartFailure/CausesAndRisksForHeartFailure/Causes-and-Risks-for-Heart-Failure_UCM_002046_Article.jsp#.V0XLnrgrLq4 (accessed 2018 Feb 1).
9. Feenstra J, Grobbee DE, Remme WJ et al. Drug-induced heart failure. *J Am Coll Cardiol.* 1999; 33:1152-62.
10. McMurray JJV, Adamopoulos S, Anker SD et al. ESC guidelines for the diagnosis and treatment of acute and chronic heart failure 2012. *Eur Heart J.* 2012; 33:1787-1847.
11. Borlaug BA. Heart failure with preserved and reduced ejection fraction: different risk profiles for different diseases. *Eur Heart J.* 2013; 34:1393-5.
12. ALLHAT Collaborative Research Group. Major cardiovascular events in hypertensive patients randomized to doxazosin vs chlorthalidone: the antihypertensive and lipid-lowering treatment to prevent heart attack trial (ALLHAT). *JAMA.* 2000; 283:1967-75.
13. Vale JA, Maclean KS. Amantadine-induced heart-failure. *Lancet.* 1977; 1:548.
14. Johansson SA. Acute right heart failure during treatment with epsilon amino caproic acid (E-ACA). *Acta Med Scand.* 1967; 182:331-4.
15. Arsura EL, Ismail Y, Freedman S et al. Amphotericin B-induced dilated cardiomyopathy. *Am J Med.* 1994; 97:560-2.
16. Danaher PJ, Cao MK, Anstead GM et al. Reversible dilated cardiomyopathy related to amphotericin B therapy. *J Antimicrob Chemother.* 2004; 53:115-7.
17. Anagrelide Study Group. Anagrelide, a therapy for thrombocythemic states: experience in 577 patients. *Am J Med.* 1992; 92:69-76.
18. Schimmel KJ, Richel DJ, van den Brink RB et al. Cardiotoxicity of cytotoxic drugs. *Cancer Treat Rev.* 2004; 30:181-91.
19. Pai VB, Nahata MC. Cardiotoxicity of chemotherapeutic agents: incidence, treatment and prevention. *Drug Saf.* 2000; 22:263-302.
20. Von Hoff DD, Layard MW, Basa P et al. Risk factors for doxorubicin-induced congestive heart failure. *Ann Intern Med.* 1979; 91:710-17.
21. Swain SM, Whaley FS, Ewer MS. Congestive heart failure in patients treated with doxorubicin: a retrospective analysis of three trials. *Cancer.* 2003; 97:2869-79.
22. Kremer LC, van Dalen EC, Offringa M et al. Frequency and risk factors of anthracycline-induced clinical heart failure in children: a systematic review. *Ann Oncol.* 2002; 13:503-12.
23. van Dalen EC, van der Pal HJH, Kok WEM et al. Clinical heart failure in a cohort of children treated with anthracyclines: a long-term follow-up study. *Eur J Cancer.* 2006; 42:3191-8.
24. Jensen BV, Skovsgaard T, Nielsen SL. Functional monitoring of anthracycline cardiotoxicity: a prospective, blinded, long-term observational study of outcome in 120 patients. *Ann Oncol.* 2002; 13:699-709.
25. Kelly RA, Smith TW. Recognition and management of digitalis toxicity. *Am J Cardiol.* 1992; 69:108G-19G.
26. Pharand C, Kluger J, O'Rangers E et al. Lidocaine prophylaxis for fatal ventricular arrhythmias after acute myocardial infarction. *Clin Pharmacol Ther.* 1995; 57:471-8.
27. Greene HL, Richardson DW, Hallstrom AP et al. Congestive heart failure after acute myocardial infarction in patients receiving antiarrhythmic agents for ventricular premature complexes (Cardiac Arrhythmia Pilot Study). *Am J Cardiol.* 1989; 63:393-8.
28. Ravid S, Podrid PJ, Lampert S et al. Congestive heart failure induced by six of the newer antiarrhythmic drugs. *J Am Coll Cardiol.* 1989; 14:1326-30.
29. Pfisterer M. Negative inotropic effects of antiarrhythmic drugs: a clinical point of view. *J Cardiovasc Pharmacol.* 1991; 17(suppl 6): S44-7.
30. Kober L, Torp-Pedersen C, McMurray JJ et al. Increased mortality after dronedarone therapy for severe heart failure. *N Engl J Med.* 2008; 358:2678-87.
31. Garcia Robles JA, Moreno Barrio F, Lombardia Prieto J et al. [Clinical study of the causes of cardiac insufficiency in 100 patients over 65 years of age]. *Rev Clin Esp.* 1988; 183:20-3.
32. Greenblatt DJ, Koch-Weser J. Adverse reactions to beta-adrenergic receptor blocking drugs: a report from the Boston Collaborative Drug Surveillance Program. *Drugs.* 1974; 7:118-29.
33. Jones TK, Lawson BM. Profound neonatal congestive heart failure caused by maternal consumption of blue cohosh herbal medication. *J Pediatr.* 1998; 132:550-2.
34. Dukes M. *Meyler's Side Effects of Drugs.* 14th ed. Amsterdam, the Netherlands: Elsevier Science; 1996.

35. Horvath J, Fross RD, Kleiner-Fisman G et al. Severe multivalvular heart disease: a new complication of the ergot derivative dopamine agonists. *Mov Disord.* 2004; 19:656-62.
36. Ling LH, Ahlskog JE, Munger TM et al. Constrictive pericarditis and pleuropulmonary disease linked to ergot dopamine agonist therapy (cabergoline) for Parkinson's disease. *Mayo Clin Proc.* 1999; 74:371-5.
37. Townsend M, MacIver DH. Constrictive pericarditis and pleuropulmonary fibrosis secondary to cabergoline treatment for Parkinson's disease. *Heart.* 2004; 90:e47.
38. Goldstein RE, Boccuzzi SJ, Cruess D et al. Diltiazem increases late-onset congestive heart failure in postinfarction patients with early reduction in ejection fraction. The Adverse Experience Committee; and the Multicenter Diltiazem Postinfarction Research Group. *Circulation.* 1991; 83:52-60.
39. Elkayam U, Amin J, Mehra A et al. A prospective, randomized, double-blind, crossover study to compare the efficacy and safety of chronic nifedipine therapy with that of isosorbide dinitrate and their combination in the treatment of chronic congestive heart failure. *Circulation.* 1990; 82:1954-61.
40. Ferlinz J, Gallo C. Responses of patients in heart failure to long-term verapamil administration. *Circulation.* 1984; 70(suppl 2):305.
41. Killian JG, Kerr K, Lawrence C et al. Myocarditis and cardiomyopathy associated with clozapine. *Lancet.* 1999; 354:1841-5.
42. Juul Povlsen U, Noring U, Fog R et al. Tolerability and therapeutic effect of clozapine: a retrospective investigation of 216 patients treated with clozapine for up to 12 years. *Acta Psychiatr Scand.* 1985; 71:176-85.
43. Leo RJ, Kreeger JL, Kim KY. Cardiomyopathy associated with clozapine. *Ann Pharmacother.* 1996; 30:603-5.
44. Phan KL, Taylor SF. Clozapine-associated cardiomyopathy. *Psychosomatics.* 2002; 43:248.
45. Sholter DE, Armstrong PW. Adverse effects of corticosteroids on the cardiovascular system. *Can J Cardiol.* 2000; 16:505-11.
46. Wei L, MacDonald TM, Walker BR. Taking glucocorticoids by prescription is associated with subsequent cardiovascular disease. *Ann Intern Med.* 2004; 141:764-70.
47. Ayash LJ, Wright JE, Tretyakov O et al. Cyclophosphamide pharmacokinetics: correlation with cardiac toxicity and tumor response. *J Clin Oncol.* 1992; 10:995-1000.
48. Manthorpe R, Svensson O. Cardiomyopathy following intravenous cyclophosphamide therapy in a patient with Wegener's granulomatosis. *Clin Exp Rheumatol.* 1996; 14:702-3.
49. Conrad ME. Cytarabine and cardiac failure. *Am J Hematol.* 1992; 41:143-4.
50. Cowan RE, Wright JT. Dapsone and severe hypoalbuminaemia in dermatitis herpetiformis. *Br J Dermatol.* 1981; 104:201-4.
51. Kwon HJ, Cote TR, Cuffe MS et al. Case reports of heart failure after therapy with a tumor necrosis factor antagonist. *Ann Intern Med.* 2003; 138:807-11.
52. Schober C, Papageorgiou E, Harstrick A et al. Cardiotoxicity of 5-fluorouracil in combination with folinic acid in patients with gastrointestinal cancer. *Cancer.* 1993; 72:2242-7.
53. Brown DL, Sather S, Cheitlin MD. Reversible cardiac dysfunction associated with foscarnet therapy for cytomegalovirus esophagitis in an AIDS patient. *Am Heart J.* 1993; 125:1439-41.
54. Mudaliar S, Henry RR. New oral therapies for type 2 diabetes mellitus: the glitazones or insulin sensitizers. *Annu Rev Med.* 2001; 52:239-57.
55. Tang WH, Francis GS, Hoogwerf BJ et al. Fluid retention after initiation of thiazolidinedione therapy in diabetic patients with established chronic heart failure. *J Am Coll Cardiol.* 2003; 41:1394-8.
56. Nesto RW, Bell D, Bonow RO et al. Thiazolidinedione use, fluid retention, and congestive heart failure: a consensus statement from the American Heart Association and American Diabetes Association. *Circulation.* 2003; 108:2941-8.
57. Wooltorton E. Rosiglitazone (Avandia) and pioglitazone (Actos) and heart failure. *CMAJ.* 2002; 166:219.
58. Wang CH, Weisel RD, Liu PP et al. Glitazones and heart failure: critical appraisal for the clinician. *Circulation.* 2003; 107:1350-4.
59. Singh S, Loke YK, Furberg CD. Long-term risk of cardiovascular events with rosiglitazone: a meta-analysis. *JAMA.* 2007; 298:1189-95.
60. Gerstein HC, Yusuf S, Bosch J et al. Effect of rosiglitazone on the frequency of diabetes in patients with impaired glucose tolerance or impaired fasting glucose: a randomised controlled trial. *Lancet.* 2006; 368:1096-1105.
61. Home PD, Pocock SJ, Beck-Nielsen H et al. Rosiglitazone evaluated for cardiovascular outcomes—an interim analysis. *N Engl J Med.* 2007; 357:28-38.
62. Lago RM, Singh PP, Nesto RW. Congestive heart failure and cardiovascular death in patients with prediabetes and type 2 diabetes given thiazolidinediones: a meta-analysis of randomised clinical trials. *Lancet.* 2007; 370:1129-36.
63. Singh S, Loke YK, Furberg CD. Thiazolidinediones and heart failure: a teleo-analysis. *Diabetes Care.* 2007; 30:2148-53.
64. Delea TE, Edelsberg JS, Hagiwara M et al. Use of thiazolidinediones and risk of heart failure in people with type 2 diabetes: a retrospective cohort study. *Diabetes Care.* 2003; 26:2983-9.
65. Dormandy JA, Charbonnel B, Eckland DJ et al. Secondary prevention of macrovascular events in patients with type 2 diabetes in the PROactive Study (PROspective pioglitAzone Clinical Trial In macroVascular Events): a randomised controlled trial. *Lancet.* 2005; 366:1279-89.
66. Lincoff AM, Wolski K, Nicholls SJ et al. Pioglitazone and risk of cardiovascular events in patients with type 2 diabetes mellitus: a meta-analysis of randomized trials. *JAMA.* 2007; 298:1180-8.
67. Quezado ZM, Wilson WH, Cunnion RE et al. High-dose ifosfamide is associated with severe, reversible cardiac dysfunction. *Ann Intern Med.* 1993; 118:31-6.
68. Kerkela R, Grazette L, Yacobi R et al. Cardiotoxicity of the cancer therapeutic agent imatinib mesylate. *Nat Med.* 2006; 12: 908-16.
69. Chung ES, Packer M, Lo KH et al. Randomized, double-blind, placebo-controlled, pilot trial of infliximab, a chimeric monoclonal antibody to tumor necrosis factor-alpha, in patients with moderate-to-severe heart failure: results of the anti-TNF Therapy Against Congestive Heart Failure (ATTACH) trial. *Circulation.* 2003; 107:3133-40.
70. Cohen MC, Huberman MS, Nesto RW. Recombinant alpha 2 interferon-related cardiomyopathy. *Am J Med.* 1988; 85:549-51.
71. Sonnenblick M, Rosenmann D, Rosin A. Reversible cardiomyopathy induced by interferon. *BMJ.* 1990; 300:1174-5.
72. Deyton LR, Walker RE, Kovacs JA et al. Reversible cardiac dysfunction associated with interferon alfa therapy in AIDS patients with Kaposi's sarcoma. *N Engl J Med.* 1989; 321:1246-9.
73. Ahmad SR, Singer SJ, Leissa BG. Congestive heart failure associated with itraconazole. *Lancet.* 2001; 357:1766-7.
74. Ferguson JE, Chalmers RJ, Rowlands DJ. Reversible dilated cardiomyopathy following treatment of atopic eczema with Chinese herbal medicine. *Br J Dermatol.* 1997; 136:592-3.
75. Oken DE. Renal and extrarenal considerations in high-dose mannitol therapy. *Ren Fail.* 1994; 16:147-59.
76. Tchekmedyian NS, Tait N, Aisner J. High-dose megestrol acetate in the treatment of postmenopausal women with advanced breast cancer. *Semin Oncol.* 1986; 13:20-5.
77. Nathan M, Rubin SA, Siemienczuk D et al. Effects of acute and chronic minoxidil administration on rest and exercise hemodynamics and clinical status in patients with severe, chronic heart failure. *Am J Cardiol.* 1982; 50:960-6.
78. Mather FJ, Simon RM, Clark GM et al. Cardiotoxicity in patients treated with mitoxantrone: Southwest Oncology Group phase II studies. *Cancer Treat Rep.* 1987; 71:609-13.

79. Heerdink ER, Leufkens HG, Herings RM et al. NSAIDs associated with increased risk of congestive heart failure in elderly patients taking diuretics. *Arch Intern Med.* 1998; 158:1108-12.
80. Bleumink GS, Feenstra J, Sturkenboom MC et al. Nonsteroidal anti-inflammatory drugs and heart failure. *Drugs.* 2003; 63:525-34.
81. Page J, Henry D. Consumption of NSAIDs and the development of congestive heart failure in elderly patients: an underrecognized public health problem. *Arch Intern Med.* 2000; 160:777-84.
82. Merlo J, Broms K, Lindblad U et al. Association of outpatient utilisation of non-steroidal anti-inflammatory drugs and hospitalised heart failure in the entire Swedish population. *Eur J Clin Pharmacol.* 2001; 57:71-5.
83. Feenstra J, Heerdink ER, Grobbee DE et al. Association of nonsteroidal anti-inflammatory drugs with first occurrence of heart failure and with relapsing heart failure: the Rotterdam Study. *Arch Intern Med.* 2002; 162:265-70.
84. Garcia Rodriguez LA, Diaz S. Nonsteroidal antiinflammatory drugs as a trigger of clinical heart failure. *Epidemiology.* 2003; 14:240-6.
85. Mamdani M, Juurlink DN, Lee DS et al. Cyclooxygenase-2 inhibitors versus non-selective non-steroidal anti-inflammatory drugs and congestive heart failure outcomes in elderly patients: a population-based cohort study. *Lancet.* 2004; 363:1751-6.
86. Hudson M, Richard H, Pilote L. Differences in outcomes of patients with congestive heart failure prescribed celecoxib, rofecoxib, or non-steroidal antiinflammatory drugs: population based study. *BMJ.* 2005; 330:1370.
87. Whelton A, White WB, Bello AE et al. Effects of celecoxib and rofecoxib on blood pressure and edema in patients > or =65 years of age with systemic hypertension and osteoarthritis. *Am J Cardiol.* 2002; 90:959-63.
88. Whelton A, Fort JG, Puma JA et al. Cyclooxygenase2–specific inhibitors and cardiorenal function: a randomized, controlled trial of celecoxib and rofecoxib in older hypertensive osteoarthritis patients. *Am J Ther.* 2001; 8:85-95.
89. Zhao SZ, Burke TA, Whelton A et al. Cost of heart failure among hypertensive users of nonspecific NSAIDs and COX-2-specific inhibitors. *Am J Manag Care.* 2002; 8(suppl 15):S414-27.
90. Jekunen A, Heikkila P, Maiche A et al. Paclitaxel-induced myocardial damage detected by electron microscopy. *Lancet.* 1994; 343:727-8.
91. Gianni L, Munzone E, Capri G et al. Paclitaxel by 3-hour infusion in combination with bolus doxorubicin in women with untreated metastatic breast cancer: high antitumor efficacy and cardiac effects in a dose-finding and sequence-finding study. *J Clin Oncol.* 1995; 13:2688-99.
92. Granberry MC, White LM, Gardner SF. Exacerbation of congestive heart failure after administration of polyethylene glycol-electrolyte lavage solution. *Ann Pharmacother.* 1995; 29:1232-5.
93. Banerjee D. Myocarditis in penicillin sensitivity. *Indian Heart J.* 1968; 20:72-5.
94. Garty BZ, Offer I, Livni E et al. Erythema multiforme and hypersensitivity myocarditis caused by ampicillin. *Ann Pharmacother.* 1994; 28:730-1.
95. Pritchett AM, Morrison JF, Edwards WD et al. Valvular heart disease in patients taking pergolide. *Mayo Clin Proc.* 2002; 77:1280-6.
96. Van Camp G, Flamez A, Cosyns B et al. Heart valvular disease in patients with Parkinson's disease treated with high-dose pergolide. *Neurology.* 2003; 61:859-61.
97. Murphy N, Mockler M, Ryder M et al. Decompensation of chronic heart failure associated with pregabalin in patients with neuropathic pain. *J Card Fail.* 2007; 13:227-9.
98. Slamon DJ, Leyland-Jones B, Shak S et al. Use of chemotherapy plus a monoclonal antibody against HER2 for metastatic breast cancer that overexpresses HER2. *N Engl J Med.* 2001; 344:783-92.
99. Vogel CL, Cobleigh MA, Tripathy D et al. Efficacy and safety of trastuzumab as a single agent in first-line treatment of HER2-overexpressing metastatic breast cancer. *J Clin Oncol.* 2002; 20:719-26.
100. Suter TM, Cook-Bruns N, Barton C. Cardiotoxicity associated with trastuzumab (Herceptin) therapy in the treatment of metastatic breast cancer. *Breast.* 2004; 13:173-83.
101. Ewer SM, Ewer MS. Cardiotoxicity profile of trastuzumab. *Drug Saf.* 2008; 31:459-67.
102. Seidman A, Hudis C, Pierri MK et al. Cardiac dysfunction in the trastuzumab clinical trials experience. *J Clin Oncol.* 2002; 20:1215-21.
103. Cobleigh MA, Vogel CL, Tripathy D et al. Multinational study of the efficacy and safety of humanized anti-HER2 monoclonal antibody in women who have HER2-overexpressing metastatic breast cancer that has progressed after chemotherapy for metastatic disease. *J Clin Oncol.* 1999; 17:2639-48.
104. Dalack GW, Roose SP, Glassman AH. Tricyclics and heart failure. *Am J Psychiatry.* 1991; 148:1601.
105. Howland JS, Poe TE, Keith JF Jr. Cardiomyopathy associated with tricyclic antidepressants. *South Med J.* 1983; 76:1455-6.
106. Jefferson JW. Cardiovascular effects and toxicity of anxiolytics and antidepressants. *J Clin Psychiatry.* 1989; 50:368-78.
107. Marti V, Ballester M, Obrador D et al. Reversal of dilated cardiomyopathy after chronic tricyclic antidepressant drug withdrawal. *Int J Cardiol.* 1995; 48:192-4.
108. Drent M, Singh S, Gorgels AP et al. Drug-induced pneumonitis and heart failure simultaneously associated with venlafaxine. *Am J Respir Crit Care Med.* 2003; 167:958-61.
109. Herskowitz A, Willoughby SB, Baughman KL et al. Cardiomyopathy associated with antiretroviral therapy in patients with HIV infection: a report of six cases. *Ann Intern Med.* 1992; 116:311-3.
110. Amabile CM, Spencer AP. Keeping your patient with heart failure safe: a review of potentially dangerous medications. *Arch Intern Med.* 2004; 164:709-20.
111. Slordal L, Spigset O. Heart failure induced by non-cardiac drugs. *Drug Saf.* 2006; 29:567-86.
112. Maxwell CB, Jenkins AT. Drug-induced heart failure. *Am J Health-Syst Pharm.* 2011; 68:1791-1804.
113. Tsuyuki RT, McKelvie RS, Arnold JM et al. Acute precipitants of congestive heart failure exacerbations. *Arch Intern Med.* 2001; 161:2337-42.
114. Rich MW, Shah AS, Vinson JM et al. Iatrogenic congestive heart failure in older adults: clinical course and prognosis. *J Am Geriatr Soc.* 1996; 44:638-43.
115. Ghali JK, Kadakia S, Cooper R et al. Precipitating factors leading to decompensation of heart failure: traits among urban blacks. *Arch Intern Med.* 1988; 148:2013-6.
116. Opasich C, Febo O, Riccardi PG et al. Concomitant factors of decompensation in chronic heart failure. *Am J Cardiol.* 1996; 78:354-7.
117. Chin MH, Goldman L. Factors contributing to the hospitalization of patients with congestive heart failure. *Am J Public Health.* 1997; 87:643-8.
118. Packer M, Carson P, Elkayam U et al. Effect of Amlodipine on the Survival of Patients With Severe Chronic Heart Failure Due to a Nonischemic Cardiomyopathy: Results of the PRAISE-2 Study (Prospective Randomized Amlodipine Survival Evaluation 2). *JACC Heart Failure.* 2013; 1:308-14.
119. Cohn JN, Ziesche S, Smith R et al. Effect of the calcium antagonist felodipine as supplementary vasodilator therapy in patients with chronic heart failure treated with enalapril: V-HeFT III. Vasodilator-Heart Failure Trial (V-HeFT) Study Group. *Circulation.* 1997; 96:856-63.
120. Kahn SE, Haffner SM, Heise MA et al. Glycemic durability of rosiglitazone, metformin, or glyburide monotherapy. *N Engl J Med.* 2006; 355:2427-43.

121. Nissen SE, Wolski K. Effect of rosiglitazone on the risk of myocardial infarction and death from cardiovascular causes. *N Engl J Med.* 2007; 356:2457-71.
122. Scirica BM, Bhatt DL, Braunwald E et al. Saxagliptin and cardiovascular outcomes in patients with type 2 diabetes mellitus. *N Engl J Med.* 2013; 369:1317-26.
123. White WB, Cannon CP, Heller SR et al. Alogliptin after acute coronary syndrome in patients with type 2 diabetes. *N Engl J Med.* 2013; 369:1327-35.
124. Green JB, Bethel MA, Armstrong PW et al. Effect of Sitagliptin on cardiovascular outcomes in type 2 diabetes. *N Engl J Med.* 2013; 369:1327-35.
125. Weir DL, McAlister FA, Senthiselvan A et al. Sitagliptin use in patients with diabetes and heart failure. *JACC: Heart Failure.* 2014; 2:573-82.
126. Li L, Li S, Liu J et al. Dipeptidyl peptidase-4 inhibitors and risk of heart failure in type 2 diabetes: systematic review and meta-analysis of randomized and observational studies. *BMJ.* 2016; 352:i61D.
127. Cathcart-Rake WF, Coker JE, Atkins FL et al. The effect of concurrent oral administration of propranolol and disopyramide on cardiac function in healthy men. *Circulation.* 1980; 61:938-45.
128. Hohnloser SH, Crijns HJ, van Eickels M et al. Effect of dronedarone on cardiovascular events in atrial fibrillation. *N Engl J Med.* 2009; 360:668-78.
129. Reed BN, Sueta CA. A practical guide for the treatment of symptomatic heart failure with reduced ejection fraction (HFrEF). *Curr Cardiol Rev.* 2015; 11:23-32.
130. January CT, Wann S, Alpert JS et al. 2014 AHA/ACC/HRS Guideline for the Management of Patients With Atrial Fibrillation: Executive Summary. *J Am Coll Cardiol.* 2014; 64:2246-80.
131. Romond EH, Perez EA, Bryant J et al. Trastuzumab plus adjuvant chemotherapy for operable HER2-positive breast cancer. *N Engl J Med.* 2005; 353:1673-84.
132. Suter TM, Procter M, van Veldhuisen DJ et al. Trastuzumab-associated cardiac adverse effects in the herceptin adjuvant trial. *J Clin Oncol.* 2007; 25:3859-65.
133. Tan-Chiu E, Yothers G, Romond E et al. Assessment of cardiac dysfunction in a randomized trial comparing doxorubicin and cyclophosphamide followed by paclitaxel, with or without trastuzumab as adjuvant therapy in node-positive, human epidermal growth factor receptor 2-overexpressing breast cancer: SABP B31. *J Clin Oncol.* 2005; 23:7811-9.
134. Piccart-Gebhart MJ, Procter M, Leyland-Jones B et al. Trastuzumab after adjuvant chemotherapy in HER2 positive breast cancer. *N Engl J Med.* 2005; 353:1659-72.
135. Joensuu H, Kellokumpu-Lehtinen PL, Bono P et al. Adjuvant docetaxel or vinorelbine with or without trastuzumab for breast cancer. *N Engl J Med.* 2006; 354:809-20.
136. Guarneri V, Lenihan DJ, Valero V et al. Long-term cardiac tolerability of trastuzumab in metastatic breast cancer: the M.D. Anderson Cancer Center experience. *J Clin Oncol.* 2006; 24:4107-15.
137. Choueiri TK, Mayer EL, Je Y et al. Congestive heart failure risk in patients with breast cancer treated with bevacizumab. *J Clin Oncol.* 2011; 29:632-8.
138. Chung ES, Packer M, Hung Lo K et al. Randomized, double-blind, placebo-controlled, pilot trial of infliximab, a chimeric monoclonal antibody to tumor necrosis factor-alpha, in patients with moderate-to-severe heart failure: results of the anti-TNF Therapy Against Congestive Heart Failure (ATTACH) trial. *Circulation.* 2003; 107:3133-40.
139. Perez EA, Koehler M, Byrne J. Cardiac safety of lapatinib: pooled analysis of 3689 patients enrolled in clinical trials. *Mayo Clin Proc.* 2008; 83:679-86.
140. Avezum A, Tsuyuki RT, Pogue J et al. Beta-blocker therapy for congestive heart failure: a systemic overview and critical appraisal of the published trials. *Can J Cardiol.* 1998; 14:1045-53.
141. Lechat P, Packer M, Chalon S et al. Clinical effects of beta-adrenergic blockade in chronic heart failure: a metaanalysis of double-blind, placebo-controlled, randomized trials. *Circulation.* 1998; 98:1184-91.
142. Tsuyuki RT, McAlister FA, Teo KK. Beta-blockers for congestive heart failure: what is the current consensus? *Drugs Aging.* 2000; 16:1-7.
143. Ko DT, Hebert PR, Coffey CS et al. Adverse effects of beta-blocker therapy for patients with heart failure: a quantitative overview of randomized trials. *Arch Intern Med.* 2004; 164:1389-94.
144. Parameshwar J, Poole-Wilson PA. The role of calcium antagonists in the treatment of chronic heart failure. *Eur Heart J.* 1993; 14(suppl A):38-44.
145. Dougall HT, McLay J. A comparative review of the adverse effects of calcium antagonists. *Drug Saf.* 1996; 15:91-106.
146. Bohm M, Schwinger RH, Erdmann E. Different cardiodepressant potency of various calcium antagonists in human myocardium. *Am J Cardiol.* 1990; 65:1039-41.
147. Karalliedde J, Buckingham R, Starkie M et al. Effect of various diuretic treatments on rosiglitazone-induced fluid retention. *J Am Soc Nephrol.* 2006; 17:3482-90.
148. Karalliedde J, Buckingham RE. Thiazolidinediones and their fluid-related adverse effects: facts, fiction and putative management strategies. *Drug Saf.* 2007; 30:741-53.
149. Page II RL, O'Bryant CL, Cheng D et al. Drugs that may cause or exacerbate heart failure: a scientific statement from the American Heart Association. *Circulation.* 2016; 134:00–00.
150. Sanon VP, Sanon S, Pham SV et al. Play of chance versus concerns regarding Dipeptidyl Peptidase-4 Inhibitors: heart failure and diabetes. *Clin Diabetes.* 2014; 32:121-6.
151. Podrid PJ. Safety and toxicity of antiarrhythmic drug therapy: benefit versus risk. *J Cardiovasc Pharmacol.* 1991; 17(suppl 6): S65-S73.
152. Frishman WH, Sung HM, Yee HC et al. Cardiovascular toxicity with cancer chemotherapy. *Curr Probl Cancer.* 1997; 21:301-60.
153. Porembka DT, Lowder JN, Orlowski JP et al. Etiology and management of doxorubicin cardiotoxicity. *Crit Care Med.* 1989; 17:569-72.
154. Saini J, Rich MW, Lyss AP. Reversibility of severe left ventricular dysfunction due to doxorubicin cardiotoxicity: report of three cases. *Ann Intern Med.* 1987; 106:814-6.
155. Octavia Y, Tocchetti CG, Gabrielson KL et al. Doxorubicin-induced cardiomyopathy: from molecular mechanisms to therapeutic strategies. *J Mol Cell Cardiol.* 2012; 52:1213-25.
156. Ewer MS, Lippman SM. Type II chemotherapy-related cardiac dysfunction: time to recognize a new entity. *J Clin Oncol.* 2005; 23:2900-2.
157. Ewer MS, Vooletich MT, Durand JB et al. Reversibility of trastuzumab-related cardiotoxicity: new insights based on clinical course and response to medical treatment. *J Clin Oncol.* 2005; 23:7820-6.
158. Guglin M, Cutro R, Mishkin JD. Trastuzumab-induced cardiomyopathy. *J Card Fail.* 2008; 14:437-44.
159. Telli ML, Hunt SA, Carlson RW et al. Trastuzumab-related cardiotoxicity: calling into question the concept of reversibility. *J Clin Oncol.* 2007; 25:3525-33.
160. Feenstra J, Grobbee DE, Mosterd A et al. Adverse cardiovascular effects of NSAIDs in patients with congestive heart failure. *Drug Saf.* 1997; 17:166-80.
161. Nurmohamed MT, van Halm VP, Dijkmans BA. Cardiovascular risk profile of antirheumatic agents in patients with osteoarthritis and rheumatoid arthritis. *Drugs.* 2002; 62:1599-609.
162. Colucci WS. Rationale for clinical trials of beta blockers in heart failure due to systolic dysfunction. 2016. https://www.uptodate.com/contents/use-of-beta-blockers-in-heart-failure-with-reduced-ejection-fraction (accessed 2018 Feb 1).
163. Rastogi P, Jeong J, Geyer CE et al. Five year update of cardiac dysfunction on NSABP B-31, a randomized trial of sequential doxorubicin/cyclophosphamide (AC)_paclitaxel (T) vs. AC_T with trastuzumab(H) (abstract). *J Clin Oncol.* 2007; 25(suppl 18): LBA513.
164. Kirman I, Whelan RL, Nielsen OH. Infliximab: mechanism of action beyond TNF-alpha neutralization in inflammatory bowel disease. *Eur J Gastroenterol Hepatol.* 2004; 16: 639-41.

165. Philbin EF, Rocco TA Jr, Lindenmuth NW et al. Clinical outcomes in heart failure: report from a community hospital-based registry. *Am J Med.* 1999; 107:549-55.
166. Canadian Diabetes Association Clinical Practice Guidelines Expert Committee. Canadian Diabetes Association 2013 clinical practice guidelines for the prevention and management of diabetes in Canada. *Can J Diabetes.* 2013; 37(suppl 1):S1-S212.
167. Standards of medical care in diabetes—2007. *Diabetes Care.* 2007; 30(suppl 1):S4-S41.
168. Scirica BM. The safety of dipeptidyl peptidase 4 inhibitors and the risk for heart failure. *JAMA Cardiology.* 2016; 1:123-5.
169. Zinman B, Wanner C, Lachin JM et al. Empagliflozin, cardiovascular outcomes, and mortality in type 2 diabetes. *N Engl J Med.* 2015; 373:2117-28.
170. Siveski-Iliskovic N, Hill M, Chow DA et al. Probucol protects against adriamycin cardiomyopathy without interfering with its antitumor effect. *Circulation.* 1995; 91:10-15.
171. Wouters KA, Kremer LC, Miller TL et al. Protecting against anthracycline-induced myocardial damage: a review of the most promising strategies. *Br J Haematol.* 2005; 131:561-78.
172. Moore N, Pollack C, Butkerait P. Adverse drug reactions and drug-drug interactions with over-the-counter NSAIDs. *Ther Clin Risk Manag.* 2015; 11:1061-75.
173. Grunbaum A. NSAIDs: The truth about cardiovascular risk. 2015. https://www.acoi.org/15Convention/Grunbaum.pdf (accessed 2018 Feb 1).
174. Lazarevic AM, Nakatani S, Neskovic AN et al. Early changes in left ventricular function in chronic asymptomatic alcoholics: relation to the duration of heavy drinking. *J Am Coll Cardiol.* 2000; 35:1599-606.
175. Piano MR. Alcohol and heart failure. *J Card Fail.* 2002; 8:239–46.
176. Klatsky AL, Chartier D, Udaltsova N et al. Alcohol drinking and risk of hospitalization for heart failure with and without associated coronary artery disease. *Am J Cardiol.* 2005; 96:346-51.
177. Djousse L, Gaziano JM. Alcohol consumption and heart failure: a systematic review. *Curr Atheroscler Rep.* 2008; 10:117-20.
178. Arnold JM, Howlett JG, Dorian P et al. Canadian Cardiovascular Society Consensus Conference recommendations on heart failure update 2007: Prevention, management during intercurrent illness or acute decompensation, and use of biomarkers. *Can J Cardiol.* 2007; 23:21-45.
179. Nicolas JM, Fernandez-Sola J, Estruch R et al. The effect of controlled drinking in alcoholic cardiomyopathy. *Ann Intern Med.* 2002; 136:192-200.
180. Koshman SL, Charrois TL, Simpson SH et al. Pharmacist care of patients with heart failure: a systematic review of randomized trials. *Arch Intern Med.* 2008; 168:687-94.
181. American Heart Association. Physical changes to report for heart failure. 2017. http://www.heart.org/HEARTORG/Conditions/HeartFailure/LivingWithHeartFailureAndAdvancedHF/Physical-Changes-to-Report-for-Heart-Failure_UCM_306356_Article.jsp#.WnNU1K6nFtQ (accessed 2018 Feb 1).
182. Heart and stroke foundation. Understanding heart failure—the basics. 2018. https://www.heartandstroke.ca/-/media/pdf-files/canada/health-failure/hs_heartfailure_thebasics_en.ashx (accessed 2018 Feb 1).
183. Ni H, Nauman D, Burgess D et al. Factors influencing knowledge of and adherence to self-care among patients with heart failure. *Arch Intern Med.* 1999; 159:1613-9.
184. Lockwood E, McAlister FA, O'Reilly K et al. Patient knowledge of self-care activities in congestive heart failure. *Clin Invest Med.* 2002; 25:200.
185. Bucolo C, Longo L, Camillieri G et al. Safety profile assessment of buflomedil: an overview of adverse reactions between 1975 and 2011. *Pharmacoepidemiol Drug Saf.* 2011; 21:1190-6.
186. Andriole GL, Bostwick DG, Brawley OW et al. Effect of dutasteride on the risk of prostate cancer. *N Engl J Med.* 2010; 362:1192-202.
187. Fichtlscherer S, Rossig L, Breuer S et al. Tumor necrosis factor antagonism with etanercept improves systemic endothelial vasoreactivity in patients with advanced heart failure. *Circulation.* 2001; 104:3023-5.
188. Coletta AP, Clark AL, Banarjee P et al. Clinical trials update: RENEWAL (RENAISSANCE and RECOVER) and ATTACH. *Eur J Heart Fail.* 2002; 4:559-61.
189. Trent JC, Patel SS, Zhang J et al. Rare incidence of congestive heart failure in gastrointestinal stromal tumor and other sarcoma patients receiving imatinib mesylate. *Cancer.* 2010; 116:184-92.
190. Mokhles MM, Trifiro G, Dieleman JP et al. The risk of new onset heart failure associated with dopamine agonist use in Parkinson's disease. *Pharmacol Res.* 2012; 65:358-64.
191. Chu TF, Rupnick MA, Dallabrida SMs et al. Cardiotoxicity associated with tyrosine kinase inhibitor sunitinib. *Lancet.* 2007; 370:2011-9.

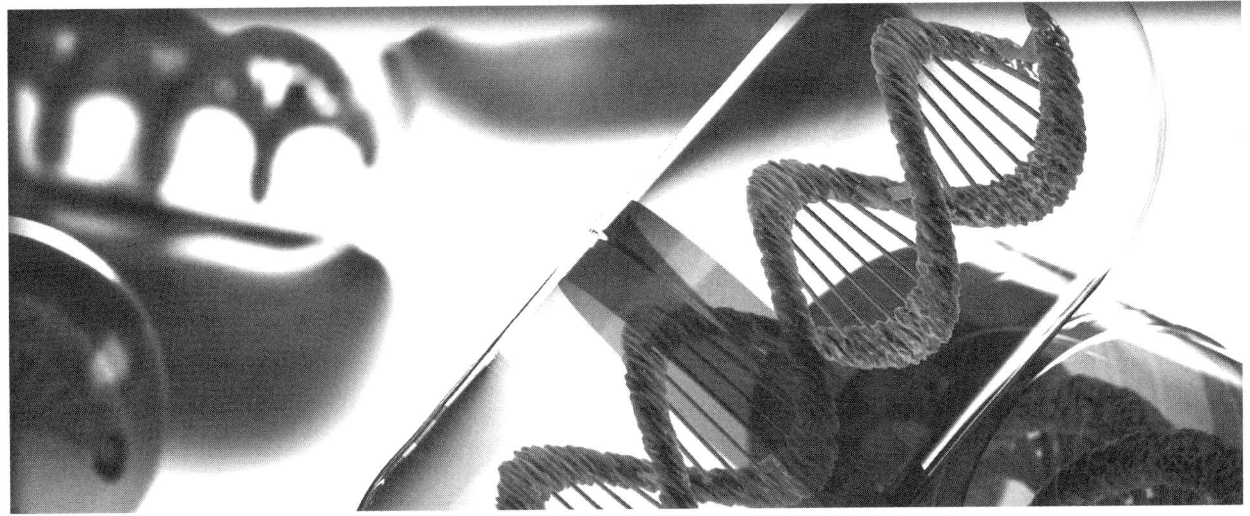

CHAPTER 25

Ventricular Arrhythmias

James E. Tisdale

Drugs may induce potentially life-threatening ventricular arrhythmias. Drug-induced ventricular arrhythmias can be divided into three categories: monomorphic ventricular tachycardia, the polymorphic ventricular tachycardia known as torsades de pointes (TdP), and drug-induced Brugada syndrome.

MONOMORPHIC VENTRICULAR TACHYCARDIA

CAUSATIVE AGENTS

Drugs that have been reported to cause or exacerbate monomorphic ventricular tachycardia are listed in **Table 25-1**.[1-177] Any of the drugs listed may cause new monomorphic ventricular tachycardia. Incessant, sinusoidal-appearing ventricular tachycardia is most often associated with the potent sodium-channel blocking agents belonging to the Vaughan Williams antiarrhythmic class IC (e.g., flecainide, propafenone), although it has also been reported in association with amiodarone. Nonsustained and sustained ventricular tachycardia have been widely reported in association with dobutamine during stress echocardiography. Although ventricular arrhythmias are a known risk associated with stress echocardiography, the incidence of ventricular tachycardia associated with dobutamine stress echocardiography is significantly higher than that associated with exercise stress echocardiography.[77,79]

EPIDEMIOLOGY

Although the overall incidence of drug-induced ventricular tachycardia is not known, the incidences associated with some specific drugs have been reported (Table 25-1). Ventricular tachycardia is recognized as a consequence of digoxin toxicity.[34-38] The incidence of ventricular tachycardia in patients taking digoxin is unknown. However, in an analysis of patients discharged from a major urban medical center with the diagnosis of digoxin intoxication, 7% had "definite" ventricular tachycardia.[35]

Table 25-1 Agents Implicated in Drug-Induced Monomorphic Ventricular Tachycardia

Drug	Incidence	Level of Evidence[a]
Aconite alkaloids[1-8]	NK	C
Acetylsalicylic acid[9,b]	NK	C
Adenosine[10-16]	Up to 5%	B
Amiodarone[17,18]	NK	C
Arsenic trioxide[19]	NK	C
Bupropion[20]	NK	C
Bupivacaine[21-25]	NK	C
Chlorpromazine[26]	NK	C
Citalopram[27,b]	NK	C
Cocaine[28-30]	NK	B
Desipramine[31-33,b]	NK	C
Digoxin[34-38]	NK	A
Dipyridamole[39-41]	0.03–0.8%	B
Disopyramide[42]	NK	C
Dobutamine[41,43-85]	0–15.7%[c]	A
Ephedrine[86,87]	NK	C
Flecainide[88-122]	0–13%	A
Gingko biloba[123]	NK	C
Ibutilide[124-131]	0–9.8%	A
Imipramine[132]	NK	C
Lacosamide[133]	NK	C
Lamotrigine[134]	NK	C
Levosimendan[135,136]	NK	A
Lithium[137,d]	NK	C
Methamphetamine[138]	NK	C
Milrinone[44,139-142]	0–9.5%	B
Niferidil[143]	3.7%	B
Procainamide[144]	NK	C
Propafenone[145-158]	0–10%	B
Ropivacaine[159,160]	NK	C
Sotalol[161]	NK	C
Terbutaline[162-164]	0–15%[e]	A
Theophylline[164-174]	NK	B
Thioridazine[32]	NK	C
Trazodone[175,176]	NK	C
Venlafaxine[134,177,b]	NK	C

NK = not known.
[a]Definitions for Levels of Evidence: Level A—evidence from one or more randomized, controlled clinical trials; Level B—evidence from nonrandomized clinical trials, prospective observational studies, cohort studies, retrospective studies, case-control studies, meta-analyses and/or postmarketing surveillance studies; and Level C—evidence from one or more published case reports or case series
[b]Primarily in overdose.
[c]Reported as high as 29% in patients with severe heart failure.
[d]Chronic toxicity.
[e]15% incidence reported in patients with a history of ventricular arrhythmias.

Table 25-2 Mechanisms of Drug-Induced Monomorphic Ventricular Tachycardia

Drug	Mechanism
Aconite alkaloids	Activate myocardial sodium channels, increasing permeability to sodium and increasing ventricular automaticity
Adenosine	Enhanced activity of the sympathetic nervous system, via increased arterial chemoreceptor and baroreceptor activity Myocardial ischemia due to coronary steal
Amiodarone Bupivacaine Chlorpromazine Desipramine Disopyramide Flecainide Imipramine Procainamide Propafenone Ropivacaine	Inhibition of sodium-channel conductance
Digoxin	Inhibition of the sodium–potassium–adenosine triphosphatase pump, leading to increased intracellular calcium concentrations, resulting in afterdepolarizations and ventricular ectopic activity
Dobutamine Terbutaline	Stimulation of β_2-receptors, leading to ventricular ectopic activity
Theophylline	Phosphodiesterase inhibition, leading to elevated concentrations of cyclic adenosine monophosphate, causing increased intracellular calcium concentrations, resulting in afterdepolarizations and ventricular ectopic activity
Ibutilide Sotalol Trazodone Venlafaxine	Unknown

MECHANISMS

Mechanisms of drug-induced monomorphic ventricular tachycardia vary depending on the causative agent(s) (**Table 25-2**). Many of the drugs that cause monomorphic ventricular tachycardia (e.g., amiodarone, chlorpromazine, disopyramide, flecainide, imipramine, procainamide, propafenone) do so as a result of potent inhibition of myocardial sodium channels, leading to a reduction in ventricular conduction velocity.[158] This changes the relationship between ventricular conduction velocity and ventricular refractoriness, which may promote the manifestation of re-entrant circuits in ventricular tissue. These drugs may particularly perturb the relationship between ventricular conduction velocity and refractoriness in patients with a history of myocardial infarction in whom alteration of electrophysiologic characteristics has already occurred in the border zone of the infarcted tissue. This is also an important proarrhythmic effect in patients with heart failure with reduced ejection fraction (HFrEF), in whom ventricular electrophysiology is altered as a result of left ventricular hypertrophy and accumulation of connective tissue in the left ventricle. In particular, potent sodium-channel inhibition caused by Vaughan Williams class IC antiarrhythmic agents (e.g., flecainide, propafenone) can lead to incessant, sinusoidal ventricular tachycardia.[178,179]

In contrast to sodium inhibition, aconite alkaloids provoke ventricular tachycardia via activation of myocardial sodium channels and increasing permeability to sodium conductance, delaying ventricular repolarization and increasing ventricular automaticity.[180,181] Adenosine may cause monomorphic ventricular tachycardia as a result of enhancement of arterial chemoreceptor and baroreceptor activity, leading to increased activity of the sympathetic nervous system or due to inducing myocardial ischemia as a result of "coronary steal," or both.[10,182] Digoxin-induced ventricular tachycardia, which is usually a manifestation of serum concentrations that are markedly elevated above the therapeutic range, occurs as a result of profound inhibition of the sodium–potassium–adenosine triphosphatase pump, leading to marked increases in intramyocyte calcium concentrations, provoking afterdepolarizations and ventricular ectopic activity.[183] Like that associated with adenosine, ventricular tachycardia induced by dipyridamole occurs as a result of induced myocardial ischemia due to the phenomenon of "coronary steal."

CLINICAL PRESENTATION AND DIFFERENTIAL DIAGNOSIS

Whether drug-induced or due to other causes, monomorphic ventricular tachycardia is defined as a series of consecutive ventricular premature depolarizations and is characterized by wide, misshapen QRS complexes on an electrocardiogram (ECG), with a heart rate >100 bpm, and sometimes as high as 150–250 bpm (**Figure 25-1**). As indicated by the term *monomorphic*, QRS complexes possess similar beat-to-beat morphologic characteristics. Potent sodium channel-blocking drugs may also cause an often incessant ventricular tachycardia characterized by wide QRS complexes with a sinusoidal appearance. This incessant, sinusoidal ventricular tachycardia is often slower than typical spontaneous ventricular tachycardia but occasionally can be quite rapid.[92]

Drug-induced monomorphic ventricular tachycardia may be nonsustained or sustained. Nonsustained ventricular tachycardia is defined as at least three consecutive beats of ventricular tachycardia, lasting ≤30 seconds and terminating spontaneously. Sustained ventricular tachycardia lasts >30 seconds and requires intervention for termination. Sinusoidal-appearing ventricular tachycardia is often sustained and is more likely to be incessant and refractory to overdrive pacing or direct current cardioversion than other monomorphic ventricular tachycardias. Occasionally, sinusoidal-appearing ventricular tachycardia is characterized by frequent nonsustained episodes that terminate spontaneously but quickly recur.[92]

Drugs may cause new ventricular tachycardia in patients who did not previously have this arrhythmia or may aggravate or worsen an underlying ventricular tachycardia. For example, specific drugs may increase the rate of a patient's pre-existing ventricular tachycardia, make it more symptomatic, more difficult to terminate, or both.[179] The symptoms of drug-induced ventricular tachycardia are related to heart rate and the resultant effect on blood pressure and cardiac output (**Table 25-3**). However, in some patients, the initial symptom of drug-induced ventricular tachycardia may be sudden cardiac death as a result of rapid degeneration of ventricular tachycardia to ventricular fibrillation.

The time from drug therapy initiation to the development of drug-induced monomorphic ventricular tachycardia is somewhat variable. In cases of drug overdose or elevated plasma drug concentrations during therapy, the arrhythmia may develop within a few minutes to several hours after the ingestion or the plasma concentration elevation.

Table 25-3 Signs and Symptoms Associated with Drug-Induced Monomorphic Ventricular Tachycardia

- Chest pain (in patients with underlying coronary artery disease)
- Dizziness
- Hypotension
- Lightheadedness
- Monomorphic ventricular tachycardia on electrocardiogram
- Near-syncope
- Palpitations
- Seizures (due to cerebral hypoxia)
- Shortness of breath
- Sinusoidal ventricular tachycardia on electrocardiogram
- Sudden cardiac death (if ventricular tachycardia is pulseless)
- Syncope
- Tachycardia

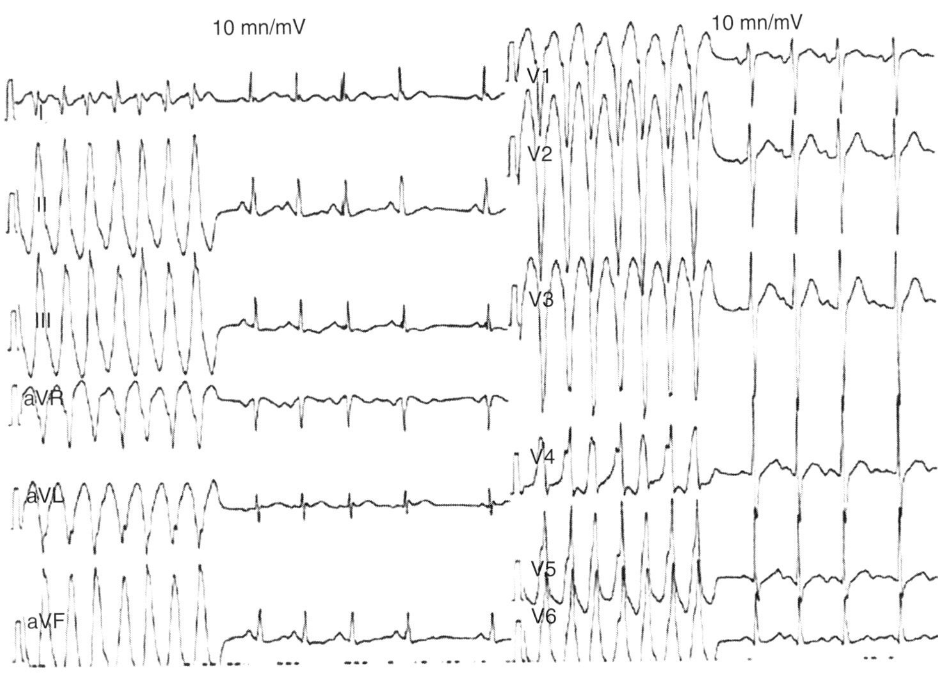

FIGURE 25-1 Monomorphic Ventricular Tachycardia Associated with Weight Loss Pills Containing Caffeine and Ephedrine

Source: Reproduced from Pareek M, Hansson NH, Grove EL. Ventricular tachycardia induced by weight loss pills. *Case Rep Med.* 2013; 2013:712383.

The majority of cases of drug-induced monomorphic ventricular tachycardia occur within hours to days after the initiation of therapy.

Drug-induced monomorphic ventricular tachycardia must be differentiated from other tachycardias (**Table 25-4**). Further, drug-induced monomorphic ventricular tachycardia must be distinguished from spontaneously occurring nondrug-induced ventricular tachycardia (**Table 25-5**). Diagnosis

Table 25-4 Conditions to Consider in the Differential Diagnosis of Drug-Induced Monomorphic Ventricular Tachycardia

- Atrial fibrillation
- Atrial flutter
- Atrial tachycardia
- Atrioventricular nodal re-entrant tachycardia
- Idioventricular tachycardia
- Junctional tachycardia
- Non-TdP polymorphic ventricular tachycardia
- Sinus tachycardia
- TdP

TdP = torsades de pointes.

Table 25-5 Differentiation of Drug-Induced Monomorphic Ventricular Tachycardia from Nondrug-Induced Ventricular Tachycardia

In patient with no history of VT

- New VT on drug therapy (VT not present before drug therapy)
- No obvious underlying cause for new VT, such as:
  - Ischemic heart disease
  - Heart failure
  - Hypokalemia
  - Hypomagnesemia

In patient with history of VT

- VT on drug therapy:
  - Has a different morphology than patient's previous clinical VT
  - Is substantially faster than patient's previous clinical VT
  - Is sustained, whereas patient previously had only nonsustained VT
  - Is sinusoidal
  - Is more difficult to terminate than patient's previous clinical VT

VT = ventricular tachycardia.

of drug-induced ventricular tachycardia is usually based on the occurrence of a new ventricular tachycardia in a patient with no history of ventricular tachycardia before the initiation of drug therapy. In addition, drug-induced ventricular tachycardia may be diagnosed in a patient with a history of nondrug-induced ventricular tachycardia if the morphology of the ventricular tachycardia that develops after the initiation of drug therapy differs from that of the ventricular tachycardia that occurred in the absence of drug therapy. The occurrence of incessant sinusoidal ventricular tachycardia may be considered a drug-induced arrhythmia, as this form of ventricular tachycardia has not been described in the absence of drug therapy and is not typical of ventricular tachycardia occurring as a result of myocardial infarction, acute coronary ischemia, left ventricular dysfunction, or other common causes of ventricular tachycardia. Drug-induced ventricular tachycardia may also be diagnosed if a patient's underlying ventricular tachycardia becomes more rapid, more symptomatic, more difficult to terminate after the initiation of therapy with a new drug, or some combination of these factors.

RISK FACTORS

Structural heart disease, particularly a history of myocardial infarction or coronary artery disease even without a history of myocardial infarction, is a major risk factor for ventricular tachycardia induced by potent sodium channel-blocking agents such as flecainide or propafenone (**Table 25-6**).[184] The Cardiac Arrhythmia Suppression Trial[185] was designed to test the hypothesis that suppression of asymptomatic ventricular ectopic activity after a myocardial infarction reduces the incidence of postinfarction mortality. In CAST, patients who had experienced a myocardial infarction within the previous 1 week to 6 months were recruited to enter a run-in study phase in which the efficacy of flecainide, encainide, and moricizine (encainide and moricizine are no longer available in the United States) were tested to determine the efficacy of each agent for the suppression of ventricular ectopic activity. Patients in whom one of these drugs was effective for the suppression of ventricular ectopic activity were then randomly assigned to the most effective (in that specific patient) of the three agents or placebo.

Table 25-6 Risk Factors for Drug-Induced Monomorphic Ventricular Tachycardia

- Coronary artery disease
- HFrEF
- History of arrhythmias (risk factor for dobutamine-induced ventricular tachycardia)
- History of ventricular arrhythmias may be a risk factor for terbutaline-induced ventricular tachycardia
- Hypokalemia, hypomagnesemia, and hypercalcemia are risk factors for ventricular tachycardia associated with digoxin
- Male sex (risk factor for dobutamine-induced ventricular tachycardia)
- Recent myocardial infarction
- Serum digoxin concentrations >2 ng/mL
- Serum theophylline concentrations >20 mcg/mL

HFrEF = heart failure with reduced ejection fraction.

The flecainide and encainide arms of the study were discontinued prematurely as a result of excess mortality in the treatment group. The arrhythmic mortality incidence in the patients who received flecainide or encainide was more than three times higher than in the placebo group.[185] The moricizine arm of the study was continued but, like the flecainide and encainide arms of the original CAST trial, was subsequently discontinued because of an increased incidence of mortality in moricizine-treated patients during the first 2 weeks of treatment.[186] Active treatment with encainide or flecainide was associated with greater mortality than placebo in the majority of subgroups, but patients with non-Q-wave myocardial infarction and frequent premature ventricular complexes were at highest risk.[184] As a result of the findings of CAST, flecainide is contraindicated in patients with a documented history of coronary artery disease. In addition, although propafenone was not included in CAST, as a Vaughan Williams class IC antiarrhythmic drug with potent sodium channel-blocking properties, it is also considered to be contraindicated in patients with a documented history of coronary artery disease, even though there are no studies specifically associating propafenone therapy with increasing mortality incidence. A subsequent meta-analysis of 138 randomized, controlled trials of antiarrhythmic agents that enrolled a total of approximately 98,000 patients with a history of myocardial infarction receiving the drugs for arrhythmia prophylaxis also reported an increased risk of mortality associated with the sodium channel-blocking antiarrhythmic agents from Vaughan Williams class IA (quinidine, procainamide, disopyramide). Although the cause of death in these studies was not documented, proarrhythmia was believed to be the major cause.[187]

HFrEF is also likely a risk factor for drug-induced monomorphic ventricular tachycardia.[188] Some risk factors are drug-specific. For example, serum digoxin concentrations >2 ng/mL—particularly in patients with hypokalemia, hypomagnesemia, or hypercalcemia—is a risk factor for monomorphic ventricular tachycardia caused by digoxin. Serum theophylline concentrations >20 mcg/mL increase the risk of theophylline-induced monomorphic ventricular tachycardia.[170] Patients with a history of ventricular arrhythmias may be at higher risk for monomorphic ventricular tachycardia induced by terbutaline.[163] A history of complex ventricular ectopic activity, HFrEF, and multivessel coronary artery disease are risk factors for dobutamine-induced ventricular tachycardia in patients with a recent myocardial infarction.[46]

MORBIDITY AND MORTALITY

There is little published information regarding the impact of drug-induced monomorphic ventricular tachycardia on hospitalization or emergency department visits, but based on the symptoms associated with this disease, it seems likely that these could be consequences. Drug-induced monomorphic ventricular tachycardia may degenerate into ventricular fibrillation and cause sudden cardiac death. Potent sodium channel-blocking drugs in Vaughan Williams antiarrhythmic classes IA and IC have been shown to increase death due to arrhythmias in patients with a history of myocardial infarction.[185-187]

Nonsustained ventricular tachycardia associated with dobutamine during stress echocardiography may have prognostic significance in patients with HFrEF. Patients without inducible ischemia who had moderately reduced left ventricular ejection fraction (LVEF) (35–45%) who experienced nonsustained ventricular tachycardia during dobutamine stress echocardiography had a significantly lower incidence of survival compared to patients with LVEF >45% during a 3-year follow-up period.[76]

Death has been reported as a result of drug-induced incessant, sinusoidal ventricular tachycardia.[189] The incidence of mortality among patients who experience drug-induced ventricular tachycardia is unknown.

PREVENTION

The risk of drug-induced ventricular tachycardia may be minimized by avoiding the use of specific causative drugs in high-risk populations and by maintaining serum potassium and magnesium concentrations at >4 and >2 mEq/L, respectively (**Table 25-7**). Flecainide and propafenone are contraindicated in patients with documented coronary artery disease. In addition, long-term use of oral quinidine and disopyramide should be avoided in patients with coronary artery disease. Drugs with substantial potential to impair myocardial contractility, including flecainide, disopyramide,

Table 25-7 Prevention of Drug-Induced Monomorphic Ventricular Tachycardia

- Appropriately adjust doses of digoxin, procainamide, and sotalol in patients with kidney disease
- Avoid use of oral Vaughan Williams class IA (quinidine, disopyramide) or class IC (flecainide, propafenone) agents in patients with coronary artery disease
- Avoid use of disopyramide, flecainide, and propafenone in patients with HFrEF
- Avoid concomitant use of hepatically metabolized drugs that may cause monomorphic ventricular tachycardia and drugs that inhibit the cytochrome P-450 enzyme system
- Maintain serum digoxin concentrations <2 ng/mL
- Maintain serum theophylline concentrations <20 mcg/mL
- Maintain serum potassium concentrations within normal range
- Maintain serum magnesium concentrations within normal range

HFrEF = heart failure with reduced ejection fraction.

procainamide, propafenone, and sotalol should be avoided in patients with HFrEF. In patients receiving digoxin, serum digoxin concentrations should be maintained at <2 ng/mL, and appropriate dose adjustment is necessary in patients with impaired digoxin clearance due to kidney disease. Similarly, patients receiving procainamide and, in particular, sotalol should undergo appropriate dose adjustment for kidney disease. Serum theophylline concentrations should be maintained at <20 mcg/mL. In patients undergoing dobutamine stress echocardiography, earlier administration of atropine (initiation prior to or at time of initiation of dobutamine) may be associated with a reduced risk of ventricular tachycardia compared with conventional timing of atropine administration (initiated near the end of the dobutamine infusion protocol).[83,84]

MANAGEMENT

In patients with drug-induced monomorphic ventricular tachycardia, the causative agent should be discontinued (**Figure 25-2**). Hemodynamically unstable drug-induced ventricular tachycardia should be terminated using synchronized direct current cardioversion, starting at 100 J monophasic or biphasic shock, and increasing to 200, 300, and 360 J if necessary.[190,191] Ventricular tachycardia is usually considered hemodynamically unstable if it results in acute impairment of vital organ function or cardiac arrest is ongoing or imminent.[181,182] Hemodynamically stable drug-induced monomorphic ventricular tachycardia may be also be treated with synchronized direct current cardioversion, at the energy levels described above, with appropriate sedation prior to shock administration.[192] Alternatively, hemodynamically stable drug-induced monomorphic ventricular tachycardia may be treated initially with intravenous procainamide, unless procainamide is believed to be the causative agent.[192] Intravenous amiodarone or intravenous sotalol may be administered if hemodynamically stable monomorphic ventricular tachycardia is refractory to procainamide.[192]

Incessant sinusoidal ventricular tachycardia is sometimes resistant to direct current cardioversion or overdrive pacing and is often resistant to antiarrhythmic drugs such as procainamide.[108] However, flecainide-induced incessant sinusoidal ventricular tachycardia has been successfully treated with intravenous lidocaine.[107] Flecainide-induced sinusoidal ventricular tachycardia has also been successfully treated using high-dose intravenous amiodarone.[108] Intravenous lipid emulsion has been used successfully for management of ventricular tachycardia associated with bupivacaine and local anesthetics.[22,23,193,194]

INFORMATION FOR PATIENTS

Patients who are taking drugs that may cause ventricular tachycardia should be told that the medication may, in rare cases, cause the heart rate (pulse) to become faster. Patients should be instructed to consult their pharmacist or physician if their heart rate increases to above 100–120 bpm or if they feel palpitations, lightheaded, dizzy, tired, weak, short of breath or experience chest pain.

TORSADES DE POINTES

TdP is a potentially life-threatening ventricular tachyarrhythmia associated with prolongation of the heart rate-corrected QT (QTc) interval.[195,196] QTc interval prolongation and TdP may be congenital or acquired. Acquired TdP is most often caused by drugs.[197]

CAUSATIVE AGENTS

Drugs that have been reported to cause TdP are presented in **Table 25-8**.[26,197-670] Up-to-date lists of drugs associated with TdP may be found at https://crediblemeds.org/index.php/login/dlcheck, a website maintained by the Arizona Center for Education and Research on Therapeutics.[197] This site categorizes QTc interval-prolonging drugs according to whether they are associated with a known risk, possible risk, or conditional risk of TdP. Known risk includes those drugs for which "substantial evidence supports the conclusion that these drugs prolong the QT interval AND are clearly associated

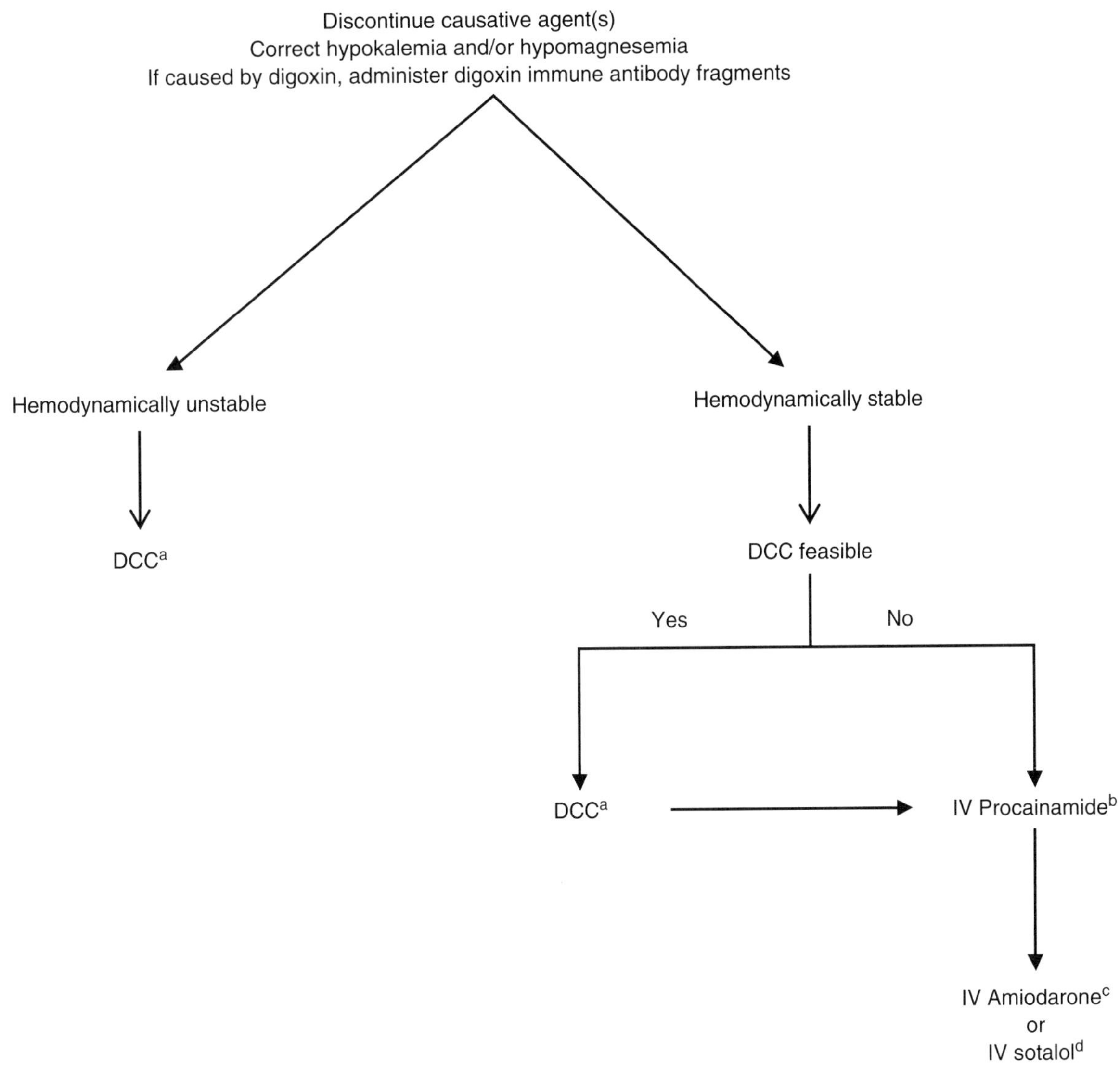

FIGURE 25-2 Management of Drug-Induced Monomorphic Ventricular Tachycardia

DCC = direct current cardioversion, IV = intravenous.

[a]100 Joules (monophasic or biphasic).

[b]10–17 mg/kg continuous intravenous infusion at a rate of 20–50 mg/min.[192]

[c]150 mg intravenously over 10 minutes, followed by continuous intravenous infusion of 1 mg/min for 6 hours, followed by continuous intravenous infusion of 0.5 mg/min for 18 hours.[192]

[d]75 mg every 12 hours.[192]

with a risk of TdP, even when taken as directed in official labeling."[197] Possible risk includes those drugs for which "substantial evidence supports the conclusion that these drugs can cause QT prolongation BUT there is insufficient evidence at this time that these drugs, when used as directed in official labeling, are associated with a risk of causing TdP."[197] Conditional risk includes those drugs for which "substantial evidence supports the conclusion that these drugs are associated with a risk of TdP BUT only under certain conditions (e.g., excessive dose, hypokalemia, congenital long QT or by causing a drug–drug interaction that results in excessive QT interval prolongation)."[197] Drugs associated with a risk of TdP are categorized in Table 25-8 based on these definitions.

Table 25-8 Agents Implicated in Drug-Induced Torsades de Pointes

Drug	Incidence	Level of Evidence[a]
KNOWN RISK OF TORSADES DE POINTES[197]		
Amiodarone[198-250]	0.7%	B
Arsenic trioxide[251-257]	2.5%	B
Azithromycin[241,258-264]	0.97%[b]	B
Chloroquine[265]	NK	C
Chlorpromazine[26,266]	NK	C
Ciprofloxacin[241,270,267-275]	NK	B
Cisapride[276-285]	0.1–5.7%	B
Citalopram[241,244,286-294]	NK	B
Clarithromycin[241,250,259,277,281,295-303]	NK	B
Cocaine[304-308]	NK	C
Disopyramide[198,241,296,298,309-321]	NK	B
Dofetilide[241,322-338]	1.5–10%[c]	A
Domperidone[339,340]	NK	C
Donepezil[241,341-343]	NK	B
Dronedarone[248,344]	NK	C
Droperidol[345-349]	<0.1%	B
Erythromycin[259,284,350-372]	0.4%	B
Escitalopram[373]	NK	C
Flecainide[205,239,241,374-382]	NK	B
Fluconazole[241,372,383-395]	NK	B
Gatifloxacin[267,396,397]	NK	B
Halofantrine[398,399]	NK	C
Haloperidol[241,400-414]	3.6%[d]	B
Ibogaine[415,416]	NK	C
Ibutilide[123-125,127,131,218,417-427]	1.2–11.5%	A
Levofloxacin[236,241,267,387,393,428-433]	0.2%	B
Levomepromazine[434]	NK	C
Methadone[241,308,337,435-472]	NK	B
Moxifloxacin[241,267,394,473-477]	NK	C
Ondansetron[478,479]	NK	C
Oxaliplatin[480-482]	NK	C
Papaverine[483,484]	NK	C
Pentamidine[485-501]	Up to 21%	B
Pimozide[299,502]	NK	C
Procainamide[199,503-509]	0–3.6%	A
Propofol[510-512]	1.93 per million	B
Quinidine[199,209,215,311,369,513-528]	2–12%	A
Roxithromycin[529-531]	NK	C
Sevoflurane[394,532-535]	NK	B
Sotalol[239,241,330,337,509,524,536-580]	0.2–5%[e]	A

Table 25-8 Agents Implicated in Drug-Induced Torsades de Pointes (continued)

Drug	Incidence	Level of Evidence[a]
Sparfloxacin[581,582]	NK	C
Sulpiride[583-585]	NK	C
Terlipressin[586,587]	NK	C
Thioridazine[588-602]	NK	C
Vandetanib[603,604]	NK	A
POSSIBLE RISK OF TORSADES DE POINTES[197]		
Aripiprazole[605]	NK	C
Buprenorphine[606]	NK	C
Clozapine[607,608]	NK	C
Dolasetron[609]	NK	C
Efavirenz[610]	NK	C
Famotidine[241,611]	NK	B
Imipramine[199,f]	NK	C
Ofloxacin[267]	NK	C
Pipamperone[612]	NK	C
Risperidone[90,613-616]	NK	B
Solifenacin[617,618]	NK	C
Tacrolimus[619,620]	NK	C
Vorinostat[621]	NK	C
CONDITIONAL RISK OF TORSADES DE POINTES[197]		
Amantadine[622-624]	NK	C
Amisulpride[625-629]	NK	C
Amitriptyline[383,630]	NK	C
Atazanavir[631]	NK	C
Chloral hydrate[632,633]	NK	C
Diphenhydramine[634,f]	NK	C
Doxepin[241,635,636]	NK	C
Fluoxetine[241,293,637-639]	NK	B
Hydroxychloroquine[640]	NK	C
Hydroxyzine[641]	NK	C
Indapamide[241,642-644]	NK	B
Itraconazole[645]	NK	C
Ivabradine[263,646]	NK	C
Ketoconazole[647]	NK	C
Lansoprazole[321]	NK	C
Loperamide[648-652]	NK	B
Metoclopramide[653,654]	NK	C
Metronidazole[231,393,655]	NK	C
Nelfinavir[393]	NK	C
Olanzapine[656]	NK	C
Pantoprazole[657]	NK	C
Posaconzaole[393,658]	NK	C

Table 25-8 Agents Implicated in Drug-Induced Torsades de Pointes (continued)

Drug	Incidence	Level of Evidence[a]
Quetiapine[241,659]	NK	B
Quinine[660,661]	NK	C
Ranolazine[337,646]	NK	C
Trazodone[235,662,663]	NK	C
Voriconazole[337,393,461,664-668]	NK	B
Ziprasidone[241,623,669,670]	NK	B

[a]Definitions for Levels of Evidence: Level A—evidence from one or more randomized, controlled clinical trials; Level B—evidence from nonrandomized clinical trials, prospective observational studies, cohort studies, retrospective studies, case-control studies, meta-analyses and/or postmarketing surveillance studies; and Level C—evidence from one or more published case reports or case series.
[b]Incidence was 0.97% of patients taking azithromycin who had QTc interval >450 msec, not 0.97% of all patients taking the drug.
[c]Incidence varies depending on the presence or absence of heart failure with reduced ejection fraction and whether or not dose is adjusted appropriately in patients with kidney disease. The incidence is as high as 10% when proper dose adjustment is not performed.
[d]Intravenous haloperidol in critically ill patients.
[e]Incidence depends on whether or not drug dose is adjusted appropriately in patients with kidney disease.
[f]In overdose.

EPIDEMIOLOGY

The incidence of drug-induced TdP in the general population is unknown. An attempt was made to determine the overall incidence of drug-induced ventricular proarrhythmia in a study conducted by the Swedish Medical Products Agency.[671] This study was conducted over a period of 28 days in 32 hospitals, with a reference population of approximately 4.2 million people. All episodes of ventricular arrhythmias that were encountered during admission to the hospital or that were tracked by ambulatory ECG recordings in the hospitals and that were considered to be associated with drugs were recorded. Fourteen cases of medium or high confidence TdP were recorded. This corresponded to an incidence of 3.3 cases per million during the 28-day period of the study, which was annualized to an incidence of 4 cases per 100,000 people annually.[627] This study was very small and of very short duration. Nonetheless, if this incidence could be extrapolated to the U.S. population, it would correspond to nearly 13,000 cases of drug-induced TdP annually. However, a more recent study conducted in Berlin estimated the annual incidence of drug-induced long QT syndrome (LQTS)/TdP in that city to be 2.5 per million in men and 4 per million in women.[672] Extrapolation of those estimates to the U.S. population suggests a lower incidence of drug-induced LQTS/TdP, about 400 cases annually in men and 660 cases per women, for an annual number of about 1,060 cases.

In another study conducted in Sweden, reports to the Swedish adverse drug reaction reporting system between 1991 and 2006 were analyzed.[673] Of 61,788 reported adverse drug reactions, 101 were drug-induced TdP. In a population-based study conducted in southwest France, drug-induced TdP was estimated to comprise 5–7% of all cases of ventricular tachycardia, ventricular fibrillation, or sudden cardiac death.[674] These studies did not attempt to determine the overall incidence of drug-induced TdP in the population. The actual incidence of drug-induced TdP in the United States remains unknown and requires further study. The incidence of TdP associated with specific agents is presented in Table 25-8.

QTc interval prolongation is common among hospitalized patients, particularly those in intensive care units (ICUs). In a study conducted in 900 consecutive patients admitted to two cardiac ICUs at a large academic medical center, QTc interval prolongation was present in 28% of patients on admission, and 18% had a QTc interval >500 msec.[675] Of these, 35% and 42%, respectively, were subsequently prescribed QT interval–prolonging drugs, despite being admitted with QTc interval prolongation.[675] In another investigation, 24% of patients in adult ICU and progressive care units developed QTc interval prolongation.[676] In a prospective cohort study of patients admitted to a mixed medical-surgical ICU, 52% had a QTc interval >500 msec during the ICU stay.[677] The prevalence of QTc interval prolongation among patients in an emergency department was 35% (95% CI 32–37%), with 8% of patients having a QTc interval >500 msec.[678]

The incidence of TdP in hospitalized patients has not been widely studied. Pickham et al. reported one case of TdP among 154 patients (0.6%) in adult ICUs and progressive care units during a 2-month period, representing 1 of 16 cardiac arrests (6%) in these units.[676]

MECHANISMS

TdP occurs in the setting of prolongation of ventricular repolarization resulting in lengthening of ventricular action potential duration, which is manifested as prolongation of the QTc interval on the ECG.[195,196,679] As a result of activation of inward depolarizing currents, action potential prolongation leads to increased susceptibility to early afterdepolarizations, which are manifested as depolarizing oscillations in membrane voltage during phase 2 or 3 of the action potential.[195] These early afterdepolarizations may result in triggered upstrokes, which, when occurring during the latter portion of phase 3 of the action potential, may initiate TdP via re-entry.[679]

Prolongation of ventricular repolarization and resulting action-potential duration lengthening may occur as a result of decreases in outward current or increases of inward current during the plateau or repolarization phase of the action potential (or both). Drugs induce TdP through inhibition of outward current through specific potassium channels, primarily the rapid component of the delayed rectifier potassium current (I_{Kr}), resulting in action potential prolongation.[195,196,679] Some drugs, such as ibutilide, also appear to prolong ventricular action potential in part through activation of slow sodium current during phase 2 of the action potential. It is believed that early afterdepolarizations that trigger TdP may be caused by increased inward calcium current through calcium channels that become reactivated as a result of prolongation in action potential duration.[195,679,680]

Although inhibition of I_{Kr} current and/or activation of late sodium current and prolongation of ventricular repolarization and the corresponding QTc interval are requisite for the development of TdP, those factors alone are not sufficient for the arrhythmia to occur. Many patients taking drugs that inhibit I_{Kr} current develop QTc interval prolongation but do not experience TdP. A major factor that is believed to increase the likelihood of TdP, and which may in part explain the lack of a direct correlation between QTc interval and the occurrence of TdP, is heterogeneity of repolarization (also referred to as dispersion of repolarization or refractoriness).[195] Action potential duration varies throughout the three primary ventricular cell types (epicardial, mid-myocardial [M cells], endocardial) as a result of variations in ion currents in the different cell types. The risk of drug-induced TdP is believed to be enhanced in patients with increased transmural dispersion of ventricular refractoriness. In addition, evidence exists to suggest that the risk of TdP may be dependent on instability of the action potential and by the degree of triangulation of the action potential. Instability of the action potential indicates rapid fluctuations in action potential duration. Triangulation of the action potential refers to the repolarization time from action potential duration at 30% repolarization to action potential duration at 90% repolarization; as this time increases, the action potential takes on a more triangular shape. In vitro and ex vivo studies have suggested that the risk of TdP is enhanced when action potential instability and triangulation are present.[681] Further study is required to better understand the conditions required for TdP to develop in patients with QTc interval prolongation.

An important concept with respect to drug-induced TdP is that of repolarization reserve.[682] Under normal conditions, there are multiple redundant mechanisms that maintain normal ventricular repolarization, which include I_{Kr} but also other repolarizing currents, including the slow component of the delayed rectifier potassium current (I_{Ks}), inward sodium current (I_{Na}), L-type inward calcium current ($I_{Ca,L}$), inward rectifier potassium current (I_{k1}), transient outward potassium current (I_{to}), sodium-potassium pump current ($I_{Na/K}$), and sodium/calcium exchange current (I_{NCX}).[683] Inhibition of I_{Kr} with a drug in the presence of fully intact repolarization reserve rarely results in TdP, as the redundancy in repolarizing currents minimizes the impact of I_{Kr} inhibition. However, in the presence of circumstances that diminish repolarization reserve, such as risk factors for TdP (discussed below), drug-induced I_{Kr} inhibition may have a much greater impact on prolonging ventricular repolarization and result in TdP.[682,683]

CLINICAL PRESENTATION AND DIFFERENTIAL DIAGNOSIS

Symptoms associated with TdP are similar to those of other tachyarrhythmias and are related to heart rate and resulting effects on blood pressure and cardiac output (**Table 25-9**). Although TdP is sometimes transient, self-limiting, and spontaneously terminating, it can degenerate into ventricular fibrillation and cause sudden cardiac death.

Table 25-9 Signs and Symptoms Associated with Drug-Induced Torsades de Pointes

- Chest pain (in patients with underlying coronary artery disease)
- Dizziness
- Hypotension
- Lightheadedness
- Near syncope
- Often a "short-long-short" initiating sequence on electrocardiogram
- Palpitations
- Seizure (due to cerebral hypoxia)
- Shortness of breath
- Syncope
- Syndrome of sudden cardiac death
- Tachycardia
- Torsades de pointes on electrocardiogram—polymorphic ventricular tachycardia in setting of prolonged QTc interval

QTc = corrected QT.

The diagnosis of TdP is dependent on the ECG. TdP is a specific polymorphic ventricular tachycardia associated with prolongation of the QTc interval in the sinus beats that precede the arrhythmia. QT interval correction is necessary because the QT interval varies depending on the heart rate; as heart rate increases, the QT interval shortens, and vice versa. There are numerous published formulas for correcting the QT interval, but that which is most commonly used in practice, and which is programmed into ECG machines, is the Bazett's correction: $QTc = QT\ interval/\sqrt{RR\ interval}$.[684]

TdP, or "twisting of the points," is characterized by the apparent twisting of the wide QRS complexes around the isoelectric baseline (**Figure 25-3**) and occurs at rates of 160–240 bpm.[685,686] A characteristic feature of TdP is a short-long-short initiating sequence (Figure 25-3), which occurs as a result of a ventricular premature beat followed by a compensatory pause that is followed by the first beat of the TdP.[687]

The onset of drug-induced TdP is variable, particularly when it is associated with oral drug therapy. TdP associated with intravenous drug therapy usually coincides with the expected time of peak concentration of the causative agent. For example, many of the cases of TdP induced by intravenous erythromycin occurred during the infusion or within 30 minutes of completion of the infusion.[350,352,355,360,362,370] TdP induced by intravenous haloperidol occurs within 15–220 minutes after the infusion.[409] Ibutilide-induced TdP occurs within 2–60 minutes after drug administration, but most often within 15 minutes.[124-126,128,417-425]

TdP induced by oral drugs may be delayed. In an analysis of 144 published articles describing 249 patients who experienced TdP associated with noncardiac drugs, only 18% of the cases occurred within 72 hours of the initiation of oral therapy; 42% occurred between 3 and 30 days after the initiation of therapy, and 40% occurred more than 30 days after the initiation of therapy.[688]

Conditions to consider in the differential diagnosis of drug-induced TdP are listed in **Table 25-10**. Other tachyarrhythmias must be excluded, through review of the ECG. If the patient has polymorphic

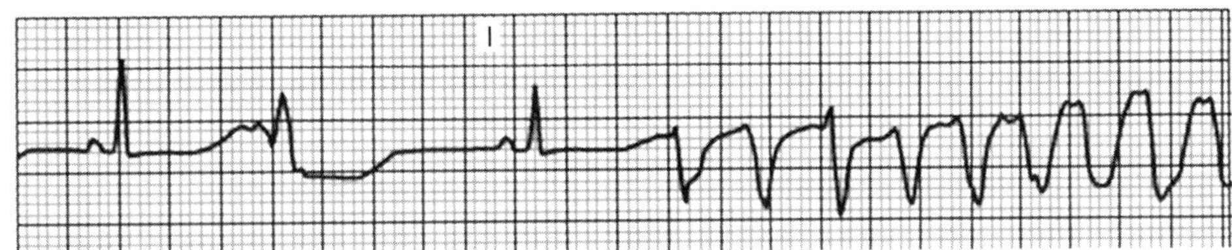

FIGURE 25-3 Torsades de Pointes Associated with Intravenous Haloperidol

Rhythm strip shows prolonged QT interval and short-long-short initiating sequence prior to arrhythmia.
Source: Reprinted with permission from Elsevier. Sharma ND, Rosman HS, Padhi ID et al. Torsades de pointes associated with intravenous haloperidol in critically ill patients. *Am J Cardiol.* 1998; 81:238.

Table 25-10 Conditions to Consider in the Differential Diagnosis of Drug-Induced Torsades de Pointes

- Atrial fibrillation
- Atrial flutter
- Atrial tachycardia
- Atrioventricular nodal re-entrant tachycardia
- Idioventricular tachycardia
- Non-TdP polymorphic ventricular tachycardia
- Sinus tachycardia
- Junctional tachycardia
- Monomorphic ventricular tachycardia
- Ventricular fibrillation

TdP = torsades de pointes.

Table 25-11 Risk Factors for Drug-Induced Torsades de Pointes

- Advanced age
- Bradycardia
- Concomitant administration of >1 agent known to cause QTc interval prolongation or TdP
- Elevated plasma concentrations of QT interval-prolonging drugs due to drug interactions or inadequate dose adjustment for organ dysfunction
- Female sex
- HFrEF
- History of drug-induced TdP
- Hypocalcemia
- Hypokalemia
- Hypomagnesemia
- Increase in QTc interval by >60 msec compared with the pretreatment value
- QTc interval >500 msec
- Rapid intravenous infusion of QTc interval-prolonging drugs
- Sepsis

HFrEF = heart failure with reduced ejection fraction, TdP = torsades de pointes.

ventricular tachycardia, TdP must be distinguished from non-TdP polymorphic ventricular tachycardia; this can be achieved by determining whether prolongation of the QTc interval is present prior to or shortly after the episode of polymorphic ventricular tachycardia. The patient's list of current medications should be reviewed to determine whether he or she is receiving a drug that has been reported to cause TdP, or at least to cause QTc interval prolongation. In addition, the patient should be evaluated for the presence of concomitant risk factors for TdP, which substantially increase the likelihood of the occurrence of the tachyarrhythmia.

RISK FACTORS

Specific risk factors for drug-induced TdP have been identified (**Table 25-11**). Prolongation of the QTc interval on the ECG has consistently been determined to be a risk factor. Evidence indicates that the risk of TdP increases markedly when the QTc interval becomes prolonged to >500 msec, and TdP is rare when the QTc interval is <500 msec.[409,689-691] The risk of TdP is also increased when the QTc interval increases >60 msec compared with pretreatment values.[690] Other TdP risk factors include female sex, advanced age, bradycardia, hypokalemia, hypomagnesemia, hypocalcemia, HFrEF, and conditions leading to elevated plasma concentrations of causative drugs, such as kidney disease, liver disease, drug interactions, or some combination of these.[195,196,691,692] A history of drug-induced

TdP likely increases the risk for TdP associated with other QT interval-prolonging drugs.[195,215]

Drug-induced TdP is exceedingly rare in patients without concomitant risk factors. An analysis of 144 published articles describing 249 patients who experienced TdP associated with noncardiac drugs revealed that nearly 100% of the patients had at least one risk factor, and 71% of the patients had at least two risk factors.[688] More than two thirds of the patients were female; 41% had heart disease (defined as myocardial infarction, heart failure, valvulopathy, or cardiomyopathy); 28% had hypokalemia; 19% had drug toxicity (defined as administration of higher-than-recommended doses or lack of dose adjustment for organ dysfunction); 18% had a familial history of long-QT syndrome, a history of previous drug-induced TdP, or a history of drug-induced QTc interval prolongation.[688] Drug interactions leading to increased plasma concentrations of the causative agent were present in 35% of the patients. These data indicate that the vast majority of patients who develop noncardiac drug-induced TdP have risk factors that are easily identifiable.

Explanations for an increased risk of drug-induced TdP in specific patient populations continue to be investigated.[693] Reasons that women are at increased risk for drug-induced TdP may involve arrhythmogenic effects of estrogen in women or protective effects of testosterone in men.[694,695] The baseline QTc interval is longer in women than in men, a difference that manifests at puberty.[696,697] In one series of 332 cases of TdP associated with antiarrhythmic agents, 70% of the cases occurred in women.[698] Other studies have documented a female predisposition to TdP associated with azimilide, dofetilide, erythromycin, ibutilide, quinidine, sotalol, and terfenadine.[333,551,691,699-702] The influence of sex hormones on ventricular repolarization and risk for TdP has been investigated and remains a subject of ongoing study. One group of investigators administered a small dose of intravenous ibutilide to healthy women during three phases of the menstrual cycle and attempted to correlate plasma concentrations of estradiol and progesterone with ibutilide-induced prolongations in the QTc interval. QTc interval prolongation was not correlated with plasma estradiol concentration but was inversely correlated with the plasma progesterone concentration and the plasma progesterone-to-estradiol ratio, suggesting that estrogen may not be proarrhythmic, but that progesterone, an androgenic compound, may be protective against drug-induced QTc interval lengthening.[703] In vitro studies have shown that dihydrotestosterone shortens basal action potential duration and diminishes the effects of potassium channel-blocking drugs on action potential duration.[704] Therefore, androgens may protect against the electrophysiologic effects of drugs with the potential to induce TdP.

HFrEF is a major risk factor for drug-induced TdP. The incidence of TdP associated with drugs such as ibutilide and dofetilide has been shown to be more than twice as high in patients with HFrEF than in patients with normal left ventricular function.[324,325,418,419] Mechanisms behind the increased risk of TdP in this population are unclear. Down-regulation of potassium channels occurs in patients with HFrEF, promoting prolongation in ventricular repolarization. Patients with HFrEF have been shown to be more sensitive to drug-induced QTc interval lengthening than those with normal left ventricular function.[705,706] In a study of ibutilide pretreatment for facilitation of direct current cardioversion of atrial fibrillation, two of 64 ibutilide-treated patients (3.1%) had TdP; both patients had a left ventricular ejection fraction <20%.[422] On the basis of this study, many recommend that QTc interval-prolonging drugs should not be administered to patients with a left ventricular ejection fraction <20%. It remains unknown whether heart failure with preserved ejection fraction is a risk factor for drug-induced TdP.

Elevated plasma concentrations of drugs known to cause TdP are an important risk factor. The majority of cases of TdP associated with erythromycin or haloperidol occurred after intravenous administration of the drug, possibly as a result of higher peak plasma concentrations.[350,352,355,359,362,365,366,370,404-407,409-412] In addition, failure to adequately adjust specific drug doses for kidney disease has resulted in TdP associated with dofetilide, levofloxacin, procainamide, and sotalol.[431,504,546,547,552,553,707] Drugs that have been reported to cause TdP that require dose adjustment in patients with kidney disease or hepatic impairment are listed in **Tables 25-12** and **25-13**, respectively.

Drug interactions are a particularly important risk factor for drug-induced TdP. Of 25 cases of TdP associated with terfenadine that were reported to the U.S. Food and Drug Administration (FDA), nine patients were receiving concomitant therapy with ketoconazole or itraconazole, which inhibit the metabolism of terfenadine.[702] Numerous reported cases of drug-induced TdP occurred as a result of drug interactions leading to elevated plasma concentrations of the offending agent.[213,277,281,284,296,299,347,358,363,369,371] Drugs associated with a risk of TdP that are substrates for the cytochrome P-450 system, and therefore subject to drug interactions when used in combination with inhibitors of enzymes of the cytochrome P-450 system, are listed in **Table 25-14**.[708]

Table 25-12 Drugs That May Induce Torsades de Pointes and Require Dose Adjustment or Are Contraindicated in Patients with Kidney Disease

• Amantadine	• Metoclopramide
• Amisulpride	• Ofloxacin
• Arsenic trioxide	• Oxaliplatin
• Chloral hydrate	• Pentamidine
• Ciprofloxacin	• Posaconazole
• Clarithromycin	• Procainamide
• Disopyramide	• Quinidine
• Dofetilide	• Quinine
• Domperidone	• Risperidone
• Famotidine	• Solifenacin
• Flecainide	• Sotalol
• Fluconazole	• Sparfloxacin
• Gatifloxacin	• Tacrolimus
• Levofloxacin	• Vandetanib
• Loratadine	

Table 25-13 Drugs That May Induce Torsades de Pointes and Require Dose Adjustment or Are Contraindicated in Patients with Liver Disease

• Atazanavir	• Nelfinavir
• Buprenorphine	• Olanzapine
• Cisapride	• Ondansetron
• Citalopram	• Quetiapine
• Domperidone	• Quinidine
• Dronedarone	• Ranolazine
• Escitalopram	• Risperidone
• Fluoxetine	• Roxithromycin
• Itraconazole	• Solifenacin
• Ivabradine	• Tacrolimus
• Levomepromazine	• Voriconazole
• Metronidazole	• Vorinostat

Bradycardia has been shown to be a risk factor for drug-induced TdP. Ventricular repolarization is dependent on heart rate; the slower the heart rate, the longer the period of ventricular repolarization.[680] The majority of drugs with the potential to cause TdP to bind to potassium channels in a manner called reverse-use-dependent (which means that the slower the heart rate, the more tightly the drug binds to the potassium channel) likely explains the higher risk of TdP at slower heart rates.[709]

Use of combinations of QT interval-prolonging drugs may increase the risk for drug-induced TdP, although conflicting data exist. Polypharmacy with QT interval-prolonging drugs and/or with interacting drugs is common. A retrospective cohort study of an outpatient prescription claims database revealed that 9.4% of approximately 1.1 million patients who filled a prescription for a QT interval-prolonging drug also filled an overlapping prescription for a second QT interval-prolonging drug or for a drug known to inhibit the clearance of the QT interval-prolonging agent.[710] In a similar study, automated drug-dispensing data from 2 million health plan members from a total of 10 health maintenance organizations were reviewed to determine the proportion of these patients who had been prescribed QT interval-prolonging drugs, and the proportion of those patients for whom a second QT interval-prolonging drug or a drug known to alter the clearance of the QT interval-prolonging medication was prescribed.[711] Of the patients from whom data were obtained, 11.4% had received prescriptions for a potentially QT interval-prolonging drug. Of the patients who received prescriptions for a QT interval-prolonging drug, 4.6% also received a prescription

Table 25-14 Drugs That May Induce Torsades de Pointes and Are Substrates for Enzymes of the Cytochrome P-450 System[708]

1A2	2B6	2C9	2C19	2D6	2E1	3A4,5,7
Amitriptyline	Methadone	Amitriptyline	Amitriptyline	Amitriptyline	Sevoflurane	Amiodarone
Clozapine		Fluoxetine	Citalopram	Aripiprazole		Aripiprazole
Haloperidol			Doxepin	Chlorpromazine		Cisapride
Imipramine			Imipramine	Donepezil		Clarithromycin
Olanzapine			Nelfinavir	Flecainide		Cocaine
Ondansetron			Pantoprazole	Fluoxetine		Domperidone
			Voriconazole	Haloperidol		Erythromycin
				Imipramine		Haloperidol
				Metoclopramide		Methadone
				Ondansetron		Nelfinavir
				Risperidone		Ondansetron
				Thioridazine		Pimozide
						Quetiapine
						Quinidine
						Quinine
						Risperidone
						Tacrolimus
						Terfenadine
						Trazodone
						Ziprasidone

Source: Adapted with permission from Flockhart DA. Drug interactions: cytochrome P450 drug interaction table. http://medicine.iupui.edu/clinpharm/ddis/main-table (accessed 2017 Dec 19).

for a potentially interacting drug that could increase the risk of TdP.[711] Approximately 15% of emergency department visits involve prescriptions of a QT interval-prolonging drug, roughly 10% of which involved prescriptions for ≥2 QT interval-prolonging agents.[712] Therefore, concomitant use of multiple QT interval-prolonging drugs is relatively common. Some evidence indicates that this practice increases the risk of QT interval prolongation and/or TdP. In an analysis of patients in cardiac critical care units, use of ≥2 QT interval-prolonging drugs was associated with an odds ratio for development of QTc interval prolongation of 2.6 (95% CI 1.9–5.6, $p = 0.02$).[692] However, other data do not indicate that combinations of QT interval-prolonging drugs increase the risk of QTc interval prolongation or TdP compared with therapy with a single QTc interval-prolonging agent. A systematic review of literature regarding antipsychotic therapy concluded that antipsychotic polypharmacy may not worsen QTc interval prolongation.[713] In a population-based cohort study of approximately 13,000 patients, the addition of a second or third QTc interval-prolonging drug to initial QTc interval-lengthening therapy exerted only a very small additional effect on QTc interval.[714] Further study is needed to ascertain the safety of use of combinations of QTc interval-prolonging drugs.

Some evidence suggests that patients in whom drug-induced TdP develops may have a genetic predisposition. Fifteen specific genetic defects have been identified that underlie the congenital long-QT interval syndromes.[715] Mutations of genes that are known to predispose to the congenital long-QT interval syndromes were shown to be present in 10–15% of patients who experience drug-induced TdP.[716] In another study, missense mutations in five long QT-interval genes were found in a small minority of patients with drug-induced TdP.[717] Itoh et al.[718] reported that 40% of 20 patients with drug-induced TdP had mutations in long-QT syndrome genes and that the incidence of mutations was higher in patients with TdP induced by nonantiarrhythmic drugs compared to antiarrhythmic drugs. The positive mutation rate in patients with drug-induced TdP was similar to that in patients with congenital long-QT syndrome. However, results from a genome-wide association study suggest that genetic polymorphisms may not contribute importantly to the risk of drug-induced TdP.[719] This study included 216 patients with TdP from Northwestern Europe and in 771 ancestry-matched controls, including treatment-tolerant patients and individuals in the general population. No single nucleotide polymorphism reached genome-wide significance, suggesting that common genomic variants do not contribute importantly to the risk of drug-induced TdP.[719]

MORBIDITY AND MORTALITY

TdP may result in clinical symptoms requiring medical attention. More importantly, TdP may result in sudden cardiac death; the incidence of sudden death due to TdP is unknown. During the past couple of decades, a number of drugs, including terfenadine, astemizole, grepafloxacin, cisapride, levomethadyl, and mesoridazine, have been removed from the U.S. market as a result of causing deaths due to TdP.

In a retrospective analysis of 205 patients with advanced HFrEF, patients with a history of drug-induced TdP had a significantly higher risk of sudden cardiac death during therapy with amiodarone as compared with amiodarone-treated patients with no history of drug-induced TdP (55% versus 15%).[720] These data suggest that drugs known to prolong the QT interval should not be administered to patients with advanced HFrEF and a history of drug-induced TdP.

Antipsychotic agents have been associated with an increased risk of sudden cardiac death, potentially as a result of TdP. The risk of sudden cardiac death associated with antipsychotic drugs was investigated in a population-based case–control study of a longitudinal database consisting of medical records from 150 general practitioners in Europe.[721] Current use of antipsychotic agents was associated with a significant increase in the risk of sudden cardiac death (OR 3.3, 95% CI 1.8–6.2). Previous use of antipsychotic drugs was not associated with an increased risk of sudden cardiac death. The risk of sudden cardiac death was highest among patients receiving butyrophenone agents (such as haloperidol).[721] The precise cause of sudden cardiac death was not documented in this study, but these drugs are known to be a cause of TdP, which may have contributed to sudden cardiac death in these patients. A retrospective cohort study of Medicaid enrollees in Tennessee also reported an increased risk of sudden cardiac death associated with both typical and atypical antipsychotic drugs.[722] In a retrospective cohort study from a large database, the adjusted relative risk of cardiac mortality associated with olanzapine was significantly elevated compared to psychiatric nonusers of olanzapine (RR 1.53, 95% CI 1.12–20.9).[723] Treatment with any antipsychotic agent and with typical antipsychotic agents was associated with significantly increased risks of out-of-hospital cardiac arrest in a study of the Danish Cardiac Arrest Register.[724] In a case-crossover study conducted using the Taiwan National Health Insurance Research Database, antipsychotic drug use was associated with a significantly increased risk of ventricular arrhythmia and/or sudden cardiac death, and antipsychotic agents with the greatest potency to inhibit I_{Kr} were associated with the highest risk of ventricular arrhythmias and/or sudden cardiac death.[725] A meta-analysis of observational studies assessing the influence of antipsychotic agents on sudden cardiac death concluded that the risk differed among different antipsychotics (thioridazine>clozapine>risperidone>haloperidol>olanzapine>quetiapine).[726]

Macrolide antibiotics have also been associated with an increased risk of sudden cardiac death. In a study of a cohort of patients identified from the Tennessee Medicaid database, the multivariate-adjusted rate of sudden death from cardiac causes was twice as high in patients currently using erythromycin as compared with that in patients who had not used the drug.[727] Further, the adjusted rate of sudden death from cardiac causes was five times higher among patients who had concurrently used drugs that inhibited activity of the cytochrome P-450 enzyme system while taking erythromycin.[727] These data indicate that erythromycin use, particularly in combination with potentially interacting drugs, may markedly increase the risk of cardiac mortality. A similar study of the Tennessee Medicaid database found that patients taking 5 days of therapy with azithromycin had an increased risk of cardiovascular death (HR 2.88, 95% CI 1.79–4.63, p <0.001) and death from any cause (HR 1.85, 95% CI 1.25–2.75, p = 0.002) compared to patients who took no antibiotics.[728] Compared to patients taking amoxicillin, those who took azithromycin for 5 days had an increased risk of cardiovascular death (HR 2.49; 95% CI 1.38–4.50, p = 0.002) and death from any cause (HR 2.02, 95% CI 1.24–3.30, p = 0.005).[728] Similarly, in a cohort study of U.S. veterans, patients receiving 5 days of azithromycin therapy had an increased risk of death (HR 1.48, 95% CI 1.05–2.09) and serious arrhythmia (HR 1.77, 95% CI 1.20–2.62) compared with patients receiving amoxicillin.[729] Clarithromycin was associated with an increased risk of cardiovascular events (defined as hospital admissions with acute coronary syndrome, decompensated heart failure, serious arrhythmia, or sudden cardiac death) in a propensity score-matched study of two prospectively collected datasets in patients with chronic obstructive pulmonary disease.[730] Conversely, however, a propensity score-matched nationwide historical cohort study of the Danish Civil Registration System found that current azithromycin use was not associated with an increased risk of cardiovascular death compared to penicillin V (rate ratio 0.93, 95% CI 0.56–1.55).[731] Cheng et al.[732] performed a meta-analysis of 33 studies involving nearly 21 million patients to assess the association between macrolide antibiotics and cardiovascular risk. Compared to those not taking macrolides, patients taking macrolides had an increased risk of sudden cardiac death or ventricular tachyarrhythmias (RR 2.42 [1.61–3.63]), sudden cardiac death (2.52 [1.91–3.31]), and cardiovascular death (1.31 [1.06–1.62]). The weight of the overall data suggests that macrolide antibiotics are associated with an increased risk of sudden cardiac death and cardiovascular death.

An analysis was performed of reports to the FDA of QTc interval prolongation and TdP associated with methadone.[443] From 1969 through October 2002, the FDA received 43 reports of TdP and 15 reports of QTc interval prolongation. Hospitalization was required in 47% of these cases, and death occurred in 8%.

In summary, drug-induced TdP may result in morbidity requiring hospitalization and mortality due to sudden cardiac death. Patients with a history of drug-induced TdP and those currently receiving typical or atypical antipsychotic agents or macrolide antibiotics have been shown to be at higher risk of cardiovascular mortality.

PREVENTION

Some methods of prevention of drug-induced TdP are listed in **Table 25-15**. Drug-induced TdP may be prevented by minimizing risk factors associated with TdP (Table 25-11). Intravenous erythromycin doses of 1 g every 6 hours should be avoided, unless *Legionella pneumophila* infection is documented. The maximum daily dose of intravenous haloperidol should not exceed 35 mg.[409]

In patients receiving drugs known to promote the development of TdP, the QTc interval should be monitored and maintained at <500 msec. Prior to initiating therapy with a drug known to cause TdP, a baseline (predrug) ECG for determination of QTc interval should be obtained wherever possible. In hospitalized patients receiving drugs known to cause TdP, QTc intervals should be monitored daily, preferably using a 12-lead ECG but at least using a lead II ECG strip. Some hospitals have the capability for fully automated QTc interval monitoring, with which an algorithm measures the QTc interval every 5 minutes, and an audible alarm sounds if there is an increase in QTc interval >60 msec from baseline or if a QTc interval >500 msec is measured for at least three consecutive measurements (i.e., 15 minutes).[686] Patients receiving long-term oral therapy with drugs known to promote the development of TdP should undergo a 12-lead ECG for the measurement of QTc intervals every 3 to 6 months depending on the presence or absence of other risk factors.

Clinical decision support tools have been developed with the objective of reducing the risk of TdP. At the Mayo Clinic, an institution-wide computer-based QT interval alert system was implemented,

Table 25-15 Prevention of Drug-Induced Torsades de Pointes

- Adjust doses of renally eliminated QTc interval-prolonging drugs in patients with kidney disease
- Adjust doses or avoid use of hepatically metabolized QTc interval-prolonging drugs in patients with liver disease
- Avoid concomitant administration of QTc interval-prolonging drugs
- Avoid drug interactions involving QTc interval-prolonging drugs that are substrates of the cytochrome P-450 enzyme system with cytochrome P-450 enzyme inhibitors
- Avoid use of QTc interval-prolonging drugs in patients who have been diagnosed with one of the congenital long QT interval syndromes
- Avoid use of QTc interval-prolonging drugs in patients with a history of drug-induced TdP
- Avoid use of QTc interval-prolonging drugs in patients with pretreatment QTc intervals >450 msec
- Discontinue QTc interval-prolonging agent if QTc increases to >500 msec
- Maintain serum calcium concentrations within normal range
- Maintain serum magnesium concentrations ≥2 mg/dL
- Maintain serum potassium concentrations ≥4 mEq/L
- Reduce dose or discontinue QTc interval-prolonging agent if QTc increases >60 msec from pretreatment value
- When possible, avoid use of QTc interval-prolonging drugs in patients with HFrEF, especially in patients with LVEF <20%

HFrEF = heart failure with reduced ejection fraction, TdP = torsades de pointes.

which screens all ECGs and alerts physicians if their patient's QTc interval is ≥500 msec.[733] Sorita et al.[734] developed and implemented a clinical decision support system integrated into the computerized physician order-entry system that identifies any attempt to order medications associated with TdP for patients with a history of QTc interval ≥500 msec and alerts the provider entering the order. This system resulted in a 13.9% reduction in administration of potentially TdP-inducing drugs to these high-risk patients. Another group of investigators developed and implemented a clinical decision support computer alert incorporating a validated risk score for QTc interval prolongation for patients in cardiac critical care units.[692,735] In this system, the computer calculates each patient's risk score for development of QTc interval prolongation. When patients are prescribed a drug with the potential to induce TdP and their QTc interval prolongation risk score is moderate or high (but not low), a computer alert appears to the pharmacist entering or reviewing the order, who can then contact the prescriber to discuss modulation of modifiable risk factors or selection of alternate drug therapy, where appropriate. Implementation of this computer alert system resulted in a significant reduction in the risk of QTc interval prolongation in these units (OR 0.65, 95% CI 0.56–0.89, p <0.0001). In addition, implementation of this alert system resulted in a significant reduction in the prescribing of noncardiovascular QTc interval-prolonging drugs.[735]

Although drugs with the potential to cause TdP should not necessarily be avoided in female patients, other risk factors associated with drug-induced TdP are easily identifiable prior to the initiation of therapy with QTc interval-prolonging drugs, and use of QTc interval-prolonging drugs in patients with these other risk factors should be avoided whenever possible.[688,692] In particular, concomitant administration of susceptible QT interval-prolonging drugs with drugs that inhibit their metabolism should be avoided, and doses of renally eliminated or hepatically metabolized QTc interval-prolonging drugs should be adequately adjusted in patients with kidney or liver disease, respectively.

Prophylactic administration of magnesium has been shown to attenuate the effects of drugs on QT interval prolongation. Administration of magnesium sulfate 2 g intravenously prior to administration of ibutilide 1 mg significantly diminished the effect of ibutilide on QT interval prolongation in patients with normal serum magnesium concentrations compared with that in a group of normomagnesemic patients who received placebo prior to ibutilide. In addition, pretreatment with magnesium significantly reduced the risk of ibutilide-induced QT interval prolongation >30 msec as compared with preibutilide values.[736] Patsilinakos et al.[131] retrospectively analyzed 476 patients who had received ibutilide for conversion of atrial fibrillation or atrial flutter to sinus rhythm during a 4-year period. All patients received ibutilide 1 mg intravenously over 10 minutes, followed by a second 1-mg dose if necessary 10 minutes following completion of the first infusion. In n = 247 patients, a 1-hour intravenous infusion of magnesium 5 g was administered prior to ibutilide, followed by a second infusion of magnesium 5 g, this time over 2 hours, without interrupting the ibutilide infusion protocol. The incidence of TdP was significantly lower in the patients who received magnesium prophylaxis compared to those that did not (0% versus 3.5%, $p = 0.009$). The incidence of all ventricular arrhythmias (sustained ventricular tachycardia, nonsustained ventricular tachycardia, and TdP) was also significantly lower in the magnesium prophylaxis group (1.2% versus 7.4%, $p = 0.002$). The two groups were similar demographically, although those in the magnesium prophylaxis group were slightly older (62 versus 58 years, $p = 0.057$). These data suggest that magnesium prophylaxis may be a reasonable strategy in patients at risk for TdP who require ibutilide therapy for atrial fibrillation or atrial flutter.

In a prospective, randomized, double-blind, placebo-controlled crossover pilot study, administration of oral progesterone 400 mg daily was found to attenuate drug-induced QTc interval lengthening in young healthy women during the menses phase of the menstrual cycle (when endogenous serum progesterone concentrations are lowest).[737] Studies are ongoing to determine whether exogenous administration of sex hormones may reduce the risk of drug-induced QTc interval prolongation in patient populations at risk.

Specific guidelines were published regarding monitoring of patients for prevention of methadone-induced TdP.[738] These guidelines recommend that all patients on methadone therapy should undergo a pretreatment ECG for determination of the QTc interval, a follow-up 12-lead ECG for determination of the QTc interval within 30 days of the initiation of methadone treatment, and a 12-lead ECG for QTc interval determination annually. More intensive QTc interval monitoring was recommended for patients who require daily methadone doses >100 mg and for those that experience unexplained syncope or seizures. Subsequent recommendations tempered the 30-day ECG suggestion on the basis of concerns regarding the resources required to implement routine ECGs and the absence of strong evidence that such routine ECG monitoring reduces the incidence of methadone-associated cardiac events.[739] These newer recommendations suggested that a baseline ECG should be performed at the time of admission into an opioid treatment program and within 30 days in patients with significant risk factors for QTc interval prolongation, and that additional ECGs should be performed annually or whenever the methadone dose exceeds 120 mg daily.[739]

MANAGEMENT

A treatment strategy for the acute management of drug-induced TdP is presented in **Figure 25-4**.[190] Management of drug-induced TdP is dependent on recognition of the arrhythmia and distinguishing it from monomorphic ventricular tachycardia or non-torsades polymorphic ventricular tachycardia. Therapy with drugs with the potential to cause TdP should be discontinued. Hypokalemia, hypomagnesemia, or hypocalcemia should be corrected with intravenous potassium, magnesium, or calcium, respectively. Patients with TdP who are hemodynamically unstable should be treated with asynchronous shocks (i.e., defibrillation).[190] Although synchronized direct current cardioversion is preferred for organized rhythms, synchronization of shocks is often not possible in patients with polymorphic ventricular tachycardias such as TdP, because the multiple QRS complex configurations and fluctuating heart rates render it very difficult, and sometimes impossible, to synchronize the delivery of the shock to a QRS complex.[190]

Several treatment options are available for patients with hemodynamically stable TdP (Figure 25-4). Intravenous magnesium has been reported to terminate TdP, irrespective of the patient's serum magnesium concentration.[199,290,458,508,521,548,561,740-747] The mechanism by which intravenous magnesium terminates TdP is not clear, but termination may occur via inhibition of early afterdepolarizations as a result of calcium-channel blockade.

Overdrive pacing via the percutaneous insertion of a temporary pacemaker is also effective for termination of TdP accompanied by bradycardia or precipitated by pauses in rhythm, as overdrive pacing leads to shortening of the QT interval.[190,312,501,536] Intravenous isoproterenol may also terminate TdP, by increasing heart rate and shortening the QT

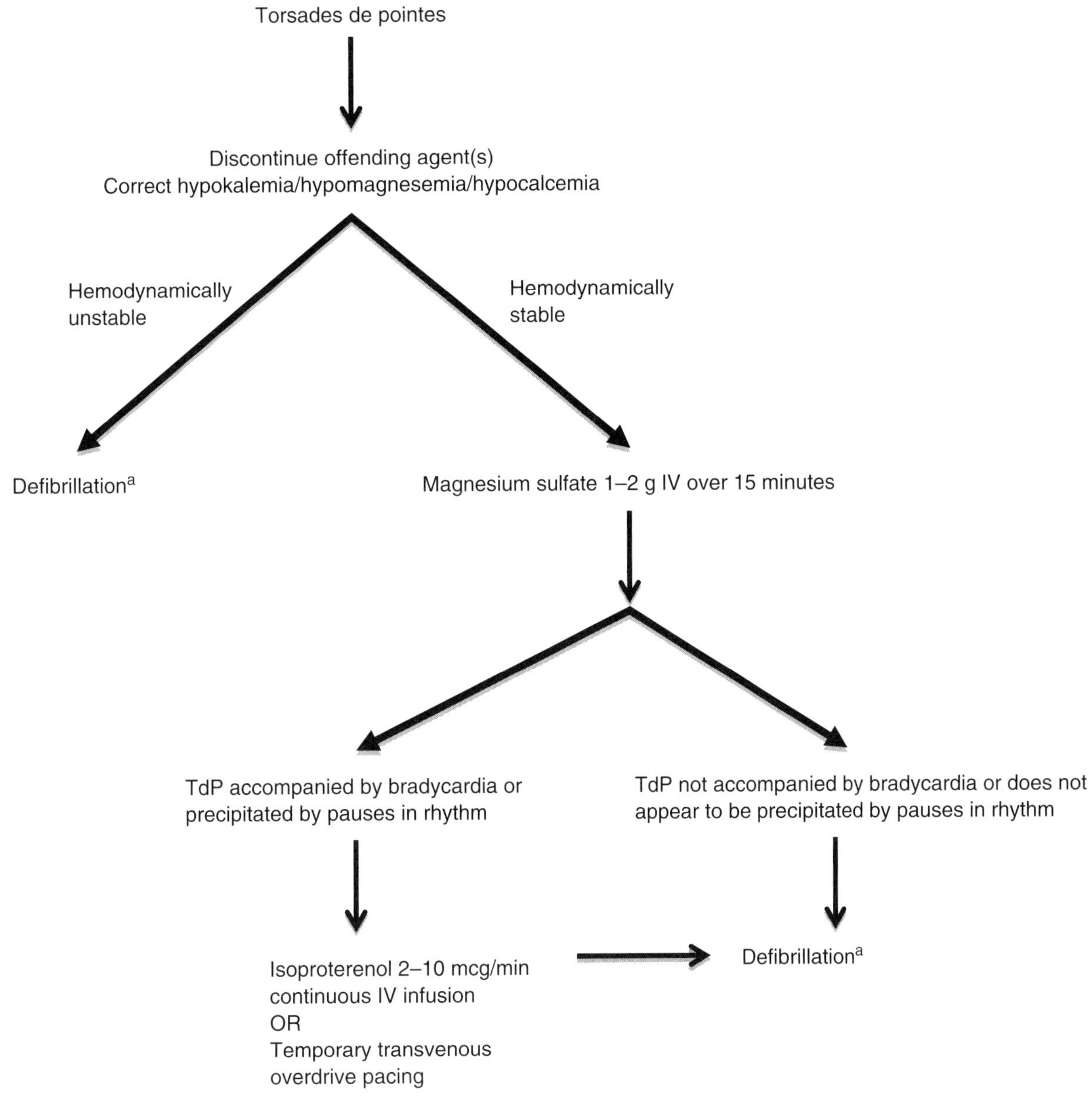

FIGURE 25-4 Management of Drug-Induced Torsades de Pointes

IV = intravenous, J = joules. [a]Biphasic shock:120–200 J; monophasic shock:360 J.

Source: Adapted with permission from Elsevier. Tisdale JE. Acute management of arrhythmias. In: Esrtad B, ed. *Critical care pharmacotherapy*. Lenexa, KS: American College of Clinical Pharmacy; 2016:1244-81.

interval.[190,191,507,748] In addition, refractory TdP associated with sotalol has been successfully managed using hemodialysis or peritoneal dialysis.[547,554,555]

INFORMATION FOR PATIENTS

Patients who are taking drugs that may cause TdP should be instructed that the drug may in rare cases cause the heart rate (pulse) to become faster. Patients should be instructed to consult their pharmacist or physician if the heart rate increases to above 100–120 bpm, or if they feel palpitations, lightheaded, dizzy, tired, weak, short of breath, or chest pain. Patients who are taking drugs that may cause TdP should be instructed not to take any nonprescription medication without first consulting their pharmacist or physician because of the possibility of interactions of potentially proarrhythmic medications with nonprescription drugs such as cimetidine. In addition, patients should make sure that their pharmacist and physician are fully aware of all medications that they are taking to avoid receiving new medications that may potentially interact with drugs that may cause TdP.

BRUGADA SYNDROME

Brugada syndrome is an inherited disorder characterized by specific ECG abnormalities not associated with myocardial ischemia, electrolyte perturbations, or structural heart disease.[749] Brugada syndrome is classified into three types, based on specific ECG abnormalities in at least two of the right chest leads (V_1–V_3): Type 1—coved ST segment elevation, J point elevation ≥2 mm, and inverted T wave; Type 2—saddle-shaped ST segments with J point elevation ≥2 mm and ST segment elevation ≥1 mm with a positive or biphasic T wave; and Type 3—saddle-shaped ST segments with J point elevation <2 mm and ST segment elevation <1 mm. In addition to the ECG abnormalities, diagnostic criteria include syncope, prior cardiac arrest, documented or inducible polymorphic ventricular tachycardia or ventricular fibrillation, a family history of sudden death <45 years of age, or Type 1 Brugada pattern and/or nocturnal agonal respiration.[750]

In the majority of cases, Brugada syndrome is caused by mutations in the gene *SCN5A*, which encodes cardiac sodium channels. Sodium channel-blocking drugs such as flecainide are often used to unmask concealed forms of the Brugada syndrome. However, a drug-induced form of Brugada syndrome has been described, in which drugs provoke Brugada syndrome ECG patterns and cause ventricular tachycardia, ventricular fibrillation, and sudden cardiac death.

CAUSATIVE AGENTS

Drugs that have been reported to exacerbate or provoke Brugada syndrome are presented in **Table 25-16.**[749,751-786] Up-to-date lists of drugs associated with Brugada syndrome may be found at Brugadadrugs.org.[787] Drugs in Table 25-16 are those with published literature supporting an association with arrhythmias and the most typical (Type 1) Brugada syndrome ECG. A list of drugs that are recommended to be avoided in patients with Brugada syndrome, but for which there is no published evidence of an association with arrhythmias, can be found at Brugadadrugs.org.[787]

EPIDEMIOLOGY

The prevalence of the Brugada syndrome is estimated to be 1–5 per 10,000 persons.[788] The prevalence is higher in countries in Southeast Asia, especially Thailand, the Philippines, and Japan, where the prevalence is roughly 0.5–1 per 1,000 persons.[750] The prevalence of Brugada syndrome is 8-10-fold higher in men than women.[788,789] The higher prevalence in males may be due to more prominent transient outward potassium current (I_{to}) and/or higher plasma testosterone concenrations.[790,791]

The overall incidence and prevalence of drug-induced Brugada syndrome are not known, and the incidence has been determined for only a small number of drugs known to exacerbate this syndrome (Table 25-16).

MECHANISMS

Brugada syndrome is inherited via autosomal dominance (with the exception of one genotype, which is inherited in an X-linked manner).[789,792] To date, 23 genotypes have been identified, which are associated with a decrease in inward sodium or calcium current or an increase in outward potassium current.[792] One genotype, caused by pathogenic variants in the *SCN5A* gene that encodes for the α subunit of the cardiac sodium channel, is responsible for 15–30% of patients with the Brugada syndrome.[789,792] The precise mechanism of the ECG abnormailities and arrhythmias associated with the Brugada syndrome is unknown. It has been proposed that the ST segment elevation associated with Brugada syndrome may be due to local conduction abnormalities, local ventricular depolarization, or an early repolarization abnormality caused by reduction in fast

Table 25-16 Agents Implicated in Drug-Induced Brugada Syndrome

Drug	Incidence	Level of Evidence[a]
Ajmaline[751-756]	0.15–1.8% (adults) 10% (children)	B
Alcohol[757-759]	NK	C
Amitriptyline[760,761]	NK	C
Bupivacaine[762]	NK	C
Cocaine[763-765]	NK	C
Desipramine[766]	NK	C
Flecainide[767-769]	NK	C
Lithium[770]	NK	C
Loxapine[771]	NK	C
Nortriptyline[772,773]	NK	C
Oxcarbazepine[774]	NK	C
Pilsicainide[775-779]	11–18%	B
Procainamide[780]	NK	C
Propafenone[781,782]	NK	C
Propofol[783-786]	NK	C
Trifluoperazine[771]	NK	C

NK = not known.
[a]Definitions for Levels of Evidence: Level A—evidence from one or more randomized, controlled clinical trials; Level B—evidence from nonrandomized clinical trials, prospective observational studies, cohort studies, retrospective studies, case-control studies, meta-analyses and/or postmarketing surveillance studies; and Level C—evidence from one or more published case reports or case series.

sodium current and/or L-type calcium current or an increase in I_{to}, which would result in shortening of the epicardial action potential.[793,794] This would produce increased dispersion of repolarization across the epicardium/endocardium. Increased dispersion of ventricular repolarization in association with extrasystoles may lead to re-entrant arrhythmias.[749] Drugs that provoke or unmask the Brugada syndrome are predominantly those that inhibit cardiac sodium channels (Table 25-16).[749,795] The mechanism of alcohol-induced Brugada syndrome is not clear, although it has been suggested that alcohol-associated enhancement of parasympathetic nervous system activity may contribute.[758]

CLINICAL PRESENTATION AND DIFFERENTIAL DIAGNOSIS

Clinical symptoms associated with drug-induced Brugada syndrome are presented in **Table 25-17**. Drug-induced Brugada syndrome manifests in relatively young individuals. In a study of the clinical characteristics and risk factors for drug-induced Brugada syndrome, the mean age of onset was 39 ± 16 years.[795] In this study, 77% of patients who developed the drug-induced Brugada syndrome ECG pattern were male, and men developed the syndrome at a younger age than women (37 ± 16 years versus 44 ± 17 years, $p = 0.07$). Symptoms associated with drug-induced Brugada syndrome include monomorphic ventricular tachycardia, idioventricular tachycardia, ventricular fibrillation or aborted sudden cardiac death, syncope, nocturnal agonal

Table 25-17 Signs and Symptoms Associated with Drug-Induced Brugada Syndrome

- Aborted sudden cardiac death
- Chest discomfort
- Idioventricular tachycardia
- Monomorphic ventricular tachycardia
- Nocturnal agonal respiration
- Palpitations
- Syncope
- Ventricular fibrillation

respiration, palpitations, and chest discomfort.[789] Ventricular fibrillation or aborted sudden cardiac death occurs more often at night than during the day. The time of onset of drug-induced Brugada syndrome after initiation of therapy with causative agents ranges from weeks to years; only a small proportion of cases occur with drug exposure <72 hours.[795]

For patients with suspected nondrug-induced Brugada syndrome, sodium channel-blocking drugs such as ajmaline, flecainide, pilsicainide, or procainamide may be administered as a component of the diagnostic process to provoke/unmask the type I ECG pattern.[789] Differential diagnosis of drug-induced Brugada syndrome includes exclusion of other arrhythmias (**Table 25-18**). In addition, other conditions that may mimic the Brugada ECG pattern include arrhythmogenic right ventricular cardiomyopathy, right ventricular ischemia or infarction, pulmonary embolism, cardiac tamponade, early repolarization syndrome, hyperkalemia, hypokalemia, hypercalcemia, or hypothermia.[750]

RISK FACTORS

Risk factors for drug-induced Brugada syndrome are presented in **Table 25-19**. As mentioned previously, male sex is a risk factor. In addition, fever is a risk factor/trigger for arrhythmias associated with drug-induced Brugada syndrome.[795] The risk of drug-induced Brugada syndrome appears to be related to drug dose, and many of the reported cases occurred in patients receiving high doses or overdoses of potentially causative agents.[759,761,763-765,768,769,772,784] In one analysis, drug toxicity was associated with 46% of 74 cases of Brugada syndrome associated with noncardiac drugs.[795]

Table 25-18 Conditions to Consider in the Differential Diagnosis of Drug-Induced Brugada Syndrome

- Atrial fibrillation
- Atrial flutter
- Atrial tachycardia
- Atrioventricular nodal re-entrant tachycardia
- Idioventricular tachycardia
- Junctional tachycardia
- Non-Brugada syndrome idioventricular tachycardia
- Non-Brugada syndrome monomorphic ventricular tachycardia
- Non-Brugada syndrome ventricular fibrillation
- Sinus tachycardia
- TdP

TdP = torsades de pointes.

Table 25-19 Risk Factors for Drug-Induced Brugada Syndrome

- Fever
- High doses/overdoses of potentially causative agents
- Male sex

MORBIDITY AND MORTALITY

Brugada syndrome is associated with sudden cardiac death. The risk of fatal or near-fatal arrhythmias in patients with Brugada syndrome who had been previously asymptomatic ranges from 1% to 8% over 30–40 months of follow-up.[789] In patients with nondrug-induced Brugada syndrome, the incidence of cardiac events (appropriate implantable cardioverter-defibrillator shocks or sudden cardiac death) was found to be 5% over a mean follow-up period of 32 months (range 14–54 months).[796] The cardiac event rate was highest in those patients who had a previous aborted episode of sudden cardiac death (7.7%) compared with those with a history of syncope (1.9%) or those who remained asymptomatic (0.5%).[796]

The incidence of lethal arrhythmias in patients with drug-induced Brugada syndrome is unknown, but fatal and near-fatal cases have been reported. In a study of 74 cases of Brugada syndrome (manifested by the classic ECG pattern) associated with noncardiac drugs, 23 patients (31%) experienced monomorphic ventricular tachycardia (4/74, 5%) or ventricular fibrillation or pulseless ventricular tachycardia (19/74, 26%).[795] The incidence of mortality was 13%.[795]

PREVENTION

Drugs that are known to provoke or unmask the Brugada syndrome should be avoided in patients with a previous diagnosis of Brugada syndrome. For patients with undiagnosed Brugada syndrome, prevention of drug-induced Brugada syndrome is difficult until the syndrome has been unmasked or provoked by drug therapy.

MANAGEMENT

In patients for whom drugs provoke or unmask Brugada syndrome, the causative agent(s) should be discontinued immediately. Intravenous procainamide should be avoided as a therapy for monomorphic ventricular tachycardia; intravenous amiodarone may be used cautiously. Although it inhibits sodium-channel conductance, amiodarone has not yet been reported to provoke or unmask Brugada syndrome, possibly because of other effects, including inhibition of potassium conductance. Alternatively, the patient can be sedated for performance of direct current cardioversion. Patients who experience ventricular fibrillation should be treated according to Advanced Cardiac Life Support guidelines.[190,191]

INFORMATION FOR PATIENTS

Patients with known Brugada syndrome who require therapy with drugs such as psychotropic agents that may cause ventricular arrhythmias by unmasking or exacerbating the syndrome should be told that the medication may, in rare cases, cause the heart rate (pulse) to become faster. These patients should be instructed to consult their pharmacist or physician if their heart rate increases to above 100–120 bpm or if they feel palpitations, lightheaded, dizzy, tired, weak, short of breath, or chest pain. Patients with known Brugada syndrome should be advised to consume alcohol in moderation, not to the point of intoxication.

REFERENCES

1. Tai YT, Lau CP, But PP et al. Bidirectional tachycardia induced by herbal aconite poisoning. *Pacing Clin Electrophysiol.* 1992; 15:831-9.
2. Tai YT, But PP, Young K et al. Cardiotoxicity after accidental herb-induced aconite poisoning. *Lancet.* 1992; 340:1254-6.
3. Dickens P, Tai YT, But PP et al. Fatal accidental aconitine poisoning following ingestion of Chinese herbal medicine: a report of two cases. *Forensic Sci Int.* 1994; 67:55-8.
4. Lin CC, Chan TY, Deng JF. Clinical features and management of herb-induced aconitine poisoning. *Ann Emerg Med.* 2004; 43:574-9.
5. Lowe L, Matteucci MJ, Schneir AB. Herbal aconite tea and refractory ventricular tachycardia. *N Engl J Med.* 2005; 353:1532.
6. Fujita Y, Terui K, Fujita M et al. Five cases of aconite poisoning: toxicokinetics of aconitines. *J Anal Toxicol.* 2007; 31:132-7.
7. Zhao Y-T, Huang YS, Yi Z. An 88-year-old man with syncope and an alternating axis. *Heart.* 2016; 102:e3.
8. Tak S, Lakhotia M, Gupta A et al. Aconite poisoning with arrhythmia and shock. *Indian Heart J.* 2016; 68(suppl 2):S207-209.
9. Kent K, Ganetsky M, Cohen J et al. Non-fatal ventricular dysrhythmias associated with severe salicylate toxicity. *Clin Toxicol.* 2008; 46:297-9.
10. Misra D, Van Tosh A, Schweitzer P. Adenosine induced monomorphic ventricular tachycardia. *Pacing Clin Electrophysiol.* 2000; 23:1044-6.
11. Tan HL, Spekhorst HH, Peters RJ et al. Adenosine induced ventricular arrhythmias in the emergency room. *Pacing Clin Electrophysiol.* 2001; 24:450-5.
12. Camaiti A, Pieralli F, Olivotto I et al. Prospective evaluation of adenosine-induced proarrhythmia in the emergency room. *Eur J Emerg Med.* 2001; 99-105.
13. Sandler DA. Adenosine-induced ventricular tachycardia. *J Cardiovasc Electrophysiol.* 2006; 17:1251.
14. Mao J, Fang K, Ananthasubramaniam K. Nonsustained polymorphic ventricular tachycardia during adenosine stress perfusion imaging in the setting of resting pre-excitation electrocardiographic pattern: should we be avoiding adenosine pharmacologic stress testing in pre-excitation syndromes? *J Nucl Cardiol.* 2008; 15:469-72.
15. Huemer M, Boldt L-H, Rolf S et al. Sustained monomorphic ventricular tachycardia after adenosine infusion (letter). *Int J Cardiol.* 2009; 131:e97-100.
16. Patel HR, Shah P, Bajaj S et al. Intracoronary adenosine-induced ventricular arrhythmias during fractional flow reserve (FFR) measurement: case series and literature review. *Cardiovasc Interv Ther.* 2017; 32:374-80.
17. Gallastegui JL, Bauman JL, Anderson JL et al. Worsening of ventricular tachycardia by amiodarone. *J Clin Pharmacol.* 1988; 28:406-11.
18. Makimoto H, Noda T, Kurita T et al. Incessant monomorphic ventricular tachycardia induced by the proarrhythmic effect of amiodarone. *Intern Med.* 2011; 50:2591-5.
19. Ducas RA, Seftel MD, Ducas J et al. Monomorphic ventricular tachycardia caused by arsenic trioxide therapy for acute promyelocytic leukaemia. *J R Coll Physicians Edinb.* 2011; 4:117-8.
20. Livshits Z, Feng Q, Chowdhury F et al. Life-threatening bupropion ingestion: is there a role for intravenous fat emulsion? *Basic Clin Pharmacol Toxicol.* 2011; 109:418-22.
21. Mallampati SR, Liu PL, Knapp RM. Convulsions and ventricular tachycardia from bupivacaine with epinephrine: successful resuscitation. *Anesth Analg.* 1984; 63:856-9.

22. Rosenblatt MA, Abel M, Fischer GW et al. Successful use of a 20% lipid emulsion to resuscitate a patient after a presumed bupivacaine-related cardiac arrest. *Anesthesiol.* 2006; 7:217-8.
23. McCutchen T, Gerancher JC. Early intralipid therapy may have prevented bupivacaine-associated cardiac arrest. *Reg Anesth Pain Med.* 2008; 33:178-80.
24. Fuzaylov G, Ying B, Tang Y et al. Successful resuscitation after inadvertent intravenous injection of bupivacaine in an adolescent. *Paediatr Anaesth.* 2010; 20:958-9.
25. Buck D, Kreeger R, Spaeth J. Case discussion and root cause analysis: bupivacaine overdose in an infant leading to ventricular tachycardia. *Anesth Analg.* 2014; 119:137-40.
26. Hoehns JD, Stanford RH, Geraets DR et al. Torsades de pointes associated with chlorpromazine: case report and review of associated ventricular arrhythmias. *Pharmacotherapy.* 2001; 21:871-83.
27. Maddry JK, Breyer K, Cook KM et al. Monomorphic ventricular tachycardia after intentional citalopram overdose. *Am J Emerg Med.* 2013; 31:447.e5-447.e8.
28. Geggel RL, McInerny J, Estes NAM. Transient neonatal ventricular tachycardia associated with maternal cocaine use. *Am J Cardiol.* 1989; 63:383-4.
29. Merigian KS. Cocaine-induced ventricular arrhythmias and rapid atrial fibrillation temporally related to naloxone administration. *Am J Emerg Med.* 1993; 11:96-7.
30. Lakkireddy D, Kanmanthareddy A, Biria M et al. Radiofrequency ablation of drug refractory ventricular tachycardia related to cocaine use: a feasibility, safety and efficacy study. *J Cardiovasc Electrophysiol.* 2014; 25:739-46.
31. Lee WR, Sheikh MU, Covarrubias EA et al. Variant ventricular tachycardia in desipramine toxicity. *South Med J.* 1981; 74:1268-9.
32. Wilens TE, Stern TA. Ventricular tachycardia associated with desipramine and thioridazine. *Psychosomatics.* 1990; 31:100-3.
33. Peters RW, Buser GA, Kim HJ et al. Tricyclic overdose causing sustained monomorphic ventricular tachycardia. *Am J Cardiol.* 1992; 70:1226-8.
34. Bigger JT Jr. Digitalis toxicity. *J Clin Pharmacol.* 1985; 25:514-21.
35. Mahdyoon H, Battilana G, Rosman H et al. The evolving pattern of digoxin intoxication: observations at a large urban hospital from 1980-1988. *Am Heart J.* 1990; 120:1189-94.
36. Valent S, Kelly P. Images in clinical medicine. Digoxin-induced bidirectional ventricular tachycardia. *N Engl J Med.* 1997; 336:550.
37. Ma G, Brady WJ, Pollack M et al. Electrocardiographic manifestations: digitalis toxicity. *J Emer Med.* 2001; 20:145-52.
38. Lee AY, Kutyifa V, Ruwald MH et al. Digoxin therapy and associated clinical outcomes in the MADIT-CRT trial. *Heart Rhythm.* 2015; 12:2010-7.
39. Lette J, Tatum JL, Fraser S et al. Safety of dipyridamole testing in 73,806 patients: the Multicenter Dipyridamole Safety Study. *J Nucl Cardiol.* 1995; 2:3-17.
40. Chang WT, Lin LC, Yen RF et al. Persistent myocardial ischemia after termination of dipyridamole-induced ventricular tachycardia by intravenous aminophylline: scintigraphic demonstration. *J Formos Med Assoc.* 2000; 99:264-6.
41. Cortigiani L, Zanetti L, Bigi R et al. Safety and feasibility of dobutamine and dipyridamole stress echocardiography in hypertensive patients. *J Hypertens.* 2002; 20:1423-9.
42. Chinushi M, Aizawa Y, Miyajima S et al. Proarrhythmic effects of antiarrhythmic drugs assessed by electrophysiologic study in recurrent sustained ventricular tachycardia. *Jpn Circ J.* 1991; 55:133-41.
43. Shehata M. Accelerated dobutamine stress testing: feasibility and safety in patients with moderate stenosis. *Egypt Heart J.* 2015; 67:107-13.
44. Biddle TL, Benotti JR, Creager MA et al. Comparison of intravenous milrinone and dobutamine for congestive heart failure secondary to either ischemic or dilated cardiomyopathy. *Am J Cardiol.* 1987; 59:1345-50.
45. Mertes H, Sawada SG, Ryan T et al. Symptoms, adverse effects, and complications associated with dobutamine stress echocardiography. Experience in 1118 patients. *Circulation.* 1993; 88:15-9.
46. Bigi R, Partesana N, Verzoni A et al. Incidence and correlates of complex ventricular arrhythmias during dobutamine stress echocardiography after acute myocardial infarction. *Eur Heart J.* 1995; 16:1819-24.
47. Previtali M, Lanzarini L, Fetiveau R et al. Dobutamine-induced and spontaneous ventricular tachycardia in recent myocardial infarction (letter). *Eur Heart J.* 1996; 17:803-4.
48. Dakik HA, Vempathy H, Verani MS. Tolerance, hemodynamic changes, and safety of dobutamine stress perfusion imaging. *J Nucl Cardiol.* 1996; 3:410-4.
49. Yeo TC, Ng WL, Ling LH et al. Dobutamine stress echocardiography in the elderly Asian patients. *Ann Acad Med Singapore.* 1997; 26:165-7.
50. Hennessy TG, Codd MB, Kane G et al. Safety of dobutamine stress echocardiography in 474 studies. *Coron Artery Dis.* 1997; 8:175-8.
51. Smart SC, Knickelbine T, Stoiber TR et al. Safety and accuracy of dobutamine-atropine stress echocardiography for the dection of residual stenosis of the infarct-related artery and multivessel disease during the first week after acute myocardial infarction. *Circulation.* 1997; 95:1394-401.
52. Secknus MA, Marwick TH. Evolution of dobutamine echocardiography protocols and indications: safety and side effects in 3,011 studies over 5 years. *J Am Coll Cardiol.* 1997; 29:1234-40.
53. Elhendy A, van Domburg RT, Roelandt JR et al. Safety and feasibility of dobutamine-atropine stress testing in hypertensive patients. *Hypertension.* 1997; 29:1232-9.
54. Hanson MW, Morris EI, Borges-Neto S et al. Analysis of cardiac arrhythmias during dobutamine pharmacologic stress testing in nuclear cardiology as related to the presence or absence of baseline arrhythmias. *J Nucl Cardiol.* 1997; 4:372-8.
55. Elhendy A, Geleijnse ML, van Domburg RT et al. Gender differences in the accuracy of dobutamine stress echocardiography for the diagnosis of coronary artery disease. *Am J Cardiol.* 1997; 80:1414-8.
56. Bremer ML, Monahan KH, Stussy VL et al. Safety of dobutamine stress echocardiography supervised by registered nurse sonographers. *J Am Soc Echocardiogr.* 1998; 11:601-5.
57. Elhendy A, Valkema R, van Domburg RT et al. Safety of dobutamine-atropine stress myocardial perfusion scintigraphy. *J Nucl Med.* 1998; 39:1662-6.
58. Elhendy A, van Domburg RT, Poldermans D et al. Safety and feasibility of dobutamine-atropine stress echocardiography for the diagnosis of coronary artery disease in diabetic patients unable to perform an exercise stress test. *Diabetes Care.* 1998; 21:1797-802.
59. Poldermans D, ten Cate FJ, Elhendy A et al. Ventricular tachycardia during dobutamine stress myocardial contrast imaging (letter). *Chest.* 1999; 115:307-8.
60. Elhendy A, van Domburg RT, Bax JJ et al. Relation between the extent of coronary artery disease and tachyarrhythmias during dobutamine stress echocardiography. *Am J Cardiol.* 1999; 83:832-5.
61. Mathias W Jr, Arruda A, Santos FC et al. Safety of dobutamine-atropine stress echocardiography: a prospective experience of 4,033 consecutive studies. *J Am Soc Echocardiogr.* 1999; 12:785-91.
62. Geleijnse ML, Elhendy A, Kasprzak JD et al. Safety and prognostic value of early dobutamine-atropine stress echocardiography in patients with spontaneous chest pain and non-diagnostic electrocardiogram. *Eur Heart J.* 2000; 21:397-406.
63. Elhendy A, van Domburg RT, Bax JJ et al. Safety, hemodynamic profile, and feasibility of dobutamine stress technetium myocardial perfusion single photon emission CT imaging for evaluation of coronary artery disease in the elderly. *Chest.* 2000; 117:649-56.
64. Lu D, Greenberg MD, Little R et al. Accelerated dobutamine stress testing: safety and feasibility in patients with known or suspected coronary artery disease. *Clin Cardiol.* 2001; 24:141-5.

65. Alhendy A, van Domburg RT, Vantrimpont P et al. Impact of heart transplantation on the safety and feasibility of the dobutamine stress test. *J Heart Lung Transplant.* 2001; 20:399-406.
66. Burger AJ, Elkayam U, Nelbaur MT et al. Comparison of the occurrence of ventricular arrhythmias in patients with acutely decompensated congestive heart failure receiving dobutamine versus nesiritide therapy. *Am J Cardiol.* 2001; 88:35-9.
67. Nijland F, Kamp O, Verhorst PMJ et al. In-hospital and long-term prognostic value of viable myocardium detected by dobutamine echocardiography early after acute myocardial infarction and its relation to indicators of left ventricular systolic dysfunction. *Am J Cardiol.* 2001; 88:949-55.
68. Joao I, Cotrim C, do Rosario L et al. Complications in stress echocardiography. *Rev Port Cardiol.* 2002; 21:871-81.
69. Burger AJ, Horton DP, LeJemtel T et al. Effect of nesiritide (B-type natriuretic peptide) and dobutamine on ventricular arrhythmias in the treatment of patients with acutely decompensated congestive heart failure: the PRECEDENT study. *Am Heart J.* 2002; 144:1102-8.
70. Wahl A, Paetsch I, Gollesch A et al. Safety and feasibility of high-dose dobutamine-atropine stress cardiovascular magnetic resonance for diagnosis of myocardial ischaemia: experience in 1000 consecutive cases. *Eur Heart J.* 2004; 25:1230-6.
71. Siddiqui TS, Stoddard MF. Safety of dobutamine stress transesophageal echocardiography in obese patients for evaluation of potential ischemic heart disease. *Echocardiography.* 2004; 21:603-8.
72. Puddu PE, Papalia U, Schiariti M et al. Dobutamine effects on spontaneous variability of ventricular arrhythmias in patients with severe chronic heart failure: the Italian Multicenter Study. *Ital Heart J.* 2004; 5:693-701.
73. Timperley J, Mitchell ARJ, Thibault H et al. Safety of contrast dobutamine stress echocardiography: a single center experience. *J Am Soc Echocardiogr.* 2005; 18:163-7.
74. Tsutsui JM, Lario FC, Fernandes DR et al. Safety and cardiac chronotropic responsiveness to the early injection of atropine during dobutamine stress echocardiography in the elderly. *Heart.* 2005; 91:1563-7.
75. Katritsis DG, Karabinos I, Papadopoulos A et al. Sustained ventricular tachycardia induced by dobutamine stress echocardiography: a prospective study. *Europace.* 2005; 7:433-9.
76. Cox DE, Farmer LD, Hoyle JR et al. Prognostic significance of nonsustained ventricular tachycardia during dobutamine stress echocardiography. *Am J Cardiol.* 2005; 96:1293-8.
77. Varga A, Rodriguez Garcia MA, Picano E et al. Safety of stress echocardiography (from the International Stress Echo Complication Registry). *Am J Cardiol.* 2006; 98:541-3.
78. San Roman JA, Sanz-Ruiz R, Ortega JR et al. Safety and predictors of complications with a new accelerated dobutamine stress echocardiography protocol. *J Am Soc Echocardiogr.* 2008; 21:53-7.
79. Kane GC, Hepinstall MJ, Kidd GM et al. Safety of stress echocardiography supervised by registered nurses: results of a 2-year audit of 15,404 patients. *J Am Soc Echocardiogr.* 2008; 21:337-41.
80. Chaowalit N, Jakrapanichakul D, Kitrattna B. Dobutamine stress echocardiography for the evaluation of coronary artery disease in Thai population: Siriraj experience. *J Med Assoc Thai.* 2007; 90(suppl 2):33-40.
81. Minardi G, Manzara C, Pulignano G et al. Feasibility, safety and tolerability of accelerated dobutamine stress echocardiography. *Cardiovasc Ultrasound.* 2007; 21:5-40.
82. Aggeli C, Giannopoulos G, Roussakis G et al. Safety of flash-contrast echocardiography in combination with dobutamine stress testing for the detection of ischaemia in 5250 studies. *Heart.* 2008; 94:1571-7.
83. Abdel-Salam Z, Nammas W. Early atropine is safer than conventional atropine administration in the elderly undergpoing dobutamine stress echocardiography. *Kardiologia Polska.* 2010; 68:422-8.
84. Shehata M. Atropine first is safer than conventional atropine administration in older people undergoing dobutamine stress echocardiography. *Ther Adv Cardiovasc Dis.* 2014; 8:176-84.
85. Rassi DD, Vieira ML, Furtado RG et al. Dobutamine stress echocardiography safety in Chagas disease patients. *Arq Bras Cardiol.* 2017; 108:122-8.
86. Rakovec P, Kozak M, Sebestjen M. Ventricular tachycardia induced by abuse of ephedrine in a young healthy woman. *Wien Klin Wochenschr.* 2006; 108:90-5.
87. Pareek M, Hansson NH, Grove EL. Ventricular tachycardia induced by weight loss pills. *Case Rep Med.* 2013; 2013:712383.
88. Muhiddin K, Nathan AW, Hellestrand KJ et al. Ventricular tachycardia associated with flecainide. *Lancet.* 1982; 2:1220-1.
89. Hohnloser S, Zeiher A, Hust MH et al. Flecainide-induced aggravation of ventricular tachycardia. *Clin Cardiol.* 1983; 6:130-5.
90. Oetgen WJ, Tibbits PA, Abt ME et al. Clinical and electrophysiologic assessment of oral flecainide acetate for recurrent ventricular tachycardia: evidence for exacerbation of electrical instability. *Am J Cardiol.* 1983; 52:746-50.
91. Spivack C, Gottlieb S, Miura DS et al. Flecainide toxicity. *Am J Cardiol.* 1984; 329-30.
92. Nathan AW, Hellestrand KJ, Bexton RS et al. Proarrhythmic effects of the new antiarrhythmic agent flecainide acetate. *Am Heart J.* 1984; 107:222-8.
93. Morganroth J, Horowitz LN. Flecainide: its proarrhythmic effect and expected changes on the surface electrocardiogram. *Am J Cardiol.* 1984; 58:89-94.
94. Sellers TD, DiMarco JP. Sinusoidal ventricular tachycardia associated with flecainide acetate. *Chest.* 1984; 85:647-9.
95. Vanhaleweyk G, Balakumaran K, Lubsen J et al. Flecainide: one-year efficacy in patients with chronic ventricular arrhythmias. *Eur Heart J.* 1984; 10:814-23.
96. Nathan AW, Hellestrand KJ, Bexton RS et al. The proarrhythmic effects of flecainide. *Drugs.* 1985; 29(suppl 4):45-53.
97. Platia EV, Estes M, Heine DL et al. Flecainide: electrophysiologic and antiarrhythmic properties in refractory ventricular tachycardia. *Am J Cardiol.* 1985; 55:956-62.
98. Muhiddin KA, Turner P, Hellestrand K et al. Evaluation of the efficacy of flecainide acetate in the treatment of ventricular premature contractions. *Postgrad Med J.* 1985; 61:489-96.
99. Wehr M, Noll B, Krappe J. Flecainide-induced aggravation of ventricular arrhythmias. *Am J Cardiol.* 1985; 55:1643-4.
100. Ward DE, Cheesman M, Dancy M. Effect of intravenous and oral flecainide on ventricular tachycardia. *Int J Cardiol.* 1986; 10:251-62.
101. Hoffmann A, Wenk M, Follath F. Exercise-induced ventricular tachycardia as a manifestation of flecainide toxicity. *Int J Cardiol.* 1986; 11:353-5.
102. Flecainide Ventricular Tachycardia Study Group. Treatment of resistant ventricular tachycardia with flecainide acetate. *Am J Cardiol.* 1986; 57:1299-304.
103. Wynn J, Fingerhood M, Keefe D et al. Refractory ventricular tachycardia with flecainide. *Am Heart J.* 1986; 112:174-5.
104. Morganroth J, Anderson JL, Gentkow GD. Classification by type of ventricular arrhythmia predicts frequency of adverse cardiac events from flecainide. *J Am Coll Cardiol.* 1986; 8:607-15.
105. Crozier IG, Ikram H, Kenealy M et al. Flecainide acetate for conversion of acute supraventricular tachycardia to sinus rhythm. *Am J Cardiol.* 1987; 59:607-9.
106. Anastasiou-Nana MI, Anderson JL, Stewart JR et al. Occurrence of exercise-induced and spontaneous wide complex tachycardia during therapy with flecainide for complex ventricular arrhythmias: a probable proarrhythmic effect. *Am Heart J.* 1987; 113:1071-7.
107. Bauman JL, Gallastegui J, Tenenbaum SR et al. Flecainide-induced sustained ventricular tachycardia successfully treated with lidocaine. *Chest.* 1987; 92:573-5.
108. Sagie A, Strasberg B, Kusniec J et al. Rapid suppression of flecainide-induced incessant ventricular tachycardia with high-dose intravenous amiodarone. *Chest.* 1988; 93:879-80.
109. Rinkenberger RL, Naccarelli GV, Berns E et al. Efficacy and safety of class IC antiarrhythmic agents for the treatment of coexisting

supraventricular and ventricular tachycardia. *Am J Cardiol.* 1988; 62:44D-55D.

110. Russell GA, Martin RP. Flecainide toxicity. *Arch Dis Child.* 1989; 64:860-2.
111. Falk RH. Flecainide-induced ventricular tachycardia and fibrillation in patients treated for atrial fibrillation. *Ann Intern Med.* 1989; 111:107-11.
112. Myerburg RJ, Kessler KM, Cox MM et al. Reversal of proarrhythmic effects of flecainide acetate and encainide hydrochloride by propranolol. *Circulation.* 1989; 80:1571-9.
113. Herre JM, Titus C, Oeff M et al. Inefficacy and proarrhythmic effects of flecainide and encainide for sustained ventricular tachycardia and ventricular fibrillation. *Ann Intern Med.* 1990; 113:671-6.
114. Gill JS, Mehta D, Ward DE et al. Efficacy of flecainide, sotalol, and verapamil in the treatment of right ventricular tachycardia in patients without overt cardiac abnormality. *Br Heart J.* 1992; 68:392-7.
115. Said SA, Somer ST, Oude Luttikhuis HA. Flecainide-induced JT prolongation, T wave inversion and ventricular tachycardia during treatment for symptomatic atrial fibrillation. *Int J Cardiol.* 1994; 44:285-7.
116. Goldman MJ, Mowry JB, Kirk MA. Sodium bicarbonate to correct widened QRS in a case of flecainide overdose. *J Emerg Med.* 1997; 15:183-6.
117. Hanley NA, Bourke JP, Gascoigne AD. Survival in a case of life-threatening flecainide overdose. *Intensive Care Med.* 1998; 24:740-2.
118. Wehling M. Meta-analysis of flecainide safety in patients with supraventricular arrhythmias. *Arzneimittelforschung.* 2002; 52:507-14.
119. Courand PY, Sibellas F, Ranc S et al. Arrhythmogenic effect of flecainide toxicity. *Cardiol J.* 2013; 20:203-5.
120. Jang DH, Hoffman RS, Nelson LS. A case of near-fatal flecainide overdose in a neonate successfully treated with sodium bicarbonate. *J Emerg Med.* 2013; 44:781-3.
121. Courand PY, Sibellas F, Ranc S et al. Arrhythmogenic effect of flecainide toxicity. *Cardiol J.* 2013; 20:203-5.
122. Barman M. Proarrhythmic effects of antiarrhythmic drugs: case study of flecainide-induced ventricular arrhythmias during treatment of atrial fibrillation. *J Atr Fibrillation.* 2015; 8:22-4.
123. Pfister O, Sticherling C, Schaer B et al. Electrical storm caused by complementary medication with ginkgo biloba extract. *Am J Med.* 2008; 121:e3-4.
124. Wood MA, Stambler BS, Ellenbogen KA et al. Suppression of inducible ventricular tachycardia by ibutilide in patients with coronary artery disease. *Am Heart J.* 1998; 135:1048-54.
125. Abi-Mansour P, Carberry PA, McCowan RJ et al. Conversion efficacy and safety of repeated doses of ibutilide in patients with atrial flutter and atrial fibrillation. *Am Heart J.* 1998; 136:632-42.
126. VanderLugt JT, Mattioni T, Denker S et al. Efficacy and safety of ibutilide fumarate for the conversion of atrial arrhythmias after cardiac surgery. *Circulation.* 1999; 100:369-75.
127. Antonicelli R, Testarmata P, Recanatini A. Ibutilide in rapid conversion of atrial flutter in octogenarians. *Drugs Aging.* 2002; 19:878-91.
128. Gowda RM, Khan IA, Punukollu G et al. Use of ibutilide for cardioversion of recent-onset atrial fibrillation and flutter in elderly. *Am J Ther.* 2004; 11:95-7.
129. Zhang N, Guo JH, Zhang HCh et al. Comparison of intravenous ibutilide vs. propafenone for rapid termination of recent onset atrial fibrillation. *Int J Clin Pract.* 2005; 59:1395-400.
130. Hoyer AW, Balaji S. The safety and efficacy of ibutilide in children and in patients with congenital heart disease. *Pacing Clin Electrophysiol.* 2007; 30:1003-8.
131. Patsilinakos S, Christou A, Kafkas N et al. Effect of high doses of magnesium on converting ibutilide to a safe and more effective agent. *Am J Cardiol.* 2010; 106:673-6.
132. Molloy DW, Penner SB, Rabson J et al. Use of sodium bicarbonate to treat tricyclic antidepressant-induced arrhythmias in a patient with alkalosis. *Can Med Assoc J.* 1984; 130:1457-9.
133. DeGiorgio AC, Desso TE, Lee L et al. Ventricular tachycardia associated with lacosamide comedication in drug-resistant epilepsy. *Epilepsy Behav Case Rep.* 2012; 1:26-8.
134. Peano C, Leikin JB, Hanashiro PK. Seizures, ventricular tachycardia, and rhabdomyolysis as a result of ingestion of venlafaxine and lamotrigine. *Ann Emerg Med.* 1997; 30:704-8.
135. Flevari P, Parissis JT, Leftheriotis D et al. Effect of levosimendan on ventricular arrhythmias and prognostic autonomic indexes in patients with decompensated advanced heart failure secondary to ischemic or dilated cardiomyopathy. *Am J Cardiol.* 2006; 98:1641-5.
136. Tuomainen PO, Magga J, Timonen P et al. Intermittent levosimendan treatment in patients with severe congestive heart failure. *Clin Res Cardiol.* 2013; 102:485-93.
137. Bosak AR, Graeme KA, Evans MD. Hemodialysis treatment of monomorphic ventricular tachycardia associated with chronic lithium toxicity. *J Med Toxicol.* 2014; 10:303-6.
138. Li J, Chen Y, Xu Y et al. Methamphetamine use associated with monomorphic ventricular tachycardia. *J Addict Med.* 2014; 8:470-3.
139. Varriale P, Ramaprasad S. Short-term intravenous milrinone for severe congestive heart failure: the good, the bad, and not so good. *Pharmacotherapy.* 1997; 17:371-4.
140. Mildred-LaForest SK, Shubert J, Mendoza B et al. Tolerability of extended duration intravenous milrinone in patients hospitalized for advanced heart failure and the usefulness of uptitration of oral angiotensin-converting enzyme inhibitors. *Am J Cardiol.* 1999; 84:894-9.
141. Smith AH, Owen J, Borgman KY et al. Relation of milrinone after surgery for congenital heart disease to significant postoperative tachyarrhythmias. *Am J Cardiol.* 2011; 108:1620-4.
142. Haglund NA, Burdorf A, Jones T et al. Inhaled milrinone after left ventricular assist device implantation. *J Card Fail.* 2015; 21:792-7.
143. Maykov EB, Yuricheva YA, Yu Mironov N et al. Efficacy of a new class III drug niferidil in cardioversion of persistent atrial fibrillation and flutter. *J Cardiovasc Pharmacol.* 2014; 64:247-55.
144. Bhandari AK, Au PK, Rahimtoola SH. Procainamide induced sustained monomorphic ventricular tachycardia in a patient with benign premature ventricular complexes. *Can J Cardiol.* 1986; 2:6-9.
145. Connolly SJ, Kates RE, Lebsack CS et al. Clinical efficacy and electrophysiology of oral propafenone for ventricular tachycardia. *Am J Cardiol.* 1983; 52:1208-13.
146. Nathan AW, Bexton RS, Hellestrand KJ et al. Fatal ventricular tachycardia in association with propafenone, a new class IC antiarrhythmic agent. *Postgrad Med J.* 1984; 60:155-6.
147. Millar RN, Lawrenson JB, Milne DA. Normal left ventricular function does not protect against propafenone-induced incessant ventricular tachycardia. *S Afr Med J.* 1993; 83:256-9.
148. Podrid PJ, Cytryn R, Lown B. Propafenone: noninvasive evaluation of efficacy. *Am J Cardiol.* 1984; 54:53D-9D.
149. Buss J, Neuss H, Bilgin Y et al. Malignant ventricular tachyarrhythmias in association with propafenone treatment. *Eur Heart J.* 1985; 6:424-8.
150. Stavens CS, McGovern B, Garan H et al. Aggravation of electrically provoked ventricular tachycardia during treatment with propafenone. *Am Heart J.* 1985; 110:24-9.
151. De Jaegere P, Huyghens L, Dewilde P. Sustained ventricular tachycardia occurring during propafenone therapy. *Ada Cardiol.* 1987; 42:207-12.
152. Scanu P, Grollier G, Guilleman D et al. Malignant ventricular tachycardia during propafenone treatment in a child with junctional automatic tachycardia: effectiveness of intravenous molar sodium lactate. *Pacing Clin Electrophysiol.* 1991; 14:783-6.
153. Kowey PR, Stohler JL, Friehling TD et al. Propafenone in the treatment of patients with malignant ventricular tachyarrhythmias. *Can J Cardiol.* 1991; 7:175-80.

154. Guccione P, Drago F, Di Donato RM et al. Oral propafenone therapy for children with arrhythmias: efficacy and adverse effects in midterm follow-up. *Am Heart J.* 1991; 122:1022-7.

155. Vignati G, Mauri L, Figini A. The use of propafenone in the treatment of tachyarrhythmias in children. *Eur Heart J.* 1993; 14:546-50.

156. Chimienti M, Cullen MT, Jr, Casadei G. Safety of flecainide versus propafenone for the long-term management of symptomatic paroxysmal supraventricular tachyarrhythmias: report from the Flecainide and Propafenone Italian Study (FAPIS) Group. *Eur Heart J.* 1995; 16:1943-51.

157. Gao E, Yang C, Li H et al. Preliminary study of the effects of metoprolol and propafenone on ventricular arrhythmia with positive ventricular late potential. *Chin Med J.* 1997; 110:723-5.

158. Janousek J, Paul T. Safety of oral propafenone in the treatment of arrhythmias in infants and children (European retrospective multicenter study): working group on Pediatric Arrhythmias and Electrophysiology of the Association of European Pediatric Cardiologists. *Am J Cardiol.* 1998; 81:1121-4.

159. Yoshida M, Matsuda H, Fukuda I et al. Sudden cardiac arrest during cesarean section due to epidural anaesthesia using ropivacaine: a case report. *Arch Gynecol Obstet.* 2008; 277:91-4.

160. Ludot H, Tharin JY, Belouadah M et al. Sucessful resuscitation after ropivacaine and lidocaine-induced ventricular arrhythmia following posterior lumbar plexus block in a child. *Anesth Analg.* 2008; 106:1572-4.

161. Krishnan SC, Galvin J, McGovern B et al. Reproducible induction of "atypical" Torsades de Pointes by programmed electrical stimulation: a novel form of sotalol-induced proarrhythmia? *J Cardiovasc Electrophysiol.* 1997; 8:1055-61.

162. Kinney EL, Trautlein JJ, Harbaugh CV et al. Ventricular tachycardia after terbutaline. *JAMA.* 1978; 240:2247.

163. Banner AS, Sunderrajan EV, Agarwal MK et al. Arrhythmogenic effects of orally administered bronchodilators. *Arch Intern Med.* 1979; 139:434-7.

164. Coleman JJ, Vollmer WM, Barker AF et al. Cardiac arrhythmias during the combined use of beta-adrenergic agonist drugs and theophylline. *Chest.* 1986; 90:45-51.

165. Poukkula A, Korhonen UR, Huikuri H et al. Theophylline and salbutamol in combination in patients with obstructive pulmonary disease and concurrent heart disease: effect on cardiac arrhythmias. *J Intern Med.* 1989; 226:229-34.

166. Cukier A, Vargas FS, Teixeira LR et al. Arrhythmogenic effects of combined orally administered theophylline and albuterol in patients with chronic obstructive pulmonary disease. *Braz J Med Biol Res.* 1994; 27:2869-77.

167. Patel AK, Skatrud JB, Thomsen JH. Cardiac arrhythmias due to oral aminophylline in patients with chronic obstructive pulmonary disease. *Chest.* 1981; 80:661-5.

168. Siemons LJ, Parizel G. Prolonged runs of ventricular tachycardia as a complication of theophylline intoxication: report of a case. *Acta Cardiol.* 1986; 41:457-64.

169. Aitken ML, Martin TR. Life-threatening theophylline toxicity is not predictable by serum levels. *Chest.* 1987; 91:10-14.

170. Taniguchi A, Ohe T, Shimorura K. Theophylline-induced ventricular tachycardia in a patient with chronic lung disease: sensitivity to verapamil. *Chest.* 1989; 96:958-9.

171. Emerman CL, Devlin C, Connors AF. Risk of toxicity in patients with elevated theophylline levels. *Ann Emerg Med.* 1990; 19:643-8.

172. Sessler CN, Cohen MD. Cardiac arrhythmias during theophylline toxicity: a prospective continuous electrocardiographic study. *Chest.* 1990; 98:672-8.

173. Chevalier B, le Heuzey JY, Colombel B et al. Ventricular tachycardia during theophylline overdose: apropos of a case of reduction by magnesium chloride. *Arch Mai Coeur Vaiss.* 1990; 83:569-73.

174. Cassel-Choudhury GN, Aydin SI, Toedt-Pingle I et al. Arrhythmias in the paediatric intensive care unit: a prospective study of the rates and predictors of arrhythmias in children without underlying cardiac disease. *Cardiol Young.* 2015; 25:1281-9.

175. Aronson MD, Hafez H. A case of trazodone-induced ventricular tachycardia. *J Clin Psychiatry.* 1986; 47:388-9.

176. Vitullo RN, Wharton JM, Allen NB et al. Trazodone-related exercise-induced nonsustained ventricular tachycardia. *Chest.* 1990; 98:247-8.

177. Mazur JE, Doty JD, Krygiel AS. Fatality related to a 30-g venlafaxine overdose. *Pharmacotherapy.* 2003; 23:1668-72.

178. Chaudhry GM, Haffajee CI. Antiarrhythmic agents and proarrhythmia. *Crit Care Med.* 2000; 28(suppl 10):N158-64.

179. McCollam PL, Parker RB, Beckman KJ et al. Proarrhythmia: a paradoxic response to antiarrhythmic agents. *Pharmacotherapy.* 1989; 9:144-53.

180. Tanz RD. Pharmacology of acotinine-induced automaticity on in vitro cat myocardial preparations. II. Efficacy of refractory period prolongation, reduced sodium and tetrodotoxin. *J Pharmacol Exp Ther.* 1974; 191:232-40.

181. Friese J, Gleitz J, Gutser UT et al. Acotinium sp. Alkaloids: the modulation of voltage-dependent Na+ channels, toxicity and antinociceptive properties. *Eur J Pharmacol.* 1997; 337:165-74.

182. Biaggioni I, Killian TJ, Mosqueda-Garcia R et al. Adenosine increases sympathetic nerve traffic in humans. *Circulation.* 1991; 83:1668-75.

183. Hauptman PJ, Kelly RA. Digitalis. *Circulation.* 1999; 99:1265-70.

184. Anderson JL, Platia EV, Hallstrom A et al. Interaction of baseline characteristics with the hazard of encainide, flecainide, and moricizine therapy in patients with myocardial infarction: a possible explanation for increased mortality in the Cardiac Arrhythmia Suppression Trial (CAST). *Circulation.* 1994; 90:2843-52.

185. Echt DS, Liebson PR, Mitchell LB et al. Mortality and morbidity in patients receiving encainide, flecainide, or placebo: The Cardiac Arrhythmia Suppression Trial. *N Engl J Med.* 1991; 324:781-8.

186. The Cardiac Arrhythmia Suppression Trial II Investigators. Effect of the antiarrhythmic agent moricizine on survival after myocardial infarction. *N Engl J Med.* 1992; 327:227-33.

187. Teo KK, Yusuf S, Furberg CD. Effects of prophylactic antiarrhythmic drug therapy in acute myocardial infarction: an overview of results from randomized controlled trials. *JAMA.* 1993; 270:1589-95.

188. Bigger JT, Sahar DI. Clinical types of proarrhythmic response to antiarrhythmic drugs. *Am J Cardiol.* 1987; 59:2E-9E.

189. Nazari J, Bauman J, Pham T et al. Exercise induced fatal sinusoidal ventricular tachycardia secondary to moricizine. *Pacing Clin Electrophysiol.* 1992; 15:1421-4.

190. Neumar RW, Otto CW, Link MS et al. Part 8: adult advanced cardiovascular life support: 2010 American Heart Association Guidelines for Cardiopulmonary Resuscitation and Emergency Cardiovascular Care. *Circulation.* 2010; 122(suppl 3):S729-67.

191. Link MS, Berkow LC, Kudenchuk PJ et al. Part 7: adult adult advanced cardiovascular life support: 2015 American Heart Association Guidelines Update for Cardiopulmonary Resuscitation and Emergency Cardiovascular Care. *Circulation.* 2015; 132(suppl 2):S444-64.

192. Al-Khatib SM, Stevenson WG, Ackerman MJ et al. 2017 AHA/ACC/HRS guideline for management of patients with ventricular arrhythmias and the prevention of sudden cardiac death: a report of the American College of Cardiology Foundation/American Heart Association Task Force on Clinical Practice Guidelines and the Heart Rhythm Society. *Circulation.* 2017; Oct 30. pii: CIR.0000000000000549.

193. Bartlett D. Intravenous lipids: antidotal therapy for drug overdose and toxic effects of local anesthetics. *Crit Care Nurse.* 2014; 34:62-7.

194. Hoegberg LC, Bania TC, Lavergne V et al. Systematic review of the effect of intravenous lipid emulsion therapy for local anesthetic toxicity. *Clin Toxicol.* 2016; 54:167-93.

195. Trinkley KE, Page II RL, Lien H et al. QT interval prolongation and the risk of torsades de pointes: essentials for clinicians. *Curr Med Res Opin.* 2013; 29:1719-26.

196. Schwartz PJ, Woosley RL. Predicting the unpredictable: drug-induced QT prolongation and torsades de pointes. *J Am Coll Cardiol.* 2016; 67:1639-50.

197. Woosley RL, Romero KA. QTdrugs list. www.Crediblemeds.org (accessed 2017 Jan 30).

198. Keren A, Tzivoni D, Gottlieb S et al. Atypical ventricular tachycardia (torsade de pointes) induced by amiodarone: arrhythmia previously induced by quinidine and disopyramide. *Chest.* 1982; 81:384-6.

199. Tzivoni D, Keren A, Cohen AM et al. Magnesium therapy for torsades de pointes. *Am J Cardiol.* 1984; 53:528-30.

200. Brown MA, Smith WM, Lubbe WF et al. Amiodarone-induced torsades de pointes. *Eur Heart J.* 1986; 7:234-9.

201. Leroy G, Haiat R, Barthelemy M et al. Torsade de pointes during loading with amiodarone. *Eur Heart J.* 1987; 8:541-3.

202. Jorens PG, van den Heuvel PA, Ranquin RE et al. Amiodarone induced torsades de pointe: report of three cases and review of literature. *Ada Cardiol.* 1989; 44:411-21.

203. Chinaglia A, Cibinel GA, Uslenghi E et al. Torsade de pointes following intravenous infusion of amiodarone. *Cardiologia.* 1989; 34:177-80.

204. Lazzara R. Amiodarone and torsade de pointes (letter). *Ann Intern Med.* 1989; 111:549-51.

205. Andrivet P, Beaslay V, Canh VD. Torsades de pointe with flecainide-amiodarone therapy. *Intensive Care Med.* 1990; 16:342-3.

206. Bajaj BP, Baig MW, Perrins EJ. Amiodarone-induced torsades de pointes: the possible lacilitatory role of digoxin. *Int J Cardiol.* 1991; 33:335-7.

207. Jorens PG, Van den Heuvel PA, Parizel GA. Amiodarone and torsades de pointes. *Am Heart J.* 1990; 120:1482.

208. Schlienger RG, Haeleli WE, Lüscher TF. Torsade de pointes during anti-arrhythmia treatment with amiodarone. *Schweiz Rundsch Med Prax.* 1993; 82:173-5.

209. Faber TS, Zehender M, Van de Loo A et al. Torsade de pointes complicating drug treatment of low-malignant forms of arrhythmia: four cases reports. *Clin Cardiol.* 1994; 17:197-202.

210. Hohnloser SH, Klingenheben T, Singh BN. Amiodarone-associated proarrhythmic effects: a review with special reference to torsade de pointes tachycardia. *Ann Intern Med.* 1994; 121:529-35.

211. Cheng TO. Amiodarone and torsade de pointes. *Ann Intern Med.* 1995; 122:553-4.

212. Mazur A, Strasberg B, Kusniec J et al. QT prolongation and polymorphous ventricular tachycardia associated with trasodone-amiodarone combination. *Int J Cardiol.* 1995; 52:27-9.

213. Faggiano P, Gardini A, D'Aloia A et al. Torsade de pointes occurring early during oral amiodarone treatment. *Int J Cardiol.* 1996; 55:205-8.

214. Skanes AC, Morton BC, Green MS et al. Torsade de pointes with amiodarone in a patient with previous torsade during beta-receptor blockade. *Can J Cardiol.* 1997; 13:383-6.

215. Tran HT, Chow MS, Kluger J. Amiodarone induced torsades de pointes with excessive QT dispersion following quinidine induced polymorphic ventricular tachycardia. *Pacing Clin Electrophysiol.* 1997; 20:2275-8.

216. Tomcsányi J, Merkely B, Tenczer J et al. Early proarrhythmia during intravenous amiodarone treatment. *Pacing Clin Electrophysiol.* 1999; 22:968-70.

217. Segura I, García-Bolao I. Meglumine antimoniate, amiodarone and torsades de pointes: a case report. *Resuscitation.* 1999; 42:65-8.

218. Glatter K, Yang Y, Chatterjee K et al. Chemical cardioversion of atrial fibrillation or flutter with ibutilide in patients receiving amiodarone therapy. *Circulation.* 2001; 103:253-7.

219. Nkomo VT, Shen WK. Amiodarone-induced long QT and polymorphic ventricular tachycardia. *Am J Emerg Med.* 2001; 19:246-8.

220. Silvetti MS, Drago F, Bevilacqua M et al. Amiodarone-induced torsade de pointes in a child with dilated cardiomyopathy. *Ital Heart J.* 2001; 2:231-6.

221. Yamada S, Kuga K, Yamaguchi I. Torsade de pointes induced by intravenous and long-term oral amiodarone therapy in a patient with dilated cardiomyopathy. *Jpn Circ J.* 2001; 65:236-8.

222. Pagano L, Delia Monica R, Malinconico M. Proarrhythmia caused by amiodarone. *Minerva Cardioangiol.* 2001; 49:421-8.

223. Makai A, Rudas L, Liszkai G et al. Torsades de pointes ventricular tachycardia induced by intravenous amiodarone. *Orv Hetil.* 2003; 144:241-7.

224. Voigt L, Coromilas J, Saul BI et al. Amiodarone-induced torsade de pointes during bladder irrigation: an unusual presentation: a case report. *Angiology.* 2003; 54:229-31.

225. Atar S, Freedberg NA, Antonelli D et al. Torsades de pointes and QT prolongation due to a combination of loratadine and amiodarone. *Pacing Clin Electrophysiol.* 2003; 26:785-6.

226. Schrickel J, Bielik H, Yang A et al. Amiodarone-associated torsade de pointes: relevance of concomitant cardiovascular medication in a patient with atrial fibrillation and structural heart disease. *Z Kardiol.* 2003; 92:889-92.

227. Díaz-Castro O, Puchol A, Almendral J et al. Predictors of in-hospital ventricular fibrillation or torsades de pointes in patients with acute symptomatic bradycardia. *J Electrocardiol.* 2004; 37:55-60.

228. Kukla P, Stowiak-Lewiftska T. Amiodarone-induced torsade de pointes: five case reports. *Kardiol Pol.* 2004; 60:365-70.

229. Lee Hwang D, Barriales Alvarez V et al. Torsade de pointes secondary to amiodarone overdose. *Med Clin (Barc).* 2004; 123:156-7.

230. Antonelli D, Atar S, Freedberg NA et al. Torsade de pointes in patients on chronic amiodarone treatment: contributing factors and drug interactions. *Isr Med Assoc J.* 2005; 7:163-5.

231. Kounas SP, Letsas KP, Sideris A et al. QT interval prolongation and torsades de pointes due to a coadministration of metronidazole and amiodarone. *Pacing Clin Electrophysiol.* 2005; 28:472-3.

232. Letsas KP, Filippatos GS, Kounas SP et al. QT interval prolongation and Torsades de Pointes in a patient receiving zolpidem and amiodarone. *Cardiology.* 2006; 105:146-7.

233. Schrickel JW, Schwab JO, Yang A et al. "Torsade de pointes" in patients with structural heart disease and atrial fibrillation treated with amiodarone, beta-blockers, and digitalis. *Pacing Clin Electrophysiol.* 2006; 29:363-6.

234. Geng DF, Jin DM, Wang JF et al. Clinical study of amiodarone-associated torsade de pointes in Chinese people. *Pacing Clin Electrophysiol.* 2006; 29:712-8.

235. Kukla P, Bryniarski L, Dragan J et al. Polymorphic ventricular tachycardia in acute myocardial infarction without ST elevation in a patient with thrombocytopenia. *Kardiol Pol.* 2006; 64:1013-4.

236. Maxa JL, Hebeler RF, Adeeko MA. Torsades de pointes following concurrent amiodarone and levofloxacin therapy. *Proc (Bayl Univ Med Cent).* 2006; 19:345-6.

237. Lim HE, Pak HN, Ahn JC et al. Torsade de pointes induced by short-term oral amiodarone therapy. *Europace.* 2006; 8:1051-3.

238. Foley P, Kalra P, Andrews N. Amiodarone-avoid the danger of Torsade de Pointes. *Resuscitation.* 2007; 76:137-41.

239. Lehtonen A, Fodstad H, Laitinen-Forsblom P et al. Further evidence of inherited long QT syndrome mutations in antiarrhythmic drug-associated torsades de pointes. *Heart Rhythm.* 2007; 4:603-7.

240. Wegener FT, Ehrlich JR, Hohnloser SH. Amiodarone-associated macroscopic T-wave alternans and torsade de pointes unmasking the inherited long QT syndrome. *Europace.* 2008; 10:112-3.

241. Poluzzi E, Raschi E, Moretti U et al. Drug-induced torsades de pointes: data mining of the public version of the FDA Adverse Event Reporting System (AERS). *Pharmacoepidemiol Drug Saf.* 2009; 18:512-8.

242. Di Micoli A, Zambruni A, Bracci E et al. "Torsade de pointes" during amiodarone infusion in a cirrhotic woman with a prolonged QT interval. *Dig Liver Dis.* 2009; 41:535-8.
243. Badshah A, Mirza B, Janjua M et al. Amiodarone-induced torsade de pointes in a patient with Wolff-Parkinson-White syndrome. *Hellenic J Cardiol.* 2009; 50:224-6.
244. Fayssoil A, Issi J, Guerbaa M et al. Torsade de pointes induced by citalopram and amiodarone. *Ann Cardiol Angeiol.* 2011; 60:165-8.
245. Digby GC, Perez Riera AR, Barbosa Barros R et al. Acquired long QT interval: a case series of multifactorial QT prolongation. *Clin Cardiol.* 2011; 34:577-82.
246. Kawaguchi T, Takasugi N, Kubota T et al. In-hospital monitoring of T-wave alternans in a case of amiodarone-induced torsades de pointes: clinical and methodologic insights. *Europace.* 2012:14; 1372-4.
247. Mukhopadhyay S, Chakraborty P, Yusuf J et al. Phenytoin in treatment of amiodarone-induced torsades de pointes. *Indian J Pharmacol.* 2012; 44:264-5.
248. Kao DP, Hiatt WR, Krantz MJ. Proarrhythmic potential of dronedarone: emerging evidence from spontaneous adverse event reporting. *Pharmacotherapy.* 2012; 32:767-71.
249. Jhuo SJ, Tang WH, Lai WT et al. Torsade de pointes induced by amiodarone in a patient with heart failure. *Kaohsiung J Med Sci.* 2014; 30:108-9.
250. Bienias P, Ciurzynski M, Paczynska M et al. Cardiac arrest and electrical storm due to recurrent torsades de pointes caused by concomitant clarithromycin, cotrimoxazole and amiodarone treatment. *Pol Merkur Lekarski.* 2014; 37:285-8.
251. Little RE, Kay GN, Cavender JB et al. Torsade de pointes and T-U wave alternans associated with arsenic poisoning. *Pacing Clin Electrophysiol.* 1990; 13:164-70.
252. Beckman KJ, Bauman JL, Pimental PA et al. Arsenic-induced torsade de pointes. *Crit Care Med.* 1991; 19:290-2.
253. Unnikrishnan D, Dutcher JP, Varshneya N et al. Torsades de pointes in 3 patients with leukemia treated with arsenic trioxide. *Blood.* 2001; 97:1514-6.
254. Soignet SL, Frankel SR, Douer D et al. United States multicenter study of arsenic trioxide in relapsed acute promyelocytic leukemia. *J Clin Oncol.* 2001; 19:3852-60.
255. Naito K, Kobayashi M, Sahara N et al. Two cases of acute promyelocytic leukemia complicated by torsade de pointes during arsenic trioxide therapy. *Int J Hematol.* 2006; 83:318-23.
256. Yamazaki K, Terada H, Satoh H et al. Arrhythmogenic effects of arsenic trioxide in patients with acute promyelocytic leukemia and an electrophysiological study in isolated guinea pig papillary muscles. *Circ J.* 2006; 70:1407-14.
257. Hai JJ, Gill H, Tse HF et al. Torsade de pointes during oral arsenic trioxide therapy for acute promyelocytic leukemia in a patients with heart failure. *Ann Hematol.* 2015; 94:501-3.
258. Arellano-Rodrigo E, García A, Mont L et al. Torsade de pointes and cardiorespiratory arrest induced by azithromycin in a patient with congenital long QT syndrome. *Med Clin.* 2001; 117:118-9.
259. Shaffer D, Singer S, Korvick J et al. Concomitant risk factors in reports of torsades de pointes associated with macrolide use: review of the United States Food and Drug Administration Adverse Event Reporting System. *Clin Infect Dis.* 2002; 35:197-200.
260. Kezerashvili A, Khattak H, Barsky A et al. Azithromycin as a cause of QT-interval prolongation and torsade de pointes in the absence of other known precipitating factors. *J Interv Card Electrophysiol.* 2007; 18:243-6.
261. Huang BH, Wu CH, Hsia CP et al. Azithromycin-induced torsade de pointes. *Pacing Clin Electrophysiol.* 2007; 30:1579-82.
262. Howard PA. Azithromycin-induced proarrhythmia and cardiovascular death. *Ann Pharmacother.* 2013; 47:1547-51.
263. Cocco G, Jerie P. Torsades de pointes induced by the concomitant use of ivabradine and azithromycin: an unexpected dangerous interaction. *Cardiovasc Toxicol.* 2015; 15:104-6.
264. Sears SP, Getz TW, Austin CO et al. Incidence of sustained ventricular tachycardia in patients with prolonged QTc after the administration of azithromycin: a retrospective study. *Drugs Real World Outcomes.* 2016; 3:99-105.
265. Demaziere J, Fourcade JM, Busseuil CT et al. The hazards of chloroquine self prescription in West Africa. *J Toxicol Clin Toxicol.* 1995; 33:369-70.
266. Ochiai H, Kashiwagi M, Usui T et al. Torsade de pointes with T wave alternans in a patient receiving moderate dose of chlorpromazine: report of a case. *Kokyu To Junkan.* 1990; 38:819-22.
267. Frothingham R. Rates of torsades de pointes associated with ciprofloxacin, ofloxacin, levofloxacin, gatifloxacin, and moxifloxacin. *Pharmacotherapy.* 2001; 21:1468-72.
268. Daya SK, Gowda RM, Khan IA. Ciprofloxacin- and hypocalcemia-induced torsade de pointes triggered by hemodialysis. *Am J Ther.* 2004; 11:77-9.
269. Flanagan MC, Mitchell ES, Haigney MC. Ciprofloxacin-induced torsade de pointes. *Int J Cardiol.* 2006; 113:239-41.
270. Kazmierczak J, Peregud-Pogorzelska M, Rzeuski R. QT Interval prolongation and torsades de pointes due to a coadministration of ciprofloxacin and azimilide in a patient with implantable cardioverter-defibrillator. *Pacing Clin Electrophysiol.* 2007; 30:1043-6.
271. Nair MK, Patel K, Starer PJ. Ciprofloxacin-induced torsades de pointes in a methadone-dependent patient. *Addiction.* 2008; 103:2062-4.
272. Barcelos AM, Teixeira MA, Maia Mda C et al. Postpartum torsades de pointes and long QT syndrome. *Arq Bras Cardiol.* 2009; 93:e58-9, e46-7.
273. Keivanidou A, Arnaoutoglou C, Krommydas A et al. Ciprofloxacin induced acquired long QT syndrome in a patient under class III antiarrhythmic therapy. *Cardiol J.* 2009; 16:172-4.
274. Salinas Acre J, Romero R, Solorzano P. A case of prolonged QT interval and torsades de pointes due to ciprofloxacin. *Rev Esp Cardiol.* 2010; 63:111-2.
275. Ibrahim M, Omar B. Ciprofloxacin-induced torsades de pointes. *Am J Emerg Med.* 2012; 30:252.e5-9.
276. Wysowski DK, Bacsanyi J. Cisapride and latal arrhythmia. *N Engl J Med.* 1996; 335:290-1.
277. Sekkarie MA. Torsades de pointes in two chronic renal failure patients treated with cisapride and clarithromycin. *Am J Kidney Dis.* 1997; 30:437-9.
278. Hill SL, Evangelista JK, Pizzi AM et al. Proarrhythmia associated with cisapride in children. *Pediatrics.* 1998; 101:1053-6.
279. Vitola J, Vukanovic J, Roden DM. Cisapride-induced torsades de pointes. *J Cardiovasc Electrophysiol.* 1998; 9:1109-13.
280. Kantoch MJ, Qurashi MM, Bulbul ZR et al. A newborn with a complex congenital heart disease, atrioventricular block, and torsade de pointes ventricular tachycardia. *Pacing Clin Electrophysiol.* 1998; 21:2664-7.
281. Piquette RK. Torsade de pointes induced by cisapride/clarithromycin interaction. *Ann Pharmacother.* 1999; 33:22-6.
282. Ng KS, Tham LS, Tan HH et al. Cisapride and torsades de pointes in a pacemaker patient. *Pacing Clin Electrophysiol.* 2000; 23:130-2.
283. Wysowski DK, Corken A, Gallo-Torres H et al. Postmarketing reports of QT prolongation and ventricular arrhythmia in association with cisapride and Food and Drug Administration regulatory actions. *Am J Gastroenterol.* 2001; 96:1698-703.
284. Kyrmizakis DE, Chimona TS, Kanoupakis EM et al. QT prolongation and torsades de pointes associated with concurrent use of cisapride and erythromycin. *Am J Otolaryngol.* 2002; 23:303-7.
285. Enger C, Cali C, Walker AM. Serious ventricular arrhythmias among users of cisapride and other QT-prolonging agents in the United States. *Pharmacoepidemiol Drug Saf.* 2002; 11:477-86.
286. Meuleman C, Jourdain P, Bellorini M et al. Citalopram and Torsades de Pointes: a case report. *Arch Mai Coeur Vaiss.* 2001; 94:1021-4.

287. Kourgiannidis G, Chierchia G-B, Wyffels E et al. A case of monomorphic ventricular tachycardia? *J Cardiovasc Electrophysiol.* 2005; 16:1014-6.
288. Kanjanauthai S, Kanluen T, Chareonthaitawee P. Citalopram induced torsade de pointes, a rare life threatening side effect. *Int J Cardiol.* 2008; 131:e33-4.
289. Blaschke D, Parwani AS, Huemer M et al. Torsade de pointes during combined treatment with risperidone and citalopram. *Pharmacopsychiatry.* 2007; 40:294-5.
290. Tarabar AF, Hoffman RS, Nelson L. Citalopram overdose: late presentation of torsades de pointes (TdP) with cardiac arrest. *J Med Toxicol.* 2008; 4:101-5.
291. de Gregorio C, Morabito G, Cerrito M et al. Citalopram-induced long QT syndrome and torsade de pointes: role for concomitant therapies and illnesses (letter). *Int J Cardiol.* 2011; 148:226-8.
292. Deshmukh A, Ulveling K, Alla V et al. Prolonged QTc interval and torsades de pointes induced by citalopram. *Tex Heart Inst J.* 2012; 39:68-70.
293. Kogut C, Crouse EB, Vieweg WV et al. Selective serotonin reuptake inhibitors and torsade de pointes: new concept and new directions derived from a series of case reports. *Ther Adv Drug Saf.* 2013; 4:189-98.
294. Kraai EP, Seifert SA. Citalopram overdose: a fatal case. *J Med Toxicol.* 2015; 11:232-6.
295. Lee KL, Jim MH, Tang SC et al. QT prolongation and torsades de pointes associated with clarithromycin. *Am J Med.* 1998; 104:395-6.
296. Hayashi Y, Ikeda U, Hashimoto T et al. Torsades de pointes ventricular tachycardia induced by clarithromycin and disopyramide in the presence of hypokalemia. *Pacing Clin Electrophysiol.* 1999; 22:672-4.
297. Kamochi H, Nii T, Eguchi K et al. Clarithromycin associated with torsades de pointes. *Jpn Circ J.* 1999; 63:421-2.
298. Choudhury L, Grais IM, Passman RS. Torsades de pointes due to drug interaction between disopyramide and clarithromycin. *Heart Dis.* 1999; 1:206-7.
299. Flockhart DA, Drici MD, Kerbusch T et al. Studies on the mechanism of a fatal clarithromycin-pimozide interaction in a patient with Tourette syndrome. *J Clin Psychopharmacol.* 2000; 20:317-24.
300. Yamaguchi S, Kaneko Y, Yamagishi T et al. Clarithromycin-induced torsades de pointes. *Nippon Naika Gakkai Zasshi.* 2003; 92:143-5.
301. Hensey C, Keane D. Clarithromycin induced torsade de pointes. *Ir J Med Sci.* 2008; 177:67-8.
302. Gysel M, Vieweg WV, Hasnain M et al. Torsades de pointes following clarithromycin treatment. *Expert Rev Cardiovasc Ther.* 2013; 11:1485-93.
303. Chang NL, Shah P, Bikkina M, Shamoon F. Clarithromycin-induced torsades de pointes. *Am J Ther.* 2016; 23:e955-6.
304. Schrem SS, Belsky P, Schwartzman D et al. Cocaine-induced torsades de pointes in a patient with the idiopathic long QT syndrome. *Am Heart J.* 1990; 120:980-4.
305. Perea M, Ortega M, Trejo O et al. Torsades de pointes induced by cocaine. *Med Clin.* 2000; 114:278.
306. Singh N, Singh HK, Singh PP et al. Cocaine-induced torsades de pointes in idiopathic long Q-T syndrome. *Am J Ther.* 2001; 8:299-302.
307. Krantz MJ, Rowan SB, Mehler PS. Cocaine-related torsade de pointes in a methadone maintenance patient. *J Addict Dis.* 2005; 24:53-60.
308. Narang A, Ozcan C. Severe torsades de pointes with acquired QT prolongation. *Eur Heart J Acute Cardiovasc Care.* 2016; May 6. pii: 2048872616649473.
309. Commerlord PJ, Beck W. Ventricular tachycardia with torsade de pointes morphology induced by oral disopyramide. *S Aft Med J.* 1980; 58:447-8.
310. Tzivoni D, Keren A, Stern S et al. Disopyramide-induced Torsade de Pointes. *Arch Intern Med.* 1981; 141:946-7.
311. Wald RW, Waxman MB, Colman JM. Torsade de pointes ventricular tachycardia: a complication of disopyramide shared with quinidine. *J Electrocardiol.* 1981; 14:301-7.
312. Schweitzer P, Mark H. Torsade de pointes caused by disopyramide and hypokalemia. *Mt Sinai J Med.* 1982; 49:110-4.
313. Riccioni N, Castiglioni M, Bartolomei C. Disopyramide-induced QT prolongation and ventricular tachyarrhythmias. *Am Heart J.* 1983; 105:870-1.
314. Azpitarte Almagro J, Casero A, Melgares R. Torsade de pointes induced by disopyramide: presentation of a case with fatal outcome. *Rev Esp Cardiol.* 1984; 37:145-8.
315. Schattner A, Gindin J, Geltner D. Fatal torsade de pointes following jaundice in a patient treated with disopyramide. *Postgrad Med J.* 1989; 65:333-4.
316. Aarskog D, Reikvam A. Torsades de pointes ventricular tachycardia induced by disopyramide at therapeutic serum concentration. *Tidsskr Nor Laegeforen.* 1992; 112:2511-3.
317. Kimura Y, Takayanagi K, Sakai Y et al. Torsades de pointes in paced patients with sick sinus syndrome after disopyramide administration. *Jpn Heart J.* 1994; 35:153-61.
318. Hirose K, Yamaguchi H, Oshima Y et al. Severe respiratory failure and torsades de pointes induced by disopyramide in a patient with myasthenia gravis. *Intern Med.* 2008; 47:1703-8.
319. Matsuhashi T, Sato T, Aizawa Y et al. Recurrent torsade de pointes during mild hypothermia therapy for a survivor of sudden cardiac arrest due to drug-induced long-QT syndrome. *J Cardiovasc Electrophysiol.* 2010; 21:462-3.
320. Miyamoto K, Kawai H, Aoyama R et al. Torsades de pointes induced by a combination of garenoxacin and disopyramide and other cytochrome P450, family 3, subfamily A polypeptide-4-influencing drugs during hypokalemia due to licorice. *Clin Exp Nephrol.* 2010; 14:164-7.
321. Asajima H, Saito N, Ohmura Y et al. Lansoprazole precipitated QT prolongation and torsade de pointes associated with disopyramide. *Eur J Clin Pharmacol.* 2012; 68:331-3.
322. Echt DS, Lee JT, Murray KT et al. A randomized, double-blind, placebo-controlled, dose-ranging study of dofetilide in patients with inducible sustained ventricular tachyarrhythmias. *J Cardiovasc Electrophysiol.* 1995; 6:687-99.
323. Bashir Y, Thomsen PE, Kingma JH et al. Electrophysiologic profile and efficacy of intravenous dofetilide (UK-68,798), a new class III antiarrhythmic drug, in patients with sustained monomorphic ventricular tachycardia: Dofetilide Arrhythmia Study Group. *Am J Cardiol.* 1995; 76:1040-4.
324. Norgaard BL, Wachtell K, Christensen PD et al. Efficacy and safety of intravenously administered dofetilide in acute termination of atrial fibrillation and flutter: a multicenter, randomized, double-blind, placebo-controlled trial: Danish Dofetilide in Atrial Fibrillation and Flutter Study Group. *Am Heart J.* 1999; 137:1062-9.
325. Torp-Pedersen C, Moller M, Bloch-Thomsen PE et al. Dofetilide in patients with congestive heart failure and left ventricular dysfunction: Danish Investigations of Arrhythmia and Mortality on Dofetilide Study Group. *N Engl J Med.* 1999; 341:857-65.
326. Bianconi L, Castro A, Dinelli M et al. Comparison of intravenously administered dofetilide versus amiodarone in the acute termination of atrial fibrillation and flutter: a multicentre, randomized, double-blind, placebo-controlled study. *Eur Heart J.* 2000; 21:1265-73.
327. Singh S, Zoble RG, Yellen L et al. Efficacy and safety of oral dofetilide in converting to and maintaining sinus rhythm in patients with chronic atrial fibrillation or atrial flutter: the Symptomatic Atrial Fibrillation Investigative Research on Dofetilide (SAFIRE-D) study. *Circulation.* 2000; 102:2385-90.
328. Kober L, Bloch Thomsen PE, Moller M et al. Effect of dofetilide in patients with recent myocardial infarction and left-ventricular dysfunction: a randomised trial. *Lancet.* 2000; 356:2052-8.

329. Moller M, Torp-Pedersen CT, Kober L. Dofetilide in patients with congestive heart failure and left ventricular dysfunction: safety aspects and effect on atrial fibrillation: the Danish Investigators of Arrhythmia and Mortality on Dofetilide (DIAMOND) Study Group. *Congest Heart Fail.* 2001; 7:146-50.
330. Boriani G, Lubinski A, Capucci A et al. A multicentre, double-blind randomized crossover comparative study on the efficacy and safety of dofetilide vs sotalol in patients with inducible sustained ventricular tachycardia and ischaemic heart disease. *Eur Heart.* 2001; 22:2180-91.
331. Nagra BS, Ledley GS, Kantharia BK. Marked QT prolongation and torsades de pointes secondary to acute ischemia in an elderly man taking dofetilide for atrial fibrillation: a cautionary tale. *J Cardiovasc Pharmacol Ther.* 2005; 10:191-5.
332. Aktas MK, Shah AH, Akiyama T. Dofetilide-induced long QT and torsades de pointes. *Ann Noninvasive Electrocardiol.* 2007; 12:197-202.
333. Pedersen HS, Elming H, Seibaek M et al. Risk factors and predictors of torsade de pointes ventricular tachycardia in patients with left ventricular systolic dysfunction receiving dofetilide. *Am J Cardiol.* 2007; 100:876-80.
334. Banchs JE, Wolbrette DL, Samii SM et al. Efficacy and safety of dofetilide in patients with atrial fibrillation and atrial flutter. *J Interv Card Electrophysiol.* 2008; 23:111-5.
335. Manocha P, Bavikati V, Langberg J et al. Coronary artery disease potentiates response to dofetilide for rhythm control of atrial fibrillation. *Pacing Clin Electrophysiol.* 2012; 35:170-3.
336. Brumberg G, Gera N, Pracy C et al. Frequency of toxicity with chemical conversion of atrial fibrillation with dofetilide. *Am J Cardiol.* 2013; 112:505-8.
337. Romero J, Baldinger SH, Goodman-Meza D et al. Drug-induced torsades de pointes in an underserved population. Methadone: is there therapeutic equipoise? *J Interv Card Electrophysiol.* 2016; 45:37-45.
338. El-Assaad I, Al-Kindi SG, Abraham J et al. Use of dofetilide in adult patients with atrial arrhythmias and congenital heart disease: a PACES collaborative study. *Heart Rhythm.* 2016; 13:2034-9.
339. Osborne RJ, Slevin ML, Hunter RW et al. Cardiotoxicity of intravenous domperidone. *Lancet.* 1985; 2:385.
340. Osborne RJ, Slevin ML, Hunter RW et al. Cardiac arrhythmias during cytotoxic chemotherapy: role of domperidone. *Human Toxicol.* 1985; 4:617-26.
341. Tanaka A, Koga S, Hiramatsu Y. Donepezil-induced adverse side effects of cardiac rhythm: 2 cases report of atrioventricular block and torsades de pointes. *Intern Med.* 2009; 48:1219-23.
342. Takaya T, Okamoto M, Yodoi K et al. Torsades de pointes with QT prolongation related to donepexil use. *J Cardiol.* 2009: 54; 507-11.
343. Kitt J, Irons R, Al-Obaidi M et al. A case of donepezil-related torsades de pointes. *BMJ Case Rep.* 2015 Oct 5; 2015. pii: bcr2015211900.
344. Huemer M, Sarganas G, Bronder E et al. Torsade de pointes tachycardia in a patient on dronedarone therapy. *Pharmacotherapy.* 2015; 35:e61-5.
345. Guy JM, André-Fouet X, Porte J et al. Torsades de pointes and prolongation of the duration of QT interval after injection of droperidol. *Ann Cardiol Angeiol.* 1991; 40:541-5.
346. Faigel DO, Metz DC, Kochman ML. Torsade de pointes complicating the treatment of bleeding esophageal varices: association with neuroleptics, vasopressin, and electrolyte imbalance. *Am J Gastroenterol.* 1995; 90:822-4.
347. Michalets EL, Smith LK, Van Tassel ED. Torsade de pointes resulting from the addition of droperidol to an existing cytochrome P450 drug interaction. *Ann Pharmacother.* 1998; 32:761-5.
348. Nuttall GA, Eckerman KM, Jacob KA et al. Does low-dose droperidol administration increase the risk of drug-induced QT prolongation and torsade de pointes in the general surgical population? *Anesthesiology.* 2007; 107:531-6.
349. Choo EK, Weber FS, Schmidt TA. Torsades de pointes after administration of droperidol for nausea and vomiting. *Prehosp Emerg Care.* 2009; 13:261-5.
350. McComb JM, Campbell NP, Cleland J. Recurrent ventricular tachycardia associated with QT prolongation after mitral valve replacement and its association with intravenous administration of erythromycin. *Am J Cardiol.* 1984; 54:922-3.
351. Gueugniaud PY, Guerin C, Mahul P et al. Torsade de pointes induced by the combination lidocaine-erythromycin and hepatic insufficiency *Presse Med.* 1985; 20:896.
352. Guelon D, Bedock B, Chartier C et al. QT prolongation and recurrent "torsades de pointes" during erythromycin lactobionate infusion (letter). *Am J Cardiol.* 1986; 58:666.
353. Kilani F, Marsepoil T. Attack of torsades de pointes induced by an intravenous injection of erythromycin lactobionate. *Ann Fr Anesth Reanim.* 1988; 7:270-1.
354. Camilleri JF, Deharo JC, Panagidès D et al. Jet intravenous injection of erythromycin lactobionate: a possible cause of the occurrence of crisis in torsade de pointe. *Ann Cardiol Angeiol.* 1989; 38:657-9.
355. Schoenenberger RA, Haefeli WE, Weiss P et al. Association of intravenous erythromycin and potentially fatal ventricular tachycardia with Q-T prolongation (torsades de pointes). *BMI.* 1990; 300:1375-6.
356. Staikowsky F, Haziza F, Guidet B et al. Access of torsades de pointes in Legionnaires' disease: an uncommon adverse effect of erythromycin. *Rev Pneumol Clin.* 1991; 47:92-4.
357. Gully C, Riem R. Torsades de pointes caused by the association of terfenadine and erythromycin. *Ann Med Interne (Paris).* 1994; 145:257-8.
358. Biglin KE, Faraon MS, Constance TD et al. Drug-induced torsades de pointes: a possible interaction of terfenadine and erythromycin. *Ann Pharmacother.* 1994; 28:282.
359. Gitler B, Berger LS, Buffa SD. Torsades de pointes induced by erythromycin. *Chest.* 1994; 105:368-72.
360. de Koning J, van der Hoeven H, Hamer B et al. Erythromycin-induced torsades de pointes and ventricular fibrillation in a patient with Legionella pneumonia. *Neth J Med.* 1994; 44:131-5.
361. Rezkalla MA, Pochop C. Erythromycin induced Torsades de Pointes: case report and review of the literature. *S D J Med.* 1994; 47:161-4.
362. Brandriss MW, Richardson WS, Barold SS. Erythromycin-induced QT prolongation and polymorphic ventricular tachycardia (torsades de pointes): case report and review. *Clin Infect Dis.* 1994; 18:995-8.
363. Paris DG, Parente TF, Bruschetta HR et al. Torsades de pointes induced by erythromycin and terfenadine. *Am J Emerg Med.* 1994; 12:636-8.
364. Orban Z, MacDonald LL, Peters MA, Guslits B. Erythromycin-induced cardiac toxicity. *Am J Cardiol.* 1995; 75:859-61.
365. Wong CB, Windle J. Erythromycin induced torsades de pointes. *Nebr Med J.* 1995; 80:285-6.
366. Oberg KC, Bauman JL. QT interval prolongation and torsades de pointes due to erythromycin lactobionate. *Pharmacotherapy.* 1995; 15:687-92.
367. Cranberry MC, Gardner SF. Erythromycin monotherapy associated with torsade de pointes. *Ann Pharmacother.* 1996; 30:777-8.
368. Hsieh MH, Chen SA, Chiang CE et al. Drug-induced torsades de pointes in one patient with congenital long QT syndrome. *Int J Cardiol.* 1996; 54:85-8.
369. Lin JC, Quasny HA. QT prolongation and development of torsades de pointes with the concomitant administration of oral erythromycin base and quinidine. *Pharmacotherapy.* 1997; 17:626-30.
370. Katapadi K, Kostandy G, Katapadi M et al. A review of erythromycin-induced malignant tachyarrhythmia—torsade de pointes: a case report. *Angiology.* 1997; 48:821-6.

371. Koh TW. Risk of torsades de pointes from oral erythromycin with concomitant carbimazole (methimazole) administration. *Pacing Clin Electrophysiol.* 2001; 24:1575-6.
372. Hinterseer M, Irlbeck M, Ney L et al. Acute respiratory distress syndrome with transiently impaired left ventricular function and Torsades de Pointes arrhythmia unmasking congenital long QT syndrome in a 25-yr-old woman. *Br J Anaesth.* 2006; 97:150-3.
373. Singh P, Maldonado-Duran JM. Drug-induced QT prolongation as a result of an escitalopram overdose in a patient with previously undiagnosed congenital long QT syndrome. *Case Rep Med.* 2014; 2014:917846.
374. Lui HK, Lee G, Dietrich P et al. Flecainide-induced QT prolongation and ventricular tachycardia. *Am Heart J.* 1982; 103:567-9.
375. Ohki R, Takahashi M, Mizuno O et al. Torsades de pointes ventricular tachycardia induced by mosapride and flecainide in the presence of hypokalemia. *Pacing Clin Electrophysiol.* 2001; 24:119-21.
376. Thevenin J, Da Costa A, Roche F et al. Flecainide induced ventricular tachycardia (torsades de pointes). *Pacing Clin Electrophysiol.* 2003; 26:1907-8.
377. Nogales Asensio JM, Moreno Sánchez N, Doncel Vecino LJ et al. Torsade-de-pointes in a patient under flecainide treatment, an unusual case of proarrhythmicity. *Int J Cardiol.* 2007; 114:E65-7.
378. van der Heide K, de Haes A, Wietasch GJ et al. Torsades de pointes during laparoscopic adrenalectomy of a pheochromocytoma: a case report. *J Med Case Rep.* 2011; 5:368.
379. Kim HS, Pak HN, Park JS et al. Flecainide-associated bradycardia-dependent torsade de pointes: another potential mechanism of proarrhythmia. *Pacing Clin Electrophysiol.* 2013; 36:e84-6.
380. Hayes K, Deshmukh A, Pant S et al. Flecainide associated torsade de pointes: a potential case of reverse use dependence. *J Res Med Sci.* 2013; 18:1108-9.
381. Oguayo KN, Oyetayo OO, Costa SM et al. An unusual case of flecainide-induced QT prolongation leading to cardiac arrest. *Pharmacotherapy.* 2014; 34:e30-3.
382. Nasser M, Idris S, Marinelli K et al. Flecainide-induced Torsades de Pointes: case report and review of the literature. *Rev Cardiovasc Med.* 2015; 16:214-20.
383. Dorsey ST, Biblo LA. Prolonged QT interval and torsades de pointes caused by the combination of fluconazole and amitriptyline. *Am J Emerg Med.* 2000; 18:227-9.
384. Wassmann S, Nickenig G, Bohm M. Long QT syndrome and torsade de pointes in a patient receiving fluconazole. *Ann Intern Med.* 1999; 131:797.
385. Tholakanahalli VN, Potti A, Hanley JF et al. Fluconazole-induced torsade de pointes. *Ann Pharmacother.* 2001; 35:432-4.
386. Khazan M, Mathis AS. Probable case of torsades de pointes induced by fluconazole. *Pharmacotherapy.* 2002; 22:1632-7.
387. Gandhi PJ, Menezes PA, Vu HT et al. Fluconazole- and levofloxacin-induced torsades de pointes in an intensive care unit patient. *Am J Health-Syst Pharm.* 2003; 60:2479-83.
388. Tatetsu H, Asou N, Nakamura M et al. Torsades de pointes upon fluconazole administration in a patient with acute myeloblastic leukemia. *Am J Hematol.* 2006; 81:366-9.
389. Pham CP, de Feiter PW, van der Kuy PH et al. Long QTc interval and torsade de pointes caused by fluconazole. *Ann Pharmacother.* 2006; 40:1456-61.
390. Esch JJ, Kantoch MJ. Torsades de pointes ventricular tachycardia in a pediatric patient treated with fluconazole. *Pediatric Cardiol.* 2008; 29:210-3.
391. McMahon JH, Grayson ML. Torsades de pointes in a patient receiving fluconazole for cerebral cryptococcosis. *Am Health-Syst Pharm.* 2008; 65:619-23.
392. Chakravarty C, Singh PM, Trikha A et al. Fluconazole-induced recurrent ventricular fibrillation leading to multiple cardiac arrests. *Anaesth Intensive Care.* 2009; 37:477-80.
393. Poluzzi E, Raschi E, Motola D et al. Antimicrobials and the risk of torsades de pointes: the contribution from data mining of the US FDA Adverse Even Reporting System. *Drug Saf.* 2010; 33:303-14.
394. Tacken MC, Bracke FA, Van Zundert AA. Torsade de pointes during sevoflurane anesthesia and fluconazole infusion in a patient with long QT syndrome. A case report. *Acta Anaesthesiol Belg.* 2011; 62:105-8.
395. Overbey AN, Austin A, Seidensticker DF et al. Overdrive pacing in a patient with incessant torsades de pointes. *BMJ Case Rep.* 2013; Oct 11:2013.
396. Bertino JS Jr, Owens RC Jr, Carnes TD et al. Gatifloxacin-associated corrected QT interval prolongation, torsades de pointes, and ventricular fibrillation in a patient with known risk factors. *Clin Infect Dis.* 2002; 34:861-3.
397. Fteha A, Fteha E, Haq S et al. Gatifloxacin induced torsades de pointes. *Pacing Clin Electrophsyiol.* 2004; 27:1449-50.
398. Toivonen L, Viitasalo M, Siikamäki H et al. Provocation of ventricular tachycardia by antimalarial drug halofantrine in congenital long QT syndrome. *Clin Cardiol.* 1994; 17:403-4.
399. Fourcade L, Hovette P, De Pina JJ et al. Prolonged QT interval and cardiac toxicity due to halofantrine. *Med Trop (Mars).* 1995; 55:182-3.
400. Zee-Cheng CS, Mueller CE, Seifert CF et al. Haloperidol and torsades de pointes. *Ann Intern Med.* 1985; 102:418.
401. Payer SA. Torsades de pointes ventricular tachyarrhythmia associated with haloperidol. *J Clin Psychopharmacol.* 1986; 6:375-6.
402. Kriwisky M, Perry GY, Tarchitsky D et al. Haloperidol-induced torsades de pointes. *Chest.* 1990; 98:482-4.
403. Henderson RA, Lane S, Henry JA. Life-threatening ventricular arrhythmia (torsades de pointes) after haloperidol overdose. *Hum Exp Toxicol.* 1991; 10:59-62.
404. Metzger E, Friedman R. Prolongation of the corrected QT and torsades de pointes cardiac arrhythmia associated with intravenous haloperidol in the medically ill. *J Clin Psychopharmacol.* 1993; 13:128-32.
405. Wilt JL, Minnema AM, Johnson RF et al. Torsade de pointes associated with the use of intravenous haloperidol. *Ann Intern Med.* 1993; 119:391-4.
406. Di Salvo TG, O'Gara PT. Torsade de pointes caused by high-dose intravenous haloperidol in cardiac patients. *Clin Cardiol.* 1995; 18:285-90.
407. Hunt N, Stern TA. The association between intravenous haloperidol and torsades de pointes: three cases and a literature review. *Psychosomatics.* 1995; 36:541-9.
408. Jackson T, Ditmanson L, Phibbs B. Torsade de pointes and low-dose oral haloperidol. *Arch Intern Med.* 1997; 157:2013-5.
409. Sharma ND, Rosman HS, Padhi ID et al. Torsades de pointes associated with intravenous haloperidol in critically ill patients. *Am J Cardiol.* 1998; 81:238-40.
410. O'Brien JM, Rockwood RP, Suh KI. Haloperidol-induced torsade de pointes. *Ann Pharmacother.* 1999; 33:1046-50.
411. Perrault LP, Denault AY, Carrier M et al. Torsades de pointes secondary to intravenous haloperidol after coronary bypass grafting surgery. *Can J Anaesth.* 2000; 47:251-4.
412. Hassaballa HA, Balk RA. Torsade de pointes associated with the administration of intravenous haloperidol. *Am J Ther.* 2003; 10:58-60.
413. Ginwalla M, Biblo LA, Paydak H. Torsade de pointes following intravenous haloperidol administration in a patient with complete heart block. *WML.* 2009; 108:48-50.
414. Meyer-Massetti C, Vaerini S, Ratz Bravo AE et al. Comparative safety of antipsychotics in the WHO pharmacovigilance database: the haloperidol case. *Int J Clin Pharm.* 2011; 33:806-14.
415. Paling FP, Andrews LM, Valk GD et al. Life-threatening complications of ibogaine: three case reports. *Neth J Med.* 2012; 70:422-4.
416. Hildyard C, Macklin P, Preendergast B et al. A case of QT prolongation and torsades de pointes caused by ibogaine toxicity. *J Emerg Med.* 2016; 50:e83-7.
417. Stambler BS, Wood MA, Ellenbogen KA et al. Efficacy and safety of repeated intravenous doses of ibutilide for rapid conversion of atrial flutter or fibrillation. Ibutilide Repeat Dose Study Investigators. *Circulation.* 1996; 94:1613-21.

418. Ellenbogen KA, Stambler BS, Wood MA et al. Efficacy of intravenous ibutilide for rapid termination of atrial fibrillation and atrial flutter: a dose-response study. *J Am Coll Cardiol.* 1996; 28:130-6.
419. Stambler BS, Beckman KJ, Kadish AH et al. Acute hemodynamic effects of intravenous ibutilide in patients with or without reduced left ventricular function. *Am J Cardiol.* 1997; 80:458-63.
420. Stambler BS, Wood MA, Ellenbogen KA. Antiarrhythmic actions of intravenous ibutilide compared with procainamide during human atrial flutter and fibrillation: electrophysiological determinants of enhanced conversion efficacy. *Circulation.* 1997; 96:4298-306.
421. Volgman AS, Carberry PA, Stambler B et al. Conversion efficacy and safety of intravenous ibutilide compared with intravenous procainamide in patients with atrial flutter or fibrillation. *J Am Coll Cardiol.* 1998; 31:1414-9.
422. Oral H, Souza JJ, Michaud GF et al. Facilitating transthoracic cardioversion of atrial fibrillation with ibutilide pretreatment. *N Engl J Med.* 1999; 340:1849-54.
423. Hennersdorf MG, Perings SM, Zuhlke C et al. Conversion of recent-onset atrial fibrillation or flutter with ibutilide after amiodarone has failed. *Intensive Care Med.* 2002; 28:925-9.
424. Das MK, Cheriparambil K, Bedi A et al. Cardioversion of atrial fibrillation with ibutilide: when is it most effective? *Clin Cardiol.* 2002; 25:411-5.
425. Gowda RM, Punukollu G, Khan IA et al. Ibutilide-induced long QT syndrome and Torsades de Pointes. *Am J Ther.* 2002; 9:527-9.
426. Gowda RM, Punukollu G, Khan IA et al. Ibutilide for pharmacological conversion of atrial fibrillation and flutter: impact of race on efficacy and safety. *Am J Ther.* 2003; 10:259-63.
427. Giudici MC, Fischer WJ III, Cervantes DC et al. Ibutilide therapy for atrial fibrillation: 5-year experience in a community hospital. *J Cardiovasc Nurs.* 2008; 23:484-8.
428. Samaha FF. QTC interval prolongation and polymorphic ventricular tachycardia in association with levofloxacin. *Am J Med.* 1999; 107:528-9.
429. Iannini PB, Doddamani S, Byazovra E et al. Risk of torsades de pointes with non-cardiac drugs. *BMJ.* 2001; 322:46-7.
430. Iannini PB. Quinolone-induced QT interval prolongation: a not-so-unexpected class effect. *J Antimicrob Chemother.* 2001; 47:893.
431. Amankwa K, Krishnan SC, Tisdale JE. Torsades de pointes associated with fluoroquinolones: importance of concomitant risk factors. *Clin Pharmacol Ther.* 2004; 75:242-7.
432. Patel PD, Afshar H, Birnbaum Y. Levofloxacin-induced torsades de pointes. *Tex Heart Inst J.* 2010; 37:216-7.
433. Stancampiano FF, Palmer WC, Betz TW et al. Rare incidence of ventricular tachycardia and torsades de pointes in hospitalized patients with prolonged QT who later received levofloxacin: a retrospective study. *Mayo Clin Proc.* 2015; 90:606-12.
434. Preβler J, Lucking M, Melter M et al. Nonsustained ventricular tachycardia in a patient with acquired long QT syndrome after levomepromazine injection. *Intensive Care Med.* 2014; 40:133-4.
435. Krantz MJ, Lewkowiez L, Hays H et al. Torsade de pointes associated with very-high-dose methadone. *Ann Intern Med.* 2002; 137:501-4.
436. Walker PW, Klein D, Kasza L. High dose methadone and ventricular arrhythmias: a report of three cases. *Pain.* 2003; 103:321-4.
437. Krantz MJ, Kutinsky IB, Robertson AD et al. Dose-related effects of methadone on QT prolongation in a series of patients with torsade de pointes. *Pharmacotherapy* 2003; 23:802-5.
438. Gil M, Sala M, Anguera I et al. QT prolongation and Torsades de Pointes in patients infected with human immunodeficiency virus and treated with methadone. *Am J Cardiol.* 2003; 92:995-7.
439. Vodoz JF, Jaquier F, Lamy O. Torsade de pointes: a severe and unknown adverse effect in a patient taking methadone. *Schweiz Rundsch Med Prax.* 2003; 92:1748-50.
440. Al-Shakarshi JS, Bent-Hansen L, Jensen GB. Life-threatening, recurrent arrhythmia in patients on high-dose methadone treatment: torsade de pointes. *Ugeskr Laeger.* 2004; 166:3104-5.
441. Almehmi A, Malas AM, Yousufuddin M et al. Methadone-induced torsade de pointes in a patient with normal baseline QT interval. *W V Med J.* 2004; 100:147-8.
442. Porter BO, Coyne PJ, Smith WR. Methadone-related torsades de pointes in a sickle cell patient treated for chronic pain. *Am J Hematol.* 2005; 78:316-7.
443. Pearson EC, Woosley RL. QT prolongation and torsades de pointes among methadone users: reports to the FDA spontaneous reporting system. *Pharmacoepidemiol Drug Saf.* 2005; 14:747-53.
444. Krantz MJ, Garcia JA, Mehler PS. Effects of buprenorphine on cardiac repolarization in a patient with methadone-related torsade de pointes. *Pharmacotherapy.* 2005; 25:611-4.
445. Sticherling C, Schaer BA, Ammann P et al. Methadone-induced torsade de pointes tachycardias. *Swiss Med Wkly.* 2005; 135:282-5.
446. Ostvold C, Topper M. Methadone-induced heart arrhythmia. *Tidsskr Nor Laegeforen.* 2005; 125:2021-2.
447. Sánchez Hernández AM, Atienza Fernández F, Arenal Maíz A et al. Torsades de pointes during methadone treatment. *Rev Esp Cardiol.* 2005; 58:1230-2.
448. Chatterjee B, Burgi U. Syncope of a drug addict—a special case. *Clin Res Cardiol.* 2006; 95:557-9.
449. Justo D, Gal-Oz A, Paran Y et al. Methadone-associated Torsades de Pointes (polymorphic ventricular tachycardia) in opioid-dependent patients. *Addiction.* 2006; 101:1333-8.
450. Lamont P, Hunt SC. A twist on torsade: a prolonged QT interval on methadone. *J Gen Intern Med.* 2006; 21:C9-12.
451. Moral Moral P, Rueda Soriano J, Tasias Pitarch M et al. Torsade de Pointes in patient infected with human immunodeficiency virus and treated with methadone. *An Med Interna.* 2006; 23:397-8.
452. Iskandar SB, Abi-Saleh BS, Mechleb BK et al. Methadone and torsade de pointes: case report and review of the literature. *Tenn Med.* 2007; 100:35-7.
453. Routhier DD, Katz KD, Brooks DE. QTc prolongation and torsades de pointes associated with methadone therapy. *J Emerg Med.* 2007; 32:275-8.
454. Luthi B, Huttner A, Speck RF et al. Methadone-induced torsade de pointes after stopping lopinavir-ritonavir. *Eur J Clin Microbiol Infect Dis.* 2007; 26:367-9.
455. George S. Methadone-associated QT prolongation and torsades de pointes. *Br J Hosp Med.* 2007; 68:221.
456. Atkinson D, Dunne A, Parker M. Torsades de pointes and self-terminating ventricular fibrillation in a prescription methadone user. *Anaesthesia.* 2007; 62:952-5.
457. Falconer M, Molloy D, Ingerhaug J et al. Methadone induced torsade de pointes in a patient receiving antiretroviral therapy. *Ir Med J.* 2007; 100:631-2.
458. Pimentel L, Mayo D. Chronic methadone therapy complicated by torsades de pointes: a case report. *J Emerg Med.* 2008; 34:287-90.
459. Esses JL, Rosman J, Do LT et al. Successful transition to buprenorphine in a patient with methadone-induced torsades de pointes. *J Interv Card Electrophysiol.* 2008; 23:117-9.
460. Reinhold JA, Sanoski CA, Russo AM et al. Torsades de pointes associated with methadone and voriconazole. *BMJ Case Rep.* 2009; 2009. pii: bcr07.2009.2119.
461. Stringer J, Welsh C, Tommasello A. Methadone-associated Q-T interval prolongation and torsades de pointes. *Am J Health-Syst Pharm.* 2009; 66:825-33.
462. Hanon S, Seewald RM, Yang F et al. Ventricular arrhythmias in patients treated with methadone for opioid dependence. *J Interv Card Electrophysiol.* 2010; 28:19-22.
463. Nordt SP, Zilberstein J, Gold B. Methadone-induced torsades de pointes. *Am J Emerg Med.* 2011; 29:476.e1-2.
464. Thanavaro KL, Thanavero JL. Methadone-induced torsades de pointes: a twist of fate. *Heart Lung.* 2011; 40:448-53.
465. Kao D, Bucher Bartelson B, Khatri V et al. Trends in reporting methadone-associated cardiac arrhythmia, 1997-2011: an analysis of registry data. *Ann Intern Med.* 2013; 158:735-40.

466. Cullington D, Dunford N, Beer S et al. Double jeopardy. *Indian Heart J.* 2013; 65:315-8.
467. Russell L, Levine D. Methadone-induced torsades de pointes. *R I Med J.* 2013; 96:20-1.
468. Katz DF, Varosy PD, Msoudi FA. Syncope. A tale of two triggers. *JAMA Intern Med.* 2013; 173:1543-4.
469. Rajpal S, Mundi AS, Reddy PC et al. Treatment of methadone-induced torsades de pointes with lidocaine. *J La State Med Soc.* 2013; 165:338-41.
470. Raina S, Paydak H, Al-Lahham T et al. Methadone induced torsades de pointes mimicking seizures in clinical presentation. *Am J Drug Alcohol Abuse.* 2014; 40:490-2.
471. Khalesi S, Shemirani H, Dehghani-Tafti F. Methadone induced torsades de pointes and ventricular fibrillation: a case review. *ARYA Atheroscler.* 2014; 10:339-42.
472. Walton G, Nolan S, Sutherland C et al. Sustained release oral morphine as an alternative to methadone for the treatment of opioid-use disorder post torsades de pointes cardiac arrest. *BMJ Case Rep.* 2015; Sep 21.
473. Dale KM, Lertsburapa K, Kluger J et al. Moxifloxacin and torsade de pointes. *Ann Pharmacother.* 2007; 41:336-40.
474. Altin T, Ozcan O, Turhan S et al. Torsade de pointes associated with moxifloxacin: a rare but potentially fatal adverse event. *Can J Cardiol.* 2007; 23:907-8.
475. Sherazi S, DiSalle M, Daubert JP et al. Moxifloxacin-induced torsades de pointes. *Cardiol J.* 2008; 15:71-3.
476. Badshah A, Janjua M, Younas F et al. Moxifloxacin-induced QT prolongation and torsades: an uncommon effect of a common drug. *Am J Med Sci.* 2009; 338:164-6.
477. Tiryakioglu SK, Tiryakioglu O, Akturk F et al. Moxifloxacin-dependent torsades de pointes. *Anadolu Kardiyol Derg.* 2011; 11:560-2.
478. Zofran® product monograph. New York: GlaxoSmithKline; 2014.
479. US Food and Drug Administration. FDA drug safety communication: new information regarding QT prolongation with ondansetron (Zofran). https://www.fda.gov/Drugs/DrugSafety/ucm310190.htm. Published June 29, 2012. (accessed 2018 Mar 4).
480. Kim HJ, An SH, Cho YH et al. Oxaliplatin-induced torsades de pointes and long QT syndrome in a patient with gastric cancer. *Acta Oncol.* 2013; 52:1223-4.
481. Chang RY, Lee MY, Kan CB et al. Oxaliplatin-induced acquired long QT syndrome with torsades de pointes and myocardial injury in a patient with dilated cardiomyopathy and rectal cancer. *J Chin Med Assoc.* 2013; 76:466-9.
482. Hancox JC, Caves RE, Choisy SC et al. QT interval prolongation and torsades de pointes with oxaliplatin. *Ther Adv Drug Saf.* 2016; 7:261-3.
483. Vrolix M, Piessens J, De Geest H. Torsades de pointes after intracoronary papaverine. *Eur Heart J.* 1991; 12:273-6.
484. Goto M, Sato M, Kitazawa H et al. Papaverine-induced QT interval prolongation and ventricular fibrillation in a patient with a history of drug-induced QT prolongation. *Intern Med.* 2014; 53:1629-31.
485. Wharton JM, Demopulos PA, Goldschlager N. Torsade de pointes during administration of pentamidine isethionate. *Am J Med.* 1987; 83:571-6.
486. Bibler MR, Chou TC, Toltzis RJ et al. Recurrent ventricular tachycardia due to pentamidine-induced cardiotoxicity. *Chest.* 1988; 94:1303-6.
487. Mitchell P, Dodek P, Lawson L et al. Torsades de pointes during intravenous pentamidine isethionate therapy. *Can Med Assoc J.* 1989; 140:173-4.
488. Green PT, Reents S, Harman E et al. Pentamidine-induced torsades de pointes in a renal transplant recipient with Pneumocystis carinii pneumonia. *South Med J.* 1990; 83:481-4.
489. Stein KM, Haronian H, Mensah GA et al. Ventricular tachycardia and torsades de pointes complicating pentamidine therapy of Pneumocystis carinii pneumonia in the acquired immunodeficiency syndrome. *Am J Cardiol.* 1990; 66:888-9.
490. Taylor AJ, Hull RW, Coyne PE et al. Pentamidine-induced torsades de pointes: safe completion of therapy with inhaled pentamidine. *Clin Pharmacol Ther.* 1991; 49:698-700.
491. Gonzalez A, Sager PT, Akil B et al. Pentamidine-induced torsade de pointes. *Am Heart J.* 1991; 122:1489-92.
492. Quadrel MA, Atkin SH, Jaker MA. Delayed cardiotoxicity during treatment with intravenous pentamidine: two case reports and a review of the literature. *Am Heart J.* 1992; 123:1377-9.
493. Engrav MB, Coodley G, Magnusson AR. Torsade de pointes after inhaled pentamidine. *Ann Emerg Med.* 1992; 21:1403-5.
494. Cortese LM, Gasser RA Jr, Bjornson DC et al. Prolonged recurrence of pentamidine-induced torsades de pointes. *Ann Pharmacother.* 1992; 26:1365-9.
495. Mani S, Kocheril AG, Andriole VT. Case report: pentamidine and polymorphic ventricular tachycardia revisited. *Am J Med Sci.* 1993; 305:236-40.
496. Harel Y, Scott WA, Szeinberg A et al. Pentamidine-induced torsades de pointes. *Pediatr Infect Dis J.* 1993; 12:692-94.
497. Farquhar Zanetti LA, Oliphant CM. Pentamidine-induced torsades de pointes. *Ann Pharmacother.* 1994; 28:282-3.
498. Eisenhauer MD, Eliasson AH, Taylor AJ et al. Incidence of cardiac arrhythmias during intravenous pentamidine therapy in HIV-infected patients. *Chest.* 1994; 105:389-95.
499. Olree K, Stein-Gocken J. Torsade de pointes and elevated magnesium and calcium requirements associated with intravenous pentamidine. *Nutr Clin Pract.* 1994; 9:191-5.
500. Otsuka M, Kanamori H, Sasaki S et al. Torsades de pointes complicating pentamidine therapy of Pneumocystis carinii pneumonia in acute myelogenous leukemia. *Intern Med.* 1997; 36:705-8.
501. Kroll CR, Gettes LS. T wave alternans and Torsades de Pointes after the use of intravenous pentamidine. *J Cardiovasc Electrophysiol.* 2002; 13:936-8.
502. Krahenbuhl S, Sauter B, Kupferschmidt H et al. Case report: reversible QT prolongation with torsades de pointes in a patient with pimozide intoxication. *Am J Med Sci.* 1995; 309:315-6.
503. Olshansky B, Martins J, Hunt S. *N*-acetylprocainamide causing torsades de pointes. *Am J Cardiol.* 1982; 50:1439-41.
504. Stratmann HG, Walter KE, Kennedy HL. Torsade de pointes associated with elevated *N*-acetylprocainamide levels. *Am Heart J.* 1985; 109:375-7.
505. Stevenson WG, Weiss J. Torsades de pointes due to *N*-acetylprocainamide. *Pacing Clin Electrophysiol.* 1985; 8:528-31.
506. Vlasses PH, Ferguson RK, Rocci ML Jr et al. Lethal accumulation of procainamide metabolite in severe renal insufficiency. *Am J Nephrol.* 1986; 6:112-6.
507. Laub GW, Muralidharan S, Janeira L et al. Refractory postoperative torsades de pointes syndrome successfully treated with isoproterenol. *J Cardiothorac Vasc Anaesth.* 1993; 7:210-2.
508. Bell D, Thoele DG, Mander G et al. Effective use of magnesium for acquired torsade de pointes in a 4-month-old infant. *Pediatr Cardiol.* 1995; 16:79-81.
509. Singh BN, Kehoe R, Woosley RL et al. Multicenter trial of sotalol compared with procainamide in the suppression of inducible ventricular tachycardia: a double-blind, randomized parallel evaluation: Sotalol Multicenter Study Group. *Am Heart J.* 1995; 129:87-97.
510. Douglas RJ, Cadogan M. Cardiac arrhythmia during propofol sedation. *Emerg Med Australas.* 2008; 20:437-40.
511. Irie T, Kaneko Y, Nakajima T et al. QT interval prolongation and torsade de pointes induced by propofol and hypoalbuminemia. *Int Heart J.* 2010; 51:365-6.
512. Abrich VA, Ramakrishna H, Mehta A et al. The possible role of propofol in drug-induced torsades de pointes: a real-world single-center analysis. *Int J Cardiol.* 2017; Jan 4. pii: S0167-5273(17)30030-X.
513. Jenzer HR, Hagemeijer R. Quinidine syncope: torsade de pointes with low quinidine plasma concentrations. *Eur J Cardiol.* 1976; 4:447-51.
514. Petelenz T, Knosata P, Iwihski J et al. Case of ventricular extrasystole of the "torsade de pointes" type after administration of quinidine. *Wiad Lek.* 1984; 37:147-9.

515. Bauman JL, Bauernfeind RA, Hoff JV et al. Torsade de pointes due to quinidine: observations in 31 patients. *Am Heart J.* 1984; 107:425-30.
516. Thomas MG, Giles TD. Mexiletine: long-term follow-up of a patient with prolonged QT interval and quinidine-induced torsades de pointes. *South Med J.* 1985; 78:205-6.
517. Maisuls E, Lorber A. Quinidine-induced torsade de pointes suppressed by paroxysmal atrial fibrillation. *Int J Cardiol.* 1987; 16:315-7.
518. Thompson KA, Murray JJ, Blair IA et al. Plasma concentrations of quinidine, its major metabolites, and dihydroquinidine in patients with torsades de pointes. *Clin Pharmacol Ther.* 1988; 43:636-42.
519. el-Sherif N, Bekheit SS, Henkin R. Quinidine-induced long QTU interval and torsade de pointes: role of bradycardia-dependent early afterdepolarizations. *J Am Coll Cardiol.* 1989; 14:252-7.
520. Ometto R, Arfiero S, Vincenzi M. Torsade de pointes induced by quinidine: a case treated successfully with verapamil. *G Ital Cardiol.* 1990; 20:431-4.
521. Gould LA, Betzu R, Vacek T et al. Magnesium treatment of torsade de pointes: a case report. *Angiology.* 1990; 41:577-81.
522. Maia IG, Sá R, Alves PA et al. Torsades de Pointes: analysis of 105 episodes. *Arq Bras Cardiol.* 1991; 56:451-6.
523. Oberg KC, O'Toole MF, Gallastegui JL et al. "Late" proarrhythmia due to quinidine. *Am J Cardiol.* 1994; 74:192-4.
524. Hohnloser SH, van de Loo A, Baedeker F. Efficacy and proarrhythmic hazards of pharmacologic cardioversion of atrial fibrillation: prospective comparison of sotalol versus quinidine. *J Am Coll Cardiol.* 1995; 26:852-8.
525. Karch M, Schmitt C, Plewan A et al. Torsade de pointes tachycardia during administration of quinidine and verapamil in atrial fibrillation. *Herz.* 1997; 22:51-6.
526. Tsai CL. Quinidine cardiotoxicity. *J Emerg Med.* 2005; 28:463-5.
527. Wroblewski HA, Kovacs RJ, Kingery JR et al. High risk of QT interval prolongation and torsades de pointes associated with intravenous quinidine used for treatment of resistant malaria or babesiosis. *Antimicrob Agents Chemother.* 2012; 56:4495-9.
528. Higgins AY, Waks JW, Josephson ME. Influence of gender on the tolerability, safety, and efficacy of quinidine used for treatment of supraventricular and ventricular arrhythmia. *Am J Cardiol.* 2015; 116:1845-51.
529. Promphan W, Khongphatthanayothin A, Horchaiprasit K et al. Roxithromycin-induced torsade de pointes in a patient with complex congenital heart disease and complete atrioventricular block. *Pacing Clin Electrophysiol* 2003; 26:1424-6.
530. Justo D, Mardi T, Zeltser D. Roxithromycin-induced torsades de pointes. *Eur J Intern Med.* 2004; 15:326-7.
531. Keskin S, Sayali E, Temeloglu E et al. QT prolongation and ventricular tachycardia due to roxithromycin. *Anadolu Kardiyol Derg.* 2005; 5:319-21.
532. Abe K, Takada K, Yoshiya I. Intraoperative torsade de pointes ventricular tachycardia and ventricular fibrillation during sevoflurane anesthesia. *Anesth Analg.* 1998; 86:701-2.
533. Saussine M, Massad I, Raczka F et al. Torsade de pointes during sevoflurane anesthesia in a child with congenital long QT syndrome. *Paediatr Anaesth.* 2006; 16:63-5.
534. Thirvenkatarajan V, Osborn KD, Van Wijk RM et al. Torsade de pointes in a patient with acute prolonged QT syndrome and poorly controlled diabetes during sevoflurane anaesthesia. *Anaesth Intensive Care.* 2010; 38:555-9.
535. Choromanski DW, Amin S, Zestos MM. Sevoflurane as a cause of torsade de pointes in patient with long QT syndrome. Case report. *Middle East J Anaesthesiol.* 2016; 23:471-4.
536. Totterman KJ, Turto H, Pellinen T. Overdrive pacing as treatment of sotalol-induced ventricular tachyarrhythmias (torsade de pointes). *Ada Med Scand.* 1982; 668:28-33.
537. Desoutter P, Medioni J, Lerasle S et al. Atrioventricular block and torsade de pointes following sotalol overdose. *Nouv Presse Med.* 1982; 11:3855.
538. Kuck KH, Kunze KP, Roewer N et al. Sotalol-induced torsade de pointes. *Am Heart J.* 1984; 107:179-80.
539. Rakovec P, Cercek B, Rode P et al. Sotalol-induced torsade de pointes. *Cathet Cardiovasc Diagn.* 1984; 10:167-70.
540. McKibbin JK, Pocock WA, Barlow JB et al. Sotalol, hypokalaemia, syncope, and torsade de pointes. *Br Heart J.* 1984; 51:157-62.
541. Beattie JM. Sotalol induced torsade de pointes. *Scott Med J.* 1984; 29:240-4.
542. Krapf R, Gertsch M. Torsade de pointes induced by sotalol despite therapeutic plasma sotalol concentrations. *Br Med J (Clin Res Ed).* 1985; 290:1784-5.
543. Bennett JM, Gourassas J, Konstantinides S. Torsade de pointes induced by sotalol and hypokalaemia. *S Afr Med J.* 1985; 68:591-2.
544. Opie LH. Torsades de pointes induced by sotalol. *Am J Cardiol.* 1987; 60:1216-7.
545. Gossinger HD, Siostrzonek P, Schmoliner R et al. Sotalol-induced torsades de pointes in a patient with pre-existent normal response to programmed ventricular stimulation. *Eur Heart J.* 1987; 8:1351-3.
546. Kehoe RF, Zheutlin TA, Dunnington CS et al. Safety and efficacy of sotalol in patients with drug-refractory sustained ventricular tachyarrhythmias. *Am J Cardiol.* 1990; 65:58A-64A.
547. Singh SN, Lazin A, Cohen A et al. Sotalol-induced torsades de pointes successfully treated with hemodialysis after failure of conventional therapy. *Am Heart J.* 1991; 121:601-2.
548. Arstall MA, Hii JT, Lehman RG et al. Sotalol-induced torsade de pointes: management with magnesium infusion. *Postgrad Med J.* 1992; 68:289-90.
549. Huynh-Do U, Wahl C, Sulzer M et al. Torsades de pointes during low-dosage sotalol therapy in haemodialysis patients. *Nephrol Dial Transplant.* 1996; 11:1153-4.
550. Feroze H, Suri R, Silverman DI. Torsades de pointes from terfenadine and sotalol given in combination. *Pacing Clin Electrophysiol.* 1996; 19:1519-21.
551. Lehmann MH, Hardy S, Archibald D et al. Sex difference in risk of torsade de pointes with d,l-sotalol. *Circulation.* 1996; 94:2535-41.
552. Basta MN, Leitch JW, Fletcher PJ. Sotalol proarrhythmia: a report of five cases and an audit of the use of a sotalol in a teaching hospital. *Aust N Z J Med.* 1996; 26:167-70.
553. Dancey D, Wullfhart Z, McEwan P. Sotalol-induced torsades de pointes in patients with renal failure. *Can J Cardiol.* 1997; 13:55-8.
554. van Uum SH, van den Merkhol LF, Lucassen AM et al. Successful haemodialysis in sotalol-induced torsade de pointes in a patient with progressive renal failure. *Nephrol Dial Transplant.* 1997; 12:331-3.
555. Tang S, Lo CY, Lo WK et al. Sotalol-induced torsade de pointes in a CAPD patient: successful treatment with intermittent peritoneal dialysis. *Perit Dial Int.* 1997; 17:207-8.
556. Gottlieb SS, Cines M, Marshall J. Torsades de pointes with administration of high-dose intravenous d-sotalol to a patient with congestive heart failure. *Pharmacotherapy.* 1997; 17:830-1.
557. Link MS, Foote CB, Sloan SB et al. Torsade de pointes and prolonged QT interval from surreptitious use of sotalol: use of drug levels in diagnosis. *Chest.* 1997; 112:556-7.
558. Haverkamp W, Martinez-Rubio A, Hiel C et al. Efficacy and safety of d,l-sotalol in patients with ventricular tachycardia and in survivors of cardiac arrest. *J Am Coll Cardiol.* 1997; 30:487-95.
559. Kuhlkamp V, Mermi J, Mewis C et al. Efficacy and proarrhythmia with the use of d,l-sotalol for sustained ventricular tachyarrhythmias. *J Cardiovasc Pharmacol.* 1997; 29:373-81.
560. Haverkamp W, Hordt M, Breithardt G et al. Torsade de pointes secondary to d,l-sotalol after catheter ablation of incessant atrioventricular reentrant tachycardia: evidence lor a significant contribution of the "cardiac memory". *Clin Cardiol.* 1998; 21:55-8.
561. Sasse M, Paul T, Bergmann P et al. Sotalol associated torsades de pointes tachycardia in a 15-month-old child: successlul therapy with magnesium aspartate. *Pacing Clin Electrophysiol.* 1998; 21:1164-6.

562. Assimes TL, Malcolm I. Torsade de pointes with sotalol overdose treated successlully with lidocaine. *Can J Cardiol.* 1998; 14:753-6.

563. Smith W. A case of sotalol associated torsades de pointes tachycardia in a 15 month old child. *Pacing Clin Electrophysiol.* 1999; 22:143.

564. Cammu G, Geelen P, Baetens P et al. Two cases of torsades de pointes caused by sotalol therapy. *Resuscitation.* 1999; 40:49-51.

565. Delacretaz E, Fuhrer J. Fatal torsade de pointes with d,l-sotalol and low potassium. *Clin Cardiol.* 1999; 22:423-4.

566. Rizza C, Valderrabano M, Singh BN. Recurrent torsades de pointes after sotalol therapy for symptomatic paroxysmal atrial fibrillation in a patient with end-stage renal disease. *J Cardiovasc Pharmacol Ther.* 1999; 4:129-34.

567. Tan HH, Hsu LF, Kam RM et al. A case series of sotalol-induced torsade de pointes in patients with atrial fibrillation: a tale with a twist. *Ann Acad Med Singapore.* 2003; 32:403-7.

568. Strohmer B, Schernthaner C, Pichler M. Nearly fatal torsade de pointes with sotalol. *Indian Pacing Electrophysiol J.* 2003; 3:268-9.

569. Süriicii H, Tatli E, Degirmenci A et al. Seventy-four defibrillations for sotalol-induced torsades de pointes. *Indian Heart J.* 2004: 56:340-2.

570. D'Aloia A, Faggiano P, Brentana L et al. Sustained torsade de pointes occurring early during oral sotalol therapy for atrial fibrillation recurrence prophylaxis in a patient without heart disease. *Int J Cardiol.* 2005; 105:337-9.

571. Singh BN, Singh SN, Reda DJ et al. Amiodarone versus sotalol lor atrial fibrillation. *N Engl J Med.* 2005; 352:1861-72.

572. Yalta K, Turgut O, Yilmaz A et al. Torsades de pointes with a severely prolonged QT interval induced by an initial low dose sotalol intake. *Int J Cardiol.* 2007; 116:e95-7.

573. Fossa AA, Wisialowksi T, Crimin K et al. Analyses of dynamic beat-to-beat QT-TQ interval (ECG restitution) changes in humans under normal sinus rhythm and prior to an event of torsades de pointes during QT prolongation caused by sotalol. *Ann Noninvasive Electrocardiol.* 2007; 12:338-48.

574. Methe H, Hinterseer M, Wilbert-Lampen U et al. Torsades de pointes: a rare complication of extra-adrenal pheochromocytoma. *Hypertens Res.* 2007; 30:1263-6.

575. Patane S, Marte F, Di Bella G. QT interval prolongation and torsade de pointes. *Int J Cardiol.* 2009; 131:e51-3.

576. Chong DW, Ankolekar SJ, McDonald J. Sotalol-induced QT prolongation and torsades de pointes. *BMJ Case Rep.* 2009; 2009. pii: bcr01.2009.1426.

577. Michiels V, Miljoen H, Vrints C. Gastroenteritis with severe consequences: a case of sotalol-induced torsades de pointes. *Acta Cardiol.* 2009; 64:839-42.

578. Wells Q, Hardin B, Raj SR et al. Sotalol-induced torsades de pointes precipitated during treatment with oseltamivir for H1N1 influenza. *Heart Rhythm.* 2010; 7:1454-7.

579. Wachowiak-Baszynska H, Straburzynska-Migaj E, Ochotny R et al. Late proarrhythmia on sotalol therapy triggered by emotional stress. *Kardiol Pol.* 2011; 69:721-3.

580. Weeke P, Delaney J, Mosley JD et al. QT variability during initial exposure to sotalol: experience based on a large electronic medical record. *Europace.* 2013; 15:1791-7.

581. Dupont H, Timsit JF, Souweine B et al. Torsades de pointes probably related to sparfloxacin. *Eur J Clin Microbiol Infect Dis.* 1996; 15:350-1.

582. Kakar A, Byotra SP. Torsade de pointes probably induced by sparfloxacin. *J Assoc Physicians India.* 2002; 50:1077-8.

583. Huang BH, Hsia CP, Chen CY. Sulpiride induced torsade de pointes. *Int J Cardiol.* 2007; 118:e100-2.

584. Chang JH, Weng TI, Fang CC. Long QT syndrome and torsades de pointes induced by acute sulpiride poisoning. *Am J Emerg Med.* 2009; 27:1016.e1-3.

585. Teng PR, Shen TY, Lai TJ. Sulpiride-associated torsade de pointes in a woman with bipolar disorder. *Psychiatry Clin Neurosci.* 2012; 66:246.

586. Urge J, Sinci F, Prochazka V et al. Terlipressin-induced ventricular arrhythmia. *Scand J Gastroenterol.* 2008; 43:1145-8.

587. Jao YT. Refractory torsade de pointes induced by terlipressin (Glypressin). *Int J Cardiol.* 2016; 222:135-40.

588. Kemper AJ, Dunlap R, Pietro DA. Thioridazine-induced torsade de pointes: successful therapy with isoproterenol. *JAMA.* 1983; 249:2931-4.

589. Liberatore MA, Robinson DS. Torsade de pointes: a mechanism lor sudden death associated with neuroleptic drug therapy? *J Clin Psychopharmacol.* 1984; 4:143-6.

590. Flugelman MY, Tal A, Pollack S et al. Psychotropic drugs and long QT syndromes: case reports. *J Clin Psychiatry.* 1985; 46:290-1.

591. Toivonen LK, Leinonen H. Limited effect of magnesium sulphate on torsades de pointes ventricular tachycardia. *Int J Cardiol.* 1986; 12:260-2.

592. Kiriike N, Maeda Y, Nishiwaki S et al. Latrogenic torsade de pointes induced by thioridazine. *Biol Psychiatry.* 1987; 22:99-103.

593. Bastecky J, Kvasnicka J, Vortel J et al. Suicidal ingestion of thioridazine as a cause of severe impairment of heart rhythm: polymorphic ventricular tachycardia. *Cesk Psychiatr.* 1990; 86:264-8.

594. Quieffin J, Brochet E, Gamerman G et al. Ventricular arrhythmia following thioridazine poisoning. *Ann Cardiol Angeiol (Paris).* 1991; 40:199-201.

595. Paoloni P, Ciliberti D, Blasi N et al. Latrogenic torsade de pointes induced by thioridazine. *Minerva Cardioangiol.* 1992; 40:245-9.

596. Donatini B, Le Blaye I, Krupp P. Transient cardiac pacing is insufficiently used to treat arrhythmia associated with thioridazine. *Cardiology.* 1992; 81:340-1.

597. Näsh O, Rydenhag A. A case report: torsades de pointes caused by overdose of thioridazine. *Lakartidningen.* 1993; 90:3677-8.

598. Le Blaye I, Donatini B, Hall M et al. Acute overdosage with thioridazine: a review of the available clinical exposure. *Vet Hum Toxicol.* 1993; 35:147-50.

599. Hulisz DT, Dasa SL, Black LD et al. Complete heart block and torsade de pointes associated with thioridazine poisoning. *Pharmacotherapy.* 1994; 14:239-45.

600. Buckley NA, Whyte IM, Dawson AH. Cardiotoxicity more common in thioridazine overdose than with other neuroleptics. *J Toxicol Clin Toxicol.* 1995; 33:199-204.

601. Liao WB, Bullard MJ, Kuo CT et al. Anticholinergic overdose induced torsade de pointes successfully treated with verapamil. *Jpn Heart J.* 1996; 37:925-31.

602. Denvir MA, Sood A, Dow R et al. Thioridazine, diarrhoea and torsades de pointe. *J R Soc Med.* 1998; 91:145-7.

603. Caprelsa prescribing information. Cambridge, UK: AstraZeneca Pharmaceuticals; 2011.

604. Loffi M, Toffetti L, Gianni C et al. Self-terminating ventricular fibrillation in vandetanib-induced torsades de pointes. *J Cardiovasc Electrophysiol.* 2015; 26:811-3.

605. Nelson S, Leung JG. Torsades de pointes after administration of low-dose aripiprazole. *Ann Pharmacother.* 2013; 47:e11.

606. Kao DP, Haigney MCP, Mehler PS et al. Arrhythmia associated with buprenorphine and methadone reported to the food and drug administration. *Addiction.* 2014; 110:1468-75.

607. Hoehns JD, Fouts MM, Kelly MW et al. Sudden cardiac death with clozapine and sertraline combination. *Ann Pharmacother.* 2001; 35:862-6.

608. Warner B, Hoffmann P. Investigation of the potential of clozapine to cause torsade de pointes. *Adverse Drug React Toxicol Rev.* 2002; 21:189-203.

609. Turner S, Mathews L, Pandharipande P et al. Dolasetron-induced torsades de pointes. *J Clin Anesth.* 2007; 19:622-5.

610. Castillo R, Pedalino RP, El-Sherif N et al. Efavirenz-associated QT prolongation and torsades de pointes arrhythmias. *Ann Pharmacother.* 2002; 36:1006-8.

611. Lee KW, Kayser SR, Hongo RH et al. Famotidine and long QT syndrome. *Am J Cardiol.* 2004; 93:1325-7.

612. Bont L, Bosker HA, Brus F et al. Torsade de pointes after pipamperone intoxication. *Pharm World Sci.* 1998; 20:137.
613. Tei Y, Morita T, Inoue S et al. Torsades de pointes caused by a small dose of risperidone in a terminally ill cancer patient. *Psychosomatics.* 2004; 45:450-1.
614. Raviña T, Raviña P, Gutierrez J. Acquired long QT svndrome: risperidone-facilitated triggered activity and torsades de pointes during complete AV block. I. *Int J Cardiol.* 2007; 116:416-20.
615. Gopal S, Hough D, Karcher K et al. Risk of cardiovascular morbidity with risperidone or paloperidone treatment: analysis of 64 randomized, double-blind trials. *J Clin Psychopharmacol.* 2013; 33:157-61.
616. Vieweg WV, Hasnain M, Hancox JC et al. Risperidone, QTc interval prolongation, and torsade de pointes: a systematic review of case reports. *Psychopharmacol.* 2013; 228:515-24.
617. Asajima H, Sekiguchi Y, Matsushima S et al. QT prolongation and torsade de pointes associated with solifenacin in an 81-year old woman. *Br J Clin Pharmacol.* 2008; 66:896-7.
618. Ozmen N, Yiginer O, Un H et al. Frequently occurring torsades de pointes attacks in an old patient on solifenacin therapy and management strategy. *Anatol J Cardiol.* 2015; 15:342-3.
619. Johnson MC, So S, Marsh JW et al. QT prolongation and Torsades de Pointes after administration of FK506. *Transplantation.* 1992; 53:929-30.
620. Hodak SP, Moubarak JB, Rodriguez I et al. QT prolongation and near fatal cardiac arrhythmia after intravenous tacrolimus administration: a case report. *Transplantation.* 1998; 66:535-7.
621. Lynch DR Jr, Washam JB, Newby LK. QT interval prolongation and torsades de pointes in a patient undergoing treatment with vorinostat: a case report and review of the literature. *Cardiol J.* 2012; 19:434-8.
622. Sartori M, Pratt CM, Young JB. Torsade de Pointe: malignant cardiac arrhythmia induced by amantadine poisoning. *Am J Med.* 1984; 77:388-91.
623. Manini AF, Raspberry D, Hoffman RS et al. QT prolongation and Torsades de Pointes following overdose of ziprasidone and amantadine. *J Med Toxicol.* 2007; 3:178-81.
624. Schwartz M, Patel M, Kazzi Z et al. Cardiotoxicity alter massive amantadine overdose. *J Med Toxicol.* 2008; 4:173-9.
625. Isbister GK, Murray L, John S et al. Amisulpride deliberate self-poisoning causing severe cardiac toxicity including QT prolongation and torsades de pointes. *Med J Aust.* 2006; 184:354-6.
626. Chung AK, Chua SE. Torsade de pointes associated with low-dose amisulpride: a case report. *J Psychopharmacol.* 2010; 24:433-5.
627. Isbister GK, Balit CR, Macleod D et al. Amisulpride overdose is frequently associated with QT prolongation and torsades de pointes. *J Clin Psychopharmacol.* 2010; 30:391-5.
628. Joy JP, Coulter CV, Duffull SB et al. Prediction of torsade de pointes from the QT interval: analysis of a case series of amisulpride overdoses. *Clin Pharmacol Ther.* 2011; 90:243-5.
629. Poluzzi E, Raschi E, Koci A et al. Antipsychotics and torsadogenic risk: signals emerging from the US FDA Adverse Event Reporting System database. *Drug Saf.* 2013; 36:467-79.
630. Davison ET. Amitriptyline-induced torsades de pointes: successful therapy with atrial pacing. *J Electrocardiol.* 1985; 18:299-301.
631. Ly T, Ruiz ME. Prolonged QT interval and torsades de pointes associated with atazanavir therapy. *Clin Infect Dis.* 2007; 44:e67-8.
632. Young JB, Vandermolen LA, Pratt CM. Torsade de pointes: an unusual manifestation of chloral hydrate poisoning. *Am Heart J.* 1986; 112:181-4.
633. Sing K, Erickson T, Amitai Y et al. Chloral hydrate toxicity from oral and intravenous administration. *J Toxicol Clin Toxicol.* 1996; 34:101-6.
634. Husain Z, Hussain K, Nair R et al. Diphenydramine induced QT prolongation and torsade de pointes: an uncommon effect of a common drug. *Cardiol J.* 2010; 17:509-11.
635. Strasberg B, Coelho A, Welch W et al. Doxepin induced torsade de pointes. *Pacing Clin Electrophysiol.* 1982; 5:873-7.
636. Alter P, Tontsch D, Grimm W. Doxepin-induced torsade de pointes tachycardia. *Ann Intern Med.* 2001; 135:384-5.
637. Appleby M, Mbewu A, Clarke B. Fluoxetine and ventricular torsade: is there a link? *Int J Cardiol.* 1995; 49:178-80.
638. Lherm T, Lottin F, Larbi D et al. Torsade de pointes after poisoning with fluoxetine alone. *Presse Med.* 2000; 29:306-7.
639. Wilting I, Smals OM, Holwerda NJ et al. QTc prolongation and torsades de pointes in an elderly woman taking fluoxetine. *Am J Psychiatry.* 2006; 163:325.
640. Chen CY, Wang FL, Lin CC. Chronic hydroxychloroquine use associated with QT prolongation and refractory ventricular arrhythmias. *Clin Toxicol.* 2006; 44:173-5.
641. Sakaguchi T, Itoh H, Ding WG et al. Hydroxyzine, a first generation H(1)-receptor antagonist, inhibits human ether-a-go-go-related gene (HERG) current and causes syncope in a patient with the HERG mutation. *J Pharmacol Sci.* 2008; 108:462-71.
642. Wang CP, Guo GB. Indapamide induced syncope in a patient with long QT syndrome. *Pacing Clin Electrophysiol.* 2002; 25:1397-9.
643. Letsas KP, Alexanian IP, Pappas LK et al. QT interval prolongation and torsade de pointes associated with indapamide. *Int J Cardiol.* 2006; 112:373-4.
644. Mok NS, Tong CK, Yuen HC. Concomitant-acquired long QT and Brugada syndromes associated with indapamide-induced hypokalemia and hyponatremia. *Pacing Clin Electrophysiol.* 2008; 31:772-5.
645. NoorZurani MH, Vicknasingam B, Narayanan S. Itraconazole-induced torsade de pointes in a patient receiving methadone substitution therapy. *Drug Alcohol Rev.* 2009; 28:688-90.
646. Mittal SR. Slow junctional rhythm, QTc prolongation and transient torsades de-pointes following combined use of ivabradine, diltiazem and ranolazine. *J Assoc Physicians India.* 2014; 62:426-7.
647. Mok NS, Lo YK, Tsui PT et al. Ketoconazole induced torsades de pointes without concomitant use of QT interval-prolonging drug. *J Cardiovasc Electrophysiol.* 2005; 16:1375-7.
648. Mukarram O, Hindi Y, Catalasan G et al. Loperamide induced torsades de pointes: a case report and review of the literature. *Case Rep Med.* 2016; 2016:4061980.
649. Vaughan P, Solik MM, Bagga S et al. Electrocardiographic abnormalities, malignant ventricular arrhythmias, and cardiomyopathy associated with loperamide abuse. *J Cardiovasc Electrophysiol.* 2016; 27:1230-3.
650. Upadhyay A, Bodar V, Malekzadegan M et al. Loperamide induced life threatening ventricular arrhythmias. *Case Rep Cardiol.* 2016: 2016:5040176.
651. Swank KA, Wu E, Kortpeter C et al. Adverse event detection using the FDA post-marketing drug safety surveillance system: cardiotoxicity associated with loperamide abuse and misuse. *J Am Pharm Assoc.* 2017; 57(2S):S63-7.
652. Kozak PM, Harris AK, McPherson JA et al. Torsades de pointes with high-dose loperamide. *J Electrocardiol.* 2017; 50:355-7.
653. Chou CC, Wu D. Torsade de pointes induced by metoclopramide in an elderly woman with preexisting complete left bundle branch block. *Chang Gung Med J.* 2001; 24:805-9.
654. Siddique SM, Shariff N, Vesuwala N et al. Metoclopramide as a possible cause of prolonged QT syndrome and torsade de pointes in a patient with heart failure and renal insufficiency (letter). *Ann Intern Med.* 2009; 150:502-4.
655. Panduranga P, Al-Mukhaini M, Rajarao MO. Multi-factorial causes of torsade de pointes in a hospitalized surgical patient. *Sultan Qaboos Univ Med J.* 2013; 13:152-5.
656. Jeon JH, Her SH, Chin JY et al. Complete atrioventricular block-induced torsade de pointes, manifested by epilepsy. *Korean J Intern Med.* 2011; 26:99-102.
657. Bibawy JN, Parikh V, Wahba J et al. Pantoprazole (proton pump inhibitor) contributing to torsades de pointes storm. *Circ Arrhthm Electrophysiol.* 2013; 6:e17-9.
658. Panos G, Velissaris D, Karamouzos V et al. Long QT syndrome leading to multiple cardiac arrests after posiconazole

administration in an immune-compromised patient with sepsis: an unusual case report. *Am J Case Rep.* 2016; 29:295-300.

659. Vieweg WV, Schneider RK, Wood MA. Torsade de pointes in a patient with complex medical and psychiatric conditions receiving low-dose quetiapine. *Ada Psychiatr Scand.* 2005; 112:318-22.
660. Bodenhamer JE, Smilkstein MJ. Delayed cardiotoxicity following quinine overdose: a case report. *J Emerg Med.* 1993; 11:279-85.
661. Sheehan ET, Frizzell JD, Gabaldon J et al. Quinine and the ABCs of long QT: a patient's misfortune with arthritis, (alcoholic) beverages, and cramps. *J Gen Intern Med.* 2016; 31:1254-7.
662. De Meester A, Carbutti G, Gabriel L et al. Fatal overdose with trazodone: case report and literature review. *Acta Clin Belg.* 2001; 56:258-61.
663. Chung KJ, Wang YC, Liu BM et al. Management of ventricular dysrhythmia secondary to trazodone overdose. *J Emerg Med.* 2008; 35:171-4.
664. Alkan Y, Haefeli WE, Burhenne J et al. Voriconazole-induced QT interval prolongation and ventricular tachycardia: a non-concentration-dependent adverse effect. *Clin Infect Dis.* 2004; 39:e49-52.
665. Philips JA, Marty FM, Stone RM et al. Torsades de pointes associated with voriconazole use. *Transpl Infect Dis.* 2007; 9:33-6.
666. Aypar E, Kendirli T, Tutar E et al. Voriconazole-induced QT interval prolongation and torsades de pointes. *Pediatr Int.* 2011; 53:761-3.
667. Elbay MA, Cil H, Onturk E et al. QTc prolongation and torsade de pointes ventricular tachycardia in a small dose voriconazole therapy. *Eur Rev Med Pharmacol Sci.* 2012; 16:100-2.
668. Brown JD, Lim LL, Koning S. Voriconazole associated torsade de pointes in two adult patients with haematological malignancies. *Med Mycol Case Rep.* 2014; 4:23-5.
669. Heinrich TW, Biblo LA, Schneider J. Torsades de pointes associated with ziprasidone. *Psychosomatics.* 2006; 47:264-8.
670. Alipour A, Cruz R, Lotts RS. Torsade de pointes after ziprasidone overdose with coingestants. *J Clin Psychopharmacol.* 2010; 30:76-7.
671. Darpö B. Spectrum of drugs prolonging QT interval and the incidence of torsades de pointes. *Eur Heart J.* 2001; 3(suppl K): K70-80.
672. Sarganas G, Garbe E, Klimpel A et al. Epidemiology of symptomatic drug-induced long QT syndrome and torsade de pointes in Germany. *Europace.* 2014; 16:101-8.
673. Aström-Lilja C, Odeberg JM, Ekman E et al. Drug-induced torsades de pointes: a review of the Swedish pharmacovigilance database. *Pharmacoepidemiol Drug Saf.* 2008; 17:587-92.
674. Molokhia M, Pathak A, Lapeyre-Mestre M et al. Case ascertainment and estimated incidence of drug-induced long-QT syndrome: study in Southwest France. *Br J Clin Pharmacol.* 2008; 66:386-95.
675. Tisdale JE, Wroblewski HA, Overholser BR et al. Prevalence of QT interval prolongation in patients admitted to cardiac care units and frequency of subsequent administration of QT-interval prolonging drugs. *Drug Saf.* 2012; 35:459-70.
676. Pickham D, Helfenbein E, Shinn JA et al. High prevalence of corrected QT interval prolongation in acutely ill patients is associated with mortality: results of the QT in Practice (QTIP) study. *Crit Care Med.* 2012; 40:394-9.
677. Hoogstraaten E, Rijkenberg S, van der Voort PHJ. Corrected QT-interval prolongation and variability in intensive care patients. *J Crit Care.* 2014; 29:835-9.
678. Seftchick MW, Adler PH, Hsieh M et al. The prevalence and factors associated with QTc prolongation among emergency department patients. *Ann Emerg Med.* 2009; 54:763-8.
679. Roden DM. Drug-induced prolongation of the QT interval. *N Engl J Med.* 2004; 350:1013-22.
680. Viskin S. Long QT syndromes and torsade de pointes. *Lancet.* 1999; 354:1625-33.
681. Hondeghem LM, Carlsson L, Duker G. Instability and triangulation of the action potential predict serious proarrhythmia, but action potential duration prolongation is antiarrhythmic. *Circulation.* 2001; 103:2004-13.
682. Kannankeril PJ, Roden DM. Drug-induced long QT and torsade de pointes: recent advances. *Curr Opin Cardiol.* 2007; 22:39-43.
683. Varro A, Baczko I. Cardiac ventricular repolarization reserve: a principle for understanding drug-related proarrhythmic risk. *Br J Pharmacol.* 2011; 164:14-36.
684. Bazett HC. An analysis of time relationships of the electrocardiogram. *Heart.* 1920; 7:353-70.
685. Dessertenne F. La tachycardie ventriculaire á deux foyers opposes variables. *Arch Mal Coeur Vaiss.* 1966; 59:263-72.
686. Drew BJ, Ackerman MJ, Funk M et al. On behalf of the American Heart Association Acute Cardiac Care Committee of the Council on Clinical Cardiology, the Council on Cardiovascular Nursing, and the American College of Cardiology Foundation. Prevention of torsade de pointes in hospital settings: a scientific statement from the American Heart Association and the American College of Cardiology Foundation. *Circulation.* 2010; 121:1047-60.
687. Yap YG, Camm AJ. Drug induced QT prolongation and torsades de pointes. *Heart.* 2003; 89:1363-72.
688. Zeltser D, Justo D, Halkin A et al. Torsade de pointes due to noncardiac drugs: most patients have easily identifiable risk factors. *Medicine.* 2003; 82:282-90
689. Moss AJ, Schwartz PJ, Crampton RS et al. The long QT syndrome. Prospective longitudinal study of 328 families. *Circulation.* 1991; 84:1136-44.
690. US Department of Health and Human Services (DHHS), Food and Drug Administration, Center for Drug Evaluation and Research *CDER), Center for Biologics Evaluation and Research (CBER). Guidance for industry. E14 clinical evaluation of QT/QTc interval prolongation and proarrhythmic potential for non-antiarrhythmic drugs. Rockville, MD: DHHS, 2005.
691. Pratt CM, Al-Khalidi HR, Brum JM et al. Cumulative experience of azimilide-associated torsades de pointes ventricular tachycardia in the 19 clinical studies comprising the azimilide database. *J Am Coll Cardiol.* 2006; 48:471-7.
692. Tisdale JE, Jaynes HA, Kingery JR et al. Development and validation of a risk score to predict QT interval prolongation in hospitalized patients. *Circ Cardiovasc Qual Outcomes.* 2013; 6:479-87.
693. Sauer AJ, Newton-Cheh C. Clinical and genetic determinants of torsade de pointes risk. *Circulation.* 2012; 125:1684-94.
694. Pham TV, Rosen MR. Sex, hormones, and repolarization. *Cardiovasc Res.* 2002; 53:740-51.
695. Hreiche R, Morissette P, Turgeon J. Drug-induced long QT syndrome in women: review of current evidence and remaining gaps. *Gend Med.* 2008; 5:124-35.
696. Ebert SN, Liu X-K, Woosley RL. Female gender as a risk factor for drug-induced cardiac arrhythmias: evaluation of clinical and experimental evidence. *J Womens Health.* 1998; 7:547-57.
697. Rautaharju PM, Zhou SH, Wong S et al. Sex differences in the evolution of the electrocardiographic QT interval with age. *Can J Cardiol.* 1992; 8:690-5.
698. Makkar RR, Fromm BS, Steinman RT et al. Female gender as a risk factor for torsades de pointes associated with cardiovascular drugs. *JAMA.* 1993; 270:2590-7.
699. Drici MD, Knollman BC, Wang W-X et al. Cardiac actions of erythromycin. Influence of female sex. *JAMA.* 1998; 280:1774-6.
700. Gowda RM, Khan IA, Punukollu G et al. Female preponderance in ibutilide-induced torsade de pointes. *Int J Cardiol.* 2004; 95:219-22.
701. Roden D, Woosley R, Primm R. Incidence and clinical features of the quinidine-associated long-QT syndrome: implications for patient care. *Am Heart J.* 1986; 111:1088-93.
702. Woosley RL, Chen Y, Freiman JP et al. Mechanisms of the cardiotoxic actions of terfenadine. *JAMA.* 1993; 269:1532-6.

703. Rodriguez I, Kilborn MJ, Liu XK et al. Drug-induced QT prolongation in women during the menstrual cycle. *JAMA*. 2001; 285:1322-6.
704. Pham TV, Sosunov EA, Anyukhovsky EP et al. Testosterone diminishes the proarrhythmic effects of dofetilide in normal female rabbits. *Circulation*. 2002; 106:2132-6.
705. Nabauer M, Kaab S. Potassium channel down-regulation in heart failure. *Cardiovasc Res*. 1998; 37:324-34.
706. Tisdale JE, Overholser BR, Sowinski KM et al. Enhanced sensitivity to drug-induced QT interval lengthening in patients with heart failure due to left ventricular systolic dysfunction. *J Clin Pharmacol*. 2012; 52:1296-305.
707. Tikosyn® package insert. New York, NY: Pfizer Labs, Division of Pfizer, Inc; 2014.
708. Flockhart DA. http://medicine.iupui.edu/clinpharm/ddis/main-table/ (accessed 2018 March 4).
709. Nattel S. The molecular and ionic specificity of antiarrhythmic drug actions. *J Cardiovasc Electrophysiol*. 1999; 10:272-82.
710. Curtis LH, Ostbye T, Sendersky V et al. Prescription of QT-prolonging drugs in a cohort of about 5 million outpatients. *Am J Med*. 2003; 114:135-41.
711. Allen LaPointe NM, Curtis LH, Chan KA et al. Frequency of high-risk use of QT-prolonging medications. *Pharmacoepidemiol Drug Saf.* 2006; 15:361-8.
712. Tay KY, Ewald MB, Bourgeois FT. Use of QT-prolonging medications in US emergency departments, 1995-2009. *Pharmacoepidemiol Drug Saf.* 2014; 23:9-17.
713. Takeuchi H, Suzuki T, Remington G et al. Antipsychotic polypharmacy and corrected QT interval: a systematic review. *Can J Psychiatr.* 2015; 60:215-22.
714. Niemeijer MN, van den Berg ME, Franco OH et al. Drugs and ventricular repolarization in a general population: the Rotterdam Study. *Pharmacoepidemiol Drug Saf.* 2015; 24:1036-41.
715. Nakano Y, Shimizu W. Genetics of long-QT syndrome. *J Hum Genet*. 2016; 61:51-5.
716. Yang P, Kanki H, Drolet B et al. Allelic variants in long-QT disease genes in patients with drug-associated torsades de pointes. *Circulation*. 2002; 105:1943-8.
717. Paulussen AD, Gilissen RA, Armstrong M et al. Genetic variations of KCNQ1, KCNH2, SCN5A, KCNE1, and KCNE2 in drug-induced long QT syndrome patients. *J Mol Med*. 2004; 82:182-8.
718. Itoh H, Sakaguchi T, Ding W-G et al. Latent genetic backgrounds and molecular pathogenesis in drug-induced long-QT syndrome. *Circ Arrhythmia Electrophysiol*. 2009; 2:511-23.
719. Behr ER, Ritchie MD, Tanaka T et al. Genome wide analysis of drug-induced torsades de pointes: lack of common variants with large effect sizes. *PLOS One*. 2013; 8:e78511.
720. Middlekauf HR, Stevenson WG, Saxon LA et al. Amiodarone and torsades de pointes in patients with advanced heart failure. *Am J Cardiol*. 1995; 76:499-502.
721. Straus SM, Bleumink GS, Dieleman JP et al. Antipsychotics and the risk of sudden cardiac death. *Arch Intern Med*. 2004; 164:1293-7.
722. Ray WA, Chung CP, Murray KT et al. Atypical antipsychotic drugs and the risk of sudden cardiac death. *N Engl J Med*. 2009; 360:225-35.
723. Jones ME, Campbell G, Patel D et al. Risk of mortality (including sudden cardiac death) and major cardiovascular events in users of olanzapine and other antipsychotics: a study with the General Practice Research Database. *Cardiovasc Psychiatry Neurol*. 2013; 2013:647476.
724. Weeke P, Jensen A, Folke F et al. Antipsychotics and associated risk of out-of-hospital cardiac arrest. *Clin Pharmacol Ther.* 2014; 96:490-7.
725. Wu CS, Tsai YT, Tsai HJ. Antipsychotic drugs and the risk of ventricular arrhythmia and/or sudden cardiac death: a nation-wide case-crossover study. *J Am Heart Assoc*. 2015; 4:e001568.
726. Salvo F, Pariente A, Shakir S et al. Sudden cardiac and sudden unexected death related to antipsychotics: a meta-analysis of observational studies. *Clin Pharmacol Ther.* 2016; 99:306-14.
727. Ray WA, Murray KT, Meredith S et al. Oral erythromycin and the risk of sudden death from cardiac causes. *N Engl J Med*. 2004; 351:1089-96.
728. Ray WA, Murray KT, Hall K et al. Azithromycin and the risk of sudden cardiac death. *N Engl J Med*. 2012; 366:1881-90.
729. Rao GA, Mann JR, Shoaibi A et al. Azithromycin and levofloxacin use and increased risk of cardiac arrhythmia and death. *Am Fam Med*. 2014; 12:121-7.
730. Schembri S, Williamson PA, Short PM et al. Cardiovascular events after clarithromycin use in lower respiratory tract infections: analysis of two prospective cohort studies. *BMJ*. 2013; 346:f1235.
731. Svanstrom H, Pasternak B, Hviid A. Use of azithromycin and death from cardiovascular causes. *N Engl J Med*. 2013; 368:1704-12.
732. Cheng JY, Nie XY, Chen XM et al. The role of macrolide antibiotics in increasing cardiovascular risk. *J Am Coll Cardiol*. 2015; 66:2173-84.
733. Haugaa KH, Bos JM, Tarrell RF et al. Institution-wide QT alert system identifies patients with a high risk of mortality. *Mayo Clin Proc*. 2013; 88:315-25.
734. Sorita A, Bos JM, Morlan BW et al. Impact of clinical decision support preventing the use of QT-prolonging medications for patients at risk for torsade de pointes. *JAMIA*. 2014; 22:e21-7.
735. Tisdale JE, Jaynes HA, Kingery JR et al. Effectiveness of a clinical decision support system for reducing the risk of QT interval prolongation in hospitalized patients. *Circ Cardiovasc Qual Outcomes*. 2014; 7:381-90.
736. Caron MF, Kluger J, Tsikouris JP et al. Effects of intravenous magnesium sulfate on the QT interval in patients receiving ibutilide. *Pharmacotherapy*. 2003; 23:296-300.
737. Tisdale JE, Jaynes HA, Overholser BR et al. Influence of oral progesterone administration on drug-induced QT interval lengthening. A randomized, placebo-controlled crossover trial. *JACC Clin Electrophysiol* 2016; 2:765-74.
738. Krantz MJ, Martin J, Stimmel B et al. QTc interval screening in methadone treatment. *Ann Intern Med*. 2009; 150:387-95.
739. Martin JA, Campbell A, Killip T et al. QT interval screening in methadone treatment: report of a SAMHSA expert panel. *J Addict Dis*. 2011; 30:283-306.
740. Perticone F, Adinolfi L, Bonaduce D. Efficacy of magnesium sulfate in the treatment of torsades de pointes. *Am Heart J*. 1986; 112:847-9.
741. Tzivoni D, Banai S, Schuger C et al. Treatment of torsades de pointes with magnesium sulfate. *Circulation*. 1988; 77:392-7.
742. Kothari SS, Krishnaswami S. Magnesium sulfate therapy in torsades de pointes. *Indian Heart J*. 1988; 40:210-1.
743. Warden T, Sacchetti A, Klodnicki WE. Magnesium sulfate termination of torsades de pointes following failure of cardioversion. *Am J Emerg Med*. 1989; 7:126-7.
744. Banai S, Schuger C, Benhorin J et al. Treatment of torsades de pointes with intravenous magnesium. *Am J Cardiol*. 1989; 63:1539-40.
745. Garcia-Rubira JC, Lopez Garcia-Aranda V, Cruz Fernandez JM. Magnesium sulphate for torsade de pointes in a patient with congenital long QT syndrome. *Int J Cardiol*. 1990; 27:282-3.
746. Hasegawa J, Takami T, Kaneda T et al. Treatment of torsade de pointes with intravenous magnesium in idiopathic long QT syndrome. *Jpn Circ J*. 1991; 55:1057-60.
747. Hasan RA, Zureikat GY, Nolan BM. Torsade de pointes associated with astemizole overdose treated with magnesium sulfate. *Pediatr Emerg Care*. 1993; 9:23-5.
748. Morrison Y, Thompson DF. Isoproterenol treatment of torsades de pointes. *Ann Pharmacother.* 1993; 27:189-90.
749. Yap YG, Behr ER, Camm AJ. Drug-induced Brugada syndrome. *Europace* 2009; 11:989-94.

750. Antzelevitch C, Brugada P, Borggrefe M et al. Brugada syndrome: report of the second consensus conference: endorsed by the Heart Rhythm Society and the European Heart Rhythm Association Brugada Syndrome: report of the second consensus conference. *Circulation*. 2005; 111:659-70.
751. Pinar Bermúdez E, García-Alberola A, Martínez Sánchez J et al. Spontaneous sustained monomorphic ventricular tachycardia after administration of ajmaline in a patient with Brugada syndrome. *Pacing Clin Electrophysiol.* 2000; 23:407-9.
752. Veltmann C, Wolpert C, Sacher F et al. Response to intravenous ajmaline: a retrospective analysis of 677 ajmaline challenges. *Europace.* 2009; 11:1345-52.
753. Sorgente A, Yazaki Y, Capulzini L et al. Accelerated idioventricular rhythm during ajmaline test: a case report. *Indian Pacing Electrophysiol J.* 2010; 10:474-8.
754. Conte G, Sieira J, Sarkozy A et al. Life-threatening ventricular arrhythmias during ajmaline challenge in patients with Brugada syndrome: incidence, clinical features, and prognosis. *Heart Rhythm.* 2013; 10:1869-74.
755. Gandjbakhch E, Fressart V, Duthoit G et al. Malignant response to ajmaline challenge in SCN5A mutation carriers: experience from a large familial study. *Int J Cardiol.* 2014; 172:256-8.
756. Conte G, Dewals W, Sieira J et al. Drug-induced brugada syndrome in children: clinical features, device-based management, and long-term follow-up. *J Am Coll Cardiol.* 2014; 63:2272-9.
757. Shimada M, Miyazaki T, Miyoshi S et al. Sustained monomorphic ventricular tachycardia in a patient with Brugada syndrome. *Jpn Circ J.* 1996; 60:364-70.
758. Ohkubo K, Nakai T, Watanabe I. Alcohol-induced ventricular fibrillation in a case of Brugada syndrome. *Europace.* 2013; 15:1058.
759. Achaiah A, Andrews N. Intoxication with alcohol: an underestimated trigger of Brugada syndrome? *JRSM Open.* 2016; 7: 2054270416640153.
760. Berbata VS, Waksman JC. Amitriptyline-induced Brugada pattern fails to respond to sodium bicarbonate. *Clin Toxicol.* 2007; 45:186-8.
761. Mooren K, Voogel AJ, Tan HL. Brugada syndrome induced by amitriptyline toxicity. *Neth J Med.* 2008; 66:358-9.
762. Vernooy K, Sicouri S, Dumaine R et al. Genetic and biophysical basis for bupivacaine-induced ST segment elevation and VT/VF. Anesthesia unmasked Brugada syndrome. *Heart Rhythm.* 2006; 3:1074-8.
763. Ortega-Carnicer J, Bertos-Polo J, Gutierrez-Tirado C. Aborted sudden death, transient Brugada pattern, and wide QRS dysrhythmias after massive cocaine ingestions. *J Electrocardiol.* 2001; 34:345-9.
764. Robertson KE, Martin TN, Rae AP. Brugada-pattern ECG and cardiac arrest in cocaine toxicity: reading between the white lines. *Heart.* 2010; 96:643-4.
765. El Mazloum R, Snehnghi R, Zorzi A et al. Out-of-hospital cardiac arrest after acute cocaine intoxication associated with Brugada ECG patterns: insights into pathophysiologic mechanisms and implications for therapy. *Int J Cardiol.* 2015; 195:245-9.
766. Chow BJW, Gollob M, Birnie D. Brugada syndrome precipitated by a tricyclic antidepressant. *Heart.* 2005; 91:651.
767. Gasparini M, Priori SG, Mantica M et al. Flecainide test in Brugada syndrome: a reproducible but risky tool. *Pacing Clin Electrophysiol.* 2003; 26:338-41.
768. Soni S, Gandhi S. Flecainide overdose causing a Brugada-type pattern on electrocardiograom in a previously well patient. *Am J Emerg Med.* 2009; 27:375.e1-375.e3.
769. Chubb H, Cooklin M, Rosenthal E. Brugada phenocopy with a flecainide overdose: a pharmacological dose effect? *J Cardiovasc Electrophsyiol.* 2014; 25:547-8.
770. Chandra PA, Chandra AB. Brugada syndrome unmasked by lithium. *South Med J.* 2009; 102:1263-5.
771. Rouleau F, Asfar P, Boulet S et al. Transient St segment elevation in right precordial leads induced by psychotropic drugs: relationship to the Brugada syndrome. *J Cardiovasc Electrophysiol.* 2001; 12:61-5.
772. Tada H, Sticherling C, Oral H et al. Brugada syndrome mimicked by tricyclic antidepressant overdose. *J Cardiovasc Electrophysiol.* 2001; 12:275.
773. Russo CR, Welch TD, Sangha RS et al. Brugada syndrome presenting as polymorphic tachycardia-ventricular fibrillation lasting 94 seconds recorded on an ambulatory monitor. *JAMA Intern Med.* 2015; 175:1951-4.
774. El-Menyar A. Oxcarbazepine-induced resistant ventricular fibrillation in an apparently healthy young man. *Am J Fam Med.* 2011; 29:693.e1-693.e3.
775. Chinushi Y, Chinushi M, Toida T et al. Class I antiarrhythmic drug and coronary vasospasm-induced T wave alternans and ventricular tachyarrhythmia in a patient with Brugada syndrome and vasospastic angina. *J Cardioavsc Electrophysiol.* 2002; 13:191-4.
776. Takagi M, Doi A, Takeuchi K et al. Pilsicainide-induced marked T wave alternans and ventricular fibrillation in a patient with Brugada syndrome. *J Cardioavsc Electrophysiol.* 2002; 13:837.
777. Chinushi M, Komura S, Izumi D et al. Incidence and initial characteristics of pilsicainide-induced ventricular arrhythmias in patients with Brugada syndrome. *Pacing Clin Elecrtophysiol.* 2007; 30:662-71.
778. Tada T, Kusano KF, Nagase S et al. Clinical significance of macroscopic T-wave alternans after sodium channel blocker administration in patients with Brugada syndrome. *J Cardiovasc Electrophysiol.* 2008; 19:56-61.
779. Ueyama T, Shimizu A, Esato M et al. Pilsicainide-induced Brugada-type ECG and ventricular arrhythmias originating from the left posterior fascicle in a case with Brugada syndrome associated with idiopathic left ventricular tachycardia. *Europace.* 2008; 10:86-90.
780. Joshi S, Raiszadeh F, Pierce W et al. Antiarrhythmic induced electrical storm in Brugada syndrome: a case report. *Ann Noninvas Electrocardiol.* 2007; 12:274-8.
781. Karaca M, Dinckal MH. Monomorphic and propafenone-induced polymorphic ventricular tachycardia in Brugada syndrome: a case report. *Acta Cardiol.* 2006; 61:481-4.
782. Shan Q, Yang B, Chen M et al. Short-term normalization of ventricular repolarization by transcatheter ablation in a patient with suspected Brugada syndrome. *J Interv Card Electrophysiol.* 2008; 21:53-7.
783. Vernooy K, Delhaas T, Cremer OL et al. Electrocardiographic changes predicting sudden death in propofol-related infusion syndrome. *Heart Rhythm.* 2006; 3:131-7.
784. Robinson JD, Melman Y, Walsh EP. Cardiac conduction disturbances and ventricular tachycardia after prolonged propofol infusion in an infant. *Pacing Clin Electrophysiol.* 2008; 31:1070-3.
785. Riezzo I, Centini F, Neri M et al. Brugada-like EKG pattern and myocardial effects in a chronic propofol abuser. *Clin Toxicol.* 2009; 47:358-63.
786. Jorens PG, Van den Eynden GG. Propfol infusion syndrome with arrhythmia, myocardial fat accumulation and cardiac failure. *Am J Cardiol.* 2009; 104:1160-2.
787. Postema PG, Neville J, de Jong JS et al. Safe drug use in long QT syndrome and Brugada syndrome: comparison of website statistics. *Europace.* 2013; 15:1042-9.
788. Benjamin EJ, Blaha MJ, Chiuve SE et al. Heart disease and stroke statistics—2017 update: a report from the American Heart Association. *Circulation.* 2017; 135:e146-603.
789. Priori SG, Wilde AA, Horie M et al. HRS/EHRA/APHRS expert consensus statement on the diagnosis and management of patients with inerited primary arrhythmia syndromes. *Heart Rhythm.* 2013; 10:1932-63.

790. Di Diego JM, Cordeiro JM, Goodrow RJ et al.Ionic and cellular basis for the predominance of the Brugada syndrome phenotype in males. *Circulation.* 2002; 106:2004-11.
791. Shimizu W, Matsuo K, Kokubo Y et al. Sex hormone and gender difference: role of testosterone on male predominance in Brugada syndrome. *J Cardiovasc Electrophysiol.* 2007; 18:415-21.
792. Brugada R, Campuzano O, Sarquella-Brugada G et al. Brugada syndrome. In: Pagon RA, Adam MP, Ardinger HH et al (eds). Gene reviews® [Internet]. https://www.ncbi.nlm.nih.gov/books/NBK1517/ (accessed 2017 Feb 18).
793. Rolf S, Bruns HJ, Wichter T et al. The ajmaline challenge in Brugada syndrome: diagnostic impact, safety, and recommended protocol. *Eur Heart J.* 2003; 24:1104-12.
794. Fish JM, Antzelevitch C. Role of sodium and calcium channel block in unmasking the Brugada syndrome. *Heart Rhythm.* 2004; 1:210-7.
795. Konigstein M, Rosso R, Topaz G et al. Drug-induced Brugada syndrome: clinical characteristics and risk factors. *Heart Rhythm.* 2016; 13:1083-7.
796. Probst V, Veltmann C, Eckardt L et al. Long-term prognosis of patients diagnosed with Brugada syndrome. Results from the FINGER Brigada syndrome registry. *Circulation.* 2010; 121:635-43.

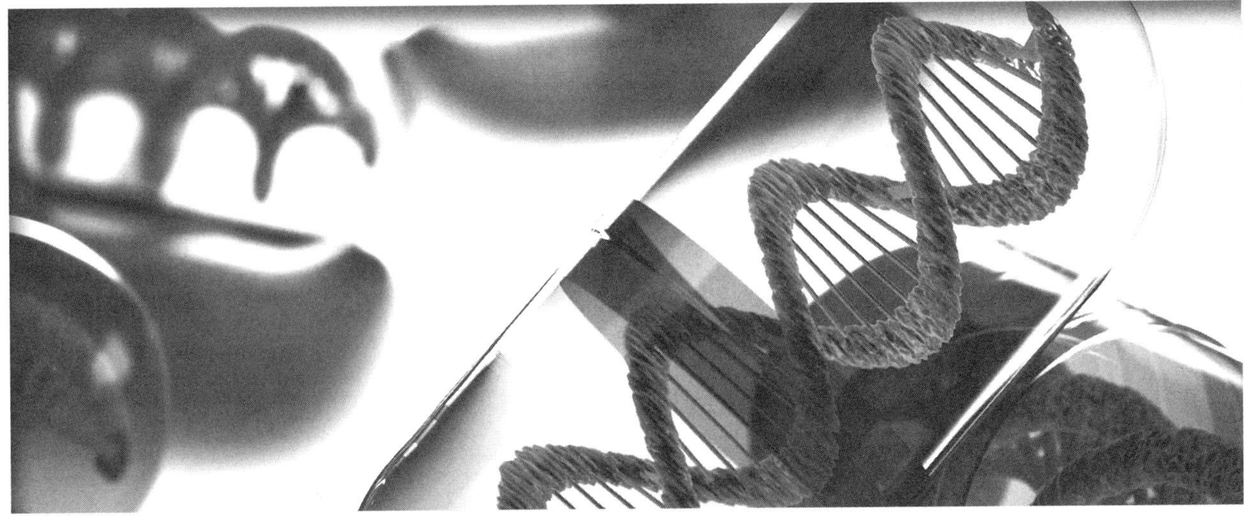

CHAPTER 26

Supraventricular Arrhythmias

James E. Tisdale

Drugs may induce a variety of supraventricular arrhythmias that may be associated with symptoms, hemodynamic instability, stroke, and, in some cases, an increased risk of death. Supraventricular arrhythmias that may be induced by drugs include sinus bradycardia, atrioventricular (AV) node block, atrial fibrillation or flutter, atrial tachycardia, and AV nodal re-entrant tachycardia.

SINUS BRADYCARDIA/ ATRIOVENTRICULAR BLOCK

Sinus bradycardia is defined as a sinus rate <60 bpm.[1] Drugs that inhibit sinus node function resulting in sinus pauses or sinus arrest are also included in this section. Sinus pauses occur when the function of the sinus node is impaired transiently, leading to "pauses" without P-waves on the electrocardiogram.[1-3] Sinus pauses are also known as periods of sinus arrest.

AV block occurs when conduction of impulses from the atria to the ventricles through the AV node is inhibited.[3] AV block is classified as first, second, or third degree. First-degree AV block is defined as prolongation of the PR interval to >0.2 seconds. Second-degree AV block is a progression of AV nodal dysfunction to the point at which some impulses are not conducted from the atria to the ventricles. Third-degree AV block, often referred to as complete heart block or AV dissociation, is defined by the absence of a relationship between atrial and ventricular depolarization. During third-degree AV block, atrial depolarization and ventricular depolarization occur independently, as a result of the complete inability of the AV node to conduct impulses.[3]

CAUSATIVE AGENTS

Sinus bradycardia with or without sinus pauses may be associated with a wide variety of drugs (**Table 26-1**).[4-522] In addition to occurring as a result of drugs administered orally or intravenously, sinus bradycardia and sinus pauses may be induced by drugs administered as eye drops. Numerous cases of sinus bradycardia associated with topical adrenergic β-receptor antagonists (β-blockers) have been reported.[523,524] The incidence of sinus bradycardia associated with topical timolol is significantly

Table 26-1 Agents Implicated in Drug-Induced Sinus Bradycardia

Drug	Incidence	Level of Evidence[a]
Adenosine[4-6]	1–8%	A
Amiodarone[7-14]	3–20%	A
Amisulpride[15]	NK	C
Baclofen[16-24,b]	NK	C
β-blockers[25-35]	0.6–25%	A
Bupivacaine[36-43]	2–32%	A
Capecitabine[44,45]	NK	C
Carbamazepine[46,47]	NK	C
Cimetidine[48-54]	NK	C
Cisplatin[55-60]	NK	B
Citalopram[61-65]	0.1–2.4%	B
Clonidine[66-99]	5–17.5%	A
Clozapine[100,101]	NK	C
Cocaine[102,103]	23–48%	B
Cytarabine[106-109]	NK	C
Dexamethasone[110-113]	NK	B
Dexmedetomidine[114-144]	4.4–55%	A
Diazepam[50,b]	NK	C
Digoxin[145-151,b]	0–7%	B
Diltiazem[152-165]	4.2–16%	A
Dipyridamole[166-172,c]	0.5–6.7%	B
Disopyramide[173-177]	0–4%	B
Donepezil[177-186]	0.6–48% HR 1.4 (95 % CI 1.1–1.6)	A
Dronedarone[187-190]	0.7–2.3% OR 1.45 (95% CI 1.02–2.08)	A
Dovitinib[191]	5%	B
Escitalopram[192-194]	NK	C
Fingolimod[195-215]	0.5–37%	A
Flecainide[216-223]	2–13.2%	B
Fludarabine[224]	NK	C
5-fluorouracil[225-227]	12%[d]	B
Fluoxetine[228-234]	NK	B
γ-hydroxybutyric acid[235-240]	NK[e]	B
Granisetron[241,242]	NK	A
Halothane[243-246]	11–24%	A
Ibutilide[247-250]	0–4.5%	B
Idarubicin[251]	NK	C
Irinotecan[252,253]	NK	C
Isradipine[254,c]	NK	C
Ivabradine[255-267]	3.7–15.7% OR 6.54 (95% CI 3.3–012.9)	A
Ketamine[268-273]	0–5.5%[f]	B

Table 26-1 Agents Implicated in Drug-Induced Sinus Bradycardia (continued)

Drug	Incidence	Level of Evidence[a]
Lidocaine[95,274-283]	0–9.3%	B
Memantine[184,284]	7%	B
Mepivacaine[285-287]	5–13%	A
Methadone[288-293]	NK	C
Methylprednisolone[111,294-307]	2.5%[g]	B
Milrinone[308]	0–13%	A
Mycophenolate[195,196]	6.4–53%	B
Neostigmine[309-321]	OR 2.7 (95% CI 1.4–5.4)	B
Nicardipine[322-325]	10–12%	A
Nitroglycerin[326-334]	0–0.7%	B
Octreotide[335-339]	NK	C
Olanzapine[340-344]	0.25%–0.7%	B
Paclitaxel[345-353]	3–29%	A
Pentazocine[354]	5%[h]	B
Prednisone[355,356]	NK	C
Pregabalin[97]	7.5%	B
Propafenone[357-362]	0.7%[i] 10%[j]	B B
Propofol[363-384]	0–50% (14.7% in analysis of combined studies)	A
Physostigmine[312,385-387]	NK	B
Pyridostigmine[312,386,388]	NK	C
Ranitidine[389-397]	NK	C
Remifentanil[398-411]	0–39%	A
Risperidone[412-414]	NK	C
Sevoflurane[244,415-428]	0–53%	A
Sotalol[429-452]	1.5–17.2%	A
Succinylcholine[453-465]	0–50%	A
Tacrolimus[466,467]	NK	C
Tetracaine[468-470]	NK	C
Thalidomide[471-484]	3.2–54%	A
Tivantinib[485]	21%	B
Tizanidine[486-489]	NK	C
Verapamil[243,490-522]	0–11%	A

CI = confidence interval, HR = hazard ratio, NK = not known, OR = odds ratio.

[a]Definitions for Levels of Evidence: Level A—evidence from one or more randomized, controlled clinical trials; Level B—evidence from nonrandomized clinical trials, prospective observational studies, cohort studies, retrospective studies, case-control studies, meta-analyses and/or postmarketing surveillance studies; and Level C—evidence from one or more published case reports or case series.

[b]Predominantly in overdose or with supratherapeutic plasma concentrations.

[c]Reported with intravenous use.

[d]Incidence associated with 5-fluorouracil-based chemotherapy regimens.

[e]Incidence in γ-hydroxybutyric acid intoxication: 6–38%.[236,239]

[f]Incidence as high as 21.1% in infants.[270]

[g]Incidence as high as 42% following pulse doses of 1,000 mg.[299]

[h]Intramuscular administration in children.

[i]Oral propafenone.

[j]Intravenous propafenone.

higher (18.4%) than that associated with topical carteolol (4.5%).[523] The lower incidence of sinus bradycardia associated with carteolol may be a result of the intrinsic sympathomimetic activity of the drug. Chronic cocaine use has been shown to increase the odds of bradycardia and severe bradycardia by factors of 3.02 and 5.11, respectively.[103] Drugs that have been reported to cause AV block are listed in **Table 26-2.**[4,5,46,148,154,158,174,176,179,198,199,202,204,207,209,212-214,216,345-347,446,519,525-679]

EPIDEMIOLOGY

The overall incidence of drug-induced sinus bradycardia or AV block is unknown. The incidence of sinus bradycardia and sinus pauses associated with specific agents, where known, is presented in Table 26-1, and the incidence of drug-induced AV block associated with specific drugs, where known, is presented in Table 26-2.

Amiodarone has been reported to cause sinus-node and AV nodal bradyarrhythmias requiring pacemaker insertion.[9] In a study of 15,824 patients with atrial fibrillation and a history of myocardial infarction who were receiving amiodarone, the incidence of pacemaker implantation was 2.2% per person-year (mean duration [±SD] of follow-up, 1.8 ± 1.5 years), and was 5.2% per person-year during the first 90 days of therapy.[9] The odds ratio for pacemaker insertion to treat bradyarrhythmias associated with amiodarone use was 2.14 (95% CI 1.30–3.54).[680] Although the incidence of sinus bradycardia associated with conventional doses of intravenous amiodarone (1–2 g/24 hr) is similar to that associated with oral amiodarone,[681] the incidence may be as high as 10% when doses of 3 g per 24 hours are administered.[682]

Sinus bradycardia or arrest or AV block may be caused by digoxin, primarily in overdose or other situations in which serum digoxin concentrations become elevated.[148] The overall incidence of sinus bradycardia or AV block associated with digoxin is unknown. In an analysis of patients with a discharge diagnosis of digoxin intoxication, "definite" sinus bradycardia and sinus pauses <2 seconds were documented in 26% and 19%, respectively, of those with digoxin intoxication.[148] In addition, "definite" second- or third-degree AV block was documented in 33% of patients with digoxin intoxication.[148] Sotalol has been reported to cause clinically important sinus bradycardia and sinus pauses in up to 17.2% of patients treated for atrial fibrillation, with 2.5% requiring permanent pacemaker implantation.[445]

Ivabradine is a recent addition to therapy for patients with heart failure with reduced ejection fraction (HFrEF) and is indicated for patients with HFrEF with heart rates >70 bpm who are on maximally tolerated doses of β-blockers or are intolerant of β-blocker therapy. Ivabradine is associated with sinus bradycardia in up to 16% of patients. A meta-analysis of placebo-controlled studies of ivabradine in patients with stable coronary artery disease with and without HFrEF reported an odds ratio for bradycardia of 6.54 (95% CI 3.30–12.9, p <0.01).[264] Fingolimod, which is indicated for relapsing forms of multiple sclerosis, is associated with sinus bradycardia in up to 37% of patients.[195]

Zeltser et al.[568] reviewed a series of 169 consecutive patients admitted or discharged with the diagnosis of second- or third-degree AV block that was not caused by acute myocardial infarction, vasovagal syncope, radiofrequency ablation, or digitalis toxicity. Of these, 54% were receiving therapy with β-blockers with or without diltiazem, diltiazem alone, or verapamil. The investigators reported that drug discontinuation was followed by resolution of AV block in 41% of patients but that 56% of these patients subsequently had recurrence of AV block in the absence of causative drugs. Based on their criteria for causation, the investigators concluded that drugs were the specific cause of AV block in only 15% of the patients who were receiving therapy with β-blockers with or without diltiazem, diltiazem alone, or verapamil.[568]

MECHANISMS

Drug-induced sinus bradycardia may be caused by inhibition of automaticity of the node, slowing of sinus node conduction, or prolongation of sinus node repolarization (**Table 26-3**). AV block may be caused by agents that inhibit AV node conduction

Table 26-2 Agents Implicated in Drug-Induced Atrioventricular Block

Drug	Incidence	Level of Evidence[a]
Aconite[525,526]	NK	C
Adenosine[4,5,527-551]	3–15% RR 7.88 (95% CI 4.15–14.9) RR 6.78 (95% CI 2.15–21.38)	A
Amiodarone[552-559]	0–14.8%	A
Amitriptyline[560,561]	NK	C
β-blockers[552,562-574]	0.15–2.4%	A
Bupivacaine[575,576]	3.5%	B
Carbamazepine[46,577-585]	NK	C
Chloroquine[586-588]	NK	C
Cimetidine[589]	NK	C
Citalopram[590]	NK	C
Clonidine[591-594]	NK	C
Cocaine[595,596]	NK	C
Digoxin[148,573,597-613]	NK	B
Diltiazem[154,158,568,614-619]	0–2%	A
Dipyridamole[620-623]	NK	C
Disopyramide[174,176,624,625]	0–2%	B
Donepezil[179,626-628]	NK	C
Etomidate[629]	NK	C
Famotidine[630]	NK	C
Fingolimod[198,199,202,204,207,209,212-214,631-636]	0.2–0.5%	A
Flecainide[216,637]	NK	C
Guanabenz[638]	NK	C
Hydroxychloroquine[639]	NK	C
Imipramine[640,641]	NK	C
Infliximab[642]	NK	C
Nicardipine[643]	NK	C
Paclitaxel[345-347,644]	0–4.4%	B
Pentamidine[645]	NK	C
Phenylpropanolamine[646,647]	NK	C
Propafenone[648-650]	0.3%	A
Propofol[651-654]	NK	C
Pyridostigmine[655]	NK	C
Remifentanil[656]	NK	C
Sotalol[446,657]	0.8–4.2%	B
Thioridazine[658,659]	NK	C
Ticagrelor[660-664]	NK	C
Verapamil[519,568,616,665-679]	0–8%	A

CI = confidence interval, NK = not known, RR = relative risk.

[a]Definitions for Levels of Evidence: Level A—evidence from one or more randomized, controlled clinical trials; Level B—evidence from nonrandomized clinical trials, prospective observational studies, cohort studies, retrospective studies, case-control studies, meta-analyses and/or postmarketing surveillance studies; and Level C—evidence from one or more published case reports or case series.

Table 26-3 Mechanisms of Drug-Induced Sinus Bradycardia

Drug	Mechanism
All drugs that may cause sinus bradycardia (except nitrates)	Inhibition of automaticity of the sinus node and/or slowing of sinus node conduction and/or prolongation of sinus node repolarization
β-blockers	Inhibit activity of sympathetic nervous system, leading to inhibition of automaticity of sinus node
Clonidine	Stimulates central α_2-receptors, reducing release of norepinephrine
Fingolimod	Modulation of the sphingosine 1-phosphate (S1P) receptors
Ivabradine	Inhibition of hyperpolarization-activated cyclic nucleotide-gated "funny" (I_f) channels in the sinus node
Neostigmine, physostigmine, pyridostigmine	Stimulate activity of the parasympathetic nervous system, leading to inhibition of automaticity of sinus node
Nitroglycerin	Stimulates peripheral sensory receptors with vagal afferents to the medulla, resulting in sympathetic nervous system inhibition via stimulation of central α_2-receptors

Table 26-4 Mechanisms of Drug-Induced Atrioventricular Block

Drug	Mechanism
All drugs that may cause AV block	Inhibition of AV node conduction
β-blockers	Inhibit activity of sympathetic nervous system, leading to inhibition of conduction through the AV node
Clonidine	Stimulates central α_2-receptors, reducing release of norepinephrine
Fingolimod	Modulation of the sphingosine 1-phosphate (S1P) receptors
Neostigmine, physostigmine, pyridostigmine	Stimulate activity of the parasympathetic nervous system, leading to inhibition of conduction through the AV node

AV = atrioventricular.

or prolong AV node repolarization (**Table 26-4**). Both the sinus node and the AV node are heavily influenced by sympathetic and parasympathetic nervous system activity. Drugs that inhibit activity of the sympathetic nervous system (e.g., β-blockers) and drugs that stimulate the parasympathetic nervous system (e.g., neostigmine, physostigmine, pyridostigmine) may cause sinus bradycardia or AV block. The action potentials of both the sinus node and the AV node depend primarily on calcium and sodium flux, and calcium or sodium channel inhibitors may cause sinus bradycardia, AV block, or both.

Nitrates may cause a syndrome associated with sinus bradycardia and hypotension.[326-334] Sinus bradycardia induced by nitrates is an idiosyncratic reaction. This syndrome resembles neurocardiogenic syncope but may occur when patients are in the supine position. The mechanism of nitrate-induced sinus bradycardia remains unclear, but evidence suggests that nitrates may stimulate peripheral sensory receptors with vagal afferents to the medulla, resulting in sympathetic nervous system inhibition via stimulation of central α_2-receptors (Table 26-3).[683]

Ivabradine is a hyperpolarization-activated cyclic nucleotide-gated "funny" channel (I_f) blocker, the primary mechanism of which is to slow heart rate in patients with HFrEF.[259,260] Sinus bradycardia is an extension of the pharmacologic effect of the drug. Fingolimod causes sinus bradycardia via modulation of the sphingosine 1-phosphate (S1P) receptors.[684] S1P contributes to regulation of heart rate and cardiac conduction via modulation of intramyocyte calcium concentrations.[685]

CLINICAL PRESENTATION AND DIFFERENTIAL DIAGNOSIS

Normal heart rate is usually defined somewhat arbitrarily as ranging between 60 and 100 bpm. However, many individuals routinely have heart rates <60 bpm and even <50 bpm without evidence of symptoms. Patients with symptomatic sinus bradycardia resulting in the need for medical attention typically have heart rates between 30 and 50 bpm, resulting in hemodynamic compromise. Signs and symptoms associated with clinically

Table 26-5 Signs and Symptoms Associated with Drug-Induced Sinus Bradycardia and Atrioventricular Block

- Dizziness
- Light-headedness
- Fatigue
- Lethargy
- Dyspnea
- Weakness
- Presyncope
- Syncope
- Chest pain
- Symptoms of heart failure

important sinus bradycardia and sinus pauses are listed in **Table 26-5.**[1,3]

First-degree AV block is a common electrocardiographic phenomenon that is almost always asymptomatic and is, therefore, not a drug-induced disease as defined in this text.[3] However, if extreme prolongation of the PR interval occurs (>0.3 sec), patients may experience symptoms during exercise due to AV dysynchrony, as the PR interval may not shorten enough as the RR interval decreases.[3] Second- and third-degree AV block can result in bradycardia, leading to symptoms that result in the need for medical attention or even requiring hospitalization.

Second-degree AV block occurs most commonly in two distinct patterns. Mobitz type I second-degree AV block (also known as Wenckebach) is characterized by progressive prolongation of the PR interval on the electrocardiogram (ECG) until a P-wave is not followed by a QRS complex.[3] Mobitz type I is usually caused by impulse conduction delay in the AV node (as opposed to further down in the bundle of His).[1] Mobitz type II second-degree AV block is typified by constant PR intervals with abrupt, intermittent absence of QRS complexes. Mobitz type II second-degree AV block often occurs in specific patterns with P-wave to QRS complex ratios such as 2:1 or 3:1. This type of second-degree AV block is likely caused by impulse-conduction delay in the bundle of His.

During third-degree AV block, the AV node is completely unable to conduct impulses, and atrial depolarization occurs independently of ventricular depolarization. Therefore, P-waves and QRS complexes are present on ECG but are unrelated to one another. Third-degree AV block can occur either in the AV node itself or further down in the bundle of His.[3]

Second- or third-degree AV block may result in bradycardia, with heart rates in the range of 40–60 bpm, and sometimes as low as 20–40 bpm. Symptoms of second- or third-degree AV block are the same as those associated with sinus bradycardia (Table 26-5).

Drug-induced sinus bradycardia or AV block must be distinguished from other causes of sinus or AV node impairment. Dysfunction of the sinus node unrelated to drug therapy is common, with a prevalence as high as 1 in 600 patients over the age of 65 years.[686] Intrinsic AV nodal abnormalities also may occur during the aging process. Transient sinus node dysfunction may occur in the setting of acute myocardial ischemia or infarction when the infarct/ischemia-related vessel is the right coronary artery or the left circumflex artery, but permanent sinus-node damage in this setting is uncommon. Myocardial infarction may result in some degree of permanent AV nodal dysfunction in some patients. Conditions to consider in the differential diagnosis of drug-induced sinus bradycardia or AV block are listed in **Table 26-6.**[1]

Drug-induced sinus or AV node dysfunction can often be distinguished from nondrug-related sinus bradycardia or AV block. When a patient with symptoms that appear to be related to sinus bradycardia/sinus pauses/sinus arrest or AV block seeks medical attention, therapy with drugs known to induce sinus or AV node dysfunction should be discontinued. If the sinus or AV node dysfunction persists after five half-lives of the respective drug(s) have passed, a drug-induced cause may be ruled out. While awaiting drug washout, evaluation and diagnostic testing for nonpharmacologic causes can be performed, including determination of serum potassium and magnesium concentrations, thyroid function tests, and assessment for myocardial ischemia or infarction. However, it may not be possible or desirable in every case to discontinue therapy with drugs suspected of causing sinus bradycardia

Table 26-6 Conditions to Consider in the Differential Diagnosis of Drug-Induced Sinus Bradycardia or Atrioventricular Block[a]

- Age-related idiopathic degenerative fibrosis of the sinus or AV node
- Myocardial ischemia/infarction (results in transient, not permanent, sinus bradycardia or AV block)
- Hypothyroidism
- Hypoxia
- Hypothermia
- Electrolyte abnormalities (hyperkalemia, hypokalemia, hypermagnesemia)
- Congenital heart disease
- Amyloidosis
- Hemochromatosis
- Sarcoidosis
- Myocarditis
- Systemic lupus erythematosus
- Scleroderma
- Rheumatoid arthritis
- Myotonic muscular dystrophy
- Surgical trauma (valve replacement, heart transplantation, correction of congenital heart disease)
- Chagas disease
- Endocarditis
- Diptheria
- Neurocardiac syncope
- Carotid sinus hypersensitivity
- Coughing
- Micturition
- Defecation
- Vomiting

AV = atrioventricular.
[a]See reference 1 for more information.

Table 26-7 Risk Factors for Drug-Induced Sinus Bradycardia or Atrioventricular Block

Sinus bradycardia[9,53,63,242,420,421,423,681-687]

- Pretreatment heart rate <60 bpm
- Underlying sinus-node dysfunction (may occur with advancing age)
- Impaired baroreflex control (risk factor for nitroglycerin-induced sinus bradycardia)
- Concomitant use of less than one sinus-node inhibiting drug
- Elevate plasma drug concentrations due to kidney or liver disease or drug interactions
- Age >65 years (citalopram-induced bradycardia)
- Amiodarone dose >200 mg daily
- Female (risk factor for pacemaker implantation due to amiodarone-induced bradycardia)
- Down syndrome (risk factor for sevoflurane-induced bradycardia)

Atrioventricular block[546,554,688]

- Concomitant use of less than one AV-blocking drug
- Pretreatment PR interval >0.2 sec
- Underlying AV nodal disease (may occur with advancing age)
- Elevated plasma drug concentration due to kidney or liver disease or drug interactions
- Hypothyroidism (may be a risk factor for amiodarone-induced AV block)
- Prior use of aspirin (adenosine-induced AV block)

AV = atrioventricular, bpm = beats per minute.

or AV block. For example, β-blocker therapy should not generally be discontinued in a patient treated for HFrEF or after myocardial infarction. Rather, therapy with the β-blocker should be continued and implantation of a permanent pacemaker considered as a means to protect against possible drug-induced sinus or AV node dysfunction.

RISK FACTORS

Risk factors for drug-induced sinus bradycardia are listed in **Table 26-7**. Higher drug doses may increase the risk for sinus bradycardia.[9] Conditions that may result in elevated plasma concentrations of drugs known to cause sinus bradycardia increase the risk. Patients with kidney disease who are receiving renally eliminated drugs that may cause sinus bradycardia (atenolol, clonidine, digoxin) are also at increased risk. Age >65 years is a risk factor for citalopram-induced bradycardia; the incidence was 2.4% in patients >65 years of age compared to 0.2% in patients younger than 65 years ($p < 0.05$).[64] Kidney disease has been identified as a risk factor for sinus bradycardia associated with clonidine.[75] Drugs that have been reported to cause sinus bradycardia or AV block that require dose adjustment in patients with kidney disease are listed in **Table 26-8**, and drugs that have been reported to cause sinus bradycardia or AV block that require dose adjustment in patients with liver disease are listed in **Table 26-9**. In addition, concomitant use of drugs that inhibit the hepatic metabolism of drugs known to induce sinus bradycardia should be avoided (**Table 26-10**).[688]

Table 26-8 Drugs Known to Cause Sinus Bradycardia or Atrioventricular Block That May Require Dose Adjustment or Are Contraindicated in Patients with Kidney Disease

- Acebutolol
- Amisulpride
- Atenolol
- Baclofen
- Betaxolol
- Capecitabine
- Carteolol
- Cimetidine
- Cisplatin (recommended to be avoided in patients with pre-existing kidney disease)
- Clonidine
- Dexmedetomidine
- Digoxin
- Disopyramide
- Famotidine
- Flecainide
- Fludarabine
- Guanabenz
- Idarubicin
- Isradipine
- Memantine
- Milrinone
- Mycophenolate
- Nadolol
- Nicardipine
- Ranitidine
- Risperidone
- Sotalol
- Tacrolimus

Other interactions may result in sinus bradycardia. Dipyridamole inhibits the cellular uptake of adenosine; therefore, patients receiving adenosine concomitantly with dipyridamole are at increased risk of adenosine-associated sinus bradycardia/sinus pauses.[6,689] A number of drugs inhibit the elimination of digoxin, particularly amiodarone, verapamil, and quinidine, and concomitant use of these drugs with digoxin increases the risk of digoxin-induced sinus bradycardia, unless appropriate digoxin dose reduction is implemented.[690-692] In addition, patients receiving therapy with more than one drug known to reduce heart rate are at increased risk.[75,309]

Table 26-9 Drugs Known to Cause Sinus Bradycardia or Atrioventricular Block That May Require Dose Adjustment or Are Contraindicated in Patients with Liver Disease

- Acebutolol
- Citalopram
- Dronedarone
- Escitalopram
- Fluoxetine
- Idarubicin
- Ivabradine
- Paclitaxel
- Propafenone
- Risperidone
- Tacrolimus

Women are at greater risk for amiodarone-induced bradycardia requiring implantation of a permanent pacemaker.[693] In a study of 1,005 patients with new-onset atrial fibrillation, the hazard ratio for amiodarone use requiring a permanent pacemaker was 4.69 (95% CI 1.99–11.05) in women, as compared with 1.05 (95% CI 0.42–2.58) in men.[693] Mechanisms for the increased risk of bradycardia requiring pacemaker implantation in women are unknown.

Down syndrome has been reported to be a risk factor for bradycardia induced by sevoflurane.[425,426,428] The mechanism of increased risk is unknown, but individuals with trisomy 21 exhibit a decreased heart rate response to orthostatic challenges, suggesting that these patients may have blunted activation of the sympathetic nervous system or impaired parasympathetic regulation of heart rate.[428]

Specific risk factors for the majority of drug-induced AV block have not been identified. In the study by Zeltser et al.[568] of 169 consecutive cases of AV block, there were no significant differences in age, male sex, or presence of hypertension or ischemic heart disease between patients receiving therapy with β-blockers with or without diltiazem or verapamil and those not receiving therapy with drugs that could induce AV block. In a retrospective analysis of 102 cardiac transplant patients

Table 26-10 Drugs Known to Cause Sinus Bradycardia or Atrioventricular Block That Are Substrates for Enzymes of the Cytochrome P-450 System[688]

1A2	2B6	2C8	2C9	2C19	2D6	2E1	3A4,5,7
Amitriptyline	Ketamine	Paclitaxel	Amitriptyline	Amitriptyline	Amitriptyline	Halothane	Carbamazepine
Clozapine	Methadone		Fluoxetine		Carvedilol	Sevoflurane	Cocaine
Olanzapine	Propofol				Clonidine		Diazepam
Propranolol					Flecainide		Diltiazem
Tizanidine					Fluoxetine		Lidocaine
Verapamil					Imipramine		Methadone
					Lidocaine		Paclitaxel
					Metoprolol		Propranolol
					Nebivolol		Quinidine
					Propafenone		Risperidone
					Propranolol		Tacrolimus
					Risperidone		Verapamil
					Timolol		

who received adenosine for stress myocardial perfusion imaging, prior use of aspirin and baseline first-degree AV block were independent risk factors for adenosine-induced second- or third-degree AV block.[546] Possible risk factors for drug-induced AV block are listed in Table 26-7. Risk factors have been identified for AV block induced by digoxin and include the drug interactions listed above, hypokalemia, hypomagnesemia, hypoxia, hypothyroidism, and inadequate dose reduction in patients with kidney disease.[694]

MORBIDITY AND MORTALITY

The incidence of morbidity, hospitalization, or death associated with drug-induced sinus bradycardia or AV block is unknown. Drug-induced sinus bradycardia or AV block may result in the need for temporary or permanent pacemaker implantation.[9,62,662,680] In a population of patients with new-onset atrial fibrillation, the adjusted hazard ratio for amiodarone use leading to a requirement for a permanent pacemaker was 2.01 (95% CI 1.08–3.76).[693] Death due to drug-induced sinus bradycardia or AV block is likely very uncommon.

PREVENTION

Drug-induced sinus or AV node dysfunction (or both) is often preventable (**Table 26-11**). When possible, drugs with the potential to inhibit sinus or AV node function should be avoided in patients with known sinus or AV node dysfunction in the absence of a functioning pacemaker. Once a pacemaker has been implanted, however, patients with sinus node dysfunction may receive sinus node-inhibiting drugs, and patients with AV node dysfunction may receive AV node-inhibiting agents. Patients who are taking drugs with the potential to cause sinus bradycardia, sinus pauses, or AV block should be taught to monitor their heart rate daily and to consult their pharmacist or physician if heart rate falls below 50 bpm or if they experience symptoms of bradycardia (Table 26-5). Combinations of drugs that may inhibit sinus or AV node function should be minimized but are not contraindicated if the benefits of such therapy outweigh the risks.

Drug-induced sinus or AV node dysfunction may be prevented by not exceeding maximum daily doses of drugs known to cause these drug-induced diseases and by appropriate dose adjustment of specific drugs

Table 26-11 Approaches to Help Prevent Drug-Induced Sinus Bradycardia and Atrioventricular Block

For all drugs that may cause sinus bradycardia, AV block, or both

- Patient should take pulse daily, report if <50 bpm
- Do not exceed maximum daily doses
- Use combinations of drugs that may cause sinus bradycardia or AV block only when necessary and when the benefits likely outweigh the risks
- Appropriately adjust drug doses for liver or kidney disease
- Avoid sinus or AV node-inhibiting drugs in patients with underlying sinus node dysfunction, unless a functioning pacemaker is present (in the case of AV node-inhibiting drugs, there must be a functioning ventricular pacemaker)

For digoxin

- *Measure serum digoxin concentrations:*
    - If kidney function is changing
    - If a drug that interacts with digoxin is added to therapy
    - Every 6 months if there is no kidney disease or concomitant use of interacting drugs

AV = atrioventricular.

to account for organ dysfunction, drug interactions, or both. Maintaining serum digoxin concentrations <2 ng/mL, and optimally <1 ng/mL, reduces the risk of digoxin-associated sinus or AV node dysfunction. In certain circumstances, substituting medications within a class may prevent drug-induced sinus or AV node dysfunction. For example, a patient with kidney disease who is receiving atenolol is at higher risk for atenolol-induced sinus bradycardia or AV block as a result of diminished atenolol clearance. In this situation, replacing atenolol with a nonrenally cleared β-blocker such as metoprolol or propanolol may reduce the likelihood of drug-induced sinus bradycardia or AV block.

Patients receiving drugs known to inhibit AV node conduction should undergo a 12-lead ECG periodically and at least every 6 months. First-degree AV block is not an absolute contraindication to receiving AV node-blocking drugs, but the PR interval should be monitored every 3–6 months to ensure that AV block is not progressing. In addition, combinations of AV node-blocking drugs are best avoided in patients with pretreatment PR intervals >0.2 seconds. If the PR interval progresses to >0.2 seconds while on AV node-blocking therapy, it is not necessary to discontinue therapy, but more frequent ECG monitoring is recommended and administration of additional AV node-blocking agents should be avoided.

MANAGEMENT

Management options for patients with drug-induced sinus bradycardia or AV block are presented in **Table 26-12**. In some cases, a reduction in dose of the offending medication may be sufficient, but in most cases in which drug-induced sinus or AV node dysfunction has resulted in a hospitalization, discontinuation of therapy is necessary. In the case of sinus bradycardia or AV block induced by adenosine, treatment is not usually required

Table 26-12 Management of Drug-Induced Sinus Bradycardia or Atrioventricular Block

- Discontinue the causative agent
- Temporary pacemaker
- *If underlying sinus or AV node dysfunction:* Permanent pacemaker may be necessary (if AV node dysfunction, must be a ventricular pacemaker)
- *In severe cases:* Atropine 0.5–1 mg q 3–5 min until heart rate increases or total dose of 1.5–3 mg is administered
- *If atropine not effective:* Epinephrine 2–10 mcg/min or dopamine 2–10 mcg/kg/min continuous IV infusion
- *If due to calcium-channel blocker or β-blocker overdose:*
    - Gastric lavage (within 1 hour of ingestion)
    - Activated charcoal 25–50 g in an aqueous slurry of 120–240 mL water (within 1 hour of ingestion)
    - Glucagon 3–10 mg (0.05–0.15 mg/kg) intravenously followed by continuous infusion of 3–5 mg/hr (β-blocker overdose only)
    - Calcium 0.3 mEq/kg intravenously, administered as calcium gluconate (10%) 0.6 mL/kg or calcium chloride (10%) 0.2 mL/kg over 5–10 minutes, followed by 0.3 mEq/kg/hr
    - *HIE:* Regular insulin 1 international unit/kg bolus followed by continuous IV infusion of 0.5–1 international unit/kg/hr
- Temporary pacemaker, if necessary

AV = atrioventricular, HIE = hyperinsulinemia/euglycemia therapy, IV = intravenous.

because the drug is metabolized very quickly (half-life = 10 seconds) and the heart rate usually returns to pretreatment values within 20–30 seconds.

Percutaneous insertion of a temporary pacemaker may be necessary. If the patient is subsequently diagnosed with underlying intrinsic sinus or AV node dysfunction, therapy with the offending medication may be reinitiated after the implantation of a permanent pacemaker. In severe cases, intravenous atropine may be administered in doses of 0.5–1 mg every 3–5 minutes to a total dose of 1.5–3 mg, the dose at which full blockade of the parasympathetic nervous system occurs in humans.[695,696] If atropine is not effective, then epinephrine (2–10 mcg/min) or dopamine (2–10 mcg/kg/min) may be administered. Transcutaneous pacing may be necessary for patients in whom pharmacotherapy is ineffective.

If the drug-induced bradycardia or AV block is a result of an overdose of verapamil, diltiazem, or a β-blocker, gastric lavage may be performed if the patient presents within 1 hour of ingestion. Activated charcoal may be administered and may be particularly useful if the drug was ingested in the form of a sustained-release preparation. For management of sinus bradycardia/AV block due to a β-blocker overdose, treatment with intravenous glucagon, calcium, and/or hyperinsulinemia-euglycemia (HIE) therapy may be initiated.[697,698] Glucagon may be administered as an intravenous bolus dose of 3–10 mg (0.05–0.15 mg/kg), followed by a continuous infusion of 3–5 mg/hr (0.05–0.10 mg/kg/hr), titrated to achieve an adequate hemodynamic response.[698] Calcium 0.3 mEq/kg may be administered, either as calcium gluconate (10%) 0.6 mL/kg or calcium chloride (10%) 0.2 mL/kg over 5–10 minutes, followed by an infusion of 0.3 mEq/kg/hr.[697] Although recommended, evidence supporting calcium infusion for β-blocker overdose is somewhat limited.[697] For patients with β-blocker overdose and sinus bradycardia/AV block refractory to other treatments, HIE may be administered as regular insulin 1 international unit/kg bolus followed by continuous infusion of 0.5–1 international unit/kg/hr. The infusion dose may be titrated every 30 minutes to achieve the desired response. Because of the potential for insulin-associated electrolyte shifts, close monitoring of serum electrolyte concentrations during HIE therapy is recommended. Intravenous dextrose 25 g may be administered with the initial insulin bolus to maintain euglycemia (blood glucose 100–250 mg/dL), followed by continuous dextrose infusion at 0.5 g/kg/hr.[697,698]

In refractory cases of β-blocker or calcium-channel blocker overdose, lipid emulsion infusions have been administered with some success.[697,699,700] The mechanism by which lipid emulsion infusions may be effective has not been elucidated completely. Lipid emulsions may act as a lipid sink, pulling lipophilic drugs away from tissue receptors into plasma, where the drug can then be bound to the emulsion.[699] Another theory suggests that lipid emulsions may enhance myocardial availability of free fatty acids, reversing the conversion from lipid to glucose metabolism that occurs in damaged heart muscle, thereby augmenting availability of substrate with which to resume normal metabolism.[699]

If sinus bradycardia/AV block is a result of a presumed or documented overdose of diltiazem or verapamil, evidence supporting the efficacy of specific antidotes is lacking.[697] Several case reports describe administration of HIE for management of calcium-channel blocker overdose and suggest that HIE, at doses described previously, is a reasonable therapeutic option.[697] More limited evidence, also from case reports, is available to support calcium administration for management of calcium-channel blocker overdose; calcium administration may be considered for patients with calcium-channel blocker overdose and shock that are refractory to other treatments.[697] Evidence is insufficient to recommend glucagon for management of calcium channel overdose.[697] In cases of β-blocker or calcium-channel blocker overdose, insertion of a temporary pacemaker may be necessary.

For patients with a history of myocardial infarction or heart failure in whom sinus bradycardia or AV block induced by β-blockers develops, implantation of a permanent pacemaker may be necessary to allow the patient to continue therapy with these agents, which have been shown to prolong survival in these specific conditions.[701-703]

INFORMATION FOR PATIENTS

Patients should be instructed that specific drug(s) may cause the heart rate (pulse) to become slower. Patients should be taught to take their pulse and to monitor their heart rate daily. Patients should be instructed to consult their pharmacist or physician if their heart rate falls below 50 bpm, or if they feel lightheaded, dizzy, tired, weak, short of breath, experience chest pain, or lose consciousness.

ATRIAL FIBRILLATION/ ATRIAL FLUTTER

Atrial fibrillation is a supraventricular arrhythmia that is characterized on ECG by an irregularly irregular pattern of narrow QRS complexes, an absence of discernible P-waves and an undulating baseline. Atrial flutter is a supraventricular arrhythmia that is characterized on ECG by a regular pattern of narrow QRS complexes, with discernible P-waves that exhibit a "sawtooth" appearance. Atrial flutter is often associated with a ratio of P-waves to QRS complexes of 4:1, 3:1, or, in some cases, 2:1.

CAUSATIVE AGENTS

Drugs that have been associated with atrial fibrillation or atrial flutter are listed in **Table 26-13**.[229,260,263,264,267,302,308,351,386,541,635,704-834] The majority of drugs that have been associated with induction of atrial fibrillation or flutter are cardiovascular agents, but drugs from other classes have been implicated as well, including alcohol, bisphosphonates, corticosteroids, and anticancer agents.[302,351,725-753,784,786,787,792-794,799-805,812,816,833-844]

EPIDEMIOLOGY

The overall incidence of drug-induced atrial fibrillation or flutter is not known, but it is likely very low. Adenosine has been reported to cause a substantial incidence of atrial fibrillation in patients undergoing treatment for AV nodal re-entrant tachycardia.[711] Although the incidence of alcohol-induced atrial fibrillation (often referred to as the "holiday heart syndrome") is unknown, in a case-control study of patients with acute idiopathic atrial fibrillation, 62% of cases were associated with heavy alcohol use.[728] In a prospective cohort study of the association between self-reported alcohol use and incident atrial fibrillation, moderate alcohol intake was not associated with new-onset atrial fibrillation. However, consumption of 35 or more drinks per week was associated with a hazard ratio for atrial fibrillation of 1.45 (95% CI 1.02–2.04) in men.[734] About 5% of cases of atrial fibrillation in men were estimated to be attributable to heavy alcohol intake. In women, consumption of two or more drinks daily was associated with an increased risk of atrial fibrillation (HR 1.60, 95% CI 1.13–2.25) in a prospective study.[735] In a large prospective study of 79,019 men and women, the risk of atrial fibrillation was increased in those who drank 15–21 drinks per week (RR 1.14 [1.01–1.28]) and >21 drinks per week (1.39 [1.22–1.58]) compared to those who drank <1 drink weekly.[746] Even comparatively small amounts of alcohol ingestion appear to increase atrial fibrillation risk; every 10 g of alcohol per day (just under 1 drink daily) is associated with a 5% higher risk of developing new-onset atrial fibrillation.[748] In an epidemiological study of hospital-based healthcare encounters conducted in Texas, residents of counties in which alcohol sales were not restricted had a significantly greater prevalence of atrial fibrillation than residents of "dry" counties, where alcohol sales were prohibited, and conversion of counties from "dry" to unrestricted alcohol sales resulted in significant increases in atrial fibrillation prevalence.[749]

In a randomized study of the prevention of fractures in postmenopausal women, the bisphosphonate drug alendronate was found to increase the risk of "serious" atrial fibrillation (1.5% versus 1% in the placebo group, relative hazard 1.51, 95% CI 0.97–2.40, p = 0.07).[750] However, alendronate did not increase the risk of "all atrial fibrillation adverse events." In addition, in a case-control study in women, a higher proportion of patients with atrial fibrillation had used alendronate as compared with those who had never used any bisphosphonate (odds ratio of atrial fibrillation 1.86, 95% CI 1.09–3.15).[751] Furthermore, another bisphosphonate drug, zoledronic acid, was reported to increase the risk of "serious" atrial fibrillation as compared with placebo (1.3% versus 0.5%, p <0.001).[833] However, zoledronic acid did not increase the risk of all atrial fibrillation events. In 2008, the FDA released a statement

Table 26-13 Agents Implicated in Drug-Induced Atrial Fibrillation or Atrial Flutter

Drug	Incidence	Level of Evidence[a]
Adenosine[541,704-720]	1–12%[b]	B
Albuterol[721-724]	NK	C
Alcohol[725-749]	OR/RR 1.51 (95% CI 1.3–17.4)[740] HR 1.60 (95% CI 1.02–2.51)[741] HR 1.14 (95% CI 1.04–1.26)[743] HR 1.29 (95% CI 1.02–1.62)[743,c]	B
Alendronate[750-753]	0.5% OR 1.86 (95% CI 1.09–3.15)[751] IR 1.58 (95% CI 1.07–2.33)[752,d] OR 1.97 (95% CI 1.59–2.43)[753]	A
Amiodarone[754-757]	NK	B
Caffeine[724,758-765]	NK	B
1,3 Dimethylamylamine[761]	NK	C
Diltiazem[766]	NK	C
Dobutamine[308,767-783]	0–18%	A
Docetaxel[784]	NK	C
Dopamine[779,785,e]	NK	B
Doxorubicin[786,787]	5.8–13.8%	B
Enoximone[778]	8.3%	A
Fingolimod[635,788]	0.5%	B
Flecainide[789,790]	NK	C
Fluoxetine[229,791]	NK	C
Interleukin-2[792-794]	3.5–4.7%	B
Ipratropium bromide[795]	NK	C
Ivabradine[260,263,264,267,796,797]	1.3% OR 1.35 (95% CI 1.19–1.53)[264] RR 1.15 (95% CI 1.07–1.24)[796] RR 1.24 (95% CI 1.08–1.42)[797]	A
Levosimendan[781]	0–9.1%	A
Loxapine[791]	NK	C
Metaproterenol[798]	2.5%	A
Methylprednisolone[302,799-805]	1.8%	B
Milrinone[308,806-811]	2.9–5%	A
Mitoxantrone[812]	1.4%	B
Morphine[813]	HR 4.37 (95% CI 3.56–5.36)	B
Ondansetron[814,815]	NK	C
Paclitaxel[351,816]	2% (atrial flutter) 1–1.7% (atrial fibrillation)	B
Physostigmine[386,817]	NK	C
Propafenone[754,790,818]	9%[f]	C
Sildenafil[819-821]	NK	C
Theophylline[721,822-827]	NK	B
Ticagrelor[828]	NK	C
Tiotropium[829]	1.7/100 person-years	B
Vardenafil[830]	NK	C

Table 26-13 Agents Implicated in Drug-Induced Atrial Fibrillation or Atrial Flutter (continued)

Drug	Incidence	Level of Evidence[a]
Verapamil[831,832]	5%	C
Zoledronic acid[833,834]	0.8–2.2%	A

CI = confidence interval, HR = hazard ratio, IR = incidence ratio, NK = not known, OR = odds ratio, RR = relative risk.
[a]Definitions for Levels of Evidence: Level A—evidence from one or more randomized, controlled clinical trials; Level B—evidence from nonrandomized clinical trials, prospective observational studies, cohort studies, retrospective studies, case-control studies, meta-analyses and/or postmarketing surveillance studies; and Level C—evidence from one or more published case reports or case series.
[b]Atrial fibrillation, 1–11%, atrial flutter, 1%.
[c]Binge drinkers.
[d]During the first 4–8 weeks of therapy.
[e]Reported following cardiac surgery only.
[f]Percent of patients with atrial fibrillation who develop new atrial flutter during propafenone therapy.[818]

regarding the cardiovascular safety of bisphosphonate drugs in which they stated there was "no clear association between overall bisphosphonate use and the rate of serious or nonserious atrial fibrillation in patients taking bisphosphonates."[845] Since that time, numerous cohort studies have been published indicating a significant association between bisphosphonate use and risk of new-onset atrial fibrillation.[752,835-837,843] In addition, several meta-analyses have reported that bisphosphonate drugs increase the risk of new-onset atrial fibrillation.[839-842,844] In contrast, however, numerous studies published since the FDA's 2008 statement have not found an association between bisphosphonate use and new-onset atrial fibrillation, and some meta-analyses have not reported an association between bisphosphonate drugs and new-onset atrial fibrillation.[846-852] In view of these discordant studies, the issue as to whether bisphosphonate drugs induced atrial fibrillation remains unresolved.

New-onset atrial flutter associated with drugs is also uncommon but has been reported to occur in patients with atrial fibrillation who are receiving Vaughan Williams class IC antiarrhythmic agents (flecainide or propafenone) or amiodarone (Table 26-13).

MECHANISMS

Mechanisms by which some drugs induce atrial fibrillation or flutter are presented in **Table 26-14**. In general, atrial fibrillation is believed to be induced by ectopic impulses originating from pulmonary veins, atria, or both and sustained via multiple atrial re-entrant wavelets.[853] Evidence indicates that the shorter the wavelength, the more likely that atrial fibrillation develops and is sustained.[854,855] Wavelength is the product of the atrial conduction velocity and the atrial effective refractory period.[854,855] Atrial flutter is generally a macro re-entrant atrial tachycardia due to a single re-entrant circuit involving the atrial septum, the lateral atrial wall, and the cavotricuspid isthmus between the annulus of the tricuspid valve and the inferior vena cava.[853]

Table 26-14 Mechanisms of Drug-Induced Atrial Fibrillation/Flutter

Drug	Mechanism
Adenosine	Promotes pulmonary vein ectopic activity Shortens atrial effective refractory period/ atrial wavelength
Alcohol	Sympathetic nervous system stimulation Shortens atrial effective refractory period Increases interatrial electromechanical delays Vagal activity
Amiodarone	Some cases likely due to thyrotoxicosis
Dobutamine	Enhances intracellular cAMP, resulting in increased myocyte cytosolic calcium, promoting depolarizations in pulmonary veins Shortens atrial effective refractory periods
Theophylline	Increases atrial automaticity
Other drugs	Unknown

cAMP = 3′–5′cyclic adenosine monophosphate.

Adenosine has been shown to induce atrial fibrillation via a direct stimulatory effect on pulmonary vein tissue, increasing pulmonary vein ectopic activity.[856] Adenosine has been also shown to shorten the atrial effective refractory period and, therefore, may promote reduction in atrial wavelength and the development of multiple re-entrant atrial wavelets.[857,858] There may be multiple mechanisms of alcohol-induced atrial fibrillation, including increased sympathetic nervous system stimulation, shortening of atrial effective refractory periods, increasing inter-atrial electromechanical delays, and/or via vagal activity.[733,742,859,860]

Mechanisms by which the bisphosphonate drugs alendronate and zoledronic acid could cause atrial fibrillation are unclear. It has been suggested that bisphosphonate drugs may cause atrial fibrillation through the release of inflammatory cytokines, which have been associated with the development of atrial fibrillation.[750,861,862] However, bisphosphonate drugs have been shown to directly shorten atrial action potential duration and effective refractory periods, suggesting that the drugs exert direct atrial electrophysiologic effects.[863] Further study is necessary to determine the mechanism of bisphosphonate-induced atrial fibrillation and to confirm that this is truly a disease that is induced by drugs from this class.

The mechanism by which ivabradine induces atrial fibrillation is unknown. Ivabradine inhibits hyperpolarization-activated cyclic nucleotide-gated (I_f) channels in the pulmonary veins, decreasing spontaneous electrical activity; this should translate to an antiaarhythmic action rather than atrial proarrhythmia.[864] Mechanisms underlying ivabradine-induced atrial fibrillation require further investigation.

Many of the drugs that have been reported to cause atrial fibrillation or atrial flutter have commonly been used for the management of these arrhythmias. Despite the fact that flecainide has been shown to be effective for the prevention and management of atrial fibrillation, data from studies in animals indicate that flecainide may shorten atrial conduction velocity and wavelength, effects which may promote the development of atrial fibrillation.[865,866] Amiodarone-induced atrial fibrillation may, at least in some cases, be due to amiodarone-induced thyrotoxicosis.[867,868] Dobutamine has been shown to shorten atrial effective refractory periods, while theophylline has been shown to increase atrial automaticity.[869,870] Mechanisms by which other drugs may induce atrial fibrillation or flutter require further study.

CLINICAL PRESENTATION AND DIFFERENTIAL DIAGNOSIS

The symptoms of drug-induced atrial fibrillation and atrial flutter are related to the degree of tachycardia and the resultant effect on blood pressure and cardiac output (**Table 26-15**). The symptoms of atrial fibrillation may be indistinguishable from those of atrial flutter, and, therefore, atrial fibrillation and atrial flutter must be distinguished from one another (and from other tachyarrhythmias) by ECG.

The onset of drug-induced atrial fibrillation or flutter is variable, depending on the inducing drug. Adenosine-induced atrial fibrillation or flutter occurs within 1 minute of administration of this extremely short-acting agent.[541] In a study of amiodarone or propafenone-induced atrial flutter, the mean (±SD) time of onset was 5 + 5.5 months after the initiation of treatment, whereas atrial flutter has been reported in association with flecainide therapy of 2 months' duration.[754,789] The duration of episodes of drug-induced atrial fibrillation or flutter is also somewhat variable; a case of albuterol-induced atrial fibrillation lasted several hours, whereas atrial flutter associated with amiodarone or

Table 26-15 Signs and Symptoms Associated with Drug-Induced Atrial Fibrillation/Flutter

- Fatigue
- Palpitations
- Dizziness
- Light-headedness
- Dyspnea
- Hypotension
- Chest pain (if underlying coronary artery disease is present)
- Heart failure symptoms
- Near-syncope
- Syncope

Table 26-16 Conditions to Consider in the Differential Diagnosis of Drug-Induced Atrial Fibrillation/Flutter

- Atrial fibrillation or flutter not induced by drugs
- Sinus tachycardia
- Atrial tachycardia
- Atrioventricular node re-entrant tachycardia
- Junctional tachycardia
- Ventricular tachycardia

propafenone may require intervention to terminate the arrhythmia.[722,754]

Sinus rhythm was the preceding rhythm in 88% of patients in whom adenosine-induced atrial fibrillation developed, whereas the remaining 12% of patients had atrial ectopic activity prior to the development of atrial fibrillation.[711] The mean ventricular rate associated with adenosine-induced atrial fibrillation was 107 + 43 bpm.[711] Adenosine-induced episodes of atrial fibrillation tend to be of short duration. The mean duration of episodes of atrial fibrillation associated with adenosine was 5.6 + 6.7 minutes (range, 8 seconds to 20.7 minutes).[711]

Conditions to consider in the differential diagnosis of drug-induced atrial fibrillation/flutter are presented in **Table 26-16**. Nondrug-induced atrial fibrillation/flutter must be considered; drug-induced atrial fibrillation/flutter is more likely in patients who are receiving drugs that have been reported to cause atrial fibrillation or flutter, particularly in patients with no known risk factors or causes for nondrug-induced atrial fibrillation/flutter, such as hypertension, ischemic heart disease, heart failure, valvular heart disease, rheumatic fever, or hyperthyroidism, or in those who have undergone thoracic surgery within the previous 2–5 days.

RISK FACTORS

Risk factors for drug-induced atrial fibrillation or flutter have not yet been fully characterized; known risk factors are presented in **Table 26-17**. Atrial fibrillation associated with adenosine does not appear to be related to sex or age and may occur in patients with no history of atrial fibrillation.[711] Atrial fibrillation induced by adenosine is not related to the type of arrhythmia being treated.[711] Premature atrial complexes occur significantly more frequently in patients who have experienced adenosine-induced atrial fibrillation (100%) compared with those who did not (58%) and, therefore, may be somewhat predictive of impending drug-induced atrial fibrillation.[711]

Table 26-17 Risk Factors for Drug-Induced Atrial Fibrillation/Flutter

Adenosine

- Premature atrial complexes

Alcohol

- Dose >30 g daily
- Withdrawal

Amiodarone

- Left atrial hypertrophy

Dobutamine

- Advancing age
- History of atrial fibrillation
- Combined history of atrial fibrillation and heart failure

Other drugs

- Unknown

Alcohol dose is a risk factor for alcohol-induced atrial fibrillation. In one study, the mean dose of alcohol consumed during the week prior to the atrial fibrillation episode was 186 g compared with 86 g in a control population in whom alcohol-induced atrial fibrillation did not develop.[732] Another study found that the risk of alcohol-induced atrial fibrillation was increased in patients who consumed more than an average of 30 g alcohol daily.[731] The risk of alcohol-induced atrial fibrillation increases with the number of drinks consumed, with the risk greatest for those patients who consume >21 drinks weekly, although as little as 1 alcoholic drink per day may increase the risk.[746,748] Alcohol withdrawal may increase the risk of alcohol-induced atrial fibrillation.[729]

In patients receiving amiodarone for treatment of atrial fibrillation, amiodarone-induced atrial flutter does not appear to be related to age, sex, presence of structural heart disease, left ventricular function, or duration of atrial fibrillation; however, left atrial enlargement (>40 mm) may be a risk factor.[754] Independent risk factors for dobutamine-induced atrial fibrillation include advancing age (OR 1.37 [95% CI 1.13–1.65]) per 10-year increase), history of atrial fibrillation (18.4 [12.2–27.7]), and combined history of atrial fibrillation and heart failure (7.98 [4.11–15.5]).[783]

MORBIDITY AND MORTALITY

Symptoms associated with drug-induced atrial fibrillation or flutter could potentially result in hospitalization or prolonged duration of stay in a hospital or critical care unit, although prolonged duration of hospital stay as a result of drug-induced atrial fibrillation or flutter has not been reported. Drug-induced atrial fibrillation could result in stroke, but this has not yet been described. Death due to drug-induced atrial fibrillation or flutter has not been reported.

PREVENTION

For the most part, specific methods of prevention of drug-induced atrial fibrillation or atrial flutter have not been determined. However, the risk of alcohol-induced atrial fibrillation can be minimized by avoiding binge drinking and excessive doses of alcohol, by consuming less than 30 g alcohol daily, and by consuming less than 15 drinks per week (**Table 26-18**).[741,742,746] Moretti et al.[801] reported the case of a patient treated with intermittent courses of high doses of intravenous methylprednisolone for multiple sclerosis in whom recurrent atrial fibrillation attributed to the corticosteroid developed. Pretreatment prophylaxis with sotalol was ineffective, but pretreatment prophylaxis with oral propafenone 300 mg three times daily was effective at preventing methylprednisolone-induced atrial fibrillation.

Table 26-18 Approaches to Help Prevent Drug-Induced Atrial Fibrillation/Flutter

Alcohol[741,742,746]

- Avoid binge drinking/excessive doses
- Consume <30 g daily
- Consume <15 drinks per week

Methylprednisolone[801]

- Propafenone 300 mg 3 times daily

Other drugs

- Administer lowest effective dose

MANAGEMENT

The causative agent should be discontinued. In a series of cases of adenosine-induced atrial fibrillation, 67% of patients converted to sinus rhythm spontaneously, whereas 33% required cardioversion.[711] Therefore, hemodynamically stable drug-induced atrial fibrillation or atrial flutter is associated with a high incidence of spontaneous conversion, and treatment may not be necessary. In patients who do not convert spontaneously to sinus rhythm, intravenous drugs for ventricular rate control should be administered (**Table 26-19**).[853] For patients with normal left ventricular function, an intravenous β-blocker or calcium-channel blocker should be administered. Diltiazem may be preferred over verapamil as a result of a lower risk of symptomatic hypotension.[871] For patients with HFrEF, intravenous calcium-channel blockers and β-blockers should be avoided because of the risk of exacerbation of heart failure; intravenous digoxin or amiodarone should be administered instead.[853] In patients with rapid heart rates that do not respond promptly to drug therapy for ventricular rate control, or in patients with atrial fibrillation/flutter in whom symptoms are unacceptable, direct-current cardioversion should be administered. However, if atrial fibrillation has been present for >48 hours, or if the duration of the episode of atrial fibrillation is unknown, patients should undergo transesophageal echocardiography to rule out an atrial thrombus before electrical or pharmacologic cardioversion is performed.

After the administration of agents to control the ventricular rate, drug-induced atrial fibrillation or flutter should be converted to sinus rhythm, using either elective direct-current cardioversion or pharmacologic cardioversion. Acceptable

Table 26-19 Treatment Options for Drug-Induced Atrial Fibrillation[853]

DISCONTINUE THE OFFENDING AGENT

Drug/Treatment	Recommended Doses
Ventricular rate control in patients with normal left ventricular function	
Esmolol	*Loading dose:* 500 mcg/kg IV over 1 minute *Maintenance infusion:* 50–300 mcg/kg/min IV
Metoprolol	2.5–5 mg IV bolus over 2 minutes; up to 3 doses at 10-minute intervals
Propranolol	1 mg IV over 1 minute; up to 3 doses at 2-minute intervals
Diltiazem	*Loading dose:* 0.25 mg/kg IV over 2 minutes *Maintenance infusion:* 5–15 mg/hr IV
Verapamil	0.075–0.15 mg/kg IV over 2 minutes If necessary, administer an additional dose of 10 mg 30 minutes later
Ventricular rate control in patients with heart failure with reduced ejection fraction	
Amiodarone	*Loading dose:* 300 mg IV over 1 hour *Maintenance infusion:* 10–50 mg/hr IV for up to 24 hours
Conversion to sinus rhythm	
Direct-current cardioversion	100 Joules, escalating if necessary
Amiodarone[a]	*Loading dose:* 150 mg IV over 10 minutes *Maintenance dose:* 1 mg/min continuous IV infusion for 6 hours, then 0.5 mg/min continuous IV infusion for 18 hours
Dofetilide	*CrCL >60 mL/min:* 500 mcg orally twice daily *CrCL 40–60 mL/min:* 250 mcg orally twice daily *CrCL 20–40 mL/min:* 125 mcg orally twice daily *CrCL <20 mL/min:* contraindicated
Flecainide[a]	200–300 mg single oral dose
Ibutilide	1 mg IV over 10 minutes; repeat with a second 1-mg dose 10 minutes after the first dose if atrial fibrillation persists
Propafenone[a]	600 mg single oral dose

CrCL = creatinine clearance, IV = intravenously.

[a]If the cause of the atrial fibrillation is a sodium channel-blocking drug (amiodarone, flecainide, propafenone), avoid the use of additional sodium channel-blocking agents and administer direct-current cardioversion or ibutilide. If the atrial fibrillation is caused by theophylline toxicity, administer activated charcoal 50–100 g, followed by 50 g q 4 hr. Alternatively, continuous hemodialysis with filtration may be performed.

agents for pharmacologic cardioversion include amiodarone, dofetilide, flecainide, ibutilide, or propafenone (Table 26-19). If the atrial fibrillation was induced by a sodium channel blocking agent, conversion to sinus rhythm should be achieved using direct-current cardioversion or ibutilide. It should be noted, however, that the effectiveness of antiarrhythmic drug therapy for drug-induced atrial fibrillation or atrial flutter has not been studied.

In patients with atrial fibrillation in whom new atrial flutter induced by amiodarone or propafenone develops, radiofrequency catheter ablation of the isthmus between the tricuspid annulus and the inferior vena cava has been used to terminate the atrial flutter while allowing patients to remain on antiarrhythmic drug therapy for the management of the atrial fibrillation.[754,755] Radiofrequency catheter ablation of drug-induced atrial flutter is successful in 90–100% of patients, and drug-induced atrial flutter did not recur in 14 of 15 patients during a 1-year follow-up period.[754]

If the drug-induced atrial fibrillation is a result of a theophylline overdose, activated charcoal may

Table 26-20 Agents Implicated in Drug-Induced Atrial Tachycardia

Drug	Incidence	Level of Evidence[a]
Albuterol[721]	NK	C
Caffeine[874-876]	NK	C
Digoxin[148,877-889]	0–4%	B
Phenylpropanolamine[875]	NK	C
Terbutaline[890]	NK	C
Theophylline[822,890-895]	0–16%[b]	B

[a]Definitions for Levels of Evidence: Level A—evidence from one or more randomized, controlled clinical trials; Level B—evidence from nonrandomized clinical trials, prospective observational studies, cohort studies, retrospective studies, case-control studies, meta-analyses and/or postmarketing surveillance studies; and Level C—evidence from one or more published case reports or case series.
[b]Incidence increases with increasing serum theophylline concentration.

be administered.[872] Alternatively, continuous hemodialysis with filtration may be performed.[827]

INFORMATION FOR PATIENTS

Patients who are taking drugs known to cause atrial fibrillation or flutter should be instructed that the medication, in rare instances, may cause the heart rate (pulse) to become faster. Patients should take their pulse daily and should be instructed to consult their pharmacist or physician if the heart rate increases to above 100–120 bpm, or if they feel palpitations, light-headed, dizzy, fatigued, weak, short of breath, or experience chest pain.

ATRIAL TACHYCARDIA

Atrial tachycardia is a supraventricular arrhythmia that is characterized on ECG by discrete P-waves and narrow or normal QRS duration, at a rate usually between 100 and 250 bpm.[873] There are two primary types of atrial tachycardia: focal atrial tachycardia (which will be referred to simply as atrial tachycardia), in which the arrhythmia is initiated at a single localized atrial focus, and multifocal atrial tachycardia, in which there are multiple atrial foci. Focal atrial tachycardia is characterized by regular intervals between QRS complexes on ECG, whereas multifocal atrial tachycardia is associated with irregular QRS intervals and three or more P-wave morphologies.[873] Atrial tachycardia may occur intermittently, which is commonly referred to as paroxysmal atrial tachycardia.

CAUSATIVE AGENTS

Drugs that have been reported to cause atrial tachycardia are listed in **Table 26-20**.[148,721,822,874-895]

EPIDEMIOLOGY

Paroxysmal atrial tachycardia is often described as a characteristic arrhythmia associated with digoxin toxicity.[885] However, at one large urban medical center, "definite" paroxysmal atrial tachycardia was documented in only 2% of 219 patients with a discharge diagnosis of digoxin intoxication.[148] In this analysis, paroxysmal atrial tachycardia occurred less frequently than any other arrhythmia associated with digoxin intoxication. Therefore, despite the commonly held belief that paroxysmal atrial tachycardia is commonly associated with digoxin toxicity, it appears to occur relatively rarely.

The incidence of multifocal atrial tachycardia associated with theophylline is dependent on serum theophylline concentrations.[895] In an analysis of 100 patients receiving theophylline, atrial tachycardia did not occur in the patients with serum theophylline concentrations <10 mcg/mL. However, in patients with serum theophylline concentrations between 10 and 20 mcg/mL, the incidence of atrial tachycardia was 8%, and the incidence rose to 16% in patients with serum theophylline concentrations >20 mcg/mL.[895]

Table 26-21 Mechanisms of Drug-Induced Atrial Tachycardia

Drug	Mechanism
Albuterol, terbutaline	Stimulation of β-receptors, leading to enhanced atrial automaticity
Caffeine, theophylline	Phosphodiesterase inhibition, leading to increased plasma concentrations of cyclic adenosine monophosphate, resulting in enhanced atrial automaticity
Digitalis glycoside toxicity	Extreme inhibition of the sodium–potassium–adenosine triphosphatase pump, leading to markedly increased myocyte concentrations of sodium, which are exchanged with calcium, ultimately resulting in markedly increased myocyte calcium concentrations, promoting enhanced atrial automaticity

MECHANISMS

Mechanisms of drug-induced atrial tachycardia are not entirely clear, but are likely related to increasing the automaticity of atrial tissue (**Table 26-21**).[873] This may occur because of β-receptor stimulation associated with drugs such as albuterol or terbutaline or through phosphodiesterase inhibition and the resulting elevated concentrations of cyclic adenosine monophosphate associated with caffeine or theophylline.

The mechanism of paroxysmal atrial tachycardia with AV nodal blockade associated with digitalis glycoside toxicity is likely related to profound inhibition of the sodium–potassium–adenosine triphosphatase pump. This leads to markedly increased myocyte sodium concentrations, which in turn are exchanged with calcium, ultimately resulting in markedly increased myocyte concentrations of calcium. This promotes enhanced atrial automaticity due to delayed phase-4 repolarization in the atrial action potential.[896]

CLINICAL PRESENTATION AND DIFFERENTIAL DIAGNOSIS

The symptoms of drug-induced atrial tachycardia are related to heart rate and the resultant effect on blood pressure and cardiac output (**Table 26-22**). The diagnosis of drug-induced atrial tachycardia must be made primarily on the basis of the appearance on ECG. Conditions to consider in the differential diagnosis of drug-induced atrial tachycardia are presented in **Table 26-23**.

Table 26-22 Signs and Symptoms Associated with Drug-Induced Atrial Tachycardia

- Palpitations
- Fatigue
- Dizziness
- Light-headedness
- Shortness of breath
- Chest pain (if underlying coronary artery disease is present)
- Near-syncope
- Syncope

Table 26-23 Conditions to Consider in the Differential Diagnosis of Drug-Induced Atrial Tachycardia

- Atrial fibrillation
- Atrial flutter
- Atrial tachycardia not induced by drugs
- Sinus tachycardia
- AV nodal re-entrant tachycardia
- Junctional tachycardia
- Ventricular tachycardia

AV = atrioventricular.

Table 26-24 Risk Factors for Drug-Induced Atrial Tachycardia

Digoxin

- Serum digoxin concentrations >2 ng/mL
- Kidney disease
- Drug interactions leading to elevated serum digoxin concentrations
- Hypomagnesemia

Theophylline

- Serum theophylline concentrations >20 mcg/mL

RISK FACTORS

Risk factors for drug-induced atrial tachycardia are presented in **Table 26-24**. Paroxysmal atrial tachycardia with AV block is extremely rare at therapeutic serum digoxin concentrations but occurs primarily when serum digoxin concentrations increase to >2 ng/mL. Therefore, risk factors for digoxin-induced paroxysmal atrial tachycardia with AV block are the same as those for digoxin toxicity. Because digoxin is cleared primarily by the kidneys, renal dysfunction is a primary risk factor for digoxin toxicity and digoxin-induced atrial tachycardia with AV block. In addition, drug interactions that result in increased serum digoxin concentrations enhance the risk of digoxin-related arrhythmias. Amiodarone, verapamil, and quinidine are known to significantly increase serum digoxin concentrations.[690-692]

Paroxysmal atrial tachycardia with AV block associated with digitalis toxicity may occur in patients across a wide range of ages. In one series, in which 31 cases of paroxysmal atrial tachycardia with AV block were reported in association with digitoxin, the age range of patients varied from 20 to 73 years (average, 52).[878] There were 15 women and 16 men, with a variety of underlying cardiovascular disorders, including valvular heart disease (n = 14), congenital heart diseases (n = 6), and ischemic heart disease (n = 1).[878] Although digoxin-induced atrial tachycardia most commonly occurs in patients with digoxin toxicity, it has been reported in patients with therapeutic serum digoxin concentrations who are hypomagnesemic.[889] As mentioned previously, elevated serum theophylline concentration is a risk factor for theophylline-induced atrial tachycardia. New supraventricular arrhythmias including multifocal atrial tachycardia were reported in seven patients with serum theophylline concentrations between 21 and 40 mcg/mL.[894]

MORBIDITY AND MORTALITY

Patients with paroxysmal atrial tachycardia with AV block may present to the emergency department and require hospitalization for management of digoxin toxicity. The incidence of mortality associated with digitalis-induced paroxysmal atrial fibrillation and AV block has not been reported, but is likely extremely low. In the series of 31 patients with digitoxin-induced paroxysmal atrial tachycardia, two patients died, but neither death appears to have been related to the arrhythmia or the digitoxin toxicity.[878] Patients with atrial tachycardia associated with other drugs may also present to the emergency department for treatment, particularly in the event of theophylline toxicity.

Table 26-25 Approaches to Help Prevent Drug-Induced Atrial Tachycardia

Digoxin

- Maintain serum digoxin concentrations <2 ng/mL
- Appropriate dose adjustment for kidney disease
- Appropriate dose adjustment in the presence of interacting drugs, particularly amiodarone, verapamil, or quinidine
- Maintain normal serum magnesium concentration

Theophylline

- Maintain serum theophylline concentrations <20 mcg/mL

PREVENTION

Digoxin-associated paroxysmal atrial tachycardia with AV nodal blockade is usually preventable by maintaining serum digoxin concentrations <2 ng/mL (**Table 26-25**). Measurement of serum digoxin concentrations is therefore recommended in patients who may be at risk for elevated concentrations, including patients with kidney disease or changing kidney function and those receiving concomitant therapy with drugs known to increase serum digoxin concentrations (particularly amiodarone, verapamil, or quinidine). In patients with kidney disease, appropriate dose adjustment should be made. In general, patients with calculated creatinine clearance ≤20 mL/min should receive an initial reduced digoxin dose of 0.125 mg daily.[897,898] In patients with calculated creatinine clearance <20 mL/min who are receiving concomitant therapy with drugs known to inhibit the elimination of digoxin, the initial digoxin dose should be 0.125 mg every other day. In patients taking digoxin, serum potassium and magnesium concentrations should be maintained within the normal range.

Atrial tachycardia associated with theophylline may be prevented by maintaining serum theophylline concentrations <20 mcg/mL.

MANAGEMENT

Treatment options for drug-induced atrial tachycardia are presented in **Table 26-26**. Digoxin-associated paroxysmal atrial tachycardia with AV nodal block should be managed by withholding digoxin therapy until

Table 26-26 Management of Drug-Induced Atrial Tachycardia

DISCONTINUE THE OFFENDING AGENT

Hemodynamic Stability	Recommended Doses
Hemodynamically unstable	Synchronized DC cardioversion (initial energy 50–100 J, focal atrial tachycardia; 120–200 J biphasic shock or 200 J monophasic shock for multifocal atrial tachycardia) *If due to digoxin toxicity:* Administer digoxin immune antibody fragments. The dose is based on the serum digoxin concentration: Number of 38-mg vials = serum digoxin concentration × weight (kg) ÷ 100. *If the arrhythmia is a result of an acute digoxin overdose and the amount of digoxin ingested is known, the dose of digoxin immune antibody fragments should be calculated as follows:* Number of 38-mg vials = mg digoxin ingested acutely × 0.8 ÷ 0.5. *If due to theophylline toxicity:* Administer activated charcoal: 50–100 g, followed by 50 g q 4 hr
Hemodynamically stable focal atrial tachycardia	Esmolol 500 mcg IV bolus over 1 minute, followed by 50–300 mcg/kg/min, with repeated boluses between each dose increase Or Metoprolol 2.5–5 mg IV bolus over 2 minutes; can repeat 2.5–5 mg IV bolus in 10 minutes, up to 3 doses Or Propranolol 1 mg IV over 1 minute; can repeat 1 mg IV at 2-minute intervals, up to 3 doses Or Diltiazem 0.25 mg/kg IV bolus over 2 minutes, followed by infusion at 5–10 mg/hr Or Verapamil 5–10 mg (0.075–0.15 mg/kg) IV bolus over 2 minutes; if no response, administer an additional 10 mg (0.15 mg/kg) 30 minutes after the first dose, then infusion at 0.005 mg/kg/min **For patients with HFrEF:** Adenosine 6 mg rapid IV injection bolus, administered over 1–2 seconds, followed by rapid saline flush; if no response within 1–2 minutes, administer 12 mg IV rapid bolus; a second 12 mg dose can be administered if necessary
Hemodynamically stable multifocal atrial tachycardia	IV metoprolol or verapamil at doses recommended above

DC = direct current, HFrEF = heart failure with reduced ejection fraction, IV = intravenous.

serum digoxin concentrations decline to <2 ng/mL. Because paroxysmal atrial tachycardia with AV block is rarely life-threatening, it is usually not necessary to administer digoxin immune antibody fragments. In the very rare event that the arrhythmia is hemodynamically unstable, synchronized direct-current cardioversion should be used to terminate the arrhythmia. Attempts to sedate the patient should be made, unless the urgency of the situation does not permit. Initial cardioversion energy should be 50–100 J for focal atrial tachycardia and 120–200 J biphasic or 200 J monophasic for multifocal atrial tachycardia. Following the conversion of hemodynamically unstable paroxysmal atrial tachycardia with AV block, digoxin immune antibody fragments should be administered to prevent recurrence of the hemodynamically unstable arrhythmia.

Hemodynamically stable drug-induced atrial tachycardia should be managed with intravenous β-blockers, diltiazem or verapamil.[873,892] Drug-induced atrial tachycardia may also be responsive to treatment with adenosine.[873] In patients with drug-induced atrial tachycardia who have HFrEF and are unresponsive to adenosine, intravenous amiodarone may be administered. If the drug-induced atrial tachycardia is a result of a theophylline overdose, activated charcoal may administered.[872] For patients with drug-induced multifocal atrial tachycardia, therapy with intravenous metoprolol or verapamil is recommended.[873]

INFORMATION FOR PATIENTS

Patients who are taking drugs that are known to cause atrial tachycardia should be instructed that the drug may in rare cases cause the heart rate (pulse) to become faster. Patients should be taught to take their pulse and to monitor their heart rate daily. Patients should be instructed to consult their pharmacist or physician if the heart rate increases above

Table 26-27 Agents Implicated in Drug-Induced Atrioventricular Node Re-entrant Tachycardia

Drug	Incidence	Level of Evidence[a]
Albuterol[721,899-908]	0–21%[b]	A
Caffeine[909-912,c]	NK	C
Carbamazepine[913]	NK	C
Clozapine[911,914,915]	NK	C
Dobutamine[771,772,782,916-929]	0–12%	A
Enoximone[916]	NK	A
Fluoxetine[930, 931]	NK	C
Furosemide[932]	NK	C
Ipratropium[933,934]	0.5%	A
Methylprednisolone[935,936]	NK	C
Phenylpropanolamine[937]	NK	C
Theophylline[721,824,892,894,899,938,939]	NK[b]	C

NK = not known.

[a]Definitions for Levels of Evidence: Level A—evidence from one or more randomized, controlled clinical trials; Level B—evidence from nonrandomized clinical trials, prospective observational studies, cohort studies, retrospective studies, case-control studies, meta-analyses and/or postmarketing surveillance studies; and Level C—evidence from one or more published case reports or case series.

[b]Incidence reported to be up to 76% in patients receiving concomitant therapy with albuterol and theophylline.

[c]Suicide attempt or overdose, 2.7–35 g caffeine ingested; one case with intravenous caffeine administration, one case with intradermal caffeine administration.

100–120 bpm or if they feel light-headed, dizzy, tired, weak, or short of breath, or experience chest pain.

AV NODE RE-ENTRANT TACHYCARDIA

AV node re-entrant tachycardia (AVNRT) is the most common form of the group of arrhythmias commonly referred to as paroxysmal supraventricular tachycardia. AVNRT is characterized on ECG by regular, narrow QRS complexes, often with an absence of discernible P-waves.[873]

CAUSATIVE AGENTS

Drugs that have been associated with AVNRT are listed in **Table 26-27**.[721,771,772,782,824,892,894,899-939]

EPIDEMIOLOGY

The incidence of drug-induced AVNRT is largely unknown. The incidences of AVNRT associated with albuterol, dobutamine, and ipratropium are presented in Table 26-27.

MECHANISMS

Mechanisms of drug-induced AVNRT are somewhat unclear. Nondrug-related AVNRT was previously thought to be caused by a re-entrant circuit involving the AV node, in which there is antegrade conduction over the slow-conducting portion of the circuit and retrograde conduction over the faster-conducting portion.[940,941] However, it is now recognized that the re-entrant circuit often is not confined to the AV node, but involves perinodal tissue.[873] AV nodal or perinodal re-entry is usually initiated by a premature atrial impulse that "uncovers" the latent re-entrant circuit by creating the circumstances required for re-entry, namely, unidirectional block in the fast pathway and further slowing of impulse conduction down the slow pathway. Therefore, it is possible that drugs that cause AVNRT do so by stimulating premature atrial depolarizations that provoke AV nodal re-entry. In cases of AVNRT that occurred in association with continuous furosemide infusions in infants or children after cardiac surgery, the authors speculated that a rapid change in intravascular volume may have contributed to the development of the arrhythmias, possibly as a result

Table 26-28 Signs and Symptoms Associated with Drug-Induced Atrioventricular Node Re-entrant Tachycardia

- Palpitations
- Dizziness
- Fatigue
- Light-headedness
- Shortness of breath
- Chest pain (if underlying coronary artery disease is present)
- Near-syncope
- Syncope

Table 26-29 Conditions to Consider in the Differential Diagnosis of Drug-Induced Atrioventricular Node Re-entrant Tachycardia

- Atrial fibrillation
- Atrial flutter
- Atrial tachycardia
- Sinus tachycardia
- Junctional tachycardia
- AV nodal re-entrant tachycardia not induced by drugs
- Ventricular tachycardia

AV = atrioventricular.

of intercompartmental electrolyte shifts.[932] Overall, the mechanisms by which drug-induced AVNRT occurs have not been determined but are likely related to stimulation of premature atrial depolarizations, alterations in AV nodal conduction velocity or repolarization, or both.

CLINICAL PRESENTATION AND DIFFERENTIAL DIAGNOSIS

The symptoms of drug-induced AVNRT are similar to those of other tachyarrhythmias (**Table 26-28**) and are related to heart rate and the resultant effect on blood pressure and cardiac output. Ventricular rates associated with drug-induced AVNRT can be quite fast, ranging from 150 to 300 bpm.[931,932,937] Conditions to consider in the differential diagnosis of drug-induced AVNRT are presented in **Table 26-29**. The diagnosis of AVNRT must be made primarily on the basis of the appearance of the rhythm on ECG.

Table 26-30 Risk Factors for Drug-Induced Atrioventricular Node Re-entrant Tachycardia

Albuterol

- Continuous intravenous infusion
- Intravenous infusion rate >60 mcg/min
- Concomitant therapy with theophylline

Dobutamine

- Male sex
- Elderly
- Myocardial infarction score on dobutamine stress test

Furosemide

- Reported only in infants or children following cardiac surgery
- Continuous infusion resulting in profound diuresis (8–10 mL/kg/hr)

Theophylline

- Serum theophylline concentrations >20 mcg/mL
- Concomitant therapy with albuterol

RISK FACTORS

Known or potential risk factors for drug-induced AVNRT are presented in **Table 26-30**. Albuterol-induced AVNRT appears to be more likely in patients receiving the drug intravenously, particularly at infusion rates >60 mcg/min.[890,900] AVNRT associated with dobutamine occurs more commonly in men than in women and in elderly patients.[774,921,922] In addition, severity of myocardial ischemia has been shown to be an independent predictor of dobutamine-induced AVNRT; in a study of 1,076 patients undergoing dobutamine stress myocardial perfusion imaging, the mean myocardial infarction score (calculated based on assessment of fixed perfusion defects during myocardial perfusion scintigraphy) was 4.4 ± 4.1 in patients with AVNRT, as compared with 2.8 ± 3.5 in those without it, and the infarction score was an independent predictor of AVNRT.[922]

All of the reported cases of AVNRT associated with continuous furosemide infusions ($n = 3$ patients) have occurred in infants or children after cardiac surgery. In these patients, the arrhythmia occurred within 3–7 hours after the initiation of a furosemide infusion of 1 mg/kg/hr. A common factor in these three patients was substantial diuresis resulting from the furosemide, in the range of

8–10 mL/kg/hr, as compared with an average fluid elimination of 2.5 mL/kg/hr in 22 other patients who had received a similar furosemide infusion.[932] Serum potassium concentration was below normal limits in one of the three patients in whom the arrhythmia developed but remained normal in the other two cases. Therefore, it is possible that a large amount of fluid loss may be a risk factor or predictor of drug-induced AVNRT in infants or children receiving a continuous infusion of furosemide after cardiac surgery. Serum theophylline concentration is a risk factor for theophylline-induced supraventricular arrhythmias; new supraventricular arrhythmias were reported in seven patients with serum theophylline concentrations between 21 and 40 mcg/mL.[894] Risk factors for AVNRT associated with other drugs have not been identified.

MORBIDITY AND MORTALITY

Drug-induced AVNRT may result in symptoms sufficient to result in presentation to the emergency department and hospitalization.[909,910,930,934] In addition, drug-induced AVNRT may result in prolongation of stays in the intensive care unit and the hospital.[931,932] Mortality associated with drug-induced AVNRT is likely quite rare.

PREVENTION

The likelihood of albuterol-induced AVNRT may be reduced by avoiding continuous intravenous infusions at doses >60 mcg/min (**Table 26-31**). Combinations of drugs that may induce AVNRT should be avoided, particularly the concomitant administration of albuterol and theophylline. In the cases of furosemide-induced AVNRT in infants and children after cardiac surgery, substantial fluid elimination appears to have been a risk factor, and in that population, avoidance of diuresis of volumes >2.5 mL/kg/hr over periods of 3–7 hours may minimize the risk.[932] Maintaining serum theophylline concentrations <20 mcg/mL reduces the risk of theophylline-induced supraventricular arrhythmias.

Table 26-31 Approaches to Help Prevent Drug-Induced Atrioventricular Node Re-entrant Tachycardia

Albuterol

- Avoid continuous intravenous infusions at rate >60 mcg/min
- Avoid concomitant therapy with theophylline

Furosemide

- Avoid diuresis of volumes >2.5 mL/kg/hr over periods of 3–7 hr in infants/children after cardiac surgery

Theophylline

- Maintain serum theophylline concentrations <20 mcg/ mL
- Avoid concomitant therapy with albuterol

MANAGEMENT

Management options for drug-induced AVNRT are presented in **Table 26-32**. As with other drug-induced arrhythmias, initial management of drug-induced AVNRT is discontinuation of therapy with the offending agent. If the patient is hemodynamically unstable, synchronized direct-current cardioversion should be administered, using an initial energy of 50–100 J.[695] Sedation of the patient is always preferred unless hemodynamic instability is so severe that there is no time for sedation.

In patients who are hemodynamically stable, drug-induced AVNRT may respond to agents typically used to treat nondrug-induced AVNRT.[873] Adenosine has been found to be effective for AVNRT associated with albuterol and may be used as a drug of first choice for hemodynamically stable AVNRT.[873,903,907] Intravenous verapamil 2.5 mg has been effective for terminating AVNRT associated with fluoxetine.[931]

INFORMATION FOR PATIENTS

Patients who are taking drugs that may cause AVNRT should be instructed that the medication may, in rare instances, cause the heart rate (pulse) to become faster. Patients should be instructed to take their pulse daily and to consult their pharmacist or

Table 26-32 Management Options for Drug-Induced Atrioventricular Node Re-entrant Tachycardia[873]

In hemodynamically unstable patients:	In hemodynamically stable patients:
Discontinue the offending agent	Discontinue the offending agent
Synchronized DC cardioversion (initial energy 50–100 J)	Vagal maneuvers (cough, carotid sinus massage, Valsalva)
	Adenosine 6 mg IV rapid bolus, followed by saline flush
	If no response within 2 minutes, adenosine 12 mg IV rapid bolus, followed by saline flush; can administer a second 12 mg dose if necessary
	If no response to adenosine and patient has LVEF >40% and/or no history of HFrEF: IV β-blocker, diltiazem or verapamil at doses listed in Table 26-26
	If no response to IV β-blocker, diltiazem or verapamil: synchronized DC cardioversion
	If no response to adenosine in patient with HFrEF: synchronized DC cardioversion

DC = direct current, HFrEF = heart failure with reduced ejection fraction, IV = intravenous, J = Joules, LVEF = left ventricular ejection fraction.

physician if the heart rate increases to above 100–120 bpm, or if they feel palpitations, light-headed, dizzy, tired, weak, or short of breath, or experience chest pain.

REFERENCES

1. Mangrum JM, DiMarco JP. The evaluation and management of bradycardia. *N Engl J Med.* 2000; 342:703-9.
2. Kaushik V, Leon AR, Forrester JS et al. Bradyarrhythmias, temporary and permanent pacing. *Crit Care Med.* 2000; 28(suppl):N121-N128.
3. Vogler JV, Breithardt G, Eckardt L. Bradyarrhythmias and conduction blocks. *Rev Esp Cardiol* 2012; 65:656-67.
4. DiMarco JP, Miles W, Akhtar M et al. Adenosine for paroxysmal supraventricular tachycardia: dose ranging and comparison with verapamil: assessment in placebo controlled, multicenter trials. *Ann Intern Med.* 1990; 113:104-10.
5. Madsen CD, Pointer JE, Lynch TG. A comparison of adenosine and verapamil for the treatment of supraventricular tachycardia in the hospital setting. *Ann Emerg Med.* 1995; 25:649-55.
6. Littmann L, Anderson JD, Monroe MH. Adenosine and Aggrenox: a hazardous combination. *Ann Intern Med.* 2002; 137:W1.
7. Roy D, Talajic M, Dorian P et al. Amiodarone to prevent recurrence of atrial fibrillation: Canadian Trial of Atrial Fibrillation Investigators. *N Engl J Med.* 2000; 342:913-20.
8. The AFFIRM First Antiarrhythmic Drug Substudy Investigators: maintenance of sinus rhythm in patients with atrial fibrillation: an AFFIRM substudy of the first antiarrhythmic drug. *J Am Coll Cardiol.* 2003; 42:20-9.
9. Essebag V, Hadjis T, Platt RW et al. Effect of amiodarone dose on the risk of permanent pacemaker insertion. *Pacing Clin Electrophysiol.* 2004; 27:1519-25.
10. Patel AA, White CM, Gillespie EL et al. Safety of amiodarone in the prevention of postoperative atrial fibrillation: a meta-analysis. *Am J Health-Syst Pharm.* 2006; 63:829-37.
11. Bongard V, Marc D, Philippe V et al. Incidence rate of adverse drug reactions during long-term follow-up of patients newly treated with amiodarone. *Am J Ther.* 2006; 13:315-9.
12. Santangeli P, Di Biase L, Burkhardt JD et al. Examining the safety of amiodarone. *Expert Opin Drug Saf.* 2012; 11:191-214.
13. Shibata SC, Uchiyama A, Ohta N et al. Efficacy and safety of landiolol compared to amiodarone for the management of postoperative atrial fibrillation in intensive care patients. *J Cardiothorac Vasc Anesth.* 2016; 30:418-22.
14. Ad N, Holmes SD, Shuman DJ et al. Amiodarone after surgical ablation for atrial fibrillation: is it really necessary? A prospective, randomized controlled trial. *J Thorac Vasc Anesth.* 2016; 151:789-803.
15. Huang LC, Huang LY, Tseng SY et al. Amisulpride and symptomatic bradycardia: a case report. *Gen Hosp Psychiatry.* 2015; 37:497.e1-2.
16. Perry HE, Wright RO, Shannon MW et al. Baclofen overdose: drug experimentation in a group of adolescents. *Pediatrics.* 1998; 101:1045-8.
17. Endmann M, Kutz R. Baclofen-intoxication in a child resulting in coma, bradycardia, and transitory defect of visual power. *Klin Padiatr.* 2005; 217:89-91.
18. Leung NY, Whyte IM, Isbister GK. Baclofen overdose: defining the spectrum of toxicity. *Emerg Med Australas.* 2006; 18:77-82.
19. Smit CAJ, Slim EJ. Heart conduction problems in a tetraplegic patients caused by a single therapeutic dosage of Baclofen. *Spinal Cord.* 2008; 46:317-8.
20. Dasarwar N, Shanbag P, Kumbhare N. Baclofen intoxication after accidental ingestion in a 3-year-old child. *Indian J Pharmacol.* 2009; 41:89-90.
21. Rifici C, D'Aleo G, D'Aleo P et al. Cardiovascular alterations heralded by intrathecal baclofen bolus. *NeuroRehabilitation.* 2011; 28:389-93.
22. Weißhaar GF, Hoemberg M, Bender K et al. Baclofen intoxication: a "fun drug" causing deep coma and nonconvulsive status epilepticus—a case report and review of the literature. *Eur J Pediatr* 2012; 171:1541-7.
23. Kiel LB, Hoegberg LC, Jansen T et al. A nationwide register-based survey of baclofen toxicity. *Basic Clin Pharmacol Toxicol.* 2015; 116:452-6.
24. Sechrist C, Kinsman S, Cain N. Profound bradycardia after intrathecal baclofen injection in a patient with hydranencephaly. *Pediatr Neurol.* 2015; 53:532-4.
25. Hjalmarson A, Goldstein S, Fagerberg B et al. Effects of controlled-release metoprolol on total mortality, hospitalizations, and

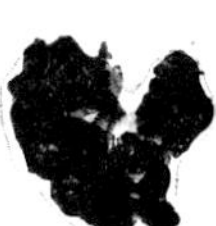

well-being in patients with heart failure: the Metoprolol CR/XL Randomized Intervention Trial in congestive heart failure (MERIT-HF): MERIT-HF Study Group. *JAMA.* 2000; 283:1295-302.

26. Ko DT, Hebert PR, Coffey CS et al. Adverse effects of β-blocker therapy for patients with heart failure: a quantitative overview of randomized trials. *Arch Intern Med.* 2004; 164:1389-94.
27. Dungen HD, Apostolovic S, Inkrot S et al. Titration to target dose of bisoprolol vs. carvedilol in elderly patients with heart failure: the CIBIS-ELD trial. *Eur J Heart Fail.* 2011; 13:670-80.
28. Barron AJ, Zaman N, Cole D et al. Systematic review of genuine versus spurious side-effects of beta-blockers in heart failure using placebo control: recommendation for patient information. *Int J Cardiol.* 2013; 168:3572-9.
29. Ptaszynski P, Kaczmarek K, Ruta J et al. Metoprolol succinate vs ivabradine in the treatment of inappropriate sinus tachycardia in patients unresponsive to previous pharmacological therapy. *Europace.* 2013; 15:116-21.
30. Roberts MA, Pilmore HL, Ierino FL et al. The β-blocker to lower cardiovascular dialysis events (BLOCADE) feasibility study: a randomized controlled trial. *Am J Kidney Dis.* 2016; 67:902-11.
31. Bateman BT, Patorno E, Desai RJ et al. Late pregnancy β blocker exposure and risks of neonatal hypoglycemia and bradycardia. *Pediatrics.* 2016; Sep;138. pii: e20160731.
32. Leaute-Labreze C, Boccara O, Degrugillier C et al. Safety of oral propranolol for the treatment of infantile hemangioma: a systematic review. *Pediatrics.* 2016; Oct;138. pii: e20160353.
33. von Alvensleben JC, LaPage MJ, Caruthers T et al. Nadolol for treatment of supraventricular tachycardia in infants and young children. *Pediatr Cardiol.* 2017; 38:525-30.
34. Jiang J, Cong H, Zhang Y et al. Effect of metoprolol succinate in patients with stable angina and elevated heart rate receiving low-dose β-blocker therapy. *Int J Med Sci.* 2017; 14:477-83.
35. Naguib M, Magboul MM, Samarkandi AH et al. Adverse effects and drug interactions associated with local and regional anaesthesia. *Drug Saf.* 1998; 18:221-50.
36. Martinek RM. Witnessed asystole during spinal anesthesia treated with atropine and ondansetron: a case report. *Can J Anaesth.* 2004; 51:226-30.
37. Fattorini F, Ricci Z, Rocco A et al. Levobupivacaine versus racemic bupivacaine for spinal anaesthesia in orthopedic major surgery. *Minerva Anestesiol.* 2006; 72:637-44.
38. Aydin F, Akan B, Susleyen C et al. Comparison of bupivacaine alone and in combination with sufentanil in patients undergoing arthroscopic knee surgery. *Knee Surg Sports Tarmatol Arthrosc.* 2011; 19:1915-9.
39. Tiwari AK, Tomar GS, Agrawal J. Intrathecal bupivacaine in comparison with a combination of nalbuphine and bupivacaine for subarachnoid block: a randomized prospective double-blind clinical study. *Am J Ther.* 2013; 20:592-5.
40. Acar NS, Uzman S, Toptas M et al. Spinal anesthesia with hyperbaric bupivacaine: a comparison of hypertensive and normotensive patients. *Med Sci Monitor.* 2013; 19:1109-13.
41. Imbelloni LE, Gouveia MA. A comparison of thoracic spinal anesthesia with low-dose isobaric and low-dose hyperbaric bupivacaine for orthopedic surgery: a randomized controlled trial. *Anesth Essays Res.* 2014; 8:26-31.
42. Tomak Y, Erdivanli B, Sen A et al. Effect of cooled hyperbaric bupivacaine on unilateral spinal anesthesia success rate and hemodynamic complications in inguinal hernia surgery. *J Anesth.* 2016; 30:26-30.
43. Bhar D, RoyBasunia S, Das A et al. Repeat spinal anesthesia in cesarean section: a comparison between 10 mg and 12 mg doses of intrathecal hyperbaric (0.05%) bupivacaine repeated after failed spinal anesthesia: a prospective, parallel group study. *Anesth Essays Res.* 2016; 10:362-9.
44. Ang C, Kornbluth K, Thirlwell MP et al. Capecitabine-induced cardiotoxicity: case report and review of the literature. *Curr Oncol.* 2010; 17:59-63.
45. Tunio MA, Hashmi A, Shoaib M. Capecitabine induced cardiotoxicity: a case report and review of the literature. *Pak J Pharm Sci.* 2012; 25:277-81.
46. Takayanagi K, Hisauchi I, Watanabe J et al. Carbamazepine-induced sinus node dysfunction and atrioventricular block in elderly women. *Jpn Heart J.* 1998; 39:469-79.
47. Kaul S, Meena NK, Murthy JM. Carbamazepine induced bradycardia. *Neurol India.* 2002; 48:403-4.
48. Reding P, Devroede C, Barbier P. Bradycardia after cimetidine. *Lancet.* 1977; 2:1227.
49. Jefferys DB, Vale JA. Cimetidine and bradycardia. *Lancet.* 1978; 1:828.
50. Hiss J, Hepler BR, Falkowski AJ et al. Fatal bradycardia after intentional overdose of cimetidine and diazepam. *Lancet.* 1982; 2:982.
51. Matthews SJ, Michelson PA, Cersosimo RJ. Cimetidine-induced sinus bradycardia. *Clin Pharm.* 1982; 1:556-8.
52. Tanner LA, Arrowsmith JB. Bradycardia and H2 antagonists. *Ann Intern Med.* 1988; 109:434-5.
53. Cohen N, Modai D, Golik A et al. Cimetidine-related cardiac conduction disturbances and confusion. *J Clin Gastroenterol.* 1989; 11:68-9.
54. Hulisz DT, Welko JR, Heiselman DE. Sinus arrest associated with continuous-infusion cimetidine. *Pharmacotherapy.* 1993; 13:64-7.
55. Schlaeffer F, Tovi F, Leiberman A. Cisplatin-induced bradycardia. *Drug Intell Clin Pharm.* 1983; 17:899-901.
56. Rowinsky EK, Gilbert MR, McGuire WP et al. Sequences of taxol and cisplatin: a phase I and pharmacologic study. *J Clin Oncol.* 1991; 9:1692-703.
57. Altundagˇ O, Celik I, Kars A. Recurrent asymptomatic bradycardia episodes after cisplatin infusion. *Ann Pharmacother.* 2001; 35:641-2.
58. Schlumbrecht MP, Hehr K. Cisplatin-induced bradycardia and the importance of the QT interval. *J Oncol Pharm Pract.* 2015; 21:157-60.
59. Darling HS. Cisplatin induced bradycardia. *Int J Cardiol.* 2015; 182:304-6.
60. Kucharz J, Michalowska-Kaczmarczyk A, Zygulska AL et al. Bradycardia as a rare symptom of cisplatin cardiotoxicity: a case report. *Oncol Lett.* 2016; 11:2297-9.
61. Favre MP, Sztajzel J, Bertschy G. Bradycardia during citalopram treatment: a case report. *Pharmacol Res.* 1999; 39:149-50.
62. Rothenhäusler HB, Hoberl C, Ehrentrout S et al. Suicide attempt by pure citalopram overdose causing long-lasting severe sinus bradycardia, hypotension and syncopes: successful therapy with a temporary pacemaker. *Pharmacopsychiatry.* 2000; 33:150-2.
63. Isbister GK, Prior FH, Foy A. Citalopram-induced bradycardia and presyncope. *Ann Pharmacother.* 2001; 35:1552-5.
64. Barak Y, Swartz M, Levy D et al. Age-related differences in the side effect profile of citalopram. *Prog Neuropsychopharmacol Biol Psychiatry.* 2003; 27:545-8.
65. Padala KP, Padala PR, Wengel SP. Dose-dependent bradycardia with citalopram in an elderly patient. *Prim Care Companion J Clin Psychiatry.* 2010; 12:PCC.09100789.
66. Pai GS, Lipsitz DJ. Clonidine poisoning. *Pediatrics.* 1976; 58:749-50.
67. MacFaul R, Miller G. Clonidine poisoning in children. *Lancet.* 1977; 1:1266-7.
68. van Etta L, Burchell H. Severe bradycardia with clonidine. *JAMA.* 1978; 240:2047.
69. Neuvonen PJ, Vilska J, Keränen A. Severe poisoning in a child caused by a small dose of clonidine. *Clin Toxicol.* 1979; 14:369-74.
70. Anderson RJ, Hart GR, Crumpler CP et al. Clonidine overdose: report of six cases and review of the literature. *Ann Emerg Med.* 1981; 10:107-12.
71. Artman M, Boerth RC. Clonidine poisoning: a complex problem. *Am J Dis Child.* 1983; 137:171-4.

72. Olsson JM, Pruitt AW. Management of clonidine ingestion in children. *J Pediatr.* 1983; 103:646-50.
73. Marruecos L, Roglan A, Frati ME et al. Clonidine overdose. *Crit Care Med.* 1983; 11:959-60.
74. Schwartz E, Friedman E, Mouallem M et al. Sinus arrest associated with clonidine therapy. *Clin Cardiol.* 1988; 11:53-4.
75. Byrd BF 3rd, Collins HW, Primm RK. Risk factors for severe bradycardia during oral clonidine therapy for hypertension. *Arch Intern Med.* 1988; 148:729-33.
76. Dawson PM, Vander Zanden JA, Werkman SL et al. Cardiac dysrhythmia with the use of clonidine in explosive disorder. *DICP.* 1989; 23:465-6.
77. Bonnet F, Boico O, Rostaing S et al. Clonidine-induced analgesia in postoperative patients: epidural versus intramuscular administration. *Anesthesiology.* 1990; 72:423-7.
78. Wiley JF 2nd, Wiley CC, Torrey SB et al. Clonidine poisoning in young children. *J Pediatr.* 1990; 116:654-8.
79. Heidemann SM, Sarnaik AP. Clonidine poisoning in children. *Crit Care Med.* 1990; 18:618-20.
80. Harris JM. Clonidine patch toxicity. *DICP.* 1990; 24:1191-4.
81. Raber JH, Shinar C, Finkelstein S. Clonidine patch ingestion in an adult. *Ann Pharmacother.* 1993; 27:719-22.
82. Rosenblum D. Clonidine-induced bradycardia in patients with spinal cord injury. *Arch Phys Med Rehabil.* 1993; 74:1206-7.
83. Golusinski LL Jr, Blount BW. Clonidine-induced bradycardia. *J Fam Pract.* 1995; 41:399-401.
84. Owen MD, Fibuch EE, McQuillan R et al. Postoperative analgesia using a low-dose, oral-transdermal clonidine combination: lack of clinical efficacy. *J Clin Anesth.* 1997; 9:8-14.
85. Van Elstraete AC, Pastureau F, Lebrun T et al. Caudal clonidine for postoperative analgesia in adults. *Br J Anaesth.* 2000; 84:401-2.
86. Nishina K, Mikawa K, Uesugi T et al. Efficacy of clonidine for prevention of perioperative myocardial ischemia: a critical appraisal and meta-analysis of the literature. *Anesthesiol.* 2002; 96:323-9.
87. Klein-Schwartz W. Trends and toxic effects from pediatric clonidine exposures. *Arch Pediatr Adolesc Med.* 2002; 156:392-6.
88. Sinha Y, Cranswick NE. Clonidine poisoning in children: a recent experience. *J Paediatr Child Health.* 2004; 40:678-80.
89. Spiller HA, Klein-Schwartz W, Colvin JM et al. Toxic clonidine ingestion in children. *J Pediatr.* 2005; 146:263-6.
90. Horowitz R, Mazor SS, Aks SE et al. Accidental clonidine patch ingestion in a child. *Am J Ther.* 2005; 12:272-4.
91. Daviss WB, Patel NC, Robb AS et al. Clonidine for attention-deficit/ hyperactivity disorder: II. ECG changes and adverse events analysis. *J Am Acad Child Adolesc Psychiatry.* 2008; 47:189-98.
92. Rangan C, Everson G, Cantrell FL. Central alpha-2 adrenergic eye drops: case series of 3 pediatric systemic poisonings. *Pediatr Emerg Care.* 2008; 24:167-9.
93. Popping DM, Elia N, Marret E et al. Clonidine as an adjuvant to local anesthetics for peripheral nerve and plexus blocks: a meta-analysis of randomized trials. *Anesthesiology.* 2009; 111:406-15.
94. Gupta K, Sharma D, Gupta PK. Oral premedication with pregabalin or clonidine for hemodynamic stability during laryngoscopy and laparoscopic cholecystectomy: a comparative evaluation. *Saudi J Anaesth.* 2011; 5:179-84.
95. Soltani Mohammadi S, Maziar A, Saliminia A. Comparing clonidine and lidocaine on attenuation of hemodynamic response to laryngoscopy and tracheal intubation in controlled hypertensive patients: a randomized, double-blinded clinical trial. *Anesth Pain Med.* 2016; 27 Mar;6:e34271. eCollection 2016 Apr.
96. Cates AL, Wheatley SM, Katz KD. Clonidine overdose in a toddler due to accidental ingestion of a compounding cream. *Pedriatr Emerg Care.* 2018; 34:e79-e81.
97. Parveen S, Negi DS, Kumar R et al. Oral clonidine vs oral pregabalin premedication to attenuate pressor response to direct laryngoscopy in patients undergoing laparoscopic cholecystectomy: a randomized double blind study. *J Clin Diagn Res.* 2016; 10:UC21-UC25.
98. Isbister GK, Heppell SP, Page CB et al. Adult clonidine overdose: prolonged bradycardia and central nervous system depression, but not severe toxicity. *Clin Toxicol.* 2017; 55:187-92.
99. Banerjee G, Nath PK, Halder R et al. Prophylactic use of intravenous clonidine compared to tramadol in prevention of intraoperative shivering under regional anesthesia. *Anesth Essays Res.* 2017; 11:477-82.
100. Pitner JK, Mintzer JE, Pennypacker LC et al. Efficacy and adverse effects of clozapine in four elderly psychotic patients. *J Clin Psychiatry.* 1995; 56:180-5.
101. Tupala E, Niskanen L, Tiihonen J. Transient syncope and ECG changes associated with the concurrent administration of clozapine and diazepam. *J Clin Psychiatry.* 1999; 60:619-20.
102. Castro VJ, Nacht R. Cocaine-induced bradyarrhythmia: an unsuspected cause of syncope. *Chest.* 2000; 117:275-7.
103. Sharma J, Rathnayaka N, Green C et al. Bradycardia as a marker of chronic cocaine use: a novel cardiovascular finding. *Behav Med.* 2016; 42:1-8.
104. Mahoney JJ 3rd, Haile CN, De La Garza L 2nd et al. Electrocardiographic characteristics in individuals with cocaine use disorder. *Am J Addict.* 2017; 26:221-7.
105. Franklin SM, Thihalolipavan S, Fontaine JM. Sinus bradycardia in habitual cocaine users. *Am J Cardiol.* 2017; 119:1611-5.
106. Stamatopoulos K, Kanellopoulou G, Vaiopoulos G et al. Evidence for sinoatrial blockade associated with high dose cytarabine therapy. *Leuk Res.* 1998; 22:759-61.
107. Cil T, Kaplan MA, Altintas A et al. Cytosine-arabinoside induced bradycardia in patient with non-Hodgkin lymphoma: a case report. *Leuk Lymphoma.* 2007; 48:1247-9.
108. Romani C, Pettinau M, Murru R et al. Sinusal bradycardia after receiving intermediate or high dose cytarabine: four cases from a single institution. *Eur J Cancer Care.* 2009; 18:320-1.
109. Wayangankar SA, Patel BC, Parekh HD et al. High-dose cytosine arabinoside-induced symptomatic bradycardia. *J Cardiovasc Med.* 2015;16(suppl 1):S38-41.
110. Ohlsson A, Heyman E. Dexamethasone-induced bradycardia (letter). *N Engl J Med.* 1988; 2:1074.
111. Mursch K, Buhre W, Behnke-Mursch J et al. Peroperative cardiovascular stability during brainstem surgery. The use of high-dose methylprednisolone compared to dexamethasone. A retrospective analysis. *Acta Anaesthesiol Scand.* 2000; 44:378-82.
112. Marinov M, Fuessel MU, Unterrainer AF. Bradycardia after dexamethasone for postoperative nausea and vomiting prophylaxis during induction of anaesthesia. *Br J Anaesth.* 2013; 111:1025-6.
113. John PR, Khaladj-Ghom A, Still KL. Bradycardia associated with steroid use for laryngeal edema in an adult: a case report and literature review. *Case Rep Cardiol.* 2016; 2016:9785467.
114. Aantaa R, Kanto J, Scheinin M. Intramuscular dexmedetomidine, a novel alpha 2-adrenoceptor agonist, as premedication for minor gynaecological surgery. *Acta Anaesthesiol Scand.* 1991; 35:283-8.
115. Aho MS, Erkola OA, Scheinin H et al. Effect of intravenously administered dexmedetomidine on pain after laparoscopic tubal ligation. *Anesth Analg.* 1991; 73:112-8.
116. Aantaa R, Jaakola ML, Kallio A et al. A comparison of dexmedetomidine, and alpha 2-adrenoceptor agonist, and midazolam as i.m. premedication for minor gynaecological surgery. *Br J Anaesth.* 1991; 67:402-9.
117. Aho M, Scheinin M, Lehtinen AM et al. Intramuscularly administered dexmedetomidine attenuates hemodynamic and stress hormone responses to gynecologic laparoscopy. *Anesth Analg.* 1992; 75:932-9.
118. Scheinin H, Jaakola ML, Sjövall S et al. Intramuscular dexmedetomidine as premedication for general anesthesia: a comparative multicenter study. *Anesthesiology.* 1993; 78:1065-75.

119. Erkola O, Korttila K, Aho M et al. Comparison of intramuscular dexmedetomidine and midazolam premedication for elective abdominal hysterectomy. *Anesth Analg.* 1994; 79:646-53.
120. Talke P, Li J, Jain U et al. Effects of perioperative dexmedetomidine infusion in patients undergoing vascular surgery: the Study of Perioperative Ischemia Research Group. *Anesthesiology.* 1995; 82:620-33.
121. Levänen J, Mäkelä ML, Scheinin H. Dexmedetomidine premedication attenuates ketamine-induced cardiostimulatory effects and postanesthetic delirium. *Anesthesiology.* 1995; 82:1117-25.
122. Lawrence CJ, De Lange S. Effects of a single pre-operative dexmedetomidine dose on isoflurane requirements and peri-operative haemodynamic stability. *Anaesthesia.* 1997; 52:736-44.
123. Berkenbosch JW, Tobias JD. Development of bradycardia during sedation with dexmedetomidine in an infant concurrently receiving digoxin. *Pediatr Crit Care Med.* 2003; 4:203-5.
124. Dasta JF, Kane-Gill SL, Durtschi AJ. Comparing dexmedetomidine prescribing patterns and safety in the naturalistic setting versus published data. *Ann Pharmacother.* 2004; 38:1130-5.
125. Karaaslan D, Peker TT, Alaca A et al. Comparison of buccal and intramuscular dexmedetomidine premedication for arthroscopic knee surgery. *J Clin Anesth.* 2006; 18:589-93.
126. Coskuner I, Tekin M, Kati I et al. Effects of dexmedetomidine on the duration of anaesthesia and wakefulness in bupivacaine epidural block. *Eur J Anaesthesiol.* 2007; 24:535-40.
127. MacLaren R, Forrest LK, Kiser TH. Adjunctive dexmedetomidine therapy in the intensive care unit: a retrospective assessment of impact on sedative and analgesic requirements, levels of sedation and analgesia, and ventilatory and hemodynamic parameters. *Pharmacotherapy.* 2007; 27:351-9.
128. Gómez-Vázquez ME, Hernández-Salazar E, Hernández-Jiménez A et al. Clinical analgesic efficacy and side effects of dexmedetomidine in the early postoperative period after arthroscopic knee surgery. *J Clin Anesth.* 2007; 19:576-82.
129. Biccard BM, Goga S, de Beurs J. Dexmedetomidine and cardiac protection for non-cardiac surgery: a metaanalysis of randomised controlled trials. *Anaesthesia.* 2008; 63:4-14.
130. Mason KP, Zurakowski D, Zgleszewski SE et al. High dose dexmedetomidine as the sole sedative for pediatric MRI. *Paediatr Anaesth.* 2008; 18:403-11.
131. Carroll CL, Krieger D, Campbell M et al. Use of dexmedetomidine for sedation of children hospitalized in the intensive care unit. *J Hosp Med.* 2008; 3:142-7.
132. Riker RR, Shehabi Y, Bokesch PM et al. Dexmedetomidine vs midazolam for sedation of critically ill patients: a randomized trial. *JAMA* 2009; 301:489-99.
133. Hosokawa K, Shime N, Kato Y et al. Dexmedetomidine sedation in children after cardiac surgery. *Pediatr Crit Care Med.* 2010; 11:39-43.
134. Jakob SM, Ruokonen E, Grounds RM et al. Dexmedetomidine vs midazolam or propofol for sedation during prolonged mechanical ventilation: two randomized controlled trials. *JAMA.* 2012; 307:1151-60.
135. Huang Z, Chen YS, Yang ZL et al. Dexmedetomidine versus midazolam for the sedation of patients with non-invasive ventilation failure. *Intern Med.* 2012; 51:2299-305.
136. Liu C, Zhang Y, She S et al. A randomized controlled trial of dexmedetomidine for suspension laryngoscopy. *Anaesthesia.* 2013; 68:60-6.
137. Ozaki M, Takeda J, Tanaka K et al. Safety and efficacy of dexmedetomidine for long-term sedation in critically ill patients. *J Anesth.* 2014; 28:38-50.
138. Mueller SW, Preslaski CR, Kiser TH et al. A randomized, double-blind, placebo-controlled dose range study of dexmedetomidine as adjunctive therapy for alcohol withdrawal. *Crit Care Med.* 2014; 42:1131-9.
139. VanderWeide LA, Foster CJ, MacLaren R et al. Evaluation of early dexmedetomidine addition to the standard of care for severe alcohol withdrawal in the ICU: a retrospective controlled cohort study. *J Intensive Care Med.* 2016; 31:198-204.
140. Lee JS, Wu R, Wong T et al. Extended sedation with continuous midazolam or dexmedetomidine infusion for young children receiving[131I]-MIBG radiopharmaceutical therapy for advanced neuroblastoma. *Pediatr Blood Cancer.* 2016; 63:471-8.
141. Pan W, Wang Y, Lin L et al. Outcomes of dexmedetomidine treatment in pediatric patients undergoing congenital heart disease surgery: a meta-analysis. *Paediatr Anaesth.* 2016; 26:239-48.
142. Jin S, Zhou X. Influence of dexmedetomidine on cardiac complications in non-cardiac surgery: a meta-analysis of randomized trials. *Int J Clin Pharm.* 2017; 39:629-40.
143. Venkatraman R, Hungerford JL, Hall MW et al. Dexmedetomidine for sedation during noninvasive ventilation in pediatric patients. *Pediatr Crit Care Med.* 2017; 18:831-7.
144. Gong Z, Ma L, Zhong YL et al. Myocardial protective effects of dexmedetomidine in patients undergoing cardiac surgery: a meta-analysis and systematic review. *Exp Ther Med.* 2017; 13:2355-61.
145. Margolis JR, Strauss HC, Miller HC et al. Digitalis and the sick sinus syndrome: clinical and electrophysiologic documentation of severe toxic effect on sinus node function. *Circulation.* 1975; 52:162-9.
146. Williams P, Aronson J, Sleight P. Is a slow pulse-rate a reliable sign of digitalis toxicity? *Lancet.*1978; 2:1340-2.
147. Rossi R, Leititis JU, Hagel KJ et al. Severe digoxin intoxication in a child treated by infusion of digoxin- specific Fab-antibody-fragments. *Eur J Pediatr.* 1984; 142:138-40.
148. Mahdyoon H, Battilana G, Rosman H et al. The evolving pattern of digoxin intoxication: observations at a large urban hospital from 1980 to 1988. *Am Heart J.* 1990; 120:1189-94.
149. Bibault P, Oubaassine R, Rahmani H et al. Emergency step-by-step specific immunotherapy in severe digoxin poisoning: an observational cohort study. *Eur J Emerg Med.* 2009; 16:145-9.
150. Pita-Fernandez S, Lombardia-Cortina M, Orozco-Cortina M et al. Clinical manifestations of elderly patients with digitalis intoxication in the emergency department. *Arch Gerontol Geriatr.* 2011; 53:e106-e110.
151. Manin AF, Nelson LS, Hoffman RS. Prognostic utility of serum potassium in chronic digoxin toxicity: a case-control study. *Am J Cardiovasc Drugs.* 2011; 11:173-8.
152. Valette H, Barnay C, Lopez M et al. Effects of intravenous diltiazem on sinus node function and atrioventricular conduction in patients. *J Cardiovasc Pharmacol.* 1983; 5:62-6.
153. Schroeder JS, Hung J, Lamb IH et al. Diltiazem and propranolol, alone and in combination, on exercise performance and left ventricular function in patients with stable effort angina: a double-blind, randomized, and placebo-controlled study. *Acta Pharmacol Toxicol.* 1985; 57(suppl 2):55-60.
154. Gibson RS, Boden WE, Theroux P et al. Diltiazem and reinfarction in patients with non-Q-wave myocardial infarction: results of a double-blind, randomized, multicenter trial. *N Engl J Med.* 1986; 315:423-9.
155. Sagie A, Strasberg B, Kusnieck J et al. Symptomatic bradycardia induced by the combination of oral diltiazem and beta blockers. *Clin Cardiol.*1991; 14:314-6.
156. Felicetta JV, Serfer HM, Cutler NR et al. A dose-response trial of once-daily diltiazem. *Am Heart J.* 1992; 123:1022-6.
157. Andrivet P, Beaslay V, Kiger JP et al. Complete sinus arrest during diltiazem therapy: clinical correlates and efficacy of intravenous calcium. *Eur Heart J.* 1994; 15:350-4.
158. Boudonas G, Lefkos N, Efthymiadis AP et al. Intravenous administration of diltiazem in the treatment of supraventricular tachyarrhythmias. *Acta Cardiol.* 1995; 50:125-34.
159. Théroux P, Grégoire J, Chin C et al. Intravenous diltiazem in acute myocardial infarction: Diltiazem as Adjunctive Therapy to Activase (DATA) trial. *J Am Coll Cardiol.* 1998; 32:620-8.
160. Edoute Y, Nagachandran P, Svirski B et al. Cardiovascular adverse drug reaction associated with combined beta-adrenergic and calcium entry-blocking agents. *J Cardiovasc Pharmacol.* 2000; 35:556-9.

161. Shapira OM, Alkon JD, Macron DS et al. Nitroglycerin is preferable to diltiazem for prevention of coronary bypass conduit spasm. *Ann Thorac Surg*. 2000; 70:883-8.
162. Amorim S, Dias P, Rocha G et al. Poisoning with calcium channel blockers: a case report and review of the literature. *Rev Port Cardiol*. 2001; 20:1249-57.
163. Punukollu G, Gowda RM, Khan IA et al. Delayed presentation of calcium channel antagonist overdose. *Am J Ther*. 2003; 10:132-4.
164. Mills TA, Kawji MM, Cataldo VD et al. Profound sinus bradycardia due to diltiazem, verapamil, and/or beta-adrenergic blocking drugs. *J La State Med Soc*. 2004; 156:327-31.
165. Fromm C, Suau SJ, Cohen V et al. Diltiazem vs. metoprolol in the management of atrial fibrillation or flutter with rapid ventricular rate in the emergency department. *J Emerg Med*. 2015; 49:175-82.
166. Pennell DJ, Underwood SR, Ell PJ. Symptomatic bradycardia complicating the use of intravenous dipyridamole for thallium-201 myocardial perfusion imaging. *Int J Cardiol*. 1992; 27:272-4.
167. Picano E, Marini C, Pirelli S et al. Safety of intravenous high-dose dipyridamole echocardiography. *Am J Cardiol*. 1992; 15:252-8.
168. Bjoernstad K, Aakhus S, Lundbom J et al. Digital dipyridamole stress echocardiography in silent ischemia after coronary artery bypass grafting and/or after healing of acute myocardial infarction. *Am J Cardiol*. 1993; 72:640-6.
169. Roach PJ, Magee MA, Freedman SB. Asystole and bradycardia during dipyridamole stress testing in patients receiving beta blockers. *Int J Cardiol*. 1993; 42:92-4.
170. Lo Mauro R, Sabella FP, Enia F. Sinus arrest associated with dipyridamole infusion. *Chest*. 1994; 105:604-5.
171. Bjørnstad K, Aakhus S, Hatle L. Digital high frame rate stress echocardiography for detection of coronary artery stenosis by high dose dipyridamole stress testing. *Int J Card Imaging*. 1995; 11:163-70.
172. Roman MR, Angelides S, Freeman AP et al. The safety of dipyridamole in patients undergoing myocardial perfusion scintigraphy prior to lung volume reduction surgery. *Eur J Nucl Med*. 2001; 28:1405-8.
173. Hayler AM, Holt DW, O'Keeffe B et al. Treatment of disopyramide overdosage. *Med J Aust*. 1979; 1:234.
174. Camm J, Ward D, Spurrell RA. The effect of intravenous disopyramide phosphate on recurrent paroxysmal tachycardias. *Br J Clin Pharmacol*. 1979; 8:441-9.
175. Warrington SJ, Hamer J. Some cardiovascular problems with disopyramide. *Postgrad Med J*. 1980; 56:229-33.
176. Desai JM, Scheinman MM, Hirschfeld D et al. Cardiovascular collapse associated with disopyramide therapy. *Chest*. 1981; 79:545-51.
177. Shepherd G, Klein-Schwartz W, Edwards R. Donepezil overdose: a tenfold dosing error. *Ann Pharmacother*. 1999; 33:812-5.
178. Relkin NR, Reichman WE, Orazem J et al. A large, community-based, open-label trial of donepezil in the treatment of Alzheimer's disease. *Dement Geriatr Cogn Disord*. 2002; 16:15-24.
179. Bordier P, Garrigue S, Barold SS et al. Significance of syncope in patients with Alzheimer's disease treated with cholinesterase inhibitors. *Europace*. 2003; 5:429-31.
180. Bordier P, Lanusse S, Garrigue S et al. Causes of syncope in patients with Alzheimer's disease treated with donepezil. *Drugs Aging*. 2005; 22:687-94.
181. Doody RS, Corey-Bloom J, Zhang R et al. Safety and tolerability of donepezil at doses up to 20 mg/day. Results from a pilot study in patients with Alzheimer's Disease. *Drugs Aging*. 2008; 25:163-74.
182. Hernandez RK, Farwell W, Cantor MD et al. Cholinesterase inhibitors and incidence of bradycardia in patients with dementia in the veterans affairs New England healthcare system. *J Am Geriatr Soc*. 2009; 57:1997-2003.
183. Rosenbloom MH, Finley R, Scheinman MM et al. Donepezil-associated bradyarrhythmia in a patient with dementia with lewy bodies (DLB). *Alzheimer Dis Assoc Disord*. 2010; 24:209-11.
184. Babai S, Auriche P, LeLouet H. Comparison of adverse drug reactions with donepezil versus memantine: analysis of the French pharmacovigilance database. *Therapie*. 2010; 65:255-9.
185. Garlich FM, Balakrishnan K, Shah SK et al. Prolonged altered mental status and bradycardia following pediatric donepezil ingestion. *Clin Toxicol*. 2014; 52:291-4.
186. Pourmand A, Shay C, Redha W et al. Cholinergic symptoms and QTc prolongation following donepezil overdose. *Am J Emerg Med*. 2017; Jun 22. pii: S0735-6757(17)30495-3.
187. Singh BN, Connolly SJ, Crijns HJ et al. Dronedarone for maintenance of sinus rhythm in atrial fibrillation or flutter. *N Engl J Med*. 2007; 357:987-99.
188. Hohnloser SH, Crijns HJ, van Eickels M et al. Effect of dronedarone on cardiovascular events in atrial fibrillation. *N Engl J Med*. 2009; 360:668-78.
189. Freemantle N, Lafuente-Lafuente C, Mitchell S et al. Mixed treatment comparison of dronedarone, amiodarone, sotalol, flecainide, and propafenone, for the management of atrial fibrillation. *Europace*. 2011; 13:329-45.
190. Immordino L, Connolly S, Crijns H et al. Effects of dronedarone started rapidly after amiodarone discontinuation. *Clin Cardiol*. 2013; 36:88-95.
191. Angevin E, Lopez-Martin JA, Lin CC et al. Phase I study of dovitinib (TKI258), an oral FGFR, VEGFR, and PDGFR inhibitor, in advanced or metastatic renal cell carcinoma. *Clin Cancer Res*. 2013; 19:1257-68.
192. Beyenburg S, Schönegger K. Severe bradycardia in a stroke patient caused by a single low dose of escitalopram. *Eur Neurol*. 2007; 57:50-1.
193. van Gorp F, Whyte IM, Isbister GK. Clinical and ECG effects of escitalopram overdose. *Ann Emerg Med*. 2009; 54:404-8.
194. Degiacomo J, Luedtke S. Neonatal toxicity from escitalopram use *in utero*: a case report. *J Pediatr Pharmacol Ther*. 2016; 21:522-6.
195. Oppenheimer F, Mulgaonkar S, Ferguson R et al. Impact of long-term therapy with FTY720 or mycophenolate on cardiac conduction and rhythm in stable adult renal transplant patients. *Transplantation*. 2007; 83:645-8.
196. Tedesco-Silva H, Szakaly P, Shoker A et al. FTY720 versus mycophenolate mofetil in de novo renal transplantation: six month results of a double-blind study. *Transplantation*. 2007; 84:885-92.
197. Kappos L, Radue E-W, O'Connor P et al. A placebo-controlled trial of oral fingolimod in relapsing multiple sclerosis. *N Engl J Med*. 2010; 362:387-401.
198. Cohen JA, Barkhof F, Comi G et al. Oral fingolimod or intramuscular interferon for relapsing multiple sclerosis. *N Engl J Med*. 2010; 362:402-15.
199. Saida T, Kikuchi S, Itoyama Y et al. A randomized, controlled trial of fingolimod (FTY720) in Japanese patients with multiple sclerosis. *Mult Scler*. 2012; 18:1269-77.
200. Ontaneda D, Hara-Cleaver C, Rudick RA et al. Early tolerability and safety of fingolimod in clinical practice. *J Neurol Sci*. 2012; 323:167-72.
201. Stephenson M, Wong A, Rotella JA et al. Deliberate fingolimod overdose presenting with delayed hypotension and bradycardia responsive to atropine. *J Med Toxicol*. 2014; 10:215-8.
202. Gold R, Comi G, Palace J et al. Assessment of cardiac safety during fingolimod treatment initiation in a real-world relapsing multiple sclerosis population: a phase 3b, open-label study. *J Neurol*. 2014; 261:267-76.
203. Calabresi PA, Radue EW, Goodin D et al. Safety and efficacy of fingolimod in patients with relapsing-remitting multiple sclerosis (FREEDOMS II): a double-blind, randomised, placebo-controlled, phase 3 trial. *Lancet Neurol*. 2014; 13:545-56.
204. Laroni A, Brogi D, Morra VB et al. Safety of the first dose of fingolimod for multiple sclerosis: results of an open-label clinical trial. *BMC Neurol*. 2014; 14:65.

205. Fragoso YD, Arruda CC, Arruda WO et al. The real-life experience with cardiovascular complications in the first dose of fingolimod for multiple sclerosis. *Arq Neuropsiquiatr.* 2014; 72:712-4.

206. Schurmann P, Basra S, Awar OG et al. Abnormal rhythms in patients without known cardic disease after a first dose of fingolimod. *Mult Scler Relat Disord.* 2014; 3:408-12.

207. Kappos L, Cohen J, Collins W et al. Fingolimod in relapsing multiple sclerosis: an integrated analysis of safety findings. *Mult Scler Relat Disord.* 2014; 3:494-504.

208. Hughes B, Cascione M, Freedman MS et al. First-dose effects of fingolimod after switching from injectable therapies in the randomized, open-label, multicenter, Evaluate Patient OutComes (EPOC) study in relapsing multiple sclerosis. *Mult Scler Relat Disord.* 2014; 3:620-8.

209. DiMarco JP, O'Connor P, Cohen JA et al. First-dose effects of fingolimod: pooled safety data from three phase 3 studies. *Mult Scler Relat Disord.* 2014; 3:629-38.

210. Ordonez-Boschetti L, Rey R, Cruz A et al. Safety and tolerability of fingolimod in Latin American patients with relapsing-remitting multiple sclerosis: the open-label FIRST LATAM study. *Adv Ther.* 2015; 32:626-35.

211. Lublin F, Miller DH, Freedman MS et al. Oral fingolimod in primary progressive multiple sclerosis (INFORMS): a phase 3, randomised, double-blind, placebo-controlled trial. *Lancet.* 2016; 387:1075-84.

212. Linker RA, Wendt G. Cardiac safety profile of first dose of fingolimod for relapsing-remitting multiple sclerosis in real-world settings: data from a German prospective multi-center observational study. *Neurol Ther.* 2016; 5:193-201.

213. Voldsgaard A, Koch-Henriksen N, Magyari M et al. Early safety and efficacy of fingolimod treatment in Denmark. *Acta Neurol Scand.* 2017; 135:129-33.

214. Limmroth V, Ziemssen T, Lang M et al. Electrocardiographic assessments and cardiac events after fingolimod first dose – a comprehensive monitoring study. *BMC Neurol.* 2017; Jan 18;17:11.

215. Abdar M, Ebrahimifar P, Etemadifar M. The outbreak fingolimod cardiovascular side effects in relapsing-remitting multiple sclerosis patient: a longitudinal study in an Iranian population. *ARYA Atheroscler.* 2016; 12:274-80.

216. Reid PR, Griffith LS, Platia EV et al. Evaluation of flecainide acetate in the management of patients at high risk of sudden cardiac death. *Am J Cardiol.* 1984; 53:108B-11B.

217. Platia EV, Estes M, Heine DL et al. Flecainide: electrophysiologic and antiarrhythmic properties in refractory ventricular tachycardia. *Am J Cardiol.* 1985; 55:956-62.

218. Crozier IG, Ikram H, Kenealy M et al. Flecainide acetate for conversion of acute supraventricular tachycardia to sinus rhythm. *Am J Cardiol.* 1987; 59:607-9.

219. Van Gelder IC, Crijns HJGM, Van Glist WH et al. Efficacy and safety of flecainide acetate in the maintenance of sinus rhythm after electrical cardioversion of chronic atrial fibrillation or atrial flutter. *Am J Cardiol.* 1989; 64:1317-21.

220. Köppel C, Oberdisse U, Heinemeyer G. Clinical course and outcome in class IC antiarrhythmic overdose. *J Toxicol Clin Toxicol.* 1990; 28:433-44.

221. Hanley NA, Bourke JP, Gascoigne AD. Survival in a case of life-threatening flecainide overdose. *Intensive Care Med.* 1998; 24:740-2.

222. Aliot E, De Roy L, Capucci A et al. Safety of a controlled-release flecainide acetate formulation in the prevention of paroxysmal atrial fibrillation in outpatients. *Ann Cardiol Angeiol.* 2003; 52:34-40.

223. D'Alessandro LC, Rieder MJ, Gloor J et al. Life-threatening flecainide intoxication in a young child secondary to medication error. *Ann Pharmacother.* 2009; 43:1522-7.

224. Chung-Lo W, Hsieh CY, Chiu CF et al. Fludarabine-induced bradycardia in a patient with refractory leukemia. *Ann Saudi Med.* 2010; 30:246-7.

225. Aziz SA, Tramboo NA, Mohi-ud-Din K et al. Supraventricular arrhythmia: a complication of 5-fluorouracil therapy. *Clin Oncol.* 1998; 10:377-8.

226. Lee AD, McKay MJ. Symptomatic 5-fluorouracil-induced sinus bradycardia. *Intern Med J.* 2011; 41:566-70.

227. Khan MA, Masood N, Husain N et al. A retrospective study of cardiotoxicities induced by 5-fluouracil (5-FU) and 5-FU based chemotherapy regimens in Pakistani adult cancer center patients at Shaukat Khanum Memorial Cancer Hospital and Research Center. *J Pak Med Assoc.* 2012; 62:430-4.

228. Ellison JM, Milofsky JE, Ely E. Fluoxetine-induced bradycardia and syncope in two patients. *J Clin Psychiatry.* 1990; 51:385-6.

229. Buff DD, Brenner R, Kirtane SS et al. Dysrhythmia associated with fluoxetine treatment in an elderly patient with cardiac disease. *J Clin Psychiatry.* 1991; 52:174-6.

230. Ahmed I, Dagincourt PG, Miller LG et al. Possible interaction between fluoxetine and pimozide causing sinus bradycardia. *Can J Psychiatry.* 1993; 38:62-3.

231. Hussein S, Kaufman BM. Bradycardia associated with fluoxetine in an elderly patient with sick sinus syndrome. *Postgrad Med J.* 1994; 70:56.

232. Anderson J, Compton SA. Fluoxetine induced bradycardia in presenile dementia. *Ulster Med J.* 1997; 66:144-5.

233. Spigset O. Adverse reactions of selective serotonin reuptake inhibitors: reports from a spontaneous reporting system. *Drug Saf.* 1999; 20:277-87.

234. Compton R, Spiller HA, Bosse GM. Fatal fluoxetine ingestion with postmortem blood concentrations. *Clin Toxicol.* 2005; 43:277-9.

235. Chin RL, Sporer KA, Cullison B et al. Clinical course of gamma-hydroxybutyrate overdose. *Ann Emerg Med.* 1998; 31:716-22.

236. Anonymous. Adverse events associated with ingestion of gamma-butyrolactone: Minnesota, New Mexico, and Texas, 1998-1999. *MMWR Morb Mortal Wkly Rep.* 1999; 48:137-40.

237. Liechti ME, Kunz I, Greminger P et al. Clinical features of gamma-hydroxybutyrate and gamma-butyrolactone toxicity and concomitant drug and alcohol use. *Drug Alcohol Depend.* 2006; 81:323-6.

238. Runnacles JL, Stroobant J. γ-hydroxybutyrate poisoning: poisoning from toy beads (letter). *BMJ.* 2008; Jan 19:336.

239. Munir VL, Hutton JE, Harney JP et al. Gamma-hydroxybutyrate: a 30 month emergency department review. *Emerg Med Australas.* 2008; 20:521-30.

240. Dutch MJ, Austin KB. Hospital in the field: prehospital management of GHB intoxication by medical assistance teams. *Prehosp Disaster Med.* 2012; 27:463-7.

241. Watanabe H, Hasegawa A, Shinozaki T et al. Possible cardiac side effects of granisetron, an antiemetic agent, in patients with bone and soft-tissue sarcomas receiving cytotoxic chemotherapy. *Cancer Chemother Pharmacol.* 1995; 35:278-82.

242. Cakir FB, Yapar O, Canpolat C et al. Cardiac effects of granisetron in a prospective crossover randomized dose comparison. *Support Care Cancer.* 2012; 20:2451-7.

243. Zuck D, Rao JJ. Profound bradycardia with verapamil and halothane. *Anaesthesia.* 1985; 40;84-5.

244. Kataria B, Epstein R, Bailey A et al. A comparison of sevoflurane to halothane in paediatric surgical patients: results of a multicentre international study. *Paediatr Anaesth.* 1996; 6:283-92.

245. Annila P, Rorarius M, Reinikainen P et al. Effect of pretreatment with intravenous atropine or glycopyrrolate on cardiac arrhythmias during halothane anaesthesia for adenoidectomy in children. *Br J Anaesth.* 1998; 80:756-60.

246. Annila P, Viitanen H, Reinikainen P et al. Induction characteristics of thiopentone/suxamethonium, propofol/alfentanil or halothane alone in children aged 1-3 years. *Eur J Anaesthesiol.* 1999; 16:359-66.

247. Amin N, Borzak S, Housholder SA et al. Multiple episodes of sinus arrest following the administration of ibutilide in a patient with underlying sinus node dysfunction. *Heart.* 1998; 79:628-9.

248. Taylor CT, Donaldson AR. Safety and effectiveness of ibutilide in a community hospital. *Pharmacotherapy.* 2001; 21:488-92.

249. Gowda RM, Khan IA, Punukollu G et al. Use of ibutilide for cardioversion of recent-onset atrial fibrillation and flutter in elderly. *Am J Ther.* 2004; 11:95-7.

250. Viktorsdottir O, Henriksdottir A, Arnar DO. Ibutilide for treatment of atrial fibrillation in the emergency department. *Emerg Med J.* 2006; 23:133-4.

251. Pratila MG, Steinherz LJ, Pratilas V. Sick sinus syndrome in a teenager treated with idarubicin. *J Cardiothorac Vasc Anesth.* 1993; 7:125-6.

252. Miya T, Fujikawa R, Fukushima J et al. Bradycardia induced by irinotecan: a case report. *Jpn J Clin Oncol.* 1998; 28:709-11.

253. Pua U. Bradycardia associated with drug-eluting beads loaded with irinotecan (DEBIR) infusion for colorectal liver metastases. *Cardiovasc Intervent Radiol.* 2013; 36:864-6.

254. Romano MJ, Gaylor A, Sang CJ Jr. Life-threatening isradipine poisoning in a child. *Pharmacotherapy.* 2002; 22:766-70.

255. Ruzyllo W, Tendera M, Ford I et al. Antianginal efficacy and safety of ivabradine compared with amlodipine in patients with stable effort angina pectoris. A 3-month randomised, double-blind, multicenter, noninferiority trial. *Drugs.* 2007; 57:393-405.

256. Lopez-Bescos L, Filipova S, Martos R. Long-term safety and efficacy of ivabradine in patients with chronic stable angina. *Cardiology.* 2007; 108:387-96.

257. Tardif JC, Ponikowski P, Kahan T. Efficacy of the I(f) current inhibitor ivabradine in patients with chronic stable angina receiving beta-blocker therapy: a 4-month, randomized, placebo-controlled trial. *Eur Heart J.* 2009; 30:540-8.

258. Danchin N. Impact of a pure reduction in heart rate for the treatment of left ventricular dysfunction: clinical benefits of ivabradine in the BEAUTIFUL trial. *Therapie.* 2009; 64:111-4.

259. Borer JS, Tardif-J-C. Efficacy of ivabradine, a selective I_f inhibitor, in patients with chronic stable angina pectoris and diabetes mellitus. *Am J Cardiol.* 2010; 05:29-35.

260. Swedberg K, Komajda M, Bohm M et al. Ivabradine and outcomes in chronic heart failure (SHIFT): a randomised placebo-controlled study. *Lancet.* 2010; 376:875-85.

261. Reil J-C, Robertson M, Ford I et al. Impact of left bundle branch block on heart rate and its relationship to treatment with ivabradine in chronic heart falure. *Eur J Heart Fail.* 2013; 15:1044-52.

262. Fox K, Ford I, Steg PG et al. Ivabradine in stable coronary artery disease without clinical heart failure. *N Engl J Med.* 2014; 371:1091-9.

263. Fox K, Ford I, Steg PG et al. Bradycardia and atrial fibrillation in patients with stable coronary artery disease treated with ivabradine: an analysis from the SIGNIFY study. *Eur Heart J.* 2015; 36:3291-6.

264. Cammarano C, Silva M, Comee M et al. Meta-analysis of ivabradine in patients with stable coronary artery disease with and without left ventricular dysfunction. *Clin Ther* 2016; 38:387-95.

265. Maskell K, Tse A, Wolf CE et al. Acute on chronic ivabradine overdose: a case report. *J Med Toxicol.* 2016; 12:189-91.

266. Romero-Leon JM, Galvez-Contreras MC, Diez-Garcia LF. Symptomatic bradycardia and heart failure triggered by ivabradine in a patient receiving antiretroviral therapy. *Rev Esp Cardiol.* 2016; 69:529-30.

267. Mengesha HG, Weldearegawi B, Petrucka P et al. Effect of ivabradine on cardiovascular outcomes in patients with stable angina: meta-analysis of randomized clinical trials. *BMC Cardiovasc Disord.* 2017; Apr 28;17:105.

268. Nettles DC, Herrin TJ, Mullen JG. Ketamine induction in poor-risk patients. *Anesth Analg.* 1973; 52:59-64.

269. Wolfson B, Kielar CM, Shenoy NR et al. Analgesic "cocktails" for pneumoencephalography: ketamine, diazepam, alphaprodine, and droperidol. *Anesth Analg.* 1974; 52:779-83.

270. Levin RM, Seleny FL, Streczyn MV. Ketamine-pancuronium-narcotic technic for cardiovascular surgery in infants: a comparative study. *Anesth Analg.* 1975; 54:800-5.

271. Radnay PA, Hollinger I, Santi A et al. Ketamine for pediatric cardiac anesthesia. *Anaesthesist.* 1976; 25:259-65.

272. Green SM, Denmark TK, Cline J et al. Ketamine sedation for pediatric critical care procedures. *Pediatr Emerg Care.* 2001; 17:244-8.

273. Sibley A, Mackenzie M, Bawden J et al. A prospective review of the use of ketamine to facilitate endotracheal intubation in the helicopter emergency medical services setting. *Emerg Med J.* 2011; 28:521-5.

274. Cheng TO, Wadhwa K. Sinus standstill following intravenous lidocaine administration. *JAMA.* 1973; 223:790-2.

275. Parameswaran R, Kahn D, Monheit R et al. Sinus bradycardia due to lidocaine: clinical-electrophysiologic correlations. *J Electrocardiol.* 1974; 7:75-8.

276. Marriott HJ, Phillips K. Profound hypotension and bradycardia after a single bolus of lidocaine. *J Electrocardiol.* 1974; 7:79-82.

277. Klein HO, Jutrin I, Kaplinsky E. Cerebral and cardiac toxicity of a small dose of lignocaine. *Br Heart J.* 1975; 37:775-8.

278. Zoll WR, Täuber M, Vorburger C. Sinus arrest after intravenous administration of lidocaine. *Schweiz Med Wochenschr.* 1979; 109:1946-8.

279. Demczuk RJ. Significant sinus bradycardia following intravenous lidocaine injection. *Anesthesiology.* 1984; 60:69-70.

280. Amornyotin S, Srikureja W, Chalayonnavin W et al. Topical viscous lidocaine solution versus lidocaine spray for pharyngeal anesthesia in unsedated esophagogastroduodenoscopy. *Endoscopy.* 2009; 41:581-6.

281. Kim KO, Chung S, Lee K et al. Profound bradycardia with lidocaine during anesthesia induction in a silent sick sinus syndrome patient. *J Clin Anesth.* 2011; 23:227-30.

282. Lundqvist M, Agren J, Hellstrom-Westas L et al. Efficacy and safety of lidocaine for treatment of neonatal seizures. *Acta Paediatr.* 2013; 102:863-7.

283. Nicholas E, Thornton MD. Lidocaine toxicity during attempted epistaxis cautery. *J Emerg Med.* 2016; 51:303-4.

284. Gallini A, Sommet A, Montastruc JL et al. Does memantine induce bradycardia? A study in the French PharmacoVigilance Database. *Pharmacoepidemiol Drug Saf.* 2008; 17:887-1.

285. Goins JR. Experience with mepivacaine paracervical block in an obstetric private practice. *Am J Obstet Gynecol.* 1992; 167:342-4.

286. Ayestaran C, Matorras R, Gomez S et al. Severe bradycardia and bradypnea following vaginal oocyte retrieval: a possible toxic effect of paracervical mepivacaine. *Eur J Obstet Gynecol Reprod Biol.* 2000; 91:71-3.

287. Pawlowski J, Orr K, Kim K et al. Anesthetic and recovery profiles of lidocaine versus mepivacaine for spinal anesthesia in patients undergoing outpatient orthopedic arthroscopic procedures. *J Clin Anesthes.* 2012; 24:109-15.

288. Karir V. Bradycardia associated with intravenous methadone administered for sedation in a patient with acute respiratory distress syndrome. *Pharmacotherapy.* 2002; 22:1196-9.

289. Ashwath ML, Ajjan M, Culclasure T. Methadone-induced bradycardia. *J Emerg Med.* 2005; 29:73-5.

290. Wheeler AD, Tobias JD. Bradycardia during methadone therapy in an infant. *Pediatr Crit Care Med.* 2006; 7:83-5.

291. Hussain T, Ewer AK. Maternal methadone may cause arrhythmias in neonates. *Acta Paediatr.* 2007; 96:768-9.

292. Buchanan D. Sinus bradycardia related to methadone in a patient with myeloma receiving thalidomide therapy. Palliat Med. 2010; 24:742-3.

293. Swenson O. Accidental methadone intoxication masquerading as asthma exacerbation with respiratory arrest in a six-year old boy. *Del Med J.* 2015; 87:147-9.

294. Tvede N, Nielsen LP, Andersen V. Bradycardia after high-dose intravenous methylprednisolone therapy. *Scand J Rheumatol.* 1986; 15:302-4.

295. Lucas KG, Howrie DL, Phebus CK. Cardiorespiratory decompensation following methylprednisolone administration. *Pediatr Hematol Oncol.* 1993; 10:249-55.

296. Küçükosmanoğlu O, Karabay A, Ozbarlas N et al. Marked bradycardia due to pulsed and oral methylprednisolone therapy in a patient with rapidly progressive glomerulonephritis. *Nephron.* 1998; 80:484.

297. Guillén EL, Ruíz AM, Bugallo JB. Hypotension, bradycardia, and asystole after high-dose intravenous methylprednisolone in a monitored patient. *Am J Kidney Dis.* 1998; 32:E4.

298. Thornton PD, Hamblin M, Treleaven JG et al. High dose methyl prednisolone in refractory chronic lymphocytic leukaemia. *Leuk Lymphoma.* 1999; 34:167-70.

299. Pudil R, Hrncir Z. Severe bradycardia after a methylprednisolone "minipulse" treatment. *Arch Intern Med.* 2001; 161:1778-9.

300. Beyan E, Urun Y, Uzuner A. Bradycardia due to methylprednisolone therapy. *J Clin Rheumatol.* 2004; 10:230.

301. Akikusa JD, Feldman BM, Gross GJ et al. Sinus bradycardia after intravenous pulse methylprednisolone. *Pediatrics.* 2007; 119:e778-82.

302. Vasheghani-Farahani A, Sahraian MA, Darabi L et al. Incidence of various cardiac arrhythmias and conduction disturbances due to high dose intravenous methylprednisolone in patients with multiple sclerosis. *J Neurol Sci* 2011; 309:75-8.

303. Darling HS, Marwah V, Rajput AK et al. Low dose methylprednisolone induced bradycardia. *J Assoc Physicians India.* 2013; 61:920-2.

304. Kundu A, Fitzgibbons TP. Acute symptomatic sinus bradycardia in a woman treated with pulse dose steroids for multiple sclerosis: a case report. *J Med Case Rep.* 2015; 9:216.

305. Yong KL, Chng CL, Htoon HM et al. Safety profile and effects of pulsed methylprednisolone on vital signs in thyroid eye disease. *Int J Endocrinol.* 2015; 2015:457123.

306. Osuagwu F, Jahnke B. Intravenous methylprednisolone-induced nocturnal sinus bradycardia in a multiple sclerosis patients. *Prim Care Companion CNS Disord.* 2016; Mar 3;18. eCollection 2016.

307. Ohshima M, Kawahata K, Kanda H et al. Sinus bradycardia after intravenous pulse methylprednisolone therapy in patients with systemic lupus erythematosus. *Mod Rheumatol.* 2017; 1:1-4.

308. Feneck RO, Sherry KM, Withington PS et al. Comparison of the hemodynamic effects of milrinone with dobutamine in patients after cardiac surgery. *J Cardiothorc Vasc Anesth.* 2001; 15:306-15.

309. Sprague DH. Severe bradycardia after neostigmine in a patient taking propranolol to control paroxysmal atrial tachycardia. *Anesthesiology.* 1975; 42:208-10.

310. Seidl DC, Martin DE. Prolonged bradycardia after neostigmine administration in a patient taking nadolol. *Anesth Analg.* 1984; 63:365-7.

311. Triantafillou AN, Tsueda K, Berg J et al. Refractory bradycardia after reversal of muscle relaxant in a diabetic with vagal neuropathy. *Anesth Analg.* 1986; 65:1237-41.

312. Arsura EL, Brunner NG, Namba T et al. Adverse cardiovascular effects of anticholinesterase medications. *Am J Med Sci.* 1987; 293:18-23.

313. Eldor J, Hoffman B, Davidson JT. Prolonged bradycardia and hypotension after neostigmine administration in a patient receiving atenolol. *Anaesthesia.* 1987; 42:1294-7.

314. Shankar KB, Moseley H, Kumar A. Prolonged bradycardia and hypotension after neostigmine administration in a patient receiving atenolol. *Anaesthesia.* 1988; 43:797-8.

315. Backman SB, Ralley FE, Fox GS. Neostigmine produces bradycardia in a heart transplant patient. *Anesthesiology.* 1993; 78:777-9.

316. Backman SB, Fox GS, Stein RD et al. Neostigmine decreases heart rate in heart transplant patients. *Can J Anaesth.* 1996; 43:373-8.

317. Backman SB, Stein RD, Ralley FE et al. Neostigmine-induced bradycardia following recent vs remote cardiac transplantation in the same patient. *Can J Anaesth.* 1996; 43:394-8.

318. Ponec RJ, Saunders MD, Kimmey MB. Neostigmine for the treatment of acute colonic pseudo-obstruction. *N Engl J Med.* 1999; 341:137-41.

319. Abeyta BJ, Albrecht RM, Schermer CR. Retrospective study of neostigmine for the treatment of acute colonic pseudo-obstruction. *Am Surg.* 2001; 67:265-8.

320. Ho KM, Ismail H, Lee KC et al. Use of intrathecal neostigmine as an adjunct to other spinal medications in perioperative and peripartum analgesia: a meta-analysis. *Anaesth Intensive Care.* 2005; 33:41-53.

321. Mouchli MA, Camilleri M, Lee T et al. Evaluating the safety and the effects of colonic compliance of meostigmine during motility testing in patients with chronic constipation. *Neurogastroenterol Motil.* 2016; 28:871-8.

322. Kross RA, Ferri E, Leung D et al. A comparative study between a calcium channel blocker (Nicardipine) and a combined alpha-beta-blocker (Labetalol) for the control of emergence hypertension during craniotomy for tumor surgery. *Anesth Analg.* 2000; 91:904-9.

323. Arima H, Sobue K, Tanaka S et al. Profound sinus bradycardia after intravenous nicardipine. *Anesth Analg.* 2002; 95:53-5.

324. Liu-Deryke X, Janisse J, Coplin WM et al. A comparison of nicardipine and labetolol for acute hypertension and management following stroke. *Neurocrit Care.* 2008; 9:167-76.

325. Abboud ME, Frasure SE. Bradycardia caused by intravenous nicardipine in an elderly patient with acute ischemic infarct. *Am J Emerg Med.* 2016; 43:761:e1-2.

326. Come PC, Pitt B. Nitroglycerin-induced severe hypotension and bradycardia in patients with acute myocardial infarction. *Circulation.* 1976; 54:624-8.

327. Ong EA, Bass S. Nitroglycerin-induced bradycardia and hypotension in acute myocardial infarction. *Chest.* 1980; 77:244.

328. Meretoja OA. Haemodynamic effects of combined nitroglycerin and dobutamine-infusions after coronary by-pass surgery: with one nitroglycerin-related complication. *Acta Anaesthesiol Scand.* 1980; 24:211-5.

329. Nemerovski M, Shah PK. Syndrome of severe bradycardia and hypotension following sublingual nitroglycerin administration. *Cardiology.* 1981; 67:180-9.

330. Khan AH, Carleton RA. Nitroglycerin-induced hypotension and bradycardia. *Arch Intern Med.* 1981; 141:984.

331. Brandes W, Santiago T, Limacher M. Nitroglycerin induced hypotension, bradycardia, and asystole: report of a case and review of the literature. *Clin Cardiol.* 1990; 13:741-4.

332. Buckley R, Roberts R. Symptomatic bradycardia following the administration of sublingual nitroglycerin. *Am J Emerg Med.* 1993; 11:253-5.

333. Wuerz R, Swope G, Meador S et al. Safety of prehospital nitroglycerin. *Ann Emerg Med.* 1994; 23:31-6.

334. Engelberg S, Singer AJ, Moldashel J et al. Effects of prehospital nitroglycerin on hemodynamics and chest pain intensity. *Prehosp Emerg Care.* 2000; 4:290-3.

335. Herrington AM, George KW, Moulds CC. Octreotide-induced bradycardia. *Pharmacotherapy.* 1998; 18:413-6.

336. Dilger JA, Rho EH, Que FG et al. Octreotide-induced bradycardia and heart block during surgical resection of a carcinoid tumor. *Anesth Analg.* 2004; 98:318-20.

337. Erem C, Ersoz HO, Ukinc K et al. Acromegaly presenting with diabetic ketoacidosis, associated with retinitis pigmentosa and octreotide-induced bradycardia: a case report and a review of the literature. *Endocrine.* 2006; 20:145-9.

338. Batra YK, Rajeev S, Samra T et al. Octreotide-induced severe paradoxical hyperglycemia and bradycardia during subtotal pancreatectomy for congenital hyperinsulinism in an infant. *Paediatr Anaesth.* 2007; 17:1117-9.

339. Kubota K, Hasumi Y, Numata A et al. Octreotide acetate administration for malignant bowel obstruction induced severe bradycardia in patients with terminal stage cancer: two case reports. *J Palliat Med.* 2013; 16:596-7.

340. Markowitz JS, DeVane CL, Boulton DW et al. Hypotension and bradycardia in a healthy volunteer following a single 5 mg dose of olanzapine. *J Clin Pharmacol.* 2002; 42:104-6.
341. Lee TW, Tsai SJ, Hwang JP. Severe cardiovascular side effects of olanzapine in an elderly patient: case report. *Int J Psychiatry Med.* 2003; 33:399-401.
342. Chen CC, Tsai JH, Yang P et al. Bradyarrhythmic shock associated with olanzapine. *Aust N Z J Psychiatry.* 2007; 41:89.
343. Escobar R, Pérez V, San L et al. Effectiveness results of olanzapine in acute psychotic patients with agitation in the emergency room setting: results from NATURA study. *Actas Esp Psiquiatr.* 2008; 36:151-7.
344. Cole JB, Moore JC, Dolan BJ et al. A prospective observational study of patients receiving intravenous and intramuscular olanzapine in the Emergency Department. *Ann Emerg Med.* 2017; 69:327-36.
345. McGuire WP, Rowinsky EK, Rosenshein NB et al. Taxol: a unique antineoplastic agent with significant activity in advanced ovarian epithelial neoplasms. *Ann Intern Med.* 1989; 111:273-9.
346. Rowinsky EK, McGuire WP, Guarnieri T et al. Cardiac disturbances during the administration of taxol. *J Clin Oncol.* 1991; 9:1704-12.
347. Arbuck SG, Strauss H, Rowinsky E et al. A reassessment of cardiac toxicity associated with Taxol. *J Natl Cancer Inst Monogr.* 1993; 15:117-30.
348. Chamberlain MC, Kormanik P. Salvage chemotherapy with paclitaxel for recurrent primary brain tumors. *J Clin Oncol.* 1995; 13:2066-71.
349. Glück S, Germond C, Lopez P et al. A phase I trial of high-dose paclitaxel, cyclophosphamide and mitoxantrone with autologous blood stem cell support for the treatment of metastatic breast cancer. *Eur J Cancer.* 1998; 34:1008-14.
350. Kanat O, Evrensel T, Baran I et al. Protective effect of amifostine against toxicity of paclitaxel and carboplatin in non-small cell lung cancer: a single center randomized study. *Med Oncol.* 2003; 20:237-45.
351. Kamineni P, Prakasa K, Hasan SP et al. Cardiotoxicities of paclitaxel in African Americans. *J Natl Med Assoc.* 2003; 95:977-81.
352. Ruiz-Casado A, Calzas J, García J et al. Life-threatening adverse drug reaction to paclitaxel: postmarketing surveillance. *Clin Transl Oncol.* 2006; 8:60-1.
353. Kietpeerakool C, Tiyayon J, Suprasert P et al. Benefit of electrocardiography during front-line combination paclitaxel and carboplatin chemotherapy for epithelial ovarian cancer. *J Med Assoc Thai.* 2006; 89:1805-10.
354. Rita L, Cox JM, Seleny FL et al. Ketamine hydrochloride for pediatric premedication: I. Comparison with pentazocine. *Anesth Analg.* 1974; 53:375-9.
355. Al Shibli A, Al Attrach I, Hamdan MA. Bradycardia following oral corticosteroid use: case report and literature review. *Arab J Nephrol Transplant.* 2012; 5:47-9.
356. Taylor MR, Gaco D. Symptomatic sinus bradycardia after a treatment course of high-dose oral prednisone. *J Emerg Med.* 2013; 45:e55-8.
357. Clémenty J, Coste P, Metzinger M. Efficacy and tolerance of propafenone in the treatment of cardiac rhythm disorders: evaluation of a multicenter open trial on 3,687 patients. *Ann Cardiol Angeiol.* 1987; 36:207-12.
358. Lee PK, Kerr CR, Vorderbrugge S et al. Symptomatic sinus node dysfunction associated with the use of propafenone. *Am J Cardiol.* 1988; 62:480-1.
359. Kerns W 2nd, English B, Ford M. Propafenone overdose. *Ann Emerg Med.* 1994; 24:98-103.
360. Mörike K, Magadum S, Mettang T et al. Propafenone in a usual dose produces severe side-effects: the impact of genetically determined metabolic status on drug therapy. *J Intern Med.* 1995; 238:469-72.
361. Ardic I, Gunebakmaz O, Yarlioglues M et al. Acute intoxication with propafenone and trimethoprim-sulfamethoxazole in a case of suicide attempt. *Turk Kardiyol Dem Ars.* 2009; 37:410-3.
362. Alsaad AA, Ortiz Gonzalez Y, Austin CO et al. Revisiting propafenone toxicity. *BMJ Case Rep.* 2017; Apr 26;2017. pii: bcr-2017-219270.
363. Thomson SJ, Yate PM. Bradycardia after propofol infusion. *Anaesthesia.* 1987; 42:430.
364. Baraka A. Severe bradycardia following propofol-suxamethonium sequence. *Br J Anaesth.* 1988; 61:482-3.
365. Saarnivaara L, Hiller A, Oikkonen M. QT interval, heart rate and arterial pressures using propofol, thiopentone or methohexitone for induction of anaesthesia in children. *Acta Anaesthesiol Scand.* 1993; 37:419-23.
366. Hug CC Jr, McLeskey CH, Nahrwold ML et al. Hemodynamic effects of propofol: data from over 25,000 patients. *Anesth Analg.* 1993; 77(suppl 4):S21-9.
367. McConaghy P, Bunting HE. Assessment of intubating conditions in children after induction with propofol and varying doses of alfentanil. *Br J Anaesth.* 1994; 73:596-9.
368. Tramèr MR, Moore RA, McQuay HJ. Propofol and bradycardia: causation, frequency and severity. *Br J Anaesth.* 1997; 78:642-51.
369. Bassett KE, Anderson JL, Pribble CG et al. Propofol for procedural sedation in children in the emergency department. *Ann Emerg Med.* 2003; 42:773-82.
370. Ulmer BJ, Hansen JJ, Overley CA et al. Propofol versus midazolam/fentanyl for outpatient colonoscopy: administration by nurses supervised by endoscopists. *Clin Gastroenterol Hepatol.* 2003; 1:425-32.
371. Taha S, Siddik-Sayyid S, Alameddine M et al. Propofol is superior to thiopental for intubation without muscle relaxants. *Can J Anaesth.* 2005; 52:249-53.
372. Wilson SE, Boyack DA, Ezeife-Ugorji OC et al. Propofol-induced bradycardia in a pediatric patient undergoing chemotherapy with the known cardiotoxic agent cytarabine. *Paediatr Anaesth.* 2006; 16:702-4.
373. Yorozu T, Iijima T, Matsumoto M et al. Factors influencing intraoperative bradycardia in adult patients. *J Anesth.* 2007; 21:136-41.
374. Sieg A. Propofol sedation in outpatient colonoscopy by trained practice nurses supervised by the gastroenterologist: a prospective evaluation of over 3000 cases. *Z Gastroenterol.* 2007; 45:697-701.
375. Poon CM, Leung TL, Wong CW et al. Safety of nurse-administered propofol sedation using PCA pump for outpatient colonoscopy in Chinese patients: a pilot study. *Asian J Surg.* 2007; 30:239-43.
376. Kongkam P, Rerknimitr R, Punyathavorn S et al. Propofol infusion versus intermittent meperidine and midazolam injection for conscious sedation in ERCP. *J Gastrointestin Liver Dis.* 2008; 17:291-7.
377. Huang J, Wilson S. Severe bradycardia after propofol induction. *AANA J.* 2008; 76:413.
378. Sundarathiti P, Sirinan C, Seangrung R et al. Selective spinal anesthesia versus intravenous propofol in transrectal ultrasound-guided prostate biopsy. *J Med Assoc Thai.* 2009; 92:920-4.
379. Kuypers MI, Menci F, Verhagen MF et al. Safety and efficacy of procedural sedation with propofol in a county with a young emergency medicine training program. *Eur J Emerg Med.* 2011; 18:162-7.
380. Correia LM, Bonilha DQ, Gomes GF et al. Sedation during upper GI endoscopy in cirrhotic outpatients: a randomized, controlled trial comparing propofol and fentanyl with midazolam and fentanyl. *Gastrointest Endosc.* 2011; 73:45-51.
381. Martinez JF, Aparicio JR, Company L et al. Safety of continuous propofol sedation for endoscopic procedures in elderly patients. *Rev Esp Enferm Dig.* 2011; 103:76-82.
382. Agostoni M, Fanti L, Gemma M et al. Adverse events during monitored anesthesia care for GI endoscopy: an 8-year experience. *Gastrointest Endosc.* 2011; 74:266-75.

383. Tschopp JM, Purek L, Frey JG et al. Titrated sedation with propofol for medical thoracoscopy: a feasibility and safety study. *Respiration.* 2011; 82:451-7.
384. Milius EM, Papademetrious TR, Heitlinger LA. Retrospective review of propofol dosing for procedural sedation in pediatric patients. *J Pediatr Pharmacol Ther.* 2012; 17:246-51.
385. Baraka A, Dajani A. Severe bradycardia following physostigmine in the presence of beta-adrenergic blockade: a case report. *Middle East J Anesthesiol.* 1984; 7:291-3.
386. Stein RD, Backman SB, Collier B et al. Bradycardia produced by pyridostigmine and physostigmine. *Can J Anesth.* 1997; 44:1286-92.
387. Zvosec DL, Smith SW, Litonjua R et al. Physostigmine for gamma-hydroxybutyrate coma: inefficacy, adverse events, and review. *Clin Toxicol.* 2007; 45:261-5.
388. Young DL, Halstead LA. Pyridostigmine for reversal of severe sequelae from botulinum toxin injection. *J Voice.* 2014; 28:830-4.
389. Camarri E, Chirone E, Fanteria G et al. Ranitidine-induced bradycardia. *Lancet.* 1984; 2:160.
390. Jack D, Richards DA, Granata F. Side-effects of ranitidine. *Lancet.* 1982; 2:264-5.
391. Shah RR. Symptomatic bradycardia in association with H2-receptor antagonists. *Lancet.* 1982; 2:1108.
392. Schifman C. Gynecomastia and bradycardia: side effects of ranitidine? *Clin Pharm.* 1983; 2:209.
393. Balestrazzi P, Gregori G, Bernasconi S et al. Bradycardia and neurologic disorders associated with ranitidine in a child. *Am J Dis Child.* 1985; 139:442.
394. Johnson WS, Miller DR. Ranitidine and bradycardia. *Ann Intern Med.* 1988; 108:493.
395. Khera DC, Smith SL, Slabic SF. Ranitidine-induced bradycardia. *Am J Gastroenterol.* 1988; 83:332-3.
396. Nahum E, Reish O, Naor N et al. Ranitidine-induced bradycardia in a neonate: a first report. *Eur J Pediatr.* 1993; 152:933-4.
397. Yang J, Russell DA, Bourdeau JE. Case report: ranitidine-induced bradycardia in a patient with dextrocardia. *Am J Med Sci.* 1996; 312:133-5.
398. Schüttler J, Albrecht S, Breivik H et al. A comparison of remifentanil and alfentanil in patients undergoing major abdominal surgery. *Anaesthesia.* 1997; 52:307-17.
399. DeSouza G, Lewis MC, TerRiet MF. Severe bradycardia after remifentanil. *Anesthesiology.* 1997; 87:1019-20.
400. Reid JE, Mirakhur RK. Bradycardia after administration of remifentanil. *Br J Anaesth.* 2000; 84:422-3.
401. Elliott P, O'Hare R, Bill KM et al. Severe cardiovascular depression with remifentanil. *Anesth Analg.* 2000; 91:5861.
402. Prys-Roberts C, Lerman J, Murat I et al. Comparison of remifentanil versus regional anaesthesia in children anaesthetised with isoflurane/nitrous oxide: International Remifentanil Paediatric Anaesthesia Study group. *Anaesthesia.* 2000; 55:870-6.
403. Chung F, Mulier JP, Scholz J et al. A comparison of anaesthesia using remifentanil combined with either isoflurane, enflurane or propofol in patients undergoing gynaecological laparoscopy, varicose vein or arthroscopic surgery. *Acta Anaesthesiol Scand.* 2000; 44:790-8.
404. Chinachoti T, Werawatganon T, Suksompong S et al. A multicenter randomized double-blind comparison of remifentanil and alfentanil during total intravenous anaesthesia for out-patient laparoscopic gynaecological procedures. *J Med Assoc Thai.* 2000; 83:1324-32.
405. Krenn H, Deusch E, Jellinek H et al. Remifentanil or propofol for sedation during carotid endarterectomy under cervical plexus block. *Br J Anaesth.* 2002; 89:637-40.
406. Nilsson LB, Viby-Mogensen J, Møller J et al. Remifentanil vs. alfentanil for direct laryngoscopy: a randomized study comparing two total intravenous anaesthesia techniques: TIVA for direct laryngoscopy. *Acta Anaesthesiol Belg.* 2002; 53:213-9.
407. Breslin DS, Farling PA, Mirakhur RK. The use of remifentanil in the anaesthetic management of patients undergoing adrenalectomy: a report of three cases. *Anaesthesia.* 2003; 58:358-62.
408. Weale NK, Rogers CA, Cooper R et al. Effect of remifentanil infusion rate on stress response to the prebypass phase of paediatric cardiac surgery. *Br J Anaesth.* 2004; 92:187-94.
409. Leidinger W, Schwinn P, Hofmann HM et al. Remifentanil for analgesia during retrobulbar nerve block placement. *Eur J Anaesthesiol.* 2005; 22:40-3.
410. Briassoulis G, Spanaki AM, Vassilaki E et al. Potentially life-threatening bradycardia after remifentanil infusion in a child. *Acta Anaesthesiol Scand.* 2007; 51:1130.
411. Shin SH, Kim HS, Lee J et al. A comparative study of two remifentanil doses for procedural pain in ventilated preterm infants: a randomized, controlled study. *Pediatr Crit Care Med.* 2014; 15:451-5.
412. Goyal RS, Goyal SB. Symptomatic bradyarrhythmia secondary to risperidone. *Am J Psychiatry.* 2003; 160:2243.
413. Tran KT, Golden P, Lark T et al. Bradycardia at low doses of risperidone. *Am J Psychiatry.* 2004; 161:2325-6.
414. Olgun H, Sepetcigil O, Karacan M et al. An unreported side effect of risperidone in children: sinus arrest with long pauses causing syncope. *Pediatr Emerg Care.* 2009; 25:465-6.
415. Raeder J, Gupta A, Pedersen FM. Recovery characteristics of sevoflurane or propofol-based anaesthesia for day-care surgery. *Acta Anaesthesiol Scand.* 1997; 41:988-94.
416. Townsend P, Stokes MA. Bradycardia during rapid inhalation induction with sevoflurane in children. *Br J Anaesth.* 1998; 80:410.
417. Gravel NR, Searle NR, Taillefer J et al. Comparison of the hemodynamic effects of sevoflurane anesthesia induction and maintenance vs TIVA in CABG surgery. *Can J Anaesth.* 1999; 46:240-6.
418. Green DH, Townsend P, Bagshaw O et al. Nodal rhythm and bradycardia during inhalation induction with sevoflurane in infants: a comparison of incremental and high-concentration techniques. *Br J Anaesth.* 2000; 85:369-70.
419. Roodman S, Bothwell M, Tobias JD. Bradycardia with sevoflurane induction in patients with trisomy 21. *Paediatr Anaesth.* 2003; 13:538-40.
420. Casati A, Aldegheri G, Vinciguerra E et al. Randomized comparison between sevoflurane anaesthesia and unilateral spinal anaesthesia in elderly patients undergoing orthopaedic surgery. *Eur J Anaesthesiol.* 2003; 20:640-6.
421. Hodgson RE, Dawson P, Hold AR et al. Anaesthesia for electroconvulsive therapy: a comparison of sevoflurane with propofol. *Anaesth Intensive Care.* 2004; 32:241-5.
422. Nagata S, Kazekawa K, Aikawa H et al. Hemodynamic stability under general anesthesia in carotid artery stenting. *Radiat Med.* 2005; 23:427-31.
423. Taylor MH, Wilton NC. Bradycardia with sevoflurane in siblings with Branchio-oto-renal syndrome. *Paediatr Anaesth.* 2007; 17:80-3.
424. Goldfinger MM, Tripi PA. Cardiac arrest in a child with cerebral palsy undergoing sevoflurane induction of anesthesia after preoperative clonidine. *Paediatr Anaesth.* 2007; 17:270-2.
425. Kraemer FW, Stricker PA, Gurnaney HG et al. Bradycardia during induction of anesthesia with sevoflurane in children with Down syndrome. *Anesth Analg.* 2010; 111:1259-63.
426. Bai W, Voepel-Lewis T, Malviya S. Hemodynamic changes in children with Down syndrome during and following inhalation of anesthesia with sevoflurane. *J Clin Anesth.* 2010; 22:592-7.
427. Boonmak P, Boonmak S, Pattanittum P. High initial concentration versus low initial concentration sevoflurane for inhalational induction of anesthesia. *Cochrane Database Syt Rev.* 2012; Sep 12: 9:CD006837.
428. Walia H, Ruda J, Tobias JD. Sevoflurane and bradycardia in infants with trisomy 21: a case report and review of the literature. *Int J Pediatr Otorhinolaryngol.* 2016; 80:5-7.
429. Latour Y, Dumont G, Brosseau A et al. Effects of sotalol in twenty patients with cardiac arrhythmias. *Int J Clin Pharmacol Biopharm.* 1977; 15:275-8.

430. Neuvonen PJ, Elonen E, Tarssanen L. Sotalol intoxication, two patients with concentration-effect relationships. *Acta Pharmacol Toxicol.* 1979; 45:52-7.
431. Gupta K. Hazards of β-blockers in the elderly: severe bradycardia due to Sotacor overdose. *Br J Clin Pract.* 1985; 39:116-7.
432. Campbell TJ, Gavaghan TP, Morgan JJ. Intravenous sotalol for the treatment of atrial fibrillation and flutter after cardiopulmonary bypass: comparison with disopyramide and digoxin in a randomised trial. *Br Heart J.* 1985; 54:86-90.
433. Edvardsson N, Varnauskas E. Clinical course, serum concentrations and elimination rate in a case of massive sotalol intoxication. *Eur Heart J.* 1987; 8:544-8.
434. Anastasiou-Nana MI, Anderson JL, Askins JC et al. Long-term experience with sotalol in the treatment of complex ventricular arrhythmias. *Am Heart J.* 1987; 114:288-96.
435. Soyka LF, Wirtz C, Spangenberg RB. Clinical safety profile of sotalol in patients with arrhythmias. *Am J Cardiol.* 1990; 65:74A-81A.
436. Obel IW, Jardine R, Haitus B et al. Efficacy of oral sotalol in reentrant ventricular tachycardia. *Cardiovasc Drugs Ther.* 1990; 4(suppl 3):613-8.
437. Tipple M, Sandor G. Efficacy and safety of oral sotalol in early infancy. *Pacing Clin Electrophysiol.* 1991; 14:2062-5.
438. Horrigan MC, Davis MJ, May C et al. Dual chamber rate responsive pacing to allow sotalol therapy for ventricular tachycardia. *Pacing Clin Electrophysiol.* 1992; 15:2108-10.
439. Winters SL, Kukin M, Pe E et al. Effect of oral sotalol on systemic hemodynamics and programmed electrical stimulation in patients with ventricular arrhythmias and structural heart disease. *Am J Cardiol.* 1993; 72:38A-43A.
440. Jacquet L, Evenepoel M, Marenne F et al. Hemodynamic effects and safety of sotalol in the prevention of supraventricular arrhythmias after coronary artery bypass surgery. *J Cardiothorac Vasc Anesth.* 1994; 8:431-6.
441. Fernandes CM, Daya MR. Sotalol-induced bradycardia reversed by glucagon. *Can Fam Physician.* 1995; 41:659-60, 663-65.
442. Halinen MO, Huttunen M, Paakkinen S et al. Comparison of sotalol with digoxin-quinidine for conversion of acute atrial fibrillation to sinus rhythm (the Sotalol-Digoxin-Quinidine Trial). *Am J Cardiol.* 1995; 76:495-8.
443. Lee SH, Chen SA, Tai CT et al. Comparisons of oral propafenone and sotalol as an initial treatment in patients with symptomatic paroxysmal atrial fibrillation. *Am J Cardiol.* 1997; 79:905-8.
444. Beaufort-Krol GC, Bink-Boelkens MT. Sotalol for atrial tachycardias after surgery for congenital heart disease. *Pacing Clin Electrophysiol.* 1997; 20:2125-9.
445. Maisel WH, Kuntz KM, Reimold SC et al. Risk of initiating antiarrhythmic drug therapy for atrial fibrillation in patients admitted to a university hospital. *Ann Intern Med.* 1997; 127:281-4.
446. Chung MK, Schweikert RA, Wilkoff BL et al. Is hospital admission for initiation of antiarrhythmic therapy with sotalol for atrial arrhythmias required? Yield of inhospital monitoring and prediction of risk for significant arrhythmia complications. *J Am Coll Cardiol.* 1998; 32:169-76.
447. Gomes JA, Ip J, Santoni-Rugiu F, Mehta D et al. Oral d,l sotalol reduces the incidence of postoperative atrial fibrillation in coronary artery bypass surgery patients: a randomized, double-blind, placebo-controlled study. *J Am Coll Cardiol.* 1999; 34:334-9.
448. Matsuura K, Takahara Y, Sudo Y et al. Effect of Sotalol in the prevention of atrial fibrillation following coronary artery bypass grafting. *Jpn J Thorac Cardiovasc Surg.* 2001; 49:614-7.
449. Celiker A, Ayabakan C, Ozer S et al. Sotalol in treatment of pediatric cardiac arrhythmias. *Pediatr Int.* 2001; 43:624-30.
450. Auer J, Weber T, Berent R et al. A comparison between oral antiarrhythmic drugs in the prevention of atrial fibrillation after cardiac surgery: the pilot study of prevention of postoperative atrial fibrillation (SPPAF), a randomized, placebo-controlled trial. *Am Heart J.* 2004; 147:636-43.
451. Connolly SJ, Dorian P, Roberts RS et al. Comparison of β-blockers, amiodarone plus β-blockers, or sotalol for prevention of shocks from implantable cardioverter defibrillators. The OPTIC study: a randomized trial. *JAMA.* 2006; 295:165-71.
452. Rao S, Boramanand NK, Burton DA et al. Atrial tachycardia in young adolescents with congenital heart disease: conversion using single dose oral sotalol. *Int J Cardiol.* 2009; 136:253-7.
453. Barreto RS. Effect of intravenously administered succinylcholine upon cardiac rate and rhythm. *Anesthesiology.* 1960; 21:401-4.
454. Craythorne NW, Turndorf H, Dripps RD. Changes in the pulse rate and rhythm associated with the use of succinylcholine in anesthetized children. *Anesthesiology.* 1960; 21:465-70.
455. Perez H. Cardiac arrhythmia after succinylcholine. *Anesth Analg.* 1970; 49:33-8.
456. Cozanitis DA, Dundee JW, Khan MM. Comparative study of atropine and glycopyrrolate on suxamethonium induced changes in cardiac rate and rhythm. *Br J Anaesth.* 1980; 52:291-3.
457. Lerman J, Chinyanga HM. The heart rate response to succinylcholine in children: a comparison of atropine and glycopyrrolate. *Can Anaesth Soc J.* 1983; 30:377-81.
458. Sørensen M, Engbaek J, Viby-Mogensen J et al. Bradycardia and cardiac asystole following a single injection of suxamethonium. *Acta Anaesthesiol Scand.* 1984; 28:232-5.
459. Green DW, Bristow AS, Fisher M. Comparison of i.v. glycopyrrolate and atropine in the prevention of bradycardia and arrhythmias following repeated doses of suxamethonium in children. *Br J Anaesth.* 1984; 56:981-5.
460. Inoue K, Reichelt W. Asystole and bradycardia in adult patients after a single dose of suxamethonium. *Acta Anaesthesiol Scand.* 1986; 30:571-3.
461. Sherman EP, Lebowitz PW, Street WC. Bradycardia following sufentanil-succinylcholine. *Anesthesiology.* 1987; 66:106.
462. Rivard JC, Lebowitz PW. Bradycardia after alfentanil: succinylcholine. *Anesth Analg.* 1988; 67:907.
463. Baraka A. Severe bradycardia following propofol-suxamethonium sequence. *Br J Anaesth.* 1988; 61:482-3.
464. Hansen D. Suxamethonium-induced cardiac arrest and death following 5 days of immobilization. *Eur J Anaesthesiol.* 1998; 15:240-1.
465. Pace SA, Fuller FP. Out-of-hospital succinylcholine-assisted endotracheal intubation by paramedics. *Ann Emerg Med.* 2000; 35:568-72.
466. Sawabe T, Mizuno S, Gondo H et al. Sinus arrest during tacrolimus (FK506) and digitalis treatment in a bone marrow transplant recipient. *Transplantation.* 1997; 64:182-3.
467. Cox TH, Baillie GM, Baliga P. Bradycardia associated with intravenous administration of tacrolimus in a liver transplant recipient. *Pharmacotherapy.* 1997; 17:1328-30.
468. Tuominen M, Pitkanen M, Doepel M et al Spinal anesthesia with hyperbaric tetracaine: effect of age and body mass. *Acta Anaesthesiol Scand.* 1987; 31:474-8.
469. Taddio A, Lee CM, Parvez B et al. Contact dermatitis and bradycardia in a preterm infant given tetracaine 4% gel. *Ther Drug Monit.* 2006; 28:291-4.
470. Maulidi H, McNair C, Seller N et al. Arrhythmia-associated with tetracaine in an extremely low birth weight premature infant. *Pediatrics.* 2012; 130:e1704-7.
471. Juliusson G, Celsing F, Turesson I et al. Frequent good partial remissions from thalidomide including best response ever in patients with advanced refractory and relapsed myeloma. *Br J Haematol.* 2000; 109:89-96.
472. Rajkumar SV, Gertz MA, Lacy MQ et al. Thalidomide as initial therapy for early-stage myeloma. *Leukemia.* 2003; 17:775-9.
473. Kaur A, Yu SS, Lee AJ et al. Thalidomide-induced sinus bradycardia. *Ann Pharmacother.* 2003; 37:1040-3.
474. Kropff MH, Lang N, Bisping G et al. Hyperfractionated cyclophosphamide in combination with pulsed dexamethasone and thalidomide (HyperCDT) in primary refractory or relapsed multiple myeloma. *Br J Haematol.* 2003; 122:607-16.
475. Coutsouvelis J, Corallo CE. Thalidomide-induced bradycardia and its management. *Med J Aust.* 2004; 180:366-7.

476. Fahdi IE, Gaddam V, Saucedo JF et al. Bradycardia during therapy for multiple myeloma with thalidomide. *Am J Cardiol.* 2004; 93:1052-5.
477. Palladini G, Perfetti V, Perlini S et al. The combination of thalidomide and intermediate-dose dexamethasone is an effective but toxic treatment for patients with primary Amyloidosis (AL). *Blood.* 2005; 105:2949-51.
478. Schütt P, Ebeling P, Buttkereit U et al. Thalidomide in combination with dexamethasone for pretreated patients with multiple myeloma: serum level of soluble interleukin-2 receptor as a predictive factor for response rate and for survival. *Ann Hematol.* 2005; 84:594-600.
479. Rajkumar SV, Blood E, Vesole D et al. Phase III clinical trial of thalidomide plus dexamethasone compared with dexamethasone alone in newly diagnosed multiple myeloma: a clinical trial coordinated by the Eastern Cooperative Oncology Group. *J Clin Oncol.* 2006; 24:431-6.
480. Meyer T, Maier A, Borisow N et al. Thalidomide causes sinus bradycardia in ALS. *J Neurol.* 2008; 255:587-91.
481. Sanborn SL, Cooney MM, Dowlati A et al. Phase I trial of docetaxel and thalidomide: a regimen based on metronomic therapeutic principles. *Invest New Drugs.* 2008; 26:355-62.
482. Yamaguchi T. Syncope and sinus bradycardia from combined use of thalidomide and beta-blocker. *Pharmacoepidemiol Drug Saf.* 2008; 17:1033-5.
483. Ali A, Hothi SS, Thompson A et al. Negative chronotropic effects and coronary ischaemic abnormalities following thalidomide therapy. *Cardiology.* 2013; 125:34-7.
484. Misawa S, Sato Y, Katayama K et al. Safety and efficacy of thalidomide in patients with POEMS syndrome: a multicenter, randomized, double-blind, placebo-controlled trial. *Lancet Neurol.* 2016; 15:1129-37.
485. Goldman JW, Laux I, Chai F et al. Phase 1 dose-escalation trial evaluating the combination of the selective MET (mesenchymal-epithelial transition factor) inhibitor tivantinib (ARQ 197) plus erlotinib. *Cancer.* 2012; 118:5903-11.
486. Kitabata Y, Orita H, Kamimura M et al. Symptomatic bradycardia probably due to tizanidine hydrochloride in a chronic hemodialysis patient. *Ther Apher Dial.* 2005; 9:74-7.
487. Publow SW, Branam DL. Hypotension and bradycardia associated with concomitant tizanidine and lisinopril therapy. *Am J Health-Syst Pharm.* 2010; 67:1606-10.
488. Cortes J, Hall B, redden D. Profound symptomatic bradycardia requiring transvenous pacing after a single dose of tizanidine. *J Emerg Med.* 2015; 48:458-60.
489. Masood U, Kahlon A, Mousa O. Clinical significant bradycardia from tizanidine. *Am J Ther.* 2018; 25:e385-6.
490. de Faire U, Lundman T. Attempted suicide with verapamil. *Eur J Cardiol.* 1977; 6:195-8.
491. de Faire U, Lundman T. Serious verapamil poisoning. *Br J Med.* 1978; 2:1574.
492. Jain SC, Bharadwaj RP, Shukla RK et al. Severe hypotension and bradycardia after suicidal consumption of 100 tablets of verapamil: a case report. *Indian Heart J.* 1982; 34:175-6.
493. Wayne VS, Harper RW, Laufer E et al. Adverse interaction between beta-adrenergic blocking drugs and verapamil: report of three cases. *Aust N Z J Med.* 1982; 12:285-9.
494. Subramanian VB, Bowles MJ, Khurmi NS et al. Randomized double-blind comparison of verapamil and nifedipine in chronic stable angina. *Am J Cardiol.* 1982; 50:696-703.
495. Crump BJ, Holt DW, Vale JA. Lack of response to intravenous calcium in severe verapamil poisoning. *Lancet.* 1982; 2:939-40.
496. Leitner RP, Hawker RE, Celermajer JM. Intravenous verapamil in the treatment of paroxysmal supraventricular tachycardia in children. *Aust Paediatr J.* 1983; 19:40-4.
497. Radford D. Side effects of verapamil in infants. *Arch Dis Child.* 1983; 58:465-6.
498. Morris DL, Goldschlager N. Calcium infusion for reversal of adverse effects of intravenous verapamil. *JAMA.* 1983; 249:3212-3.
499. Subramanian VB, Bowles MJ, Khurmi NS et al. Evaluation of verapamil and high dose nifedipine in patients with chronic stable angina with objective methods. *Acta Med Scand.* 1984; 681;61-73.
500. Passal DB, Crespin FH Jr. Verapamil poisoning in an infant. *Pediatrics.* 1984; 73:543-5.
501. Zatuchni J. Bradycardia and hypotension after propranolol HCl and verapamil. *Heart Lung.* 1985; 14:9495.
502. Winniford MD, Fulton KL, Corbett JR et al. Propranolol-verapamil versus propranolol-nifedipine in severe angina pectoris of effort: a randomized, double-blind, crossover study. *Am J Cardiol.* 1985; 55:281-5.
503. Purnell RJ. Bradycardia after verapamil and spinal analgesia. *Anaesthesia.* 1985; 40:1245.
504. Pennock GD, Dalton WS, Roeske WR et al. Systemic toxic effects associated with high-dose verapamil infusion and chemotherapy administration. *J Natl Cancer Inst.* 1991; 83:105-10.
505. Quezado Z, Lippmann M, Wertheimer J. Severe cardiac, respiratory, and metabolic complications of massive verapamil overdose. *Crit Care Med.* 1991; 19:436-8.
506. Watson NA, FitzGerald CP. Management of massive verapamil overdose. *Med J Aust.* 1991; 155:124-5.
507. Arstall MA, Beltrame JF, Mohan P et al. Incidence of adverse events during treatment with verapamil for suspected acute myocardial infarction. *Am J Cardiol.* 1992; 70:1611-2.
508. Doyon S, Roberts JR. The use of glucagon in a case of calcium channel blocker overdose. *Ann Emerg Med.* 1993; 2:1229-33.
509. Howarth DM, Dawson AH, Smith AJ et al. Calcium channel blocking drug overdose: an Australian series. *Hum Exp Toxicol.* 1994; 13:161-6.
510. Ashraf M, Chaudhary K, Nelson J et al. Massive overdose of sustained-release verapamil: a case report and review of literature. *Am J Med Sci.* 1995; 310:258-3.
511. Van Mieghem W, Tits G, Demuynck K et al. Verapamil as prophylactic treatment for atrial fibrillation after lung operations. *Ann Thorac Surg.* 1996; 61:1083-5.
512. Pahor M, Manto A, Pedone C et al. Age and severe adverse drug reactions caused by nifedipine and verapamil: Gruppo Italiano di Farmacovigilanza nell' Anziano (GIFA). *J Clin Epidemiol.* 1996; 49:921-8.
513. Brass BJ, Winchester-Penny S, Lipper BL. Massive verapamil overdose complicated by noncardiogenic pulmonary edema. *Am J Emerg Med.* 1996; 14:459-61.
514. Yörükog˘lu D, Göktug A, Alanog˘lu Z et al. Comparison of intravenous metoprolol, verapamil and diltiazem on the attenuation of haemodynamic changes associated with tracheal extubation. *Eur J Anaesthesiol.* 1999; 16:462-7.
515. Yuan TH, Kerns WP 2nd, Tomaszewski CA et al. Insulin-glucose as adjunctive therapy for severe calcium channel antagonist poisoning. *J Toxicol Clin Toxicol.* 1999; 37:463-74.
516. Kuhlmann U, Schoenemann H, Müller T et al. Plasmapheresis in life-threatening verapamil intoxication. *Artif Cells Blood Substit Immobil Biotechnol.* 2008; 28:429-40.
517. White WB, Johnson MF, Anders RJ et al. Safety of controlled-onset extended-release verapamil in middle-aged and older patients with hypertension and coronary artery disease. *Am Heart J.* 2001; 142:1010-5.
518. Kato M, Dote K, Sasaki S et al. Intracoronary verapamil rapidly terminates reperfusion tachyarrhythmias in acute myocardial infarction. *Chest.* 2004; 126:702-8.
519. Patel NP, Pugh ME, Goldberg S et al. Hyperinsulinemic euglycemia therapy for verapamil poisoning: case report. *Am J Crit Care.* 2007; 16:518-9.
520. Osthoff M, Bernsmeier C, Marsch SC et al. Levosimendan as treatment option in severe verapamil intoxication: a case report and review of the literature. *Case Rep Med.* 2010; 2010:pii:546904.

521. Fu Q, Lu W, Huang YJ et al. Verapamil reverses myocardial no-reflow after primary percutaneous coronary intervention in patients with acute myocardial infarction. *Cell Biochem Biophys.* 2013; 67:911-4.
522. Mandigers L, Bollen PD, Bijlstra PJ et al. Severe verapamil intoxication despite correct use of low-dose verapamil. *Drug Metabol Personal Ther.* 2016; 31:55-8.
523. Netland PA, Weiss HS, Stewart WC et al. Cardiovascular effects of topical carteolol hydrochloride and timolol maleate in patients with ocular hypertension and primary open-angle glaucoma: Night Study Group. *Am J Ophthalmol.* 1997; 123:465-77.
524. Williams T, Ginther WH. Hazard of ophthalmic timolol. *N Engl J Med.* 1982; 306:1485-6.
525. Guha S, Dawn B, Dutta G et al. Bradycardia, reversible panconduction defect and syncope following self-medication with a homeopathic medicine. *Cardiology.* 1999; 91:268-71.
526. Chan TY. Aconite poisoning. *Clin Toxicol.* 2009; 47:279-85.
527. DiMarco JP, Sellers TD, Berne RM et al. Adenosine: electrophysiologic effects and therapeutic use for terminating paroxysmal supraventricular tachycardia. *Circulation.* 1983; 68:1254-63.
528. Tajima T, Muramatsu T, Kanaka S et al. Electrophysiologic effects of intravenous adenosine triphosphate disodium on the paroxysmal supraventricular tachycardias. *Jpn Heart J.* 1985; 26:33-43.
529. diMarco JP, Sellers TD, Lerman BB et al. Diagnostic and therapeutic use of adenosine in patients with supraventricular tachyarrhythmias. *J Am Coll Cardiol.* 1985; 6:417-25.
530. Watt AH, Routledge PA. Transient bradycardia and subsequent sinus tachycardia produced by intravenous adenosine in healthy adult subjects. *Br J Clin Pharmacol.* 1986; 21:533-6.
531. Sylvén C, Jonzon B, Brandt R et al. Adenosine-provoked angina pectoris-like pain: time characteristics, influence of autonomic blockade and naloxone. *Eur Heart J.* 1987; 8:738-43.
532. Sylvén C, Jonzon B, Edlund A. Angina pectoris-like pain provoked by i.v. bolus of adenosine: relationship to coronary sinus blood flow, heart rate and blood pressure in healthy volunteers. *Eur Heart J.* 1989; 10:48-54.
533. Till J, Shinebourne EA, Rigby ML et al. Efficacy and safety of adenosine in the treatment of supraventricular tachycardia in infants and children. *Br Heart J.* 1989; 62:204-11.
534. Rossen JD, Quillen JE, Lopez AG et al. Comparison of coronary vasodilation with intravenous dipyridamole and adenosine. *J Am Coll Cardiol.* 1991; 18:485-91.
535. Abreu A, Mahmarian JJ, Nishimura S et al. Tolerance and safety of pharmacologic coronary vasodilation with adenosine in association with thallium-201 scintigraphy in patients with suspected coronary artery disease. *J Am Coll Cardiol.* 1991; 18:730-5.
536. Lee J, Heo J, Ogilby JD et al. Atrioventricular block during adenosine thallium imaging. *Am Heart J.* 1992; 123:1569-74.
537. Anderson TJ, Ryan TJ Jr, Mudge GH et al. Sinoatrial and atrioventricular block caused by intracoronary infusion of adenosine early after heart transplantation. *Heart Lung Transplant.* 1993; 12:522-4.
538. Toft J, Mortensen J, Hesse B. Risk of atrioventricular block during adenosine pharmacologic stress testing in heart transplant recipients. *Am J Cardiol.* 1998; 82:696-7.
539. Alkoutami GS, Reeves WC, Movahed A. The safety of adenosine pharmacologic stress testing in patients with first-degree atrioventricular block in the presence and absence of atrioventricular blocking medications. *J Nucl Cardiol.* 1999; 6:495-7.
540. Alkoutami GS, Reeves WC, Movahed A. The frequency of atrioventricular block during adenosine stress testing in young, middle-aged, young-old, and old-old adults. *Am J Geriatr Cardiol.* 2001; 10:159-61.
541. Camaiti A, Pieralli F, Olivotto I et al. Prospective evaluation of adenosine-induced proarrhythmia in the emergency room. *Eur J Emerg Med.* 2001; 8:99-105.
542. Treuth MG, Reyes GA, He ZX et al. Tolerance and diagnostic accuracy of an abbreviated adenosine infusion for myocardial scintigraphy: a randomized, prospective study. *J Nucl Cardiol.* 2001; 8:548-54.
543. Makaryus JN, Catanzaro JN, Friedman ML et al. Persistent second-degree atrioventricular block following adenosine infusion for nuclear stress testing. *J Cardiovasc Med.* 2008; 9:304-7.
544. Karamitsos TD, Arnold JR, Pegg TJ et al. Tolerance and safety of adenosine stress perfusion cardiovascular magnetic resonance imaging in patients with severe coronary artery disease. *Int J Cardiovasc Imaging.* 2009; 25:277-83.
545. Karamitsos TD, Ntusi NA, Francis JM et al. Feasibility and safety of high-dose adenosine perfusion cardiovascular magnetic resonance. *J Cardiovasc Magn Reson.* 2020; 12:66.
546. Al-Mallah MH, Arida M, Garcia-Sayan E et al. Safety of adenosine pharmacologic stress myocardial perfusion imaging in orthotopic cardiac transplant recipients: a single center experience of 102 transplant patients. *Int J Cardiovasc Imaging.* 2011; 27:1105-11.
547. Singh M, Shah T, Khosla K et al. Safety and efficacy of intracoronary adenosine administration in patients with acute myocardial infarction undergoing primary percutaneous coronary intervention: a meta-analysis of randomized controlled trials. *Ther Adv Cardiovasc Dis.* 2012; 6:101-14.
548. Seo MK, Koo BK, Kim JH et al. Comparison of hyperemic efficacy between central and peripheral venous adenosine infusion for fractional flow reserve measurement. *Circ Cardiovas Interv.* 2012; 5:401-5.
549. Su Q, Nyi TS, Li L. Adenosine and verapamil for no-reflow during primary percutaneous coronary intervention in people with acute myocardial infarction. *Cochrane Database Syst Rev.* 2015; May 18; 5:CD009503.
550. Wang X, Li S, Zhao X et al. Effects of intracoronary sodium nitroprusside compared with adenosine on fractional flow reserve measurement. *J Invasive Cardiol* 2014; 26:119-122.
551. Sun H, Tian Y, Zheng L et al. Electrocardiographic profile of adenosine pharmacological stress testing. *Exp Ther Med.* 2015; 9:1178-84.
552. Nägele H, Bohlmann M, Eck U et al. Combination therapy with carvedilol and amiodarone in patients with severe heart failure. *Eur J Heart Fail.* 2000; 2:71-9.
553. Morady F, Scheinman MM, Shen E et al. Intravenous amiodarone in the acute treatment of recurrent symptomatic ventricular tachycardia. *Am J Cardiol.* 1983; 51:156-9.
554. Mangiardi L, Gaita F, Brun S et al. Atrioventricular block complicating amiodarone-induced hypothyroidism in a patient with preexcitation and rate-dependent bilateral bundle branch block. *J Am Coll Cardiol.* 1986; 7:180-4.
555. Raviña T, Gutierrez J. Amiodarone-induced AV block and ventricular standstill: a forme fruste of an idiopathic long QT syndrome. *Int J Cardiol.* 2000; 75:105-8.
556. McMahon CJ, Laird WP, Fenrich AL. Amiodarone-induced 2 to 1 atrioventricular block in association with prolongation of the QT interval. *Cardiol Young.* 2003; 13:305-7.
557. Saul JP, Scott WA, Brown S et al. Intravenous amiodarone for incessant tachyarrhythmias in children: a randomized, double-blind, antiarrhythmic drug trial. *Circulation.* 2005; 112:3470-7.
558. Sato Y, Dohi K, Kusuki H et al. Heart failure exacerbation associated with newly developed atrioventricular dyssynchrony after chemical conversion to a sinus rhythm in a patients receiving cardiac resynchromization therapy. *Intern Med.* 2013; 52:1359-63.
559. Sequeira OR, Aquino NJ, Gomez NB et al. Amiodarone-induced third degree atrioventricular block and extreme QT prolongation generating torsade des pointes in paroxysmal atrial fibrillation. *J Atr Fibrillation.* 2016; 9:1502.
560. Smith RB, Rusbatch BJ. Amitriptyline and heart block. *Br Med J.* 1967; 3:311.
561. Lappa A, Castagna A, Imperiale C et al. Near fatal case of atrioventricular block induced by amitriptyline at therapeutic dose. *Intensive Care Med.* 2000; 26:1399.

562. Ilyas M. Intermittent atrioventricular block after propranolol. *N Engl J Med.* 1972; 286:376-7.
563. Zeis PM, Thanopoulos B, Pierroutsakos IN et al. Complete atrioventricular block associated with propranolol therapy. *J Pediatr.* 1981; 98:326-7.
564. García-Rubira JC, Pavón M, Romero-Chacón D. Syncope induced by propranolol in hypertrophic cardiomyopathy. *Int J Cardiol.* 1991; 31:358-61.
565. Kelkar PN. Atenolol induced high grade AV block. *J Assoc Physicians India.* 1998; 46:748-51.
566. Krum H, Shusterman N, MacMahon S et al. Efficacy and safety of carvedilol in patients with chronic heart failure receiving concomitant amiodarone therapy: Australia/New Zealand Heart Failure Research Collaborative Group. *J Cardiac Fail.* 1998; 4:281-8.
567. Ruiz-Ruiz FJ, Perez-Calvo JI, Sanjuan-Cuartero R. Topical beta blockers and atrioventricular block in the elderly. *J Postgrad Med.* 2002; 48:327-8.
568. Zeltser D, Justo D, Halkin A et al. Drug-induced atrioventricular block: prognosis after discontinuation of the culprit drug. *J Am Coll Cardiol.* 2004; 44:105-8.
569. Tarantini L, Cioffi G, Opasich C et al. Pre-discharge initiation of beta-blocker therapy in elderly patients hospitalized for acute decompensation of chronic heart failure: an effective strategy for the implementation of beta-blockade in heart failure. *Ital Heart J.* 2004; 5:441-9.
570. Onalan O, Cumurcu BE, Bekar L. Complete atrioventricular block associated with concomitant use of metoprolol and paroxetine. *Mayo Clin Proc.* 2008; 83:595-9.
571. Hunag M, Zhang X, Chen S et al. The effect of carvedilol treatment on chronic heart failure in pediatric patients with dilated cardiomyopathy: a prospective, randomized-controlled study. *Pediatr Cardiol.* 2013; 34:680-5.
572. Kassamali RH, Kim DH, Patel H et al. Safety of an i.v. β-adrenergic blockade protocol for heart rate optimization before coronary CT angiography. *Am J Roentgenol.* 2014; 203:759-62.
573. Knudsen MB, Thogersen AM, Hjortshoj SP et al. The impact of drug discontinuation in patients treated with temporary pacemaker due to atrioventricular block. *J Cardiovasc Electrophysiol.* 2013; 24:1255-8.
574. Ozcan KS, Gungor B, Osmonov D et al. Management and outcome of topical beta-blocker-induced atrioventricular block. *Cardiovasc J Afr.* 2015; 26:210-3.
575. Timour Q, Freysz M, Couzon P et al. Possible role of drug interactions in bupivacaine-induced problems related to intraventricular conduction disorders. *Reg Anesth.* 1990; 15:180-5.
576. Shen CL, Ho YY, Hung YC et al. Arrhythmias during spinal anesthesia for Cesarean section. *Can J Anaesth.* 2000; 47:393-7.
577. Beermann B, Edhag O, Vallin H. Advanced heart block aggravated by carbamazepine. *Br Heart J.* 1975; 37:668-71.
578. Ladefoged SD, Møgelvang JC. Total atrioventricular block with syncopes complicating carbamazepine therapy. *Acta Med Scand.* 1982; 212:185-6.
579. Boesen F, Andersen EB, Jensen EK et al. Cardiac conduction disturbances during carbamazepine therapy. *Acta Neurol Scand.* 1983; 68:49-52.
580. Labrecque J, Coté MA, Vincent P. Carbamazepine-induced atrioventricular block. *Am J Psychiatry.* 1992; 149:572-3.
581. Hantson P, Ilunga K, Martin N et al. Cardiac conduction abnormalities during carbamazepine therapy for neuralgia following Guillain-Barré syndrome. *Acta Neurol Belg.* 1993; 93:40-3.
582. Ide A, Kamijo Y. Intermittent complete atrioventricular block after long term low-dose carbamazepine therapy with a serum concentration less than the therapeutic level. *Intern Med.* 2007; 46:627-9.
583. Koutsampasopoulos K, Zotos A, Papamichalis M et al. Carbamazepine induced atrial tachycardia with complete AV block. *Hippokratia.* 2014; 18:185-6.
584. Celik IE, Akyel A, Colgecen M et al. A rare cause of 2:1 atrioventricular block: carbamazepine. *Am J Emerg Med.* 2015; 33:1541.e3-4.
585. Can I, Tholakanahalli V. Carbamazepine-induced atrioventricular block in an elderly woman. *Turk Kardiyol Dern Ars.* 2016; 44:68-70.
586. Guedira N, Hajjaj-Hassouni N, Srairi JE et al. Third degree atrioventricular block in a patient under chloroquine therapy. *Rev Rhum Engl Ed.* 1998; 65:58-62.
587. Reuss-Borst M, Berner B, Wulf G et al. Complete heart block as a rare complication of treatment with chloroquine. *J Rheumatol.* 1999; 26:1394-5.
588. Teixeira RA, Martinelli Filho M, Benvenuti LA et al. Cardiac damage from chronic use of chloroquine: a case report and review of the literature. *Arg Bras Cardiol.* 2002; 79:85-8.
589. Tordjman T, Korzets A, Kotas R et al. Complete atrioventricular block and long-term cimetidine therapy. *Arch Intern Med.* 1994; 144:861.
590. Gambassi G, Incalzi RA, Gemma A. Atrioventricular blocks associated with citalopram. *Am J Geriatr Psychiatry.* 2005; 13:918-9.
591. Williams PL, Krafcik JM, Potter BB et al. Cardiac toxicity of clonidine. *Chest.*1977; 72:784-5.
592. Abiuso P, Abelow G. Atrioventricular dissociation in a patient receiving clonidine. *JAMA.* 1978; 240:108-9.
593. Ciaccheri M, Dolara A, Manetti A et al. A-V block by an overdose of Clonidine. *Acta Cardiol.* 1983; 38:233-6.
594. Jaffe R, Livshits T, Bursztyn M. Adverse interaction between clonidine and verapamil. *Ann Pharmacother.* 1994; 28:881-3.
595. Om A, Ellenbogen KA, Vetrovec GW. Cocaine-induced bradyarrhythmias. *Am Heart J.* 1992; 124:232-4.
596. Hall PS, Nazer B, Lee RJ. Reversible high-grade atrioventricular block associated with cocaine use. *JAMA Intern Med.* 2015; 175:1965-7.
597. Smith TW, Haber E. Digoxin intoxication: the relationship of clinical presentation to serum digoxin concentration. *J Clin Invest.* 1970; 49:2377-86.
598. Duke M. Atrioventricular block due to accidental digoxin ingestion treated with atropine. *Am J Dis Child.* 1972; 124:754-56.
599. Smith TW, Haber E, Yeatman L et al. Reversal of advanced digoxin intoxication with Fab fragments of digoxin-specific antibodies. *N Engl J Med.* 1976; 294:797-800.
600. Chan W, Ikram H. A case of self-induced digoxin poisoning: with His bundle studies of the site of heart block. *N Z Med J.* 1976; 84:443-6.
601. Rostás L, Tarján J. Wenckebach type H-V block induced by digitalis intoxication. *Z Kardiol.* 1980; 69:779-81.
602. Goren C, Denes P. The role of Holter monitoring in detecting digitalis-provoked arrhythmias. *Chest.* 1981; 79:555-8.
603. Rossi R, Leititis JU, Hagel KJ et al. Severe digoxin intoxication in a child treated by infusion of digoxin-specific Fab-antibody-fragments. *Eur J Pediatr.* 1984; 142:138-40.
604. Smolarz A, Roesch E, Lenz E et al. Digoxin specific antibody (Fab) fragments in 34 cases of severe digitalis intoxication. *J Toxicol Clin Toxicol.* 1985; 23:327-40.
605. Moorman JR. Digitalis toxicity at Duke Hospital, 1973-1984. *South Med J.* 1985; 78:561-4.
606. Lai KN, Swaminathan R, Pun CO et al. Hemofiltration in digoxin overdose. *Arch Intern Med.* 1986; 146:1219-20.
607. Lewander WJ, Gaudreault P, Einhorn A et al. Acute pediatric digoxin ingestion: a ten-year experience. *Am J Dis Child.* 1986; 140:770-3.
608. Kearns GL, Moss MM, Clayton BD et al. Pharmacokinetics and efficacy of digoxin specific Fab fragments in a child following massive digoxin overdose. *J Clin Pharmacol.* 1989; 29:901-8.
609. Woolf AD, Wenger T, Smith TW et al. The use of digoxin-specific Fab fragments for severe digitalis intoxication in children. *N Engl J Med.* 1992; 326:1739-44.

610. Wofford JL, Hickey AR, Ettinger WH et al. Lack of age-related differences in the clinical presentation of digoxin toxicity. *Arch Intern Med.* 1992; 152:2261-4.

611. Abad-Santos F, Carcas AJ, Ibáñez C et al. Digoxin level and clinical manifestations as determinants in the diagnosis of digoxin toxicity. *Ther Drug Monit.* 2000; 22:163-8.

612. Spodick DH. Well concealed atrial tachycardia with Wenckebach (Mobitz I) atrioventricular block: digitalis toxicity. *Am J Geriatr Cardiol.* 2001; 10:59.

613. Juneja D, Singh O, Bhasin A et al. Severe suicidal digoxin toxicity managed with resin hemoperfusion: a case report. *Indian J Crit Care Med.* 2012; 16:231-3.

614. Hossack KF. Conduction abnormalities due to diltiazem. *N Engl J Med.* 1982; 307:953-4.

615. Bessho F, Kinumaki H, Kobayashi M et al. Treatment of children with refractory acute lymphocytic leukemia with vincristine and diltiazem. *Med Pediatr Oncol.* 1985; 13:199-202.

616. Ramoska EA, Spiller HA, Winter M et al. A one-year evaluation of calcium channel blocker overdoses: toxicity and treatment. *Ann Emerg Med.* 1993; 22:196-200.

617. Fugit MD, Rubal BJ, Donovan DJ. Effects of intracoronary nicardipine, diltiazem and verapamil on coronary blood flow. *J Invasive Cardiol.* 2000; 12:80-5.

618. Wills BK, Liu JM, Wahl M. Third-degree AV block from extended-release diltiazem ingestion in a nine-month-old. *J Emerg Med.* 2010; 38:328-31.

619. Brenes JA, Cha YM. Diltiazem-induced transient complete atrioventricular block in an elderly patient with acute on chronic renal failure. *Open Cardiovasc Med J.* 2013; 7:23-6.

620. Shammas RL, DeAntonio HJ, Movahed A. High-grade atrioventricular block during dipyridamole stress testing. *Int J Cardiol.* 1994; 46:279-282.

621. Preumont N, Velez Roa S, Berkenboom G et al. Transient second-degree heart block during dipyridamole myocardial perfusion imaging. *Acta Cardiol.* 1998; 53:275-7.

622. Alakhras M, Baldari D, El-Sherif N et al. Location and clinical implications of high-degree atrioventricular block during dipyridamole infusion: a case report. *Ann Noninvasive Electrocardiol.* 2002; 7:174-6.

623. Massalha S, Reizberg I, Israel O et al. Conduction abnormalities during dipyridamole stress testing. *J Nucl Cardiol.* 2017; 24:405-9.

624. Rothman MT. Prolonged QT interval, atrioventricular block, and torsade de pointes after antiarrhythmic therapy. *Br J Med.* 1980; 280:922-33.

625. Bergfeldt L, Rosenqvist M, Vallin H et al. Disopyramide induced second and third degree atrioventricular block in patients with bifascicular block: an acute stress test to predict atrioventricular block progression. *Br Heart J.* 1985; 53:328-34.

626. Suleyman T, Tevfik P, Abdulkadir G et al. Complete atrioventricular block and ventricular tachyarrhythmia associated with donepezil. *Emerg Med J.* 2006; 23:641-2.

627. Tanaka A, Koga S, Hiramastu Y. Donepezil-induced adverse side effects of cardiac rhythm: 2 cases report of atrioventricular block and Torsade de Pointes. *Intern Med* 2009; 48:1219-23.

628. Hundae A, Afzal A, Assar MD et al. Syncope secondary to second-degree atrioventricular block with donepezil use. *Proc (Bayl Univ Med Cent).* 2014; 27:325-6.

629. Combeer A. Complete atrioventricular block following etomidate. *Eur J Anaesthesiol.* 2007; 24:1067-8.

630. Schoenwald PK, Sprung J, Abdelmalak B et al. Complete atrioventricular block and cardiac arrest following intravenous famotidine administration. *Anesthesiology.* 1999; 90:623-6.

631. Voon V, Saiva L, O'Kelly S et al. Fingolimod-induced atrioventricular conduction defects in a young lady with multiple sclerosis—insights into possible drug mechanism. *Eur J Clin Pharmacol.* 2014; 70:373-5.

632. Hojer J, Olsson E. AV block II in a toddler after ingestion of a single tablet fingolimod. *Clin Toxicol.* 2014; 52:644.

633. Gialafos E, Gerakoulis S, Grigoriou A et al. Intermittent atrioventricular block following fingolimod initiation. *Case Rep Neurol Med.* 2014; 2014:191305.

634. Rosini JM, Rajasimhan S, Fellows SE et al. Delayed cardiac dysrhythmias after fingolimod administration. *Am J Merg Med.* 2015; 33:987. e1-3.

635. Paolicelli D, Manni A, Direnzo V et al. Long-term cardiac safety and tolerability of fingolimod in multiple sclerosis: a Postmarketing study. *J Clin Pharmacol.* 2015; 55:1131-6.

636. Sacca F, Puorro G, Marsili A et al. Mobitz type I and II atrioventricular blocks during fingolimod therapy. *Neurol Sci.* 2016; 37:1557-9.

637. Hanley NA, Bourke JP, Gascoigne AD. Survival in a case of life-threatening flecainide overdose. *Intensive Care Med.* 1998; 24:740-2.

638. LaRusso P, Jessup SA, Rogers FJ et al. Sinoatrial and atrioventricular dysfunction associated with the use of guanabenz acetate. *Can J Cardiol.* 1988; 4:146-8.

639. Comin-Colet J, Sanchez-Corral MA, Alegre-Sancho JJ et al. Complete heart block in an adult with systemic lupus erythematosus and recent onset of hydroxychloroquine therapy. *Lupus.* 2001; 10:59-62.

640. Kantor SJ, Bigger JT Jr, Glassman AH et al. Imipramine-induced heart block: a longitudinal case study. *JAMA.* 1975; 231:1364-6.

641. Martin CI. Imipramine-induced heart block. *JAMA.* 1975; 234:383.

642. Sofos S, Savoye G, Ramirez S et al. Transient type III atrioventricular block after infliximab infusion in a fistulizing perianal Crohn's disease patient. *Am J Gastroenterol.* 2007; 102:217-9.

643. Ibanez L, Laporte JR, Carne X. Adverse drug reactions leading to hospital admission. *Drug Saf.* 1991; 6:450-9.

644. Wheeler DW, Liew TV, Bailey AR. Peri-operative atrioventricular block as a result of chemotherapy with epirubicin and paclitaxel. *Anaesthesia.* 2007; 62:186-9.

645. Antoniou T, Gough KA. Early-onset pentamidine-associated second-degree heart block and sinus bradycardia: case report and review of the literature. *Pharmacotherapy.* 2005; 25:899-903.

646. Burton BT, Rice M, Schmertzler LE. Atrioventricular block following overdose of decongestant cold medication. *J Emerg Med.* 1985; 2:415-9.

647. Woo OF, Benowitz NL, Bialy FW et al. Atrioventricular conduction block caused by phenylpropanolamine. *JAMA.* 1985; 253:2646-7.

648. Libersa C, Caron J, Pladys A et al. Propafenone versus disopyramide: a double-blind randomized crossover trial in patients presenting chronic ventricular arrhythmias. *Clin Cardiol.* 1987; 10:405-10.

649. Kerns W 2nd, English B, Ford M. Propafenone overdose. *Ann Emerg Med.* 1994; 24:98-103.

650. Janousek J, Paul T. Safety of oral propafenone in the treatment of arrhythmias in infants and children (European retrospective multicenter study): Working Group on Pediatric Arrhythmias and Electrophysiology of the Association of European Pediatric Cardiologists. *Am J Cardiol.* 1998; 81:1121-4.

651. James MF, Reyneke CJ, Whiffler K. Heart block following propofol: a case report. *Br J Anaesth.* 1989; 62:213-5.

652. Ganansia MF, Francois TP, Ormezzano X et al. Atrioventricular Mobitz I block during propofol anesthesia for laparoscopic tubal ligation. *Anesth Analg.* 1989; 69:524-5.

653. Sochala C, Deenen D, Ville A et al. Heart block following propofol in a child. *Paediatr Anaesth.* 1999; 9:349-51.

654. Noh JI, Lee JH, Woo SY et al. Complete atrioventricular nodal block after propofol administration in an elderly patient undergoing total knee replacement arthroplasty—a case report. *Korean J Anesthesiol.* 2013; 64:363-5.

655. Gehi A, Benatar M, Langberg J. Treatment of pyridostigmine-induced AV block with hyoscyamine in a patient with myasthenia gravis. *J Cardiovasc Electrophysiol.* 2008; 19:214-6.

656. Taghavi Gilani M, Razavi M. Mobitz Type II atrioventricular block followed by remifentanil in a patient with severe aortic stenosis. *Case Rep Anesthesiol* 2013; 2013:852143.
657. Pfammatter JP, Paul T, Lehmann C et al. Efficacy and proarrhythmia of oral sotalol in pediatric patients. *J Am Coll Cardiol.* 1995; 26:1002-7.
658. Donatini B, Le Blaye I, Krupp P. Transient cardiac pacing is insufficiently used to treat arrhythmia associated with thioridazine. *Cardiology.* 1992; 81:340-1.
659. Hulisz DT, Dasa SL, Black LD et al. Complete heart block and torsade de pointes associated with thioridazine poisoning. *Pharmacotherapy.* 1994; 14:239-45.
660. Teng R, Butler K. Safety, tolerability, pharmacokinetics and pharmacodynamics of high single-ascending doses of ticagrelor in healthy volunteers. *Int J Clin Pharmacol Ther.* 2013; 51:795-806.
661. Goldberg A, Rosenfeld I, Nordkin I et al. Life-threatening complete atrioventricular block associated with ticagrelor therapy. *Int J Cardiol.* 2015; 182:379-80.
662. Unlu M, Demirkol S, Yildirim AO et al. Atrioventricular block associated with ticagrelor therapy may require permanent pacemaker. *Int J Cardiol.* 2016; 202:946-7.
663. Baker NC, Nadour W, Friehling M. Clinically significant ticagrelor induced conduction abnormalities following percutaneous coronary intervention. *Int J Cardiol.* 2016; 214:21-2.
664. De Maria E, Borghi A, Modonesi L et al. Ticagrelor therapy and atrioventricular block: do we need to worry? *World J Clin Cases.* 2017; 5:178-82.
665. de Faire U, Lundman T. Attempted suicide with verapamil. *Eur J Cardiol.* 1977; 6:195-8.
666. Chimienti M, Previtali M, Medicia A et al. Acute verapamil poisoning: successful treatment with epinephrine. *Clin Cardiol.* 1982; 5:219-22.
667. Perrot B, Danchin N, Terrier de la Chaise A. Verapamil: a cause of sudden death in a patient with hypertrophic cardiomyopathy. *Br Heart J.* 1984; 51:352-4.
668. Danish Multicenter Study Group on Verapamil in Myocardial Infarction. Verapamil in acute myocardial infarction. *Am J Cardiol.* 1984; 54:24E-8E.
669. Spiller HA, Meyers A, Ziemba T et al. Delayed onset of cardiac arrhythmias from sustained-release verapamil. *Ann Emerg Med.* 1991; 20:201-3.
670. Pritza DR, Bierman MH, Hammeke MD. Acute toxic effects of sustained-release verapamil in chronic renal failure. *Arch Intern Med.* 1991; 151:2081-4.
671. Ramoska EA, Spiller HA, Winter M et al. A one-year evaluation of calcium channel blocker overdoses: toxicity and treatment. *Ann Emerg Med.* 1993; 22:196-200.
672. Barrow PM, Houston PL, Wong DT. Overdose of sustained-release verapamil. *Br J Anaesth.* 1994; 72:361-5.
673. Martín-Gago J, Pascual J, Rodríguez-Palomares JR et al. Complete atrioventricular blockade secondary to conventional-release verapamil in a patient on hemodialysis. *Nephron.* 1999; 83:89-90.
674. Goldschmidt N, Azaz-Livshits T, Gotsman et al. Compound cardiac toxicity of oral erythromycin and verapamil. *Ann Pharmacother.* 2001; 35:1396-9.
675. Werner GS, Lang K, Kuehnert H et al. Intracoronary verapamil for reversal of no-reflow during coronary angioplasty for acute myocardial infarction. *Catheter Cardiovasc Interv.* 2002; 57:444-51.
676. Vijayalakshmi K, Whittaker VJ, Kunadian B et al. Prospective, randomised, controlled trial to study the effect of intracoronary injection of verapamil and adenosine on coronary blood flow during percutaneous coronary intervention in patients with acute coronary syndromes. *Heart.* 2006; 92:1278-84.
677. Letavernier E, Couzi L, Delmas Y et al. Verapamil and mild hyperkalemia in hemodialysis patients: a potentially hazardous association. *Hemodial Int.* 2006; 10:170-2.
678. Cohen AS, Matharu MS, Goadsby PJ. Electrocardiographic abnormalities in patients with cluster headache on verapamil therapy. *Neurology.* 2007; 69:668-75.
679. Tanzilli G, Greco C, Pasceri V et al. Dipyridamole versus verapamil for treatment of no-reflow during primary angioplasty. *Catheter Cardiovasc Interv.* 2010; 76:787-93.
680. Essebag V, Hadjis T, Platt RW et al. Amiodarone and the risk of bradyarrhythmia requiring permanent pacemaker in elderly patients with atrial fibrillation and prior myocardial infarction. *J Am Coll Cardiol.* 2003; 41:249-54.
681. Lee SH, Chang CM, Lu MJ et al. Intravenous amiodarone for prevention of atrial fibrillation after coronary artery bypass grafting. *Ann Thorac Surg.* 2000; 70:157-61.
682. Cotter G, Blatt A, Kaluski E et al. Conversion of recent onset paroxysmal atrial fibrillation to normal sinus rhythm: the effect of no treatment and high-dose amiodarone: a randomized, placebo-controlled study. *Eur Heart J.* 1999; 20:1833-42.
683. Ma S, Long JP. Hypotensive and bradycardiac responses to reflex sympathetic inhibition produced by nitroglycerin in rats with sinoaortic deafferentation. *J Cardiovasc Pharmacol.* 1993; 21:136-43.
684. Cohen JA, Chun J. Mechanisms of fingolimod's efficacy and adverse effects in multiple sclerosis. *Ann Neurol.* 2011; 69:759-77.
685. Peters LM, Alewijnse AE. Sphingosine-1-phosphate signaling in the cardiovascular system. *Curr Opin Pharmacol.* 2007; 7:186-92.
686. Bernstein AD, Parsonnet V. Survey of cardiac pacing in the United States in 1989. *Am J Cardiol.* 1992; 69:331-8.
687. Melenovsky V, Wichterle D, Malik J et al. Nitroglycerin induced syncope occurs in subjects with delayed phase shift of baroreflex action. *PACE.* 2002; 25:828-32.
688. Flockhart DA. Drug Interactions: Cytochrome P450 Drug Interaction Table. http://medicine.iupui.edu/clinpharm/ddis/main-table/ (accessed 2017 Jul 17).
689. Knabb RM, Gidday GM, Ely SW. Effects of dipyridamole on myocardial adenosine on active hyperemia. *Am J Physiol.* 1984; 247:804-10.
690. Fenster PE, White NW Jr, Hanson CD. Pharmacokinetic evaluation of the digoxin-amiodarone interaction. *J Am Coll Cardiol.* 1985; 5:108-12.
691. Klein HO, Lang R, Weiss E et al. The influence of verapamil on serum digoxin concentration. *Circulation.* 1982; 65:998-1003.
692. Chen TS, Friedman HS. Alteration of digoxin pharmacokinetics by a single dose of quinidine. *JAMA.* 1980; 244:669-72.
693. Essebag V, Reynolds MR, Hadjis T et al. Sex differences in the relationship between amiodarone use and the need for permanent pacing in patients with atrial fibrillation. *Arch Intern Med.* 2007; 167:1648-53.
694. Surawicz B. Factors affecting tolerance to digoxin. *J Am Coll Cardiol.* 1985; 5:69A-81A.
695. Neumar RW, Otto CW, Link MS et al. Part 8: Adult advanced cardiovascular life support: 2010 American Heart Association guidelines for cardiopulmonary resuscitation and emergency cardiovascular care. *Circulation.* 2010; 122(suppl 2):S729-67.
696. Link MS, Berkow LC, Kudenchuk PJ et al. Part 7: Adult advanced cardiovascular life support. 2015 American Heart Association guidelines update for cardiopulmonary resuscitation and emergency cardiovascular care. *Circulation.* 2015; 132(suppl 2):S444-64.
697. Vanden Hoek TL, Morrison LJ, Shuster M et al. Part 12: Cardiac arrest in special situations. 2010 American Heart Association guidelines for cardiopulmonary resuscitation and emergency cardiovascular care. *Circulation.* 2010; 122(suppl):S829-61.
698. Kerns W II. Management of β-adrenergic blocker and calcium channel antagonist toxicity. *Emerg Med Clin North Am.* 2007; 25:309-31.
699. Barton CA, Johnson NB, Mah ND et al. Successful treatment of a massive metoprolol overdose using intravenous lipid emulsion and hyperinsulinemia/euglycemia therapy. *Pharmacotherapy.* 2015; 35:e56-60.
700. Sebe A, Dişel NR, Akpinar AA et al. Role of intravenous lipid emulsions in the management of calcium channel blocker and β-blocker overdose: 3 years experience of a university hospital. *Postgrad Med.* 2015; 127:119-24.

701. Epstein AE, DiMarco JP, Ellenbogen KA et al. ACCF/AHA/HRS focused update incorporated into the 2008 guidelines for device-based therapy of cardiac rhythm abnormalities: a report of the American College of Cardiology Foundation/American Heart Association Task Force on Practice Guidelines and the Heart Rhythm Society. *J Am Coll Cardiol.* 2012; 61:e6-75.

702. Amsterdam EA, Wenger NK, Brindis RG et al. 2014 ACC/AHA guideline for the management of patients with non-ST-elevation acute coronary syndromes: a report of the American College of Cardiology/ American Heart Association Task Force on Practice Guidelines. *Circulation.* 2014; 130:e344-426.

703. Yancy CW, Jessup M, Bozkurt B et al. 2013 ACCF/AHA guideline for the management of heart failure: a report of the American College of Cardiology Foundation/American Heart Association Task Force on Practice Guidelines. *Circulation.* 2013; 128:e240-327.

704. Belhassen B, Pelleg A, Shoshani D et al. Atrial fibrillation induced by adenosine triphosphate. *Am J Cardiol.* 1984; 53:1405-6.

705. Garratt CJ, Antoniou A, Griffith MJ et al. Use of intravenous adenosine in sinus rhythm as a diagnostic test for latent preexcitation. *Am J Cardiol.* 1990; 65:868-73.

706. Meurer MK. A 21-year-old woman with rapid atrial fibrillation after adenosine administration. *J Emerg Nurs.* 1991; 17:135-6.

707. Cowell RP, Paul VE, Ilsley CD. Haemodynamic deterioration after treatment with adenosine. *Br Heart J.* 1994; 71:569-71.

708. Crosson JE, Etheridge SP, Milstein S et al. Therapeutic and diagnostic utility of adenosine during tachycardia evaluation in children. *Am J Cardiol.* 1994; 74:155-60.

709. Tebbenjohanns J, Pfeiffer D, Schumacher B et al. Intravenous adenosine during atrioventricular reentrant tachycardia: induction of atrial fibrillation with rapid conduction over an accessory pathway. *Pacing Clin Electrophysiol.* 1995; 18:743-6.

710. Silverman AJ, Machado C, Baga JJ et al. Adenosine-induced atrial fibrillation. *Am J Emerg Med.* 1996; 14:300-1.

711. Strickberger SA, Man KC, Daoud EG et al. Adenosine-induced atrial arrhythmia: a prospective analysis. *Ann Intern Med.* 1997; 127:417-22.

712. Kaplan IV, Kaplan AV, Fisher JD. Adenosine induced atrial fibrillation precipitating polymorphic ventricular tachycardia. *Pacing Clin Electrophysiol.* 2000; 23:140-1.

713. Israel C, Klingenheben T, Grönefeld G et al. Adenosine-induced atrial fibrillation. *J Cardiovasc Electrophysiol.* 2000; 11:825.

714. Kaltman JR, Tanel RE, Shah MJ et al. Induction of atrial fibrillation after the routine use of adenosine. *Pediatr Emerg Care.* 2006; 22:113-5.

715. Cummings M, Raza J, Movahed A. Atrial fibrillation during adenosine pharmacologic stress testing. *J Nucl Cardiol.* 2006; 13:576-81.

716. Stuber T, Lim PB, O'Neill MD et al. Ultra rapid local activity in adenosine-induced atrial fibrillation. *J Cardiovasc Electrophysiol.* 2008; 19:566-7.

717. Kanei Y, Hanon S, Van-Tosh A et al. Adenosine-induced atrial fibrillation during pharmacologic stress testing: report of eight cases and review of the literature. *Int J Cardiol.* 2008; 129:e15-7.

718. Turley AJ, Murray S, Thambyrajah J. Preexcited atrial fibrillation triggered by intravenous adenosine: a commonly used drug with potentially life-threatening adverse effects. *Emerg Med J.* 2008; 25:46-8.

719. Park E, Price A, Vidovich MI. Adenosine-induced atrial fibrillation during fractional flow reserve measurement. *Cardiol J.* 2012; 19:650-1.

720. Hoyt WJ Jr, Thomas PE, Snyder CS. Induction of atrial fibrillation with adenosine during a transesophageal electrophysiology study to risk stratify a patient with asymptomatic ventricular preexcitation. *Congenit Heart Dis.* 2013; 8:E99-101.

721. Poukkula A, Korhonen UR, Huikuri H et al. Theophylline and salbutamol in combination in patients with obstructive pulmonary disease and concurrent heart disease: effect on cardiac arrhythmias. *J Intern Med.* 1989; 226:229-34.

722. Breeden CC, Safirstein BH. Spacer-induced atrial fibrillation. *N J Med.* 1990; 87:113-4.

723. Breeden CC, Safirstein BH. Albuterol and spacer-induced atrial fibrillation. *Chest.* 1990; 98:762-3.

724. Patane S, Marte F, La Rosa FC et al. Atrial fibrillation associated with chocolate intake abuse and chronic salbutamol inhalation abuse (letter). *Int J Cardiol.* 2010; 145:e74-6.

725. Ettinger PO, Wu CF, De La Cruz C Jr et al. Arrhythmias and the "Holiday Heart": alcohol-associated cardiac rhythm disorders. *Am Heart J.* 1978; 95:555-62.

726. Thornton JR. Atrial fibrillation in healthy non-alcoholic people after an alcoholic binge. *Lancet.* 1984; 2:1013-5.

727. Nissen MB, Lemberg L. The "Holiday Heart" syndrome. *Heart Lung.* 1984; 13:89-92.

728. Rich EC, Siebold C, Campion B. Alcohol-related acute atrial fibrillation: a case-control study and review of 40 patients. *Arch Intern Med.* 1985; 145:830-3.

729. Watt AH. Atrial fibrillation and alcohol. *Lancet.* 1985; 1:162.

730. Sipila R. Atrial fibrillation precipitated by alcohol. *Lancet.* 1985; 1:391-2.

731. Koskinen P, Kupari M, Leinonen H et al. Alcohol and new onset atrial fibrillation: a case-control study of a current series. *Br Heart J.* 1987; 57:468-73.

732. Koskinen P, Kupari M, Leinonen H. Role of alcohol in recurrences of atrial fibrillation in persons <65 years of age. *Am J Cardiol.* 1990; 66:954-8.

733. Maki T, Toivonen L, Koskinen P et al. Effect of ethanol drinking, hangover, and exercise on adrenergic activity and heart rate variability in patients with a history of alcohol-induced atrial fibrillation. *Am J Cardiol.* 1998; 82:317-22.

734. Mukamal KJ, Tolstrup JS, Friberg J et al. Alcohol consumption and risk of atrial fibrillation in men and women: the Copenhagen City Heart Study. *Circulation.* 2005; 112:1736-42.

735. Conen D, Tedrow UB, Cook NR et al. Alcohol consumption and risk of incident atrial fibrillation in women. *JAMA.* 2008; 300:2489-96.

736. Minami M, Kobayashi Y, Toyokawa S et al. Risk factors for new-onset atrial fibrillation during routine medical checkups of Japanese male workers. *Int Heart J.* 2009; 50:457-64.

737. Krishnamoorthy S, Lip GY, Lane DA. Alcohol and illicit drug use as precipitants of atrial fibrillation in young adults: a case series and literature review. *Am J Med.* 2009; 122:851-6.

738. Falcone AM, Schussler JM. Sudden atrial fibrillation associated with acute alcohol ingestion and cor triatriatum. *Proc (Bayl Univ Med Cent).* 2009; 22:335-6.

739. Samokhvalov AV, Irving HM, Rehm J. Alcohol consumption as a risk factor for atrial fibrillation: a systematic review and meta-analysis. *Eur J Cardiovasc Prev Rehabil.* 2010; 17:706-12.

740. Kodama S, Saito K, Tanaka S et al. Alcohol consumption and risk of atrial fibrillation: a meta-analysis. *J Am Coll Cardiol.* 2011; 57:427-36.

741. Ariansen I, Reims HM, Gjesdal K et al. Impact of alcohol habits and smoking on the risk of new-onset atrial fibrillation in hypertensive patients with ECG left ventricular hypertrophy: the LIFE study. *Blood Press.* 2012; 21:6-11.

742. Mandyam MC, Vedantham V, Scheinman MM et al. Alcohol and vagal tone as triggers for paroxysmal atrial fibrillation. *Am J Cardiol.* 2012; 110:364-8.

743. Linag Y, Mente A, Yusuf S et al. Alcohol consumption and the risk of incident atrial fibrillation among people with cardiovascular disease. *CMAJ.* 2012; 184:E857-66.

744. Li Y, Wu YF, Chen KP et al. Prevalence of atrial fibrillation in China and its risk factors. *Biomed Environ Sci.* 2013; 26:709-16.

745. San F, Ohira T, Kitamura A et al. Heavy alcohol consumption and risk of atrial fibrillation. The Circulatory Risk in Communities Study (CIRCS). *Circ J.* 2014; 78:955-61.

746. Larsson SC, Drca N, Wolk A. Alcohol consumption and risk of atrial fibrillation: a prospective study and dose-response meta-analysis. *J Am Coll Cardiol.* 2014; 64:281-9.

747. Tolstrup JS, Wium-Anderson MK, Orsted DD et al. Alcohol consumption and risk of atrial fibrillation: observational and genetic estimates of association. *Eur J Prev Cardiol.* 2016; 23:1514-23.

748. McManus DD, Yin X, Gladstone R et al. Alcohol consumption, left atrial diameter, and atrial fibrillation. *J Am Heart Assoc.* 2016; Sep 14; 5(9):pii:e004060.

749. Dukes JW, Dewland TA, Vittinghoff E et al. Access to alcohol and heart disease among patients in hospital: observational cohort study using differences in alcohol sales laws. *BMJ.* 2016; Jun 14;353:i2714.

750. Cummings SR, Schwartz AV, Black DM. Alendronate and atrial fibrillation. *N Engl J Med.* 2007; 356:1895-6.

751. Heckbert SR, Li G, Cummings SR et al. Use of alendronate and risk of incident atrial fibrillation in women. *Arch Intern Med.* 2008; 168:826-31.

752. Grosso A, Douglas I, Hingorani A et al. Oral bisphosphonates and risk of atrial fibrillation and flutter in women: a self-controlled case-series safety analysis. *PLoS One.*2009; 4:e4720.

753. Herrera L, Leal I, Lapi F et al. Risk of atrial fibrillation among bisphosphonate users: a multicenter, population-based, Italian study. *Osteoporos Int.* 2015; 26:1499-506.

754. Tai CT, Chiang CE, Lee SH et al. Persistent atrial flutter in patients treated for atrial fibrillation with amiodarone and propafenone: electrophysiologic characteristics, radiofrequency catheter ablation, and risk prediction. *J Cardiovasc Electrophysiol.* 1999; 10:1180-7.

755. Reithmann C, Hoffmann E, Spitzlberger G et al. Catheter ablation of atrial flutter due to amiodarone therapy for paroxysmal atrial fibrillation. *Eur Heart J.* 2000; 21:565-72.

756. Schreiber DH, DeFreest MS. Paroxysmal atrial fibrillation precipitated by amiodarone-induced thyrotoxicosis five months after cessation of therapy. *J Emerg Med.* 2006; 31:61-4.

757. Kurt IH, Yigit T, Karademir BM. Atrial fibrillation due to late amiodarone-induced thyrotoxicosis. *Clin Drug Investig.* 2008; 28:527-31.

758. Mattioli AV, Bonatti S, Zennaro M et al. Effect of coffee consumption, lifestyle and acute life stress in the development of acute lone atrial fibrillation. *J Cardiovasc Med.* 2008; 9:794-8.

759. Artin B, Singh M, Richeh C et al. Caffeine-related atrial fibrillation. *Am J Ther.* 2010; 17:e169-71.

760. Di Rocco JR, During A, Morelli PJ et al. Atrial fibrillation in healthy adolescents after highly caffeinated beverage consumption: two case reports. *J Med Case Rep.* 2011; 5:18.

761. Armstrong M. Atrial fibrillation with rapid ventricular response following use of dietary supplement containing 1,3 dimethylamylamine and caffeine. *J Spec Oper Med.* 2012; 12:1-4.

762. Ciszowski K, Biedron W, Gomolka E. Acute caffeine poisoning resulting in atrial fibrillation after guarana extract overdose. *Przegl Lek.* 2014; 71:495-8.

763. Thyagarajan B, Alagusundaramoorthy SS, Agrawal A. Atrial fibrillation due to over the counter stimulant drugs in a young adult. *J Clin Diagn Res.* 2015; 9:OD05-7.

764. Mattioli AV, Pennella S. Energy drink overconsumption can trigger atrial fibrillation. *J Cardiovasc Med.* 2016; 17:902-4.

765. Mattioli AV, Pennella S, Farinetti A et al. Energy drinks and atrial fibrillation in young adults. *Clin Nutr.* 2017 May 6; pii:S0261-5614(17)30162-0.

766. Doiuchi J, Hamada M, Ochi T et al. Adverse effects of atrial fibrillation and syncope induced by calcium channel blockers in hypertrophic cardiomyopathy. *Clin Cardiol.* 1985; 8:176-9.

767. Baig MW, Sheard K, Thorley PJ et al. The use of dobutamine stress thallium scintigraphy in the diagnosis of syndrome X. *Postgrad Med J.* 1992; 68(suppl 2):S20-4.

768. Poldermans D, Fioretti PM, Boersma E et al. Safety of dobutamine-atropine stress echocardiography in patients with suspected or proven coronary artery disease. *Am J Cardiol.* 1994; 73:456-9.

769. Poldermans D, Fioretti PM, Boersma E et al. Dobutamine-atropine stress echocardiography in elderly patients unable to perform an exercise test: hemodynamic characteristics, safety, and prognostic value. *Arch Intern Med.* 1994; 154:2681-6.

770. Wirtz CE. Sustained atrial fibrillation after dobutamine stress echocardiography in an older patient with left atrial enlargement. *West J Med.* 1995; 162:268-9.

771. Cornel JH, Balk AH, Boersma E et al. Safety and feasibility of dobutamine-atropine stress echocardiography in patients with ischemic left ventricular dysfunction. *J Am Soc Echocardiogr.* 1996; 9:2732.

772. Yeo TC, Ng WL, Ling LH et al. Dobutamine stress echocardiography in the elderly Asian patients. *Ann Acad Med Singapore.* 1997; 26:165-7.

773. Pezzano A, Gentile F, Mantero A et al. RITED (Registro Italiano Test Eco-Dobutamina): side effects and complications of echo-dobutamine stress test in 3041 examinations. *G Ital Cardiol.* 1998; 28:102-11.

774. Elhendy A, van Domburg RT, Bax JJ et al. Safety, hemodynamic profile, and feasibility of dobutamine stress technetium myocardial perfusion single-photon emission CT imaging for evaluation of coronary artery disease in the elderly. *Chest.* 2000; 117:649-56.

775. Coisne D, Donal E, Torremocha F et al. Dobutamine stress echocardiography response of asymptomatic patients with diabetes. *Echocardiography.* 2001; 18:373-9.

776. Cortigiani L, Zanetti L, Bigi R et al. Safety and feasibility of dobutamine and dipyridamole stress echocardiography in hypertensive patients. *J Hypertens.* 2002; 20:1423-9.

777. Wahl A, Paetsch I, Gollesch A et al. Safety and feasibility of high-dose dobutamine-atropine stress cardiovascular magnetic resonance for diagnosis of myocardial ischaemia: experience in 1000 consecutive cases. *Eur Heart J.* 2004; 25:1230-6.

778. Onorati F, Renzulli A, De Feo M et al. Perioperative enoximone infusion improves cardiac enzyme release after CABG. *J Cardiothorac Vasc Anesth.* 2004; 18:409-14.

779. Salaria V, Mehta NJ, Abdul-Aziz S et al. Role of postoperative use of adrenergic drugs in occurrence of atrial fibrillation after cardiac surgery. *Clin Cardiol.* 2005; 28:131-5.

780. Carasso S, Sandach A, Kuperstein R et al. Atrial fibrillation in dobutamine stress echocardiography. *Int J Cardiol.* 2006; 111:53-8.

781. Mebazaa A, Nieminen MS, Packer M et al. Levosimendan vs dobutamine for patients with acute decompensated heart failure: the SURVIVE Randomized Trial. *JAMA.* 2007; 297;1883-91.

782. Kane GC, Hepinstall MJ, Kidd GM et al. Safety of stress echocardiography supervised by registered nurses: results of a 2-year audit of 15,404 patients. *J Am Soc Echocardiogr.* 2008; 21:337-41.

783. Sheldon SH, Askew JW 3rd, Klarich KW et al. Occurrence of atrial fibrillation during dobutamine stress echocardiography: incidence, risk factors, and outcomes. *J Am Soc Echocardiogr.* 2011; 24:86-90.

784. Palma M, Mancuso A, Grifaalchi F et al. Atrial fibrillation during adjuvant chemotherapy with docetaxel: a case report. *Tumori.* 2002; 88:527-9.

785. Argalious M, Motta P, Khandwala F et al. "Renal dose" dopamine is associated with the risk of new-onset atrial fibrillation after cardiac surgery. *Crit Care Med.* 2005; 33:1327-32.

786. Numico G, Castiglione F, Granetto C et al. Single-agent pegylated liposomal doxorubicin (Caelix) in chemotherapy pretreated non-small cell lung cancer patients: a pilot trial. *Lung Cancer.* 2002; 35:59-64.

787. Kilickap S, Barista I, Akgul E et al. Early and late arrhythmogenic effects of doxorubicin. *South Med J.* 2007; 100:262-5.

788. Rolf L, Muris AH, Damoiseaux J et al. Paroxysmal atrial fibrillation after initiation of fingolimod for multiple sclerosis treatment. *Neurology.* 2014; 82:1008-9.

789. Feld GK, Chen PS, Nicod P et al. Possible atrial proarrhythmic effects of class 1C antiarrhythmic drugs. *Am J Cardiol.* 1990; 66:378-83.

790. Nabar A, Rodriguez LM, Timmermans C et al. Class IC antiarrhythmic drug induced atrial flutter: electrocardiographic and

electrophysiological findings and their importance for long term outcome after right atrial isthmus ablation. *Heart.* 2001; 85:424-9.

791. Roberge RJ, Martin TG. Mixed fluoxetine/loxapine overdose and atrial flutter. *Ann Emerg Med.* 1994; 23:586-90.
792. White RL Jr, Schwartzentruber DJ, Guleria A et al. Cardiopulmonary toxicity of treatment with high dose interleukin-2 in 199 consecutive patients with metastatic melanoma of renal cell carcinoma. *Cancer.* 1994; 74:3212-22.
793. Citterio G, Fragasso G, Rossetti E et al. Isolated left ventricular filling abnormalities may predict interleukin-2-induced cardiovascular toxicity. *J Immunother Emphasis Tumor Immunol.* 1996; 19:134-41.
794. Koulova L, Novik Y, Caliendo G et al. A phase 2 study of moderate dose interleukin-2 and granulocyte-macrophage colony-stimulating factor in patients with metastatic or unresectable renal cell carcinoma. *J Immunother.* 2005; 28:576-81.
795. O'Driscoll BR. Supraventricular tachycardia caused by nebulised ipratropium bromide. *Thorax.* 1989; 44:312.
796. Martin RI, Pogoryelova O, Koref MS et al. Atrial fibrillation associated with ivabradine treatment: meta-analysis of randomised controlled trials. *Heart.* 2014; 100:1506-10.
797. Tanboga IH, Topcu S, Aksakal E et al. The risk of atrial fibrillation with ivabradine treatment: a meta-analysis with trial sequential analysis of more than 40000 patients. *Clin Cardiol.* 2016; 39:615-20.
798. McDermott MF, Nasr I, Rydman RJ et al. Comparison of two regimens of beta-adrenergics in acute asthma. *J Med Syst.* 1999; 23:269-79.
799. Ueda N, Yoshikawa T, Chihara M et al. Atrial fibrillation following methylprednisolone pulse therapy. *Pediatr Nephrol.* 1988; 2:29-31.
800. McLuckie AE, Savage RW. Atrial fibrillation following pulse methylprednisolone therapy in an adult. *Chest.* 1993; 104:622-3.
801. Moretti R, Torre P, Antonello RM et al. Recurrent atrial fibrillation associated with pulse administration of high doses of methylprednisolone: a possible prophylactic treatment. *Eur J Neurol.* 2000; 7:130.
802. Aslam AK, Vasavada BC, Sacchi TJ et al. Atrial fibrillation associated with systemic lupus erythematosus and use of methylprednisolone. *Am J Ther.* 2001; 8:303-5.
803. Dogukan A, Ilkay E, Poyrazoglu OK et al. Atrial fibrillation due to oral methylprednisolone in a patient with membranoproliferative glomerulonephritis. *Acta Medica.* 2008; 51:63-4.
804. Iqbal FM, Beeharilal PS, Sadat K et al. Steroid induced atrial fibrillation. *Compr Ther.* 2008; 34:111-4.
805. Yamamura K, Ohga S, Nishiyama K et al. Recurrent atrial fibrillation after high-dose methylprednisolone therapy in a girl with lupus-associated hemophagocytic syndrome. *Lupus.* 2011; 20:871-5.
806. Wright EM, Sherry KM. Clinical and haemodynamic effects of milrinone in the treatment of low cardiac output after cardiac surgery. *Br J Anaesth.* 1991; 67:585-90.
807. Feneck RO. Intravenous milrinone following cardiac surgery: I. Effects of bolus infusion followed by variable dose maintenance infusion: the European Milrinone Multicentre Trial Group. *J Cardiovasc Thorac Anesth.* 1992; 6:554-62.
808. Cuffe MS, Califf RM, Adams KF Jr et al. Outcomes of a Prospective Trial of Intravenous Milrinone for Exacerbations of Chronic Heart Failure (OPTIME-CHF) Investigators: short-term intravenous milrinone for acute exacerbation of chronic heart failure: a randomized controlled trial. *JAMA.* 2002; 287:1541-7.
809. Fleming GA, Murray KT, Yu C et al. Milrinone use is associated with postoperative atrial fibrillation after cardiac surgery. *Circulation.* 2008; 118:1619-25.
810. Smith AH, Owen J, Borgman KY et al. Relation to milrinone after surgery for congenital heart disease to significant postoperative tachyarrhythmias. *Am J Cardiol.* 2011; 108:1620-4.
811. Acharya D, Sanam K, Revilla-Martinez M et al. Infections, arrhythmias, and hospitalizations on home intravenous inotropic therapy. *Am J Cardiol.* 2016; 117:952-6.
812. Zingler VC, Nabauer M, Jahn K et al. Assessment of potential cardiotoxic side effects of mitoxantrone in patients with multiple sclerosis. *Eur Neurol.* 2005; 54:2833.
813. Lee CW, Muo CH, Liang JA et al. Atrial fibrillation is associated with morphine treatment in female breast cancer patients: a retrospective population-based time-dependent cohort study. *Medicine.* 2016; Mar;95:e3102.
814. Kasinath NS, Malak O, Tetzlaff J. Atrial fibrillation after ondansetron for the prevention and treatment of postoperative nausea and vomiting: a case report. *Can J Anaesth.* 2003; 50:229-31.
815. Havrilla PL, Kane-Gill SL, Verrico MM et al. Coronary vasospasm and atrial fibrillation associated with ondansetron therapy. *Ann Pharmacother.* 2009; 43:532-36.
816. Lombardi D, Crivellari D, Scuderi C et al. Long-term, weekly one-hour infusion of paclitaxel in patients with metastatic breast cancer: a phase II monoinstitutional study. *Tumori.* 2004; 90:285-8.
817. Maister AH. Atrial fibrillation following physostigmine. *Can Anaesth Soc J.* 1983; 30:419-21.
818. Murdock CJ, Kyles AE, Yeung-Lai-Wah JA et al. Atrial flutter in patients treated for atrial fibrillation with propafenone. *Am J Cardiol.* 1990; 66:755-7.
819. Hayashi K, Minezaki KK, Narukawa M et al. Atrial fibrillation and continuous hypotension induced by sildenafil in an intermittent WPW syndrome patient. *Jpn Heart J* 1999; 40:827-30.
820. Awan GM, Calderon E, Dawood G et al. Acute, symptomatic atrial fibrillation after sildenafil citrate therapy in a patient with hypertrophic obstructive cardiomyopathy. *Am J Med Sci.* 2000; 320:69-71.
821. Hahn I-H, Hoffman RS. Aroused to atrial fibrillation? (letter). *Am J Emerg Med.* 2000; 18:842.
822. Patel AK, Skatrud JB, Thomsen JH. Cardiac arrhythmias due to oral aminophylline in patients with chronic obstructive pulmonary disease. *Chest.* 1981; 80:661-5.
823. Richardson JP. Theophylline toxicity associated with the administration of ciprofloxacin in a nursing home patient. *J Am Geriatr Soc.* 1990; 38:236-8.
824. Henderson A, Wright DM, Pond SM. Management of theophylline overdose patients in the intensive care unit. *Anaesth Intensive Care.* 1992; 20:56-62.
825. Varriale P, Ramaprasad S. Aminophylline induced atrial fibrillation. *Pacing Clin Electrophysiol.* 1993; 16:1953-5.
826. Chazan R, Karwat K, Tyminska K et al. Cardiac arrhythmias as a result of intravenous infusions of theophylline in patients with airway obstruction. *Int J Clin Pharmacol Ther.* 1995; 33:170-5.
827. Okada S, Teramoto S, Matsuoka R. Recovery from theophylline toxicity by continuous hemodialysis with filtration. *Ann Intern Med.* 2000; 133:922.
828. Zhang N, Chen K-Y, Zhao J et al. Another side effect of ticagrelor: atrial fibrillation. *Int J Cardiol.* 2016; 212:242-4.
829. Jara M, Lanes SF, Wentworth III C et al. Comparative safety of long-acting inhaled bronchodilators. A cohort study using the UK THIN primary care database. *Drug Saf.* 2007; 30:1151-60.
830. Veloso HH, de Paola AA. Atrial fibrillation after vardenafil therapy. *Emerg Med J.* 2005; 22:823.
831. Falk RH, Knowlton AA, Manaker S. Verapamil-induced atrial fibrillation. *N Engl J Med.* 1980; 318:640-1.
832. Garratt C, Linker N, Griffith M et al. Comparison of adenosine and verapamil for termination of paroxysmal junctional tachycardia. *Am J Cardiol.* 1989; 64:1310-6.
833. Black DM, Delmas PD, Eastell R et al. Once-yearly zoledronic acid for treatment of postmenopausal osteoporosis. *N Engl J Med.* 2007; 356:1809-22.
834. Konsta M, Bournia V-K, Dania V, Iliopoulos A. Atrial fibrillation following intravenous zoledronic acid for osteoporosis (letter). *J Clin Rheumatol.* 2014; 20:239-40.
835. Abrahamsen B, Eiken P, Brixen K. Atrial fibrillation in fracture patients treated with oral bisphosphonates. *J Intern Med.* 2009; 265:581-92.

836. Erichsen R, Christiansen CF, Frøslev T et al. Intravenous bisphosphonate therapy and atrial fibrillation risk in cancer patients: a nationwide cohort study. *Br J Cancer.* 2011; 105:881-3.
837. Wilkinson GS, Baillargeon J, Kuo YF et al. Atrial fibrillation and stroke associated with intravenous bisphosphonate therapy in older patients with cancer. *J Clin Oncol.* 2010; 28:4898-905.
838. Rhee CW, Lee J, Oh S et al. Use of bisphosphonate and risk of atrial fibrillation in older women with osteoporosis. *Osteoporos Int.* 2012; 23:247-54.
839. Loke YK, Jeevanantham V, Singh S. Bisphosphonates and atrial fibrillation: systematic review and meta-analysis. *Drug Saf.* 2009; 32:219-28.
840. Bhuriya R, Singh M, Molnar J et al. Bisphosphonate use in women and the risk of atrial fibrillation: a systematic review and meta-analysis. *Int J Cardiol.* 2010; 142:213-7.
841. Sharma A, Chatterjee S, Arbab-Zadeh A et al. Risk of serious atrial fibrillation and stroke with use of bisphosphonates. Evidence from a meta-analysis. *Chest.* 2013; 144:1311-22.
842. Sharma A, Einstein AJ, Vallakati A et al. Risk of atrial fibrillation with use of oral and intravenous bisphosphonates. *Am J Cardiol.* 2014; 113:1815-21.
843. Herrera L, Leal I, Lapi F et al. Risk of atrial fibrillation among bisphosphonate users: a multicenter, population-based, Italian study. *Osteoporos Int.* 2015; 26:1499-506.
844. Kim DH, Rogers JR, Fulchino LA et al. Bisphosphonates and risk of cardiovascular events: a meta-analysis. *PLoS One.* 2015; 10:e0122646.
845. http://www.fda.gov/Drugs/DrugSafety/PostmarketDrugSafetyInformationforPatientsandProviders/DrugSafetyInformationforHeathcareProfessionals/ucm136201.htm (accessed 2017 Nov 3).
846. Bunch TJ, Anderson JL, May HT et al. Relation of bisphosphonate therapies and risk of developing atrial fibrillation. *Am J Cardiol.* 2009; 103:824-8.
847. Huang WF, Tsai YW, Wen YW et al. Osteoporosis treatment and atrial fibrillation: alendronate versus raloxifene. *Menopause.* 2010; 17:57-63.
848. Vestergaard P, Schwartz K, Pinholt EM et al. Risk of atrial fibrillation associated with use of bisphosphonates and other drugs against osteoporosis: a cohort study. *Calcif Tissue Int.* 2010; 86:335-42.
849. Pazianas M, Cooper C, Wang Y et al. Atrial fibrillation and the use of oral bisphosphonates. *Ther Clin Risk Manag.* 2011; 7:131-44.
850. Mak A, Cheung MW, Ho RC et al. Bisphosphonates and atrial fibrillation: Bayesian meta-analyses of randomized controlled trials and observational studies. *BMC Musculoskelet Disord.* 2009; 10:113.
851. Kim SY, Kim MJ, Cadarette SM et al. Bisphosphonates and risk of atrial fibrillation: a meta-analysis. *Arthritis Res Ther.* 2010; 12:R30.
852. Barrett-Connor E, Swern AS, Hustad CM et al. Alendronate and atrial fibrillation: a meta-analysis of randomized placebo-controlled clinical trials. *Osteoporosis Int.* 2012; 23:233-45.
853. January CT, Wann LS, Alpert JS et al. 2014 AHA/ACC/HRS guideline for the management of patients with atrial fibrillation: a report of the American College of Cardiology/American Heart Association Task Force on Practice Guidelines and the Heart Rhythm Society. *J Am Coll Cardiol.* 2014; 64:e1-76.
854. Smeets JL, Allessie MA, Lammers WJ et al. The wavelength of the cardiac impulse and reentrant arrhythmias in isolated rabbit atrium: the role of heart rate, autonomic transmitters, temperature, and calcium. *Circ Res.* 1986; 58:96-108.
855. Rensma PL, Allessie MA, Lammers WJ et al. The length of the excitation wave and susceptibility to reentrant arrhythmias in normal conscious dogs. *Circ Res.* 1988; 62:395-410.
856. Ip JE, Chung JH, Liu CF et al. Adenosine-induced atrial fibrillation. Insights into mechanisms. *Circ Arrhytm Electrophysiol.* 2013; 6:e34-7.
857. O'Nunain S, Garratt C, Paul V et al. Effect of intravenous adenosine on human atrial and ventricular repolarisation. *Cardiovasc Res.* 1992; 26:939-1043.
858. O'Nunain S, Jennison S, Bashir Y et al. Effects of adenosine on atrial repolarization in the transplanted human heart. *Am J Cardiol.* 1993; 71:248-51.
859. Marcus GM, Smith LM, Whiteman D et al. Alcohol intake is significantly associated with atrial flutter in patients under 60 years of age and a shorter right atrial effective refractory period. *Pacing Clin Electrophysiol.* 2008; 31:266-72.
860. Sengul C, Cevik C, Ozveren O et al. Acute alcohol consumption is associated with increased interatrial electromechanical delay in healthy men. *Cardiol J.* 2011; 18:682-6.
861. Hewitt RE, Lissina A, Green AE et al The bisphosphonate acute phase response: rapid and copious production of proinflammatory cytokines by peripheral blood gd T cells in response to aminobisphosphonates is inhibited by statins. *Clin Exp Immunol.* 2005; 139:101-11.
862. Aviles RJ, Martin DO, Apperson-Hansen C et al. Inflammation as a risk factor for atrial fibrillation. *Circulation.* 2003; 108:3006-10.
863. Tisdale JE, Allen MR, Overholser BR et al. Influence of zoledronic acid on atrial electrophysiological parameters and electrocardiographic measurements. *J Cardiovasc Electrophysiol.* 2015; 26:671-7.
864. Suenari K, Cheng C-C, Chen Y-C et al. Effects of ivabradine on the pulmonary vein electrical activity and modulation of pacemaker currents and calcium homeostasis. *J Cardiovasc Electrophysiol.* 2012; 23:200-6.
865. Wijffels MC, Dorland R, Allessie MA. Pharmacologic cardioversion of chronic atrial fibrillation in the goat by class IA, IC, and III drugs: a comparison between hydroquinidine, cibenzoline, flecainide, and d-sotalol. *J Cardiovasc Electrophysiol.* 1999; 10:178-93.
866. Wijffels MC, Dorland R, Mast F et al. Widening of the excitable gap during pharmacological cardioversion of atrial fibrillation in the goat: effects of cibenzoline, hydroquinidine, flecainide, and d-sotalol. *Circulation.* 2000; 102:260-7.
867. Schreiber DH, DeFreest MS. Paroxysmal atrial fibrillation precipitated by amiodarone-induced thyrotoxicosis five months after cessation of therapy. *J Emerg Med.* 2006; 31:61-4.
868. Kurt IH, Yigit T, Karademir BM. Atrial fibrillation due to late amiodarone-induced thyrotoxicosis. *Clin Drug Invest.* 2008; 28:527-31.
869. Masoni A, Alboni P, Malacarne C et al. Effects of dobutamine on electrophysiological properties of the specialized conduction system in man. *J Electrocardiol.* 1979; 12:361-70.
870. Lin CI, Chuang IN, Cheng KK et al. Arrhythmogenic effects of theophylline in human atrial tissue. *Int J Cardiol.* 1987; 17:289-97.
871. Phillips BG, Gandhi AJ, Sanoski CA et al. Comparison of intravenous diltiazem and verapamil for the acute treatment of atrial fibrillation and atrial flutter. *Pharmacotherapy.* 1997; 17:1238-45.
872. Minton NA, Henry JA. Treatment of theophylline overdose. *Am J Emerg Med.* 1996; 14:606-12.
873. Page RL, Joglar JA, Caldwell MA et al. 2015 ACC/AHA/HRS Guideline for the management of adult patients with supraventricular tachycardia. *J Am Coll Cardiol.* 2016; 67:e27-115.
874. Josephson GW, Stine RJ. Caffeine intoxication: a case of paroxysmal atrial tachycardia. *JACEP.* 1976; 5:776-8.
875. Clark JE, Simon WA. Cardiac arrhythmias after phenylpropanolamine ingestion. *Drug Intell Clin Pharm.* 1983; 17:737-8.
876. Kinugawa T, Kurita T, Nohara R et al. A case of atrial tachycardia sensitive to increased caffeine intake. *Int Heart J.* 2011; 52:398-400.
877. Somani PN, Jhingran SG. A case of paroxysmal atrial tachycardia with block due to digitalis overdosage. *Indian Heart J.* 1965; 17:85-90.
878. Storstein O, Rasmussen K. Digitalis and atrial tachycardia with block. *Br Heart J.* 1974; 36:171-6.

879. Rose MR, Glassman E, Spencer FC. Arrhythmias following cardiac surgery: relation to serum digoxin levels. *Am Heart J.* 1975; 89:288-94.

880. Storstein O, Hansteen V, Hatle L et al. Studies on digitalis: XIII. A prospective study of 649 patients on maintenance treatment with digitoxin. *Am Heart J.* 1977; 93:434-43.

881. Bramlet DA, From AH. Double tachycardias associated with digitalis intoxication. *Chest.* 1980; 78:324-6.

882. Goren C, Denes P. The role of Holter monitoring in detecting digitalis-provoked arrhythmias. *Chest.* 1981; 79:555-8.

883. Chowdhry IH, Hariman RJ, Gomes JA et al. Transient digitoxic double tachycardia. *Chest.* 1983; 83:686-7.

884. Moorman JR. Digitalis toxicity at Duke Hospital, 1973-1984. *South Med J.* 1985; 78:561-4.

885. Bigger JT Jr. Digitalis toxicity. *J Clin Pharmacol.* 1985; 25:514-21.

886. Desantola JR, Marchlinski FE. Response of digoxin toxic atrial tachycardia to digoxin-specific Fab fragments. *Am J Cardiol.* 1986; 58:1109-10.

887. Miura T, Kojima R, Sugiura Y et al. Effect of aging on the incidence of digoxin toxicity. *Ann Pharmacother.* 2000; 34:427-32.

888. Rajpal S, Beedupalli J, Reddy P. Recrudescent digoxin toxicity treated with plasma exchange: a case report and review of literature. *Cardiovasc Toxicol.* 2012; 12:363-8.

889. Raja Rao MP, Panduranga P, Sulaiman K et al. Digoxin toxicity with normal digoxin and serum potassium levels: beware of magnesium, the hidden malefactor. *J Emerg Med.* 2013; 45:e31-4.

890. Laaban JP, Iung B, Chauvet JP et al. Cardiac arrhythmias during the combined use of intravenous aminophylline and terbutaline in status asthmaticus. *Chest.* 1988; 94:496-502.

891. Levine JH, Michael JR, Guarnieri T. Multifocal atrial tachycardia: a toxic effect of theophylline. *Lancet.* 1985; 1:12-4.

892. Marchlinski FE, Miller JM. Atrial arrhythmias exacerbated by theophylline. Response to verapamil and evidence for triggered activity in man. *Chest.* 1985; 88:931-4.

893. Sessler CN, Cohen MD. Cardiac arrhythmias during theophylline toxicity: a prospective continuous electrocardiographic study. *Chest.* 1990; 98:672-8.

894. Emerman CL, Devlin C, Connors AF. Risk of toxicity in patients with elevated theophylline levels. *Ann Emerg Med.* 1990; 19:643-8.

895. Bittar G, Friedman HS. The arrhythmogenicity of theophylline: a multivariate analysis of clinical determinants. *Chest.* 1991; 99:1415-20.

896. Hoffman BF, Bigger JT. Digitalis and allied cardiac glycosides. In: Gilman AG, Goodman LS, Gilman A, eds. *Goodman and Gilman's the pharmacological basis of therapeutics.* 6th ed. New York, NY: MacMillan Publishing Co Inc; 1985:729-60.

897. Cockcroft DW, Gault MH. Prediction of creatinine clearance from serum creatinine. *Nephron.* 1976; 16:31-41.

898. Schentag JJ, Bang AJ, Kozinski-Tober JL. Digoxin. In: Burton ME, Shaw LM, Schentag JJ et al, eds. *Applied pharmacokinetics and pharmacodynamics.* 4th ed. Philadelphia, PA: Lippincott Williams and Wilkins; 2006:410-39.

899. Eidelman DH, Sami MH, McGregor M et al. Combination of theophylline and salbutamol for arrhythmias in severe COPD. *Chest.* 1987; 91:808-12.

900. Rotstein Z, Battler A, Rath S et al. Acute hemodynamic and arrhythmogenic effects of high-dose intravenous salbutamol in patients with chronic left ventricular dysfunction. *Clin Cardiol.* 1990; 13:468-72.

901. Franklin WH, Dietrich AM, Hickey RW et al. Anomalous left coronary artery masquerading as infantile bronchiolitis. *Pediatr Emerg Care.* 1992; 8:338-41.

902. Lin RY, Smith AJ, Hergenroeder P. High serum albuterol levels and tachycardia in adult asthmatics treated with high-dose continuously aerosolized albuterol. *Chest.* 1993; 103:221-5.

903. Cook P, Scarfone RJ, Cook RT. Adenosine in the termination of albuterol-induced supraventricular tachycardia. *Ann Emerg Med.* 1994; 24:316-9.

904. Keller KA, Bhisitkul DM. Supraventricular tachycardia: a complication of nebulized albuterol. *Pediatr Emerg Care.* 1995; 11:98-9.

905. Duane M, Chandran L, Morelli PJ. Recurrent supraventricular tachycardia as a complication of nebulized albuterol treatment. *Clin Pediatr.* 2000; 39:673-7.

906. Habashy D, Lam LT, Browne GJ. The administration of beta2-agonists for paediatric asthma and its adverse reaction in Australian and New Zealand emergency departments: a cross-sectional survey. *Eur J Emerg Med.* 2003; 10:219-24.

907. Trachsel D, Newth CJ, Hammer J. Adenosine for salbutamol-induced supraventricular tachycardia. *Intensive Care Med.* 2007; 33:1676.

908. Wills BK, Kwan C, Bailey M et al. Recalcitrant supraventricular tachycardia: occult albuterol toxicity due to a factitious disorder. *J Emerg Med.* 2015; 49:436-8.

909. Zimmerman PM, Pulliam J, Schwengels J et al. Caffeine intoxication: a near fatality. *Ann Emerg Med.* 1985; 14:1227-9.

910. Price KR, Fligner DJ. Treatment of caffeine toxicity with esmolol. *Ann Emerg Med.* 1990; 19:44-6.

911. Beale MD, Pritchett JT, Kellner CH. Supraventricular tachycardia in a patient receiving ECT, clozapine, and caffeine. *Convuls Ther.* 1994; 10:228-31.

912. Vukcevic NP, Babic G, Segrt Z et al. Severe acute caffeine poisoing due to intradermal injections: a mesotherapy hazard. *Vojnosanit Pregl.* 2012; 69:707-13.

913. Takayanagi K, Yamaguchi H, Hayashi T et al. Carbamazepine-induced bradycardia-tachycardia syndrome with pharmacological analysis and concurrent ECG monitoring. *J Electrocardiol.* 1990; 23:85-8.

914. Kupchik M, Spivak B, Mester R et al. Combined electroconvulsive-clozapine therapy. *Clin Neuropharmacol.* 2000; 23:14-6.

915. Settem JV, Trivedi S, Kamath G et al. Clozapine-induced supraventricular tachycardia and its treatment with verapamil. *Indian J Psychol Med.* 2015; 37:358-9.

916. Caldicott LD, Hawley K, Heppell R et al. Intravenous enoximone or dobutamine for severe heart failure after acute myocardial infarction: a randomized double-blind trial. *Eur Heart J.* 1993; 14:696-700.

917. Picano E, Mathias W Jr, Pingitore A et al. Safety and tolerability of dobutamine-atropine stress echocardiography: a prospective, multicentre study: Echo Dobutamine International Cooperative Study Group. *Lancet.* 1994; 344:1190-2.

918. Weissman NJ, Rose GA, Foster GP et al. Effects of prolonging peak dobutamine dose during stress echocardiography. *J Am Coll Cardiol.* 1997; 29:526-30.

919. Hennessy TG, Codd MB, Kane G et al. Safety of dobutamine stress echocardiography in 474 consecutive studies. *Coron Artery Dis.* 1997; 8:175-8.

920. Secknus MA, Marwick TH. Evolution of dobutamine echocardiography protocols and indications: safety and side effects in 3,011 studies over 5 years. *J Am Coll Cardiol.* 1997; 29:1234-40.

921. Elhendy A, Geleijnse ML, van Domburg RT et al. Gender differences in the accuracy of dobutamine stress echocardiography for the diagnosis of coronary artery disease. *Am J Cardiol.* 1997; 80:1414-8.

922. Elhendy A, Valkema R, van Domburg RT et al. Safety of dobutamine-atropine stress myocardial perfusion scintigraphy. *J Nucl Med.* 1998; 39:1662-6.

923. Elhendy A, van Domburg RT, Poldermans D et al. Safety and feasibility of dobutamine-atropine stress echocardiography for the diagnosis of coronary artery disease in diabetic patients unable to perform an exercise stress test. *Diabetes Care.* 1998; 21:1797-1802.

924. Elhendy A, van Domburg RT, Bax JJ et al. Relation between the extent of coronary artery disease and tachyarrhythmias during dobutamine stress echocardiography. *Am J Cardiol.* 1999; 83:832-5.

925. Lu D, Greenberg MD, Little R et al. Accelerated dobutamine stress testing: safety and feasibility in patients with known or suspected coronary artery disease. *Clin Cardiol.* 2001; 24:141-5.
926. Bountioukos M, Kertai MD, Schinkel AF et al. Safety of dobutamine stress echocardiography in patients with aortic stenosis. *J Heart Valve Dis.* 2003; 12:441-6.
927. Timperley J, Mitchell AR, Thibault H et al. Safety of contrast dobutamine stress echocardiography: a single center experience. *J Am Soc Echocardiogr.* 2003; 18:63-7.
928. Tsutsui JM, Elhendy A, Xie F et al. Safety of dobutamine stress real-time myocardial contrast echocardiography. *J Am Coll Cardiol.* 2005; 45:1235-42.
929. Chaowalit N, Jakrapanichakul D, Udol K et al. Dobutamine stress echocardiography for the evaluation of coronary artery disease in Thai population: Siriraj experience. *J Med Assoc Thail* 2007; 90(suppl 2):33-40.
930. Gardner SF, Rutherford WF, Munger MA et al. Drug-induced supraventricular tachycardia: a case report of fluoxetine. *Ann Emerg Med.* 1991; 20:194-7.
931. Allhof T, Bender S, Banger M et al. Atrial arrhythmia in a woman treated with fluoxetine: is there a causal relationship? *Ann Emerg Med.* 2001; 37:116-7.
932. Wilson NJ, Adderley RJ, McEniery JA. Supraventricular tachycardia associated with continuous furosemide infusion. *Can J Anaesth.* 1991; 38:502-5.
933. O'Driscoll BR. Supraventricular tachycardia caused by nebulised ipratropium bromide. *Thorax.* 1989; 44:312.
934. Anthonisen NR, Connett JE, Enright PL et al. Hospitalizations and mortality in the Lung Health Study. *Am J Respir Crit Care Med.* 2002; 166:333-9.
935. Smith RS, Warren DJ. Effects of high-dose intravenous methylprednisolone on circulation in humans. *Transplantation.* 1983; 35:349-51.
936. Kumari R, Uppal SS. First report of supraventricular tachycardia after intravenous pulse methylprednisolone therapy, with a brief review of the literature. *Rheumatol Int.* 2005; 26:70-3.
937. Conway EE Jr, Walsh CA, Palomba AL. Supraventricular tachycardia following the administration of phenylpropanolamine in an infant. *Pediatr Emerg Care.* 1989; 5:173-4.
938. Loughnan PM, McNamara JM. Paroxysmal supraventricular tachycardia during theophylline therapy in a premature infant. *J Pediatr.* 1978; 92:1016-8.
939. Fisher J, Graudins A. Intermittent haemodialysis and sustained low-efficiancy dialysis (SLED) for acute theophylline toxicity. *J Med Toxicol.* 2015; 11:359-63.
940. Ganz LI, Friedman PL. Supraventricular tachycardia. *N Engl J Med.* 1995; 332:162-73.
941. Ferguson JD, DiMarco JP. Contemporary management of paroxysmal supraventricular tachycardia. *Circulation.* 2003; 107:1096-9.

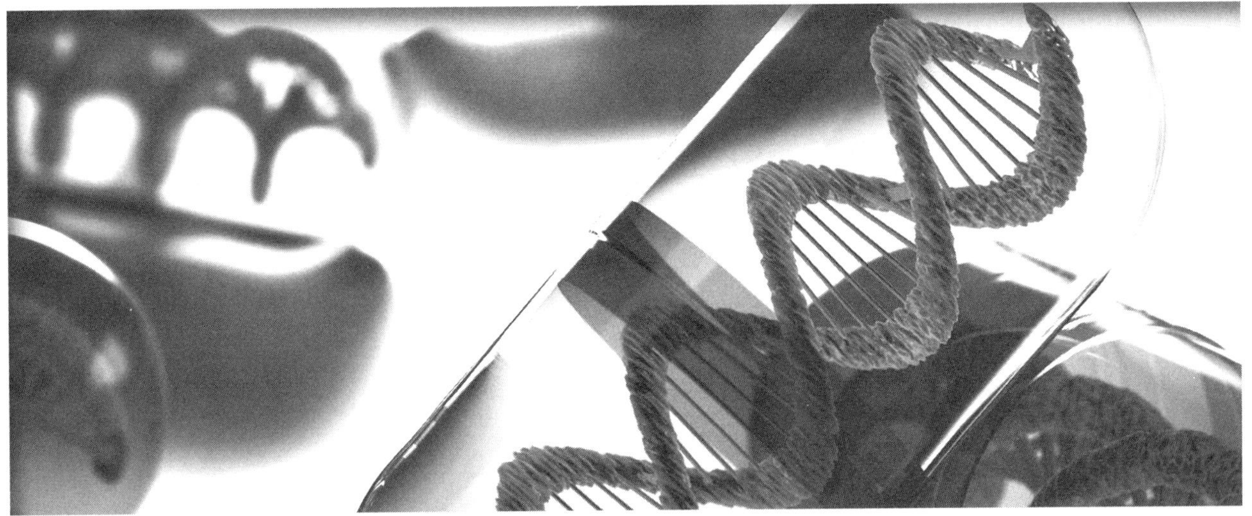

CHAPTER 27

Hypertension

Liza W. Claus and Joseph J. Saseen

More than 80 million Americans have hypertension, or approximately one out of three adults.[1] Hypertension is a chronic medical condition that is characterized by persistent increases in systolic or diastolic blood pressure, or both. The term *elevated blood pressure* has replaced the category formerly known as prehypertension and is used to identify patients with blood pressures higher than normal but not yet to the threshold diagnostic for hypertension.[2] Hypertension is elevated blood pressure nearly always asymptomatic. Target organ damage (e.g., coronary artery disease, chronic kidney disease/failure, ischemic stroke), commonly presenting as a cardiovascular event, is the primary cause of associated morbidity and mortality in patients with hypertension.[2] Most patients (90–95%) with hypertension have primary (also known as essential) hypertension. The remainder have secondary hypertension, which includes patients with drug-induced causes.

CAUSATIVE AGENTS

Drug-induced hypertension is defined as high blood pressure caused by using (or discontinuing the use of) a chemical substance, drug, or medication.[3] Expert reviews of drug-induced hypertension are available, but do not thoroughly evaluate published literature to support the association between a comprehensive list of cited drugs and drug-induced hypertension.[4,5] Drugs that have been reported to cause hypertension are listed in **Table 27-1**.[6-108] Drugs on this list are also identified as potential causes of resistant hypertension.[109] There are some limitations to this list. Adverse drug effect reporting often identifies increases in blood pressure, not always drug-induced hypertension per se. Therefore, for many drugs that have been reported to increase blood pressure, the incidence of drug-induced hypertension may be unknown. This list also represents agents that are used primarily for chronic conditions or that are used for a prolonged period of time. These medications may cause hypertension, exacerbate previously well-controlled hypertension, or antagonize the effects of antihypertensive pharmacotherapy.

EPIDEMIOLOGY

Hypertension is one of the most common chronic medical conditions. Despite increased public awareness, the prevalence of hypertension is not

Table 27-1 Agents Implicated in Drug-Induced Hypertension

Drug	Incidence[a]	Level of Evidence[b]
Amphetamines[6,7]	NK	A
Antihypertensive agents[8-27,c]	NK	B
Bevacizumab[28-32]	8–18%	A
Bupropion[33-35]	2–6.1%	B
Caffeine[36]	NK	B
Celecoxib[37-42]	2.4–12.5%	A
Cocaine[43]	NK	C
Corticosteroids[44-49]	NK	A
Cyclosporine[50-56]	11.2–50%	A
Darbepoetin-α[57]	23%	A
Desvenlafaxine[58]	1.3–2.3%	A
Ephedra alkaloids[59-61]	NK	B
Ergot alkaloids[62]	NK	C
Erythropoetin-α[63,64]	24%	A
Estrogen-containing oral contraceptives[65-71]	5%	A
Ivabradine[72]	8.9%	A
Licorice[73-75]	NK	C
Monoamine oxidase inhibitors[76,77,d]	NK	C
NSAIDs[78-83]	NK	A
Phenylephrine[84,85]	NK	C
Pseudoephedrine[86-90]	NK	A
Sibutramine[91-96]	NK	A
Sorafenib[97,98]	17%	A
Sunitinib[99-101]	15–30%	A
Tacrolimus[102-104]	47–50%	A
Testosterone[105,106]	3%	A
Venlafaxine[107,108]	3–13%	A

NK = not known, NSAID = nonsteroidal anti-inflammatory drug.

[a]Based on reported incidence of hypertension or persistent blood pressure elevation, not just increase in blood pressure, from product information or literature (not placebo-corrected).

[b]Definitions for Levels of Evidence: Level A—evidence from one or more randomized, controlled clinical trials; Level B—evidence from nonrandomized clinical trials, prospective observational studies, cohort studies, retrospective studies, case-control studies, meta-analyses and/or postmarketing surveillance studies; and Level C—evidence from one or more published case reports or case series.

[c]When therapy is abruptly discontinued.

[d]Result of a drug–food interaction with tyramine-containing foods or a drug–drug interaction.

declining. Over 30% of the American population has hypertension.[110] With the introduction of the 2017 American College of Cardiology (ACC)/American Heart Association (AHA)/American Academy of Physician Assistants (AAPA)/Association of Black Cardiologists (ABC)/American College of Preventive Medicine (ACPM)/American Geriatrics Society (AGS)/American Pharmacists Association (APhA)/American Society of Hypertension (ASH)/American Society for Preventive Medicine (ASPM)/National Medical Association (NMA)/Preventive Cardiovascular Nurses Association (PCNA) Guideline for the Prevention, Detection, Evaluation, and Management of High

Table 27-2 Blood Pressure Classification According to the 2017 ACC/AHA/AAPA/ABC/ACPM/AGS/APhA/ASH/ASPC/NMA/PCNA Guideline for the Prevention, Detection, Evaluation, and Management of High Blood Pressure in Adults to Detect Drug-Induced Hypertension[2]

Classification	Systolic Blood Pressure (mm Hg)		Diastolic Blood Pressure (mm Hg)
Normal	<120	and	<80
Elevated	120–129	and	<80
Stage 1 hypertension	130–139	or	80–89
Stage 2 hypertension	≥140	or	≥90

ACC/AHA = American College of Cardiology/American Heart Association.[2]

Blood Pressure in Adults and its lower blood pressure thresholds (**Table 27-2**), it is now estimated that a substantially higher number of patients will be diagnosed with hypertension.[2,111] Although most patients who truly have hypertension are aware of their condition (greater than 80%), only two-thirds of these patients are treated for hypertension, and just over half have controlled blood pressure values.[1] When considering these statistics, the potential impact of drug-induced hypertension is significant, as many patients in whom drug-induced hypertension develops may not be identified or appropriately treated. Although the precise incidence of drug-induced hypertension in the general population is unknown, it is reasonable to assume that drugs may cause some undiagnosed cases of hypertension. The prevalence of drug-induced hypertension is possibly very low, but drug-induced exacerbations of hypertension are likely more common.

The 2017 ACC/AHA Hypertension Guideline identifies medications that can cause hypertension.[2] This chapter expands on the list provided by the 2017 ACC/AHA/AAPA/ABC/ACPM/AGS/APhA/ASH/ASPC/NMA/PCNA Guideline for the Prevention, Detection, Evaluation, and Management of High Blood Pressure in Adults to include additional drugs.[2] These agents may either cause hypertension or be a reason for resistant hypertension.[109] Estimated incidences of drug-induced hypertension associated with specific agents are also presented in Table 27-1. The exact incidence of drug-induced hypertension associated with several agents is unknown; however, these medications have been shown to increase blood pressure.

MECHANISMS

Arterial blood pressure is regulated by several factors: the adrenergic nervous system, the renin–angiotensin–aldosterone system, kidney function and blood flow, hormonal regulatory systems (adrenal cortical hormones, vasopressin, thyroid, insulin), and the vascular endothelium (nitric oxide, bradykinin, prostacyclin, endothelin).[5,112] Drug-induced alterations of these systems may explain persistent increases in blood pressure associated with certain agents. The various mechanisms by which drugs may induce hypertension (**Table 27-3**) are broadly categorized as stimulation of sympathetic nervous system activity, fluid-volume expansion, interference with the action of antihypertensive drugs, paradoxical responses to antihypertensive agents, and unknown mechanisms.[5]

SYMPATHETIC NERVOUS SYSTEM STIMULATION

Certain drugs (e.g., cocaine, amphetamines, ephedra, some antidepressants) can activate the sympathetic nervous system through norepinephrine or norepinephrine-like stimulation. Stimulation of peripheral adrenergic α-receptors causes vasoconstriction, while stimulation of myocardial adrenergic β-receptors increases heart rate and contractility, both of which can increase blood pressure. Under normal circumstances, compensatory mechanisms are triggered that decrease total peripheral resistance, which usually maintains normal blood pressure. However, drugs that cause hypertension may blunt or impair this compensatory response.

Table 27-3 Mechanisms of Drug-Induced Hypertension

Drug	Mechanism
Amphetamines Caffeine Cocaine Desvenlafaxine Ergot alkaloids (ergonovine, methysergide) Phenylephrine–ophthalmic Pseudoephedrine Sibutramine Venlafaxine	Increased stimulation of sympathetic nervous system activity
Antivascular endothelin growth factor agents	Possible mechanism: endothelin damage secondary to decreased nitric oxide release and release of growth factors that stimulate the renin–angiotensin–aldosterone system
β-blockers Centrally acting α-agonists	Abrupt discontinuation, causing overstimulation of α- and/or β-receptors
Calcineurin inhibitors (cyclosporine, tacrolimus)	Increased prostaglandin production resulting in decreases in sodium, water, and potassium excretion, causing increased fluid-volume expansion
Corticosteroids Licorice	Stimulation of the mineralocorticoid receptor, causing increased fluid-volume expansion
Erythropoiesis-stimulating agents	Supratherapeutic effects of increasing blood cell production, causing increased fluid volume
Estrogen-containing oral contraceptives	Increased hepatic production of angiotensinogen, causing stimulation of the renin–angiotensin–aldosterone system
Monoamine oxidase inhibitors	Overall stimulation of sympathetic nervous system activity by increased production of adrenergic substances secondary to ingesting tyramine-containing foods or a drug interaction
NSAIDs and COX-2 inhibitors	Inhibition of prostaglandins, causing vasoconstriction and stimulation of the renin–angiotensin–aldosterone system, resulting in increased fluid-volume expansion
Testosterone	Increased fluid-volume expansion; stimulation of sympathetic nervous system activity

COX = cyclooxygenase, NSAID = nonsteroidal anti-inflammatory drug.

FLUID-VOLUME EXPANSION

The renin–angiotensin–aldosterone system functions with the kidneys to regulate arterial blood pressure. Decreases in blood pressure or kidney blood flow, volume depletion, or sodium depletion all increase renin secretion from the kidney. Renin mediates the transformation of angiotensinogen to angiotensin I, which is converted by angiotensin-converting enzyme to angiotensin II. Angiotensin II is a potent direct vasoconstrictor that stimulates production of aldosterone, which causes sodium and water retention. Several drugs (e.g., nonsteroidal anti-inflammatory drugs [NSAIDs], including the cyclooxygenase-2 [COX-2] selective inhibitor celecoxib, certain immunosuppressants) can indirectly trigger renin release, primarily by decreasing kidney perfusion.[113,114] In premenopausal women, estrogens have been shown to stimulate the renin–angiotensin–aldosterone system by increasing hepatic production of angiotensinogen.[115,116] These effects are normally overcome by negative-feedback mechanisms that prevent excessive renin release. However, this may not occur in patients taking drugs known to induce hypertension or in patients with chronic kidney disease or cardiovascular risk factors. Generalized vasoconstriction, especially in the kidney, is the hypothesized cause of cyclosporine-induced hypertension.[50,117]

Certain drugs that alter hormonal regulation (e.g., oral contraceptives, corticosteroids) can cause hypertension. The estrogen component of oral contraceptives is primarily responsible for blood-pressure elevation, but the mechanism is unclear. In premenopausal women, oral contraceptive use results in serum estrogen and progestin concentrations that are higher than those that result from endogenous hormone production. This is in sharp contrast to the use of estrogen-replacement therapy (ERT) or hormone-replacement therapy (HRT) in postmenopausal women, during which serum estrogen and progestin concentrations are lower than those associated with premenopausal endogenous hormone production. Clinical trials have shown that the use of either ERT or HRT in both premenopausal and postmenopausal women increases the risk of cardiovascular events.[118-121] However, ERT or HRT do not cause drug-induced hypertension in postmenopausal women.[122]

Hormonal dysregulation can cause hypertension by inducing insulin resistance (the metabolic syndrome), sodium and water retention, or myriad other effects. Other miscellaneous agents cause hypertension via unique mechanisms not related to these neurohumoral effects. Both erythropoietin-α and darbepoetin-α can cause dose-dependent increases in blood pressure.[123] Possible mechanisms include increased hematocrit and erythrocyte mass, changes in the production or sensitivity of endogenous vasopressor and vasodilatory factors, alterations in vascular smooth muscle, direct vasoconstriction, and arterial remodeling by stimulation of vascular cell growth.[124] However, the exact mechanism is unknown.

REBOUND HYPERTENSION

The adrenergic antihypertensive agents, β-blockers and centrally acting α-receptor agonists, can cause rebound hypertension when therapy is abruptly discontinued.[8-27] Long-term exposure to β-blocking agents causes upregulation and increased expression of β-receptors. When β-blocker therapy is abruptly discontinued, excessive stimulation of these additional β-receptors occurs, potentially resulting in increases in blood pressure and heart rate, leading to rebound hypertension. Cardioselective β-blockers or those with intrinsic sympathomimetic activity have been touted as not being associated with rebound hypertension, but this has not been proven. The mechanism by which rebound hypertension occurs in association with central α-agonists has not been fully established, but is believed to be similar to that of β-blockers. When exposed to long-term central α-agonist therapy, α-receptor density, sensitivity, or both can increase.[5] Abrupt discontinuation of therapy with central α-agonists leads to elevated plasma norepinephrine concentrations, peripheral α-receptor stimulation, and increased blood pressure. This occurs in association with both oral and transdermal administration.

CLINICAL PRESENTATION AND DIFFERENTIAL DIAGNOSIS

The classification of blood pressure is based on systolic and diastolic blood pressure values (Table 27-2).[2] This classification includes normal blood pressure, elevated blood pressure, stage 1 hypertension, and stage 2 hypertension. Elevated blood pressure and the development of hypertension are nearly always asymptomatic. Therefore, assessing patients for the presence of signs and symptoms of drug-induced hypertension (**Table 27-4**) is not very helpful. When blood pressure elevations are extreme (usually much higher than 200/110 mm Hg), symptoms consistent with hypertensive emergency (e.g., anxiety, chest pain, confusion, excessive perspiration, nausea/vomiting, pale or red skin, visual changes) are more likely to be present but are still not common.

The clinical significance of elevated blood pressure associated with the use of a drug varies, depending on an individual's baseline blood pressure. Moreover, the precise time of onset for

Table 27-4 Signs and Symptoms Associated with Drug-Induced Hypertension

- No symptoms usually reported by patients
- Increase in blood pressure
- In patients with a history of treated hypertension, requirement for increased doses of antihypertensive medications
- In patients with a history of treated hypertension, need for additional antihypertensive agents to maintain blood pressure goal
- Rarely, hypertensive emergency: neurologic deficits, anxiety, nausea, vomiting, chest discomfort, back pain, dyspnea, visual changes

drug-induced hypertension is unknown and likely highly variable and dependent on the particular mechanism of drug-induced hypertension. For the purposes of this chapter, drug-induced hypertension will be defined as blood pressure increases from baseline that confer stage 1 hypertension or higher. The threshold blood pressure for the diagnosis of hypertension is 130/80 mm Hg.

Drug-induced blood pressure elevations, if persistent, may be clinically significant even if the blood pressure is not increased to above an individual's goal value. Many drugs have been reported to induce statistically significant blood pressure increases, some as small as 2–4 mm Hg.[6-108] The clinical significance of these small increases is debatable. However, data from observational studies and randomized trials suggest that a 2 mm Hg reduction in diastolic blood pressure correlates with a 17% decrease in the prevalence of hypertension, a 6% reduction in the risk of coronary heart disease (CHD), and a 15% reduction in the risk of stroke and transient ischemic attacks.[125-127] It has been documented that patients with blood pressure in the stage 1 hypertension range have a higher risk of cardiovascular events than patients with normal blood pressure (see Morbidity and Mortality section, below).[128] Therefore, depending on a patient's baseline blood pressure, small but persistent blood pressure increases may be clinically significant.

Several other conditions should be considered in patients with suspected drug-induced hypertension (**Table 27-5**). The possibility of new-onset primary (essential) hypertension must always be considered. The patient's blood pressure history and a comprehensive medical examination are necessary components for this evaluation. Other origins of secondary hypertension in addition to drug-induced causes should also be ruled out. Additional diagnostic tests such as laboratory evaluations, polysomnography, and aortic and kidney imaging may be required for a comprehensive evaluation.

Table 27-5 Conditions to Consider in the Differential Diagnosis of Drug-Induced Hypertension

Primary hypertension

- New onset
- Undiagnosed
- Previously diagnosed but not at goal blood pressure

Secondary hypertension

- Alcohol abuse
- Cancer
- Chronic kidney disease
- Coarctation of the aorta
- Cushing syndrome
- Hyperparathyroidism
- Pheochromocytoma
- Polycystic kidney disease
- Primary aldosteronism
- Renovascular disease
- Sleep apnea
- Thyroid disease

RISK FACTORS

Patient-specific risk factors for drug-induced hypertension are listed in **Table 27-6**. Perhaps the most relevant is a history of increased blood pressure, either significant enough to fulfill the diagnostic criteria for hypertension or high enough to be classified as elevated blood pressure. A history of drug-induced hypertension or drug-induced increases in blood pressure is also noteworthy. There are many major cardiovascular risk factors that increase the risk of target organ damage associated with hypertension. One prospective cohort study evaluating oral contraceptive–induced hypertension showed that the relative risk for hypertension increased from 1.5 to 1.8 when other hypertension risk factors were considered.[66] Therefore, major cardiovascular risk factors should

Table 27-6 Risk Factors for Drug-Induced Hypertension

- Elevated blood pressure in the past
- History of hypertension or elevated blood pressure
- Previous history of drug-induced hypertension
- Decreased glomerular filtration rate (especially <60 mL/min/1.73 m^2)
- Metabolic syndrome
- Advanced age
- Persistent use of high-dose NSAID therapy

NSAID = nonsteroidal anti-inflammatory drug.

be considered when evaluating a patient's overall risk of drug-induced hypertension.

Age has been identified as a risk factor for several forms of cardiovascular disease.[5] NSAID-induced elevations in blood pressure are especially prominent in the elderly population.[78] Data from a case-control study of 9,411 elderly patients in whom antihypertensive therapy was initiated revealed that chronic NSAID users had a higher risk of initiating antihypertensive therapy than nonusers (OR 1.66, 95% CI 1.54–1.80).[80] A dose-dependent relationship with regard to risk was also revealed in this database. These findings suggest that age and dose, at least with persistent NSAID therapy, are both risk factors for drug-induced hypertension.

MORBIDITY AND MORTALITY

Morbidity and mortality, manifesting as cardiovascular disease, are clearly increased in patients with primary hypertension. However, the exact association between drug-induced hypertension and morbidity and mortality is unknown. A reasonable assumption is that prolonged drug-induced hypertension would result in a similar increase in risk of cardiovascular disease as compared with primary hypertension. Approximately 85 million Americans have some form of cardiovascular disease.[1] CHD is a long-term complication of hypertension that is the largest contributor to hypertension-related morbidity and mortality. It is often the fatal event related to cardiovascular mortality. Estimates have identified CHD as the most costly physical health condition in the United States.[129] Moreover, cardiovascular disease is the primary cause of death in the United States.[1]

Hypertension-related complications manifest as target organ damage. The various forms of target organ damage include heart disease (left ventricular hypertrophy, CHD [angina, myocardial infarction, acute coronary syndrome], heart failure), cerebrovascular disease (ischemic stroke, transient ischemic attacks), chronic kidney disease, peripheral arterial disease, and retinopathy. Observational data have established a direct correlation between blood pressure elevation and risk of target organ damage in patients of all ages with hypertension.[127,130] Randomized, double-blind, placebo-controlled clinical trials have also clearly demonstrated reduced morbidity and mortality associated with blood pressure reduction in patients with hypertension, even in the very elderly.[2,131-137] Therefore, persistent drug-induced hypertension may be associated with long-term increased risk of target organ damage.

A consistent, continuous, and independent relationship between blood pressure and risk of cardiovascular disease and other target organ damage is present in patients with elevated blood pressure that is not sufficiently high to be classified as hypertension.[2,128] Starting at a blood pressure of 115/75 mm Hg, the risk of future cardiovascular disease doubles with every 20 mm Hg increase in systolic blood pressure and 10 mm Hg increase in diastolic blood pressure.[130] Therefore, drug-induced increases in blood pressure, even within the normal or elevated blood pressure range, may be associated with a long-term increased risk of morbidity and mortality.

PREVENTION

Strategies for prevention of drug-induced hypertension are listed in **Table 27-7**. Drug-induced hypertension is ideally detected by closely monitoring blood pressure. Clinic-based blood pressure measurements should be obtained 2–4 weeks after initiating therapy with a drug known to increase blood pressure. Home or ambulatory blood pressure monitoring may be helpful but is not essential.[138-140] Moreover, both home and ambulatory blood pressure values are lower than those measured in the clinic. Average home blood pressure measurements are typically 5 mm Hg lower than clinic values, and 24-hour ambulatory blood pressure measurements in individuals with hypertension are typically 10 mm Hg lower.[140] However, clinic-based blood pressure measurements are sufficient for detecting drug-induced hypertension.

The most effective prevention strategy is avoiding the use of agents known to cause drug-induced hypertension. This is especially important

Table 27-7 Approaches to Help Prevent Drug-Induced Hypertension

- Avoid use of agents reported to cause drug-induced hypertension in high-risk patients
- For patients taking medications known to cause drug-induced hypertension:
    - Avoid tyramine-containing foods in patients taking monoamine oxidase inhibitors
    - Use minimum effective dose of NSAIDs, including celecoxib
    - Measure blood pressure at least every 2–4 weeks
    - Evaluate for symptoms of hypertension-related target organ damage periodically
- Engage in lifestyle modifications:
    - Weight reduction: Maintain normal body weight and body-mass index, 18.5–24.9 kg/m^2
    - Adopt the DASH eating plan: consume a diet rich in fruits, vegetables and low-fat dairy products with a reduced content of saturated and total fat
    - Reduce dietary sodium intake to 1.5 g sodium daily
    - Engage in regular aerobic physical activity (at least 30 minutes/day, most days of the week)
    - Moderate alcohol consumption: limit consumption to ≤2 drinks/day in most men and ≤1 drink/day in women and lighter-weight persons

DASH = dietary approaches to stop hypertension, NSAID = nonsteroidal anti-inflammatory drug.

in patients with either established cardiovascular disease or multiple risk factors for drug-induced hypertension or cardiovascular disease (Table 27-6). For women requiring oral contraceptive therapy, preparations with low estrogen (≤30 mcg ethinyl estradiol) and progestin (≤1 mg norethindrone) content appear to be associated with the lowest risk of hypertension.

Lifestyle modifications that lower cardiovascular risk and blood pressure should be recommended for all patients, especially those using drugs known to increase blood pressure.[141,142] These modifications include diet and exercise recommendations. The Dietary Approaches to Stop Hypertension (DASH) diet is rich in vegetables, fruits, and low-fat dairy products and has been proven to lower blood pressure.[142] Other methods, such as weight reduction, dietary sodium restriction, moderate and regular aerobic activity, and moderation of alcohol consumption are also effective in lowering blood pressure.

MANAGEMENT

Management of drug-induced hypertension depends on differentiating drug-induced from either primary or other secondary causes of hypertension. When drug-induced hypertension is strongly suspected, the offending agent should be discontinued when possible (**Table 27-8**). Blood pressure should then return to baseline values within 2–4 weeks under most circumstances. If the blood pressure remains consistently elevated after discontinuing therapy with the offending agent, further investigation to evaluate primary hypertension or other secondary causes is needed. The offending agent should not be reintroduced. However, if no reasonable treatment alternative can be identified, a reintroduction of therapy with a reduced dose and blood pressure monitoring may be attempted. Lifestyle modifications to lower blood pressure, as previously discussed, should be implemented in these patients.

CALCINEURIN INHIBITORS

When therapy with certain offending agents must be continued, specific management approaches may be considered (Table 27-8). Cyclosporine and tacrolimus, which are calcineurin inhibitors, are immunosuppressant agents that are used in patients after solid organ transplantation and to treat a variety of other conditions.[51-53,102] Due to their crucial role in therapy, calcineurin inhibitors usually cannot be discontinued. Therefore, managing the drug-induced hypertension is the primary goal in these patients.

Table 27-8 Management of Drug-Induced Hypertension

Drug	Management
Most agents	Discontinue offending agent when possible
Cyclosporine	• If stage 1 hypertension, decrease dose by 25% • If stage 2 hypertension, decrease dose by 50%, and consider antihypertensive therapy • Dihydropyridine calcium channel blockers are preferred antihypertensive agents
Erythropoietin and darbepoetin	• Use the lowest effective dose: decrease dose if hemoglobin concentration approaches 12 g/dL or if hemoglobin increase is >1 g/dL in a 2-week period; hold dose if hemoglobin concentration exceeds 13 g/dL • Subcutaneous administration is preferred over intravenous to minimize abrupt increases in blood pressure
Oral contraceptives	• Monitor blood pressure for up to 3 months after discontinuation of therapy • When no other form of contraception is feasible, use the lowest estrogen/progestin-content product and treat with antihypertensive therapy
Rebound hypertension from discontinuation of therapy with β-blockers or central α-agonists	• Reinitiate therapy with agent at previous long-term dose • Gradually taper if therapy is to be discontinued

A consensus guideline based on reports from clinical trials and from clinical experience using cyclosporine in patients with rheumatoid arthritis was published in 1999.[143] When patients taking cyclosporine have stage 1 hypertension on at least two consecutive visits, the cyclosporine dose should be reduced by 25%. The dose should be reduced by 50% in those in whom stage 2 hypertension develops, and initiation of antihypertensive pharmacotherapy may be necessary. If blood pressure remains elevated despite initial dose reductions, additional reductions and initiation of antihypertensive pharmacotherapy should be considered. Persistent blood pressure elevation may require cyclosporine discontinuation if an acceptable alternative agent can be used.

Dihydropyridine calcium-channel blockers (e.g., amlodipine, felodipine) are preferred agents for the treatment of cyclosporine-induced hypertension.[117,143] These agents do not interact with cyclosporine and promote vasodilation of the afferent and efferent renal arterioles. Pharmacologically, this mechanism of action is ideal for managing cyclosporine-induced hypertension. Nondihydropyridine calcium-channel blockers (i.e., diltiazem, verapamil) increase serum cyclosporine concentrations and are less desirable pharmacotherapy options for cyclosporine-induced hypertension. Patients with pre-existing hypertension treated with a β-blocker can remain on this therapy. However, diuretics, angiotensin-converting enzyme inhibitors, or angiotensin-II receptor blockers are not highly effective for managing this type of hypertension, and their use as first-line agents for cyclosporine-induced hypertension is discouraged.[116,143]

Guidelines for management of tacrolimus-induced hypertension have not been published. An approach similar to that recommended for cyclosporine-induced hypertension is reasonable. However, manufacturers' recommendations are to control blood pressure "with any of the common" antihypertensive agents.[102] These recommendations state that because tacrolimus may cause hyperkalemia, potassium-sparing diuretics should be avoided. As with cyclosporine, certain calcium-channel blockers (diltiazem, verapamil) can increase serum tacrolimus concentrations and should be avoided or used with extreme caution.

ORAL CONTRACEPTIVES

Women who are treated with estrogen-containing oral contraceptive agents should have their blood pressure measured within the first month of treatment, then after 3, 6, and 12 months. If oral contraceptive-induced hypertension occurs, the drug should be discontinued and replaced with an alternative form of contraception. Blood pressure should return to pretreatment values within 3 months after discontinuation of therapy. If it does not, additional evaluation for primary hypertension or other secondary forms of hypertension is necessary. If an alternative form of contraception cannot be used and other secondary forms of hypertension are ruled out, an oral contraceptive agent with a low estrogen (≤30 mcg ethinyl estradiol) and progestin (≤1 mg norethindrone) content may be used. Lifestyle modifications should be implemented, with the addition of antihypertensive drug therapy when necessary.

According to the American College of Obstetricians and Gynecologists, women with pre-existing and well-controlled hypertension who are younger than 35 years of age may initiate a trial of combined oral contraceptives if the woman is otherwise healthy, exhibits no evidence of end-organ vascular disease, and does not smoke cigarettes. Careful monitoring should be performed for several months following initiation of the combined oral contraceptive.[144] If blood pressure remains controlled, therapy may be continued. If hypertension occurs, progestin-only or nonhormonal contraceptives should be used as an alternative method.

ERYTHROPOIESIS-STIMULATING AGENTS

Erythropoietin-α and darbepoetin-α are erythropoiesis-stimulating agents that are indicated for the treatment of anemia associated with chronic kidney disease, human immunodeficiency virus infection and cancer chemotherapy, and for reduction of the need for allogeneic blood transfusion in surgery.[57,63,64] These drugs can enhance quality of life and improve cardiac function. Discontinuing therapy is not always a feasible option to manage hypertension induced by these drugs. Although lifestyle modifications might minimize blood pressure increases, close monitoring of serum hemoglobin concentration during therapy is essential to avoid excessive therapeutic effects that can result in blood pressure elevations. The dose of these agents should be reduced if serum hemoglobin concentrations approach 12 g/dL or if increases in serum hemoglobin concentration exceed 1 g/dL in a 2-week period. Therapy should be withheld if serum hemoglobin concentrations exceed 13 g/dL.[57,63,64]

Use of erythropoiesis-stimulating agents in patients with chronic kidney disease undergoing dialysis treatment requires close monitoring for the development of drug-induced hypertension. The need for dialysis alone increases the risk of hypertension or worsening of hypertension. Optimizing dialysis treatments in patients with kidney disease, closely monitoring and managing volume status when needed, and using subcutaneous administration to ensure gradual red blood cell increases are additional strategies that may minimize the risk of blood pressure elevations.[145]

REBOUND HYPERTENSION

When rebound hypertension occurs after abrupt discontinuation of a β-blocker or a centrally acting α-receptor agonist, therapy with the drug should be reinitiated at the previous long-term dose. If discontinuation of therapy with the offending agent is intended, therapy can be reinitiated, with the dose subsequently gradually decreased, followed by discontinuation. There are no guidelines regarding the optimal manner in which to gradually discontinue therapy with such medications. However, the dosing schedule should be individualized based on the dose of the drug that caused the rebound hypertension. A 50% dose decrease for 3–7 days is considered a tapering step. If a patient experiences rebound hypertension on a low-to-moderate dose of a drug, one tapering step may be sufficient to treat rebound hypertension, whereas two or more tapering steps may be needed for patients receiving higher doses.

INFORMATION FOR PATIENTS

Patients taking drugs that are known to cause drug-induced hypertension should be made aware of the potential risks. Patients should be counseled that their blood pressure may increase to the point of a diagnosis of hypertension. They should be instructed to comply with medical visits to detect elevations in blood pressure. Patients should also be encouraged to periodically monitor and document their blood pressure values outside of their prescribing practitioner's office (e.g., at home, in a community pharmacy). If persistent increases in systolic or diastolic blood pressure values are detected (even if small) or blood pressure increases to above their goal value (Table 27-2), patients should consult a healthcare professional (e.g., pharmacist, physician). If symptoms consistent with hypertensive emergency develop (e.g., chest pain, unilateral weakness, severe headache, shortness of breath), patients should be instructed to seek immediate emergency care.

Lifestyle modifications (Table 27-7) should be encouraged in all patients at risk for hypertension, especially those receiving drugs that may cause hypertension. Patients using β-blockers or centrally acting α-receptor agonists should be educated regarding potential rebound hypertension and instructed not to abruptly discontinue therapy with these agents. Use of any nonprescription medication without first consulting a pharmacist or other healthcare professional should be discouraged. Lastly, patients should be encouraged to ensure that all healthcare professionals involved with providing their care are fully aware of all current medications and risk factors for hypertension so that new medications that may potentially interact with drugs or further increase the risk of hypertension can be avoided.

REFERENCES

1. Mozaffarian D, Benjamin E, Go A et al. Heart disease and stroke statistics—2015 update: a report from the American Heart Association. *Circulation*. 2015; 131:e29-e322.
2. Whelton PK, Carey RM, Aronow WS et al. ACC/AHA/AAPA/ABC/ACPM/AGS/APhA/ASH/ASPC/NMA/PCNA guideline for the prevention, detection, evaluation, and management of high blood pressure in adults: a report of the American College of Cardiology/American Heart Association Task Force on Clinical Practice Guidelines. *J Am Coll Cardiol*. 2018; 71:e127-248.
3. US National Library of Medicine and the National Institutes of Health. Medline Plus Health Information. Medical Encyclopedia. Drug-Induced Hypertension. November 25, 2014. Available at: http://www.nlm.nih.gov/medlineplus/ency/article/000155.htm (accessed 2018 Apr 10).
4. Grossman A, Messerli FH, Grossman E. Drug induced hypertension—an unappreciated cause of secondary hypertension. *Eur J Pharmacol*. 2015; 763(Pt A):15-22.
5. Kaplan NM, Victor RG. *Kaplan's Clinical Hypertension,* 11th ed. Philadelphia, PA: Wolters Kluwer; 2015:1-461.
6. Samuels JA, Franco K, Wan F et al. Effect of stimulants on 24-h ambulatory blood pressure in children with ADHD: a double-blind, randomized, cross-over trial. *Pediatr Nephrol*. 2006; 21:92-5.
7. Lester SJ, Baggott M, Welm S et al. Cardiovascular effects of 3,4-methylenedioxymethamphetamine: a doubleblind, placebo-controlled trial. *Ann Intern Med*. 2000; 133:969-73.
8. Lewis MJ, Ross PJ, Henderson AH. Rebound effect after stopping beta-blockers. *BMJ*. 1979; 2:606.
9. Shiroff RA, Mathis J, Zelis R et al. Propranolol rebound—a retrospective study. *Am J Cardiol*. 1978; 41:778-80.
10. Weber MA. Blood pressure rebound following withdrawal of antihypertensive treatment. *JAMA*. 1978; 239:833.
11. Backo AL, Clause SL, Triller DM et al. Clonidine-induced hypertension in a patient with a spinal lesion. *Ann Pharmacother*. 2002; 36:1396-8.
12. England JF. Clonidine rebound hypertension. *Med J Aust*. 1977; 1:756-7.
13. Ferguson RP, Alvino E. Rebound hypertension after low-dose clonidine withdrawal. *South Med J*. 1983; 76:98.
14. Fitzgibbon D, Rapp S, Butler S et al. Rebound hypertension and withdrawal associated with discontinuation of an infusion of epidural clonidine. *Anesthesiology*. 1996; 84:729-31.
15. Hauger-Klevene JH. Treatment of clonidine rebound syndrome with sublingual captopril. *N Engl J Med*. 1986; 314:181-2.
16. Hong E, Moreno JA, Nava-Felix P. Characterization of the rebound hypertension following withdrawal of clonidine treatment. *Proc West Pharmacol Soc*. 1985; 28:23-5.
17. Kushins L. Clonidine withdrawal, propranolol, and rebound hypertension. *Anesthesiology*. 1980; 53:178-9.
18. Leckman JF, Ort S, Caruso KA et al. Rebound phenomena in Tourette's syndrome after abrupt withdrawal of clonidine. Behavioral, cardiovascular, and neurochemical effects. *Arch Gen Psychiatry*. 1986; 43:1168-76.
19. Mehta JL, Lopez LM. Rebound hypertension following abrupt cessation of clonidine and metoprolol: treatment with labetalol. *Arch Intern Med*. 1987; 147:389-90.
20. Metz S, Klein C, Morton N. Rebound hypertension after discontinuation of transdermal clonidine therapy. *Am J Med*. 1987; 82:17-9.
21. Rupp H, Maisch B, Brilla CG. Drug withdrawal and rebound hypertension: differential action of the central antihypertensive drugs moxonidine and clonidine. *Cardiovasc Drugs Ther*. 1996; 10(suppl 1):251-62.
22. Schmidt GR, Schuna AA. Rebound hypertension after discontinuation of transdermal clonidine. *Clin Pharm*. 1988; 7:772-4.
23. Stewart M, Burris JF. Rebound hypertension during initiation of transdermal clonidine. *Drug Intell Clin Pharm*. 1988; 22:573-4.
24. White TM, Guidry JR. Rebound hypertension associated with transdermal clonidine and contact dermatitis. *West J Med*. 1986; 145:104.
25. Burden AC, Alexander CP. Rebound hypertension after acute methyldopa withdrawal. *BMJ*. 1976; 1:1056-7.
26. Frewin DB, Penhall RK. Rebound hypertension after sudden discontinuation of methyldopa therapy. *Med J Aust*. 1977; 1:659.
27. Vanholder R, Carpentier J, Schurgers M et al. Rebound phenomenon during gradual withdrawal of clonidine. *BMJ*. 1977; 1:1138.
28. Avastin package insert. South San Francisco, CA: Genentech, Inc; 2008.
29. Pande A, Lombardo J, Spangenthal E et al. Hypertension secondary to anti-angiogenic therapy: experience with bevacizumab. *Anticancer Res*. 2007; 27:3465-70.
30. Rasier R, Artunay O, Yuzbasioglu E et al. The effect of intravitreal bevacizumab (Avastin) administration on systemic hypertension. *Eye*. 2009; 23:1714-8.
31. Rosiak J, Sadowski L. Hypertension associated with bevacizumab. *Clin J Oncol Nurs*. 2005; 9:407-11.

32. Zhu X, Wu S, Dahut WL et al. Risks of proteinuria and hypertension with bevacizumab, an antibody against vascular endothelial growth factor: systematic review and meta-analysis. *Am J Kidney Dis.* 2007; 49:186-93.
33. Roose SP, Dalack GW, Glassman AH et al. Cardiovascular effects of bupropion in depressed patients with heart disease. *Am J Psychiatry.* 1991; 148:512-6.
34. Wellbutrin XL package insert. Research Triangle, NC: GlaxoSmithKline; 2008.
35. Zyban package insert. Greenville, NC: GlaxoSmithKline; 2008.
36. Noordzij M, Uiterwaal CS, Arends LR et al. Blood pressure response to chronic intake of coffee and caffeine: a meta-analysis of randomized controlled trials. *J Hypertens.* 2005; 23:921-8.
37. Whelton A, Schulman G, Wallemark C et al. Effects of celecoxib and naproxen on renal function in the elderly. *Arch Intern Med.* 2000; 160:1465-70.
38. Whelton A, White WB, Bello AE et al. Effects of celecoxib and rofecoxib on blood pressure and edema in patients > or =65 years of age with systemic hypertension and osteoarthritis. *Am J Cardiol.* 2002; 90:959-63.
39. Weaver A, Alderman M, Sperling R. Blood pressure control and rates of edema following the administration of the cyclooxygenase-2 specific inhibitors celecoxib versus rofecoxib in patients with systemic hypertension and osteoarthritis. *Am J Cardiol.* 2003; 91:1291-2.
40. Celebrex package insert. New York, NY: G.D. Searle, LLC Division of Pfizer Inc; 2008.
41. Wolfe F, Zhao S, Pettitt D. Blood pressure destabilization and edema among 8538 users of celecoxib, rofecoxib, and nonselective nonsteroidal antiinflammatory drugs (NSAID) and nonusers of NSAID receiving ordinary clinical care. *J Rheumatol.* 2004; 31:1143-51.
42. Solomon SD, McMurray JJ, Pfeffer MA et al. Cardiovascular risk associated with celecoxib in a clinical trial for colorectal adenoma prevention. *N Engl J Med.* 2005; 352:1071-80.
43. Nzerue CM, Hewan-Lowe K, Riley LJ Jr. Cocaine and the kidney: a synthesis of pathophysiologic and clinical perspectives. *Am J Kidney Dis.* 2000; 35:783-95.
44. Hussain RM, McIntosh SJ, Lawson J et al. Fludrocortisone in the treatment of hypotensive disorders in the elderly. *Heart.* 1996; 76:507-9.
45. Chobanian AV, Volicer L, Tifft CP et al. Mineralocorticoid-induced hypertension in patients with orthostatic hypotension. *N Engl J Med.* 1979; 301:68-73.
46. Sherwood H, Epstein J, Maurer ML et al. Intramuscular triamcinolone acetonide for the treatment of allergic and cutaneous diseases: report of 582 patients. *Curr Ther Res Clin Exp.* 1967; 9:114-30.
47. Hari P, Bagga A, Mantan M. Short term efficacy of intravenous dexamethasone and methylprednisolone therapy in steroid resistant nephrotic syndrome. *Indian Pediatr.* 2004; 41:993-1000.
48. Ferrari P. Cortisol and the renal handling of electrolytes: role in glucocorticoid-induced hypertension and bone disease. *Best Pract Res Clin Endocrinol Metab.* 2003; 17:575-89.
49. Whitworth JA. Mechanisms of glucocorticoid-induced hypertension. *Kidney Int.* 1987; 31:1213-24.
50. Bennett WM, Porter GA. Cyclosporine-associated hypertension. *Am J Med.* 1988; 85:131-3.
51. Gengraf package insert. North Chicago, IL: Abbott Laboratories; 2006.
52. Neoral package insert. East Hanover, NJ: Novartis Pharmaceuticals Corp; 2005.
53. Sandimmune package insert. East Hanover, NJ: Novartis Pharmaceuticals Corp; 2007.
54. Vercauteren SB, Bosmans JL, Elseviers MM et al. A metaanalysis and morphological review of cyclosporine induced nephrotoxicity in auto-immune diseases. *Kidney Int.* 1998; 54:536-45.
55. Charnick SB, Nedelman JR, Chang CT et al. Description of blood pressure changes in patients beginning cyclosporin A therapy. *Ther Drug Monit.* 1997; 19:17-24.
56. Fung JJ, Todo S, Jain A et al. Conversion from cyclosporine to FK 506 in liver allograft recipients with cyclosporine-related complications. *Transplant Proc.* 1990; 22:6-12.
57. Aranesp package insert, Thousand Oaks, CA; Amgen Manufacturing, Limited; 2008.
58. Pristiq package insert. Philadelphia, PA: Wyeth Pharmaceuticals Inc; 2009.
59. Fugh-Berman A. Herb-drug interactions. *Lancet.* 2000; 355:134-8.
60. Haller CA, Benowitz NL. Adverse cardiovascular and central nervous system events associated with dietary supplements containing ephedra alkaloids. *N Engl J Med.* 2000; 343:1833-8.
61. Samenuk D, Link MS, Homoud MK et al. Adverse cardiovascular events temporally associated with ma huang, an herbal source of ephedrine. *Mayo Clin Proc.* 2002; 77:12-16.
62. Joyce DA, Gubbay SS. Arterial complications of migraine treatment with methysergide and parenteral ergotamine. *Br Med J (Clin Res Ed).* 1982; 285:260-1.
63. Epogen package insert. Thousand Oaks, CA: Amgen Manufacturing Limited; 2008.
64. Procrit package insert. Raritan, NJ: Ortho Biotech Products, L.P.; 2008.
65. Heintz B, Schmauder C, Witte K et al. Blood pressure rhythm and endocrine functions in normotensive women on oral contraceptives. *J Hypertens.* 1996; 14:333-9.
66. Chasan-Taber L, Willett WC, Manson JE et al. Prospective study of oral contraceptives and hypertension among women in the United States. *Circulation.* 1996; 94:483-9.
67. Laragh JH, Sealey JE, Ledingham JG et al. Oral contraceptives: renin, aldosterone, and high blood pressure. *JAMA.* 1967; 201:918-22.
68. Woods JW. Oral contraceptives and hypertension. *Hypertension.* 1988; 11:II11-II15.
69. Woods JW. Oral contraceptives and hypertension. *Lancet.* 1967; 2:653.
70. Kubba A, Guillebaud J, Anderson RA et al. Contraception. *Lancet.* 2000; 356:1913-19.
71. Lim KG, Isles CG, Hodsman GP et al. Malignant hypertension in women of childbearing age and its relation to the contraceptive pill. *Br Med J (Clin Res Ed).* 1987; 294:1057-59.
72. Corlanor package insert. Thousand Oaks, CA: Amgen Inc; 2015.
73. Bernardi M, D'Intino PE, Trevisani F et al. Effects of prolonged ingestion of graded doses of licorice by healthy volunteers. *Life Sci.* 1994; 55:863-72.
74. Farese RV Jr, Biglieri EG, Shackleton CH et al. Licorice induced hypermineralocorticoidism. *N Engl J Med.* 1991; 325:1223-7.
75. Walker BR, Edwards CR. Licorice-induced hypertension and syndromes of apparent mineralocorticoid excess. *Endocrinol Metab Clin North Am.* 1994; 23:359-77.
76. Fallon B, Foote B, Walsh BT et al. "Spontaneous" hypertensive episodes with monoamine oxidase inhibitors. *J Clin Psychiatry.* 1988; 49:163-5.
77. Gunn J, Hamilton MM, Boyle RM. Hypertensive crisis and broad complex bradycardia after a single dose of monoamine oxidase inhibitor. *BMJ.* 1989; 298:964.
78. Johnson AG. NSAIDs and blood pressure: clinical importance for older patients. *Drugs Aging.* 1998; 12:17-27.
79. Johnson AG, Nguyen TV, Day RO. Do nonsteroidal anti-inflammatory drugs affect blood pressure? A meta-analysis. *Ann Intern Med.* 1994; 121:289-300.
80. Gurwitz JH, Avorn J, Bohn RL et al. Initiation of antihypertensive treatment during nonsteroidal anti-inflammatory drug therapy. *JAMA.* 1994; 272:781-6.

81. MacFarlane LL, Orak DJ, Simpson WM. NSAIDs, antihypertensive agents and loss of blood pressure control. *Am Fam Physician.* 1995; 51:849-56.
82. Mene P, Pugliese F, Patrono C. The effects of nonsteroidal anti-inflammatory drugs on human hypertensive vascular disease. *Semin Nephrol.* 1995; 15:244-52.
83. US Food and Drug Administration Center for Drug Evaluation and Research. Medication Guide for Non-Steroidal Anti-Inflammatory Drugs (NSAIDs). May 2016. http://www.fda.gov/downloads/Drugs/DrugSafety/UCM387559.pdf (accessed 2017 Jan 30).
84. Lai YK. Adverse effect of intraoperative phenylephrine 10%: case report. *Br J Ophthalmol.* 1989; 73:468-9.
85. Fraunfelder FW, Fraunfelder FT, Jensvold B. Adverse systemic effects from pledgets of topical ocular phenylephrine 10%. *Am J Ophthalmol.* 2002; 134:624-5.
86. Chua SS, Benrimoj SI, Gordon RD et al. A controlled clinical trial on the cardiovascular effects of single doses of pseudoephedrine in hypertensive patients. *Br J Clin Pharmacol.* 1989; 28:369-72.
87. Rutstein HR. Ingestion of pseudoephedrine. *Arch Otolaryngol.* 1963; 77:145-7.
88. Salerno SM, Jackson JL, Berbano EP. Effect of oral pseudoephedrine on blood pressure and heart rate: a meta-analysis. *Arch Intern Med.* 2005; 165:1686-94.
89. Coates ML, Rembold CM, Farr BM. Does pseudoephedrine increase blood pressure in patients with controlled hypertension? *J Fam Pract.* 1995; 40:22-6.
90. Bradley JG, Kallail KJ, Dorsch JN et al. The effects of pseudoephedrine on blood pressure in patients with controlled, uncomplicated hypertension: a randomized, double-blind, placebo-controlled trial. *J Am Board Fam Pract.* 1991; 4:201-6.
91. Jordan J, Scholze J, Matiba B et al. Influence of sibutramine on blood pressure: evidence from placebo controlled trials. *Int J Obes (Lond).* 2005; 29:509-16.
92. Kim SH, Lee YM, Jee SH et al. Effect of sibutramine on weight loss and blood pressure: a meta-analysis of controlled trials. *Obes Res.* 2003; 11:1116-23.
93. Sharma AM, Caterson ID, Coutinho W et al. Blood pressure changes associated with sibutramine and weight management—an analysis from the 6-week lead-in period of the sibutramine cardiovascular outcomes trial (SCOUT). *Diabetes Obes Metab.* 2008.
94. Lean ME. Sibutramine—a review of clinical efficacy. *Int J Obes Relat Metab Disord.* 1997; 21(suppl 1):S30-6; discussion 37-9.
95. Meridia package insert. North Chicago, IL: Abbott Laboratories; 2007.
96. Perrio MJ, Wilton LV, Shakir SA. The safety profiles of orlistat and sibutramine: results of prescription-event monitoring studies in England. *Obesity.* 2007; 15:2712-22.
97. Nexavar package insert. Wayne, NJ: Bayer HealthCare Pharmaceuticals, Inc; 2007.
98. Wu S, Chen JJ, Kudelka A et al. Incidence and risk of hypertension with sorafenib in patients with cancer: a systematic review and meta-analysis. *Lancet Oncol.* 2008; 9:117-23.
99. Sutent package insert. New York, NY: Pfizer Labs Division of Pfizer Inc; 2008.
100. Kapiteijn E, Brand A, Kroep J et al. Sunitinib induced hypertension, thrombotic microangiopathy and reversible posterior leukencephalopathy syndrome. *Ann Oncol.* 2007; 18:1745-7.
101. Zhu X, Stergiopoulos K, Wu S. Risk of hypertension and renal dysfunction with an angiogenesis inhibitor sunitinib: systematic review and meta-analysis. *Acta Oncol.* 2009; 48:9-17.
102. Prograf package insert. Deerfield, IL: Astellas Pharma US Inc; 2008.
103. Pham SM, Kormos RL, Hattler BG et al. A prospective trial of tacrolimus (FK 506) in clinical heart transplantation: intermediate-term results. *J Thorac Cardiovasc Surg.* 1996; 111:764-72.
104. Jain A, Reyes J, Kashyap R et al. Liver transplantation under tacrolimus in infants, children, adults, and seniors: long-term results, survival, and adverse events in 1000 consecutive patients. *Transplant Proc.* 1998; 30:1403-4.
105. Androjel package insert. Marietta, GA: Solvay Pharmaceuticals, Inc; 2007.
106. Tangredi JF, Buxton IL. Hypertension as a complication of topical testosterone therapy. *Ann Pharmacother.* 2001; 35:1205-7.
107. Effexor XR package insert. Philadelphia, PA: Wyeth Pharmaceuticals Inc; 2008.
108. Thase ME. Effects of venlafaxine on blood pressure: a meta-analysis of original data from 3744 depressed patients. *J Clin Psychiatry.* 1998; 59:502-8.
109. Calhoun DA, Jones D, Textor S et al. Resistant hypertension: diagnosis, evaluation, and treatment: a scientific statement from the American Heart Association Professional Education Committee of the Council for High Blood Pressure Research. *Circulation.* 2008; 117:e510-26.
110. National Center for Health Statistics. *Health, United States, 2014: With Special Feature on Adults Aged 55–64.* Hyattsville, MD; 2015.
111. Muntner P, Carey RM, Gidding S et al. Potential US population impact of the 2017 ACC/AHA high blood pressure guideline. *Circulation.* 2018; 137:109-18.
112. Frohlich ED. Mechanisms contributing to high blood pressure. *Ann Intern Med.* 1983; 98:709-14.
113. Cheng HF, Harris RC. Cyclooxygenases, the kidney, and hypertension. *Hypertension.* 2004; 43:525-30.
114. Howard PA, Delafontaine P. Nonsteroidal anti-Inflammatory drugs and cardiovascular risk. *J Am Coll Cardiol.* 2004; 43:519-25.
115. Ribstein J, Halimi JM, du Cailar G et al. Renal characteristics and effect of angiotensin suppression in oral contraceptive users. *Hypertension.* 1999; 33:90-5.
116. Goldhaber SZ, Hennekens CH, Spark RF et al. Plasma renin substrate, renin activity, and aldosterone levels in a sample of oral contraceptive users from a community survey. *Am Heart J.* 1984; 107:119-22.
117. Cifkova R, Hallen H. Cyclosporin-induced hypertension. *J Hypertens.* 2001; 19:2283-5.
118. Effects of estrogen or estrogen/progestin regimens on heart disease risk factors in postmenopausal women. The Postmenopausal Estrogen/Progestin Interventions (PEPI) Trial. The Writing Group for the PEPI Trial. *JAMA.* 1995; 273:199-208.
119. Rossouw JE. Effect of postmenopausal hormone therapy on cardiovascular risk. *J Hypertens Suppl.* 2002; 20:S62-5.
120. Rossouw JE, Anderson GL, Prentice RL et al. Risks and benefits of estrogen plus progestin in healthy postmenopausal women: principal results from the Women's Health Initiative randomized controlled trial. *JAMA.* 2002; 288:321-33.
121. Baillargeon JP, McClish DK, Essah PA et al. Association between the current use of low-dose oral contraceptives and cardiovascular arterial disease: a meta-analysis. *J Clin Endocrinol Metab.* 2005; 90:3863-70.
122. Scuteri A, Bos AJ, Brant LJ et al. Hormone replacement therapy and longitudinal changes in blood pressure in postmenopausal women. *Ann Intern Med.* 2001; 135:229-38.
123. Ifudu O, Dawood M, Homel P. Erythropoietin-induced elevation in blood pressure is immediate and dose dependent. *Nephron.* 1998; 79:486-7.
124. Vaziri ND. Mechanism of erythropoietin-induced hypertension. *Am J Kidney Dis.* 1999; 33:821-8.
125. Cook NR, Cohen J, Hebert PR et al. Implications of small reductions in diastolic blood pressure for primary prevention. *Arch Intern Med.* 1995; 155:701-9.
126. Collins R, Peto R, MacMahon S et al. Blood pressure, stroke, and coronary heart disease. Part 2: Short-term reductions in blood pressure: overview of randomized drug trials in their epidemiological context. *Lancet.* 1990; 335:827-38.

127. MacMahon S, Peto R, Cutler J et al. Blood pressure, stroke, and coronary heart disease. Part 1: Prolonged differences in blood pressure: prospective observational studies corrected for the regression dilution bias. *Lancet.* 1990; 335:765-74.
128. Vasan RS, Larson MG, Leip EP et al. Impact of high normal blood pressure on the risk of cardiovascular disease. *N Engl J Med.* 2001; 345:1291-7.
129. Centers for Disease Control and Prevention. Chronic disease prevention and health promotion. Chronic disease overview. August 26, 2015. Available at: http://www.cdc.gov/chronicdisease/overview/#ref16 (accessed 2018 Apr 10).
130. Lewington S, Clarke R, Qizilbash N et al. Age-specific relevance of usual blood pressure to vascular mortality: a meta-analysis of individual data for one million adults in 61 prospective studies. *Lancet.* 2002; 360:1903-13.
131. Rosendorff C, Black HR, Cannon CP et al. Treatment of hypertension in the prevention and management of ischemic heart disease: a scientific statement from the American Heart Association Council for High Blood Pressure Research and the Councils on Clinical Cardiology and Epidemiology and Prevention. *Circulation.* 2007; 115:2761-88.
132. Effects of treatment on morbidity in hypertension: results in patients with diastolic blood pressures averaging 115 through 129 mm Hg. *JAMA.* 1967; 202:1028-34.
133. Dahlof B, Lindholm LH, Hansson L et al. Morbidity and mortality in the Swedish Trial in Old Patients with Hypertension (STOP-Hypertension). *Lancet.* 1991; 338:1281-5.
134. MRC Working Party. Medical Research Council trial of treatment of hypertension in older adults: principal results. *BMJ.* 1992; 304:405-12.
135. SHEP Cooperative Research Group. Prevention of stroke by antihypertensive drug treatment in older persons with isolated systolic hypertension: final results of the Systolic Hypertension in the Elderly Program (SHEP). *JAMA.* 1991; 265:3255-64.
136. Staessen JA, Fagard R, Thijs L et al. Randomised doubleblind comparison of placebo and active treatment for older patients with isolated systolic hypertension. The Systolic Hypertension in Europe (Syst-Eur) Trial Investigators. *Lancet.* 1997; 350:757-64.
137. Beckett NS, Peters R, Fletcher AE et al. Treatment of hypertension in patients 80 years of age or older. *N Engl J Med.* 2008; 358:1887-98.
138. Pickering TG, Hall JE, Appel LJ et al. Recommendations for blood pressure measurement in humans and experimental animals. Part 1: blood pressure measurement in humans: a statement for professionals from the Subcommittee of Professional and Public Education of the American Heart Association Council on High Blood Pressure Research. *Circulation.* 2005; 111:697-716.
139. Pickering TG, Miller NH, Ogedegbe G et al. Call to action on use and reimbursement for home blood pressure monitoring: executive summary: a joint scientific statement from the American Heart Association, American Society of Hypertension, and Preventive Cardiovascular Nurses Association. *Hypertension.* 2008; 52:1-9.
140. Pickering TG, White WB. ASH Position Paper: Home and ambulatory blood pressure monitoring: when and how to use self (home) and ambulatory blood pressure monitoring. *J Clin Hypertens (Greenwich).* 2008; 10:850-5.
141. Lichtenstein AH, Appel LJ, Brands M et al. Diet and lifestyle recommendations revision 2006: a scientific statement from the American Heart Association Nutrition Committee. *Circulation.* 2006; 114:82-96.
142. Appel LJ, Brands MW, Daniels SR et al. Dietary approaches to prevent and treat hypertension: a scientific statement from the American Heart Association. *Hypertension.* 2006; 47:296-308.
143. Cush JJ, Tugwell P, Weinblatt M et al. US consensus guidelines for the use of cyclosporin A in rheumatoid arthritis. *J Rheumatol.* 1999; 26:1176-86.
144. ACOG practice bulletin. No. 73: Use of hormonal contraception in women with coexisting medical conditions. *Obstet Gynecol.* 2006; 107:1453-72.
145. Luft FC. Erythropoietin and arterial hypertension. *Clin Nephrol.* 2000; 53:S61-4.

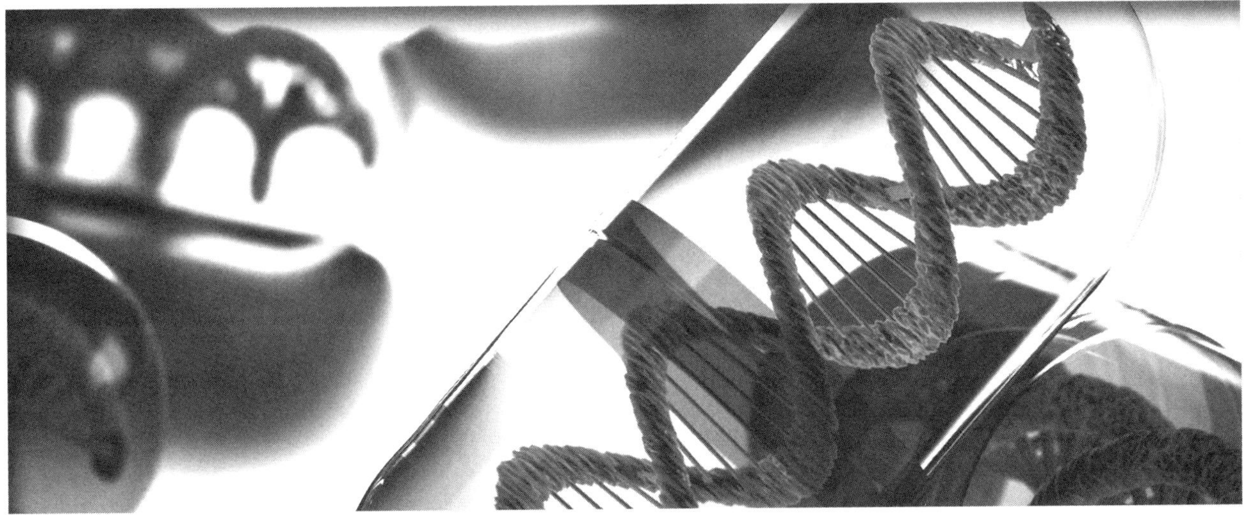

CHAPTER 28

Hypotension

Katy E. Trinkley and Robert L. Page II

Drug-induced hypotension is a clinically important and potentially disabling problem, which can lead to syncope, falls and injury, or sustained lack of organ perfusion resulting in ischemia, infarction, or both. These hypotension-related complications can be the result of either chronic hypotension, acute hypotension in the institutionalized setting, or orthostatic hypotension. Chronic hypotension describes the situation when the blood pressure is consistently low, regardless of posture, whereas orthostatic hypotension describes a decline in blood pressure upon assuming an upright position. The majority of drug-induced hypotension episodes are the result of orthostatic hypotension, also referred to as postural hypotension. Orthostatic hypotension is a reduction in systolic blood pressure of at least 20 mm Hg or a reduction in diastolic pressure of at least 10 mm Hg within 3 minutes of standing or during a head-up tilt test of at least 60 degrees.[1-4]

Drug-induced orthostatic hypotension is primarily due to autonomic failure in which the causative agent affects central or peripheral autonomic pathways.[5] However, orthostatic hypotension can also result from neurally mediated syncope.[5] Autonomic failure involves chronic debilitation of sympathetic efferent activity such that vasoconstriction is impeded. Upon standing, blood pressure precipitously falls and presyncope or syncope develops. In neurally mediated orthostatic hypotension, the typical pattern of autonomic outflow that preserves blood pressure in the standing position is acutely reversed in response to a trigger.

CAUSATIVE AGENTS

Drugs that cause hypotension can be separated into two groups: those for which hypotension is an extension of the drug's therapeutic effect (e.g., antihypertensives) and those for which hypotension is not an extension of the drug's therapeutic effect. Examples of drugs that may cause orthostatic hypotension include phenothiazines, tricyclic antidepressants, anxiolytics, and levodopa/carbidopa. **Table 28-1** lists drugs that have been reported to cause hypotension and their respective incidences.[6-248]

EPIDEMIOLOGY

Drug-induced chronic hypotension is less common than drug-induced orthostatic hypotension,

Table 28-1 Agents Implicated in Drug-Induced Hypotension

Drug	Incidence	Level of Evidence[a]
ANTIHYPERTENSIVES		
ACE INHIBITORS[b,c,d]		
Benazepril[6]	0.3–0.4%	A
Captopril[7,8]	3.6%	A
Enalapril (particularly with IV administration)[9]	0.9–6.7%	A
Fosinopril[10]	2.4–4.4%	A
Lisinopril[11]	Up to 11%	A
Moexipril[12]	0.5%	A
Perindopril[13]	0.3–0.8%	A
Ramipril[14]	2–11%	A
Quinapril[15]	2.9%	A
Trandolapril[16]	0.6–11%	A
ANGIOTENSIN-RECEPTOR BLOCKERS[b,c,d]		
Azilsartan[17]	0.4%	A
Candesartan[18]	18.8%	A
Eprosartan[19]	<1%	A
Irbesartan[20]	0.1–5.4%	A
Losartan[21,22]	0.5–7%	A
Olmesartan[23]	0.1%	A
Telmisartan[19]	<1%	B
Valsartan[24,25]	6.9%	A
PERIPHERAL α-BLOCKERS[c,d]		
Alfuzosin[26]	0.4–2%	A
Doxazosin[27,28]	0.3–10%	A
Prazosin[29,30]	1–4%	A
Tamsulosin[31]	0.2–0.4%	A
Terazosin[32,33]	1.3–7%	A
β-ADRENERGIC BLOCKERS (PARTICULARLY WITH IV ADMINISTRATION)		
Acebutolol[34,35]	2%	B
Atenolol[36,c]	4–25%	A
Betaxolol[37,c]	<2%	A
Bisoprolol[38]	Up to 12%	A
Carvedilol (particularly immediate-release)[39,b]	2–20%	A
Esmolol[40,41]	20–50%	A
Propranolol[42,43]	NK	A
Labetalol[44,45]	Oral 1%, IV 5%	A
Metoprolol (particularly immediate-release)[46,b]	27.4%	A
Nadolol[47]	1%	A
Pindolol[48,49]	2%	A
Nebivolol[50]	0.5%	A
CALCIUM-CHANNEL BLOCKERS		
Amlodipine[51,c]	<1%	A

Table 28-1 Agents Implicated in Drug-Induced Hypotension (continued)

Drug	Incidence	Level of Evidence[a]
Diltiazem (particularly with IV administration)[52,53]	6–11%	A
Felodipine[54]	0.5–1.5%	A
Isradipine[55]	NK	C
Nicardipine (particularly with IV administration)[56]	0.9–5.6%	A
Nifedipine (particularly immediate-release)[57]	0.5–5%	A
Nimodipine[58,59]	Up to 8.1%	A
Nisoldipine[60]	<1%	A
Verapamil (particularly with IV administration)[61,62]	1–3%	B
CENTRALLY ACTING α-ADRENERGIC AGONISTS[c]		
Clonidine (lowest with patch, highest with IV administration)[63]	Up to 44.8%	A
Guanfacine[64,65]	15%	A
Guanabenz[66,67]	<1%	A
Methyldopa[68]	NK	B
Reserpine[69,70]	16%	A
PERIPHERAL-ACTING ARTERIAL VASODILATORS		
Diazoxide[71,72]	NK	B
Hydralazine (particularly with IV administration)[71-76]	NK	B
Minoxidil[77,78]	NK	B
Nitroglycerin[406-408]	4%	A
Nitroprusside[79]	NK	B
DIURETICS[b,c]		
Amiloride[80,81]	<1%	B
Bumetanide[82]	0.8%	A
Chlorothiazide[83]	NK	B
Chlorthalidone[84]	2.2%	A
Ethacrynic acid[85]	NK	B
Furosemide[86,87]	20%	A
Hydrochlorothiazide[87,88]	12.5–60%	A
Indapamide[89]	<5%	A
Metolazone[90,91]	NK	B
Torsemide[92,93]	0–7%	A
DOPAMINE AGONISTS		
Fenoldopam[94,95,c,e]	2–18.5%	A
RENIN INHIBITORS		
Aliskiren[96]	0.1%	A
NONANTIHYPERTENSIVES		
ANGIOTENSIN-RECEPTOR NEPRILYSIN INHIBITOR		
Sacubitril/Valsartan[409]	18%	A
ALZHEIMER DISEASE AGENTS		
Galantamine[97,98,c,d]	1–3.6%	A
Donepezil[99,100,c,d]	1–3%	A

Table 28-1 Agents Implicated in Drug-Induced Hypotension (continued)

Drug	Incidence	Level of Evidence[a]
ANESTHETIC AGENTS		
Bupivacaine[101,102,c]	NK	B
Halothane[103,104,c]	NK	B
Isoflurane[105,106,c]	NK	B
Propofol[107,108,c]	3–10%	A
ANTIANGINAL AGENTS		
Amyl nitrate[109,110]	NK	C
Isosorbide dinitrate[111,112]	16%	A
Isosorbide mononitrate[113]	<5%	A
Nitroglycerin[114,115,c,d]	1–48%	A
ANTIARRHYTHMIC AGENTS		
Amiodarone (IV only)[116,117]	10–20%	A
Bretylium[118,119,e]	50%	A
Ibutilide[120,121]	2%	A
Mexiletine[122,f]	<1%	C
Procainamide (IV only)[123,124]	NK	C
Quinidine[125,126,d,e,f]	NK	C
Sotalol[127,128]	5–9%	A
Tocainide[129]	3%	A
Vernakalant[130,131,e]	5–6%	A
ANTIDIABETIC AGENTS		
Dapagliflozin[410]	0.6–0.8%	A
ANTIDEPRESSANTS		
Amitriptyline[132,133,c,f]	5–20%	A
Clomipramine[134,c,f]	4–6%	B
Doxepin[135,136,c]	3–4%	B
Desipramine[133,137-139,c,f]	Up to 15%	A
Imipramine[133,139-144,c,f]	20–37%	A
Trazodone[145,c]	3.8–7%	B
ANTIEMETICS		
Droperidol[146,d]	NK	B
Prochlorperazine[147,148,d]	1.2%	B
Promethazine[149,e]	NK	B
ANTIEPILEPTIC DRUGS		
Phenytoin (IV only)[150,151]	4.9%	A
Fosphenytoin (IV only)[152,d,e]	7.7%	A
ANTIHISTAMINIC AGENTS		
Diphenhydramine[153,f]	NK	C
ANTIMICROBIAL AGENTS		
Pentamidine (IV and IM only)[154,155]	1.7–5%	B

Table 28-1 Agents Implicated in Drug-Induced Hypotension (continued)

Drug	Incidence	Level of Evidence[a]
Levofloxacin (IV only)[156,e]	NK	C
Vancomycin (IV only)[157,158,e]	0–63%	A
ANTIPARKINSONIAN AGENTS		
Bromocriptine[159,160,c,d]	0.2–0.7%	A
Carbidopa plus levodopa[161,162,c,d]	1%	A
Pergolide[163,c]	2.1%	A
Pramipexole[164,165,c]	<5%	A
Ropinirole[166,167,c]	2–25%	A
Selegiline[168,c]	9.8%	A
Rasagiline[169,c]	7–44%	A
Entacapone[170,c]	1.2%	A
Tolcapone[171,c]	13–14%	A
ANTIPSYCHOTIC AGENTS		
Aripiprazole[172,173,c]	0.2–4%	A
Aripiprazole lauroxil[411]	0.2–0.5%	A
Brexpiprazole[412]	0.1–0.4%	A
Chlorpromazine (particularly IV)[413,c]	0–10%	A
Clozapine[174,175,c,d]	9–13%	A
Haloperidol[176,177,c]	0–2%	A
Loxapine[178,179,c,d]	0.4–3%	A
Lurasidone[180]	0.3–2.1%	A
Olanzapine[181,c]	2%	A
Quetiapine[182,183,c]	Up to 7%	A
Pimozide[184-186,c]	NK	C
Risperidone[187-189,c]	Oral 1–2%, IM: <4%	A
Thioridazine[190,191,c]	16%	A
Thiothixene[178,192]	4%	A
Trifluoperazine[176]	NK	C
Ziprasidone[176,193,194,c,d]	1.3–18%	A
β-ADRENERGIC AGONISTS		
High-dose dobutamine[195-197,d]	20%	A
BIOLOGIC AGENTS		
Interleukin-2[198,d]	71%	A
Muromonab-CD3[199,200]	25%	A
Defibrotide[414]	37%	A
CHEMOPROTECTANT AGENTS		
Amifostine[201-203,d,e]	3–62%	A
CANCER CHEMOTHERAPY AGENTS		
Cabozantinib[415]	7%	A
Carmustine[204,205,d]	NK	B

Table 28-1 Agents Implicated in Drug-Induced Hypotension (continued)

Drug	Incidence	Level of Evidence[a]
Dinutuximab[416]	60%	A
Dacarbazine[206,d]	NK	B
Etoposide[207,208,e]	1–2%	A
Fludarabine[209,210]	1–2%	A
Vinblastine[211,c]	NK	B
Vincristine[212,213,c,d]	4%	A
ENDOTHELIN MODIFIERS		
Bosentan[214]	7%	A
Treprostinil[215]	4%	A
Magnesium[216,217,d]	4%	A
NATRIURETIC PEPTIDES		
Nesiritide[218-220,d,e]	4–17%	A
NEUROMUSCULAR BLOCKING AGENTS		
Atracurium[221,d]	NK	A
Mivacurium[221,222,d,e]	NK	A
Succinylcholine[223]	NK	A
d-tubocurare[224]	NK	C
OPIATES		
Codeine (particularly with IV administration)[225-227,d]	NK	C
Fentanyl (particularly with IV administration)[228,229,e]	2.8–4%	A
Hydromorphone[230,231,e]	IV 20%, oral <2%	A
Morphine (particularly with IV administration)[232-234,e]	NK	A
OSMOTIC DIURETICS		
Mannitol[235,236,c,d]	NK	C
PHOSPHODIESTERASE INHIBITORS		
Milrinone[237]	2.9%	A
Vardenafil[238,239]	<2%	A
Sildenafil[240,241]	<2%	A
Tadalafil[242]	2%	A
PROSTAGLANDINS		
Epoprostenol[243-245,d,e]	13–16%	A
Iloprost[246-248]	11–76%	A
SOLUBLE GUANYLATE CYCLASE STIMULATORS		
Riociguat[417]	10%	A

ACE = angiotensin-converting enzyme, IM = intramuscular, IV = intravenous, NK = not known.

[a]Definitions for Levels of Evidence: Level A—evidence from one or more randomized, controlled clinical trials; Level B—evidence from nonrandomized clinical trials, prospective observational studies, cohort studies, retrospective studies, case-control studies, meta-analyses and/or postmarketing surveillance studies; and Level C—evidence from one or more published case reports or case series.

[b]Higher incidence in patients with heart failure.

[c]May also cause orthostatic hypotension.

[d]Dose-related.

[e]Administration rate-related.

[f]In overdose.

because causes of drug-induced chronic hypotension, such as over-intensive antihypertensive therapy, are generally more easily correctable. As a result, the prevalence of drug-induced chronic hypotension is unknown. Orthostatic hypotension from all causes has been estimated to occur in 0.5% of individuals in the general population, with older adults and acutely ill patients at greater risk. Approximately 5% of individuals under 50 years of age experience orthostatic hypotension, which increases to a prevalence of 30% in individuals over 70 years of age.[3] In acute care settings, 17% of patients experience orthostatic hypotension,[5] while the prevalence of orthostatic hypotension among patients presenting with syncope to the emergency department ranges from 21–64%.[249,250]

MECHANISMS

Mean arterial pressure is determined by heart rate, stroke volume, and total peripheral resistance. When a person changes from a supine to an upright position, orthostatic hypotension results from a profound and immediate shift of blood volume primarily to the lower extremities. Within 10–15 minutes of a posture change, stroke volume may decline by 15%, and roughly 1 L of blood may pool in capacitance vessels below the diaphragm.[251,252] The resultant reduction in venous return and decreases in cardiac output and blood pressure stimulate arterial baroreceptors, which trigger intricate compensatory mechanisms. Centrally mediated activation of sympathetic efferent neurons increases vascular tone, myocardial contractility, and heart rate. Cardiopulmonary volume receptors cause vasopressin release, which also leads to arteriolar vasoconstriction and water conservation by the kidney. All of these reflex mechanisms limit the potentially adverse hemodynamic effects of an upright posture; however, should any one or a combination of these mechanisms fail, orthostatic hypotension may result.[253]

Orthostatic hypotension can be the direct result of chronic autonomic failure from neurodegenerative conditions such as Parkinson disease, or it can be secondary to conditions such as diabetes, which is associated with higher-risk neurological conditions.[3] Conditions or situations that impair diastolic filling such as blood loss, dehydration, and excessive diuresis may also lead to orthostatic hypotension. One example is splanchnic blood pooling that occurs after eating, which can lead to a decrease in blood pressure.[254]

In healthy patients of any age, orthostatic hypotension occurs infrequently. However, as patients age, changes in cardiovascular physiology, concomitant diseases, and exposure to medications that may reduce blood pressure increase the risk of orthostatic hypotension. Physiologic changes that may contribute to orthostatic hypotension include alterations in baroreceptor activity, parasympathetic activity, arterial and cardiac compliance, renal sodium conservation, vasopressin response, plasma renin activity, plasma angiotensin and aldosterone concentrations, and plasma volume.[255]

The administration of drugs that interfere with the cardiovascular reflex response can unmask or exacerbate orthostatic hypotension. For example, antihypertensive agents may produce hypotension by decreasing sympathetic outflow through central and peripheral vasodilatory actions or by depleting intravascular volume. There are many drugs that cause direct vasodilation resulting in drug-induced hypotension. Drugs can induce hypotension through many different mechanisms (**Table 28-2**).[5,34,36-40,43,49-51,69,70,74-78,94,98,109,110,114-117,124,150-153,195-197,212-214,219-221,232,233,235,236,243,246-248,256-296]

CLINICAL PRESENTATION AND DIFFERENTIAL DIAGNOSIS

Orthostatic hypotension may manifest with symptoms as mild as light-headedness or as severe as presyncope or syncope (**Table 28-3**).[3,253,297,298] Although presyncope is less severe than syncope, it may be a part of a continuum that leads to syncope, which is a sudden loss of consciousness and postural tone usually lasting no more than 15 seconds.[297] The "common faint," or neurocardiogenic syncope (also called vasovagal syncope), is most common, in which the triggering of a neural reflex results in a usually self-limited episode of systemic hypotension characterized by both bradycardia and peripheral

Table 28-2 Mechanisms of Drug-Induced Hypotension

Drug	Mechanism
Benazepril Captopril Enalapril Fosinopril Lisinopril Moexipril Perindopril Ramipril Quinapril Trandolapril	Inhibition of angiotensin II with increase in bradykinin concentrations[256]
Aliskiren	Inhibition of renin[256]
Candesartan Eprosartan Irbesartan Losartan Olmesartan Telmisartan Valsartan	Inhibition of angiotensin II at the receptor level[257]
Acebutolol Atenolol Betaxolol Bisoprolol Esmolol Propranolol Metoprolol Nadolol Pindolol Nebivolol	Blockade of β-adrenoreceptors[34,36-38,40,43,49,50]
Carvedilol Labetalol	Blockade of β- and α_1-adrenoreceptors[39,258]
Amiloride Bumetanide Chlorothiazide Chlorthalidone Ethacrynate Furosemide Hydrochlorothiazide Indapamide Metolazone Torsemide	Inhibition of renal sodium reabsorption thereby leading to intravascular volume depletion[259-261]
Mannitol	Intravascular volume depletion[235,236]
Atracurium Codeine d-tubocurare Hydromorphone Fentanyl Mivacurium Morphine Succinylcholine Vancomycin	Release of histamine[221,232,233,262-265]

Table 28-2 Mechanisms of Drug-Induced Hypotension (continued)

Drug	Mechanism
Alfuzosin Aripiprazole Chlorpromazine Clozapine Doxazosin Haloperidol Loxapine Lurasidone Olanzapine Pimozide Prazosin Quetiapine Risperidone Tamsulosin Terazosin Thioridazine Thiothixene Trifluoperazine Ziprasidone	Blockade of central and/or peripheral[5,266,267] α-adrenoreceptors[5,266,267]
Dobutamine, high-dose	The following mechanisms may be responsible[195-197]: • Inadequate increase in cardiac output due to impaired systolic reserve • Marked prolongation of isovolumic relaxation time due to induced myocardial ischemia • Marked isolated reduction in systemic vascular resistance • Decrease in cardiac output associated with cavity obliteration and reflex bradycardia
Clonidine Guanfacine Guanabenz Methyldopa	Direct stimulation of α-receptors in the vasomotor center of the medulla leading to[268]: • Reduction in peripheral vascular resistance • Decreased heart rate (secondary to increased vagal tone)
Reserpine	Depletion of catecholamine and 5-hydroxytryptophan in the central nervous system resulting in[69,70]: • Decreased peripheral resistance • Reduced cardiac output
Chlorpromazine Prochlorperazine Promethazine	• Calmodulin-mediated inhibition of phosphodiesterase • Relaxation of vascular smooth muscle[5]
Amitriptyline Clomipramine Desipramine Doxepin Imipramine Trazodone	Reduced systemic vascular resistance due to α-adrenoreceptor blockade[269,270]
Amlodipine Diltiazem Felodipine Isradipine Nicardipine Nifedipine Nimodipine Nisoldipine Verapamil	Blockade of L-type calcium channel[51,271]

Table 28-2 Mechanisms of Drug-Induced Hypotension (continued)

Drug	Mechanism
Pentamidine, intravenous	Vasomotor reaction[153]
Interleukin-2	Increased capillary permeability; decreased peripheral vascular resistance[273]
Amifostine Diazoxide Epoprostenol Hydralazine Iloprost Minoxidil	Direct arteriolar vasodilation[74-78,243,246-248,274,275]
Nitroprusside	Director arteriolar and venous vasodilation[79]
Bosentan Treprostinil	Inhibition of endothelin-1[214,276,277]
Milrinone	Inhibition of phosphodiesterase type III[278,279]
Nesiritide	Stimulates guanylate cyclase-linked natriuretic peptide A/B receptors[220]
Diphenhydramine	Inhibition of fast sodium channels Inhibition of potassium channels in overdose[280]
Dacarbazine	Calcium chelation by citric acid in the preparation[281]
Carmustine	Vasodilation due to alcohol content of the diluent[282,283]
Vincristine	Neurotoxicity Inhibition of norepinephrine secretion[212,213]
Vinblastine	Neurotoxicity[211]
Magnesium	Opposition of calcium-dependent arterial constriction[284] Improves endothelial function
Amiodarone Etoposide	Vasoactive solvents in the intravenous formulation[117,285]
Amyl nitrate Isosorbide dinitrate Isosorbide mononitrate Nitroglycerin	Increase intracellular cyclic guanosine monophosphate concentrations[109,110,114-116,219,286-288]
Procainamide, intravenous	Ganglionic blockade Central nervous system sympathetic inhibition[124]
Vardenafil Sildenafil Tadalafil	Inhibition of vascular phosphodiesterase type V[289]
Phenytoin Fosphenytoin	Vasodilation from the propylene glycol content (phenytoin only); unknown for fosphenytoin[150-152,290,291]
Bromocriptine Carbidopa–levodopa Entacapone Pergolide Pramipexole Rasagiline Ropinirole Selegiline Tolcapone	Increased dopamine, which exerts hypotension through the following:[292-295] Systemic, mesenteric, and renal vasodilation mediated by dopamine receptors Displacement of norepinephrine from nerve terminals Decreased renin and aldosterone secretion Reduction in sympathetic outflow
Fenoldopam	Systemic, mesenteric, and renal vasodilation mediated by dopamine receptor activation[94]
Donepezil Galantamine	Overactivation of muscarinic and nicotinic sites of autonomic and somatic nerves[98]
Propofol[180]	Direct vasodilation of venous smooth muscle[296]
Fludarabine Levofloxacin	Unknown

Table 28-3 Signs and Symptoms Associated with Drug-Induced Hypotension

Most common

- Decline in systolic blood pressure ≥20 mm Hg or diastolic blood pressure ≥10 mm Hg within 1–3 minutes of standing, or during head-up tilt test of ≥60 degrees
- Lightheadedness
- Presyncope
- Syncope
- Blurry vision
- Weakness
- Buckling of legs
- Cognitive slowing
- Headache
- Neck pain
- Chest pain (in patients with underlying coronary artery disease)
- Seizure or clonic jerks (due to cerebral hypoxia)
- Dizziness
- Tachycardia
- Postprandial angina pectoris

vasodilation.[250,253] If syncope occurs as a result of neurocardiogenic syncope, hypoperfusion-related symptoms typically resolve immediately when supine.[298] The syncope associated with orthostatic hypotension is generally differentiated from other causes such as seizures by a lack of postictal confusion or drowsiness. Symptoms of syncope are most commonly documented in the morning, after medication administration or following meals. Focal neurologic findings, if present, may suggest concomitant cerebrovascular disease.[277] Although there is not a clear rationale for each, common signs and symptoms associated with orthostatic hypotension include mild anemia, hypohidrosis, a Parkinsonian-like syndrome, recurrent urinary tract infection, bladder dysfunction, sleep apnea, hoarseness, nasal stuffiness, impotence, constipation, or diarrhea.[253] Anemia is believed to be due to decreased erythropoietin release related to reduced β_2 adrenoceptor stimulation, while bladder dysfunction or urinary tract infections may lead to dehydration and ultimately orthostatic hypotension, which could also be related to an underlying neurogenic condition.[299]

Given that only 2% of elderly patients with orthostatic hypotension are symptomatic, proactive screening is important to identify those who may remain undiagnosed, in view of the fact that orthostatic hypotension increases morbidity and mortality.[3,300] A detailed medication history, including a review of prescription and nonprescription medications and supplements, a medical history, a thorough physical exam, and in some cases, specific diagnostic tests should be used to rule out other possible causes of hypotension. Conditions to consider in the differential diagnosis of drug-induced hypotension are presented in **Table 28-4**.[3,254,255,280,297,298] To evaluate a patient for possible orthostatic hypotension, blood pressure and heart rate should be measured at three different times: after the patient has rested in the supine position for 5 minutes, immediately after the patient stands, and 1–2 minutes after standing. If the heart rate does not increase in the presence of orthostatic hypotension, then baroreceptor reflex dysfunction may be implicated. Heart rate responses to deep breathing and to the Valsalva maneuver may also aid in differentiating between autonomic impairment and other causes of orthostatic hypotension. As the time of day, ingestion of medications, and food consumption can influence orthostatic hypotension, the use of an ambulatory blood pressure monitor and a patient's corresponding log or diary of events may be necessary. Early morning measurements, especially after a high-carbohydrate meal, are helpful to identify symptoms from postprandial hypotension that may be contributing to drug-induced orthostatic hypotension. In the absence of an ambulatory blood pressure monitor, patients should be instructed to keep a detailed log with times and measurements of their blood pressure before breakfast, after taking their medications, after meals, and before bedtime.[255]

RISK FACTORS

Risk factors for drug-induced hypotension are presented in **Table 28-5**.[255] As mentioned previously, elderly patients are at increased risk for drug-induced orthostatic hypotension. The risk of orthostatic hypotension associated with some drugs may increase based on specific patient and drug characteristics. Patients at highest risk of amifostine-induced hypotension are those who

Table 28-4 Conditions to Consider in the Differential Diagnosis of Drug-Induced Hypotension[3,254,255,280,297,298]

Autonomic neuropathies

- Primary
  - Bradbury–Eggleston syndrome
  - Shy–Drager syndrome
  - Riley–Day syndrome
  - Dopamine-β-hydroxylase deficiency
  - Parkinson disease
  - Lewy body dementia
  - Idiopathic
- Secondary
  - Diabetes mellitus
  - Uremia
  - Guillain–Barré syndrome
  - Amyloidosis
  - Porphyria
  - Kidney disease
  - β_1-receptor polymorphisms
  - Spinal cord injury

Endocrine disorders

- Pheochromocytoma
- Hypoaldosteronism
- Renal vascular hypertension

Hypovolemic disorders

- Anemia
- Decreased plasma volume
- Hemorrhage
- Anorexia nervosa
- Diarrhea
- Overdialysis
- Overdiuresis

Transient neurogenic syncope

- Micturition syncope
- Carotid sinus syncope
- Vasovagal syncope
- Bezold–Jarisch reflex activation
- Glossopharyngeal neuralgia

Vascular insufficiency/vasodilation

- Varicose veins
- Arteriovenous malformations
- Absent venous valves
- Carcinoid syndrome
- Cardiogenic shock
- Mastocytosis
- Hyperbradykininism

Miscellaneous

- Anaphylaxis
- Nutritional deficiencies (vitamin B_{12}, folate)
- Pregnancy
- Space flight

Table 28-5 Risk Factors for Drug-Induced Hypotension[255]

- Alcohol use
- Cardiovascular disease
- Concurrent use of more than one drug associated with hypotension
- Decreased hepatic drug metabolism
- Fever
- Hot baths/showers
- Hot weather
- Hyperventilation
- Hyponatremia, hypokalemia
- Intravascular volume depletion
- Isometric exercise
- Large meals
- Overdiuresis
- Poor hepatic blood flow
- Prolonged recumbency
- Rapid ascent to high altitude
- Standing still
- Straining to urinate or defecate
- β_1-receptor polymorphisms

receive doses in excess of 910 mg/m^2; have infusion times of 15 minutes or longer; have head and neck, esophageal, or lung cancer; have undergone neck irradiation; or have carotid artery disease or hypercalcemia.[201,218,301] Hypotension associated with intravenous opiates occurs primarily in hypovolemic patients; therefore, these agents should be avoided in patients with shock or reduced blood volumes. The risk of sildenafil-induced hypotension is greater in patients with spinal cord injuries, specifically cervical-level injuries.[302] Spinal cord injuries have not been established as a risk factor for hypotension with other phosphodiesterase type-5 inhibitors. Concurrent use of any phosphodiesterase type-5 inhibitor and nitrates should be avoided to prevent hypotension.[238,240,242,303] The frequency of orthostatic hypotension caused by tricyclic antidepressants and antipsychotic agents increases in patients with advancing age and those with overt cardiovascular disease, particularly in those with left ventricular dysfunction or autonomic disease.[5,304,305]

Patients receiving angiotensin-converting enzyme (ACE) inhibitors are at risk for hypotension if they are receiving high doses of diuretics, have a low serum sodium concentration (<130 mEq/L), have a serum creatinine concentration

>1.7 mg/dL or have cardiovascular disease.[11,256,306] Hypotension associated with β-adrenergic-receptor blocking agents is more likely in patients with pretreatment systolic blood pressure <90 mm Hg, heart rate <60 beats/min, depressed left ventricular ejection fraction, or changes in fluid status.[307,308] The risk of hypotension associated with diuretics is increased in patients with generalized disability, dehydration, intravascular volume depletion, or concomitant use of vasodilating agents such as nitrates, alcohol, barbiturates, or narcotics.[309]

Genomic factors may also play a role in the development of orthostatic hypotension. Although results are conflicting, a single-nucleotide polymorphism with a glycine to arginine switch at position 389 of the β_1-adrenergic receptor has been found to significantly lower contractile responsiveness to catecholamines, thus increasing susceptibility to orthostatic hypotension.[280,310-312]

MORBIDITY AND MORTALITY

Drug-induced orthostatic hypotension may lead to falls, myocardial infarction, transient ischemic attack, stroke, and organ damage and may be particularly hazardous in the elderly population. Othostatic hypotension results in increased healthcare utilization, with an estimated 233 persons per 100,000 hospitalized for orthostatic hypotension and an average length of stay of 3 days.[313] Fifty percent of admissions due to an injury from a fall result in a discharge to a nursing home.[314] Of those admitted for orthostatic hypotension, nearly 1% die while hospitalized. Orthostatic hypotension is associated with an increased risk of mortality and cardiovascular morbidity and is an independent predictor of mortality and falls in the elderly. In community-dwelling elderly who sustain a fall, 5–10% suffer a serious injury such as a fracture, head trauma, or serious laceration.[315-318] These injuries can lead to considerable long-term mortality. In the older population, 1% of falls result in a hip fracture; within 1 year, these fractures are associated with a mortality rate of 20–30%.[314,319-321] The most severe consequences of drug-induced orthostatic hypotension are cerebrovascular accident, myocardial infarction, and death.[322-325] It is unknown whether death is directly owing to orthostatic hypotension or secondary to stroke or myocardial infarction, but there appears to be a clear relationship between orthostatic hypotension and death.[322,326,327]

Table 28-6 Approaches to Help Prevent Drug-Induced Hypotension[3,254,255,298]

- Avoid concurrent use of nitrates and phosphodiesterase type-5 inhibitors
- Elevate the head of the bed to a 5–20° angle
- Encourage mild-to-moderate exercise
- Initiate therapy with the lowest possible dose, administering the first dose at bedtime, and increasing the dose slowly
- Instruct the patient to arise slowly upon waking, allowing the feet to dangle over the side of the bed for a few seconds to minutes, before rising to a completely elevated stance
- Instruct the patient to avoid consuming large meals
- Instruct the patient to avoid situations that may potentially induce orthostatic hypotension (Table 28-5)
- Instruct the patient to consume 200–250 mg of caffeine (2 cups of coffee) with a meal
- Instruct the patient to eat low-carbohydrate foods
- Instruct the patient to eat sodium-containing foods and increase water intake
- Instruct the patient to minimize alcohol intake
- Obtain an extensive medical and medication history
- Use Jobst stockings, waist-high custom-fitted elastic stockings, and knee-length elastic stockings with an abdominal binder

PREVENTION

Strategies for prevention of drug-induced orthostatic hypotension are presented in **Table 28-6**.[3,254,255,298]

PHARMACOLOGIC STRATEGIES

In patients with one or more risk factors for drug-induced hypotension, there are certain measures that can minimize the risk. The drug with the lowest risk of orthostatic hypotension should be chosen and initiated at the lowest dose possible, with slow dose titration, and ideally administered at bedtime. Furthermore, for patients with multiple comorbidities, such as automonic dysfunction, heart failure, or diabetes, who are a fall risk or have multiple risk factors, then the first dose of the potentially causative drug should be administered in a controlled setting.

In patients receiving drugs that are associated with orthostatic hypotension, the risk can be reduced with drug-specific measures. If a diuretic is to be administered concomitantly with another antihypertensive agent, administration of the two drugs should be separated as much as possible.[328] In patients who experience histamine-related hypotension associated with vancomycin or the opioid derivatives, prophylactic administration of oral or intravenous histamine-1 receptor blockers may help prevent future episodes. Methylprednisolone may be administered 1 hour before the first and second doses of thymoglobulin to prevent cytokine-mediated hypotension.[272] Doses of atracurium and mivacurium should be divided or administered over 1–2 minutes, or both, to decrease the risk of histamine-related hypotension.[262] To reduce the risk of ACE inhibitor-induced hypotension, the initial dose of these drugs should be reduced by 50% if the pretreatment systolic blood pressure is ≤100 mm Hg; however, if the pretreatment systolic blood pressure is <90 mm Hg, therapy with an ACE inhibitor should be initiated only with caution and with careful monitoring.[307,308]

Within the inpatient setting, patients may experience acute hypotension associated with the use of intravenous vasodilatory inotropes such as milrinone, direct vasodilators such as hydralazine or nicardipine or mixed arterial/venous vasodilators such as nitroprusside or nesiritide. Kidney function should be taken into account when selecting initial doses of intravenous vasodilators that are eliminated renally, such as milrinone and nitroprusside. If symptomatic hypotension develops, doses of these intravenous agents should be titrated as low as possible to restore adequate hemodynamics, or therapy should be discontinued. Invasive blood pressure monitoring with an arterial catheter should be used to assess hemodynamic parameters and adjust doses of vasoactive agents if the patient develops cardiogenic shock.

NONPHARMACOLOGIC STRATEGIES

Other strategies to minimize the risk of drug-induced hypotension include elevating the head of the patient's bed to a 5–20° angle. This helps activate the renin-angiotensin-aldosterone system and reduces nocturnal diuresis while preserving interstitial fluid in the extremities.[42] Patients should arise slowly upon waking, allowing their feet to dangle over the side of the bed for a few seconds to minutes before rising to a completely elevated position. Situations that may potentially induce orthostatic hypotension should be avoided (Table 28-5).[255] If drug-induced hypotension is exacerbated by postprandial hypotension, symptoms can be minimized by reducing alcohol intake, eating low-carbohydrate foods, and avoiding large meals. By blocking adenosine receptors, consumption of two cups of coffee (200–250 mg of caffeine) with breakfast and lunch can increase systolic pressure by about 12 mm Hg and diastolic pressure by about 6 mm Hg.[329,330] Drinking caffeinated beverages around the clock increases the risk of tolerance to the caffeine; thus, consumption of caffeinated beverages are recommended in the morning and midday only. Exercise may be helpful in patients with poor orthostatic tolerance. Mild exercise may improve symptoms with minimal effects on resting blood pressure. Postural maneuvers may also be used to increase blood pressure. Leg crossing and squatting may allow patients to increase their blood pressure by as much as 13–44 mm Hg.[254,255,280,297,298]

Compression stockings, waist-high custom-fitted elastic stockings, and knee-length elastic stockings with an abdominal binder may help decrease venous pooling of blood. In patients with no contraindications, water and foods containing sodium can be consumed liberally.[254,255,298,331] As little as 240 mL of water may exert a pressor effect, resulting in seated blood pressure increasing within 5 minutes, peaking within 35 minutes, and persisting for 60 minutes or longer.[332-334]

MANAGEMENT

When possible, contributing factors should be eliminated, and the offending medication should be identified, discontinued, and replaced with another medication with a lower risk of hypotension. Because drug-induced hypotension may be directly related to a high therapeutic dose, overdose, or administration rate, management varies depending on the precipitant medication. **Table 28-7**

Table 28-7 Medication-Specific Management for Drug-Induced Hypotension

Medication	Recommendation
ACE inhibitors[256]	Reduce or briefly discontinue diuretic and/or ACE inhibitor; restart at 50% of the dose
Amiodarone[116,335]	Reduce rate of IV infusion; may consider use of fluids or vasopressor or inotrope
Amifostine[202]	Place patient in the Trendelenburg position, discontinue amifostine, and initiate fluid infusion (saline); infusion duration >15 minutes is associated with a higher incidence of adverse effects
Antipsychotic agents[336-338]	Discontinue agent; restart at 25–50% of initial dose; in severe cases, begin fluid resuscitation or vasopressors (i.e., dopamine, epinephrine, norepinephrine)
Centrally acting α-adrenergic agonists[308,336]	Slowly decrease dose and discontinue agent; in severe cases, begin fluid resuscitation, vasopressors (i.e., epinephrine), or naloxone, or all of these
Direct-acting arterial vasodilators[309,336]	If severe, consider fluid resuscitation and/or vasopressors (i.e., dopamine)
Dopamine agonists[176,185]	Reduce dose
β-blockers[309,336]	Reduce dose of β-blocker, adjust dose of ACE inhibitor and diuretic, or both; if severe, consider fluid resuscitation and/or vasopressors (epinephrine or norepinephrine)
Epoprostenol[243,339]	Discontinue infusion and hypotension should resolve within 5 minutes; begin again at a slower rate
Etoposide[273]	If hypotension occurs, discontinue the infusion and, if necessary, administer fluids; infuse etoposide over at least 30–60 minutes
Fenoldopam[340]	Discontinue IV infusion and restart at slower rate and lower dose
Interleukin-2[273]	Use IV fluids judiciously; vasopressors such as dopamine or phenylephrine may be required
Levofloxacin[156]	Discontinue IV infusion and restart at slow rate (over 60 to 90 minutes)
Milrinone[237,341]	Consider fluid resuscitation, vasopressors (i.e., dopamine, norepinephrine, phenylephrine), or vasopressin (0.03–0.07 units/min)
Nesiritide[220]	Discontinue nesiritide and observe patient; once stabilized, restart therapy with no bolus at 30% of initial dose
Nitrates[309,336]	For IV, discontinue infusion and restart at a lower dose
Opiates[309,336]	Discontinue IV infusion and begin at a slower rate; pretreat with histamine antagonists; for severe hypotension, administer naloxone; avoid use of IV codeine
Pentamidine[154,155]	Patients should be supine and blood pressure monitored closely during and following administration until stable
Phenytoin[150-152,290,291] Fosphenytoin[150-152,290,291]	Reduce rate of IV infusion or discontinue the drug
Procainamide[124]	Reduce rate of IV infusion, lower the dose, or both
Tricyclic antidepressants[269,342]	Slowly decrease dose, then discontinue; consider alternative agent such as SSRI or nortriptyline; if severe, begin fluid resuscitation or vasopressors (i.e., dopamine, epinephrine)
Vancomycin[157,158,265,343,344]	Discontinue IV infusion and restart at slower rate; infuse over more than 1 hour; fluids, antihistamines, or corticosteroids may also be considered

ACE = angiotensin-converting enzyme, IV = intravenous, SSRI = selective serotonin reuptake inhibitor.

provides specific recommendations for managing hypotension caused by specific drugs.[116,124,150-152,154-158,176,185,202,220,237,243,256,265,269,273,290,291,308,309,335-344]

If the initial management measures listed in Table 28-7 do not sufficiently correct hypotension, then drug treatment may be considered (**Table 28-8**).[340,345-382] With one exception noted below, drug treatment has not been studied in the setting of drug-induced hypotension.

Although fludrocortisone has not been directly evaluated for the treatment of drug-induced orthostatic hypotension, it is considered a treatment of choice for orthostatic hypotension.[383,384] Fludrocortisone is a potent mineralocorticoid with minimal glucocorticoid effects. Fludrocortisone may increase blood volume by stimulating renal sodium retention and vascular sensitivity to norepinephrine and by raising peripheral vascular resistance via

Table 28-8 Drug Therapy Regimens Used to Treat Orthostatic Hypotension

Medication	Dose	Level of Evidence[a]
Atenolol[345,346]	50 mg PO daily	A
Atomoxetine[347]	18 mg PO daily	A
Clonidine[357,382,398,399]	0.4 mg PO twice daily	B
Desmopressin[348]	4 mcg IM at bedtime	B
Dihydroergotamine[349,350]	0.5–1 mg IM twice daily	A
Droxidopa[351-354]	100–600 mg PO 3 times daily	A
Ergotamine tartrate[355]	1–3 mg PO daily or twice daily	C
Ergotamine[356,357]	0.36–0.72 mg inhalation 2 or 3 times daily	A
Epoetin alpha[358-361]	25–75 units/kg sub-Q 3 times weekly	B
Fludrocortisone[362,363,b]	0.1–0.3 mg PO daily	A
Fluoxetine[364,365]	20 mg PO daily	B
Flurbiprofen[366,367]	50–200 mg PO 2–3 times daily	B
Indomethacin[368,369]	25–50 mg PO 3 times daily	B
Metoprolol[370]	50–100 mg PO twice daily	A
Midodrine[371,372,b]	2.5–10 mg PO 3 times daily	A
Paroxetine[375]	20 mg PO daily	A
Pindolol[376,377]	5 mg PO 3 times daily	B
Propranolol[340,378]	40–240 mg PO daily in 3–4 divided doses	C
Pyridostigmine[379]	60 mg PO daily	A
Yohimbine[380,381]	5 mg PO 2–3 times daily	B

IM = intramuscularly, PO = oral, sub-Q = subcutaneous.

[a]Definitions for Levels of Evidence: Level A—evidence from one or more randomized, controlled clinical trials; Level B—evidence from nonrandomized clinical trials, prospective observational studies, cohort studies, retrospective studies, case-control studies, meta-analyses and/or post-marketing surveillance studies; and Level C—evidence from one or more published case reports or case series.

[b]Preferred therapy. Other drugs listed in this table reserved for hypotension refractory to fludrocortisone or midrodine.

enhancement of catecholamine release. The initial dose is 0.1 mg orally once daily, and the dose should be titrated upward based on efficacy every 1–2 weeks to a maximum dose of 1 mg/day; total daily doses exceeding 0.3 mg daily may not provide added benefit. The full therapeutic effect may require up to 1–2 weeks. Adverse effects include hypokalemia and hypomagnesemia, which may occur within the first 2 weeks of therapy. Headache, edema, weight gain, and supine hypertension may also occur. Despite the fact that fludrocortisone is used commonly for orthostatic hypotension, limited data exist regarding its efficacy, and some studies have questioned its value as compared with placebo.[362,363,385,386] If fludrocortisone is not tolerated or does not eliminate orthostatic symptoms, midodrine can be added in place of, or as adjunctive therapy to, fludrocortisone.[1,383]

Midodrine, a prodrug of desglymidorine, is a peripherally acting α-adrenergic agonist that constricts both the arterial and venous vasculature. This was the first U.S. Food and Drug Administration (FDA)-approved agent for the treatment of orthostatic hypotension and has demonstrated efficacy in small randomized, controlled trials.[371,372,387-391] However, in view of limited postmarketing effectiveness data, in 2012 the FDA requested the manufacturer of midodrine to conduct two trials, the results of which are pending.[392] The initial dose is typically 2.5 mg two to three times daily, which may be titrated upward by 2.5 mg three times daily at weekly intervals to a maximum total daily dose of 30 mg. The drug should be administered two or three times daily, with the last dose given 4 hours before bedtime to avoid supine hypertension. Other adverse effects include piloerection, pruritus, and tingling of the scalp.

Droxidopa, a synthetic norepinephrine precursor, is the second FDA-approved drug for the treatment of orthostatic hypotension, supported by evidence from several studies.[351-354] Most studies of droxidopa are in the setting of severe orthostatic hypotension often associated with autonomic disorders, such as Parkinson disease. The initial dose of droxidopa is 100 mg three times daily, titrated by 100 mg increments to achieve effect, or a maximum total daily dose of 1,800 mg. Adverse effects are mostly limited to supine hypertension; thus, the last dose should be administered 5 hours before bedtime.[393]

Pyridostigmine is a cholinesterase inhibitor that improves autonomic neurotransmission. The initial and maintenance dose of immediate-release pyridostigmine for orthostatic hypotension is 60 mg daily. Pyridostigmine has demonstrated efficacy as monotherapy or in combination with midodrine 2.5–5 mg once daily without increasing supine hypertension.[379] Pyridostigmine has also been studied in combination with yohimbine, but synergistic effects were not demonstrated.[394] Adverse effects associated with pyridostigmine include diaphoresis, hypersalivation, nausea, emesis, and diarrhea.

The ergot alkaloids ergotamine and dihydroergotamine administered parenterally, orally as a solid dosage form or via inhalation have shown some promise in improving blood pressure or venous pooling defects.[349,350,355,356,395] Dihydroergotamine has also demonstrated improvements specifically for drug-induced orthostatic hypotension resulting from antihypertensives and psychotropics.[396,397] In patients with refractory or severe orthostatic hypotension, therapy with the central α_2-adrenergic receptor agonist clonidine, the peripheral α_2-adrenergic receptor antagonist yohimbine, or the norepinephrine transporter blocker atomoxetine may be considered.[347,357,380-382,398-400] Although clonidine is generally thought to increase the risk of orthostatic hypotension, small studies suggest it may assist in raising blood pressure in patients with hypoadrenergic orthostatic hypotension by causing pronounced vasoconstriction.[382]

For patients with orthostatic hypotension and concurrent anemia, epoetin alpha may be a therapeutic option.[299,358-361] Epoetin alpha increases blood pressure, hematocrit, blood volume, and viscosity. Epoetin is especially helpful for patients with underlying anemia. Epoetin alpha is administered at a dose of 25–75 units per kilogram subcutaneously three times weekly with oral iron. Although there is no target hematocrit for the management of orthostatic hypotension, it is not recommended to exceed the normal ranges based on sex. It can be used as monotherapy or as an adjunct to other therapies. A risk and mitigation strategy (REMS) is no longer required for epoetin alpha, but possible adverse effects include edema, nausea, vomiting, and myalgia.[401]

Other adjunctive therapies include nonsteroidal anti-inflammatory drugs (NSAIDs). However, this approach is controversial. Although the true mechanism is unknown, NSAIDs are postulated to inhibit vasodilatory prostanoids and enhance vascular sensitivity to angiotensin II, thereby increasing peripheral vascular resistance. In addition, these agents cause sodium retention, thus increasing intravascular volume. Indomethacin 50 mg orally three times daily and flurbiprofen 50–200 mg orally two to three times daily, either alone or in combination with fludrocortisone, have each been shown to relieve symptoms of orthostatic hypotension and increase blood pressure.[366-369] However, indomethacin should be avoided, when possible, because of the increased risk of confusion. Further, chronic use of all NSAIDs should be used with caution in all patients because of the risk of cardiovascular, gastrointestinal, and renal adverse effects.

Oral propranolol or pindolol may reestablish sympathetic homeostasis in patients with low plasma catecholamine concentrations and impaired baroreceptor function.[340,376-378,402] Inhibiting α-adrenergic receptors allows plasma catecholamines to exhibit predominant effects on the vasoconstrictive β-adrenergic receptors. The efficacy of using β_1 selective β-blockers remains unclear.[345,346,370,403,404]

It has also been reported that 5-hydroxytriptamine (serotonin) may play an important role in the modulation of central nervous system blood pressure and heart rate regulation; thus, fluctuations in central serotonin concentrations could play a role in the pathogenesis of neurocardiogenic vasovagal syncope. Robust data support the efficacy of paroxetine for improvement of symptoms in patients with vasovagal syncope who are unresponsive to or intolerant of traditional medications.[375] Fluoxetine has also demonstrated efficacy in treating refractory orthostatic hypotension.[364,365]

In summary, treatment of drug-induced orthostatic hypotension should begin with conservative, nonpharmacologic measures and resort to drug treatment only when necessary. With the exception of dihydroergotamine, drug treatments for drug-induced orthostatic hypotension have not been studied. However, extrapolating the body of evidence for treatment of orthostatic hypotension, fludrocortisone remains the initial choice for drug treatment for most patients with drug-induced orthostatic hypotension.

INFORMATION FOR PATIENTS

Patients susceptible to drug-induced hypotension and their care providers should be educated regarding the proper technique for measurement of blood pressure in both the supine and upright positions, acceptable blood pressure ranges, and medications that may cause hypotension.[3] Patients should be instructed that simply sitting or lying down quickly may alleviate symptoms of orthostatic hypotension. However, patients should be warned not to lie down for several hours after taking short-acting pressor agents. Patients taking antihypertensive medications should be instructed to always change their posture gradually, pausing for 10–30 seconds before arising from a seated position. If orthostatic hypotension develops in a seated position, patients should place their feet on a footrest. Several smaller meals rather than larger meals should be ingested to decrease the risk of postprandial hypotension. Patients should avoid excessive alcohol consumption, exposure to extended periods of heat, and remain well hydrated at all times. Because physical deconditioning may worsen orthostatic hypotension, healthcare providers may wish to encourage mild-to-moderate physical activity. Patient education handouts with patient-friendly information can also be useful.[405]

REFERENCES

1. Shibao C, Lipsitz LA, Biaggioni I. ASH Position Paper: evaluation and treatment of orthostatic hypotension. *J Clin Hypertens.* 2013; 15:147-53.
2. Freeman R, Wieling W, Axelrod FB et al. Consensus statement on the definition of orthostatic hypotension, neurally mediated syncope and the postural tachycardia syndrome. *Auton Neurosci.* 2011; 161:69-72.
3. Ricci F, De Caterina R, Fedorowski A. Orthostatic hypotension: epidemiology, prognosis, and treatment. *J Am Coll Cardiol.* 2015; 66:848-60.
4. Consensus statement on the definition of orthostatic hypotension, pure autonomic failure, and multiple system atrophy. *J Neurol Sci.* 1996; 144:218-9.
5. Buckley NA, Sanders P. Cardiovascular adverse effects of antipsychotic drugs. *Drug Saf.* 2000; 23:215-28.
6. Benazepril Hydrochloride package insert. Suffern, NY: Novartis Pharmaceuticals Corp; 2007.
7. Captopril package insert. Broomfield, CO: Sandoz Inc; 2003.
8. Oral captopril versus placebo among 13,634 patients with suspected acute myocardial infarction: interim report from the Chinese Cardiac Study (CCS-1). *Lancet (London, England).* 1995;345:686-7.
9. Vasotec Oral Tablets, Enalapril Maleate Oral Tablets package insert. Bridgewater, NJ: BTA Pharmaceuticals; 2008.
10. Monopril Oral Tablet, Fosinopril Sodium Oral Tablet package insert. Princeton, NJ: Bristol-Myers Squibb Company; 2008.
11. Zestril Oral Tablets, Lisinopril Oral Tablets package insert. Wilmington, DE: AstraZeneca Pharmaceuticals LP; 2014.
12. Univasc Oral Tablets, Moexipril HCl Oral Tablets package insert. Smyrna, GA: Schwarz Pharma LLC; 2010.
13. Aceon Oral Tablet, Perindopril Erbumine Oral Tablet package insert. North Chicago, IL: Abbott Laboratories; 2010.
14. Altace Oral Capsules, Ramipril Oral Capsules package insert. Bristol, TN: King Pharmaceuticals; 2010.
15. Accupril Oral Tablets, Quinapril HCl Oral Tablets package insert. Collegeville, PA: Pfizer Pharms; 2015.
16. Mavik Oral Tablets, Trandolapril Oral Tablets package insert. North Chicago, IL: Abbott Laboratories; 2012.
17. EDARBI Oral Tablets, Azilsartan Medoxomil Oral Tablets package insert. Deerfield, IL: Takeda Pharmaceuticals America Inc; 2011.
18. Atacand Oral Tablets, Candesartan Cilexetil Oral Tablets package insert. Wilmington, DE: AstraZeneca Pharmaceuticals LP; 2015.
19. Brabant SM, Bertrand M, Eyraud D et al. The hemodynamic effects of anesthetic induction in vascular surgical patients chronically treated with angiotensin II receptor antagonists. *Anesth Analg.* 1999; 89:1388-92.
20. Avapro Oral Tablets, Irbesartan Oral Tablets package insert. Bridgewater, NJ: Sanofi-Aventis US LLC; 2014.
21. Cozaar Oral Tablets, Losartan Potassium Oral Tablets package insert. Whitehouse Station, NJ: Merck Sharp and Dohme Corp; 2011.
22. Weber MA, Byyny RL, Pratt JH et al. Blood pressure effects of the angiotensin II receptor blocker, losartan. *Arch Intern Med.* 1995; 155:405-11.
23. Brunner HR. Olmesartan medoxomil: current status of its use in monotherapy. *Vasc Health Risk Manag.* 2006; 2:327-40.
24. Captopril Multicenter Research Group. A placebo-controlled trial of captopril in refractory chronic congestive heart failure. *J Am Coll Cardiol.* 1983; 2:755-63.
25. Diovan, Valsartan Capsules package insert. East Hanover, NJ: Novartis Pharmaceuticals Corporation; 2002.
26. Uroxatral Oral Extended-Release Tablets, Alfuzosin HCl Oral Extended-Release Tablets package insert. Cary, NC: Covis Pharmaceuticals Inc; 2014.
27. Young RA, Brogden RN. Doxazosin. A review of its pharmacodynamic and pharmacokinetic properties, and therapeutic efficacy in mild or moderate hypertension. *Drugs.* 1988; 35:525-41.
28. Cardura XL Oral Extended-Release Tablets, Doxazosin Mesylate Oral Extended-Release Tablets package insert. New York, NY: Roerig; 2011.

29. Moulds RJ, Jauernig RA. Mechanism of prazosin collapse. *Lancet (London, England)*. 1977; 1:200-1.
30. Minipress Oral Capsules, Prazosin HCl Oral Capsules package insert. New York, NY: Pfizer Labs; 2009.
31. Flomax Oral Capsules, Tamsulosin HCl Oral Capsules package insert. Ridgefield, CT: Boehringer Ingelheim Pharmaceuticals Inc; 2011.
32. Hytrin Oral Tablets, Terazosin HCl Oral Tablets package insert. North Chicago, IL: Abbott Laboratories; 2009.
33. Lepor H, Jones K, Williford W. The mechanism of adverse events associated with terazosin: an analysis of the Veterans Affairs Cooperative Study. *J Urol*. 2000; 163:1134-7.
34. Sectral Oral Capsules, Acebutolol HCl Oral Capsules package insert. Manati, PR: Mova Pharmaceutical; 2007.
35. Biron P, Proulx A, Lapointe L et al. Properties of acebutolol in twenty patients with cardiac arrhythmias. *Eur J Clin Pharmacol*. 1975; 8:11-4.
36. Tenormin Oral Tablets, Atenolol Oral Tablets package insert. Wilmington, DE: AstraZeneca Pharmaceuticals LP; 2008.
37. Kerlone Oral Tablets, Betaxolol HCl Oral Tablets package insert. Bridgewater, NJ: Sanofi-Aventis US LLC; 2008.
38. McGavin JK, Keating GM. Bisoprolol: a review of its use in chronic heart failure. *Drugs*. 2002; 62:2677-96.
39. Coreg Oral Tablets, Carvedilol Oral Tablets package insert. Research Triangle Park, NC: GlaxoSmithKline; 2008.
40. Brevibloc Intravenous Injection, Esmolol HCl Intravenous Injection product insert. Deerfield, IL: Baxter Healthcare Corporation; 2014.
41. Morganroth J, Horowitz LN, Anderson J et al. Comparative efficacy and tolerance of esmolol to propranolol for control of supraventricular tachyarrhythmia. *Am J Cardiol*. 1985; 56:33F-39F.
42. Zacharias FJ, Cowen KJ. Controlled trial of propranolol in hypertension. *Br Med J*. 1970; 1:471-4.
43. Fulco CS, Cymerman A, Reeves JT et al. Propranolol and the compensatory circulatory responses to orthostasis at high altitude. *Aviat Space Environ Med*. 1989; 60:1049-55.
44. Breckenridge A, Orme M, Serlin MJ, Maciver M. Labetalol in essential hypertension. *Br J Clin Pharmacol*. 1982; 13(suppl 1):37S-39S.
45. Labetalol HCl Oral Tablet package insert. Verna, Salcette Goa, India: Watson Pharma Private Limited; 2008.
46. Lopressor Oral Tablets, IV Injection; Metoprolol Tartrate Oral Tablets, IV Injection package insert. Suffren, NY: Novartis Pharmaceuticals Corporation; 2009.
47. Corgard Oral Tablets, Nadolol Oral Tablets package insert. Bristol, TN: King Pharmaceuticals Inc; 2007.
48. Gonasun LM, Langrall H. Adverse reactions to pindolol administration. *Am Heart J*. 1982; 104(2 pt 2):482-6.
49. Visken Oral Tablets, Pindolol Oral Tablets package insert. Dorval, Quebec, Canada: Novartis Pharmaceuticals Canada Inc; 2007.
50. Flather MD, Shibata MC, Coats AJ et al. Randomized trial to determine the effect of nebivolol on mortality and cardiovascular hospital admission in elderly patients with heart failure (SENIORS). *Eur Heart J*. 2005; 26:215-25.
51. Norvasc Oral Tablets, Amlodipine Besylate Oral Tablets package insert. New York, NY: Pfizer Labs; 2010.
52. Magometschnigg D, Bonelli J, Gassner A et al. Cardiovascular effects of diltiazem in healthy volunteers at rest, supine and erect, and during physical and mental stress. *Int J Clin Pharmacol Ther Toxicol*. 1981; 18:514-8.
53. Salerno DM, Dias VC, Kleiger RE et al. Efficacy and safety of intravenous diltiazem for treatment of atrial fibrillation and atrial flutter. The Diltiazem-Atrial Fibrillation/Flutter Study Group. *Am J Cardiol*. 1989; 63:1046-51.
54. Chan JC, Critchley JA, Lappe JT et al. Randomised, double-blind, parallel study of the anti-hypertensive efficacy and safety of losartan potassium compared with felodipine ER in elderly patients with mild to moderate hypertension. *J Hum Hypertens*. 1995; 9:765-71.
55. Dynacirc CR Controlled Release Oral Tablets, Isradipine Controlled Release Oral Tablets package insert. Research Triangle Park, NC: GlaxoSmithKline; 2009.
56. Cardene Premixed Intravenous Injection, Nicardipine Hydrochloride Premixed Intravenous Injection package insert. Bedminster, NJ: EKR Therapeutics; 2009.
57. PROCARDIA Oral Capsules, Nifedipine Oral Capsules package insert. New York, NY: Pfizer Labs; 2015.
58. Nimodipine Oral Capsules package insert. Detroit, MI: Caraco Pharmaceutical Laboratories Ltd; 2012.
59. NYMALIZE Oral Solution, Nimodipine Oral Solution package insert. Atlanta, GA: Arbor Pharmaceuticals Inc; 2013.
60. Friedel HA, Sorkin EM. Nisoldipine: a preliminary review of its pharmacodynamic and pharmacokinetic properties, and therapeutic efficacy in the treatment of angina pectoris, hypertension and related cardiovascular disorders. *Drugs*. 1988; 36:682-731.
61. Epstein SE, Rosing DR. Verapamil: its potential for causing serious complications in patients with hypertrophic cardiomyopathy. *Circulation*. 1981; 64:437-41.
62. Rankin AC, Rae AP, Cobbe SM. Misuse of intravenous verapamil in patients with ventricular tachycardia. *Lancet*. 1987; 2:472-4.
63. Duraclon Intravenous Injection, Clonidine Hydrochloride Intravenous Injection package insert. Newport, KY: Xanodyne Pharmaceuticals Inc; 2009.
64. Jerie P, Lasance A. Long-term efficacy and tolerance of the antihypertensive agent guanfacine. *J Clin Pharmacol Ther Toxicol*. 1984; 22:170-4.
65. Jerie P. Clinical experience with guanfacine in long-term treatment of hypertension. Part II: adverse reactions to guanfacine. *Br J Clin Pharmacol*. 1980; 10(suppl 1):157S-164S.
66. McMahon FG, Ryan JR, Jain AK et al. Guanabenz in essential hypertension. *Clin Pharmacol Ther*. 1977; 21:272-7.
67. Walker BR, Deitch MW, Schneider BE et al. Long-term therapy of hypertension with guanabenz. *Clin Ther*. 1981; 4:217-28.
68. Merki W. Erfahrungen mit alpha-methyl-dopa (Aldomet) in der hypertonie-sprechstunde-behandlung. *Schweiz Med Wochenschr*. 1966; 95:25.
69. Krämer KD, Vogt W, Ghabussi P, Hochrein H. Effects and complications of antihypertensive combined therapy with furosemid-reserpin. *Med Klin*. 1973; 68:1303-8.
70. Acevedo A, Reginato AJ, Schnell AM. Effect of intraarterial reserpine in patients suffering from Raynaud's phenomenon. *J Cardiovasc Surg (Torino)*. 1978; 19:77-84.
71. Magee LA, Cham C, Waterman EJ et al. Hydralazine for treatment of severe hypertension in pregnancy: meta-analysis. *BMJ*. 2003; 327:955-60.
72. Smith WM, Damato AN, Galluzzi NJ et al. The evaluation of antihypertensive therapy cooperative clinical trial method I double-blind control comparisonof chlorothiazide, rauwolfia serpentina, and hydralazine. *Ann Intern Med*. 1964; 61:829-46.
73. Silas JH, Ramsay LE, Freestone S. Hydralazine once daily in hypertension. *Br Med J (Clin Res Ed)*. 1982; 284:1602-4.
74. Romberg GP, Lordon RE. Hypotensive sequelae of diazoxide and hydralazine therapy. *JAMA*. 1977; 238:1025.
75. Mizroch S, Yurasek M. Hypotension and bradycardia following diazoxide and hydralazine therapy. *JAMA*. 1977; 237:2471-2.
76. Henrich WL, Cronin R, Miller PD et al. Hypotensive sequelae of diazoxide and hydralazine therapy. *JAMA*. 1977; 237:264-5.
77. Allon M, Hall WD, Macon EJ. Prolonged hypotension after initial minoxidil dose. *Arch Intern Med*. 1986; 146:2075-6.
78. Noel HC. Orthostatic hypotension occurring after discontinuation of long-term minoxidil therapy. *Nurse Pr*. 1988; 13:25, 28, 30-2.
79. Jack RD. Toxicity of sodium nitroprusside. *Br J Anaesth*. 1974; 46:952.
80. Rosenfeld JB. Comparative evaluation of the antihypertensive effect of moduretic and thiazides. *Schweiz Med Wochenschr*. 1980; 110:1498-1501.

81. Amiloride HCl Oral Tablets package insert. Spring Valley, NY: Par Pharmaceutical Inc; 2009.
82. Bumetanide Oral Tablet package insert. Princeton, NJ: Sandoz Inc; 2010.
83. Jones B, Nanra RS. Double-blind trial of antihypertensive effect of chlorothiazide in severe renal failure. *Lancet*. 1979; 2:1258-60.
84. Prevention of stroke by antihypertensive drug treatment in older persons with isolated systolic hypertension. Final results of the Systolic Hypertension in the Elderly Program (SHEP). SHEP Cooperative Research Group. *JAMA*. 1991; 265:3255-64.
85. Hilton JG, Kessler E. Toxic reactions to ethacrynic acid, a new oral diuretic. *J New Drugs*. 1964; 4:93-7.
86. Mehagnoul-Schipper DJ, Colier WN, Hoefnagels WH et al. Effects of furosemide versus captopril on postprandial and orthostatic blood pressure and on cerebral oxygenation in patients > or = 70 years of age with heart failure. *Am J Cardiol*. 2002; 90:596-600.
87. Heseltine D, Bramble MG. Loop diuretics cause less postural hypotension than thiazide diuretics in the frail elderly. *Curr Med Res Opin*. 1988; 11:232-5.
88. Vardan S, Hill NE, Mehrotra KG et al. Hemodynamic response to orthostatic stress in the elderly with systolic systemic hypertension before and after long-term thiazide therapy. *Am J Cardiol*. 1993; 71:582-6.
89. Indapamide Oral Film Coated Tablets package insert. Rockford, Il: UDL Laboratories Inc; 2010.
90. Fotiu S, Mroczek WJ, Davidov M et al. Antihypertensive efficacy of metolazone. *Clin Pharmacol Ther*. 1974; 16:318-21.
91. Dornfeld L KR, Dornfeld L, Kane RE. Metolazone in essential hypertension: the long-term clinical efficacy of a new diuretic. *Curr Ther Res Clin Exp*. 1975; 18:527-33.
92. Fowler SF, Murray KM. Torsemide: a new loop diuretic. *Am J Health-Syst Pharm*. 1995; 52:1771-80.
93. Broekhuysen J, Deger F, Douchamps J et al. Torasemide, a new potent diuretic. Double-blind comparison with furosemide. *Eur J Clin Pharmacol*. 1986; 31(suppl):29-34.
94. Munger MA, Rutherford WF, Anderson L et al. Assessment of intravenous fenoldopam mesylate in the management of severe systemic hypertension. *Crit Care Med*. 1990; 18:502-4.
95. Bednarczyk EM, White WB, Munger MA et al. Comparative acute blood pressure reduction from intravenous fenoldopam mesylate versus sodium nitroprusside in severe systemic hypertension. *Am J Cardiol*. 1989; 63:993-6.
96. Tekturna Oral Tablets, Aliskiren Oral Tablets product insert. East Hanover, NJ: Novartis Pharmaceuticals Corporation; 2014.
97. Jones RW, Soininen H, Hager K et al. A multinational, randomised, 12-week study comparing the effects of donepezil and galantamine in patients with mild to moderate Alzheimer's disease. *Int J Geriatr Psychiatry*. 2004; 19:58-67.
98. Fisher AA, Davis MW. Prolonged QT interval, syncope, and delirium with galantamine. *Ann Pharmacother*. 2008; 42:278-83.
99. Bordier P, Lanusse S, Garrigue S et al. Causes of syncope in patients with Alzheimer's disease treated with donepezil. *Drugs Aging*. 2005; 22:687-94.
100. Black S, Roman GC, Geldmacher DS et al. Efficacy and tolerability of donepezil in vascular dementia: positive results of a 24-week, multicenter, international, randomized, placebo-controlled clinical trial. *Stroke*. 2003; 34:2323-30.
101. Moore DC, Bridenbaugh LD, Bridenbaugh PO et al. Bupivacaine: a review of 2,077 cases. *JAMA*. 1970; 214:713-8.
102. Sinclair CJ, Scott DB, Edström HH. Effect of the trendelenberg position on spinal anaesthesia with hyperbaric bupivacaine. *Br J Anaesth*. 1982; 54:497-500.
103. Rao TL, Jacobs K, Salem MR et al. Deliberate hypotension and anesthetic requirements of halothane. *Anesth Analg*. 1981; 60:513-6.
104. Enderby GE. Halothane and hypotension. *Anaesthesia*. 1960; 15:25-32.
105. Lam AM, Gelb AW. Cardiovascular effects of isoflurane-induced hypotension for cerebral aneurysm surgery. *Anesth Analg*. 1983; 62:742-8.
106. Newman B, Gelb AW, Lam AM. The effect of isofluraneinduced hypotension on cerebral blood flow and cerebral metabolic rate for oxygen in humans. *Anesthesiology*. 1986; 64:307-10.
107. Cummings GC, Dixon J, Kay NH et al. Dose requirements of ICI 35,868 (propofol, "Diprivan") in a new formulation for induction of anaesthesia. *Anaesthesia*. 1984; 39:1168-71.
108. Claeys MA, Gepts E, Camu F. Haemodynamic changes during anaesthesia induced and maintained with propofol. *Br J Anaesth*. 1988; 60:3-9.
109. Ma S LJ, Ma S, Long JP. Central noradrenergic activity and the cardiovascular effects of nitroglycerin and amyl nitrate. *J Cardiovasc Pharmacol*. 1992; 20:826-36.
110. James JS. Viagra warning re "poppers" and notice re protease inhibitors. *AIDS Treat News*. 1998; 294:1.
111. Aronow WS, Chesluk HM. Evaluation of nitroglycerin in angina in patients on isosorbide dinitrate. *Circulation*. 1970; 42:61-3.
112. Häussinger G, Bachmann K. Nitrate-induced orthostatic hypotension and long-term circulatory adaptation. *Z Kardiol*. 1983; 72(suppl 3):255-8.
113. Isosorbide Mononitrate Extended-Release Oral Tablets package insert. St. Louis, MO: Ethex Corporation; 2008.
114. Ferguson JJ, Diver DJ, Boldt M et al. Significance of nitroglycerin-induced hypotension with inferior wall acute myocardial infarction. *Am J Cardiol*. 1989; 64:311-4.
115. Thadani U, Ripley TL. Side effects of using nitrates to treat heart failure and the acute coronary syndromes, unstable angina and acute myocardial infarction. *Expert Opin Drug Saf*. 2007; 6:385-96.
116. Kowey PR, Marinchak RA, Rials SJ et al. Pharmacologic and pharmacokinetic profile of class III antiarrhythmic drugs. *Am J Cardiol*. 1997; 80:16G-23G.
117. Somberg JC, Timar S, Bailin SJ et al. Lack of a hypotensive effect with rapid administration of a new aqueous formulation of intravenous amiodarone. *Am J Cardiol*. 2004; 93:576-81.
118. Alfery DD, Denlinger JK. Profound hypotension following a "test dose" of bretylium tosylate. *Anesth Analg*. 1979; 58:516-8.
119. Sanna G, Arcidiacono R. Chemical ventricular defibrillation of the human heart with bretylium tosylate. *Am J Cardiol*. 1973; 32:982-7.
120. Abi-Mansour P, Carberry PA, McCowan RJ et al. Conversion efficacy and safety of repeated doses of ibutilide in patients with atrial flutter and atrial fibrillation. Study Investigators. *Am Heart J*. 1998; 136(4 pt 1):632-42.
121. Stambler BS, Wood MA, Ellenbogen KA et al. Efficacy and safety of repeated intravenous doses of ibutilide for rapid conversion of atrial flutter or fibrillation. Ibutilide Repeat Dose Study Investigators. *Circulation*. 1996; 94:1613-21.
122. Mexiletine HCl Oral Capsules package insert. Sellersville, PA: Teva Pharmaceuticals USA; 2015.
123. Giardina EG, Heissenbuttel RH, Bigger JT. Intermittent intravenous procaine amide to treat ventricular arrhythmias: correlation of plasma concentration with effect on arrhythmia, electrocardiogram, and blood pressure. *Ann Intern Med*. 1973; 78:183-93.
124. Rea RF, Hamdan M, Schomer SJ et al. Inhibitory effects of procainamide on sympathetic nerve activity in humans. *Circ Res*. 1991; 69:501-8.
125. Maisel AS, Motulsky HJ, Insel PA. Hypotension after quinidine plus verapamil. Possible additive competition at alpha-adrenergic receptors. *N Engl J Med*. 1985; 312:167-70.
126. Kinney EL. Orthostatic hypotension due to quinidine and propranolol. *Am J Med*. 1987; 82:1276-7.
127. Gomes JA, Ip J, Santoni-Rugiu F et al. Oral d,l sotalol reduces the incidence of postoperative atrial fibrillation in coronary artery bypass surgery patients: a randomized, double-blind, placebo-controlled study. *J Am Coll Cardiol*. 1999; 34:334-9.

128. Sotalol HCl IV Injection package insert. Lake Bluff, IL: Academic Pharmaceutical Inc; 2009.

129. Bastian BC, Macfarlane PW, McLauchlan JH et al. A prospective randomized trial of tocainide in patients following myocardial infarction. *Am Heart J.* 1980; 100(6 pt 2):1017-22.

130. Cheng JW. Vernakalant in the management of atrial fibrillation. *Ann Pharmacother.* 2008;42:533-42.

131. Brinaness IV Injection Concentrated Solution, Vernakalant HCl IV Injection Concentrated Solution product insert. Middlesex, United Kingdom: Cardiome UK Limited; 2015.

132. Joubert PH, Starke DD, VanReener O et al. A comparison of the cardiovascular effects and subjective tolerability of binedaline and amitriptyline in healthy volunteers. *Eur J Clin Pharmacol.* 1985; 27:667-70.

133. Marshall JB, Forker AD. Cardiovascular effects of tricyclic antidepressant drugs: therapeutic usage, overdose, and management of complications. *Am Heart J.* 1982;103:401-14.

134. Anafranil Oral Capsules, Clomipramine HCl Oral Capsules package insert. Hazelwood, MO: Mallinckrodt Inc; 2007.

135. Roose SP, Dalack GW, Glassman AH et al. Is doxepin a safer tricyclic for the heart? *J Clin Psychiatry.* 1991; 52:338-41.

136. Pitts N. The clinical evaluation doxepin—a new psychotherapeutic agent. *Psychosomatics.* 1969; 10:164-71.

137. Nelson JC, Jatlow PI, Bock J et al. Major adverse reactions during desipramine treatment: relationship to plasma drug concentrations, concomitant antipsychotic treatment, and patient characteristics. *Arch Gen Psychiatry.* 1982; 39:1055-61.

138. Max MB, Kishore-Kumar R, Schafer SC et al. Efficacy of desipramine in painful diabetic neuropathy: a placebo-controlled trial. *Pain.* 1991; 45:3-9.

139. Pacher P, Kecskemeti V. Cardiovascular side effects of new antidepressants and antipsychotics: new drugs, old concerns? *Curr Pharm Des.* 2004; 10:2463-75.

140. Brown TC, Leversha A. Comparison of the cardiovascular toxicity of three tricyclic antidepressant drugs: imipramine, amitriptyline, and doxepin. *Clin Toxicol.* 1979; 14:253-6.

141. Glassman AH, Bigger JT Jr, Giardina EV et al. Clinical characteristics of imipramine-induced orthostatic hypotension. *Lancet.* 1979;1:468-72.

142. Glassman AH, Roose SP. Tricyclic drugs in the treatment of depression. *Med Clin North Am.* 1982; 66:1037-45.

143. Koehl GW, Wenzel JE. Severe postural hypotension due to imipramine therapy. *Pediatrics.* 1971; 47:132-4.

144. Roose SP, Glassman AH, Siris SG et al. Comparison of imipramine- and nortriptyline-induced orthostatic hypotension: a meaningful difference. *J Clin Psychopharmacol.* 1981; 1:316-9.

145. Poon IO, Braun U. High prevalence of orthostatic hypotension and its correlation with potentially causative medications among elderly veterans. *J Clin Pharm Ther.* 2005; 30:173-8.

146. Droperidol IM Injection, Droperidol IV Injection package insert. Shirley, NY: American Reagent Inc; 2009.

147. Prochlorperazine Oral Tablets package insert. Salisbury, MD: Jubilant Cadista Pharmaceuticals Inc; 2011.

148. Jones J, Sklar D, Dougherty J et al. Randomized double-blind trial of intravenous prochlorperazine for the treatment of acute headache. *JAMA.* 1989; 261:1174-6.

149. Kovak AL. Prevention and treatment of postoperative nausea and vomiting. *Drugs.* 2000; 59:213-43.

150. Binder L, Trujillo J, Parker D et al. Association of intravenous phenytoin toxicity with demographic, clinical, and dosing parameters. *Am J Emerg Med.* 1996; 14:398-401.

151. Leppik IE, Boucher BA, Wilder BJ et al. Pharmacokinetics and safety of a phenytoin prodrug given i.v. or i.m. in patients. *Neurology.* 1990; 40(3 pt 1):456-60.

152. Cerebyx IV Injection, Fosphenytoin Na IV Injection package insert. New York, NY: Pfizer Labs; 2015.

153. Thakur AC, Aslam AK, Aslam AF et al. QT interval prolongation in diphenhydramine toxicity. *Int J Cardiol.* 2005; 98:341-3.

154. Mallory DL, Parrillo JE, Bailey KR et al. Cardiovascular effects and safety of intravenous and intramuscular pentamidine isethionate. *Crit Care Med.* 1987; 15:503-5.

155. Western KA, Perera DR SM, Western KA, Perera DR, Schultz MG. Pentamidine isethionate in the treatment of Pneumocystis carinii pneumonia. *Ann Intern Med.* 1970; 73:695-702.

156. Levofloxacin package insert. Raritan, NJ: Ortho-McNeil Pharmaceuticals; 2014.

157. Garrelts JC, Peterie JD. Vancomycin and the "red man's syndrome". *N Engl J Med.* 1985; 312:245.

158. Romanelli VA, Howie MB, Myerowitz PD et al. Intraoperative and postoperative effects of vancomycin administration in cardiac surgery patients: a prospective, double-blind, randomized trial. *Crit Care Med.* 1993; 21:1124-31.

159. Franks S, Horrocks PM, Lynch SS et al. Treatment of hyperprolactinaemia with pergolide mesylate: acute effects and preliminary evaluation of long-term treatment. *Lancet.* 1981; 2:659-61.

160. Van Loon GR. Bromocriptine-induced orthostatic hypotension. *Clin Invest Med.* 1979; 2:131-4.

161. Carbidopa-Levodopa package insert. Whitehouse Station, NJ: Merck and Co; 2002.

162. Irwin RP, Nutt JG, Woodward WR, Gancher ST. Pharmacodynamics of the hypotensive effect of levodopa in parkinsonian patients. *Clin Neuropharmacol.* 1992; 15:365-74.

163. Permax Oral Tablets, Pergolide Oral Tablets package insert. Costa Mesa, CA: Valeant Pharmaceuticals International; 2006.

164. Hubble JP, Koller WC, Cutler NR et al. Pramipexole in patients with early Parkinson's disease. *Clin Neuropharmacol.* 1995; 18:338-47.

165. Pramipexole package insert. Ridgefield, CT: Boehringer Ingelheim; 2007.

166. Requip Oral Tablets, Ropinirole Oral Tablets package insert. Research Triangle Park, NC: GlaxoSmithKline; 2014.

167. Requip XL Oral Extended-Release Tablets, Ropinirole Oral Extended-Release Tablets package insert. Research Triangle Park, NC: GlaxoSmithKline; 2014.

168. Emsam Transdermal Patch, Selegiline Transdermal Patch package insert. Basking Ridge, NJ: Mylan Specialty LP; 2012.

169. Azilect Oral Tablets, Rasagiline Mesylate Oral Tablets package insert. North Wales, PA: Teva Pharmaceuticals; 2014.

170. Comtan Oral Tablets, Entacapone Oral Tablets package insert. East Hanover, NJ: Novartis Pharmaceuticals Corporation; 2014.

171. Tasmar Oral Tablets, Tolcapone Oral Tablets package insert. Bridgewater, NJ: Valeant Pharmaceuticals North America LLC; 2013.

172. Abilify Discmelt Oral Disintegrating Tablet, Aripiprazole Oral Disintegrating Tablet package insert. Rockville, MD: Otsuka Pharmaceutical Co Ltd; 2013.

173. Abilify Maintena IM Injection Extended-Release Suspension, Aripiprazole IM Injection Extended-Release Suspension package insert. Rockville, MD: Otsuka America Pharmaceutical Inc; 2014.

174. Versacloz Oral Suspension, Clozapine Oral Suspension package insert. Palo Alto, CA: Jazz Pharmaceuticals Inc; 2013.

175. Fazaclo Orally Disintegrating Tablets, Clozapine, USP Orally Disintegrating Tablets package insert. Philadelphia, PA: Azur Pharma Inc; 2010.

176. Stanniland C, Taylor D. Tolerability of atypical antipsychotics. *Drug Saf.* 2000; 22:195-214.

177. Arvanitis LA, Miller BG. Multiple fixed doses of "Seroquel" (quetiapine) in patients with acute exacerbation of schizophrenia: a comparison with haloperidol and placebo. The Seroquel Trial 13 Study Group. *Biol Psychiatry.* 1997; 42:233-46.

178. Vianna Filho U, Versiani Caldeira V, Romildo Bueno J. The efficacy and safety of loxapine succinate in the treatment of

schizophrenia: a comparative study with thiothixene. *Curr Ther Res Clin Exp*. 1975; 18:476-90.

179. Adasuve Oral Inhalation Powder, Loxapine Oral Inhalation Powder package insert. Mountain View, CA: Alexza Pharmaceuticals Inc; 2012.
180. LATUDA Oral Tablets, Lurasidone HCl Oral Tablets. package insert. Marlborough, MA: Sunovion Pharmaceuticals Inc; 2013.
181. Zyprexa Oral Tablets, IM Injection, Olanzapine Oral Tablets, IM Injection package insert. Indianapolis, IN: Eli Lilly and Company; 2010.
182. Seroquel XR Oral Extended-Release Tablets, Quetiapine Fumarate Oral Extended-Release Tablets package insert. Wilmington, DE: Pharmaceuticals LP; 2013.
183. Seroquel Oral Tablets, Quetiapine Fumarate Oral Tablets package insert. Wilmington, DE: AstraZeneca Pharmaceuticals LP; 2013.
184. Kopera H. Anticholinergic and blood pressure effects of mianserin, amitriptyline and placebo. *Br J Clin Pharmacol*. 1978; 5 (suppl 1):29S-34S.
185. Mackin P. Cardiac side effects of psychiatric drugs. *Hum Psychopharmacol*. 2008; 23 (suppl 1):3-14.
186. Pinder RM, Brogden RN, Swayer R et al. Pimozide: a review of its pharmacological properties and therapeutic uses in psychiatry. *Drugs*. 1976; 12:1-40.
187. Risperdal Consta IM Injection, Risperidone IM Injection package insert. Titusville, NJ: Janssen Ortho LLC; 2010.
188. Risperdal Oral Tablets, Oral Solution, Risperidone Oral Tablets, Oral Solution package insert. Titusville, NJ: Janssen Pharmaceuticals Inc; 2012.
189. Risperdal M-Tab Oral Disintegrating Tablets, Risperidone Oral Disintegrating Tablets package insert. Titusville, NJ: Janssen Pharmaceuticals Inc; 2012.
190. Hindmarch I, Tiplady B. A comparison of the psychometric effects of remoxipride with those of haloperidol, thioridazine, and lorazepam in healthy volunteers. *Hum Psychopharmacol Clin Exp*. 1994; 9:43-9.
191. Swift CG, Lee DR, Maskrey VL et al. Single dose pharmacodynamics of thioridazine and remoxipride in healthy younger and older volunteer. *J Psychopharmacol*. 1999; 13:159-65.
192. Morales Belda FJ, De Haro T. Clinical trial with thiothixene parenteral in agitated schizophrenic patients. *Curr Ther Res Clin Exp*. 1969; 11:599-602.
193. Miceli JJ, Wilner KD, Hansen RA et al. Single-and multiple-dose pharmacokinetics of ziprasidone under non-fasting conditions in healthy male volunteers. *Br J Clin Pharmacol*. 2000; 49 (suppl 1):5S-13S.
194. Daniel DG, Zimbroff DL, Potkin SG et al. Ziprasidone 80 mg/day and 160 mg/day in the acute exacerbation of schizophrenia and schizoaffective disorder: a 6-week placebo-controlled trial. Ziprasidone Study Group. *Neuropsychopharmacology*. 1999; 20:491-505.
195. Wang CH, Cherng WJ, Hung MJ. Dobutamine-induced hypotension is an independent predictor for mortality in patients with left ventricular dysfunction following myocardial infarction. *Int J Cardiol*. 1999; 68:297-302.
196. Tanimoto M, Pai RG, Jintapakorn W et al. Mechanisms of hypotension during dobutamine stress echocardiography in patients with coronary artery disease. *Am J Cardiol*. 1995; 76:26-30.
197. Marcovitz PA, Bach DS, Mathias W et al. Paradoxic hypotension during dobutamine stress echocardiography: clinical and diagnostic implications. *J Am Coll Cardiol*. 1993; 21:1080-6.
198. Proleukin IV Injection, Aldesleukin IV Injection package insert. San Diego, CA: Prometheus Laboratories Inc; 2011.
199. Orthoclone OKT 3 IV Injection, Muromonab-CD3 IV Injection package insert. Raritan, NJ: Ortho Biotech Products LP; 2004.
200. Norman DJ, Chatenoud L, Cohen D et al. Consensus statement regarding OKT3-induced cytokine-release syndrome and human antimouse antibodies. *Transpl Proc*. 1993; 25(2 suppl 1): 89-92.
201. Glover D, Grabelsky S, Fox K et al. Clinical trials of WR-2721 and cis-platinum. *Int J Radiat Oncol Biol Phys*. 1989; 16:1201-4.
202. Ethyol IV Injection, Amifostine IV Injection package insert. Bedford, OH: MedImmune Pharma BV; 2008.
203. Budd GT, Ganapathi R, Bauer L et al. Phase I study of WR-2721 and carboplatin. *Eur J Cancer*. 1993; 29A:1122-7.
204. Henner WD, Peters WP, Eder JP et al. Pharmacokinetics and immediate effects of high-dose carmustine in man. *Cancer Treat Rep*. 1986; 70:877-80.
205. Jones AL, O'Brien ME, Lorentzos A et al. A randomised phase II study of carmustine alone or in combination with tumour necrosis factor in patients with advanced melanoma. *Cancer Chemother Pharmacol*. 1992; 30:73-6.
206. Cocconi G, Bella M, Calabresi F et al. Treatment of metastatic malignant melanoma with dacarbazine plus tamoxifen. *N Engl J Med*. 1992; 327:516-23.
207. Rozencweig M, Von Hoff DD, Henney JE et al. VM 26 and VP 16-213: a comparative analysis. *Cancer*. 1977; 40:334-42.
208. Cohen MH, Broder LE, Fossieck BE et al. Phase II clinical trial of weekly administration of VP-16-213 in small cell bronchogenic carcinoma. *Cancer Treat Rep*. 1977; 61:489-90.
209. Byrd JC, Peterson BL, Morrison VA et al. Randomized phase 2 study of fludarabine with concurrent versus sequential treatment with rituximab in symptomatic, untreated patients with B-cell chronic lymphocytic leukemia: results from Cancer and Leukemia Group B 9712 (CALGB 9712). *Blood*. 2003; 101:6-14.
210. Byrd JC, Rai K, Peterson BL et al. Addition of rituximab to fludarabine may prolong progression-free survival and overall survival in patients with previously untreated chronic lymphocytic leukemia: an updated retrospective comparative analysis of CALGB 9712 and CALGB 9011. *Blood*. 2005; 105:49-53.
211. Young JA, Howell SB, Green MR. Pharmacokinetics and toxicity of 5-day continuous infusion of vinblastine. *Cancer Chemother Pharmacol*. 1984; 12:43-5.
212. Carmichael SM, Eagleton L, Ayers CR et al. Orthostatic hypotension during vincristine therapy. *Arch Intern Med*. 1970; 126:290-3.
213. DiBella NJ. Vincristine-induced orthostatic hypotension: a prospective clinical study. *Cancer Treat Rep*. 1980; 64:359-6.
214. Tracleer Oral Tablets, Bosentan Oral Tablets package insert. South San Francisco, CA: Actelion Pharmaceuticals US Inc; 2009.
215. Remodulin Injection, Treprostinil Injection package insert. Research Triangle Park, NC: United Therapeutics Corp; 2010.
216. Magnesium in Coronaries trial investigators. Early administration of intravenous magnesium to high-risk patients with acute myocardial infarction in the Magnesium in Coronaries (MAGIC) Trial: a randomised controlled trial. *Lancet*. 2002; 360:1189-96.
217. Bourgeois FJ, Thiagarajah S, Harbert GM Jr et al. Profound hypotension complicating magnesium therapy. *Am J Obs Gynecol*. 1986; 154:919-20.
218. Turrisi AT, Glover DJ, Hurwitz S et al. Final report of the phase I trial of single-dose WR-2721 [S-2-(3-aminopropylamino)ethylphosphorothioic acid]. *Cancer Treat Rep*. 1986; 70:1389-93.
219. El-Sayed YY, Riley ET, Holbrook RH Jr et al. Randomized comparison of intravenous nitroglycerin and magnesium sulfate for treatment of preterm labor. *Obs Gynecol*. 1999; 93:79-83.
220. Colucci WS, Elkayam U, Horton DP et al. Intravenous nesiritide, a natriuretic peptide, in the treatment of decompensated congestive heart failure. *N Engl J Med*. 2000; 343:246-53.
221. Naguib M, Samarkandi AH, Bakhamees HS et al. Histamine-release haemodynamic changes produced by rocuronium, vecuronium, mivacurium, atracurium and tubocurarine. *Br J Anaesth*. 1995; 75:588-92.
222. Ali HH, Savarese JJ, Embree PB et al. Clinical pharmacology of mivacurium chloride (BW B1090U) infusion: comparison with vecuronium and atracurium. *Br J Anaesth*. 1988; 61:541-6.

223. Williams CH, Deutsch S, Linde HW et al. Effects of intravenously administered succinyldicholine on cardiac rate, rhythm, and arterial blood pressure in anesthetized man. *Anesthesiology*. 1961; 22:947-54.

224. Murray MJ, Cowen J, DeBlock H et al. Clinical practice guidelines for sustained neuromuscular blockade in the adult critically ill patient. *Crit Care Med*. 2002; 30:142-56.

225. Parke TJ, Nandi PR, Bird KJ et al. Profound hypotension following intravenous codeine phosphate: three case reports and some recommendations. *Anaesthesia*. 1992; 47:852-4.

226. Cox RG. Hypoxaemia and hypotension after intravenous codeine phosphate. *Can J Anaesth*. 1994; 41:1211-3.

227. Shanahan EC, Marshall AG, Garrett CP. Adverse reactions to intravenous codeine phosphate in children: a report of three cases. *Anaesthesia*. 1983; 38:40-3.

228. Joshi GP, Warner DS, Twersky RS et al. A comparison of the remifentanil and fentanyl adverse effect profile in a multicenter phase IV study. *J Clin Anesth*. 2002; 14:494-9.

229. Twersky RS, Jamerson B, Warner DS et al. Hemodynamics and emergence profile of remifentanil versus fentanyl prospectively compared in a large population of surgical patients. *J Clin Anesth*. 2001; 13:407-16.

230. Sarhill N, Walsh D, Nelson KA. Hydromorphone: pharmacology and clinical applications in cancer patients. *Support Care Cancer*. 2001; 9:84-96.

231. Exalgo Oral Extended-Release Tablets, Hydromorphone HCl Oral Extended-Release Tablets package insert. Hazelwood, MO: Mallinckrodt Brand Pharmaceuticals Inc; 2014.

232. Fahmy NR, Sunder N, Soter NA. Role of histamine in the hemodynamic and plasma catecholamine responses to morphine. *Clin Pharmacol Ther*. 1983; 33:615-20.

233. Lowenstein E, Hallowell P, Levine FH et al. Cardiovascular response to large doses of intravenous morphine in man. *N Engl J Med*. 1969; 281:1389-93.

234. Mildh LH, Tuomisto LM, Scheinin M et al. Morphine-induced cardiovascular stimulation: the effects of two doses on healthy subjects. *Anesth Analg*. 2000; 91:51-7.

235. James JW, Evans RA. Use of oral mannitol in the oedematous patient. *Br Med J*. 1970; 1:463-5.

236. Domaingue CM, Nye DH. Hypotensive effect of mannitol administered rapidly. *Anaesth Intens Care*. 1985; 13:134-6.

237. Primacor Injection, Milrinone Lactate Injection package insert. Bridgewater, NJ: Sanofi-Aventis US LLC; 2007.

238. Levitra Oral Tablets, Vardenafil Oral Tablets package insert. Research Triangle Park, NC: GlaxoSmithKline; 2015.

239. Kloner RA. Cardiovascular effects of the 3 phosphodiesterase-5 inhibitors approved for the treatment of erectile dysfunction. *Circulation*. 2004; 110:3149-55.

240. Revatio Oral Tablets, IV Injection, Sildenafil Oral Tablets, IV Injection package insert. New York, NY: Pfizer Labs; 2010.

241. Zusman RM, Morales A, Glasser DB et al. Overall cardiovascular profile of sildenafil citrate. *Am J Cardiol*. 1999; 83:35C-44C.

242. CIALIS Oral Tablets, Tadalafil Oral Tablets package insert. Indianapolis, IN: Lilly USA LLC; 2011.

243. Flolan IV Injection Powder, Epoprostenol Sodium IV Injection Powder package insert. Research Triangle Park, NC: GlaxoSmithKline; 2011.

244. Veletri IV Powder for Injection, Epoprostenol IV Powder for Injection package insert. South San Francisco, CA: Actelion Pharmaceuticals US Inc; 2011.

245. Paramothayan NS, Lasserson TJ, Wells AU et al. Prostacyclin for pulmonary hypertension. *Cochrane Database Syst Rev*. 2003; (2) CD002994.

246. Upward JW, Strong HA, George CF et al. Hypotension in response to iloprost, a prostacyclin analogue. *Br J Clin Pharmacol*. 1986; 21:241-3.

247. Swedberg K, Held P, Wadenvik H, Kutti J. Central haemodynamic and antiplatelet effects of iloprost—a new prostacyclin analogue—in acute myocardial infarction in man. *Eur Heart J*. 1987; 8:362-8.

248. Ylitalo P, Kaukinen S, Reinikainen P et al. A randomized, double-blind, crossover comparison of iloprost with dextran in patients with peripheral arterial occlusive disease. *Int J Clin Pharmacol Ther Toxicol*. 1990; 28:197-204.

249. Gorelik O, Fishlev G, Litvinov V et al. First morning standing up may be risky in acutely ill older inpatients. *Blood Press*. 2005; 14:139-43.

250. Sarasin FP, Louis-Simonet M, Carballo D et al. Prevalence of orthostatic hypotension among patients presenting with syncope in the ED. *Am J Emerg Med*. 2002; 20:497-501.

251. Jacob G, Ertl AC, Shannon JR et al. Effect of standing on neurohumoral responses and plasma volume in healthy subjects. *J Appl Physiol*. 1998; 84:914-21.

252. Youmans JB, Wells HS, Donley D et al. The effect of posture (standing) on the reum protein concentration and colloid osmotic pressure of blood from the foot in relation to the formation of edema. *Clin Invest*. 1934; 13:447-59.

253. Medow MS, Stewart JM, Sanyal S et al. Pathophysiology, diagnosis, and treatment of orthostatic hypotension and vasovagal syncope. *Cardiol Rev*. 2008; 16:4-20.

254. Naschitz JE, Rosner I. Orthostatic hypotension: framework of the syndrome. *Postgrad Med J*. 2007; 83:568-74.

255. Gupta V, Lipsitz LA. Orthostatic hypotension in the elderly: diagnosis and treatment. *Am J Med*. 2007; 120:841-7.

256. ASHP therapeutic guidelines on angiotensin-converting-enzyme inhibitors in patients with left ventricular dysfunction. This official ASHP practice standard was developed through the ASHP Commission on Therapeutics and approved by the ASHP Board of Directo. *Am J Health-Syst Pharm*. 1997; 54:299-313.

257. Ellis ML, Patterson JH. A new class of antihypertensive therapy: angiotensin II receptor antagonists. *Pharmacotherapy*. 1996; 16:849-60.

258. Labetalol HCl Intravenous Injection package insert. Paramus, NJ: Mayne Pharma (USA) Inc; 2004.

259. Kleyman TR, Cragoe EJ Jr. Amiloride and its analogs as tools in the study of ion transport. *J Membr Biol*. 1988; 105:1-21.

260. Kleyman TR, Cragoe EJ Jr. The mechanism of action of amiloride. *Semin Nephrol*. 1988; 8:242-8.

261. Wilcox CS. Metabolic and adverse effects of diuretics. *Semin Nephrol*. 1999; 19:557-68.

262. Fisher D. Clinical pharmacology of neuromuscular blocking agents. *Am J Health-Syst Pharm*. 1999; 56(11 suppl 1):S4-9.

263. Rosow CE, Moss J, Philbin DM et al. Histamine release during morphine and fentanyl anesthesia. *Anesthesiology*. 1982; 56:93-6.

264. Orebaugh SL. Succinylcholine: adverse effects and alternatives in emergency medicine. *Am J Emerg Med*. 1999; 17:715-21.

265. Renz CL, Thurn JD, Finn HA et al. Oral antihistamines reduce the side effects from rapid vancomycin infusion. *Anesth Analg*. 1998; 87:681-5.

266. de Mey C. Cardiovascular effects of alpha-blockers for the treatment of symptomatic BPH. *Eur Urol*. 1998; 34(suppl 2):18-28; discussion 47.

267. Drici M-D, Priori S. Cardiovascular risks of atypical antipsychotic drug treatment. *Pharmacoepidemiol Drug Saf*. 2007; 16:882-90.

268. Leary WP, Asmal AC, Williams PC. Evaluation of the efficacy and safety of guanabenz versus clonidine. *S Afr Med J*. 1979; 55:83-5.

269. Thanacoody HK, Thomas SH. Tricyclic antidepressant poisoning: cardiovascular toxicity. *Toxicol Rev*. 2005; 24:205-14.

270. Spivak B, Radvan M, Shine M. Postural hypotension with syncope possibly precipitated by trazodone. *Am J Psychiatry*. 1987; 144:1512-3.

271. Henneman A, Thornby KA. Risk of hypotension with concomitant use of calcium-channel blockers and macrolide antibiotics. *Am J Health-Syst Pharm*. 2012; 69:1038-43.

272. Lindenfeld J, Miller GG, Shakar SF et al. Drug therapy in the heart transplant recipient: part I: cardiac rejection and immunosuppressive drugs. *Circulation*. 2004; 110:3734-40.
273. Perry MC. *The chemotherapy source book*. 3rd ed. Baltimore, MD: Williams and Wilkins; 2001.
274. Santini G, Coser P, Congiu AM et al. VACOP-B, high-dose cyclophosphamide and high-dose therapy with peripheral blood progenitor cell rescue for aggressive non-Hodgkin's lymphoma with bone marrow involvement: a study by the non-Hodgkin's Lymphoma Co-operative Study Group. *Haematologica*. 2000; 85:160-6.
275. Bryan RK, Hoobler SW, Rosenzweig J et al. Effect of minoxidil on blood pressure and hemodynamics in severe hypertension. *Am J Cardiol*. 1977; 39:796-801.
276. Kaufmann H. Treatment of patients with orthostatic hypotension and syncope. *Clin Neuropharmacol*. 2002; 25:133-41.
277. Freeman R. Neurogenic orthostatic hypotension. *N Engl J Med*. 2008; 358:615-24.
278. Gold JA, Cullinane S, Chen J et al. Vasopressin as an alternative to norepinephrine in the treatment of milrinone-induced hypotension. *Crit Care Med*. 2000; 28:249-52.
279. Gold J, Cullinane S, Chen J et al. Vasopressin in the treatment of milrinone-induced hypotension in severe heart failure. *Am J Cardiol*. 2000; 85:506-8, A11.
280. Márquez MF, Hernández-Pacheco G, Hermosillo AG et al. The Arg389Gly beta1-adrenergic receptor gene polymorphism and susceptibility to faint during head-up tilt test. *Europace*. 2007; 9:585-8.
281. Buesa JM, Gracia M, Valle M et al. Phase I trial of intermittent high-dose dacarbazine. *Cancer Treat Rep*. 1984; 68:499-504.
282. Kanj SS, Sharara AI, Shpall EJ et al. Myocardial ischemia associated with high-dose carmustine infusion. *Cancer*. 1991; 68:1910-2.
283. Weiss RB, Issell BF. The nitrosoureas: carmustine (BCNU) and lomustine (CCNU). *Cancer Treat Rev*. 1982; 9:313-30.
284. Frohlich EP. Profound hypotension complicating magnesium therapy. *Am J Obstet Gynecol*. 1987; 157:513.
285. Siderov J, Prasad P, De Boer R et al. Safe administration of etoposide phosphate after hypersensitivity reaction to intravenous etoposide. *Br J Cancer*. 2002; 86:12-3.
286. Publication Committee for the VMAC Investigators (Vasodilation in the Management of Acute CHF). Intravenous nesiritide vs nitroglycerin for treatment of decompensated congestive heart failure: a randomized controlled trial. *JAMA*. 2002; 287:1531-40.
287. Alpert JS. Nitrate therapy in the elderly. *Am J Cardiol*. 1990; 65:23J-27J.
288. Kelly JG, O'Malley K. Nitrates in the elderly: pharmacological considerations. *Drugs Aging*. 1992; 2:14-9.
289. Brant WO, Bella AJ, Lue TF. Treatment options for erectile dysfunction. *Endocrinol Metab Clin North Am*. 2007; 36:465-79.
290. Cranford RE, Leppik IE, Patrick B et al. Intravenous phenytoin: clinical and pharmacokinetic aspects. *Neurology*. 1978; 28(9 pt 1):874-80.
291. Durelli L, Mutani R, Sechi GP et al. Cardiac side effects of phenytoin and carbamazepine. A dose-related phenomenon? *Arch Neurol*. 1985; 42:1067-8.
292. Johns DW, Ayers CR, Carey RM. The dopamine agonist bromocriptine induces hypotension by venous and arteriolar dilation. *J Cardiovasc Pharmacol*. 1984; 6:582-7.
293. Kujawa K, Leurgans S, Raman R et al. Acute orthostatic hypotension when starting dopamine agonists in Parkinson's disease. *Arch Neurol*. 2000; 57:1461-3.
294. Bhattacharya KF, Nouri S, Olanow CW et al. Selegiline in the treatment of Parkinson's disease: its impact on orthostatic hypotension. *Parkinsonism Relat Disord*. 2003; 9:221-4.
295. Kaakkola S. Clinical pharmacology, therapeutic use and potential of COMT inhibitors in Parkinson's disease. *Drugs*. 2000; 59:1233-50.
296. Muzi M, Berens RA, Kampine JP et al. Venodilation contributes to propofol-mediated hypotension in humans. *Anesth Analg*. 1992; 74:877-83.
297. Strickberger SA, Benson DW, Biaggioni I et al. AHA/ACCF Scientific Statement on the evaluation of syncope: from the American Heart Association Councils on Clinical Cardiology, Cardiovascular Nursing, Cardiovascular Disease in the Young, and Stroke, and the Quality of Care and Outcomes Research Interdisciplinary Working Group; and the American College of Cardiology Foundation: in collaboration with the Heart Rhythm Society: endorsed by the American Autonomic Society. *Circulation*. 2006; 113:316-27.
298. Tan MP, Parry SW. Vasovagal syncope in the older patient. *J Am Coll Cardiol*. 2008; 51:599-606.
299. Biaggioni I, Robertson D, Krantz S et al. The anemia of primary autonomic failure and its reversal with recombinant erythropoietin. *Ann Intern Med*. 1994; 121:181-6.
300. Rutan GH, Hermanson B, Bild DE et al. Orthostatic hypotension in older adults. The Cardiovascular Health Study. CHS Collaborative Research Group. *Hypertension*. 1992; 19(6 pt 1):508-19.
301. Glover D, Fox KR, Weiler C et al. Clinical trials of WR-2721 prior to alkylating agent chemotherapy and radiotherapy. *Pharmacol Ther*. 1988; 39:3-7.
302. Ethans KD, Casey AR, Schryvers OI et al. The effects of sildenafil on the cardiovascular response in men with spinal cord injury at or above the sixth thoracic level. *J Spinal Cord Med*. 2003; 26:222-6.
303. Stendra Oral Tablets, Avanafil Oral Tablets package insert. Mountain View, CA: VIVUS Inc; 2014.
304. Glassman AH. Cardiovascular effects of antidepressant drugs: updated. *Int Clin Psychopharmacol*. 1998; 13(suppl 5):S25-30.
305. Glassman AH, Preud'homme XA. Review of the cardiovascular effects of heterocyclic antidepressants. *J Clin Psychiatry*. 1993; 54(suppl):16-22.
306. Benazepril Hydrochloride package insert. Suffren, NY: Novartis Pharmaceuticals Corp; 2007.
307. Executive Summary: HFSA 2006 Comprehensive Heart Failure Practice Guideline. *J Card Fail*. 2006; 12:10-38.
308. Hunt SA. ACC/AHA 2005 guideline update for the diagnosis and management of chronic heart failure in the adult: a report of the American College of Cardiology/American Heart Association Task Force on Practice Guidelines (Writing Committee to Update the 2001 Guidelines). *J Am Coll Cardiol*. 2005; 46:e1-82.
309. Schoenberger JA. Drug-induced orthostatic hypotension. *Drug Saf*. 1991; 6:402-7.
310. Gao Y, Lin Y, Sun K et al. Orthostatic blood pressure dysregulation and polymorphisms of β-adrenergic receptor genes in hypertensive patients. *J Clin Hypertens (Greenwich)*. 2014; 16:207-13.
311. Sorrentino S, Forleo C, Iacoviello M et al. Lack of association between genetic polymorphisms affecting sympathetic activity and tilt-induced vasovagal syncope. *Auton Neurosci*. 2010; 155:98-103.
312. Zelazowska M, Lelonek M, Fendler W et al. Arg389Gly β_1-adrenergic receptor polymorphism and susceptibility to syncope during tilt test. *Arch Med Sci*. 2014; 10:240-5.
313. Shibao C, Grijalva CG, Raj SR et al. Orthostatic hypotension-related hospitalizations in the United States. *Am J Med*. 2007; 120:975-80.
314. Sattin RW, Lambert Huber DA, DeVito CA et al. The incidence of fall injury events among the elderly in a defined population. *Am J Epidemiol*. 1990; 131:1028-37.
315. Ricci F, Fedorowski A, Radico F et al. Cardiovascular morbidity and mortality related to orthostatic hypotension: a meta-analysis of prospective observational studies. *Eur Heart J*. 2015; 36:1609-17.
316. Luukinen H, Koski K, Laippala P et al. Prognosis of diastolic and systolic orthostatic hypotension in older persons. *Arch Intern Med*. 1999; 159:273-80.
317. Gangavati A, Hajjar I, Quach L et al. Hypertension, orthostatic hypotension, and the risk of falls in a community-dwelling elderly population: the maintenance of balance, independent living, intellect, and zest in the elderly of Boston study. *J Am Geriatr Soc*. 2011; 59:383-9.

318. Ooi WL, Hossain M, Lipsitz LA. The association between orthostatic hypotension and recurrent falls in nursing home residents. *Am J Med.* 2000; 108:106-11.
319. Magaziner J, Simonsick EM, Kashner TM et al. Predictors of functional recovery one year following hospital discharge for hip fracture: a prospective study. *J Gerontol.* 1990; 45:M101-7.
320. Nevitt MC, Cummings SR, Hudes ES. Risk factors for injurious falls: a prospective study. *J Gerontol.* 1991; 46:M164-70.
321. Tinetti ME, Doucette J, Claus E et al. Risk factors for serious injury during falls by older persons in the community. *J Am Geriatr Soc.* 1995; 43:1214-21.
322. Eigenbrodt ML, Rose KM, Couper DJ et al. Orthostatic hypotension as a risk factor for stroke: the atherosclerosis risk in communities (ARIC) study, 1987-1996. *Stroke.* 2000; 31:2307-13.
323. Fischberg GM, Lozano E, Rajamani K et al. Stroke precipitated by moderate blood pressure reduction. *J Emerg Med.* 2000; 19:339-46.
324. Grossman E, Messerli FH, Grodzicki T et al. Should a moratorium be placed on sublingual nifedipine capsules given for hypertensive emergencies and pseudoemergencies? *JAMA.* 1996; 276:1328-31.
325. Boutitie F, Gueyffier F, Pocock S et al. J-shaped relationship between blood pressure and mortality in hypertensive patients: new insights from a meta-analysis of individual-patient data. *Ann Intern Med.* 2002; 136:438-48.
326. Masaki KH, Schatz IJ, Burchfiel CM et al. Orthostatic hypotension predicts mortality in elderly men: the Honolulu Heart Program. *Circulation.* 1998; 98:2290-5.
327. Räihä I, Luutonen S, Piha J et al. Prevalence, predisposing factors, and prognostic importance of postural hypotension. *Arch Intern Med.* 1995; 155:930-5.
328. Executive Summary of the Third Report of The National Cholesterol Education Program (NCEP) Expert Panel on Detection, Evaluation, And Treatment of High Blood Cholesterol in Adults (Adult Treatment Panel III). *JAMA.* 2001; 285:2486-97.
329. Hoeldtke RD, Cavanaugh ST, Hughes JD et al. Treatment of orthostatic hypotension with dihydroergotamine and caffeine. *Ann Intern Med.* 1986; 105:168-73.
330. Onrot J, Goldberg MR, Biaggioni I et al. Hemodynamic and humoral effects of caffeine in autonomic failure. *N Engl J Med.* 1985; 313:549-54.
331. Smeenk HE, Koster MJ, Faaij RA et al. Compression therapy in patients with orthostatic hypotension: a systematic review. *Neth J Med.* 2014; 72:80-5.
332. Jordan J, Shannon JR, Black BK et al. The pressor response to water drinking in humans: a sympathetic reflex? *Circulation.* 2000; 101:504-9.
333. Jordan J, Shannon JR, Grogan E et al. A potent pressor response elicited by drinking water. *Lancet.* 1999; 353:723.
334. Frishman WH, Azer V, Sica D. Drug treatment of orthostatic hypotension and vasovagal syncope. *Hear Dis.* 2003; 5:49-64.
335. Kowey PR, Marinchak RA, Rials SJ et al. Intravenous amiodarone. *J Am Coll Cardiol.* 1997; 29:1190-8.
336. Verhaeverbeke I, Mets T. Drug-induced orthostatic hypotension in the elderly: avoiding its onset. *Drug Saf.* 1997; 17:105-18.
337. Lader M. Some adverse effects of antipsychotics: prevention and treatment. *J Clin Psychiatry.* 1999; 60(suppl 1):18-21.
338. Udabe RU. Clinical experience with a new psychotropic drug, trazodone: a review of literature. *Curr Ther Res Clin Exp.* 1973; 15:755-63.
339. Paramothayan NS, Lasserson TJ, Wells AU, Walters EH. Prostacyclin for pulmonary hypertension in adults. *Cochrane Database Syst Rev.* 2005; (2):CD002994.
340. Brevetti G, Chiariello M, Giudice P et al. Effective treatment of orthostatic hypotension by propranolol in the Shy-Drager syndrome. *Am Heart J.* 1981; 102:938-41.
341. Cuffe MS, Califf RM, Adams KF et al. Short-term intravenous milrinone for acute exacerbation of chronic heart failure: a randomized controlled trial. *JAMA.* 2002; 287:1541-7.
342. Bradberry SM, Thanacoody HKR, Watt BE et al. Management of the cardiovascular complications of tricyclic antidepressant poisoning: role of sodium bicarbonate. *Toxicol Rev.* 2005; 24:195-204.
343. Newfield P, Roizen MF. Hazards of rapid administration of vancomycin. *Ann Intern Med.* 1979; 91:581.
344. Renz C, Lynch J, Thurn J et al. Histamine release during rapid vancomycin administration. *Inflamm Res.* 1998; 47(suppl 1): S69-70.
345. Madrid AH, Ortega J, Rebollo JG et al. Lack of efficacy of atenolol for the prevention of neurally mediated syncope in a highly symptomatic population: a prospective, double-blind, randomized and placebo-controlled study. *J Am Coll Cardiol.* 2001; 37:554-9.
346. Mahanonda N, Bhuripanyo K, Kangkagate C et al. Randomized double-blind, placebo-controlled trial of oral atenolol in patients with unexplained syncope and positive upright tilt table test results. *Am Heart J.* 1995; 130:1250-3.
347. Shibao C, Raj SR, Gamboa A et al. Norepinephrine transporter blockade with atomoxetine induces hypertension in patients with impaired autonomic function. *Hypertension.* 2007; 50:47-53.
348. Mathias CJ, Fosbraey P, da Costa DF et al. The effect of desmopressin on nocturnal polyuria, overnight weight loss, and morning postural hypotension in patients with autonomic failure. *Br Med J (Clin Res Ed).* 1986; 293:353-4.
349. Krüger K, Neff K. Dihydroergotamine (Dihydergot) in the treatment of orthostatic circulatory disorders: a double-blind comparison with placebo. *J Med.* 1973; 4:106-17.
350. Nordenfelt I, Mellander S. Central haemodynamic effects of dihydroergotamine in patients with orthostatic hypotension. *Acta Med Scand.* 1972; 191:115-20.
351. Kaufmann H, Freeman R, Biaggioni I et al. Droxidopa for neurogenic orthostatic hypotension: a randomized, placebo-controlled, phase 3 trial. *Neurology.* 2014; 83:328-35.
352. Kaufmann H, Saadia D, Voustianiouk A et al. Norepinephrine precursor therapy in neurogenic orthostatic hypotension. *Circulation.* 2003; 108:724-8.
353. Mathias CJ, Senard JM, Braune S et al. L-threo-dihydroxyphenylserine (L-threo-DOPS; droxidopa) in the management of neurogenic orthostatic hypotension: a multi-national, multi-center, dose-ranging study in multiple system atrophy and pure autonomic failure. *Clin Auton Res.* 2001; 11:235-42.
354. Freeman R, Landsberg L, Young J. The treatment of neurogenic orthostatic hypotension with 3,4-DL-threo-dihydroxyphenylserine: a randomized, placebo-controlled, crossover trial. *Neurology.* 1999; 53:2151-7.
355. Toh V, Duncan E, Lewis N et al. Ergotamine use in severe diabetic autonomic neuropathy. *Diabet Med.* 2006; 23:574-6.
356. Siminoski K, Lukinuk C, Armstrong PW. Treatment of postural hypotension with aerosol ergotamine. *CMAJ.* 1988; 139:51-2.
357. Brahmbhatt R, Baggaley P, Hockings B. Normalization of blood pressure in a patient with severe orthostatic hypotension and supine hypertension using clonidine. *Hypertension.* 2001; 37:E24.
358. Hoeldtke RD, Streeten DH. Treatment of orthostatic hypotension with erythropoietin. *N Engl J Med.* 1993; 329:611-5.
359. Winkler AS, Landau S, Watkins P et al. Observations on haematological and cardiovascular effects of erythropoietin treatment in multiple system atrophy with sympathetic failure. *Clin Auton Res.* 2002; 12:203-6.
360. Winkler AS, Landau S, Watkins PJ. Erythropoietin treatment of postural hypotension in anemic type 1 diabetic patients with autonomic neuropathy: a case study of four patients. *Diabetes Care.* 2001; 24:1121-3.
361. Kanjwal K, Saeed B, Karabin B et al. Erythropoietin in the treatment of postural orthostatic tachycardia syndrome. *Am J Ther.* 2012; 19:92-5.
362. Rowe PC, Calkins H, DeBusk K et al. Fludrocortisone acetate to treat neurally mediated hypotension in chronic fatigue syndrome: a randomized controlled trial. *JAMA.* 2001; 285:52-9.

363. Salim MA, Di Sessa TG. Effectiveness of fludrocortisone and salt in preventing syncope recurrence in children: a double-blind, placebo-controlled, randomized trial. *J Am Coll Cardiol.* 2005; 45:484-8.
364. Montastruc JL, Pelat M, Verwaerde P et al. Fluoxetine in orthostatic hypotension of Parkinson's disease: a clinical and experimental pilot study. *Fundam Clin Pharmacol.* 1998; 12:398-402.
365. Grubb BP, Samoil D, Kosinski D et al. Fluoxetine hydrochloride for the treatment of severe refractory orthostatic hypotension. *Am J Med.* 1994; 97:366-8.
366. Perkins CM, Lee MR. Flurbiprofen and fludrocortisone in severe autonomic neuropathy. *Lancet (London, England).* 1978; 2:1058.
367. Watt SJ, Tooke JE, Perkins CM et al. The treatment of idiopathic orthostatic hypotension: a combined fludrocortisone and flurbiprofen regime. *Q J Med.* 1981; 50:205-12.
368. Imaizumi T, Takeshita A, Ashihara T et al. Increase in reflex vasoconstriction with indomethacin in patients with orthostatic hypotension and central nervous system involvement. *Br Heart J.* 1984; 52:581-4.
369. Abate G, Polimeni RM, Cuccurullo F et al. Effects of indomethacin on postural hypotension in Parkinsonism. *Br Med J.* 1979; 2:1466-8.
370. Sheldon R. Prevention of Syncope Trial (POST): a randomized, placebo-controlled study of metoprolol in the prevention of vasovagal syncope. *Circulation.* 2006; 113:1164-70.
371. Perez-Lugones A, Schweikert R, Pavia S et al. Usefulness of midodrine in patients with severely symptomatic neurocardiogenic syncope: a randomized control study. *J Cardiovasc Electrophysiol.* 2001; 12:935-8.
372. Samniah N, Sakaguchi S, Lurie KG et al. Efficacy and safety of midodrine hydrochloride in patients with refractory vasovagal syncope. *Am J Cardiol.* 2001; 88:A7, 80-3.
373. Hoeldtke RD, Israel BC. Treatment of orthostatic hypotension with octreotide. *J Clin Endocrinol Metab.* 1989; 68:1051-9.
374. Hoeldtke RD, Horvath GG, Bryner KD et al. Treatment of orthostatic hypotension with midodrine and octreotide 1. *J Clin Endocrinol Metab.* 1998; 83:339-43.
375. Di Girolamo E, Di Iorio C, Sabatini P et al. Effects of paroxetine hydrochloride, a selective serotonin reuptake inhibitor, on refractory vasovagal syncope: a randomized, double-blind, placebo-controlled study. *J Am Coll Cardiol.* 1999; 33:1227-30.
376. Frewin DB, Leonello PP, Penhall RK et al. Pindolol in orthostatic hypotension: possible therapy? *Med J Aust.* 1980; 1:128.
377. Nair N, Padder FA, Kutalek SP et al. Usefulness of pindolol for treatment of neurocardiogenic syncope. *Am J Cardiol.* 2004; 94:1189-91.
378. Chobanian AV, Volicer L, Liang CS et al. Use of propranolol in the treatment of idiopathic orthostatic hypotension. *Trans Assoc Am Physicians.* 1977; 90:324-34.
379. Singer W, Sandroni P, Opfer-Gehrking TL et al. Pyridostigmine treatment trial in neurogenic orthostatic hypotension. *Arch Neurol.* 2006; 63:513-8.
380. Biaggioni I, Robertson RM, Robertson D. Manipulation of norepinephrine metabolism with yohimbine in the treatment of autonomic failure. *J Clin Pharmacol.* 1994; 34:418-23.
381. Onrot J, Goldberg MR, Biaggioni I et al. Oral yohimbine in human autonomic failure. *Neurology.* 1987; 37:215-20.
382. Victor RG, Talman WT. Comparative effects of clonidine and dihydroergotamine on venomotor tone and orthostatic tolerance in patients with severe hypoadrenergic orthostatic hypotension. *Am J Med.* 2002; 112:361-8.
383. Lanier JB, Mote MB, Clay EC. Evaluation and management of orthostatic hypotension. *Am Fam Physician.* 2011; 84:527-36.
384. Briasoulis A, Silver A, Yano Y et al. Orthostatic hypotension associated with baroreceptor dysfunction: treatment approaches. *J Clin Hypertens (Greenwich).* 2014; 16:141-8.
385. Campbell IW, Ewing DJ, Clarke BF. Therapeutic experience with fludrocortisone in diabetic postural hypotension. *Br Med J.* 1976; 1:872-4.
386. Chobanian AV, Volicer L, Tifft CP et al. Mineralocorticoid-induced hypertension in patients with orthostatic hypotension. *N Engl J Med.* 1979; 301:68-73.
387. Low PA, Gilden JL, Freeman R et al. Efficacy of midodrine vs placebo in neurogenic orthostatic hypotension. A randomized, double-blind multicenter study. Midodrine Study Group. *JAMA.* 1997; 277:1046-51.
388. Jankovic J, Gilden JL, Hiner BC et al. Neurogenic orthostatic hypotension: a double-blind, placebo-controlled study with midodrine. *Am J Med.* 1993; 95:38-48.
389. Wright RA, Kaufmann HC, Perera R et al. A double-blind, dose-response study of midodrine in neurogenic orthostatic hypotension. *Neurology.* 1998; 51:120-4.
390. Fouad-Tarazi FM, Okabe M, Goren H. Alpha sympathomimetic treatment of autonomic insufficiency with orthostatic hypotension. *Am J Med.* 1995; 99:604-10.
391. Ward CR, Gray JC, Gilroy JJ et al. Midodrine: a role in the management of neurocardiogenic syncope. *Heart.* 1998; 79:45-9.
392. Mitka M. Trials to address efficacy of midodrine 18 years after it gains FDA approval. *JAMA.* 2012; 307:1124-7.
393. Biaggioni I. New developments in the management of neurogenic orthostatic hypotension. *Curr Cardiol Rep.* 2014; 16:542.
394. Shibao C, Okamoto LE, Gamboa A et al. Comparative efficacy of yohimbine against pyridostigmine for the treatment of orthostatic hypotension in autonomic failure. *Hypertension.* 2010; 56:847-51.
395. Biaggioni I, Zygmunt D, Haile V et al. Pressor effect of inhaled ergotamine in orthostatic hypotension. *Am J Cardiol.* 1990; 65:89-92.
396. Conte J, Ader JL, Suc JM. [Treatment of orthostatic hypotension due to major hypotensive drugs (exception of ganglioplegics). Trial of dihydroergotamine]. *La Nouv Press médicale.* 1973; 2:1761-4.
397. Thulesius O, Berlin E. Dihydroergotamine therapy in orthostatic hypotension due to psychotropic drugs. *Int J Clin Pharmacol Ther Toxicol.* 1986; 24:465-7.
398. Robertson D, Goldberg MR, Hollister AS et al. Clonidine raises blood pressure in severe idiopathic orthostatic hypotension. *Am J Med.* 1983; 74:193-200.
399. Gaffney FA, Lane LB, Pettinger W et al. Effects of long-term clonidine administration on the hemodynamic and neuroendocrine postural responses of patients with dysautonomia. *Chest.* 1983; 83(suppl 2):436-8.
400. Mosqueda-Garcia R, Fernandez-Violante R, Tank J et al. Yohimbine in neurally mediated syncope. Pathophysiological implications. *J Clin Invest.* 1998; 102:1824-30.
401. US Food and Drug Administration. FDA Drug Safety Communication: erythropoiesis-stimulating agents (ESAs): Procrit, Epogen and Aranesp (February 2010). https://www.fda.gov/Drugs/DrugSafety/PostmarketDrugSafetyInformationforPatientsandProviders/ucm200297.htm (accessed 2018 Jun 5).
402. Man in 't Veld AJ, Schalekamp MA. Pindolol acts as beta-adrenoceptor agonist in orthostatic hypotension: therapeutic implications. *Br Med J (Clin Res Ed).* 1981; 282:929-31.
403. Dendi R, Goldstein DS. Meta-analysis of nonselective versus beta-1 adrenoceptor-selective blockade in prevention of tilt-induced neurocardiogenic syncope. *Am J Cardiol.* 2002; 89:1319-21.
404. Alegria JR, Gersh BJ, Scott CG et al. Comparison of frequency of recurrent syncope after beta-blocker therapy versus conservative management for patients with vasovagal syncope. *Am J Cardiol.* 2003; 92:82-4.
405. Orthostatic hypotension. *Am Fam Physician.* 2011; 84:537.
406. Nitroglycerin Transdermal System, Nitroglycerin Transdermal System package insert. Mequon, WI: Kremers Urban LLC; 2005.
407. GONITRO Sublingual Powder, Nitroglycerin Sublingual Powder package insert. Jacksonville, FL: Espero Pharmaceuticals Inc; 2016.

408. RECTIV Intra-Anal Ointment, Nitroglycerin 0.4% Intra-Anal Ointment package insert. Bedminster, NJ: ProStrakan Inc; 2011.
409. Entresto Oral Tablets, Sacubitril/valsartan package insert. East Hanover, NJ: Novartis Pharmaceuticals Corp; 2016.
410. FARXIGA Oral Tablets, Dapagliflozin Oral Tablets. Princeton, NJ: Bristol-Myers Squibb Company; 2014.
411. ARISTADA Intramuscular Extended-Release Injection, Aripiprazole Lauroxil Intramuscular Extended-Release Injection. Waltham, MA: Alkermes Inc; 2015.
412. REXULTI Oral Tablets, Brexpiprazole Oral Tablets. Rockville, MD: Otsuka America Pharmaceutical Inc; 2015.
413. Swett C Jr, Cole JO, Hartz SC et al. Hypotension due to chlorpromazine. Relation to cigarette smoking, blood pressure, and dosage. *Arch Gen Psychiatry*. 1977; 34:661-3.
414. DEFITELIO Intravenous Injection, Defibrotide Sodium Intravenous Injection. Palo Alto, CA: Jazz Pharmaceuticals; 2016.
415. OMETRIQ Oral Capsules, Cabozantinib Oral Capsules. South San Francisco, CA: Exelixis Inc; 2012.
416. UNITUXIN Intravenous Injection, Dinutuximab Intravenous Injection. Silver Spring, MD: United Therapeutics Corp; 2015.
417. Adempas Oral Tablets, Riociguat Oral Tablets. Whippany, NJ: Bayer Healthcare Pharmaceuticals Inc; 2013.

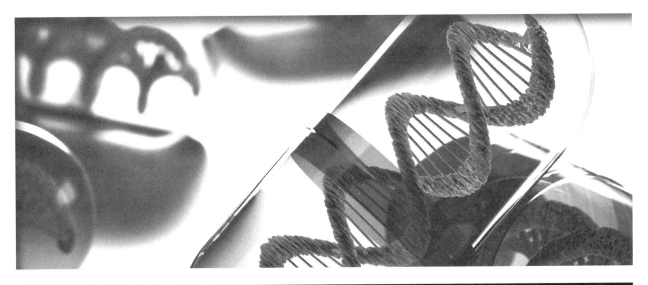

CHAPTER 29

Valvular and Pericardial Heart Disease

Sarah A. Spinler and Frank E. Silvestry

Although cardiovascular disease is the leading cause of death in the United States, valvular and pericardial disease remain relatively uncommon as compared with other cardiovascular diseases such as hypertension and ischemic heart disease. Valvular heart disease accounts for approximately 3.1% of all cardiovascular deaths in the United States.[1] Pericarditis is responsible for approximately 5% of emergency department visits for chest pain and results in 0.1% of hospital admissions.[2] Drug therapy may result in a wide variety of cardiovascular complications, including valvular heart disease and pericardial disease. Although more commonly a result of degenerative or rheumatic processes, valvular heart disease (which includes aortic, mitral, and tricuspid regurgitation) has been reported to occur in association with or as a result of drug therapy. Pericardial disease associated with drug therapy includes pericarditis due to drug-induced systemic lupus erythematosus (SLE)-like syndrome (with or without cardiac tamponade), acute pericarditis, constrictive pericarditis, and hemopericardium. This chapter will review the manifestations of drug-induced valvular and pericardial heart disease.

CAUSATIVE AGENTS

Drugs that have been reported to induce valvular or pericardial heart disease are listed in **Table 29-1**.[3-156] Three main drug classes that have been associated with the development of new valvular or pericardial heart disease are: ergot alkaloids (for migraine headache), ergot-derived dopamine agonists (for Parkinson disease), and 5-hydroxytryptamine (5-HT or serotonin) uptake regulators/inhibitors for weight loss. The earliest reports of drug-induced valvular heart disease appeared in the 1960s, in association with the ergot alkaloids ergotamine and methysergide.[16,17,23,62,63] The anorectic agents fenfluramine and its D-isomer dexfenfluramine, as well as fenfluramine in combination with phentermine, a combination commonly referred to as "fen-phen," have been associated with left-sided regurgitant valvular lesions.[4-15,18-21] Both fenfluramine and dexfenfluramine were withdrawn from the U.S. market in 1997, after reports of valvular heart disease associated with these agents began to appear.[8,19] The ergot-derived dopamine agonists bromocriptine, cabergoline, and pergolide, used to treat Parkinson disease, have

Table 29-1 Agents Implicated in Drug-Induced Valvular and Pericardial Heart Disease

Drug	Incidence	Level of Evidence[a]
AORTIC REGURGITATION		
Bromocriptine[3,97,125]	NK	B
Cabergoline[77,79,80,86-91,97,126,127]	16.7–68.8%	B
Dexfenfluramine[4-15]	6.6–38%	B
Dexfenfluramine in combination with phentermine[4-15]	6.6–38%	B
Ergotamine[16,17]	NK	C
Fenfluramine[4-15,18-21]	6.6–38%	B
Fenfluramine in combination with phentermine[5-15,18-21]	6.6–38%	B
MDMA[98]	14%	B
Methysergide[59,62,63]	0.02%	B
Pergolide[22,76-78,80,81,82-88,90-97,127]	0.005–67%	B
MITRAL REGURGITATION		
Bromocriptine[3,97,125]	NK	C
Cabergoline[77,80,86-91,97,126,127]	28.6–68.8%	B
Dexfenfluramine[4-15]	1.3–3.5%	B
Dexfenfluramine in combination with phentermine[4-15]	1.3–3.5%	B
Ergotamine[16,17,23]	NK	C
Fenfluramine[4-15,18-21]	1.3–3.5%	B
Fenfluramine in combination with phentermine[4-15,18-21]	1.3–3.5%	B
MDMA[98]	14%	B
Methysergide[59,62,63]	0.02%	B
Pergolide[22,76-78,80-88,90-97,127]	0.005–75%	B
TRICUSPID REGURGITATION		
Bromocriptine[3,97,125]	NK	C
Cabergoline[80,88,126,127]	NK	B
Ergotamine[16,23]	NK	C
MDMA[98]	NK	C
Methysergide[59,62,63]	0.02%	B
Pergolide[22,76-78,80-88,90-97,127]	0.005–78%	B
MITRAL STENOSIS		
Ergotamine[16,17,23]	NK	C
Methysergide[59,62,63]	NK	B
ACUTE EFFUSIVE PERICARDITIS		
Adalimumab[155,156]	NK	C
Azactidine[124]	NK	C
Balsalazide[137,138]	NK	C
Busulfan[24,25]	NK	C
Clozapine[99-109,156-159]	NK	B
Cromolyn sodium[26]	NK	C
Cyclophosphamide[24,27,28,141]	NK	C
Cytarabine[24,29-31]	NK	C
Dantrolene sodium[32,33]	NK	C

Table 29-1 Agents Implicated in Drug-Induced Valvular and Pericardial Heart Disease (continued)

Drug	Incidence	Level of Evidence[a]
ACUTE EFFUSIVE PERICARDITIS (Continued)		
Daunorubicin[24,34]	NK	C
Doxorubicin[24,34]	NK	C
5-flurouracil[144,145]	NK	C
Hydralazine (secondary to SLE-like syndrome)[35-37]	2%	C
Isoniazid (secondary to SLE-like syndrome)[38,39,128]	30%	C
Methyldopa (secondary to SLE-like syndrome)[40]	NK	C
Mesalazine (mesalamine)[75,112-122,134-136]	NK	C
Methotrexate[110,111,130,131]	NK	C
Minoxidil[41-44]	3.8–20%	C
Phenylbutazone[45]	NK	C
Phenytoin (secondary to SLE-like syndrome)[35]	NK	C
Procainamide (secondary to SLE-like syndrome)[48-53]	18–57%	C
Sulfasalazine[112,123]	NK	C
Tretinoin[24,54]	NK	C
CONSTRICTIVE PERICARDITIS		
Cyclophosphamide[55]	NK	C
Cytarabine[56]	NK	C
Ergotamine[57]	NK	C
Methysergide[58-63]	0.02%	C
Procainamide (secondary to SLE-like syndrome)[48]	NK	C
HEMOPERICARDIUM		
Apixaban[148]	NK	C
Busulfan[64]	NK	C
Dabigatran[149-152]	NK	C
Fibrinolytics[65-71]	8.75–42%	C
Rivaroxaban[153-154]	NK	C
Vitamin K antagonists (oral)[72-74]	NK	C

MDMA = methylenedioxymethamphetamine, NK = not known, SLE = systemic lupus erythematosus.
[a]Definitions for Levels of Evidence: Level A—evidence from one or more randomized, controlled clinical trials; Level B—evidence from nonrandomized clinical trials, prospective observational studies, cohort studies, retrospective studies, case-control studies, meta-analyses and/or postmarketing surveillance studies; and Level C—evidence from one or more published case reports or case series.

also been reported to result in both left- and right-sided valvular disease.[3,22,76-88,90-97,125-127] In 2006, the U.S. Food and Drug Administration (FDA) ordered the inclusion of a black box warning in pergolide's labeling regarding the potential for valvular heart disease. The drug was voluntarily withdrawn from the U.S. market in 2007 amid continuing reports of this drug-induced disease. Cabergoline, when used at lower doses for the treatment of prolactinoma and acromegaly, has not been associated with valvulopathy.[157-165] A multicountry nested case-control study found that pergolide and cabergoline were both associated with significant valvulopathy in patients with Parkinson disease but not when used for treatment of hyperprolactinemia.[163] This may be due to lower weekly and cumulative doses used in the treatment of hyperprolactinomas.[161] In 2007, the European Medicines Agency added a warning about valvulopathy to the labeling of all ergot alkaloids and restricted the maximum dose of cabergoline and bromocriptine to 3 mg/day and 30 mg/day, respectively.[166-168] In August 2011, the FDA added a cardiac valvulopathy warning to the product labeling of cabergoline.[169,170] The product label recommends a maximum dose of 1 mg twice weekly for treatment of prolactinomas and baseline echocardiography to exclude significant valvular disease (a contraindication to use) as well as echocardiograms every 6–12 months and diagnostic monitoring using chest x-ray and computed tomography (CT) scan if clinical signs and symptoms such as edema, new cardiac murmur, dyspnea, or heart failure appear.

Acute pericarditis has been associated with a wide variety of drugs (Table 29-1), including those that may induce the syndrome resembling SLE (hydralazine, isoniazid, methyldopa, phenytoin, procainamide), cancer chemotherapy drugs (busulfan cyclophosphamide, cytarabine, methotrexate,-doxorubicin, daunorubicin, tretinoin, 5-flurouracil, azacitidine), and other drugs including mesalazine (mesalamine), sulfasalazine, balsalazide, infliximab, adalimumab, minoxidil, dantrolene sodium, phenylbutazone, cromolyn sodium, and interferon alpha.[4,24-54,75,109-122,124,128-143,155,156] Clozapine has been associated with pericarditis, often in conjunction with myocarditis.[99-109,144-147] Constrictive pericarditis has been reported in association with ergotamine, methysergide, cyclophosphamide, cytarabine, and procainamide.[48,55-63] Finally, hemopericardium, with or without pericarditis, has been described after fibrinolytic therapy for acute myocardial infarction or stroke, during busulfan therapy (in conjunction with severe thrombocytopenia), during therapy with vitamin K antagonist anticoagulants such as warfarin, and more recently with the direct-acting oral anticoagulants apixaban, dabigatran, and rivaroxaban.[64-74,148-154]

EPIDEMIOLOGY

There are no available estimates of the overall incidence or frequency of drug-induced valvular or pericardial diseases. However, incidences of pericardial effusion due to minoxidil, pericarditis in patients with drug-induced SLE, valvular disease with long-term ergot alkaloid therapy, hemopericardium after fibrinolysis for myocardial infarction, and regurgitant valvular disease induced by anorectic agents have all been described relatively well.

The incidence of pericardial effusion occurring during minoxidil therapy ranges from 3.8% (73 of 1,919 patients) to 20% (1 of 5) depending on the population studied, with a higher frequency in patients with kidney disease.[41,43] The prevalence of acute pericarditis in those with idiopathic SLE ranges from 30% to 45%.[48] Reported rates of acute pericarditis complicating drug-induced SLE are similar to those associated with idiopathic SLE; the incidences of acute pericarditis associated with isoniazid and procainamide are approximately 30% and 18–57%, respectively.[48] Pericarditis in patients with SLE-like syndrome secondary to hydralazine and methyldopa is relatively uncommon.[37,40] Cardiac tamponade occurring in patients with idiopathic or drug-induced SLE is rare.[36,37]

Although the vascular complications associated with ergot alkaloid treatment have been known for well over a century, the frequency of valvular disease is less well characterized. Early reports relied on auscultatory findings, which are less sensitive than echocardiography in the detection of valvular disease. Graham and colleagues[62,63] estimated that the incidence of methysergide-associated valvular disease is 1 in 5,000 patients treated.

The incidence of echocardiographically detected pericardial effusion and hemopericardium after fibrinolysis is highly variable, ranging from 8.75% in 80 consecutive patients treated with streptokinase to 24% in 112 patients treated with alteplase.[69,71] In a study of 192 patients who underwent serial echocardiography on days 1, 5, 10, and 21 and then annually for 3 years, pericardial effusion was detected at least once in 43% of patients, and the incidence was similar in those who received fibrinolytics (42%) and those who did not (50%).[70] The frequency of pericardial effusion varies depending on the duration of echocardiographic follow-up, with an increasing frequency occurring during the first 5 days after myocardial infarction, regardless of whether fibrinolytic drugs were administered.[70]

The best-studied example of drug-induced valvular heart disease is that of mitral and aortic regurgitation caused by the anorexiant agents fenfluramine and dexfenfluramine. In 1997, the FDA defined anorexiant drug–related cardiac valvulopathy as moderate or greater mitral regurgitation, mild or greater aortic regurgitation, or both detected on a standard echocardiogram, in the absence of other known causes of valvular disease. Patients with these drug-related findings are defined as FDA-positive.[8] Using that definition, the reported prevalence of fenfluramine-associated and dexfenfluramine-associated valvular disease ranged from <0.1% to 38%, depending on the population studied and method used.[8,9] Assessing data only from controlled studies, the incidence of FDA-positive valvular heart disease associated with anorexiant drugs varies from 1% to 15%, which is still significantly higher than that reported in controls (3–6%).[5,6,171,172] Aortic regurgitation occurs more frequently than mitral regurgitation.[6,77,78] A prospective study did not find an association between phentermine (when taken without fenfluramine or dexfenfluramine) and valvulopathy, and as a result, phentermine remains currently used as monotherapy.[5,10] Moderate-to-severe cardiac valvular regurgitation associated with ergot alkaloids in patients with Parkinson disease has also been well studied. Case-control studies comparing the frequency of cardiac valvular disease with ergot drugs (pergolide, cabergoline) to either nonergot drugs (such as ropinirole or pramipexole) or controls report a frequency of 18–37% in ergot-treated patients, 0–25% in non-ergot-treated patients and 4–18% in controls, with ergot-treated patients at increased risk of valvular heart disease.[79-81,83,84,87,93,94,126,127]

MECHANISMS

There are a number of proposed mechanisms for drug-induced valvular and pericardial heart disease (**Table 29-2**). A common link between valvular regurgitation after ergotamine, methysergide, fenfluramine, and dexfenfluramine is that these agents (and their metabolites) are similar structurally to serotonin and are potent agonists of the 5-hydroxytryptamine $(HT)_{2B}$ subtype of serotonin receptor, which promotes serotonin release.[5,7,173-175] 5-HT exerts a direct mitogenic transcriptionally controlled proliferative effect on cardiac valve vascular interstitial cells.[176,177] Excessive cell division and proliferation leads to cell overgrowth resulting in valve dysfunction.

Table 29-2 Mechanisms of Drug-Induced Valvular and Pericardial Heart Disease

Drug	Mechanism
Alteplase, reteplase, streptokinase, tenecteplase (hemopericardium)	Fibrinolytic effect coupled with pericarditis caused by myocardial infarction
Fenfluramine, dexfenfluramine (valvulopathy) Ergotamine (valvulopathy) Pergolide (valvulopathy) Cabergoline (valvulopathy) MDMA (valvulopathy)	Activation of the 5-HT_{2B} subtype of serotonin receptor, which promotes serotonin release

HT = hydroxytryptamine, MDMA = methylenedioxymethamphetamine.

The type of valvular lesions observed in association with these agents is similar to that observed in patients with carcinoid heart syndrome, which is also associated with high concentrations of circulating serotonin.[5] Human cardiac valves express large numbers of 5-HT_{2B} receptors and no appreciable 5-HT_{2C} receptors.[80] Examination of affected native valves excised after valve-replacement surgery reveals glistening white leaflets and chordae covered with a thick coating; however, underlying structures in the valves are preserved. On histologic examination, there is a proliferation of myofibroblasts with deposition of abundant extracellular matrix. Echocardiography has defined diastolic doming and anterior leaflet thickening with affected mitral valves. Leaflet mobility is preserved in the anterior leaflets but is impaired in the posterior leaflets.[6,16] Animal models suggest that activation of the 5-HT_{2B} receptor and decreased 5-HT transporter gene activity (resulting in reduced 5-HT clearance and processing at the receptor) are associated with valvulopathy. Pergolide, cabergoline, and bromocriptine are derivatives of ergotamine and are also 5-HT_{2B} receptor agonists.[178-180] Bromocriptine has a lower receptor-binding affinity and is a partial agonist of the 5-HT_{2B} receptor, which may be the reason that there are fewer and only inconsistent reports of valvulopathy associated with this drug.[77,79,97,180]

Lorcaserin, a weight-loss medication that is a specific agonist of 5-HT_{2C}, has not been associated with valvulopathy.[176,181] For unknown reasons, the valvulopathy observed with methysergide, ergotamines, fenfluramine, and dexfenfluramine is more often left-sided, while that associated with pergolide and cabergoline is right-sided.[178] Drugs with serotonergic activity but lacking activation of the 5-HT_{2B} receptor, such as selective serotonin-reuptake inhibitors, triptans (5-HT_{1B} and 5-HT_{1D} receptor antagonist), or ondansetron (5-HT_3 antagonist), have not been associated with cardiac valvulopathy.[178]

Interestingly, 3,4-methylenedioxymethamphetamine (MDMA, or "ecstasy") also binds to and stimulates serotonin 5-HT_{2B} receptors, producing an in vitro mitogenic response in cardiac valvular interstitial cells that is identical to that induced by fenfluramine.[175] One case-control echocardiographic study comparing the frequency of valvular heart disease using the FDA criteria for appetite-suppressant-induced valvular heart disease in users of MDMA (mean duration of use, 6.1 years) found an alarming incidence of 28% (8 of 29) in these young adults, as compared with 0% (0 of 28) among nonuser controls.[98] There has been a single published case report of pulmonary hypertension and severe mitral stenosis and regurgitation requiring valve replacement in a patient reporting chronic ecstasy use.[182]

Acute pericarditis and pericardial effusion occurring in patients with drug-induced SLE-like syndrome are pathologically indistinguishable from those occurring in association with idiopathic SLE. A more detailed discussion of the proposed mechanisms of drug-induced SLE-like syndrome may be found in Chapter 7. Pericarditis associated with mesalamine therapy has been postulated to be a type IV hypersensitivity reaction; there is an anamnestic response to re-exposure with recurrence on subsequent exposure to sulfasalazine.[75] The association of dantrolene with development of concomitant pleural and pericardial effusions and eosinophilia also suggests an allergic-type reaction.[32] Pericarditis and pericardial effusion associated with cancer chemotherapy in the absence of pericardial metastases are believed to be caused by an inflammatory reaction secondary to direct cytotoxicity, an immune-mediated hypersensitivity process, or both.[24,29,34]

Hemopericardium in patients with acute myocardial infarction who are treated with fibrinolytics is believed to be due to the antithrombotic effect of the fibrinolytic agent coupled with pericarditis caused by the myocardial infarction. However, at least one case of fibrinolytic-associated hemopericardium with cardiac tamponade has been reported after treatment of acute ischemic stroke with alteplase in the absence of myocardial infarction.[68] Hemopericardium associated with administration of the oral vitamin K antagonist warfarin occurs most often, but not exclusively, in the setting of underlying pericarditis or after cardiac surgery and is believed to be due to the drug's anticoagulant effect.[72,74]

CLINICAL PRESENTATION AND DIFFERENTIAL DIAGNOSIS

Symptoms associated with drug-induced valvular and pericardial heart disease are similar to those of nondrug-induced disease and may occur at any time after initiation of therapy (**Table 29-3**). Patients with drug-induced valvular disease may present with a murmur on auscultation, signs of atrial or ventricular enlargement or dysfunction, fatigue, exercise intolerance, dyspnea on exertion, peripheral or pulmonary edema, as well as other signs of acute or chronic heart failure.[178,183,184] Many patients have no symptoms or obvious physical findings. Those with tricuspid regurgitation present with right-sided heart failure, symptoms of peripheral edema, ascites, hepatomegaly, jugular venous distention, or any combination of these.[184] Patients with drug-induced valvular disease may also present with endocarditis.[183,184] Individuals with drug-induced pericarditis may present with an enlarged cardiac silhouette, suggesting pericardial effusion on chest radiography, a characteristic pericardial friction rub on auscultation, dyspnea, pulsus paradoxus, cough, abdominal distention secondary to hepatic congestion, and a characteristic pleuritic chest pain that radiates to the scapula or jaw, worsens on inspiration or when laying supine and improves when leaning forward.[2] A 12-lead electrocardiogram (ECG) may reveal PR segment depression (except in lead aVR, where the PR segment

Table 29-3 Signs and Symptoms Associated with Valvular and Pericardial Heart Disease

Valvular heart disease

- Atrial and ventricular enlargement on physical examination, echocardiogram, or both
- Dyspnea at rest or on exertion
- Murmur characteristic of the involved valve(s) detected on auscultation
- Signs and symptoms of endocarditis
- Signs and symptoms of heart failure, including peripheral edema, ascites, hepatomegaly, venous distention, rales

Acute and constrictive pericarditis

- Abdominal distention
- Chest pain
- Concomitant pleural effusion
- Cough
- Dyspnea
- Pericardial friction rub on auscultation
- PR segment depression (except in lead aVR, where PR segment may be elevated) and diffuse ST segment elevation on 12-lead electrocardiogram
- Pulsus paradoxus
- Retroperitoneal fibrosis (ergotamine, methysergide, pergolide, cabergoline)
- Signs and symptoms of systemic lupus erythematosus-like syndrome

Pericardial tamponade

- Cardiac arrest with pulseless electrical activity
- Diffuse low voltage on 12-lead electrocardiogram
- Feeling of apprehension
- Pericardial effusion
- Pulsus paradoxus
- Signs of hemodynamic compromise such as hypotension or cardiogenic shock
- Tachycardia
- Tachypnea

may be elevated) and diffuse concave upward ST-segment elevation, as is observed in patients with other causes of acute pericarditis. Pleural effusion may also accompany pericardial effusion. Markers of inflammation such as C-reactive protein, erythrocyte sedimentation rate, and white blood cell count may also be elevated. If concomitant myocarditis is present, serum troponin concentrations may also be increased.[2] Cardiac magnetic resonance imaging (MRI) should be performed in patients with suspected concomitant myocarditis.[2] Other causes of pericarditis, such as infection, autoimmune disorders (e.g., SLE, sarcoidosis or amyloidosis) or malignancy, may be excluded using cardiac MRI, pericardiocentesis, and cell cytology. Percutaneous pericardial biopsy is often performed in conjunction with pericardiocentesis and reveals fibrosis and nonspecific inflammation. Patients with pericarditis and pericardial effusion secondary to SLE-like syndrome may also present with signs and symptoms of SLE, which are described in more detail in Chapter 7. Those with ergot-induced valvular or pericardial heart disease may also present with concomitant retroperitoneal fibrosis.[58,89,185] Patients with cardiac tamponade typically present with tachycardia, tachypnea, pericardial effusion, pulsus paradoxus, diffuse low voltage on 12-lead ECG, and clinical signs of hemodynamic compromise, such as hypotension. In addition, they may present with cardiogenic shock or cardiac arrest with pulseless electrical activity.[2]

All patients with suspected drug-induced valvular or pericardial disease should undergo full transthoracic echocardiography with Doppler interrogation of the valves. Transesophageal echocardiography may be used if the transthoracic study is nondiagnostic because of technical limitations. Calcification, stenosis, and rheumatic thickening of the valves are generally absent. Examples of echocardiographic findings in patients with anorexiant-associated valvulopathy are shown in **Figure 29-1**, **Figure 29-2**, and **Figure 29-3**, and cardiac tamponade associated with drug-induced SLE-like syndrome is shown in **Figure 29-4** and **Figure 29-5**.

Conditions to consider in the differential diagnosis of drug-induced valvular or pericardial disease are presented in **Table 29-4**. All patients presenting with suspected drug-induced valvular disease should undergo evaluation to exclude the diagnosis of carcinoid tumor using a 24-hour urine collection for determination of 5-hydroxy-indolacetic acid excretion, serum analysis of chromogranin A, as well as radiologic imaging to exclude the presence of a primary tumor or liver metastases.[3,186] Alternative causes of mitral regurgitation should be excluded, including myxomatous degeneration of the mitral

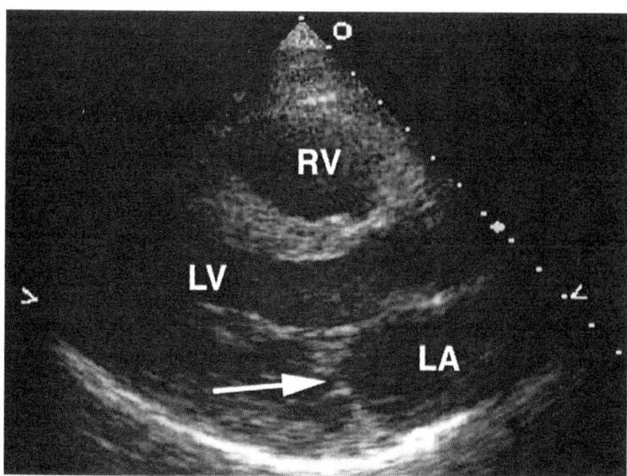

FIGURE 29-1 Transthoracic Echocardiogram from the Parasternal Window in the Long Axis

Demonstrating a normal left atrium (LA), left ventricle (LV), and right ventricle (RV) with mild thickening and restriction of the posterior mitral-valve leaflet (arrow). A finding that is typical of anorexiant-induced valvulopathy.

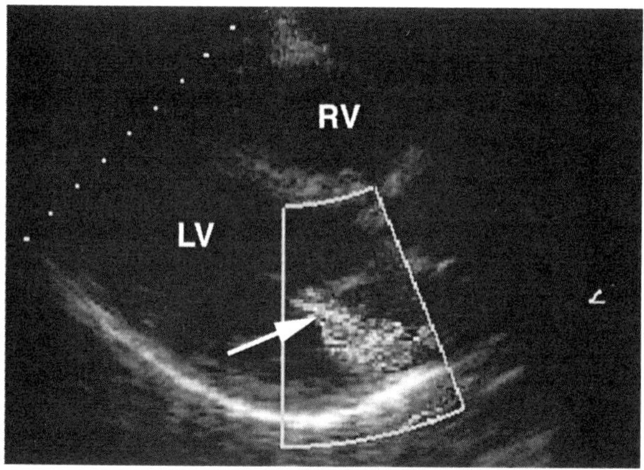

FIGURE 29-2 Transthoracic Echocardiogram with Doppler Map from the Parasternal Window in the Long Axis of the Same Patient as in Figure 29-1

Demonstrating a jet of moderate mitral regurgitation (arrow) directed slightly posteriorly, due to mild restriction of the posterior leaflet, as is characteristic of anorexiant-induced valvulopathy. LV = left ventricle, RV = right ventricle. (See color section.)

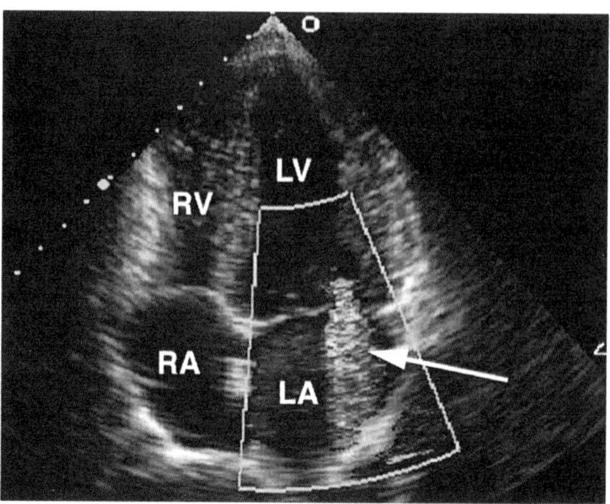

FIGURE 29-3 Apical 4-Chamber View from a Transthoracic Echocardiogram from the Same Patient as in Figures 29-1 and 29-2

Demonstrating a jet of moderate mitral regurgitation (arrow) directed slightly posteriorly and laterally, due to mild restriction of the posterior leaflet, characteristic of anorexiant-induced valvulopathy. LA = left atrium, LV = left ventricle, RA = right atrium, RV = right ventricle. (See color section.)

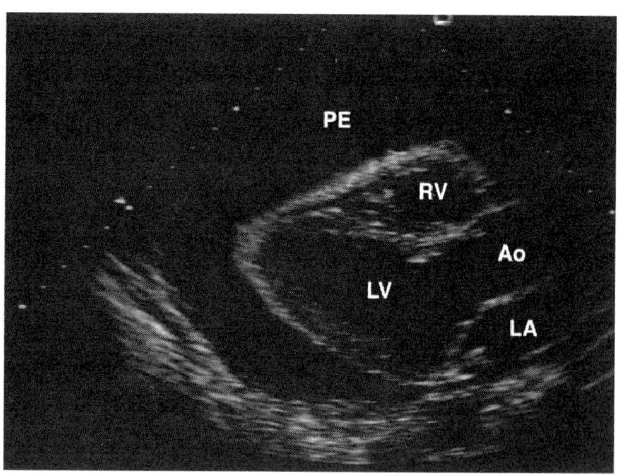

FIGURE 29-4 Transthoracic Echocardiogram from the Parasternal Window Demonstrating a Large Circumferential Pericardial Effusion (PE) Surrounding the Heart

In a patient with a drug-induced syndrome resembling systemic lupus erythematosus and who subsequently progressed to massive pericardial effusion with tamponade. Note the small and underfilled left atrium (LA), left ventricle (LV), and right ventricle (RV). Ao = aorta.

valve, infective endocarditis, rheumatic heart disease, idiopathic SLE, amyloidosis, congenital heart disease, papillary muscle rupture, Marfan syndrome, and hypertrophic cardiomyopathy.[183-185,187] Other causes of aortic regurgitation should be excluded, including congenital abnormality of the aortic valve, calcific degeneration, rheumatic disease, myxomatous proliferation, infective endocarditis, aortic dissection, Marfan syndrome, and traumatic injury.[183-185,187]

Table 29-4 Conditions to Consider in the Differential Diagnosis of Drug-Induced Valvular and Pericardial Heart Disease

All valvular heart disease

- Carcinoid syndrome

Mitral regurgitation

- Amyloidosis
- Congenital heart disease
- Hypertrophic cardiomyopathy
- Infective endocarditis
- Marfan syndrome
- Myxomatous degeneration
- Papillary muscle rupture
- Rheumatic heart disease
- Systemic lupus erythematosus

Aortic regurgitation

- Aortic dissection
- Calcific degeneration
- Congenital heart disease
- Infective endocarditis
- Marfan syndrome
- Myxomatous proliferation
- Rheumatic heart disease
- Traumatic injury

Tricuspid regurgitation

- Cardiac tumor
- Collagen vascular disease
- Congenital heart disease
- Fabry disease
- Gout
- Heart failure with preserved ejection fraction
- Heart failure with reduced ejection fraction
- Intrinsic pulmonary disease
- Left ventricular dysfunction
- Mitral stenosis
- Mucopolysaccharidosis
- Pulmonary hypertension
- Rheumatic heart disease
- Rheumatoid arthritis
- Whipple disease

Pericardial tamponade

- Acute or constrictive pericarditis
- Bacterial infection
- Fungal infection
- Malignancy
- Myocardial infarction
- Neoplasm
- Trauma
- Tuberculosis
- Uremia
- Viral infection
- Collagen vascular disease

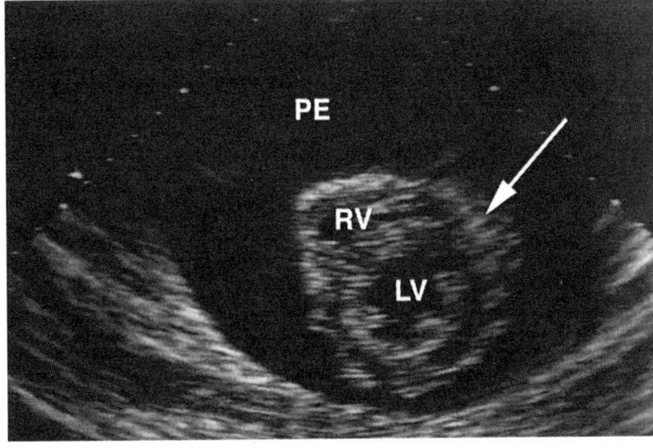

FIGURE 25-5 Transthoracic Echocardiogram from the Parasternal Window of the Heart in Short Axis

Demonstrating a Large Circumferential Pericardial Effusion (PE) Surrounding the Right Ventricle (RV) and Left Ventricle (LV). In a patient with a drug-induced syndrome resembling systemic lupus erythematosus and who subsequently progressed to massive pericardial effusion with tamponade. Note the thickened visceral pericardium (arrow), which is typical of patients with inflammatory PE.

Other diseases causing tricuspid regurgitation that should be considered include left ventricular dysfunction, heart failure (either with reduced ejection fraction or with preserved ejection fraction), cardiac tumors, pulmonary hypertension, mitral stenosis, congenital heart diseases such as Ebstein's anomaly, rheumatic heart disease, collagen vascular diseases, and pulmonary diseases such as chronic obstructive pulmonary disease.[183-185,187] Patients with mitral stenosis should be evaluated for rheumatic heart disease and other degenerative valvular diseases in addition to carcinoid syndrome, including Fabry disease, mucopolysaccharidosis, Whipple disease, gout, and rheumatoid arthritis.[183,187] The diagnoses of malignancy, trauma, and uremia should be considered in patients presenting with cardiac tamponade.[183,187,188] Viral, bacterial, and fungal infections, as well as tuberculosis, uremia, myocardial infarction, neoplasm, trauma, and collagen vascular disease should be considered in patients presenting with acute or constrictive pericarditis.[183,187]

RISK FACTORS

Risk factors for certain types of drug-induced valvular and pericardial heart disease have been identified (**Table 29-5**). Risk factors for the development of mitral or aortic regurgitation associated with fenfluramine and dexfenfluramine include duration of therapy, dose, older age, and female sex.[6,189] Exposure to fenfluramine or dexfenfluramine for <3 months is associated with a lower incidence of valvulopathy than that associated with treatment durations >6 months.[13,21,171,190] Doses of either fenfluramine or dexfenfluramine >60 mg/day have also been associated with the development of valvular regurgitation.[21] Continuous use of methysergide or ergotamine for >9 months, rather than episodic use, has been associated with the development of valvulopathy.[23,58] Larger doses of ergotamine (>6 mg/day) and methysergide (>8 mg/day) have been associated with the development of valvular heart disease.[23,57,58] In a transthoracic echocardiographic study of 78 patients with Parkinson disease, the incidence of valvulopathy was higher in those who received cumulative doses of pergolide of 4,400 g compared with patients who received cumulative doses of 2,200 g.[76] Another case-control analysis suggested that even lower cumulative doses of either pergolide or cabergoline were associated with left-sided valvulopathy.[77] In that study, age, male sex, history of hypertension, and duration of use of either pergolide or cabergoline were risk factors.[77] Several other case-control studies[79,80,84,87,91-93] have found a positive relationship between either cumulative dose or duration of therapy with pergolide or cabergoline and risk of valvulopathy, although conflicting data exist.[85,90,94] When cabergoline is used for treating prolactinomas, doses are approximately one-tenth those used to treat Parkinson disease, and valvulopathy has not been observed.[157-165] Male sex, older age, and hypertension were found to be risk factors for the development of drug-induced valvulopathy in patients with Parkinson disease.[191]

Single doses or initial courses of cancer chemotherapy with any of the agents listed in Table 29-1 may cause pericarditis occurring early (within hours to 1 month) after initial treatment. Higher doses of cancer chemotherapy agents are associated with a greater risk of cardiotoxicity.[11,24,25,28,31,55] Mean total cyclophosphamide doses of 174 mg/kg were associated with a higher rate of pericarditis compared with that associated with a cumulative dose of 87 mg/kg.[28] High doses of cytarabine (≥3 g/m^2) have been associated with pericarditis and heart failure symptoms occurring as early as after the first dose.[24]

Table 29-5 Risk Factors for Drug-Induced Valvular and Pericardial Heart Disease

Valvular heart disease associated with fenfluramine and dexfenfluramine

- Doses >60 mg
- Duration of use >3 months
- Female sex
- Older age

Valvular heart disease associated with ergotamine and methysergide

- Continuous use rather than episodic use
- Ergotamine dose >6 mg/day
- Methysergide dose >8 mg/day
- Duration of use >9 months

Valvular heart disease associated with pergolide and cabergoline

- Cabergoline dose >2 mg/day
- Cumulative dose >1,000 mg (applies to both pergolide and cabergoline)
- Hypertension
- Longer duration of use
- Male sex

Pericarditis associated with chemotherapy

- High doses
  - Cyclophosphamide cumulative dose ≥174 mg/kg
  - Cytarabine dose ≥3 g/m^2

Pericardial effusion associated with minoxidil

- Chronic kidney disease

Hemopericardium associated with fibrinolytic therapy and vitamin k antagonists

- Excessive anticoagulation (dose)
- Presence of pericarditis or pericardial effusion
- Recent cardiothoracic surgery

Minoxidil-associated pericardial effusion has been reported more frequently in patients with chronic kidney disease than in those with normal kidney function.[41]

Risk factors for the development of hemopericardium after fibrinolytic therapy include concomitant underlying pericarditis and pericardial effusion.[65] Pericarditis, excessive anticoagulation, and recent cardiac surgery are risk factors for the development of hemopericardium associated with oral vitamin K antagonist therapy.[72,74]

MORBIDITY AND MORTALITY

After cessation of therapy with fenfluramine and dexfenfluramine, approximately 50% of valve lesions stabilize, approximately 30% improve, and <10% worsen over a subsequent 6-month to 1-year period.[4-6,14,18,107,192] In the largest reported case series to date, Dahl et al. reported the outcomes of 5,743 previous fenfluramine users. In their single-center study, aortic regurgitation stabilized in 63%, worsened in 15%, and improved in 22% while mitral regurgitation stabilized in 47%, worsened in 25%, and improved in 28% of patients monitored during a mean follow-up of 30 months.[190] Outcomes after discontinuation of therapy with ergot derivatives in patients with Parkinson disease are not well studied, and no conclusions can be made.[76,192]

Most cases of drug-induced pericarditis are self-limited and resolve within 2–4 weeks after discontinuation of therapy with the offending agent. Although extremely rare, death may occur secondary to cardiogenic shock in patients with drug-induced cardiac tamponade as well as after valve-replacement surgery in patients with drug-induced valvular disease.[8,24,43]

PREVENTION

There are no specific recommendations to prevent drug-induced valvular or pericardial heart disease. Some general suggestions for the prevention of valvular or pericardial heart disease are listed in **Table 29-6**. Fenfluramine and dexfenfluramine have been removed from the U.S. and European markets, and ergot therapy for migraine has been supplanted by selective 5-HT_1 receptor agonist therapy. When possible, selective 5-HT_1 receptor agonists should be selected for treatment. Pergolide has been removed from the U.S. market. Nonergot dopamine agonists, either ropinirole or pramipexole, should be selected to treat Parkinson disease, as those agents do not bind substantially to the 5-HT_{2B} receptor.[180] Patients receiving cabergoline for prolactinoma should undergo a baseline echocardiogram, with repeat echocardiograms every 6–12 months or when symptoms occur.[170] Patients with kidney disease taking minoxidil should be monitored more closely for clinical signs of pericarditis. The diagnosis of pericarditis should be excluded clinically before the administration of fibrinolytic agents, and anticoagulant doses should be monitored carefully, especially in patients undergoing cardiothoracic surgery, to prevent hemopericardium.

Table 29-6 Approaches to Help Prevent Drug-Induced Valvular and Pericardial Heart Disease

- Cabergoline (valvulopathy)—limit dose to <2 mg/day (maximum 1 mg twice weekly recommended for treatment of prolactinoma)
- Ergotamine (valvulopathy)—administer episodically and limit treatment duration to <9 months
- Fibrinolytic therapy (hemopericardium)—exclude the diagnosis of pericarditis before administering to patients with acute myocardial infarction
- Minoxidil (pericarditis/pericardial effusion)—monitor closely for signs and symptoms of pericarditis in patients with kidney disease

MANAGEMENT

Management of drug-induced valvular or pericardial heart diseases should be individualized based on the specific type and severity of cardiac disease. Treatment options for the management of drug-induced valvular and pericardial diseases are presented in **Table 29-7**.

Whether all patients who are exposed to a drug with the potential to induce valvular heart disease require an initial screening echocardiogram is not known. It is prudent for clinicians to maintain a high index of suspicion and to screen patients carefully

Table 29-7 Treatment Options for Management of Drug-Induced Valvular and Pericardial Heart Disease

Management of valvular heart disease
• Administer antimicrobial prophylaxis against endocarditis before invasive procedures
• Discontinue therapy with the offending agent
• Obtain baseline and serial echocardiograms
• Treat heart failure symptoms with diuretics and vasodilators
• Valve replacement or repair for severe symptomatic disease
Management of pericarditis
• Bed rest
• Corticosteroids for patients with drug-induced SLE-like syndrome
• Discontinue the offending agent
• Management of large pericardial effusion or hemopericardium and cardiac tamponade
• NSAID and/or colchicine with supplemental narcotic analgesia if needed
• Pericardiocentesis
• Surgical pericardectomy for severe constrictive pericarditis
• Surgical pericardiotomy
Management of large pericardial effusion or hemopericardium and cardiac tamponade
• Discontinue therapy with the offending agent
• Pericardiocentesis
• Surgical pericardiotomy

NSAID = nonsteroidal anti-inflammatory drug, SLE = systemic lupus erythematosus.

for potential cardiac symptoms, cardiac murmurs on auscultation, or ECG abnormalities. If drug-associated valvulopathy is suspected, therapy with the suspected culprit agent should be discontinued. Serial echocardiography should be performed every 6–12 months to monitor for progression of valvular disease if significant disease is identified at the time of the baseline exam.[9] The most recent valvular heart disease guidelines from the American College of Cardiology/American Heart Association are not specific regarding diagnosis or monitoring of suspected drug-associated valvular heart disease.[187] It seems prudent to perform echocardiography in all patients who have received therapy with fenfluramine, dexfenfluramine, pergolide, or cabergoline. Routine follow-up echocardiography is not recommended for patients classified as having trivial disease or in those without valvular abnormalities on the initial echocardiogram.[187] Either transthoracic or transesophageal echocardiography may be used for initial diagnosis and serial evaluations for patients with suspected drug-induced valvulopathy.[189] Symptomatic severe valvular regurgitation may necessitate valve replacement or repair based on standard criteria.[187] Heart failure symptoms should be treated with diuretics and vasodilators. Patients with valvular heart disease due to drug therapy should receive antimicrobial prophylaxis against endocarditis before undergoing invasive procedures with the potential to result in bacteremia.[187]

Patients with pericarditis should be placed on bed rest, receive nonsteroidal anti-inflammatory drugs (e.g., aspirin, ibuprofen, or colchicine), and, in severe cases of SLE-associated pericardial disease, should receive therapy with systemic corticosteroids.[2] Colchicine is used for recurrent or persistent pericarditis and has also been used for acute pericarditis associated with cancer chemotherapy.[188,193] Surgical pericardectomy may be required for constrictive pericarditis.[179] Patients with cardiac tamponade and some patients with large pericardial effusion or hemopericardium require pericardiocentesis or surgical pericardiotomy.[2]

INFORMATION FOR PATIENTS

Patients taking drugs known to cause valvular or pericardial heart disease should be instructed to report symptoms of heart failure to their healthcare provider. Patients taking drugs associated with pericarditis should be directed to immediately report symptoms of dyspnea, chest pain, or peripheral edema. Those taking agents associated with drug-induced SLE-like syndrome should be advised of the symptoms of this condition. All patients exposed to drugs associated with valvular or pericardial disease should be screened carefully, and appropriate diagnostic testing should be initiated if any abnormalities are detected by history, physical exam, or ECG.

REFERENCES

1. Mozaffarian D, Benjamin EJ, Go AS et al. Heart and stroke disease statistics-2016 update: a report from the American Heart Association. *Circulation.* 2016; 133:e38-e360.
2. Adler Y, Charron P, Imazio M et al. 2015 ESC guidelines for the diagnosis and management of pericardial disease of the European Society of Cardiology (ESC). *Eur Heart J.* 2015; 36:2921-64.
3. Serratrice J, Disdier P, Habib G et al. Fibrotic valvular heart disease subsequent to bromocriptine treatment. *Cardiol Rev.* 2002: 10:334-6.
4. Weissman NJ, Panza JA, Tiche JF Jr et al. Natural history of valvular regurgitation 1 year after discontinuation of dexfenfluramine therapy: a randomized, double-blind, placebo-controlled trial. *Ann Intern Med.* 2001; 134:267-73.
5. Weissman NJ. Appetite suppressants and valvular heart disease. *Am J Med Sci.* 2001; 321:285-91.
6. Gross SB, Lepor NE. Anorexigen-related cardiopulmonary toxicity. *Rev Cardiovasc Med.* 2000; 1:80-9.
7. Rothman RB, Baumann MH. Therapeutic and adverse actions of serotonin transporter substrates. *Clin Pharmacol Ther.* 2002; 95:73-8.
8. Bowen R, Glicklich A, Khan M et al. Cardiac valvulopathy associated with exposure to fenfluramine or dexfenfluramine: US Department of Health and Human Services Interim Public Health Recommendations, November 1997. *MMWR Morb Mortal Wkly Rep.* 1997; 46:1061-6.
9. Bonow RO, Carabello B, McKay CR et al. ACC/AHA guidelines for the management of patients with valvular heart disease: a report of the American College of Cardiology/American Heart Association Task Force on Practice Guidelines (Committee on Management of Patients with Valvular Heart Disease). *J Am Coll Cardiol.* 1998; 32:1486-1588.
10. Jick H, Vasilakis C, Weinrauch LA et al. A population-based study of appetite-suppressant drugs and the risk of cardiac-valve regurgitation. *N Engl J Med.* 1998; 339:719-24.
11. Khan MA, Herzog CA, St. Peter JV et al. The prevalence of cardiac valvular insufficiency assessed by transthoracic echocardiography in obese patients treated with appetite-suppressant drugs. *N Engl J Med.* 1998; 339:713-8.
12. Palmieri V, Arnett DK, Roman MJ et al. Appetite suppressants and valvular heart disease in a population-based sample: the HyperGEN study. *Am J Med.* 2002; 112:710-5.
13. Jollis JG, Landolfo CK, Kisslo J et al. Fenfluramine and phentermine and cardiovascular findings: effect of treatment duration on prevalence of valve abnormalities. *Circulation.* 2000; 101:2071-7.
14. Mast ST, Jollis JG, Ryan T et al. The progression of fenfluramine-associate valvular heart disease assessed by echocardiography. *Ann Intern Med.* 2001; 134:261-6.
15. Hopkins PN, Polukoff GI. Risk of valvular disease associated with use of fenfluramine. *BMC Cardiovasc Disord.* 2003; 3:5.
16. Hauck AJ, Edwards WD, Danielson GK et al. Mitral and aortic valve disease associated with ergotamine therapy for migraine: report of two cases and review of literature. *Arch Pathol Lab Med.* 1990; 114:62-4.
17. Hendrikx M, Van Dorpe J, Flameng W et al. Aortic and mitral valve disease induced by ergotamine therapy for migraine: a case report and review of the literature. *J Heart Valve Dis.* 1996; 5:235-7.
18. Hensrud DD, Connolly HM, Grogan M et al. Echocardiographic improvement over time after cessation of use of fenfluramine and phentermine. *Mayo Clin Proc.* 1999; 74:1191-7.
19. Connolly HM, Crary JL, McGoon MD et al. Valvular heart disease associated with fenfluramine-phentermine. *N Engl J Med.* 1997; 337:581-8.
20. Burger AJ, Sherman HB, Charlamb MJ et al. Low prevalence of valvular heart disease in 226 phentermine-fenfluramine protocol subjects prospectively followed for up to 30 months. *J Am Coll Cardiol.* 1999; 34:1153-8.
21. Lepor NE, Gross SB, Daley WL et al. Dose and duration of fenfluramine-phentermine therapy impacts the risk of significant valvular heart disease. *Am J Cardiol.* 2000; 86:107-10.
22. Pritchett AM, Morrison JF, Edwards WD et al. Valvular heart disease in patients taking pergolide. *Mayo Clin Proc.* 2002; 77:1280-6.
23. Austin SM, El-Hayek A, Comianos M et al. Mitral valve disease associated with long-term ergotamine use. *South Med J.* 1993; 86:1179-81.
24. Pai VB, Nahata MC. Cardiotoxicity of chemotherapeutic agents: incidence, treatment and prevention. *Drug Saf.* 2000; 22:263-302.
25. Angelucci E, Mariotto E, Lucarelli G et al. Sudden cardiac tamponade after chemotherapy for marrow transplantation in thalassaemia. *Lancet.* 1992; 339:287-9.
26. Slater EE. Cardiac tamponade and peripheral eosinophilia in a patient receiving cromolyn sodium. *Chest.* 1978; 73:878-9.
27. Yamamoto R, Kanda Y, Matsuyama T et al. Myopericarditis caused by cyclophosphamide used to mobilize peripheral blood stem cells in a myeloma patient with renal failure. *Bone Marrow Transplant.* 2000; 26:685-8.
28. Braverman AC, Antin JH, Plappert MT et al. Cyclophosphamide cardiotoxicity in bone marrow transplantation: a prospective evaluation of new dosing regimens. *J Clin Oncol.* 1991; 9:1215-23.
29. Gahler A, Hitz F, Hess U et al. Acute pericarditis and pleural effusion complicating cytarabine therapy. *Onkologie.* 2003; 26:348-50.
30. Reykdal S, Sham R, Kouides P. Cytarabine-induced pericarditis: a case report and review of the literature of the cardio-pulmonary complications of cytarabine therapy. *Leuk Res.* 1995; 19:141-4.
31. Vaickus L, Letendre L. Pericarditis induced by high-dose cytarabine. *Arch Intern Med.* 1984; 144:1868-9.
32. Petusevsky ML, Faling J, Ricklin RE et al. Pleuropericardial reaction to treatment with dantrolene. *JAMA.* 1979; 242:2772-4.
33. Miller DH, Haas JF. Pneumonitis, pleural effusion and pericarditis following treatment with dantrolene. *J Neurol Neurosurg Psychiatr.* 1984; 47:553-4.
34. Bristow MR, Thompson PD, Martin RP et al. Early anthracycline cardiotoxicity. *Am J Med.* 1978; 65:823-32.
35. Alarcon-Sergovia D. Drug-induced systemic lupus erythematosus. *Mayo Clin Proc.* 1969; 44:664-81.
36. Aylward PE, Tonkin AM, Bune A. Cardiac tamponade in hydralazine-induced systemic lupus erythematosus. *Aust N Z J Med.* 1982; 12:546-9.
37. Carey RM, Coleman M, Feder A. Pericardial tamponade: a major presenting manifestation of hydralazine-induced lupus syndrome. *Am J Med.* 1973; 54:84-7.
38. Greenberg JH, Lutcher CL. Drug-induced systemic lupus erythematosus: a case with life-threatening pericardial tamponade. *JAMA.* 1972: 222:191-3.
39. Siddiqui M, Khan IA. Isoniazid-induced lupus erythematosus presenting with cardiac tamponade. *Am J Ther.* 2002; 9:163-5.
40. Harrington TM, Davis DE. Systemic lupus-like syndrome induced by methyldopa therapy. *Chest.* 1981; 79:696-7.
41. Houston MC, McChesney JA, Chatterjee K. Pericardial effusion associated with minoxidil therapy. *Arch Intern Med.* 1981; 141:69-71.
42. Webb DB, Whale RJ. Pleuropericardial effusion associated with minoxidil administration. *Postgrad Med J.* 1982; 58:319-20.
43. Kadir S, Osinfade K, Lawal SO. Pericardial effusion associated with minoxidil therapy: case reports. *West Afr J Med.* 1992; 11:79-81.
44. Shirwany A, D'Cruz IA, Munir A. Very large pericardial effusion attributable to minoxidil: resolution without drainage of fluid. *Echocardiography.* 2002; 19:513-6.
45. Ford MJ, Prescott LF. Phenylbutazone pericarditis. *Scott Med J.* 1982; 27:252-3.
46. Trimble GX. Phenylbutazone-induced pericarditis. *Br Med J.* 1965; 5471:1184.
47. Shafar J. Phenylbutazone-induced pericarditis. *Br Med J.* 1965; 5465:795-7.

48. Sunder SK, Shah A. Constrictive pericarditis in procainamide-induced lupus erythematosus syndrome. *Am J Cardiol.* 1975: 36:960-2.

49. Stein HB, Dodek A, Lawson L et al. Procainamide-induced lupus erythematosus: report of a case with a large pericardial effusion and fluid analysis. *J Rheumatol.* 1979; 6:543-8.

50. Donlan CJ Jr, Forker AD. Cardiac tamponade in procainamide induced lupus erythematosus. *Chest.* 1972; 61:685-6.

51. Dubois EL. Procainamide induction of a systemic lupus erythematosus-like syndrome. *Medicine.* 1969; 48:217-28.

52. Fakhro AM, Ritchie RF, Lown B. Lupus-like syndrome induced by procainamide. *Am J Cardiol.* 1967; 20:367-73.

53. Swarbrick ET, Gray IR. Systemic lupus erythematosus during treatment with procainamide. *Br Heart J.* 1972: 34:284-8.

54. Larrea L, de la Rubia J, Jimenez C et al. Cardiac tamponade and cardiogenic shock as a manifestation of all-trans retinoic acid syndrome: an associate not previously reported. *Haematologica.* 1997; 82:463-4.

55. Tulleken JE, Kooiman CG, van der Werf TS et al. Constrictive pericarditis after high-dose chemotherapy. *Lancet.* 1997: 350:1601.

56. Woods T, Vidarsson B, Mosher D et al. Transient effusive-constrictive pericarditis due to chemotherapy. *Clin Cardiol.* 1999; 22:316-8.

57. Robert M, Derbaudrenghien JP, Blampain JP et al. Fibrotic processes associated with long-term ergotamine therapy. *N Engl J Med.* 1984; 311:601-2.

58. Silberstein SD. Methysergide. *Cephalalgia.* 1998; 18:421-35.

59. Bana DS, MacNeal PS, LeCompte PM et al. Cardiac murmurs and endocardial fibrosis associated with methysergide therapy. *Am Heart J.* 1974; 88:640-55.

60. Meeran MK, Ahmed AH, Parsons FM et al. Constrictive pericarditis due to methysergide therapy. *South Afr Med J.* 1976; 50:1595-7.

61. Greenberg BH, Suros J, Nunn SL et al. Partial pericardial defect with constrictive pericarditis. *Chest.* 1970; 57:383-6.

62. Graham JR, Suby HI, LeCompte PR et al. Fibrotic disorders associated with methysergide therapy for headache. *N Engl J Med.* 1966; 274:360-8.

63. Graham JR. Cardiac and pulmonary fibrosis during methysergide therapy for headache. *Am J Med Sci.* 1967; 254:1-12.

64. Mohapatra MK, Das SP, Mohanty NC et al. Hemopericardium with cardiac tamponade and pleural effusion in chronic myeloid leukemia. *Indian Heart J.* 2000; 52:209-11.

65. Aydinalp AA, Wishniak A, van den Akker-Berman L et al. Pericarditis and pericardial effusion in acute ST-elevation myocardial infarction in the fibrinolytic era. *Israel Med Assoc J.* 2002; 4:181-3.

66. Renkin J, de Bruyne B, Benit E et al. Cardiac tamponade early after thrombolysis for acute myocardial infarction: a rare but not reported hemorrhagic complication. *J Am Coll Cardiol.* 1991: 17:280-5.

67. Tilley WS, Harston WE. Inadvertent administration of streptokinase to patients with pericarditis. *Am J Med.* 1986; 81:541-4.

68. Kasner S, Villar-Cordova CE, Tong D et al. Hemopericardium and cardiac tamponade after thrombolysis for acute ischemic stroke. *Neurology.* 1998; 50:1857-9.

69. Otasevic P, Neskovic AN, Bojic M et al. Pericardial effusion after streptokinase for acute myocardial infarction: an echocardiographic 1-year follow-up study. *Cardiology.* 1997; 88:544-7.

70. Widimsky P, Pavel G. Pericardial involvement during the course of myocardial infarction: a long-term clinical and echocardiographic study. *Chest.* 1995; 108:89-93.

71. Belkin RN, Mark DB, Aronson L et al. Pericardial effusion after intravenous recombinant tissue-type plasminogen activator for acute myocardial infarction. *Am J Cardiol.* 1991; 67:496-500.

72. Miller RL. Hemopericardium with use of oral anticoagulant therapy. *JAMA.* 1969; 209:1362-4.

73. Fell SC, Rubin IL, Enselberg CD et al. Anticoagulant-induced hemopericardium with tamponade. *N Engl J Med.* 1965: 272:670-4.

74. Malouf JF, Gharzeddine W, Stefadouros MA. The role of anticoagulation in the development of pericardial effusion and late tamponade after cardiac surgery. *Eur Heart J.* 1993; 14:1451-7.

75. Sentongo TAS, Piccoli DA. Recurrent pericarditis due to mesalamine hypersensitivity: a pediatric case report and review of the literature. *J Pediatr Gastroenterol Nutr.* 1998; 27:344-7.

76. Van Camp G, Flamez A, Cosyns B et al. Treatment of Parkinson's disease with pergolide and relation to restrictive valvular heart disease. *Lancet.* 2004; 363:1179-83.

77. Oeda T, Masaki M, Yamamoto K et al. High-risk factors for valvular heart disease from dopamine agonists in patients with Parkinson's Disease. *J Neural Transm.* 2009; 116:171-8.

78. Dupuy D, Lesbre JP, Gerard P et al. Valvular heart disease in patients with Parkinson's disease treated with pergolide. *J Neurol.* 2008; 255:1045-58.

79. Yamashiro K, Komine-Kobayashi M, Hatano T et al. The frequency of cardiac valvular regurgitation in Parkinson's disease. *Mov Disord.* 2008; 23:935-41.

80. Zanettini R, Antonini A, Gatto G et al. Valvular heart disease and the use of dopamine agonists for Parkinson's disease. *N Engl J Med.* 2007; 356:39-46.

81. Zadikoff C, Duong-hua M, Sykora K et al. Pergolide associated cardiac valvulopathy based on Ontario administrative data. *Can J Neurol Sci.* 2008; 35:173-8.

82. Dewey RB Jr, Reinold S, O'Suilleabhain P. Cardiac valve regurgitation with pergolide compared with nonergot agonists in Parkinson's disease. *Arch Neurol.* 2007; 64:377-80.

83. Peralta C, Wolf E, Alber H et al. Valvular heart disease in Parkinson's disease vs controls: an echocardiographic study. *Mov Disord.* 2006; 21:1109-13.

84. Corvol J-C, Anzouan-Kacou J-B, Fauveay E et al. Heart valve regurgitation, pergolide use and Parkinson's disease. *Arch Neurol.* 2007; 64:1721-6.

85. Ruzicka E, Linkova H, Penicka M et al. Low incidence of restrictive valvulopathy in patients with Parkinson's disease on moderate dose of pergolide. *J Neurol.* 2007; 254:1575-8.

86. Simonis G, Fuhrmann J, Stasser RH. Meta-analysis of heart valve abnormalities in Parkinson's disease patients treated with dopamine agonists. *Mov Disord.* 2007; 22:1936-42.

87. Yamamoto M, Uesugi T, Nakayama T. Dopamine agonists and cardiac valvulopathy in Parkinson's disease: a case control study. *Neurology.* 2006; 67:1225-9.

88. Kenangil G, Ozekmekci S, Koldas K et al. Assessment of valvulopathy in Parkinson's disease patients on pergolide and/or cabergoline. *Clin Neurol Neurosurg.* 2007; 109:350-3.

89. Dhawan V, Medcalf P, Stegie F et al. Retrospective evaluation of cardio-pulmonary fibrotic side effects in symptomatic patients from a group of 234 Parkinson's disease patients treated with cabergoline. *J Neurol Transm.* 2005; 112:661-8.

90. Junghanns S, Fuhrmann JT, Simonis G et al. Valvular heart disease in Parkinson's disease patients treated with dopamine agonists: a reader-blinded monocenter echocardiography study. *Mov Disord.* 2007; 22:234-8.

91. Schade R, Andersohn F, Suissa S et al. Dopamine agonists and the risk of cardiac-valve regurgitation. *N Engl J Med.* 2007; 356:29-38.

92. Kim JY, Chung EJ, Park SW et al. Valvular heart disease in Parkinson's disease treated with ergot derivative dopamine agonists. *Mov Disord.* 2006; 21:1261-4.

93. Waller EA, Kaplan J, Heckman MG. Valvular heart disease in patients taking pergolide. *Mayo Clin Proc.* 2005; 80:1016-20.

94. Baseman DG, O'Suilleabhain PE, Reimold SC et al. Pergolide use in Parkinson disease is associated with cardiac valve regurgitation. *Neurology.* 2004; 63:310-4.

95. Steiger M, Jost W, Grandas F. Risk of valvular heart disease associated with the use of dopamine agonist in Parkinson's disease: a systematic review. *J Neural Transm.* 2009; 116:179-91.

96. Rasmussen VG, Poulsen SH, Dupont E et al. Heart valve disease associated with treatment with ergot-derived dopamine agonists: a clinical and echocardiographic study of patients with Parkinson's disease. *J Intern Med.* 2007; 263:90-8.
97. Tan LC, Ng KK, Au WL et al. Bromocriptine use and the risk of valvular heart disease. *Mov Disord.* 2008; 24:344-9.
98. Droogmans S, Cosyns B, D'haenen H et al. Possible association between 3,4-methylenedioxymethamphetamine abuse and valvular heart disease. *Am J Cardiol.* 2007; 100:1442-5.
99. Kay SE, Doery J, Sholl D. Clozapine associated pericarditis and elevated troponin I. *Aust N Z J Psychiatry.* 2002; 36:143-4.
100. Murko A, Clarke S, Black DW. Clozapine and pericarditis with pericardial effusion. *Am J Psychiatry.* 2002; 159:494.
101. Branik E, Nitschke M. Pericarditis and polyserositis as a side effect of clozapine in an adolescent girl. *J Child Adolesc Psychopharmacol.* 2004; 14:311-4.
102. Rathore S, Masani ND, Callaghan PO. Clozapine-induced effuso-constrictive pericarditis. *Cardiology.* 2007; 108:183-5.
103. Catalano G, Catalano MC, Frankel Wetter RL. Clozapine induced polyserositis. *Clin Neuropharmacol.* 1997; 20:353-6.
104. Daly JM, Goldberg RJ, Braman SS. Polyserositis associated with clozapine treatment. *Am J Psychiatry.* 1992; 149:1274-5.
105. Boot E, de Haan L, Guzelcan Y et al. Pericardial and bilateral pleural effusion associated with clozapine treatment. *Eur Psychiatry.* 2004; 19:65.
106. Wehmeier PM, Heiser P, Remschmidt H. Pancreatitis followed by pericardial effusion in an adolescent treated with clozapine. *J Clin Psychopharmacol.* 2003; 23:102-3.
107. Bhattacharyya S, Constantin C, Davar J et al. Longitudinal effects of fenfluramine phentermine use. *Angiology.* 2008; 58:772-3.
108. Kortner K, Neuhaus AH, Schurer F et al. Eosinophilia indicating subclinical clozapine-induced pericarditis. *J Clin Psychiatry.* 2007; 68:1147-8.
109. Bhatti MA, Zander J, Reeve E. Clozapine-induced pericarditis, pericardial tamponade, polyserositis, and rash. *J Clin Psychiatry.* 2005; 66:1490-1.
110. Forbat LN, Hancock BW, Gershlick AH. Methotrexate-induced pericarditis and pericardial effusion: first reported case. *Postgrad Med J.* 1995; 71:244-5.
111. Mohyuddin T, Elyan M, Kushner I. Pericarditis: a rare complication of methotrexate therapy. *Clin Rheumatol.* 2007; 26:2157-8.
112. Hermida J-S, Six I, Jarry G. Drug-induced pericarditis mimicking Brugada syndrome. *Europace.* 2007; 9:66-8.
113. Garcia-Moran S, Saez-Royeila F, Perez-Alvarez J-C et al. Myopericarditis and mitral insufficiency associated with ulcerative colitis treated with mesalazine. *Inflamm Bowel Dis.* 2006; 12:334-5.
114. Doganay L, Akinci B, Pekel N et al. Mesalazine-induced myopericarditis in a patient with ulcerative colitis. *Int J Colorectal Dis.* 2006; 21:199-200.
115. Waite RA, Malinowski JM. Possible mesalamine-induced pericarditis: case report and literature review. *Pharmacother.* 2002; 22:391-4.
116. Kaiser GC, Milov DE, Erhart NA et al. Massive pericardial effusion in a child following the administration of mesalamine. *J Pediatr Gastroenterol Nutr.* 1997; 25:435-8.
117. Food and Drug Administration. Rate adverse reactions with Rowasa. *FDA Drug Bull.* 1989; 19:17-8.
118. Jenss H, Becker WE, Weber P. Pericardial effusions during treatment with 5-aminosalicylic acid in a patient with Crohn's disease. *Am J Gastroenterol.* 1990; 85:332-3.
119. Pent MT, Ganapathy S, Holdsworth CD et al. Mesalamine-induced lupus-like syndrome. *BMJ.* 1992; 305:159.
120. Lim AG, Hine KR. Fever vasculitic rash, arthritis, pericarditis and pericardial effusion after mesalazine. *BMJ.* 1994; 308:113.
121. Gujral N, Friedenberg F, Freidenberg J et al. Pleuropericarditis related to the use of mesalamine. *Dig Dis Sci.* 1996; 41:634-6.
122. Inaquinto G, Sorrentini I, Petillo FE et al. Pleuropericarditis in a patient with ulcerative colitis in longstanding 5-aminosalicylic acid therapy. *Ital J Gastroenterol.* 1994; 26:145-7.
123. Perrot S, Aslangul E, Szwebel T et al. Sulfasalazine-induced pericarditis in a patient with ulcerative colitis without recurrence when switching to mesalazine. *Int J Colorectal Dis.* 2007; 22:1119-21.
124. Newman M, Malla M, Gojo I. Azacitidine-induced pericarditis: a case series. *Pharmacotherapy.* 2016; 36:443-8.
125. Cautres T, Cautres M, Mohty D. Multiple valvular regurgitation associated with bromocriptine therapy. *Arch Cardiovasc Dis.* 2014; 107:579-80.
126. De Vecchis R, Esposito C, Ariano C. Cabergoline use and risk of fibrosis and insufficiency of cardiac valves. Meta-analysis of observational studies. *Herz.* 2013; 38:868-80.
127. Rasmussen VG, Ostergaard K, Dupont E et al. The risk of valvular regurgitation in patients with Parkinson's disease treated with dopamine receptor agonists. *Mov Disord.* 2011; 26:801-6.
128. Kubo S, Yamaoka K, Saito K et al. Pericarditis induced by prophylactic administration of isoniazid in a patient with rheumatoid arthritis. *Joint Bone Spine.* 2011; 78:99-100.
129. Katayama M, Imai Y, Hashimoto H et al. Fulminant fatal cardiotoxicity following cyclophosphamide therapy. *J Cardiol.* 2009; 54:330-4.
130. Cudzilo C, Aragaki A, Guitron J et al. Methotrexate-induced pleuropericarditis and eosinophilic pleural effusion. *J Bronchology Interv Pulmonol.* 2014; 21:90-2.
131. Savoia F, Gaddoni G, Casadio C et al. A case of aseptic pleuropericarditis in a patient with chronic plaque psoriasis under methotrexate therapy. *Dermatol Online J.* 2010; 16:13.
132. Killu A, Madhavan M, Prasad A et al. 5-flurouracil induced pericarditis. *BMJ Case Rep.* 2011; Apr 15 2011. pii: bcr0220113883.
133. Saif MW, Shah MM, Shah AR. Fluropyrimadine-associated cardiotoxicity: revisited. *Expert Opin Drug Saf.* 2009; 8:191-202.
134. Kiyomatsu H, Kawai K, Tanaka T et al. Mesalazine-induced pleuropericarditis in a patient with Crohn's disease. *Intern Med.* 2015; 54:1605-8.
135. Park EH, Kim BJ, Huh JK et al. Recurrent mesalazine-induced myopericarditis in a patient with ulcerative colitis. *J Cardiovasc Ultrasound.* 2012; 29:154-6.
136. Sposato B, Allegri MP, Riccardi MP et al. Mesalazine-induced multi-organ hypersensitivity. *Clin Drug Investig.* 2010; 30;413-7.
137. Coman RM, Glover SC, Gjymishka A. Febrile pleuropericarditis, a potentially life-threatening adverse effect of balsalazide-case report and review of the side effects of 5-aminosalicylates. *Expert Rev Clin Immunol.* 2014; 19:667-75.
138. Adhiyaman V, Vaishnavi A, Froese S. Drug points: hypersensitivity reaction to balsalazide. *BMJ.* 2001; 323:489.
139. Burke JP, Kelleher B, Ramadan S et al. Pericarditis as a complication of infliximab therapy in Crohn's disease. *Inflamm Bowel Dis.* 2008; 14:428-9.
140. Devasahayam J, Pillai U, Lacasse A. A rare case of pericarditis, complication of infliximab treatment for Crohn's disease. *J Crohns Colitis.* 2012; 6:730-1.
141. Nishio K, Konndo T, Okada S et al. Pericarditis and chronic inflammatory demyelinating polyneuropathy during therapy with pegylated interferon alfa-2a for chronic hepatitis C. *World J Hepatol.* 2010; 2:358-61.
142. Popescu C, Arama V, Gliga S. Acute pericarditis due to pegylated interferon alpha therapy for chronic HCV hepatitis-case report. *BMC Gastroenterol.* 2011; 11:30.
143. Gressens B, Gohy P. Pericarditis due to interferon-alpha therapy during treatment for chronic hepatitis C. *Acta Gastroenterol Belg.* 2004; 67:301-2.
144. Cadeddu G, Deidda A, Stochino ME et al. Clozapine toxicity due to a multiple drug interaction: a case report. *J Med Case Rep.* 2015; 2:77.

145. De Berardis D, Campanella D, Serroni N et al. Clozapine-related pericarditis during titration phase in a patient with resistant schizophrenia and concomitant valproate treatment: a case report. *J Clin Psychopharmacol.* 2014; 34:649-51.
146. Markovic J, Momcilov-Popin T, Mitrovic D et al. Clozapine-induced pericarditis. *Afr J Psychiatry (Johannesbg).* 2011; 14:236-8.
147. Crews MP, Dhillon GS, MacCabe JH. Clozapine rechallenge following clozapine-induced pericarditis. *J Clin Psychiatry.* 2010; 71:959-61.
148. Sigawy C, Apter S, Vine J et al. Spontaneous hemopericardium in a patient receiving apixaban therapy: first case report. *Pharmacotherapy.* 2015; 35:e115-7.
149. Stollberger C, Heger M, Finsterer J. Hemopericardium under dabigatran for stroke prevention in atrial fibrillation. *Blood Coagul Fibrinolysis.* 2017; 28:185-8.
150. Kizilirmak F, Gunes HM, Guler E et al. Hemopericardium and cardiac tamponade in a patient treated with dabigatran etexilate. *Korean Circ J.* 2016; 46:99-101.
151. Abdallah M, Abdallah T, Abi RN et al. A sanguineous pleuro pericardial effusion in a patient recently treated with dabigatran. *Heart Lung.* 2015; 44:209-11.
152. Barton CA, McMillian WD, Raza SS et al. Hemopericardium in a patient treated with dabigatran etexilate. *Pharmacotherapy.* 2012; 32:e103-7.
153. Shivamurthy P, Brar N, Therrien ML. Isolated hemopericardium associated with rivaroxaban. *Pharmacotherapy.* 2014; 34:e169-72.
154. Boone S. Cardiac tamponade associated with rivaroxaban. *Del Med J.* 2015; 87:206-7.
155. Ozkan H, Cetinkaya AS, Yildiz T et al. A rare side effect due to TNF-alpha blocking agent: acute pleuropericarditis with adalimumab. *Case Rep Rheumatol.* 2013; 2013:985914.
156. Soh MC, Hart HH, Corkill M. Pericardial effusion with tamponade and visceral construction in patients with rheumatoid arthritis on tumour necrosis factor (TNF)-inhibitor therapy. *Int J Rheum Dis.* 2009; 12:74-7.
157. Kars M, Pereira AM, Bax JJ et al. Cabergoline and cardiac valve disease in prolactinoma patients: additional studies during long-term treatment are required. *Eur J Endocrinol.* 2008; 159:363-7.
158. Wakil A, Rigby AS, Clark AL et al. Low dose cabergoline for hyperprolactinaemia is not associated with clinically significant valvular heart disease. *Eur J Endocrinol.* 2008; 59:R11-4.
159. Lancellotti P, Livadariu E, Markov M et al. Cabergoline and the risk of valvular lesions in endocrine disease. *Eur J Endocrinol.* 2008; 159:1-5.
160. Vallette S, Serri K, Rivera J et al. Long-term cabergoline therapy is not associated with valvular heart disease in patients with prolactinomas. *Pituitary.* 2009; 12:153-7.
161. Auriemma RS, Pivonello R, Ferreri L et al. Cabergoline use for pituitary tumors and valvular disorders. *Endocrinol Metab Clin North Am.* 2015; 44:89-97.
162. Tan T, Cabrita IZ, Hensman D et al. Assessment of cardiac valve dysfunction in patients receiving cabergoline treatment for hyperprolactinemia. *Clin Endocrinol (Oxf).* 2010; 73:369-74.
163. Trifiro G, Mokhles MM, Dieleman JP et al. Risk of cardiac valve regurgitation with dopamine agonist use in Parkinson's disease and hyperprolactinaemia: a multi-country, nested case-control study. *Drug Saf.* 2012; 35:159-71.
164. Cabergoline use for pituitary tumors and valvular disorders. *Endocrinol Metab Clin North Am.* 2015; 44:89-97.
165. Delgado V, Biermasz NR, van Thiel SW et al. Changes in heart valve structure and function in patients treated with dopamine agonists for prolactinomas, a 2-year follow-up study. *Clin Endocrinol (Oxf).* 2012; 77:99-105.
166. European Medicines Agency. Ergot-derived dopamine agonists. http://www.ema.europa.eu/ema/index.jsp?curl=pages/medicines/human/referrals/Ergot_derived_dopamine_agonists/human_referral_000107.jsp (accessed 2018 Mar 26).
167. European Medicines Agency. ANNEX II. Scientific conclusions and grounds for amendment of the summaries of product characteristics and package leaflets presented by the EMEA. Scientific conclusions overall summary of the scientific evaluation of cabergoline and pergolide and associated names (see ANNEX I). http://www.ema.europa.eu/docs/en_GB/document_library/Referrals_document/Ergot_derived_dopamine_agonists_31/WC500011459.pdf (accessed 2018 Mar 26).
168. European Medicines Agency. ANNEX II. Scientific conclusions and grounds for amendment of the summaries of product characteristics and package leaflets presented by the EMEA. Scientific conclusions. Overall summary of the scientific evaluation of bromocriptine dihydroergocryptine and lisuride and associated names (see ANNEX I). http://www.ema.europa.eu/docs/en_GB/document_library/Referrals_document/Ergot_derived_dopamine_agonists_31/WC500011459.pdf (accessed 2018 Mar 26).
169. Cabergoline. FDA prescribing information. http://www.drugs.com/pro/cabergoline.html (accessed 2018 Mar 26).
170. Dostinex (Cabergoline) Food and Drug Administration supplemental new drug approval letter. https://www.accessdata.fda.gov/drugsatfda_docs/appletter/2011/020664s011ltr.pdf (accessed 2018 Mar 26).
171. Loke YK, Derry S, Pritchard-Copley A. Appetite suppressants and valvular heart disease: a systematic review. *BMC Clin Pharmacol.* 2002; 2:6.
172. Sachdev M, Miller WC, Ryan T et al. Effect of fenfluramine derivative diet pills on cardiac valves: a meta-analysis of observational studies. *Am Heart J.* 2002; 144:1065-73.
173. Rothman RB, Baumann MH, Savage JE et al. Evidence for possible involvement of 5-HT2B receptors in the cardiac valvulopathy associated with fenfluramine and other serotonergic medications. *Circulation.* 2000; 102:2836-41.
174. Fitzgerald LW, Burn TC, Brown BS et al. Possible role of valvular serotonin 5-HT(2B) receptors in the cardiopathy associated with fenfluramine. *Mol Pharmacol.* 2000; 57:75-81.
175. Setola V, Hufeisen SJ, Grande-Allen J et al. 3,4-Methylenedioxymethamphetamine (MDMA, "ecstasy") induces fenfluramine-like proliferative actions on human cardiac valvular interstitial cells in vitro. *Mol Pharmacol.* 2003; 63:1223-9.
176. Meltzer HY, Roth BL. Locaserin and pimavanserin: emerging selectivity of serotonin receptor subtype-targeted drugs. *J Clin Invest.* 2013; 123:4986-91.
177. Elangban CS. Drug-induced valvulopathy: an update. *Toxicol Pathol.* 2010; 38:837-48.
178. Smith SA, Waggoner AD, de las Fuentes L et al. Role of serotoninergic pathways in drug-induced valvular heart disease and diagnostic features by echocardiography. *J Am Soc Echocardiogr.* 2009; 22:883-9.
179. Roth B. Drugs and valvular heart disease. *N Engl J Med.* 2007; 356:6-9.
180. Kvernmo T, Hartter S, Burger E. A review of the receptor-binding and pharmacokinetic properties of dopamine agonists. *Clin Ther.* 2006; 28:1065-78.
181. Weissman NJ, Sanchez M, Koch GC et al. Echocardiographic assessment of cardiac valvular regurgitation with lorcaserin from analysis of 3 phase 3 clinical trials. *Circ Cardiovasc Imaging.* 2013; 6:560-7.
182. Montastruc F, Montastruc G, Vigreux P et al. Valvular heart disease in a patient taking 3,4-methylenedioxymethamphetamine (MDMA, 'ecstasy'). *Br J Clin Pharmacol.* 2012; 74:547-8.
183. Alpert JS, Aurigemma GP, Balady GJ et al. *The AHA clinical cardiac consult.* 2nd ed. Philadelphia, PA: Lippincott Williams and Wilkins; 2001.
184. Topol EJ. *Textbook of cardiovascular medicine.* Philadelphia, PA: Lippincott Williams and Wilkins; 2007.
185. Agarwal P, Fahn S, Frucht SJ. Diagnosis and management of pergolide-induced fibrosis. *Mov Disord.* 2004; 19:611-3.

186. Pinchot SN, Holen K, Sippel RS et al. Carcinoid tumors. *Oncologist*. 2008; 13:1255-69.

187. Nishimura RA, Otto CM, Bonow RO et al. 2014 ACC/AHA guideline for the management of patients with valvular heart disease: a report of the American College of Cardiology/American Heart Association Task Force on Practice Guidelines. *J Am Coll Cardiol*. 2014; 63:2438-88.

188. Lee GY, Ahn KT, Jung CW et al. Recurrent pericarditis after chemotherapy for acute myeloid leukemia: a case report and a modern approach to chemotherapy-induced pericarditis. *Cardiology*. 2011; 120:130-4.

189. Porter TR, Shillcutt SK, Adams MS et al. Guidelines for the use of echocardiography as a monitor for therapeutic intervention in adults: a report of the American Society of Echocardiography. *J Am Soc Echocardiogr*. 2015; 28:40-56.

190. Dahl CF, Allen MR, Urie PM et al. Valvular regurgitation and surgery associated with fenfluramine use: an analysis of 5743 individuals. *BMC Med*. 2008; 6:34.

191. Oeda T, Masaki M, Yamamoto K et al. High risk factors for valvular heart disease from dopamine agonists in patients with Parkinson's disease. *J Neural Transm (Vienna)*. 2009; 116:171-8.

192. Zanenttini R, Antonini A, Gatto G et al. Regression of cardiac valvulopathy related to ergot-derived dopamine agonists. *Cardiovasc Ther*. 2011; 29:404-10.

193. LeWinter MM. Clinical practice. Acute pericarditis. *N Engl J Med*. 2014; 371:2410-6.

SECTION VII

DRUG-INDUCED ENDOCRINE DISEASES

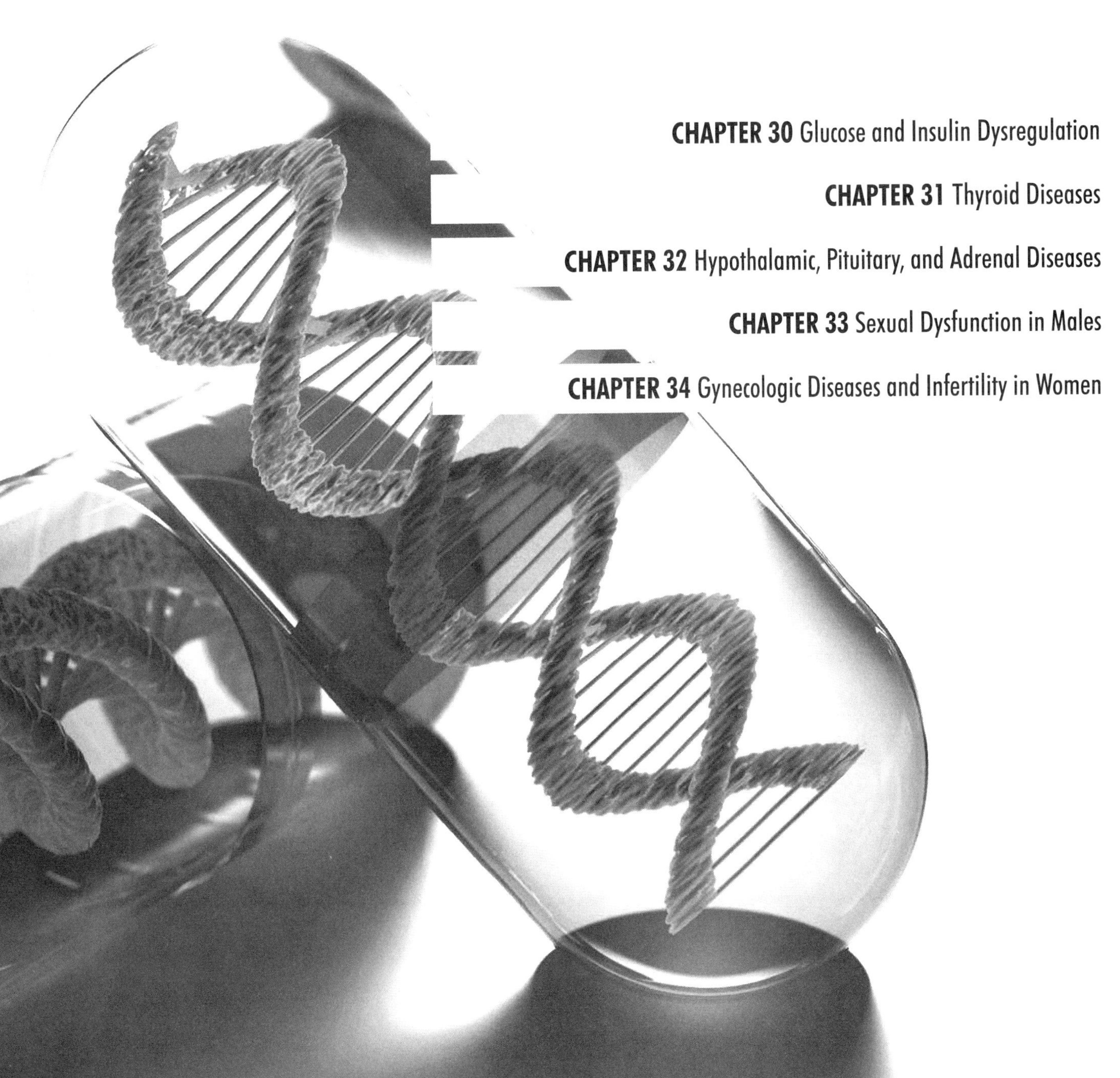

CHAPTER 30 Glucose and Insulin Dysregulation

CHAPTER 31 Thyroid Diseases

CHAPTER 32 Hypothalamic, Pituitary, and Adrenal Diseases

CHAPTER 33 Sexual Dysfunction in Males

CHAPTER 34 Gynecologic Diseases and Infertility in Women

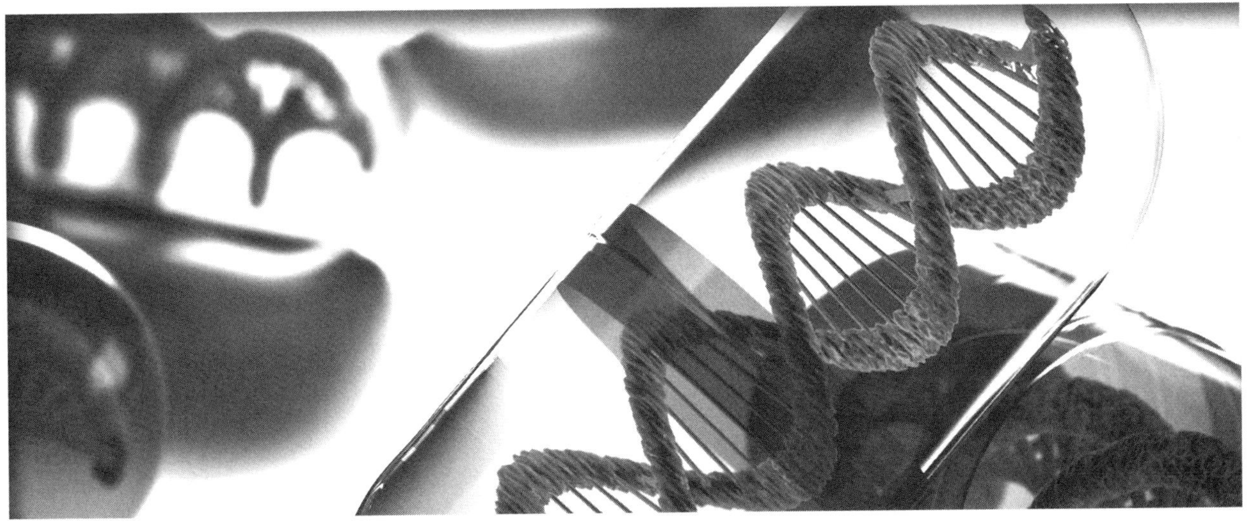

CHAPTER 30

Glucose and Insulin Dysregulation

Devra K. Dang, Frank Pucino, Jr., Charles D. Ponte, and Karim Anton Calis

Glucose homeostasis is regulated by the complex interplay of insulin, hepatic glucose production, peripheral glucose utilization, and counterregulatory mechanisms. Insulin is secreted by pancreatic β cells in response to an increase in plasma glucose concentration and promotes glucose uptake by the liver, muscle, and adipose tissue. Insulin stimulates glycogen synthesis, lipogenesis, and protein synthesis and inhibits lipolysis and hepatic gluconeogenesis. In healthy individuals, a normal plasma glucose concentration is needed to maintain physiological function and meet the energy needs of the brain and various tissues. Insulin secretion is reduced as plasma glucose concentrations decline. When plasma glucose concentrations decrease below the physiological range, counterregulatory hormones are secreted, including glucagon, adrenaline (epinephrine), growth hormone, and cortisol. These hormones restore plasma glucose concentrations to the physiological range through various effects, including stimulation of gluconeogenesis and glycogenolysis, inhibition of insulin secretion and peripheral glucose utilization, and stimulation of lipolysis. Hyperglycemia and hypoglycemia both result from an imbalance between plasma glucose and insulin concentration. Drugs may induce hyper- or hypoglycemia through a variety of mechanisms, including alterations of insulin secretion and sensitivity, changes in gluconeogenesis, and direct cytotoxic effects on pancreatic β cells. Drug-induced hyper- or hypoglycemia can lead to significant consequences, including diabetes mellitus, severe hypoglycemia, coma, and death. However, these events can be prevented and/or minimized with awareness of the problem, close monitoring, and judicious use of the suspect drug(s).

CAUSATIVE AGENTS

Table 30-1 and **Table 30-2** list the medications that have been associated with hyperglycemia and hypoglycemia, respectively. Although sporadic reports of glucose and insulin dysregulation associated with many drugs appear in the literature, only those drugs reported to cause these diseases in one or more clinical trials or observational studies or in multiple case reports will be discussed in this chapter. Glucocorticoids, protease inhibitors, atypical antipsychotics, niacin, pentamidine, and diazoxide are among the agents that have been consistently associated with

Table 30-1 Agents Implicated in Drug-Induced Hyperglycemia

Drug or Drug Class	Incidence[a]	Level of Evidence[b]
Antidepressants[34,35,c]	Variable	B
Atypical antipsychotics[4,15,36-42]	NK Highest incidence with olanzapine and clozapine	B
β-adrenergic receptor blockers[43-46]	NK Incidence higher with nonselective β blockers Vasodilating β blockers (carvedilol, nebivolol, and labetalol) do not affect glycemic control	B
Calcium channel blockers[47-50]	Rare (most reports with high doses of diltiazem and verapamil; a few case reports with nifedipine)	C
Chlorpromazine[51,52]	NK	C
Cyclosporine[53-56]	New-onset PTDM: 4–11% in kidney transplant patients	B
Diazoxide[57-60]	NK	B
Thiazide and thiazide-like diuretics[10,22,61-66]	NK Incidence is lower with doses <25 mg of HCTZ equivalent	A
Fish oil[67-71,d]	NK	B
HMG CoA reductase inhibitors[28,30,72,73,e]	Variable	A
Glucocorticoids[9,10,74-81]	<1–46% for new-onset diabetes Incidence varies depending on dose, duration, and route of administration Lower incidence with inhaled formulations	A
Gonadotropin-releasing hormone agonists[82-84]	<5%–10.9%	B
Recombinant human growth hormone[54,85,86]	NK	C
Interferons[87-89]	NK	C
l-asparaginase[54,90-95]	NK	B
Mammalian target of rapamycin (mTOR) inhibitors[96-99]	13–55% with everolimus, 18–22% with sirolimus, 26% with temsirolimus Data for sirolimus are with concomitant administration with cyclosporine, mycophenolate tacrolimus, or azathioprine	A
Megestrol acetate[54,100-106]	NK	B
Niacin (nicotinic acid)[54,107-109]	NK	A
Nucleoside reverse transcriptase inhibitors[54,110-119]	NK More commonly associated with stavudine, zidovudine, and didanosine	B
Oral contraceptives[120-124]	NK More common with formulations containing high-dose estrogen (>35 mcg ethinyl estradiol or equivalent) or second-generation progestin	B
Pentamidine[125-132]	NK	B
Phenytoin[133-136]	Rare	B
Protease inhibitors [32,137-144]	5% for new-onset diabetes mellitus; up to 40% for impaired glucose tolerance	B
Rifampin[145]	NK	B
Ritodrine[146-148]	NK	C
Somatostatin analogs[149-152]	14% with lanreotide; 40% pasireotide; 16–27% with octreotide For octreotide: 16% in acromegaly patients, 27% in carcinoid patients with the depot version	A

Table 30-1 Agents Implicated in Drug-Induced Hyperglycemia (continued)

Drug or Drug Class	Incidence[a]	Level of Evidence[b]
Tacrolimus[56,153-157]	Variable New-onset insulin-dependent PTDM: 20% (kidney transplant patients), 11–18% (liver transplant patients) Hyperglycemia: 22% (kidney transplant patients), 33–47% (liver transplant patients) Patients received concomitant corticosteroid therapy Lower incidence 1 year post-transplant Higher incidence with tacrolimus than with cyclosporine	A
Terbutaline[158-160]	NK	A
Thalidomide[161,162]	NK	B
Tyrosine kinase inhibitors[99,163-174]	36% with alectinib, 28% with axitinib, 37% with cabozantinib, 49% with ceritinib, 13–57% with dabrafenib, 9.8% with imatinib, NK for lenvatinib, 50% with nilotinib, 41% with pazopanib, 58% with ponatinib, 23–71% with sunitinib, 27–65% with trametinib (combination therapy with dabrafenib) Has not been reported for all agents within the drug class	A

HCTZ = hydrochlorothiazide, HMG CoA = 3-hydroxy-3-methylglutaryl-coenzyme A, NK = not known, PTDM = post-transplant diabetes mellitus.

[a]Incidence may be related to drug dose.

[b]Definitions for Levels of Evidence: Level A—evidence from one or more randomized, controlled clinical trials; Level B—evidence from nonrandomized clinical trials, prospective observational studies, cohort studies, retrospective studies, case-control studies, meta-analyses and/or postmarketing surveillance studies; and Level C—evidence from one or more published case reports or case series.

[c]Controversial: data mostly from observational studies, with some showing no association with hyperglycemia/diabetes. Many studies did not differentiate between antidepressant drug classes and those that did found differing results. Association with diabetes confounded by concomitant depression.

[d]Usually only occurs in patients with impaired glucose tolerance or diabetes mellitus. Risk is usually associated with doses >3 g/day. A 2008 Cochrane meta-analysis concluded that there were no significant changes in fasting glucose or hemoglobin A1C in randomized, placebo-controlled trials conducted in patients with type 2 diabetes.[69]

[e]Risk appears to be higher with higher potency statins and doses (highest risk with rosuvastatin). A 2013 meta-analysis calculated that the increased risk for new-onset diabetes, compared with placebo, is 25% with rosuvastatin 20 mg/day, 15% with atorvastatin 80 mg/day, and 7% with pravastatin 40 mg/day.[73]

hyperglycemia and diabetes mellitus. Agents commonly implicated in drug-induced hypoglycemia include insulin, sulfonylureas, and ethanol alone or taken concomitantly. These agents accounted for more than 70% of 1418 cases of severe hypoglycemia in a report spanning the years 1940–1989.[1] In children 2 years of age or younger, salicylate poisoning was reported to cause the majority of cases of drug-induced hypoglycemia.[1]

EPIDEMIOLOGY

The true incidence of glucose and insulin dysregulation associated with most drugs is unknown. This is due, in large part, to a lack of data from controlled clinical trials, underreporting of postmarketing events, and failure to establish causality. For some medications, the incidence of drug-induced hyperglycemia or hypoglycemia may also vary depending on the dose, frequency, and/or duration of drug administration as well as the patient's underlying disease states. For example, in the Diabetes Control and Complications Trial, the incidence of severe hypoglycemia requiring assistance associated with insulin administration was threefold higher in the intensively-treated group (insulin pump or ≥3 daily insulin injections) compared to the conventionally-treated group (1–2 daily insulin injections).[2,3] Within a specific drug class, the incidence of drug-induced hyper- or hypoglycemia also may vary. Hyperglycemia and diabetes mellitus occur more commonly in association with

Table 30-2 Agents Implicated in Drug-Induced Hypoglycemia

Drug or Drug Class	Incidence[a]	Level of Evidence[b]
Angiotensin-converting enzyme inhibitors[24,175-177]	NK	A
β-adrenergic receptor blockers[1,24,44,178-183]	NK, but likely rare Effects more commonly associated with nonselective β blockers	C
Bitter melon (*Momordica charantia*) (also commonly known as karela)[184-190]	NK	B
Dipeptidyl peptidase 4 inhibitors[191]	Rare as monotherapy, increased risk when combined with insulin or insulin secretagogue	A
Disopyramide[192-196]	NK	B
Ethanol[1,24,178,197]	NK	C
Fenugreek (*Trigonella foenum graecum*)[189,198-200]	NK	B[d]
Fluoroquinolones[201-207]	NK	B
Ginseng[189,208-211]	NK	B[c]
Glucagon-like peptide 1 receptor agonists[212]	Up to 15.9% with monotherapy Up to 42% in combination with a sulfonylurea	A
Insulin[2,25,213]	Variable: 2.76–62 episodes per 100 patient-years for severe hypoglycemia requiring assistance Higher incidence in patients with type 1 versus type 2 diabetes.	A
Ivy gourd (*Coccinia indica*)[189,214]	NK	B[c]
L-carnitine[189,215-217]	NK	B
Nonsulfonylurea secretagogues[218-220]	NK; lower incidence compared to sulfonylureas	A
Pentamidine[8,128,129,131,221-223]	6–40% with intravenous or intramuscular formulations, 1% or less with nebulized formulation	B
Pramlintide[224-226,d]	0.6–16.8% Does not cause hypoglycemia when used alone but increases risk of insulin-induced hypoglycemia (can be severe) when combined with insulin Higher incidence in patients with type 1 (5.2–16.8%) versus type 2 (0.4–8.2%) diabetes Incidence is lowered (0.9–5.7%) when the dose of preprandial insulin is decreased by 50% when initiating pramlintide	A
Quinine[178,227-232]	NK	B
Quinidine[178,227,233]	NK	B
Salicylates[1,18,178,234]	NK More common in children compared to adults Most common cause of severe hypoglycemia in children ≤2 years	B
Sodium-glucose cotransporter 2 inhibitors[235-237]	Low as monotherapy, increased risk when combined with insulin or insulin secretagogue	A
Somatostatin analogs[149-152]	9% in a study with pasireotide 2–4% with octreotide	A
Sulfamethoxazole[238-242]	NK Rare reaction with kidney disease and/or high doses	C

Table 30-2 Agents Implicated in Drug-Induced Hypoglycemia (continued)

Drug or Drug Class	Incidence[a]	Level of Evidence[b]
Sulfonylureas[1,6,213,243,e]	Variable 1.8% per year for recorded hypoglycemia, 1.23 per 100 person-years or 3.3% for severe hypoglycemia requiring medical attention	A
Tyrosine kinase inhibitors[99,165,166,172,173,244,245]	Lenvatinib >5%, 2–10% with sunitinib, 17% with pazopanib, 24% with ponatinib, 24% with vandetanib Reported but incidence not known with dasatinib, imatinib, nilotinib, and sorafenib Has not been reported for all agents within the drug class	A (lenvatinib, nilotinib, pazopanib, sunitinib, vandetanib) C (dasatinib, imatinib, and sorafenib)

NK = not known.
[a]Incidence may be related to drug dose.
[b]Definitions for Levels of Evidence: Level A—evidence from one or more randomized, controlled clinical trials; Level B—evidence from nonrandomized clinical trials, prospective observational studies, cohort studies, retrospective studies, case-control studies, meta-analyses and/or postmarketing surveillance studies; and Level C—evidence from one or more published case reports or case series.
[c]Even though there are one or more randomized, controlled clinical trials demonstrating the glucose-lowering effect of this herbal agent, a B rating for level of evidence is given because the overall effect is inconclusive.
[d]Severe hypoglycemia, if occurs, onset is usually within 2–3 hours after administration of pramlintide.
[e]Higher incidence reported with chlorpropamide and glyburide.

olanzapine and clozapine than with the other atypical antipsychotic drugs.[4,5] However, an increased background risk for diabetes mellitus associated with schizophrenia, in addition to the rising incidence of diabetes in the general population, complicate determination of precise risk estimates. The incidence of treatment-related hyperglycemia also may be higher if the patient has predisposing risk factors for diabetes mellitus, such as obesity or a family history. Hypoglycemia is more common in association with long-acting (e.g., chlorpropamide and glyburide) than shorter-acting sulfonylureas (e.g., tolbutamide).[6,7] The reported incidence of drug-induced hypoglycemia may also vary depending on the specific definition of hypoglycemia used. Additionally, factors such as the presence of active drug metabolites and the presence of other risk factors for hypoglycemia also account for the difference in reported incidences of hypoglycemia among various drugs. Finally, the route of administration and systemic availability of a drug may also influence the incidence of drug-induced hyper- or hypoglycemia. For example, inhalation of corticosteroids or pentamidine infrequently causes alterations in glucose homeostasis compared to administration via the oral or parenteral routes.[8,9]

MECHANISMS

Drugs can induce hyper- or hypoglycemia through multiple mechanisms, including alteration of insulin secretion or clearance, changes in insulin sensitivity (either directly at the receptor level or by indirect effects on weight or adiposity), changes in gluconeogenesis or glucose metabolism, and direct cytotoxic effects on pancreatic β cells. Mechanisms by which specific drugs are believed to alter glucose or insulin regulation are listed in **Table 30-3** and **Table 30-4**. With some medications, it is not clear if hyperglycemia is a direct effect of the drug itself or if the drug is simply a contributing factor, as occurs in cases when a drug unmasks a patient's pre-existing diabetes.[10]

CLINICAL PRESENTATION AND DIFFERENTIAL DIAGNOSIS

The signs and symptoms of drug-induced hyperglycemia and diabetes mellitus are listed in **Table 30-5**. The diagnosis of diabetes mellitus can be made if a patient's glycosylated hemoglobin (A1C) is ≥6.5%, the fasting plasma glucose concentration is

Table 30-3 Mechanisms of Drug-Induced Hyperglycemia[4,9,10,15,22,28,30,34-174]

Drug or Drug Class	Proposed Mechanism(s)
Antidepressants	Weight gain, ↑ cortisol, inhibits insulin signaling, inhibits insulin secretion, ↑ gluconeogenesis and glycogenolysis
Atypical antipsychotics	↓ peripheral insulin sensitivity, ↓ insulin secretion (inhibition of β-cell responsiveness via antagonism of the 5-HT_{1A} receptor), promote weight gain; may also cause hyperglycemia through drug-induced pancreatitis
β-adrenergic receptor blockers	↓ insulin secretion, ↓ insulin sensitivity; effects attenuated but not abolished with cardioselective β blockers
Calcium channel blockers[48]	↓ insulin secretion
Cyclosporine	↓ insulin production, inhibits insulin secretion, ↓ β-cell volume and function, ↑ insulin resistance
Diazoxide	↓ insulin secretion, may also ↑ glucose production and ↓ insulin sensitivity
Fish oil	Unknown
HMG CoA reductase inhibitors	↑ insulin resistance, ↓ insulin secretion
Glucocorticoids[79]	↑ gluconeogenesis, ↑ insulin resistance, ↓ insulin secretion
Gonadotropin-releasing hormone agonists	↓ testosterone concentrations leading to ↑ fat mass and ↑ insulin resistance
Growth hormone	Causes insulin resistance
Interferons	Formation of islet cell antibodies
l-asparaginase	↓ insulin synthesis
Mammalian target of rapamycin (mTOR) inhibitors	↑ insulin resistance, ↑ gluconeogenesis, chronic administration leads to pancreatic β-cell apoptosis
Megestrol acetate	↓ insulin sensitivity and promotes weight gain; binds to glucocorticoid receptor
Niacin (nicotinic acid)	↓ insulin sensitivity, ↑ hepatic gluconeogenesis
Nucleoside reverse transcriptase inhibitors	↑ insulin resistance, promote lipodystrophy; can also cause pancreatitis (more common with didanosine and stavudine) leading to β-cell injury; didanosine postulated to inhibit insulin release secondary to hypokalemia
Oral contraceptives	Estrogen-induced ↓ peripheral insulin sensitivity
Pentamidine	Direct cytolytic effects on pancreatic β cells; causes hypoglycemia initially; effect may be irreversible; can also cause pancreatitis
Phenytoin	↓ insulin secretion, may also ↓ insulin sensitivity
Protease inhibitors	↑ insulin resistance directly or indirectly, promote lipodystrophy, ↓ insulin secretion
Recombinant human growth hormone	Causes insulin resistance
Rifampin	Unknown, may ↑ intestinal absorption of glucose
Ritodrine	↑ hepatic gluconeogenesis
Somatostatin analogs	Inhibits secretion of insulin; pasireotide also ↓ GLP-1 and GIP
Tacrolimus	↓ insulin secretion, ↓ insulin sensitivity; may cause pancreatic islet cell toxicity; hyperglycemia and diabetes mellitus reported without use of concomitant corticosteroids
Terbutaline	↑ gluconeogenesis and glycogenolysis, ↓ peripheral insulin sensitivity
Thalidomide	↓ insulin-stimulated glucose uptake and glycogen synthesis
Thiazide and thiazide-like diuretics	↓ insulin release secondary to hypokalemia (hyperglycemia may be preventable through correction/prevention of hypokalemia); other mechanisms, including a direct inhibition of insulin release, ↓ insulin sensitivity, ↑ hepatic gluconeogenesis, a direct toxic effect on pancreatic β cells from increased free fatty acids, and increased sympathetic nervous system activity (contributing to hypokalemia) have also been proposed
Tyrosine kinase inhibitors	↑ insulin resistance, inhibits glycogen synthesis, activates glycogenolysis

↑ = increases, ↓ = decreases, GLP-1 = glucagon-like peptide-1, GIP = glucose-dependent insulinotropic polypeptide, HMG CoA = 3-hydroxy-3-methylglutaryl-coenzyme A, HT = hydroxytryptamine.

Table 30-4 Mechanisms of Drug-Induced Hypoglycemia[1,2,8,18,24,25,44,99,129,131,175-245]

Drug or Drug Class	Proposed Mechanism(s)
Angiotensin-converting enzyme inhibitors[177]	↑ peripheral insulin sensitivity
β-adrenergic receptor blockers	May ↑ peripheral glucose uptake and indirectly ↓ gluconeogenesis; can delay recovery from hypoglycemia; also mask many autonomic hypoglycemic symptoms
Bitter melon (*Momordica charantia*) (also commonly known as karela)	Proposed: components of extracts structurally similar to animal insulin, ↑ insulin secretion, ↑ tissue glucose uptake, ↑ hepatic glycogen synthesis, ↑ peripheral glucose oxidation in erythrocytes and adipocytes, ↓ hepatic gluconeogenesis
Dipeptidyl peptidase-4 inhibitors	Inhibit degradation of the incretin hormones GIP and GLP-1, which ↑ glucose-dependent insulin synthesis and release; GLP-1 also ↓ glucagon secretion from alpha cells in the pancreas
Disopyramide[194,196]	↑ insulin secretion
Ethanol	Inhibits hepatic gluconeogenesis, impairs activation of the HPA axis' hormonal response to hypoglycemia, and can potentiate hypoglycemic effects of other drugs; more problematic when glycogen stores are low
Fenugreek (*Trigonella foenum graecum*)	Proposed: slows carbohydrate absorption, inhibits glucose transport
Fluoroquinolones[204,207]	Unknown, may be due to stimulation of pancreatic insulin secretion and/or interaction with antidiabetic agents; most reports with gatifloxacin; resistant hypoglycemia (resolves with discontinuation only) may occur
Ginseng	Proposed: ↓ rate of carbohydrate absorption into portal hepatic circulation, ↑ glucose transport and uptake mediated by nitric oxide, ↑ glycogen storage, modulation of insulin secretion; most clinical trials done using American ginseng (*Panax quiquefoliu*)
Glucagon-like peptide 1 receptor agonists	Stimulates glucose-dependent insulin release, suppresses glucagon secretion
Insulin	↑ glucose utilization
Ivy gourd (*Coccinia indica*)	Insulin-mimetic
L-carnitine[215-217]	↑ glucose uptake and storage
Nonsulfonylurea secretagogues	↑ pancreatic insulin secretion
Pentamidine[131]	↑ insulin release through direct cytotoxic effects to pancreatic β cells
Pramlintide	Suppresses postprandial glucagon secretion, slows gastric emptying
Quinine	↑ pancreatic insulin secretion, usually with high doses or rapid IV infusion; *Plasmodium falciparum* infection itself is associated with hypoglycemia
Quinidine	↑ pancreatic insulin secretion; see quinine
Salicylates[18]	↑ pancreatic insulin secretion, ↑ peripheral glucose utilization, ↓ gluconeogenesis; usually occurs only with anti-inflammatory doses
Sodium-glucose cotransporter 2 inhibitors	Inhibits renal reabsorption of filtered glucose leading to increased urinary glucose excretion
Somatostatin analogs	Inhibits secretion of glucagon
Sulfamethoxazole	↑ pancreatic insulin secretion
Sulfonylureas	↑ pancreatic insulin secretion
Tyrosine kinase inhibitors	Unknown

↑ = increases, ↓ = decreases, GIP = glucose-dependent insulinotropic polypeptide (GIP), GLP-1 = glucagon-like peptide-1, HPA = hypothalamic-pituitary-adrenal, IV = intravenous, NK = not known.

Table 30-5 Signs and Symptoms Associated with Drug-Induced Hyperglycemia

Mild-to-moderate hyperglycemia

- Blurred vision
- Fatigue/weakness
- Polydipsia
- Polyphagia
- Polyuria
- Unexplained weight loss

Severe hyperglycemia

- Abdominal pain
- Coma
- Dehydration
- Hypokalemia
- Hypotension
- Kussmaul respiration and breath with fruity odor
- Lethargy
- Metabolic acidosis
- Muscle cramping
- Nausea and vomiting
- Obtundation

Table 30-6 Signs and Symptoms Associated with Drug-Induced Hypoglycemia

Mild-to-moderate hypoglycemia

- Dizziness
- Headache
- Hunger
- Shakiness/tremors
- Sweating/diaphoresis
- Tachycardia
- Weakness/fatigue

Severe hypoglycemia

- Behavioral changes such as anxiety and irritability
- Blurred vision
- Coma
- Confusion and difficulty concentrating
- Loss of consciousness
- Seizure

≥126 mg/dL, or the patient is found to have a plasma glucose concentration of ≥200 mg/dL 2 hours after a 75-g oral glucose load. A positive result on any of these tests should be confirmed on a separate occasion unless there is unequivocal hyperglycemia. A diagnosis can also be made if the patient has classic symptoms of diabetes and a random plasma glucose concentration of ≥200 mg/dL.[11] Depending on the causative agent, drug-induced hyperglycemia can appear within hours or weeks to months after initiation of therapy. Hyperglycemia may be severe in some cases, manifesting as diabetic ketoacidosis and hyperglycemic coma.

Although there is considerable interindividual variation, the typical signs and symptoms associated with hypoglycemia are presented in **Table 30-6**. The glycemic threshold at which patients experience hypoglycemic symptoms varies. Symptoms commonly manifest when the plasma glucose concentration falls below 60 mg/dL. However, factors such as prolonged hyperglycemia, caffeine use, or frequent episodes of hypoglycemia may shift this threshold in either direction. Patients who experience repeated episodes of hypoglycemia over a short period of time may become unaware of these events. These patients do not experience typical hypoglycemic symptoms and may fail to take corrective action as a result of central nervous system impairment.[12] Severe hypoglycemia can lead to cognitive dysfunction, mental status changes, seizures, coma, or even death.

Before implicating a drug as the cause of glucose or insulin dysregulation, other possible etiologies must be ruled out (**Table 30-7**). Hyperglycemia may occur during periods of physiologic stress such as surgery, infection, or trauma. Elevations in serum glucose concentrations associated with Cushing syndrome may result either from exogenous administration or endogenous overproduction of glucocorticoids. When assessing possible causes of hypoglycemia, intentional self-administration of hypoglycemic drugs, usually insulin or a sulfonylurea (i.e., factitious hypoglycemia), and iatrogenic causes (including medication dispensing errors) should be considered.[13] Hypoglycemia also occurs in patients with acute illness. Uncommon causes of hypoglycemia include insulin-producing tumors (e.g., an insulinoma) and several other rare disorders (**Table 30-7**). To adequately assess drug-induced causality, it is important to consider such variables as temporal sequence, biologic plausibility, and whether hyper- or hypoglycemia is a known class or drug effect in the absence of other potential confounders (e.g., concomitant diseases or medications).

Table 30-7 Conditions to Consider in the Differential Diagnoses of Drug-Induced Glucose and Insulin Dysregulation

Differential diagnoses for drug-induced hyperglycemia

- Acromegaly
- Cushing syndrome
- Diabetes mellitus
- Kidney disease
- Liver cirrhosis
- Metabolic acidosis
- Metabolic syndrome
- Pancreatitis
- Parenteral nutrition therapy (dextrose administration)
- Stress hyperglycemia

Differential diagnoses for drug-induced hypoglycemia[33,246]

- Acute kidney injury or chronic kidney disease
- Adrenal insufficiency (e.g., Addison disease, adrenal crisis)
- Alcoholism
- Beckwith-Wiedemann syndrome
- Carnitine deficiency
- Congenital hyperinsulinemic hypoglycemia of infancy
- Defective type 1 glucose transporter in the brain
- Erythroblastosis fetalis
- Factitious or iatrogenic hypoglycemia
- Galactosemia
- Glycogen storage disease
- Heart failure
- Hepatic failure
- Hereditary fructose intolerance
- Hypopituitarism
- Insulin-binding antibodies disorder
- Insulinoma
- Isolated adrenocorticotropic hormone deficiency
- Isolated growth hormone deficiency
- Lactic acidosis
- Large non- β-cell tumor
- Noninsulinoma pancreatogenous hypoglycemia syndrome
- Pancreatic islet cell hyperplasia/nesidioblastosis
- Persistent hyperinsulinemic hypoglycemia of infancy
- Postoperative following removal of pheochromocytoma
- Pseudohypoglycemia (i.e., in vitro glycolysis resulting in artifactually low glucose concentrations as observed with leukemias, polycythemia and hemolytic anemia)
- Reye syndrome
- Roux-en-Y gastric bypass (leading to pancreatic islet nesidioblastosis or insulinoma)
- Sepsis
- Small size for gestational age infants

Table 30-8 Risk Factors for Drug-Induced Hyperglycemia

- Patients with underlying risk factors for type 2 diabetes mellitus[11]
    - Age ≥45 years
    - Diagnosis of prediabetes (as per hemoglobin A1C, impaired fasting glucose, or impaired glucose tolerance)
    - First-degree relative with diabetes
    - High-density lipoprotein cholesterol <35 mg/dL (0.90 mmol/L) and/or a triglyceride concentration >250 mg/dL (2.82 mmol/L)
    - History of gestational diabetes mellitus
    - History of cardiovascular disease
    - Hypertension (≥140/90 mm Hg or on treatment for hypertension)
    - Other clinical conditions associated with insulin resistance such as severe obesity or acanthosis nigricans
    - Overweight (BMI ≥25 kg/m^2 or BMI ≥23 kg/m^2 in Asian Americans)
    - Physical inactivity
    - Polycystic ovary syndrome
    - Race/ethnicity (e.g., African-American, Latino, Native American, Asian-American, and Pacific Islander)
- Higher doses (e.g., thiazide diuretics or corticosteroids) or misuse of suspected drug
- Concomitant use of more than one drug that can induce hyperglycemia
- Drug interactions (use of drugs that may increase the plasma concentration and/or hyperglycemic effect of offending drug)

BMI = body mass index.

RISK FACTORS

Risk factors for drug-induced hyperglycemia and hypoglycemia are listed in **Table 30-8** and **Table 30-9**, respectively. Patients with type 2 diabetes mellitus or those predisposed to it (e.g., individuals with metabolic syndrome) may be at particular risk for drug-induced hyperglycemia due to worsening of pre-existing insulin resistance and β cell dysfunction. Patients with other underlying disease states also may be at increased risk. For example, hypertension and schizophrenia are associated with a higher incidence of diabetes mellitus and therefore may confound the diagnosis of drug-induced hyperglycemia.[14,15] Polymedication is another important risk factor, because the concomitant use of multiple medications associated with glucose or insulin

Table 30-9 Risk Factors for Drug-Induced Hypoglycemia

- Advanced age
- Concomitant use of more than one drug that can induce hypoglycemia
- Decreased carbohydrate intake (e.g., overnight fast, missed meals)
- Hepatic dysfunction (decreased gluconeogenesis)
- Higher doses or misuse of offending drug
- History of hypoglycemia
- Hospitalization within past 30 days
- Increased carbohydrate utilization (e.g., exercise) or reduced stores (e.g., malnutrition)
- Pharmacodynamic or pharmacokinetic interactions (e.g., increased response and/or plasma concentration of suspected drug)
- Recent or excessive alcohol intake
- Renal dysfunction (decreased insulin clearance)
- Tight glycemic control in patients with diabetes

dysregulation may lead to additive pharmacokinetic and/or pharmacodynamic effects. For example, the combined use of sulfonylureas and nonsteroidal anti-inflammatory drugs, including ibuprofen and aspirin, may lead to an increased risk of hypoglycemia due in part to decreased sulfonylurea metabolism or increased insulin release.[16-18]

MORBIDITY AND MORTALITY

Drug-induced hyperglycemia may be transient or may result in permanent changes in glucose regulation. Similar to other causes of diabetes mellitus, drug-induced hyperglycemia is believed to increase the risk of microvascular (retinopathy, neuropathy, and nephropathy) and macrovascular (atherosclerotic cardiovascular disease, cerebrovascular disease, and peripheral vascular disease) complications, delayed wound healing and resolution of infections, hyperosmolar coma, and death. Cases of diabetic ketoacidosis and death have been reported in association with many of the drugs listed in Table 30-1. Diabetic nephropathy, sensorimotor peripheral neuropathy, ketoacidosis, hyperosmolar coma or precoma, myocardial infarction, and stroke were reported in a cohort of kidney transplant recipients (followed on average for 9.3 years) who developed post-transplant diabetes mellitus. The immunosuppressive regimen prescribed for these patients consisted of cyclosporine and corticosteroids, which are known to be associated with hyperglycemia.[19] New-onset diabetes after transplantation is known to be associated with decreased graft and patient survival, and increased risk of infection and cardiovascular disease.[20,21] However, drug-induced hyperglycemia may not always lead to the development of macrovascular complications. This was evident in the Antihypertensive and Lipid-Lowering Treatment to Prevent Heart Attack Trial, a large, randomized controlled study of older hypertensive patients with and without metabolic syndrome.[22] Although the incidence of newly-diagnosed diabetes was greater in chlorthalidone-treated patients compared to those treated with either lisinopril or amlodipine, the risk of developing coronary heart disease, stroke, end-stage renal disease, and all-cause mortality did not differ significantly among groups. The systolic blood pressure was 0.8-mm Hg and 2-mm Hg lower in the chlorthalidone group compared to the amlodipine and lisinopril group, respectively.[23]

Although drug-induced hypoglycemia typically produces transient, mild-to-moderate symptoms, some patients may experience discomfort and reduced quality of life and consequently discontinue treatment due to fear of recurrent episodes. Severe hypoglycemic episodes can lead to mental status changes, seizures, loss of consciousness, permanent neurological damage, and death. Sulfonylurea-induced hypoglycemia has resulted in permanent neurological deficits in 5% of survivors and has a reported mortality rate of 10%. Furthermore, insulin-induced hypoglycemia may be responsible for approximately 2–4% of deaths reported in patients with type 1 diabetes.[24,25]

In addition to substantial morbidity and mortality, drug-induced glucose and insulin dysregulation also carries a significant economic burden. Hospitalizations and urgent care visits related to drug-induced hyper- or hypoglycemia can substantially increase healthcare costs.[26,27] Healthcare expenditures include not only direct treatment costs, but also costs associated with the investigations required to rule out nondrug-related etiologies.

Relative risks and benefits of administering medications known to cause hyper- or hypoglycemia must be weighed. For example, a meta-analysis calculated that the use of 3-hydroxy-3-methylglutaryl coenzyme A (HMG CoA) reductase inhibitors (also known as statins) may cause one new case of diabetes for every 255 patients treated for 4 years. However, 5.4 major coronary events (coronary heart disease death and nonfatal myocardial infarction) are prevented.[28] Statin therapy is recommended in patients with diabetes by both the 2017 American Diabetes Association's *Standards of Medical Care in Diabetes* guideline and the 2017 American Association of Clinical Endocrinologists and American College of Endocrinology's *Comprehensive Type 2 Diabetes Management Algorithm* to prevent atherosclerotic cardiovascular disease (ASCVD).[11,29] For patients with prediabetes, both guidelines only provide a general recommendation that the same treatment recommendations for the general population to prevent ASCVD also apply to these patients.[11,29] The Justification for the Use of Statins in Prevention: an Intervention Trial Evaluating Rosuvastatin investigated the effects of rosuvastatin 20 mg daily on the development of first major cardiovascular events. An exclusion criterion at study entry was diagnosed diabetes. The authors calculated that in patients with one or more major diabetes risk factors, for every 54 new cases of diabetes, 134 total cardiovascular events or deaths were avoided. In patients without a major diabetes risk factor, no new case of diabetes was diagnosed, and 86 total cardiovascular events or deaths were avoided.[30]

PREVENTION

Approaches for preventing drug-induced glycemic changes are listed in **Table 30-10**. Although not always possible, avoiding potentially causative drugs in high-risk patients is the best preventive strategy. The relative risks and benefits of drug therapy must be considered on a case-by-case basis. Close monitoring for signs and symptoms of abnormalities in blood glucose concentrations is essential for patients receiving drugs that may alter glucose or insulin regulation. Healthcare professionals should always inquire about their patients' use of nonprescription medications and dietary supplements, as some of these have been linked to changes in glycemic control (Tables 30-1 and 30-2). Depending on risk assessment, blood glucose concentrations should be obtained before initiating therapy with drugs known to cause glucose or insulin dysregulation and periodically thereafter. The frequency of blood glucose monitoring should be dependent upon several factors including the patient's risk for, or overt manifestations of, hypo- or hyperglycemia, provider assessment, and the availability of published guidelines from drug manufacturers or other sources. Monitoring for changes in blood glucose concentrations and clinical manifestations of hypo- or hyperglycemia also is recommended following discontinuation of medications known to induce glucose and/or insulin dysregulation.

Table 30-10 Approaches to Help Prevent Drug-Induced Glucose and Insulin Dysregulation

- Avoid or minimize concomitant administration of drugs that may have pharmacokinetic or pharmacodynamic drug interactions with potentially causative drug
- Avoid or minimize concomitant administration of more than one drug that can induce glucose and/or insulin dysregulation
- Inquire about symptoms of hyperglycemia and hypoglycemia at each office visit
- Monitor fasting plasma glucose concentration within the first few weeks after initiating high-risk drugs and regularly thereafter, especially in the presence of weight changes or pre-existing disorders of glucose metabolism; for patients taking glucocorticoids, consider also monitoring postprandial plasma glucose concentration, given the onset of action of prednisone
- Monitor weight at each office visit
- Obtain baseline fasting plasma glucose concentration prior to initiation of potentially causative drugs, particularly in patients with risk factors
- Use lowest effective dose for the shortest duration of administration if possible

MANAGEMENT

Strategies for managing drug-induced glucose and insulin dysregulation are presented in **Table 30-11**. Although discontinuation of therapy with the

Table 30-11 Management of Drug-Induced Glucose and Insulin Dysregulation

Hyperglycemia

- Administer antidiabetic medications if patient develops diabetes mellitus
- Assess glycemic control (e.g., home blood glucose monitoring, hemoglobin A1C) as appropriate
- Discontinue or reduce dose of offending drug if possible
- Implement appropriate dietary and lifestyle changes, including increased physical activity
- Use offending drug for shortest duration possible at the lowest effective dose

Hypoglycemia

- Administer treatment to reverse hypoglycemia as appropriate (e.g., glucose, dextrose, glucagon, diazoxide)
- Assess glycemic control (e.g., fasting plasma glucose concentration) as appropriate
- Discontinue or reduce dose of offending drug if possible
- Implement dietary changes (e.g., frequent, small meals)
- Use offending drug for shortest duration possible at the lowest effective dose

offending agent usually reverses the drug-induced hypo- or hyperglycemia, this strategy may not always be possible. It may not be feasible to discontinue therapy with protease inhibitors, atypical antipsychotics, or tacrolimus, for example. In some of these cases, modifying therapy to a drug less likely to affect blood glucose can be considered. For example, Spivak et al. reported a case of olanzapine-induced diabetes mellitus that resolved after therapeutic substitution with ziprasidone.[31] Also, short-term improvements in insulin resistance have been reported when a non-nucleoside reverse transcriptase inhibitor or abacavir were substituted for a protease inhibitor in patients infected with human immunodeficiency virus-1.[32]

The time required for improvement of signs and symptoms and/or return to baseline of glycemic status following discontinuation of the causative drug depends on its pharmacokinetic and/or pharmacodynamic properties. In most cases, drug-induced hyperglycemia is reversible within days, but recovery may take longer with drugs such as atypical antipsychotics, protease inhibitors, or corticosteroids that cause hyperglycemia via weight gain or peripheral insulin resistance. In some cases, the effects may be irreversible (e.g., pentamidine-induced destruction of pancreatic β cells). For agents that exhibit a dose-dependent effect on plasma glucose concentrations (e.g., corticosteroids), reducing the dose may ameliorate or reverse the drug-induced disease.

Approaches specific to the management of drug-induced glucose abnormalities have not been studied systematically and patients with drug-induced hyper- or hypoglycemia are typically managed similarly to those with diabetes or hypoglycemia, by following accepted clinical practice guidelines and/or recommendations for these conditions.[11,25,33] Patients with pre-existing diabetes may require an adjustment to their antidiabetic medications to compensate for drug-induced changes in glycemic control. Initiation or discontinuation of therapy with antidiabetic agents also may be required.

INFORMATION FOR PATIENTS

Patients receiving medications known to cause hypoglycemia or hyperglycemia should be educated regarding the associated signs and symptoms, the importance of follow-up testing, and the need for careful management and close medical supervision. Those who already have a diagnosis of diabetes should be informed that they may need to monitor their blood glucose concentrations more frequently and may require adjustments to their antidiabetic regimen. Patients should be educated about the risks and benefits of using medications known to induce glucose or insulin dysregulation and should be counseled to discontinue a potentially causative medication only under medical supervision. Patients should be further advised to inform each of their healthcare professionals about all medication use, including nonprescription medications and dietary supplements.

REFERENCES

1. Seltzer HS. Drug-induced hypoglycemia: a review of 1418 cases. *Endocrinol Metab Clin North Am.* 1989; 18:163-83.
2. The Diabetes Control and Complications Trial Research Group. The effect of intensive treatment of diabetes on the development and progression of long-term complications in insulin-dependent diabetes mellitus. *N Engl J Med.* 1993; 329:977-86.
3. The Diabetes Control and Complications Trial Research Group. Hypoglycemia in the Diabetes Control and Complications Trial. *Diabetes.* 1997; 46:271-86.

4. Fuller MA, Shermock KM, Secic M, Grogg AL. Comparative study of the development of diabetes mellitus in patients taking risperidone and olanzapine. *Pharmacotherapy*. 2003; 23:1037-43.
5. Haupt DW, Newcomer JW. Hyperglycemia and antipsychotic medications. *J Clin Psychiatry*. 2001; 62(suppl 27):15-26; discussion 40-1.
6. Krentz AJ, Ferner RE, Bailey CJ. Comparative tolerability profiles of oral antidiabetic agents. *Drug Saf*. 1994; 11:223-41.
7. Shorr RI, Ray WA, Daugherty JR, Griffin MR. Individual sulfonylureas and serious hypoglycemia in older people. *J Am Geriatr Soc*. 1996; 44:751-5.
8. Pentamidine. Micromedex 2018. http://www.micromedexsolutions.com (accessed 2018 Feb 28).
9. Keenan GF. Management of complications of glucocorticoid therapy. *Clin Chest Med*. 1997; 18:507-20.
10. Luna B, Feinglos MN. Drug-induced hyperglycemia. *JAMA*. 2001; 286:1945-8.
11. Standards of Medical Care in Diabetes-2017. *Diabetes Care*. 2017; 40(suppl 1):S1-135.
12. Cryer PE. Symptoms of hypoglycemia, thresholds for their occurrence, and hypoglycemia unawareness. *Endocrinol Metab Clin North Am*. 1999; 28:495-500, v-vi.
13. Marks V, Teale JD. Hypoglycemia: factitious and felonious. *Endocrinol Metab Clin North Am*. 1999; 28:579-601.
14. American Diabetes Association. Screening for type 2 diabetes. *Diabetes Care*. 2004; 27(suppl 1):S11-4.
15. Lindenmayer JP, Nathan AM, Smith RC. Hyperglycemia associated with the use of atypical antipsychotics. *J Clin Psychiatry*. 2001; 62(suppl 23):30-8.
16. Li J, Zhang N, Ye B et al. Non-steroidal anti-inflammatory drugs increase insulin release from beta cells by inhibiting ATP-sensitive potassium channels. *Br J Pharmacol*. 2007; 151:483-93.
17. Sone H, Takahashi A, Yamada N. Ibuprofen-related hypoglycemia in a patient receiving sulfonylurea. *Ann Intern Med*. 2001; 134:344.
18. Vierhapper H, Bratusch-Marrain P, Waldhausl W et al. type II diabetics treated with acetyl-salicylic acid. *Clin Endocrinol (Oxf)*. 1983; 18:613-9.
19. Miles AM, Sumrani N, Horowitz R et al. Diabetes mellitus after renal transplantation: as deleterious as non-transplant-associated diabetes? *Transplantation*. 1998; 65:380-4.
20. Lane JT, Dagogo-Jack S. Approach to the patient with new-onset diabetes after transplant (NODAT). *J Clin Endocrinol Metab*. 2011; 96:3289-97.
21. Wilkinson A, Davidson J, Dotta F et al. Guidelines for the treatment and management of new-onset diabetes after transplantation. *Clin Transplant*. 2005; 19:291-8.
22. Black HR, Davis B, Barzilay J et al. Metabolic and clinical outcomes in nondiabetic individuals with the metabolic syndrome assigned to chlorthalidone, amlodipine, or lisinopril as initial treatment for hypertension: a report from the Antihypertensive and Lipid-Lowering Treatment to Prevent Heart Attack Trial (ALLHAT). *Diabetes Care*. 2008; 31:353-60.
23. Major outcomes in high-risk hypertensive patients randomized to angiotensin-converting enzyme inhibitor or calcium channel blocker vs diuretic: The Antihypertensive and Lipid-Lowering Treatment to Prevent Heart Attack Trial (ALLHAT). *JAMA*. 2002; 288:2981-97.
24. Chan JC, Cockram CS, Critchley JA. Drug-induced disorders of glucose metabolism. Mechanisms and management. *Drug Saf*. 1996; 15:135-57.
25. Cryer PE, Davis SN, Shamoon H. Hypoglycemia in diabetes. *Diabetes Care*. 2003; 26:1902-12.
26. Heaton A, Martin S, Brelje T. The economic effect of hypoglycemia in a health plan. *Manag Care Interface*. 2003; 16:23-7.
27. Leese GP, Wang J, Broomhall J et al. Frequency of severe hypoglycemia requiring emergency treatment in type 1 and type 2 diabetes: a population-based study of health service resource use. *Diabetes Care*. 2003; 26:1176-80.
28. Sattar N, Preiss D, Murray HM et al. Statins and risk of incident diabetes: a collaborative meta-analysis of randomised statin trials. *Lancet*. 2010; 375:735-42.
29. American Association of Clinical Endocrinologists. https://www.aace.com/sites/all/files/diabetes-algorithm-executive-summary.pdf (accessed 2017 Mar 15).
30. Ridker PM, Pradhan A, MacFadyen JG et al. Cardiovascular benefits and diabetes risks of statin therapy in primary prevention: an analysis from the JUPITER trial. *Lancet*. 2012; 380:565-71.
31. Spivak B, Alamy SS, Jarskog LF et al. Ziprasidone alternative for olanzapine-induced hyperglycemia. *Am J Psychiatry*. 2002; 159:1606.
32. Schambelan M, Benson CA, Carr A et al. Management of metabolic complications associated with antiretroviral therapy for HIV-1 infection: recommendations of an International AIDS Society-USA panel. *J Acquir Immune Defic Syndr*. 2002; 31:257-75.
33. Cryer PE, Axelrod L, Grossman AB et al. Evaluation and management of adult hypoglycemic disorders: an Endocrine Society Clinical Practice Guideline. *J Clin Endocrinol Metab*. 2009; 94:709-28.
34. Barnard K, Peveler RC, Holt RI. Antidepressant medication as a risk factor for type 2 diabetes and impaired glucose regulation: systematic review. *Diabetes Care*. 2013; 36:3337-45.
35. Yoon JM, Cho EG, Lee HK, Park SM. Antidepressant use and diabetes mellitus risk: a meta-analysis. *Korean J Fam Med*. 2013; 34:228-40.
36. Bettinger TL, Mendelson SC, Dorson PG, Crismon ML. Olanzapine-induced glucose dysregulation. *Ann Pharmacother*. 2000; 34:865-7.
37. DuMouchel W, Fram D, Yang X et al. Antipsychotics, glycemic disorders, and life-threatening diabetic events: a Bayesian data-mining analysis of the FDA adverse event reporting system (1968–2004). *Ann Clin Psychiatry*. 2008; 20:21-31.
38. Hedenmalm K, Hagg S, Stahl M et al. Glucose intolerance with atypical antipsychotics. *Drug Saf*. 2002; 25:1107-16.
39. Henderson DC. Atypical antipsychotic-induced diabetes mellitus: how strong is the evidence? *CNS Drugs*. 2002; 16:77-89.
40. Koller EA, Doraiswamy PM. Olanzapine-associated diabetes mellitus. *Pharmacotherapy*. 2002; 22:841-52.
41. Logue DD, Gonzalez N, Heligman SD et al. Hyperglycemia in a 7-year-old child treated with aripiprazole. *Am J Psychiatry*. 2007; 164:173.
42. Yang SH, McNeely MJ. Rhabdomyolysis, pancreatitis, and hyperglycemia with ziprasidone. *Am J Psychiatry*. 2002; 159:1435.
43. Gress TW, Nieto FJ, Shahar E et al. Hypertension and antihypertensive therapy as risk factors for type 2 diabetes mellitus: Atherosclerosis Risk in Communities Study. *N Engl J Med*. 2000; 342:905-12.
44. Majumdar SR. Beta-blockers for the treatment of hypertension in patients with diabetes: exploring the contraindication myth. *Cardiovasc Drugs Ther*. 1999; 13:435-9.
45. Wicklmayr M, Rett K, Dietze G, Mehnert H. Effects of beta-blocking agents on insulin secretion and glucose disposal. *Horm Metab Res*. 1990; 22:29-33.
46. Fonseca VA. Effects of beta-blockers on glucose and lipid metabolism. *Curr Med Res Opin*. 2010; 26:615-29.
47. Bhatnagar SK, Amin MM, Al-Yusuf AR. Diabetogenic effects of nifedipine. *Br Med J (Clin Res Ed)*. 1984; 289:19.
48. Hedner T, Samuelsson O, Lindholm L. Effects of antihypertensive therapy on glucose tolerance: focus on calcium antagonists. *J Intern Med Suppl*. 1991; 735:101-11.
49. Roth A, Miller HI, Belhassen B, Laniado S. Slow-release verapamil and hyperglycemic metabolic acidosis. *Ann Intern Med*. 1989; 110:171-2.
50. Levine M, Boyer EW, Pozner CN et al. Assessment of hyperglycemia after calcium channel blocker overdoses involving diltiazem or verapamil. *Crit Care Med*. 2007; 35:2071-5.
51. Bhattacharyya J, Das KP. Aggregation of insulin by chlorpromazine. *Biochem Pharmacol*. 2001; 62:1293-7.

52. Erle G, Basso M, Federspil G et al. Effect of chlorpromazine on blood glucose and plasma insulin in man. *Eur J Clin Pharmacol.* 1977; 11:15-8.
53. Boudreaux JP, McHugh L, Canafax DM et al. The impact of cyclosporine and combination immunosuppression on the incidence of posttransplant diabetes in renal allograft recipients. *Transplantation.* 1987; 44:376-81.
54. Comi RJ. Drug-induced diabetes mellitus. In: Olefsky JM, ed. *Diabetes mellitus: a fundamental and clinical text.* Baltimore, MD: Lippincott Williams and Wilkins, 2000:582-8.
55. Jindal RM, Sidner RA, Milgrom ML. Post-transplant diabetes mellitus. The role of immunosuppression. *Drug Saf.* 1997; 16:242-57.
56. Vanrenterghem YF. Which calcineurin inhibitor is preferred in renal transplantation: tacrolimus or cyclosporine? *Curr Opin Nephrol Hypertens.* 1999; 8:669-74.
57. Altszuler N, Moraru E, Hampshire J. On the mechanism of diazoxide-induced hyperglycemia. *Diabetes.* 1977; 26:931-5.
58. Charles MA, Danforth E Jr. Nonketoacidotic hyperglycemia and coma during intravenous diazoxide therapy in uremia. *Diabetes.* 1971; 20:501-3.
59. Fajans SS, Floyd JC Jr, Thiffault CA et al. Further studies on diazoxide suppression of insulin release from abnormal and normal islet tissue in man. *Ann N Y Acad Sci.* 1968; 150:261-80.
60. Updike SJ, Harrington AR. Acute diabetes ketoacidosis—a complication of intravenous diazoxide treatment for refractory hypertension. *N Engl J Med.* 1969; 280:768.
61. Amery A, Berthaux P, Bulpitt C et al. Glucose intolerance during diuretic therapy: results of trial by the European Working Party on Hypertension in the Elderly. *Lancet.* 1978; 1:681-3.
62. Barzilay JI, Davis BR, Cutler JA et al. Fasting glucose levels and incident diabetes mellitus in older nondiabetic adults randomized to receive 3 different classes of antihypertensive treatment: a report from the Antihypertensive and Lipid-Lowering Treatment to Prevent Heart Attack Trial (ALLHAT). *Arch Intern Med.* 2006; 166:2191-201.
63. Fonseca V, Phear DN. Hyperosmolar non-ketotic diabetic syndrome precipitated by treatment with diuretics. *Br Med J (Clin Res Ed).* 1982; 284:36-7.
64. Rowe PA, Mather HG. Hyperosmolar non-ketotic diabetes mellitus associated with metolazone. *Br Med J (Clin Res Ed).* 1985; 291:25-6.
65. Carter BL, Einhorn PT, Brands M et al. Thiazide-induced dysglycemia: call for research from a working group from the national heart, lung, and blood institute. *Hypertension.* 2008; 52:30-6.
66. Zillich AJ, Garg J, Basu S et al. Thiazide diuretics, potassium, and the development of diabetes: a quantitative review. *Hypertension.* 2006; 48:219-24.
67. Friday KE, Childs MT, Tsunehara CH et al. Elevated plasma glucose and lowered triglyceride levels from omega-3 fatty acid supplementation in type II diabetes. *Diabetes Care.* 1989; 12:276-81.
68. Glauber H, Wallace P, Griver K at al. Adverse metabolic effect of omega-3 fatty acids in non-insulin-dependent diabetes mellitus. *Ann Intern Med.* 1988; 108:663-8.
69. Hartweg J, Perera R, Montori V et al. Omega-3 polyunsaturated fatty acids (PUFA) for type 2 diabetes mellitus. *Cochrane Database Syst Rev.* 2008:CD003205.
70. Kris-Etherton PM, Harris WS, Appel LJ. Fish consumption, fish oil, omega-3 fatty acids, and cardiovascular disease. *Circulation.* 2002; 106:2747-57.
71. Stacpoole PW, Alig J, Ammon L, Crockett SE. Dose-response effects of dietary marine oil on carbohydrate and lipid metabolism in normal subjects and patients with hypertriglyceridemia. *Metabolism.* 1989; 38:946-56.
72. Chogtu B, Magazine R, Bairy KL. Statin use and risk of diabetes mellitus. *World J Diabetes.* 2015; 6:352-7.
73. Navarese EP, Buffon A, Andreotti F et al. Meta-analysis of impact of different types and doses of statins on new-onset diabetes mellitus. *Am J Cardiol.* 2013; 111:1123-30.
74. Prednisone. Micromedex 2018. http://www.micromedexsolutions.com (accessed 2018 Feb 28).
75. Braithwaite SS, Barr WG, Rahman A, Quddusi S. Managing diabetes during glucocorticoid therapy. How to avoid metabolic emergencies. *Postgrad Med.* 1998; 104:163-6, 171, 175-6.
76. Faul JL, Tormey W, Tormey V, Burke C. High dose inhaled corticosteroids and dose dependent loss of diabetic control. *BMJ.* 1998; 317:1491.
77. Gurwitz JH, Bohn RL, Glynn RJ et al. Glucocorticoids and the risk for initiation of hypoglycemic therapy. *Arch Intern Med.* 1994; 154:97-101.
78. Hoogwerf B, Danese RD. Drug selection and the management of corticosteroid-related diabetes mellitus. *Rheum Dis Clin North Am.* 1999; 25:489-505.
79. Schacke H, Docke WD, Asadullah K. Mechanisms involved in the side effects of glucocorticoids. *Pharmacol Ther.* 2002; 96:23-43.
80. Sobngwi E, Lubin V, Ury P et al. Adrenal insufficiency and diabetes mellitus secondary to the use of topical corticosteroids for cosmetic purpose. *Ann Endocrinol (Paris).* 2003; 64:202-4.
81. Blackburn D, Hux J, Mamdani M. Quantification of the risk of corticosteroid-induced diabetes mellitus among the elderly. *J Gen Intern Med.* 2002; 17:717-20.
82. Zoladex [package insert]. Wilmington, DE: AstraZeneca Pharmaceuticals LP; February 2016.
83. Keating NL, O'Malley A, Freedland SJ, Smith MR. Diabetes and cardiovascular disease during androgen deprivation therapy: observational study of veterans with prostate cancer. *J Natl Cancer Inst.* 2012; 104:1518-23.
84. Keating NL, O'Malley AJ, Freedland SJ, Smith MR. Diabetes and cardiovascular disease during androgen deprivation therapy: observational study of veterans with prostate cancer. *J Natl Cancer Inst.* 2010; 102:39-46.
85. Botero D, Danon M, Brown RS. Symptomatic non-insulin-dependent diabetes mellitus during therapy with recombinant human growth hormone. *J Pediatr.* 1993; 123:590-2.
86. Schauster AC, Geletko SM, Mikolich DJ. Diabetes mellitus associated with recombinant human growth hormone for HIV wasting syndrome. *Pharmacotherapy.* 2000; 20:1129-34.
87. INTRON [package insert]. A solution for injection, interferon alfa-2b recombinant solution for injection. Kenilworth, NJ: Schering Corporation; 2007.
88. Campbell S, McLaren EH, Danesh BJ. Rapidly reversible increase in insulin requirement with interferon. *BMJ.* 1996; 313:92.
89. Lopes EP, Oliveira PM, Silva AE et al. Exacerbation of type 2 diabetes mellitus during interferon-alfa therapy for chronic hepatitis B. *Lancet.* 1994; 343:244.
90. Cetin M, Yetgin S, Kara A et al. Hyperglycemia, ketoacidosis and other complications of L-asparaginase in children with acute lymphoblastic leukemia. *J Med.* 1994; 25:219-29.
91. Dacou-Voutetakis C, Palis J, Haidas S et al. Abnormal glucose tolerance in children with acute leukemia. Effect of induction chemotherapy including L-asparaginase. *Am J Pediatr Hematol Oncol.* 1983; 5:139-46.
92. Jaffe N. Diabetes mellitus secondary to L-asparaginase therapy. *J Pediatr.* 1972; 81:1220-1.
93. Pui CH, Burghen GA, Bowman WP, Aur RJ. Risk factors for hyperglycemia in children with leukemia receiving L-asparaginase and prednisone. *J Pediatr.* 1981; 99:46-50.
94. Rovira A, Cordido F, Vecilla C et al. Study of beta-cell function and erythrocyte insulin receptors in a patient with diabetic ketoacidosis associated with L-asparaginase therapy. *Acta Paediatr Scand.* 1986; 75:670-1.
95. Uysal K, Uguz A, Olgun N et al. Hyperglycemia and acute parotitis related to L-asparaginase therapy. *J Pediatr Endocrinol Metab.* 1996; 9:627-9.
96. Afinitor [package insert]. East Hanover, NJ: Novartis Pharmaceuticals Corporation; June 2016.

97. Johnston O, Rose CL, Webster AC, Gill JS. Sirolimus is associated with new-onset diabetes in kidney transplant recipients. *J Am Soc Nephrol.* 2008; 19:1411-8.
98. Torisel [package insert]. New York: Pfizer; February 2015.
99. Verges B, Walter T, Cariou B. Endocrine side effects of anti-cancer drugs: effects of anti-cancer targeted therapies on lipid and glucose metabolism. *Eur J Endocrinol.* 2014; 170:R43-55.
100. Gonzalez Del Valle L, Herrero Ambrosio A, Martinez Hernandez P et al. Hyperglycemia induced by megestrol acetate in a patient with AIDS. *Ann Pharmacother.* 1996; 30:1113-4.
101. Henry K, Rathgaber S, Sullivan C, McCabe K. Diabetes mellitus induced by megestrol acetate in a patient with AIDS and cachexia. *Ann Intern Med.* 1992; 116:53-4.
102. Jain P, Girardi LS, Sherman L et al. Insulin resistance and development of diabetes mellitus associated with megestrol acetate therapy. *Postgrad Med J.* 1996; 72:365-7.
103. Kilby JM, Tabereaux PB. Severe hyperglycemia in an HIV clinic: preexisting versus drug-associated diabetes mellitus. *J Acquir Immune Defic Syndr Hum Retrovirol.* 1998; 17:46-50.
104. Mann M, Koller E, Murgo A et al. Glucocorticoidlike activity of megestrol. A summary of Food and Drug Administration experience and a review of the literature. *Arch Intern Med.* 1997; 157:1651-6.
105. Panwalker AP. Hyperglycemia induced by megestrol acetate. *Ann Intern Med.* 1992; 116:878.
106. Salinas I, Lucas A, Clotet B. Secondary diabetes induced by megestrol acetate therapy in a patient with AIDS-associated cachexia. *AIDS.* 1993; 7:894.
107. Garg A, Grundy SM. Nicotinic acid as therapy for dyslipidemia in non-insulin-dependent diabetes mellitus. *JAMA.* 1990; 264:723-6.
108. Grundy SM, Vega GL, McGovern ME et al. Efficacy, safety, and tolerability of once-daily niacin for the treatment of dyslipidemia associated with type 2 diabetes: results of the assessment of diabetes control and evaluation of the efficacy of Niaspan trial. *Arch Intern Med.* 2002; 162:1568-76.
109. Schwartz ML. Severe reversible hyperglycemia as a consequence of niacin therapy. *Arch Intern Med.* 1993; 153:2050-2.
110. De Wit S, Sabin CA, Weber R et al. Incidence and risk factors for new-onset diabetes in HIV-infected patients: the Data Collection on Adverse Events of Anti-HIV Drugs (D:A:D) study. *Diabetes Care.* 2008; 31:1224-9.
111. Albrecht H, Stellbrink HJ, Arasteh K. Didanosine-induced disorders of glucose tolerance. *Ann Intern Med.* 1993; 119:1050.
112. Garcia-Benayas T, Rendon AL, Rodriguez-Novoa S et al. Higher risk of hyperglycemia in HIV-infected patients treated with didanosine plus tenofovir. *AIDS Res Hum Retroviruses.* 2006; 22:333-7.
113. Munshi MN, Martin RE, Fonseca VA. Hyperosmolar nonketotic diabetic syndrome following treatment of human immunodeficiency virus infection with didanosine. *Diabetes Care.* 1994; 17:316-7.
114. Brambilla AM, Novati R, Calori G et al. Stavudine or indinavir-containing regimens are associated with an increased risk of diabetes mellitus in HIV-infected individuals. *AIDS.* 2003; 17:1993-5.
115. Ertekin V, Selimoglu MA, Orbak Z. Effects of lamivudine therapy on the glucose metabolism in children with chronic hepatitis B: first year follow-up results. *Eur J Gastroenterol Hepatol.* 2005; 17:655-9.
116. Hammer SM, Squires KE, Hughes MD et al. A controlled trial of two nucleoside analogues plus indinavir in persons with human immunodeficiency virus infection and CD4 cell counts of 200 per cubic millimeter or less. AIDS Clinical Trials Group 320 Study Team. *N Engl J Med.* 1997; 337:725-33.
117. Leow MK, Addy CL, Mantzoros CS. Clinical review 159: Human immunodeficiency virus/highly active antiretroviral therapy-associated metabolic syndrome: clinical presentation, pathophysiology, and therapeutic strategies. *J Clin Endocrinol Metab.* 2003; 88:1961-76.
118. Modest GA, Fuller J. Abacavir and diabetes. *N Engl J Med.* 2001; 344:142-4.
119. Panel on Antiretroviral Guidelines for Adults and Adolescents. Guidelines for the use of antiretroviral agents in HIV-1-infected adults and adolescents. Department of Health and Human Services. http://www.aidsinfo.nih.gov/ContentFiles/AdultandAdolescentGL.pdf (accessed 2018 Jan 23).
120. Chasan-Taber L, Willett WC, Stampfer MJ et al. A prospective study of oral contraceptives and NIDDM among US women. *Diabetes Care.* 1997; 20:330-5.
121. Godsland IF, Crook D, Simpson R et al. The effects of different formulations of oral contraceptive agents on lipid and carbohydrate metabolism. *N Engl J Med.* 1990; 323:1375-81.
122. Godsland IF, Walton C, Felton C et al. Insulin resistance, secretion, and metabolism in users of oral contraceptives. *J Clin Endocrinol Metab.* 1992; 74:64-70.
123. Kim C, Siscovick DS, Sidney S et al. Oral contraceptive use and association with glucose, insulin, and diabetes in young adult women: the CARDIA Study. Coronary Artery Risk Development in Young Adults. *Diabetes Care.* 2002; 25:1027-32.
124. Rimm EB, Manson JE, Stampfer MJ et al. Oral contraceptive use and the risk of type 2 (non-insulin-dependent) diabetes mellitus in a large prospective study of women. *Diabetologia.* 1992; 35:967-72.
125. Assan R, Perronne C, Assan D et al. Pentamidine-induced derangements of glucose homeostasis. Determinant roles of renal failure and drug accumulation. A study of 128 patients. *Diabetes Care.* 1995; 18:47-55.
126. Chen JP, Braham RL, Squires KE. Diabetes after aerosolized pentamidine. *Ann Intern Med.* 1991; 114:913-4.
127. Coyle P, Carr AD, Depczynski BB, Chisholm DJ. Diabetes mellitus associated with pentamidine use in HIV-infected patients. *Med J Aust.* 1996; 165:587-8.
128. Herchline TE, Plouffe JF, Para MF. Diabetes mellitus presenting with ketoacidosis following pentamidine therapy in patients with acquired immunodeficiency syndrome. *J Infect.* 1991; 22:41-4.
129. Perronne C, Bricaire F, Leport C et al. Hypoglycaemia and diabetes mellitus following parenteral pentamidine mesylate treatment in AIDS patients. *Diabet Med.* 1990; 7:585-9.
130. Shen M, Orwoll ES, Conte JE Jr, Prince MJ. Pentamidine-induced pancreatic beta-cell dysfunction. *Am J Med.* 1989; 86:726-8.
131. Uzzan B, Bentata M, Campos J et al. Effects of aerosolized pentamidine on glucose homeostasis and insulin secretion in HIV-positive patients: a controlled study. *AIDS.* 1995; 9:901-7.
132. Zuger A, Wolf BZ, el-Sadr W et al. Pentamidine-associated fatal acute pancreatitis. *JAMA.* 1986; 256:2383-5.
133. al-Rubeaan K, Ryan EA. Phenytoin-induced insulin insensitivity. *Diabet Med.* 1991; 8:968-70.
134. Banner W Jr, Johnson DG, Walson PD, Jung D. Effects of single large doses of phenytoin on glucose homeostasis—a preliminary report. *J Clin Pharmacol.* 1982; 22:79-81.
135. Carter BL, Small RE, Mandel MD, Starkman MT. Phenytoin-induced hyperglycemia. *Am J Hosp Pharm.* 1981; 38:1508-12.
136. Fariss BL, Lutcher CL. Diphenylhydantoin-induced hyperglycemia and impaired insulin release. Effect of dosage. *Diabetes.* 1971; 20:177-81.
137. Gomez-Vera J, de Alarcon A, Jimenez-Mejias ME et al. Hyperglycemia associated with protease inhibitors in HIV-1-infected patients. *Clin Microbiol Infect.* 2000; 6:391-4.
138. Justman JE, Benning L, Danoff A et al. Protease inhibitor use and the incidence of diabetes mellitus in a large cohort of HIV-infected women. *J Acquir Immune Defic Syndr.* 2003; 32:298-302.
139. Kaufman MB, Simionatto C. A review of protease inhibitor-induced hyperglycemia. *Pharmacotherapy.* 1999; 19:114-7.
140. Koster JC, Remedi MS, Qiu H et al. HIV protease inhibitors acutely impair glucose-stimulated insulin release. *Diabetes.* 2003; 52:1695-700.

141. Mehta SH, Moore RD, Thomas DL et al. The effect of HAART and HCV infection on the development of hyperglycemia among HIV-infected persons. *J Acquir Immune Defic Syndr.* 2003; 33:577-84.
142. Noor MA, Lo JC, Mulligan K et al. Metabolic effects of indinavir in healthy HIV-seronegative men. *AIDS.* 2001; 15:F11-8.
143. Noor MA, Seneviratne T, Aweeka FT et al. Indinavir acutely inhibits insulin-stimulated glucose disposal in humans: a randomized, placebo-controlled study. *AIDS.* 2002; 16:F1-8.
144. Tsiodras S, Mantzoros C, Hammer S, Samore M. Effects of protease inhibitors on hyperglycemia, hyperlipidemia, and lipodystrophy: a 5-year cohort study. *Arch Intern Med.* 2000; 160:2050-6.
145. Takasu N, Yamada T, Miura H et al. Rifampicin-induced early phase hyperglycemia in humans. *Am Rev Respir Dis.* 1982; 125:23-7.
146. Mordes D, Kreutner K, Metzger W, Colwell JA. Dangers of intravenous ritodrine in diabetic patients. *JAMA.* 1982; 248:973-5.
147. Richards SR, Klingelberger CE. Intravenous ritodrine as a possibly provocative predictive test in gestational diabetes. A case report. *J Reprod Med.* 1987; 32:798-800.
148. Steel JM, Parboosingh J. Insulin requirements in pregnant diabetics with premature labour controlled by ritodrine. *Br Med J.* 1977; 1:880.
149. Somatuline Depot [package insert]. Basking Ridge, NJ: Ipsen Biopharmaceuticals Inc; December 2014.
150. Signifor [package insert]. East Hanover, NJ: Novartis Pharmaceuticals Corporation; December 2012.
151. Sandostatin [package insert]. East Hanover, NJ: Novartis Pharmaceuticals Corporation; March 2012.
152. Sandostatin LAR Depot [package insert]. East Hanover, NJ: Novartis Pharmaceuticals Corporation; 2013.
153. Dmitrewski J, Krentz AJ, Mayer AD et al. Metabolic and hormonal effects of tacrolimus (FK506) or cyclosporin immunosuppression following renal transplantation. *Diabetes Obes Metab.* 2001; 3:287-92.
154. Gonwa T, Johnson C, Ahsan N et al. Randomized trial of tacrolimus + mycophenolate mofetil or azathioprine versus cyclosporine + mycophenolate mofetil after cadaveric kidney transplantation: results at three years. *Transplantation.* 2003; 75:2048-53.
155. Mayer AD, Dmitrewski J, Squifflet JP et al. Multicenter randomized trial comparing tacrolimus (FK506) and cyclosporine in the prevention of renal allograft rejection: a report of the European Tacrolimus Multicenter Renal Study Group. *Transplantation.* 1997; 64:436-43.
156. Pirsch JD, Miller J, Deierhoi MH et al. A comparison of tacrolimus (FK506) and cyclosporine for immunosuppression after cadaveric renal transplantation. FK506 Kidney Transplant Study Group. *Transplantation.* 1997; 63:977-83.
157. Weir MR, Fink JC. Risk for posttransplant diabetes mellitus with current immunosuppressive medications. *Am J Kidney Dis.* 1999; 34:1-13.
158. Peterson A, Peterson K, Tongen S et al. Glucose intolerance as a consequence of oral terbutaline treatment for preterm labor. *J Fam Pract.* 1993; 36:25-31.
159. Regenstein AC, Belluomini J, Katz M. Terbutaline tocolysis and glucose intolerance. *Obstet Gynecol.* 1993; 81:739-41.
160. Smigaj D, Roman-Drago NM, Amini SB et al. The effect of oral terbutaline on maternal glucose metabolism and energy expenditure in pregnancy. *Am J Obstet Gynecol.* 1998; 178:1041-7.
161. Iqbal N, Zayed M, Boden G. Thalidomide impairs insulin action on glucose uptake and glycogen synthesis in patients with type 2 diabetes. *Diabetes Care.* 2000; 23:1172-6.
162. Pathak RD, Jayaraj K, Blonde L. Thalidomide-associated hyperglycemia and diabetes: case report and review of literature. *Diabetes Care.* 2003; 26:1322-3.
163. Tafinlar [package insert]. East Hanover, NJ: Novartis Pharmaceuticals Corporation; June 2016.
164. Villadolid J, Ersek JL, Fong MK et al. Management of hyperglycemia from epidermal growth factor receptor (EGFR) tyrosine kinase inhibitors (TKIs) targeting T790M-mediated resistance. *Transl Lung Cancer Res.* 2015; 4:576-83.
165. Sutent [package insert]. New York: Pfizer Inc; April 2015.
166. Tasigna [package insert]. East Hanover, NJ: Novartis Pharmaceuticals Corporation; January 2015.
167. Alecensa [package insert]. San Francisco: Genenetch Inc; December 2015.
168. Inlyta [package insert]. New York: Pfizer; August 2014.
169. Carbometyx [package insert]. San Francisco, CA: Exelixis Inc; April 2016.
170. Zykadia [package insert]. East Hanover, NJ: Novartis Pharmaceuticals Corporation; July 2015.
171. Gleevec [package insert]. East Hanover, NJ: Novartis Pharmaceuticals Corporation; January 2015.
172. Lenvima [package insert]. Woodcliff Lake, NJ: Eisai Inc; May 2016.
173. Iclusig [package insert]. Cambridge, MA: ARIAD Pharmaceuticals Inc; August 2016.
174. Mekinist [package insert]. Research Triangle Park, NC: GlaxoSmithKline; November 2015.
175. Herings RM, de Boer A, Stricker BH et al. Hypoglycaemia associated with use of inhibitors of angiotensin converting enzyme. *Lancet.* 1995; 345:1195-8.
176. Morris AD, Boyle DI, McMahon AD et al. ACE inhibitor use is associated with hospitalization for severe hypoglycemia in patients with diabetes. DARTS/MEMO Collaboration. Diabetes Audit and Research in Tayside, Scotland. Medicines Monitoring Unit. *Diabetes Care.* 1997; 20:1363-7.
177. Vuorinen-Markkola H, Yki-Jarvinen H. Antihypertensive therapy with enalapril improves glucose storage and insulin sensitivity in hypertensive patients with non-insulin-dependent diabetes mellitus. *Metabolism.* 1995; 44:85-9.
178. Marks V, Teale JD. Drug-induced hypoglycemia. *Endocrinol Metab Clin North Am.* 1999; 28:555-77.
179. Mills GA, Horn JR. Beta-blockers and glucose control. *Drug Intell Clin Pharm.* 1985; 19:246-51.
180. Shorr RI, Ray WA, Daugherty JR, Griffin MR. Antihypertensives and the risk of serious hypoglycemia in older persons using insulin or sulfonylureas. *JAMA.* 1997; 278:40-3.
181. Brown DR, Brown MJ. Hypoglycemia associated with preoperative metoprolol administration. *Anesth Analg.* 2004; 99:1427-8; table of contents.
182. Bush GH, Steward DJ. Severe hypoglycaemia associated with preoperative fasting and intraoperative propranolol. A case report and discussion. *Paediatr Anaesth.* 1996; 6:415-7.
183. McLindon JP, Babbs C, Gordon C et al. Profound hypoglycaemia induced by propranolol in a patient with hepatic cirrhosis and severe hyperandrogenaemia. *Ann Clin Biochem.* 1995; 32(pt 3): 334-6.
184. Aslam M, Stockley IH. Interaction between curry ingredient (karela) and drug (chlorpropamide). *Lancet.* 1979; 1:607.
185. Basch E, Gabardi S, Ulbricht C. Bitter melon (Momordica charantia): a review of efficacy and safety. *Am J Health-Syst Pharm.* 2003; 60:356-9.
186. Leatherdale BA, Panesar RK, Singh G et al. Improvement in glucose tolerance due to Momordica charantia (karela). *Br Med J (Clin Res Ed).* 1981; 282:1823-4.
187. Pitchumoni CS. Karela and blood sugar. *Lancet.* 1979; 1:924-5.
188. Welihinda J, Karunanayake EH, Sheriff MH, Jayasinghe KS. Effect of Momordica charantia on the glucose tolerance in maturity onset diabetes. *J Ethnopharmacol.* 1986; 17:277-82.
189. Yeh GY, Eisenberg DM, Kaptchuk TJ, Phillips RS. Systematic review of herbs and dietary supplements for glycemic control in diabetes. *Diabetes Care.* 2003; 26:1277-94.

190. Dans AM, Villarruz MV, Jimeno CA et al. The effect of Momordica charantia capsule preparation on glycemic control in type 2 diabetes mellitus needs further studies. *J Clin Epidemiol.* 2007; 60:554-9.
191. Januvia [package insert]. Whitehouse Station, NJ: Merck and Co; August 2015.
192. Cacoub P, Deray G, Baumelou A et al. Disopyramide-induced hypoglycemia: case report and review of the literature. *Fundam Clin Pharmacol.* 1989; 3:527-35.
193. Hasegawa J, Mori A, Yamamoto R et al. Disopyramide decreases the fasting serum glucose level in man. *Cardiovasc Drugs Ther.* 1999; 13:325-7.
194. Hayashi S, Horie M, Tsuura Y et al. Disopyramide blocks pancreatic ATP-sensitive K+ channels and enhances insulin release. *Am J Physiol.* 1993; 265:C337-42.
195. Reynolds RM, Walker JD. Hypoglycaemia induced by disopyramide in a patient with Type 2 diabetes mellitus. *Diabet Med.* 2001; 18:1009-10.
196. Smith RC, Sullivan M, Geller J. Inadequate adrenergic response to disopyramide-induced hypoglycemia. *Ann Pharmacother.* 1992; 26:490-1.
197. Jain H, Beriwal S, Singh S. Alcohol induced ketoacidosis, severe hypoglycemia and irreversible encephalopathy. *Med Sci Monit.* 2002; 8:CS77-9.
198. Madar Z, Abel R, Samish S, Arad J. Glucose-lowering effect of fenugreek in non-insulin dependent diabetics. *Eur J Clin Nutr.* 1988; 42:51-4.
199. Sharma RD, Raghuram TC, Rao NS. Effect of fenugreek seeds on blood glucose and serum lipids in type I diabetes. *Eur J Clin Nutr.* 1990; 44:301-6.
200. Gupta A, Gupta R, Lal B. Effect of Trigonella foenum-graecum (fenugreek) seeds on glycaemic control and insulin resistance in type 2 diabetes mellitus: a double blind placebo controlled study. *J Assoc Physicians India.* 2001; 49:1057-61.
201. Mehlhorn AJ, Brown DA. Safety concerns with fluoroquinolones. *Ann Pharmacother.* 2007; 41:1859-66.
202. Tequin [package insert]. Princeton, NJ: Bristol-Myers Squibb Company; July 2003.
203. Baker SE, Hangii MC. Possible gatifloxacin-induced hypoglycemia. *Ann Pharmacother.* 2002; 36:1722-6.
204. Gajjar DA, LaCreta FP, Kollia GD et al. Effect of multiple-dose gatifloxacin or ciprofloxacin on glucose homeostasis and insulin production in patients with noninsulin-dependent diabetes mellitus maintained with diet and exercise. *Pharmacotherapy.* 2000; 20:76S-86S.
205. LeBlanc M, Belanger C, Cossette P. Severe and resistant hypoglycemia associated with concomitant gatifloxacin and glyburide therapy. *Pharmacotherapy.* 2004; 24:926-31.
206. Roberge RJ, Kaplan R, Frank R, Fore C. Glyburide-ciprofloxacin interaction with resistant hypoglycemia. *Ann Emerg Med.* 2000; 36:160-3.
207. Saraya A, Yokokura M, Gonoi T, Seino S. Effects of fluoroquinolones on insulin secretion and beta-cell ATP-sensitive K(+) channels. *Eur J Pharmacol.* 2004; 497:111-7.
208. Sotaniemi EA, Haapakoski E, Rautio A. Ginseng therapy in non-insulin-dependent diabetic patients. *Diabetes Care.* 1995; 18:1373-5.
209. Vuksan V, Sievenpiper JL, Koo VY et al. American ginseng (Panax quinquefolius L) reduces postprandial glycemia in nondiabetic subjects and subjects with type 2 diabetes mellitus. *Arch Intern Med.* 2000; 160:1009-13.
210. Vuksan V, Sievenpiper JL, Wong J et al. American ginseng (Panax quinquefolius L.) attenuates postprandial glycemia in a time-dependent but not dose-dependent manner in healthy individuals. *Am J Clin Nutr.* 2001; 73:753-8.
211. Vuksan V, Stavro MP, Sievenpiper JL et al. Similar postprandial glycemic reductions with escalation of dose and administration time of American ginseng in type 2 diabetes. *Diabetes Care.* 2000; 23:1221-6.
212. Trujillo JM, Nuffer W, Ellis SL. GLP-1 receptor agonists: a review of head-to-head clinical studies. *Ther Adv Endocrinol Metab.* 2015; 6:19-28.
213. Shorr RI, Ray WA, Daugherty JR, Griffin MR. Incidence and risk factors for serious hypoglycemia in older persons using insulin or sulfonylureas. *Arch Intern Med.* 1997; 157:1681-6.
214. Khan AK, S AK, Mahtab H. Treatment of diabetes mellitus with Coccinia indica. *Br Med J.* 1980; 280:1044.
215. Capaldo B, Napoli R, Di Bonito P et al. Carnitine improves peripheral glucose disposal in non-insulin-dependent diabetic patients. *Diabetes Res Clin Pract.* 1991; 14:191-5.
216. De Gaetano A, Mingrone G, Castagneto M, Calvani M. Carnitine increases glucose disposal in humans. *J Am Coll Nutr.* 1999; 18:289-95.
217. Mingrone G, Greco AV, Capristo E et al. L-carnitine improves glucose disposal in type 2 diabetic patients. *J Am Coll Nutr.* 1999; 18:77-82.
218. Davies MJ. Insulin secretagogues. *Curr Med Res Opin.* 2002; 18(suppl 1):s22-30.
219. Hirshberg B, Skarulis MC, Pucino F et al. Repaglinide-induced factitious hypoglycemia. *J Clin Endocrinol Metab.* 2001; 86:475-7.
220. Nagai T, Imamura M, Iizuka K, Mori M. Hypoglycemia due to nateglinide administration in diabetic patient with chronic renal failure. *Diabetes Res Clin Pract.* 2003; 59:191-4.
221. Karboski JA, Godley PJ. Inhaled pentamidine and hypoglycemia. *Ann Intern Med.* 1988; 108:490.
222. O'Brien JG, Dong BJ, Coleman RL et al. A 5-year retrospective review of adverse drug reactions and their risk factors in human immunodeficiency virus-infected patients who were receiving intravenous pentamidine therapy for *Pneumocystis carinii pneumonia. Clin Infect Dis.* 1997; 24:854-9.
223. Waskin H, Stehr-Green JK, Helmick CG, Sattler FR. Risk factors for hypoglycemia associated with pentamidine therapy for Pneumocystis pneumonia. *JAMA.* 1988; 260:345-7.
224. SYMLIN injection, pramlintide acetate injection [package insert]. San Diego: Amylin Pharmaceuticals. 2005.
225. Ratner RE, Dickey R, Fineman M et al. Amylin replacement with pramlintide as an adjunct to insulin therapy improves long-term glycaemic and weight control in Type 1 diabetes mellitus: a 1-year, randomized controlled trial. *Diabet Med.* 2004; 21:1204-12.
226. Rodriguez LM, Mason KJ, Haymond MW, Heptulla RA. The role of prandial pramlintide in the treatment of adolescents with type 1 diabetes. *Pediatr Res.* 2007; 62:746-9.
227. Davis TM, Karbwang J, Looareesuwan S et al. Comparative effects of quinine and quinidine on glucose metabolism in healthy volunteers. *Br J Clin Pharmacol.* 1990; 30:397-403.
228. Harats N, Ackerman Z, Shalit M. Quinine-related hypoglycemia. *N Engl J Med.* 1984; 310:1331.
229. Limburg PJ, Katz H, Grant CS, Service FJ. Quinine-induced hypoglycemia. *Ann Intern Med.* 1993; 119:218-9.
230. Okitolonda W, Delacollette C, Malengreau M, Henquin JC. High incidence of hypoglycaemia in African patients treated with intravenous quinine for severe malaria. *Br Med J (Clin Res Ed).* 1987; 295:716-8.
231. White NJ. The treatment of malaria. *N Engl J Med.* 1996; 335:800-6.
232. White NJ, Warrell DA, Chanthavanich P et al. Severe hypoglycemia and hyperinsulinemia in falciparum malaria. *N Engl J Med.* 1983; 309:61-6.
233. Phillips RE, Looareesuwan S, White NJ et al. Hypoglycaemia and antimalarial drugs: quinidine and release of insulin. *Br Med J (Clin Res Ed).* 1986; 292:1319-21.
234. Aspirin. Micromedex 2018. http://www.micromedexsolutions.com (accessed 2018 Feb 28).
235. Invokana [package insert]. Titusville, NJ: Janssen Pharmaceuticals; May 2016.

236. Farxiga [package insert]. Wilmington, DE: AstraZeneca Pharmaceuticals; December 2015.
237. Jardiance [package insert]. Ridgefield, CT; Boehringer Ingelheim Pharmaceuticals; March 2016.
238. Frankel MC, Leslie BR, Sax FL, Soave R. Trimethoprim–sulfamethoxazole-related hypoglycemia in a patient with renal failure. *NY State J Med.* 1984; 84:30-1.
239. Johnson JA, Kappel JE, Sharif MN. Hypoglycemia secondary to trimethoprim/sulfamethoxazole administration in a renal transplant patient. *Ann Pharmacother.* 1993; 27:304-6.
240. Lee AJ, Maddix DS. Trimethoprim/sulfamethoxazole-induced hypoglycemia in a patient with acute renal failure. *Ann Pharmacother.* 1997; 31:727-32.
241. Mathews WA, Manint JE, Kleiss J. Trimethoprim–sulfamethoxazole-induced hypoglycemia as a cause of altered mental status in an elderly patient. *J Am Board Fam Pract.* 2000; 13:211-2.
242. Schattner A, Rimon E, Green L et al. Hypoglycemia induced by co-trimoxazole in AIDS. *BMJ.* 1988; 297:742.
243. van Staa T, Abenhaim L, Monette J. Rates of hypoglycemia in users of sulfonylureas. *J Clin Epidemiol.* 1997; 50:735-41.
244. Caprelsa [package insert]. Wilmington, DE: AstraZeneca Pharmaceuticals; March 2014.
245. Agostino NM, Chinchilli VM, Lynch CJ et al. Effect of the tyrosine kinase inhibitors (sunitinib, sorafenib, dasatinib, and imatinib) on blood glucose levels in diabetic and nondiabetic patients in general clinical practice. *J Oncol Pharm Pract.* 2011; 17:197-202.
246. Service FJ. Classification of hypoglycemic disorders. *Endocrinol Metab Clin North Am.* 1999; 28:501-17, vi.

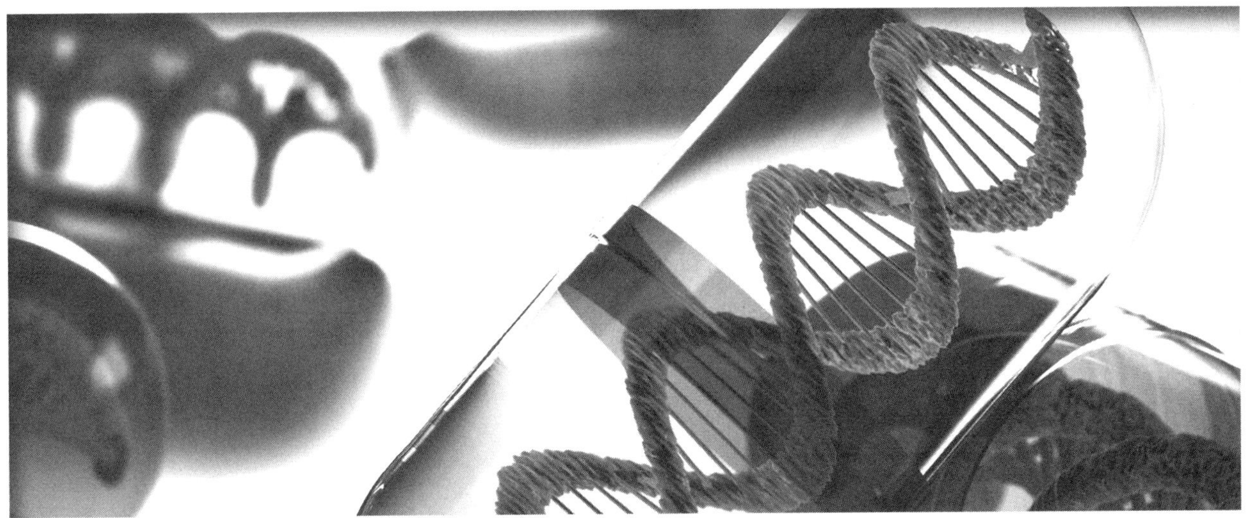

CHAPTER 31

Thyroid Diseases

Genevieve Lynn Ness, Judy T. Chen, Betty J. Dong, Frank Pucino, Jr., and Karim Anton Calis

The thyroid gland affects virtually every organ system. Thyroid hormones regulate the metabolic rate and affect the growth and function of systems throughout the body. Many drugs, including those used to treat nonthyroid disorders, may affect thyroid function. Drug-induced thyroid disorders occur as a result of changes in thyroid hormone synthesis, transport, metabolism, secretion, or function (**Figure 31-1**).[1-3] Thyroid dysfunction may also result from alterations in the synthesis or release of thyroid stimulating hormone (TSH or thyrotropin) from the pituitary gland or dysregulation of thyroid releasing hormone (TRH) at the level of the hypothalamus. The clinical significance of drug-induced thyroid abnormalities ranges from negligible to potentially life-threatening. Medications that have the potential to induce clinically significant thyroid disorders are the focus of this chapter.

Thyroid hormone synthesis is dependent on dietary iodine, which is transported into thyroid follicular cells and incorporated into thyroglobulin via thyroid peroxidases. The process of organification produces mono-iodotyrosines and di-iodotyrosines, which are bound to thyroglobulin. The follicular cells secrete thyroglobulin, which serves as a storage form for thyroid hormone precursors. TSH stimulates iodotyrosines to combine to form thyroxine (T_4) and tri-iodothyronine (T_3) through a process known as coupling. Once released into the circulation, both T_4 and T_3 are highly bound to thyroid-binding globulin and other plasma proteins. Intrinsically, T_3 is more potent than T_4, with approximately 80% of T_3 derived from the peripheral conversion of T_4 by 5'-monodeiodinase.

CAUSATIVE AGENTS

Medications have the potential to induce hypothyroidism, hyperthyroidism, and goiter. Agents most commonly associated with drug-induced thyroid disorders are listed in **Table 31-1**.[4-45] Causality has been assessed for drugs included in this table.[46] Each of these agents has been implicated as the cause of drug-induced thyroid disease in at least

Note: The authors wish to acknowledge the work of Dr. Nayahmka McGriff-Lee, who authored this chapter in a previous edition.

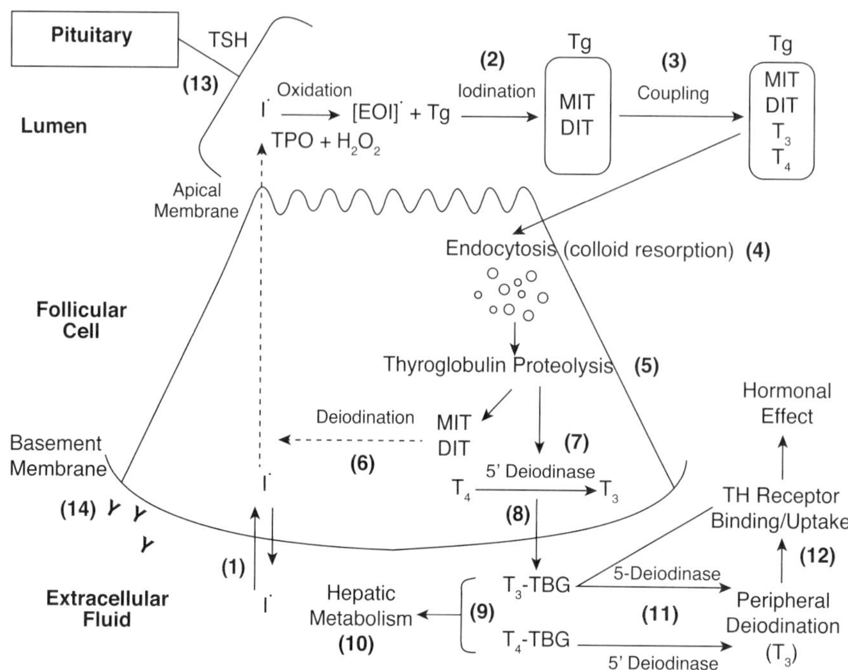

FIGURE 31-1 Steps of Thyroid Hormone Biosynthesis and Secretion and the Sites for Drug-Induced Changes
(1) Iodide is first trapped and actively transported into the follicular cell by a sodium/iodide symporter in the basement membrane. (2) Thyroid peroxidase (TPO) then catalyzes the formation of an active iodinated species [enzyme-bound hypoiodite (EOI)] important for iodination of thyroglobulin (Tg) in the follicular lumen, resulting in the formation of mono-iodotyrosine (MIT) and di-iodotyrosine (DIT). (3) The oxidized form of TPO (compound I) then initiates the coupling reaction, generating liothyronine (T_3) and levothyroxine (T_4) through combining DIT with MIT or DIT, respectively. (4) Tg is then internalized from the lumen by endocytosis. (5) Hormone release occurs after proteolysis in the endosome and lysosome system. (6) Deiodination generates iodide from free MIT and DIT, which is then recirculated, and (7) also results in the formation of T_3 from T_4. (8) Thyroid hormone is subsequently released into the circulation, (9) extensively bound to serum proteins, primarily thyroxine binding globulin (TBG) for transport. It may then undergo (10) hepatic metabolism (glucuronidation, sulfation, deiodination), (11) peripheral deiodination (activation through T_4 conversion to T_3 or inactivation of T_3 and T_4), or (12) bind to thyroid hormone (TH) receptors to elicit a pharmacodynamic response. (13) Release of thyrotropin [thyroid stimulating hormone (TSH)] from the anterior pituitary (adenohypophysis) in response to thyrotropin-releasing hormone (TRH) from the hypothalamus has a stimulatory effect on most steps of iodine metabolism and hormone synthesis and release. Drug and chemical compounds are known to alter the function of each of these steps, result in goiter, and/or (14) initiate an immune reaction resulting in thyroiditis. See Table 31-2[47-61] for a listing of specific drug actions. Adapted with permission from Taurog AM. Hormone synthesis: thyroid iodine metabolism. In: Braverman LE, Utiger RD, eds. *The thyroid: a fundamental and clinical text.* Philadelphia, PA: Lippincott Williams and Wilkins; ©2000:61-85.

Table 31-1 Agents Implicated in Drug-Induced Thyroid Disorders[4-45]

Drug	Incidence	Level of Evidence[a]
HYPOTHYROIDISM		
Abiraterone[297]	NK	B
Adalimumab[212]	NK	C
Aldesleukin[4-9]	9%	B[b]
Alemtuzumab[210]	6.9%	A
Aloe[10]	NK	C
Amiodarone[11-13,249,251,252,254,298-302]	4.3–36%	A[c]
Axitinib[191-193,303-306]	6–92%	A
Bevacizumab[271]	23%	B[d]
Bexarotene[14-16]	6–40%	A
Cabozantinib[307,308]	15–78.8%	A

Table 31-1 Agents Implicated in Drug-Induced Thyroid Disorders[4-45] (continued)

Drug	Incidence	Level of Evidence[a]
Carbamazepine[309,310]	NK	C
Cediranib[311,312]	13–56%	B
Dasatinib[190]	50%	B
Erlotinib[313]	NK	C
Escitalopram[221]	NK	C
Ethionamide[17-19,314]	NK	C
Imatinib[190]	13%	B
Infliximab[315,316]	NK	C
Interferon α[20-26,317-321]	2–84.6%	A[e]
Interferon β[27-34,322]	0.8–33%	B[e]
Iodinated compounds[35-39]	NK	A[f]
Ipilimumab[323,324]	1.5–1.6%	A
Kelp[40,41]	NK	B
Lenalidomide[269,325-330]	3.5–10%	B
Leuprolide acetate[42-44]	NK	C
Linifanib[331-333]	4.5–44%	A
Lithium[86,87,89,150,256,334-341]	1.5–35.4%	B
Motesanib[167,342,343]	5–41%	A
Nilotinib[190,344]	22%	B
Octreotide[345,346,347]	4%	B
Oxcarbazepine[310,348]	NK	C
Paroxetine[349]	NK	C
Pazopanib[194,350-353]	<10–62%	A
Pegylated interferon α[354-358]	6–12.8%	B[e]
Quetiapine[359-362]	NK	B[g]
Regorafenib[363]	31.4%	B
Rifampin[364-366]	NK	C
Sertraline[219]	NK	C
Sorafenib[138,140,174,303,305,370,379-382]	7–67.7%	A
Sunitinib[133,134,157,158,163,174-177,185,187,317,367-378]	3.4–85%	A
Thalidomide[383,384]	14%	B
Tivozanib[382,385]	22–30%	A
Vatalanib[386]	2%	B
Valproate[309,310,387]	NK	B
HYPERTHYROIDISM		
Adalimumab[388]	NK	C
Alemtuzumab[210,389,390]	14.8–33%	A
Amiodarone[11-13,249,251,252,254,299-302,391-394]	1.4–64%	A
Axitinib[191]	83%	C
Cabozantinib[308,395]	17.2%	C
Cyclosporin[396]	NK	C
Dasatinib[190]	20%	B

Table 31-1 Agents Implicated in Drug-Induced Thyroid Disorders[4-45] (continued)

Drug	Incidence	Level of Evidence[a]
Epoprostenol[397]	6.7%	B
Everolimus[398]	NK	C
Nafarelin[399]	NK	C
Imatinib[190]	13%	B[h]
Infliximab[400,401]	NK	C
Interferon α[20-26,318,320,321,402]	5.8–15.3%	A[e]
Interferon β[27-34]	0.8–33%	B[c]
Iodinated compounds[35-39,104,403-405]	NK	A[f]
Ipilimumab[406]	NK	C
Lenalidomide[45,269,327,329]	2.35–2.7%	B
Leuprolide acetate[42-44]	NK	C
Leuprorelin[399]	NK	C
Lithium[86,87,89,150,293,334-339,407,408]	0.1–1.7%	B
Minocycline[214,215]	NK	C
Nilotinib[190,409]	33%	B
Pazopanib[194]	1%	B
Pegylated interferon α[354-358,410,411]	6–12.8%	B[e]
Pegylated interferon α-2a[412]	NK	C
Radioiodine[413-416]	2%	B[i]
Sibutramine[417]	NK	C[j]
Sorafenib[140,368,379]	3–5%	B
Sunitinib[134,163,368,418,419]	10–24%	B

NK = not known (case reports only).

[a]Definitions for Levels of Evidence: Level A—evidence from one or more randomized, controlled clinical trials; Level B—evidence from nonrandomized clinical trials, prospective observational studies, cohort studies, retrospective studies, case-control studies, meta-analyses and/or postmarketing surveillance studies; and Level C—evidence from one or more published case reports or case series.

[b]Thyroid dysfunctions have been reported in a randomized controlled trial evaluating aldesleukin in combination with antitumor vaccines.[8,420] Weill et al. reported thyroid abnormalities with aldesleukin in combination with lymphokine-activated killer cells.

[c]Connolly et al. reported thyroid abnormalities in an amiodarone plus β-blocker group; no thyroid abnormalities were reported with β-blocker monotherapy.[12]

[d]Study was conducted in pediatric patients who were receiving radiation therapy in combination with bevacizumab.[271]

[e]Thyroid abnormalities with interferon have been reported as monotherapy[21-34,354-358] or in combination with ribavirin.[20,411]

[f]This category comprises over 50 drug entities, including iodinated glycerol, potassium iodide, and povidone iodine (Table 33-3). Despite great variability in the quality of published reports for specific agents, the overall body of evidence suggests a consistent "class effect." As such, iodinated compounds are classified here according to the highest level of evidence available for iodine rather than for individual agents.

[g]Although quetiapine does not meet the strict criteria for level B, a higher risk of hypothyroidism compared to placebo (OR 1.75, 95% CI 0.89–3.44) that required thyroid hormone replacement was observed in ~23% of patients suggests a higher level of causality.[362]

[h]One study conducted in 68 patients assessing the TSH levels before and after imatinib therapy found that imatinib does not impact thyroid function.[421]

[i]Jarvis et al. reported a prospective study conducted in a iodine-deficient region assessing the occurrence of iodine-induced thyrotoxicosis after iodinated contrast for CT and found that 2% of patients experienced subclinical hyperthyroidism.[416] Case reports identified a worsening in hyperthyroidism or autoimmune hyperthyroidism after administration of radioiodine.[413-415]

[j]Case report of a patient experiencing thyrotoxicosis and thyroiditis due to a sibutramine overdose.[417]

one published case report in which a patient exhibited signs or symptoms of disease in addition to any laboratory abnormalities that may have been present. Some agents alter thyroid function tests without causing substantial clinical effects (i.e., they may cause subclinical hypothyroidism or hyperthyroidism). For example, subclinical hypothyroidism is an elevated serum TSH concentration, while free T_3 (FT_3) and free T_4 (FT_4) concentrations remain within the normal reference ranges in a patient with no symptoms or with mild, nonspecific symptoms. Similarly, subclinical hyperthyroidism (associated with low serum TSH and normal FT_3 and FT_4 concentrations) is also a biochemical definition because hyperthyroid symptoms are often absent or nonspecific. Proposed mechanisms of drug-induced thyroid disorders are summarized in **Table 31-2**.[47-61] Drugs known to cause analytical interference with thyroid laboratory tests are not addressed in this chapter.

Drug-induced thyroid disorders have been reported mostly in adults. However, a number of thyroid abnormalities have been reported in association with drugs used in the treatment of children.[62-74]

Patients infected with human immunodeficiency virus (HIV) and those with advanced acquired immunodeficiency syndrome are commonly affected with thyroid abnormalities.[75] Controversy exists regarding the association of highly active antiretroviral therapy (HAART) with the

Table 31-2 Proposed Mechanisms of Drug-Induced Thyroid Disorders[47-61,134,195,199,211-213,242,316,390,413,422-430]

Drug	Mechanism(s)
Acetylsalicylic acid (aspirin)	Decreased TSH release and/or response to TRH
Activated charcoal	Decreased TH bioavailability
Adalimumab[212]	Thyroid peroxidase antibody formation
Alemtuzumab[213,390]	Self-tolerance deficit in immune reconstitution occurring after lymphopenia, autoimmunity
Aluminum hydroxide	Decreased TH bioavailability
Amiodarone	Inhibit iodide binding/transport, inhibit iodination, inhibit endocytosis, inhibit proteolysis, inhibit intra-thyroidal deiodination of T_4, inhibit TH secretion, inhibit peripheral deiodination, inhibit TH receptor binding/uptake/action, increased TSH release and/or response to TRH, decreased thyrotropin receptor response, increased autoimmunity, dilatation of thyroid follicles with colloid, follicular cells having many residual bodies flattening
Amphetamines	Increased TSH release and/or response to TRH
Androgens (danazol)	Decreased TBG
Antipyrine	Inhibit iodination, inhibit coupling
Bexarotene	Inhibit TH receptor binding/uptake/action, decrease TSH secretion[199,211]
Bromine	Inhibit iodide binding/transport
Bromocriptine	Decreased TSH release and/or response to TRH
Calcium carbonate[51]	Decreased TH bioavailability
Carbamazepine	Increased hepatic metabolism
Chlorpromazine	Increased TSH release and/or response to TRH
Cholestyramine	Decreased TH bioavailability
Chromium	Decreased TH bioavailability
Cimetidine	Increased TSH release and/or response to TRH
Clofibrate	Increased TBG
Clomiphene	Increased TSH release and/or response to TRH
Clomipramine	Inhibit intra-thyroidal deiodination of T_4, inhibit peripheral deiodination
Colchicine	Inhibit endocytosis
Colestipol	Decreased TH bioavailability
Diazepam	Displacement from protein binding sites
Dietary/environmental goitrogens	Goitrogens
Dopamine/dopaminergics	Decreased TSH release and/or response to TRH

Table 31-2 Proposed Mechanisms of Drug-Induced Thyroid Disorders[47-61,134,195,199,211-213,242,316,390,413,422-430] (continued)

Drug	Mechanism(s)
Estrogens (conjugated estrogen, ethinyl estradiol)	Increased TBG
Ethionamide[199]	Inhibit iodide binding/transport
Ferrous sulfate	Decreased TH bioavailability
Fluorine	Inhibit iodide binding/transport
Fluorouracil	Increased TBG
Free fatty acids (lipid emulsions in TPN)	Displacement from protein binding sites
Furosemide (>80 mg)	Displacement from protein binding sites, inhibit TH receptor binding/uptake/action
Glucocorticoids (dexamethasone)	Inhibit intra-thyroidal deiodination of T_4, decreased TBG, inhibit peripheral deiodination, decreased TSH release and/or response to TRH
Growth hormone (somatropin)	Decreased TSH release and/or response to TRH
Haloperidol	Increased TSH release and/or response to TRH
Heparins (fractionated and unfractionated)	Displacement from protein binding sites
Heroin	Increased TBG, decreased TSH release and/or response to TRH
Imatinib[195]	Increased hepatic metabolism
Infliximab[316]	Autoimmunity
Interferon α[54,211,242,425]	Destruction of thyroid cells, immune responses due to HLA overexpression, increased autoimmunity
Interferon γ[58]	Increased autoimmunity
Interleukin-1[58]	Inhibit iodination, inhibit TH secretion, modify the making of thyroglobulin and thyrocytes
Interleukin-2[199,211]	Induce inflammatory cytokines which can increase HLA-II and antigens on thyrocytes leading to autoimmune thyroiditis; increase thyroid antibodies and lymphocyte permeation in the thyroid, increase TSH secretion
Interleukin-6[199]	Decreased TSH secretion
Iodine-containing compounds (e.g., contrast agents)	Inhibit iodide binding/transport, inhibit iodination, inhibit endocytosis, inhibit proteolysis, inhibit intra-thyroidal deiodination of T_4, inhibit TH secretion, inhibit peripheral deiodination, increased TSH release and/or response to TRH, decreased thyrotropin receptor response
Isotretinoin[426]	Autoimmune thyroiditis
Ketoconozole	Inhibit coupling
L-asparaginase	Decreased TBG
Lenalidomide/thalidomide[211]	Decreased iodine uptake and thyroid hormone secretion interference, antiangiogenic activity
Levodopa/carbidopa	Decreased TSH release and/or response to TRH
Lithium	Inhibit iodide binding/transport, inhibit iodination, inhibit endocytosis, inhibit TH secretion, increased TSH release and/or response to TRH, increased autoimmunity, goitrogens
Metformin[61]	Decreased TSH release
Methadone	Increased TBG
Metoclopramide	Increased TSH release and/or response to TRH
Mifepristone[56,57]	Inhibit iodide binding/transport
Minerals (bromine, calcium, fluorine, nitrate, rubidium)	Goitrogens
Mitotane	Increased TBG

Table 31-2 Proposed Mechanisms of Drug-Induced Thyroid Disorders[47-61,134,195,199,211-213,242,316,390,413,422-430] (continued)

Drug	Mechanism(s)
Nicotinic acid	Decreased TBG
NSAIDs (salicylates)	Displacement from protein binding sites, inhibit TH receptor binding/uptake/action
Octreotide	Decreased TSH release and/or response to TRH
Omeprazole[60]	Decreased TH bioavailability
Opiates (morphine)	Decreased TSH release and/or response to TRH
Orphenadrine	Displacement from protein binding sites
Pegylated interferon α[211]	Production of thyroid antibodies
Perchlorate[199]	Inhibit iodide binding/transport
Perphenazine	Increased TBG
Phenobarbital	Increased hepatic metabolism
Phentolamine	Decreased TSH release and/or response to TRH
Phenytoin	Displacement from protein binding sites, increased hepatic metabolism, inhibit TH receptor binding/uptake/action, decreased TSH release and/or response to TRH, phenytoin toxicity[a,430]
Pimozide	Decreased TSH release and/or response to TRH
Propranolol	Inhibit intra-thyroidal deiodination of T_4, inhibit peripheral deiodination
Propylthiouracil	Inhibit intra-thyroidal deiodination of T_4, inhibit peripheral deiodination
Radioiodine[413]	Increase thyroid antigens and radiation thyroiditis
Raloxifene[52]	Decreased TH bioavailability
Rifampin	Increased hepatic metabolism
Ritonavir[199]	Increase TSH secretion
Salicylamides (*p*-aminosalicylic acid, *p*-aminobenzoic acid)	Inhibit iodide binding/transport, inhibit iodination, inhibit coupling, displacement from protein binding sites, goitrogens
Serotonin antagonist (cyproheptadine, metergoline, methysergide)	Decreased TSH release and/or response to TRH
Sertraline	Increased hepatic metabolism
Sevelamer	Decreased TH bioavailability
Sodium polystyrene sulfonate	Decreased TH bioavailability
Spironolactone	Increased TSH release and/or response to TRH
St. John's Wort[199]	Increased TSH secretion
Sucralfate	Decreased TH bioavailability
Sulfonamides	Inhibit iodide binding/transport, inhibit iodination, inhibit coupling
Sulfonylureas (chlorpropamide, tolbutamide)[50]	Inhibit iodide binding/transport, inhibit iodination, inhibit coupling, displacement from protein binding sites
Sunitinib[134,427-429]	Iodine uptake inhibition, destructive thyroiditis, peroxidase inhibition, autoimmunity
Tamoxifen	Increased TBG
Thioamides (propylthiouracil, carbimazole, methimazole)	Inhibit coupling
Thioridazine	Decreased TSH release and/or response to TRH
Thyroid hormones (levothyroxine)	Decreased TSH release and/or response to TRH
Tumor necrosis factor α[58]	Inhibit iodination, inhibit TH secretion, modify the making of thyroglobulin and thyrocytes

NSAID = nonsteroidal anti-inflammatory drug, TBG = thyroid-binding globulin, TH = thyroid hormone, TRH = thyrotropin-releasing hormone, TSH = thyroid-stimulating hormone, TPN = total parenteral nutrition.
[a]Case report of a patient with phenytoin toxicity experiencing hypothyroidism while receiving thyroid replacement.

development of thyroid abnormalities in HIV-infected patients. Antiretroviral therapy has been associated with subclinical hypothyroidism, particularly after stavudine therapy.[75-77] In a cohort study of 350 HIV-infected patients, use of stavudine was associated with subclinical hypothyroidism in one subgroup of patients and with low serum FT_4 concentrations in another subgroup.[77] Graves disease also has been reported after immune restoration with HAART.[75] However, HIV-infected persons usually are clinically asymptomatic, and recommendations for routine thyroid screening remain controversial due to the absence of supporting evidence.[75]

EPIDEMIOLOGY

According to the 1999–2002 National Health and Nutrition Examination Survey (NHANES), the prevalence of hypothyroidism in the United States is 3.7% (overt 0.3%, mild 3.4%).[78] Females have a higher prevalence of hypothyroidism (4.2%) compared to males (3.1%). In contrast, only 0.5% (overt 0.2%, mild 0.3%) of the U.S. population has hyperthyroidism, with a higher incidence in females (0.8%) compared to males (0.1%). A 20-year follow-up study of 2,779 adults in Whickham, England, reported an annual incidence of overt hypothyroidism of 3.5 and 0.6 cases per 1,000 in women and men, respectively.[79] In women 75–80 years of age, the annual incidence increased to 14 cases per 1,000. With increased use of sensitive TSH assays, the diagnosis of subclinical thyroid disease has become more prevalent. In the United States, the prevalence of both hypothyroidism and hyperthyroidism appear to increase with age.[78] In the Whickham study, the annual incidence of hyperthyroidism was 0.8 cases per 1,000 women.[79] The prevalence of subclinical hyperthyroidism in the general population is 2–16%.[80] In women with underlying multinodular goiter, the prevalence of subclinical hyperthyroidism is 20%.[81]

The overall incidence of drug-induced thyroid disorders has not been clearly elucidated. The incidence of thyroid disorders associated with specific agents is listed in Table 31-1.[4-45]

Thyroid disorders associated with amiodarone and lithium are the most extensively documented. Amiodarone contains 37.3% iodine by weight; however, global variations in iodine intake influence the epidemiology of amiodarone-induced thyroid dysfunction.[82] In countries such as the United States and the United Kingdom where iodine intake is adequate, the incidence of amiodarone-induced hyperthyroidism and hypothyroidism is 1.7–3% and 13–22%, respectively.[80,83] In areas with inadequate iodine intake, however, hyperthyroidism occurs in 10–12% of amiodarone-treated patients, whereas only 6.4% have hypothyroidism.[80,83,84]

The epidemiology of lithium-induced thyroid dysfunction has also been well described, with hypothyroidism and goiter observed in 4–34% of patients exposed to the drug.[85-89] Exposure to lithium has also been implicated in the development of thyroid carcinoma, but the exact incidence remains unknown.[90-92] Published data concerning thyroid abnormalities associated with lithium therapy consist mostly of case reports, prevalence studies, retrospective studies, and small or short-term prospective studies. A 15-year evaluation of thyroid function in 150 patients using lithium reported a relative risk of clinical hypothyroidism of 8.4 in patients with antithyroid antibodies.[87]

Tyrosine kinase inhibitors have been associated with drug-induced hypothyroidism and hyperthyroidism at a rate of 38.5–68% and 20%, respectively.[93,94] Studies have reported improved survival in patients with metastatic renal cell carcinoma who developed hypothyroidism in association with tyrosine kinase inhibitor therapy.[94,95]

MECHANISMS

Specific mechanisms of drug-induced thyroid disorders include changes in autoregulation, inflammatory and autoimmune thyroiditis, and *de novo* development of increased levels of thyroid antibodies. Many mechanisms have not been fully elucidated, and some medications may have multiple thyroid-related effects. Most notable among the medications with relatively well-described mechanisms are iodides, amiodarone, lithium, interferon α, and tyrosine kinase inhibitors (e.g., sunitinib). Possible mechanisms by which drugs affect the thyroid gland are presented in Figure 31-1[96] and Table 31-2.[47-61]

DRUG-INDUCED HYPERTHYROIDISM

Iodine is a required substrate for thyroid hormone synthesis. Iodide enters the thyroid and becomes oxidized via thyroid peroxidase. The oxidized iodine atom is then added to selected tyrosyl residues within thyroglobulin. This process is referred to as organification. The optimal iodine intake is 150–250 mcg/day; consumption of 1,000 mcg or more per day is considered toxic.[97] In the presence of excess iodine, the thyroid normally inhibits organification, which is called the Wolff–Chaikoff effect.[37,98] This is a method of autoregulation that prevents excessive hormone production in response to an increase in the intrathyroidal iodine content. In individuals with a normal thyroid, the gland eventually escapes from this inhibitory effect and iodide organification resumes; nonetheless, the suppressive action of high intrathyroidal iodide content may persist in patients with underlying autoimmune thyroid disease. Patients residing in iodine-deficient areas often have multinodular goiter with loss of the Wolff–Chaikoff effect and autoregulation. Thus, iodine-induced hyperthyroidism, or Jod-Basedow phenomenon, occurs when patients, particularly those with multinodular goiters, increase their iodine intake or exposure.[38,99,100]

Medications with high iodine content include amiodarone, radiographic contrast media (e.g., diatrizoate), iodinated glycerol, and certain nonprescription preparations such as kelp tablets, Triiodine, and Iodoral.[101] A number of case reports have described iodine-induced hyperthyroidism from iodine-containing antiseptic solutions, contrast agents, and povidone-iodine soaked abdominal packs.[102,103] One report described the occurrence of subclinical hyperthyroidism in patients receiving iodinated radiographic contrast media for coronary angiography.[104] A list of iodine-containing medications is presented in **Table 31-3**.[38,105-107]

Each 200-mg amiodarone tablet contains 75 mg of iodine and releases approximately 6 mg of free iodine, exceeding the recommended daily intake, optimal daily allowance, and the toxic dosage range. In addition to its iodine content, the effects of amiodarone on the thyroid may be related to its structural homology with thyroid hormones. Thyroid dysfunction associated with amiodarone has been reported in pediatric and adult patients.[108-110] There are several proposed mechanisms for amiodarone-induced hyperthyroidism. Type 1 is related to the drug's high iodine content, and most often occurs in patients with pre-existing or underlying risk factors for thyroid disorders (e.g., autoimmune thyroid disease, multinodular goiter).[93,111-114] Type 2 results from a destructive inflammatory type of thyroiditis, causing excessive release of stored thyroid hormone into the systemic circulation.[113,114] This typically occurs in patients with ostensibly normal thyroid glands.[112,115-118] The inflammatory process is postulated to be caused by either the large iodine burden or, more likely, by a direct toxic effect of the drug.[119] Type 3 is known as a mixed form encompassing characteristics of both type 1 and type 2.[93,113,114] The time to onset of amiodarone-induced hyperthyroidism is quite variable and may range from 1 to 24 months after initiation of therapy.[120,121]

Interferon α has been associated with two types of drug-induced hyperthyroidism, a Graves-like immune disorder or an inflammatory destructive thyroiditis similar to that associated with amiodarone. Hashitoxicosis, an autoimmune thyroid disease in which patients present with hyperthyroidism followed by hypothyroidism, is more common than the Graves disease-like hyperthyroidism induced by interferon α.[122,123] Typically, the pattern of thyroid dysfunction with interferon α is biphasic, presenting as initial hyperthyroidism followed by hypothyroidism. A prospective observational study found that the average onset of drug-induced thyroid disease in hepatitis C patients taking interferon α was approximately 10 weeks.[124] In some cases, thyroid abnormalities may persist even after discontinuation of interferon α. In a prospective study of 201 patients with hepatitis C receiving interferon α, 11 patients developed biphasic

Table 31-3 Iodine Content of Selected Medications and Dietary Supplements[38,105-107]

Medication	Route	Iodine Content (mcg)
Amiodarone	Oral	75,000/tablet
Calcium iodide	Oral	26,000/mL
Clioquinol (iodochlorhydroxyquin)	Topical	12 mg/g
Diatrizoate meglumine	Parenteral/urogenital	85,000–358,000/mL
Diatrizoate meglumine/sodium	Oral/parenteral	292,00–370,000/mL
Diatrizoate and iodipamide meglumine	Parenteral	380,000/mL
Diatrizoate sodium	Oral/parenteral/rectal/urogenital	600,000/g, 120,000–300,000/mL
Echothiophate iodide	Ophthalmic	5–41/drop
Ethiodized oil	Parenteral	370,000/mL
Hydriodic acid syrup	Oral	13,000–15,000/mL
Idoxuridine	Ophthalmic	358/mL
Iocetamic acid	Oral	465,000/mL
Iodamide meglumine	Parenteral	300,000/mL
Iodinated glycerol	Oral	15,000/tablet 6,000–25,000/mL
Iodine-containing vitamins (various)	Oral	54–200/tablet
Iodine Gel Gel pad Ointment Solution Tincture	Topical	9,000/g 9,000/g 47,000/g 20,000/mL 20,000–70,000/mL
Iodine and potassium iodide Lugol's solution, strong iodine tincture (various)	Topical	108,225–126,450/mL
Iodine and sodium iodide Iodine tincture (various)	Topical	40,321/mL
Iodipamide meglumine	Parenteral	257,000/mL
Iodixanol	Parenteral	270,000–320,000/mL
Iodized organic oils	Nasal	5,000–7,000/mL
Iodized salt	Oral	67/1.5 g (1 serving)
Iodoform gauze	Topical	4,800/100 mg
Iodoquinol	Oral Topical	134,274–415,610/tablet 6,000/g
Iohexol	Parenteral	140,000–350,000/mL
Iopamidol	Parenteral	250,000–370,000/mL
Iopromide	Parenteral	150,000–370,000/mL
Iothalamate meglumine	Parenteral/urogenital	81,000–282,000/mL
Iothalamate meglumine/sodium	Parenteral	400,000/mL
Iothalamate sodium	Parenteral	325,000–400,000/mL
Ioversol	Parenteral	160,000–350,000/mL
Ioxaglate meglumine/sodium	Parenteral	320,000/mL
Isopropamide iodide	Oral	1,321–1,800/tablet
Kelp (various)	Oral	100–4,200/g

Table 31-3 Iodine Content of Selected Medications and Dietary Supplements[38,105-107] (continued)

Medication	Route	Iodine Content (mcg)
Levothyroxine	Oral/parenteral	63/100 mcg
Liothyronine	Oral/parenteral	15/25 mcg
Liotrix	Oral	39/60–65 mg
Metrizamide (subarachnoid)	Parenteral	170,000–300,000/mL
Potassium iodide (Iosat, Thyro-Block) (Pima) (SSKI)	Oral	 99,385/tablet 49,692/mL 764,500/mL
Potassium iodide and nicotinamide hydroiodide	Oral	115,000/tablet
Povidone-iodine 0.5–10% (various)	Topical	500–10,000/mL
Sodium iodide	Parenteral	85,000/mL
Thyroid, dessicated	Oral	29/65 mg
Tyropanoate sodium	Oral	430,000/capsule

Source: Adapted with permission from Roti E, Uberti ED. Iodine excess and hyperthyroidism. *Thyroid.* 2001; 11:493-500. The publisher for this copyrighted material is Mary Ann Liebert, Inc.

thyroiditis.[125] All 11 patients achieved a sustained virologic response (SVR) or cure of their hepatitis C; however a meta-analysis did not find a positive correlation between the thyroiditis and SVR results. In addition, a case report described the development of thyroid peroxidase antibodies and biphasic thyroid disorder of hyperthyroidism and hypothyroidism following the use of pegylated interferon and ribavirin.[126]

Chronic lithium therapy has been associated with silent thyroiditis causing hyperthyroidism.[127,128] Silent thyroiditis, an inflammation of the thyroid gland, is often a self-limiting disorder characterized by transient thyrotoxicosis and subsequent hypothyroidism.[129] A retrospective review of 400 patients with thyroid disease reported a 4.7-fold increase in the likelihood of lithium exposure for patients with silent thyroiditis compared with Graves disease.[127] Lithium may also cause hyperthyroidism by acting as an immunomodulator. One study reported that 20% of patients receiving lithium therapy were found positive for thyroid microsomal and/or thyroglobulin antibodies that can lead to autoimmune thyroid disease.[130] In addition, one case report described thyroid storm from chronic lithium therapy.[131] The time to onset for lithium-induced hyperthyroidism is variable and not well defined.[127,128,131]

Recently, tyrosine kinase inhibitors, specifically sunitinib and sorafenib, have been shown to induce hyperthyroidism.[132] Some studies have reported initial hyperthyroidism before the onset of hypothyroidism.[133-137] One study reported development of sorafenib-induced hyperthyroidism in 23.9% of patients, which was characterized by suppressed TSH concentrations and increased free T_3/T_4 for a median duration of 2.3 months before ensuing hypothyroidism.[138] In a retrospective study, 4 of 15 patients developed sunitinib-induced hyperthyroidism. Three of these patients had elevated TSH concentrations before treatment, suggesting that patients with hypothyroidism may be at greater risk of sunitinib-induced hyperthyroidism.[139] Another study reported the onset of sorafenib-induced hyperthyroidism in 1 of 39 patients approximately 6 weeks after starting therapy.[140] A case report described a similar scenario of thyroid storm occurring 8 weeks after initiation of sorafenib therapy.[141] Following discontinuation of sorafenib, TSH concentrations increased but remained marginally suppressed. Additionally, a case report described a patient with sorafenib-induced thyrotoxicosis, which resolved with continued therapy and the addition of prednisone.[132] Symptoms of hyperthyroidism can also occur with excessive doses of thyroid hormone therapy (e.g., levothyroxine).[142]

DRUG-INDUCED HYPOTHYROIDISM

Excess iodine ingestion can also cause hypothyroidism. Iodide administration inhibits thyroid hormone synthesis and release and decreases iodide trapping.[143,144] Iodide-induced hypothyroidism ensues when the gland is unable to escape from the Wolff–Chaikoff effect. Iodine excess may also result in impaired TSH response, inhibition of proteolytic enzymes responsible for cleaving T_3 and T_4 from thyroglobulin before release, and inhibition of peripheral 5'-monodeiodinase conversion of T_4 to T_3.[2] Patients most susceptible to iodide-induced hypothyroidism include those with undiagnosed Hashimoto thyroiditis and those with a history of autoimmune thyroiditis not receiving thyroxine replacement. Consumption of an iodine-rich seaweed (kelp) diet has been associated with hypothyroidism and goiter in regions of Japan.[40,41,145,146] However, a short-term prospective clinical trial of euthyroid patients supplemented with kelp for 4 weeks found no clinical consequences of thyroid abnormalities despite evidence of chemical hypothyroidism.[147] With amiodarone, the Wolff–Chaikoff effect persists, resulting in a continuous decline in T_4 production. In addition, amiodarone may also inhibit thyroid hormone cellular uptake, pituitary and peripheral deiodination, and binding to thyroid receptor sites.[3] Amiodarone-induced hypothyroidism has been reported to occur during the first 3 to 18 months of therapy.[11,121]

Lithium impairs thyroid hormone synthesis by inhibiting iodide release from the thyroid tissue.[88,148-151] The resulting decrease in hormone production induces sustained TSH release, which can lead to development of a simple nontoxic goiter. The reported annual incidence of lithium-induced goiter is up to 50%.[152,153] However, regression of goiter was observed during a 15-year follow-up study in patients who continued to receive lithium treatment, and the proportion of palpable goiter decreased from 53% to 29%.[87] Lithium also may reduce iodine-concentrating capacity and inhibit synthesis of iodotyrosine and iodothyronines.[2] Lithium-induced hypothyroidism has been reported to occur within the first few months and up to 18 months of therapy.[154] One study reported the onset separated by sex.[150] Lithium-induced hypothyroidism occurred within the first 24 months of treatment in the female cohort and 59 months in the male cohort.[150]

Interferon α–induced hypothyroidism is more common than hyperthyroidism and typically follows episodes of hyperthyroidism. One study reported an association between the absence of SVR and the occurrence of central hypothyroidism in patients taking interferon α for hepatitis C.[155] The onset of hypothyroidism associated with interferon α has not been clearly elucidated, and, because symptoms of hypothyroidism are often attributed to the condition this drug is commonly used to treat (i.e., hepatitis C), the diagnosis of hypothyroidism in these patients may be delayed.[156]

The mechanism of tyrosine kinase inhibitor-induced hypothyroidism (specifically sunitinib) is postulated to involve impaired iodine uptake, partial inhibition of thyroid peroxidase, antiangiogenic effects (resulting in decreased blood flow and inhibition of vascular endothelial growth factor [VEGF] signals to the thyroid gland), destructive thyroiditis, capillary regression and/or constriction causing a decrease in vascularity, decrease in thyroid gland volume, thyroid hormone plasma membrane transport inhibition, and/or RET/PTC (rearranged in transformation/papillary thyroid carcinomas) kinase inhibition.[134,157-166] In addition, the mechanism by which motesanib causes hypothyroidism is thought to be due to changes in the metabolism or absorption of thyroxine.[167] Studies are underway to elucidate these mechanisms.[168] Additionally, a single-center Phase II study suggested that sorafenib may decrease the clearance of TSH, resulting in supranormal TSH concentrations.[169] The risk of hypothyroidism is positively correlated with the duration of treatment.[170] On average, the onset of symptoms was reported after 50 weeks of therapy.[134] Progressive worsening of pre-existing hypothyroidism is observed in most cases, but sudden development of severe hypothyroidism also has been described.[157] The literature hypothesizes that sunitinib causes more thyroid dysfunction compared to the other tyrosine kinase inhibitors due to its ability to target platelet-derived growth factor receptor (PDGFR) as well as vascular endothelial growth factor receptors 1 and 2 (VEGFR1 and VEGFR2).[171] Clinically significant thyroid dysfunction has also been reported with sorafenib, although not as frequently as with sunitinib.[140,172] However, a study of Japanese patients with metastatic renal cell carcinoma reported hypothyroidism in 46 (67.7%) patients treated with sorafenib.[138] In a 26-week Phase II study, levothyroxine requirements increased from 2.48 mcg/kg to 2.71 mcg/kg after sorafenib administration.[173] Another study reported 20.5% and 42.1% of patients taking sunitinib and sorafenib, respectively developed TSH concentrations higher than 3.77 μM/mL during the first month of therapy.[174] During the second month of treatment, 27.3% and 46.2% of patients receiving sunitinib and sorafenib, respectively, maintained elevated TSH concentrations. In a prospective study, thyroid replacement was required in 27% (16/59) of patients with sunitinib-induced hypothyroidism.[175] Eighty-five percent of patients taking sunitinib for metastatic renal cell carcinoma experienced hypothyroidism.[176] Additionally, of 80 patients receiving sunitinib in prospective clinical trials, 14 (18%) developed hypothyroidism.[177] The onset of sunitinib-induced hypothyroidism occurred within 10 weeks of therapy.[178] A retrospective study reported a high incidence of hypothyroidism in patients receiving axitinib (6 of 6 patients), sunitinib (9 of 15 patients), and sorafenib (6 of 12 patients).[139]

The occurrence of hypothyroidism in patients taking sunitinib and sorafenib for renal cell carcinoma may serve as a biomarker of efficacy, but the evidence is conflicting.[133,159,174,179-188] A retrospective study conducted in Brazil found an improvement in the overall response rate of patients with metastatic renal cell carcinoma who developed hypothyroidism during treatment compared to those who remained euthyroid (90% versus 20%, respectively, $p < 0.0001$).[188] In contrast, a meta-analysis conducted in more than 500 patients did not find an association between hypothyroidism and improved survival in tyrosine kinase inhibitor–treated patients with metastatic renal cell carcinoma.[189]

Second-generation tyrosine kinase inhibitors (i.e., imatinib, nilotinib, dasatinib) have also been reported to cause thyroid dysfunction in patients with Philadelphia chromosome-positive chronic myeloid leukemia.[190] Other observational studies suggest an association of axitinib with hypothyroidism; however, the sample sizes in these studies were relatively small.[191-193] Pazopanib has been reported to increase TSH concentrations above 5 milliunits/L in 29% of patients.[194] Imatinib and vandetanib have been associated with increased dosage requirements in thyroidectomized patients receiving thyroid hormone replacement therapy.[195,196,197]

Recently, a drug safety communication issued by the U.S. Food and Drug Administration (FDA) described the association of underactive thyroid in infants following exposure to iodinated contrast media.[198] This occurred in infants with serious medical conditions or that were premature. The FDA stated that this is a rare temporary occurrence and typically resolves without treatment or long-term effects.

ANTIBODY FORMATION

Thyroid autoantibodies, antithyroid peroxidase, and antithyroglobulin autoantibodies have been observed in patients with autoimmune thyroid diseases.[199] However, TSH receptor antibodies and thyroid-stimulating immunoglobulins that stimulate the TSH receptor are only seen in patients with hyperthyroidism. Antithyroid peroxidase antibodies are often present in patients experiencing hypothyroidism secondary to lithium or interferon α.[25,88] However, a 15-year follow-up study of 150 patients reported a 1.7% annual rate of new-onset autoimmunity associated with lithium therapy, a rate similar to that found in the general population.[79,87] Antithyroid peroxidase antibodies develop in 15% of patients receiving interferon α and have been reported in up to 53.3% of patients.[20,25,200-207] The link between interferon β-1b and antithyroid antibodies is less well defined. In a cohort of 156 patients using interferon β-1b, *de novo* antithyroid antibodies developed in six patients but persisted in only two patients.[31] Interpretation is confounded by the patients' underlying conditions (e.g., chronic hepatitis C, multiple sclerosis) that also have been associated with autoimmune complications and make it difficult to establish causality.[31,208,209]

Ninety-six percent of patients receiving alemtuzumab for the treatment of multiple sclerosis experienced thyroid dysfunction associated with thyroid autoantibodies.[210] Thyroid dysfunction has not been observed in patients taking alemtuzumab for cancer.[211] One case report found an increase in thyroid peroxidase antibodies after the administration of adalimumab for Crohn disease.[212] Compared to interferon β-1a, alemtuzumab was associated with a higher incidence of hyperthyroidism (0.9% versus 14.8%, respectively) and hypothyroidism (0.9% versus 6.9%, respectively).[210] The mechanism of alemtuzumab-induced thyroid autoimmunity is thought to be due to the self-tolerance deficit in immune reconstitution occurring after lymphopenia.[213]

It has been postulated that minocycline causes hyperthyroidism due to antibody formation or damage to thyroid follicular cells.[214,215] Thyroid peroxidase antibodies have also been associated with amiodarone-induced thyroid dysfunction.[216] One study found that antibody concentrations were higher in patients exposed to amiodarone for more than 24 months compared to shorter treatment exposures.[216]

OTHER MECHANISMS

The mechanism of HAART-induced hypothyroidism is not known. HIV infection has been associated with autoimmunity, and it is difficult to determine whether thyroid abnormalities found in HIV-infected patients are related to progression of the underlying disease or exposure to HAART.[75] Nevertheless, case reports suggest that protease inhibitors may accelerate glucuronidation of levothyroxine, thereby necessitating an increased dosage of thyroid hormone for replacement therapy.[217]

Sertraline may increase serum T_3 concentrations in the presence of normal TSH and T_4 concentrations.[218] One report noted that sertraline increased serum TSH concentrations in patients with hypothyroidism receiving levothyroxine therapy, although the mechanism was not established.[219] Additional case reports have described patients who experienced hypothyroidism with the combination of aripiprazole and sertraline as well as with escitalopram alone.[220,221]

The precise mechanism of central hypothyroidism induced by bexarotene is not clearly understood. Central hypothyroidism is a rare cause of hypothyroidism characterized by insufficient thyroid-hormone production resulting from impaired hypothalamic or pituitary function. Patients with central hypothyroidism often present with low FT_4 serum concentrations while TSH concentrations may be low, normal, or mildly elevated. A study that evaluated healthy individuals who received a single dose of bexarotene 400 mg/m^2 found that there was a rapid suppression of TSH without significant effects on serum prolactin, cortisol, glucose, insulin, triglyceride, or free fatty acids.[222] Bexarotene has been postulated to increase clearance of TSH independently of the effects of thyroid hormones.[222,223] Thyroid hormone replacement has been required in approximately 37% of the patients receiving bexarotene, with higher replacement needs in those receiving increased bexarotene doses.[16] Bexarotene-induced central hypothyroidism is often associated with a suppressed TSH and subsequent reduction in FT_4 serum concentrations. Clinical symptoms of hypothyroidism reverse within weeks of stopping therapy.[15,224]

Antitubercular medications have also been associated with hypothyroidism.[18,225-227] Ethionamide can inhibit thyroid-hormone synthesis, most likely because of its structural similarity to methimazole. This drug-induced hypothyroidism appears to be reversible with discontinuation of therapy.[18] Ethionamide use led to hypothyroidism in 6 of 207 patients, necessitating discontinuation of the medication.[227] A retrospective study of 186 patients in Lesotho with multidrug-resistant tuberculosis receiving combination therapy (ethionamide and para-aminosalicylic acid) reported hypothyroidism (TSH >10 milli-international units/L) occurring in 69% of the patients.[225] Similar results were reported with para-aminosalicylic acid and prothionamide (a thiocarbamide chemically related to ethionamide).[226] The mechanism by which these medications cause hypothyroidism is postulated to be due to the inhibition of iodine binding in the synthesis of thyroid hormone.[17,226,228,229]

Table 31-4 Signs and Symptoms Associated with Drug-Induced Thyroid Disorders[230,231]

Hypothyroidism	Hyperthyroidism
• Ataxia	• Alteration in appetite
• Bradycardia	• Atrial fibrillation
• Coarseness or loss of hair	• Changes in vision, photophobia, eye irritation, diplopia
• Constipation	• Decreased menstrual flow
• Cool peripheral extremities	• Exertional intolerance and dyspnea
• Delayed tendon reflex relaxation	• Exophthalmos
• Depression	• Fatigue and muscle weakness
• Dry skin and cold intolerance	• Frequent bowel movement or diarrhea
• Dyspnea	• Heat intolerance and sweating
• Fatigue and weakness	• Impaired fertility
• Goiter	• Lid retraction or lag
• Hoarse voice	• Mental disturbances
• Hyperlipidemia	• Nervousness and irritability
• Hypothermia	• Palpitations
• Impaired hearing	• Peripheral edema
• Irregular or heavy menses and infertility	• Pretibial myxedema
• Memory and mental impairment	• Sleep disturbances (including insomnia)
• Myalgias	• Sudden paralysis
• Paresthesias	• Tachycardia
• Puffy face, hands and feet (myxedema)	• Thyroid enlargement
• Weight gain from fluid retention	• Tremor
• Yellow skin	• Weight loss or gain

CLINICAL PRESENTATION AND DIFFERENTIAL DIAGNOSIS

The clinical features associated with drug-induced hyperthyroidism and drug-induced hypothyroidism are often related to accelerated or impaired metabolism, respectively, or to an underlying autoimmune process. Specific signs and symptoms are presented in **Table 31-4**.[199,230,231] The severity, duration, and extent of illness may vary greatly from patient to patient.

Unfortunately, the association between drug dose and duration and dose response and the development of hypo- or hyperthyroidism is not well established for many of the agents implicated in these drug-induced diseases. Possible risk factors that should be evaluated include the patient's age, sex, thyroid hormone status, iodine status, overall nutritional status, and other coexisting medical conditions (e.g., previous thyroid disease, diabetes, rheumatoid arthritis, pernicious anemia). In countries where the population receives adequate iodine supplementation, such as the United States, it is generally reasonable to assume that iodine deficiency is not a factor.

In patients presenting with symptoms of hyperthyroidism, primary causes of the disease should be excluded. These include Graves disease, toxic multinodular goiter, subacute thyroiditis, toxic adenoma, and thyrotoxicosis factitia. Common causes that should be considered in the differential diagnosis of hyperthyroidism are included in **Table 31-5**. Some patients may present with new-onset or worsening heart failure, atrial fibrillation, or angina. In elderly patients with unexplained weight loss, an evaluation for possible malignancies is indicated.

Individuals with symptoms of hypothyroidism should be evaluated for primary causes such as Hashimoto thyroiditis, dyshormonogenesis, iodine deficiency, infiltrative diseases (e.g., amyloidosis, sarcoidosis), and transient subacute thyroiditis. Central hypothyroidism associated with secondary (i.e., hypopituitarism) and tertiary

Table 31-5 Conditions to Consider in the Differential Diagnosis of Drug-Induced Thyroid Disorders

Hypothyroidism

- Autoimmune thyroiditis (e.g., Hashimoto disease)
- Congenital cretinism (maternal induced)
- Dyshormonogenesis (e.g., defect in hormone synthesis/transport/action)
- Deficiency of TSH (e.g., pituitary or hypothalamic dysfunction)
- Goitrogens (e.g., cabbage/rutabagas/turnips)
- Iatrogenic thyroid gland destruction (e.g., surgery/radiation)
- Idiopathic atrophy
- Iodine deficiency

Hyperthyroidism

- Choriocarcinoma[231]
- Functional thyroid cancer metastases[231]
- Graves disease[231]
- Pituitary resistance to thyroid hormone
- Thyroiditis[231]
- Thyrotoxicosis factitia (self-administered thyroid hormone)[231]
- Toxic multinodular goiter
- Toxic uninodular goiter (Plummer disease)
- TSH-producing adenoma[231]
- Tumors (e.g., thyroid/pituitary/trophoblastic tumors/struma ovarii)[231]

TSH = thyroid-stimulating hormone.

(i.e., hypothalamic disease) causes also should be excluded. Early symptoms such as constipation, fatigue, weight gain, and dry skin may be incorrectly attributed to aging. Common causes that should be considered in the differential diagnosis of hypothyroidism are included in Table 31-5.

Laboratory evaluation of thyroid function is also required for patients with suspected drug-induced thyroid disease. A serum TSH concentration is the single most important diagnostic test.[199,231] A suppressed or undetectable serum TSH concentration along with elevated thyroid hormones is indicative of hyperthyroidism, whereas a suppressed or undetectable serum TSH concentration with a normal T_3 and FT_4 suggest subclinical hyperthyroidism.[231] Conversely, an elevated serum TSH and a low serum FT_4 concentration indicate hypothyroidism, while an elevated serum TSH and a normal serum FT_4 concentration without symptoms signifies subclinical hypothyroidism.[199] Thyroid diagnostic tests should be interpreted with caution in patients with unstable thyroid function or in the presence of hypothalamic-pituitary-thyroid axis abnormalities.[199] Before a diagnosis of drug-induced thyroid disease can be confirmed, nonthyroidal systemic illnesses and other causes associated with alterations in thyroid function tests must be excluded. A number of conditions can result in altered thyroid hormone metabolism and may even be present in patients who appear clinically euthyroid. The euthyroid sick syndrome is characterized by alterations in thyroid laboratory parameters without clinical disease. Such conditions may include malnutrition, fasting, infectious diseases, malignancy, surgery, chronic diseases (cardiac, pulmonary, renal, hepatic), acute psychiatric illness, and metabolic disorders (e.g., diabetes). Interpretation of laboratory findings in such settings may be difficult, and treatment should be directed at correction of the underlying illness.

In circumstances in which serum TSH and FT_4 results are equivocal for the definitive diagnosis of hyperthyroidism, evaluation of serum total T_3 and FT_3 concentrations may be helpful. Medications that modify TSH secretion, alter thyroid-binding globulin (TBG), displace thyroid hormone from protein-binding sites, increase hepatic metabolism, decrease T_4-to-T_3 conversion, or impair T_4 absorption (Table 31-2) may confound interpretation of laboratory findings. In addition to medications, certain disease states can alter serum TBG concentrations. For example, patients with nephrotic syndrome may present with low total serum T_4 concentrations due to lowered serum TBG concentrations, but serum FT_4 and TSH concentrations often remain normal.[232]

Subclinical disease should always be considered in the differential diagnosis of drug-induced thyroid dysfunction. Management of subclinical hypothyroidism is controversial because the risks and benefits of treatment are not well understood.[199] Nonetheless, progression to overt hypothyroidism, can lead to significant health risks, such as hyperlipidemia and associated atherosclerotic complications.[233] Patients with subclinical hyperthyroidism, especially the elderly, may be at increased risk of cardiovascular complications (e.g., atrial fibrillation) and osteoporosis.[199]

It can be difficult to differentiate between the types of amiodarone-induced hyperthyroidism. In general, serum TSH concentrations are suppressed and serum FT_4 concentrations are elevated. In type 1 amiodarone-induced thyrotoxicosis, increased thyroidal blood flow and hypervascularity are present on color-flow Doppler sonography. In contrast, type 2 amiodarone-induced thyrotoxicosis is characterized by decreased or normal thyroidal blood flow on sonography.[234] A combination of type 1 and type 2 amiodarone-induced thyrotoxicosis can also occur, thereby making the diagnosis challenging. Elevations in serum interleukin-6 concentrations also have been reported in type 2 disease, but changes are negligible in type 1.[235] The time to onset of amiodarone-induced hyperthyroidism is quite variable and may range from 1 to 24 months after initiation of therapy.[120,121]

Lithium-induced thyroid changes may occur within a few weeks of therapy initiation but are most often observed after prolonged treatment.[87,88,150] However, one study found no correlation between thyroid dysfunction and duration of treatment (i.e., thyroid function was similar in patients taking lithium for 10–20 years and for more than 20 years).[236]

RISK FACTORS

Risk factors for drug-induced thyroid dysfunction are listed in **Table 31-6.**[237] A personal or family history of thyroid disease or presence of thyroid antibodies is associated with an increased risk of drug-induced thyroid illness. Without normal thyroid adaptive mechanisms, excess iodine intake may result in hyperthyroidism, hypothyroidism, or goiter. The clinical presentation of drug-induced thyroid dysfunction is generally more severe in patients who already have an underlying thyroid condition. Autoimmune thyroiditis, such as Hashimoto disease, has been implicated as a risk factor.[238] Women are considered to be at greater risk for thyroid disease and drug-induced thyroid dysfunction. Partial thyroidectomy, pre-existing or new thyroid autoimmunity, a history of radioactive iodine administration, postpartum thyroid disease, and previous thyroid damage have been identified as risk factors for the development of drug-induced thyroid disease.

Table 31-6 Risk Factors for Drug-Induced Thyroid Disorders[237]

- **Current Thyroid Abnormality**
  - Hashimoto thyroiditis
  - Thyroid autoimmunity
  - Partial thyroidectomy
- **Previous Thyroid Abnormality**
  - Previous thyroid disease
  - History of radioactive iodine administration
  - History of postpartum thyroid disease
- **Family History of Thyroid Disease**
- **Female Sex**

Studies assessing risk factors for interferon α–induced thyroid dysfunction confirmed that female sex, white race, nonsmokers, presence of thyroid peroxidase antibodies before treatment, and patients with a history of thyroid disease are at the greater risk.[239-245] Also, patients taking interferon α for hepatitis C are more likely to develop thyroid dysfunction compared to those with hepatitis B.[246,247]

Patients <62 years old may also be at increased risk of developing amiodarone-induced thyrotoxicosis.[248-252] Additionally, patients with congenital heart disease taking amiodarone were more likely to experience amiodarone-induced thyrotoxicosis if their body mass index (BMI) was <21 or if a goiter was present.[253] Female sex and the presence of antithyroid peroxidase antibodies also have been associated with an increased risk of amiodarone-induced hypothyroidism.[254,255]

Additional studies in lithium-treated patients found that female sex, use of antidepressants and valproate sodium, younger age (<60 years), as well as elevated lithium serum concentrations may increase the risk of hypothyroidism.[256,257]

Nutritional deficiencies, malnutrition, and dietary goitrogens are other potential risk factors for the development of thyroid abnormalities. Foods that may be goitrogenic include chou moellier, cassava, sorghum, corn, millet, cabbage, kale, Brussel sprouts, cauliflower, kohlrabi, turnip, rutabaga, mustard, and horseradish.

Iodine deficiency is the leading cause of goiter. National iodine supplementation programs are designed to protect populations against chronic iodine deficiency. Most industrialized countries provide dietary iodine supplements, and the World Health Organization has been active in promoting universal supplementation programs. Because of the possible effects of selenoenzymes on control of thyroid hormone metabolism, a diet low in selenium may be associated with increased serum T_3, resulting in subclinical hyperthyroidism.[258] In addition to thyroid disease associated with nutritional deficiencies, endemic goiter may result from consumption of foods rich in antithyroid substances such as cyanogenic glucosides, thioglucosides, thiocyanate, or goitrin. Goiter has occurred as a result of excessive direct or indirect (typically transferred through cow's milk) exposure to these compounds.

MORBIDITY AND MORTALITY

Drug-induced thyroid disease may result in clinical manifestations of hypothyroidism, hyperthyroidism, or goiter. Left untreated, overt hyperthyroidism may result in serious medical complications, including structural thyroid gland changes, osteoporosis, exaggerated hyperthyroidism symptoms, and cardiac complications such as dysrhythmias and heart failure, which may be associated with substantial morbidity and mortality. Severe, uncontrolled hypothyroidism can result in a decompensated thyroid state leading to hypothermia, biochemical abnormalities, respiratory failure, cardiovascular collapse, and myxedema coma, which can be fatal. A goiter, when substantially enlarged, may be cosmetically unacceptable and lead to respiratory distress and swallowing difficulties that, in some cases, can be relieved only by surgical intervention.

PREVENTION

Baseline laboratory tests and physical examination, including examination of the thyroid gland, should be performed in all patients receiving a drug with the potential to cause thyroid dysfunction (Table 31-1).[4-45] Except in patients who have an abnormal hypothalamic-pituitary-adrenal axis (e.g., those with Cushing syndrome or Addison disease), a baseline serum TSH concentration (and possibly a serum FT_4 determination) should suffice. In patients with pre-existing thyroid dysfunction, a risk-benefit assessment should be performed to determine the appropriateness of initiating therapy with any drug known to cause thyroid disease. During therapy, laboratory evaluation should be performed periodically, with the frequency based on the patient's risk factors for thyroid disease and the likely seriousness of drug-induced thyroid disease should it occur.

Patients receiving bexarotene therapy may benefit from monitoring of FT_4 for management of central hypothyroidism because serum TSH alone cannot reliably be used as an indicator of thyroid status.[15] A cohort study of patients with multiple sclerosis taking interferon β, reported an increased incidence of thyroid dysfunction and thyroid autoimmunity within the first year of treatment; therefore, monitoring during the first year is advised.[259] In addition, thyroid function should be assessed for at least 6 months after the discontinuation of interferon-based therapy.[260]

In patients receiving therapy with amiodarone, interferon α, or lithium, laboratory tests (e.g., TSH, FT_4, thyroid antibodies) should be done at baseline and at 3- to 6-month intervals, and if symptoms occur or dosages are modified.[58,156,231,261] A case series reported six patients who experienced thyrotoxicosis more than 60 days after discontinuation of amiodarone, four of which received amiodarone for short-term therapy.[262] Additionally, one report noted amiodarone-induced thyrotoxicosis 6 months after treatment discontinuation.[263] These studies suggest the need for long-term monitoring of thyroid function tests even after withdrawal of therapy.[264] When amiodarone-induced hyperthyroidism occurs, the American Thyroid Association and the American Association of Clinical Endocrinologists recommend conducting follow-up tests to determine if type 1 (iodine-induced) or type 2 (thyroiditis) hyperthyroidism is present.[231] A retrospective study also suggested the use of radioiodine (800 MBq [22 mCi]) as a preventative therapy for euthyroid patients who were hyperthyroid prior to starting amiodarone.[265,266] Although serum interleukin-6 concentrations may be elevated with destructive

Table 31-7 Approaches to Help Prevent Drug-Induced Thyroid Disorders

- Avoid drugs known to cause thyroid disorders
- Avoid goitrogens
- Consume a sufficient amount of iodine to prevent a low iodine state
- Consume an adequate amount of selenium
- Correct underlying thyroid abnormalities
- Educate patients and families on the possible symptoms associated with drug-induced thyroid disease and need to promptly inform their healthcare providers of symptom occurrence
- Screen for thyroid abnormalities before initiating therapy and periodically thereafter
- Use alternative therapies that are not associated with thyroid disease in high-risk patients when possible

Table 31-8 Management of Drug-Induced Thyroid Disorders

Hypothyroidism

- Thyroid replacement (e.g., levothyroxine)

Hyperthyroidism

- Adrenergic β-receptor blockers
- Calcium-channel blockers
- Glucocorticoids
- Iodides
- Iodinated contrast media
- Thioamides (e.g., methimazole, propylthiouracil)
- Thyroidectomy

thyroid disease (e.g., type 2 amiodarone-induced hyperthyroidism), this test is not readily available or consistently helpful.

Patients receiving alemtuzumab therapy should have laboratory assessments at baseline, every 2–3 months, or if the patient is symptomatic.[213] To detect hypothyroidism earlier, thyroid function should be monitored at the beginning of each sunitinib treatment cycle.[162,183] Regular thyroid function monitoring in patients taking lenalidomide is recommended monthly or every 2 months.[267-269] In addition, patients taking carbamazepine should have thyroid function assessed monthly for the first 4 months and every 6–12 months thereafter.[270] Thyroid hormone concentrations should be monitored every 6–8 weeks in patients taking bevacizumab.[271]

A conservative approach to minimize the risk of potential complications is to use the lowest effective dose of drugs that may cause thyroid disorders for the shortest time possible. Because the onset of drug-induced thyroid disease is highly variable, routine laboratory monitoring, patient education, and vigilance for symptom onset are important components of disease surveillance. Specific strategies for prevention are summarized in **Table 31-7**.

MANAGEMENT

In a patient with new-onset thyroid dysfunction, drugs with the potential to cause thyroid irregularities should be discontinued, if feasible. Resolution of the thyroid abnormality may require several months and, in some cases, the condition may be irreversible. Rechallenge with the offending agent should not be attempted unless medically necessary. If the drug cannot be discontinued or if the condition does not resolve after discontinuation, appropriate antithyroid therapy or thyroid hormone replacement may be required (**Table 31-8**).

Drug-induced hypothyroidism is best treated with levothyroxine. The initial dose should be 1.6–1.7 mcg/kg/day, and the dose should be titrated upward, as necessary, every 4–6 weeks until the patient is clinically and chemically euthyroid. Lower initial doses (e.g., 25 mcg) and a more gradual dosage escalation (12.5–25 mcg every 6–8 weeks) may be necessary in the elderly and in those with clinically significant cardiovascular disease (e.g., angina, palpitations). Serum TSH and FT_4 concentrations should be determined after levothyroxine has reached a steady state (approximately 6–8 weeks after the initiation of therapy).

For patients with amiodarone-induced hypothyroidism, levothyroxine requirements may be higher than usual due to inhibition of pituitary and peripheral conversion of T_4 to T_3.[118] Managing amiodarone-induced hyperthyroidism is more complex because it is often difficult to distinguish between the two types of thyrotoxicosis. Antithyroid medications, such as methimazole or propylthiouracil, combined with potassium perchlorate often are used for the treatment of type 1 amiodarone-induced hyperthyroidism as its underlying pathogenesis is related to the drug's high iodine content, which results in excessive thyroid-hormone synthesis.[231,272,231,273] In contrast, type 2 amiodarone-induced hyperthyroidism is often unresponsive to the thioamides, and treatment with corticosteroids is most effective because of the underlying inflammatory process.[117,272,231,273,274] The dose of prednisone (or equivalent doses of other corticosteroids) can range from 30 mg daily for 2 weeks followed by gradual tapering and discontinuation after 3 months of therapy to doses of 0.5 mg/kg/day until euthyroidism is restored.[117,275] Baseline FT_4 and thyroid volume (measured by ultrasonography) appear to be independently useful in identifying patients at risk for delayed treatment response with corticosteroids.[275] Because of the potential for additive cardiac effects with amiodarone, adrenergic β-receptor blockers or calcium-channel blockers are typically not recommended for control of hyperthyroid symptoms.

Results from studies of patients with amiodarone-induced hyperthyroidism suggest that there is no difference in the duration of thyrotoxicosis between patients who continue or temporarily discontinued amiodarone therapy.[274,276-278] This suggests that amiodarone may be continued in cases in which withdrawal could result in detrimental cardiac consequences, and the use of alternative antiarrhythmic agents is contraindicated.[276] Discontinuation of amiodarone does not result in complete resolution of thyroid abnormalities, and cases of amiodarone-induced hyperthyroidism have been reported several months after cessation of therapy.[279,280] In patients who require continued amiodarone therapy or who are nonresponsive to medical therapy, thyroidectomy can be considered for cosmetic or medical reasons, particularly dysphagia, respiratory difficulty, or voice alterations.[112,114,231,281-285] A case report also described the use of therapeutic apheresis prior to thyroidectomy to reduce thyroid hormone concentrations.[286]

Radioactive iodine is typically not recommended because the gland is already iodine-loaded, thereby interfering with uptake and retention of radioactive iodine. In a recent study, the efficacy of radioiodine (RAI, 131-I) therapy for the management of type 2 amiodarone-induced thyrotoxicosis was compared between patients with a high or normal radioiodine uptake who received amiodarone in the past and patients with low radioiodine uptake currently taking amiodarone.[287] This study found 131-I (22 mCi) to be an effective alternative option for patients unable to undergo thyroidectomy. However, death occurred in 10% of patients who had received amiodarone in the past compared to 44% in those with low radioiodine uptake who were currently receiving the drug. Several other studies that evaluated the use of radioiodine therapy for amiodarone-induced thyrotoxicosis in patients with low radioiodine uptake reported clinical benefit without any reported deaths.[288,289] A case report described a patient with Eisenmenger syndrome who developed amiodarone-induced thyrotoxicosis and was successfully treated with 131-I (22 mCi) despite continuation of amiodarone therapy.[290] In a second report involving another patient with Eisenmenger syndrome, total thyroidectomy resulted in rapid resolution of thyrotoxicosis and an uncomplicated recovery, so that surgery was suggested as a treatment option for amiodarone-induced thyrotoxicosis.[291] Conversely, a retrospective analysis of amiodarone-induced thyrotoxicosis in patients with congenital heart disease found that thyrotoxicosis, particularly in asymptomatic individuals, often can be managed without the need for surgical or medical intervention.[277]

β-blockers can be administered if needed for symptomatic relief in patients with interferon β–induced hyperthyroidism, although the disorder typically resolves spontaneously within weeks to several months after drug discontinuation. Clinical practice guidelines recommend attempting to identify the etiology of the interferon α or interleukin-2-induced hyperthyroidism (e.g., thyroiditis versus Graves disease) and to treat the patient accordingly.[231] Interferon α–induced hypothyroidism is usually transient, resolving spontaneously within weeks to several months after drug discontinuation.[124] In patients with interferon α–induced hypothyroidism who are asymptomatic, T_4 therapy is often not necessary. If levothyroxine treatment is initiated, it should be discontinued 6 months after the cessation of interferon α therapy and thyroid status reevaluated to determine the need for continued replacement. Case reports have described the use of radioactive iodine as a treatment option for patients with interferon α–induced hyperthyroidism with mild Graves ophthalmopathy in which β-blockers and antithyroid medications are ineffective.[242,292]

Iodine-induced hyperthyroidism should be treated with β-blockers either as monotherapy or as combination therapy with methimazole.[231]

During the occurrence of lithium-induced thyrotoxicosis, discontinuation of lithium is not recommended due to the potential for further exacerbation of thyrotoxicosis.[293,294] However, several case reports have described patients experiencing resolution of thyrotoxicosis following lithium withdrawal.[293,295]

INFORMATION FOR PATIENTS

Individuals with a history of thyroid disease appear to be at increased risk for developing drug-induced thyroid complications. Patients who receive medications known to be associated with thyroid abnormalities should be taught to recognize and instructed to report symptoms of hypothyroidism, hyperthyroidism, or gland enlargement. Specifically, they should be advised to consult their primary healthcare providers if they experience fatigue, constipation, palpitations, nervousness, heat or cold intolerance, or any other new or unusual symptoms (Table 31-4).[199,230] Certain weight-loss preparations may contain thyroid hormones or excessive amounts of iodine.[296] Given that these preparations as well as some herbal and other alternative therapies have the potential to induce thyroid dysfunction or interfere with thyroid-related medications, their use without medical supervision should be discouraged.

REFERENCES

1. Davies PH, Franklyn JA. The effects of drugs on tests of thyroid function. *Eur J Clin Pharmacol.* 1991; 40:439-51.
2. Gittoes NJ, Franklyn JA. Drug-induced thyroid disorders. *Drug Saf.* 1995; 13:46-55.
3. Meier CA, Burger AG. Effects of pharmacologic agents on thyroid hormone homeostasis. In: Braverman LE, Utiger RD, eds. *The thyroid: a fundamental and clinical text.* Philadelphia, PA: Lippincott-Raven; 1996:276-86.
4. Angevin E, Valteau-Couanet D, Farace F et al. Phase I study of prolonged low-dose subcutaneous recombinant interleukin-2 (IL-2) in patients with advanced cancer. *J Immunother Emphasis Tumor Immunol.* 1995; 18:188-95.
5. Meloni G, Trisolini SM, Capria S et al. How long can we give interleukin-2? Clinical and immunological evaluation of AML patients after 10 or more years of IL2 administration. *Leukemia.* 2002; 16:2016-8.
6. Krouse RS, Royal RE, Heywood G et al. Thyroid dysfunction in 281 patients with metastatic melanoma or renal carcinoma treated with interleukin-2 alone. *J Immunother.* 1996; 18:272-8.
7. Schwartzentruber DJ, White DE, Zweig MH et al. Thyroid dysfunction associated with immunotherapy for patients with cancer. *Cancer.* 1991; 68:2384-90.
8. Weijl NI, Van der Harst D, Brand A et al. Hypothyroidism during immunotherapy with interleukin-2 is associated with antithyroid antibodies and response to treatment. *J Clin Oncol.* 1993; 11:1376-83.
9. Vialettes B, Guillerand MA, Viens P et al. Incidence rate and risk factors for thyroid dysfunction during recombinant interleukin-2 therapy in advanced malignancies. *Acta Endocrinol* 1993; 129:31-8.
10. Pigatto PD, Guzzi G. Aloe linked to thyroid dysfunction. *Arch Med Res.* 2005; 36:608.
11. Batcher EL, Tang XC, Singh BN et al. Thyroid function abnormalities during amiodarone therapy for persistent atrial fibrillation. *Am J Med.* 2007; 120:880-5.
12. Connolly SJ, Dorian P, Roberts RS et al. Comparison of beta-blockers, amiodarone plus beta-blockers, or sotalol for prevention of shocks from implantable cardioverter defibrillators: the OPTIC Study: a randomized trial. *JAMA.* 2006; 295:165-71.
13. Greene HL. The CASCADE Study: randomized antiarrhythmic drug therapy in survivors of cardiac arrest in Seattle. CASCADE Investigators. *Am J Cardiol.* 1993; 72:70F-74F.
14. Esteva FJ, Glaspy J, Baidas S et al. Multicenter phase II study of oral bexarotene for patients with metastatic breast cancer. *J Clin Oncol.* 2003; 21:999-1006.
15. Duvic M, Martin AG, Kim Y et al. Phase 2 and 3 clinical trial of oral bexarotene (Targretin capsules) for the treatment of refractory or persistent early-stage cutaneous T-cell lymphoma. *Arch Dermatol.* 2001; 137:581-93.
16. Targretin package insert. San Diego, CA: Eisai, Inc; 2007.
17. Drucker D, Eggo MC, Salit IE, Burrow GN. Ethionamide-induced goitrous hypothyroidism. *Ann Intern Med.* 1984; 100:837-9.
18. McDonnell ME, Braverman LE, Bernardo J. Hypothyroidism due to ethionamide. *N Engl J Med.* 2005; 352:2757-9.
19. Moulding T, Fraser R. Hypothyroidism related to ethionamide. *Am Rev Respir Dis.* 1970; 101:90-4.
20. Dalgard O, Bjoro K, Hellum K et al. Thyroid dysfunction during treatment of chronic hepatitis C with interferon alpha: no association with either interferon dosage or efficacy of therapy. *J Intern Med.* 2002; 251:400-6.
21. Reichen J, Bianchi L, Frei PC et al. Efficacy of steroid withdrawal and low-dose interferon treatment in chronic active hepatitis B. Results of a randomized multicenter trial. Swiss Association for the Study of the Liver. *J Hepatol.* 1994; 20:168-74.
22. Baudin E, Marcellin P, Pouteau M et al. Reversibility of thyroid dysfunction induced by recombinant alpha interferon in chronic hepatitis C. *Clin Endocrinol.* 1993; 39:657-61.
23. Kuloglu Z, Kansu A, Berberoglu M et al. The incidence and evolution of thyroid dysfunction during interferon-alpha therapy in children with chronic hepatitis B infection. *J Pediatr Endocrinol Metab.* 2007; 20:237-45.
24. Benelhadj S, Marcellin P, Castelnau C et al. Incidence of dysthyroidism during interferon therapy in chronic hepatitis C. *Horm Res.* 1997; 48:209-14.
25. Tsuboi K, Katayama M, Yuasa R et al. Interferon-alpha-induced thyroid dysfunction in patients with chronic active hepatitis C: a transient, reversible and self-limited dysfunction. *Intern Med.* 1998; 37:27-31.

26. Durelli L, Bongioanni MR, Ferrero B et al. Long term recombinant interferon alpha treatment in MS with special emphasis to side effects. *Mult Scler.* 1996; 1:366-71.
27. Abdalla JA. Thyroid abnormalities related to interferon beta-1a therapy. *Neurology.* 2002; 58(suppl 3):A459.
28. Amenomori M, Mori T, Fukuda Y et al. Incidence and characteristics of thyroid dysfunction following interferon therapy in patients with chronic hepatitis C. *Intern Med.* 1998; 37:246-52.
29. Monzani F, Caraccio N, Meucci G et al. Effect of 1-year treatment with interferon-beta1b on thyroid function and autoimmunity in patients with multiple sclerosis. *Eur J Endocrinol.* 1999; 141:325-31.
30. Durelli L, Ferrero B, Oggero A et al. Autoimmune events during interferon beta-1b treatment for multiple sclerosis. *J Neurol Sci.* 1999; 162:74-83.
31. Durelli L, Ferrero B, Oggero A et al. Thyroid function and autoimmunity during interferon beta-1b treatment: a multicenter prospective study. *J Clin Endocrinol Metab.* 2001; 86:3525-32.
32. Rotondi M, Oliviero A, Profice P et al. Occurrence of thyroid autoimmunity and dysfunction throughout a nine-month follow-up in patients undergoing interferon-beta therapy for multiple sclerosis. *J Endocrinol Invest.* 1998; 21:748-52.
33. Monzani F, Meucci G, Caraccio N et al. Discordant effect of IFN-beta1a therapy on anti-IFN antibodies and thyroid disease development in patients with multiple sclerosis. *J Interferon Cytokine Res.* 2002; 22:773-81.
34. Kreisler A, de Seze J, Stojkovic T et al. Multiple sclerosis, interferon beta and clinical thyroid dysfunction. *Acta Neurol Scand.* 2003; 107:154-7.
35. Kahaly G, Dienes HP, Beyer J, Hommel G. Randomized, double blind, placebo-controlled trial of low dose iodide in endemic goiter. *J Clin Endocrinol Metab.* 1997; 82:4049-53.
36. Kahaly GJ, Dienes HP, Beyer J, Hommel G. Iodide induces thyroid autoimmunity in patients with endemic goitre: a randomised, double-blind, placebo-controlled trial. *Eur J Endocrinol.* 1998; 139:290-7.
37. Markou K, Georgopoulos N, Kyriazopoulou V, Vagenakis AG. Iodine-induced hypothyroidism. *Thyroid.* 2001; 11:501-10.
38. Roti E, Uberti ED. Iodine excess and hyperthyroidism. *Thyroid.* 2001; 11:493-500.
39. Braga M, Cooper DS. Clinical review 129: Oral cholecystographic agents and the thyroid. *J Clin Endocrinol Metab.* 2001;86:1853-60.
40. Suzuki H, Higuchi T, Sawa K et al. "Endemic coast goitre" in Hokkaido, Japan. *Acta Endocrinol.* 1965; 50:161-76.
41. Konno N, Makita H, Yuri K et al. Association between dietary iodine intake and prevalence of subclinical hypothyroidism in the coastal regions of Japan. *J Clin Endocrinol Metab.* 1994; 78:393-7.
42. Amino N, Hidaka Y, Takano T et al. Possible induction of Graves' disease and painless thyroiditis by gonadotropin-releasing hormone analogues. *Thyroid.* 2003; 13:815-8.
43. Eyal O, Rose SR. Autoimmune thyroiditis during leuprolide acetate treatment. *J Pediatr.* 2004; 144:394-6.
44. Kasayama S, Miyake S, Samejima Y. Transient thyrotoxicosis and hypothyroidism following administration of the GnRH agonist leuprolide acetate. *Endocr J.* 2000; 47:783-5.
45. Stein EM, Rivera C. Transient thyroiditis after treatment with lenalidomide in a patient with metastatic renal cell carcinoma. *Thyroid.* 2007; 17:681-3.
46. Naranjo CA, Busto U, Sellers EM et al. A method for estimating the probability of adverse drug reactions. *Clin Pharmacol Ther.* 1981; 30:239-45.
47. Cavalieri RR. The effects of nonthyroid disease and drugs on thyroid function tests. *Med Clin North Am.* 1991; 75:27-39.
48. De Groot LJ. Dangerous dogmas in medicine: the nonthyroidal illness syndrome. *J Clin Endocrinol Metab.* 1999; 84:151-64.
49. Fontanilla JC, Schneider AB, Sarne DH. The use of oral radiographic contrast agents in the management of hyperthyroidism. *Thyroid.* 2001; 11:561-7.
50. Hershman JM, Craane TJ, Colwell JA. Effect of sulfonylurea drugs on the binding of triiodothyronine and thyroxine to thyroxine-binding globulin. *J Clin Endocrinol Metab.* 1968; 28:1605-10.
51. Singh N, Weisler SL, Hershman JM. The acute effect of calcium carbonate on the intestinal absorption of levothyroxine. *Thyroid.* 2001; 11:967-71.
52. Siraj ES, Gupta MK, Reddy SS. Raloxifene causing malabsorption of levothyroxine. *Arch Intern Med.* 2003; 163:1367-70.
53. Surks MI, DeFesi CR. Normal serum free thyroid hormone concentrations in patients treated with phenytoin or carbamazepine. A paradox resolved. *JAMA.* 1996; 275:1495-8.
54. Surks MI, Sievert R. Drugs and thyroid function. *N Engl J Med.* 1995; 333:1688-94.
55. Wenzel KW. Disturbances of thyroid function tests by drugs. *Acta Med Austriaca.* 1996; 23:57-60.
56. Spitz IM, Grunberg SM, Chabbert-Buffet N et al. Management of patients receiving long-term treatment with mifepristone. *Fertil Steril.* 2005; 84:1719-26.
57. Takiyama Y, Tanaka H, Takiyama Y, Makino I. The effects of hydrocortisone and RU486 (mifepristone) on iodide uptake in porcine thyroid cells in primary culture. *Endocrinology.* 1994; 135:1972-9.
58. George J, Joshi SR. Drugs and thyroid. *J Assoc Physicians India.* 2007; 55:215-23.
59. John-Kalarickal J, Pearlman G, Carlson HE. New medications which decrease levothyroxine absorption. *Thyroid.* 2007; 17:763-5.
60. Centanni M, Gargano L, Canettieri G et al. Thyroxine in goiter, Helicobacter pylori infection, and chronic gastritis. *N Engl J Med.* 2006; 354:1787-95.
61. Meng X, Xu S, Chen G et al. Metformin and thyroid disease. *J Endocrinol.* 2017; 233:R43-51.
62. Lombard F, Dalla-Vale F, Veyrac C et al. Severe hypothyroidism after contrast enema in premature infants. *Eur J Pediatr.* 2009; 168:499-500.
63. Thaker VV, Leung AM, Braverman LE et al. Iodine-induced hypothyroidism in full-term infants with congenital heart disease: more common than currently appreciated? *J Clin Endocrinol Metab.* 2014; 99:3521-6.
64. Pinsker JE, McBayne K, Edwards M et al. Transient hypothyroidism in premature infants after short-term topical iodine exposure: an avoidable risk? *Pediatr Neonatol.* 2013; 54:128-31.
65. Teleanu RI, Matei M, Sandu M, Nita S. Valproate induced subclinical hypothyroidism in children with epilepsy. *Romanian J Neurology/ Revista Romana de Neurologie.* 2013; 12:183-4.
66. Batra CM, Gupta V, Gupta N, Menon PSN. Fetal hyperthyroidism: intrauterine treatment with carbimazole in two siblings. *Indian J Pediatr.* 2015; 82:962-4.
67. Ares SS, de Pipaón Marcos MS, Ruiz-Díaz AI et al. Hypothyroidism and high plasma and urine iodine levels related to the use of gastrografin. *Curr Pediatr Rev.* 2008; 4:194-7.
68. Rohrs IHJ, Silverstein JH, Weinstein DA et al. Thyroid storm following radioactive iodine (RAI) therapy for pediatric Graves' disease. *Am J Case Rep.* 2014; 15:212-5.
69. Kim SH, Chung HR, Kim SH et al. Subclinical hypothyroidism during valproic acid therapy in children and adolescents with epilepsy. *Neuropediatrics.* 2012; 43:135-9.
70. Sahu JK, Gulati S, Kabra M et al. Evaluation of subclinical hypothyroidism in ambulatory children with controlled epilepsy on valproate monotherapy. *J Child Neurol.* 2012; 27:594-7.
71. Moayeri H, Hemati A, Bidad K, Dalili H. Effects of growth hormone replacement therapy on thyroid function tests in growth hormone deficient children. *Acta Medica Iranica.* 2008; 46:473-6.

72. Aitken J, Williams FL. A systematic review of thyroid dysfunction in preterm neonates exposed to topical iodine. *Arch Dis Child Fetal Neonatal Ed.* 2014; 99:F21-8.

73. Emder PJ, Jack MM. Iodine-induced neonatal hypothyroidism secondary to maternal seaweed consumption: a common practice in some Asian cultures to promote breast milk supply. *J Paediatr Child Health.* 2011; 47:750-2.

74. Yilmaz U, Yilmaz TS, Akinci G et al. The effect of antiepileptic drugs on thyroid function in children. *Seizure.* 2014; 23:29-35.

75. Hoffmann CJ, Brown TT. Thyroid function abnormalities in HIV-infected patients. *Clin Infect Dis.* 2007; 45:488-94.

76. Madeddu G, Spanu A, Chessa F et al. Thyroid function in human immunodeficiency virus patients treated with highly active antiretroviral therapy (HAART): a longitudinal study. *Clin Endocrinol.* 2006; 64:375-83.

77. Beltran S, Lescure FX, El Esper I et al. Subclinical hypothyroidism in HIV-infected patients is not an autoimmune disease. *Horm Res.* 2006; 66:21-6.

78. Aoki Y, Belin RM, Clickner R et al. Serum TSH and total T4 in the United States population and their association with participant characteristics: National Health and Nutrition Examination Survey (NHANES 1999-2002). *Thyroid.* 2007; 17:1211-23.

79. Vanderpump MP, Tunbridge WM, French JM et al. The incidence of thyroid disorders in the community: a twenty-year follow-up of the Whickham Survey. *Clin Endocrinol.* 1995; 43:55-68.

80. Hanna FW, Lazarus JH, Scanlon MF. Controversial aspects of thyroid disease. *BMJ.* 1999; 319:894-9.

81. Marqusee E, Haden ST, Utiger RD. Subclinical thyrotoxicosis. *Endocrinol Metab Clin North Am.* 1998; 27:37-49.

82. Cordarone package insert. Philadelphia, PA: Wyeth Laboratories; 2008.

83. Martino E, Bartalena L, Bogazzi F, Braverman LE. The effects of amiodarone on the thyroid. *Endocr Rev.* 2001; 22:240-54.

84. Goichot B, Grunenberger F, Schlienger JL. Amiodarone-induced hyperthyroidism. *Arch Intern Med.* 2001; 161:295.

85. Hullin R. The place of lithium in biological psychiatry. In: Johnson FN, Johnson S, eds. *Lithium in medical practice.* Lancaster, PA: MTP Press; 1978:433.

86. Yassa R, Saunders A, Nastase C, Camille Y. Lithium-induced thyroid disorders: a prevalence study. *J Clin Psychiatry.* 1988; 49:14-6.

87. Bocchetta A, Cocco F, Velluzzi F et al. Fifteen-year follow-up of thyroid function in lithium patients. *J Endocrinol Invest.* 2007; 30:363-6.

88. Lazarus JH. The effects of lithium therapy on thyroid and thyrotropin-releasing hormone. *Thyroid.* 1998; 8:909-13.

89. Schou M, Amdisen A, Eskjaer Jensen S, Olsen T. Occurrence of goitre during lithium treatment. *Br Med J.* 1968; 3:710-3.

90. Aksoy S, Kilickap S, Erman M. Lithium-associated hypothyroidism and thyroid papillary carcinoma: a case report. *South Med J.* 2006; 99:279-81.

91. Brownlie BE, Turner JG, Millner GM et al. Lithium associated thyroid cancer. *Aust N Z J Med.* 1980; 10:62-3.

92. McHenry CR, Rosen IB, Rotstein LE et al. Lithiumogenic disorders of the thyroid and parathyroid glands as surgical disease. *Surgery.* 1990; 108:1001-5.

93. Hubalewska-Dydejczyk A. Thyroid dysfunction associated with the administration of medications, including amiodarone and tyrosine kinase inhibitors. *Endokrynologia Polska.* 2012; 63:168-9.

94. Bailey EB, Tantravahi SK, Poole A et al. Correlation of degree of hypothyroidism with survival outcomes in patients with metastatic renal cell carcinoma receiving vascular endothelial growth factor receptor tyrosine kinase inhibitors. *Clinical Genitourinary Cancer.* 2015; 13:e131-7.

95. Bailey EB, Tantravahi SK, Wells CE et al. Incidence and severity of hypothyroidism and survival outcomes in patients (pts) with metastatic renal cell carcinoma (mRCC) treated with vascular endothelial growth factor (VEGF) tyrosine kinase inhibitors (TKIs). *Journal of Clinical Oncology.* 2014; 32.

96. Taurog AM. Hormone synthesis: thyroid iodine metabolism. In: Braverman LE, Utiger RD, eds. *The thyroid: a fundamental and clinical text.* Philadelphia, PA: Lippincott Williams and Wilkins; 2000:61-85.

97. Zimmermann MB. Iodine deficiency. *Endocr Rev.* 2009; 30:376-408.

98. Lee K, Bradley R, Dwyer J, Lee SL. Too much versus too little: the implications of current iodine intake in the United States. *Nutr Rev.* 1999; 57:177-81.

99. Woeber KA. Iodine and thyroid disease. *Med Clin North Am.* 1991; 75:169-78.

100. Laurberg P, Pedersen KM, Vestergaard H, Sigurdsson G. High incidence of multinodular toxic goitre in the elderly population in a low iodine intake area vs. high incidence of Graves' disease in the young in a high iodine intake area: comparative surveys of thyrotoxicosis epidemiology in East-Jutland Denmark and Iceland. *J Intern Med.* 1991; 229:415-20.

101. Hoang TD, Mai VQ, Clyde PW, Shakir MKM. Over-the-counter-drug-induced thyroid disorders. *Endocr Pract.* 2013; 19:268-74.

102. Brotfain E, Koyfman L, Frenkel A et al. Iodine-induced hyperthyroidism—an old clinical entity that is still relevant to daily ICU practice: a case report. *Case Rep Endocrinol.* 2013; 2013:792745.

103. Patil VP, Kulkarni AP, Jacques T. Iodine induced thyrotoxicosis following povidine-iodine dressings: a case report. *Crit Care Resusc.* 2003; 5:186-8.

104. Özkan S, Oysu AS, Kayataş K et al. Thyroid functions after contrast agent administration for coronary angiography: a prospective observational study in euthyroid patients. *Anadolu Kardiyoloji Dergisi.* 2013; 13:363-9.

105. Lexi-Comp ONLINE with AHFS® [online database]. Bethesda, MD: ASHP; 2008. Updated May 29, 2008.

106. *Drug facts and comparisons.* St. Louis: Facts and Comparisons; 2008.

107. Beers MH, Porter RS, eds. *The Merck manual.* Whitehouse Station, NJ: Merck and Co Inc; 2006.

108. Trudel K, Sanatani S, Panagiotopoulos C. Severe amiodarone-induced hypothyroidism in an infant. *Pediatr Crit Care Med.* 2011; 12:e43-5.

109. Hacihamdioglu B, Berberoglu M, Siklar Z et al. Amiodarone-induced thyrotoxicosis in children and adolescents is a possible outcome in patients with low iodine intake. *J Pediatr Endocrinol Metab.* 2010; 23:363-8.

110. Nikitina I, Vasichkina E, Artemeva I et al. Influence of amiodarone on thyroid function in children. *Horm Res Paediatr.* 2014; 82:317.

111. Danzi S, Klein I. Amiodarone-induced thyroid dysfunction. *J Intensive Care Med.* 2015; 30:179-85.

112. Jabrocka-Hybel A, Bednarczuk T, Bartalena L et al. Amiodarone and the thyroid. *Endokrynologia Polska.* 2015; 66:176-96.

113. Barvalia U, Amlani B, Pathak R. Amiodarone-induced thyrotoxic thyroiditis: a diagnostic and therapeutic challenge. *Case Rep Med.* 2014; 2014:231651.

114. Bogazzi F, Bartalena L, Martino E. Approach to the patient with amiodarone-induced thyrotoxicosis. *J Clin Endocrinol Metab.* 2010; 95:2529-35.

115. Bartalena L, Bogazzi F, Martino E. Amiodarone-induced thyrotoxicosis: a difficult diagnostic and therapeutic challenge. *Clin Endocrinol.* 2002; 56:23-4.

116. Bartalena L, Brogioni S, Grasso L et al. Treatment of amiodarone-induced thyrotoxicosis, a difficult challenge: results of a prospective study. *J Clin Endocrinol Metab.* 1996; 81:2930-3.

117. Bogazzi F, Bartalena L, Cosci C et al. Treatment of type II amiodarone-induced thyrotoxicosis by either iopanoic acid or glucocorticoids: a prospective, randomized study. *J Clin Endocrinol Metab.* 2003; 88:1999-2002.

118. Bouvy ML, Heerdink ER, Hoes AW, Leufkens HG. Amiodarone-induced thyroid dysfunction associated with cumulative dose. *Pharmacoepidemiol Drug Saf.* 2002; 11:601-6.

119. Benbassat CA, Mechlis-Frish S, Cohen M, Blum I. Amiodarone-induced thyrotoxicosis type 2: a case report and review of the literature. *Am J Med Sci.* 2000; 320:288-91.
120. Nademanee K, Piwonka RW, Singh BN, Hershman JM. Amiodarone and thyroid function. *Prog Cardiovasc Dis.* 1989; 31:427-37.
121. Trip MD, Wiersinga W, Plomp TA. Incidence, predictability, and pathogenesis of amiodarone-induced thyrotoxicosis and hypothyroidism. *Am J Med.* 1991; 91:507-11.
122. Ross DS. Disorders that cause hyperthyroidism. In: Post TW, ed. UpToDate [online database]. Waltham, MA: Wolters Kluwer. http://www.uptodate.com. Updated September 12, 2017 (accessed 2018 Mar 1).
123. Czarnywojtek A, Zgorzalewicz-Stachowiak M et al. Patients with chronic hepatitis type C and interferon-alpha-induced hyperthyroidism in two-years clinical follow-up. *Neuro Endocrinol Lett.* 2013; 34:154-61.
124. Tran HA, Jones TL, Ianna EA, Reeves GE. The natural history of interferon-α induced thyroiditis in chronic hepatitis c patients: a long term study. *Thyroid Res.* 2011; 4:2.
125. Tran HA, Malcolm Reeves GE, Gibson R, Attia JR. Development of thyroid diseases in the treatment of chronic hepatitis C with alpha-interferon may be a good prognosticator in achieving a sustained virological response: a meta-analysis. *J Gastroenterol Hepatol.* 2009; 24:1163-8.
126. Geantă GR, Streinu-Cercel A, Moţoi MM, Neguţ A. Unusual evolution of a patient with autoimmune thyroiditis related to interferon therapy. *J Gastrointestin Liver Dis.* 2012; 21:58.
127. Miller KK, Daniels GH. Association between lithium use and thyrotoxicosis caused by silent thyroiditis. *Clin Endocrinol.* 2001; 55:501-8.
128. Pearce EN, Farwell AP, Braverman LE. Thyroiditis. *N Engl J Med.* 2003; 348:2646-55.
129. Kar N, Hullumane SR, Williams C. Thyrotoxicosis followed by hypothyroidism in a patient on lithium. *Mental Illness.* 2014; 6:38-9.
130. Maddu N, Raghavendra PB. Review of lithium effects on immune cells. *Immunopharmacol Immunotoxicol.*2015;37:111-25.
131. Fridman A, Nguyen Q, Plummer E. A case of lithium-induced polyendocrinopathy including thyroid storm. *Endocrinologist.* 2010; 20:131-3.
132. Barbaro D. Sorafenib and thyrotoxicosis. *J Endocrinol Invest.* 2010; 33:436-436.
133. Shinohara N, Takahashi M, Kamishima T et al. The incidence and mechanism of sunitinib-induced thyroid atrophy in patients with metastatic renal cell carcinoma. *Br J Cancer.* 2011; 104:241-7.
134. Desai J, Yassa L, Marqusee E et al. Hypothyroidism after sunitinib treatment for patients with gastrointestinal stromal tumors. *Ann Intern Med.* 2006; 145:660-4.
135. Jazvić M, Prpić M, Jukić T et al. Sunitinib-induced thyrotoxicosis—a not so rare entity. *Anticancer Res.* 2015; 35:481-5.
136. Sakurai K, Fukazawa H, Arihara Z, Yoshida K. Sunitinib-induced thyrotoxicosis followed by persistent hypothyroidism with shrinkage of thyroid volume. *Tohoku J Exp Med.* 2010; 222:39-44.
137. van Doorn L, Eskens FA, Visser TJ et al. Sorafenib induced thyroiditis in two patients with hepatocellular carcinoma. *Thyroid.* 2011; 21:197-202.
138. Miyake H, Kurahashi T, Yamanaka K et al. Abnormalities of thyroid function in Japanese patients with metastatic renal cell carcinoma treated with sorafenib: a prospective evaluation. *Urol Oncol.* 2010; 28:515-9.
139. Daimon M, Kato T, Kaino W et al. Thyroid dysfunction in patients treated with tyrosine kinase inhibitors, sunitinib, sorafenib and axitinib, for metastatic renal cell carcinoma. *Jpn J Clin Oncol.* 2012; 42:742-7.
140. Tamaskar I, Bukowski R, Elson P et al. Thyroid function test abnormalities in patients with metastatic renal cell carcinoma treated with sorafenib. *Ann Oncol.* 2008; 19:265-8.
141. Haraldsdottir S, Li Q, Villalona-Calero MA et al. Case of sorafenib-induced thyroid storm. *J Clin Oncol.* 2013; 31:e262-4.
142. Levothyroxine Sodium package insert. Lake Zurich, IL: Fresenius Kabi USA, LLC; 2013.
143. Daniels GH. Amiodarone-induced thyrotoxicosis. *J Clin Endocrinol Metab.* 2001; 86:3-8.
144. Ingbar SH. Autoregulation of the thyroid. Response to iodide excess and depletion. *Mayo Clin Proc.* 1972; 47:814-23.
145. Crawford BA, Cowell CT, Emder PJ et al. Iodine toxicity from soy milk and seaweed ingestion is associated with serious thyroid dysfunction. *Med J Aust.* 2010; 193:413-5.
146. Leung AM, Braverman LE. Iodine-induced thyroid dysfunction. *Curr Opin Endocrinol Diabetes Obes.* 2012; 19:414-9.
147. Clark CD, Bassett B, Burge MR. Effects of kelp supplementation on thyroid function in euthyroid subjects. *Endocr Pract.* 2003; 9:363-9.
148. Caykoylu A, Capoglu I, Unuvar N et al. Thyroid abnormalities in lithium-treated patients with bipolar affective disorder. *J Int Med Res.* 2002; 30:80-4.
149. Dang AH, Hershman JM. Lithium-associated thyroiditis. *Endocr Pract.* 2002; 8:232-6.
150. Johnston AM, Eagles JM. Lithium-associated clinical hypothyroidism. Prevalence and risk factors. *Br J Psychiatry.* 1999; 175:336-9.
151. Kleiner J, Altshuler L, Hendrick V, Hershman JM. Lithium-induced subclinical hypothyroidism: review of the literature and guidelines for treatment. *J Clin Psychiatry.* 1999; 60:249-55.
152. Lazarus JH. Lithium and thyroid. *Best Pract Res Clin Endocrinol Metab.* 2009; 23:723-33.
153. Perrild H, Hegedüs L, Baastrup PC et al. Thyroid function and ultrasonically determined thyroid size in patients receiving long-term lithium treatment. *Am J Psychiatry.* 1990; 147:1518-21.
154. Chakrabarti S. Thyroid functions and bipolar affective disorder. *J Thyroid Res.* 2011; 2011.
155. Zantut-Wittmann DE, Pavan MH, Pavin EJ, Goncales FL Jr. Central hypothyroidism in patients with chronic hepatitis C and relation with interferon-alpha treatment. *Endocr Regul.* 2011; 45:157-61.
156. Mandac JC, Chaudhry S, Sherman KE, Tomer Y. The clinical and physiological spectrum of interferon-alpha induced thyroiditis: toward a new classification. *Hepatology.* 2006; 43:661-72.
157. Mannavola D, Coco P, Vannucchi G et al. A novel tyrosine-kinase selective inhibitor, sunitinib, induces transient hypothyroidism by blocking iodine uptake. *J Clin Endocrinol Metab.* 2007; 92:3531-4.
158. Wong E, Rosen LS, Mulay M et al. Sunitinib induces hypothyroidism in advanced cancer patients and may inhibit thyroid peroxidase activity. *Thyroid.* 2007; 17:351-5.
159. Aparicio-Gallego G, Blanco M, Figueroa A et al. New insights into molecular mechanisms of sunitinib-associated side effects. *Molecular Cancer Therapeutics.* 2011; 10:2215-23.
160. Jebreel Ae, England J, Bedford K et al. Vascular endothelial growth factor (VEGF), VEGF receptors expression and microvascular density in benign and malignant thyroid diseases. *Int J Exp Pathol.* 2007; 88:271-7.
161. Yamada E, Yamazaki K, Takano K, Obara T, Sato K. Iodide inhibits vascular endothelial growth factor-A expression in cultured human thyroid follicles: a microarray search for effects of thyrotropin and iodide on angiogenesis factors. *Thyroid.* 2006; 16:545-54.
162. Torino F, Corsello SM, Longo R et al. Hypothyroidism related to tyrosine kinase inhibitors: an emerging toxic effect of targeted therapy. *Nat Rev Clin Oncol.* 2009; 6:219-28.
163. Grossmann M, Premaratne E, Desai J, Davis ID. Thyrotoxicosis during sunitinib treatment for renal cell carcinoma. *Clin Endocrinol.* 2008; 69:669-72.
164. Makita N, Miyakawa M, Fujita T, Iiri T. Sunitinib induces hypothyroidism with a markedly reduced vascularity. *Thyroid.* 2010; 20:323-6.

165. Rogiers A, Wolter P, Op de Beeck K et al. Shrinkage of thyroid volume in sunitinib-treated patients with renal-cell carcinoma: a potential marker of irreversible thyroid dysfunction? *Thyroid.* 2010; 20:317-22.
166. Braun D, Kim TD, le Coutre P et al. Tyrosine kinase inhibitors noncompetitively inhibit MCT8-mediated iodothyronine transport. *J Clin Endocrinol Metab.* 2012; 97:E100-5.
167. Sherman SI, Wirth LJ, Droz J-P et al. Motesanib diphosphate in progressive differentiated thyroid cancer. *New Engl J Med.* 2008; 359:31-42.
168. Salem AK, Fenton MS, Marion KM, Hershman JM. Effect of sunitinib on growth and function of FRTL-5 thyroid cells. *Thyroid.* 2008; 18:631-5.
169. Verloop H, Smit JWA, Dekkers OM. Sorafenib therapy decreases the clearance of thyrotropin. *Eur JEndocrinol.* 2013; 168:163-7.
170. Faris JE, Moore AF, Daniels GH. Sunitinib (sutent)-induced thyrotoxicosis due to destructive thyroiditis: a case report. *Thyroid.* 2007; 17:1147-9.
171. Makita N, Iiri T. Tyrosine kinase inhibitor-induced thyroid disorders: a review and hypothesis. *Thyroid.* 2013; 23:151-9.
172. Iavarone M, Perrino M, Viganò M et al. Sorafenib-induced destructive thyroiditis. *Thyroid.* 2010; 20:1043-4.
173. Abdulrahman RM, Verloop H, Hoftijzer H et al. Sorafenib-induced hypothyroidism is associated with increased type 3 deiodination. *J Clin Endocrinol Metab.* 2010; 95:3758-62.
174. Schmidinger M, Vogl UM, Bojic M et al. Hypothyroidism in patients with renal cell carcinoma. *Cancer.* 2011; 117:534-44.
175. Wolter P, Stefan C, Decallonne B et al. The clinical implications of sunitinib-induced hypothyroidism: a prospective evaluation. *Br J Cancer.* 2008; 99:448-54.
176. Rini BI, Tamaskar I, Shaheen P et al. Hypothyroidism in patients with metastatic renal cell carcinoma treated with sunitinib. *J Natl Cancer Inst.* 2007; 99:81-3.
177. Feldman DR, Martorella AJ, Robbins RJ, Motzer RJ. Re: Hypothyroidism in patients with metastatic renal cell carcinoma treated with sunitinib. *J Natl Cancer Inst.* 2007; 99:974-5.
178. Kappers MH, van Esch JH, Smedts FM et al. Sunitinib-induced hypothyroidism is due to induction of type 3 deiodinase activity and thyroidal capillary regression. *J Clin Endocrinol Metab.* 2011; 96:3087-94.
179. Sabatier R, Gravis G, Deville J et al. Hypothyroidism and survival during sunitinib therapy in metastatic renal cell cancer: a prospective observational analysis. Paper presented at: Proceedings of the 2009 Genitourinary Cancers Symposium, Orlando, Florida, 2009.
180. Bladou F, Gravis G, Sabatier R et al. Hypothyroidism and survival during sunitinib therapy in metastatic renal cell carcinoma (mRCC): a prospective observational analysis. Paper presented at: ASCO Annual Meeting Proceedings 2010.
181. Dienstmann R, Braña I, Rodon J, Tabernero J. Toxicity as a biomarker of efficacy of molecular targeted therapies: focus on EGFR and VEGF inhibiting anticancer drugs. *The Oncologist.* 2011; 16:1729-40.
182. Wolter P, Stefan C, Decallonne B et al. Evaluation of thyroid dysfunction as a candidate surrogate marker for efficacy of sunitinib in patients (pts) with advanced renal cell cancer (RCC). Paper presented at: ASCO Annual Meeting Proceedings 2008.
183. Bianchi L, Rossi L, Tomao F et al. Thyroid dysfunction and tyrosine kinase inhibitors in renal cell carcinoma. *Endocrine-Related Cancer.* 2013; 20:R233-45.
184. Riesenbeck LM, Bierer S, Hoffmeister I et al. Hypothyroidism correlates with a better prognosis in metastatic renal cancer patients treated with sorafenib or sunitinib. *World J Urol.* 2011; 29:807-13.
185. Baldazzi V, Tassi R, Lapini A et al. The impact of sunitinib-induced hypothyroidism on progression-free survival of metastatic renal cancer patients: a prospective single-center study. *Urol Oncol.* 2012; 30:704-10.
186. Baldazzi V, Tassi R, Caruso S et al. TSH elevation as markers of efficacy in mRCC patient treated with Sunitinib. *Tumor Biol.* 2011; 32:S71-2.
187. Gonçalves B, Pinto L, Paulo J et al. The effect of sunitinib-induced hypothyroidism in the outcome of mRCC patients. *Eur Urol, Supplements.* 2014; 13:160.
188. Ismael Pinto FA, Rodrigues Pereira AA, Formiga MN et al. Association of hypothyroidism with improved outcomes in first-line treatment of renal cell carcinoma with sunitinib. *J Clin Oncol.* 2012; 30.
189. Nearchou AD, Valachis A, Lind P et al. Acquired hypothyroidism as a predictive marker of outcome in patients with metastatic renal cell carcinoma (mRCC) treated with tyrosine-kinase inhibitors (TKIs): a literature-based meta-analysis. *J Clinl Oncol.* 2014; 32.
190. Kim TD, Schwarz M, Nogai H et al. Thyroid dysfunction caused by second-generation tyrosine kinase inhibitors in Philadelphia chromosome-positive chronic myeloid leukemia. *Thyroid.* 2010; 20:1209-14.
191. Ohba K, Takayama T, Matsunaga H et al. Inappropriate elevation of serum thyrotropin levels in patients treated with axitinib. *Thyroid.* 2013; 23:443-8.
192. Fujiwara Y, Kiyota N, Chayahara N et al. Management of axitinib (AG-013736)-induced fatigue and thyroid dysfunction, and predictive biomarkers of axitinib exposure: results from phase I studies in Japanese patients. *Invest New Drugs.* 2012; 30:1055-64.
193. Mukohara T, Nakajima H, Mukai H et al. Effect of axitinib (AG-013736) on fatigue, thyroid-stimulating hormone, and biomarkers: A phase I study in Japanese patients. *Cancer Science.* 2010; 101:963-8.
194. Wolter P, McCann L, Sternberg C et al. Incidence of thyroid dysfunction in renal cell carcinoma (RCC) patients treated with pazopanib in prospective clinical trials. Paper presented at: ASCO Annual Meeting Proceedings 2011.
195. de Groot JW, Zonnenberg BA, Plukker JT et al. Imatinib induces hypothyroidism in patients receiving levothyroxine. *Clin Pharmacol Ther.* 2005; 78:433-8.
196. De Groot J, Zonnenberg B, van Ufford-Mannesse PQ et al. A phase II trial of imatinib therapy for metastatic medullary thyroid carcinoma. *J Clin Endocrinol Metab.* 2007; 92:3466-9.
197. Robinson BG, Paz-Ares L, Krebs A et al. Vandetanib (100 mg) in patients with locally advanced or metastatic hereditary medullary thyroid cancer. *J Clin Endocrinol Metab.* 2010; 95:2664-71.
198. FDA Drug Safety Communication: FDA advises of rare cases of underactive thyroid in infants given iodine-containing contrast agents for medical imaging. 2015; http://www.fda.gov/Drugs/DrugSafety/ucm472782.htm?source=govdelivery&utm_medium=email&utm_source=govdelivery. Updated January 15, 2016 (accessed 2018 Mar 1).
199. Garber JR, Cobin RH, Gharib H et al. Clinical practice guidelines for hypothyroidism in adults: cosponsored by the American Association of Clinical Endocrinologists and the American Thyroid Association. *Endocr Pract.* 2012; 18:988-1028.
200. Carella C, Mazziotti G, Morisco F et al. Long-term outcome of interferon-α-induced thyroid autoimmunity and prognostic influence of thyroid autoantibody pattern at the end of treatment. *J Clin Endocrinol Metab.* 2001; 86:1925-9.
201. Custro N, Montalto G, Scafidi V et al. Prospective study on thyroid autoimmunity and dysfunction related to chronic hepatitis C and interferon therapy. *J Endocrinol Invest.* 1997; 20:374-80.
202. Dobhan R. Thymic hyperplasia associated with alpha interferon therapy. *Am J Gastroenterol.* 2000; 95:2570.
203. Fernandez-Soto L, Gonzalez A, Escobar-Jimenez F et al. Increased risk of autoimmune thyroid disease in hepatitis C vs hepatitis B before, during, and after discontinuing interferon therapy. *Arch Intern Med.* 1998; 158:1445-8.
204. Koh LK, Greenspan FS, Yeo PP. Interferon-alpha induced thyroid dysfunction: three clinical presentations and a review of the literature. *Thyroid.* 1997; 7:891-6.
205. Marazuela M, Garcia-Buey L, Gonzalez-Fernandez B et al. Thyroid autoimmune disorders in patients with chronic hepatitis C before and during interferon-α therapy. *Clin Endocrinol.* 1996; 44:635-42.

206. Wong V, Fu AX, George J, Cheung NW. Thyrotoxicosis induced by alpha-interferon therapy in chronic viral hepatitis. *Clin Endocrinol.* 2002; 56:793-8.

207. Lichiardopol C, Moţa M. The thyroid and autoimmunity. *Romanian J Int Med.* 2009; 47:207-15.

208. Okanoue T, Sakamoto S, Itoh Y et al. Side effects of high-dose interferon therapy for chronic hepatitis C. *J Hepatol.* 1996; 25:283-91.

209. Watanabe U, Hashimoto E, Hisamitsu T et al. The risk factor for development of thyroid disease during interferon-alpha therapy for chronic hepatitis C. *Am J Gastroenterol.* 1994; 89:399-403.

210. Coles AJ, Compston DAS, Selmaj KW et al. Alemtuzumab vs. interferon beta-1a in early multiple sclerosis. *New Engl J Med.* 2008; 359:1786-801.

211. Torino F, Barnabei A, Paragliola R et al. Thyroid dysfunction as an unintended side effect of anticancer drugs. *Thyroid.* 2013; 23:1345-66.

212. Brahmbhatt P, Atia A, Hasan A et al. A novel case of thyroid dysfunction associated with adalimumab use for crohn's disease. *Am J Gastroenterol.* 2013; 108:S424.

213. Hamnvik O-PR, Larsen PR, Marqusee E. Thyroid dysfunction from antineoplastic agents. *J Natl Cancer Inst.* 2011; 103:1572-87.

214. Benjamin RW, Calikoglu AS. Hyperthyroidism and lupus-like syndrome in an adolescent treated with minocycline for acne vulgaris. *Pediatr Dermatol.* 2007; 24:246-9.

215. Tacon L, Tan CTK, Alvarado R et al. Drug-induced thyroiditis and papillary carcinoma in a minocycline-pigmented black thyroid gland. *Thyroid.* 2008; 18:795-7.

216. Aleksic Z, Aleksic A, Mitov V et al. Amiodaron treatment and thyroid autoimmunity markers. *Hell J Nucl Med.* 2008; 11:105-9.

217. Touzot M, Le Beller C, Touzot F et al. Dramatic interaction between levothyroxine and lopinavir/ritonavir in a HIV-infected patient. *AIDS.* 2006; 20:1210-2.

218. Sagud M, Pivac N, Muck-Seler D et al. Effects of sertraline treatment on plasma cortisol, prolactin and thyroid hormones in female depressed patients. *Neuropsychobiology.* 2002; 45:139-43.

219. McCowen KC, Garber JR, Spark R. Elevated serum thyrotropin in thyroxine-treated patients with hypothyroidism given sertraline. *N Engl J Med.* 1997; 337:1010-1.

220. Church CO, Callen EC. Myxedema coma associated with combination aripiprazole and sertraline therapy. *Ann Pharmacother.* 2009; 43:2113-6.

221. Mazokopakis EE, Karefilakis CM, Starakis IK. Escitalopram-induced subclinical hypothyroidism. A case report. *Hormones (Athens).* 2012; 11:101-3.

222. Golden WM, Weber KB, Hernandez TL et al. Single-dose rexinoid rapidly and specifically suppresses serum thyrotropin in normal subjects. *J Clin Endocrinol Metab.* 2007; 92:124-30.

223. Smit JW, Stokkel MP, Pereira AM, Romijn JA, Visser TJ. Bexarotene-induced hypothyroidism: bexarotene stimulates the peripheral metabolism of thyroid hormones. *J Clin Endocrinol Metab.* 2007; 92:2496-9.

224. Sherman SI, Gopal J, Haugen BR et al. Central hypothyroidism associated with retinoid X receptor-selective ligands. *N Engl J Med.* 1999; 340:1075-9.

225. Satti H, Mafukidze A, Jooste PL et al. High rate of hypothyroidism among patients treated for multidrug-resistant tuberculosis in Lesotho. *Int J Tuberc Lung Dis.* 2012; 16:468-72.

226. Gupta J, Breen RAM, Milburn HJ. Drug-induced hypothyroidism in patients receiving treatment for multidrug-resistant tuberculosis in the UK. *Int J Tuberc Lung Dis.* 2012; 16:1278-1278.

227. Bhushan B, Chander R, Kajal N et al. Profile of adverse drug reactions in drug resistant tuberculosis from Punjab. *Indian J Tuberc.* 2014; 61:318-24.

228. Macgregor AG, Somner AR. The anti-thyroid action of para-aminosalicylic acid. *Lancet (London).* 1954; 267:931-6.

229. Edwards DA, Rowlands EN, Trotter WR. The mechanism of the goitrogenic action of p-aminosalicylic acid. *Lancet (London).* 1954; 267:1051-2.

230. AACE Thyroid Task Force. American Association of Clinical Endocrinologists medical guidelines for clinical practice for the evaluation and treatment of hyperthyroidism and hypothyroidism. *Endocr Pract.* 2002; 8:457-69.

231. Bahn RS, Burch HB, Cooper DS et al. Hyperthyroidism and other causes of thyrotoxicosis: management guidelines of the American Thyroid Association and American Association of Clinical Endocrinologists. *Endocr Pract.* 2011; 17:456-520.

232. Gregerman RI. Thyroid disorders. In: Barker LR, Burton JR, Zieve PD, eds. *Principles of ambulatory medicine.* Baltimore, MD: Williams and Wilkins; 1999:1066-95.

233. Cooper DS. Clinical practice: subclinical hypothyroidism. *N Engl J Med.* 2001; 345:260-5.

234. Loy M, Perra E, Melis A et al. Color-flow Doppler sonography in the differential diagnosis and management of amiodarone-induced thyrotoxicosis. *Acta Radiol.* 2007; 48:628-34.

235. Bartalena L, Grasso L, Brogioni S et al. Serum interleukin-6 in amiodarone-induced thyrotoxicosis. *J Clin Endocrinol Metab.* 1994; 78:423-7.

236. Kraszewska A, Chlopocka-Wozniak M, Abramowicz M et al. A cross-sectional study of thyroid function in 66 patients with bipolar disorder receiving lithium for 10-44 years. *Bipolar Disorders.* 2015; 17:375-80.

237. Dong BJ. How medications affect thyroid function. *West J Med.* 2000; 172:102-6.

238. Bogazzi F, Bartalena L, Gasperi M et al. The various effects of amiodarone on thyroid function. *Thyroid.* 2001; 11:511-9.

239. Mammen JS, Ghazarian SR, Rosen A, Ladenson PW. Patterns of interferon-alpha-induced thyroid dysfunction vary with ethnicity, sex, smoking status, and pretreatment thyrotropin in an international cohort of patients treated for hepatitis C. *Thyroid.* 2013; 23:1151-8.

240. Jamil KM, Leedman PJ, Kontorinis N et al. Interferon-induced thyroid dysfunction in chronic hepatitis C. *J Gastroenterol Hepatol.* 2009; 24:1017-23.

241. Yan Z, Fan K, Fan Y et al. Thyroid dysfunction in Chinese patients with chronic hepatitis C treated with interferon alpha: incidence, long-term outcomes and predictive factor. *Hepatitis Monthly.* 2012; 12.

242. Maiga I, Valdes-Socin H, Thiry A et al. [Alpha interferon induced hyperthyroidism: a case report and review of the literature]. *Rev Med Liege.* 2015; 70:390-4.

243. Nadeem A, Aslam M. Association of interferon-alpha and ribavirin-induced thyroid dysfunction with severity of disease and response to treatment in pakistani asian patients of chronic hepatitis C. *Hepat Res Treat.* 2012; 2012:864315.

244. Nadeem A, Aslam M, Khan DA et al. Effects of combined interferon alpha and ribavirin therapy on thyroid functions in patients with chronic hepatitis C. *J Coll Physicians Surg Pak.* 2009; 19:86-9.

245. Nadeem A, Hussain MM, Aslam M, Hussain T. Interferon-alpha induced and ribavirin induced thyroid dysfunction in patients with chronic hepatitis C. *Hepat Mon.* 2010; 10132-40.

246. Ziaee A, Esfehanian F, Alavian SM, Sarreshtedari M. Thyroid dysfunction in patients with chronic viral hepatitis B and C during alpha interferon therapy. *Hepat Mon.* 2009; 9:110-3.

247. Kozielewicz D, Zalesna A, Dybowska D. Can pegylated interferon alpha 2a cause development of thyroid disorders in patients with chronic hepatitis B? *Expert Opin Drug Saf.* 2014; 13:1009-14.

248. Uchida T, Kasai T, Takagi A et al. Prevalence of Amiodarone-induced thyrotoxicosis and associated risk factors in japanese patients. *Int J Endocrinol.* 2014; 2014.

249. Ahmed S, Van Gelder IC, Wiesfeld AC et al. Determinants and outcome of amiodarone-associated thyroid dysfunction. *Clin Endocrinol (Oxf).* 2011; 75:388-94.

250. Huang CJ, Chen PJ, Chang JW et al. Amiodarone-induced thyroid dysfunction in Taiwan: a retrospective cohort study. *Int J Clin Pharm.* 2014; 36:405-11.

251. Lee KF, Lee KM, Fung TT. Amiodarone-induced thyroid dysfunction in the Hong Kong Chinese population. *Hong Kong Med J.* 2010; 16:434-9.

252. Zosin I, Balas M. Amiodarone-induced thyroid dysfunction in an iodine-replete area: epidemiological and clinical data. *Endokrynol Pol.* 2012; 63:2-9.

253. Stan MN, Ammash NM, Warnes CA et al. Body mass index and the development of amiodarone-induced thyrotoxicosis in adults with congenital heart disease—a cohort study. *Int J Cardiol.* 2013; 167:821-6.

254. Farhan H, Albulushi A, Taqi A et al. Incidence and pattern of thyroid dysfunction in patients on chronic amiodarone therapy: experience at a tertiary care centre in Oman. *Open Cardiovasc Med J.* 2013; 7:122-6.

255. Aleksic Z, Aleksic A. Incidence of amiodarone-induced thyroid dysfunction and predictive factors for their occurrence. *Med Pregl.* 2011; 64:533-8.

256. Tsui KYQ. The impact of Lithium on thyroid function in Chinese psychiatric population. *Thyroid Research.* 2015; 8.

257. Shine B, McKnight RF, Leaver L, Geddes JR. Long-term effects of lithium on renal, thyroid, and parathyroid function: a retrospective analysis of laboratory data. *Lancet.* 2015; 386:461-8.

258. Hawkes WC, Keim NL. Dietary selenium intake modulates thyroid hormone and energy metabolism in men. *J Nutr.* 2003; 133:3443-8.

259. Frisullo G, Calabrese M, Tortorella C et al. Thyroid autoimmunity and dysfunction in multiple sclerosis patients during long-term treatment with interferon beta or glatiramer acetate: an Italian multicenter study. *Mult Scler J.* 2014; 20:1265-8.

260. Tran HA, Reeves GEM. The spectrum of autoimmune thyroid disease in the short to medium term following interferon-therapy for chronic hepatitis C. *Int J Endocrinol.* 2009; 2009.

261. Goldschlager N, Epstein AE, Naccarelli GV et al. A practical guide for clinicians who treat patients with amiodarone: 2007. *Heart Rhythm.* 2007; 4:1250-9.

262. Middeldorp ME, Mahajan R, Pathak R, Sanders P. Thyrotoxicosis occurring after the cessation of amiodarone: a need for ongoing survelience. *Heart Rhythm.* 2013; 10:S51-2.

263. Kurt IH, Yigit T, Karademir BM. Atrial fibrillation due to late amiodarone-induced thyrotoxicosis. *Clin Drug Investig.* 2008; 28:527-31.

264. Yagishita A, Hachiya H, Kawabata M et al. Amiodarone-induced thyrotoxicosis late after amiodarone withdrawal. *Circ J.* 2013; 77:2898-903.

265. Czarnywojtek A, Wolinski K, Czepczynski R et al. Amiodarone induced thyrotoxicosis—the dilemma to treat or not to treat by radioiodine. *Eur J Nucl Med Mol Imaging.* 2014; 41:S568.

266. Czarnywojtek A, Zgorzalewicz-Stachowiak M, Woliński K et al. Results of preventive radioiodine therapy in euthyroid patients with history of hyperthyroidism prior to administration of amiodarone with permanent atrial fibrillation—a preliminary study. *Endokrynologia Polska.* 2014; 65:269-74.

267. Giagounidis A, Fenaux P, Mufti GJ et al. Practical recommendations on the use of lenalidomide in the management of myelodysplastic syndromes. *Ann Hematol.* 2008; 87:345-52.

268. Menon S, Habermann T, Witzig T. Lenalidomide-associated hypothyroidism. *Leukemia & Lymphoma.* 2007; 48:2465.

269. Figaro MK, Clayton W Jr, Usoh C et al. Thyroid abnormalities in patients treated with lenalidomide for hematological malignancies: results of a retrospective case review. *Am J Hematol.* 2011; 86:467-70.

270. Friedman ES. Medical monitoring in patients with bipolar disorder: clinical recommendations. *J Clin Psych.* 2009; 70:e27-e27.

271. Reismüller B, Azizi AA, Peyrl A et al. Feasibility and tolerability of bevacizumab in children with primary CNS tumors. *Pediatr Blood Cancer.* 2010; 54:681-6.

272. Eskes SA, Wiersinga WM. Amiodarone and thyroid. *Best Pract Res Clin Endocrinol Metab.* 2009; 23:735-51.

273. Tsang W, Houlden RL. Amiodarone-induced thyrotoxicosis: a review. *Can J Cardiol.* 2009; 25:421-4.

274. Cai X, Bhushan S. Amiodarone induced toxicity. *J Gen Int Med.* 2015; 30:S356.

275. Bogazzi F, Bartalena L, Tomisti L et al. Glucocorticoid response in amiodarone-induced thyrotoxicosis resulting from destructive thyroiditis is predicted by thyroid volume and serum free thyroid hormone concentrations. *J Clin Endocrinol Metab.* 2007; 92:556-62.

276. Uzan L, Guignat L, Meune C et al. Continuation of amiodarone therapy despite type II amiodarone-induced thyrotoxicosis. *Drug Saf.* 2006; 29:231-6.

277. Stan MN, Sathananthan M, Warnes C et al. Amiodarone-induced thyrotoxicosis in adults with congenital heart disease—clinical presentation and response to therapy. *Endocr Pract.* 2014; 20:33-40.

278. Bogazzi F, Bartalena L, Tomisti L et al. Continuation of amiodarone delays restoration of euthyroidism in patients with type 2 amiodarone-induced thyrotoxicosis treated with prednisone: a pilot study. *J Clin Endocrinol Metab.* 2011; 96:3374-80.

279. Gough J, Gough IR. Total thyroidectomy for amiodarone-associated thyrotoxicosis in patients with severe cardiac disease. *World J Surg.* 2006; 30:1957-61.

280. Schreiber DH, DeFreest MS. Paroxysmal atrial fibrillation precipitated by amiodarone-induced thyrotoxicosis five months after cessation of therapy. *J Emerg Med.* 2006; 31:61-4.

281. Goldschlager N, Epstein AE, Naccarelli G et al. Practical guidelines for clinicians who treat patients with amiodarone. *Arch Intern Med.* 2000; 160:1741-8.

282. Ishay A, Carmeli J, Rozner E, Luboshitzky R. Refractory amiodarone-induced thyrotoxicosis: the surgical option. *World J Endocr Surg.* 2013; 5:21-4.

283. Birkedal C, Touliatos J, Gaskin T, Spence RK. Surgical considerations for treatment of amiodarone-induced thyrotoxicosis. *Curr Surg.* 2001; 58:478-80.

284. Hashimoto K, Ota M, Irie T et al. A case of type 2 amiodarone-induced thyrotoxicosis that underwent total thyroidectomy under high-dose steroid administration. *Case Rep Endocrinol.* 2015; 2015:416145.

285. Patel N, Inder WJ, Sullivan C, Kaye G. An audit of amiodarone-induced thyrotoxicosis—do anti-thyroid drugs alone provide adequate treatment? *Heart Lung Circ.* 2014; 23:549-54.

286. Yamamoto J, Dostmohamed H, Schacter I et al. Preoperative therapeutic apheresis for severe medically refractory amiodarone-induced thyrotoxicosis: a case report. *J Clin Apher.* 2014; 29:168-70.

287. Czarnywojtek A, Warmuz-Stangierska I, Wolinski K et al. Radioiodine therapy in patients with type II amiodarone-induced thyrotoxicosis. *Polskie Archiwum Medycyny Wewnetrznej.* 2014; 124:695-703.

288. Czarnywojtek A, Czepczynski R, Ruchala M et al. Radioiodine therapy in patients with amiodarone-induced thyrotoxicosis (AIT). *Neuro Endocrinol Lett.* 2009; 30:209-14.

289. Gursoy A, Tutuncu NB, Gencoglu A et al. Radioactive iodine in the treatment of type-2 amiodarone-induced thyrotoxicosis. *J Natl Med Assoc.* 2008; 100:716-9.

290. Czarnywojtek A, Wolinski K, Wasko R et al. Amiodarone-induced thyrotoxicosis in a case of Eisenmenger's syndrome. *Neuro Endocrinol Lett.* 2013; 34:767-72.

291. Pratap R, Qayyum A, Ahmad N, Jani P. Surgical management of amiodarone-induced thyrotoxicosis in a patient with Eisenmenger's syndrome: literature review and case report. *J Laryngol Otol.* 2009; 123:1276-9.

292. Czarnywojtek A, Waligorska-Stachura J, Szczepanek E et al. A rare case of interferon-alpha-induced hyperthyroidism in patients with a chronic hepatitis C with granulocytopenia and transaminasemia treated successfully with radioiodine. *Neuro Endocrinol Lett.* 2012; 33:268-72.
293. Jorge G, Queirós J, Nogueira C et al. Lithium associated thyrotoxicosis: a bipolar diagnosis. *Eur Thyroid J.* 2011: 150.
294. Sato Y, Taki K, Honda Y et al. Lithium toxicity precipitated by thyrotoxicosis due to silent thyroiditis: cardiac arrest, quadriplegia, and coma. *Thyroid.* 2013; 23:766-70.
295. Siyam FF, Deshmukh S, Garcia-Touza M. Lithium-associated hyperthyroidism. *Hosp Pract (1995).* 2013; 41:101-4.
296. Ohye H, Fukata S, Kanoh M et al. Thyrotoxicosis caused by weight-reducing herbal medicines. *Arch Intern Med.* 2005; 165:831-4.
297. Heidegger I, Nagele U, Pircher A et al. Latent hypothyreosis as a clinical biomarker for therapy response under abiraterone acetate therapy. *Anticancer Res.* 2014; 34:307-11.
298. Ghiculescu RA, Martin J. Rapidly progressive severe amiodarone-induced hypothyroidism in an elderly female. *J Pharm Pract Res.* 2009; 39:140-1.
299. Hofmann A, Nawara C, Ofluoglu S et al. Incidence and predictability of amiodarone-induced thyrotoxicosis and hypothyroidism. *Wien Klin Wochenschr.* 2008; 120:493-8.
300. Preda C, Aprotosoaie AC, Petris A, Costache, II. Amiodarone-induced thyroid dysfunction—clinical picture. Study on 215 cases. *Rev Med Chir Soc Med Nat Iasi.* 2014; 118:359-63.
301. Takeuchi D, Honda K, Shinohara T et al. Incidence, clinical course, and risk factors of amiodarone-induced thyroid dysfunction in Japanese adults with congenital heart disease. *Circ J.* 2015; 79:1828-34.
302. Yiu KH, Jim MH, Siu CW et al. Amiodarone-induced thyrotoxicosis is a predictor of adverse cardiovascular outcome. *J Clin Endocrinol Metab.* 2009; 94:109-14.
303. Rini BI, Escudier B, Tomczak P et al. Comparative effectiveness of axitinib versus sorafenib in advanced renal cell carcinoma (AXIS): a randomised phase 3 trial. *Lancet (London).* 2011; 378:1931-9.
304. Tomita Y, Uemura H, Fujimoto H et al. Key predictive factors of axitinib (AG-013736)-induced proteinuria and efficacy: a phase II study in Japanese patients with cytokine-refractory metastatic renal cell Carcinoma. *Eur J Cancer (Oxford, Eng.: 1990).* 2011; 47:2592-602.
305. Motzer RJ, Escudier B, Tomczak P et al. Axitinib versus sorafenib as second-line treatment for advanced renal cell carcinoma: overall survival analysis and updated results from a randomised phase 3 trial. *Lancet. Oncol.* 2013; 14:552-62.
306. Kindler HL, Ioka T, Richel DJ et al. Axitinib plus gemcitabine versus placebo plus gemcitabine in patients with advanced pancreatic adenocarcinoma: a double-blind randomised phase 3 study. *Lancet. Oncol.* 2011; 12:256-62.
307. Smith DC, Smith MR, Sweeney C et al. Cabozantinib in patients with advanced prostate cancer: results of a phase II randomized discontinuation trial. *J Clin Oncology.* 2013; 31:412-9.
308. Yavuz S, Apolo AB, Kummar S et al. Cabozantinib-induced thyroid dysfunction: a review of two ongoing trials for metastatic bladder cancer and sarcoma. *Thyroid.* 2014; 24:1223-31.
309. Krysiak R, Stojko R. Transient hypothyroidism induced by anticonvulsant agents. *Neuro Endocrinol Lett.* 2014; 35:183-5.
310. Lai EC, Yang YH, Lin SJ, Hsieh CY. Use of antiepileptic drugs and risk of hypothyroidism. *Pharmacoepidemiol Drug Saf.* 2013; 22:1071-9.
311. Matulonis UA, Berlin S, Ivy P et al. Cediranib, an oral inhibitor of vascular endothelial growth factor receptor kinases, is an active drug in recurrent epithelial ovarian, fallopian tube, and peritoneal cancer. *J Clin Oncol.* 2009; 27:5601-6.
312. Garland LL, Chansky K, Wozniak AJ et al. Phase II Study of AZD2171 in patients with malignant pleural mesothelioma: SWOG S0509. *J Thorac Ooncol.* 2011; 6:1938.
313. Kastoon T, Stump CS, Thomson SP, Yassine H. Erlotinib-associated exacerbation of hypothyroidism with pericardial tamponade. *Endocr Pract.* 2012; 18:e111-3.
314. Mallela AR, Koya R, Nagari SK, Mohapatra AK. Ethionamide: unusual cause of hypothyroidism. *JJ Clin Diagn Res.* 2015; 9:OD08-9.
315. Ozkan C, Altinova AE, Cerit ET et al. Destructive thyroiditis followed by hypothyroidism associated with infliximab therapy. *Endocr Pract.* 2014; 20:e207-10.
316. Cerniglia B, Judson MA. Infliximab-Induced hypothyroidism: a novel case and postulations concerning the mechanism. *Case Rep Med.* 2013; 2013:216939.
317. Motzer RJ, Hutson TE, Tomczak P et al. Overall survival and updated results for sunitinib compared with interferon alfa in patients with metastatic renal cell carcinoma. *J Clin Oncol.* 2009; 27:3584-90.
318. Gardezi MAI, Ali A, Malik SH et al. Assessment of thyroid dysfunction in chronic hepatitis c patients treated with interferon alpha and ribavirin therapy. *Pakistan J Med Hlth Sci.* 2012; 6:872-4.
319. Santos SRX, Ferreira MS, Borges AS et al, Thyroid disorders in hepatitis c patients treated or not with α-interferon and ribavirin. *Endocrinologist.* 2010; 20:122-4.
320. Masood N, Ghori R, Memon A et al. Frequency of thyroid disorders during interferon and ribavirin therapy in chronic hepatitis C infection. *J Coll Physicians Surg Pak.* 2008; 18:347-51.
321. Chutto MA, Chand H, Gurbakshani AL et al. Frequency of thyroid dysfunction following interferon therapy in patients with chronic hepatitis C. *Pakistan J Med Hlth Sci.* 2010; 4:165-8.
322. Nonchev B, Trenova A, Pavlov P et al. Autoimmune thyroiditis in patients with multiple sclerosis treated with interferon-beta. *Eur Thyroid J.* 2013; 2:155.
323. Hodi FS, O'Day SJ, McDermott DF et al. Improved survival with ipilimumab in patients with metastatic melanoma. *New Engl J Med.* 2010; 363:711-23.
324. Min L, Vaidya A, Becker C. Thyroid autoimmunity and ophthalmopathy related to melanoma biological therapy. *Eur J Endocrinol.* 2011; 164:303-7.
325. List A, Kurtin S, Roe DJ et al. Efficacy of lenalidomide in myelodysplastic syndromes. *New Engl J Med.* 2005; 352:549-57.
326. Dispenzieri A, Lacy MQ, Zeldenrust SR et al. The activity of lenalidomide with or without dexamethasone in patients with primary systemic amyloidosis. *Blood.* 2007; 109:465-70.
327. Krejci M, Adam Z, Pour L et al. Combination of lenalidomide, dexamethasone and cyclophosphamide as treatment for the first relapse of multiple myeloma: efficacy, toxicity and occurance of thyroid abnormalities. *Blood.* 2013; 122.
328. Trask LE, Bauman A, Comi RJ. Lenalidomide-exacerbated hypothyroidism: a case report. *Endocr Rev.* 2011; 32.
329. Muoio A, Leone MC, Galimberti D et al. Drug induced thyrotoxic storm: a misleading presentation. *Ital J Med.* 2014; 8:89.
330. Iams WT, Hames ML, Tsai JP et al. Increased serum tumor necrosis factor alpha levels in patients with lenalidomide-induced hypothyroidism. *Exp Hematol.* 2015; 43:74-8.
331. Tan E-H, Goss GD, Salgia R et al. Phase 2 trial of linifanib (ABT-869) in patients with advanced non-small cell lung cancer. *J Thorac Oncol.* 2011; 6:1418-25.
332. Toh HC, Chen PJ, Carr BI et al. Phase 2 trial of linifanib (ABT-869) in patients with unresectable or metastatic hepatocellular carcinoma. *Cancer.* 2013; 119:380-7.
333. Asahina H, Tamura Y, Nokihara H et al. An open-label, phase 1 study evaluating safety, tolerability, and pharmacokinetics of linifanib (ABT-869) in Japanese patients with solid tumors. *Cancer Chemother Pharmacol.* 2012; 69:1477-86.
334. Shulman KI, Sykora K, Gill SS et al. New thyroxine treatment in older adults beginning lithium therapy: implications for clinical practice. *Am J Geriatr Psychiatry.* 2005; 13:299-304.
335. Aliasgharpour M, Abbassi M, Shafaroodi H, Razi F. Subclinical hypothyroidism in lithium-treated psychiatric patients in Tehran, Islamic Republic of Iran. *East Mediterr Health J.* 2005; 11:329-33.

336. Barclay ML, Brownlie BE, Turner JG, Wells JE. Lithium associated thyrotoxicosis: a report of 14 cases, with statistical analysis of incidence. *Clin Endocrinol.* 1994; 40:759-64.
337. Fagiolini A, Kupfer DJ, Scott J et al. Hypothyroidism in patients with bipolar I disorder treated primarily with lithium. *Epidemiol Psichiatr Soc.* 2006; 15:123-7.
338. Ahmadi-Abhari SA, Ghaeli P, Fahimi F et al. Risk factors of thyroid abnormalities in bipolar patients receiving lithium: a case control study. *BMC Psychiatry.* 2003; 3:4.
339. Lee S, Chow CC, Wing YK, Shek CC. Thyroid abnormalities during chronic lithium treatment in Hong Kong Chinese: a controlled study. *J Affect Disord.* 1992; 26:173-8.
340. Mir SA, Wani AI, Masoodi SR et al. Lithium toxicity and myxedema crisis in an elderly patient. *Indian J Endocrinol Metab.* 2013; 17(suppl 3):S654-6.
341. van Melick EJ, Wilting I, Meinders AE, Egberts TC. Prevalence and determinants of thyroid disorders in elderly patients with affective disorders: lithium and nonlithium patients. *Am J Geriatr Psychiatry.* 2010; 18:395-403.
342. Schlumberger MJ, Elisei R, Bastholt L et al. Phase II study of safety and efficacy of motesanib in patients with progressive or symptomatic, advanced or metastatic medullary thyroid cancer. *J Clin Oncol.* 2009; 27:3794-801.
343. Blumenschein G, Kabbinavar F, Menon H et al. A phase II, multicenter, open-label randomized study of motesanib or bevacizumab in combination with paclitaxel and carboplatin for advanced nonsquamous non-small-cell lung cancer. *Ann Oncol.* 2011: mdq731.
344. Yoshizato T, Nannya Y, Yoshiki Y et al. Nilotinib-induced hypothyroidism in a patient with chronic myeloid leukemia. *Int J Hematol.* 2011; 93:400-2.
345. Newman CB, Melmed S, Snyder PJ et al. Safety and efficacy of long-term octreotide therapy of acromegaly: results of a multicenter trial in 103 patients—a clinical research center study. *J Clin Endocrinol Metab.* 1995; 80:2768-75.
346. Sandostatin package insert. East Hanover, NJ: Novartis Pharmaceuticals Corporation; 2005.
347. Maayan-Metzger A, Sack J, Mazkereth R et al. Somatostatin treatment of congenital chylothorax may induce transient hypothyroidism in newborns. *Acta Paediatr.* 2005; 94:785-9.
348. Miller J, Carney P. Central hypothyroidism with oxcarbazepine therapy. *Pediatr Neurol.* 2006; 34:242-4.
349. Takahashi M, Sawayama E, Sawayama T, Miyaoka H. Reversible paroxetine-induced symptomatic hypothyroidism. *Pharmacopsychiatry.* 2007; 40:201-2.
350. Motzer RJ, Hutson TE, Cella D et al. Pazopanib versus sunitinib in metastatic renal-cell carcinoma. *New Engl J Med.* 2013; 369:722-31.
351. Sternberg CN, Davis ID, Mardiak J et al. Pazopanib in locally advanced or metastatic renal cell carcinoma: results of a randomized phase III trial. *J Clin Oncol.* 2010; 28:1061-8.
352. Bible KC, Suman VJ, Molina JR et al. Efficacy of pazopanib in progressive, radioiodine-refractory, metastatic differentiated thyroid cancers: results of a phase 2 consortium study. *Lancet. Oncol.* 2010; 11:962-72.
353. Matrana MR, Duran C, Shetty A et al. Outcomes of patients with metastatic clear-cell renal cell carcinoma treated with pazopanib after disease progression with other targeted therapies. *Eur J Cancer (Oxford, Eng.: 1990).* 2013; 49:3169-75.
354. Castera L, Constant A, Henry C et al. Impact on adherence and sustained virological response of psychiatric side effects during peginterferon and ribavirin therapy for chronic hepatitis C. *Aliment Pharmacol Ther.* 2006; 24:1223-30.
355. Gehring S, Kullmer U, Koeppelmann S et al. Prevalence of autoantibodies and the risk of autoimmune thyroid disease in children with chronic hepatitis C virus infection treated with interferon-alpha. *World J Gastroenterol.* 2006; 12:5787-92.
356. Kee KM, Lee CM, Wang JH et al. Thyroid dysfunction in patients with chronic hepatitis C receiving a combined therapy of interferon and ribavirin: incidence, associated factors and prognosis. *J Gastroenterol Hepatol.* 2006; 21(1 Pt 2):319-26.
357. Minelli R, Valli MA, Di Secli C et al. Is steroid therapy needed in the treatment of destructive thyrotoxicosis induced by alpha-interferon in chronic hepatitis C? *Horm Res.* 2005; 63:194-9.
358. Hasan F, Asker H, Al-Khaldi J et al. Peginterferon alfa-2b plus ribavirin for the treatment of chronic hepatitis C genotype 4. *Am J Gastroenterol.* 2004; 99:1733-7.
359. Feret BM, Caley CF. Possible hypothyroidism associated with quetiapine. *Ann Pharmacother.* 2000; 34:483-6.
360. Liappas J, Paparrigopoulos T, Mourikis I, Soldatos C. Hypothyroidism induced by quetiapine: a case report. *J Clin Psychopharmacol.* 2006; 26:208-9.
361. Ramaswamy S, Siddiqui Z, Saharan S et al. Quetiapine-induced hypothyroidism. *J Psychiatry Neurosci.* 2005; 30:57.
362. Seroquel package insert. Wilmington, DE: AstraZeneca; 2008.
363. Sugita K, Kawakami K, Yokokawa T et al. Investigation of regorafenib-induced hypothyroidism in patients with metastatic colorectal cancer. *Anticancer Res.* 2015; 35:4059-62.
364. Takasu N, Kinjou Y, Kouki T et al. Rifampin-induced hypothyroidism. *J Endocrinol Invest.* 2006; 29:645-9.
365. Takasu N, Takara M, Komiya I. Rifampin-induced hypothyroidism in patients with Hashimoto's thyroiditis. *N Engl J Med.* 2005; 352:518-9.
366. Kim DL, Song KH, Lee JH et al. Rifampin-induced hypothyroidism without underlying thyroid disease. *Thyroid.* 2007; 17:793-5.
367. Collinson FJ, Vasudev NS, Berkin L et al. Sunitinib-induced severe hypothyroidism with cardiac compromise. *Med Oncol (Northwood, London, Eng.).* 2011; 28(suppl 1):S699-701.
368. Ahmadieh H, Salti I. Tyrosine kinase inhibitors induced thyroid dysfunction: a review of its incidence, pathophysiology, clinical relevance, and treatment. *Biomed Res Inl.* 2013; 2013: 725410-725410.
369. Sabatier R, Eymard J, Walz J et al. Could thyroid dysfunction influence outcome in sunitinib-treated metastatic renal cell carcinoma? *Ann Oncol.* 2012; 23:714-21.
370. Clemons J, Gao D, Naam M et al. Thyroid dysfunction in patients treated with sunitinib or sorafenib. *Clin Genitourin Cancer.* 2012; 10:225-31.
371. Raymond E, Dahan L, Raoul J-L et al. Sunitinib malate for the treatment of pancreatic neuroendocrine tumors. *New Engl J Med.* 2011; 364:501-13.
372. Chu TF, Rupnick MA, Kerkela R et al. Cardiotoxicity associated with tyrosine kinase inhibitor sunitinib. *Lancet (London, Eng.).* 2007; 370:2011-9.
373. Motzer RJ, Hutson TE, Olsen MR et al. Randomized phase II trial of sunitinib on an intermittent versus continuous dosing schedule as first-line therapy for advanced renal cell carcinoma. *J Clin Oncol.* 2012; 30:1371-7.
374. Demetri GD, Garrett CR, Schöffski P et al. Complete longitudinal analyses of the randomized, placebo-controlled, phase III trial of sunitinib in patients with gastrointestinal stromal tumor following imatinib failure. *Clin Cancer Res.* 2012; 18:3170-9.
375. Barrios CH, Liu M-C, Lee SC et al. Phase III randomized trial of sunitinib versus capecitabine in patients with previously treated HER2-negative advanced breast cancer. *Breast Cancer Res. Treat.* 2010; 121:121-31.
376. Del Fabbro E, Dev R, Cabanillas ME et al. Extreme hypothyroidism associated with sunitinib treatment for metastatic renal cancer. *J Chemotherapy (Florence, Italy).* 2012; 24:221-5.
377. Petrova M, Hristozov K, Konsoulova A, Kalev D. Sunitinib-induced hypothyroidism. *Eur Thyroid J.* 2011; 181.
378. Presotto F, Vastola F, Schiesaro MG, Bonciarelli G. Sunitinib-induced thyroid dysfunction: An emerging side-effect? *Italian J Med.* 2011; 5:89.
379. Clement P, Wolter P, Stefan C et al. Thyroid dysfunction in patients (pts) with metastatic renal cell cancer (RCC) treated with sorafenib. Paper presented at: ASCO Annual Meeting Proceedings 2008.

380. Ahmed M, Barbachano Y, Riddell A et al. Analysis of the efficacy and toxicity of sorafenib in thyroid cancer: a phase II study in a UK based population. *Eur J Endocrinol.* 2011; 165:315-22.
381. Schneider T, Abdulrahman R, Corssmit EP et al. Long-term analysis of the efficacy and tolerability of sorafenib in advanced radio-iodine refractory differentiated thyroid carcinoma: final results of a phase II trial. *Eur J Endocrinol.* 2012; 167:643-50.
382. Motzer RJ, Nosov D, Eisen T et al. Tivozanib versus sorafenib as initial targeted therapy for patients with metastatic renal cell carcinoma: results from a phase III trial. *J Clin Oncol.* 2013: JCO. 2012.2047. 4940.
383. Badros AZ, Siegel E, Bodenner D et al. Hypothyroidism in patients with multiple myeloma following treatment with thalidomide. *Am J Med.* 2002; 112:412-3.
384. de Savary N, Lee R, Vaidya B. Severe hypothyroidism after thalidomide treatment. *J R Soc Med.* 2004; 97:443-443.
385. Niwakawa M, Yamaguchi R, Onozawa Y et al. Phase I study of highly selective inhibitor of VEGFR tyrosine kinase, tivozanib, in Japanese patients with solid tumors. *Cancer Science.* 2013; 104:1039-44.
386. Joensuu H, De Braud F, Grignagni G et al. Vatalanib for metastatic gastrointestinal stromal tumour (GIST) resistant to imatinib: final results of a phase II study. *Br J Cancer.* 2011; 104:1686-90.
387. Mishra H, Rai YK, Mishra A, Singh V. Valproate-induced subclinical hypothyroidism. *Indian J Forensic Med Toxicol.* 2011; 5:110-2.
388. Chiriac A, Foia L, Chiriac AE, Solovan C. A case of sub acute thyroiditis in a patient on adalimumab for treatment of refractory palmo-plantar psoriasis. *J Eur Acad Dermatol Venereol.* 2013; 27:37.
389. Tsourdi E, Gruber M, Rauner M et al. Graves' disease after treatment with Alemtuzumab for multiple sclerosis. *Hormones.* 2015; 14:148-53.
390. Aranha AA, Amer S, Reda ES et al. Autoimmune thyroid disease in the use of alemtuzumab for multiple sclerosis: a review. *Endocr Pract.* 2013; 19:821-8.
391. Tohooloo B, Jhummon NP, Qu S. Amiodarone-induced thyrotoxicosis after administration of an intravenous infusion of amiodarone. *Cardiovasc Endocrinol.* 2013; 2:63-5.
392. Inaba H, Suzuki S, Takeda T et al. Amiodarone-induced thyrotoxicosis with thyroid papillary cancer in multinodular goiter: case report. *Med Princ Pract.* 2012; 21:190-2.
393. Khan A, Puttanna A, Raskauskiene D. Amiodarone-induced thyrotoxicosis: type 1 or type 2? *BMJ Case Rep.* 2014; 2014.
394. Liang YL, Huang SM, Peng SL et al. Amiodarone-induced thyrotoxicosis in a patient with autonomously functioning nodular goiter. *Ann Pharmacother.* 2009; 43:134-8.
395. Yavuz S, Apolo AB, Madan RA et al. The combined use of ultrasound and 99mTc scan in the evaluation of tyrosine kinase inhibitor-induced subacute thyroiditis with severe thyrotoxicosis. *Endocr Rev.* 2013; 34.
396. Shin JI, Park JM, Lee JS et al. Development of Graves' disease during cyclosporin treatment for severe Henoch-Schonlein nephritis. *Nephrol Dial Transplant.* 2005; 20:2014-5.
397. Chadha C, Pritzker M, Mariash CN. Effect of epoprostenol on the thyroid gland: enlargement and secretion of thyroid hormone. *Endocr Pract.* 2009; 15:116-21.
398. Assi HNA, Perkins JM. Hyperthyroidism associated with the use of everolimus in the treatment of metastatic renal cell carcinoma: The first reported case in the literature. *Endocr Rev.* 2011; 32.
399. Nakashima A, Nakagawa K, Ohgi S et al. Transient thyrotoxicosis following prolonged use of gonadotropin-releasing hormone agonist in women with endometriosis—a case report. *Arch Med Sci.* 2008; 4:200-3.
400. Kawashima J, Naoe H, Sasaki Y, Araki E. A rare case showing subacute thyroiditis-like symptoms with amyloid goiter after antitumor necrosis factor therapy. *Endocrinol Diabetes Metab Case Rep.* 2015; 2015.
401. Yarlo1lueş H, Cüce I, Akgül Ö et al. Hyperthyroidism in a patient with ankylosing spondylitis in association with the use of tumor necrosis factor-alpha. *Turkiye Fiziksel Tip ve Rehabilitasyon Dergisi.* 2013; 59:484.
402. Martin CS, Ionescu LN, Barbu CG et al. Takotsubo cardiomyopathy and transient thyrotoxicosis during combination therapy with interferon-alpha and ribavirin for chronic hepatitis C. *BMC Endocr Disord.* 2014; 14.
403. Higgs M, Hull E, Lujan E. A case report of post-operative jöd-basedow phenomennon following oral and IV iodine contrast administration. *Case Rep Endocrinol.* 2014; 2014.
404. Rhee CM, Bhan I, Alexander EK, Brunelli SM. Association between iodinated contrast media exposure and incident hyperthyroidism and hypothyroidism. *Arch Intern Med.* 2012; 172:153-9.
405. Calvi L, Daniels GH. Acute thyrotoxicosis secondary to destructive thyroiditis associated with cardiac catheterization contrast dye. *Thyroid.* 2011; 21:443-9.
406. Yu C, Chopra IJ, Ha E. A novel melanoma therapy stirs up a storm: ipilimumab-induced thyrotoxicosis. *Endocrinol Diabetes Metab Case Rep.* 2015; 2015:140092.
407. El-Bakush A, Fuller A, Tello W, Nugent K. Diverse complications in a patient with lithium toxicity. *J Invest Med.* 2014; 62:430.
408. Nefzi R, Abid Y, Ouanes S, Johnson I, Ghachem R. Lithium associated hyperthyroidism. *Eur Psychiatr.* 2015; 30:1598.
409. Bakerywala S, Schwarcz MD, Goldberg MD et al. Nilotinib-associated destructive thyroiditis. *Case Rep Endocrinol.* 2015; 2015:736092.
410. Lowndes SA, Asher R, Middleton MR. Thyrotoxicosis with pegylated interferon alfa-2b. *Arch Dermatol.* 2010; 146:1273-5.
411. Yagyu H, Okada K, Sato S et al. Pegylated interferon-alpha2b and ribavirin combination therapy induces Hashitoxicosis followed by type 1 diabetes mellitus. *Diabetes Res Clin Pract.* 2012; 95:e52-4.
412. Kwon SY, Choe WH, Kim JH, Kim HJ. Pegylated interferon-induced autoimmune thryoiditis and agraulocytosis by anti-thyroid drug: a case report. *Hepatology Int.* 2013; 7:S405.
413. Oo YH, Winer N. Delayed presentation of thyroid storm after radioiodine therapy. *Gazz Med Ital.* 2014; 173:365-8.
414. Bulzico DA, Cabizuca CA, De Mello RCR, Vaisman M. Radioiodine-induced autoimmune hyperthyroidism: case report. *Endocrinologist.* 2008; 18:124-5.
415. Haenel LCt, Gordon BM, Sagel J. Radioiodine-induced thyrotoxicosis and thyroiditis after ablative therapy for papillary carcinoma: a case discussion and literature review. *Clin Nucl Med.* 1999; 24:741-3.
416. Jarvis C, Simcox K, Tamatea JA et al. A low incidence of iodine-induced hyperthyroidism following administration of iodinated contrast in an iodine-deficient region. *Clin Endocrinol (Oxf).* 2015.
417. Kim SK, Lee SM, Yoo SS et al. Transient thyrotoxicosis from thyroiditis induced by sibutramine overdose: a case report. *Hum Exp Toxicol.* 2013; 32:890-2.
418. Wildiers H, Fontaine C, Vuylsteke P et al. Multicenter phase II randomized trial evaluating antiangiogenic therapy with sunitinib as consolidation after objective response to taxane chemotherapy in women with HER2-negative metastatic breast cancer. *Breast Cancer Res. Treat.* 2010; 123:463-9.
419. Trifanescu R, Trifanescu OG, Carsote M, Poiana C. Sunitinib-induced transient thyrotoxicosis in a patient with renal cell carcinoma. *Eur Thyroid J.* 2014; 3:139.
420. Chianese-Bullock KA, Woodson EM, Tao H et al. Autoimmune toxicities associated with the administration of antitumor vaccines and low-dose interleukin-2. *J Immunother.* 2005; 28:412-9.
421. Dora JM, Leie MA, Netto B et al. Lack of imatinib-induced thyroid dysfunction in a cohort of non-thyroidectomized patients. *Eur J Endocrinol.* 2008; 158:771-2.

422. Barbesino G. Drugs affecting thyroid function. *Thyroid.* 2010; 20:763-70.
423. Raggatt P, Wilkins M, Hoskins R, Park G. The effects of dopamine, dopexamine and dobutamine on TSH secretion in healthy subjects. *Clin Intensive Care.* 1999; 10:233-40.
424. Nakazawa T, Murata S-i, Kondo T et al. Histopathology of the thyroid in amiodarone-induced hypothyroidism. *Pathol Int.* 2008; 58:55-8.
425. Tomer Y, Menconi F. Interferon induced thyroiditis. *Best Pract Res Clin Endocrinol Metab.* 2009; 23:703-12.
426. Gursoy H, Cakmak I, Yildirim N, Basmak H. Presumed isotretinoin-induced, concomitant autoimmune thyroid disease and ocular myasthenia gravis: a case report. *Case Rep Dermatol.* 2012; 4:256-60.
427. Babacan T, Sevinc A, Akarsu E, Balakan O. Sunitinib-induced autoimmune thyroiditis in a patient with metastatic renal cell carcinoma: a case report. *Chemotherapy.* 2012; 58:142-5.
428. Karagöz B, Bilgi O, Özgün A et al. Autoimmunity and thyroid dysfunction during sunitinib treatment in metastatic renal cell carcinoma. *Endocrinologist.* 2009; 19:224- 5.
429. Sato S, Muraishi K, Tani J et al. Clinical characteristics of thyroid abnormalities induced by sunitinib treatment in Japanese patients with renal cell carcinoma. *Endocr J.* 2010; 57:873-80.
430. Betteridge T, Fink J. Phenytoin toxicity and thyroid dysfunction. *N Z Med J.* 2009; 122:102-4.

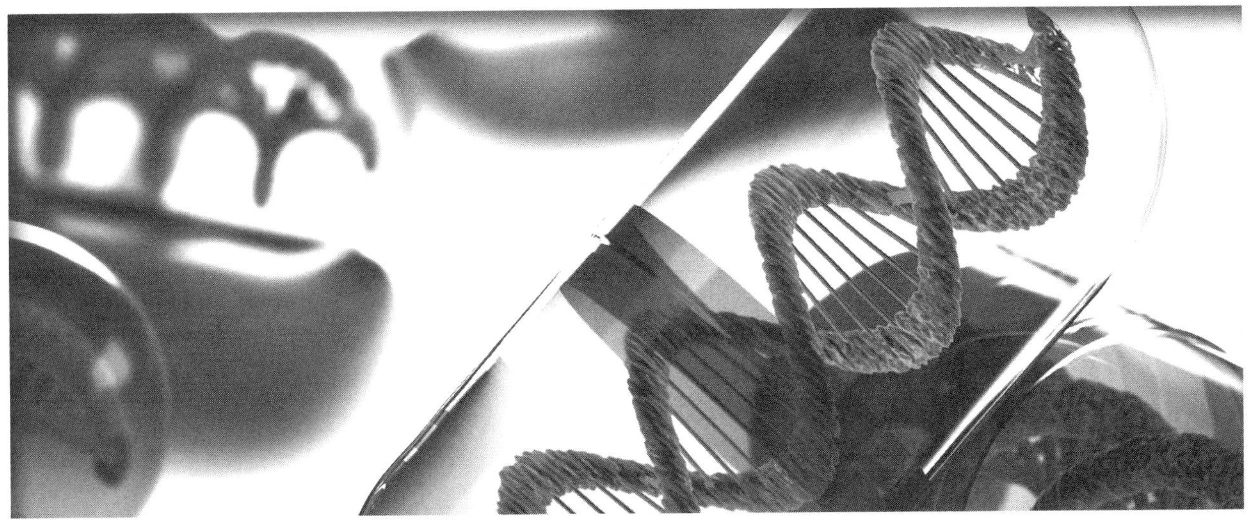

CHAPTER 32

Hypothalamic, Pituitary, and Adrenal Diseases

Andrew Y. Hwang, Steven M. Smith, and John G. Gums

Drug-induced disorders of the hypothalamus, pituitary, and adrenal glands are difficult to classify because of the complex interrelationship of the various endocrine glands. Nonetheless, the most commonly reported are those caused by adrenocortical dysfunction and excess prolactin secretion by the anterior pituitary. Adrenal glands are responsible for the secretion of catecholamines and three hormones responsible for the regulation of some of the most vital processes in the body. Aldosterone, the main end product of mineralocorticoid production, is secreted preferentially by the zona glomerulosa and is responsible for electrolyte and volume homeostasis. The zona fasciculata is primarily responsible for glucocorticoid production, mainly cortisol, and controls fat, protein, and glucose metabolism. The zona reticularis is primarily responsible for production of the sex steroids (estrogen and testosterone) that control the development of primary and secondary sex characteristics.

The pituitary gland, also known as the hypophysis, is under the control of the hypothalamus through direct nerve stimulation (posterior lobe) and by the actions of inhibitory and stimulating hormones (anterior lobe) such as thyrotropin-releasing hormone and corticotropin-releasing hormone (CRH). The anterior lobe of the pituitary gland is responsible for the synthesis of growth hormone (GH), prolactin, luteinizing hormone, follicle-stimulating hormone, thyroid-stimulating hormone, and adrenocorticotropic hormone (ACTH). In addition, vasopressin, also known as antidiuretic hormone, and oxytocin are synthesized in neurons of the hypothalamus, stored in the posterior lobe of the pituitary, and released upon direct nerve stimulation. The complex interplay between the hypothalamus, pituitary, and adrenal glands is commonly referred to as the hypothalamic–pituitary–adrenal (HPA) axis (**Figure 32-1**).

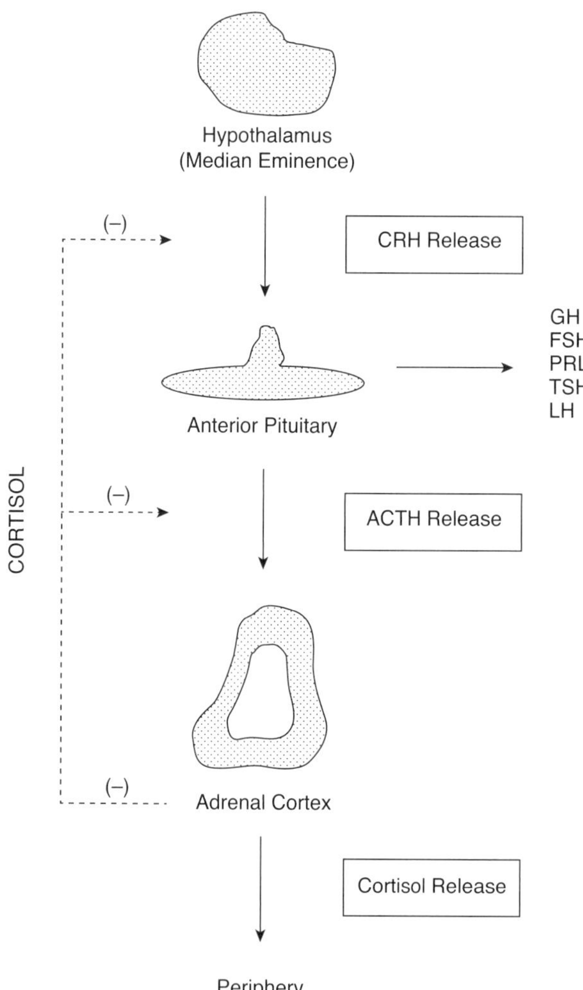

FIGURE 32-1 Hypothalamus

ACTH = adrenocorticotropin, CRH = corticotropin-releasing hormone, GH = growth hormone, FSH = follicle-stimulating hormone, LH = luteinizing hormone, PRL = prolactin, TSH = thyroid-stimulating hormone.

GLUCOCORTICOID EXCESS (CUSHING SYNDROME)

In 1932, Cushing first described a syndrome of pituitary basophilism that attracted national attention. Until that time, no definitive diagnosis was available for patients with unexplained central obesity, striae, osteoporosis, weakness, hypertension, and diabetes mellitus. Daughaday discovered elevated steroids in the urine of patients with this clinical presentation, and the syndrome was at last correctly explained as an excess of cortisol in the plasma (hypercortisolism).

CAUSATIVE AGENTS

Specific drugs that have been reported to induce Cushing syndrome are listed in **Table 32-1**.[1-40] Prolonged or excessive administration of corticosteroids is the most common cause of drug-induced Cushing syndrome; these drug-induced cases can occur following administration of virtually any corticosteroid by any route.[1-24,41-43] Other drug-induced causes include progestins and ACTH administration.

EPIDEMIOLOGY

The incidence of drug-induced Cushing syndrome in the general population is unknown, although it likely substantially exceeds the estimated 1 to 3 cases per million person-years observed in persons with Cushing syndrome secondary to pituitary tumors or adrenal adenomas and carcinomas (collectively referred to as endogenous Cushing syndrome).[44,45] Approximately 2–5% of obese patients with uncontrolled type 2 diabetes and hypertension screen positive for Cushing syndrome, although scarce data exist to help differentiate the drug-induced disease from other causes. Nevertheless, the vast majority of Cushing syndrome cases are thought to be drug-induced, and the syndrome has been recognized with increased frequency as the use of glucocorticoids for a wide range of nonendocrine diseases has expanded.

MECHANISMS

Mechanisms for drug-induced Cushing syndrome are listed in **Table 32-2**. In vivo, glucocorticoid drugs resemble the naturally occurring glucocorticoid, cortisol, and bind with high affinity to specific cytoplasmic glucocorticoid receptors (GRs) found in virtually all tissues of the body. This binding induces a response by modifying transcription and ultimately by causing changes in protein synthesis that can produce adverse physiologic effects similar to those seen in classic Cushing syndrome (hypercortisolism secondary to a pituitary tumor). Increased sensitivity to glucocorticoids may play a role in some cases of drug-induced Cushing syndrome, especially when the route of administration

Table 32-1 Agents Implicated in Drug-Induced Cushing Syndrome

Drug	Incidence[a]	Level of Evidence[b]
ORAL GLUCOCORTICOIDS		
Budesonide[38]	NK	C
Prednisolone[1]	5%	A
INHALED GLUCOCORTICOIDS		
Beclomethasone dipropionate[3,4]	NK	B
Budesonide[3,9]	NK	B
Fluticasone propionate[2-7,10,11,39]	NK	B
Mometasone furoate[7]	NK	B
Triamcinolone acetonide[3]	NK	B
NASAL GLUCOCORTICOIDS		
Fluticasone propionate[5,8]	NK	C
Fluticasone furoate[11]	NK	C
TOPICAL GLUCOCORTICOIDS		
Betamethasone[18]	NK	C
Clobetasol propionate[13,14,16]	NK	C
Dexamethasone[15]	NK	C
Hydrocortisone butyrate[17]	NK	C
Prednisolone acetate[23,24]	NK	C
Triamcinolone acetonide[12]	NK	C
INJECTABLE GLUCOCORTICOIDS		
Triamcinolone acetonide[19-22,40]	NK	C
PROGESTINS		
Medroxyprogesterone acetate[26-28]	NK	C
Megestrol acetate[29-31]	NK	C
OTHERS		
Corticotropin or adrenocorticotropic hormone[32-37,c]	NK	A
γ-hydroxybutyric acid[25]	NK	C

NK = not known.
[a]Incidence depends on dose and duration of exposure.
[b]Definitions for Levels of Evidence: Level A—evidence from one or more randomized, controlled clinical trials; Level B—evidence from nonrandomized clinical trials, prospective observational studies, cohort studies, retrospective studies, case-control studies, meta-analyses and/or postmarketing surveillance studies; and Level C—evidence from one or more published case reports or case series.
[c]Used as a confirmatory test to stimulate cortisol release.

Table 32-2 Mechanisms of Drug-Induced Cushing Syndrome

Drug	Mechanism
Adrenocorticotropin hormone (corticotropin, ACTH)[41]	Stimulates cortisol release from the zona fasciculata of the adrenal cortex
γ-hydroxybutyric acid[25]	Stimulates ACTH release from the pituitary gland
Glucocorticoids[46]	Resemble the naturally occurring glucocorticoid, cortisol, and bind with high affinity to specific cytoplasmic glucocorticoid receptors Binding modifies transcription and causes changes in protein synthesis that can produce adverse physiologic effects
Progestins[29]	Possess glucocorticoid-like activity and can bind to the glucocorticoid receptors

ACTH = adrenocorticotropic hormone.

is expected to result in minimal systemic exposure.[46] However, drug–drug interactions causing inhibition of the metabolism of glucocorticoids—particularly those with high first-pass metabolism such as fluticasone, budesonide, and mometasone—also may precipitate Cushing syndrome.[5-11] Medroxyprogesterone acetate (MPA) and megestrol acetate possess glucocorticoid-like activity and appear to induce Cushing syndrome through their ability to bind to GRs.[26-31,41,42] ACTH or drugs that stimulate ACTH release from the pituitary (e.g., γ-hydroxybutyric acid) may also contribute through the direct stimulation of the adrenal glands to release endogenous glucocorticoids.[25,41]

CLINICAL PRESENTATION AND DIFFERENTIAL DIAGNOSIS

Signs and symptoms of drug-induced Cushing syndrome are summarized in **Table 32-3**.[41,43,44] Common findings include progressive adiposity, dermopathies, myopathy, hypertension, insulin resistance (and corresponding elevations in glucose), hyperlipidemia, psychiatric changes, osteoporosis, gonadal and thyroid dysfunction, and growth deceleration in children.[41,43,44] Some features, such as increased intraocular pressure, cataracts, osteoporosis, and pancreatitis may be more prevalent with drug-induced Cushing syndrome; while other features such as hypertension, hirsutism, and amenorrhea may be more prevalent with the other etiologies.[47]

The biochemical diagnosis of Cushing syndrome relies on two steps: (1) confirming the presence of hypercortisolism and (2) identifying the underlying etiology of hypercortisolism. Hypercortisolism can be established using one or more of the following: the 24-hour urinary free cortisol test, the midnight serum cortisol test, the late-night salivary cortisol test, or the low-dose dexamethasone-suppression test.[32-37] Elevated urinary free cortisol values four times the upper limit of normal, late-night salivary cortisol >250 ng/dL, midnight serum cortisol >7.5 mcg/dL, or morning serum cortisol after low-dose dexamethasone suppression test >1.8 mcg/dL strongly suggest Cushing syndrome.[32-37] Midnight serum cortisol is often considered to be a second-line test, because admission to the hospital for 48 hours prior to testing may be necessary to help avoid false positive responses secondary to the stress of hospitalization. An additional confirmatory test is the determination of the plasma ACTH concentration, where values <5 pg/mL confirm drug-induced Cushing syndrome.[32-37]

Table 32-3 Signs and Symptoms Associated with Drug-Induced Cushing Syndrome

Signs and Symptoms	Incidence[a]
Central obesity	95%
Moon-shaped face	90%
Thin skin	85%
Oligomenorrhea or amenorrhea	80%
Hirsutism	75%
Hypertension	75%
Psychiatric mood changes	70%
Easy bruising	65%
Diabetes	60%
Glucose intolerance	60%
Proximal muscle weakness	60%
Osteopenia or osteoporosis	50%
Acne	NK
Buffalo hump	NK
Glaucoma, increased ocular pressure	NK
Kyphosis	NK
Pancreatitis	NK
Striae	NK

NK = not known.
[a]Prevalence related to general Cushing syndrome.

The clinical manifestation of drug-induced hypercortisolism is often quite similar to endogenous causes of hypercortisolism, such as Cushing syndrome, thus requiring a careful history in combination with dynamic testing of the integrity of the HPA axis to arrive at a correct diagnosis. Drugs, stress, renal insufficiency, alcohol ingestion, obesity, pregnancy, sleep disorders, and psychiatric illness can interfere with the diagnostic tests, making it challenging to differentiate between the causes (**Table 32-4**).[32,36] Patients with drug-induced Cushing syndrome typically present with low 24-hour urinary free cortisol concentration, low serum cortisol concentration, and suppressed ACTH levels.[47] Other significant laboratory findings in these

Table 32-4 Conditions to Consider in the Differential Diagnosis of Drug-Induced Cushing Syndrome

- Alcohol abuse
- Diabetes mellitus (Type 2)
- Metabolic syndrome
- Nondrug-induced Cushing syndrome (e.g., Cushing syndrome)
- Obesity
- Pregnancy
- Psychiatric illness
- Renal insufficiency
- Sleep disorders
- Stress

Table 32-5 Risk Factors for Drug-Induced Cushing Syndrome

- Administration of drugs that inhibit the metabolism of glucocorticoids
- Administration of high doses of offending agent
- Prolonged duration of therapy
- Use of high-potency glucocorticoids
- Use of topical glucocorticoids in patients with broken or atrophic skin and in infants

patients may include presence of synthetic glucocorticoids in the urine, elevation of total cholesterol, high concentrations of very-low-density lipoprotein and triglycerides, hypokalemia, and low bone density as measured by dual x-ray absorptiometry.[33,47]

RISK FACTORS

Risk factors for drug-induced Cushing syndrome are presented in **Table 32-5**.[43] Prolonged use, especially at a high dose, of any drug(s) that can cause Cushing syndrome is a known risk factor. Although inhaled, nasal, and topical glucocorticoids are intended to minimize systemic absorption, high doses and incorrect administration may result in increased absorption sufficient to cause Cushing syndrome.[1-18,43] High doses of drugs that possess glucocorticoid-like activity may enhance GR binding, as seen with oral progestins (e.g., 200–400 mg of MPA or 160 mg of megestrol acetate).[26-31] Additional risk factors for increased absorption of topical glucocorticoids include a broader area of coverage, high frequency of application, older patient age, and compromised skin integrity.[17,43,48]

Administration of high-potency glucocorticoids or drugs with a high affinity for GRs is another known risk factor for drug-induced Cushing syndrome. Of the available inhaled corticosteroids (ICS), fluticasone is considered the most potent, exhibiting prolonged drug retention at receptors in both blood and systemic tissues.[2,5] Clobetasol is one of the most potent topical glucocorticoids and, when used in high doses and for prolonged periods, has been reported to induce Cushing syndrome.[48,49]

Coadministration of potent inhibitors of the Cytochrome P450 (CYP450) isoenzyme family with glucocorticoids metabolized by these isoenzymes can lead to hypercortisolism via increased binding to the GRs. Cases of drug-induced Cushing syndrome have been reported when normal doses of inhaled fluticasone are coadministered with ritonavir and itraconazole, known inhibitors of fluticasone metabolism.[5,6,8-11] Cushingoid features also may develop in poor metabolizers of corticosteroids even when administering normal doses.[46]

MORBIDITY AND MORTALITY

Persons with overt but incompletely controlled endogenous Cushing syndrome have a fivefold increased risk of mortality relative to those with controlled Cushing syndrome.[45] Although the incidence of death due to drug-induced Cushing syndrome, per se, is unknown, it likely carries a lower risk than endogenous Cushing syndrome given that most cases are reversible following discontinuation of the causative agent. Cardiovascular complications have traditionally been regarded as the major contributor to morbidity and mortality in patients with Cushing syndrome and usually stem from uncontrolled blood pressure, glucose concentrations, and weight gain.[32,44] However, osteoporosis, fractures, thromboembolic events, and psychiatric illnesses are also common if hypercortisolism is not corrected.[32,44]

PREVENTION

Approaches to help prevent drug-induced Cushing syndrome are presented in **Table 32-6**. Minimizing

Table 32-6 Approaches to Help Prevent Drug-Induced Cushing Syndrome

- Avoid drug–drug interactions (e.g., CYP inhibitors) that will increase plasma concentrations of the offending agent
- Use alternative route of administration to minimize systemic absorption
- Use lowest effective dose and avoid prolonged use of offending agent

the risk factors presented in Table 32-5 may prevent drug-induced Cushing syndrome.[43] When administering agents with the potential to induce Cushing syndrome, practitioners should make every effort to use the lowest effective dose for the shortest period of time. In addition, concurrent administration of agents that reduce glucocorticoid metabolism should be avoided.

Inhaled and intranasal glucocorticoid administration can minimize systemic absorption and may help prevent Cushing syndrome. Topical glucocorticoids can produce desired pharmacologic effects without associated systemic adverse effects, although caution is advised in patients with broken skin or when occlusive dressings are required. The administration of glucocorticoids in the form of enemas may obviate the need for systemic glucocorticoids in patients with inflammatory bowel disease. Practitioners should be aware of these and other alternatives to systemic glucocorticoid therapy.

MANAGEMENT

The first and most important step in managing drug-induced Cushing syndrome is discontinuation of the offending agent when feasible. If the patient has been receiving a supra-physiologic dose of glucocorticoids (>7.5 mg daily of prednisone or its equivalent), that dose must be slowly tapered to a physiologic dose, often over months, to avoid precipitating adrenal insufficiency. After a physiologic dose has been achieved, the patient should continue to have the dose slowly tapered until the HPA axis has returned to normal function, which may take up to 1 year. Morning serum cortisol may be used to test for HPA axis integrity. Glucocorticoid replacement may be discontinued when cortisol plasma concentration is >20 mcg/dL. In cases in which alternative therapy is not an option and continued steroid treatment is required, strategies to reduce inhibition of the HPA axis should be considered, including the use of alternate-day dosing schedules (e.g., alternating between "on" and "off" days), the use of a less potent glucocorticoid, and nonsystemic routes of administration.[30,32]

INFORMATION FOR PATIENTS

Patients receiving long-term glucocorticoid therapy by any route of administration should be informed about the signs and symptoms of Cushing syndrome and advised to contact their pharmacist or physician if any of these develop. Because development of Cushingoid features is often insidious, periodic review and comparison between old and new photographs can be helpful in identifying physical changes when Cushing syndrome is suspected. The potential dangers of using higher doses than prescribed should also be discussed with patients in an effort to prevent supra-physiologic concentrations of glucocorticoids. Patients should also be instructed not to abruptly discontinue glucocorticoid therapy to avoid occurrence of adrenal crisis that can be a life-threatening problem in patients who have suppression of the HPA axis. Appropriate medication administration instructions should also be provided to patients taking or using any corticosteroid preparation to help minimize systemic exposure. Consultation points can include proper inhaler technique and avoidance of applying topical corticosteroids to nonintact skin.

SECONDARY ADRENAL INSUFFICIENCY

Hypocortisolism is the hallmark of adrenal insufficiency, which can be separated into two categories: primary and secondary. Primary adrenal insufficiency, commonly referred to as Addison disease, is caused by the inability of the adrenal cortex to produce cortisol, aldosterone, and androgens while the preceding components of the HPA axis remain functional. Because of the reduced negative feedback on the hypothalamus and pituitary, CRH and

ACTH plasma concentrations are elevated in primary adrenal insufficiency. Secondary adrenal insufficiency (SAI) often results from exogenous glucocorticoid use, which suppresses the HPA axis, decreases ACTH release, and impairs cortisol and androgen production. In SAI, CRH and ACTH concentrations are usually low and aldosterone production is typically preserved.

Primary and secondary adrenal insufficiency share many clinical features related to hypocortisolism. In primary adrenal insufficiency, increased CRH stimulates release of melanocyte-stimulating hormone. Both melanocyte-stimulating hormone and ACTH cause melanocytes to form melanin in the skin's epidermis, leading to hyperpigmentation, a characteristic trait of Addison disease. In addition, patients with primary adrenal insufficiency more commonly experience electrolyte abnormalities, especially hyperkalemia. These clinical findings are usually absent in drug-induced SAI.

CAUSATIVE AGENTS

Drugs that have been reported to suppress the HPA axis and cause SAI on discontinuation are listed in **Table 32-7**.[5,15-17,21,22,27-30,39-41,43,50-77] The most common cause of drug-induced SAI is exogenous glucocorticoid, with clinical manifestations of the disorder occurring on abrupt withdrawal of these agents. Medications used for the treatment of Cushing syndrome, including ketoconazole, etomidate, and mitotane, have also been implicated in drug-induced SAI.

EPIDEMIOLOGY

SAI has an overall estimated prevalence of 150–280 cases per 1 million persons.[78] Excessive glucocorticoid therapy induces atrophy of pituitary corticotroph cells and is thought to be the primary cause of this disorder, with an estimated prevalence of 20–50% among patients taking exogenous glucocorticoids for longer than 1 year.[79,80] Drug-induced SAI is usually only clinically relevant during or after glucocorticoid withdrawal, although a few other mechanisms have been identified (see below). Higher glucocorticoid doses administered over longer periods (>7.5 mg of prednisone or equivalent for >3 weeks) are often implicated in SAI, but patient response is highly variable, and HPA axis suppression may occur with any dose or duration of therapy.[43] As with Cushing syndrome, glucocorticoid administration via virtually any route may suppress the HPA axis.[5,15-17,21,22,41,43,50-58] In most patients, adrenal function returns to normal within 14 days after glucocorticoid withdrawal.[81] In a minority of patients with drug-induced SAI due to corticosteroid use, normalization of the adrenal gland may take up to 1 year.[43,82] In other drug-induced causes where the adrenocortical tissue is destroyed, hypofunction of the adrenal glands may be permanent.

MECHANISMS

Mechanisms of drug-induced SAI are listed in **Table 32-8**. Drug-induced SAI is characterized by a reduction in ACTH secretion from the pituitary gland, resulting in atrophy of the adrenal cortex. A low endogenous cortisol concentration is not clinically manifest if glucocorticoid activity is supplemented through exogenous glucocorticoid administration. However, when exogenous glucocorticoid therapy is abruptly stopped or when the patient is exposed to stressful stimuli (e.g., surgery, trauma, infection), adrenal suppression becomes clinically apparent because of the inability of the adrenal cortex to mount a sufficient cortisol response.

Sustained negative feedback activity on GRs in the anterior pituitary gland and hypothalamus, as occurs with high-dose and prolonged exogenous glucocorticoid administration, may lead to prolonged suppression of CRH, which in turn, suppresses ACTH release from the anterior pituitary and results in a lack of adrenal secretion of cortisol.[41,78,83]

Numerous studies have documented the ability of inhaled and nasal glucocorticoids to suppress the HPA axis, especially when administered in high doses or when combined with inhibitors of CYP450 3A4.[5,50-57,84] At recommended doses, however, inhaled and nasal glucocorticoids rarely suppress adrenal function. Topical, intra-articular, intradermal, intramuscular, intralesional, and paraspinal administration of glucocorticoids have also been implicated in SAI.[15-17,21,22,58] Patients with compromised skin integrity who use high-potency topical

Table 32-7 Agents Implicated in Drug-Induced Adrenal Insufficiency

Drug	Incidence[a]	Level of Evidence[b]
ORAL GLUCOCORTICOIDS		
Dexamethasone[50]	83%	A
Prednisone[50]	80%	A
INHALED GLUCOCORTICOIDS		
Beclomethasome dipropionate[3,53]	NK	B
Budesonide[3,51]	NK	B
Fluticasone propionate[3,5,6,39,46]	NK	B
Mometasone furoate[7]	NK	B
Triamcinolone acetonide[3]	NK	B
NASAL GLUCOCORTICOIDS		
Beclomethasome dipropionate[56]	NK	C
Fluticasone propionate[5,50]	NK	C
TOPICAL GLUCOCORTICOIDS		
Betamethasone[18]	NK	C
Clobetasol propionate[13,14,16]	NK	C
Dexamethasone[15]	NK	C
Hydrocortisone butyrate[17]	NK	C
Prednisolone acetate[24]	NK	C
Triamcinolone acetonide[12]	NK	C
INJECTABLE GLUCOCORTICOIDS		
Triamcinolone acetonide[21,22,40]	NK	C
PROGESTINS		
Medroxyprogesterone acetate[27,59,60]	NK	C
Megestrol acetate[30,61,62]	NK	C
OTHERS		
Etomidate[66,67,c]	NK	B
Fentanyl[74]	NK	C
Flunitrazepam[75,d]	NK	C
Hydromorphone[73]	NK	C
Ketoconazole[63-65,c]	NK	B
Mirtazapine[72]	NK	B
Mitotane[68,c]	NK	C
Rifampin[70,71]	NK	C

NK = not known.
[a]Incidence depends on dose and duration of exposure.
[b]Definitions for Levels of Evidence: Level A—evidence from one or more randomized, controlled clinical trials; Level B—evidence from nonrandomized clinical trials, prospective observational studies, cohort studies, retrospective studies, case-control studies, meta-analyses and/or postmarketing surveillance studies; and Level C—evidence from one or more published case reports or case series.
[c]Used as medical treatment for hypercortisolism.
[d]Not approved for use in the United States, but it is sometimes acquired illegally for recreational use.

glucocorticoids (e.g., clobetasol propionate) may be at higher risk for SAI.[15-17,49,58]

When administered at high doses, progestins or progestin analogs also may suppress the HPA axis. These agents, specifically MPA and megestrol acetate, possess glucocorticoid-like activity thought to be due to existing cross-reactivity within this family of steroid receptors.[27,30,59-62] Ketoconazole,

Table 32-8 Mechanisms of Drug-Induced Secondary Adrenal Insufficiency

Drug	Mechanism
Etomidate[66]	Inhibits 17α-hydroxylase and 11α-hydroxylase, resulting in reduced cortisol synthesis
Fentanyl[74] Flunitrazepam[75]	Inhibit pituitary response to CRH
Glucocorticoids[78,83]	Sustained stimulation of the negative feedback effect on GRs in the anterior pituitary gland and hypothalamus leads to prolonged suppression of CRH, which in turn suppresses ACTH release from the anterior pituitary and results in a lack of adrenal secretion of cortisol. This process is also referred to as suppression of the HPA axis.
Hydromorphone[73]	Inhibits CRH release through binding to hypothalamic 6- and n-opiate receptors
Ketoconazole[63,64]	Inhibits cholesterol side-chain cleavage and cytochrome P450 enzymes, 17α-hydroxylase and 17,20-lyase, resulting in reduced cortisol synthesis
Mirtazapine[72]	Antagonizes central 5-hydroxytryptamine$_2$ and/or histamine$_1$ receptors, resulting in decreased CRH release, ACTH secretion, and cortisol release
Mitotane[41,68]	Inhibits 11α-hydroxylase, 18-hydroxylase, 3α-hydroxylase, and cholesterol side-chain cleavage, resulting in reduced cortisol synthesis Degenerates cells within the zona fasciculata and reticularis; the zona glomerulosa can be affected with long-term treatment
Progestins[59,61]	Suppress HPA through their ability to bind to the GR
Rifampin[70,71]	Induces cytochrome P450 isoenzymes responsible for cortisol metabolism

ACTH = adrenocorticotropic hormone, CRH = corticotropin-releasing hormone, GR = glucocorticoid receptor, HPA = hypothalamic–pituitary–adrenal.

etomidate, mitotane, and other agents used to treat Cushing syndrome interfere with cortisol synthesis leading to lower circulating endogenous cortisol.[41,63-69] Mitotane also possesses cytotoxic properties and can cause atrophy of the adrenal cortex, mostly affecting the zona fasciculata and zona reticularis.[41] Thus, production of endogenous cortisol and sex hormones may be affected, while production of aldosterone is usually spared.[85] Rifampin, phenytoin, and phenobarbital may suppress the axis by inducing CYP450 isozymes responsible for cortisol metabolism.[41,70,71] Mirtazapine appears to cause adrenal suppression by antagonizing central 5-hydroxytryptamine$_2$ receptors responsible for the stimulation of cortisol secretion.[72] Opioids inhibit CRH release by binding to hypothalamic δ- and κ-opiate receptors.[73,74] Certain benzodiazepines may inhibit pituitary response to CRH.[75]

CLINICAL PRESENTATION AND DIFFERENTIAL DIAGNOSIS

Signs and symptoms associated with drug-induced SAI are presented in **Table 32-9**.[77,78,82,83,86] Patients may present with abnormal laboratory values such as hyponatremia, hypoglycemia, mild normocytic anemia, lymphocytosis, and mild eosinophilia. **Table 32-10** lists conditions that must be considered in the differential diagnosis of drug-induced SAI.[78] Rarely, acute adrenal insufficiency may be life-threatening. Patients with this disorder may exhibit severe hypotension or hypovolemic shock, hypoglycemia, acute abdominal pain, vomiting, and fever.[82,86]

The laboratory diagnosis of adrenal insufficiency involves measurement of early morning plasma cortisol concentration as well as dynamic testing.[77-79,82,86] Adrenal insufficiency can be ruled out by measuring a plasma cortisol concentration between 7 and 9 a.m. A concentration of <3 mcg/dL (100 nmol/L) is indicative of adrenal insufficiency, and a concentration of >18 mcg/dL (500 nmol/L) rules out the disorder.[77,78,87] Dynamic testing is required for patients with a cortisol concentration between 3 and 18 mcg/dL and can be useful in determining the cause of the disease. Dynamic tests include the insulin-tolerance test, metyrapone test, ACTH stimulation test, and CRH stimulation test.[77-79,82,83,86,88]

The insulin-tolerance test is considered the standard for the evaluation of SAI because hypoglycemia

Table 32-9 Signs and Symptoms Associated with Drug-Induced Secondary Adrenal Insufficiency

Signs and Symptoms	Incidence[a]
Weakness or fatigue	100%
Weight loss or anorexia	100%
Hypotension or postural hypotension	88–94%
Gastrointestinal symptoms (abdominal cramps, nausea, diarrhea, vomiting)	92%
Hyponatremia	88%
Myalgia or arthralgia	6–13%
Anemia, lymphocytosis, eosinophilia	NK
Hypoglycemia	NK
Vitiligo	NK

NK = not known.
[a]Prevalence related to general adrenal insufficiency.

Table 32-10 Conditions to Consider in the Differential Diagnosis of Drug-Induced Secondary Adrenal Insufficiency

- Addison disease
- Anemia
- Chronic fatigue syndrome
- Chronic heart failure
- Liver disease
- Myopathies
- Neuropsychiatric weakness
- Pigmentation disorders
- Syndrome of inappropriate antidiuretic hormone

in normal subjects results in rapid activation of the HPA axis.[77,78,83,88] This test is labor-intensive, with patients requiring constant supervision by a medical professional because a serum glucose of <40 mg/dL and symptoms of hypoglycemia are required elements of the test. The insulin-tolerance test is contraindicated in patients >60 years of age, those with cardiovascular disease, and those with a history of seizures.[77,78] An ACTH stimulation test is often preferred because of its ease of use and relatively high correlation with the insulin-tolerance test. Patients are given 250 mcg of synthetic ACTH (cosyntropin) intravenously or intramuscularly, and serum cortisol concentrations are measured at baseline and 60–90 minutes after the injection. An increase in the cortisol concentration to >18 mcg/dL at 60–90 minutes rules out adrenal insufficiency. In several studies, doses of 0.5 mcg or 1 mcg instead of the customary 250 mcg dose of synthetic ACTH have been effective in stimulating a cortisol response and are associated with higher sensitivity in identifying patients with subtle SAI. Because cortisol secretion can vary throughout the day, the test should ideally be done in the morning to ensure optimal sensitivity and specificity.[89] Studies also suggest that cortisol concentrations should be obtained at 30–60 minutes for the low-dose test.[77-79,82,83] The CRH stimulation test also correlates well with the insulin-tolerance test in patients with SAI, but it is less standardized and is costly.[77-79,82,83]

RISK FACTORS

Specific risk factors associated with drug-induced SAI are presented in **Table 32-11**.[3,41,43,49,82,90] Because this disorder is often a result of the exogenous administration of glucocorticoids, risk factors for SAI and Cushing syndrome are very similar; however, differences exist in terms of the precipitating event (e.g., continued use versus abrupt withdrawal of corticosteroids) that leads to the clinical syndrome.

In contrast to the use of standard doses, administration of high doses of inhaled and intranasal glucocorticoids have been associated with a higher incidence of adrenal suppression.[4,51,52,55-57] Specifically, ICSs such as beclomethasone dipropionate, budesonide, and triamcinolone acetonide at doses >1.5 mg/day and fluticasone propionate at a dose >0.75 mg/day caused marked adrenal suppression.[3]

Likewise, topical glucocorticoids administered at high doses are associated with a higher risk of adrenal suppression.[49]

High levels of systemic absorption can contribute to adrenal suppression with glucocorticoids, and the degree of CRH suppression is proportional to the amount of circulating cortisol or cortisol-like compounds. Because of rapid and extensive systemic absorption, the long-term (>3 week) use of oral glucocorticoids may induce significant adrenal suppression regardless of the dose administered.[43,49,82] ICSs are intended to limit systemic absorption through local deposition in the lung and high first-pass metabolism of any swallowed drug. However, 60% to 90% of the ICS dose may be swallowed and available for gastrointestinal absorption, and systemic absorption of small ICS particles may occur via lung alveoli.[91] Therefore, the risk of SAI from ICSs with high first-pass metabolism (e.g., fluticasone, mometasone) may be increased with drugs that inhibit the metabolism of glucocorticoids (e.g., ketoconazole, ritonavir) and when step-down therapy is not practiced following the reversal of airflow obstruction and inflammation.

Table 32-11 Risk Factors for Drug-Induced Secondary Adrenal Insufficiency

- In the setting of abrupt glucocorticoid withdrawal
  - Administration of high doses
  - Prolonged duration of therapy
  - Use of high-potency glucocorticoids
  - Administration of drugs that inhibit the metabolism of endogenous and exogenous glucocorticoids
- Concomitant diseases (e.g., hypothyroidism, acquired immunodeficiency syndrome)
- Physical stress (stressful situation, surgery, infection, trauma)

Use of high-potency glucocorticoids increases the risk of drug-induced SAI. A list of commonly used orally administered glucocorticoids, according to relative potency, can be found in **Table 32-12**. In a meta-analysis of 21 studies examining ICS potencies, inhaled fluticasone exhibited significantly greater dose-related adrenal suppression as compared with inhaled beclomethasone, budesonide, or triamcinolone.[3] In another study, inhaled mometasone showed similar adrenal suppression at medium and high doses as compared with inhaled fluticasone.[92] Levin and Maibach identified the use of high-potency topical glucocorticoids such as clobetasol propionate as a risk factor for mild or reversible adrenal suppression.[58] Other risk factors for SAI associated with topical administration of glucocorticoids include prolonged duration of treatment, use on thin or damaged skin, and use in children and infants.[58]

Most cases of adrenal crisis in those with chronic SAI occur because of reduction of the glucocorticoid dose or as a result of failure to adjust

Table 32-12 Pharmacologic Characteristics of Orally Administered Glucocorticoids

Glucocorticoid	Relative Anti-inflammatory Potency	Dose Equivalent (mg)	Approximate Half-Life (min)
LOW POTENCY			
Cortisone	0.8	25	30
Hydrocortisone	1	20	90
MEDIUM POTENCY			
Prednisone	3.5	5	60
Prednisolone	4	5	200
Triamcinolone	5	4	300
Methylprednisolone	5	4	180
HIGH POTENCY			
Betamethasone	25	0.6	100–300
Dexamethasone	30	0.75	100–300

Table 32-13 Approaches to Help Prevent Drug-Induced Adrenal Insufficiency

- Avoid abrupt withdrawal of glucocorticoids (e.g., nonadherence, quick dose tapers upon discontinuation)
- Avoid drug–drug interactions (e.g., CYP inducers) that will decrease concentrations in patients on therapy with corticosteroids
- Double or triple oral glucocorticoid dose during times of severe physical stress (e.g., febrile illness or injury, surgery)
- Use topical or inhaled agents, as appropriate to minimize glucocorticoid systemic absorption
- Use a spacer to minimize swallowed glucocorticoid after metered-dose inhaler
- Use lowest effective dose of offending agent
- Use step-down therapy with inhaled corticosteroid after pulmonary obstruction and inflammation subside

Table 32-14 Management of Drug-Induced Secondary Adrenal Insufficiency

- Discontinue offending agent and initiate appropriate therapeutic alternative
- Taper slowly, if necessary, depending on agent being discontinued (e.g., glucocorticoids, progestins)
- If glucocorticoid replacement is required, the usual dose of hydrocortisone is 15–20 mg/day and that of prednisone 5–7.5 mg/day (one half to two thirds of the dose may be given in the morning)

glucocorticoid-replacement doses properly in the presence of stressors.[78] Concomitant diseases (e.g., hypothyroidism, acquired immunodeficiency syndrome) may impair the central response to stress and cortisol secretion and are also risk factors for the development of adrenal insufficiency.[86]

MORBIDITY AND MORTALITY

As discussed above, drug-induced SAI is accompanied by a constellation of nonspecific and usually non-life-threatening symptoms such as fatigue, anorexia, asthenia, weight loss, abdominal pain, nausea, vomiting, and weakness. However if unrecognized and untreated, SAI can be a fatal disorder because of the risk of circulatory collapse.[86]

PREVENTION

Methods to prevent drug-induced secondary adrenal insufficiency are presented in **Table 32-13.** Drug-induced SAI may be prevented by minimizing the risk factors associated with drug-induced adrenal insufficiency (Table 32-11). Practitioners should make an effort to use the lowest possible dose of agents that are known to suppress the HPA axis. This can be accomplished by using a step-down approach when symptoms resolve and by not exceeding the dose limits for the selected agent.

Because glucocorticoid requirements are increased during times of stressful events, patients should be instructed to double or triple their oral glucocorticoid dose during febrile illness or injury. Patients may also be supplied with and instructed regarding the proper use of hydrocortisone intramuscular injections for emergency use. In some nonsevere cases where patients are experiencing nausea or vomiting, the glucocorticoid can be given in the form of rectal suppositories.[78,93]

The use of a spacer attached to a metered-dose inhaler may reduce the amount of drug that is swallowed and therefore decrease gastrointestinal absorption,[89] particularly for ICSs with lower first-pass metabolism. For higher-potency ICSs (e.g., fluticasone), appropriate administration, use of a spacer, and using the lowest possible maintenance dose may help reduce the risk of SAI.[91]

MANAGEMENT

Because drug-induced SAI is often due to the inappropriate withdrawal of glucocorticoids, replacement with glucocorticoids is generally the treatment of choice to correct the resultant adrenal crisis. In other cases of drug-induced SAI, identification of the offending medication is usually the first step, and discontinuation of the offending medication or substitution of an appropriate therapeutic alternative should be considered. In patients with chronic SAI or in those where discontinuation of the offending medication is not possible, treatment should be guided by replacement with physiological doses of glucocorticoids (**Table 32-14**).

Glucocorticoid replacement usually involves the administration of two or three daily doses.

On average, the healthy adult produces approximately 10–30 mg of cortisol per day, with the peak concentration occurring around 8:00 a.m. This cortisol concentration is equivalent to approximately 15–20 mg of hydrocortisone or 5–7.5 mg of prednisone every day. One half to two thirds of the dose may be given in the morning to mimic the normal diurnal variation of cortisol.[78,92] Hydrocortisone and prednisone are preferred over agents with longer half-lives, such as prednisolone, triamcinolone, dexamethasone, and betamethasone, because the former agents may allow the HPA axis more opportunity to recover and appropriately release CRH and ACTH based on the body's need for cortisol.[43,78,82,86]

Minor abnormalities discovered on dynamic testing should be treated only in the presence of symptomatic adrenal insufficiency. Testing should be performed on any patient who reports suggestive symptoms or on any child whose growth velocity is slowed. The lowest effective dose of glucocorticoid should be used, and dosing should be guided by symptomatic management of fatigue and other symptoms as described in Table 32-9.[77,78,93]

Because suppression of the HPA axis is a major concern only when exogenous glucocorticoids are withdrawn, practitioners should avoid abruptly stopping oral glucocorticoids taken for longer than 14 days. A variety of recommendations for steroid tapering are available; however, no consensus exists regarding the best approach.[41,43] In general, for patients who have been taking long-term steroid therapy, the steroid should be gradually withdrawn toward physiologic doses over months. As the steroid dose approaches physiologic levels, the taper should be slowed and the patient monitored for HPA axis function. The primary modes to test HPA axis integrity are the ACTH test, either high- or low-dose, or measurement of a morning serum cortisol level.[41,43] A normal morning serum cortisol concentration (>20 mcg/dL) or a normal ACTH test indicates that daily steroid maintenance therapy is not needed. If the morning serum cortisol concentration is between 3 and 20 mcg/dL, an ACTH test or an CRH stimulation test may be useful in the assessment of pituitary–adrenal function.[43] A morning cortisol concentration <3 mcg/dL indicates axis suppression and the need for continued replacement therapy. Caution should be used to prevent disease exacerbation during the steroid taper and the resultant need to treat the patient with another course of high-dose corticosteroids.[41]

Adrenal crisis has been reported after the discontinuation of MPA and megestrol acetate; therefore, tapering is also recommended for patients receiving these agents. Although adrenal suppression can occur in patients receiving inhaled, intranasal, and topical glucocorticoids, supplementation during periods of stress and/or tapering of doses prior to complete discontinuation is usually not needed.[58] Due to the direct cytotoxic effects on the adrenal cortex, therapy with mitotane may require replacement with both glucocorticoids and sex hormones, although data regarding management of mitotane-induced adrenal insufficiency are sparse.[85]

INFORMATION FOR PATIENTS

Patients receiving long-term inhaled, topical, and oral glucocorticoids should be educated regarding the signs and symptoms associated with SAI and instructed to contact their healthcare provider if these develop. The importance of adherence to long-term therapy with glucocorticoids should be addressed with patients in an effort to prevent any abrupt withdrawal leading to adrenal crisis. Patients should carry an information card with details about their current treatment and instructions for emergency treatment, including instructions on doubling or tripling the glucocorticoid dose during febrile illness or injury and using alternative routes of administration during vomiting.[77,78,93] Patients should be instructed to rinse their mouth after administration of an ICS to minimize side effects (e.g., thrush, hoarseness) as well as to decrease systemic absorption from oropharyngeal deposition. Lastly, patients should be educated to not use topical glucocorticoids on thin skin areas (e.g., eyelid, scrotum), on broken skin, or over large surface areas.

DRUG-INDUCED HYPERPROLACTINEMIA

The regulation of prolactin is unique among the anterior pituitary hormones. Prolactin is regulated through hypothalamic inhibition, with dopamine as the main inhibitory factor. As a result, drug-induced hyperprolactinemia may occur with any drug that inhibits the action of dopamine in the central nervous system.

CAUSATIVE AGENTS

Specific drugs that have been reported to induce hyperprolactinemia are listed in **Table 32-15**.[94-147] Conventional first-generation antipsychotics have been frequently associated with drug-induced hyperprolactinemia. Atypical, or second-generation, antipsychotics were developed to minimize side effects seen with first-generation antipsychotics; however, these medications are still associated with some risk for hyperprolactinemia. Risperidone is known to cause hyperprolactinemia more frequently than other atypical antipsychotics. Additional medications that have been implicated in causing hyperprolactinemia include antidepressants, antihypertensive agents, and gastrointestinal motility drugs.

EPIDEMIOLOGY

Hyperprolactinemia is the most common endocrine disorder of the HPA axis, with an estimated prevalence of 0.4% in the normal adult population and as high as 9% among women with amenorrhea.[148] The prevalence is approximately 5% among men presenting with impotence. The highest prevalence is among women with amenorrhea and galactorrhea, at 70%.[148] The incidence of drug-induced hyperprolactinemia is unknown.

MECHANISMS

Mechanisms of drug-induced hyperprolactinemia are listed in **Table 32-16**. Prolactin secretion by the lactotroph cells of the anterior pituitary is controlled by the inhibitory effect of the hypothalamus through one or more prolactin inhibitory factors (PIFs). Dopamine is the main physiologic PIF; therefore, any drug that is associated with inhibition of dopamine release or action can induce hyperprolactinemia. Antipsychotics and antiemetics with strong dopamine-receptor (D_2) blockade such as the phenothiazine derivatives, haloperidol, and metoclopramide work through this mechanism and have traditionally been reported to cause hyperprolactinemia.[94-97,107-109,116-125,136,147,149]

Serotonin is a strong stimulator of prolactin secretion; therefore, antidepressants that inhibit the reuptake or breakdown of serotonin can increase prolactin concentration.[94-106,147] Antihypertensives such as methyldopa and reserpine stimulate prolactin secretion by negating dopaminergic inhibition, whereas hormones such as estrogen appear to promote prolactin secretion by stimulating lactotroph growth.[94-97,110,111,126] Verapamil is believed to cause hyperprolactinemia by decreasing dopaminergic activity through blockade of N-type calcium channels in the cell membranes of neurons in the tuberoinfundibular dopaminergic tract.[94,97,113,145] Although protease inhibitors have been identified as a possible direct cause of hyperprolactinemia, the condition is most likely due to concomitant use of antiemetics or the presence of infection in patients receiving protease inhibitors.[134-137]

CLINICAL PRESENTATION AND DIFFERENTIAL DIAGNOSIS

The most common symptoms associated with hyperprolactinemia typically are related to sexual dysfunction and may be difficult to recognize.[150] In men, these symptoms may include decreased libido, impotence, and erectile dysfunction; whereas in women, symptoms include menstrual disorders and galactorrhea.[97,148-151] Sustained hyperprolactinemia can also be associated with increased risk of pituitary tumors and breast cancer, although the exact causal relationship is currently unknown.[149,150] Due to prolonged disruption of the hypothalamic-pituitary-gonadal axis, chronic hyperprolactinemia may also lead to decreased bone mineral density.[149,150] Signs

Table 32-15 Agents Implicated in Drug-Induced Hyperprolactinemia

Drug	Incidence	Level of Evidence[a]
ANTIDEPRESSANTS		
Amitriptyline[104,145,146]	NK	C
Amoxapine[105,145]	NK	B
Citalopram[101,145,146]	NK	B
Clomipramine[104,145,146]	1≤10%	C
Duloxetine[103,145]	NK	C
Fluoxetine[98,145,146]	4.5% in men 22% in women	B
Fluvoxamine[100,145]	NK	B
Moclobemide[106,145,b]	NK	B
Paroxetine[99,145,146]	≥0.01%	C
Sertraline[102,145,146]	NK	C
Venlafaxine[103,145,146]	NK	C
ANTIEMETICS		
Domperidone[108,109,145,b]	NK	A
Metoclopramide[107,108,145]	NK	A
ANTIHYPERTENSIVES		
Atenolol[115]	NK	C
Labetalol (intravenous)[114]	NK	C
Methyldopa[110,111,145]	NK	B
Reserpine[112]	NK	B
Verapamil[113,145]	8.5%	B
ANTIPSYCHOTICS		
Butyrophenones (i.e., haloperidol)[118,147]	40–90%[c]	A
Conventional[116,145]	48% in women[c] 29% in men[c]	B
Miscellaneous (i.e., loxapine[121], pimozide[122])	NK	A
Molindone[125]	NK	C
Olanzapine[119,147]	36%[c]	A
Phenothiazines (i.e., chlorpromazine, thioridazine, perphenazine)[117,145,147]	40–90%[c]	A
Quetiapine[124,147]	NK	C
Risperidone[116,147]	88% in women[c] 70% in men[c]	B
Thioxanthenes (i.e., thiothixene)[120,147]	NK	C
Ziprasidone[123,147]	NK	C
HORMONES		
Estrogen[126,145]	12–30%	B
Gonadotropin-releasing hormone analogs[127,128]	3.8%	B
HISTAMINE$_2$-RECEPTOR ANTAGONISTS		
Cimetidine[129,130]	NK	C
Famotidine[131]	NK	C
OPIATES AND OPIOIDS		
Methadone[133]	NK	B
Morphine and morphine analogs[132]	NK	B

Table 32-15 Agents Implicated in Drug-Induced Hyperprolactinemia (continued)

Drug	Incidence	Level of Evidence[a]
ANTIRETROVIRALS		
Nevirapine[137]	NK	C
Protease inhibitors[134-136,145]	NK	C
MISCELLANEOUS		
Alcohol[138]	NK	C
Azathioprine[140]	NK	C
Cisplatin[141]	NK	C
Cocaine[142]	NK	B
Cyclosporine[143]	NK	C
Cyproterone acetate[139]	NK	C
Tetrahydrocannabinol[144]	NK	C

NK = not known.

[a]Definitions for Levels of Evidence: Level A—evidence from one or more randomized, controlled clinical trials; Level B—evidence from nonrandomized clinical trials, prospective observational studies, cohort studies, retrospective studies, case-control studies, meta-analyses and/or postmarketing surveillance studies; and Level C—evidence from one or more published case reports or case series.

[b]Not approved for use in the United States.

[c]Incidence depends on dose.

Table 32-16 Mechanisms of Drug-Induced Hyperprolactinemia

Drug	Mechanism
Alcohol[138]	Stimulates the release of prolactin possibly through a decreased inhibitory effect of dopamine
Antidepressants[100,101,147]	Serotonin is a strong stimulator of prolactin secretion Antidepressants inhibit the reuptake or breakdown of serotonin
Antiemetics[94,97,107,147] Antipsychotics[94,97,116,147] Methyldopa[94,97,110,147] Reserpine[94,97,112]	Prolactin's secretion is controlled by the inhibitory effect of the hypothalamus through one or more prolactin inhibitory factors Dopamine is the main physiologic prolactin inhibitory factor Any drug that is associated with inhibition of dopamine production (e.g., methyldopa), release (e.g., reserpine), or action (e.g., antiemetics, antipsychotics) can induce hyperprolactinemia
Antiretrovirals[134,135]	Most likely due to concomitant antiemetics or concurrent infection
Estrogens[94,97,126,145]	Increase the number of prolactin-secreting cells in the pituitary
Gonadotropin-releasing hormone analogs[127,128]	Decrease in the release of hypothalamic prolactin inhibitory factors
H_2-receptor antagonists[130,131]	Unknown centrally mediated prolactin release
Opioids[132,133,145]	Bind to μ-opioid receptors that may inhibit hypothalamic dopamine secretion
Tetrahydrocannabinol[144]	Stimulates the release of prolactin possibly through a decreased inhibitory effect of dopamine
Verapamil[94,97,113,145]	Decreases dopaminergic activity by blocking N-type calcium channels

and symptoms associated with hyperprolactinemia are presented in **Table 32-17**.[92,97,148-152]

The diagnosis of hyperprolactinemia requires two or more serum prolactin concentrations above 20 mcg/L (424 mU/L) in males and 25 mcg/L (530 mU/L) in females in combination with symptoms. However, as in drug-induced Cushing syndrome, determining the cause can prove challenging. A thorough and careful medication history will help identify possible drug-related causes of hyperprolactinemia, and an evaluation of thyroid, kidney, and liver function is essential to rule out elevated prolactin concentrations secondary to organ dysfunction (**Table 32-18**).[96,97,148,151] The severity of hyperprolactinemia also can be useful in determining the

Table 32-17 Signs and Symptoms Associated with Drug-Induced Hyperprolactinemia

Signs and Symptoms	Incidence
MEN	
Gynecomastia	1–11%
Erectile dysfunction	NK
Decreased body hair	NK
WOMEN	
Oligomenorrhea or amenorrhea	40–50%
Hirsutism	NK
MEN AND WOMEN	
Osteoporosis	57% men, 32% women
Galactorrhea	20%
Decreased libido	NK
Infertility	NK
Weight gain	NK

NK = not known.

Table 32-18 Conditions to Consider in the Differential Diagnosis of Drug-Induced Hyperprolactinemia

- Acromegaly
- Breast stimulation
- Chest wall trauma and surgery
- Cirrhosis
- Excessive exercise
- Hypothyroidism
- Macroprolactinemia
- Nonfasting blood sample used for determination of prolactin concentration
- Polycystic ovarian syndrome
- Postictal (1–2 hours after seizure) prolactin elevation
- Pregnancy or postpartum prolactin elevation
- Prolactin-secreting adenomas
- Renal failure
- Sexual activity

Table 32-19 Risk Factors for Drug-Induced Hyperprolactinemia and Growth Hormone Deficiency

Hyperprolactinemia

- Administration of high doses of offending agent
- Female sex
- Use of potent D_2-receptor antagonists

Growth hormone deficiency

- Development of Cushing syndrome (see Table 32-5)
- Family history

cause. In drug-related hyperprolactinemia, serum prolactin concentrations rarely exceed 100 mcg/L, whereas serum prolactin concentrations exceeding 200 mcg/L are almost always associated with pituitary macroadenomas.[96,97,148,151] An elevated prolactin concentration can also be seen in the presence of macroprolactinemia, an immune complex formed by immunoglobulin G and prolactin.[152] This condition must be ruled out, as this abnormality is found in 10% of patients with hyperprolactinemia.[96] Macroprolactinemia is often asymptomatic, and the need for treating asymptomatic patients is controversial.[153]

RISK FACTORS

Risk factors associated with drug-induced hyperprolactinemia are presented in **Table 32-19**.[94,96,97,148,149,151] The highest risk for developing drug-induced hyperprolactinemia is associated with the use of potent D_2 receptor antagonists such as conventional antipsychotics, risperidone, and the antiemetics—metoclopramide and domperidone.[97,149,152] Although the dose of antipsychotic drugs has been correlated with prolactin levels in some studies, others have shown a tolerance to drug effects over time with normalizing prolactin levels.[149] Higher doses of drugs that potentiate prolactin via alternative mechanisms (e.g., estrogen, antidepressants) are probably needed to induce hyperprolactinemia.[97,151]

MORBIDITY AND MORTALITY

The incidence of death due to drug-induced hyperprolactinemia is unknown. Spontaneous galactorrhea, amenorrhea, gynecomastia in men, and sexual dysfunction may lead to embarrassment and reduced quality of life.[97,150] Osteoporosis is a long-term consequence that may lead to fracture, and certain fractures (e.g., hip) may increase the risk of death. Other potential long-term consequences of drug-induced hyperprolactinemia include pituitary tumors, breast cancer, venous thromboembolism, and depression.[97,149,150] Most, if not all, symptoms resolve when prolactin levels return to normal.[97]

PREVENTION

Methods to prevent drug-induced hyperprolactinemia are presented in **Table 32-20**. Drug-induced hyperprolactinemia may be prevented by minimizing the risk factors associated with hyperfunction of the hypothalamus, adrenal, or pituitary glands. When agents that can potentially induce hyperprolactinemia must be used, practitioners should make an effort to use the lowest effective dose of these agents, particularly with the D_2 antagonists. Effective therapy can be achieved by using a stepwise approach in the management and administration of these agents, starting with a low dose and titrating up to the desired effect or decreasing the dose if adverse effects occur. In addition, agents that interact pharmacokinetically (e.g., inhibit metabolism) with drugs known to cause hyperprolactinemia should be avoided.

Table 32-20 Approaches to Help Prevent Drug-Induced Hyperprolactinemia

- Avoid drug interactions that increase plasma concentrations of the offending agent
- Avoid drugs that exert potent D_2-receptor antagonism
- Use lowest effective dose of offending agent

MANAGEMENT

Management of drug-induced hyperprolactinemia requires recognition of the causative agent(s). Once a drug has been identified as the cause, the logical first step is to attempt to discontinue the offending medication and replace it with an appropriate alternative. Problems can arise, however, when the patient is well controlled with the offending agent and alternatives are not available, which is often the case with conventional or first-generation antipsychotics. In these cases, changing to an antipsychotic with less potential to cause drug-induced hyperprolactinemia (e.g., olanzapine, quetiapine, aripiprazole, clozapine) is perhaps the most appropriate option, as administration of a dopamine agonist may worsen psychiatric symptoms.[97,149] If maintaining the offending agent is the only option, initiating a dopamine agonist and, in those who require it (e.g., patient with estrogen deficiency), sex-steroid replacement are options.[94,97,148,149,153] Pharmacologic sex-steroid monotherapy may be the safest option for patients treated with antipsychotics.

The greatest evidence for the effectiveness of dopamine agonist use in patients with hyperprolactinemia exists for the ergot derivatives, such as bromocriptine and cabergoline.[153] However, these agents may increase the risk of exacerbation of underlying psychosis and should be used cautiously in patients managed with antipsychotics.[145,150] Risk of cardiac valvulopathy is also a concern with these ergot derivatives; however, this risk is most evident during the treatment of Parkinson disease, where larger doses are typically used.[154] Pramipexole and ropinirole are nonergot derivatives that may possess a safer cardiac profile; however, very limited data exist for their use in the treatment of hyperprolactinemia.[153] Treatment options for hyperprolactinemia are presented in **Table 32-21**.

INFORMATION FOR PATIENTS

Patients receiving antipsychotic therapy should be provided information regarding the risks of elevated prolactin such as osteoporosis, reduced fertility, and sexual dysfunction.[155] Patients' concerns may be alleviated through appropriate education

Table 32-21 Management of Drug-Induced Hyperprolactinemia

- Discontinue offending agent
- Initiate appropriate therapeutic alternative
- Consider initiation of dopamine agonist
  - Bromocriptine (2.5–10 mg/day)[a]
  - Cabergoline (0.25–1 mg/wk)[a]
  - Pramipexole[b]
  - Ropinirole[b]
  - Pergolide[c]
- Consider sex-steroid replacement in patients who require it
  - Testosterone
  - Estrogen
- Consider a bisphosphonate if low bone mineral density is found

[a]U.S. Food and Drug Administration–approved indication for hyperprolactinemia.
[b]Limited evidence of effectiveness.
[c]Not approved for use in the United States.

that these side effects typically subside once the offending agent is discontinued or switched to an acceptable alternative agent. When discontinuing the offending antipsychotic or initiating treatment with dopamine agonists, patients should be aware that their psychotic symptoms may worsen, and closer monitoring may be warranted during this period. Women should also be informed that dopamine agonists may restore fertility and appropriate contraceptive precautions should be used if pregnancy is not desired.[97,151] Finally, patients should be warned of common adverse effects associated with dopamine agonists, including nausea, insomnia, somnolence, peripheral edema, and orthostatic hypotension.[153]

GROWTH HORMONE DEFICIENCY

Growth hormone (GH) is synthesized, stored, and released from somatotropes located in the anterior pituitary. GH secretion is mainly under the control of two hypothalamic peptides: GH-releasing hormone (GHRH) and somatostatin, also known as somatotropin-release–inhibiting factor (SRIF) or GH-inhibiting hormone (GHIH).[156,157] The secretion of GH is different from that of most other hormones in that it is released in a pulsatile fashion. This timing of release often complicates the diagnosis of GH deficiency, and provocative testing is required for accurate diagnosis.

CAUSATIVE AGENTS

Specific drugs that have been reported to cause GH deficiency are listed in **Table 32-22**.[41,156-168] Glucocorticoids play a prominent role in the regulation of GH secretion and thus may be the most common agents implicated in drug-induced GH deficiency. Other drugs that have been found to cause GH deficiency include phentolamine, isoproterenol, somatostatin analogs such as octreotide, and tyrosine kinase (TK) inhibitors such as imatinib.

EPIDEMIOLOGY

The frequency of drug-induced GH deficiency in the general population is unknown but is assumed to be rare. The average annual incidence of GH deficiency from any cause is approximately 1.76 per 100,000 persons as reported in a nationwide study from Denmark.[169] The most common cause of GH deficiency is a pituitary adenoma.[169,170]

MECHANISMS

Mechanisms for drug-induced GH deficiency are listed in **Table 32-23**. Inhibition of GH secretion by α- and β-adrenergic agonists may be mediated by an increase in SRIF secretion; however, β-adrenergic agonists may also reduce the GH response to GHRH.[156,158] Glucocorticoid excess increases hypothalamic secretion of somatostatin by enhancing responsiveness, thus inhibiting GH release from the pituitary.[167,171] In addition, chronic use of glucocorticoids can decrease the number of GH receptors leading to reduced tissue response to GH.[162,171] Gonadotropin-releasing hormone agonists used to treat precocious puberty and hormone-responsive cancers decrease hormone release from the pituitary.[161,165] Gonadotropin-releasing hormone is normally released in a pulsatile fashion; however, continuous administration of these hormone agonists downregulates pituitary

Table 32-22 Agents Implicated in Drug-Induced Growth Hormone Deficiency

Drug	Incidence[a]	Level of Evidence[b]
Amphetamine derivatives[c]		
Methylphenidate[163]	NK	C
Dextroamphetamine[164]	NK	C
Glucocorticoids[159,171]	Variable	B
GnRH agonists[161,d]	NK	B
Isoproterenol[158]	NK	B
Phentolamine[158]	NK	B
Somatostatin analogs[160]	NK[e]	B
Tyrosine kinase inhibitors[168]	NK	C

GnRH = gonadotropin-releasing hormone, NK = not known.
[a]Incidence depends on dose and duration of exposure.
[b]Definitions for Levels of Evidence: Level A—evidence from one or more randomized, controlled clinical trials; Level B—evidence from nonrandomized clinical trials, prospective observational studies, cohort studies, retrospective studies, case-control studies, meta-analyses and/or postmarketing surveillance studies; and Level C—evidence from one or more published case reports or case series.
[c]Studies report inhibition, no change, and even stimulation of GH secretion.
[d]After repeated dosing.
[e]Unknown incidence due to use in patients with growth hormone excess.

Table 32-23 Mechanisms of Drug-Induced Growth Hormone Deficiency

Drug	Mechanism
α-adrenergic antagonists[156,158]	May decrease secretion of GH-releasing factor
Amphetamine derivatives[157]	Possibly decreases GH release through dopaminergic effects May decrease sleep-related GH release
β-adrenergic agonists[156,158]	May increase secretion of somatostatin or GH-inhibiting factor May also reduce the GH response to GH-releasing hormone
Glucocorticoids[162,166,167,171]	Increase hypothalamic secretion of somatostatin by enhancing β-adrenergic responsiveness, thus inhibiting GH release from the pituitary Reduce the number of GH receptors in tissue
GnRH agonists[161,165]	Continuous administration downregulates pituitary receptors ultimately decreasing GH release
Somatostatin analogs[156,157]	Directly inhibit GH release from the pituitary
Tyrosine kinase inhibitors[168]	May inhibit release of GH from somatotropes in the anterior pituitary May also attenuate response of GH on peripheral tissues

GH = growth hormone, GnRH = gonadotropin-releasing hormone.

receptors, ultimately decreasing sex hormone and GH release.[41] Methylphenidate has a potent effect to alter the dopaminergic pathways involved in the regulation of GH secretion.[172] However, the effect of methylphenidate and amphetamines on the GH axis has been a matter of controversy, with some studies reporting inhibition, some no change, and some even reporting stimulation of GH secretion.[163] TK is involved in the complex signal transduction for GHRH in somatotropes to promote the secretion of GH.[173] In the peripheral tissues, TK also assists in the activation of cellular pathways to promote the actions of GH.[174]

CLINICAL PRESENTATION AND DIFFERENTIAL DIAGNOSIS

Signs and symptoms associated with GH deficiency are presented in **Table 32-24.**[41,175,176] Children with GH deficiency often present with short stature,

Table 32-24 Signs and Symptoms Associated with Drug-Induced Growth Hormone Deficiency

Children

- Reduced growth velocity
- Short stature

Adults

- Central obesity
- Decreased lean muscle mass
- Decreased well-being
- Difficulty forming relationships
- Dyslipidemia
- Emotional lability
- Impaired socioeconomic performance
- Increased homeostasis model assessment
- Low bone mineral density
- Reduced energy
- Reduced muscle strength
- Social isolation

plump physique, and a round immature-looking face. When compared with the general population, adults with GH deficiency have increased fat mass, reduced muscle mass and strength, and lower bone density.[176,177]

The diagnosis of drug-induced GH deficiency is based on signs and symptoms of disease combined with documented low GH under provocative testing (e.g., an insulin tolerance test) and use of an agent known to cause the disease. Low serum GH concentration alone is not conclusive because GH secretion is pulsatile.[178] A diagnosis of GH deficiency can be made if the serum GH concentration in response to insulin-induced hypoglycemia is ≤5 mcg/L or ≤4 mcg/L using the GHRH–arginine stimulation test as measured by radioimmunoassay in adults.[178] In children and adolescents, the diagnosis is made if the serum GH concentration after provocative testing is <10 mcg/L.[175] The standard provocation used to stimulate GH is the insulin-induced hypoglycemia stimulation test, but the GHRH–arginine stimulation test provides a safer alternative in children and in patients with a history of seizure disorder and cardiovascular disease.[178] Alternative causes, such as pituitary adenoma, genetic GH deficiency, abuse/neglect, and diabetes, must still be ruled out (**Table 32-25**).

Table 32-25 Conditions to Consider in the Differential Diagnosis of Drug-Induced Growth Hormone Deficiency

- Brain tumor (craniopharyngioma)
- Central nervous system surgery or radiation
- Cushing syndrome
- Genetic growth hormone deficiency
- Hypothyroidism
- Idiopathic growth hormone deficiency
- Metabolic disturbances (e.g., uncontrolled diabetes)
- Noonan syndrome, Turner syndrome
- Prepubertal
- Short stature associated with abuse or neglect

RISK FACTORS

The main risk factor associated with GH deficiency is the presence of Cushing syndrome, which usually manifests as weight gain and is frequently associated with growth failure. The severity of growth impairment is directly related to the age at onset and the duration of hypercortisolemia.[179] Patients with Cushing syndrome can have persistent impairment of GH secretion long after correction of hypercortisolism. Several factors may play a role in this phenomenon, including delayed remission of hypercortisolism and, in cases of surgically treated Cushing syndrome, damage to the pituitary gland. Sustained hypercortisolism for long periods has also been suggested to impair the physiological function of somatotropes.[171] Therefore, any drug that may induce Cushing syndrome or cause sustained hypercortisolism (e.g., long-term administration of glucocorticoids) should be considered a risk factor (Table 32-19).

MORBIDITY AND MORTALITY

The risk of death from drug-induced GH deficiency is unknown, but data suggest that adults with GH deficiency from other causes have reduced life expectancy.[177] Increased mortality is mostly attributed to premature cardiovascular disease, possibly due to dyslipidemia and insulin resistance, and may be more pronounced in childhood-onset GH deficiency and in females.[180]

Table 32-26 Approaches to Help Prevent Drug-Induced Growth Hormone Deficiency

- Avoid drug–drug interactions that will increase plasma concentrations of the offending agent
- Close monitoring of signs and symptoms during treatment with known causative agent (e.g., growth velocity in children)
- Use alternative route of administration to minimize systemic absorption
- Use lowest effective dose and avoid prolonged use of offending agent

PREVENTION

General strategies to prevent drug-induced GH deficiency are presented in **Table 32-26**. In children, the growth velocity should be closely monitored throughout treatment with a known causative agent and timely diagnostic testing should be performed if GH deficiency is suspected. Because Cushing syndrome is a risk factor for GH deficiency, patients presenting with Cushingoid symptoms should be evaluated for evidence of concomitant GH deficiency. When feasible, use of nonsystemic corticosteroids, or corticosteroids with lower potency, may reduce the risk of developing GH deficiency.

MANAGEMENT

Management of drug-induced GH deficiency is dependent on recognition of the offending drug. Whenever possible, the offending medication should be discontinued in favor of an appropriate therapeutic alternative. In children whose growth has been impaired by persistent hypercortisolism, GH therapy should be initiated as soon as cortisol has normalized because a limited window of opportunity exists to promote increased linear growth. Additionally, GH therapy has been shown to improve body composition in the majority of children.[171] On the other hand, the role of GH replacement in adults has been controversial. GH replacement may be considered for symptomatic relief as well as to increase muscle mass, decrease fat mass, and increase bone mineral density.[32,176,181]

Dosing of recombinant GH is individualized to patient need. In general, premenopausal women and women taking estrogen therapy require higher doses than men because of reduced GH response in the periphery due to estrogen.[178] Children typically require much higher doses than adults. Somatropin should be started at low doses (e.g., 200–300 mcg/day) and slowly titrated upward by 100–200 mcg/day every 1–2 months in adults. Somatropin is routinely started at 20 mcg/kg/week for children.[175,178] Subcutaneous injections may be administered at various intervals (e.g., nightly, every other night, or once per week at night). Clinical response, adverse effects, and the measurement of insulin-like growth factor 1 concentrations guide therapy in adults.[178] In children, height and height velocity are the main therapeutic outcomes, with normalization of growth the goal of therapy.[175] Somatropin may be discontinued in children when growth normalizes and full somatic development (i.e., maximal bone and muscle mass) is achieved.[175] Normalization of GH sensitivity in adults may take up to 2 years.[32] Limited data exist on the benefits of somatropin in drug-induced GH deficiency; however, studies in adults with GH deficiency have shown reductions in cardiovascular disease and risk of fractures.[182,183] Indefinite GH replacement may be considered if the offending agent must be continued. **Table 32-27** summarizes management strategies.

Table 32-27 Management of Drug-Induced Growth Hormone Deficiency

- Discontinue offending agent or initiate appropriate therapeutic alternative
- Children
  - Initiate growth hormone (somatropin) at 20 mcg/kg/wk; height and height velocity guide therapy
  - Goal: growth normalization
- Adults
  - Initiate growth hormone (200–300 mcg/day) for symptomatic relief and to increase muscle mass, decrease fat mass, and increase bone mineral density
  - Titrate dose by 100–200 mcg every 1–2 months; clinical response, adverse effects, and insulin-like growth factor 1 concentrations guide therapy
  - Goal: Normalization of growth hormone sensitivity

INFORMATION FOR PATIENTS

Patients receiving recombinant GH should be informed that slow titration over months is necessary to reduce adverse effects associated with treatment. Common dose-dependent adverse effects include fluid retention, arthralgia, myalgia, headache, nausea, and vomiting. Injection site reactions are also common and dose-dependent. GH requirements change with age and can be affected by sex hormone replacement. Testosterone sensitizes tissues, whereas oral estrogen causes a reduced response to GH. If transdermal estrogen is used to replace oral estrogen, a lower dose of GH may be needed.[178]

HYPOALDOSTERONISM AND HYPERALDOSTERONISM

Hypoaldosteronism is rare and usually not related to medications. Nevertheless, generalized secondary adrenal insufficiency may be responsible for a subset of patients with nonselective hypoaldosteronism.[41] Likewise, most cases of hyperaldosteronism are primary and are often due to physiologic abnormalities that arise in the adrenal cortex.[41,184] A small number of patients may present with secondary hyperaldosteronism that occurs as a result of overstimulation of the zona glomerulosa by the renin–angiotensin–aldosterone system. Excess potassium intake and use of oral contraceptives may also contribute. Signs and symptoms include hypokalemia, hypertension, and possibly evidence of end-organ damage. Correction of the extra-adrenal stimulation of aldosterone secretion usually resolves this disorder. Normalizing serum potassium, considering alternative forms of contraception, and therapy with spironolactone should also be considered.

REFERENCES

1. Wassenberg S, Rau R, Steinfeld et al. Very low-dose prednisolone in early rheumatoid arthritis retards radiographic progression over two years. *Arthritis Rheum.* 2005; 52:3371-80.
2. Wilson AM, Blumsohn A, Jung RT et al. Asthma and Cushing's syndrome. *Chest.* 2000; 117:593-4.
3. Lipworth BJ. Systemic adverse effects of inhaled corticosteroid therapy: a systematic review and metaanalysis. *Arch Intern Med.* 1999; 159:941-55.
4. Yiallouros PK, Milner AD, Conway E et al. Adrenal function and high dose inhaled corticosteroids for asthma. *Arch Dis Child.* 1997; 76:405-10.
5. St. Germain RM, Yigit S, Wells L et al. Cushing syndrome and severe adrenal suppression caused by fluticasone and protease inhibitor combination in an HIV-infected adolescent. *AIDS Patient Care STDs.* 2007; 21:373-7.
6. Pessanha TM, Campos JMS, Barros ACM et al. Iatrogenic Cushing's syndrome in a adolescent with AIDS on ritonavir and inhaled fluticasone: case report and literature review. *AIDS.* 2007; 21:529-38.
7. Fardon, TC, Lee DKC, Haggart K et al. Adrenal suppression with dry powder formulations of fluticasone propionate and mometasone furoate. *Am J Respir Crit Care Med.* 2004; 170:960-6.
8. Hillebrand-Haverkort ME, Prummel MF, ten Veen JH. Ritonavir-induced Cushing's syndrome in a patient treated with nasal fluticasone. *AIDS.* 1999; 13:1803.
9. Bolland MJ, Bagg W, Thomas MG et al. Cushing's syndrome due to interaction between inhaled corticosteroids and itraconazole. *Ann Pharmacother.* 2004: 38:46-9.
10. Woods DR, Arun CS, Corris PA et al. Cushing's syndrome without excess cortisol. *BMJ.* 2006; 332:469-70.
11. Azevedo L, Pego H, Souto Moura T, Germano I. Iatrogenic Cushing's syndrome and osteoporosis due to an interaction between fluticasone and ritonavir. *BMJ Case Rep.* 2015.
12. May P, Stein EJ, Ryter RJ et al. Cushing syndrome from percutaneous absorption of triamcinolone cream. *Arch Intern Med.* 1976; 136:612-3.
13. Gen R, Akbay E, Sezer K. Cushing syndrome caused by topical corticosteroid: a case report. *Am J Med Sci.* 2007; 333:173-4.
14. Druce M, Goldstone AP, Tan TMM et al. The pursuit of beauty. *Lancet.* 2008; 371:596.
15. Oldenburg-Ligtenberg PC, van der Westerlaken MML. A woman with Cushing's syndrome after use of an Indonesian herb: a case report. *Neth J Med.* 2007; 65:150-2.
16. Atabek ME, Pirgon O, Unal E. Pituitary-adrenal axis suppression due to topical steroid administration in an infant. *Pediatr Int.* 2007; 49:242-4.
17. Halverstam CP, Vachharajani A, Mallory SB. Cushing syndrome from percutaneous absorption of 1% hydrocortisone ointment in Netherton syndrome. *Pediatr Dermatol.* 2007; 24:42-5.
18. Tsuruoka S, Sugimoto K, Fujimura A. Drug-induced Cushing syndrome in a patient with ulcerative colitis after betamethasone enema: evaluation of plasma drug concentration. *Ther Drug Monit.* 1998; 20:387-9.
19. Lavin PJ, Workman R. Cushing syndrome induced by serial occipital nerve blocks containing corticosteroids. *Headache.* 2001; 41:902-4.
20. Liu MF, Yencha M. Cushing's syndrome secondary to intralesional steroid injections of multiple keloid scars. *Otolaryngol Head Neck Surg.* 2006; 135:960-1.
21. Hameed R, Zacharin MR. Cushing syndrome, adrenal suppression and local corticosteroid use. *J Pediatr Child Health.* 2006; 42:392-4.
22. Iglesias P, Gonzalez J, Diez JJ. Acute and persistent iatrogenic Cushing's syndrome after a single dose of triamcinolone acetonide. *J Endocrinol Invest.* 2005; 28:1019-23.
23. Ozerdem U, Levi L, Cheng LY et al. Systemic toxicity of topical and periocular corticosteroid therapy in a 11-year-old male with posterior uveitis. *Am J Ophthalmol.* 2000; 130:240-1.
24. Chiang MYM, Sarkar M, Koppens JM et al. Exogenous Cushing's syndrome and topical ocular steroids. *Eye.* 2006; 20:725-7.
25. Razenberg AJ, Elte JW, Rietveld AP et al. A smart type of Cushing's syndrome. *Eur J Endocrinol.* 2007; 157:779-81.
26. Grenfell A, Rudenski A, Watts M et al. Cushing's syndrome and medroxyprogesterone acetate. *Lancet.* 1990; 336:256.
27. Dux S, Bishara J, Marom D et al. Medroxyprogesterone acetate-induced secondary adrenal insufficiency. *Ann Pharmacother.* 1998; 32:134.
28. Krueger RB, Hembree W, Hill M. Prescription of medroxyprogesterone acetate to a patient with pedophilia resulting in Cushing's syndrome and adrenal insufficiency. *Sex Abuse.* 2006; 18:227-8.

29. Mann M, Koller E, Murgo A et al. Glucocorticoid-like activity of megestrol: a summary of Food and Drug Administration experience and a review of the literature. *Arch Intern Med.* 1997; 157:1651-6.
30. Goodman A, Cagliero E. Megestrol-induced clinical adrenal insufficiency. *Eur J Gynaecol Oncol.* 2000; 21:117-8.
31. Caparrós GC, Zambrana JL, Delgado-Fernandez M et al. Megestrol-induced Cushing syndrome. *Ann Pharmacother.* 2001; 35:1208-10.
32. Arnaldi G, Angeli A, Atkinson AB et al. Diagnosis and complications of Cushing's syndrome: a consensus statement. *J Clin Endocrinol Metab.* 2003; 88:5593-602.
33. Findling JW, Raff H. Screening and diagnosis of Cushing's syndrome. *Endocrinol Metab Clin N Am.* 2005; 34:385-402.
34. Nieman LK, Ilias I. Evaluation and treatment of Cushing's syndrome. *Am J Med.* 2005; 118:1340-6.
35. de Castro M, Moreira AC. Screening and diagnosis of Cushing's syndrome. *Arq Bras Endocrinol Metab.* 2007; 51:1191-8.
36. Vilar L, Freitas MC, Faria M et al. Pitfalls in the diagnosis of Cushing's syndrome. *Arq Bras Endocrinol Metab.* 2007; 51:1207-16.
37. Gross BA, Mindea SA, Pick AJ et al. Diagnostic approach to Cushing disease. *J Neurosurg Focus.* 2007; 23:1-7.
38. Jones W, Chastain CA, Wright PW. Iatrogenic Cushing syndrome secondary to probable interaction between voriconazole and budesonide. *Pharmacotherapy.* 2014; 34:e116-9.
39. Tsoukas MA, Krishnamoorthy P, Richards BJ et al. Adrenal suppression with cushingoid features from inhaled corticosteroid therapy in an adult asthmatic patient. *Am J Med.* 2014; 127e1-2.
40. Schwarze-Zander C, Klingmuller D, Klumper J et al. Triamcinolone and ritonavir leading to drug-induced Cushing syndrome and adrenal suppression: description of a new case and review of the literature. *Infection* 2013; 41:1183-7.
41. DiPiro JT, Talbert RL, Yee GC et al., eds. *Pharmacotherapy: a pathophysiologic approach.* 9th ed. Stamford, CT: McGraw-Hill; 2014.
42. McEvoy GK, ed. *American hospital formulary service (AHFS) drug information.* Bethesda, MD: American Society of Hospital Pharmacists; 2015.
43. Hopkins RL, Leinung MC. Exogenous Cushing's syndrome and glucocorticoid withdrawal. *Endocrinol Metab Clin North Am.* 2005; 34:371-84.
44. Newell-Price J, Bertagna X, Grossman AB et al. Cushing's syndrome. *Lancet.* 2006; 367:1605-17.
45. Lindholm J, Juul S, Jorgensen JO et al. Incidence and late prognosis of Cushing's syndrome: a population-based study. *J Clin Endocrinol Metab.* 2001; 86:117-23.
46. Vassiliadi D, Tsagarakis S. Unusual causes of Cushing's syndrome. *Arg Bras Endocrinol Metab.* 2007: 51:1245-52.
47. Raveendran AV. Inhalational steroids and Iatrogenic Cushing's syndrome. *Open Respir Med J.* 2014; 8:74-84.
48. Tempark T, Phatarakijnirund V, Chatproedprai S et al. Exogenous Cushing's syndrome due to topical corticosteroid application: a case report and review of literature. *Endocr.* 2010; 38:328-34.
49. Hengge UR, Ruzicka T, Schwartz RA, Cork MJ. Adverse effects of topical glucocorticosteroids. *J Am Acad Dermatol.* 2006; 54:1-15.
50. Einaudi S, Bertorello N, Masera N et al. Adrenal axis function after high-dose steroid therapy for childhood acute lymphoblastic leukemia. *Pediatr Blood Cancer.* 2008; 50:537-41.
51. Wong J, Black P. Acute adrenal insufficiency associated with high dose inhaled steroids. *BMJ.* 1992; 304:1415.
52. Todd GR, Acerini CL, Buck JJ et al. Acute adrenal crisis in asthmatics treated with high-dose fluticasone propionate. *Eur Respir J.* 2002; 19:1207-9.
53. Shenoy SD, Swift PG, Cody D. Growth impairment and adrenal suppression on low-dose inhaled beclomethasone. *J Paediatr Child Health.* 2006; 42:143-4.
54. Gordon AC, McDonald CF, Thomson SA et al. Dose of inhaled budesonide required to produce clinical suppression of plasma cortisol. *Eur J Respir Dis.* 1987; 71:10-4.
55. Sizonenko PC. Effects of inhaled or nasal glucocorticosteroids on adrenal function and growth. *J Pediatr Endocrinol Metab.* 2002; 15:5-26.
56. Licata AA. Systemic effects of fluticasone nasal spray: report of 2 cases. *Endocr Pract.* 2005; 11:194-6.
57. Sorkin S, Warren D. Probable adrenal suppression from intranasal beclomethasone. *J Fam Pract.* 1986; 22:449-50.
58. Levin C, Maibach HI. Topical corticosteroid-induced adrenocortical insufficiency: clinical implications. *Am J Clin Dermatol.* 2002; 3:141-7.
59. Hellman L, Yoshida K, Zumoff B et al. The effect of medroxyprogesterone acetate on the pituitary-adrenal axis. *J Clin Endocrinol Metab.* 1976; 42:912-7.
60. Hug V, Kau S, Hortobagyi GN, Jones L. Adrenal failure in patients with breast carcinoma after long-term treatment of cyclic alternating oestrogen progesterone. *Br J Cancer.* 1991; 63:454-7.
61. Stoffer SS, Krakauer JC. Induction of adrenal suppression by megestrol acetate. *Ann Intern Med.* 1996; 124:613-4.
62. Dev R, Del Fabbro E, Bruera E. Association between megestrol acetate treatment and symptomatic adrenal insufficiency with hypogonadism in male patients with cancer. *Cancer.* 2007; 110:1173-7.
63. Pont A, Williams PL, Loose DS et al. Ketoconazole blocks adrenal steroid synthesis. *Ann Intern Med.* 1982; 97:370-2.
64. Best TR, Jenkins JK, Murphy FY et al. Persistent adrenal insufficiency secondary to low-dose ketoconazole therapy. *Am J Med.* 1987; 82:676-80.
65. Khosla S, Wolfson JS, Demerjian Z et al. Adrenal crisis in the setting of high-dose ketoconazole therapy. *Arch Intern Med.* 1989; 149:802-4.
66. Wagner RL, White PF, Kan PB et al. Inhibition of adrenal steroidogenesis by the anesthetic etomidate. *N Engl J Med.* 1984; 310:1415-21.
67. Lundy JB, Slane ML, Frizzi JD. Acute adrenal insufficiency after a single dose of etomidate. *J Intensive Care Med.* 2007; 22:111-7.
68. Robinson BG, Hales IB, Henniker AJ et al. The effect of o,p'-DDD on adrenal steroid replacement therapy requirements. *Clin Endocrinol (Oxf).* 1987; 27:437-44.
69. Russell CA, Green SJ, O'Sullivan J et al. Megestrol acetate and aminoglutethimide/hydrocortisone in sequence or in combination as second-line endocrine therapy of estrogen receptor-positive metastatic breast cancer: a Southwest Oncology Group phase III trial. *J Clin Oncol.* 1997; 15:2494-501.
70. Elansary EH, Earis JE. Rifampicin and adrenal crisis. *BMJ.* 1983; 286:1861-2.
71. Ediger SK, Isley WL. Rifampicin-induced adrenal insufficiency in the acquired immunodeficiency syndrome: difficulties in diagnosis and treatment. *Postgrad Med J.* 1988; 64:405-6.
72. Schule C, Baghai T, Bidlingmaier M et al. Endocrinological effects of mirtazapine in healthy volunteers. *Prog Neuropsychopharmacol Biol Psychiatry.* 2002; 26:1253-61.
73. Müssig K, Knaus-Dittmann D, Schmidt H et al. Secondary adrenal failure and secondary amenorrhoea following hydromorphone treatment. *Clin Endocrinol (Oxf).* 2007; 66:604-5.
74. Oltmanns KM, Fehm HL, Peters A. Chronic fentanyl application induces adrenocortical insufficiency. *J Intern Med.* 2005; 257:478-80.
75. Müssig K, Friess E, Wudy SA et al. Secondary adrenal failure due to long-term treatment with flunitrazepam. *Clin Endocrinol (Oxf).* 2006; 65:549-50.
76. Ten S, New M, Maclaren N. Addison's disease 2001. *J Clin Endocrinol Metab.* 2001; 86:2909-22.
77. Salvatori R. Adrenal insufficiency. *JAMA.* 2005; 294:2481-8.

78. Arlt W, Allolio B. Adrenal insufficiency. *Lancet.* 2003; 361:1881-93.
79. Dorin RI, Qualls CR, Crapo LM. Diagnosis of adrenal insufficiency. *Ann Intern Med.* 2003; 139:194-204.
80. Broersen LH, Pereira AM, Jorgensen JO, Dekkers OM. Adrenal Insufficiency in corticosteroids use: systematic review and meta-analysis. *Endocrinol Metab.* 2015; 100:2171-80.
81. Henzen C, Suter A, Lerch E et al. Suppression and recovery of adrenal response after short-term, high-dose glucocorticoid treatment. *Lancet.* 2000; 355:542-5.
82. Asare K. Diagnosis and treatment of adrenal insufficiency in the critically ill patient. *Pharmacotherapy.* 2007; 27:1512-28.
83. Zollner EW. Hypothalamic-pituitary-adrenal axis suppression in asthmatic children on inhaled corticosteroids: Part 1. Which test should be used? *Pediatr Allergy Immunol.* 2007; 18:401-9.
84. Foisy MM, Yakiwchuk EMK, Chiu I, Singh AE. Adrenal suppression and Cushing's syndrome secondary to an interaction between ritonavir and fluticasone: a review of the literature. *HIV Med.* 2008; 9:389-96.
85. Daffara F, Francia SD, Reimondo G et al. Prospective evaluation of mitotane toxicity in adrenocortical cancer patients treated adjuvantly. *Endocr Relat Cancer.* 2008; 15:1043-53.
86. Bouillon R. Acute adrenal insufficiency. *Endocrinol Metab Clin North Am.* 2006; 35:767-75.
87. Charmandari E, Nicolaides NC, Chrousos GP. Adrenal insufficiency. *Lancet.* 2014; 383:2152-61.
88. Raff H, Sharma ST, Nieman LK. Physiological basis for etiology, diagnosis, and treatment of adrenal disorders: Cushing's syndrome, adrenal insufficiency, and congenital adrenal hyperplasia. *Compr Physiol.* 2014; 4:739-69.
89. Ahmet A, Kim H, Spier S. Adrenal suppression: a practical guide to the screening and management of this under-recognized complication of inhaled corticosteroid therapy. *Allergy Asthma Clin Immunol.* 2011; 7:13.
90. Zollner EW. Hypothalamic-pituitary-adrenal axis suppression in asthmatic children on inhaled corticosteroids: Part 2. The risk as determined by gold standard adrenal function tests: a systemic review. *Pediatr Allergy Immunol.* 2007; 18:469-74.
91. Barnes NC. The properties of inhaled corticosteroids: similarities and differences. *Prim Care Resp J.* 2007; 16:149-54.
92. Fardon TC, Lee DK, Haggart K et al. Adrenal suppression with dry powder formulations of fluticasone propionate and mometasone furoate. *Am J Respir Crit Care Med.* 2004; 170:960-6.
93. Shulman DI, Palmert MR, Kemp SF. Adrenal insufficiency: still a cause of morbidity and death in childhood. *Pediatrics.* 2007; 119:e484-94.
94. Molitch ME. Medication-induced hyperprolactinemia. *Mayo Clin Proc.* 2005; 80:1050-7.
95. Ma RCW, Kong APS, Chan N et al. Drug-induced endocrine and metabolic disorders. *Drug Saf.* 2007; 30:215-45.
96. Cortet-Rudelli C, Sapin R, Bonneville JF, Brue T. Etiological diagnosis of hyperprolactinemia. *Ann Endocrinol.* 2007; 68:98-105.
97. Bandyopadhyay P. Drug-induced hyperprolactinemia. *Drugs Today.* 2006; 42:103-19.
98. Papakostas GI, Miller KK, Petersen T et al. Serum prolactin levels among outpatients with major depressive disorder during the acute phase of treatment with fluoxetine. *J Clin Psychiatry.* 2006; 67:952-7.
99. González E, Minguez L, Sanguino RM. Galactorrhea after paroxetine treatment. *Pharmacopsychiatry.* 2000; 33:118.
100. Spigset O, Mjorndal T. The effect of fluvoxamine on serum prolactin and serum sodium concentrations: relation to platelet 5-HT2A receptor status. *J Clin Psychopharmacol.* 1997; 17:292-7.
101. Seifritz E, Baumann P, Müller MJ et al. Neuroendocrine effects of a 20-mg citalopram infusion in healthy males. A placebo-controlled evaluation of citalopram as 5-HT function probe. *Neuropsychopharmacology.* 1996; 14:253-63.
102. Lesaca TG. Sertraline and galactorrhea. *J Clin Psychopharmacol.* 1996; 16:333-4.
103. Ashton AK, Longdon MC. Hyperprolactinemia and galactorrhea-induced by serotonin and norepinephrine reuptake inhibiting antidepressants. *Am J Psychiatry.* 2007; 164:1121-2.
104. Egberts AC, Meyboom RH, De Koning FH et al. Non-puerperal lactation associated with antidepressant drug use. *Br J Clin Pharmacol.* 1997; 44:277-81.
105. Gelenberg AJ, Wojcik JD, Lydiard RB et al. Double-blind comparison of amoxapine and imipramine in the treatment of depressed patients. *J Clin Psychiatry.* 1984; 45:54-9.
106. Juruena MF, Pires ML, Calil HM. Moclobemide effects on prolactin plasma levels in healthy individuals: the hormonal increase induced by a single dose is maintained during a 4-week period of drug intake. *Int Clin Psychopharmacol.* 1997; 12:317-21.
107. Madani S, Tolia V. Gynecomastia with metoclopramide use in pediatric patients. *J Clin Gastroenterol.* 1997; 24:79-81.
108. Maddern GJ, Kiroff GK, Leppard PI et al. Domperidone, metoclopramide, and placebo: all give symptomatic improvement in gastroesophageal reflux. *J Clin Gastroenterol.* 1986; 8:135-40.
109. De S, Taylor CM. Domperidone toxicity in an infant on maintenance haemodialysis. *Pediatr Nephrol.* 2007; 22:161-2.
110. Baldini M, Cornelli U, Molinari M, Cantalamessa L. Effect of methyldopa on prolactin serum concentration: comparison between normal and sustained-release formulations. *Eur J Clin Pharmacol.* 1988; 34:513-5.
111. Arze RS, Ramos JM, Rashid HU et al. Amenorrhoea, galactorrhoea, and hyperprolactinaemia induced by methyldopa. *Br Med J (Clin Res Ed).* 1981; 283:194.
112. Asnis GM, Sachar EJ, Halbreich U et al. The prolactin-stimulating potency of reserpine in man. *Psychiatry Res.* 1981; 5:39-45.
113. Romeo JH, Dombrowski R, Kwak YS et al. Hyperprolactinaemia and verapamil: prevalence and potential association with hypogonadism in men. *Clin Endocrinol (Oxf).* 1996; 45:571-5.
114. Barbieri C, Larovere MT, Mariotti G et al. Prolactin stimulation by intravenous labetalol is mediated inside the central nervous system. *Clin Endocrinol (Oxf).* 1982; 16:615-9.
115. Kelleher JA. Atenolol-induced breast pain in a woman with hypertension. *Ann Pharmacother.* 2006; 40:990-2.
116. Kinon BJ, Gilmore JA, Liu H, Halbreich UM. Hyperprolactinemia in response to antipsychotic drugs: characterization across comparative clinical trials. *Psychoneuroendocrinology.* 2003; 28:69-82.
117. Kane JM, Meltzer HY, Carson WH Jr et al. Aripiprazole for treatment-resistant schizophrenia: results of a multicenter, randomized, double-blind, comparison study versus perphenazine. *J Clin Psychiatry.* 2007; 68:213-23.
118. Tollefson GD, Beasley CM Jr, Tran PV et al. Olanzapine versus haloperidol in the treatment of schizophrenia and schizoaffective and schizophreniform disorders: results of an international collaborative trial. *Am J Psychiatry.* 1997; 154:457-65.
119. Tran PV, Hamilton SH, Kuntz AJ et al. Double-blind comparison of olanzapine versus risperidone in the treatment of schizophrenia and other psychotic disorders. *J Clin Psychopharmacol.* 1997; 17:407-18.
120. Ash PR, Bouma D. Exaggerated hyperprolactinemia in response to thiothixene. *Arch Neurol.* 1981; 38:534-5.
121. Gruen PG, Sachar EJ, Altman N et al. Relation of plasma prolactin to clinical response in schizophrenic patients. *Arch Gen Psychiatry.* 1978; 35:1222-7.
122. The Scottish First Episode Schizophrenia Study. II. Treatment: pimozide versus flupenthixol. The Scottish Schizophrenia Research Group. *Br J Psychiatry.* 1987; 150:334-8.
123. Saldana SN, Delgado SV. Ziprasidone-associated galactorrhea in an adolescent female. *J Child Adolescent Psychopharmacol.* 2007; 17:259-60.
124. Gupta M. Low dose quetiapine induced galactorrhoea: a case report. *Clin Pract Epidemiol Ment Health.* 2007; 3:12.

125. Pandurangi AK, Narasimhachari N, Blackard WG, Landa BS. Relation of serum molindone levels to serum prolactin levels and antipsychotic response. *J Clin Psychiatry.* 1989; 50:379-81.
126. Luciano AA, Sherman BM, Chapler FK et al. Hyperprolactinemia and contraception: a prospective study. *Obstet Gynecol.* 1985; 65:506-10.
127. Siegel YI, Korczak D, Lindner A. Serum prolactin levels in patients treated with a gonadotropin-releasing hormone analogue for adenocarcinoma of the prostate. *Eur Urol.* 1991; 19:16-8.
128. Massart F, Parrino R, Placidi G et al. Prolactin secretion before, during, and after chronic gonadotropin-releasing hormone agonist treatments in children. *Fertil Steril.* 2005; 84:719-24.
129. Delle Fave GF, Tamburrano G, de Magistris L et al. Gynaecomastia with cimetidine. *Lancet.* 1977; 1:13-9.
130. Majumdar SK, Thomson AD, Shaw GK. Cimetidine and serum prolactin. *BMJ.* 1978; 1:409.
131. Delpre G, Lapidot M, Lipchitz A et al. Hyperprolactinaemia during famotidine therapy. *Lancet.* 1993; 342:868.
132. Zis AP, Haskett RF, Albala AA et al. Morphine inhibits cortisol and stimulates prolactin secretion in man. *Psychoneuroendocrinology.* 1984; 9:423-7.
133. Bart G, Borg L, Schluger JH et al. Suppressed prolactin response to dynorphin A1–13 in methadone-maintained versus control subjects. *J Pharmacol Exp Ther.* 2003; 306:581-7.
134. Hutchinson J, Murphy M, Harries R et al. Galactorrhea and hyperprolactinemia associated with protease inhibitors. *Lancet.* 2000; 356:1003-4.
135. Montero A, Bottasso OA, Luraghi MR et al. Galactorrhoea, hyperprolactinaemia, and protease inhibitors. *Lancet.* 2001; 357:473-4.
136. Luzzati R, Crosato IM, Mascioli M et al. Galactorrhea and hyperprolactinemia associated with HIV postexposure chemoprophylaxis. *AIDS.* 2002; 16:1306-7.
137. Duval X, Larger E, Longuet P et al. Galactorrhoea, hyperprolactinaemia, and protease inhibitors. *Lancet.* 2001; 357:475.
138. Farré M, de la Torre R, González ML et al. Cocaine and alcohol interactions in humans: neuroendocrine effects and cocaethylene metabolism. *J Pharmacol Exp Ther.* 1997; 283:164-76.
139. Fonzo D, Angeli A, Sivieri R et al. Hyperprolactinemia in girls with idiopathic precocious puberty under prolonged treatment with cyproterone acetate. *J Clin Endocrinol Metab.* 1977; 45:164-8.
140. Uygur-Bayramicli O, Aydin D, Ak O et al. Hyperprolactinemia caused by azathioprine. *J Clin Gastroenterol.* 2003; 36:79-80.
141. Siimes MA, Ropponen P, Aalberg V et al. Prolactinemia in adolescent males surviving malignancies in childhood: impaired dating activity. *J Adolesc Health.* 1993; 14:543-7.
142. Lee MA, Bowers MM, Nash JF et al. Neuroendocrine measures of dopaminergic function in chronic cocaine users. *Psychiatry Res.* 1990; 33:151-9.
143. Iaria G, Urbani L, Catalano G et al. Switch to tacrolimus for cyclosporine-induced gynecomastia in liver transplant recipients. *Transplant Proc.* 2005; 37:2632-3.
144. Olusi SO. Hyperprolactinaemia in patients with suspected cannabis-induced gynaecomastia. *Lancet.* 1980; 1:255.
145. Molitch ME. Drugs and prolactin. *Pituitary.* 2008; 11:209-18.
146. Coker F, Taylor D. Antidepressant-induced hyperprolactinaemia: incidence, mechanisms, and management. *CNS Drugs.* 2010; 24:563-74.
147. Madhusoodanan S, Parida S, Jimenez C. Hyperprolactinemia associated with psychotropics—a review. *Hum Psychopharmacol Clin Exp.* 2010; 25:281-97.
148. Serri O, Chik CL, Ur E, Ezzat S. Diagnosis and management of hyperprolactinemia. *CMAJ.* 2003; 169:575-81.
149. Byerly M, Suppes T, Tran QV, Baker RA. Clinical implications of antipsychotic-induced hyperprolactinemia in patients with schizophrenia spectrum or bipolar spectrum disorders. *J Clin Psychopharmacol.* 2007; 27:639-61.
150. Ajmal A, Joffe H, Nachtigall LB. Psychotropic-induced hyperprolactinemia: a clinical review. *Psychosomatics.* 2014; 55:29-36.
151. Brue T, Delemer B. Diagnosis and management of hyperprolactinemia: expert consensus—French Society of Endocrinology. *Ann Endocrinol.* 2007; 68:58-64.
152. Inder WJ, Castla D. Antipsychotic-induced hyperprolactinaemia. *Aust N Z Psychiatry.* 2011; 45:830-7.
153. Bankowski BJ, Zacur HA. Dopamine agonist therapy for hyperprolactinemia. *Clin Obstet Gynecol.* 2003; 46:349-62.
154. Zanettini R, Antonini A, Gatto G et al. Valvular heart disease and the use of dopamine agonists for Parkinson's disease. *N Engl J Med.* 2007; 356:39-46.
155. Peveler RC, Branford D, Citrome L et al. Antipsychotics and hyperprolactinaemia: clinical recommendations. *J Psychopharmacol.* 2008; 22(suppl 2):98-103.
156. Cuttler L. The regulation of growth hormone secretion. *Endocrinol Metab Clin North Am.* 1996; 25:541-71.
157. Goldenberg N, Barkan A. Factors regulating growth hormone secretion in humans. *Endocrinol Metab Clin North Am.* 2007; 36:37-55.
158. Imura H, Kato Y, Ikeda M et al. Effect of adrenergic blocking or stimulating agents on plasma growth hormone, immunoreactive insulin, and blood free fatty acid levels in man. *J Clin Invest.* 1971; 50:1069-79.
159. Kaufmann S, Jones KL, Wehrenberg WB. Inhibition by prednisone of growth hormone response to GHRHa in normal men. *J Clin Endocrinol Metab.* 1988; 67:1258-61.
160. Mulligan T, Jaen-Vinuales A, Godschalk M et al. Synthetic somatostatin analog (octreotide) suppresses daytime growth hormone secretion equivalently in young and older men: preserved pituitary responsiveness to somatostatin's inhibition in aging. *J Am Geriatr Soc.* 1999; 47:1422-4.
161. Thomas BC, Stanhope R, Leiper AD. Gonadotropin releasing hormone analogue and growth hormone therapy in precocious and premature puberty following cranial irradiation for acute lymphoblastic leukaemia. *Horm Res.* 1993; 39:25-9.
162. Mauras N. Growth hormone therapy in the glucocorticosteroid-dependent child: metabolic and linear growth effects. *Horm Res.* 2001; 56:13-8.
163. Holtkamp K, Peters-Wallraf B, Wuller S et al. Methylphenidate-related growth impairment. *J Child Adolesc Psychopharmacol.* 2002; 12:55-61.
164. Dommisse CS, Schulz SC, Narasimhachari N et al. The neuroendocrine and behavioral response to dextroamphetamine in normal individuals. *Biol Psychiatry.* 1984; 19:1305-15.
165. Oberg K. Established clinical use of octreotide and lanreotide in oncology. *Chemotherapy.* 2001; 47:40-53.
166. Rose SR, Vogiatzi MG, Copeland KC. A general pediatric approach to evaluating a short child. *Pediatr Rev.* 2005; 26:410-20.
167. Lima L, Arce V, Diaz MJ et al. Glucocorticoids may inhibit growth hormone release by enhancing betaadrenergic responsiveness in hypothalamic somatostatin neurons. *J Clin Endocrinol Metab.* 1993; 76:439-44.
168. Hobernicht SL, Schweiger B, Zeitler P et al. Acquired growth hormone deficiency in a girl with chronic myelogenous leukemia treated with tyrosine kinase inhibitor therapy. *Pediatr Blood Cancer.* 2011; 56:671-3.
169. Stochholm K, Gravholt CH, Laursen T et al. Incidence of GH deficiency—a nationwide study. *Eur J Endocrinol.* 2006; 155:61-71.
170. Schneider HJ, Aimaretti G, Kreitschmann-Andermahr I et al. Hypopituitarism. *Lancet.* 2007; 369:1461-70.
171. Mazziotti G, Giustina A. Glucocorticoids and the regulation of growth hormone secretion. *Nat Rev Endocrinol.* 2013; 9:265-76.
172. Renes JS, Ridder MAJ, Breukhoven PE et al. Methylphenidate and the response to growth hormone treatment in short children born small for gestational age. *PLoS ONE.* 2012; 7:e53164.

173. Anderson L, Jeftinija S, Scanes C. Growth hormone secretion: molecular and cellular mechanism and in vivo approaches. *Exp Biol Med.* 2004; 229:291-302.

174. Bougneres P, Goffin V. The growth hormone receptor in growth. *Endocrinol Metab Clin N Am.* 2007; 36:1-16.

175. Growth Hormone Research Society. Consensus guidelines for the diagnosis and treatment of growth hormone (GH) deficiency in childhood and adolescence: summary statement of the GH Research Society. GH Research Society. *J Clin Endocrinol Metab.* 2000; 85:3990-3.

176. Nilsson AG, Svensson J, Johannsson G. Management of growth hormone deficiency in adult. *Growth Horm IGF Res.* 2007; 17:441-62.

177. Stochholm K, Christiansen J, Laursen T et al. Mortality and reduced growth hormone secretion. *Horm Res.* 2007; 68(suppl 5):173-6.

178. Molitch ME, Clemmons DR, Malozowski S et al. Evaluation and treatment of adult growth hormone deficiency: an Endocrine Society Clinical Practice Guideline. *Clin Endocrinol Metab.* 2011; 96:1587-1609.

179. Lebrethon MC, Grossman AB, Afshar F et al. Linear growth and final height after treatment for Cushing's disease in childhood. *J Clin Endocrinol Metab.* 2000; 85:3262-5.

180. Stochholm K, Gravholt CH, Laursen T et al. Mortality in growth hormone deficiency—a nationwide study. *Eur J Endocrinol.* 2007; 157:9-18.

181. Johannssonn G. Management of adult growth hormone deficiency. *Endocrinol Metab Clin North Am.* 2007; 36:203-20.

182. van Bunderen CC, van Varsseveld NC, Erfurh EM et al. Efficacy and safety of growth hormone treatment in adults with growth hormone deficiency: a systematic review of studies on morbidity. *Clin Endocrinol.* 2014; 81:1-14.

183. Gazzaruso C, Gola M, Karamouzis I et al. Cardiovascular risk in adult patients with growth hormone (GH) deficiency and following substitution with GH—an update. *J Clin Endocrinol Metab.* 2014; 99:18029.

184. Rossi GP, Pessina AC, Heagerty AM. Primary aldosteronism: an update on screening, diagnosis, and treatment. *J Hypertens.* 2008; 26:613-21.

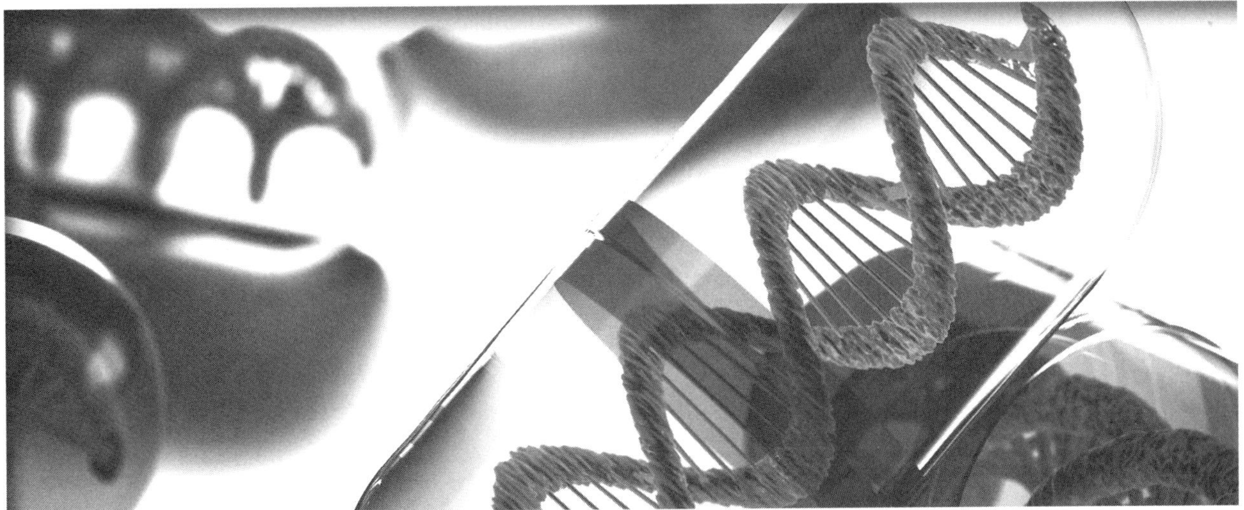

CHAPTER 33

Sexual Dysfunction in Males

Mary Lee and Roohollah Sharifi

Sexual dysfunction in males can be broadly classified into five major types: disorders of libido (increased or decreased sexual drive), erectile dysfunction (penile impotence), ejaculatory disorders (premature ejaculation, delayed ejaculation, emission failure or anejaculation, decreased ejaculation volume, or retrograde ejaculation), priapism (prolonged, painful erection), and infertility. Although some patients suffer from only one type of sexual dysfunction, others may experience more than one. In some cases, a patient may suffer from one disorder, and then secondarily another type of sexual dysfunction develops. For example, an elderly menopausal male patient may experience decreased libido, and then erectile dysfunction develops secondary to the lack of sexual drive. Some drugs have the potential to cause several types of sexual dysfunction. For example, phenothiazine antipsychotic agents may cause decreased libido, erectile dysfunction, or priapism, which may occur together in some patients or separately in others.

CAUSATIVE AGENTS

Table 33-1, **Table 33-2**, **Table 33-3**, **Table 33-4**, and **Table 33-5** list the many drugs that have been commonly reported to cause various types of sexual dysfunction in males. Many of the published references used to create these tables are observational studies, case reports, or case series. Thus, a cause-effect relationship has not been established for many of the drugs. An effort was made to include drugs for which a proposed mechanism for the drug-induced disease could be described based on the drug's pharmacologic effects. Thus, Tables 33-1 to 33-5 should not be considered exhaustive lists.

Key to the interpretation of the published literature on drug-induced sexual dysfunction is the fact that, in some cases, the disease for which the offending drug was prescribed is, itself, a risk factor for sexual dysfunction. For example, diuretics are a common cause of erectile dysfunction. However, diuretics are commonly prescribed for hypertension,

Table 33-1 Agents Implicated in Drug-Induced Decrease in Libido

Drug	Incidence	Level of Evidence
5α-reductase inhibitors[1-3]	6.4%, up to 94%[1]	A,B
Anabolic steroids[4]	25%	A,B
Antidepressants, tricyclic[5]	NK[a]	C
Antidepressants, selective serotonin reuptake inhibitors[6]	1–12%	A
Antidepressants, other[5]	4%	A
Atypical antipsychotics[7,8]	0.1–5%, up to 60%	A
β-adrenergic antagonists[9]	NK	C
Carbamazepine[10]	22–67%	B
Cimetidine[11,12]	1–4%[b]	C
Cocaine[13]	NK	C
Digoxin[14]	NK	C
Estrogens[15]	8%	B
Ethanol[16]	NK[c]	C
Gonadotropin-releasing hormone agonists[15]	NK[d]	A
Gonadotropin-releasing hormone antagonists[17]	NK	C
Haloperidol[15]	NK	C
HMG CoA reductase inhibitors[18,19]	NK	C
Hypnotics, benzodiazepines[15]	NK	C
Isotretinoin[20]	NK	C
Ketoconazole[16,21]	NK	B
Levetiracetam[22]	NK	C
Lithium[23]	NK	C
Metoclopramide[15]	NK	C
Opiates (natural and synthetic)[24-28]	19%[e]	B,C
Phenothiazines[29]	NK[f]	B
Proton pump inhibitors[30]	NK	C
Spironolactone[13]	NK[g]	B

NK = not known.
[a]Most common with tertiary amines, as these have the highest incidence of sedative adverse effects.
[b]Uncommon. Most often reported with high-dose parenteral drug treatment.
[c]Common with high doses of ethanol. Low doses may improve libido.
[d]Common after the first 2–3 wk of the start of treatment. This adverse effect is likely underreported because patients who receive this medication may not be sexually active.
[e]Associated with morphine doses of 100 mg orally/day or its equivalent.
[f]Common with highly sedating phenothiazines. Less common with less-sedating agents: thiothixene, haloperidol, or loxapine.
[g]Common in patients treated with large daily doses (e.g., those with hyperaldosteronism).

Table 33-2 Agents Implicated in Drug-Induced Erectile Dysfunction

Drug	Incidence	Level of Evidence
α-adrenergic antagonists[2]	0–2.8%	A
5α-reductase inhibitors[1,2,32-36]	8.1–18.5%	A
Amiodarone[9,37]	NK	C
Antiandrogen (e.g., flutamide, ketoconazole)[37]	NK	C
Antihistamines[13]	NK[a]	C
Antiparkinsonian agents[13]	NK	C
Antidepressants, norepinephrine and serotonin reuptake inhibitors[38]	1–5%	A
Antidepressants, selective serotonin reuptake inhibitors[38,39]	0–13%[b]	B, C
Antidepressants, tetracyclic[29]	0.1–1%	A
Antidepressants, tricyclic[13]	NK	B
Antidepressants, other[38]	3.4%[b]	A
Antipsychotics, first generation (e.g., chlorpromazine, thioridazine, etc.)[6,8]	NK[c]	C
Antipsychotics, atypical[23]	0.1–1%[d]	A
β-adrenergic antagonists[9,31,41,42]	6–40%[e,f]	C
Baclofen[43,44]	0.2–1.6%	A
Benzodiazepines[45,60]	NK	C
Busulfan[37]	NK	C
Calcium-channel antagonists[41,46]	<1%	A
Celecoxib[47]	NK	C
Cocaine[37]	NK	C
Central α-adrenergic agonists[48]	3–7%, up to 24%	A
Cyclophosphamide[37]	NK	C
Digoxin[37]	NK	C
Disopyramide[13-15]	1–3%	A
Diuretics, thiazides[13-15,31,42,48]	10–20%[f]	B
Diuretics, loop[13-15,42,48]	NK[f]	C
Estrogens[15]	12%	A
Ethanol[37]	NK	C
Gabapentin[49-51]	1.5%	A
Gemfibrozil[13,52]	NK	C
Gonadotropin-releasing hormone agonists[53]	4%[g]	A
Gonadotropin-releasing hormone antagonists[17]	NK[g]	C
Guanethidine[48]	54%	B
Haloperidol[33,40]	NK	C
Histamine H_2-receptor antagonists (e.g., cimetidine)[45]	NK	C
HMG-CoA reductase inhibitors[52,54-58]	Variable	B,C
Lithium carbonate[15,40,59,60]	NK	C
Marijuana[37,61]	Variable	C
Methyldopa[48]	36%[f,h]	B
Monoamine oxidase inhibitors[13,40]	NK	C
Nonsteroidal anti-inflammatory agents[45,47,62,63]	9.7%	B

Table 33-2 Agents Implicated in Drug-Induced Erectile Dysfunction (continued)

Drug	Incidence	Level of Evidence
Omeprazole[64-66]	NK	C
Opiates[67]	Up to 50%[h]	B
Phenothiazines[6,13-15]	N[c,h]	B
Pregabalin[68]	71%	A
Protease inhibitors[69]	6%	B
Reserpine[13-15]	NK[h]	C
Spironolactone[13-15]	4–30%[h]	C
Topiramate[70-72]	≥1%	A

NK = not known.
[a]Frequency is highest with drugs with the greatest anticholinergic or sedative adverse effects.
[b]Frequency is lower with antidepressants with lower anticholinergic adverse effects and lower serotoninergic effects (e.g., bupropion, nefazodone, vilazodone, mirtazapine).[40,79,157,175]
[c]Frequency is highest with thioridazine, which has the greatest anticholinergic potency as compared with other agents. Some literature suggests using prolactin-sparing agents (e.g., aripiprazole, clozapine, olanzapine, quetiapine, and ziprasidone), but this has variable results.[6]
[d]Of these agents, risperidone has been reported to cause the highest incidence (>5%).
[e]Frequency is highest with lipophilic drugs, which cross the blood–brain barrier.
[f]Antihypertensives with a lower prevalence of erectile dysfunction include angiotensin-converting enzyme inhibitors, angiotensin II antagonists, and calcium-channel antagonists.
[g]Because these medications lower serum testosterone to castration levels, the incidence is probably much higher. However, patients receiving this medication may not report this adverse effect because they are not sexually active.
[h]Frequency is dose-related.

Table 33-3 Agents Implicated in Drug-Induced Ejaculation Disorders

Drug	Incidence	Level of Evidence
α-adrenergic antagonists[73,74,76,77]	9.7–28.1%[a,b]	A,B
5α-reductase inhibitors[1,2,32-35,76]	0.1–7.2%[c]	A
Antidepressants, selective serotonin reuptake inhibitors[29,40,78-83]	6–28%[d]	A
Antidepressants, tricyclic[79,81,82]	NK	C
Antidepressants, tetracyclic[82,84]	<0.1%	A
Antidepressants, norepinephrine and serotonin reuptake inhibitors[82,85]	2–3%	A
Antidepressants, triazolopyridine[82,86]	NK	C
Antidepressants, other[87]	0.1–1%	C
Antipsychotics, atypical[6,88-91]	0–5%	A
Baclofen[92]	NK	A
Haloperidol[6,91]	NK	C
Monoamine oxidase inhibitors[6,38,82]	NK	C
Naproxen[91]	NK	C
Phenothiazines[78]	NK	C
Thiazide diuretics[42]	NK[e]	C
Topiramate[90,92]	1–3%	C

NK = not known.
[a]Highest incidences reported with tamsulosin 0.8 mg per day and silodosin (90%).[2,7,75,76]
[b]Combination of α-adrenergic antagonist and 5α-reductase inhibitor is associated with threefold increase in ejaculation disorders compared to either drug alone.[76]
[c]Variable incidence rates reported. Rates as high as 20% reported.[33]
[d]Occurs in up to 50% of patients treated with paroxetine. Paroxetine is associated with the highest incidence as compared with other agents in this class.
[e]Incidence of ejaculation disorders is much lower than those of erectile dysfunction and decreased libido.

Table 33-4 Agents Implicated in Drug-Induced Priapism

Drug	Incidence	Level of Evidence
Adalimumab[93]	NK	C
α-adrenergic antagonists[94-96]	<1%	A
Alprostadil[97,98]	0.4%[a]	A
Antianxiety agents	NK	C
Antidepressants[29,40]	NK	C
Antidepressants, selective serotonin reuptake inhibitors[40,99-102]	NK	C
Antidepressants, triazolopyridine (e.g., trazodone)[38,40,103,104]	NK	C
Antipsychotics, atypical[6,105-113]	0.1–1%	A
Atomoxetine[114]	NK	C
Buspirone[115]	NK	C
Cocaine[116]	NK	C
Ethanol[115]	NK	C
Fat emulsion, intravenous[117]	NK	C
Heparin[118-120]	NK	C
Hydralazine[118]	NK	C
Hydroxyzine[115]	NK	C
Lithium[121]	NK	C
Marijuana[61,115]	NK	C
Methylphenidate[122,123]	NK	C
Olanzapine[124]	NK	C
Paliperidone[125]	NK	C
Papaverine[126,127]	NK[b]	C
Phenothiazines[6,128]	NK[c]	C
Phentolamine[115]	NK[b]	C
Phosphodiesterase type 5 inhibitors (e.g., sildenafil)[115,129-131]	NK[d]	C
Quetiapine[121,132,133]	NK	C
Sodium valproate[134]	NK	C
Warfarin[118,120,135]	NK	C

NK = not known.
[a]Usually occurs when administered intracavernosally or intraurethrally in large doses, or when used along with other erectogenic drugs.
[b]Usually occurs when administered in large doses intracavernosally or when used along with other erectogenic drugs.
[c]This drug category is one of the most common causes of priapism in clinical practice.
[d]Usually when used in excessive doses or when combined with other erectogenic agents.

which itself may cause erectile dysfunction. Also, sexual dysfunction is generally an underreported adverse effect. Many patients are uncomfortable sharing information about this and some healthcare providers do not routinely question patients about this adverse drug reaction.

EPIDEMIOLOGY

Up to 25% of cases of erectile dysfunction may be drug induced, and the most common offending agents are thiazide diuretics, β-blockers, antipsychotic agents, and antidepressants. According to the Massachusetts Male Aging Study, which was conducted in male outpatients aged 40 to 70 years, up to 51% of men had some degree of erectile dysfunction.[16,149] Erectile dysfunction was more common in men who were taking antihypertensive drugs, oral hypoglycemic agents, vasodilators, or cardiac medications. In the 4-year Treatment of Mild Hypertension Study, patients responded to an annual survey of sexual function. At the 2-year point, the incidence of the

Table 33-5 Agents Implicated in Drug-Induced Infertility

Drug	Incidence	Level of Evidence
Anabolic steroids[4,136]	NK[a]	C
Antidepressants, selective serotonin reuptake inhibitors[137,138]	NK[b]	B
Antineoplastic agents, alkylating[23,139,140]	Up to 100%[a,c]	B
Carbamazepine[141]	NK	C
Cimetidine[23,118]	NK	C
Cisplatin[139,140]	Up to 100%[d]	B
Corticosteroids	100%[e]	B
Erythromycin[142]	NK	C
Escitalopram[143]	NK[b]	C
Estrogens[23]	NK[f]	C
Ethanol, chronic use[144]	NK[f]	C
Gonadotropin-releasing hormone agonists[145]	NK[f]	B
Ketoconazole[146]	NK[a,g]	C
Nitrofurantoin[146,147]	NK[a,g]	C
Phenothiazines[23]	NK	C
Spironolactone[23]	NK[a]	C
Sulfasalazine[118]	NK	C
Testosterone undecanoate[148]	NK[h]	C

NK = not known.
[a]Frequency is dose-related.
[b]Has been shown to decrease sperm concentration and motility or to increase the concentration of sperm with abnormal morphology.[137,138]
[c]Incidence increases with dose and duration of treatment, and if chemotherapy is administered with radiation therapy or in combination with other chemotherapy known to affect spermatogenesis.
[d]Up to 100% of patients become infertile when cisplatin is used to treat testicular cancer. When dose is 0.6 g/m^2 or higher, azoospermia develops in most patients.
[e]This applies to patients treated with corticosteroids in pharmacologic doses in combination with antineoplastic chemotherapy regimens.
[f]Probably common; however, incidence not studied.
[g]Not reported with usual therapeutic doses; occurs with large doses.
[h]This is based on high-dose testosterone supplementation for an infertile couple.

inability to achieve an erection was 2.8%, 15.7%, and 4.9% in the doxazosin, chlorthalidone, and placebo groups, respectively.[31] In contrast, the incidences of drug-induced disorders of libido, ejaculation, priapism, or fertility are not as well studied, and therefore, less data are available.

A wide range of prevalence rates has been reported for sexual dysfunction associated with specific drugs. This is related to methodological limitations in study design, including the absence of validated sexual dysfunction survey tools used at baseline and during the trial to assess the presence of disorders, and the lack of objective assessments to confirm a patient's self-reported complaints.[40] In addition, patient factors directly influence the frequency of reported sexual dysfunction, including the willingness of the patient to report the adverse effect, persistence of the healthcare provider in questioning the patient about the adverse effect, patient's age and general health status, whether or not the patient is a smoker or uses recreational drugs, dosage regimen of the offending agent, use of the offending agent in combination with other drugs that could also cause sexual dysfunction, and concurrent medical illnesses that could contribute to sexual dysfunction.[150,151]

MECHANISMS

Mechanisms of drug-induced sexual dysfunction are dependent on the type of dysfunction (**Table 33-6**). A normal male libido is mediated by serum androgen concentrations. Testosterone is the chief male androgen, comprising 90% of circulating androgens, and is produced by the testes. Serum testosterone concentrations are responsible for male sexual drive.[150,164] The role of dihydrotestosterone, the chief active metabolite of testosterone, in maintaining libido is not clear. In patients with

Table 33-6 Mechanisms of Drug-Induced Sexual Dysfunction in Males

Drug	Mechanism
DRUG-INDUCED DECREASED LIBIDO	
5-α reductase inhibitors	Decrease dihydrotestosterone in the central nervous system[1,34,35]
Anabolic steroids	Suppress hypothalamic–pituitary–gonadal axis[4]
Antidepressants	Cause sedation, which depresses libido[5,40]
Antipsychotics	Cause sedation, which depresses libido[6,7]
β-adrenergic antagonists	Cause sedation, particularly the lipophilic agents (e.g., propranolol)[152]
Carbamazepine	Increases sex hormone–binding globulin, which decreases serum free (active) testosterone levels[153,154]
Cimetidine	Increases prolactin, which depresses androgen production; may be an androgen receptor antagonist[11-15]
Clofibrate	Reduces cholesterol, a precursor for androgen synthesis[9,13-16]
Digoxin	(Metabolite) Competes with androgen at receptors[13-16]
Estrogens	Decrease pituitary LH secretion and testicular testosterone production
Ethanol, high doses	Causes sedation, which depresses libido[13-16]
Gemfibrozil	Reduces cholesterol, a precursor for androgen synthesis[13-16]
Gonadotropin-releasing hormone agonists	Decrease pituitary LH secretion and testicular testosterone production[50]
Gonadotropin-releasing hormone antagonists	Decrease pituitary LH secretion and testicular testosterone production[155]
HMG-CoA inhibitors	Decrease serum testosterone[17,18,19,52]
Hypnotics	Cause sedation, which depresses libido[13-15]
Ketoconazole	Inhibits adrenal and testicular testosterone production[21]
Methadone	Increases serum prolactin, which depresses androgen production[156]
Metoclopramide	Increases prolactin, which depresses androgen production[13-15]
Opiates	Suppress hypothalamic–pituitary–gonadal axis and decrease pulsatile release of luteinizing hormone[24-27,67]
Phenobarbital	Increases sex hormone–binding globulin, which decreases serum free (active) testosterone levels[153,154]
Phenothiazines	Increase prolactin, which depresses androgen production; has sedative effects[6-8]
Phenytoin	Increases sex hormone–binding globulin, which decreases serum free (active) testosterone levels[46,153,154]
Spironolactone	Competes with androgen at receptor (metabolite) Inhibits testosterone synthesis[13,14]
DRUG-INDUCED ERECTILE DYSFUNCTION	
5-α reductase inhibitors	Decrease dihydrotestosterone, which may result in decreased smooth muscle in cavernosal tissue and apoptosis of cells[1,2,36,159]

Table 33-6 Mechanisms of Drug-Induced Sexual Dysfunction in Males (continued)

Drug	Mechanism
Anticonvulsants	Sedative adverse effects decrease libido; patients may develop erectile dysfunction secondary to decreased libido.[15,16] Some agents with potent hepatic microsomal enzyme-inducing properties (e.g., phenytoin, carbamazepine) may increase sex hormone–binding globulin, thereby decreasing free (active) testosterone.[153,154]
Antidepressants	Sedative adverse effects decrease libido; patients may develop erectile dysfunction secondary to decreased libido; anticholinergic effects decrease arterial blood flow into and filling of corpora cavernosa.[5] Also, antidepressants with strong serotoninergic properties (e.g., fluoxetine, paroxetine, citalopram, or sertraline) are associated with the higher prevalence of sexual dysfunction than agents that have less potent serotoninergic effects (e.g., bupropion, mirtazapine, nefazodone, vilazodone).[40,157,158] Selective serotonin reuptake inhibitors activate central serotonin receptors, which inhibit neurotransmission of norepinephrine and dopamine.[40]
Antihistamine	Sedative adverse effects cause decreased libido; patients develop erectile dysfunction secondary to decreased libido.
Anticholinergic-antiparkinsonian agents (e.g., benztropine)	Anticholinergic effects decrease arterial blood flow into and filling of corpora cavernosa.[13-15]
Antipsychotics (phenothiazines, atypical antipsychotics)	Sedative adverse effects cause decreased libido; patients develop erectile dysfunction secondary to decreased libido. Anticholinergic effects decrease arterial blood flow into and filling of corpora cavernosa; in addition, some antipsychotic agents antagonize dopamine, which results in increased prolactin[167]; increased prolactin is also associated with decreased testicular testosterone production.[6,160]
β-adrenergic antagonists	Decrease systemic blood pressure resulting in decreased blood flow to corpora cavernosa, may decrease libido and cause erectile dysfunction secondarily, decrease central sympathetic outflow Prevalence may be greater with lipophilic agents.[13-15]
Digoxin	Blocks smooth muscle relaxation of corpora cavernosa, which inhibits blood filling[9]
Diuretics, thiazide or loop Centrally acting sympatholytics (e.g., clonidine)	Decrease systemic blood pressure resulting in decreased blood flow to corpora cavernosa[13-15,42]
Estrogens Gonadotropin-releasing hormone agonists Gonadotropin-releasing hormone antagonists	Decreased serum testosterone concentrations causing decreased libido and secondary erectile dysfunction[50,53,155]
Ethanol, high doses Hypnotics	Sedative adverse effects cause decreased libido; patients develop erectile dysfunction secondary to decreased libido.[13-15]
Haloperidol	Blocks D_1 and D_2 receptors in the central nervous system[6]
Pregabalin	Decreases release of neurotransmitters (e.g., glutamate, substance P, and calcitonin gene-related peptide)[161]
Topiramate	Interferes with blood flow to corpora cavernosa[70]
DRUG-INDUCED EJACULATION DISORDERS	
α-adrenergic antagonists	Relaxation of bladder neck during coitus leads to retrograde or delayed emission.[6,73,76,77,87-89,162]
Antipsychotics, atypical Phenothiazines	Inhibit α-adrenergic receptors at the bladder neck, leading to retrograde or delayed ejaculation[7,90]
5α-reductase inhibitors	Decrease in prostate volume leads to decrease in ability of prostate to produce prostatic secretions; decreased semen volume results.[163]

Table 33-6 Mechanisms of Drug-Induced Sexual Dysfunction in Males (continued)

Drug	Mechanism
Anticholinergic agents Phenothiazines[40,80] Tricyclic antidepressants[38,80]	Anticholinergic effects lead to delayed emission.[78,80]
Guanethidine	Blocks contraction of vas deferens, which results in delayed emission[48]
Antidepressants, selective serotonin reuptake inhibitors[29,40,78-83]	Stimulate central 5-HT_2 receptors, which leads to emission failure
Trazodone	Stimulate central serotonin receptors and causes peripheral α-adrenergic blockade, which leads to an ejaculation[82,86]
DRUG-INDUCED PRIAPISM	
Fat emulsion, intravenous Heparin[119] Warfarin[18]	Cause a hypercoagulable state[117]
Aripiprazole[107] Phenothiazines[6,128] Clozapine[108] Quetiapine[110,132] Risperidone[105,112,113]	α-adrenergic blockade prevents detumescence of the penis.
Bupropion[40] Antidepressants, selective serotonin reuptake inhibitors[40] Trazodone[103,104]	α-adrenergic blockade prevents detumescence of the penis. Central serotonin stimulation may also lead to low-flow priapism. α-adrenergic blockade prevents detumescence of the penis.
Hydralazine α-adrenergic antagonists[94-96]	Arteriolar vasodilation increases blood flow to corpora cavernosa.[9,97]
Alprostadil[97,98] Papaverine[126,127]	Increase cyclic AMP in cavernosal tissue, which increases blood filling of sinusoidal tissue
Phosphodiesterase type 5 inhibitors (e.g., sildenafil, vardenafil, tadalafil, avanafil)	When used in excessive doses or when combined with other erectogenic drugs, they increase cyclic GMP in cavernosal tissue, which increases blood filling of sinusoidal tissue.[130,131]
DRUG-INDUCED INFERTILITY	
Anabolic steroids	Suppress hypothalamic–pituitary gonadal axis[4]
Antineoplastic agents	Damage germinal epithelium in testes; sperm production is impaired.[23,139,140]
Estrogens Gonadotropin-releasing hormone superagonists Ketoconazole Spironolactone	Decrease serum testosterone concentration or block testosterone at receptors, which interfere with maturation of spermatogonia[23,145,146]
Cimetidine	Blocks androgen receptor, which interferes with maturation of spermatogonia[23,118]
Erythromycin	Decreases sperm motility and sperm number[142]
Ethanol, chronic	Decreases testosterone production, which interferes with sperm maturation[144]
Nitrofurantoin	Inhibits sperm maturation and protein synthesis, which interferes with sperm motility[147]
Sulfasalazine	Decreases sperm production, maturation, and motility[118]
Testosterone undecanoate	Suppresses FSH and LH, which decreases sperm production and maturation[148]

AMP = adenosine monophosphate, FSH = follicle-stimulating hormone, GMP = guanosine monophosphate, HT = hydroxytryptamine, LH = luteinizing hormone.

primary hypogonadism who have serum testosterone concentrations that are below the normal range, exogenous administration of testosterone replacement agents restores libido.[165]

The hypothalamic–pituitary–gonadal–adrenal axis controls testicular testosterone production. Increased release of luteinizing hormone-releasing hormone or gonadotropin-releasing hormone from the hypothalamus stimulates pituitary release of luteinizing hormone. Luteinizing hormone stimulates the production of testosterone in Leydig cells. Therefore, drugs that suppress hypothalamic release of luteinizing hormone-releasing hormone or pituitary release of luteinizing hormone, or that directly suppress testicular testosterone production,[166] may suppress libido. Similarly, drugs that increase serum prolactin concentrations, which results in a decrease in testicular androgen production, can indirectly suppress libido.[167] In addition to the stimulatory effect of testosterone on libido, males must be conscious and receptive to sexual stimuli, which can be visual, auditory, olfactory, tactile, or gustatory. As these stimuli are processed in the brain, drugs that cause sedation or depress the sensorium can suppress libido.[166]

Theoretically, it follows then that supraphysiologic serum testosterone concentrations may enhance male sexual drive in elderly patients. However, this has not been demonstrated clinically. Administration of excessive doses of testosterone to elderly male patients, resulting in supraphysiologic serum testosterone concentrations, is not associated with increased libido.[165,168] The mechanism for increased sexual drive is poorly understood and may be due to a combination of causes, including a supratentorial component.

In order for a penile erection to occur, a patient must have intact penile vascular and neurologic systems. The penis is composed of three vascular bodies: two dorsal corpora cavernosa and one corpus spongiosum. During an erection, the corpora fill with arterial blood, which must be trapped within the corpora. Thus, arterial blood flow must be adequate and the degree of arterial inflow must exceed the degree of venous outflow for penile tumescence to occur. When compounded by contraction of the ischiocavernosus muscles surrounding the bulbous urethra, these effects produce a long, hard, penile shaft suitable for vaginal penetration. Thus, systemic antihypertensive agents, which decrease peripheral blood pressure, or diuretics, which decrease blood volume, may compromise arterial blood flow and cause erectile dysfunction.[169]

Both the central and peripheral nervous systems can mediate a penile erection. With visual, olfactory, auditory, tactile, or gustatory sexual stimulation, the brain sends nerve impulses down the spinal cord. Preganglionic sympathetic nerve fibers emerge from the spinal cord at the thoracolumbar vertebra T11-L2; postganglionic neurotransmission to the corpora is mediated by parasympathetic pathways in the pelvic plexus. Tactile stimulation of the genitalia can also stimulate a somatic reflex nerve arc at the level of the sacral vertebrae S2 to S4. In either case, acetylcholine is the primary neurotransmitter responsible for penile tumescence. Acetylcholine probably works through noncholinergic, nonadrenergic neurotransmitters, such as nitric oxide, and secondary messengers, such as cyclic adenosine monophosphate and cyclic guanine monophosphate, to mediate corporal relaxation and blood filling of cavernosal tissue sinuses. Therefore, drugs that antagonize acetylcholine at its receptor, producing anticholinergic effects, can cause erectile dysfunction.[169]

In male patients with normal sexual function, antegrade ejaculation of seminal fluids out of the urethra occurs at climax. Antegrade ejaculation requires emission (or the movement of seminal fluids from the prostate, seminal vesicles, and vas deferens into the proximal urethra); contraction of the bladder neck sphincter (to prevent the retrograde flow of seminal fluids into the bladder); and contraction of periurethral skeletal muscles to propel the ejaculate out of the urethra. Emission and bladder neck closure are sympathetically mediated by norepinephrine.[170] Thus, postsynaptic α-adrenergic receptor antagonists (e.g., tamsulosin) block norepinephrine at its receptor and may lead to retrograde ejaculation or emission failure.[170] The antegrade propulsion of ejaculate from the posterior urethra and out of the patient's body is parasympathetically mediated. Thus, drugs with anticholinergic effects may cause delayed ejaculation.[40,78,80,91] In addition, stimulation of central serotonin receptors appears to inhibit ejaculation. Thus, selective serotonin reuptake inhibitors are associated with anejaculation.[171]

The ejaculate is composed of three major components: sperm-containing fluid from the vas deferens, fructose-containing fluid from the seminal vesicles, and prostatic secretions from the prostate. A normal ejaculate volume is 2 to 6 mL. Contributors of ejaculate volume include the seminal vesicles (75–80% of the total volume) and prostate (10% of the total volume), both of which are androgen-dependent tissues. Thus, medications that interfere with testosterone stimulation of these target tissues (e.g., finasteride) can decrease ejaculate volume.[78]

Following climax and ejaculation, the penis returns to a flaccid state. For detumescence to occur, venous outflow must exceed arterial inflow. Detumescence is sympathetically mediated. Therefore, norepinephrine normally causes arteriolar vasoconstriction, thereby decreasing arteriolar inflow and causing cavernosal vasoconstriction. This improves venous outflow, and the penis eventually becomes flaccid. β_2-adrenergic stimulation of peripheral blood vessels causes venodilation, which improves venous outflow and blood emptying from the corpora cavernosa. When detumescence does not occur, and the penile erection is sustained in the absence of sexual stimulation, priapism can develop. Penile pain may result from blood sludging within and hypoxia of cavernosal tissue. Permanent cavernosal injury may develop if priapism does not resolve on its own or is not treated appropriately.

The mechanism of drug-induced priapism is poorly understood. Priapism may result from drug-induced increased arteriolar inflow to the cavernosa (e.g., hydralazine), drug-induced decreased venous outflow mediated by inhibition of α-adrenergic tone (e.g., phentolamine, phenothiazines, trazodone), blood sludging in the corpora because of platelet or clotting factor dysfunction (e.g., heparin, warfarin), or some other mechanism.[172]

The fertility of a male is dependent on multiple physiologic functions: adequate quantitative and qualitative production of sperm and effective emission of sperm into the prostatic urethra. Luteinizing hormone and follicle-stimulating hormone (FSH) are essential for the induction of sperm production at puberty. After puberty, maintenance of spermatogenesis is dependent on FSH stimulation of Sertoli cells and the presence of adequate concentrations of testosterone in the seminiferous tubules so that spermatogonia can undergo differentiation and maturation into spermatozoa.[173] Normal semen parameters include a semen volume of 2 to 6 mL, a sperm concentration of at least 20 million per mL, at least 50% to 60% motile sperm, and at least 30% of sperm with normal morphology.[173] Although variably defined, infertility refers to the inability of the female partner to become pregnant after 1 year or more of purposeful attempts to conceive.[173,174] Infertility can be due to an inadequate number of sperm in the semen; abnormal sperm morphology, which interferes with their motility; or their ability to penetrate an egg. Thus, drug-induced infertility can result from damage to the Sertoli cells (e.g., antineoplastic alkylating agents, radiation therapy), interference with the maturation of sperm (e.g., antiandrogens), or motility of sperm (e.g., sulfasalazine, vaginal spermicides).[23] The extent of damage to the germinal epithelium by antineoplastic agents is dependent on the pharmacologic class of agent used (alkylating agents are the most potent, followed by antimetabolites, vinca alkaloids, procarbazine, and cisplatin), dose used (higher doses cause worse damage than lower doses), combined use of alkylating agents (combination therapy causes worse damage than monotherapy), age of the patient (prepubertal males tend to be more resistant to the effects of antineoplastic chemotherapy than adult patients), and combined use with radiation (worse than with chemotherapy alone).[140]

CLINICAL PRESENTATION AND DIFFERENTIAL DIAGNOSIS

Symptoms of drug-induced sexual dysfunction in males are similar to those of patients with sexual dysfunction due to other causes (**Table 33-7**). With decreased libido, patients may report no desire for or interest in sexual intercourse. Patients commonly profess to be busy with work, engaged in other activities, or to not feel well and use these as excuses

Table 33-7 Signs and Symptoms Associated with Drug-Induced Sexual Dysfunction in Males

Decreased libido

- Decreased or absent desire for sexual intercourse, depressed mood
- Gynecomastia, small testicles, decreased muscle mass, and decreased axillary and pubic body hair, decreased spontaneous erections, hot flashes, low bone mineral density, and subphysiologic serum testosterone concentrations
- Patient may not complain of this adverse effect if he is not sexually active.
- Symptoms are temporally related to start of causative drug, although onset may be variable after the causative medication is started.
- Usually adverse effect resolves after the causative medication is discontinued.

Erectile dysfunction

- Absence of penile curvature or palpable plaques
- Erectile dysfunction is temporally related to start of causative drug, although onset may be variable after the causative medication is started.
- Erectile dysfunction may persist even after discontinuation of the suspected causative medication.
- Inability to achieve a penile erection sufficient for successful intercourse; partner may express dissatisfaction or frustration with patient.
- Inability to achieve a penile erection with stimulation; patient may have a medical illness that also causes erectile dysfunction for which the causative drug is being taken; for example, the patient may suffer from depression and need to take an antidepressant.
- No signs of infection
- Patient may not complain of this adverse effect if he is not sexually active.
- Usually adverse effect resolves after the causative medication is discontinued.

Ejaculation disorder

- Absent, decreased, or delayed ejaculation; patient reports dry sex or lack of sexual satisfaction/enjoyment during climax; if retrograde ejaculation, patient reports cloudy urine immediately after intercourse; if premature ejaculation, patient reports ejaculation before intercourse or before climax is reached; partner may express dissatisfaction or frustration with patient.
- Ejaculation disorder may persist even after discontinuation of the suspected causative medication.
- Ejaculation disorders are temporally related to start of causative drug, although onset may be variable after the causative medication is started.
- If decreased ejaculation, semen volume is <1.5–2 mL.
- If retrograde ejaculation, microscopic examination of urine after intercourse shows sperm.
- Patient may not complain of this adverse effect if he is not sexually active.

Priapism

- Physical exam shows a rigid, hard dorsal surface of penis and a soft ventral surface.
- Priapism is temporally related to start of the causative drug, although onset may be variable after the causative medication is started.
- Priapism may result in permanent erectile dysfunction if not treated promptly.
- Prolonged erection (>4 hr) in the absence of sexual stimulation; penis is painful and may be bluish in color.
- This is considered a urologic urgency/emergency; patient needs to seek medical attention for this.

Infertility

- Female partner is unable to conceive despite 1 yr of trying.
- Infertility due to radiation therapy and antineoplastic chemotherapy may take 1–10 yr to recover after the causative agent is discontinued; in some patients, drug-induced infertility is irreversible.
- Infertility is temporally related to start of the causative drug, although onset may be variable after the causative medication is started; with antineoplastic chemotherapy, the onset of infertility is commonly 8–12 wk after the start of treatment.
- Semen analysis shows an abnormality: if volume is <1.5–2 mL, <50–60% of sperm are motile; if sperm concentration is <20 million/mL, <30% of sperm have normal morphology; increased serum concentrations of follicle-stimulating hormone.

for having no desire. Decreased libido often results from a recent history of divorce, separation from a loved one, death of a spouse, sudden job loss, or performance anxiety. Patients with increased libido usually do not come to the attention of a clinician unless the patient's sexual desires are inappropriate, such as in precocious puberty.[165]

Patients with erectile dysfunction present with failure to achieve a penile erection sufficient for vaginal penetration. Although periodic erectile dysfunction is generally acceptable, a patient who experiences erectile dysfunction in more than 50% of attempts at sexual intercourse should seek medical treatment if he wishes to be sexually active.[16,37,175]

Patients with ejaculatory dysfunction may present with a variety of symptoms, including premature ejaculation, reduced ejaculation volume, retrograde ejaculation, delayed ejaculation, anejaculation (no ejaculation), or emission failure. With premature ejaculation, the patient ejaculates within one minute of vaginal penetration or before climax is reached, often rapidly followed by detumescence.[171] A chief problem is spousal dissatisfaction with the patient's sexual performance. Alternatively, some patients report reduced ejaculatory volume. Confirmation of the existence of the problem requires measurement of ejaculatory volume prior to and after the supposed disorder developed, which is rarely performed in clinical practice. Thus, this is more often a subjective report by the patient. On the other hand, in patients with retrograde ejaculation, the patient usually reports "dry sex" and no antegrade flow of seminal fluid during climax. Instead, during the first urine voiding after intercourse, the patient may produce cloudy urine, which indicates the presence of seminal fluid in the urine. The presence of sperm in the urine can be confirmed by microscopic examination of a postejaculation urine sample. Anejaculation is a failure to ejaculate, which may be due to a disorder of emission or a delay in emission. The patient complains of "dry sex."[91]

Patients with priapism often have a sickle cell anemia or chronic granulocytic leukemia, use combinations or large doses of erectogenic drugs, or have a history of unusually prolonged sexual activity or drug abuse. Because of a persistent painful erection for several hours, the patient will present for urgent or emergency care. Priapism more commonly involves the corpora cavernosa as opposed to the corpus spongiosum. Thus, the dorsal surface of the penis will be hard, but not the ventral surface.[172]

In a patient with infertility, the failure to successfully impregnate his female partner after 1 year's time is obvious. However, the diagnostic assessment to determine the cause generally requires an extensive workup, as the cause could be multifactorial.

In the diagnostic evaluation of patients with sexual dysfunction, it is important to take a careful history of present illnesses, past medical problems and surgical procedures, and concurrent medications. In many cases, information should also be obtained from the spouse or significant other so that sensitive data collected from the patient regarding the nature of the sexual dysfunction can be corroborated. Knowledge of past medical problems and concurrent prescription and nonprescription medications is key to rule out diseases or other drugs or drug combinations that could be contributing to the patient's current symptoms.[29] Conditions to consider in the differential diagnosis of drug-induced sexual dysfunction are listed in **Table 33-8**. These medical conditions may cause sexual dysfunction or contribute to drug-induced sexual dysfunction. Therefore, if the latter is suspected, treatment of the underlying medical condition may correct the patient's sexual dysfunction. In addition, patients with erectile dysfunction should be asked to complete a standardized, validated, self-assessment survey of sexual function, such as the International Index of Erectile Function or Brief Sexual Function Inventory.[176] This should be done at baseline and after a corrective measure has been instituted. Physical examination should include gross examination of the external genitalia and assessment of pelvic nerve function, including assessment of genitoperineal pain sensation, the bulbocavernosal reflex, and anal sphincter tone.[151]

Patients evaluated for drug-induced diminished libido should undergo two serial measurements of serum testosterone concentrations, obtained in the morning at the same time each day. Repeated morning measurements are recommended because of the circadian pattern of endogenous testosterone secretion and because of substantial variability in serum testosterone concentrations throughout the day. In addition, the patient should be checked for physical signs of hypogonadism, including gynecomastia, decreased muscle mass, and undersized testes.

In patients with erectile dysfunction, no specific diagnostic tests are usually performed. With the availability of phosphodiesterase inhibitors (e.g., sildenafil), which are effective in the majority of patients with erectile dysfunction independent of the cause, diagnostic testing is not necessary. Nocturnal penile tumescence testing, penile Doppler ultrasound, cavernosography, and cavernosometry are generally reserved for patients with no response to phosphodiesterase inhibitors or when

Table 33-8 Conditions to Consider in the Differential Diagnosis of Drug-Induced Sexual Dysfunction in Males

Decreased libido

- End-stage renal disease
- Hyperprolactinemia
- Moderate-severe chronic obstructive pulmonary disease
- Primary hypogonadism due to testes removal (postorchiectomy) or injury (e.g., mumps orchitis)
- Secondary hypogonadism due to hypothalamic or pituitary disorder or tumor

Erectile dysfunction

- Hormonal disorders (e.g., primary or secondary hypogonadism, hyperprolactinemia[a])
- Penile disorders (e.g., Peyronie disease, penile trauma, previous priapism, congenital penile anomalies, such as hypospadias)
- Psychiatric disorders (e.g., depression, schizophrenia, performance anxiety)
- Neurologic disorders (e.g., diabetes mellitus, spinal cord injury, stroke, postradical prostatectomy, postpelvic trauma with pelvic nerve injury, chronic alcoholism, peripheral neuropathy, Parkinson disease)
- Vascular disorders (e.g., hypertension, arteriosclerotic cardiovascular disease, peripheral vascular disease)

Ejaculation disorder

- If anejaculation, long-standing diabetes mellitus, radical prostatectomy[92]
- If premature or delayed ejaculation, performance anxiety
- If retrograde ejaculation, prostatectomy, surgical injury to the bladder neck or diabetes mellitus, pelvic surgery (e.g., aorto-iliac reconstruction, colorectal excision), neurologic illness (e.g., multiple sclerosis, autonomic neuropathy, spinal cord injury)

Priapism

- Chronic granulocytic leukemia
- Coagulopathy
- Drug abuse
- Excessive sexual activity
- Fat embolus during intravenous hyperalimentation
- Glucose-6-phosphate dehydrogenase deficiency
- Hemodialysis
- Infections mediated by toxins (e.g., scorpion sting, spider bite, rabies, malaria)
- Multiple myeloma
- Neoplasms
- Sickle cell disease
- Spinal cord injury
- Thalassemia

Infertility

- Absent or nonfunctional testes
- Cryptorchidism
- Extensive radiation therapy to pelvis
- Hyperprolactinemia
- Obstruction of epididymis or vas deferens (e.g., congenital cystic fibrosis)
- Presence of antisperm antibodies, sperm dysfunction, or decreased sperm count
- Primary or secondary hypogonadism
- Testicular cancer
- Testicular infection
- Testicular trauma

[a]These disorders produce decreased libido and secondary erectile dysfunction.

specific surgically correctable organic causes of sexual dysfunction are suspected.

Patients with ejaculatory dysfunction should be requested to provide two semen samples under controlled conditions in the clinic. Each sample should be collected on a different day, and sample collection should be preceded by 3 days of sexual abstinence. The specimen should be checked for ejaculate volume and sperm motility and morphology. If retrograde ejaculation is suspected, a post-ejaculation urine specimen should also be evaluated for the presence of sperm.

Patients with infertility are diagnosed with semen analysis and FSH serum concentrations. Patients with drug-induced infertility due to testicular damage present with increased FSH, azoospermia/oligospermia, decreased semen volume, abnormal sperm motility and morphology, or all of these. Antineoplastic chemotherapy is one of the most common causes of infertility. The usual onset is 8–12 weeks after the start of chemotherapy. The incidence and duration of infertility are greater with the use of alkylating agents in high doses in repeated cycles, which are associated with extensive damage to spermatogonia.[174] Recovery of fertility is dependent on the number of remaining functional spermatogonia after chemotherapy. Significant delays in recovery, up to several years after the last dose of chemotherapy, are due to extensive reduction in the numbers of spermatogonia and stem cells.[140]

RISK FACTORS

Specific risk factors for drug-induced sexual dysfunction in males have been proposed but not confirmed. Possible risk factors for drug-induced sexual dysfunction in males are listed in **Table 33-9**. Several factors associated with diminished sexual function include age >40 years, smoking, drinking excessive amounts of alcohol, cardiovascular disease, hypertension, diabetes mellitus, spinal cord injury, stroke, cancer, and mental depression or other psychiatric illness.[177,178] In addition, the risk of drug-induced sexual dysfunction is greater in patients taking combinations of drugs known to cause sexual dysfunction. In all patients with sexual dysfunction, independent of the etiology, elimination of these risk factors and/or treatment of underlying diseases that could contribute to sexual dysfunction is always recommended.

Table 33-9 Risk Factors for Drug-Induced Sexual Dysfunction in Males[13,150,169,177-179]

Vascular risk factors

- Arteriosclerotic cardiovascular disease
- Hyperlipidemia
- Hypertension
- Peripheral vascular disease
- Sickle cell anemia
- Smoking

Neurologic risk factors

- Chronic alcohol use
- Diabetes mellitus
- Parkinson disease, various causes
- Pelvic trauma with nerve injury
- Postradical prostatectomy or retroperitoneal surgery
- Spinal cord injury
- Stroke

Hormonal risk factors

- Hyperprolactinemia
- Hyperthyroidism
- Hypothyroidism
- Primary or secondary hypogonadism

Psychogenic risk factors

- Anxiety disorder
- Depression
- Psychosis
- Strained relationship with significant other

Other risk factors

- Cancer
- Kidney failure
- Liver failure
- Obesity
- Penile disorder (e.g., Peyronie disease, penile injury, penile fracture)
- Poor physical health
- Recreational drug abuse
- Respiratory failure

MORBIDITY AND MORTALITY

Except for priapism, drug-induced sexual dysfunction is largely a benign disease.[179] Patient morbidity is largely related to the negative impact of drug-induced sexual dysfunction on the quality of life of affected patients and their partners.[180,181] Depression, performance anxiety, and lack of self-confidence or diminished self-esteem can result. Priapism can be painful.

Decreased libido, erectile dysfunction, and ejaculatory disorders do not result in mortality. Some patients may not seek medical treatment for sexual dysfunction, as they attribute these disorders to the natural aging process, are not sexually active or do not have a sexual partner, are embarrassed to seek treatment, or do not think the adverse effect is important (e.g., a 65-year-old male who already has many children may not be concerned about infertility).

Untreated priapism or priapism that responds poorly to drug or surgical intervention may result in penile fibrosis, which can lead to irreversible erectile dysfunction. In one rare case of papaverine-induced priapism, a pulmonary embolus developed.[172]

PREVENTION

Minimizing risk factors associated with drug-induced sexual dysfunction may prevent the disease (Table 33-9). Drugs known to cause sexual dysfunction should be avoided in young, sexually active males, if possible. If this is not possible, these drugs should be used at the lowest effective dose for the shortest period of time.

Comorbid conditions that have been associated with sexual dysfunction should be treated optimally (Table 33-8). Lifestyle modifications, such as smoking cessation, weight loss, and avoidance of excessive alcohol use (which decreases libido and secondarily produces erectile dysfunction) should be implemented, if necessary. Often, optimal treatment of an underlying condition that could be contributing to erectile dysfunction can help reduce the sexual disorder.[182] Taking complete and careful medical and medication histories is important so that unnecessary medications can be discontinued. This should be followed by evaluation of pertinent physical examination findings. Laboratory tests, such as measurement of serum testosterone concentrations and semen analyses, should not be obtained routinely in patients for whom a drug is prescribed that has been associated with sexual dysfunction; such laboratory tests should be obtained only if the patient has a medical history and symptoms that are consistent with drug-induced sexual dysfunction. **Table 33-10** describes a general approach to prevent drug-induced sexual dysfunction and infertility.

Table 33-10 Approaches to Help Prevent Drug-Induced Sexual Dysfunction in Males

- Maintain heart-healthy lifestyle: do not smoke, avoid excessive alcohol, maintain ideal body weight, and exercise regularly.[150,177,178]
- If patient has hypertension, diabetes mellitus, or depression, he should optimize treatment of these conditions.
- If the patient is older than 50 yr of age, he should undergo an annual urologic evaluation to check for genitourinary tract disorders (e.g., benign prostatic hypertrophy, prostate cancer) that could affect sexual function.
- If the patient will need to take a medication that may cause sexual dysfunction or infertility, the healthcare professional should consider any of the following measures: if possible, to minimize the risk of drug-induced sexual dysfunction: use the lowest effective dose of the medication, change the timing of the medication so that the peak serum concentration does not occur when the patient wants to be sexually active (this works for medications with short half-lives or that cause sedation), or switch the patient from a medication with a higher prevalence of sexual dysfunction to a medication with a lower prevalence of sexual dysfunction.

It has been suggested that prescribers can choose medications that are less likely to cause sexual dysfunction for sexually active patients. Published literature is available for a limited number of pharmacologic categories of medications. For example, among the antipsychotic agents, olanzapine, aripiprazole, and quetiapine appear to cause less sexual dysfunction than risperidone.[91,191] Among the antihypertensives, angiotensin II-receptor antagonists, angiotensin-converting enzyme inhibitors, and calcium antagonists appear to cause less sexual dysfunction than thiazide diuretics, sympatholytics, and β-adrenergic antagonists.[194] Among the antidepressants, bupropion, mirtazapine, nefazodone, and vilazodone appear to cause less sexual dysfunction than sertraline, venlafaxine, citalopram, paroxetine, fluoxetine, imipramine, phenelzine, duloxetine, escitalopram, and fluvoxamine.[40,79,157,175] Among the anticonvulsants, levetiracetam and topiramate appear to cause less sexual dysfunction than other agents.[50] However, it is important to recognize that literature comparing the frequency of sexual dysfunction among agents in the same pharmacologic category includes many poorly designed research studies; most are not randomized controlled trials, standardized definitions of sexual dysfunction were not used, patient sample sizes are small, and study results often conflict with one another. Also, in some patient cases, choosing an agent with a lower propensity to cause sexual dysfunction may not be possible, as the patient's underlying medical illness may not respond to the medication.

MANAGEMENT

Treatment options for the management of drug-induced sexual dysfunction are presented in **Table 33-11**. When drug-induced sexual dysfunction occurs and the patient seeks treatment, it is recommended that the causative agent be discontinued or stopped temporarily (drug holiday). After an adequate washout period, the patient should be reassessed to determine whether sexual dysfunction is still present. If the offending agent cannot be discontinued, dose reduction is often helpful. Alternatively, replacing the causative agent with a drug that is associated with a lower likelihood of causing sexual dysfunction could be considered.[190,191] However, as mentioned in the section "Prevention,"

Table 33-11 Approaches to Manage Drug-Induced Sexual Dysfunction in Males

In all cases of drug-induced sexual dysfunction, management should include the following:

- Temporarily holding (drug holiday), discontinuing, or reducing dose of offending agent, if possible
- Switching to another drug that does not cause or is less likely to cause sexual dysfunction, if possible
- Initiating a specific drug to treat sexual dysfunction only if first two steps do not work or cannot be implemented

Type of Dysfunction	Additional Management Approaches
Decreased libido	• Psychotherapy or counseling • If patient has low serum testosterone concentration, consider testosterone supplementation (e.g., testosterone cypionate or testosterone enanthate 200 mg intramuscularly q 3–4 wk), provided the patient has no contraindications.[150,165]
Erectile dysfunction	• Initiate a phosphodiesterase type 5 inhibitor (e.g., sildenafil 50–100 mg orally 1 hr before sexual intercourse; vardenafil 10–20 mg orally [Levitra] or 10 mg on the tongue [Staxyn] 1 hr before sexual intercourse; tadalafil 10–20 mg orally 30 min before sexual intercourse or 2.5–5 mg daily; or avanafil 100–200 mg orally 15 min before sexual intercourse). • If oral agents are unsuccessful or contraindicated, initiate intracavernosal alprostadil (e.g., alprostadil 10 mcg intracavernosally 30 min before intercourse) or intraurethral alprostadil 125–250 mcg 30–60 min before intercourse. • If oral agents are unsuccessful or contraindicated, initiate use of a vacuum erection device. • Surgical implantation of a penile prosthesis is a treatment of last resort; it is highly effective but is associated with more potential adverse effects than medical treatments. • The American Urological Association has published guidelines on management of erectile dysfunction[183]; other management guidelines have been published.[175,179,184]
Ejaculation disorder	• If retrograde ejaculation or emission failure, initiate imipramine 25–50 mg daily for 7 days prior to planned sexual activity, or pseudoephedrine 60 mg 1 hr prior to planned sexual activity.[91,92] • For anejaculation, penile vibratory stimulation, rectal probe electroejaculation, or direct microsurgical sperm harvesting has been employed.[92] • If premature ejaculation, psychotherapy or other self-control techniques may be useful. Alternatively, manual squeezing of the glans penis to stop ejaculation may be helpful[174]; alternatively, application of 2% lidocaine jelly or lidocaine 2.5%/prilocaine 2.5% cream (EMLA) to the glans penis 20–30 min before coitus may decrease sensitivity of penis to tactile stimulation; however, a condom should be applied after topical application to prevent inadvertent exposure to female partner[186]; administration of sertraline 25–200 mg orally daily, paroxetine 10–40 mg orally daily, fluoxetine 5–20 mg orally daily, or clomipramine 25–50 mg orally daily for 1 or 2 wk, which produces anejaculation, has been used with some success[6,91,157,185]; these agents have also been dosed as an episodic regimen, several hours before sexual intercourse, instead of daily.[186] The American Urological Association has published guidelines on management for premature ejaculation[186]; other published recommendations are available for ejaculation disorders.[80,91,92,187]
Priapism	• Sedate patient to reduce central nervous system stimulation that might be causing or exacerbating priapism. • Put the patient in a quiet, darkened room. • Apply ice packs to the penis. • Aspirate and irrigate sludged blood from corpora, if necessary. • If due to excessive use of intracavernosal alprostadil, can use intracavernosal phenylephrine (100–500 mcg/mL) 1 mL q 3–5 min until detumescence occurs. • Initiate surgical arteriovenous shunts of the corpora as a treatment of last resort. • The American Urological Association has published guidelines on management of priapism[188]; other published recommendations are available.[115,172,192]

Table 33-11 Approaches to Manage Drug-Induced Sexual Dysfunction in Males (continued)

Infertility	• Reassure the patient that after a significant time after the last dose of chemotherapy, fertility may return; however, the time to recovery is highly dependent on the degree of damage to the germinal cells; if the patient is receiving antineoplastic chemotherapy for cancer, the benefit of continuing treatment outweighs the risk of this adverse effect.[174] • Sometimes, this adverse effect can be minimized by using lower doses of drugs in combination and using combinations of drugs with a lower potential to cause infertility. • Although a variety of hormonal therapies have been tried (e.g., testosterone supplements, clomiphene citrate, human chorionic gonadotropin), none has been uniformly effective. • The American Urological Association has published guidelines on the diagnosis and management of infertility[189]; other published recommendations are available.[173,174]

this strategy may not be effective and could compromise treatment of an underlying medical condition that requires treatment. For certain types of drug-induced sexual dysfunction, specific treatments have been described in the literature. However, in many cases, no direct comparison studies have been performed to determine whether one specific treatment is more effective than another. In addition, implementation of drug therapy to treat a disease caused by another drug is never a preferred management approach, as it adds to the patient's drug costs and is usually associated with additional adverse effects. Pharmacotherapy for the purpose of treating sexual dysfunction induced by another drug should be implemented only when other measures fail or are not feasible.

INFORMATION FOR PATIENTS

Practitioners who counsel patients with drug-induced sexual dysfunction should have a clear understanding of the categories of sexual dysfunction so that there is no confusion in discussing the specific problem with the patient.[29] Patients should be advised that drug-induced sexual dysfunction (with the exception of alkylating agent-induced infertility) is usually reversible following discontinuation of the culprit drug. Patients who are taking drugs that may cause sexual dysfunction should be counseled regarding the specific type(s) of dysfunction that could occur and the specific symptoms that may result. Patients should be advised to implement lifestyle changes (e.g., quitting smoking, reducing alcohol consumption, losing weight if obese) that may minimize the risk of drug-induced sexual dysfunction. Patients should be instructed to consult their healthcare provider if sexual dysfunction that interferes with their lifestyle or negatively impacts their quality of life occurs. Patients should be instructed to avoid using nonprescription medications, illicit drugs, and some herbal medicines, including those that may cause sedation, produce anticholinergic effects, have antiandrogenic effects, or inhibit hepatic metabolism of the offending drug, as these factors can worsen the degree of drug-induced sexual dysfunction. In addition, patients should inform the healthcare provider of any new medications so that these can be checked for interactions with existing medications that may cause or exacerbate drug-induced sexual dysfunction. If the patient has risk factors for priapism (e.g., the patient has sickle cell anemia or is using erectogenic drugs), he should be instructed to seek medical attention immediately if an erection persists for 4 hours or more. Because extensive radiation therapy and chemotherapy for cancer may cause irreversible damage to the testes and infertility, patients should be advised to bank semen before chemotherapy. After chemotherapy, to minimize teratogenic effects due to persistent drug-induced mutations to sperm, patients should be advised to delay conception for 6 months to 2 years after the last dose of chemotherapy.[174,193]

Practitioners caring for patients with drug-induced sexual dysfunction should talk to these patients, respond to their questions, and anticipate their concerns. These cases must be handled with the utmost confidentiality. Counseling should take place in a quiet, secure area. The practitioner should project an attitude of caring and respect and be non-judgmental in handling the patient's issues.

Some patients find it difficult to discuss their concerns regarding drug-induced sexual dysfunction. Practitioners can be helpful and proactive. For example, pharmacists can initiate a follow-up consultation session when refilling a prescription by stating, "This medication may cause changes to your sexual function when used in usual doses. Has this been a problem for you?" Such a statement immediately puts the patient at ease because the patient is reminded up front that the problem is not unique and occurs commonly. Also, some patients who experience drug-induced sexual dysfunction may refuse to continue to take necessary medications. In this case, the pharmacist should discuss the benefits and risks of taking the medication, notify the prescriber of the problem, and offer options for management of the patient's primary problem and for his drug-induced sexual dysfunction.

REFERENCES

1. Irwig MS, Kolukula S. Persistent sexual side effects of finasteride for male pattern hair loss. *J Sex Med.* 2011; 8:1747-53.
2. LaTorre A, Giupponi G, Duffy D et al. Sexual dysfunction related to drugs: a critical review. Part V: α-blocker and 5-ARI drugs. *Pharmacopsychiatry.* 2016; 49:3-13.
3. Toren P, Margel D, Kulkarni G et al. Effect of dutasteride on clinical progression of benign prostatic hyperplasia in asymptomatic men with enlarged prostate: a post hoc analysis of the Reduce Study. *BMJ.* 2013; 346:f2109.
4. Rahnema CD, Lipshultz LI, Crosnoe LE et al. Anabolic steroid-induced hypogonadism: diagnosis and treatment. *Fertil Steril.* 2014; 101:1271-9.
5. Montejo AL, Llorca G, Izquierdo JA et al. Incidence of sexual dysfunction associated with antidepressant agents: a prospective multicenter study of 1022 outpatients. Spanish Working Group for the Study of Psychotropic-Related Sexual Dysfunction. *J Clin Psychiatry.* 2001; 62(suppl 3):10-21.
6. LaTorre A, Conca A, Duffy D et al. Sexual dysfunction related to psychotropic drugs: a critical review-Part II: Antipsychotics. *Pharmacopsychiatry.* 2013; 46:201-8.
7. Bobes J, Garcia-Portilla MP, Rjas J et al. Frequency of sexual dysfunction and other reproductive side effects in patients with schizophrenia treated with risperidone, olanzapine, quetiapine, or haloperidol: the results of the EIRE study. *J Sex Marital Ther.* 2003; 29:125-47.
8. Knegtering H, van der Moolen AE, Castelein S et al. What are the effects of antipsychotics on sexual dysfunction and endocrine functioning? *Psychoneuroendocrinology.* 2003; 28(suppl 2):109-23.
9. LaTorre A, Giupponi G, Duffy D et al. Sexual dysfunction related to drugs: a critical review. Part IV: Cardiovascular drugs. *Pharmacopsychiatry.* 2015; 48:1-6.
10. Bauer J, Blumenthal S, Reuber M et al. Epilepsy syndrome, focus location, and treatment choice affect testicular function in men with epilepsy. *Neurology.* 2004; 62:243-6.
11. Winters SJ, Banks JL, Loreaux DL. Cimetidine is an antiandrogen in the rat. *Gastroenterology.* 1979; 76:504-8.
12. Jensen RT, Collen MJ, Pandol ST et al. Cimetidine-induced impotence and breast changes in patients with gastric hypersecretory states. *N Engl J Med.* 1983; 308:883-7.
13. Keene LC, Davies PH. Drug-related erectile dysfunction. *Adverse Drug React Toxicol Rev.* 1999; 18:5-24.
14. McWaine DE, Procci WR. Drug-induced sexual dysfunction. *Med Toxicol Adverse Drug Exp.* 1988; 3:289-306.
15. Brock GB, Lue TF. Drug-induced male sexual dysfunction. *Drug Saf.* 1993; 8:414-26.
16. Lue TF. Erectile dysfunction. *N Engl J Med.* 2000; 342:1802-13.
17. Xu Y, Jiang YF, Wu B. New agonist- and antagonist-based treatment approaches for advanced prostate cancer. *J Int Med Res.* 2012; 40:1217-26.
18. deGraaf L, Brouwers AH, Diemont WL. Is decreased libido associated with the use of HMG-CoA reductase inhibitors? *Br J Clin Pharmacol.* 2004; 58:326-8.
19. Corona G, Boddi V, Balercia G et al. The effect of statin therapy on testosterone levels in subjects consulting for erectile dysfunction. *J Sex Med.* 2010; 7(4 part 1):1547-56.
20. Hogan C, LeNoury J, Hely D et al. One hundred and twenty cases of enduring sexual dysfunction following treatment. *Int J Risk Saf Med.* 2014; 26:109-16.
21. Evans KC, Peterson AC, Ruiz HE et al. Use of oral ketoconazole to prevent postoperative erections following penile surgery. *Int J Impot Res.* 2004; 16:346-9.
22. Calabro RS, Italiano D, Militi D et al. Levetiracetam-associated loss of libido and anhedonia. *Epilepsy Behav.* 2012; 24:283-4.
23. Nudel M, Monoski MM, Lipshultz LI. Common medications and drugs: how they affect male fertility. *Urol Clin North Am.* 2002; 29:965-73.
24. Mendelson JG, Mendelson JE, Patch VD. Plasma testosterone levels in heroin addiction and during methadone maintenance. *J Pharmacol Exp Ther.* 1975; 192:211-7.
25. Murphy EN, Miranda R. Doubts about treating hypogonadism due to long-term opioid use with testosterone therapy. *JAMA Int Med.* 2014; 174:1892-3.
26. Brennan MJ. The use of opioid therapy on endocrine function. *Am J Med.* 2013; 126(3 suppl 1):S12-8.
27. Smith HS, Elliott JA. Opioid-induced androgen deficiency. *Pain Physician.* 2012; 15(suppl 3):ES145-56.
28. Ramsey S. Opioids for back pain are linked to increased risk of erectile dysfunction. *BMJ.* 2013; 346:f3223.
29. Stimmel GL, Gutierrez MA. Counseling patients about sexual issues. *Pharmacotherapy.* 2006; 26:1608-15.
30. Rosenshein B, Flockhart DA, Ho H. Induction of testosterone metabolism by esomeprazole in a CYP2C19*2 heterozygote. *Am J Med Sci.* 2004; 327:289-93.
31. Grimm RH, Grandits GA, Prineas RJ et al. Long-term effects on sexual function of five antihypertensive drugs and nutritional hygienic treatment in hypertensive men and women. Treatment of Mild Hypertension Study (TOMHS). *Hypertension.* 1997; 29(1 part 1):8-14.
32. Wessells H, Roy J, Bannow J et al. Incidence and severity of sexual adverse experiences in finasteride and placebo-treated men with benign prostatic hyperplasia. *Urology.* 2003; 61:579-84.
33. Gur S, Kadowitz PJ, Hellstrom WJG. Effects of 5-alpha reductase inhibitors on erectile function, sexual desire and ejaculation. *Expert Opin Drug Saf.* 2013; 12:81-90.
34. Chiriaco G, Cauci S, Maxxon G et al. An observational retrospective evaluation of 79 young men with long-term adverse effects after use of finasteride against androgenetic alopecia. *Andrology.* 2016; 4:245-50.

35. Corona G, Rastrelli G, Maseroli E et al. Inhibitors of 5α-reductase–related side effects in patients seeking medical care for sexual dysfunction. *J Endocrinol Invest.* 2012; 35:915-20.
36. Irwig MS. Safety concerns regarding 5α reductase inhibitors for the treatment of androgenetic alopecia. *Curr Opin Endocrinol Diabetes Obes.* 2015; 22:248-53.
37. Shamloul R, Ghanem H. Erectile dysfunction. *Lancet.* 2013; 381:153-65.
38. Segraves RT. Sexual dysfunction associated with antidepressant therapy. *Urol Clin North Am.* 2007; 34:575-9.
39. Balon R. SSRI-associated sexual dysfunction. *Am J Psychiatry.* 2006; 163:1504-9.
40. LaTorre A, Giuppoi G, Duffy D et al. Sexual dysfunction related to psychotropic drugs: a critical review-Part I: Antidepressants. *Pharmacopsychiatry.* 2013; 46:191-9.
41. Derby CA, Barbour MM, Hume AL et al. Drug therapy and prevalence of erectile dysfunction in the Massachusetts male aging study cohort. *Pharmacotherapy.* 2001; 21:676-83.
42. Chang SW, Fine R, Siegel D et al. The impact of diuretic therapy on reported sexual function. *Arch Intern Med.* 1991; 151:2402-8.
43. Denys P, Mane M, Azouvi P et al. Side effects of chronic intrathecal baclofen on erection and ejaculation in patients with spinal cord lesions. *Arch Phys Med Rehabil.* 1998; 79:494-6.
44. Calabro RS, D'Aleo G, Sessa E et al. Sexual dysfunction induced by intrathecal baclofen administration: is this the price to pay for severe spasticity management? *J Sex Med.* 2014; 11:1807-15.
45. Kupelian V, Hall SA, McKinlay JB. Common prescription medication use and erectile dysfunction. Results from the Boston Area Community Health (BACH) Survey. *BJU Int.* 2013; 112:1178-87.
46. Dombrowski RC, Romeo JH, Aron DC. Verapamil-induced hyperprolactinaemia complicated by a pituitary incidentaloma. *Ann Pharmacother.* 1995; 29:999-1001.
47. Dhikav V, Gupta S, Anand KS. Erectile dysfunction induced probably by celecoxib. *Pharmacoepidemiol Drug Saf.* 2008; 17:211-2.
48. Croog SH, Levine S, Sudilovsky A et al. Sexual symptoms in hypertensive patients. A clinical trial of antihypertensive medications. *Arch Intern Med.* 1988; 148:788-94.
49. Dalal A, Shou L. Gabapentin and sexual dysfunction: report of two cases. *Neurologist.* 2008; 14:50-1.
50. Fusco F, Franco M, Longo N et al. The impact of non-urologic drugs on sexual function in men. *Arch Ital Urol Androl.* 2014; 8:50-5.
51. Kaufman KR, Struck PJ. Gabapentin-induced sexual dysfunction. *Epilepsy Behav.* 2011; 21:324-6.
52. Rizvi K, Hampson JP, Harvey JN. Do lipid-lowering drugs cause erectile dysfunction? A systematic review. *Fam Pract.* 2002; 19:95-8.
53. Holzbeierlein JM, Castle EP, Trasher JB. Complications of androgen-deprivation therapy for prostate cancer. *Clin Prostate Cancer.* 2003; 2:147-52.
54. Davis R, Reveles KR, Ali SK et al. Statins and male sexual health: a retrospective cohort analysis. *J Sex Med.* 2015; 12:158-67.
55. Bruckert E, Giral P, Hishmati HM et al. Men treated with hypolipidaemic drugs complain more frequently of erectile dysfunction. *J Clin Pharm Ther.* 1996; 21:89-94.
56. Do C, Huyghe E, Lapeyre-Mestre M et al. Statins and erectile dysfunction. Results of a case/non-case study using the French Pharmacovigilance System Database. *Drug Saf.* 2009; 32:591-7.
57. Kostis JB, Dobrzynski JM. The effect of statins on erectile dysfunction: a meta analysis of randomized trials. *J Sex Med.* 2014; 11:1626-35.
58. Davis R, Reveles KR, Ali SK et al. Statins and male sexual health: a retrospective cohort analysis. *J Sex Med.* 2015; 12:158-67.
59. Buffum J. Pharmacosexology update: prescription drugs and sexual function. *J Psychoactive Drugs.* 1986; 18:97-106.
60. Ghardirian AM, Annable L, Belanger MC. Lithium, benzodiazepines, and sexual function in bipolar patients. *Am J Psychiatry.* 1992: 149:801-5.
61. Shamloul R, Bella AJ. Impact of cannabis use on male sexual health. *J Sex Med.* 2011; 8:971-5.
62. Gleason JM, Slezak JM, Jung H et al. Regular nonsteroidal anti-inflammatory drug use and erectile dysfunction. *J Urol.* 2011; 185:1388-93.
63. Shiri R, Koskimaki J, Hakkinen J et al. Effect of nonsteroidal anti-inflammatory drug use on the incidence of erectile dysfunction. *J Urol.* 2006; 175:1812-5.
64. Lindquist M, Edwards IR. Endocrine adverse effects of omeprazole. *BMJ.* 1992; 305:451-2.
65. Santucci L, Faroni F, Fiorucci S et al. Gynecomastia during omeprazole therapy. *N Engl J Med.* 1991; 324:635.
66. Convens C, Verhelst J, Mahler C. Painful gynecomastia during omeprazole therapy. *Lancet.* 1991; 338:1153.
67. Gudin JA, Latiman A, Nalamachu S. Opioid related endocrinopathy. *Pain Med.* 2015; 16(suppl 1):S9-15.
68. Bozkurt M, Gocmez C, Soylemez H et al. Association between neuropathic pain, pregabalin treatment and erectile dysfunction. *J Sex Med.* 2014; 11:1816-22.
69. Colebunders R, Smets E, Verdonck K et al. Sexual dysfunction with protease inhibitors. *Lancet.* 1999; 353:1802.
70. Civardi C, Collini A, Gontero P et al. Vasogenic erectile dysfunction: topiramate-induced. *Clin Neurol Neurosurg.* 2012; 114:70-1.
71. Hung LC, Chow JC, Chang CY et al. Topiramate-related reversible erectile dysfunction in temporal lobe epilepsy. *Neurol Sci.* 2012; 33:331-3.
72. Keller J, Chen YK, Lin HC. Association between epilepsy and erectile dysfunction: evidence from a population-based study. *J Sex Med.* 2012; 9:2248-55.
73. Bozkurt O, Demir O, Sen V et al. Silodosin causes impaired ejaculation and enlargement of seminal vesicles in sexually active men treated for lower urinary tract symptoms suggestive of benign prostatic hyperplasia. *Urology.* 2015; 85:1085-9.
74. Novara G, Tubaro A, Sanseverino R et al. Systematic review and meta-analysis of randomized controlled trials evaluating silodosin in the treatment of non-neurogenic male lower urinary tract symptoms suggestive of benign prostatic enlargement. *World J Urol.* 2013; 31:997-1008.
75. Yokoyama T, Hara R, Fukumoto K et al. Effects of three types of alpha-1 adrenoceptor blockers on lower urinary tract symptoms and sexual function in males with benign prostatic hyperplasia. *Int J Urol.* 2011; 18:225-30.
76. Gacci M, Ficarra V, Sebastianelli A et al. Impact of medical treatments for male lower urinary tract symptoms due to benign prostatic hyperplasia on ejaculatory function: a systematic review and meta analysis. *J Sex Med.* 2014; 11:1554-66.
77. Kobayashi K, Masumori N, Hisasue S et al. Inhibition of seminal emission is the main cause of anejaculation induced by a highly selective alpha1A-blocker in normal volunteers. *J Sex Med.* 2008; 5:2185-90.
78. Waldinger MD. Premature ejaculation—definition and drug treatment. *Drugs.* 2007; 67:547-68.
79. Serretti A, Chiesa A. Treatment-emergent sexual dysfunction related to antidepressants: a meta analysis. *J Clin Psychopharmacol.* 2009; 29:259-66.
80. Stimmel GL, Gutierrez MA. Sexual dysfunction and psychotropic medication. *CNS Spectr.* 2006; 11(8 suppl 9):24-30.
81. Sovner R. Anorgasmia associated with imipramine but not desipramine: case report. *J Clin Psychiatry.* 1983; 44:345-6.
82. Pollack MH, Reiter S, Hammerness P. Genitourinary and sexual adverse effects of psychotropic medication. *Int J Psychiatry Med.* 1992; 22:305-27.
83. Waldinger MD, Berendsen HH, Block BF et al. Premature ejaculation and serotoninergic antidepressant-induced delayed ejaculation: the involvement of the serotoninergic system. *Behav Brain Res.* 1998; 92:111-8.
84. Remeron package insert. Roseland, NJ: Organon USA, Inc; 2012.
85. Cymbalta package insert. Indianapolis, IN: Lilly; 2015.

86. Kaufman KR, Marin H, Menza M. Trazodone and ejaculatory inhibition. *J Sex Marital Ther.* 2007; 33:225-30.
87. Wellbutrin package insert. Research Triangle Park, NC: GlaxoSmithKline; 2014.
88. Clozaril package insert. Suffern, NY: Novartis Pharmaceuticals Corporation; 2015.
89. Seroquel package insert. Wilmington, DE: AstraZeneca Pharmaceuticals LP; 2013.
90. Chen LW, Chen MY, Chen KY et al. Topiramate-associate sexual dysfunction: a systematic review. *Epilepsy Behav.* 2017; 73:10-17.
91. Schmidt HM, Hagen M, Kriston L et al. Management of sexual dysfunction due to antipsychotic drug therapy. *Cochrane Database Syst Rev.* 2012; 11:CD003546.
92. Phillips E Carpenter C, Oates RD. Ejaculatory dysfunction. *Urol Clin North Am.* 2014; 41:115-28.
93. Kreitenberg AJ, Ortiz EC, Arkfeld DG. Priapism after tumor necrosis factor alpha inhibitor use. *Clin Rheumatol.* 2015; 34:801-2.
94. Qazi HA, Ananthakrishnan K, Mandikandan R et al. Stuttering priapism after ingestion of alfuzosin. *Urology.* 2006; 68:890.e5-6.
95. Sadeghi-Nejad H, Jackson I. New-onset priapism associated with ingestion of terazosin in an otherwise healthy man. *J Sex Med.* 2007; 4:1766-8.
96. Dodds PR, Batter SJ, Serels SR. Priapism following ingestion of tamsulosin. *J Urol.* 2003; 169:2302.
97. Perimenis P, Athanasopoulos A, Geramoutsos I et al. The incidence of pharmacologically induced priapism in the diagnostic and therapeutic management of 685 men with erectile dysfunction. *Urol Int.* 2001; 66:27-9.
98. Bettocchi C, Ashford L, Pryor JP et al. Priapism alter transurethral alprostadil. *Br J Urol.* 1998; 81:926.
99. Samuel RZ. Priapism associated with venlafaxine use. *J Am Acad Child Adolesc Psychiatry.* 2000; 39:16-7.
100. Javed MA. Priapism associated with fluoxetine therapy: a case report. *J Pak Med Assoc.* 1996; 46:45-6.
101. Rand EH. Priapism in a patient taking sertraline. *J Clin Psychiatry.* 1998; 59:538.
102. Mendelson WB, Franko T. Priapism with sertraline and lithium. *J Clin Psychopharmacol.* 1994; 14:434-5.
103. Pecknold JC, Langer SF. Priapism: trazodone versus nefazodone. *J Clin Psychiatry.* 1999; 57:547-8.
104. Kem DL, Posey DJ, McDougle CJ. Priapism associated with trazodone in an adolescent with autism. *J Am Acad Child Adolesc Psychiatry.* 2002; 41:758.
105. Wang CS, Kao WT, Chen CD et al. Priapism associated with typical and atypical antipsychotics. *Int Clin Psychopharmacol.* 2006; 21:245-8.
106. Sood S, James W, Bailon MJ. Priapism associated with atypical antipsychotic medications: a review. *Int Clin Psychopharmacol.* 2008; 23:9-17.
107. Mago R, Anolik R, Johnson RA et al. Recurrent priapism associated with use of aripiprazole. *J Clin Psychiatry.* 2006; 67:1471-2.
108. Moinfar N, Goad S, Brink DD et al. Clozapine-related priapism. *Hosp Community Psychiatry.* 1995: 45:1044.
109. Songer DA, Barclay JC. Olanzapine-induced priapism. *Am J Psychiatry.* 2001; 158:2087-8.
110. Harrison G, Dilley JW, Loeb L et al. Priapism and quetiapine: a case report. *Psychopharmacol Bull.* 2006; 39:117-9.
111. Davol P, Rukstalis D. Priapism associated with routine use of quetiapine: case report and review of the literature. *Urology.* 2005; 66:880.
112. Prabhuswamy M, Srinath S, Girimaji S et al. Risperidone-induced priapism in a 12 year old boy with schizophrenia. *J Child Adolesc Psychopharmacol.* 2007; 17:539-40.
113. Makesar D, Thome J. Risperidone-induced priapism. *World J Biol Psychiatry.* 2007; 8:45-7.
114. Eiland LS, Bell EA, Erramouspe J. Priapism associated with the use of stimulant medications and atomoxetine for attention-deficit/hyperactivity disorder in children. *Ann Pharmacother.* 2014; 48:1350-5.
115. Salonia A, Eardley I, Giuliano F et al. European Association of Urology Guidelines on Priapism. *Eur Urol.* 2014; 65:480-9.
116. Altman AL, Seftel AD, Brown SL et al. Cocaine associated priapism. *J Urol.* 1999; 161:1817-8.
117. Klein EA, Montague DK, Steiger E. Priapism associated with the use of intravenous fat emulsion: case reports and postulated pathogenesis. *J Urol.* 1985; 133:857-9.
118. Thomas A, Woodward C, Rovner ES et al. Urologic complications of nonurologic medications. *Urol Clin North Am.* 2003; 30:123-31.
119. Bschleipfer TH, Hauck EW, Diemer TH et al. Heparin-induced priapism. *Int J Impot Res.* 2001; 13:357-9.
120. Nagathan DS, Pahwa HS, Kumar A et al. Anticoagulant-induced priapism progressing to penile gangrene: a devastating complication. *BMJ Case Rep.* 2012:bcr2012007073. Published online 2012 Nov 21.
121. Wysokinski A. Persistent penile erection association with quetiapine and lithium. *J Neuropsychiatry Clin Neurosci.* 2015 Winter; 27:e77.
122. US Food and Drug Administration. FDA drug safety communications: FDA warns of rare risk of long-lasting erections in males taking methylphenidate ADHD medications and has approved label changes. www.fda.gov/Drugs/Drugsafety/ucm375796.htm (accessed 2018 Aug 9).
123. Kelly BD, Lundon DJ, McGuinness D et al. Methylphenidate-induced erections in a prepubertal child. *J Pediatr Urol.* 2013; 9: e 1-2.
124. Shahani L, Olanzepine-induced priapism. *J Neuropsychiatry Clin Neurosci.* 2012; 24:e28.
125. Wearne D. A case of priapism associated with paliperidone. *Aust N Z J Psychiatry.* 2014; 48:962.
126. Hashmat AI, Abrahams J, Fani K et al. A lethal complication of papaverine-induced priapism. *J Urol.* 1991; 145:146-7.
127. Prasad K, el-Sherif A. Priapism following ingestion of papaverine tablets. *Scand J Urol Nephrol.* 1996; 30:515-6.
128. Kotin J, Wilber DE, Verburg D. Thioridazine and sexual dysfunction. *Am J Psychiatry.* 1976; 133:82-5.
129. Sur RL, Kane CJ. Sildenafil citrate-associated priapism. *Urology.* 2000; 55:950.
130. King SH, Hallock M, Strote J et al. Tadalafil-associated priapism. *Urology.* 2005; 66:432.
131. Kassim AA, Fabry ME, Nagel RL. Acute priapism associated with the use of sildenafil in a patient with sickle cell trait. *Blood.* 2000; 95:1878-9.
132. Maakaron JE, Matta BN, Rebeiz J et al. Idiosyncratic intermittent nocturnal priapism occurring after quetiapine dose reduction. *Aust N Z J Psychiatry.* 2013; 47:1087.
133. Tsai AC. A case of recurrent priapism in the context of quetiapine use, discontinuation and rechallenge. *J Clin Psychopharmacol.* 2011; 31:235-6.
134. Bansal S, Gupta SK. Sodium valproate induced priapism in an adult with bipolar affective disorder. *Indian J Pharmacol.* 2013; 45:629-30.
135. Zimbelman J, Lefkowitz J, Schaeffer C et al. Unusual complications of warfarin therapy: skin necrosis and priapism. *J Pediatr.* 2000; 137:266-8.
136. Drife JO. The effect of drugs on sperm. *Drugs.* 1987; 33:610-22.
137. Koyuncu H, Serefoglu EC, Ozdemir AT et al. Deleterious effects of selective serotonin reuptake inhibitor treatment on semen parameters in patients with lifelong premature ejaculation. *Int J Impot Res.* 2012; 24:171-3.
138. Anon. Semen abnormalities with SSRI antidepressants. *Prescrire Int.* 2015; 24:16-7.

139. Schrader M, Muller M, Straub B et al. The impact of chemotherapy on male fertility: a survey of the biologic basis and clinical aspects. *Reprod Toxicol.* 2001; 15:611-7.
140. Pectasides D, Pectasides E, Papaxoinis G et al. Testicular function in poor-risk seminomatous germ cell tumors treated with methotrexate, paclitaxel, ifosfamide, and cisplatin combination chemotherapy. *J Androl.* 2009; 30:280-6.
141. Isojarvi JI, Lofgren E, Juntunen KS et al. Effect of epilepsy and antiepileptic drugs on male reproductive health. *Neurology.* 2004; 62:247-53.
142. White IG. The toxicity of some antibacterials for bull, ram, rabbit and human spermatozoa. *Aust J Exp Biol Med Sci.* 1954; 32:41-8.
143. Koyuncu H, Serofoglu EC, Yencilek E et al. Escitalopram treatment for premature ejaculation has a negative effect on semen parameters. *Int J Impot Res.* 2011; 23:257-61.
144. Villalta J, Ballesca JL, Nicolas JM et al. Testicular function in asymptomatic chronic alcoholics: relation to ethanol intake. *Alcohol Clin Exp Res.* 1997; 21:128-33.
145. Doelle GC, Alexander AN, Evans RM et al. Combined treatment with an LHRH agonist and testosterone in man: reversible oligospermia without impotence. *J Androl.* 1983; 4:298-302.
146. Millsop JW, Heller MM, Eliason MJ et al. Dermatological medication effects on male fertility. *Dermatol Ther.* 2013; 26:337-46.
147. Albert PS, Mininberg DT, Davis JE. The nitrofurans as sperm immobilizing agents: their tissue toxicity and their clinical application. *Br J Urol.* 1975; 47:459-62.
148. Bang JK, Lim JJ, Choi J et al. Reversible infertility associated with testosterone therapy for symptomatic hypogonadism in infertile couples. *Yonsei Med J.* 2013; 54:702-6.
149. Johannes CB, Araujo AB, Feldman HA et al. Incidence of erectile dysfunction in men 40-69 years old: longitudinal results from the Massachusetts Male Aging Study. *J Urol.* 2000; 163:460-3.
150. Corona G, Rastrelli G, Maseroli E et al. Sexual function of the ageing male. *Best Pract Res Clin Endocrinol Metab.* 2013; 27:581-601.
151. McVary KT. Erectile dysfunction. *N Engl J Med.* 2007; 357:2472-81.
152. Ferrario CM, Levy P. Sexual dysfunction in patients with hypertension: implications for therapy. *J Clin Hypertens.* 2002; 4:424-32.
153. Silvaraaman K, Mintzer S. Hormonal consequences of epilepsy and its treatment in men. *Curr Opin Endocrinol Diabetes Obes.* 2011; 18:204-9.
154. Herzog AG, Drislane FW, Schomer DL et al. Differential effects of antiepileptic drugs on sexual function and hormones in men with epilepsy. *Neurology.* 2005; 65:1016-23.
155. Klotz L. Pharmacokinetic and pharmacodynamics profile of degarelix for prostate cancer. *Expert Opin Drug Metab Toxicol.* 2015; 11:1795-1802.
156. Trajanovska AS, Vujovic V, Ignjatova L et al. Sexual dysfunction as a side effect of hyperprolactinemia in methadone maintenance therapy. *Med Arch.* 2013; 67:48-50.
157. Clayton AH, Croft HA, Handiwala L. Antidepressants and sexual dysfunction: mechanisms and clinical implications. *Postgrad Med.* 2014; 126:91-9.
158. LaTorre A, Giupponi G, Duffy DM et al. Sexual dysfunction related to psychotropic drugs: a critical review. Part III. Mood stabilizers and anxiolytic drugs. *Pharmacopsychiatry.* 2014; 47:1-6.
159. Canguyen O, Burnett AL. The effect of 5 alpha-reductase inhibitors on erectile function. *J Androl.* 2008; 29:514-23.
160. Malik P. Sexual dysfunction in schizophrenia. *Curr Opin Psychiatry.* 2007; 20:138-42.
161. Micheva KD, Taylor CP, Smith SJ. Pregabalin reduces the release of synaptic vesicles from cultured hippocampal neurons. *Mol Pharmacol.* 2006; 70:467-76.
162. Hisasue S, Suruya R, Itoh N et al. Ejaculatory disorder caused by alpha-1-adrenoreceptor antagonists is not retrograde ejaculation but a loss of seminal emission. *Int J Urol.* 2006; 13:1311-6.
163. Amory JK, Anawalt BD, Matsumoto AM et al. The effect of 5alpha-reductase inhibition with dutasteride and finasteride on bone mineral density, serum lipoproteins, hemoglobin, prostate specific antigen, and sexual functions in healthy young men. *J Urol.* 2008; 179:2333-8.
164. Buena F, Swerdloff RS, Steiner BS et al. Sexual function does not change when serum testosterone levels are pharmacologically varied within the normal male range. *Fertil Steril.* 1993; 59:1118-23.
165. Bhasin S, Cunningham GR, Hayes FJ et al. Testosterone therapy in adult men with androgen deficiency syndromes: an Endocrine Society Practice Guideline. *J Clin Endocrinol Metab.* 2010; 95:2536-59.
166. Sansone A, Romanelli F, Gianfrilli D et al. Endocrine evaluation of erectile dysfunction. *Endocrine.* 2014; 46:423-30.
167. Davis PH. Drug-related hyperprolactinemia. *Adverse Drug React Toxicol Rev.* 1997; 16:83-94.
168. Cunningham GR, Stephens-Shields AJ, Rosen RC et al. Association of sex hormones with sexual function, vitality, and physical function of symptomatic older men with low testosterone levels at baseline in the testosterone trials. *J Clin Endocrinol Metab.* 2015; 100:1146-55.
169. Lewis RW, Fugl-Meyer KS, Corona G et al. Definitions/epidemiology/risk factors for sexual dysfunction. *J Sex Med.* 2010; 7(4 part 2):1598-607.
170. Hellstrom WJ, Sikka SC. Effects of acute treatment with tamsulosin versus alfuzosin on ejaculatory function in normal volunteers. *J Urol.* 2006; 176(4 part 1):1529-33.
171. Schuster TG, Ohl DA. Diagnosis and treatment of ejaculatory dysfunction. *Urol Clin North Am.* 2002; 29:939-48.
172. Banos JE, Bosch F, Farre M. Drug-induced priapism: its aetiology, incidence and treatment. *Med Toxicol Adverse Drug Exp.* 1989; 4:46-58.
173. Brugh VM, Lipshultz LI. Male factor infertility: evaluation and management. *Med Clin North Am.* 2004; 88:367-85.
174. Puscheck E, Philip PA, Jeyendran RS. Male fertility preservation and cancer treatment. *Cancer Treat Rev.* 2004; 30:173-80.
175. Perelman MA. Erectile dysfunction and depression: screening and treatment. *Urol Clin North Am.* 2011; 38:125-39.
176. Rosen RC, Riley A, Wagner G et al. The International Index of Erectile Dysfunction: a multidimensional scale for assessment of erectile dysfunction. *Urology.* 1997; 49:822-30.
177. Vlachopoulos C, Jackson G, Stefanadis C et al. Erectile dysfunction in the cardiovascular patient. *Eur Heart J.* 2013; 34:2034-46.
178. Glina S, Sharlip ID, Hellstrom WJG. Modifying risk factors to prevent and treat erectile dysfunction. *J Sex Med.* 2013; 10:115-9.
179. Porst H, Burnett A, Brock G et al. SOP conservative (medical and mechanical) treatment of erectile dysfunction. *J Sex Med.* 2013; 10:130-71.
180. Litwin, MS, Nied RJ, Dhanani N. Health-related quality of life in men with erectile dysfunction. *J Gen Intern Med.* 1998; 13:159-66.
181. Ventegodt S. Sex and the quality of life in Denmark. *Arch Sex Behav.* 1998; 27:295-307.
182. Glina S, Roehrborn CG, Esen A et al. Sexual function in men with lower urinary tract symptoms and prostatic enlargement secondary to benign prostatic hyperplasia: results of a 6-month, randomized, double-blind, placebo-controlled study of tadalafil coadministered with finasteride. *J Sex Med.* 2015; 12:129-38.
183. Burnett AL, Nehra A, Breau RH et al. American Urological Association Guideline 2018: Erectile Dysfunction. www.auanet.org/guidelines/male-sexual-dysfunction-erectile-dysfunction-(2018) (accessed 2018 Aug 9).
184. McMahon CG. Erectile dysfunction. *Int Med J.* 2014; 44:18-26.
185. Althof SE, Levin SB, Corty EW et al. A double blind crossover trial of clomipramine for rapid ejaculation in 15 couples. *J Clin Psychiatry.* 1995; 56:401-7.

186. Montague DK, Jarow J, Broderick G et al. American Urological Association Guideline on the Pharmacologic Management of Premature Ejaculation. Published 2004; reviewed and validity confirmed 2010. www.auanet.org/guidelines/male-sexual-dysfunction-premature-ejaculation-(2004-reviewed-for-currency-2010) (accessed 2018 Aug 9).

187. Jenkins LC, Mulhall JP. Delayed orgasm and anorgasmia. *Fertil Steril.* 2015; 104:1082-8.

188. Montague DK, Jarow J, Broderick G et al. American Urological Association Guideline on the Management of Priapism. Published 2003; reviewed and validity confirmed 2010. www.auanet.org/guidelines/male-sexual-dysfunction-priapism-(2003-reviewed-for-currency-2010) (accessed 2018 Aug 9).

189. Jarow J, Sigman M, Kolettis PN et al. AUA Best Practice Statement: Optimal Evaluation of the Infertile Male. Reviewed and validity confirmed 2011. www.auanet.org/guidelines/male-infertility-optimal-evaluation-(reviewed-and-validity-confirmed-2011) (accessed 2018 Aug 9).

190. Montorsi F, Adaikan G, Bechler E et al. Summary of the recommendations on sexual dysfunction in men. *J Sex Med.* 2010; 7:3572-88.

191. Nunes LV, Moreira HC, Razzouk D et al. Strategies for the treatment of antipsychotic-induced sexual dysfunction and/or hyperprolactinemia among patients of the schizophrenia spectrum: a review. *J Sex Marital Ther.* 2012; 38:281-301.

192. Kovac JR, Mak SK, Garcia MM et al. A pathophysiology-based approach to the management of early priapism. *Asian J Androl.* 2013; 15:20-6.

193. Hayghe E, Matsuda T, Daudin M et al. Fertility after testicular cancer treatments: results of a large multicenter study. *Cancer.* 2004; 100:732-7.

194. Handler J. Managing erectile dysfunction in hypertensive patients. *J Clin Hypertens.* 2011; 13:450-4.

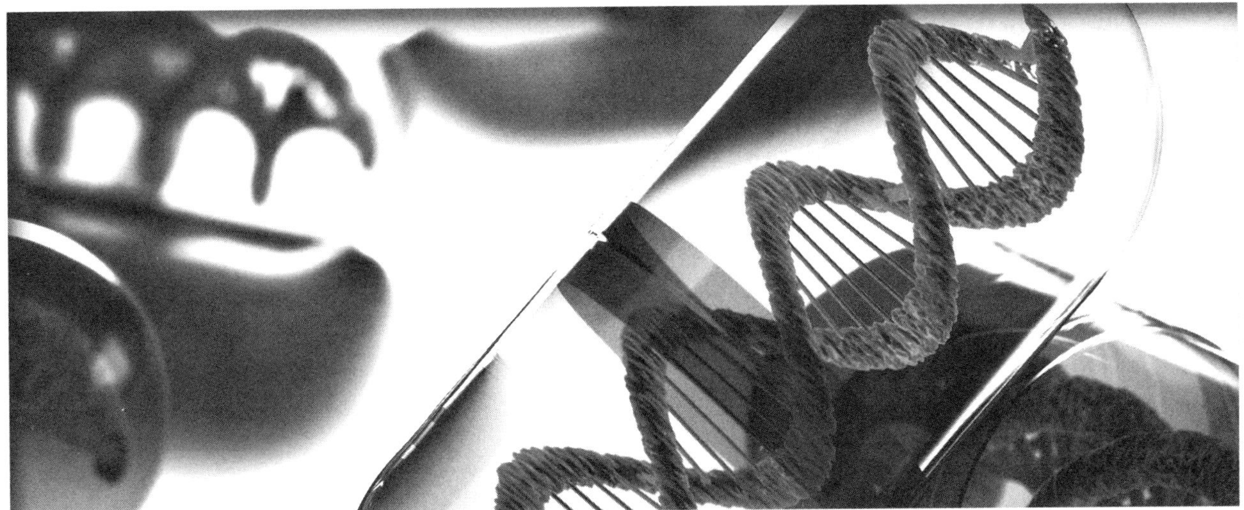

CHAPTER 34

Gynecologic Diseases and Infertility in Women

Judith A. Smith

Drug-induced gynecologic diseases and infertility in women can have an enormous impact on the quality of life for those afflicted. The true incidence of drug-induced gynecologic diseases, dysfunctions, and disorders is difficult to estimate because of significant underreporting. The drug-induced gynecologic diseases have an insidious and inconsistent onset that can make prevention and diagnosis a challenge. Moreover, women often do not identify the relationship between the use of the offending agent and the onset of the gynecologic disease, dysfunction, or condition. Although appropriate interventions often can successfully manage and relieve the symptoms associated with the various drug-induced gynecologic diseases discussed in this chapter, some will result in irreversible outcomes such as sexual dysfunction or infertility. There is a need to continue research in the women's health arena particularly to advance the management and prevention of the drug-induced gynecologic disorders addressed in this chapter.

OVARIAN HYPERSTIMULATION

CAUSATIVE AGENTS

Drug-induced ovarian hyperstimulation occurs after repeated or prolonged use of ovulation-induction agents such as antiestrogens (clomiphene citrate or tamoxifen), gonadotropins (gonadorelin, human chorionic gonadotropin [hCG]), or gonadotropin-releasing agonists (goserelin acetate). Drugs implicated in ovarian hyperstimulation are listed in **Table 34-1**.[1-36]

EPIDEMIOLOGY

Ovulation-induction medications were introduced over 40 years ago. Drug-induced ovarian hyperstimulation has been reported to occur in up to 27.7% of

Table 34-1 Agents Implicated in Drug-Induced Gynecologic Diseases and Infertility in Women

Drug	Incidence	Level of Evidence[a]
OVARIAN HYPERSTIMULATION[1-36,b]		
Clomiphene citrate	NK	B
Gonadotropins	NK	B
Gonadotropin-releasing agonists	NK	B
Tamoxifen	NK	C
VULVOVAGINAL CANDIDIASIS[37-42,c]		
Antibiotics (systemic)	NK	B
Corticosteroids	NK	C
Hormone-replacement therapy	NK	C
Oral contraceptives	NK	C
Tamoxifen	NK	C
VAGINAL BLEEDING DISORDERS: AMENORRHEA/OLIGOMENORRHEA[55-61]		
Antiepileptic drugs	12–59%	B
Antihypertensive agents	NK	C
Platinum analogues	>60%	B
Chlorambucil	NK	C
Alkylating agents	>60%	A
Danazol	>50%	C
Doxorubicin	>60%	B
Estrogen	NK	C
Etoposide	>60%	B
Goserelin	NK	C
Medroxyprogesterone	NK	C
Methyldopa	NK	C
Oral contraceptives	NK	C
Progesterone	NK	C
Spironolactone	NK	C
Tamoxifen	NK	C
Thalidomide	NK	C
VAGINAL BLEEDING DISORDERS: MENORRHAGIA/MENOMETRORRHAGIA[81-88]		
Ginseng	NK	C
Human relaxin	NK	C
Levonorgestrol–intrauterine contraceptive devices	2–4%	A
Methadone	>50%	B
Selective serotonin reuptake inhibitors	<1%	B
VAGINAL BLEEDING DISORDERS: DYSMENORRHEA[102,d]		
Estrogen	NK	C
Oxytocin	NK	C
Progesterone	NK	C
Vasopressin	NK	C

Table 34-1 Agents Implicated in Drug-Induced Gynecologic Diseases and Infertility in Women (continued)

Drug	Incidence	Level of Evidence[a]
SEXUAL DYSFUNCTION[109-112,117-122]		
Antiepileptic drugs	NK	C
Antihypertensive agents	11%	B
Antidepressants	16–57%	B
Antipsychotics	28–93%	B
Amphetamines	NK	C
Baclofen	NK	C
Bromocriptine	NK	C
Cimetidine	NK	C
Digoxin	NK	C
Granisetron	NK	C
Indinavir	40%	C
Ketamine	NK	C
Methadone	NK	C
Methazolamide	NK	C
Naproxen	NK	C
Norethandrolone	NK	C
INFERTILITY[131-144]		
Alkylating agents	<60%	A
Antiepileptic drugs	12–59%	B
Anthracyclines	<60%	B
Bleomycin	<60%	C
Caffeine	NK, dose-dependent	A
Etoposide	<60%	B
Fluorouracil	<60%	B
Methotrexate	<60%	A
Platinum analogues	<60%	B
Thalidomide	<60%	A
Vinca alkaloids	<60%	C

NK = not known.
[a]Definitions for Levels of Evidence: Level A—evidence from one or more randomized, controlled clinical trials; Level B—evidence from nonrandomized clinical trials, prospective observational studies, cohort studies, retrospective studies, case-control studies, meta-analyses and/or postmarketing surveillance studies; and Level C—evidence from one or more published case reports or case series.
[b]Occurs in up to 27.7% of patients receiving ovulation-induction drugs, with severe cases occurring in less than 2% of patients.
[c]Approximately 17–39% of gynecologic office visits are associated with cases of vulvovaginal candidiasis.
[d]The incidence of dysmenorrhea in menstruating women ranges from 3–90%.

patients receiving ovulation-induction drugs, with severe cases occurring in <2% of patients.[3-6]

MECHANISMS

Gonadotropins or gonadotropin-releasing agonists are used in the follicular phase of the ovarian cycle to increase serum concentrations of follicle-stimulating hormone (FSH) and luteinizing hormone (LH), for the purpose of increasing the maturation of multiple ovarian follicles resulting in multiple ovulations.[7] Antiestrogen agents interact with estrogen receptors at the hypothalamus, displacing endogenous estrogen, thereby disrupting the endogenous estrogen negative feedback loop effect.[7] Ultimately, this results in stimulation of the release of FSH and LH, increasing the maturation of multiple ovarian follicles, producing multiple ovulations. Endogenous and exogenous hCG (or both) also likely contribute to the pathogenesis of ovarian hyperstimulation.[8] It is believed that hCG stimulates continuous ovulation, and it may also increase ovarian capillary permeability.[8] Mechanisms of drug-induced ovarian hyperstimulation are described in **Table 34-2**.

CLINICAL PRESENTATION AND DIFFERENTIAL DIAGNOSIS

Signs and symptoms associated with ovarian hyperstimulation are listed in **Table 34-3**. This drug-induced disease may occur either early (within 7 days) or late (within 7–14 days) after initiation of drug therapy. The primary sign of ovarian hyperstimulation is significant enlargement of the ovary that leads to the leakage of protein-rich fluid from ovarian capillaries into the peritoneal space.[9] Drug-induced ovarian hyperstimulation may be associated with multiple nonspecific symptoms related to the accumulation of this peritoneal fluid and including abdominal distention, pain or a pulling sensation in the pelvis, nausea, vomiting, diarrhea, pleural effusions, dyspnea, or chest pain.[4] In addition to ovary enlargement, specific signs suggestive of ovarian hyperstimulation include ascites, oliguria, tachycardia, and, in severe cases, pleural effusion.[6,11] These signs and symptoms of drug-induced ovarian hyperstimulation must be differentiated from other conditions that may result in similar symptoms, such as gastrointestinal complications of ovarian cysts, endometriosis, and ectopic pregnancy. Conditions to consider in the differential diagnosis of ovarian hyperstimulation are presented in **Table 34-4**.

RISK FACTORS

Specific risk factors for the development of drug-induced ovarian hyperstimulation are not well established. Those that are known are listed in **Table 34-5**. Younger patients tend to be at higher risk because they have a larger number of recruitable follicles and gonadotropin receptors.[11,12] Although some data suggest that women with a history of polycystic ovarian syndrome may have an increased risk for drug-induced ovarian hyperstimulation, in most cases this drug-induced disease is not predictable.[13-16] Repeated or prolonged cycles of clomiphene citrate and gonadotropins as well as high doses contribute to an increased risk of drug-induced ovarian hyperstimulation.[17-21]

MORBIDITY AND MORTALITY

Early or mild drug-induced ovarian hyperstimulation typically resolves without intervention and with no significant sequelae. However, severe cases of drug-induced ovarian hyperstimulation or cases that are diagnosed late can be life-threatening.[4] In the short term, the fluid shifts can result in significant ascites, intravascular volume depletion, and pleural effusion that may lead to significant breathing difficulties and, in rare cases, acute respiratory distress syndrome. Ascitic fluid can put pressure on the inferior vena cava and lead to decreased cardiac output.[4] Severe cases of drug-induced ovarian hyperstimulation have been associated with significant thromboembolic events.[5,6] In addition, patients are at risk of ovarian torsion or cyst rupture that may potentially lead to hemorrhage with fatal outcomes.[5,6] Finally, although it is controversial if a truly causative relationship, ovarian hyperstimulation from use of fertility drugs has been associated with the development of ovarian cancer.[18-29]

PREVENTION

A few measures may prevent drug-induced ovarian hyperstimulation, including suspending the treatment cycle of the offending agent, extending the interval between treatments with the offending agent, planning early follicular aspiration, or administration of albumin or concomitant progesterone therapy (**Table 34-6**).[3,5,6] Patients should be monitored closely while undergoing any type of ovarian stimulation therapy with serum estradiol concentrations obtained prior to initiating each new cycle of treatment as well as after completion of each cycle and ultrasound performed at baseline and at least once after each treatment

Table 34-2 Mechanisms of Drug-Induced Gynecologic Diseases and Infertility in Women

Drug	Mechanism
OVARIAN HYPERSTIMULATION[1-36]	
Clomiphene citrate	Disrupts endogenous estrogen negative feedback loop at the hypothalamic level by blocking estrogen receptors inducing ovulation
Gonadotropins	Increase FSH and LH inducing multiple ovulations
Gonadotropin-releasing agonists	Increase FSH and LH inducing multiple ovulations
Tamoxifen	Disrupts endogenous estrogen negative feedback loop at the hypothalamic level by blocking estrogen receptors inducing ovulation
VULVOVAGINAL CANDIDIASIS[37-46]	
Antibiotics (systemic)	Alter normal flora (lactobacilli) of vagina resulting in overgrowth of *Candida*
Corticosteroids	Increase glycogen content, increasing pH and promoting growth of *Candida*
Hormone-replacement therapy	Increases glycogen content, increasing pH and promoting growth of *Candida*
Oral contraceptives	Increase glycogen content, increasing pH and promoting growth of *Candida*
Tamoxifen	Increases glycogen content, increasing pH and promoting growth of *Candida*
VAGINAL BLEEDING DISORDERS: AMENORRHEA/OLIGOMENORRHEA[55-61]	
Antiepileptic drugs	Increase hormone-binding globulin, resulting in decreased binding of estradiol leading to ovarian dysfunction
Antihypertensive agents	Microvascular instability inducing breakthrough bleeding
Alkylating agents and platinum analogues	Direct toxic effects on oocytes that halts ovulation, inducing amenorrhea
Chlorambucil	Direct toxic effects on oocytes that halts ovulation, inducing amenorrhea
Danazol	Indirect inhibition of negative feedback loop of the hypothalamic–pituitary pathway, decreasing FSH/LH release and altering ovarian function
Doxorubicin	Direct toxic effects on oocytes that halts ovulation, inducing amenorrhea
Estrogen	Indirect inhibition of negative feedback loop of the hypothalamic–pituitary pathway, decreasing FSH/LH release and altering ovarian function
Etoposide	Direct toxic effects on oocytes that halts ovulation, inducing amenorrhea
Goserelin	Indirect inhibition of negative feedback loop of the hypothalamic–pituitary pathway, decreasing FSH/LH release and altering ovarian function
Medroxyprogesterone	Direct effect on uterine lining
Methyldopa	Increases prolactin concentrations; indirect effect on LH secretion
Oral contraceptives	Indirect inhibition of negative feedback loop of the hypothalamic–pituitary pathway, decreasing FSH/LH release and altering ovarian function
Progesterone	Indirect inhibition of negative feedback loop of the hypothalamic–pituitary pathway, decreasing FSH/LH release and altering ovarian function
Spironolactone	Microvascular instability, inducing breakthrough bleeding
Tamoxifen	Indirect inhibition of negative feedback loop of the hypothalamic–pituitary pathway, decreasing FSH/LH release and altering ovarian function
Thalidomide	Direct toxic effects on oocytes that halts ovulation, inducing amenorrhea
VAGINAL BLEEDING DISORDERS: MENORRHAGIA/MENOMETRORRHAGIA[81-88]	
Ginseng	Unknown
Human relaxin	Induction of vascular endothelial growth factor receptor
Levonorgestrol–intrauterine contraceptive devices	Unknown; possible changes in prostaglandin concentrations in uterine tissue
Methadone	Unknown
Selective serotonin reuptake inhibitors	Decreased clotting function

Table 34-2 Mechanisms of Drug-Induced Gynecologic Diseases and Infertility in Women (continued)

Drug	Mechanism
VAGINAL BLEEDING DISORDERS: DYSMENORRHEA[102]	
Estrogen	Rapid fluctuations in serum hormone concentrations; activation of inflammation cascade leading to pelvic swelling and pain
Oxytocin	Antidiuretic effect that alters uterine contractions to dysrhythmic and painful pattern
Progesterone	Rapid fluctuations in serum hormone concentrations; activation of inflammation cascade leading to pelvic swelling and pain
Vasopressin	Antidiuretic effect that alters uterine contractions to dysrhythmic and painful pattern
SEXUAL DYSFUNCTION[109-112,117-122]	
Antiepileptic drugs	Increase serum concentrations of hormone-binding globulin, decreasing estradiol binding and altering the hypothalamic–pituitary axis regulation of hormone release
Antihypertensive agents	Decrease vaginal lubrication; decrease libido via antiandrogenic and antidopaminergic activity
Antidepressants	Loss of libido and orgasm dysfunction by altering central serotonergic activity that disrupts hypothalamic–pituitary axis regulation of hormone release
Antipsychotics	Elevate prolactin concentrations via inhibition of dopamine-2 receptors, which decreases libido and disrupts orgasms
Amphetamines	Loss of libido and orgasm dysfunction by altering central serotonergic and dopaminergic activity and, indirectly, hypothalamic–pituitary axis regulation of hormone release
Baclofen	Proposed to be associated with inhibitory effects of $GABA_B$ receptors
Bromocriptine	Elevates prolactin concentrations, which decreases libido and disrupts orgasms
Cimetidine	Antiandrogenic effects
Digoxin	Disrupts hypothalamic–pituitary axis regulation of hormone release
Granisetron	Unknown
Indinavir	Unknown
Ketamine	Unknown; possible dissociation effects, altered muscle tone
Methadone	Decrease in lutenizing hormone production and subsequent testosterone concentrations
Methazolamide	Unknown
Naproxen	Unknown
Norethandrolone	Disrupts hypothalamic–pituitary axis regulation of hormone release
INFERTILITY[131-144]	
Alkylating agents	Direct toxic effect on oocytes, permanently halt ovulation
Antiepileptic drugs	Increase serum concentrations of hormone binding globulin decreasing estradiol binding and decreasing/ halting ovarian function
Anthracyclines	Direct toxic effect on oocytes, permanently halts ovulation
Bleomycin	Direct toxic effect on oocytes, permanently halts ovulation
Caffeine	Unknown
Etoposide	Direct toxic effect on oocytes, permanently halts ovulation
Fluorouracil	Direct toxic effect on oocytes, permanently halts ovulation
Methotrexate	Direct toxic effect on oocytes, permanently halts ovulation
Platinum analogues	Direct toxic effect on oocytes, permanently halts ovulation
Thalidomide	Direct toxic effect on oocytes, permanently halts ovulation
Vinca alkaloids	Direct toxic effect on oocytes, permanently halts ovulation

LH = luteinizing hormone, FSH = follicle-stimulating hormone.

Table 34-3 Signs and Symptoms Associated with Drug-Induced Gynecologic Diseases and Infertility in Women

Ovarian hyperstimulation

- Abdominal distention
- Ascites
- Chest pain
- Diarrhea
- Dyspnea
- Enlargement of ovary
- Nausea and vomiting
- Pelvic pain

Vulvovaginal candidiasis

- Dyspareunia
- Vaginal erythema
- Vaginal pruritus
- Vaginal swelling (edema)
- White, curd-like vaginal discharge

Vaginal bleeding disorders

- Amenorrhea and oligomenorrhea
  - Decreased cervical mucus
  - Dyspareunia
  - Irregular menses
  - Irritability
  - Mood swings
  - No menses
  - Vaginal dryness
  - Vaginal wall thinning
- Menorrhagia and menometrorrhagia
  - Heavy menses (>80 mL)
  - Irregular menses
  - Prolonged menses
  - Uterine fibroids
  - Uterine polyps
- Dysmenorrhea
  - Abdominal cramping
  - Backache
  - Bloating
  - Breast tenderness
  - Fatigue
  - Headache
  - Mood changes
  - Nausea
  - Pelvic pain
  - Syncope
  - Vomiting

Sexual dysfunction

- Anger or fear
- Anxiety
- Dyspareunia
- Fatigue
- Loss of libido or desire (may present as depression)
- Vaginismus
- Frequent/recurrent miscarriages
- Inability to conceive
- Irregular menses
- No menses

Infertility

- Frequent/recurrent miscarriages
- Inability to conceive
- Irregular menses
- No menses

cycle. If serum estradiol concentrations increase rapidly at any time during the treatment or if ultrasound reveals massive follicle recruitment, one of the interventions described above should be undertaken to prevent the development of drug-induced ovarian hyperstimulation.[30] In patients at increased risk for drug-induced ovarian hyperstimulation, a lower dose of hCG (5,000 international units instead of the standard 10,000 international units) may be administered. Alternatively, exogenous progesterone (50 mg intramuscularly, 100 mg intravaginal suppository, or 8% intravaginal gel) may be administered in place of additional doses of hCG to support the luteal phase.[30,31] Another option is the intravenous administration of 25% albumin during follicular aspiration; however, the effectiveness of this approach for prevention of drug-induced ovarian hyperstimulation has been variable.[30,32-34]

MANAGEMENT

Treatment options for drug-induced ovarian hyperstimulation are described in **Table 34-7**. Mild cases in which patients present with some discomfort and for which the only physical finding is mild abdominal distention will resolve without any intervention.[4] Fluid shifts can occur because of significant ascites, intravascular volume depletion, and pleural effusions. To help prevent progression and adverse sequelae related to these fluid shifts, patients should be instructed to increase fluid intake. Patients with moderate drug-induced ovarian hyperstimulation

Table 34-4 Conditions to Consider in the Differential Diagnosis of Drug-Induced Gynecologic Diseases and Infertility in Women

Ovarian hyperstimulation

- Endometriosis
- Ectopic pregnancy
- Ovarian cysts

Vulvovaginal candidiasis

- Bacterial vaginosis
- Chlamydia
- Gonorrhea
- Trichomoniasis
- Urinary tract infection

Vaginal bleeding disorders

- Amenorrhea and oligomenorrhea
  - Anorexia nervosa
  - Endocrine disorders
  - Excessive physiological stress
  - Excessive psychological/emotional stress
  - Hypothalamus tumor
  - Metabolic disorders
  - Pituitary tumor
- Menorrhagia and menometrorrhagia
  - Abnormal endometrial hyperplasia
  - Endometrial cancer
  - Endometriosis
  - Fibroids
  - Uterine polyps
- Dysmenorrhea
  - Premenstrual syndrome

Sexual dysfunction

- Anxiety/anger or fear
- Depression
- Dyspareunia
- Fatigue

Infertility

- Early menopause
- Endocrine disorder
- Metabolic disorder

Table 34-5 Risk Factors for Drug-Induced Gynecologic Diseases and Infertility in Women

Ovarian hyperstimulation

- Polycystic ovarian syndrome
- Younger age

Vulvovaginal candidiasis

- Diabetes
- Heat/moisture
- History of vulvovaginal candidiasis
- Obesity
- Pregnancy
- Tight clothing

Vaginal bleeding disorders

- Amenorrhea and oligomenorrhea
  - Advancing age
  - Anorexia
  - Excessive exercise
  - Perimenopause
  - Poor nutritional status
  - Psychological (i.e., work/family/school) stress
- Menorrhagia and menometrorrhagia
  - Unknown
- Dysmenorrhea
  - Early menarche
  - Family history
  - Heavy menses
  - High omega-6 fatty acid diets

Sexual dysfunction

- Depression
- Hypogonadism
- Hypothyroidism
- Hysterectomy
- Oophorectomy
- Schizophrenia
- Vulvovaginal resection

Infertility

- Autoimmune diseases
- Endocrine disorders
- Epilepsy
- Older age

often present with increasing abdominal girth, pain, nausea and vomiting, diarrhea, shortness of breath, or any combination of these. Moderate ovarian hyperstimulation can be treated on an outpatient basis, but close monitoring and follow-up are required. These patients should be instructed to increase oral hydration and may benefit from a short course of intravenous hydration. Outpatients with moderate drug-induced ovarian hyperstimulation should be on strict bed rest and should

Table 34-6 Approaches to Help Prevent Drug-Induced Gynecologic Diseases and Infertility in Women

Ovarian hyperstimulation

- Add progesterone to treatment cycle
- Extend interval between treatment cycles
- Monitor serum estradiol concentrations
- Perform pelvic ultrasound
- Plan early follicular aspiration
- Suspend treatment cycle

Vulvovaginal candidiasis

- Consume acidophilus/yogurt with activated cultures
- Take prophylactic antifungal treatment when taking systemic antibiotics
- Wear loose clothing and cotton undergarments
- Wipe away from vulvovaginal area after bowel movement

Vaginal bleeding disorders

- Amenorrhea and oligomenorrhea
  - Eat a well-balanced diet and exercise
  - Monitor the duration and frequency of menses episodes
  - Preserve ovarian function during cytotoxic exposure (i.e., oral contraceptives)
- Menorrhagia and menometrorrhagia
  - Avoid aspirin use
  - Monitor for early indirect signs/symptoms
  - Anemia
  - Monitor for low hemoglobin
  - Monitor serum iron concentrations
  - Use iron-replacement therapy
  - Increasing duration of menses
  - Consider use of oral contraceptives to reduce irregular bleeding
- Dysmenorrhea
  - Avoid uterine stimulants (oxytocin, vasopressin)
  - Prophylactic use of anti-inflammatory agents (nonsteroidal anti-inflammatory drugs, cyclooxygenase-2 inhibitors)

Sexual dysfunction

- Identify and manage contributing symptoms (i.e., vaginal dryness)
- Offer alternative drug therapy options
- Provide education to prepare patient
- Provide resources for development of communication/coping skills for couples

Infertility

- Counsel patient and provide support resources
- Decrease consumption of caffeine-containing beverages
- Offer interventions prior to initiation of offending agent
  - Oocyte collection
  - Frozen embryos
  - Provide patient education
  - Consider use of oral contraceptives to halt ovulation during treatment with offending agent

monitor oral intake, weight, and urine output. Short-term use of antiemetic agents and analgesics can be used to alleviate nausea and mild pelvic pain. The administration of a gonadotropin-releasing–hormone agonist (intramuscular leuprolide 7.5 mg once monthly) has been reported to be successful for the treatment of tamoxifen-induced ovarian hyperstimulation.[35]

Patients with life-threatening cases of ovarian hyperstimulation present with significant ascites, intravascular volume depletion, possible pleural effusions, severe hemoconcentration, potential renal failure, risk for acute respiratory distress syndrome, or thromboembolic events. Hospital admission with immediate intervention is required. Aggressive intravenous fluid hydration is needed in patients with severe cases of drug-induced ovarian hyperstimulation characterized by dehydration with a hematocrit >45%.[4] The rate of infusion should be adjusted to maintain urine output >30 mL/hr. All diuretics, antihistamines, angiotensin-converting enzyme inhibitors, and nonsteroidal anti-inflammatory drugs (NSAIDs) should be discontinued or avoided to prevent future volume depletion. Once the patient's condition has been stabilized, paracentesis is used, if necessary, to remove ascites fluid to alleviate pelvic pain and dyspnea. Because these patients are at risk for thromboembolic events, anticoagulation therapy with heparin (5,000 units subcutaneously every 12 hours) or low-molecular-weight heparin (e.g., enoxaparin 40 mg subcutaneously once daily) with or without sequential compression device therapy should be considered for the duration of the patient's confinement to bed. Surgical interventions such as unilateral oophorectomy or removal of cysts may be required to prevent ovarian torsion or cyst rupture that may lead to intraperitoneal hemorrhage.[4]

Table 34-7 Management of Drug-Induced Gynecologic Diseases and Infertility in Women

Ovarian hyperstimulation	*Vulvovaginal candidiasis*	*Vaginal bleeding disorders*	*Sexual dysfunction*	*Infertility*
IV fluids as appropriate • Diuretics (e.g., furosemide 20–40 mg PO/IV) • Antihistamines (e.g., diphenhydramine 50 mg IV q 4 hr as needed) • Bed rest • Antiemetic of choice (e.g., ondansetron 8 mg IV q 8 hr) • Analgesics (e.g., acetaminophen 500 mg q 6 hr as needed) • Gonadotropin-releasing–hormone agonist (leuprolide 7.5 mg IM once monthly) • Anticoagulation therapy (heparin 5,000 units sub-Q q 12 hr or enoxaparin 40 mg sub-Q once daily)	**Topical (intravaginal)** *Miconazole* • 2% cream 5 g daily × 7 days • 100 mg supp daily × 7 days • 200 mg supp daily × 3 days *Clotrimazole* • 1% cream 5 g daily × 7–14 days • 100 mg vaginal tablet daily × 7 days • 2–100 mg vaginal tablets daily × 3 days • 500 mg vaginal tablet × 1 day *Tioconazole* • 6.5 % ointment 5 g × 1 dose *Terconazole* • 0.4% cream 5 g daily × 7 days • 0.8 % cream 5 g daily × 3 days • 80 mg supp daily × 3 days **Oral** *Fluconazole* • 150 mg orally × 1 dose	**Amenorrhea and oligomenorrhea** • Combination oral contraceptives of preference (e.g., 35–50 mcg ethinyl estradiol with 0.5–1 mg norethindrone) **Menorrhagia and menometrorrhagia** • Combination oral contraceptives of preference (e.g., 35–50 mcg ethinyl estradiol with 0.5–1 mg norethindrone) • SSRI of choice (e.g., fluoxetine 20 mg daily or sertraline 50–100 mg daily) **Dysmenorrhea** • NSAID of choice (i.e., ibuprofen 400–800 mg q 6 hr with food or naproxen 250–500 mg twice daily as needed for pain) • Celecoxib 200 mg once daily	**Topical estrogen (intravaginal)** • Estropipate cream (0.15%) 2–4 g once daily × 21 days, 1 week off • Estradiol vaginal cream (0.01%) 2–4 g once daily × 2 wk, 2 weeks off • Conjugated estrogens cream (0.0625%) 0.5–2 g once daily × 21 days, 1 week off • Dienestrol cream (0.01%) 2–4 g once daily × 2 weeks, then 1 g 3 × weekly • Estradiol vaginal ring 0.05–0.1 mg per day; replace every 3 mo • Vaginal lubricants or moisturizers as needed • Sildenafil citrate 50 mg orally ~60 min prior to activity • Vibrator or mechanical stimulation	• Gonadotropin-releasing–hormone agonist (e.g., leuprolide 3.75 mg IM once monthly) • Oral contraceptives • Cryopreservation ○ Embryo freezing ○ Oocyte freezing ○ Ovarian cortex freezing ○ Follicle freezing

IM = intramuscular, IV = intravenous, PO = by mouth, NSAID = nonsteroidal anti-inflammatory drug, SSRI = selective serotonin reuptake inhibitor, sub-Q = subcutaneous.

When drug-induced ovarian hyperstimulation is detected early and interventions and treatment can be performed on an outpatient basis, symptoms usually resolve within 1 week.[6] In moderate-to-severe cases when the patients typically require hospitalization, complete symptom resolution may take 10 days or more.[6,36]

INFORMATION FOR PATIENTS

When planning ovarian-stimulation therapy, patients should be informed that they will need to be closely monitored. Patients should be told that if symptoms such as abdominal discomfort, shortness of breath, diarrhea, nausea, or vomiting occur, they should seek medical attention immediately.

VULVOVAGINAL CANDIDIASIS

CAUSATIVE AGENTS

Drug-induced vulvovaginal candidiasis most often results from the use of systemic antibiotics causing an alteration in the normal flora of the vaginal canal and allowing for an overgrowth of *Candida* species.

Drugs associated with drug-induced vulvovaginal candidiasis are listed in Table 34-1.[37-41]

EPIDEMIOLOGY

Vaginal symptoms are one of the most common reports of women during annual gynecologic office visits.[42] Approximately 17% to 39% of these office visits are associated with cases of vulvovaginal candidiasis.[43,44] The majority of women (>75%) experience at least one case of vulvovaginal candidiasis during their lifetime, and many (up to 50%) suffer from recurrent or persistent cases of vulvovaginal candidiasis.[42,45]

MECHANISMS

An overgrowth of *Candida albicans, C. tropicalis, C. glabrata,* or *C. parapsilosis* resulting from environmental changes in the vagina that alter the natural flora causes vulvovaginal candidiasis, which is a common fungal infection.[37,44] Drug-induced vulvovaginal candidiasis results from change in the normal flora of the vaginal canal most often from the use of systemic antibiotics that causes an overgrowth of *Candida* species (Table 34-2).[37-46] Oral contraceptives, corticosteroids, and hormone-replacement therapy can increase the pH and glycogen content of the vaginal secretions, favoring *Candida* infections.[47] Retinoids such as acitretin also may alter vaginal secretions and indirectly change the natural flora of the vaginal canal.[48]

CLINICAL PRESENTATION AND DIFFERENTIAL DIAGNOSIS

Physical symptoms of vulvovaginal candidiasis range from absent to severe. Symptoms in patients presenting with drug-induced vulvovaginal candidiasis are no different from those in patients presenting with spontaneous cases of vulvovaginal candidiasis (Table 34-3). The most common presenting symptom is vaginal pruritus, which may or may not be accompanied by a white, curd-like, thick vaginal discharge often described by patients as "cottage cheese-like." The infection typically originates in the vaginal canal and spreads to the vulva. The vulva and vaginal tissue may develop erythema, edema, or both because of local irritation and inflammation. The onset of signs or symptoms of drug-induced vulvovaginal candidiasis varies. As the infection progresses, symptoms increase and patients may report burning, soreness, and dyspareunia.

When a patient presents with these vaginal symptoms, a vaginal smear (culture) should be obtained to determine whether the symptoms are a result of bacterial vaginosis, trichomoniasis, or candidiasis.[51] Urinary tract infections should also be ruled out. Patients are often tested for gonorrhea or chlamydia, although neither has been closely associated with vaginal discharge.[50,51] Table 34-4 describes the conditions that should be considered in the differential diagnosis of drug-induced vulvovaginal candidiasis.

RISK FACTORS

A number of factors have been identified that predispose women to drug-induced vulvovaginal candidiasis (Table 34-5). These include younger age (<40 years), comorbid diseases or conditions, including diabetes, obesity, and pregnancy.[46,52] Environmental factors such as increased moisture and heat or tight clothing such as panty hose or use of panty liners or continuous use of cranberry juice may alter vaginal pH or acidophilus-containing products may alter vaginal normal flora and also increase a women's risk of drug-induced vulvovaginal candidiasis.[52] Sexual intercourse has not been reported as a means of transmission of vulvovaginal candidiasis.[45]

MORBIDITY AND MORTALITY

The majority of episodes of drug-induced vulvovaginal candidiasis are classified as "uncomplicated" and characterized by sporadic or infrequent episodes, mild symptoms, most likely caused by *Candida albicans* infection, and without any medical comorbities/complications. In these cases, symptoms typically resolve within 48–72 hours following initiation of appropriate therapy. Uncomplicated vulvovaginal candidiasis is not associated with morbidity. However, approximately 10% of cases of vulvovaginal candidiasis are more complicated and are associated with recurrent infections, significant symptoms (erythema, edema, pruritus, and dyspareunia), likely to be non-*Candida albicans* infection, and occur in the presence of significant comorbidities such as diabetes, immunosuppression, or severe medical conditions.

PREVENTION

Methods to prevent drug-induced vulvovaginal candidiasis are described in Table 34-6. Behavior modification, such as wearing loose clothing and cotton undergarments and wiping away from the vulvovaginal area after bowel movements, can help prevent episodes of drug-induced disease.[52] It has been suggested that consuming yogurt with "activated cultures" or taking *lactobacillus acidophilus* capsules to maintain the balance of the normal flora in the vaginal tract may prevent drug-induced vulvovaginal candidiasis infections when consumed short-term during a course of antibiotics.[41] Therapy with vitamin C (250 mg intravaginally for 6 days), which is available by prescription, may increase vaginal secretions and reduce infection and may help prevent drug-induced vulvovaginal candidiasis.[53] Douching with vinegar and water, yogurt, or potassium sorbate may help prevent reinfection by restoring the acidic pH to the vulvovaginal canal.[41]

For patients who routinely experience episodes of vulvovaginal candidiasis when taking systemic antibiotics, prophylactic antifungal treatment should be considered. Preventive treatment should be initiated simultaneously with the first dose of antibiotics.[45] A topical azole drug (miconazole, clotrimazole, ticonazole, terconazole) may be administered for 3–7 days as indicated, or two doses of fluconazole 150 mg may be administered 72 hours apart.[47] Measures for prevention of drug-induced vulvovaginal candidiasis may improve adherence to and completion of prescribed antibiotic regimens.[44,52]

MANAGEMENT

Drug-induced vulvovaginal candidiasis can be effectively treated with antifungal topical cream or vaginal suppositories administered for 1, 3, 7, or up to 14 days in severe cases when symptoms do not resolve after one course of treatment (Table 34-7).[45] The most common topical antifungal agents used to treat vulvovaginal candidiasis include miconazole and clotrimazole, both of which are available without a prescription in the United States, and terconazole, which is still only available by prescription in the United States.[47] For both prescription and nonprescription topical regimens, the recommended duration of treatment ranges from 1 to 7 days, depending on the dose and strength of the agent selected. The treatment cycle may be repeated if symptoms persist after one course. For complicated infections, the most effective option is a single 150 mg oral dose of fluconazole with the dose repeated after 3 days.[47] This treatment approach also requires a prescription in the United States.[45] The strategies discussed above for prevention of drug-induced vulvovaginal candidiasis may also have some benefit for treatment.

Patients with significant erythema, edema, and local irritation may require more prolonged treatment (up to 14 days) to achieve a complete response and eradication of all symptoms.[45,51] Although topical therapy provides more immediate relief of symptoms as compared with oral treatment, either route will successfully eradicate vulvovaginal candidiasis.[45,51,54]

INFORMATION FOR PATIENTS

Wearing loose clothing and cotton undergarments to limit excessive moisture to the vulva area will help reduce patients' risk of drug-induced vulvovaginal candidiasis.[51] Exposure to the *Candida* organisms can be minimized if patients remember to wipe away from the vulva area after a bowel movement.[51] Patients should seek medical attention for diagnosis of the first vulvovaginal candidiasis infection.[44,45] However, patients with recurrent drug-induced vulvovaginal candidiasis infections should learn to recognize the symptoms and begin early self-treatment with nonprescription medications.[41,44] Patients that receive fluconazole for treatment need to be reminded not to consume alcohol for a least 7 days after completing treatment.

VAGINAL BLEEDING DISORDERS

AMENORRHEA AND OLIGOMENORRHEA

CAUSATIVE AGENTS

Agents that alter hormone balance directly or indirectly are associated with drug-induced amenorrhea (cessation of menses), oligomenorrhea (irregular menses), or intermenstrual bleeding.[55-61] Drugs that are known to be toxic to actively dividing cells may induce premature or temporary ovarian failure that presents as drug-induced amenorrhea/oligomenorrhea.[56] For example, drug-induced amenorrhea is an unfortunate long-term consequence of chemotherapy used to treat cancer and autoimmune disorders such as systemic lupus erythematosus.[62-67] Other agents may affect microvascular stability or hormone production/release, causing drug-induced amenorrhea/oligomenorrhea (Table 34-1).[55-61]

EPIDEMIOLOGY

A persistent menstruation disorder is often the primary reason for a woman to seek medical attention. Both amenorrhea and oligomenorrhea are often symptoms of more complex endocrine, gynecologic, or metabolic disorders.[70] *Intermenstrual bleeding*, often described as *breakthrough bleeding*, is bleeding that occurs between regular menses and is usually associated with nonadherence with oral contraceptives or inadequate doses of oral contraceptives based on endogenous, baseline hormone concentrations that may vary between individuals.[70,71]

Antiepileptic drugs such as phenytoin, valproic acid, and carbamazepine alter various aspects of endocrine function, although endocrine dysfunction has itself been associated with epilepsy. From 12% to 59% of women receiving antiepileptic drugs experience amenorrhea/oligomenorrhea.[75] More than 60% of women receiving cytotoxic chemotherapy have experienced one or more symptoms of ovarian failure.[64] The incidence of amenorrhea/oligomenorrhea associated with other drugs is unknown, as the evidence is published primarily in the form of case reports.

MECHANISMS

Drugs can affect uterine function through direct effects on the endometrium, such as causing microvascular instability that leads to breakthrough bleeding.[71] Antineoplastic drugs exert a direct toxic effect on oocytes, decreasing follicular formation and halting ovulation, leading to amenorrhea.[56] Drugs can also indirectly inhibit the negative feedback loop of the hypothalamic–pituitary pathway via modulation of serum hormone concentrations. This leads to decreased FSH and LH release, resulting in decreased ovarian function and induction of amenorrhea/oligomenorrhea.[68-74]

Antiepileptic drugs such as phenytoin and carbamazepine have been reported to increase serum concentrations of hormone-binding globulin, resulting in increased binding of estradiol and thus less free/active circulating estradiol resulting in amenorrhea/oligomenorrhea.[75-79] The mechanism of valproic acid–induced amenorrhea is not well understood, but it is thought to be related to weight gain, elevated serum insulin concentrations, and decreased serum concentrations of insulin-like growth factor I, leading to decreased ovarian androgen synthesis.[75,79-81] Mechanisms of drug-induced amenorrhea and oligomenorrhea are described in Table 34-2.[55-61]

CLINICAL PRESENTATION AND DIFFERENTIAL DIAGNOSIS

Patients with drug-induced amenorrhea/oligomenorrhea often will present with either no menses or irregular bleeding. These symptoms may occur at any time after therapy with the causative drug is initiated. Amenorrhea is a common presenting symptom of ovarian failure and is typically not the only symptom that patients may experience related to the hormonal imbalances. Other symptoms include mood swings, irritability, vaginal dryness, dyspareunia, decreased cervical mucus, and thinning of the vaginal mucosa (Table 34-3).[53]

Drug-induced amenorrhea/oligomenorrhea must be differentiated from other causes, including endocrine disorders, metabolic disorders, anorexia nervosa, pituitary or hypothalamus tumors, or excessive psychological or emotional stress (Table 34-4).[60]

RISK FACTORS

Women who have advanced in age to the perimenopausal stage are more susceptible to drug-induced amenorrhea/oligomenorrhea.[55] The probability of permanent chemotherapy-induced amenorrhea or menopause increases proportionally with advancing age.[55] Poor nutritional status caused by crash diets or anorexia nervosa can also influence the susceptibility to drug-induced amenorrhea/oligomenorrhea.[60] Physiologic stress such as excessive exercise (e.g., marathon training programs) and psychological stress (e.g., anxiety, work/school/family pressure) also increases the risk of drug-induced amenorrhea/oligomenorrhea (Table 34-5).[60]

MORBIDITY AND MORTALITY

Drug-induced amenorrhea/oligomenorrhea is not associated with increased mortality but can significantly impact quality of life. Drug-induced amenorrhea/oligomenorrhea may interfere with the ability to plan conception as well as to conceive and can be associated with numerous other undesirable symptoms that interfere with daily activities and relationships, including vaginal dryness, moodiness, and painful intercourse.[53,60,70] Drug-induced amenorrhea/oligomenorrhea may disguise underlying gynecologic and endocrine conditions requiring medical evaluation, including polycystic ovarian syndrome and hypothyroidism.[60,82]

PREVENTION

No specific studies have addressed the prevention of drug-induced amenorrhea/oligomenorrhea. Oral contraceptives and gonadotropin-releasing hormone (GnRH)–agonists inhibit ovarian function, primarily ovulation, which may decrease susceptibility to the gonadotoxic effects of chemotherapy.[60,61,64,83] The use of oral contraceptives or GnRH-agonists during courses of cytotoxic chemotherapy has demonstrated some benefit in the prevention of drug-induced ovarian failure/amenorrhea; this preventive strategy is successful primarily in younger patients.[60,61,80] Use of GnRH agonists has shown limited benefit for the prevention of chemotherapy-induced amenorrhea/ovarian failure in perimenopausal women.[60,61] Maintenance of a well-balanced diet with regular exercise may help reduce the risk of developing drug-induced amenorrhea/oligomenorrhea (Table 34-6).

MANAGEMENT

Treatment options for drug-induced amenorrhea/oligomenorrhea vary depending on the causative agent. Drug-induced amenorrhea/oligomenorrhea associated with the use of progesterone implants can be reversed, if the patient desires, by discontinuing the implant and selecting an alternative contraceptive agent, such as oral contraceptives, or using alternative modes of contraception such as barrier methods.[66,72] Breakthrough bleeding can be decreased by encouraging better patient adherence or use/changing hormone concentration of the oral contraceptive product (OCP). If breakthrough bleeding is occurring early in the menstrual cycle, an OCP with higher estrogen content (up to 50-mcg ethinyl estradiol) may help or, if later in the cycle, an OCP with higher progesterone content may help.[60]

Once the causative agent is discontinued or doses modified, drug-induced amenorrhea/oligomenorrhea usually resolves within 4–6 weeks (Table 34-7). GnRH agonists (e.g., leuprolide 3.75 mg intramuscularly once monthly) may promote the reversal of chemotherapy-induced amenorrhea/ovarian failure in some younger patients.[61,64,80] However, because chemotherapy-induced amenorrhea (ovarian failure) is often permanent, in most cases it is advisable to discuss alternative options to compensate for future infertility, such as cryopreservation of embryos, unfertilized ova, or ovary cortex tissue (contains primordial follicles) before chemotherapy administration.[60]

INFORMATION FOR PATIENTS

Patients receiving drugs that may induce amenorrhea or oligomenorrhea should be counseled that amenorrhea is the absence of menstrual bleeding and oligomenorrhea is the presence of infrequent/irregular menstrual cycles, and that if either occurs a healthcare provider needs to evaluate the patient. Patients who will be receiving cancer chemotherapy agents that may cause drug-induced amenorrhea and ovarian failure should be informed of the potential for occurrence of this drug-induced disease. Healthcare providers should discuss the potential impact on fertility and options for future childbearing with the patient before chemotherapy administration.[64,65,80,81]

MENORRHAGIA AND MENOMETRORRHAGIA

Menorrhagia, also described as heavy menstrual bleeding, is prolonged menses or excessive bleeding that occurs at regular intervals. *Menometrorrhagia*, also described as intermenstrual bleeding, is prolonged menses or excessive bleeding that occurs at irregular intervals.

CAUSATIVE AGENTS

Drug-induced menorrhagia has been reported with the use of selective serotonin reuptake inhibitors (SSRIs), hormones (estrogen and progesterone), intrauterine contraceptive devices (IUDs), and prostaglandins (Table 34-1).[81-88] Drug-induced menometrorrhagia has been found to be associated with the oral and topical use of ginseng and the investigational agent recombinant human relaxin, which is a disease-modifying agent that has demonstrated benefit in the treatment of scleroderma.[87,88]

EPIDEMIOLOGY

The incidences of drug-induced menorrhagia or menometrorrhagia have not been clearly determined. There are few case reports or reviews that describe the risk.[70,89-91] In one large study evaluating the associated risk of bleeding caused by SSRIs, the incidence of drug-induced menorrhagia or menometrorrhagia was <1%.[92] As many as 50% of women receiving maintenance therapy with methadone experience drug-induced menorrhagia or menometrorrhagia.[70] Historically, menorrhagia and menometrorrhagia are among the most common reasons for discontinuing IUD use, as the incidence of these diseases increases by 70–100% in association with the insertion of copper-containing IUDs. However, the incidence of menorrhagia or menometrorrhagia is only approximately 2–4% in patients using the levonorgestrel-releasing IUD.[72]

MECHANISMS

Serotonin receptors, those specific for 5-hydroxytryptamine$_{2a}$, are expressed on platelets. Serotonin is released during platelet activation and binds to these receptors, contributing to platelet aggregation and thrombus formation. Administration of SSRIs results in a relative decrease in clotting function, resulting in potential episodes of drug-induced menorrhagia.[81,82] The cause of increased blood loss in association with IUDs is unclear. When exposed to IUDs, concentrations of hydrogen peroxide and prostaglandins in uterine tissue increase, but whether or not this is related to menorrhagia is unclear.[83,89]

The mechanism of ginseng-induced menometrorrhagia is not known. Relaxin-induced menometrorrhagia results from the induction of vascular endothelial growth factor receptor expression in the endometrial cell.[85] Table 34-2 describes the mechanisms for drug-induced menorrhagia and menometrorrhagia.

CLINICAL PRESENTATION AND DIFFERENTIAL DIAGNOSIS

Patients with drug-induced menorrhagia present with a chief symptom of heavy or prolonged menstrual cycles that may occur at any time after the initiation of treatment with the culprit agent (Table 34-3). Drug-induced menorrhagia or menometrorrhagia may lead to the development of anemia and fatigue.

Drug-induced menorrhagia or menometrorrhagia must be distinguished from nondrug-induced causes, including common uterine complications such as fibroids or polyps or endometriosis.[93-97] Patients with menorrhagia or menometrorrhagia should undergo a complete physical exam and an endometrial biopsy to determine the primary cause. Endometrial biopsy can detect abnormal hyperplasia or cancer but cannot differentiate between a drug-induced and a nondrug-induced cause (Table 34-4).

RISK FACTORS

There are no known risk factors for drug-induced menorrhagia or menometrorrhagia.

MORBIDITY AND MORTALITY

If drug-induced menorrhagia or menometrorrhagia is left untreated, it may lead to more significant health complications, including anemia, thrombocytopenia, shortness of breath, altered nutritional status, and episodes of syncope. The majority of these symptoms can be directly associated with blood loss. Diminished nutritional status is an indirect result of fatigue associated with anemia that leads to decreased appetite and weight loss.

PREVENTION

Oral contraceptive therapy may be instituted prophylactically in patients undergoing treatment with SSRIs to prevent the development of menorrhagia.[86,96] Oral contraceptives may also help prevent recurrent episodes of bleeding in patients with a history of menorrhagia/menometrorrhagia.[98] Avoidance of other platelet-inhibiting agents such as aspirin may decrease the risk of drug-induced menorrhagia or menometrorrhagia (Table 34-6).[97,99]

MANAGEMENT

Drug-induced menorrhagia is usually effectively treated with combination oral contraceptive therapy. Product selection is generally based on patient and prescriber preference.[86,96,99] Patients who have had menorrhagia for an extended time may also require iron-replacement therapy until the hemoglobin concentration returns to normal. In patients with IUDs, therapy with the antioxidant vitamin E (100 international units once every other day for 14 days) has been successful in attenuating menorrhagia.[83] Drug-induced menometrorrhagia can be effectively treated with GnRH agonists such as leuprolide (3.75 mg intramuscularly once monthly) or goserelin (3.6 mg intramuscularly once monthly).[94,96] When a patient is experiencing drug-induced menorrhagia or menometrorrhagia, the risks and benefits of discontinuation of the causative agent should be weighed. If the causative agent is discontinued, it may take up to 3 months for symptoms to resolve completely.

INFORMATION FOR PATIENTS

Patients receiving drugs that may cause menorrhagia or menometrorrhagia should be counseled that heavy or prolonged menstrual cycles (at regular or irregular intervals) may occur and that this should prompt them to seek medical attention.

DYSMENORRHEA

CAUSATIVE AGENTS

Drug-induced dysmenorrhea is associated with known uterine stimulants such as oxytocin and known vasoconstrictors such as vasopressin (antidiuretic hormone) (Table 34-1).[102] Estrogen and progesterone are also believed to be associated with some cases of drug-induced dysmenorrhea.[100,101]

EPIDEMIOLOGY

Dysmenorrhea is one of the most common gynecologic symptoms of menstruating women, with an incidence ranging from 3% to 90%.[101] The incidence and magnitude of drug-induced dysmenorrhea is unknown. It is possible that dysmenorrhea has been overlooked as a drug-induced condition, and occurrences therefore may be underreported.

MECHANISMS

Dysmenorrhea occurs often with normal ovulation because release of arachidonic acid promotes the release and elevated serum concentrations of prostaglandin-2α that mediates vasoconstriction and leukotrienes initiating the inflammation that produces cramps, bloating, and abdominal discomfort.[102] Drug-induced dysmenorrhea associated with the administration of the combination of oxytocin and vasopressin occurs as a result of vasopressin-related antidiuretic effects that alter the uterine contractions stimulated by oxytocin into a dysrhythmic and painful pattern (Table 34-2).[101]

The mechanism of estrogen- and progesterone-induced dysmenorrhea is not well understood. It has been suggested that the rapid fluctuations in serum hormone concentrations, primarily progesterone withdrawal, activates the inflammation cascade, causing pelvic congestion (swelling) and contributing to the development of dysmenorrhea (Table 34-2).[103,104]

CLINICAL PRESENTATION AND DIFFERENTIAL DIAGNOSIS

Dysmenorrhea is a pelvic pain that occurs in relationship to menses. It is associated with a variety of symptoms, including nausea, vomiting, diarrhea, bloating, headache, backache, syncope, dizziness, breast tenderness, abdominal cramping, mood changes, nervousness, and fatigue (Table 34-3). Symptoms typically present within 24–48 hours before menstruation begins and usually continue for 48–72 hours after menstruation commences.[101] Drug-induced dysmenorrhea must be distinguished from other causes of dysmenorrhea. Pelvic pain with menses can be a natural physiologic occurrence in association with ovulation or premenstrual syndrome or may have other primary or secondary causes, including adverse effects of drugs (Table 34-4).[101,102]

RISK FACTORS

Diets high in omega-6 fatty acids, including most Western diets, increase the release of arachidonic acid after progesterone withdrawal and may result in inflammation and cramping (Table 34-5).[101] Early menarche and heavier menstrual blood flow are both associated with an increased risk of drug-induced dysmenorrhea.[103,104] Individuals who have more than one first-degree relative with dysmenorrhea have a higher risk of drug-induced dysmenorrhea.[101,105]

MORBIDITY AND MORTALITY

Dysmenorrhea is one of the most common gynecologic symptoms associated with repeated absenteeism from school or work.[102] Although dysmenorrhea has significant impact on quality of life, it is not associated with mortality.

PREVENTION

Drug-induced dysmenorrhea can be prevented by avoiding the use of uterine-stimulating drugs in women predisposed to the disorder. In women with a history of dysmenorrhea, prophylactic use of NSAIDs (e.g., ibuprofen 400 mg orally every 6 hours or 800 mg orally every 8 hours or cyclooxygenase [COX]-2 inhibitors such as celecoxib 200 mg orally once daily) often is effective to decrease and limit the symptoms of drug-induced dysmenorrhea (Table 34-6).[102,103,106]

MANAGEMENT

Management of drug-induced dysmenorrhea should be individualized to the patient's pain threshold, contraception goals, and overall health status. Hot or cold compresses may help provide some temporary relief. NSAIDs (e.g., ibuprofen 400 mg orally every 6 hours or 800 mg orally every 8 hours) or COX-2 inhibitors (e.g., celecoxib 200 mg orally once daily) are effective for alleviation of pain, and therapy should be continued until the end of menses (Table 34-7).[102,105] In patients with lower pain thresholds, short-term use of combination opioid products might be considered.[103,105] Acetaminophen alone is not as effective as NSAIDs in controlling the inflammation and symptoms associated with dysmenorrhea.[106]

INFORMATION FOR PATIENTS

Patients taking medications that may cause dysmenorrhea should be informed of the possibility and should be instructed to take anti-inflammatory medications at the first symptoms. Prompt treatment will help control the pain and can prevent the development or more significant discomfort. Patients should take NSAIDs with food to avoid development of gastrointestinal distress. Patients with sulfa allergies should avoid the use of COX-2 inhibitors.

SEXUAL DYSFUNCTION

Human sexual response can be classified into five phases: desire, excitement, plateau, orgasm, and resolution.[107] Sexual desire is an innate component of human social well-being. Any impairment or abnormality in the human sexual response is defined as sexual dysfunction.

CAUSATIVE AGENTS

Drug-induced sexual dysfunction often contributes to patient nonadherence to important medications, including antihypertensives, antidepressants, antipsychotics, sedatives, antiretroviral agents, androgen antagonists, and narcotics.[107-111] Alcohol may also interfere with sexual function. Sexual dysfunction can be classified into two categories: disorders of libido and disorders of excitement and orgasm. Disorders of libido are generally mediated by neuronal factors, whereas disorders of excitement and orgasm generally involve the genital organs. Drugs associated with sexual dysfunction in women are listed in Table 34-1.[101-112,117-122]

EPIDEMIOLOGY

Drug-induced sexual dysfunction in women is often underreported but is one of the contributing factors to nonadherence to prescribed pharmacotherapy and decreased quality of life.[111] It is difficult to distinguish drug-induced sexual dysfunction from the effects of specific diseases on sexual function. This is especially true with psychiatric disorders, where the disease itself has profound effects on social and sexual function.[112] Since the success of sildenafil and similar drugs for the treatment of erectile dysfunction, there has been increased attention to the incidence of drug-induced sexual dysfunction.[112] Antidepressants have been associated with decreased libido and sexual dysfunction, with an incidence in women ranging from 16.3% to 57%.[113-115] Antipsychotic agents such as haloperidol, risperidone, and thioridazine have been associated with a 28–93% incidence of drug-induced sexual dysfunction in women.[116-121] Antiretroviral agents are associated with an incidence of drug-induced sexual dysfunction of 40%.[110] The incidence of drug-induced sexual dysfunction associated with the use of antihypertensive agents in women is approximately 11%.[122]

MECHANISMS

Drug-induced sexual dysfunction is often associated with agents that affect the autonomic and central nervous systems and with agents that elevate serum prolactin concentrations (Table 34-2). For example, antipsychotic agents are known to elevate serum prolactin concentrations via inhibition of dopamine-2 receptors that are responsible for blocking prolactin secretion.[123-125] The mechanism by which prolactin diminishes libido and causes orgasm disturbances is not well understood.[110,111,116,122,125] Elevated serum prolactin concentrations have been associated with decreasing serum testosterone concentrations, which may contribute to diminished libido.[126]

Drug-induced sexual dysfunction, primarily loss of libido and orgasm dysfunction, has been associated with all classes of antidepressant agents.[112,125,127] Although the mechanism involved is not well understood, antidepressants may cause sexual dysfunction by altering central serotonergic activity and indirectly influencing adrenergic activity. Alterations in central serotonergic activity may disrupt hypothalamic–pituitary axis regulation of hormone release, including the release of testosterone. Indirect effects on adrenergic activity may contribute to direct effects on gonads, leading to decreases in muscle tension, vaginal lubrication, or both.

Antihypertensive agents are more often associated with erectile dysfunction and diminished libido in men. However, these drugs may also decrease libido in women via antiandrogenic and antidopaminergic activity. The mechanism by which antiretroviral agents induce sexual dysfunction is not well understood. It has been shown that serum hormone concentrations are not altered in patients receiving antiretroviral agents, suggesting that the mechanism of antiretroviral-induced sexual dysfunction involves a yet to be determined nonhormone-related pathway.[110]

CLINICAL PRESENTATION AND DIFFERENTIAL DIAGNOSIS

Identifying individuals who have drug-induced sexual dysfunction can be difficult because patients are often embarrassed and hesitant to report sexual complications to the healthcare team.[128] Healthcare providers should specifically ask questions regarding sexual activity and relations and should volunteer information to dispel misconceptions that patients may have about sexuality to alleviate fear, guilt, or frustration regarding sexual dysfunction.

Once comfortable, patients may begin to volunteer information regarding symptoms they are experiencing. These may include vaginismus, dyspareunia, or loss of libido or orgasm dysfunction (Table 34-3). Dyspareunia can often be attributed to physical disorders of the vagina, such as decreased lubrication, infections, or local irritation. Patients with loss of libido or orgasm dysfunction often present with other psychological symptoms, including depression, fatigue, anxiety, anger, or fear (Table 34-4). Again, extensive counseling and discussion is necessary to sort through the vague symptoms. A close evaluation of the medication history is necessary to determine whether sexual dysfunction can be attributed to a drug. Drug-induced sexual dysfunction usually occurs within 2 weeks of initiating therapy with the culprit agent, although SSRI-induced sexual dysfunction may take longer to manifest.

RISK FACTORS

Specific disease-related factors may increase the risk of drug-induced sexual dysfunction. These include endocrine disorders associated with hormone imbalances such as hypogonadism or hypothyroidism; neurologic/psychiatric impairments such as schizophrenia or depression; surgery such as hysterectomy, oophorectomy, or vulvovaginal resections; or pelvic irradiation that directly alters ovarian function or the structure or function of the vagina.[129] Anxiety, stress, depression, or substance abuse may compound the patient's psychological ability to tolerate and discuss symptoms associated with sexual dysfunction (Table 34-5).

Drug-induced sexual dysfunction is not always dose-related, but in some cases, especially those caused by antihypertensive agents or SSRIs, using lower doses or instituting "drug holidays" may help minimize symptoms.[112,122] Of course, the risk versus benefit would need to be part of this decision process before implementing a drug holiday or using lower doses.

MORBIDITY AND MORTALITY

The physical complications of drug-induced sexual dysfunction are not life-threatening. However, the psychological stress generated from these complications can significantly impact mental health (depression, anxiety, disposition) and quality of life and have negative impact on relationships with partners, family, and friends.

PREVENTION

Education is the most important component of prevention and may help lead to acceptance and improve the ability of the patient to communicate her concerns regarding sexual dysfunction. Counseling should include education regarding the potential for sexual complications associated with prescribed therapy and possible treatment options for symptom management. The risk of drug-induced sexual dysfunction should be weighed against the prescribed drug's potential therapeutic benefit and the availability of alternative treatment options. Avoidance of agents known to be associated with sexual dysfunction is recommended if and when acceptable alternative agents for treatment are available (Table 34-6).

MANAGEMENT

The first step in the management of drug-induced sexual dysfunction is completion of a thorough physical examination to determine any possible physical causes that could be contributing to symptoms. The patient's medication history should be closely evaluated to identify drugs that may be causing sexual dysfunction. Once a drug is identified as the likely source of sexual complications, alternative medical treatment options should be considered. It is sometimes reasonable to substitute therapy with other agents within the same class to determine whether symptoms improve. Although symptoms generally improve within 2 weeks after discontinuation of the causative agent, in some cases sexual function may not completely return to normal without additional interventions to treat the sexual dysfunction. This is often the case with sexual dysfunction associated with antipsychotic agents, where treatment of the drug-induced disease may be confounded by the underlying psychiatric disorder.[125]

Topical estrogen (estradiol 0.05–0.1 mg vaginal ring inserted once every 3 months, or estradiol

0.01% cream vaginally 2–4 g once daily for 2 weeks followed by once-weekly maintenance) may help improve arousal dysfunction by increasing vaginal secretions and engorgement.[128] Other pharmacotherapy to increase libido could include phosphodiesterase-5 inhibitors such as sildenafil citrate (50 mg orally 1 hour before sexual activity). In addition, vaginal lubricants and moisturizers may be used to relieve vaginal dryness and improve genital arousal (Table 34-7).[128] Mechanical stimulatory devices, such as vibrators, that increase blood flow to the vaginal muscle can be used in conjunction with pharmacologic interventions to optimize relief of symptoms.[128]

When treating a patient with drug-induced sexual dysfunction, it is extremely important to be sensitive and supportive. Psychological support and assurance can be extremely effective in alleviating the stress and anxiety experienced by patients with drug-induced sexual dysfunction.[129]

INFORMATION FOR PATIENTS

Sexual function is an important component of adult relationships. Patients who are taking antipsychotic agents, antidepressants, antihypertensive agents, or other drugs associated with sexual dysfunction should be counseled regarding the potential for occurrence of this drug-induced disease and should be instructed to discuss symptoms such as painful intercourse, vaginal dryness, lack of or decreased orgasm, or diminished libido with their healthcare provider.

INFERTILITY IN WOMEN

CAUSATIVE AGENTS

Drug-induced infertility is a tragic yet predictable outcome associated with treatment with cytotoxic chemotherapy agents. Although there is potential for drug-induced infertility after treatment with any cytotoxic agent, the most common classes of agents that cause infertility include the alkylating agents, platinum analogues, antitumor antibiotics, antimetabolites, and vinca alkaloids (Table 34-1).[130-144] Even patients who may resume normal menses after completion of cytotoxic chemotherapy may not have a viable ovarian follicular reserve.[132] Whereas cytotoxic agents are associated with permanent infertility, caffeine is associated with a reversible or transient infertility.[133-137] Caffeine is found in many beverages and is an additive in both prescription and nonprescription medications. In addition to infertility, caffeine has also been associated with a dose-related increased risk of miscarriage in the first trimester.[138] Many antiepileptic drugs have been associated with endocrine dysfunction and drug-induced infertility that is reversible once medication is stopped.[78-80,88,139-144]

EPIDEMIOLOGY

Women with cancer are most often afflicted with drug-induced infertility after completion of a cytotoxic chemotherapy regimen. However, lower doses of these same cytotoxic agents are used in treatment of systemic lupus erythematosus or other autoimmune disorders and can cause drug-induced infertility in these situations as well. In addition, the very prevalent use of caffeine today could put many women at risk for reversible drug-induced infertility.

MECHANISMS

Antineoplastic drugs have a direct toxic effect on oocytes, decreasing follicular formation and halting ovulation resulting in permanent drug-induced infertility.[56] This also leads to decreased FSH and LH release, resulting in decreased ovarian function and induction of infertility.[68-74] Antiepileptic drugs have also been reported to increase the serum concentration of hormone-binding globulin, resulting in decreased binding of estradiol, which can result in drug-induced infertility.[75-79] The mechanism of drug-induced infertility is not as well understood for caffeine (Table 34-2).

CLINICAL PRESENTATION AND DIFFERENTIAL DIAGNOSIS

Drug-induced infertility associated with cytotoxic agents is fairly easy to recognize because most of these drugs cause infertility. Conversely, the diagnosis of reversible drug-induced infertility associated with caffeine is more difficult to establish and requires a detailed medication and diet history. The obvious and primary symptoms of drug-induced infertility include inability to conceive and/or frequent miscarriages (Table 34-3). Patients may also have cessation of menses or irregular menses. Underlying or contributing endocrine or metabolic conditions should be ruled out as well as possible early menopause. Conditions to consider in the differential diagnosis of drug-induced infertility are presented in Table 34-4.

RISK FACTORS

The probability of permanent drug-induced infertility after chemotherapy increases proportionally with advancing age.[144,145] In patients with autoimmune disorders, there are specific disease-related factors that may increase the risk of drug-induced infertility, including the presence of antiovarian antibodies, polyglandular insufficiency, and viral infections.[146-148] Epilepsy also has been associated with an increased risk for endocrine disorders resulting in infertility (Table 34-5).[149]

MORBIDITY AND MORTALITY

As with drug-induced sexual dysfunction, the physical complications of drug-induced infertility are not life-threatening. However, finite and predictable infertility can be associated with significant psychological stress reflected in a diminished mental health (i.e., depression, reduced self-esteem), a decreased quality of life, and a negative impact on relationships with partners, family, and friends.

PREVENTION

Instructing patients to reduce or to eliminate the frequent consumption of caffeine-containing beverages and medications from their diet can prevent caffeine-induced infertility. Patients will find that fertility is regained within months after the discontinuation of caffeine consumption. Efforts to prevent drug-induced infertility associated with other agents may not be as successful. Some studies have suggested the use of oral contraceptives during chemotherapy in younger patients may help prevent permanent drug-induced infertility by temporarily halting ovulation, which may protect oocytes from exposure to offending chemotherapy.[144] Another pharmacologic option that has been proposed, although still controversial, is the prophylactic use of GnRH agonists to also temporarily halt ovulation, which may protect oocytes from exposure to offending chemotherapy to prevent permanent drug-induced infertility (Table 34-6).[61,150,151]

MANAGEMENT

Management strategies for drug-induced infertility are listed in Table 34-7. Prior to receiving cytotoxic chemotherapy, patients need to be made aware of the high risk and likelihood of drug-induced infertility, which in most cases will be permanent. These patients need to consider multiple options for cryopreservation of eggs or embryos to preserve fertility options once treatment is completed. Factors that can influence this decision include time restraints (how quickly treatment needs to be initiated), the type of cancer or disease being treated (specifically if estrogen-sensitive), whether or not the patient has a partner, desire to have (more) children, and the patient's age. For those with a partner and enough time before cytotoxic therapy begins, cryopreservation of embryos is preferred and has the highest success rate.[152] Other cryopreservation options include freezing of oocytes, ovarian cortex, or follicles.[152,153] Although these options do not require a partner and can be accomplished in less time than cryopreservation of embryos, the potential of achieving viable pregnancies is less than with cryopreservation of embryos.

For patients receiving antiepileptic drugs, infertility is often, but not always, reversible once the culprit agent is removed and endocrine function is allowed to normalize. Unfortunately, the option to discontinue medications is generally available only for patients whose seizure disorder can be managed effectively by an alternative, newer antiepileptic agent.[149]

INFORMATION FOR PATIENTS

Infertility is a highly sensitive and emotional topic for most women and couples. In some cases, fertility is the essence of a women's identity. Patients about to receive cytotoxic chemotherapy need to be educated regarding the multiple methods available to preserve fertility options after completion of treatment. Once treatment is completed and residual treatment-related toxicities have resolved, patients should be encouraged to exercise fertility options at that time to avoid additional complications with pregnancy. In patients receiving antiepileptic drugs, the potential for infertility should be discussed prospectively and alternative agents should be considered. Patients should understand that there is no guarantee that fertility will return after removal of the offending agent. Finally, patients with drug-induced infertility associated with caffeine intake should be counseled on the benefits of the short-term cessation of all caffeine products and caffeine-containing medications. Patients should be reminded that caffeine withdrawal side effects are temporary and resolve quickly and that the potential benefit of regaining fertility and the prevention of miscarriages outweighs any short-term discomfort.

REFERENCES

1. Artini PG, Fasciani A, Cela V et al. Fertility drugs and ovarian cancer. *Gynecol Endocrinol.* 1997; 11:59-68.
2. Tucker KE. Reproductive toxicity of ovulation induction. *Semin Reprod Endocrinol.* 1996; 14:345-53.
3. Delvigne A, Rozenberg S. Epidemiology and prevention of ovarian hyperstimulation syndrome (OHSS): a review. *Hum Reprod Update.* 2002; 8:559-77.
4. Mitchell SY, Fletcher HM, Williams E. Ovarian hyperstimulation syndrome associated with clomiphene citrate. *West Indian Med J.* 2001; 50:227-29.
5. Dourron NE, Williams DB. Prevention and treatment of ovarian hyperstimulation syndrome. *Semin Reprod Endocrinol.* 1996; 14:355-65.
6. Brinsden PR, Wada I, Tan SL et al. Diagnosis, prevention and management of ovarian hyperstimulation syndrome. *Br J Obstet Gynaecol.* 1995; 102:767-72.
7. Derman SG, Adashi EY. Adverse effects of fertility drugs. *Drug Saf.* 1994; 11:408-21.
8. Elchalal U, Schenker JG. The pathophysiology of ovarian hyperstimulation syndrome: views and ideas. *Hum Reprod.* 1997;12: 1129-37.
9. Rutkowski A, Dubinsky I. Ovarian hyperstimulation syndrome: imperatives for the emergency physician. *J Emerg Med.* 1999; 17:669-72.
10. Thakur R, EL-Menabawey M. Combined intra-uterine and extra-uterine pregnancy associated with mild hyperstimulation syndrome after clomiphene ovulation induction. *Hum Reprod.* 1996; 11:1583-4.
11. Navot D, Relou A, Birkenfeld A et al. Risk factors and prognostic variables in the ovarian hyperstimulation syndrome. *Am J Obstet Gynecol.* 1988; 159:210-5.
12. Delvigne A, Demoulin A, Smitz J et al. The ovarian hyperstimulation syndrome in in-vitro fertilization: a Belgian multicentric study: I. Clinical and biological features. *Hum Reprod.* 1993; 8:1353-60.
13. Cremisi HD, Mitch WE. Profound hypotension and sodium retention with the ovarian hyperstimulation syndrome. *Am J Kidney Dis.* 1994; 24:854-7.
14. Buyalos RP, Lee CT. Polycystic ovary syndrome: pathophysiology and outcome with in vitro fertilization. *Fertil Steril.* 1996; 65:1-10.
15. MacDougall MJ, Tan SL, Jacobs HS. In vitro fertilization and the ovarian hyperstimulation syndrome. *Hum Reprod.* 1992; 7:597-600.
16. Navot D, Bergh PA, Laufer N. Ovarian hyperstimulation syndrome in novel reproductive technologies: prevention and treatment. *Fertil Steril.* 1992; 58:249-51.
17. Salle B, de Saint Hilaire P, Devouassoux M et al. Another two cases of ovarian tumors in women who had undergone multiple ovulation induction cycles. *Hum Reprod.* 1997; 12: 1732-5.
18. Grimbizis G, Tarlatzis BC, Bontis J et al. Two cases of ovarian tumors in women who had undergone multiple ovarian stimulation attempts. *Hum Reprod.* 1995; 10:520-3.
19. Hull ME, Kriner M. Schneider E et al. Ovarian cancer after successful ovulation induction: a case report. *J Reprod Med.* 1996; 41:52-4.
20. Adewole IF, Babarnisa IA, Thomas JO et al. Ovarian cancer associated with ovulation induction: a case report. *Afr J Med Sci.* 1997; 26:203-4.
21. Weissman A, Barash A, Shapiro H et al. Ovarian hyperstimulation following the sole administration of agonistic analogues of gonadotropin releasing hormone. *Hum Reprod.* 1998; 13:3421-4.
22. Klip H, Burger CW, Kenemans P et al. Cancer risk associated with subfertility and ovulation induction: a review. *Cancer Causes Control.* 2000; 11:319-44.
23. Anderson SM, Dimitrievich E. Ovulation induction for infertility is it safe or not? *SD J Med Pharm.* 1996; 49:419-21.
24. Fathalla MF. Incessant ovulation: a factor in ovarian cancer? *Lancet.* 1971; 2:163.
25. Spinillo A, Capuzzo E, Acciano S et al. Effect of antibiotic use on the prevalence of symptomatic vulvovaginal candidiasis. *Am J Obstet Gynecol.* 1999; 180:14-7.
26. Check JH, Check ML. A case report demonstrating that follicle maturing drugs may create an adverse uterine environment even when not used for controlled ovarian hyperstimulation. *Clin Exp Obstet Gynecol.* 2001; 28:217-8.
27. Bristow RE, Karlan BY. Ovulation induction, infertility, and ovarian cancer risk. *Fertil Steril.* 1996; 66:499-507.

28. Shushan A, Paltiel O, Schenker JG. Induction of ovulation and borderline ovarian cancer: the hormonal connection? *Eur J Obstet Gynecol.* 1999; 85:71-4.
29. Kashyap S, Moher D, Fung MFK. Assisted reproductive technology and the incidence of ovarian cancer: a meta analysis. *Obstet Gynecol.* 2004; 103:785-94.
30. Whelan JG, Vlahos NF. The ovarian hyperstimulation syndrome. *Fertil Steril.* 2000; 73:883-96.
31. Forman RG, Fyrdman R, Egan D et al. Severe ovarian hyperstimulation syndrome using agonists of gonadotropins-releasing hormone for in vitro fertilization: a European series and a proposal for prevention. *Fertil Steril.* 1990; 53:502-9.
32. Asch RH, Ivery G, Goldsman M et al. The use of intravenous albumin in patients at high risk for severe ovarian hyperstimulation syndrome. *Hum Reprod.* 1993; 8:1015-20.
33. Shoham Z, Weissman A, Barsh A et al. Intravenous albumin for the prevention of severe ovarian hyperstimulation syndrome in an in vitro fertilization program: a prospective, randomized, placebo-controlled study. *Fertil Steril.* 1994; 62:137-42.
34. Shalev E, Giladi Y, Matilsky M et al. Decreased incidence of severe ovarian hyperstimulation syndrome in high risk in vitro fertilization patients receiving intravenous albumin: a prospective study. *Hum Reprod.* 1995; 10:1373-6.
35. Turan C, Unal O, Dansuk R et al. Successful management of an ovarian enlargement resembling ovarian hyperstimulation in a premenopausal breast cancer patient receiving tamoxifen with cotreatment of GnRH-agonist. *Eur J Obstet Gynecol Reprod Biol.* 2001; 97:105-7.
36. American Society for Reproductive Medicine. Ovarian hyperstimulation syndrome. *Fertil Steril.* 2003; 80:1309-14.
37. Wilton L, Kollarova M, Heeley E, Shakir S. Relative risk of vaginal candidias after use of antibiotics compared with antidepressants in women: postmarketing surveillance data in England. *Drug Saf.* 2003; 26:589-97.
38. Dan M, Kaneti N, Levin D et al. Vaginitis in a gynecologic practice in Israel: causes and risk factors. *Isr Med Assoc J.* 2003; 5:629-32.
39. Nyirjesy P, Sobel JD. Vulvovaginal candidiasis. *Obstet Gynecol Clin North Am.* 2003; 30:671-84.
40. Parmet S, Cassio MA, Glass RM. Vaginal symptoms. *JAMA.* 2004; 291:1406-7.
41. Pirotta MV, Gunn JM, Chondros P. "Not thrush again!" Women's experience of post-antibiotic vulvovaginitis. *Med J Aust.* 2003; 179:43-6.
42. Xu J, Schwartz K, Bartoces M et al. Effect of antibiotics on vulvovaginal candidiasis: a MetroNet study. *J Am Board Fam Med.* 2008; 21:261-8.
43. Carlson P, Richardson M, Paavonen J. Evaluation of the Oricult-N dipslide for laboratory diagnosis of vaginal candidiasis. *J Clin Microbiol.* 2000; 38:1063-5.
44. Bro F. The diagnosis of candidal vaginitis in general practice. *Scand J Prim Health Care.* 1989; 7:19-22
45. Centers for Disease Control and Prevention. Sexually transmitted disease treatment guidelines 2002. *MMWR Recomm Rep.* 2002; 51:45-7.
46. Wilton LV, Kollarova M, Heeley E et al. Relative risk of vaginal candidiasis after the use of antibiotics compared with antidepressants in women. *Drug Saf.* 2003; 26:589-97.
47. ACOG Practice Bulletin. Clinical management guidelines for obstetrician-gynecologists. *Obstet Gynecol.* 2006; 72:1-12.
48. Sturkenboom MCJM, Middelbeek A, De Jong Van Den berg LTW et al. Vulvo-vaginal candidiasis associated with acitretin. *J Clin Epidemiol.* 1995; 48:991-7.
49. Carcio HA, Clark-Secor RM. Vulvovaginal candidiasis: a current update. *Nurse Pract Forum.* 1992; 3:135.
50. Burstein GR, Murray PJ. Diagnosis and management of sexually transmitted diseases among adolescents. *Pediatr Rev.* 2003; 24:119-27.
51. Ryan CA, Courtois BN, Haules SE et al. Risk assessment, symptoms and signs as predictors of vulvovaginal and cervical infections in an urban US STD clinic: implications for use of STD algorithms. *Sex Transm Infect.* 1998; 74(suppl 1):559-76.
52. Patel DA, Gillespie B, Sobel JD et al. Risk of factors for recurrent vulvovaginal candidiasis in women receiving maintenance antifungal therapy: results of a prospective cohort study. *Am J Obstet Gynecol.* 2004; 190:644-53.
53. Petersen EE, Magnani P. Efficacy and safety of vitamin C vaginal tablets in treatment of non-specific vaginitis: a randomized, double-blind placebo-controlled study. *Eur J Obstet Gynecol Reprod Biol.* 2004; 117:70-5.
54. Anderson MR, Klink K, Cohrssen A. Evaluation of vaginal complaints. *JAMA.* 2004; 291:1368-79.
55. Datey S, Gaur LN, Saxena BN. Vaginal bleeding patterns of women using different contraceptive methods (implants, injectables, IUDs, oral pills): an Indian experience. *Contraception.* 1995; 51:155-65.
56. Minton SE, Munster PN. Chemotherapy induced amenorrhea and fertility in women undergoing adjuvant treatment for breast cancer. *Cancer Control.* 2002; 9:466-72.
57. Hipkin LJ. The induction of amenorrhea. *J R Army Med Corps.* 1992; 138:15-8.
58. Contreras G, Pardo V, Leclercq B et al. Sequential therapies for proliferative lupus nephritis. *N Engl J Med.* 2004; 350:971-80.
59. Hickey M, d'Arcangues C. Vaginal bleeding disturbances and implantable contraceptives. *Contraception.* 2002; 65:75-84.
60. Practice Committee, American Society for Reproduction Medicine. Ovarian tissue cryopreservation: a committee opinion. *Fertil Steril.* 2014; 101:1237-43.
61. Blumenfeld Z, Shapiro D, Shteinberg M et al. Preservation of fertility and ovarian function and minimizing gonadotoxicity in young women with systemic lupus erythematosus treated by chemotherapy. *Lupus.* 2000; 9:401-5.
62. Schilsky RL, Sherins RJ, Hubbard SM et al. Long-term follow up of ovarian function in women treated with MOPP chemotherapy for Hodgkin's disease. *Am J Med.* 1981; 71:552-6.
63. McDermott EM, Powerll RJ. Incidence of ovarian failure in systemic lupus erythematosus after treatment with pulse cyclophosphamide. *Ann Rheum Dis.* 1996; 55:224-9.
64. Blumenfeld, Z. Gynaecologic concerns for young women exposed to gonadotoxic chemotherapy. *Curr Opin Obstet Gynecol.* 2003; 15:359-70.
65. Whitehead E, Shalet SM, Blackledge G et al. The effect of combination chemotherapy on ovarian function in women treated for Hodgkin's disease. *Cancer.* 1983; 52:988-93.
66. Dana-Haeri J, Oxely J, Richens A. Reductions of free testosterone by antiepileptic drugs. *BMJ.* 1982; 284:85-6.
67. Potter C, Willis D, Sharp HL et al. Primary and secondary amenorrhea with spironolactone therapy in chronic liver disease. *J Pediatr.* 1992; 121:141-3.
68. Arnold BJ, Cumming CE, Lees AW et al. Tamoxifen in breast cancer: symptom reporting. *Breast J.* 2001; 2001:97-100.
69. Edmonds SEF, Montgomery JC. Reversible ovarian failure induced by a Chinese herbal medicine: lei gong teng. *Br J Obstet Gynaecol.* 2003; 110:77-8.
70. Nygren KG, Rybo G. Prostaglandins and menorrhagia. *Acta Obstet Gynecol Scand Suppl.* 1983; 113:101-3.
71. Malo JW, Bezdicek BJ. Secondary amenorrhea: a protocol for pinpointing the underlying cause. *Postgrad Med.* 1986; 79:86-95.
72. Sarkola T, Makisalo H, Fukunaga T et al. Acute effect of alcohol on estradiol, estrone, progesterone, prolactin, cortisol, and luteinizing hormone in premenopausal women. *Alcohol Clin Exp Res.* 1999; 23:976-82.
73. Lappohn RE, van de Wiel HB, Brownell J. The effect of two dopaminergic drugs on menstrual function and psychological state in hyperprolactinemia. *Fertil Steril.* 1992; 58:321-7.

74. Faundes A, Alvrez-Sanchez F, Brache V et al. Hormonal changes associated with bleeding during low dose progestogen contraception delivered by norplant subdermal implants. *Adv Contracept*. 1991; 7:85-94.
75. Isojarvi J. Reproductive dysfunction in women with epilepsy. *Neurology*. 2003; 61(suppl 2):S27-34.
76. Beastall GH, Cowan RA, Gray JMB et al. Hormone binding globulins and anticonvulsant therapy. *Scott Med J*. 1985; 30:101-5.
77. Murialdo G, Galimberti CA, Gianelli MV et al. Effects of valproate, phenobarbital and carbamazepine on sex steroid setup in women with epilepsy. *Clin Neuropharmacol*. 1998; 21:52-8.
78. Victor A, Lundberg PO, Johansson EDB. Induction of sex hormone binding globulin by phenytoin. *BMJ*. 1977; 2:934-5.
79. Isojarvi JIT, Laatikainen TJ, Knip M et al. Obesity and endocrine disorders in women taking valproate for epilepsy. *Ann Neurol*. 1996; 39:579-84.
80. Giudice LC. Insulin-like growth factors and ovarian follicular development. *Endocr Rev*. 1992; 13:641-9.
81. Conover CA, Phillip DKL, Kanaley JA et al. Insulin regulation of insulin-like growth factor binding protein-1 in obese and nonobese humans. *J Clin Endocrinol Metab*. 1992; 74:1355-60.
82. Dasgupta PR, Dutta S, Banerjee P et al. Vitamin E (alpha tocopherol) in the management of menorrhagia associated with the use of intrauterine contraceptive devices (IUCD). *Int J Fertil*. 1983; 28:55-6.
83. Blumenfield Z, Dann E, Aviv I et al. Fertility after treatment for Hodgkin's disease. *Ann Oncol*. 2002; 13(suppl 1):138-47.
84. Oktay K, Kan MT, Rosenwaks Z. Recent progress in oocyte and ovarian tissue cryopreservation and transplantation. *Curr Opin Obstet Gynecol*. 2001; 13:263-8.
85. Layton D, Clark DWJ, Pearce GL et al. Is there an association between selective serotonin reuptake inhibitors and risk of abnormal bleeding? *Eur J Clin Pharmacol*. 2001; 57:167-76.
86. Murialdo G, Galimberti CA, Magri F et al. Menstrual cycle and ovary alterations in women with epilepsy on antileptic therapy. *J Endocrinol Invest*. 1997; 20:519-26.
87. Larsen EC, Muller J, Schmiegelow K et al. Reduced ovarian function in long term survivors of radiation- and chemotherapy-treated childhood cancer. *J Clin Endocrinol Metab*. 2003; 88:5307-14.
88. Wathen PI, Henderson MC, Witz CA. Abnormal uterine bleeding. *Med Clin North Am*. 1995; 79:329-44.
89. Kabalak AA, Soyal OB, Urfalioglu A et al. Menometrorrhagia and tachyarrhythmia after using oral and topical ginseng. *J Womens Health*. 2004; 13:830-3.
90. Seibold JR, Korn JH, Simms R et al. Recombinant human relaxin in the treatment of scleroderma: a randomized, double-blind, placebo-controlled trial. *Ann Intern Med*. 2000; 132:871-9.
91. Nielson H. Hypermenorrhoea associated with ritonavir. *Lancet*. 1999; 353:811-2.
92. Santen FJ, Sofsky J, Bilic N et al. Mechanism of action of narcotics in the production of menstrual dysfunction in women. *Fertil Steril*. 1975; 26:538-48.
93. Bilan X. Intrauterine devices. *Best Pract Res Clin Obstet Gynecol*. 2002; 16:155-68.
94. Unemori EN, Erikson ME, Rocco SE et al. Relaxin stimulated expression of vascular endothelial growth factor in normal human endometrial cells in vitro and is associated with menometrorrhagia in women. *Hum Reprod*. 1999; 14:800-6.
95. Rivera R, Rountree W. Characteristics of menstrual problems associated with Norplant discontinuation: results of multinational study. *Contraception*. 2003; 67:373-7.
96. Donnez J, Schrurs B, Gillerot S et al. Treatment of uterine fibroids with implants of gonadotropins-releasing hormone agonist: assessment by hysterography. *Fertil Steril*. 1989; 51: 947-50.
97. Child TJ, Tan SL. Endometriosis: aetiology, pathogenesis and treatment. *Drugs*. 2001; 61:1735-50.
98. Shaw RW. Assessment of medical treatments for menorrhagia. *Br J Obstet Gynaecol*. 1994; 101(suppl 11):15-8.
99. Field CS. Dysfunctional uterine bleeding. *Prim Care*. 1988; 15:561-74.
100. Wiegratz I, Kuhl H. Long-cycle treatment with oral contraceptives. *Drugs*. 2004; 64:2447-62.
101. Deligeoroglou E. Dysmenorrhea. *Ann N Y Acad Sci*. 2000; 900:237-44.
102. Harel A. Cyclooxygenase-2 specific inhibitors in the treatment of dysmenorrhea. *J Pediatr Adolesc Gynecol*. 2004; 17:75-9.
103. Klein JR, Litt IF. Epidemiology of adolescent dysmenorrheal. *Pediatrics*. 1981; 68:661.
104. Alvin PE, Litt IF. Current status of etiology and management of dysmenorrhea in adolescents. *Pediatrics*. 1982; 70:516.
105. Smith RP. Cyclic pelvic pain and dysmenorrhea. *Obstet Gynecol Clin North Am*. 1993; 20:753-64.
106. DiGirolamo G, Sanchez AJ, De Los Santos AR et al. Is acetaminophen, and its combination with pamabrom, an effective therapeutic option in primary dysmenorrhoea? *Expert Opin Pharmacother*. 2004; 5:561-70.
107. Schiavi RC, Segraves RT. The biology of sexual dysfunction. *Psychiatr Clin North Am*. 1995; 18:7-23.
108. Nelson EB, Shah VN, Welge JA et al. A placebo-controlled, crossover trial of granisetron in SRI-induced sexual dysfunction. *J Clin Psychiatry*. 2001; 62:469-73.
109. Drugs that cause sexual dysfunction: an update. *Med Lett Drugs Ther*. 1992; 34:73-8.
110. Collazos J, Mayo J, Martinez E et al. Association between sexual disturbances and sexual hormones with specific antiretroviral drugs. *AIDS*. 2002; 16:1294-5.
111. Rosenberg KP, Bleiberg KL, Koscis J et al. A survey of sexual side effects among severely mentally ill patients taking psychotropic medications: impact on compliance. *J Sex Marital Ther*. 2003; 29:289-96.
112. Montgomery SA, Baldwin DS, Riley A. Antidepressant medications: a review of the evidence for drug-induced sexual dysfunction. *J Affect Disord*. 2002; 69:119-40.
113. Ashton AK, Hamer R, Rosen RC. Serotonin reuptake inhibitor-induced sexual dysfunction and its treatment: a large-scale retrospective study of 596 outpatients. *J Sex Marital Ther*. 1997; 23:165-76.
114. Balon R, Yeragani VK, Pohl R et al. Sexual dysfunction during antidepressant treatment. *J Clin Psychiatry*. 1993; 54:209-12.
115. Zajecka J, Mitchell S, Fawcett J. Treatment-emergent changes in sexual function with selective serotonin reuptake inhibitors as measured with the Rush Sexual Inventory. *Psychopharmacology*. 1997; 33:755-60.
116. Bobes J, Gare A-Portilla MP, Rejas J et al. Frequency of sexual dysfunction and other reproductive side-effects in patients with schizophrenia treated with risperidone, olanzapine, quetiapine, or haloperidol: the results of the EIRE study. *J Sex Marital Ther*. 2003; 29:125-47.
117. LaTorre A, Conca A, Duffy D et al. Sexual dysfunction relatated to psychotropic durgs: a critical review part II: antipsychotics. *Pharmacopsychiarty*. 2013; 46:201-8.
118. Ghadirian A, Chouinard G, Annable L. Sexual dysfunction and plasma prolactin levels in neuroleptic-treated schizophrenic outpatients. *J Nerv Ment Dis*. 1982; 170:463-7.
119. Kotin J, Wilbert DE, Verburg D et al. Thioridazine and sexual dysfunction. *Am J Psychiatry*. 1976; 133:82-5.
120. Shader R, Grinspoon L. Schizophrenia, oligospermia, and the phenothiazines. *Dis Nerv Syst*. 1967; 28:240-4.
121. Saval A, Chiodo AE. Sexual dysfunction associated with intrathecal baclofen use; a report of two cases. *J Spinal Cord Med*. 2008; 31:103-5.

122. Grimm RH Jr, Grandits GA, Prineas RJ et al. Long-term effects on sexual function of five antihypertensive drugs and nutritional hygienic treatment in hypertensive men and women: treatment of mild hypertension study (TOMHS). *Hypertension.* 1997; 29:8-14.
123. Hummer M, Kemmler G, Kurz M et al. Sexual disturbances during clozapine and haloperidol treatment for schizophrenia. *Am J Psychiatry.* 1999; 156:631-3.
124. Halbreich U, Kinon BJ, Gilmore JA et al. Elevated prolactin levels in patients with schizophrenia: mechanisms and related adverse effects. *Psychoneuroendocrinology.* 2003; 28:53-67.
125. Culter AJ. Sexual dysfunction and antipsychotic treatment. *Psychoneuroendocrinology.* 2003; 28:69-82.
126. Barnes TRE, Harvey CA. Psychiatric drugs and sexuality. In: Riley AJ, Peet M, Wilson C, eds. *Sexual pharmacology.* Oxford, England: Oxford Medical Publications; 1993:176-96.
127. Schiavi RC, Segraves RT. The biology of sexual function. *Psychiatr Clin North Am.* 1995; 18:7-23.
128. LaTorrw A, Giupponi G, Duffy D, Conca A. Sexual dysfunction related to psychotropic drugs: a critical review—Part I: antidepressants. *Pharmacopsychiatry.* 2013; 46:191-9.
129. Carmack Taylor CL, Basen-Engquist K, Shinn EH et al. Predictors of sexual functioning in ovarian cancer patients. *J Clin Oncol.* 2004; 22:881-9.
130. Meirow D. Reproduction post-chemotherapy in young cancer patients. *Mol Cell Endocrinol.* 2000; 169:123-31.
131. Maltaris T, Seufert R, Fischl R et al. The effect of cancer treatment on female fertility and strategies for preserving fertility. *Eur J Obstet Gynecol Reprod Biol.* 2007; 130:148-55.
132. Meirow D, Epstein M, Lewis H et al. Administration of cyclophosphamide at different stages of follicular maturation in mice: effects on reproductive performance and fetal malformations. *Hum Reprod.* 2001; 16:632-7.
133. Wilcox A, Weinberg C, Baird D. Caffeinated beverages and decreased fertility. *Lancet.* 1988; 2:1453-6.
134. Christianson RE, Oechsli FW, van den Berg BJ. Caffeinated beverages and decreased fertility. *Lancet.* 1989; 1:378.
135. Williams MA, Monson RR, Goldman MB et al. Coffee and delayed conception. *Lancet.* 1990; 335:1603.
136. Hatch EE, Bracken MB. Association of delay conception with caffeine consumption. *Am J Epidemiol.* 1993; 138:1082-92.
137. Williams MS, Mittendorf R, Stubblefield PG et al. Cigarettes, coffee, and preterm premature rupture of the membranes. *Am J Epidemiol.* 1992; 135:895-903.
138. Weng X, Odouli R, Li DK. Maternal caffeine consumption during pregnancy and the risk of miscarriage: a prospective cohort study. *Am J Obstet Gynecol.* 2008; 198:279.e1-8.
139. Isojarvi JIT, Laatikainen TJ, Pakarinen AJ et al. Polycystic ovaries and hyperandrogenism in women taking valproate for epilepsy. *N Engl J Med.* 1993; 329:1383-8.
140. Oppenheimer JH, Fischer LV, Nielson KM et al. Depression of the serum protein-bound iodine level by diphenylhydantoin. *J Clin Endocrinol Metab.* 1961; 21:252-62.
141. Isojarvi JIT. Serum steroid hormones and pituitary function in female epileptic patients during carbazepine. *Arch Neurol.* 1989; 46:1175-8.
142. Isojarvi JIT, Laatikainen TJ, Pakarinen AJ et al. Menstrual disorders in women with epilepsy receiving carbamazepine. *Epilepsia.* 1995; 36:676-81.
143. Isojarvi JIT, Tauboll E, Pakarinen AH et al. Altered ovarian function and cardiovascular risk factors in valproate-treated women. *Am J Med.* 2001; 111:290-6.
144. Meirow D, Nugent D. The effects of radiotherapy and chemotherapy on female reproduction. *Hum Reprod Update.* 2001; 7:535-43.
145. Behringer K, Breuer K, Reineke T et al. A report from the German Hodgkin's Lymphoma Study Group: secondary amenorrhea after Hodgkin's lymphoma is influenced by age at treatment, stage of disease, chemotherapy regimen and the use of oral contraceptives during therapy. *J Clin Oncol.* 2005; 23:7555-64.
146. Moncayo-Naveda H, Moncayo R, Benz R et al. Organ-specific antibodies against ovary in patients with systemic lupus erythematosus. *Am J Obstet Gynecol.* 1989; 160:1227-9.
147. Pasto SG, Viana VST, Mendonca BB et al. Anti-corpus luteum antibody: a novel serological marker for ovarian dysfunction in systemic lupus erythematosus? *J Rheumatology.* 1999; 26:1087-93.
148. Lieman H, Santoro N. Premature ovarian failure: a modern approach to diagnosis and treatment. *Endocrinology.* 1997; 7:314-21.
149. Isojarvi JIT. Reproductive dysfunction in women with epilepsy. *Neurology.* 2003; 61(suppl 2):S27-34.
150. Pereya PB, Mendez Ribas JM, Milone G et al. Use of GnRH analogs for functional protection of the ovary and preservation of fertility during cancer treatment in adolescents: a preliminary report. *Gynecol Oncol.* 2001; 81:391-7.
151. Blumenfield Z, Avivi I, Linn S et al. Prevention of irreversible chemotherapy-induced ovarian damage in young women with lymphoma by a gonadotropin-releasing hormone agonist in parallel to chemotherapy. *Hum Reprod.* 1996; 11:1620-6.
152. Sim AA. Fertility preservation in female cancer patients: current developments and future directions. *Fertil Steril.* 2006; 85:1-11.
153. Maltaris T, Seufert R, Fischl F et al. The effect of cancer treatment on female fertility and strategies for preserving fertility. *Eur J Obstet Gynecol.* 2007; 130:148-55.

SECTION VIII

DRUG-INDUCED GASTROINTESTINAL DISEASES

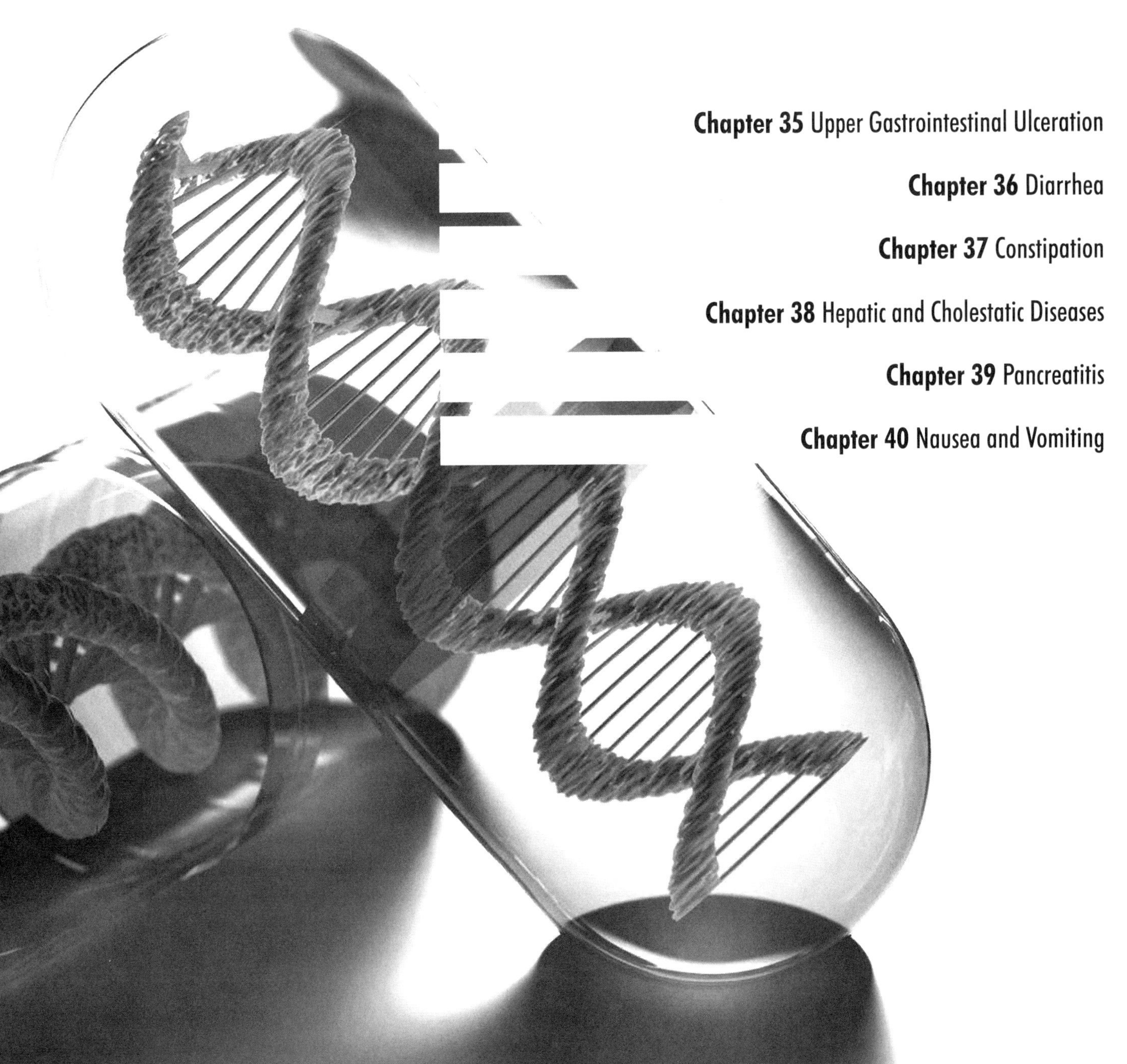

Chapter 35 Upper Gastrointestinal Ulceration

Chapter 36 Diarrhea

Chapter 37 Constipation

Chapter 38 Hepatic and Cholestatic Diseases

Chapter 39 Pancreatitis

Chapter 40 Nausea and Vomiting

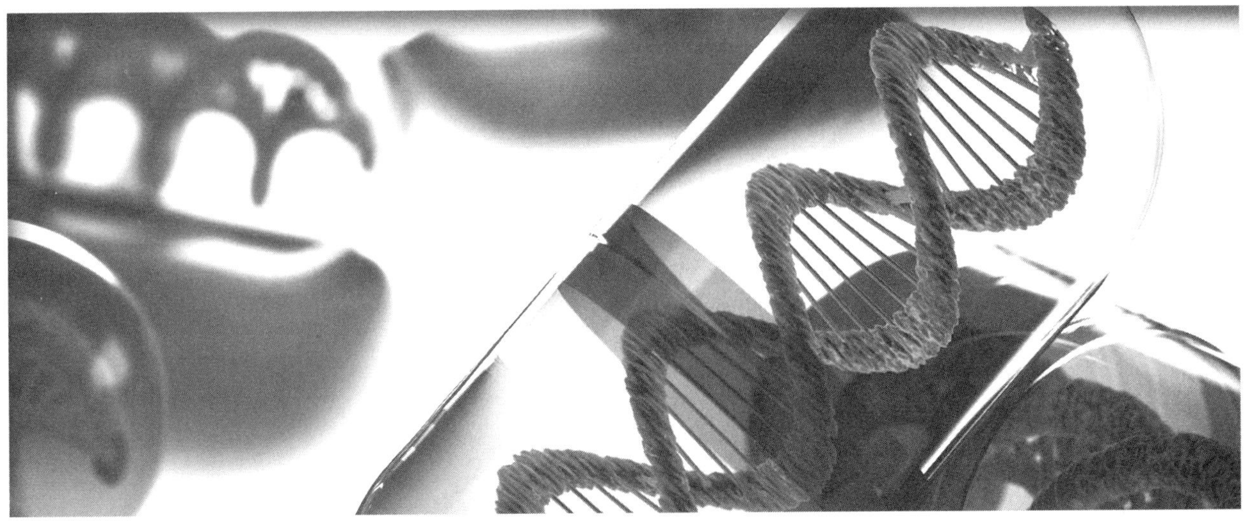

CHAPTER 35

Upper Gastrointestinal Ulceration

Dianne W. May, Micaela Carroll, and J. Russell May

The upper gastrointestinal (GI) tract consists of the mouth, pharynx, esophagus, stomach, and duodenum. The ligament of Treitz, or the suspensory muscle of the duodenum, is found at the duodenojejunal flexure and is typically used as a landmark to differentiate between the upper and lower GI tract.[1] Any injury that occurs before the ligament of Treitz would be considered an upper GI event. Drug-induced ulcerations of the upper GI tract can occur anywhere in this region before the jejunum, but the esophagus and stomach are primary targets. Patients may present with signs and symptoms that range from benign lesions with no sequelae to serious complications including GI bleeding, strictures, perforation, and obstruction. Distinguishing characteristics of drug-induced mucosal damage of the upper GI tract are typically evident on endoscopy. Understanding the mechanisms and risk factors for drug-induced upper GI ulceration can help healthcare providers minimize and manage the complications that may occur.

CAUSATIVE AGENTS

Medications that have been reported to cause upper GI ulceration are listed in **Table 35-1**.[2-19] Overall, nonsteroidal anti-inflammatory drugs (NSAIDs), including aspirin, are the most common causative agents. The risk of gastrointestinal toxicity with NSAIDs is not specific to route used. Gastrointestinal toxicity is seen with the oral route as well as the intravenous route.[20] Other medications that are commonly associated with upper GI ulceration include ferrous sulfate, quinidine, doxycycline, selective serotonin reuptake inhibitors (SSRIs), and corticosteroids (especially when used in combination with other medications that can cause ulceration).

The mucosa of the esophagus is particularly vulnerable to the direct mucosal injury that can occur with many medications. Over 70 medications have been associated with esophageal damage, including certain bisphosphonates (e.g., alendronate), potassium chloride (oral), aspirin, clindamycin, ferrous sulfate, quinidine, valproic acid (sustained-release), and tetracyclines.[2,10] Many β-lactams, including penicillin, ampicillin, amoxicillin, and cloxacillin have been implicated in causing pill-induced esophagitis. The gelatin capsule of many antibiotics is sticky and, therefore, makes the capsule prone to esophageal retention.[21] Esophageal perforation has been reported with sustained-release valproic acid,

Table 35-1 Agents Implicated in Drug-Induced Upper Gastrointestinal Ulceration

Drug	Incidence	Level of Evidence[a]
Ascorbic acid[2,3]	NK	C
Aspirin[4,5]	10–15%	A
Bisphosphonates (oral)[3,6,7,8]	0.2–0.4%	A
Ciprofloxacin,[9] clindamycin[10]	NK	C
Clopidogrel[11]	NK	B
Corticosteroids[6,12]	0.4%	B
Dabigatran[13,14]	NK	C
Erythromycin[6]	NK	C
Ferrous sulfate[2,3]	5%	B
Nonselective NSAIDs[15,16]	10–25%	A
Potassium chloride (oral)[2,3]	8–19%	A
Quinidine[2,3]	NK	C
Selective COX-2 NSAIDs[17]	5–8%	A
Selective serotonin reuptake inhibitors[18,19]	NK	B
Sulfasalazine[6]	NK	C
Tetracyclines[2,6]	NK	B
Valproic acid[2]	NK	C

COX = cyclooxygenase, NK = not known, NSAIDs = nonsteroidal anti-inflammatory drugs.
[a]Definitions for Levels of Evidence: Level A—evidence from one or more randomized, controlled clinical trials; Level B—evidence from nonrandomized clinical trials, prospective observational studies, cohort studies, retrospective studies, case-control studies, meta-analyses and/or postmarketing surveillance studies; and Level C—evidence from one or more published case reports or case series.

aspirin-caffeine products, and sustained-release ferrous sulfate.[2] Although anticoagulant and antiplatelet medications may increase the risk of bleeding, they are not generally considered major culprits in upper GI ulceration. The exception is dabigatran, a direct thrombin inhibitor, which has been associated with symptomatic esophagitis.[13]

EPIDEMIOLOGY

The true incidence of drug-induced upper GI ulceration is difficult to determine because of possible under-reporting or misdiagnosis. Many patients self-medicate, making it impossible to know actual exposure rates. In addition, some patients in whom ulceration develops have minimal sequelae or are asymptomatic. Dyspepsia, for example, is present in <50% of patients taking NSAIDs who present with life-threatening complications such as GI bleeding or perforation.[15] Additionally, event rates often change over time; recent data showed that rates of GI adverse events in women taking bisphosphonate therapy increased from 16.1%, to 25.6%, to 38.9% at 3, 6, and 12 months, respectively.[22] Another factor that complicates the collection and interpretation of incidence data is the use of differing definitions for the diagnosis of drug-induced upper GI ulceration that appear in published literature. Knowing the criteria that were used to define ulceration is important when attempting to compare study results.

Notwithstanding the difficulties described above, NSAIDs, which includes aspirin, appear to be the most common cause of upper GI ulceration.[16] Endoscopic surveys of patients receiving ≤325 mg aspirin daily reported gastroduodenal ulcers in 11% of patients.[23] More serious GI complications may also develop in patients receiving NSAIDs including bleeding, stricture formation, and perforation.[6,15] The incidence of hospitalization for NSAID-induced upper GI bleeding has been reported to be as high as 2.2% annually in patients with rheumatoid arthritis.[16]

The highest risk for upper GI ulceration in patients receiving NSAIDs appears to occur when these agents are used in combination with other medications also known to cause GI ulceration. When combined with even low doses of aspirin (<325 mg/day), the risk of upper GI bleeding in patients receiving other NSAIDs may be increased as much as 12-fold. The presence of *Helicobacter pylori* (*H. pylori*) infection has also been shown to increase the risk of upper GI ulceration in those taking NSAIDs, including low-dose aspirin, and also in those taking thienopyridines. Peptic ulcers were identified on endoscopy in 10.7% of elderly patients on aspirin doses of 75–325 mg per day. Interestingly, eradicating *H. pylori* infection prior to starting low-dose aspirin was not associated with an increased risk of upper GI ulceration. With NSAIDs other than aspirin, the presence of *H. pylori* infection is an independent risk factor for NSAID-induced ulcers. Fortunately, eradicating *H. pylori* infection prior to initiating NSAID therapy decreases that risk by up to 57%. The benefit of eradicating *H. pylori* in chronic NSAID users is less clear.[24]

Although the incidence of drug-induced upper GI ulceration is relatively low in patients receiving corticosteroids and selective serotonin reuptake inhibitors alone, the combination of these drugs with an NSAID increases the risk for ulceration considerably. Patients taking a selective serotonin reuptake inhibitor concurrently with an NSAID had as much as a 3.6-fold increase in the risk of upper GI bleeding.[18] The incidence of ulceration appears to be least common with ibuprofen, especially at doses <1,200 mg/24 hours. Selective cyclooxygenase (COX)-2 NSAIDs also are associated with a lower incidence of drug-induced ulceration ranging from 5% to 8%.[25]

Although GI damage due to NSAIDs is most common at sites distal to the esophagus, they can cause esophageal damage as well. One review of medications associated with drug-induced esophageal injury showed NSAIDs to be responsible for 40% of cases. This was followed by tetracyclines (22%), potassium chloride (10%), and bisphosphonates (9%). Antimicrobials, quinidine, and ascorbic acid were responsible for the remainder of cases.[2] Dabigatran, a direct thrombin inhibitor that was approved in 2010, has also been implicated in several cases of symptomatic esophagitis.[13] With both dabigatran and rivaroxaban, another direct thrombin inhibitor, lower GI bleeding reported in clinical trials was more common than upper gastrointestinal bleeding.[26]

MECHANISMS

Various mechanisms are responsible for drug-induced upper GI ulceration, ranging from simple direct irritation of the GI lining to more complex interactions with mucosal cells and prostaglandin inhibition. Because ulceration can occur in the absence of direct contact with the GI tract, no route of administration can be considered completely safe with respect to this drug-induced disease. An understanding of mechanisms is important in preventing or minimizing adverse effects in patients at greatest risk. **Table 35-2** lists causative agents with their proposed mechanism(s). With some medications, more than one mechanism may be involved.[1-3,6,9-11,13,14,18,19]

NSAIDs have long been thought to cause upper GI ulceration through their inhibition of COX, a major enzyme needed for the synthesis of prostaglandins.

Table 35-2 Mechanism(s) of Drug-Induced Upper Gastrointestinal Ulceration

Drug	Mechanism(s)
Aspirin[6]	COX inhibition, platelet effects, direct irritant
Bisphosphonates (oral)[2,6]	Direct irritant
Ciprofloxacin[9]	Chemical injury
Clindamycin[10]	Direct irritant
Clopidogrel[11]	Platelet effects
Corticosteroids[6]	Impair mucosal healing
Dabigatran[13,14]	Direct irritant
Erythromycin[6]	Direct irritant
Ferrous sulfate[1]	Direct irritant
Nonsteroidal anti-inflammatory drugs[6]	COX inhibition, platelet effects, direct irritant
Potassium chloride[3,6]	Direct irritant
Selective serotonin reuptake inhibitors[18,19]	Platelet effects
Tetracyclines[2,6]	Direct irritant

COX = cyclooxygenase.

Prostaglandins have a strong cytoprotective effect on the GI mucosa. They help maintain mucosal blood flow, increase secretion of mucus and bicarbonate, and augment epithelial defense against cytotoxic injury.[2] There are at least two subtypes of the COX enzyme, COX-1 and COX-2. COX-1 is the predominant subtype found in the stomach. NSAIDs that preferentially inhibit COX-2, therefore, might be expected to cause fewer adverse GI effects than those that inhibit COX-1. Indeed, when COX-1 inhibitors were directly compared with COX-2 inhibitors, patients experienced fewer minor GI problems with the COX-2 inhibitors.[17] Importantly, the risk of adverse GI effects is not completely eliminated with the use of these selective agents.[27] Celecoxib, for example, has been shown to increase the risk of GI toxicity compared with placebo.[28] Additionally, the long-term use of COX-2 inhibitors is limited because they have been associated with greater cardiovascular toxicity. Nonacetylated salicylates, such as salsalate, are weaker inhibitors of COX activity and therefore less damaging to the GI tract. NSAIDs also have a direct cytotoxic effect on GI mucosal cells that is independent of COX activity and can result in lesions and necrotic injury.[29]

As previously noted, the relationship between *H. pylori* positivity and the incidence of NSAID-induced GI ulceration appears to depend on when the NSAID therapy was started. New users of NSAIDs have been shown to have fewer ulcers and ulcer-associated complications if they are *H. pylori*-negative at time of initiation.[24,30] Whether the presence of one affects the mechanism of ulceration of the other is unknown. Clearly, *H. pylori* is an independent risk factor for NSAID-induced ulceration and ulcer bleeding.[24,31]

Corticosteroids have been implicated in GI ulceration, but the exact mechanism is unclear. These medications may impair mucosal healing through the reduction of epithelial regeneration.[32] Corticosteroids may pose a greater risk to the lower GI tract than to the upper GI tract.[2] Studies have failed to confirm the mechanism or quantify the actual risk.[12]

Pill-induced esophagitis, a localized ulcer of variable depth, can occur when capsules or tablets do not clear the esophagus in a timely manner. Gelatin capsules can become sticky and lodge in the esophagus if not taken with adequate water. In addition, tablets may be difficult to swallow or contain a caustic coating that causes direct mucosal irritation. The pH and concentration of the medication may also be contributing factors. Pill-induced esophagitis occurs commonly with oral bisphosphonates, such as alendronate. Even patients who strictly adhere to the recommended directions for use can experience esophagitis that is often exudative in nature and resolves with discontinuation of the medication. Oral potassium chloride may induce irritation in a localized area of the esophagus or stomach because of the high salt concentration. The slow-release, wax matrix formulations are more likely to cause damage than the microencapsulated forms. Liquid forms of potassium supplementation are much less likely to cause ulceration or other injury.[33] In most cases the esophageal injury is caused by the prolonged contact of medication, resulting in direct damage to the esophageal wall.[34] This also applies to dabigatran-induced esophagitis, with the tartaric acid contained within the capsules playing a role in causing tissue damage.[13]

A number of other mechanisms for drug-induced upper GI bleeding exist. Vascular shunting due to an increased osmotic load of sorbitol has led to ischemic necrosis in patients taking sodium polystyrene.[35] Clopidogrel may cause re-bleeding in patients with a history of bleeding because of its antiplatelet effect.[11] There is some evidence suggesting that selective serotonin reuptake inhibitors increase the risk of upper GI bleeding by possibly decreasing platelet serotonin and interfering with platelet aggregation.[19] This effect is potentiated when selective serotonin reuptake inhibitors are administered with NSAIDs, including low-dose aspirin.[18]

CLINICAL PRESENTATION AND DIFFERENTIAL DIAGNOSIS

Patients with drug-induced GI ulceration may be asymptomatic or may present with life-threatening complications including bleeding, perforation, and strictures. The most common signs and symptoms of upper GI ulceration are listed in **Table 35-3**.[2,3] Heartburn, dyspepsia, cramps, and abdominal pain are

Table 35-3 Signs and Symptoms Associated with Drug-Induced Upper Gastrointestinal Ulceration[2,3]

- Abdominal pain or tenderness
- Burning in the back or stomach
- Cramps
- Dyspepsia
- Heartburn
- Hematemesis
- Hematochezia
- Indigestion
- Nausea/vomiting
- Odynophagia

Table 35-4 Conditions to Consider in the Differential Diagnosis of Drug-Induced Upper Gastrointestinal Ulceration[2]

- Chest pain secondary to cardiovascular disease
- Crohn disease
- Esophageal stricture
- Gastric outlet obstruction
- Infectious cause of esophagitis (herpes, candida, HIV, cytomegalovirus)
- Malignancy
- Nasogastric intubation
- Peptic ulcer disease
- Perforation
- Reflux esophagitis
- Sclerotherapy
- Stevens–Johnson syndrome

HIV = human immunodeficiency virus.

common, but do not always correlate with ulceration. As previously noted, dyspepsia was reported by <50% of patients presenting with life-threatening bleeding due to NSAID use in one series.[15] Hematemesis and/or black, tarry stools may be signs of bleeding and should be carefully evaluated. Likewise, dysphagia, odynophagia, weight loss, or severe abdominal pain may be indicative of severe complications or other diseases (e.g., malignancy) and warrant careful evaluation.

NSAIDs most commonly cause ulceration in the stomach. Ulceration of the small intestines is less common, and esophageal ulceration is the least common of the three sites. Of note, indomethacin, diclofenac, piroxicam, and aspirin have been shown to induce esophageal injury.[10] There appears to be a correlation between NSAID use and the development of esophagitis and esophageal strictures.[36] Although esophageal injury may not be as common with NSAIDs, when it occurs it can have serious consequences, including bleeding and stricture formation.

Patients with pill-induced esophagitis, as occurs with doxycycline or alendronate, may present with sudden, painful swallowing shortly after the offending agent is taken. It can also be described as a dull aching pain in the shoulder or chest.[3] Sequelae from this type of injury can include severe ulceration and strictures. Hemorrhage is rare, although patients may occasionally present with melena caused by esophageal bleeding.[37] Symptoms generally resolve within 7–10 days following discontinuation of the culprit drug.[3] Pill-induced esophagitis should be suspected whenever patients present with the above symptoms and especially in those without previous esophageal symptoms.

Patients with pill-induced esophageal injury due to oral solid dosage forms of potassium chloride tend to have progressive dysphagia with little pain.[10] The connection between drug and injury can be difficult to recognize, as symptoms may progress over months or even years. In many cases, strictures develop because of the chronic nature of injury. Healthcare providers should be alert for pill-induced esophagitis or gastritis in elderly patients who require oral potassium chloride supplements while being treated with diuretics for heart failure. Quinidine may cause production of an exudate and edema in the upper GI tract that must be distinguished from carcinoma.[10]

Lack of awareness of drug-induced GI injury can lead to persistent exposure to causative medications, resulting in severe complications. Many of the signs and symptoms associated with upper GI ulceration are also common with other diseases. It is important, therefore, to distinguish drug-induced upper GI ulceration from other ulcerative, erosive, or inflammatory conditions, as well as trauma, tumors, or other diseases. **Table 35-4** lists conditions that should be considered in the differential diagnosis of drug-induced upper GI ulceration.[2]

Patients presenting with weight loss, recurrent emesis, and dyspepsia may have gastric outlet obstruction. Patients who present with chest pain or pain that radiates to the shoulder should be evaluated for cardiovascular causes. Dysphagia, odynophagia, and weight loss may be indicative of carcinoma and patients with these symptoms require careful evaluation.

It is difficult to distinguish pill-induced esophagitis from herpes esophagitis, because both may present radiographically as shallow ulcerations in the mid or distal esophagus. Differentiation can sometimes be made by determining the presence or absence of a temporal relationship between medication ingestion and the onset of symptoms. Patients with pill-induced esophagitis may experience an abrupt onset of odynophagia, dysphagia, or retrosternal burning pain within a few moments of taking the causative medication.[37] Patients with herpes-induced ulcers are usually immunocompromised, and their esophageal lesions tend to be more widely distributed than those in patients with pill-induced esophagitis.[10] Reflux esophagitis generally causes ulcers in the more distal segment of the esophagus.

There are several characteristic morphologic and pathophysiologic changes that can help differentiate drug-induced GI ulceration from other conditions.[35] Candidal esophagitis is characterized by its "shaggy" appearance due to plaque formation.[10] Crohn disease is usually distinguished by evidence of the disease in multiple parts of the GI tract, including the small and large bowel.[10] In pill-induced esophagitis, inflammatory markers are a common finding. Infiltration of macrophages, T lymphocytes, and intraepithelial mast cells and eosinophils can often be seen.[38] An exudative, ulcerative esophagitis may develop specifically in patients receiving alendronate. This exudate shows translucent crystalline material, with multinucleated giant cells seen in as many as 30% of cases, a process indicative of pill-induced esophagitis. In addition, alendronate-induced esophagitis may also manifest as strictures. Esophageal injury caused by dabigatran has been reported as both an exfoliative esophagitis and as esophageal ulceration.[14]

Iron-induced GI injury occurs most commonly in the esophagus, but the stomach may also be affected.[35] The injury manifests as a chemical burn with erosive injury and is characterized by brown-black crystalline material within the epithelium.[35] Less commonly, endoscopic examination can reveal impacted pill fragments, or remnants of drug coating.[37] Elderly patients are at increased risk for impacted pill fragments or drug coating remnants because of low saliva production. They also tend to consume more medications including bisphosphonates or NSAIDs.[37] Any patient who is in a recumbent position for extended periods is also at risk for iron-induced GI injury. Iron can also deposit in the stomach epithelium, causing damage.

Patients with uremia are very susceptible to vascular shunting because of the sorbitol osmotic load in sodium polystyrene. Basophilic crystalline material may be evident on morphologic evaluation. Ischemic necrosis has been reported. Most upper GI lesions due to sodium polystyrene are reversible and do not generally lead to serious sequelae.[35]

RISK FACTORS

Knowledge of the risk factors associated with GI bleeding caused by NSAIDs and those for bisphosphonate-induced esophageal damage provide excellent guidance when considering the risk associated with any of the medications described in this chapter. Risk factors for drug-induced upper GI ulceration are listed in **Table 35-5**.[2,6]

Factors that increase the risk for GI bleeding with aspirin specifically include dose, history of ulcer or upper GI bleeding, age >70 years, and concomitant use of other NSAIDs.[4] Other risk factors for GI bleeding with aspirin, even low-dose aspirin, are the concomitant use of corticosteroids or anticoagulants.[5]

A history of GI complications is the most important predictor of NSAID-induced GI toxicity.[39,40] Other risk factors include a history of uncomplicated peptic ulcer; age >75 years; concomitant use of corticosteroids, warfarin, or other NSAID, including aspirin; the dose of NSAID; a history of dyspepsia; and the disease being treated (e.g., due to the side effect profile of the medications used for

Table 35-5 Risk Factors for Drug-Induced Upper Gastrointestinal Ulceration[2,6]

- Concomitant anticoagulation
- Concomitant corticosteroid use
- Concomitant use of two NSAIDs (including low-dose aspirin)
- *Helicobacter pylori* infection
- High NSAID dose
- History of gastrointestinal bleeding
- History of ulceration
- Increasing age
- Prolonged NSAID use
- Specific risks for pill-induced esophagitis:
    - Decreased saliva production
    - Fasting
    - Inadequate fluid intake
    - Returning to a supine position too soon after medication administration
    - Swallowing abnormalities (e.g., stroke, dysmotility, anatomic abnormalities)

NSAID = nonsteroidal anti-inflammatory drug.

treatment, patients with rheumatoid arthritis have higher prevalence of GI events than those treated for osteoarthritis).[39] The duration of NSAID use may also be an important factor in the development of GI toxicity. Short-term use (<1 week) in healthy patients is unlikely to be problematic; however, longer-term use is associated with increased GI toxicity. GI complications are most common within the first 3 months of the initiation of NSAID therapy.

Because COX-1 produces prostaglandins that are known to protect the GI mucosa, it is thought that NSAIDs with greater COX-1 inhibitory activity would present a greater risk of GI toxicity. This idea is supported by evidence that ketorolac, the NSAID with the greatest COX-1 inhibitory effects, produces the highest risk for GI bleeding of all the medications in this class.[41,42] COX-2 inhibiting agents (e.g., celecoxib) have a minimal effect on COX-1 and theoretically present a lower risk of GI bleeding. However, no NSAID is completely free of ulceration risks and associated complications. Most of the factors that raise the risk for GI complications in patients taking NSAIDs also increase the likelihood of GI complications in non-NSAID-treated patients.[25] As a result, patients may be at continued risk for GI complications even after switching to alternative medications. In addition, the incidence of cardiovascular toxicities has been shown to be higher with COX-2 inhibitors, so proper patient selection following evaluation of the risks and benefits is extremely important.

Patients who have undergone renal transplantation have multiple risk factors for GI ulceration, including the stress of surgery, use of NSAIDs and corticosteroids, and increased gastric acid secretion during dialysis postrenal transplantation.[43] Also contributing is the possible impairment of native GI cytoprotection due to azathioprine or mycophenolate-induced slowing of intestinal cell turnover. Ulcers can be asymptomatic with the symptoms masked by the use of corticosteroids. Risk factors for bleeding following transplantation include NSAID use for at least 1 week post-transplantation, high-dose intravenous corticosteroids used for acute rejection, and cyclosporine use.[43]

Patients with a history of GI bleeding may also be at increased risk of rebleeding when taking clopidogrel.[11] Nine of 70 such patients (14%) had significant GI bleeding after a median follow-up of 1 year. All except one lesion was identical to the previous lesion, suggesting that clopidogrel causes rebleeding only in patients with underlying mucosal defects or scarring. Pre-existing mucosal breaks, caused by esophagitis or peptic ulcers, can be aggravated by the antiplatelet effects of thienopyridines, promoting bleeding.[44] Healthcare providers should be alert to the fact that patients with a history of aspirin-induced GI bleeding are at high risk for the development of the same outcome with clopidogrel, which has been reported to have a favorable GI safety profile as compared with aspirin, although patients who were studied received only 325 mg doses of nonbuffered and nonenteric-coated aspirin. In addition, healthcare providers were permitted to exclude any patient they defined as aspirin-intolerant.[45]

Patients at risk for pill-induced esophagitis are those who do not take enough fluids with their medications, those with swallowing abnormalities due to stroke or esophageal dysmotility, and those with anatomic abnormalities such as strictures.[3] Other risk factors include fasting, decreased production of saliva, age >70 years, and polypharmacy.[10] Patients with left atrial enlargement are predisposed because the left atrium can compress the esophagus.[46] In most case reports of bisphosphonate-related ulcerative esophagitis or esophageal stricture, the patient took alendronate with little to no water or returned to a supine position too soon after swallowing the tablet.[7] Women with a history of upper GI disease or patients with gastroesophageal reflux disease also appear to be at greater risk for esophageal complications from bisphosphonates.[8] When used in combination, NSAIDs and bisphosphonates appear to have a synergistic effect on the risk for the development of gastric ulceration.[47]

MORBIDITY AND MORTALITY

Although some drug-induced upper GI ulceration may be relatively insignificant and transient, there is always a risk of severe complications including perforation, penetration of an ulcer from the stomach or duodenum into an adjacent organ, GI obstruction, and bleeding. Any of these complications can necessitate hospitalization with possible surgical intervention and can be life-threatening.

The highest rates of complication are associated with NSAIDs. Problems range from minor but common side effects such as dyspepsia and abdominal pain to the more severe complications of ulceration, perforation, and bleeding. Although the more serious complications are relatively uncommon, they are a major public concern because of the large numbers of patients who are exposed each year to aspirin and other NSAIDs. With an estimated 111 million Americans taking NSAIDs, the reported 2–4.5% rate of significant upper GI events results in a large number of patients requiring care.[44,48,49] Although estimates vary, NSAID-related mortality has been reported to be as high as 16,500 per year in the United States.[16] When nonaspirin NSAIDs are used concomitantly with aspirin, the annual risk of upper GI events increases to 5.6%.[44]

Studies have attempted to determine hospitalization rates due to NSAID-induced complications. Patients with upper GI symptoms who were admitted through emergency departments were more likely to be NSAID users as compared with controls (odds ratio = 2.4).[50] Blood transfusion requirements were also higher in the NSAID user group. Another population-based study reported a hospitalization rate of 2% over a 3-year period among NSAID users >50 years old.[51] Eighteen hospitals in Spain and Italy participated in a study of risk for upper GI bleeding in which the incidence of upper GI bleed was 401.4 per million inhabitants aged 18 and older, with 38% of the cases attributable to NSAIDs.[52] An observational study of NSAID-related GI complications and death included patients in more than 200 hospitals in the Spanish National Health System that provides care for 80% of the country.[53] The mortality was reported to be 15.3 deaths per 100,000 NSAID users.

PREVENTION

Approaches to help prevent drug-induced upper GI ulceration are listed in **Table 35-6**.[2,3,6,18,19] The first and most important step is to avoid agents

Table 35-6 Approaches to Help Prevent Drug-Induced Upper Gastrointestinal Ulceration

Aspirin[2,6]

- Use lowest possible dose; avoid other ulcerogenic medications

Bisphosphonates[3,6]

- Take with 8 ounces of water; remain upright for at least 30 minutes after taking medication

Corticosteroids[3]

- Avoid concomitant use of nonsteroidal anti-inflammatory drugs or aspirin, if possible

Nonsteroidal anti-inflammatory drugs (NSAIDs)[3,6]

- Use lowest possible dose; use least ulcerogenic nonsteroidal anti-inflammatory drug
- Consider addition of proton pump inhibitor or misoprostol
- Avoid other ulcerogenic medications
- Treat *Helicobacter pylori* if found

Potassium chloride (oral)[6]

- Use preferred microencapsulated or liquid formulation; avoid slow-release, wax-matrix formulations

Selective serotonin reuptake inhibitors[18,19]

- Use alternative class of antidepressant; avoid concomitant use of NSAIDs, if possible

Tetracyclines[3]

- Use tablet formulation rather than capsule formulation

known to increase the risk of disease in patients who already have known risk factors. Whenever possible, an alternative medication with little or no risk for upper GI ulceration should be used in these patients. An example might be using acetaminophen instead of aspirin to treat osteoarthritis in an elderly patient.

When the use of a medication known to cause upper GI ulceration cannot be avoided, using the lowest possible dose is helpful. Several strategies are available to help minimize upper GI injury in patients who require NSAID therapy. Eradication of *H. pylori* infection before starting NSAID therapy reduces the risk of ulceration and related bleeding. Randomized controlled trials, however, indicate that *H. pylori* eradication does not reduce the incidence of new peptic ulcers in chronic NSAID users.[24] In low-risk patients (those having no known risk factors), using the lowest dose possible and avoiding concomitant use of other agents known to cause upper GI ulceration is recommended.[40] An increased risk of GI toxicity has been seen when aspirin (even low-dose aspirin) is combined with other NSAIDs. Likewise, corticosteroids have a low incidence of GI ulceration when used alone; however, the incidence increases significantly when combined with NSAIDs.

In patients at moderate risk (one or two risk factors), concomitant treatment with acid suppression therapy, such as a proton pump inhibitor (PPI) or misoprostol, should be considered.[40] There is a large body of evidence to support the use of these agents, but it is estimated that over 50% of NSAID users with an increased risk for GI complications do not receive a gastroprotective therapy.[28] PPIs prevent upper GI toxicity associated with NSAIDs and are generally well tolerated. They are considered effective in terms of acid suppression and prevention of peptic ulcers when coadministered with NSAIDs.[29] PPIs may be especially important for patients with a true need for aspirin therapy, such as those at risk for a secondary cardiovascular event. In these patients, PPIs have been shown to reduce rates of aspirin discontinuation by decreasing the incidence of upper GI tract adverse events.[23] Misoprostol is effective in increasing mucosal blood flow and stimulating mucus and bicarbonate production in the upper GI tract, and has been shown to reduce NSAID-induced GI ulceration considerably.[29] However, it is associated with numerous adverse effects, such as diarrhea, which can limit its routine use. The use of a selective COX-2 inhibitor, such as celecoxib, may be considered in some patients. Selective COX-2 inhibitors reduce the incidence of GI toxicity as compared with traditional NSAIDs while still maintaining the anti-inflammatory properties. However, other toxicities, such as cardiovascular risk, associated with COX-2 selective inhibitors must be weighed against the potential benefit. Other options include using NSAIDs that undergo less enterohepatic circulation, such as nabumetone or etodolac.

High-risk patients (greater than three risk factors or concomitant use of aspirin, corticosteroids, or warfarin) may benefit from the addition of a PPI or misoprostol.[40] In the highest-risk patients (history of recent ulcer complications), it is best to avoid NSAIDs altogether. If avoidance is not possible, these patients should also receive a PPI or misoprostol.[40] It is recommended that patients at high risk for ulcer-related bleeding from NSAIDs should take a PPI for as long as they continue to take NSAIDs. For patients who are able to discontinue the offending agents, short-term therapy with PPIs is preferred over longer-term therapy.[54]

When PPI therapy is indicated to either treat or to provide prophylaxis against NSAID-induced ulceration, the risks and benefits should be considered. PPIs have been associated with *Clostridium difficile* infection, acute kidney injuries, and increased risk of bone fractures. There is evidence to suggest they may also be linked to dementia, small intestine bacterial overgrowth, pneumonia, and micronutrient deficiencies. Risks of these adverse effects are greatest during long-term therapy. When long-term therapy is indicated, as with the high-risk patients mentioned above, the dose should be evaluated periodically so that the lowest effective dose can be prescribed.[54]

With other medications that cause upper GI ulceration, changing to an agent less likely to cause injury may be an option. In patients requiring oral potassium supplementation, switching to a microencapsulated form may be preferable to a slow-release, wax-matrix form. If patients are able to tolerate the taste, liquid formulations of potassium are also less likely to cause injury. Patients requiring a bisphosphonate for osteoporosis may tolerate risedronate better than alendronate, because it appears to be less ulcerogenic.

Education is important for prevention of pill-induced esophagitis. Patients should sit or stand upright and take medications with ample fluids. They should remain upright for at least 15 minutes after taking the medication. Careful selection of the dosage form of the medication may also help prevent mucosal injury. Liquid or tablet formulations may be less problematic than capsules.

In addition to the steps outlined above, patients at risk for upper GI ulceration should be educated regarding important lifestyle modifications, including avoidance of acidic beverages (e.g., citrus juices) and irritating foods (e.g., onions, spicy foods).

MANAGEMENT

The first step in the management of drug-induced upper GI ulceration is to reassess the need for the offending agent. Changing to an alternative medication is often ideal; however, if this is not possible, the lowest possible dose of the offending agent should be used. Gastric ulceration should be confirmed via endoscopy and, when present, treated with acid-suppressing therapy such as a PPI. Treatment of *H. pylori* infections should be considered as eradication can reduce the risk for further complications, such as bleeding.[29] Surgery may be necessary to treat strictures. The addition of a PPI to a patient's therapy may permit re-challenge with a medication that has previously caused GI ulceration.[55]

With pill-induced esophagitis, discontinuation of the offending agent is often the best treatment option. Symptoms usually improve within 2–6 days after stopping the medication. Antacids may provide rapid relief of pain and a topical anesthetic (e.g., viscous lidocaine) can also provide relief.[10,46] Acid suppressing therapy (e.g., PPI) may be used as an adjunct in treating esophageal damage and is beneficial if gastroesophageal reflux is present, as the refluxed material may worsen esophagitis.[10] Sucralfate may also be an option to reduce exposure of the injured mucosa to refluxed acids.[46] Avoiding foods or beverages (e.g., citrus, alcohol) that might exacerbate symptoms may also be helpful in selected patients.[10] Drinking plenty of water is also helpful in preventing tablets or capsules from adhering to the mucosa and causing damage.

INFORMATION FOR PATIENTS

Patient consultation is essential to help ensure the safe use of the medications known to cause upper GI ulceration. As previously noted, one of the biggest risk factors for drug-induced upper GI ulceration is the concomitant use of NSAIDs, including low-dose aspirin, with any other medication known to cause upper GI ulceration. Because many NSAIDs are available over the counter under a variety of brand names and as combination products, an informed patient may be the best protection against these adverse events. Patients should be reminded to carefully read labels of nonprescription medications to avoid inadvertently purchasing products containing NSAIDs. A discussion of potentially harmful nonprescription medications should be conducted with all patients receiving a prescription for any of the causative drugs. Patients should also be instructed to always use one pharmacy so that any potential interactions or additive toxicities are brought to the pharmacist's attention.

For NSAIDs, patients should take the recommended dose for the indicated length of time. If prescribed for a chronic condition, patients should be regularly reminded of the warning signs of ulceration. They should report any nausea, abdominal pain or tenderness, or coffee-ground or bloody emesis or stools immediately to their healthcare provider. Patients must realize that even low-dose aspirin can result in complications. When treating patients with acute pain, the benefits of analgesia from NSAIDs must be weighed against the aforementioned risks. Although patients and providers are often wary of the risk of developing addiction and substance abuse disorder, therapy with opioids may be more appropriate than NSAIDs in the short term in many cases.

Patients taking bisphosphonates should strictly adhere to recommendations regarding administration, including taking the medication first thing in the morning at least 30 minutes before eating or drinking anything, taking the medication with a full glass of water, and staying in a sitting or standing position for at least 30 minutes following ingestion. Patients should also be educated as to the temporal relationship that often exists between taking the medication and the onset of symptoms, so they may realize the cause and seek medical attention more quickly. Any medication known to cause pill-induced esophagitis should be taken with sufficient fluid every time a dose is administered.

REFERENCES

1. Cappell MS, Friedel D. Initial management of acute upper gastrointestinal bleeding: from initial evaluation up to gastrointestinal endoscopy. *Med Clin N Am.* 2008; 92:491-509.
2. Shih AR, Misdraji J. Drug-induced pathology of the upper gastrointestinal tract. Mini-symposium: upper gastrointestinal tract pathology. *Diagnostic Histopathology.* 2017; 23:84-95.
3. Tolstoi LG. Drug-induced gastrointestinal disorders. *Medscape Pharmacotherapy.* 2002; 4:1-9.
4. Hsu PI, Tsai TJ. Epidemiology of upper gastrointestinal damage associated with low-dose aspirin. *Current Pharmaceutical Design.* 2015; 21:5049-55.
5. Lin KJ, De Caterina R, Rodriguez LAG. Low-dose aspirin and upper gastrointestinal bleeding in primary versus secondary cardiovascular prevention: a population-based, nested case-control study. *Circulation: Cardiovascular Quality and Outcomes.* 2014; 7:70-7.
6. Fortun P, Hawkey CJ. Drug induced gastrointestinal disorders. *Medicine.* 2007; 35:210-5.
7. Orozco C, Maalouf NM. Safety of bisphosphonates. *Rheumatic Disease Clinics of North America.* 2012; 38:681-705.
8. Cryer B, Bauer D. Oral bisphosphonates and upper gastrointestinal tract problems: what is the evidence? *Mayo Clinic Proc.* 2002; 77:1031-43.
9. Santos VM, Carneiro LR, Paixao GTG. Drug-induced esophageal lesions and use of ciprofloxacin. *An Sist Sanit Navar.* 2012; 35:127-31.
10. Grossi L, Ciccaglione AF, Marzio L. Esophagitis and its causes: who is "guilty" when acid is found "not guilty"? *World J Gastroenterol.* 2017; 23):3011-16.
11. Yasuda H, Matsuo Y, Sato Y et al. Treatment and prevention of gastrointestinal bleeding in patients receiving antiplatelet therapy. *World J Crit Care Med.* 2015; 4:40-6.
12. Carpani DK, Rentsch R, Levi S et al. Corticosteroids reduce regenerative repair of epithelium in experimental gastric ulcers. *Gut.* 1995; 37:613-6.
13. Toya, Y, Nakamura S, Tomita K et al. Dabigatran-induced esophagitis: the prevalence and endoscopic characteristics. *J Gastroenterol Hepatol.* 2016; 31:610-4.
14. Okada M, Okada K. Exfoliative esophagitis and esophageal ulcer induced by dabigatran. *Endoscopy.* 2012; 44:E23-24.
15. MacDonald TM. Epidemiology and pharmacoeconomic implications of nonsteroidal anti-inflammatory drug-associated gastrointestinal toxicity. *Rheumatology.* 2000; 39(suppl 2):13-20.
16. Singh G, Triadafilopoulos G. Epidemiology of NSAID induced gastrointestinal complications. *J Rheumatol.* 1999; 26(suppl 56): 18-24.
17. Fitzgerald GA, Patrono C. The coxibs, selective inhibitors of cyclooxygenase-2. *N Engl J Med.* 2001; 345:433-42.
18. Dalton SO, Johansen C, Mellemkjaer L et al. Use of selective serotonin reuptake inhibitors and risk of upper gastrointestinal tract bleeding: a population-based cohort study. *Arch Intern Med.* 2003; 163:59-64.
19. Andrade C, Sharma E. Serotonin reuptake inhibitors and risk of abnormal bleeding. *Psychiatric Clinics of North America.* 2016; 39:413-26.
20. Ong CKS, Lirk P, Tan CH, Seymour RA. An evidence-based update on nonsteroidal anti-inflammatory drugs. *Clinical Medicine and Research.* 2007; 5:19-34.
21. Zezos P, Harel Z, Saibil F. Cloxacillin: a new cause of pill-induced esophagitis. *Can J Gastroenterol Hepatol.* 2016; 2904256:1-2.
22. Modi A, Saijan S, Lewiecki EM et al. Relationship between gastrointestinal events and compliance with osteoporosis therapy: an administrative claims analysis of the US managed care population. *Clin Ther.* 2016; 38:1074-80.
23. Lavie CJ, Howden CW, Scheiman J, Tursi J. Upper gastrointestinal toxicity associated with long-term aspirin therapy: Consequences and prevention. *Curr Probl Cardiol.* 2017; 42:146-64.
24. Chey WD, Leontiadis GI, Howden CW, Moss SF. ACG Clinical Guideline: Treatment of Helicobacter pylori infection. *Am J Gastroenterol.* 2017; 112:212-39.
25. Goldstein JL, Cryer B. Gastrointestinal injury associated with NSAID use: a case study and review of risk factors. *Drug, Healthcare, and Patient Safety.* 2015; 7:31-41.
26. Desai J, Kolb JM, Weitz JI et al. Gastrointestinal bleeding with the new anticoagulants—defining the issues and the management strategies. *Thromb Haemost.* 2013; 110:205-12.
27. Rafaniello C, Ferrajolo C, Sullo MG et al. Risk of gastrointestinal complications associated to NSAIDs, low-dose aspirin and their combinations: results of a pharmacovigilance reporting system. *Pharmacol Res.* 2016; 104:108-14.
28. Bakhriansyah M, Souverein PC, de Boer A et al. Gastrointestinal toxicity among patients taking selective COX-2 inhibitors or conventional NSAIDs, alone or combined with proton pump inhibitors: a case-control study. *Pharmacoepidemiol Drug Saf.* 2017; 26:1141-8.
29. Sinha M, Gautam L, Shukla PK et al. Current perspectives in NSAID-induced gastropathy. *Mediators Inflamm.* 2013; 2013:258209.
30. Chan FK, To KF, Wu JC et al. Eradication of Helicobacter pylori and risk of peptic ulcers in patients starting long-term treatment with non-steroidal anti-inflammatory drugs: a randomized trial. *Lancet.* 2002; 359:9-13.
31. Huang JQ, Sridhar S, Hunt RH. Role of *Helicobacter pylori* infection and non-steroidal anti-inflammatory drugs in peptic ulcer disease: a meta-analysis. *Lancet.* 2002; 359:14-22.
32. Gore RM, Levine MS, Ghahremani GG. Drug-induced disorders of the stomach and duodenum. *Abdom Imaging.* 1999; 24:9-16.
33. McMahon FG, Ryan JR, Akdamar K, Ertan A. Effect of potassium chloride supplements on upper gastrointestinal mucosa. *Clin Pharmacol Ther.* 1984; 35:852-5.
34. Boyce HW. Drug-induced esophageal damage: diseases of medical progress. *Gastrointest Endosc.* 1998; 47:547-50.
35. Parfitt JR, Driman DK. Pathological effects of drugs on the gastrointestinal tract: a review. *Hum Pathol.* 2007; 38:527-36.
36. Panarelli NC. Other forms of esophagitis. *Surgical Pathology Clinics.* 2017; 4:765-79.
37. Kim S Jeong J, Kim J et al. Clinical and endoscopic characteristics of drug-induced esophagitis. *World J Gastroenterol.* 2014; 20:10994-9.

38. Kim JW, Kim BG, Kim SH et al. Histomorphological and immunophenotypic features of pill-induced esophagitis. *PLOS One.* 2015; 10:e0128110.

39. Lanas A, Hunt R. Prevention of anti-inflammatory drug-induced gastrointestinal damage: benefits and risks of therapeutic strategies. *Ann Med.* 2006; 38:415-28.

40. Chan FK, Graham DY. Review article: prevention of non-steroidal anti-inflammatory drug gastrointestinal complications-review and recommendations based on risk assessment. *Aliment Pharmacol Ther.* 2004; 19: 1051-61.

41. Bruno A, Tacconelli S, Patrignani P. Variability in the response to non-steroidal anti-inflammatory drugs: mechanisms and perspectives. *Basic Clin Pharmacol Toxicol.* 2014; 114:56-63.

42. Llorente MJ, Tenias JM, Zaragoza A. Comparative incidence of upper gastrointestinal bleeding associated with individual non-steroidal anti-inflammatory drugs. *Rev Esp Enferm Dig.* 2002; 94:7-18.

43. Helderman JH, Goral S. Gastrointestinal complications of transplant immunosuppression. *J Am Soc Nephrol.* 2002; 13:277-87.

44. Bhatt DL, Scheiman J, Abraham NS et al. ACCF/ACG/AHA 2008 expert consensus document on reducing the gastrointestinal risks of antiplatelet therapy and NSAID use: a report of the American College of Cardiology Foundation Task Force on Clinical Expert Consensus Documents. *Circulation.* 2008; 118:1894-909.

45. CAPRIE Steering Committee. A randomized, blinded, trial of clopidogrel versus aspirin in patients at risk of ischemic events (CAPRIE). *Lancet.* 1996; 348:1329-39.

46. Andrade C. Learning from history: how to swallow a pill. *J Clin Psychiatry.* 2013; 74:e949-51.

47. Graham D, Malatya H. Alendronate and naproxen are synergistic for the development of gastric ulcers. *Arch Intern Med.* 2001; 161:107-10.

48. Dai C, Stafford RS, Alexander GC. National trends in cyclooxygenase-2 inhibitor use since market release: non-selective diffusion of a selectively cost-effective innovation. *Arch Intern Med.* 2005; 165:171-7.

49. Silverstein FE, Faich G, Goldstein JL et al. Gastrointestinal toxicity with celecoxib versus nonsteroidal anti-inflammatory drugs for osteoarthritis and rheumatoid arthritis: the CLASS study: a randomized controlled trial. *JAMA.* 2000; 284:1247-55.

50. Blower AL, Brooks A, Fenn GC et al. Emergency admissions for upper gastrointestinal disease and their relation to NSAID use. *Aliment Pharmacol Ther.* 1997; 11:283-91.

51. MacDonald TM, Morant SV, Robinson GC et al. Association of upper gastrointestinal toxicity of non-steroidal anti-inflammatory drugs with continued exposure: cohort study. *BMJ.* 1997; 315:1333-7.

52. Laporte JR, Lbanez L, Vidal X et al. Upper gastrointestinal bleeding associated with the use of NSAIDs. *Drug Saf.* 2004; 27:411-20.

53. Lanas A, Perez-Asia MA, Feu F et al. A nationwide study of mortality associated with hospital admission due to severe gastrointestinal events and those associated with nonsteroidal anti-inflammatory drug use. *Am J Gastroenterol.* 2005; 100:1685-93.

54. Freedberg DE, Kim LS, Yang YX. The risks and benefits of long-term use of proton pump inhibitors: Expert review and best practice advice from the American Gastroenterological Association. *Gastroenterology.* 2017; 152:706-15.

55. Dall M, Christensen RD, Schaddalitzky de Muckadell OB et al. Re-prescribing of causative drugs in persons discharged after serious drug-induced upper gastrointestinal bleeding. *Aliment Pharmacol Ther.* 2012 35:948-54.

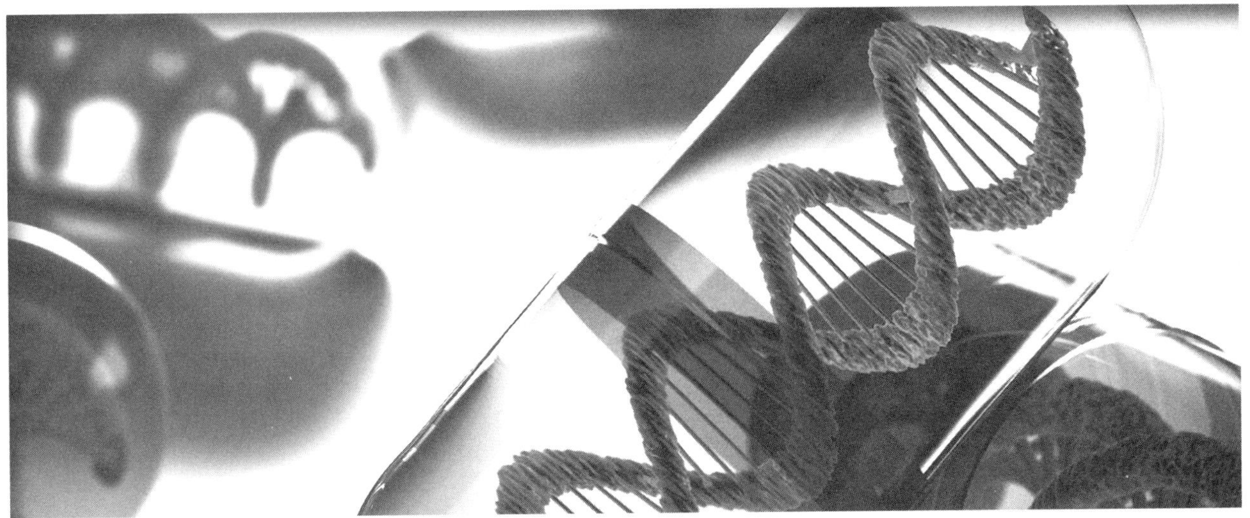

CHAPTER 36

Diarrhea

Sarah A. Nisly and Alison M. Walton

Diarrhea is a relatively frequent adverse drug effect. Symptoms may be mild and transient, disappearing within days, or severe and life-threatening, causing electrolyte disturbances and dehydration. Because even healthy individuals may experience symptoms of diarrhea from time to time, the identification of drug-induced diarrhea can be challenging. In addition, drug-induced diarrhea may present after months of routine drug use, further complicating its recognition.

CAUSATIVE AGENTS

Drug classes and specific agents with a >10% incidence of diarrhea are listed in **Table 36-1**.[1-120] However, this list should not be interpreted as exhaustive, because diarrhea can be a side effect of a multitude of drugs. Agents from the following drug classes are common culprits: antibiotics, antidepressants, antihyperglycemic agents, and antineoplastics.[2-47,49-87]

Antineoplastics represent an important class of drugs associated with a high incidence of drug-induced diarrhea, referred to as cancer treatment–induced diarrhea (CTID).[121-123] The actual incidence of diarrhea associated with individual antineoplastic drugs is difficult to determine because most chemotherapeutic regimens use combination therapies; however, it is reported that between 50% and 80% of patients experience diarrhea during treatment.[123] The potential for CTID increases with the number of antineoplastic agents administered and when radiation therapy is used.[121-123]

Antibiotics also represent a class of drugs with a high incidence (>20%) of drug-induced diarrhea, referred to as antibiotic-associated diarrhea (AAD).[124-126] The incidence of AAD is similar with oral and parenteral antibiotic administration.[127] AAD can be due to a secondary *Clostridium difficile* infection (CDI) or may be a manifestation of alterations in colonic flora.[124,127] Pseudomembraneous colitis, attributed to CDI, specifically describes the formation and proliferation of membranous exudates in the colon resulting in diarrhea. Clindamycin, β-lactams, and fluoroquinolones are most frequently associated with

Note: The authors wish to acknowledge the work of Dr. Jane M. Gervasio, who authored this chapter in a previous edition.

Table 36-1 Agents Implicated in Drug-Induced Diarrhea

Drug Class	Incidence	Level of Evidence[a]
ANTIBIOTICS		
Carbapenems[2-4]	3–10%	A
Cephalosporins[5-14]	10–30%	A
Clindamycin[15-20]	2–31%	A
Fluoroquinolones[21-22]	5–10%	A
Macrolides[23-28]	5–11.6%	A
Penicillins[23,29-41]	5–29%	A
ANTIDEPRESSANTS		
Selective serotonin reuptake inhibitors[21,42-44]	11–18%	A
Serotonin/norepinephrine reuptake inhibitors[42,45-47]	7–13%	A
ANTIHYPERGLYCEMIC AGENTS		
α-glucosidase inhibitors[49-53]	15–49%	A
Biguanides[54-55]	12.5–30%	A
Glucagon-like peptide-1 receptor agonists[56-58]	3–18%	A
ANTINEOPLASTIC AGENTS		
Monoclonal antibodies[59-67]	20–50%	A
Immune checkpoint inhibitors[68-69]	8–44%	A
Topoisomerase inhibitors[21,70-75]	20–90%	A
Tyrosine kinase inhibitors[76-89]	30–50%	A
MISCELLANEOUS		
Erythropoietin-stimulating agents[90-92]	10–20%	A
Interferon α-2B[93-94]	2–45%	A
Misoprostol[95-96]	15–50%	A
Mycophenolic acid[97-101]	27.6–51.3%	A
Orlistat[102-107]	11–20%	A
Protease inhibitors[108-116]	15–60%	A
Peginterferon α-2a[116-119]	19–31%	A

[a]Definitions for Levels of Evidence: Level A—evidence from one or more randomized, controlled clinical trials; Level B—evidence from nonrandomized clinical trials, prospective observational studies, cohort studies, retrospective studies, case-control studies, meta-analyses and/or postmarketing surveillance studies; and Level C—evidence from one or more published case reports or case series.

CDI, often resulting in hospitalization and, if untreated, death.[124,126-128]

Herbal agents are also known to induce diarrhea and must be considered when evaluating a patient with this disorder. Commonly used herbal products associated with diarrhea include chondroitin, glucosamine, ginkgo, and saw palmetto.[129-132] Although limited research makes it difficult to determine the exact incidence of diarrhea associated with the use of herbal products, it may help to consult a natural medicine database.[133] Careful attention must also be paid to over-the-counter (OTC) products containing magnesium, sorbitol, and lactulose as each of these ingredients may lead to osmotic diarrhea. Likewise, agents used to treat or prevent constipation (e.g., mineral oil, bulk forming laxatives) may overcorrect and lead to diarrhea.[21]

EPIDEMIOLOGY

The epidemiology of diarrhea differs in developed versus developing countries. In the United States, it is estimated that 375 million episodes of acute diarrhea occur annually, with the highest prevalence in children younger than 5 years of age. Worldwide, diarrhea is reported as the second leading cause of death in children under 5 years of age.[134]

Elderly individuals are also at an increased risk, due to declining gastrointestinal (GI) tract function. Approximately 10% of individuals over 65 years of age report routine diarrhea.[135] Overall, drug-induced diarrhea accounts for approximately 7% of all adverse drug events. More than 700 drugs are associated with diarrhea, and about 25% of those are antibiotics.[114]

MECHANISMS

Diarrhea arises from various mechanisms including decreased absorption of water, electrolytes, or nutrients, active secretion into the GI tract, increased GI motility, or infection.[21,114,123,127,134] Mechanisms for drug-induced diarrhea are listed in **Table 36-2**.

Decreased absorption of water may occur in association with drug-induced osmotic and secretory diarrhea. Drugs commonly used to treat constipation, such as lactulose and magnesium, affect the lumen of the gut and promote retention of water and electrolytes. Drug-induced secretory diarrhea occurs when a medication increases secretions or decreases absorption of large amounts of water and electrolytes in the gut lumen.[136] Drug-induced diarrhea has also been attributed to fat malabsorption (termed *steatorrhea*). Drugs can prevent absorption of fatty acids in the small intestine. When nonabsorbed fatty acids reach the colon, they inhibit fluid absorption and diarrhea ensues. Orlistat, a gastrointestinal lipase inhibitor, uses this principle to inhibit absorption of dietary fats for the purpose of weight loss.[100-105]

Table 36-2 Mechanisms of Drug-Induced Diarrhea[8,69,118,125,129,136,139]

Drug	Mechanism
α-glucosidase inhibitors	Osmotic
Antibiotics Antineoplastics Biguanides Calcitonin Colchicine Misoprostol Olsalazine Theophylline	Secretory
Erythromycin Cisapride Metoclopramide	Motility
Antibiotics Antineoplastics	Exudative (increased active secretion)
Antibiotics (aminoglycosides, tetracyclines) Antiretroviral therapy Biguanides Cholestyramine Colchicine Orlistat	Malabsorption of fat (steatorrhea)
Antibiotics Antineoplastics Immunosuppressive agents Nonsteroidal anti-inflammatory drugs	Microbial proliferation

An increase in active secretion is associated with drugs that destroy the mucosa of the small and large intestine.[121-123] This exudative process causes discharge of mucus, serum proteins, and blood into the gut, altering water and electrolyte absorption. Irinotecan is a common antineoplastic agent associated with intestinal damage leading to increased colonic exudate.[123]

Drugs that increase GI motility (thereby decreasing the amount of time chyme is exposed to intestinal epithelium) cause abnormal absorption and secretion that can result in diarrhea. Prokinetic medications including metoclopramide and the macrolide antibiotic, erythromycin, are associated with this type of direct effect on the intestine.[21,114,127,136]

AAD occurs as a result of the disruption in the delicate organism balance throughout the GI tract.[137] Antibiotic exposure may result in the overgrowth of antibiotic-resistant bacteria, fungi, or toxin-producing *Clostridium difficile. C. difficile* secretes enterotoxin A and cytotoxin B. Enterotoxin A adheres to the brush-border membrane of enterocytes, inducing lesions and an inflammatory response. Cytotoxin B may also cause GI mucosal damage. Both toxins are necessary for the characteristic tissue damage associated with CDI.[21,138,139]

CLINICAL PRESENTATION AND DIFFERENTIAL DIAGNOSIS

Diarrhea is defined as an increased frequency of bowel movements (≥3 per 24 hours), decreased stool consistency, and/or increased stool weight (>200 g per 24 hours).[134,140] Because bowel habits, stool characteristics, and daily stool output vary considerably among individuals and populations, diarrhea, including drug-induced diarrhea, should always be evaluated in light of the patient's age, weight, and comorbid conditions. Patients with prolonged, voluminous, bloody diarrhea or severe abdominal pain from diarrhea should be carefully evaluated. A patient may present with weight loss, weakness, orthostatic hypotension, tachycardia, electrolyte imbalances and acid–base disturbances.[134,140] Signs and symptoms of drug-induced diarrhea are listed in **Table 36-3**.

The clinical presentation of diarrhea may be acute or chronic, and drugs have been recognized as a cause in both. Diarrhea subsiding within 72 hours is usually considered acute; although episodes of acute diarrhea can persist for up to 14 days.[141] Patients with acute diarrhea may also experience abrupt onset of nausea, vomiting, abdominal pain, headache, fever, chills, and malaise. There may be generalized or local abdominal tenderness with hyperactive bowel sounds. Bowel movements are frequent and usually not bloody.[134,140] Patients seeking medical attention should be screened for dehydration and electrolyte imbalances. Infectious etiologies may require evaluation, although symptoms are typically self-resolving. A complete blood count to assess for leukocytosis and eosinophilia may be warranted if the patient has risk factors for a parasitic infection (e.g., recent travel).[141]

Table 36-3 Signs and Symptoms Associated with Drug-Induced Diarrhea[136,142]

- Abdominal pain
- Acid–base disorders
- Chills
- Cramping
- Dehydration
- Dizziness
- Electrolyte imbalance
- Fever
- Headache
- Hyperactive bowel sounds
- Hypotension
- Malaise
- Nausea/vomiting
- Tachycardia
- Thirst
- Weakness
- Weight loss

Diarrhea lasting 30 days or longer is considered chronic.[141] Chronic diarrhea involves frequent attacks over extended periods, making its cause more difficult to identify. With chronic diarrhea, patients are more likely to seek medical attention and diagnostic tests become more important.[40] A more thoughtful and systematic evaluation for possible malabsorption, food allergies, inflammatory bowel disease, and drug causes is necessary.[142] Flexible sigmoidoscopy, colonoscopy, and abdominal computed tomography may all be useful in determining abnormalities and alternate causes for chronic diarrhea (e.g., Crohn disease).[141,142]

Malabsorption of fat results in pale and voluminous stool with a stool fat content >6 g per day and a stool weight >200 g per day.[142] A stool sample is necessary to determine stool fat content and weight. If possible, sample collection over 3–5 days is preferred to reduce errors and variability, because slight increases in fecal fat not associated with fat malabsorption have been identified in patients with diarrhea. Because of the difficulty in obtaining a 3–5 day collection of stool, other diagnostic tests are often used. The Sudan III stain, acid steatocrit, and the near infrared reflectance analysis offer accurate and simplified alternatives for diagnosing steatorrhea.[143-146]

Food allergies often must be ruled out when evaluating patients for possible drug-induced diarrhea. However, this can be difficult and time-consuming, requiring a thorough patient history, stool samples, laboratory testing, and invasive procedures (e.g., colonoscopy).[147] Having a patient avoid high-risk foods on a trial basis is often an initial diagnostic approach because it is relatively easy and frequently successful. Typically gluten is the first to be removed from the diet, evaluating patient response after 2–8 weeks.[147,148] Aggressive diet restrictions may also be attempted, slowly adding back foods after symptoms resolve. Serum IgE or IgA antitissue transglutaminase (TTG) antibody testing, under the care and direction of an allergist, may also be done to identify specific food allergies.[148,149] In the case of celiac disease, the IgA TTG demonstrates a 95% specificity and sensitivity.[147]

Antineoplastic agents are well-recognized causes of drug-induced diarrhea.[123] Two National Cancer Institute–sponsored cooperative group trials of irinotecan plus high-dose fluorouracil and leucovorin for advanced colorectal cancer led to the recognition of a life-threatening GI syndrome, with symptoms including severe diarrhea, nausea, vomiting, anorexia, and abdominal cramping.[72,73,150] These symptoms were associated with severe dehydration, neutropenia, fever, and electrolyte imbalance. Severe abdominal cramping appeared to be an important early warning sign of imminent diarrhea.

Immune checkpoint inhibitors, such as cytotoxic T-lymphocyte antigen-4 and programmed cell death protein-1 antibodies, are commonly associated with diarrhea. Patients typically report an onset of diarrhea at 7 weeks with ipilimumab and nivolumab, while pembrolizumab-induced diarrhea typically occurs at 6 months. Beyond diarrhea, these agents are associated with a high incidence of enterocolitis, defined by abdominal pain, rectal bleeding, and colonic inflammation. Irrespective of the agent responsible, early detection and treatment of diarrhea is imperative to prevent life-threatening complications.[66,67,150]

AAD and CDI may occur from a few days after initiation of antibiotic therapy to 8 weeks after discontinuation of the drug.[139] Patients with CDI present with profuse diarrhea (rarely with blood) consisting of mucoid, greenish, foul-smelling, watery stools, abdominal pain, bloating, low-grade fever, and leukocytosis. Stool culture remains the gold standard for diagnosing CDI; however, testing is difficult to perform and time-consuming, and results take 24–48 hours to finalize. Rapid diagnostic testing can be used to identify the presence of *C. difficile* and associated toxins. Initial testing done using glutamate dehydrogenase (GDH) demonstrated variable sensitivity (~90%) and specificity (~91%). Development of the nucleic acid amplification test and polymerase chain reaction allowed for high sensitivity (~90%) and specificity (~97%), replacing the GDH in practice.[138,151] Use of rapid diagnostic testing allows for quicker diagnosis and treatment, often within the same day. It is important to note that no diagnostic test available can ascertain the difference between colonization with *C. difficile* and true infection.

Differentiating between drug-induced diarrhea and other forms of diarrhea can be challenging. Practitioners should seek to identify any changes in diet (including alcohol) or drug therapy that have occurred recently and any new drugs (prescription, OTC, illicit) or herbal and nutritional supplements to which the patient has been exposed.[140] Because diarrhea may result from drug therapy started as long as 4 weeks prior to the onset of symptoms and 8 weeks following discontinuation, the temporal relationship between onset and changes in drug therapy must be carefully and thoroughly explored. Additive or synergistic effects from possible drug–drug interactions must also be considered. To help rule out common nondrug causes of diarrhea, eating habits, alcohol and caffeine consumption, and illicit drug use as well as psychosocial factors that might be affecting the patient all must be considered. Any environmental changes in the patient's home or office, recent travel or exposure to possible sources of bacterial or viral pathogens, disease processes, or comorbid complications must all be identified. Conditions to consider in the differential diagnosis of drug-induced diarrhea are listed in **Table 36-4**.

RISK FACTORS

General risk factors for diarrhea are listed in **Table 36-5**. Although specific risk factors for drug-induced diarrhea have not been identified, it can reasonably be assumed that patients are at increased risk for drug-induced diarrhea when one or more of the general risk factors are present or if multiple agents known to cause diarrhea are used concomitantly. Furthermore, because changes in bowel function or a developing GI tract put the elderly and pediatric populations at increased risk for diarrhea, healthcare providers must recognize that the potential for drug-induced diarrhea is increased in these populations as well.[123,134-136]

Table 36-4 Conditions to Consider in the Differential Diagnosis of Drug-Induced Diarrhea[21,116,123,126,136]

- Celiac disease
- Crohn disease
- Diverticulitis
- Gastroenteritis
- Infectious diarrhea/traveler's diarrhea
    - *Campylobacter*
    - *Cryptosporidium*
    - *Cyclospora*
    - Enterotoxigenic *Escherichia coli*
    - *Giardia lamblia*
    - *Microsporidia*
    - *Plesiomonas shigelloides*
    - *Rotavirus*
    - *Salmonella*
    - *Shigella*
- Irritable bowel syndrome
- Ischemic bowel disease
- Malabsorption syndrome
- Psychiatric disease
- Psychosocial/psychological disorders
- Ulcerative colitis

Table 36-5 Risk Factors for Drug-Induced Diarrhea[136-138]

- Age (pediatric and elderly)
- Diet (high-fat, high-fiber)
- Female sex
- Malnutrition
- Pain
- Unsanitary conditions

MORBIDITY AND MORTALITY

The morbidity and mortality of drug-induced diarrhea is largely unknown. Severe diarrhea may result in dehydration, electrolyte abnormalities, and shock, leading to hospitalization and even death. Worldwide, diarrhea is reported as the second leading cause of death in children under 5 years of age.[134] CDIs during hospitalization doubled between 2001 and 2010.[151] In 2009, the 30-day readmission rate for patients with *C. difficile* was 12.8%.[152] Two National Cancer Institute–sponsored cooperative group studies reported mortality rates of 0.6% and 1.9% due to severe diarrhea and subsequent complications secondary to the use of irinotecan, fluorouracil, and leucovorin in cancer patients.[68-69]

PREVENTION

Techniques for decreasing the risk of drug-induced diarrhea are listed in **Table 36-6**. Although proper diet and adequate fluid intake should be always be encouraged, implementing specific preventive measures in all patients receiving a drug with the potential to induce diarrhea may be overzealous. It is more effective for healthcare providers to implement preventive measures in patients with a history of intolerance to medications or in patients receiving medications associated with a high incidence of diarrhea. Whenever possible, healthcare providers should attempt to minimize drug-induced diarrhea in their patients by avoiding the use of medications with high sorbitol content or high tonicity,[153] using alternative medications with lower incidences of causing diarrhea, using low doses and slowly

Table 36-6 Approaches to Help Prevent Drug-Induced Diarrhea[139,155,162]

- Adjust dosage to patient-specific parameters (e.g., age, weight, renal/hepatic function)
- Avoid foods with artificial sweeteners (e.g., sorbitol, mannitol, fructose)
- Encourage fluid and proper diet
- Encourage rational antibiotic use; prescribe antibiotics only when necessary; reserve broad-spectrum antibiotics where possible
- Identify any drug intolerance or allergy previously experienced
- Identify liquid medications with high sorbitol content and substitute the tablet/capsule form when possible
- Implement probiotic therapy (further investigation necessary; see text)
- Instruct patient to eat low-residual diet (e.g., bananas, rice, applesauce, toast)
- Instruct patients to consume low-fat meals (e.g., with orlistat)
- Instruct patients to eat frequent, small meals
- Instruct patients to take medication with meals (if not contraindicated)
- Slowly increase dosage of potential offending agent (if able)
- Use alternative medications with a lower risk of diarrhea when available

increasing the dose of drugs known to cause diarrhea, and judiciously prescribing antibiotics.

In addition to general measures, drug-specific preventive measures are sometimes available. Patients may decrease the incidence of orlistat-induced diarrhea by consuming low-fat meals. Patients experiencing GI cramping and diarrhea associated with iron therapy or multivitamins may benefit from taking these preparations with meals. Patients with chemotherapy-induced diarrhea may benefit from smaller, more frequent meals, avoiding certain foods known to contribute to their diarrhea, and increasing intake of oral fluids.[123]

Probiotics are commonly promoted as being effective in strengthening the immune system and/or recolonizing the gut. Patients with AAD may express interest in using probiotics or have specific questions regarding product selection.[154] The use of probiotics in the prevention and treatment of AAD has been studied. Unfortunately, the evidence is insufficient to determine which probiotics have the greatest efficacy or which antibiotic-treated AAD patients receive the greatest benefit.[155]

Probiotics have also been suggested and evaluated for use in prevention of CDI.[156-158] A Cochrane Review that pooled the findings of 23 randomized clinical trials suggested that probiotics, when given simultaneously with antibiotics, reduced the risk of CDI.[157] However, given the difficulty with interpretation from meta-analyses. Evidence remains insufficient to recommend probiotics for the prevention of CDI.[139] Probiotic use is likely safe if recommended in otherwise healthy patients. Caution should be used in patients with risk factors for probiotic sepsis, including those with immune compromise.[158]

MANAGEMENT

Approximately 90% of cases of acute diarrhea are self-limiting and require no intervention.[159] Drug-induced diarrhea usually spontaneously resolves within a few days following withdrawal of the drug and, in some cases, resolves even with continued use of the causative agent.[114] When diarrhea persists, identification of the offending agent is

Table 36-7 Antidiarrheal Agents Utilized in Drug-Induced Diarrhea[125,140,141]

Cause	Antidiarrheal Drug
Cancer treatment–induced diarrhea	Loperamide
	Octreotide
	Tincture of opium (persistent symptoms)
Clostridium difficile–associated diarrhea	Bismuth subsalicylate
	Cholestyramine (persistent symptoms)

imperative to direct appropriate therapy. Patients should be asked specifically about new or recently discontinued drugs (prescription, OTC, or illicit) or herbal and nutritional supplements as well as changes in eating habits and alcohol or caffeine intake.[140]

Whenever possible, the culprit drug should be discontinued or changed to an agent less likely to cause diarrhea. Solid oral dosage forms may be considered when sorbitol-containing liquid medications or high-tonicity formulations are associated with diarrhea. Another option, if a formulation change is not feasible, is to dilute the liquid medication with water. When therapy with the offending agent must be continued, some of the preventive measures described in Table 36-6 may be helpful. With a few exceptions, antidiarrheal medications should not be thought of as first-line therapy for drug-induced diarrhea; however, if the culprit drug cannot be changed or discontinued and preventive measures do not resolve the diarrhea, antidiarrheal drugs may be used. The selection of the antidiarrheal drug depends on the cause of the drug-induced diarrhea (**Table 36-7**).[123,138,139]

CANCER TREATMENT–INDUCED DIARRHEA

Patients with CTID are a population in which antidiarrheal medications may be indicated as first-line therapy, especially in situations in which it would be detrimental to discontinue or lower the dose of the culprit chemotherapeutic agent. CTID has been recognized as a severe and life-threatening complication

Table 36-8 Criteria for Grading Severity of Diarrhea[123-125]

	Grade 1	Grade 2	Grade 3	Grade 4
Patients without a colostomy	Increase of <4 stools/day over pretreatment No other symptoms	Increase of 4–6 stools/day or nocturnal stools Moderate cramping, not interfering with normal activity	Increase of ≥7 stools/day Severe cramping and incontinence, interfering with daily activities	>10 stools/day Grossly bloody diarrhea and need for parenteral support
Patients with a colostomy	Mild increase in loose, watery colostomy output compared with pretreatment	Moderate increase in loose, watery colostomy output compared with pretreatment, but not interfering with normal activity	Severe increase in loose, watery colostomy output compared with pretreatment, interfering with normal activity	Physiologic consequences requiring intensive care; hemodynamic collapse

for which vigilant monitoring and aggressive therapy is warranted.[121-123,160-162] Patients with uncomplicated, grade 1 or 2 CTID (**Table 36-8**) should be treated with loperamide 4 mg initially followed by 2 mg every 4 hours or after every unformed stool to a maximum of 16 mg daily. Patients should be reassessed after 12–24 hours, and, if diarrhea persists, the loperamide dose should be increased to 2 mg every 2 hours and therapy with an oral antibiotic (e.g., fluoroquinolone) initiated. For patients with unresolved diarrhea after an additional 12- to 24-hour period, loperamide should be discontinued and octreotide 100–150 mcg should be given subcutaneously three times daily. The optimum dose of octreotide has not been determined; doses may be increased up to 500 mcg three times daily until symptoms are controlled with expected response within 4 days. Tincture of opium is another potential second-line antidiarrheal agent to consider in patients who do not respond to other treatment approaches. Patients presenting with grade 3 or 4 CTID should be admitted to the hospital and given intravenous fluids and antibiotics (e.g., fluoroquinolone). Octreotide in subcutaneous doses as outlined above or intravenously in a dose of 25–50 mcg per hour should be administered. Cytotoxic chemotherapy should be discontinued until all symptoms have resolved; afterward, chemotherapy should be reinstituted at reduced dosages.[121-123]

Oral antibiotics (e.g., fluoroquinolone) are used in CTID to prevent superinfection from widespread necrosis of crypt stem cells, especially in patients with immunosuppression or neutropenia. Superinfection can worsen diarrhea via direct secretory effects on the intestinal mucosa and destruction of the intestinal epithelium. Antibiotic therapy should be targeted at opportunistic pathogens, including *C. difficile*, *Clostridium perfringens*, *Bacillus cereus*, *Giardia lamblia*, *Cryptosporidium*, *Salmonella*, *Shigella*, and *Campylobacter* and guided by local patterns of sensitivity and resistance.[122]

CLOSTRIDIUM DIFFICILE–ASSOCIATED DIARRHEA

In patients with CDI, the culprit antimicrobial agent(s) should be stopped as soon as possible.[138-139] Oral metronidazole and vancomycin are first-line antibiotics used to treat patients with *C. difficile* and resulting CDI. For mild-to-moderate CDI, oral metronidazole is preferred initially based on equal efficacy and decreased cost in comparison to oral vancomycin. Metronidazole should be given orally in doses of 500 mg three times a day.[139] Although oral metronidazole is preferred, intravenous metronidazole may be considered when the oral route is not available. Vancomycin therapy delivered via enema may be another appropriate option for patients in whom oral antibiotics cannot reach a segment of the colon. For severe CDI, patients should be treated with oral vancomycin 125 mg four times a day. Oral vancomycin is also recommended for patients who do not respond to initial metronidazole treatment within 5–7 days, for patients with intolerance or allergy to metronidazole, and for pregnant or breastfeeding women. Intravenous vancomycin is not indicated in treatment of CDI. In patients with severe and complicated CDI (e.g., those with hypotension or shock, ileus, megacolon), a combination regimen of oral vancomycin 500 mg four times daily in addition to intravenous metronidazole 500 mg every 8 hours may be warranted. If ileus is present, one should consider adding a vancomycin retention enema (500 mg in 500 mL normal saline) administered every 6 hours. The American College of Gastroenterology guidelines recommend a treatment duration of 10 days for initial CDI, although the Society for Healthcare Epidemiology of America and the Infectious Diseases Society of America guidelines include a range of 10–14 days.[138,139] Fidaxomicin (200 mg orally twice daily for 10 days) is an alternative antibiotic approved for the treatment of mild-to-moderate CDI; however, the cost of the agent is significantly higher than vancomycin, the efficacy is similar, and clinical practice guidelines urge caution with its use until additional data are available.[138,139,162,163] There are no convincing efficacy data to support use of other antibiotics, including rifampin, rifaximin, nitazoxanide, or tigecycline.[138,139]

Recurrence is a common challenge in the management of CDI.[139] The first recurrence of CDI should be managed with the same regimen used in the initial episode unless the disease is severe, in which case vancomycin should be used. The second recurrence should be managed with a tapered, pulsed vancomycin regimen, such as 125 mg orally four times daily for 10 days followed by 125 mg orally three times a week for 10 doses. For a third recurrence, fecal transplant should be considered.[139]

Although antibiotics are the focus in CDI management, other treatment modalities have been studied. Case reports and small case series have described use of intravenous immunoglobulin (IVIG) to bolster the immune response to *C. difficile* toxins.[139] The dosing regimen of IVIG is 300–500 mg/kg daily until resolution or to a maximum of six doses. IVIG should only be considered in select patients as an adjunct to antibiotic therapy in severe refractory or recurrent CDI.[139,164,165] Treatment directed at binding the *C. difficile* toxin has included use of the bile acid–binding resin cholestyramine. Studies, however, have failed to show a high success rate with cholestyramine, and it has been relegated to adjunct treatment status for patients who do not respond adequately to antibiotics.[164,165]

In patients with CDI, antidiarrheal medications that inhibit peristalsis (e.g., diphenoxylate) should be limited or avoided, because these agents can mask symptoms, prevent toxin elimination potentially prolonging the course of illness, and have been associated with the serious complication of toxic megacolon.[138,139] Agents such as bismuth subsalicylate are preferred in CDI if antidiarrheal treatment is necessary. Probiotics have also been studied for the treatment of CDI.[166,167] A systematic review and meta-analysis of *Saccharomyces boulardii* concluded that the evidence for efficacy in the treatment of CDI as an adjunct to antibiotics is weak.[167] The use of adjunct probiotics is not recommended for initial treatment based on limited efficacy data, high costs, potential risks, and product variability.[138,139]

REHYDRATION MANAGEMENT

The most common complication of severe diarrhea is dehydration.[134] Patients with mild or moderate dehydration can nearly always be rehydrated with oral rehydration solution (ORS). An appropriate ORS contains sodium, potassium, chloride, citrate, and glucose to address electrolyte and bicarbonate losses. The rehydration volume for dehydrated patients is approximately 50–100 mL/kg. Additional volumes may be necessary to account for continuing stool losses.[134]

Intravenous fluid is recommended for patients with severe dehydration or when oral rehydration is contraindicated.[134] Volumes of 100 mL/kg of body weight or more may be required for rehydration. Rapid replacement of fluid and electrolyte losses is necessary to prevent shock and subsequent death. A polyelectrolyte solution such as Ringer's lactate is considered appropriate for this purpose. Normal saline is a poorer choice for rehydration in these patients because it does not correct the acidosis or hypokalemia that may result from severe diarrhea.[134]

INFORMATION FOR PATIENTS

Patients prescribed drugs that may cause clinically relevant diarrhea should be warned of the potential for this adverse effect prior to the initiation of therapy. A detailed list of potential adverse effects with a timeline should be communicated and strategies to combat symptoms that arise discussed. To help anticipate and avoid complications, patients should always be carefully questioned regarding any adverse drug reactions previously experienced.

Adequate fluid intake and a proper diet should be recommended for any patient who might experience drug-induced diarrhea. Use of OTC agents to alleviate diarrhea may be appropriate. Patients with CDI should be cautioned to avoid antidiarrheals, as use can retain toxins produced by *C. difficile* within the colon. Probiotics may be useful in AAD, and it is reasonable to recommend a product in an otherwise healthy patient.

Patients should be aware that most incidences of drug-induced diarrhea are self-limiting and resolve within a few days. However, if symptoms are chronic, lasting more than 30 days, or severe (e.g., presence of blood, existence of fever, excruciating pain), the patient should notify the healthcare provider immediately.

REFERENCES

1. Truven Health Analytics, Inc. Micromedex solutions 2018. http://www.micromedexsolutions.com/micromedex2/librarian (accessed 2018 Mar 6).
2. Shiber S, Yahav D, Avni T et al. B-lactam/B-lactamase inhibitors versus carbapenems for the treatment of sepsis: systematic review and meta-analysis of randomized controlled trials. *J Antimicrob Chemother.* 2015; 70:41-7.
3. Zhanel GC, Wiebe R, Dilay L et al. Comparative review of the carbapenems. *Drugs.* 2007; 67:1027-52.
4. Calandra GB, Brown KR, Grad LC et al. Review of adverse experiences and tolerability in the first 2,516 patients treated with imipenem/cilastatin. *Am J Med.* 1985; 78:73-8.
5. Settle CD, Wilcox MH, Fawley WN et al. Prospective study of the risk of Clostridium difficile diarrhoea in elderly patients following treatment with cefotaxime or piperacillin-tazobactam. *Aliment Pharmacol Ther.* 1998; 12:1217-23.
6. Gales MA, Gales BJ. Recognition of severe cefixime-induced diarrhea. *Clin Pharm.* 1993; 12:881.
7. Gooch WM III, Philips A, Rhoades R et al. Comparison of the efficacy, safety and acceptability of cefixime and amoxicillin/clavulanate in acute otitis media. *Pediatr Infect Dis J.* 1997; 16:S21-4.
8. Asmar BI, Dajani AS, Del Beccaro MA et al. Comparison of cefpodoxime proxetil and cefixime in the treatment of acute otitis media in infants and children. Otitis Study Group. *Pediatrics.* 1994; 94:847-52.
9. Harrison CJ, Chartrand SA, Pichichero ME. Microbiologic and clinical aspects of a trial of once daily cefixime compared with twice daily cefaclor for treatment of acute otitis media in infants and children. *Pediatr Infect Dis J.* 1993; 12:62-9.
10. Osier T, Lott D, Bordley J et al. Cefazolin induced pseudomembranous colitis resulting in perforation of the sigmoid colon. *Dis Colon Rectum.* 1986; 29:140-3.
11. Saito A. Cefmetazole postmarketing surveillance in Japan. *J Antimicrob Chemother.* 1989; 23:131-9.
12. Meyers BR. Comparative toxicities of third-generation cephalosporins. *Am J Med.* 1985; 79:96-103.
13. Bartlett JG, Willey SH, Chang TW et al. Cephalosporin-associated pseudomembranous colitis due to clostridium difficile. *JAMA.* 1979; 242:2683-5.
14. Hutcheon DF, Milligan FD, Yardley JH et al. Cephalosporin-associated pseudomembranous colitis. *Dig Dis.* 1978; 23:321-6.
15. Kelly CP, Pothoulakis C, LaMont JT. Clostridium difficile colitis. *N Engl J Med.* 1994; 330:257.
16. Schwartzberg JE, Maresca RM, Remington JS. Gastrointestinal side effects associated with clindamycin. 1000 consecutive patients. *Arch Intern Med.* 1976; 136:876-9.
17. Mahakit P, Vicente JG, Butt DI et al. Oral clindamycin 300 mg BID compared with oral amoxicillin/clavulanic acid 1 g BID in the outpatient treatment of acute recurrent pharyngotonsillitis caused by group a beta-hemolytic streptococci: an international, multicenter, randomized, investigator-blinded, prospective trial in patients between the ages of 12 and 60 years. *Clin Ther.* 2006; 28:99-109.
18. Jacobson MA, Besch CL, Child C et al. Toxicity of clindamycin as prophylaxis for AIDS-associated toxoplasmic encephalitis. Community Programs for Clinical Research on AIDS. *Lancet.* 1992; 339:333-4.
19. Wilson WR, Cockerill FR 3rd. Tetracyclines, chloramphenicol, erythromycin, and clindamycin. *Mayo Clin Proc.* 1987; 62:906-15.
20. Davis JS. Severe colitis following lincomycin and clindamycin therapy. *Am J Gastroenterol.* 1974; 62:16.
21. Chassany O, Michaux A, Bergmann J. Drug induced diarrhea. *Drug Safety.* 2000; 22:53-72.
22. Angel CA, Green J, Swischuk L et al. Severe ciprofloxacin-associated pseudomembranous colitis in an eight-year-old child. *J Pediatr Surg.* 2004; 39:1590-2.
23. Arguedas A, Emparanza P, Schwartz RH et al. A randomized, multicenter, double blind, double dummy trial of single dose azithromycin versus high dose amoxicillin for treatment of uncomplicated acute otitis media. *Pediatr Infect Dis J.* 2005; 24:153-61.
24. Akhyani M, Ehsani AH, Ghiasi M et al. Comparison of efficacy of azithromycin vs. doxycycline in the treatment of rosacea: a randomized open clinical trial. *Int J Dermatol.* 2008; 47:284-8.
25. Block SL, Cifaldi M, Gu Y et al. A comparison of 5 days of therapy with cefdinir or azithromycin in children with acute otitis media: a multicenter, prospective, single-blind study. *Clin Ther.* 2005; 27:786-94.
26. Langley JM, Halperin SA, Boucher FD, Smith B. Pediatric Investigators Collaborative Network on Infections in Canada (PICNIC). Azithromycin is as effective as and better tolerated than erythromycin estolate for the treatment of pertussis. *Pediatrics.* 2004; 114:e96-101.
27. Damrongmanee A, Ukarapol N. Incidence of antibiotic-associated diarrhea in a pediatric ambulatory care setting. *J Med Assoc Thai.* 2007; 90:513-7.
28. Brook I, Aronovitz GH, Pichichero ME. Open-Label, parallel-group, multicenter, randomized study of cefprozil versus erythromycin in children with group A streptococcal pharyngitis/tonsillitis. *Clin Ther.* 2001; 23:1889-900.

29. Eppes SC, Childs JA. Comparative study of cefuroxime axetil versus amoxicillin in children with early Lyme disease. *Pediatrics.* 2002; 109:1173-7.
30. Bartlett JG. Antimicrobial agents implicated in clostridium difficile toxin associated diarrhea or colitis. *Johns Hopkins Med J.* 1981; 1490:6-9.
31. Roddis MJ. Antibiotic-associated colitis: a retrospective study of fifteen cases. *Age Ageing.* 1978; 7:182-8.
32. Léophonte P, File T, Feldman C. Gemifloxacin once daily for 7 days compared to amoxicillin/clavulanic acid thrice daily for 10 days for the treatment of community-acquired pneumonia of suspected pneumococcal origin. *Respir Med.* 2004; 98:708-20.
33. Henry DC, Riffer E, Sokol WN et al. Randomized double-blind study comparing 3- and 6-day regimens of azithromycin with a 10-day amoxicillin-clavulanate regimen for treatment of acute bacterial sinusitis. *Antimicrob Agents Chemother.* 2003; 47:2770-4.
34. Bucher HC, Tschudi P, Young J et al. Effect of amoxicillin-clavulanate in clinically diagnosed acute rhinosinusitis: a placebo-controlled, double-blind, randomized trial in general practice. *Arch Intern Med.* 2003; 163:1793-8.
35. Iravani A, Richard GA. Amoxicillin-clavulanic acid versus cefaclor in the treatment of urinary tract infections and their effects on the urogenital and rectal flora. *Antimicrob Agents Chemother.* 1986; 29:107-11.
36. Gold JA, Hegarty CP, Deitch MW et al. Double-blind clinical trials of oral cyclacillin and ampicillin. *Antimicrob Agents Chemother.* 1979; 15:55-8.
37. Gotz V, Romankiewicz JA, Moss J et al. Prophylaxis against ampicillin-associated diarrhea with a lactobacillus preparation. *Am J Hosp Pharm.* 1979; 36:754-7.
38. Van der Auwera P, D'Haens J, Noterman J. Pseudomembranous colitis associated with oxacillin therapy. *Ada Clin Belg.* 1982; 37:116-7.
39. Friedman RJ, Mayer IE, Galambos JT et al. Oxacillin-induced pseudomembranous colitis. *Am J Gastroenterol.* 1980; 73:445-7.
40. Jaccard C, Troillet N, Harbarth S et al. Prospective randomized comparison of imipenem-cilastatin and piperacillin-tazobactam in nosocomial pneumonia or peritonitis. *Antimicrob Agents Chemother.* 1998; 42:2966-72.
41. Sweet RL, Roy S, Faro S et al. Piperacillin and tazobactam versus clindamycin and gentamicin in the treatment of hospitalized women with pelvic infection. The Piperacillin/tazobactam Study Group. *Obstet Gynecol.* 1994; 83:280-6.
42. Vanderkooy JD, Kennedy SH, Bagby RM. Antidepressant side effects in depression patients treated in a naturalistic setting: a study of bupropion, moclobemide, paroxetine, sertraline, and venlafaxine. *Can J Psychiatry.* 2002; 47:174-80.
43. Haffmans PM, Timmerman L, Hoogduin CA. Efficacy and tolerability of citalopram in comparison with fluvoxamine in depressed outpatients: a double-blind, multicentre study. The LUCIFER Group. *Int Clin Psychopharmacol.* 1996; 11:157-64.
44. Leonard BE. Pharmacological differences of serotonin reuptake inhibitors and possible clinical relevance. *Drugs.* 1992; 43:3-9.
45. Raskin J, Wiltse CG, Dinkel JJ et al. Safety and tolerability of duloxetine at 60 mg once daily in elderly patients with major depressive disorder. *J Clin Psychopharmacol.* 2008; 28:32-8.
46. Hurley DJ, Turner CL, Yalcin I et al. Duloxetine for the treatment of stress urinary incontinence in women: an integrated analysis of safety. *Eur J Obstet Gynecol Reprod Biol.* 2006; 125:120-8.
47. Detke MJ, Wiltse CG, Mallinckrodt CH et al. Duloxetine in the acute and long-term treatment of major depressive disorder: a placebo- and paroxetine-controlled trial. *Eur Neuropsychopharmacol.* 2004; 14:457-70.
48. Singh KP, Periyandavar I, Rajadhyaksha GC et al. Evaluation of the efficacy, safety and tolerability of miglitol in adult Indian patients with uncomplicated type 2 diabetes mellitus. *Indian Med Assoc.* 2007; 105:344,346,350.
49. Johnston PS, Lebovitz HE, Coniff RF et al. Advantages of alpha-glucosidase inhibition as monotherapy in elderly type 2 diabetic patients. *J Clin Endocrinol Metab.* 1998; 83:1515-22.
50. Johnston PS, Feig PU, Coniff RF et al. Long-term titrated-dose alpha-glucosidase inhibition in non-insulin-requiring Hispanic NIDDM patients. *Diabetes Care.* 1998; 21:409-15.
51. Federlin KF, Mehlburger L, Hillebrand I et al. The effect of two new glucosidase inhibitors on blood glucose in healthy volunteers and in type 2 diabetics. *Ada Diabetol Lat.* 1987; 24:213-21.
52. Hollander P. Safety profile of acarbose, an alpha-glucosidase inhibitor. *Drugs.* 1992; 44:47-53.
53. Schweizer A, Couturier A, Foley JE et al. Comparison between vildagliptin and metformin to sustain reductions in HbA(lc) over 1 year in drug-naïve patients with Type 2 diabetes. *Diabet Med.* 2007; 24:955-61.
54. Josephkutty S, Potter JM. Comparison of tolbutamide and metformin in elderly diabetic patients. *Diabet Med.* 1990; 7:510-4.
55. Tella SH, Rendell MS. Glucagon-like polypeptide agonists in type 2 diabetes mellitus: efficacy and tolerability, a balance. *Ther Adv Endocrinol Metab.* 2015; 6:109-34.
56. Heine RJ, Van Gaal LF, Johns D et al. Exenatide versus insulin glargine in patients with suboptimally controlled type 2 diabetes: a randomized trial. *Ann Intern Med.* 2005; 143:559-69.
57. Bukowski RM, Kabbinavar FF, Figlin RA et al. Randomized phase II study of erlotinib combined with bevacizumab compared with bevacizumab alone in metastatic renal cell cancer. *J Clin Oncol.* 2007; 25:4536-41.
58. Miller KD, Chap LI, Holmes FA et al. Randomized phase III trial of capecitabine compared with bevacizumab plus capecitabine in patients with previously treated metastatic breast cancer. *J Clin Oncol.* 2005; 23:792-9.
59. Schoffski P, Lutz C-H, Folprecht G et al. Cetuximab (C225Erbitux) in combination with irinotecan, infusional 5-fluoro-uracil and folinic acid is safe and active in patients with metastatic colorectal cancer expressing epidermal growth factor receptor. Results of a phase I study. *Eur J Cancer.* 2002; 38:S148-9.
60. Raoul JL, Van Laethem JL, Mitry E et al. Phase II study of cetuximab combined with FOLFIRI (bi-weekly irinotecan plus infusional 5-FU and folinic acid (FA)) in patients (pts) with metastatic, Epidermal Growth Factor Receptor (EGFR) expressing colorectal cancer (CRC). *Eur J Cancer Suppl.* 2003; 1:S89.
61. Cascinu S, Berardi R, Labianca R et al. Cetuximab plus gemcitabine and cisplatin compared with gemcitabine and cisplatin alone in patients with advanced pancreatic cancer: a randomised, multicentre, phase II trial. *Lancet Oncol.* 2008: 9:39-44.
62. Hecht JR, Patnaik A, Berlin J et al. Panitumumab monotherapy in patients with previously treated metastatic colorectal cancer. *Cancer.* 2007; 110:980-8.
63. Rowinsky EK, Schwartz GH, Gollob JA et al. Safety, pharmacokinetics, and activity of ABX-EGF, a fully human anti-epidermal growth factor receptor monoclonal antibody in patients with metastatic renal cell cancer. *J Clin Oncol.* 2004; 22:3003-15.
64. Slamon DJ, Leyland-Jones B, Shak S et al. Use of chemotherapy plus a monoclonal antibody against HER2 for metastatic breast cancer that overexpresses HER2. *N Engl J Med.* 2001; 344:783-92.
65. Marty M, Cognetti F, Maraninchi D et al. Randomized phase II trial of the efficacy and safety of trastuzumab combined with docetaxel in patients with human epidermal growth factor receptor 2-positive metastatic breast cancer administered as first-line treatment: the M77001 study group. *J Clin Oncol.* 2005; 23:4265-74.
66. Spain L, Diem S, Larkin J. Management of toxicities of immune checkpoint inhibitors. *Cancer Treatment Reviews.* 2016; 14:51-60.
67. Gupta A, De Felice KM, Loftus EV et al. Systemic review: colitis associated with anti-CTLA-4 therapy. *Aliment Pharmacol Ther.* 2015; 42:406-17.
68. Rothenberg ML, Meropol NJ, Poplin EA et al. Mortality associated with irinotecan plus bolus fluorouracil/leucovorin: summary findings of an independent panel. *J Clin Oncol.* 2001; 19:3801-7.

69. Saltz LB, Cox JV, Blanke C et al. Irinotecan plus fluorouracil and leucovorin for meta-static colorectal cancer: Irinotecan Study Group. *N Engl J Med.* 2000; 343:905-14.
70. Faivre S, Delbaldo C, Boige V et al. Safety of repeated administrations of ixabepilone given as a 3-hour infusion every other week in combination with irinotecan in patients with advanced malignancies. *Eur J Cancer.* 2008; 44:674-82.
71. Feldman EJ, Seiter K, Damon L et al. A randomized trial of high- vs standard-dose mitoxantrone with cytarabine in elderly patients with acute myeloid leukemia. *Leukemia.* 1997; 11:485-9.
72. Eckardt JR, von Pawel J, Pujol JL et al. Phase III study of oral compared with intravenous topotecan as second-line therapy in small-cell lung cancer. *J Clin Oncol.* 2007; 25:2086-92.
73. O'Brien ME, Ciuleanu TE, Tsekov H et al. Phase III trial comparing supportive care alone with supportive care with oral topotecan in patients with relapsed small-cell lung cancer. *J Clin Oncol.* 2006; 24:5441-7.
74. Heymach JV, Johnson BE, Prager D et al. Randomized, placebo-controlled phase II study of vandetanib plus docetaxel in previously treated non small-cell lung cancer. *J Clin Oncol.* 2007; 25:4270-7.
75. Shepherd FA, Rodrigues Pereira J, Ciuleanu T. Erlotinib in previously treated non-small-cell lung cancer. *N Engl J Med.* 2005; 353:123-32.
76. Herbst RS, Prager D, Hermann R et al. TRIBUTE: a phase III trial of erlotinib hydrochloride (OSI-774) combined with carboplatin and paclitaxel chemotherapy in advanced non-small-cell lung cancer. *J Clin Oncol.* 2005; 23:5892-9.
77. Fukuoka M, Yano S, Giaccone G et al. Multi-institutional randomized phase II trial of gefitinib for previously treated patients with advanced non-small-cell lung cancer (the IDEAL 1 trial). *J Clin Oncol.* 2003; 21:2237-46.
78. Herbst RS, Giaccone G, Schiller JH et al. Gefitinib in combination with paclitaxel and carboplatin in advanced non-small-cell lung cancer: a phase III trial-INTACT 2. *J Clin Oncol.* 2004; 22:785-94.
79. Burrhis HA 3rd, Hurwitz HL, Dees EC et al. Phase 1 safety, pharmacokinetics, and clinical activity study of lapatinib (GW572016), a reversible dual inhibitor of epidermal growth factor receptor tyrosine kinases in heavily pretreated patients with metastatic carcinomas. *J Clin Oncol.* 2005; 5305-13.
80. le Coutre P, Ottmann OG, Giles F et al. Nilotinib (formerly AMN107), a highly selective BCR-ABL tyrosine kinase inhibitor, is active in patients with imatinib-resistant or -intolerant accelerated-phase chronic myelogenous leukemia. *Blood.* 2008; 111:1834-9.
81. Kantarjian HM, Giles F, Gattermann N et al. Nilotinib (formerly AMN107), a highly selective BCR-ABL tyrosine kinase inhibitor, is effective in patients with Philadelphia chromosome-positive chronic myelogenous leukemia in chronic phase following imatinib resistance and intolerance. *Blood.* 2007; 110:3540-6.
82. Demetri GD, von Mehren M, Blanke CD et al. Efficacy and safety of imatinib mesylate in advanced gastrointestinal stromal tumors. *N Engl J Med.* 2002; 347:472-80.
83. Geyer CE, Forster J, Lindquist D et al. Lapatinib plus capecitabine for HER2-positive advanced breast cancer. *N Engl J Med.* 2006; 355:2733-43.
84. Escudier B, Lassau N, Angevin E et al. Phase I trial of sorafenib in combination with IFN alpha-2a in patients with unresectable and/or metastatic renal cell carcinoma or malignant melanoma. *Clin Cancer Res.* 2007; 13:1801-9.
85. Motzer RJ, Rini BI, Bukowski RM et al. Sunitinib in patients with metastatic renal cell carcinoma. *JAMA.* 2006; 295:2516-24.
86. Motzer RJ, Hutson TE, Tomczak P et al. Sunitinib versus interferon alfa in metastatic renal-cell carcinoma. *N Engl J Med.* 2007; 356:115-24.
87. Demetri GD, van Oosterom AT, Garrett CR et al. Efficacy and safety of sunitinib in patients with advanced gastrointestinal stromal tumour after failure of imatinib: a randomised controlled trial. *Lancet.* 2006; 368:1329-38.
88. Hedenus M, Adriansson M, San Miguel J et al. Efficacy and safety of darbepoetin alfa in anaemic patients with lymphoproliferative malignancies: a randomized, double-blind, placebo-controlled study. *Br J Haematol.* 2003; 122:394-403.
89. Case DC Jr, Bukowski RM, Carey RW et al. Recombinant human erythropoietin therapy for anemic cancer patients on combination chemotherapy. *J Natl Cancer Inst.* 1993; 85:801-6.
90. Canaud B, Mingardi G, Braun J et al. Intravenous C.E.R.A. maintains stable haemoglobin levels in patients on dialysis previously treated with darbepoetin alfa: results from STRIATA, a randomized phase III study. *Nephrol Dial Transplant.* 2008; 23:3654-61.
91. Kosmidis PA, Tsavaris N, Skarlos D et al. Fluorouracil and leucovorin with or without interferon alfa-2b in advanced colorectal cancer: analysis of a prospective randomized phase III trial. Hellenic Cooperative Oncology Group. *J Clin Oncol.* 1996; 14:2682-7.
92. Köhne CH, Wilke H, Hecker H et al. Interferon-alpha does not improve the antineoplastic efficacy of high-dose infusional 5-fluorouracil plus folinic acid in advanced colorectal cancer. First results of a randomized multicenter study by the Association of Medical Oncology of the German Cancer Society (AIO). *Ann Oncol.* 1995; 6:461-6.
93. Ackerman Z, Cominelli F, Reynolds TB. Effect of misoprostol on ibuprofen-induced renal dysfunction in patients with decompensated cirrhosis: results of a double-blind placebo-controlled parallel group study. *Am J Gastroenterol.* 2002; 97:2033-9.
94. Ching CK, Lam SK. A comparison of two prostaglandin analogues (enprostil vs misoprostol) in the treatment of acute duodenal ulcer disease. *J Gastroenterol.* 1995; 30:607-14.
95. Eisen HJ, Kobashigawa J, Keogh A et al. Three-year results of a randomized, double-blind, controlled trial of mycophenolate mofetil versus azathioprine in cardiac transplant recipients. *J Heart Lung Transplant.* 2005; 24:517-25.
96. Ensley RD, Bristow MR, Olsen SL et al. The use of mycophenolate mofetil (RS-61443) in human heart transplant recipients. *Transplantation.* 1993; 56:75-82.
97. Deierhoi MH, Kauffman RS, Hudson SL et al. Experience with mycophenolate mofetil (RS61443) in renal transplantation at a single center. *Ann Surg.* 1993; 217:476-84.
98. Goldblum R. Therapy of rheumatoid arthritis with mycophenolate mofetil. *Clin Exp Rheumatol.* 1993; 11:S117-9.
99. Sollinger HW, Belzer FO, Deierhoi MH et al. RS-61443 (mycophenolate mofetil): a multicenter study for refractory kidney transplant rejection. *Ann Surg.* 1992; 216:513-9.
100. Torgerson JS, Hauptman J, Boldrin MN et al. XENical in the prevention of diabetes in obese subjects (XENDOS) study: a systemic randomized study of orlistat as an adjunct to lifestyle changes for the prevention of type 2 diabetes in obese patients. *Diabetes Care.* 2004; 27:155-61.
101. Hanefeld M, Sachse G. The effects of orlistat on body weight and glycaemic control in overweight patients with type 2 diabetes: a randomized, placebo-controlled trial. *Diabetes Obes Metab.* 2002; 4:415-23.
102. Didangelos TP, Thanopoulou AK, Bousboulas SH et al. The ORLIstat and CArdiovascular risk profile in patients with metabolic syndrome and type 2 DIAbetes (ORLICARDIA) Study. *Curr Med Res Opin.* 2004; 20:1393-1401.
103. Davidson MH, Hauptman J, DiGirolamo M et al. Weight control and risk factor reduction in obese subjects treated for 2 years with orlistat: a randomized controlled trial. *JAMA.* 1999; 281:235-42.
104. Chanoine JP, Hampl S, Jensen C et al. Effect of orlistat on weight and body composition in obese adolescents: a randomized controlled trial. *JAMA.* 2005; 293:2873-83.
105. Kiortsis DN, Filippatos TD, Elisaf MS. The effects of orlistat on metabolic parameters and other cardiovascular risk factors. *Diabetes Metab.* 2005; 31:15-22.
106. Katlama C, Esposito R, Gatell JM et al. Efficacy and safety of TMC114/ritonavir in treatment-experienced HIV patients: 24-week results of POWER 1. *AIDS.* 2007; 21:395-402.

107. Molina JM, Cohen C, Katlama C et al. Safety and efficacy of darunavir (TMC114) with low-dose ritonavir in treatment-experienced patients: 24-week results of POWER 3. *J Acquir Immune Defic Syndr.* 2007; 46:24-31.
108. Rachlis A, Gill J, Baril JG et al. Effectiveness of step-wise intervention plan for managing nelfinavir-associated diarrhea: a pilot study. *HIV Clin Trials.* 2005; 6:203-12.
109. Gathe JC Jr, Ive P, Wood R et al. SOLO: 48-week efficacy and safety comparison of once-daily fosamprenavir/ritonavir versus twice-daily nelfinavir in naive HIV-1-infected patients. *AIDS.* 2004; 18:1529-37.
110. Rodriguez-French A, Boghossian J, Gray GE et al. The NEAT study: a 48-week open-label study to compare the antiviral efficacy and safety of GW433908 versus nelfinavir in antiretroviral therapy-naive HIV-1-infected patients. *J Acquir Immune Defic Syndr.* 2004; 35:22-32.
111. Sanne I, Piliero P, Squires K et al. Results of a phase 2 clinical trial at 48 weeks (AI424-007): a dose-ranging, safety, and efficacy comparative trial of atazanavir at three doses in combination with didanosine and stavudine in antiretroviral-naive subjects. *J Acquir Immune Defic Syndr.* 2003; 32:18-29.
112. Markowitz M, Slater LN, Schwartz R et al. Long-term efficacy and safety of tipranavir boosted with ritonavir in HIV-1-infected patients failing multiple protease inhibitor regimens: 80-week data from a phase 2 study. *J Acquir Immune Defic Syndr.* 2007; 45:401-10.
113. Walmsley SL, Katlama C, Lazzarin A et al. Pharmacokinetics, safety, and efficacy of tipranavir boosted with ritonavir alone or in combination with other boosted protease inhibitors as part of optimized combination antiretroviral therapy in highly treatment-experienced patients (BI Study 1182.51). *J Acquir Immune Defic Syndr.* 2008; 47:429-40.
114. Abraham B, Sellin JH. Drug-induced diarrhea. *Curr Gastroenterol Rep.* 2007; 9:365-72.
115. Heathcote EJ, Shiftman ML, Cooksley WG et al. Peginterferon alfa-2a in patients with chronic hepatitis C and cirrhosis. *N Engl J Med.* 2000; 343:1673-80.
116. Reddy KR, Wright TL, Pockros PJ et al. Efficacy and safety of pegylated (40-kd) interferon alpha-2a compared with interferon alpha-2a in noncirrhotic patients with chronic hepatitis C. *Hepatology.* 2001; 33:433-8.
117. Zeuzem S, Feinman SV, Rasenack J et al. Peginterferon alfa-2a in patients with chronic hepatitis C. *N Engl J Med.* 2000; 343:1666-72.
118. Piper DW. A comparative overview of the adverse effects of antiulcer drugs. *Drug Saf.* 1995; 12:120-38.
119. Yen L. Cimetidine-induced diarrhea. *Drug Intell Clin Pharm.* 1985; 19:185.
120. Beaugerie L, Patey N, Brousse N. Ranitidine, diarrhea, and lymphocytic colitis. *Gut.* 1995; 37:708-11.
121. Kornblau S, Benson AB, Catalono R et al. Management of cancer treatment-related diarrhea: issues and therapeutic strategies. *J Pain Symptom Manage.* 2000; 19:118-29.
122. Benson AB, Ajani JA, Catalano RB et al. Recommended guidelines for the treatment of cancer treatment-induced diarrhea. *J Clin Oncol.* 2004; 22:2918-26.
123. Stein A, Voigt W, Jordan K. Chemotherapy-induced diarrhea: pathophysiology, frequency, and guideline-based management. *Ther Adv Med Onc.* 2010: 2:51-63.
124. Bartlett JG. Antibiotic-associated diarrhea. *N Engl J Med.* 2002; 346:334-9.
125. Wistrom J, Norrby SR, Myhre EB. Frequency of antibiotic-associated diarrhea in 2462 antibiotic-treated hospitalized patients: a prospective study. *J Antimicrob Chemother.* 2001; 47:43-50.
126. Montoya M, DeTorres O. Antimicrobial selection and its impact on the incidence of *Clostridium difficile*-associated diarrhea. *J Pharm Pract.* 2013; 26:483-7.
127. Hogenauer C, Hammer H, Krejs G et al. Mechanisms and management of antibiotic associated diarrhea. *CID.* 1998; 27:702-10.
128. Piacenti F, Leuthner K. Antimicrobial stewardship and *Clostridium difficile*-associated diarrhea. *J Pharm Pract.* 2013; 26:506-13.
129. Sherman A, Ojeda-Correal G, Mena J. Use of glucosamine and chondroitin in persons with osteoarthritis. *PM R* 2012; 4(suppl 5): S110-6.
130. Singh V, Singh SP, Chan K. Review and meta-analysis of usage of ginkgo as an adjunct therapy in chronic schizophrenia. *Int J Neuropsychopharmacol.* 2010; 13:257-71.
131. Langmead L, Rampton D. Review article: herbal treatment in gastrointestinal and liver disease—benefits and dangers. *Aliment Pharmacol Ther.* 2001; 15:1239-52.
132. Agbabiaka T, Pittler M, Wider B, Ernst E. Serenoa repens (saw palmetto) a systematic review of adverse events. *Drug Safety* 2009; 32:637-47.
133. Natural Medicines [online database]. Somerville, MA: Therapeutic Research Center; 2015. https://naturalmedicines.therapeuticresearch.com/ (accessed 2018 Feb 12).
134. Farthing M, Salam M, Lindberg G et al. Acute diarrhea in adults and children: a global perspective. *J Clin Gastroenterol.* 2013; 47:12-20.
135. Pilotto A, Franceschi M, Vitale D et al. The prevalence of diarrhea and its association with drug use in elderly outpatients: a multicenter study. *Am J Gastroenterol.* 2008; 103:2816-23.
136. Parfitt J, Driman D. Pathological effect of drugs on the gastrointestinal tract: a review. *Human Pathology.* 2007; 38:527-36.
137. Varughese C, Vakil N, Phillips K. Antibiotic-associated diarrhea: a refresher on causes and possible prevention with probiotics—continuing education article. *J Pharm Pract.* 2013; 26:476-82.
138. Cohen AH, Gerding DN, Johnson S et al. Clinical practice guidelines for *Clostridium difficile* infections in adults: 2010 update by the Society for Healthcare Epidemiology of America (SHEA) and the Infectious Diseases Society of America (IDSA). *Infect Control Hosp Epidemiol.* 2010; 31:431-55.
139. Surawicz CM, Brandt LJ, Binion DG et al. Guidelines for the diagnosis, treatment, and prevention of *Clostridium difficile* infections. *Am J Gastroenterol.* 2013; 108:478-98.
140. Barr W, Smith A. Acute diarrhea in adults. *Am Fam Phy.* 2014; 89:180-9.
141. DuPont H. Acute infectious diarrhea in immunocompetent adults. *N Engl J Med* 2014; 370:1532-40.
142. Schiller L. Definitions, pathophysiology, and evaluation of chronic diarrhoea. *Best Practice & Research Clinical Gastroenterology.* 2012; 26:551-62.
143. Fine KD, Ogunji F. A new method of quantitative fecal fat microscopy and its correlation with chemically measured fecal fat output. *Am J Clin Pathol.* 2000; 113:528-34.
144. Simko V. Fecal fat microscopy: acceptable predictive value in screening for steatorrhea. *Am J Gastroenterol.* 1981; 75:204-8.
145. Amann ST, Josephson SA, Toskes PP. Acid steatocrit: a simple, rapid gravimetric method to determine steatorrhea. *Am J Gastroenterol.* 1997; 92:2280-4.
146. Peled Y, Doron O, Laufer H et al. D-xylose absorption test: urine or blood? *Dig Dis Sci.* 1991; 36:188-92.
147. Elli L, Branchi F, Tomba C et al. Diagnosis of gluten related disorders: Celiac disease, wheat allergy, and non-celiac gluten sensitivity. *World J Gastroenterol.* 2015; 21:7110-9.
148. Boyce JA, Assa'ad A, Burks AW et al. Guidelines for the diagnosis and management of food allergy in the United States: report of the NIAID-sponsored expert panel. *J Allergy Clin Immunol.* 2010; 126(suppl 6):S1-58.
149. Rubio-Tapia A, Hill I, Kelly C et al. ACG clinical guidelines: diagnosis and management of celiac disease. *Am J Gastroenterol.* 2013; 108:656-76.
150. Merrouche Y, Extra JM, Abigerges D et al. High dose-intensity of irinotecan administered every 3 weeks in advanced cancer patients: a feasibility study. *J Clin Oncol.* 1997; 15:1080-6.

151. Bagdasarian N, Rao K, Malani PN. Diagnosis and treatment of Clostridium difficile in adults: a systematic review. *JAMA.* 2015; 313:398-408.

152. Elixhauser A (AHRQ), Steiner C (AHRQ), Gould C (CDC). Readmissions following hospitalizations with Clostridium difficile infections, 2009. HCUP Statistical Brief #145. December 2012. Agency for Healthcare Research and Quality, Rockville, MD. http://www.hcup-us.ahrq.gov/reports/statbriefs/sb145.pdf (accessed 2018 Feb 12).

153. Johnston KR, Govel LA, Andritz MH. Gastrointestinal effects of sorbitol as an additive in liquid medications. *Am J Med.* 1994; 97:185-91.

154. Therapeutic Research Center. Pharmacist's Letter/Prescriber's Letter, July 2015. PL Detail-Document #310709. Comparison of common probiotic products. Stockton, CA: Therapeutic Research Center; July 2015.

155. Hempel S, Newberry SJ, Maher AR et al. Probiotics for the prevention and treatment of antibiotic-associated diarrhea: a systematic review and meta-analysis. *JAMA.* 2012; 307:1959-69.

156. Allen S. The potential of probiotics to prevent *clostridium difficile* infection. *Infect Dis Clin N Am.* 2015; 29:135-44.

157. Goldenberg JZ, Ma SS, Saxton JD et al. Probiotics for the prevention of *Clostridium difficile*-associated diarrhea in adults and children. *Cochrane Database Syst Rev.* 2013; (5):CD006095.

158. Boyle RJ, Robins-Browne RM, Tang MK. Probiotic use in clinical practice: what are the risks? *Am J Clin Nutr.* 2006; 83:1256-64.

159. Guerrant RL, Van Gilder T, Steiner TS et al. Practice guidelines for the management of infectious diarrhea. *Clin Infect Dis.* 2001; 32:331-51.

160. Maroun JA, Anthony LB, Blais N et al. Prevention and management of chemotherapy-induced diarrhea in patients with colorectal cancer: a consensus statement by the Canadian working group on chemotherapy-induced diarrhea. *Curr Oncol.* 2007; 14:13-20.

161. Walder S, Bensen AB 3rd, Engelking C et al. Recommended guidelines for the treatment of chemotherapy-induced diarrhea. *J Clin Oncol.* 1998; 16:3169-78.

162. Louie TJ, Miller MA, Mullane KM et al. Fidaxomicin versus vancomycin for *Clostridium difficile* infection. *N Engl J Med.* 2011; 364:422-31.

163. Cornely OA, Crook DW, Esposito R et al. Fidaxomicin versus vancomycin for infection with Clostridium difficile in Europe, Canada, and the USA: a double-blind, non-inferiority, randomised controlled trial. *Lancet Infect Dis.* 2012; 12:281-9.

164. Leffler DA, Lamont JT. Treatment of Clostridium difficile-associated disease. *Gastroenterology.* 2009; 136:1899-912.

165. Hookman P, Barkin JS. Clostridium difficile associated infection, diarrhea, and colitis. *World J Gastroenterol.* 2009; 15:1554-80.

166. McFarland LV. Systematic review and meta-analysis of Saccharomyces boulardii in adult patients. *World J Gastroenterol.* 2010; 16:2202-22.

167. McFarland LV. Meta-analysis of probiotics for the prevention of antibiotic associated diarrhea and the treatment of Clostridium difficile disease. *Am J Gastroenterol.* 2006; 101:812-22.

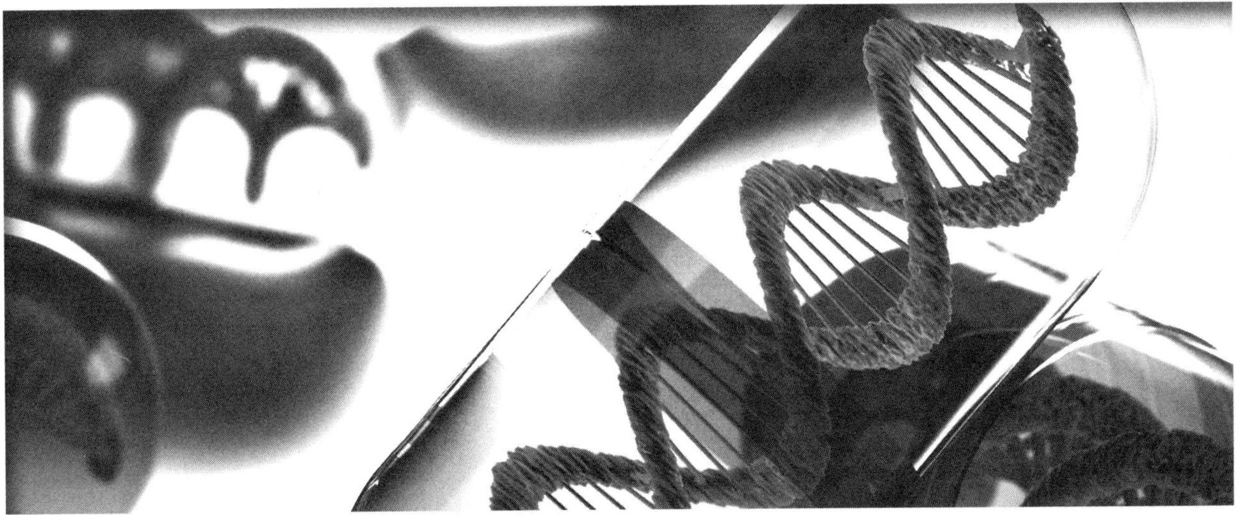

CHAPTER 37

Constipation

Sarah A. Nisly and Carolyn M. Jung

Constipation is a common gastrointestinal disorder and is frequently drug induced. Signs and symptoms vary considerably between patients. Although constipation is often relatively mild and interferes only slightly with a patient's quality of life, it can, at times, necessitate discontinuation of essential drug therapy, increase the cost of care, and even prove to be life threatening. Identification of drug-induced constipation is difficult due to a number of confounders which may contribute to or exacerbate the problem. In addition, there is significant variation among both patients and health professionals in defining what actually constitutes constipation.

CAUSATIVE AGENTS

Commonly used drugs known to be associated with a 10% or greater incidence of causing constipation are listed in **Table 37-1**.[1-57] Constipation is commonly listed as an adverse effect for both prescription and nonprescription medications; thus, this list should not be considered all-encompassing. Opioids and antineoplastic agents are two of the most common classes of medications known to cause constipation.[20-29,46-55] Any medication with anticholinergic properties, including antidepressants and antipsychotics, has the potential to cause constipation as well.[4-13,32-38] Medication classes with lower incidences of constipation include anticonvulsants, antihistamines, nondihydropyridine calcium channel blockers, diuretics, calcium supplements, and aluminum-containing antacids.[58-66] Some medications within these classes may have higher incidences of constipation similar to those of opioids. Herbal preparations including chondroitin sulfate, glucosamine sulfate, *Echinacea*, and saw palmetto have also been reported to cause constipation.[67-80]

EPIDEMIOLOGY

The reported prevalence of constipation due to any cause varies considerably among published studies. A systematic review of published literature on

Note: The authors wish to acknowledge the work of Dr. Jane M. Gervasio, who authored this chapter in a previous edition.

Table 37-1 Agents Implicated in Drug-Induced Constipation

Drug Class	Example(s) (% incidence)	Level of Evidence[a]
Antibiotics	Dalbavancin[2] (18.2%)	A
Anticholinergic agents	Solifenacin[3] (13–16%)	A
Antidepressants	Bupropion[4,5] (5–10%) Duloxetine[6,7] (5–15%) Fluoxetine[8,9] (4–17.9%) Imipramine[10,11] (20%) Paroxetine[4,11,12] (18–25%) Venlafaxine[4,13] (15%)	A A A A A A
Antihypertensives	Clonidine[14,15] (1–10%) Guanfacine[17] (10–15%) Verapamil[18,19] (7.3–42%)	A A A
Antineoplastic agents	Abiraterone[20] (23%) Ado-Trastuzumab[21] (26.5%) Axatinib[22] (20%) Bevacizumab[23] (29–40%) Bicalutamide[24-26] (22%) Decitabine[27] (11%) Doxorubicin[28] (41%) Temsirolimus[29] (20%) Thalidomide[30-31] (54%)	A A A A A A A A A
Antipsychotics	Aripiprazole[32-34] (8–13%) Clozapine[35,36] (14%) Olanzapine[35,36] (5–15%) Quetiapine[37,38] (8–10%)	A A A A
Bile acid sequestrants	Colesevelam[39] (8.7–11%) Colestipol[40] (10%)	A A
Bisphosphonates	Zoledronic acid[41,42] (6–27%)	B
Diuretics	Furosemide[16] (29.2%)	B
HMG-CoA reductase inhibitors	Atorvastatin[16] (21.4%)	B
Immunologic agents	Belatacept[43] (33%)	A
Iron preparations	Various salts[44,45] (15.6%)	A
NSAIDs	Ibuprofen[16] (19.4%)	B
Opioids	Codeine[46-48] (10–21%) Fentanyl[49,50] (8–26%) Hydrocodone[48,51] (10–29%) Hydromorphone[52] (29%) Methadone[53] (20%) Morphine[50,54,55] (5.1–57%)	A A A A A A
5-HT_3 antagonists	Alosetron[56] (32%) Granisetron[57] (3–18%)	A A
Miscellaneous	Ursodiol[1] (9.7–26.4%)	B

NSAID = nonsteroidal anti-inflammatory drug.
[a]Definitions for Levels of Evidence: Level A—evidence from one or more randomized, controlled clinical trials; Level B—evidence from nonrandomized clinical trials, prospective observational studies, cohort studies, retrospective studies, case-control studies, meta-analyses and/or postmarketing surveillance studies; and Level C—evidence from one or more published case reports or case series.

constipation found a median prevalence of 16% in North America, but ranges between 2.5% and 79% worldwide.[81] Females experience constipation more commonly than males, with a median ratio of 1.5:1 cases.[81,82] Females are also more likely to seek medical care for constipation and receive treatment, as opposed to males. The prevalence of constipation increases with age, with 33.5% of adults ages 60–101 affected.[81] Within the geriatric population, nursing home residents experience constipation more often than the general community. Lastly, ethnicity may play a role with nonwhites more likely to be affected by constipation than whites.[81,82] Although drugs are well recognized as a potential cause of constipation, the incidence of drug-induced constipation is unknown. Opioid-induced constipation, a subset of drug-induced constipation, occurs in 17–67% of patients in the United States according to survey and medical chart review data.[83]

MECHANISMS

Chronic constipation is differentiated into five types and mechanisms vary with each type. Primary constipation disorders include normal transit constipation (NTC), slow transit constipation (STC), pelvic floor dysfunction or defecatory disorders, and combination disorders. Colonic motility disorders such as NTC or STC are associated with decreased function of the colon, although many of the changes that occur with STC cause or are a consequence of chronic constipation.[84] Defecatory or pelvic floor disorders result from structural abnormalities within the colon or rectum.[82,85] Drug-induced constipation, as well as mechanical obstruction and constipation due to systemic disease, are all considered secondary constipation disorders. Mechanisms of drug-induced constipation differ based on the implicated drug class. Opioid-induced constipation results in decreased gastrointestinal motility both through effects on the central nervous system and binding of opioid receptors in the intestines.[86] In contrast, furosemide is thought to mediate constipation through simple dehydration.[16] Common mechanisms for drug-induced constipation are listed in **Table 37-2**.[16,82,85,86]

CLINICAL PRESENTATION AND DIFFERENTIAL DIAGNOSIS

Bowel symptoms such as hard or infrequent stools or incomplete rectal evacuation constitute the syndrome of constipation. Patients and practitioners may describe constipation with additional symptoms such as the inability to defecate at will, excessive straining, bloating, and abdominal pain or distention.[82,87] The Rome III symptom criteria for chronic constipation take into consideration the variety of symptoms with which patients may present. Symptoms must be present for at least 6 months prior to diagnosis and two or more symptoms must occur in a quarter of defecation episodes in the past 3 months. Symptoms include straining, lumpy or hard stools, sensation of incomplete evacuation, feeling of anorectal obstruction, use of manual maneuvers to stimulate defecation, less than three bowel movements per week, and absence of loose stools with lack of diagnostic criteria for irritable bowel syndrome.[87] Signs and symptoms associated with drug-induced constipation are presented in **Table 37-3**.[82,87] The onset of drug-induced constipation is highly variable.

Differentiating between drug-induced constipation and other potential causes is important to the determination of appropriate treatment and/or methods of prevention.[85] **Table 37-4** lists conditions to consider in the differential diagnosis of drug-induced constipation. A detailed history including bowel habits and the onset of constipation with relation to any risk factors should be obtained from the patient. Patients should be encouraged to complete a stool diary and chart dietary habits and medications

Table 37-2 Mechanisms of Drug-Induced Constipation

Drug	Mechanism
Diuretics	Decreased fluid secretion
Drugs with anticholinergic properties (examples include antihistamines, antidepressants)	Parasympatholytic actions affecting innervation of many regions of the gastrointestinal tract
Opioids and related compounds	Inhibition of acetylcholine release from the central nervous system Prolongation of intestinal transient time (reduced peristalsis) Increased electrolyte and water reabsorption

to help in the identification of any potential correlations. The medication history should document the patient's use of prescription drugs, nonprescription drugs, and nutritional supplements. Also, a temporal relationship between changes in therapy and onset of symptoms should be carefully explored. Additive or synergistic effects of medications to which the patient has been exposed must be considered and ruled out as a possible cause of constipation. Assessment of the patient's hydration status and mobility can help rule out other common causes of constipation. Psychosocial factors, changes in the home or office environment, other disease processes or comorbid conditions can also lead to constipation and should be assessed.[85]

Severe abdominal pain, unintended weight loss (>10 lb), hematochezia, positive occult-blood test, unexplained anemia, sudden change in stools (e.g., changes in consistency, color, or appearance), a family history of colorectal cancer, or a combination of any of these, should be considered alarm symptoms and receive careful attention during the evaluation.[82] Gastrointestinal endoscopy or imaging via computerized tomography scan should be considered to help rule out malignancy in patients presenting with these symptoms. A rectal examination can help identify some anatomical complications (e.g., pelvic floor dysfunction) associated with constipation.[82]

Table 37-3 Signs and Symptoms Associated with Drug-Induced Constipation[a]

- Abdominal pain
- Anal or perianal pain
- Anal prolapse/hemorrhoids
- Anorexia
- Bloating
- Cramping
- Discomfort
- Feeling of fullness
- Hypoperistalsis
- Ineffective straining
- Infrequent bowel movements
- Lack of bowel sounds
- Local distention
- Nausea/vomiting
- No urge to defecate
- Sense of incomplete evacuation
- Sense of anal blockage/obstruction
- Stools difficult to pass (small, hard, dry)
- Weight loss

[a]Severe abdominal pain, weight loss >10 lb, hematochezia, positive fecal occult test, unexplained anemia or sudden change in stools constitute "Alarm Symptoms" and these patients should be referred immediately to a proper source of care.

Table 37-4 Conditions to Consider in the Differential Diagnosis of Drug-Induced Constipation

- Dehydration
- Diabetes mellitus
- Disorders of bowel structure/function
- Diverticulitis
- Hypercalcemia
- Hypothyroidism
- Irritable bowel syndrome
- Ischemic bowel disease
- Malignancy
- Mechanical obstruction
- Neuropathic diseases
- Pregnancy
- Psychiatric disease
- Psychosocial/psychological disorders

RISK FACTORS

Patient parameters and comorbid disease states that place patients at increased risk for constipation are listed in **Table 37-5**.[61,82,88] Certain drugs are notorious for causing constipation (e.g., opioids).[88] Opioid-induced constipation (OIC) is associated with longer durations of therapy and concurrent use of multiple opioids.[89,90] The incidence of drug-induced constipation may be increased in the

Table 37-5 Risk Factors for Drug-Induced Constipation

- Age (elderly)
- Concurrent medications which may provide an additive effect
- Dehydration
- Female sex
- Inactivity
- Poor diet
- Pregnancy

elderly because of an associated decline in bowel function (e.g., decreased transit time).[91]

MORBIDITY AND MORTALITY

Constipation drastically alters quality of life, affecting mood, mobility, work, recreation, and enjoyment of life.[92-94] Constipation associated with opioid use has been reported in 40% and 60% of opioid users for noncancer and cancer pain, respectively.[95,96] Severe constipation may result in small bowel obstruction, impaction, gastrointestinal perforation, and death. Chronic constipation has also been associated with an increased mortality and decreased quality of life.[97,98] The advent of new and novel treatment options for constipation has led to an increased cost for treatment; however, up to 56% of patients remain unsatisfied with their treatment regimen.[96] Reports suggest there are over 6 million ambulatory care visits annually due to constipation, leading to estimated direct costs of $1.6 billion.[99] Additionally, over $800 million is spent annually within the United States on over-the-counter treatment of constipation.[100] In one 12-month analysis, OIC was associated with a 109% increase in overall healthcare costs.[89]

PREVENTION

Techniques for decreasing the risk of drug-induced constipation are listed in **Table 37-6.**[91,101-103] Patients may decrease risk by staying active, maintaining a routine bowel habit schedule, drinking plenty of fluids, and eating a balanced, high-fiber diet. Healthcare providers may further decrease or prevent drug-induced constipation in their patients by adjusting doses of causative agents with respect to specific patient parameters, using the lowest possible effective dose of the drug to treat the patient, slowly escalating the doses of medications to allow for better tolerance, and using alternative medications with a lower risk of constipation. In patients beginning chronic opioid therapy, careful attention must be paid to the possibility of OIC. Initiation of a prophylactic bowel regimen, using a stimulant laxative alone or in combination, is appropriate in high-risk patients or those anticipated to receive long-term opioid therapy.[91,101-103]

Table 37-6 Approaches to Help Prevent Drug-Induced Constipation

- Adjust dosage to patient specific parameters (e.g., age, weight, renal/hepatic function)
- Encourage activity (exercise, especially aerobic)
- Encourage fluids and high-fiber diet (25–35 g/day of fiber for adults)
- Encourage patients to avoid postponing defecation
- Identify any intolerance already experienced to drugs
- Maintain a routine bowel habit schedule
- Slowly escalate doses to allow for better patient tolerance
- Use alternative medications with a lower risk of constipation

MANAGEMENT

Patients presenting with chronic constipation, severe pain, hematochezia, or fever should be evaluated for small-bowel obstruction, impaction, or gastrointestinal perforation.[87] Whenever possible and appropriate, the culprit drug should be discontinued and an alternative agent less likely to cause constipation substituted.[91,101] When that is not possible, lowering the dose of the drug may help relieve symptoms. Lifestyle modifications, including dietary changes (increasing consumption of fruits, vegetables, and other dietary sources of fiber), increasing fluid consumption, and increasing physical activity, can sometimes also be helpful. Removal of the offending agent and/or implementation of lifestyle changes may take weeks to relieve constipation. Providing thorough patient education and creating realistic patient expectations are keys to successful treatment of this drug-induced disease.[91,101] Discontinuation of agents inducing constipation is not always feasible, and patients may need to weigh the benefits of that agent (e.g., pain control) with the ongoing risk of persistent constipation and quality of life indicators.

Pharmacotherapy may be implemented if dietary and lifestyle modifications do not relieve the constipation.[90,96,101,104-106] **Table 37-7** lists possible agents for use and the corresponding mechanisms

Table 37-7 Drugs Used to Treat Drug-Induced Constipation

Agent	Generic Name	Mechanism of Action
Emollient laxative	Docusate sodium	Soften stool Stimulate net intestinal secretion Surfactant properties
Fiber, bulk-forming laxatives	Methylcellulose Calcium polycarbophil Psyllium	Increase stool weight Modify stool consistency
Lubricant laxatives	Mineral oil	Facilitates transit by coating feces
Miscellaneous	Lubiprostone Prucalopride Tegaserod	Increases intestinal fluid secretion via activation of the chloride channel Stimulates intestinal secretions and peristalsis through activation of the 5-HT_4 receptor
Nonselective opioid antagonist	Naloxone Nalmefene	Opioid receptor antagonist in the gastrointestinal tract Crosses the blood–brain barrier and may reverse opioid analgesic effects
Osmotic laxatives	Glycerin Lactulose Phosphate salts Polyethylene glycol	Attract and retain water in intestinal lumen Increases intraluminal pressure Exert an osmotic effect Stimulate colonic motility (lactulose)
PAMORA	Alvimopan Methylnaltrexone Naloxegol	Antagonize opioid receptors in the gastrointestinal tract. Do not cross the blood–brain barrier; do not reverse opioid analgesic effects.
Saline laxative	Magnesium salts	Fluid osmotically drawn into small intestine; cholecystokinin-stimulated
Stimulants	Bisacodyl Senna	Stimulate intestinal motor activity Stimulate net intestinal secretion Increase stool volume/weight Induces urge to defecate

5-HT_4 = 5-hydroxytryptamine (4), PAMORA = peripheral acting mu-opioid receptor antagonist.

of action. Bulk-forming agents, emollient laxatives, osmotic laxatives, and saline laxatives modify the characteristics of stool to increase bulk, decrease consistency, or facilitate passage through the digestive tract and anus. Stimulant laxatives and chloride channel agonists accelerate transit time and facilitate evacuation of stool from the rectal vault. Agent selection should be carefully matched to the root drug cause of constipation and anticipated duration of therapy.[90,96,101,104-106]

Bulk-forming agents and osmotic laxatives are generally used first-line; however, stimulant laxatives may be used when patients do not respond adequately to bulk or osmotic laxatives given alone.[96,101,104] Exaggerated concerns regarding stimulant laxative abuse have led to hesitation on the part of healthcare providers to use this class of laxatives. Caution should be exercised when a valid concern for abuse or misuse exists (e.g., anorexic patients).

Peripheral acting mu-opioid receptor antagonists (PAMORA), developed specifically for the treatment of OIC, include alvimopan, methylnaltrexone, and naloxegol.[90,96,105] These agents work to target opioid receptors specific to the gastrointestinal tract, thus blocking the constipating effects of systemic opioids. This mechanism is more specific than that of naloxone or nalmefene, which reverse both peripheral and central opioid effects, thereby relieving symptoms of OIC but also potentially reversing the intended opioid analgesic effects.[107,108] Lubiprostone is an additional agent used for OIC and is considered a PAMORA, although the mechanism is through chloride channel activation.[109] Axelopran and sustained-release naloxone are two new PAMORAs in clinical trials for OIC.[109] Successful bowel evacuation is reported to occur in up to 35% of patients receiving one of the newer PAMORA agents.[96,109] Flatulence and diarrhea are the most common adverse events with PAMORA, although abdominal pain can occur. Dosage forms and agent-specific safety concerns should be considered when evaluating treatment options. Methylnaltrexone, for example, is only available as a subcutaneous injection, making this agent less advantageous for routine outpatient use.[96] Alvimopan carries a U.S. Food and Drug Administration "black box warning" for risk of myocardial infarction and has restricted distribution requirements.[109]

INFORMATION FOR PATIENTS

Fluids and a proper diet, including fiber consumption of at least 25 g/day, should be recommended for any patient at risk for drug-induced constipation. Patients should be instructed to maintain regular bowel habits and not to ignore the urge to defecate. Increased activity and exercise should be encouraged. Continued evaluation of the appropriateness of the offending medication is warranted and initiation of drug therapy treatment may be necessary if and when lifestyle and dietary measures do not resolve constipation. If symptoms of abdominal distention, severe pain, hematochezia, unintentional weight loss >10 pounds, or fever occur, the patient should notify a healthcare provider immediately for evaluation and assistance.

REFERENCES

1. Truven Health Analytics, Inc. Micromedex solutions 2018. http://www.micromedexsolutions.com/micromedex2/librarian (accessed 2018 Mar 6).
2. Seltzer E, Dorr MB, Goldstein BP et al. Once-weekly dalbavancin versus standard-of-care antimicrobial regimens for treatment of skin and soft-tissue infections. *Clin Infect Dis*. 2003; 37:1298-303.
3. Yamaguchi O, Marui E, Kakizaki H et al. Randomized, double-blind, placebo- and propiverine-controlled trial of the once-daily antimuscarinic agent solifenacin in Japanese patients with overactive bladder. *BJU Int*. 2007; 100:579-87.
4. Vanderkooy JD, Kennedy SH, Bagby RM. Antidepressant side effects in depression patients treated in a naturalistic setting: a study of bupropion, moclobemide, paroxetine, sertraline, and venlafaxine. *Can J Psychiatry*. 2002; 47:174-80.
5. Semenchuk MR, Sherman S, Davis B. Double-blind, randomized trial of bupropion SR for the treatment of neuropathic pain. *Neurology*. 2001; 57:1583-8.
6. Detke MJ, Lu Y, Goldstein DJ et al. Duloxetine 60 mg once daily dosing versus placebo in the acute treatment of major depression. *J Psychiatr Res*. 2002; 36:383-90.
7. Steers WD, Herschorn S, Kreder KJ et al. Duloxetine compared with placebo for treating women with symptoms of overactive bladder. *BJU Int*. 2007; 100:337-45.
8. Beasley CM Jr, Holman SL, Potvin JH. Fluoxetine compared with imipramine in the treatment of inpatient depression: a multicenter trial. *Ann Clin Psychiatry*. 1993; 5:199-207.
9. Chouinard G, Saxena B, Bélanger MC et al. A Canadian multicenter, double-blind study of paroxetine and fluoxetine in major depressive disorder. *J Affect Disord*. 1999; 54:39-48.
10. Versiani M, Amrein R, Stabl M. Moclobemide and imipramine in chronic depression (dysthymia): an international double-blind, placebo-controlled trial. International Collaborative Study Group. *Int Clin Psychopharmacol*. 1997; 12:183-93.
11. Cohn JB, Crowder JE, Wilcox CS et al. A placebo- and imipramine-controlled study of paroxetine. *Psychopharmacol Bull*. 1990; 26:185-9.
12. Bielski RJ, Bose A, Chang CC. A double-blind comparison of escitalopram and paroxetine in the long-term treatment of generalized anxiety disorder. *Ann Clin Psychiatry*. 2005; 17:65-9.
13. Thase ME, Shelton RC, Khan A. Treatment with venlafaxine extended release after SSRI nonresponse or intolerance: a randomized comparison of standard- and higher-dosing strategies. *J Clin Psychopharmacol*. 2006; 26:250-8.
14. Goldberg RM, Loprinzi CL, O'Fallon JR et al. Transdermal clonidine for ameliorating tamoxifen-induced hot flashes. *J Clin Oncol*. 1994; 12:155-8.
15. Distler A, Kirch W, Lüth B. Antihypertensive effect of guanfacine: a double-blind cross-over trial compared with clonidine. *Br J Clin Pharmacol*. 1980; 10:49S-53S.
16. Fosnes GS, Lydersen S, Farup PG. Constipation and diarrhea—common adverse drug reactions? A cross sectional study in the general population. *BMC Clin Pharmacol*. 2011; 11(2).
17. Roeckel A, Heidland A. Comparative studies of guanfacine and methyldopa. *Br J Clin Pharmacol*. 1980; 10:55S-59S.
18. Rosei EA, Dal Palù C, Leonetti G et al. Clinical results of the verapamil in hypertension and atherosclerosis study. VHAS Investigators. *J Hypertens*. 1997; 15:1337-44.
19. Cutler NR, Anders RJ, Jhee SS et al. Placebo-controlled evaluation of three doses of a controlled-onset, extended-release formulation of verapamil in the treatment of stable angina pectoris. *Am J Cardiol*. 1995; 75:1102-6.
20. Ryan CJ, Smith MR, deBono JS et al. Abiraterone in metastatic prostate cancer without previous chemotherapy. *N Engl J Med*. 2013; 368:138-48.
21. Kadcyla [package insert]. South San Francisco, CA: Genentech Inc; 2013.
22. Rini BI, Escudier B, Tomczak P et al. Comparative effectiveness of axitinib versus sorafenib in advanced renal cell carcinoma (AXIS): a randomized phase 3 trial. *Lancet*. 2011; 378:1931-9.
23. Avastin [package insert]. South San Francisco, CA: Genentech Inc; 2015.
24. Wirth M, Tyrrell C, Delaere K et al. Bicalutamide (Casodex) 150 mg plus standard care in early non-metastatic prostate cancer: results from Early Prostate Cancer Trial 24 at a median 7 years' follow-up. *Prostate Cancer Prostatic Dis*. 2007; 10:87-93.
25. Tyrrell CJ, Iversen P, Tammela T et al. Tolerability, efficacy and pharmacokinetics of bicalutamide 300 mg, 450 mg or 600 mg as monotherapy for patients with locally advanced or metastatic prostate cancer, compared with castration. *BJU Int*. 2006; 98:563-72.

26. See WA, Tyrrell CJ; CASODEX Early Prostate Cancer Trialists' Group. The addition of bicalutamide 150 mg to radiotherapy significantly improves overall survival in men with locally advanced prostate cancer. *J Cancer Res Clin Oncol.* 2006; 132:S7-16.
27. Steensma DP, Baer MR, Slack JL et al. Multicenter study of decitabine administered daily for 5 days every 4 weeks to adults with myelodysplastic syndromes: the alternative dosing for outpatient treatment (ADOPT) trial. *J Clin Oncol.* 2009; 27:23:3842-8.
28. Coleman RE, Biganzoli L, Canney P et al. A randomised phase II study of two different schedules of pegylated liposomal doxorubicin in metastatic breast cancer (EORTC-10993). *Eur J Cancer.* 2006; 42:882-7.
29. Hudes G, Carducci M, Tomczak P et al. Temsirolimus, interferon alfa, or both for advanced renal-cell carcinoma. *N Engl J Med.* 2007; 356:2271-81.
30. Chiou TJ, Wang TH, Chao TY et al. Randomized Phase II trial of thalidomide alone versus thalidomide plus interferon alpha in patients with refractory multiple myeloma. *Cancer Invest.* 2007; 25:140-7.
31. Zervas K, Mihou D, Katodritou E et al. VAD-doxil versus VAD-doxil plus thalidomide as initial treatment for multiple myeloma: results of a multicenter randomized trial of the Greek Myeloma Study Group. *Ann Oncol.* 2007; 18:1369-75.
32. Marcus RN, McQuade RD, Carson WH et al. The efficacy and safety of aripiprazole as adjunctive therapy in major depressive disorder: a second multicenter, randomized, double-blind, placebo-controlled study. *J Clin Psychopharmacol.* 2008; 28:156-5.
33. Thase ME, Jonas A, Khan A et al. Aripiprazole monotherapy in nonpsychotic bipolar I depression: results of 2 randomized, placebo-controlled studies. *J Clin Psychopharmacol.* 2008; 28:13-20.
34. Anton RF, Kranzler H, Breder C et al. A randomized, multicenter, double-blind, placebo-controlled study of the efficacy and safety of aripiprazole for the treatment of alcohol dependence. *J Clin Psychopharmacol.* 2008; 28:5-12.
35. Kelly DL, Richardson CM, Yu Y et al. Plasma concentrations of high-dose olanzapine in a double-blind crossover study. *Hum Psychopharmacol.* 2006; 21:393-8.
36. Tollefson GD, Birkett MA, Kiesler GM et al. Double-blind comparison of olanzapine versus clozapine in schizophrenic patients clinically eligible for treatment with clozapine. *Biol Psychiatry.* 2001; 49:52-63.
37. Potkin SG, Gharabawi GM, Greenspan AJ et al. A double-blind comparison of risperidone, quetiapine and placebo in patients with schizophrenia experiencing an acute exacerbation requiring hospitalization. *Schizophr Res.* 2006; 85:254-65.
38. Thase ME, Macfadden W, Weisler RH et al. Efficacy of quetiapine monotherapy in bipolar I and II depression: a double-blind, placebo-controlled study (the BOLDER II study). *J Clin Psychopharmacol.* 2006; 26:600-9.
39. Zieve FJ, Kalin MF, Schwartz SL et al. Results of the glucose-lowering effect of WelChol study (GLOWS): a randomized, double-blind, placebo-controlled pilot study evaluating the effect of colesevelam hydrochloride on glycemic control in subjects with type 2 diabetes. *Clin Ther.* 2007; 29:74-83.
40. Spence JD, Huff MW, Heidenheim P et al. Combination therapy with colestipol and psyllium mucilloid in patients with hyperlipidemia. *Ann Intern Med.* 1995; 123:493-9.
41. Berenson JR, Vescio RA, Rosen LS et al. A phase I dose-ranging trial of monthly infusions of zoledronic acid for the treatment of osteolytic bone metastases. *Clin Cancer Res.* 2001; 7:478-5.
42. Berenson JR, Vescio R, Henick K et al. A Phase I, open label, dose ranging trial of intravenous bolus zoledronic acid, a novel bisphosphonate, in cancer patients with metastatic bone disease. *Cancer.* 2001; 91:144-54.
43. Nulojix [package insert]. Princeton, NJ: Bristol-Myers Squibb; 2014.
44. Liguori L. Iron protein succinylate in the treatment of iron deficiency: controlled, double-blind, multicenter clinical trial on over 1,000 patients. *Int J Clin Pharmacol Ther Toxicol.* 1993; 31:103-23.
45. Coplin M, Schuette S, Leichtmann G et al. Tolerability of iron: a comparison of bis-glycino iron II and ferrous sulfate. *Clin Ther.* 1991; 13:606-12.
46. Bourne MH, Rosenthal NR, Xiang J et al. Tramadol/acetaminophen tablets in the treatment of postsurgical orthopedic pain. *Am J Orthop.* 2005; 34:592-7.
47. Smith AB, Ravikumar TS, Kamin M et al. Combination tramadol plus acetaminophen for postsurgical pain. *Am J Surg.* 2004;187:521-7.
48. Rodriguez RF, Castillo JM, Del Pilar Castillo M et al. Codeine/acetaminophen and hydrocodone/acetaminophen combination tablets for the management of chronic cancer pain in adults: a 23-day prospective, double-blind, randomized, parallel-group study. *Clin Ther.* 2007; 29:581-7.
49. Allan L, Richarz U, Simpson K et al. Transdermal fentanyl versus sustained release oral morphine in strong-opioid naïve patients with chronic low back pain. *Spine.* 2005; 30:2484-90.
50. van Seventer R, Smit JM, Schipper RM et al. Comparison of TTS-fentanyl with sustained-release oral morphine in the treatment of patients not using opioids for mild-to-moderate pain. *Curr Med Res Opin.* 2003; 19:457-69.
51. Marco CA, Plewa MC, Buderer N et al. Comparison of oxycodone and hydrocodone for the treatment of acute pain associated with fractures: a double-blind, randomized, controlled trial. *Acad Emerg Med.* 2005; 12:282-8.
52. Hale M, Tudor IC, Khanna S et al. Efficacy and tolerability of once-daily OROS hydromorphone and twice-daily extended-release oxycodone in patients with chronic, moderate to severe osteoarthritis pain: results of a 6-week, randomized, open-label, noninferiority analysis. *Clin Ther.* 2007; 29:874-88.
53. Johnson RE, Chutuape MA, Strain EC et al. A comparison of levomethadyl acetate, buprenorphine, and methadone for opioid dependence. *N Engl J Med.* 2000; 343:1290-97.
54. Allan L, Richarz U, Simpson K et al. Transdermal fentanyl versus sustained release oral morphine in strong-opioid naïve patients with chronic low back pain. *Spine.* 2005; 30:2484-90.
55. Nicholson B, Ross E, Sasaki J et al. Randomized trial comparing polymer-coated extended-release morphine sulfate to controlled-release oxycodone HC1 in moderate to severe nonmalignant pain. *Curr Med Res Opin.* 2006; 22:1503-14.
56. Wolfe SG, Chey WY, Washington MK et al. Tolerability and safety of alosetron during long-term administration in female and male irritable bowel syndrome patients. *Am J Gastroenterol.* 2001; 96:803-11.
57. Sigsgaard T, Herrstedt J, Andersen LJ et al. Granisetron compared with prednisolone plus metopimazine as anti-emetic prophylaxis during multiple cycles of moderately emetogenic chemotherapy. *Br J Cancer.* 1999; 80:412-8.
58. Herndon CM, Jackson KC, Hallin PA. Management of opioid-induced gastrointestinal effects in patients receiving palliative care. *Pharmacotherapy.* 2002; 22:240-50.
59. Staats PS, Markowitz J, Schein J. Incidence of constipation associated with long-acting opioid therapy: a comparative study. *South Med J.* 2004; 97:129-34.
60. Donatelle EP. Constipation: pathophysiology and treatment. *Am Fam Physician.* 1990; 42:1335-42.
61. Talley NJ, Jones M, Nuyts G et al. Risk factors for chronic constipation based on a general practice sample. *Am J Gastroenterol.* 2003; 98:1107-11.
62. Opie LH. Calcium channel antagonists. Part III: use and comparative efficacy in hypertension and supraventricular arrhythmias. Minor indications. *Cardiovasc Drugs Ther.* 1988; 1:625-56.
63. Opie LH. Calcium channel antagonists. Part IV: side effects and contraindications drug interactions and combinations. *Cardiovasc Drugs Ther.* 1988; 2:177-89.
64. Dougall HT, McLay J. A comparative review of the adverse effects of calcium antagonists. *Drug Saf.* 1996; 15:91-106.
65. Findling R, Frishman W, Javed MT et al. Calcium channel blockers and the gastrointestinal tract. *Am J Ther.* 1996; 3:383-408.

66. Chang JY, Locke GR, Schleck CD et al. Risk factors for chronic constipation and a possible role of analgesics. *Neurogastroenterol Motil.* 2007; 19:905-11.
67. Leeb BF, Schweitzer H, Montag K et al. A meta-analysis of chondroitin sulfate in the treatment of osteoarthritis. *J Rheumatol.* 2000; 27:205-11.
68. McAlindon TE, LaValley MP, Gulin JP et al. Glucosamine and chondroitin for treatment of osteoarthritis a systematic quality assessment and meta-analysis. *JAMA.* 2000; 283:1469-75.
69. Kudolo GB. The effect of 3-month ingestion of Ginkgo biloba extract on pancreatic beta-cell function in response to glucose loading in normal glucose tolerant individuals. *J Clin Pharmacol.* 2000; 40:647-54.
70. Diamond BJ, Shiflett SC, Reiwel N et al. Ginkgo biloba extract: mechanisms and clinical indications. *Arch Phys Med Rehabil.* 2000; 81:668-778.
71. Cesarani A, Meloni F, Alpini D et al. Ginkgo biloba (EGb 761) in the treatment of equilibrium disorders. *Adv Ther.* 1998; 15:291-304.
72. Mullins RJ, Heddle R. Adverse reactions associated with *Echinacea:* the Australian experience. *Ann Allergy Asthma Immunol.* 2002; 88:42-51.
73. Yale SH, Liu K. *Echinacea purpurea* therapy for the treatment of the common cold: a randomized, double-blind, placebo-controlled clinical trial. *Arch Intern Med.* 2004; 164:1237-41.
74. Sperber SJ, Shah LP, Gilbert RD et al. Echinacea purpurea for prevention of experimental rhinovirus colds. *Clin Infect Dis.* 2004; 38:1367-71.
75. Goel V, Lovlin R, Barton R et al. Efficacy of a standardized echinacea preparation (Echinilin) for the treatment of the common cold: a randomized, double-blind, placebo-controlled trial. *J Clin Pharm Ther.* 2004; 29:75-83.
76. Huntley AL, Thompson Coon J, Ernst E. The safety of herbal medicinal products derived from *Echinacea* species: a systematic review. *Drug Saf.* 2005; 28:387-400.
77. Braeckman J. The extract of serenoa repens in the treatment of benign prostatic hyperplasia: a multicenter open study. *Curr Ther Res.* 1994; 55:776-85.
78. Reece-Smith H, Memon A, Smart CJ et al. The value of permixon in benign prostatic hypertrophy. *Br J Urol.* 1986; 58:36-40.
79. Wilt T, Ishani A, Stark G et al. Serenoa repens for benign prostatic hyperplasia. *Cochrane Database Syst Rev.* 2000; 2:CD01423.
80. Kaplan SA, Volpe MA, Te AE. A prospective, 1-year trial using saw palmetto versus finasteride in the treatment of category III prostatitis/chronic pelvic pain syndrome. *J Urol.* 2004; 171:284-8.
81. Mugie SM, Benninga MA, DiLorenzo C. Epidemiology of constipation in children and adults: a systematic review. *Best Prac Res Clin Gastroenterol.* 2011; 25:3-18.
82. Bharucha AE, Dorn SD, Lembo A, Pressman A. American Gastroenterological Association Medical Position Statement on Constipation. *Gastroenterology.* 2013; 144:211-7.
83. LoCasale RJ, Datto C, Wilson H et al. The burden of opioid-induced constipation: discordance between patient and health care provider reports. *J Manag Care Spec Pharm.* 2016; 22:236-45.
84. Brenner DM, Shah M. Chronic constipation. *Gastroenterol Clin N Am.* 2016; 45:205-16.
85. Shah BJ, Rughwani N, Rose S. In the clinic: constipation. *Ann Intern Med.* 2015; 162: ITC1.
86. Lat I, Foster DR, Erstad B. Drug-induced acute liver failure and gastrointestinal complications. *Crit Care Med.* 2010; 38:S175-187.
87. Bharucha AE, Pemberton JH, Locke GR. American Gastroenterological Association technical review on constipation. *Gastroenterology.* 2013; 144:218-38.
88. Staats PS, Markowitz J, Schein J. Incidence of constipation associated with long-acting opioid therapy: a comparative study. *South Med J.* 2004; 97:129-34.
89. Candrilli SD, Davis, KL, Iyer S. Impact of constipation on opioid use patterns, health care resource utilization, and costs in cancer patients on opioid therapy. *J Pain Palliat Care Pharmacother.* 2009; 23:231-41.
90. Szigethy E, Schwartz M, Drossman D. Narcotic bowel syndrome and opioid-induced constipation. *Curr Gastroenterol Rep.* 2014; 16:410-20.
91. Roque M, Bouras EP. Epidemiology and management of chronic constipation in elderly patients. *Clin Interv Aging.* 2015; 10:919-30.
92. Higgins PD, Johanson JF. Epidemiology of constipation in North America: a systematic review. *Am J Gastorenterol.* 2004; 99:750-9.
93. Schmidt FM, Santos VL. Prevalence of constipation in the general adult population: an integrative review. *J Wound Ostomy Continence Nurs.* 2014; 41:70-6.
94. Sanchez MI, Bercik P. Epidemiology and burden of chronic constipation. *Can J Gastroenterol.* 2011; 25:11B-15.
95. Herndon CM, Jackson KC, Hallin PA. Management of opioid-induced gastrointestinal effects in patients receiving palliative care. *Pharmacotherapy.* 2002; 22:240-50.
96. Siemens W, Gaertner J, Becker G. Advances in pharmacotherapy for opioid-induced constipation-a systematic review. *Expert Opin Pharmacother.* 2015; 16:515-32.
97. Koloski NA, Jones M, Wai R et al. Impact of persistent constipation on health-related quality of life and mortality in older community-dwelling women. *Am J Gastroenterol* 2013; 108:1152-8.
98. Johnson DA, Argoff CE. Management of opioid-induced constipation. *J Fam Pract.* 2015; 64:S4-9. Review.
99. Choung RS, Branda ME, Chitkara D et al. Longitudinal direct medical costs associated with constipation in women. *Aliment Pharmacol Ther.* 2011; 33:251-60.
100. Rao S, Rattanakovit K, Patcharatrakul. Diagnosis and management of chronic constipation in adults. *Nat Rev Gastroenterol Hepatol.* 2016; 13:295-305.
101. Dorn S, Lembo A, Cremonini F. Opioid-induced bowel dysfunction: epidemiology, pathophysiology, diagnosis, and initial therapeutic approach. *Am J Gastroenterol.* 2014; 2:31-7.
102. Locke GR, Pemberton JH, Phillips SF. AGA technical review on constipation. *Gastroenterology.* 2000; 119:1766-78.
103. Johanson JF. Review of the treatment options for chronic constipation. *Med Gen Med.* 2007; 9:25-40.
104. Wald A. Constipation: pathophysiology and management. *Curr Opin Gastroenterol* 2015; 31:45-9.
105. Ford AC, Suares NC. Effect of laxatives and pharmacological therapies in chronic idiopathic constipation: systematic review and meta-analysis. *Gut* 2011; 60:209-18.
106. Camilleri M. New treatment options for chronic constipation: mechanisms, efficacy, and safety. *Can J Gastroenterol.* 2011; (suppl B):29B-35.
107. Handal KA, Schauben JL, Salamone FR. Naloxone. *Ann Emerg Med.* 1983; 12:438-45.
108. Meissner W, Schmidt U, Hartmann M et al. Oral naloxone reverses opioid-associated constipation. *Pain.* 2000; 84:105-9.
109. Holder RM, Rhee D. Novel oral therapies for opioid-induced bowel dysfunction in patients with chronic noncancer pain. *Pharmacotherapy* 2016; 36:287-99.

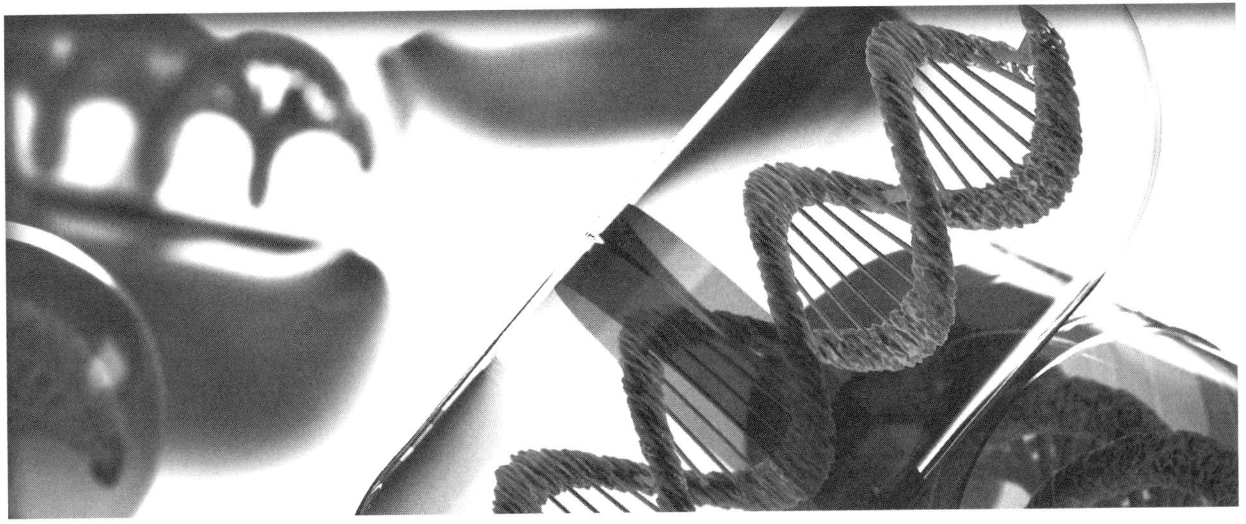

CHAPTER 38

Hepatic and Cholestatic Diseases

Scott S. Malinowski and Daniel M. Riche

The liver is the body's most important organ in terms of metabolism and elimination of drugs and other chemical substances. The nature of these functions makes the liver inherently susceptible to toxicity from foreign substances (xenobiotics). In light of this and because of its many other critical functions, damage to the liver carries significant risk for morbidity and mortality. Hepatic and cholestatic (hepatocholestatic) injury is a well-documented result of many drugs taken or administered in excessive quantities but can also occur with some drugs at usual or even low therapeutic doses (idiosyncratic reactions). Although pharmaceutical agents are the focus of this chapter, herbal and natural products, illicit drugs, and other environmental chemicals are discussed where appropriate.

CAUSATIVE AGENTS

Over 1,100 chemical agents are associated with the potential to cause significant hepatocholestatic injury. **Table 38-1** lists medicinal and illicit drugs, herbal products, and chemical agents implicated in drug-induced hepatocholestatic diseases.[1-48] An excellent public domain online resource is the LiverTox Database (www.livertox.nih.gov), sponsored by the National Institute of Diabetes and Digestive and Kidney Diseases and the National Library of Medicine. This searchable website provides up-to-date information on medications and dietary supplements associated with drug-induced liver disease.[49]

The predominant pathologic pattern of injury serves as the basis for the categorization of the various types of drug-induced hepatocholestatic diseases. The categories of injury are hepatocellular (which is also called cytoxic and includes necrosis, apoptosis, and steatosis), cholestatic, vascular, and neoplastic. The pathophysiologies of these categories are discussed in further detail in the Mechanisms section of this chapter. Agents and classes of agents corresponding with each category are described in **Table 38-2**.[1-14,17-21,25,33,43,47,50-58]

EPIDEMIOLOGY

As the availability and use of drugs and herbal remedies increase, so too does the risk and incidence of drug-induced hepatocholestatic disease. Hepatotoxicity is a common reason for withdrawal of drugs from the market and, due largely to the inability of premarketing trials to detect rare events, is usually discovered during postmarketing

Table 38-1 Agents Implicated in Drug-Induced Hepatic and Cholestatic Diseases

Drug	Incidence	Level of Evidence[a]
ANALGESICS/ANTI-INFLAMMATORY AGENTS		
Acetaminophen[1-16]	NK	B
Aspirin[1-18]	NK	C
Bromfenac[19]	NK	C
Celecoxib[15,16,20,21]	NK	C
Diclofenac[1-16,22,23]	0.001–0.005%	B
Etodolac[1-16]	NK	C
Ibuprofen[1-16,20,21]	NK	C
Indomethacin[22]	NK	C
Ketorolac[22]	NK	C
Leflunamide[1-16]	4.4%	A
Naproxen[20,21]	NK	C
Nimesulide[1-16]	NK	C
Oxaprozin[1-16]	NK	C
Phenylbutazone[1-14,20,21,24]	NK	C
Piroxicam[1-18]	NK	C
Propoxyphene[1-14,17,18]	NK	C
Propionic acid derivatives[1-18]	NK	B
Sulindac[15,20,21,24]	NK	C
Tolmetin[1-18]	NK	C
ANTIMICROBIAL AGENTS		
Amoxicillin[25]	0.003%	C
Ampicillin[1-14,20-22,27,28]	NK	C
Amoxicillin–clavulanate[1-14,20-22,26-28]	0.0099–0.017%	C
Amphotericin[1-14,26-28]	NK	C
Antimonial antiparasitics[1-14,17,18,27,28]	NK	C
Azole antifungals[1-14,20-22,27,28]	0.2%	C
Azole antiparasitics[1-14,27,28]	5%	B
Carbapenems[20,21,27,28]	NK	C
Caspofungin[1-14,27,28]	NK	C
Ceftriaxone[20,21,27,28]	NK	C
Chloramphenicol[1-14,20,21,27,28]	NK	C
Chloroquine[1-14,17,18,27,28]	NK	C
Clindamycin[1-14,20,21,27,28]	NK	C
Cloxacillin/nafcillin[1-14,27,28]	≤0.01%	C
Cotrimoxazole[1-14,17,18,20,21,27,28]	NK	C
Dapsone[1-14,20,21,27,28]	≤1.3%	C
Erythromycin[15,20,21,24]	NK	C
Ethionamide[1-14,26-30]	NK	C
Flucloxacillin[31]	0.0018–0.0036%	C
Flucytosine[1-14,20,21,27,28]	NK	C
Fluoroquinolones[1-14,23,27,28]	≤0.0001%	C

Table 38-1 Agents Implicated in Drug-Induced Hepatic and Cholestatic Diseases (continued)

Drug	Incidence	Level of Evidence[a]
Fusidic acid[20,21]	NK	C
Griseofulvin[20,21]	NK	C
Hydroxychloroquine[1-14,22,27,28]	NK	C
Isoniazid[1-14,26-30]	1%	B
NNRTIs[1-14,17,18,23,26-29,32]	<15%	B
NRTIs[1-15,20,21,23,30,32,35,45]	<16%	A
Nitrofurantoin[1-14,20,21,27,28]	0.03%	B
Pentamidine[1-14,27,28]	NK	C
Protease inhibitors[1-14,17,18,29,23,26,27,28,32]	<3%	B
Pyrazinamide[1-14,26-30]	NK	C
Ribavirin[1,22]	NK	C
Rifampin[1-14,20,21,26-30]	1.4%	B
Sulfonamides[1-14,20,21,27,28]	NK	C
Telithromycin[1-14,27-29]	NK	C
Terbinafine[1-14,17,18,24,25]	0.02%	C
Tetracyclines[1-18,20,24,25]	NK	B
Thiabendazole[17,18]	NK	C
CARDIOVASCULAR AGENTS		
ACE inhibitors[1-15,20-22]	NK	C
Ajmaline[20,21]	NK	C
Aprindine[20,21]	NK	C
Amiodarone[1-15,17,18,22,26,29]	0.6–3%	B
Angiotensin-receptor blockers[1-15,20-22]	NK	C
β-blockers[1-15,17,18,20,21]	NK	C
Calcium-channel blockers[1-15,17,18,20,21]	NK	C
Disopyramide[15,20,21]	NK	C
Hydralazine[1-15,20,21]	NK	C
Loop diuretics[1-15]	NK	C
Methyldopa[1-15,20,21]	<0.1%	B
Procainamide[15,20,21]	NK	C
Propafenone[15,20,21]	NK	C
Quinidine[1-15,20,21]	2%	B
Spironolactone[1-15]	NK	C
Thiazide diuretics[15,20,21]	NK	C
CHEMOTHERAPEUTIC AGENTS		
Actinomycin[1-14]	NK	C
Aminoglutethimide[20,21]	NK	C
Amsacrine[1-14,20,21]	NK	C
Asparaginase[1-4,17,18]	NK	C
BCNU/CCNU[1-14]	NK	C
Bleomycin[1-14]	NK	C
Bortezomib[29]	NK	C

Table 38-1 Agents Implicated in Drug-Induced Hepatic and Cholestatic Diseases (continued)

Drug	Incidence	Level of Evidence[a]
Busulfan[1-14]	NK	C
Capecitabine[1-14]	NK	C
Carboplatin[1-14]	NK	C
Carmustine[1-14]	NK	C
Chlorambucil[1-14]	NK	C
Cisplatin[1-14]	NK	C
Cyclophosphamide[1-14]	NK	C
Cyclosporine[1-14,20,21,26]	NK	C
Cyproterone acetate[1-14,22]	NK	C
Cytarabine[1-14,20,21]	NK	C
Dacarbazine[1-14]	NK	C
Daunorubicin[1-14]	NK	C
Doxorubicin[1-14]	NK	C
Etoposide[1-14]	NK	C
Floxuridine[20,21]	NK	C
Fluorouracil[29,33]	30–47%	C
Flutamide[1-14,22,29]	NK	C
Gemcitabine[1-14,20,21]	NK	C
Hydroxyurea[1-14]	NK	C
Interleukin-2[20,21]	NK	C
Irinotecan[33]	NK	C
Mercaptopurine[1-14,20,21,23,29]	NK	C
Mitomycin[1-14,17,18]	NK	C
Procarbazine[1-14]	NK	C
Riluzole[1-14,17,18]	NK	C
Streptozocin[1-14]	NK	C
Tamoxifen[17,18,20-22,26]	7%	B
Temozolomide[29]	NK	C
Teniposide[1-14]	NK	C
Thalidomide[22]	NK	C
Thioguanine[1-14,22,26]	NK	C
Thiotepa[1-14]	NK	C
Topotecan[1-14]	NK	C
Toremifene[1-14]	NK	C
Tyrosine kinase inhibitors[29,34]	2%	C
Vinca alkaloids[1-14]	NK	C
ENDOCRINE AGENTS		
Alendronate[29]	NK	C
Androgens[20,21]	NK	C
Carbimazole[22]	NK	C
Corticosteroids[17,18]	NK	C
Cyclofenil[1-14]	NK	C

Table 38-1 Agents Implicated in Drug-Induced Hepatic and Cholestatic Diseases (continued)

Drug	Incidence	Level of Evidence[a]
Danazol[1-14]	NK	C
Estrogens[25,31]	<1%	C
Fenofibrate[1-15,22,26,35]	NK	C
Gemfibrozil[22]	NK	C
Levothyroxine[29]	NK	C
Lomitapide[33]	NK	C
Metformin[1-15,20,21,35]	NK	C
Methimazole[20,21]	NK	C
Mipomersen[33]	NK	C
Niacin[1-15,22,29,35]	NK	C
Orlistat[1-15]	NK	C
Propylthiouracil[1-15,26]	NK	C
Repaglinide[1-15]	NK	C
Sex steroids[17,18,20,21]	0.025%	C
Sibutramine[26]	NK	C
Statins[1-15,20,21,23,27,35,36]	<0.0003%	B
Sulfonylureas[1-15,20,21,35]	NK	C
Thiazolidinediones[1-15,22-24,26,29,35,37]	NK	B
Voglibose[20,21]	NK	C
ENVIRONMENTAL CHEMICALS		
Aflatoxin[1-14,20,21]	NK	C
Allyl compounds[1-14]	NK	C
Amanitin[17,18]	NK	C
Aniline derivatives[20,21]	NK	C
Arsenicals[20,21]	NK	C
Beryllium[1-14]	NK	C
Carbon tetrachloride[1-14,17,18]	NK	C
Chloroform[17,18]	NK	C
Chromium[17,18]	NK	C
Cycad nut[1-14]	NK	C
Dichloroethylate[17,18]	NK	C
Dimethylacetaminde[1-14]	NK	C
Dimethylformamide[1-14]	NK	C
Dioxane[1-14]	NK	C
Ethionine[117,18]	NK	C
Ethyl bromide/chloride, methyl bromide/chloride/dichloride[117,18]	NK	C
Hexachlorethane[22]	NK	C
Nitroaliphatic compounds[1-14]	NK	C
Nitroaromatic compounds[1-14]	NK	C
Orotic acid[17,18]	NK	C
Paraquat[20,21]	NK	C
Phosphorus[1-4,17,18]	NK	C

Table 38-1 Agents Implicated in Drug-Induced Hepatic and Cholestatic Diseases (continued)

Drug	Incidence	Level of Evidence[a]
Selenium[17,18]	NK	C
Tannic acid[17,18]	NK	C
Tetrachloroethylene/trichloroethylene[17,18]	NK	C
Tripelennamine[20,21]	NK	C
Uranium[17,18]	NK	C
Urethane[1-14]	NK	C
Vinyl chloride[1-14]	NK	C
GASTROINTESTINAL AGENTS		
Alverine[1-14]	NK	C
Histamine$_2$-receptor antagonists[1-14,20-22]	NK	C
Mesalamine[20,21]	NK	C
Octreotide[1-14]	NK	C
para-aminosalicylic acid[1-14]	NK	C
Proton pump inhibitors[1-14,26]	NK	C
Sulfasalazine[1-14]	NK	C
GENERAL ANESTHETICS		
Desflurane[26,29]	NK	C
Enflurane[1-14]	NK	C
Halothane[1-14,61]	0.03–0.01%	B
Isoflurane[1-14,22]	NK	C
Sevoflurane[26,29]	NK	C
HERBAL AGENTS		
Aloe vera[29]	NK	C
β-carotene[20,21]	NK	C
Black cohosh[1-14,21,22,26,38-41]	NK	C
Cade oil[26]	NK	C
Camellia senesis[42]	NK	C
Camphor[1-14,17,18,38-41]	NK	C
Carp capsules (cyprinol)[1-14,22,38-41]	NK	C
Cascara sagrada[20,21]	NK	C
Celandine[20,21]	NK	C
Chaparral leaf[1-14,20,21,38-41]	NK	C
Chaso[1-14,38-41]	NK	C
Colpachi[29]	NK	C
Comfrey[38-41]	NK	C
Garlic[22]	NK	C
Garcinia cambogia[42]		
Germander[1-14,38-41]	NK	C
Glue thistle (*Atractylis gummifera*)[34,43]	NK	C
Gordoloba tea[38-41]	NK	C
Impila[1-14,38-41]	NK	C
Ju bu huan[1-14,20,21,38-41]	NK	C

Table 38-1 Agents Implicated in Drug-Induced Hepatic and Cholestatic Diseases (continued)

Drug	Incidence	Level of Evidence[a]
Kava[1-14,38-41]	NK	C
Lantana camara[29]	NK	C
Linghzi[20,21]	NK	C
Lipokinetix[1-14,38-41]	NK	C
Ma huang[1-14,38-41]	NK	C
Margosa oil[17,18,26]	NK	C
Mediterranean glue thistle[1-14,38-41]	NK	C
Mistletoe[1-14,38-41]	NK	C
Noni juice[22,26]	NK	C
Oil of cloves[1-14,38-41]	NK	C
Pennyroyal oil[1-14,38-41]	NK	C
Prostata[1-14,38-41]	NK	C
Sairei-to[29]	NK	C
Sassafras[38-41]	NK	C
Saw palmetto[34]	NK	C
Senna[23,26,34]	NK	C
Shark cartilage[1-14,38-41]	NK	C
Shen-min[22]	NK	C
Sho-saiko-to[1-14,17,18,20,21,38-41]	NK	C
Skull cap[38-41]	NK	C
Teucrium polium[29]	NK	C
Usnic acid[42]	NK	C
Valerian root[1-14,38-41]	NK	C
Venencapsan[17,18]	NK	C
ILLICIT AGENTS		
Amphetamines (including MDMA)[1-14]	NK	C
Cocaine[1-14,17,18]	NK	C
Mushroom poisoning[1-14]	NK	C
Phencyclidine[1-14]	NK	C
NEUROPSYCHIATRIC AGENTS		
Amantadine[17,18]	NK	C
Barbiturates[20,21]	NK	C
Benzodiazepines[1-14]	NK	C
Carbamazepine[1-14,20,21]	0.03%	B
Chlormethiazole[1-14]	NK	C
Chlopromazine[17,18,20,21]	1%	C
Clozapine[1-14,20,21]	0.001%	B
Dantrolene[1-14]	0.5%	B
Disulfiram[1-14,22]	NK	C
Duloxetine[22]	NK	C
Felbamate[1-14]	NK	C
Fluphenazine[20,21]	NK	C

Table 38-1 Agents Implicated in Drug-Induced Hepatic and Cholestatic Diseases (continued)

Drug	Incidence	Level of Evidence[a]
Gabapentin[20,21]	NK	C
Haloperidol[20,21]	NK	C
Lamotrigine[1-14]	NK	C
Loxapine[20,21]	NK	C
Monoamine oxidase inhibitors[1-14,44-46]	NK	C
Methylphenidate[1-14]	NK	C
Molindone[20,21]	NK	C
Nefazodone[1-14,29,44-46]	NK	C
Olanzapine[1-14,22]	NK	C
Pemoline[1-14]	NK	C
Phenytoin[1-14,20-22]	0.03%	B
Prochlorperazine[20,21]	NK	C
Promazine[20,21]	NK	C
Riluzole[17,18]	NK	C
Risperidone[20,21]	NK	C
Selective serotonin reuptake inhibitors[1-14,20,21,23,29,44-46]	NK	C
Tacrine[1-14,17,18]	2–25%	A
Thioridazine[17,18,20,21]	NK	C
Tolcapone[1-14,29]	NK	B
Topiramate[1-14,22]	NK	C
Trazodone[1-14,20,21,44-46]	NK	C
Tricyclic antidepressants[17,18,20,21,44-46]	1%	C
Valproic acid[1-14,17,18,22,23]	NK	B
Venlafaxine[1-14,22,44-46]	NK	C
TUMOR NECROSIS FACTOR α-ANTAGONISTS		
Adalimumab[25,34,47]	NK	C
Etanercept[25,34,47]	NK	C
Infliximab[25,34,47]	NK	C
OTHERS		
Allopurinol[20,21]	NK	C
Azathioprine[20,21]	NK	C
Bosentan[1-14,26]	3–7%	A
Cetirizine[23]	NK	C
Chlorpheniramine[17,18]	NK	C
Clopidogrel[1-15,22,23,26]	NK	C
Colchicine[23]	NK	C
Cyclizine[17,18]	NK	C
Cyproheptadine[20,21]	NK	C
Ethanol[17,18]	NK	B
Etretinate[1-14]	<1%	B
Fenfluramine[17,18]	NK	C
Ferrous salts[1-14]	NK	C

Table 38-1 Agents Implicated in Drug-Induced Hepatic and Cholestatic Diseases (continued)

Drug	Incidence	Level of Evidence[a]
Gold[20,21]	NK	C
Interferon[1-14,22]	NK	C
Loratadine[1-14]	NK	C
Methotrexate[17,18]	NK	C
Montelukast[1-14,48]	NK	C
Parenteral lipid[17,18]	NK	B
Penicillamine[20,21]	NK	C
Pentoxifylline[1-15]	NK	C
Probenecid[1-14]	NK	C
Ritodrine[1-14]	NK	C
Sirolimus[23,26]	NK	C
Tacrolimus[20,21]	NK	C
Terbutaline[1-14]	NK	C
Terfenadine[20,21]	NK	C
Ticlopidine[17,18,20,21,29]	NK	C
Tiopronin[20,21]	NK	C
Trimethobenzamide[20,21]	NK	C
Vitamin A[17,18]	NK	B
Warfarin[17,18,26]	NK	C
Zafirlukast[1-14,48]	NK	C

ACE = angiotensin-converting enzyme, BCNU = bischloroethylnitrosourea, CCNU = 1-(2-chloroethyl)-3-cyclohexyl-1-nitrosourea, MDMA = 3,4-methylenedioxymethamphetamine, NNRTIs = nonnucleoside reverse-transcriptase inhibitors, NRTI = nucleoside reverse-transcriptase inhibitor, NK = not known.

[a]Definitions for Levels of Evidence: Level A—evidence from one or more randomized, controlled clinical trials; Level B—evidence from nonrandomized clinical trials, prospective observational studies, cohort studies, retrospective studies, case-control studies, meta-analyses and/or postmarketing surveillance studies; and Level C—evidence from one or more published case reports or case series.

surveillance. Accurately determining the incidence of drug-induced liver injury has been problematic due to a number of factors, including unknown numbers of overall populations exposed, lack of simple objective diagnostic tests, difficulty in attributing causation to a single drug for people taking multiple medications, and a lack of systematic reporting.[34]

The incidence of drug-induced liver injury (excluding acetaminophen toxicity) has been estimated at 19.1 cases per 100,000 inhabitants per year in a population-based cohort in Iceland. In this population, the injury was caused by a single drug in 75% of the cases (most commonly amoxicillin–clavulanate) and attributed to multiple agents in 9% of cases. Dietary supplements accounted for 16% of all cases of drug-induced hepatic disease. The age-standardized incidence in this population increased dramatically with increasing age.[60] These incidences are likely similar in other populations of European descent.

Hepatotoxicity accounts for approximately 6% of all reported adverse drug reactions, and drug-induced liver injury is responsible for 13% of cases of acute liver failure not caused by acetaminophen toxicity.[59,62] Acetaminophen has been implicated in 39–51% of cases of acute liver failure, and remains a common reason for liver transplantation.[62,63]

Ten percent of cases of acute hepatitis are related to drug toxicity. In patients >50 years of age, 40% of cases of hepatotoxicity are due to medicinal agents. With idiosyncratic drug-induced hepatotoxicity, an individual's particular susceptibility is influenced by both acquired and genetic factors. The risk of hepatotoxicity from drugs ranges from 1 in 10,000 to 1 in 100,000 persons exposed.[59]

Table 38-2 Mechanisms of Drug-Induced Hepatic and Cholestatic Diseases

Predominant Injury	Agents or Class of Agents
HEPATOCELLULAR[1-14,17,18,25,47,50-54]	
Cytotoxic	ACE inhibitors (primarily captopril, enalapril, lisinopril), acetaminophen, actinomycin, adalimumab, aflatoxin (found in foods such as nuts), afluzosin, alendronate, allyl compounds, aloe vera, alverine, amiodarone, amoxicillin, ampicillin, amphetamines (including MDMA), amphotericin (primarily lipid-based), amsacrine, angiotensin-receptor blockers (primarily irbesartan, losartan), azole antifungals (primarily ketoconazole), azole antiparasitics (albendazole, mebendazole, ornidazole), β blockers (primarily propranolol, metoprolol, acebutalol, labetolol), BCNU/CCNU, benzodiazepines, beryllium, black cohosh, bleomycin, bortezomib, bosentan, cade oil, camphor, capecitabine, carbamazepine, carboplatin, carmustine, carp capsules (cyprinol), caspofungin, calcium channel blockers, carbon tetrachloride, cetirizine, chaparral leaf, chaso, chlorambucil, chloramphenicol, chlormethiazole, cisplatin, clindamycin, cloxacillin/nafcillin, clopidogrel, clozapine, cocaine, colchicine, colpachi, cotrimoxazole, cycad nut, cyclofenil, cyclophosphamide, cyclosporine, cyproterone acetate, cytarabine, dacarbazine, danazol, dantrolene, dapsone, desflurane, diclofenac, daunorubicin, dimethylacetaminde, dioxane, disulfiram, doxorubicin, duloxetine, enflurane, ertotinib, etanercept, ethionamide, etodolac, etoposide, etretinate, felbamate, fenofibrate, ferrous salts, flutamide, fluoroquinolones (primarily ciprofloxacin, trovafloxacin), flucytosine, fluorouracil, garlic, gemcitabine, germander, halothane, hexachloroethane, histamine$_2$-receptor antagonists, hydralazine, hydroxychloroquine, hydroxyurea, ibuprofen, imatinib mesylate, indomethacin, infliximab, interferons, isoflurane, isoniazid, jin bu huan (tetrahydropalmatine), kava, lamotrigine, lantana camara, leflunamide, lipokinetix, loop diuretics (primarily furosemide), loratadine, ma huang, monoamine oxidase inhibitors, Mediterranean glue thistle, mercaptopurine, metformin, methyldopa, methylphenidate, minocycline, mistletoe, mitomycin, montelukast, mushroom poisoning, nefazodone, niacin, nimesulide, nitroaliphatic compounds, nitroaromatic compounds, NNRTIs (primarily nevirapine, abacavir), noni, NRTIs (primarily zidovudine, didanosine, stavudine), nitrofurantoin, octreotide, oil of cloves, olanzapine, orlistat, oxaprozin, *para*-aminosalicylic acid, pemoline, pennyroyal oil, pentamidine, pentoxifylline, phencyclidine, phenylbutazone, phenytoin, phosphorus, piroxicam, proton pump inhibitors (primarily omeprazole, rabeprazole), probenecid, procarbazine, propionic acid derivatives (bromfenac, fenoprofen, ketoprofen), propylthiouracil, protease inhibitors (primarily ritonavir, indinavir), pyrazinamide, quinidine, repaglinide, rifampin, riluzole, ritodrine, saireito, senna fruit, sevoflurane, shark cartilage, shen-min, sho-saiko-to, sirolimus, spironolactone, SSRIs (primarily fluoxetine, fluvoxamine, sertraline), statins (primarily atorvastatin and simvastatin), streptozocin, sulfasalazine, sulfonamides, sulfonylureas (primarily acetohexamide, gemfibrozil, gliclazide), tacrine, telithromycin, temozolomide, teniposide, terbinafine, terbutaline, teucrium polium, thalidomide, thiazolidinediones (primarily pioglitazone, rosiglitazone, troglitazone), thioguanine, thiotepa, tienilic acid, tolcapone, topiramate, topotecan, trazodone, urethane, valerian root, valproic acid, venlafaxine, vinca alkoloids, zafirlukast
STEATOSIS[1-3,17,18,33,55]	
Microvesicular	Aflatoxin (a contaminant produced by molds), aminosalicylates, amiodarone, antimony antiparasitics, asparaginase, aspirin, camphor, cocaine, didanosine, diltiazem, dimethylformamide, ibuprofen, margosa oil, naproxen, NNRTIs, NRTIs, piroxicam, protease inhibitors (primarily ritonavir and indinavir), riluzole, selenium, sho-saiko-to, tetrabamate, tolmetin, tetracyclines (primarily minocycline), ticlopidine, valproic acid, venencapsan, vinyl chloride, vitamin A, zidovudine
Macrovesicular	Alcohol, amanitin, amiodarone, asparaginase, calcium-channel blockers, carbon tetrachloride, chloroform, chromium, corticosteroids, dichloroethylate, estrogens, ethanol, ethionine, ethyl bromide/chloride, fluorouracil, glucocorticoids, methotrexate, methyl bromide/chloride/dichloride, mitomycin, orotic acid, parenteral lipid, phosphorus, sex steroids, tamoxifen, tannic acid, tetrachloroethylene/trichloroethylene, toremifene, uranium, warfarin, zidovudine
Phospholipidosis	Amantadine, amiodarone, chloroquine, chlorpheneramine, chlorpromazine, cotrimoxazole, cyclizine, fenfluramine, perhexiline maleate, propranolol, sex steroids, tacrine, TCAs, thioridazine, tripelennamine

Table 38-2 Mechanisms of Drug-Induced Hepatic and Cholestatic Diseases (continued)

Predominant Injury	Agents or Class of Agents
CHOLESTASIS[20,21,56-58]	
Pure cholestasis	Anabolic steroids, azathioprine, cyclosporine, cytarabine, fosinopril, infliximab, mercaptopurine, sex steroids, tamoxifen
Canalicular	ACE inhibitors (primarily captopril), allopurinol, aminoglutethimide, amoxicillin–clavulanate, anabolic steroids, aniline derivatives, arsenicals, atenolol, azathioprine, barbiturates, carbamazepine, carbapenems, carbimazole, ceftriaxone, chloramphenicol, chlorpropamide, citalopram, clindamycin, cotrimoxazole, cyclosporine, cyproheptadine, cytarabine, diltiazem, disopyramide, flucytosine, fusidic acid, glibenclamide, glipizide, glyburide, gold compounds, griseofulvin, haloperidol, histamine$_2$-receptor antagonists, hydralazine, irbesartan, ketorolac, methyldopa, naproxen, penicillamine, phenytoin, propafenone, propoxyphene, rifampin, risperidone, sex steroids, sho-saiko-to, sulindac, tacrolimus, tricyclic antidepressants, terfenadine, thiazide diuretics, ticlopidine, trazodone, trimethobenzamide, tripelennamine, voglibose
Hepatocanalicular	ACE inhibitors, acetohexamide, amsacrine, azathioprine, β-carotene, carbamazepine, carbimazole, cephalosporins, cascara sagrada, celandine, cetirizine, chaparral leaf, chlorpromazine, clozapine, dapsone, erythromycins (primarily estolate salt), floxuridine, fluphenazine, gabapentin, gemcitabine, gemfibrozil, glimepiride, infliximab, interleukin-2, jin bu huan, linhgzi, loxapine, mercaptopurine, metformin, methimazole, methyldopa, molindone, nitrofurantoin, phenylbutazone, phenytoin, procainamide, prochlorperazine, promazine, quinidine, risperidone, sertraline, statins (primarily cerivastatin, pravastatin), thioridazine, tolazamide, tolbutamide
Cholangiodestructive	Ajmaline, amoxicillin–clavulanate, aprindine, azathioprine, barbiturates, chlorpromazine, chlorpropamide, cimetidine, clindamycin, cotrimoxazole, COX-2 inhibitors (primarily celecoxib), cyproheptadine, flucloxacillin, fluoroquinolones, glibenclamide, glyburide, gold compounds, ibuprofen, mesalamine, nitrofurantoin, paraquot, penicillamine, phenytoin, prochlorperazine, semisynthetic penicillins, sex steroids, sulfonamides, tricyclic antidepressants (primarily amitriptyline, imipramine), terbinafine, tetracycline, thiabendazole, thiazide diuretics, ticlopidine, tiopronin, tolazamide, tolbutamide
VASCULAR[1-14,19,43,50-54]	
Hepatic vein thrombosis	Contraceptive hormones, comfrey, dacarbazine, gordolobo tea, parenteral lipid
Sinusoidal obstruction syndrome (veno-occlusive disease)	Actinomycin, arsenic, azathioprine, busulfan, carmustine, comfrey, cyclophosphamide, cytarabine, dacarbazine, daunorubicin, floxuridine, gordolobo tea, insecticides, mitomycin, nitrosoureas, oxaliplatin, pyrrolizidine alkaloids, skullcap, thioguanine, thorium dioxide, trovafloxacin, urethane, vinca alkaloids, vinyl chloride
Peliosis hepatis	Anabolic steroids, arsenicals, azathioprine, sex steroids, tamoxifen, thioguanine, vitamin A
NEOPLASM[1-3,50-52]	
Benign (adenoma)	Anabolic steroids, antineoplastic agents, octreotide, sex steroids, sassafras
Malignant	Anabolic steroids, sex steroids, vinyl chloride (carcinoma)

ACE = angiotensin-converting enzyme, BCNU = bischloroethylnitrosourea, CCNU = 1-(2-chloroethyl)-3-cyclohexyl-1-nitrosourea, COX-2 = cyclooxygenase-2 inhibitor, MDMA = 3,4-methylenedioxymethamphetamine, NNRTI = nonnucleoside reverse-transcriptase inhibitor, NRTI = nucleoside reverse-transcriptase inhibitor, SSRI = selective serotonin-reuptake inhibitor.

MECHANISMS

Drug-induced liver injury occurs with a wide range of dosages and lengths of exposure. Resultant injuries may involve one or a combination of the pathologic categories (e.g., a patient can suffer from both hepatocellular and cholestatic disease at the same time). The wide variety of pathological manifestations are a function of the mechanism of hepatotoxicity, the drug itself, amount and duration of exposure, and the inherent susceptibility of the individual taking the drug.[59]

Toxicity from drugs or their metabolites that cause direct damage to cellular components and biochemical processes or elicit immune responses is the foundation for the pathogenesis of the drug-induced liver diseases. The resultant damage and cell death ultimately lead to the clinical manifestation of hepatitis. Injuries are typically categorized by their predominant mechanism: hepatocellular or cytotoxic injury, cholestasis, vascular injury, or neoplasms (Table 38-2).[1-14,17-21,25,33,43,47,50-58] Drugs can cause more than one type of injury, either concurrently or at different points in time.

HEPATOCELLULAR INJURY

Acetaminophen and methotrexate are the most common examples of drugs known to cause direct hepatotoxicity. This injury results from either metabolic derangements or a triggering of an immune response, or, in some cases and to varying degrees, a combination of these. Metabolic injury is typically caused by covalent binding of the drug or its metabolite to intracellular proteins, the mutation of lipid peroxidation by free radicals, the depletion of protective substances such as glutathione, or the loss of ionic gradients and ion homeostasis (particularly calcium). Damage to intracellular structures, organelles, and nuclear DNA can lead to necrosis. Mitochondrial damage and the resultant inability to synthesize ATP can be particularly devastating. The downstream production of reactive oxygen species and free radicals that cause significant oxidative stress by overwhelming antioxidants and other host cell defense mechanisms influence much of this pathogenesis. The subsequent structural and functional damage leads to actin disruption, cell swelling and rupture, and, eventually, cell death.[1,64]

Acetaminophen is responsible for 39–51% of all acute liver failure cases.[62] It is predominantly metabolized by glucuronidation and sulfation, with approximately 10% being converted to the reactive metabolite *N*-acetyl-*p*-benzoquinone imine (NAPQI) via the CYP enzyme system. NAPQI is responsible for acetaminophen-associated hepatotoxicity. This metabolite is formed by CYP2E1 through a direct two-electron oxidation of acetaminophen and is rapidly detoxified by glutathione when acetaminophen is ingested in typical therapeutic amounts.[65] Glutathione is an antioxidant that protects important cellular components from damage caused by reactive oxygen species such as free radicals. When too much acetaminophen is ingested (e.g., from intentional or unintentional overdose), the sulfation and glucuronidation pathway becomes saturated, resulting in a shunting to the CYP system and the production of large amounts of NAPQI, which binds and depletes liver reserves of glutathione.[66] NAPQI is toxic to cellular components if not detoxified by conjugation with glutathione. NAPQI reacts with protein sulfhydryl groups in the hepatocyte mitochondria. Resultant mitochondrial damage includes collapse of the membrane potential (mediated by triggering the opening of the mitochondrial permeability transition pore), release of endonuclease G and apoptosis-inducing factor (both of which translocate to the cell nucleus and cause extensive DNA fragmentation), and inhibition of ATP synthesis.[66-68]

Mitochondrial oxidative stress from NAPQI results in the production of superoxide anion and subsequently peroxynitrite (both of which are deleterious to many intracellular components, particularly DNA and proteins). Peroxynitrite can also inactivate superoxide dismutase 2 (a process normally blocked by glutathione). These processes lead to further production of reactive oxygen species which in turn activates the redox-sensitive mitogen-activated protein kinase c-Jun N-terminal kinase 1/2, which translocates into the mitochondria, thereby creating an amplification loop that further increases mitochondrial oxidative stress. Translocation of mitochondrial proteins such as apoptosis-inducing factor and endonuclease G into the nucleus results in DNA fragmentation and oncotic necrosis.[68] Recent research has described the role of additional kinases such as receptor-interacting protein kinases 1 and 3 in promoting hepatocellular mitochondrial fission and oxidant stress.[66] The combination of mitochondrial damage and nuclear disintegration ultimately leads to widespread hepatocellular necrosis. In fact, all signaling pathways ultimately result in cellular necrosis.[66] Apoptosis is no longer considered to be a relevant mechanism of acetaminophen-associated hepatotoxicity.[69] Further investigation is needed to determine the role of inflammatory mediators, the innate immune system, Kupffer cells, non-Kupffer cells, neutrophils, and macrophages in the development and propagation of hepatocellular injury related to acetaminophen overdose.[65]

Immune-mediated hepatotoxicity is another form of direct liver injury but compared with the dose-dependent cytotoxicity tends to be idiosyncratic in nature. Idiosyncratic drug-induced liver disease is most commonly immune-mediated. The inherently unpredictable nature of idiosyncratic reactions poses a particular challenge to the clinician. Largely related to individual susceptibility, these reactions vary widely in latency, presentation, and course. This form of drug-induced liver injury involves sensitization of hepatocytes to cytokines by way of haptenization (covalent binding of the drug or metabolite to a cellular protein). This promotes the formation of antigen-recognizing helper and cytotoxic T cells via the major histocompatibility complex type II. Interaction with major histocompatibility complex type I leads to activation of humoral and cellular immune responses. Damage to hepatocytes leads to cell destruction and apoptosis.[3]

Examples of identified antibodies include antiliver/kidney microsomal antibody that specifically targets CYP2C9 of the liver and kidney; antiliver microsomal antibody (e.g., as induced by carbamazepine) that targets CYP1A2, an isoenzyme not found in the kidney; antimitochondrial antibody (e.g., as induced by isoniazid); antimicrosomal epoxide hydrolase (e.g., as induced by germander); anti-CYP 1A2 (e.g., as induced by hydralazine); and anti-CYP 2E1 (e.g., as induced by halothane). The inflammatory reaction is mediated by inflammatory cytokines, including interleukin-1, tumor necrosis factor (TNF), nitric oxide, and interferon.[13,50-54,70-73]

Hepatic steatosis is histologically defined as a deposition of triglycerides within the hepatocyte. Intrahepatocyte triglycerides are the product of glycerol and free fatty acid metabolism, and inappropriate accumulation is usually due to increased uptake from peripheral tissue or dietary sources, increased de novo lipogenesis within the hepatocyte, reduced utilization (β-oxidation), or reduced elimination (export of triglyceride in the form of very-low-density lipoprotein [VLDL]). Steatohepatitis is steatosis accompanied by inflammation and hepatocyte injury (ballooning), with or without fibrosis.[55,74]

Drug-induced steatosis is further categorized by the predominant steatotic feature: macrovesicular steatosis (peripheral displacement of the cell nucleus), microvesicular steatosis, and steatohepatitis.[75] Some drugs (e.g., tamoxifen and amiodarone) can accumulate in the mitochondria of hepatocytes. This accumulation can interfere with the mitochondrial electron transport chain and β-oxidation. Blocking the flow of electrons through the electron transport chain leads to an accumulation of electrons that can directly interact with oxygen to promote the formation of reactive oxygen species. This, along with ATP depletion and inflammation, ultimately result in cellular necrosis.[55] Other medications (e.g., troglitazone and salicylate) inhibit the entry of long-chain fatty acids into the mitochondrial matrix, leading to their accumulation in the cytosol and subsequent conversion (esterification) into triglycerides. This by itself can lead to triglyceride accumulation within the hepatocyte, while other drugs (e.g., tetracycline) inhibit the export and transport of triglycerides as VLDL.[55]

If the drug-induced steatosis does not progress to steatohepatitis or cirrhosis, it is generally reversible. Some individuals may be more susceptible to drug-induced hepatic steatosis due to risk factors (e.g., obesity and metabolic syndrome), comorbidities, or genetic predisposition. Steatosis may increase the liver's vulnerability to injury, particularly from other drugs known to interfere with mitochondrial function. Because steatosis associated with nonalcoholic fatty liver disease is becoming increasingly prevalent in Western populations, there is concern that consumption of drugs with the potential for inducing steatosis could increase risk for progression to steatohepatitis. A steatotic liver may also lead to impairment of CYP enzymatic function and altered metabolism of substrates.[33,55]

Other mechanisms that appear to play a role in drug-induced hepatic steatosis and are being investigated include increased expression levels of fatty acid translocase via increased peroxisome proliferator-activated receptor alpha, increased expression of sterol regulatory element-binding protein-1c, and decreased adenosine monophosphate-activated protein kinase.[33]

CHOLESTATIC INJURY

Cholestasis is defined clinically as stagnant bile or the failure of bile to reach the small intestine and is the result of impaired bile acid secretion by hepatocytes or obstruction of bile flow through intra- or extrahepatic bile ducts.[31] Drug-induced hepatocholestasis tends to be an idiosyncratic reaction and is classified as either acute or chronic. Acute hepatocholestasis is more common and occurs primarily as a result of alterations in bile secretion into the canaliculus. This can occur either with hepatocellular injury and inflammation or without (known as bland cholestasis). Injury to the hepatocyte is caused by an accumulation of bile acids within the cell causing mitochondrial damage and ultimately resulting in apoptosis and necrosis.[76] After some drugs (e.g., cyclosporine) are detoxified via Phase 1 and II reactions in the hepatocyte, their metabolites are transported (effluxed) into hepatic canaliculi for biliary excretion. Canalicular transporters, known as multidrug-resistance proteins, facilitate the efflux of bile acids from the hepatocyte into the canaliculus. Drugs and metabolites that induce hepatocholestasis by disrupting bile acid homeostasis typically do so via inhibition of bile acid transport across the canalicular membrane (the rate-limiting step in bile formation). This disruption occurs either through the direct inhibition of transport proteins, indirectly, through internalization and degradation of the transporter protein, or through altered gene expression for these proteins. The bile salt export pump (BSEP) is thought to be the most common transporter inhibited by drugs that induce hepatocholestasis, particularly in individuals with the V444A polymorphism of BSEP.[31]

Chronic hepatocholestasis is a result of direct injury to the bile ducts or ductules (vanishing bile duct syndrome) and can occur more than 6 months after the initial cholestatic insult. It can also appear as sclerosing cholangitis. Direct injury to bile ductular cells is a result of exposure to the offending drug or metabolite during canalicular excretion, either by direct toxic effects or immune sensitizing effects.[10]

VASCULAR INJURY

Certain drugs (particularly antineoplastics) can cause injury to hepatic stellate cells and endothelial cells lining the hepatic sinusoids. This results in endothelial swelling and thrombosis within the small hepatic venules, leading to venous outflow obstruction (due to luminal occlusion), sinusoidal dilatation, congestion, hepatocellular necrosis, and possibly centrilobular fibrosis. This condition is known as sinusoidal obstruction syndrome, or veno-occlusive disease. Other drugs can cause the development of peliosis hepatis, in which the hepatic parenchyma develops multiple blood-filled cavities without an endothelial lining. This is hypothesized to result from either sinusoidal endothelial cell injury, increased sinusoidal pressure due to blood outflow obstruction, or hepatocellular necrosis. Rupture of these blood-filled cavities can result in severe peritoneal hemorrhage.[43]

A rare drug-induced vascular abnormality is hepatic vein thrombosis, which occludes the hepatic vein and presents clinically as Budd–Chiari syndrome. Injury to endothelial cells of both sinusoids and small hepatic venules activates the coagulation cascade and formation of a thrombus. This thrombosis then occludes the hepatic vein, leading to increased portal vein and hepatic sinusoid pressures and the formation of ascites and esophageal varices.[43,77]

NEOPLASTIC INJURY

Neoplastic lesions of the liver such as focal nodular hyperplasia, hepatocellular adenoma, hepatocellular carcinoma, and angiosarcoma have been linked to several drugs. Most neoplasms are benign and are typically associated with prolonged exposure. The pathologic mechanisms explaining drug-induced liver neoplasms have not been fully elucidated, but are likely related to alterations in DNA.[43,78]

CLINICAL PRESENTATION AND DIFFERENTIAL DIAGNOSIS

There are no standard diagnostic criteria for drug-induced liver injury, and a diagnosis is typically one of exclusion. Diagnosis is a challenge due to lack of standardized diagnostic criteria, broad heterogeneity of clinical presentation, delays in patient presentation, and difficulty in determining a specific culprit in cases of polypharmacy. The diagnosis of drug-induced liver injury is often based on clinical suspicion and how well the symptoms and signs correlate with information from similar case reports. This emphasizes the importance of obtaining a thorough medication history including use of prescription and nonprescription drugs as well as exposure to recreational drugs, dietary supplements, herbal and natural products, alternative and complimentary therapies, chemicals, and toxins. Integrating the exposure history, the dose and duration of use of the suspected agent, presenting signs and symptoms, and pathologic and histologic patterns is paramount in formulating a diagnosis.

To assist with the diagnostic differentiation between the major types of drug-induced liver disease, a method using biochemical patterns has been described. It determines the ratio of alanine aminotransferase (ALT) to alkaline phosphatase (ALP) relative to their respective upper limits of normal (ULN). The R (ratio) value is calculated according to the formula R = ALT/ULN ÷ ALP/ULN. An R value ≥5 indicates hepatocellular liver injury, and a value ≤2 indicates cholestatic injury. Values between 2 and 5 characterize the mixed form of drug-induced liver injury.[31,79-81] **Table 38-3** presents the typical biochemical patterns observed with each mechanistic category of drug-induced liver disease.[1-14,17,18,21,56,82-86]

Several scales and algorithms have been developed to help assess causality in cases of suspected drug-induced liver injury. The most widely used scale is the Roussel Uclaf Causality Assessment Method (RUCAM).[80,81] This method assigns a categorical likelihood of causality to a given drug and liver injury situation. It incorporates data from seven domains: (1) time to onset of the injury after initiation of the suspected agent, (2) progression and course of the reaction after suspected drug discontinuation, (3) risk factors, (4) concomitant drugs, (5) nondrug causes of liver injury, (6) previous information on the hepatotoxic potential of the drug, and (7) response to rechallenge. The RUCAM scale has demonstrated 86% sensitivity, 89% specificity, and positive and negative predictive values of 93% and 78%, respectively. The likelihood categories determined are highly probable, probable, possible, unlikely, and excluded.[80,81] **Table 38-4** provides situations in which a drug or other xenobiotic could be a likely cause of liver injury.[1-58,82-86]

Table 38-3 Patterns of Biochemical Features of Acute Hepatocholestatic Injuries as Fold Deviations from Baseline

Pathologic Injury	ALP	5NC	GGT	AST	ALT	ALT/ULN ÷ ALP/ULN (R value)	LDH	Tbili	Ibili	Dbili
CYTOTOXIC[1-14,17,18,82-86]										
Necrosis/apoptosis	1–2×	1–2×	1–2×	10–500×	10–500×	≥5	10–500×	1–10×	1–10×	Normal
Steatosis										
Microvesicular	1–2×	1–2×	1–2×	5–20×	5–20×	≥5	5–20×	1–10×	1–10×	Normal
Macrovesicular	1–2×	1–2×	1–2×	2–5×	2–5×	Variable	2–5×	1–3×	1–3×	Normal
CHOLESTASIS[21,56,82-86]										
Pure cholestasis	3–20×	3–20×	3–20×	1–2×	1–2×	≤2	1–4×	2–20×	1–2×	2–20×
Canalicular	3–20×	3–20×	3–20×	1–4×	1–4×	≤2	1–4×	2–20×	1–2×	2–20×
Hepatocanalicular	3–20×	3–20×	3–20×	10–100×	10–100×	2–5	1–20×	2–20×	1–10×	2–20×
Cholangiodestructive	3–10×	3–10×	3–10×	1–4×	1–4×	≤2	1–4×	2–20×	1–2×	2–20×
Vascular[1-14,82-86]	1–5×	1–5×	1–5×	2–100×	2–100×	Variable, but often ≥5	2–100×	1–5×	1–5×	1–2×
NEOPLASM[1-14,82-86]	1–2×	1–2×	1–2×	2–10×	2–10×	Variable	2–10×	1–3×	1–3×	1–2×

ALP = alkaline phosphatase (normal range, 38–126 units/L), ALT = alanine aminotransferase (normal range, 7–53 units/L), AST = aspartate aminotransferase (normal range, 11–47 units/L), Dbili = direct (conjugated) bilirubin (normal range, 0–0.2 mg/dL), 5NC = 5′-nucleotidase (normal range, 2–16 units/L), GGT = γ-glutamyltransferase (normal range, 12–76 units/L), Ibili = indirect (unconjugated) bilirubin (normal range, 0–1.1 mg/dL), LDH = lactate dehydrogenase (normal range, 90–280 units/L), Tbili = total bilirubin (normal range, 0.2–1.3 mg/dL), ULN = upper limit of the normal range.

Table 38-4 Situations Indicating Xenobiotics as a Likely Cause of Hepatocholestatic Disease[1-58,82-86]

- Abnormal results on liver tests in complex medical situations
- Acute hepatitis or cholestasis not readily accounted for by other causes, such as viruses, other infections, gallstones, alcohol, metabolic or immunologic disorders
- Atypical features of liver disease are present, such as mixed hepatocholestatic injury or microvesicular steatosis
- Cholestasis with normal bile duct caliber on imaging
- Chronic hepatitis without autoantibodies or hyperglobulinemia
- Histologic features representative of drug-induced hepatic injury (see text)
- Indication by a questionnaire or algorithm designed to determine likelihood of an adverse effect (e.g., Naranjo Scale >8)
- Obscure or poorly explained liver disease among those taking long-term steroids (anabolic or sex steroids), immunosuppressive agents, or other drugs (including dietary supplements)
- Presence of extrahepatic manifestations, especially rash, lymphadenopathy, eosinophilia
- The patient has recently started a new medication or dietary supplement

Patients experiencing drug-induced liver injury usually present with either hepatitis-like symptoms (nausea, vomiting, lethargy, jaundice, abdominal discomfort, pruritus) or elevated liver enzymes. Most cases of drug-induced liver disease occur within 1 week to 3 months following initial exposure to the agent.[2] **Table 38-5** provides a detailed list of signs and symptoms that have been associated with drug-induced hepatocholestatic diseases.[1-14,17-21,31,56,60]

Drug-induced hepatic injury mimics many other liver disorders, making diagnosis challenging. It can be difficult to distinguish the clinical presentation from viral hepatitis, cholangitis, and autoimmune hepatitis. This underscores the importance of obtaining a detailed history of the presenting illness, recent travel, therapeutic drug and dietary supplement use, and illicit drug use.[31] **Table 38-6** lists the various conditions to consider in the differential diagnosis of drug-induced liver disease.[1-14,17,18,20,21,56] **Table 38-7** describes extrahepatic syndromes associated with drug-induced hepatocholestatic diseases.[1-14,17,18,20,21,56]

Table 38-5 Signs and Symptoms Associated with Hepatic and Cholestatic Diseases[1-14,17-21,31,56,60]

- Abdominal pain
- Anemia
- Anorexia, weight loss, fatigue, malaise
- Ascites
- Asterixis
- Caput medusae
- Coagulopathy
- Decreased albumin
- Encephalopathy
- Eosinophilia
- Epigastric valvular murmur (Cruveilhier–Baumgarten syndrome)
- Fetor hepaticus (sweet-pungent smell on breath)
- Fever
- Finger clubbing
- Gynecomastia, loss of hair in males
- Hepatomegaly
- Hepatopulmonary syndrome
- Hepatorenal syndrome
- Hypoglycemia or hyperglycemia
- Hypogonadism
- Hyponatremia
- Increased 5′-nucleotidase
- Increased ALP/GGT
- Increased AST/ALT
- Increased bilirubin
- Jaundice
- Lactic acidosis
- Nodular liver
- Palmar erythema
- Presence of autoimmune serum markers (e.g., antinuclear antibody, antismooth muscle antibody, lupus erythematosus, antimitochondrial antibody)
- Presence of liver-specific antibodies (e.g., LKM, LM)
- Pruritus
- Rash
- Scleral icterus
- Spider angioma
- Splenomegaly
- Steatorrhea
- Thrombocytopenia and leukopenia
- Varices
- Weight gain
- White nails

ALP = alkaline phosphatase, ALT = alanine aminotransferase, AST = aspartate aminotransferase, GGT = γ-glutamyl transferase, LKM = antiliver/kidney microsomal antibody, LM = antiliver microsomal antibody.

Table 38-6 Conditions to Consider in the Differential Diagnosis of Drug-Induced Hepatic and Cholestatic Diseases[1-14,17,18,20,21,56]

Cytotoxic pattern of damage

- Autoimmune disorders
- Epstein–Barr virus
- Heat stroke
- Ischemic liver
- Leukemia/lymphoma
- Neoplasms
- Pregnancy
- Reye syndrome
- Sea anemone stings
- Trauma
- Varicella zoster
- Viral hepatitis
- Wilson disease

Cholestasic pattern of damage

- Acquired immunodeficiency syndrome
- Allograft rejection
- Autoimmune cholangiopathic disorders
- Bacterial infections
- Bile duct strictures
- Biliary atresia
- Cholangitis
- Cholecystitis
- Cholestatic liver disease
- Congenital abnormalities (e.g. porphyrias, Byler syndrome, α_1-antitrypsin deficiency)
- Cystic fibrosis
- Graft-versus-host disease
- Lymph node compression (lymphoma)
- Neoplasms
- Pancreatitis
- Portal vein thrombosis
- Postoperative cholestasis
- Viral hepatitis

Vascular damage

- Behçet disease
- Budd–Chiari syndrome
- Cirrhosis
- Collagen vascular diseases
- Constrictive pericarditis
- Hypercoagulation states
- Infections
- Inflammatory bowel disease
- Myeloproliferative disorders, sarcoidosis
- Polycystic liver disease
- Pregnancy
- Systemic lupus erythematosus
- Total-body irradiation
- Trauma

Neoplasm formation

- Metastatic neoplasms
- Primary neoplasm of liver, pancreas, gastrointestinal tract

Table 38-7 Extrahepatic Syndromes Associated with Drug-Induced Hepatic and Cholestatic Diseases[1-14,17,18,20,21,56]

Drug	Syndrome
Amoxicillin–clavulanate, chlorpromazine, erythromycin estolate	Obstructive jaundice
Anticonvulsants, chloramphenicol, gold salts, propylthiouracil, phenylbutazone	Associated bone marrow injury
Carbamazepine, phenytoin	Fever, rash, atypical lymphocytosis, lymphadenopathy
Clofibrate	Mylagias, stiffness, weakness, elevated creatine kinase
Dapsone	Fever, jaundice, rash, anemia (sulfone syndrome)
Dapsone, carbamazepine, minocycline, phenytoin, sulfonamides	Fever, rash, perspiration, lymphadenopathy (mononucleosis syndrome)
Gold salts, methoxyflurane, paraquat, penicillamine	Associated renal injury
Intravenous tetracycline, valproic acid	Anorexia, nausea, vomiting, somnolence, encephalopathy resembling fatty liver of pregnancy
Methyldopa, oxyphenisatin	Autoimmune hemolysis
Nitrofurantoin, amiodarone	Associated pulmonary injury
Phenytoin, *para*-aminosalicylate, sulfonamides	Fever, rash, lymphadenopathy, arthralgias (serum sickness syndrome)

HEPATOCELLULAR INJURY

Signs and symptoms of hepatocellular injury can occur within days after exposure but most commonly (with the exception of acetaminophen) take a week or more to develop. The clinical presentation typically includes malaise, abdominal pain, and jaundice. These findings along with coagulopathy (indicated by an elevated prothrombin time or international normalized ratio [INR]) and encephalopathy indicate particularly severe liver injury.[4] Marked elevations in ALT and aspartate aminotransferase (AST), usually preceding increases in total bilirubin levels, and only modest increases in ALP are characteristic of hepatocyte damage. Immune-mediated cytotoxicity is frequently associated with fever, rash, arthralgia, and eosinophilia.

Drug-induced hepatic steatosis is usually asymptomatic, so diagnosis is often delayed. The disorder may be discovered when liver enzymes are measured as part of routine screening or work-up for an unrelated medical problem and found to be elevated. Fatigue and right upper quadrant discomfort may be the only presenting symptoms. Patients with steatohepatitis may report abdominal fullness or discomfort. If the disease is more severe, patients may present with nausea, vomiting, steatorrhea, abdominal pain, pruritus, and fatigue. ALT increases are variable. Histologic examination can provide a definitive diagnosis of steatosis and steatohepatitis, but even then, establishing causality with a specific drug is challenging.[43,55,75]

CHOLESTATIC INJURY

Drug-induced cholestatic injury is typically seen within 4 weeks following drug initiation but can also occur even after the drug has been discontinued. Although the clinical presentation is nonspecific and variable, it is commonly characterized by jaundice and pruritus. Additional signs and symptoms may include fatigue, malaise, anorexia, and nausea. Patients may also be asymptomatic. For a diagnosis of cholestatic injury, patients must have an ALP greater than twice the ULN and/or an R value of less than 2. ALP elevations usually precede increases in ALT. Elevations of gamma-glutamyl transferase have also been observed. Fever and rash are characteristic of drug-induced hypersensitivity reactions.[31] Most acute cases resolve shortly after discontinuation of the offending agent. Patients with chronic cholestasis initially present with elevated ALP and jaundice, which can sometimes last several months to years. These patients can also experience protracted pruritus and fatigue and may develop xanthomas. Although uncommon, pain may occur with intrahepatic cholestasis and can mimic that associated with acute cholecystitis, cholangitis, or choledocholithiasis.[31]

VASCULAR INJURY

Sinusoidal obstruction syndrome usually manifests within 1–3 weeks following initial drug exposure, but a chronic form of this disorder can present months to years afterward. Presenting signs and symptoms typically include some combination of rapid weight gain, ascites, jaundice, right upper-quadrant pain, portal hypertension (as evidenced by varices, ascites, and edema and occasionally encephalopathy, muscle wasting, and weakness), and varying degrees of ALT and AST elevation. The histologic pattern reflects sinusoid obstruction in central areas with hepatocyte necrosis and hemorrhage.[19]

The clinical presentation of other drug-induced hepatic vascular injuries, such as peliosis hepatis (a rare condition of multiple blood-filled cavities throughout the liver), are nonspecific and can include epigastric pain and nausea. It is not uncommon for these injuries to be found as incidental findings on abdominal imaging.[87] Hepatic vein thrombosis presents clinically as Budd–Chiari syndrome, featuring hepatomegaly, abdominal pain, and ascites.[77]

NEOPLASTIC INJURY

Drug-induced hepatic neoplasms may be benign or malignant. The most common signs and symptoms include fatigue, anorexia and weight loss, presence of a palpable mass, and abdominal pain or discomfort.

RISK FACTORS

Table 38-8 lists the various risk factors (and examples of associated medications) for drug-induced hepatic and cholestatic diseases.[34,59,85,88-91] Both nonmodifiable (genetic predisposition, sex, age)

Table 38-8 Risk Factors for Drug-Induced Hepatic and Cholestatic Diseases[34,59,85,88-91,a]

Factor	Medications
Age	
Older	Acetaminophen, amoxicillin–clavulanate, isoniazid, halothane, nitrofurantoin, troglitazone
Younger	Erythromycin, salicylates, valproic acid
Gender	
Male	Amoxicillin–clavulanate, azathioprine
Female	Diclofenac, halothane, isoniazid, methyldopa, minocycline, nitrofurantoin, sulindac, propoxyphene, erythromycin
Obesity	Halothane, methotrexate, tamoxifen
Diabetes mellitus	Methotrexate
Autoimmune/Immune-mediated disorders	Salicylates, TNFα inhibitors, azathioprine, 6-mercaptopurine
Pregnancy	Acetaminophen, isoniazid, tetracycline
Renal dysfunction	Allopurinol, intravenous tetracycline, methotrexate
Cancer chemotherapy	Tyrosine kinase inhibitors, interleukin 2, monoclonal antibodies, cisplatin, oxaliplatin, etoposide, vinca alkaloids, doxorubicin, daunorubicin, azathioprine, fluorodeoxyuridine, thioguanine, 6-mercaptopurine
Dyslipidemia	Statins, niacin
Acquired immune deficiency syndrome	Trimethoprim–sulfamethozazole, dapsone, isoniazid
Underlying liver disease	
Chronic hepatitis B or C	Flutamide, ibuprofen, isoniazid, ritonavir, methotrexate
Nonalcoholic fatty liver disease	Steroids, methotrexate, tamoxifen, tetracycline, irinotecan, nucleoside reverse transcriptase inhibitors
Fasting, malnutrition	Acetaminophen, methimazole, rifampin
Alcohol consumption	Acetaminophen, halothane, isoniazid, methotrexate, vitamin A
Cumulative dose	Amiodarone, bromfenac, methotrexate, oral contraceptives
Increased dose	Acarbose, acetaminophen, cocaine, cyclophosphamide, cyclosporine, methotrexate, niacin, perhexiline, phencyclidine, salicylates, tacrine, tetracycline, valproic acid, vitamin A
Pharmacokinetic interaction	Phenobarbital or phenytoin enhances valproic acid toxicity; isoniazid enhances acetaminophen toxicity
Pharmacodynamic interaction	Pyrazinamide or isoniazid enhances rifampin toxicity; acetaminophen and pennyroyal oil enhance toxicity of one another; valproic acid and chlorpromazine enhance toxicity of one another; isoniazid, zidovudine, cotrimoxazole, phenytoin, carbamazepine, barbiturates enhance acetaminophen toxicity
Genetic predisposition	
CYP2C19 deficiency	Phenobarbital carbonate derivatives
CYP2E1 or CYP1A2 deficiency	Isoniazid, sulfonamides
N-acetyltransferase 2 deficiency	Hydralazine, isoniazid, sulfonamides
Sulfoxidation deficiency	Chlorpromazine
Epoxide hydrolase inhibition or deficiency	Carbamazepine, halothane, phenobarbital, phenytoin
Glutathione synthetase or transferase deficiency	Acetaminophen, tacrine, troglitazone, amoxicillin–clavulanate
Glucuronosyl transferase deficiency	Diclofenac, tolcapone
Human leukocyte antigen allele association	Antituberculosis medications, carbamazepine, amoxicillin-clavulanate, nevirapine, lapatinib, lumiracoxib, ticlopidine
Manganese superoxide dismutase variation	Antituberculosis medications
ATP-binding cassette transporter association	Diclofenac, nevirapine

ATP = adenosine triphosphate, CYP = cytochrome P450 enzyme system, TNF = tumor necrosis factor.

[a]The National Institutes of Health provides a repository of information on herbal and dietary supplements associated with drug-induced liver injury (http://www.livertox.nih.gov).[49]

and modifiable (alcohol consumption, malnutrition, medications) factors play important roles in drug-induced liver disease. Drug-induced hepatic injuries are sometimes reasonably predictable. For example, hepatic injury might be expected following a large single dose of acetaminophen or excessive cumulative doses of amiodarone or methotrexate. Also, patients with chronic viral infections (e.g., human immunodeficiency virus) may be predisposed to immune-mediated cytotoxicity from some medications (e.g., isoniazid).[50-54] Illicit drug use, including cocaine and 3,4-methylenedioxymethamphetamine ("Ecstasy"), are directly linked to fulminant hepatic failure. Psilocybin mushrooms (used illicitly) usually cause hepatotoxicity only upon repeated use, whereas ingestion of toxic (poisonous) mushrooms can lead to fulminant hepatic failure. Pharmacokinetic or pharmacodynamic interactions may enhance susceptibility to idiosyncratic hepatocholestatic injuries. Exposure to some foods and chemical agents associated with construction, agriculture, horticulture, printing, plastic fabrication, plumbing, dry cleaning, and laboratory techniques may independently produce hepatic dysfunction.[59,86]

Although some evidence exists for cross-sensitivity between medications within a given class, there are only a few concrete examples, including the antiepileptics (phenytoin and carbamazepine), inhaled anesthetics (isoflurane, halothane, and enflurane), and the histamine$_2$-receptor antagonists.[59,86]

Growing evidence suggests that high daily dose, regardless of the medication itself, is associated with increased mortality and should be considered a modifiable risk factor.[34] As an example, the use of oral contraceptives has been described as a cumulative dose-dependent risk factor for veno-occlusive hepatic dysfunction.

In general, patients with mild-to-moderate chronic liver disease are not at increased risk of idiosyncratic drug-induced liver diseases.[1-3] Exceptions include patients who receive methotrexate, tolcapone, pemoline, or niacin. Patients with severe liver disease or cirrhosis have altered pharmacokinetic profiles (absorption, metabolism, volume of distribution) increasing the risk of drug-induced liver injury. Injury may not ensue, however, because several enzyme systems, particularly Phase 2 conjugation reactions, are often preserved. Patients with diabetes, obesity, or hyperlipidemia are at increased risk of steatohepatitis, which may increase the susceptibility to various types of liver injury.[17,18,92] It is prudent to consider dose adjustment for any medication implicated in drug-induced hepatic and cholestatic diseases (Table 38-1) based on severity of liver disease.[93]

The study of genetic variations on drug-induced liver injury has led to the conclusion that liver injury due to medication varies by genetic susceptibility. Further work in this field may have lasting impact on the incidence of drug-induced liver injury.

An understanding of the risk factors associated with acetaminophen toxicity provides insight into the complexities of drug-induced liver disease. As noted above, approximately 10% of ingested acetaminophen undergoes biotransformation to the toxic metabolite NAPQI, which, under normal circumstances, is immediately inactivated by conjugation with glutathione. CYP2E1 is the enzyme primarily responsible for the production of NAPQI; therefore, increasing CYP2E1 activity can increase concentrations of NAPQI, as is the case with chronic alcohol ingestion, which results in a twofold increase in CYP2E1 concentrations.[50,51,53] In addition to enzymatic impact on NAPQI production, concomitant medications can significantly impact the CYP system. Inducers of bioactivating enzymes of acetaminophen may increase the acetaminophen bioactive dose and, therefore, toxicity. For example, tobacco use is an independent risk factor for mortality following acetaminophen exposure, presumably because tobacco smoke contains inducers of CYP1A2.[50,51,53] Isoniazid induces CYP2E1 and antiepileptics (phenytoin, carbamazepine, barbiturates) induce CYP3A4, which may lead to an increase in acetaminophen and NAPQI concentrations. Individuals treated with zidovudine for human immunodeficiency virus infection or co-trimoxazole for urinary tract or skin and soft tissue infection may have increased acetaminophen toxicity due to shunting more of the drug to the CYP system from competitive inhibition for glucuronyl transferase.[50,51,53] Poor nutritional status contributes to diminished glucuronidation, induction of CYP2E1, and glutathione depletion, possibly enhancing acetaminophen toxicity. And, finally, the existence of genetic polymorphisms may influence the metabolism of acetaminophen and alter the risk of toxicity.[50,51,53] In summary, risk assessment of drug-induced liver disease is complex and typically multifactorial.

MORBIDITY AND MORTALITY

The majority of patients with drug-induced hepatic injury will completely recover after removal of the offending medication. However, this drug-induced disease accounts for 2–3% of all hospital admissions and only 20–25% of patients with acute idiosyncratic fulminant hepatic failure survive 3 weeks without liver transplantation.[62,94] The most likely causes of death in these patients include cerebral edema, sepsis, multiorgan failure, cardiac arrhythmia/arrest, and respiratory failure.[62] Although mild-to-moderate liver dysfunction can cause significant morbidity (Table 38-5), mortality is not common.[1-14,17,18,20,21,56] Factors related to an increased risk for mortality include pre-existing liver disease; elevated serum creatinine or the need for hemodialysis; jaundice (bilirubin >2× ULN) with aminotransferase concentrations >3× ULN (Hy's Law); occurrence in childhood (particularly in children taking antiepileptic drugs); and higher daily medication doses.[34,95-98] In general, extended exposure to the hepatotoxin will also worsen the prognosis. Jaundice can persist for several months after resolution of acute liver injury. Elevated AST or bilirubin, female sex, and increased age are associated with higher mortality in patients who experience hepatocellular reactions, whereas only elevated bilirubin is predictive of mortality in patients with cholestatic injuries.[96-98]

PREVENTION

Table 38-9 lists approaches to help prevent drug-induced hepatic and cholestatic diseases.[1-9,94,99] Early recognition of signs and symptoms of hepatic injury and rapid discontinuation of the causative agent are the best approaches to prevent serious sequelae. Patients with known risk factors should not receive

Table 38-9 Approaches to Help Prevent Drug-Induced Hepatic and Cholestatic Diseases[1-9,94,99]

Global

- Postmarketing surveillance and reporting
- Preclinical drug testing in animals
- Restricted availability (e.g., blister packaging of nonprescription medication)
- Serial biochemical assessment during clinical studies

Patient-specific

- Adherence to dosing guidelines
- Appropriate patient education on the medication expectations and signs/symptoms of hepatic injury (Table 38-5)
- Appropriate use of the medication
- Avoid polypharmacy and herbal medicines
- Avoid use of agents in patients with known risk factors (Table 38-8)
- Control other disease states (e.g., hyperthyroidism, diabetes mellitus, and hyperlipidemia)
- Genomic testing for potential susceptibility, if applicable/suspected
- Maintain nutrition
- Minimize alcohol consumption, occupational exposures, and illicit drug use
- Rapid recognition of injury and associated extrahepatic syndromes (Table 38-7)
- Serial biochemical monitoring in high-risk patients or with agents known to cause injury

hepatotoxic agents if alternative treatment methods are available. Manufacturers of some medications with known hepatotoxic potential provide specific recommendations for biochemical monitoring that can be followed and some professional organizations have published guidelines for monitoring use of potential hepatotoxins. For medications known to induce serious liver injury in 1–2% of exposures, monthly biochemical monitoring may be cost-effective. This has not been found to be true, however, for medications that are less frequently associated with severe drug-induced liver disease.[59]

MANAGEMENT

Most cases of drug-induced hepatocholestatic dysfunction can be treated by discontinuing the offending medication. In general, discontinuation results in rapid reversal of signs and symptoms if the injury is mild-to-moderate. A 50% reduction of hepatic-associated serum enzymes can be expected within 1 week if the injury is hepatocellular, but this degree of improvement may take 6 months or longer if the injury is cholestatic.[1-14,16,17,20,21,56,96-98] Recovery following discontinuation of drugs with longer half-lives may be prolonged or incomplete.

Cautious rechallenge may be considered only after all signs and symptoms of drug-induced hepatocholestatic injury have resolved and only when other nonhepatotoxic alternative therapies are unavailable. The rechallenge dose may be reduced by at least one-half and titrated upward to a desired dose over several months, if tolerated.[1-14,16,17,20,21,56,93,94,99] Serum aminotransferase concentrations should be monitored frequently (i.e., at least weekly) during rechallenge.

A culprit medication should be permanently discontinued if fulminant hepatocholestatic injury or immune-mediated hepatic injury has occurred. To prevent further injury, medications with dose-dependent toxicity should be removed rapidly from the patient's system by aspiration, activated charcoal, or dialysis. Determination of serum concentration of the offending medication can help gauge the success of removal strategies. These concentrations should be obtained daily, but more frequent monitoring may be necessary in cases of severe hepatotoxicity or as required by institutional protocol.

In most cases, management of patients with drug-induced liver disease is limited to supportive care. **Table 38-10** describes management of drug-induced hepatocholestatic diseases and associated complications.[94,99-186,192,193] There are very few rescue treatments for drug-induced liver disease, and some potential rescue treatments are not available for human use in the United States. Mevalonic acid, for example, could help prevent and/or ameliorate cholestatic injury due to hydroxymethylglutaryl coenzyme A reductase inhibitors (statins).[100] Other rescue options are time-sensitive. Folic acid, for example, is protective against methotrexate-induced hepatotoxicity when given within 24 hours of exposure.[193]

A rescue treatment proven effective for acetaminophen-induced hepatitis is *N*-acetylcysteine (NAC). Although NAC is typically administered within 24 hours of acetaminophen ingestion, a randomized, placebo-controlled study showed that NAC infusions of 6.25 mg/kg/hr reduced mortality, the incidence of cerebral edema, and vasopressor requirements in patients with acetaminophen-induced fulminant liver failure who presented >24 hours after ingestion.[101] All patients had undetectable serum acetaminophen concentrations when NAC was initiated, suggesting that NAC may have therapeutic effects other than its glutathione-replenishing ability (via providing the precursor L-cysteine). Pennyroyal oil and carbon tetrachloride can deplete glutathione, and some evidence suggests that administering NAC shortly after exposure to these agents is beneficial.[102-106] Case reports also indicate that NAC may be beneficial in the treatment of acute hepatic failure caused by valproic acid and sulfasalazine.[107,108]

In theory, NAC may be beneficial for other drug-induced causes of direct hepatotoxicity because it facilitates the replenishment of glutathione, acts as an antioxidant, decreases inflammation by reducing leukocyte chemotaxis and suppressing the expression of nuclear factor-κB, and enhances the synthesis of nitric oxide to increase oxygen delivery.[109,110] Studies have demonstrated benefits of treatment in certain cases of nonacetaminophen drug-induced hepatic injury.[111-113] However, until more evidence is available, intravenous NAC should generally be reserved for use in the situations described previously.

Corticosteroids reduce the inflammatory response to toxic stimuli. Prednisone 10–80 mg daily may reduce the inflammatory reaction associated with immune-mediated hypersensitivity reactions. Azathioprine 50–150 mg daily may be substituted or added.[115,116] Because corticosteroids are possibly effective for alcohol-induced hepatitis, several studies have investigated their clinical use for other causes of hepatitis.[117-120] Unfortunately, no trial has specifically studied the effectiveness of corticosteroids in patients with drug-induced hepatitis. The results of a multicenter study that enrolled

Table 38-10 Management of Drug-Induced Hepatic and Cholestatic Diseases and Associated Complications[94,99-186,192,193]

Agent or Symptom	Management
Acetaminophen toxicity (unintentional or chronic), carbon tetrachloride, pennyroyal oil, other cytotoxic agents (case-specific)[100-112]	NAC intravenously 150 mg/kg (MAX: 15,000 mg) over 1 hr, then 50 mg/kg (MAX: 5,000 mg) over 4 hr, then 6.25 mg/kg/hr (MAX: 10,000 mg) for 16 hr, may continue until resolution if clinically indicated or NAC enterally 140 mg/kg loading dose, then 70 mg/kg every 4 hr for 17 additional doses
Alcoholic hepatitis[99,114]	Prednisolone 40 mg enterally daily for 4–6 weeks or pentoxifylline 400 mg enterally 3 times daily for 4 weeks
Ascites[145-150,156-162]	Fluid restriction 1–2 L/day and sodium restriction 1–2 g/day and furosemide 40 mg intravenously or enterally daily and spironolactone 100 mg enterally daily (diuretics titrated to remove 0.5–2 kg/day) ± large-volume paracentesis if diuretic- refractory, abdominal pain, or breathing difficulties
Cerebral edema with increased intracranial pressure[145-150,176-182]	Minimize agitation, hyperthermia, pain, hypoxia, and acidosis ± mannitol 25–50 g intravenously as needed for intracranial pressure >20 mm Hg and serum osmolarity <320 mOsm/kg (or hypertonic saline to keep serum sodium 145–155 mEq/L) ± hyperventilation for pCO_2 near 35 mm Hg ± pentobarbital or thiopental 250 mg intravenously as needed for intracranial pressure >20 mm Hg ± hypothermia 32–35°C
Cholestasis[128-132]	Ursodiol 300–600 mg daily enterally daily until resolution
Coagulopathy (INR >1.5)[141-154]	Vitamin K 10 mg intravenously or enterally daily ± fresh-frozen plasma ± platelets (to keep platelet count >50×10^9/L) ± desmopressin acetate 0.4 mcg/kg intravenously ± factor VIIa 10–100 mcg/kg intravenously (usually reserved for refractory hemorrhage)
Electrolytes[133]	Correct hypokalemia, hypomagnesemia, and hypophosphatemia
Encephalopathy[167-175]	Lactulose enterally or rectally 30 mL as needed to produce 2 stools daily ± enteral antibiotic (rifaximin 200–400 mg 3 times daily or metronidazole 500 mg 2–4 times daily)
Hepatorenal syndrome[133,187-192]	Renal replacement therapy ± vasopressin 0.1–0.4 units/min (or midodrine 2.5–10 mg enterally 3 times daily + octreotide)
Hyperglycemia[145-150]	Short-acting (regular) insulin intravenously or subcutaneously
Hypoglycemia[145-150]	Dextrose 50% (*w/v*) intravenously
Immune-mediated hypersensitivity reaction (case-specific)[115-123]	Prednisone 10–80 mg enterally daily for 4–6 weeks ± azathioprine 50–150 mg enterally daily
Pruritus[140]	Cholestyramine 4 g enterally twice daily or colestipol 5 g enterally twice daily (titrate to relief or diarrhea) ± rifampin 600 mg enterally daily ± phenobarbital 60–120 mg enterally daily ± chlorpromazine 150–300 mg orally daily ± naloxone 20 mg subcutaneously daily ± ondansetron 8 mg intravenously or enterally once
Spontaneous bacterial peritonitis[156-166]	Antibiotic (third-generation cephalosporin, fluoroquinolone, or extended-spectrum penicillin) for 5–7 days, and albumin 1.5 g/kg intravenously at diagnosis then 1 g/kg intravenously 3 days later
Valproic acid toxicity[124-127]	L-carnitine 50–300 mg/kg intravenously daily until resolution
Variceal hemorrhage[161-163,183-185,186]	Hemodynamic resuscitation and endoscopy (banding preferred) and octreotide 50 mcg intravenously, then 25–50 mcg/hr for 72 hr ± transjugular intrahepatic portosystemic shunt
Veno-occlusive or veno-thrombotic disease[134-139]	Stent placement or angioplasty ± thrombolysis (rTPA 2 mg then 0.5–1 mg/hr infused locally for 24 hr) ± anticoagulation ± transjugular intrahepatic portosystemic shunt

NAC = *N*-acetylcysteine, INR = international normalized ratio, pCO_2 = partial pressure of arterial carbon dioxide, rTPA = recombinant tissue plasminogen activator.

62 patients with acute hepatic failure found that 9 of 10 patients with drug-induced liver failure (6 due to halothane, 2 due to methyldopa, 1 due to isoniazid, and 1 due to propylthiouracil) died despite daily therapy with hydrocortisone 40–800 mg.[121] Until additional studies are conducted, corticosteroids cannot be routinely recommended for the treatment of drug-induced hepatitis. Corticosteroids may have a role in certain case-specific scenarios, including use in patients with lesions resembling immune-mediated hypersensitivity reactions or macrovesicular steatosis caused by agents other than alcohol, including methotrexate, parenteral lipids, and warfarin.[122] Another potential role for corticosteroids is in patients demonstrating hypersensitivity with extrahepatic manifestations (Table 38-7).

Several other agents have reported potential in treating multiple etiologies of hepatitis, including colchicine, gemfibrozil, betaine glucuronate, ursodiol, pentoxifylline, α-tocopherol, nitric oxide, methionine, vitamin E, L-carnitine, and silymarin (milk thistle).[123,124] Only L-carnitine and silymarin have been studied for reversal of drug-induced liver dysfunction.

L-carnitine induces ureagenesis, facilitates fatty acyl transport, and reduces inflammation by inhibiting TNF. The results of a retrospective study of 92 patients with apparent fulminant liver failure secondary to valproic acid showed that L-carnitine therapy at unspecified doses improved survival from 10% to 48%.[125,126] It should be noted, however, that specific data describing the patients, severity of liver injury, and morphologic and histologic pathologies were not presented. The typical dose of intravenous L-carnitine is 50–100 mg/kg/day given in divided doses every 6–8 hours, and therapy should be initiated as soon as possible after suspected/confirmed exposure.

Silymarin, also known as milk thistle, is an herbal supplement used sometimes by patients to "protect the liver" when taking agents with hepatotoxic potential. Silymarin is reported to possess antioxidant, anti-inflammatory, and antifibrotic properties that protect hepatocytes from lipid peroxidation. Unfortunately, beneficial effects have not been substantiated. A meta-analysis of 14 trials of silymarin used in patients with chronic liver disease (two studies of drug-induced liver diseases) found that ALT was reduced by only 9 international units per liter ($p = 0.05$).[127] AST, albumin, and prothrombin time were not significantly affected. Although silymarin was thought to have potential to inhibit hepatitis C virus (HCV) replication, a randomized, controlled trial evaluating high-dose oral silymarin administration was unable to show improvement in concentrations of ALT or HCV RNA in patients with HCV unsuccessfully treated with interferon therapy.[194] As a result, silymarin cannot be recommended in the treatment or prevention of drug-induced hepatotoxicity or other types of hepatic disease.

Patients with drug-induced cholestasis may require long-term daily treatment with ursodiol 300–600 mg/day to dissolve cholesterol gallstones and inhibit apoptosis.[21,56,128-132] Anticoagulation therapy, thrombolytic therapy, or both should be considered after stent placement or angioplasty for drug-induced veno-occlusive or venothrombotic diseases.[134-139] If there is evidence of hepatic impairment or ascites, patients with veno-occlusive or venothrombotic disorders should receive minimal sodium (<2 g/day) and may require diuretics for the removal of accumulated fluid, similar to the treatment of ascites with other etiologies.[134-139]

Ultimately, patients with fulminant liver failure who do not respond to the measures described above will likely require liver transplantation to survive. Unfortunately, only 50% of patients with drug-induced liver failure receive a liver transplant, primarily due to the limited availability of organs and patients' relatively short survival time.[62,195] The use of liver-assist devices or hepatic regeneration therapy with agents such as malotilate is not common, and most data supporting their use are from case reports.[187,191] Extracorporeal liver-assist devices may be artificial or cell-based.[189] Artificial devices use either conventional dialysis along with hemodialysis with a 5–10% albumin dialysate solution over an albumin-impermeable membrane or a fractionated plasma separation technique that uses a membrane with a 250-kDa cutoff between circuits, thereby making the membrane permeable to albumin.[189] Cell-based devices incorporate hepatocytes from various sources and have the theoretical advantage of not only providing blood purification through dialysis but also providing hepatocyte-specific functions (e.g., protein synthesis, ureagenesis, gluconeogenesis, and detoxification through CYP activity).[189] A meta-analysis suggests that liver-assist devices may reduce the incidence of encephalopathy by 33% but do not alter mortality.[187] These devices may, however, improve the likelihood that a patient will survive until transplantation is possible.[188] Devices are not currently available clinically, but represent avenues of future research. In patients with portal hypertension and refractory bleeding or refractory ascites, transjugular intrahepatic portosystemic shunt may be considered to provide time until a liver transplantation can be performed. This approach, however, is associated with worsening encephalopathy.[186]

Liver dysfunction may be associated with pruritus, coagulopathy, malabsorption of fat-soluble vitamins (vitamins A, D, E, K), glycemic dysregulation, ascites, spontaneous bacterial peritonitis (SBP) or other infectious processes, encephalopathy with increased intracranial pressure (ICP), variceal hemorrhage, hepatorenal syndrome, electrolyte abnormalities, metabolic acidosis, and cardiovascular collapse. Biliary dysfunction may cause osteoporosis and hypercholesterolemia. The majority of these are chronic manifestations seen in patients with cirrhosis.

Pruritus in patients with liver dysfunction is likely due to the accumulation of bile acids, even though the concentration of bile acids in the skin does not correlate with the degree of pruritus.[140] Management of this condition is difficult because traditional histamine$_1$-receptor antagonists (e.g., promethazine) typically offer little relief from itching. First-line treatment is the administration of a bile acid sequestrant (e.g., cholestyramine or colestipol).[140] Doses are initially low (cholestyramine 4 g or colestipol 5 g daily or twice daily) and increased over a period of several weeks until symptomatic relief is achieved or constipation develops. Both of these agents may bind and reduce the gastrointestinal absorption of other drugs. Consequently, dosing schedules should be adjusted so that other drugs are given at least 1 hour before or 4 hours after the sequestrant. In cases in which the bile-acid sequestrant is ineffective or not tolerated, therapy with rifampin in a dose of 600 mg daily may be tried.[140] Symptomatic relief usually occurs within 1–3 weeks of initiating rifampin, likely due to enzyme induction and enhanced clearance of bile acids. Caution is necessary when rifampin is used in this patient population. Serum concentrations of liver enzymes and bilirubin should be obtained within 2 weeks of initiating therapy to ensure that the drug is not worsening hepatic disease. Phenobarbital may alleviate pruritus and also provides sedation. Chlorpromazine 25–100 mg every 6 hours produces variable results. As with rifampin, serum concentrations of liver enzymes and bilirubin should be determined within 2 weeks of initiating therapy with chlorpromazine. Daily subcutaneous administration of naloxone has been shown to be effective.[140] A single intravenous dose of ondansetron 8 mg has been shown to alleviate pruritus within 24 hours of administration in one case series, presumably by blocking serotonin (5-hydroxytryptamine type 3) receptors on sensory nerve endings.[140]

Hepatic dysfunction alters coagulation and fibrinolysis through several mechanisms, including reducing concentrations of coagulation factors V, VII, IX, X, XI, prothrombin, thrombin-activated fibrinolysis inhibitor, endogenous anticoagulants (proteins C, S, Z; heparin cofactor II; Z-dependent protease inhibitor; antithrombin), producing defective vitamin K-dependent coagulation factors (VII, IX, X, prothrombin) and increasing concentrations of tissue plasminogen activator, plasminogen activator inhibitor, and von Willebrand factor.[141,142] Renal dysfunction frequently accompanies hepatic dysfunction and usually increases bleeding risk due to acquired platelet dysfunction and abnormal platelet–vessel wall interaction.[141,142] Hepatic injury prevents efficient use of vitamin K, and a dose of 10 mg of vitamin K can reverse coagulopathy to some extent in many patients with mild-to-moderate liver dysfunction.[143-150] The treatment of coagulopathy secondary to drug-induced hepatic dysfunction frequently necessitates the administration of exogenous clotting factors (e.g., fresh-frozen plasma or cryoprecipitate).[145-150] Exogenous platelets should be administered only when life-threatening thrombocytopenia is present.[151] Intravenous desmopressin acetate at maximum doses of 0.4 mcg/kg promotes the release of factor VIII from platelets and reverses coagulopathy with variable success.[151] Intravenous recombinant factor VIIa in a dose of 10–100 mcg/kg rapidly reverses coagulopathy and may alleviate hemorrhagic episodes; but these effects last less than 6 hours so this treatment is usually reserved for cases of refractory hemorrhage.[152,153] Higher doses of recombinant factor VIIa may be associated with thrombosis.[154] In general, the INR should be maintained at a value <1.5 and the platelet count ≥50,000 per cubic millimeter. However, reversing coagulopathy may require substantial fluid administration that can induce ascites and intracranial hypertension, negating the ability to use coagulopathy as a prognostic marker.[145-150] Although the production of endogenous thrombopoietin is frequently diminished in patients with severe liver dysfunction, there is no evidence supporting the routine use of exogenous thrombopoietin.[151]

Fat-soluble vitamins (A, D, E, K) should be administered with careful attention to the dose of vitamin A because it may induce liver failure at high doses or worsen existing injury at therapeutic doses. In these situations, vitamin A induces hepatic inflammation and diminishes the antioxidant capacity of the liver.[155]

Hypoglycemia is a common manifestation of liver dysfunction because the production of glucagon is impaired and hepatic glycogen stores are minimal.[145-150] Patients with fulminant liver dysfunction are often hypervolemic; therefore, the intravenous administration of high concentrations of dextrose (50% *w/v*) may be needed to correct hypoglycemia without adding volume. Patients may develop hyperglycemia due to peripheral insulin resistance and the inability of the liver to convert glucose to glycogen.[145-150] Subcutaneous or intravenous insulin can be used to control hyperglycemia.

Portal hypertension and arterial vasodilation produce ascites by activating the renin–angiotensin–aldosterone–vasopressin system to increase intravascular blood volume. Peritoneal fluid collects when an elevated hepatosplanchnic pressure forces the passage of fluid from the sinusoidal lumen into the interstitial spaces because the endothelial cells that line the sinusoids are compromised.[156-162] Therefore, ascites should be treated with fluid restriction (1–2 L/day), sodium restriction (1–2 g/day), and the administration of diuretics, preferably furosemide and spironolactone in doses of 40 mg/day and 100 mg/day, respectively.[145,150,156-162] These doses may be titrated over time to 160 mg/day and 400 mg/day, respectively. The goal of diuretic therapy is to remove fluid at a rate of 0.5 kg/day in patients without peripheral edema and 2 kg/day in patients with peripheral edema. Large-volume paracentesis (>5 L) may be performed if the patient has severe abdominal pain or breathing difficulty.[156-162] Albumin (8 g for each liter of ascitic fluid removed) administered during or immediately after paracentesis can help prevent circulatory and renal dysfunction.[145-150,157-162]

Small-volume paracentesis (<2 L) is used to evaluate patients with new-onset ascites for the presence of SBP, and an ascitic fluid polymorphonuclear count of ≥250 cells per cubic millimeter is considered diagnostic.[156-165] SBP occurs when bacteria translocate from the intestinal tract to the peritoneum via the mesenteric lymphatic system. This complication of hepatic disease is secondary to impaired gastrointestinal motility, damage to the intestinal mucosa, gastrointestinal bacterial overgrowth, low concentrations of protein and complement in the ascitic fluid, impaired activity of the reticuloendothelial system including Kupffer cells, and reduced neutrophil function.[164,165] Antibiotic therapy for 5–7 days is indicated for the treatment of patients with SBP.[156-165] Therapy should be designed to cover the most likely organisms and penetrate the ascitic fluid. Coverage for *Escherichia coli*, *Streptococcus pneumoniae*, *Klebsiella* species, and other enteric gram-negative organisms should be provided. Third-generation cephalosporins (cefotaxime, ceftriaxone), extended-spectrum penicillins (ampicillin–sulbactam), and fluoroquinolones (ciprofloxacin) are all effective in eradicating these organisms, with resolution rates generally ≥90%.[165] Empiric selection of initial antibiotic therapy should consider the local antimicrobial resistance patterns. Albumin in a dose of 1.5 g/kg given at the time of diagnosis and 1 g/kg given 3 days later has been shown to reduce the incidence of renal impairment and hospital mortality in patients with SBP.[166] Prophylactic antibiotics for the prevention of SBP in patients with ascites may be warranted when fulminant liver failure is present.[160-165]

Encephalopathy is a metabolic disorder of mental activity, neuromuscular function, and consciousness associated with hepatic disease. It is believed to be caused by the accumulation of substances (e.g., ammonia) that are efficiently metabolized/eliminated under normal conditions but accumulate with liver dysfunction.[167-169] Single measurements of serum ammonia concentrations do not reflect the degree of encephalopathy, but trends in serial measurements correlate with the progression or reversal of encephalopathy.[167-169] Initial treatment of encephalopathy should include the reversal of precipitating factors (including hemorrhage, excess dietary protein, azotemia, infection, constipation, and metabolic/electrolyte disturbances) and the discontinuation of central nervous system depressants.[167-169] Pharmacotherapy of encephalopathy may be initiated with enteral or rectal lactulose (30 mL as often as hourly until stool is produced and then 3–4 times daily as needed to produce two to three soft stools per day) and enteral rifaximin (200–400 mg 3 times daily) or metronidazole (500 mg 2–4 times daily).[145-150,167-170] Meta-analysis has shown that lactulose improves encephalopathy.[171] Neomycin (1–2 g 4 times daily) is used for encephalopathy in rare cases, and caution is warranted as it is associated with nephrotoxicity.[170] Protein restriction is not recommended unless other treatment modalities fail to control symptoms, and nutritional products containing branched-chain amino acids may reduce the degree of encephalopathy, although major outcomes, such as returning to baseline mental status, length of hospital stay, and survival do not improve.[172-174]

Altered mental status should be investigated using computed tomography to rule out intracranial hemorrhage. Insertion of an ICP monitoring device may be considered but may constitute an unacceptable risk for the patient when coagulopathy is present.[176,177] The use of an ICP monitor is associated with hemorrhage and 30-day survival after liver transplantation has been found to be similar in both monitored and nonmonitored patients.[178] Treatment of increased ICP should include minimizing agitation with short-acting benzodiazepine agents, providing analgesia with short-acting opioid agents, controlling hyperthermia, and minimizing acidosis and hypoxia.[145-150,176,177] Cerebral edema and increased ICP may be treated with intravenous mannitol 25–50 g as needed to keep the ICP <20 mm Hg and the serum osmolality between 310–320 mOsm/kg.[167-169,176,177] Mannitol may accumulate in astrocytes if renal failure is present and may cause rebound cerebral edema. Hypertonic saline (3% *w/v*) administered to a target serum sodium concentration of 145–155 mEq/L may be used as an alternative to mannitol but can contribute to serum sodium irregularities.[179]

Hyperventilation to maintain the partial pressure of arterial carbon dioxide near 35 mm Hg should reduce ICP without substantially compromising cerebral blood flow, but this effect is limited to several hours.[145-150,180] Intravenous thiopental or pentobarbital may be used if mannitol is unsuccessful or contraindicated.[145-150,176,177] Mild hypothermia (32–35°C) is also used in the treatment of elevated ICP. This therapy maintains hepatic function by decreasing ischemia-reperfusion injury and the inflammatory response; however; it is associated with coagulopathy, electrolyte abnormalities, altered hemodynamics, variable glucose control, and rebound intracranial hypertension during rewarming.[181,182]

Variceal hemorrhage and hepatorenal syndrome are rarely associated with idiosyncratic drug reactions. Varices are caused by portal hypertension and develop when the portal pressure gradient exceeds 10 mm Hg, resulting in the development of portosystemic collateral circulation.[161-163,183,184] A variceal hemorrhage should be treated with endoscopic procedures (banding is preferred) followed by the administration of octreotide (50 mcg bolus followed by intravenous infusion of 25 or 50 mcg/hr for 3–5 days).[161-163,183,184] Octreotide reduces the rate of rebleeding and transfusion requirements.[185] In some countries, terlipressin (a vasopressin analogue) is available and has demonstrated improved survival.[183] Acute renal failure may require renal dialysis, but hepatorenal syndrome may be temporarily alleviated by intravenous vasopressin infusion (0.1–0.4 units/minute) or the combination of octreotide and midodrine (2.5–10 mg 3 times daily).[192]

Common electrolyte abnormalities associated with liver dysfunction include hypophosphatemia, hypokalemia, and hypomagnesemia. Electrolyte replacement may be required. Hypervolemic hyponatremia is common and usually asymptomatic even when sodium concentrations are profoundly low; however, it may indicate the onset of hepatorenal syndrome or increase the predictive mortality potential for Model for End-stage Liver Disease scoring in cirrhosis.[133] The benefits of raising serum sodium concentrations in severe hyponatremia are controversial in patients with severe hepatic dysfunction (e.g., cirrhosis). Diuretic therapy combined with fluid restriction can improve serum sodium concentrations.[133] Intravenous sodium chloride should be administered only when patients are symptomatic (e.g., when seizures are present), as increases in serum sodium concentrations are transient and the excess fluid may precipitate ascites.

Vasopressin receptor antagonists (e.g., conivaptan and tolvaptan) are a novel class of diuretics used to correct hyponatremia. Unlike loop diuretics, vasopressin receptor antagonists increase urine flow and decrease urine osmolality while increasing plasma osmolality without increasing the renal elimination of sodium. All vasopressin receptor antagonists are contraindicated in severe hepatic impairment, and tolvaptan should generally be avoided with any underlying liver disease.[196,197] Following liver transplantation, the restoration of hepatic function and isotonic fluids received during surgery will induce rapid correction of hyponatremia. However, if baseline sodium concentrations are too low, this correction may be rapid enough to induce osmotic demyelination syndrome. Osmotic demyelination syndrome can occur with rapid rises in sodium concentrations (>9 mEq/L in 24 hours and ≥18 mEq/L in 48 hours), which can be associated with cerebral edema and severe neurologic complications.[198,199] Therefore, in patients with a serum sodium concentration <130 mEq/L awaiting liver transplant, administration of hypertonic saline for slow correction of hyponatremia prior to transplantation may help prevent this potential complication.[198]

Systemic complications (e.g., metabolic acidosis and cardiovascular collapse) may cause acute hypoperfusion of the liver, commonly called shock liver or ischemic hepatitis. Treating the underlying cause of shock liver generally leads to resolution of hepatic injury. If long-term complications of biliary dysfunction occur (e.g., osteoporosis or hypercholesterolemia), treatment should be implemented according to current practice guidelines, with special consideration for dose adjustments for hepatic impairment.

INFORMATION FOR PATIENTS

Patients taking agents that may cause hepatocholestatic injury should be instructed to consult their healthcare provider if they experience nausea, vomiting, unexplained weight loss, decreased appetite, or abdominal pain that lasts several days and cannot be attributed to other causes. Patients with altered mental status, increased abdominal girth, peripheral edema, bleeding episodes, protracted pruritus, jaundice, or reduced urine production should receive immediate medical attention. In some cases, no symptoms may be present and medical tests (imaging, biopsy, and/or bloodwork) may be required. Patients should be instructed not to take any nonprescription medications or herbal products without first consulting their healthcare provider. Patients should inform their healthcare provider of all medications (including herbal remedies and dietary supplements) they are taking to avoid drug–drug interactions. All patients should be educated about their medications and risk factors, including alcohol, illicit drugs, and other environmental exposures. It is important to emphasize to patients that they should only take their medications in doses recommended or prescribed by their healthcare provider. This may help avoid toxicity, but some medications can cause toxicity even at recommended doses (idiosyncratic reactions).

Toxicity may occur within days or months of starting a medication. The most effective treatment for drug-induced liver toxicity is stopping or avoiding the offending medication. In most cases, the liver repairs itself but may take several months to heal. In severe cases (e.g., liver failure or cirrhosis), liver transplantation may be needed.

REFERENCES

1. Lee WM. Drug-induced hepatotoxicity. *N Engl J Med.* 2003; 349:474-85.
2. Lewis JH. Drug-induced liver disease. *Med Clin North Am.* 2000; 84:1275-311.
3. Bliebel W, Kim S, D'Silva K et al. Drug-induced liver injury: review article. *Dig Dis Sci.* 2007; 52:2463-71.
4. Navarro VJ, Senior JR. Drug-related hepatotoxicity. *N Engl J Med.* 2006; 354:731-9.
5. Hussaini SH, Farrington EA. Idiosyncratic drug-induced liver injury: an overview. *Expert Opin Drug Saf.* 2007; 6:673-84.
6. Halegoua-De Marzio D, Navarro VJ. Drug-induced hepatotoxicity in humans. *Curr Opin Drug Discov Devel.* 2008; 11:53-9.
7. Chang CY, Schiand TD. Review article: drug hepatotoxicity. *Aliment Pharmacol.* 2007; 25:1135-51.
8. Larrey D, Pageaux GR. Drug-induced acute liver failure. *Eur J Gastroenterol Hepatol.* 2005; 17:141-3.
9. Kaplowitz N. Drug-induced liver injury. *Clin Infect Dis.* 2004; 38(suppl 2):S44-8.
10. Abboud G, Kaplowitz N. Drug-induced liver injury. *Drug Saf.* 2007; 30:277-94.
11. Nathwani RA, Kaplowitz N. Drug hepatotoxicity. *Clin Liver Dis.* 2006; 10:207-17.
12. Kaplowitz N. Idiosyncratic drug hepatotoxicity. *Nat Rev Drug Discov.* 2005; 4:489-99.
13. Andrade RJ, Robles M, Fernandez-Castaner A et al. Assessment of drug-induced hepatotoxicity in clinical practice: a challenge for gastroenterologists. *World J Gastroenterol.* 2007; 13:329-40.
14. Maddrey WC. Drug-induced hepatotoxicity. *J Clin Gastroenterol.* 2005; 39:S83-9.
15. Chitturi S, George J. Hepatotoxicity of commonly used drugs; nonsteroidal anti-inflammatory drugs, antihypertensives, antidiabetic agents, anticonvulsants, lipid-lowering agents, psychotropic drugs. *Semin Liver Dis.* 2002; 22:169-84.
16. Teoh NC, Farrell GC. Hepatotoxicity associated with nonsteroidal anti-inflammatory drugs. *Clin Liver Dis.* 2003; 7:401-13.
17. Stravitz RT, Sanyal AJ. Drug-induced steatohepatitis. *Clin Liver Dis.* 2003; 7:435-51.
18. Farrell GC. Drugs and steatohepatitis. *Semin Liver Dis.* 2002; 22:169-84.
19. Giordano CM, Zervos XB. Clinical manifestations and treatment of drug-induced hepatotoxicity. *Clin Liver Dis.* 2013; 17:565-73.
20. Fernandez TP, Lopez Serrano P, Tomas E et al. Diagnostic and therapeutic approach to cholestatic liver disease. *Rev Esp Enferm Dig.* 2004; 96:60-73.
21. Levy C, Lindor KD. Drug-induced cholestasis. *Clin Liver Dis.* 2003; 7:311-30.
22. Arundel C, Lewis JH. Drug-induced liver diseases in 2006. *Curr Opin Gastroenterol.* 2007; 23:244-54.
23. Lazerow SK, Abdi MS, Lewis JH. Drug-induced liver disease in 2004. *Curr Opin Gastroenterol.* 2005; 21:283-92.
24. Scheen AJ. Hepatotoxicity with thiazolidinediones: is it a class effect? *Drug Saf.* 2001; 24:873-8.
25. Fisher K, Vuppalanchi R, Saxena R. Drug-induced liver injury. *Arch Pathol Lab Med.* 2015; 139:876-87.
26. Lewis JH, Ahmed M, Shobassy A et al. Drug-induced liver disease. *Curr Opin Gastroenterol.* 2006; 22:223-33.
27. Brown SJ, Desmond PV. Hepatotoxicity of antimicrobial agents. *Semin Liver Dis.* 2002; 22:157-68.
28. Thiim M, Friedman LS. Hepatotoxicity of antibiotics and antifungals. *Clin Liver Dis.* 2003; 7:381-99.
29. Norris W, Paredes AH, Lewis JH. Drug-induced liver injury in 2007. *Curr Opin Gastroenterol.* 2008; 24:287-97.
30. Tostmann A, Boeree MJ, Aarnouste RE et al. Antituberculosis drug-induced hepatotoxicity: concise up-to-date review. *J Gastroenterol Hepatol.* 2008; 23:192-202.
31. Bhamidimarri KR, Schiff E. Drug-induced cholestatis. *Clin Liver Dis.* 2013; 17:519-31.
32. Ogedegbe AO, Sulkowski MS. Antiretroviral-associated liver injury. *Clin Liver Dis.* 2003; 7:475-99.
33. Amacher DE, Chalasani N. Drug-induced hepatic steatosis. *Semin Liver Dis.* 2014; 34:205-14.
34. Leise MD, Poterucha JJ, Talwalkar JA. Drug-induced liver injury. *Mayo Clin Proc.* 2014; 89:95-106.
35. Parra JL, Reddy KR. Hepatotoxicity of hypolipidemic drugs. *Clin Liver Dis.* 2003; 7:415-33.
36. de Denus S, Spinler SA, Miller K et al. Statins and liver toxicity: a meta-analysis. *Pharmacotherapy.* 2004; 24:584-91.
37. Tolman KG, Chandramouli J. Hepatotoxicity of the thiazolidinediones. *Clin Liver Dis.* 2003; 7:369-79.
38. Stedman C. Herbal hepatotoxicity. *Semin Liver Dis.* 2002; 22:195-206.
39. Pittler MH, Ernst E. Systematic review: hepatotoxic events associated with herbal medicinal products. *Aliment Pharmacol Ther.* 2003; 18:451-71.
40. Schiano TD. Hepatotoxicity and complementary and alternative medicines. *Clin Liver Dis.* 2003; 7:453-73.
41. Willett KL, Roth RA, Walker L. Workshop overview: hepatotoxicity assessment for botanical dietary supplements. *Toxicol Sci.* 2004; 79:4-9.
42. Zheng EX, Navarro VJ. Liver injury from herbal, dietary, and weight loss supplements: a review. *J Clin Transl Hepatol.* 2015; 3:93-8.
43. Ramachandran R, Kakar S. Histological patterns in drug-induced liver disease. *J Clin Pathol.* 2009; 62:481-92.
44. Lucena MI, Carvajal A, Andrade RJ et al. Antidepressant-induced hepatotoxicity. *Expert Opin Drug Saf.* 2003; 2:249-62.
45. DeSanty KP, Amabile CM. Antidepressant-induced liver injury. *Ann Pharmacother.* 2007; 41:1201-11.
46. Carvajal GP, Garcia D, Sanchez SA et al. Hepatotoxicity associated with the new antidepressants. *J Clin Psychiatry.* 2002; 63:135-7.
47. Ghabril M, Bonkovsky HL, Kum C et al. Liver injury from tumor necrosis factor-α antagonists: analysis of thirty-four cases. *Clin Gastroenterol Hepatol.* 2013; 11:558-64.
48. Davern TJ, Bass NM. Leukotriene antagonists. *Clin Liver Dis.* 2003; 7;501-12.
49. National Institutes of Health. LiverTox: Clinical and Research Information on Drug-Induced Liver Injury [online database]. https://livertox.nlm.nih.gov (accessed 2018 Mar 15).
50. Gunawan BK, Kaplowitz N. Mechanisms of drug-induced liver disease. *Clin Liver Dis.* 2007; 11:459-75.
51. Holt MP, Ju C. Mechanisms of drug-induced liver injury. *AAPS J.* 2006; 8:E48-54.
52. Marschall HU, Wagner M, Zollner G et al. Clinical hepatotoxicity: regulation, and treatment with inducers of transport and cofactors. *Mol Pharm.* 2007; 4:895-910.
53. Ganey PE, Luyendyk JP, Maddox JF et al. Adverse hepatic drug reactions: inflammatory episodes as consequence and contributor. *Chem Biol Interact.* 2004; 150:35-51.

54. Castell JV, Castell M. Allergic hepatitis induced by drugs. *Curr Opin Allergy Clin Immunol.* 2006; 6:258-65.
55. Patel V, Sanyal AJ. Drug-induced steatophepatitis. *Clin Liv Dis.* 2013; 17:533-46.
56. Chitturi S, Farrell GC. Drug-induced cholestasis. *Semin Gastrointest Dis.* 2001; 12:113-24.
57. Pauli-Magnus C, Meier PJ. Hepatobiliary transporters and drug-induced cholestasis. *Hepatology.* 2006; 44:778-87.
58. Mohi-ud-din R, Lewis JH. Drug- and chemical-induced cholestasis. *Clin Liver Dis.* 2004; 8:95-132.
59. Larrey D. Epidemiology and individual susceptibility to adverse drug reactions affecting the liver. *Semin Liver Dis.* 2002; 22:145-56.
60. Bjornsson ES, Bergmann OM, Bjornsson HK et al. Incidence, presentation, and outcomes in patients with drug-induced liver injury in the general population of Iceland. *Gastroenterology.* 2013; 144:1419-25.
61. Friis H, Andreasen PB. Drug-induced hepatic injury: an analysis of 1100 cases reported to the Danish Committee on Adverse Drug Reactions between 1978 and 1987. *J Intern Med.* 1992; 232:133-8.
62. Ostapowicz G, Fontana RJ, Schiodt FV et al. Results of a prospective study of acute liver failure at 17 tertiary care centers in the United States. *Ann Intern Med.* 2002; 137:947-54.
63. Larson AM, Polson J, Fontana RJ et al. Acetaminophen-induced acute liver failure: results of a United States multicenter, prospective study. *Hepatology.* 2005; 42:1364-72.
64. Larrey D. Drug-induced liver diseases. *J Hepatol.* 2000; 32(suppl 1):77-88.
65. Hinson JA, Roberts DW, James LP. Mechanisms of acetaminophen-induced liver necrosis. *Handb Exp Pharmacol.* 2010; 196:369-405.
66. Jaeschke H. Acetaminophen: dose-dependent drug hepatotoxicity and acute liver failure in patients. *Dig Dis.* 2015; 33:464-71.
67. McGill MR, Jaeschke H. Metabolism and disposition of acetaminophen: recent advances in relation to hepatotoxicity and diagnosis. *Pharm Res.* 2013; 30:2174-87.
68. Jaeschke H, McGill MR, Ramachandran A. Oxidant stress, mitochondria, and cell death mechanisms in drug-induced liver injury: lessons learned from acetaminophen hepatotoxicity. *Drug Metab Rev.* 2012; 44:88-106.
69. Gujral JS, Knight TR, Farhood A et al. Mode of cell death after acetaminophen overdose in mice: apoptosis or oncotic necrosis? *Toxicol Sci.* 2002; 67:322-8.
70. Lee WM. Drug-induced hepatotoxicity. *N Engl Med.* 1995; 333:1118-27.
71. Kaplowitz N. Biochemical and cellular mechanisms of toxic liver injury. *Semin Liver Dis.* 2002; 22:137-44.
72. Jaeschke H, Gores GJ, Cederbaum AI et al. Mechanisms of hepatotoxicity. *Toxicol Sci.* 2002; 65:166-76.
73. Kass GE. Mitochondrial involvement in drug-induced hepatic injury. *Chem Biol Interact.* 2006; 163:145-59.
74. Chalasani N, Younossi Z, Lavine JE et al. The diagnosis and management of non-alcoholic fatty liver disease: practice guideline by the American Association for the Study of Liver Diseases, American College of Gastroenterology, and the American Gastroenterological Association. *Hepatology.* 2012; 55:2005-23.
75. Rabinowich L, Shibolet O. Drug induced steatohepatitis: an uncommon culprit of a common disease. *Biomed Res Int.* 2015; 2015:168905.
76. Yang K, Kock K, Sedykh A, Tropsha A, Brouwer KLR. An updated review on drug-induced cholestasis: mechanisms and investigation of physicochemical properties and pharmacokinetic parameters. *J Pharm Sci.* 2013; 102:3037-57.
77. Senzolo M, Riggio O, Primignani M. Vascular disorders of the liver: recommendations from the Italian Association for the Study of the Liver (AISF) ad hoc committee. *Dig Liver Dis.* 2011; 43:503-14.
78. Lee FI, Smith PM, Bennett B, Williams DMJ. Occupationally related angiosarcoma of the liver in the United Kingdom 1972-1994. *Gut.* 1996; 39:312-8.
79. Benichou C, Uclaf R. Criteria of drug-induced liver disorders: report of an international consensus meeting. *J Hepatol.* 1990; 11:272-6.
80. Benichou C, Danan G, Flahault A. Causality assessment of adverse reactions to drugs-II. An original model for validation of drug causality assessment methods: case reports with positive rechallenge. *J Clin Epidemiol.* 1993; 46:1331-6.
81. Danan G, Benichou C. Causality assessment of adverse reactions to drugs-I. A novel method based on the conclusions of international consensus meetings: application to drug-induced liver injuries. *J Clin Epidemiol.* 1993; 46:1323-30.
82. Standardization of definitions and criteria of causality assessment of adverse drug reactions, drug-induced liver disorders: report of an international consensus meeting. *Int J Clin Pharmacol Ther Toxicol.* 1990; 28:317-22.
83. Tandon BN, Bernauau J, O'Grady J et al. Recommendations of the International Association for the Study of the Liver Subcommittee on Nomenclature of Acute and Subacute Liver Failure. *J Gastroenterol Hepatol.* 1999; 14:403-4.
84. Sakka SG. Assessing liver function. *Curr Opin Crit Care.* 2007; 13:207-14.
85. Ramaiah SK. A toxicologist guide to the diagnostic interpretation of hepatic biochemical parameters. *Food Chem Toxicol.* 2007; 45:1551-7.
86. Shapiro MA, Lewis JH. Causality assessment of drug-induced hepatotoxicity: promises and pitfalls. *Clin Liv Dis.* 2007; 11:477-505.
87. Kootte AM, Siegel AM, Koorenhof M. Generalised peliosis hepatis mimicking metastases after long-term use of oral contraceptives. *Neth J Med.* 2015; 73:41-3.
88. Khoury T, Rmeileh AA, Yosha L et al. Drug-induced liver injury: review with a focus on genetic factors, tissue diagnosis, and treatment options. *J Clin Transl Hepatol.* 2015; 3:99-108.
89. Huang YS, Su WJ, Huang YH et al. Genetic polymorphisms of manganese superoxide dismutase, NAD(P)H:quinone oxidoreductase, glutathione S-transferase M1 and T1, and the susceptibility to drug-induced liver injury. *J Hepatol.* 2007; 47:128-34.
90. Urban TJ, Daly AK, Aithal GP. Genetic basis of drug-induced liver injury: present and future. *Semin Liver Dis.* 2014; 34:123-33.
91. Bahirwani R, Reddy KR. Drug-induced liver injury due to cancer chemotherapeutic agents. *Semin Liver Dis.* 2014; 34:162-71.
92. Malinowski SS, Byrd JS, Bell AM et al. Pharmacologic therapy for nonalcoholic fatty liver disease in adults. *Pharmacotherapy.* 2013; 33:223–42.
93. Spray JW, Willett K, Chase D et al. Dosage adjustment for hepatic dysfunction based on Child-Pugh scores. *Am J Health-Syst Pharm.* 2007; 64:690-3.
94. Dossing M, Sonne J. Drug-induced hepatic disorders: incidence, management, and avoidance. *Drug Saf.* 1993; 9:441-9.
95. Reuben A. Hy's law. *Hepatology.* 2004; 39:574-8.
96. Andrade RJ, Lucena MI, Fernandez MC et al. Drug-induced liver injury: an analysis of 461 incidences submitted to the Spanish registry over a 10 year period. *Gastroenterology.* 2005; 129:512-21.
97. Andrade RJ, Lucena MI, Kaplowitz N et al. Outcome of acute idiosyncratic drug-induced injury: long-term follow-up in a hepatotoxicity registry. *Hepatology.* 2006; 44:1581-8.
98. Bjornsson E, Olsson R. Outcome and prognostic markers in severe drug-induced liver disease. *Hepatology.* 2005; 42:481-9.
99. Marino G, Zimmerman HJ, Lewis JH. Management of drug-induced liver disease. *Curr Gastroenterol Rep.* 2001; 3:38-48.
100. Kornbrust DJ, MacDonald JS, Peter CP et al. Toxicity of the HMG-Coenzyme A reductase inhibitor, lovastatin, to rabbits. *J Pharmacol Exp Ther.* 1989; 248:498-505.
101. Keays R, Harrison PM, Wendon JA et al. Intravenous acetylcysteine in paracetamol induced fulminant hepatic failure: a prospective controlled trial. *BMJ.* 1991; 303:1026-9.
102. Mathieson PW, Williams G, Mac Sweeney JE. Survival after massive ingestion of carbon tetrachloride treated by intravenous infusion of acetylcysteine. *Hum Toxicol.* 1985; 4:627-31.

103. Anderson IB, Mullen WH, Meeker JE et al. Pennyroyal toxicity: measurement of toxic metabolite levels in two cases and review of the literature. *Ann Intern Med.* 1996; 124:726-34.
104. Valles EG, de Castro CR, Castro JA. *N*-acetylcysteine in an early but also a late preventative agent against carbon tetrachloride-induced liver necrosis. *Toxicol Lett.* 1994; 71:87-95.
105. Simko V, Michael S, Katz J et al. Protective effects of oral acetylcysteine against hepatorenal toxicity of carbon tetrachloride potentiated by ethyl alcohol. *Alcohol Clin Exp Res.* 1992; 16:795-9.
106. Sklar GE, Subramaniam M. Acetylcysteine treatment for non-acetaminophen-induced acute liver failure. *Ann Pharmacother.* 2004; 38:498-501.
107. Gabay C, De Bandt M, Palazzo E. Sulphasalazine-related life-threatening side effects: is *N*-acetylcysteine of therapeutic value? *Clin Exp Rheumatol.* 1993; 11:417-20.
108. Gopaul SV, Farrell K, Abbott FS. Identification and characterization of *N*-acetylcysteine conjugates of valproic acid in humans and animals. *Drug Metab Dispos.* 2000; 28:823-32.
109. Harrison PM, Wendon JA, Gimson AE et al. Improvement by acetylcysteine of hemodynamics and oxygen transport in fulminant hepatic failure. *N Engl J Med.* 1991; 324:1852-7.
110. Devlin J, Ellis AE, McPeake J et al. *N*-acetylcysteine improves indocyanine green extraction and oxygen transport during hepatic dysfunction. *Crit Care Med.* 1997; 25:236-42.
111. Ben-Ari Z, Vaknin H, Tur-Kaspa R. *N*-acetylcysteine in acute hepatic failure (non-paracetamol-induced). *Hepatogastroenterology.* 2000; 47:786-9.
112. Kortsalioudaki C, Taylor RM, Cheeseman P et al. Safety and efficacy of *N*-acetylcysteine in children with non-acetaminophen-induced acute liver failure. *Liver Transpl.* 2008; 14:25-30.
113. Lee WM, Hynan LS, Rossaro L et al. Intravenous *N*-acteylcysteine improves transplant-free survival in early stage non-acetaminophen acute liver failure. *Gastroenterology.* 2009; 137:856-64.
114. Thursz MR, Richardson P, Allison M et al. Prednisolone or pentoxifylline for alcoholic hepatitis. *N Engl J Med.* 2015; 372:1619-28.
115. Czaja AJ. Emerging treatments for autoimmune hepatitis. *Curr Drug Targets Inflamm Allergy.* 2002; 1:317-26.
116. Czaja AJ. Drug therapy in the management of type 1 autoimmune hepatitis. *Drugs.* 1999; 57:49-68.
117. Christensen E, Gluud C. Glucocorticoids are ineffective in alcoholic hepatitis: a meta-analysis adjusting for confounding variables. *Gut.* 1995; 37:113-8.
118. Imperiale TF, McCullough AJ. Do corticosteroids reduce mortality from alcoholic hepatitis? A meta-analysis of the randomized trials. *Ann Intern Med.* 1990; 113:299-307.
119. Mathurin P, Mendenhall CL, Carithers RL Jr et al. Corticosteroids improve short-term survival in patients with severe alcoholic hepatitis (AH): individual data analysis of the last three randomized placebo controlled double blind trials of corticosteroids in severe AH. *J Hepatol.* 2002; 36:480-7.
120. Phillips M, Curtis H, Portmann B et al. Antioxidants versus corticosteroids in the treatment of severe alcoholic hepatitis - a randomised clinical trial. *J Hepatol.* 2006; 44:784-90.
121. Rakela J, Mosley JW, Edwards VM et al. A double-blinded, randomized trial of hydrocortisone in acute hepatic failure. The Acute Hepatic Failure Study Group. *Dig Dis Sci.* 1991; 36:1223-8.
122. O'Beirne J, Holmes M, Agarwal B et al. Adrenal insufficiency in liver disease - what is the evidence? *J Hepatol.* 2007; 47:418-23.
123. Akriviadis E, Botla R, Briggs W et al. Pentoxifylline improves short-term survival in severe acute alcoholic hepatitis: a double-blind, placebo-controlled trial. *Gastroenterology.* 2000; 119:1637-48.
124. Muriel P, Rivera-Espinoza Y. Beneficial drugs for liver diseases. *J Appl Toxicol.* 2008; 28:93-103.
125. Bohan TP, Helton E, McDonald I et al. Effect of L-carnitine treatment for valproate-induced hepatotoxicity. *Neurology.* 2001; 56:1405-9.
126. Winter SC. Treatment of carnitine deficiency *J Inherit Metab Dis.* 2003; 26:171-80.
127. Jacobs BP, Dennehy C, Ramirez G et al. Milk thistle for the treatment of liver disease: a systematic review and meta-analysis. *Am J Med.* 2002; 113:506-15.
128. Cicognani C, Malavolti M, Morselli-Labate AM et al. Flutamide-induced toxic hepatitis. Potential utility of ursodeoxycholic acid administration in toxic hepatitis. *Dig Dis Sci.* 1996; 41:2219-21.
129. Lazaridis KN, Gores GJ, Lindor KD. Ursodeoxycholic acid and mechanisms of action and clinical use in hepatobiliary disorders. *J Hepatol.* 2001; 35:134-46.
130. Kumar D, Tandon RK. Use of ursodeoxycholic acid in liver disease. *J Gastroenterol Hepatol.* 2001; 16:3-14.
131. Trauner M, Graziadei IW. Review article: mechanisms of action and therapeutic applications of ursodeoxycholic acid in chronic liver diseases. *Aliment Pharmacol Ther.* 1999; 13:979-96.
132. Pust T, Beuers U. Ursodeoxycholic acid treatment of vanishing bile duct syndromes. *World J Gastroenterol.* 2006; 12:3487-95.
133. Martin-Llahi M, Guevara M, Gines P. Hyponatremia in cirrhosis: clinical features and management. *Gastroenterol Clin Biol.* 2006; 30:1144-51.
134. Willner IR. Veno-occlusive disease. *Curr Treat Options Gastroenterol.* 2002; 5:465-9.
135. Slakey DP, Klein AS, Venbrux AC et al. Budd-Chiari Syndrome: current management options. *Ann Surg.* 2001; 233:522-7.
136. Sharma S, Texeira A, Texeira P et al. Pharmacological thrombolysis in Budd-Chiari syndrome: a single centre experience and review of the literature. *J Hepatol.* 2004; 40:172-80.
137. Zimmerman MA, Cameron AM, Ghobrial RM. Budd-Chiari syndrome. *Clin Liver Dis.* 2006; 10:259-73.
138. Menon KV, Shah V, Kamath PS. The Budd-Chiari syndrome. *N Engl J Med.* 2004; 350:578-85.
139. Malkowski P, Pawlak J, Michalowicz B et al. Thrombolytic treatment of portal thrombosis. *Hepatogastroenterology.* 2003; 50:2098-100.
140. Franco J. Pruritus. *Curr Treat Options Gastroenterol.* 1999; 2:451-6.
141. Caldwell SH, Hoffman M, Lisman T et al. Coagulation disorders and hemostasis in liver disease: pathophysiology and critical assessment of current management. *Hepatology.* 2006; 44:1039-46.
142. Lisman T, Leebeek FW. Hemostatic alterations in liver disease: a review on pathophysiology, clinical consequences, and treatment. *Dig Surg.* 2007; 24:250-8.
143. Thalheimer U, Triantos CK, Samonakis N et al. Infection, coagulation, and variceal bleeding in cirrhosis. *Gut.* 2005; 54:556-63.
144. MacLaren R, Wilson SJ, Campbell A et al. Evaluation and survey of intravenous vitamin K1 for treatment of coagulopathy in critically ill patients. *Pharmacotherapy.* 2001; 21:175-82.
145. Rahman T, Hodgson. Clinical management of acute hepatic failure. *Intensive Care Med.* 2001; 27:467-76.
146. Marrero J, Martinez FJ, Hyzy R. Advances in critical care hepatology. *Am J Respir Crit Care Med.* 2003; 168:1421-6.
147. Rinella ME, Sanyal A. Intensive management of hepatic failure. *Semin Respir Crit Care Med.* 2006; 27:241-61.
148. Stravitz RT, Kramer AH, Davern T et al. Intensive care of patients with acute liver failure: recommendations of the US acute liver failure study group. *Crit Care Med.* 2007; 35:2488-508.
149. Han MK, Hyzy R. Advances in critical management of hepatic failure and insufficiency. *Crit Care Med.* 2006; 34:S226-31.
150. Jalan R. Acute liver failure: current management and future prospects. *J Hepatol.* 2005; 42:S115-23.
151. Peck-Radosavljevic M. Thrombocytopenia in liver disease. *Can J Gastroenterol.* 2000; 14:60D-6D.
152. Bosch J, Thabut D, Albillos A et al. Recombinant factor VIIa for variceal bleeding in patients with advanced cirrhosis: a randomized, controlled trial. *Hepatology.* 2008; 47:1604-14.

153. Shami VM, Caldwell SH, Hespenheide EE et al. Recombinant factor VIIa for coagulopathy in fulminant hepatic failure compared with conventional therapy. *Liver Transpl.* 2003; 9:138-43.
154. O'Connell KA, Wood JJ, Wise PR et al. Thromboembolic adverse events after use of recombinant human coagulation factor VIIa. *JAMA.* 2006; 295:293-8.
155. Russell RM. The vitamin A spectrum: from deficiency to toxicity. *Am J Clin Nutr.* 2000; 71:878-84.
156. Runyon BA. Care of patients with ascites. *N Engl J Med.* 1994; 330:337-42.
157. Kuiper JJ, de Man RA, van Buuren HR. Review article: management of ascites and associated complications in patients with cirrhosis. *Aliment Pharmacol Ther.* 2007; 26(suppl 2):183-93.
158. Moore KP, Wong F, Gines P et al. The management of ascites in cirrhosis: report on the Consensus Conference of the International Ascites Club. *Hepatology.* 2003; 38:258-66.
159. Choudhury J, Sanyal AJ. Treatment of ascites. *Curr Treat Options Gastroenterol.* 2003; 6:481-91.
160. Sandhu BS, Sanyal AJ. Management of ascites in cirrhosis. *Clin Liver Dis.* 2005; 9:715-32.
161. Dib N, Oberti F, Cales P. Current management of the complications of portal hypertension. *CMAJ.* 2006; 174:1433-43.
162. Sanyal AJ, Bosch J, Blei A et al. Portal hypertension and its complications. *Gastroenterology.* 2008; 134:1715-28.
163. Blei AT. Portal hypertension and its complications. *Curr Opin Gastroenterol.* 2007; 23:275-82.
164. Hillebrand DJ. Spontaneous bacterial peritonitis. *Curr Treat Options Gastroenterol.* 2002; 5:479-89.
165. Koulaouzidis A, Bhat S, Karagiannidis A et al. Spontaneous bacterial peritonitis. *Postgrad Med J.* 2007; 83:379-83.
166. Sort P, Navasa M, Arroyo V et al. Effect of intravenous albumin in renal replacement impairment and mortality in patients with cirrhosis and spontaneous bacterial peritonitis. *N Engl J Med.* 1999; 341:403-9.
167. Mas A. Hepatic encephalopathy: from pathophysiology to treatment. *Digestion.* 2006; 73:86-93.
168. Morgan MY, Blei A, Grungreiff K et al. The treatment of hepatic encephalopathy. *Metab Brain Dis.* 2007; 22:389-405.
169. Bass NM. Review article: the current pharmacological therapies for hepatic encephalopathy. *Aliment Pharmacol Ther.* 2007; 25:23-31.
170. Festi D, Vestito A, Mazzella G et al. Management of hepatic encephalopathy: focus on antibiotic therapy. *Digestion.* 2006; 73:94-101.
171. Als-Nielsen B, Gluud LL, Gluud C. Nonadsorbable disaccharides for hepatic encephalopathy. *Cochrane Database Syst Rev.* 2004; 2:CD003044.
172. Als-Nielsen B, Koretz RL, Kjaergard LL et al. Branched-chain amino acids for hepatic encephalopathy. *Cochrane Database Syst Rev.* 2003; 2:CD001939.
173. Plauth M, Cabré E, Riggio O et al. ESPEN guidelines on enteral nutrition: liver disease. *Clin Nutr.* 2006; 25:285-94.
174. Schulz GJ, Campos AC, Coelho JC. The role of nutrition in hepatic encephalopathy. *Curr Opin Clin Nutr Metab Care.* 2008; 11:275-80.
175. Als-Nielsen B, Gluud LL, Gluud C. Benzodiazepine receptor antagonists for hepatic encephalopathy. *Cochrane Database Syst Rev.* 2004; 4:CD002798.
176. Detry O, De Roover A, Honore P et al. Brain edema and intracranial hypertension in fulminant hepatic failure: pathophysiology and management. *World J Gastroenterol.* 2006; 12:7405-12.
177. Blei A. Brain edema in acute liver failure. *Crit Care Clin.* 2008; 24:99-114.
178. Vaquero J, Fontana RJ, Larson AM et al. Complications and use of intracranial pressure monitoring in patients with acute liver failure and severe encephalopathy. *Liver Transpl.* 2005; 11:1581-9.
179. Himmelseher S. Hypertonic saline solutions for treatment of intracranial hypertension. *Curr Opin Anaesthesiol.* 2007; 20:414-26.
180. Strauss GI. The effect of hyperventilation upon cerebral blood flow and metabolism in patients with fulminant hepatic failure. *Dan Med Bull.* 2007; 54:99-111.
181. Jalan R, Rose C. Hypothermia in acute liver failure. *Metab Brain Dis.* 2004; 19:215-21.
182. Vaquero J, Blei AT. Mild hypothermia for acute liver failure. *J Clin Gastroenterol.* 2005; 39:S147-57.
183. Abraldes JG, Bosch J. The treatment of acute variceal bleeding. *J Clin Gastroenterol.* 2007; 41:S312-7.
184. Lata J, Hulek P, Vanasek T. Management of acute variceal bleeding. *Dig Dis.* 2003; 21:6-15.
185. Gotzsche PC, Hrobjartsson A. Somatostatin analogues for acute bleeding oesophageal varices. *Cochrane Database Syst Rev.* 2005; 1:CD000193.
186. Colombato L. The role of transjugular intrahepatic portosystemic shunt (TIPS) in the management of portal hypertension. *J Clin Gastroenterol.* 2007; 41:S344-51.
187. Kjaergard LL, Liu J, Als-Nielsen B et al. Artificial and bioartificial support systems for acute and acute-on-chronic liver failure: a systematic review. *JAMA.* 2003; 289:217-22.
188. Lee KH, Lee MK, Sutedja DS et al. Outcome from molecular adsorbent recirculating system (MARS) liver dialysis following drug-induced liver failure. *Liver Int.* 2005; 25:973-7.
189. Stadlbauer V, Davies N, Sen S et al. Artificial liver support systems in the management of complications of cirrhosis. *Semin Liver Dis.* 2008; 28:96-109.
190. Saliba F. The Molecular Adsorbent Recirculating System (MARS) in the intensive care unit: a rescue therapy for patients with hepatic failure. *Crit Care.* 2006; 10:118.
191. Karvellas CJ, Gibney N, Kutsogiannis D et al. Bench-to-bedside review: current evidence for extracorporeal albumin dialysis systems in liver failure. *Crit Care.* 2007; 11:215.
192. Wadei HM, Mai ML, Ahsan N et al. Hepatorenal syndrome: pathophysiology and management. *Clin J Am Soc Nephrol.* 2006; 1:1066-79.
193. van Ede AE, Laan RF, Rood MJ et al. Effect of folic or folinic acid supplementation on the toxicity and efficacy of methotrexate in rheumatoid arthritis: a forty-eight week, multicenter, randomized, double-blind, placebo-controlled study. *Arthritis Rheum.* 2001; 44:1515-24.
194. Fried MW, Navarro VJ, Afdhal N et al. Effect of silymarin (milk thistle) on liver disease in patients with chronic hepatitis C unsuccessfully treated with interferon therapy: a randomized controlled trial. *JAMA.* 2012; 308:274-82.
195. Lee WM. Acute liver failure in the United States. *Semin Liver Dis.* 2003; 23:217-26.
196. SAMSCA (tolvaptan) package insert. Rockville, MD: Otsuka America Pharmaceutical, Inc; February 2014. http://www.samsca.com/prescribing-information-samsca.pdf (accessed 2018 Feb 12).
197. Vaprisol (conivaptan hydrochloride) package insert. Deerfield, IL: Astellas Pharma US, Inc; October 2012. https://www.astellas.us/docs/vaprisol.pdf (accessed 2018 Feb 12).
198. Yun BC, Kim WR, Benson JT et al. Impact of pretransplant hyponatremia on outcome following liver transplantation. *Hepatology.* 2009; 49:1610-5.
199. King JD, Rosner MH. Osmotic demyelination syndrome. *Am J Med Sci.* 2010; 339:561-7.

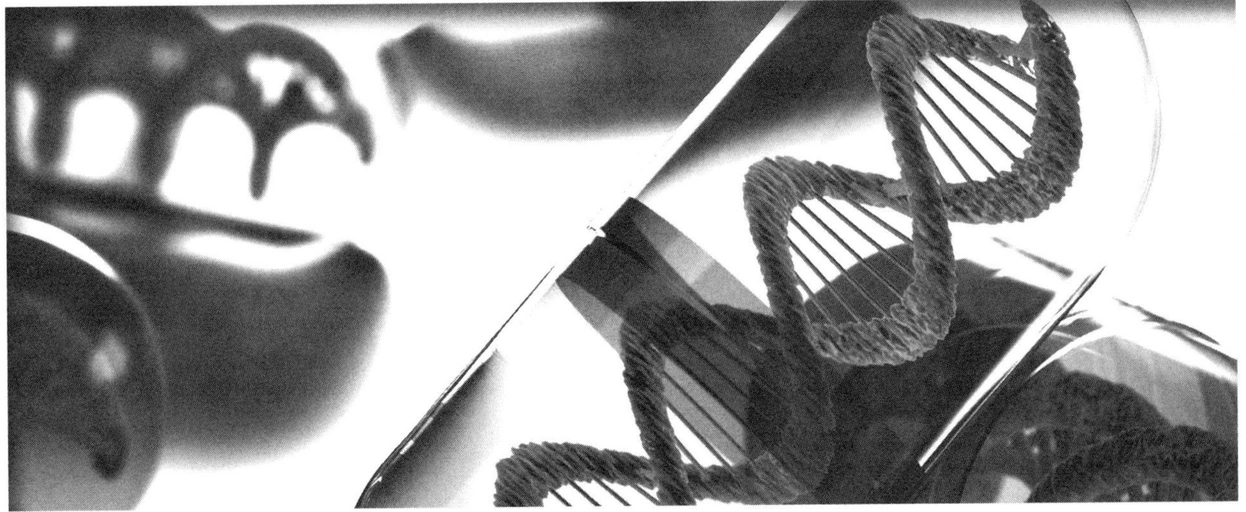

CHAPTER 39

Pancreatitis

Pramodini B. Kale-Pradhan and Sheila M. Wilhelm

Pancreatitis, an inflammatory process of the pancreas, may be described as either acute, in which the normal function of the pancreas returns, or chronic, in which the damage to pancreatic function is irreversible.[1] Although a number of drugs have been reported to cause pancreatitis, the cause-and-effect relationship is often difficult to verify. It is unclear how drugs cause pancreatitis, although several mechanisms have been hypothesized, including immune-mediated, direct pancreatic toxicity, pancreatic duct constriction, thrombosis, and metabolic effects.

CAUSATIVE AGENTS

Table 39-1 lists the agents implicated in drug-induced pancreatitis. Typically, drugs are associated with acute pancreatitis although there are some reports of drug-induced chronic pancreatitis as well. One review reported that 44 of the top 100 most frequently prescribed medications in the United States have been associated with acute pancreatitis.[2] Drug-induced pancreatitis has no features that allow it to be differentiated from other forms of the disorder.[3] Mallory and Kern classified drugs that may cause pancreatitis into three groups: those with a definite association, those with a probable association, and those with a questionable association.[4] Drugs are classified as having a definite association if the disease develops during treatment with the drug, disappears after the drug is withdrawn, and returns when the patient is rechallenged. Drugs are classified as having a probable association with pancreatitis if an association is thought to be likely and one or two of the definite association criteria are met. Drugs are classified as having a questionable association if the supporting evidence is inadequate or contradictory. In addition to the Mallory and Kern system, two additional classification systems have been proposed and are also frequently cited in the literature. Trivedi and Pitchumoni proposed a system that modified the three-group classification system giving more weight to the number of cases reported and positive rechallenge.[2] Badalov's system categorizes drug-induced pancreatitis using five classes.[5] Class Ia includes drugs with at least one case report, evidence of a positive rechallenge, and exclusion of other causes of acute pancreatitis. Class Ib is similar to class Ia, but in this class, other causes of acute pancreatitis could not be ruled out.

Table 39-1 Agents Implicated in Drug-Induced Pancreatitis[1-7,11,23,38,43,67,68,170,544]

Drug	Incidence	Level of Evidence[a]
DEFINITE ASSOCIATION		
5-ASA[112,198,199,201,202,204-217,496]	NK	B
ACE inhibitors (benazepril, enalapril, lisinopril, captopril, quinapril, ramipril)[16,44-54,57,58,61-65,67,510,511,538,545,546]	0.3–1.07%	B
Amiodarone[483-486]	0.01–0.02%	B
Asparaginase[131-135,138-140,142-147,149-152,155-159,161-163,165-169,503]	2–18%	B
Azathioprine[10,12,16,103-107,109-111,113,116,117,120-123]	4.5–5.3%	B
Bortezomib[409-412]	NK	C
Carbamazepine[379-382]	NK	C
Cisplatin[225-227]	NK	C
Codeine[547,548]	NK	C
Corticosteroids[2,11,244,245,519,549-560]	NK	C
Cytarabine[218,221,223,224]	NK	C
Didanosine[20,21,25-28,30-37,39-41,561,562]	1.5–9%	C
Estrogen[303-309,311,312]	NK	C
Furosemide[313-320]	NK	C
Interferon α[418-426]	NK	B
Isoniazid[287-298]	NK	C
6-mercaptopurine[102,114,115,119,120]	3.3%	C
Methyldopa[299-302]	NK	C
Metronidazole[77-86]	NK	C
Pentamidine[268-283,494]	NK	C
Pentavalent antimonials (sodium stibogluconate, meglumine antimoniate)[563-572]	NK	C
Sorafenib[400-404,407,408]	NK	C
Statins (atorvastatin, fluvastatin, lovastatin pravastatin, simvastatin)[87-98,573,574]	NK	B
Sulfonamide (sulfamethoxazole)[203,247-249]	NK	C
Sulindac[178-183,186,187,497]	NK	C
Tetracycline[251-256,261]	NK	B
Thiazides (chlorthalidone, chlorothiazide, hydrocholorthiazide)[323,324,326,327,330,332-335]	NK	C
Tigecycline[263-267,575]	NK	B
Valproic acid[338-342,344-358,360-376]	0.0025%	B
PROBABLE ASSOCIATION		
Acetaminophen[188-197]	4% (overdose)	B
Ampicillin[284,325]	NK	C
Angiotensin receptor blockers (losartan, irbesartan)[55,56,576,577]	NK	C
Bezafibrate[578]	NK	C
Brentuximab vedotin[413-415]	NK	C
Bumetanide[321]	NK	C
Calcium[173-175,177,530,532,534]	7–11%	C
Cimetidine[69-74]	NK	C
Clozapine[383-391]	NK	C

Table 39-1 Agents Implicated in Drug-Induced Pancreatitis[1-7,11,23,38,43,67,68,170,544] (continued)

Drug	Incidence	Level of Evidence[a]
Dipeptidyl peptidase 4 (DPP-4) inhibitors (sitagliptin, saxagliptin, linagliptin, alogliptin, vildagliptin)[430,440,443-448,450,453,455-459,461,466-468,470,471,473-475,478-480]	NK	B
Doxycycline[259-261]	NK	B
Erythromycin[579-581]	NK	C
Ethacrynic acid[322]	NK	C
Glucagon-like peptide 1 (GLP-1) receptor agonists (exenatide, liraglutide, albiglutide, dulaglutide)[430-442,449,453,455-458,460,462-469,471-473,476,481]	NK	B
Ifosfamide[219,582,583]	NK	C
Itraconazole[584]	NK	C
Lamivudine[562,585]	<0.5%	C
Minocycline[257,258,261]	NK	B
Olanzapine[586-589]	NK	C
Omeprazole[74,75]	NK	C
Orlistat[443,590-592]	NK	C
Piroxicam[178,513]	NK	C
Procainamide[593]	NK	C
Ribavirin[37,424,426,429]	NK	C
Stavudine[562,594,595]	NK	C
Vinblastine[231]	NK	C
Vincristine[231]	NK	C
Zalcitabine[562,596]	<1%	C

[a]Definitions for Levels of Evidence: Level A—evidence from one or more randomized, controlled clinical trials; Level B—evidence from nonrandomized clinical trials, prospective observational studies, cohort studies, retrospective studies, case-control studies, meta-analyses and/or postmarketing surveillance studies; and Level C—evidence from one or more published case reports or case series.

Criteria for Class II drugs include at least four case reports with a consistent latency period for at least 75% of the cases. Class III drugs have at least two case reports but do not have rechallenge data or a consistent latency period. Finally, Class IV drugs have one case report without rechallenge data.

EPIDEMIOLOGY

Drugs are found responsible for pancreatitis in approximately 0.1–5.3% of patients who are diagnosed with the disease.[6-12] Drugs are the cause in 13–30% of pancreatitis cases in children.[13-15] Pediatric patients with drug-induced pancreatitis have longer hospital stays and are more likely to require parenteral nutrition than those where the etiology is not drug-related.[15] The incidence of acute drug-induced pancreatitis is higher in patients with disease states that predispose to the development of pancreatitis, including infection with the human immunodeficiency virus (HIV), acquired immune deficiency syndrome (AIDS), renal transplantation (immunocompromised patients), and inflammatory bowel disease (autoimmune diseases).[9,11] Other subgroups with higher incidences include the very young or very old and females.[10-12]

A case-control study was conducted at a network of 51 hospitals in Berlin from 2002 to 2011.[16] During this time, 64 of 102 cases of acute pancreatitis were determined to be possibly related to drugs, including fenofibrate, formoterol and budesonide, ramipril and hydrochlorothiazide, lisinopril, and azathioprine.

There is a much higher incidence of drug-induced pancreatitis in patients who are HIV positive and treated with didanosine.[17-22] In contrast, the incidence of didanosine-induced pancreatitis is substantially lower in patients without HIV.[23-25] Pancreatitis develops 10–20 weeks after initiation of didanosine with an incidence of up to 9%.[20,21,23,25-41]

Angiotensin-converting enzyme (ACE) inhibitors were implicated as the cause of pancreatitis in 209 of 2,749 reports of drug-induced pancreatitis that the World Health Organization (WHO) received from 1968 to 1993.[42] More recently, over 300 cases of drug-induced pancreatitis were associated with enalapril or captopril.[43] The estimated incidence of ACE inhibitor-associated pancreatitis ranges from 0.3% to 1.07%.[44] A retrospective cohort study of 174,824 elderly patients prescribed ACE inhibitors reported an incidence of nine per 10,000 person-years, which was not significantly different from control groups.[45] Several cases of ACE inhibitor and angiotensin II receptor antagonist-induced pancreatitis have been reported.[46-62] Pancreatitis may develop several months after initiation of ACE inhibitor therapy and may recur with rechallenge with a latency period ranging from 4 to 26 months.[63-65] Acute necrotizing pancreatitis developed in a patient receiving sulindac and hydrochlorothiazide for more than 6 years and lisinopril for 1 year and progressed to chronic pancreatitis possibly due to repeated subclinical drug-induced acute pancreatitis and a third insult involving lisinopril.[66] ACE inhibitors are associated with an increased risk of acute pancreatitis, particularly in the first 6 months of therapy, and the risk increases as the daily dose increases.[67]

From 1968 to 1993, the WHO received 127 case reports of pancreatitis associated with histamine H_2 receptor antagonists.[68] The association between cimetidine and pancreatitis is probable, and there are numerous published reports.[69-74] There is a small number of case reports of pancreatitis associated with the use of proton pump inhibitors. At least one case report of omeprazole-induced pancreatitis has been published.[75,76] However, a retrospective case-control study of more than 180,000 subjects did not find an increased risk.[74]

There are at least eight well-documented cases of metronidazole-induced pancreatitis.[77-84] In these cases, the onset of symptoms ranged from 12 hours to 7 days after initiation of therapy and resolved after discontinuation of the drug. Several patients experienced recurrence with rechallenge of metronidazole.[77-79,83-85] In addition, a population-based case-control study reported a threefold increased risk of acute pancreatitis in patients treated with metronidazole.[86]

There are numerous reports of 3-hydroxy-3-methyl-glutaryl-CoA (Hmg-CoA) reductase inhibitor- or statin-induced pancreatitis in the literature.[87-98] Meta-analyses demonstrate conflicting results.[88,99] The risk for pancreatitis does not appear to be dose-related.[100] In several case reports, patients receiving statins experienced other adverse effects including myalgia or rhabdomyolysis before the onset of acute pancreatitis.[101] Drug interactions mediated through CYP3A4 have been hypothesized to contribute to the development of statin-induced pancreatitis; therefore, statins not metabolized by CYP3A4, such as pravastatin, may present a lower risk for drug-induced acute pancreatitis than other statins. Pancreatitis can occur at any time but may be more likely after many months of treatment with statins.[101]

Azathioprine and 6-mercaptopurine are potent immunosuppressive agents associated with pancreatitis with an incidence of 3.3–5.3%.[102-120] Several epidemiological studies have identified azathioprine as one of the most frequent causes of drug-induced acute pancreatitis.[10,12,16] The median time to onset of pancreatitis after initiation of therapy was 21 days with females at higher risk.[120-123] Case series have documented successful treatment with 6-mercaptopurine after azathioprine had been discontinued as a result of acute pancreatitis.[124,125] A meta-analysis determined that approximately one-third of patients are able to tolerate mercaptopurine following an episode of azathioprine-induced pancreatitis.[126] A small, prospective, open-label study of patients resistant and intolerant to azathioprine and mercaptopurine concluded that thioguanine may be an alternative treatment as patients who had experienced an episode of pancreatitis with azathioprine or 6-mercaptopurine did not develop pancreatitis while receiving thioguanine.[127] Genomic studies have attempted to identify genetic variants useful in predicting patients at risk for thiopurine-induced pancreatitis. One genome-wide study reported an association within the class II HLA region with almost twice the risk for homozygotes compared to heterozygotes.[128] No association was found between pancreatitis and thiopurine methyltransferase polymorphisms.[128,129] A variant allele that codes for the enzyme xanthine dehydrogenase was potentially associated with an increased risk of pancreatitis compared to the standard genotype.[130]

L-asparaginase induces pancreatitis in 2–18% of patients.[131-134] There are numerous case reports of L-asparaginase-induced pancreatitis with and without fatalities.[135-151] Two other preparations have largely replaced L-asparaginase: erwinia carotovora-derived L-asparaginase (erwinia L-asparaginase) and polyethylene glycol-L-asparaginase (PEG-asparaginase, Oncaspar). The available literature is inconsistent and has not established a clear difference in incidence of pancreatitis among the three preparations. Some early studies suggested that erwinia L-asparaginase was associated with a lower incidence of pancreatitis when compared to L-asparaginase, although other studies found no difference.[151-157] The incidence of pancreatitis associated with PEG-asparaginase is similar to that of L-asparaginase, but a few studies suggested that the rate of pancreatitis may be higher with PEG-asparaginase.[156,158-165] The variation in rates across studies may be due to differences in criteria used to define and classify acute pancreatitis, variation in number of doses, or differences in chemotherapy regimens.[134,151,156] However, these factors have not been found to be predictive of the risk of asparaginase-induced pancreatitis.[134,151,156,163,165-167] Pancreatitis induced by preparations of asparaginase usually occurs during administration of the drug, often after just one or a few doses.[133,138,149,166-169] Pancreatitis may occur during any phase of chemotherapy, and cases of pancreatitis have been reported as long as 16 weeks after therapy has been discontinued.[4,131,134,156,166] Fatalities have been rarely reported as a result of asparaginase-associated pancreatitis in recent studies, which may reflect improved supportive care measures.[134,167] Rates of recurrence with rechallenge have ranged from 0% to 63%.[134,156,157,167]

Pancreatitis secondary to hypercalcemia occurs in up to 7% of patients.[170,171] Pancreatitis has been associated with intravenous calcium administration, total parenteral nutrition, and over-the-counter antacids containing calcium carbonate.[172-176] Hypercalcemia-related pancreatitis is more common in patients who have undergone renal transplantation, with an approximate incidence of 11%.[177]

The incidence of pancreatitis induced by nonsteroidal anti-inflammatory drugs (NSAIDs) appears low. In a population-based study of over 100,000 users of piroxicam, naproxen, or diclofenac, only one case of pancreatitis occurred (in a patient receiving piroxicam).[178] In contrast, there are numerous reports of sulindac-induced pancreatitis, including reports of recurrence after rechallenge.[179-186] Reports suggest pancreatitis develops within 2 weeks to 9 months following initiation of sulindac therapy; however, a latency period of up to 5 years also has been reported.[66,186,187]

Rare, acute pancreatitis has been reported with acetaminophen overdose.[188-196] In a retrospective review of 814 acetaminophen overdoses, hyperamylasemia was frequent, but acute pancreatitis rarely occurred.[197] A poor prognosis was associated with higher serum amylase concentrations.

Salicylate-induced pancreatitis has been reported, particularly in association with poisoning or aspirin desensitization.[198-200] Pancreatitis has been reported in association with the salicylate derivatives sulfapyridine and sulfasalazine.[201-215] In a retrospective analysis of serious adverse events, pancreatitis was reported seven times more frequently with mesalamine than sulfasalazine.[216] In a retrospective study, inflammatory bowel disease patients who received mesalamine and sulfasalazine did not show an increased risk of pancreatitis.[217]

Cisplatin, cytarabine, ifosfamide, paclitaxel, docetaxel, oxaliplatin, capecitabine, and the vinca alkaloids have been associated with pancreatitis, but the incidence is unknown.[218-242] Many cases of drug-induced pancreatitis have been reported during concurrent cytarabine and L-asparaginase administration. In one study, pancreatitis developed within 10 days of cytarabine and recurred with a rechallenge.[224] The lack of data from case-control studies or population-based studies makes it difficult to estimate the incidence of pancreatitis associated with these chemotherapeutic agents.[11]

In the 1950s, corticosteroids became the first drugs to be implicated in drug-induced pancreatitis. Steroids and adrenocorticotropic hormone (ACTH) accounted for 45.5% of the cases of reported drug-induced pancreatitis in the literature as of 1977.[171] Recurrences of pancreatitis have been reported following patients' re-exposure to steroids, including cases in which patients received intra-articular corticosteroid injections.[243,244] A population-based case-control study demonstrated an increased risk of acute pancreatitis in patients receiving oral glucocorticoids and suggested the risk is highest 4–14 days after the drug is dispensed.[245]

In 1963, the first case of sulfonamide-induced pancreatitis was reported.[246] More recently, there have been three reported cases of pancreatitis secondary to trimethoprim–sulfamethoxazole in which the disease developed within 5 days to 10 weeks after the initiation of therapy.[23,203,247-249]

Tetracycline-induced pancreatitis has been reported in patients with and without underlying liver disease.[250-256] Two reports of minocycline-induced pancreatitis and two reports of doxycycline-induced pancreatitis have been published.[257-260] A population-based case-control study identified a 60% increased risk of acute pancreatitis among current users of tetracycline antibiotics with doxycycline being the most commonly prescribed.[261] Tigecycline, an agent related to the tetracyclines, has been implicated in drug-induced pancreatitis in four case reports with the onset ranging from 7 to 14 days.[262-266] A retrospective cohort study of the U.S. Food and Drug Administration (FDA) Adverse Event Reporting System (FAERS) identified 62 cases of tigecycline-associated pancreatitis with females being at higher risk.[267]

A number of cases—the majority in the HIV/AIDS population—of aerosolized and injectable pentamidine-induced pancreatitis have been documented, including a report of recurrence after rechallenge.[23,268-283] Pancreatitis secondary to pentamidine typically occurs in the second week of treatment and resolves within 10 days after discontinuation, although there have been some reports of persistent pancreatitis following discontinuation. This may be explained by the lipophilic properties of pentamidine and/or a cumulative dose effect on the pancreas.[274,276] In a report of five cases of pentamidine-induced pancreatitis, all patients experienced episodes of hypo- or hyperglycemia, and four of the five also developed sepsis.[276] Glucose abnormalities, renal insufficiency, nonspecific abdominal pain, and nausea/vomiting after initiation of pentamidine may be early warning signs of pancreatitis.[268]

At least one case report supports a probable association between pancreatitis and ampicillin.[284] The patient developed pancreatitis 6 days after initiation of therapy, recovered 5 days after discontinuation, and relapsed 4 days after ampicillin therapy was reinstituted.

One case report of ciprofloxacin, potentially involving recurrent episodes 18 months apart, has been published.[285] In a single-center study, 3.1% of patients developed acute pancreatitis within an average of 5.5 days of receiving ciprofloxacin.[286]

Isoniazid-induced pancreatitis has been reported in 12 cases, eight of which were confirmed by rechallenge.[287-298] Isoniazid-associated acute pancreatitis typically has a median onset of 16 days after starting therapy and consistently recurs earlier, with a median onset of 9.4 days after rechallenge.[288]

The incidence of methyldopa-induced pancreatitis is unknown. Symptoms of methyldopa-induced pancreatitis generally occur within 1 week after initiation of therapy.[299-302] Patients typically recover without sequelae; however, a patient in one report developed chronic pancreatitis.[5,302]

There are numerous reports of estrogen-induced pancreatitis (with and without concomitant progesterone therapy).[303-309] Estrogen-induced pancreatitis begins 2–78 weeks after the initiation of therapy, and symptoms usually resolve approximately 10 days after discontinuation of estrogen.[23] Additionally, there is at least one case report of clomiphene (an estrogen agonist/antagonist) -induced pancreatitis in the literature.[310] Despite the case reports of estrogen-induced pancreatitis, a population-based case-control study did not find an association between pancreatitis and postmenopausal hormone therapy.[311] However, a retrospective study of 70 women found that estrogen use was associated with increased risk of pancreatitis.[312]

Several cases of furosemide-induced pancreatitis have been reported.[313-320] Doses ranged from 40 mg to 1,000 mg daily, and symptoms typically occurred within 2–5 weeks after initiation of therapy.[23] Additionally, other loop diuretics (bumetanide and ethacrynic acid) have been associated with pancreatitis.[317,321,322]

Chlorothiazide, hydrochlorothiazide, and chlorothalidone have all been reported to cause pancreatitis, which has developed from 2 weeks up to 1 year or more after initiation of therapy.[323-337]

Acute pancreatitis associated with valproic acid was first recognized in 1979, and since then there have been many case reports involving both adults and children.[338-374] The estimated incidence is one in 40,000.[375] The onset of pancreatitis with valproic acid may occur as early as 1 week or as long as several years after therapy has been initiated, although it most commonly occurs during the first year of therapy.[359] In a retrospective case-controlled trial, the risk of pancreatitis with valproic acid was similar to the risk with other antiepileptic agents.[376] Valproic acid-induced pancreatitis is more common in patients requiring higher doses, those receiving polytherapy, and those with chronic encephalopathies or on hemodialysis.[373] Fatalities secondary to valproic acid-induced pancreatitis in children have been reported.[377]

There are at least five case reports of drug-induced pancreatitis associated with carbamazepine.[378-382] In one of the reports, an initial episode of pancreatitis occurred 6 weeks after initiating therapy with carbamazepine, resolved when carbamazepine was discontinued, and recurred within 48 hours of a rechallenge.[379]

There are at least seven case reports of drug-induced pancreatitis with clozapine.[383-389] In two of these reports, pancreatitis resolved when the drug was withdrawn and recurred when therapy was reinitiated.[385,388] Other reports describe a syndrome of "asymptomatic pancreatitis" (characterized by hyperamylasemia) and eosinophilia induced by clozapine (although asymptomatic hyperamylasemia is usually not considered diagnostic for pancreatitis).[390,391]

There are at least eight reports of acute pancreatitis associated with tamoxifen.[392-399] Five reports noted that patients had a history of dyslipidemia.[393-395,397,398] Because hypertriglyceridemia is associated with pancreatitis, tamoxifen's effect on triglycerides may contribute to pancreatitis risk. In one report, a patient who experienced pancreatitis while receiving tamoxifen alone was restarted on tamoxifen with a concomitant fibrate and did not experience recurrence during 3 years of follow-up.[395] The development of pancreatitis is delayed and variable ranging from 4 to 24 months.

Reports have associated tyrosine kinase inhibitors, sorafenib, axitinib, sunitinib, and nilotinib with drug-induced pancreatitis.[400-408] One report describes a patient who experienced acute pancreatitis 10 days after initiating sorafenib therapy.[400] After the drug was discontinued and the patient recovered from the acute episode, therapy with sunitinib was initiated. The patient remained on sunitinib without recurrence of pancreatitis for 20 months before being lost to follow-up.[400]

There are at least four case reports of patients experiencing drug-induced pancreatitis within 2–7 days after receiving bortezomib.[409-412] In two of these cases, rechallenge resulted in recurrence within hours.[411,412]

Pancreatitis has been reported to develop 2 weeks after administration of vermurafenib with recurrence following rechallenge.[413] In an open-label, multicenter study of 3,222 patients, three patients developed pancreatitis judged to be caused by vemurafenib.[414] In 2015, Health Canada approved updated labeling for vemurafenib to include a warning regarding the risk of pancreatitis.[415] The agency further reported that the cases generally occurred in the first 2 weeks of treatment.

There are at least nine reports of pancreatitis associated with brentuximab vedotin in the literature.[416,417] Two fatalities were reported as a result of progressive multiorgan dysfunction as a consequence of pancreatitis.[417] The median time to onset of pancreatitis was 26 days from initiation of therapy and 12 days from the most recent dose, with all cases occurring by the third cycle of therapy. One of three patients rechallenged with brentuximab vedotin experienced a recurrent episode of pancreatitis.[416,417] In one case, an additional six cycles of therapy were administered without recurrence.[416]

Case reports have associated pancreatitis with interferon alfa, both the standard and pegylated preparations, when used as monotherapy and in combination with ribavirin.[418-425] Two of these case reports describe recurrence of pancreatitis after rechallenge with interferon alfa-2b.[419] A retrospective review of 1,706 chronic hepatitis C-infected patients treated with interferon-alfa and ribavirin found that acute pancreatitis occurred in seven patients after a median duration of therapy of 12 weeks.[426] Pancreatitis resolved rapidly in all seven patients, and none had recurrent pancreatitis during a median follow-up of 18 months. The package inserts for pegylated interferon alfa-2a, pegylated interferon alfa-2b, and ribavirin contain warnings about the risk of pancreatitis and advise withholding or discontinuing therapy in cases of suspected pancreatitis.[427-429] The package inserts for both pegylated interferon formulations note that pancreatitis, including fatal cases, has been observed.[427,428]

Although there are numerous reports of drug-induced pancreatitis associated with the incretin-based therapies including the glucagon-like peptide 1 (GLP-1) receptor agonists and the dipeptidyl peptidase 4 (DPP-4) inhibitors used to treat type 2 diabetes mellitus, the association is controversial due to conflicting published information and because patients with type 2 diabetes mellitus have up to a threefold higher risk of developing acute pancreatitis compared to nondiabetic contols.[430]

There are at least 19 case reports in the literature of pancreatitis associated with incretin-based therapies.[431-448] In 2007 and 2008, the FDA issued alerts concerning postmarketing reports of 30 cases of acute pancreatitis and six cases of hemorrhagic or necrotizing pancreatitis in patients taking exenatide.[449] In 2009, the FDA issued an alert regarding 88 cases of acute pancreatitis including two cases of hemorrhagic or necrotizing pancreatitis in patients taking sitagliptin. As a result, the FDA encouraged manufacturers to warn about the risk of pancreatitis.[450-452]

In one analysis of reports in the FAERS, pancreatitis was found to occur greater than six times more frequently in patients receiving exenatide (OR 10.68, 95% CI 7.75–15.1, $p < 10^{-16}$) or sitagliptin (OR 6.74, 95% CI 4.61–10.0, $p < 10^{-16}$) than those receiving other antidiabetic therapies.[453] The Institute for Safe Medication Practices conducted another analysis of the FAERS data and also reported an increased risk with incretin-based therapies compared to other antidiabetic agents used to treat type 2 diabetes.[454] An analysis of the Italian Spontaneous ADR (adverse drug reaction) database likewise noted a higher incidence of pancreatitis associated with incretin-based therapies compared to other hypoglycemic agents (excluding insulin).[455] Conversely, at least 12 observational studies of data extracted from large insurance claims databases and national registries conducted to date failed to identify an increased risk of pancreatitis associated with the use of incretin-based therapies, and multiple meta-analyses have assessed the available literature and not identified an increased risk of pancreatitis associated with incretin-based therapies compared to control populations receiving placebo or other antidiabetic therapies.[430,456-476]

A population-based matched case-control study using a large administrative database in the United States found that the risk of hospitalization for acute pancreatitis was increased with current or recent past exposure to exenatide or sitagliptin.[477] Three large randomized controlled studies evaluated pancreatitis as a safety outcome in more than 18,000 patients exposed to the DPP-4 inhibitors saxagliptin, alopgliptin, and sitagliptin.[478-480] These studies showed that cases of acute pancreatitis were rare; however, they generally occurred more often in the exposed groups, but the differences were not significant. In a 56-week trial of 3,731 patients without type 2 diabetes, 0.4 pancreatitis events per 100 patient/years at risk was reported in the liraglutide group and <0.1 pancreatitis events per 100 patient/years at risk was reported in the placebo group.[481] There is the potential for confounding factors, including the presence of gallstones in 55% of the cases.

In 2014, FDA and the European Medicines Agency released a joint report that causal association between incretin-based drugs and pancreatitis is inconsistent with the current data; however, a final conclusion had not been reached.[482] Notwithstanding this joint report, pancreatitis will continue to be considered a risk associated with these drugs and that risk is reflected in the current product information and labeling. All incretin-based therapies currently on the market contain warnings pertaining to pancreatitis, recommend immediate discontinuation of treatment when pancreatitis is suspected, and cautious use (or use of alternative therapy) in patients with a history of pancreatitis.[451,452]

There are isolated reports of amiodarone-induced pancreatitis.[483-485] A recent nested case-control study using a large database of U.S. health insurance claims found an association between amiodarone (but not other antiarrhythmic agents) and increased risk of acute pancreatitis in patients treated for nonvalvular atrial fibrillation.[486] The greatest risk was detected in the first 12 months after therapy was initiated.

There are at least four case reports of pancreatitis induced by the thioamide drugs methimazole and carbimazole, a prodrug of methimazole available outside of the United States.[487-490] All cases reported onset of symptoms within the first month of therapy. Rechallenge was attempted in three cases and recurrence of symptoms with an onset within 24 hours was noted each time.[487,489,490] In two of the four reports, the patients presented with concomitant mild cholestatic hepatitis, and in one of the cases the patient was further diagnosed with erythema nodosum.[488,489]

MECHANISMS

Drugs may induce pancreatitis through several possible mechanisms, including pancreatic duct hypertension secondary to intraluminal or extraluminal duct blockage and increased viscosity of pancreatic fluid leading to peripheral duct rupture and proenzyme release.[3] In addition, animal data have shown that reduced exocytosis and premature fusion of zymogen granules to lysosomes in pancreatic exocrine cells may activate pancreatic proenzymes and lead to cellular autodigestion. Drugs could play a role in this process. Predisposition to infection through immunosuppression may also be involved in pancreatitis caused by drugs such as corticosteroids and other immunosuppressants.[3] **Table 39-2** lists additional mechanisms that have been proposed for drugs known to be associated with pancreatitis.

ANTIMICROBIAL AGENTS

Metronidazole-induced pancreatitis may occur as a result of a redox cycling reaction that occurs under aerobic conditions and yields hydrogen peroxide and other oxygen-free radicals.[81,83,84,491,492] These redox active compounds are toxic to pancreatic β-cells and cause pancreatitis in animal models. Other suggested mechanisms for metronidazole-induced pancreatitis include an immune-mediated inflammatory response, pancreatic duct constriction, and metabolic effects.[81,83] The mechanism of tetracycline-induced pancreatitis is not completely understood; however, it may be related to a toxic metabolite of tetracycline, tetracycline-induced hypertriglyceridemia, or a high biliary concentration.[261,264,265,493] The precise mechanism of pentamidine-induced pancreatitis is not known, but animal studies suggest a direct toxic effect on the pancreas.[494] Pentamidine is known to cause both hypoglycemia and hyperglycemia, which is possibly due to damaged pancreatic β-cells.[23]

ESTROGEN

A possible mechanism of estrogen-induced pancreatitis is hyperlipidemia, a well-known cause of pancreatitis. Glueck et al. reported that 12 of 31 women with hypertriglyceridemia were receiving estrogen replacement therapy, and four of these 12 developed pancreatitis.[303] However, patients without elevated serum lipid concentrations receiving estrogens have also developed pancreatitis, suggesting that hypertriglyceridemia may not be the only factor in estrogen-induced pancreatitis.[304] Another proposed mechanism involves pancreatic necrosis induced by a hypercoagulable state.[101]

Table 39-2 Mechanisms of Drug-Induced Pancreatitis

Drug	Mechanism(s)
ACE inhibitors (captopril, enalapril lisinopril)	Bradykinin-induced inflammation; autoantibodies
5-acetylsalicylic acid	Immune-mediated reaction
Asparginase	Inhibition of protein synthesis through the hydrolysis of the amino acid L-asparagine
Azathioprine/6-mercaptopurine (MP)	Allergic reaction (type II or type IV to 6MP) and/or direct toxic effect
Brentuximab vedotin	Potentially unintended targeting of low-level pancreatic CD30
Codeine	Unknown (potentially constriction of the sphincter of Oddi)
Didanosine	Hypersensitivity or mitochondrial toxicity
Erythromycin	May cause spasm of the sphincter of Oddi, leading to abrupt pancreatic-duct hypertension and pancreatitis
Estrogen	Unknown (potentially hyperlipidemia or pancreatic necrosis induced by a hypercoagulable state)
Furosemide	Direct toxic effect, diuretic-induced pancreatic stimulation, hypersensitivity from an immunologic response against a drug-protein adduct, and/or ischemia related to impaired pancreatic blood flow due to volume contraction
Hydrochlorothiazide	Increased serum calcium leads to calculi in the pancreatic ducts; direct toxic effect secondary to increased parathyroid hormone levels or increased calcium levels may accelerate the conversion of trypsinogen to trypsin causing pancreatitis; and/or thiazides lead to hypotension and pancreatic ischemia
Interferon α	Unknown (potentially immune system stimulation leading to autoimmune destruction of the pancreas)
Isoniazid	Unknown (potentially hypersensitivity)
Methyldopa	Unknown
Metronidazole	Undergoes redox cycling reaction yielding hydrogen peroxide and other oxygen-free radicals—toxic to pancreas Other suggested mechanisms: immune-mediated inflammatory response, pancreatic duct constriction, metabolic effects
Pentamidine	Direct toxic effect on the pancreas
Statins (atorvastatin, fluvastatin, lovastatin, pravastatin, simvastatin)	Immune-mediated inflammatory response, metabolic effect, or direct cellular toxicity Other suspected mechanisms: associated with rhabdomyolysis, myalgia, and/or metabolism or drug interactions through cytochrome P-450 3A4
Sulfonamide (sulfamethoxazole)	Hypersensitivity
Sulindac	Hypersensitivity
Tamoxifen	Increased triglycerides, cytotoxic injury
Tetracycline	Unknown (potentially toxic metabolite, hypertriglyceridemia, high biliary concentration)
Tyrosine kinase inhibitors	Effects on vascular endothelial growth factor; decreased gastrointestinal motility
Valproic acid	Hypersensitivity
Vemurafenib	Possibly induces proliferation of cells leading to obstructive pancreatitis

THIAZIDE DIURETICS

Thiazides may have a direct toxic effect on the pancreas.[324] Additionally, thiazides are known to cause hypercalcemia and hypophosphatemia, conditions present in patients with primary hyperparathyroidism, which is a disease known to increase the risk of pancreatitis.[323] Increased serum concentrations of parathyroid hormone may be present in patients treated with thiazide diuretics and can result in pancreatitis.[324,325] Additionally, elevated serum calcium concentrations may lead to calculi within the pancreatic ducts and/or may accelerate the conversion of trypsinogen to trypsin, causing pancreatitis.[495] It has also been suggested that thiazides may cause pancreatitis as a result of thiazide-induced hyperlipidemia[325] or that thiazide-induced reductions in blood pressure may lead to pancreatic ischemia.[1]

ANTI-INFLAMMATORY AGENTS

Sulfasalazine-induced pancreatitis may occur due to an immune-mediated or allergic reaction.[496,497]

VALPROIC ACID

Pancreatitis associated with valproic acid may be related to a hypersensitivity reaction and recurs after rechallenge with the drug.[338-342] It has been theorized that valproic acid may cause depletion of the free-radical scavengers superoxide dismutase (SOD), catalase (CAT), and glutathione peroxidase, resulting in an excess of free radicals that may promote endothelial permeability and lipid peroxidation, ultimately leading to tissue damage.[498-500]

L-ASPARAGINASE

L-asparaginase–induced pancreatitis may occur as a result of inhibition of protein synthesis through hydrolysis of the amino acid L-asparagine.[166,501-503] Organs with high protein synthesis rates, such as the liver and pancreas, are more severely affected. The presence of glutaminase or an endotoxin cannot be excluded as a mechanism because L-asparaginase is extracted from *Escherichia coli*.[504,505] Genetic predispositions are likely to play a role.

ACE INHIBITORS

ACE inhibitors increase serum bradykinin concentrations, and bradykinin acts as a mediator of inflammation that may lead to localized angioedema and obstruction of pancreatic ducts.[101,506] Bradykinin has also been found to increase vascular permeability in early-stage pancreatitis induced by cerulein.[507] Bradykinin antagonists such as HOE-140 have been shown to have a protective role in pancreatitis.[508] Drugs may cause local pancreatic angioedema, obstructing the pancreatic duct and causing enzymes and other toxic substances to be trapped within the pancreas. This leads to tissue damage and is a likely cause of acute pancreatitis that occurs rapidly after drug initiation.[101,509] Other possible mechanisms are ACE inhibitor-induced hypoglycemia resulting in toxic effects on the pancreas and the effects of combined toxins, including ACE inhibitors and alcohol.[46,510,511]

Animal studies suggest that ACE inhibitors may increase pancreatic secretion as a possible or contributing mechanism.[47] Another theory is that ACE inhibitors induce the formation of autoantibodies, which then attack pancreatic cells.[46] Both captopril and enalapril have been found to induce the production of autoantibodies in many tissues, including the pancreas.[512]

CLOZAPINE

The mechanism by which clozapine induces acute pancreatitis is unknown. Clozapine may have exocrine and possibly toxic effects on the pancreatic and salivary tissues, or clozapine-induced pancreatitis may occur as a result of an allergic reaction.[384,385]

HISTAMINE-2 (H_2) RECEPTOR ANTAGONISTS

This class of drugs may affect pancreatic secretory stimuli through reduction of gastric and duodenal acidity and/or may cause pancreatitis through an idiosyncratic reaction.[3,68]

NSAIDs AND ACETYLSALICYLIC ACID

The probable mechanism of acetylsalicylic acid (ASA)- or NSAID-related pancreatitis is inhibition of prostaglandins that may cause pancreatic duct constriction.[3,513] Aspirin has been shown to increase pancreatic duct permeability in animals.[514,515] Administration of intravenous aspirin increases calcium secretion from the pancreas, which is considered a marker of pancreatic damage.[516] Experimental studies suggest that prostaglandins may have a protective effect on pancreatic cells. Administration of prostaglandin E_2 in a mouse model of experimental pancreatitis was associated with an improved survival rate compared with the 100% mortality reported in controls. Membrane stabilization of pancreatic cells may be the mechanism behind the cytoprotection conferred by prostaglandins.[517] A proposed mechanism for sulindac-induced pancreatitis is metabolite deposition in biliary epithelial cells and inhibition of canalicular bile transport, leading to hypercholoresis.[66]

CALCIUM

It is possible that hypercalcemia induces chronic pancreatic exocrine secretion changes that may affect ductal epithelium.[171] Intracellular calcium in pancreatic zymogen granules is important in the maintenance of granule stability, and factors disrupting this delicate balance may contribute to calcium-induced pancreatitis.[518]

CORTICOSTEROIDS

Corticosteroids may induce pancreatitis through toxic effects, immune suppression, or increased viscosity of pancreatic fluids.[171] The viscosity of pancreatic secretions was greater in steroid-treated glands in an ex vivo study of perfused canine pancreas exposed to high doses of methylprednisolone.[519] Steroids stimulate both exocrine and endocrine pancreatic secretions, which may contribute to the development of drug-induced pancreatitis.[520]

STATINS

The exact mechanism of statin-induced pancreatitis is unclear. Some hypothesized mechanisms include immune-mediated inflammatory response, a metabolic effect, and direct cellular toxicity.[88] The propensity of the statins to cause pancreatitis may differ based on their inhibitory effects on cytochrome P450 and their lipophilicity. Other possible mechanisms of statin-induced acute pancreatitis involve rhabdomyolysis and drug interactions or changes in metabolism that may alter the pharmacokinetics of the agents.[101]

TYROSINE KINASE INHIBITORS

The mechanism of tyrosine kinase inhibitor-induced acute pancreatitis is not well understood, but possible explanations include effects on vascular endothelial growth factor (VEGF) and gastrointestinal motility.[400,403] The inhibition of VEGF may cause ischemia of the pancreatic tissue, increasing the risk of pancreatitis.[521] VEGF may also play a role in regulating the cell cycle of acinar cells; therefore, inhibition of VEGF may lead to acinar cell apoptosis and the release of autodigestive enzymes.[400,403] Tyrosine kinase inhibitors may decrease gastrointestinal motility, leading to reflux of the duodenal contents into the pancreatic duct and premature activation of pancreatic acinar cell digestive enzymes, leading to autodigestion.[400,403]

TAMOXIFEN

The exact mechanism for tamoxifen-induced pancreatitis is unclear but may be related to increased synthesis of triglycerides, leading to the presence of numerous chylomicrons in the blood that may obstruct capillaries, leading to pancreatic ischemia. Additionally, the degradation of triglycerides to free fatty acids by pancreatic lipases may lead to cytotoxic injuries that increase inflammatory mediators.[392]

INCRETIN-BASED THERAPIES

The mechanism of pancreatitis induced by incretin-based therapies is unknown. One theoretical model has proposed that the agents could have effects on the exocrine pancreas resulting in amplification of pancreatic ductal replication. This could lead to overgrowth of cells lining the smaller ducts and a resultant partial obstruction, which increases the risk for low-grade pancreatitis and may predispose the patient to acute pancreatitis.[472]

THIOAMIDES

The mechanism of thioamide-induced pancreatitis is unknown and hypersensitivity reactions, direct toxic effects, and autoimmune reactions have all been considered.[487] The development of pancreatitis within 1 month of therapy initiation and rapid recurrence with rechallenge supports a hypersensitivity mechanism possibly due to the sulfhydryl group.[488-490]

CLINICAL PRESENTATION AND DIFFERENTIAL DIAGNOSIS

The clinical presentation of drug-induced pancreatitis is similar to that of acute pancreatitis secondary to other causes.[3] **Table 39-3** summarizes the usual signs and symptoms associated with

Table 39-3 Signs and Symptoms Associated with Drug-Induced Pancreatitis[1]

- Abdominal distention (75%)
- Abdominal pain (95%)
- Hypotension (30%)
- Jaundice (20%)
- Low-grade fever (75%)
- Mental aberrations (25%)
- Nausea/vomiting (80%)
- Pain radiating to back (50%)

drug-induced pancreatitis. Typically, patients with acute pancreatitis present with abdominal pain, nausea, vomiting, abdominal distention, and low-grade fever. The presentation may also include pain that radiates to the back, hypotension, mental aberrations, and jaundice. Complications may include the development of pancreatic abscess, pseudocyst formation, and the development of subcutaneous fat necrosis and bluish discoloration of the abdominal wall.[522]

Diagnosis is usually based on clinical and laboratory data. Laboratory parameter abnormalities that may occur in patients with drug-induced pancreatitis include leukocytosis, hyperglycemia, hypoalbuminemia, mild hyperbilirubinemia, elevated blood urea nitrogen and serum creatinine concentrations, elevated hemoglobin, elevated hematocrit, hypocalcemia, thrombocytopenia, and prolongation of prothrombin time and international normalized ratio (INR).[1] Serum amylase concentrations usually increase within 24 hours of the onset of symptoms and will return to normal over a period of several days. Persistent elevation in serum amylase concentrations is suggestive of extensive pancreatic necrosis and/or related complications. Serum amylase concentrations do not correlate with severity of disease or etiology. In contrast, lipase originates in the pancreas, making it a more specific marker for pancreatitis than serum amylase. Elevations in serum lipase concentrations persist longer than those of serum amylase concentrations. Imaging techniques such as ultrasound may be indicated in patients with suspected biliary involvement. Contrast-enhanced computerized tomography (CECT) may be useful in determining severity of the inflammatory process, and it also provides an estimate of risk for systemic and local complications.[523,524] Some literature has asserted that a mean peak C-reactive protein value is significantly lower in drug-induced acute pancreatitis than in pancreatitis from other causes; therefore, careful search for an adverse drug reaction is appropriate in patients with acute pancreatitis of unknown cause and a low peak C-reactive protein level.[525]

Table 39-4 Conditions to Consider in the Differential Diagnosis of Drug-Induced Pancreatitis[526]

- Abdominal trauma
- Cholelithiasis
- Drugs
- Endoscopic retrograde cholangiopancretography
- Hyperlipidemia
- Infection
- Pancreatic tumor
- Surgery
- Toxins

As the clinical presentation of drug-induced pancreatitis is similar to that of pancreatitis due to other causes, drug-induced pancreatitis is usually diagnosed after other more common etiologies have been ruled out. A careful medication history including prescription and nonprescription medications as well as herbal supplements should always be done and will be helpful in differential diagnosis. Most commonly, acute pancreatitis occurs secondary to alcohol ingestion or cholelithiasis. Less common etiologies include abdominal trauma, toxins, hyperlipidemia, pancreatic tumor, complications of surgery, infection, and vascular abnormalities.[526] Endoscopic retrograde cholangiopancreatography (ERCP), which is used to diagnose pancreatitis, can also, ironically, cause pancreatitis in up to 40% of patients who undergo the procedure.[527] A recent single-center cohort of 318 patients undergoing ERCP procedures evaluated risk factors for post-ERCP pancreatitis and found that use of Badalov Class I or II drugs during the prior month was associated with an increased risk of post-ERCP pancreatitis.[528] **Table 39-4** lists conditions to consider in the differential diagnosis of drug-induced pancreatitis.

With drug-induced pancreatitis, the time from initiation of therapy to the onset of pancreatitis symptoms varies depending on the causative drug. No generalizations can be made, and for most drugs, pancreatitis can occur from within a short time after administration of the first dose to years after therapy begins.

RISK FACTORS

Risk factors for drug-induced pancreatitis are presented in **Table 39-5**. Any disease state that predisposes patients to hypercalcemia, such as hyperparathyroidism, malignancy, thyrotoxicosis, or multiple myeloma, as well as circumstances such as hard-water syndrome, tumor lysis syndrome, and cholecalciferol overdose increase the risk of drug-induced pancreatitis.[230,529-534] In addition, the risk for drug-induced pancreatitis is increased in patients receiving a drug with a definite or probable association with pancreatitis for management of a disease state that is also independently associated with pancreatitis.[535] For example, immunosuppression increases the risk of infection, infectious processes are often associated with pancreatitis, and patients with disease states associated with immunosuppression, such as renal transplantation or HIV/AIDS, have an increased incidence of drug-induced pancreatitis.[3] Autoimmune diseases such as inflammatory bowel disease have also been linked to pancreatitis, and patients with these conditions are at increased risk of developing drug-induced pancreatitis when treated with drugs that have definite or probable associations with the disease.[9,536]

Table 39-5 Risk Factors for Drug-Induced Pancreatitis

- Autoimmune disease
  - Crohn disease
- Drug-induced
  - Idiosyncratic reaction—large number of risk factors are unknown
- Female sex
- Hypercalcemia
  - Cholecalciferol overdose
  - Hard-water syndrome
  - Hyperparathyroidism
  - Malignancy
  - Multiple myeloma
  - Thyrotoxicosis
  - Tumor lysis syndrome
- Hyperlipidemias
  - Concurrent estrogen therapy
- Immunosuppression
  - HIV/AIDS
  - Renal transplantation
- Pediatric patients

AIDS = acquired immunodeficiency syndrome, HIV = human immunodeficiency virus.

Specific risk factors for didanosine-associated pancreatitis in the AIDS population have been identified. These include severity of HIV disease (CD4 count <200 cells/μL), didanosine dose >9.6 mg/kg/d, drug-related hyperlipidemia, therapy >10 weeks in duration, previous history of pancreatitis, concomitant alcohol use, and concomitant use of pentamidine.[20,25,537] Additionally, concomitant use of other drugs known to cause pancreatitis, particularly pentamidine, hydroxyurea, or stavudine increases the risk of didanosine-induced pancreatitis.[32,33,35] Ribavirin should be used with extreme caution in patients receiving didanosine due to the risk of fatal lactic acidosis and pancreatitis.[37] Previous exposure to didanosine is a risk factor for developing pentamidine-induced pancreatitis.[282]

MORBIDITY AND MORTALITY

Drug-induced pancreatitis may be mild to severe. The majority of patients recover without any long-term morbidity, but 5–15% of patients experience life-threatening complications, with a majority of severe complications occurring within 48 hours of onset.[3] Approximately 3–13% of acute pancreatitis cases develop into chronic pancreatitis.[101] A retrospective study including data from 43 German centers of gastroenterology found that the majority of drug-induced pancreatitis cases run a benign course; no patients experienced pseudocyst development or required mechanical ventilation.[9] However, the mean hospital stay was 25.5 days. Of all cases of suspected drug-induced pancreatitis reported to the Danish Committee on Adverse Drug Reactions from 1968 to 1999, 68% required hospitalization for treatment, with a 9%

Table 39-6 Severity of Pancreatitis Based on Ranson's Criteria[101,522]

At Hospital Admission or Diagnosis[a]	During First 48 Hours After Admission or Diagnosis[a]
• Age >55 years	• Fall in hematocrit of >10% (absolute %)
• WBC >16,000 cells/mm^3	• Rise in BUN of >5 mg/dL
• Blood glucose >200 mg/dL	• Serum calcium <8 mg/dL
• Serum LDH >350 units/L	• Arterial oxygen pressure of <60 mm Hg
• Serum aspartate aminotransferase >250 units/dL	• Base deficit of >4 mEq/L • Estimated fluid sequestration of >6 L

BUN = blood urea nitrogen, LDH = lactic dehydrogenase, WBC = white blood cell.
[a]The presence of three or more of these criteria indicates a more severe disease with a higher risk of mortality.

mortality rate.[6] Another Dutch study reported a 15% mortality rate associated with drug-induced pancreatitis.[68]

Ranson's criteria may be used to assess the severity of an episode of drug-induced pancreatitis and may be used to predict mortality (**Table 39-6**).[101,522] The presence of three or more of these criteria indicates a more severe disease with a higher risk of mortality. Severe acute pancreatitis is associated with an Acute Physiology and Chronic Health Status Evaluation (APACHE) score >8, associated organ failure, or >30% pancreatic necrosis viewed on computerized tomography scan, and with a Ranson's score >3.[537] There have been fatalities in case reports of pancreatitis associated with many drugs, with a seemingly higher incidence of mortality in patients with pancreatitis due to azathioprine, didanosine, furosemide, or hydrochlorothiazide. Many fatal cases with azathioprine occur after renal transplantation, and most didanosine-related cases occur in AIDS patients, in which the incidence of pancreatitis is greater.[9] In severe cases, circulatory, pulmonary, and renal complications may occur and ultimately result in death.[522]

PREVENTION

Drug-induced pancreatitis is a relatively rare, idiosyncratic disease. It is important for clinicians to be aware of this potential adverse event and to consider medications as potentially causative when other etiologies of pancreatitis are not present. Prevention strategies for specific agents and drug categories are summarized in **Table 39-7**. Measurement of serum lipase and amylase concentrations should be performed in patients who develop abdominal discomfort and who are taking medications associated with pancreatitis.[44,281,390,537] Indications for monitoring serum amylase and lipase concentrations in the absence of symptoms are less clear. One group of authors suggests monitoring serum amylase and lipase in patients taking ACE inhibitors.[538] Some have recommended routine monitoring of serum amylase and lipase concentrations during mirtazapine treatment and, in particular, when upward dose adjustments are made. This recommendation, however, is based on only one confirmed case of pancreatitis and two other reports that describe only asymptomatic elevations in serum lipase and amylase concentrations.[539] Serial serum amylase concentration monitoring and sonograms are not helpful in making an early diagnosis of pancreatitis

Table 39-7 Approaches to Help Prevent Drug-Induced Pancreatitis

- Azathioprine, 6-mercaptopurine, mesalamine, corticosteroids, metronidazole for inflammatory bowel disease
  - For patients with abdominal pain, consider pancreatitis as part of the differential diagnosis
- Didanosine
  - Adjust dose for weight <60 kg
  - Avoid alcohol or other drugs that can cause pancreatitis
  - Avoid use with *Pneumocystis jiroveci* therapy
- Hypercalcemia
  - Treat underlying condition (hyperparathyroidism, malignancy, thyrotoxicosis)
- Immunosuppressive agents
  - Use lowest effective dose of immunosuppressive agents (tacrolimus, cyclosporine, sirolimus)

in patients receiving L-asparaginase therapy.[137,540-542] In patients with a pre-existing pancreatic disorder, L-asparaginase is contraindicated because of its well-known pancreatic toxicity.[543]

The National Institute of Allergy and Infectious Diseases recommends screening all patients for a history of pancreatitis before initiating therapy with didanosine. Patients taking didanosine should avoid alcohol and other drugs known to cause pancreatitis. Didanosine therapy should be discontinued during and for 1 week after treatment with pentamidine or sulfonamides for *Pneumocystis jiroveci* pneumonia. The dose of didanosine should be reduced from 400 mg to 250 mg in patients that weigh <60 kg.[37,39]

Clinical judgment should be used when deciding whether or not to monitor serum pancreatic enzyme concentrations. In most cases, routine monitoring of serum amylase and lipase concentrations is not warranted unless symptoms suggestive of pancreatitis develop. This is due to the low incidence of drug-induced pancreatitis and often asymptomatic (and thus clinically unimportant) hyperamylasemia that occurs in association with many drugs. If abdominal pain, nausea, and vomiting occur in patients being treated with drugs known to cause pancreatitis, prompt laboratory evaluation of serum pancreatic enzyme concentrations and other diagnostics should be initiated.

MANAGEMENT

If drug-induced pancreatitis is suspected, prompt discontinuation of the suspect agent is necessary. Traditional therapeutic management of pancreatitis should be initiated, including administration of intravenous fluids, administering nothing by mouth, advancing the diet as tolerated, and providing adequate analgesia.[3]

INFORMATION FOR PATIENTS

Patients taking medications with a definite or probable association with pancreatitis should be instructed to report the onset of acute abdominal pain to their healthcare provider immediately. Some clinicians recommend advising patients to immediately discontinue the suspected causative drug and seek medical attention if they experience abdominal pain, nausea, or vomiting. If possible, patients should avoid drugs that caused pancreatitis for them in the past.

REFERENCES

1. Bolesta S, Montgomery P. Pancreatitis. In: DiPiro J, Talbert R, Yee G et al., eds. *Pharmacotherapy: a pathophysiologic approach.* 9th ed. New York: McGraw-Hill; 2014:721-36.
2. Trivedi CD, Pitchumoni CS. Drug-induced pancreatitis: an update. *J Clin Gastroenterol.* 2005; 39:709-16.
3. Banerjee AK, Patel KJ, Grainger SL. Drug-induced acute pancreatitis. A critical review. *Med Toxicol Adverse Drug Exp.* 1989; 4:186-98.
4. Mallory A, Kern F Jr. Drug-induced pancreatitis: a critical review. *Gastroenterology.* 1980; 78:813-20.
5. Badalov N, Baradarian R, Iswara K et al. Drug-induced acute pancreatitis: an evidence-based review. *Clin Gastroenterol Hepatol.* 2007; 5:648-61; quiz 644.
6. Andersen V, Sonne J, Andersen M. Spontaneous reports on drug-induced pancreatitis in Denmark from 1968 to 1999. *Eur J Clin Pharmacol.* 2001; 57:517-21.
7. Wilmink T, Frick TW. Drug-induced pancreatitis. *Drug Saf.* 1996; 14:406-23.
8. Thomson SR, Hendry WS, McFarlane GA, Davidson AI. Epidemiology and outcome of acute pancreatitis. *Br J Surg.* 1987; 74:398-401.
9. Lankisch PG, Droge M, Gottesleben F. Drug induced acute pancreatitis: incidence and severity. *Gut.* 1995; 37:565-7.
10. Barreto SG, Tiong L, Williams R. Drug-induced acute pancreatitis in a cohort of 328 patients. A single-centre experience from Australia. *JOP.* 2011; 12:581-5.
11. Nitsche C, Maertin S, Scheiber J et al. Drug-induced pancreatitis. *Curr Gastroenterol Rep.* 2012; 14:131-8.
12. Vinklerova I, Prochazka M, Prochazka V, Urbanek K. Incidence, severity, and etiology of drug-induced acute pancreatitis. *Dig Dis Sci.* 2010; 55:2977-81.
13. Mader TJ, McHugh TP. Acute pancreatitis in children. *Pediatr Emerg Care.* 1992; 8:157-61.
14. Jordan SC, Ament ME. Pancreatitis in children and adolescents. *J Pediatr.* 1977; 91:211-6.
15. Bai HX, Ma MH, Orabi AI et al. Novel characterization of drug-associated pancreatitis in children. *J Pediatr Gastroenterol Nutr.* 2011; 53:423-8.
16. Douros A, Bronder E, Andersohn F et al. Drug-induced acute pancreatitis: results from the hospital-based Berlin case-control surveillance study of 102 cases. *Aliment Pharmacol Ther.* 2013; 38:825-34.
17. Cappell MS, Marks M. Acute pancreatitis in HIV-seropositive patients: a case control study of 44 patients. *Am J Med.* 1995; 98:243-8.
18. Clas D, Falutz J, Rosenberg L. Acute pancreatitis associated with HIV infection. *CMAJ.* 1989; 140:823.
19. Schwartz MS, Brandt LJ. The spectrum of pancreatic disorders in patients with the acquired immune deficiency syndrome. *Am J Gastroenterol.* 1989; 84:459-62.
20. Butler KM, Husson RN, Balis FM et al. Dideoxyinosine in children with symptomatic human immunodeficiency virus infection. *N Engl J Med.* 1991; 324:137-44.

21. Maxson CJ, Greenfield SM, Turner JL. Acute pancreatitis as a common complication of 2',3'-dideoxyinosine therapy in the acquired immunodeficiency syndrome. *Am J Gastroenterol.* 1992; 87:708-13.
22. Aboulafia DM. Acute pancreatitis. A fatal complication of AIDS therapy. *J Clin Gastroenterol.* 1997; 25:640-5.
23. Underwood TW, Frye CB. Drug-induced pancreatitis. *Clin Pharm.* 1993; 12:440-8.
24. Yarchoan R, Pluda JM, Thomas RV et al. Long-term toxicity/activity profile of 2',3'-dideoxyinosine in AIDS or AIDS-related complex. *Lancet.* 1990; 336:526-9.
25. Rozencweig M, McLaren C, Beltangady M et al. Overview of phase I trials of 2',3'-dideoxyinosine (ddI) conducted on adult patients. *Rev Infect Dis.* 1990; 12(suppl 5):S570-5.
26. Butler KM, Venzon D, Henry N et al. Pancreatitis in human immunodeficiency virus-infected children receiving dideoxyinosine. *Pediatrics.* 1993; 91:747-51.
27. Cina SJ, Conradi SE. Acute pancreatitis in a prisoner with AIDS. Bugs or drugs? *Am J Forensic Med Pathol.* 1994; 15:28-31.
28. Pelucio MT, Rothenhaus T, Smith M, Ward DJ. Fatal pancreatitis as a complication of therapy for HIV infection. *J Emerg Med.* 1995; 13:633-7.
29. Levin TL, Berdon WE, Seigle RR, Nash MA. Valproic-acid-associated pancreatitis and hepatic toxicity in children with end-stage renal disease. *Pediatr Radiol.* 1997; 27:192-3.
30. Allaouchiche B, Duflo F, Cotte L et al. Acute pancreatitis with severe lactic acidosis in an HIV-infected patient on didanosine therapy. *J Antimicrob Chemother.* 1999; 44:137-8.
31. Lederman JC, Nawaz H. Toxic interaction of didanosine and acetaminophen leading to severe hepatitis and pancreatitis: a case report and review of the literature. *Am J Gastroenterol.* 2001; 96:3474-5.
32. Longhurst HJ, Pinching AJ. Drug points: pancreatitis associated with hydroxyurea in combination with didanosine. *BMJ.* 2001; 322:81.
33. Moore RD, Keruly JC, Chaisson RE. Incidence of pancreatitis in HIV-infected patients receiving nucleoside reverse transcriptase inhibitor drugs. *AIDS.* 2001; 15:617-20.
34. Sarner L, Fakoya A. Acute onset lactic acidosis and pancreatitis in the third trimester of pregnancy in HIV-1 positive women taking antiretroviral medication. *Sex Transm Infect.* 2002; 78:58-9.
35. Callens S, De Schacht C, Huyst V, Colebunders R. Pancreatitis in an HIV-infected person on a tenofovir, didanosine and stavudine containing highly active antiretroviral treatment. *J Infect.* 2003; 47:188-9.
36. Blanchard JN, Wohlfeiler M, Canas A et al. Pancreatitis with didanosine and tenofovir disoproxil fumarate [corrected]. *Clin Infect Dis.* 2003; 37:e57-62.
37. Butt AA. Fatal lactic acidosis and pancreatitis associated with ribavirin and didanosine therapy. *AIDS Read.* 2003; 13:344-8.
38. Glesby MJ, Gerber JG. Editorial comment: drug-drug interactions, hepatitis C, and mitochondrial toxicity. *AIDS Read.* 2003; 13:346-7.
39. Dolin R, Lambert JS, Morse GD et al. 2',3'-Dideoxyinosine in patients with AIDS or AIDS-related complex. *Rev Infect Dis.* 1990; 12(suppl 5):S540-9; discussion S549-51.
40. Yarchoan R, Mitsuya H, Pluda JM et al. The National Cancer Institute phase I study of 2',3'-dideoxyinosine administration in adults with AIDS or AIDS-related complex: analysis of activity and toxicity profiles. *Rev Infect Dis.* 1990; 12(suppl 5):S522-33.
41. NIAID updates dideoxyinosine toxicity profile, suggests ways to reduce risk of pancreatitis. *Clin Pharm.* 1990; 9:832, 838.
42. Bergholm U, Langman MJ, Rawlins MD et al. Drug induced acute pancreatitis. *Pharmacoepidemiol Drug Saf.* 1995; 4:329-34.
43. Lancashire RJ, Cheng K, Langman MJ. Discrepancies between population-based data and adverse reaction reports in assessing drugs as causes of acute pancreatitis. *Aliment Pharmacol Ther.* 2003; 17:887-93.
44. Standridge JB. Fulminant pancreatitis associated with lisinopril therapy. *South Med J.* 1994; 87:179-81.
45. Cheng RM, Mamdani M, Jackevicius CA, Tu K. Association between ACE inhibitors and acute pancreatitis in the elderly. *Ann Pharmacother.* 2003; 37:994-8.
46. Tilkemeier P, Thompson PD. Acute pancreatitis possibly related to enalapril. *N Engl J Med.* 1988; 318:1275-6.
47. Niebergall-Roth E, Teyssen S, Weber T, Singer MV. Effect of 8-week administration of enalapril plus additional 2-week administration of furosemide on heart rate and exocrine pancreas secretion in dogs. *Berl Munch Tierarztl Wochenschr.* 1996; 109:414-8.
48. Pedro-Botet J, Miralles R, Coll J, Rubies-Prat J. Captopril versus enalapril: cough versus pancreatitis. *DICP.* 1990; 24:438-9.
49. Maringhini A, Termini A, Patti R, Ciambra M et al. Enalapril-associated acute pancreatitis: recurrence after re-challenge. *Am J Gastroenterol.* 1997; 92:166-7.
50. Madsen JS, Jacobsen IA. Angiotensin converting enzyme inhibitor therapy and acute pancreatitis. *Blood Press.* 1995; 4:369-71.
51. Australian Adverse Drug Reaction Advisory Committee. Pancreatitis and ACE-inhibitors. *Australian Adverse Drug Reactions Bulletin.* August 1989.
52. Martin T, Taupignon A, Graf E et al. Pancreatitis and hepatitis in a patient treated with enalapril maleate, a case report. *Therapie.* 1989; 44:449-50.
53. Gonzalez Ramallo VJ, Muino Miguez A, Torres Segovia FJ. Necrotizing pancreatitis and enalapril. *Eur J Med.* 1992; 1:123.
54. Carnovale A, Esposito P, Bassano P et al. Enalapril-induced acute recurrent pancreatitis. *Dig Liver Dis.* 2003; 35:55-7.
55. Fisher AA, Bassett ML. Acute pancreatitis associated with angiotensin II receptor antagonists. *Ann Pharmacother.* 2002; 36:1883-6.
56. Famularo G, Minisola G, Nicotra GC, De Simone C. Acute pancreatitis associated with irbesartan therapy. *Pancreas.* 2005; 31:294-5.
57. Maliekal J, Drake CF. Acute pancreatitis associated with the use of lisinopril. *Ann Pharmacother.* 1993; 27:1465-6.
58. Marinella MA, Billi JE. Lisinopril therapy associated with acute pancreatitis. *West J Med.* 1995; 163:77-8.
59. Roush MK, McNutt RA, Gray TF. The adverse effect dilemma: quest for accessible information. *Ann Intern Med.* 1991; 114:298-9.
60. Can B, Sali M, Batman A et al. Valsartan-induced acute pancreatitis. *Internal medicine (Tokyo, Japan).* 2014; 53:703-5.
61. Muchnick JS, Mehta JL. Angiotensin-converting enzyme inhibitor-induced pancreatitis. *Clin Cardiol.* 1999;22:50-1.
62. Arjomand H, Kemp DG. Quinapril and pancreatitis. *Am J Gastroenterol.* 1999; 94:290-1.
63. Kanbay M, Selcuk H, Yilmaz U, Boyacioglu S. Recurrent acute pancreatitis probably secondary to lisinopril. *South Med J.* 2006; 99:1388-9.
64. Kanbay M, Korkmaz M, Yilmaz U et al. Acute pancreatitis due to ramipril therapy. *Postgrad Med J.* 2004; 80:617-8.
65. Bracamonte JD, Underhill M, Sarmiento P. Acute pancreatitis associated with lisinopril and olanzapine. *Am J Health-Syst Pharm.* 2010; 67:214-6.
66. Lee SC, Dalia SM. Drug-induced chronic pancreatitis. *Med Health R I.* 2012; 95:19-20.
67. Eland IA, Sundstrom A, Velo GP et al. Antihypertensive medication and the risk of acute pancreatitis: the European case-control study on drug-induced acute pancreatitis (EDIP). *Scand J Gastroenterol.* 2006; 41:1484-90.
68. Eland IA, van Puijenbroek EP, Sturkenboom MJ et al. Drug-associated acute pancreatitis: twenty-one years of spontaneous reporting in The Netherlands. *Am J Gastroenterol.* 1999; 94:2417-22.
69. Wilkinson ML, O'Driscoll R, Kiernan TJ. Cimetidine and pancreatitis. *Lancet.* 1981; 1(Part 1):610-1.
70. Nott DM, de Sousa BA. Suspected cimetidine-induced acute pancreatitis. *Br J Clin Pract.* 1989; 43:264-5.

71. Arnold F, Doyle PJ, Bell G. Acute pancreatitis in a patient treated with cimetidine. *Lancet.* 1978; 1:382-3.
72. Seo JH, Lee da Y, Hong CW et al. Severe lactic acidosis and acute pancreatitis associated with cimetidine in a patient with type 2 diabetes mellitus taking metformin. *Intern Med.* 2013; 52:2245-8.
73. Boehm KM, Gunaga S. Cimetidine-induced lactic acidosis and acute pancreatitis. *South Med J.* 2010; 103:849.
74. Eland IA, Alvarez CH, Stricker BH, Rodriguez LA. The risk of acute pancreatitis associated with acid-suppressing drugs. *Br J Clin Pharmacol.* 2000; 49:473-8.
75. Youssef SS, Iskandar SB, Scruggs J, Roy TM. Acute pancreatitis associated with omeprazole. *Int J Clin Pharmacol Ther.* 2005; 43:558-61.
76. Das S, Ganguly A, Ghosh A et al. Oral pantoprazole-induced acute pancreatitis in an 11-year-old child. *Ther Drug Monit.* 2012; 34:242-4.
77. Plotnick BH, Cohen I, Tsang T, Cullinane T. Metronidazole-induced pancreatitis. *Ann Intern Med.* 1985; 103(Part 1):891-2.
78. Sanford KA, Mayle JE, Dean HA, Greenbaum DS. Metronidazole-associated pancreatitis. *Ann Intern Med.* 1988; 109:756-7.
79. Celifarco A, Warschauer C, Burakoff R. Metronidazole-induced pancreatitis. *Am J Gastroenterol.* 1989; 84:958-60.
80. Corey WA, Doebbeling BN, DeJong KJ, Britigan BE. Metronidazole-induced acute pancreatitis. *Rev Infect Dis.* 1991; 13:1213-5.
81. Sura ME, Heinrich KA, Suseno M. Metronidazole-associated pancreatitis. *Ann Pharmacother.* 2000; 34:1152-5.
82. Feola DJ, Thornton AC. Metronidazole-induced pancreatitis in a patient with recurrent vaginal trichomoniasis. *Pharmacotherapy.* 2002; 22:1508-10.
83. Nigwekar SU, Casey KJ. Metronidazole-induced pancreatitis. A case report and review of literature. *JOP.* 2004; 5:516-9.
84. O'Halloran E, Hogan A, Mealy K. Metronidazole-induced pancreatitis. *HPB Surg.* 2010; 2010:523468.
85. Tsesmeli NE, Giannoulis KE, Savopoulos CG et al. Acute pancreatitis as a possible consequence of metronidazole during a relapse of ulcerative colitis. *Eur J Gastroenterol Hepatol.* 2007; 19:805-6.
86. Norgaard M, Ratanajamit C, Jacobsen J et al. Metronidazole and risk of acute pancreatitis: a population-based case-control study. *Aliment Pharmacol Ther.* 2005; 21:415-20.
87. Tsigrelis C, Pitchumoni CS. Pravastatin: a potential cause for acute pancreatitis. *World J Gastroenterol.* 2006; 12:7055-7.
88. Singh S, Loke YK. Statins and pancreatitis: a systematic review of observational studies and spontaneous case reports. *Drug Saf.* 2006; 29:1123-32.
89. Couderc M, Blanc P, Rouillon JM et al. A new case of simvastatin induced pancreatitis. *Gastroenterol Clin Biol.* 1991; 15:986-7.
90. Ramdani M, Schmitt AM, Liautard J. Simvastatin induced acute pancreatitis (two cases). *Gastroenterol Clin Biol.* 1991; 15:986.
91. Belaiche G, Ley G, Slama JL. Acute pancreatitis associated with atorvastatin therapy. *Gastroenterol Clin Biol.* 2000; 24:471-2.
92. McDonald KB, Garber BG, Perreault MM. Pancreatitis associated with simvastatin plus fenofibrate. *Ann Pharmacother.* 2002; 36:275-9.
93. Lons T, Chousterman M. Simvastatin: a new drug responsible for acute pancreatitis? *Gastroenterol Clin Biol.* 1991; 15:93-4.
94. Anagnostopoulos GK, Tsiakos S, Margantinis G et al. Acute pancreatitis due to pravastatin therapy. *JOP.* 2003; 4:129-32.
95. Tysk C, Al-Eryani AY, Shawabkeh AA. Acute pancreatitis induced by fluvastatin therapy. *J Clin Gastroenterol.* 2002; 35:406-8.
96. Plunhar W. A case of possible lovastatin induced pancreatitis in concomitant Gilbert Syndrome. *Wien Klin Wochenschr.* 1989; 101:551-4.
97. Abdul-Ghaffar NU, el-Sonbaty MR. Pancreatitis and rhabdomyolysis associated with lovastatin-gemfibrozil therapy. *J Clin Gastroenterol.* 1995; 21:340-1.
98. Van Woerkom RC, Adler DG. Report of simultaneous acute pancreatitis and acute hepatitis in a patient taking ezetimibe/simvastatin. *J Clin Lipidol.* 2010; 4:314-5.
99. Preiss D, Tikkanen MJ, Welsh P et al. Lipid-modifying therapies and risk of pancreatitis: a meta-analysis. *JAMA.* 2012; 308:804-11.
100. Thisted H, Jacobsen J, Munk EM et al. Statins and the risk of acute pancreatitis: a population-based case-control study. *Aliment Pharmacol Ther.* 2006; 23:185-90.
101. Jones MR, Hall OM, Kaye AM, Kaye AD. Drug-induced acute pancreatitis: a review. *Ochsner J.* 2015; 15:45-51.
102. Haber CJ, Meltzer SJ, Present DH, Korelitz BI. Nature and course of pancreatitis caused by 6-mercaptopurine in the treatment of inflammatory bowel disease. *Gastroenterology.* 1986; 91:982-6.
103. Herskowitz LJ, Olansky S, Lang PG. Acute pancreatitis associated with long-term azathioprine therapy. Occurrence in a patient with systemic lupus erythematosus. *Arch Dermatol.* 1979; 115:179.
104. Sturdevant RA, Singleton JW, Deren JL et al. Azathioprine-related pancreatitis in patients with Crohn's disease. *Gastroenterology.* 1979; 77(Part 2):883-6.
105. Kawanishi H, Rudolph E, Bull FE. Azathioprine-induced acute pancreatitis. *N Engl J Med.* 1973; 289:357.
106. Paloyan D, Levin B, Simonowitz D. Azathioprine-associated acute pancreatitis. *Am J Dig Dis.* 1977; 22:839-40.
107. Niederle B, Bartos V, Hrodek O, Hyniova H. Acute pancreatitis after imuran in a patient with autoimmune haemolytic anaemia. *Mater Med Pol.* 1978; 10:60-2.
108. Simons-Ling N, Schachner L, Penneys N et al. Childhood systemic lupus erythematosus. Association with pancreatitis, subcutaneous fat necrosis, and calcinosis cutis. *Arch Dermatol.* 1983; 119:491-4.
109. Tragnone A, Bazzocchi G, Aversa G et al. Acute pancreatitis after azathioprine treatment for ulcerative colitis. *Ital J Gastroenterol.* 1996; 28:102-4.
110. Siwach V, Bansal V, Kumar A et al. Post-renal transplant azathioprine-induced pancreatitis. *Nephrol Dial Transplant.* 1999; 14:2495-8.
111. Castiglione F, Del Vecchio Blanco G, Rispo A, Mazzacca G. Prevention of pancreatitis by weekly amylase assay in patients with Crohn's disease treated with azathioprine. *Am J Gastroenterol.* 2000; 95:2394-5.
112. Toubanakis C, Batziou E, Sipsas N et al. Acute pancreatitis after long-term therapy with mesalazine, and hyperamylasaemia associated with azathioprine in a patient with ulcerative colitis. *Eur J Gastroenterol Hepatol.* 2003; 15:933-4.
113. Floyd A, Pedersen L, Nielsen GL, Tet al. Risk of acute pancreatitis in users of azathioprine: a population-based case-control study. *Am J Gastroenterol.* 2003; 98:1305-8.
114. Bank L, Wright JP. 6-mercaptopurine-related pancreatitis in 2 patients with inflammatory bowel disease. *Dig Dis Sci.* 1984; 29:357-9.
115. Willert JR, Dahl GV, Marina NM. Recurrent mercaptopurine-induced acute pancreatitis: a rare complication of chemotherapy for acute lymphoblastic leukemia in children. *Med Pediatr Oncol.* 2002; 38:73-4.
116. Weersma RK, Peters FT, Oostenbrug LE et al. Increased incidence of azathioprine-induced pancreatitis in Crohn's disease compared with other diseases. *Aliment Pharmacol Ther.* 2004; 20:843-50.
117. Nogueira JR, Freedman MA. Acute pancreatitis as a complication of Imuran therapy in regional enteritis. *Gastroenterology.* 1972; 62:1040-1.
118. Lai SW, Wang YC, Wang CH, Huang TY. Acute pancreatitis and erythema nodosum associated with azathioprine. *QJM.* 2012; 105:363-4.
119. Halalsheh H, Bazzeh F, Alkayed K et al. 6-mercaptopurine-induced recurrent acute pancreatitis in children with acute lymphoblastic leukemia/lymphoma. *J Pediatr Hematol Oncol.* 2013; 35:470-2.

120. Chaparro M, Ordas I, Cabre E et al. Safety of thiopurine therapy in inflammatory bowel disease: long-term follow-up study of 3931 patients. *Inflamm Bowel Dis.* 2013; 19:1404-10.
121. Bermejo F, Lopez-Sanroman A, Taxonera C et al. Acute pancreatitis in inflammatory bowel disease, with special reference to azathioprine-induced pancreatitis. *Aliment Pharmacol Ther.* 2008; 28:623-8.
122. Rasmussen HH, Fonager K, Sorensen HT et al. Risk of acute pancreatitis in patients with chronic inflammatory bowel disease. A Danish 16-year nationwide follow-up study. *Scand J Gastroenterol.* 1999; 34:199-201.
123. van Geenen EJ, de Boer NK, Stassen P et al. Azathioprine or mercaptopurine-induced acute pancreatitis is not a disease-specific phenomenon. *Aliment Pharmacol Ther.* 2010; 31:1322-9.
124. Alexander S, Dowling D. Azathioprine pancreatitis in inflammatory bowel disease and successful subsequent treatment with mercaptopurine. *Intern Med J.* 2005; 35:570-1.
125. Ledder OD, Lemberg DA, Ooi CY, Day AS. Are thiopurines always contraindicated after thiopurine-induced pancreatitis in inflammatory bowel disease? *J Pediatr Gastroenterol Nutr.* 2013; 57:583-6.
126. Kennedy NA, Rhatigan E, Arnott ID et al. A trial of mercaptopurine is a safe strategy in patients with inflammatory bowel disease intolerant to azathioprine: an observational study, systematic review and meta-analysis. *Aliment Pharmacol Ther.* 2013; 38:1255-66.
127. Bonaz B, Boitard J, Marteau P et al. Tioguanine in patients with Crohn's disease intolerant or resistant to azathioprine/mercaptopurine. *Aliment Pharmacol Ther.* 2003; 18:401-8.
128. Heap GA, Weedon MN, Bewshea CM et al. HLA-DQA1-HLA-DRB1 variants confer susceptibility to pancreatitis induced by thiopurine immunosuppressants. *Nat Genet.* 2014; 46:1131-4.
129. Dong XW, Zheng Q, Zhu MM et al. Thiopurine S-methyltransferase polymorphisms and thiopurine toxicity in treatment of inflammatory bowel disease. *World J Gastroenterol.* 2010; 16:3187-95.
130. Wroblova K, Kolorz M, Batovsky M et al. Gene polymorphisms involved in manifestation of leucopenia, digestive intolerance, and pancreatitis in azathioprine-treated patients. *Dig Dis Sci.* 2012; 57:2394-401.
131. Weetman RM, Baehner RL. Latent onset of clinical pancreatitis in children receiving L-asparaginase therapy. *Cancer.* 1974; 34:780-5.
132. Haskell CM, Canellos GP, Leventhal BG et al. L-asparaginase: therapeutic and toxic effects in patients with neoplastic disease. *N Engl J Med.* 1969; 281:1028-34.
133. Land VJ, Sutow WW, Fernbach DJ et al. Toxicity of L-asparginase in children with advanced leukemia. *Cancer.* 1972; 30:339-47.
134. Raja RA, Schmiegelow K, Albertsen BK et al. Asparaginase-associated pancreatitis in children with acute lymphoblastic leukaemia in the NOPHO ALL2008 protocol. *Br J Haematol.* 2014; 165:126-33.
135. Greenstein R, Nogeire C, Ohnuma T, Greenstein A. Management of asparaginase induced hemorrhagic pancreatitis complicated by pseudocyst. *Cancer.* 1979; 43:718-22.
136. Kurtzberg J. Asparaginase. In: Holland JF, Fre E, Bast Jr RC et al., eds. *Cancer Medicine.* 4th ed. Baltimore: Williams and Wilkins; 1997:1027-35.
137. Pratt CB, Simone JV, Zee P et al. Comparison of daily versus weekly L-asparaginase for the treatment of childhood acute leukemia. *J Pediatr.* 1970; 77:474-83.
138. Shaw MT, Barnes CC, Madden FJ, Bagshawe KD. L-asparaginase and pancreatitis. *Lancet.* 1970; 2:721.
139. Tan CL, Chiang SP, Wee KP. Acute haemorrhagic pancreatitis following L-asparaginase therapy in acute lymphoblastic leukaemia—a case report. *Singapore Med J.* 1974; 15:278-82.
140. Koniver GA, Scott JE. Pancreatitis with pseudocyst: a complication of L-asparaginase therapy for leukemia. *Del Med J.* 1978; 50:330-2.
141. Jain R, Ramanan SV. Latrogenic pancreatitis. A fatal complication in the induction therapy for acute lymphocytic leukemia. *Arch Intern Med.* 1978; 138:1726.
142. Yang CM, Hsieh YL, Hwang B. Acute pancreatitis in association with L-asparaginase therapy: report of one case. *Zhonghua Yi Xue Za Zhi (Taipei).* 1993; 51:74-7.
143. Sadoff J, Hwang S, Rosenfeld D et al. Surgical pancreatic complications induced by L-asparaginase. *J Pediatr Surg.* 1997; 32:860-3.
144. Cheung YF, Lee CW, Chan CF et al. Somatostatin therapy in L-asparaginase-induced pancreatitis. *Med Pediatr Oncol.* 1994; 22:421-4.
145. Sahu S, Saika S, Pai SK, Advani SH. L-asparaginase (Leunase) induced pancreatitis in childhood acute lymphoblastic leukemia. *Pediatr Hematol Oncol.* 1998; 15:533-8.
146. Garrington T, Bensard D, Ingram JD, Silliman CC. Successful management with octreotide of a child with L-asparaginase induced hemorrhagic pancreatitis. *Med Pediatr Oncol.* 1998; 30:106-9.
147. Hsu YJ, Chen YC, Ho CL et al. Diabetic ketoacidosis and persistent hyperglycemia as long-term complications of L-asparaginase-induced pancreatitis. *Zhonghua Yi Xue Za Zhi (Taipei).* 2002; 65:441-5.
148. [No authors listed]. Latrogenic pancreatitis. *Br Med J.* 1977; 2:1043.
149. Jaffe N, Traggis D, Das L et al. Comparison of daily and twice-weekly schedule of L-asparaginase in childhood leukemia. *Pediatrics.* 1972; 49:590-5.
150. Larsen CC, Laursen CB, Dalby K, Graumann O. Splenic artery pseudoaneurysm due to acute pancreatitis in a 6-year-old boy with acute lymphoblastic leukaemia treated with L-aspariginase. *BMJ Case Rep.* 2014; 2014. pii: bcr2013202298.
151. Treepongkaruna S, Thongpak N, Pakakasama S et al. Acute pancreatitis in children with acute lymphoblastic leukemia after chemotherapy. *J Pediatr Hematol Oncol.* 2009; 31:812-5.
152. Eden OB, Shaw MP, Lilleyman JS, Richards S. Non-randomised study comparing toxicity of Escherichia coli and Erwinia asparaginase in children with leukaemia. *Med Pediatr Oncol.* 1990; 18:497-502.
153. Oncaspar-pegasparagase package insert. Collegeville, PA: Rhone-Poulenc Rorer Pharmaceuticals; 1994.
154. Ridgway D, Neerhout RC, Bleyer A. Attenuation of asparaginase-induced hyperglycemia after substitution of the Erwinia carotovora for the *Escherichia coli* enzyme preparation. *Cancer.* 1989; 63:561-3.
155. Raja RA, Schmiegelow K, Frandsen TL. Asparaginase-associated pancreatitis in children. *Br J Haematol.* 2012; 159:18-27.
156. Samarasinghe S, Dhir S, Slack J et al. Incidence and outcome of pancreatitis in children and young adults with acute lymphoblastic leukaemia treated on a contemporary protocol, UKALL 2003. *Br J Haematol.* 2013; 162:710-3.
157. Vrooman LM, Supko JG, Neuberg DS et al. Erwinia asparaginase after allergy to E. coli asparaginase in children with acute lymphoblastic leukemia. *Pediatr Blood Cancer.* 2010; 54:199-205.
158. Ettinger LJ, Kurtzberg J, Voute PA et al. An open-label, multicenter study of polyethylene glycol-L-asparaginase for the treatment of acute lymphoblastic leukemia. *Cancer.* 1995; 75:1176-81.
159. Asselin B, Gever R, Sallan S. Relative toxicity of E. coli L-asparaginase and pegasparagase in newly diagnosed childhood acute lymphoblastic leukemia. *Blood.* 1995; 86(suppl 1):177a.
160. Manuel SM. 1994 biotechnology drug approvals. *Am PharmNS.* 1995; 35:12-3.
161. Douer D, Cohel LJ, Periclou LA et al. PEG L-asparaginase: pharmacokinetics and clinical response in newly diagnosed adults with acute lymphoblastic leukemia treated with multiagent chemotherapy. *Blood.* 1997; 10(suppl 1):334a.
162. Frankel SR, Kurtzberg J, De Oliveira D et al. Toxicity and pharmacokinetics of PEG-asparaginase in newly diagnosed adult acute lymphoblastic leukemia. *Blood.* 1997; 10(suppl 1):334a.

163. Alvarez OA, Zimmerman G. Pegaspargase-induced pancreatitis. *Med Pediatr Oncol.* 2000; 34:200-5.

164. Buie LW, Moore J, van Deventer H. Successful use of octreotide as a chemoprotectant for prevention of PEG-asparaginase-induced pancreatitis. *Pharmacotherapy.* 2014; 34:e149-51.

165. Knoderer HM, Robarge J, Flockhart DA. Predicting asparaginase-associated pancreatitis. *Pediatr Blood Cancer.* 2007; 49:634-9.

166. Flores-Calderon J, Exiga-Gonzalez E, Moran-Villota S et al. Acute pancreatitis in children with acute lymphoblastic leukemia treated with L-asparaginase. *J Pediatr Hematol Oncol.* 2009; 31:790-3.

167. Kearney SL, Dahlberg SE, Levy DE et al. Clinical course and outcome in children with acute lymphoblastic leukemia and asparaginase-associated pancreatitis. *Pediatr Blood Cancer.* 2009; 53:162-7.

168. Oettgen HF, Stephenson PA, Schwartz MK et al. Toxicity of E. coli L-asparaginase in man. *Cancer.* 1970; 25:253-78.

169. Zubrod CG. The clinical toxicities of L-asparaginase in treatment of leukemia and lymphoma. *Pediatrics.* 1970; 45:555-9.

170. Runzi M, Layer P. Drug-associated pancreatitis: facts and fiction. *Pancreas.* 1996; 13:100-9.

171. Nakashima Y, Howard JM. Drug-induced acute pancreatitis. *Surg Gynecol Obstet.* 1977; 145:105-9.

172. Fernandez-del Castillo C, Harringer W, Warshaw AL et al. Risk factors for pancreatic cellular injury after cardiopulmonary bypass. *N Engl J Med.* 1991; 325:382-7.

173. Hochgelerent EL, David DS. Acute pancreatitis secondary to calcium infusion in a dialysis patient. *Arch Surg.* 1974; 108:218-9.

174. Izsak EM, Shike M, Roulet M, Jeejeebhoy KN. Pancreatitis in association with hypercalcemia in patients receiving total parenteral nutrition. *Gastroenterology.* 1980; 79:555-8.

175. Manson RR. Acute pancreatitis secondary to iatrogenic hypercalcemia: implications of hyperalimentation. *Arch Surg.* 1974; 108:213-5.

176. Nykamp D, Kraus EJ. Antacid-induced acute pancreatitis. *Consult Pharm.* 2013; 28:247-51.

177. Frick TW, Fryd DS, Sutherland DE et al. Hypercalcemia associated with pancreatitis and hyperamylasemia in renal transplant recipients. Data from the Minnesota randomized trial of cyclosporine versus antilymphoblast azathioprine. *Am J Surg.* 1987; 154:487-9.

178. Jick H, Derby LE, Garcia Rodriguez LA et al. Nonsteroidal anti-inflammatory drugs and certain rare, serious adverse events: a cohort study. *Pharmacotherapy.* 1993; 13:212-7.

179. Goldstein J, Laskin DA, Ginsberg GH. Sulindac associated with pancreatitis. *Ann Intern Med.* 1980; 93:151.

180. Siefkin AD. Sulindac and pancreatitis. *Ann Intern Med.* 1980; 93:932-3.

181. Lilly EL. Pancreatitis after administration of sulindac. *JAMA.* 1981; 246:2680.

182. Memon AN. Pancreatitis and sulindac. *Ann Intern Med.* 1982; 97:139.

183. Klein SM, Khan MA. Hepatitis, toxic epidermal necrolysis and pancreatitis in association with sulindac therapy. *J Rheumatol.* 1983; 10:512-3.

184. Clark BG, Vestal RE. Adverse drug reactions in the elderly: case studies. *Geriatrics.* 1984; 39:53-4, 60-3, 66.

185. Detlefs RL. Drug-induced pancreatitis presenting as subcutaneous fat necrosis. *J Am Acad Dermatol.* 1985; 13(Part 1):305-7.

186. Sugerman HJ. Sulindac-induced acute pancreatitis mimicking gallstone pancreatitis. *Am Surg.* 1989; 55:536-8.

187. Zygmunt DJ, Williams HJ, Bienz SR. Acute pancreatitis associated with long-term sulindac therapy. *West J Med.* 1986; 144:461-2.

188. Coward RA. Paracetamol-induced acute pancreatitis. *Br Med J.* 1977; 1:1086.

189. Gilmore IT, Tourvas E. Paracetamol-induced acute pancreatitis. *Br Med J.* 1977; 1:753-4.

190. Caldarola V, Hassett JM, Hall AH et al. Hemorrhagic pancreatitis associated with acetaminophen overdose. *Am J Gastroenterol.* 1986; 81:579-82.

191. Mofenson HC, Caraccio TR, Nawaz H, Steckler G. Acetaminophen induced pancreatitis. *J Toxicol Clin Toxicol.* 1991; 29:223-30.

192. Igarashi H, Ito T, Yoshinaga M et al. Acetaminophen-induced acute pancreatitis. A case report. *JOP.* 2009; 10:550-3.

193. Farrell J, Schmitz PG. Paracetamol-induced pancreatitis and fulminant hepatitis in a hemodialysis patient. *Clin Nephrol.* 1997; 48:132-3.

194. Yang CC, Deng JF, Lin TJ. Pancytopenia, hyperglycemia, shock, coma, rhabdomyolysis, and pancreatitis associated with acetaminophen poisoning. *Vet Hum Toxicol.* 2001; 43:344-8.

195. Fernandes R. Acute pancreatitis following paracetamol overdose. *BMJ case reports.* 2009; 2009.

196. Cavanaugh Z, Naut ER. Acetaminophen-induced pancreatic pseudocyst: first case report. *Conn Med.* 2014; 78:37-9.

197. Schmidt LE, Dalhoff K. Hyperamylasaemia and acute pancreatitis in paracetamol poisoning. *Aliment Pharmacol Ther.* 2004; 20:173-9.

198. Cabooter M, Elewaut A, Barbier F. Salicylate-induced pancreatitis. *Gastroenterology.* 1981; 80:214.

199. Sussman S. Severe salicylism and acute pancreatitis. *Calif Med.* 1963; 99:29-32.

200. Hoyte FC, Weber RW, Katial RK. Pancreatitis as a novel complication of aspirin therapy in patients with aspirin-exacerbated respiratory disease. *J Allergy Clin Immunol.* 2012; 129:1684-6.

201. Block MB, Genant HK, Kirsner JB. Pancreatitis as an adverse reaction to salicylazosulfapyridine. *N Engl J Med.* 1970; 282:380-2.

202. Chiba M, Horie Y, Ishida H et al. A case of salicylazosulfapyridine (Salazopyrin)-induced acute pancreatitis with positive lymphocyte stimulation test (LST). *Gastroenterol Jpn.* 1987; 22:228-33.

203. Brazer SR, Medoff JR. Sulfonamide-induced pancreatitis. *Pancreas.* 1988; 3:583-6.

204. Meyers S. Disodium azodisalicylate and sulfasalazine. *Am J Gastroenterol.* 1988; 83:1187.

205. Rubin R. Sulfasalazine-induced fulminant hepatic failure and necrotizing pancreatitis. *Am J Gastroenterol.* 1994; 89:789-91.

206. Garau P, Orenstein SR, Neigut DA, Kocoshis SA. Pancreatitis associated with olsalazine and sulfasalazine in children with ulcerative colitis. *J Pediatr Gastroenterol Nutr.* 1994; 18:481-5.

207. Sachedina B, Saibil F, Cohen LB, Whittey J. Acute pancreatitis due to 5-aminosalicylate. *Ann Intern Med.* 1989; 110:490-2.

208. Isaacs KL, Murphy D. Pancreatitis after rectal administration of 5-aminosalicylic acid. *J Clin Gastroenterol.* 1990; 12:198-9.

209. Erdkamp F, Houben M, Ackerman E et al. Pancreatitis induced by mesalamine. *Neth J Med.* 1992; 41:71-3.

210. Radke M, Bartolomaeus G, Muller M, Richter I. Acute pancreatitis in Crohn's disease due to 5-ASA therapy. *J Pediatr Gastroenterol Nutr.* 1993; 16:337-9.

211. Abdullah AM, Scott RB, Martin SR. Acute pancreatitis secondary to 5-aminosalicylic acid in a child with ulcerative colitis. *J Pediatr Gastroenterol Nutr.* 1993; 17:441-4.

212. Fernandez J, Sala M, Panes J et al. Acute pancreatitis after long-term 5-aminosalicylic acid therapy. *Am J Gastroenterol.* 1997; 92:2302-3.

213. Adachi E, Okazaki K, Matsushima Y et al. Acute pancreatitis secondary to 5-aminosalicylic acid therapy in a patient with ulcerative colitis. *Int J Pancreatol.* 1999; 25:217-21.

214. Paul AC, Oommen SP, Angami S, Moses PD. Acute pancreatitis in a child with idiopathic ulcerative colitis on long-term 5-aminosalicylic acid therapy. *Indian J Gastroenterol.* 2000; 19:195-6.

215. Ouakaa-Kchaou A, Gargouri D, Kochlef A et al. Acute pancreatitis secondary to long-term 5-aminosalicylic acid therapy in a patient with ulcerative colitis: a case-report. *La Tunisie medicale.* 2014; 92:423.

216. Ransford RA, Langman MJ. Sulphasalazine and mesalazine: serious adverse reactions re-evaluated on the basis of suspected adverse reaction reports to the Committee on Safety of Medicines. *Gut.* 2002; 51:536-9.
217. Munk EM, Pedersen L, Floyd A et al. Inflammatory bowel diseases, 5-aminosalicylic acid and sulfasalazine treatment and risk of acute pancreatitis: a population-based case-control study. *Am J Gastroenterol.* 2004; 99:884-8.
218. McBride CE, Yavorski RT, Moses FM et al. Acute pancreatitis associated with continuous infusion cytarabine therapy: a case report. *Cancer.* 1996; 77:2588-91.
219. Izraeli S, Adamson PC, Blaney SM, Balis FM. Acute pancreatitis after ifosfamide therapy. *Cancer.* 1994; 74:1627-8.
220. Puckett JB, Butler WM, McFarland JA. Pancreatitis and cancer chemotherapy. *Ann Intern Med.* 1982; 97:453.
221. Altman AJ, Dinndorf P, Quinn JJ. Acute pancreatitis in association with cytosine arabinoside therapy. *Cancer.* 1982; 49:1384-6.
222. Newman CE, Ellis DJ. Pancreatitis during combination chemotherapy. *Clin Oncol.* 1979; 5:83-4.
223. Siemers RF, Friedenberg WR, Norfleet RG. High-dose cytosine arabinoside-associated pancreatitis. *Cancer.* 1985; 56:1940-2.
224. McGrail LH, Sehn LH, Weiss RB et al. Pancreatitis during therapy of acute myeloid leukemia: cytarabine related? *Ann Oncol.* 1999; 10:1373-6.
225. Calvo DB, 3rd, Patt YZ, Wallace S et al. Phase I-II trial of percutaneous intra-arterial cis-diamminedichloro platinum (II) for regionally confined malignancy. *Cancer.* 1980; 45:1278-83.
226. Bunin N, Meyer WH, Christensen M, Pratt CB. Pancreatitis following cisplatin: a case report. *Cancer Treat Rep.* 1985; 69:236-7.
227. Stewart DJ, Feun LG, Maor M et al. Weekly cisplatin during cranial irradiation for malignant melanoma metastatic to brain. *J Neurooncol.* 1983; 1:49-51.
228. Socinski MA, Garnick MB. Acute pancreatitis associated with chemotherapy for germ cell tumors in two patients. *Ann Intern Med.* 1988; 108:567-8.
229. Yeung KY, Haidak DJ, Brown JA, Anderson D. Metastasis-induced acute pancreatitis in small cell bronchogenic carcinoma. *Arch Intern Med.* 1979; 139:552-4.
230. Spiegel RJ, Magrath IT. Tumor lysis pancreatitis. *Med Pediatr Oncol.* 1979; 7:169-72.
231. Nevalainen TJ. Cytotoxicity of vinblastine and vincristine to pancreatic acinar cells. *Virchows Arch B Zellpathol.* 1975; 18:119-127.
232. Ben Kridis W, Khanfir A, Frikha M. Acute pancreatitis induced by anticancer chemotherapy. *Acta Clin Belg.* 2013; 68:309-10.
233. Garg R, Agarwala S, Bhatnagar V. Acute pancreatitis induced by ifosfamide therapy. *J Pediatr Surg.* 2010; 45:2071-3.
234. Kumar DM, Sundar S, Vasanthan S. A case of paclitaxel-induced pancreatitis. *Clin Oncol (R Coll Radiol).* 2003; 15:35.
235. Hoff PM, Valero V, Holmes FA et al. Paclitaxel-induced pancreatitis: a case report. *J Natl Cancer Inst.* 1997; 89:91-3.
236. Hudis C, Riccio L, Holmes F et al. Phase II study of semisynthetic paclitaxel in metastatic breast cancer. *Eur J Cancer.* 1997; 33:2198-202.
237. Butt W, Saadati H, Saif MW. Oxaliplatin-induced pancreatitis: a case series. *Anticancer Res.* 2010; 30:5113-5.
238. Chan HY, Ng CM, Tiu SC et al. Hypertriglyceridaemia-induced pancreatitis: a contributory role of capecitabine? *Hong Kong Med J.* 2012; 18:526-9.
239. Yucel H, Warmerdam LV. Capecitabine-induced pancreatitis. *J Oncol Pharm Pract.* 2010; 16:133-4.
240. Jones KL, Valero V. Capecitabine-induced pancreatitis. *Pharmacotherapy.* 2003; 23:1076-8.
241. Gurzu S, Jung I, Comsulea M et al. Lethal cardiotoxicity, steatohepatitis, chronic pancreatitis, and acute enteritis induced by capecitabine and oxaliplatin in a 36-year-old woman. *Diagn Pathol.* 2013; 8:150.
242. Singh V, Devata S, Cheng YC. Carboplatin and docetaxel-induced acute pancreatitis: brief report. *Int J Clin Oncol.* 2010; 15:642-4.
243. Khanna S, Kumar A. Acute pancreatitis due to hydrocortisone in a patient with ulcerative colitis. *J Gastroenterol Hepatol.* 2003; 18:1110-1.
244. Ungprasert P, Permpalung N, Summachiwakij S, Manatsathit W. A case of recurrent acute pancreatitis due to intra-articular corticosteroid injection. *JOP.* 2014; 15:208-9.
245. Sadr-Azodi O, Mattsson F, Bexlius TS et al. Association of oral glucocorticoid use with an increased risk of acute pancreatitis: a population-based nested case-control study. *JAMA Intern Med.* 2013; 173:444-9.
246. Barrett PV, Thier SO. Meningitis and pancreatitis associated with sulfamethizole. *N Engl J Med.* 1963; 268:36-7.
247. Antonow DR. Acute pancreatitis associated with trimethoprim-sulfamethoxazole. *Ann Intern Med.* 1986; 104:363-5.
248. Alberti-Flor JJ, Hernandez ME, Ferrer JP et al. Fulminant liver failure and pancreatitis associated with the use of sulfamethoxazole-trimethoprim. *Am J Gastroenterol.* 1989; 84:1577-9.
249. Bartels RH, van der Spek JA, Oosten HR. Acute pancreatitis due to sulfamethoxazole-trimethoprim. *South Med J.* 1992; 85:1006-7.
250. Ober WB, Lecompte PM. Acute fatty metamorphosis of the liver associated with pregnancy; a distinctive lesion. *Am J Med.* 1955; 19:743-58.
251. Schultz JC, Adamson JS Jr, Workman WW, Norman TD. Fatal liver disease after intravenous administration of tetracycline in high dosage. *N Engl J Med.* 1963; 269:999-1004.
252. Kunelis CT, Peters JL, Edmondson HA. Fatty liver of pregnancy and its relationship to tetracycline therapy. *Am J Med.* 1965; 38:359-77.
253. Peters RL, Edmondson HA, Mikkelsen WP, Tatter D. Tetracycline-induced fatty liver in nonpregnant patients. A report of six cases. *Am J Surg.* 1967; 113:622-32.
254. Torosis J, Vender R. Tetracycline-induced pancreatitis. *J Clin Gastroenterol.* 1987; 9:580-1.
255. Elmore MF, Rogge JD. Tetracycline-induced pancreatitis. *Gastroenterology.* 1981; 81:1134-6.
256. Nicolau DP, Mengedoht DE, Kline JJ. Tetracycline-induced pancreatitis. *Am J Gastroenterol.* 1991; 86:1669-71.
257. Boudreaux JP, Hayes DH, Mizrahi S et al. Fulminant hepatic failure, hepatorenal syndrome, and necrotizing pancreatitis after minocycline hepatotoxicity. *Transplant Proc.* 1993; 25:1873.
258. Boyle MP. Minocycline-induced pancreatitis in cystic fibrosis. *Chest.* 2001; 119:1283-5.
259. Ocal S, Selcuk H, Korkmaz M et al. Acute pancreatitis following doxycycline and ornidazole coadministration. *JOP.* 2010; 11:614-6.
260. Wachira JK, Jensen CH, Rhone K. Doxycycline-induced pancreatitis: a rare finding. *S D Med.* 2013; 66:227-9.
261. Ljung R, Lagergren J, Bexelius TS et al. Increased risk of acute pancreatitis among tetracycline users in a Swedish population-based case-control study. *Gut.* 2012; 61:873-6.
262. Gilson M, Moachon L, Jeanne L et al. Acute pancreatitis related to tigecycline: case report and review of the literature. *Scand J Infect Dis.* 2008; 40:681-3.
263. Lipshitz J, Kruh J, Cheung P, Cassagnol M. Tigecycline-induced pancreatitis. *J Clin Gastroenterol.* 2009; 43:93.
264. Hung WY, Kogelman L, Volpe G et al. Tigecycline-induced acute pancreatitis: case report and literature review. *Int J Antimicrob Agents.* 2009; 34:486-9.
265. Marshall R. Tigecycline-induced pancreatitis. *I Int J Antimicrob Agents.* 2009; 44:239-41.
266. Prot-Labarthe S, Youdaren R, Benkerrou M et al. Pediatric acute pancreatitis related to tigecycline. *Pediatr Infect Dis J.* 2010; 29:890-1.
267. Okon E, Engell C, van Manen R, Brown J. Tigecycline-related pancreatitis: a review of spontaneous adverse event reports. *Pharmacotherapy.* 2013; 33:63-8.
268. Murphey SA, Josephs AS. Acute pancreatitis associated with pentamidine therapy. *Arch Intern Med.* 1981; 141:56-8.

269. Salmeron S, Petitpretz P, Katlama C et al. Pentamidine and pancreatitis. *Ann Intern Med.* 1986; 105:140-1.
270. Zuger A, Wolf BZ, el-Sadr W et al. Pentamidine-associated fatal acute pancreatitis. *JAMA.* 1986; 256:2383-5.
271. Herer B, Chinet T, Labrune S et al. Pancreatitis associated with pentamidine by aerosol. *BMJ.* 1989; 298:605.
272. Kumar S, Schnadig VJ, MacGregor MG. Fatal acute pancreatitis associated with pentamidine therapy. *Am J Gastroenterol.* 1989; 84:451-3.
273. Schwartz MS, Cappell MS. Pentamidine-associated pancreatitis. *Dig Dis Sci.* 1989; 34:1617-20.
274. Hart CC. Aerosolized pentamidine and pancreatitis. *Ann Intern Med.* 1989; 111:691.
275. Pauwels A, Eliaszewicz M, Larrey D et al. Pentamidine-induced acute pancreatitis in a patient with AIDS. *J Clin Gastroenterol.* 1990; 12:457-9.
276. O'Neil MG, Selub SE, Hak LJ. Pancreatitis during pentamidine therapy in patients with AIDS. *Clin Pharm.* 1991; 10:56-9.
277. Wood G, Wetzig N, Hogan P, Whitby M. Survival from pentamidine induced pancreatitis and diabetes mellitus. *Aust N Z J Med.* 1991; 21:341-2.
278. Villamil A, Hammer RA, Rodriguez FH. Edematous pancreatitis associated with intravenous pentamidine. *South Med J.* 1991; 84:796-8.
279. Millard PS, van der Horst C. Reversible diabetes mellitus after intravenous pentamidine. *Am J Med.* 1991; 91:442.
280. Klatt EC. Pathology of pentamidine-induced pancreatitis. *Arch Pathol Lab Med.* 1992; 116:162-4.
281. Sauleda J, Gea JG, Aguar MC et al. Probable pentamidine-induced acute pancreatitis. *Ann Pharmacother.* 1994; 28:52-3.
282. Foisy MM, Slayter KL, Hewitt RG, Morse GD. Pancreatitis during intravenous pentamidine therapy in an AIDS patient with prior exposure to didanosine. *Ann Pharmacother.* 1994; 28:1025-8.
283. Singh G, el-Gadi SM, Sparks RA. Pancreatitis associated with aerosolised pentamidine. *Genitourin Med.* 1995; 71:130-1.
284. Hanline MH Jr. Acute pancreatitis caused by ampicillin. *South Med J.* 1987; 80:1069.
285. Mann S, Thillainayagam A. Is ciprofloxacin a new cause of acute pancreatitis? *J Clin Gastroenterol.* 2000; 31:336.
286. Sung HY, Kim JI, Lee HJ et al. Acute pancreatitis secondary to ciprofloxacin therapy in patients with infectious colitis. *Gut and Liver.* 2014; 8:265-70.
287. Yi PH, Veltre DR, Kuttab JS et al. Acute groove pancreatitis due to isoniazid. *Neth J Med.* 2013; 71:104.
288. Mattioni S, Zamy M, Mechai F et al. Isoniazid-induced recurrent pancreatitis. *JOP.* 2012; 13:314-6.
289. Pandey AS, Surana A. Isoniazid-induced recurrent acute pancreatitis. *Trop Doct* 2011; 41:249-50.
290. Rabassa AA, Trey G, Shukla U et al. Isoniazid-induced acute pancreatitis. *Ann Intern Med.* 1994; 121:433-4.
291. Stephenson I, Wiselka MJ, Qualie MJ. Acute pancreatitis induced by isoniazid in the treatment of tuberculosis. *Am J Gastroenterol.* 2001; 96:2271-2.
292. Chan KL, Chan HS, Lui SF, Lai KN. Recurrent acute pancreatitis induced by isoniazid. *Tuber Lung Dis.* 1994; 75:383-5.
293. Chow KM, Szeto CC, Leung CB, Li PK. Recurrent acute pancreatitis after isoniazid. *Neth J Med.* 2004; 62:172-4.
294. Kvale PA, Parks RD. Acute abdomen. An unusual reaction to isoniazid. *Chest.* 1975; 68:271-2. Letter.
295. Jin CF, Sable R. Isoniazid-induced acute hepatitis and acute pancreatitis in a patient during chemoprophylaxis. *J Clin Gastroenterol.* 2002; 35:100-1.
296. Saleem AF, Arbab S, Naz FQ. Isoniazid induced acute pancreatitis in a young girl. *J Coll Physicians Surg Pak.* 2015; 25:299-300.
297. Izzedine H, Launay-Vacher V, Storme T, Deray G. Acute pancreatitis induced by isoniazid. *Am J Gastroenterol.* 2001; 96:3208-9.
298. Dickson I. Acute pancreatitis following administration of isonicotinic acid hydrazide; report of a case. *Br J Tuberc Dis Chest.* 1956; 50:277-8.
299. Rominger JM, Gutierrez JG, Curtis D, Chey WY. Methyldopa-induced pancreatitis. *Am J Dig Dis.* 1978; 23:756-8.
300. Warren SE, Mitas JA, 2nd, Swerdlin AH. Pancreatitis due to methyldopa: case report. *Mil Med.* 1980; 145:399-400.
301. Van der Heide H, Ten Haaft MA, Stricker BH. Pancreatitis caused by methyldopa. *Br Med J (Clin Res Ed).* 1981; 282:1930-1.
302. Ramsay LE, Wakefield VA, Harris EE. Methyldopa-induced chronic pancreatitis. *Practitioner.* 1982; 226:1166-9.
303. Glueck CJ, Scheel D, Fishback J, Steiner P. Estrogen-induced pancreatitis in patients with previously covert familial type V hyperlipoproteinemia. *Metabolism.* 1972; 21:657-66.
304. Blake WE, Pitcher ME. Estrogen-related pancreatitis in the setting of normal plasma lipids: case report. *Menopause.* 2003; 10:99-101.
305. Davidoff F, Tishler S, Rosoff C. Marked hyperlipidemia and pancreatitis associated with oral contraceptive therapy. *N Engl J Med.* 1973; 289:552-5.
306. Editorial: Pancreatitis from oral contraceptives. *Br Med J.* 1973; 4:688-9.
307. Parker WA. Estrogen-induced pancreatitis. *Clin Pharm.* 1983; 2:75-9.
308. Isley WL, Oki J. Estrogen-induced pancreatitis after discontinuation of concomitant medroxyprogesterone therapy. *Am J Med.* 1997; 102:416-7.
309. Ruman J, Brenner S, Sauer MV. Severe hypertriglyceridemia and pancreatitis following hormone replacement prior to cryothaw transfer. *J Assist Reprod Genet.* 2002; 19:94-7.
310. Keskin M, Songur Y, Isler M. Clomiphene-induced acute pancreatitis without hypertriglyceridemia. *Am J Med Sci.* 2007; 333:194-6.
311. Tetsche MS, Jacobsen J, Norgaard M et al. Postmenopausal hormone replacement therapy and risk of acute pancreatitis: a population-based case-control study. *Am J Gastroenterol.* 2007; 102:275-8.
312. Lieb JG, 2nd, Toskes PP. A pilot retrospective study of the relationship between estrogen use and pancreatitis/pancreatic function in women with chronic abdominal pain. *JOP.* 2013; 14:237-42.
313. Wilson AE, Mehra SK, Gomersall CR, Davies DM. Acute pancreatitis associated with frusemide therapy. *Lancet.* 1967; 1:105.
314. Strunge P. Frusemide-induced pancreatitis? *Br Med J.* 1975; 3:434. Letter.
315. Jones PE, Oelbaum MH. Frusemide-induced pancreatitis. *Br Med J.* 1975; 1:133-4.
316. Call T, Malarkey WB, Thomas FB. Acute pancreatitis secondary to furosemide with associated hyperlipidemia. *Am J Dig Dis.* 1977; 22:835-8.
317. Stenvinkel P, Alvestrand A. Loop diuretic-induced pancreatitis with re-challenge in a patient with malignant hypertension and renal insufficiency. *Acta Med Scand.* 1988; 224:89-91.
318. Juang P, Page RL, 2nd, Zolty R. Probable loop diuretic-induced pancreatitis in a sulfonamide-allergic patient. *Ann Pharmacother.* 2006; 40:128-34.
319. Buchanan N, Cane RD. Frusemid-induced pancreatitis. *Br Med J.* 1977; 2:1417.
320. Chao CT, Chao JY. Case report: furosemide and pancreatitis: Importance of dose and latency period before reaction. *Can Fam Physician.* 2013; 59:43-5.
321. Lynggaard F, Bjorndal N. Bumetanide-induced hyperamylaseaemia in patients with renal insufficiency. *Lancet.* 1977; 2:1355.
322. Schmidt P, Friedman IS. Adverse effects of ethacrynic acid. *N Y State J Med.* 1967; 67:1438-42.
323. Pickleman J, Straus FH, 2nd, Paloyan E. Pancreatitis associated with thiazide administration. A role for the parathyroid glands? *Arch Surg.* 1979; 114:1013-6.

324. Weaver GA, Bordley Jt, Guiney WB, D'Accurzio A. Chronic pancreatitis with cyst formation after prednisone and thiazide treatment. *Am J Gastroenterol.* 1982; 77:164-8.
325. Sammett D, Greben C, Sayeed-Shah U. Acute pancreatitis caused by penicillin. *Dig Dis Sci.* 1998; 43:1778-83.
326. Ances IG, McClain CA. Acute pancreatitis following the use of thiazide in pregnancy. *South Med J.* 1971; 64:267-9.
327. Diamond MT. Hyperglycemic hyperosmolar coma associated with hydrochlorothiazide and pancreatitis. *N Y State J Med.* 1972; 72:1741-2.
328. Cohen L, Sandbank U, Rosenfeld JB. Silent acute pancreatitis with encephalomalacia mimicking hepatic coma. *Am J Gastroenterol.* 1975; 63:75-8.
329. Fuchs JE Jr. Keith MR, Galanos AN. Probable metolazone-induced pancreatitis. *DICP.* 1989; 23:711.
330. Eckhauser ML, Dokler M, Imbembo AL. Diuretic-associated pancreatitis: a collective review and illustrative cases. *Am J Gastroenterol.* 1987; 82:865-70.
331. Anderson PE, Ellis GG Jr. Austin SM. Case report: metolazone-associated hypercalcemia and acute pancreatitis. *Am J Med Sci.* 1991; 302:235-7.
332. Rion RJ. Recurrent pancreatitis after treatment with hydrochlorothiazide. *J Am Board Fam Pract.* 1994; 7:74-6.
333. Bedrossian S, Vahid B. A case of fatal necrotizing pancreatitis: complication of hydrochlorothiazide and lisinopril therapy. *Dig Dis Sci.* 2007; 52:558-60.
334. Jones MF, Caldwell JR. Acute hemorrhagic pancreatitis associated with administration of chlorthalidone. Report of a case. *N Engl J Med.* 1962; 267:1029-31.
335. Prigogine TH, Futeral B, Kraytman M. Acute hemorrhagic pancreatitis associated with chlorthalidone therapy. *Acta Clinica Belgica.* 1978; 33:272.
336. Ibanez L, Laporte JR, Carne X. Adverse drug reactions leading to hospital admission. *Drug Saf.* 1991; 6:450-9.
337. Bruijn JA, van Albada-Kuipers GA, Smit VT, Eulderink F. Acute pancreatitis in systemic lupus erythematosus. *Scand J Rheumatol.* 1986; 15:363-7.
338. Batalden PB, Van Dyne BJ, Cloyd J. Pancreatitis associated with valproic acid therapy. *Pediatrics.* 1979; 64:520-2.
339. Camfield PR, Bagnell P, Camfield CS, Tibbles JA. Pancreatitis due to valproic acid. *Lancet.* 1979; 1:1198-9.
340. Coulter DL, Allen RJ. Pancreatitis associated with valproic acid therapy for epilepsy. *Ann Neurol.* 1980; 7:92.
341. Parker PH, Helinek GL, Ghishan FK, Greene HL. Recurrent pancreatitis induced by valproic acid. A case report and review of the literature. *Gastroenterology.* 1981; 80:826-8.
342. Evans RJ, Miranda RN, Jordan J, Krolikowski FJ. Fatal acute pancreatitis caused by valproic acid. *Am J Forensic Med Pathol.* 1995; 16:62-5.
343. Mangini RJ. Drug-induced pancreatitis—additional review. *Gastroenterology.* 1980; 79:605.
344. Allen RJ, Coulter DL. Valproic acid induced pancreatitis in children. *Pediatrics.* 1980; 65:1194-5.
345. Ng JY, Disney AP, Jones TE, Purdie G. Acute pancreatitis and sodium valproate. *Med J Aust.* 1982; 2:362.
346. Williams LH, Reynolds RP, Emery JL. Pancreatitis during sodium valproate treatment. *Arch Dis Child.* 1983; 58:543-4.
347. Rosenberg HK, Ortega W. Hemorrhagic pancreatitis in a young child following valproic acid therapy. Clinical and ultrasonic assessment. *Clin Pediatr (Phila).* 1987; 26:98-101.
348. Wyllie E, Wyllie R, Cruse RP et al. Pancreatitis associated with valproic acid therapy. *Am J Dis Child.* 1984; 138:912-4.
349. Lott JA, Bond LW, Bobo RC et al. Valproic acid-associated pancreatitis: report of three cases and a brief review. *Clin Chem.* 1990; 36:395-7.
350. Binek J, Hany A, Heer M. Valproic-acid-induced pancreatitis. Case report and review of the literature. *J Clin Gastroenterol.* 1991; 13:690-3.
351. Pezzilli R, Billi P, Melandri R et al. Anticonvulsant-induced chronic pancreatitis. A case report. *Ital J Gastroenterol.* 1992; 24:245-6.
352. Talwar D. Valproate-associated acute pancreatitis in a child with neuronal ceroid lipofuscinosis. *J Child Neurol.* 1994; 9:36-7.
353. Fecik SE, Stoner SC, Raphael J, Lindsey C. Recurrent acute pancreatitis associated with valproic acid use for mood stabilization. *J Clin Psychopharmacol.* 1999; 19:483-4.
354. Moreiras Plaza M, Rodriguez Goyanes G, Cuina L, Alonso R. On the toxicity of valproic-acid. *Clin Nephrol.* 1999; 51:187-9.
355. Chapman SA, Wacksman GP, Patterson BD. Pancreatitis associated with valproic acid: a review of the literature. *Pharmacotherapy.* 2001; 21:1549-60.
356. Mileusnic D, Donoghue ER, Lifschultz BD. Pathological case of the month: sudden death in a child as a result of pancreatitis during valproic acid therapy. *Pediatr Pathol Mol Med.* 2002; 21:477-84.
357. Yazdani K, Lippmann M, Gala I. Fatal pancreatitis associated with valproic acid: review of the literature. *Medicine (Baltimore).* 2002; 81:305-10.
358. Pellock JM, Wilder BJ, Deaton R, Sommerville KW. Acute pancreatitis coincident with valproate use: a critical review. *Epilepsia.* 2002; 43:1421-4.
359. Depakote (divalproex sodium) package insert. Abbott Park, IL: Abbott Laboratories; 2000.
360. Grosse P, Rusch L, Schmitz B. Pancreatitis complicating treatment with intravenous valproic acid. *J Neurol.* 2002; 249:484-5.
361. Cooper MA, Groll A. A case of chronic pancreatic insufficiency due to valproic acid in a child. *Can J Gastroenterol.* 2001; 15:127-30.
362. Taira N, Nishi H, Mano M et al. Pancreatitis induced by valproic acid: report of a case. *Surg Today.* 2001; 31:1027-31.
363. Torelli D, Galeone D, Lamontanara G. Serum amylase in patients treated with sodium valproate. *Acta Neurol (Napoli).* 1982; 4:455-9.
364. Phillips RA, Nadel ES, Brown DF. Epigastric pain. *J Emerg Med.* 2006; 30:81-4.
365. Ozaydin E, Yukselgungor H, Kose G. Acute hemorrhagic pancreatitis due to the use of valproic acid in a child. *Eur J Paediatr Neurol.* 2008; 12:141-3.
366. Gerstner T, Bauer MO, Longin E et al. Reversible hepatotoxicity, pancreatitis, coagulation disorder and simultaneous bone marrow suppression with valproate in a 2-year-old girl. *Seizure.* 2007; 16:554-6.
367. Grauso-Eby NL, Goldfarb O, Feldman-Winter LB, McAbee GN. Acute pancreatitis in children from Valproic acid: case series and review. *Pediatr Neurol.* 2003; 28:145-8.
368. Houben ML, Wilting I, Stroink H, van Dijken PJ. Pancreatitis, complicated by a pancreatic pseudocyst associated with the use of valproic acid. *Eur J Paediatr Neurol.* 2005; 9:77-80.
369. Yaman A, Kendirli T, Odek C et al. Valproic acid-induced acute pancreatitis and multiorgan failure in a child. *Pediatr Emerg Care.* 2013; 29:659-61.
370. Veri K, Uibo O, Talvik I, Talvik T. Valproic acid-induced pancreatitis in a 15-year-old boy with juvenile myoclonic epilepsy. *Medicina (Kaunas, Lithuania).* 2013; 49:487-9.
371. Capolongo G, Zacchia M, Pollastro RM et al. A case of valproic acid-induced acute pancreatitis in tuberous sclerosis coexisting with end-stage renal disease. *J Nephrol.* 2013; 26:412-6.
372. Dinopoulos A, Karapanou O, Alexopoulou E et al. VPA-induced recurrent pancreatitis in a cystic fibrosis carrier. *Eur J Paediatr Neurol.* 2011; 15:453-5.
373. Santos BL, Fernandes RM, Neves FF. Valproic acid-induced pancreatitis in an adult. *Arq Neuropsiquiatr.* 2010; 68:135-6.
374. Guevara-Campos J, Gonzalez-Guevara L, Vacaro-Bolivar I, Rojas JM. Acute pancreatitis associated to the use of valproic acid. *Arq Neuropsiquiatr* 2009; 67:513-5.

375. Zaccara G, Franciotta D, Perucca E. Idiosyncratic adverse reactions to antiepileptic drugs. *Epilepsia.* 2007; 48:1223-44.
376. Norgaard M, Jacobsen J, Ratanajamit C et al. Valproic acid and risk of acute pancreatitis: a population-based case-control study. *Am J Ther.* 2006; 13:113-7.
377. Star K, Edwards IR, Choonara I. Valproic acid and fatalities in children: a review of individual case safety reports in VigiBase. *PloS one.* 2014; 9:e108970.
378. Storer A. A 54-year-old woman with a rare case of drug-induced pancreatitis. *Adv Emerg Nurs J.* 2011; 33:23-8.
379. Laczek JT, Shrestha M, Kortan ND, Lake JM. Carbamazepine-induced pancreatitis with positive re-challenge. *J Clin Gastroenterol.* 2010; 44:153-4.
380. Forte A, Gallinaro L, Montesano G et al. A possible case of carbamazepine induced pancreatitis. *Riv Eur Sci Med Farmacol.* 1996; 18:187-9.
381. Soman M, Swenson C. A possible case of carbamazepine-induced pancreatitis. *Drug Intell Clin Pharm.* 1985; 19:925-7.
382. Tsao CY, Wright FS. Acute chemical pancreatitis associated with carbamazepine intoxication. *Epilepsia.* 1993; 34:174-6.
383. Jubert P, Fernandez R, Ruiz A. Clozapine-related pancreatitis. *Ann Intern Med.* 1994; 121:722-3.
384. Martin A. Acute pancreatitis associated with clozapine use. *Am J Psychiatry.* 1992; 149:714.
385. Frankenburg FR, Kando J. Eosinophilia. Clozapine, and pancreatitis. *Lancet.* 1992; 340:251.
386. Wehmeier PM, Heiser P, Remschmidt H. Pancreatitis followed by pericardial effusion in an adolescent treated with clozapine. *J Clin Psychopharmacol.* 2003; 23:102-3.
387. Gatto EM, Castronuovo AP, Uribe Roca MC. Clozapine and pancreatitis. *Clin Neuropharmacol.* 1998; 21:203.
388. Huang YJ, Lane HY, Liao CH, Huang CC. Recurrent pancreatitis without eosinophilia on clozapine re-challenge. *Prog Neuropsychopharmacol Biol Psychiatry.* 2009; 33:1561-2.
389. Chengappa KN, Pelucio M, Baker RW, Cole D. Recurrent pancreatitis on clozapine re-challenge. *J Psychopharmacol.* 1995; 9:381-2.
390. Garlipp P, Rosenthal O, Haltenhof H, Machleidt W. The development of a clinical syndrome of asymptomatic pancreatitis and eosinophilia after treatment with clozapine in schizophrenia: implications for clinical care, recognition and management. *J Psychopharmacol.* 2002; 16:399-400.
391. Bergemann N, Ehrig C, Diebold K et al. Asymptomatic pancreatitis associated with clozapine. *Pharmacopsychiatry.* 1999; 32:78-80.
392. Sakhri J, Ben Salem C, Harbi H et al. Severe acute pancreatitis due to tamoxifen-induced hypertriglyceridemia with positive rechallenge. *JOP.* 2010; 11:382-4.
393. Alagozlu H, Cindoruk M, Unal S. Tamoxifen-induced severe hypertriglyceridaemia and acute pancreatitis. *Clin Drug Investig.* 2006; 26:297-302.
394. Lin HH, Hsu CH, Chao YC. Tamoxifen-induced severe acute pancreatitis: a case report. *Dig Dis Sci.* 2004; 49:997-9.
395. Athyros VG, Giouleme OI, Nikolaidis NL et al. Long-term follow-up of patients with acute hypertriglyceridemia-induced pancreatitis. *J Clin Gastroenterol.* 2002; 34:472-5.
396. Artac M, Sari R, Altunbas H, Karayalcin U. Asymptomatic acute pancreatitis due to tamoxifen-induced severe hypertriglyceridemia in a patient with diabetes mellitus and breast cancer. *J Chemother.* 2002; 14:309-11.
397. Elisaf MS, Nakou K, Liamis G, Pavlidis NA. Tamoxifen-induced severe hypertriglyceridemia and pancreatitis. *Ann Oncol.* 2000; 11:1067-9.
398. Colls BM, George PM. Severe hypertriglyceridaemia and hypercholesterolaemia associated with tamoxifen use. *Clin Oncol (R Coll Radiol).* 1998; 10:270-1.
399. Noguchi M, Taniya T, Tajiri K et al. Fatal hyperlipaemia in a case of metastatic breast cancer treated by tamoxifen. *Br J Surg.* 1987; 74:586-7.
400. Sevin A, Chen A, Atkinson B. Tyrosine kinase inhibitor induced pancreatitis. *J Oncol Pharm Pract.* 2013; 19:257-60.
401. Kobayashi Y, Kanemitu T, Kamoto A et al. Painless acute pancreatitis associated with sorafenib treatment: a case report. *Med Oncol.* 2011; 28:463-5.
402. Saadati H, Saif MW. Sorafenib-induced acute pancreatitis. *JOP.* 2010; 11:283-4.
403. Li M, Srinivas S. Acute pancreatitis associated with sorafenib. *South Med J.* 2007; 100:909-11.
404. Amar S, Wu KJ, Tan WW. Sorafenib-induced pancreatitis. *Mayo Clin Proc.* 2007; 82:521.
405. Peron J, Khenifer S, Potier V et al. Axitinib-induced acute pancreatitis: a case report. *Anti-cancer Drugs.* 2014; 25:478-9.
406. Engel T, Justo D, Amitai M et al. Nilotinib-associated acute pancreatitis. *Ann Pharmacother.* 2013; 47:e3.
407. Strumberg D, Richly H, Hilger RA et al. Phase I clinical and pharmacokinetic study of the Novel Raf kinase and vascular endothelial growth factor receptor inhibitor BAY 43-9006 in patients with advanced refractory solid tumors. *J Clin Oncol.* 2005; 23:965-72.
408. Pezzilli R, Corinaldesi R, Morselli-Labate AM. Tyrosine kinase inhibitors and acute pancreatitis. *JOP.* 2010; 11:291-3.
409. Wang HH, Tsui J, Wang XY et al. Bortezomib-induced acute pancreatitis in a patient with multiple myeloma. *Leuk Lymphoma.* 2014; 55:1404-5.
410. Solakoglu T, Akyol P, Guney T et al. Acute pancreatitis caused by bortezomib. *Pancreatology.* 2013; 13:189-90.
411. Elouni B, Ben Salem C, Zamy M et al. Bortezomib-induced acute pancreatitis. *JOP.* 2010; 11:275-6.
412. Solakoglu T, Akar M, Aktan Kosker Tet al. Is bortezomib a rare cause of acute pancreatitis? *JOP.* 2013; 14:682-3.
413. Muluneh B, Buie LW, Collichio F. Vemurafenib-associated pancreatitis: case report. *Pharmacotherapy.* 2013; 33:e43-4.
414. Larkin J, Del Vecchio M, Ascierto PA et al. Vemurafenib in patients with BRAF(V600) mutated metastatic melanoma: an open-label, multicentre, safety study. *Lancet Oncol.* 2014; 15:436-44.
415. Health Canada. Recalls and safety alerts: skin-cancer drug Zelboraf (vemurafenib): new warning on the risk of pancreatitis. http://healthycanadians.gc.ca/recall-alert-rappel-avis/hc-sc/2015/43697a-eng.php?_ga=2.247290756.1690533576.1520344904-444226074.1520344904 (accessed 2018 Mar 6).
416. Urru SA, Mariotti E, Carta P et al. Acute pancreatitis following brentuximab vedotin therapy for refractory Hodgkin lymphoma: a case report. *Drugs R D.* 2014; 14:9-11.
417. Gandhi MD, Evens AM, Fenske TS et al. Pancreatitis in patients treated with brentuximab vedotin: a previously unrecognized serious adverse event. *Blood.* 2014; 123:2895-7.
418. Sotomatsu M, Shimoda M, Ogawa C, Morikawa A. Acute pancreatitis associated with interferon-alpha therapy for chronic myelogenous leukemia. *Am J Hematol.* 1995; 48:211-2.
419. Eland IA, Rasch MC, Sturkenboom MJ et al. Acute pancreatitis attributed to the use of interferon alfa-2b. *Gastroenterology.* 2000; 119:230-3.
420. Tannir NM, Talpaz M, Ghazal H et al. Acute pancreatitis associated with interferon alpha therapy for chronic myelogenous leukemia. *Leuk Lymphoma.* 2000; 39:647-50.
421. Cecchi E, Forte P, Cini E et al. Pancreatitis induced by pegylated interferon alfa-2b in a patient affected by chronic hepatitis C. *Emerg Med Australas.* 2004; 16:473-5.
422. Ozdogan O, Tahan V, Cincin A et al. Acute pancreatitis associated with the use of peginterferon. *Pancreas.* 2007; 34:485-7.
423. Tahan V, Tahan G, Dane F et al. Acute pancreatitis attributed to the use of pegylated interferon in a patient with chronic hepatitis C. *J Gastrointestin Liver Dis.* 2007; 16:224-5.
424. Kim SR, Imoto S, Mita K et al. Pegylated interferon plus ribavirin combination therapy for chronic hepatitis C with high viral load of serum hepatitis C virus RNA, genotype 1b, discontinued on attaining sustained virological response at week 16 after onset of acute pancreatitis. *Digestion.* 2009; 79:36-9.

425. Vignon RK, Seddik H, Rouibaa F et al. Acute pancreatitis during pegylated interferon therapy in a patient with chronic hepatitis B. *J Gastrointestin Liver Dis.* 2009; 18:512.
426. Chaudhari S, Park J, Anand BS et al. Acute pancreatitis associated with interferon and ribavirin therapy in patients with chronic hepatitis C. *Dig Dis Sci.* 2004; 49:1000-6.
427. INTRON A, interferon alfa-2b, recombinant for injection [product information]. Kenilworth, NJ: Merck and Company; 2015.
428. PEGASYS (peginterferon alfa-2a) [product information]. Highlights of prescribing information. South San Francisco, CA: Genentech; 2015.
429. COPEGUS (ribavirin) [product information]. Highlights of prescribing information. South San Francisco, CA: Genentech; 2011.
430. Wang T, Wang F, Gou Z et al. Using real-world data to evaluate the association of incretin-based therapies with risk of acute pancreatitis: a meta-analysis of 1,324,515 patients from observational studies. *Diabetes Obes Metab.* 2015; 17:32-41.
431. Denker PS, Dimarco PE. Exenatide (exendin-4)-induced pancreatitis: a case report. *Diabetes Care.* 2006; 29:471.
432. Cure P, Pileggi A, Alejandro R. Exenatide and rare adverse events. *N Engl J Med.* 2008; 358:1969-1970; discussion 1971-1962.
433. Tripathy NR, Basha S, Jain R et al. Exenatide and acute pancreatitis. *J Assoc Physicians India.* 2008; 56:987-8.
434. Ayoub WA, Kumar AA, Naguib HS, Taylor HC. Exenatide-induced acute pancreatitis. *Endocr Pract.* 2010; 16:80-3.
435. Iyer SN, Drake AJ, 3rd, West RL et al. Case report of acute necrotizing pancreatitis associated with combination treatment of sitagliptin and exenatide. *Endocr Pract.* 2012; 18:e10-3.
436. Lee PH, Stockton MD, Franks AS. Acute pancreatitis associated with liraglutide. *Ann Pharmacother.* 2011; 45:e22.
437. Knezevich E, Crnic T, Kershaw S, Drincic A. Liraglutide-associated acute pancreatitis. *Am J Health-Syst Pharm.* 2012; 69:386-9.
438. Famularo G, Gasbarrone L, Minisola G. Pancreatitis during treatment with liraglutide. *JOP.* 2012; 13:540-1.
439. Bourezane H, Kastler B, Kantelip JP. Late and severe acute necrotizing pancreatitis in a patient with liraglutide. *Therapie.* 2012; 67):539-43.
440. Nakata H, Sugitani S, Yamaji S et al. Pancreatitis with pancreatic tail swelling associated with incretin-based therapies detected radiologically in two cases of diabetic patients with end-stage renal disease. *Intern Med.* 2012; 51:3045-9.
441. Artero A, Bourguet M, Lorente RI, Real JT. [Acute pancreatitis in a patient treated with liraglutide]. *Med Clin (Barc).* 2013; 141:368-9.
442. Jeyaraj S, Shetty AS, Kumar CR et al. Liraglutide-induced acute pancreatitis. *J Assoc Physicians India.* 2014; 62:64-6.
443. Garg R, Hussey C, Ibrahim S. Pancreatitis associated with the use of sitagliptin and orlistat combination: a case report. *Diabet Med.* 2010; 27:485-6.
444. Sue M, Yoshihara A, Kuboki K et al. A case of severe acute necrotizing pancreatitis after administration of sitagliptin. *Clin Med Insights Case Rep.* 2013; 6:23-27.
445. Lee CF, Sun MS, Tai YK. Saxagliptin-induced recurrent acute pancreatitis. *Intl Med.* 2014; 53:1351-4.
446. Girgis CM, Champion BL. Vildagliptin-induced acute pancreatitis. *Endocr Pract.* 2011; 17:e48-50.
447. Saraogi R, Mallik R, Ghosh S. Mild acute pancreatitis with vildagliptin use. *Indian J Endocrinol Metab.* 2012; 16(suppl 2): S480-2.
448. Kunjathaya P, Ramaswami PK, Krishnamurthy AN, Bhat N. Acute necrotizing pancreatitis associated with vildagliptin. *JOP.* 2013; 14:81-4.
449. US Food and Drug Administration. Information for Healthcare Professionals: Exenatide (marketed as Byetta) - 8/2008 Update. 2008. http://www.fda.gov/Drugs/DrugSafety/PostmarketDrugSafetyInformationforPatientsandProviders/ucm124713.htm (accessed 2017 May 16).
450. Department of Health and Human Services, US Food and Drug Administration, Center for Drug Evaluation and Research. Application Number 21-919. Summary review. https://www.accessdata.fda.gov/drugsatfda_docs/nda/2009/021919s000sumr.pdf (accessed 2018 Mar 6).
451. Neumiller JJ. Incretin-based therapies. *Med Clin North Am.* 2015; 99:107-29.
452. de Heer J, Goke B. Are incretin mimetics and enhancers linked to pancreatitis and malignant transformations in pancreas? *Expert Opin Drug Saf.* 2014; 13:1469-81.
453. Elashoff M, Matveyenko AV, Gier B et al. Pancreatitis, pancreatic, and thyroid cancer with glucagon-like peptide-1-based therapies. *Gastroenterol.* 2011; 141:150-6.
454. Cohen D. Reports of pancreatitis are 20–30 times more likely with GLP-1 drugs, analysis finds. *BMJ.* 2013; 346:f2607.
455. Delfino M, Motola D, Benini A et al. Incretin-mimetics associated pancreatitis: evidence from the spontaneous adverse drug reactions reporting in Italy. *Expert Opin Drug Saf.* 2014; 13:151-6.
456. Li X, Zhang Z, Duke J. Glucagon-like peptide 1-based therapies and risk of pancreatitis: a self-controlled case series analysis. *Pharmacoepidemiol Drug Saf.* 2014; 23:234-9.
457. Giorda CB, Picariello R, Nada E et al. Incretin therapies and risk of hospital admission for acute pancreatitis in an unselected population of European patients with type 2 diabetes: a case-control study. *Lancet Diabetes Endocrinol.* 2014; 2:111-5.
458. Faillie JL, Azoulay L, Patenaude V et al. Incretin based drugs and risk of acute pancreatitis in patients with type 2 diabetes: cohort study. *BMJ.* 2014; 348:g2780.
459. Chou HC, Chen WW, Hsiao FY. Acute pancreatitis in patients with type 2 diabetes mellitus treated with dipeptidyl peptidase-4 inhibitors: a population-based nested case-control study. *Drug Saf.* 2014; 37:521-8.
460. Funch D, Gydesen H, Tornoe K et al. A prospective, claims-based assessment of the risk of pancreatitis and pancreatic cancer with liraglutide compared to other antidiabetic drugs. *Diabetes Obes Metab.* 2014; 16:273-5.
461. Eurich DT, Simpson S, Senthilselvan A et al. Comparative safety and effectiveness of sitagliptin in patients with type 2 diabetes: retrospective population based cohort study. *BMJ.* 2013; 346:f2267.
462. Dore DD, Hussein M, Hoffman C et al. A pooled analysis of exenatide use and risk of acute pancreatitis. *Curr Med Res Opin.* 2013; 29:1577-86.
463. Wenten M, Gaebler JA, Hussein M et al. Relative risk of acute pancreatitis in initiators of exenatide twice daily compared with other anti-diabetic medication: a follow-up study. *Diabet Med.* 2012; 29:1412-8.
464. Romley JA, Goldman DP, Solomon M et al. Exenatide therapy and the risk of pancreatitis and pancreatic cancer in a privately insured population. *Diabetes Technol. Ther.* 2012; 14:904-11.
465. Dore DD, Bloomgren GL, Wenten M et al. A cohort study of acute pancreatitis in relation to exenatide use. *Diabetes Obes Metab.* 2011; 13:559-66.
466. Garg R, Chen W, Pendergrass M. Acute pancreatitis in type 2 diabetes treated with exenatide or sitagliptin: a retrospective observational pharmacy claims analysis. *Diabetes Care.* 2010; 33:2349-54.
467. Dore DD, Seeger JD, Arnold Chan K. Use of a claims-based active drug safety surveillance system to assess the risk of acute pancreatitis with exenatide or sitagliptin compared to metformin or glyburide. *Curr Med Res Opin.* 2009; 25:1019-27.
468. Monami M, Dicembrini I, Nardini C et al. Glucagon-like peptide-1 receptor agonists and pancreatitis: a meta-analysis of randomized clinical trials. *Diabetes Res Clin Pract.* 2014; 103:269-75.
469. Monami M, Dicembrini I, Mannucci E. Dipeptidyl peptidase-4 inhibitors and pancreatitis risk: a meta-analysis of randomized clinical trials. *Diabetes Obes Metab.* 2014; 16:48-56.
470. Li L, Shen J, Bala MM et al. Incretin treatment and risk of pancreatitis in patients with type 2 diabetes mellitus: systematic review and meta-analysis of randomised and non-randomised studies. *BMJ.* 2014; 348:g2366.

471. Alves C, Batel-Marques F, Macedo AF. A meta-analysis of serious adverse events reported with exenatide and liraglutide: acute pancreatitis and cancer. *Diabetes Res Clin Pract.* 2012; 98:271-84.
472. Meier JJ, Nauck MA. Risk of pancreatitis in patients treated with incretin-based therapies. *Diabetologia.* 2014; 57:1320-4.
473. Engel SS, Williams-Herman DE, Golm GT et al. Sitagliptin: review of preclinical and clinical data regarding incidence of pancreatitis. *Int J Clin Pract.* 2010; 64:984-90.
474. Ligueros-Saylan M, Foley JE, Schweizer A et al. An assessment of adverse effects of vildagliptin versus comparators on the liver, the pancreas, the immune system, the skin and in patients with impaired renal function from a large pooled database of Phase II and III clinical trials. *Diabetes Obes Metab.* 2010; 12:495-509.
475. Macconell L, Brown C, Gurney K, Han J. Safety and tolerability of exenatide twice daily in patients with type 2 diabetes: integrated analysis of 5594 patients from 19 placebo-controlled and comparator-controlled clinical trials. *Diabetes Metab Syndr Obes.* 2012; 5:29-41.
476. MacConell L, Gurney K, Malloy J et al. Safety and tolerability of exenatide once weekly in patients with type 2 diabetes: an integrated analysis of 4,328 patients. *Diabetes Metab Syndr Obes.* 2015; 8:241-53.
477. Singh S, Chang HY, Richards TM et al. Glucagonlike peptide 1-based therapies and risk of hospitalization for acute pancreatitis in type 2 diabetes mellitus: a population-based matched case-control study. *JAMA Intern Med.* 2013; 173:534-9.
478. Raz I, Bhatt DL, Hirshberg B et al. Incidence of pancreatitis and pancreatic cancer in a randomized controlled multicenter trial (SAVOR-TIMI 53) of the dipeptidyl peptidase-4 inhibitor saxagliptin. *Diabetes Care.* 2014; 37:2435-41.
479. White WB, Cannon CP, Heller SR et al. Alogliptin after acute coronary syndrome in patients with type 2 diabetes. *N Engl J Med.* 2013; 369:1327-35.
480. Green JB, Bethel MA, Armstrong PW et al. Effect of sitagliptin on cardiovascular outcomes in type 2 diabetes. *N Engl J Med.* 2015; 373:232-42.
481. Pi-Sunyer X, Astrup A, Fujioka K et al. A randomized, controlled trial of 3.0 mg of liraglutide in weight management. *N Engl J Med.* 2015; 373:11-22.
482. Egan AG, Blind E, Dunder K et al. Pancreatic safety of incretin-based drugs—FDA and EMA assessment. *N Engl J Med.* 2014; 370:794-7.
483. Bosch X, Bernadich O. Acute pancreatitis during treatment with amiodarone. *Lancet.* 1997; 350:1300.
484. Chen YY, Chen CY, Leung KK. Acute pancreatitis and amiodarone: a case report. *World J Gastroenterol.* 2007; 13:975-7.
485. Famularo G, Minisola G, Nicotra GC, De Simone C. Acute pancreatitis caused by amiodarone. *Eur J Emerg Med.* 2004; 11:305-6.
486. Alonso A, MacLehose RF, Lutsey PL et al. Association of amiodarone use with acute pancreatitis in patients with atrial fibrillation: a nested case-control study. *JAMA Int Med.* 2015; 175:449-50.
487. Yang M, Qu H, Deng HC. Acute pancreatitis induced by methimazole in a patient with Graves' disease. *Thyroid.* 2012; 22:94-6.
488. Chng CL, Kek PC, Khoo DH. Carbimazole-induced acute pancreatitis and cholestatic hepatitis. *Endocr Pract.* 2011; 17:960-1.
489. Marazuela M, Sanchez de Paco G, Jimenez I et al. Acute pancreatitis, hepatic cholestasis, and erythema nodosum induced by carbimazole treatment for Graves' disease. *Endocr J.* 2002; 49:315-8.
490. Taguchi M, Yokota M, Koyano H et al. Acute pancreatitis and parotitis induced by methimazole in a patient with Graves' disease. *Clin Endocrinol (Oxf).* 1999; 51:667-70.
491. Rutledge PL, Saluja AK, Powers RE, Steer ML. Role of oxygen-derived free radicals in diet-induced hemorrhagic pancreatitis in mice. *Gastroenterology.* 1987; 93:41-7.
492. Blind PJ, Marklund SL, Stenling R, Dahlgren ST. Parenteral superoxide dismutase plus catalase diminishes pancreatic edema in sodium taurocholate-induced pancreatitis in the rat. *Pancreas.* 1988; 3:563-7.
493. Steinberg WM. Acute drug and toxin induced pancreatitis. *Hosp Pract (Off Ed).* 1985; 20:95-102.
494. Murphy RL, Noskin GA, Ehrenpreis ED. Acute pancreatitis associated with aerosolized pentamidine. *Am J Med.* 1990; 88:53N-6N.
495. Ludwig GD, Chaykin LD. Pancreatitis associated with primary hyperparathyroidism. *Med Clin North Am.* 1966; 50:1403-18.
496. Debongnie JC, Dekoninck X. Sulfasalazine. 5-ASA and acute pancreatitis in Crohn's disease. *J Clin Gastroenterol.* 1994; 19:348-9.
497. Lerche A, Vyberg M, Kirkegaard E. Acute cholangitis and pancreatitis associated with sulindac (clinoril). *Histopathology.* 1987; 11:647-53.
498. Sanfey H, Bulkley GB, Cameron JL. The role of oxygen-derived free radicals in the pathogenesis of acute pancreatitis. *Ann Surg.* 1984; 200:405-13.
499. Pippenger CD, Meng X, Van Lente F, Rothner AD. Valproate therapy depresses free radical scavenging enzyme activity: a probable mechanism for induction of acute pancreatitis or hepatotoxicity. *Neurology.* 1989; 39(suppl 1):214.
500. Asconape JJ, Penry JK, Dreifuss FE et al. Valproate-associated pancreatitis. *Epilepsia.* 1993; 34:177-83.
501. Whitecar JP Jr, Bodey GP, Harris JE, Freireich EJ. L-asparaginase. *N Engl J Med.* 1970; 282:732-4.
502. Dolowy WC, Henson D, Cornet J, Sellin H. Toxic and antineoplastic effects of L-asparaginase. Study of mice with lymphoma and normal monkeys and report on a child with leukemia. *Cancer.* 1966; 19:1813-9.
503. Earl M. Incidence and management of asparaginase-associated adverse events in patients with acute lymphoblastic leukemia. *Clin Adv Hematol Oncol.* 2009; 7:600-6.
504. Carbone PP, Haskell CM, Leventhal BGet al. Clinical experience with L-asparaginase. *Recent Results Cancer Res.* 1970; 33:236-43.
505. Gailani S, Nussbaum A, Onuma T, Freeman A. Diabetes in patients treated with asparaginase. *Clin Pharmacol Ther.* 1971; 12:487-90.
506. Hoffmann TF, Waldner H, Messmer K. The bradykinin antagonist CP-0597 can limit the progression of postischemic pancreatitis. *Immunopharmacology.* 1996; 33:243-6.
507. Sunamura M, Yamauchi J, Shibuya K et al. Pancreatic microcirculation in acute pancreatitis. *J Hepatobiliary Pancreat Surg.* 1998; 5:62-8.
508. Griesbacher T, Lembeck F. Effects of the bradykinin antagonist, HOE 140, in experimental acute pancreatitis. *Br J Pharmacol.* 1992; 107:356-60.
509. Dabaghi S. ACE inhibitors and pancreatitis. *Ann Intern Med.* 1991; 115:330-1.
510. Gershon T, Olshaker JS. Acute pancreatitis following lisinopril re-challenge. *Am J Emerg Med.* 1998; 16:523-4.
511. Miller LG, Tan G. Drug-induced pancreatitis (lisinopril). *J Am Board Fam Pract.* 1999; 12:150-3.
512. Bi CK, Soltani K, Sloan JB et al. Induction of tissue specific autoantibodies by captopril. *Clin Res.* 1988; 36:633A.
513. Haye OL. Piroxicam and pancreatitis. *Ann Intern Med.* 1986; 104:895.
514. Wedgwood KR, Adler G, Kern H, Reber HA. Effects of oral agents on pancreatic duct permeability. A model of acute alcoholic pancreatitis. *Dig Dis Sci.* 1986; 31:1081-8.
515. Mosley JG, Fox JN, Reber HA. Aspirin secretion by the pancreas: effect on the pancreatic duct mucosal barrier. *Surgery.* 1979; 86:17-22.
516. Mentes A, Batur Y, Bayol U. Salycylate–induced pancreatic injury in the cat: a preliminary study. *Rom J Gastroenterol.* 2002; 11:309-12.

517. Standfield NJ, Kakkar VV. Prostaglandins and acute pancreatitis—experimental and clinical studies. *Br J Surg.* 1983; 70:573-6.
518. Steer ML, Meldolesi J. The cell biology of experimental pancreatitis. *N Engl J Med.* 1987; 316:144-50.
519. Kimura T, Zuidema GD, Cameron JL. Steroid administration and acute pancreatitis: studies with an isolated, perfused canine pancreas. *Surgery.* 1979; 85:520-4.
520. Dreiling DA, Janowitz HD, Rolbin H. Effect of ACTH and adrenocortical steroids on external pancreatic secretion in man. *N Engl J Med.* 1958; 258:603-5.
521. Pezzilli R, Fabbri D, Imbrogno A, Corinaldesi R. Tyrosine kinase inhibitors, pancreatic hyperenzymemia and acute pancreatitis: a review. *Recent Pat Inflamm Allergy Drug Discov.* 2011; 5:165-8.
522. Ranson JH, Rifkind KM, Roses DF et al. Prognostic signs and the role of operative management in acute pancreatitis. *Surg Gynecol Obstet.* 1974; 139:69-81.
523. Grendell JH. Acute pancreatitis. *Clin Perspect Gastroenterol.* 2000; 3:327-33.
524. Somogyi L, Martin SP, Venkatesan T, Ulrich CD, 2nd. Recurrent acute pancreatitis: an algorithmic approach to identification and elimination of inciting factors. *Gastroenterology.* 2001; 120:708-17.
525. Ksiadzyna D. Drug-induced acute pancreatitis related to medications commonly used in gastroenterology. *Eur J Case Rep Intern Med.* 2011; 22:20-5.
526. Steinberg W, Tenner S. Acute pancreatitis. *N Engl J Med.* 1994; 330:1198-1210.
527. Cooper ST, Slivka A. Incidence, risk factors, and prevention of post-ERCP pancreatitis. *Gastroenterol Clin North Am.* 2007; 36:259-76, vii-viii.
528. Sigounas DE, Christodoulou DK, Tatsioni A et al. Pancreatitis potentially associated drugs as a risk factor for post-endoscopic retrograde cholangiopancreatography pancreatitis: a prospective cohort study. *Pancreas.* 2013; 42:601-6.
529. Mixter CJ, Keynes M, Cope O. Further experience with pancreatitis as a diagnostic clue to hyperparathyroidism. *N Engl J Med.* 1962; 266:265-272.
530. Gafter U, Mandel EM, Har-Zahav L, Weiss S. Acute pancreatitis secondary to hypercalcemia. Occurrence in a patient with breast carcinoma. *JAMA.* 1976; 235:2004-5.
531. May P, Levy RP. Thyrotoxicosis associated with renal tubular acidosis and acute pancreatitis: a case report. *Ann Intern Med.* 1976; 84:569-70. Letter.
532. Meltzer LE, Palmon FP Jr, Paik YK, Custer RP. Acute pancreatitis secondary to hypercalcemia of multiple myeloma. *Ann Intern Med.* 1962; 57:1008-12.
533. Evans DB, Slapak M. Pancreatitis in the hard water syndrome. *Br Med J.* 1975; 3:748.
534. Waele BD, Smitz J, Willems G. Recurrent pancreatitis secondary to hypercalcemia following vitamin D poisoning. *Pancreas.* 1989; 4:378-80.
535. Moir DC. Drug-associated acute pancreatitis. *Lancet.* 1978; 2:369-70.
536. Tromm A, Huppe D, Micklefield GH et al. Acute pancreatitis complicating Crohn's disease: mere coincidence or causality? *Gut.* 1992; 33:1289-91.
537. McArthur KE. Review article: drug-induced pancreatitis. *Aliment Pharmacol Ther.* 1996; 10:23-38.
538. Borgia MC, Celestini A, Caravella P, Catalano C. Angiotensin-converting-enzyme inhibitor administration must be monitored for serum amylase and lipase in order to prevent an acute pancreatitis: a case report. *Angiology.* 2001; 52:645-7.
539. Lankisch PG, Werner HM. Mirtazapine: another drug responsible for drug-induced acute pancreatitis? A letter of warning. *Pancreas.* 2003; 26:211.
540. Cooney DA, Handschumacher RE. L-asparaginase and L-asparagine metabolism. *Annu Rev Pharmacol.* 1970; 10:421-40.
541. Samuels BI, Culbert SJ, Okamura J, Sullivan MP. Early detection of chemotherapy-related pancreatic enlargement in children using abdominal sonography: a preliminary report. *Cancer.* 1976; 38:1515-23.
542. Nguyen DL, Wilson DA, Engelman ED et al. Serial sonograms to detect pancreatitis in children receiving L-asparaginase. *South Med J.* 1987; 80:1133-6.
543. Elspar-asparaginase package insert. West Point, PA: Merck and Company; 2000.
544. Frick TW, Speiser DE, Bimmler D, Largiader F. Drug-induced acute pancreatitis: further criticism. *Dig Dis.* 1993; 11:113-32.
545. Jeandidier N, Klewansky M, Pinget M. Captopril-induced acute pancreatitis. *Diabetes Care.* 1995; 18:410-1.
546. Iliopoulou A, Giannakopoulos G, Pagoy H et al. Acute pancreatitis due to captopril treatment. *Dig Dis Sci.* 2001; 46:1882-3.
547. Hastier P, Longo F, Buckley M et al. Pancreatitis induced by codeine: a case report with positive re-challenge. *Gut.* 1997; 41:705-6.
548. Hastier P, Buckley MJ, Peten EP et al. A new source of drug-induced acute pancreatitis: codeine. *Am J Gastroenterol.* 2000; 95:3295-8.
549. Kaplan MH, Dreiling DA. Steroids revisited. II. Was cortisone responsible for the pancreatitis? *Am J Gastroenterol.* 1977; 67:141-7.
550. Schrier RW, Bulger RJ. Steroid-induced pancreatitis. *JAMA.* 1965; 194:564-5.
551. Levine RA, McGuire RF. Corticosteroid-induced pancreatitis: a case report demonstrating recurrence with re-challenge. *Am J Gastroenterol.* 1988; 83:1161-4.
552. Barr HS, Wolff OH. Pancreatic necrosis in cortisone-treated children. *Lancet.* 1957; 272:812-5.
553. Bourne MS, Dawson H. Acute pancreatitis complicating prednisolone therapy. *Lancet.* 1958; 2:1209-10.
554. Nelp WB. Acute pancreatitis associated with steroid therapy. *Arch Intern Med.* 1961; 108:702-10.
555. Cortese AF, Glenn F. Hypocalcemia and tetany with steroid-induced acute pancreatitis. *Arch Surg.* 1968; 96:119-22.
556. Riemenschneider TA, Wilson JF, Vernier RL. Glucocorticoid-induced pancreatitis in children. *Pediatrics.* 1968; 41:428-37.
557. Goldberg BH, Bergstein JM. Acute respiratory distress in a child after steroid-induced pancreatitis. *Pediatrics.* 1978; 61:317-8.
558. Carone FA, Liebow AA. Acute pancreatic lesions in patients treated with ACTH and adrenal corticoids. *N Engl J Med.* 1957; 257:690-7.
559. [No authors listed]. Pancreatitis in children on steroid therapy. *Br Med J.* 1968; 4:533-4.
560. Oppenheimer EH, Boitnott JK. Pancreatitis in children following adrenal corticosteroid therapy. *Bull Johns Hopkins Hosp.* 1960; 107:297-306.
561. Levin TL, Berdon WE, Tang HB, Haller JO. Dideoxyinosine-induced pancreatitis in human immunodeficiency virus-infected children. *Pediatr Radiol.* 1997; 27:189-91.
562. Bush ZM, Kosmiski LA. Acute pancreatitis in HIV-infected patients: are etiologies changing since the introduction of protease inhibitor therapy? *Pancreas.* 2003; 27:e1-5.
563. McCarthy AE, Keystone JS, Kain KC. Pancreatitis occurring during therapy with stibogluconate: two case reports. *Clin Infect Dis.* 1993; 17:952-3.
564. Halim MA, Alfurayh O, Kalin ME et al. Successful treatment of visceral leishmaniasis with allopurinol plus ketoconazole in a renal transplant recipient after the occurrence of pancreatitis due to stibogluconate. *Clin Infect Dis.* 1993; 16:397-9.
565. Donovan KL, White AD, Cooke DA, Fisher DJ. Pancreatitis and palindromic arthropathy with effusions associated with sodium stibogluconate treatment in a renal transplant recipient. *J Infect.* 1990; 21:107-10.

566. McBride MO, Linney M, Davidson RN, Weber JN. Pancreatic necrosis following treatment of leishmaniasis with sodium stibogluconate. *Clin Infect Dis.* 1995; 21:710.

567. Reymond JM, Desmeules J. Sodium stibogluconate (pentostan) overdose in a patient with acquired immunodeficiency syndrome. *Ther Drug Monit.* 1998; 20:714-6.

568. Lambertucci JR, Franca BM, Queiroz Ede M. Acute pancreatitis caused by meglumine antimoniate given for the treatment of visceral leishmaniasis. *Rev Soc Bras Med Trop.* 2004; 37:74-5.

569. Kuyucu N, Kara C, Bakirtac A, Tezic T. Successful treatment of visceral leishmaniasis with allopurinol plus ketoconazole in an infant who developed pancreatitis caused by meglumine antimoniate. *Pediatr Infect Dis J.* 2001; 20:455-7.

570. Gasser RA Jr, Magill AJ, Oster CN et al. Pancreatitis induced by pentavalent antimonial agents during treatment of leishmaniasis. *Clin Infect Dis.* 1994; 18:83-90.

571. de Lalla F, Pellizzer G, Gradoni L et al. Acute pancreatitis associated with the administration of meglumine antimonate for the treatment of visceral leishmaniasis. *Clin Infect Dis.* 1993; 16:730-1.

572. Domingo P, Ferrer S, Kolle L et al. Acute pancreatitis associated with sodium stibogluconate treatment in a patient with human immunodeficiency virus. *Arch Intern Med.* 1996; 156:1029, 1032.

573. Hunninghake D, Bakker-Arkema RG, Wigand JP et al. Treating to meet NCEP-recommended LDL cholesterol concentrations with atorvastatin, fluvastatin, lovastatin, or simvastatin in patients with risk factors for coronary heart disease. *J Fam Pract.* 1998; 47:349-56.

574. Wong PW, Dillard TA, Kroenke K. Multiple organ toxicity from addition of erythromycin to long-term lovastatin therapy. *South Med J.* 1998; 91:202-5.

575. Gilson M, Moachon L, Jeanne L et al. Acute pancreatitis related to tigecycline: case report and review of the literature. *Scand J Infect Dis.* 2008; 40:681-3.

576. Bosch X. Losartan-induced acute pancreatitis. *Ann Intern Med.* 1997; 127:1043-4.

577. Birck R, Keim V, Fiedler F, van der Woude FJ, Rohmeiss P. Pancreatitis after losartan. *Lancet.* 1998; 351:1178.

578. Gang N, Langevitz P, Livneh A. Relapsing acute pancreatitis induced by re-exposure to the cholesterol lowering agent bezafibrate. *Am J Gastroenterol.* 1999; 94:3626-8.

579. Fang CC, Wang HP, Lin JT. Erythromycin-induced acute pancreatitis. *J Toxicol Clin Toxicol.* 1996; 34:93-5.

580. Gumaste VV. Erythromycin-induced pancreatitis. *Am J Med.* 1989; 86(Part 1):725.

581. Hawksworth CR. Acute pancreatitis associated with infusion of erythromycin lactobionate. *BMJ.* 1989; 298:190.

582. Hung MC, Hung GY, Lin PC et al. Acute pancreatitis associated with ifosfamide. *J Chin Med Assoc.* 2007; 70:176-9.

583. Gerson R, Serrano A, Villalobos A et al. Acute pancreatitis secondary to ifosfamide. *J Emerg Med.* 1997; 15:645-7.

584. Passier JL, van Puijenbroek EP, Jonkers GJ, van Grootheest AC. Pancreatitis associated with the use of itraconazole. *Neth J Med.* 2010; 68:285-9.

585. EPIVIR-HBV (lamivudine) package insert. Research Triangle Park, NC: GlaxoSmithKline LLC; 2009.

586. Woodall BS, DiGregorio RV. Comment: olanzapine-induced acute pancreatitis. *Ann Pharmacother.* 2001; 35:506-8.

587. Hagger R, Brown C, Hurley P. Olanzapine and pancreatitis. *Br J Psychiatry.* 2000; 177:567.

588. Doucette DE, Grenier JP, Robertson PS. Olanzapine-induced acute pancreatitis. *Ann Pharmacother.* 2000; 34:1128-31.

589. Gupta A, Ghoshal UC, Mohindra S, Saraswat VA. Acute necrotizing pancreatitis following olanzapine therapy. *Tropical Gastroenterology: Official Journal of the Digestive Diseases Foundation.* 2014; 35:132-4.

590. Kose M, Emet S, Akpinar TS et al. An unexpected result of obesity treatment: Orlistat-related acute pancreatitis. *Case Rep Gastroenterol.* 2015; 9:152-5.

591. Napier S, Thomas M. 36- year-old man presenting with pancreatitis and a history of recent commencement of Orlistat case report. *Nutr J.* 2006; 5:19.

592. Ahmad FA, Mahmud S. Acute pancreatitis following orlistat therapy: report of two cases. *JOP.* 2010; 11:61-3.

593. Falko JM, Thomas FB. Acute pancreatitis due to procainamide-induced lupus erythematosus. *Ann Intern Med.* 1975; 83:832-3. Letter.

594. ZERIT (stavudine) package insert. Princeton, NJ: Bristol-Myers Squibb Company; 2010.

595. Riedel DJ, Gebo KA, Moore RD, Lucas GM. A ten-year analysis of the incidence and risk factors for acute pancreatitis requiring hospitalization in an urban HIV clinical cohort. *AIDS Patient Care STDS.* 2008; 22:113-21.

596. HIVID (zalcitabine) tablets package insert. Nutley, NJ: Roche Laboratories; 2000.

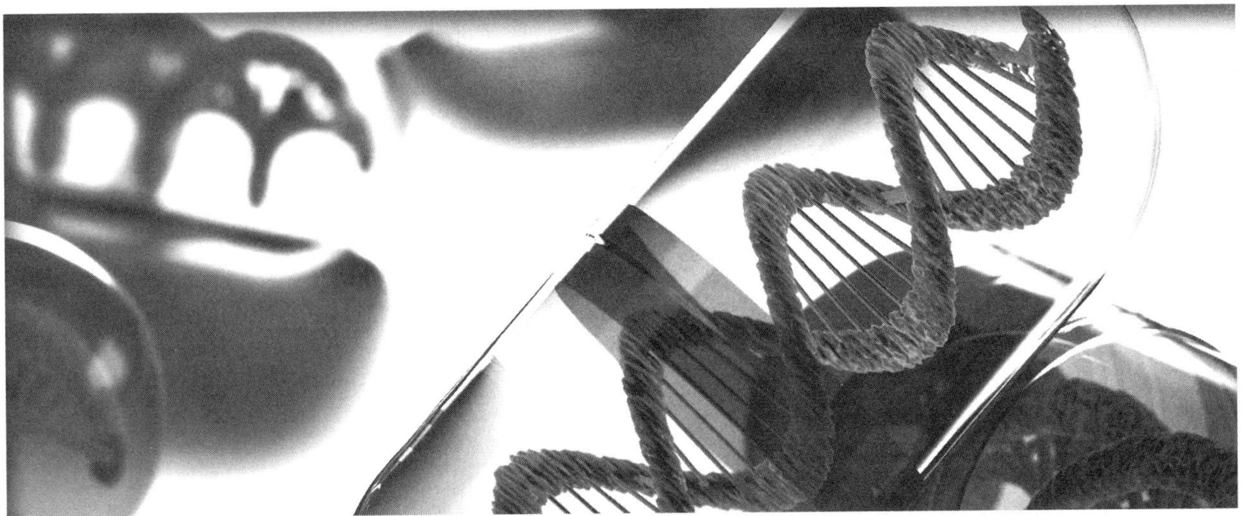

CHAPTER 40

Nausea and Vomiting

Saeed K. Alzghari, Bonnie A. Labdi, and Jon D. Herrington

Nausea and vomiting account for the majority of medication-related gastrointestinal (GI) maladies.[1] Although any drug, including placebos, can potentially induce nausea and vomiting, some classes of medications are more likely to cause these effects than others.[2] Drug-induced nausea and vomiting can adversely affect quality of life, and patients who experience significant symptoms may stop taking the culprit drug as prescribed, thus compromising their own treatment. If therapy is continued, symptoms can become severe enough to interfere with normal daily activities, and, if left untreated, vomiting can lead to serious health risks, including esophageal tears and malnutrition, requiring additional medical attention.

Nausea is a subjective feeling and a singular symptom. It may or may not be followed by vomiting, although both are thought to be components of the same reflex.[3,4] The term itself is derived from the Greek word *naus,* meaning ship, alluding to the way one feels when seasick.[5] Nausea is most easily defined as an inclination to vomit, or the way one feels when vomiting is imminent.

Practically any drug can cause nausea, vomiting, or both via one of several mechanisms, and many can cause nausea and vomiting through a combination of mechanisms. Three classes of drugs known to cause nausea and vomiting in a significant percentage of patients—the opioids, the anesthetics and related drugs, and the chemotherapeutic agents—will be discussed in detail in this chapter. Other miscellaneous agents will be discussed where information exists.

CAUSATIVE AGENTS

Agents commonly associated with nausea and vomiting are listed in **Table 40-1**. References cited are from controlled trials of single agents administered without prophylactic antiemetics.[6-115] Because of the large number of agents reported to cause nausea and vomiting and wide interindividual variability, this list should not be regarded as comprehensive.

Note: The authors wish to acknowledge the work of Dr. Erika N. Brown, who authored this chapter in a previous edition.

Table 40-1 Agents Implicated in Drug-Induced Nausea and Vomiting

Drug	Incidence	Level of Evidence[a]
OPIOIDS		
Alfentanil[6]	N = 19% V = 9%	A
Buprenorphine[7]	V = 20%	A
Butorphanol IV[8,9]	V = 14% N/V = 13%	A
Codeine[10,11]	N = 41% V = 24% N/V = 44%	A
Diamorphine[7]	V = 12%	A
Dihydrocodeine[12]	N = 15–27% V = 10–12%	A
Fentanyl IV[6,13]	N = 19–32% V = 10–20%	A
Hydrocodone[10]	N = 29% V = 10%	A
Hydromorphone[14]	N = 35% V = 17%	A
Meperidine[15]	N/V = 13%	B
Methadone[16]	N = 50% V = 24%	B
Morphine[13,17,18]	N = 20–52% V = 15–36%	A
Nalbuphine[18]	N = 4% V = 4%	A
Oxycodone[14]	N = 30% V = 12%	A
Oxymorphone[19]	N = 39% V = 24%	A
Piritramide[17]	N = 30% V = 19%	A
Propoxyphene[11]	N/V = 38%	A
Remifentanil[13]	N = 20% V = 8%	A
Sufentanil[6]	N = 19% V = 7%	A
Tapentadol (75 mg)[20]	N = 21% V = 14%	A
Tramadol[10,11]	N = 39% V = 16% N/V = 39%	A
INHALED ANESTHETICS		
Desflurane[21]	N/V = 11%	A
Enflurane[22]	V = 41%	A
Halothane[22]	V = 46%	A
Isoflurane[22]	V = 36%	A

Table 40-1 Agents Implicated in Drug-Induced Nausea and Vomiting (continued)

Drug	Incidence	Level of Evidence[a]
Nitrous oxide[23]	N = 44% V = 15%	A
Sevoflurane[21,24]	N = 32% V = 17%	A
IV ANESTHETICS		
Etomidate[25]	V = 13%	A
Ketamine[26,27]	N = 22% V= 18%	A
Methohexital[28,29]	N = 13% V = 0–1%	A
Propofol[24,30]	N = 6% V = 0–3%	A
Thiopental[31]	N = 35% V = 25%	A
NEUROMUSCULAR BLOCKING AGENTS		
Pancuronium[32]	N = 17% V = 9%	A
Rocuronium[32]	N = 9% V = 9%	A
CHEMOTHERAPY AGENTS		
Actinomycin D[33]	N = 85% V = 46%	B
Amifostine (≥450 mg/m^2)[34,35]	N = <100% V = 14–100%	B
Aldesleukin (≥25 million units/m^2)[36]	N = 35% V = 24%	B
Altretamine[37]	N = 63% V = 54%	B
Arsenic trioxide[38,39]	N = 75% V = 58% N/V = 50%	B
Azacitidine[40]	N = 70% V = 54%	C
Bendamustine[41,42]	N = 20–72% V = 16–41%	B
Bosutinib[43]	N = 32% V = 33%	A
Busulfan[44] (3.2 mg/kg of body weight per day IV)	N = 92% V = 43%	C
Carboplatin[45-47]	V = 55–65% N/V = 86%	B
Carmustine (200 mg/m^2 to 1,050 mg/m^2)[48]	N = 76% V = 32% N/V = 28%	A
Ceritinib[49]	N = 82% V = 65%	B
Cisplatin (50–120 mg/m^2)[50,51]	V = 87–100%	A

Table 40-1 Agents Implicated in Drug-Induced Nausea and Vomiting (continued)

Drug	Incidence	Level of Evidence[a]
Clofarabine[52]	N = 41% V = 22%	C
Crizotinib[53]	N = 56% V = 39%	B
Cyclophosphamide (40–75 mg/kg)[54,55] (1,500 mg/m^2)[56]	N = 92% V = 92% N/V = 89–100%	A
Cyclophosphamide (oral)[57,58]	N = 40% V = 18–20%	A
Cytarabine (1,000 mg/m^2)[59-61]	N = 75% N/V = 64–100%	A
Dacarbazine[62]	V = 49% N/V = 14%	A
Daunorubicin[63]	N = 55% V = 45%	A
Docetaxel[64]	N/V = 15%	B
Doxorubicin (40–75 mg/m^2)[65-69]	N/V = 32–95% V = 71%	A
Eribulin[70]	N = 41% V = 12%	B
Etoposide[71]	N/V = 42%	B
Epirubicin[67]	V = 53%	A
Idarubicin[72]	N/V = 35%	B
Ifosfamide[73-75]	N/V = 50–100%	A
Imatinib[43]	N = 36% V = 16%	A
Irinotecan[76]	N/V = 53%	B
Lenvatinib[77]	N = 41% V = 28%	A
Lomustine[48,78]	V = 31% N/V =38%	A
Mechlorethamine[79]	N/V = 93%	B
Methotrexate (40–60 mg/m^2)[80]	N = 37% V = 34%	B
Mitoxantrone[68]	N/V = 48%	A
Oxaliplatin[81]	N/V = 95%	B
Paclitaxel (40 mg/m^2)[82]	N/V = 10%	B
Nab-paclitaxel[83]	N = 38% V = 11%	B
Pazopanib[84]	N = 25–54% V = 21–33%	A
Pemetrexed[85]	N/V = 24%	B
Pralatrexate[86]	N = 54%	B
Procarbazine[78,87]	N = 34% V = 27–32%	A
Sorafenib[84]	N = 11–19% V = 5–12%	A
Sunitinib[84]	N = 24–45% V = 15–34%	A

Table 40-1 Agents Implicated in Drug-Induced Nausea and Vomiting (continued)

Drug	Incidence	Level of Evidence[a]
Streptozocin[78,88,89]	V = 70% N/V = 83–87%	A
Temozolomide[90]	N = 80% V = 73%	B
Topotecan (10 mg/m^2)[91]	N/V = 8%	B
ANTI-INFECTIVES		
Abacavir[92]	N/V = 35%	A
Erythromycin[93]	N/V = 53%	A
Metronidazole[94]	N = 27–56% V = 22–23%	A
Tigecycline[95,96]	N = 25–31% V = 12–26%	A
Trimethoprim–sulfamethoxazole[97,98]	N = 7–58% V = 5–25%	A
Imipenem–cilastatin[95]	N = 25% V = 19%	A
Ritonavir[99]	N = 30% V = 15%	A
Zidovudine[100]	N = 47–58% V = 10–11%	B
PSYCHOTROPICS		
Bupropion[101,102]	N/V = 13%	A
Fluoxetine[103,104]	N = 17–24% N/V = 20%	A
Lithium[105]	N = 17% V = 13%	A
Paroxetine[102]	N = 13%	A
IRON SUPPLEMENTS		
Ferrous gluconate[106]	N/V = 13–36%	A
Ferrous sulfate[107]	N = 14–18% V = 10–21%	A
MISCELLANEOUS		
Ethinyl estradiol–levonorgestrel[108]	N = 43–54% V = 8–16%	A
Ethinyl estradiol–norethindrone[108]	N = 53% V = 15%	A
Exenatide (10 mcg sub-Q)[109-111]	N = 45–51% V = 12–13%	A
Liraglutide (1.2 mg sub-Q)[112,113]	N = 10–29% V = 4–7%	A
Metformin[114]	N/V = 8–9%	A
Theophylline[115]	N = 19%	A

IV = intravenous, N = nausea, N/V = report does not differentiate between the occurrence of nausea and vomiting, V = vomiting, sub-Q = subcutaneous.

[a]Definitions for Levels of Evidence: Level A—evidence from one or more randomized, controlled clinical trials; Level B—evidence from nonrandomized clinical trials, prospective observational studies, cohort studies, retrospective studies, case-control studies, meta-analyses and/or postmarketing surveillance studies; and Level C—evidence from one or more published case reports or case series.

OPIOIDS

All opioid receptor agonists may cause nausea and vomiting. In general, when compared at equianalgesic doses, opioids are similar in their likelihood to induce nausea and vomiting.[116,117]

PERIOPERATIVE AGENTS

The majority of the studies included in Table 40-1 are from randomized, placebo-controlled trials in which patients did not receive other agents known to be emetogenic or to possess antiemetic effects (e.g., propofol, ondansetron). For those that included multiple emetogenic agents, the groups were similar except for the study agent. In many postoperative nausea and vomiting (PONV) trials, patients receive a host of drugs for supportive care, making data interpretation challenging.

CHEMOTHERAPY

Emetogenicity varies between chemotherapy agents and can also depend on the number of agents administered on the same day. Whenever possible, references included in Table 40-1 represent reports in which patients received single agents without prophylactic antiemetic therapy.

EPIDEMIOLOGY

OPIOIDS

It has been estimated that 10–40% of ambulatory patients experience nausea and 15–40% experience vomiting on the initiation of opioid therapy.[118]

PERIOPERATIVE AGENTS

The overall incidence of PONV has been estimated to be 10–80%, depending on the number of patient-specific risk factors present, type of surgery, choice of anesthesia, and age and sex of the patient.[119-123]

CHEMOTHERAPY

The expected incidence of emesis associated with chemotherapy without the use of antiemetics is included in Table 40-1. In 1981, insight into chemotherapy-induced nausea and vomiting (CINV) was provided in a study of patients receiving high-dose cisplatin. Patients were randomly assigned to receive placebo (n = 10) or high-dose metoclopramide (n = 11).[51] In the high-dose metoclopramide group, a median of 1 emetic episode (range, 0–9) occurred in a 24-hour period as compared with 10.5 episodes (range, 5–25) in the placebo group. All placebo-treated patients vomited, as compared with 7 of 11 metoclopramide-treated patients. Although this was a small study, it helped to clearly demonstrate the necessity of prophylactic antiemetic therapy in patients receiving chemotherapy.

When antiemetic drugs (5-hydroxytryptamine-3 [5-HT_3] receptor antagonist plus dexamethasone) are administered before emetogenic chemotherapy, the incidence of vomiting varies from 20% to 75%, and the incidence of nausea is as high as 96%.[124] With the use of newer antiemetics, the presence of nausea is still problematic; however, the intensity of the nausea episodes has decreased.[125]

MISCELLANEOUS AGENTS

The expected incidence of nausea and vomiting associated with a variety of medication classes is listed in Table 40-1. As noted above, virtually any drug is capable of causing nausea or vomiting or both, and the list, therefore, is not exhaustive.

Some drugs cause nausea and vomiting when administered in normal therapeutic doses while with others nausea and vomiting can be a sign of toxicity. For example, nausea and vomiting is a classic finding in patients with digoxin toxicity. In a review of elderly patients with a mean digoxin serum concentration >6 ng/mL, 47% were found to have nausea and vomiting.[126]

MECHANISMS

The mechanisms of drug-induced nausea and vomiting are described in **Table 40-2.**[117,121,127-149] Nausea with or without subsequent vomiting is thought to be the result of a centrally controlled protective mechanism involving the GI tract.[4,5,127,148] The sensation of nausea and the act of vomiting serve to discourage the ingestion and/or absorption of toxic substances or to indicate that a portion of the GI tract is not functioning properly.[149,150] Nausea and

Table 40-2 Mechanisms of Drug-Induced Nausea and Vomiting

Drugs	Mechanism
Bromocriptine[144]	• Causes CTZ stimulation by dopamine
Chemotherapy[135,136]	• Has direct CTZ stimulation by neurotransmitters (e.g., dopamine, serotonin, substance P, histamine, norepinephrine) • Damages GI mucosa and allows release of 5-HT_3, which stimulates the vagal afferent nerve and thus activates CTZ and emetic center, the nucleus tractus solitarius • Has indirect or direct effects on the cerebral cortex • Vestibular alterations • Causes taste and olfactory changes, which enhance the gag, nausea, and vomiting reflexes
Digoxin[144,145]	• Stimulates CTZ
Estrogens[145]	• Stimulate CTZ
Erythromycin[137-140]	• Motilin agonist • 5-HT_3, cholinergic agonist • Disruption of interdigestive migrating motor complex
GLP-1 receptor agonists[159]	• Increase glucose-dependent insulin secretion • Decrease glucagon secretion • Delay gastric emptying
Inhaled anesthetic agents[121,131-133]	• Stimulate CTZ • Cause afferent sensory input from higher cortical centers, the vestibular nucleus • Directly stimulate serotoninergic receptors in the GI tract
Levodopa[146]	• Causes CTZ stimulation by dopamine
Metronidazole[141-143]	• Causes taste alterations • Causes monoamine release
Neuromuscular-blocking agents[131]	• Block acetylcholine receptors in muscle
Nitrous oxide[131,132]	• Stimulates the release of dopamine in the medulla • Changes middle ear pressure, resulting in stimulation of the vestibular apparatus • Abdominal distention during mask ventilation, leading to direct activation of the nociceptors • Causes hypoxia, which has been correlated with PONV • Stimulates opioid receptors
Opioids[117,127-130]	• Stimulate CTZ • Decrease neural activity in the GI tract, leading to a decrease in motility and a decrease in pyloric tone • Increase vestibular sensitivity via histaminergic and muscarinic pathways
Serotonin reuptake inhibitors[147]	• Cause CTZ stimulation by serotonin
Spinal anesthesia[134]	• Blocks sympathetic nerves leading to an increase in vagal tone • Decreases in cerebral blood flow with subsequent hypoxia caused by reductions in blood pressure

5-HT_3 = 5-hydroxytryptamine$_3$, CTZ = chemoreceptor trigger zone, GI = gastrointestinal.

vomiting may also occur during periods of stress secondary to decreased activity of the parasympathetic nervous system.[149]

The signs and symptoms of nausea and vomiting can be quite dramatic and troublesome for any patient (**Table 40-3**). Emesis, or the act of vomiting, may be divided into three distinct phases: pre-ejection, ejection, and postejection.[148] Nausea, which often (but not always) precedes vomiting, is included in the pre-ejection phase and is often accompanied by other symptoms, such as pallor, salivation, shivering, tachycardia, and gastric stasis.[127,128,148,151]

Table 40-3 Signs and Symptoms Associated with Drug-Induced Nausea and Vomiting

- Abdominal muscle contraction
- Confusion
- Deep breath
- Dizziness
- Feeling cold or hot
- Feeling sick
- Gastric stasis
- Loss of appetite
- Loss of taste
- Orthostatic hypotension
- Pallor
- Retching
- Salivation
- Sweating
- Tachycardia
- Vomiting

Retching marks the beginning of the ejection phase of emesis and involves the coordinated rhythmic contraction of the diaphragm, the abdominal muscles, and the external intercostal muscles.[3,127,148,152] During this phase, the glottis remains closed. With each retch, the esophageal pressure decreases while the intra-abdominal pressure increases. Emesis occurs when the contracting abdominal muscles cause an increase in esophageal pressure, forcing the glottis open and allowing the contents of the upper GI tract to be expelled.[127,148] Lethargy and muscle weakness mark the beginning of the postejection phase and are a direct result of emesis. Depending on the circumstances, an individual may experience additional episodes of retching or vomiting or both, and this cycle may be repeated several times.[148]

Nausea and vomiting are centrally mediated responses to the presence of chemicals, toxins, or stressors.[3,4,148-150] The vomiting center, located in the medulla, is thought to initiate the vomiting reflex after receiving afferent sensory input from other areas, including the GI tract, cerebral cortex, and the chemoreceptor trigger zone (CTZ).[127] The CTZ, the emetic or vomiting center, and the GI tract possess a variety of neurotransmitter receptors. The primary receptors involved with emesis are dopamine subtype 2 (D_2) and 5-HT_3 receptors. Other receptors thought to be involved in nausea and vomiting include the prostaglandin, opiate, cannabinoid, muscarine subtype 1 (M1), histamine subtype 1 (H1), and neurokinin (NK-1) receptors.[127,129] The CTZ can be stimulated by a wide variety of neurotransmitters, chemicals, and toxins found in the blood and in the cerebrospinal fluid.[129] Upon stimulation, the CTZ, located in the area postrema, sends afferent impulses to the vomiting center, nucleus tractus solitarius, which in turn sends efferent impulses to the respiratory and salivary centers, cranial nerves, and the abdominal muscles.[127]

Neuronal pathways originating in the GI tract can also directly activate the vomiting center.[151] Drugs or chemicals that irritate or damage the lining of the GI tract are thought to cause nausea and vomiting via these pathways.[128] In addition, the release of 5-HT_3 from the enterochromaffin cells located throughout the GI tract can induce vomiting via serotoninergic afferent pathways to the vomiting center.[129] **Figure 40-1** depicts the afferent pathways involved in the act of vomiting and nausea.[153]

Anticipatory nausea and vomiting are thought to be the result of afferent impulses originating in the cerebral cortex, whereas the nausea associated with motion sickness is attributed to stimulation of the vestibular apparatus.[128] Regardless of the origin of the stimulus, the end result is the same; the vomiting center initiates the act of emesis in response to afferent input.[129,151]

OPIOIDS

Opioids are thought to induce nausea and vomiting via several mechanisms. First, opioid analgesics stimulate the CTZ, resulting in activation of the vomiting center.[127,128] Second, opioids decrease neural activity in the GI tract, leading to a decrease in motility and a decrease in pyloric tone, both of which can induce nausea or vomiting or both.[117,130] Third, opioids are thought to increase vestibular sensitivity via histaminergic and muscarinic pathways.[117,129]

PERIOPERATIVE AGENTS

Because of the number of different agents that are used before, during, and immediately after surgery, it is often difficult to determine which drug(s)

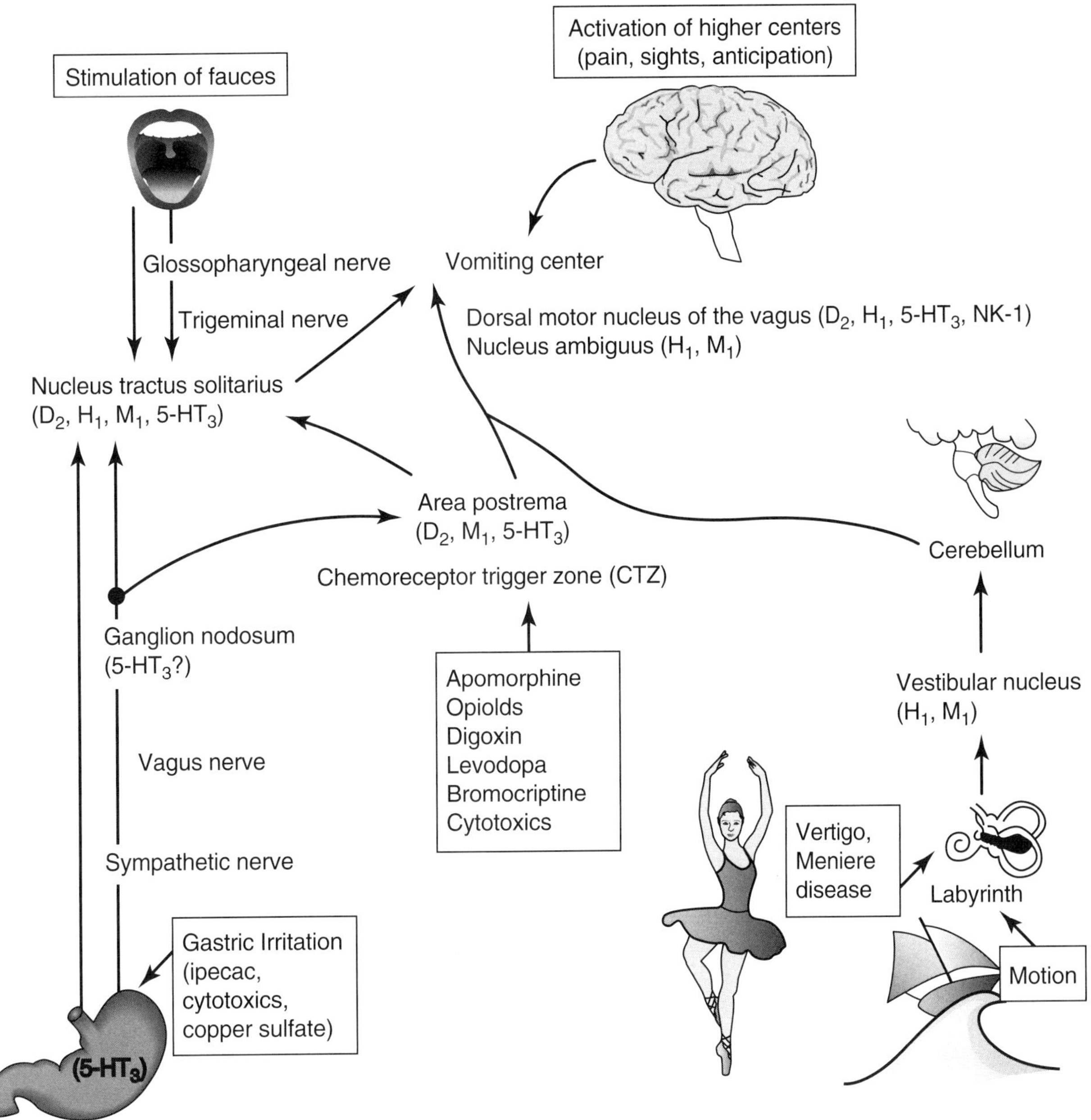

FIGURE 40-1 Afferent Pathways Involved in the Act of Vomiting

5-HT_3,= 5-hydroxytryptamine$_3$ (serotonin), D_2 = dopamine subtype 2, H_1 = histamine subtype 1, M_1 = muscarine subtype 1, NK-1 = neurokinin.

Source: Reprinted with permission from F Mitchelson. Pharmacological agents affecting emesis. A review (Part I). *Drugs.* 1992; 43:295-315 (figure 1, p. 298) ©1992, Springer International Publishing. All rights reserved.

are responsible for PONV. Opioids are frequently administered perioperatively and can be a cause of nausea and vomiting, as described above.

The mechanism by which inhaled anesthetic agents cause nausea and vomiting has not been elucidated. Like the opioid agonists, the inhaled anesthetics are thought to induce nausea and vomiting via stimulation of the CTZ, which in turn causes activation of the vomiting center.[121] Afferent sensory input from higher cortical centers may also contribute to PONV.[121,131,132] The vestibular nucleus is thought to play an important role in the nausea associated with anesthesia. Direct stimulation of serotoninergic receptors in the GI tract is also thought to contribute to PONV from the inhaled anesthetic agents.[133] After receiving and integrating the afferent input from the sources listed above, the vomiting center sends efferent signals to the respiratory and salivary centers and to the muscles directly involved in the act of emesis.[127]

Nitrous oxide is thought to produce nausea and vomiting via several separate mechanisms. It is believed that nitrous oxide stimulates the release of dopamine in the medulla.[131] In addition, nitrous oxide diffuses into the middle ear, resulting in pressure changes within the ear and stimulation of the vestibular apparatus.[154] Nitrous oxide can also produce abdominal distention during mask ventilation, leading to direct activation of the nociceptors and subsequent nausea and vomiting.[131,132] Finally, nitrous oxide exerts its analgesic effects via stimulation of opioid receptors in the central nervous system. This opioid-like activity is also thought to contribute to the emetogenic effects of nitrous oxide.[131]

During spinal anesthesia, the sympathetic nerves are essentially blocked, leading to an unopposed increase in vagal tone, which many think is a cause of PONV.[134] Others believe that the decrease in cerebral blood flow and subsequent hypoxia caused by reductions in blood pressure contribute to the nausea and vomiting associated with the administration of spinal anesthesia.[134]

The neuromuscular blocking agents produce nausea by blocking acetylcholine receptors found in muscle.[131] Although the mechanisms by which ketamine and many of the other perioperative agents induce nausea or vomiting or both are not well understood, one or more of the aforementioned mechanisms is likely involved.

CHEMOTHERAPY

Previously, direct stimulation of the CTZ was thought to be the main mechanism for chemotherapy-induced vomiting. Although CTZ stimulation is an important element, it is now known that the primary initial mechanism is direct damage to the GI mucosa and subsequent stimulation of GI neurotransmitter 5-HT_3 receptors. Once stimulated, the impulse is directed through the CTZ or directly to the emetic center. Other mechanisms involved include psychogenic stimulation through indirect or direct effects on the cerebral cortex, vestibular alterations, and taste and olfactory changes.[135] It is important to note that while 5-HT_3 receptor antagonists and NK-1 receptor antagonists (NK-1 RAs) can play an important role in the prevention of chemotherapy-induced emesis, there has been minor progress in the pharmacologic prevention of nausea.[135]

There are three distinct patterns of chemotherapy-related emesis: acute, delayed, and anticipatory. Acute emesis is mediated primarily by the release of serotonin within the first 8–12 hours after chemotherapy with drugs such as cisplatin.[136] With delayed vomiting, the primary mediator is substance P, which interacts preferentially with the NK-1 receptor.[136] It has been shown that substance P levels tend to trend upward 48 hours after the administration of cisplatin chemotherapy.[155] However, not all agents produce a significant release of substance P. Even cisplatin has a varying release of substance P at different doses. For example, cisplatin doses >75 mg/m^2 produced more substance P than cisplatin doses of <75 mg/m^2.[156] Delayed nausea and emesis can be quite debilitating for patients and may last for up to 1 week after chemotherapy. In addition to the role of substance P, there have been many other mechanisms describing the pathophysiology of delayed emesis. One theory holds that disruption of the blood–brain barrier occurs; this increases the risk of cerebral edema, which increases intracranial pressure. Other possible causes of delayed emesis include the interaction of serotonin with 5-HT_4 receptors and the development of hypomotility of the GI tract or gastroparesis.

Anticipatory nausea and emesis develop as a result of a classical conditioning (or Pavlovian) response to certain stimuli. Anticipatory effects do not occur unless a conditioned response develops as a result of previous adverse symptoms of chemotherapy.

MISCELLANEOUS AGENTS

The mechanisms responsible for nausea and vomiting associated with each of the miscellaneous agents listed in Table 40-1 vary, but typically involve one or more of the mechanisms described above. In addition, direct gastric or esophageal irritation, or both, is a mechanism of drug-induced nausea and vomiting that may occur with vitamins, minerals, and preparations used for electrolyte replacement.

Metronidazole may cause nausea and vomiting through several possible mechanisms. The development of an altered taste, often metallic, can lead to nausea.[141] When metronidazole is taken concurrently with ethanol, a disulfiram-like reaction consisting of flushing, nausea, vomiting, and tachycardia may occur.[141] It has been proposed that metronidazole, like disulfiram, inhibits hepatic aldehyde dehydrogenase, leading to an accumulation of acetaldehyde following the ingestion of ethanol.[142] However, in a double-blind, placebo-controlled study, 12 healthy male volunteers received 5 days of therapy with metronidazole or placebo plus ethanol 0.4 g/kg. Blood samples were taken every 20 minutes for 4 hours, and blood acetaldehyde and ethanol concentrations were measured. Volunteers were assessed for signs and symptoms of disulfiram-like reaction. Metronidazole did not affect blood acetaldehyde concentrations or lead to any objective or subjective adverse effects when used with ethanol in these subjects.[157]

An animal study also failed to find a correlation between the concomitant administration of metronidazole and ethanol and the development of high acetaldehyde concentrations.[143] An interesting observation, however, was that treated animals had an increase in brain serotonin concentrations after the use of metronidazole. The authors postulated that the mechanism of the metronidazole–alcohol interaction is a "toxic serotonin syndrome" and not an increase in acetaldehyde concentrations. Further study will be needed to elucidate the exact mechanism or mechanisms involved in the interaction between metronidazole and alcohol.

Erythromycin is notorious for its ability to induce nausea and vomiting, and several mechanisms are possibly involved. Erythromycin has been described as a motilin agonist that stimulates the contraction of the stomach and small intestines. It also is believed to induce the interdigestive migratory motor complex located in the stomach and proximal duodenum.[138] Disturbing this complex has been linked to vomiting, and effects have continued for up to 3 hours in a canine model.[139,140]

The mechanism of trimethoprim–sulfamethoxazole (TMP/SMX)-induced nausea and vomiting is unknown, although a disulfiram-like reaction (flushing, sweating, palpitations, drowsiness) has been described. Two patients receiving TMP/SMX double-strength were reported to have experienced a disulfiram-type reaction after the ingestion of 24–36 ounces of beer. One of the patients was rechallenged with TMP/SMX the next day after ingesting 6 ounces of beer, and a similar reaction developed. It is possible that TMP/SMX inhibits aldehyde dehydrogenase or the elimination of acetaldehyde via the cytochrome P-450 (CYP 450) hepatic pathway.[158]

Glucagon-like peptide (GLP-1) receptor agonists, such as exenatide and liraglutide, can induce nausea and vomiting by increasing glucose-dependent insulin secretion and decreasing glucagon secretion leading to delayed gastric emptying.[159]

CLINICAL PRESENTATION AND DIFFERENTIAL DIAGNOSIS

Signs and symptoms associated with drug-induced nausea and vomiting are listed in Table 40-3. Conditions to consider in the differential diagnoses are presented in **Table 40-4**.[129,151,152,160,161]

OPIOIDS

Nausea and vomiting associated with opioid use normally occur immediately upon initiation of therapy and can last anywhere from a few days to a week or longer while the patient is taking the drug.[162-164] The majority of patients beginning opioid treatment experience a reduction or resolution of nausea and vomiting within the first week of therapy. A distinction should be made between nausea and vomiting caused by the opioid itself and that which occurs because of opioid-induced constipation. Patients usually develop a tolerance to the emetogenic effects of the opioid, but not to constipation.[116]

PERIOPERATIVE AGENTS

PONV associated with the use of the inhaled anesthetics most often occurs during the first 2 hours after surgery. Nausea and vomiting occurring

Table 40-4 Conditions to Consider in the Differential Diagnosis of Nausea and Vomiting

- Alcoholism
- Bacterial enterotoxins
- Bacterial or viral gastroenteritis
- Bulimia
- Cholecystitis
- Crohn disease
- Gastroparesis
- Hepatitis
- Increased intracranial pressure
- Irritable bowel syndrome
- Malignancy
- Mechanical obstruction
- Metabolic abnormalities
- Myocardial infarction
- Pancreatitis
- Peptic or gastric ulcer
- Postoperative nausea and vomiting
- Pregnancy
- Psychiatric disorders
- Radiation therapy
- Vestibular dysfunction

Table 40-5 Onset and Duration of Emesis Associated with Antineoplastic Agents with >30% Emesis Frequency

Agent	Onset (hr)	Emesis Duration (hr)
Carboplatin	2–6	1–48
Carmustine	2–6	4–24
Cisplatin	1–6	>24
Cyclophosphamide	6–12	6–36
Cytarabine ≥1,000 mg/m^2	6–12	3–5
Dacarbazine	2–6	6–24
Dactinomycin	2–6	12–24
Daunorubicin	2–6	<24
Doxorubicin ≥20 mg/m^2	2–6	6–24
Ifosfamide	3–6	6–12
Irinotecan	2–6	6–12
Lomustine	3–6	6–12
Mechlorethamine	0.5–2	6–24
Methotrexate ≥250 mg/m^2	4–12	3–12
Streptozocin	2–6	12–24

2–24 hours postoperatively have been associated with other factors, including opioid use, increased physical activity after surgery, and insufficient supplemental hydration.[165-167] Nausea and vomiting occurring at any time following surgery may be caused by any of several other factors unrelated to anesthesia, including decreased GI motility, anxiety, and uncontrolled pain.[168]

CHEMOTHERAPY

Chemotherapy-related emesis occurs with an acute, delayed, or anticipatory onset. **Table 40-5** describes the usual time of onset and duration of emesis associated with chemotherapy.[160] Delayed nausea and vomiting occurs more than 24 hours after the administration of chemotherapy although this phase may begin as early as 16 hours after cisplatin administration.[161] The development of anticipatory vomiting may occur in patients whose nausea and vomiting have not been well controlled during previous chemotherapy treatments. By the fourth treatment cycle, approximately 25% of patients have anticipatory nausea or vomiting or both.[125] In addition, more intense prior symptoms increase the likelihood that patients will have a conditioned or anticipatory response.[125] A patient who has severe chemotherapy-related nausea and emesis may remember the surroundings (including the healthcare providers present) during the event. The patient may subsequently associate the emesis with those surroundings or providers and may have anticipatory nausea or vomiting or both by just seeing or hearing the voice of those individuals.

MISCELLANEOUS AGENTS

Other drugs that cause clinical presentation and differential diagnosis of nausea and vomiting are similar to those described above. It should be noted, however, that it can be more difficult for healthcare providers to identify nausea and vomiting as being drug-induced when caused by agents infrequently associated with these effects. Under these circumstances, proper diagnosis can be delayed.

RISK FACTORS

OPIOIDS

Risk factors associated with the development of opioid-induced nausea and vomiting are listed in **Table 40-6**.[163] A retrospective study involving over 8,800 participants found that those 80 years of age or older were less likely to have opioid-induced nausea and vomiting than those between the ages of 16 and 45.[163] In addition, men were found to be less likely to experience opioid-induced nausea and vomiting than women. Race was also found to be a factor, with a higher risk of developing opioid-induced nausea and vomiting in whites than in blacks. The route of administration appears to affect the risk for developing nausea and vomiting in patients receiving parenteral opioids, with the intravenous (IV) route conferring a higher risk than the intramuscular (IM) or subcutaneous (sub-Q) routes. As would be expected, increasing the opioid dose increases the likelihood of nausea and vomiting.[163] Reasons for the majority of these risk factors are not known, but may be related to peak opioid concentrations.

PERIOPERATIVE AGENTS

The various risk factors associated with an increased incidence of drug-induced PONV are listed in **Table 40-7**.[122,123,165-167] No single factor is of primary importance in accurately predicting which patients will experience PONV, although female sex has shown to be the most predictive. This can be appreciated by reviewing the simple models available to aid clinicians in predicting the PONV risk in adults and children (**Table 40-8**).[122,123] The primary PONV risk factors have been shown to include female sex, nonsmoking status, previous history of PONV or motion sickness, childhood to young adulthood ages, long duration of surgery, and the use of volatile anesthetics, nitrous oxide, or perioperative opioids. The specific type of surgical procedure also affects the risk of PONV, with gynecological and abdominal surgeries conferring a higher risk of PONV.[169]

Table 40-6 Risk Factors for Opioid-Induced Nausea and Vomiting

- Concomitant administration of other potentially emetogenic agents
- Dose (higher dose is greater than lower dose)
- Opioid exposure (patient with no previous opioid exposure is greater than patient with previous opioid exposure)
- Oral doses taken without food
- Race (whites greater than blacks)
- Route of administration (intravenous > intramuscular and subcutaneous)
- Sex (females greater than males)
- Younger age (patients 16–45 yr of age are at higher risk than those ≥80 yr)

Table 40-7 Risk Factors for Postoperative Nausea and Vomiting

Anesthesia related

- Experience level of anesthesiologist
  - Less experienced is greater than more experienced
- Type of anesthesia
  - General is greater than spinal is greater than peripheral block
- Use of nitrous oxide

Other factors

- Eating or drinking too soon after surgery
- Increased postoperative movement
- Perioperative administration of opioids
- Presence of postoperative pain

Patient related

- Age
  - Children (6–16 yr) greater than adults greater than infants (<12 mo)
- Female sex
- Nonsmoker
- Presence of delayed gastric emptying
  - Obstruction
  - Pregnancy
  - Diabetes
- Prior history of PONV or motion sickness

Surgery related

- Decrease in systolic blood pressure by ≥35% during surgery or induction of anesthesia
- Increased duration of surgery
  - Each 30-minute surgery increment increases PONV risk by 60%
- Type of surgery
  - Laparoscopy, laparotomy, breast, strabismus, plastic surgery, maxillofacial, gynecologic, abdominal, neurologic, ophthalmologic, urologic

PONV = postoperative nausea and vomiting.

Table 40-8 Assessing Risk for Postoperative Nausea and Vomiting

ADULT PONV RISK SCORE PREDICTORS

One point for each risk factor: female sex, nonsmoker, history of PONV, postoperative opioids

No. of Points	Approximate Risk of PONV (%)
0	10
1	20
2	40
3	60
4	80

CHILDREN PONV RISK SCORE PREDICTORS

One point for each risk factor: surgery lasting ≥30 minutes, age ≥3 years, strabismus surgery, personal or family history of PONV

No. of Points	Approximate Risk of PONV (%)
0	10
1	10
2	30
3	55
4	70

PONV = postoperative nausea and vomiting.

Patients who are ultrarapid metabolizers of *CYP2D6*, which codes for a CYP isozyme important in drug metabolism, may be less likely to respond as expected to agents used to control PONV. All 5-HT_3 receptor antagonists except granisetron are substrates for *CYP2D6* and may be susceptible to increased metabolism and clearance in patients who are *CYP2D6* ultrarapid metabolizers. This relationship was studied in 250 patients receiving ondansetron 4 mg IV for PONV prevention.[168] The incidence of vomiting in poor, intermediate, extensive, and ultrarapid metabolizers was found to be 1 in 12 (8%), 5 in 30 (17%), 26 in 176 (15%), and 5 in 11 (45%), respectively. There was no difference in the incidence of nausea between groups.

Another study compared granisetron 1 mg intravenously and dolasetron 12.5 mg IV in a prospective, randomized, double-blind study of 150 adult patients.[170] Because *CYP2D6* does not metabolize granisetron, it was theorized it would be more effective than dolasetron in rapid metabolizers. Overall, a complete response (no vomiting or rescue medication required) occurred more frequently in the granisetron group (54.7%) as compared with the dolasetron group (38.7%). Ultrarapid metabolizers who received dolasetron (n = 6) experienced more vomiting episodes than those (n = 4) who received granisetron (six episodes versus one episode, respectively).

CHEMOTHERAPY

The most common risk factors for CINV are listed in **Table 40-9**.[125,135,160,171-173] As with PONV, CYP metabolizer status is an area of interest as it relates to

Table 40-9 Risk Factors for Chemotherapy-Induced Nausea and Vomiting

Chemotherapy-specific factors

- Administration of multiple agents on the same day
- Circadian cycle with cisplatin (morning administration is greater than evening)
- Emetogenicity of agent
- High dose
- Infusion rate (bolus is greater than continuous infusion)
- Lack of maintenance antiemetics after chemotherapy

History

- Emesis from chemotherapy
- Hyperemesis with pregnancy
- Motion sickness

Patient-specific factors

- Age (<50 yr)
- Anxiety
- Enhanced cytochrome P450 2D6 activity
  - Ultrarapid metabolizers of 5-HT_3 receptor antagonists (except granisetron)
- Feeling hot or warm after chemotherapy
- Female sex
- History of minimal long-term alcohol consumption
- Poor performance status

Risk factors for delayed nausea and emesis

- Female sex
- Poor control in the acute phase (0–24 hr after chemotherapy)
- Poor control with first cycle
- Use of certain chemotherapy agents
  - Anthracyclines
  - Carboplatin
  - Cisplatin, especially with dose >90 mg/m^2
  - Cyclophosphamide

the effectiveness of antiemetics in preventing CINV. All 5-HT_3 receptor antagonists except granisetron are substrates for *CYP2D6*. In a study to investigate the efficacy of ondansetron and tropisetron based on *CYP2D6* genotype, patients who were ultrarapid metabolizers had greater intensity of vomiting and nausea as well as lower antiemetic serum concentrations as compared with poor metabolizers.[173] It was determined that approximately 50 subjects would have to be genotyped to protect one patient from severe emesis. The feasibility of identifying patients' *CYP2D6* genotype and thereby assisting health professionals in adjusting antiemetic regimens is unclear.

MISCELLANEOUS AGENTS

General risk factors for nausea and vomiting associated with other agents include a recent increase in medication dose, a change in the patient's underlying renal or hepatic function resulting in a higher drug concentration, and drug–food, drug–drug, and drug–disease interactions. Patients with a history of multiple drug allergies or side effects typically have a higher incidence of nausea and vomiting when exposed to new drugs.

MORBIDITY AND MORTALITY

OPIOIDS

Nausea and vomiting associated with any drug can lead to a decreased adherence to prescribed therapy. With opioid-induced nausea and vomiting, decreased adherence can lead to uncontrolled pain and severely compromise the patient's quality of life. Nausea and vomiting may also prevent patients from eating, resulting in nutritional deficiencies that can exacerbate other underlying medical conditions. In severe cases of drug-induced emesis, dehydration with subsequent electrolyte disturbances can occur, leading to potentially life-threatening complications.

PERIOPERATIVE AGENTS

PONV causes significant morbidity. Even minor episodes of nausea and vomiting can lead to delays in eating, drinking, and walking postoperatively thus retarding recovery. In addition, nausea and vomiting may prevent patients from taking oral medications. If vomiting is severe, dehydration and electrolyte disturbances such as hyponatremia and hypokalemia can occur. Forceful retching can cause Mallory-Weiss tears in the esophagus as well as abdominal wound dehiscence.[174] In addition, the risk for aspiration of GI contents is increased with protracted postoperative emesis. PONV may delay the patient's transfer from the postanesthesia care unit, which could result in an increased length of hospital stay.[174,175] Patients who undergo outpatient surgery and experience significant PONV may have to be admitted to the hospital.

CHEMOTHERAPY

The incidence of mortality related to CINV is unknown. However, the incidence of morbidity related to CINV has been evaluated. In a longitudinal secondary analysis performed on data from a prospective, observational quality-of-life study involving 200 newly diagnosed cancer patients who underwent chemotherapy, 62% of patients experienced nausea and 27% experienced vomiting; furthermore, patients with nausea experienced significant quality-of-life impairment and psychological distress compared to those unaffected in the areas of physical, role and social functioning, fatigue, appetite loss, overall physical health, and overall quality of life.[176] Similarly, patients with vomiting experienced significant quality-of-life impairment and psychological stress compared to those unaffected in the areas of physical, role and social functioning, fatigue, appetite loss, sleep disturbance, overall physical health, and cancer distress.[176] The sequelae can be quite dramatic and may lead to dissatisfaction with the healthcare system and nonadherence to the treatment plan. In a trial comparing metoclopramide and placebo in patients receiving high-dose cisplatin, placebo-treated patients experienced an average of 10.5 emetic episodes in a 24-hour period and had nausea and vomiting lasting over 3.6 hours.[51] This type of unrelenting nausea and vomiting can lead to metabolic imbalances, diminished quality of life and functional ability, nutritional deficiencies, anorexia, decreased performance and psychological status, wound dehiscence, and esophageal tears and can ultimately lead to withdrawal from cancer treatment programs.[161,177]

In a retrospective study to ascertain the impact of therapy-related nausea and vomiting on the outcomes of patients receiving cisplatin for lung, ovarian, and testicular cancer, an association was found between the incidence of vomiting and the length of hospital stay per cycle of chemotherapy.[178] Patients with lung cancer who did not have emesis had an average hospitalization of 2.1 days, versus 4.2 days if they experienced emesis. Patients with testicular cancer receiving a 3-day chemotherapy regimen had an average of 5.5 versus 4.2 days of hospitalization if they experienced emesis versus no emesis. In the lung cancer group, 2.5% of patients stopped therapy for reasons related to poorly controlled emesis; however, survival was not affected by this choice. No patient in the ovarian or testicular cancer groups withdrew from the study because of vomiting. Even though most patients received prophylactic 5-HT_3 receptor antagonists, the development of nausea and vomiting was still found to prolong hospitalization.

MISCELLANEOUS AGENTS

Tigecycline, an antibiotic related to minocycline, can induce nausea and vomiting. In a large randomized study, 1% of patients treated with tigecycline stopped taking the drug because of nausea and vomiting versus none in the vancomycin and aztreonam groups.[96] In another study, 2.5% of the patients treated with tigecycline discontinued therapy early because of nausea or vomiting or both.[95]

Up to 24% of patients receiving fluoxetine for depression may experience treatment-related nausea.[103,104] Fortunately, only 8% or fewer discontinue therapy as a result.[103,104]

Adherence problems caused by drug-induced nausea and vomiting can affect the morbidity and mortality of patients with human immunodeficiency virus infection who take complicated regimens such as highly active antiretroviral therapy (HAART). A study evaluated the self-reported adverse effects of patients taking HAART for at least 1 month and whether or not these adverse effects had an impact on adherence.[179] A total of 358 patients were evaluated. Nonadherence in the past 3 days was reported by 22% of patients and 25% reported not refilling their medications in a timely fashion. Those with nausea had a 4.47 times greater risk of poor adherence. However, it is unknown if nonadherence affected their overall morbidity or mortality.

Erythromycin has a significant GI adverse effect profile. In a randomized controlled trial, therapy with IV erythromycin had to be discontinued in 10% of patients because of severe GI toxicity.[93]

It is well known that oral iron preparations can cause a variety of GI symptoms. In a study evaluating the relationship of nausea and vomiting to adherence with iron therapy in higher and lower socioeconomic groups, it was found that adherence decreased from 82% to 48% in members of the lower socioeconomic group in whom nausea and vomiting developed.[107] In the higher socioeconomic group, however, adherence rates remained similar in patients with or without nausea and vomiting.

PREVENTION

General guidelines to help prevent drug-induced nausea and vomiting are listed in **Table 40-10**.

OPIOIDS

Nausea and vomiting following the initiation of opioid therapy is relatively common and should be anticipated. Patients should be informed of the potential for this effect before the initiation of therapy. In addition, appropriate antiemetic therapy should be available in case nausea or vomiting occurs. Any conditions or medications that could exacerbate the adverse GI effects of opioid analgesics should be identified and steps taken to remove them if possible.

Starting at a lower dose and titrating upward may help minimize some of the emetogenic effects of opioid therapy. When patients require continuing therapy with opioids, a bowel regimen containing a stimulant laxative should be initiated to help prevent the constipation that is common with this class of drugs. Oral opioid analgesics may be taken with meals to help decrease local gastric emetogenic

Table 40-10 Approaches to Help Prevent Drug-Induced Nausea and Vomiting

- If possible, avoid agents with high emetogenic potential
- For opioid-induced nausea and vomiting:
  - Use lowest effective dose
  - Take oral opioids with food to minimize nausea and vomiting

For PONV

- Ensure that patient is fully hydrated and that pain is controlled before surgery
- Avoid inhaled anesthetics
- For the patient at risk for PONV, administer antiemetic perioperatively
- Minimize motion and activity after surgery
- Minimize eating and drinking up to 8 hr after surgery

For chemotherapy-induced nausea and vomiting

- Assess risk factors and adjust antiemetics as necessary
- Patients need to be protected throughout full period of risk with highly emetogenic agents (at least 3 days) and moderately emetogenic agents (at least 2 days)
- For highly and moderately emetogenic agents, use a 5-HT_3–receptor antagonist and dexamethasone
- For those at risk for delayed nausea and vomiting, use a NK-1 antagonist or olanzapine in combination with a 5-HT_3 receptor antagonist and dexamethasone
- For low emetogenic agents, use dexamethasone, metoclopramide, prochlorperazine, or a 5-HT_3–receptor antagonist
- For minimally emetogenic agents, no routine prophylaxis recommended
- Follow established, peer-reviewed guidelines for the prevention of postoperative and chemotherapy-induced nausea and vomiting
- Identify high-risk individuals and use prophylactic antiemetics according to guidelines
- Adjust antiemetics as necessary for patients in whom previous antiemetic regimens have failed
- Eating small, frequent meals, choosing healthful foods, controlling amount of food consumed, and eating food at room temperature may help alleviate nausea/vomiting.

PONV = postoperative nausea and vomiting.

effects. A study evaluating the effect of food on an oral, extended-release formulation of hydrocodone in healthy volunteers showed that food did not affect plasma concentration over time; however, 50% of volunteers experienced nausea in the fasting state while only 25% experienced nausea in the fed state.[180] In hospitalized patients, switching from oral to parenteral administration may be useful; local effects on the GI tract may be decreased, although the central emetogenic effects of the opioid will remain. In patients who experience significant nausea or vomiting, a switch to a different opioid analgesic may be helpful. There is no clinical evidence supporting the use of prophylactic antiemetic agents in all patients beginning opioid therapy.[162,181,182]

PERIOPERATIVE AGENTS

The incidence of PONV has decreased dramatically since the development of newer inhaled anesthetics, the increasing use of IV anesthesia, and the advent of ultra-short-acting neuromuscular blocking agents.[131,132] Before any surgical procedure, a thorough preoperative history and physical examination should be conducted.[174] Patient-specific risk factors for PONV should be identified, along with risk factors associated with the type of surgery and the type and duration of anesthesia planned. A comprehensive preoperative evaluation is the most important step in reducing the likelihood of intraoperative and postoperative complications.[183]

Several steps can help reduce a patient's risk for PONV. Rather than using anesthetic agents known to cause nausea and vomiting, those with less emetogenic potential can be used. Propofol has been found to cause significantly less nausea and vomiting when used during induction and during maintenance of anesthesia as compared with many of the more traditional inhaled or IV agents.[184-189] Nitrous oxide causes nausea and vomiting in a significant number of patients.[183,185] In patients at high risk for PONV or those in whom postoperative vomiting may hinder recovery, the risks of using nitrous oxide may outweigh any potential benefit. Perioperative opioid use should be minimized in patients at high risk for PONV. However, because uncontrolled postoperative pain can itself lead to PONV, adjustment of the opioid dose should be done cautiously.

Patients should be instructed not to eat or drink anything immediately before their surgery. In addition, discouraging eating and drinking within the first 8 hours postoperatively can decrease the risk of PONV. Patients should not be moved unnecessarily in the immediate hours following surgery, as sudden movements and positional changes can precipitate nausea.[120] Techniques that have been shown beneficial in reducing the incidence of PONV include the administration of supplemental IV fluids preoperatively, maintenance of blood pressure and increased oxygenation intraoperatively, and frequent nasogastric suctioning postoperatively.[121,132,165]

Patients at high risk for PONV (e.g., those who have experienced nausea, vomiting, or both after previous surgical procedures) and those in whom PONV is likely to significantly delay or complicate recovery (e.g., patients undergoing open abdominal surgery) may benefit from prophylactic antiemetic therapy.[174,190,191] Prophylactic antiemetic administration in patients with no history of PONV or in those with no identifiable risk factors is not warranted. In these patients, the PONV risk is estimated to be only 10%.[119]

Several antiemetic agents have been shown to be particularly effective in PONV prevention, including promethazine, droperidol, granisetron, dolasetron, ondansetron, palonosetron, dexamethasone, scopolamine, and aprepitant.[175,189,192-194] The usual dose of promethazine for the PONV prevention is 25 mg administered orally (PO), rectally (PR), IM, or IV. However, a retrospective analysis showed no difference in complete response (no PONV and no further rescue) between 6.25 mg of promethazine and higher doses.[195] Promethazine frequently causes drowsiness, especially when given with opioid analgesics or other sedating agents. In addition, promethazine can occasionally cause extrapyramidal symptoms.[189] In 2004, the U.S. Food and Drug Administration (FDA) required the addition of a black box warning to the labeling for promethazine that included a contraindication for use in children <2 years of age and a cautionary warning regarding use in children >2 years of age.[196]

Droperidol should be administered in doses of 0.625–1.25 mg IM or slow IV push for PONV prevention. The use of droperidol has been associated with prolongation of the QT interval and ventricular tachycardia, including torsades de pointes. Droperidol is contraindicated in patients with QT interval prolongation and should be used with caution in patients at risk for cardiac arrhythmias. Like promethazine, droperidol can cause extrapyramidal symptoms.[121]

Ondansetron, a 5-HT_3 receptor antagonist, has been shown to be effective for PONV prevention and treatment in doses of 4 mg IV or 8 mg PO.[197-203] A single 4-mg IV dose has been shown to be effective in preventing and treating postoperative emesis for up to 24 hours.[204-206] It should be noted that ondansetron and the other 5-HT_3 receptor antagonists are more effective in preventing vomiting than they are in preventing nausea.[192] A 4-mg IV dose has a number needed to treat (NNT) of 6 for prevention of vomiting and a NNT of 7 for prevention of nausea.[192] Ondansetron is associated with relatively few adverse effects as compared to many of the other antiemetics, although some studies have shown QT interval prolongation in patients receiving this agent.[189]

Palonosetron has also been used successfully in PONV prevention. Over 500 patients were randomly assigned to receive palonosetron 0.025 mg, 0.05 mg, or 0.075 mg or placebo IV prior to anesthesia.[207] The incidence of complete response (no vomiting and no rescue antiemetics required) was evaluated during the period after surgery (0 to 72 hours). Of 138 patients treated with 0.075 mg palonosetron and evaluated for 24 hours after surgery, 43% had a complete response versus 26% in the placebo group. For 24–72 hours after surgery, there was no significant difference between palonosetron and placebo with respect to reducing PONV. Over the 72-hour period, the nausea intensity improved with palonosetron but was not statistically different as compared with placebo. The other 5-HT_3 receptor antagonists, dolasetron and granisetron, had similar efficacy in PONV prevention.

Dexamethasone has been used for the prevention of chemotherapy-induced emesis for many years, and it is now used for PONV prevention. The mechanism of action of corticosteroids, including dexamethasone, for the prevention of nausea and vomiting is not clearly understood but may involve the inhibition of prostaglandin and cytokine release.[141,208] Dexamethasone interacts with glucocorticoid receptors found in different areas of the brain such as the nucleus tractus solitarius and the area postrema, which may contribute to its antiemetic effects. Dexamethasone doses of 8 mg

IV or 10 mg PO have been shown to be effective in reducing the incidence of nausea and vomiting to 8–20% versus 36–40% compared with placebo after surgery.[208] Dexamethasone should be administered before the induction of anesthesia for maximal benefit. Dexamethasone, like other corticosteroids, has many adverse effects; however, administration of single doses minimizes this possibility.[192,208]

A multicenter, randomized, placebo-controlled study of over 5,100 patients found similar rates of efficacy in decreasing the incidence of PONV with prophylactic administration of droperidol (1.25 mg IV), dexamethasone (4 mg IV), or ondansetron (4 mg IV).[200] Overall, 54.5% of the patients in this study had a history of PONV or motion sickness, known risk factors for PONV. Over 78% of the patients received opioids postoperatively, further increasing the PONV risk. Thirty-four percent of the patients had at least one episode of postoperative nausea or vomiting or both. As expected, patients who had received inhaled anesthetics, nitrous oxide, or both had a higher incidence of PONV as compared with those who received propofol anesthesia. Patients who received propofol had a 19% lower incidence of PONV as compared with those who received inhaled anesthetics. Those who received oxygen and nitrous oxide had a 12% higher incidence of PONV as compared with those who received oxygen and nitrogen. Without prophylactic antiemetics, 52% experienced PONV, as compared with 37%, 28%, and 22% when one, two, and three antiemetic agents, respectively, were given. The authors suggest that single-agent prophylaxis with dexamethasone, droperidol, or ondansetron is equally effective. In patients at high risk for PONV or in those in whom postoperative vomiting may be detrimental, a combination prophylactic antiemetic regimen may be warranted.[200]

The NK-1 RA aprepitant is one of the most recent agents to demonstrate efficacy for PONV prevention. A large study compared aprepitant to ondansetron for PONV prevention.[194] Over 800 patients were randomly assigned to receive either a single dose of aprepitant 40 mg PO, aprepitant 125 mg PO, or ondansetron 4 mg IV preoperatively. The primary outcome was the incidence of complete response (no vomiting and no rescue antiemetics required) in the 24 hours after surgery. There were no significant differences among the three groups, with complete response reported in 45%, 43%, and 42% of patients, respectively. However, when evaluating vomiting only, 90% and 95% of patients in the aprepitant groups had not vomited in the 24 hours after surgery as compared with 74% in the ondansetron group. This beneficial effect carried over for 48 hours after surgery. In terms of need for rescue antiemetics and nausea control, there were no differences among the groups. As with other aprepitant trials, greater benefit was demonstrated in the prevention of vomiting than in the control of nausea.

Two other frequently used antiemetic agents, metoclopramide and prochlorperazine, have been shown to be of benefit for prophylaxis in PONV in some clinical trials but no more effective than placebo at preventing PONV in others.[209-212] Drugs and doses for the prophylaxis of PONV in adults are listed in **Table 40-11**.[141,160,192] Appropriate dose adjustments are required for pediatric use.[160]

Recent data suggest that gabapentin may decrease PONV. A single oral dose of 600 mg given 1 to 2 hours preoperatively in addition to a standard multimodal antiemetic regimen has shown to result in a significant reduction in the incidence of nausea and vomiting, thereby decreasing the need for rescue antiemetics in the postoperative setting when compared to the standard regimen alone.[213] The majority of the clinical trials conducted utilizing gabapentin as an adjunct in various preoperative regimens focused on its efficacy in reducing postoperative pain. The drug's activity in reducing PONV was discovered serendipitously.[213,214] There are a very small number of trials that focus on gabapentin's reduction in the incidence of PONV as a primary endpoint; the ones which exist also suggest that a single dose of the drug, when given in combination with the standard preoperative antiemetic agents, results in a reduction in PONV incidence.[214,215] It should be noted that in most of these trials, the patients studied received general anesthesia.[215]

The exact mechanism by which gabapentin exerts its antiemetic effect is not known. One proposed mechanism involves gabapentin causing a decrease in calcium signaling in the area postrema. Another

Table 40-11 Pharmacotherapy to Help Prevent Drug-Induced Postoperative Nausea and Vomiting

Drugs	Dose	Timing with Respect to Anesthesia/Surgery
Aprepitant	40 mg PO	At induction
Dexamethasone	4–8 mg IV	At induction
Dimenhydrinate	1 mg/kg (maximum, 100 mg) IV	Before induction
Dolasetron	12.5 mg IV	At end of surgery
Droperidol	0.625–1.25 mg IV	At end of surgery
Ephedrine	0.5 mg/kg IM	At end of surgery
Granisetron	0.35–1.5 mg IV	At end of surgery
Haloperidol	0.5–2 mg IV/IM	At end of surgery
Methylprednisolone	40 mg IV	At induction
Ondansetron	4 mg IV	At end of surgery
Palonosetron	0.075 mg IV	Before induction
Prochlorperazine	5–10 mg IV/IM	At end of surgery
Promethazine	6.25–25 mg IV	At induction
Scopolamine	Transdermal patch	Evening before or 2 hr before induction
Tropisetron	2 mg IV	At end of surgery

IM = intramuscular, IV = intravenous, PO = oral.

possible mechanism involves a decrease in tachykinin neurotransmission, while yet another implicates postoperative anti-inflammatory effects.[216,217] A more simple explanation involves the drug's established activity in reducing postoperative pain, which may lead to a reduction in perioperative opioid requirements and their associated nausea and vomiting.[218] It is likely that a combination of these as well as other, yet undiscovered, mechanisms leads to gabapentin's reduction in PONV.[216-218]

Ginger (*Zingiber officinale*) has been used as a medicinal agent for nearly 2,500 years. The mechanism of a reported antiemetic effect with ginger is unknown but studies suggest that phytochemicals contained in the root may function as a 5-HT_3 antagonist and a NK-1 RA.[219] Evidence for the use of ginger for the prevention of PONV has been equivocal. A meta-analysis of six randomized placebo-controlled trials that included 538 patients comparing doses of ginger ranging from 100 mg to 1 g found no difference in the pooled relative risk in preventing PONV 24 hours after surgery (RR 0.84, 95% CI 0.69–1.03).[220] However, a subsequent meta-analysis comparing five randomized placebo-controlled trials that included 363 patients and a fixed dose of 1 g of ginger found a difference in the pooled relative risk favoring ginger in preventing PONV 24 hours after surgery (RR 0.65, 95% CI 0.51–0.84).[221] Ginger may play a role in PONV, but further studies need to be conducted elucidating which phytochemical in ginger is responsible for this effect.

CHEMOTHERAPY

Prevention of CINV is an important goal, and several national and international oncology groups have published recommendations to assist with this objective.[161,222-224] **Table 40-12** provides detailed information regarding pharmacotherapy for the prevention of acute and delayed CINV.[161,222,223] Although there has been good success in preventing emesis in the majority of patients, a similar reduction in the incidence of nausea has not been achieved.

Most protocols for the prevention CINV include a 5-HT_3 receptor antagonist and dexamethasone. The 5-HT_3 receptor antagonists have all been considered clinically equivalent for the prevention of acute nausea and vomiting; however, palonosetron is the preferred 5-HT_3 receptor antagonist for

Table 40-12 Approaches to Prevent Chemotherapy-Induced Nausea and Vomiting

- Ascertain acute and delayed nausea and vomiting risk factors and adjust antiemetics as necessary
- Multiple-day chemotherapy regimens may require additional days of antiemetic prophylaxis
- 5-HT_3–receptor antagonists are typically given as a single dose before the emetogenic agent
- To improve antiemetic response, corticosteroids should be administered with the 5-HT_3–receptor antagonist
- Lorazepam or another benzodiazepine may be administered to reduce anxiety during the chemotherapy regimens
- H2 blockers or proton pump inhibitors may be added to prevent dyspepsia
- For patients receiving a highly emetogenic agent:
    - On day 1, 5-HT_3–receptor antagonist[a], NK-1 antagonist[b], and steroid[c]
    - On days 2–3, if aprepitant given, aprepitant 80 mg PO and dexamethasone 8 mg PO/IV days 2–4; otherwise, dexamethasone 8 mg PO/IV on day 2 then 8 mg PO/IV BID days 2–4; if fosaprepitant given day 1 or dexamethasone, 8 mg PO/IV BID days 2–4 if rolapitant given
- For patients receiving a moderately emetogenic agent:
    - On day 1, 5-HT_3–receptor antagonist[a] and dexamethasone 12 mg PO/IV plus aprepitant[d] 125 mg PO or fosaprepitant 150 mg IV, or rolapitant 180 mg PO in select patients at high risk of delayed nausea and vomiting
    - On days 2–3, if aprepitant given, aprepitant 80 mg PO daily with or without dexamethasone 8 mg PO daily; if fosaprepitant or rolapitant, with or without dexamethasone, 8 mg PO/IV daily
- For patients at lower risk of delayed emesis, administer a 5-HT_3–receptor antagonist plus dexamethasone on day 1 with or without dexamethasone on days 2–3
- For patients receiving low emetogenic agent:
    - Dexamethasone 12 mg PO/IV, prochlorperazine 10 mg PO/IV, and then q 6 hr PRN, metoclopramide 10–40 mg PO/IV then either q 4–6 hr PRN, or serotonin 5-HT_3–receptor antagonist[e]
- For patients receiving a minimal-risk agent:
    - No routine prophylaxis

IV = intravenous, PO = oral; PRN = as needed.
[a]Palonosetron 0.25 mg IV (preferred only when not combined with a NK-1 RA); ondansetron 8–16 mg IV or 16–24 mg PO; granisetron 0.01 mg/kg (1 mg max) IV or 2 mg PO or transdermal patch (3.1 mg/24 hr) applied 24–48 hr before first dose of chemotherapy; dolasteron 100 mg PO.
[b]Aprepitant 125 mg PO; fosaprepitant 150 mg IV; rolapitant 180 mg PO.
[c]Dexamethasone 12 mg PO/IV if aprepitant or fosaprepitant given; dexamethasone 20 mg PO/IV if rolapitant given.
[d]Data from large randomized trials with aprepitant support use in patients receiving cisplatin (70 mg/m^2) or anthracycline–cyclophosphamide combination regimens for breast cancer.
[e]Dolasteron 100 mg PO; granisetron 1–2 mg PO; ondansetron 8–16 mg PO.

preventing acute nausea and vomiting if/when a NK-1 RA is not to be used in combination.[161,222] For the prevention of acute emesis in patients receiving highly emetogenic chemotherapy, the use of a corticosteroid such as dexamethasone in combination with a 5-HT_3 receptor blocker and NK-1 RAs should be considered unless contraindicated. For patients receiving cisplatin chemotherapy, the dose of dexamethasone should be at least 12 mg but preferably 20 mg/day, based on findings of the Italian Group for Antiemetic Research.[225] This group also evaluated dexamethasone use in patients receiving anthracyclines, carboplatin, or cyclophosphamide.[226] Their results demonstrated that lower doses of dexamethasone (a single 8-mg IV dose) were as effective as higher doses (24 mg) for the prevention of acute emesis in this patient population.

Palonosetron, a 5-HT_3 receptor antagonist with a longer half-life (approximately 40 hours) and higher 5-HT_3–receptor binding as compared with other 5-HT_3 receptor antagonists, is used for the prevention of acute and delayed nausea and vomiting from highly and moderately emetogenic chemotherapy.[207] A study evaluating single-dose palonosetron versus ondansetron (both without dexamethasone) demonstrated efficacy (no emesis and no rescue medication required) of palonosetron as compared with ondansetron during the first day (81% versus 69%), days 2 to 5 (74% versus 55%), and over the entire period of 1 to 5 days (69% versus 50%) of chemotherapy.[227] The proportion of nausea-free patients was similar between the groups on days 1 to 2, while palonosetron-treated patients had significantly less nausea on days 3 to 5.

Aprepitant and the IV formulation fosaprepitant are NK-1 RAs and are important agents in the prevention of acute and delayed nausea and vomiting from highly (e.g., cisplatin) and moderately (e.g., anthracycline-cyclophosphamide combinations) emetogenic chemotherapy.[228] A study evaluating an aprepitant regimen versus standard therapy in the prevention of CINV in patients receiving cisplatin showed that a regimen including aprepitant, ondansetron, and dexamethasone was more effective than a regimen of ondansetron and dexamethasone.[229] In days 1 to 5 after cisplatin, 73% of aprepitant recipients versus 52% of patients in the control group had a complete response (no emesis and no rescue medications required). In terms of nausea control, there were no significant differences between the groups during the acute and delayed phases or overall.

In another study, patients receiving anthracycline–cyclophosphamide regimens were randomly assigned to receive oral ondansetron and dexamethasone with or without aprepitant on day 1.[230] On days 2 to 3, patients received either aprepitant or placebo with no additional dexamethasone. Overall, patients who received aprepitant had a better complete response (no emesis and no rescue medications required) than the placebo group (51% versus 42%). When the effects were evaluated in each phase separately, patients taking aprepitant achieved a better complete response during the acute phase (76% versus 69%); however, there was no significant difference in the delayed phase. Also, as in other trials, there was little or no impact on nausea in either group.

In an attempt to define the smallest aprepitant dose needed to effectively prevent CINV, a study was completed evaluating a single 125-mg dose of aprepitant. This randomized, double-blind, placebo-controlled trial evaluated palonosetron 0.25 mg IV, aprepitant 125 mg PO, and dexamethasone PO versus the standard 3-day aprepitant (125 mg on day 1 and 80 mg on days 2 and 3) regimen.[231] Overall, during days 1 to 5 both groups displayed similar effectiveness in the prevention of emesis (93%) and similar outcomes in the control of nausea and complete response (no emesis and no rescue antiemetics required). Further studies will be necessary to verify these findings. The idea of a single oral aprepitant dose is solidified with the FDA approval of a single IV dose of fosaprepitant.[232]

Netupitant–palonosetron (NEPA) is the first antiemetic combination agent for CINV. In three pivotal clinical trials, NEPA plus dexamethasone demonstrated improvement over oral palonosetron plus dexamethasone for acute and delayed nausea and vomiting for cisplatin-based highly emetogenic chemotherapy (overall: 89.6% versus 76.5%, respectively) or anthracycline–cyclophosphamide chemotherapy (overall: 74.3% versus 66.6%, respectively).[233] NEPA plus dexamethasone also showed significant improvement in nausea in both the delayed and acute settings over oral palonosetron plus dexamethasone for cisplatin-based highly emetogenic chemotherapy (overall: 89.6% versus 79.4%, respectively) or anthracycline-cyclophosphamide-based chemotherapy (overall: 74.6% versus 69.1%, respectively).[233]

Rolapitant is a highly selective oral NK-1 RA utilized in the prevention of acute and delayed nausea and vomiting from highly and moderately emetogenic chemotherapy. Three studies have shown, after cycle 1, that rolapitant combined with granisetron and dexamethasone was significantly more effective than granisetron and dexamethasone during the delayed phase of CINV (70.1–72.7% versus 58.4–61.9%, respectively).[233]

Olanzapine has been evaluated as first-line prophylaxis of CINV. An olanzapine/5-HT_3 receptor antagonist/dexamethasone combination regimen showed superior delayed and overall complete response rates compared to 5-HT_3 receptor antagonist/dexamethasone combination regimen in a phase III trial.[233] Another phase III trial compared olanzapine and aprepitant, both in combination with dexamethasone and palonosetron.[234] Complete response rates were comparable for the olanzapine and aprepitant regimens (97% acute, 77% delayed, 77% overall phases versus 87% acute, 73% delayed, 73% overall phases, respectively). Furthermore, patients without nausea in the olanzapine group were 87% acute, 69% delayed, and 69% overall compared to 87% acute, 38% delayed, and 38% overall for the aprepitant group.[234]

In patients who experience breakthrough nausea and emesis, changes should be made to the prophylactic regimen prior to the next chemotherapy session. When an antiemetic regimen fails, replacing the 5-HT_3 receptor blocker with another appears to benefit approximately 50% of patients.[235-237] If patients are experiencing delayed vomiting, adding NK-1 RAs or changing the 5-HT_3 receptor blocker to palonosetron or both are appropriate choices. The addition of a benzodiazepine may assist patients with anxiety problems. For those patients experiencing nausea, the use of olanzapine with a 5-HT_3 receptor blocker and dexamethsone has been shown to help prevent nausea.[161]

Despite the existence of published guidelines, it should be noted that patients have unique nausea and emesis risk factors and may respond differently to both chemotherapy agents and antiemetics. Therefore, individualization of the antiemetic regimens is necessary to provide optimal emetic control.

MISCELLANEOUS AGENTS

Drugs known to induce nausea and vomiting should be avoided if there are equally effective alternative agents available. Unfortunately, it is difficult to predict which patients will experience nausea or vomiting because these adverse events occur sporadically. Taking an oral medication with food may decrease nausea and vomiting in some cases and with some agents; however, drug–food interactions should be considered and avoided. Prophylactic use of an antiemetic may be necessary and appropriate in some situations. Ginger has also been evaluated in the prevention of CINV. A systematic review found seven studies that were mixed in their support of ginger for CINV, including three studies demonstrating a positive effect, two in favor but with caveats, and two trials with no effect on CINV.[238] Therefore, the use of ginger for CINV is equivocal, and further studies are required before recommending ginger for clinical use.

MANAGEMENT

OPIOIDS

Nausea and vomiting are common in patients beginning opioid therapy and generally resolve within the first several days of initiation. Often, having the patient take the opioid agent with food can minimize nausea and vomiting. Decreasing the dose or switching to a different opioid drug is another option. Patients who experience severe or repeated episodes of nausea or vomiting or both despite these interventions may benefit from scheduled doses of an antiemetic agent. The patient should be evaluated to rule out other causes of the GI symptoms. **Table 40-13** lists agents commonly used in the treatment of opioid-induced nausea and vomiting.[116,117]

In general, drugs useful in the treatment of opioid-induced nausea and vomiting include dopamine receptor antagonists, anticholinergic agents, and 5-HT_3–receptor antagonists.[153,239-241] Nausea and vomiting accompanied by abdominal distention or occurring immediately after meals may be attributed to opioid-induced gastroparesis, which may respond to metoclopramide administration before each meal and at bedtime. If the nausea and vomiting are associated with movement or are accompanied by dizziness, an anticholinergic agent or an antihistamine would be a more appropriate option.[162]

Ondansetron has been compared to metoclopramide for the management of opioid-induced emesis after surgery. In a study of over 1,000 patients, ondansetron 8 mg IV, ondansetron 16 mg IV, and metoclopramide 10 mg IV were evaluated for the

Table 40-13 Agents for the Management of Opioid-Induced Nausea and Vomiting

Class	Drugs
Anticholinergic	Scopolamine
Antihistamine	Diphenhydramine
Benzodiazepine	Midazolam
Corticosteroid	Dexamethasone
DOPAMINE ANTAGONISTS	
5-HT_3–receptor antagonist	Ondansetron
Substituted benzamide	Metoclopramide[a]
Butyrophenones	Droperidol, haloperidol
Opioid antagonist[b]	Naloxone
Phenothiazines	Prochlorperazine, promethazine[c]

[a]Also possesses peripheral activity at 5-HT_3 and 5-HT_4 receptors.
[b]When administered systemically in very low doses; may counteract analgesia.
[c]Also possesses antihistaminic and anticholinergic activity.

treatment of opioid-induced emesis.[241] Control of emesis was achieved in 63%, 61%, and 48% of patients, respectively; however, there was no significant difference in nausea scores among groups. This finding is similar to other trials. Overall, it appears that ondansetron 8 mg IV is effective for the management of opioid-induced vomiting.

Methylnaltrexone, a peripheral opioid antagonist, may have the potential to treat opioid-induced nausea and vomiting. A small double-blind, randomized, placebo-controlled trial of 12 participants receiving morphine with placebo or morphine with methylnaltrexone showed that patients in the methylnaltrexone arm had a significant reduction in delayed gastric emptying as well as significantly reduced opioid subjective effects including nausea.[242] Larger, randomized controlled trials will need to be performed to address methylnaltrexone's role in treating or preventing opioid-induced nausea and vomiting.

Table 40-14 Agents for the Management of Postoperative Nausea and Vomiting

Drug	Dose
Dexamethasone	2–4 mg IV
Dolasetron	12.5 mg IV
Droperidol[a,b]	0.625–1.25 mg IM/IV; may give additional 1.25 mg as needed
Granisetron	0.1 mg IV
Metoclopramide[b]	10 mg IV q 4–6 hr as needed
Ondansetron	1–4 mg IV
Prochlorperazine[b]	5–10 mg IM/IV; may repeat once if needed
Promethazine[b]	6.25–25 mg IM/IV; may repeat once if needed
Tropisetron	0.5 mg IV

IM = intramuscular, IV = intravenous.
[a]Caution should be exercised when giving additional doses because of the risk of inducing cardiac arrhythmias.
[b]Repeated doses may increase the risk of extrapyramidal symptoms.

PERIOPERATIVE AGENTS

Patients who experience PONV should limit movement and position changes, because excessive motion may exacerbate the condition. In general, any food or fluid intake by mouth should be discouraged for the first 8 hours postoperatively in patients experiencing PONV.[120] Patients who did not receive prophylactic therapy with a 5-HT_3–receptor antagonist should be treated with one of these agents postoperatively at the onset of PONV. Repeating the antiemetic used for PONV prophylaxis within 6 hours after the patient leaves the postanesthesia care unit offers no additional benefit. Instead, an antiemetic from another class should be tried. If more than 6 hours have elapsed, repeating the dose of the 5-HT_3–receptor antagonist or droperidol can be attempted; however, limited data support this practice.[192]

The effectiveness of granisetron or ondansetron for breakthrough PONV following prophylactic ondansetron has been evaluated.[243] In this trial, there were no significant differences between the granisetron and ondansetron groups in the 4-hour postoperative period. Up to a 68% complete response rate (resolution of PONV with no additional rescue medication required) was reported. A randomized, placebo-controlled trial of ondansetron 4 mg IV was conducted to evaluate PONV treatment in over 400 patients receiving inhaled anesthesia. All patients received preoperative prophylactic ondansetron. Complete response (no emesis and no rescue medication required) was similar for both the ondansetron and placebo groups at 2 hours (34% and 43%, respectively) and 24 hours (28% and 32%, respectively) after anesthesia. Patients who received repeated ondansetron doses for postoperative emesis or nausea had effects similar to those who received placebo.[244] **Table 40-14** lists antiemetic agents and their recommended doses for PONV treatment.[141,192]

CHEMOTHERAPY

Prevention is the best management strategy for chemotherapy-induced nausea and vomiting. Although the oncology literature is replete with information regarding prevention of this drug-induced disease, data regarding the effectiveness of various management strategies are sparse. Several national groups have developed guidelines for the treatment of CINV.[160,161,237,245] The drugs and doses commonly used are listed in **Table 40-15**. If breakthrough emesis develops despite adequate prophylaxis with a 5-HT_3 antagonist combined with

Table 40-15 Agents for the Management of Chemotherapy-Induced Nausea and Vomiting

For treatment of breakthrough nausea and vomiting despite the use of prophylactic antiemetics:

- Dexamethasone 12 mg IV/PO
- Dolasetron 100 mg PO
- Dronabinol 5–10 mg PO
- Granisetron 1–2 mg PO or 0.01 mg/kg (max 1 mg) IV
- Haloperidol 0.5–2 mg PO/IV
- Lorazepam 0.5–2 mg PO/ SL/IV
- Metoclopramide 10–40 mg IV
- Nabilone 1–2 mg PO
- Olanzapine 5–10 mg PO
- Ondansetron 16–24 mg PO or 8–16 mg IV
- Prochlorperazine 10 mg PO/IV or 25 mg PR
- Promethazine 12.5–25 mg PO/IV or 25 mg PR
- Scopalamine transdermal patch q 72 hr

IV = intravenous, PO = oral, PR = rectal, SL = sublingual.

dexamethasone, therapy with an agent from a different drug class should be initiated. A single dose of a 5-HT$_3$ antagonist is expected to occupy the receptor site and maintain effectiveness for up to 24 hours, thereby obviating the need for repeat dosing.

Choice of a specific drug to treat CINV depends on the patient's prophylactic regimen and his or her ability to tolerate potential adverse effects of the agent selected. Many drugs, including lorazepam, phenothiazines, metoclopramide, corticosteroids, butyrophenones, and dronabinol, have been used for the treatment of chemotherapy-induced emesis. Oral cannabinoids (i.e., dronabinol, nabilone) have also been shown to be effective in relieving CINV. Smoked marijuana, although highly touted as an effective treatment, has not been thoroughly evaluated in patients who are undergoing chemotherapy. A small, double-blind, placebo-controlled trial compared ondansetron and smoked marijuana in 13 patients who ingested ipecac syrup.[246] Ondansetron was significantly more effective than either smoked marijuana or placebo for the prevention of nausea and emesis. There was no difference in the incidence of nausea in patients treated with marijuana versus those who received placebo. Several states allow the use of marijuana for medicinal purposes. Although distributors and users can still be prosecuted under federal law, enforcement hasn't occurred in recent years. The American Cancer Society supports the need for more scientific research on cannabinoids in patients with cancer.[247]

If a patient received a 5-HT$_3$–receptor antagonist for prophylaxis, dopamine receptor inhibitors such as phenothiazines, metoclopramide, or butyrophenones can be administered for breakthrough nausea and vomiting.[160,161,237] Olanzapine, at a dose of 10 mg orally for 3 days, has been compared to metoclopramide for breakthrough nausea and vomiting where a higher proportion of patients had no significant vomiting (70% versus 31%) and no significant nausea (68% versus 23%) with olanzapine than metoclopramide, respectively.[248] These agents should be used cautiously, however, in patients at risk for extrapyramidal effects (e.g., pediatric and young adult patients and those with underlying Parkinson disease).[249] If a patient did not receive a 5-HT$_3$ antagonist as prophylaxis, then postchemotherapy nausea and vomiting may be treated with one of these drugs. Before the next chemotherapy cycle, the patient's antiemetic regimen should be altered to include a 5-HT$_3$–receptor antagonist and dexamethasone with the addition of NK-1 RA or olanzapine if the patient experienced delayed nausea and vomiting.

MISCELLANEOUS AGENTS

A study of patients with acquired immunodeficiency syndrome (AIDS) who were newly diagnosed with *Pneumocystis (carinii) jiroveci* pneumonia evaluated the role of ondansetron in the treatment of TMP/SMX-induced nausea and vomiting.[250] Sixteen patients were treated with 1,120 mg of the trimethoprim component of parenteral TMP/SMX with plans to switch to two oral TMP/SMX double-strength tablets four times a day for a total of 21 days. Patients received ondansetron 8 mg PO every 8 hours for 25 days. Only 7 patients completed all of the planned TMP/SMX treatment. Therapy was discontinued in the others for a variety of reasons. Overall, for 16 patients who initially received TMP/SMX, 69% had a "good emetic response," defined as two or fewer emetic episodes, and 44% experienced a "good nausea response," defined as no or mild nausea. Six patients were switched to a trimethoprim–dapsone regimen and did not experience any additional emesis. It is obvious from this trial that nausea and vomiting may develop in AIDS patients receiving high-dose TMP/SMX and that it can require switching therapy or the addition of antiemetics. It is unclear what impact ondansetron provided, because there was no control group.

Erythromycin can induce nausea and vomiting in a substantial number of patients. One study evaluated the role of glycopyrrolate and longer erythromycin infusion times on the incidence of nausea and vomiting.[93] This randomized, double-blind, placebo-controlled trial studied 51 patients receiving erythromycin 500 mg IV every 6 hours infused over either 30 or 60 minutes. Patients were randomly assigned to receive either glycopyrrolate 0.1 mg IV or placebo. Nausea and vomiting were significantly reduced in patients who received the 60-minute infusion and pretreatment with glycopyrrolate.

When nausea and vomiting are due to high serum concentrations of a drug, as with digoxin, for example, it is often necessary to temporarily discontinue the medication to allow the drug concentration to decrease before restarting therapy at a lower dose.

INFORMATION FOR PATIENTS

OPIOIDS

Patients started on therapy with opioid analgesics should be warned of the likely occurrence of nausea with or without vomiting. Patients should be informed that these symptoms are generally transient and will usually subside after the first few days of therapy. The exception is nausea and vomiting that occur as a result of opioid-induced constipation, to which tolerance will not develop. Patients who will receive long-term opioid therapy should take an appropriate stimulant laxative to prevent constipation and its associated problems, including nausea and vomiting. These patients should be informed that the bowel regimen should be continued throughout the duration of opioid treatment. Patients should be told that they can take the opioid analgesic with meals to help lessen gastric irritation that can often lead to nausea, vomiting, and abdominal pain.

Patients beginning opioid therapy should be counseled regarding the specific antiemetic agent to be used if nausea, vomiting, or both occur, and a prescription for an appropriate rescue antiemetic should be provided. Patients should also be instructed to seek medical attention if the nausea and vomiting become severe or if these symptoms are accompanied by others, such as abdominal pain or fever.

PERIOPERATIVE AGENTS

Patients should be informed during the preoperative interview that the overall risk of PONV ranges from 10% to 80%. In patients with no identifiable risk factors, the PONV probability is approximately 10%. Patients should be made aware of the risk factors associated with PONV and should be questioned about their previous experiences with general anesthesia. In addition, any prior adverse drug reactions or drug-induced diseases should be documented during the preoperative evaluation.

Patients should be instructed not to eat or drink anything during the specified preoperative period (anesthesiologists have preferences regarding the specific duration of time based on the type of surgery, type and duration of anesthesia, and patient-related risk factors for PONV). Questions that the patient may have regarding the surgery should be answered, and any concerns should be addressed. Preoperative anxiety has been linked to PONV, so anything that can alleviate the patient's anxiety may reduce that risk.[120]

CHEMOTHERAPY

CINV can be a distressing drug-induced disease that can significantly affect quality of life. Clinicians and patients must understand that there are no available drugs that are effective for the prevention or treatment of nausea and vomiting in all cases. If a patient has a prescription for a scheduled antiemetic therapy at home, he or she should be advised to take that medication as instructed. Many patients feel well immediately following chemotherapy and do not have prescriptions filled promptly; others cannot afford the medications. In either case, patients may find themselves unprepared to deal with delayed nausea and vomiting if and when it occurs. Patients with persistent nausea and vomiting that interferes with oral intake should be instructed to contact their healthcare professional. Patients should be advised to seek immediate medical attention if severe symptoms of dehydration (e.g., dizziness, confusion) occur and should be advised to maintain adequate fluid intake to prevent dehydration. Good communication between the patient and healthcare provider(s) is essential to the maintenance of effective antiemetic therapy. Patients in whom nausea develops should be instructed to eat small meals and choose bland foods (crackers, flat soda, etc.) and should avoid fatty, fried, very spicy, or sweet foods. To prevent nausea, patients should be encouraged to eat foods that are cold or at room temperature, because the aroma of warm or hot foods can increase nausea.

MISCELLANEOUS AGENTS

Anyone beginning therapy with a new medication may experience nausea and vomiting. Patients should routinely be instructed to contact their healthcare providers to discuss alternative therapeutic approaches if they are unable to tolerate the new agent. In some cases, the strategies to control nausea and vomiting described above may be helpful and necessary.

REFERENCES

1. Berman PM, Kirsner JB. Recognizing and avoiding adverse gastrointestinal effects of drugs. *Geriatrics.* 1974; 29:59-62.
2. Reuter U, Sanchez del Rio M, Carpay JA et al. Placebo adverse events in headache trials: headache as an adverse event of placebo. *Cephalalgia.* 2003; 23:496-503.
3. Carpenter DO. Neural mechanisms of emesis. *Can J Physiol Pharmacol.* 1990; 68:230-6.
4. Haubrich WS. Nausea and vomiting. In: Berk JE, Haubrich WS, Eds. *Gastrointestinal symptoms: clinical interpretation.* Philadelphia: BC Decker; 1991:91-103.
5. Bruppacher R, Gyr N, Fisch T. Abdominal pain, indigestion, anorexia, nausea and vomiting. *Baillières Clin Gastroenterol.* 1988; 2:275-92.
6. Langevin S, Lessard MR, Trépanier CA et al. Alfentanil causes less postoperative nausea and vomiting than equipotent doses of fentanyl or sufentanil in outpatients. *Anesthesiology.* 1999; 91:1666-73.
7. Hayes MJ, Fraser AR, Hampton JR. Randomised trial comparing buprenorphine and diamorphine for chest pain in suspected myocardial infarction. *Br Med J.* 1979; 2:300-2.
8. Splinter WM, O'Brien HV, Komocar L. Butorphanol: an opioid for day-care paediatric surgery. *Can J Anaesth.* 1995; 42:483-6.
9. Stadol package insert. Princeton, NJ: Bristol-Myers Squibb; 1996.
10. Rodriguez RF, Bravo LE, Castro F et al. Incidence of weak opioids adverse events in the management of cancer pain: a double-blind comparative trial. *J Palliat Med.* 2007; 10:56-60.
11. Crighton IM, Hobbs GJ, Wrench IJ. Analgesia after day case laparoscopic sterilisation. A comparison of tramadol with paracetamol/dextropropoxyphene and paracetamol/codeine combinations. *Anaesthesia.* 1997; 52:649-52.
12. McQuay HJ, Carroll D, Guest PG et al. A multiple dose comparison of ibuprofen and dihydrocodeine after third molar surgery. *Br J Oral Maxillofac Surg.* 1993; 31:95-100.
13. Gurbet A, Goren S, Sahin S et al. Comparison of analgesic effects of morphine, fentanyl, and remifentanil with intravenous patient-controlled analgesia after cardiac surgery. *J Cardiothorac Vasc Anesth.* 2004; 18:755-8.
14. Hale M, Tudor IC, Khanna S et al. Efficacy and tolerability of once-daily OROS hydromorphone and twice-daily extended-release oxycodone in patients with chronic, moderate to severe osteoarthritis pain: results of a 6-week, randomized, open-label, noninferiority analysis. *Clin Ther.* 2007; 29:874-88.
15. Silverman ME, Shih RD, Allegra J. Morphine induces less nausea than meperidine when administered parenterally. *J Emerg Med.* 2004; 27:241-3.
16. Murphy GS, Szokol JW, Avram MJ et al. Intraoperative methadone for the prevention of postoperative pain: a randomized, double-blinded clinical trial in cardiac surgical patients. *Anesthesiology.* 2015; 122:1112-22.
17. Breitfeld C, Peters J, Vockel T et al. Emetic effects of morphine and piritramide. *Br J Anaesth.* 2003; 91:218-23.
18. Minai FN, Khan FA. A comparison of morphine and nalbuphine for intraoperative and postoperative analgesia. *J Pak Med Assoc.* 2003; 53:391-6.
19. Kivitz A, Ma C, Ahdieh H et al. A 2-week, multicenter, randomized, double-blind, placebo-controlled, dose-ranging, phase III trial comparing the efficacy of oxymorphone extended release and placebo in adults with pain associated with osteoarthritis of the hip or knee. *Clin Ther.* 2006; 28:352-64.
20. Hartrick C, Van Hove I, Stegmann JU et al. Efficacy and tolerability of tapentadol immediate release and oxycodone HCl immediate release in patients awaiting primary joint replacement surgery for end-stage joint disease: a 10-day, phase III, randomized, double-blind, active- and placebo-controlled study. *Clin Ther.* 2009; 31:260-71.
21. Saros GB, Doolke A, Anderson RE et al. Desflurane vs. sevoflurane as the main inhaled anaesthetic for spontaneous breathing via a laryngeal mask for varicose vein day surgery: a prospective randomized study. *Acta Anaesthesiol Scand.* 2006; 50:549-52.
22. van den Berg AA, Honjol NM, Mphanza T et al. Vomiting, retching, headache and restlessness after halothane-, isoflurane- and enflurane-based anaesthesia. An analysis of pooled data following ear, nose, throat and eye surgery. *Acta Anaesthesiol Scand.* 1998; 42:658-63.
23. Bloomfield E, Porembka D, Grimes-Rice M. Avoidance of nitrous oxide and increased isoflurane during alfentanil based anesthesia decreases the incidence of postoperative nausea. *Anesth Prog.* 1997; 44:27-31.
24. Smith I, Terhoeve PA, Hennart D et al. A multicentre comparison of the costs of anaesthesia with sevoflurane or propofol. *Br J Anaesth.* 1999; 83:564-70.

25. Jacoby J, Heller M, Nicholas J et al. Etomidate versus midazolam for out-of-hospital intubation: a prospective, randomized trial. *Ann Emerg Med.* 2006; 47:525-30.
26. Launo C, Bassi C, Spagnolo L et al. Preemptive ketamine during general anesthesia for postoperative analgesia in patients undergoing laparoscopic cholecystectomy. *Minerva Anestesiol.* 2004; 70:727-34.
27. Roback MG, Wathen JE, MacKenzie T et al. A randomized, controlled trial of i.v. versus i.m. ketamine for sedation of pediatric patients receiving emergency department orthopedic procedures. *Ann Emerg Med.* 2006; 48:605-12.
28. Yee JB, Schafer PG, Crandall AS et al. Comparison of methohexital and alfentanil on movement during placement of retrobulbar nerve block. *Anesth Analg.* 1994; 79:320-3.
29. Austin T, Vilke GM, Nyheim E et al. Safety and effectiveness of methohexital for procedural sedation in the emergency department. *J Emerg Med.* 2003; 24:315-8.
30. Luntz SP, Janitz E, Motsch J et al. Cost-effectiveness and high patient satisfaction in the elderly: sevoflurane versus propofol anaesthesia. *Eur J Anaesthesiol.* 2004; 21:115-22.
31. Crawford ME, Carl P, Bach V et al. A randomized comparison between midazolam and thiopental for elective cesarean section anesthesia. I. Mothers. *Anesth Analg.* 1989; 68:229-33.
32. Murphy GS, Szokol JW, Franklin M et al. Postanesthesia care unit recovery times and neuromuscular blocking drugs: a prospective study of orthopedic surgical patients randomized to receive pancuronium or rocuronium. *Anesth Analg.* 2004; 98:193-200.
33. Ross GT, Stolbach LL, Hertz R. Actinomycin D in the treatment of methotrexate-resistant trophoblastic disease in women. *Cancer Res.* 1962; 22:1015-7.
34. Woolley PV 3rd, Ayoob MJ, Smith FP et al. Clinical trial of the effect of S-2-(3-aminopropylamino)-ethylphosphorothioic acid (WR-2721) (NSC 296961) on the toxicity of cyclophosphamide. *J Clin Oncol.* 1983; 1:198-203.
35. Turrisi AT, Glover DJ, Hurwitz S et al. Final report of the phase I trial of single-dose WR-2721 [S-2-(3-aminopropylamino)ethylphosphorothioic acid]. *Cancer Treat Rep.* 1986; 70:1389-93.
36. Atkins MB, Gould JA, Allegretta M et al. Phase I evaluation of recombinant interleukin-2 in patients with advanced malignant disease. *J Clin Oncol.* 1986; 4:1380-91.
37. Rustin GJ, Nelstrop AE, Crawford M et al. Phase II trial of oral altretamine for relapsed ovarian carcinoma: evaluation of defining response by serum CA125. *J Clin Oncol.* 1997; 15:172-6.
38. Ohnishi K, Yoshida H, Shigeno K et al. Arsenic trioxide therapy for relapsed or refractory Japanese patients with acute promyelocytic leukemia: need for careful electrocardiogram monitoring. *Leukemia.* 2002; 16:617-22.
39. Trisenox package insert. Frazer, PA: Cephalon; 2006.
40. Vidaza package insert. Boulder, CO: Pharmion Corporation; 2007.
41. Treanda package insert. Frazer, PA: Cephalon; 2008.
42. Friedberg JW, Cohen P, Chen L et al. Bendamustine in patients with rituximab-refractory indolent and transformed non-Hodgkin's lymphoma: results from a phase II multicenter, single-agent study. *J Clin Oncol.* 2008; 26:204-10.
43. Gambacorti-Passerini C, Cortes JE, Lipton JH et al. Safety of bosutinib versus imatinib in the phase 3 BELA trial in newly diagnosed chronic phase chronic myeloid leukemia. *Am J Hematol.* 2014; 89:947-53.
44. Busulfex package insert. Rockville, MD: Otsuka America Pharmaceutical, Inc; 2008.
45. Curt GA, Grygiel JJ, Corden BJ et al. A phase I and pharmacokinetic study of diamminecyclobutane-dicarboxylatoplatinum (NSC 241240). *Cancer Res.* 1983; 43:4470-73.
46. Smith IE, Harland SJ, Robinson BA et al. Carboplatin: a very active new cisplatin analog in the treatment of small cell lung cancer. *Cancer Treat Rep.* 1985; 69:43-6.
47. Joss RA, Kaplan S, Goldhirsch A et al. A phase I trial of cis-diammine-1,1-cyclobutane dicarboxylate platinum II (Carboplatin, CBDCA, JM-8) with a single dose every five week-schedule. *Invest New Drugs.* 1984; 2:297-304.
48. Hansen HH, Selawry OS, Pajak TF et al. The superiority of CCNU in the treatment of advanced Hodgkin's disease: Cancer and Leukemia Group B Study. *Cancer.* 1981; 47:14-8.
49. Shaw AT, Kim DW, Mehra R et al. Ceritinib in ALK-rearranged non-small-cell lung cancer. *N Engl J Med.* 2014; 370:1189-97.
50. Hong WK, Schaefer S, Issell B et al. A prospective randomized trial of methotrexate versus cisplatin in the treatment of recurrent squamous cell carcinoma of the head and neck. *Cancer.* 1983; 52:206-10.
51. Gralla RJ, Itri LM, Pisko SE et al. Antiemetic efficacy of high-dose metoclopramide: randomized trials with placebo and prochlorperazine in patients with chemotherapy-induced nausea and vomiting. *N Engl J Med.* 1981; 305:905-9.
52. Arranon package insert. Research Triangle Park, NC: GlaxoSmithKline; 2006.
53. Camidge DR, Bang YJ, Kwak EL et al. Activity and safety of crizotinib in patients with ALK-positive non-small-cell lung cancer: updated results from a phase 1 study. *Lancet Oncol.* 2012; 13:1011-9.
54. Carmo-Pereira J, Costa FO, Henriques E et al. Advanced ovarian carcinoma: a prospective and randomized clinical trial of cyclophosphamide versus combination cytotoxic chemotherapy (Hexa-CAF). *Cancer.* 1981; 48:1947-51.
55. Fetting JH, Grochow LB, Folstein MF et al. The course of nausea and vomiting after high-dose cyclophosphamide. *Cancer Treat Rep.* 1982; 66:1487-93.
56. Mendelson D, Block JB, Serpick AA. Effect of large intermittent intravenous doses of cyclophosphamide in lymphoma. *Cancer.* 1970; 25:715-20.
57. Brincker H, Mouridsen HT, Andersen KW. Adjuvant chemotherapy with cyclophosphamide or CMF in premenopausal women with stage II breast cancer. *Breast Cancer Res Treat.* 1983; 3:91-5.
58. Cole MP, Todd ID, Wilkinson PM. Cyclophosphamide and nandrolone decanoate in the treatment of advanced carcinoma of the breast—results of a comparative controlled trial of the agents used singly and in combination. *Br J Cancer.* 1973; 27:396-9.
59. Vogler WR, Preisler HD, Winton EF et al. Randomized trial of high-dose cytarabine versus amsacrine in acute myelogenous leukemia in relapse: a Leukemia Intergroup Study. *Cancer Treat Rep.* 1986; 70:455-9.
60. Early AP, Preisler HD, Slocum H et al. A pilot study of high-dose 1-beta-D-arabinofuranosylcytosine for acute leukemia and refractory lymphoma: clinical response and pharmacology. *Cancer Res.* 1982; 42:1587-94.
61. Pommier Y, Pochat L, Marie JP et al. High-dose cytarabine in acute leukemia: toxicity and pharmacokinetics. *Cancer Treat Rep.* 1983; 67:371-3.
62. Costanza ME, Nathanson L, Costello WG et al. Results of a randomized study comparing DTIC with TIC mustard in malignant melanoma. *Cancer.* 1976; 37:1654-9.
63. Wiernik PH, Serpick AA. A randomized clinical trial of daunorubicin and a combination of prednisone, vincristine, 6-mercaptopurine, and methotrexate in adult acute nonlymphocytic leukemia. *Cancer Res.* 1972; 32:2023-6.
64. Extra JM, Rousseau F, Bruno R et al. Phase I and pharmacokinetic study of Taxotere (RP 56976; NSC 628503) given as a short intravenous infusion. *Cancer Res.* 1993; 53:1037-42.
65. Falkson G, Moertel CG, Lavin P et al. Chemotherapy studies in primary liver cancer: a prospective randomized clinical trial. *Cancer.* 1978; 42:2149-56.
66. Creagan ET, Hahn RG, Ahmann DL et al. A clinical trial adriamycin (NSC 123127) in advanced sarcomas. *Oncology.* 1977; 34:90-1.

67. Brambilla C, Rossi A, Bonfante V et al. Phase II study of doxorubicin versus epirubicin in advanced breast cancer. *Cancer Treat Rep.* 1986; 70:261-6.
68. Neidhart JA, Gochnour D, Roach R et al. A comparison of mitoxantrone and doxorubicin in breast cancer. *J Clin Oncol.* 1986; 4:672-7.
69. Chang P, Wiernik PH. Combination chemotherapy with adriamycin and streptozotocin. I. Clinical results in patients with advanced sarcoma. *Clin Pharmacol Ther.* 1976; 20:605-10.
70. Goel S, Mita AC, Mita M et al. A phase I study of eribulin mesylate (E7389), a mechanistically novel inhibitor of microtubule dynamics, in patients with advanced solid malignancies. *Clin Cancer Res.* 2009; 15:4207-12.
71. Bennett CL, Sinkule JA, Schilsky RL et al. Phase I clinical and pharmacological study of 72-hour continuous infusion of etoposide in patients with advanced cancer. *Cancer Res.* 1987; 47:1952-6.
72. Daghestani AN, Arlin ZA, Leyland-Jones B et al. Phase I and II clinical and pharmacological study of 4-demethoxydaunorubicin (idarubicin) in adult patients with acute leukemia. *Cancer Res.* 1985; 45:1408-12.
73. Bramwell VH, Mouridsen HT, Santoro A et al. Cyclophosphamide versus ifosfamide: preliminary report of a randomized phase II trial in adult soft tissue sarcomas. *Cancer Chemother Pharmacol.* 1986; 18(suppl 2):S13-6.
74. De Forges A, Droz JP, Ghosn M et al. Phase II trial of ifosfamide/mesna in metastatic adult renal carcinoma. *Cancer Treat Rep.* 1987; 71:1103.
75. Costanzi JJ, Gagliano R, Loukas D et al. Ifosfamide in the treatment of recurrent or disseminated lung cancer: a phase II study of two dose schedules. *Cancer.* 1978; 41:1715-9.
76. Negoro S, Fukuoka M, Masuda N et al. Phase I study of weekly intravenous infusions of CPT-11, a new derivative of camptothecin, in the treatment of advanced non-small-cell lung cancer. *J Natl Cancer Inst.* 1991; 83:1164-8.
77. Schlumberger M, Tahara M, Wirth LJ et al. Lenvatinib versus placebo in radioiodine-refractory thyroid cancer. *N Engl J Med.* 2015; 372:621-30.
78. Horton J, Mittelman A, Taylor SG et al. Phase II trials with procarbazine (NSC-77213), streptozotocin (NSC-85998), 6-thioguanine (NSC-752), and CCNU (NSC-79037) in patients with metastatic cancer of the large bowel. *Cancer Chemother Rep.* 1975; 59(2 Pt 1):333-40.
79. Dameshek W, Weisfuse L, Stein T. Nitrogen mustard therapy in Hodgkin's disease; analysis of 50 consecutive cases. *Blood.* 1949; 4:338-79.
80. Leone LA, Albala MM, Rege VB. Treatment of carcinoma of the head and neck with intravenous methotrexate. *Cancer.* 1968; 21:828-37.
81. Extra JM, Espie M, Calvo F et al. Phase I study of oxaliplatin in patients with advanced cancer. *Cancer Chemother Pharmacol.* 1990; 25:299-303.
82. Legha SS, Tenney DM, Krakoff IR. Phase I study of taxol using a 5-day intermittent schedule. *J Clin Oncol.* 1986; 4:762-6.
83. Sasaki Y, Nishina T, Yasui H et al. Phase II trial of nanoparticle albumin-bound paclitaxel as second-line chemotherapy for unresectable or recurrent gastric cancer. *Cancer Sci.* 2014; 105:812-7.
84. Santoni M, Conti A, De Giorgi U et al. Risk of gastrointestinal events with sorafenib, sunitinib and pazopanib in patients with solid tumors: a systematic review and meta-analysis of clinical trials. *Int J Cancer.* 2014; 135:763-73.
85. Rinaldi DA, Burris HA, Dorr FA et al. Initial phase I evaluation of the novel thymidylate synthase inhibitor, LY231514, using the modified continual reassessment method for dose escalation. *J Clin Oncol.* 1995; 13:2842-50.
86. Krug LM, Azzoli CG, Kris MG et al. 10-propargyl-10-deazaa minopterin: an antifolate with activity in patients with previously treated non-small cell lung cancer. *Clin Cancer Res.* 2003; 9:2072-8.
87. Yung WK, Albright RE, Olson J et al. A phase II study of temozolomide vs. procarbazine in patients with glioblastoma multiforme at first relapse. *Br J Cancer.* 2000; 83:588-93.
88. Moertel CG, Hanley JA, Johnson LA. Streptozocin alone compared with streptozocin plus fluorouracil in the treatment of advanced islet-cell carcinoma. *N Engl J Med.* 1980; 303:1189-94.
89. Schein PS, O'Connell MJ, Blom J et al. Clinical antitumor activity and toxicity of streptozotocin (NSC-85998). *Cancer.* 1974; 34:993-1000.
90. Brada M, Judson I, Beale P et al. Phase I dose-escalation and pharmacokinetic study of temozolomide (SCH 52365) for refractory or relapsing malignancies. *Br J Cancer.* 1999; 81:1022-30.
91. Kantarjian HM, Beran M, Ellis A et al. Phase I study of topotecan, a new topoisomerase I inhibitor, in patients with refractory or relapsed acute leukemia. *Blood.* 1993; 81:1146-51.
92. Staszewski S, Katlama C, Harrer T et al. A dose-ranging study to evaluate the safety and efficacy of abacavir alone or in combination with zidovudine and lamivudine in antiretroviral treatment-naive subjects. *AIDS.* 1998; 12:F197-202.
93. Bowler WA, Hostettler C, Samuelson D et al. Gastrointestinal side effects of intravenous erythromycin: incidence and reduction with prolonged infusion time and glycopyrrolate pretreatment. *Am J Med.* 1992; 92:249-53.
94. Lloyd CJ, Earl PD. Metronidazole: two or three times daily—a comparative controlled clinical trial of the efficacy of two different dosing schedules of metronidazole for chemoprophylaxis following third molar surgery. *Br J Oral Maxillofac Surg.* 1994; 32:165-7.
95. Oliva ME, Rekha A, Yellin A et al. A multicenter trial of the efficacy and safety of tigecycline versus imipenem/cilastatin in patients with complicated intra-abdominal infections [Study ID Numbers: 3074A1-301-WW; ClinicalTrials.gov Identifier: NCT00081744]. *BMC Infect Dis.* 2005; 5:88.
96. Breedt J, Teras J, Gardovskis J et al. Safety and efficacy of tigecycline in treatment of skin and skin structure infections: results of a double-blind phase 3 comparison study with vancomycin-aztreonam. *Antimicrob Agents Chemother.* 2005; 49:4658-66.
97. Talan DA, Stamm WE, Hooton TM et al. Comparison of ciprofloxacin (7 days) and trimethoprim-sulfamethoxazole (14 days) for acute uncomplicated pyelonephritis pyelonephritis in women: a randomized trial. *JAMA.* 2000; 283:1583-90.
98. Joos B, Blaser J, Opravil M et al. Monitoring of co-trimoxazole concentrations in serum during treatment of *pneumocystis carinii* pneumonia. *Antimicrob Agents Chemother.* 1995; 39:2661-6.
99. Markowitz M, Saag M, Powderly WG et al. A preliminary study of ritonavir, an inhibitor of HIV-1 protease, to treat HIV-1 infection. *N Engl J Med.* 1995; 333:1534-9.
100. Lee LM, Henderson DK. Tolerability of postexposure antiretroviral prophylaxis for occupational exposures to HIV. *Drug Saf.* 2001; 24:587-97.
101. Settle EC, Stahl SM, Batey SR et al. Safety profile of sustained-release bupropion in depression: results of three clinical trials. *Clin Ther.* 1999; 21:454-63.
102. Weihs KL, Settle EC Jr, Batey SR et al. Bupropion sustained release versus paroxetine for the treatment of depression in the elderly. *J Clin Psychiatry.* 2000; 61:196-202.
103. De Wilde J, Spiers R, Mertens C et al. A double-blind, comparative, multicentre study comparing paroxetine with fluoxetine in depressed patients. *Acta Psychiatr Scand.* 1993; 87:141-5.
104. Beasley CM Jr, Koke SC, Nilsson ME et al. Adverse events and treatment discontinuations in clinical trials of fluoxetine in major depressive disorder: an updated meta-analysis. *Clin Ther.* 2000; 22:1319-30.
105. Li H, Ma C, Wang G et al. Response and remission rates in Chinese patients with bipolar mania treated for 4 weeks with either quetiapine or lithium: a randomized and double-blind study. *Curr Med Res Opin.* 2008; 24:1-10.
106. Rimon E, Kagansky N, Kagansky M et al. Are we giving too much iron? Low-dose iron therapy is effective in octogenarians. *Am J Med.* 2005; 118:1142-7.

107. Hyder SM, Persson LA, Chowdhury AM et al. Do side-effects reduce compliance to iron supplementation? A study of daily- and weekly-dose regimens in pregnancy. *J Health Popul Nutr.* 2002; 20:175-9.
108. Ellertson C, Webb A, Blanchard K et al. Modifying the Yuzpe regimen of emergency contraception: a multicenter randomized controlled trial. *Obstet Gynecol.* 2003; 101:1160-7.
109. Buse JB, Henry RR, Han J et al. Effects of exenatide (exendin-4) on glycemic control over 30 weeks in sulfonylurea-treated patients with type 2 diabetes. *Diabetes Care.* 2004; 27:2628-35.
110. DeFronzo RA, Ratner RE, Han J et al. Effects of exenatide (exendin-4) on glycemic control and weight over 30 weeks in metformin-treated patients with type 2 diabetes. *Diabetes Care.* 2005; 28:1092-1100.
111. Kendall DM, Riddle MC, Rosenstock J et al. Effects of exenatide (exendin-4) on glycemic control over 30 weeks in patients with type 2 diabetes treated with metformin and a sulfonylurea. *Diabetes Care.* 2005; 28:1083-91.
112. Marre M, Shaw J, Brändle M et al. Liraglutide, a once-daily human GLP-1 analogue, added to a sulphonylurea over 26 weeks produces greater improvements in glycaemic and weight control compared with adding rosiglitazone or placebo in subjects with Type 2 diabetes (LEAD-1 SU). *Diabet Med.* 2009; 26:268-78.
113. Zinman B, Gerich J, Buse JB et al. Efficacy and safety of the human glucagon-like peptide-1 analog liraglutide in combination with metformin and thiazolidinedione in patients with type 2 diabetes (LEAD-4 Met+TZD). *Diabetes Care.* 2009; 32:1224-30.
114. Fujioka K, Brazg RL, Raz I et al. Efficacy, dose-response relationship and safety of once-daily extended-release metformin (Glucophage XR) in type 2 diabetic patients with inadequate glycaemic control despite prior treatment with diet and exercise: results from two double-blind, placebo-controlled studies. *Diabetes Obes Metab.* 2005; 7:28-39.
115. Marlin GE, Butcher MA, Klumpp JA et al. Serum level monitoring of a new slow release theophylline formulation in patients with chronic lung disease. *Br J Clin Pharmacol.* 1980; 10:265-71.
116. Zuckerman LA, Ferrante FM. Nonopioid and opioid analgesics. In: Ashburn MA, Rice LJ, eds. *The Management of pain.* New York, NY: Churchill Livingstone; 1998:111141.
117. Nicholson B. Responsible prescribing of opioids for the management of chronic pain. *Drugs.* 2003; 63:17-32.
118. Coyle N, Cherny N, Portenoy RK. Pharmacological management of cancer pain. In: McGuire DB, Yarbro CH, Ferrell BR, eds. *Cancer pain management.* 2nd ed. Boston, MA: Jones and Bartlett; 1995:89-130.
119. Rollins G. Guidelines outline strategies to reduce post-operative nausea and vomiting. *Rep Med Guidel Outcomes Res.* 2002; 13:9-10, 12.
120. Arif AS, Kaye AD, Frost E. Postoperative nausea and vomiting—a review. *Middle East J Anaesthesiol.* 2001; 16:127-54.
121. Royston D, Cox F. Anaesthesia: the patient's point of view. *Lancet.* 2003; 362:1648-58.
122. Apfel CC, Läärä E, Koivuranta M et al. A simplified risk score for predicting postoperative nausea and vomiting: conclusions from cross-validations between two centers. *Anesthesiology.* 1999; 91:693-700.
123. Eberhart LH, Geldner G, Kranke P et al. The development and validation of a risk score to predict the probability of postoperative vomiting in pediatric patients. *Anesth Analg.* 2004; 99:1630-7.
124. Osoba D, Zee B, Pater J et al. Determinants of postchemotherapy nausea and vomiting in patients with cancer. Quality of Life and Symptom Control Committees of the National Cancer Institute of Canada Clinical Trials Group. *J Clin Oncol.* 1997; 15:116-23.
125. Morrow GR, Rosenthal SN. Models, mechanisms and management of anticipatory nausea and emesis. *Oncology.* 1996; 53(suppl 1):4-7.
126. Wofford JL, Hickey AR, Ettinger WH et al. Lack of age-related differences in the clinical presentation of digoxin toxicity. *Arch Intern Med.* 1992; 152:2261-4.
127. Taylor AT. Nausea and vomiting. In: Dipiro JT, Talbert RL, Yee GC et al, eds. *Pharmacotherapy: a pathophysiologic approach.* 5th ed. New York, NY: McGraw-Hill; 2002:641653.
128. Pasricha PJ. Prokinetic agents, antiemetics, and agents used in irritable bowel syndrome. In: Hardman JG, Limbird LE, eds. *Goodman and Gilman's the pharmacological basis of therapeutics.* 10th ed. New York, NY: McGraw-Hill; 2001:1021-36.
129. Hasler WL. Approach to the patient with nausea and vomiting. In: Yamada T, ed. *Textbook of gastroenterology.* Vol. 1, 3rd ed. Philadelphia, PA: Lippincott Williams and Wilkins; 1999:775-94.
130. Kurz A, Sessler DI. Opioid-induced bowel dysfunction: pathophysiology and potential new therapies. *Drugs.* 2003; 63:649-71.
131. Watcha MF. Postoperative nausea and emesis. *Anesthesiol Clin North America.* 2002; 20:709-22.
132. Watcha MF, White PF. Postoperative nausea and vomiting. Its etiology, treatment, and prevention. *Anesthesiology.* 1992; 77:162-84.
133. Aitkenhead AR. Anaesthesia and the gastro-intestinal system. *Eur J Anaesthesiol.* 1988; 5:73-112.
134. Carpenter RL, Caplan RA, Brown DL et al. Incidence and risk factors for side effects of spinal anesthesia. *Anesthesiology.* 1992; 76:906-16.
135. Berger AM, Clark-Snow RA. Adverse effects of treatment. In: DeVita VT, Jr, Hellman S, Rosenberg SA, eds. *Cancer: principles & practices of oncology.* 7th ed. Philadelphia, PA: Lippincott Williams and Wilkins; 2005:2515-22.
136. Hesketh PJ, Van Belle S, Aapro M et al. Differential involvement of neurotransmitters through the time course of cisplatin-induced emesis as revealed by therapy with specific receptor antagonists. *Eur J Cancer.* 2003; 39:1074-80.
137. Weber FH, Jr, Richards RD, McCallum RW. Erythromycin: a motilin agonist and gastrointestinal prokinetic agent. *Am J Gastroenterol.* 1993; 88:485-90.
138. Qin XY, Pilot MA, Thompson H et al. Effects of cholinoceptor and 5-hydroxytryptamine3 receptor antagonism on erythromycin-induced canine intestinal motility disruption and emesis. *Br J Pharmacol.* 1993; 108:44-9.
139. Zara GP, Thompson HH, Pilot MA et al. Effects of erythromycin on gastrointestinal tract motility. *J Antimicrob Chemother.* 1985; 16(suppl A):175-9.
140. Itoh Z, Suzuki T, Nakaya M et al. Gastrointestinal motor-stimulating activity of macrolide antibiotics and analysis of their side effects on the canine gut. *Antimicrob Agents Chemother.* 1984; 26:863-9.
141. Micromedex(r) Healthcare Series [online database]. Metronidazole. http://www.micromedexsolutions.com/micromedex2/librarian/CS/B01B5B/ND_PR/evidencexpert/ND_P/evidencexpert/DUPLICATIONSHIELDSYNC/1AA678/ND_PG/evidencexpert/ND_B/evidencexpert/ND_AppProduct/evidencexpert/ND_T/evidencexpert/PFActionId/evidencexpert.DoIntegratedSearch?SearchTerm=metronidazole&UserSearchTerm=metronidazole&SearchFilter=filterNone&navitem=searchALL# (accessed 2018 Mar 13).
142. Mays DC, Nelson AN, Benson LM et al. Photolysis of sulfiram: a mechanism for its disulfiram-like reaction. *Biochem Pharmacol.* 1994; 48:1917-25.
143. Karamanakos PN, Pappas P, Boumba VA et al. Pharmaceutical agents known to produce disulfiram-like reaction: effects on hepatic ethanol metabolism and brain monoamines. *Int J Toxicol.* 2007; 26:423-32.
144. Borison HL, Borison R, McCarthy LE. Role of the area postrema in vomiting and related functions. *Fed Proc.* 1984; 43:2955-8.
145. Bateman DN, Aziz EE. Gastrointestinal disorders. In: Davies DM, Ferner RE, de Glanville H, eds. *Davies's textbook of adverse drug reactions.* 5th ed. London, England: Chapman and Hall Medical; 1998:259-74.
146. Morris JG. A review of some aspects of the pharmacology of levodopa. *Clin Exp Neurol.* 1978; 15:24-50.

147. Fujiwara-Sawada M, Imanishi T, Yoshida A et al. Possible involvement of peripheral serotonin 5-HT$_3$ receptors in fluvoxamine-induced emesis in Suncus murinus. *J Pharm Pharmacol.* 2003; 55:271-4.
148. Andrews PL, Hawthorn J. The neurophysiology of vomiting. *Baillières Clin Gastroenterol.* 1988; 2:141-68.
149. Stern RM. The psychophysiology of nausea. *Acta Biol Hung.* 2002; 53:589-99.
150. Spiller RC. ABC of the upper gastrointestinal tract: anorexia, nausea, vomiting, and pain. *BMJ.* 2001; 323:1354-7.
151. Lee M. Nausea and vomiting. In: Feldman M, Friedman LS, Sleisenger MH, eds. *Sleisenger & Fordtran's gastrointestinal and liver disease: pathophysiology/diagnosis/management.* Vol. 1, 7th ed. Philadelphia, PA: Saunders; 2002:119-30.
152. Hanson JS, McCallum RW. The diagnosis and management of nausea and vomiting: a review. *Am J Gastroenterol.* 1985; 80:210-8.
153. Mitchelson F. Pharmacological agents affecting emesis. A review (Part I). *Drugs.* 1992; 43:295-315.
154. Davis E. Nitrous oxide use during general anaesthesia for general surgical cases. *Br J Hosp Med (Lond).* 2015; 76:178.
155. Higa GM, Auber ML, Altaha R et al. Concordance between substance P levels and antiemetic guidelines. *J Support Oncol.* 2009; 7:138-42.
156. Higa GM, Auber ML, Altaha R et al. 5-Hydroxyindoleacetic acid and substance P profiles in patients receiving emetogenic chemotherapy. *J Oncol Pharm Pract.* 2006; 12:201-9.
157. Visapää JP, Tillonen JS, Kaihovaara PS et al. Lack of disulfiram-like reaction with metronidazole and ethanol. *Ann Pharmacother.* 2002; 36:971-4.
158. Heelon MW, White M. Disulfiram-cotrimoxazole reaction. *Pharmacotherapy.* 1998; 18:869-70.
159. Trujillo JM, Nuffer W, Ellis SL. GLP-1 receptor agonists: a review of head-to-head clinical studies. *Ther Adv Endocrinol Metab.* 2015; 6:19-28.
160. ASHP therapeutic guidelines on the pharmacologic management of nausea and vomiting in adult and pediatric patients receiving chemotherapy or radiation therapy or undergoing surgery. *Am J Health-Syst Pharm.* 1999; 56:729-64.
161. National Comprehensive Cancer Network [online database]. Antiemesis. https://www.nccn.org/professionals/physician_gls/pdf/antiemesis.pdf (accessed 2018 Mar 13).
162. Portenoy RK. Management of common opioid side effects during long-term therapy of cancer pain. *Ann Acad Med Singapore.* 1994; 23:160-70.
163. Cepeda MS, Farrar JT, Baumgarten M et al. Side effects of opioids during short-term administration: effect of age, gender, and race. *Clin Pharmacol Ther.* 2003; 74:102-12.
164. Bohn LM, Raehal KM. Opioid receptor signaling: relevance for gastrointestinal therapy. *Curr Opin Pharmacol.* 2006; 6:559-63.
165. Apfel CC, Kranke P, Katz MH et al. Volatile anaesthetics may be the main cause of early but not delayed postoperative vomiting: a randomized controlled trial of factorial design. *Br J Anaesth.* 2002; 88:659-68.
166. Kenny GN. Risk factors for postoperative nausea and vomiting. *Anaesthesia.* 1994; 49(suppl):6-10.
167. Ali SZ, Taguchi A, Holtmann B et al. Effect of supplemental preoperative fluid on postoperative nausea and vomiting. *Anaesthesia.* 2003; 58:780-4.
168. Morgan GE, Mikhail MS, Murray MJ et al. Postanesthesia care. In: Morgan GE, Mikhail MS, Murray MJ et al, eds. *Clinical anesthesiology.* 3rd ed. New York, NY: Lange Medical Books; 2002:936-50.
169. Apfel CC, Heidrich FM, Jukar-Rao S et al. Evidence-based analysis of risk factors for postoperative nausea and vomiting. *Br J Anaesth.* 2012; 109:742-53.
170. Janicki PK, Schuler HG, Jarzembowski TM et al. Prevention of postoperative nausea and vomiting with granisetron and dolasetron in relation to CYP2D6 genotype. *Anesth Analg.* 2006; 102:1127-33.
171. Roila F, Donati D, Tamberi S et al. Delayed emesis: incidence, pattern, prognostic factors and optimal treatment. *Support Care Cancer.* 2002; 10:88-95.
172. Jacobsen PB, Andrykowski MA, Redd WH et al. Nonpharmacologic factors in the development of posttreatment nausea with adjuvant chemotherapy for breast cancer. *Cancer.* 1988; 61:379-85.
173. Kaiser R, Sezer O, Papies A et al. Patient-tailored antiemetic treatment with 5-hydroxytryptamine type 3 receptor antagonists according to cytochrome P-450 2D6 genotypes. *J Clin Oncol.* 2002; 20:2805-11.
174. Kovac AL. Prevention and treatment of postoperative nausea and vomiting. *Drugs.* 2000; 59:213-43.
175. Gan TJ, Meyer TA, Apfel CC et al. Society for Ambulatory Anesthesia guidelines for the management of postoperative nausea and vomiting. *Anesth Analg.* 2007; 105:1615-28.
176. Pirri C, Bayliss E, Trotter J et al. Nausea still the poor relation in antiemetic therapy? The impact on cancer patients' quality of life and psychological adjustment of nausea, vomiting and appetite loss, individually and concurrently as part of a symptom cluster. *Support Care Cancer.* 2013; 21:735-48.
177. Mitchell EP. Gastrointestinal toxicity of chemotherapeutic agents. *Semin Oncol.* 1992; 19:566-79.
178. Neymark N, Crott R. Impact of emesis on clinical and economic outcomes of cancer therapy with highly emetogenic chemotherapy regimens: a retrospective analysis of three clinical trials. *Support Care Cancer.* 2005; 13:812-8.
179. Ammassari A, Murri R, Pezzotti P et al. Self-reported symptoms and medication side effects influence adherence to highly active antiretroviral therapy in persons with HIV infection. *J Acquir Immune Defic Syndr.* 2001; 28:445-9.
180. Farr SJ, Robinson CY, Rubino CM. Effects of food and alcohol on the pharmacokinetics of an oral, extended-release formulation of hydrocodone in healthy volunteers. *Clin Pharmacol.* 2015; 7:1-9.
181. Paoloni R, Talbot-Stern J. Low incidence of nausea and vomiting with intravenous opiate analgesia in the ED. *Am J Emerg Med.* 2002; 20:604-8.
182. Talbot-Stern J, Paoloni R. Prophylactic metoclopramide is unnecessary with intravenous analgesia in the ED. *Am J Emerg Med.* 2000; 18:653-7.
183. Morgan GE, Mikhail MS, Murray MJ et al. The practice of anesthesiology. In: Morgan GE, Mikhail MS, Murray MJ et al., eds. *Clinical anesthesiology.* 3rd ed. New York, NY: Lange Medical Books; 2002:1-14.
184. Visser K, Hassink EA, Bonsel GJ et al. Randomized controlled trial of total intravenous anesthesia with propofol versus inhalation anesthesia with isoflurane-nitrous oxide: postoperative nausea with vomiting and economic analysis. *Anesthesiology.* 2001; 95:616-26.
185. Mathias JM. New anesthetics have fewer side effects. *OR Manager.* 1995; 11:16-9.
186. White PF, Watcha MF. Pharmacoeconomics in anaesthesia: what are the issues? *Eur J Anaesthesiol Suppl.* 2001; 23:10-15.
187. Sneyd JR, Carr A, Byrom WD et al. A meta-analysis of nausea and vomiting following maintenance of anaesthesia with propofol or inhalational agents. *Eur J Anaesthesiol.* 1998; 15:433-45.
188. Fleischmann E, Akça O, Wallner T et al. Onset time, recovery duration, and drug cost with four different methods of inducing general anesthesia. *Anesth Analg.* 1999; 88:930-5.
189. Sung YF. Risks and benefits of drugs used in the management of postoperative nausea and vomiting. *Drug Saf.* 1996; 14:181-97.
190. Akhtar TM, Kerr WJ, Kenny GN. Effect of nitrous oxide on postoperative nausea and vomiting during propofol anaesthesia for short surgical operations. *Eur J Anaesthesiol.* 1993; 10:337-41.
191. Boucher BA, Witt WO, Foster TS. The postoperative adverse effects of inhalational anesthetics. *Heart Lung.* 1986; 15:63-9.
192. Gan TJ, Diemunsch P, Habib AS et al. Consensus guidelines for the management of postoperative nausea and vomiting. *Anesth Analg.* 2014; 118:85-113.

193. Blanc VF, Ruest P, Milot J et al. Antiemetic prophylaxis with promethazine or droperidol in paediatric outpatient strabismus surgery. *Can J Anaesth*. 1991; 38:54-60.
194. Gan TJ, Apfel CC, Kovac A et al. A randomized, double-blind comparison of the NK1 antagonist, aprepitant, versus ondansetron for the prevention of postoperative nausea and vomiting. *Anesth Analg*. 2007; 104:1082-9.
195. Habib AS, Reuveni J, Taquchi A et al. A comparison of ondansetron with promethazine for treating postoperative nausea and vomiting in patients who received prophylaxis with ondansetron: a retrospective database analysis. *Anesth Analg*. 2007; 104:548-51.
196. Starke PR, Weaver J, Chowdhury BA. Boxed warning added to promethazine labeling for pediatric use. *N Engl J Med*. 2005; 352:2653.
197. McKenzie R, Kovac A, O'Connor T et al. Comparison of ondansetron versus placebo to prevent postoperative nausea and vomiting in women undergoing ambulatory gynecologic surgery. *Anesthesiology*. 1993; 78:21-8.
198. Sung YF, Wetchler BV, Duncalf D et al. A double-blind, placebo-controlled pilot study examining the effectiveness of intravenous ondansetron in the prevention of postoperative nausea and emesis. *J Clin Anesth*. 1993; 5:22-9.
199. Khalil SN, Kataria B, Pearson K et al. Ondansetron prevents postoperative nausea and vomiting in women outpatients. *Anesth Analg*. 1994; 79:845-51.
200. Apfel CC, Korttila K, Abdalla M et al. A factorial trial of six interventions for the prevention of postoperative nausea and vomiting. *N Engl J Med*. 2004; 350:2441-51.
201. Scuderi P, Wetchler B, Sung YF et al. Treatment of postoperative nausea and vomiting after outpatient surgery with the 5-HT_3 antagonist ondansetron. *Anesthesiology*. 1993; 78:15-20.
202. Rodrigo MR, Campbell RC, Chow J et al. Ondansetron for prevention of postoperative nausea and vomiting following minor oral surgery: a double-blind randomized study. *Anaesth Intensive Care*. 1994; 22:576-9.
203. Furst SR, Rodarte A. Prophylactic antiemetic treatment with ondansetron in children undergoing tonsillectomy. *Anesthesiology*. 1994; 81:799-803.
204. Carroll NV, Miederhoff P, Cox FM et al. Postoperative nausea and vomiting after discharge from outpatient surgery centers. *Anesth Analg*. 1995; 80:903-9.
205. Claybon L. Single dose intravenous ondansetron for the 24-hour treatment of postoperative nausea and vomiting. *Anaesthesia*. 1994; 49(suppl):24-9.
206. Pearman MH. Single dose intravenous ondansetron in the prevention of postoperative nausea and vomiting. *Anaesthesia*. 1994; 49(suppl):11-15.
207. Aloxi package insert. Bloomington, MN: MGI Pharma, Inc; 2007.
208. Henzi I, Walder B, Tramèr MR. Dexamethasone for the prevention of postoperative nausea and vomiting: a quantitative systematic review. *Anesth Analg*. 2000; 90:186-94.
209. Cohen SE, Woods WA, Wyner J. Antiemetic efficacy of droperidol and metoclopramide. *Anesthesiology*. 1984; 60:67-9.
210. Korttila K, Kauste A, Auvinen J. Comparison of domperidone, droperidol, and metoclopramide in the prevention and treatment of nausea and vomiting after balanced general anesthesia. *Anesth Analg*. 1979; 58:396-400.
211. Cramb R, Fargas-Babjak A, Hirano G. Intraoperative prochlorperazine for prevention of post-operative nausea and vomiting. *Can J Anaesth*. 1989; 36:565-7.
212. Patterson KW, Armstrong C, Timon D et al. Buccal prochlorperazine as an antiemetic for day care surgery. *Ir Med J*. 1993; 86:186-8.
213. Pandey CK, Navkar DV, Giri PJ et al. Evaluation of the optimal preemptive dose of gabapentin for postoperative pain relief after lumbar diskectomy: a randomized, double-blind, placebo-controlled study. *J Neurosurg Anesthesiol*. 2005; 17:65-8.
214. Khan ZH, Rahimi M, Makarem J et al. Optimal dose of pre-incision/post-incision gabapentin for pain relief following lumbar laminectomy: a randomized study. *Acta Anaesthesiol Scand*. 2011; 55:306-12.
215. Heidari M, Honarmand A, Safavi M et al. Geranisetron versus gabapentin in preventing postoperative nausea and vomiting after middle ear surgery in adults: a double-blinded randomized clinical trial study. *Adv Biomed Res*. 2015; 4:22.
216. Maneuf YP, Hughes J, McKnight AT. Gabapentin inhibits the substance P-facilitated K(+)-evoked release of [(3)H]glutamate from rat caudial trigeminal nucleus slices. *Pain*. 2001; 93:191-6.
217. Fehrenbacher JC, Taylor CP, Vasko MR. Pregabalin and gabapentin reduce release of substance P and CGRP from rat spinal tissues only after inflammation or activation of protein kinase C. *Pain*. 2003; 105:133-41.
218. Achuthan S, Singh I, Varthya SB et al. Gabapentin prophylaxis for postoperative nausea and vomiting in abdominal surgeries: a quantitative analysis of evidence from randomized controlled clinical trials. *Br J Anaesth*. 2015; 114:588-97.
219. Abdel-Aziz H, Windeck T, Ploch M et al. Mode of action of gingerols and shogaols on 5-HT_3 receptors: binding studies, cation uptake by the receptor channel and contraction of isolated guinea-pig ileum. *Eur J Pharmacol*. 2006; 530:136-43.
220. Morin AM, Betz O, Kranke P et al. [Is ginger a relevant antiemetic for postoperative nausea and vomiting?]. *Anästhesiol Intensivmed Notfallmedizin Schmerzther*. 2004; 39:281-5.
221. Chaiyakunapruk N, Kitikannakorn N, Nathisuwan S et al. The efficacy of ginger for the prevention of postoperative nausea and vomiting: a meta-analysis. *Am J Obstet Gynecol*. 2006; 194:95-9.
222. Basch E, Prestrud AA, Hesketh PJ et al. Antiemetics: American Society of Clinical Oncology clinical practice guideline update. *J Clin Oncol*. 2011; 29:4189-98.
223. Herrstedt J. Antiemetics: an update and the MASCC guidelines applied in clinical practice. *Nat Clin Pract Oncol*. 2008; 5:32-43.
224. Navari RM, Reinhardt RR, Gralla RJ et al. Reduction of cisplatin-induced emesis by a selective neurokinin-1-receptor antagonist. L-754,030 Antiemetic Trials Group. *N Engl J Med*. 1999; 340:190-5.
225. Double-blind, dose-finding study of four intravenous doses of dexamethasone in the prevention of cisplatin-induced acute emesis. Italian Group for Antiemetic Research. *J Clin Oncol*. 1998; 16:2937-42.
226. Italian Group for Antiemetic Research. Randomized, double-blind, dose-finding study of dexamethasone in preventing acute emesis induced by anthracyclines, carboplatin, or cyclophosphamide: *J Clin Oncol*. 2004; 22:725-9.
227. Gralla R, Lichinitser M, Van Der Vegt S et al. Palonosetron improves prevention of chemotherapy-induced nausea and vomiting following moderately emetogenic chemotherapy: results of a double-blind randomized phase III trial comparing single doses of palonosetron with ondansetron. *Ann Oncol*. 2003; 14:1570-7.
228. Emend package insert. Whitehouse Station, NJ: Merck; 2008.
229. Hesketh PJ, Grunberg SM, Gralla RJ et al. The oral neurokinin-1 antagonist aprepitant for the prevention of chemotherapy-induced nausea and vomiting: a multinational, randomized, double-blind, placebo-controlled trial in patients receiving high-dose cisplatin—the Aprepitant Protocol 052 Study Group. *J Clin Oncol*. 2003; 21:4112-9.
230. Warr DG, Hesketh PJ, Gralla RJ et al. Efficacy and tolerability of aprepitant for the prevention of chemotherapy-induced nausea and vomiting in patients with breast cancer after moderately emetogenic chemotherapy. *J Clin Oncol*. 2005; 23:2822-30.
231. Herrington JD, Jaskiewicz AD, Song J. Randomized, placebo-controlled, pilot study evaluating aprepitant single dose plus palonosetron and dexamethasone for the prevention of acute and delayed chemotherapy-induced nausea and vomiting. *Cancer*. 2008; 112:2080-7.

232. Grunberg S, Chua D, Maru A et al. Single-dose fosaprepitant for the prevention of chemotherapy-induced nausea and vomiting associated with cisplatin therapy: randomized, double-blind study protocol—EASE. *J Clin Oncol.* 2011; 29:1495-1501.

233. Jordan K, Jahn F, Aapro M. Recent developments in the prevention of chemotherapy-induced nausea and vomiting (CINV): a comprehensive review. *Ann Oncol.* 2015; 26:1081-90.

234. Navari RM, Gray SE, Kerr AC. Olanzapine versus aprepitant for the prevention of chemotherapy-induced nausea and vomiting: a randomized phase III trial. *J Support Oncol.* 2011; 9:188-95.

235. de Wit R, de Boer AC, vd Linden GH et al. Effective cross-over to granisetron after failure to ondansetron, a randomized double blind study in patients failing ondansetron plus dexamethasone during the first 24 hours following highly emetogenic chemotherapy. *Br J Cancer.* 2001; 85:1099-1101.

236. Carmichael J, Keizer HJ, Cupissol D et al. Use of granisetron in patients refractory to previous treatment with antiemetics. *Anticancer Drugs.* 1998; 9:381-5.

237. Aapro MS, Perugia Consensus, Antiemetic Subcommittee of the Multinational Association of Supportive Care in Cancer (MASCC). How do we manage patients with refractory or breakthrough emesis? *Support Care Cancer.* 2002; 10:106-9.

238. Marx WM, Teleni L, McCarthy AL et al. Ginger (Zingiber officinale) and chemotherapy-induced nausea and vomiting: a systematic literature review. *Nutr Rev.* 2013; 71:245-54.

239. Scuderi PE. Pharmacology of antiemetics. *Int Anesthesiol Clin.* 2003; 41:41-66.

240. Maxwell LG, Kaufmann SC, Bitzer S et al. The effects of a small-dose naloxone infusion on opioid-induced side effects and analgesia in children and adolescents treated with intravenous patient-controlled analgesia: a double-blind, prospective, randomized, controlled study. *Anesth Analg.* 2005; 100:953-8.

241. Chung F, Lane R, Spraggs C et al. Ondansetron is more effective than metoclopramide for the treatment of opioid-induced emesis in post-surgical adult patients. Ondansetron OIE Post-Surgical Study Group. *Eur J Anaesthesiol.* 1999; 16:669-77.

242. Yuan CS, Wei G, Foss JF et al. Effects of subcutaneous methylnaltrexone on morphine-induced peripherally mediated side effects: a double-blind randomized placebo-controlled trial. *J Pharmacol Exp Ther.* 2002; 300:118-23.

243. Candiotti KA, Nhuch F, Kamat A et al. Granisetron versus ondansetron treatment for breakthrough postoperative nausea and vomiting after prophylactic ondansetron failure: a pilot study. *Anesth Analg.* 2007; 104:1370-3.

244. Kovac AL, O'Connor TA, Pearman MH et al. Efficacy of repeat intravenous dosing of ondansetron in controlling postoperative nausea and vomiting: a randomized, double-blind, placebo-controlled multicenter trial. *J Clin Anesth.* 1999; 11:453-9.

245. De Mulder PH, Roila F, Kris MG et al. Consensus regarding multiple day and rescue antiemetic therapy. *Support Care Cancer.* 1998; 6:248-52.

246. Söderpalm AH, Schuster A, de Wit H. Antiemetic efficacy of smoked marijuana: subjective and behavioral effects on nausea induced by syrup of ipecac. *Pharmacol Biochem Behav.* 2001; 69:343-50.

247. Marijuana and Cancer. American Cancer Society. http://www.cancer.org/treatment/treatmentsandsideeffects/physicalsideeffects/chemotherapyeffects/marijuana-and-Cancer (accessed 2018 Feb 12).

248. Navari RM, Nagy CK, Gray SE. The use of olanzapine versus metoclopramide for the treatment of breakthrough chemotherapy-induced nausea and vomiting in patients receiving highly emetogenic chemotherapy. *Support Care Cancer.* 2013; 21:1655-63.

249. Holloman LC, Marder SR. Management of acute extrapyramidal effects induced by antipsychotic drugs. *Am J Health-Syst Pharm.* 1997; 54:2461-77.

250. Gompels M, McWilliams S, O'Hare M et al. Ondansetron usage in HIV positive patients: a pilot study on the control of nausea and vomiting in patients on high dose co-trimoxazole for pneumocystis carinii pneumonia. *Int J STD AIDS.* 1993; 4:293-6.

SECTION IX

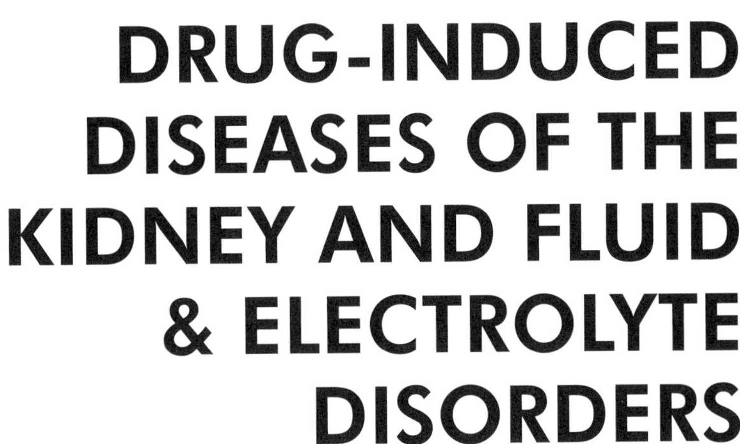

DRUG-INDUCED DISEASES OF THE KIDNEY AND FLUID & ELECTROLYTE DISORDERS

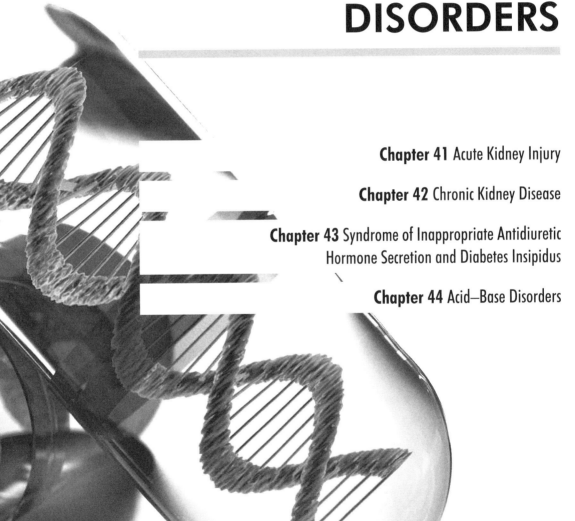

Chapter 41 Acute Kidney Injury

Chapter 42 Chronic Kidney Disease

Chapter 43 Syndrome of Inappropriate Antidiuretic Hormone Secretion and Diabetes Insipidus

Chapter 44 Acid–Base Disorders

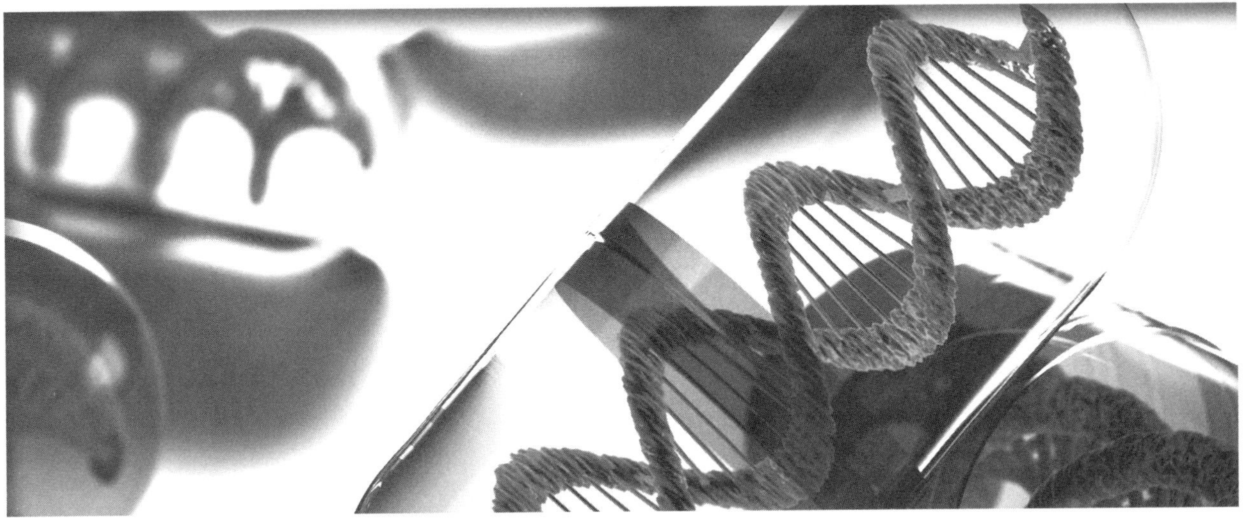

CHAPTER 41

Acute Kidney Injury

Amy Barton Pai and Nicole M. Wegrzyn

The kidneys are a primary pathway for the elimination of drugs and toxins, and they receive 25% of cardiac output, thus increasing their exposure to circulating drugs. In addition, renal hemodynamics may be altered by drugs. These factors result in enhanced susceptibility to drug-induced injury by enhancing potential for proximal tubule cell uptake and by reducing glomerular capillary pressure.[1] Although there is no universal definition of acute kidney injury (AKI), an increase in serum creatinine concentration of 25–30% above baseline values is a useful working definition. Newer definitions exist, but are not yet universally used in the literature.[2,3] AKI occurs in up to 5% of hospitalized patients, and it has been estimated that approximately 20% of these cases are drug induced.[4] In an analysis of adverse events in hospitalized patients, kidney dysfunction accounted for 6.7% of drug-related complications.[5] The true incidence of drug-induced AKI is difficult to determine due to the lack of consistency in defining the condition.[6]

To help distinguish between differing etiologies and outcomes, AKI can be categorized as either community-acquired (CA-AKI) or hospital-acquired (HA-AKI). Common causes of HA-AKI include sepsis or other critical illnesses and exposure to contrast media or nephrotoxic medications commonly used in inpatient care. CA-AKI is characterized by a rapid decline in kidney function that occurs in the outpatient setting and is typically caused by disease and by medications that alter renal hemodynamics and reduce effective perfusion. Because of the rapid onset of AKI, uremia and fluid overload are often worse than seen in patients with chronic kidney disease. Early symptoms reported by patients include fatigue, reduced urine output, and edema, especially in the lower extremities.[7]

Recent analyses have shown that the incidence of CA-AKI is higher than the incidence of HA-AKI. Approximately 80% of those hospitalized and discharged with the AKI International Classification of Diseases (ICD)-9 fit criteria for CA-AKI.[8] Duration of hospitalization and mortality rate are lower among CA-AKI patients than in those with HA-AKI. Recovery of kidney function is incomplete in those with CA-AKI, and data show similar long-term outcomes on kidney function to patients who experience HA-AKI, with nearly 40% developing new-onset or progression of chronic kidney disease (CKD).[9-12] A recent cohort analysis of Veterans

Affairs (VA) hospital patients in upstate New York found the incidence of CA-AKI to be 3.5 times higher than HA-AKI.[8] In a large cohort study performed in the United Kingdom, significantly more patients with CA-AKI received a new diagnosis of CKD within 14 months of the CA-AKI episode versus those with HA-AKI. Approximately 15% of patients with CA-AKI had no notation of renal impairment or planned follow-up at discharge.[12] A retrospective analysis of AKI admissions (335 CA-AKI and 87 HA-AKI) at a VA hospital in Kentucky found that documented outpatient nonsteroidal anti-inflammatory drug (NSAID) use was higher in the CA-AKI group than the HA-AKI (64 versus 10 patients).[10] Potential biomarkers of AKI and kidney failure are being identified and evaluated and may in the future refine our ability to predict and prevent drug-induced AKI.[13,14]

Drug-induced AKI can result from renal hemodynamic alterations leading to reduced renal perfusion, from direct toxicity to the renal tubule cells (acute tubular necrosis), from tubulointerstitial inflammation secondary to an allergic reaction (acute interstitial nephritis), from precipitation of drug crystals resulting in obstruction (nephrolithiasis), or from an immune-mediated reaction resulting in damage to the glomerulus (glomerulonephritis). The sections that follow provide additional detail regarding the agents known to cause AKI by each of these mechanisms.

HEMODYNAMIC-MEDIATED AKI

Hemodynamic-mediated AKI manifests primarily as prerenal azotemia and is the most frequently reported cause of CA-AKI.[15] Dilation of the efferent arteriole or constriction of the afferent arteriole reduces the effective perfusion of the glomerulus, thus decreasing filtration.

CAUSATIVE AGENTS

Any agent that decreases intravascular volume and renal perfusion (e.g., diuretics), constricts the afferent arteriole (e.g., NSAIDs, cyclooxygenase-2 [COX-2] inhibitors, cyclosporine) or dilates the efferent arteriole (e.g., angiotensin-converting enzyme inhibitors [ACEIs], angiotensin receptor blockers [ARBs], direct renin inhibitors) can induce hemodynamically mediated AKI when predisposing factors are present. The drugs most frequently associated with alteration of intrarenal hemodynamics are the ACEIs and NSAIDs.[16] These and other agents implicated in drug-induced AKI are included in **Table 41-1**.

EPIDEMIOLOGY

ACEIs and ARBs are frequently used to treat hypertension, reduce ventricular remodeling, and prevent progression of proteinuric kidney disease.[17] According to one report, an acute rise in serum creatinine concentration greater than three times baseline occurred in 38% of patients with unilateral renal artery stenosis who received captopril.[17] In a series of patients with no known renal artery stenosis, 6% receiving captopril had a rise in serum creatinine that warranted discontinuation of the drug.[18] Aliskiren is a direct renin inhibitor that has been investigated as an antihypertensive and renoprotective agent.[88,89] Short-term studies (2–6 months) have not demonstrated increased risk of elevation of serum creatinine concentrations with aliskiren combined with losartan or ramipril versus losartan or ramipril alone.[89,90] However, in a large multicenter trial of patients with diabetic nephropathy, two patients in the aliskiren plus losartan combination group developed acute kidney failure, versus none who received the ARB alone.[90]

NSAIDs are used extensively worldwide. An estimated 36 million Americans use nonprescription analgesics on a daily basis.[21,91] NSAIDs and COX-2 inhibitors are among the most frequently prescribed agents in the United States.[92,93] Adverse kidney effects secondary to NSAID use occur in 1–5% of patients and account for an estimated 37% of drug-associated AKI cases.[16,21] COX-2 inhibitor–induced AKI has been documented in approximately 240 reports to the U.S. Food and Drug Administration and in 20 published case reports.[22,94-96] A study completed while rofecoxib was still available in the United States examined the incidence of adverse

Table 41-1 Agents Implicated in Drug-Induced Acute Kidney Injury

Drug	Incidence	Level of Evidence[a]
ACUTE INTERSTITIAL NEPHRITIS		
Allopurinol[1]	NK	C
5-aminosalicylic acids[64]	NK	C
β-lactam antibiotics[1]	NK	C
Ciprofloxacin[65]	NK	C
Erythromycin[66]	NK	C
H_2-receptor antagonists[1]	NK	C
Lithium[67]	NK	B
Loop diuretics[1]	NK	C
NSAIDs[1,68]	NK	C
Phenytoin[69]	NK	C
Proton pump inhibitors[70]	NK	C
Rifampin[71]	NK	B
Thiazide diuretics[72]	NK	C
Valproic acid[73]	NK	C
ACUTE TUBULAR NECROSIS		
Aminoglycosides[28-32]	5–25%	A
Amphotericin B desoxycholate[27,33-37]	20–65%	A
Amphotericin B lipid-based formulations[38,39]	15–25%[b]	A
Carboplatin[45]	6%	C
Cisplatin[58-60]	10–30%[c]	A
Colistin[173,174]	43–45%	A
Ifosfamide[61-63]	6%	A
Radiocontrast media[40-57]		
No diabetes or pre-existing chronic kidney disease	0–10%	A
Diabetes	8–20%	A
Pre-existing chronic kidney disease	15–55%	A
Pre-existing chronic kidney disease and diabetes	27–81%	A
GLOMERULONEPHRITIS		
Allopurinol[1]	NK	B
Ampicillin	NK	C
Gold[83]	NK	C
Hydralazine[84]	NK	C
Lithium[70]	NK	B
NSAIDs[16]	NK	B
Penicillamine[85]	NK	C
Phenytoin[86]	NK	C
Propylthiouracil[87]	NK	C
Rifampin[71]	NK	C
HEMODYNAMIC-MEDIATED		
ACEI and ARBs[17-19]	6–38%[d]	B
Cyclosporine[20]	25–38%	A

Table 41-1 Agents Implicated in Drug-Induced Acute Kidney Injury (continued)

Drug	Incidence	Level of Evidence[a]
Diuretics (loop diuretics such as furosemide have a greater risk than hydrochlorothiazide)[15]	5–12%	B
NSAIDs and COX-2 inhibitors[21-27]	1–7%	A
NEPHROLITHIASIS		
Acyclovir[74]	NK	C
Allopurinol[75]	NK	C
Foscarnet[76]	1–5%	A
Furosemide[77]	14%	B
Indinavir[78,79]	12.4%	A
Topiramate[80]	1–3%[c]	A
Sulfonamides[81]	29%	B
Zonisamide[82]	1.9–4%	B

ACEI = angiotensin-converting enzyme inhibitor, ARB = angiotensin receptor blocker, COX-2 = cyclooxygenase-2, NK = not known, NSAID = nonsteroidal anti-inflammatory drug.

[a]Definitions for Levels of Evidence: Level A—evidence from one or more randomized, controlled clinical trials; Level B—evidence from nonrandomized clinical trials, prospective observational studies, cohort studies, retrospective studies, case-control studies, meta-analyses and/or postmarketing surveillance studies; and Level C—evidence from one or more published case reports or case series.

[b]Incidence is higher when contemporary definitions of AKI are applied.

[c]Incidence is dose-dependent.

[d]Patients with unilateral renal artery constriction.

kidney experiences with that agent when used for osteoarthritis versus ibuprofen, diclofenac, and nabumetone.[97] The incidence of adverse renovascular events, including the development of edema, heart failure, hypertension, and elevated serum creatinine were similar between drugs, with no reported cases of fulminant AKI. However, this trial excluded high-risk patients with CKD. There have been no prospective studies linking NSAID use to AKI or other renal complications. The majority of data have been from large cohort studies in the United Kingdom, Europe, and Canada—countries that have nationalized healthcare and database infrastructure that allows linkage of outpatient and inpatient data. All of the existing literature has examined prescription NSAID use, which underscores the need to capture nonprescription NSAID exposure as well. Previous studies have also relied on accurate coding of AKI admissions which likely limits assessment of CA-AKI because patients may not be admitted.[98,99] Studies evaluating estimated glomerular filtration rate decline are limited by inclusion of relatively young patients with intact kidney function.[100,101] Because the major causes of CA-AKI are hypovolemia and clinical situations or medications that can affect renal blood flow, an understanding of the relationships between NSAID use and drug-induced hemodynamic changes is important in the identification of at-risk populations and the design of effective methods to minimize NSAID exposure. Several authors have identified varying levels of risk for AKI associated with what has been referred to as the "triple whammy" (concomitant exposure to diuretics, renin angiotension system inhibitors, and NSAIDs).[102-104] A nested case-control study utilizing Tennessee Medicaid enrollees represents the only published U.S. data to date.[27] The study evaluated the association of NSAID use on ICD-9 coded AKI hospitalizations and serum creatinine parameters. NSAID use was higher among AKI cases versus population controls. Use of NSAIDs increased the risk of AKI by 58% (RR 1.58, 95% CI 1.34–1.86), and the authors specifically reported that higher doses of ibuprofen (defined as doses greater than or equal to the maximum recommended starting dose) were associated with higher risk of developing AKI.[27]

MECHANISMS

Mechanisms of drug-induced AKI are listed in **Table 41-2**. ACEIs and ARBs affect renal hemodynamics by selectively dilating the efferent arteriole.

Table 41-2 Mechanisms of Drug-Induced Acute Kidney Injury

Drug	Mechanism
ACEI, ARBs[17-19]	Efferent arteriole vasodilation especially when renin-angiotensin-aldosterone system–dependent vasoconstriction is present
Acyclovir,[74] sulfadiazine,[81] indinavir[78,79]	Supersaturation of the urine with solute, resulting in crystal formation
Aminoglycosides[28-32]	Saturable accumulation of aminoglycosides in the S1 and S2 segments of the proximal tubule, leading to inhibition of phospholipases and tubular cell death
Amphotericin B[28,33-37]	Afferent arteriole vasoconstriction and altered tubule cell permeability leading to cell lysis
Cisplatin[58-60]	Tubular cell toxicity secondary to binding to mitochondrial DNA, impairing cellular function and inducing apoptosis
Lithium[70]	Development of minimal-change disease and focal segmental glomerulosclerosis
NSAIDs, COX-2 inhibitors[21-27]	Hemodynamic: Inhibition of prostaglandin-dependent afferent arteriole vasodilation Acute interstitial nephritis: T cells infiltrate the kidney interstitium, imitating an immunologic response
Radiocontrast media[40-57]	Afferent arteriole vasoconstriction and reactive oxygen species–mediated tubular toxicity

ACEI = angiotensin-converting enzyme inhibitor, ARB = angiotensin receptor blocker, COX-2 = cyclooxygenase-2, DNA = deoxyribonucleic acid, NSAID = nonsteroidal anti-inflammatory drug.

In patients with adequate renal perfusion and no disease-specific risks, dilation of the efferent arteriole rarely compromises the GFR.[105] However, in the setting of reduced renal perfusion, as might occur in patients with hypovolemia or heart failure, adequate glomerular filtration is maintained by activation of the renin–angiotensin–aldosterone system (RAAS). The resultant constriction of the efferent arteriole allows glomerular capillary pressure to be maintained. In these "renin-dependent" states, inhibition of the RAAS by ACEIs or ARBs may result in a precipitous drop in glomerular filtration. In addition, decreasing renal perfusion increases the risk of kidney ischemia and necrosis.[106]

COX-2 inhibitors and nonselective NSAIDs inhibit the enzymatic activity of COX, blocking the formation of autocoid prostaglandins from arachidonic acid. Two isoforms of COX have been identified.[24] COX-1 is constitutively expressed and mediates homeostatic functions such as gastrointestinal cytoprotection, platelet aggregation, and renal perfusion.[24] COX-2 is considered to be an inducible isoform that channels the production of prostaglandins responsible for pain and inflammation.[21] Conventional NSAIDs inhibit the activity of both COX-1 and COX-2 isoforms. The COX-2 inhibitors specifically block the enzymatic activity of the inducible COX-2 isoform of COX. The therapeutic benefits of the NSAIDs are attributed to COX-2 inhibition, whereas the adverse gastrointestinal, platelet, and kidney effects are attributed to COX-1 inhibition.[21,24] The primary kidney effects of nonselective COX inhibition are vasoconstriction of the afferent arteriole, increased sodium reabsorption, and decreased potassium excretion.[25] Data from human and animal studies confirm that COX-2 is constitutively expressed in the kidney and its expression is increased in states of sodium restriction.[21,107,108] Current data suggest that COX-2 is essential to the maintenance of renal hemodynamics because of prostaglandin-mediated vasodilation of the afferent arteriole.[109] COX-2 expression also appears to be mediated by angiotensin II.[26] The renal effects of COX-2 inhibitors appear to be similar to those of NSAIDs and, in high-risk patients can lead to AKI, necessitating cautious use in certain populations.[25,97,110]

CLINICAL PRESENTATION AND DIFFERENTIAL DIAGNOSIS

Signs and symptoms associated with AKI are included in **Table 41-3**. Patients with AKI secondary to ACEI or ARB therapy frequently have experienced an acute hypovolemic insult with an associated rise in serum creatinine concentration.[111] Patients

Table 41-3 Signs and Symptoms Associated with Drug-Induced Acute Kidney Injury

General

- Costovertebral-angle tenderness
- Edema
- Elevated serum creatinine concentration
- Fever
- Hypertension
- Malaise
- Rapid weight gain

Acute interstitial nephritis

- Arthralgias
- Eosinophilia
- Eosinophiluria
- Proteinuria
- Pyuria
- Skin rash

Acute tubular necrosis

- Magnesium wasting (cisplatin/carboplatin-induced)
- Oliguria

Glomerulonephritis

- Foamy urine
- Marked facial and lower extremity pitting edema
- Oliguria
- Proteinuria
- Skin rash

Nephrolithiasis

- Hematuria
- Renal colic

Table 41-4 Conditions to Consider in the Differential Diagnosis of Drug-Induced Acute Kidney Injury

For patients with suspected drug-induced AKI

- Autoimmune glomerular disease
- Chronic kidney disease
- Cirrhosis
- Heart failure exacerbation
- Hypovolemia
- Infection
- Sepsis

For patients with suspected drug-induced nephrolithiasis

- Abdominal aortic aneurysm
- Appendicitis
- Ectopic pregnancy
- Pyelonephritis

AKI = acute kidney injury.

may have laboratory findings consistent with prerenal azotemia but rarely present with symptoms of fulminant uremia. Kidney dysfunction due to an ACEI or ARB is commonly identified during routine laboratory monitoring in the outpatient setting. Elevations in serum creatinine concentration typically occur within 2 weeks after the initiation of these drugs and can be more pronounced in patients with known risk factors (see below).[112] Differential diagnosis includes other causes of prerenal azotemia, including hypovolemia (e.g., excessive diuresis, vomiting, diarrhea), heart failure, cirrhosis, or sepsis (**Table 41-4**). Acute renal compromise can occur with a single dose of an NSAID, and the risk has been shown to escalate with increasing doses and duration of use.[25,27,113] Patients typically present with elevated serum creatinine and blood urea nitrogen concentrations, weight gain, and diminished urine output. Patients receiving NSAIDs may also present with kidney dysfunction following any event that compromises renal blood flow (e.g., heart failure, gastroenteritis). NSAIDs inhibit prostaglandin-mediated renin release, impairing the excretion of potassium, and thus hyperkalemia is also commonly found in patients presenting with NSAID-induced AKI.[113] Irreversible kidney failure due to prolonged renal ischemia can occur in high-risk patients in whom kidney dysfunction is not recognized.[114]

Patients with COX-2 inhibitor–induced AKI present with a clinical picture similar to NSAID-induced AKI. Hyperkalemia, volume overload, and hyponatremia are common features of COX-2 inhibitor–induced AKI.[95] The duration of COX2–inhibitor use before presenting with AKI has varied within the range of 6–21 days.[95]

RISK FACTORS

Table 41-5 and **Table 41-6** provide an overview of risk factors for drug-induced AKI. Acute hypovolemia secondary to vomiting, diarrhea, or excessive diuresis are common precipitating events for the development of AKI secondary to ACEI or ARB therapy, especially in patients over the age

Table 41-5 Drug-Specific Risk Factors for Acute Kidney Injury

Risk Factor	ACEI	NSAID	AMG	AmB	CM
Diabetes mellitus	D	D	NK	NK	D
Dose/duration of therapy	P	D	D	D	P
Elderly	D	D	D	P	D
Hypoperfusion	D	D	D	D	D
Pre-existing chronic kidney disease	D	D	D	D	D

ACEI = angiotensin-converting enzyme inhibitor, AmB = amphotericin B, AMG = aminoglycoside, CM = contrast media, D = definite risk factor, NSAID = nonsteroidal anti-inflammatory drug, NK = not known if risk factor, P = probable risk factor.

Table 41-6 Risk Factors for Drug-Induced Acute Kidney Injury

- Concomitant administration of nephrotoxins
- Elderly
- Hemodynamic dose-dependent effects
- Known allergic response to agent (acute interstitial nephritis)
- Pre-existing chronic kidney disease
- Prolonged therapy with nephrotoxins
- Renin-dependent disease states
  - Cirrhosis
  - Heart failure
  - Hypovolemia
  - Overdiuresis

of 80 years.[105,112,115] The risk of an acute increase in serum creatinine concentration >30% above baseline with renin–angiotensin system blockade is markedly increased in patients with CKD and in conditions in which reduced effective plasma volume leads to renal hypoperfusion including, most commonly, volume depletion, heart failure, or cirrhosis.[106] In patients with severe atherosclerotic cardiovascular disease or those who are heavy smokers, bilateral renal artery stenosis should be considered as a potential cause of hemodynamic-mediated AKI when other more obvious causes are not present.[97] Concomitant therapy with NSAIDs, diuretics, or both has been identified as a predisposing factor for ACEI–induced AKI.[105,116] Longer-acting ACEIs (e.g., lisinopril) have been associated with a higher incidence of AKI, as compared with shorter-acting agents (e.g., captopril).[19]

Prostaglandin inhibition by nonselective NSAIDs and COX-2 inhibitors rarely compromises kidney function in healthy patients receiving therapeutic doses of these agents on a short-term basis (e.g., 7–10 days).[117] Patients at risk for AKI are those with disease states that reduce renal perfusion and require a compensatory increase in renal prostaglandins to promote vasodilation of the afferent arteriole and maintain adequate glomerular capillary pressure and filtration.[118] Elderly patients with age-related CKD are at high risk for drug-induced AKI, and the use of NSAIDs may increase the risk by up to 58% in patients older than 65 years.[27] A greater risk of AKI has also been associated with total daily doses of ibuprofen >1,200 mg.[27] Reported risk factors for COX2 inhibitor–induced AKI are similar to those of NSAID-induced AKI, including age >60 years, CKD, and concomitant therapy with loop diuretics.[95] ACE inhibition up-regulates COX-2 expression, and patients dependent on angiotensin II for glomerular perfusion may be at increased risk for AKI when receiving concomitant ACEI therapy.[26] The development of kidney failure may also be associated with doses exceeding the labelling recommendation for COX-2 inhibitors.[23]

MORBIDITY AND MORTALITY

Mortality secondary to AKI induced by an ACEI or ARB alone is low. Morbidity has not been well characterized but may be substantial given the high prevalence of ACEI and ARB use in high-risk populations such as those with CKD and heart failure.[112] Analysis of the Studies of Left Ventricular Dysfunction data demonstrated a 4% greater risk of decreased kidney function (defined as a serum creatinine concentration increase ≥0.5 mg/dL from baseline) in patients receiving enalapril 2.5–10 mg twice daily as compared with a placebo-treated group.[119]

The majority of NSAID-induced AKI cases resolve promptly after discontinuation of the offending agent; however, hospitalization may be necessary to provide supportive management, particularly if volume overload or hyperkalemia is present. Rarely, hemodynamic-mediated deterioration of kidney function can lead to irreversible, long-term kidney failure, necessitating dialysis.[25] The majority of reported cases of COX-2–induced AKI have resolved within 2–8 days after discontinuing the offending agent.[22,95] Some patients have required short-term hemodialysis to manage hyperkalemia and volume overload.[95]

PREVENTION

Approaches to help prevent drug-induced AKI are outlined in **Table 41-7**. With ACEIs and ARBs, the primary strategy for preventing acute elevations in serum creatinine concentration is to ensure that patients have an adequate plasma volume before initiating therapy. Diuretics should be withheld or the dose reduced before initiating therapy with an ACEI or ARB.[105] Therapy should be initiated at low doses, which can then be slowly titrated upward after evaluation of serum creatinine concentration. Serum creatinine concentration should be monitored every 2 weeks until it stabilizes and after any dose increase.[105]

Avoiding NSAID use in patients with CKD and in other high-risk populations prevents most cases of AKI associated with these drugs. A serum creatinine concentration >1.7 mg/dL has been identified as a significant risk factor for the development of AKI.[16] If NSAIDs must be used in these populations, minimum effective doses for short durations (3–5 days) should be used or alternative agents (e.g., acetaminophen or narcotic analgesics) should be considered.[120] If NSAIDs are used for longer periods, monitoring should include measurement of serum sodium, potassium, blood urea nitrogen, and creatinine concentrations within 1–3 weeks of therapy initiation and then every 3–6 months thereafter.[120] NSAIDs should be promptly discontinued if elevations in serum creatinine, blood urea nitrogen, or potassium concentration occurs. Concomitant therapy with other agents affecting renal hemodynamics including diuretics, ACEIs, and ARBs should be avoided.[105] Patients using nonprescription NSAIDs should be counseled regarding risk factors for NSAID-induced AKI.

Table 41-7 Approaches to Help Prevent Drug-Induced Acute Kidney Injury

- Avoid use of drugs associated with AKI in patients with risk factors listed in Tables 41-5 and 41-6
- Avoid concurrent use of other agents that affect renal hemodynamics
- Avoid overdiuresis
- Avoid concomitant exposure to nephrotoxins
- Consider once-daily dosing with aminoglycosides (amikacin, gentamicin, tobramycin)
- Counsel patients regarding increased risk if volume depletion occurs and need to maintain adequate fluid intake
- Consider preferential use of lipid-based products (amphotericin B)
- Consider preferential use of nonionic, iso-osmolar radio contrast media
- Dose reduction (drugs with hemodynamic effects)
- Limit duration of therapy for drugs associated with AKI, when possible
- Maintain adequate hydration
- Monitor kidney function closely in high-risk patients
- Prophylaxis with *N*-acetylcysteine or isotonic sodium bicarbonate infusion in patients at high risk for radiocontrast media-induced AKI
- Start at lowest dose (drugs with hemodynamic effects)

AKI = acute kidney injury.

MANAGEMENT

Initiation of therapy with an ACE inhibitor or ARB is frequently associated with an increase in serum creatinine concentration, especially in patients with CKD. This rise is most likely due to reversal of glomerular hyperfiltration by the remnant nephrons and subsequent reduced glomerular capillary pressure from dilation of the efferent arteriole.[112] If the rise in serum creatinine concentration is <30% of baseline, the ACEI or ARB can be continued. A rise in serum creatinine concentration >30% above baseline can initially be managed by attempting a 50% dose reduction of the ACEI or ARB. If the patient is already receiving the lowest dose of the drug and the rise in serum creatinine concentration persists for more than 4 weeks, the ACEI should be discontinued and the patient should be treated with other antihypertensive agents.[97] AKI associated with ACEIs and ARBs is rapidly reversible, provided that blood flow to the kidney was not impaired long enough to cause irreversible ischemic injury.[105] NSAIDs and other agents that affect renal hemodynamics should be withheld, and supportive measures, such as volume repletion, should be initiated when patients first present. Instituting these measures promptly will typically reverse kidney dysfunction within 72–96 hours; however, resolution may take up to 1 week.[25] Hyperkalemia may also be present in patients with ACEI- or ARB-induced AKI, especially in older patients with CKD, and should resolve spontaneously after fluid resuscitation and restoration of glomerular filtration.[116,121] Concurrent therapy with potassium supplements, potassium-sparing diuretics, or NSAIDs increases the risk of hyperkalemia.[121] Patients with serum potassium concentrations >5.5 mEq/L who have not responded to fluid resuscitation may require treatment with sodium polystyrene sulfonate (15–60 g repeated every 4 hours if needed) to enhance gastrointestinal potassium elimination. ACEIs or ARBs may be restarted at low doses in patients who have recovered from AKI when there is a compelling indication.[122] Serum creatinine and potassium concentrations should be re-evaluated 1–2 weeks after resuming therapy with the ACEIs or ARBs.

The primary management for NSAID-induced AKI is discontinuation of the culprit agent. Administration of intravenous or oral fluids can hasten recovery of renal perfusion. Nonemergent hyperkalemia (serum potassium concentration <6 mEq/L) can be managed with oral potassium exchange resins. If hyperkalemia becomes symptomatic (e.g., electrocardiogram changes) or symptomatic uremia develops, the patient should be hospitalized for acute treatment.

INFORMATION FOR PATIENTS

Patients with known risk factors for AKI, including CKD, age >80 years, heart failure, or any combination of these should be instructed to notify their healthcare provider should they notice reduced urine output or edema after therapy with an ACEI or ARB is begun or after an increase in dose.[108] Patients should also be advised to notify their healthcare provider if any intercurrent illness develops that may decrease circulatory volume (i.e., vomiting, diarrhea, heart failure exacerbation), as these reduce effective perfusion of the kidney.

Patients with CKD or other risk factors for AKI should be advised to avoid NSAIDs and COX-2 inhibitors, and alternative therapies should be discussed. If alternatives cannot be used and NSAID or COX-2 inhibitor therapy is initiated, patients should limit use to the shortest duration at the lowest possible dose. Patients should further be advised to have serum creatinine concentrations measured within 1–3 weeks and to monitor weight and blood pressure. Patients should be counseled to notify a healthcare professional if hypertension develops or worsens or if they experience weight gain, edema, or decreased urine output.

ACUTE TUBULAR NECROSIS

Acute tubular necrosis (ATN) can be caused by prolonged renal ischemia or by direct toxicity to the renal tubules. Drug-induced decreases in renal perfusion, as described previously, can lead to ischemia and ATN if not recognized or treated promptly.[123] Drugs can also cause direct toxicity to the renal tubules through a variety of mechanisms, including alteration of cellular function, hyperosmotic fluid shifts, and disruption of the cell membrane.[6]

CAUSATIVE AGENTS

Many drugs can induce direct tubular toxicity through a variety of mechanisms. Aminoglycosides are frequently administered antimicrobials associated with ATN, and amphotericin B (desoxycholate or conventional) is a polyene antifungal agent also associated with a high incidence of nephrotoxicity. Delivery of amphotericin B in lipid-based systems has been used to limit amphotericin B–induced ATN. Current lipid-based amphotericin

B products include amphotericin B lipid complex, liposomal amphotericin B, and amphotericin B colloidal dispersion.

In patients with kidney impairment, high-osmolality contrast media have been shown to be more nephrotoxic than low-osmolality products.[42,124] Nonionic, monomeric low-osmolality contrast media do not appear to improve kidney tolerance as compared with ionic low-osmolality contrast media.[30] In nondiabetic patients with normal kidney function, low-osmolality contrast media do not offer a clinical advantage over high-osmolality contrast media and are significantly more expensive.[42]

Cisplatin is a chemotherapeutic agent used in oncology regimens for numerous malignancies and is associated with dose-dependent ATN. Colistin, a polymyxin antibiotic, has historically been implicated in ATN, leading to diminished popularity between the 1970s and 1990s. Emergence of extensively drug-resistant bacteria has prompted a resurgence of colistin use.[125]

Table 41-1 provides additional information regarding drugs known to cause ATN.

EPIDEMIOLOGY

Aminoglycoside-induced ATN is reported to occur in 5–25% of treated patients.[28] Variability in the reported incidence is likely the result of variation in the definition of nephrotoxicity, patient population studied, and duration of therapy.[118]

Nephrotoxicity (defined as a doubling of serum creatinine concentration) is a serious, dose-limiting adverse event associated with the use of conventional amphotericin B. The incidence of nephrotoxicity is reported to be as high as 65%.[126] In contrast, the incidence of nephrotoxicity is estimated to be 15–25% with newer lipid-based amphotericin B formulations.[126] Contemporary definitions of AKI detect more potential cases, yielding a higher incidence of liposomal amphotericin-B induced AKI than previously thought (54.8%).[127]

Two types of radiocontrast media, high osmolality and low osmolality, are currently marketed. High-osmolality contrast media are associated with greater reduction in renal blood flow and glomerular filtration rate than the low-osmolality preparations.[40] The incidence of contrast media-induced nephrotoxicity in patients without risk factors is reported to be 0–10%.[41,42] In patients with CKD, the risk is much higher, ranging from 40% to 50%.[41,43] The true incidence in high-risk populations is difficult to establish because diagnostic criteria are not well defined and vary significantly between studies.[44]

Nephrotoxicity related to cisplatin and other platin-containing compounds is dose related. Initial experiences with single doses of cisplatin resulted in the development of azotemia in approximately 25% of patients.[45] Since then, nephrotoxicity rates have been reduced to approximately 10% by lowering doses and slowing infusion rates. High-dose cisplatin (200 mg/m^2) is associated with nephrotoxicity rates approaching 30%.[45] Carboplatin is associated with less nephrotoxicity because the drug is more soluble, chemically stable, and binds more slowly to plasma proteins.[45] The incidence of AKI and associated rise in serum creatinine concentration in patients receiving carboplatin is approximately 6%. The incidence of nephrotoxicity associated with colistin is 43–45%.[173,174] Development of acute renal insufficiency occurs in a dose-dependent manner.[173]

MECHANISMS

In animal models, aminoglycosides have been shown to accumulate by a saturable process within endosomal and lysosomal vacuoles in epithelial cells lining the S1 and S2 segments of the proximal tubule.[29] This lysosomal accumulation inhibits phospholipases, causing formation of phospholipid-protein aggregates known as myeloid bodies, which contribute to cell death and tubular necrosis.[124]

The pathophysiology of amphotericin B-induced nephrotoxicity includes renal arterial vasoconstriction and a direct interaction with the epithelial cell membrane of the distal tubule. Several in vitro experiments revealed that amphotericin B alters cell permeability, allowing leakage of cellular constituents, followed by cell lysis and death. Infusion of amphotericin B through a peripheral vein or directly into the renal artery of animals resulted in an increase in vascular resistance and reduction in renal blood flow. These mechanisms lead to a decrease in the glomerular filtration rate as well as tubular dysfunction.[33]

Compromised renal hemodynamics and direct proximal tubular toxicity are the primary mechanisms for contrast media-induced nephrotoxicity.[42,44] Intrakidney perfusion is reduced after exposure to contrast media, and several known mediators of vasoconstriction are released, including calcium, adenosine, endothelin, and oxygen-free radicals.[68] Direct tubular toxicity has been associated with proximal tubule cell uptake of contrast media by lysosomal vacuolization.[42,44,46]

The primary mechanism of cisplatin-induced nephrotoxicity is proximal tubule cell damage and necrosis as a result of binding to mitochondrial DNA and impaired cellular energy functions.[47]Apoptosis has been identified as another potential mechanism for cell death associated with cisplatin.[128]

CLINICAL PRESENTATION AND DIFFERENTIAL DIAGNOSIS

Aminoglycoside-induced nephrotoxicity manifests clinically as nonoliguric kidney failure, with an average rise in serum creatinine concentration of 2 mg/dL and a hypo-osmolar urinary output typically occurring after 5–7 days of treatment.[28,129,130] Urinary markers such as β_2-microglobulin are sensitive indicators of aminoglycoside-induced nephrotoxicity, but patients with urinary β_2-microglobulin may not have clinically relevant toxicity.[165] Conditions to consider in the differential diagnosis of aminoglycoside-induced nephrotoxicity should include sepsis and exposure to other nephrotoxic agents.

An extensive retrospective analysis of amphotericin B-induced nephrotoxicity in adult patients with normal baseline kidney function has been published.[34] The median interval from drug exposure to nephrotoxicity was 7 days. Thirteen percent of patients had mild nephrotoxicity (defined as a 50% increase in serum creatinine concentration), 12% had moderate-to-severe nephrotoxicity (defined as a doubling of serum creatinine concentration to ≥2 mg/dL), and 3% had severe nephrotoxicity (defined as a tripling of serum creatinine concentration to ≥3 mg/dL).[34] As with aminoglycoside-induced nephrotoxicity, conditions to consider in the differential diagnosis of amphotericin-induced nephrotoxicity include sepsis and exposure to other nephrotoxic agents.[35]

Contrast media-induced nephrotoxicity—most frequently defined as a 25% or greater increase in serum creatinine concentration from baseline that occurs within 24–72 hours after the administration of contrast media—is typically nonoliguric and reversible.[46,50,51] Serum creatinine concentrations typically reach peak values at 3–5 days, depending on baseline kidney function.[42,44,46,51] Conditions to consider in the differential diagnosis of contrast media-induced nephrotoxicity should include exposure to other nephrotoxic agents (e.g., aminoglycosides, ACEIs, or ARBs), hypotension, and renal artery thrombosis after an invasive procedure has been performed.

Treatment with cisplatin commonly results in a 20–40% reduction in the glomerular filtration rate.[58] Serum creatinine concentrations typically peak within 10 days after the administration of cisplatin and may remain elevated for up to 3 weeks.[45] Magnesium wasting and hypomagnesemia occur in up to 50% of patients with cisplatin-induced nephrotoxicity and may persist after the cessation of therapy.[59] Conditions to consider in the differential diagnosis should include exposure to other drugs with direct tubular toxicity (e.g., aminoglycosides) and tumor lysis syndrome.

RISK FACTORS

Risk factors associated with aminoglycoside-induced nephrotoxicity include age >50 years, pre-existing kidney dysfunction, volume depletion, hypotension, cirrhosis, diabetes, treatment duration ≥3 days, and concomitant use of other nephrotoxic agents.[131] Serum concentrations of aminoglycosides are not predictive for the development of aminoglycoside-induced nephrotoxicity.[30] Measurement of peak serum concentrations is commonly used to ensure adequate antibacterial efficacy for this concentration-dependent class of antibiotics. Trough serum concentrations reflect the adequacy of renal elimination, with high concentrations reflective of impaired clearance requiring an extension of the dosing interval.[28]

Risk factors for amphotericin B-induced nephrotoxicity include mean daily doses ≥35 mg for at least 7 days, male sex, weight ≥90 kg, CKD, increasing age, use of ACEI, use of diuretics, and the concomitant use of other nephrotoxic agents.[34,127]

The most prominent risk factor for contrast media-induced nephrotoxicity is pre-existing reduced kidney function.[42,46] Patients with diabetes mellitus and reduced kidney function have the highest risk of contrast media-induced nephrotoxicity with an incidence as high as 50% in some studies.[43,44] The risk in patients with diabetes mellitus and normal kidney function has been reported to be only slightly higher (8–16% incidence) than in nondiabetic patients.[43,46] The volume of contrast media administered has been correlated with the development of contrast media-induced nephrotoxicity, especially in patients with diabetes mellitus and CKD, and efforts should be made to minimize the volume of contrast media administered to these patients.[40,50] Other potential risk factors that have not been as well established include concurrent use of drugs that affect renal hemodynamics (e.g., NSAIDs and ACEIs), intravascular volume depletion, heart failure, multiple contrast procedures, and multiple myeloma.[40,46,50,51]

The primary risk factor for cisplatin-induced nephrotoxicity is the dose of drug administered. Doses ranging from 50 mg/m^2 to 75 mg/m^2 are generally associated with reversible kidney dysfunction, whereas doses ≥100 mg/m^2 are frequently associated with AKI and marked ATN.[59] Ultrafilterable platinum concentration is positively correlated with intensity of renal dysfunction.[166,167]

MORBIDITY AND MORTALITY

Progression of aminoglycoside-induced nephrotoxicity to dialysis-dependent kidney failure is rare, and tubular injury is usually reversible after discontinuing therapy.[31] In one retrospective review of patients treated with an aminoglycoside, 7.3% were found to have aminoglycoside-induced nephrotoxicity and 0.2% had significant nephrotoxicity requiring hemodialysis.[32]

The incidence of mortality with amphotericin B-induced nephrotoxicity is three times higher in patients requiring hemodialysis as compared with those not requiring hemodialysis.[35] In a retrospective review of patients receiving amphotericin B for suspected or proven aspergillosis, a doubling of serum creatinine concentration was noted in 53% of patients and hemodialysis was initiated in 15% of patients.[35] The incidence of nephrotoxicity is consistently higher in bone marrow and solid organ transplant recipients. Only patients receiving cyclosporine, aminoglycosides, foscarnet, or other nephrotoxins concomitantly with amphotericin B required hemodialysis.[36]

Permanent kidney impairment, evidenced by serum creatinine concentrations that do not return to baseline, occurs in 30% of patients with amphotericin B-induced nephrotoxicity. Approximately 10–15% of patients with contrast media-induced nephrotoxicity require long-term dialysis.[52,126]

AKI secondary to cisplatin is generally reversible with supportive care, including vigorous hydration and intermittent dialysis as necessary.[59] Chronic kidney disease associated with cisplatin may occur and is characterized by polyuria and hypomagnesemia.[124] Repeated courses of cisplatin therapy can also result in irreversible kidney failure.[59]

PREVENTION

AMINOGLYCOSIDES

Although administration of aminoglycosides in a once-daily dose was thought to decrease the risk of tubular aminoglycoside accumulation, meta-analyses of clinical trials have failed to demonstrate increased safety with this approach.[132,133] Some data highlight the importance of circadian variation in the glomerular filtration rate and subsequent exposure of tubular cells to aminoglycoside.[134] Administration of gentamicin between midnight and 7 a.m. was more likely to cause nephrotoxicity than administration during other times. Coadministration of polyaspartic acid, pentoxifylline, daptomycin, and various antioxidants with aminoglycosides has been shown to decrease aminoglycoside-induced nephrotoxicity in animals, but there has been no clinical validation in humans.[31]

AMPHOTERICIN B

The successful treatment of certain invasive fungal infections requires the use of high doses of amphotericin B over prolonged periods. Drug dose and duration of treatment are independently associated with increased risk of amphotericin B-induced nephrotoxicity. The lipid-based formulations including amphotericin B lipid complex, amphotericin B colloidal complex, and liposomal amphotericin B are associated with lower incidences of nephrotoxicity and allow the delivery of larger doses of the drug for longer periods.[38,135] The beneficial effects of lipid-based formulations are thought to be related to an increased reticuloendothelial system clearance of amphotericin B and consequent reduced delivery to the kidney. Administration of 150–250 mEq of sodium (1–1.6 L normal saline) per day has been shown to minimize azotemia associated with amphotericin B by altering the tubuloglomerular feedback response.[39,171]

RADIOCONTRAST MEDIA

Numerous prophylactic interventions have been proposed to prevent contrast media-induced nephrotoxicity. Hydration with 0.45% sodium chloride solution at a rate of 100 mL/hr for 4 hours before and 8–12 hours after the administration of contrast media is recommended.[46,50] All medications known to adversely affect renal hemodynamics, including NSAIDs, ACEIs, ARBs, and diuretics should be discontinued 24–72 hours before the procedure, whenever possible.[50] Mannitol and loop diuretics have been considered for prophylaxis because of their ability to increase urinary flow rates and possibly limit contact of contrast media with the tubules. However, these agents have been associated with an increased risk of contrast media-induced nephrotoxicity, as compared with hydration alone, and are not recommended for prophylaxis.[54]

Studies investigating the potential nephroprotective effect of theophylline, an adenosine antagonist, are equivocal.[136,137] A study of 39 patients, including 17 with CKD, randomly assigned subjects to receive theophylline 5 mg/kg or placebo (normal saline) given 45 minutes before the administration of contrast media.[136] In patients with CKD, the glomerular filtration rate decreased significantly in the placebo group but not in the theophylline-treated group. Another study examined the effects of theophylline (as aminophylline) and dopamine on the prevention of contrast media-induced nephrotoxicity (defined as an increase in serum creatinine concentration >25% above baseline) after coronary angioplasty in patients with CKD.[137] Sixty patients were randomly assigned to receive either saline hydration, aminophylline 4 mg/kg followed by a continuous infusion of 0.4 mg/kg/hr plus saline hydration, or dopamine 2.5 mcg/kg/min plus saline hydration. No significant difference in the incidence of contrast media-induced nephrotoxicity was found among the three groups.

Calcium-channel blockers have been shown to reverse hemodynamic changes induced by contrast media.[55] A clinical trial of nitrendipine, a dihydropyridine calcium-channel blocker, reported improved renal blood flow and reduction in tubular enzymes measured in urine when 20 mg was administered 1 day before and 2 days after the administration of contrast media; however, a single dose of nitrendipine 10–20 mg 1 hour before the administration of contrast media offered no benefit.[138,139]

Although dopamine is a nonselective dopaminergic agonist at low doses (2–2.5 mcg/kg/min), it selectively activates the D-1 receptor, thus promoting dilation of the renal arteries and increasing renal blood flow. Investigation of this agent for prevention of contrast media-induced nephrotoxicity has yielded conflicting results, and therefore the use of prophylactic low-dose dopamine is not recommended.[43,137,140] Fenoldopam is a newer, selective D-1 agonist.[57] A study in dogs showed that fenoldopam administered via the renal artery before a high-osmolality contrast media (diatrizoate) prevented decreases in renal blood flow and glomerular filtration rate.[56] In small studies and retrospective analyses in humans, fenoldopam administered at 0.1 mcg/kg/min 1–2 hours before the administration of contrast media and up to 4 hours after has been shown to reduce the incidence of contrast media-induced nephrotoxicity.[117,141,142] However, these data need to be confirmed by a large, controlled trial and pharmacoeconomic factors need to be evaluated before fenoldopam's role in the prophylaxis of contrast media-induced nephrotoxicity can be defined.

When patients at relatively low risk for contrast media-induced nephrotoxicity were given *N*-acetylcysteine (NAC) 600 mg orally twice daily on the day before and the day of contrast media administration, only 2% had nephrotoxicity (defined as a 0.5 mg/dL increase in serum creatinine concentration within 48 hours of the administration of contrast media), as compared to 21% in a control group.[143] The same benefit has not been confirmed by other studies, however, and one study in which NAC was given to high-risk patients who received contrast media for coronary angiography failed to show a decreased risk of nephrotoxicity.[144-146]

Prophylactic intermittent hemodialysis after the administration of contrast media has not been shown to reduce the incidence of nephrotoxicity.[57] However, two studies that investigated the role of prophylactic continuous venovenous hemofiltration (CVVH) versus intravenous hydration in patients with a baseline serum creatinine concentration of >2 mg/dL found a significantly lower incidence of AKI in the CVVH group.[145,146] When performed after exposure to contrast media, 6-hour CVVH was able to remove an amount of contrast media similar to that removed by the kidneys in 12 hours.[172] These data should be interpreted cautiously, however, because hemofiltration itself affects serum creatinine concentrations. Nevertheless, CVVH was associated with lower in-hospital mortality (2% versus 14%).

Sodium bicarbonate alkalinizes the urine and has been shown to inhibit free radical formation in animal models. In a prospective, randomized trial to study the effectiveness of sodium bicarbonate in preventing contrast media induced nephrotoxicity, patients received either intravenous normal saline or sodium bicarbonate. Eight patients in the normal saline group had contrast media-induced nephrotoxicity versus only one patient in the sodium bicarbonate group ($p = 0.02$).[57]

HMG-CoA reductase inhibitors (statins) may be beneficial in statin-naïve patients undergoing coronary angiography given their pleiotropic properties. A meta-analysis of 13 randomized controlled trials demonstrated that pretreatment with high-dose statin therapy in combination with a hydration protocol reduced the risk of contrast-induced AKI by 53% compared to placebo. Several studies included in this analysis used concomitant prophylactic measures such as NAC or sodium bicarbonate.[147]

Clinical applicability of the data regarding prevention of contrast-induced AKI is hindered by study design limitations such as enrolling too few subjects, using surrogate and inconsistent primary endpoints, and including low-risk patients. These key methodological issues informed the design of the Prevention of Serious Adverse Events following Angiography trial, an ongoing randomized prospective study comparing the effectiveness of sodium bicarbonate, sodium chloride, and NAC.[148]

CISPLATIN

Cisplatin-induced nephrotoxicity is best prevented by dose reduction and aggressive hydration.[35] Infusion of 1–4 L of normal saline within 24 hours of cisplatin therapy is recommended to maintain urine flow rates of 125 mL/hr.[58] Hypertonic saline has also been used to increase chloride concentrations and reduce conversion of cisplatin to reactive platinum species.[59] The use of hypertonic saline (3%) as a vehicle for cisplatin doses >100 mg/m^2 may reduce nephrotoxicity.[58] Hypertonic saline must be used very cautiously in patients at risk for adverse effects, including those with underlying heart failure. Mannitol has been used to enhance dilution of drug within the tubules; however, some clinical trials have found no benefit.[58] The protective effect of furosemide is controversial because of the prerenal effects of diuretics. However, loop diuretics are frequently administered to maintain adequate diuresis in patients at risk for heart failure secondary to hydration.[58] Amifostine is a prodrug that is metabolized to a sulfhydryl donor and can reduce kidney toxicities related to cisplatin therapy. Amifostine should be administered before the initiation of cisplatin therapy to patients at high risk for drug-induced nephrotoxicity. Doses of amifostine ranging from 710 mg to 1,000 mg administered 15 minutes before cisplatin have been shown to significantly reduce nephrotoxicity.[58,60]

MANAGEMENT

Clinicians should consider discontinuing aminoglycosides and using an alternative agent, if possible, when a decline in kidney function occurs during therapy. Spontaneous recovery of kidney function usually occurs within a few days after drug discontinuation.[28] If kidney function does not improve, other causes of nephrotoxicity should be considered. In situations in which aminoglycoside therapy cannot be discontinued, aminoglycoside doses may be continued with a reported recovery of kidney function in some patients.[149-151] A review of six patients with gram-negative osteomyelitis managed with gentamicin for 5–7 weeks demonstrated that aminoglycoside-induced nephrotoxicity occurred with a peak rise in serum creatinine concentration and stabilization of values after approximately 30 days of treatment. Continuation of gentamicin therapy after individualized adjustment of the dosing interval to yield targeted trough concentrations of <2 mcg/ml did not cause additional increases in serum creatinine concentration and was associated with a 50% reduction in serum creatinine concentration in three of the cases.[151]

Amphotericin B should be discontinued in patients in whom nephrotoxicity develops, and therapy with an alternative antifungal agent or a lipid-based product initiated. Substitution of a lipid-based amphotericin B product has resulted in improved kidney function in patients in whom amphotericin B-induced nephrotoxicity developed.[37]

Patients with contrast media-induced nephrotoxicity should receive supportive care. Adequate hydration with 0.45% saline solution and the avoidance of other nephrotoxins may help hasten kidney recovery.[41] Infusion rates of intravenous fluids should be titrated to maintain positive fluid balance and high urine output.[50]

Management of AKI secondary to cisplatin therapy is typically supportive and should include aggressive hydration. Electrolyte wasting, especially the loss of magnesium, is a frequent manifestation of cisplatin-induced AKI. Supplementation with intravenous magnesium (0.5 mEq/kg/day given as a continuous infusion) is indicated in patients with serum magnesium concentrations <1 mEq/mL to prevent adverse neurologic and cardiac effects.[58] Patients with serum magnesium concentrations >1 mEq/L can be treated with oral magnesium oxide. Hypokalemia and hypocalcemia can also occur and may be refractory to treatment if hypomagnesemia is not corrected.

INFORMATION FOR PATIENTS

Patients scheduled for elective procedures requiring iodinated contrast media should be counseled regarding the possibility of acute kidney dysfunction, especially if they are diabetic and have pre-existing kidney disease. Patients and providers should be advised to hold medications that affect renal hemodynamics. Patients should be counseled regarding the potential risk of AKI with cisplatin therapy and should be advised of the preventive measures required (e.g., hydration and amifostine, if indicated) to minimize the risk of chemotherapy-related kidney problems. Kidney function should be evaluated after completion of the chemotherapy cycles, and patients should be advised to notify their healthcare provider if they notice symptoms of frequent urination, low serum magnesium (muscle weakness, tremors, agitation, confusion, fainting), low serum calcium (muscle twitching, paresthesia), or low serum potassium (muscle weakness or cramps).

ACUTE INTERSTITIAL NEPHRITIS

Acute interstitial nephritis (AIN) is most commonly caused by hypersensitivity to a drug that results in infiltration of the tubulointerstitium by inflammatory cells, including T cells, monocytes, and eosinophils.

CAUSATIVE AGENTS

The agents most frequently associated with AIN are antibiotics and NSAIDs.[1,61] Methicillin, rifampin, and fenoprofen are among the agents most frequently implicated.[150] Table 41-1 lists other causative agents.

EPIDEMIOLOGY

AIN is a relatively rare complication of drug therapy. AIN attributed to various causes, including drugs, was present in 2–3% of biopsies reviewed in two case series.[61,62] AIN is associated with many classes of drugs but the incidence can be higher for some agents within a given class.[63] For example, β-lactams are known to be associated with AIN; however, methicillin was found to be associated with a much higher incidence than other β-lactams, resulting in its removal from the U.S. market. The reason for the increased incidence is not clear but may be due to haptenic dimethoxyphenylpenicilloyl groups.

MECHANISMS

AIN is a hypersensitivity reaction with kidney manifestations. There are four principal mechanisms by which drugs may induce AIN: (1) the drug binds to the tubular basement membrane, acting as a hapten; (2) the drug may be structurally similar to an antigen that is normally present in the tubular basement membrane resulting in inappropriate immune complex formation; (3) the drug may bind to the tubular basement membrane itself, inducing an antibody response; and (4) the drug may elicit an antibody response and circulating immune complexes may deposit in the tubular interstitium.[63,149]

CLINICAL PRESENTATION AND DIFFERENTIAL DIAGNOSIS

Although the rise in serum creatinine and blood urea nitrogen concentrations associated with AIN may not occur for several weeks after a patient's initial exposure to a causative agent, increases may be seen within 3–5 days of a second exposure.[149] Systemic manifestations of hypersensitivity may be present, including low-grade fever (30–50%), maculopapular rash (33–50%), and eosinophilia (16–33%).[61-63,152,153] Urinalysis may reveal eosinophiluria (40–90%), hematuria (48–60%), proteinuria (16–60%), or pyuria (50–53%).[61-64,152,153] The only definitive diagnostic test for AIN is kidney biopsy, which typically reveals patchy or diffuse inflammatory infiltrates consisting predominantly of lymphocytes and plasma cells within the interstitium.[63,64,149] However, biopsies are not frequently performed unless the injury does not resolve after the offending drug is discontinued. Differential diagnosis includes other potential causes of intrinsic kidney injury including nondrug-related AIN and glomerulonephritis if large amounts of protein are present in the urine.

RISK FACTORS

AIN is idiopathic and there are no well-established risk factors. AIN is not dose-related.[149] Previous exposure to some agents such as rifampin has been associated with the development of AIN on subsequent exposure.[150]

MORBIDITY AND MORTALITY

AIN is frequently reversible when the suspect drug is identified and discontinued.[63,149] Dialysis may be required temporarily if kidney recovery is slow and the patient has clinical signs of uremia, emergent hyperkalemia (serum concentration >6 mEq/L or electrocardiographic changes), or volume overload.[153] In cases of progressive AIN (involving a majority of the interstitium), kidney function may not return to baseline. The prognosis is worse when diffuse versus patchy infiltrates are found on kidney biopsy. AIN that persists for >3 weeks is also associated with a poor prognosis.[154] Approximately 33% of patients require short-term dialysis.[63]

PREVENTION

AIN is rare, and there are no known predictors of the disease. In general, a patient should not be re-challenged with a drug that has caused AIN or another drug from the same class of agents. The occurrence of drug-induced AIN should be carefully documented in the patient's medical record to help prevent future exposures.

MANAGEMENT

The primary management of AIN involves discontinuation of the suspect drug or drugs.[152] Although administration of corticosteroids is sometimes recommended, there have been no controlled studies to determine the benefit of this intervention. Doses of 1 mg/kg/day of prednisolone or prednisone given orally for 1 week have been used with or without intravenous methylprednisolone pulses; however, this treatment has not been shown to correlate well with resolution of AIN.[61,64,155,156]

INFORMATION FOR PATIENTS

Patients should be advised to consult with their healthcare provider if fever, rash, edema, or reduced urine output develops while taking an agent known to cause AIN. Patients who have a history of AIN should be cautioned to avoid future exposure to the causative agent or drugs within the same class.

NEPHROLITHIASIS

Nephrolithiasis is most commonly caused by precipitation of drug crystals in the ureter, resulting in obstruction of urine flow.[157,158]

CAUSATIVE AGENTS

Table 41-1 lists the drugs most frequently reported to cause nephrolithiasis. The drugs most commonly associated with this disorder have acidic pKa values (e.g., sulfadiazine, pKa = 6.5) and are more likely to supersaturate at acidic urinary pH (normal urine pH ranges from 4.5 to 7.8).

EPIDEMIOLOGY

Although approximately 3–5% of people experience nephrolithiasis, drug-induced nephrolithiasis is a rare condition, accounting for only 0.8–2.5% of all cases.[159,160]

MECHANISMS

Crystal formation occurs due to supersaturation of the urine with solute, resulting in the formation of calculi or stones in the ureter.[159] Depending on the salt form of the drug, crystal formation is enhanced under either alkaline or acidic conditions.[159] Indinavir (pKa 6.2), for example, is more soluble at an acidic pH and stone formation and the risk of nephrolithiasis may increase when the urine pH is above 5.[157] pKa of other agents associated with nephrolithiasis are as follows: acyclovir (9.25), allopurinol (7.83), foscarnet (7.27), furosemide (7.5), topiramate (8.6), and zonisamide (10.2). Drugs that increase urinary calcium or uric acid may enhance the risk of stone formation.[161]

CLINICAL PRESENTATION AND DIFFERENTIAL DIAGNOSIS

The majority of patients with nephrolithiasis present with renal colic resulting from crystals lodging in the ureter.[157] The hallmark is severe flank pain unrelieved by change in position.[157] Other symptoms may include pain radiating to the groin, fever, and nausea and vomiting.[157,161] Nonspecific findings on urinalysis may include the presence of red or white cells and fractional excretion of sodium >1%. If the stone is passed, it can frequently be identified by microscopic examination, and further examination with techniques such as x-ray diffractometry and infrared spectroscopy is sometimes carried out. Drugs can produce crystals with characteristic structure. Indinavir, for example, produces crystals that appear as tangled rods and needle-shaped crystals within a protein matrix.[161] Conditions to consider in the differential diagnosis of drug-induced nephrolithiasis include abdominal aortic aneurysm, appendicitis, ectopic pregnancy, pyelonephritis and nephrolithiasis secondary to calcium oxalate or uric acid crystal formation. Definitive diagnosis of drug-induced nephrolithiasis is made by intravenous pyelography or ultrasound and microscopic examination of the passed stone.[157,161]

RISK FACTORS

Decreased fluid intake is a potential risk factor for drug-induced nephrolithiasis as it can increase stasis in the ureter. Longer duration of therapy with drugs known to cause nephrolithiasis may be associated with an increased risk of stone formation. In addition, the risk of nephrolithiasis appears to increase with increasing doses of drugs such as felbamate and indinavir.[78,157]

PREVENTION

Increasing urine flow rates may decrease the risk of crystallization. Increasing the urine output to 150 mL/hr by increasing fluid intake for 3 hours after an oral dose of indinavir has been recommended.[157]

MANAGEMENT

Management of nephrolithiasis and renal colic should include aggressive diuresis to encourage spontaneous passage of the stone and pain management, most commonly with narcotic analgesics or ketorolac.[79,157] Meperidine and morphine should not be used for pain management if significant kidney impairment is present and an extended duration of therapy (>3 days) is expected. Both agents have renally excreted metabolites that are associated with adverse neurologic (meperidine) and central nervous system (morphine) effects in the presence of kidney dysfunction. If the stone is passed spontaneously, it should be sent for analysis to confirm the diagnosis.

INFORMATION FOR PATIENTS

Patients who have been prescribed drugs known to cause nephrolithiasis should be advised to maintain adequate fluid intake, especially after drug administration, and to notify a healthcare professional if they have symptoms of renal colic.

GLOMERULONEPHRITIS

Drug-induced glomerulonephritis is immune-mediated and causes damage to the glomerular basement membrane. This damage compromises filtration and increases permeability, allowing protein to pass into the urine.[162]

CAUSATIVE AGENTS

Table 41-1 lists the drugs reported to cause glomerulonephritis. These drugs are diverse in their structure and pharmacology; however, all can cause immune-mediated damage to the glomerulus.

EPIDEMIOLOGY

Drug-induced glomerulonephritis is a rare complication of drug therapy, and most of the available data regarding its occurrence come from published case reports. Although a number of agents have been implicated, the disease is most frequently associated with NSAIDs.

MECHANISMS

Drug-induced glomerulonephritis is typically immune-mediated. Similar to the pathogenic mechanisms in AIN, the causative drugs may act as haptens, result in immune complex formation, or stimulate production of autoantibodies against glomerular structures.[162] Drug-induced glomerular damage can also occur because of acute vasculitis, in which glomerular capillaries are damaged by inflammatory reactions to circulating immune complexes.[68]

CLINICAL PRESENTATION AND DIFFERENTIAL DIAGNOSIS

Drug-induced glomerulonephritis typically presents as nephrotic syndrome, which is defined as proteinuria >3.5 g/day. Other clinical manifestations may include reduced urine output and edema of the lower extremities and possibly the face. When drug-induced glomerulonephritis is associated with a severe hypersensitivity reaction, fever, rash, and eosinophilia may also be present.[68] Definitive diagnosis is made by kidney biopsy, and three associated lesions have been identified: membranous nephropathy, minimal-change nephropathy, and focal segmental glomerulosclerosis.[68,163] Glomerular injury from drug therapy is relatievely rare compared to other etiologies of drug-induced kidney injury. A consensus report sought to define a phenotype for glomerular disorders. Because of the low incidence and overlap with other kidney injury diagnoses, one of the primary criteria for the phenotype was biopsy-proven drug-induced glomerular disease. The consensus report further indicates that the biopsy should be done while the patient is receiving the drug or within 4 weeks of stopping.[170]

Membranous nephropathy is the most common lesion that occurs in patients with drug-induced glomerulonephritis.[162] It is characterized by immune complex deposition in the glomerular basement membrane. The membranous deposits are more widely spaced and focally distributed in patients with drug-induced disease than those in idiopathic membranous nephropathy.[162] Drugs most commonly associated with membranous drug-induced glomerulonephritis include NSAIDs, gold, and penicillamine.[83,162] Because of the idiopathic nature of drug-induced glomerulonephritis, time to onset is not well-documented for most drugs. A review of the literature focused on NSAID-induced membranous nephropathy reported a median onset of 43 weeks after initiation with a range of 4 weeks to 3 years.[168]

In patients with minimal-change nephropathy, glomeruli appear normal and no deposits are visible with immunofluorescence microscopy or electron microscopy; however, patients typically have nephrotic-range proteinuria. Minimal-change nephropathy is commonly associated with AIN and has been reported to occur with NSAIDs, rifampin, phenytoin, and ampicillin.[162]

Focal segmental glomerulosclerosis is characterized by areas of sclerosis in <50% of the glomeruli. This lesion is commonly associated with heroin abuse and has also been reported with lithium therapy.[164]

RISK FACTORS

Drug-induced glomerulonephritis is idiopathic, and there are no well-established risk factors. The presence of the human leukocyte antigens DR3 and B8 appear to be associated with increased susceptibility to gold-induced glomerulonephritis.[162] A review of reports of NSAID-induced glomerulonephritis identified an association between duration of therapy and the severity of the glomerular lesion.[68] Patients with minimal-change disease were more likely to have an underlying rheumatologic disease. The risk for drug-induced glomerulonephritis has not been associated with drug dose.

MORBIDITY AND MORTALITY

Drug-induced glomerulonephritis typically resolves after discontinuation of the causative agent. Follow-up evaluation of 72 patients with NSAID-induced glomerulonephritis found that 68 who had discontinued NSAIDs had improved kidney function, with 57 returning to their baseline kidney function.[68] A renal biopsy is typically not performed unless proteinuria and kidney function fail to improve after stopping the drug.

PREVENTION

Drug-induced glomerulonephritis is rare and idiopathic, and there is little information available regarding risk factors or prevention. Gold therapy should be avoided in patients with human leukocyte antigens DR3 or B8.

MANAGEMENT

The primary management strategy for drug-induced glomerulonephritis is discontinuation of the suspected causative agent. Corticosteroids may be initiated in severe cases; however, the value of this treatment has not been demonstrated conclusively. The dose of corticosteroid is not well established; traditional aggressive regimens used for nondrug-related glomerulonephritis can be used (e.g., 1 g of methylprednisolone) or a more conservative approach similar to doses used in AIN can be initiated.[169] Diuretics may be required to manage severe edema. Dialysis is indicated only if the patient has kidney insufficiency associated with clinical signs of uremia or hyperkalemia that does not respond to other treatment.

INFORMATION FOR PATIENTS

Patients receiving drugs known to cause glomerulonephritis should be advised to consult their healthcare provider if they develop fever, rash, edema, or reduced urine output. If the patient has a history of drug-induced glomerulonephritis, he or she should be cautioned to avoid future therapy with the causative agent or related drugs.

REFERENCES

1. Paller MS. Drug-induced nephropathies. *Med Clin North Am.* 1990;74:909-17.
2. Bellomo R, Kellum J, Ronco C. Acute renal failure: time for consensus. *Intensive Care Med.* 2001; 27:1685-8.
3. Acute Kidney Injury Work Group. Kidney disease: improving global outcomes (KDIGO)—KDIGO clinical practice guideline for acute kidney injury. *Kidney Int.* 2012; 2:1-138.
4. Hou SH, Bushinsky DA, Wish JB et al. Hospital acquired chronic kidney disease. *Am J Med.* 1983; 74:243-8.
5. Leape LL, Brennan TA, Laird N. The nature of adverse events in hospitalized patients. *N Engl J Med.* 1991; 324:377-84.
6. Thadhani R, Pascual M, Bonventre JV. ARF. *N Engl J Med.* 1996; 334:1448-60.
7. Mehta RL, Kellum JA, Shah SV et al. Acute Kidney Injury Network: report of an initiative to improve outcomes in acute kidney injury. *Crit Care.* 2007; 11:R31.
8. Der Mesropian PJ, Kalamaras JS, Eisele G et al. Long-term outcomes of community-acquired versus hospital-acquired acute kidney injury: a retrospective analysis. *Clin Nephrol.* 2014; 81:174-84.
9. Chawla LS, Kimmel PL. Acute kidney injury and chronic kidney disease: an integrated clinical syndrome. *Kidney Int.* 2012; 82:516-24.
10. Schissler MM, Zaidi S, Kumar H et al. Characteristics and outcomes in community-acquired versus hospital-acquired acute kidney injury. *Nephrology (Carlton).* 2013; 18:183-7.
11. Triverio PA, Martin PY, Romand J et al. Long-term prognosis after acute kidney injury requiring renal replacement therapy. *Nephrol Dial Transplant.* 2009; 24: 2186-9.
12. Wonnacott A, Meran S, Amphlett B et al. Epidemiology and outcomes in community-acquired versus hospital-acquired AKI. *Clin J Am Soc Nephrol.* 2014; 9:1007-14.
13. Chen L-X, Koyner JL. Biomarkers in acute kidney injury. *Crit Care Clin.* 2015; 31:633-48.
14. Mårtensson J1, Martling CR, Bell M. Novel biomarkers of acute kidney injury and failure: clinical applicability. *Br J Anaesth.* 2012; 109:843-50.
15. Kaufman J, Dhakal M, Patel B et al. Community acquired renal failure. *Am J Kidney Dis.* 1991;17:191-8.
16. Kleinknect D, Landais P, Goldfarb B et al. Analgesic and nonsteroidal anti inflammatory drug-associated ARF: a prospective collaborative study. *Clin Nephrol.* 1986; 25:275-81.
17. Jackson B, Matthews PG, McGrath BP et al. Angiotensin converting enzyme inhibition in renovascular hypertension: frequency of reversible renal failure. *Lancet.* 1984; 1:225-6.
18. Hollenberg NK. Medical therapy of renovascular hypertension: efficacy and safety of captopril in 269 patients. *Cardiovasc Rev Rep.* 1983; 4:852-76.
19. Mason NA. Angiotensin-converting enzyme inhibitors and renal function. *Ann Pharmacother.* 1990; 24:496-505.
20. de Mattos AM, Olyaei AJ, Bennett WM. Nephrotoxicity of immunosuppressive drugs: long-term consequences and challenges for the future. *Am J Kidney Dis.* 2000; 35:333-46.
21. Whelton A, Hamilton C. Non-steroidal anti inflammatory drugs: effects on kidney function. *J Clin Pharmacol.* 1991; 31:588-98.
22. Graham MG. ARF related to high dose celecoxib. *Ann Intern Med.* 2001; 135:69-70.
23. Ahmad SR, Kortepeter C, Brinker A et al. Renal failure associated with the use of celecoxib and rofecoxib. *Drug Saf.* 2002; 25:537-44.
24. Whelton A. Nephrotoxicity of non-steroidal anti inflammatory drugs: physiologic foundations and clinical implications. *Am J Med.* 1999; 106:13S-24S.
25. Brater DC. Effects of non-steroidal anti inflammatory drugs on renal function: focus on COX-2 selective inhibition. *Am J Med.* 1999; 107:65S-71S.
26. Cheng H, Wang J, Zhang MZ et al. Angiotensin II attenuates renal cortical cyclooxygenase-2 expression. *J Clin Invest.* 1999; 103:953-61.
27. Griffin MR, Yared A, Ray WA. Non-steroidal anti inflammatory drugs and AKI in elderly persons. *Am J Epidemiol.* 2000; 151:488-96.
28. Swan SK. Aminoglycoside nephrotoxicity. *Semin Nephrol.* 1997; 17:27-33.
29. Vandewalle A, Farman N, Morin JP et al. Gentamicin incorporation along the nephron: autoradiographic study on isolated tubules. *Kidney Int.* 1981; 19:529-39.
30. McCormack JP, Jewesson PJ. A critical reevaluation of the "therapeutic range of aminoglycosides." *Clin Infect Dis.* 1992; 14:320-39.
31. Mingeot-Leclerco MP, Tulkens PM. Aminoglycosides: nephrotoxicity. *Antimicrob Agents Chemother.* 1999; 43:1003-12.
32. Eisenberg JM, Koffer H, Glick HA et al. What is the cost of nephrotoxicity associated with aminoglycosides? *Ann Intern Med.* 1987; 107:900-9.
33. Sabra R, Branch RA. Amphotericin B nephrotoxicity. *Drug Saf.* 1990; 5:94-108.
34. Harbarth S, Pestotnik SL, Lloyd JF et al. The epidemiology of nephrotoxicity associated with conventional amphotericin B therapy. *Am J Med.* 2001; 111:528-34.
35. Wingard JR, Kubilis P, Lee L. Clinical significance of nephrotoxicity in patients treated with amphotericin B for suspected or proven Aspergillosis. *Clin Infect Dis.* 1999; 29:1402-7.
36. Pathak A, Pien FD, Carvalho L. Amphotericin B use in a community hospital, with special emphasis on side effects. *Clin Infect Dis.* 1998; 26:334-38.
37. Nagata MP, Gentry CA, Hampton EM. Is there a therapeutic or pharmacokinetic rationale for amphotericin B dosing in systemic Candida infections? *Ann Pharmacother.* 1996; 30:811-8.
38. Dupont B. Overview of the lipid formulations of amphotericin B. *J Antimicrob Chemother.* 2002; 49(suppl 1):31-6.
39. Walsh TJ, Hiemenz JW, Seibel NL et al. Amphotericin B lipid complex for invasive fungal infections: analysis of safety and efficacy in 556 cases. *Clin Infect Dis.* 1998; 26:1383-96.
40. Rudnick MR, Berns JS, Cohen RM et al. Contrast media-associated nephrotoxicity. *Semin Nephrol.* 1997; 17:15-26.
41. Morcos SK. Contrast media-induced nephrotoxicity-questions and answers. *Br J Rad.* 1998; 71:357-65.
42. Rudnick MR, Goldfarb S, Wexler L et al. Nephrotoxicity of ionic and nonionic contrast media in 1196 patients a randomized trial. *Kidney Int.* 1995; 47:254-61.
43. Weisberg LS, Kurnik PB, Burnik BRC. Risk of radiocontrast nephropathy in patients with and without diabetes mellitus. *Kidney Int.* 1994; 45:259-65.
44. Gerlach AT, Pickworth KP. Contrast medium-induced nephrotoxicity: pathophysiology and prevention. *Pharmacotherapy.* 2000; 20:540-8.
45. Briguori C, Manganelli E, Scarpato F et al. Acetylcysteine contrast agent-associated nephropathy. *J Am Coll Cardiol.* 2002; 40:298-303.

46. Berg KJ. Nephrotoxicity related to contrast media. *Scan J Urol.* 2000; 34:317-22.
47. Diaz-Sandoval LJ, Kosowsky BD, Losordo DW. Acetylcysteine to prevent angiography related renal tissue injury (the APART trial). *Am J Cardiol.* 2002; 40:298-303.
48. Barrett BJ, Carlisle EJ. Meta analysis of the relative nephrotoxicity of high and low-osmolality iodinated contrast media. *Radiology.* 1993; 186:183-7.
49. Deray G, Jacobs C. Renal tolerance of nonionic dimmers. *Invest Radiol.* 1996; 31:372-7.
50. Waybill MM, Waybill PN. Contrast media-induced nephrotoxicity: identification of patients at risk and algorithms for prevention. *Vasc Interv Radiol.* 2001; 12:3-9.
51. Morcos SK, Thomsen HS, Webb JAW. Contrast-media-induced nephrotoxicity: a consensus report. *Eur Radiol.* 1999; 9:1602-13.
52. Lepor NE. A review of contemporary prevention strategies for radiocontrast nephropathy: a focus on fenoldopam and *N*-acetylcysteine. *Rev Cardiovasc Med.* 2003; 4:S15-20.
53. Deray G. Amphotericin B nephrotoxicity. *J Antimicrob Chemother.* 2002; 49 (suppl 1):37-41.
54. Solomon R, Werner C, Mann D et al. Effects of saline, mannitol and furosemide on acute decreases in renal function by radiocontrast agents. *N Engl J Med.* 1994; 331:1416-20.
55. Esnault VLM. Radiocontrast media-induced nephrotoxicity in patients with renal failure: rationale for a new double-blind, prospective, randomized trial testing calcium channel antagonists. *Nephrol Dial Transplant.* 2002; 17:1362-4.
56. Bakris GL, Lass NA, Glock D. Renal hemodynamics in radiocontrast medium-induced renal dysfunction: a role for dopamine-1 receptors. *Kidney Int.* 1999; 56:206-10.
57. Merten GJ, Burgess PW, Gray LV et al. Prevention of contrast-induced nephropathy with sodium bicarbonate: a randomized controlled trial. *JAMA.* 2004; 291:2328-34.
58. Cornelison TL, Reed E. Nephrotoxicity and hydration management for cisplatin, carboplatin and ormaplatin. *Gynecol Oncol.* 1993; 50:147-58.
59. Safirstein R, Winston J, Golstein M et al. Cisplatin nephrotoxicity. *Am J Kidney Dis.* 1986; 5:356-67.
60. Lau AH. Apoptosis induced by cisplatin nephrotoxic injury. *Kidney Int.* 1999; 56:1295-8.
61. Kintzel PE. Anticancer drug-induced kidney disorders. *Drug Saf.* 2001; 24:19-38.
62. Ries F, Klatersky J. Nephrotoxicity induced by cancer chemotherapy with special emphasis on cisplatin. *Am J Kidney Dis.* 1986; 8:368-79.
63. Hartmann JT, Knop S, Fels LM et al. The use of reduced doses of amifostine to ameliorate nephrotoxicity of cisplatin/ifosfamide-based chemotherapy in patients with solid tumors. *Anticancer Drugs.* 2000; 11:1-6.
64. Praga M, Sevillano A, Auñón P, González E. Changes in the aetiology, clinical presentation and management of acute interstitial nephritis, an increasingly common cause of acute kidney injury. *Nephrol Dial Transplant.* 2015; 30:1472-9.
65. Bailey JR, Trott SA, Philbrick JT. Ciprofloxacin-induced acute interstitial nephritis. *Am J Nephrol.* 1992; 12:271-3.
66. Rosenfeld J, Gura V, Boner G et al. Interstitial nephritis with acute renal failure after erythromycin. *Br Med J (Clin Res Ed).* 1983; 286:938-9.
67. Bendz H: Kidney function in lithium-treated patients. *Acta Psychiatr Scand.* 1983; 68:303-24.
68. Ravnskov U. Glomerular, tubular and interstitial nephritis associated with non-steroidal anti inflammatory drugs: evidence of a common mechanism. *Br J Clin Pharmacol.* 1999; 47:203-10.
69. Hoffman EW. Phenytoin-induced interstitial nephritis. *South Med J.* 1981; 74:1160-1.
70. Ruffenach SJ, Siskind MS, Lien YH. Acute interstitial nephritis due to omeprazole. *Am J Med.* 1992; 93:472-3.
71. Muthukumar T, Jayakumar M, Fernando EM et al. Acute renal failure due to rifampicin: a study of 25 patients. *Am J Kidney Dis.* 2002; 40:690-6.
72. Magil AB, Ballon HS, Cameron EC et al. Acute interstitial nephritis associated with thiazide diuretics. *Am J Med.* 1980; 69:939-43.
73. Lin CY, Chiang H. Sodium-valproate-induced interstitial nephritis. *Nephron.* 1988; 48:43-6.
74. Rashed A, Azadeh B, Abu Romeh SH. Acyclovir-induced acute tubulo-interstitial nephritis. *Nephron.* 1990; 56:436-8.
75. Potter JL, Silvidi AA. Xanthine lithiasis, nephrocalcinosis, and renal failure in a leukemia patient treated with allopurinol. *Clin Chem.* 1987; 33:2314-16.
76. Cacoub P, Deray G, Baumelou A. Acute renal failure induced by foscarnet: 4 cases. *Clin Nephrol.* 1988; 29:315-8.
77. Saarela T, Lanning P, Koivisto M et al. Nephrocalcinosis in full-term infants receiving furosemide treatment for congestive heart failure: a study of the incidence and 2-year follow up. *Eur J Pediatr.* 1999; 158:668-72.
78. Martinez F, Mommeja-Marin H, Estepa-Maurice L et al. Indinavir crystal deposits associated with tubulointerstitial nephropathy. *Nephrol Dial Transplant.* 1998; 13:750-3.
79. Wu D, Stoller ML. Indinavir urolithiasis. *Curr Opin Urol.* 2000; 10:557-61.
80. Lamb EJ, Stevens PE, Nashef L. Topiramate increases biochemical risk of nephrolithiasis. *Ann Clin Biochem.* 2004; 41(pt 2):166-9.
81. Sasson JP, Dratch PL, Shortsleeve MJ. Renal US findings in sulfadiazine-induced crystalluria. *Radiology.* 1992; 185:739-40.
82. Kubota M, Nishi-Nagase M, Sakakihara Y et al. Zonisamide-induced urinary lithiasis in patients with intractable epilepsy. *Brain Dev.* 2000; 22:230-3.
83. Hall CL. Gold nephropathy. *Nephron.* 1988; 50:265-72.
84. Björck S, Westberg G, Svalander C et al. Rapidly progressive glomerulonephritis after hydralazine. *Lancet.* 1983; 2:42.
85. Habib GS, Saliba W, Nashashibi M et al. Penicillamine and nephrotic syndrome. *Eur J Intern Med.* 2006; 17:343-8.
86. Messiaen TG, Plaisier EM, Rossert J et al. Heavy proteinuria, podocyte hypertrophy and severe systemic manifestations in a patient on phenytoin therapy. *Nephrol Dial Transplant.* 1997; 12:2723-5.
87. Fujieda M, Nagata M, Akioka Y et al. Antineutrophil cytoplasmic antibody-positive crescentic glomerulonephritis associated with propylthiouracil therapy. *Acta Paediatr Jpn.* 1998; 40:286-9.
88. Sepehrdad R, Frishman WH, Stier CT et al. Direct inhibition of renin as a cardiovascular pharmacotherapy. *Cardiol Rev.* 2007; 15:242-56.
89. Uresin Y, Taylor AA, Kilo C et al. Efficacy and safety of the direct renin inhibitor aliskiren and ramipril or in combination in patients with diabetes and hypertension. *J Renin Angiotensin Aldosterone Syst.* 2007; 8:190-8.
90. Parving HH, Persson F, Lewis JB et al. Aliskiren combined with losartan in Type 2 Diabetes and nephropathy. *N Engl J Med.* 2008; 358:2433-46.
91. Hersh EV, Pinto A, Moore PA. Adverse drug interactions involving common prescription and over-the-counter analgesic agents. *Clin Ther.* 2007; 29(Suppl):2477-97.
92. Buttar NS, Wang KK. The "aspirin" of the new millennium: cyclooxygenase-2 inhibitors. *Mayo Clin Proc.* 2000; 75:1027-38.
93. Rxlist. The internet drug index. www.rxlist.com (accessed 2017 Jun 5).
94. Harris RC. COX-2 and the kidney. *J Cardiovasc Pharmacol.* 2006; 47(suppl 1):S37-42.
95. Perazella MA, Eras J. Are COX-2 inhibitors nephrotoxic? *Am J Kidney Dis.* 2000; 35:937-40.
96. Perazella MA, Tray K. Selective cyclooxygenase-2 inhibitors: a pattern of nephrotoxicity similar to traditional non-steroidal anti inflammatory drugs. *Am J Med.* 2001; 111:64-7.

97. Gertz BJ, Krupa D, Bolognese JA et al. A comparison of adverse renovascular experiences among steoarthritis patients treated with rofecoxib and comparator non-selective non-steroidal anti inflammatory agents. *Curr Med Res Opin*. 2002; 18:82-91.
98. Evans JMM, McGeregor AD, McMahon MM et al. Non-steroidal anti-inflammatory drugs and hospitalization for acute renal failure. *Q J Med*. 1995; 88:551-7.
99. Pérez Gutthann S, García Rodríguez LA, Raiford DS et al. Nonsteroidal anti-inflammatory drugs and the risk of hospitalization for acute renal failure. *Arch Intern Med*. 1996; 156:2433-9.
100. Gooch K, Culleton BF, Manns BJ et al. NSAID use and progression of chronic kidney disease. *Am J Med*. 2007; 120:280, e1-7.
101. Nderitu P, Doos L, Strauss VY et al. Dose prescribing and estimated glomerular filtration rate decline: a general practice database linkage cohort study. *BMJ Open*. 2014; 4:e005581.
102. Fournier JP, Sommet A, Durrieu G et al. More on the "Triple Whammy:" antihypertensive drugs, non-steroidal anti-inflammatory agents and acute kidney injury—a case/non-case study in the French pharmacovigilance database. *Ren Fail*. 2014; 36:1166-8.
103. Lapi F, Azoulay L, Yin H, Nessim SJ et al. Concurrent use of diuretics, angiotensin converting enzyme inhibitors, and angiotensin receptor blockers with non-steroidal anti-inflammatory drugs and risk of acute kidney injury: nested case-control study. *BMJ*. 2013; 346:e8525.
104. Dreischulte T, Morales DR, Bell S et al. Combined use of non-steroidal anti-inflammatory drugs with diuretics and/or renin-angiotensin system inhibitors in the community increases the risk of acute kidney injury. *Kidney Int*. 2015; 88:396-403.
105. Thomas MC. Diuretics ACE inhibitors and NSAIDs: the triple whammy. *Med J Aust*. 2000; 172:184-5.
106. Hricik DE, Dunn MJ. Angiotensin-converting enzyme inhibitor-induced renal failure: causes consequences and diagnostic uses. *J Am Soc Nephrol*. 1990; 1:845-8.
107. Crofford LJ, Wilder RL, Ristamaki AP et al. Cyclooxygenase-1 and -2 expression in rheumatoid synovial issues: effects of interleukin-1 beta, phorbol ester, and corticosteroids. *J Clin Invest*. 1994; 93:1095-1101.
108. Komhoff M, Hermann-Josef G, Klein T et al. Localization of cyclooxygenase-1 and -2 in adult and fetal human kidney: implication for renal function. *Renal Physiol*. 1997; 41:F460-8.
109. Swan SK, Rudy DW, Lasseter KC. Effects of cyclooxygenase-2 inhibition on renal function in elderly persons eceiving a low-salt diet: a randomized controlled trial. *Ann Intern Med*. 2000; 133:1-9.
110. Scwartz JI, Vandomael K, Malice MP et al. Comparison of rofecoxib, celecoxib and naproxen on renal unction in elderly subjects receiving a normal salt diet. *Clin Pharmacol Ther*. 2002; 72:50-61.
111. Anandh U, Renuka S, Somiah S et al. ARF in the tropics: emerging trends from a tertiary care hospital in South India. *Clin Nephrol*. 2003; 59:341-4.
112. Bakris G, Weir M. Angiotensin-converting enzyme inhibitor-associated elevations in serum creatinine. *Arch Intern Med*. 2000; 160:685-93.
113. Bennett WM, Henrich WL, Stoff JS. The renal effects of non-steroidal anti inflammatory drugs. *Am J Kidney Dis*. 1996; 28:S56-S62.
114. Pazmino PA, Pazmino PB. Ketoprofen-induced irreversible renal failure. *Nephron*. 1988; 50:70-1.
115. Saine DR, Ahrens ER. Renal impairment associated with losartan. *Ann Intern Med*. 1996; 124:775.
116. Farrugia E. Drug-induced renal toxicity: diagnosis and prevention. *Hosp Med*. 1998; 59:140-44.
117. Dishart MK, Kellum JA. An evaluation of pharmacological strategies for the prevention and treatment of AKI. *Drugs*. 2000; 59:79-91.
118. Clive DM, Stoff JS. Renal syndromes associated with non-steroidal anti inflammatory drugs. *N Engl J Med*. 1984; 310:563-72.
119. Schoolwerth AC, Sica DA, Ballermann BJ et al. Renal considerations in angiotensin converting enzyme inhibitor therapy: a statement for healthcare professionals from the Council on the Kidney in Cardiovascular Disease and the Council for High Blood Pressure Research of the American Heart Association. *Circulation*. 2001; 104:1985-91.
120. Bush TM, Shlotzhauer TL, Imai K. Nonsteroidal anti inflammatory drugs proposed guidelines for monitoring for toxicity. *West J Med*. 1991; 155:39-42.
121. Reardon LC, Macpherson DS. Hyperkalemia in outpatients using angiotensin-converting enzyme inhibitors. *Arch Intern Med*. 1998; 158:26-32.
122. Alderman CP. Adverse effects of the angiotensin converting enzyme inhibitors. *Ann Pharmacother*. 1996; 30:55-61.
123. Cameron JS. ARF: the continuing challenge. *Q J Med*. 1986; 59:337-43.
124. Appelkvist EL, Soderstrom M., Nassberger C et al. Characterization of the lipid and protein contents of myelin bodies isolated from the renal cortex of gentamicin-treated rats. *Biochem Biophys Res Commun*. 1991; 181:894-901.
125. Lim LM, Ly N, Anderson D, Yang JC et al. Resurgence of colistin: a review of resistance, toxicity, pharmacodynamics, and dosing. *Pharmacotherapy*. 2010; 30:1279-91.
126. Deray G, Jacobs C. Radiocontrast nephrotoxicity: a review. *Invest Radiol*. 1995; 30:221-5.
127. Rocha PN, Kobayashi CD, de Carvalho AL et al. Incidence, predictors, and impact of hospital mortality on amphotericin B nephrotoxicity defined using newer acute kidney injury diagnostic criteria. *Antimicrob Agents Chemother*. 2015; 59:4759-69.
128. Durham JD, Caputo C, Dokko J et al. A Randomized controlled trial of *N*-acetylcysteine to prevent contrast nephropathy in cardiac angiography. *Kidney Int*. 2002; 62:2202-7.
129. Oliveira JFP, Silva CA, Barbieri CD et al. Prevalence and risk factors for aminoglycoside nephrotoxicity in intensive care units. *Antimicrob Agents Chemother*. 2009; 53:2887-91.
130. Picard W, Bazin F, Clouzeau B et al. Propensity-based study of aminoglycoside nephrotoxicity in patients with svere sepsis or septic shock. *Antimicrob Agents Chemother*. 2014; 58:7468-74.
131. Moore RD, Smith CR, Lipsky JJ et al. Risk factors for nephrotoxicity in patients treated with aminoglycosides. *Ann Intern Med*. 1984; 100:352-7.
132. Hatala R, Dinh T, Cook DJ. Once-daily aminoglycoside dosing in immunocompetent adults: a meta-analysis. *Ann Intern Med*. 1996; 124:717-25.
133. Ali MZ, Goetz MB. A meta-analysis of the relative efficacy and toxicity of single daily dosing versus multiple aily dosing of aminoglycosides. *Clin Infect Dis*. 1997; 24:796-809.
134. Rougier F, Claude D, Maurin M et al. Aminoglycoside nephrotoxicity: modeling, simulation, and control. *Antimicrob Agents Chemother*. 2003; 47:1010-16.
135. Mistro S, Maciel Ide M, de Menezes RG et al. Does lipid emulsion reduce amphotericin B nephrotoxicity? A systematic review and meta-analysis. *Clin Infect Dis*. 2012; 54:1774-7.
136. Erley CM, Duda SH, Schlepkow S et al. Adenosine antagonist theophylline prevents reduction of glomerular filtration rate after contrast media application. *Kidney Int*. 1994; 45:1425-31.
137. Abizaid AS, Clark CE, Mintz GS et al. Effects of dopamine and aminophylline on contrast-induced AKI after coronary angioplasty in patients with preexisting chronic kidney disease. *Am J Cardiol*. 1999; 83:260-3.
138. Neumayer HH, Junge W, Kufner A et al. Prevention of radiocontrast media-induced nephrotoxicity by the calcium channel blocker nitrendipine: a prospective randomized clinical trial. *Nephrol Dial Transplant*. 1989; 4:1030-6.
139. Carraro M, Mancini W, Artero M et al. Dose effect of nitrendipine on urinary enzymes and microproteins following non-ionic radiocontrast administration. *Nephrol Dial Transplant*. 1996; 11:444-8.

140. Hall KA, Wong RW, Hunter RW et al. Contrast-induced nephrotoxicity: the effects of vasodilator therapy. *Surg Res.* 1992; 53:317-20.
141. Halpenny M, Lakshmi S, O'Donnell A. Fenoldopam: renal and splanchnic effects in undergoing coronary artery bypass grafting. *Anesthesia.* 2001; 56:953-60.
142. Madyoon H, Croushore L, Weaver D et al. Use of Fenoldopam to prevent radiocontrast nephropathy in high risk patients. *Catheter Cardiovasc Interv.* 2001; 53:341-5.
143. Tepel M, van der Giet M, Schwarzfeld C et al. Prevention of radiocontrast agent-induced reductions in renal function by acetylcysteine. *N Engl J Med.* 2000; 343:180-4.
144. Vogt B, Ferrari P, Schonholzer C et al. Prophylactic hemodialysis after radiocontrast media in patients with renal insufficiency is potentially harmful. *Am J Med.* 2001; 111:692.
145. Marenzi G, Lauri G, Campodonico J et al. Comparison of two hemofiltration protocols for prevention of contrast-induced nephropathy in high-risk patients. *Am J Med.* 2006; 119:155-62.
146. Marenzi G, Marana I, Lauri G et al. The prevention of radiocontrast-agent-induced nephropathy by hemofiltration. *N Engl J Med.* 2003; 349:1333-40.
147. Lee JM, Park J, Jeon K-H et al. Efficacy of short-term high-dose statin pretreatment in prevention of contrast-induced acute kidney injury: updated study-level meta-analysis of 13 randomized controlled trials. *PLoS One.* 2014; 9:1-12.
148. Weisbord SD, Gallagher M, Kaufman J et al. Prevention of contrast-induced AKI: a review of published trials and the design of the Prevention of Serious Adverse Events following Angiography (PRESERVE) trial. *Clin J Am Soc Nephrol.* 2013; 8:1618-31.
149. Alexopoulos E. Drug-induced acute interstitial nephritis. *Ren Fail.* 1998; 20:809-19.
150. Buysen JGM. Acute interstitial nephritis: a clinical and morphological study in 27 patients. *Nephrol Dial Transplant.* 1990; 5:94-9.
151. Trollfors B. Gentamicin-associated changes in renal function reversible during continued treatment. *J Antimicrob Chemother.* 1983; 12:285-7.
152. Davison AM, Jones CH. Acute interstitial nephritis in the elderly: a report from the UK MRC Glomerulonephritis Register and a review of the literature. *Nephrol Dial Transplant.* 1998; 13(suppl 7):12-6.
153. Rossert J. Drug-induced interstitial nephritis. *Kidney Int.* 2001; 60:804-17.
154. Cameron JS. Allergic interstitial nephritis: clinical features and pathogenesis. *Q J Med.* 1988; 250:97-115.
155. Clarkson MR, Giblin L, O'Connell FP et al. Acute interstitial nephritis: clinical features and response to corticosteroid therapy. *Nephrol Dial Transplant.* 2004; 19: 2778-83.
156. Ten RM, Torres VE, Milliner DS et al. Acute interstitial nephritis: immunologic and clinical aspects. *Mayo Clin Proc.* 1988; 63:921-30.
157. Manthey DE, Teichman J. Nephrolithiasis. *Emerg Med Clin North Am.* 2001; 19:633-54.
158. Sparagana SP, Strand WR, Adams RC. Felbamate urolithiasis. *Epilepsia.* 2001; 42:682-5.
159. Murray KM, Keane WR. Review of drug-induced acute interstitial nephritis. *Pharmacotherapy.* 1992; 12:462-7.
160. Laberke HG. Acute interstitial nephritis: correlations between clinical and morphological findings. *Clin Nephrol.* 1980; 14:263-73.
161. Rapardo A, Traba ML, Caycho C et al. Drug-induced renal stones: incidence, clinical expression and stone analysis. *Contrib Nephrol.* 1987; 58:25-9.
162. Antonovych TT. Drug-induced nephropathies. *Pathol Ann.* 1984; 19:165-96.
163. ten Holder SM, Joy MS, Falk RJ. Cutaneous and systemic manifestations of drug-induced vasculitis. *Ann Pharmacother.* 2002; 36:130-47.
164. Santella RN, Rimmer JH, MacPherson BR. Focal segmental glomerulosclerosis in patients receiving lithium carbonate. *Am J Med.* 1988; 84:951-4.
165. Herget-Rosenthal S, Poppen D, Hüsing J et al. Prognostic value of tubular proteinuria and enzymuria in nonoliguric acute tubular necrosis. *Clin Chem.* 2004; 50:552-8.
166. Lagrange JL, Médecin B, Etienne MC et al. Cisplatin nephrotoxicity: a multivariate analysis of potential predisposing factors. *Pharmacotherapy.* 1997; 17:1246-53.
167. Reece PA, Stafford I, Russell J et al. Creatinine clearance as a predictor of ultrafilterable platinum disposition in cancer patients treated with cisplatin: relationship between peak ultrafilterable plantium plasma levels and nephrotoxicity. *J Clin Oncol.* 1987; 5:304-9.
168. Radford MG Jr, Holley KE, Grande JP et al. Reversible membranous nephropathy associated with the use of nonsteroidal anti-inflammatory drugs. *JAMA.* 1996; 14:276:466-9.
169. Ponticelli C, Glassock RJ. Glomerular diseases: membranous nephropathy—a modern view. *Clin J Am Soc Nephrol.* 2014; 9:609-16.
170. Mehta RL, Awdishu L, Davenport A et al. Phenotype standardization for drug-induced kidney disease. *Kidney Int.* 2015; 88:226-34.
171. Branch RA. Prevention of amphotericin B-induced renal impairment: a reviw on the use of sodium supplementation. *Arch Intern Med.* 1988; 148:2389-94.
172. Guastoni C, Bellotti N, Poletti F et al. Continuous venovenous hemofiltration after coronary procedures for the prevention of contrast-induced acute kidney injury in patients with severe chronic renal failure. *Am J Cardiol.* 2014; 113:588-92.
173. Pogue JM, Lee J, Marchaim D et al. Incidence of and risk factors for colistin-associated nephrotoxicity in a large academic health system. *Clin Infect Dis.* 2011; 53:879-84.
174. Hartzell JD, Neff R, Ake J et al. Nephrotoxicity associated with intravenous colistin (colistimethate sodium) treatment at a tertiary care medical center. *Clin Infect Dis.* 2009; 48:1724-8.

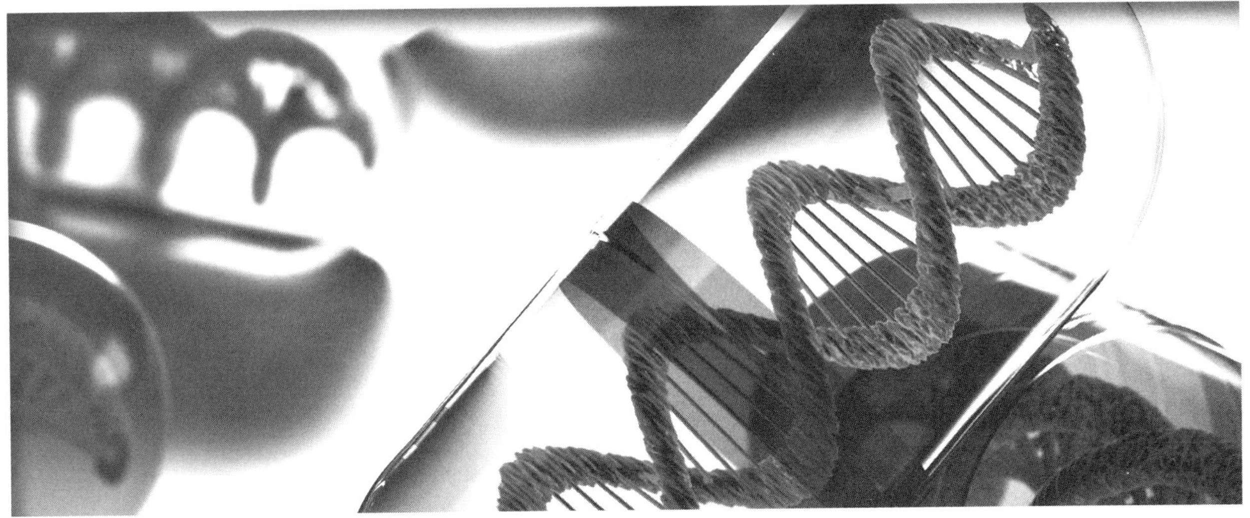

CHAPTER 42

Chronic Kidney Disease

Mary K. Stamatakis

Drugs can adversely affect kidney structure and function, leading to acute or chronic nephrotoxicity. Although acute kidney injury (AKI) is commonly recognized as a consequence of drug therapy, drugs have also been associated with chronic kidney disease (CKD), which is defined as an abnormality of kidney structure or function of at least 3 months' duration with implications for health.[1] Criteria for CKD are a glomerular filtration rate (GFR) of <60 mL/min/1.73 m^2 and/or the presence of markers of kidney damage, such as albuminuria or electrolyte abnormalities due to tubular disorders. The term *end-stage renal disease* (ESRD) is typically used to describe the final stage of CKD characterized by a GFR of <15 mL/min/1.73 m^2 requiring renal replacement therapy (e.g., dialysis, kidney transplantation).[1] This chapter summarizes the pathophysiology and treatment of drug-induced CKD.

CAUSATIVE AGENTS

A variety of drugs have been associated with CKD (**Table 42-1**).[2-54] Drugs frequently reported to cause CKD include tacrolimus, cyclosporine, lithium, and combination analgesics (containing at least two antipyretic analgesics, often with the addition of caffeine and/or codeine). CKD is also reported in association with Chinese herbal supplements containing aristolochic acid. Many of the drugs implicated in causing CKD also cause other types of renal diseases. For example, cyclosporine and tacrolimus cause a common dose-related, hemodynamically mediated AKI.[16] Nonsteroidal anti-inflammatory drugs (NSAIDs) can cause hemodynamically mediated AKI as well as acute interstitial nephritis.[55] In addition, drug-induced AKI, such as that associated with aminoglycosides, amphotericin B, and contrast dye, can progress to CKD in some patients.

PROTON PUMP INHIBITORS

Recently, proton pump inhibitors (PPIs), such as omeprazole, esomeprazole, and pantoprazole, were linked to CKD in a population-based observational study of more than 10,000 patients.[47] After 13.9 years of study, researchers found a 50% higher risk of CKD in patients who self-reported use of PPIs. The risk was similar when adjusted for patient variables such as obesity, diabetes, and hypertension. No association was found with self-reported use of H_2 receptor antagonists and CKD. The data

Table 42-1 Agents Implicated in Drug-Induced Chronic Kidney Disease

Drug	Incidence	Level of Evidence[a]
Adefovir[48,49,52]	1–12%[b]	B
Aristolochic acid (Chinese herbs)[2-6]	NK	C
Antipyretic analgesics[7-10,c]	0.8–9%	B
Cidofovir[15]	NK	C
Cisplatin[11,13,35]	10–80%	B
Cyclosporine[16-29]	NK[d,e]	A
Entecavir[53]	<1%	C
Gold salts[30,31]	1–5%[e]	B
Ifosfamide[11,13,32-35]	20–60%	B
Lithium[36-43]	0.2–21%	B
Nitrosoureas (streptozocin, carmustine, lomustine)[14]	10%	C
D-penicillamine[44]	NK	C
Propylthiouracil[45]	NK	C
Proton pump inhibitors[47] (omeprazole, esomeprazole, pantoprazole, rabeprazole, lansoprazole, dexlansoprazole)	NK	B
Tacrolimus[16,18,26,46]	NK[d]	A
Tenofovir[53]	<1%	C

NK = not known, information in the literature is conflicting, or information varies substantially based on indication or dose.
[a]Definitions for Levels of Evidence: Level A—evidence from one or more randomized, controlled clinical trials; Level B—evidence from nonrandomized clinical trials, prospective observational studies, cohort studies, retrospective studies, case-control studies, meta-analyses and/or postmarketing surveillance studies; and Level C—evidence from one or more published case reports or case series.
[b]10 mg QD dose, rates of 13–50% at higher doses.
[c]Chronic consumption of a combination of at least two antipyretic analgesics, and usually caffeine or codeine or both.
[d]Incidence varies widely based on dose and indication. Average serum creatinine concentration is elevated, glomerular filtration rate is decreased, or both in studies evaluating the long-term safety of calcineurin inhibitors.
[e]In one study, CKD developed in 18% of liver transplant recipients.

were replicated in a cohort of patients receiving care in the Geisinger Health System of Pennsylvania.[47] Although these results do not prove causality, they do raise concern because PPIs are commonly prescribed or self-administered, often with no clear indication. A recent meta-analysis of five studies demonstrated a 1.3-fold increased risk of CKD in patients treated with PPIs.[56] Prospective studies are needed to determine causality as well as understand the potential mechanism of kidney injury and risk factors.

ANTIVIRAL AGENTS

Adefovir dipivoxil is a nucleotide analog reverse transcriptase inhibitor indicated for the treatment of chronic hepatitis B (CHB). Adefovir was initially used to treat human immunodeficiency virus (HIV); however, nephrotoxicity was a rate-limiting side effect at the high doses necessary for HIV treatment.[50] The incidence of nephrotoxicity is low at currently recommended doses of 10 mg/day in CHB; however, routine monitoring of serum creatinine is recommended when treatment duration is >1 year as the likelihood of CKD increases with duration of therapy. Every 3-month monitoring is recommended in patients at risk of CKD, including the elderly and those with pre-existing renal disease, diabetes, or hypertension.[51] Entecavir and tenofovir are first-line nucleotide inhibitors used preferentially over adefovir in CHB. Kidney manifestations with entecavir and tenofovir are infrequent, with AKI and hypophosphatemia most frequently observed with tenofovir.[53] The American Association for the Study of Liver Diseases 2016 treatment guidelines of CHB recommend yearly monitoring of serum creatinine in patients treated with entecavir and tenofovir. More frequent monitoring is warranted in patients with pre-existing kidney disease or at risk for its development.[53]

Tenofovir is also administered to patients with HIV as part of a multidrug combination, typically as the tenofovir disoproxil prodrug. AKI and Fanconi syndrome are the most frequently reported kidney manifestations, but CKD may also occur.[54] Tenofovir alafenamide is a new prodrug of tenofovir that maintains antiviral efficacy with smaller doses and has the potential for reduced kidney and bone toxicity. Whether this prodrug will result in less CKD remains to be determined. Other antiviral drugs, such as acyclovir and indinavir, primarily result in AKI, which may rarely progress to ESRD.

This chapter focuses primarily on tacrolimus, cyclosporine, lithium, combination analgesics, and Chinese herbs, the agents most commonly associated with drug-induced CKD.

EPIDEMIOLOGY

TACROLIMUS/CYCLOSPORINE

Tacrolimus and cyclosporine are calcineurin inhibitors that are administered in combination with other immunosuppressive medications to prevent rejection in solid organ transplantation and for prevention and treatment of graft-versus-host disease. These drugs may also be used for the management of autoimmune disorders such as psoriasis, rheumatoid arthritis, ulcerative colitis, Crohn disease, and atopic dermatitis. Tacrolimus and cyclosporine cause both AKI and CKD. Tacrolimus- or cyclosporine-induced AKI typically occurs within 6–12 months after the organ transplantation and is often reversible with dose reduction, whereas drug-induced CKD is progressive, often occurring after 6–12 months of treatment, and may culminate in chronic allograft loss.[16] Tacrolimus and cyclosporine contribute to chronic renal allograft nephropathy to a similar degree and have similar risk factors and clinical presentations. In one early study, CKD (defined as a serum creatinine concentration >2.5 mg/dL) occurred in 18% of liver transplant patients receiving cyclosporine or tacrolimus within 13 years after transplantation; half of those patients experienced progression to ESRD.[26] In heart transplant recipients, the incidence of renal insufficiency, defined as a GFR <60 mL/min/1.73 m^2, increased from 28.8% at baseline to 59.6% at 36 months post-transplantation.[58] In patients receiving cyclosporine for treatment of psoriasis, creatinine clearance declined at a rate of 3.1 mL/min/yr and was associated with interstitial fibrosis and tubular atrophy.[59]

The incidence of drug-induced nephrotoxicity is more difficult to determine in patients who undergo kidney transplantation because chronic rejection, recurring renal disease, and drug-induced nephrotoxicity all can play a role in progressive loss of kidney function. In an early retrospective study of more than 1,600 kidney transplant patients receiving cyclosporine, the average serum creatinine concentration 3 years after transplantation was 1.9 mg/dL.[60] More recent studies have evaluated the incidence of calcineurin inhibitor nephrotoxicity at lower doses. More than 1,600 kidney transplant recipients treated with low-dose tacrolimus in combination with daclizumab induction, mycophenolate, and corticosteroids had a GFR of 65.4 mL/min 12 months post-transplantation, a value which was higher than with patients receiving regimens of standard dose cyclosporine, low-dose cyclosporine, or a calcineurin-free regimen (56–59 mL/min).[28]

Despite numerous studies that have evaluated the chronic nephrotoxicity of these medications, there is a growing body of evidence to support a variety of causes of CKD in the kidney transplant population, with only one component being exposure to calcineurin inhibitors. Results from the Long-term Deterioration of Kidney Allograft Function study of patients with late graft dysfunction and kidney biopsy data showed evidence of antibody-mediated kidney injury in 57% of patients with new-onset late kidney allograft dysfunction.[61] In a study evaluating the causes of kidney allograft loss in more than 1,300 kidney transplant patients, calcineurin inhibitor toxicity alone caused 0.6% of grafts lost, although the authors speculate that the drugs may have contributed to the development or progression of fibrosis and atrophy in about 30% of the grafts lost.[62] Thus, the role of calcineurin inhibitors in overall chronic kidney allograft damage required further study.

LITHIUM

Several renal complications are reported as a consequence of chronic lithium therapy. Well-known manifestations include polyuria, polydipsia, and nephrogenic diabetes insipidus (defined as an inability to concentrate the urine despite normal or increased concentrations of the antidiuretic hormone arginine vasopressin).[42,63] A causal relationship between lithium therapy and CKD has not been conclusively established. Numerous retrospective and cross-sectional studies have described an association between lithium therapy and impaired kidney function, particularly in patients receiving long-term (e.g., 10–20 years) therapy. However, significant variability is reported in the literature, with an incidence ranging from <1% to as high as 21%, and with progression to ESRD occurring rarely.[36-43] Other studies have found no association between lithium intake and reduction in GFR.[64-66] Poor quality of published data, small sample sizes, and exclusion of patients with a history of lithium intoxication limit extrapolation of the results. A meta-analysis of studies published from the 1960s to the present involving patients with mood disorders treated with lithium found only a small risk of renal failure secondary to lithium treatment (overall reduction in GFR of 6.2 mL/min).[65] Other factors such as age, concomitant medications, and occurrence of lithium intoxication may play a role. Thus, the incidence of lithium-induced CKD is not clear. The prevailing consensus is that lithium rarely causes CKD, and its occurrence appears to be related primarily to the duration of administration and cumulative dose.[42]

ANALGESICS

Analgesic nephropathy is defined as CKD resulting from long-term intake (more than 1 year) of two or more antipyretic analgesics, often in combination with substances with potential dependence (e.g., caffeine, codeine).[69] It is estimated that analgesic nephropathy is the cause of kidney failure in <1% of cases in the United States, but it may account for 3–9% of all cases of kidney failure in Europe and Australia, where combination analgesic products have been available without a prescription for longer than in the United States.[7] Analgesics reported to cause CKD include acetaminophen, aspirin, NSAIDs, pyrazolones, and phenacetin.[70] An association between analgesic use and renal failure was first identified in patients consuming phenacetin-containing analgesics.[9,71,72] As a result, phenacetin use has been restricted around the world, and it was removed from the U.S. market in 1983.[73,74] Although these restrictions were followed by a decrease in the incidence of kidney failure secondary to analgesic nephropathy, the overall incidence of drug-induced CKD increased in some regions possibly due to other combinations of analgesics, including those containing acetaminophen.[73]

Acetaminophen is a metabolite of phenacetin, and it has been speculated that acetaminophen could similarly induce CKD, particularly when consumed as part of analgesic combinations. Heavy consumption of acetaminophen has been associated with a dose-dependent increased risk of kidney failure in some studies, although it is not entirely clear in these reports whether patients consumed single-entity or combination products.[9,10,75] In addition, other studies did not find a decrease in GFR following normal or high-dose acetaminophen therapy.[75-77]

The Nurses' Health Study evaluated self-reported lifetime use of acetaminophen, aspirin, and NSAIDs and change in GFR over an 11-year period (1989–2000) in 1,697 women.[74] Acetaminophen, but not aspirin or NSAIDs, was associated with an increased risk of kidney failure and a 30% reduction in GFR. However, other studies have not found a correlation between acetaminophen consumption and kidney failure, particularly at lower acetaminophen doses. The National Kidney Foundation expert panel on analgesic nephropathy issued a consensus statement that the habitual use of combination antipyretic analgesics is associated with an increased prevalence of CKD, whereas the use of single-entity products (aspirin, acetaminophen, NSAIDs) appears to carry a lower risk for analgesic nephropathy.[69] Further, the panel's statement indicates that acetaminophen remains the non-narcotic analgesic of choice in patients with kidney failure, although habitual consumption is not recommended.[69] In summary, there is little convincing evidence that acetaminophen causes analgesic nephropathy when used alone and at recommended doses.

Conflicting data also exist regarding NSAID use and worsening CKD. High-dose NSAIDs may accelerate progression of CKD, although chronic consumption of regular-dose NSAIDs does not appear to have the same effect. In addition, NSAIDs may worsen hypertension, lead to hyperkalemia, and may cause a prostaglandin-mediated decrease in renal blood flow resulting in AKI. Therefore, routine monitoring of kidney function is required with use of NSAIDs, particularly in individuals with reduced GFR and in the elderly.

DIETARY SUPPLEMENTS CONTAINING ARISTOLOCHIC ACID

Nephropathy associated with Chinese herbs was first identified in the early 1990s in Belgium after kidney failure developed in nine patients from the same weight loss clinic in association with weight reduction regimens containing Chinese herbs.[6] It was subsequently confirmed that weight reduction regimens from this clinic inadvertently contained plant material from species of *Aristolochia*.[3] *Aristolochia* contains aristolochic acids I and II, which are known nephrotoxins.[78] One cross-sectional survey in adult Chinese participants found an association between aristolochic acid intake and GFR <60 mL/min/1.73 m^2 and albuminuria.[79] Originally termed *Chinese herb nephropathy*, the condition has been renamed *aristolochic acid nephropathy* (AAN) because exposure has occurred secondary to food contamination and in the manufacturing of dietary supplements.[80] Although the incidence is not known, nephropathy associated with Chinese herbs has been reported worldwide. Urinary tract cancer has also been associated with aristolochic acid, which resulted in its classification as a carcinogen by the International Agency for Research on Cancer. Since the early 1990s, many countries have banned the use of *Aristolochia* species. In 2001, the U.S. Food and Drug Administration (FDA) issued an alert indicating that dietary supplements are unsafe if they contain (or there is even a suspicion that they contain) aristolochic acids.[81] Manufacturers have been warned to remove aristolochic acid from their products, and any products containing aristolochic acid are considered unsafe and adulterated.[82] However, even with these warnings, cases of AAN continue to be reported around the world, and the product may be available online.[78]

MECHANISMS

TACROLIMUS/CYCLOSPORINE

CKD induced by tacrolimus and cyclosporine typically presents as chronic tubulointerstitial nephritis, characterized on renal biopsy as interstitial fibrosis appearing in a "striped" pattern, widespread tubular atrophy, and to a lesser extent, glomerulosclerosis. Renal arteriolar hyalinosis is a primary manifestation thought to be indicative of cyclosporine- or tacrolimus-induced CKD.[17] Glomerular changes may be absent or may occur only in more advanced stages of CKD. Direct vascular toxicity and direct tubular toxicity have also been suggested as mechanisms for chronic kidney injury.[17] Direct vascular toxicity of endothelial cells and release of vasoactive substances, cytokines, and growth factors lead to tubulointerstitial fibrosis and glomerulosclerosis. In addition, direct tubular toxicity may occur after long-term exposure to calcineurin inhibitors because of the induction of apoptosis and inhibition of P-glycoprotein, thus allowing intracellular calcineurin inhibitor accumulation.[84] Biopsies from patients who received kidney-pancreas transplants demonstrated severe chronic allograft nephropathy in 58.4% of patients and glomerulosclerosis in 37.3%.[20] Mechanisms of CKD are described in **Table 42-2**.

LITHIUM

Lithium-induced CKD presents as chronic tubulointerstitial nephritis, characterized on renal biopsy as interstitial fibrosis and inflammation, widespread tubular atrophy, and glomerulosclerosis. Distal tubular dilation, glycogen deposition,

Table 42-2 Mechanisms of Drug-Induced Chronic Kidney Disease

Drug	Mechanism
Adefovir/cidofovir/entecavir/tenofovir[15,49-50]	Proximal renal tubular injury, tubular atrophy
Aristolochic acid (Chinese herbs)[4,5]	Interstitial fibrosis, tubular atrophy
Antipyretic analgesics[8,a]	Papillary necrosis, interstitial nephritis
Cisplatin[12,14]	Interstitial fibrosis, tubular atrophy
Cyclosporine[17,84]	Interstitial fibrosis, tubular atrophy, afferent arteriolopathy
Gold salts[30,31]	Proteinuria, membranous glomerulonephritis, minimal-change disease, immune complex mesangial glomerulonephritis
Ifosfamide[13-14]	Interstitial fibrosis, tubular atrophy
Lithium[83,85-86]	interstitial fibrosis, tubular atrophy, tubular cysts
Nitrosoureas (streptozocin, carmustine, lomustine)[14]	Glomerulosclerosis, interstitial fibrosis, tubular atrophy
D-penicillamine[44]	Proteinuria, membranous nephropathy, immune complex mesangial glomerulonephritis, rapidly progressive crescentic glomerulonephritis
Propylthiouracil[45]	Glomerulonephritis, tubulointerstitial nephritis
Tacrolimus[17,84]	Interstitial fibrosis, tubular atrophy, afferent arteriolopathy

[a]Chronic consumption of a combination of at least two antipyretic analgesics, and usually caffeine or codeine or both.

and microcyst formation have been reported in lithium-treated patients with CKD.[83,85,86] The mechanism of lithium-induced CKD is not known but has been speculated to be decreased intracellular formation of cyclic adenosine monophosphate or inhibition of water transport in the cortical collecting duct.[67]

ANALGESICS

Papillary necrosis associated with calcification is a hallmark feature of analgesic nephropathy and often precedes the development of cortical changes.[8] A potential mechanism for the toxicity of combination analgesics has been suggested.[8] Acetaminophen and phenacetin are primarily removed from the body by renal excretion of glucuronides. However, acetaminophen is also oxidized to *N*-acetylbenzoquinoneimine, a highly reactive intermediate, which accumulates in the papillae of the kidney. Reduced glutathione can quickly react with and decrease free radical toxicity; however, concomitant ingestion of salicylates depletes renal medullary glutathione, thus enabling the reactive metabolites to cause papillary necrosis. In addition, decreased synthesis of vasodilatory prostaglandins by NSAIDs and salicylates can cause renal ischemia.[8]

DIETARY SUPPLEMENTS CONTAINING ARISTOLOCHIC ACID

Pathologic features associated with AAN include extensive interstitial fibrosis and tubular atrophy, with the most significant lesions in the superficial cortex.[4] Glomerulosclerosis is more limited and is often secondary to tubular and interstitial damage. Thickening of Bowman's capsule and swelling of interlobar and afferent arteriole walls may also be present.[4] Because the cortex is most severely damaged, it has been speculated that direct proximal-tubule epithelial cell damage is the most likely mechanism.[5] It has also been suggested that the primary lesion occurs in small arterial walls, leading to ischemia and interstitial fibrosis, or that interstitial fibroblasts are stimulated directly.[5]

CLINICAL PRESENTATION AND DIFFERENTIAL DIAGNOSIS

Patients with drug-induced CKD typically present with nonspecific symptoms attributed to kidney failure. **Table 42-3** lists signs and symptoms commonly associated with CKD, including drug-induced causes. In addition to drugs, a variety of

Table 42-3 Signs and Symptoms Associated with Drug-Induced Chronic Kidney Disease

Water and sodium imbalance

- Elevated blood pressure
- Nocturia
- Peripheral edema
- Pulmonary edema
- Weight gain

Hematologic

- Anemia
- Bleeding
- Dizziness
- Fatigue
- Headache
- Shortness of breath

Hyperphosphatemia

- Persistent itching

Urinary

- Decreased urine output
- Blood in urine
- Protein in urine

Hyperkalemia

- Palpitations or irregular heartbeat
- Numbness or tingling

Cardiovascular

- Chest pain
- Dizziness
- Edema
- Fatigue
- Headache
- Hypertension
- Nervousness

Neurologic

- Fatigue
- Insomnia and sleep disturbances
- Malaise
- Paresthesias
- Restless legs
- Seizures
- Weakness

Gastrointestinal

- Diarrhea or constipation
- Nausea, vomiting, anorexia
- Unpleasant taste

Metabolic/endocrine

- Bone fractures
- Bone pain
- Glucose intolerance
- Gout
- Growth retardation
- Sexual dysfunction

Nutritional

- Anorexia
- Decreased muscle mass
- Weight loss
- Proteinuria (gold salts, D-penicillamine, nonsteroidal anti-inflammatory agents)

Psychological

- Anxiety
- Depression
- Psychosis

Dermatologic

- Pigmentation
- Pruritus

medical conditions can lead to CKD. **Table 42-4** lists conditions to be considered in the differential diagnosis of drug-induced CKD.

TACROLIMUS/CYCLOSPORINE

CKD induced by tacrolimus or cyclosporine occurs insidiously, usually beginning after at least 6–12 months of therapy. Patients have an increase in serum creatinine and blood urea nitrogen (BUN) concentrations and often present with hypertension. Differentiating chronic organ rejection from drug-induced nephrotoxicity is difficult, especially in kidney transplant recipients.[16] Kidney biopsy findings

Table 42-4 Conditions to Consider in the Differential Diagnosis of Drug-Induced Chronic Kidney Disease

- Chronic rejection of a transplanted kidney
- Cystic kidney disease
- Diabetic nephropathy
- Glomerulonephritis
- Hereditary (e.g., Alport disease)
- Hypertensive nephrosclerosis
- Obstructive uropathy
- Pyelonephritis
- Renal vascular disease

associated with chronic cyclosporine or tacrolimus nephrotoxicity include nodular arterial hyalinosis, tubular atrophy, glomerulosclerosis, and tubulointerstitial fibrosis in a "striped" pattern.[57,87-89] Manifestations of cyclosporine- or tacrolimus-associated CKD are similar to those of other causes of CKD (e.g., fluid overload, anemia, electrolyte abnormalities). Recent evidence suggests that calcineurin inhibitor use may not be a major factor in late graft loss, and that immune injury from donor antibodies may play a prominent role.[90]

LITHIUM

Patients with lithium-induced CKD present with an insidious increase in serum creatinine and BUN concentrations, often after decades or more of treatment.[91] Patients may present rarely with hypertension and proteinuria. In most reported cases of lithium-induced CKD, reduction in renal function was mild (creatinine clearance >50 mL/min). Progression of CKD to ESRD is uncommon.[43]

ANALGESICS

Patients with analgesic-induced nephropathy develop an insidious increase in BUN and serum creatinine concentrations.[92] Symptoms of renal failure secondary to analgesic nephropathy are nonspecific. Patients may rarely report renal colic and hematuria secondary to excreting necrotic papilla in the urine.[8] A careful medication history is needed to determine a pattern of analgesic use that lists lifetime usage of prescription and nonprescription medications, including those that are no longer commercially available. Daily consumption of analgesic combinations for more than 1 year is highly indicative of abuse.[69] In suspected cases, a computed tomography (CT) scan without contrast medium is indicated. In patients with analgesic-induced nephropathy, the CT scan reveals decreased bilateral renal mass in addition to bumpy contours of the kidney, papillary calcifications, or both.[70]

DIETARY SUPPLEMENTS CONTAINING ARISTOLOCHIC ACID

Patients with AAN typically present with nonspecific findings attributed to CKD, although anemia may be more pronounced than expected based on the stage of CKD.[92] In addition, mild proteinuria and glycosuria may be present.[93] An accurate medication history to confirm ingestion of Chinese herbs is critical to the diagnosis. Aristolochic acid was found not only in dietary supplements but also in supplements for arthritis, pain, and hepatitis.[2] Kidney size is decreased, and diagnosis may be confirmed with a kidney biopsy, which reveals extensive interstitial fibrosis.[92] In addition, urothelial lesions or urothelial transitional cell carcinoma may also be present.[94] Progression to ESRD occurs rapidly.[78]

RISK FACTORS

Although risk factors for CKD induced by calcineurin inhibitors and analgesics have been identified (**Table 42-5**), risk factors for CKD caused by other drugs are not well defined.

Table 42-5 Risk Factors for Drug-Induced Chronic Kidney Disease

Cyclosporine/tacrolimus

- Age >50 years
- Diminished pretreatment renal function
- Higher cumulative dose
- Increased duration of exposure
- Number of episodes of acute renal failure secondary to cyclosporine or tacrolimus
- Number of rejection episodes
- Poor kidney function in the first 3–12 months after surgery
- Postoperative acute renal failure

Lithium (risk factors not well established, but may include the following)

- Concurrent treatment with other psychotropic drugs
- Episodes of acute lithium intoxication
- Higher cumulative doses
- Longer durations of exposure
- Occurrence of nephrogenic diabetes insipidus
- Serum creatinine concentration ≥2.5 mg/dL at diagnosis

Antipyretic analgesics (long-term use, usually in combination with caffeine or codeine or both)

- ≥1 g daily for ≥1 year
- Cumulative doses of 1–3 kg

Aristolochic acid

- Risk factors not established; dose and duration of therapy have been speculated to be risk factors

TACROLIMUS/CYCLOSPORINE

Some risk factors for developing tacrolimus- or cyclosporine-induced CKD have been more clearly elucidated than others. Potential risk factors include increased length of exposure (minimum duration 6–12 months), higher cumulative dose, poor kidney function during the first 3–12 months after transplantation, episodes of cyclosporine- or tacrolimus-induced AKI, at least one acute rejection episode, diminished pretreatment renal function (GFR <70 mL/min/1.73 m^2), postoperative AKI, and age >50 years.[16,17,23,95-99] Diabetes and hypertension may have a role.[23] There is no consistent correlation between trough cyclosporine or tacrolimus concentrations and the development of chronic nephropathy.[100]

LITHIUM

The most consistent risk factor for lithium-induced CKD is duration of therapy.[43] One study found a decrease in GFR of 0.64 mL/min/yr of lithium treatment.[101] Other risk factors have not been clearly identified. It has been speculated that episodes of acute lithium intoxication and nephrogenic diabetes insipidus may contribute to development of CKD.[37] Long-term concurrent treatment with other psychotropic drugs is another potential risk factor.[37] Daily lithium dose and serum lithium concentrations do not appear to be risk factors, although once-daily dosing has been speculated to pose less risk than multiple-daily dosing due to tubular regeneration with once-daily administration.[102] It is unknown whether pre-existing CKD is a risk factor for renal toxicity. Increased individual sensitivity to lithium has not been demonstrated, but lithium sensitivity could explain why CKD develops in some patients but not others.

ANALGESICS

The primary risk factor for analgesic nephropathy is long-term consumption of antipyretic analgesics. Consumption of these drugs in doses of ≥1 g daily for 1 year or more are at increased risk, as are individuals consuming cumulative amounts of 1 to 3 kg or more.[72,103] It has been suggested that analgesics containing caffeine may increase the risk of nephropathy, but the role of caffeine in analgesic-induced CKD has not been clearly elucidated.[104] Caffeine may inhibit prostaglandin synthesis via suppression of cyclooxygenase-2, decrease medullary oxygen supply, or promote analgesic dependence.[104] There is limited evidence that long-term consumption of acetaminophen alone leads to analgesic nephropathy, although its role as a cause of this drug-induced disease cannot be excluded completely.

DIETARY SUPPLEMENTS CONTAINING ARISTOLOCHIC ACID

Risk factors for AAN have not been well established. It has been speculated that dose, duration of therapy, and concurrent ingestion of dexfenfluramine, phentermine, or both may increase the risk.[92] In addition, most cases of AAN have occurred in women. However, women are more likely to consume weight-loss products than men and may therefore have increased risk of exposure to Chinese herbs. Whether female sex is a risk factor for nephropathy induced by Chinese herbs is not known.

MORBIDITY AND MORTALITY

TACROLIMUS/CYCLOSPORINE

Chronic allograft nephropathy is a term that was used historically to characterize the syndrome that encompasses both chronic kidney rejection and calcineurin toxicity in kidney transplant recipients.[90] However, morbidity and mortality risk associated with the drugs needs to be further elucidated given the uncertainty about whether the kidney injury is solely attributable to calcineurin use as recent evidence suggests that calcineurin inhibitor nephrotoxicity may not be the major factor in late graft failure and that antibody-mediated rejection may predominate.[90]

Chronic allograft nephropathy resulting in graft loss has been reported to occur in approximately 10–40% of heart transplant recipients.[58] In lung transplant recipients, kidney failure developed in 15% of tacrolimus-treated patients at 1 year.[46]

In a study of heart transplant recipients receiving cyclosporine, there was a 12% probability of developing stage 5 CKD at 10 years postoperative.[27]

LITHIUM

Lithium-induced CKD results in mild reduction in renal function. Studies have reported a yearly decrease in GFR ranging from 0.64 mL/min to 2.29 mL/min.[42,101] In a study of 61 patients receiving lithium for an average of 15.6 years, estimated GFR was 66.1 mL/min compared to 75 mL/min in the control group.[105] Rarely does lithium-induced CKD progress to ESRD and necessitate dialysis.

ANALGESICS

Progression to kidney failure is likely if chronic analgesic consumption continues. Discontinuation of analgesics may slow progression, but renal function is not likely to improve.

DIETARY SUPPLEMENTS CONTAINING ARISTOLOCHIC ACID

Progression to kidney failure occurs at a very rapid rate, typically within 1–7 years.[80] There is some evidence that high cumulative exposure causes faster progression to ESRD.[80] Progression of CKD may continue even after discontinuation of the herb-containing supplement.[92]

PREVENTION

Prevention of drug-induced CKD includes routine monitoring of kidney function and evaluation of patients for signs and symptoms associated with CKD (**Table 42-6**).

Table 42-6 Approaches to Help Prevent Drug-Induced Chronic Kidney Disease

Cyclosporine

- Avoid concurrent nephrotoxic medications
- Minimize dose and duration of use
- Assess renal function up to twice weekly in new transplant recipients; with decreasing frequency in individuals with stable kidney function (monthly to yearly evaluation)

Lithium

- Avoid acute lithium intoxication
- Avoid elevated serum lithium concentrations
- Consider withdrawal of lithium to minimize length and total drug exposure in patients with decreased kidney function suspected to be due to lithium (based on risk–benefit assessment determined on an individual basis)
- Assess renal function every 6–12 months

Antipyretic analgesics

- Completely preventable by avoidance
- Institute interventions to curb analgesic abuse

Chinese herbs (aristolochic acid)

- Completely preventable by avoidance
- Glucocorticoids may delay progression to ESRD[3]

ESRD = end-stage renal disease.

TACROLIMUS/CYCLOSPORINE

Whether it is possible to prevent development of chronic nephrotoxicity from calcineurin inhibitors is a subject of much debate. Increased duration of exposure and increased cumulative drug exposure have been postulated to cause chronic renal damage, but an association between blood cyclosporine concentrations and CKD has not been established.[17,96] Thus, routine monitoring of trough blood cyclosporine concentrations does not aid in preventing CKD as it does in AKI. Eliminating or reducing patient exposure to calcineurin inhibitors has been one strategy to prevent development of CKD. Although some studies found lower mean serum creatinine concentrations with regimens not containing calcineurin inhibitors compared to regimens containing the combination of mycophenolate and steroids with calcineurin inhibitors, other studies found decreased allograft survival when tacrolimus and cyclosporine are excluded.[106,107] Total avoidance of calcineurin inhibitors result in reduced graft survival in liver transplant recipients.[21] One study using data from the Scientific Registry of Renal Transplant Recipients demonstrated decreased allograft survival when tacrolimus and cyclosporine are excluded (64% allograft survival) compared to regimens containing cyclosporine or tacrolimus (78% allograft survival).[107] Other protocols that discontinued calcineurin inhibitors in patients who had initially received them demonstrated mixed results.[100]

The National Kidney Foundation and the Kidney Disease Outcomes Quality Initiative Clinical Practice Guidelines recommend initial therapy with tacrolimus compared to a calcineurin-free regimen in kidney transplantation. In cases where chronic allograft injury develops, dose reduction followed by calcineurin withdrawal can be considered.[29,108]

LITHIUM

Elevated serum lithium concentrations may predispose patients to lithium-related adverse effects. In addition, some evidence suggests that episodes of acute intoxication or the occurrence of nephrogenic diabetes insipidus can predispose a patient to CKD.[37] Thus, it is recommended to maintain serum lithium concentrations as low as clinically feasible. It is also important to rule out other causes of renal failure (e.g., diabetes, hypertension) and to establish the relative contribution of each risk factor. Whether discontinuation of lithium leads to improvement in the GFR is not clear. Kidney function should be assessed every 2–3 months during the first 6 months of lithium treatment and at least yearly in stable patients; more frequent monitoring is indicated in higher-risk patients (e.g., increased age, occurrence of lithium intoxication).[109]

ANALGESICS

Analgesic nephropathy is one of the few preventable causes of CKD. Because the primary risk factor is long-term consumption of non-narcotic analgesics, identification of analgesic abuse and interventions to curb abuse may prevent progression to ESRD. Discontinuation of analgesics may stabilize kidney function, but kidney function is not likely to return to baseline.[110] More importantly, limiting the sale of combination analgesics can decrease the prevalence of analgesic-induced CKD. The National Kidney Foundation recommends that the "availability of analgesic mixtures as an over-the-counter (OTC) product should cease" and prescription products should bear a warning of the association between kidney disease and the habitual consumption of analgesic mixtures.[69] However, combination OTC analgesic products remain commercially available.

DIETARY SUPPLEMENTS CONTAINING ARISTOLOCHIC ACID

Avoiding the use of *Aristolochia* species prevents AAN. In 2001, the FDA issued an alert stating that dietary supplements are unsafe if they contain (or if there is even a suspicion that they may contain) aristolochic acids.[81] Manufacturers of dietary supplements must ensure the safety of their products with strict manufacturing procedures that ensure that these products do not contain aristolochic acid. Despite this warning, products containing aristolochic acids may still be available over the Internet.[111] In one study, aristolochic acids I and II were found in 20% and 7%, respectively, of 30 herbal products marketed in the United States via the Internet.[112] Practitioners must consider the potential role of dietary supplements when evaluating new patients presenting with kidney disease. The public also needs to be made aware of the potential dangers associated with such herbal products.

MANAGEMENT

Management of drug-induced CKD is largely supportive. General recommendations for managing complications associated with CKD are presented in **Table 42-7**.

TACROLIMUS/CYCLOSPORINE

There is presently no effective treatment for tacrolimus- or cyclosporine-induced chronic nephrotoxicity.[113] Withdrawal of therapy or substitution of alternative immunosuppressive agents (e.g., sirolimus) may slow the rate of loss of renal function or lead to improvements in GFR.[114] However, the benefits of continued therapy in terms of graft survival must be weighed against the risk of drug-induced CKD. Routine monitoring of renal function is required in all patients treated with cyclosporine or tacrolimus.

LITHIUM

Although there are multiple treatment options for lithium-induced polyuria (e.g., thiazides, amiloride, indomethacin), less is known about effective treatment for lithium-induced CKD. Minimizing progression with an angiotensin-converting enzyme

Table 42-7 Treatment Options for the Management of Drug-Induced Chronic Kidney Disease

- Discontinue the offending agent (may lead to reversal or halt progression of CKD) and administer less nephrotoxic medication
- Dialysis or kidney transplantation (if progression to end-stage renal disease)
- Treatment of common complications of CKD:
  - Anemia—erythropoietin or darbepoetin; iron
  - Bleeding—red-cell transfusion, DDAVP, conjugated estrogens, erythropoietin
  - Hyperkalemia—dietary potassium restriction, sodium polystyrene sulfonate, intravenous calcium, intravenous insulin and glucose, intravenous sodium bicarbonate
  - Hyperlipidemia—bile acid sequestrants, nicotinic acid, statins, gemfibrozil, clofibrate, probucol
  - Hyperphosphatemia/secondary hyperparathyroidism—dietary phosphorus restriction, phosphate binders, calcium supplements, vitamin D analogs, calcimimetics, parathyroidectomy
  - Hypertension—All classes of antihypertensives can be used; multidrug regimens may be needed; select therapy based on concomitant medical needs
  - Malnutrition—vitamin and nutritional supplements
  - Water and sodium imbalance—sodium restriction, diuretics

CKD = chronic kidney disease, DDAVP = 1-deamino-8-D-arginine vasopressin.

inhibitor, normalizing blood pressure, and avoiding other nephrotoxic medications have been suggested.[115] Whether discontinuation of lithium therapy decreases progression of lithium-induced CKD remains controversial. Because rate of progression to CKD is slow, lithium could be tapered slowly while alternative treatment is titrated upward.[68]

ANALGESICS

Discontinuation of analgesic consumption is a primary treatment goal, as this may prevent progression of CKD.[116] In patients with established nephropathy, complications of CKD should be treated and dialysis initiated as indicated.

DIETARY SUPPLEMENTS CONTAINING ARISTOLOCHIC ACID

There is no specific treatment for AAN. In rare cases, CKD is reversible with discontinuation of treatment.[117] However, in at least 70% of cases, patients progress to stage 5 CKD and require either dialysis or kidney transplantation.[81] One small study found that corticosteroids slowed progression to kidney failure.[118]

INFORMATION FOR PATIENTS

Patients receiving medications such as cyclosporine, tacrolimus, and lithium (Table 42-1) should be instructed that routine blood work for assessment of renal function is essential, because patients remain asymptomatic until creatinine clearance is significantly reduced (<30 mL/min). Patients should be counseled regarding the signs and symptoms associated with CKD (Table 42-3) and should be instructed to seek medical attention if any of these occur.

In addition, patients must recognize that nonprescription medications can cause nephrotoxicity. Acetaminophen remains the non-narcotic analgesic of choice in individuals with CKD. However, patients should be informed that acetaminophen is not intended for long-term consumption and that any long-term use should be undertaken with the supervision of the patient's healthcare providers. In addition, patients should be educated about the association of kidney injury with long-term consumption of combination analgesics, and chronic use should be strongly discouraged. Patients should be informed that the FDA regulates dietary supplements as foods rather than drugs, and therefore products are not required to undergo the same rigorous clinical testing and quality control as drugs. Caution in using these products is advised. Importantly, patients should be instructed that diet aids containing aristolochic acid can lead to development of CKD and that their use must be immediately discontinued.

REFERENCES

1. Kidney Disease: Improving Global Outcomes (KDIGO) CKD Work Group. KDIGO 2012 Clinical Practice Guideline for the Evaluation and Management of Chronic Kidney Disease. *Kidney Int Suppl.* 2013; 3:1-150.
2. Debelle FD, Vanherweghem JL, Nortier JL. Aristolochic acid nephropathy: a worldwide problem. *Kidney Int.* 2008; 74:158-69.
3. Luciano RL, Perazella MA. Aristolochic acid nephropathy: epidemiology, clinical presentation, and treatment. *Drug Saf.* 2015: 38:55-64.

4. Chen D, Tang Z, Chen H et al. Clinical and pathological spectrums of aristolochic acid nephropathy. *Clin Nephrol.* 2012; 78:54-60.
5. Jadot I, Decleves AE, Nortier J et al. An integrative view of aristolochic acid nephropathy: update of the literature. *Int J Mol Sci.* 2017; 18:pii:E297.
6. Vanherweghem JL, Depierreux M, Tielemans C et al. Rapidly progressive interstitial renal fibrosis in young women: association with slimming regimen including Chinese herbs. *Lancet.* 1993; 341:387-91.
7. De Broe ME, Elseviers MM. Analgesic nephropathy. *N Engl J Med.* 1998; 338:446-52.
8. Elseviers MM, De Broe ME. Analgesic nephropathy: is it caused by multi-analgesic abuse or single substance use? *Drug Saf.* 1999; 20:15-24.
9. De Broe ME, Elseviers MM. Over-the-counter analgesic use. *J Am Soc Nephrol.* 2009; 20:2098-103.
10. Segasothy M, Suleiman AB, Puvaneswary M et al. Paracetamol: a cause for analgesic nephropathy and end-stage renal disease. *Nephron.* 1988; 50:50-4.
11. Mulder RL, Knijnenburg SL, Geskus RB et al. Glomerular function time trends in long-term survivors of childhood cancer: a longitudinal study. *Cancer Epidemiol Biomarkers Prev.* 2013: 22:1736-46.
12. Launay-Vacher V, Rey JB, Isnard-Bagnis C et al. Prevention of cisplatin nephrotoxicity: state of the art and recommendations from the European Society of Clinical Pharmacy Special Interest Group on Cancer Care. *Cancer Chemother Pharmacol.* 2008; 61:903-9.
13. Lameire N, Kruse V, Rottey S. Nephrotoxicity of anticancer drugs—an underestimated problem? *Acta Clin Belg.* 2011; 66:337-45.
14. Perazella MA, Moeckel GW. Nephrotoxicity from chemotherapeutic agents: clinical manifestations, pathobiology, and prevention/therapy. *Semin Nephrol.* 2010; 30:570-81.
15. Meier P, Dautheville-Guibal S, Ronco PM et al. Cidofovir-induced end-stage renal failure. *Nephrol Dial Transplant.* 2002; 17:148-9.
16. de Matto AM, Olyaei AJ, Bennett WM. Nephrotoxicity of immunosuppressive drugs: long-term consequences and challenges for the future. *Am J Kidney Dis.* 2000; 35:333-46.
17. Stratta P, Canavese C, Quaglia M et al. Posttransplantation chronic renal damage in nonrenal transplant recipients. *Kidney Int.* 2005; 68:1453-63.
18. Lynn M, Abreo K, Zibari G et al. End-stage renal disease in liver transplants. *Clin Transplant.* 2001; 15(suppl 6):S66-69.
19. Burdmann EA, Andoh TF, Yu L et al. Cyclosporine nephrotoxicity. *Semin Nephrol.* 2003; 23:465-76.
20. Nankivell BJ, Borrows RJ, Fung CL et al. The natural history of chronic allograft nephropathy. *NEJM.* 2003; 349:2326-33.
21. Zhang W, Fung J. Limitations of current liver transplant immunosuppressive regimens: renal considerations. *Hepatobiliary Pancreat Dis Int.* 2017; 16:27-32.
22. Ben Hmida M, Baumelou A, Desruesnnes M et al. Long term nephrotoxicity of low doses of cyclosporine in heart transplant recipients. *Transplantation Proc.* 1995; 27:2725-7.
23. Lachance K, White M, de Denus S. Risk factors for chronic renal insufficiency following cardiac transplantation. *Ann Transplant.* 2015; 20:576-87.
24. Costanzo MR, Dipchand A, Starling R et al. The International Society of Heart and Lung Transplantation Guidelines for the care of heart transplant recipients. *J Heart Lung Transplant.* 2010; 29:914-56.
25. Soleymani T, Vassantachart JM, Wu JJ. Comparison of guidelines for the use of cyclosporine for psoriasis: a critical appraisal and comprehensive review. *J Drugs Dermatol.* 2016; 15:293-301.
26. Gonwa TA, Mai ML, Melton LB et al. End-stage renal disease (ESRD) after orthotopic liver transplantation (OLTX) using calcineurin-based immunotherapy: risk of development and treatment. *Transplantation.* 2001; 72:1934-9.
27. Hamour IM, Omar F, Lyster HS et al. Chronic kidney disease after heart transplantation. *Nephrol Dial Transplant.* 2009; 24:1655-62.
28. Ekberg H, Tedesco-Silva H, Demirbas A et al. Reduced exposure to calcineurin inhibitors in renal transplantation. *NEJM.* 2007; 357:2562-75.
29. Kasiske BL, Zeier MG, Chapman JR et al. KDIGO clinical practice guidelines for the care of kidney transplant recipients: a summary. *Kidney Int.* 2010; 77:299-311.
30. Kvien TK, Zeidler HK, Hannonen P et al. Long term efficacy and safety of cyclosporin versus parenteral gold in early rheumatoid arthritis: a three year study of radiographic progression, renal function, and arterial hypertension. *Ann Rheum Dis.* 2002; 61:511-6.
31. Sander O, Herborn G, Bock E et al. Prospective six year follow up of patients withdrawn from a randomised study comparing parenteral gold salt and methotrexate. *Ann Rheum Dis.* 1999; 58:281-7.
32. Farry JK, Flombaum CD, Latcha S. Long term renal toxicity of ifosfamide in adult patients—5 year data. *Eur J Cancer.* 2012; 48:1326-31.
33. Skinner R, Cotterill SJ, Stevens MCG. Risk factors for nephrotoxicity after ifosfamide treatment in children: a UKCCSG Late Effects Group Study. *Br J Cancer.* 2000; 82:1636-45.
34. Skinner R. Chronic ifosfamide nephrotoxicity in children. *Med Pediatr Oncol.* 2003; 41:190-7.
35. Skinner R. Late renal toxicity of treatment for childhood malignancy: risk factors, long-term outcomes, and surveillance. *Pediatr Nephrol.* 2018; 33:215-25.
36. Bendz H, Aurell M, Lanke J. A historical cohort study of kidney damage in long-term lithium patients: continued surveillance needed. *Eur Psychiatry.* 2001; 16:199-206.
37. Bendz H, Aurell M, Balldin J et al. Kidney damage in long-term lithium patients: a cross-sectional study of patients with 15 years or more on lithium. *Nephrol Dial Transplant.* 1994; 9:1250-4.
38. Aiff H, Attman PO, Aufell M et al. End-stage renal disease associated with prophylactic lithium treatment. *Eur Neuropsychopharmacol.* 2014; 24:540-4.
39. Azab AN, Shnaider A, Osher Y et al. Lithium nehrotoxicity. *Int J Bipolar Disord.* 2015; 3:3-9.
40. Bocchetta A, Cabras F, Pinna M et al. An observational study of 110 elderly lithium-treated patients followed up for 6 years with particular reference to renal function. *Int J Bipolar Disord.* 2017; 5:1-7.
41. McCann SM, Daly J, Kelly CB. The impact of long-term lithium treatment on renal function in an outpatient population. *Ulster Med J.* 2008; 77:102-5.
42. Presne C, Fakhouri F, Noel LH et al. Lithium-induced nephropathy: rate of progression and prognostic factors. *Kidney Int.* 2003; 64:585-92.
43. Bendz H, Schon S, Attman PO, Aurell M. Renal failure occurs in chronic lithium treatment but is uncommon. *Kidney Int.* 2010; 77:219-24.
44. Karpinski J, Jothy S, Radoux V et al. D-penicillamine-induced crescentic glomerulonephritis and antimyeloperoxidase antibodies in a patient with scleroderma. Case report and review of the literature. *Am J Nephrol.* 1997; 17:528-32.
45. Chen Y, Bao H, Liu Z et al. Clinico-pathological features and outcomes of patients with propylthiouracil-associated ANCA vasculitis with renal involvement. *J Nephrol.* 2014; 27:159-64.
46. Sikma MA, Hunault CC, van de Graaf EA et al. High tacrolimus blood concentrations early after lung transplantation and the risk of kidney injury. *Eur J Clin Pharmacol.* 2017; 73:573-80.
47. Lazarus B, Chen Y, Wilson FP et al. Proton pump inhibitor use and the risk of chronic kidney disease. *JAMA Intern Med.* 2016; 176:238-46.
48. Luo Q, Deng Y, Cheng F et al. Relationship between nephrotoxicity and long-term adefovir dipivoxil therapy for chronic hepatitis B: a meta-analysis. *Medicine (Baltimore).* 2016; 95:e5578.
49. Murakami C, Melda Urekli H, Atta MG. Antiviral medications for the treatment of hepatitis B and C infection and their effects on kidney function. *Minerva Gastroenterol Dietol.* 2014; 60:177-89.

50. Fung J, Seto WK, Lai CL et al. Extrahepatic effects of nucleoside and nucleotide analogues in chronic hepatitis B treatment. *J Gastroenterol Hepatol.* 2013; 29:428-34.

51. Vigano M, Lampertico P, Colombo M. Drug safety evaluation of adefovir in HBV infection. *Expert Opin Drug Saft.* 2011; 10:809-18.

52. Yang Q, Shi Y, Yang Y et al. Association between adefovir dipivoxil treatment and the risk of renal insuffiency in patients with chronic hepatitis B: a meta-analysis. *Biomedical Reports.* 2015; 3:269-75.

53. Terrault NA, Bzowej NH, Chang KM et al. ASSLD guidelines for treatment of chronic hepatitis B. *Hepatol.* 2016; 63:261-83.

54. Tourret J, Deray G, Isnard-Bagnis C. Tenofovir effect on the kidneys of HIV-infected patients: a double-edged sword? *J Am Soc Nephrol.* 2013; 24:1519-27.

55. Harirforoosh S, Jamali F. Renal adverse effects of nonsteroidal anti-inflammatory drugs. *Expert Opin Drug Saf.* 2009; 8:669-81.

56. Wijarnpreecha K, Thongprayoon C, Chesdachai S et al. Associations of proton-pump inhibitors and H2 receptor antagonists with chronic kidney disease: a meta-analysis. *Dig Dis Sci.* 2017; 62:2821-7.

57. Bennett WM, DeMattos A, Meyer MM et al. Chronic cyclosporine nephropathy: the Achilles' heel of immunosuppressive therapy. *Kidney Int.* 1996; 50:1089-100.

58. Janus N, Launay-Vacher V, Sebbag L et al. Renal insufficiency, mortality, and drug management in heart transplant. Results of the CARIN study. *Transplant Int.* 2014; 27:931-8.

59. Young EW, Ellis CN, Messana JM et al. A prospective study of renal structure and function in psoriasis patients treated with cyclosporin. *Kidney Int.* 1994; 46:1216-22.

60. Burke JF, Pirsch JD, Ramos EL et al. Long-term efficacy and safety of cyclosporine in renal-transplant recipients. *N Engl J Med.* 1994;331:358-63.

61. Gaston RS, Cecka JM, Kasiske BL et al. Evidence for antibody-mediated injury as a major determinant of late kidney allograft failure. *Transplantation.* 2010; 90:68-74.

62. El-Zoghby ZM, Stegall MD, Lager DJ et al. Identifying specific causes of kidney allograft loss. *Am J Transplantation.* 2009; 9:527-35.

63. Deen PM, Marr N, Kamsteeg EJ et al. Nephrogenic diabetes insipidus. *Curr Opin Nephrol Hypertens.* 2000; 9:591-5.

64. Paul R, Minay J, Cardwell C et al. Meta-analysis of the effects of lithium usage on serum creatinine levels. *J Psychopharmacol.* 2010; 24:1425-31.

65. McKnight RF, Adida M, Budge K et al. Lithium toxicity profile: a systematic review and meta-analysis. *Lancet.* 2012; 379:721-8.

66. Clos S, Rauchhaus P, Severn A et al. Long-term effect of lithium maintenance therapy on estimated glomerular filtration rate in patients with affective disorders: a population-based cohort study. *Lancet Psychiatry.* 2015; 2:1075-83.

67. Boton R, Gaviria M, Batlle DC. Prevalence, pathogenesis, and treatment of renal dysfunction associated with chronic lithium therapy. *Am J Kidney Dis.* 1987; 10:329-45.

68. Gitlin M. Lithium side effects and toxicity: prevalence and management strategies. *Int J Bipolar Disord.* 2016; 4:27.

69. Henrich WL, Agodoa LE, Barrett B et al. Analgesics and the kidney: summary and recommendations to the Scientific Advisory Board of the National Kidney Foundation from an Ad Hoc Committee of the National Kidney Foundation. *Am J Kidney Dis.* 1996; 27:162-5.

70. De Broe ME, Elseviers MM, Bengtsson U et al. Analgesic nephropathy. *Nephrol Dial Transplant.* 1996; 11:2407-8.

71. Dubach UC, Rosner B, Sturmer T. An epidemiologic study of abuse of analgesic drugs: effects of phenacetin and salicylate on mortality and cardiovascular morbidity (1968-1987). *N Engl J Med.* 1991; 324:155-60.

72. Dubach UC, Rosner B, Pfister E. Epidemiologic study of abuse of analgesics containing phenacetin: renal morbidity and mortality (1968–1979). *N Engl J Med.* 1983; 308:357-62.

73. Buckalew VM. Habitual use of acetaminophen as a risk factor for chronic renal failure: a comparison with phenacetin. *Am J Kidney Dis.* 1996; 28(1 suppl 1):S7-13.

74. Curhan GC, Knight EL, Rosner B et al. Lifetime nonnarcotic analgesic use and decline in renal function in women. *Arch Intern Med.* 2004; 164;1519-24.

75. Perneger TV, Whelton PK, Klag MJ. Risk of kidney failure associated with the use of acetaminophen, aspirin, and nonsteroidal anti-inflammatory drugs. *N Engl J Med.* 1994; 331:1675-9.

76. Nderitu P, Doos L, Strauss VY et al. Analgesia dose prescribing and estimated glomerular filtration rate decline: a general practice database linkage cohort study. *BMJ Open.* 2014 Aug 19; 4:e005581.

77. Mihatsch MJ, Khaniari B, Brunner FP. Obituary to analgesic nephropathy – an autopsy study. *Nephrol Dial Transplant.* 2006; 21:3139-45.

78. Gokmen MR, Cosyns JP, Arlt VM et al. The epidemiology, diagnosis, and management of aristolochic acid nephropathy: a narrative review. *Ann Intern Med.* 2013; 158:469-77.

79. Zhang J, Zhang L, Wang W et al. Association between aristolochic acid and CKD: a cross-sectional survey in China. *Am J Kidney Dis.* 2013; 61:918-22.

80. Yang HY, Chen PC, Wang JD. Chinese herbs containing aristolochic acid associated with renal failure and urothelial carcinoma: a review from epidemiologic observations to causal inference. *Biomed Res Int.* 2014; 2014:569325.

81. US Food and Drug Administration. Aristolochic acid: FDA warns consumers to discontinue use of botanical products that contain aristolochic acid. http://www.fda.gov/Food/RecallsOutbreaksEmergencies/SafetyAlertsAdvisories/ucm096388.htm (accessed 2017 Dec 18).

82. US Food and Drug Administration. Letter to industry associations regarding safety concerns related to the use of botanical products containing aristolochic acid. http://www.fda.gov/Food/RecallsOutbreaksEmergencies/SafetyAlertsAdvisories/ucm096374.htm (accessed 2017 Dec 18).

83. Fogo AB, Lusco MA, Andeen NK et al. *AJKD* atlas of renal pathology: lithium nephrotoxicity. *Am J Kidney Dis.* 2017; 69:e1-2.

84. Campistol JM, Grinyo JM. Exploring treatment options in renal transplantation: the problems of chronic allograft dysfunction and drug-related nephrotoxicity. *Transplantation.* 2001; 71:SS45-51.

85. Markowitz GS, Radhakrishnan J, Kambham N et al. Lithium nephrotoxicity: a progressive combined glomerular and tubulointerstitial nephropathy. *J Am Soc Nephrol.* 2000; 11:1439-48.

86. Karaosmanoglu AD, Butros SR, Arellano R. Imaging findings of renal toxicity in patients on chronic lithium therapy. *Diagn Interv Radiol.* 2013; 19:299-303.

87. Neau-Cransac M, Morel D, Bernard PH et al. Renal failure after liver transplantation: outcome after calcineurin inhibitor withdrawal. *Clin Transplant.* 2002; 16:368-73.

88. Mihatsch MJ, Antonovych T, Bohman SO et al. Cyclosporin A nephropathy: standardization of the evaluation of kidney biopsies. *Clin Nephrol.* 1994; 41:23-32.

89. Nankivell BJ, P'Ng CH, O'Connell PJ et al. Calcineurin inhibitor nephrotoxicity through the lens of longitudinal hisology: comparison of cyclosporine and tacrolimus. *Transplantation.* 2016; 100:1723-31.

90. Camilleri B, Bridson JM, Halawa A. Calcineurin inhibitor-sparing strategies in renal transplantation. Where are we? A comprehensive review of the current literature. *Exp Clin Transplant.* 2016; 14:471-83.

91. Alsady M, Baumgarten R, Deen PMT et al. Lithium in the kidney: friend and foe? *J Am Soc Nephrol.* 2016; 27:1587-95.

92. Reginster F, Jadoul M, van Ypersele de Strihou C. Chinese herbs nephropathy presentation, natural history and fate after transplantation. *Nephrol Dial Transplant.* 1997; 12:81-6.

93. Stefanović V, Polenaković M. Fifty years of research in Balkan endemic nephropathy: where are we now? *Nephron Clin Pract.* 2009; 112:c51-6.

94. Cosyns JP, Jadoul M, Squifflet JP et al. Urothelial lesions in Chinese-herb nephropathy. *Am J Kidney Dis.* 1999; 33:1011-7.
95. Gonzalez-Vilchez F, Vazquez de Prada JA. Chronic renal insufficiency in heart transplant recipients: risk factors and management options. *Drugs.* 2014; 74:1481-94.
96. Robinson PD, Shroff RC, Spencer H. Renal complications following lung and heart-lung transplantation. *Pediatr Nephrol.* 2013; 28:375-86.
97. Ojo AO, Held PJ, Port FK et al. Chronic renal failure after transplantation of a nonrenal organ. *N Engl J Med.* 2003; 349:931-40.
98. Pawarode A, Fine DM, Thuluvath PJ. Independent risk factors and natural history of renal dysfunction in liver transplant recipients. *Liver Transplant.* 2003; 9:741-7.
99. Webster AC, Woodroffe RC, Taylor RS et al. Tacrolimus versus ciclosporin as primary immunosuppression for kidney transplant recipients: meta-analysis and meta-regression of randomised trial data. *BMJ.* 2005; 331:810.
100. Issa N, Kukla A, Ibrahim HN. Calcineurin inhibitor nephrotoxicity: a review and perspective of the evidence. *Am J Nephrol.* 2013; 37:602-12.
101. Bocchetta A, Ardau R, Carta P et al. Duration of lithium treatment is a risk factor for reduced glomerular function: a cross-sectional study. *BMC Medicine.* 2013; 11:33.
102. Oliveira JL, Silva Junior GB, Abreu KL et al. Lithium nephrotoxicity. *Rev Assoc Med Bras.* 2010; 56:600-6.
103. Delzell E, Shapiro S. A review of epidemiological studies of nonnarcotic analgesics and chronic renal disease. *Medicine (Baltimore).* 1998; 77:102-21.
104. Zhang W. A benefit-risk assessment of caffeine as an analgesic adjuvant. *Drug Saf.* 2001; 24:1127-42.
105. Tredget J, Kirov A, Kirov G. Effects of chronic lithium treatment on renal function. *J Affect Disord.* 2010; 126:436-40.
106. Flechner SM, Goldfarb D, Modlin C et al. Kidney transplantation without calcineurin inhibitor drugs: a prospective, randomized trial of sirolimus versus cyclosporine. *Transplantation.* 2002; 74:1070-6.
107. Srinivas TR, Schold JD, Guerra G et al. Mycophenolate mofetil/sirolimus compared to other common immunosuppressive regimens in kidney transplantation. *Am J Transplant.* 2007; 7:586-94.
108. Bia M, Adey DB, Bloom RD et al. KDOQI US commentary on the 2009 KDIGO clinical practice guideline for the care of kidney transplant recipients. *Am J Kidney Dis.* 2010; 56:189-218.
109. Jefferson JW. A clinician's guide to monitoring kidney function in lithium-treated patients. *J Clin Psychiatry.* 2010; 71:1153-7.
110. Gault MH, Barrett BJ. Analgesic nephropathy. *Am J Kidney Dis.* 1998; 32:351-60.
111. Debelle FD, Vanherweghem JL, Nortier JL. Aristolochic acid nephropathy: a worldwide problem. *Kidney Int.* 2008; 74:158-69.
112. Vaclavik L, Krynitsky AJ, Rader JI. Quantification of aristolochic acids I and II in herbal dietary supplements by ultra-high-performance liquid chromatography-multistage fragmentation mass spectrometry. *Food Addit Contam Part A Chem Anal Control Expo Risk Assess.* 2014; 31:784-91.
113. Flechner SM. Minimizing calcineurin inhibitor drugs in renal transplantation. *Transplant Proc.* 2003; 35(3 suppl):S118-121.
114. Ducloux D. Is cyclosporine withdrawal a therapeutic option in renal transplant recipients with chronic allograft dysfunction? *Minerva Urol Nefrol.* 2003; 55:81-9.
115. Alexander MP, Farag YMK, Mittal BV et al. Lithium toxicity: a double-edged sword. *Kidney Int.* 2008; 73:233-7.
116. Mackinnon B, Boulton-Jones M, McLaughlin K. Analgesic-associated nephropathy in the West of Scotland: a 12-year observational study. *Nephrol Dial Transplant.* 2003; 18:1800-5.
117. Krumme B, Endmeir R, Vanhaelen M et al. Reversible Fanconi syndrome after ingestion of a Chinese herbal 'remedy' containing aristolochic acid. *Nephrol Dial Transplant.* 2001; 16:400-2.
118. Vanherweghem JL. Nephropathy and herbal medicine. *Am J Kidney Dis.* 2000; 35:330-2.

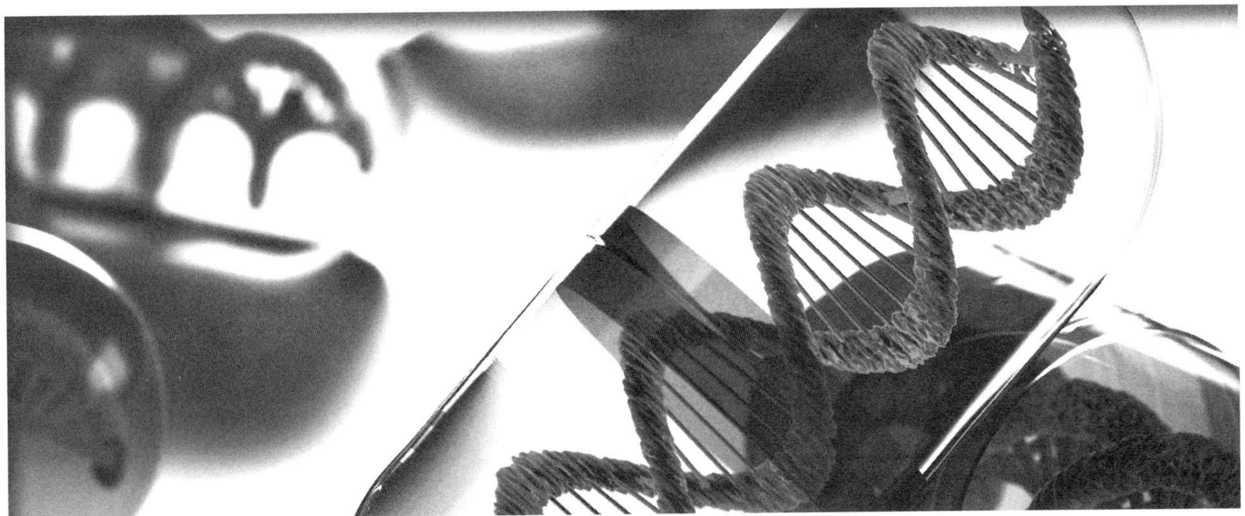

CHAPTER 43

Syndrome of Inappropriate Antidiuretic Hormone Secretion and Diabetes Insipidus

Mark A. Malesker and Daniel E. Hilleman

The syndrome of inappropriate antidiuretic hormone secretion (SIADH) and diabetes insipidus (DI) are conditions of altered water balance related to the abnormal secretion and/or action of antidiuretic hormone (ADH), also known as arginine vasopressin (AVP). ADH is produced in the posterior pituitary gland and acts to increase cellular permeability to water in the distal tubule and the collecting duct of the nephron, thus increasing water reabsorption. SIADH causes reabsorption of water in the nephron that is inappropriate for the patient's serum osmolality, and this results in hyponatremia. Conversely, DI causes hypernatremia due to the loss of large amounts of dilute urine. DI can be either central (reduced secretion of ADH) or nephrogenic (reduced sensitivity to ADH in the nephron) in origin.[1-6] There are many causes of SIADH and DI and both can be drug-induced.

SIADH

CAUSATIVE AGENTS

Drugs that have been reported to cause SIADH are listed in **Table 43-1**.[7-252] Antidepressants (in particular the selective serotonin reuptake inhibitors or SSRIs); the serotonin–norepinephrine reuptake inhibitors (SNRIs) venlafaxine and duloxetine; chemotherapy agents including vinca alkaloids, cisplatin, and cyclophosphamide; the anticonvulsants carbamazepine and oxcarbazepine; and the sulfonylureas are the agents most strongly associated with SIADH. Methylenedioxymetham-phetamine (MDMA or "ecstasy")-induced SIADH has been widely reported in the literature. Other medications that have been implicated in SIADH, but are less well studied, include the angiotensin–converting enzyme inhibitors and amiodarone.

Note: The authors wish to acknowledge the work of Edward F. Foote, who authored this chapter in a previous edition.

Table 43-1 Agents Implicated in Drug-Induced Syndrome of Inappropriate Antidiuretic Hormone Secretion

Drug	Incidence	Level of Evidence[a]
SSRIs[b]		
Citalopram[7-19]	NK	C
Escitalopram[20-23]	NK	C
Fluoxetine[24-40]	NK	C
Fluvoxamine[41,42]	NK	C
Levomilnacipran[43]	NK	C
Paroxetine[29,41,44-60]	12%	B
Sertraline[24,30,31,57,61-76]	0–17.5%	B
Vortioxetine[77]	NK	C
TRICYCLIC ANTIDEPRESSANTS		
Amitriptyline[78-83]	NK	C
Amoxipine[84-85]	<1%	B
Clomipramine[86-88]	NK	C
Desipramine[89,90]	NK	C
Doxepine[84]	NK	C
Imipramine[33,91-94]	NK	C
Nortriptyline[95]	NK	C
Protriptyline[96]	NK	C
Trimipramine[97]	NK	C
OTHER ANTIDEPRESSANTS		
Bupropion[94,98]	NK	C
Duloxetine[19,99-101]	NK	C
Desvenlafaxine[102]	NK	C
Isocarboxazid[103]	NK	C
Mirtazapine[18,90,104-106]	NK	C
Phenelzine[107]	NK	C
Tranylcypromine[108]	NK	C
Trazodone[109]	NK	C
Venlafaxine[14,51,90,100-116]	NK	C
Vilazodone[117]	NK	C
ANTIPSYCHOTIC AGENTS		
Aripiprazole[118,119]	NK	C
Chlorpromazine[120]	NK	C
Clozapine[121]	NK	C
Fluphenazine[122]	NK	C
Haloperidol[123,124]	NK	C
Olanzapine[125]	NK	C
Perphenazine[126]	NK	C
Pimozide[127,128]	NK	C
Quetiapine[129]	NK	C
Risperidone[130,131]	NK	C

Table 43-1 Agents Implicated in Drug-Induced Syndrome of Inappropriate Antidiuretic Hormone Secretion (continued)

Drug	Incidence	Level of Evidence[a]
Thioridazine[78,132,133]	NK	C
Trifluoperazie[82,134]	NK	C
Thiothixene[133]	NK	C
CANCER CHEMOTHERAPY AGENTS		
Aminoglutethimide[135]	NK	C
Bortezomib[136]	NK	C
Carboplatin[137]	NK	C
Chlorambucil[138]	NK	C
Cisplatin[139-143]	NK	C
Cyclophosphamide (intravenous)[144-147]	NK	C
Docetaxel[148]	NK	C
Etoposide[149]	NK	C
Ifosfamide[36,150,151]	NK	C
Levamisole[152]	NK	C
Melphalan[153]	NK	C
Thiotepa[154]	NK	C
Vinblastine[155-158]	NK	C
Vincristine[159-161]	NK	C
Vinorelbine[67,162]	NK	C
ANTIEPILEPTIC DRUGS		
Carbamazepine[163-170]	2.8–40%	B
Felbamate[171]	NK	C
Lamotrigine[172]	NK	C
Levetiracetam[173]	NK	C
Oxcarbazepine[163,170,174-179]	12.4–29.9%	B
Valproic acid[180-182]	NK	C
ORAL HYPOGLYCEMIC AGENTS		
Chlorpropamide[183-187]	2–7%	B
Glimepiride[188]	NK	C
Glipizide[189]	NK	C
Glyburide[190]	NK	C
Rosiglitazone[191]	NK	C
Tolbutamide[187]	NK	C
ANGIOTENSIN-CONVERTING ENZYME INHIBITORS		
Enalapril[192-194]	NK	C
Lisinopril[195]	NK	C
Ramipril[196]	NK	C
MISCELLANEOUS		
Alemtuzumab[197]	NK	C
Amiodarone[198-202]	NK	C
Amantadine[203-205]	NK	C

Table 43-1 Agents Implicated in Drug-Induced Syndrome of Inappropriate Antidiuretic Hormone Secretion (continued)

Drug	Incidence	Level of Evidence[a]
Atomoxetine[206]	NK	C
Azithromycin[207]	NK	C
Ciprofloxacin[208]	NK	C
Clonidine[209]	NK	C
Cyclobenzaprine[210]	<1%	B
Diclofenac[211]	NK	C
Dinutuximab[212]	NK	C
Esomeprazole[213]	NK	C
Fentanyl[214]	NK	C
Foscarnet[215]	<1%	B
Ganciclovir[216]	NK	C
Ibuprofen[217]	NK	C
Imatinib[218]	NK	C
L-dopamine[203,219]	NK	C
Lopinavir–ritonavir[220]	NK	C
Lorazepam[221]	NK	C
Memantine[222]	NK	C
Methadone[223]	NK	C
Methyldopa[224]	NK	C
MDMA (ecstasy)[225-235]	0–34.5%	B
Morphine[236]	NK	C
Moxifloxacin[237]	NK	C
Nicotine patch[238]	NK	C
Omeprazole[239]	NK	C
Oxycodone[240]	NK	C
Pentamidine[241]	NK	C
Pentostatin[242]	NK	C
Polyethylene glycol bowel preparation[243]	NK	C
Propafenone[244]	NK	C
Quinupristin–dalfopristin[245]	NK	C
Rifabutin[246]	NK	C
Ropinirole[247]	NK	C
Theophylline[248]	NK	C
Thiazide diuretics[249]	NK	C
Tolterodine[250]	NK	C
Trihexyphenidyl[204]	NK	C
Trimethoprim[251]	NK	C

NK = not known, MDMA = methylenedioxymethamphetamine, SSRI = selective serotonin reuptake inhibitor.

[a]Definitions for Levels of Evidence: Level A—evidence from one or more randomized, controlled clinical trials; Level B—evidence from nonrandomized clinical trials, prospective observational studies, cohort studies, retrospective studies, case-control studies, meta-analyses and/or postmarketing surveillance studies; and Level C—evidence from one or more published case reports or case series.

[b]The overall incidence of drug-induced SIADH with SSRIs was reported to be as high as 39% in one case-control study.[252]

EPIDEMIOLOGY

The exact incidence of drug-induced SIADH is not known but is likely very low. The incidence is difficult to determine because most studies are small and retrospective. In addition, most studies use hyponatremia rather than urine electrolyte concentrations and osmolality as criteria for diagnosing SIADH. Urine electrolyte concentrations and osmolality are much better indicators of SIADH, although they are rarely reported. Additionally, varying definitions of hyponatremia have been used in case reports and studies and during postmarketing surveillance. Some studies, for example, have used mild hyponatremia (e.g., serum sodium <135 mEq/L) as the sole marker for SIADH. This approach may result in a higher reported incidence of SIADH associated with a given drug, even though relatively small decreases in serum sodium concentrations likely have negligible clinical significance.

Most of the clinical studies of drug-induced SIADH involve antidepressants, in particular the SSRIs, and are primarily retrospective, case-control studies conducted in psychiatric inpatients.[56,114,252,254,256] In one such study, 39% of elderly psychiatric inpatients receiving an SSRI or venlafaxine (a norepinephrine–serotonin reuptake inhibitor) had hyponatremia (defined as serum sodium concentrations <135 mEq/L), as compared with an incidence of 10% in controls.[252] In a retrospective case study, the incidence of symptomatic SIADH due to SSRIs was 12.5%; however, this incidence may be overstated due to the retrospective nature of the trial and because patients were identified through hospital admissions and may not represent an otherwise "healthy" population.[255] No cases of hyponatremia were found in a retrospective review of 246 primarily male patients receiving sertraline, while a prospective trial noted an incidence of 17.2%.[114,256] A prospective study of paroxetine in 75 patients (age 63–90 years) in an ambulatory psychiatric clinic revealed an incidence of hyponatremia (defined as serum sodium concentration <135 mEq/L) of 12%.[56] Venlafaxine has been associated with an even higher risk of hyponatremia in psychiatric inpatients.[252]

Although many case reports have associated antipsychotics with SIADH, a retrospective study of 328 patients being treated for schizophrenia failed to find such a relationship. The authors suggest that schizophrenia itself (or perhaps other factors), and not the drugs used to treat the disease, is the cause of hyponatremia in this patient population.[257]

Carbamazepine is well known to cause SIADH. The reported incidence varies from 4.8% to 40%.[170,258] Oxcarbazepine is a 10-keto analog of carbamazepine that may be associated with a higher incidence of hyponatremia secondary to SIADH.[170,177,259] Hyponatremia (serum sodium concentrations <135 mEq/L) has been estimated to occur in as many as 25% to 29.9% of patients receiving oxcarbazepine.[170,259] In a cross-sectional study of 548 patients, the incidence of hyponatremia (with serum sodium concentrations <128 mEq/L) associated with carbamazepine and oxcarbazepine was 2.8% and 12.4%, respectively.[170] In one study, approximately 40% of patients experienced a reduction in serum sodium concentration when carbamazepine was replaced with oxcarbazepine, although most changes were mild and probably of no clinical significance.[177]

Chlorpropamide has frequently been associated with SIADH, but is no longer widely prescribed in the United States for diabetes management. Two percent of patients receiving chlorpropamide were found to experience hyponatremia with a serum sodium concentration of <130 mEq/L, while 7% experienced hyponatremia with concentrations in the range of 130–134 mEq/L.[183] Hyponatremia or SIADH associated with the newer-generation sulfonylureas has been recognized in postmarketing surveillance.[188-190]

A retrospective review of 1,436 MDMA (ecstasy) intoxication cases in California revealed a 34.5% incidence of hyponatremia (serum sodium concentration <130 mEq/L) among the 188 patients who had serum sodium concentrations reported.[260] This incidence is likely higher than what would be seen in the general population of MDMA users, as patients who presented with significant mental-status changes were probably more likely to have had a serum sodium concentration measured.

MECHANISMS

The precise mechanisms of drug-induced SIADH are not well understood. The disorder occurs as a result of either an increase in central ADH production (as occurs with cyclophosphamide, carbamazepine, vinca alkaloids, antidepressants, and antipsychotics) or an increased sensitivity to ADH at the level of the nephron (as occurs with chlorpropamide, carbamazepine, and cyclophosphamide).[5]

Animal models suggest that 5-hydroxytryptophan (HT or serotonin) stimulates ADH release.[261-263] Specifically, 5-HT_{2C}, 5-HTs_4, and 5-HT_7 receptors are implicated in the pathogenesis of drug-induced SIADH.[261] MDMA is known to have serotoninergic activity, and the likely mechanism for MDMA-induced SIADH, therefore, is increased ADH release.[226] A small prospective study of eight healthy volunteers showed that even small doses of MDMA could cause increased secretion of ADH, most likely due to central serotoninergic stimulation.[233] This effect may be attributed to both the parent compound and its metabolites.[264]

A study in patients with epilepsy and healthy volunteers assessed water disposition before and after oxcarbazepine administration. Oxcarbazepine exposure resulted in reductions in serum sodium concentrations and osmolality after water loading in both groups. There was no difference in serum ADH concentrations before or after oxcarbazepine exposure, suggesting that the hyponatremia might be due to increased sensitivity to ADH or even a direct antidiuretic effect rather than inappropriate secretion of ADH.[265] However, because the variation in ADH serum concentrations that may normally occur within a given range of serum osmolality is not known and serum ADH concentrations are not a routine part of the diagnostic workup for SIADH, this study cannot be considered conclusive. More studies will be needed before the exact mechanism(s) of oxcarbazepine-induced SIADH is understood.

CLINICAL PRESENTATION AND DIFFERENTIAL DIAGNOSIS

SIADH is associated with a decreased volume of inappropriately highly concentrated urine (e.g., urinary sodium >40 mEq/L and urinary osmolality >100 mOsm/kg water). If fluid intake is not significantly reduced, the increased water reabsorption in the nephron leads to a dilutional hyponatremia. Patients with SIADH present with normal volume status (euvolemia) because the excess water distributes throughout the body's fluid compartments. Because sodium and its associated anions are the primary contributors to extracellular tonicity, hypotonicity ensues. Symptoms of hyponatremia are related to the degree of serum hypotonicity and the time frame over which hypotonicity occurs. Signs and symptoms of hyponatremia are listed in **Table 43-2**. The most important manifestations of hypotonicity involve the central nervous system, because serum hypotonicity causes water to move into cells, resulting in cerebral cellular swelling. Hyponatremia caused by SIADH is generally not acute, usually developing over >48 hours. As a result, patients may experience only mild symptoms or may be completely asymptomatic. If hyponatremia is acute and serum sodium concentrations are <120 mEq/L, patients can present with symptoms such as headache, nausea, vomiting, muscle weakness, or mental-status changes. Serum sodium concentrations <110 mEq/L can be associated with more severe symptoms, including gait disturbances and potential falls, stupor, coma, seizures, and, rarely, death.[1-3,266]

Table 43-2 Signs and Symptoms Associated with Drug-Induced Syndrome of Inappropriate Antidiuretic Hormone Secretion (Hyponatremia)[1-3,a]

Moderate

- Anorexia
- Headache
- Malaise
- Mental status changes
- Muscle weakness and cramps
- Nausea
- Vomiting

Severe

- Coma
- Gait disturbances
- Seizure
- Stupor

[a]Signs and symptoms associated with hyponatremia due to SIADH are often mild or absent, because hyponatremia often occurs over a long period of time.

Analyses of reported cases of SSRI-associated SIADH reveal that hyponatremia occurs 3–120 days after the initiation of therapy, with a median time to onset of 13–15 days.[267,268] In a prospective study, the mean time from the start of therapy to the onset of hyponatremia was 9.3 days, with a range of 1–14 days.[56] Venlafaxine-induced SIADH may occur within 3–5 days following initiation of drug therapy.[114] Oxcarbazepine-induced SIADH usually develops within the first 3 months of therapy.[176] Hyponatremia has been detected within 3–10 days after exposure to the vinca alkaloids.[67,155,160]

Hyponatremia appears to occur much more quickly in association with MDMA than with other drugs known to cause SIADH. Patients generally present with symptoms within 12–24 hours after drug ingestion. The rapid onset of symptoms is probably partially due to MDMA users often concomitantly ingesting large amounts of nonalcoholic or alcoholic beverages, which compounds the inadequate renal response to water loading caused by the drug. In one published case series, 17 patients with MDMA-induced SIADH and hyponatremia presented with a constellation of symptoms including vomiting, behavioral changes, drowsiness, agitation, and (in 11 of 17 cases), seizures.[227] Another larger review of 553 documented cases of exposure to MDMA reported symptoms of tachycardia, agitation, and seizures.[260] Rhabdomyolysis has also been reported.[225] Hyponatremia has been documented in patients taking as little as "one-half tablet" of the drug (tablets of ecstasy usually contain 50–150 mg of MDMA).[227] Serum sodium concentrations tend to normalize within 24 hours after the initial presentation, although symptoms including drowsiness and disorientation may persist for several days.[227]

To diagnose SIADH the clinician must exclude other causes of hyponatremia. As described above, patients with SIADH present with a euvolemic, hypotonic hyponatremia. Serum concentrations of ADH are inappropriately high for the patient's serum osmolality. As a result, the urine is inappropriately concentrated, with urine osmolality >100 mOsm/kg water and sodium >40 mEq/L with a normal sodium intake. To make a definitive diagnosis of SIADH, the patient must also have normal renal, adrenal, and thyroid function, as abnormalities in these systems can also cause a euvolemic hyponatremia.[1,3,266]

Most cases of SIADH are not drug-related, and clinicians must be alert to other potential causes so that a drug is not incorrectly identified as the culprit.[3,5] Conditions to consider in the differential diagnosis of drug-induced SIADH are listed in **Table 43-3**.

When evaluating a patient with hyponatremia, the clinician must also exclude many common causes of non-SIADH hyponatremia, including the patient's use of thiazide diuretics; volume depletion caused by vomiting, diarrhea, or laxative abuse; and volume expansion that may occur in patients with cirrhosis, heart failure, and the nephritic syndrome.

Table 43-3 Conditions to Consider in the Differential Diagnosis of Drug-Induced Syndrome of Inappropriate Antidiuretic Hormone Secretion[3,6]

- Alcohol withdrawal
- Acquired immunodeficiency syndrome
- Endocrine disorders
  - Glucocorticoid deficiency
  - Hypothyroidism
- Hereditary SIADH
- Idiopathic SIADH
- Malignant tumors
  - Bladder, ureter
  - Duodenum
  - Ovary
  - Pancreas
  - Small-cell lung
- Neuropsychiatric disorders
  - Head trauma
  - Infections
  - Neoplasms
  - Psychosis
  - Stroke, vascular
- Pain
- Postoperative state
- Pulmonary disorders
  - Functional (asthma, acute respiratory failure, mechanical ventilation)
  - Infection
- Severe nausea

Although psychogenic polydipsia can also cause euvolemic hyponatremia and patients may present very much like those with SIADH, urinalysis in these patients reveals an appropriately dilute urine.

RISK FACTORS

Risk factors for drug-induced SIADH are presented in **Table 43-4**. Risk factors identified for hyponatremia due to the SSRIs include older age, concurrent diuretic use, high serum potassium concentration, female sex, lower baseline serum sodium concentration (<139 mEq/L), thiazide use, salt-restricted diet, and lower body-mass index.[15,56,114,252,267-270] At least one study failed to detect a relationship between plasma paroxetine concentrations and serum sodium concentrations.[56] Advanced age is a very important risk factor. One review of published case reports and individual reports to the U.S. Food and Drug Administration (FDA) identified 70 cases of hyponatremia associated with the SSRIs.[268] Eighty-four percent of these patients were elderly (>65 years), with a mean age of 70 years. Elevated serum potassium concentration was identified as a risk factor for SIADH in one study.[252] The majority of cases of SIADH associated with SSRIs occur in women, but it is unclear whether this is due simply to an increased exposure to the drug class as compared with men. The risk for SIADH appears to be highest in the first few weeks of therapy.[271,272] SSRIs appear to be associated with a higher risk of hyponatremia as compared with the older antidepressant agents. The risk of SIADH associated with the SSRIs has been reported to be 3.3–3.5 times greater than that with other antidepressants, although one of the trials included venlafaxine with the SSRIs in the analysis.[252,253] It has been suggested that SSRI-associated SIADH may be attributed to high serum drug concentrations.[25] However, there does not appear to be a relationship between the rate of drug metabolism or serum drug concentration and the severity of hyponatremia.[273]

Table 43-4 Risk Factors for Drug-Induced Syndrome of Inappropriate Antidiuretic Hormone Secretion

For patients taking selective serotonin-reuptake inhibitors

- Advanced age (≥65 yr)
- Baseline serum sodium concentration <139 mEq/L
- Concomitant diuretic administration
- Concomitant use of thiazide diuretics
- Elevated serum potassium concentration
- Female sex
- Lower body-mass index
- Salt-restricted diet

For patients taking carbamazepine or oxcarbazepine

- Advanced age
- Concomitant use of levetiracetam (oxcarbazepine)
- Elevated serum concentrations (carbamazepine)
- Higher doses (carbamazepine)

For patients taking vincristine, vinblastine

- Asian race

Hyponatremia due to carbamazepine may be related to higher doses and elevated serum concentrations, as doses >30 mg/kg/day have been associated with a higher incidence of hyponatremia.[164,259] Hyponatremia occurred in a patient previously stable on carbamazepine when clarithromycin was prescribed.[169] Presumably, the clarithromycin increased serum carbamazepine concentrations, causing hyponatremia, further supporting a concentration-related effect. Concomitant use of levetiracetam may increase the risk for hyponatremia with oxcarbazepine, while sex likely is not a risk factor.[170] It has been reported that hyponatremia due to oxcarbazepine occurs more commonly in patients older than 65 years of age (7.3%) as compared with children younger than 17 years of age (0.4%).[259] However, one noncontrolled trial indicated that 26.6% of children and adolescents experience hyponatremia (with serum sodium concentrations <135 mEq/L) in association with oxcarbazepine. Hyponatremia with serum sodium concentrations <125 mEq/L occurred in 2.6% of the patients.[163]

A review of the manufacturer's database of adverse drug reactions suggests that Asians may be at higher risk for SIADH induced by vincristine; of the 39 cases that included information on race, 35 patients were Asian. A similar relationship between Asian race and SIADH was found with vinblastine.[159]

Many of the initial case reports of hyponatremia associated with MDMA occurred in women, leading some to suggest that women may be at higher risk.[225] Although one series of case reports found an equal distribution between men and women, a more recent, larger study suggested that women are more likely to experience hyponatremia after MDMA ingestion.[227,260]

MORBIDITY AND MORTALITY

Many patients with drug-induced SIADH probably have mild hyponatremia that is asymptomatic and goes undetected. The published reports include more severe cases, in which patients experience symptoms including encephalopathy and seizures.[40,167,182] Most patients with drug-induced SIADH recover fully, but at least six deaths due to MDMA-induced hyponatremia have been reported.[227,229,274] In 545 cases of MDMA intoxication reported to a poison control center in California, 13 patients died.[260] Deaths due to SIADH associated with cyclophosphamide and carbamazepine have also been reported.[146,275]

PREVENTION

Although there are no universally accepted recommendations for prevention of drug-induced SIADH, some strategies that may help are listed in **Table 43-5**. It is always wise to use the lowest possible therapeutic dose of drugs with the potential to induce SIADH. Specific guidelines for monitoring serum sodium concentrations are not available. It has been suggested, however, that patients with risk factors for SSRI-induced hyponatremia (Table 43-4) should have serum sodium concentrations measured 1 and 2 weeks after the initiation of treatment.[56]

Table 43-5 Approaches to Help Prevent Drug-Induced Syndrome of Inappropriate Antidiuretic Hormone Secretion

- Use lowest possible dose of drugs with potential to induce SIADH
- Patients at risk should have serum sodium determinations 1 and 2 weeks after initiation of treatment

MANAGEMENT

Treatment strategies for drug-induced SIADH are presented in **Table 43-6**. If drug-induced SIADH is suspected, the offending agent should be discontinued whenever possible. Most patients with drug-induced SIADH have chronic, asymptomatic hyponatremia, and in this situation, water restriction (500–1,000 mL/day) should be initiated. This may allow the serum sodium concentration to normalize. Furosemide (20–40 mg orally or intravenously every 12–24 hours) can be used to increase free water excretion; simultaneous replacement of salt and volume should be performed as needed using 0.9% sodium chloride solution. Although central nervous system symptoms are fairly rare in drug-induced SIADH, when present, treatment should be initiated with hypertonic saline to raise the serum sodium concentration. The goal of therapy is to reverse neurologic symptoms and raise the serum sodium concentration by 1–2 mEq/L/hr. The use of hypertonic saline requires close monitoring and infusion should be discontinued when the serum sodium concentration increases by 10–12 mEq/L or to 130 mEq/L.[266,276] If hyponatremia correction is too rapid, osmotic demyelination may occur.[266]

Vasopressin-receptor antagonists offer a relatively new approach in the management of hyponatremia, including that which occurs as a result of SIADH. Antagonism of the arginine vasopressin receptor V_2 results in increased renal elimination of free water, with a resultant increase in the serum sodium concentration. Conivaptan is an FDA-approved intravenous

Table 43-6 Treatment Options for Drug-Induced Syndrome of Inappropriate Antidiuretic Hormone Secretion

- Demeclocycline (150–300 mg 3 times daily)
- Discontinue offending agent
- Hypertonic saline (symptomatic hyponatremia only)
- Isotonic saline
- Loop diuretic (furosemide 20–40 mg orally or intravenously every 12–24 hours)
- Vasopressin antagonists (conivaptan or tolvaptan)
- Water restriction (500–1,000 mL/day)

vasopressin-receptor antagonist for the treatment of euvolemic hyponatremia in hospitalized patients, including those with SIADH, hypothyroidism, adrenal disorders, and pulmonary disorders.[277] Tolvaptan is an orally administered vasopressin-receptor antagonist that received FDA approval for use in the treatment of euvolemic or hypervolemic (i.e., heart failure) hyponatremia. Although these medications are effective in SIADH, they have not been studied specifically for the treatment of drug-induced SIADH, and the role of these agents is likely limited. Most patients respond well to discontinuation of the offending agent; in addition, the high cost of the vasopressin antagonists will likely deter their use.

Expert panels have published recommendations for the treatment of hyponatremia.[278,279] A panel supported by Otsuka, the manufacturer of tolvaptan, supports the use of vasopressin antagonists in patients with SIADH in situations where fluid restriction has failed. A second expert panel (the European Practice Guideline)[280] does not recommend the use of the vasopressin antagonists in euvolemic patients with SIADH and noted the paucity of survival benefit with the vasopressin antagonists.[281]

In cases of SSRI-induced SIADH, it is probably not appropriate to substitute a different drug within the same class, as cross-sensitivity has been documented.[24,29,41] It is unknown whether dose reduction is beneficial. Venlafaxine should not be used in these patients, as this drug has been reported to cause hyponatremia in a patient with previously diagnosed SSRI-induced SIADH.[14,52] Recurrence of hyponatremia has also been reported with switches from citalopram to mirtazapine and from citalopram to duloxetine although a switch from citalopram to mirtazapine proved to be safe.[9,18,19] Bupropion-induced SIADH has been reported in a patient who previously experienced imipramine-induced SIADH.[94] However, bupropion was used safely in another patient with a history of SSRI-induced SIADH.[90] Hyponatremia did not recur when doxepin was administered to a patient with imipramine-induced SIADH.[92]

Although haloperidol has been reported to cause SIADH, it was administered safely to a patient who had previously experienced risperidone-induced SIADH.[123,124,130] Clozapine has been reported to cause hyponatremia, although SIADH was not definitively diagnosed.[121] Of note, clozapine has been used effectively to manage hyponatremia associated with psychogenic polydipsia, presumably by managing the underlying psychological disorder.[282,283]

A 12-year-old girl who developed symptomatic hyponatremia after exposure to oxcarbazepine did not experience recurrence of hyponatremia when carbamazepine was substituted.[284] Nevertheless, careful monitoring of serum sodium concentrations is warranted if carbamazepine is to be used in a patient who has had oxcarbazepine-induced SIADH.

Demeclocycline (oral: 600–1,200 mg/day) has been used for chronic SIADH, and both doxycycline (100 mg orally twice daily) and demeclocycline (300 mg orally twice daily for 3–5 days then 600 mg twice daily) have been used to treat hyponatremia associated with carbamazepine.[2,162,285] Demeclocycline has been found to be effective for the prevention of vinorelbine-induced SIADH.[67] Despite these successes, there is a paucity of clinical and economic evidence to support the use of demeclocycline for hyponatremia secondary to SIADH.[286]

INFORMATION FOR PATIENTS

Although SIADH is relatively rare, medications including psychotropics, antihypertensives, chemotherapy agents, and anticonvulsants can cause SIADH. Patients at risk for the development of SIADH, particularly the elderly, should be advised to avoid excessive intake of fluids when starting therapy with a drug known to cause this drug-induced disease. Individuals who use MDMA (ecstasy) tend to have more acute episodes of hyponatremia because they sometimes "water-load" to prevent hyperthermia associated with this drug. Unfortunately, water loading leads to more serious episodes of hyponatremia. Consequently, individuals who use MDMA should avoid ingesting excessive amounts of fluid.

DRUG-INDUCED DIABETES INSIPIDUS

CAUSATIVE AGENTS

Nephrogenic diabetes insipidus is manifested by diminished ability to concentrate the urine resulting from resistance to AVP. Except in the case of olanzapine, drug-induced diabetes insipidus (DI) is always nephrogenic.[2] Although lithium is the most important cause of drug-induced DI, other agents implicated are included in **Table 43-7**. In three patients in whom amphotericin B–induced DI developed, the disease did not recur when liposomal amphotericin therapy was substituted.[288,290] However, the first report of a DI related to liposomal amphotericin involved a patient who was not previously receiving conventional amphotericin therapy.[291] In the cases of mesalamine-induced and rifampin-induced DI, an acute interstitial nephritis was also present.[325] Although 10 reports of clozapine-induced nephrogenic DI were identified from the World Health Organization's database of adverse drug reactions, none have been reported in the literature.[294,330]

EPIDEMIOLOGY

By far, the most common culprit in drug-induced DI is lithium. The incidence of DI in patients receiving lithium has been estimated at 15–87%.[294] A retrospective study of 142 patients receiving long-term lithium therapy found an incidence of DI of 12%.[310] Limited case reports of DI caused by drugs other than lithium don't permit estimates of incidence.

MECHANISMS

Drug-induced nephrogenic DI is caused by inhibition of the opening of aquaporins (water-transport channels) in nephrons, with resultant polyuria. The exact mechanism is complex and not completely understood. In rat models, lithium administration has been associated with a reduced expression of the aquaporin-2 receptor. The specific action of lithium on the aquaporins may be related to antagonism of adenylate cyclase and cyclic adenosine monophosphate.[338] Central DI is caused by impaired production of AVP and may be acquired (head trauma) or congenital (hereditary).

Table 43-7 Agents Implicated in Drug-Induced Diabetes Insipidus

Drug	Incidence	Level of Evidence[a]
Amiodarone[287]	NK	C
Amphotericin B[288-290]	NK	C
Amphotericin (liposomal)[291,292]	NK	C
Cidofovir[293]	NK	C
Clozapine[294]	NK	C
Colchicine[295]	NK	C
Cyclophosphamide[296]	NK	C
Demeclocyline[297]	NK	C
Didanosine[298]	NK	C
Efavirenz/emtricitabine/tenofovir[299]	NK	C
Emtricitabine/rilpivirine/tenofovir[300]	NK	C
Emtricitabine/tenofovir[301]	NK	C
Foscarnet[302-304]	NK	C
Fosphenytoin[305,306]	0.1–1%	B
Ifosfamide[307]	NK	C
Lithium[294,308-324]	12–87%	B
Mesalamine[325]	NK	C
Ofloxacin[326]	NK	C
Octreotide[327]	NK	C
Olanzapine[328,b]	NK	C
Phenytoin[329]	NK	C
Rifampin[330]	NK	C
Riluzole[331]	<0.1%	B
Streptomycin[332]	NK	C
Temozolomide[333]	NK	C
Tenofovir[334,335]	NK	C
Triamterene/hydrochlorothiazide[336]	NK	C
Voriconazole[337]	<2%	B

[a]Definitions for Levels of Evidence: Level A—evidence from one or more randomized, controlled clinical trials; Level B—evidence from nonrandomized clinical trials, prospective observational studies, cohort studies, retrospective studies, case-control studies, meta-analyses and/or postmarketing surveillance studies; and Level C—evidence from one or more published case reports or case series.
[b]Presents as central diabetes insipidus.

CLINICAL PRESENTATION AND DIFFERENTIAL DIAGNOSIS

Both central and nephrogenic DI are characterized by the production of inappropriately large amounts of dilute urine (urinary osmolality <250 mOsm/kg water). Polyuria results in increased thirst (polydipsia). If there is not appropriate access to or administration of free water, hypernatremia and dehydration occur within hours. Symptoms of hypernatremia are related to cellular dehydration because of the movement of water out of cells and, like those of hyponatremia, are primarily neurologic and include altered mental status, weakness, lethargy, and occasionally coma or seizures (**Table 43-8**). Severe acute hypernatremia can result in death.[1-3] Although generally reversible, some permanent urine-concentrating defects can occur after prolonged exposure to lithium.[339] DI can occur at any time after lithium initiation but generally occurs after long-term exposure (>15 years).

As with SIADH, DI is diagnosed by excluding other causes of disordered sodium homeostasis. If adequate fluid intake is not maintained, patients with central or nephrogenic DI present with a euvolemic, hypertonic hypernatremia. The urine is inappropriately dilute (urine osmolality <250 mOsm/kg water) given the hypertonicity of the plasma. The diagnosis of DI can be made by measuring the urine-concentrating ability of the kidney during a water-deprivation test.[294] After 3–6 hours of water deprivation, patients with DI continue to produce large amounts of dilute urine (urine osmolality <400 mOsm/kg water). During this test, central and nephrogenic DI can generally be differentiated by patients' response to desmopressin (1-deamino-8-D-arginine vasopressin). In patients with nephrogenic DI, desmopressin administration (5 units of aqueous vasopressin subcutaneously or 10 mcg of intranasal desmopressin) does not result in the production of a concentrated urine, in contrast to patients with central DI. Hypernatremia due to DI must be distinguished from other causes, such as insensible water loss and gastrointestinal and renal losses. Patients with insensible water loss or gastrointestinal or renal losses generally are hypovolemic. In addition, these patients usually have maximally concentrated urine, owing to an appropriate action of ADH in the nephron. Conditions to consider in the differential diagnosis of drug-induced DI are listed in **Table 43-9**.

Table 43-8 Signs and Symptoms Associated with Drug-Induced Diabetes Insipidus (Hypernatremia)[1-3]

- Altered mental status
- Coma
- Fever
- Focal neurologic deficits
- Nausea
- Neuromuscular irritability
- Seizures
- Thirst
- Vomiting
- Weakness

RISK FACTORS

Proposed risk factors for lithium-induced nephrogenic DI are presented in **Table 43-10** and include chronic kidney disease (estimated creatinine

Table 43-9 Conditions to Consider in the Differential Diagnosis of Diabetes Insipidus

Central diabetes insipidus

- Head trauma
- Hypoxic or ischemic encephalopathy
- Idiopathic diabetes insipidus
- Neoplasm
- Neurosurgery
- Miscellaneous (histiocytosis X, sarcoidosis, anorexia nervosa, cerebral aneurysm, encephalitis, meningitis)

Nephrogenic diabetes insipidus

- Amyloidosis
- Congenital diabetes insipidus
- Hypercalcemia
- Hypokalemia
- Osmotic diuresis (glucose, mannitol)
- Pregnancy
- Renal failure
- Sickle-cell anemia
- Sjögren syndrome

Table 43-10 Risk Factors for Lithium-Induced Diabetes Insipidus

- Chronic kidney disease (estimated creatinine clearance <60 mL/min)
- Higher trough serum lithium concentrations
- Long treatment durations (>15 yr)
- Multiple daily doses (vs. a once-daily regimen)

clearance <60 mL/min), multiple daily doses (versus a once-daily regimen), long treatment durations (>15 years), and higher trough serum lithium concentrations.[294,340-342] It should be noted, however, that many of the studies used to define these risk factors were relatively small and some produced contradictory information.

MORBIDITY AND MORTALITY

Impaired urinary concentrating ability can occur in up to 20% of patients receiving chronic lithium therapy. Drug-induced SI is often reversible. Although the impact of drug-induced DI on health and quality of life can be significant, there have been only three case reports of death due to lithium-induced nephrogenic DI.[229,294]

PREVENTION

Some general strategies to reduce the likelihood of lithium-induced DI are listed in **Table 43-11**. Use of the lowest possible dose is critical to reducing the risk of lithium-induced DI. Trough serum lithium concentrations should be 0.6–1.0 mEq/L, and serum concentrations >1 mEq/L should definitely be avoided.[294] Administration of lithium as a once-daily regimen, administration of lower total daily doses, or both can reduce the risk of lithium-induced DI.[341]

MANAGEMENT

Strategies for the treatment of drug-induced nephrogenic DI are outlined in **Table 43-12**. The offending agent should be discontinued if possible. The polyuria associated with lithium usually resolves within a few weeks after discontinuation, although nonreversible DI is a possibility.[294,311] If patients have access to water and are neurologically competent, hypernatremia will not occur, as patients will drink to quench thirst. Mild cases of nephrogenic DI can be managed with sufficient adequate water intake. Low-sodium diet may reduce water excretion. In some cases, a reduction of the lithium dose may control the polyuria; however, discontinuation of lithium and initiation of an alternative therapy may be necessary.[294] The potassium-sparing diuretic amiloride, at doses of 10–20 mg daily, has been shown to reduce urinary output in patients with lithium-induced DI.[308,317] Amiloride may be preferable to hydrochlorothiazide because of its potassium-sparing effect and reduced propensity to cause volume depletion (which can induce or exacerbate lithium toxicity).[294] In one case of foscarnet-induced DI, treatment with amiloride was not successful in reducing polyuria.[303] Lithium-induced DI has been managed with indomethacin (50 mg every 8 hours).[311,313,315,316] It should be noted, however, that indomethacin can impair kidney function.[313]

Table 43-11 Approaches to Help Prevent Lithium-Induced Diabetes Insipidus

- Administer once daily
- Trough serum concentrations should be 0.4–0.6 mEq/L Avoid serum concentrations >1 mEq/L
- Use lowest possible dose

Table 43-12 Treatment Options for Drug-Induced Diabetes Insipidus

- Amiloride (10–20 mg daily)
- Discontinue offending agent
- Hydrochlorothiazide (25 mg once or twice daily)
- Indomethacin (50 mg every 8 hours)
- Water administration (allow free access)

INFORMATION FOR PATIENTS

Patients receiving therapy with lithium and their caregivers should be informed regarding the need to monitor for increased urinary output and excessive thirst. Patients should be instructed to report excessive urination and urine volumes to their healthcare provider.

REFERENCES

1. Mount DB. Fluid and electrolyte disturbances. In: Kasper D, Fauci A, Hauser S et al., *Harrison's principles of internal medicine.* 19th ed. New York, NY: McGraw-Hill; 2014. http://accessmedicine.mhmedical.com/content.aspx?bookid=1130§ionid=79726591 (accessed 2017 May 19).
2. Robertson GL. Disorders of the neurohypophysis. In: Kasper D, Fauci A, Hauser S et al., eds. *Harrison's principles of internal medicine.* 19th ed. New York, NY: McGraw-Hill; 2014. http://accessmedicine.mhmedical.com/content.aspx?bookid=1130§ionid=79751712 (accessed 2017 May 19).
3. Sterns RH. Renal function and disorders of water and sodium balance. In: Dale DC, Federman DD, eds. *Scientific American medicine.* New York, NY: WebMD Inc; 2003:1874-90.
4. Berl T, Schrier RW. Disorders of water homeostasis. In: Schrier RW, ed. *Renal and electrolyte disorders.* 7th ed. Philadelphia, PA: Wolters Kluwer/Lippincott Williams and Wilkins; 2010:1-44.
5. Rose BD. Hypoosmolal states—hyponatremia. In: Rose BD, Post TW, eds. *Clinical physiology of acid-base and electrolyte disorders.* 5th ed. New York, NY: McGraw-Hill Companies, Inc; 2001:696-744.
6. Adrogue HJ, Madias NE. Hyponatremia. *N Engl J Med.* 2000; 342:1581-9.
7. Fisher A, Davis M, Croft-Baker J et al. Citalopram induced severe hyponatraemia with coma and seizure: case report with literature and spontaneous reports review. *Adverse Drug React Toxicol Rev.* 2002; 21:179-87.
8. Hull M, Kottlors M, Braune S. Prolonged coma caused by low sodium and hypo-osmolarity during treatment with citalopram. *J Clin Psychopharmacol.* 2002; 22:337-8.
9. Barclay TS, Lee AJ. Citalopram-associated SIADH. *Ann Pharmacother.* 2002; 36:1558-63.
10. Bourgeois JA, Babine SE, Bahadur N. A case of SIADH and hyponatremia associated with citalopram. *Psychosomatics.* 2002; 43:241-2.
11. Odeh M, Beny A, Oliven A. Severe symptomatic hyponatremia during citalopram therapy. *Am J Med Sci.* 2001; 321:159-60.
12. Zullino D, Brauchli S, Horvath A et al. Inappropriate antidiuretic hormone secretion and rhabdomyolysis associated with citalopram. *Therapie.* 2000; 55:651-2.
13. Spigset O, Adielsson G. Combined serotonin syndrome and hyponatraemia caused by a citalopram-buspirone interaction. *Int Clin Psychopharmacol.* 1997; 12:61-3.
14. Romero S, Pintor L, Serra M et al. Syndrome of inappropriate secretion of antidiuretic hormone due to citalopram and venlafaxine. *Gen Hosp Psychiatry.* 2007; 29:81-4.
15. Bez Y, Aktolga S, Balci M et al. Citalopram-induced SIADH in a hypertensive patient on salt restricted diet. *J Psychopharmacol.* 2007; 21:665-7.
16. Miehle K, Paschke R, Koch CA. Citalopram therapy as a risk factor for symptomatic hyponatremia caused by the syndrome of inappropriate secretion of antidiuretic hormone (SIADH): a case report. *Pharmacopsychiatry.* 2005; 38:181-2.
17. Iraqi A, Baickle E. A case report of hyponatremia with citalopram use. *J Am Med Dir Assoc.* 2004; 5:64-5.
18. Bavbek N, Kargili A, Akcay A et al. Recurrent hyponatremia associated with citalopram and mirtazapine. *Am J Kidney Dis.* 2006; 48:e61-2.
19. Dirks AC, van Hyfte DM. Recurrent hyponatremia after substitution of citalopram with duloxetine. *J Clin Psychopharmacol.* 2007; 27:313.
20. Nahshoni E, Weizman A, Shefet D et al. A case of hyponatremia associated with escitalopram. *J Clin Psychiatry.* 2004; 65:1722.
21. Nirmalani A, Stock SL, Catalano G. Syndrome of inappropriate antidiuretic hormone associated with escitalopram therapy. *CNS Spectr.* 2006; 11:429-32.
22. Grover S, Biswas P, Bhateja G et al. Escitalopram-associated hyponatremia. *Psychiatry Clin Neurosci.* 2007; 61:132-3.
23. Covyeou JA, Jackson CW. Hyponatremia associated with escitalopram. *N Engl J Med.* 2007; 356:94-5.
24. Raphael K, Tokeshi J. Hyponatremia associated with sertraline and fluoxetine: a case report. *Hawaii Med J.* 2002; 61:46-7.
25. Girault C, Richard JC, Chevron V et al. Syndrome of inappropriate secretion of antidiuretic hormone in two elderly women with elevated serum fluoxetine. *J Toxicol Clin Toxicol.* 1997; 35:93-5.
26. ten Holt WL, van Iperen CE, Schrijver G et al. Severe hyponatremia during therapy with fluoxetine. *Arch Intern Med.* 1996; 156:681-2.
27. Schattner A, Skurnik Y. Fluoxetine-induced SIADH. *J Am Geriatr Soc.* 1996; 44:1413.
28. Burke D, Fanker S. Fluoxetine and the syndrome of inappropriate secretion of antidiuretic hormone (SIADH). *Aust N Z J Psychiatry.* 1996; 30:295-8.
29. Flint AJ, Crosby J, Genik JL. Recurrent hyponatremia associated with fluoxetine and paroxetine. *Am J Psychiatry.* 1996; 153:134.
30. Taylor IC, McConnell JG. Severe hyponatraemia associated with selective serotonin reuptake inhibitors. *Scott Med J.* 1995; 40:147-8.
31. Jackson C, Carson W, Markowitz J et al. SIADH associated with fluoxetine and sertraline therapy. *Am J Psychiatry.* 1995; 152:809-10.
32. Pillans PI, Coulter DM. Fluoxetine and hyponatraemia: a potential hazard in the elderly. *N Z Med J.* 1994; 107:85-6.
33. Blacksten JV, Birt JA. Syndrome of inappropriate secretion of antidiuretic hormone secondary to fluoxetine. *Ann Pharmacother.* 1993; 27:723-4.
34. Vishwanath BM, Navalgund AA, Cusano W et al. Fluoxetine as a cause of SIADH. *Am J Psychiatry.* 1991; 148:542-3.
35. Marik PE, van Heerden W, Steenkamp V. Fluoxetine induced syndrome of inappropriate antidiuretic hormone excretion. *S Afr Med J.* 1990; 78:760-1.
36. Staab JP, Yerkes SA, Cheney EM et al. Transient SIADH associated with fluoxetine. *Am J Psychiatry.* 1990; 147:1569-70.
37. Gommans JH, Edwards RA. Fluoxetine and hyponatraemia. *N Z Med J.* 1990; 103:106.
38. Cohen BJ, Mahelsky M, Adler L. More cases of SIADH with fluoxetine. *Am J Psychiatry.* 1990; 147:948-9.
39. Hwang AS, Magraw RM. Syndrome of inappropriate secretion of antidiuretic hormone due to fluoxetine. *Am J Psychiatry.* 1989; 146:399.
40. Twardowschy CA, Bertolucci CB, Gracia CM et al. Severe hyponatremia and the syndrome of inappropriate secretion of antidiuretic hormone (SIADH) associated with fluoxetine: case report. *Arq Neuropsiquiatr.* 2006; 64:142-5.
41. Arinzon ZH, Lehman YA, Fidelman ZG et al. Delayed recurrent SIADH associated with SSRIs. *Ann Pharmacother.* 2002; 36:1175-7.
42. Baliga RR, McHardy KC. Syndrome of inappropriate antidiuretic hormone secretion due to fluvoxamine therapy. *Br J Clin Pract.* 1993; 47:62-3.
43. Fetzima (levomilnacipran) extended-release capsules package insert. St. Louis, MO: Forest Laboratories, Inc; 2014 Jul.
44. Corrington KA, Gatlin CC, Fields KB. A case of SSRI- induced hyponatremia. *J Am Board Fam Pract.* 2002; 15:63-5.
45. Schouten WE, Sepers JM. Hyponatraemia associated with the use of a selective serotonin-reuptake inhibitor in an older patient. *Age Ageing.* 2001; 30:94.
46. Monmany J, Vazquez G, Rodriguez J et al. Syndrome of inappropriate secretion of antidiuretic hormone induced by paroxetine. *Arch Intern Med.* 1999; 159:2089-90.
47. Madhusoodanan S, Brenner R, Brafman I et al. Hyponatremia associated with paroxetine use. *South Med J.* 1999; 92:843.

48. Odeh M, Seligmann H, Oliven A. Severe life-threatening hyponatremia during paroxetine therapy. *J Clin Pharmacol.* 1999; 39:1290-1.
49. Leung VP, Chiu HF, Lam LC. Hyponatremia associated with paroxetine. *Pharmacopsychiatry.* 1998; 31:32-4.
50. Paul S, Sankaran SK. An unusually rapid onset of hyponatraemia following paroxetine. *Aust N Z J Med.* 1998; 28:840.
51. van der Klooster JM, Peters R, Ashruf RZ et al. Hyponatraemia and the syndrome of inappropriate antidiuretic hormone secretion with convulsions, coma and pulmonary oedema in a patient using paroxetine. *Neth J Med.* 1997; 51:237-9.
52. Meynaar IA, Peeters AJ, Mulder AH et al. Syndrome of inappropriate ADH secretion attributed to the serotonin re-uptake inhibitors, venlafaxine and paroxetine. *Neth J Med.* 1997; 50:243-5.
53. van Campen JP, Voets AJ. SIADH caused by paroxetine. *Ann Pharmacother.* 1996; 30:1499.
54. Ayonrinde OT, Reutens SG, Sanfilippo FM. Paroxetine induced SIADH. *Med J Aust.* 1995; 163:390.
55. Chua TP, Vong SK. Paroxetine and hyponatraemia. *Br J Clin Pract.* 1994; 48:49.
56. Fabian TJ, Amico JA, Kroboth PD et al. Paroxetine induced hyponatremia in older adults: a 12-week prospective study. *Arch Intern Med.* 2004; 164:327-32.
57. Malik AR, Wolf PK, Ravasia S. Recurrent paroxetine induced hyponatremia. *Can J Psychiatry.* 2004; 49:785.
58. Chuang YF, Chiu YL, Hwang TJ et al. Delirium and multiple electrolyte abnormalities associated with high dose paroxetine exposure. *Psychiatry Clin Neurosci.* 2006; 60:642-3.
59. Kubota T, Miyata A. Syndrome of inappropriate secretion of antidiuretic hormone associated with paroxetine. *J Anesth.* 2006; 20:126-8.
60. Wakita M, Matsuoka H, Hamada R et al. Hyponatremia upon resumption of paroxetine therapy. *Intern Med.* 2005; 44:240-2.
61. Lowenthal MN. Sertraline-induced hyponatremia in an older patient. *J Am Geriatr Soc.* 1999; 47:1274.
62. Belton K, Thomas SH. Drug-induced syndrome of inappropriate antidiuretic hormone secretion. *Postgrad Med J.* 1999; 75:509-10.
63. Levsky ME, Schwartz JB. Sertraline-induced hyponatremia in an older patient. *J Am Geriatr Soc.* 1998; 46:1582-3.
64. Bouman WP, Johnson H, Trescoli-Serrano C et al. Recurrent hyponatremia associated with sertraline and lofepramine. *Am J Psychiatry.* 1997; 154:580.
65. Catalano G, Kanfer SN, Catalano MC et al. The role of sertraline in a patient with recurrent hyponatremia. *Gen Hosp Psychiatry.* 1996; 18:278-83.
66. Bradley ME, Foote EF, Lee EN et al. Sertraline-associated syndrome of inappropriate antidiuretic hormone: case report and review of the literature. *Pharmacotherapy.* 1996; 16:680-3.
67. Garrett CA, Simpson TA Jr. Syndrome of inappropriate antidiuretic hormone associated with vinorelbine therapy. *Ann Pharmacother.* 1998; 32:1306-9.
68. Goldstein L, Barker M, Segall F et al. Seizure and transient SIADH associated with sertraline. *Am J Psychiatry.* 1996; 153:732.
69. Leung M, Remick R. Sertraline-associated hyponatremia. *Can J Psychiatry.* 1995; 40:497-8.
70. Bluff DD, Oji N. SIADH in a patient receiving sertraline. *Ann Intern Med.* 1995; 123:811.
71. Thornton SL, Resch DS. SIADH associated with sertraline therapy. *Am J Psychiatry.* 1995; 152:809.
72. Llorente MD, Gorelick M, Silverman MA. Sertraline as the cause of inappropriate antidiuretic hormone secretion. *J Clin Psychiatry.* 1994; 55:543-4.
73. Doshi D, Borison R. Association of transient SIADH with sertraline. *Am J Psychiatry.* 1994; 151:779-80.
74. Crews JR, Potts NL, Schreiber J et al. Hyponatremia in a patient treated with sertraline. *Am J Psychiatry.* 1993; 150:1564.
75. Agrawal NK, Rastogi A, Goyal R et al. Sertraline-induced hyponatremia in the elderly. *CJEM.* 2007; 9:415.
76. Papelbaum M, Aguiar MC. Sertraline-induced hyponatraemia. *Rev Bras Psiquiatr.* 2006; 28:256.
77. Brintellix (vortioxetine tablets) package insert. Deerfield, IL: Takeda Pharmaceuticals America, Inc; 2014 Jul.
78. Ananth J, Lin KM. SIADH: a serious side effect of psychotropic drugs. *Int J Psychiatry Med.* 1986; 16:401-7.
79. Henkin Y, Kaplan Z, Alkan M. Psychiatric presentation of hyponatremia associated with the use of amitriptyline: a report of two cases. *Isr J Med Sci.* 1989; 25:587-9.
80. Madhusoodanan S, Osnos R. Amitriptyline induced hyponatremia: a case report. *Mt Sinai J Med.* 1981; 48:431-3.
81. Solammadevi SV. Inappropriate antidiuresis during amitriptyline therapy. *South Med J.* 1981; 74:775-6.
82. Hamburger S, Langley H, Bowers G. The syndrome of inappropriate secretion of antidiuretic hormone associated with amitriptyline or trifluoperazine administration. *J Kans Med Soc.* 1980; 81:469-70.
83. Beckstrom D, Reding R, Cerletty J. Syndrome of inappropriate antidiuretic hormone secretion associated with amitriptyline administration. *JAMA.* 1979; 241:133.
84. Abbott R. Hyponatremia due to antidepressant medications. *Ann Emerg Med.* 1983; 12:708-10.
85. Amoxapine package insert. Corona, CA: Watson Laboratories, Inc; 2014 Jun.
86. Sommer BR. Syndrome of inappropriate antidiuretic hormone (SIADH) in an 80-year-old woman given clomipramine. *Am J Geriatr Psychiatry.* 1997; 5:268-9.
87. Spigset O, Hedenmalm K. Hyponatremia during treatment with clomipramine, perphenazine, or clozapine: study of therapeutic drug monitoring samples. *J Clin Psychopharmacol.* 1996; 16:412-4.
88. Pledger DR, Mathew H. Hyponatraemia and clomipramine therapy. *Br J Psychiatry.* 1989; 154:263-4.
89. Bretzel RG, Bollen CC, Maeser E et al. Nephroprotective effects of nitrendipine in hypertensive type I and type II diabetic patients. *Am J Kidney Dis.* 1993; 21:53-64.
90. Blass DM, Pearson VE. SIADH with multiple antidepressants in a geriatric patient. *J Clin Psychiatry.* 2000; 61:448-9.
91. Adlakha A, Manocha AP, Bechard DL. Imipramine induced syndrome of inappropriate antidiuretic hormone secretion. *South Med J.* 1991; 84:1507-9.
92. Mitsch RA, Lee AK. Syndrome of inappropriate antidiuretic hormone with imipramine. *Drug Intell Clin Pharm.* 1986; 20:787-9.
93. Parker WA. Imipramine-induced syndrome of inappropriate antidiuretic hormone secretion. *Drug Intell Clin Pharm.* 1984; 18:890-4.
94. Liskin B, Walsh BT, Roose SP et al. Imipramine-induced inappropriate ADH secretion. *J Clin Psychopharmacol.* 1984; 4:146-7.
95. Miller MG. Tricyclics as a possible cause of hyponatremia in psychiatric patients. *Am J Psychiatry.* 1989; 146:807.
96. Vivactil (protriptyline) package insert. East Hanover, NJ: Odyssey Pharmaceuticals, Inc; 2014 Jul.
97. Surmontil (trimipramine maleate) package insert. East Hanover, NJ: Odyssey Pharmaceuticals, Inc; 2014 Jul.
98. Bagley SC, Yaeger D. Hyponatremia associated with bupropion, a case verified by rechallenge. *J Clin Psychopharmacol.* 2005; 25:98-9.
99. Safdieh JE, Rudominer R. A case of hyponatremia induced by duloxetine. *J Clin Psychopharmacol.* 2006; 26:675-6.
100. Maramattom BV. Duloxetine-induced syndrome of inappropriate antidiuretic hormone secretion and seizures. *Neurology.* 2006; 66:773-4.
101. Kruger S, Lindstaedt M. Duloxetine and hyponatremia: a report of 5 cases. *J Clin Psychopharmacol.* 2007; 27:101-4.

102. Lee GTH, Leung JLM, Syndrome of inappropriate secretion of antidiuretic hormone due to desvenlafaxine. *General Hospital Psychiatry.* 2013; 35:574.e1-574.e3.

103. Marplan (isocarboxazid) package insert. Parsippany, NJ: Validus Pharmaceuticals; 2012 March.

104. Roxanas MG. Mirtazapine-induced hyponatraemia. *Med J Aust.* 2003; 179:453-4.

105. Jagsch C, Marksteiner J, Seiringer E et al. Successful mirtazapine treatment of an 81-year-old patient with syndrome of inappropriate antidiuretic hormone secretion. *Pharmacopsychiatry.* 2007; 40:129-31.

106. Ladino M, Guardiola VD, Paniagua M. Mirtazapine induced hyponatremia in an elderly hospice patient. *J Palliat Med.* 2006; 9:258-60.

107. Giese AA, Leibenleft E, Green S et al. Phenelzine-associated inappropriate ADH secretion. *J Clin Psychopharmacol.* 1989; 9:309-10.

108. Parnate (tranylcypromine) package insert. Research Triangle Park, NC: GlaxoSmithKline; 2012 Jun.

109. Vanpee D, Laloyaux P, Gillet JB. Seizure and hyponatraemia after overdose of trazadone. *Am J Emerg Med.* 1999; 17:430-1.

110. Izzedine H, Launay-Vacher V, Ciroldi M et al. Fanconi and inappropriate secretion of antidiuretic hormone syndromes secondary to venlafaxine therapy. *Nephron.* 2002; 92:944-6.

111. Boyd IW. Comment: hyponatremia with venlafaxine. *Ann Pharmacother.* 1998; 32:981-2.

112. Masood GR, Karki SD, Patterson WR. Hyponatremia with venlafaxine. *Ann Pharmacother.* 1998; 32:49-51.

113. Gupta AK, Saravay SM. Venlafaxine-induced hyponatremia. *J Clin Psychopharmacol.* 1997; 17:223-5.

114. Roxanas M, Hibbert E, Field M. Venlafaxine hyponatraemia: incidence, mechanism and management. *Aust N Z J Psychiatry.* 2007; 41:411-8.

115. Egger C, Muehlbacher M, Nickel M et al. A case of recurrent hyponatremia induced by venlafaxine. *J Clin Psychopharmacol.* 2006; 26:439.

116. Bourgeois JA. Reversible hyponatremia and venlafaxine. *Psychosomatics.* 2005; 46:495-6.

117. Viibryd (vilazodone) package insert. St. Louis, MO: Forest Pharmaceuticals, Inc; 2015 Mar.

118. Bachu K, Godkar D, Gasparyan A et al. Aripiprazole-induced syndrome of inappropriate antidiuretic hormone secretion (SIADH). *Am J Ther.* 2006; 13:370-2.

119. Behere RV, Venkatasubramanian G, Naveen MN et al. Aripiprazole-induced hyponatremia: a case report. *J Clin Psychiatry.* 2007; 68:640-1.

120. Tildesley HD, Toth E, Crockford PM. Syndrome of inappropriate secretion of antidiuretic hormone in association with chlorpromazine ingestion. *Can J Psychiatry.* 1983; 28:487-8.

121. Ogilvie AD, Croy MF. Clozapine and hyponatraemia. *Lancet.* 1992; 340:672.

122. Kosten TR, Camp W. Inappropriate secretion of antidiuretic hormone in a patient receiving piperazine phenothiazines. *Psychosomatics.* 1980; 21:351-5.

123. Husband C, Mai FM, Carruthers G. Syndrome of inappropriate secretion of anti-diuretic hormone in a patient treated with haloperidol. *Can J Psychiatry.* 1981; 26:196-7.

124. Peck V, Shenkman L. Haloperidol-induced syndrome of inappropriate secretion of antidiuretic hormone. *Clin Pharmacol Ther.* 1979; 26:442-4.

125. Dudeja S. Olanzapine induced hyponatraemia. *Ulster Med J.* 2010 May; 79:104–5.

126. Perphenazine package insert. Princeton, NJ: Sandoz Inc; 2010 Sept.

127. Leclercq P, Canivet JL, Damas P et al. A case of severe hyponatremia under pimozide (Orap) administration. [French]. *Rev Med Liege.* 1995; 50:151-2.

128. Koide H. Three cases of hyponatremia during administration of pimozide. [Japanese]. *No to Hattatsu.* 1991; 23:502-5.

129. Atalay A, Turhan N, Aki OE. A challenging case of syndrome of inappropriate secretion of antidiuretic hormone in an elderly patient secondary to quetiapine. *South Med J.* 2007; 100:832-3.

130. Collins A, Anderson J. SIADH induced by two atypical antipsychotics. *Int J Geriatr Psychiatry.* 2000; 15:282-3.

131. Whitten JR, Ruehter VL. Risperidone and hyponatremia: a case report. *Ann Clin Psychiatry.* 1997; 9:181-3.

132. Caron C, Shooner K, Martineau M et al. Water intoxication in a schizophrenic patient under treatment with thioridazine: study of the physiopathological mechanisms involved. [French]. *Union Med Can.* 1979; 108:1078-82.

133. Ajlouni K, Kern MW, Tures JF et al. Thiothixene-induced hyponatremia. *Arch Intern Med.* 1974; 134:1103-5.

134. Kennedy MJ, Shelley RK, Daly PA. Potentiation of small cell lung cancer-related SIADH by trifluoperazine. *Eur J Respir Dis.* 1987; 71:450-4.

135. Box M, Saltissi D, Fawcett D. Inappropriate secretion of antidiuretic hormone following aminoglutethimide therapy. *Br J Urol.* 1986; 58:724-5.

136. Brodmann S, Gyr KE, Cathomas R et al. Severe hyponatremia in a patient with mantle cell lymphoma treated with bortezomib: a case report and review of the literature. *Onkologie.* 2007; 30:651-4.

137. Yokoyama Y, Shigeto T, Futagami M et al. Syndrome of inappropriate secretion of anti-diuretic hormone following carboplatin-paclitaxel administration in a patient with recurrent ovarian cancer. *Eur J Gynaecol Oncol.* 2005; 26:531-2.

138. Wagner AM, Brunet S, Puig J et al. Chlorambucil-induced inappropriate antidiuresis in a man with chronic lymphocytic leukemia. *Ann Hematol.* 1999; 78:37-8.

139. Ishii K, Aoki Y, Sasaki M et al. Syndrome of inappropriate secretion of antidiuretic hormone induced by intraarterial cisplatin chemotherapy. *Gynecol Oncol.* 2002; 87:150-1.

140. Kagawa K, Fujitaka K, Isobe T et al. Syndrome of inappropriate secretion of ADH (SIADH) following cisplatin administration in a pulmonary adenocarcinoma patient with a malignant pleural effusion. *Intern Med.* 2001; 40:1020-3.

141. Boku N, Ohtsu A, Nagashima F et al. Retrospective study of hyponatremia in gastric cancer patients treated with a combination chemotherapy of 5-fluorouracil and cisplatin: a possible warning sign of severe hematological toxicities? *Jpn J Clin Oncol.* 2001; 31:382-7.

142. Otsuka F, Hayashi Y, Ogura T et al. Syndrome of inappropriate secretion of antidiuretic hormone following intra-thoracic cisplatin. *Intern Med.* 1996; 35:290-4.

143. Littlewood TJ, Smith AP. Syndrome of inappropriate antidiuretic hormone secretion due to treatment of lung cancer with cisplatin. *Thorax.* 1984; 39:636-7.

144. Spital A, Ristow S. Cyclophosphamide induced water intoxication in a woman with Sjogren's syndrome. *J Rheumatol.* 1997; 24:2473-5.

145. Bressler RB, Huston DP. Water intoxication following moderate-dose intravenous cyclophosphamide. *Arch Intern Med.* 1985; 145:548-9.

146. Harlow PJ, DeClerck YA, Shore NA et al. A fatal case of inappropriate ADH secretion induced by cyclophosphamide therapy. *Cancer.* 1979; 44:896-8.

147. Lazarevic V, Hagg E, Wahlin A. Hiccups and severe hyponatremia associated with high-dose cyclophosphamide in conditioning regimen for allogeneic stem cell transplantation. *Am J Hematol.* 2007; 82:88.

148. Langer-Nitsche C, Luck HJ, Heilmann M. Severe syndrome of inappropriate antidiuretic hormone secretion with docetaxel treatment in metastatic breast cancer. *Acta Oncologica.* 2000; 39:1001.

149. Kleta R, Wagner A, Jurgens H. Recurrence of SIADH after a high-dose regimen of thiotepa, carboplatin, and etoposide phosphate. *Med Pediatr Oncol.*1998; 31:129.

150. Kirch C, Gachot B, Germann N et al. Recurrent ifosfamide-induced hyponatraemia. *Eur J Cancer.* 1997; 33:2438-9.

151. Izquierdo R, Leinung M. Hyponatraemia secondary to administration of ifosfamide. *Eur J Cancer.* 1993; 29A:2072-3.

152. Tweedy CR, Silverberg DA, Scott L. Levamisole-induced syndrome of inappropriate antidiuretic hormone. *N Engl J Med.* 1992; 326:1164.

153. Greenbaum-Lefkoe B, Rosenstock JG, Belasco JB et al. Syndrome of inappropriate antidiuretic hormone secretion: a complication of high-dose intravenous melphalan. *Cancer.* 1985; 55:44-6.

154. Sica S, Cicconi S, Sora F et al. Inappropriate antidiuretic hormone secretion after high-dose thiotepa. *Bone Marrow Transplant.* 1999; 24:571-2.

155. Fraschini G, Recchia F, Holmes FA. Syndrome of inappropriate antidiuretic hormone secretion associated with hepatic arterial infusion of vinblastine in three patients with breast cancer. *Tumori.* 1987; 73:513-6.

156. Ravikumar TS, Grage TB. The syndrome of inappropriate ADH secretion secondary to vinblastine-bleomycin therapy. *J Surg Oncol.* 1983; 24:242-5.

157. Stahel RA, Oelz O. Syndrome of inappropriate ADH secretion secondary to vinblastine. *Cancer Chemother Pharmacol.* 1982; 8:253-4.

158. Antony A, Robinson WA, Roy C et al. Inappropriate antidiuretic hormone secretion after high dose vinblastine. *J Urol.* 1980; 123:783-4.

159. Hammond IW, Ferguson JA, Kwong K et al. Hyponatremia and syndrome of inappropriate antidiuretic hormone reported with the use of Vincristine: an over-representation of Asians? *Pharmacoepidemiol Drug Saf.* 2002; 11:229-34.

160. Escuro RS, Adelstein DJ, Carter SG. Syndrome of inappropriate secretion of antidiuretic hormone after infusional vincristine. *Cleve Clin J Med.* 1992; 59:643-4.

161. Tomiwa K, Mikawa H, Hazama F et al. Syndrome of inappropriate secretion of antidiuretic hormone caused by vincristine therapy: a case report of the neuropathology. *J Neurol.* 1983; 229:267-72.

162. Canzler U, Schmidt-Gohrich UK, Bergmann S et al. Syndrome of inappropriate antidiuretic hormone secretion (SIADH) induced by vinorelbine treatment of metastatic breast cancer. *Onkologie.* 2007; 30:455-6.

163. Holtmann M, Krause M, Opp J et al. Oxcarbazepine-induced hyponatremia and the regulation of serum sodium after replacing carbamazepine with oxcarbazepine in children. *Neuropediatrics.* 2002; 33:298-300.

164. Kelly BD, Hillery J. Hyponatremia during carbamazepine therapy in patients with intellectual disability. *J Intellect Disabil Res.* 2001; 45:2-6.

165. Boutros NN, Guerra BM, Votolato NA et al. Carbamazepine-induced hyponatremia resolved with doxycycline. *J Clin Psychiatry.* 1995; 56:377-8.

166. Huang SC, Tsai SJ. Hyponatremia and Stevens-Johnson syndrome in a patient receiving carbamazepine. *Gen Hosp Psychiatry.* 1995; 17:458-60.

167. Holtschmidt-Taschner B, Soyka M. Hyponatremia-induced seizure during carbamazepine treatment. *World J Biol Psychiatry.* 2007; 8:51-3.

168. Kuz GM, Manssourian A. Carbamazepine-induced hyponatremia: assessment of risk factors. *Ann Pharmacother.* 2005; 39:1943-6.

169. Kanbay M, Alkis M, Turgut F et al. Hyponatremia due to an additive effect of carbamazepine and clarithromycin. *South Med J.* 2007; 100:222.

170. Dong X, Leppik IE, White J et al. Hyponatremia from oxcarbazepine and carbamazepine. *Neurology.* 2005; 65:1976-8.

171. Felbatol (felbamate tablets and oral suspension) package insert. Somerset, NJ: Meda Pharmaceuticals, Inc; 2011 July.

172. Huseyin K, Barış E, Yakup E et al. Lamotrigine-induced SIADH in a child with central diabetes insipidus. *J Pediatr Neurosci.* 2011 Jan-Jun; 6:89-90.

173. Nasrallah K, Silver B. Hyponatremia associated with repeated use of levetiracetam. *Epilepsia.* 2005; 46:972-3.

174. Sand PG, Atzinger AK, Buwe A. SNRI and hyponatremia. *Int J Geriatr Psychiatry.* 2002; 17:491-2.

175. Cilli AS, Algun E. Oxcarbazepine-induced syndrome of inappropriate secretion of antidiuretic hormone. *J Clin Psychiatry.* 2002; 63:742.

176. Smith PE, The UK Oxcarbazepine Advisory Board. Clinical recommendations for oxcarbazepine. *Seizure.* 2001; 10:87-91.

177. Isojarvi JI, Huuskonen UE, Pakarinen AJ et al. The regulation of serum sodium after replacing carbamazepine with oxcarbazepine. *Epilepsia.* 2001; 42:741-5.

178. Oxcarbazepine: hyponatraemia and skin reactions. *Prescrire Int.* 2007; 16:18.

179. Paliwal V, Garg RK, Kar AM et al. Oxcarbazepine induced hyponatremic coma. *Neurol India.* 2006; 54:214-5.

180. Miyaoka T, Seno H, Itoga M et al. Contribution of sodium valproate to the syndrome of inappropriate secretion of antidiuretic hormone. *Int Clin Psychopharmacol.* 2001; 16:59-61.

181. Branten AJ, Wetzels JF, Weber AM et al. Hyponatremia due to sodium valproate. *Ann Neurol.* 1998; 43:265-7.

182. Siniscalchi A, Mancuso F, Scornaienghi D et al. Acute encephalopathy induced by oxcarbazepine and furosemide. *Ann Pharmacother.* 2004; 38:509-10.

183. Hirokawa CA, Gray DR. Chlorpropamide-induced hyponatremia in the veteran population. *Ann Pharmacother.* 1992; 26:1243-4.

184. Ravat HK, Joshi VR. Chlorpropamide induced syndrome of inappropriate secretion of antidiuretic hormone. *J Assoc Physicians India.* 1991; 39:645-6.

185. Tanay A, Firemann Z, Yust I et al. Chlorpropamide-induced syndrome of inappropriate antidiuretic hormone secretion. *J Am Geriatr Soc.* 1981; 29:334-6.

186. Fonseca VA, Deb M, Gokani SS et al. Chlorpropamide induced syndrome of inappropriate antidiuretic hormone secretion. *J Postgrad Med.* 1980; 26:127-30.

187. Moore TD, Bechtel TP. Hyponatremia secondary to tolbutamide and chlorothiazide. *Am J Hosp Pharm.* 1979; 36:1107-10.

188. Amaryl (glimepiride) package insert. Bridgewater, NJ: Sanofi-Aventis; 2013 Jan.

189. Glucotrol (glipizide) package insert. New York, NY; Pfizer Pharmaceuticals; 2011 Feb.

190. Diabeta (glyburide) package insert. Bridgewater, NJ: Sanofi-Aventis; 2009 Feb.

191. Berker D, Aydin Y, Arduc, A et al. Severe hyponatremia due to rosiglitazone use in an elderly woman with diabetes mellitus: a rare cause of syndrome of inappropriate antidiuretic hormone secretion. *Endocr Pract* 2008; 14:1017-9.

192. Izzedine H, Fardet L, Launay-Vacher V et al. Angiotensin-converting enzyme inhibitor-induced syndrome of inappropriate secretion of antidiuretic hormone: case report and review of the literature. *Clin Pharmacol Ther.* 2002; 71:503-7.

193. Gonzalez-Martinez H, Gaspard JJ, Espino DV. Hyponatremia due to enalapril in an elderly patient: a case report. *Arch Fam Med.* 1993; 2:791-3.

194. Castrillon JL, Mediavilla A, Mendez MA et al. Syndrome of inappropriate antidiuretic hormone secretion (SIADH) and enalapril. *J Intern Med.* 1993; 233:89-91.

195. Shaikh ZH, Taylor HC, Maroo PV et al. Syndrome of inappropriate antidiuretic hormone secretion associated with lisinopril. *Ann Pharmacother.* 2000; 34:176-9.

196. Tilly-Gentric A. Severe hyponatremia associated with ramipril therapy in an old woman. *J Am Geriatr Soc.* 1995; 43:1448-9.

197. Kunz JS, Bannerji R. Alemtuzumab-induced syndrome of inappropriate anti-diuretic hormone. *Leuk Lymphoma.* 2005; 46:635-7.

198. Patel GP, Kasiar JB. Syndrome of inappropriate antidiuretic hormone-induced hyponatremia associated with amiodarone. *Pharmacotherapy.* 2002; 22:649-51.
199. Ikegami H, Shiga T, Tsushima T et al. Syndrome of inappropriate antidiuretic hormone secretion (SIADH) induced by amiodarone: a report on two cases. *J Cardiovasc Pharmacol Ther.* 2002; 7:25-8.
200. Odeh M, Schiff E, Oliven A. Hyponatremia during therapy with amiodarone. *Arch Intern Med.* 1999; 159:2599-600.
201. Shavit E, Sherer Y. Hyponatremia induced by amiodarone therapy. *Isr Med Assoc J.* 2007; 9:564-5.
202. Aslam MK, Gnaim C, Kutnick J et al. Syndrome of inappropriate antidiuretic hormone secretion induced by amiodarone therapy. *Pacing Clin Electrophysiol.* 2004; 27:831-2.
203. Lammers GJ, Roos RA. Hyponatraemia due to amantadine hydrochloride and L-dopa/carbidopa. *Lancet.* 1993; 342:439.
204. van Laar T, Lammers GJ, Roos RA et al. Antiparkinsonian drugs causing inappropriate antidiuretic hormone secretion. *Mov Disord.* 1998; 13:176-8.
205. Alonso Navarro H, Sánz-Aiz A, Izquierdo L et al. Syndrome of inappropriate antidiuretic hormone secretion possibly associated with amantadine therapy in Parkinson disease. *Clin Neuropharmacol.* 2009 May-Jun; 32:167-8.
206. Singh T. Atomoxetine-induced hyponatremia. *Aust N Z J Psychiatry.* 2007; 41:458.
207. Cadle RM, Darouiche RO, Ashton CM. Symptomatic syndrome of inappropriate antidiuretic hormone secretion associated with azithromycin. *Ann Pharmacother.* 1997; 31:1308-10.
208. Babar SM. SIADH associated with ciprofloxacin. *Ann Pharmacother.* 2013 Oct; 47:1359-63.
209. Burrows AW, Gribbin B. Clonidine-induced dilutional hyponatraemia. *Postgrad Med J.* 1979; 55:42-3.
210. Amrix (cyclobenzaprine hydrochloride) capsule, extended release package insert. North Wales, PA: Teva Pharmaceuticals USA, Inc; 2013 Jun.
211. Cheung NT, Coley S, Sheeran T et al. Syndrome of inappropriate secretion of antidiuretic hormone induced by diclofenac. *BMJ.* 1993; 306:186.
212. Unituxin (dinutuximab) injection package insert. Silver Spring, MD: United Therapeutics Corp; 2015 Mar.
213. Mennecier D, Ceppa F, Gidenne S et al. Hyponatremia with consciousness disturbance associated with esomeprazole. *Ann Pharmacother.* 2005; 39:774-5.
214. Kokko H, Hall PD, Afrin LB. Fentanyl-associated syndrome of inappropriate antidiuretic hormone secretion. *Pharmacotherapy.* 2002; 22:1188-92.
215. Foscavir (foscarnet) package insert. Lake Forest, IL: Hospira, Inc; 2014 Nov.
216. Cytovene IV (ganciclovir) package insert. South San Francisco, CA: Genentech USA, Inc; 2010 Feb.
217. Rault RM. Case report: hyponatremia associated with nonsteroidal anti-inflammatory drugs. *Am J Med Sci.* 1993; 305:318-20.
218. Liapis K, Apostolidis J, Charitaki E et al. Syndrome of inappropriate secretion of antidiuretic hormone associated with imatinib. *Ann Pharmacother.* 2008 Dec; 42:1882-6.
219. Larner AJ. Hyponatraemia and dopaminergic agents. *Postgrad Med J.* 1994; 70:310-1.
220. Roberts MT, Aliyu SH. Hyponatraemia associated with lopinavir–ritonavir? *Int J Infect Dis.* 2007; 11:83-4.
221. Engel WR, Grau A. Inappropriate secretion of antidiuretic hormone associated with lorazepam. *BMJ.* 1988; 297:858.
222. Namenda (memantine) package insert. St. Louis, MO: Forest Pharmaceuticals; 2014 Aug.
223. Methadone tablets for oral suspension (Methadone Diskets). Columbus, OH: Boehringer Ingelheim Roxane Laboratories; 2013 Sept.
224. Varkel Y, Braester A, Nusem D et al. Methyldopa-induced syndrome of inappropriate antidiuretic hormone secretion and bone marrow granulomatosis. *Drug Intell Clin Pharm.* 1988; 22:700-1.
225. Sue YM, Lee YL, Huang JJ. Acute hyponatremia, seizure, and rhabdomyolysis after ecstasy use. *J Toxicol Clin Toxicol.* 2002; 40:931-2.
226. Traub SJ, Hoffman RS, Nelson LS. The "ecstasy" hangover: hyponatremia due to 3,4 methylenedioxymethamphetamine. *J Urban Health.* 2002; 79:549-55.
227. Hartung TK, Schofield E, Short AI et al. Hyponatraemic states following 3,4-methylenedioxymethamphetamine (MDMA, 'ecstasy') ingestion. *QJM.* 2002; 95:431-7.
228. Gomez-Balaguer M, Pena H, Morillas C et al. Syndrome of inappropriate antidiuretic hormone secretion and "designer drugs" (ecstasy). *J Pediatr Endocrinol Metab.* 2000; 13:437-8.
229. O'Connor A, Cluroe A, Couch R et al. Death from hyponatraemia-induced cerebral oedema associated with MDMA ("Ecstasy") use. *N Z Med J.* 1999; 112:255-6.
230. Holmes SB, Banerjee AK, Alexander WD. Hyponatraemia and seizures after ecstasy use. *Postgrad Med J.* 1999; 75:32-3.
231. Ajaelo I, Koenig K, Snoey E. Severe hyponatremia and inappropriate antidiuretic hormone secretion following ecstasy use. *Acad Emerg Med.* 1998; 5:839-40.
232. Magee C, Staunton H, Tormey W et al. Hyponatraemia, seizures and stupor associated with ecstasy ingestion in a female. *Irish Med J.* 1998; 91:178.
233. Henry JA, Fallon JK, Kicman AT et al. Low-dose MDMA ("ecstasy") induces vasopressin secretion. *Lancet.* 1998; 351:1784.
234. Brvar M, Kozelj G, Osredkar J et al. Polydipsia as another mechanism of hyponatremia after 'ecstasy' (3,4 methyldioxymethamphetamine) ingestion. *Eur J Emerg Med.* 2004; 11:302-4.
235. Kalantar-Zadeh K, Nguyen MK, Chang R et al. Fatal hyponatremia in a young woman after ecstasy ingestion. *Nat Clin Pract Nephrol.* 2006; 2:283-8, quiz.
236. Kadian (morphine sulfate extended-release capsules) package insert. Parnippany, NJ: Actavis Pharma, Inc; 2014 Apr.
237. Yam FK, Erally SA. Syndrome of inappropriate antidiuretic hormone associated with moxifloxacin. *Am J Health-Syst Pharm.* 2012; 69:217-20.
238. Finch CK1, Andrus MR, Curry WA. Nicotine replacement therapy-associated syndrome of inappropriate antidiuretic hormone. *South Med J.* 2004 Mar; 97:322-4.
239. Durst RY, Pipek R, Levy Y. Hyponatremia caused by omeprazole treatment. *Am J Med.* 1994; 97:400-1.
240. OxyContin (oxycodone HCl extended-release) package insert. Stamford, CT: Purdue Pharma L.P.; 2015 Aug.
241. NebuPent (pentamidine isethionate) inhalation package insert. Schaumburg, IL: APP Pharmaceuticals, LLC; 2010 Dec.
242. Bruno JJ, Canada TW. Possible pentostatin-induced symptomatic hyponatremia. *Pharmacotherapy.* 2007; 27:164-9.
243. Ko SH, Lim CH, Kim JY et al. Case of inappropriate ADH syndrome: hyponatremia due to polyethylene glycol bowel preparation. *World J Gastronenterol* 2014; 20:12350-4.
244. Dirix LY, Moeremans C, Fierens H et al. Symptomatic hyponatremia related to the use of propafenone. *Acta Clin Belg.* 1988; 43:143-5.
245. Cole RP, Roberts WD, Cheng MD. Hyponatremia associated with quinupristin–dalfopristin. *Ann Intern Med.* 2000; 133:485.
246. Chitre MM, Berenson CS. Idiosyncratic rifabutin-induced leukopenia and SIADH: case report and review. *Pharmacotherapy.* 2001; 21:493-7.
247. Requip (ropinirole hydrochloride) package insert. Research Triangle Park, NC: GlaxoSmithKline; 2014 Aug.
248. Liberopoulos EN, Alexandridis GH, Christidis DS et al. SIADH and hyponatremia with theophylline. *Ann Pharmacother.* 2002; 36:1180-2.
249. Hamburger S, Koprivica B, Ellerbeck E et al. Thiazide-induced syndrome of inappropriate secretion of antidiuretic hormone: time course of resolution. *JAMA.* 1981; 246:1235-6.

250. Juss JK, Radhamma AK, Forsyth DR. Tolterodine-induced hyponatraemia. *Age Ageing.* 2005; 34:524-5.
251. Babayev R, Terner S, Chandra S et al. Trimethoprim-associated hyponatremia. *Am J Kidney Dis.* 2013; 62:1188-92.
252. Kirby D, Harrigan S, Ames D. Hyponatraemia in elderly psychiatric patients treated with selective serotonin reuptake inhibitors and venlafaxine: a retrospective controlled study in an inpatient unit. *Int J Geriatr Psychiatry.* 2002; 17:231-7.
253. Movig KL, Leufkens HG, Lenderink AW et al. Association between antidepressant drug use and hyponatraemia: a case-control study. *Br J Clin Pharmacol.* 2002; 53:363-9.
254. Strachan J, Shepherd J. Hyponatraemia associated with the use of selective serotonin re-uptake inhibitors. *Aust N Z J Psychiatry.* 1998; 32:295-8.
255. Bouman WP, Pinner G, Johnson H. Incidence of selective serotonin reuptake inhibitor (SSRI) induced hyponatraemia due to the syndrome of inappropriate antidiuretic hormone (SIADH) secretion in the elderly. *Int J Geriatr Psychiatry.* 1998; 13:12-5.
256. Catalano MC, Catalano G, Kanfer SN et al. The effect of sertraline on routine blood chemistry values. *Clin Neuropharmacol.* 2000; 23:267-70.
257. Jessani M, Montgomery J, Fedde JD et al. Lack of association between antipsychotics and hyponatremia in chronic schizophrenia. *Schizophr Res.* 2006; 83:307-9.
258. Van Amelsvoort T, Bakshi R, Devaux CB et al. Hyponatremia associated with carbamazepine and oxcarbazepine therapy: a review. *Epilepsia.* 1994; 35:181-8.
259. Glauser TA. Oxcarbazepine in the treatment of epilepsy. *Pharmacotherapy.* 2001; 21:904-19.
260. Rosenson J, Smollin C, Sporer KA et al. Patterns of ecstasy-associated hyponatremia in California. *Ann Emerg Med.* 2007; 49:164-71, 171.e1.
261. Jorgensen H, Riis M, Knigge U et al. Serotonin receptors involved in vasopressin and oxytocin secretion. *J Neuroendocrinol.* 2003; 15:242-9.
262. Anderson IK, Martin GR, Ramage AG. Central administration of 5-HT activates 5-HT1A receptors to cause sympathoexcitation and 5-HT2/5-HT1C receptors to release vasopressin in anaesthetized rats. *Br J Pharmacol.* 1992; 107:1020-8.
263. Brownfield MS, Greathouse J, Lorens SA et al. Neuropharmacological characterization of serotoninergic stimulation of vasopressin secretion in conscious rats. *Neuroendocrinology.* 1988; 47:277-83.
264. Fallon JK, Shah D, Kicman AT et al. Action of MDMA (ecstasy) and its metabolites on arginine vasopressin release. *Ann N Y Acad Sci.* 2002; 965:399-409.
265. Sachdeo RC, Wasserstein A, Mesenbrink PJ et al. Effects of oxcarbazepine on sodium concentration and water handling. *Ann Neurol.* 2002; 51:613-20.
266. Ellison DH, Berl T. Clinical practice: the syndrome of inappropriate antidiuresis. *N Engl J Med.* 2007; 356:2064-72.
267. Liu BA, Mittmann N, Knowles SR et al. Hyponatremia and the syndrome of inappropriate secretion of antidiuretic hormone associated with the use of selective serotonin reuptake inhibitors: a review of spontaneous reports. *CMAJ.* 1996; 155:519-27.
268. Madhusoodanan S, Bogunovic OJ, Moise D et al. Hyponatraemia associated with psychotropic medications: a review of the literature and spontaneous reports. *Adverse Drug React Toxicol Rev.* 2002; 21:17-29.
269. Finfgeld DL. SSRI-related hyponatremia among aging adults. *J Psychosoc Nurs Ment Health Serv.* 2003; 41:12-6.
270. Rosner MH. Severe hyponatremia associated with the combined use of thiazide diuretics and selective serotonin reuptake inhibitors. *Am J Med Sci.* 2004; 327:109-11.
271. Movig KL, Leufkens HG, Lenderink AW et al. Serotonergic antidepressants associated with an increased risk for hyponatraemia in the elderly. *Eur J Clin Pharmacol.* 2002; 58:143-8.
272. Wilkinson TJ, Begg EJ, Winter AC et al. Incidence and risk factors for hyponatraemia following treatment with fluoxetine or paroxetine in elderly people. *Br J Clin Pharmacol.* 1999; 47:211-7.
273. Stedman CA, Begg EJ, Kennedy MA et al. Cytochrome P450 2D6 genotype does not predict SSRI (fluoxetine or paroxetine) induced hyponatraemia. *Hum Psychopharmacol.* 2002; 17:187-90.
274. Parr MJ, Low HM, Botterill P. Hyponatraemia and death after "ecstasy" ingestion. *Med J Aust.* 1997; 166:136-7.
275. Kloster R, Borresen HC, Hoff-Olsen P. Sudden death in two patients with epilepsy and the syndrome of inappropriate antidiuretic hormone secretion (SIADH). *Seizure.* 1998; 7:419-20.
276. Chan TY. Drug-induced syndrome of inappropriate antidiuretic hormone secretion: causes, diagnosis and management. *Drugs Aging.* 1997; 11:27-44.
277. Walter KA. Conivaptan: new treatment for hyponatremia. *Am J Health-Syst Pharm.* 2007; 64:1385-95.
278. Nagler EV, Vanmassenhove J, van der Veer S et al. Diagnosis and treatment of hyponatremia: a systematic review of clinical practice guidelines and consensus statements. *BMC Medicine.* 2014; 12:231.
279. Berl T. Vasopressin antagonists. *N Engl J Med.* 2015; 72:2207-16.
280. Verbalis JG, Goldsmith SR, Greenberg A et al. Diagnosis, evaluation, and treatment of hyponatremia: expert panel recommendations. *Am J Med.* 2013; 126(suppl 1):S1-42.
281. Spasovski G, Vanholder R, Allolio B et al. Clinical practice guideline on diagnosis and treatment of hyponatremia. *European Journal of Endocrinology.* 2014; 170:G1-47.
282. Canuso CM, Goldman MB. Clozapine restores water balance in schizophrenic patients with polydipsia-hyponatremia syndrome. *J Neuropsychiatry Clin Neurosci.* 1999; 11:86-90.
283. Spears NM, Leadbetter RA, Shutty MS Jr. Clozapine treatment in polydipsia and intermittent hyponatremia. *J Clin Psychiatry.* 1996; 57:123-8.
284. Borusiak P, Korn-Merker E, Holert N et al. Hyponatremia induced by oxcarbazepine in children. *Epilepsy Res.* 1998; 30:241-6.
285. Brewerton TD, Jackson CW. Prophylaxis of carbamazepine-induced hyponatremia by demeclocycline in six patients. *J Clin Psychiatry.* 1994; 55:249-51.
286. Miell J, Dhanjal P, Jamookeeah C. Evidence for the use of demeclocycline in the treatment of hyponatremia secondary to SIADH: a systemic review. *Int J Clin Pract.* 2015; 69:1396-417.
287. Palakurthy PR, Iyer V, Klein J. Amiodarone induced encephalopathy and diabetes insipidus. *J Ky Med Assoc.* 1987; 85:373-4.
288. Smith OP, Gale R, Hamon M et al. Amphotericin B-induced nephrogenic diabetes insipidus: resolution with its liposomal counterpart. *Bone Marrow Transplant.* 1994; 13:107-8.
289. Hopp L, Bernardi J, Reeves G. Amphotericin B-induced partial nephrogenic diabetes insipidus in a child. *Pediatr Nephrol.* 2001; 16:594-7.
290. Spath-Schwalbe E, Koschuth A, Dietzmann A et al. Successful use of liposomal amphotericin B in a case of amphotericin B-induced nephrogenic diabetes insipidus. *Clin Infect Dis.* 1999; 28:680-1.
291. Canada TW, Weavind LM, Augustin KM. Possible liposomal amphotericin B-induced nephrogenic diabetes insipidus. *Ann Pharmacother.* 2003; 37:70-3.
292. Fujita Y, Kasahara K, Uno K et al. Amphotericin B-induced nephrogenic diabetes insipidus in a case of cryptococcemia. *Intern Med.* 2005; 44:458-61.
293. Schliefer K, Rockstroh JK, Spengler U et al. Nephrogenic diabetes insipidus in a patient taking cidofovir. *Lancet.* 1997; 350:413-4.
294. Bendz H, Aurell M. Drug-induced diabetes insipidus: incidence, prevention and management. *Drug Saf.* 1999; 21:449-56.
295. Usalan C, Altun B, Ulusoy S et al. Hypernatraemia and polyuria due to high-dose colchicine in a suicidal patient. *Nephrol Dial Transplant.* 1999; 14:1556-7.
296. Finn G, Denning D. Transient nephrogenic diabetes insipidus following high-dose cyclophosphamide chemotherapy and

autologous bone marrow transplantation. *Cancer Treat Rep.* 1987; 71:220-1.

297. Hayek A, Ramirez J. Demeclocycline-induced diabetes insipidus. *JAMA.* 1974; 229:676-7.
298. D'Ythurbide G, Goujard C, Méchaï F et al. Fanconi syndrome and nephrogenic diabetes insipidus associated with didanosine therapy in HIV infection: a case report and literature review. *Nephrol Dial Transplant.* 2007 Dec; 22:3656-9.
299. Atripla (efavirenz; emtricitabine; tenofovir) package insert. Foster City, CA: Bristol-Myers Squibb, Gilead Sciences, LLC; 2015 Jan.
300. Complera (emtricitabine; rilpivirine; tenofovir) package insert. Foster City, CA: Gilead Sciences, Inc; 2015 May.
301. Truvada (emtricitabine; tenofovir) package insert. Foster City, CA: Gilead Sciences, Inc; 2013 Oct.
302. Navarro JF, Quereda C, Quereda C et al. Nephrogenic diabetes insipidus and renal tubular acidosis secondary to foscarnet therapy. *Am J Kidney Dis.* 1996; 27:431-4.
303. Farese RV Jr, Schambelan M, Hollander H et al. Nephrogenic diabetes insipidus associated with foscarnet treatment of cytomegalovirus retinitis. *Ann Intern Med.* 1990; 112:955-6.
304. Conn J, Colman P, Brown G et al. Nephrogenic diabetes insipidus associated with foscarnet—a case report. *J Antimicrob Chemother.* 1996; 37:1179-81.
305. Cerebyx (fosphenytoin sodium) package insert. New York, NY: Pfizer Labs; 2015 Jun.
306. Govind E, Naik R, Srinivas BJ, Meddi I. Case of fosphenytoin induced acute cerebellar dysfunction and pituitary bleed causing central diabetes insipidus in a case of AML M2 during allogenic hematopoietic stem cell transplant. *Int J Pharmacol and Clin Sci.* 2012; 1:111-4.
307. Negro A, Regolisti G, Perazzoli F et al. Ifosfamide-induced renal Fanconi syndrome with associated nephrogenic diabetes insipidus in an adult patient. *Nephrol Dial Transplant.* 1998; 13:1547-9.
308. Finch CK, Kelley KW, Williams RB. Treatment of lithium-induced diabetes insipidus with amiloride. *Pharmacotherapy.* 2003; 23:546-50.
309. Bendz H, Aurell M, Lanke J. A historical cohort study of kidney damage in long-term lithium patients: continued surveillance needed. *Eur Psychiatry.* 2001; 16:199-206.
310. Bendz H, Aurell M, Balldin J et al. Kidney damage in long-term lithium patients: a cross-sectional study of patients with 15 years or more on lithium. *Nephrol Dial Transplant.* 1994; 9:1250-4.
311. Martinez EJ, Sinnott JT, Rodriguez-Paz G et al. Lithium-induced nephrogenic diabetes insipidus treated with indomethacin. *South Med J.* 1993; 86:971-3.
312. Martin A. Clinical management of lithium-induced polyuria. *Hosp Comm Psychiatry.* 1993; 44:427-8.
313. Weinstock RS, Moses AM. Desmopressin and indomethacin therapy for nephrogenic diabetes insipidus in patients receiving lithium carbonate. *South Med J.* 1990; 83:1475-7.
314. Vierhapper H. Indomethacin in the treatment of lithium-induced nephrogenic diabetes insipidus. *Arch Intern Med.* 1990; 150:2420.
315. Allen HM, Jackson RL, Winchester MD et al. Indomethacin in the treatment of lithium-induced nephrogenic diabetes insipidus. *Arch Intern Med.* 1989; 149:1123-6.
316. Grindlinger GA, Boylan MJ. Amelioration by indomethacin of lithium-induced polyuria. *Crit Care Med.* 1987; 15:538-9.
317. Kosten TR, Forrest JN. Treatment of severe lithium-induced polyuria with amiloride. *Am J Psychiatry.* 1986; 143:1563-8.
318. Leeman MF, Vuylsteke A, Ritchie AJ. Lithium-induced nephrogenic diabetes insipidus after coronary artery bypass. *Ann Thorac Surg.* 2007; 84:656-7.
319. Sze L, Ulrich B, Brandle M. Severe hypernatraemia due to nephrogenic diabetes insipidus. *Exp Clin Endocrinol Diabetes.* 2006; 114:596-8.
320. Kamijo Y, Soma K, Hamanaka S et al. Dural sinus thrombosis with severe hypernatremia developing in a patient on long-term lithium therapy. *J Toxicol Clin Toxicol.* 2003; 41:359-62.
321. Shen HC, Li JY, Lo YK. Lithium intoxication-induced acute parkinsonism complicated with hyperparathyroidism and nephrogenic diabetes insipidus: report of a case. *Acta Neurol Taiwan.* 2007; 16:231-3.
322. Dalan R, Leow MK, Jong M. Multiple endocrinopathies associated with lithium therapy. *Endocr Pract.* 2007; 13:758-63.
323. Paw H, Slingo ME, Tinker M. Late onset nephrogenic diabetes insipidus following cessation of lithium therapy. *Anaesth Intensive Care.* 2007; 35:278-80.
324. Imam SK, Hasan A, Shahid SK. Lithium-induced nephrogenic diabetes insipidus. *J Pak Med Assoc.* 2005; 55:125-7.
325. Masson EA, Rhodes JM. Mesalazine associated nephrogenic diabetes insipidus presenting as weight loss. *Gut.* 1992; 33:563-4.
326. Bharani A, Kumar H. Drug points: diabetes inspidus induced by ofloxacin. *BMJ.* 2001; 323:547.
327. Sandostatin (octreotide) package insert. Stein, Switzerland: Novartis Pharma Stein AG Corporation; 2012 Mar.
328. Etienne L, Wittebole X, Liolios A et al. Polyuria after olanzapine overdose. *Am J Psychiatry.* 2004; 161:1130.
329. Misra S, Chakraborty S, Gangopadhyay P et al. Phenytoin sodium induced diabetes insipidus. *J Assoc Physicians India.* 1999; 47:456.
330. Quinn BP, Wall BM. Nephrogenic diabetes insipidus and tubulointerstitial nephritis during continuous therapy with rifampin. *Am J Kidney Dis.* 1989; 14:217-20.
331. Rilutek (riluzole) package insert. Cary, NC: Covis Pharmaceuticals, Inc; 2013 April.
332. Zanosar (streptozocin) package insert. Irvine, CA: Teva Parenteral Medicines, Inc; 2007 May.
333. Temodar (temozolomide) capsules and injection package insert. Whitehouse Station, NJ: Merck and Co, Inc; 2015 Sept.
334. Costa M, Teixeira C, Costa CM et al. Nephrogenic diabetes insipidus associated with tenofovir administration: report of a pediatric case. *Port J Nephrol Hypert.* 2012; 26:171-3.
335. Karras A, Lafaurie M, Furco A et al. Tenofovir-related nephrotoxicity in human immunodeficiency virus-infected patients: three cases of renal failure, Fanconi syndrome, and nephrogenic diabetes insipidus. *Clin Infect Dis.* 2003; 36:1070-3.
336. Macleod MD, Bell GM, Irvine WJ. Nephrogenic diabetes insipidus associated with Dyazide (triamterenehydrochlorothiazide). *BMJ.* 1981; 283:1155-6.
337. VFEND (voriconazole) tablets, suspension, and injection package insert. New York, NY: Pfizer, Inc; 2015 Feb.
338. Nguyen MK, Nielsen S, Kurtz I. Molecular pathogenesis of nephrogenic diabetes insipidus. *Clin Exp Nephrol.* 2003; 7:9-17.
339. Rose BD, Post TW. Hyperosmolal states—hypernatremia. In: Rose BD, Post TW, eds. *Clinical physiology of acid-base and electrolyte disorders.* 5th ed. New York, NY: McGraw-Hill Companies, Inc; 2001:746-93.
340. Neithercut WD, Spooner RJ, Hendry A et al. Persistent nephrogenic diabetes insipidus, tubular proteinuria, aminoaciduria, and parathyroid hormone resistance following longterm lithium administration. *Postgrad Med J.* 1990; 66:479-82.
341. Bowen RC, Grof P, Grof E. Less frequent lithium administration and lower urine volume. *Am J Psychiatry.* 1991; 148:189-92.
342. Mellerup ET, Dam H, Plenge P et al. Serum lithium minimum and diuresis. *Psychiatry Res.* 1985; 14:309-13.

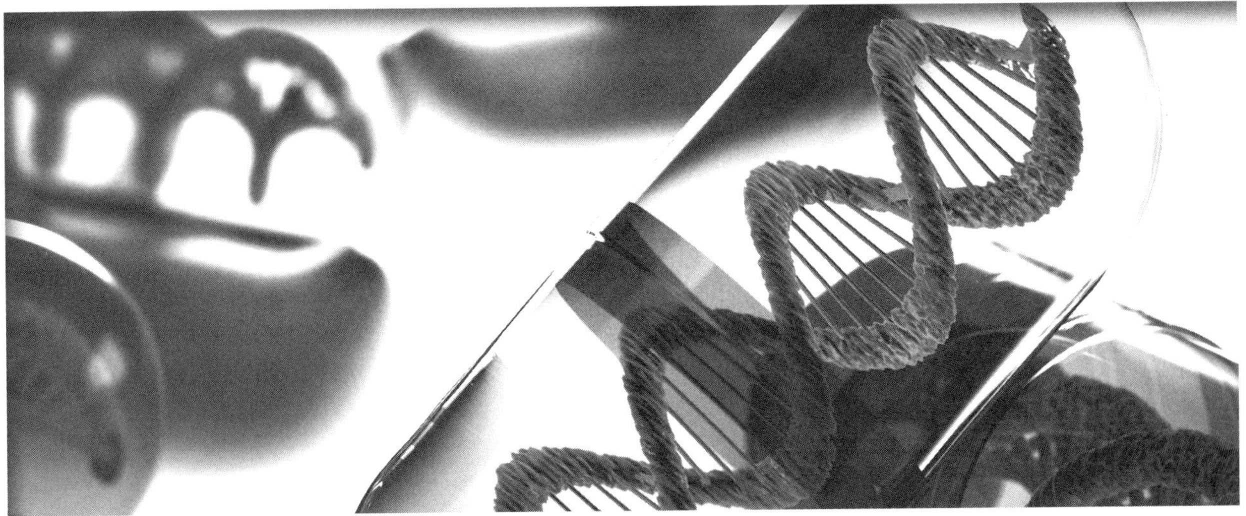

CHAPTER 44

Acid–Base Disorders

Lori D. Wazny, J. Christine Davis, and Robert E. Ariano

Acid–base balance can be defined as homeostasis of body fluids at a normal arterial blood pH between 7.35 and 7.45. Clinicians must be able to anticipate and help avoid or minimize the clinical consequences of drug-induced acid–base disorders, and, when that is not possible, they must be able to design appropriate treatment regimens to correct the abnormality.[1] A skilled clinician can play a significant role in the prevention, identification, and management of potentially life-threatening drug-induced disturbances in acid–base balance.

ACIDOSIS

CAUSATIVE AGENTS

Drugs that have been reported to cause metabolic or respiratory acidosis are listed in **Table 44-1.** Drug-induced metabolic acidosis is caused by acid accumulation from increased acid production or acid ingestion; decreased acid excretion; or gastrointestinal (GI) or renal bicarbonate loss. Drug-induced respiratory acidosis is caused by either depression of the central respiratory center leading to decreased ventilation and accumulation of carbon dioxide (CO_2) or increased CO_2 production as might occur, for example, with overfeeding during nutritional support.

EPIDEMIOLOGY

Overall, the incidence of drug-induced acidosis is largely unknown, with the majority of evidence limited to case reports, case series, or open-label studies. Unintentional overdosage of central respiratory depressants may occur in the hospital setting, but published reports on the frequency of this complication or the number of patients in whom a clinically significant respiratory acidosis develops as a result are not available.

MECHANISMS

Mechanisms of drug-induced acidosis, where known, are noted in Table 44-1 and described in **Table 44-2**. Metabolic acidosis is caused by acid accumulation from increased acid production or acid ingestion, decreased acid excretion, or GI or renal bicarbonate loss. Acidemia (arterial

Table 44-1 Agents Implicated in Drug-Induced Acidosis

Drug	Incidence	Level of Evidence[a]
ELEVATED ANION-GAP METABOLIC ACIDOSIS		
Lactic Acidosis		
Amygdalin[39,40]	NK	C
Antibacterial-induced D-lactic acidosis (tetracycline, metronidazole) in patients post intestinal bypass surgery or small bowel resection[41,42]	NK	C
β_2 agonists (albuterol, salbutamol, theophylline)[43-47]	NK	C
Biguanides: metformin,[b] phenformin,[b] buformin[42]	3–10 per 100,000 patient years for metformin, higher incidences for phenformin and buformin[48-50]	B
Catecholamines (epinephrine, norepinephrine)[51,52]	NK	C
Isoniazid overdose >30 mg/kg[53,54]	NK	C
Linezolid[55,56]	NK	C
Nalidixic acid overdose[57]	NK	C
Niacin[42]	NK	C
Nitroprusside[58]	NK	C
Nucleoside reverse transcriptase inhibitors (didanosine, lamivudine, stavudine, zidovudine)[42]	1.3–10 cases/1,000 patient years Didanosine>stavudine>zidovudine[59]	B
Propylene glycol containing IV medications (Table 44-7)	NK	C
Propofol[60,61]	24%[42]	B
Rhabdomyolysis induced by statins, fibric acids, or neuroleptic malignant syndrome[42]	NK	C
Sorbitol and xylitol[62,63]	NK	C
Topical emollients containing lactic acid[64]	NK	C
Ketoacidosis		
Atypical antipsychotics (aripiprazole, clozapine, olanzapine, risperidone, quetiapine)[65,66]	NK	C
Salicylate overdose (mixed disorder: metabolic acidosis + respiratory alkalosis)[67,68]	NK	C
Sodium-glucose cotransporter 2 (SGLT2) inhibitors (canagliflozin, dapagliflozin, empagliflozin)[69]	NK	C
Addition of Unmeasured Anions		
Acetaminophen[70,71]	NK	C
Sodium thiosulfate[72]	NK	C
Other		
Ibuprofen overdose[73]	NK	C
Iron overdose[1]	NK	C
Papaverine[74]	NK	C
NORMAL ANION-GAP METABOLIC ACIDOSIS		
Cholestyramine (GI HCO_3 loss)[75,76]	NK	C
Laxative abuse-induced diarrhea (GI HCO_3 loss)[77]	NK	C
Sevelamer hydrochloride (not carbonate)[78,79]	22%	C
Rapid 0.9% NaCl administration[80] (dilutional acidosis)	NK	C

Table 44-1 Agents Implicated in Drug-Induced Acidosis (continued)

Drug	Incidence	Level of Evidence[a]
PROXIMAL (TYPE II) RENAL TUBULAR ACIDOSIS		
Aminoglycosides[42]	NK	C
Carbonic anhydrase inhibitors (e.g., acetazolamide, brinzolamide eye drop, topiramate, zonisamide)[42]	Up to 55% with acetazolamide[42]; up to 48% with topiramate[42]	C
Cidofovir[81]	1%	B
Ifosfamide[42,82]	7–14%	C
Leflunomide[42]	NK	C
Mercaptopurine[42]	NK	C
Nucleoside reverse transcriptase inhibitors (abacavir, adefovir [high doses], didanosine, tenofovir)[42]	48% with tenofovir; 27–50% with adefovir	A
Oxaliplatin[83]	NK	C
Ranitidine[42]	NK	C
Sulfamethoxazole[84]	NK	C
Streptozocin[85]	NK	C
Tetracycline, expired[86,87]	NK	C
Valproic acid[42]	NK	C
TYPE I DISTAL RENAL TUBULAR ACIDOSIS		
Amphotericin B[84]	1%	C
Cisplatin[88]	NK	C
Foscarnet[42]	NK	C
Lithium[89]	NK	C
TYPE IV DISTAL RENAL TUBULAR ACIDOSIS		
Impaired renin release (NSAIDs, cyclosporine, tacrolimus)[42]	NK	B
RAAS blockade (ACEI, ARBs, direct renin inhibitors, e.g., aliskiren)[42]	NK	C
Impaired aldosterone metabolism (heparin)[42]	NK	C
Aldosterone antagonists (spironolactone, eplerenone)[42]	NK	C
K+ sparing diuretics (amiloride, triamterene)[42]	NK	C
Trimethoprim[84]	NK	C
RESPIRATORY ACIDOSIS[5,90]		
Central Respiratory Depression		
Anesthetics	NK	C
Barbiturates	NK	B
Benzodiazepines	NK	B
Narcotics	NK	B
Increased CO_2 Production		
Parenteral or enteral nutrition (if excessive calories)	NK	B

IV = intravenous, NK = not known.

[a]Definitions for Levels of Evidence: Level A—evidence from one or more randomized, controlled clinical trials; Level B—evidence from nonrandomized clinical trials, prospective observational studies, cohort studies, retrospective studies, case-control studies, meta-analyses and/or postmarketing surveillance studies; and Level C—evidence from one or more published case reports or case series.

[b]Available in countries outside of the United States.

Table 44-2 Mechanisms of Drug-Induced Acidosis[42]

Cause	Mechanism
ELEVATED ANION GAP	
Addition of unmeasured anions	Acetaminophen: accumulation of pyroglutamic acid (5-oxoproline) Sodium thiosulfate: thiosulfuric acid produced when dissolved in aqueous solution
Ketoacidosis	Increased metabolism of fatty acids leading to increased ketone (acetoacetate, β-hydroxybutyrate) synthesis in the liver
Lactic acidosis	Increased lactate production due to either altered pyruvate conversion to lactate, increased pyruvate production, or impaired pyruvate utilization or removal Serum lactate concentrations >5 mEq/L
NORMAL ANION GAP	
Distal type I renal tubular acidosis	Selective deficiency of H^+ secretion in the distal tubule; commonly associated with hypokalemia due to renal potassium wasting
Distal type IV renal tubular acidosis	Aldosterone deficiency or antagonism impairs distal renal Na^+ reabsorption and K^+ and H^+ excretion leading to acidosis; the resulting hyperkalemia may worsen the acidosis as K^+ moves into cells and H^+ moves out
Gastrointestinal bicarbonate loss	Cholestyramine binds intestinal bicarbonate in exchange for chloride Laxative-induced diarrhea causes significant bicarbonate loss through the stool
Proximal (type II) renal tubular acidosis	Selective defect in the proximal tubule to adequately reabsorb filtered bicarbonate The bicarbonate defect may occur alone or as part of Fanconi syndrome whereby proximal tubule reabsorption of phosphate, glucose, amino acids, and uric acid is also impaired
Rapid 0.9% NaCl administration (dilutional acidosis)[80]	Nonalkali-containing IV fluids result in dilution of bicarbonate in the ECF; the condition corrects itself as the kidneys generate bicarbonate and reduce the ECF
Sevelamer hydrochloride salt	Exchanges hydrochloride for bicarbonate
RESPIRATORY ACIDOSIS	
Acute respiratory acidosis due to ↓ respiratory drive	Exposure to central nervous system depressing drugs or ↑ production of CO_2 from overfeeding during nutritional support

CO_2 = carbon dioxide, ECF = extracellular fluid, H = hydrogen, IV = intravenous, K = potassium, Na = sodium, NaCl = sodium chloride.

pH <7.35) results when respiratory compensation (i.e., removal of CO_2 via the lungs) is overwhelmed. Determination of the anion gap (AG) is useful in distinguishing the type of metabolic acidosis. It is calculated by subtracting the sum of the serum chloride (Cl^-) and bicarbonate (HCO_3^-) concentrations from the serum sodium (Na^+) concentration:

$$AG = ([Na^+]) - ([Cl^-] + [HCO_3^-])$$

The normal range for the AG may differ among laboratories, and clinicians should consider their particular laboratory's reference range when assessing this value. In general, an elevated AG is >12 mEq/L.

Metabolic acidosis with an elevated AG can be caused by endogenous (lactate, ketones, myoglobin, uremia) or exogenous (methanol, ethylene glycol, propylene glycol, salicylates) substances. The majority of elevated AG metabolic acidoses due to prescription drugs are a result of lactic acidosis, although some drugs (e.g., acetaminophen, sodium thiosulfate) cause acidosis by adding unmeasured anions.

Metabolic acidosis with a normal AG is caused either by gastrointestinal loss of bicarbonate or by renal loss of bicarbonate (e.g., renal tubular acidosis [RTA]). RTA is a defect of urinary acidification occurring in either the proximal or the distal renal tubule. Proximal (Type II) RTA involves a failure in proximal tubule reabsorption of filtered bicarbonate; distal RTA is characterized by impaired acid excretion. Distal RTA is subdivided into that associated with hypokalemia (Type I) and that associated with hyperkalemia (Type IV). Drugs may be implicated as causative agents in any of these RTA types, but the mechanism by which drugs cause RTA in most cases is either not known or incompletely understood. Readers are referred to the references listed in Table 44-1 for more specific details regarding the proposed mechanisms behind a specific drug-induced RTA.

Respiratory acidosis is the result of an accumulation of CO_2 in the blood. Accumulation may occur for several reasons: (1) decreased excretion by a depressed respiratory drive, abnormal neuromuscular transmission, or muscle dysfunction all resulting in alveolar hypoventilation; (2) decreased removal of CO_2 as is seen with obstructive pulmonary disorders or ventilation–perfusion mismatches; and/or, (3) an increased production of CO_2. Irrespective of the etiology, the accumulation of CO_2 within plasma water promptly forms carbonic acid and subsequent acidemia.

Respiratory acidosis may be classified as either acute or chronic. The absence of normal physiologic compensation defines an acute process. The normal compensatory response to respiratory acidosis requires the metabolic system (i.e., the kidney) to retain bicarbonate to partially correct the acidemia. Renal compensation for respiratory acidosis is slow, however, (taking hours to days) so the hallmarks of this acid–base disorder include an acidemia (pH <7.35) with an elevated carbon dioxide ($paCO_2$) above the reference range of 45 mm Hg and a serum bicarbonate level within the normal range (22–28 mEq/L). In contrast, patients with chronic respiratory acidosis will present with an acidemia >24 hours in duration, an elevated $paCO_2$, and a significantly elevated serum bicarbonate level (>30 mEq/L).[2] Elevated $paCO_2$ mediates bicarbonate retention through the renal production of ammonia. Generated ammonia binds and titrates down serum chloride to form ammonium chloride, which is then excreted renally causing hypochloremia. There is renal retention of bicarbonate and sodium as a consequence of urinary ammonium chloride losses. Thus the acidemia from respiratory acidosis is partially corrected by the slow retention of bicarbonate.[3]

Acute respiratory acidosis may be the result of reduced respiratory drive from central nervous system–depressing drugs like narcotics and sedatives or from overfeeding during nutritional support. It may also arise from neuromuscular weakness disorders (myasthenia gravis, acute Guillain-Barré syndrome, or high cervical cord lesions) and from acute cardiopulmonary disorders such as exacerbations of chronic obstructive pulmonary disease (COPD), pulmonary edema, and acute respiratory distress syndrome.[4] Generally, drug-induced respiratory acidosis is an acute process.

Patients with acute respiratory acidosis typically present with ventilatory failure leading to hypercapnea and hypoxemia. A useful method to determine whether or not acute hypoxemia is due to reduced respiratory drive is to measure the alveolar–arterial oxygen gradient [$P(A\text{-}a)O_2$]. The $P(A\text{-}a)\ O_2$ gradient is helpful in assessing the efficiency of alveolar-capillary gas exchange. An elevated $P(A\text{-}a)\ O_2$ gradient suggests parenchymal lung disease with either a ventilation–perfusion imbalance or intrapulmonary shunting. Drug-induced acute respiratory acidosis commonly presents with a normal $P(A\text{-}a)\ O_2$ gradient.

An increased production of CO_2 may be the result of hypercatabolic states such as sepsis or malignant hyperthermia or the result of overfeeding during nutritional support. Carbohydrate overfeeding has often been identified as a cause of hypercapnia and respiratory acidosis.[5] Evidence has shown, however, that it is not actually high carbohydrate administration that increases CO_2 production, rather it is the total calories delivered. CO_2 increases when the caloric intake exceeds the rate of carbohydrate metabolism, and CO_2 production remains constant when the proportion of total calories delivered as carbohydrates is reduced.[6] Excessive CO_2 production from overfeeding is associated with prolonged weaning from mechanical ventilation, especially when the ventilatory rate is fixed.[7]

CLINICAL PRESENTATION AND DIFFERENTIAL DIAGNOSIS

General features of metabolic acidosis include an increase in ventilation, a decrease in central and pulmonary vascular compliance predisposing to pulmonary edema with even minimal volume overload, and depression of central nervous function. Acidosis is usually first suspected as a result of the discovery of abnormalities in arterial blood gases or electrolytes, which then leads to evaluation of the AG.[8] Screening to identify drug-induced metabolic acidosis should include a thorough medication history to uncover evidence of exposure to potential causative agents and, in patients who present with an elevated AG, determination of the serum lactate concentration.

Signs and symptoms associated with drug-induced metabolic acidosis are listed in **Table 44-3**. Mild acidemia is generally asymptomatic; however, as acidemia becomes more severe, patients may experience nausea, vomiting, loss of appetite, and abdominal pain. These symptoms may appear at higher pH if acidosis develops rapidly. The most characteristic sign is hyperpnea, which leads to Kussmaul breathing, a deep and labored breathing pattern reflecting a compensatory increase in alveolar ventilation. Severe, acute acidosis predisposes to reduced cardiac output, hypotension and shock, ventricular arrhythmias, and coma. Chronic acidosis can cause bone demineralization and osteoporosis.

Table 44-3 Signs and Symptoms Associated with Drug-Induced Acidosis[1,91]

Signs	*Symptoms*
MILD TO MODERATE METABOLIC ACIDOSIS (pH 7.1–7.35)	
• Hyperkalemia • Serum lactate concentration ≥5 mEq/L (lactic acidosis) • Tachycardia	• Abdominal pain • Flushing • Hyperventilation/ Kussmaul respirations • Loss of appetite • Nausea and Vomiting
SEVERE METABOLIC ACIDOSIS (pH <7.1)	
• Hyperglycemia • Hypotension • Multisystem organ failure	• Obtundation and coma
ACUTE RESPIRATORY ACIDOSIS	
• Asterixis • Coma • Combativeness • Congestive heart failure/ cardiogenic shock (if severe hypercapnia develops) • Increased intracranial pressure (pseudotumor cerebri) • Myoclonic jerks • Seizures • Stupor • Tremor	• Disorientation • Drowsiness • Severe breathlessness • Confusion • Headache • Anxiety

Conditions to consider in the differential diagnosis of metabolic acidosis are listed in **Table 44-4**. The differential diagnosis of metabolic acidosis in patients with a normal AG includes GI bicarbonate loss and renal tubular acidification defects. Calculation of the urine anion gap (UAG) is helpful in distinguishing between bicarbonate loss occurring via the GI tract or via the kidneys:

$$UAG = [Urine_{Na} + Urine_{K}] - Urine_{Cl}$$

When bicarbonate is lost via the GI tract, the UAG is negative. When the kidneys are unable to generate sufficient amounts of ammonium or when loss of bicarbonate through the kidney occurs, the UAG is zero or positive.[8] Calculation of fractional bicarbonate excretion (FE-HCO_3) can help differentiate between distal and proximal RTA. FE-HCO_3 is calculated as:

$$\text{FE-}HCO_3 = (uHCO_3 \times sCr) / (sHCO_3 \times uCr)$$

where $uHCO_3$ is urine bicarbonate concentration, $sHCO_3$ is serum bicarbonate concentration, uCr is urine creatinine concentration, and sCr is serum creatinine concentration.

An FE–HCO_3 <0.05 indicates distal RTA, whereas an FE–HCO_3 >0.15 is indicative of proximal RTA, assuming in both instances that serum bicarbonate is >20 mEq/L.

Signs and symptoms of respiratory acidosis (Table 44-3) vary depending on the rate and degree of CO_2 increase and are typically the result of high CO_2 concentrations in the central nervous system and hypoxemia, if present. Acute respiratory acidosis may cause headache, confusion, anxiety, drowsiness, seizure, and stupor. Patients with respiratory acidosis that develops slowly over time typically display minimal symptoms but may experience memory loss, sleep disturbances, excessive daytime sleepiness, and personality changes. Conditions to consider in the differential diagnosis

Table 44-4 Conditions to Consider in the Differential Diagnosis of Drug-Induced Acidosis[2,91-93,a]

Anion gap metabolic acidosis

Diabetic or alcoholic ketoacidosis
Ethylene glycol
Lactic acidosis
Methanol
Uremia

Non-anion-gap metabolic acidosis

Diarrhea
Pancreatic fistula
Parenteral hyperalimentation
Renal tubular acidosis (RTA)
Ureteroenterostomy

Respiratory acidosis—acute and chronic

Depressed central respiratory drive

- Brain-stem lesion, or tumor
- Central sleep apnea (C)
- Cerebral edema
- Cerebrovascular accident
- Encephalitis
- Head trauma
- Hypothyroidism (C)
- Obesity hypoventilation syndrome

Abnormal neuromuscular transmission

- Amytrophic lateral sclerosis (C)
- Guillain–Barré syndrome
- Multiple sclerosis (C)
- Muscle dysfunction
- Muscular dystrophy (C)
    - Fatigue
    - Hyperkalemia
    - Hypokalemia
- Myasthenia gravis
- Polymyositis (C)
- Status epilepticus

Enhanced ventilatory demand

- Failure of CO_2 transport
    - Pulmonary embolism
    - Cardiac arrest
- High caloric intake
- Increased dead space ventilation

Ventilation/perfusion mismatch

- Acute lung injury/acute respiratory distress syndrome
- Angioedema
- Augmented airway flow resistance
- Chronic obstructive pulmonary disease
- Emphysema (C)
- Pulmonary fibrosis (C)
- Severe pneumonia
- Status asthmaticus
- Upper airway obstruction

Pleural/chest wall/lung stiffness

- Abdominal distension
- Atelectasis
- Chest wall trauma with flail chest
- Kyphoscoliosis (C)
- Obesity (C)
- Pneumothorax

[a](C) defines chronic respiratory acidosis etiologies only. All others may present either acutely or chronically.

of drug-induced respiratory acidosis are listed in Table 44-4. Patient evaluation should include a careful medication history, examination of the arterial blood gases, hematocrit measurement, chest x-ray, an assessment of the upper airways, and evaluation of respiratory and neuromuscular function.

RISK FACTORS

Table 44-5 lists risk factors for drug-induced acidosis. Drug-induced respiratory depression is typically dose-related, and higher doses lead to increased risk of respiratory acidosis, but the data supporting dose-dependency primarily derive from the literature with respect to narcotics.[9]

MORBIDITY AND MORTALITY

The risk of morbidity and mortality associated with drug-induced metabolic or respiratory acidosis has not been quantified in most cases. However, mortality data are available for metabolic acidosis, specifically lactic acidosis, induced by nucleoside reverse-transcriptase inhibitors (NRTIs) (33–57% mortality), metformin (45–50% mortality), and propofol (65% mortality).[10-14]

PREVENTION

General strategies for the prevention of drug-induced acidosis are listed in **Table 44-6**. Overall, strategies are aimed at identifying patients at risk

Table 44-5 Risk Factors for Drug-Induced Acidosis[42,76,94]

Metabolic acidosis

General risks

- Cirrhosis
- Diabetes
- Extracellular fluid volume depletion
- Heart failure
- Renal dysfunction

Drug risks

- Acetaminophen: Renal or hepatic insufficiency, alcoholism, female sex, chronic ingestion
- Aminoglycosides: High doses, prolonged administration
- Amphotericin B: Cumulative doses of >2–3 g
- Cholestyramine: Renal insufficiency, volume depletion, combination with spironolactone; co-administration of more than one drug implicated in drug-induced acidosis
- Ifosfamide: Total dose >100 g/m^2, administration with other nephrotoxic drugs
- Metformin: Renal insufficiency (eGFR <30 mL/min/1.73 m^2), hepatic insufficiency, history of lactic acidosis, hypoxia or serious illness, cardiovascular or pulmonary dysfunction, IV contrast agent exposure
- Niacin: High doses, co-ingestion with alcohol
- NRTI-induced lactic acidosis: Co-infection with hepatitis B or C, more than one antiretroviral drug, more than one drug known to cause lactic acidosis, female sex, renal insufficiency, low CD4 count, obesity, pregnancy
- Propofol: Infusion rates >4 mg/kg/hr, duration of infusion >48 hr, concomitant use of catecholamines or corticosteroids, age <18 years, sepsis, head injury
- Propylene glycol–containing drugs: Renal or hepatic insufficiency, alcoholism, age <4 years or elderly, pregnancy, less than one propylene glycol–containing drug
- Statins: Thiamine deficiency, hepatic insufficiency
- Topiramate: Dose-dependent, renal insufficiency

Respiratory acidosis

General risks

- Patients with sepsis or on a ventilator with fixed settings receiving enteral or parenteral nutrition
- Patients with underlying chronic respiratory acidosis (e.g., brainstem infarct, obesity-hypoventilation syndrome, tumors, poliomyelitis, multiple sclerosis, diaphragmatic paralysis, COPD, kyphoscoliosis, interstitial pulmonary disease)

Drug risks

- High doses of respiratory depressants (dose-related effect)
- Overdose of any agent with sedative properties
- Total calories delivered through enteral or parenteral solutions

CD4 = cluster of differentiation 4, COPD = chronic obstructive pulmonary disease, eGFR = estimated glomerular filtration rate, IV = intravenous, NRTI = nucleoside reverse-transcriptase inhibitor.

Table 44-6 Approaches to Help Prevent Drug-Induced Acidosis and Alkalosis

- Counsel about the early signs and symptoms of acidosis or alkalosis if the patient receiving a high-risk drug or has underlying risk factors
- Identify and minimize use of high-risk drugs
- Preventive monitoring using laboratory tests is not recommended

Table 44-7 Intravenous Medications Containing Propylene Glycol[42,95-97]

- Chlordiazepoxide
- Diazepam
- Digoxin
- Esmolol
- Etomidate
- Hydralazine
- Lorazepam
- Multivitamims
- Nitroglycerin
- Pentobarbital
- Phenobarbital
- Phenytoin
- Trimethoprim–sulfamethoxazole

and educating both patients and heathcare professionals to help promote early recognition. More specific preventative measures have been suggested for lactic acidosis due to propylene glycol and propofol. Patients receiving continuous intravenous infusions of products containing propylene glycol (**Table 44-7**) for more than 2–5 days should be carefully monitored. Serum osmolality should be measured twice weekly (propylene glycol contributes to osmolality), and alternative therapeutic agents should be considered when the serum osmolality is >320 mOsm/kg.[15] Propofol infusion rates of >4–5 mg/kg/hr for longer than 48 hours should also be avoided.[13,14]

MANAGEMENT

Treatment of drug-induced metabolic acidosis involves prompt identification and discontinuation of the offending agent. Other important aspects of treatment include ensuring adequate oxygen supply to tissues through proper ventilation and reducing oxygen demand by using sedation when indicated.[16] Intravenous bicarbonate therapy is reserved for more severe cases (i.e., pH <7.1) because this therapy carries the potential for fluid overload and hypernatremia and because the effect on plasma bicarbonate concentration may be only temporary.[16,17] Specific treatment measures are outlined in **Figure 44-1**. The goal of sodium bicarbonate therapy is to return the blood pH to a safer level (pH 7.15–7.2) or to increase the plasma bicarbonate to 8–10 mEq/L.

Thiamine, riboflavin, and L-carnitine have been used to treat patients with NRTI-induced acidosis because these agents are necessary enzyme cofactors in the mitochondrial respiratory chain. Thiamine (100–200 mg daily), riboflavin (50 mg daily), and L-carnitine (1,000 mg twice daily) have been used together and individually (orally and intravenously)

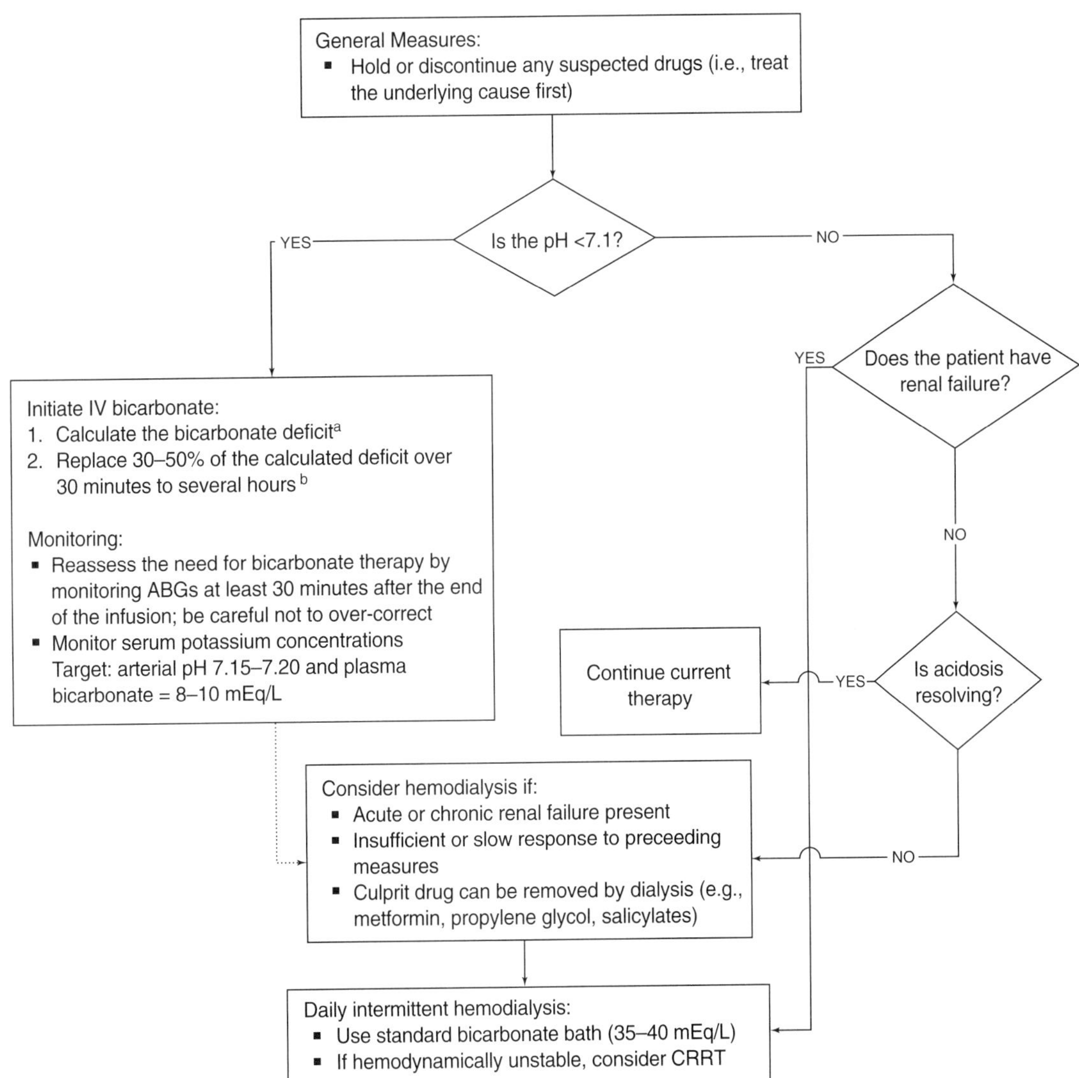

FIGURE 44-1 Treatment of Metabolic Acidosis (excluding RTA)

ABG = arterial blood gas, CRRT = continuous renal replacement therapy, RTA = renal tubular acidosis.

[a]Bicarbonate deficit (mEq) = 0.5 L/kg × weight (kg) × [HCO_3] desired – [HCO_3] observed, where 0.5 L/kg = volume of distribution of bicarbonate, HCO_3 = plasma bicarbonate concentration.

[b]Usual dose 100–150 mEq (2–3 ampules) $NaHCO_3$ in 0.9% NaCl, D5W, or other compatible fluid.

Source: Adroque HJ, Madias NE. Management of life-threatening acid-base disorders. *N Engl J Med.* 1998; 338:26-34.

in the treatment of NRTI-induced lactic acidosis.[18,19] Current guidelines recommend changing to an NRTI-sparing regimen after patients completely recover from NRTI-induced lactic acidosis.[20]

Continuous or intermittent hemodialysis may be used in the treatment of metformin-, propylene glycol-, and propofol-induced metabolic acidosis to facilitate removal of metformin, propylene glycol, and the metabolic acids and lipids that accumulate with propofol infusion syndrome. Hemodialysis can also correct acidosis through bicarbonate supplementation and removal of lactate from the circulation.[21-23]

Drug-induced RTA is generally reversible upon discontinuation of the drug. If the acidosis does not improve within 1–3 days or the patient is symptomatic, oral alkali therapy may be considered. Treatment of proximal (Type II) RTA requires large doses of alkali because of the significant excretion of bicarbonate. Potassium citrate or combinations of potassium and sodium citrate are used, because low serum potassium concentrations due to distal potassium wasting are a consistent finding in proximal RTA. Classical distal (Type I) RTA responds to treatment with oral sodium bicarbonate. Reduction of serum potassium concentrations to within the normal range may reverse acidosis in patients with hyperkalemic (Type IV) distal RTA. **Table 44-8** lists the available options for oral alkali replacement therapy and **Figure 44-2** provides an algorithm for treatment of RTA.

The immediate restoration of normal alveolar gas exchange is the most important feature in the treatment of acute respiratory acidosis. **Table 44-9** reviews treatment options for drug-induced acute respiratory acidosis. Successful management of chronic respiratory acidosis relies on the prompt recognition and treatment of the underlying conditions, such as for COPD or sepsis. Bicarbonate administration is rarely necessary, and rapid correction of respiratory acidosis with bicarbonate may eliminate the patient's respiratory drive or precipitate an acute metabolic alkalosis.[1] Sodium bicarbonate infusions used to treat respiratory acidosis can buffer hydrogen ions; however, dissociation can also lead to unwanted formation of CO_2. The effects of sodium bicarbonate overall on correcting the pH then become dependent on the patient's ability to eliminate that CO_2. Tracheal intubation with mechanical ventilation is key at this point and should continue until the underlying cause of acidosis is resolved. In addition to the extracellular effects of bicarbonate administration, generated CO_2 passively diffuses into cells where carbonic acid is formed. This can worsen intracellular acidosis.[24] Tris-hydroxymethyl aminomethane (THAM) may be considered as an alternative to bicarbonate administration because it buffers respiratory acidosis and, unlike bicarbonate, easily enters cells to buffer pH and reduce CO_2 levels. THAM may more effectively correct pH and mitigate adverse effects of the acidosis in

Table 44-8 Oral Alkali Replacement Products

Generic Name	Brand Name	mEq Bicarbonate
Potassium bicarbonate–potassium citrate	K-lyte	25 mEq bicarbonate/tablet (25 mEq K/tablet)
	K-lyte DS	50 mEq bicarbonate/tablet (50 mEq K/tablet)
Potassium citrate	Urocit-K	5 mEq, 10 mEq, or 15 mEq bicarbonate/tablet (5 mEq, 10 mEq, 15 mEq K/tablet)
Potassium citrate–citric acid	Polycitra K	2 mEq bicarbonate/mL (2 mEq K/mL)
Sodium bicarbonate	Various	325 mg tablet = 3.9 mEq bicarbonate (3.9 mEq Na) 650 mg tablet = 7.8 mEq bicarbonate (7.8 mEq Na)
Sodium citrate–citric acid	Shohl's solution, Bicitra	1 mEq bicarbonate/mL (1 mEq Na/mL)
Sodium citrate–potassium citrate–citric acid	Polycitra	2 mEq bicarbonate/mL (1 mEq K/mL and 1 mEq Na/mL)

K = potassium, Na = sodium.

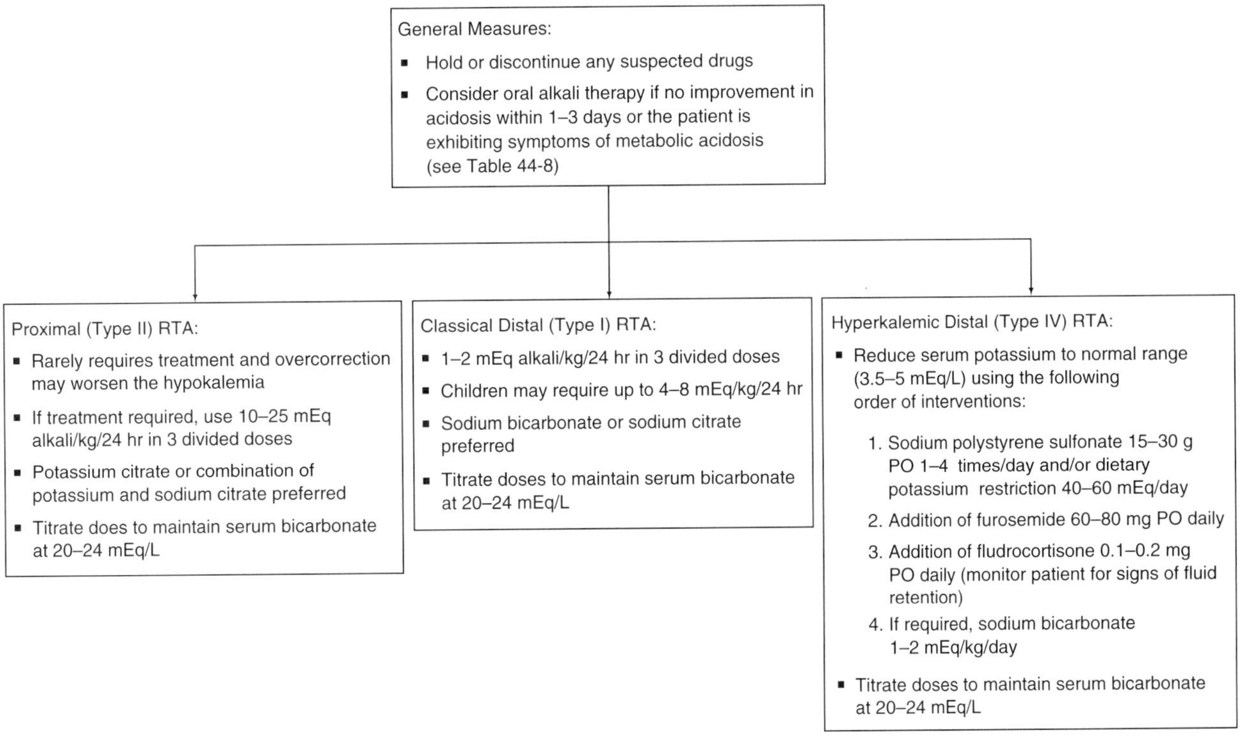

General Measures:

- Hold or discontinue any suspected drugs
- Consider oral alkali therapy if no improvement in acidosis within 1–3 days or the patient is exhibiting symptoms of metabolic acidosis (see Table 44-8)

Proximal (Type II) RTA:

- Rarely requires treatment and overcorrection may worsen the hypokalemia
- If treatment required, use 10–25 mEq alkali/kg/24 hr in 3 divided doses
- Potassium citrate or combination of potassium and sodium citrate preferred
- Titrate does to maintain serum bicarbonate at 20–24 mEq/L

Classical Distal (Type I) RTA:

- 1–2 mEq alkali/kg/24 hr in 3 divided doses
- Children may require up to 4–8 mEq/kg/24 hr
- Sodium bicarbonate or sodium citrate preferred
- Titrate doses to maintain serum bicarbonate at 20–24 mEq/L

Hyperkalemic Distal (Type IV) RTA:

- Reduce serum potassium to normal range (3.5–5 mEq/L) using the following order of interventions:
  1. Sodium polystyrene sulfonate 15–30 g PO 1–4 times/day and/or dietary potassium restriction 40–60 mEq/day
  2. Addition of furosemide 60–80 mg PO daily
  3. Addition of fludrocortisone 0.1–0.2 mg PO daily (monitor patient for signs of fluid retention)
  4. If required, sodium bicarbonate 1–2 mEq/kg/day
- Titrate doses to maintain serum bicarbonate at 20–24 mEq/L

FIGURE 44-2 Treatment of Renal Tubular Acidosis

Table 44-9 Treatment Options for the Management of Acute Drug-Induced Respiratory Acidosis

- Hold or discontinue any respiratory depressant drugs
- Reverse effects of respiratory depressants, if present:
  - For opiates: Give naloxone 0.04–0.4 mg IV/IM. Sub-Q may provide more gradual reversal than IV. Naloxone may be administered via nebulization or by endotracheal tube. Response should be observed within 1–2 minutes after IV dose; duration of naloxone action is variable from 0.5–3 hours; and repeated administration may be required. Naloxone may also be administered as a continuous IV infusion (0.4–0.8 mg/hr in 5% dextrose). Guidelines recommend using the lowest effective dose of naloxone to prevent respiratory acidosis and minimize the risk of withdrawal in opiate-dependent patients.[98,122]
  - For benzodiazepines: give flumazenil 0.2 mg IV q 1 min as needed (maximum, 5 doses per series; may repeat series at 20-minute intervals up to 5-mg total dose); obtain arterial blood gases every 2–4 hours initially then every 12–24 hours as acidosis improves; flumazenil is not recommended in the absence of specific knowledge of a benzodiazepine overdose as its administration may precipitate seizures in patients with tricyclic antidepressant overdose[98]

IM = intramuscular, IV = intravenous, sub-Q = subcutaneous.

patients with severe cardiovascular and hemodynamic instability.[24]

INFORMATION FOR PATIENTS

Patients receiving drugs known to cause acidosis should be aware that associated symptoms are not specific and may include epigastric pain, nausea, vomiting, lethargy, somnolence, and diarrhea. Many patients who have experienced NRTI-induced lactic acidosis describe a 2- to 4-week prodrome that has included nausea, vomiting, weight loss, and abdominal pain and distention.[10] The occurrence of any of these symptoms should be reported to a healthcare provider.

Patients receiving large doses of central respiratory depressants and their caregivers should be cautioned to be alert to the signs and symptoms of respiratory acidosis, including altered mental status and abnormal behavior.

ALKALOSIS

CAUSATIVE AGENTS

Metabolic alkalosis is a primary increase in serum bicarbonate concentration and occurs as a consequence of a loss of hydrogen ions or/and a gain in bicarbonate. Patients with metabolic alkalosis present with an elevated arterial pH, increased plasma bicarbonate concentration, and a compensatory decrease in lung ventilation (hypoventilation) resulting in an increased partial pressure of CO_2. Hypochloremia and/or hypokalemia may also be present.[8] Because the kidney under normal circumstances is able to excrete a significant alkali load, evaluation of patients with metabolic alkalosis must include both an assessment of the process initially responsible for the acid–base abnormality as well as the alterations in renal function that are preventing prompt correction of the alkalemic state.

Respiratory alkalosis is a condition of elevated arterial pH and hyperventilation resulting in a low partial pressure of CO_2 with a compensatory decrease in plasma bicarbonate concentration. Similar to respiratory acidosis, respiratory alkalosis can be classified as acute or chronic depending on the degree of bicarbonate compensation observed. Drugs reported to cause metabolic or respiratory alkalosis are listed in **Table 44-10**.

EPIDEMIOLOGY

Metabolic alkalosis is a common acid–base disorder, accounting for a large proportion of all acid–base disorders.[25] The high incidence is attributed to the frequency of vomiting and the use of diuretics and nasogastric suction in hospitalized patients. Respiratory alkalosis is the most common acid–base abnormality observed in critically ill patients because it is associated with numerous illnesses and is a common finding in patients on mechanical ventilation.[8] However, the incidence of drug-induced respiratory alkalosis is not well defined.

MECHANISMS

Table 44-11 lists the mechanisms of metabolic and respiratory drug-induced alkalosis. The development and continuation of metabolic alkalosis requires both an elevation in the plasma bicarbonate concentration and a decrease in renal bicarbonate excretion. There are three major mechanisms of metabolic alkalosis. The first involves extracellular fluid (ECF) volume contraction, low blood pressure, potassium deficiency, and secondary hyperaldosteronism. ECF volume contraction leads to an increased plasma bicarbonate concentration, whereas low blood pressure decreases glomerular filtration rate in the kidneys, leading to decreased renal bicarbonate excretion. Secondary hyperaldosteronism occurs and is an attempt to correct the volume contraction and low blood pressure, and hypokalemia is the result of aldosterone's effect on potassium excretion. Hyperaldosteronism and hypokalemia both directly increase renal bicarbonate reabsorption and lead to an increased plasma bicarbonate concentration. Treatment with diuretics may produce hypochloremia, which reduces bicarbonate excretion by increasing renal distal tubule reabsorption and reducing renal distal tubule secretion of bicarbonate. It has been suggested that this type of metabolic alkalosis would more accurately be termed *chloride depletion alkalosis*. Animal models and a study in healthy human volunteers found that metabolic alkalosis can be corrected with chloride repletion alone (without volume expansion), whereas volume expansion without chloride administration does not correct the alkalosis.[26] When volume deficits exist in patients with alkalosis, they are typically corrected with solutions of 0.9% sodium chloride.

The second major mechanism of metabolic alkalosis involves ECF volume expansion, hypertension, hypokalemia, and mineralocorticoid excess. Drugs with mineralocorticoid activity produce aldosterone-like effects. The resulting increased absorption of sodium and water leads to ECF volume expansion and hypertension, and the increased potassium excretion leads to hypokalemia. The net result is that aldosterone-like effects and

Table 44-10 Agents Implicated in Drug-Induced Alkalosis

Drug	Incidence	Level of Evidence[a]
METABOLIC ALKALOSIS		
Acetate[98]	NK	C
Anions—nonreabsorbable, large doses (Penicillins,[99,100] Carbapenems)[101,102]	NK	C
Aminoglycosides[103-106]	NK	C
Calcium carbonate (calcium-alkali syndrome, reported with doses 4–60 g/day, may occur with lower doses)[35,36]	NK	C
Cisplatin[107]	NK	C
Citrate (from transfused blood, fresh-frozen plasma, or citrate anticoagulation in continuous renal replacement therapies)	NK	C
Diuretics (loop and thiazide)[108,109]	NK	B
Fludrocortisone[110]	NK	C
Glycyrrhizic acid (found in genuine black licorice, chewing tobacco, herbal products containing licorice)[37,111]	NK	C
Laxative abuse[77]	NK	B
Sodium bicarbonate—excessive administration (found in nonprescription antacids, IV sodium bicarbonate, baking soda)[38,112-115]	NK	B
Sodium polystyrene sulfonate combined with aluminum or magnesium hydroxide[116,117]	NK	C
Stanozolol[118]	NK	C
RESPIRATORY ALKALOSIS		
Amphetamines	NK	C
Catecholamines[91]	NK	C
Doxapram[28,29,118]	NK	A
Loratadine (overdose)[121]	NK	C
Nicotine	NK	C
Progesterone[119]	NK	A
Quetiapine[30]	NK	C
Salicylate (overdose—mixed disorder: metabolic acidosis and respiratory alkalosis)[68]	NK	B
Theophylline (overdose)[120]	NK	B

IV = intravenous, NK = not known.

[a]Definitions for Levels of Evidence: Level A—evidence from one or more randomized, controlled clinical trials; Level B—evidence from nonrandomized clinical trials, prospective observational studies, cohort studies, retrospective studies, case-control studies, meta-analyses and/or postmarketing surveillance studies; and Level C—evidence from one or more published case reports or case series.

hypokalemia increase bicarbonate reabsorption and lead to the development of metabolic alkalosis.

The third major mechanism involves exogenous alkali loading. Sustained metabolic alkalosis usually occurs in patients who have underlying risk factors (e.g., renal dysfunction) and receive large doses of alkali-containing drugs such as antacids, sodium bicarbonate (e.g., baking soda), or bicarbonate precursors (citrate, acetate).

Drug-induced respiratory alkalosis occurs as a result of stimulation of the central respiratory center and the subsequent increase in minute ventilation and reduction in the partial pressure of CO_2. Progesterone exerts this effect and rising endogenous progesterone concentrations may in fact be responsible for inducing respiratory alkalosis in pregnant women. Medroxyprogesterone has been shown to induce small but sustained decreases in the partial pressure of CO_2 and increases in serum bicarbonate concentrations and has been used to treat patients with central hypoventilation.[27] Doxapram increases respiratory rate and can cause

Table 44-11 Mechanisms of Drug-Induced Alkalosis

Drug	Mechanism
METABOLIC ALKALOSIS	
Aminoglycosides	Bartter-like syndrome
Cisplatin Large doses of nonreabsorbable anion Loop and thiazide diuretics	ECF volume contraction (renal origin), normotension, hypokalemia, and secondary hyperaldosteronism
Combined administration of sodium polystyrene sulfonate and aluminum or magnesium hydroxide Laxative abuse	ECF volume contraction (gastrointestinal origin), normotension, hypokalemia, and secondary hyperaldosteronism
Fludrocortisone Glycyrrhizic acid (found in genuine black licorice, chewing tobacco, herbal products containing licorice) Stanozolol	ECF volume expansion, hypertension, hypokalemia, and mineralocorticoid excess
Acetate Calcium carbonate (calcium-alkali syndrome) Citrate (from transfused blood, fresh-frozen plasma, or citrate anticoagulation in renal replacement therapies) Excessive sodium bicarbonate injection/administration (found in over-the-counter antacids, intravenous sodium bicarbonate, baking soda)	Exogenous alkali load
RESPIRATORY ALKALOSIS	
Amphetamines	Central respiratory stimulation
Doxapram	Central respiratory stimulation
Loratadine overdose	Central respiratory stimulation
Progesterone	Central respiratory stimulation
Quetiapine	Hyperventilation secondary to peripheral serotonin depletion
Salicylate overdose (mixed disorder: metabolic acidosis and respiratory alkalosis)	Central respiratory stimulation
Theophylline overdose	Central respiratory stimulation

ECF = extracellular fluid.

respiratory alkalosis. It has been used for patients in intensive care units to help obviate the need for intubation and mechanical ventilation, although its use is limited by its propensity to induce cardiac arrhythmia.[28,29] Quetiapine has been associated with hyperventilation and respiratory alkalosis possibly secondary to peripheral serotonin depletion.[30] Serotonin is known to be involved in the regulation of ventilation. It has been hypothesized that hyperventilation results from serotonin depletion at vagal receptor sites in the airway and lungs.[30]

CLINICAL PRESENTATION AND DIFFERENTIAL DIAGNOSIS

Mild-to-moderate metabolic alkalosis, with serum bicarbonate levels <40 mEq/L, is usually asymptomatic. Often it is the electrolyte abnormalities, such as hypokalemia, that lead to signs and symptoms such as paresthesias, muscle cramping, tetany, and cardiac arrhythmias. When serum bicarbonate levels exceed 45 mEq/L, hypoxemia secondary to compensatory hypoventilation may occur, especially in patients with COPD. Mental status changes, seizures, and coma may occur with serum bicarbonate levels >50 mEq/L.[31]

The cause of metabolic alkalosis can often easily be discerned with careful medical and medication histories and physical examination. However, without arterial blood gas measurements, metabolic alkalosis may be difficult to distinguish from respiratory acidosis, as the signs and symptoms are similar (Table 44-3 and **Table 44-12**). Patients presenting with metabolic alkalosis associated with ECF volume contraction may exhibit orthostatic hypotension, tachycardia, and other features of reduced circulatory volume. Unless they are receiving diuretic therapy and have associated chloride depletion, these patients generally have intense chloride conservation, with urinary concentrations <10 mEq/L. In metabolic alkalosis associated with ECF volume expansion and mineralocorticoid excess, patients tend to present with hypertension and urinary chloride concentrations >30 mEq/L. Urine chloride concentrations between 10 and 30 mEq/L are associated with various causes such as severe hypokalemia, diuretic-induced volume depletion, Bartter and Gitelman syndromes, or alkali ingestion. Therefore, results within this range are not helpful in determining the cause of metabolic alkalosis.[31] Urinary potassium concentrations >30 mEq/L in the presence of hypokalemia indicate renal potassium wasting, often from diuretic therapies.[32] Conditions to consider in the differential diagnosis of metabolic alkalosis are listed in **Table 44-13**.

The clinical features of respiratory alkalosis are listed in Table 44-12. In addition to a physical examination and medication history, the diagnostic workup should include arterial blood gases to avoid possible misdiagnosis as metabolic acidosis. Conditions to consider in the differential diagnosis of drug-induced respiratory alkalosis are listed in Table 44-13.

Table 44-12 Signs and Symptoms Associated with Alkalosis[98]

Signs and symptoms
MILD TO MODERATE METABOLIC ALKALOSIS (pH 7.5–7.6)
• Extracellular fluid volume depletion and postural hypotension • Hypokalemia • Muscle weakness
SEVERE METABOLIC ALKALOSIS (pH >7.6)
• Cardiac arrhythmias • Confusion • Hyperactive reflexes or tetany • Hypoxemia stimulated tachypnea • Muscle cramping • Paresthesia
RESPIRATORY ALKALOSIS
• Arrhythmias • Confusion • Neuromuscular irritability • Seizures • Decreased cardiac output • Dizziness • Ischemic ECG changes • Hyponatremia • Hypokalemia • Hyperchloremia ◦ Hyponatremia ◦ Hypokalemia ◦ Hyperchloremia

ECG = electrocardiogram.

RISK FACTORS

Patients with underlying medical causes of hydrochloric acid loss, such as vomiting or nasogastric suction, or reduced renal bicarbonate excretion due to low effective blood volume may be at higher risk of experiencing drug-induced metabolic alkalosis. Patients with renal dysfunction are more likely to develop metabolic alkalosis with large doses of alkali-containing drugs. With primary respiratory alkalosis, the elevation in pH and decrease in pCO_2 occur as the result of any disorder that increases respiratory drive. Risk factors for metabolic and respiratory alkalosis are presented in **Table 44-14**.

MORBIDITY AND MORTALITY

Although specific rates of morbidity and mortality for patients with drug-induced alkalosis are not known, mortality rates for alkalosis of all types

Table 44-13 Conditions to Consider in the Differential Diagnosis of Drug-Induced Alkalosis[8,31,91]

Metabolic alkalosis	Respiratory alkalosis

Exogenous bicarbonate administration
• Alkali administration
• Milk-alkali syndrome
ECF volume contraction, hypokalemia, and secondary hyperaldosteronism
• Gastrointestinal losses
  ○ Congenital chloridorrhea
  ○ High-volume ileostomy losses
  ○ Nasogastric suction
  ○ Villous adenoma
  ○ Vomiting
• Renal losses
  ○ Bartter syndrome (inherited defect in TALH characterized by alkalosis, hypokalemia, and normal-to-low blood pressure)
  ○ Gitelman syndrome (loss of function mutation in Na^+–Cl^- cotransporter in DCT)
  ○ Hypercalcemia/hypoparathyroidism
  ○ Hypokalemia
  ○ Magnesium deficiency
  ○ Posthypercapnic state
  ○ Recovery from lactic acidosis or ketoacidosis
ECF volume expansion, hypertension, hypokalemia, and mineralocorticoid excess
• Secondary hyperaldosteronism (high renin)
  ○ Accelerated hypertension
  ○ Renal artery stenosis
  ○ Renin-secreting tumor
• Low renin
  ○ Cushing syndrome or disease
  ○ Primary aldosteronism
  ○ Adrenal enzyme defects
    –11β-hydroxylase deficiency
    –17α-hydroxylase deficiency
• Liddle syndrome—Genetic disorder associated with increased function of renal sodium channel resulting in ECFV expansion, hypertension, K^+ deficiency, and hyporeninemic-hypoaldosteronism
	Central nervous system stimulation
	• Anxiety-hyperventilation syndrome
	• Cerebrovascular accident
	• Fever
	• Meningoencephalitis
	• Pain
	• Psychosis
	• Trauma
	• Tumor
	Hypoxemia or tissue hypoxia
	• Aspiration
	• High altitude
	• Pneumonia
	• Pulmonary edema
	• Severe anemia
	Stimulation of chest wall receptors
	• Acute respiratory distress syndrome
	• Asthma
	• Cardiac failure
	• Flail chest
	• Hemothorax
	• Pneumonia
	• Pneumothorax
	• Pulmonary embolism
	Miscellaneous
	• Heat exposure
	• Hepatic failure
	• Mechanical hyperventilation
	• Pregnancy (progesterone)
	• Recovery from metabolic acidosis
	• Septicemia

DCT = distal convoluted tubule, ECFV = extracellular fluid volume, TALH = thick ascending limb of Henle's loop.

have been published. Patients with arterial blood pH of 7.55 have been found to have a mortality rate of 45% and mortality increases to 80% when pH is >7.65.[33] Hospitalized patients with respiratory alkalosis and a partial pressure of arterial CO_2 <15 mm Hg have a mortality rate of approximately 90%.[34]

MANAGEMENT

There are two goals in the treatment of metabolic alkalosis: (1) correct the existing deficit, and (2) prevent continuing bicarbonate gains by discontinuing the causative agent. Metabolic alkalosis associated with ECF volume contraction can be

Table 44-14 Risk Factors for Drug-Induced Alkalosis[1,8]

Metabolic alkalosis

- Hemodynamic disturbances that impair bicarbonate excretion
- Renal dysfunction
- Vomiting or nasogastric suction

Respiratory alkalosis

- Altitude
- Anxiety
- Asthma
- Brain tumors, vascular accidents
- Carbon monoxide intoxication
- Fever
- Gram-negative sepsis
- Head trauma
- Heart failure
- Hepatic cirrhosis
- Hyperventilation (mechanical or voluntary)
- Hypotension
- Pain
- Pneumonia
- Pregnancy
- Pulmonary emboli
- Pulmonary shunts

effectively treated with an infusion of 0.9% sodium chloride. This will correct both the volume and the chloride deficits. Patients with overt signs of volume contraction usually require a minimum of 3–5 L. As the chloride deficit is corrected, an alkaline diuresis will occur, with plasma bicarbonate decreasing toward normal.[32] Other treatment measures are outlined in **Figure 44-3**.

The only effective therapy in patients with respiratory alkalosis is elimination of the underlying cause of hyperventilation. If a medication is suspected, its use should be discontinued. Management of salicylate and theophylline overdose includes supportive care and administration of activated charcoal to reduce absorption. Intravenous sodium bicarbonate is used to alkalinize the urine and to enhance urinary excretion of salicylates. Whole bowel irrigation may be used to enhance elimination of sustained-release theophylline. Hemodialysis or hemoperfusion is recommended to enhance elimination in severe cases of salicylate or theophylline overdose. Oxygen therapy should be initiated in all patients with severe hypoxemia (partial pressure of oxygen <40 mm Hg), and patients with life-threatening alkalosis (pH >7.6) may require mechanical ventilation to control hyperventilation.[1] **Table 44-15** summarizes the treatment options available for drug-induced respiratory alkalosis.

INFORMATION FOR PATIENTS

Patients exposed to drugs that can induce metabolic alkalosis should be instructed to report muscle weakness or cramping (hypokalemia), tetany (hypocalcemia), or postural dizziness (ECF volume depletion) promptly to their healthcare provider. To avoid development of calcium-alkali syndrome in patients with risk factors for metabolic alkalosis, intake of calcium supplements should be limited to no more than 1.2–1.5 g per day of elemental calcium (includes total from diet and supplements). This is especially important in patients exposed to other sources of alkali or when there is concomitant use of agents associated with drug-induced alkalosis.[35,36] An indication of possible diuretic or laxative abuse may be identified by clinicians during a review of a patient's purchase or refill history, and these patients should be cautioned regarding the risks associated with this practice. Patients should also be warned about the use of herbal supplements with mineralocorticoid activity (e.g., natural licorice) and overuse of baking soda as a home remedy.[37,38]

Patients should be advised to take medications known to cause respiratory alkalosis exactly as directed to prevent unintentional overdose. Patients receiving large doses of aspirin for treatment of arthritis or other conditions should be made aware of, and advised to avoid, other salicylate-containing medications to prevent accidental overdose. Patients should also be instructed to promptly report symptoms of light-headedness, confusion, syncope, or seizures to their healthcare provider.

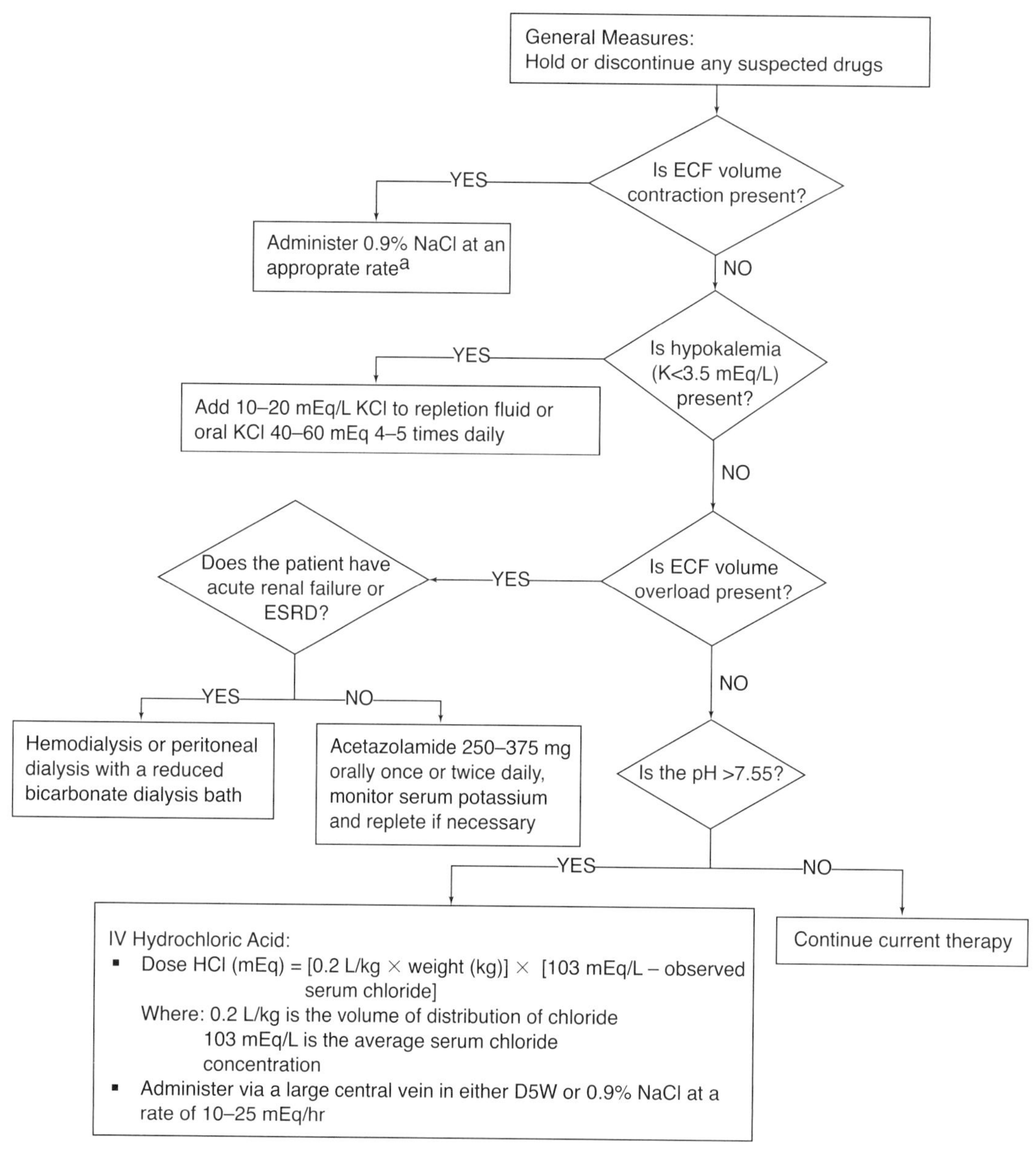

FIGURE 44-3 Treatment of Metabolic Alkalosis

ECF = extracellular fluid, ESRD = end-stage renal disease, HCl = hydrochloric acid, KCl = potassium chloride, NaCl = sodium chloride.
[a]For severe dehydration, administer 1 L 0.9% NaCl over 30 minutes followed by a second liter over the next hour. Repeat physical examination and electrolytes to determine subsequent rate of administration.

Table 44-15 Treatment Options for Management of Drug-Induced Respiratory Alkalosis[98]

- Hold or discontinue any suspected drugs
- Initiate oxygen therapy in patients with severe hypoxemia (partial pressure of oxygen <40 mm Hg)
- Rebreathing techniques are effective in patients with hyperventilation due to anxiety
- Treat theophylline and salicylate overdoses appropriately

REFERENCES

1. Devlin J, Matzke G. Acid-base disorders. In: Dipiro J, Talbert R, Yee G et al., eds. *Pharmacotherapy: a pathophysiologic approach.* 9th ed. New York, NY: McGraw-Hill Education; 2014:797-816.
2. Byrd RP. Respiratory acidosis. Medscape. http://emedicine.medscape.com/article/301574-overview (accessed 2018 Mar 6).
3. Seifter JL. Integration of acid-base and electrolyte disorders. *N Engl J Med.* 2014; 371:1821-31.
4. Raoof S, George L, Saleh A, Sung A. Manual of critical care. In: Saydain G, Feinfeld DA, eds. *Acid-base disorders.* New York, NY: McGraw-Hill; 2009:494-7.

5. Btaiche IF, Khalidi N. Metabolic complications of parenteral nutrition in adults, part 1. *Am J Health-Syst Pharm.* 2004; 61:1938-49.
6. Talpers SS, Romberger DJ, Bunce SB, Pingleton SK. Nutritionally associated increased carbon dioxide production. Excess total calories vs high proportion of carbohydrate calories. *Chest.* 1992; 102:551-5.
7. Klein CJ, Stanek GS, Wiles CE. Overfeeding macronutrients to critically ill adults: Metabolic complications. *J Am Diet Assoc.* 1998; 98:795-806.
8. Dubose TD. Acidosis and alkalosis. In: Kasper D, Fauci A, Hauser S et al., *Harrison's principles of internal medicine.* 19th ed. New York, NY: McGraw-Hill Education; 2015.
9. Dahan A. Opioid-induced respiratory effects: New data on buprenorphine. *Palliat Med.* 2006; 20(suppl 1):s3-8.
10. Ogedegbe AE, Thomas DL, Diehl AM. Hyperlactataemia syndromes associated with HIV therapy. *Lancet Infect Dis.* 2003; 3:329-37.
11. Sirtori CR, Pasik C. Re-evaluation of a biguanide, metformin: Mechanism of action and tolerability. *Pharmacological Research.* 1994; 30:187-228.
12. Lalau JD, Race JM. Lactic acidosis in metformin-treated patients. Prognostic value of arterial lactate levels and plasma metformin concentrations. *Drug Saf.* 1999; 20:377-84.
13. Kam PC, Cardone D. Propofol infusion syndrome. *Anaesthesia.* 2007; 62:690-701.
14. Corbett SM, Montoya ID, Moore FA. Propofol-related infusion syndrome in intensive care patients. *Pharmacotherapy.* 2008; 28:250-8.
15. Neale BW, Mesler EL, Young M et al. Propylene glycol-induced lactic acidosis in a patient with normal renal function: A proposed mechanism and monitoring recommendations. *Ann Pharmacother.* 2005; 39:1732-6.
16. Forsythe SM, Schmidt GA. Sodium bicarbonate for the treatment of lactic acidosis. *Chest.* 2000; 117:260-7.
17. Adrogue HJ, Madias NE. Management of life-threatening acid-base disorders. First of two parts. *N Engl J Med.* 1998; 338:26-34.
18. Arici C, Tebaldi A, Quinzan GP et al. Severe lactic acidosis and thiamine administration in an HIV-infected patient on HAART. *Int J STD AIDS.* 2001; 12:407-9.
19. Dalton SD, Rahimi AR. Emerging role of riboflavin in the treatment of nucleoside analogue-induced type B lactic acidosis. *AIDS Patient Care & Stds.* 2001; 15:611-4.
20. Gunthard HF, Aberg JA, Eron JJ et al. Antiretroviral treatment of adult HIV infection: 2014 recommendations of the International Antiviral Society-USA panel. *JAMA.* 2014; 312:410-25.
21. Parker MG, Fraser GL, Watson DM, Riker RR. Removal of propylene glycol and correction of increased osmolar gap by hemodialysis in a patient on high dose lorazepam infusion therapy. *Intensive Care Med.* 2002; 28:81-4.
22. Akoglu H, Akan B, Piskinpasa S et al. Metformin-associated lactic acidosis treated with prolonged hemodialysis. *Am J Emerg Med.* 2011; 29:575.e3-575.e5.
23. Laforest C, Saint-Marcoux F, Amiel JB et al. Monitoring of metformin-induced lactic acidosis in a diabetic patient with acute kidney failure and effect of hemodialysis. *Int J Clin Pharmacol Ther.* 2013; 51:147-51.
24. Marhong J, Fan E. Carbon dioxide in the critically ill: Too much or too little of a good thing? *Respir Care.* 2014; 59:1597-605.
25. Hodgkin JE, Soeprono FF, Chan DM. Incidence of metabolic alkalemia in hospitalized patients. *Crit Care Med.* 1980; 8:725-8.
26. Luke RG, Galla JH. It is chloride depletion alkalosis, not contraction alkalosis. *J Am Soc Nephrol.* 2012; 23:204-7.
27. Foster GT, Vaziri ND, Sassoon CS. Respiratory alkalosis. *Respir Care.* 2001; 46:384-91.
28. Greenstone M, Lasserson TJ. Doxapram for ventilatory failure due to exacerbations of chronic obstructive pulmonary disease. *Cochrane Database Syst Rev.* 2003; CD000223.
29. Moser KM, Luchsinger PC, Adamson JS et al. Respiratory stimulation with intravenous doxapram in respiratory failure. A double-blind co-operative study. *N Engl J Med.* 1973; 288:427-31.
30. Shelton PS, Barnett FL, Krick SE. Hyperventilation associated with quetiapine. *Ann Pharmacother.* 2000; 34:335-7.
31. Soifer JT KH. Approach to metabolic alkalosis. *Emerg Med Clin North Am.* 2014; 32:453-63.
32. Galla JH. Metabolic alkalosis. *J Am Soc Nephrol.* 2000; 11:369-75.
33. Anderson LE, Henrich WL. Alkalemia-associated morbidity and mortality in medical and surgical patients. *South Med J.* 1987; 80:729-33.
34. Dafnis E, Sabatini S. Respiratory alkalosis and acidosis. In: Massry SG, Glassock RJ, eds. *Massry & Glassock's textbook of nephrology.* 4th ed. Philadelphia, PA: Lippincott Williams and Wilkins; 2000.
35. Patel AM, Goldfarb S. Got calcium? Welcome to the calcium-alkali syndrome. *J Am Soc Nephrol.* 2010; 21:1440-3.
36. Arroyo M, Fenves AZ, Emmett M. The calcium-alkali syndrome. *Proceedings of Baylor University Medical Centre.* 2013; 26:179-81.
37. Johns C. Glycyrrhizic acid toxicity caused by consumption of licorice candy cigars. *Can J Emerg Med.* 2009; 11:94-6.
38. Yi J, Han S, Song J, Kim H. Metabolic alkalosis from unsuspected ingestion: use of urine pH and anion gap. *Am J Kidney Dis.* 2012; 59:577-81.
39. Bromley J, Hughes BG, Leong DC, Buckley NA. Life-threatening interaction between complementary medicines: cyanide toxicity following ingestion of amygdalin and vitamin C. *Ann Pharmacother.* 2005; 39:1566-9.
40. Kalyanaraman UP, Kalyanaraman K, Cullinan SA, McLean JM. Neuromyopathy of cyanide intoxication due to "laetrile" (amygdalin). A clinicopathologic study. *Cancer.* 1983; 51:2126-33.
41. Coronado BE, Opal SM, Yoburn DC. Antibiotic-induced D-lactic acidosis. *Ann Intern Med.* 1995; 122:839-42.
42. Liamis G, Milionis HJ, Elisaf M. Pharmacologically-induced metabolic acidosis: a review. *Drug Saf.* 2010; 33:371-91.
43. Dodda VR, Spiro P. Can albuterol be blamed for lactic acidosis? *Respir Care.* 2012; 57:2115-8.
44. Liem EB, Mnookin SC, Mahla ME. Albuterol-induced lactic acidosis. *Anesthesiology.* 2003; 99:505-6.
45. Saxena R, Marais G. Salbutamol: beware of the paradox! *BMJ Case Reports.* 2010.
46. Koh YI, Choi IS. Lactic acidosis associated with the usual theophylline dose in a patient with asthma. *Korean J Intern Med.* 2002; 17:147-9.
47. Kovacevic A, Schwahn B, Schuster A. Hyperlactic acidosis as metabolic side-effect of albuterol and theophylline in acute severe asthma. *Klin Padiatr.* 2010; 222:271-2.
48. Ching CK, Lai CK, Poon WT et al. Hazards posed by a banned drug—phenformin is still hanging around. *Hong Kong Medical Journal.* 2008; 14:50-4.
49. Krishnamurthy M, Sahouria JJ, Desai R, Caguiat J. Buformin-induced lactic acidosis—a symptom of modern healthcare malady. *J Am Geriatr Soc.* 2004; 52:1785.
50. Inzucchi SE, Lipska KJ, Mayo H et al. Metformin in patients with type 2 diabetes and kidney disease: a systematic review. *JAMA.* 2014; 312:2668-75.
51. James JH, Fischer JE. Epinephrine and gut lactate production. *Crit Care Med.* 2001; 29:454-5.
52. Totaro RJ, Raper RF. Epinephrine-induced lactic acidosis following cardiopulmonary bypass. *Crit Care Med.* 1997; 25:1693-9.
53. Uzman S, Uludag Yanaral T, Toptas M et al. Acute isoniazid intoxication: an uncommon cause of convulsion, coma and acidosis. *Tuberk Toraks.* 2013; 61:50-3.
54. Gokhale YA, Vaidya MS, Mehta AD, Rathod NN. Isoniazid toxicity presenting as status epilepticus and severe metabolic acidosis. *J Assoc Physicians India.* 2009; 57:70-1.
55. Hsu SN, Shih MF, Yang CW et al. Severe linezolid-induced lactic acidosis in a cirrhosis patient. *Nephrology.* 2015; 20:47-8.

56. Sawyer AJ, Haley HL, Baty SR et al. Linezolid-induced lactic acidosis corrected with sustained low-efficiency dialysis: a case report. *Am J Kid Dis*. 2014; 64:457-9.
57. Eizadi-Mood N. Nalidixic acid overdose and metabolic acidosis. *CJEM*. 2006; 8:78.
58. MacRae WR. Nitroprusside-induced metabolic acidosis. *Anesthesiology*. 1976; 45:578-9.
59. International Study Group. Risk factors for lactic acidosis and severe hyperlactataemia in HIV-1-infected adults exposed to antiretroviral therapy. *AIDS*. 2007; 21:2455-64.
60. Deters D, Metzler M, Morgan M et al. Propofol infusion syndrome associated with large-dose infusion for treatment of seizure activity. *DCCN - Dimensions of Critical Care Nursing*. 2013; 32:118-22.
61. Testerman GM, Chow TT, Easparam S. Propofol infusion syndrome: an algorithm for prevention. *Am Surg*. 2011; 77:1714-5.
62. Buijs EJ, van Zuylen HJ. Metabolic consequences of a sorbitol overdose during neurosurgery. *J Neurosurg Anesthesiol*. 1997; 9:17-20.
63. Thomas DW, Gilligan JE, Edwards JB, Edwards RG. Lactic acidosis and osmotic diuresis produced by xylitol infusion. *Med J Aust*. 1972; 1:1246-8.
64. Ramirez ME, Youseef WF, Romero RG et al. Acute percutaneous lactic acid poisoning in a child. *Pediatr Dermatol*. 2006; 23:282-5.
65. Madsen KR. Fatal hypertriglyceridaemia, acute pancreatitis and diabetic ketoacidosis possibly induced by quetiapine. *BMJ Case Reports*. 2014 Jan 8;2014. pii: bcr2013202039.
66. Heal DJ, Gosden J, Jackson HC et al. Metabolic consequences of antipsychotic therapy: preclinical and clinical perspectives on diabetes, diabetic ketoacidosis, and obesity. *Handb Exp Pharmacol*. 2012: 135-64.
67. Hodgman MJ, Horn JF, Stork CM et al. Profound metabolic acidosis and oxoprolinuria in an adult. *J Med Toxicol*. 2007; 3:119-24.
68. Ellenhorn MJ. Salicylates. In: Ellenhorn MJ, ed. *Ellenhorn's medical toxicology: diagnosis and treatment of human poisoning*. 2nd ed. Baltimore, MD: Lippincott Williams and Wilkins; 1997.
69. US Food and Drug Administration. Drug safety communication: FDA revises labels of SGLT2 inhibitors for diabetes to include warnings about too much acid in the blood and serious urinary tract infections Dec. 4, 2015. https://www.fda.gov/downloads/drugs/drugsafety/ucm475487.pdf (accessed 2018 Mar 6).
70. Emmett M. Acetaminophen toxicity and 5-oxoproline (pyroglutamic acid): a tale of two cycles, one an ATP-depleting futile cycle and the other a useful cycle. *Clin J Am Soc Nephrol*. 2014; 9:191-200.
71. Abkur TM, Mohammed W, Ali M, Casserly L. Acetaminophen-induced anion gap metabolic acidosis secondary to 5-oxoproline: a case report. *J Med Case Rep*. 2014; 8:409.
72. Selk N, Rodby RA. Unexpectedly severe metabolic acidosis associated with sodium thiosulfate therapy in a patient with calcific uremic arteriolopathy. *Semin Dial*. 2011; 24:85-8.
73. Page CB, Wilson PA, Foy A et al. Life-threatening hypokalaemia associated with ibuprofen-induced renal tubular acidosis. *Med J Aust*. 2011; 194:614.
74. Vaziri ND, Stokes J, Treadwell TR. Lactic acidosis, a complication of papaverine overdose. *Clin Toxicol*. 1981; 18:417-23.
75. Zapater P, Alba D. Acidosis and extreme hyperkalemia associated with cholestyramine and spironolactone. *Ann Pharmacother*. 1995; 29:199-200.
76. Scheel PJ, J., Whelton A, Rossiter K, Watson A. Cholestyramine-induced hyperchloremic metabolic acidosis. *J Clin Pharmacol*. 1992; 32:536-8.
77. Roerig JL, Steffen KJ, Mitchell JE, Zunker C. Laxative abuse: epidemiology, diagnosis and management. *Drugs*. 2010; 70:1487-503.
78. Pai AB, Shepler BM. Comparison of sevelamer hydrochloride and sevelamer carbonate: risk of metabolic acidosis and clinical implications. *Pharmacotherapy*. 2009; 29:554-61.
79. Sonikian MA, Pani IT, Iliopoulos AN et al. Metabolic acidosis aggravation and hyperkaliemia in hemodialysis patients treated by sevelamer hydrochloride. *Ren Fail*. 2005; 27:143-7.
80. Ho AM, Karmakar MK, Contardi LH et al. Excessive use of normal saline in managing traumatized patients in shock: a preventable contributor to acidosis. *J Trauma*. 2001; 51:173-7.
81. Kay TD, Hogan PG, McLeod SE, Johnson DW. Severe irreversible proximal renal tubular acidosis and azotaemia secondary to cidofovir. *Nephron*. 2000; 86:348-9.
82. Lehrich RW, Moll S, Luft FC. Evaluating a critically ill patient with metabolic acidosis: the ifosfamide paradigm. *Nephrol Dial Transplant*. 1999; 14:226-30.
83. Negro A, Grasselli C, Galli P. Oxaliplatin-induced proximal renal tubular acidosis. *Intern Emerg Med*. 2010; 5:267-8.
84. Hemstreet BA. Antimicrobial-associated renal tubular acidosis. *Ann Pharmacother*. 2004; 38:1031-8.
85. Fennell JS, Falls WF Jr. Streptozotocin nephrotoxicity: studies on the defect in renal tubular acidification. *Clin Nephrol*. 1981; 15:97-101.
86. Chusil S, Tungsanga K, Wathanavaha A, Pansin P. Hypouricemia, hypokalemia, proximal and distal tubular acidification defect following administration of outdated tetracycline: a case report. *J Med Assoc Thai*. 1994; 77:98-102.
87. Montoliu J, Carrera M, Darnell A, Revert L. Lactic acidosis and Fanconi's syndrome due to degraded tetracycline. *Br Med J (Clin Res Ed)*. 1981; 283:1576-7.
88. Kondo K, Fujiwara M, Murase M et al. Severe acute metabolic acidosis and Wernicke's encephalopathy following chemotherapy with 5-fluorouracil and cisplatin: case report and review of the literature. *Jpn J Clin Oncol*. 1996; 26:234-6.
89. Jefferson JW. Lithium and metabolic acidosis. *Ann Intern Med*. 1978; 88:434.
90. Epstein SK, Singh N. Respiratory acidosis. *Respir Care*. 2001; 46:366-83.
91. Madias NE, Adrogue HJ. Respiratory acid-base disorders. In: Seldin DW, Giebisch G, eds. *The kidney: physiology and pathophysiology*. 5th ed. New York, NY: Elsevier Academic Press; 2013:2113-36.
92. Casaletto JJ. Differential diagnosis of metabolic acidosis. *Emerg Med Clin North Am*. 2005; 23:771-87, ix.
93. Roussos C, Koutsoukou A. Respiratory failure. *Eur Respir J Suppl*. 2003; 47:3s-14s.
94. Kazazis C. A case of lactic acidosis (LA) after administration of tenofovir and metformin in a diabetic patient with recently diagnosed HIV infection. *J Ren Care*. 2011; 37:174.
95. Miller MA, Forni A, Yogaratnam D. Propylene glycol-induced lactic acidosis in a patient receiving continuous infusion pentobarbital. *Ann Pharmacother*. 2008; 42:1502-6.
96. Glover ML, Reed MD. Propylene glycol: the safe diluent that continues to cause harm. *Pharmacotherapy*. 1996; 16:690-3.
97. Demey HE, Daelemans RA, Verpooten GA et al. Propylene glycol-induced side effects during intravenous nitroglycerin therapy. *Intensive Care Med*. 1988; 14:221-6.
98. Varon J, Acosta P. *Handbook of critical and intensive care medicine*. 2nd ed. New York, NY: Springer; 2010.
99. Andreoli SP, Kleiman MB, Glick MR, Bergstein JM. Nafcillin, pseudoproteinuria, and hypokalemic alkalosis. *J Pediatr*. 1980; 97:841-2.
100. Brunner FP, Frick PG. Hypokalaemia, metabolic alkalosis, and hypernatraemia due to "massive" sodium penicillin therapy. *Br Med J*. 1968; 4:550-2.
101. Panda PS, Dube SK, Sarkar S, Singh DK. Metabolic alkalosis: a less appreciated side effect of imipenem-cilastatin use. *Indian J Crit Care Med*. 2013; 17:263-4.
102. Bhagwat A, Goel N, Sharma R et al. Meropenem: a unusual cause of metabolic alkalosis in critical care patients. *Anaesth Intensive Care*. 2008; 36:745-6.

103. Chou CL, Chen YH, Chau T, Lin SH. Acquired Bartter-like syndrome associated with gentamicin administration. *Am J Med Sci.* 2005; 329:144-9.

104. Chen YS, Fang HC, Chou KJ et al. Gentamicin-induced Bartter-like syndrome. *Am J Kidney Dis.* 2009; 54:1158-61.

105. Chrispal A, Boorugu H, Prabhakar AT, Moses V. Amikacin-induced type 5 Bartter-like syndrome with severe hypocalcemia. *J Postgrad Med.* 2009; 55:208-10.

106. Geara AS, Parikh A, Rekhtman Y, Rao MK. The case mid R: metabolic alkalosis in a patient with cystic fibrosis. *Kidney Int.* 2012; 81:421-2.

107. Panichpisal K, Angulo-Pernett F, Selhi S, Nugent KM. Gitelman-like syndrome after cisplatin therapy: a case report and literature review. *BMC Nephrol.* 2006; 7:10.

108. Field MJ, Lawrence JR. Complications of thiazide diuretic therapy: an update. *Med J Aust.* 1986; 144:641-4.

109. Bohmig GA, Schmaldienst S, Horl WH, Mayer G. Iatrogenic hypercalcaemia, hypokalaemia and metabolic alkalosis in a lady with vena cava thrombosis—beware of overzealous diuretic treatment. *Nephrol Dial Transplant.* 1999; 14:782-4.

110. Burns A, Brown TM, Semple P. Extreme metabolic alkalosis with fludrocortisone therapy. *Postgrad Med J.* 1983; 59:506-7.

111. Ishiguchi T, Mikita N, Iwata T et al. Myoclonus and metabolic alkalosis from licorice in antacid. *Intern Med.* 2004; 43:59-62.

112. Gawarammana IB, Coburn J, Greene S et al. Severe hypokalaemic metabolic alkalosis following ingestion of gaviscon. *Clin Toxicol.* 2007; 45:176-8.

113. Okada H, Inoue T, Takahira S et al. Daytime hypertension, sleep apnea and metabolic alkalosis in a haemodialysis patient—the result of sodium bicarbonate abuse. *Nephrol Dial Transplant.* 1999; 14:452-4.

114. Sahani MM, Brennan JF, Nwakanma C et al. Metabolic alkalosis in a hemodialysis patient after ingestion of a large amount of an antacid medication. *Artif Organs.* 2001; 25:313-5.

115. Al-Abri SA, Olson KR. Baking soda can settle the stomach but upset the heart: case files of the medical toxicology fellowship at the University of California, San Francisco. *J Med Toxicol.* 2013; 9:255-8.

116. Ziessman HA. Alkalosis and seizure due to a cation-exchange resin and magnesium hydroxide. *South Med J.* 1976; 69:497-9.

117. Fernandez PC, Kovnat PJ. Metabolic acidosis reversed by the combination of magnesium hydroxide and a cation-exchange resin. *N Engl J Med.* 1972; 286:23-4.

118. Maini AA, Maxwell-Scott H, Marks DJ. Severe alkalosis and hypokalemia with stanozolol misuse. *Am J Emerg Med.* 2014; 32:196.e3-196.e4.

119. Orr-Walker BJ, Horne AM, Evans MC et al. Hormone replacement therapy causes a respiratory alkalosis in normal postmenopausal women. *J Clin Endocrinol Metab.* 1999; 84:1997-2001.

120. Hall KW, Dobson KE, Dalton JG et al. Metabolic abnormalities associated with intentional theophylline overdose. *Ann Intern Med.* 1984; 101:457-62.

121. Gokel Y, Satar S, Sebe A. Loratadine toxicity. *Am J Emerg Med.* 2000; 18:639-40.

122. Lynn RR, Galinkin JL. Naloxone dosage for opioid reversal: current evidence and clinical implications. *Ther Adv Drug Saf.* 2018; 9:63-88.

SECTION X

DRUG-INDUCED HEMATOLOGICAL DISORDERS

Chapter 45 Bleeding Disorders

Chapter 46 Thrombocytopenia

Chapter 47 Thromboembolic Diseases

Chapter 48 Neutropenia and Agranulocytosis

Chapter 49 Anemias

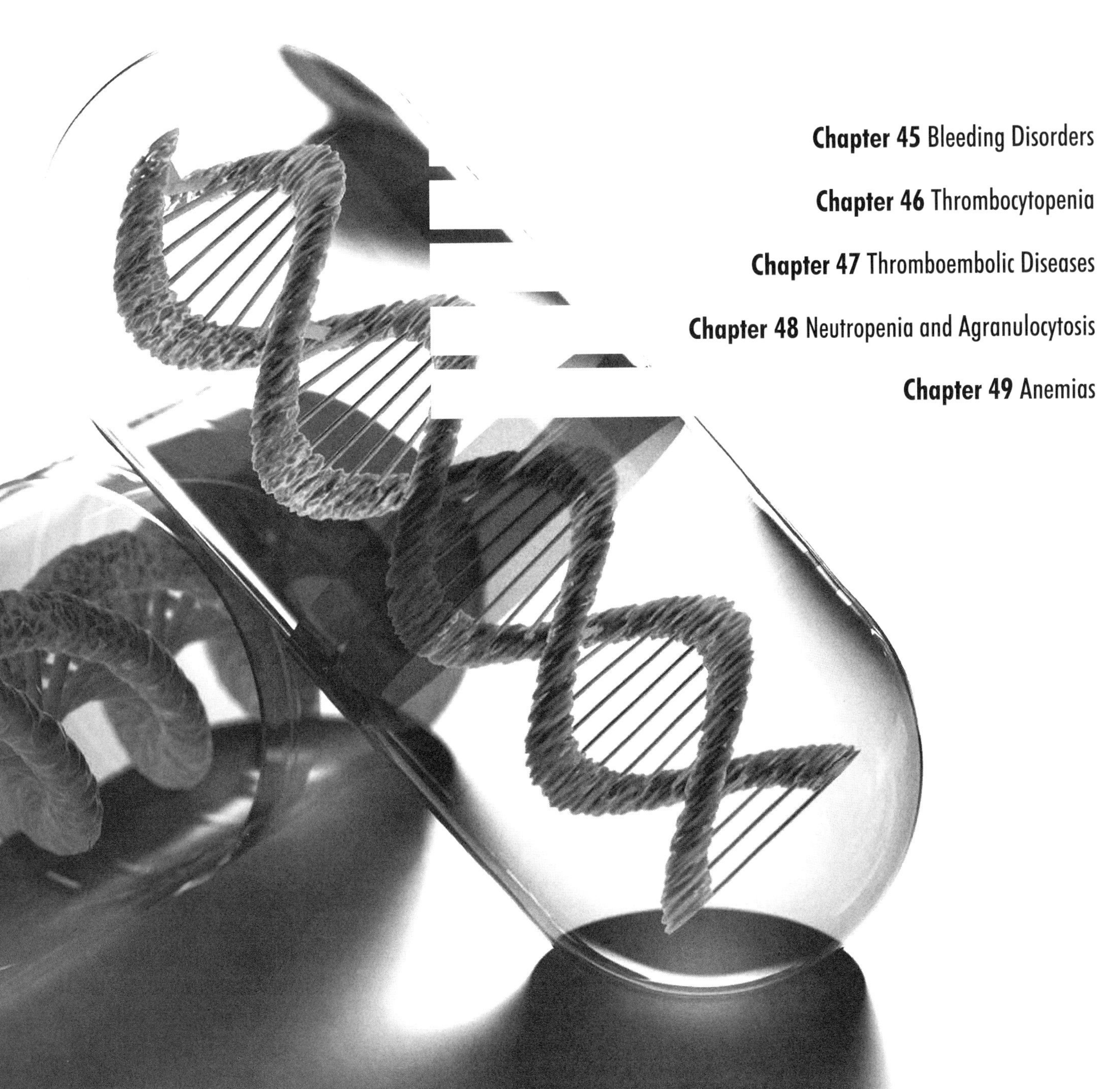

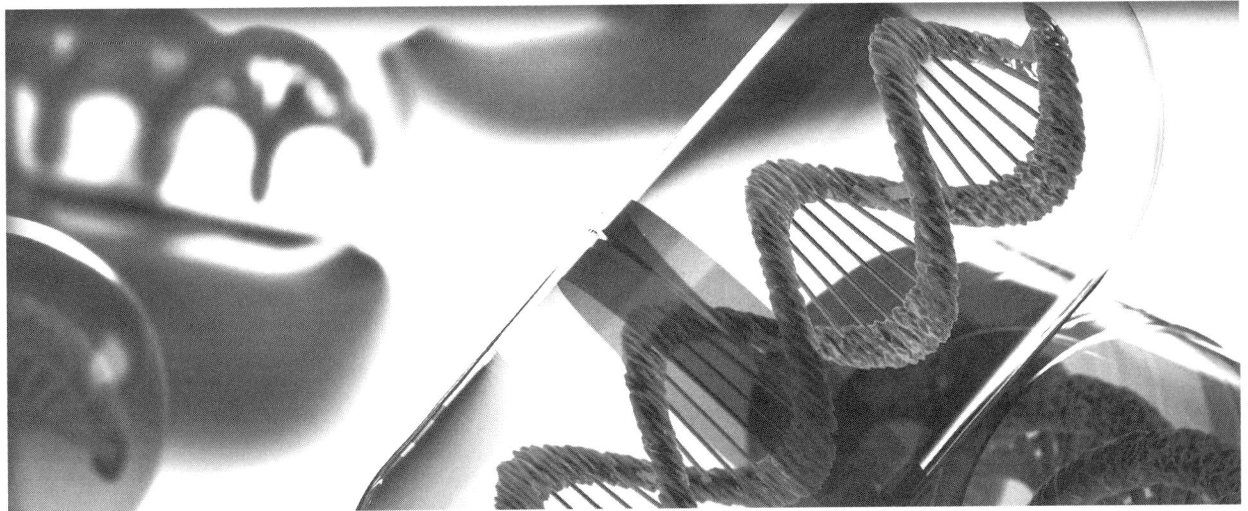

CHAPTER 45

Bleeding Disorders

Tiffany Pon and Jaekyu Shin

Drug-induced bleeding is a common problem. In this chapter, we use the term *drug-induced* to describe situations in which drugs cause, exacerbate, or increase the risk of bleeding. As anticoagulant and antiplatelet therapies have become the mainstay of treatment for various cardiovascular diseases, the utilization of drugs that increase bleeding risk has grown. From 1995 to 2002, the percentage of patients with atrial fibrillation who received an anticoagulant increased from 40.3% to 49.1%.[1] Furthermore, patients may take multiple drugs that increase bleeding risk, and polypharmacy greatly increases the risk of drug-induced bleeding as many agents are prone to drug–drug interactions and have narrow therapeutic indices. Drug-induced bleeding events not only lead to morbidity and mortality but they are also costly. In one study, mean unadjusted all-cause health costs in the first year after warfarin initiation for atrial fibrillation was approximately $42,000 for patients with at least one intracranial bleed compared with $24,000 for patients without bleeding.[2] As a result, many of the drugs discussed in this chapter are considered high-alert medications by the Institute for Safe Medication Practices, and clinicians should be aware of how to prevent, recognize, and manage drug-induced bleeding.

CAUSATIVE AGENTS

Drugs associated with bleeding can be divided primarily into two groups: those that affect hemostasis through inhibition of the coagulation cascade and platelet aggregation pathways and those that exert direct toxicity (**Table 45-1**).[3-152]

Drugs that impair hemostasis include anticoagulants, thrombolytics, and antiplatelet agents, and they are intended to treat or prevent thrombosis. Thus, while they do not directly cause bleeding, they can exacerbate or increase the risk of bleeding from other causes. In contrast, nonsteroidal anti-inflammatory drugs (NSAIDs) primarily increase bleeding risk by inhibiting prostaglandin synthesis in the upper gastrointestinal mucosa, causing direct damage.[153]

Aspirin falls into both groups because it exerts similar direct gastrointestinal toxicity as NSAIDs, but it also affects hemostasis through inhibition of platelet aggregation.[154] Finally, selective serotonin reuptake inhibitors (SSRIs) are thought to increase bleeding risk through inhibition of platelet

Table 45-1 Agents Implicated in Drug-Induced Bleeding

Drug	Incidence	Level of Evidence[a]
ANTICOAGULANTS		
Direct oral thrombin inhibitors[10,11,37-40]	9.7–16.1% (all[b]); 0.–1.4% (major[c])	A
Direct oral Xa inhibitors[6,9,12-28]	4.9–21.7% (all); <0.1%–0.8% (major)	A
Fondaparinux[29-36]	1.0–5.3% (all); 0.1–2.2% (major)	A
IV direct thrombin inhibitors[41-59]	3.2–12.5% (all); 0–13.8 (major)	A, B
Low-molecular-weight heparin[5,7,25,27,28,32-35,58,60-80]	0.6–25.4% (all); 0–9.1% (major)	A
Unfractionated heparin[31,32,36,65,69-75,77,78,80,81]	2.1–18.4% (all); 0.1–8.3% (major)	A
Vitamin K antagonists[3-12]	13.2–25.8%/yr (all); 2.2–3.43% (major)	A
ANTIPLATELET DRUGS		
Anagrelide[128,129]	11.3–18.9% (all); 4.1% (major)	A, B
Aspirin[62,82-90]	1.8–16.1% (all);1.3%/yr–3.9% (major)	A
Aspirin plus dipyridamole[88,89,91]	1.19%/yr; 0.09%/yr–4.1% (major)	A
Cilostazole[122-125]	0.7–4% (all); 0% (major)	A
Dipyridamole[88-89]	15.1% (all); 2.6% (major)	A
GPIIb/IIIa inhibitors[106-121]	3–23.5% (all); 0.2–10.6% (major)	A
IV P2Y12 receptor antagonists[102-105]	0.3–11.8% (all); 0.1–0.4% (major)	A
Oral P2Y12 receptor antagonists[84-87,89,92-101]	0.1–11.4% (all); 0.1–7.9% (major)	A
OTHER AGENTS		
Defibrotide[150,d]	1% (all)	A
NSAIDs[130-134]	6.0% (all); 0.4–4.9% (GI bleed)	A, B
SSRIs[151,152]	0.4–0.6% (GI bleed)	B
Thrombolytics[135-149]	20.3–32% (all); 2.7–10% (major)	A
Vorapaxar[126,127,e]	2.8–3.2 (major)	A

GI = gastrointestinal, GPIIb/IIIa inhibitors = glycoprotein IIb/IIIa inhibitors, IV = intravenous, NSAID = nonsteroidal anti-inflammatory drug, SSRI = selective serotonin reuptake inhibitor.

[a]Definitions for Levels of Evidence: Level A—evidence from one or more randomized, controlled clinical trials; Level B—evidence from nonrandomized clinical trials, prospective observational studies, cohort studies, retrospective studies, case-control studies, meta-analyses and/or postmarketing surveillance studies; and Level C—evidence from one or more published case reports or case series.

[b]All-cause bleeding.

[c]Major bleeding.

[d]Incidences of major bleeding were not reported.

[e]Incidences of all-cause bleeding were not reported.

aggregation; however, there is also evidence that they may directly increase gastric acidity, which increases the risk of ulceration and gastrointestinal bleeding.[155,156]

EPIDEMIOLOGY

The incidence of drug-induced bleeding has been reported in multiple randomized clinical trials, and risk differs by drug class (Table 45-1). The site of bleeding is often also a function of drug class. Vitamin K antagonists (VKAs) are more likely to cause intracranial hemorrhage (ICH) than direct oral anticoagulants (DOACs), whereas DOACs are more likely to cause gastrointestinal bleeding than VKAs, and upper gastrointestinal bleeding is highly associated with aspirin and NSAIDs.[6,9,11,12,90,130,131] Moreover, drug-induced bleeding may differ by ethnicity, with Caucasians possibly having a lower risk of drug-induced bleeding.[157-159]

The true incidence of drug-induced bleeding, however, is not completely clear because it is impacted by several factors. Some factors relate to study design (e.g., inconsistent bleeding classifications and definitions, varying study durations, and different statistical methods), and other factors include concomitant medication use and continuously evolving practice standards.

Classifications of bleeding have included major, fatal, life-threatening, serious, excessive, clinically significant, overt, trivial, minor, nuisance bleeding events, and more, and the definitions of these classifications have also differed among trials. Criteria used in selected clinical trials involving nonsurgical patients are listed in **Table 45-2**.

Clinical trials of longer duration typically report a higher incidence of bleeding compared to trials of shorter duration, and this may be due to the use of different methods to calculate the incidence of bleeding events. Although percent incidence is most commonly used to describe risk, percent per year and incidence rates such as person-years have also been used.

Concomitant use of multiple medications that can induce or exacerbate bleeding also confounds determination of the true incidence of bleeding for each individual drug. Virtually all trials evaluating clopidogrel in acute coronary syndrome included patients who also took aspirin, and patients who were assigned to a glycoprotein (GP) IIb/IIIa inhibitor often received unfractionated heparin (UFH) at the same time.

Table 45-2 Bleeding Definitions

Criteria	Bleeding Definition
Thrombolysis in Myocardial Infarction (TIMI)[160]	• Major: ○ Any intracranial bleeding (excluding hemorrhages <10 mm evident only on gradient-echo magnetic resonance imaging scan) ○ Clinically overt signs of hemorrhage associated with a drop in hemoglobin of ≥5 g/dL ○ Fatal bleeding (bleeding that directly results in death within 7 days) • Minor: Clinically overt, resulting in hemoglobin drop of 3–5 g/dL • Requiring medical attention: Any overt sign of hemorrhage that meets one of the following criteria and does not meet criteria for a major or minor bleeding event, as defined above: ○ Requiring intervention (medical practitioner-guided medical or surgical treatment to stop or treat bleeding, including temporarily or permanently discontinuing or changing the dose of a medication or study drug) ○ Leading to or prolonging hospitalization ○ Prompting evaluation (leading to an unscheduled visit to a healthcare professional and diagnostic testing, either laboratory or imaging)
Global Use of Strategies to Open Occluded Arteries (GUSTO)[160]	• Severe or life-threatening bleeding: ○ Intracerebral hemorrhage ○ Resulting in substantial hemodynamic compromise requiring treatment • Moderate: Requiring blood transfusion but not resulting in hemodynamic compromise • Mild: Bleeding that does not meet above criteria
International Society on Thrombosis and Haemostasis (ISTH)[161,162]	• Major bleeding: ○ Fatal bleeding, and/or ○ Symptomatic bleeding in a critical area or organ, such as intracranial, intraspinal, intraocular, retroperitoneal, intraarticular or pericardial, or intramuscular with compartment syndrome, and/or ○ Bleeding causing a fall in hemoglobin level of 2 g/dL or more, or leading to transfusion of two or more units of whole blood or red cells • Clinically relevant nonmajor bleeding: ○ Any sign or symptom of hemorrhage (e.g., more bleeding than would be expected for a clinical circumstance, including bleeding found by imaging alone) that does not fit the criteria for the ISTH definition of major bleeding but does meet at least one of the following criteria: ▪ Requiring medical intervention by a healthcare professional ▪ Leading to hospitalization or increased level of care ▪ Prompting a face-to-face (i.e., not just a telephone or electronic communication) evaluation

In addition to combination therapy, clinical trial protocols may not represent current clinical practice, and this can also confound determination of true bleeding incidence. The majority of trials testing GPIIb/IIIa inhibitors, for example, did not use a P2Y12 antagonist during percutaneous coronary intervention (PCI) despite this being a current standard of practice, and many venous thromboembolism (VTE) trials assessing UFH used a different dose than that used currently in most practices.[77,78,163] As a result, it is difficult to compare the incidence of bleeding events between the trials.

MECHANISMS

The coagulation cascade pathway involves a series of serine proteases leading to the eventual generation of fibrin (**Figure 45-1**). The platelet aggregation pathway provides platelet plugs via the following events: adhesion of platelets, change in platelet shape, release of stimulators from granules such as adenosine diphosphate (ADP) and thromboxane A2 (TXA2), recruitment of additional platelets, and aggregation of platelets. Importantly, these two pathways are interconnected. For example, thrombin, which cleaves fibrinogen to fibrin in the coagulation cascade pathway, is a powerful stimulator of platelet aggregation.[164] In addition, the activation of the coagulation cascade largely takes place on the surface of activated platelets.[164]

ANTICOAGULANTS

Anticoagulants inhibit the activity or production of one or more serine proteases in the coagulation cascade pathway and can be divided into two groups: (1) drugs that directly block the activity of the pre-existing coagulation factors and (2) drugs that inhibit the production of coagulation factors (Table 45-3).

In the first group, some drugs inhibit one specific coagulation factor whereas others block multiple factors. Direct factor Xa inhibitors (apixaban, rivaroxaban, and edoxaban) inhibit only factor Xa. Low-molecular-weight heparins (LMWHs) block both factor Xa and thrombin, although they have a higher affinity for factor Xa.[165] UFH and LMWHs require an endogenous molecule, antithrombin, for full anticoagulation activity; antithrombin is necessary for these agents to inhibit both thrombin and factor Xa and provide an anticoagulant effect.[165]

The second group includes VKAs. Vitamin K is an essential cofactor for the posttranslational γ-carboxylation of glutamyl residues on the vitamin-K–dependent coagulation factors (II, VII, IX, and X). VKAs also target vitamin K epoxide reductase, a substance involved in the process of vitamin K recycling.[166,167] As a result, VKAs reduce the production of functional vitamin-K–dependent coagulation factors.

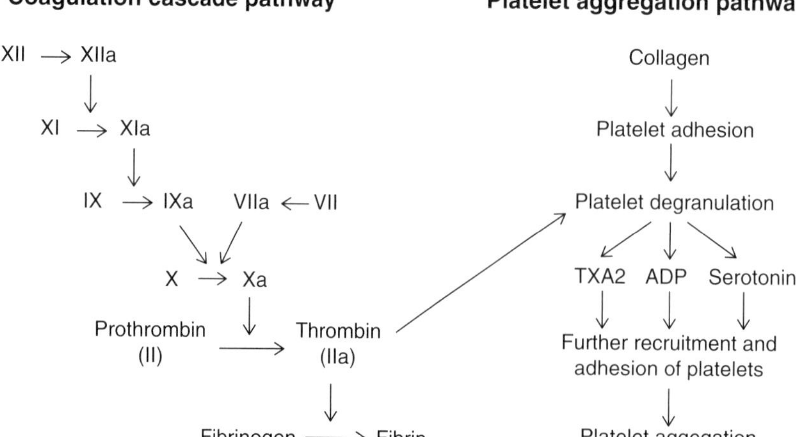

FIGURE 45-1 Coagulation Cascade and Platelet Aggregation Pathways

ADP = adenosine diphosphate, TXA2 = thromboxane A2.

ANTIPLATELET DRUGS

Antiplatelet drugs can be divided into two groups according to their site of action in the platelet aggregation pathway. Agents in the first group antagonize stimulators of platelet aggregation, and those in the second group interfere with the binding of stimulated platelets to each other (Table 45-3).

Aspirin, clopidogrel, prasugrel, ticagrelor, cangrelor, ticlopidine, dipyridamole, vorapaxar, and cilostazole belong to the first group. Aspirin inhibits cyclooxygenase (COX), an enzyme important in generating TXA2, a stimulator of platelet aggregation. P2Y12 antagonists block the binding of ADP, another stimulator of platelet aggregation, to its receptors on platelets. Dipyridamole does not antagonize platelet receptors, but instead interferes with uptake of ADP into platelets. Thrombin stimulates the platelet aggregation pathway; it does this by binding to protease activated receptors (PAR) on platelets. Vorapaxar antagonizes PAR on platelets. Cilostazol is a phosphodiesterase III inhibitor that increases the concentration of cyclic adenosine monophosphate, a secondary messenger important in preventing platelet aggregation. The second group, GPIIb/IIIa receptor antagonists, directly antagonizes the binding of fibrinogen to GPIIb/IIIa receptors on platelets, a critical step in platelet plug formation.

Table 45-3 Mechanism of Drug-Induced Bleeding

Drugs	Mechanism
ANTICOAGULANTS	
Direct factor Xa inhibitors (apixaban, edoxaban, fondaparinux, rivaroxaban)	Inhibition of factor Xa
Direct thrombin inhibitors (argatroban, bivalirudin, dabigatran)	Inhibition of thrombin (factor II)
Low-molecular-weight heparin (e.g., dalteparin, enoxaparin, tinzaparin, etc.)	Inhibition of both thrombin and factor Xa
Unfractionated heparin	Inhibition of both thrombin and factor Xa
Vitamin K antagonists (acenocoumarol, fluindione, phenprocoumon, warfarin)	Depletion of coagulation factors II, VII, IX, and X
ANTIPLATELET DRUGS	
Anagrelide	Interference with maturation of megakaryocytes
Aspirin	Inhibition of production of TXA2 by inhibiting COX
Cilostazol	Inhibition of phosphodiesterase III
Dipyridamole	Inhibition of uptake of adenosine by platelets
Glycoprotein IIb/IIIa inhibitors (abciximab, eptifibatide, tirofiban)	Prevention of fibrinogen from binding by blocking glycoprotein IIb/IIIa receptors on platelets
P2Y12 receptor antagonists (cangrelor, clopidogrel, prasugrel, ticagrelor, ticlopidine)	Inhibition of adenosine diphosphate receptors on platelets
OTHER AGENTS	
Defibrotide	Increasing tissue-type plasminogen activator function and decreasing plasminogen activator inhibitor-1 activity
NSAIDs	Inhibition of production of TXA2 by blocking COX
SSRIs	Inhibition of serotonin uptake by platelets
Thrombolytics (alteplase, reteplase, tenecteplase)	Degradation of fibrin by activating plasminogen to plasmin
Vorapaxar	Prevention of thrombin from binding to protease-activated receptors on platelets

COX = cyclooxygenase, NSAID = nonsteroidal anti-inflammatory drug, SSRI = selective serotonin reuptake inhibitor, TXA2 = thromboxane A2.

NSAIDs

Like aspirin, NSAIDs inhibit COX, reducing the production of TXA2.[168] Unlike aspirin, which is an irreversible COX inhibitor, NSAIDs are reversible inhibitors. As a result, their antiplatelet effect depends, in part, on their half-lives, and NSAIDs with short half-lives (e.g., ibuprofen) do not have sustained antiplatelet effects. As COX-1 is more responsible for generating TXA2, NSAIDs with a higher specificity for COX-2 (e.g., celecoxib) may have reduced antiplatelet effect compared to those without COX-2 selectivity.[169] Additionally, by inhibiting COX, aspirin and NSAIDs prevent the synthesis of prostaglandins and inhibit their mucosal-protective effects most notably in the gastrointestinal tract.[170]

SSRIs

SSRIs also exhibit an antiplatelet effect. Serotonin stimulates platelet aggregation. By inhibiting the uptake of serotonin into platelets, SSRIs interfere with this process. The antiplatelet effects of SSRIs may be weak because serotonin is a weak stimulator of platelet aggregation.[156]

THROMBOLYTICS

Thrombolytics are analogs of human tissue plasminogen activator (t-PA). Plasmin, an enzyme degrading fibrin, is converted from a precursor, plasminogen, and this conversion is facilitated by t-PA. Thrombolytics facilitate the degradation of fibrin.[171] Among the drug classes listed in Table 45-1, thrombolytics are generally considered to have the highest bleeding risk followed by anticoagulants, although direct comparison is lacking.

CLINICAL PRESENTATION AND DIFFERENTIAL DIAGNOSIS

Abnormal laboratory values, changes in vital signs, and other physical findings (**Table 45-4**) can suggest the presence of bleeding. Decreased hemoglobin and hematocrit levels are common signs of bleeding and sudden drops in hemoglobin and hematocrit in a patient receiving a drug known to cause or exacerbate bleeding may indicate drug-induced bleeding.[160] Activated partial thromboplastin time (aPTT), prothrombin time (PT), and international normalized ratio (INR) can be elevated, particularly in patients receiving anticoagulants. A substantial loss of blood can compromise hemodynamics, resulting in hemorrhagic shock.[172]

Table 45-4 Signs and Symptoms Associated with Drug-Induced Bleeding

- Bruises, ecchymosis
- Decrease in blood pressure, increase in heart rate
- Decrease in hemoglobin and hematocrit levels
- Decreased or hazy vision, floating objects in the vision, blindness (bleeding in the eye)
- Dizziness, lightheadedness, fainting, loss of consciousness
- Elevation of coagulation test results (e.g., activated partial thromboplastin time, prothrombin time, international normalized ratio) in patients on an anticoagulant
- Fatigue, lethargy, coma
- Hematemesis, melena, hematochezia
- Hematuria
- Pain, swelling in the area of bleeding
- Positive guaiac test
- Symptoms of stroke (inability to speak, facial droop, inability to move part of body, nausea, vomiting, seizure)

Other signs and symptoms of bleeding may be site specific. A patient with gastrointestinal bleeding may present with melena and a positive guaiac test result, whereas a patient with intracranial bleeding may show symptoms of stroke (e.g., facial droop, inability to speak).[173,174] Pain can also occur if a hemotoma compresses an organ or nerve ending.

A careful medication history can help clinicians identify the most likely culprit drug(s) and the possible site(s) of bleeding. Additional laboratory tests (e.g., occult blood) and/or imaging modalities (e.g., computed tomography) can then be used to confirm the diagnosis.

Many disease states can cause signs and symptoms similar to those seen with drug-induced bleeding (**Table 45-5**), and some diseases can cause bleeding themselves. Iron-deficiency anemia and anemia of chronic disease, for example, decrease hemoglobin levels, and patients with end-stage liver disease typically have elevated INR values. In addition, ischemic

Table 45-5 Conditions to Consider in the Differential Diagnosis of Drug-Induced Bleeding

- Anemia
- Cancer (bladder, colon, rectal)
- Esophageal variceal bleeding
- Hypotension
- Liver cirrhosis, end-stage liver disease
- Shock
- Stroke
- Syncope
- Trauma
- Tuberculosis

stroke can cause symptoms that may be indistinguishable from those of drug-induced hemorrhagic stroke. Liver cirrhosis can lead to esophageal variceal bleeding by increasing portal vein pressure gradient, and bladder cancer can cause hematuria. Careful medical and medication histories as well as appropriate laboratory tests and imaging are essential to differentiate among the various causes and to arrive at a timely and accurate diagnosis.

RISK FACTORS

Bleeding risk factors are summarized in **Table 45-6**. Common risk factors include older age, female sex, small body habitus, excessive anticoagulation, polypharmacy, prior history of bleeding, anemia, and liver or kidney disease.[175-177] With respect to invasive procedures, the duration of the procedure itself, the choice of access site (e.g., selection of the femoral versus radial artery during PCI), and the use of open versus laparoscopic/arthroscopic procedures can influence bleeding risk.[177-179]

Drug-specific bleeding risk factors include genetic polymorphisms and drug–drug interactions. Drugs have unique metabolic pathways, and genetic polymorphisms and concomitant administration of other drugs may influence a medication's metabolic pathway in ways that increase bleeding risk. Warfarin is metabolized by cytochrome P450 (CYP) 2C9. Carriers of a dysfunctional *CYP2C9* allele, such as *CYP2C9*2* and **3,* have an increased risk of bleeding compared with *CYP2C9*1/*1* (wild-type allele).[185,189]

Table 45-6 Risk Factors for Drug-Induced Bleeding

Common risk factors

- Age[175,177,180]
- Anemia[176]
- Body size (e.g., weight)
- Combination antithrombotic therapy (e.g., coadministration of antiplatelet drugs, NSAIDs, and/or anticoagulants)[178,179]
- Diabetes mellitus[183]
- Excessive alcohol intake[180]
- Hepatic dysfunction[180]
- History of bleeding[176,180]
- Hypertension[180]
- Initiation of an anticoagulant[175]
- Intensity of anticoagulation[175]
- Malignancy[180]
- Non-Caucasians[181]
- Previous stroke[97,180]
- Renal insufficiency[176,177]
- Sex[176,177]
- Thrombocytopenia[180,182]

Drug-specific risk factors

- Drug interactions increasing anticoagulation effect[184]

<u>Warfarin:</u>

- *CYP2C9* reduced functional allele (e.g., **2, *3*)[185,186]
- Decreased dietary intake of vitamin K (for VKA)
- Labile INR[187]

<u>Clopidogrel:</u>

- *CYP2C19* gain-of-function allele (e.g.,**17*)[188]

INR = international normalized ratio, NSAID = nonsteroidal anti-inflammatory drug, VKA = vitamin K antagonist.

Drugs that inhibit CYP2C9, such as fluconazole, metronidazole, amiodarone, and sulfamethoxazole–trimethoprim, can also increase the risk of bleeding in patients taking warfarin. Additionally, clopidogrel, a prodrug, is activated by CYP2C19. Carriers of the gain of function *CYP2C19*17* allele may have an increased risk of clopidogrel-associated bleeding compared with noncarriers of the allele because *CYP2C19*17* increases conversion of the inactive prodrug to active clopidogrel.[190]

Many risk assessment tools (e.g., HAS-BLED, HEMORR2HAGES, ATRIA) have been developed to stratify the risk of bleeding.[180,187,191] These tools have been validated in patients with atrial fibrillation; however, they may also prove useful in other situations such as in patients being treated for

Table 45-7 HAS-BLED Risk Assessment Scoring Systems[187]

Hypertension	1 point
Abnormal kidney or liver function	1 point for each (2 max)
Stroke	1 point
Bleeding (history, anemia, predisposition)	1 point
Labile INR	1 point
Elderly (≥65 yr)	1 point
Drugs and alcohol	1 point (antiplatelet treatment) 1 point (≥8 drinks/wk) 2 points for both
A score of 3 or above indicates a high bleeding risk	

VTE.[180,187,191,192] Each tool utilizes a scoring system to assign a value to each risk factor, the summed total providing an assessment of overall bleeding risk, which can be labeled as low, intermediate, or high. For example, HAS-BLED, which predicts 1-year risk of major bleeding, assigns 1 point for the presence of a risk factor listed in **Table 45-7**. Patients with a score ≥3 are considered to be at high bleeding risk.

Which tool provides the best assessment of risk is currently unknown.[193-195] In addition, many of the risk factors incorporated into the tools are also risk factors for thrombosis (and are also included in tools used to stratify the risk of thrombosis). For example, the CHA2DS2VASc score, a tool used to predict the risk of ischemic stroke in patients with atrial fibrillation, includes blood pressure, history of previous stroke, and age in its risk assessment.[196] A patient who is predicted to have a high risk of thrombosis based on the CHA2DS2VASc score, therefore, would also likely have a high risk of bleeding using HAS-BLED, HEMORR2HAGE, or ATRIA scores. Clinicians should be aware of these limitations when using these tools.

MORBIDITY AND MORTALITY

Hemorrhage is the most common and significant adverse event associated with anticoagulants, antiplatelet drugs, NSAIDs, and thrombolytics; however, morbidity and mortality vary among the different classes and incidences are not well established. Bleeding morbidity and mortality associated with SSRIs is even less well characterized, but their common concomitant use with anticoagulants, antiplatelet drugs, and NSAIDs can affect these outcomes.[197-200]

ANTICOAGULANTS

Anticoagulants are widely accepted as high-risk drugs with respect to medication errors that can cause morbidity and mortality.[201] Major bleeding associated with therapeutic anticoagulation has been linked to increased length of hospital stay, higher total hospitalization costs, and higher costs for outpatient medical service and emergency department claims.[202] Intravenous (IV) UFH infusions in particular come with a high propensity for error and high mortality rates when compared to warfarin and LMWH.[201] Bivalirudin has been associated with a lower incidence of bleeding than UFH (used alone or with GPIIb/IIIa inhibitor) when used for PCI; however, the effect on mortality is not clear.[56,57,203] Major bleeding secondary to therapeutic parenteral anticoagulation with UFH or LMWH in the intensive care unit (ICU) has been shown to increase length of ICU stay, overall hospital stay, and in-hospital mortality.[204,205]

Warfarin consistently tops the list of medications implicated in adverse drug event-related emergency department visits and admissions.[206,207] The bleeding frequency associated with warfarin is approximately 15% to 20% per year, with life-threatening bleeds occurring at a rate of 1% to 3% annually.[208,209] Major bleeding mortality associated with warfarin has been reported as high as 15%.[210] Warfarin-associated ICH is especially serious because of its significant morbidity and mortality.[211] In a prospective study of patients admitted for ICH, patients receiving warfarin had earlier and higher rates of mortality than others, and those who survived the bleeding event had significantly higher costs and increased lengths of hospital stay.[212] There are likely many factors that influence mortality with warfarin. One study demonstrated warfarin use increased the incidence of ICH with age and INR >3.5 associated with a significant increase in mortality.[213]

Compared to warfarin, DOACs are associated with reduced all-cause, vascular, and bleeding mortality.[214] This benefit of reduced bleeding mortality, however, does not appear to apply to patients age 75 years or older.[215] In a single-center prospective cohort study of patients seen in the emergency department for severe bleeding from dabigatran, rivaroxaban, or apixaban, 83% were hospitalized with an average length of stay >1 week. Almost 30% of patients required an ICU level of care and 20% required reversal of the anticoagulant; 30-day mortality was 24% overall.[216] The costs associated with DOAC-related bleeding have not been well defined.[217] One study found DOAC-related bleeding was associated with shorter length of hospital stay compared to warfarin-related bleeding, a factor that could reduce the cost of treatment.[218] Nevertheless, the actual costs of treating DOAC-related bleeding are unknown because relatively few antidotes are available and experience with them is relatively limited.[219-221]

ANTIPLATELET DRUGS

Major bleeding post-PCI is associated with increased mortality and major adverse cardiovascular events, and bleeding secondary to the combination of antithrombotic medications used for acute coronary syndrome has been linked to increased mortality, nonfatal myocardial infarction, and stent thrombosis.[160,222] The concomitant use of GPIIb/IIIa inhibitors with UFH for PCI is correlated with more post-PCI bleeding than UFH or bivalirudin alone; however, bivalirudin has been associated with more ischemic events.[55] There is conflicting evidence regarding bleeding mortality associated with GPIIb/IIIa inhibitors for PCI, with some trials suggesting no increased risk over anticoagulation alone and others reporting significantly increased risk.[223,224]

With respect to oral antiplatelet therapy, prasugrel and ticagrelor are more potent than clopidogrel and have a higher association with bleeding.[97-100,225] However, the impact of these factors on morbidity and mortality is not well established. One study evaluated patients undergoing PCI for acute coronary syndrome and found no difference in in-hospital bleeding leading to prolonged hospital stay among clopidogrel, prasugrel, and ticagrelor. However, patients were followed for only 30 days post-PCI.[226] Cangrelor, an IV P2Y12 inhibitor, is associated with a higher risk of bleeding than clopidogrel; however, associated morbidity and mortality are unknown.[227] Further studies are needed to characterize the morbidity and mortality associated with the oral P2Y12 inhibitors.

NSAIDs AND ASPIRIN

The incidence of NSAID-induced bleeding depends on the drug and the dose. Higher risk of upper gastrointestinal bleeding is seen when daily doses of 2,400 mg ibuprofen, 100 mg diclofenac, 1,000 mg naproxen, and 20 mg piroxicam are used.[228] In patients who experience upper gastrointestinal bleeding secondary to NSAIDs (including aspirin), mortality is estimated at 20%.[229] Additionally, NSAIDs were associated with approximately 30% of hospitalizations due to adverse drug reactions in one study, with aspirin-related reactions accounting for the majority of cases.[230]

Aspirin use in the United States is widespread, with over 30% of adults age 40 years or older reporting taking preventive aspirin.[231] Aspirin can induce bleeding at any dose, and aspirin-induced moderate and major bleeding has been associated with increased all-cause mortality, which includes bleeding and cardiovascular related mortality.[232-234] Aspirin is commonly used concomitantly with other antiplatelet agents (e.g., GPIIb/IIIa inhibitors, P2Y12 inhibitors), and, although the combination increases the risk of bleeding and mortality, the extent of that effect has not been well defined.[235,236]

THROMBOLYTICS

Thrombolytic therapy is indicated for treatment of ischemic stroke, ST-segment elevation myocardial infarction (STEMI), and acute pulmonary embolism (PE); morbidity and mortality varies with indication. The rates of ICH associated with thrombolysis for stroke, STEMI, and acute PE are approximately 7%, 1%, and 1.5%, respectively.[237-240] Thrombolytic-associated ICH is best characterized in the stroke population where the mortality rate appears to range from 30% to 50%.[241,242] The average total cost of care for stroke in patients who receive thrombolysis ranges between $70,000–80,000, but the specific cost of managing thrombolytic complications and the impact on aspects such as hospital length of stay is unclear.[240]

SSRIs

Morbidity and mortality from bleeding associated with SSRIs are mostly described in patient populations with significant comorbidities (e.g., stroke, coronary artery bypass graft surgery, ICU admission), and outcomes vary from study to study.[199,200,243] One study suggested patients taking SSRIs prior to experiencing hemorrhagic stroke have increased stroke severity and mortality, and another study linked initiating SSRI therapy in patients admitted for peptic ulcer bleed to increased mortality.[197,199,200,243] More research is warranted to elucidate the actual impact of SSRI-associated bleeding.

PREVENTION

Prevention of drug-associated bleeding is multifaceted; general prevention strategies are included in **Table 45-8**. A key step in the prevention of drug-associated bleeding is to carefully weigh a patient's risk for bleeding (Table 45-6) against his or her risk for experiencing a thrombotic event prior to initiating therapy with a medication known to carry a risk of hemorrhage.

Appropriate laboratory monitoring is also important. Activated partial thromboplastin time is most commonly used to monitor IV UFH and direct thrombin inhibitor (DTI) therapy. Target aPTT values for UFH monitoring vary based on indication and type of reagent used in the laboratory; for DTI therapy, a target aPTT from 1.5 to 3 times the control is typically used.[249-251] A customary protocol for monitoring aPTT would include collection at the time of initiation of the infusion, 6 hours after initiation, 6 hours after any dosing rate changes, and then at least once daily if the patient remains at a constant drip rate.[250] Antifactor Xa can also be used to monitor IV UFH but is more typically used as a parameter to measure the anticoagulant effect of LMWH in special populations (e.g., patients with obesity).[252] The goal antifactor Xa range in adult patients is 0.6–1 anti-Xa units/mL for twice daily enoxaparin and >1 anti-Xa units/mL for once daily enoxaparin and dalteparin.[165,252]

Table 45-8 Approaches to Prevent Drug-Associated Bleeding

- Gastroprotective therapy (e.g., proton pump inhibitors are preferred over histamine receptor antagonists) is indicated in the following scenarios to prevent GI bleeding:[246-248]
  - Dual antiplatelet therapy + history of GI ulcer or bleed
  - Dual antiplatelet therapy + multiple risk factors for GI bleed (multiple concomitant NSAIDs, high-dose NSAIDs, concomitant anticoagulant, age >75, corticosteroid use, hemodialysis)
- Institutional order sets and protocols should be implemented for initiation, titration, and laboratory monitoring of continuous IV infusion unfractionated heparin or direct thrombin inhibitors
- Medications should be reviewed for renal dosing adjustments or contraindications to renal insufficiency (e.g., DOACs, parenteral DTIs, eptifibatide, tirofiban, NSAIDs)
- Patients receiving warfarin or DOACs should be educated regarding the indication/duration of therapy, monitoring, drug–drug interactions, drug–nutrition interactions, and signs and symptoms of bleeding
- Patients treated with LMWH should be educated on proper administration technique and, if appropriate, bridging instructions
- Polypharmacy should be avoided if possible (e.g., patients receiving warfarin therapy who undergo PCI may not need triple antithrombotic therapy with warfarin, aspirin, and clopidogrel[179,244,245])

DOAC = direct-acting oral anticoagulant, DTI = direct thrombin inhibitor, GI = gastrointestinal, IV = intravenous, LMWH = low-molecular-weight heparin, NSAID = nonsteroidal anti-inflammatory drug, PCI = percutaneous coronary intervention.

INR, which is derived from PT, is the gold standard for monitoring VKA therapy. Indication determines the desired target INR, and INR should be monitored regularly.[253-255] In the hospital, patients on warfarin should receive daily INR monitoring until therapeutic for at least two consecutive results.[253] Once this is achieved and the patient is on a stable dose, less frequent monitoring can be employed. In the outpatient setting, monitoring is more frequent for patients starting therapy (e.g., once every few days) and can be less frequent for patients who are stable (e.g., every 4–6 weeks).[256]

Although DOACs are marketed as not requiring any coagulation laboratory monitoring, some situations (e.g., need for emergent surgical procedures or concern regarding possible overanticoagulation) require measurements to be made. In the RE-LY trial, steady-state trough concentrations for patients taking dabigatran 150 mg twice daily ranged from approximately 40 ng/mL to 215 ng/mL; however, these concentrations have not been correlated with clinical outcomes to permit use in therapeutic monitoring.[257] PT and INR are increased by dabigatran but are insensitive to high concentrations.[258-260] Diluted thrombin clotting time and ecarin clotting time correlate linearly to dabigatran concentrations but are not yet widely available.[259,260] Specific anticoagulation laboratory parameters have been investigated for factor Xa inhibitor monitoring. Chromogenic antifactor Xa assays correlate linearly with direct Xa inhibitor plasma concentrations and utility may increase as more data accumulate.[261,262] Unfortunately, none of these laboratory values or assays has been clinically proved to predict therapeutic effectiveness or incidence of bleeding. As a result, to help optimize safety, clinicians should be familiar with DOACs pharmacokinetic properties (**Table 45-9**). For example, all DOACs are excreted

Table 45-9 Dosing and Pharmacokinetic Properties of DOACSs

	Dabigatran	Rivaroxaban	Apixaban	Edoxaban
Typical standard dose	150 mg twice daily	20 mg daily (15 mg twice daily for first 3 weeks of VTE treatment)	5 mg twice daily	60 mg daily
Half-life (h)	12–17	5–9 11–13 (elderly)	12	10–14
Time to peak plasma concentration (h)	2	2–5	1–3	1.5
Urinary excretion (%)	80	35	27	50
Renal dosing adjustment	75 mg twice daily for CrCl 15–30 mL/min	15 mg daily for CrCl 15–50 mL/min	2.5 mg twice daily if two risk factors: age ≥80, body weight 60 kg, SCr ≥1.5 mg/dL, concomitant CYP3A4 and P-gp inhibitors	• Avoid for CrCl >95 mL/min • 30 mg daily for CrCl 15–50 mL/min
Protein binding	35%	92–95%	87%	55%
Drug interactions requiring dose adjustment	• Concomitant P-gp inducer (rifampin), contraindicated VTE Indication • Any P-gp inhibitor,[a] avoid use AF Indication • Dronedarone or ketoconazole and CrCl 30–50 mL/min and atrial fibrillation indication, reduce dose to 75 mg twice daily • Any P-gp inhibitor[a] and CrCl <30 mL/min; avoid use	Concomitant strong P-gp and CYP3A4 inhibitors[b]; avoid use	Concomitant strong P-gp and CYP3A4 inhibitors[c]; reduce apixaban dose by 50% (to 2.5 mg twice daily)	Concomitant P-gp inhibitor,[d] reduce dose to 30 mg

AF = atrial fibrillation, CrCl = creatinine clearance, DOAC = direct-acting oral anticoagulant, P-gp = P-glycoprotein, VTE = venous thromboembolism.

[a]Amiodarone, clarithromycin, dronedarone, quinidine, verapamil.

[b]Ketoconazole, itraconazole, posaconazole, ritonavir.

[c]Clarithromycin, ketoconazole, itraconazole, ritonavir.

[d]Verapamil, quinidine; the short-term use of azithromycin, clarithromycin, erythromycin, oral itraconazole, oral ketoconazole.

to some extent by the kidney, so creatinine clearance can be used to help anticipate and avoid drug accumulation. Additionally, an understanding of the metabolism of these medications can help clinicians identify and avoid potential interacting medications that can increase anticoagulant effect.

There are no specific therapeutic drug-monitoring parameters for antiplatelet drugs, thrombolytics, or SSRIs; however, standard hematology laboratory values (e.g., hemoglobin, hematocrit, platelets, etc.) should be assessed. Renal function should also be evaluated at baseline and periodically for patients on regular NSAID therapy.

There are a number of prophylactic measures that can be effectively used to minimize bleeding risk. Medication regimens that increase the risk of gastrointestinal bleeding may necessitate the addition of gastroprotective therapy. Patients requiring DAT following myocardial infarction should receive gastroprotective therapy with a proton pump inhibitor (PPI) if they have a history of gastrointestinal bleeding, concomitant anticoagulant therapy, and/or chronic NSAID or corticosteroid use.[247,263] PPIs have been shown to have better protective effects than the histamine receptor antagonists.[247,264] There is, however, controversial evidence that PPIs interact with antiplatelet regimens by decreasing the antithrombotic effects and increasing the risk for cardiovascular events.[263,265-267]

MANAGEMENT

Management of drug-induced bleeding requires both nonpharmacological and pharmacological measures to achieve hemostasis and/or reversal of anticoagulant effect. Nonpharmacological measures are listed in **Table 45-10**.

ANTICOAGULANTS

Hemostasis is most rapidly achieved via administration of hemostatic agents (e.g., prothrombin complex concentrates [PCCs], fresh-frozen plasma [FFP]) and, if available, targeted reversal agents (e.g., idarucizumab, vitamin K, and protamine). Severity, site of hemorrhage, and time frame for achieving hemostasis should guide reversal strategy; not all bleeding requires administration of hemostatic agents, and caution should be exercised given the risk of thrombotic adverse events associated with some agents.[269-271] **Table 45-11** lists characteristics of reversal agents, and **Figures 45-2** and **45-3** describe anticoagulant reversal strategies.

Table 45-10 Nonpharmacological Measures for Management of Drug-Associated Bleeding[268,269]

- Apply pressure to the source of bleeding, if possible, and stop the offending agent
- Assess hepatic and renal function; estimate half-life and time to washout of offending agent
- Obtain information regarding timing and amount of last dose of offending agent
- Order complete blood cell count and other pertinent anticoagulation laboratory values (e.g., aPTT, PT/INR, antifactor Xa) as appropriate to assess level of antithrombotic effect
- Plan for radiological interventions, endoscopy, or surgery as appropriate

aPTT = activated partial thromboplastin time, INR = international normalized ratio, PT = prothrombin time.

For heparin-related hemorrhage, protamine is the agent of choice; however, protamine should only be used to reverse therapeutic doses of UFH or LMWH.[274] When managing bleeding associated with IV UFH, the length of time the patient has been receiving the infusion, whether or not therapeutic aPTT values have been achieved, and when the infusion was stopped should be considered. Additionally, clinicians must account for the amount of UFH infused over the 2–3 hours preceding discontinuation of the drip. The maximum dose of protamine is 50 mg due to a paradoxical anticoagulant effect that can occur at high doses.[275,276] It is important to note that protamine only partially reverses LMWHs.[277] The timing of the last LMWH dose must be determined because protamine should only be used within 8 hours of the last enoxaparin dose or within 24 hours of last dalteparin dose.[274]

Vitamin K is central to the management of warfarin-associated bleeding. It is available in oral, subcutaneous, and IV formulations. Oral vitamin K

Table 45-11 Characteristics of Reversal Agents and Hemostatic Agents

Agent	Mechanism	Dose	Kinetics
REVERSAL AGENTS			
Idarucizumab	Monoclonal antibody directly neutralizes the effects of dabigatran	2.5 g × 2 IV boluses (5 g total) within 15 minutes of each other	Onset: • Immediate Duration: • Up to 24 hours
Protamine	Binds heparin molecules to form inactive salt	For IV unfractionated heparin: 1 mg protamine per 100 units of heparin, (max dose 50 mg) • Must account for UFH infused over preceding 2–3 hours • Use 0.5 mg/100 units IF drip is held >60 minutes • Use 0.25 mg/100 units IF drip held >2 hours For LMWH: 1 mg/100 anti-Xa units within 8 hours of last enoxaparin dose or 24 hours of dalteparin dose	Onset: • ~5 minutes
Vitamin K (phytonadione)	Cofactor for hepatic production of factors II, VII, IX and X	Variable: • 2–2.5 mg PO vitamin K is recommended for INR >10 without bleeding • Low doses of IV vitamin K (e.g., 0.5–1 mg) are effective in causing partial reversal at 24–48 hours	Onset: • PO 12–24 hours • IV 4–12 hours
HEMOSTATIC AGENTS			
3-factor prothrombin complex concentrate (PCC-3)	Replaces coagulation factors II, IX, and X, in concentrations 25 times that of FFP	For warfarin: • INR <2: 20 units/kg • INR 2–4: 30 units/kg • INR >4: 50 units/kg For dabigatran or factor Xa inhibitor: Up to 50 units/kg	Onset: • ~5–15 minutes Duration: 12–24 hours
4-factor prothrombin complex concentrate (PCC-4)	Replaces coagulation factors II, VII, IX, and X, in concentrations 25 times that of FFP	For warfarin: • INR 2 to <4: 25 units/kg (maximum dose 2,500 units) • INR 4–6: 35 units/kg (maximum dose 3,500 units) • INR >6: 50 units/kg (maximum dose 5,000 units) For dabigatran or factor Xa inhibitor: • Up to 50 units/kg	Onset: • ~5–15 minutes Duration: • 12–24 hours
Activated PCC (e.g. factor eight inhibitor bypass activity [FEIBA])	Replaces coagulation factors II, IX, X, and activated VII	8–25 units/kg[273]	Onset: • ~5–15 minutes Duration: • 8–12 hours
Fresh-frozen plasma (FFP)	Replaces coagulation factors lowered by warfarin (II, VII, IX, and X) at lower concentration than PCCs	5–20 mL/kg IV (~10 mL/min)	Onset: • ~1–4 hours Duration: • ≤6 hours
Recombinant activated factor VII (rFVIIa)	Replaces activated factor VII	2nd-line therapy for fondaparinux: 90 mcg/kg[a]	Onset: • ~5–10 minutes Duration: • 4–6 hours

INR = international normalized ratio, IV = intravenous, LMWH = low-molecular-weight heparin, PCC = prothrombin complex concentrate, UFH = unfrationated heparin.
[a]Doses of 1 mg IV are typically sufficient.[272]

is preferred for nonemergent, minor bleeding or for patients presenting without bleeding but with an INR >10.[278] Because oral vitamin K has a slower onset of action and subcutaneous vitamin K has erratic absorption properties, IV vitamin K is preferred for the management of emergent, major bleeding.[274,278,279] The dose of IV vitamin K typically ranges from 0.5 mg to 10 mg, with larger doses associated with a longer duration of action but not a greater INR reduction.[280] For management of warfarin-associated ICH, an IV dose of 10 mg is recommended.[274] Because vitamin K does not have an immediate onset, it should be used with a hemostatic agent to manage emergent, major bleeding. Prothrombin complex concentrates are considered first line for warfarin-associated ICH and are dosed based on INR.[274] FFP should only be used if PCCs are not available or are contraindicated.

Idarucizumab is the first-line agent for treating dabigatran-associated ICH.[274] It is a monoclonal antibody that directly binds dabigatran, and dabigatran's affinity for idarucizumab is approximately 350 times greater than its affinity for thrombin. It is administered in two 2.5-g bolus doses (total dose 5 g) that should be given no more than 15 minutes apart. Idarucizumab should be given within 3–5 half-lives (approximately 24 hours) of the last dabigatran dose in patients with normal renal function. For patients with renal insufficiency, idarucizumab can be given without regard to the last dabigatran dose. If idarucizumab is not available or is contraindicated, activated PCC (aPCC) or 4-factor PCC (PCC-4) can be utilized. Because dabigatran is not highly protein bound, it can be removed via hemodialysis. However, prolonged hemodialysis is required to avoid rebound anticoagulant effect.[281] In addition, insertion of a dialysis catheter may increase a patient's risk for further bleeding.

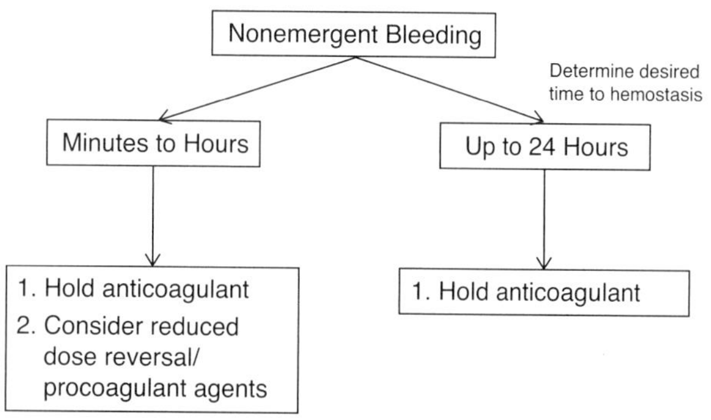

FIGURE 45-2 Oral Anticoagulant Reversal Algorithm: Nonemergent Bleeding

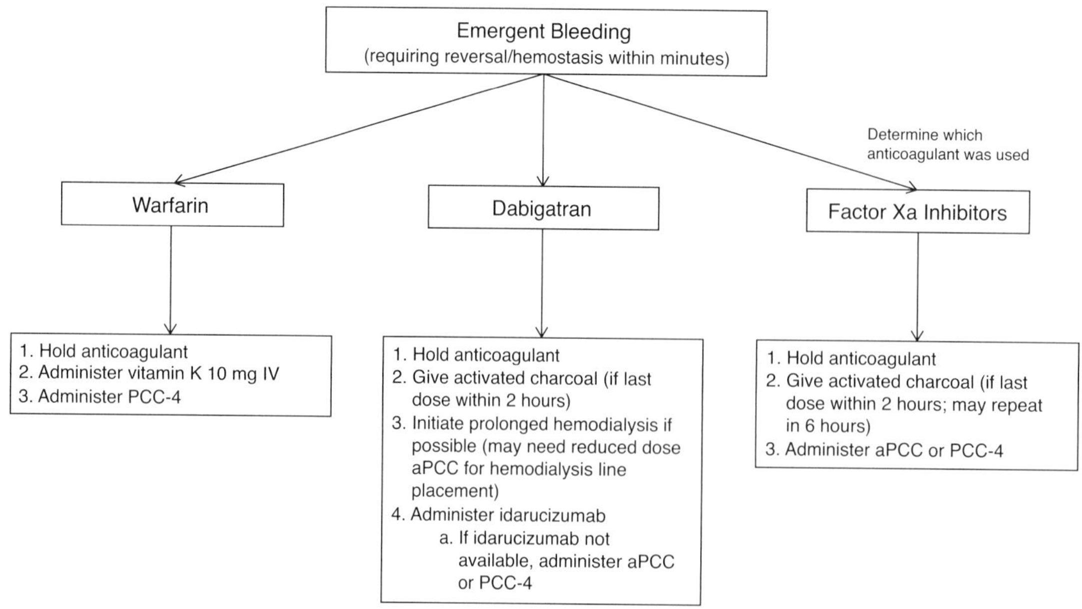

FIGURE 45-3 Oral Anticoagulant Reversal Algorithm: Emergent Bleeding

aPCC = activated prothrombin complex concentrate, IV = intravenous, PCC-4 = 4-factor prothrombin complex concentrate.

Both aPCC and PCC-4 are considered first-line agents for managing factor Xa inhibitor-associated ICH and, like idarucizumab for dabigatran, should be given only within 3–5 half-lives of the last factor Xa inhibitor dose.[274] Activated charcoal is also recommended if the last dose of dabigatran or factor Xa inhibitor was within 2 hours.

Prior to the availability of PCC-4, recombinant activated factor VII (rFVIIa) was recommended for reversal of warfarin-associated bleeding. However, given its higher associated risk of myocardial infarction and thrombosis, its use in managing anticoagulant-associated bleeding is limited to second-line therapy for fondaparinux-related bleeding.[274] First-line therapy for fondaparinux-associated ICH is aPCC. Additionally, rFVIIa can also be considered for reversal of parenteral DTI-associated bleeding, although given the relatively short half-life of these agents, simply stopping the infusion may be sufficient in achieving hemostasis.[274,282]

As previously described, hemostatic agents may increase the risk for thrombotic events, and reversing the effects of anticoagulant agents will also increase a patient's risk for thrombosis. Furthermore, all DOACs have a boxed warning for premature, abrupt discontinuation leading to increased risk of thrombotic event.[283,284] Thus, when managing anticoagulant-associated bleeding, clinicians should continue to consider patients' risks for thrombosis and factor restarting anticoagulation therapy into treatment plans.

ANTIPLATELET DRUGS, ASPIRIN, AND NSAIDs

Strategies to manage antiplatelet-associated bleeding include general nonpharmacologic measures, and in cases of critical bleeding, platelet transfusion.[268,274] To avoid pharmacologic inhibition of transfused platelets, transfusion should occur 3–5 half-lives after the last antiplatelet dose. Desmopressin can be considered and is administered intravenously as a single dose of 0.4 mcg/kg.[274]

It should be noted that platelet transfusion is ineffective at reversing GpIIb/IIIa inhibitors, but because of their short half-lives, management of GpIIb/IIIa-associated bleeding typically requires only discontinuation of the agent and supportive care. Similarly, NSAID-associated hemorrhage is managed primarily by discontinuation of the offending agent along with nonpharmacologic and supportive measures.

THROMBOLYTICS

Several mechanisms are involved with fibrinolytic/thrombolytic-associated bleeding, so management strategies employ several different agents. Institutional protocols typically include the use of FFP, cryoprecipitate (10 units), vitamin K, platelets, and antifibrinolytics (aminocaproic acid 4–5 g or tranexamic acid 10–15 mg/kg).[268,274,285-288]

INFORMATION FOR PATIENTS

Patient education is crucial to the prevention of drug-associated bleeding. Patients should be familiar with how the various medications will impact their activities of daily living and should be taught to detect signs and symptoms of major or minor bleeding. It is imperative that patients understand when to seek medical treatment. For patients receiving anticoagulation therapy, providers can consider recommending patients follow up at an anticoagulation clinic. Education programs are key elements of these clinics, and anticoagulation clinic patients receiving warfarin experience fewer adverse events.[289-291]

Providers should discuss the risks of polypharmacy with patients. Patients should be encouraged to share updated medication lists (including nutritional supplements and over-the-counter medications) with all healthcare professionals involved in their care.

REFERENCES

1. Rowan SB, Bailey DN, Bublitz CE, Anderson RJ. Trends in anticoagulation for atrial fibrillation in the US: an analysis of the national ambulatory medical care survey database. *J Am Coll Cardiol.* 2007; 49:1561-5.
2. Ghate SR, Biskupiak J, Ye X et al. All-cause and bleeding-related health care costs in warfarin-treated patients with atrial fibrillation. *J Manag Care Pharm.* 2011; 17:672-84.
3. Verhoef TI, Ragia G, de Boer A et al. A randomized trial of genotype-guided dosing of acenocoumarol and phenprocoumon. *New Engl J Med.* 2013; 369:2304-12.
4. Leroyer C, Bressollette L, Oger E et al. Early versus delayed introduction of oral vitamin K antagonists in combination with low-molecular-weight heparin in the treatment of deep vein

thrombosis. A randomized clinical trial. The ANTENOX Study Group. *Haemostasis.* 1998; 28:70-7.

5. Lopez-Beret P, Orgaz A, Fontcuberta J et al. Low molecular weight heparin versus oral anticoagulants in the long-term treatment of deep venous thrombosis. *J Vasc Surg.* 2001; 33:77-90.
6. Patel MR, Mahaffey KW, Garg J et al. Rivaroxaban versus warfarin in nonvalvular atrial fibrillation. *N Engl J Med.* 2011; 365:883-91.
7. Lee AY, Kamphuisen PW, Meyer G et al. Tinzaparin vs warfarin for treatment of acute venous thromboembolism in patients with active cancer: a randomized clinical trial. *JAMA.* 2015; 314:677-86.
8. Connolly S, Pogue J, Hart R et al. Clopidogrel plus aspirin versus oral anticoagulation for atrial fibrillation in the Atrial fibrillation Clopidogrel Trial with Irbesartan for prevention of Vascular Events (ACTIVE W): a randomised controlled trial. *Lancet.* 2006; 367:1903-12.
9. Granger CB, Alexander JH, McMurray JJ et al. Apixaban versus warfarin in patients with atrial fibrillation. *N Engl J Med.* 2011; 365:981-92.
10. Eikelboom JW, Connolly SJ, Brueckmann M et al. Dabigatran versus warfarin in patients with mechanical heart valves. *N Engl J Med.* 2013; 369:1206-14.
11. Connolly SJ, Ezekowitz MD, Yusuf S et al. Dabigatran versus warfarin in patients with atrial fibrillation. *N Engl J Med.* 2009; 361:1139-51.
12. Giugliano RP, Ruff CT, Braunwald E et al. Edoxaban versus warfarin in patients with atrial fibrillation. *N Engl J Med.* 2013; 369:2093-104.
13. Goldhaber SZ, Leizorovicz A, Kakkar AK et al. Apixaban versus enoxaparin for thromboprophylaxis in medically ill patients. *N Engl J Med.* 2011; 365:2167-77.
14. Lassen MR, Raskob GE, Gallus A et al. Apixaban or enoxaparin for thromboprophylaxis after knee replacement. *N Engl J Med.* 2009; 361:594-604.
15. Lassen MR, Raskob GE, Gallus A et al. Apixaban versus enoxaparin for thromboprophylaxis after knee replacement (ADVANCE-2): a randomised double-blind trial. *Lancet.* 2010; 375:807-15.
16. Lassen MR, Gallus A, Raskob GE et al. Apixaban versus enoxaparin for thromboprophylaxis after hip replacement. *N Engl J Med.* 2010; 363:2487-98.
17. Agnelli G, Buller HR, Cohen A et al. Oral apixaban for the treatment of acute venous thromboembolism. *N Engl J Med.* 2013; 369:799-808.
18. Agnelli G, Buller HR, Cohen A et al. Apixaban for extended treatment of venous thromboembolism. *N Engl J Med.* 2013; 368:699-708.
19. Raskob G, Cohen AT, Eriksson BI et al. Oral direct factor Xa inhibition with edoxaban for thromboprophylaxis after elective total hip replacement. A randomised double-blind dose-response study. *Thromb Haemost.* 2010; 104:642-9.
20. Buller HR, Decousus H, Grosso MA et al. Edoxaban versus warfarin for the treatment of symptomatic venous thromboembolism. *N Engl J Med.* 2013; 369:1406-15.
21. Fuji T, Wang CJ, Fujita S et al. Safety and efficacy of edoxaban, an oral factor Xa inhibitor, versus enoxaparin for thromboprophylaxis after total knee arthroplasty: the STARS E-3 trial. *Thromb Res.* 2014; 134:1198-204.
22. Buller HR, Prins MH, Lensin AW et al. Oral rivaroxaban for the treatment of symptomatic pulmonary embolism. *N Engl J Med.* 2012; 366:1287-97.
23. Bauersachs R, Berkowitz SD, Brenner B et al. Oral rivaroxaban for symptomatic venous thromboembolism. *N Engl J Med.* 2010; 363:2499-510.
24. Cohen AT, Spiro TE, Buller HR et al. Rivaroxaban for thromboprophylaxis in acutely ill medical patients. *N Engl J Med.* 2013; 368:513-23.
25. Eriksson BI, Borris LC, Friedman RJ et al. Rivaroxaban versus enoxaparin for thromboprophylaxis after hip arthroplasty. *N Engl J Med.* 2008; 358:2765-75.
26. Kakkar AK, Brenner B, Dahl OE et al. Extended duration rivaroxaban versus short-term enoxaparin for the prevention of venous thromboembolism after total hip arthroplasty: a double-blind, randomised controlled trial. *Lancet.* 2008; 372:31-9.
27. Lassen MR, Ageno W, Borris LC et al. Rivaroxaban versus enoxaparin for thromboprophylaxis after total knee arthroplasty. *N Engl J Med.* 2008; 358:2776-86.
28. Turpie AG, Lassen MR, Davidson BL et al. Rivaroxaban versus enoxaparin for thromboprophylaxis after total knee arthroplasty (RECORD4): a randomised trial. *Lancet.* 2009; 373:1673-80.
29. Cohen AT, Davidson BL, Gallus AS et al. Efficacy and safety of fondaparinux for the prevention of venous thromboembolism in older acute medical patients: randomised placebo controlled trial. *BMJ.* 2006; 332:325-9.
30. Decousus H, Prandoni P, Mismetti P et al. Fondaparinux for the treatment of superficial-vein thrombosis in the legs. *N Engl J Med.* 2010; 363:1222-32.
31. Buller HR, Davidson BL, Decousus H et al. Subcutaneous fondaparinux versus intravenous unfractionated heparin in the initial treatment of pulmonary embolism. *New Engl J Med.* 2003; 349:1695-702.
32. Eriksson BI, Bauer KA, Lassen MR, Turpie AG. Fondaparinux compared with enoxaparin for the prevention of venous thromboembolism after hip-fracture surgery. *N Engl J Med.* 2001; 345:1298-304.
33. Bauer KA, Eriksson BI, Lassen MR, Turpie AG. Fondaparinux compared with enoxaparin for the prevention of venous thromboembolism after elective major knee surgery. *N Engl J Med.* 2001; 345:1305-10.
34. Buller HR, Davidson BL, Decousus H et al. Fondaparinux or enoxaparin for the initial treatment of symptomatic deep venous thrombosis: a randomized trial. *Ann Intern Med.* 2004; 140:867-73.
35. Yusuf S, Mehta SR, Chrolavicius S et al. Comparison of fondaparinux and enoxaparin in acute coronary syndromes. *N Engl J Med.* 2006; 354:1464-76.
36. Yusuf S, Mehta SR, Chrolavicius S et al. Effects of fondaparinux on mortality and reinfarction in patients with acute ST-segment elevation myocardial infarction: the OASIS-6 randomized trial. *JAMA.* 2006; 295:1519-30.
37. Schulman S, Kearon C, Kakkar AK et al. Dabigatran versus warfarin in the treatment of acute venous thromboembolism. *N Engl J Med.* 2009; 361:2342-52.
38. Eriksson BI, Dahl OE, Rosencher N et al. Dabigatran etexilate versus enoxaparin for prevention of venous thromboembolism after total hip replacement: a randomised, double-blind, non-inferiority trial. *Lancet.* 2007; 370:949-56.
39. Eriksson BI, Dahl OE, Huo MH et al. Oral dabigatran versus enoxaparin for thromboprophylaxis after primary total hip arthroplasty (RE-NOVATE II*). A randomised, double-blind, non-inferiority trial. *Thromb Haemost.* 2011; 105:721-9.
40. Schulman S, Kearon C, Kakkar AK et al. Extended use of dabigatran, warfarin, or placebo in venous thromboembolism. *N Engl J Med.* 2013; 368:709-18.
41. Rossig L, Genth-Zotz S, Rau M et al. Argatroban for elective percutaneous coronary intervention: the ARG-E04 multi-center study. *Int J Cardiol.* 2011; 148:214-9.
42. Doepker B, Mount KL, Ryder LJ et al. Bleeding risk factors associated with argatroban therapy in the critically ill. *Thromb Haemost.* 2012; 34:491-8.
43. Lewis BE, Wallis DE, Hursting MJ et al. Effects of argatroban therapy, demographic variables, and platelet count on thrombotic risks in heparin-induced thrombocytopenia. *Chest.* 2006; 129:1407-16.
44. Begelman SM, Baghdasarian SB, Singh IM et al. Argatroban anticoagulation in intensive care patients: effects of heart failure

and multiple organ system failure. *Intensive Care Med.* 2008; 23:313-20.

45. Yeh RW, Baron SJ, Healy JL et al. Anticoagulation with the direct thrombin inhibitor argatroban in patients presenting with acute coronary syndromes. *Catheter Cardiovasc Interv.* 2009; 74:359-64.
46. Stone GW, McLaurin BT, Cox DA et al. Bivalirudin for patients with acute coronary syndromes. *N Engl J Med.* 2006; 355:2203-16.
47. Han Y, Guo J, Zheng Y et al. Bivalirudin vs heparin with or without tirofiban during primary percutaneous coronary intervention in acute myocardial infarction: the BRIGHT randomized clinical trial. *JAMA.* 2015; 313:1336-46.
48. Steg PG, van 't Hof A, Hamm CW et al. Bivalirudin started during emergency transport for primary PCI. *N Engl J Med.* 2013; 369:2207-17.
49. Shahzad A, Kemp I, Mars C et al. Unfractionated heparin versus bivalirudin in primary percutaneous coronary intervention (HEAT-PPCI): an open-label, single centre, randomised controlled trial. *Lancet.* 2014; 384:1849-58.
50. Kiser TH, Burch JC, Klem PM, Hassell KL. Safety, efficacy, and dosing requirements of bivalirudin in patients with heparin-induced thrombocytopenia. *Pharmacotherapy.* 2008; 28:1115-24.
51. Stone GW, Witzenbichler B, Guagliumi G et al. Bivalirudin during primary PCI in acute myocardial infarction. *N Engl J Med.* 2008; 358:2218-30.
52. Kastrati A, Neumann FJ, Mehilli J et al. Bivalirudin versus unfractionated heparin during percutaneous coronary intervention. *N Engl J Med.* 2008; 359:688-96.
53. Kastrati A, Neumann FJ, Schulz S et al. Abciximab and heparin versus bivalirudin for non-ST-elevation myocardial infarction. *N Engl J Med.* 2011; 365:1980-9.
54. Valgimigli M, Frigoli E, Leonardi S et al. Bivalirudin or unfractionated heparin in acute coronary syndromes. *N Engl J Med.* 2015; 373:997-1009.
55. Navarese EP, Schulze V, Andreotti F et al. Comprehensive meta-analysis of safety and efficacy of bivalirudin versus heparin with or without routine glycoprotein IIb/IIIa inhibitors in patients with acute coronary syndrome. *JACC Cardiovasc Interv.* 2015; 8(1 Part B):201-13.
56. Bangalore S, Toklu B, Kotwal A et al. Anticoagulant therapy during primary percutaneous coronary intervention for acute myocardial infarction: a meta-analysis of randomized trials in the era of stents and P2Y12 inhibitors. *BMJ.* 2014; 349:g6419.
57. Cavender MA, Sabatine MS. Bivalirudin versus heparin in patients planned for percutaneous coronary intervention: a meta-analysis of randomised controlled trials. *Lancet.* 2014; 384:599-606.
58. Eriksson BI, Wille-Jorgensen P, Kalebo P et al. A comparison of recombinant hirudin with a low-molecular-weight heparin to prevent thromboembolic complications after total hip replacement. *N Engl J Med.* 1997; 337:1329-35.
59. Cooper T, White CL, Taber D et al. Safety and effectiveness outcomes of an inpatient collaborative drug therapy management service for direct thrombin inhibitors. *Am J Health-Syst Pharm.* 2012; 69:1993-8.
60. Douketis JD, Spyropoulos AC, Kaatz S et al. Perioperative bridging anticoagulation in patients with atrial fibrillation. *N Engl J Med.* 2015; 373:823-33.
61. Lee AY, Levine MN, Baker RI et al. Low-molecular-weight heparin versus a coumarin for the prevention of recurrent venous thromboembolism in patients with cancer. *N Engl J Med.* 2003; 349:146-53.
62. Anderson DR, Dunbar MJ, Bohm ER et al. Aspirin versus low-molecular-weight heparin for extended venous thromboembolism prophylaxis after total hip arthroplasty: a randomized trial. *Ann Intern Med.* 2013; 158:800-6.
63. Hull RD, Pineo GF, Francis C et al. Low-molecular-weight heparin prophylaxis using dalteparin extended out-of-hospital vs in-hospital warfarin/out-of-hospital placebo in hip arthroplasty patients: a double-blind, randomized comparison. North American Fragmin Trial Investigators. *Arch Intern Med.* 2000; 160:2208-15.
64. Hull RD, Pineo GF, Francis C et al. Low-molecular-weight heparin prophylaxis using dalteparin in close proximity to surgery vs warfarin in hip arthroplasty patients: a double-blind, randomized comparison. The North American Fragmin Trial Investigators. *Arch Intern Med.* 2000; 160:2199-207.
65. Cook D, Meade M, Guyatt G et al. Dalteparin versus unfractionated heparin in critically ill patients. *N Engl J Med.* 2011; 364:1305-14.
66. Low molecular weight heparinoid, ORG 10172 (danaparoid), and outcome after acute ischemic stroke: a randomized controlled trial. The Publications Committee for the Trial of ORG 10172 in Acute Stroke Treatment (TOAST) Investigators. *JAMA.* 1998; 279:1265-72.
67. Gent M, Hirsh J, Ginsberg JS et al. Low-molecular-weight heparinoid organ is more effective than aspirin in the prevention of venous thromboembolism after surgery for hip fracture. *Circulation.* 1996; 93:80-4.
68. de Valk HW, Banga JD, Wester JW et al. Comparing subcutaneous danaparoid with intravenous unfractionated heparin for the treatment of venous thromboembolism. A randomized controlled trial. *Ann Intern Med.* 1995; 123:1-9.
69. Blazing MA, de Lemos JA, White HD et al. Safety and efficacy of enoxaparin vs unfractionated heparin in patients with non-ST-segment elevation acute coronary syndromes who receive tirofiban and aspirin: a randomized controlled trial. *JAMA.* 2004; 292:55-64.
70. Stellbrink C, Nixdorff U, Hofmann T et al. Safety and efficacy of enoxaparin compared with unfractionated heparin and oral anticoagulants for prevention of thromboembolic complications in cardioversion of nonvalvular atrial fibrillation: the Anticoagulation in Cardioversion using Enoxaparin (ACE) trial. *Circulation.* 2004; 109:997-1003.
71. Cohen M, Demers C, Gurfinkel EP et al. A comparison of low-molecular-weight heparin with unfractionated heparin for unstable coronary artery disease. Efficacy and Safety of Subcutaneous Enoxaparin in Non-Q-Wave Coronary Events Study Group. *N Engl J Med.* 1997; 337:447-52.
72. Antman EM, Morrow DA, McCabe CH et al. Enoxaparin versus unfractionated heparin with fibrinolysis for ST-elevation myocardial infarction. *N Engl J Med.* 2006; 354:1477-88.
73. Silvain J, Beygui F, Barthelemy O et al. Efficacy and safety of enoxaparin versus unfractionated heparin during percutaneous coronary intervention: systematic review and meta-analysis. *BMJ.* 2012; 344:e553.
74. Ferguson JJ, Califf RM, Antman EM et al. Enoxaparin vs unfractionated heparin in high-risk patients with non-ST-segment elevation acute coronary syndromes managed with an intended early invasive strategy: primary results of the SYNERGY randomized trial. *JAMA.* 2004; 292:45-54.
75. Kearon C, Ginsberg JS, Julian JA et al. Comparison of fixed-dose weight-adjusted unfractionated heparin and low-molecular-weight heparin for acute treatment of venous thromboembolism. *JAMA.* 2006; 296:935-42.
76. Camporese G, Bernardi E, Prandoni P et al. Low-molecular-weight heparin versus compression stockings for thromboprophylaxis after knee arthroscopy: a randomized trial. *Ann Intern Med.* 2008; 149:73-82.
77. Koopman MM, Prandoni P, Piovella F et al. Treatment of venous thrombosis with intravenous unfractionated heparin administered in the hospital as compared with subcutaneous low-molecular-weight heparin administered at home. The Tasman Study Group. *N Engl J Med.* 1996; 334:682-7.
78. Hull RD, Raskob GE, Brant RF et al. Low-molecular-weight heparin vs heparin in the treatment of patients with pulmonary embolism. American-Canadian Thrombosis Study Group. *Arch Intern Med.* 2000; 160:229-36.

79. Michalis LK, Katsouras CS, Papamichael N et al. Enoxaparin versus tinzaparin in non-ST-segment elevation acute coronary syndromes: the EVET trial. *Amer Heart J.* 2003; 146:304-10.
80. Simonneau G, Sors H, Charbonnier B et al. A comparison of low-molecular-weight heparin with unfractionated heparin for acute pulmonary embolism. The THESEE Study Group. Tinzaparine ou Heparine Standard: Evaluations dans l'Embolie Pulmonaire. *N Engl J Med.* 1997; 337:663-9.
81. Steg PG, Jolly SS, Mehta SR et al. Low-dose vs standard-dose unfractionated heparin for percutaneous coronary intervention in acute coronary syndromes treated with fondaparinux: the FUTURA/OASIS-8 randomized trial. *JAMA.* 2010; 304:1339-49.
82. Ogawa H, Nakayama M, Morimoto T et al. Low-dose aspirin for primary prevention of atherosclerotic events in patients with type 2 diabetes: a randomized controlled trial. *JAMA.* 2008; 300:2134-41.
83. Ikeda Y, Shimada K, Teramoto T et al. Low-dose aspirin for primary prevention of cardiovascular events in Japanese patients 60 years or older with atherosclerotic risk factors: a randomized clinical trial. *JAMA.* 2014; 312:2510-20.
84. Connolly SJ, Pogue J, Hart RG et al. Effect of clopidogrel added to aspirin in patients with atrial fibrillation. *N Engl J Med.* 2009; 360:2066-78.
85. A randomised, blinded, trial of clopidogrel versus aspirin in patients at risk of ischaemic events (CAPRIE). CAPRIE Steering Committee. *Lancet.* 1996; 348:1329-39.
86. Bhatt DL, Fox KA, Hacke W et al. Clopidogrel and aspirin versus aspirin alone for the prevention of atherothrombotic events. *N Engl J Med.* 2006; 354:1706-17.
87. Yusuf S, Zhao F, Mehta SR et al. Effects of clopidogrel in addition to aspirin in patients with acute coronary syndromes without ST-segment elevation. *N Engl J Med.* 2001; 345:494-502.
88. Halkes PH, van Gijn J, Kappelle LJ et al. Aspirin plus dipyridamole versus aspirin alone after cerebral ischaemia of arterial origin (ESPRIT): randomised controlled trial. *Lancet.* 2006; 367:1665-73.
89. Sacco RL, Diener HC, Yusuf S et al. Aspirin and extended-release dipyridamole versus clopidogrel for recurrent stroke. *N Engl J Med.* 2008; 359:1238-51.
90. Jankowski J, Attwood S, deCaestecker J, Barr H. Aspirin in the primary prevention of vascular disease. *Lancet.* 2009; 374:877-8; 879.
91. Dixon BS, Beck GJ, Vazquez MA et al. Effect of dipyridamole plus aspirin on hemodialysis graft patency. *N Engl J Med.* 2009; 360:2191-201.
92. Bertrand ME, Rupprecht HJ, Urban P, Gershlick AH. Double-blind study of the safety of clopidogrel with and without a loading dose in combination with aspirin compared with ticlopidine in combination with aspirin after coronary stenting: the clopidogrel aspirin stent international cooperative study (CLASSICS). *Circulation.* 2000; 102:624-9.
93. Steinhubl SR, Berger PB, Mann JT, 3rd et al. Early and sustained dual oral antiplatelet therapy following percutaneous coronary intervention: a randomized controlled trial. *JAMA.* 2002; 288:2411-20.
94. Diener HC, Bogousslavsky J, Brass LM et al. Aspirin and clopidogrel compared with clopidogrel alone after recent ischaemic stroke or transient ischaemic attack in high-risk patients (MATCH): randomised, double-blind, placebo-controlled trial. *Lancet.* 2004; 364:331-7.
95. Montalescot G, Bolognese L, Dudek D et al. Pretreatment with prasugrel in non-ST-segment elevation acute coronary syndromes. *N Engl J Med.* 2013; 369:999-1010.
96. Roe MT, Armstrong PW, Fox KA et al. Prasugrel versus clopidogrel for acute coronary syndromes without revascularization. *N Engl J Med.* 2012; 367:1297-309.
97. Wiviott SD, Braunwald E, McCabe CH et al. Prasugrel versus clopidogrel in patients with acute coronary syndromes. *N Engl J Med.* 2007; 357:2001-15.
98. Montalescot G, van 't Hof AW, Lapostolle F et al. Prehospital ticagrelor in ST-segment elevation myocardial infarction. *N Engl J Med.* 2014; 371:1016-27.
99. Bonaca MP, Bhatt DL, Cohen M et al. Long-term use of ticagrelor in patients with prior myocardial infarction. *N Engl J Med.* 2015; 372:1791-800.
100. Wallentin L, Becker RC, Budaj A et al. Ticagrelor versus clopidogrel in patients with acute coronary syndromes. *N Engl J Med.* 2009; 361:1045-57.
101. Leon MB, Baim DS, Popma JJ et al. A clinical trial comparing three antithrombotic-drug regimens after coronary-artery stenting. Stent Anticoagulation Restenosis Study Investigators. *N Engl J Med.* 1998; 339:1665-71.
102. Angiolillo DJ, Firstenberg MS, Price MJ et al. Bridging antiplatelet therapy with cangrelor in patients undergoing cardiac surgery: a randomized controlled trial. *JAMA.* 2012; 307:265-74.
103. Bhatt DL, Lincoff AM, Gibson CM et al. Intravenous platelet blockade with cangrelor during PCI. *N Engl J Med.* 2009; 361:2330-41.
104. Harrington RA, Stone GW, McNulty S et al. Platelet inhibition with cangrelor in patients undergoing PCI. *N Engl J Med.* 2009; 361:2318-29.
105. Bhatt DL, Stone GW, Mahaffey KW et al. Effect of platelet inhibition with cangrelor during PCI on ischemic events. *N Engl J Med.* 2013; 368:1303-13.
106. Bertrand OF, De Larochelliere R, Rodes-Cabau J et al. A randomized study comparing same-day home discharge and abciximab bolus only to overnight hospitalization and abciximab bolus and infusion after transradial coronary stent implantation. *Circulation.* 2006; 114:2636-43.
107. Brasselet C, Tassan S, Nazeyrollas P et al. Randomised comparison of femoral versus radial approach for percutaneous coronary intervention using abciximab in acute myocardial infarction: results of the FARMI trial. *Heart.* 2007; 93:1556-61.
108. Mehilli J, Kastrati A, Schulz S et al. Abciximab in patients with acute ST-segment-elevation myocardial infarction undergoing primary percutaneous coronary intervention after clopidogrel loading: a randomized double-blind trial. *Circulation.* 2009; 119:1933-40.
109. Ellis SG, Tendera M, de Belder MA et al. Facilitated PCI in patients with ST-elevation myocardial infarction. *N Engl J Med.* 2008; 358:2205-17.
110. Stone GW, Maehara A, Witzenbichler B et al. Intracoronary abciximab and aspiration thrombectomy in patients with large anterior myocardial infarction: the INFUSE-AMI randomized trial. *JAMA.* 2012; 307:1817-26.
111. Kastrati A, Mehilli J, Schuhlen H et al. A clinical trial of abciximab in elective percutaneous coronary intervention after pretreatment with clopidogrel. *N Engl J Med.* 2004; 350:232-8.
112. Kastrati A, Mehilli J, Neumann FJ et al. Abciximab in patients with acute coronary syndromes undergoing percutaneous coronary intervention after clopidogrel pretreatment: the ISAR-REACT 2 randomized trial. *JAMA.* 2006; 295:1531-8.
113. Giugliano RP, White JA, Bode C et al. Early versus delayed, provisional eptifibatide in acute coronary syndromes. *N Engl J Med.* 2009; 360:2176-90.
114. [No authors listed]. Novel dosing regimen of eptifibatide in planned coronary stent implantation (ESPRIT): a randomised, placebo-controlled trial. *Lancet.* 2000; 356:2037-44.
115. Zeymer U, Margenet A, Haude M et al. Randomized comparison of eptifibatide versus abciximab in primary percutaneous coronary intervention in patients with acute ST-segment elevation myocardial infarction: results of the EVA-AMI Trial. *J Am Coll Cardiol.* 2010; 56:463-9.
116. Kirtane AJ, Piazza G, Murphy SA et al. Correlates of bleeding events among moderate- to high-risk patients undergoing percutaneous coronary intervention and treated with eptifibatide: observations from the PROTECT-TIMI-30 trial. *J Am Coll Cardiol.* 2006; 47:2374-9.
117. Platelet Glycoprotein IIb/IIIa in Unstable Angina: Receptor Suppression Using Integrilin Therapy (PURSUIT) Trial Investigators. Inhibition of platelet glycoprotein IIb/IIIa with eptifibatide

in patients with acute coronary syndromes. *N Engl J Med.* 1998; 339:436-43.

118. Valgimigli M, Campo G, Percoco G et al. Comparison of angioplasty with infusion of tirofiban or abciximab and with implantation of sirolimus-eluting or uncoated stents for acute myocardial infarction: the MULTISTRATEGY randomized trial. *JAMA.* 2008; 299:1788-99.
119. Van't Hof AW, Ten Berg J, Heestermans T et al. Prehospital initiation of tirofiban in patients with ST-elevation myocardial infarction undergoing primary angioplasty (On-TIME 2): a multicentre, double-blind, randomised controlled trial. *Lancet.* 2008; 372:537-46.
120. Platelet Receptor Inhibition in Ischemic Syndrome Management (PRISM) Study Investigators. A comparison of aspirin plus tirofiban with aspirin plus heparin for unstable angina. *N Engl J Med.* 1998; 338:1498-505.
121. Topol EJ, Moliterno DJ, Herrmann HC et al. Comparison of two platelet glycoprotein IIb/IIIa inhibitors, tirofiban and abciximab, for the prevention of ischemic events with percutaneous coronary revascularization. *N Engl J Med.* 2001; 344:1888-94.
122. Han Y, Li Y, Wang S et al. Cilostazol in addition to aspirin and clopidogrel improves long-term outcomes after percutaneous coronary intervention in patients with acute coronary syndromes: a randomized, controlled study. *Am Heart J* 2009; 157:733-9.
123. Douglas JS Jr, Holmes DR Jr, Kereiakes DJ et al. Coronary stent restenosis in patients treated with cilostazol. *Circulation.* 2005; 112:2826-32.
124. Park SW, Lee CW, Kim HS et al. Comparison of cilostazol versus ticlopidine therapy after stent implantation. *Am J Cardiol.* 1999; 84:511-4.
125. Yoon Y, Shim WH, Lee DH et al. Usefulness of cilostazol versus ticlopidine in coronary artery stenting. *Am J Cardiol.* 1999; 84:1375-80.
126. Morrow DA, Braunwald E, Bonaca MP et al. Vorapaxar in the secondary prevention of atherothrombotic events. *N Engl J Med.* 2012; 366.1404-13.
127. Tricoci P, Huang Z, Held C et al. Thrombin-receptor antagonist vorapaxar in acute coronary syndromes. *N Engl J Med.* 2012; 366:20-33.
128. Gisslinger H, Gotic M, Holowiecki J et al. Anagrelide compared with hydroxyurea in WHO-classified essential thrombocythemia: the ANAHYDRET Study, a randomized controlled trial. *Blood.* 2013; 121:1720-8.
129. Steurer M, Gastl G, Jedrzejczak WW et al. Anagrelide for thrombocytosis in myeloproliferative disorders: a prospective study to assess efficacy and adverse event profile. *Cancer.* 2004; 101:2239-46.
130. Silverstein FE, Faich G, Goldstein JL et al. Gastrointestinal toxicity with celecoxib vs nonsteroidal anti-inflammatory drugs for osteoarthritis and rheumatoid arthritis: the CLASS study: a randomized controlled trial. Celecoxib Long-term Arthritis Safety Study. *JAMA.* 2000; 284:1247-55.
131. Chan FK, Hung LC, Suen BY et al. Celecoxib versus diclofenac and omeprazole in reducing the risk of recurrent ulcer bleeding in patients with arthritis. *N Engl J Med.* 2002; 347:2104-10.
132. Laine L, Connors LG, Reicin A et al. Serious lower gastrointestinal clinical events with nonselective NSAID or coxib use. *Gastroenterology.* 2003; 124:288-92.
133. Schnitzer TJ, Burmester GR, Mysler E et al. Comparison of lumiracoxib with naproxen and ibuprofen in the Therapeutic Arthritis Research and Gastrointestinal Event Trial (TARGET), reduction in ulcer complications: randomised controlled trial. *Lancet.* 2004; 364:665-74.
134. Solomon DH, Rassen JA, Glynn RJ et al. The comparative safety of analgesics in older adults with arthritis. *Arch Intern Med.* 2010; 170:1968-76.
135. Zinkstok SM, Roos YB. Early administration of aspirin in patients treated with alteplase for acute ischaemic stroke: a randomised controlled trial. *Lancet.* 2012; 380:731-7.
136. Enden T, Haig Y, Klow NE et al. Long-term outcome after additional catheter-directed thrombolysis versus standard treatment for acute iliofemoral deep vein thrombosis (the CaVenT study): a randomised controlled trial. *Lancet.* 2012; 379:31-8.
137. Wang C, Zhai Z, Yang Y et al. Efficacy and safety of low dose recombinant tissue-type plasminogen activator for the treatment of acute pulmonary thromboembolism: a randomized, multicenter, controlled trial. *Chest.* 2010; 137:254-62.
138. Administration of Alteplase (COBALT) Investigators. A comparison of continuous infusion of alteplase with double-bolus administration for acute myocardial infarction. The Continuous Infusion versus Double-Bolus. *N Engl J Med.* 1997; 337:1124-30.
139. Hacke W, Kaste M, Bluhmki E et al. Thrombolysis with alteplase 3 to 4.5 hours after acute ischemic stroke. *N Engl J Med.* 2008; 359:1317-29.
140. The GUSTO Investigators. An international randomized trial comparing four thrombolytic strategies for acute myocardial infarction. *N Engl J Med.* 1993; 329:673-82.
141. Broderick JP, Palesch YY, Demchuk AM et al. Endovascular therapy after intravenous t-PA versus t-PA alone for stroke. *N Engl J Med.* 2013; 368:893-903.
142. Hemmelgarn BR, Moist LM, Lok CE et al. Prevention of dialysis catheter malfunction with recombinant tissue plasminogen activator. *N Engl J Med.* 2011; 364:303-12.
143. Ciccone A, Valvassori L, Nichelatti M et al. Endovascular treatment for acute ischemic stroke. *N Engl J Med.* 2013; 368:904-13.
144. The Global Use of Strategies to Open Occluded Coronary Arteries (GUSTO III) Investigators. A comparison of reteplase with alteplase for acute myocardial infarction. *N Engl J Med.* 1997; 337:1118-23.
145. Topol EJ. Reperfusion therapy for acute myocardial infarction with fibrinolytic therapy or combination reduced fibrinolytic therapy and platelet glycoprotein IIb/IIIa inhibition: the GUSTO V randomised trial. *Lancet.* 2001; 357:1905-14.
146. Van De Werf F, Adgey J, Ardissino D et al. Single-bolus tenecteplase compared with front-loaded alteplase in acute myocardial infarction: the ASSENT-2 double-blind randomised trial. *Lancet.* 1999; 354:716-22.
147. Giugliano RP, Roe MT, Harrington RA et al. Combination reperfusion therapy with eptifibatide and reduced-dose tenecteplase for ST-elevation myocardial infarction: results of the integrilin and tenecteplase in acute myocardial infarction (INTEGRITI) Phase II Angiographic Trial. *J Am Coll Cardiol.* 2003; 41:1251-60.
148. Meyer G, Vicaut E, Danays T et al. Fibrinolysis for patients with intermediate-risk pulmonary embolism. *N Engl J Med.* 2014; 370:1402-11.
149. Armstrong PW, Gershlick AH, Goldstein P et al. Fibrinolysis or primary PCI in ST-segment elevation myocardial infarction. *N Engl J Med.* 2013; 368:1379-87.
150. Corbacioglu S, Cesaro S, Faraci M et al. Defibrotide for prophylaxis of hepatic veno-occlusive disease in paediatric haemopoietic stem-cell transplantation: an open-label, phase 3, randomised controlled trial. *Lancet.* 2012; 379:1301-9.
151. Dalton SO, Johansen C, Mellemkjaer L et al. Use of selective serotonin reuptake inhibitors and risk of upper gastrointestinal tract bleeding: a population-based cohort study. *Arch Intern Med.* 2003; 163:59-64.
152. Coupland C, Dhiman P, Morriss R et al. Antidepressant use and risk of adverse outcomes in older people: population based cohort study. *BMJ.* 2011; 343:d4551.
153. Russell RI. Non-steroidal anti-inflammatory drugs and gastrointestinal damage-problems and solutions. *Postgrad Med J.* 2001; 77:82-8.
154. Doery JC, Hirsh J, De Grouchy GC. Aspirin: its effect on platelet glycolysis and release of adenosine diphosphate. *Science.* 1968; 165:65-7.
155. Jiang HY, Chen HZ, Hu XJ et al. Use of selective serotonin reuptake inhibitors and risk of upper gastrointestinal bleeding: a

systematic review and meta-analysis. *Clin Gastroenterol Hepatol.* 2015; 13:42-50.e43.

156. Li N, Wallen NH, Ladjevardi M, Hjemdahl P. Effects of serotonin on platelet activation in whole blood. *Blood Coagul Fibrinolysis.* 1997; 8:517-23.
157. Mak KH, Bhatt DL, Shao M et al. Ethnic variation in adverse cardiovascular outcomes and bleeding complications in the Clopidogrel for High Atherothrombotic Risk and Ischemic Stabilization, Management, and Avoidance (CHARISMA) study. *Am Heart J.* 2009; 157:658-65.
158. Wang TY, Chen AY, Roe MT et al. Comparison of baseline characteristics, treatment patterns, and in-hospital outcomes of Asian versus non-Asian white Americans with non-ST-segment elevation acute coronary syndromes from the CRUSADE quality improvement initiative. *Am J Cardiol.* 2007; 100:391-6.
159. Shen AY, Yao JF, Brar SS et al. Racial/ethnic differences in the risk of intracranial hemorrhage among patients with atrial fibrillation. *J Am Coll Cardiol.* 2007; 50:309-15.
160. Mehran R, Rao SV, Bhatt DL et al. Standardized bleeding definitions for cardiovascular clinical trials: a consensus report from the Bleeding Academic Research Consortium. *Circulation.* 2011; 123:2736-47.
161. Kaatz S, Ahmad D, Spyropoulos AC, Schulman S. Definition of clinically relevant non-major bleeding in studies of anticoagulants in atrial fibrillation and venous thromboembolic disease in non-surgical patients: communication from the SSC of the ISTH. *J Thromb Haemost.* 2015; 13:2119-26.
162. Schulman S, Kearon C. Definition of major bleeding in clinical investigations of antihemostatic medicinal products in non-surgical patients. *J Thromb Haemost.* 2005; 3:692-4.
163. Levine GN, Bates ER, Blankenship JC et al. 2011 ACCF/AHA/SCAI guideline for percutaneous coronary intervention. A report of the American College of Cardiology Foundation/American Heart Association Task Force on Practice Guidelines and the Society for Cardiovascular Angiography and Interventions. *J Am Coll Cardiol.* 2011; 58:e44-122.
164. De Caterina R, Husted S, Wallentin L et al. General mechanisms of coagulation and targets of anticoagulants (Section I). Position Paper of the ESC Working Group on Thrombosis—Task Force on Anticoagulants in Heart Disease. *Thromb Haemost* 2013; 109:569-79.
165. Garcia DA, Baglin TP, Weitz JI, Samama MM. Parenteral anticoagulants: antithrombotic therapy and prevention of thrombosis, 9th ed: American College of Chest Physicians Evidence-Based Clinical Practice Guidelines. *Chest.* 2012; 141(suppl 2):e24S-43S.
166. Li T, Chang CY, Jin DY et al. Identification of the gene for vitamin K epoxide reductase. *Nature.* 2004; 427:541-4.
167. Rost S, Fregin A, Ivaskevicius V et al. Mutations in VKORC1 cause warfarin resistance and multiple coagulation factor deficiency type 2. *Nature.* 2004; 427:537-41.
168. Schafer AI. Effects of nonsteroidal antiinflammatory drugs on platelet function and systemic hemostasis. *J Clin Pharmacol.* 1995; 35:209-19.
169. McAdam BF, Catella-Lawson F, Mardini IA et al. Systemic biosynthesis of prostacyclin by cyclooxygenase (COX)-2: the human pharmacology of a selective inhibitor of COX-2. *Proc Natl Acad Sci USA.* 1999; 96:272-7.
170. Cryer B, Feldman M. Cyclooxygenase-1 and cyclooxygenase-2 selectivity of widely used nonsteroidal anti-inflammatory drugs. *Am J Med.* 1998; 104:413-21.
171. Llevadot J, Giugliano RP, Antman EM. Bolus fibrinolytic therapy in acute myocardial infarction. *JAMA.* 2001; 286:442-9.
172. Gutierrez G, Reines HD, Wulf-Gutierrez ME. Clinical review: hemorrhagic shock. *Crit Care.* 2004; 8:373-81.
173. Kerlin MP, Tokar JL. Acute gastrointestinal bleeding. *Ann Intern Med.* 2013; 159:793-4.
174. Smucker WD, Disabato JA, Krishen AE. Systematic approach to diagnosis and initial management of stroke. *Am Fam Physician.* 1995; 52:225-34.
175. Hylek EM, Evans-Molina C, Shea C et al. Major hemorrhage and tolerability of warfarin in the first year of therapy among elderly patients with atrial fibrillation. *Circulation.* 2007; 115:2689-96.
176. Goodman SG, Wojdyla DM, Piccini JP et al. Factors associated with major bleeding events: insights from the ROCKET AF trial (rivaroxaban once-daily oral direct factor Xa inhibition compared with vitamin K antagonism for prevention of stroke and embolism trial in atrial fibrillation). *J Am Coll Cardiol.* 2014; 63:891-900.
177. Hochholzer W, Wiviott SD, Antman EM et al. Predictors of bleeding and time dependence of association of bleeding with mortality: insights from the Trial to Assess Improvement in Therapeutic Outcomes by Optimizing Platelet Inhibition With Prasugrel-Thrombolysis in Myocardial Infarction 38 (TRITON-TIMI 38). *Circulation.* 2011; 123:2681-9.
178. Dans AL, Connolly SJ, Wallentin L et al. Concomitant use of antiplatelet therapy with dabigatran or warfarin in the Randomized Evaluation of Long-Term Anticoagulation Therapy (RE-LY) trial. *Circulation.* 2013; 127:634-40.
179. Dewilde WJ, Oirbans T, Verheugt FW et al. Use of clopidogrel with or without aspirin in patients taking oral anticoagulant therapy and undergoing percutaneous coronary intervention: an open-label, randomised, controlled trial. *Lancet.* 2013; 381:1107-15.
180. Gage BF, Yan Y, Milligan PE et al. Clinical classification schemes for predicting hemorrhage: results from the National Registry of Atrial Fibrillation (NRAF). *Am Heart J.* 2006; 151:713-9.
181. Mehta RH, Cox M, Smith EE et al. Race/Ethnic differences in the risk of hemorrhagic complications among patients with ischemic stroke receiving thrombolytic therapy. *Stroke.* 2014; 45:2263-9.
182. Slichter SJ. Relationship between platelet count and bleeding risk in thrombocytopenic patients. *Transfus Med Rev.* 2004; 18:153-67.
183. Peng YL, Leu HB, Luo JC et al. Diabetes is an independent risk factor for peptic ulcer bleeding: a nationwide population-based cohort study. *J Gastroenterol Hepatol.* 2013; 28:1295-9.
184. Gasse C, Hollowell J, Meier CR, Haefeli WE. Drug interactions and risk of acute bleeding leading to hospitalisation or death in patients with chronic atrial fibrillation treated with warfarin. *Thromb Haemost.* 2005; 94:537-43.
185. Limdi NA, McGwin G, Goldstein JA et al. Influence of CYP2C9 and VKORC1 1173C/T genotype on the risk of hemorrhagic complications in African-American and European-American patients on warfarin. *Clin Pharmacol Ther.* 2008; 83:312-21.
186. Sanderson S, Emery J, Higgins J. CYP2C9 gene variants, drug dose, and bleeding risk in warfarin-treated patients: a HuGEnet systematic review and meta-analysis. *Genet Med.* 2005; 7:97-104.
187. Pisters R, Lane DA, Nieuwlaat R et al. A novel user-friendly score (HAS-BLED) to assess 1-year risk of major bleeding in patients with atrial fibrillation: the Euro Heart Survey. *Chest.* 2010; 138:1093-100.
188. Li Y, Tang HL, Hu YF, Xie HG. The gain-of-function variant allele CYP2C19*17: a double-edged sword between thrombosis and bleeding in clopidogrel-treated patients. *J Thromb Haemost.* 2012; 10:199-206.
189. Higashi MK, Veenstra DL, Kondo LM et al. Association between CYP2C9 genetic variants and anticoagulation-related outcomes during warfarin therapy. *JAMA.* 2002; 287:1690-8.
190. Sibbing D, Koch W, Gebhard D et al. Cytochrome 2C19*17 allelic variant, platelet aggregation, bleeding events, and stent thrombosis in clopidogrel-treated patients with coronary stent placement. *Circulation.* 2010; 121:512-8.
191. Fang MC, Go AS, Chang Y et al. A new risk scheme to predict warfarin-associated hemorrhage: The ATRIA (Anticoagulation and Risk Factors in Atrial Fibrillation) Study. *J Am Coll Cardiol* 2011; 58:395-401.
192. Kooiman J, van Hagen N, Iglesias Del Sol A et al. The HAS-BLED Score identifies patients with acute venous thromboembolism at high risk of major bleeding complications during the first six months of anticoagulant treatment. *PloS one.* 2015; 10:e0122520.
193. Apostolakis S, Lane DA, Guo Y et al. Performance of the HEMORR(2)HAGES, ATRIA, and HAS-BLED bleeding risk-prediction

scores in patients with atrial fibrillation undergoing anticoagulation: the AMADEUS (evaluating the use of SR34006 compared to warfarin or acenocoumarol in patients with atrial fibrillation) study. *J Am Coll Cardiol.* 2012; 60:861-7.

194. Roldan V, Marin F, Fernandez H et al. Predictive value of the HAS-BLED and ATRIA bleeding scores for the risk of serious bleeding in a "real-world" population with atrial fibrillation receiving anticoagulant therapy. *Chest.* 2013; 143:179-84.
195. Kiviniemi T, Puurunen M, Schlitt A et al. Performance of bleeding risk-prediction scores in patients with atrial fibrillation undergoing percutaneous coronary intervention. *J Am Coll Cardiol.* 2014; 113:1995-2001.
196. January CT, Wann LS, Alpert JS et al. 2014 AHA/ACC/HRS guideline for the management of patients with atrial fibrillation: a report of the American College of Cardiology/American Heart Association Task Force on practice guidelines and the Heart Rhythm Society. *Circulation.* 2014; 130:e199-267.
197. Gasse C, Christensen S, Riis A et al. Preadmission use of SSRIs alone or in combination with NSAIDs and 30-day mortality after peptic ulcer bleeding. *Scand J Gastroenterol.* 2009; 44:1288-95.
198. Lopponen P, Tetri S, Juvela S et al. Association between warfarin combined with serotonin-modulating antidepressants and increased case fatality in primary intracerebral hemorrhage: a population-based study. *J Neurosurg.* 2014; 120:1358-63.
199. Singh I, Achuthan S, Chakrabarti A et al. Influence of preoperative use of serotonergic antidepressants (SADs) on the risk of bleeding in patients undergoing different surgical interventions: a meta-analysis. *Pharmacoepidemiol Drug Saf.* 2015; 24:237-45.
200. Tully PJ, Cardinal T, Bennetts JS, Baker RA. Selective serotonin reuptake inhibitors, venlafaxine and duloxetine are associated with in hospital morbidity but not bleeding or late mortality after coronary artery bypass graft surgery. *Heart Lung Circ.* 2012; 21:206-14.
201. [No authors listed]. Preventing errors relating to commonly used anticoagulants. *Sentinel Event Alert.* 2008:1-4.
202. Amin A, Bruno A, Trocio J et al. Incremental health care burden of bleeding among patients with venous thromboembolism in the United States. *J Manag Care Spec Pharm.* 2015; 21:965-72.
203. Bertrand OF, Jolly SS, Rao SV et al. Meta-analysis comparing bivalirudin versus heparin monotherapy on ischemic and bleeding outcomes after percutaneous coronary intervention. *J Am Cardiol.* 2012; 110:599-606.
204. Ayas NT, Dodek PM, Wang H et al. Attributable length of stay and mortality of major bleeding as a complication of therapeutic anticoagulation in the intensive care unit. *J Patient Saf.* 2015; 11:23-7.
205. Lauzier F, Arnold DM, Rabbat C et al. Risk factors and impact of major bleeding in critically ill patients receiving heparin thromboprophylaxis. *Intensive Care Med.* 2013; 39:2135-43.
206. Budnitz DS, Lovegrove MC, Shehab N, Richards CL. Emergency hospitalizations for adverse drug events in older Americans. *N Engl J Med.* 2011; 365:2002-12.
207. Budnitz DS, Shehab N, Kegler SR, Richards CL. Medication use leading to emergency department visits for adverse drug events in older adults. *Ann Intern Med.* 2007; 147:755-65.
208. Fihn SD, Callahan CM, Martin DC et al. The risk for and severity of bleeding complications in elderly patients treated with warfarin. The National Consortium of Anticoagulation Clinics. *Ann Intern Med.* 1996; 124:970-9.
209. Zareh M, Davis A, Henderson S. Reversal of warfarin-induced hemorrhage in the emergency department. *West J Emerg Med.* 2011; 12:386-92.
210. Hylek EM, Held C, Alexander JH et al. Major bleeding in patients with atrial fibrillation receiving apixaban or warfarin: The ARISTOTLE Trial (Apixaban for Reduction in Stroke and Other Thromboembolic Events in Atrial Fibrillation): predictors, characteristics, and clinical outcomes. *J Am Coll Cardiol.* 2014; 63:2141-7.
211. The Stroke Prevention in Atrial Fibrillation Investigators. Bleeding during antithrombotic therapy in patients with atrial fibrillation. *Arch Intern Med.* 1996; 156:409-16.
212. Kam JK, Chen Z, Liew D, Yan B. Does warfarin-related intracerebral haemorrhage lead to higher costs of management? *Clin Neurol Neurosurg.* 2014; 126:38-42.
213. Witt DM, Delate T, Hylek EM et al. Effect of warfarin on intracranial hemorrhage incidence and fatal outcomes. *ThrombRes.* 2013; 132:770-5.
214. Liew A, O'Donnell M, Douketis J. Comparing mortality in patients with atrial fibrillation who are receiving a direct-acting oral anticoagulant or warfarin: a meta-analysis of randomized trials. *J Thromb Haemost.* 2014; 12:1419-24.
215. Sharma M, Cornelius VR, Patel JP et al. Efficacy and harms of direct oral anticoagulants in the elderly for stroke prevention in atrial fibrillation and secondary prevention of venous thromboembolism: systematic review and meta-analysis. *Circulation.* 2015; 132:194-204.
216. Bouget J, Oger E. Emergency admissions for major haemorrhage associated with direct oral anticoagulants. *Thromb Res.* 2015; 136:1190-4.
217. Chai-Adisaksopha C, Hillis C, Isayama T et al. Mortality outcomes in patients receiving direct oral anticoagulants: a systematic review and meta-analysis of randomized controlled trials. *J Thromb Haemost.* 2015; 13:2012-20.
218. Charlton B. Length of hospital stay and mortality for bleeding among adults with atrial fibrillation treated with warfarin, dabigatran, or rivaroxaban. *AHA.* 2015; Abstract S40842015.
219. Ansell JE. Universal, class-specific and drug-specific reversal agents for the new oral anticoagulants. *J Thromb Thrombolysis.* 2016; 41:248-52.
220. Pollack CV Jr, Reilly PA, Eikelboom J et al. Idarucizumab for dabigatran reversal. *N Engl J Med.* 2015; 373:511-20.
221. Siegal DM, Curnutte JT, Connolly SJ et al. Andexanet alfa for the reversal of factor Xa inhibitor activity. *N Engl J Med.* 2015; 373:2413-24.
222. Kwok CS, Rao SV, Myint PK et al. Major bleeding after percutaneous coronary intervention and risk of subsequent mortality: a systematic review and meta-analysis. *Open Heart.* 2014; 1:e000021.
223. Ferguson JJ, Antman EM, Bates ER et al. Combining enoxaparin and glycoprotein IIb/IIIa antagonists for the treatment of acute coronary syndromes: final results of the National Investigators Collaborating on Enoxaparin-3 (NICE-3) study. *Am Heart J.* 2003; 146:628-34.
224. Howard JP, Jones DA, Gallagher S et al. Glycoprotein IIb/IIIa inhibitors use and outcome after percutaneous coronary intervention for non-ST elevation myocardial infarction. *Biomed Res Int.* 2014; 2014:643981.
225. Bavishi C, Panwar S, Messerli FH, Bangalore S. Meta-analysis of comparison of the newer oral P2Y12 Inhibitors (prasugrel or ticagrelor) to clopidogrel in patients with non-ST-elevation acute coronary syndrome. *Am J Coll Cardiol.* 2015; 116:809-17.
226. Yudi MB, Clark DJ, Farouque O et al. Clopidogrel, prasugrel or ticagrelor in patients with acute coronary syndromes undergoing percutaneous coronary intervention. *Intern Med J.* 2016; 46:559-65.
227. Serebruany VL, Aradi D, Kim MH, Sibbing D. Cangrelor infusion is associated with an increased risk for bleeding: meta-analysis of randomized trials. *Int J Cardiol.* 2013; 169:225-8.
228. Moore RA, Derry S, Simon LS, Emery P. Nonsteroidal anti-inflammatory drugs, gastroprotection, and benefit-risk. *Pain Pract.* 2014; 14:378-95.
229. Straube S, Tramer MR, Moore RA et al. Mortality with upper gastrointestinal bleeding and perforation: effects of time and NSAID use. *BMC Gastroenterol.* 2009; 9:41.
230. Pirmohamed M, James S, Meakin S et al. Adverse drug reactions as cause of admission to hospital: prospective analysis of 18 820 patients. *BMJ.* 2004; 329:15-19.

231. Gu Q, Dillon CF, Eberhardt MS et al. Preventive aspirin and other antiplatelet medication use among US adults aged ≥ 40 years: data from the National Health and Nutrition Examination Survey, 2011–2012. *Public Health Rep.* 2015; 130:643-54.
232. Soni A. Aspirin use among the adult US noninstitutionalized population, with and without indicators of heart disease, 2005. *AHRQ Statistical Brief #179.* 2007.
233. Berger JS, Bhatt DL, Steg PG et al. Bleeding, mortality, and antiplatelet therapy: results from the Clopidogrel for High Atherothrombotic Risk and Ischemic Stabilization, Management, and Avoidance (CHARISMA) trial. *Am Heart J.* 2011; 162:98-105.e101.
234. Campbell CL, Smyth S, Montalescot G, Steinhubl SR. Aspirin dose for the prevention of cardiovascular disease: a systematic review. *JAMA.* 2007; 297:2018-24.
235. Benavente OR, Hart RG, McClure LA et al. Effects of clopidogrel added to aspirin in patients with recent lacunar stroke. *N Engl J Med.* 2012; 367:817-25.
236. Palacio S, Hart RG, Pearce LA, Benavente OR. Effect of addition of clopidogrel to aspirin on mortality: systematic review of randomized trials. *Stroke.* 2012; 43:2157-62.
237. Chatterjee S, Chakraborty A, Weinberg I et al. Thrombolysis for pulmonary embolism and risk of all-cause mortality, major bleeding, and intracranial hemorrhage: a meta-analysis. *JAMA.* 2014; 311:2414-21.
238. Daley MJ, Murthy MS, Peterson EJ. Bleeding risk with systemic thrombolytic therapy for pulmonary embolism: scope of the problem. *Ther Adv Drug Saf.* 2015; 6:57-66.
239. Marti C, John G, Konstantinides S et al. Systemic thrombolytic therapy for acute pulmonary embolism: a systematic review and meta-analysis. *Eur Heart J.* 2015; 36:605-14.
240. George BP, Asemota AO, Dorsey ER et al. United States trends in thrombolysis for older adults with acute ischemic stroke. *Clin Neurol Neurosurg.* 2015; 139:16-23.
241. Wardlaw JM, Murray V, Berge E, del Zoppo GJ. Thrombolysis for acute ischaemic stroke. *The Cochrane Database of Systematic Reviews.* 2014; 7:Cd000213.
242. The National Institute of Neurological Disorders and Stroke rt-PA Stroke Study Group. Tissue plasminogen activator for acute ischemic stroke. *N Engl J Med.* 1995; 333:1581-7.
243. Mortensen JK, Larsson H, Johnsen SP, Andersen G. Post stroke use of selective serotonin reuptake inhibitors and clinical outcome among patients with ischemic stroke: a nationwide propensity score-matched follow-up study. *Stroke.* 2013; 44:420-6.
244. Oyetayo OO, Slicker K, De La Rosa L et al. Dual antiplatelet compared to triple antithrombotic therapy in anterior wall acute myocardial infarction complicated by depressed left ventricular ejection fraction. *Proc (Bayl Univ Med Cent).* 2015; 28:445-9.
245. Staudacher DL, Kaiser M, Hehrlein C et al. Triple antithrombotic therapy after percutaneous coronary intervention (pci) in patients with indication for oral anticoagulation: data from a single center registry. *PloS One.* 2015; 10:e0140101.
246. Abraham NS, Hlatky MA, Antman EM et al. ACCF/ACG/AHA 2010 expert consensus document on the concomitant use of proton pump inhibitors and thienopyridines: a focused update of the ACCF/ACG/AHA 2008 expert consensus document on reducing the gastrointestinal risks of antiplatelet therapy and NSAID use: a report of the American College of Cardiology Foundation Task Force on Expert Consensus Documents. *Circulation.* 2010; 122:2619-33.
247. Bhatt DL, Scheiman J, Abraham NS et al. ACCF/ACG/AHA 2008 expert consensus document on reducing the gastrointestinal risks of antiplatelet therapy and NSAID use: a report of the American College of Cardiology Foundation Task Force on Clinical Expert Consensus Documents. *J Am Coll Cardiol.* 2008; 52:1502-17.
248. Parekh PJ, Oldfield EC, Johnson DA. Current strategies to reduce gastrointestinal bleeding risk associated with antiplatelet agents. *Drugs.* 2015; 75:1613-25.
249. Vandiver JW, Vondracek TG. Antifactor Xa levels versus activated partial thromboplastin time for monitoring unfractionated heparin. *Pharmacotherapy.* 2012; 32:546-58.
250. Fruge KS, Lee YR. Comparison of unfractionated heparin protocols using antifactor Xa monitoring or activated partial thrombin time monitoring. *Am J Health-Syst Pharm.* 2015; 72(suppl 2): S90-7.
251. Gosselin RC, King JH, Janatpour KA et al. Comparing direct thrombin inhibitors using aPTT, ecarin clotting times, and thrombin inhibitor management testing. *Ann Pharmacother.* 2004; 38:1383-8.
252. Smythe MA, Priziola J, Dobesh PP et al. Guidance for the practical management of the heparin anticoagulants in the treatment of venous thromboembolism. *J Thromb Thrombolysis.* 2016; 41:165-86.
253. Kearon C, Akl EA, Comerota AJ et al. Antithrombotic therapy for VTE disease: antithrombotic therapy and prevention of thrombosis, 9th ed: American College of Chest Physicians Evidence-Based Clinical Practice Guidelines. *Chest.* 2012; 141 (suppl 2):e419S-94S.
254. Whitlock RP, Sun JC, Fremes SE et al. Antithrombotic and thrombolytic therapy for valvular disease: antithrombotic therapy and prevention of thrombosis, 9th ed: American College of Chest Physicians Evidence-Based Clinical Practice Guidelines. *Chest.* 2012; 141(suppl 2):e576S-600S.
255. You JJ, Singer DE, Howard PA et al. Antithrombotic therapy for atrial fibrillation: antithrombotic therapy and prevention of thrombosis, 9th ed: American College of Chest Physicians Evidence-Based Clinical Practice Guidelines. *Chest.* 2012; 141 (suppl 2):e531S-75S.
256. Ageno W, Gallus AS, Wittkowsky A et al. Oral anticoagulant therapy: antithrombotic therapy and prevention of thrombosis, 9th ed: American College of Chest Physicians Evidence-Based Clinical Practice Guidelines. *Chest.* 2012; 141(suppl 2):e44S-88S.
257. Reilly PA, Lehr T, Haertter S et al. The effect of dabigatran plasma concentrations and patient characteristics on the frequency of ischemic stroke and major bleeding in atrial fibrillation patients: the RE-LY Trial (Randomized Evaluation of Long-Term Anticoagulation Therapy). *J Am Coll Cardiol.* 2014; 63:321-8.
258. Lindahl TL, Baghaei F, Blixter IF et al. Effects of the oral, direct thrombin inhibitor dabigatran on five common coagulation assays. *Thromb Haemost.* 2011; 105:371-8.
259. Sarma A, Giugliano RP. Current and developing strategies for monitoring and reversing direct oral anticoagulants in patients with non-valvular atrial fibrillation. *Hosp Pract. (1995).* 2015; 43:258-67.
260. van Ryn J, Stangier J, Haertter S et al. Dabigatran etexilate—a novel, reversible, oral direct thrombin inhibitor: interpretation of coagulation assays and reversal of anticoagulant activity. *J Thromb Haemost.* 2010; 103:1116-27.
261. Gosselin RC, Francart SJ, Hawes EM et al. Heparin-calibrated chromogenic anti-Xa activity measurements in patients receiving rivaroxaban: can this test be used to quantify drug level? *Ann Pharmacother.* 2015; 49:777-83.
262. Samama MM. Which test to use to measure the anticoagulant effect of rivaroxaban: the anti-factor Xa assay. *J Thromb Haemost.* 2013; 11:579-80.
263. Moukarbel GV, Bhatt DL. Antiplatelet therapy and proton pump inhibition: clinician update. *Circulation.* 2012; 125:375-80.
264. Lanas A, Garcia-Rodriguez LA, Arroyo MT et al. Effect of antisecretory drugs and nitrates on the risk of ulcer bleeding associated with nonsteroidal anti-inflammatory drugs, antiplatelet agents, and anticoagulants. *Am J Gstroenterol.* 2007; 102:507-15.
265. Bhatt DL, Cryer BL, Contant CF et al. Clopidogrel with or without omeprazole in coronary artery disease. *N Engl J Med.* 2010; 363:1909-17.
266. Cardoso RN, Benjo AM, DiNicolantonio JJ et al. Incidence of cardiovascular events and gastrointestinal bleeding in patients receiving clopidogrel with and without proton pump inhibitors: an updated meta-analysis. *Open Heart.* 2015; 2:e000248.

267. Scott SA, Owusu Obeng A, Hulot JS. Antiplatelet drug interactions with proton pump inhibitors. *Expert Opin Drug Metab Toxicol.* 2014; 10:175-89.
268. Makris M, Van Veen JJ, Tait CR et al. Guideline on the management of bleeding in patients on antithrombotic agents. *Br J Haematol.* 2013; 160:35-46.
269. Sartori MT, Prandoni P. How to effectively manage the event of bleeding complications when using anticoagulants. *Expert Rev Hematol.* 2016; 9:37-50.
270. Miller MP, Trujillo TC, Nordenholz KE. Practical considerations in emergency management of bleeding in the setting of target-specific oral anticoagulants. *Am J Emerg Med.* 2014; 32:375-82.
271. Nutescu EA, Dager WE, Kalus JS et al. Management of bleeding and reversal strategies for oral anticoagulants: clinical practice considerations. *Am J Health-Syst Pharm.* 2013; 70:1914-29.
272. Sarode R, Matevosyan K, Bhagat R et al. Rapid warfarin reversal: a 3-factor prothrombin complex concentrate and recombinant factor VIIa cocktail for intracerebral hemorrhage. *J Neurosurg.* 2012; 116:491-7.
273. Dager WE, Gosselin RC, Roberts AJ. Reversing dabigatran in life-threatening bleeding occurring during cardiac ablation with factor eight inhibitor bypassing activity. *Crit Care Med.* 2013; 41:e42-6.
274. Frontera JA, Lewin JJ III, Rabinstein AA et al. Guideline for reversal of antithrombotics in intracranial hemorrhage: a statement for healthcare professionals from the Neurocritical Care Society and Society of Critical Care Medicine. *Neurocrit Care.* 2016; 24:6-46.
275. Bolliger D, Szlam F, Azran M et al. The anticoagulant effect of protamine sulfate is attenuated in the presence of platelets or elevated factor VIII concentrations. *Anesth Analg.* 2010; 111:601-8.
276. Nielsen VG. Protamine enhances fibrinolysis by decreasing clot strength: role of tissue factor-initiated thrombin generation. *Ann Thorac Surg.* 2006; 81:1720-7.
277. Crowther MA, Berry LR, Monagle PT, Chan AK. Mechanisms responsible for the failure of protamine to inactivate low-molecular-weight heparin. *Br J Haematol.* 2002; 116:178-86.
278. Holbrook A, Schulman S, Witt DM et al. Evidence-based management of anticoagulant therapy: antithrombotic therapy and prevention of thrombosis, 9th ed: American College of Chest Physicians Evidence-Based Clinical Practice Guidelines. *Chest.* 2012; 141(suppl 2):e152S-84S.
279. Dezee KJ, Shimeall WT, Douglas KM et al. Treatment of excessive anticoagulation with phytonadione (vitamin K): a meta-analysis. *Arch Intern Med.* 2006; 166:391-7.
280. Tsu LV, Dienes JE, Dager WE. Vitamin K dosing to reverse warfarin based on INR, route of administration, and home warfarin dose in the acute/critical care setting. *Ann Pharmacother.* 2012; 46:1617-26.
281. Chang DN, Dager WE, Chin AI. Removal of dabigatran by hemodialysis. *Am J Kidney Dis.* 2013; 61:487-9.
282. Young G, Yonekawa KE, Nakagawa PA et al. Recombinant activated factor VII effectively reverses the anticoagulant effects of heparin, enoxaparin, fondaparinux, argatroban, and bivalirudin ex vivo as measured using thromboelastography. *Blood Coagul Fibrinolysis.* 2007; 18:547-53.
283. Reynolds MR. Discontinuation of rivaroxaban: filling in the gaps. *J Am Coll Cardiol.* 2013; 61:659-60.
284. Haynes LM, Orfeo T, Mann KG. Rivaroxaban delivery and reversal at a venous flow rate. *Arterioscler Thromb Vasc Biol.* 2012; 32:2877-83.
285. French KF, White J, Hoesch RE. Treatment of intracerebral hemorrhage with tranexamic acid after thrombolysis with tissue plasminogen activator. *Neurocrit Care.* 2012; 17:107-11.
286. Goldstein JN, Marrero M, Masrur S et al. Management of thrombolysis-associated symptomatic intracerebral hemorrhage. *Arch Neurol.* 2010; 67:965-9.
287. O'Carroll CB, Aguilar MI. Management of postthrombolysis hemorrhagic and orolingual angioedema complications. *Neurohospitalist.* 2015; 5:133-41.
288. Yaghi S, Eisenberger A, Willey JZ. Symptomatic intracerebral hemorrhage in acute ischemic stroke after thrombolysis with intravenous recombinant tissue plasminogen activator: a review of natural history and treatment. *JAMA Neurol.* 2014; 71:1181-5.
289. Bungard TJ, Gardner L, Archer SL et al. Evaluation of a pharmacist-managed anticoagulation clinic: improving patient care. *Open Med.* 2009; 3:e16-21.
290. Rudd KM, Dier JG. Comparison of two different models of anticoagulation management services with usual medical care. *Pharmacotherapy.* 2010; 30:330-8.
291. Witt DM, Humphries TL. A retrospective evaluation of the management of excessive anticoagulation in an established clinical pharmacy anticoagulation service compared to traditional care. *J Thromb Thrombolysis.* 2003; 15:113-8.

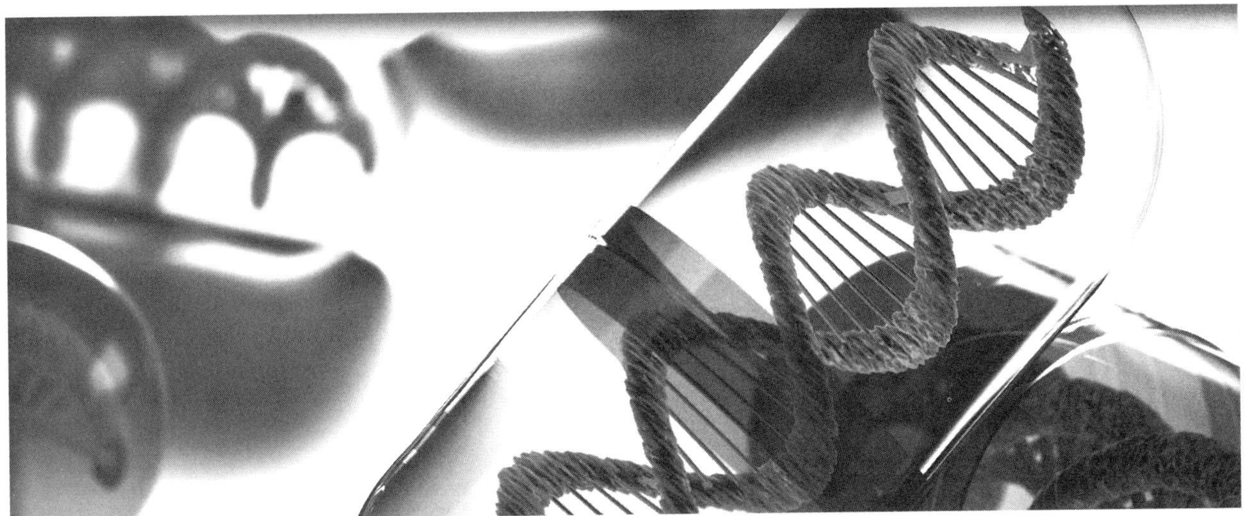

CHAPTER 46

Thrombocytopenia

Kellie Jones Weddle and Patrick J. Kiel

Thrombocytopenia is typically defined as a platelet count <150,000/mm^3 or a >50% decrease in the count from baseline.[1] Thrombocytopenia is considered to be moderate when the platelet count is 20,000–150,000/mm^3 and severe when the platelet count falls to <20,000/ mm^3. Patients with severe thrombocytopenia risk serious bleeding and even death.

Drug-induced thrombocytopenia is often a diagnosis of exclusion. Laboratory confirmation of drug-induced thrombocytopenia is an unusually difficult task because of the unavailability of drug-dependent antiplatelet antibodies for testing. Nondrug causes (e.g., viruses, intravascular coagulation disorders, or autoimmune disorders) must always be ruled out and pseudothrombocytopenia and dilutional thrombocytopenia should be excluded as potential causes as well.[2] A careful review of the patient's medication history (including current medications and any recent changes as well as nonprescription medications, herbal and/or nutritional supplements) is essential to help identify and address all potential causes of drug-induced thrombocytopenia. Although thrombocytopenia is listed as a possible adverse effect of many medications, it is actually considered a rare event.

CAUSATIVE AGENTS

There are many nondrug causes of thrombocytopenia, including human immunodeficiency virus, disseminated intravascular coagulation, blood transfusions, lupus, and sepsis.[3] In addition, many herbal supplements have been documented to cause precipitous drops in platelet counts. Although discussion of these conditions and agents is beyond the scope of this chapter, all should be considered as possible causes in any patient with thrombocytopenia. Numerous commonly prescribed drugs have been associated with thrombocytopenia and, in 1998, George and colleagues published an extensive review of drugs known to cause this disorder.[4] This database has continually been updated to include newer drugs, with the last update published in 2012.[5] Classes of medications known to cause thrombocytopenia include the cinchona alkaloids, antimicrobial agents, platelet inhibitors, antirheumatic agents, anticonvulsants, analgesics, heparins, chemotherapeutic agents, and immunosuppressants.[6] **Table 46-1** lists agents implicated in drug-induced thrombocytopenia. Many chemotherapeutic agents also cause thrombocytopenia, although, in contrast to the agents listed in Table 46-1, the thrombocytopenia that occurs during chemotherapy is generally predictable and represents an expected consequence of therapy.

EPIDEMIOLOGY

Although the exact incidence of drug-induced thrombocytopenia is not known, it is estimated to be approximately 10 cases per 1 million people per year.[3,6] The risk of thrombocytopenia in patients receiving trimethoprim–sulfamethoxazole is reported to be 38 occurrences per 1 million users

Table 46-1 Agents Implicated in Drug-Induced Thrombocytopenia

Drug	Incidence	Level of Evidence[a]
Abciximab[74]	0.5–1%: first exposure 10–14%: second exposure	A
Acetaminophen[4]	NK	C
Adefovir dipivoxil[5]	NK	C
Alfuzocin[5]	NK	C
Alprenolol[4]	NK	C
Aminoglutethimide[4]	NK	C
Amiodarone[4]	NK	C
Aminosalicylic acid[4]	NK	C
Amphotericin B[4]	NK	C
Ampicillin[4]	NK	C
Captopril[4]	NK	C
Carbamazepine[4]	NK	C
Chlordiazepoxide–clidinium bromide[75]	NK	C
Chlorothiazide[4]	NK	C
Chlorpromazine[4]	NK	C
Chlorpropamide[4]	NK	C
Cimetidine[4]	NK	C
Danazol[4]	NK	C
Diazepam[4]	NK	C
Diatrizoate meglumine[76]	<1%	C
Diazoxide[4]	NK	C
Deferoxamine[4]	NK	C
Diclofenac[4]	<1%	C
Digoxin[4]	NK	C
Efalizumab[77]	0.3%	A
Ethambutol[4]	NK	C
Etretinate[5]	NK	C
Eptifibatide[74]	0.2–0.5%	A
Famotidine[5]	NK	C
Fenofibrate[83]	NK	C
Fluconazole[4]	NK	C
Glyburide[3]	NK	C
Gold salts[4]	1–2%	C

Table 46-1 Agents Implicated in Drug-Induced Thrombocytopenia (continued)

Drug	Incidence	Level of Evidence[a]
Haloperidol[14]	NK	C
Heparin[6]	3–6%	A
Hydrochlorothiazide[4]	NK	C
Interferon α[4]	NK	C
Ibuprofen[6]	<1%	C
Iloprost[5]	NK	C
Isoniazid[4]	NK	C
Linezolid[54]	21%	C
Levamisole[4]	NK	C
Lopinavir/ritonavir[5]	NK	C
Methyldopa[4]	NK	C
Minoxidil[4]	NK	C
Meloxicam[82]	NK	C
Moxifloxacin[81]	NK	C
Nalidixic acid[4]	NK	C
Naphazoline[4]	NK	C
Naproxen[74]	<1%	C
Nitroglycerin[4]	NK	C
Octreotide[74]	NK	C
Oxprenolol[4]	NK	C
Pentoxifylline[84]	NK	C
Phenytoin[4]	NK	C
Piperacillin[4]	NK	C
Procainamide[6]	1%	C
Quinidine[4]	<1%	C
Quinine[4]	<1%	C
Ranitidine[4]	NK	C
Rifampin[4]	NK	C
Simvastatin[78]	<0.1%	C
Sulfasalazine[79]	<1%	C
Sulindac[4]	<1%	C
Tamoxifen[4]	NK	C
Terbinafine[75]	NK	C
Thiothixene[4]	NK	C
Tirofiban[75]	0.2–0.5%	A
Tolmentin[4]	<1%	C
Trimethoprim–sulfamethoxazole[4]	NK	C
Sulfisoxazole[4]	NK	C
Valproate[53]	20%	C
Vancomycin[80]	NK	A

NK = not known.

[a]Definitions for Levels of Evidence: Level A—evidence from one or more randomized, controlled clinical trials; Level B—evidence from nonrandomized clinical trials, prospective observational studies, cohort studies, retrospective studies, case-control studies, meta-analyses and/or postmarketing surveillance studies; and Level C—evidence from one or more published case reports or case series.

and in patients receiving quinine or quinidine, the risk is reported to be 26 occurrences for every 1 million users.[6]

MECHANISMS

Mechanisms of drug-induced thrombocytopenia are diverse and can involve both immunologic and nonimmunologic processes (**Table 46-2**).

DRUGS AS HAPTENS

Covalent bonding between drug molecules (haptens) and autologous proteins has been implicated in the production of drug-protein–specific antibodies.[7-9] Evidence is insufficient to support this as the mechanism responsible for drug-induced thrombocytopenia, however, except in the cases of mild hemolytic anemia and rare instances of penicillin-induced thrombocytopenia.[10] In general, antibodies are not directed toward a drug (hapten) that is covalently bound to platelets. The "innocent bystander hypothesis," which suggests that an antibody directed toward a drug molecule somehow cross-reacts with platelets resulting in thrombocytopenia has largely been refuted.[11]

COMPOUND EPITOPE FORMATION

Quinine, quinidine, sulfonamide antibiotics, and nonsteroidal anti-inflammatory drugs or all their respective metabolites may induce thrombocytopenia through the formation of new epitope (part drug, part protein) compound.[6,12] Over a century ago, quinine was the first drug recognized to cause severe thrombocytopenia. Initially used for the treatment of malaria, quinine can also be found in common tonic water, which may be consumed alone or mixed with alcohol for consumption. Quinine is also sometimes used to treat nocturnal leg cramps, although this use is not approved by the U.S. Food and Drug Administration (FDA) due to the risk of adverse reactions.[13]

Quinine is thought to cause glycoprotein (GP) structural modifications via one of two possible mechanisms. First, the soluble drug may react with the GP in a complementary manner with respect to charge or hydrophobic domain.[6,14] An antibody may then interact with the drug and adjacent peptides, resulting in platelet destruction.[11] A second widely accepted possible mechanism is that drug binding occurring at one locus induces a structural modification on a GP at another locus, leading to antibody binding and subsequent lysis.[11] It is known that the fragment antigen binding (Fab) region of the antibody is responsible for drug-dependent antibody binding.[15] The epitopes targeted by these antibodies include GPIIb/IIIa or GPIb/V/IX complexes.[10,14,16]

DRUG-INDUCED AUTOANTIBODIES

Rarely, autoantibodies are capable of destroying platelets after drug exposure. Such is the case in approximately 1–3% of patients receiving gold therapy for rheumatoid arthritis. The onset of

Table 46-2 Mechanisms of Drug-Induced Thrombocytopenia

Drug	Mechanism
Abciximab, eptifibatide, tirofiban[6,25]	Drug-dependent antibody recognition of Fab fragment and glycoprotein IIb/IIIa neoepitope
Chloramphenicol,[54] linezolid[54]	Mitochondrial respiration suppression
Gold salts, procainamide[6,17,18]	Autoantibodies
Heparin, low-molecular-weight heparin[6,21-24]	Antibodies targeting epitope formation of heparin and Platelet Factor 4
Penicillins, cephalosporins and respective metabolites[6-8]	Hapten formation
Quinine, quinidine, sulfonamides[6,12] Nonsteroidal anti-inflammatory drugs, acetaminophen (paracetamol)	Compound epitope formation
Valproic acid, amiodarone[52,53]	Nonidiosyncratic concentration-dependent
Vancomycin[80]	Vancomycin-dependent antibodies against glycoprotein IIb/IIIa and unknown glycoproteins

gold-induced thrombocytopenia can be either rapid or delayed.[17] Patients may present with a sudden drop in platelets, or the platelet count may gradually decline over weeks to months. Delayed onset may be associated with pancytopenia. Sudden thrombocytopenia has been likened to idiopathic thrombocytopenia purpura (ITP), in which there is acute onset of immune-mediated platelet destruction with normal megakaryocytes found on bone marrow biopsy.[17] Through an unknown mechanism, gold stimulates immunoglobulin G (IgG) to target glycoprotein V on platelets.[10,18] This autoimmune-mediated reaction is independent of gold serum concentrations and may temporarily persist even after the drug is discontinued.[18] Similar occurrences have been described with procainamide but without known GP targets.[19,20]

HEPARIN-INDUCED THROMBOCYTOPENIA

Type II heparin-induced thrombocytopenia (HIT) is a result of antibodies targeting the epitope formation of heparin and platelet factor 4 (PF4), as opposed to HIT Type I which is benign and nonimmune mediated.[21,22] PF4 is a cytokine found in platelet α-granules and is released in response to platelet aggregation. It is thought that PF4 is involved in coagulation, inflammation, and chemotaxis and occurs in 1–3% of patients exposed to heparin products.[22] Heparin forms a complex with PF4, leading antibodies to recognize this entity as a new epitope.[22-24] Heparin may also cause conformational changes on PF4, where antibodies might be recognized as "foreign," or vice versa.[22] It is known that IgG, IgM, and IgA antibodies are responsible for HIT, with IgG being the most prevalent.[22,24] Although patients with HIT have circulating immunoglobulins for the heparin–PF4 complex, there are patients with the same immunoglobulins who do not present with HIT.[22] Thrombosis results from PF4 binding to glycosaminoglycan on endothelial cells, leading to the initiation of HIT antibodies targeting those cells. The apoptosis of endothelial cells leads to subsequent platelet activation and procoagulant reactions.[22] Platelet activation leads to microparticle release and further thrombosis stimulation. HIT can occur regardless of the dose, route, or frequency of administration of heparin products.

FIBRINOGEN INHIBITORS

Abciximab, tirofiban, and eptifibatide antagonize fibrinogen at GPIIb/IIIa, thereby inhibiting platelet–fibrinogen interactions and subsequent thrombus formation.[25] These agents are used in patients undergoing percutaneous transluminal coronary angioplasty to prevent restenosis.[26-29] Fibrinogen inhibitors cause thrombocytopenia within hours of administration in approximately 1% of patients after first exposure and in 4% after second exposure.[27,29]

Abciximab is a chimeric Fab fragment derived from a murine monoclonal antibody, 7E3. Acute thrombocytopenia, characterized by a decrease in platelet count that develops within hours after drug administration, is thought to be caused by preexisting antibodies directed toward murine components of abciximab.[6,29] Compared with other fibrinogen inhibitors, abciximab is associated with a more severe thrombocytopenia, with platelet counts decreasing to <10,000/mm^3. Delayed thrombocytopenia is characterized by a decrease in platelet count that develops within a week after drug administration and may occur upon re-exposure via newly induced IgG or IgM antibodies that possibly recognize epitopes on abciximab-coated platelets.[26,29]

A number of factors have been associated with an increased risk of thrombocytopenia in patients receiving a fibrinogen inhibitor, including the concomitant administration of aspirin or heparin and the use of intra-aortic balloon pumps.[30,31] Tirofiban and eptifibatide bind to the Arg-Gly-Asp recognition sites on GPIIb/IIIa, thereby antagonizing fibrinogen binding and subsequent platelet aggregation via platelet–fibrinogen–platelet interactions.[25] Specific antibodies recognizing drug binding at GPIIb/IIIa have not been identified as a definitive pathogenesis. Drug-dependent antibodies may recognize several epitopes because of conformational changes conferred from tirofiban or eptifibatide binding.[25,27] Nonimmune-mediated thrombocytopenia has also been discussed as a possible cause, but exact mechanisms have not been identified.[25]

HISTAMINE-RECEPTOR ANTAGONISTS

Case reports have implicated histamine-receptor antagonists as a possible trigger for thrombocytopenia.[32] Most reported cases occurred in intensive care units when the agents were used for stress-related mucosal injury prophylaxis. Proposed mechanisms include bone-marrow suppression via inhibition of stem-cell differentiation and formation of IgG antibodies.[32] However, well-designed retrospective and prospective studies have failed to confirm that histamine-receptor antagonists are a cause of thrombocytopenia in critically ill patients.[33,34]

THROMBOTIC THROMBOCYTOPENIC PURPURA

Thrombotic thrombocytopenic purpura–hemolytic uremic syndrome (TTP-HUS) is an inclusive term used to describe multiple causes of a clinicopathologic disorder with a fatality rate of 90%. This disorder is characterized by microangiopathic hemolytic anemia, erythrocyte fragmentation (schistocytes), thrombocytopenia, and other clinical features.[35,36] Ensuing complications include renal failure, neurologic abnormalities, bleeding, and fever. TTP-HUS can occur as a result of von Willebrand factor–cleaving protease deficiency, infections with *Escherichia coli* O157:H7, hematopoietic stem-cell transplantation, and certain drugs.[35,37-39] Evidence for drug-induced TTP-HUS exists for mitomycin C, cyclosporine, tacrolimus, sirolimus, quinine, ticlodipine, clopidogrel, and simvastatin.[35,36,40-45]

Drug-induced TTP has been postulated to occur via endothelial damage leading to subsequent platelet aggregation, such as with mitomycin C, cyclosporine, tacrolimus, and sirolimus.[36,43] In addition, these agents are thought to cause TTP in a dose-dependent manner.[36] In contrast, quinine-induced TTP is thought to be mediated by antibodies in the presence of soluble drug.[40] Quinine-induced TTP has been described after brief and even single exposures and is thought to be antibody-mediated, although antibodies directed toward von Willebrand factor–cleaving protease have not been reported.[36,38,40] Ticlopidine- and clopidogrel-induced TTP are somewhat paradoxical; case reports suggest an association with TTP, but mechanisms have not been elucidated.[42,44,45] Also, the reported incidence of TTP associated with these drugs appears to be similar to the incidence of TTP found in the general population (<1%).[36]

CLINICAL PRESENTATION AND DIFFERENTIAL DIAGNOSIS

Usually patients presenting with drug-induced thrombocytopenia have been exposed to the culprit agent for approximately 1–2 weeks; however, symptoms may develop immediately after exposure (**Table 46-3**). Patients may present with petechiae, ecchymosis, and purpura. With more severe

Table 46-3 Signs and Symptoms Associated with Drug-Induced Thrombocytopenia[6,22,52]

Systemic symptoms

- Chills
- Dizziness
- Fatigue
- Fever
- Nausea/vomiting

Moderate thrombocytopenia (20,000–150,000 platelets/mm³)

- Ecchymosis
- Microscopic hematuria
- Petechiae
- Purpura

Severe thrombocytopenia (<20,000 platelets/mm³)

- Central nervous system hemorrhage
- Epistaxis
- Florid purpura
- Gingival bleeding
- Gross hematuria
- Hematochezia
- Menorrhagia
- Retroperitoneal bleeding

Heparin-induced thrombocytopenia–specific symptoms

- Anaphylaxis
- Gangrene
- Skin necrosis
- Upper and lower extremity deep-vein thrombosis or pulmonary embolism

thrombocytopenia, patients may experience epistaxis, hematuria, gingival bleeding, and hematochezia. Standardized scoring systems may be helpful to estimate the likelihood of HIT. The 4T score can be utilized to evaluate the following potential indicators of HIT: (1) relative platelet count fall, (2) timing of the onset of the platelet count fall, (3) presence or absence of thrombosis, or (4) likelihood of another cause. Each indicator is scored on a scale of 0 to +2. The higher the resultant score, the higher the likelihood of having HIT.[22]

Differentiating between decreased platelet production, increased platelet destruction, splenic sequestration of platelets and hemodilution as well as a review of a blood smear can help the clinician rule in or exclude various possible causes of thrombocytopenia. An abrupt decrease in platelet count usually signifies an acute destructive process via immune or nonimmune processes. Decreased megakaryocytes on bone-marrow biopsy and pancytopenia are indicative of thrombocytopenia due to decreased production. Splenomegaly can lead to thrombocytopenia secondary to platelet redistribution in splenic vascular beds. Hemodilution may result from the administration of crystalloids, colloids, or even platelet-deprived blood products and can result in a relative thrombocytopenia. In addition to drugs, one must consider many nondrug causes of thrombocytopenia in the differential diagnosis (**Table 46-4**).

Ethylenediamine tetra-acetic acid, an in vitro calcium-chelating anticoagulant used for laboratory processing, reacts with GPIIb/IIIa-reactive autoantibodies and can cause an electronic particle counter to falsely read blood samples as thrombocytopenia.[46] This pseudothrombocytopenia is estimated to occur in approximately 0.1% of analyzed blood samples and can be avoided by using sodium citrate or heparin anticoagulant-treated collection tubes.

With HIT, platelet counts rarely decrease to <10,000/mm^3.[47] Onset of thrombocytopenia in a patient not previously exposed to heparin typically occurs after 5–10 days of exposure as compared with hours for previously exposed patients.[48] HIT, unlike other drug-induced thrombocytopenias, carries a risk of venous thromboembolism rather than petechiae and hemorrhage.[21,22,49] In addition,

Table 46-4 Conditions to Consider in the Differential Diagnosis of Drug-Induced Thrombocytopenia[22,34,52]

- Acute lymphoid leukemia
- Acute myeloid leukemia
- Alcohol consumption
- Antineoplastic chemotherapy
- Aplastic anemia
- Chronic hepatic failure
- Chronic leukemia
- Disrupted hematopoiesis
- Disseminated intravascular coagulation
- Exposure to blood products
- Hepatic disease
- Human immunodeficiency virus
- Immune (idiopathic) thrombocytopenic purpura
- Insertion of pulmonary artery catheter
- Lymphomas
- Metastatic cancer
- Myelodysplastic syndromes
- Myeloproliferative neoplasia
- Myeloproliferative syndromes
- Pregnancy
- Prosthetic valves
- Pseudothrombocytopenia (platelet clumping)
- Sepsis
- Splenomegaly
- Thrombotic thrombocytopenic purpura
- Vasculitis

low-molecular-weight heparins (LMWHs) such as enoxaparin and dalteparin can be responsible for HIT. Although anecdotal case reports exist, fondaparinux, which binds directly to antithrombin, is considered to have a low potential for HIT.[22,50,51]

Heparin is considered one of the most thrombogenic drugs, and patients may present with upper-extremity deep-vein thrombosis, lower-extremity deep-vein thrombosis, or a pulmonary embolism.[48] Patients may also present with heparin-induced skin necrosis, gangrene, or anaphylaxis.[21,22]

A careful medical and medication history should be obtained for patients presenting with thrombocytopenia. The medication history should include details regarding recent medication changes and use of complementary and alternative medicines. The laboratory evaluation of patients with suspected drug-induced thrombocytopenia may include GP-specific platelet antibody assays and an evaluation of drug-dependent increases in platelet-associated IgG.[52] Specifically for HIT, C-serotonin platelet release assay, PF4/heparin enzyme-linked immunosorbent assay (ELISA), or both may be used, with a positive predictive value of 89–100% and 10–93%, respectively.[21,52] The negative predictive value of a serotonin assay and ELISA are approximately 80% and 95%, respectively.[21]

RISK FACTORS

Drug-induced thrombocytopenia is a rare event, and general risk factors other than recent drug exposure are unknown. With cyclosporine, tacrolimus, sirolimus, and valproic acid, there appears to be a relationship between higher serum concentrations and a risk for thrombocytopenia.[36,43] With valproic acid, a daily dose exceeding 1,000 mg, concurrent use of aspirin, and advanced age appear to confer higher risk.[53] Therapy with linezolid for >2 weeks has been associated with drug-induced thrombocytopenia.[54] Past use of heparin and LMWHs (especially within the past 100 days) places individuals at an increased risk for drug-induced thrombocytopenia (**Table 46-5**).[22,48,52,55]

MORBIDITY AND MORTALITY

A review by George and colleagues suggests that patients presenting with definite or probable drug-induced thrombocytopenia (nonheparin-related) have a 9% risk of major bleeding and an associated mortality rate of 0.8%.[4,5] HIT may occur in 1–3% of patients receiving treatment, and the typical onset is 5–14 days. HIT is associated with a 50% cumulative risk of thrombosis over 30 days.[55] Venous thrombotic events are more common than arterial events in HIT, and practitioners must recognize that pulmonary embolism may be more prevalent than deep-vein thrombosis, with risk persisting even weeks after platelet recovery.[21,55]

Thrombotic thrombocytopenic purpura is associated with cerebral and myocardial infarctions and renal failure, resulting in a mortality rate of 90% in patients not receiving treatment.[35,36] It is estimated that plasma exchange in quinine-induced TTP has increased survival from 25% without treatment to 100% with treatment.[44] However, neurologic sequelae and chronic renal failure may persist despite treatment and cessation of quinine therapy.[40]

Table 46-5 Risk Factors for Drug-Induced Thrombocytopenia

Heparin, low-molecular-weight heparins[22,48,52,55]

- History of heparin-induced thrombocytopenia
- Previous exposure to heparin or low-molecular-weight heparin (especially within the past 100 days)

Valproic acid[53]

- Advanced age
- Concurrent use of aspirin
- High-serum valproic acid concentrations

Linezolid[54]

- >2 weeks of treatment

PREVENTION

Many commonly prescribed drugs can cause thrombocytopenia and, given the unpredictable nature of this drug-induced disease, prevention is challenging. In contrast to most drugs, thrombocytopenia secondary to many of the chemotherapy agents is predictable, and clinicians can often make dosing adjustments to help minimize this effect (**Table 46-6**). For patients who experience severe chemotherapy-associated thrombocytopenia, oprelvekin can be used.[56,57] Oprelvekin promotes growth and maturation of megakaryocytes. The adult dose is 50 mcg/kg/day given subcutaneously for 10–21 days after chemotherapy. Treatment should be started at least 24 hours after chemotherapy and should be discontinued at least 48 hours before the next cycle. Oprelvekin is associated with significant toxicity. Many of the side effects mimic capillary-leak syndrome, with patients having fluid retention, dyspnea, tachycardia, atrial arrhythmias, syncope, headache, fever, nausea, anemia, arthralgias, myalgias, and pleural effusions. Clinicians must weigh the risk of these adverse effects against the benefits of treatment.

Routine monitoring of platelet counts is necessary for many patients who receive unfractionated heparin or LMWH, and the American College of

Table 46-6 Early Detection and Prevention of Drug-Induced Thrombocytopenia[58]

For patients starting unfractionated heparin or LMWH
(if exposed to heparin in the past 100 days or if exposure history is uncertain)

- Baseline platelet count
- Platelet count within 24 hours

For patients receiving therapeutic-dose unfractionated heparin

- Baseline platelet count
- Platelet count at least every 2–3 days on days 4–14 of therapy
- Monitoring can be stopped at discontinuation of heparin therapy or after 14 days of therapy (whichever comes first)

For patients receiving postoperative antithrombotic prophylaxis with unfractionated heparin

- Every-other-day platelet count monitoring on postoperative days 4–14
- Monitoring can be stopped at discontinuation of heparin therapy or after 14 days of therapy (whichever comes first)

For medical or obstetrical patients receiving prophylactic-dose unfractionated heparin or LMWH after first receiving unfractionated heparin; for postoperative patients receiving prophylactic-dose LMWH or intravascular catheter unfractionated heparin "flushes"

- Platelet count monitoring at least every 2–3 days on days 4–14
- Monitoring can be stopped at discontinuation of heparin therapy or after 14 days of therapy (whichever comes first)

For detection of chemotherapy-related thrombocytopenia

- Platelet count prior to initial chemotherapy
- Platelet count prior to next cycle
- If complications occur, check the platelet count

LMWH = low-molecular-weight heparin.

Chest Physicians has published recommendations to help guide clinicians.[21,58] For patients who are starting unfractionated heparin or LMWH treatment and who have received unfractionated heparin within the past 100 days, or for those in whom exposure history is uncertain, a baseline platelet count and then a repeat platelet count within 24 hours of starting heparin is recommended. For patients who are receiving therapeutic dose unfractionated heparin, platelet count monitoring at least every 2–3 days from days 4–14 (or until heparin is stopped, whichever occurs first) is recommended.

Patients who are receiving postoperative antithrombotic prophylaxis with unfractionated heparin are at highest risk for HIT. In these patients, every-other-day platelet count monitoring between postoperative days 4 and 14 (or until unfractionated heparin is stopped, whichever occurs first) is recommended. Specific recommendations regarding monitoring of individual fibrinogen inhibitors/GPIIb/IIIa are also available.[30]

Medical or obstetrical patients who are receiving prophylactic-dose unfractionated heparin, postoperative patients receiving prophylactic-dose LMWH, postoperative patients receiving intravascular catheter unfractionated heparin "flushes," or medical or obstetrical patients receiving LMWH after first receiving unfractionated heparin are at relatively low risk for HIT. In these patients, platelet count monitoring at least every 2–3 days from day 4 to day 14 (or until heparin is stopped, whichever occurs first), when practical, is recommended.

HIT is rare in medical and obstetrical patients who are receiving only LMWH, and medical patients who are receiving only intravascular catheter unfractionated heparin flushes. In these patients, routine platelet count monitoring is not recommended.

MANAGEMENT

The most obvious primary treatment for drug-induced thrombocytopenia is discontinuation of the offending agent. In most cases, the platelet count returns to pretreatment levels relatively quickly, with a median time to platelet recovery of approximately 7 days (range of 1–30 days).[4] In patients with HIT, management must include the removal of all sources of heparin, including heparin flushes. The ultimate goal of therapy for patients with HIT is to prevent thrombosis, because these patients have a 30-fold increased risk of suffering a thrombotic event. Management includes decreasing both platelet activation and thrombin generation, and this is typically accomplished by using alternative anticoagulation therapy such as a direct thrombin inhibitor.[59]

Warfarin and other anticoagulants (e.g., LMWH) should not be prescribed in patients with HIT. Individuals receiving LMWH have a high cross reactivity with PF4 heparin antibodies.[22,58] Patients with HIT who are treated with warfarin usually develop an international normalized ratio >4. This occurs because of the reduction of protein C and persistent thrombin generation. Once thrombin generation is controlled with a direct thrombin inhibitor and thrombocytopenia has resolved (i.e., platelets >150,000/mm^3), warfarin can be given safely. If HIT is not resolved before initiating warfarin, fulminant venous limb gangrene can occur.[22,52,60,61]

Two drug classes available for the treatment of HIT are the direct thrombin inhibitors and heparinoids. Direct thrombin inhibitors include lepirudin, bivalirudin, and argatroban. Danaparoid is a representative heparinoid. These agents directly bind to and inactivate thrombin and do not require antithrombin.[21] There is no cross-reactivity between heparin and the direct thrombin inhibitors and all of the products have short half-lives (25–80 minutes).[22,52]

Lepirudin is a recombinant hirudin derivative (i.e., leech protein). It is approved by the FDA for use in the treatment of HIT and associated thromboembolic diseases to prevent further thromboembolic complications. This agent is metabolized by the kidneys and its use should be avoided in patients with renal failure. Although current recommendations suggest that an initial bolus dose is not necessary, in life-threatening situations a bolus dose of 0.2 mg/kg may be used. The highest infusion rate recommended during initiation of therapy is 0.10 mg/kg. The target activated partial thromboplastin time (aPTT) is 1.5–2 times baseline. The aPTT should be checked every 4 hours initially and then less often once steady state has been achieved.[22,58]

Studies have demonstrated reduction in composite end points (i.e., new thrombosis, limb amputation, and mortality from all causes) when lepirudin was used.[62,63] In an analysis of three of these studies, the incidence of death, amputation, and thrombosis was decreased to 20.3% in patients treated with lepirudin from 43% in controls.[64] Patients treated with lepirudin experienced more bleeding (17.6% versus 5.8% in the control group). There have been reports of the development of antibodies to lepirudin with repeated exposure and after the administration of even a single bolus dose. Antibody formation has been associated with fatal anaphylactic reactions; therefore, lepirudin should not be used more than once in a given patient.[64]

Bivalirudin, a synthetic thrombin inhibitor modeled after hirudin, is approved for use in percutaneous coronary intervention in patients who have or are at risk for HIT. The half-life is shorter than that of lepirudin (25 minutes versus 80 minutes) and it undergoes enzymatic metabolism, so only minor dose adjustments are needed in patients with renal insufficiency.[21,22,52] No bolus administration is required for use in HIT, and initial infusion rates range from 0.15 to 0.2 mg/kg/hr. If a patient has renal dysfunction, the infusion rate should be reduced from 0.03 to 0.1 mg/kg/hr.[65] The aPTT should be monitored, with target values 1.5–2.5 times baseline.

Argatroban is also a direct thrombin inhibitor that binds reversibly to thrombin. It is approved for use in the treatment and prevention of thrombosis in HIT. No bolus dose is needed, and the initial infusion rate is 2 mcg/kg/min. To achieve target aPTT levels, doses can range from 0.5 to 2 mcg/kg/min. Unlike the other direct thrombin inhibitors, argatroban is metabolized by the liver. In patients with moderate hepatic impairment (Child-Pugh score of 7–11), the dose should be reduced to 0.5 mcg/kg/min. The drug should not be used at all in patients who have alanine aminotransferase or aspartate aminotransferase values >3 times the upper limit of normal.[66-68] A baseline aPTT should be determined and values then monitored to maintain an aPTT of 1.5–3 times the baseline. The incidence of composite end points (death, amputation, thrombosis) has been reported to decrease from 43% in controls to 35% with argatroban treatment, and the major improvement noted was a significant decrease in the risk of thrombotic events (10–14% with argatroban versus 25% in controls).[22,67,68]

Danaparoid, which is classified as a heparinoid, represents another class of drugs used for the treatment of HIT. This agent works by inhibiting the activation of factor X via antithrombin. It is the only agent that has compared favorably with direct thrombin inhibitors; however, it is not currently available for use in the United States.

Direct-acting oral anticoagulants are approved for various indications, including nonvalvular atrial fibrillation, deep-vein thrombosis, pulmonary embolism, and postoperative venous thromboprophylaxis. With regard to HIT, data are limited to case reports and case series, and there is insufficient clinical experience to recommend them as a treatment option.[69]

Thrombocytopenia is a well-known adverse effect associated with cancer chemotherapy. Depending on the chemotherapy regimen and the number of previous chemotherapy cycles, platelet counts typically return to normal over time. In certain situations, however, a decision to administer a platelet transfusion may be warranted. This decision is based on the presence or absence of bleeding and a patient's platelet count. Guidelines have been established to help clinicians decide when to administer platelet transfusions and when it is appropriate to wait.[70,71] Based on guidelines published by the American Society of Clinical Oncology, a platelet transfusion is recommended for patients with no evidence of active bleeding when the platelet count decreases to <10,000/mm^3. Data derived from patients with leukemia who have chemotherapy-induced thrombocytopenia showed that this approach conserved healthcare resources and did not place the patient at increased risk for bleeding.[70] There are situations in which a platelet transfusion is recommended despite a platelet count >10,000 mm^3, including cancers associated with necrotic tumors such as gynecologic, colorectal, and bladder cancers, as well as melanoma. Patients who are to undergo surgery should have platelet counts of at least 40,000–50,000/mm^3 to ensure safety.[71] The use of platelet transfusions in patients with HIT is not recommended.[58]

Although these various recommendations have been established to help guide clinicians in the appropriate use of platelet transfusions, patients should be evaluated on a case-by-case basis. Platelet transfusions are not without risk, and patients can experience fever, allergic reactions, alloimmunization, and infection.[70]

Steroids and high-dose intravenous immunoglobulin have also been used to treat drug-induced thrombocytopenia, although their utility and benefit have not been clearly demonstrated.[72] Different steroid agents and dose ranges have been suggested. Prednisolone 15–160 mg daily, methylprednisolone 1 mg/kg every 8 hours, or oral prednisone up to 1 mg/kg/day have been used.[1,72] It is often difficult to differentiate between ITP and drug-induced thrombocytopenia. Because corticosteroids have proven beneficial in the treatment of ITP, these agents should be used when ITP is suspected and at least until ITP can be ruled out.[3] Similarly, intravenous immunoglobulin in a dose of 1 g/kg/day for 2 consecutive days, may be considered in patients in whom ITP is suspected.[73] Thrombopoietin mimetics, such as romiplostim or eltrombopag, which regulate megakaryocyte and platelet production, have been studied for use in patients with thrombocytopenia. However, benefit of use specifically in drug-induced thrombocytopenia is not established. These agents are FDA-labeled for chronic immune-mediated thrombocytopenia.

INFORMATION FOR PATIENTS

Patients should be adequately counseled when prescribed any agent that could potentially induce thrombocytopenia. Education should include signs and symptoms of bleeding, including unusual bruising, heavy or prolonged menses, prolonged bleeding of the gums after brushing or flossing, or even prolonged bleeding from a minor cut. Patients should be advised to contact their healthcare provider immediately if any of these occur. Once a drug-induced thrombocytopenia has been diagnosed, it is important to ensure that this information is added to the patient's medical records to help prevent recurrent events.

REFERENCES

1. Wazny LD, Ariano RE. Evaluation and management of drug-induced thrombocytopenia in the acutely ill patient. *Pharmacotherapy.* 2000; 23:292-307.
2. Patnode NM, Gandhi PJ. Drug-induced thrombocytopenia in the coronary care unit. *J Thromb Thrombolysis.* 2000; 10:155-67.
3. Van den Bemt PMLA, Meyboom RHB. Drug-induced immune thrombocytopenia. *Drug Saf.* 2004; 27:1243-52.
4. George JN, Raskob GE, Shah SR et al. Drug-induced thrombocytopenia: a systematic review of published case reports. *Ann Intern Med.* 1998; 129:886-90.
5. Al-Nouri ZL, George JN. Drug-induced thrombocytopenia. An updated systematic review, 2012. *Drug Saf.* 2012; 35:693-4.
6. Curtis BR. Drug-induced immune thrombocytopenia: incidence, clinical features, laboratory testing, and pathogenic mechanisms. *Immunohematology.* 2014; 30:55-65.
7. Salamon DJ, Nusbacher J, Stroupe T et al. Red cell and platelet-bound IgG penicillin antibodies in a patient with thrombocytopenia. *Transfusion.* 1984; 24:395-8.
8. Murphy MF, Riordan T, Minchinton RM et al. Demonstration of an immune mediated mechanism of penicillin-induced neutropenia and thrombocytopenia. *Br J Haematol.* 1983; 55:155-60.
9. Parker CW. Hapten immunology and allergic reactions in humans. *Arthritis Rheum.* 1981;24:1024-1036.
10. Aster RH. Drug-induced immune thrombocytopenia: an overview of pathogenesis. *Semin Hematol.* 1999; 36(1 suppl 1):2-6.
11. Bougie DW, Wilker PR, Aster RH. Patients with quinine- induced immune thrombocytopenia have both "drug- dependent" and "drug-specific" antibodies. *Blood.* 2006; 108:922-7.
12. Bougie D, Aster R. Immune thrombocytopenia resulting from sensitivity to metabolites of naproxen and acetaminophen. *Blood.* 2001; 97:3846-50.
13. Reddy JC, Shuman MA, Aster RH. Quinine/quinidine-induced thrombocytopenia: a great imitator. *Arch Intern Med.* 2004; 164:218-20.
14. Visentin GP, Newman PJ, Aster RH. Characteristics of quinine- and quinidine-induced antibodies specific for platelet glycoproteins IIb and IIIa. *Blood.* 1991; 77:2668-76.
15. Christie DJ, Mullen PC, Aster RH. Fab-mediated binding of drug-dependent antibodies to platelets in quinidine- and quinine-induced thrombocytopenia. *J Clin Invest.* 1985; 75:310-4.
16. Asvadi P, Ahmadi Z, Chong BH. Drug-induced thrombocytopenia: localization of the binding site of GPIX-specific quinine-dependent antibodies. *Blood.* 2003; 102:1670-7.
17. von dem Borne AE, Pegels JG, van der Stadt RJ et al. Thrombocytopenia associated with gold therapy: a drug- induced autoimmune disease? *Br J Haematol.* 1986; 63:509-16.
18. Garner SF, Campbell K, Metcalfe P et al. Glycoprotein V: the predominant target antigen in gold-induced autoimmune thrombocytopenia. *Blood.* 2002; 100:344-6.
19. Landrum EM, Siegert EA, Hanlon JT et al. Prolonged thrombocytopenia-associated with procainamide in an elderly patient. *Ann Pharmacother.* 1994; 28:1172-6.
20. Rosenstein R, Kosfeld RE, Leight L et al. Procainamide-induced thrombocytopenia. *Am J Hematol.* 1984; 16:181-3.
21. Arepally GM, Ortel TL. Heparin-induced thrombocytopenia. *N Engl J Med.* 2006; 355:809-17.
22. Greinacher A. Heparin-Induced Thrombocytopenia. *N Engl J Med.* 2015; 373:252-62.
23. Amiral J, Bridey F, Dreyfus M et al. Platelet factor 4 complexed to heparin is the target for antibodies generated in heparin-induced thrombocytopenia. *Thromb Haemost.* 1992; 68:95-6.
24. Visentin GP, Ford SE, Scott JP et al. Antibodies from patients with heparin-induced thrombocytopenia/thrombosis are specific for platelet factor 4 complexed with heparin or bound to endothelial cells. *J Clin Invest.*1994; 93:81-8.
25. Aster RH. Immune thrombocytopenia caused by glycoprotein IIb/IIIa inhibitors. *Chest.* 2005; 127(2 suppl):53S-59S.
26. Curtis BR, Divgi A, Garritty M et al. Delayed thrombocytopenia after treatment with abciximab: a distinct clinical entity associated with the immune response to the drug. *J Thromb Haemost.* 2004; 2:985-92.
27. Bougie DW, Wilker PR, Wuitschick ED et al. Acute thrombocytopenia after treatment with tirofiban or eptifibatide is associated with antibodies specific for ligand-occupied GPIIb/IIIa. *Blood.* 2002; 100:2071-6.
28. Peter K, Straub A, Kohler B et al. Platelet activation as a potential mechanism of GP IIb/IIIa inhibitor-induced thrombocytopenia. *Am J Cardiol.* 1999; 84:519-24.
29. Curtis BR, Swyers J, Divgi A et al. Thrombocytopenia after second exposure to abciximab is caused by antibodies that recognize abciximab-coated platelets. *Blood.* 2002; 99:2054-9.
30. Matthai WH. Thrombocytopenia in cardiovascular patients. *Chest.* 2005; 127:46S-52S.
31. Dasgupta H, Blankenship JC, Wood CG et al. Thrombocytopenia complicating treatment with intravenous glycoprotein IIb/IIIa receptor inhibitors: a pooled analysis. *Am Heart J.* 2000; 140:206-11.
32. Wade EE, Rebuck JA, Healy MA et al. H2 Antagonist- induced thrombocytopenia: is this a real phenomenon? *Intensive Care Med.* 2002; 28:459-65.
33. Baughman RP, Lower EE, Flessa H et al. Thrombocytopenia in the intensive care unit. *Chest.* 1993; 104:1243-7.
34. Shalansky SJ, Verma AK, Levine M et al. Risk markers for thrombocytopenia in critically ill patients: a prospective analysis. *Pharmacotherapy.* 2002; 33:803-13.
35. George JN. Clinical practice. Thrombotic thrombocytopenic purpura. *N Engl J Med.* 2006; 354:1927-35.
36. Reese JA, Bougie DW, Curtis BR et al. Drug-induced thrombotic microangiopathy: Experience of the Oklahoma Registry and the Blood Center of Wisconsin. *Am J Hematol.* 2015; 90:2406-10.
37. Furlan M, Robles R, Galbusera M et al. von Willebrand factor-cleaving protease in thrombotic thrombocytopenic purpura and the hemolytic-uremic syndrome. *N Engl J Med.* 1998; 339:1578-84.
38. Tsai HM, Lian EC. Antibodies to von Willebrand factor- cleaving protease in acute thrombotic thrombocytopenic purpura. *N Engl J Med.* 1998; 339:1585-94.
39. Levy GG, Nichols WC, Lian EC et al. Mutations in a member of the ADAMTS gene family cause thrombotic thrombocytopenic purpura. *Nature.* 2001; 413:488-94.
40. McCarthy LJ, Porcu P, Fausel CA et al. Thrombotic thrombocytopenic purpura and simvastatin. *Lancet.* 1998; 352:1284-5.
41. Kojouri K, Vesely SK, George JN. Quinine-associated thrombotic thrombocytopenic purpura-hemolytic uremic syndrome: frequency, clinical features, and long-term outcomes. *Ann Intern Med.* 2001; 135:1047-51.
42. Manor SM, Guillory GS, Jain SP. Clopidogrel-induced thrombotic thrombocytopenic purpura-hemolytic uremic syndrome after coronary artery stenting. *Pharmacotherapy.* 2004; 24:664-7.
43. Crew RJ, Radhakrishnan J, Cohen DJ et al. De novo thrombotic microangiopathy following treatment with sirolimus: report of two cases. *Nephrol Dial Transplant.* 2005; 20:203-9.
44. Zakarija A, Bandarenko N, Pandey DK et al. Clopidogrel- associated TTP: an update of pharmacovigilance efforts conducted by independent researchers, pharmaceutical suppliers, and the Food and Drug Administration. *Stroke.* 2004; 35:533-7.
45. Bennett CL, Weinberg PD, Rozenberg-Ben-Dror K et al. Thrombotic thrombocytopenic purpura associated with ticlopidine: a review of 60 cases. *Ann Intern Med.* 1998; 128:541-4.
46. Casonato A, Bertomoro A, Pontara E et al. EDTA dependent pseudothrombocytopenia caused by antibodies against the cytoadhesive receptor of platelet gpIIB-IIIA. *J Clin Pathol.* 1994;4 7:625.

47. Warkentin TE, Kelton JG. Temporal aspects of heparin- induced thrombocytopenia. *N Engl J Med.* 2001; 344:1286-92.
48. Warkentin TE, Levine MN, Hirsh J et al. Heparin- induced thrombocytopenia in patients treated with low molecular-weight heparin or unfractionated heparin. *N Engl J Med.* 1995; 332:1330-5.
49. Aster RH. Heparin-induced thrombocytopenia and thrombosis. *N Engl J Med.* 1995; 332:1374-6.
50. Warkentin TE, Cook RJ, Marder VJ et al. Anti-platelet factor 4/heparin antibodies in orthopedic surgery patients receiving antithrombotic prophylaxis with fondaparinux or enoxaparin. *Blood.* 2005; 106:3791-6.
51. Rota E, Bazzan M, Fantino G. Fondaparinux-related thrombocytopenia in a previous low-molecular-weight heparin-induced thrombocytopenia. *Thromb Haemost.* 2008; 99:779-81.
52. Warkentin TE, Kelton JC. Thrombocytopenia due to platelet destruction and hypersplenism. In: Hoffman R, ed. *Hematology Basic Principles and Practice.* Philadelphia, PA: Churchill Livingston; 2009; 2113-31.
53. Conley EL, Coley KC, Pollock BG et al. Prevalence and risk of thrombocytopenia with valproic acid: experience at a psychiatric teaching hospital. *Pharmacotherapy.* 2001; 21:1325-30.
54. Bernstein WB, Trotta RF, Rector JT et al. Mechanisms for linezolid-induced anemia and thrombocytopenia. *Ann Pharmacother.* 2003; 37:517-20.
55. Warkentin TE, Kelton JG. A 14-year study of heparin- induced thrombocytopenia. *Am J Med.* 1996; 101:502, 507.
56. Wilde MI, Faulds D. Oprelvekin: a review of its pharmacology and therapeutic potential in chemotherapy-induced thrombocytopenia. *BioDrugs.* 1998; 10:159-71.
57. Demetri GD. Pharmacologic treatment options in patients with thrombocytopenia. *Semin Hematol.* 2000; 37(suppl 4):11-8.
58. Linkins LA, Dans AL, Moores LK et al. Treatment and prevention of heparin-induced thrombocytopenia: American College of Chest Physicians Evidence-Based Clinical Practice Guidelines. *Chest.* 2012; 141:e495S-e530S.
59. Girolami B, Prandoni P, Stefani PM et al. The incidence of heparin-induced thrombocytopenia in hospitalized medical patients treated with subcutaneous unfractionated heparin: A prospective cohort study. *Blood.* 2003; 101:2955-9.
60. Smythe MA, Warkentin TE, Stephens JL et al. Venous limb gangrene during overlapping therapy with warfarin and a direct thrombin inhibitor for immune heparin induced thrombocytopenia. *Am J Hematol.* 2002; 71:50-2.
61. Sinivasan AF, Rice L, Bartholomew JR et al. Warfarin- induced skin necrosis and venous limb gangrene in the setting of heparin-induced thrombocytopenia. *Arch Int Med.* 2004; 164:66-70.
62. Greinacher A, Eichler P, Lubenow N et al. Heparin- induced thrombocytopenia with thromboembolic complications: meta-analysis of two prospective trials to assess the value of parental treatment with lepirudin and its therapeutic aPTT range. *Blood.* 2000; 96:846-51.
63. Eichler P, Lubenow N, Greinacher A. Results of the third prospective study of treatment with lepirudin in patients with heparin-induced thrombocytopenia (HIT) abstract. *Blood.* 2002; 100(suppl 1):704a.
64. Lubenow N, Eichler P, Liety T et al. Lepirudin in patients with heparin-induced thrombocytopenia: results of the third prospective study (HAT-3) and a combined analysis of HAT-1, HAT-2, and HAT-3. *J Thromb Haemost.* 2005; 3:2428-36.
65. Kiser TH, Burch J, Klem P et al. Safety, efficacy, and dosing requirements of bivalirudin in patients with heparin-induced thrombocytopenia. *Pharmacotherapy.* 2008; 28:1115-24.
66. Beiderlinden M, Treschan TA, Gorlinger K et al. Argatroban anticoagulation in critically ill patients. *Ann Pharmacother.* 2007; 41:749-54.
67. Lewis BE, Wallis DE, Leya F et al. Argatroban anticoagulant therapy in patients with heparin-induced thrombocytopenia. *Circulation.* 2001;103:1838-1843.
68. Lewis BE, Wallis DE, Leya F et al. Argatroban anticoagulation in patients with heparin-induced thrombocytopenia. *Arch Intern Med.* 2003; 163:1849-56.
69. Miyares MA, Davis KA. Direct-acting oral anticoagulants as emerging treatment options for Heparin-Induced Thrombocytopenia. *Annals of Pharmacother.* 2015; 49:735-39.
70. Benjamin RJ, Anderson KC. What is the proper threshold for platelet transfusion in patients with chemotherapy- induced thrombocytopenia? *Crit Rev Oncol Hematol.* 2002; 42:163-71.
71. Schiffer CA, Anderson KC, Bennett CL et al. Platelet transfusion for patients with cancer: Clinical Practice Guidelines of the American Society of Clinical Oncology. *J Clin Oncol.* 2001; 19:1519-38.
72. Pedersen BV, Anderson M, Hansen PB. Drug-induced thrombocytopenia: clinical data on 309 cases and the effect of corticosteroid therapy. *Eur J Clin Pharmacol.* 1997; 52:183-9.
73. Greinacher A, Eichler P, Lubenow N et al. Drug-induced and drug dependent immune thrombocytopenia. *Rev Clin Exp Hematol.* 2001; 5:166-200.
74. Hibbard AB, Medina PJ, Vesely SK. Reports of drug- induced thrombocytopenia. *Ann Intern Med.* 2003; 138:239.
75. Li X, Hunt L, Vesely SK. Drug-induced thrombocytopenia: an updated systematic review. *Ann Intern Med.* 2005; 142:475.
76. Hypaque-cysto (Diatrizoate meglumine) [package insert]. Princeton, NJ: Amersham Health; 2003.
77. Raptiva (Efalizumab) [package insert]. San Francisco, CA: Genetech; 2005.
78. Yamada T, Shinohara K, Katsuki K. Severe thrombocytopenia caused by simvastatin in which thrombocyte recovery was initiated after severe bacterial infection. *Clin Drug Invest.* 1998; 16:172-4.
79. Farr M, Scott DGI, Bacon PA. Side effect profile of 200 patients with inflammatory arthritides treated with sulfasalazine. *Drugs.* 1986; 32(suppl 1):49-53.
80. Von Drygalski A, Curtis BR, Bougie DW et al. Vancomycin-induced immune thrombocytopenia. *N Engl J Med.* 2007; 356:904-10.
81. Mailman JF, Stigant C, Martinusen D. Moxifloxacin-induced immune-mediated thrombocytopenia in a chronic kidney disease patient receiving hemodialysis. *Annal Pharmacother.* 2014; 48:191-22.
82. Ranieri MM, Bradley EF, Simon AB. Meloxicam-induced thrombocytopenia. *Pharmacotherapy.* 2014; 34:e14-17.
83. Agapakis DI, Massa EV. A case of fenofibrate-induced immune thrombocytopenia: first report. *P R Health Sci J.* 2015; 34:170-3.
84. Tan MW, Sklar GE. Pentoxifylline-induced thrombocytopenia: a case report. *J Pharm Pract.* 2015; 28:572-6.

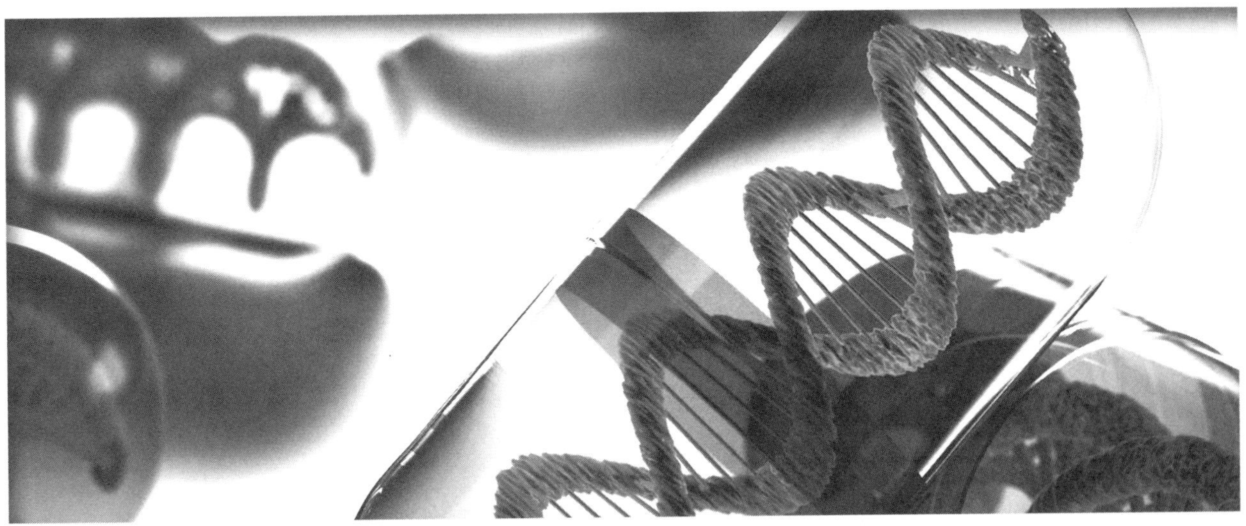

CHAPTER 47

Thromboembolic Diseases

Candice L. Garwood

Thromboembolic disease is one of the most common cardiovascular disorders, characterized by blood clot formation known as thrombosis. Although thrombosis may occur almost anywhere within the vascular system, the most common presentation involves deep vein thrombosis (DVT), which develops in the venous circulation, with the possible complication of pulmonary embolism (PE). DVT and PE are distinct but related manifestations of the same disease process known as venous thromboembolism (VTE). Typically, DVT develops within the large deep veins of the calf. About 10–20% of distal DVT extend proximally. DVT may also develop elsewhere, such as the upper extremity, mesenteric, renal, or cerebral veins. About 1–5% of thrombi are dislodged, travelling through the vasculature, also known as an embolus. The most common site for emboli to lodge is a vessel of the lung, forming a PE. VTE can be provoked by immobility, trauma, or may result from drug or disease factors. However, VTE may also be idiopathic, without a specific known predisposing factor. In general, development of VTE is multifactorial, making it difficult to identify a primary cause.[1] This chapter will focus on drug-induced thromboembolic disease.

CAUSATIVE AGENTS

Table 47-1 lists agents, grouped by drug class, that have been reported to cause thromboembolism.[2-227] Drugs that interact with and reduce the effectiveness of anticoagulants are not included if they have not been directly associated with thromboembolic development (e.g., rifampin inducing the metabolism of warfarin).

EPIDEMIOLOGY

The overall incidence of drug-induced thromboembolism is unknown because of the multifactorial pathogenesis of this disease. Furthermore many patients have clinically silent disease or go undiagnosed.[228] The incidence and level of supportive evidence associated with some specific drugs are reported in Table 47-1. When examining the rate of objectively diagnosed VTE, the annual incidence is estimated at 2–3/1,000. The rate of VTE increases with advancing age, such that the incidence doubles each decade of life after age 50 years, reaching a rate of 8/1,000 in those over 80 years. With an aging

Table 47-1 Agents Implicated in Drug-Induced Thromboembolic Diseases Agents Implicated in Drug-Induced Thromboembolic Diseases

Drug	Incidence	Level of Evidence[a]
HEMOSTATIC AGENTS		
Aminocaproic acid[2-5]	NK	C
Aprotinin[6-9]	1%	B
Cyanoacrylate[10-12]	NK	C
Desmopressin[13,14]	NK	C
Eptifibitide[15,16]	NK	C
Protamine sulfate[17]	NK	B
Activated prothrombin complex concentrate[18]	NK	B
3-factor prothrombin complex concentrate[19]	0.7%	B
4-factor prothrombin complex concentrate[19]	1.8%	B
Recombinant factor VIIa[20-23]	7–9.4%	A
Tranexamic acid[24,25]	NK	C
ANTICOAGULANTS		
Heparin[26-30]	1–5% develop HIT, 25–50% of those develop HITT	B[a]
Low-molecular-weight heparin[26,27]	2.2%	B[a]
Pentosan[31-33]	NK	B
Streptokinase[34-36]	NK	C
Urokinase[37]	NK	C
Warfarin (coumarin derivatives)[38-40]	NK	B
HEMATOPOIETIC AGENTS		
Darbepoetin[41-45]	3.3–8%	A
Erythropoietin[43-48]	3.3–26.7%	A
G-CSF[49,50]	NK	B
GM-CSF[49,51]	NK	B
ESTROGEN-CONTAINING AGENTS		
Diethylstilbestrol[52,53]	6.8–7%	A
Oral contraceptives[54-58]	6 times the risk of nonusers; 1–2/10,000 woman-year	A
Hormone replacement[57,59-61]	0.2–5.9/100 woman-year	A
ANTIANDROGENS		
Cyproterone[62-64]	5.23 increased odds	B
Flutamide[65]	5%	B[a]
Goserelin[66]	1–5%	B
Leuprolide[67-69]	16.7%	A
SELECTIVE ESTROGEN-RECEPTOR MODULATORS		
Raloxifene[57,70]	9.5/100 woman-year	A
Tamoxifene[57,71-74]	3.6–12/100 woman-year	A
Toremifene[75]	1.5%	B
AROMATASE INHIBITORS		
Anastrozole[76-79]	1–2.2%	A
Letrazole[80]	NK	C

Table 47-1 Agents Implicated in Drug-Induced Thromboembolic Diseases Agents Implicated in Drug-Induced Thromboembolic Diseases (continued)

Drug	Incidence	Level of Evidence[a]
ANDROGENIC AGENTS		
Danazol[81,82]	NK	C
Nandrolone[83,84]	NK	C
Megestrol[85,86]	4.9%	B[a]
FOLLICLE-STIMULATING HORMONE		
Follitropin alfa[87-89]	NK	C
ANTINEOPLASTIC AGENTS		
Aldsleukin[90,91]	<1%	B
Asparaginase[92-96]	11–36.7%	A
Basiliximab[97]	3–10%	B
Bevicizumab[98-100]	4.4–5%	A
Bleomycin[101,102]	NK	B
Carboplatin[103,104]	NK	B
Cisplatin[101,102,105-108,112,113]	0.67%	B
Dacarbazine[109,110]	NK	C
Denileukin[111]	11%	B[a]
Docetaxel[114-116]	8.8%	A
Estramustine[116-120]	0 ≥20%	A
Etoposide[102,120]	NK	A
Fluorouracil[121-123]	NK	B
Gemcitabine[112]		
Imatinib[116,124,125]	NK	B
Irinotecan[100,126]	12.5%	B
Lenalidomide[127-131]	8%	A
Paclitaxel[120,132-134]	NK	B
Ponatinib[135,136]	NK	A
Ranibizumab[137,138]	NK	B
Rituximab[139]	NK	B
Soraftnanib[140]	NK	B
Thalidomide[43,130,131,141-146]	3.4–26%	A
IMMUNOLOGIC AGENTS		
Cyclosporine[147-151]	NK	B
Dexamethasone[93,142,152]	NK	A
Foscarnet[153]	NK	C
Infliximab[154-156]	NK	B
Immunoglobins[157-161]	3–3.8%	A
Interferon gamma[162,163]	NK	B
Interferon alfa-2a[164,165]	NK	B
Interferon alfa-2b[166-168]	NK	C
Interferon beta[169,170]	NK	C
Interleukin-3[171]	NK	C

Table 47-1 Agents Implicated in Drug-Induced Thromboembolic Diseases Agents Implicated in Drug-Induced Thromboembolic Diseases (continued)

Drug	Incidence	Level of Evidence[a]
Methylprednisolone[172]	NK	B
Muromonab[150,172,173]	<1%	B[a]
Prednisone[93,152,174]	NK	A
Sirolimus[175,176]	NK	B
Tacrolimus[147-149,151]	NK	B
ANTIPSYCHOTIC AGENTS		
Chlorpromazine[177-181]	NK	B
Clozapine[182,183]	1.35%	B
Olanzapine[182,184,185]	1.17%	B
Quetiapine[182]	1.35%	B
Risperidone[177,182]	1.25%	B
Thioridazine[181,186]	NK	B
OTHER PSYCHOTROPIC AGENTS		
Clomipramine[187]	NK	C
Escitalopram[188]	NK	C
Lithium[189-191]	NK	C
CONTRAST AGENTS		
Iohexol[192-194]	22.2%	B
Iomeprol[195]	0.8–4.2%	B[a]
Iopamidol[196]	9–22.2%	B[a]
Iothalamate[197,198]	8–28.6%	B
Ioxaglate[192,193,195,196,199]	2.7–4.8%	B[a]
MISCELLANEOUS		
Acetohydroxamic acid[200]	NK	B
Botulinin toxin[202,203]	NK	C
Bromocriptine[203-205]	NK	C
Calcium gluconate[206]	NK	C
Cocaine[207-209]	NK	C
Dihydroergotamine[210-212]	NK	C
Ecstasy (3,4-methylenedioxymethamphetamine; MDMA)[213,214]	NK	C
Ergotamine[210,215-217]	NK	C
Metolazone[218]	NK	C
Papaverine[219]	NK	B
Procainamide[220,221]	NK	C
Sildenafil[222-224]	NK	C
Topiramate[225]	6.1%	A
Tretinoin[226,227]	NK	B

G-CSF = granulocyte colony-stimulating factor, GM-CSF = granulocyte /macrophage colony-stimulating factor, HIT = heparin-induced thrombocytopenia, HITT = heparin-induced thrombocytopenia and thrombosis, NK = not known.

[a]Definitions for Levels of Evidence: Level A—evidence from one or more randomized, controlled clinical trials; Level B—evidence from nonrandomized clinical trials, prospective observational studies, cohort studies, retrospective studies, case-control studies, meta-analyses and/or postmarketing surveillance studies; and Level C—evidence from one or more published case reports or case series.

population, it is expected that the incidence of DVT and PE will rise.[229]

Oral contraceptives are perhaps the best-recognized class of agents known to cause VTE. A meta-analysis of 26 studies identified a 3.5-fold increased relative risk of VTE with use of oral contraceptives compared with nonuse. The relative risk of VTE for combined oral contraceptives with 30–35 mcg ethinyl estradiol and either a third- or fourth-generation progestin (gestodene, desogestrel, cyproterone acetate, or drospirenone) were about 50–80% higher than for combined oral contraceptives with levonorgestrel, with higher doses associated with higher thrombosis risk.[230] However, other reports raise questions about the increased thromboembolic risk associated with newer generation progestins.[231,232] The reported incidence of VTE with other drugs varies widely, from <1% in patients receiving the antineoplastic agent aldesleukin and up to 26% in patients treated with thalidomide.[90,91,130]

MECHANISMS

Hemostasis is dependent on a delicate balance in the complex relationship between thrombogenic and antithrombotic factors. A disruption in this equilibrium may lead to inappropriate clot formation and the possibility of embolization to a distant vascular bed. Any circumstance resulting in venous stasis, vascular injury, or hypercoagulability, factors known as Virchow's triad, may lead to VTE.[233-236] Venous stasis occurs with a slowed rate of blood flow. The most common site for venostasis is the large venous sinuses of the thigh or calf, where pooling of blood can be precipitated by periods of physical immobility such as bed rest and air travel. Vascular injury can be a result of trauma or surgical procedures. In addition, vascular injury may be caused by pooling of blood that causes distention of the vessel where resultant damage to the endothelium can activate the coagulation system.[237]

Hypercoagulability is the result of an inherited defect or the presence of an acquired, often transient, risk factor such as a drug. Although venous thromboemboli generally originate in the lower-extremity venous pathways, they may also occur in other regions, such as renal veins, pelvic veins, upper-extremity veins, or the cerebral venous sinuses.[233] The most common location for embolization to occur is the lung.[233] The proposed mechanisms for agents known to cause VTE are described in **Table 47-2**.[5,9-11,13,14,17,23,24,32,34,49,50,57,58,92,106,107,114,122,125,130,135,145,151,165,167,170,178,188,189,200,210,215,222,226,227,238-266]

Hemostatic agents that inhibit fibrinolysis may prevent the lysing of previously formed clots and predispose patients to VTE. Drugs including aminocaproic acid, aprotinin, desmopressin, and tranexamic acid have been associated with VTE, likely via this mechanism.[2-9,13,14,24,25] Other drugs, including antipsychotic agents and contrast media can create a hypercoagulable state through platelet activation and aggregation that can lead to VTE.[177,179,181,182 192,195-197,199] Some studies suggest that ionic contrast media (e.g., iothalamate, ioxaglate) are less thrombogenic than the nonionic forms (e.g., iopamidol).[196]

Although uncommon, anticoagulation therapy itself may cause VTE by creating a hypercoagulable state. Warfarin can cause thrombosis in the microvasculature, which is known as skin necrosis. This appears to be caused by the drug's early inhibition of vitamin K–dependent anticoagulant proteins C and S and a slower onset of the complete inhibition of vitamin K–mediated clotting factors necessary for warfarin's full anticoagulation effect. The potential for warfarin-induced hypercoagulability is primarily associated with a known protein C deficiency. Hypercoagulability has been reported less commonly with protein S deficiency and also can occur in nondeficient individuals.[242] For this reason, it is prudent to begin heparin therapy prior to or concurrent with the start of warfarin in patients with acute VTE who will be anticoagulated with warfarin.[242,267,268] Heparin can cause thrombosis by inducing formation of antibodies in a syndrome known as heparin-induced thrombocytopenia (HIT). Low-molecular-weight heparins (LMWHs) have also been reported to cause HIT, but at a much lower rate than heparin.[241] Pentosan, a heparin analog, also has the ability to induce antibodies causing thrombosis.[31,32]

Hormonal and other agents that affect the endocrine system exhibit a diverse spectrum of

Table 47-2 Mechanisms of Drug-Induced Thromboembolic Diseases

Drug	Mechanism
HEMOSTATIC AGENTS	
Aminocaproic acid[5]	Inhibits fibrinolysis
Aprotinin[9]	High doses inhibit kallikrein and protein C; inhibits fibrinolysis
Cyanoacrylate[10,11,238]	Endothelial damage, embolization
Desmopressin[13,14]	Increases plasminogen-activator activity; inhibits fibrinolysis
Eptifibitide[15,16]	Induced thrombocytopenia and disseminated intravascular coagulation
Protamine sulfate[17]	Platelet-activating, anti-protamine-heparin antibodies
Activate prothrombin complex concentrate[239]	Concentrated active clotting factor repletion
3-factor prothrombin complex concentrate[239]	Concentrated clotting factor repletion
4-factor prothrombin complex concentrate[239]	Concentrated clotting factor repletion
Tranexamic acid[24,240]	Inhibits fibrinolysis
Recombinant factor VIIa[23,239]	Increased clotting-factor activity; dose-related
ANTICOAGULANTS	
Heparin/low-molecular-weight heparin[241]	Platelet activation secondary to antibody formation
Pentosan[32,33]	Platelet aggregation; heparin analog with potential to cause HIT
Streptokinase[34]	Antibody-induced platelet aggregation
Urokinase	NK
Warfarin (coumarin derivatives)[242]	Inhibits proteins C and S activity, potential for temporary hypercoagulability
HEMATOPOIETIC AGENTS	
Darbepoetin[243]	Increases endothelial-cell activity and increases platelet reactivity; dose-related
Erythropoietin[243]	Increases endothelial cell activity and platelet reactivity; dose-related
G-CSF[49,50]	Uncertain; increases platelet adhesion, fibrinogen, and clotting factors; decreases proteins C and S activity
GM-CSF[49,50]	Uncertain; increases platelet adhesion; increases fibrinogen and clotting factors; decreases proteins C and S activity
ESTROGEN-CONTAINING AGENTS	
Diethylstilbestrol	NK
Oral contraceptives[57,58]	Acquired resistance to activated protein C
Hormone replacement[57]	Acquired resistance to activated protein C
ANTIANDROGENS	
Cyproterone	NK
Flutamide	NK
Goserelin	NK
Leuprolide	NK
SELECTIVE ESTROGEN-RECEPTOR MODULATORS	
Raloxifene[57]	Uncertain; decreases antithrombin III, proteins C and S
Tamoxifen[57]	Uncertain; decreases antithrombin III, proteins C and S
Toremifene[57]	Uncertain; decreases antithrombin III, proteins C and S
AROMATASE INHIBITORS	
Anastrozole	NK
Letrazole	NK
ANDROGENIC AGENTS	
Danazol	NK

Table 47-2 Mechanisms of Drug-Induced Thromboembolic Diseases (continued)

Drug	Mechanism
Nandrolone	NK
Megestrol[244]	Increases prothrombin, fibrin, and plasmin–antiplasmin complex
FOLLICLE-STIMULATING HORMONE	
Follitropin alfa[245]	Ovarian hyperstimulation syndrome leading to elevated estrogen concentrations and hypercoagulability
ANTINEOPLASTIC AGENTS	
Aldesleukin[246]	Induces antiphospholipid antibodies
Asparaginase[92,247]	Hyperfibrinogenemia Decreases anti-plasmin and plasminogen concentrations and increases thrombin
Basiliximab[248]	Uncertain; endothelial-cell apoptosis and dysfunction
Bevacizumab[248,249]	Uncertain; endothelial-cell apoptosis and dysfunction
Bleomycin[250]	Uncertain; thrombotic microangiopathy
Carboplatin[251]	Increase procoagulant activity via isomerase decryption of tissue factor
Cisplatin[106,107,251]	Endothelial damage, platelet aggregation; increase procoagulant activity via isomerase decryption of tissue factor; possible increase vonWillebrand factor.
Dacarbazine	NK
Denileukin	NK
Docetaxel[114]	Uncertain; up regulation of thrombomodulin
Estramustine[252]	Uncertain; estrogenic component may cause acquired resistance to activated protein C
Fluorouracil[122,253,254]	Left ventricular dyskinesia leading to apical thrombus; disruption of folate synthesis leading to hyperhomocysteinemia; vascular injury
Gemcitibine[251]	Increase procoagulant activity via isomerase decryption of tissue factor
Imatinib[125]	Induces thrombotic thrombocytopenic purpura
Irinotecan	NK
Lenalidomide [130]	Uncertain; platelet hyperactivity
Paclitaxel[251]	Increase procoagulant activity via isomerase decryption of tissue factor
Ponitanib[135]	Platelet activation; increased platelet aggregation
Ranibizumab[249]	Uncertain; endothelial-cell apoptosis and dysfunction
Rituximab	NK
Soraftanib[249]	Uncertain; endothelial-cell apoptosis and dysfunction
Thalidomide[130,145]	Uncertain; platelet hyperactivity; activated protein C resistance
IMMUNOLOGIC AGENTS	
Cyclosporine[151]	Increases factor VIII, fibrinogen, and von Willebrand factor
Dexamethasone[255]	Decreases fibrinolysis due to inhibitory effects of PAI-1 on plasminogen activator; increases p-selectin and von Willebrand factor
Foscarnet	NK
Infliximab[256]	Induces antibodies, including antiphospholipid antibodies
Immunoglobulins[257]	Red cell aggregation; dose-related
Interferon gamma[258]	Modulates fibrinolytic effect of endothelial cells; increases plasma-activated complement
Interferon alfa-2a[165]	Procoagulant antibodies; increases plasma-activated complement
Interferon alfa-2b[167]	Procoagulant antibodies; increases plasma-activated complement

Table 47-2 Mechanisms of Drug-Induced Thromboembolic Diseases (continued)

Drug	Mechanism
Interferon beta[170]	Procoagulant antibodies; increases plasma-activated complement
Interleukin-3	NK
Methylprednisolone[255]	Decreases fibrinolysis due to inhibitory effects of PAI-1 on plasminogen activator; increased p-selectin and von Willebrand factor
Muromonab[259,260]	Increases platelet activity and endothelial activity
Prednisone[255]	Decreases fibrinolysis due to inhibitory effects of PAI-1 on plasminogen activator; increases p-selectin and von Willebrand factor
Sirolimus[261]	Vascular endothelial growth factor upregulation resulting in disruption of vessel network
Tacrolimus [261]	Vascular endothelial growth factor upregulation resulting in disruption of vessel network
ANTIPSYCHOTIC AGENTS	
Chlorpromazine[178]	Hyperprolactinemia-increased platelet activity; induces anticardiolipin antibodies
Clozapine[262]	Hyperprolactinemia-increased platelet activity
Olanzapine[262]	Hyperprolactinemia-increased platelet activity
Quetiapine[262]	Hyperprolactinemia-increased platelet activity
Risperidone[262]	Hyperprolactinemia-increased platelet activity
Thioridazine[262]	Hyperprolactinemia-increased platelet activity
OTHER PSYCHOTROPIC AGENTS	
Clomipramine[188]	Uncertain; increased serotonin concentrations cause an increase in platelet aggregation
Escitalopram[188]	Uncertain; increased serotonin concentrations cause an increase in platelet aggregation
Lithium[189]	Uncertain; induces dehydration
CONTRAST AGENTS	
Iohexol[263,264]	Platelet aggregation and activation
Iomeprol[263,264]	Platelet aggregation and activation
Iopamidol[263,264]	Platelet aggregation and activation
Iothalamate[263,264]	Platelet aggregation and activation
Ioxaglate[263,264]	Platelet aggregation and activation
MISCELLANEOUS	
Acetohydroxamic acid[200]	Increases thrombin and platelets
Botulinum toxin	NK
Bromocriptine	NK
Calcium gluconate	NK
Cocaine[265]	Increases platelet activation
Dihydroergotamine[210,215]	Uncertain; ergotism, ischemia, venous stasis
Ecstasy (3,4-methylenedioxyethamphetamine; MDMA)	NK
Ergotamine[210,215]	Uncertain; ergotism, ischemia, venous stasis
Metolazone	NK
Papaverine	NK
Procainamide[266]	Induces antiphospholipid antibodies

Table 47-2 Mechanisms of Drug-Induced Thromboembolic Diseases (continued)

Drug	Mechanism
Sildenafil[222]	Uncertain; decreases blood flow to microcirculation; decreases antithrombin III and protein S
Topiramate	Unknown
Tretinoin[226,227]	Releases plasminogen activators and lysosomal neutrophil enzymes leading to diffuse intravascular coagulation

G-CSF = granulocyte colony-stimulating factor, GM-CSF = granulocyte/macrophage colony-stimulating factor, HIT = heparin-induced thrombocytopenia, HITT = heparin-induced thrombocytopenia and thrombosis, PAI = plasminogen-activator inhibitor, NK = not known.

mechanisms for inducing thromboembolic disease. Estrogen-containing agents increase factor II, VII, VIII, and fibrinogen levels. There are reductions in natural anticoagulants, antithrombin III, and protein S. In addition, estrogens are known to cause resistance to activated protein C. This is especially problematic in patients with factor V Leiden mutation, as these patients possess an inherited resistance to activated protein C. The cumulative effect of estrogen's induced hypercoagulability can lead to thrombosis.[57,230] The antiandrogens may increase platelet aggregation and alter the fibrinolytic system. Finally, selective estrogen-receptor modulators are thought to reduce the concentrations of antithrombin, protein C, and protein S, causing venous thrombosis.[57]

Although the mechanism for drug-induced thromboembolism associated with the antineoplastic agents is not precisely known, it is likely that a combination of factors is involved. The drugs themselves may cause hypercoagulability, or drug-induced endothelial damage may occur propagating clot formation. The patient's disease state and the presence of catheters also likely play a role in the development of VTE in patients receiving antineoplastic agents.

CLINICAL PRESENTATION AND DIFFERENTIAL DIAGNOSIS

The signs and symptoms of VTE are outlined in **Table 47-3**. There is often a great deal of interindividual variability in the presenting signs and symptoms of VTE as well as in the time-to-initial presentation. Clinical manifestations of drug-induced VTE are generally not distinct from those of VTE due to any other cause. DVT of the thigh or calf is associated with warmth, redness, and swelling that is generally unilateral. Skin discoloration may also occur, and palpation may reveal a nickel-sized or cord-like obstruction. PE should be suspected whenever a patient has dyspnea without another apparent cause, pleuritic pain, circulatory

Table 47-3 Signs and Symptoms Associated with Drug-Induced Thromboembolic Diseases

Pulmonary embolism

- Accentuated second heart sounds and fourth heart sound
- Cough
- Cyanosis
- Dyspnea
- Hemoptysis
- Hypoxemia (i.e., abnormal arterial blood gases or pulse oximetry)
- Palpitations
- Pleuritic chest pain
- Rales
- Syncope
- Tachycardia
- Tachypnea

Deep vein thrombosis

- Pain or tenderness
- Palpation of a nickel-sized or cord-like obstruction
- Positive Homan's sign
- Skin discoloration (i.e., pallor, cyanosis, or erythema)
- Unilateral warmth, redness, or swelling

collapse with no apparent cause, hemoptysis, or syncope.[233] In addition, patients presenting acutely with PE may have sinus tachycardia, gallop rhythm, and elevated jugular venous pressure.

The diagnosis of DVT or PE can be challenging, as signs and symptoms are sometimes subtle and nonspecific, and patient presentation can vary substantially. Conditions to consider in the differential diagnoses of DVT include muscular injuries, superficial thromboses, lymphedema, and cellulitis (**Table 47-4**). On physical examination, calf pain resulting from dorsiflexion of the ankle while the knee is in a flexed position (positive Homans sign) is consistent with DVT.[269] The Wells criteria have been created for determining the probability of DVT and PE (**Table 47-5**).[270,271] Each of these criteria has been validated and are commonly used; however, clinical assessment should be used only in conjunction with objective testing.[272] D-dimer is a degradation product of a cross-linked fibrin blood clot. Although the D-dimer test cannot be used to affirmatively diagnose VTE, it has a relatively high negative predictive value, especially in younger patients without associated comorbidity. The American College of Chest Physicians (ACCP) Expert Panel Report makes recommendations about the diagnosis of DVT.[273] In patients found to have a low pretest probability of first extremity DVT or PE as determined by the Wells criteria, a high-sensitivity D-dimer test should be used to rule out VTE. Ultrasonography has high sensitivity and specificity for diagnosis of symptomatic proximal DVT of the lower extremity. Sensitivity of this test decreases, however, in patients who are asymptomatic or have DVT in the calf.[274] Patients with moderate pretest probability are recommended to receive D-dimer testing, proximal compression ultrasonography, or

Table 47-4 Conditions to Consider in the Differential Diagnosis of Drug-Induced Thromboembolic Diseases

Pulmonary embolism

- Exacerbation of heart failure
- Exacerbation of other pulmonary disease
- Musculoskeletal pain
- Myocardial infarction
- Pneumonia
- Pneumothorax

Deep vein thrombosis

- Baker's cyst
- Cellulitis
- Drug-induced edema
- Knee injury/abnormality
- Leg swelling in a paralyzed limb
- Lymph obstruction
- Muscle strain/tear
- Superficial thrombophlebitis
- Venous insufficiency

Table 47-5 Wells Criteria for Predicting Pretest Probability of Deep-Vein Thrombosis and Pulmonary Embolism[270,271]

Clinical Characteristic	Points
DEEP-VEIN THROMBOSIS[a]	
Active cancer	1
Calf swelling at least 3 cm larger than on the asymptomatic side	1
Collateral superficial veins (nonvaricose)	1
Entire leg swollen	1
Localized tenderness along the distribution of the deep venous system	1
Paralysis, paresis, or recent plaster immobilization of the lower extremities	1
Pitting edema confined to the symptomatic leg	1
Previously documented DVT	1
Recently bedridden for 3 days or more, or major surgery within the previous 12 weeks requiring general or local anesthesia	1
Alternative diagnosis at least as likely as DVT	-2
PULMONARY EMBOLISM[b]	
An alternative diagnosis is less likely than PE	3
Clinical signs and symptoms of DVT	3
Heart rate >100 bpm	1.5
Immobilization or surgery in the previous 4 weeks	1.5
Previous DVT or PE	1.5
Active cancer	1
Hemoptysis	1

DVT = deep-vein thrombosis, PE = pulmonary embolism.

[a]A score ≥2 indicates a high probability of DVT; a score <2 indicates a low probability of DVT.

[b]A score <2 indicates a low probability of PE; a score of 2–6 indicates a moderate probability of PE; and a score >6 indicates a high probability of PE.

whole leg ultrasound.[273] D-dimer can be used to rule out DVT if a negative ultrasound occurs.[274] Those with high pretest probability are recommended to receive proximal compression or whole leg ultrasonography. Again, D-dimer can be used to rule out a negative result.[274] Contrast venography is the most definitive test for DVT, but it is expensive and requires venous access. For these reasons, lower-extremity ultrasound is preferred.[273]

Conditions to consider in the differential diagnoses of PE include pneumonia, pneumothorax, acute myocardial infarction, and exacerbation of other pulmonary diseases. Patients with PE may have abnormal arterial blood gases and nonspecific electrocardiographic changes. As with DVT, a whole-blood D-dimer assay may be useful to rule out PE in those with low pretest probability using the Wells criteria for PE. However, imaging is essential to diagnose PE in patients with intermediate-to-high pretest probability. Imaging options include a ventilation/perfusion (V/Q) lung scan, helical computed tomography (CT), or multidetector CT angiography. Multidetector CT angiography is most commonly utilized and is the diagnostic test of choice for PE in the United States. It may be used in patients with PE and a positive D-dimer assay result or in those who have a high pretest probability of PE regardless of D-dimer result. In patients with negative CT but high pretest probability, follow-up ultrasound of the lower extremities or pulmonary angiography may be warranted.[274]

RISK FACTORS

Risk factors for drug-induced thromboembolic events do not differ from those for VTE of any other cause. The use of drugs associated with VTE in patients with other risk factors often compounds the risk. **Table 47-6** lists the most important acquired and hereditary risk factors.[233] These risk factors are additive. In some cases, patient risk factors are readily identified or easily calculated using clinical predictive assessment tools.[275,276] A prior history of VTE is perhaps the strongest risk factor for recurrent VTE, presumably because of damage to venous valves and obstruction of blood flow caused by the initial event.[237] Age and sex must both be considered in evaluating relative risk. Women have a higher incidence of VTE during their childbearing years. The incidence of VTE nearly doubles in each decade of life over the age of 50 and is slightly higher in men.[237] Over 80% of patients with VTE have at least one risk factor, whereas many patients possess a combination of factors of Virchow's triad.[234-236]

Table 47-6 Risk Factors for Drug-Induced Thromboembolic Diseases

Acquired

- Age
- Antiphospholipid syndrome
- Heart failure
- Heparin-induced thrombocytopenia
- History of VTE
- Immobilization via institutionalization, long-distance travel, or paralysis
- Indwelling venous catheters
- Inflammatory bowel disease
- Liver disease
- Malignancy
- Myeloproliferative disorders
- Nephrotic syndrome
- Neurologic disease
- Obesity
- Pregnancy/postpartum
- Secondary hyperhomocysteinemia
- Sickle-cell anemia
- Smoking
- Sticky-platelet syndrome
- Superficial vein thrombosis
- Surgery
- Transvenous pacemakers
- Trauma

Hereditary

- Antithrombin deficiency
- Dysfibrinogenemia
- Factor V Leiden/activated protein C resistance gene mutation
- Factor VIII overactivity
- Factor XII deficiency
- Heparin cofactor II deficiency
- Plasminogen activator inhibitor-1 excess
- Primary hyperhomocysteinemia
- Protein C deficiency
- Protein S deficiency
- Prothrombin *20210A* gene mutation

VTE = venous thromboembolism.

Recent surgery imparts a great VTE risk to patients. Orthopedic surgery and trauma surgery confer especially high risks of associated VTE. In addition, there is an increased vulnerability seen in patients who have undergone neurovascular or cardiovascular surgery, renal transplantation, or major surgery for malignancy of the leg, pelvis, abdominal, or thoracic areas.[277-279]

Recent trauma or injury imparts a high risk of VTE. Specifically, there is a high association between DVT and spinal injury, head trauma, and fractures of the pelvis, tibia, and femur. Situations involving prolonged periods of immobilization, such as long-distance travel, total or partial paralysis, and institutionalization (e.g., long-term care facility or hospital) create potential danger for patients because of decreased blood flow in the extremities. The presence of malignancy increases the risk of thromboembolic events. There are several reasons for this, including direct vein compression or invasion by the tumor, increased concentrations of procoagulants such as fibrinogen in the malignant state, and the use of cytotoxic chemotherapy for the treatment of the primary disease.[237]

Varicose veins, obesity, and tobacco smoking are weakly associated VTE risk factors. However, previous DVT or superficial thrombosis are known to increase the odds of developing a new VTE. Other independent risk factors include the presence of central venous catheters or transvenous pacemakers, liver disease, and pregnancy.[237]

MORBIDITY AND MORTALITY

Thromboembolic disease can cause significant morbidity and mortality. Mortality rates can mostly be attributed to PE, in which approximately a quarter of cases present as sudden death.[237] An estimated 2 million people in the United States develop VTE each year, of whom 600,000 are hospitalized and 60,000 die.[280,281] Rate of recurrence following a first episode of VTE is 7.8/100 person-years in 1-year follow-up, and the recurrence rate in the years following is 3/100 person-years.[282] VTE-associated morbidity is most commonly related to development of post-thrombotic syndrome (PTS) in which patients experience pain and chronic swelling, tenderness, skin discoloration, or even skin ulceration long after the initial event. Within 2 years of a symptomatic DVT, PTS will be present in 23–60% of patients and 10% will develop venous ulcers in that time frame. PTS is associated with a high burden of direct and indirect costs. It is estimated that the U.S. average annual per person costs for someone with PTS is $7,000.[283] Morbidity may also arise from the development of chronic thromboembolic pulmonary hypertension (CTEPH), following PE. Most often CTEPH develops as a result of obstruction of the pulmonary vascular bed due to nonresolving PEs. Despite adequate anticoagulation, CTEPH develops in 1–3.8% of patients within 2 years of a PE.[284,285] Symptoms include shortness of breath, especially on exertion, and fatigue. In severe cases, abdominal and peripheral edema may occur. Without intervention, the prognosis of patients with CTEPH is poor and depends on the severity of pulmonary hypertension. Intervention can be medical or surgical, and costs can be quite high.[286,287] The incidence of morbidity and mortality specifically due to drug-induced VTE is unknown.

PREVENTION

Many VTE risk factors (Table 47-6) are unavoidable. Prevention strategies, therefore, are aimed at minimizing patients' exposure to drugs or combinations of drugs known to increase the risk of VTE (Table 47-1) and closely monitoring patients who have known risk factors. **Table 47-7** provides recommendations for the prevention of drug-induced thromboembolic disease.[94,237,241,242,252,268,288-297]

Patients with a history of VTE or known hypercoagulability should be advised to avoid use of estrogen-containing products, such as oral contraceptives, hormone-replacement therapy, and raloxifene or tamoxifen. In addition, oral contraceptives should be used cautiously in women over 35 years of age and in women of any age who smoke. Whenever possible, oral contraceptives, hormone-replacement therapy, and raloxifene should be discontinued at least 4 weeks (72 hours for raloxifene) prior to surgery. In addition, these agents should be withheld for 2 weeks after surgery and during and after prolonged immobilization.[288,298] Oral contraceptives

Table 47-7 Approaches to Help Prevent Drug-Induced Thromboembolic Diseases

Oral contraceptives, hormone-replacement therapy[237,288,289,305]

- Ambulate periodically during long episodes of travel or flight
- Estrogen-containing products are contraindicated in patients with acute VTE, history of VTE, or known hypercoagulability
- Discontinue drug 4 weeks in advance of surgery or immobile period; resume 2 weeks after procedure or after mobile
- May use progestin-only pills, medroxyprogesterone, progesterone implant, or IUD in those with history of VTE
- Use gestodene and drosperinone in combination with the lowest dose of ethinyl estradiol (<30 mcg daily) in patients without VTE history

Raloxifene, tamoxifen[291,298]

- Contraindicated in patients with previous VTE or known hypercoagulability
- Discontinue drug at least 72 hours in advance of surgery or immobile period, resume after mobile

Heparin products[241]

- Add heparins to patient allergy list
- Avoid all heparin products in the future
- In patients who develop HIT or HITT or who have a history of HIT or HITT, discontinue heparin products and use alternative anticoagulant acutely and for long-term anticoagulant needs

Warfarin[242,268]

- In patients with skin necrosis, discontinue warfarin and start heparin
- Overlap heparin or LMWH and warfarin for at least 7 days and until INR is ≥2 in those with known protein C or S deficiency or cancer

Erythropoietin, darbopoietin[292,293]

- Adjust dose such that rate of hemoglobin rise does not exceed 1 g/dL over a 2-week period
- Do not initiate treatment if hemoglobin concentration is ≥10 mg/dL
- Maintain hemoglobin concentrations <12 mg/dL in treating patients with anemia
- Use with caution in patients with previous VTE or known hypercoagulability

Thalidomide and lenalidomide[294]

- Patients with multiple myeloma and concurrently receiving chemotherapy and/or dexamethasone should receive prophylactic dose LMWH (enoxaparin 40 mg q 24 hr) or warfarin (INR 2–3), or aspirin 81–325 mg daily, depending on number of VTE risk factors present

Recombinant factor VIIa[295,296]

- Avoid in geriatric patients, those with current or recent VTE, severe atherosclerosis, crush injuries, disseminated intravascular coagulation, or sepsis

Asparaginase[94]

- Consider prophylaxis with LMWH

Estramustine[252]

- Consider use of low-dose warfarin or aspirin 325 mg for prophylaxis

Contrast dye[297]

- Avoid if possible; consider heparin-saline flush after use in venography

DES = diethylstilbestrol, HIT = heparin-induced thrombocytopenia, HITT = heparin-induced thrombocytopenia and thrombosis, IUD = intrauterine device, LMWH = low-molecular-weight heparin, VTE = venous thromboembolism.

should be started no earlier than 4–6 weeks after the postpartum period.[288] Patients taking estrogens should ambulate and perform exercises during periods of temporary immobility, such as long car rides or air travel. Estrogen as a component of oral contraceptives should be dosed at 10–35 mcg of ethinyl estradiol per day to minimize thrombosis risk. It is controversial as to whether combined hormonal contraceptives containing desogestrel, gestodene (not available in United States) or drospirenone increase the risk of VTE to a greater extent than products with other progestins. Thus, they should probably be avoided in patients at risk for VTE.[50,231,232,299]

Practitioners should complete a careful risk–benefit analysis before prescribing any agent known to induce VTE. This is especially important when the patient has known VTE risk factors. Prophylactic anticoagulation with warfarin, direct oral anticoagulants (DOACs), LMWH, or aspirin is typically not recommended, but may be considered for some patients who require therapy with drugs known to cause VTE or if the patient also has known VTE risk factors. Decisions regarding the use of prophylactic anticoagulation should be made on an individual basis. Risk-factor modification, when possible, should be pursued in all patients.

MANAGEMENT

Anticoagulation is the primary treatment for VTE, whether or not it is drug-induced. Because DVT and PE are manifestations of the same disease process, their treatments are virtually identical. The therapeutic goals are to prevent clot extension and embolization, reduce recurrence, and prevent long-term complications such as PTS.

The ACCP Expert Panel Report set guidelines for the treatment of VTE.[268] Recommended treatment includes the initial administration of subcutaneous LMWH, subcutaneous or intravenous unfractionated heparin (UFH), subcutaneous fondaparinux or DOACs (dabigatran, rivaroxaban, apixaban, and edoxaban).[300-303] When using LMWH, weight-based therapeutic doses can be given once or twice daily and will depend on the agent selected. Intravenous UFH is initiated as a bolus (80 units/kg or 5,000 units), followed by continuous infusion (18 units/kg/hr) and adjusted to achieve an activated partial thromboplastin time (aPTT) corresponding to an anti-factor Xa activity of 0.3–0.7 unit/mL. If monitored subcutaneous UFH is chosen, then an initial dose of 17,500 units or 250 units/kg twice daily should be selected with the same aPTT target as for intravenous UFH. Fondaparinux is dosed at 5 mg daily for a patient weighing <50 kg, 7.5 mg daily for patients weighing 50–100 kg, or 10 mg daily for patients weighing >100 kg. It is recommended that LMWH or UFH or fondaparinux be overlapped with warfarin for at least 5 days, then discontinued when the international normalized ratio (INR) is 2 for 24 hours. In patients with either DVT or PE, warfarin should be dosed to maintain an INR of 2–3.[268] The DOAC class has been studied and approved for use in the treatment of acute VTE and prevention of VTE recurrence. When one of the DOACs is used for acute VTE treatment, the need for pretreatment with UFH or LMWH will depend on the agent selected. Patients prescribed apixaban or rivaroxaban can start therapy immediately upon VTE diagnosis, without need for parenteral pretreatment.[300,303] However, dabigatran and edoxaban both require pretreatment with UFH or LMWH for 5–10 days.[301,302] Dosing for the DOAC agents is dependent on renal function. Despite U.S. labeling, the DOACs ideally should be avoided in populations that were excluded from clinical trials (patients with creatinine clearance below 30 mL/min and, in the case of apixaban, those with a creatinine clearance <25 mL/min).[300-303] **Table 47-8** lists dosing recommendations for VTE treatment and reduction of VTE recurrence with DOACs.[298-301]

Patients experiencing a first episode of VTE due to a transient risk factor (such as drug-induced VTE) should undergo anticoagulation for 3 months.[268] If the provoking risk factor remains present (such as a case in which a culprit drug cannot be discontinued), the patient should remain on anticoagulation therapy until the risk factor is no longer present. Patients with a first episode of unprovoked VTE, inherited hypercoagulability, or antiphospholipid syndrome should receive anticoagulation for at least 3 months. After 3 months, therapy should be re-evaluated and risk-benefit considerations should be weighed to decide whether or not to employ extended duration therapy. Extended therapy is recommended for patients with a second occurrence of unprovoked VTE and the continuing use of treatment should be reassessed periodically (e.g., annually). Patients with cancer and a VTE should receive LMWH for the first 3 months, followed by therapy with either LMWH or warfarin until the cancer is resolved.[268] In rare circumstances, thrombectomy or thrombolysis may be considered. Inferior vena cava interruption using a filter is also an option for those with contraindications to anticoagulation therapy. The ACCP does not recommend routine use of either thrombolysis, thrombectomy, or vena cava interruption.[268]

Heparin should be discontinued in patients who experience thrombotic complications related to that drug and an alternative, nonheparin anticoagulant should be substituted. A direct thrombin inhibitor should be used initially for the treatment of patients with HIT or HIT and thrombosis (HITT).[241] Further studies evaluating the role of fondaparinux and the DOACs in the treatment of HIT are needed.[241]

When acute thrombotic complications secondary to warfarin occur, the drug should be immediately discontinued and UFH, LMWH, or fondaparinux should be initiated. Warfarin should be reinitiated only with extreme caution after the resolution of the thrombosis, with very slow dose titration and careful

Table 47-8 DOAC U.S. Labelled Dosing Recommendations for VTE Treatment and Reduction of VTE Recurrence

Drug	Dosage Recommendations	Recommended Pretreatment with UFH or LMWH
Dabigatran[301]	150 mg BID Renal dose adjustment CrCl ≤30 mL/min or on dialysis: Avoid use CrCl <50 mL/min with concomitant use of strong P-gp inhibitors: Avoid use	5–10 days parenteral pretreatment required
Rivaroxaban[300]	15 mg BID × 21 days; then 20 mg daily. May reduce to 10 mg daily for extended treatment after 6 months of therapy Renal dose adjustment CrCl <30 mL/min or on dialysis: Avoid use Concomitant use of strong dual inhibitors of P-gp and CYP3A4: Avoid use	No parenteral pretreatment required
Apixaban[303]	10 mg BID × 7 days; then 5 mg BID May reduce to 2.5 mg BID for extended treatment after 6 months of therapy Renal dose adjustment No recommendations for dose adjustment in renal impairment Concomitant use of strong dual inhibitors of P-gp and CYP3A4: Reduce dose by 50% if taking 10 mg or 5 mg dose; avoid use if taking 2.5-mg dose	No parenteral pretreatment required
Edoxaban[302]	CrCl >50 mL/min: 60 mg daily CrCl 15–50 mL/min: 30 mg daily Weight ≤60 kg: 30 mg daily Concomitant use of strong P-gp inhibitor: 30 mg daily Renal dose adjustment CrCl <15 mL/min or on dialysis: Avoid use	5–10 days parenteral pretreatment required

BID = twice daily, DOAC = direct acting oral anticoagulant, VTE = venous thromboembolism, UFH = unfractionated heparin, LMWH = low-molecular-weight heparin.

patient monitoring. Overlap of warfarin with therapeutic doses of the parenteral agent is necessary over 1 or more weeks until INR is >2.[242]

When a patient experiences drug-induced VTE, the culprit agent should be discontinued, when possible, and, in most instances, therapy with that drug should not be reinstituted. In cases in which the causative drug cannot be discontinued (e.g., in a patient with cancer who is responding appropriately to chemotherapy), anticoagulation should be initiated and continued for as long as therapy with the culprit drug is required. Hormonal therapy is not associated with an increased risk of recurrent VTE in women receiving therapeutic anticoagulation.[304] In such cases, the risks and benefits of drug continuation and anticoagulation must be carefully weighed and decisions made on a case-by-case basis.

INFORMATION FOR PATIENTS

Patients receiving drugs known to cause VTE should know the signs and symptoms of DVT and PE and should be instructed to contact their primary care provider if they experience unilateral pain, tenderness, or swelling, especially in lower limbs, or if they experience sudden shortness of breath or chest pain. In addition, patients should be counseled about decreasing preventable risk factors, including smoking and obesity. Women receiving any type of estrogen therapy should be advised to discontinue treatment before, during, and after significant periods of immobilization. Extensive education regarding anticoagulant use, drug interactions, and monitoring is essential for patients treated for VTE. Finally, patients should be advised to keep all their healthcare providers apprised regarding their use of prescription and nonprescription medications and changes in drug therapy.

REFERENCES

1. Turpie AG, Chin BS, Lip GY. Venous thromboembolism: pathophysiology, clinical features, and prevention. *BMJ*. 2002; 325:887-90.
2. Fanashawe MP, Shore-Lesserson L, Reich DL. Two cases of fatal thrombosis after aminocaproic acid therapy and deep hypothermic circulatory arrest. *Anesthesiology*. 2001; 95:1525-7.
3. Achiron A, Gornish M, Melamed E. Cerebral sinus thrombosis as a potential hazard of antifibrinolytic treatment in menorrhagia. *Stroke*. 1990; 21:817-9.
4. Wymenga LF, van der Boon WJ. Obstruction of the renal pelvis due to an insoluble blood clot after epsilon-aminocaproic acid therapy: resolution with intraureteral streptokinase instillations. *J Urol*. 1998; 159:490-2.
5. Hocker JR, Saving KL. Fatal aortic thrombosis in a neonate during infusion of epsilon-aminocaproic acid. *J Pediatr Surg*. 1995; 30:1490-2.
6. Ellenberger C, Mentha G, Giostra E, Licker M. Cardiovascular collapse due to massive pulmonary thromboembolism during orthotopic liver transplantation. *J Clin Anesth*. 2006; 18:367-71.
7. Ramsay MA, Randall HB, Burton EC. Intravascular thrombosis and thromboembolism during liver transplantation: antifibrinolytic therapy implicated? *Liver Transpl*. 2004; 10:310-4.
8. Van der Meer J, Hillege HL, Ascoop CA et al. Aprotinin in aortocoronary bypass surgery: increased risk of vein-graft occlusion and myocardial infarction? Supportive evidence from a retrospective study. *Thromb Haemost*. 1996; 75:1-3.
9. Shore-Lesserson L, Reich DL. A case of severe diffuse venous thromboembolism associated with aprotinin and hypothermic circulatory arrest in a cardiac surgical patient with factor V Leiden. *Anesthesiology*. 2006; 105:219-21.
10. Upadhyay AP, Ananthasivan R, Radhakrishnan S, Zubaidi G. Cortical blindness and acute myocardial infarction following injection of bleeding gastric varices with cyanoacrylate glue. *Endoscopy*. 2005; 37:1034.
11. Roesch W, Rexroth G. Pulmonary, cerebral and coronary emboli during bucrylate injection of bleeding fundic varices. *Endoscopy*. 1998; 30:S89-90.
12. Nakajima N, Nagahiro S, Matsubara S, Satoh K. Ruptured de novo thrombotic giant aneurysm induced by ethyl 2-cyanoacrylate: case report. *Surg Neurol*. 2004; 62:346-51; discussion 51-2.
13. Albert SG, Salvato-Lechner V, Joist JH. Venous thromboembolism and transient thrombocytopenia in a patient with diabetes insipidus treated with desmopressin acetate (DDAVP). *Thromb Res*. 1988; 50:695-705.
14. Byrnes JJ, Larcada A, Moake JL. Thrombosis following desmopressin for uremic bleeding. *Am J Hematol*. 1988; 28:63-5.
15. Tempelhof MW, Benzuly KH, Fintel D, Krichavsky MZ. Eptifibatide-induced thrombocytopenia: with thrombosis and disseminated intravascular coagulation immediately after left main coronary artery percutaneous coronary angioplasty. *Tex Heart Inst J*. 2012; 39:86-91.
16. Yang EH, Perez E, Zhiroff KA, Burstein S. Left main stent thrombosis: Complicated by eptifibatide-induced acute thrombocytopenia. *Tex Heart Inst J*. 2011; 38:174-8.
17. Bakchoul T, Zollner H, Amiral J et al. Anti-protamine-heparin antibodies: incidence, clinical relevance, and pathogenesis. *Blood*. 2013; 121:2821-7.
18. Wojcik C, Schymik ML, Cure EG. Activated prothrombin complex concentrate factor VIII inhibitor bypassing activity (FEIBA) for the reversal of warfarin-induced coagulopathy. *Int J Emerg Med*. 2009; 2:217-25.
19. Dentali F, Marchesi C, Giorgi Pierfranceschi M et al. Safety of prothrombin complex concentrates for rapid anticoagulation reversal of vitamin K antagonists. A meta-analysis. *Thromb Haemost*. 2011; 106:429-38.
20. Thomas GO, Dutton RP, Hemlock B et al. Thromboembolic complications associated with factor VIIa administration. *J Trauma*. 2007; 62:564-9.
21. Raivio P, Suojaranta-Ylinen R, Kuitunen AH. Recombinant factor VIIa in the treatment of postoperative hemorrhage after cardiac surgery. *Ann Thorac Surg*. 2005; 80:66-71.
22. O'Connell KA, Wood JJ, Wise RP et al. Thromboembolic adverse events after use of recombinant human coagulation factor VIIa. *JAMA*. 2006; 295:293-8.
23. Mayer SA, Brun NC, Begtrup K et al. Recombinant activated factor VII for acute intracerebral hemorrhage. *New Engl J Med*. 2005; 352:777-85.
24. Fodstad H, Liliequist B. Spontaneous thrombosis of ruptured intracranial aneurysms during treatment with tranexamic acid (AMCA). Report of three cases. *Acta Neurochir (Wien)*. 1979; 49:129-44.
25. Woo KS, Tse LK, Woo JL, Vallance-Owen J. Massive pulmonary thromboembolism after tranexamic acid antifibrinolytic therapy. *Br J Clin Pract*. 1989; 43:465-6.
26. Lindhoff-Last E, Nakov R, Misselwitz F et al. Incidence and clinical relevance of heparin-induced antibodies in patients with deep vein thrombosis treated with unfractionated or low-molecular-weight heparin. *Br J Haematol*. 2002; 118:1137-42.
27. Warkentin TE, Levine MN, Hirsh J et al. Heparin-induced thrombocytopenia in patients treated with low-molecular-weight heparin or unfractionated heparin. *New Engl J Med*. 1995; 332:1330-5.
28. Warkentin TE, Kelton JG. A 14-year study of heparin-induced thrombocytopenia. *Am J Med*. 1996; 101:502-7.
29. Ganzer D, Gutezeit A, Mayer G et al. Prevention of thromboembolism as a cause of thromboembolic complications. A study of the incidence of heparin-induced thrombocytopenia type II. *Z Orthop Ihre Grenzgeb*. 1997; 135:543-9.
30. Ohman EM, Granger CB, Rice L et al. Identification, diagnosis and treatment of heparin-induced thrombocytopenia and thrombosis: a registry of prolonged heparin use and thrombocytopenia among hospitalized patients with and without cardiovascular disease. The Complication After Thrombocytopenia Caused by Heparin (CATCH) Registry steering committee. *J Thromb Thrombolysis*. 2005; 19:11-9.
31. Losonczy H, David M, Nagy I. Effect of pentosan polysulfate on activated partial thromboplastin time, thrombin time, euglobulin clot lysis, and on tissue-type plasminogen activator and plasminogen activator inhibitor activities in patients with thromboembolic disease. *Semin Thromb Hemost*. 1991; 17:394-8.
32. Tardy-Poncet B, Tardy B, Grelac F et al. Pentosan polysulfate-induced thrombocytopenia and thrombosis. *Am J Hematol*. 1994; 45:252-7.
33. Rice L, Kennedy D, Veach A. Pentosan-induced cerebral sagittal sinus thrombosis: a variant of heparin induced thrombocytopenia. *J Urol*. 1998; 160:2148.
34. Vaughan DE, Kirshenbaum JM, Loscalzo J. Streptokinase-induced, antibody-mediated platelet aggregation: a potential cause of clot propagation in vivo. *J Am Coll Cardiol*. 1988; 11:1343-8.
35. Sugarman DI, Solomon DA. Recurrent pulmonary thromboembolism after initiating fibrinolytic therapy: a therapeutic dilemma. *South Med J*. 1983; 76:1044-5.
36. Dejaeger P, Van de Werf F, Vermylen J, De Geest H. Thromboembolic complication after streptokinase therapy of pulmonary emboli. *Acta Cardiol*. 1988; 43:61-5.

37. Hassall E, Ulich T, Ament ME. Pulmonary embolus and Malassezia pulmonary infection related to urokinase therapy. *J Pediatr.* 1983; 102:722-5.
38. AbuRahma AF, Stickler DL, Robinson PA. A prospective controlled study of the efficacy of short-term anticoagulation therapy in patients with deep vein thrombosis of the lower extremity. *J Vasc Surg.* 1998; 28:630-7.
39. Kurt M, Shorbagi A, Aksu S et al. Warfarin-induced skin necrosis and leukocytoclastic vasculitis in a patient with acquired protein C and protein S deficiency. *Blood Coagul Fibrinolysis.* 2007; 18:805-6.
40. Rafiei N, Tabandeh H, Hirschbein M. Warfarin-induced skin necrosis of the eyelids. *Arch Ophthalmol.* 2007; 125:421.
41. Charu V, Belani CP, Gill AN et al. Efficacy and safety of every-2-week darbepoetin alfa in patients with anemia of cancer: a controlled, randomized, open-label phase II trial. *Oncologist.* 2007; 12:727-37.
42. Bohlius J, Wilson J, Seidenfeld J et al. Recombinant human erythropoietins and cancer patients: updated meta-analysis of 57 studies including 9353 patients. *J Natl Cancer Inst.* 2006; 98:708-14.
43. Bennett CL, Silver SM, Djulbegovic B et al. Venous thromboembolism and mortality associated with recombinant erythropoietin and darbepoetin administration for the treatment of cancer-associated anemia. *JAMA.* 2008; 299:914-24.
44. Ross SD, Allen IE, Henry DH et al. Clinical benefits and risks associated with epoetin and darbepoetin in patients with chemotherapy-induced anemia: a systematic review of the literature. *Clin Ther.* 2006; 28:801-31.
45. Palmer SC, Saglimbene V, Mavridis D et al. Erythropoiesis-stimulating agents for anaemia in adults with chronic kidney disease: a network meta-analysis. *Cochrane Database Syst Rev.* 2014; 12:CD010590.
46. Besarab A, Bolton WK, Browne JK et al. The effects of normal as compared with low hematocrit values in patients with cardiac disease who are receiving hemodialysis and epoetin. *New Engl J Med.* 1998; 339:584-90.
47. Corwin HL, Gettinger A, Fabian TC et al. Efficacy and safety of epoetin alfa in critically ill patients. *New Engl J Med.* 2007; 357:965-76.
48. Wright JR, Ung YC, Julian JA et al. Randomized, double-blind, placebo-controlled trial of erythropoietin in non-small-cell lung cancer with disease-related anemia. *J Clin Oncol.* 2007; 25:1027-32.
49. Barbui T, Finazzi G, Grassi A, Marchioli R. Thrombosis in cancer patients treated with hematopoietic growth factors—a meta-analysis. On behalf of the Subcommittee on Haemostasis and Malignancy of the Scientific and Standardization Committee of the ISTH. *Thromb Haemost.* 1996; 75:368-71.
50. Sohngen D, Wienen S, Siebler M et al. Analysis of rhG-CSF-effects on platelets by in vitro bleeding test and transcranial Doppler ultrasound examination. *Bone Marrow Transplant.* 1998; 22:1087-90.
51. Tolcher AW, Giusti RM, O'Shaughnessy JA, Cowan KH. Arterial thrombosis associated with granulocyte-macrophage colony-stimulating factor (GM-CSF) administration in breast cancer patients treated with dose-intensive chemotherapy: a report of two cases. *Cancer Invest.* 1995; 13:188-92.
52. Leaf AN, Propert K, Corcoran C et al. Phase III study of combined chemohormonal therapy in metastatic prostate cancer (ECOG 3882): an Eastern Cooperative Oncology Group study. *Med Oncol.* 2003; 20:137-46.
53. Bosset PO, Albiges L, Seisen T et al. Current role of diethylstilbestrol in the management of advanced prostate cancer. *BJU Int.* 2012; 110:E826-9.
54. Jick H, Kaye JA, Vasilakis-Scaramozza C, Jick SS. Risk of venous thromboembolism among users of third generation oral contraceptives compared with users of oral contraceptives with levonorgestrel before and after 1995: cohort and case-control analysis. *BMJ.* 2000; 321:1190-5.
55. Kemmeren JM, Algra A, Grobbee DE. Third-generation oral contraceptives and risk of venous thrombosis: meta-analysis. *BMJ.* 2001; 323:131-4.
56. Hennessy S, Berlin JA, Kinman JL et al. Risk of venous thromboembolism from oral contraceptives containing gestodene and desogestrel versus levonorgestrel: a meta-analysis and formal sensitivity analysis. *Contraception.* 2001; 64:125-33.
57. Romero A, Alonso C, Rincon M et al. Risk of venous thromboembolic disease in women A qualitative systematic review. *Eur J Obstet Gynecol Reprod Biol.* 2005; 121:8-17.
58. Vandenbroucke JP, Koster T, Briet E et al. Increased risk of venous thrombosis in oral-contraceptive users who are carriers of factor V Leiden mutation. *Lancet.* 1994; 344:1453-7.
59. Rossouw JE, Anderson GL, Prentice RL et al. Risks and benefits of estrogen plus progestin in healthy postmenopausal women: principal results From the Women's Health Initiative randomized controlled trial. *JAMA.* 2002; 288:321-33.
60. Rossouw JE, Manson JE, Kaunitz AM, Anderson GL. Lessons learned from the Women's Health Initiative trials of menopausal hormone therapy. *Obstet Gynecol.* 2013; 121:172-6.
61. Hulley S, Furberg C, Barrett-Connor E et al. Noncardiovascular disease outcomes during 6.8 years of hormone therapy: Heart and Estrogen/progestin Replacement Study follow-up (HERS II). *JAMA.* 2002; 288:58-66.
62. Vasilakis-Scaramozza C, Jick H. Risk of venous thromboembolism with cyproterone or levonorgestrel contraceptives. *Lancet.* 2001; 358:1427-9.
63. Seaman HE, de Vries CS, Farmer RD. The risk of venous thromboembolism in women prescribed cyproterone acetate in combination with ethinyl estradiol: a nested cohort analysis and case-control study. *Hum Reprod.* 2003; 18:522-6.
64. Seaman HE, Langley SE, Farmer RD, de Vries CS. Venous thromboembolism and cyproterone acetate in men with prostate cancer: a study using the General Practice Research Database. *BJU Int.* 2007; 99:1398-403.
65. Chang A, Yeap B, Davis T et al. Double-blind, randomized study of primary hormonal treatment of stage D2 prostate carcinoma: flutamide versus diethylstilbestrol. *J Clin Oncol.* 1996; 14:2250-7.
66. Asbury RF, Brunetto VL, Lee RB et al. Goserelin acetate as treatment for recurrent endometrial carcinoma: a Gynecologic Oncology Group study. *Am J Clin Oncol.* 2002; 25:557-60.
67. Covens A, Thomas G, Shaw P et al. A phase II study of leuprolide in advanced/recurrent endometrial cancer. *Gynecol Oncol.* 1997; 64:126-9.
68. Federici TJ. Leuprolide acetate and central retinal vein occlusion. *Ophthalmic Surg Lasers Imaging.* 2007; 38:497-9.
69. Sharifi R, Lee M, Ojeda L et al. Comparison of leuprolide and diethylstilbestrol for stage D2 adenocarcinoma of prostate. *Urology.* 1985; 26:117-24.
70. Cummings SR, Eckert S, Krueger KA et al. The effect of raloxifene on risk of breast cancer in postmenopausal women: results from the MORE randomized trial. Multiple Outcomes of Raloxifene Evaluation. *JAMA.* 1999; 281:2189-97.
71. Cuzick J, Forbes J, Edwards R et al. First results from the International Breast Cancer Intervention Study (IBIS-I): a randomised prevention trial. *Lancet.* 2002; 360:817-24.
72. Cuzick J, Forbes JF, Sestak I et al. Long-term results of tamoxifen prophylaxis for breast cancer—96-month follow-up of the randomized IBIS-I trial. *J Natl Cancer Inst.* 2007; 99:272-82.
73. Powles T, Eeles R, Ashley S et al. Interim analysis of the incidence of breast cancer in the Royal Marsden Hospital tamoxifen randomised chemoprevention trial. *Lancet.* 1998; 352:98-101.
74. Veronesi U, Maisonneuve P, Costa A et al. Prevention of breast cancer with tamoxifen: preliminary findings from the Italian randomised trial among hysterectomised women. Italian Tamoxifen Prevention Study. *Lancet.* 1998; 352:93-7.
75. Harvey HA, Kimura M, Hajba A. Toremifene: an evaluation of its safety profile. *Breast.* 2006; 15:142-57.
76. Baum M, Budzar AU, Cuzick J et al. Anastrozole alone or in combination with tamoxifen versus tamoxifen alone for adjuvant treatment of postmenopausal women with early breast cancer: first results of the ATAC randomised trial. *Lancet.* 2002; 359:2131-9.

77. Baum M, Buzdar A, Cuzick J et al. Anastrozole alone or in combination with tamoxifen versus tamoxifen alone for adjuvant treatment of postmenopausal women with early stage breast cancer: results of the ATAC (Arimidex, Tamoxifen Alone or in Combination) trial efficacy and safety update analyses. *Cancer.* 2003; 98:1802-10.
78. Bonneterre J, Buzdar A, Nabholtz JM et al. Anastrozole is superior to tamoxifen as first-line therapy in hormone receptor positive advanced breast carcinoma. *Cancer.* 2001; 92:2247-58.
79. Rose PG, Brunetto VL, VanLe L et al. A phase II trial of anastrozole in advanced recurrent or persistent endometrial carcinoma: a Gynecologic Oncology Group study. *Gynecol Oncol.* 2000; 78:212-6.
80. Oyan B, Altundag K, Ozisik Y. Does letrozole have any place in adjuvant setting in breast cancer patients with documented hypercoagulability? *Am J Clin Oncol.* 2004; 27:210-1.
81. Alvarado RG, Liu JY, Zwolak RM. Danazol and limb-threatening arterial thrombosis: two case reports. *J Vasc Surg.* 2001; 34:1123-6.
82. Corno M, Vallar G, Scarlato G, Meola G. Danazol and internal carotid artery thrombosis. *Eur Neurol.* 1989; 29:235-7.
83. Sahraian MA, Mottamedi M, Azimi AR, Moghimi B. Androgen-induced cerebral venous sinus thrombosis in a young body builder: case report. *BMC Neurol.* 2004; 4:22.
84. Huie MJ. An acute myocardial infarction occurring in an anabolic steroid user. *Med Sci Sports Exerc.* 1994; 26:408-13.
85. Thurlimann B, Castiglione M, Hsu-Schmitz SF et al. Formestane versus megestrol acetate in postmenopausal breast cancer patients after failure of tamoxifen: a phase III prospective randomised cross over trial of second-line hormonal treatment (SAKK 20/90). Swiss Group for Clinical Cancer Research (SAKK). *Eur J Cancer.* 1997; 33:1017-24.
86. Loprinzi CL, Kugler JW, Sloan JA et al. Randomized comparison of megestrol acetate versus dexamethasone versus fluoxymesterone for the treatment of cancer anorexia/cachexia. *J Clin Oncol.* 1999; 17:3299-306.
87. Espensen MK, Baggesen KL. Ischemic cerebral infarction in a young woman undergoing gonadotropin treatment for infertility. *Ugeskr Laeger.* 2005; 167:2901-3.
88. Loret de Mola JR, Kiwi R, Austin C, Goldfarb JM. Subclavian deep vein thrombosis associated with the use of recombinant follicle-stimulating hormone (Gonal-F) complicating mild ovarian hyperstimulation syndrome. *Fertil Steril.* 2000; 73:1253-6.
89. Germond M, Wirthner D, Thorin D et al. Aorto-subclavian thromboembolism: a rare complication associated with moderate ovarian hyperstimulation syndrome. *Hum Reprod.* 1996; 11:1173-6.
90. Kerst JM, Bex A, Mallo H et al. Prolonged low dose IL-2 and thalidomide in progressive metastatic renal cell carcinoma with concurrent radiotherapy to bone and/or soft tissue metastasis: a phase II study. *Cancer Immunol Immunother.* 2005; 54:926-31.
91. Eastman ME, Khorsand M, Maki DG et al. Central venous device-related infection and thrombosis in patients treated with moderate dose continuous-infusion interleukin-2. *Cancer.* 2001; 91:806-14.
92. Appel IM, Hop WC, Pieters R. Changes in hypercoagulability by asparaginase: a randomized study between two asparaginases. *Blood Coagul Fibrinolysis.* 2006; 17:139-46.
93. Athale UH, Siciliano SA, Crowther M et al. Thromboembolism in children with acute lymphoblastic leukaemia treated on Dana-Farber Cancer Institute protocols: effect of age and risk stratification of disease. *Br J Haematol.* 2005; 129:803-10.
94. Meister B, Kropshofer G, Klein-Franke A et al. Comparison of low-molecular-weight heparin and antithrombin versus antithrombin alone for the prevention of symptomatic venous thromboembolism in children with acute lymphoblastic leukemia. *Pediatr Blood Cancer.* 2008; 50:298-303.
95. Mitchell LG, Andrew M, Hanna K et al. A prospective cohort study determining the prevalence of thrombotic events in children with acute lymphoblastic leukemia and a central venous line who are treated with L-asparaginase: results of the Prophylactic Antithrombin Replacement in Kids with Acute Lymphoblastic Leukemia Treated with Asparaginase (PARKAA) Study. *Cancer.* 2003; 97:508-16.
96. Ross CS, Brown TM, Kotagal S, Rodriguez V. Cerebral venous sinus thrombosis in pediatric cancer patients: long-term neurological outcomes. *J Pediatr Hematol Oncol.* 2013; 35:299-302.
97. Clark G, Walsh G, Deshpande P, Koffman G. Improved efficacy of basiliximab over antilymphocyte globulin induction therapy in paediatric renal transplantation. *Nephrol Dial Transplant.* 2002; 17:1304-9.
98. Cohen MH, Gootenberg J, Keegan P, Pazdur R. FDA drug approval summary: bevacizumab (Avastin) plus Carboplatin and Paclitaxel as first-line treatment of advanced/metastatic recurrent nonsquamous non-small cell lung cancer. *Oncologist.* 2007; 12:713-8.
99. Chen HX, Mooney M, Boron M et al. Phase II multicenter trial of bevacizumab plus fluorouracil and leucovorin in patients with advanced refractory colorectal cancer: an NCI Treatment Referral Center Trial TRC-0301. *J Clin Oncol.* 2006; 24:3354-60.
100. Shah MA, Ilson D, Kelsen DP. Thromboembolic events in gastric cancer: high incidence in patients receiving irinotecan- and bevacizumab-based therapy. *J Clin Oncol.* 2005; 23:2574-6.
101. Weijl NI, Rutten MF, Zwinderman AH et al. Thromboembolic events during chemotherapy for germ cell cancer: a cohort study and review of the literature. *J Clin Oncol.* 2000; 18:2169-78.
102. Yanazume S, Tsuji T, Matsuo T et al. Systemic thromboembolism after anti-cancer chemotherapy in a woman with ovarian germ cell tumor. *J Obstet Gynaecol Res.* 2013; 39:742-5.
103. Flaig TW, Barqawi A, Miller G et al. A phase II trial of dexamethasone, vitamin D, and carboplatin in patients with hormone-refractory prostate cancer. *Cancer.* 2006; 107:266-74.
104. Karim M, Vaux E, Davies DR, Mason PD. Renal failure due to scleroderma with thrombotic microangiopathy developing in a woman treated with carboplatin for ovarian cancer. *Clin Nephrol.* 2002; 58:384-8.
105. Eisen T, Smith IE, Johnston S et al. Randomized phase II trial of infusional fluorouracil, epirubicin, and cyclophosphamide versus infusional fluorouracil, epirubicin, and cisplatin in patients with advanced breast cancer. *J Clin Oncol.* 1998; 16:1350-7.
106. Grenader T, Shavit L, Ospovat I et al. Aortic occlusion in patients treated with Cisplatin-based chemotherapy. *Mt Sinai J Med.* 2006; 73:810-2.
107. Ohashi S, Yazumi S, Nishio A et al. Acute cerebral infarction during combination chemotherapy with s-1 and cisplatin for a young patient with a mucin-producing adenocarcinoma of the stomach. *Intern Med.* 2006; 45:1049-53.
108. Jacobson GM, Kamath RS, Smith BJ, Goodheart MJ. Thromboembolic events in patients treated with definitive chemotherapy and radiation therapy for invasive cervical cancer. *Gynecol Oncol.* 2005; 96:470-4.
109. Camci C, Sari R, Sevinc A, Buyukberber S. Dacarbazine-induced carotid artery and deep venous thrombosis in a patient with leiomyosarcoma: case report. *J Chemother.* 2001; 13:206-9.
110. Ceci G, Bella M, Melissari M et al. Fatal hepatic vascular toxicity of DTIC. Is it really a rare event? *Cancer.* 1988; 61:1988-91.
111. Olsen E, Duvic M, Frankel A et al. Pivotal phase III trial of two dose levels of denileukin diftitox for the treatment of cutaneous T-cell lymphoma. *J Clin Oncol.* 2001; 19:376-88.
112. Nakazawa S, Uemura M, Matsuzaki K et al. Cardiorespiratory arrest due to acute pulmonary thromboembolism during chemotherapy for female urothelial carcinoma of urethra: a case report. *Hinyokika Kiyo.* 2013; 59:287-92.
113. Proverbs-Singh T, Chiu SK, Liu Z et al. Arterial thromboembolism in cancer patients treated with cisplatin: a systematic review and meta-analysis. *J Natl Cancer Inst.* 2012; 104:1837-40.
114. Gonzalez-Martin A, Fernandez E, Vaz MA et al. Long-term outcome of a phase II study of weekly docetaxel with a short course of estramustine and enoxaparine in hormone-resistant prostate cancer patients. *Clin Transl Oncol.* 2007; 9:323-8.

115. Beer TM, Venner PM, Ryan CW et al. High dose calcitriol may reduce thrombosis in cancer patients. *Br J Haematol.* 2006; 135:392-4.
116. Lin AM, Rini BI, Derynck MK et al. A phase I trial of docetaxel/estramustine/imatinib in patients with hormone-refractory prostate cancer. *Clin Genitourin Cancer.* 2007; 5:323-8.
117. Galsky MD, Small EJ, Oh WK et al. Multi-institutional randomized phase II trial of the epothilone B analog ixabepilone (BMS-247550) with or without estramustine phosphate in patients with progressive castrate metastatic prostate cancer. *J Clin Oncol.* 2005; 23:1439-46.
118. Lundgren R, Sundin T, Colleen S et al. Cardiovascular complications of estrogen therapy for nondisseminated prostatic carcinoma. A preliminary report from a randomized multicenter study. *Scand J Urol Nephrol.* 1986; 20:101-5.
119. Clark PE, Peereboom DM, Dreicer R et al. Phase II trial of neoadjuvant estramustine and etoposide plus radical prostatectomy for locally advanced prostate cancer. *Urology.* 2001; 57:281-5.
120. Rosenthal SA, Bae K, Pienta KJ et al. Phase III multi-institutional trial of adjuvant chemotherapy with paclitaxel, estramustine, and oral etoposide combined with long-term androgen suppression therapy and radiotherapy versus long-term androgen suppression plus radiotherapy alone for high-risk prostate cancer: preliminary toxicity analysis of RTOG 99-02. *Int J Radiat Oncol Biol Phys.* 2009; 73:672-8.
121. van Riel JM, van Groeningen CJ, Albers SH et al. Hepatic arterial 5-fluorouracil in patients with liver metastases of colorectal cancer: single-centre experience in 145 patients. *Ann Oncol.* 2000; 11:1563-70.
122. Leitman M, Baram S, Sidenko S et al. Transient left ventricular and right atrial thrombosis after 5-fluorouracil therapy. *J Am Soc Echocardiogr.* 2004; 17:778-9.
123. Yoon S, Schmassmann-Suhijar D, Zuber M et al. Chemotherapy with bevacizumab, irinotecan, 5-fluorouracil and leucovorin (IFL) associated with a large, embolizing thrombus in the thoracic aorta. *Ann Oncol.* 2006; 17:1851-2.
124. Beumer JH, Natale JJ, Lagattuta TF, Raptis A et al. Disposition of imatinib and its metabolite CGP74588 in a patient with chronic myelogenous leukemia and short-bowel syndrome. *Pharmacotherapy.* 2006; 26:903-7.
125. Al Aly Z, Philoctete Ashley JM, Gellens ME, Gonzalez EA. Thrombotic thrombocytopenic purpura in a patient treated with imatinib mesylate: true association or mere coincidence? *Am J Kidney Dis.* 2005; 45:762-8.
126. Goel A, Grossbard ML, Malamud S et al. Pooled efficacy analysis from a phase I-II study of biweekly irinotecan in combination with gemcitabine, 5-fluorouracil, leucovorin and cisplatin in patients with metastatic pancreatic cancer. *Anticancer Drugs.* 2007; 18:263-71.
127. Mansfield JC, Parkes M, Hawthorne AB et al. A randomized, double-blind, placebo-controlled trial of lenalidomide in the treatment of moderately severe active Crohn's disease. *Aliment Pharmacol Ther.* 2007; 26:421-30.
128. Palumbo A, Falco P, Corradini P et al. Melphalan, prednisone, and lenalidomide treatment for newly diagnosed myeloma: a report from the GIMEMA—Italian Multiple Myeloma Network. *J Clin Oncol.* 2007; 25:4459-65.
129. Richardson PG, Blood E, Mitsiades CS et al. A randomized phase 2 study of lenalidomide therapy for patients with relapsed or relapsed and refractory multiple myeloma. *Blood.* 2006; 108:3458-64.
130. Wiley KE. Multiple myeloma and treatment-related thromboembolism: oncology nurses' role in prevention, assessment, and diagnosis. *Clin J Oncol Nurs.* 2007; 11:847-51.
131. Bennett CL, Angelotta C, Yarnold PR et al. Thalidomide- and lenalidomide-associated thromboembolism among patients with cancer. *JAMA.* 2006; 296:2558-60.
132. Chiappino I, Destefanis P, Addeo A et al. Activity of weekly paclitaxel in advanced hormone-refractory prostate cancer. *Am J Clin Oncol.* 2007; 30:234-8.
133. Pather S, Quinn MA. Clear-cell cancer of the ovary-is it chemosensitive? *Int J Gynecol Cancer.* 2005; 15:432-7.
134. Sutton G, Blessing JA, Ball H. Phase II trial of paclitaxel in leiomyosarcoma of the uterus: a gynecologic oncology group study. *Gynecol Oncol.* 1999; 74:346-9.
135. Loren CP, Aslan JE, Rigg RA et al. The BCR-ABL inhibitor ponatinib inhibits platelet immunoreceptor tyrosine-based activation motif (ITAM) signaling, platelet activation and aggregate formation under shear. *Thromb Res.* 2015; 135:155-60.
136. Ariad suspends ponatinib sales. *Cancer Discov.* 2014; 4:6-7.
137. Schmidt-Erfurth U. Clinical safety of ranibizumab in age-related macular degeneration. *Expert Opin Drug Saf.* 2010; 9:149-65.
138. Campbell RJ, Gill SS, Bronskill SE et al. Adverse events with intravitreal injection of vascular endothelial growth factor inhibitors: nested case-control study. *BMJ.* 2012; 345:e4203.
139. Oki Y, Westin JR, Vega F et al. Prospective phase II study of rituximab with alternating cycles of hyper-CVAD and high-dose methotrexate with cytarabine for young patients with high-risk diffuse large B-cell lymphoma. *Br J Haematol.* 2013; 163:611-20.
140. Nishiofuku H, Tanaka T, Anai H et al. Hepatic arterial thrombosis: a critical complication during combination therapy of arterial chemoinfusion and sorafenib. *Anticancer Res.* 2012; 32:4121-4.
141. Altintas A, Ayyildiz O, Atay AE et al. Thalidomide-associated arterial thrombosis: two case reports. *Ann Acad Med Singapore.* 2007; 36:304-6.
142. Rajkumar SV, Blood E, Vesole D et al. Phase III clinical trial of thalidomide plus dexamethasone compared with dexamethasone alone in newly diagnosed multiple myeloma: a clinical trial coordinated by the Eastern Cooperative Oncology Group. *J Clin Oncol.* 2006; 24:431-6.
143. Rus C, Bazzan M, Palumbo A et al. Thalidomide in front line treatment in multiple myeloma: serious risk of venous thromboembolism and evidence for thromboprophylaxis. *Thromb Haemost.* 2004; 2:2063-5.
144. Zangari M, Anaissie E, Barlogie B et al. Increased risk of deep-vein thrombosis in patients with multiple myeloma receiving thalidomide and chemotherapy. *Blood.* 2001; 98:1614-5.
145. Zangari M, Barlogie B, Anaissie E et al. Deep vein thrombosis in patients with multiple myeloma treated with thalidomide and chemotherapy: effects of prophylactic and therapeutic anticoagulation. *Br J Haematol.* 2004; 126:715-21.
146. Zangari M, Barlogie B, Cavallo F et al. Effect on survival of treatment-associated venous thromboembolism in newly diagnosed multiple myeloma patients. *Blood Coagul Fibrinolysis.* 2007; 18:595-8.
147. Kuypers DR, Malaise J, Claes K et al. Secondary effects of immunosuppressive drugs after simultaneous pancreas-kidney transplantation. *Nephrol Dial Transplant.* 2005; 20(suppl 2):ii33-9, ii62.
148. Malaise J, Kuypers DR, Claes K et al. Immunosuppressive drugs after simultaneous pancreas-kidney transplantation. *Transplant Proc.* 2005; 37:2840-2.
149. Malaise J, Saudek F, Boucek P et al. Tacrolimus compared with cyclosporine microemulsion in primary simultaneous pancreas-kidney transplantation: the EURO-SPK 3-year results. *Transplant Proc.* 2005; 37:2843-5.
150. Stratta RJ, Gaber AO, Shokouh-Amiri MH et al. A 9-year experience with 126 pancreas transplants with portal enteric drainage. *Arch Surg.* 2001; 136:1141-9.
151. White M, Ross H, Haddad H et al. Subclinical inflammation and prothrombotic state in heart transplant recipients: impact of cyclosporin microemulsion vs. tacrolimus. *Transplantation.* 2006; 82:763-70.
152. Nowak-Gottl U, Ahlke E, Fleischhack G et al. Thromboembolic events in children with acute lymphoblastic leukemia (BFM protocols): prednisone versus dexamethasone administration. *Blood.* 2003; 101:2529-33.
153. Calligaro KD, Stern J, DeLaurentis DA. Foscarnet: a possible cause of ulnar artery thrombosis in a patient with AIDS. *J Vasc Surg.* 1994; 20:1007-8.

154. Nosbaum A, Goujon C, Fleury B et al. Arterial thrombosis with anti-phospholipid antibodies induced by infliximab. *Eur J Dermatol.* 2007;17:546-7.
155. Ruyssen-Witrand A, Gossec L, Salliot C et al. Complication rates of 127 surgical procedures performed in rheumatic patients receiving tumor necrosis factor alpha blockers. *Clin Exp Rheumatol.* 2007; 25:430-6.
156. Grange L, Nissen MJ, Garambois K et al. Infliximab-induced cerebral thrombophlebitis. *Rheumatology. (Oxford).* 2005; 44:260-1.
157. Min J, Bhatt A, Aburashed R, Burton S. Cerebral venous and sinus thrombosis associated with subcutaneous immunoglobulin injection and oral contraceptive use. *Neurol Sci.* 2012; 33:627-9.
158. Hommes OR, Sorensen PS, Fazekas F et al. Intravenous immunoglobulin in secondary progressive multiple sclerosis: randomised placebo-controlled trial. *Lancet.* 2004; 364:1149-56.
159. Dalakas MC. High-dose intravenous immunoglobulin and serum viscosity: risk of precipitating thromboembolic events. *Neurology.* 1994; 44:223-6.
160. Marie I, Maurey G, Herve F et al. Intravenous immunoglobulin-associated arterial and venous thrombosis; report of a series and review of the literature. *Br J Dermatol.* 2006; 155:714-21.
161. White DA, Leonard MC. Acute stroke with high-dose intravenous immune globulin. *Am J Health-Syst Pharm.* 2007; 64:1611-4.
162. Khorana AA, Rosenblatt JD, Sahasrabudhe DM et al. A phase I trial of immunotherapy with intratumoral adenovirus-interferon-gamma (TG1041) in patients with malignant melanoma. *Cancer Gene Ther.* 2003; 10:251-9.
163. Bouros D, Antoniou KM, Siafakas NM. Deep venous thrombosis as a possible complication of interferon-gamma treatment. *Sarcoidosis Vasc Diffuse Lung Dis.* 2001; 18:201.
164. Tilg H, Vogelsang H, Ludwiczek O et al. A randomised placebo controlled trial of pegylated interferon alpha in active ulcerative colitis. *Gut.* 2003; 52:1728-33.
165. Zandieh I, Adenwalla M, Cheong-Lee C et al. Retinal vein thrombosis associated with pegylated-interferon and ribavirin combination therapy for chronic hepatitis C. *World J Gastroenterol.* 2006; 12:4908-10.
166. Deutsch M, Manesis EK, Hadziyannis E et al. Thrombotic thrombocytopenic purpura with fatal outcome in a patient with chronic hepatitis C treated with pegylated interferon-a/2b. *Scand J Gastroenterol.* 2007; 42:408-9.
167. Okuse C, Adachi K, Katakura Y et al. A case of deep venous thrombosis associated with pegylated interferon alpha2b plus ribavirin treatment of chronic hepatitis C. *J Gastroenterol.* 2006; 41:1231-6.
168. Rubio JE Jr, Charles S. Interferon-associated combined branch retinal artery and central retinal vein obstruction. *Retina.* 2003; 23:546-8.
169. Wells J, Kossard S, McGrath M. Abdominal wall ulceration and mucinosis secondary to recombinant human interferon-beta-1b. *Australas J Dermatol.* 2005; 46:202-4.
170. Casoni F, Merelli E, Bedin R et al. Necrotizing skin lesions and NABs development in a multiple sclerosis patient treated with IFNbeta 1b. *Mult Scler.* 2003; 9:420-3.
171. Theodossiou C, Kroog G, Ettinghausen S et al. Acute arterial thrombosis in a patient with breast cancer after chemotherapy with 5-fluorouracil, doxorubicin, leucovorin, cyclophosphamide, and interleukin-3. *Cancer.* 1994; 74:2808-10.
172. Abramowicz D, De Pauw L, Le Moine A et al. Prevention of OKT3 nephrotoxicity after kidney transplantation. *Kidney Int Suppl.* 1996; 53:S39-43.
173. Vela C, Cristol JP, Chong G et al. Antilymphocyte globulins versus OKT3 as prophylactic treatment in highly sensitized renal transplant recipients. *Transpl Int.* 1994; 7(suppl 1):S259-62.
174. Montagnino G, Sandrini S, Casciani C et al. A randomized trial of steroid avoidance in renal transplant patients treated with everolimus and cyclosporine. *Transplant Proc.* 2005; 37:788-90.
175. Pelle G, Xu Y, Khoury N et al. Thrombotic microangiopathy in marginal kidneys after sirolimus use. *Am J Kidney Dis.* 2005; 46:1124-8.
176. Hachem RR, Yusen RD, Chakinala MM et al. Thrombotic microangiopathy after lung transplantation. *Transplantation.* 2006; 81:57-63.
177. Kamijo Y, Soma K, Nagai T et al. Acute massive pulmonary thromboembolism associated with risperidone and conventional phenothiazines. *Circ J.* 2003; 67:46-8.
178. Ducloux D, Florea A, Fournier V et al. Inferior vena cava thrombosis in a patient with chlorpromazine-induced anticardiolipin antibodies. *Nephrol Dial Transplant.* 1999; 14:1335-6.
179. Metzer WS, Canoso RT, Newton JE. Anticardiolipin antibodies in a sample of chronic schizophrenics receiving neuroleptic therapy. *South Med J.* 1994; 87:190-2.
180. Matsumoto T, Azekawa T, Yamaguchi A et al. Habitual self-mutilation in Japan. *Psychiatry Clin Neurosci.* 2004; 58:191-8.
181. Zornberg GL, Jick H. Antipsychotic drug use and risk of first-time idiopathic venous thromboembolism: a case-control study. *Lancet.* 2000; 356:1219-23.
182. Liperoti R, Pedone C, Lapane KL et al. Venous thromboembolism among elderly patients treated with atypical and conventional antipsychotic agents. *Arch Intern Med.* 2005; 165:2677-82.
183. Gallien S, Rollot F, Caron B et al. Pulmonary embolism and deep jugular venous thrombosis resulting from compression by a lipoma. *Dermatol Online J.* 2006; 12:13.
184. Bhanji NH, Chouinard G, Hoffman L, Margolese HC. Seizures, coma, and coagulopathy following olanzapine overdose. *Can J Psychiatry.* 2005; 50:126-7.
185. Hagg S, Tatting P, Spigset O. Olanzapine and venous thromboembolism. *Int Clin Psychopharmacol.* 2003; 18:299-300.
186. Parkin L, Skegg DC, Herbison GP, Paul C. Psychotropic drugs and fatal pulmonary embolism. *Pharmacoepidemiol Drug Saf.* 2003; 12:647-52.
187. Eikmeier G, Kuhlmann R, Gastpar M. Thrombosis of cerebral veins following intravenous application of clomipramine. *J Neurol Neurosurg Psychiatry.* 1988; 51:1461.
188. Kurne A, Ertugrul A, Anil Yagcioglu AE, Yazici KM. Venous thromboembolism and escitalopram. *Gen Hosp Psychiatry.* 2004; 26:481-3.
189. Kamijo Y, Soma K, Hamanaka S et al. Dural sinus thrombosis with severe hypernatremia developing in a patient on long-term lithium therapy. *J Toxicol Clin Toxicol.* 2003; 41:359-62.
190. Lyles MR. Deep venous thrombophlebitis associated with lithium toxicity. *J Natl Med Assoc.* 1984; 76:633-4.
191. Wasay M, Bakshi R, Kojan S et al. Superior sagittal sinus thrombosis due to lithium: local urokinase thrombolysis treatment. *Neurology.* 2000; 54:532-3.
192. Sato E, Saito I. Risk of clot formation with ionic and nonionic contrast media in cerebral angiography. Tama Contrast Media Study Group. *Acad Radiol.* 1996; 3:925-8.
193. Qureshi NR, den Heijer P, Crijns HJ. Percutaneous coronary angioscopic comparison of thrombus formation during percutaneous coronary angioplasty with ionic and nonionic low osmolality contrast media in unstable angina. *Am J Cardiol.* 1997; 80:700-4.
194. Esplugas E, Cequier A, Gomez-Hospital JA et al. Comparative tolerability of contrast media used for coronary interventions. *Drug Saf.* 2002; 25:1079-98.
195. Schrader R, Esch I, Ensslen R et al. A randomized trial comparing the impact of a nonionic (Iomeprol) versus an ionic (Ioxaglate) low osmolar contrast medium on abrupt vessel closure and ischemic complications after coronary angioplasty. *J Am Coll Cardiol.* 1999; 33:395-402.
196. Malekianpour M, Bonan R, Lesperance J et al. Comparison of ionic and nonionic low osmolar contrast media in relation to thrombotic complications of angioplasty in patients with unstable angina. *Am Heart J.* 1998; 135:1067-75.
197. Bettmann MA, Robbins A, Braun SD et al. Contrast venography of the leg: diagnostic efficacy, tolerance, and complication rates with ionic and nonionic contrast media. *Radiology.* 1987; 165:113-6.

198. Walters HL, Clemenson J, Browse NL, Thomas ML. 125I-fibrinogen uptake following phlebography of the leg. Comparison of ionic and nonionic contrast media. *Radiology.* 1980; 135:619-21.
199. Dieu V, Joffre F, Krause D et al. A comparison of the efficacy and safety of ioxaglate and iobitridol in renal angioplasty. *Cardiovasc Intervent Radiol.* 2000; 23:91-6.
200. Rodman JS, Williams JJ, Jones RL. Hypercoagulability produced by treatment with acetohydroxamic acid. *Clin Pharmacol Ther.* 1987; 42:346-50.
201. Fernandez Lopez F, Conde Freire R, Rios Rios A et al. Botulinum toxin for the treatment of anal fissure. *Dig Surg.* 1999; 16:515-8.
202. Jost WH, Schanne S, Mlitz H, Schimrigk K. Perianal thrombosis following injection therapy into the external anal sphincter using botulin toxin. *Dis Colon Rectum.* 1995; 38:781.
203. Dargaud Y, Pariset C, Pinede L et al. Multiple arterial thromboses in a patient with primary antiphospholipid syndrome receiving a bromocriptine therapy. *Lupus.* 2004; 13:957-60.
204. Loewe C, Dragovic LJ. Acute coronary artery thrombosis in a postpartum woman receiving bromocriptine. *Am J Forensic Med Pathol.* 1998; 19:258-60.
205. Nagaki Y, Hayasaka S, Hiraki S, Yamada Y. Central retinal vein occlusion in a woman receiving bromocriptine. *Ophthalmologica.* 1997; 211:397-8.
206. Chen SC, Chang JM, Wang CS et al. Upper limb deep vein thrombosis following calcium gluconate injection. *Nephrology (Carlton).* 2009; 14:621.
207. Meyer G, Marjanovic Z, Valcke J et al. Comparison of low-molecular-weight heparin and warfarin for the secondary prevention of venous thromboembolism in patients with cancer: a randomized controlled study. *Arch Intern Med.* 2002; 162:1729-35.
208. Villota JN, Rubio LF, Fores JS et al. Cocaine-induced coronary thrombosis and acute myocardial infarction. *Int J Cardiol.* 2004; 96:481-2.
209. Zoghby Z, Sekhon IS, Miller DV, Sethi S. Cocaine, loin pain, and renal vein thrombosis. *Am J Kidney Dis.* 2007; 49:859-61.
210. Bongard O, Bounameaux H. Severe iatrogenic ergotism: incidence and clinical importance. *Vasa.* 1991; 20:153-6.
211. Evans MS, Naritoku DK, Couch JR, Ghobrial MW. Onset of neurologic deficits after treatment with dihydroergotamine in a patient with sagittal sinus thrombosis. *Clin Neuropharmacol.* 1996; 19:177-84.
212. Iaquinto G, Ambrosone L, Rotiroti D et al. A case of portal thrombosis arisen after treatment with dihydroergotamine. *Ital J Gastroenterol.* 1991;23:219-21.
213. Goldstein LH, Mordish Y, Abu-Kishak I et al. Acute paralysis following recreational MDMA (Ecstasy) use. *Clin Toxicol (Phila).* 2006; 44:339-41.
214. Lai TI, Hwang JJ, Fang CC, Chen WJ. Methylene 3, 4 dioxymethamphetamine-induced acute myocardial infarction. *Ann Emerg Med.* 2003; 42:759-62.
215. Lenger R. Ergot poisoning in paraplegia. *Paraplegia.* 1984; 22:42-4.
216. Lindboe CF, Dahl T, Rostad B. Fatal stroke in migraine: a case report with autopsy findings. *Cephalalgia.* 1989; 9:277-80.
217. Mintz U, Bar-Meir S, De Vries A. Ergotamine-induced venous thrombosis. *Postgrad Med J.* 1974; 50:244-6.
218. Green ST, Ng JP, Callaghan M. Metolazone and axillary vein thrombosis. *Scott Med J.* 1988; 33:211-2.
219. Likosky DS, Donegan DJ, Groom RC et al. Embolic activity subsequent to injection of the internal mammary artery with papaverine hydrochloride. *Heart Surg Forum.* 2005; 8:E434-6.
220. List AF, Doll DC. Thrombosis associated with procainamide-induced lupus anticoagulant. *Acta Haematol.* 1989; 82:50-2.
221. Li GC, Greenberg CS, Currie MS. Procainamide-induced lupus anticoagulants and thrombosis. *South Med J.* 1988; 81:262-4.
222. Rufa A, Cerase A, Monti L et al. Recurrent venous thrombosis including cerebral venous sinus thrombosis in a patient taking sildenafil for erectile dysfunction. *J Neurol Sci.* 2007; 260:293-5.
223. Saha SA, O'Cochlain B, Singh A, Khosla S. Sildenafil-associated coronary thrombosis in a patient with angiographically normal coronary arteries: a case report with review of literature. *Am J Ther.* 2006; 13:378-84.
224. Gedik S, Yilmaz G, Akova YA. Sildenafil-associated consecutive nonarteritic anterior ischaemic optic neuropathy, cilioretinal artery occlusion, and central retinal vein occlusion in a haemodialysis patient. *Eye.* 2007; 21:129-30.
225. Cudkowicz ME, Shefner JM, Schoenfeld DA et al. A randomized, placebo-controlled trial of topiramate in amyotrophic lateral sclerosis. *Neurology.* 2003; 61:456-64.
226. Escudier SM, Kantarjian HM, Estey EH. Thrombosis in patients with acute promyelocytic leukemia treated with and without all-trans retinoic acid. *Leuk Lymphoma.* 1996; 20:435-9.
227. Torromeo C, Latagliata R, Avvisati G et al. Coronaric thrombotic events in acute promyelocytic leukemia during all-trans retinoic acid treatment: a role for adhesion molecules overexpression? *Leukemia.* 1999; 13:312-3.
228. Spencer FA, Emery C, Lessard D et al. The Worcester Venous Thromboembolism study: a population-based study of the clinical epidemiology of venous thromboembolism. *J Gen Intern Med.* 2006; 21:722-7.
229. Reitsma PH, Versteeg HH, Middeldorp S. Mechanistic view of risk factors for venous thromboembolism. *Arterioscler Thromb Vasc Biol.* 2012; 32:563-8.
230. de Bastos M, Stegeman BH, Rosendaal FR et al. Combined oral contraceptives: venous thrombosis. *Cochrane Database Syst Rev.* 2014; 3:CD010813.
231. Sidney S, Cheetham TC, Connell FA et al. Recent combined hormonal contraceptives (CHCs) and the risk of thromboembolism and other cardiovascular events in new users. *Contraception.* 2013; 87:93-100.
232. Han L, Jensen JT. Does the Progestogen Used in Combined Hormonal Contraception Affect Venous Thrombosis Risk? *Obstet Gynecol Clin North Am.* 2015; 42:683-98.
233. Kroegel C, Reissig A. Principle mechanisms underlying venous thromboembolism: epidemiology, risk factors, pathophysiology and pathogenesis. *Respiration.* 2003; 70:7-30.
234. Chung I, Lip GY. Virchow's triad revisited: blood constituents. *Pathophysiol Haemost Thromb.* 2003; 33:449-54.
235. Blann AD. How a damaged blood vessel wall contributes to thrombosis and hypertension. *Pathophysiol Haemost Thromb.* 2003; 33:445-8.
236. Lowe GD. Virchow's triad revisited: abnormal flow. *Pathophysiol Haemost Thromb.* 2003; 33:455-7.
237. Heit JA. Risk factors for venous thromboembolism. *Clin Chest Med.* 2003; 24:1-12.
238. Gallet B, Zemour G, Saudemont JP et al. Echocardiographic demonstration of intracardiac glue after endoscopic obturation of gastroesophageal varices. *J Am Soc Echocardiogr.* 1995; 8:759-61.
239. Suryanarayan D, Schulman S. Potential antidotes for reversal of old and new oral anticoagulants. *Thrombosis Res.* 2014; 133(suppl 2):S158-66.
240. Hunt BJ. The current place of tranexamic acid in the management of bleeding. *Anaesthesia.* 2015; 70:e18-53.
241. Linkins LA, Dans AL, Moores LK et al. Treatment and prevention of heparin-induced thrombocytopenia: antithrombotic therapy and prevention of thrombosis (9th ed): American College of Chest Physicians Evidence-Based Clinical Practice Guidelines. *Chest.* 2012; 141:e495S-530S.
242. Ageno W, Gallus AS, Wittkowsky A et al. Oral anticoagulant therapy: antithrombotic therapy and prevention of thrombosis (9th ed): American College of Chest Physicians Evidence-Based Clinical Practice Guidelines. *Chest.* 2012; 141:e44S-88S.
243. Steurer M, Sudmeier I, Stauder R, Gastl G. Thromboembolic events in patients with myelodysplastic syndrome receiving thalidomide in combination with darbepoietin-alpha. *Br J Haematol.* 2003; 121:101-3.

244. Oberhoff C, Hoffmann O, Winkler UH, Schindler AE. Hemostatic effects of high-dose megestrol acetate therapy in patients with advanced gynecological cancer. *Gynecol Endocrinol.* 2001; 15:341-8.
245. Baumann P, Diedrich K. Thromboembolic complications associated with reproductive endocrinologic procedures. *Hematol Oncol Clin North Am.* 2000; 14:431-43.
246. Becker JC, Winkler B, Klingert S, Brocker EB. Antiphospholipid syndrome associated with immunotherapy for patients with melanoma. *Cancer.* 1994; 73:1621-4.
247. Imamura T, Morimoto A, Kato R et al. Cerebral thrombotic complications in adolescent leukemia/lymphoma patients treated with L-asparaginase-containing chemotherapy. *Leuk Lymphoma.* 2005; 46:729-35.
248. van Heeckeren WJ, Sanborn SL, Narayan A et al. Complications from vascular disrupting agents and angiogenesis inhibitors: aberrant control of hemostasis and thrombosis. *Curr Opin Hematol.* 2007; 14:468-80.
249. Keefe D, Bowen J, Gibson R et al. Noncardiac vascular toxicities of vascular endothelial growth factor inhibitors in advanced cancer: a review. *Oncologist.* 2011; 16:432-44.
250. Nadir Y, Hoffman R, Brenner B. Drug-related thrombosis in hematologic malignancies. *Rev Clin Exp Hematol.* 2004; 8:E4.
251. Lysov Z, Swystun LL, Kuruvilla S et al. Lung cancer chemotherapy agents increase procoagulant activity via protein disulfide isomerase-dependent tissue factor decryption. *Blood Coagul Fibrinolysis.* 2015; 26:36-45.
252. Lubiniecki GM, Berlin JA, Weinstein RB, Vaughn DJ. Thromboembolic events with estramustine phosphate-based chemotherapy in patients with hormone-refractory prostate carcinoma: results of a meta-analysis. *Cancer.* 2004; 101:2755-9.
253. Tham J, Albertsson M. Upper extremity deep venous thrombosis in patients with 5-fluorouracil-containing adjuvant chemotherapy--three case reports and a review. *Acta Oncol.* 2004; 43:108-12.
254. Schiavon G, Vincenzi B, Santini D et al. Recurrent thrombophlebitis in a colon cancer patient with C677T heterozygous genotype for MTHFR treated with 5-fluorouracil-based adjuvant chemotherapy. *Chemotherapy.* 2004; 50:194-5.
255. Patrassi GM, Sartori MT, Rigotti P et al. Reduced fibrinolytic potential one year after kidney transplantation. Relationship to long-term steroid treatment. *Transplantation.* 1995; 59:1416-20.
256. Ferraccioli G, Gremese E. Thrombogenicity of TNF alpha in rheumatoid arthritis defined through biological probes: TNF alpha blockers. *Autoimmun Rev.* 2004; 3:261-6.
257. Ben-Ami R, Barshtein G, Mardi T et al. A synergistic effect of albumin and fibrinogen on immunoglobulin-induced red blood cell aggregation. *Am J Physiol Heart Circ Physiol.* 2003; 285:H2663-9.
258. Arnman V, Stemme S, Rymo L, Risberg B. Interferon-gamma modulates the fibrinolytic response in cultured human endothelial cells. *Thromb Res.* 1995; 77:431-40.
259. Deira J, Alberca I, Lerma JL et al. Changes in coagulation and fibrinolysis in the postoperative period immediately after kidney transplantation in patients receiving OKT3 or cyclosporine A as induction therapy. *Am J Kidney Dis.* 1998; 32:575-81.
260. Lozano M, Oppenheimer F, Cofan F et al. Platelet procoagulant activity induced in vivo by muromonab-CD3 infusion in uremic patients. *Thromb Res.* 2001; 104:405-11.
261. Guba M, Yezhelyev M, Eichhorn ME et al. Rapamycin induces tumor-specific thrombosis via tissue factor in the presence of VEGF. *Blood.* 2005; 105:4463-9.
262. Axelsson S, Hagg S, Eriksson AC et al. In vitro effects of antipsychotics on human platelet adhesion and aggregation and plasma coagulation. *Clin Exp Pharmacol Physiol.* 2007; 34:775-80.
263. Van Beek EJ, Levi M, Reekers JA et al. Increased plasma levels of PAI-1 after administration of nonionic contrast medium in patients undergoing pulmonary angiography. *Radiology.* 1994; 193:821-3.
264. Ogawa T, Fujii S, Urasawa K, Kitabatake A. Effects of nonionic contrast media on platelet aggregation: assessment by particle counting with laser-light scattering. *Jpn Heart J.* 2001; 42:115-24.
265. Heesch CM, Wilhelm CR, Ristich J et al. Cocaine activates platelets and increases the formation of circulating platelet containing microaggregates in humans. *Heart.* 2000; 83:688-95.
266. Merrill JT, Shen C, Gugnani M et al. High prevalence of antiphospholipid antibodies in patients taking procainamide. *J Rheumatol.* 1997; 24:1083-8.
267. Ballard JO. Anticoagulant-induced thrombosis. *JAMA.* 1999; 282:310-2.
268. Kearon C, Akl EA, Ornelas J et al. Antithrombotic therapy for VTE Disease: CHEST Guideline and Expert Panel Report. *Chest.* 2016; 149:315-52.
269. Urbano FL. Homan's sign in the diagnosis of deep venous thrombosis. *Hosp Physician.* 2001; 37:22-4.
270. Wells PS, Anderson DR, Rodger M et al. Evaluation of D-dimer in the diagnosis of suspected deep-vein thrombosis. *New Engl J Med.* 2003; 349:1227-35.
271. Wells PS, Anderson DR, Rodger M et al. Derivation of a simple clinical model to categorize patients probability of pulmonary embolism: increasing the models utility with the SimpliRED D-dimer. *Thromb Haemost.* 2000; 83:416-20.
272. Wells PS, Anderson DR, Bormanis J et al. Value of assessment of pretest probability of deep-vein thrombosis in clinical management. *Lancet.* 1997; 350:1795-8.
273. Bates SM, Jaeschke R, Stevens SM et al. Diagnosis of DVT: Antithrombotic Therapy and prevention of thrombosis (9th ed): American College of Chest Physicians Evidence-Based Clinical Practice Guidelines. *Chest.* 2012; 141:e351S-418S.
274. Wilbur J, Shian B. Diagnosis of deep venous thrombosis and pulmonary embolism. *Am Fam Physician.* 2012; 86:913-9.
275. Barbar S, Noventa F, Rossetto V et al. A risk assessment model for the identification of hospitalized medical patients at risk for venous thromboembolism: the Padua Prediction Score. *Thromb Haemost.* 2010; 8:2450-7.
276. Bahl V, Hu HM, Henke PK et al. A validation study of a retrospective venous thromboembolism risk scoring method. *Ann Surg.* 2010; 251:344-50.
277. Falck-Ytter Y, Francis CW, Johanson NA et al. Prevention of VTE in orthopedic surgery patients: antithrombotic therapy and prevention of thrombosis (9th ed): American College of Chest Physicians Evidence-Based Clinical Practice Guidelines. *Chest.* 2012; 141:e278S-325S.
278. Gould MK, Garcia DA, Wren SM et al. Prevention of VTE in nonorthopedic surgical patients: antithrombotic therapy and prevention of thrombosis (9th ed): American College of Chest Physicians Evidence-Based Clinical Practice Guidelines. *Chest.* 2012; 141:e227S-77S.
279. Kahn SR, Lim W, Dunn AS et al. Prevention of VTE in nonsurgical patients: antithrombotic therapy and prevention of thrombosis (9th ed): American College of Chest Physicians Evidence-Based Clinical Practice Guidelines. *Chest.* 2012; 141:e195S-226S.
280. Lilienfeld DE, Chan E, Ehland J et al. Mortality from pulmonary embolism in the United States: 1962 to 1984. *Chest.* 1990; 98:1067-72.
281. Lilienfeld DE. Decreasing mortality from pulmonary embolism in the United States, 1979–1996. *Int J Epidemiol.* 2000; 29:465-9.
282. Arshad N, Bjori E, Hindberg K et al. Recurrence and mortality after first venous thromboembolism in a large population-based cohort. *Thromb Haemost.* 2017; 15:295-303.
283. [No authors listed]. Neuroleptics: increased rate of venous thromboembolic events. *Prescrire Int.* 2006; 15:224.
284. Becattini C, Agnelli G, Pesavento R et al. Incidence of chronic thromboembolic pulmonary hypertension after a first episode of pulmonary embolism. *Chest.* 2006; 130:172-5.
285. Pengo V, Lensing AW, Prins MH et al. Incidence of chronic thromboembolic pulmonary hypertension after pulmonary embolism. *New Engl J Med.* 2004; 350:2257-64.
286. Riedel M, Stanek V, Widimsky J, Prerovsky I. Longterm follow-up of patients with pulmonary thromboembolism. Late prognosis

and evolution of hemodynamic and respiratory data. *Chest.* 1982; 81:151-8.

287. Lewczuk J, Piszko P, Jagas J et al. Prognostic factors in medically treated patients with chronic pulmonary embolism. *Chest.* 2001; 119:818-23.

288. US Food and Drug Administration; Center for Drug Evaluation and Research. Guidance for industry labeling for combined oral contraceptives: draft guidance (2004). https://www.fda.gov/downloads/ScienceResearch/SpecialTopics/WomensHealthResearch/UCM133346.pdf (accessed 2018 Feb 26).

289. Prempro, conjugated estrogens/medroxyprogesterone acetate [package insert]. Philadelphia: Wyeth Pharmaceuticals; 2008.

290. Evista [package insert]. Indianapolis, IN: Eli Lilly; 2001.

291. Nolvadex, tamoxifen [package insert]. Wilmington, DE: AstraZeneca; 2004.

292. Epogen, epoetin alpha [package insert]. Thousand Oaks, CA: Amgen; 2008.

293. Aranesp, darbepoetin alpha [package insert]. Thousand Oaks, CA: Amgen; 2008.

294. National Comprehensive Cancer Network. NCCN clinical practice guidelines in oncology (version 1.2015): cancer associated venous thromboembolic disease. http://www.triadhealthcarenetwork.com/wp-content/uploads/2016/04/2015-nccn-vte.pdf (accessed 2018 Feb 26).

295. Johnson SJ, Ross MB, Moores KG. Dosing factor VIIa (recombinant) in nonhemophiliac patients with bleeding after cardiac surgery. *Am J Health-Syst Pharm.* 2007; 64:1808-12.

296. Novoseven, recombinant Factor VIIa [package insert]. Bagsværd, Denmark: Novo Nordisk; 1999.

297. Blumgart RL, Immelman EJ, Jeffery PC, Lipinski JK. Thrombotic side-effects of lower limb venography. The use of heparin-saline flush. *S Afr Med J.* 1991; 79:88-9.

298. Evista [package insert]. Indianapolis, IN: Eli Lilly; 2011.

299. Lidegaard O, Nielsen LH, Skovlund CW et al. Risk of venous thromboembolism from use of oral contraceptives containing different progestogens and oestrogen doses: Danish cohort study, 2001–2009. *BMJ.* 2011; 343:d6423.

300. Xarelto [package insert]. Titusville, NJ: Janssen Pharmaceuticals; 2011.

301. Pradaxa [package insert]. Ridgefield, CT: Boehringer Ingelheim; 2015.

302. Savaysa [package insert]. Parsippany, NJ: Daiichai Sankyo; 2015.

303. Eliquis [package insert]. Princeton, MJ: Bristol-Myers Squibb; 2015.

304. Martinelli I, Lensing AW, Middeldorp S et al. Recurrent venous thromboembolism and abnormal uterine bleeding with anticoagulant and hormone therapy use. *Blood.* 2016; 127:1417-25.

305. Curtis KM, Tepper NK, Jatlaoui TC et al. US Medical Eligibility Criteria for Contraceptive Use, 2016. *MMWR Recomm Rep.* 2016; 65(no. RR-3):1-104.

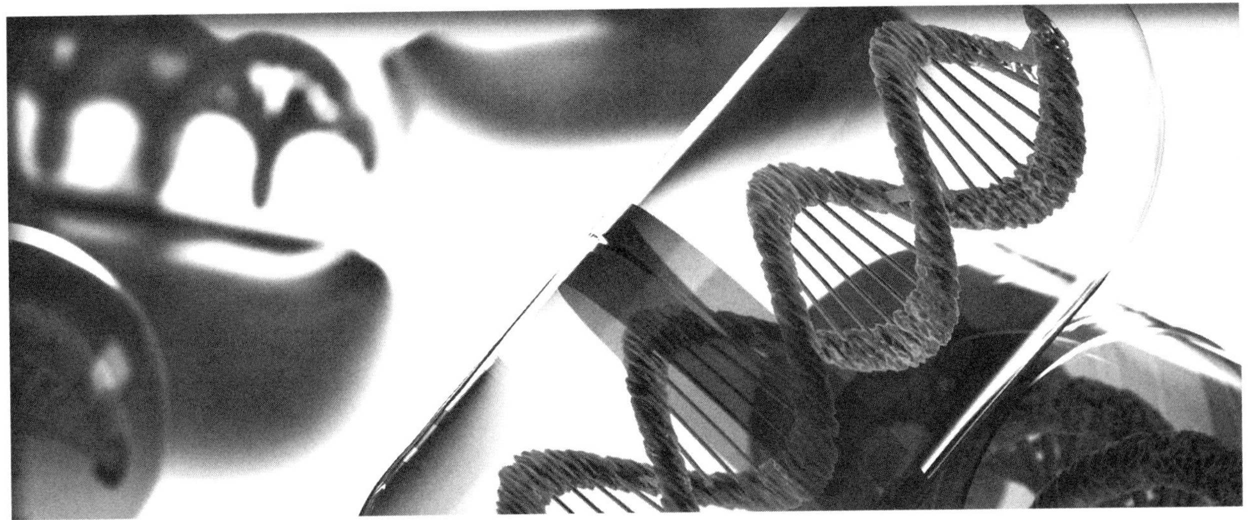

CHAPTER 48

Neutropenia and Agranulocytosis

Teresa C. Thakrar and Christopher A. Fausel

Neutropenia has been generally defined as an absolute neutrophil count (ANC) of <500 cells/mm^3 or <1,000 cells/mm^3 with an expected decline to <500 cells/mm^3.[1] The Infectious Diseases Society of America also defines neutropenia as an ANC of <500 cells/mm^3 or an anticipated decrease of the ANC to <500 cells/mm^3 but adds that the decline must be anticipated within the next 48 hours.[2] Neutropenia is classified as either acquired or intrinsic. Drug-induced neutropenia is an acquired neutropenia that is potentially life-threatening.[3,4] It occurs most commonly as an expected untoward effect associated with antineoplastic drugs. When noncytotoxic drugs cause a precipitous decline in neutrophil count, the condition is called agranulocytosis, and this disorder is well documented.[5,6] Agranulocytosis has been defined as a drug-mediated reduction in the peripheral ANC to <500 cells/mm^3 due to immunologic or cytotoxic mechanisms.[7]

CAUSATIVE AGENTS

It is common clinical practice in hematology/oncology to administer chemotherapy drugs in combination to treat the disease. The risk of myelosuppression with cytotoxic chemotherapy generally increases with an increasing number of agents per regimen, increasing drug dose, frequency, and duration of exposure.[8] Conventional cytotoxic chemotherapy drugs include the alkylating agents, antimetabolites, anthracyclines, topoisomerase inhibitors, taxanes, and vinca alkaloids; all may cause neutropenia when used alone or in combination chemotherapy regimens. Most molecular-targeted antineoplastic drugs cause a much lower incidence of neutropenia than conventional cytotoxic agents. Select tyrosine kinase inhibitors such as imatinib, dasatinib, nilotinib, bosutinib, and ponatinib cause neutropenia in patients with Philadelphia chromosome-positive (Ph+) acute and chronic leukemia, especially in those with more advanced disease. An in-depth discussion of specific chemotherapy regimens used in clinical practice and their risk for causing neutropenia is beyond the scope of this chapter, and the reader is referred to specialized sources for that specific information.[9,10]

Commonly used classes of drugs reported to cause agranulocytosis include nonsteroidal anti-inflammatory drugs (NSAIDs), antibiotics, antiplatelet, antithyroid, antirheumatic, antiarrhythmic, and antipsychotic agents.[10,11] In an extensive review of the medical literature published between 1966 and 2006, investigators found 980 cases of reported agranulocytosis. The authors evaluated each of these cases for causality and defined 6% as definite, 44% as probable, 49% as possible, and 1% as unlikely, using World Health Organization causality assessment criteria. A total of 125 drugs were found to be either definitely or probably causative.[12] A more recent surveillance study conducted in Berlin between 2000 and 2010 identified clozapine, sulfasalazine, methimazole, and thiamazole as the drugs with the highest probability of causing agranulocytosis, which is consistent with previous case-control studies. This indicates a relatively unchanged spectrum of causative agents, despite introduction of newly approved drugs.[13] **Table 48-1** lists drugs that have been reported to cause agranulocytosis.[12-32]

EPIDEMIOLOGY

Neutropenia is considered to be a dose-limiting toxicity for cancer treatments, and accordingly, documentation of this effect is meticulous in phase I, II, and III oncology trials.[33] Treatment of malignancies such as acute leukemia or procedures such as hematopoietic stem cell transplantation use drug doses and schedules to intentionally destroy the normal and diseased bone marrow cells to eradicate the primary disease. This strategy is illustrated by remission-induction therapy for acute leukemia, in which a state of aplasia persisting for several weeks is induced, followed by bone marrow recovery.[34] High-dose chemotherapy requiring an outside stem cell replacement source (allogeneic) used in bone marrow transplant procedures typically results in a 2- to 4-week period with bone marrow aplasia preceding engraftment of the transplanted bone marrow.[35]

The overall incidence of agranulocytosis has been reported in three large epidemiologic studies. A study conducted in Europe and Israel documented an incidence of agranulocytosis of 3.4 cases per million population per year.[36] This estimate is derived from data collected from hospitals by the International Aplastic Anemia and Agranulocytosis Study (IAAAS) over a 7-year period. The incidence of agranulocytosis in the United States was studied using computerized Medicaid billing data from three states from 1980 through 1985.[37] The overall incidence was 7.2 cases (range, 2.4–15.4) per million population per year. The Dutch healthcare system conducted a population-based, case-cohort study to determine the risk of agranulocytosis as a reason for hospital admission.[24] Review of hospital discharge data with subsequent case reviews yielded a mean incidence of 2 per million per year over 4 years.

The most recent epidemiologic data set consists of 17 hematology units in Europe contributing to case–control surveillance for agranulocytosis and aplastic anemia. The incidence of community-acquired agranulocytosis was 3.4 cases per million population per year with a mortality rate of 0.24 per million population per year and a case fatality rate of 7%.[17]

The risk of agranulocytosis associated with specific drug classes has been studied. A population-based, case-control study was performed with Medicaid claim data from six states to determine the association between NSAID use and agranulocytosis.[27] The odds ratio was found to be 3.3. No specific NSAID was associated with a higher risk, leading the authors to conclude that the low incidence does not necessitate establishing usage restrictions for any specific agent(s). These findings were similar to those of a previous IAAAS study.[15]

The epidemiology of agranulocytosis induced by cardiovascular drugs has also been evaluated, and an increased risk of agranulocytosis in patients treated for at least 1 week with propranolol, digoxin, dipyridamole, and procainamide was found.[23] IAAAS and others have documented an increased risk of agranulocytosis associated with trimethoprim–sulfamethoxazole and with the macrolide, β-lactam, and cephalosporin antibiotics.[18,19] Studies have been conducted to document the association of agranulocytosis with other drugs, including antithyroid agents, sulfonamides, sulfasalazine, and carbonic anhydrase inhibitors.[16,20,28,29,31]

The atypical antipsychotic drug clozapine is known to cause agranulocytosis. The manufacturer has instituted a stringent registration program for patients in which weekly white cell count monitoring is required before a drug supply is dispensed.

Table 48-1 Agents Implicated in Drug-Induced Neutropenia and Agranulocytosis

Drug	Incidence	Level of Evidence[a]
Abacavir[13]	NK	C
Acetaminophen[14]	NK	C
Acetazolamide[15]	NK	C
Allopurinol[11]	NK	C
Aminoglutethimide[11]	NK	C
Amoxapine[11]	NK	C
Aspirin[16]	NK	C
Auranofin[11]	NK	C
β-Lactam antibiotics[11,17,18]	NK	C
Brompheniramine[13]	NK	C
Captopril[11]	NK	C
Carbamazepine[11]	NK	C
Carbimazole[19,b]	0.2–0.5%	C
Cephalosporins[11,17]	NK	C
Clindamycin[17]	NK	C
Chloramphenicol[17,18]	NK	C
Chlordiazepoxide[13]	NK	C
Chlorpheniramine[13]	NK	C
Chlorpropamide[11]	NK	C
Chloroquine[17]	NK	C
Cimetidine[11]	NK	C
Clomipramine[13]	NK	C
Clozapine[20,21,b]	0.7–0.8%	B
Colchicine[13]	NK	C
Dapsone[13,b]	NK	C
Desipramine[11]	NK	C
Digoxin[22]	NK	C
Dipyridamole[22]	NK	C
Erythromycin[23]	NK	C
Ethosuximide[13]	NK	C
Etanercept[24]	NK	C
Famotidine[11]	NK	C
Flucytosine[17]	NK	C
Furosemide[13]	NK	C
Ganciclovir[25]	NK	C
Gentamicin[17]	NK	C
Griseofulvin[17]	NK	C
Hydralazine[13]	NK	C
Hydrochlorothiazide[13]	NK	C
Hydroxychloroquine[13]	NK	C
Imipramine[11]	NK	C
Infliximab[11]	NK	C

Table 48-1 Agents Implicated in Drug-Induced Neutropenia and Agranulocytosis (continued)

Drug	Incidence	Level of Evidence[a]
Isoniazid[17]	NK	C
Levodopa[13]	NK	C
Mebendazole[17]	NK	C
Meprobamate[11]	NK	C
Metoclopramide[13]	NK	C
Methimazole[19,b]	0.2–0.5%	B
Methyldopa[22]	NK	C
Nifedipine[22]	NK	C
Nitrofurantoin[17]	NK	C
NSAIDs[14,16,26]	NK	C
Olanzapine[13]	NK	C
Penicillamine[11]	NK	C
Phenothiazines[11]	NK	C
Phenytoin[11]	NK	C
Potassium perchlorate[13]	NK	C
Procainamide[22,b]	0.56%	C
Propafenone[22]	NK	C
Propranolol[22]	NK	C
Propylthiouracil[19,b]	0.2–0.5%	C
Pyrimethamine[17]	NK	C
Quinacrine[17]	NK	C
Quinidine[22]	NK	C
Quinine[13]	NK	C
Ranitidine[11]	NK	C
Rituximab[11,a]	NK	C
Spironolactone[22]	NK	C
Streptomycin[17]	NK	C
Sulfasalazine[27,28,b]	0.6%	B
Tamoxifen[13]	NK	C
Ticlopidine[29,b]	2.4%	B
Tocainide[22]	NK	C
Trimethoprim–sulfamethoxazole[30]	NK	C
Valganciclovir[31]	NK	C
Valproic acid[13]	NK	C
Vancomycin[11]	NK	C
Zidovudine[11]	NK	C

NK = not known, NSAID = nonsteroidal anti-inflammatory drug.

[a]Definitions for Levels of Evidence: Level A—evidence from one or more randomized, controlled clinical trials; Level B—evidence from nonrandomized clinical trials, prospective observational studies, cohort studies, retrospective studies, case-control studies, meta-analyses and/or postmarketing surveillance studies; and Level C—evidence from one or more published case reports or case series.

[b]Ten or more published cases where agranulocytosis was deemed to be probably or definitely related to the drug.

Two large pharmacovigilance studies have examined the incidence of clozapine-induced agranulocytosis based on the registry data. In over 11,000 patients in the United States, the cumulative incidence of agranulocytosis at 1 year was 0.8%. These findings were corroborated by a European study that reported a cumulative incidence of clozapine-induced agranulocytosis of 0.73% in 12,760 patients.[21,22]

MECHANISMS

Neutropenia secondary to chemotherapy occurs as a direct result of the cytotoxic effects of these agents on the bone marrow progenitor cells. The principal action of most antineoplastic agents is the disruption of cell proliferation, especially relating to cell division and deoxyribonucleic acid (DNA) synthesis.[38] These drugs all have the propensity to damage DNA during replication, particularly in rapidly growing tissues such as the bone marrow. Alkylating agents, antimetabolites, antimitotic drugs, anthracyclines, and topoisomerase inhibitors appear to cause neutropenia via this mechanism.[39] Newer immune-based therapies and molecular targeted drugs may also cause neutropenia; however, the mechanism involved is less clearly understood.[40]

Mechanisms of agranulocytosis may be divided into three broad categories: type I, immune-mediated; type II, direct toxicity; or type III, a combination of types I and II. Mechanisms of agranulocytosis, where known, are summarized in **Table 48-2**.[30,41-52] In type I agranulocytosis, assays such as leukoagglutination or enzyme-linked immunosorbent assay testing may be used to confirm the presence of antibodies directed against granulocytes.[53] Chlorpropamide has been shown to induce production of specific antibodies that inhibit granulocytic precursor cells in a dose-dependent manner.[54] Methimazole and propylthiouracil are associated with the formation of antibodies to neutrophils.[41,43,55] Procainamide-associated agranulocytosis is believed to result from an immune mechanism distinct from the one responsible for the systemic lupus erythematosus–like syndrome associated with this drug.[44]

Type II agranulocytosis is due to direct damage to myeloid precursor cells, leading to cell death. Cimetidine and quinidine have been reported to induce dose-dependent suppression of the bone marrow cells in vitro.[45,46] The suspected mechanism of ticlopidine-induced agranulocytosis involves a reactive metabolite interfering with normal neutrophil formation.[30,47] Activation of reactive metabolites via neutrophil myeloperoxidase mediates *N*-chlorination of sulfonamides, yielding direct neutrophil toxicity.[48]

Type III agranulocytosis may involve hapten formation, which has been linked to drugs such as flecainide and the penicillins.[49,50] There are cases in which multiple mechanisms appear to be involved with individual drugs. For example, clozapine-induced agranulocytosis may not be due solely to an immune-mediated process.[51] Accumulation of a nitrenium-containing metabolite of clozapine results in depletion of glutathione and adenosine triphosphate that results in apoptosis of neutrophils.[52] More evidence supporting this theory is that there is typically a delay of 14 weeks between clozapine rechallenge and neutrophil disappearance. This delay is inconsistent with a normal immune response.

Table 48-2 Mechanisms of Drug-Induced Neutropenia and Agranulocytosis

Drug	Mechanism
Antithyroid agents, β-lactam antibiotics, procainamide[40-43]	Immune-mediated, with antibody formation against granulocytes and granulocyte precursors
Cimetidine, cytotoxic chemotherapy, quinine, quinidine sulfonamides, ticlopidine[29,44-47]	Direct damage to myeloid precursors
Clozapine[49,50]	Metabolite-mediated depletion of adenosine triphosphate and glutathione-inducing apoptosis secondary to oxidative stress
Flecainide[48]	Hapten formation

CLINICAL PRESENTATION AND DIFFERENTIAL DIAGNOSIS

The evaluation of patients with suspected drug-induced neutropenia and agranulocytosis requires a careful history and physical examination. In addition, a complete blood count with differential should be obtained; however, extensive laboratory evaluation or diagnostic procedures are generally not warranted on initial presentation, particularly if the ANC is >1,000 cells/mm^3. Signs and symptoms in patients with neutropenia and agranulocytosis are generally related to infectious complications (**Table 48-3**).[56] Without antibiotics or other treatment, patients commonly present with septicemia, but may also present with subtle symptoms of pneumonia, cellulitis, or oropharyngeal, periodontal, or perianal infection.[11] Patients with an ANC <500 cells/mm^3 are at risk for bacteremia from either the bowel or skin flora. Signs and symptoms of infection are typically blunted as a consequence of the inability to mount an adequate inflammatory response, especially when antibiotics are preemptively administered. In the absence of overt abnormal findings on physical examination, the clinician must rely on the presence of fever as the only reliable indicator of an active infectious process.[57]

The timing of a neutropenic episode in relation to chemotherapy depends on the chemotherapy regimen administered; however, the ANC nadir during most myelosuppressive chemotherapy regimens occurs within 7–10 days of initiation of the most recent treatment cycle. Myeloablative and high-dose chemotherapy regimens may result in ANC nadirs within several days following the start of chemotherapy.[9,10]

Patients presenting with neutropenia who have not received cytotoxic chemotherapy require a thorough review of systems for evidence of a recent viral infection and a careful medication history that includes a review of the use of prescription and nonprescription medications and herbal supplements. The typical time course for the onset of agranulocytosis is 7–14 days following exposure to the causative drug. Once the causative agent has been discontinued, bone marrow recovery can typically be expected within 10–14 days if the neutropenia is secondary to a drug/antibody effect directed at mature cells or if neutrophil maturation has merely been halted. However, insult to myeloid precursors will likely cause delayed recovery of more than 14 days.[11] A more extensive diagnostic workup to rule out malignancy—particularly leukemia or lymphoma, human immunodeficiency virus, or idiopathic neutropenia—may be undertaken in cases in which cause is not established (**Table 48-4**). Anemia and thrombocytopenia were associated with neutropenia in 30% and 10%, respectively, of elderly patients who presented with more severe symptoms

Table 48-3 Signs and Symptoms Associated with Drug-Induced Neutropenia and Agranulocytosis

- Bronchitis
- Chills
- Fever
- Gingivitis/thrush
- Lethargy
- Myalgias
- Pharyngitis
- Sepsis
- Sinusitis
- Stomatitis
- Weakness

Table 48-4 Conditions to Consider in the Differential Diagnosis of Drug-Induced Neutropenia and Agranulocytosis

- Aplastic anemia
- Autoimmune neutropenia
- Chronic idiopathic neutropenia
- Collagen vascular disorder
- Cyclic neutropenia
- Human immunodeficiency virus
- Hypersplenism
- Leukemia
- Myelodysplastic syndrome
- Pure white cell aplasia
- Radiation therapy
- Recent serious infection such as viral syndrome or sepsis
- Sjögren syndrome
- Toxic environmental exposure

(i.e., sepsis and/or septic shock). Bone marrow aspiration and biopsy with immunologic and cytogenetic evaluation is indicated for these patients and those with neutropenia with an undefined cause to rule out other underlying pathology. Other clinically relevant causes of neutropenia to consider are sepsis, myelodysplastic syndromes, and hypersplenism.[11]

RISK FACTORS

Risk factors for chemotherapy-induced neutropenia include advanced age, previous exposure to chemotherapy or radiation therapy, poor nutrition, and end-organ dysfunction (**Table 48-5**). Factors known to increase the risk of infection in patients with neutropenia include the degree and duration of neutropenia, phagocytic function, compromise in cellular and humoral immunity, alteration in skin and mucosal physical defense barriers, and the patient's endogenous flora or nosocomial colonization.[58]

More intensive chemotherapy treatment programs coupled with the greater prevalence of indwelling central venous catheters have increased the number of portals of entry for bacteria with the resultant disruption of skin and gastrointestinal barriers.[59] Chemotherapy or antecedent diseases such as myelodysplastic disorders impair the remaining vestiges of phagocytic defense in patients with neutropenia.[60] The increasing incidence of resistant gram-positive and gram-negative bacteria places patients with neutropenia at greater risk for morbidity and mortality from bacterial sepsis.[61]

Methods to stratify the risk of infection in febrile patients with neutropenia have been published.[62,63] A practical approach is to designate patients as either low-risk or high-risk for infection. Neutropenia with duration of <7–10 days has been defined as low-risk and typically occurs in patients treated for solid tumor malignancies. Neutropenia with duration >10 days is defined as high-risk and most commonly occurs in patients treated for acute leukemia or undergoing stem cell transplantation. As the duration of neutropenia increases, the risk of invasive fungal infection increases. Patients who have had neutropenia for 14 days have been found to have an increased incidence of invasive aspergillosis or candidiasis.[64]

Advanced age, female sex, mononucleosis, renal insufficiency, autoimmune disease, certain drug combinations, and genetic predisposition have all been associated with an increased risk for agranulocytosis (Table 48-5).[36] IAAAS noted that more than half of reported cases of agranulocytosis occurred in patients older than 50 years of age. The incidence of agranulocytosis in women is twice that reported in men. A higher incidence of agranulocytosis in older patients and in women was confirmed with analysis of the clozapine registry data in the United States.[21] The use of particular drugs in patients with specific disease states, such as the use of captopril in patients with renal failure, may increase the risk of agranulocytosis. In addition, case reports suggest that the concomitant use of captopril and probenecid or interferon may also increase the risk of agranulocytosis.[65] Genetic predisposition to agranulocytosis induced by drugs such as methimazole or clozapine may be present in patients with similar histocompatibility antigens within certain racial populations or with underlying immune disorders.[66,67] A recent study confirmed the role of the previously implicated *HLA-DQB1* variant in clozapine-associated neutropenia and further established the relationship between clozapine-associated neutropenia and genetic variants in members of a family of hepatic transporters, SLCO1B3 and SLCO1B7.[68] Dosing and duration of treatment may also play a role in

Table 48-5 Risk Factors for Drug-Induced Neutropenia and Agranulocytosis

- Advanced age
- Autoimmune disease
- Concurrent or previous treatment with radiation
- Female sex
- Genetic predisposition
- Infection preceding agranulocytosis
- Jewish ancestry (clozapine)
- Leukopenia during initiation of therapy (clozapine)
- Mononucleosis
- Multiagent chemotherapy regimens
- Polypharmacy
- Poor nutrition
- Prior treatment with chemotherapy
- Renal insufficiency or other end-organ dysfunction

frequency of drug-induced agranulocytosis. A retrospective study found that methimazole 30 mg daily was associated with a significantly higher incidence of agranulocytosis compared to those who received 15 mg daily (0.814% versus 0.219%, respectively).[69] Duration-dependent neutropenia was studied in β-lactam antibiotic usage in an analysis of published reports, where the incidence of neutropenia was found to differ significantly based on the duration of β-lactam antibiotic use. The incidence of neutropenia in patients treated with β-lactam antibiotics for 10 days or greater ranged from 5% to over 15%; whereas, the incidence of neutropenia in patients treated with <10 days of antibiotics was as low as 0.1%.[70]

MORBIDITY AND MORTALITY

Approximately half of patients with neutropenia who become febrile have an established apparent or occult infection. The risk is even greater when the ANC falls below 100 cells/mm^3, where 20% of febrile patients will have a potentially life-threatening bacteremia.[71] The morbidity and mortality associated with neutropenic fever has decreased as a result of prompt recognition, improved antibacterial prophylaxis and therapy, and the availability of colony stimulating factor support. Organisms such as *Pseudomonas aeruginosa, Staphylococcus aureus,* and *Streptococcus viridans* pose a mortal threat to patients with neutropenia.[72-74] In addition, invasive fungal infections, particularly *Candida* and *Aspergillus* species, are associated with a mortality risk of 90% or more in highly vulnerable populations, such as recipients of allogeneic stem cell transplants.[75]

In a study published in 1991, prognostic factors were evaluated in 168 episodes of agranulocytosis in which the overall mortality rate was 16%.[76] In a univariate analysis, the presence of renal failure, bacteremia, shock, advanced age, low lymphocyte count, low percentage of myeloid precursors, and high percentage of bone marrow plasma cells were significant indicators of poor survival. Bacteremia, renal insufficiency, and shock remained significantly correlated with a fatal outcome with multivariate analysis. More recently, the mortality rate has dropped to between 2.5% and 10% with advancements in therapeutic management of acute agranulocytosis and its complications.[77]

Mortality rates due to clozapine-induced agranulocytosis have been reported to be 0.016% to 0.017% in two studies that included over 24,000 patients.[21,22] A French database of 102 cases of agranulocytosis collected over a 15-year period revealed that 1 of 21 patients with antibiotic-induced agranulocytosis died.[19] The Swedish Drug Monitoring System reported mortality in 5 of 19 patients with sulfasalazine-induced agranulocytosis over a 6-year period.[29] A literature review cited 10% mortality in patients with agranulocytosis who had an ANC <100 cells/mm^3, and 3% in patients with an ANC >100 cells/mm^3.[12] Mortality increased from 14% in patients with agranulocytosis and no symptoms of infection to 29% in patients with symptoms of infection, regardless of neutrophil count.

PREVENTION

Prevention of neutropenia associated with cytotoxic chemotherapy can be optimized with two basic strategies. First, the dose of chemotherapy may be reduced in patients who have had a documented episode of neutropenia caused by a previous cycle of chemotherapy. This option is often pursued in patients receiving palliative chemotherapy. The second approach is to stimulate myeloid cell production with either filgrastim (granulocyte colony-stimulating factor [G-CSF]), pegfilgrastim (pegylated granulocyte colony-stimulating factor), or sargramostim (granulocyte macrophage colony-stimulating factor [GM-CSF]). The 2015 American Society of Clinical Oncology practice guideline makes practical recommendations for use of white blood cell growth factors in patients receiving chemotherapy.[78] This group recommended use of colony-stimulating factors if the chemotherapy regimen is associated with a documented incidence of febrile neutropenia of ≥20%; in patients who experienced neutropenic fever with a previous cycle of chemotherapy (secondary prophylaxis); after remission induction therapy for acute leukemia; and after high-dose chemotherapy to accelerate engraftment after stem cell transplantation.

Table 48-6 Approaches to Help Prevent Drug-Induced Neutropenia and Agranulocytosis

Neutropenia due to cytotoxic chemotherapy

- Dose modification
- Prophylactic administration of filgrastim (or equivalent) or sargramostim

Agranulocytosis (general)

- Avoid drugs in the same class as an agent that previously caused agranulocytosis

Agranulocytosis due to clozapine

- Weekly monitoring of white cell count as recommended by manufacturer

Given the relatively low incidence of agranulocytosis, a practical method for early detection or prevention of this drug-induced disease has not been identified. There is no reliable, inexpensive assay or test available to identify the rare patient who may be at risk for agranulocytosis. Monitoring programs like the one implemented for patients receiving clozapine may lead to early detection of a declining white cell count. However, the high cost of implementing and administering such a comprehensive monitoring program makes it an impractical approach, except in very special circumstances. **Table 48-6** lists approaches to help prevent drug-induced neutropenia and agranulocytosis.

MANAGEMENT

Neutropenia can lead to potentially life-threatening complications. As with other drug-induced diseases, discontinuation of the culprit agent(s) must always be a first consideration when patients present with drug-induced neutropenia or agranulocytosis. Drug-induced febrile neutropenia is considered a medical emergency and requires immediate evaluation and treatment. Because currently available diagnostic tests are not sufficiently rapid, sensitive, or specific for identifying or excluding specific microbial causes of a febrile episode, prompt administration of broad-spectrum antibacterial therapy is warranted after blood cultures have been obtained. Initial antibacterial therapy is directed at common organisms found in the gastrointestinal tract and on the skin. Broad-spectrum antibacterial therapy with reliable activity against *P. aeruginosa* is standard; the selection of specific antibiotics should be tailored based on local susceptibility patterns. Initial therapy with vancomycin may be instituted in clinical scenarios such as sepsis, mucositis, colonization with methicillin-resistant *S. aureus* or penicillin-resistant pneumococci, recent treatment with a fluoroquinolone antibiotic, or obvious catheter-related infections. Invasive fungal infection should be suspected in patients with neutropenia who have a fever that persists despite treatment with broad-spectrum antibiotics for 3–7 days. Institution of empirical antifungal therapy is standard practice in these cases. Patients with neutropenia in whom fever or other signs of infection develop should be treated quickly, following established treatment protocols. The Infectious Diseases Society of America has published guidelines for the management of neutropenic fever.[2]

The principal determinant of successful reversal of agranulocytosis is rapid recognition and immediate discontinuation of the causative agent. In some cases, the antineutrophil antibody test and a bone marrow biopsy and aspiration can help confirm a diagnosis of agranulocytosis. After the causative drug is discontinued, recovery of neutrophils generally occurs within two weeks. Specific guidelines for monitoring white cell counts in patients receiving clozapine have been developed to facilitate early detection of agranulocytosis. Given the rare occurrence of agranulocytosis with most drugs, however, the benefit of routinely monitoring blood counts in the general population is low relative to associated cost.

There is a large body of literature regarding the use of myeloid colony-stimulating factors to facilitate neutrophil recovery in agranulocytosis, although most are case reports or series or meta-analyses.[79-83] These agents support the survival and stimulate the proliferation of bone marrow progenitor cells, thereby increasing neutrophil counts.[84] G-CSF and GM-CSF are administered subcutaneously in doses of 5 mcg/kg/day and 250 mcg/kg/day, respectively. The pegylated formulation of G-CSF (pegfilgrastim) is administered subcutaneously at a fixed one-time dose of 6 mg. These agents are costly, but relatively well tolerated; the adverse effects are generally limited to bone pain, fever, and injection-site reactions. Given the rarity of agranulocytosis, it is unlikely that an adequately powered, randomized trial designed to evaluate the benefit of these agents in patients with agranulocytosis will be carried out. There are, however, several published reports describing the utility of colony-stimulating factors in patients with this drug-induced disease.[25,26,32,85] A cohort of 145 consecutive cases of agranulocytosis has been reported.[86] G-CSF 300 mcg/day was administered to 101 of these patients. Although no significant difference in mortality was noted in treated patients, G-CSF was found to decrease the median period of recovery to an ANC of 1,000 cells/mm^3 from 7 to 5 days. In a review of published case reports of patients with agranulocytosis, Andersohn and colleagues found that those treated with G-CSF or GM-CSF had a shorter median duration of neutropenia (8 days versus 9 days) and among asymptomatic patients at diagnosis, had a lower proportion of infectious or fatal complications than untreated patients (14% versus 29%).[12] In addition to a reduction in duration of neutropenia, Andres and colleagues also reported benefits of G-CSF through decreased length of hospital stay and antibiotic duration, particularly in patients who presented with poor prognostic factors.[77,87]

INFORMATION FOR PATIENTS

Patients undergoing cytotoxic chemotherapy should be counseled regarding the risk of neutropenia, the symptoms associated with this drug-induced disease, and the importance of seeking prompt medical attention when these symptoms occur. Clear written and verbal instructions should be provided outlining information such as when to measure temperatures, what constitutes a fever, when to have a complete blood count checked, and who to call or where to seek treatment if a fever occurs. Patients should be informed that symptoms such as cough, mouth sores, sore throat, and shortness of breath necessitate immediate medical attention. Given the complexity of modern chemotherapy regimens and the risk for drug interactions with chemotherapy agents, antiemetics, and other supportive medications, the patient should ensure that the primary oncology providers are aware of all drugs being used and screen all new prescription and nonprescription drugs and herbal supplements for safety.

Patients who have experienced agranulocytosis should be advised to avoid other drugs within the same structural class when possible. If patients are to receive a myeloid colony-stimulating factor to accelerate neutrophil recovery, they must be taught the proper technique for subcutaneous injection and counseled regarding the risk of injection site reactions, fever, and bone pain. Because these agents are expensive, patients may need special assistance to find ways to offset the cost.

REFERENCES

1. Pizzo P. Management of fever in patients with cancer and treatment-induced neutropenia. *N Engl J Med.* 1993; 328:1323-32.
2. Freifeld AG, Bow EJ, Sepkowitz KA et al. Clinical practice guideline for the use of antimicrobial agents in neutropenic patients with cancer: 2010 update by the infectious diseases society of America. *Clin Infect Dis.* 2011; 52:e56-93.
3. Pisciotta V. Drug-induced agranulocytosis. *Drugs.* 1978; 15:132-43.
4. Pisciotta AV. Drug-induced leukopenia and aplastic anemia. *Clin Pharmacol Ther.* 1971; 12:13-43.
5. Pisciotta AV. Drug-induced agranulocytosis. *Haematologica.* 1982; 67:292-318.
6. Young GA, Vincent PC. Drug-induced agranulocytosis. *Clin Haematol.* 1980; 9:483-504.
7. Pisciotta AV. Drug-induced agranulocytosis: peripheral destruction of polymorphonuclear leukocytes and their marrow precursors. *Blood Rev.* 1990; 4:226-37.
8. Einhorn LH. Curing metastatic germ cell tumors. *Proc Natl Acad Sci U S A.* 2002; 99:4592-5.
9. Shayne M, Culakova E, Poniewierski MS et al. Dose intensity and hematologic toxicity in older cancer patients receiving systemic chemotherapy. *Cancer.* 2007; 110:1611-20.
10. Crawford J, Dale DC, Kuderer NM et al. Risk and timing of neutropenic events in adult cancer patients receiving chemotherapy: the results of a prospective nationwide study of oncology practice. *J Natl Compr Canc Netw.* 2008; 6:109-18.
11. Andres E, Maloisel F. Idiosyncratic drug-induced agranulocytosis or acute neutropenia. *Curr Opin Hematol.* 2008; 15:15-21.
12. Andersohn F, Konzen C, Garbe E. Systematic review: agranulocytosis induced by non-chemotherapy drugs. *Ann Intern Med.* 2007; 146:657-65.
13. Huber M, Andersohn F, Bronder E et al. Drug-induced agranulocytosis in the Berlin case-control surveillance study. *Eur J Clin Pharmacol.* 2014; 70:339-45.
14. Andres E, Maloisel F. Idiosyncratic drug-induced agranulocytosis or acute neutropenia. *Curr Opin Hematol.* 2008; 15:15-21.
15. The International Agranulocytosis and Aplastic Anemia Study. Risks of agranulocytosis and aplastic anemia: a first report of their relation to drug use with special reference to analgesics. *JAMA.* 1986; 256:1749-57.

16. Fraunfelder FT, Meyer SM, Bagby GC et al. Hematologic reactions to carbonic anhydrase inhibitors. *Am J Ophthalmol.* 1985; 100:79-81.
17. Ibanez L, Vidal X, Ballarin E et al. Population-based drug-induced agranulocytosis. *Arch Intern Med.* 2005; 165:869-74.
18. The International Agranulocytosis and Aplastic Anemia Study. Anti-infective drug use in relation to the risk of agranulocytosis and aplastic anemia. *Arch Intern Med.* 1989; 149:1036-40.
19. Andres E, Maloisel F. Antibiotic-induced agranulocytosis: a monocentric study of 21 cases. *Arch Intern Med.* 2001; 161:2619.
20. The International Agranulocytosis and Aplastic Anemia Study. Risk of agranulocytosis and aplastic anemia in relation to use of antithyroid drugs. *Br Med J.* 1988; 297:262-5.
21. Ma J, Alvir J, Lieberman JA et al. Clozapine-induced agranulocytosis: incidence and risk factors in the United States. *N Engl J Med.* 1993; 329:162-7.
22. Munro J, O'Sullivan D, Andrews C et al. Active monitoring of 12,760 clozapine recipients in the UK and Ireland: beyond pharmacovigilance. *Br J Psychol.* 1999; 175:576-80.
23. Kelly JP, Kaufman DW, Shapiro S. Risks of agranulocytosis and aplastic anemia in relation to the use of cardiovascular drugs: the International Agranulocytosis and Aplastic Anemia Study. *Clin Pharmacol Ther.* 1991; 49:330-41.
24. Van der Klauw MM, Goudsmit R, Halie MR et al. A population-based case-cohort study of drug-associated agranulocytosis. *Arch Intern Med.* 1999; 159:369-74.
25. Wenham C, Gadsby K, Deighton C. Three significant cases of neutropenia with etanercept. *Rheumatology.* 2008; 46:376-7.
26. Salzberger B, Bowden RA, Hackman RC et al. Neutropenia in allogeneic marrow transplant recipients receiving ganciclovir for prevention of cytomegalovirus disease: risk factors and outcome. *Blood.* 1997; 90:2502-8.
27. Strom BL, Carson JL, Schinnar R et al. Nonsteroidal anti-inflammatory drugs and neutropenia. *Arch Intern Med.* 1993; 153:2119-24.
28. Derry CL, Schwinghammer TL. Agranulocytosis associated with sulfasalazine. *Drug Intell Clin Pharm.* 1988; 22:139-42.
29. Keisu M, Ekman E. Sulfasalazine associated agranulocytosis in Sweden 1972–1989: clinical features and estimation of its incidence. *Eur J Clin Pharmacol.* 1992; 43:215-8.
30. Kazutoshi O, Kurohara K, Yoshihara M et al. Agranulocytosis caused by ticlopidine and its mechanism. *Am J Hematol.* 1991; 37:239-42.
31. Keishu M, Ekman E, Wilhom BE. Comparing risk estimates of sulfonamide-induced agranulocytosis from the Swedish Drug Monitoring System and a case-control system. *Eur J Clin Pharmacol.* 1992; 43:211-4.
32. Hartmann EL, Gatesman M, Roskopf-Somerville J et al. Management of leukopenia in kidney and pancreas transplant recipients. *Clin Transplant.* 2008; 22:822-8.
33. Schwartsmann G, Wanders J, Koier IJ et al. EORTC New Drug Development Office coordinating and monitoring programme for phase I and II trials with new anticancer agents. *Eur J Cancer.* 1991; 27:1162-8.
34. Burnett AK, Eden OB. The treatment of acute leukaemia. *Lancet.* 1997; 349:270-5.
35. Cassileth PA, Harrington DP, Appelbaum FR et al. Chemotherapy compared with autologous or allogeneic bone marrow transplantation in the management of acute myeloid leukemia in first remission. *N Engl J Med.* 1998; 339:1649-56.
36. Young NS. Agranulocytosis. *JAMA.* 1994; 271;935-8.
37. Strom BL, Carson JL, Schinnar R et al. Descriptive epidemiology of agranulocytosis. *Arch Intern Med.* 1992; 152:1475-80.
38. Schein PS, Winkour SH. Immunosuppressive and cytotoxic chemotherapy: long-term complications. *Ann Intern Med.* 1975; 82:84-95.
39. Pisciotta AV. Immune and toxic mechanisms in drug- induced agranulocytosis. *Hematology.* 1973; 10:279-310.
40. Druker BJ, Talpaz M, Resta DJ et al. Efficacy and safety of a specific inhibitor of the BCR-ABL tyrosine kinase in chronic myeloid leukemia. *N Engl J Med.* 2001; 344:1031-7.
41. Fibbe WE, Claas FHJ, Van der Star-Dijkstra W et al. Agranulocytosis induced by propylthiouracil: evidence of a drug dependent antibody reacting with granulocytes, monocytes and haematopoietic progenitor cells. *Br J Haematol.* 1986; 64:363-73.
42. Guffy MM, Goeken NE, Burns CP. Granulocytotoxic antibodies in a patient with propylthiouracil-induced agranulocytosis. *Arch Intern Med.* 1984; 144:1687-88.
43. Toth EL, Mant MJ, Shivji S et al. Propylthiouracil-induced agranulocytosis: an unusual presentation and a possible mechanism. *Am J Med.* 1988; 85:725-7.
44. Starkebaum G, Kenyon CM, Simrell CR et al. Procainamide-induced agranulocytosis differs serologically and clinically from procainamide-induced lupus. *Clin Immunol Immunopathol.* 1996; 112-9.
45. Fitchen JH, Koeffler HP. Cimetidine and granulopoiesis: bone marrow culture studies in normal man and patients with cimetidine-associated neutropenia. *Br J Haematol.* 1980; 46:361-6.
46. Ascensao JL, Flynn PJ, Slungaard A et al. Quinidine induced neutropenia: report of a case with drug- dependent inhibition of granulocyte colony generation. *Acta Haematol.* 1984; 72:349-54.
47. Lui ZC, Uetrecht JP. Metabolism of ticlopidine by activated neutrophils: implications for ticlopidine induced agranulocytosis. *Drug Metab Dispos.* 2000; 28:726-30.
48. Uetrecht JP, Shear NH, Zahid N et al. N-chlorination of sulfamethoxazole and dapsone by the myeloperoxidase system. *Drug Metab Dispos.* 1993; 21:830-4.
49. Samlowski WE, Frame RN, Logue GL. Flecainide-induced immune neutropenia: documentation of a hapten-mediated mechanism of cell destruction. *Arch Intern Med.* 1987; 147:383-4.
50. Weitzman SA, Stossel TP. Drug-induced immunological neutropenia. *Lancet.* 1978; 311:1068-72.
51. Uetrecht JP. Metabolism of clozapine by neutrophils: possible implications for clozapine-induced agranulocytosis. *Drug Saf.* 1992; 7(suppl 1):51-6.
52. Williams DP, Pirmohamad M, Naisbitt DJ et al. Induction of metabolism-dependent and independent neutrophil apoptosis by clozapine. *Mol Pharmacol.* 2000; 58:207-16.
53. Heit WF. Hematologic effects of antipyretic analgesics: drug-induced agranulocytosis. *Am J Med.* 1983; 75:65-8.
54. Levitt LJ. Chlorpropamide-induced pure white blood cell aplasia. *Blood.* 1987; 69:394-400.
55. Wall JR, Fang SL, Kuroki T et al. In vitro immunoreactivity to propylthiouracil, methimazole and carbimazole in patients with Graves' disease: a possible cause of antithyroid drug-induced agranulocytosis. *J Clin Endocrinol Metab.* 1984; 58:868-72.
56. Talcott JA, Finberg R, Mayer R et al. The medical course of cancer patients with fever and neutropenia. *Arch Intern Med.* 1988; 148:2561-68.
57. Sickles EA, Greene WH, Wiernik PH. Clinical presentation of infection in granulocytopenic patients. *Arch Intern Med.* 1975; 135:715-9.
58. Hughes WT, Armstrong D, Bodey GP et al. 1997 Guidelines for the use of antimicrobial agents in neutropenic patients with unexplained fever. *Clin Infect Dis.* 1997; 25:551-73.
59. Mueller BU, Skelton J, Callender DP et al. A prospective randomized trial comparing the infectious and noninfectious complications of externalized catheter versus a subcutaneously implanted device in cancer patients. *J Clin Oncol.* 1992; 10:1943-8.
60. Heany ML, Golde DW. Myelodysplasia. *N Engl J Med.* 1999; 340:1649-60.
61. Johnson MP, Ramphal R. Beta-lactam-resistant Enterobacter bacteremia in febrile neutropenia patients receiving monotherapy. *J Infect Dis.* 1990; 162:981-3.
62. Talcott JA, Siegel RD, Finberg R et al. Risk assessment in cancer patients with fever and neutropenia: a prospective, two-center validation of a prediction rule. *J Clin Oncol.* 1992; 10:316-22.

63. Klastersky J, Paesmans M, Rubenstein EB et al. The Multinational Association for Supportive Care in Cancer risk index: a multinational scoring system for identifying low-risk febrile neutropenic cancer patients. *J Clin Oncol.* 2000; 18:3038-51.
64. Gerson SL, Talbot GH, Hurwitz S et al. Prolonged granulocytopenia: the major risk factor for invasive Aspergillus in patients with acute leukemia. *Ann Intern Med.* 1984; 100:345-8.
65. Sinhvi SM, Duchin KL, Willard DL et al. Renal handling of captopril: effect of probenecid. *Clin Pharmacol Ther.* 1982; 32:182-9.
66. Tamai H, Sudo T, Kimura A et al. Association between the DRB108032 histocompatibility antigen and methimazole-induced agranulocytosis in Japanese patients with Graves' disease. *Ann Intern Med.* 1996; 124:490-4.
67. Dettling M, Cascorbi I, Roots I et al. Genetic determinants of clozapine-induced agranulocytosis: recent results of HLA subtyping in a non-Jewish Caucasian sample. *Arch Gen Psychiatry.* 2001; 158:93-4.
68. Legge SE, Hamshere ML, Ripke S et al. Genome-wide common and rare variant analysis provides novel insights into clozapine-associated neutropenia. *Mol Psychiatry.* 2018; 23:162-3.
69. Takata K, Kubota S, Fukata S et al. Methimazole-induced agranulocytosis in patients with Graves' disease is more frequent with an initial dose of 30 mg daily than with 15 mg daily. *Thyroid.* 2009; 19:559-63.
70. Klaus A, Hauser SP, Muller MR. Inhibition of granulopoiesis in vivo and in vitro by β-lactam antibiotics. *J Infect Dis.* 1985; 152:90-8.
71. Bodey GP, Buckley M, Sathe YS et al. Quantitative relationship between circulating leukocytes and infection in patients with acute leukemia. *Ann Intern Med.* 1966; 64:328.
72. Ladisch SL, Pizzo PA. Staphylococcus aureus sepsis in children with cancer. *Pediatrics.* 1978; 61:231-4.
73. Bodey GP, Jadeja L, Elting L. Pseudomonas bacteremia: retrospective analysis of 410 episodes. *Arch Intern Med.* 1985; 145:1621-9.
74. Dybedal I, Lamvik J. Respiratory insufficiency in acute leukemia following treatment with cytosine arabinoside and septicemia with streptococcus viridans. *Eur J Haematol.* 1989; 42:405-6.
75. Burch PA, Karp JE, Merz WG et al. Favorable outcome of invasive aspergillosis in patients with acute leukemia. *J Clin Oncol.* 1987; 5:1985-93.
76. Julia A, Olona M, Bueno J et al. Drug-induced agranulocytosis: prognostic factors in a series of 168 patients. *Br J Haematol.* 1991; 79:366-71.
77. Andres E, Maloisel F, Zimmer J. The role of haematopoietic growth factors granulocyte colony-stimulating factor and granulocyte-macrophage colony-stimulating factor in the management of drug-induced agranulocytosis. *Br J Haematol.* 2010; 150:3-8.
78. Smith TJ, Bohlke K, Lyman GH et al. Recommendations for the use of WBC growth factors: American Society of Clinical Oncology clinical practice guideline update. *J Clin Oncol.* 2015; 33:3199-212.
79. Kuipers EJ, Vellenga E, de Wolf JT et al. Sulfasalazine induced agranulocytosis treated with granulocyte-macrophage colony stimulating factor. *J Rheumatol.* 1992; 19:621-2.
80. Tajiri J, Noguchi S, Okamura S et al. Granulocyte colony-stimulating factor treatment of antithyroid drug-induced granulocytopenia. *Arch Intern Med.* 1993; 153:509-14.
81. Bradford CR, Ong EL, Hendrick DJ et al. Use of colony stimulating factors for the treatment of drug-induced agranulocytosis. *Br J Haematol.* 1993; 84:182-3.
82. Sprikkelman A, de Wolf JT, Vellenga E. The application of hematopoietic growth factors in drug-induced agranulocytosis: a review of 70 cases. *Leukemia.* 1994; 8:2031-6.
83. Pasquale D, Newton M, Goss JB et al. Granulocyte colony-stimulating factor treatment of clozapine-induced agranulocytosis. *Am J Psychol.* 1996; 153:1503-4.
84. Kaushansky K. Lineage-specific colony stimulating factors. *N Engl J Med.* 2006; 354:2043-5.
85. Hermans P. Hematopoietic growth factors as supportive therapy in HIV-infected patients. *AIDS.* 1995; 9(suppl 2):S9-14.
86. Ibanez L, Sabate M, Ballarin E et al. Use of granulocyte colony-stimulating factor and outcome in patients with non-chemotherapy agranulocytosis. *Pharmacoepidemiol Drug Saf.* 2008; 17:224-8.
87. Andres E, Kurtz JE, Martin-Hunyadi C et al. Nonchemotherapy drug-induced agranulocytosis in elderly patients: the effects of granulocyte colony-stimulating factor. *Am J Med.* 2002; 112:460-4.

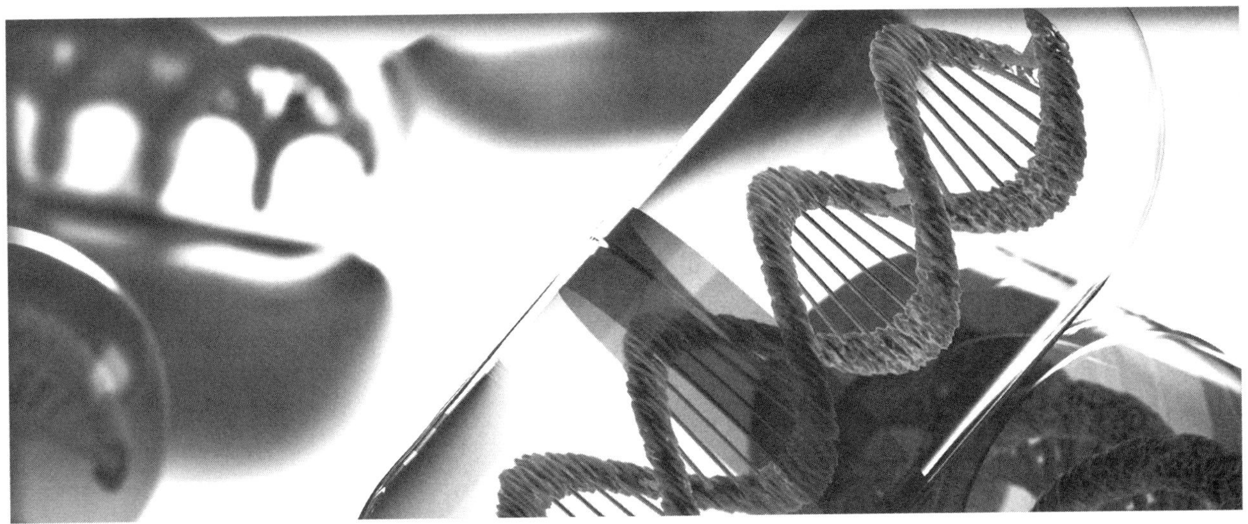

CHAPTER 49

Anemias

LeAnn B. Norris and Charles L. Bennett

Hematologic complications including anemia are an unfortunate consequence of modern pharmacotherapy. Most drug-induced anemias are well documented, and 20–25% are allergic or idiosyncratic.[1] Idiosyncratic reactions can be difficult to recognize and assign causality and may not be directly related to the culprit drug's pharmacology. Aplastic anemia, hemolytic anemia, megaloblastic anemia, and chemotherapy-induced anemia are the most common drug-related anemias.[2] Drug-induced anemias can lead to fatal outcomes and reported mortality rates range from 4% to 70%.[3]

The World Health Organization defines *anemia* as a hemoglobin (Hgb) <13 g/dL (130 g/L; <8.07 mmol/L) in men or <12 g/dL (<120 g/L; <7.45 mmol/L) in women.[4] A decrease in oxygenation secondary to anemia can result in a variety of symptoms, including fatigue, shortness of breath, skin pallor, and dizziness. Significant cardiovascular sequelae including arrhythmias and heart failure may occur in severe cases and when anemia occurs rapidly. The most common causes of anemia include blood loss, decreased production of red blood cells (RBCs) due to nutritional deficiencies (iron, folate, vitamin B_{12}), or increased destruction of RBCs (hemolytic anemia). These common causes of anemia must be ruled out prior to attributing anemia to drugs alone. A comprehensive medication history (current prescription and nonprescription medications, illicit drugs, herbal/nutritional supplements, and any medication exposures or changes that have occurred in the last 6 months) should be completed as part of the investigation into the cause(s) of anemia. The initial work-up for suspected drug-induced anemias should include a count of RBCs, white blood cells (WBCs) (with differential), and platelets as well as measurement of Hgb concentration, hematocrit (HCT), and mean corpuscular volume (MCV).

Risk factors for drug-induced anemias are not well defined and have not been well studied. In a study of over 600 cases, Bottiger et al.[5] determined the risk of drug-induced anemias increases with advancing age and the incidence is higher in women than in men. Genetic factors are perhaps the best understood risk factors for drug-induced anemias. Patients with glucose-6-phosphate dehydrogenase (G6PD) deficiency are at risk for hemolytic anemia when exposed to certain drugs or chemicals. G6PD is the rate-limiting enzyme in the pathway that is responsible for maintaining adequate concentrations of nicotinamide adenine dinucleotide phosphate (NADPH), which maintains glutathione in its reduced form by reducing free radical formation. Oxidative stress in patients with G6PD deficiency denatures hemoglobin and causes hemolysis.[2] Glutathione deficiency, peroxidase deficiency, and β-thalassemia are other genetic disorders known to increase a patient's risk for drug-induced anemias.

APLASTIC ANEMIA

Aplastic anemia is a deficiency in RBCs, WBCs, and platelets (pancytopenia). It results in a hypoplastic bone marrow caused by the decrease in hematopoietic stem cells.[6,7]

CAUSATIVE AGENTS

Drugs found to have at least a moderate association with causing drug-induced aplastic anemia are listed in **Table 49-1**. The most common drug classes include anticonvulsants (carbamazepine and phenytoin), antibiotics (sulfonamides and linezolid), anti-inflammatory agents (nonsteroidal anti-inflammatory drugs), and chemotherapy agents.

EPIDEMIOLOGY

Accurate prospective data regarding the incidence of aplastic anemia in the United States are lacking. The estimated incidence is approximately 0.6–0.61 cases per million population, although this is mostly based on retrospective, historical data and death registries.[5] This rate could be lower now as some of the older causative agents are no longer available or are not used as frequently. Epidemiologic studies suggest the incidence in Europe is 2 cases per million population.[64,65] Aplastic anemia is thought to be more common in Asia, with an estimated 4–6 cases per million population. This difference may be due to increased exposure to environmental factors, including toxic chemicals (benzene, pesticides, or insecticides) or viruses.[66]

Table 49-1 Agents Associated with Drug-Induced Aplastic Anemia

Drug	Incidence	Level of Evidence[a]
Acetazolamide[8]	1 case per 18,000 patient-years	B
Captopril[9-11]	NK	C
Carbamazepine[12-14]	3–4 cases per 100,000 years	B
Chloramphenicol[15-18]	NK[b]	B
Felbamate[19,20]	127 cases per 1 million users	B
Furosemide[21]	NK	C
Gold salts[22-25]	NK[c]	B
Imatinib[26-28]	NK	C
Linezolid[29-32]	1 case per 2,900 users	B
Mesalamine[56-58]	NK	C
Methimazole[33-36]	NK	C
NONSTEROIDAL ANTI-INFLAMMATORY DRUGS		
Diclofenac[37-41]	NK	C
Etodolac[42]	NK	C
Ibuprofen[43]	NK	C
Indomethacin[44]	NK	C
Salicylates[23]	NK	C
Sulindac[45]	NK	C
Phenytoin[46-52]	NK	C
Sulfonamides[5,23,53]	NK	C
Sulfisoxazole[18]	NK	C
Sulfasalazine[54,55]	NK	C
Temozolomide[59]	NK	C
ANTIPLATELET DRUGS		
Clopidogrel[60]	NK	C
Ticlopidine[61-63]	NK	C

NK = not known.

[a]Definitions for Levels of Evidence: Level A—evidence from one or more randomized, controlled clinical trials; Level B—evidence from nonrandomized clinical trials, prospective observational studies, cohort studies, retrospective studies, case-control studies, meta-analyses and/or postmarketing surveillance studies; and Level C—evidence from one or more published case reports or case series.

[b]Incidence of death is reported to be 1 per 21,000–36,000 users.

[c]Incidence of death is reported to be 1.5 per 10,000 prescriptions.

MECHANISMS

There are two main types of aplastic anemia: inherited and acquired. Drug-induced aplastic anemia is thought to be acquired, although like other autoimmune disorders, genetic factors may predispose some patients to acquire aplastic anemia.[67,68] Three mechanisms are thought to cause damage to the pluripotent hematopoietic stem cells in acquired aplastic anemia.[69] The first mechanism, dose-dependent drug toxicity, most often caused by chemotherapy or radiotherapy, induces transient marrow failure due to suppression of proliferating cell lines. Hematopoietic suppression may also occur with continued dose escalation. The second mechanism is an idiosyncratic reaction where toxic metabolites of the parent drug cause the anemia. The third mechanism is immune-related and occurs when drug metabolites form complexes with cellular proteins within bone marrow cells. The hapten–protein complex formed due to an exposure to an inciting antigen (drug) activates cells and cytokines of the immune system, leading to the death of stem cells.[69] **Table 49-2** further describes potential mechanisms of the drug-induced anemias.

CLINICAL PRESENTATION AND DIFFERENTIAL DIAGNOSIS

The clinical presentation of aplastic anemia may include the typical symptoms of anemia such as weakness, fatigue, headache, lethargy, palpitations, and shortness of breath (**Table 49-3**). Neutropenia typically occurs first followed by thrombocytopenia. Anemia usually occurs last due to the longer life span of RBCs.[100] Abnormal bleeding including mucosal or gingival bleeding may be present in addition to petechial rashes secondary to thrombocytopenia. Patients may develop infections, fever, and pharyngeal ulcerations although data suggest that fever may not always be present.[101] The average onset of symptoms is 6.5 weeks; however, symptoms have been reported to appear as early as days and as long as months following exposure to the offending drug.[102] An extensive work-up should be conducted

Table 49-2 Mechanisms of Drug-Induced Anemia

Anemia Type	Mechanism(s)
APLASTIC ANEMIA	
Chemotherapy platinum-based therapies[70-75]	Immunologic response—drug metabolites form complexes with cellular proteins and ultimately stimulate T-cell autoimmune destruction of hematopoietic precursors
HEMOLYTIC ANEMIA	
Cefazolin[76,77] Cefotaxime[78] Cefotetan[79-82] Cefoxitin[83] Ceftizoxime[84,85] Ceftriaxone[86-90] Cefuroxime[91] Cephalothin[77,92] Quinidine[75] Quinine[75] Melthydopa[93,94]	Drug absorption-cell-bound—nonimmune drug adsorption modifies red blood cell membrane and nonimmunologic protein binding Neoantigen—antibody binds drug and red cells Autoimmune—induces a drug-independent immune response
MACROCYTIC ANEMIA	
Phenytoin[14,46-52,95,96] Zidovudine[97-99]	Inhibition of DNA synthesis and replication, which leads to abnormal erythrocytosis and the production of megaloblasts, which are larger than normal erythrocytes
CHEMOTHERAPY-INDUCED ANEMIA	
Chemotherapy[26-28,70-75] (antimicrotubular agents, alkylating agents, camptothecins, platinum-based therapies, tyrosine kinase inhibitors)	Myelosuppressive chemotherapy destroys precursors, red cells, which results in a hypoproliferative state and eventually anemia; direct cytotoxicity stops DNA synthesis and/or replication leading to apoptosis of hematopoietic stem cells

DNA = deoxyribonucleic acid.

Table 49-3 Signs and Symptoms of Drug-Induced Anemia

Aplastic anemia

- Fatigue
- Headache
- Lethargy
- Neutropenia
  - Fever
  - Chills
  - Infection
- Tachycardia
- Thrombocytopenia
  - Easy bruisability
  - Petechiae
  - Bleeding
- Weakness

Hemolytic anemia, macrocytic anemia, and chemotherapy-induced anemia

- Fatigue
- Headache
- Lethargy
- Tachycardia
- Weakness

Table 49-4 Conditions to Consider in the Differential Diagnosis of Drug-Induced Anemia

Microcytic anemia

- Anemia of chronic disease
- Inherited disorders of iron metabolism or hemoglobin synthesis
  - Thalassemias
- Iron-deficiency anemia
- Lead intoxication
- Sideroblastic anemias

Normocytic anemia

- Acute bleeding
- Anemia of chronic disease
- Anemia of chronic kidney disease
- Anemia of chronic liver disease
- Aplastic anemia
- Leukemias and lymphomas
- Hypothyroidism
- Hemolytic anemia
  - Autoimmune
- Myelodysplasia

Macrocytic anemia

- Megaloblastic
  - Vitamin B_{12} deficiency
  - Folate deficiency
  - Inherited disorders of DNA synthesis
- Nonmegaloblastic
  - Alcoholism
  - Chronic obstructive pulmonary disease
  - Inherited disorders
  - Refractory anemias
    - Aplastic anemia
    - Myelodysplasia

DNA = deoxyribonucleic acid.

including complete blood count (CBC) and a bone marrow biopsy. Chemical and medical drug exposures should be discussed as part of the patient interview and are considered an essential part of the differential diagnosis, although causality is often difficult to determine. The patient's past medical history including any earlier blood counts should be reviewed and knowledge of a personal or family history of pulmonary or hepatic diseases or any other single-lineage cytopenias may be helpful in narrowing the differential diagnosis.[101] Additional conditions to consider in the differential diagnosis for drug-induced anemia are listed in **Table 49-4**. A diagnosis of aplastic anemia can be made by the presence of two of the following criteria: a WBC count of 3,500 cells/mm^3 or less, a platelet count of 55,000 cells/mm^3 or less, or a hemoglobin value of 10 g/dL or less with a reticulocyte count of 30,000 cells/mm^3 or less.[103] Aplastic anemia is classified as severe when at least two of three peripheral blood smears show a neutrophil count of <500 cells/mm^3, platelet count of <20,000 cells/mm^3, and anemia with a corrected reticulocyte index of <1%.[3,104]

RISK FACTORS

Aplastic anemia is rare and drug-induced aplastic anemia is very rare. As a result, risk factors are not well defined. Risk factors for all drug-induced anemias can be found in **Table 49-5**.[3]

MORBIDITY AND MORTALITY

Aplastic anemia is the most serious of the drug-induced blood dyscrasias. Morbidity and mortality in patients with aplastic anemia typically occur as a result of infection and bleeding.[105] The average

Table 49-5 Risk Factors for Drug-Induced Anemias

Aplastic anemia

- Exposure to pesticides and chemicals
  - Benzene
  - Pesticides
  - Insecticides
- Occupational radiation exposure
- Viral exposure (e.g., hepatitis A)

Hemolytic anemia

- Infections
- Malaria
- Plasmodium
- Presence of rare inherited disorders
  - G6PD
  - Hereditary spherocytosis
  - Sickle cell anemia
  - Thalassemias
- Exposure to traumatic and microangiographic conditions
  - Valve replacement
  - Graft rejection

Macrocytic anemia

- Abdominal or intestinal surgery
- Diet low in vitamin B_{12}
- Chronic alcoholism
- Crohn disease
- Intestinal malabsorption syndromes
- Pernicious anemia

Chemotherapy-induced anemia

- Patient-related factors
  - Extent and type of cancer
  - Prior myelosuppressive chemotherapy
  - Prior skeletal radiation
- Regimen-related factors
  - Combination chemotherapy
  - Dose and schedule
  - Duration
- Specific agent administered
  - Platinum-based therapy
    - Cisplatin
    - Carboplatin
    - Oxaliplatin
  - Camptothecins
    - Topotecan
    - Irinotecan
  - Antimicrotubular agents
    - Docetaxel
    - Paclitaxel
    - Vinorelbine
  - Alkylating agents
    - Doxorubicin
    - Gemcitabine
    - Mitomycin C
  - Tyrosine kinase inhibitor
    - Imatinib

G6PD = glucose-6-phosphate dehydrogenase deficiency.

mortality rate is 50% and rises to >70% in severe cases with supportive care alone.[3]

PREVENTION

Prevention is challenging because drug-induced anemia is rare and unpredictable. Avoidance of drugs associated with aplastic anemia is recommended whenever alternatives are available. Regular hematologic monitoring is suggested when offending agents can't be avoided. Patient education and counseling may also play a role in prevention. Approaches to help prevent drug-induced anemia are outlined in **Table 49-6**.

MANAGEMENT

Due to the high mortality rate, diagnosis and treatment should be initiated quickly. Goals for therapy include improving blood counts, decreasing the need for blood transfusions, eliminating symptoms, and minimizing the risk for infections. The first step is removal of the suspected agent. Supportive care strategies may also be necessary, including transfusion support, antibiotic use, and iron chelation therapy if iron overload is suspected from frequent transfusions. Additional treatment modalities are based on the disease severity. For nonsevere disease, removal of the offending agent

Table 49-6 Approaches to Prevent Drug-Induced Anemia

- Careful documentation and patient education to prevent rechallenge when drug-induced anemias have occurred
- Consider modifying the chemotherapy regimen to a less myelosuppressive dose schedule or agent in patients with risk factors for developing chemotherapy-induced anemia
- Genetic testing (e.g., G6PD)
- Hematologic monitoring for drugs with higher risk of anemia

G6PD = glucose-6-phosphate dehydrogenase deficiency.

and supportive care may be sufficient to reverse cytopenias. In more severe cases, immunosuppression or hematopoietic stem cell transplant (HSCT) may be required. Allogenic HSCT from a human-leukocyte-antigen (HLA)-matched sibling donor is the treatment of choice in patients <40 years of age. The 5-year survival rate in adults and children under the age of 18 years is 77% and 90%, respectively.[106,107] Not all patients have an HLA-matched sibling, and therefore allogeneic HSCT from an unrelated donor should be considered after a trial of immunosuppressive therapy. For patients who are not HSCT candidates or are older than 40 years of age, immunosuppressive therapy is recommended. Combination therapy with antithymocyte globulin (ATG) and cyclosporine has been shown to achieve 5-year survival rates of 75–85%.[108] Other agents have been evaluated, but none have shown to be superior to ATG and cyclosporine.[106]

INFORMATION FOR PATIENTS

Patients should be educated on the importance of recognizing signs and symptoms of drug-induced anemia whenever they are prescribed medications with known risk. Immediate reporting of symptoms to a medical professional is imperative and routine monitoring of CBC over the course of therapy is recommended. For patients receiving long-term immunosuppressive therapy, education about the potential for infection and other known complications is necessary. Patients should understand the need for monitoring drug levels to ensure safety and efficacy while taking immunosuppressives.

HEMOLYTIC ANEMIA

Hemolytic anemia, a normocytic anemia, is a result of premature RBC destruction, or hemolysis. Hemolysis may occur either from changes in the intravascular environment or defective RBCs, both of which may be induced by exposure to various drugs. Hemolytic anemia can be immune-related or metabolic. The direct Coombs test (also known as a direct antiglobulin test) may be used to detect the presence of antibodies on red cells and determine if the hemolytic anemia is immune-related. If the test is negative, the cells are normal, and other secondary causes need to be ruled out.

CAUSATIVE AGENTS

Drugs found to have an association with drug-induced hemolytic anemia are listed in **Table 49-7**. Cases of drug-induced hemolytic anemia have been reported with cephalosporin and fluoroquinolone antibiotics. Other implicated drugs include H_2 antagonists, antihypertensives, and anti-inflammatory agents.

EPIDEMIOLOGY

As with other drug-induced anemias, establishing a clear causal relationship between a drug and hemolytic anemia can be difficult. Although rare, drug-induced hemolytic anemia does occur more frequently than drug-induced aplastic anemia. The estimated incidence of drug-induced hemolytic anemia has been reported as approximately 1 in 1.2 million individuals.[143]

MECHANISMS

Four mechanisms have been described for drug-induced hemolytic anemia. In the hapten mechanism, the body makes an antibody against the drug.[144] When exposure to the drug occurs again, the drug–antidrug complex forms, attaches to the RBC, activates the complement and leads to cell destruction.[78,145] Penicillin and cephalosporins, when given in high doses, are associated with this type of immune reaction. The onset of effects can occur over a week, and it may take several weeks for counts to normalize once the offending drug has been removed. Other agents associated with this type of hemolytic anemia include minocycline and streptomycin.[146]

With the immune bystander mechanism or the innocent bystander phenomenon, the drug binds to an antibody (e.g., IgG) to form an immune complex that attaches to the RBC, activates the complement, and leads to intravascular hemolysis.[78] Once the complement is activated, the complex (neoantigen) detaches itself and may bind to other RBCs,

Table 49-7 Agents Associated with Drug-Induced Hemolytic Anemia

Drug	Incidence	Level of Evidence[a]
Acetaminophen[109]	NK	C
Ascorbic acid[110]	NK	C
Captopril[111]	NK	C
Carbamazepine[12-14]	3–4 blood dyscrasias per 100,000 prescriptions	B
Dapsone[112]	NK	C
CEPHALOSPORINS		
Cefazolin[75-77]	NK	C
Cefotaxime[75,113]	NK	C
Cefotetan[75,78-82]	NK	C
Cefoxitin[75,83]	NK	C
Ceftizoxime[84,85]	NK	C
Ceftriaxone[78,86-90]	NK	C
Cefuroxime[75,91]	NK	C
Cephalothin[77,92]	NK	C
Ceftazidime[75]	NK	C
Erythromycin[114]		
FLUOROQUINOLONES		
Ciprofloxacin[115]	NK	C
Levofloxacin[116]	NK	C
H_2-ANTAGONISTS		
Cimetidine[15,16,117,118]	NK	C
Famotidine[118]	NK	C
Ranitidine[118,119]	NK	C
Nizatidine[118]	NK	C
Interferon alfa[65,120,121]	NK	C
Isoniazid[46,122-127]	NK	C
Metformin[128,129]	NK	C
Methyldopa[93,94,130]	NK	C
Methylene blue[131]	NK	C
Nitrofurantoin[132]	NK	C
NONSTEROIDAL ANTI-INFLAMMATORY DRUGS		
Diclofenac[38-41,104]	NK	C
Etodolac[42]	NK	C
Ibuprofen[43]	NK	C
Indomethacin[44,104]	NK	C
Salicylates[23,104]	NK	C
Sulindac[45]	NK	C
Tolmetin[75]	NK	C
Piperacillin–tazobactam[75]	NK	C
Phenazopyridine[133,134]	NK	C
Probenecid[75]	NK	C
Quinidine[18,75]	NK	C
Quinine[18,75,100]	NK	C
Rasburicase[135,136]	NK	C

Table 49-7 Agents Associated with Drug-Induced Hemolytic Anemia (continued)

Drug	Incidence	Level of Evidence[a]
Ribavirin[120,137]	NK	C
Rifampin[138,139]	NK	C
Sulfacetamide[140]	NK	C
Sulfamethoxazole[141,142]	NK	C

NK = not known.

[a]Definitions for Levels of Evidence: Level A—evidence from one or more randomized, controlled clinical trials; Level B—evidence from nonrandomized clinical trials, prospective observational studies, cohort studies, retrospective studies, case-control studies, meta-analyses and/or postmarketing surveillance studies; and Level C—evidence from one or more published case reports or case series.

WBCs, and platelets. Only a small amount of drug is needed to cause this reaction, but this mechanism is often severe and may lead to hemoglobinuria and renal failure. The RBCs act as "innocent bystanders" in this type of immunologic reaction.[78] Quinine and several sulfonamides have been associated with this mechanism.

Production of RBC autoantibodies is the third mechanism and has mostly been associated with methyldopa-induced hemolytic anemia.[93] Autoantibodies can be identified even in the absence of the offending drug or its metabolites. The mechanism by which methyldopa produces autoantibodies is not completely known. Approximately 10–20% of patients receiving methyldopa will develop a positive Coombs test; however, <1% of these patients will experience hemolysis. Hemolysis may occur from 4 months up to 2 years after initiation of methyldopa therapy.[94,147] Cladribine and fludarabine have also been associated with autoantibody production.[148]

The final mechanism for hemolytic anemia is nonimmunologic protein adsorption. This occurs when a drug binds to the RBC membrane followed by the binding of other proteins. These other proteins are not necessarily antibodies, but the net effect is modification of the RBC membrane.

CLINICAL PRESENTATION AND DIFFERENTIAL DIAGNOSIS

Symptoms of drug-induced hemolytic anemia can present within 7–10 days or as long as months or even years after drug exposure. The Coombs test detects the presence of antibodies on RBCs and may be used as a confirmatory test and/or to rule out drug-induced causes.[117] The onset of symptoms may be directly related to the mechanism involved. Fatigue, malaise, pallor, and shortness of breath are all symptoms associated with hemolytic anemia (Table 49-3). Additional diseases that should be considered in the differential for hemolytic anemia can be found in Table 49-4.

RISK FACTORS

G6PD deficiency is the most common hereditary risk factor for drug-induced hemolytic anemia. Other associated abnormalities include thalassemias, hereditary spherocytosis, and sickle cell anemia. Additional risk factors are listed in Table 49-5.

MORBIDITY AND MORTALITY

Symptoms from drug-induced hemolytic anemia, especially severe symptoms, can increase morbidity. Mortality is low if the true offending drug is discontinued immediately. A case series suggests that mortality from drug-induced hemolytic anemia is approximately 4%.[149]

PREVENTION

Due to the unpredictability of drug-induced hemolytic anemia, prevention of this disease can be difficult. G6PD deficiency screening is a good prevention strategy in patients where initiating therapies associated with hemolytic anemia is imperative. Agents known to be associated with drug-induced hemolytic anemia should be avoided when possible. If the use of these agents is necessary, routine monitoring of CBC and other hematologic laboratory values is recommended. Patients should be educated about the signs and symptoms of hemolytic anemia. Additional prevention strategies can be found in Table 49-6.

MANAGEMENT

Treatment required for drug-induced hemolytic anemia is largely dependent on the severity of disease. Regardless of severity, however, identification and removal of the offending drug is the first step. Supportive care strategies should be implemented, including blood transfusions where necessary. Hemodialysis may be necessary in severe cases. Glucocorticoids may be utilized to treat autoimmune hemolytic anemia after the offending agent has been removed.[150] Both chimeric anti-CD20 monoclonal antibody rituximab and IgG treatments have been studied for treatment of drug-induced hemolytic anemia, but more data are needed before routine use can be recommended.[151,152] Patients who experience drug-induced hemolytic anemia should never be rechallenged with the offending agent.

INFORMATION FOR PATIENTS

Patients should be educated regarding the importance of recognizing signs and symptoms of drug-induced hemolytic anemia if and when they are prescribed medications known to carry that risk. Immediate reporting of symptoms of anemia to a healthcare professional is imperative, and routine monitoring of the CBC is recommended while receiving offending agents. Patients with hereditary risks (e.g., G6PD deficiency) should be alerted to the prescription and nonprescription medications that should be avoided to prevent drug-induced hemolytic anemia.

MACROCYTIC ANEMIA

Macrocytic anemias are characterized by an increase in the average volume of the RBC (an increased MCV) and increase in the diameter and thickness of the erythrocyte. Megaloblasts are large, immature, and dysfunctional RBCs, and macrocytic anemia can be megaloblastic or nonmegaloblastic. Nonmegaloblastic macrocytic anemias are most commonly associated with alcoholism or liver disease. Megaloblastic anemias are produced by disorders of deoxyribonucleic acid (DNA) synthesis, most commonly a result of folic acid and vitamin B_{12} deficiencies. Both dietary vitamin B_{12} and folic acid are necessary for DNA synthesis; in their absence DNA synthesis is halted, but ribonucleic acid (RNA) synthesis continues, leading to protein production and ultimately resulting in formation of megaloblasts and macrocytosis. Drugs may cause macrocytic anemia by interfering with DNA synthesis and replication leading to abnormal erythrocytosis and the production of megaloblasts.

CAUSATIVE AGENTS

A list of drugs found to have an association with drug-induced macrocytic anemia can be found in **Table 49-8**. Sulfonamides, metformin, phenytoin, zidovudine, and methotrexate are the most common agents with documented case reports of macrocytic anemia.

EPIDEMIOLOGY

The incidence of drug-induced macrocytic anemia is not well documented. Antimetabolites that inhibit DNA synthesis, such as methotrexate and hydroxyurea, often cause clinically insignificant macrocytosis. Methotrexate-associated macrocytic anemia occurs in approximately 3–9% of patients.[165] Zidovudine-induced macrocytosis has been reported as high as 80% in patients with human immunodeficiency virus (HIV) and may or may not lead to clinically significant anemia.[163,164]

MECHANISMS

Folate and vitamin B_{12} are essential to DNA synthesis. When there is a deficiency in either folate or vitamin B_{12}, DNA synthesis is halted but RNA synthesis continues, leading to an increase in megaloblasts and macrocytosis.[166] Mechanisms for disruption of DNA synthesis often vary by drug. Dihydrofolate reductase inhibition by either trimethoprim or methotrexate may cause macrocytic anemia. Phenytoin has been shown to decrease the absorption of folate or facilitate its clearance.[95] Zidovudine interferes with the heme protein by inhibiting DNA polymerase.[167]

Table 49-8 Agents Associated with Macrocytic Anemia

Drug	Incidence	Level of Evidence[a]
Azathioprine[46,153-156]	NK	C
Leflunomide[157]	NK	C
Mesalamine[56-58]	NK	C
Metformin[158,159]	NK	C
Nitrofurantoin[160,161]	NK	C
Phenytoin[14,46-52,95,96]	NK	C
SULFONAMIDES	NK	C
Sulfisoxazole[53]	NK	C
Sulfasalazine[18,54,55]	NK	C
Trimethoprim–sulfamethoxazole[142,162]	NK	C
Zidovudine[97-99,163,164]	NK	C

NK = not known.

[a]Definitions for Levels of Evidence: Level A—evidence from one or more randomized, controlled clinical trials; Level B—evidence from nonrandomized clinical trials, prospective observational studies, cohort studies, retrospective studies, case-control studies, meta-analyses and/or postmarketing surveillance studies; and Level C—evidence from one or more published case reports or case series.

Metformin inhibits the absorption of vitamin B_{12}. Additional mechanisms for drug-induced macrocytic anemia can be found in Table 49-2.

CLINICAL PRESENTATION AND DIFFERENTIAL DIAGNOSIS

In the presence of low hemoglobin, an increased MCV is indicative of macrocytic anemia. Patients may experience common signs and symptoms of anemia, including fatigue, shortness of breath, and skin pallor. Additional signs and symptoms of drug-induced macrocytic anemia are listed in Table 49-3. Prior to a diagnosis of drug-induced anemia, nutritional deficiencies (e.g., folate and vitamin B_{12}) and malabsorption syndromes must be ruled out. Clinicians should consider documenting patients' baseline folate and vitamin B_{12} levels prior to initiating therapy with agents having high risk for causing drug-induced anemia.

RISK FACTORS

Risk factors for drug-induced macrocytic anemia are listed in Table 49-5. Conditions that result in a diet low in vitamin B_{12} as well as the presence of malabsorption syndromes and chronic alcoholism may increase a patient's risk of drug-induced macrocytic anemia.

MORBIDITY AND MORTALITY

Macrocytic anemia is not associated with significant morbidity or mortality. In severe cases, neurologic complications may occur, but these are reversible if caught early and properly treated.

PREVENTION

Avoidance of drugs that may be associated with macrocytic anemia is recommended. Regular hematologic monitoring is suggested when agents are known to cause macrocytic anemia can't be avoided. Patient education can also be important to prevention. Approaches to help prevent drug-induced anemia are listed in Table 49-6.

MANAGEMENT

Discontinuation of the offending drug is usually recommended in the treatment of drug-induced macrocytic anemia. When drug-induced macrocytic anemia occurs secondary to chemotherapy, it is typically considered an expected side effect of therapy and patients are treated symptomatically while therapy is continued. Supplementation of folic acid or vitamin B_{12} may be considered if their use won't alter the effectiveness of the treatment. Patients receiving trimethoprim–sulfamethoxazole may be given folinic acid, 5–10 mg up to 4 times a day, to correct macrocytic anemia.[168,169] Folic acid may be considered in patients receiving chronic methotrexate therapy to decrease side effects associated with that drug. Daily supplementation of folic acid (1 mg) may be utilized to correct drug-induced anemia caused by phenytoin or phenobarbital, although it may decrease the effectiveness of the seizure medications.[96]

INFORMATION FOR PATIENTS

Patients should be taught about the importance of recognizing signs and symptoms of drug-induced macrocytic anemia when they are prescribed medications known to increase risk. Immediate reporting of symptoms to a healthcare professional is important, and routine monitoring of CBC is recommended while patients are receiving drugs known to cause this disorder. For patients who are receiving long-term folic acid therapy, education about the reason for and the importance of supplementation is necessary.

CHEMOTHERAPY-INDUCED ANEMIA

Anemia occurs in 30–90% of all cancer patients.[170] Causes of anemia in cancer patients are often multifactorial, and the etiology can be difficult to determine. Other causes of anemia should be ruled out prior to diagnosing and treating a patient for chemotherapy-induced anemia (CIA).[171]

CAUSATIVE AGENTS

Chemotherapy agents associated with a relatively high incidence of mild-moderate anemia are listed in **Table 49-9**. Multiple drug classes, including alkylating agents (cyclophosphamide, carboplatin, cisplatin), antimetabolites (fluorouracil, gemcitabine, capecitabine, pemetrexed), topoisomerase inhibitors (doxorubicin, irinotecan, etoposide), and taxanes (paclitaxel and docetaxel), are associated with CIA. Other agents have been associated with different types of anemia: imatinib with bone marrow aplasia and oxaliplatin with hemolytic anemia.[26-28,172,173]

EPIDEMIOLOGY

Depending on the tumor type, between 32% and 49% of patients are anemic at the time of cancer diagnosis. Rates of CIA are difficult to determine because patients with cancer can have multiple anemia etiologies.[180,181] The myelosuppressive effects of chemotherapy are thought to be cumulative; therefore, the incidence of anemia may steadily increase with additional cycles of chemotherapy.[182]

Table 49-9 Agents Associated with Chemotherapy-Induced Anemia

Drug	Incidence	Level of Evidence[a]
Cancer chemotherapy[70-74,171,174] (single agents and combination platinum-based therapies, camptothecins, antimicrotubular agents, alkylating agents)	37–41% of all cancer patients and as high as 50–60% of all solid tumor patients; grade 3 or 4 anemia in as high as 40–55% in cisplatin-based therapies	B
Capecitabine[175]	NK	C
Erlotinib[176]	NK	C
Imatinib[26-28]	NK	C
Lapatinib[175]	NK	C
Nilotinib[177]	NK	C
Oxaliplatin[172,173]	NK	C
Sunitinib[178]	NK	C
Sorafenib[178]	NK	C
Vemurafenib[179]	NK	C

NK = not known.
[a]Definitions for Levels of Evidence: Level A—evidence from one or more randomized, controlled clinical trials; Level B—evidence from nonrandomized clinical trials, prospective observational studies, cohort studies, retrospective studies, case-control studies, meta-analyses and/or postmarketing surveillance studies; and Level C—evidence from one or more published case reports or case series.

MECHANISMS

Chemotherapy impairs hematopoiesis and disrupts RBC precursors' synthesis.[183] The exact mechanism of chemotherapy-induced anemia can be multifactorial, including a decrease in RBC production and a decreased erythropoietin production or decreased responsiveness to endogenous erythropoietin. Agents that cause nephrotoxicity, including cisplatin, also inhibit erythropoiesis by affecting erythropoietin production in the kidney. Anemia from underlying comorbidities, chronic blood loss, the cancer itself, or a combination of these factors may exacerbate the anemia.[184,185] Cancer cells can also suppress hematopoiesis through bone marrow infiltration and increased cytokine release that decreases the production and survival of RBCs.[181] Nutritional deficiencies, hemolysis, and coagulopathies may also contribute to anemia in cancer patients. Additional mechanisms are listed in Table 49-2.

CLINICAL PRESENTATION AND DIFFERENTIAL DIAGNOSIS

Signs and symptoms of CIA are listed in Table 49-3 and are similar to those found in patients with other causes of anemia. According to guidelines for patients with cancer, a Hgb level of 11 g/dL or below should prompt an evaluation of anemia. In patients with a baseline Hgb >11 g/dL, a drop in Hgb of 2 g/dL or more in a relatively short period of time is a cause for concern and assessment.[181] Initial assessments should include a CBC with differential, iron studies, folate, vitamin B_{12}, and a detailed history and physical exam including onset of symptoms, comorbidities, and any exposure to chemotherapy agents or radiation. If a deficiency in iron, folate, or vitamin B_{12} is found, the deficiency should be treated accordingly. Any other cause of anemia that may be rectified independent of cancer therapy should also be treated as indicated. When no such etiology is identified, the myelosuppressive chemotherapy should be considered the cause of anemia.[181]

RISK FACTORS

Risk factors for CIA can be divided into two categories: patient-related risk factors and regimen-related risks (Table 49-5). Individual characteristics that increase the incidence of bone marrow suppression or predispose the patient to becoming symptomatic with anemia are considered patient-related risks. Radiation therapy, especially to the bones, can increase the risk of RBCs. Patients with a history of receiving chemotherapy may have ongoing anemia of chronic disease. Cancer that infiltrates the bone marrow may also increase the risk of CIA due to weakened erythropoiesis. Patients with significant cardiovascular, pulmonary, or cerebral vascular disease may also have an increased risk of CIA due to lower baseline levels of Hgb. Regimen-related risks include the regimen's anemic potential, length of therapy, the use of combination versus single-agent therapy, dosage, and administration schedule.

MORBIDITY AND MORTALITY

CIA can significantly affect patients' quality of life, due either to the symptoms of anemia or the treatment required to treat the anemia. Prior to initiating therapy, the risks of treatment must be weighed against the benefits. Prior to the use of blood transfusion, documented complications (e.g., transfusion-related reactions, transfusion-associated circulatory overload, bacterial contamination, viral infections, and iron overload) should be considered.[181] Although they may help reduce the need for RBC transfusions, erythrocyte stimulating agents (ESAs) are associated with significant risks including venous thromboembolism (VTE), tumor progression, and death.[181,186] For this reason, ESA therapy for chemotherapy-induced anemia is only recommended in patients who have a noncurable, nonmyeloid cancer who are actively receiving chemotherapy.

PREVENTION

A thorough assessment should be conducted at the onset of chemotherapy to determine if the patient may be at risk for CIA. Evaluation of underlying risk factors, the type of tumor the patient has, and the chemotherapy regimen being utilized is appropriate. If the patient's risk of CIA is high, the healthcare team may want to consider an alternative treatment regimen. When treating with curative intent, however, substituting treatment regimens simply to avoid CIA may not be appropriate.

MANAGEMENT

Prior to initiating treatment for CIA, a risk assessment based on the causative agent(s), the patient's past medical history, and baseline laboratory values will help determine the initial intervention plan. A decision to use blood transfusions should be based on the patient's symptoms (onset, severity, and duration) and comorbidities rather than on Hgb alone.[181] If a rapid correction in Hgb is needed, a blood transfusion is the only option. Administration of 1 unit of packed red blood cells (PRBC) is estimated to increase a patient's hemoglobin by 1 g/dL nonbleeding.

ESAs approved for use for CIA include epoetin alfa and darbepoetin alfa. Unlike blood transfusions, ESAs can take several weeks to trigger a hemoglobin response. The National Comprehensive Cancer Network (NCCN) guidelines recommend specific dosing strategies to ensure appropriate treatment and to minimize side effects.[181] Risks versus benefits should be discussed with the patient prior to initiation. Studies have demonstrated a decrease in survival and tumor progression in patients receiving ESA therapy. VTE and hypertension are significant effects that may also occur and should be monitored. As a result, the U.S. Food and Drug Administration (FDA) has added a boxed warning to ESA labeling highlighting the side effects. To minimize complications when ESA therapy is deemed necessary, the lowest dose required to avoid the need for blood transfusions should be used.[187,188] ESA should also be discontinued within 6 weeks if chemotherapy is no longer used. Patients who have a curable cancer should not be treated with ESA therapy. Recommended dosing of ESAs in provided in **Table 49-10**.

INFORMATION FOR PATIENTS

Patients should be educated to recognize the signs and symptoms of anemia if they are to receive chemotherapy. Immediate reporting of symptoms to a healthcare professional is imperative and routine monitoring of CBC is recommended while the patient is exposed to possible causative agents. The potential risks and benefits of ESA therapy must be discussed with patients prior to the use of those agents, and the FDA requires informed consent under the Risk Evaluation and Mitigation Strategy (REMS) program. A medication guide must also be provided to patients prior to initiation of therapy to ensure understanding of the risks and benefits of using ESAs.

Table 49-10 Dosing of Erythropoiesis-Stimulating Agents[181]

Agent	Starting Dosage	Dosage Increase	Dosing Parameters
Erythropoietin (Procrit, Epogen)	150 units/kg sub-Q 3 times/week 40,000 units sub-Q weekly	300 units/kg sub-Q 3 times/week 60,000 units sub-Q weekly	Hemoglobin must be <10 g/dL to initiate and continue therapy Evaluate after 4 weeks and increase dosage if rise is <1 g/dL Decrease by ~25% if rapid rise in hemoglobin Discontinue therapy if no response after 8 weeks
Darbepoetin (Aranesp)	2.25 mcg/kg sub-Q weekly 500 mcg every 3 weeks	4.5 mcg/kg sub-Q weekly Not applicable	Hemoglobin must be <10 g/dL to initiate and continue therapy Evaluate after 6 weeks and increase dosage if rise is <1 g/dL Decrease by ~40% if rapid rise in hemoglobin Discontinue therapy if no response after 8 weeks

Sub-Q = subcutaneous.

REFERENCES

1. Executive summary of disease management of drug hypersensitivity: a practice parameter. Joint Task Force on Practice Parameters, the American Academy of Allergy, Asthma and Immunology, and the Joint Council of Allergy, Asthma and Immunology. *Ann Allergy Asthma Immunol.* 1999; 83:665-700.
2. Rao KV. Drug-induced hematologic disorders. In: Dipiro JT, Talbert RL, Yee GC et al., eds. *Pharmacotherapy: a pathophysiologic approach* (internet). 9th ed. http://accesspharmacy.mhmedical.com/content.aspx?bookid=689§ionid=48811451.
3. Camitta BM, Thomas ED, Nathan DG et al. A prospective study of androgens and bone marrow transplantation for treatment of severe aplastic anemia. *Blood.* 1979; 53:504-14.
4. McLean E, Cogswell M, Egli I et al. Worldwide prevalence of anaemia, WHO Vitamin and Mineral Nutrition Information System, 1993–2005. *Public Health Nutr.* 2009; 12:444-54.
5. Bottiger LE, Furhoff AK, Holmberg L. Drug-induced blood dyscrasias. A ten-year material from the Swedish Adverse Drug Reaction Committee. *Acta Med Scand.* 1979; 205:457-61.
6. Dolberg OJ, Levy Y. Idiopathic aplastic anemia: diagnosis and classification. *Autoimmun Rev.* 2014; 13:569-73.
7. Kaufman D KJ et al. *The drug etiology of agranulocytosis and aplastic anemia.* New York: Oxford University Press; 1991:259.
8. Keisu M, Wiholm BE, Ost A, Mortimer O. Acetazolamide-associated aplastic anaemia. *J Intern Med.* 1990; 228:627-32.
9. Hirakata H, Onoyama K, Iseki K et al. Worsening of anemia induced by long-term use of captopril in hemodialysis patients. *Am J Nephrol.* 1984; 4:355-60.
10. Israeli A, Or R, Leitersdorf E. Captopril-associated transient aplastic anemia. *Acta Haematol.* 1985; 73:106-7.
11. Kim CR, Maley MB, Mohler ER Jr. Captopril and aplastic anemia. *Ann Intern Med.* 1989; 111:187-8.
12. Sobotka JL, Alexander B, Cook BL. A review of carbamazepine's hematologic reactions and monitoring recommendations. *Dicp.* 1990; 24:1214-9.
13. Moore NC, Lerer B, Meyendorff E, Gershon S. Three cases of carbamazepine toxicity. *Am J Psychiatry.* 1985; 142:974-5.
14. Blackburn SC, Oliart AD, Garcia Rodriguez LA, Perez Gutthann S. Antiepileptics and blood dyscrasias: a cohort study. *Pharmacotherapy.* 1998; 18:1277-83.
15. Farber BF, Brody JP. Rapid development of aplastic anemia after intravenous chloramphenicol and cimetidine therapy. *South Med J.* 1981; 74:1257-8.
16. West BC, DeVault GA Jr, Clement JC, Williams DM. Aplastic anemia associated with parenteral chloramphenicol: review of 10 cases, including the second case of possible increased risk with cimetidine. *Rev Infect Dis.* 1988; 10:1048-51.
17. Wallerstein RO, Condit PK, Kasper CK et al. Statewide study of chloramphenicol therapy and fatal aplastic anemia. *JAMA.* 1969; 208:2045-50.
18. Danielson DA, Douglas SW III, Herzog P et al. Drug-induced blood disorders. *JAMA.* 1984; 252:3257-60.
19. Kaufman DW, Kelly JP, Anderson T et al. Evaluation of case reports of aplastic anemia among patients treated with felbamate. *Epilepsia.* 1997; 38:1265-9.
20. Pennell PB, Ogaily MS, Macdonald RL. Aplastic anemia in a patient receiving felbamate for complex partial seizures. *Neurology.* 1995; 45:456-60.
21. Kelly JP, Kaufman DW, Shapiro S. Risks of agranulocytosis and aplastic anemia in relation to the use of cardiovascular drugs: The International Agranulocytosis and Aplastic Anemia Study. *Clin Pharmacol Ther.* 1991; 49:330-41.
22. Rawson NS, Harding SR, Malcolm E, Lueck L. Hospitalizations for aplastic anemia and agranulocytosis in Saskatchewan: incidence and associations with antecedent prescription drug use. *J Clin Epidemiol.* 1998; 51:1343-55.
23. Mary JY, Guiguet M, Baumelou E. Drug use and aplastic anaemia: the French experience. French Cooperative Group for the Epidemiological Study of Aplastic Anaemia. *Eur J Haematol Suppl.* 1996; 60:35-41.
24. Gibson J, McGirr EE, York J, Kronenberg H. Aplastic anemia in association with gold therapy for rheumatoid arthritis. *Aust N Z J Med.* 1983; 13:130-4.
25. Hansen RM, Csuka ME, McCarty DJ, Saryan LA. Gold induced aplastic anemia. Complete response to corticosteroids, plasmapheresis, and *N*-acetylcysteine infusion. *J Rheumatol.* 1985; 12:794-7.
26. Cervetti G, Carulli G, Galimberti S et al. Transitory marrow aplasia during Imatinib therapy in a patient with chronic myeloid leukemia. *Leuk Res.* (England). 2008; 32:194-5.
27. LeMarbre G, Schinstock C, Hoyer R et al. Late onset aplastic anemia during treatment of chronic myeloid leukemia with imatinib mesylate. *Leuk Res.* (England). 2007; 31:414-415.
28. Srinivas U, Pillai LS, Kumar R et al. Bone marrow aplasia—a rare complication of imatinib therapy in CML patients. *Am J Hematol.* 2007; 82:314-6.
29. Kuter DJ, Tillotson GS. Hematologic effects of antimicrobials: focus on the oxazolidinone linezolid. *Pharmacotherapy.* 2001; 21:1010-3.
30. Bernstein WB, Trotta RF, Rector JT et al. Mechanisms for linezolid-induced anemia and thrombocytopenia. *Ann Pharmacother.* 2003; 37:517-20.
31. Green SL, Maddox JC, Huttenbach ED. Linezolid and reversible myelosuppression. *JAMA.* 2001; 285:1291.
32. Waldrep TW, Skiest DJ. Linezolid-induced anemia and thrombocytopenia. *Pharmacotherapy.* 2002; 22:109-12.
33. Biswas N, Ahn YH, Goldman JM, Schwartz JM. Aplastic anemia associated with antithyroid drugs. *Am J Med Sci.* 1991; 301:190-4.
34. Moreb J, Shemesh O, Shilo S et al. Transient methimazole-induced bone marrow aplasia: in vitro evidence for a humoral mechanism of bone marrow suppression. *Acta Haematol.* 1983; 69:127-31.
35. Bishara J, Dux S, Pitlik SV. Methimazole-induced aplastic anemia? *Ann Pharmacother.* 1996; 30:684.
36. Mezquita P, Luna V, Munoz-Torres M et al. Methimazole-induced aplastic anemia in third exposure: successful treatment with recombinant human granulocyte colony-stimulating factor. *Thyroid.* 1998; 8:791-4.
37. Eustace S, O'Neill T, McHale S, Molony J. Fatal aplastic anaemia following prolonged diclofenac use in an elderly patient. *Ir J Med Sci.* 1989; 158:217.
38. Kramer MR, Levene C, Hershko C. Severe reversible autoimmune haemolytic anaemia and thrombocytopenia associated with diclofenac therapy. *Scand J Haematol.* 1986; 36:118-20.
39. Meyer O, Hoffmann T, Aslan T et al. Diclofenac-induced antibodies against RBCs and platelets: two case reports and a concise review. *Transfusion.* 2003; 43:345-9.
40. Bougie D, Johnson ST, Weitekamp LA, Aster RH. Sensitivity to a metabolite of diclofenac as a cause of acute immune hemolytic anemia. *Blood.* 1997; 90:407-13.
41. Ahrens N, Genth R, Kiesewetter H, Salama A. Misdiagnosis in patients with diclofenac-induced hemolysis: new cases and a concise review. *Am J Hematol.* 2006; 81:128-31.
42. Cunha PD, Lord RS, Johnson ST et al. Immune hemolytic anemia caused by sensitivity to a metabolite of etodolac, a nonsteroidal anti-inflammatory drug. *Transfusion.* 2000; 40:663-8.
43. Guidry JB, Ogburn CL Jr, Griffin FM Jr. Fatal autoimmune hemolytic anemia associated with ibuprofen. *JAMA.* 1979; 242:68-9.
44. Kornberg A, Rachmilewitz EA. Aplastic anemia after prolonged ingestion of indomethacin. *Acta Haematol.* 1982; 67:136-8.
45. Angeles ML, Reid ME, Yacob UA et al. Sulindac-induced immune hemolytic anemia. *Transfusion.* 1994; 34:255-8.
46. Thompson DF, Gales MA. Drug-induced pure red cell aplasia. *Pharmacotherapy.* 1996; 16:1002-8.

47. Gerson WT, Fine DG, Spielberg SP, Sensenbrenner LL. Anticonvulsant-induced aplastic anemia: increased susceptibility to toxic drug metabolites in vitro. *Blood.* 1983; 61:889-93.
48. Shalev O, Gilon D, Nubani NH. Masked phenytoin-induced megaloblastic anemia in beta-thalassemia minor. *Acta Haematol.* 1987; 77:186-7.
49. Dessypris EN, Redline S, Harris JW, Krantz SB. Diphenylhydantoin-induced pure red cell aplasia. *Blood.* 1985; 65:789-94.
50. Huijgens PC, Thijs LG, den Ottolander GJ. Pure red cell aplasia, toxic dermatitis and lymphadenopathy in a patient taking diphenylhydantoin. *Acta Haematol.* 1978; 59:31-6.
51. Pritchard KI, Quirt IC, Simpson WJ, Fleming JF. Phenytoin-associated reversible red cell aplasia. *Can Med Assoc J.* 1979; 121:1491-3.
52. Jeong YG, Jung Y, River GL. Pure RBC aplasia and diphenylhydantoin. *JAMA.* 1974; 229:314-5.
53. Adams JG, Heller P, Abramson RK, Vaithianathan T. Sulfonamide-induced hemolytic anemia and hemoglobin Hasharon. *Arch Intern Med.* 1977; 137:1449-51.
54. Nurmohamed MT, Soesan M, van Oers MH et al. Cyclosporin for sulphasalazine-induced aplastic anaemia in a patient with early rheumatoid arthritis. *Rheumatology (Oxford).* 2000; 39:1431-3.
55. Schneider R, Beeley L. Megaloblastic anaemia associated with sulphasalazine treatment. *Br Med J.* 1977; 2:580.
56. Otsubo H, Kaito K, Sekita T et al. Mesalazine-associated severe aplastic anemia successfully treated with antithymocyte globulin, cyclosporine and granulocyte colony-stimulating factor. *Int J Hematol.* 1998; 68:445-8.
57. Abboudi ZH, Marsh JC, Smith-Laing G, Gordon-Smith EC. Fatal aplastic anaemia after mesalazine. *Lancet.* 1994; 343:542.
58. Laidlaw ST, Reilly JT. Antilymphocyte globulin for mesalazine-associated aplastic anaemia. *Lancet.* 1994; 343:981-2.
59. Jalali R, Singh P, Menon H, Gujral S. Unexpected case of aplastic anemia in a patient with glioblastoma multiforme treated with Temozolomide. *J Neurooncol.* 2007; 85:105-7.
60. Meyer B, Staudinger T, Lechner K. Clopidogrel and aplastic anaemia. *Lancet.* 2001; 357:1446-7.
61. Bahng H, Lee JH, Suh C et al. Severe aplastic anemia induced by ticlopidine: report of two cases. *J Korean Med Sci.* 1998; 13:541-4.
62. Yeh SP, Hsueh EJ, Wu H, Wang YC. Ticlopidine-associated aplastic anemia. A case report and review of literature. *Ann Hematol.* 1998; 76:87-90.
63. Symeonidis A, Kouraklis-Symeonidis A, Seimeni U et al. Ticlopidine-induced aplastic anemia: two new case reports, review, and meta-analysis of 55 additional cases. *Am J Hematol.* 2002; 71:24-32.
64. Marsh JC, Ball SE, Darbyshire P et al. Guidelines for the diagnosis and management of acquired aplastic anaemia. *Br J Haematol.* 2003; 123:782-801.
65. Gonzalez-Casas R, Garcia-Buey L, Jones EA et al. Systematic review: hepatitis-associated aplastic anaemia—a syndrome associated with abnormal immunological function. *Aliment Pharmacol Ther.* 2009; 30:436-43.
66. Miano M, Dufour C. The diagnosis and treatment of aplastic anemia: a review. *Int J Hematol.* 2015; 101:527-35.
67. Nimer SD, Ireland P, Meshkinpour A, Frane M. An increased HLA DR2 frequency is seen in aplastic anemia patients. *Blood.* 1994; 84:923-7.
68. Poonkuzhali B, Shaji RV, Salamun DE et al. Cytochrome P4501A1 and glutathione S transferase gene polymorphisms in patients with aplastic anemia in India. *Acta Haematol.* 2005; 114:127-32.
69. Young NS, Maciejewski J. The pathophysiology of acquired aplastic anemia. *N Engl J Med.* 1997; 336:1365-72.
70. Osterborg A, Brandberg Y. Relationship between changes in hemoglobin level and quality of life during chemotherapy in anemic cancer patients receiving epoetin alfa therapy. *Cancer.* 2003; 97:3126-7.
71. Cella D, Dobrez D, Glaspy J. Control of cancer-related anemia with erythropoietic agents: a review of evidence for improved quality of life and clinical outcomes. *Ann Oncol.* 2003; 14:511-9.
72. Groopman JE, Itri LM. Chemotherapy-induced anemia in adults: incidence and treatment. *J Natl Cancer Inst.* 1999; 91:1616-34.
73. Mercadante S, Gebbia V, Marrazzo A, Filosto S. Anaemia in cancer: pathophysiology and treatment. *Cancer Treat Rev.* 2000; 26:303-11.
74. Kuhn JG. Chemotherapy-associated hematopoietic toxicity. *Am J Health-Syst Pharm.* 2002; 59(suppl 4):S4-7.
75. Johnson ST, Fueger JT, Gottschall JL. One center's experience: the serology and drugs associated with drug-induced immune hemolytic anemia—a new paradigm. *Transfusion.* 2007; 47:697-702.
76. Cerynik DL, Lee GC, Fayssoux R, Amin NH. Case report: cefazolin-induced hemolytic anemia. *Clin Orthop Relat Res.* 2007; 459:260-2.
77. Moake JL, Butler CF, Hewell GM et al. Hemolysis induced by cefazolin and cephalothin in a patient with penicillin sensitivity. *Transfusion.* 1978; 18:369-73.
78. Garratty G. Immune hemolytic anemia associated with drug therapy. *Blood Rev.* 2010; 24:143-50.
79. Moes GS, MacPherson BR. Cefotetan-induced hemolytic anemia: a case report and review of the literature. *Arch Pathol Lab Med.* 2000; 124:1344-6.
80. Chenoweth CE, Judd WJ, Steiner EA, Kauffman CA. Cefotetan-induced immune hemolytic anemia. *Clin Infect Dis.* 1992; 15:863-5.
81. Franchini M, Piccoli PL, Gandini G et al. Clinical and laboratory study of an episode of cefotetan-induced severe hemolytic anemia. *Hematology.* 2004; 9:65-9.
82. Stroncek D, Procter JL, Johnson J. Drug-induced hemolysis: cefotetan-dependent hemolytic anemia mimicking an acute intravascular immune transfusion reaction. *Am J Hematol.* 2000; 64:67-70.
83. DeTorres OH. Hemolytic anemia and pancytopenia induced by cefoxitin. *Drug Intell Clin Pharm.* 1983; 17:816-8.
84. Endoh T, Yagihashi A, Sasaki M, Watanabe N. Ceftizoxime-induced hemolysis due to immune complexes: case report and determination of the epitope responsible for immune complex-mediated hemolysis. *Transfusion.* 1999; 39:306-9.
85. Shammo JM, Calhoun B, Mauer AM et al. First two cases of immune hemolytic anemia associated with ceftizoxime. *Transfusion.* 1999; 39:838-44.
86. Longo F, Hastier P, Buckley MJ et al. Acute hepatitis, autoimmune hemolytic anemia, and erythroblastocytopenia induced by ceftriaxone. *Am J Gastroenterol.* 1998; 93:836-7.
87. Bell MJ, Stockwell DC, Luban NL et al. Ceftriaxone-induced hemolytic anemia and hepatitis in an adolescent with hemoglobin SC disease. *Pediatr Crit Care Med.* 2005; 6:363-6.
88. Demirkaya E, Atay AA, Musabak U et al. Ceftriaxone-related hemolysis and acute renal failure. *Pediatr Nephrol.* 2006; 21:733-6.
89. Meyer O, Hackstein H, Hoppe B et al. Fatal immune haemolysis due to a degradation product of ceftriaxone. *Br J Haematol.* 1999; 105:1084-5.
90. Mattis LE, Saavedra JM, Shan H et al. Life-threatenting ceftriaxone-induced immune hemolytic anemia in a child with Crohn's disease. *Clin Pediatr (Phila).* 2004; 43:175-8.
91. Malloy CA, Kiss JE, Challapalli M. Cefuroxime-induced immune hemolysis. *J Pediatr.* 2003; 143:130-2.
92. Jeannet M, Bloch A, Dayer JM et al. Cephalothin-induced immune hemolytic anemia. *Acta Haematol.* 1976; 55:109-17.
93. Dacie SJ. The immune haemolytic anaemias: a century of exciting progress in understanding. *Br J Haematol.* 2001; 114:770-85.
94. Carstairs KC, Breckenridge A, Dollery CT, Worlledge SM. Incidence of a positive direct coombs test in patients on alphamethyldopa. *Lancet.* 1966; 2:133-5.

95. Scott JM, Weir DG. Drug-induced megaloblastic change. *Clin Haematol.* 1980; 9:587-606.

96. Rivey MP, Schottelius DD, Berg MJ. Phenytoin-folic acid: a review. *Drug Intell Clin Pharm.* 1984; 18:292-301.

97. Richman DD, Fischl MA, Grieco MH et al. The toxicity of azidothymidine (AZT) in the treatment of patients with AIDS and AIDS-related complex. A double-blind, placebo-controlled trial. *N Engl J Med.* 1987; 317:192-7.

98. Walker RE, Parker RI, Kovacs JA et al. Anemia and erythropoiesis in patients with the acquired immunodeficiency syndrome (AIDS) and Kaposi sarcoma treated with zidovudine. *Ann Intern Med.* 1988; 108:372-6.

99. Koduri PR, Parekh S. Zidovudine-related anemia with reticulocytosis. *Ann Hematol.* 2003; 82:184-5.

100. Vandendries ER, Drews RE. Drug-associated disease: hematologic dysfunction. *Crit Care Clin.* 2006; 22:347-55, viii.

101. Scheinberg P, Young NS. How I treat acquired aplastic anemia. *Blood.* 2012; 120:1185-96.

102. Shadduck R. Aplastic anemia. In: Williams W, ed. *Hematology.* New York: McGraw-Hill; 1995:238-51.

103. Heimpel H. Epidemiology and etiology of aplastic anemia. In: Schrezenmeier H, Bacigalupo A, eds. *Aplastic anemia: pathophysiology and treatment.* Cambridge, UK: Cambridge University Press; 1999:97-116.

104. Risks of agranulocytosis and aplastic anemia. A first report of their relation to drug use with special reference to analgesics. The International Agranulocytosis and Aplastic Anemia Study. *JAMA.* 1986; 256:1749-57.

105. Bacigalupo A, Brand R, Oneto R et al. Treatment of acquired severe aplastic anemia: bone marrow transplantation compared with immunosuppressive therapy—The European Group for Blood and Marrow Transplantation experience. *Semin Hematol.* 2000; 37:69-80.

106. Young NS, Calado RT, Scheinberg P. Current concepts in the pathophysiology and treatment of aplastic anemia. *Blood.* 2006; 108:2509-19.

107. Horowitz MM. Current status of allogeneic bone marrow transplantation in acquired aplastic anemia. *Semin Hematol.* 2000; 37:30-42.

108. Peinemann F, Grouven U, Kroger N et al. Unrelated donor stem cell transplantation in acquired severe aplastic anemia: a systematic review. *Haematologica.* 2009; 94:1732-42.

109. Sklar GE. Hemolysis as a potential complication of acetaminophen overdose in a patient with glucose-6-phosphate dehydrogenase deficiency. *Pharmacotherapy.* 2002; 22:656-8.

110. Ibrahim IH, Sallam SM, Omar H, Rizk M. Oxidative hemolysis of erythrocytes induced by various vitamins. *Int J Biomed Sci.* 2006; 2:295-8.

111. Trimble MA, Sketch MH Jr, Mehta RH. Hemolytic anemia: a rare but potentially serious adverse effect of captopril. *Herz.* 2007; 32:62-4.

112. Jollow DJ, Bradshaw TP, McMillan DC. Dapsone-induced hemolytic anemia. *Drug Metab Rev.* 1995; 27:107-24.

113. Shulman IA, Arndt PA, McGehee W, Garratty G. Cefotaxime-induced immune hemolytic anemia due to antibodies reacting in vitro by more than one mechanism. *Transfusion.* 1990; 30:263-6.

114. Del Vasto F, Pinta MF, Marchese L et al. [Drug-induced immune hemolytic anemia in an 18-month-old patient. Responsible agent: erythromycin]. *Pediatr Med Chir.* 1990; 12:275-6.

115. Lim S, Alam MG. Ciprofloxacin-induced acute interstitial nephritis and autoimmune hemolytic anemia. *Ren Fail.* 2003; 25:647-51.

116. Oh YR, Carr-Lopez SM, Probasco JM, Crawley PG. Levofloxacin-induced autoimmune hemolytic anemia. *Ann Pharmacother.* 2003; 37:1010-3.

117. Petz LD, Gitlin N, Grant K et al. Cimetidine-induced hemolytic anemia: the fallacy of clinical associations. *J Clin Gastroenterol.* 1983; 5:405-9.

118. Aymard JP, Aymard B, Netter P et al. Haematological adverse effects of histamine H2-receptor antagonists. *Med Toxicol Adverse Drug Exp.* 1988; 3:430-48.

119. Pixley JS, MacKintosh FR, Sahr EA, Zanjani ED. Mechanism of ranitidine associated anemia. *Am J Med Sci.* 1989; 297:369-71.

120. Sykia A, Gigi E, Sinakos E et al. Severe autoimmune hemolytic anemia complicated with liver decompensation and invasive aspergillosis in a patient with chronic hepatitis C during treatment with peg-interferon-a and ribavirin. *J Gastrointestin Liver Dis.* 2009; 18:118-9.

121. Oliveira TL, Caetano AZ, Belem JM et al. Interferon-alpha induced psoriatic arthritis and autoimmune hemolytic anemia during chronic hepatitis C treatment. *Acta Reumatol Port.* 2014; 39:327-30.

122. Lewis CR, Manoharan A. Pure red cell hypoplasia secondary to isoniazid. *Postgrad Med J.* 1987; 63:309-10.

123. Veale KS, Huff ES, Nelson BK, Coffman DS. Pure red cell aplasia and hepatitis in a child receiving isoniazid therapy. *J Pediatr.* 1992; 120:146-8.

124. Marseglia GL, Locatelli F. Isoniazid-induced pure red cell aplasia in two siblings. *J Pediatr.* 1998; 132:898-900.

125. Hoffman R, McPhedran P, Benz EJ Jr, Duffy TP. Isoniazid-induced pure red cell aplasia. *Am J Med Sci.* 1983; 286:2-9.

126. Claiborne RA, Dutt AK. Isoniazid-induced pure red cell aplasia. *Am Rev Respir Dis.* 1985; 131:947-9.

127. Robinson MG, Foadi M. Hemolytic anemia with positive Coombs' test. Association with isoniazid therapy. *JAMA.* 1969; 208:656-8.

128. Ruggiero NA, Kish TD, Lee ML. Metformin-induced hemolytic anemia in a patient with glucose-6-phosphate dehydrogenase deficiency. *Am J Ther.* 2016; 23:e575-8.

129. Kirkiz S, Yarali N, Arman Bilir O, Tunc B. Metformin-induced hemolytic anemia. *Med Princ Pract.* 2014; 23:183-5.

130. Aldomet (methyldopa) prescribing information. Whitehouse Station, NJ: Merck and Co Inc; 1998. https://gp2u.com.au/static/pdf/A/ALDOMET-PI.pdf.

131. Sills MR, Zinkham WH. Methylene blue-induced Heinz body hemolytic anemia. *Arch Pediatr Adolesc Med.* 1994; 148:306-10.

132. van de Mheen L, Smits SM, Terpstra WE et al. Haemolytic anaemia after nitrofurantoin treatment in a pregnant woman with G6PD deficiency. *BMJ Case Rep.* 2014; Apr 30:2014.

133. Chang LC, Kuo CW, Chau T, Lin SH. Phenazopyridine-induced hemolytic anemia in advanced kidney disease. *J Am Geriatr Soc.* 2014; 62:2464-6.

134. Siddiqui MA. Chronic severe hemolytic anemia from phenazopyridine. *Ann Intern Med.* 1995; 122:157.

135. Hrisinko MA, Chen YH. Rasburicase-induced Heinz body hemolytic anemia in a patient with chronic lymphocytic leukemia. *Blood.* 2015; 126:826.

136. Nguyen AP, Ness GL. Hemolytic anemia following rasburicase administration: a review of published reports. *J Pediatr Pharmacol Ther.* 2014; 19:310-6.

137. Itoh Y, Okanoue T. Ribavirin-induced hemolytic anemia in chronic hepatitis C patients. *J Gastroenterol.* 2004; 39:704-5.

138. Neunert CE, Paranjape GS, Cameron S, Rogers ZR. Intravascular hemolysis following low dose daily rifampin. *Pediatr Blood Cancer.* 2008; 51:821-3.

139. Bodmer M, Haschke M, Ratz Bravo AE, Liechti ME. [Renal failure and hemolytic anemia. Rifampicin associated interstitial nephropathy with immune hemolytic anemia]. *Praxis (Bern 1994).* 2009; 98:179-85.

140. de Leeuw N, Shapiro L, Lowenstein L. Drug-induced hemolytic anemia. *Ann Intern Med.* 1963; 58:592-607.

141. Arndt PA, Garratty G, Wolf CF, Rivera M. Haemolytic anaemia and renal failure associated with antibodies to trimethoprim and sulfamethoxazole. *Transfus Med.* 2011; 21:194-8.

142. Taraszewski R, Harvey R, Rosman P. Death from drug-induced hemolytic anemia. *Postgrad Med.* 1989; 85:79-80, 84.

143. Petz LD, Garratty G. *Immune hemolytic anemias.* 2nd ed. Philadelphia, PA: Churchill Livingston; 2004.

144. Meyer D, Schiller C, Westermann J et al. FcYRIII (CD16)-deficient mice show IgG isotype-dependent protection to experimental autoimmune hemolytic anemia. *Blood.* 1998; 92: 3997-4002.

145. Ackroyd JF. The immunological basis of purpura due to drug hypersensitivity. *Proc R Soc Med.* 1962; 55:30-6.
146. Thomas A. Autoimmune hemolytic anemias. In: Lee GR Foerster J, Lukens J et al., eds. *Wintrobe's clinical hematology*, 10th ed. Baltimore, MD: Williams and Wilkins, 1999: 1233–63.
147. Aldomet (methyldopa) prescribing information. Canonsburg, PA: Mylan Pharmaceuticals Inc; 1998.
148. Borthakur G, O'Brien S, Wierda WG et al. Immune anaemias in patients with chronic lymphocytic leukaemia treated with fludarabine, cyclophosphamide and rituximab—incidence and predictors. *Br J Haematol.* 2007; 136:800-5.
149. Patton WN, Duffull SB. Idiosyncratic drug-induced haematological abnormalities. Incidence, pathogenesis, management and avoidance. *Drug Saf.* 1994; 11:445-62.
150. Gehrs BC, Friedberg RC. Autoimmune hemolytic anemia. *Am J Hematol.* 2002; 69:258-71.
151. Ahrens N, Kingreen D, Seltsam A, Salama A. Treatment of refractory autoimmune haemolytic anaemia with anti-CD20 (rituximab). *Br J Haematol (England).* 2001; 114 :244-5.
152. Flores G, Cunningham-Rundles C, Newland AC, Bussel JB. Efficacy of intravenous immunoglobulin in the treatment of autoimmune hemolytic anemia: results in 73 patients. *Am J Hematol.* 1993; 44:237-42.
153. Creemers GJ, van Boven WP, Lowenberg B, van der Heul C. Azathioprine-associated pure red cell aplasia. *J Intern Med.* 1993; 233:85-7.
154. Kim CJ, Park KI, Inoue H et al. Azathioprine-induced megaloblastic anemia with pancytopenia 22 years after living-related renal transplantation. *Int J Urol.* 1998; 5:100-2.
155. Old CW, Flannery EP, Grogan TM et al. Azathioprine-induced pure red blood cell aplasia. *JAMA.* 1978; 240:552-4.
156. Lennard L, Murphy MF, Maddocks JL. Severe megaloblastic anaemia associated with abnormal azathioprine metabolism. *Br J Clin Pharmacol.* 1984; 17:171-2.
157. Toyokawa Y, Kingetsu I, Yasuda C et al. Pancytopenia, including macrocytic anemia, associated with leflunomide in a rheumatoid arthritis patient. *Mod Rheumatol.* 2007; 17:436-40.
158. Callaghan TS, Hadden DR, Tomkin GH. Megaloblastic anaemia due to vitamin B_{12} malabsorption associated with long-term metformin treatment. *Br Med J.* 1980; 280:1214-5.
159. Filioussi K, Bonovas S, Katsaros T. Should we screen diabetic patients using biguanides for megaloblastic anaemia? *Aust Fam Physician.* 2003; 32:383-4.
160. Morris JS. Nitrofurantoin and peripheral neuropathy with megaloblastic anaemia. *J Neurol Neurosurg Psychiatry.* 1966; 29:224-8.
161. Peaston MJ. Nitrofurantoin and megaloblastic anaemia. *Lancet.* 1964; 1:1161-2.
162. Blackwell EA, Hawson GA, Leer J, Bain B. Acute pancytopenia due to megaloblastic arrest in association with co-trimoxazole. *Med J Aust.* 1978; 2:38-41.
163. Snower DP, Weil SC. Changing etiology of macrocytosis. Zidovudine as a frequent causative factor. *Am J Clin Pathol.* 1993; 99:57-60.
164. Romanelli F, Empey K, Pomeroy C. Macrocytosis as an indicator of medication (zidovudine) adherence in patients with HIV infection. *AIDS Patient Care STDS.* 2002; 16:405-11.
165. Weinblatt ME. Toxicity of low dose methotrexate in rheumatoid arthritis. *J Rheumatol Suppl.* 1985; 12(suppl 12):35-9.
166. Hesdorffer CS, Longo DL. Drug-induced megaloblastic anemia. *N Engl J Med.* 2015; 373:1649-58.
167. Brinkman K, ter Hofstede HJ, Burger DM et al. Adverse effects of reverse transcriptase inhibitors: mitochondrial toxicity as common pathway. *Aids.* 1998; 12:1735-44.
168. Kobrinsky NL, Ramsay NK. Acute megaloblastic anemia induced by high-dose trimethoprim-sulfamethoxazole. *Ann Intern Med.* 1981; 94:780-1.
169. Magee F, O'Sullivan H, McCann SR. Megaloblastosis and low-dose trimethoprim-sulfamethoxazole. *Ann Intern Med.* 1981; 95:657.
170. Knight K, Wade S, Balducci L. Prevalence and outcomes of anemia in cancer: a systematic review of the literature. *Am J Med.* 2004; 116(suppl 7A):11s-26s.
171. Rizzo JD, Brouwers M, Hurley P et al. American Society of Clinical Oncology/American Society of Hematology clinical practice guideline update on the use of epoetin and darbepoetin in adult patients with cancer. *J Oncol Pract.* 2010 Nov; 6:317-20.
172. Chen VM, Thrift KM, Morel-Kopp MC et al. An immediate hemolytic reaction induced by repeated administration of oxaliplatin. *Transfusion.* 2004; 44:838-43.
173. Cobo F, De Celis G, Pereira A et al. Oxaliplatin-induced immune hemolytic anemia: a case report and review of the literature. *Anticancer Drugs.* 2007; 18:973-6.
174. Lyman GH, Berndt ER, Kallich JD et al. The economic burden of anemia in cancer patients receiving chemotherapy. *Value Health.* 2005; 8:149-56.
175. Sideris S, Loizidou A, Georgala A et al. Autoimmune haemolytic anaemia in a patient treated with capecitabine. *Acta Clin Belg.* 2013; 68:135-7.
176. Sakhri L, Mennecier B, Quoix A. [Hemolytic anemia under erlotinib treatment]. *Rev Pneumol Clin.* 2013; 69:345-50.
177. Song MK, Choi YJ, Seol YM et al. Nilotinib-induced bone marrow aplasia. *Eur J Haematol.* 2009; 83:161-2.
178. Berchem G, Dewilde S, Mahassen P. A case of acute haemolysis with 2 different multi target thyrosine kinase inhibitors in a patient with renal cancer. *Bull Soc Sci Med Grand Duche Luxemb.* 2009; (1):7-9.
179. Fusi A, Hodgetts J, Dennis M, Lorigan P. Vemurafenib-induced nonautoimmune haemolytic anaemia. *Melanoma Res.* 2014; 24:418-9.
180. Marks PW, Rosenthal DS. Hematologic manifestations of systemic disease: infection, chronic inflammation, and cancer. In: Hoffman R, Benz EJ Jr, Shattil SJ et al, eds. *Hematology: basic principles and practice.* 5th ed. Philadelphia, PA: Churchill Livingstone Elsevier. 2009; 2309-19.
181. National Comprehensive Cancer Network. National Comprehensive Cancer Network Guidelines for cancer and chemotherapy induced anemia. https://www.nccn.org/professionals/physician_gls/pdf/anemia.pdf (accessed 2018 Apr 24).
182. Ludwig H, Van Belle S, Barrett-Lee P et al. The European Cancer Anaemia Survey (ECAS): a large, multinational, prospective survey defining the prevalence, incidence, and treatment of anaemia in cancer patients. *Eur J Cancer.* 2004; 40:2293-306.
183. Wilson J, Yao GL, Raftery J et al. A systematic review and economic evaluation of epoetin alpha, epoetin beta and darbepoetin alpha in anaemia associated with cancer, especially that attributable to cancer treatment. *Health Technol Assess.* 2007; 11:1-202, iii-iv.
184. Schwartz RN. Anemia in patients with cancer: incidence, causes, impact, management, and use of treatment guidelines and protocols. *Am J Health-Syst Pharm.* 2007; 64(3 suppl 2):S5-13; quiz S28-30.
185. Steensma DP. Is anemia of cancer different from chemotherapy-induced anemia? *J Clin Oncol.* 2008; 26:1022-4.
186. Bennett CL, Silver SM, Djulbegovic B et al. Venous thromboembolism and mortality associated with recombinant erythropoietin and darbepoetin administration for the treatment of cancer-associated anemia. *JAMA.* 2008; 299:914-24.
187. US Food and Drug Administration. Epoetin alfa label. https://www.accessdata.fda.gov/drugsatfda_docs/label/2010/103234s5199lbl.pdf (accessed 2018 Apr 24).
188. US Food and Drug Administration. Darbepoetin alfa label. https://www.accessdata.fda.gov/drugsatfda_docs/label/2010/103234s5199lbl.pdf (accessed 2018 Apr 24).

SECTION XI

DRUG-INDUCED BONE, JOINT, AND MUSCLE DISEASES

Chapter 50 Osteoporosis and Osteomalacia

Chapter 51 Gout and Hyperuricemia

Chapter 52 Myopathy

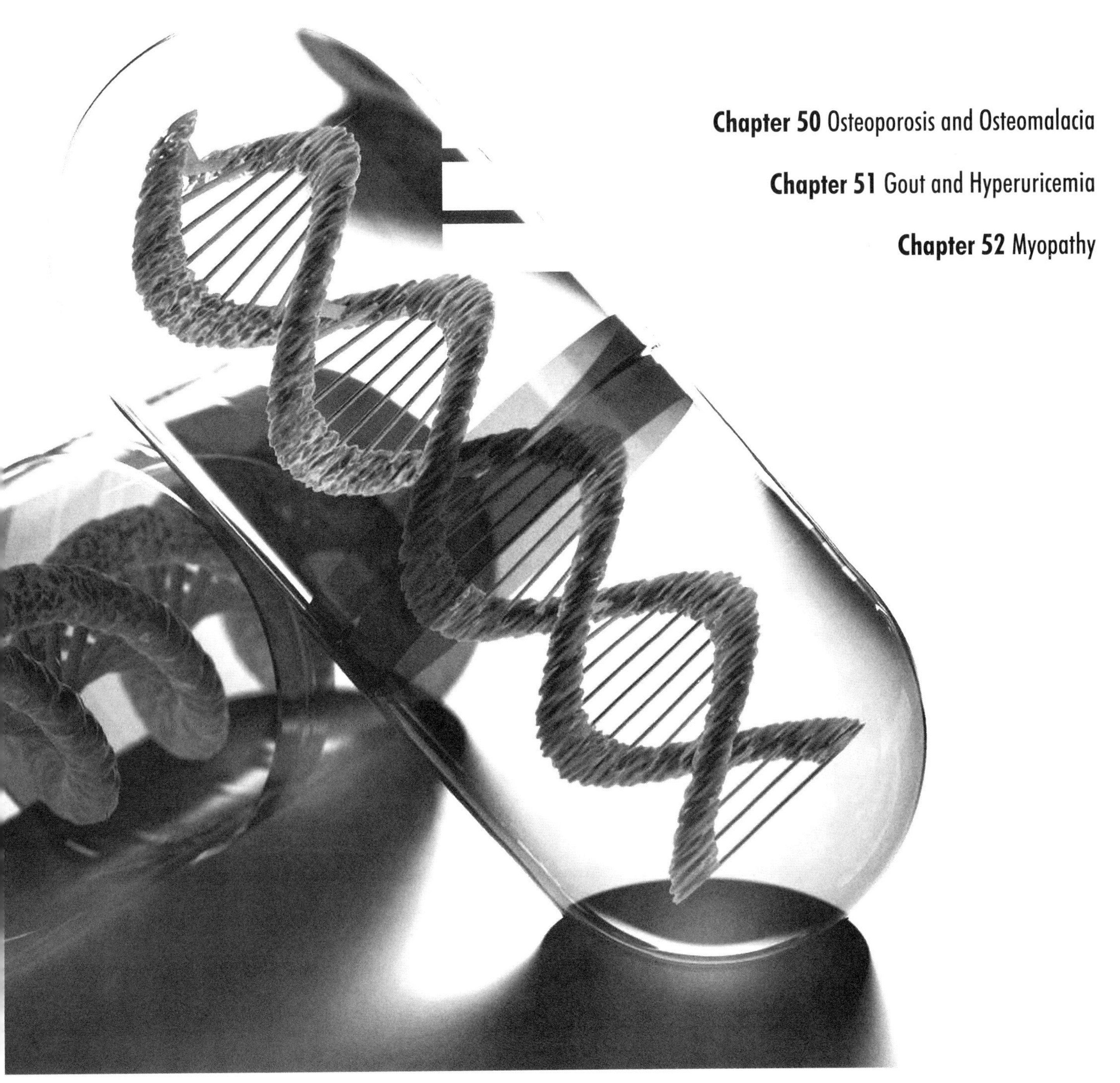

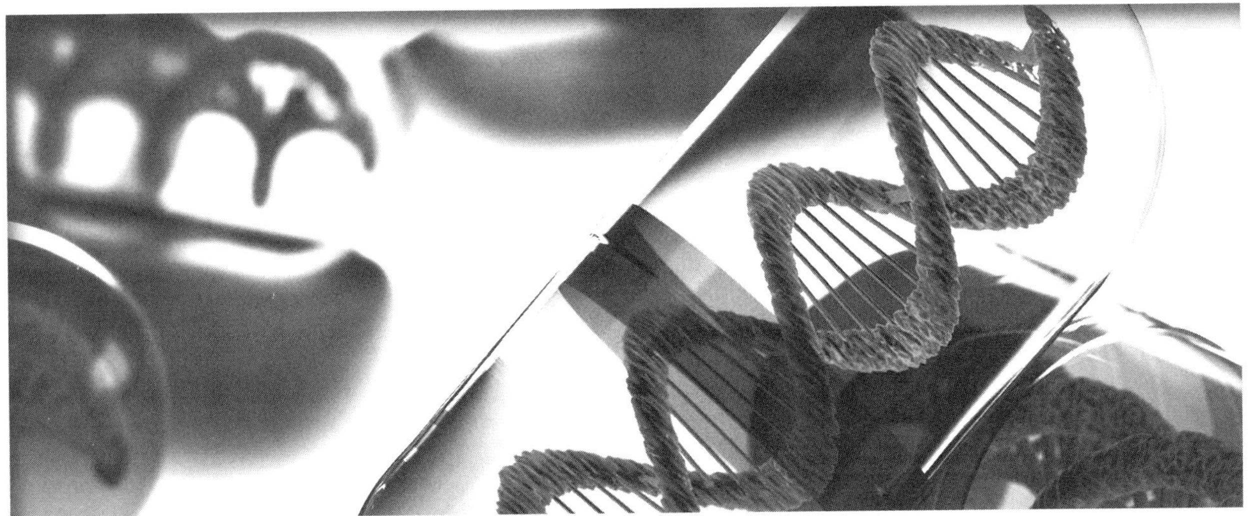

CHAPTER 50

Osteoporosis and Osteomalacia

Laura M. Borgelt and Danielle R. Fixen

The United States Bone and Joint Initiative, as part of the Global Alliance for Musculoskeletal Health, is the U.S. National Action Network of the Global Bone and Joint Decade.[1] It is a group of patient and healthcare professional organizations, medical schools, government agencies, health-system providers, and industry established to improve prevention of bone and joint disorders and the quality of life for those affected by these conditions. The primary goal of this initiative is to advance care and reduce the burden of disease for individuals with various musculoskeletal conditions. Other goals include increasing awareness and educating the world on the increasing societal impact of musculoskeletal injuries and disorders, empowering patients to participate in decisions about their care and treatment, increase global funding for prevention activities and treatment research, and continually seeking and promoting cost-effective prevention and treatment of musculoskeletal injuries and disorders. Although many musculoskeletal conditions are incorporated into its aims, osteoporosis is recognized as a significant contributor to the healthcare burden worldwide. The spirit of this initiative suggests that all healthcare providers should increase attention to screening patients, provide education, perform research, and work to help ensure proper management and follow-up of patients diagnosed with these and related disorders as a way to help prevent the devastating consequences of fracture and its potential complications of chronic pain, disability, and death.[1] This includes evaluation of medications that may cause musculoskeletal conditions such as osteoporosis and osteomalacia.

Deterioration of bone mass not associated with other chronic illness is referred to as primary osteoporosis and is related to aging and decreased gonadal function. Secondary osteoporosis can be viewed as low bone mineral density or increased risk of fragility fracture caused by any factor other than aging or postmenopausal status, such as medical disorders or medication exposures.[2] Differentiating between primary osteoporosis and the various causes of secondary osteoporosis can be challenging due to the many disease states and drugs that may be involved. Individuals with secondary osteoporosis experience bone loss greater than that caused by aging and menopause in primary osteoporosis, and it is especially important, therefore, to identify, accurately evaluate, and appropriately treat these patients.[2]

Osteomalacia is a softening of the bones, typically due to vitamin D deficiency and less commonly due to hypophosphatemia or hypocalcemia. In children, this condition is called rickets. Osteomalacia can cause fatigue, bone pain, muscle weakness, and difficulty walking and result in bone fracture.[3] Drugs that may affect vitamin D metabolism should be cautiously prescribed in patients at risk for the development of osteomalacia.

CAUSATIVE AGENTS

Medications commonly associated with osteoporosis or osteomalacia are listed in **Table 50-1**.[4-59] The impact of each of the medications on bone mineral density (BMD) or fracture incidence (or both) is presented where data are available.

Glucocorticoids are the most common cause of drug-induced osteoporosis, and their effects appear to be dose- and duration-dependent.[2,45] An increased risk of fracture has been reported for patients taking prednisone 2.5 mg or more daily; national recommendations indicate prednisone ≥5 mg/day (or equivalent exposure to other glucocorticoids) for ≥3 months may result in low bone mass or bone loss.[60] Approximately 30–50% of patients receiving long-term glucocorticoid therapy will experience a fracture.[47,48]

EPIDEMIOLOGY

It is estimated that over 200 million people worldwide suffer from osteoporosis.[61] Approximately 10 million Americans have osteoporosis and an additional 43 million have low bone mass or osteopenia as defined by the World Health Organization (WHO).[60,62] This accounts for approximately 55% of people age 50 years and older in the United States. More than 2 million fractures were attributed to osteoporosis in 2005 and this number is expected to exceed 3 million by 2025.[63] Fracture rates in other countries tend to vary. For example, wrist and hip fracture in the United Kingdom occurs at a rate about 30% lower than that in the United States and hip fracture incidence differs among various Asian countries.[64] Although secondary osteoporosis is known to be common, precise data regarding its incidence are not available. More than two thirds of men, more than half of premenopausal women, and approximately one third of postmenopausal women with osteoporosis have a disease state or drug therapy contributing to their bone loss.[65] The incidence of drug-induced bone loss or increased bone fragility is difficult to quantify, as medications usually contribute to an increased risk of osteoporosis rather than represent its sole cause. Table 50-1 provides information regarding the risks for bone loss and fractures with drug use.

Vitamin D deficiency is one of the most common secondary causes for bone loss and fractures, especially in the elderly. Prolonged, severe vitamin D deficiency can lead to poor bone mineralization and osteomalacia. The overall incidence of vitamin D–induced osteomalacia is not precisely known, but it appears to be lower in the United States than in many other countries because of fortification of milk with vitamin D.

MECHANISMS

The process through which bone undergoes repair and readjustment is called bone remodeling, and there are three main cells involved in this process: osteoblasts, osetocytes, and osteoclasts. Osteoblasts are derived from a mesenchymal stem cell precursor and are responsible for synthesizing the organic bone matrix (osteoid) and mineralizing the bone. Osteocytes, which are retired osteoblasts trapped in bone, are considered the communication cells and help coordinate the remodeling cycle at a particular site. Osteoclasts are derived from hematopoietic precursors of the monocyte–macrophage lineage and are responsible for bone resorption.

The remodeling process begins when the receptor activator of nuclear factor kappa-B ligand (RANKL), which is secreted from the osteoblast precursor cells, binds to its receptor activator of nuclear factor kappa-B (RANK) on the surface of the osteoclast precursor cells. This leads to the differentiation and activation of mature osteoclasts, which in turn resorb bone through the degradation of the protein matrix and demineralization. Once bone resorption is complete at that site, cytokines and growth factors that are involved in chemotaxis, proliferation, and

Table 50-1 Agents Implicated in Drug-Induced Osteoporosis and Osteomalacia

Drug	Incidence	Level of Evidence[a]
Antiepileptics[4-7,b]	BMD: 0.35–1.8% bone loss Fracture: RR 2.18; 95% CI 1.94–2.45	B
Antineoplastic agents[8,9]	BMD: 6.08–7.24% bone loss Fracture: OR 1.49; 95% CI 1.25–1.77	B
Antiretroviral therapy[10-13]	BMD: 1–6% bone loss; patients receiving antiretroviral therapy with osteoporosis—OR 2.38; 95% CI 1.20–4.75; patients receiving PI with osteoporosis—OR 1.57; 95% CI 1.05–2.34 Fracture: Not known	B
Aromatase inhibitors[14-19]	BMD: 2.5–5% bone loss in spine and 1.5–5% in hip (average 2% bone loss per year) Fracture: 7.1% with anastrozole; 5.7% with letrozole	B
Canagliflozin[20,21]	BMD: Decreases bone mineral density in total hip Fracture: 2.7%; difference versus noncanagliflozin 0.8%; 95% CI 1–1.74	B
Cyclosporine[22]	Not known—usually confounded by concomitant glucocorticoid use	C
Depot medroxyprogesterone[23-27,c]	BMD: 2–8% bone loss Fracture: Incidence rate ratio versus nonusers 1.41 (95% CI 1.35–1.47)	B
Furosemide[28,29]	BMD: Bone loss may increase by 0.3% per year of treatment Fracture: RR 3.9; 95% CI 1.5–10.4	B
Gonadotropin-releasing hormone agonists[30,31]	BMD: 6–7% hip bone loss; 5–10% trabecular bone loss Fracture: Vertebral RR 1.45; 95% CI 1.19–1.75; hip RR 1.3; 95% CI 1.1–1.53	B
Methotrexate (high dose)[32-35]	BMD: Bone loss 0.2–1.6% Fracture: 12–45%	C
Levothyroxine (oversupplementation)[36-39]	BMD: 10–12% bone loss Fracture: HR 1.56; 95% CI 1.03–2.37 (highest with doses >150 mcg/day)	B
Proton pump inhibitors[40,41]	BMD: Not known Fracture: HR 1.28; 95% CI 1.13–1.44	B
Selective serotonin reuptake inhibitors[42,43]	BMD: 4.4–6.2% bone loss Fracture: RR 1.61; 95% CI 1.49–1.74	B
Systemic glucocorticoids[44-48]	BMD: Density consistently lower than that expected for group of similar age and sex Fracture: 30–50%; major fracture RR 1.25; 95% CI 1.07–1.45 and hip fracture RR 1.61; 95% CI 1.18–2.20	A
Thiazolidinediones[49-51]	BMD: Accelerated bone loss by 0.6–1.2%/yr Fracture: Up to 9% Women: OR 1.94; 95% CI 1.60–2.35; p <0.001 Men: OR 1.02; 95% CI 0.83–1.27; p = 0.83	B
Unfractionated heparin and low-molecular-weight heparin[52-55,d]	BMD: Up to 30% bone loss Fracture: 2.2–3.6%	B
Vitamin A (dose >1.5 mg/day of retinol form)[56-59]	BMD: 10–14% bone loss Fracture: Increased RR	B

BMD = bone mineral density, CI = confidence interval, OR = odds ratio, RR = relative risk, PI = protease inhibitor.

[a]Definitions for Levels of Evidence: Level A—evidence from one or more randomized, controlled clinical trials; Level B—evidence from nonrandomized clinical trials, prospective observational studies, cohort studies, retrospective studies, case-control studies, meta-analyses and/or postmarketing surveillance studies; and Level C—evidence from one or more published case reports or case series.

[b]Most evidence with phenytoin and phenobarbital (limited or conflicting data with carbamazepine and valproic acid).

[c]Evidence of at least partial recovery after discontinuation.

[d]Most data related to long-term heparin use (≥15,000 units for ≥6 months) rather than low-molecular-weight heparins.

differentiation of osteoblasts are released. Osteoprotegerin (OPG), a soluble decoy protein, is secreted by the osteoblast precursor cells and competes with RANKL for RANK. This leads to inhibition of the differentiation and activation of osteoclasts, thus stopping bone resorption at that site. Mature osteoblasts form new bone by first laying down collagen and other noncollagenous proteins to create the osteoid and then mineralize it. When bone formation is complete, mature osteoblasts become either lining cells or osteocytes or undergo apoptosis. That section of bone is now in the resting phase, called quiescence, until a new remodeling cycle is activated.

Under normal circumstances, bone remodeling should not lead to a net loss of bone. However, after peak bone mass is achieved (typically between 18–25 years of age), physiologic changes occur that result in bone resorption exceeding bone formation (typically around 40 years of age).[60] During perimenopause and for up to 5–7 years after menopause, women can experience an accelerated rate of bone loss due to a drop in circulating estrogen, leading to an increase in osteoclastic activity and heightened bone resorption. In the elderly, bone loss at a rate of approximately 0.5–1% per year is caused by a combination of an accelerated rate of bone resorption and a reduced rate of bone formation. Decreased calcium absorption and sex hormone concentrations and impaired osteoblast function appear to be the largest contributors to bone loss in the elderly.

Drugs can contribute to bone loss in patients of any age by interfering with various steps in the bone remodeling process. The most common mechanism involves increased osteoclast maturation and function leading to accelerated bone resorption. Several drugs increase bone resorption by reducing sex hormone production. Suppressed osteoblast activity, increased bone resorption, and impaired bone mineralization can also be caused by medications.[20,66] Glucocorticoid use is the most common secondary cause of osteoporosis and the third most common cause of osteoporosis overall.[67] Glucocorticoids are extremely damaging to bone tissue because they can negatively affect all aspects of bone remodeling. They decrease bone formation through effects on osteoblasts.[67,68] These drugs can interfere with natural repair mechanisms through increased apoptosis of osteocytes.[67] They increase bone resorption by increasing the expression of RANKL and decreasing the expression of OPG, reducing sex hormone production, and causing a negative calcium balance through a decrease in calcium absorption and an increase in urinary calcium excretion.[67-69]

Endogenous production of cholecalciferol (vitamin D_3) from exposure to ultraviolet B (UVB) light is the primary source of vitamin D. Activation of cholecalciferol occurs in the liver and the kidney. Synthesis can be reduced by factors that interfere with the penetration of UVB light into the skin or impair the various steps in its conversion. The diet is a secondary source for vitamin D, although there are very few foods that have naturally high vitamin D content. Vitamin D is important for calcium homeostasis. Adequate concentrations of vitamin D are needed to ensure appropriate intestinal calcium absorption and adequate concentrations of calcium are needed for proper mineralization of bone. Inadequate body stores of vitamin D can lead to insufficient calcium absorption and decreased serum calcium concentrations, which can lead to secondary hyperparathyroidism. Parathyroid hormone decreases calcium excretion by the kidney and increases bone resorption to mobilize calcium stores, thus increasing serum calcium concentrations. Increased bone turnover with bone loss and poor bone mineralization are consequences of severe vitamin D deficiency. Vitamin D deficiency has also been associated with muscle weakness and an increased risk for falls.[70] Antiepileptic medications including phenytoin, carbamazepine, and phenobarbital have been implicated in contributing to severe vitamin D deficiency and osteomalacia. Interference with vitamin D metabolism and subsequent hypocalcemia is the most common mechanism for drug-induced osteomalacia. Less common mechanisms include hypophosphatemia and a direct effect on mineralization.[71] **Table 50-2** describes mechanisms of drug-induced osteoporosis and osteomalacia.

Table 50-2 Mechanisms of Drug-Induced Osteoporosis and Osteomalacia

Drug	Mechanism
Antiepileptics: phenytoin, carbamazepine, phenobarbital[71-73]	May cause severe vitamin D deficiency and osteomalacia; may induce the cytochrome P-450 enzyme system leading to inactivation of vitamin D, which decreases calcium uptake
Valproic acid[66]	Osteomalacia possibly due to increased renal excretion of calcium and phosphorus
Antiretroviral therapy[74] Nucleoside reverse-transcriptase inhibitors: tenofovir, zidovudine, didanosine, lamivudine[75] Protease inhibitors: nelfinavir > indinavir > saquinavir > ritonavir[76] Nelfinavir, lopinavir,[76] indinavir	Increase osteoclastogenesis (in vivo) Increase osteoclast activity (ex vivo data) Decrease expression of OPG (ex vivo data) Attenuate the function and recruitment of osteoblasts (in vivo)
Antineoplastic agents: bicalutamide, busulfan, cyclophosphamide, ifosfamide[71]	Bone loss secondary to inhibitory effects on gonadal function May cause renal phosphate wasting leading to osteomalacia and bone loss
Aromatase inhibitors (letrozole, anastrozole)[14]	Inhibit peripheral conversion of androgens to estrogens, leading to lower estrogen levels
Canagliflozin[77]	Increases serum phosphate concentration causing increased PTH concentration leading to bone resorption
Cyclosporine[22]	Accelerates bone turnover
Depot medroxyprogesterone[26]	Suppresses the hypothalamic-pituitary-ovarian axis leading to reduced estrogen
Furosemide[28]	Inhibits the sodium–potassium–chloride cotransporter in the thick ascending limb of Henle leading to renal calcium excretion; bone loss appears to be minimized by increases in PTH and 1,25-dihydroxyvitamin D concentrations and a subsequent increase in intestinal calcium absorption
GnRH agonists (e.g., leuprolide, goserelin)[31]	Decrease production of sex hormones
Methotrexate (high dose)[78]	Increases apoptosis of osteocytes and number of osteoclasts
Levothyroxine (oversupplementation)[79,80]	Possibly increases bone resorption
Proton pump inhibitors	Cause calcium malabsorption secondary to acid suppression
Selective serotonin reuptake inhibitors[42,43]	May inhibit serotonin transporter system in osteoblasts leading to reduced activity and bone formation
Systemic glucocorticoids[67-69]	Decrease bone formation: • Decrease proliferation and differentiation of osteoblastic cells and enhance apoptosis of osteoblasts • Interfere with the bone's natural repair mechanism through increased apoptosis of osteocytes (bone's communication cells) Increase bone resorption: • Increase the expression of RANKL and decrease the expression of OPG, its soluble decoy receptor, both of which will increase osteoclastogenesis • Reduce estrogen and testosterone concentrations by decreasing the production of luteinizing hormone from the pituitary and through adrenal suppression • Cause a negative calcium balance by decreasing calcium absorption and increasing urinary calcium excretion

Table 50-2 Mechanisms of Drug-Induced Osteoporosis and Osteomalacia (continued)

Drug	Mechanism
Thiazolidinediones (pioglitazone, rosiglitazone)[49,81,82]	Reduce osteoblastic bone formation by increasing adipogenesis and decreasing osteoblastogenesis
Unfractionated heparin/low-molecular-weight heparin[83]	Decreases bone formation and increases bone resorption by inhibiting the expression of OPG
Vitamin A (large amounts of retinol form)[84,85]	Increases osteoclastic activity and decreases osteoblastic activity leading to increased bone resorption; possible interference with vitamin D function

GnRH = gonadotropin-releasing hormone, PTH = parathyroid hormone, OPG = osteoprotegerin, RANKL = receptor activator of nuclear factor kappa-B ligand.

CLINICAL PRESENTATION AND DIFFERENTIAL DIAGNOSIS

The clinical presentation of patients with drug-induced osteoporosis is not generally different from that of patients presenting with osteoporosis from other causes (**Tables 50-3** and **50-4**).

Table 50-3 Signs and Symptoms Associated with Drug-Induced Osteoporosis and Osteomalacia[60,87]

Osteoporosis

- Acute or chronic pain, or no pain (vertebral fracture)
- Acute pain (nonvertebral fracture)
- Decreased bone mineral density (T-score −2.5 and below or Z-score −2 and below[a])
- Kyphosis (Dowager's hump)
- Low trauma fractures

Osteomalacia

- Decreased bone mineral density
- Diffuse skeletal pain
- Hyperparathyroidism
- Hypocalcemia
- Hypophosphatemia
- Low trauma fractures
- Muscle weakness
- Vitamin D deficiency
- "Waddling" gait

[a]T-score represents number of standard deviations below or above the mean bone mineral density for a healthy, sex- and race-matched, young adult (20–29 years) reference population; Z-score represents number of standard deviations below or above the mean bone mineral density for an age-, sex-, and race-matched reference population.

Table 50-4 Conditions to Consider in the Differential Diagnosis of Drug-Induced Osteoporosis and Osteomalacia[2]

- Alcoholism
- Anorexia nervosa
- End-organ failure and transplantation
- Endocrine disorders (e.g., hyperparathyroidism, Cushing syndrome, hyperthyroidism, growth hormone deficiency, acromegaly, male hypogonadism, hyperprolactinemia including drug-induced hyperprolactinemia, diabetes mellitus, vitamin D deficiency)
- Gastrointestinal disorders (e.g., celiac disease, inflammatory bowel disease, bariatric surgery)
- Genetic disorders (e.g., Ehlers–Danlos syndrome, hemochromatosis, Marfan syndrome, porphyria)
- Hematologic/oncologic disorders (e.g., multiple myeloma, sickle cell disease, thalassemia major, systemic mastocytosis)
- Idiopathic hypercalciuria
- Immobility
- Infectious diseases (e.g., human immunodeficiency virus)
- Neurologic disorders (e.g., spinal cord injury/immobilization, Parkinson disease, multiple sclerosis)
- Nutritional deficiencies (e.g., calcium, magnesium, vitamin D)
- Pulmonary disorders (e.g., chronic obstructive pulmonary disease)
- Rheumatologic disorders (e.g., rheumatoid arthritis, ankylosing spondylitis, systemic lupus erythematosus)
- Transplantation

Asymptomatic patients typically are identified through routine BMD testing, and T-scores and Z-scores are used to determine whether or not bone disease exists. The T-score represents the number of standard deviations below or above the mean BMD for a healthy, sex- and race-matched young adult

(20–29 years) reference population. A Z-score represents the number of standard deviations below or above the mean BMD for an age-, sex-, and race-matched reference population.

Dual-energy x-ray absorptiometry measurements of the hip and spine are used to establish or confirm a diagnosis of osteoporosis.[60] For postmenopausal women and men 50 years of age or over, a normal BMD is defined as a T-score of −1 and above; low bone mass or osteopenia is defined as a T-score between −1 and −2.5; and osteoporosis is defined as a T-score at or below −2.5.[60] For premenopausal women and men younger than 50 years of age with a suspected secondary cause, a Z-score of −2 or below is considered "below the expected range for age" and is indicative of osteoporosis.[86] When any Z-score is −2 or worse, secondary causes of osteoporosis (including drug-induced) should be ruled out, regardless of age.

The decision to perform bone density assessment should be based on individual fracture risk and skeletal health. BMD testing is indicated in adults taking a medication (e.g., glucocorticoids in a daily dose of ≥5 mg of prednisone or equivalent for ≥3 months) associated with low bone mass or bone loss.[60,87] The WHO fracture risk assessment model incorporates various risk factors along with hip BMD results to assess an individual's risk of future fractures. This tool describes the probability of fracture in the next 10 years and can provide guidance regarding treatment.[87]

The National Osteoporosis Foundation and the International Society of Clinical Densitometry recommends BMD testing for adults taking medications such as glucocorticoids that are associated with bone loss. Central dual-energy x-ray absorptiometry screening should be performed as part of the treatment strategy for these patients. Most experts agree that a clinical diagnosis of osteoporosis can be made without further testing in any patient who has a suspected secondary cause for osteoporosis and presents with a low trauma fracture.

Suspicion of drug-induced osteoporosis is typically higher when the disease is identified in individuals in whom it would not typically be expected (e.g., men under age 50 or premenopausal women). However, drugs should always be suspected as a possible cause of osteoporosis or osteomalacia in any patient receiving agents associated with bone loss and fractures. Other secondary causes of osteoporosis to consider include lifestyle factors such as excessive alcohol consumption, genetic disorders, hypogonadal states, human immunodeficiency virus, endocrine disorders, gastrointestinal disorders, and hematologic disorders. Table 50-4 lists conditions to consider in the differential diagnosis of drug-induced osteoporosis.

There is no current consensus regarding what constitutes appropriate and cost-effective evaluation of patients with suspected secondary osteoporosis. In addition to a complete history and physical examination, the National Osteoporosis Foundation (NOF) recommends assessing liver enzymes, thyroid-stimulating hormone, parathyroid hormone, total testosterone and gonadotropin, serum 25-hydroxyvitamin D, and serum and urine calcium.[60] The American Association of Clinical Endocrinologists recommends a complete blood count and measuring serum calcium, phosphorus, total protein, albumin, creatinine, liver enzymes, alkaline phosphatase, electrolytes, and urinary calcium excretion.[88] Additional laboratory tests may be necessary, and their use will vary depending on the suspected cause.

Signs and symptoms of drug-induced osteomalacia often develop slowly, and the presentation is generally not different from that of patients with osteomalacia from other causes.[71] Typical symptoms include generalized bone pain and muscle weakness, which can lead to a characteristic waddling gait. Patients with osteomalacia may also present with fractures and with osteopenia or osteoporosis. Abnormal laboratory findings in these patients might include hypocalcemia, hypophosphatemia, hypovitaminosis D, and increased serum parathyroid hormone or alkaline phosphatase concentrations, or both.[71]

RISK FACTORS

Many patients with drug-induced osteoporosis have other risks that increase the likelihood of bone loss and fractures. It is frequently the combination of the drug and the underlying risks that lead to osteoporosis. General risk factors for the development of osteoporosis include potentially modifiable adverse lifestyle practices such as low calcium intake, consumption of three or more alcoholic beverages per day, smoking, and inadequate physical activity. Advanced age, female sex, history of falls or fractures (or both), low body weight or body-mass index, hypogonadism (postmenopausal status), and family history of fracture all significantly increase fracture risk and may or may not be modifiable. Several of these risk factors are included in the WHO Fracture Risk Assessment Model.

Several diseases and the drugs used in their treatment have been associated with adverse bone effects. It is often difficult to separate the effects of the drugs on bone remodeling from the effects of the disease state for which the drug is being used. For example, a systematic review identified that patients with chronic obstructive pulmonary disease (COPD) were at high risk for osteopenia and osteoporosis, with a reported prevalence ranging from 9% to 69% and 27% to 67%, respectively.[89] This review also found low body mass index correlates to osteoporosis and/or low BMD. Measures of body composition, disease severity, and the use of corticosteroids in COPD make it difficult to prove causality of these individual effects on bone health. Similarly, patients undergoing solid-organ transplantation are at high risk for osteoporosis due in part to the effects antirejection medications have on bone remodeling, even though the effect of the underlying organ failure on bone remodeling may be more important.

Certain patients are at an increased risk for drug-induced vitamin D deficiency and osteomalacia. Patients who are institutionalized, live in extreme northern latitudes, are elderly, have malabsorptive disease states, have cultural or religious beliefs that require full body coverage with clothing, or who belong to ethnic and racial groups with darkly pigmented skin are all at increased risk for low vitamin D concentrations.[90,91] The elderly are especially at risk because of a combination of factors including inadequate exposure to sunlight, a reduced skin conversion of 7-dehydrocholesterol to vitamin D_3, and impaired calcium absorption secondary to decreased intestinal responsiveness to vitamin D. Risk factors for drug-induced osteoporosis and osteomalacia are presented in **Table 50-5**.

MORBIDITY AND MORTALITY

Fractures are the most disconcerting consequence of drug-induced osteoporosis or osteomalacia. In 2000, there were an estimated 9 million new osteoporotic fractures worldwide, of which 1.6 million were at the hip, 1.7 million were at the forearm,

Table 50-5 Risk Factors for Drug-Induced Osteoporosis and Osteomalacia[60,66]

- Advanced age
- Alcohol intake >2 servings per day
- Current cigarette smoking
- Female sex
- History of falls
- History of low trauma fracture in a parent or sibling
- Inadequate calcium intake
- Low body weight/body-mass index
- Low-trauma fracture as an adult
- Physical inactivity

Selected disease states associated with bone loss and fractures

- Chronic liver or kidney disease
- Chronic obstructive pulmonary disease
- Depression
- Diabetes mellitus (types 1 and 2)
- History of thyrotoxicosis
- Hypogonadism
- Inflammatory bowel disease
- Multiple sclerosis
- Rheumatoid arthritis
- Solid-organ transplant
- Vitamin D deficiency

Drug-specific risk factors

- Antiepileptic agents: Immobility, handicapped patients, combination of agents, higher doses, long-term use, factors that contribute to vitamin D deficiency such as darkly pigmented skin, institutionalization, limited sunlight exposure, malabsorptive states
- Heparin: High-dose, long-term
- Systemic glucocorticoids: Dose- and duration-dependent; higher cumulative exposure
- Thyroid hormone: Oversuppression of thyroid-stimulating hormone to <0.1 milli-international units/L
- Vitamin A: High doses (at least 2 times the recommended daily allowance)

and 1.4 million were clinical vertebral fractures.[92] Most of these fractures (51%) occurred in Europe and the Americas; the rest occurred in the Western Pacific region and Southeast Asia. Furthermore, one in three women over 50 years will experience osteoporotic fractures, as will one in five men over 50 years. By 2050, the worldwide incidence of hip fracture is projected to increase by 240% in women and 310% in men.[93] Most fractures in older adults are due in part to low bone mass, which can be drug-induced. Fractures can also impact morbidity by causing psychological symptoms, especially depression, reduced self-esteem, anxiety, fear, and anger as patients struggle with pain, physical limitations, and lifestyle and cosmetic changes.[60] Approximately 60% of patients with hip fracture lose their prefracture level of independence, which may strain interpersonal relationships and social roles for patients and their families. Furthermore, about 20% of patients with a hip fracture require long-term nursing home care.[1] Although many patients with fractures go on to full recovery, others may experience chronic pain, disability, and even death.

Hip fractures increase the risk of mortality within 1 year after the injury by 8–36% and are associated with a 2.5-fold increased risk of future fractures.[94,95] Mortality is also increased after vertebral fractures, which can cause back pain, height loss, and kyphosis.[60] The postural changes that occur with kyphosis may limit activity (e.g., bending and reaching). Vertebral fractures may result in restrictive lung disease and/or altered abdominal anatomy, which may lead to constipation, abdominal pain, distention, reduced appetite, and premature satiety. Vertebral fractures are also major predictors of future fractures with up to a 5-fold increased risk for subsequent vertebral fractures and a 2- to 3-fold increased risk for fractures at other sites.[60]

The exact incidence of morbidity and mortality secondary to drug-induced osteoporosis is not known. Glucocorticoids are the most common cause of drug-induced osteoporosis, and it is estimated that 0.2–0.5% of the general population receives systemic glucocorticoids and that 30–50% of patients receiving long-term glucocorticoid therapy will experience a fracture.[47,48]

Fracture risk increases in the first 3 months after glucocorticoid initiation and decreases after discontinuing glucocorticoid therapy; however, the risk appears never to return to baseline.[96]

PREVENTION

All persons starting or continuing therapy with a medication known to have bone-damaging effects should be assessed for the presence of other possible causes of and risk factors for bone loss and fracture. Exposure to potential culprit agents should be minimized by using the lowest dose and shortest treatment duration possible. Sometimes it is possible to substitute other drugs or routes of administration with similar efficacy but a lower risk profile. For example, inhaled glucocorticoids at usual doses are not thought to cause appreciable bone loss as compared to systemic glucocorticoids and should be used preferentially whenever possible in patients with respiratory diseases such as COPD and asthma.[96] Although data are inconclusive regarding the effects of inhaled corticosteroids on bone density, a trend toward decreased BMD and increased fracture risk in patients using long-term moderate- to high-dose inhaled corticosteroids has been demonstrated.[96,97] In patients who have undergone transplantation, use of immunosuppressive agents such as rapamycin, tacrolimus, or mycophenolate mofetil, which are less likely to cause osteoporosis than cyclosporine, may be considered. Newer antiepileptic drugs such as lamotrigine, topiramate, and levetiracetam are less likely than phenytoin, carbamazepine, or phenobarbital to cause osteomalacia and osteoporosis. Ritonavir, a protease inhibitor often used to boost antiretroviral therapy, has been shown to inhibit osteoclast maturation and function leading to reduced bone resorption and may be a bone-sparing alternative for patients with human immunodeficiency virus receiving highly active antiretroviral therapy.[98,99] Raltegravir or abacavir may be better options than tenofovir disoproxil for patients at high risk of osteopenia or osteoporosis.[11,100] Consideration of these types of lower-risk alternative therapies is especially important in patients with multiple underlying risk factors for bone loss and fractures.

An important first step in preventing drug-induced osteoporosis is educating the patient regarding a bone-healthy lifestyle. Patients should be counseled on smoking cessation and limiting alcohol and caffeine consumption.[60] Regular weight-bearing and muscle-strengthening exercises should be encouraged to help maintain bone mass and reduce the risk of falls. Other fall-prevention strategies should be discussed with patients at high risk for falling. Methods to achieve adequate intake of calcium and vitamin D should be reviewed. **Table 50-6** describes approaches to help prevent drug-induced osteoporosis and osteomalacia.

Table 50-6 Approaches to Help Prevent Drug-Induced Osteoporosis and Osteomalacia[60,69,91,101,102]

General strategies

- Identify and manage other secondary causes and risk factors
- Use an alternative therapy with a lower risk, if possible
- Use therapy for the shortest time possible and at the lowest effective dose

Drug-specific

- 2,000–4,000 units/day of oral cholecalciferol (vitamin D_3) or 50,000 units of oral ergocalciferol (vitamin D_2) every 1–4 weeks may be needed in patients receiving enzyme-inducing antiepileptic drugs
- Consider low-molecular-weight heparin instead of unfractionated heparin in patients who require long-term anticoagulation and in whom warfarin is contraindicated (e.g., pregnancy)
- Use inhaled glucocorticoids in place of systemic drugs when possible for the treatment of respiratory diseases such as asthma and chronic obstructive pulmonary disease
- Use H_2 blockers instead of proton pump inhibitor for gastroesophageal reflux disease when possible in patients taking a bisphosphonate
- Use multivitamin supplements that contain no more than the recommended dietary allowance of 700 mcg/day (adult female) to 900 mcg/day vitamin A; upper tolerable limit (adults) = 3,000 mcg/day
- Use steroid-sparing therapies for rheumatoid arthritis, inflammatory bowel disease, and organ transplantation when possible

Bone-healthy lifestyle

- Adequate calcium intake[a]:

Age (yr)	Recommendation
1–3	500 mg
4–8	800 mg
9–18	1,300 mg
19–49	1,000 mg
≥50	1,200 mg

- Adequate vitamin D intake[a,b]:

Age (yr)	Recommendation
1–18	400 units
19–49	400–800 units
≥50	800–1,000 units
Pregnant or lactating	400–800 units

- Alcohol intake ≤1 serving/day (women) and ≤2 servings/day (men)
- Caffeine intake ≤2 servings/day
- Reduce fall risk
- Resistance/strengthening exercises (free weights, resistance bands, weight machines) for 20–30 min/day, 2–3 days/wk
- Smoking cessation
- Weight-bearing exercise of moderate intensity for at least 30 min most days of the week

[a]1,500 mg of calcium and 800 international units of vitamin D are recommended in patients receiving glucocorticoids at a dose of ≥5 mg prednisone or equivalent for ≥3 months.

[b]Higher intake of vitamin D may be needed in patients with vitamin D concentrations in the deficient range (25-hydroxy vitamin D concentration <12 ng/mL).

MANAGEMENT

Treatment strategies for drug-induced osteoporosis or osteomalacia are similar to those used in the management of primary osteoporosis and osteomalacia and are presented in **Table 50-7**.

When a drug is believed to be contributing to bone loss, discontinuation of the suspected agent or a reduction in dose, when possible, is an important first step. Although specific guidelines exist for some medications known to cause secondary osteoporosis (e.g., glucocorticoids), even in the absence of specific guidelines, most experts agree that bisphosphonates and other approved agents for primary osteoporosis are reasonable treatment options for patients with drug-induced osteoporosis.[69] In all cases, counseling patients about the importance of calcium, vitamin D, exercise, and other healthy bone lifestyle practices should be incorporated as a part of the treatment plan.[60]

The NOF recommends consideration of treatment for postmenopausal women and men age 50 years and older with the following presentation(s)[60]:

- A hip or vertebral (clinical or found on vertebral imaging) fracture
- T-score ≤−2.5 at the femoral neck, total hip, or lumbar spine after appropriate evaluation to exclude secondary causes

Table 50-7 Approaches to the Treatment of Drug-Induced Osteoporosis

Antiresorptive Therapy	Fracture Reduction—Key Clinical Trials
BISPHOSPHONATES	
Alendronate[a] (10 mg orally daily or 70 mg orally weekly)[103,104]	Vertebral: RR 0.45; 95% CI 0.27–0.72; $p = 0.001$ Hip: RR 0.49; 95% CI 0.23–0.99; $p = 0.047$ Glucocorticoid-induced osteoporosis (vertebral fractures): 0.7% versus 6.8% ($p = 0.026$) alendronate-treated versus placebo, respectively.
Ibandronate (2.5 mg daily or 150 mg orally monthly or 3 mg IV every 3 months)[105]	Vertebral: RR 0.38; 95% CI 0.25–0.59; $p = 0.0001$ Hip: NS
Risedronate[a] (5 mg orally daily or 35 mg orally weekly or 150 mg orally monthly)[106-108]	Vertebral: RR 0.59; 95% CI 0.43–0.82; $p = 0.003$ Hip: RR 0.7; 95% CI 0.6–0.9; $p = 0.02$ Glucocorticoid-induced osteoporosis (vertebral fractures): 16% versus 5% ($p = 0.01$)
Zoledronic acid[a] (5 mg IV once yearly)[109]	Vertebral: RR 0.30; 95% CI 0.24–0.38; $p <0.001$ Hip: RR 0.59; 95% CI 0.42–0.83; $p = 0.002$
MONOCLONAL ANTIBODY	
Denosumab (60 mg sub-Q every 6 months)[110,111]	Vertebral: RR 0.38; 95% CI 0.19–0.78; $p = 0.006$ Hip: No data
SELECTIVE ESTROGEN RECEPTOR MODULATORS	
Raloxifene (60 mg/day)[112]	Vertebral: RR 0.7; 95% CI 0.5–0.8 Hip: NS
OTHER	
Calcitonin nasal (200 international units/day)[113]	Vertebral: RR 0.67; 95% CI 0.47–0.97; $p = 0.03$ Hip: NS
ANABOLIC THERAPY	
Teriparatide (20 mcg sub-Q daily)[104,114-116]	Vertebral: RR 0.35; 95% CI 0.22–0.55; $p \leq 0.001$ Hip: NS Glucocorticoid-induced osteoporosis (vertebral fractures, teriparatide versus alendronate): 0.6% versus 6.1% ($p = 0.004$)

CI = confidence interval, IV = intravenous, NS = not significant, RR = relative risk, sub-Q = subcutaneous.

[a]Approved by the U.S. Food and Drug Administration for glucocorticoid-induced osteoporosis.

- Low bone mass (T-score between −1 and −2.5 at the femoral neck or spine) and a 10-year probability of a hip fracture ≥3% or a 10-year probability of a major osteoporosis-related fracture ≥20% based on the U.S.-adapted WHO algorithm

Unfortunately, these intervention thresholds do not take into account the added risks associated with the use of drugs known to predispose to osteoporosis or osteomalacia. The FRAX fracture risk assessment tool may be helpful to determine appropriate treatment; however, it should be noted that the model is constructed from population-based cohorts with a limited age range, specifically women and men >50 years of age.[87] The FRAX tool was not intended for younger women and men. Prophylactic treatment with a bisphosphonate should be carefully considered in patients at risk for drug-induced osteoporosis or osteomalacia when the T-score is below −1 at the spine or hip.[69]

Alendronate, risedronate, zoledronic acid, and teriparatide are approved for use in the United States for glucocorticoid-induced osteoporosis; teripartide appears to be the most effective of these agents.[115,116] Ibandronate and denosumab are not approved for this indication, but have been shown to significantly reduce fractures in patients with osteoporosis.[105,111] Other medications that may be considered for the treatment of drug-induced osteoporosis include calcitonin and raloxifene (in women); however, fracture prevention data with these agents are not as strong as for other treatment options.[112,113]

Treatment strategies for drug-induced osteomalacia primarily focus on the causative agent, the vitamin D deficiency, or both. When possible, the culprit drug should be discontinued and vitamin D therapy initiated if concentrations are found to be insufficient.[71] Vitamin D is considered sufficient if the serum 25-hydroxyvitamin D concentration is ≥30 ng/mL.[91] High-dose vitamin D supplementation may be needed if deficiency is present. A cost-effective method of correcting vitamin D deficiency and maintaining adequate concentrations is to give patients 50,000 international units of vitamin D_2 orally once a week for 8 weeks followed by 50,000 units of vitamin D_2 every 2–4 weeks thereafter.[91] In addition, correction of hypophosphatemia may be necessary and should be considered in patients with drug-induced osteomalacia. Bisphosphonates and other approved agents for primary osteoporosis are also reasonable treatment options for patients with osteomalacia and a high risk or history of fracture.

INFORMATION FOR PATIENTS

Patients receiving medications that may cause drug-induced osteoporosis or osteomalacia should be made aware of the potential and extent of risk caused by the given agent(s). Patients should be encouraged to engage in lifestyle activities that promote bone health, such as weight-bearing exercise, avoidance of tobacco and excessive alcohol and caffeine consumption, consumption of adequate calcium and vitamin D, and participation in fall risk assessments. Healthcare providers should guide their patients in making appropriate decisions about when to perform BMD testing and when treatment may be necessary to prevent or treat drug-induced osteoporosis or osteomalacia.

If treatment with a bisphosphonate is warranted, the patient's ability to swallow the medication, renal function, and calcium and vitamin D status should be evaluated. When an oral bisphosphonate is to be prescribed, the patient should be counseled regarding proper use. Bisphosphonates should be taken 30 minutes (60 minutes for ibandronate) before the first food or drink of the day. The dose should be swallowed with the patient in an upright position and taken with a full glass of water. Patients should not lie down for 30 minutes after taking the medication. Bisphosphonates should not be taken with any other medication. Premenopausal women should be made aware that bisphosphonates are pregnancy category C/D and contraceptive measures should be recommended as appropriate. Zoledronic acid and ibandronate have intravenous formulations for patients who have difficulty swallowing or remembering to take their medication weekly.

REFERENCES

1. United States Bone and Joint Initiative. About Us. http://www.usbji.org (accessed 2017 Jun 1).
2. Emkey GR, Epstein S. Secondary osteoporosis: pathophysiology and diagnosis. *Best Pract Res Clin Endocrinol Metab.* 2014; 28:911-35.
3. Bhan A, Rao AD, Rao DS. Osteomalacia as a result of vitamin D deficiency. *Endocrinol Metab Clin North Am.* 2010; 39:321-31.
4. Vestergaard P. Epilepsy, osteoporosis and fracture risk—a meta-analysis. *Acta Neurol Scand.* 2005; 112:277-86.
5. Ensrud KE, Walczak TS, Blackwell T et al. Antiepileptic drug use increases rates of bone loss in older women: a prospective study. *Neurology.* 2004; 62:2051-7.
6. Ensrud KE, Walczak TS, Blackwell TL et al. Antiepileptic drug use and rates of hip bone loss in older men: a prospective study. *Neurology.* 2008; 71:723-30.
7. Andress DL, Ozuna J, Tirschwell D et al. Antiepileptic drug-induced bone loss in young male patients who have seizures. *Arch Neurol.* 2002; 59:781-6.
8. Eastell R, Adams JE, Coleman RE et al. Effect of anastrozole on bone mineral density: 5-year results from the anastrozole, tamoxifen, alone or in combination trial 18233230. *J Clin Oncol.* 2008; 26:1051-7.
9. Howell A, Cuzick J, Baum M et al. Results of the ATAC (Arimidex, Tamoxifen, Alone or in Combination) trial after completion of 5 years' adjuvant treatment for breast cancer. *Lancet.* 2005; 365:60-2.
10. Moyle GJ, Hardy H, Farajallah A et al. Changes in bone mineral density after 96 weeks of treatment with atazanavir/ritonavir or lopinavir/ritonavir plus tenofovir DF/emtricitabine in treatment-naive patients with HIV-1 infection: the CASTLE body composition substudy. *J Acquir Immune Defic Syndr.* 2015; 68:40-5.
11. Brown TT, Moser C, Currier JS et al. Changes in bone mineral density after initiation of antiretroviral treatment with tenofovir disoproxil fumarate/emtricitabine plus atazanavir/ritonavir, darunavir/ritonavir, or raltegravir. *J Infect Dis.* 2015; 212:1241-9.
12. Mulligan K, Glidden DV, Anderson PL et al. Effects of emtricitabine/tenofovir on bone mineral density in HIV-negative persons in a randomized, double-blind, placebo-controlled trial. *Clin Infect Dis.* 2015; 61:572-80.
13. Brown TT, Qaqish RB. Antiretroviral therapy and the prevalence of osteopenia and osteoporosis: a meta-analytic review. *AIDS.* 2006; 20:2165-74.
14. Hadji P. Aromatase inhibitor-associated bone loss in breast cancer patients is distinct from postmenopausal osteoporosis. *Crit Rev Oncol Hematol.* 2009; 69:73-82.
15. Goss PE, Ingle JN, Martino S et al. A randomized trial of letrozole in postmenopausal women after five years of tamoxifen therapy for early-stage breast cancer. *N Engl J Med.* 2003; 349:1793-802.
16. Baum M, Buzdar A, Cuzick J et al. Anastrozole alone or in combination with tamoxifen versus tamoxifen alone for adjuvant treatment of postmenopausal women with early-stage breast cancer: results of the ATAC (Arimidex, Tamoxifen Alone or in Combination) trial efficacy and safety update analyses. *Cancer.* 2003; 98:1802-10.
17. Breast International Group (BIG) 1-98 Collaborative Group 1; Thürlimann B, Keshaviah A, Coates AS et al. A comparison of letrozole and tamoxifen in postmenopausal women with early breast cancer. *N Engl J Med.* 2005; 353:2747-57.
18. Yonehara Y, Iwamoto I, Kosha S et al. Aromatase inhibitor-induced bone mineral loss and its prevention by bisphosphonate administration in postmenopausal breast cancer patients. *J Obstet Gynaecol Res.* 2007; 33:696-9.
19. Chien AJ, Goss PE. Aromatase inhibitors and bone health in women with breast cancer. *J Clin Oncol.* 2006; 24:5305-12.
20. Bode B, Stenlof K, Harris S et al. Long-term efficacy and safety of canagliflozin over 104 weeks in patients aged 55-80 years with type 2 diabetes. *Diabetes Obes Metab.* 2015; 17:294-303.
21. Watts NB, Bilezikian JP, Usiskin K et al. Effects of canagliflozin on fracture risk in patients with type 2 diabetes mellitus. *J Clin Endocrinol Metab.* 2016;1:157-66.
22. Shimizu C, Fujita T, Fuke Y et al. Effects of cyclosporine on bone mineral density in patients with glucocorticoid-dependent nephrotic syndrome in remission. *Int Urol Nephrol.* 2013; 45:803-8.
23. Lanza LL, McQuay LJ, Rothman KJ et al. Use of depot medroxyprogesterone acetate contraception and incidence of bone fracture. *Obstet Gynecol.* 2013; 121:593-600.
24. Curtis KM, Martins SL. Progestogen-only contraception and bone mineral density: a systematic review. *Contraception.* 2006; 73:470-87.
25. Cromer BA, Bonny AE, Stager M et al. Bone mineral density in adolescent females using injectable or oral contraceptives: a 24-month prospective study. *Fertil Steril.* 2008; 90:2060-7.
26. Committee Opinion No. 602: Depot medroxyprogesterone acetate and bone effects. *Obstet Gynecol.* 2014; 123:1398-402.
27. Modesto W, Bahamondes MV, Bahamondes L. Prevalence of low bone mass and osteoporosis in long-term users of the injectable contraceptive depot medroxyprogesterone acetate. *J Womens Health (Larchmt).* 2015; 24:636-40.
28. Rejnmark L, Vestergaard P, Heickendorff L et al. Effects of long-term treatment with loop diuretics on bone mineral density, calcitropic hormones and bone turnover. *J Intern Med.* 2005; 257:176-84.
29. Heidrich FE, Stergachis A, Gross KM. Diuretic drug use and the risk for hip fracture. *Ann Intern Med.* 1991; 115:1-6.
30. Diamond T, Campbell J, Bryant C, Lynch W. The effect of combined androgen blockade on bone turnover and bone mineral densities in men treated for prostate carcinoma: longitudinal evaluation and response to intermittent cyclic etidronate therapy. *Cancer.* 1998; 83:1561-6.
31. Smith MR, Lee WC, Brandman J et al. Gonadotropin-releasing hormone agonists and fracture risk: a claims-based cohort study of men with nonmetastatic prostate cancer. *J Clin Oncol.* 2005; 23:7897-903.
32. Lems WF. Are glucocorticoids harmful to bone in early rheumatoid arthritis? *Ann N Y Acad Sci.* 2014; 1318:50-4.
33. Ragab AH, Frech RS, Vietti TJ. Osteoporotic fractures secondary to methotrexate therapy of acute leukemia in remission. *Cancer.* 1970; 25:580-5.
34. Schwartz AM, Leonidas JC. Methotrexate osteopathy. *Skeletal Radiol.* 1984; 11:13-6.
35. Stanisavljevic S, Babcock AL. Fractures in children treated with methotrexate for leukemia. *Clin Orthop Relat Res.* 1977: 139-44.
36. Ko YJ, Kim JY, Lee J et al. Levothyroxine dose and fracture risk according to the osteoporosis status in elderly women. *J Prev Med Public Health.* 2014; 47:36-46.
37. Paul TL, Kerrigan J, Kelly AM et al. Long-term L-thyroxine therapy is associated with decreased hip bone density in premenopausal women. *JAMA.* 1988; 259:3137-41.
38. Faber J, Galloe AM. Changes in bone mass during prolonged subclinical hyperthyroidism due to L-thyroxine treatment: a meta-analysis. *Eur J Endocrinol.* 1994; 130:350-6.
39. Sheppard MC, Holder R, Franklyn JA. Levothyroxine treatment and occurrence of fracture of the hip. *Arch Intern Med.* 2002; 162:338-43.
40. Yang YX, Lewis JD, Epstein S, Metz DC. Long-term proton pump inhibitor therapy and risk of hip fracture. *JAMA.* 2006; 296:2947-53.
41. van der Hoorn MMC, Tett SE, de Vries OJ et al. The effect of dose and type of proton pump inhibitor use on risk of fractures and osteoporosis treatment in older Australian women: a prospective cohort study. *Bone.* 2015; 81:675-82.
42. Williams LJ, Henry MJ, Berk M et al. Selective serotonin reuptake inhibitor use and bone mineral density in women with a history of depression. *Int Clin Psychopharmacol.* 2008; 23:84-7.

43. Rabenda V, Nicolet D, Beaudart C et al. Relationship between use of antidepressants and risk of fractures: a meta-analysis. *Osteoporos Int*. 2013; 24:121-37.
44. Majumdar SR, Morin SN, Lix LM, Leslie WD. Influence of recency and duration of glucocorticoid use on bone mineral density and risk of fractures: population-based cohort study. *Osteoporos Int*. 2013; 24:2493-8.
45. Van Staa TP, Leufkens HG, Abenhaim L et al. Use of oral corticosteroids and risk of fractures. *J Bone Miner Res*. 2000; 15:993-1000.
46. van Staa TP, Leufkens HG, Cooper C. The epidemiology of corticosteroid-induced osteoporosis: a meta-analysis. *Osteoporos Int*. 2002; 13:777-87.
47. Angeli A, Guglielmi G, Dovio A et al. High prevalence of asymptomatic vertebral fractures in post-menopausal women receiving chronic glucocorticoid therapy: a cross-sectional outpatient study. *Bone*. 2006; 39:253-9.
48. Steinbuch M, Youket TE, Cohen S. Oral glucocorticoid use is associated with an increased risk of fracture. *Osteoporos Int*. 2004; 15:323-8.
49. Zhu ZN, Jiang YF, Ding T. Risk of fracture with thiazolidinediones: an updated meta-analysis of randomized clinical trials. *Bone*. 2014; 68:115-23.
50. Schwartz AV, Sellmeyer DE, Vittinghoff E et al. Thiazolidinedione use and bone loss in older diabetic adults. *J Clin Endocrinol Metab*. 2006; 91:3349-54.
51. Grey A. Skeletal consequences of thiazolidinedione therapy. *Osteoporos Int*. 2008; 19:129-37.
52. Mazziotti G, Canalis E, Giustina A. Drug-induced osteoporosis: mechanisms and clinical implications. *Am J Med*. 2010; 123:877-84.
53. Pettila V, Leinonen P, Markkola A et al. Postpartum bone mineral density in women treated for thromboprophylaxis with unfractionated heparin or LMW heparin. *Thromb Haemost*. 2002; 87:182-6.
54. Rodger MA, Kahn SR, Cranney A et al. Long-term dalteparin in pregnancy not associated with a decrease in bone mineral density: substudy of a randomized controlled trial. *J Thromb Haemost*. 2007; 5:1600-6.
55. Douketis JD, Ginsberg JS, Burrows RF et al. The effects of long-term heparin therapy during pregnancy on bone density. A prospective matched cohort study. *Thromb Haemost*. 1996; 75:254-7.
56. Joo NS, Yang SW, Song BC, Yeum KJ. Vitamin A intake, serum vitamin D and bone mineral density: analysis of the Korea National Health and Nutrition Examination Survey (KNHANES, 2008-2011). *Nutrients*. 2015; 7:1716-27.
57. Promislow JH, Goodman-Gruen D, Slymen DJ, Barrett-Connor E. Retinol intake and bone mineral density in the elderly: the Rancho Bernardo Study. *J Bone Miner Res*. 2002; 17:1349-58.
58. Michaelsson K, Holmberg L, Mallmin H et al. Diet and hip fracture risk: a case-control study. Study Group of the Multiple Risk Survey on Swedish Women for Eating Assessment. *Int J Epidemiol*. 1995; 24:771-82.
59. Melhus H, Michaelsson K, Kindmark A et al. Excessive dietary intake of vitamin A is associated with reduced bone mineral density and increased risk for hip fracture. *Ann Intern Med*. 1998; 129:770-8.
60. Cosman F, de Beur SJ, LeBoff, MS et al. Clinician's guide to prevention and treatment of osteoporosis. *Osteoporos Int*. 2014; 25:2359-81.
61. Reginster JY, Burlet N. Osteoporosis: a still increasing prevalence. *Bone*. 2006; 38:S4-9.
62. Wright NC, Looker AC, Saag KG et al. The recent prevalence of osteoporosis and low bone mass in the United States based on bone mineral density at the femoral neck or lumbar spine. *J Bone Miner Res*. 2014; 29:2520-6.
63. Burge R, Dawson-Hughes B, Solomon DH et al. Incidence and economic burden of osteoporosis-related fractures in the United States, 2005-2025. *J Bone Miner Res*. 2007; 22:465-75.
64. International Osteoporosis Foundation. Facts and Statistics. http://www.iofbonehealth.org/facts-statistics (accessed 2017 Jun 1).
65. Kelman A, Lane NE. The management of secondary osteoporosis. *Best Pract Res Clin Rheumatol*. 2005; 19:1021-37.
66. Tannirandorn P, Epstein S. Drug-induced bone loss. *Osteoporos Int*. 2000; 11:637-59.
67. Weinstein RS. Glucocorticoid-induced osteoporosis and osteonecrosis. *Endocrinol Metab Clin North Am*. 2012; 41:595–611.
68. Delany AM, Pereira RM, Pereira RC, Canalis E. The cellular and molecular basis of glucocorticoid actions in bone. *Front Horm Res*. 2002; 30:2-12.
69. Grossman JM, Gordon R, Ranganath VK et al. American College of Rheumatology 2010 recommendations for the prevention and treatment of glucocorticoid-induced osteoporosis. *Arthritis Care Res* (Hoboken). 2010; 62:1515-26.
70. Pasco JA, Henry MJ, Kotowicz MA et al. Seasonal periodicity of serum vitamin D and parathyroid hormone, bone resorption, and fractures: the Geelong Osteoporosis Study. *J Bone Miner Res*. 2004; 19:752-8.
71. Lips P, van Schoor NM, Bravenboer N. Vitamin D-related disorder. In: Rosen C, ed. *Primer on the metabolic bone diseases and disorders of mineral metabolism*. 8th ed. Ames, IA: Wiley and Sons, Inc; 2013:613-9.
72. Pack AM, Morrell MJ, Randall A et al. Bone health in young women with epilepsy after one year of antiepileptic drug monotherapy. *Neurology*. 2008; 70:1586-93.
73. Petty SJ, O'Brien TJ, Wark JD. Anti-epileptic medication and bone health. *Osteoporos Int*. 2007; 18:129-42.
74. Pan G, Yang Z, Ballinger SW, McDonald JM. Pathogenesis of osteopenia/osteoporosis induced by highly active anti-retroviral therapy for AIDS. *Ann N Y Acad Sci*. 2006; 1068:297-308.
75. Pan G, Kilby M, McDonald JM. Modulation of osteoclastogenesis induced by nucleoside reverse transcriptase inhibitors. *AIDS Res Hum Retroviruses*. 2006; 22:1131-41.
76. Jain RG, Lenhard JM. Select HIV protease inhibitors alter bone and fat metabolism ex vivo. *J Biol Chem*. 2002; 277:19247-50.
77. Taylor SI, Blau JE, Rother KI. Possible adverse effects of SGLT2 inhibitors on bone. *Lancet Diabetes Endocrinol*. 2015; 3:8-10.
78. Wissing MD. Chemotherapy- and irradiation-induced bone loss in adults with solid tumors. *Curr Osteoporos Rep*. 2015; 13:140-5.
79. Belaya ZE, Melnichenko GA, Rozhinskaya LY et al. Subclinical hyperthyroidism of variable etiology and its influence on bone in postmenopausal women. *Hormones (Athens)*. 2007; 6:62-70.
80. Schneider R, Reiners C. The effect of levothyroxine therapy on bone mineral density: a systematic review of the literature. *Exp Clin Endocrinol Diabetes*. 2003; 111:455-70.
81. Meier C, Kraenzlin ME, Bodmer M et al. Use of thiazolidinediones and fracture risk. *Arch Intern Med*. 2008; 168:820-5.
82. Soroceanu MA, Miao D, Bai XY et al. Rosiglitazone impacts negatively on bone by promoting osteoblast/osteocyte apoptosis. *J Endocrinol*. 2004; 183:203-16.
83. Rajgopal R, Bear M, Butcher MK, Shaughnessy SG. The effects of heparin and low molecular weight heparins on bone. *Thromb Res*. 2008; 122:293-8.
84. Jackson HA, Sheehan AH. Effect of vitamin A on fracture risk. *Ann Pharmacother*. 2005; 39:2086-90.
85. Binkley N, Krueger D. Hypervitaminosis A and bone. *Nutr Rev*. 2000; 58:138-44.
86. The International Society for Clinical Densitometry. 2015 ISCD Official Positions—Adult. http://www.iscd.org/official-positions/2015-iscd-official-positions-adult/ (accessed 2018 Aug 31).
87. FRAX WHO Fracture Risk Assessment Tool. Welcome to FRAX. https://www.shef.ac.uk/FRAX/ (accessed 2018 Aug 31).
88. Watts NB, Bilezikian JP, Camacho PM et al. American Association of Clinical Endocrinologists Medical Guidelines for Clinical Practice for the diagnosis and treatment of postmenopausal osteoporosis: executive summary of recommendations. *Endocr Pract*. 2010; 16:1016-9.

89. Graat-Verboom L, Wouters EF, Smeenk FW et al. Current status of research on osteoporosis in COPD: a systematic review. *Eur Respir J*. 2009; 34:209-18.
90. Martin CA, Gowda U, Renzaho AM. The prevalence of vitamin D deficiency among dark-skinned populations according to their stage of migration and region of birth: a meta-analysis. *Nutrition*. 2016; 32:21-32.
91. Holick MF. Vitamin D deficiency. *N Engl J Med*. 2007; 357:266-81.
92. Johnell O, Kanis JA. An estimate of the worldwide prevalence and disability associated with osteoporotic fractures. *Osteoporos Int*. 2006; 17:1726-33.
93. Gullberg B, Johnell O, Kanis JA. World-wide projections for hip fracture. *Osteoporos Int*. 1997; 7:407-13.
94. Abrahamsen B, van Staa T, Ariely R et al. Excess mortality following hip fracture: a systematic epidemiological review. *Osteoporos Int*. 2009; 20:1633-50.
95. Colon-Emeric C, Kuchibhatla M, Pieper C et al. The contribution of hip fracture to risk of subsequent fractures: data from two longitudinal studies. *Osteoporos Int*. 2003; 14:879-83.
96. Buehring B, Viswanathan R, Binkley N, Busse W. Glucocorticoid-induced osteoporosis: an update on effects and management. *J Allergy Clin Immunol*. 2013; 132:1019-30.
97. Scanlon PD, Connett JE, Wise RA et al. Loss of bone density with inhaled triamcinolone in Lung Health Study II. *Am J Respir Crit Care Med*. 2004; 170:1302-9.
98. Brown TT. Challenges in the management of osteoporosis and vitamin D deficiency in HIV infection. *Top Antivir Med*. 2013; 21:115-8.
99. Wang MW, Wei S, Faccio R et al. The HIV protease inhibitor ritonavir blocks osteoclastogenesis and function by impairing RANKL-induced signaling. *J Clin Invest*. 2004; 114:206-13.
100. Bernardino JI, Mocroft A, Mallon PW et al. Bone mineral density and inflammatory and bone biomarkers after darunavir-ritonavir combined with either raltegravir or tenofovir-emtricitabine in antiretroviral-naive adults with HIV-1: a substudy of the NEAT001/ANRS143 randomised trial. *Lancet HIV*. 2015; 2:e464-73.
101. Lock CA, Lecouturier J, Mason JM, Dickinson HO. Lifestyle interventions to prevent osteoporotic fractures: a systematic review. *Osteoporos Int*. 2006; 17:20-8.
102. Panday K, Gona A, Humphrey MB. Medication-induced osteoporosis: screening and treatment strategies. *Ther Adv Musculoskelet Dis*. 2014; 6:185-202.
103. Black DM, Cummings SR, Karpf DB et al. Randomised trial of effect of alendronate on risk of fracture in women with existing vertebral fractures. Fracture Intervention Trial Research Group. *Lancet*. 1996; 348:1535-41.
104. Adachi JD, Saag KG, Delmas PD et al. Two-year effects of alendronate on bone mineral density and vertebral fracture in patients receiving glucocorticoids: a randomized, double-blind, placebo-controlled extension trial. *Arthritis Rheum*. 2001; 44:202-11.
105. Chesnut CH 3rd, Skag A, Christiansen C et al. Effects of oral ibandronate administered daily or intermittently on fracture risk in postmenopausal osteoporosis. *J Bone Miner Res*. 2004; 19:1241-9.
106. Harris ST, Watts NB, Genant HK et al. Effects of risedronate treatment on vertebral and nonvertebral fractures in women with postmenopausal osteoporosis: a randomized controlled trial. Vertebral Efficacy With Risedronate Therapy (VERT) Study Group. *JAMA*. 1999; 282:1344-52.
107. McClung MR, Geusens P, Miller PD et al. Effect of risedronate on the risk of hip fracture in elderly women. Hip Intervention Program Study Group. *N Engl J Med*. 2001; 344:333-40.
108. Wallach S, Cohen S, Reid DM et al. Effects of risedronate treatment on bone density and vertebral fracture in patients on corticosteroid therapy. *Calcif Tissue Int*. 2000; 67:277-85.
109. Lyles KW, Colon-Emeric CS, Magaziner JS et al. Zoledronic acid and clinical fractures and mortality after hip fracture. *N Engl J Med*. 2007; 357:1799-809.
110. Smith MR, Egerdie B, Hernandez Toriz N et al. Denosumab in men receiving androgen-deprivation therapy for prostate cancer. *N Engl J Med*. 2009; 361:745-55.
111. Papapoulos S, Chapurlat R, Libanati C et al. Five years of denosumab exposure in women with postmenopausal osteoporosis: results from the first two years of the FREEDOM extension. *J Bone Miner Res*. 2012; 27:694-701.
112. Ettinger B, Black DM, Mitlak BH et al. Reduction of vertebral fracture risk in postmenopausal women with osteoporosis treated with raloxifene: results from a 3-year randomized clinical trial. Multiple Outcomes of Raloxifene Evaluation (MORE) Investigators. *JAMA*. 1999; 282:637-45.
113. Chesnut CH 3rd, Silverman S, Andriano K et al. A randomized trial of nasal spray salmon calcitonin in postmenopausal women with established osteoporosis: the prevent recurrence of osteoporotic fractures study. PROOF Study Group. *Am J Med*. 2000; 109:267-76.
114. Neer RM, Arnaud CD, Zanchetta JR et al. Effect of parathyroid hormone (1-34) on fractures and bone mineral density in postmenopausal women with osteoporosis. *N Engl J Med*. 2001; 344:1434-41.
115. Saag KG, Shane E, Boonen S et al. Teriparatide or alendronate in glucocorticoid-induced osteoporosis. *N Engl J Med*. 2007; 357:2028-39.
116. Glüer CC1, Marin F, Ringe JD et al. Comparative effects of teriparatide and risedronate in glucocorticoid-induced osteoporosis in men: 18-month results of the EuroGIOPs trial. *J Bone Miner Res*. 2013 Jun; 28:1355-68.

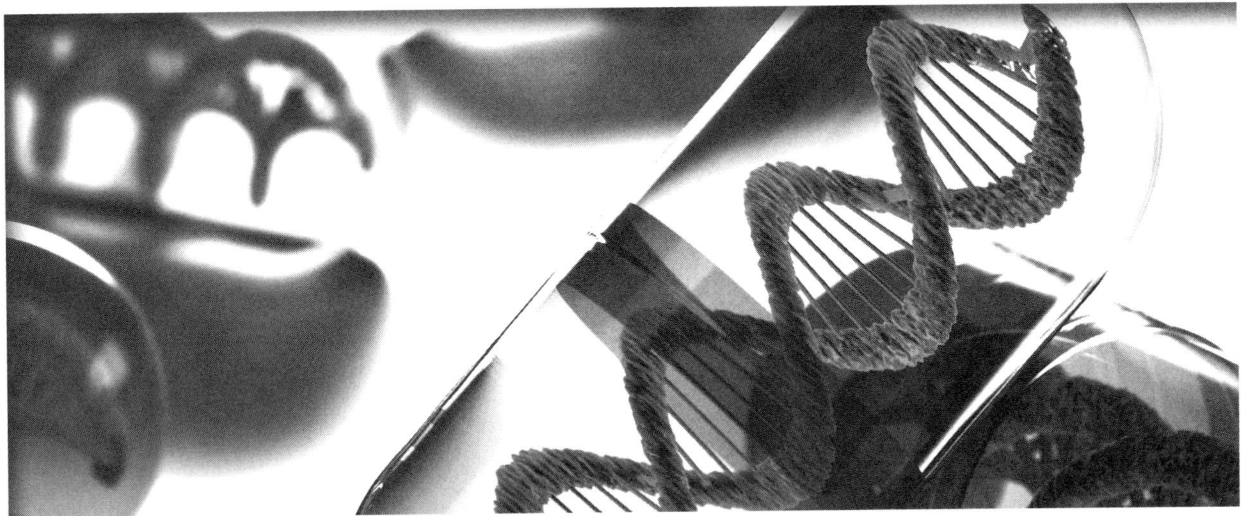

CHAPTER 51

Gout and Hyperuricemia

Jasmine D. Gonzalvo

Gout is an inflammatory disease induced by monosodium urate crystals that precipitate in joints and soft tissues, causing an intense inflammatory reaction. A number of drugs may alter urate excretion or increase uric acid production and predispose patients to hyperuricemia with or without gout. Hyperuricemia, defined as a serum urate concentration >6.8–7 mg/dL, may contribute to renal, cardiovascular, and metabolic risk. In general, pharmacotherapy is not recommended for patients with asymptomatic hyperuricemia.[1,2]

CAUSATIVE AGENTS

Agents implicated in drug-induced gout and hyperuricemia are listed in **Table 51-1**.[1-84] Reports suggest a variety of contributory mechanisms for each of these agents' ability to increase uric acid concentrations. Hyperuricemia, rather than acute attacks or an established diagnosis of gout, is more commonly associated with each of these agents.

EPIDEMIOLOGY

In the United States, gout occurs in approximately 3.9% of the general population and is more common in men.[3] A high intake of red meat or alcohol, older age, chronic kidney disease, and the presence of the metabolic syndrome (hypertension, diabetes, dyslipidemia, and truncal obesity) are all recognized risk factors for the development of hyperuricemia and gout.[1] Although the prevalence and incidence of gout have risen over several decades, the prevalence and incidence of drug-induced hyperuricemia and gout are not well documented. The incidence of drug-induced gout and hyperuricemia varies greatly among the causative agents.

MECHANISMS

Several mechanisms for drug-induced hyperuricemia and gout have been identified (**Table 51-2**). The most common mechanism is interference with uric acid excretion leading to accumulation in serum. The urate–anion exchanger, urate transporter-1 (URAT1),

Table 51-1 Agents Implicated in Drug-Induced Gout and Hyperuricemia

Drug	Incidence	Level of Evidence[a]
Allopurinol[53]	NK	B
Aspirin—low dose[9]	NK	B
Cyclosporine[1,10-24]	1–10%	B
Cytotoxic agents[13,25,53]	NK	B
Diuretics[35-40]	NK	A
Ethambutol[53-59]	66%	A
Ethanol[60-65,67]	1.5%	B
Febuxostat[5,6,53]	NK	B
Levodopa[68-71]	48.8%	B
Nicotinic acid[53]	NK	B
Pyrazinamide[30,53,76,77]	NK	C
Tacrolimus[78-81]	42%	B
Teriparatide[83,84]	3%	B
Uricosuric agents[5,6,53]	NK	B

NK = not known.

[a]Definitions for Levels of Evidence: Level A—evidence from one or more randomized, controlled clinical trials; Level B—evidence from nonrandomized clinical trials, prospective observational studies, cohort studies, retrospective studies, case-control studies, meta-analyses and/or postmarketing surveillance studies; and Level C—evidence from one or more published case reports or case series.

at the apical brush-border membrane of renal proximal tubular epithelial cells plays a role in uric acid reabsorption and can predispose to drug-induced hyperuricemia and gout. Drugs that cause cellular death (e.g., antitumor drugs) may induce gout by dramatically increasing uric acid concentrations resulting from increased protein catabolism.

ALLOPURINOL, FEBUXOSTAT, AND URICOSURIC AGENTS

Although the xanthine oxidase inhibitors allopurinol and febuxostat and uricosuric agents such as probenecid and fenofibrate have been effective in the prevention of gout attacks, these medications paradoxically induce attacks in some individuals soon after initiation of urate-lowering therapy.[3] These attacks may be due to remodeling of articular urate crystal deposits following rapid and substantial lowering of urate concentrations.[3] It is recommended that allopurinol be started at a dose of no greater than 100 mg daily and that the daily dose be increased by 100 mg every 2–5 weeks to help avoid a rapid drop in serum urate concentrations sometimes associated with precipitation of acute gout. For patients with stage 4 or worse chronic kidney disease, the dose of allopurinol should start at 50 mg daily.[3] Febuxostat should be initiated at 40 mg daily and increased to 80 mg daily if serum uric concentrations do not reach <6 mg/dL after 2 weeks of treatment.[4] A similar titration strategy should be used when initiating therapy with uricosuric

Table 51-2 Mechanisms of Drug-Induced Gout and Hyperuricemia

Drug	Mechanism
Allopurinol[53]	Not well elucidated
Aspirin—low dose[9,30]	Decreases renal uric acid excretion
Cyclosporine[10,30]	Increases renal tubular uric acid reabsorption, particularly through decreased glomerular filtration, increased blood pressure, and interstitial nephropathy
Cytotoxic agents[53]	Release large amounts of uric acid following rapid and frequent cell turnover
Diuretics[30,53]	Increase renal tubular reabsorption of uric acid
Ethambutol[30]	Decreases renal uric acid excretion
Ethanol[60-64]	Decreases uric acid excretion through competition with lactic acid; increases uric acid production through rapid hepatic breakdown of adenosine triphosphate or anti-diuretic hormone inhibition and transient dehydration
Febuxostat[53]	Not well elucidated
Levodopa[68-79]	Not well elucidated
Nicotinic acid[30]	Stimulates absorption of luminal urate through urate transporter-1
Pyrazinamide[30]	Stimulates absorption of luminal urate through urate transporter-1
Tacrolimus[30]	Increases renal tubular uric acid reabsorption, particularly through decreased glomerular filtration, increased blood pressure, and interstitial nephropathy
Teriparatide[100]	Likely related to increased serum concentrations of parathyroid hormone
Uricosuric agents[53]	Not well elucidated

agents. Individuals treated with these agents should maintain adequate hydration, and therapy should begin with low doses and the dose increased slowly over several weeks to avoid excessive uricosuria and possible kidney stone formation. Although fenofibrate has demonstrated benefit for the treatment of hyperuricemia through its uricosuric properties, it has not been associated with precipitation of acute gout attacks.[5-7]

Patients receiving long-term treatment with allopurinol or uricosuric agents are also at risk for gout with sporadic medication adherence. Extra efforts to thoroughly educate patients as to why the prescribed medication is beneficial and important and to encourage adherence to prescribed regimens is advised.

ASPIRIN—LOW DOSE

In doses <2 g daily, aspirin has been shown to cause uric acid retention and hyperuricemia due to *trans*-stimulation of URAT1.[8] Higher doses of aspirin are uricosuric due to the *cis*-inhibition of URAT1.[8] The effect of minidose aspirin on urate excretion was examined in 49 elderly patients.[9] A 6% increase in serum urate concentration and a 23% decrease in urate clearance was seen during the first week of aspirin therapy, but these values returned to baseline by week 3, even though the dose of aspirin was increased from 75–325 mg daily. Urate clearance and creatinine clearance were reduced in parallel. The hyperuricemic effects of aspirin were more pronounced in patients also taking diuretics and those with hypoalbuminemia.[9] In a large, prospective case-crossover study in a population of patients diagnosed with gout, aspirin daily doses of <325 mg were associated with an almost twofold increased risk of recurrent attacks of gout as compared to daily aspirin doses >325 mg.[8] However, this study examined aspirin use only in the prior 2 days and did not follow patients for a longer time period to identify longer-term trends.

Most clinicians would not withhold low-dose aspirin therapy in patients at high risk for cardiovascular disease who also have gout, as the cardiovascular benefits likely outweigh the risk of an increased frequency of gout attacks. Thorough patient education regarding the risks and benefits of low-dose aspirin therapy along with regular serum urate monitoring may be warranted in patients with pre-existing gout. If the decision is made to initiate treatment for hyperuricemia or gout in patients receiving low-dose aspirin, xanthine oxidase inhibitors or uricosuric agents may be considered.[8]

CYCLOSPORINE

Cyclosporine, an immunosuppressive agent commonly used to prevent rejection in patients with solid organ transplants, is associated with hyperuricemia. This effect is due to alteration of renal tubular handling of uric acid leading to decreased urate excretion.[10] It is estimated that hyperuricemia develops in up to 80% of patients receiving cyclosporine.[1,11] Gout has been reported to develop in 4–24% of patients who have undergone transplantation and are receiving cyclosporine.[11] Burack and colleagues reported hyperuricemia in 72% of males and 81% of females treated with cyclosporine following heart or heart–lung transplantation.[10] In another study, 42% of patients receiving cyclosporine required allopurinol therapy for hyperuricemia as compared with only 9% of those who did not receive cyclosporine.[12]

Although hyperuricemia appears to be quite common in patients who have undergone renal transplantation, nephrolithiasis is unusual and renal failure is extremely rare. Nonetheless, the American Society of Nephrology recommends measuring the serum urate concentration within the first 2–3 months of cyclosporine therapy.[13-24]

CYTOTOXIC AGENTS

Drug-induced hyperuricemia associated with cytotoxic drugs can lead to significant renal compromise. Cytotoxic drugs may induce tumor lysis syndrome, a condition that occurs following chemotherapy with a high cell kill. Tumors most likely to be associated with tumor lysis syndrome include mature B-cell and T-cell lymphomas such as Burkitt lymphoma, lymphoblastic lymphoma, and some acute leukemias, although breast and lung tumors have also been implicated.[25] The rapid and frequent cell turnover associated with cytotoxic agents can result in the release of intracellular contents into the blood, including large quantities of potassium, phosphorus, and uric acid. Uric acid nephropathy develops as a result of the precipitation of uric acid crystals in the kidney. High-risk patients routinely receive prophylactic therapy for tumor lysis syndrome consisting of pretreatment with hydration, urine alkalinization, and allopurinol. Rasburicase can be considered as an alternative to allopurinol. Advantages of rasburicase include a faster onset of action and increased ability to lower uric acid as compared with oral allopurinol. Disadvantages include hypersensitivity reactions and hemolytic anemia, although these are rare.[13]

DIURETICS

Diuretics, commonly used for the treatment of hypertension, increase serum urate concentrations in a dose-dependent manner by directly increasing proximal tubular reabsorption of uric acid and through volume depletion and resultant increased urate reabsorption by the proximal tubule. Research has explored pharmacogenomic associations with diuretic-induced hyperuricemia, although definitive conclusions have yet to be determined.[26,27] Hypertension itself has been independently associated with the development of gout.[28,29] However, a connection between use of diuretics and an increased risk of gout in hypertensive patients is controversial.[30-34] In a trial involving 3,693 patients with hypertension who were treated with thiazide diuretics, investigators found an association between diuretic therapy and elevated serum uric acid concentrations but concluded that these elevations did not correlate with kidney damage or significant increases in the frequency of gout.[35] A case-control study reported no relationship between the use of diuretics and an increased risk of gout.[36] Conversely, Choi and colleagues[37] have suggested that diuretics increase the relative risk of gout by almost 80% with an absolute incidence of gout in individuals treated with diuretics around 3%. Moreover, a study of 197 patients who had experienced a gout attack within the past year revealed a significantly increased risk of recurrent gout attacks attributed to the use of thiazide diuretics.[38] A retrospective population-based case-control study in a population of 91,350 patients with a first-time diagnosis of gout found an increased risk of gout with the use of loop, thiazide, and thiazide-like diuretics but not with potassium-sparing diuretics.[39]

Diuretics, along with angiotensin-converting enzyme inhibitors (ACEIs), angiotensin II receptor blockers (ARBs), and calcium channel blockers, are considered to be preferred drugs for the initial treatment of hypertension as they are highly effective and work well in combination with other classes of antihypertensives.[40] Concern about the possible precipitation of gout should not keep patients with hypertension and asymptomatic hyperuricemia from receiving diuretic therapy, although caution should be used with these agents in patients with gout. Of note, gout is unlikely to occur with hydrochlorothiazide doses <50 mg daily or chlorthalidone doses <25 mg daily.[40] Some evidence also exists suggesting that ACEIs, β-blockers, and nonlosartan ARBs are associated with an increased risk of gout.[28,39,41,42] Losartan and calcium channel blockers have been associated with a decreased risk of developing gout.[28,39,43-49]

ETHAMBUTOL

Ethambutol, an antitubercular agent, has been shown to decrease renal uric acid excretion.[30,50] Increased uric acid levels have been noted as early as 24 hours and as late as 90 days after initiation of ethambutol treatment.[51] In one study, investigators evaluated 131 patients treated for active tuberculosis. One group received ethambutol, streptomycin, and isoniazid, while the control group received streptomycin, isoniazid, and thiacetazone. Increased serum uric acid concentrations were found in 66% of patients in the ethambutol group, whereas patients in the control group experienced no significant change.[52] Of note, only two cases of gout were reported in the trial.[53,54] A second study of 14 patients with tuberculosis and a history of gout also documented an increase in serum uric acid concentrations after ethambutol treatment.[55] However, none of the patients progressed to have acute attacks of gout. Louthrenoo and colleagues[50] also found a minor, reversible increase in uric acid levels in a small population of 16 patients with tuberculosis treated with ethambutol or pyrazinamide.

Ethambutol must typically be used in combination with pyrazinamide to effectively treat tuberculosis. Close monitoring for signs and symptoms of gout is warranted in these patients because the concomitant use of these two agents may impart greater risk than the use of either agent alone.[54,56-59]

ETHANOL

Gout has been noted in association with excess ethanol consumption for centuries. Touted as "the disease of kings," gout was first reported after royal feasts at which large amounts of ethanol and meats were consumed. It is now known that ethanol can lead to hyperuricemia through both decreased uric acid excretion and increased uric acid production.[60-64] When consumed in excess, ethanol causes the rapid hepatic breakdown of adenosine triphosphate and increases urate production. Excessive ethanol consumption may also induce lactic acidosis. Lactic acid competes with urate for excretion through the kidney. Alcohol-induced inhibition of antidiuretic hormone may lead to transient dehydration, which can temporarily increase serum uric acid concentrations.[62] Secondarily, excess ethanol consumption may lead to long-term obesity, which has been associated with underexcretion of uric acid. A correlation between beer consumption and relative risk for developing hyperuricemia has been established, although moderate wine consumption does not appear to increase the risk of gout.[65,66] A related prospective study from Choi and colleagues[64] recognized alcohol consumption as an independent risk factor for gout. Patients with gout should be advised to limit alcohol consumption, especially beer.[3]

LEVODOPA

Levodopa use has been associated with an increase in serum uric acid concentration.[68-70] In one retrospective review, 48% of the 86 patients treated with an average of 4.3 g of levodopa per day developed elevated serum uric acid concentrations. The incidence of clinically evident gout was not reported.[71] Conversely, in a small, case-control study by Andreadou and colleagues,[72] an inverse relationship between levodopa dose and uric acid levels was found. Patients with concurrent diagnoses of gout and Parkinson disease treated with levodopa should be monitored for symptoms of gout. Risks and benefits should be evaluated when determining the most appropriate treatment for patients who have both gout and Parkinson disease. When levodopa is determined to be the drug of choice, the risks and benefits of prophylactic therapy for gout should also be evaluated.

NICOTINIC ACID

Nicotinic acid, a drug used to treat dyslipidemia, stimulates the absorption of uric acid through URAT1, which is located at the apical brush-border membrane of renal proximal tubular epithelial cells and is responsible for local uric acid reabsorption. Increased nicotinic acid concentrations stimulate URAT1-dependent anion exchange with uric acid, which may result in hyperuricemia.[30]

One study reported a decrease in uric acid excretion of up to 75% when nicotinic acid was given in doses up to 4.5 g daily (a much higher dose than usually tolerated by patients because of flushing).[53] Another study reported that nicotinic acid in doses of 1 g daily reduced the excretion of uric acid by 62%.[53] Serum uric acid levels may increase by 5–15% in patients receiving nicotinic acid, but for most patients these elevations are clinically inconsequential.[73] Depending on the primary lipid target, multiple classes of medications may be substituted to achieve desired effects while reducing the risk of drug-induced hyperuricemia and gout. When possible, patients with a predisposition for gout should be maintained on agents other than niacin to decrease cardiovascular risk.

PYRAZINAMIDE

Pyrazinamide, a drug chemically related to nicotinic acid, is primarily indicated for the treatment of tuberculosis. Like nicotinic acid, pyrazinamide stimulates the absorption of uric acid through the urate–anion exchanger URAT1.

A major metabolite of pyrazinamide, pyrazinoic acid, inhibits the renal tubular secretion of uric acid also contributing to hyperuricemia.[74] As many as 43–100% of individuals treated with pyrazinamide, alone or in combination, experience hyperuricemia.[74] One retrospective epidemiological survey of 226 patients treated with pyrazinamide at an average dose of 1.18 g daily found peak uric acid levels between 10–11.9 mg/dL in males and 8–9.9 mg/dL in females, although, no acute attacks of gout occurred.[75] Patients treated with pyrazinamide must be monitored for the development of gout and, because adherence to multiple drug therapy is a significant concern with tuberculosis treatment, attacks must be managed appropriately so that antitubercular therapy can continue uninterrupted.[76,77]

TACROLIMUS

Limited conclusive data exist regarding the potential for hyperuricemia in patients treated with tacrolimus, a calcineurin inhibitor associated with impaired uric acid excretion.[78] A retrospective medical record review of recipients of liver transplants revealed that 42% of 43 patients treated with tacrolimus experienced hyperuricemia.[79] Similarly, a study comparing cyclosporine and tacrolimus in stable recipients of renal transplants found significant elevations in serum uric acid concentrations for both groups.[80] In addition, switching patients from cyclosporine to tacrolimus was not associated with a significant decrease in uric acid concentrations, although this approach had previously been proposed as a method to control cyclosporine-induced hyperuricemia.[81] Switching from a twice daily to a once daily formulation of tacrolimus also did not result in an improvement in tacrolimus-induced hyperuricemia.[82]

TERIPARATIDE

The parathyroid analog hormone teriparatide has been associated with dose-dependent elevations of uric acid.[83] Increases in serum uric acid concentration to above 9 mg/dL have been associated with doses ranging from 20 to 40 mcg daily.[83,84] To date, acute gout attacks have not been associated with teriparatide therapy; therefore, increased monitoring and prophylactic therapy are not warranted in most cases.

CLINICAL PRESENTATION AND DIFFERENTIAL DIAGNOSIS

Signs and symptoms associated with drug-induced gout and hyperuricemia are listed in **Table 51-3**. The clinical presentation of drug-induced gout does not differ from that of gout associated with other causes. A patient presenting with gout should have a careful medication history taken to identify drugs that could be contributing to the disease. Patients with acute gout present with pain, swelling, and erythema, often involving just one or a few joints. An increased skin temperature is often noted over the affected joints and is associated with the inflammation. The onset of symptoms is abrupt in most patients. Acute attacks commonly occur overnight, as the affected joint space becomes saturated with monosodium urate following water reabsorption at the site.

Unlike most other inflammatory arthritic conditions, most patients have no symptoms between attacks. This characteristic can be useful in differentiating gout from other arthritic conditions. Some patients may have involvement of associated tendons and present with more diffuse swelling, a condition called tenosynovitis. Over a period of days, sloughing of superficial skin layers may occur and this is associated with intense inflammation. The most frequently involved joint is the first metatarsal joint at the base of the first toe (gouty inflammation in this location is sometimes called podagra),

Table 51-3 Signs and Symptoms Associated with Drug-Induced Gout and Hyperuricemia[96,101,102]

- Abrupt onset of attacks, usually lasting 5–10 days
- Asymmetric swelling within a joint on radiograph
- Involvement of one or more joints
- Joint fluid culture negative for organisms during attack
- Pain, erythema, swelling over joints
- Subcortical cysts without erosions on radiograph
- Symptom presentation at night
- Tophi

although any joint may be affected. Distribution is more common in the distal portion of the lower extremities. Extreme pain over the affected joint is usually noted. Characteristically, patients report pain so severe that they do not wear shoes and cannot even tolerate the weight of bedcovers over the involved joint. Pain associated with minor stimuli is called allodynia.

Gout may present at any age, but the incidence peaks between the ages of 50 and 70 for men and between the ages of 50 and 90 for women. Earlier presentation is more likely to be associated with enzyme defects, renal disease, drugs, or toxins. Initially, patients typically experience rare, intermittent attacks involving one or a few joints. Over time, attacks may become more frequent and are more likely to be polyarticular. Eventually, patients may have a chronic, polyarticular arthritis, which may be difficult to distinguish from rheumatoid arthritis.

A key diagnostic finding that occurs in some patients is the presence of gouty tophi, which are subcutaneous deposits of uric acid in a nodule. These may occur anywhere, but are frequently found on fingers, elbows, and ankles and over the metatarsal joints. The outer helix of the ear may also be involved. Tophi are painless and may have a characteristic yellow color. In some cases they drain chalky white material, which is found to contain uric acid crystals when examined microscopically under polarized light. Other diseases, such as rheumatoid arthritis, which may cause rheumatoid nodules, and hyperlipidemia, which may cause xanthomas, should be considered in the differential diagnosis of patients with nodules (**Table 51-4**). Needle aspiration is a fairly simple test that may be performed

Table 51-4 Conditions to Consider in the Differential Diagnosis of Drug-Induced Gout and Hyperuricemia[101,102]

- Cellulitis
- Fractures
- Infectious arthritis
- Palindromic rheumatism
- Pseudogout (calcium pyrophosphate deposition disease)
- Rheumatoid arthritis

to assist in differentiation. In most patients, gout is recognized long before the development of tophi, and appropriate treatment to lower serum uric acid concentrations prevents the development of these lesions.

A definitive diagnosis of gout may be made by the identification of intracellular uric acid crystals in synovial fluid neutrophils obtained on aspiration of an inflamed joint. Examination under a polarized light microscope is necessary to properly identify these crystals. Measurement of serum uric acid concentration may be of some value, although patients can have normal serum concentrations during acute attacks.[85] In the absence of crystal diagnosis, the presence of the following criteria permits a presumptive diagnosis: (1) hyperuricemia, (2) history of acute attacks of arthritis with asymptomatic periods between attacks, and (3) the ability of colchicine or nonsteroidal anti-inflammatory drugs (NSAIDs) to abort an attack. Historically, the criteria for the accurate classification of gout have lacked specificity and sensitivity. With the advent of advanced imaging techniques, in combination with other subjective and objective signs and symptoms, the classification of gout has become more standardized, specific, and sensitive. **Table 51-5** outlines the American College of Rheumatology/European League Against Rheumatism collaborative initiative classification criteria for gout. A cumulative score ≥8 using this tool is consistent with gout.[86]

Other potential causes of episodic arthritis must also be considered in evaluating patients for gout. Pseudogout is a disease caused by calcium pyrophosphate deposition and may be the most difficult to differentiate from gout. Calcium pyrophosphate crystals have morphology and polarizing characteristics that are different from those of uric acid crystals, so analysis of synovial fluid may be the best method to differentiate between gout and pseudogout. The presence of calcification of synovial cartilage (chondrocalcinosis) on a radiograph may also be helpful in differentiation, as this is found in patients with pseudogout but not gout. Septic arthritis, cellulitis, fractures, and a rare condition called palindromic rheumatism are other medical problems that may mimic gout and should be considered in the differential diagnosis.

Table 51-5 The American College of Rheumatology/European League Against Rheumatism Gout Classification Criteria[86,a]

	Categories	Score
Step 1: Entry criterion (only apply criteria in Step 3 to those meeting this entry criterion	At least one episode of swelling, pain, or tenderness in a peripheral joint or bursa	
Step 2: Sufficient criterion (if met, can classify as gout without applying criteria below)	Presence of monosodium urate monohydrate crystals in a symptomatic joint or bursa (i.e., in synovial fluid) or tophus	
Step 3: Criteria (below) to be used if sufficient criterion (Step 2) are not met:		
CLINICAL		
Pattern of joint/bursa involvement during symptomatic episode(s) ever[b]	Ankle or mid-foot (as part of monoarticular or oligoarticular episode without involvement of the first metatarsophalangeal joint) Involvement of the first metatarsophalangeal joint (as part of monoarticular or oligoarticular episode)	1 2
Characteristics of symptomatic episode(s) ever • Erythema overlying affected joint (patient reported or physician observed) • Can't bear touch or pressure to affected joint • Great difficulty with walking or inability to use affected joint	One characteristic Two characteristics Three characteristics	1 2 3
Time course of episode(s) ever Presence (ever) of ≥2, irrespective of anti-inflammatory treatment: • Time to maximal pain <24 hours • Resolution of symptoms in ≤14 days • Complete resolution (to baseline) level between symptomatic episodes	One typical episode Recurrent typical episodes	1 2
Clinical evidence of tophus Draining or chalk-like substance nodule under transparent skin, often with overlying vascularity, located in typical locations: joints, ears, olecranon bursae, finger pads, tendons (e.g., Achilles)	Present	4
Laboratory Serum urate: Measured by the uricase method Ideally should be scored at a time when the patient was not receiving urate-lowering treatment and it was >4 weeks from the start of an episode (i.e., during the intercritical period); if practicable, retest under those conditions; the highest value irrespective of timing should be scored Synovial fluid analysis of a symptomatic joint or bursa (should be assessed by a trained observer)[d]	• <4 mg/dL[c] • 6 to <8 mg/dL • 8 to <10 mg/dL • ≥10 mg/dL Monosodium urate crystal negative	−4 2 3 4 −2
Imaging[e] Imaging evidence of urate deposition in symptomatic joint or bursa: ultrasound evidence of double-contour sign[f] or dual energy computed tomography scanner demonstrating urate deposition[g] Imaging evidence of gout-related joint damage: conventional radiography of the hands and/or feet demonstrates at least one erosion[h]	Present (either modality) Present	4 4

Table 51-5 The American College of Rheumatology/European League Against Rheumatism Gout Classification Criteria[86,a] (continued)

[a]A web-based calculator can be accessed at http://goutclassificationcalculator.auckland.ac.nz, and through the American College of Rheumatology (ACR) and European League Against Rheumatism (EULAR) websites.
[b]Symptomatic episodes are periods of symptoms that include any swelling, pain, and/or tenderness in a peripheral joint or bursa.
[c]If serum urate level is <4 mg/dL (<0.24 mmol/L), subtract 4 points; if serum urate level is ≥4–6 mg/dL (≥0.24 – <0.36 mmol/L), score this item as 0.
[d]If polarizing microscopy of synovial fluid from a symptomatic joint or bursa by a trained examiner fails to show monosodium urate monohydrate (MSU) crystals, subtract 2 points. If synovial fluid was not assessed, score this item as 0.
[e]If imaging is not available, score these items as 0.
[f]Hyperechoic irregular enhancement over the surface of the hyaline cartilage that is independent of the insonation angle of the ultrasound beam (note: false-positive double-contour sign [artifact] may appear at the cartilage surface but should disappear with a change in the insonation angle of the probe).
[g]Presence of color-coded urate at articular or periarticular sites. Images should be acquired using a dual-energy computed tomography (DECT) scanner, with data acquired at 80 kV and 140 kV and analyzed using gout-specific software with a 2-material decomposition algorithm that color-codes urate. A positive scan is defined as the presence of color-coded urate at articular or periarticular sites. Nailbed, submillimeter, skin, motion, beam hardening, and vascular artifacts should not be interpreted as DECT evidence of urate deposition.
[h]Erosion is defined as a cortical break with sclerotic margin and overhanging edge, excluding distal interphalangeal joints and gull-wing appearance.
Source: Reprinted with permission from Neogi T, Jansen TL, Dalbeth N et al. 2015 gout classification criteria: an American College of Rheumatology/European League against rheumatism collaborative initiative. *Ann Rheum Dis.* 2015; 74:1789-98.

RISK FACTORS

The risk factors for drug-induced hyperuricemia and gout (**Table 51-6**) are identical to those for patients with nondrug causes. Male sex increases risk, and gout is 7 times more likely to develop in men than in women. High baseline serum uric acid concentrations increase the risk. Healthy men with serum uric acid concentrations of ≥9 mg/dL are 10 times more likely to have gout than those with concentrations 7–8.9 mg/dL and 50 times more likely than those with concentrations <7. The risk in patients with uric acid concentrations >9 mg/dL is roughly 5% annually. Other factors known to increase risk are a history of hypertension, diet, and obesity.[60,63,87,88] Diets rich in beef, pork, lamb, or seafood, which contain high amounts of purines, can contribute to hyperuricemic states.[89] Conversely, consumption of large amounts of low-fat dairy products is associated with a decreased risk of the development of hyperuricemia and gout.[89] Patients who have a combination of the aforementioned risk factors are at an especially increased risk for drug-induced hyperuricemia and gout.[1] Genetic variations have been explored as causative factors of hyperuricemia and gout, but the clinical relevance of these variations has yet to be determined.[90]

Table 51-6 Risk Factors for Drug-Induced Gout and Hyperuricemia[1]

- Alcohol consumption
- Decreased renal function
- Dehydration
- Elevated baseline serum uric acid concentration
- History of hypertension
- Hyperparathyroidism
- Ketoacidosis or lactic acidosis
- Lead nephropathy
- Lymphoproliferative and myeloproliferative disorders
- Obesity
- Psoriasis
- Sex (male >female)

MORBIDITY AND MORTALITY

Gout as the primary cause of death is extremely rare.[91] As compared to men without gout, an increased risk of all-cause mortality and cardiovascular disease mortality has been found in men with gout.[92] Although acute gout can be severe and lead to clinic or emergency department visits, the condition is generally self-limiting and resolves rapidly with appropriate treatment.

Gout accounted for about 2.3 million ambulatory care visits annually from 2001 through 2005 and was approximately 1.5% of the 1.17 million nonfederal, short-stay hospitalizations in 2007.[93] The estimated medical expenditures attributable to gout were $2,805 per person or $7.7 billion overall.[94]

PREVENTION

Approaches to help prevent drug-induced gout and hyperuricemia are listed in **Table 51-7**. Overall, healthy diets rich in vegetables and low-fat or nonfat dairy products have been associated with a reduced

Table 51-7 Approaches to Help Prevent Drug-Induced Gout and Hyperuricemia

Ethanol

- Reduced consumption of beer, in particular, but also wine and spirits

Nicotinic acid

- Use another class of lipid-lowering drugs when appropriate according to primary lipid target

Diuretics

- Hydrochlorothiazide doses <50 mg daily and chlorthalidone doses <25 mg daily when clinically appropriate, possibly in combination with other antihypertensives[40]; losartan and calcium channel blockers have shown some benefit in reducing diuretic-induced hyperuricemia[28,39,43-49]

Cytotoxic agents

- Pretreat with hydration, urine alkalinization, and allopurinol or urate[13]
- Allopurinol, febuxostat, and uricosuric agents
- Slowly titrate dose upward following initiation of therapy; encourage strict compliance and avoid unwarranted interruptions in therapy[53]

risk of gout.[95] Routine monitoring of serum uric acid concentrations is not currently recommended, as it is not thought to be helpful in predicting risk of gout in an individual patient, and evidence of adverse consequences associated with asymptomatic hyperuricemia is limited at this time. Many patients, even those with hyperuricemia, will not develop gout when given drugs with the potential to precipitate attacks. In most cases, the benefits of drug therapy outweigh the risks associated with an acute gout attack, particularly when one considers the ability to successfully treat the patient should an attack occur and the self-limiting nature of the disease.

Patients receiving drugs with the potential to cause gout should be monitored for symptoms that might suggest the onset of disease. From a practical standpoint, however, the severity of pain associated with an attack is such that most patients readily volunteer that information or present for care when an attack occurs.

MANAGEMENT

Decisions regarding whether or not to discontinue drugs that may be precipitating gout must be based on an assessment of risk and benefit.[96] When alternative therapy is available, a change to a drug less likely to cause hyperuricemia may be rational, although this strategy may not ensure prevention of future attacks. In some cases, drugs simply unmask patients already predisposed to the disease. These patients are at increased risk for future attacks even without further exposure to the suspect drug. In cases in which a suspect agent is deemed essential to a patient's treatment, prophylactic therapy to help prevent future attacks may be considered.

Hyperuricemia has been associated with renal, cardiovascular, and metabolic risk.[3] However, treatment of asymptomatic hyperuricemia is not recommended, as drug cost and potential toxicity outweigh known therapeutic benefit, although further studies may eventually support the need to treat the disorder to help prevent other complications. Nonpharmacologic and pharmacologic treatment is recommended for individuals who experience signs and symptoms of hyperuricemia and gout.

Limiting the consumption of purine-rich meats (beef, lamb, and pork) and seafood (sardines and shellfish), high fructose corn syrup–sweetened beverages and foods, salty condiments and foods, and alcohol (especially beer) may be of benefit to patients with gout.[3] Consuming low or nonfat dairy products is also encouraged. Dietary changes have been suggested to decrease serum urate by about 10–18%, which may prove beneficial for individuals with hyperuricemia albeit with limited efficacy for those with uric acid levels well above 7 mg/dL.

For individuals with hyperuricemia and at risk for acute attacks of gout, if a decision is made to initiate prophylactic therapy to help alleviate patient discomfort, patients with mild disease may be managed effectively with colchicine or NSAIDs. Similarly, acute breakthrough attacks of gout can generally be treated with NSAIDs or colchicine, particularly when symptoms are recognized early and treated promptly. Patients who experience continued breakthrough attacks despite prophylactic treatment may be candidates for urate-lowering therapy. Allopurinol or febuxostat are recommended first-line treatment agents for individuals who require urate-lowering therapy. The main goals of treatment should be resolution of signs and symptoms and a serum uric acid concentration of 6 mg/dL or less.[3] **Figure 51-1** outlines treatment strategies for gout.

Prophylactic treatment with colchicine or anti-inflammatory drugs is recommended during the initiation of therapy with any of the uricosuric agents to help reduce the likelihood of gout attacks during that time. Colchicine in doses of 0.6 mg 1–2 times daily is recommended as first-line prophylaxis against acute attacks.[96] Alternatively, low-dose NSAIDs such as ibuprofen 200–400 mg once or twice daily or naproxen 250 mg twice daily may also be used.

Xanthine oxidase is important in the metabolism of azathioprine and 6-mercaptopurine, and patients should have azathioprine doses reduced by 75% when allopurinol is administered concomitantly.[98] Even with dose reduction, patients receiving the combination are at increased risk for bone marrow suppression. Azathioprine and cyclosporine are frequently used together in transplant-rejection regimens and, because cyclosporine is associated with gout and hyperuricemia, allopurinol may be prescribed. Caution in determining azathioprine dose is warranted in these situations.[99]

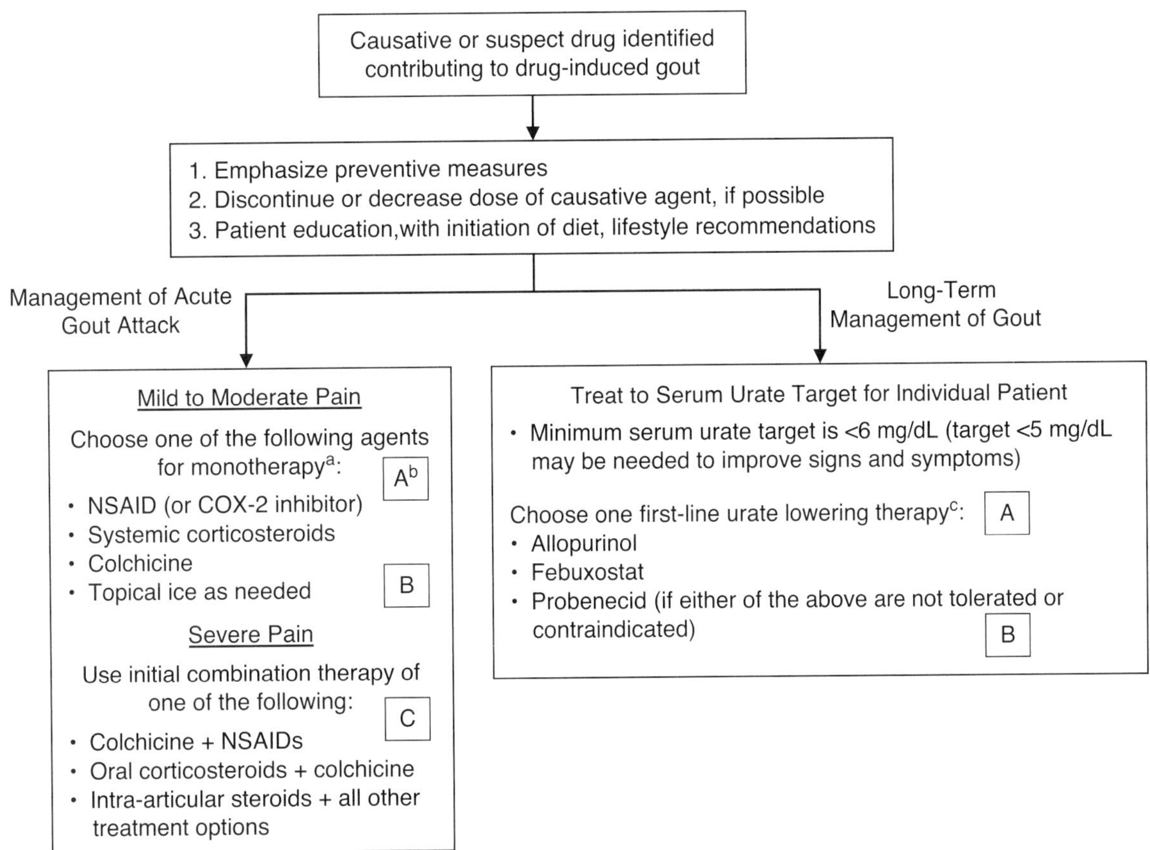

FIGURE 51-1 Treatment Strategies for Drug-Induced Gout[3,97]

[a]Switch to alternate monotherapy or add-on combination therapy if inadequate response from initial choice. Inadequate response is defined as <20% improvement in pain score within 24 hours OR <50% at 24 hours (evidence grade C).
[b]Evidence Grades for Recommendations: Level A—supported by multiple randomized clinical trials or meta-analyses; Level B—derived from single randomized trial or nonrandomized studies; and Level C—consensus opinion of experts, case studies, or standard-of-care.
[c]Increase dose of urate-lowering therapy if serum urate target is not achieved.
NSAID = nonsteroidal anti-inflammatory drug.

INFORMATION FOR PATIENTS

Patients who receive medications known to increase the risk of hyperuricemia and gout should be warned about the possibility of this disease developing and should be familiar with its common symptoms. Patients should be informed that the risk of gout is quite small and that the condition is self-limiting and relatively easy to manage, particularly when treatment is initiated soon after the onset. Patients receiving prophylactic therapy for gout should understand the importance of continuing therapy as prescribed and should be warned that attacks can be precipitated if medications are stopped and restarted. Patients should also be advised to limit alcohol intake and informed about the benefits of increasing the amount of low-fat dairy products in the diet.[3]

REFERENCES

1. Luk A, Simkin P. Epidemiology of hyperuricemia and gout. *Am J Manag Care.* 2005; 11:S435-42.
2. Bach MH, Simkin PA. Uricosuric drugs: the once and future therapy for hyperuricemia? *Curr Opin Rheumatol.* 2014; 26:169-75.
3. Khanna D, FitzGerald JD, Khanna PP et al. 2012 American College of Rheumatology guidelines for management of gout part I: systematic non-pharmacological and pharmacologic therapeutic approaches to hyperuricemia. *Arthritis Care Res (Hoboken).* 2012; 64: 1431-46.
4. Uloric package insert. Deerfield, IL: Takeda Pharmaceuticals America Inc; 2009.
5. Noguchi Y, Tatsuno I, Suyama K et al. Effect of fenofibrate on uric acid metabolism in Japanese hyperlipidemic patients. *J Atheroscler Thromb.* 2004; 11:335-40.
6. Hepburn A, Kaye S, Feher M. Long-term remission from gout associated with fenofibrate therapy. *Clin Rheumatol.* 2003; 22:73-6.
7. Feher M, Hepburn A, Hogarth M et al. Fenofibrate enhances urate reduction in men treated with allopurinol for hyperuricaemia and gout. *Rheumatology.* 2003; 42:321-5.
8. Zhang Y, Neogi T, Chen C et al. Low-dose aspirin use and recurrent gout attacks. *Ann Rheum Dis.* 2014; 73:385-90.
9. Caspi D, Lubart E, Graff E et al. The effect of mini-dose aspirin on renal function and uric acid handling in elderly patients. *Arthritis Rheum.* 2000; 43:103-8.
10. Burack DA, Griffith BP, Thompson ME et al. Hyperuricemia and gout among heart transplant recipients receiving cyclosporine. *Am J Med.* 1992; 92:141-6.
11. Kasiske BL, Vazquez MA, Harmon WE et al. Recommendations for the outpatient surveillance of renal transplant recipients. *J Am Soc Nephrol.* 2000; 11(suppl 15):S1-86.
12. Thiel G, Bock A, Spondlin M et al. Long-term benefits and risks of cyclosporin A (sandimmun)—an analysis at 10 years. *Transplant Proc.* 1994; 26:2493-8.
13. Mahmoud HH, Leverger G, Patte C et al. Advances in the management of malignancy-associated hyperuricaemia. *Br J Cancer.* 1998; 77(suppl 4):18-20.
14. Abdelrahman M, Rafi A, Ghacha R et al. Hyperuricemia and gout in renal transplant recipients. *Renal Fail.* 2002; 24:361-7.
15. Baethge BA, Work J, Landreneau MD et al. Tophaceous gout in patients with renal transplants treated with cyclosporine A. *J Rheumatol.* 1993; 20:718-20.
16. Ben Hmida M, Hachicha J, Bahloul Z et al. Cyclosporine-induced hyperuricemia and gout in renal transplants. *Transplant Proc.* 1995; 27:2722-4.
17. Clive DM. Renal transplant-associated hyperuricemia and gout. *J Am Soc Nephrol.* 2000; 11:974-9.
18. Delaney V, Sumrani N, Daskalakis P et al. Hyperuricemia and gout in renal allograft recipients. *Transplant Proc.* 1992; 24:1773-4.
19. Kelleher SP, Davis WR, Paraskevopoulos N. Gout, bradycardia, and hypercholesterolemia after renal transplantation. *South Med J.* 2001; 94:732-4.
20. Gores PF, Fryd DS, Sutherland DE et al. Hyperuricemia after renal transplantation. *Am J Surg.* 1988; 156:397-400.
21. Lin HY, Rocher LL, McQuillan MA et al. Cyclosporine-induced hyperuricemia and gout. *N Engl J Med.* 1989; 321:287-92.
22. Marcen R, Gallego N, Orofino L et al. Impairment of tubular secretion of urate in renal transplant patients on cyclosporine. *Nephron.* 1995; 70:307-13.
23. Noordzij TC, Leunissen KM, Van Hooff JP. Renal handling of urate and the incidence of gouty arthritis during cyclosporine and diuretic use. *Transplantation.* 1991; 52:64-7.
24. West C, Carpenter BJ, Hakala TR. The incidence of gout in renal transplant recipients. *Am J Kidney Dis.* 1987; 10:369-72.
25. Jeha S. Tumor lysis syndrome. *Semin Hematol.* 2001; 38:4-8.
26. Vandell AG, McDonough CW, Gong Y et al. Hydrochlorothiazide-induced hyperuricaemia in the pharmacogenomic evaluation of antihypertensive responses study. *J Intern Med.* 2014; 276:486-97.
27. McAdams-Demarco MA, Maynard JW, Baer AN et al. *Ann Rheum Dis.* 2013; 72:701-6.
28. Choi HK, SorianoLC, Zhang Y et al. Antihypertensive drugs and risk of incident gout among patients with hypertension: population based case-control study. *BMJ* 2012; 344:d8190.
29. El-Sheikh AA, van den Heuvel JJ, Koenderink JB et al. Effect of hypouricaemic and hyperuricaemic drugs on the renal urate efflux transporter, multidrug resistance protein 4. *Br J Pharmacol.* 2008; 155:1066.
30. Choi H, Mount D, Reginato A. Pathogenesis of gout. *Ann Intern Med.* 2005; 143:499-516.
31. Hueskes BA, Roovers EA, Janssen M. Use of diuretics and the risk of gouty arthritis: a systematic review. *Semin Arthritis Rheum.* 2012; 41:879-89.
32. Medical Research Council Working Party. Adverse reactions to bendrofluazide and propranolol for the treatment of mild hypertension: report of Medical Research Council Working Party on mild to moderate hypertension. *Lancet.* 1981; 318:539-43.
33. Staessen J. The determinants and prognostic significance of serum uric acid in elderly patients of the European Working Party on high blood pressure in the elderly trial. *Am J Med.* 1991; 90:50-4S.
34. Gurwitz JH, Kalish SC, Bohn RL et al. Thiazide diuretics and the initiation of anti-gout therapy. *J Clin Epidemiol.* 1997; 50:953-9.
35. Langford HG, Blaufox MD, Borhani NO et al. Is thiazide produced uric acid elevation harmful? Analysis of data from the Hypertension Detection and Follow-up Program. *Arch Intern Med.* 1987; 147:645-9.
36. Janssens H, van de Lisdank E, Janssen M et al. Gout, not induced by diuretics? A case-control study from primary care. *Ann Rheum Dis.* 2006; 65:1080-3.
37. Choi HK, Atkinson K, Karlson EW et al. Obesity, weight change, hypertension, diuretic use, and risk of incident gout in men: the health professionals follow-up study. *Arch Intern Med.* 2005; 165:742-8.
38. Hunter D, York M, Chaisson C et al. Recent diuretic use and the risk of recurrent gout attacks: the online case crossover gout study. *J Rheumatol.* 2006; 33:1341-5.

39. Bruderer S, Bodmer M, Jick S et al. Use of diuretics and risk of incident gout. *Arthritis Rheumatol.* 2014; 66:185-96.
40. James PA, Oparil S, Carter BL et al. 2014 Evidence-based guideline for the management of high blood pressure in adults report from the panel members appointed to the eighth joint national committee (JNC 8) *JAMA.* 2014; 311:507-20.
41. Tikkanen I, Omvik P, Jensen HA. Comparison of the angiotensin II antagonist losartan with the angiotensin converting enzyme inhibitor enalapril in patients with essential hypertension. *J Hypertens.* 1995; 13:1343.
42. Wurzner G, Gerster JC, Chiolero A et al. Comparative effects of losartan and irbesartan on serum uric acid in hypertensive patients with hyperuricaemia and gout. *J Hypertens.* 2001; 19:1855-60.
43. Ruilope LM, Kirwan BA, de Brouwer S et al. Uric acid and other renal function parameters in patients with stable angina pectoris participating in the ACTION trial: impact of nifedipine GITS (gastro-intestinal therapeutic system) and relation to outcome. *J Hypertens.* 2007; 25:1711-8.
44. Chanard J, Toupance O, Lavaud S et al. Amlodipine reduces cyclosporin-induced hyperuricaemia in hypertensive renal transplant recipients. *Nephrol Dial Transplant.* 2003; 18:2147-53.
45. Burnier M, Waeber B, Brunner HR. Clinical pharmacology of the angiotensin II receptor antagonist losartan potassium in healthy subjects. *J Hypertens Suppl.* 1995; 13:S23-8.
46. Burnier M, Roch-Ramel F, Brunner HR. Renal effects of angiotensin II receptor blockade in normotensive subjects. *Kidney Int.* 1996; 49:1787-90.
47. Shahinfar S, Simpson RL, Carides AD et al. Safety of losartan in hypertensive patients with thiazide-induced hyperuricemia. *Kidney Int.* 1999; 56:1879-85.
48. Hoieggen A, Alderman MH, Kjeldsen SE et al. The impact of serum uric acid on cardiovascular outcomes in the LIFE study. *Kidney Int.* 2004; 65:1041-9.
49. Alderman M, Aiyer KJ. Uric acid: role in cardiovascular disease and effects of losartan. *Curr Med Res Opin.* 2004; 20:369-79.
50. Louthrenoo W, Hongsangkiat S, Kasitanon N et al. Effect of antituberculous drugs on serum uric acid and urine uric acid excretion. *J Clin Rheumatol.* 2015; 21: 346–8.
51. Postlethwaite AE, Bartel AG, Kelley WN. Hyperuricemia due to ethambutol. *N Engl J Med.* 1972; 286:761-2.
52. American Thoracic Society; CDC; Infectious Diseases Society of America. Treatment of tuberculosis. *MMWR.* 2003; 52:1-77.
53. Scott JT. Drug-induced gout. *Baillieres Clin Rheumatol.* 1991; 5:39-60.
54. Self TH, Fountain FF, Taylor WJ et al. Acute gouty arthritis associated with the use of ethambutol. *Chest.* 1977; 71:561-2.
55. Khanna B, Gupta V, Singh M. Ethambutol-induced hyperuricaemia (abstract). *Tubercle* 1984; 65:195-9.
56. Rao TP, Schmitt JK. Gout secondary to pyrazinamide and ethambutol. *VA Med Q.* 1996; 123:271.
57. Postlethwaite AE, Kelley WN. Studies on the mechanism of ethambutol-induced hyperuricemia. *Arthritis Rheum.* 1972; 15:403-9.
58. Khanna BK. Acute gouty arthritis following ethambutol therapy. *Br J Dis Chest.* 1980; 74:409-10.
59. Postlethwaite AE, Bartel AG, Kelley WN. Hyperuricemia induced by ethambutol. *Adv Exp Med Biol.* 1974; 41:763-7.
60. Lin KC, Lin HY, Chou P. The interaction between uric acid level and other risk factors on the development of gout among asymptomatic hyperuricemic men in a prospective study. *J Rheumatol.* 2000; 27:1501-5.
61. Rodnan GP. Invitation to the gout: a consideration of the role of various predisposing and provocative factors in the genesis of acute gouty arthritis. *Trans Stud Coll Physicians Phila.* 1967; 35:47062.
62. Sharpe CR. A case-control study of alcohol consumption and drinking behaviour in patients with acute gout. *CMAJ.* 1984; 131:563-7.
63. Waller PC, Ramsay LE. Predicting acute gout in diuretic treated hypertensive patients. *J Hum Hypertens.* 1989; 3:457-61.
64. Choi H, Atkinson K, Karlson E. Alcohol intake and risk of incident gout in men: a prospective study. *Lancet.* 2004; 363:1277-81.
65. Choi H, Curhan G. Beer, liquor, and wine consumption and serum uric acid level: the third national health and nutrition examination survey. *Arthritis Rheum.* 2004; 51:1023-9.
66. Yu KH, See LC, Huang YC et al. Dietary factors associated with hyperuricemia in adults. *Semin Arthritis Rheum.* 2008; 37:243-50.
67. Emmerson BT. The management of gout. *N Engl J Med.* 1996; 334:445-51.
68. Calne DB, Fermaglich J. Gout induced by L-dopa and decarboxylase inhibitors. *Postgrad Med J.* 1976; 52:232-3.
69. Honda H, Gindin RA. Gout while receiving levodopa for Parkinsonism. *JAMA.* 1972; 219:55-7.
70. al-Hujaj M, Schonthal H. Hyperuricemia and levodopa. *N Engl J Med.* 1971; 285:859-60.
71. Barbeau A. L-dopa therapy in Parkinson's disease: critical review of nine years' experience. *CMAJ.* 1969; 101:59-68.
72. Andreadou E, Nikolaou C, Gournaras F et al. Serum uric acid levels in patients with Parkinson's disease: their relationship to treatment and disease duration. *Clin Neurol Neurosurg.* 2009 Nov; 111:724-8.
73. Guyton JR, Bays HE. Safety considerations with niacin therapy. *Am J Cardiol.* 2007; 99(suppl):22C-31C.
74. Gerdan G, Nurullah A, Ucan ES et al. Paradoxical increase in uric acid level with allopurinol use in pyrazinamide-induced hyperuricemia. *Singapore Med J.* 2013; 54 e125-6.
75. Taki H, Ogawa K, Murakami T et al. Epidemiological survey of hyperuricemia as an adverse reaction to antituberculous therapy with pyrazinamide. *Kekkaku* 2008; 83:497-501.
76. Amodio MI, Bengualid V, Lowy FD. Development of acute gout secondary to pyrazinamide in a patient without a prior history of gout. *DICP.* 1990; 24:1115-6.
77. Emmerson BT, Mirosch W, Douglas JB. The relative contributions of tubular reabsorption and secretion to urate excretion in lead nephropathy. *Aust NZ J Med.* 1971; 1:353-62.
78. Gerster J, Dudler M, Halkic N et al. Gout in liver transplant patients receiving tacrolimus. *Ann Rheum Dis* 2004; 63:894-5.
79. Neal D, Tom B, Gimson A et al. Hyperuricemia, gout, and renal function after liver transplantation. *Transplantation.* 2001; 72:1689-91.
80. Kanbay M, Akcay A, Huddam C et al. Influence of cyclosporine and tacrolimus on serum uric acid levels in stable kidney transplant patients. *Transplant Proc.* 2005; 37:3119-20.
81. Pilmore HL, Faire B, Dittmer I. Tacrolimus for the treatment of gout in renal transplantation: two case reports and review of the literature. *Transplantation.* 2001; 72:1703-5.
82. Thorat A, Chou HS, Lee CF et al. Effects of converting tacrolimus formulation from twice daily to once daily in liver transplantation recipients. *Biomed Res Int.* 2014; 2014:265658.
83. Miller PD, Schwartz EN, Chen P et al. Teriparatide in postmenopausal women with osteoporosis and mild or moderate renal impairment. *Osteoporos Int.* 2007; 18:59-68.
84. Boonen S, Marin F, Mellstrom D et al. Safety and efficacy of teriparatide in elderly women with established osteoporosis: bone anabolic therapy from a geriatric perspective. *J Am Geriatr Soc.* 2006; 54:782-9.
85. Schlesinger N, Norquist J, Watson D. Serum urate during acute gout. *J Rheumatol.* 2009; 36:1287-9.
86. Neogi T, Jansen TL, Dalbeth N et al. 2015 Gout classification criteria: an American College of Rheumatology/European League against rheumatism collaborative initiative. *Ann Rheum Dis.* 2015; 74:1789-98.
87. Campion EW, Glynn RJ, DeLabry LO. Asymptomatic hyperuricemia: risks and consequences in the Normative Aging Study. *Am J Med.* 1987; 82:421-6.

88. Lin KC, Lin HY, Chou P. Community based epidemiological study on hyperuricemia and gout in Kin Hu, Kinmen. *J Rheumatol.* 2000; 27:1045-50.
89. Choi H, Atkinson K, Karlson E et al. Purine-rich foods, dairy and protein intake, and the risk of gout in men. *N Engl J Med.* 2004; 350:1093-1103.
90. Reginato AM, Mount DB, Yang I et al. The genetics of hyperuricaemia and gout. *Nat Rev Rheumatol.* 2012; 8:610-21.
91. Sacks JJ, Helmick CG, Langmaid G. Deaths from arthritis and other rheumatic conditions, United States, 1979–1998. *J Rheumatol.* 2004; 31:1823-8.
92. Choi HK and Curhan G. Independent impact of gout on mortality and risk for coronary heart disease. *Circulation.* 2007; 116:894-900.
93. United States Bone and Joint Decade. *The Burden of Musculoskeletal Diseases in the United States.* Rosemont, IL: American Academy of Orthopaedic Surgeons; 2008. Chapter 4. Arthritis and related conditions.
94. Cisternas MG , Murphy LB, Pasta DJ et al. Annual medical care expenditures among US adults with gout, 2005–2011. *Arthritis Rheum.* 2014; 66:S888.
95. Mayo Clinic. Gout diet: what's allowed and what's not. http://www.mayoclinic.org/healthy-lifestyle/nutrition-and-healthy-eating/in-depth/gout-diet/art-20048524100 (accessed 2017 Jun 5).
96. Underwood M. Diagnosis and management of gout. *BMJ.* 2006; 332:1315-9.
97. Khanna D, Khanna PP, FitzGerald JD et al. 2012 American College of Rheumatology guidelines for management of gout. Part 2: therapy and anti-inflammatory prophylaxis of acute gouty arthritis. *Arthritis Care Res (Hoboken).* 2012; 64:1447-61.
98. Drug Interactions. Micromedex Healthcare Series. Greenwood Village, CO: Thomson Micromedex (accessed 2017 Jun 5).
99. Wluka AE, Ryan PF, Miller AM et al. Post-cardiac transplantation gout: incidence of therapeutic complications. *J Heart Lung Transplant.* 2000; 19:951-6.
100. Scott J, Dixon S, Bywaters E. Association of hyperuricaemia and gout with hyperparathyroidism. *BMJ.* 1964; 1:1070-3.
101. Hainer BL, Matheson E, Wilkes RT. Diagnosis, treatment, and prevention of gout. *Am Fam Physician.* 2014; 90:831-6.
102. Harris M, Siegel L, Alloway J. Gout and hyperuricemia. *Am Fam Physician.* 1999; 59:925-34.

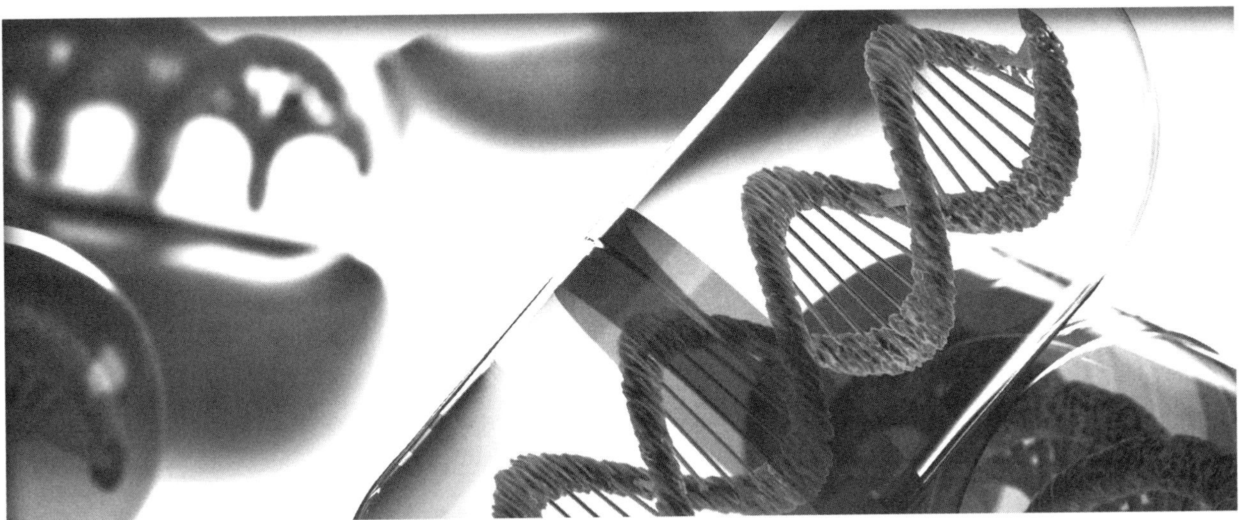

CHAPTER 52

Myopathy

Craig Williams

Over 150 marketed drugs have been associated with myopathy.[1] Although many cases are asymptomatic and self-limiting, the most severe forms can be fatal.[2] The initial diagnosis is usually made clinically, and because appropriate management includes cessation of the causative agent, it is imperative for clinicians to be aware of the drugs commonly associated with myopathy and the presenting signs and symptoms of this drug-induced disease.

Although myopathies are sometimes reported as being painful, they most often present as weakness without pain.[2,3] Patients with weakness may use descriptors such as numbness or fatigue and may describe a general discomfort which is not truly painful. It is, therefore, important to get the patient's accurate history, including a careful description of symptoms. In many cases, elevations in serum creatine kinase (CK) concentration indicate extensive myocyte death, but symptomatic myopathy and weakness may be present without an elevated CK. Because of the varied clinical presentation, the descriptive terminology of myopathy is important. For consistency, the following definitions will be used for this chapter (adapted from a clinical advisory from the National Heart Lung Blood Institute[4]):

- *Myopathy*—a general term referring to any disease of the muscles. Myopathy encompasses all of the following, more specific definitions:
    - *Myalgia*—muscular pain and/or weakness in the absence of elevations of CK.
    - *Myositis*—elevated CK with or without muscular pain or weakness (typically >2 times the upper limit of normal [ULN] which is approximately 200 units/L).
    - *Rhabdomyolysis*—muscular pain and/or weakness with CK elevation (at least >2 times and often >10 times the ULN) and evidence of acute renal disease (myoglobinuria and often, but not necessarily, elevated serum creatinine).

Myopathy associated with substance abuse or toxicity (e.g., ethanol, acetaminophen) or severe hypersensitivity reactions (malignant hyperthermia and toxic epidermal necrolysis) are not addressed in this chapter.

CAUSATIVE AGENTS

Definitive associations with some medications have been established while many others are linked only through case reports (**Table 52-1**).[5-55] Drugs may cause painful or painless myopathies.

Painful myopathies include necrotizing myopathy, mitochondrial myopathy, polymyositis or dermatomyositis, and neuromyopathies.[23,27,39] Mitochondrial myopathy is clearly associated with zidovudine.[45,46-48] D-penicillamine is most commonly associated with polymyositis, but more recently

Table 52-1 Agents Implicated in Drug-Induced Myopathy

Drug	Incidence	Level of Evidence[a]
Aminocaproic acid[5]	NK	C
Amiodarone[6]	<1%	C
Chloroquine[7,52]	3–5%	C
Clofibrate[8]	5–40%	B
Colchicine[9-11]	NK	B
Corticosteroids (systemic)[12-17,21,b]	1–5%[a]	A
Cyclosporine[18,c]	NK	B
Diuretics[2,19,20]	NK	B
D-penicillamine[21,22]	1%	B
Etretinate[19,23]	NK	C
Ezetimibe[24,d]	NK	C
Fibrates[8,25]	2–35%	B
Finasteride[9,26]	NK	C
Hydroxychloroquine[19,27]	1–3%	C
Interferon[28]	2–5%	B
Ipecac[2,19,29,30]	3%	B
Labetolol[31,32]	NK	C
Laxatives[19,27,33]	NK	B
Leuprolide[34]	NK	C
Procainamide[35]	NK	C
Proton-pump inhibitors[36,37,e]	<1%	C
Rifampin[19,20,38]	NK	C
Statins[4,25,39-43,53-55]	1–30%	A
Tenofovir[26,33]	NK	C
Terbinafine[51]	NK	C
Teriparatide[50]	NK	C
Tetracycline[44]	NK	C
Vincristine[19]	NK	B
Zidovudine[45-49]	10–15%	C

NK = not known.

[a]Definitions for Levels of Evidence: Level A—evidence from one or more randomized, controlled clinical trials; Level B—evidence from nonrandomized clinical trials, prospective observational studies, cohort studies, retrospective studies, case-control studies, meta-analyses and/or postmarketing surveillance studies; and Level C—evidence from one or more published case reports or case series.

[b]Incidence much higher with higher doses and with fluorinated steroids.

[c]More common when administered concomitantly with other drugs, especially statins.

[d]More common in patients with previous statin myopathy.

[e]More case reports implicating omeprazole likely reflect greater usage of that agent within the class.

the proton-pump inhibitors have also been implicated.[27,36,37] Painful neuromyopathies have been reported in association with amiodarone and vincristine and have also been described in patients with electrolyte disturbances caused by drugs such as diuretics, aluminum- or magnesium-containing antacids, isotonic glucose solutions, and licorice.[19,23,26]

Painless myopathies include corticosteroid myopathy, painless neuromyopathies, and some myopathies secondary to drug-induced electrolyte disturbances, particularly hypokalemia and hypermagnesemia.[13,27,31]

EPIDEMIOLOGY

The true incidence of drug-induced myopathy is unknown, but it is likely more common than generally appreciated as many cases are self-limited and unreported.[21,27,31] The incidence varies greatly between causative agents and is based on dose, duration of exposure, risk factors present in the population being treated, and the definition of myopathy applied.

In a 1-year prospective trial reviewing cases of myositis in a large university hospital system, serially measured CK values resulted in an estimated rate of drug-induced myositis of 7.2 per 10,000 inpatients and 9.3 per 10,000 outpatients. Lipid-lowering medications (fibrates and statins) were the causative agents in nearly 60% of the cases, with antiretrovirals accounting for another 14%.[56]

Reports of statin-induced myopathy offer an excellent example of how incidence can vary based on the definition of myopathy used. In the 5-year, 20,536-patient Heart Protection Study (HPS), subjective myalgias were reported in 33% of both the statin- and placebo-treated groups while myositis occurred in only 1.3% of each group and rhabdomyolysis occurred in only 5 patients receiving simvastatin (<0.1%) and 3 patients receiving placebo (<0.1%).[57] Based on these data, it would seem reasonable to expect that case series that include myalgia in the definition of myopathy will report a higher rate of myopathy than those that restrict the definition of myopathy to CK-positive events.

The low incidence of rhabdomyolysis and the relatively high incidence of myalgias reported in the HPS trial are both supported by other research with statins.[40,58] It should be kept in mind, however, that higher-risk patients (e.g., those with chronic renal failure or age >75 years) are often excluded from randomized studies, which can result in an underestimation in the risk of drug-induced myopathies that can occur with more common usage patterns in clinical practice.[43]

Corticosteroid-induced myopathy has been identified as one of the main causes of iatrogenic proximal myopathies and has an estimated prevalence of 3–60%.[12,15,19,26,27] The onset of steroid-induced myopathy is rare within 30 days of initiation.[3] This can be helpful in trying to determine whether the cause of the myopathy is due to the steroid or to the underlying condition for which the steroid is used. The incidence of D-penicillamine–induced myopathy is approximately 1%, and treatment with antimalarial agents has been associated with an incidence of myopathy of 1 per 100 patient-years.[19,59] Myopathy develops in approximately 15% to 20% of patients receiving zidovudine.[23]

MECHANISMS

Drug-induced myopathy can be broadly classified as an endocrine or toxic myopathy which results from disrupted cellular function. Skeletal muscle is a complex, heterogeneous mix of cell types that comprises 40% of adult body mass.[60] Its complexity is due in part to the physiologic complexity of transitioning millions of cells from a resting to a working state and back again within seconds. In the working state, the high energy needs of myocytes are generally met by glycogen, but in the fasting state or states of prolonged work, glycogen depletion leads to the use of free fatty acids as an alternative fuel source.[60,61]

Efficiency is achieved through division of labor with some myocytes (type I) designed to sustain slow, prolonged work and others (type II) designed for quick bursts. Cells that provide prolonged work rely heavily on a constant mitochondrial supply of energy with which some drugs can interfere.[61]

Generating muscle contractions involves the propagation of an action potential. Drugs that directly or indirectly affect electrolyte concentrations can affect the ability of myocytes to initiate or maintain contraction, leading primarily to painless myopathies characterized by weakness. The exact mechanisms by which most drugs cause myopathies are unknown, but some broad categories have been described based on histopathologic and clinical findings (**Table 52-2**).

NECROTIZING MYOPATHY

Necrotizing myopathy, also known as metabolic myopathy, is associated with underlying abnormalities in energy production that can ultimately lead to myocyte death. It is most frequently associated with statins and fibrates, although there is some evidence linking nicotinic acid, aminocaproic acid, and high-dose vitamins A and E to this disorder as well.[39,42] The mechanism of statin-induced necrotizing myopathy is unknown. However, it likely involves interference with cellular metabolism either directly by interfering with the production of important intracellular proteins or mitochondrial function or indirectly by reducing the availability of fatty acids as a fuel source to working skeletal muscle.[3,27,62] Other possible mechanisms for statin-induced myopathy include disruption of glycoprotein synthesis in muscle membrane, a decrease in chloride channels in the muscle membrane, increases in intracellular calcium concentration, and decreased cell membrane fluidity.[39,43]

MITOCHONDRIAL MYOPATHY

Zidovudine is one agent that is most commonly associated with mitochondrial myopathy.[27,45,47] A direct toxic effect of the drug on muscle mitochondria is believed to be involved. Drug-induced vascular damage or dysfunction leading to muscle ischemia is also suspected.[20] Dalakas et al.[45] determined that zidovudine causes abnormal mitochondrial function by inhibiting γ-deoxyribonucleic

Table 52-2 Mechanisms of Drug-Induced Myopathy

Drug	Mechanism
PAINFUL NEUROPATHIES	
Aminocaproic acid[5] Clofibrate[8,54,55] Etretinate[19] Ezetimibe[24] Fenofibrate[8,25,54] Gemfibrozil[8,25,54] Statins[25,40,41,43,53,57,58]	<u>Necrotizing:</u> Necrosis of muscle fibers with myophagocytosis and typically marked elevation of CK
Ipecac[2,19] Zidovudine[45-49]	<u>Mitochondrial:</u> Impaired mitochondrial function often secondary to inhibition of mitochondrial DNA polymerase
D-penicillamine[21,22] Proton-pump inhibitors[36,37]	<u>Polymyositis/dermatomyositis:</u> Inflammatory reaction; may involve eosinophil infiltration
Amiodarone[6]	<u>Lysosomal:</u> Accumulation in intracellular lysosomes disrupts normal lysosomal function and impairs vacuolar clearance of cell debris; vacuole accumulation causes cell dysfunction
PAINLESS MYOPATHIES	
Corticosteroids[12-15]	Enhanced intracellular protein breakdown and altered calcium homeostasis; CK may or may not be elevated
Chloroquine[30,52,59] Diuretics[2,19] Hydroxychloroquine[19,59] Laxatives[19,33]	<u>Neuromyopathy:</u> Deranged ion transport impairs neuromuscular signaling; may become painful if prolonged Some evidence of impaired glycogen production and storage
Colchicine[9-11]	<u>Antimicrotubular:</u> Binding to intracellular tubulin leads to altered microtubular function resulting in altered peripheral nerve conduction and changes in muscle cell structure

CK = creatine kinase, DNA = deoxyribonucleic acid.

acid (DNA) polymerase, an enzyme found exclusively in the mitochondrial matrix. Inhibition of this enzyme results in interference with the replication of mitochondrial DNA and leads to abnormal accumulation of lipid and glycogen in the muscle cells. The authors found that some subjects improved with the addition of prednisone to their medication regimen, suggesting that an inflammatory process may also be involved.[45]

POLYMYOSITIS AND DERMATOMYOSITIS

Drug-induced polymyositis and dermatomyositis are manifestations of autoimmune microvascular injury most often involving autoantibodies directed at endothelium in connective tissue. It has been classically associated with D-penicillamine, which exerts complex effects on cellular and humoral immune mechanisms, including reducing serum concentrations of Immunoglobulin M rheumatoid factor and depressing T-cell activity. These effects may be desirable for the treatment of rheumatoid arthritis, in which immunoregulatory alterations may be beneficial because of the nature of the disease. However, it is possible that the immunoregulatory disturbances created by D-penicillamine may lead to a loss of tolerance to muscle antigens, resulting in an immune response, manifested by inflammation and subsequently an inflammatory and autoimmune myopathy.[27,29,62] Polymyositis and dermatomyositis may also result from drug-induced necrosis, regeneration, and inflammation of muscle fibers.[31] The incidence of polymyositis and dermatomyositis with newer, more targeted immunotherapies such as infliximab and rituximab is extremely low with a rate in clinical trials that is not different from placebo.[63]

ELECTROLYTE DISTURBANCES

Myopathies may be induced by drugs through indirect mechanisms as may occur with diuretic-induced hypokalemia, hypophosphatemia, or by hypermagnesemia induced by overuse of magnesium-containing antacids.[19,26,27] Hypokalemia may result in reduction of cell membrane excitability, leading to decreased neuromuscular transmission.[29] Hypophosphatemia may cause myopathy via depletion of adenosine triphosphate in muscle cells.[26] Hypermagnesemia may cause myopathy by interfering with neuromuscular transmission through inhibition of the release of acetylcholine.[26]

PAINLESS MYOPATHY

The mechanism by which chloroquine and hydroxychloroquine induce myotoxicity is not definitively known, but may be due to drug accumulation in lysosomes, resulting in decreased lysosomal activity and subsequent cellular accumulation of phospholipids and glycogen.[52,64] Colchicine-induced neuromyopathy is thought to result from microtubule damage, leading to altered peripheral nerve conduction and eventual changes in muscle cell structure that are related to intracellular lysosome movement.[10]

CORTICOSTEROID MYOPATHY

The mechanism of corticosteroid-induced myopathy has been debated, and several potential mechanisms exist. Corticosteroids exert a catabolic effect on muscle and may cause atrophy of the type II muscle fibers.[23,26] Corticosteroids also impair glucose uptake and increase protein catabolism, resulting in muscle atrophy.[13] Reduced protein synthesis associated with long-term exposure to corticosteroids can also play a role in the negative protein balance induced by these drugs.[2,12,16] In addition, corticosteroids may cause mitochondrial injury, leading to muscle necrosis.[23]

CLINICAL PRESENTATION AND DIFFERENTIAL DIAGNOSIS

The presentation of drug-induced myopathy is varied, and common signs and symptoms are listed in **Table 52-3**. Although necrotizing myopathies more commonly occur early in the course of therapy (<6 months after the start of therapy), the time to onset is variable.[27] Drug-induced myopathies that occur after a long period of uncomplicated drug therapy may be caused by patient-specific factors such as changing renal or hepatic function or the recent addition of an interacting drug. Clinicians should be alert to these types of changes whenever

Table 52-3 Signs and Symptoms of Drug-Induced Myopathy[18,20,22,25,26,28,30,32]

Less severe disease

- Decreased or absent reflexes
- Fatigue
- Muscle pain or tenderness
- Muscle weakness
- Normal creatine kinase (<200 units/L)
- Shortness of breath
- Weight loss

More severe disease

- Decreased urine production
- Discolored urine
- Dysphagia
- Dyspnea
- Elevated serum creatine kinase concentration (>400 units/L)

Table 52-4 Conditions to Consider in the Differential Diagnosis of Drug-Induced Myopathy[2,18,32,61,62]

- Cushing syndrome
- Heart failure
- Hypothyroidism
- Infection: treponemal (syphilis), mycobacterial (tuberculosis), viral (cytomegalovirus, human immunodeficiency virus, Epstein–Barr, adenoviruses)
- New neuromuscular condition such as amyotrophic lateral sclerosis, muscular dystrophy, or myasthenia gravis
- New or worsening rheumatologic condition such as polymyalgia rheumatica, arthritis, fibromyalgia, systemic lupus erythematosus, or sarcoidosis
- Simple muscle strain or sprain

a patient presents with signs and symptoms consistent with myopathy that may be caused by a medication that has been used without difficulty for over a year. Myopathy caused by electrolyte disturbances typically has a rapid onset.[27,29] However, because drug-induced disturbances of serum electrolyte concentrations can have a highly variable time to onset, the temporal relationship between initiation of therapy with these agents (e.g., diuretics) and onset of myopathy is also highly variable.

Identification of a causal relationship between a new myopathy and drug therapy is important, as most drug-induced myopathies are reversible upon discontinuation of the causative agent. Symptomatic relief upon cessation of therapy is also an important aspect of the diagnosis.[65] Although a rechallenge often offers the best chance of a definitive diagnosis, it may or may not be indicated based on the initial severity of the myopathy. Other potential causes of muscle symptoms should always be kept in mind (**Table 52-4**). Changes may be present on electromyography or tissue histology, but these tests are usually performed only in more refractory cases to help with the differential diagnosis.[2]

Often, patients with drug-induced myopathy present with vague or simple muscle pain, which may evolve to muscle tenderness and/or weakness, typically of the proximal muscles (shoulders, upper arms, thighs, and pelvis).[19] In some cases, CK is elevated and electromyography may reveal myopathic changes.[8] The most severe presentation is rhabdomyolysis in which massive loss of peripheral muscle cells leads to release of intracellular contents. The urine darkens because of myoglobinuria, CK is markedly elevated (often defined as >10 times the ULN, but this is somewhat arbitrary), and urine production may decrease if acute renal failure occurs.

Necrotizing myopathy may present with acute or subacute muscle symptoms.[19] Typically, muscle pain, tenderness, and weakness are present in the proximal limbs, although a more generalized presentation is also possible.[2] Histopathologic examination may reveal mitochondrial changes.[2,27]

As previously discussed, mitochondrial myopathies are most frequently linked to antiretroviral drugs, particularly zidovudine. Complicating the diagnosis of zidovudine-associated myopathy is the natural progression of infection with the human immunodeficiency virus (HIV). Patients infected with HIV often have myopathy as part of the disease process. Zidovudine-induced myopathy may be differentiated from that caused by HIV infection by establishing a temporal relationship between initiation of antiretroviral drug therapy and the onset of symptoms of myopathy and by the resolution of symptoms after discontinuation of therapy.[23] Mitochondrial myopathies are usually painful, with pronounced wasting and tenderness.[19] Muscle biopsy in patients with zidovudine-induced myopathy often reveals abnormal mitochondria of varying size and shape. The mitochondria appear disorganized; necrosis, ragged fibers, and inflammatory infiltrates may be observed on microscopic examination.[23] CK may be normal or moderately elevated.[19]

Like necrotizing myopathy, polymyositis and dermatomyositis may present acutely or subacutely; the presentation may also be insidious. Many nonspecific symptoms may be present including fatigue, weight loss, myalgias, or arthralgias. Muscle involvement is usually, but not always, symmetrical. Proximal muscles are often affected, and patients may report pain in the shoulder, the pelvic girdle, or both.[19] Muscle biopsies in patients with dermatomyositis or polymyositis reveal a mononuclear cell infiltrate that begins in blood vessels and extends into the myofibers.[21] Patients with dermatomyositis also have a rash, which is often edematous, symmetrically involving the periorbital area and upper eyelids.[21] CK may be moderately elevated.[31]

Painful neuromyopathies have been associated with vincristine and amiodarone. Patients with vincristine-induced myopathy typically present with proximal weakness, pain, and atrophy, with absent reflexes.[33] The electromyogram is often normal, and muscle biopsy may show necrosis and regeneration.[31] Amiodarone may cause a peripheral neuromyopathy that is associated with peripheral neuropathy, weakness, and muscle pain. The CK is often high, and electromyography may reveal slowing of nerve conduction velocity. Muscle biopsy demonstrates vacuolar myopathy and no inflammation.[33]

Patients with drug-induced electrolyte disturbances resulting in myopathies may present with muscle fatigue or sudden onset of motor deficit with pain, hypotonia, and decreased or absent reflexes.[19,26] CK may be significantly elevated in some cases.[23] In the case of hypokalemic myopathy, muscle weakness is often generalized, and pain may be present or absent.[29]

Painless myopathies often present insidiously, with muscle weakness in the proximal lower limbs, which may subsequently progress to the upper limbs and trunk.[11,19] Peripheral neuropathy may accompany the weakness of the limbs. Facial muscles may also be affected. CK may be normal or elevated to slightly above normal. Electromyography reveals slowing of nerve conduction.[11,19]

Corticosteroid myopathy may develop after long-term therapy or may occur more acutely.[12,14,33] Most commonly, corticosteroid myopathy presents as an insidious process during long-term therapy and mainly involves the proximal muscle groups, particularly in the lower limbs.[19,26,31,33] Because corticosteroids may be used to treat rheumatologic conditions that may themselves be associated with myopathy, it is important to distinguish drug-induced myopathy from that associated with progression of the disease.

Acute corticosteroid myopathy may occur as the result of therapy with high-dose intravenous corticosteroids administered in an acute care setting. The presence of concomitant therapy with a neuromuscular blocking agent increases the risk of occurrence.[16,27] In this setting, myopathy typically presents acutely, with generalized muscle involvement. Respiratory muscles may be affected and serum CK concentrations may be markedly elevated.[27,62]

In patients with corticosteroid-induced myopathy related to long-term therapy, CK is usually not elevated, but urine creatine excretion is increased.[26,33] Muscle biopsy often reveals nonspecific type II muscle fiber atrophy.[26,33] Reflexes are typically preserved, and electromyography reveals myopathic changes.[31] Phosphate depletion secondary to excessive antacid consumption may result in myopathy in patients with concurrent gastrointestinal disease who are taking corticosteroids.[23] In these settings, it is difficult to determine whether the myopathy is secondary to hypophosphatemia or to corticosteroid therapy.[19,23]

In summary, many drugs have been associated with myalgias, which may be related to one of the myopathic processes discussed previously or to other types of drug-induced rheumatic disorders or hypersensitivity reactions.[19] Patients with drug-induced myalgia present with muscle pain that improves after drug discontinuation.

RISK FACTORS

General risk factors for drug-induced myopathy are listed in **Table 52-5** and typically include higher doses of the causative agent, longer duration of exposure, presence of drug interactions, prolonged and vigorous exercise, and genetic predisposition.

Table 52-5 Risk Factors for the Development of Drug-Induced Myopathy[13,22,25,26,32,51]

- Autoimmune disease (specifically, systemic lupus erythematosus and rheumatoid arthritis)
- Concurrent thyroid disorder
- Duration of therapy (longer duration > shorter duration)
- Genetic predisposition
- Hepatic impairment
- High dose of a potential causative agent
- Hypoalbuminemia
- In corticosteroid-induced myopathy—use of fluorinated versus nonfluorinated corticosteroid
- Kidney disease
- Pharmacodynamic interactions
    - Statins plus nicotinic acid or fibrates or ezetimibe (especially in patients with prior statin myopathy)
- Pharmacokinetic drug interactions
    - Neuromuscular blockers plus corticosteroids
    - Statins plus fibrates
    - Statins plus cytochrome P-450 3A4 inhibitors
- Vigorous or prolonged periods of exercise

Drug interactions leading to myopathy can be pharmacodynamic as well as pharmacokinetic. Examples of pharmacodynamic drug interactions include the neuromuscular blocking agents when given with corticosteroids and fenofibrate when given with statins.[25,27,42] The cellular mechanism of these pharmacodynamic interactions are not clear. Pancuronium possesses a bis-quaternary ammonium corticosteroid structure, which may potentiate glucocorticoid toxicity via a common corticosteroid receptor.[27] Fenofibrate, although relatively devoid of the kinetic interaction with statins that gemfibrozil possesses, reduces circulating triglyceride concentrations and may worsen cellular energy metabolism by further reducing delivery of fatty acids to skeletal muscle in patients taking a statin.[42]

Pharmacokinetic interactions account for part of the increased risk of statin-induced myopathy when administered concomitantly with gemfibrozil or inhibitors of the cytochrome P-450 3A4 (CYP 3A4) isozyme.[8,43] The pharmacokinetic interaction with gemfibrozil appears to involve reduced statin glucuronidation.[41] The prevalence of CK >10 times the ULN associated with the combined administration of statins and fibrates has been reported to be 0.12%.[66] Myopathy associated with the combination of a fibrate and statin is more frequent with gemfibrozil but is reported with all fibrates.[25,40,54,66] Case reports of myopathy occurring during combined therapy with niacin and a statin have also been published.[66] Higher doses of drugs that can cause myopathy, particularly zidovudine, corticosteroids, epsilon aminocaproic acid, and statins, increase the risk of this adverse effect.[14,27,45] Dalakas et al.[45] examined muscle biopsy specimens from 20 patients with documented HIV infections in whom myopathy developed. The majority of these patients had been treated with zidovudine at doses ranging from 800 to 1,200 mg daily for a treatment period of 6–11 months. The authors reported that patients taking higher doses of zidovudine for a longer duration are at greater risk for myopathy.

The risk of corticosteroid-induced myopathy appears to increase in patients receiving the equivalent of prednisone doses >40 mg daily.[14,19,23] Myopathy associated with lower prednisone doses appears to be uncommon.[19] Patients requiring more frequent courses of corticosteroid therapy or continuous corticosteroid therapy are also at greater risk for corticosteroid-induced myopathy as are those in whom corticosteroid use extends beyond 4 weeks.[19,23] Excessive, prolonged use of antacids may be associated with electrolyte disturbances resulting in myopathy.[19,26] Long-term use of colchicine has also been associated with myopathy.[10]

Kidney failure has been identified as a risk factor for myopathies secondary to hypermagnesemia. Magnesium is renally eliminated, and patients with impaired kidney function are at much greater risk for myopathies resulting from therapy with magnesium-containing drugs.[26] Kidney failure has also been noted as a risk factor for myopathy associated with fibrates and colchicine.[19]

GENETICS AND GENOMICS

The clear genetic susceptibility to myopathy from anesthetic-induced malignant hyperthermia helped open up investigation into other areas of genetic risk for drug-induced myopathies.[55,62,67] The contribution of genetics can be either pharmacodynamic or pharmacokinetic, including drug transport as well as metabolism. One area of recent discoveries in this field has been with the statins. As of 2007, at least 12 candidate genes had been identified for statin-induced myopathy.[67] Although work in this area continues, the clinical application of these findings remain unclear. As of 2017, no specific genetic tests are recommended to be performed in patients prior to beginning statin therapy.

In a study of 137 patients who experienced myositis while taking atorvastatin, an allele in the *CYP 3A4* gene was found to be associated with severity of myopathy.[68] In another trial of 110 patients with statin myopathy, 10% were found to harbor abnormal genes for proteins related to cellular energy metabolism, particularly carnitine palmitoyltransferase II.[55] The population frequency for the same genetic polymorphisms in unaffected control patients was 2%.

In 2008, an analysis of the myositis cases in the ongoing 12,000-patient Study of the Effectiveness of Additional Reductions in Cholesterol and Homocysteine (SEARCH) trial was conducted.[69] Among the 6,031 patients who received an 80-mg daily dose of simvastatin, 98 cases of myositis had occurred after an average follow-up of about 6 years. A genome-wide analysis revealed a strong association of myositis with a single nucleotide polymorphism located within the gene that encodes for organic anion-transporting polypeptide (OATP)1B1. The OATP transporter is known to be involved in hepatic uptake of some statins, and polymorphisms affect serum concentrations. Patients homozygous for the less active allele had a 17-fold higher risk of myopathy while receiving 80 mg of simvastatin daily.[69]

The discovery of the importance of OATP1B1 illustrates the role that genetics is likely to play in helping to prevent drug-induced myopathies. Approximately 60% of the myositis cases in SEARCH were attributable to the genetic polymorphism in *OATP1B1*. Although about 30% of the population carries this polymorphism, only about 2% of the population is homozygous for the allele. Avoiding high-dose statins in those patients would prevent about 25% of the observed cases of statin-induced myositis. That may be a reasonable trade-off if alternative therapies can be used or if the reaction that can be avoided is particularly severe. Thus, while genetics is unlikely to offer novel therapies for managing drug-induced myopathies in the near future, it could play a key role in identifying high-risk individuals in whom certain therapies should be avoided. Efforts to make the genetic test for OATP1B1 available commercially are underway.

MORBIDITY AND MORTALITY

Because the precise incidence of drug-induced myopathies is unknown, it is difficult to determine the overall incidence of morbidity and mortality associated with this drug-induced disease. In many patients with myopathy, discomfort and difficulty with the activities of daily living are encountered secondary to muscle weakness. Patients may experience difficulty walking up stairs or difficulty rising from a seated position because of proximal muscle weakness. This has the potential to lead to a significant burden on society in terms of increased healthcare costs because of the more frequent visits to healthcare providers associated with muscle pain or weakness in addition to missed days from work.

Because serious clinical sequelae may develop, it is important to recognize and treat this condition as early as possible. Myopathy may rarely result in myoglobinuria and rhabdomyolysis. These myopathic complications may result in death due to kidney failure.

PREVENTION

Although prevention of drug-induced myopathies is difficult, general preventive measures are listed in **Table 52-6**. When drugs known to cause myopathy cannot be avoided, the best strategy is to use the lowest dose possible, avoid or minimize concomitant risk factors, and monitor carefully for onset of symptoms. In general, combinations of drugs listed in Table 52-1, should be avoided whenever possible, especially in high-risk patients.[19,41,43]

Moderate amounts of exercise and physical activity may help prevent corticosteroid-induced myopathy.[13,70] Physical therapy and exercise may help counteract corticosteroid-induced muscle fiber atrophy. However, extremely vigorous or prolonged

Table 52-6 Approaches to Help Prevent Drug-Induced Myopathy[2,18,22,25,26,30,32,51,59,63,64]

- Avoid combining drugs when each has a risk of myopathy, when possible:
    - Statins and fibrates
    - Statins and cyclosporine
    - Use treatment regimens for the human immunodeficiency virus that avoid zidovudine and protease inhibitor therapy
- Avoid higher-risk drugs in patients with cirrhosis and hypoalbuminemia
- Be aware of drugs that can cause myopathy and that have a significant component of renal clearance; adjust dose or avoid use in patients with chronic kidney disease
- Consider genetic screening when drug-induced myopathy occurs; disorders for which genetic testing is available include the following:
    - Carnitine deficiency states
    - Glycogen metabolism defects
    - Ion channelopathy
    - Lipid storage disease
    - Mitochondrial myopathies
- Consider measuring a baseline CK in patients with multiple risk factors or those receiving multiple medications with a known risk of causing myopathy
- Educate patients regarding signs and symptoms:
    - Discolored urine
    - Symptoms in more than one muscle system
    - Weakness in addition to pain
- Make sure patients know whom to contact in case one or more of the above symptoms occur
- For statins: ensure euthyroid state and monitor periodically during therapy, especially in patients >60 years of age
- Use the lowest effective dose of corticosteroids for the shortest possible time

CK = creatine kinase.

periods of exercise may paradoxically increase the risk for drug-induced myopathies.[4] In one small study, "supranutritional" doses of antioxidant vitamins were shown to reduce the risk of zidovudine-related myopathy; however, no large-scale trials have been performed regarding the potential effectiveness of this preventive strategy.[46]

For necrotizing myopathy where a nutritional deficiency may be playing a causative role, data for supplementation are lacking. Perhaps best studied is the possible role for coenzyme Q10 in preventing statin-associated myopathy. Although many studies are small and suffer from design flaws including under-dosing of coenzyme Q10 and poor patient selection, a recent study of patients carefully selected to show clear myopathic symptoms with simvastatin found no benefit from 600 mg of coenzyme Q10 compared to placebo.[71]

It is reasonable to measure baseline CK when therapy with a drug known to cause myopathy is started, and particularly when the patient has risk factors for this drug-induced disease.[4,27] An elevated baseline CK (>200 units/L) that cannot be explained by recent, vigorous exercise or injury should prompt reconsideration of the risk and benefit of starting the medication until the CK is reduced to within a normal range. However, routine monitoring of CK is not recommended because there is no evidence that such monitoring is effective for myopathy prevention. Some patients with drug-induced myopathy present without elevations in CK, and concentrations can become elevated from causes other than a drug-induced effect. Therefore, determination of CK is only routinely recommended once a patient has symptoms.[4,19,23]

MANAGEMENT

Beyond discontinuation of the offending agent, there are few treatment strategies for drug-induced myopathy. Reductions in dose can be effective in cases of mild myopathy without marked elevations in CK. This has been best documented for corticosteroids and statins.[3,17,40] In cases of myopathy with marked elevations of CK, management focuses primarily on supportive care when needed and trying to prevent or minimize the renal complications of rhabdomyolysis.

When a drug-induced myopathy is suspected, evaluation of current and recent past medications is critical. Temporal relationships between drug initiation and the onset of myopathic symptoms should be determined. The potentially causative drug should be discontinued. In the majority of patients with drug-induced disease, symptom resolution occurs, in some cases almost immediately, after drug discontinuation. However, complete resolution or maximal improvement of symptoms may not occur for several weeks after discontinuation of the causative drug.[33] In some cases, particularly in patients with mitochondrial myopathy or polymyositis, a short course of therapy with a corticosteroid such as prednisone may be helpful. Specific recommendations regarding dose and duration of corticosteroid treatment vary; higher doses of prednisone are typically recommended for initial treatment, followed by tapering of the dose.[43] One recommendation for management of drug-induced polymyositis is prednisone 50–100 mg daily for up to 7 days or until acute symptoms resolve, followed by tapering of the dose over a period of months. More rapid tapering may be tolerated, but caution is advised with tapers of <1 month due to risk of polymyositis reactivation. After resolution of the myopathy, it is typically best to avoid future use of the offending agent or to use lower doses if treatment with the drug is absolutely necessary. Changing agents within a class of drugs can often be helpful, but the clinician should be alert for symptom recurrence. In a trial of 45 patients with statin-associated myopathy, 43% tolerated a different agent.[53]

Pascuzzi outlined suggestions for the treatment of patients with HIV infections who present with myopathy.[26] If the patient has been taking high-dose zidovudine for a prolonged period, therapy should be discontinued. This is not difficult in the modern era of HIV therapies where many alternate treatment options now exist. If the myopathic symptoms were due to zidovudine, improvement should be seen over 4–8 weeks. If the patient's symptoms do not improve within this time, a muscle biopsy may be performed; if inflammatory changes are present, temporary treatment with corticosteroids may be helpful. If the patient has myopathy in the absence of therapy with zidovudine, the myopathy is likely related to the disease, and treatment with appropriate antiretroviral therapy may help. Finally, if the patient has acute, fulminant myalgias or weakness, muscle biopsy should be performed to investigate the possibility of an opportunistic infection within the muscle.

The management of corticosteroid-induced myopathy typically requires discontinuation of the causative medication. Following discontinuation, many patients experience complete resolution or significant improvement in symptoms. In others, however, only partial symptom relief may occur. If it is not possible to permanently discontinue corticosteroid therapy following resolution of myopathy without recurrence of the patient's primary disease, treatment may be restarted at a lower dose. Using doses of prednisone <40 mg daily (or equivalent doses of other corticosteroids) may help prevent myopathy recurrence.[3,23]

In patients with myopathy due to drug-induced electrolyte abnormalities, discontinuation of the offending agent usually results in symptom improvement. Occasionally, potassium supplementation may be necessary for the correction of hypokalemia.[23] If drug-induced hypermagnesemia causes myopathy, discontinuation of the causative drug is necessary, and administration of calcium gluconate or, in severe cases (i.e., serum magnesium concentration >14 mEq/L), hemodialysis may be necessary.[26]

In patients who develop symptoms of myopathy while receiving statin therapy, a CK should be determined.[58] If the CK is <5 times the ULN, statin therapy may be continued, and the CK should be determined again 1 week later. However, if the initial CK is >5 times the ULN, statin therapy should be withheld and CK monitored weekly to monthly until values return to the normal range. It should be noted that product labeling for statins recommends discontinuation when CK reaches 10 times the ULN. However, severe reactions can progress when initial elevations are in the range of 3–10 times the ULN, and withholding the drug when CK elevates to 5 times the ULN appears to be a reasonable clinical approach.[4,27]

Regardless of the etiology, once CK is markedly elevated (>10,000 units/L) in the setting of rhabdomyolysis, aggressive hydration is indicated to reduce the risk of permanent renal damage. Although there is no universal protocol, intravenous hydration at a rate of 3–5 mL/kg/hr is reasonable and should be targeted to a rate of urine output of 2–3 mL/kg/hr. Monitoring of urine pH and using sodium bicarbonate to alkalinize urine is poorly supported and is unnecessary. Aggressive hydration can be stopped once serum CK has dropped below 10,000 units/L.

INFORMATION FOR PATIENTS

Although it may not be practical or desirable to warn every patient about the potential for myopathy with every drug listed in Table 52-1, a warning seems appropriate for patients prescribed a drug for which strong evidence of causation exists (i.e., drugs in Table 52-1 with level of evidence A or B). These patients should be counseled to recognize symptoms of muscle pain or weakness, particularly in the proximal muscles, and instructed to contact a healthcare provider if such symptoms occur. Patients should also be warned about the possible significance of darkened urine, especially if accompanied by a reduction in urine output. The patient should be advised to maintain a complete and accurate list of medications and to share this list with providers at each encounter to help minimize the risk of drug interactions that can increase the risk of myopathy. Patients should also be aware that, in some cases, the development of myopathy may be a secondary complication of a specific disease process, and other medical conditions can increase their risk for drug-induced myopathies.

REFERENCES

1. Micromedex Solutions. https://www.micromedexsolutions.com/home/dispatch/ssl/true (accessed 2018 Feb 28).
2. Wortmann R. Metabolic diseases of muscle. In: *Diseases of skelatal muscle*. Wortmann R, ed. Philadelphia: Lippincott Williams and Wilkins; 2000:157-87.
3. Argov Z, Mastaglia F. Endocrine and toxic myopathies. In: *Disorders of voluntary muscle*. Karparti G, Hilton-Jones. D, Bushby K, Griggs RC, eds. London: Cambridge University Press; 2010: 471-83).
4. Pasternak RC, Smith SC Jr, Bairey-Merz CN et al. ACC/AHA/NHLBI clinical advisory on the use and safety of statins. *J Am Coll Cardiol*. 2002; 40:567-72.
5. Biswas CK, Milligan DA, Agte SD et al. Acute renal failure and myopathy after treatment with aminocaproic acid. *Br Med J*. 1980; 281:115-6.
6. Clouston PD, Donnelly PE. Acute necrotising myopathy associated with amiodarone therapy. *Aust N Z J Med*. 1989; 19:483-5.
7. Parodi A, Regesta G, Rebora A. Chloroquine-induced neuromyopathy—report of a case. *Dermatologica*. 1986; 171:203-5.
8. Hodel C. Myopathy and rhabdomyolysis with lipid-lowering drugs. *Toxicol Lett*. 2002; 128:159-68.
9. Dupont P, Hunt I, Goldberg L, Warrens A. Colchicine myoneuropathy in a renal transplant patient. *Transpl Int*.2002; 15:374-6.
10. Kuncl RW, Duncan G, Watson D et al. Colchicine myopathy and neuropathy. *N Engl J Med*. 1987; 316:1562-8.
11. Tanios MA, El Gamal H, Epstein SK, Hassoun PM. Severe respiratory muscle weakness related to long-term colchicine therapy. *Respir Care*. 2004; 49:189-91.
12. Batchelor TT, Taylor LP, Thaler HT et al. Steroid myopathy in cancer patients. *Neurology*. 1997; 48:1234-8.
13. LaPier TK. Glucocorticoid-induced muscle atrophy. The role of exercise in treatment and prevention. *J Cardiopulm Rehabil*. 1997; 17:76-84.
14. Shee CD. Risk factors for hydrocortisone myopathy in acute severe asthma. *Respir Med*. 1990; 84:229-33.
15. Covar RA, Leung DY, McCormick D et al. Risk factors associated with glucocorticoid-induced adverse effects in children with severe asthma. *J Allergy Clin Immunol*. 2000; 106:651-9.
16. Polsonetti BW, Joy SD, Laos LF. Steroid-induced myopathy in the ICU. *Ann Pharmacother*. 2002; 36:1741-4.
17. Sury MR, Russell GN,Heaf DP. Hydrocortisone myopathy. *Lancet*. 1988; 2:515.
18. Fernandez-Sola J, Campistol J, Casademont J et al. Reversible cyclosporin myopathy. *Lancet*. 1990; 335:362-3.
19. Bannwarth B. Drug-induced myopathies. *Expert Opin Drug Saf*. 2002; 1:65-70.
20. Brenner J, Solitar BM, Golden BD. Rheumatic manifestations of current pharmacopeia. *Curr Rheumatol Rep*. 2000; 2:151-5.
21. Yazici Y, Kagen LJ. Clinical presentation of the idiopathic inflammatory myopathies. *Rheum Dis Clin North Am*. 2002; 28:823-32.22.
22. Chappel R, Willems J. D-penicillamine-induced myositis in rheumatoid arthritis. *Clin Rheumatol*. 1996; 15:86-7.
23. Zuckner J. Drug-related myopathies. *Rheum Dis Clin North Am*. 1994; 20:1017-32.
24. Fux R, Morike K, Gundel UF et al. Ezetimibe and statin-associated myopathy. *Ann Intern Med*. 2004; 140:671-2.
25. Jacob SS, Jacob S, Williams C, Deeg MA. Simvastatin, fenofibrate, and rhabdomyolysis. *Diabetes Care*. 2005; 28:1258.
26. Pascuzzi RM. Drugs and toxins associated with myopathies. *Curr Opin Rheumatol*. 1998; 10:511-20.
27. Sieb JP. Myopathies due to drugs, toxins and nutritional deficienies. In: *Myology*. Engel AG, Franzini-Armstrong C, eds. New York: McGraw-Hill; 2004:1693-712.
28. Arai H, Tanaka M, Ohta K et al. Symptomatic myopathy associated with interferon therapy for chronic hepatitis C. *Lancet*. 1995; 345:582.
29. Mastaglia FL. Adverse effects of drugs on muscle. *Drugs*. 1982; 24:304-21.
30. Kuntzer T, Bogousslavsky J, Deruaz JP et al. Reversible emetine-induced myopathy with ECG abnormalities: a toxic myopathy. *J Neurol*. 1989; 236:246-8.
31. Lane RJ, Mastaglia FL. Drug-induced myopathies in man. *Lancet*. 1978; 2:562-6.
32. Teicher A, Rosenthal T, Kissin E, Sarova I. Labetalol-induced toxic myopathy. *Br Med J (Clin Res Ed)*. 1981; 282:1824-5.
33. Le Quintrec JS, Le Quintrec JL. Drug-induced myopathies. *Baillieres Clin Rheumatol*. 1991; 5:21-38.
34. Crayton H, Bohlmann T, Sufit R, Graziano FM. Drug induced polymyositis secondary to leuprolide acetate (Lupron) therapy for prostate carcinoma. *Clin Exp Rheumatol*. 1991; 9: 525-8.
35. Lewis CA, Boheimer N, Rose P, Jackson G. Myopathy after short term administration of procainamide. *Br Med J (Clin Res Ed)*. 1986; 292:593-4.
36. Garrote FJ, Lacambra C, del Ser T et al. Subacute myopathy during omeprazole therapy. *Lancet*. 1992; 340:672.
37. Clark DW, Strandell J. Myopathy including polymyositis: a likely class adverse effect of proton pump inhibitors? *Eur J Clin Pharmacol*. 2006; 62:473-9.
38. Jenkins P, Emerson PA. Myopathy induced by rifampicin. *Br Med J (Clin Res Ed)*. 1981; 8:105-6.

39. Ucar M, Mjorndal T, Dahlqvist R. HMG-CoA reductase inhibitors and myotoxicity. *Drug Saf.* 2000; 22:441-57.

40. Thompson PD, Clarkson P, Karas RH. Statin-associated myopathy. *JAMA.* 2003; 289:1681-90.

41. Bruckert E, Hayem G, Dejager S et al. Mild to moderate muscular symptoms with high-dosage statin therapy in hyperlipidemic patients—the PRIMO study. *Cardiovasc Drugs Ther.* 2005; 19:403-14.

42. Prueksaritanont T, Tang C, Qiu Y et al. Effects of fibrates on metabolism of statins in human hepatocytes. *Drug Metab Dispos.* 2002; 30:1280-7.

43. Antons KA, Williams CD, Baker SK, Phillips PS. Clinical perspectives of statin-induced rhabdomyolysis. *Am J Med.* 2006; 119:400-9.

44. Sinclair D, Phillips C. Transient myopathy apparently due to tetracycline. *N Engl J Med.* 1982; 307:821-2.

45. Dalakas MC, Illa I, Pezeshkpour GH et al. Mitochondrial myopathy caused by long-term zidovudine therapy. *N Engl J Med.* 1990; 322:1098-105.

46. de la Asuncion JG, del Olmo ML, Sastre J et al. AZT treatment induces molecular and ultrastructural oxidative damage to muscle mitochondria. Prevention by antioxidant vitamins. *J Clin Invest.* 1998; 10:4-9.

47. Mhiri C, Baudrimont M, Bonne G et al. Zidovudine myopathy: a distinctive disorder associated with mitochondrial dysfunction. *Ann Neurol.* 1991; 29:606-4.

48. Helbert M, Fletcher T, Peddle B et al. Zidovudine-associated myopathy. *Lancet.* 1988; 2:689-90.

49. Daniels DG, McCormack SM, McLean KA et al. Zidovudine-related myopathy. *Lancet.* 1990; 336:1256.

50. Luigetti M, Capone F, Monforte M, Di Lazzaro V. Muscle cramps and weakness after teriparatide therapy: a new drug-induced myopathy? *Muscle Nerve.* 2013; 47:615.

51. Magro CM, Schaefer JT, Waldman J et al. Terbinafine-induced dermatomyositis: a case report and literature review of drug-induced dermatomyositis. *J Cutan Pathol.* 2008; 35:74-81.

52. Estes ML, Ewing-Wilson D, Chou SM et al. Chloroquine neuromyotoxicity. Clinical and pathologic perspective. *Am J Med.* 1987; 8:447-55.

53. Hansen KE, Hildebrand JP Ferguson EE, Stein JH. Outcomes in 45 patients with statin-associated myopathy. *Arch Intern Med.* 2005; 165:2671-6.

54. Shek A, Ferrill MJ. Statin-fibrate combination therapy. *Ann Pharmacother.* 2001; 35:908-17.

55. Vladutiu GD, Simmons Z, Isackson PJ et al. Genetic risk factors associated with lipid-lowering drug-induced myopathies. *Muscle Nerve.* 2006; 34:153-62.

56. Dugue A, Bagheri H, Lapeyre-Mestre M et al. Detection and incidence of muscular adverse drug reactions: a prospective analysis from laboratory signals. *Eur J Clin Pharmacol.* 2004; 60:285-92.

57. Collins R, Armitage J, Parish S et al.; Heart Protection Study Collaborative. MRC/BHF Heart Protection Study of cholesterol lowering with simvastatin in 20,536 high-risk individuals: a randomised placebo-controlled trial. *Lancet.* 2002; 360:7-22.

58. Ballantyne CM, Corsini A, Davidson MH et al. Risk for myopathy with statin therapy in high-risk patients. *Arch Intern Med.* 2003; 163: 553-64.

59. Avina-Zubieta JA, Johnson ES, Suarez-Almazor ME, Russell AS. Incidence of myopathy in patients treated with antimalarials. A report of three cases and a review of the literature. *Br J Rheumatol.* 1995; 34:166-70.

60. Bossen E. Muscle structure and development. In: *Diseases of skeletal muscle.* Wortmann R, ed. Philadelphia: Lippincott Williams and Wilkins; 2000:127-42.

61. Wortmann R. Skeletal muscle biology, physiology and biochemistry. In: *Disease of skeletal muscle.* Wortmann R, ed. Philadelphia: Lippincott, Williams and Wilkins; 2000:45-61.

62. Guis S, Mattei JP, Liote F. Drug-induced and toxic myopathies. *Best Pract Res Clin Rheumatol.* 2003; 17:877-907.

63. Maini R, St Clair EW, Breedveld F et al. Infliximab (chimeric anti-tumour necrosis factor alpha monoclonal antibody) versus placebo in rheumatoid arthritis patients receiving concomitant methotrexate: a randomised phase III trial. ATTRACT Study Group. *Lancet.* 1999; 354:1932-9.

64. Stein M, Bell MJ, Ang LC. Hydroxychloroquine neuromyotoxicity. *J Rheumatol.* 2000; 27:2927-31.

65. Rendt K. Inflammatory myopathies: narrowing the differential diagnosis. *Cleve Clin J Med.* 2001; 68:505, 509-14, 517-9.

66. Bellosta S, Paoletti R, Corsini A. Safety of statins: focus on clinical pharmacokinetics and drug interactions. *Circulation.* 2004; 109:III50-57.

67. Wilke RA, Lin DW, Roden DM et al. Identifying genetic risk factors for serious adverse drug reactions: current progress and challenges. *Nat Rev Drug Discov.* 2007; 6:904-16.

68. Wilke RA, Moore JH, Burmester JK. Relative impact of CYP3A genotype and concomitant medication on the severity of atorvastatin-induced muscle damage. *Pharmacogenet Genomics.* 2005; 15:415-21.

69. SEARCH Collaborative Group. SLCO1B1 variants and statin-induced myopathy—a genomewide study. *N Engl J Med.* 2008; 359:789-99.

70. Mahowald ML. Dykstra DD. Rehabilitation of patients with muscle weakness. In: *Diseases of skeletal muscle.* Wortmann RL, ed. Philadelphia: Lippincott Williams and Wilkins; 2000:349-63.

71. Taylor BA, Lorson L, White CM, Thompson PD. A randomized trial of coenzyme Q10 in patients with confirmed statin myopathy. *Atherosclerosis.* 2015; 238:329-35.

SECTION XII

MISCELLANEOUS DRUG-INDUCED DISEASES

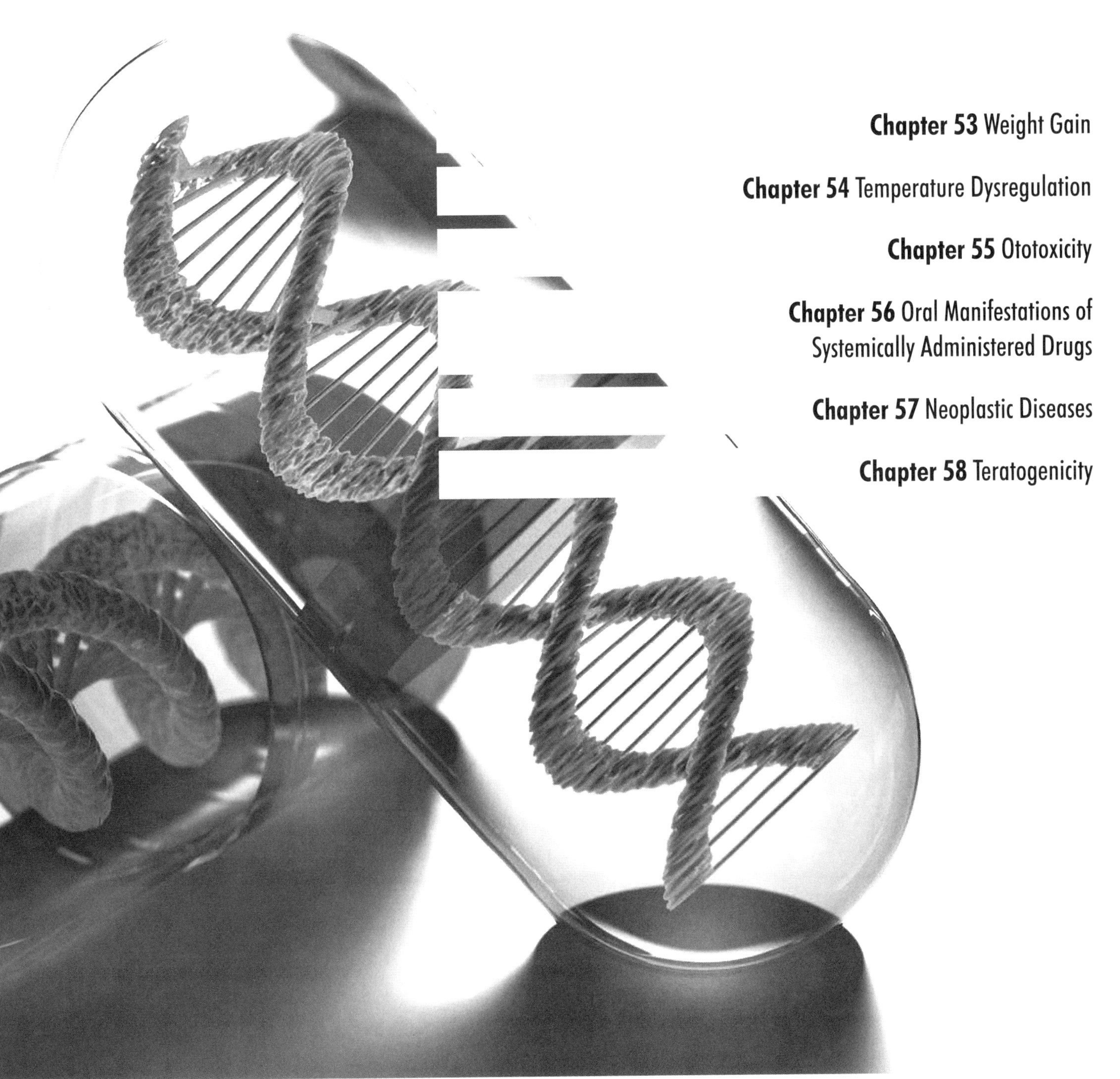

Chapter 53 Weight Gain

Chapter 54 Temperature Dysregulation

Chapter 55 Ototoxicity

Chapter 56 Oral Manifestations of Systemically Administered Drugs

Chapter 57 Neoplastic Diseases

Chapter 58 Teratogenicity

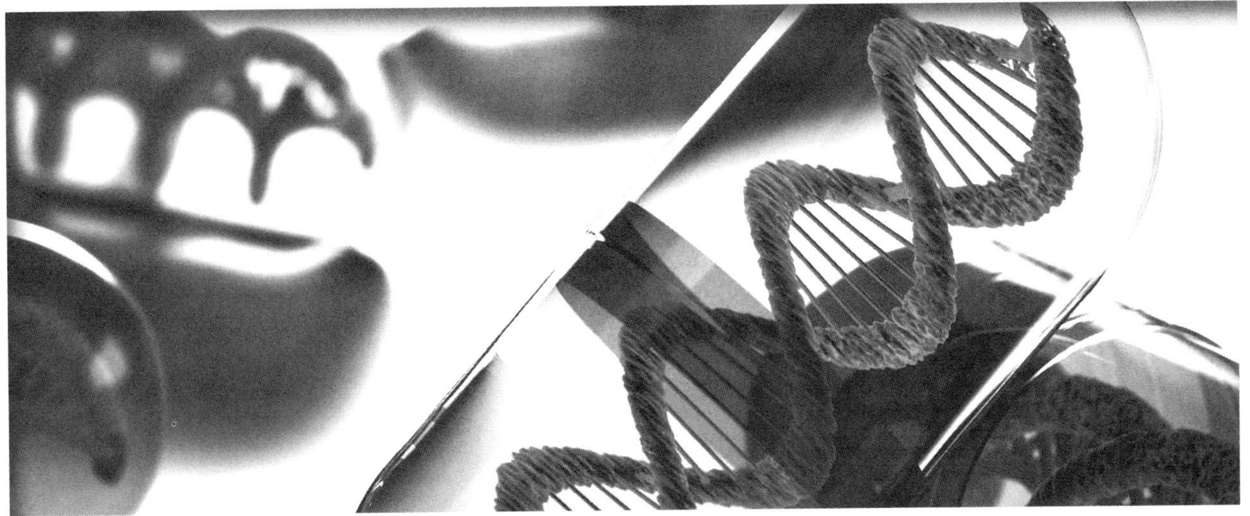

CHAPTER 53

Weight Gain

Amy Heck Sheehan

Weight gain is a complex process involving environmental and genetic factors that ultimately contribute to a metabolic imbalance between caloric intake and energy expenditure. Although weight gain is most commonly associated with lifestyle factors, it also may occur as an unintended response to drug therapy. Drug-induced weight gain increases obesity-related health risks and may compromise patient adherence to drug therapy. Observational studies have reported that a modest weight gain of ≥5 kg in healthy adults is associated with a significant increase in the risk for hypertension, type 2 diabetes, and coronary heart disease.[1-4] For adults who are already overweight or obese, increases in body mass index (BMI) are associated with greater risks of fatal and nonfatal coronary heart disease, fatal and nonfatal stroke, diabetes, and all-cause mortality.[5,6]

CAUSATIVE AGENTS

Drugs that have been reported to cause clinically relevant weight gain—defined as weight gain of ≥5 kg—are listed in **Table 53-1**.[7-275] Drugs listed in this table include only those associated with unintended weight gain. Drugs that are used to promote weight gain are not included.

EPIDEMIOLOGY

According to current guidelines, a BMI (the weight in kilograms divided by the square of the height in meters) ≥25 defines overweight, and obesity is defined as a BMI ≥30.[6] The number of overweight and obese individuals in the United States has increased significantly over the past several decades, and the latest epidemiologic data estimate that approximately 69% of the U.S. adult population is overweight or obese.[276]

The exact incidence of clinically relevant drug-induced weight gain is unknown. Estimating the incidence is complicated because body weight fluctuations are multifactorial and can depend on variables such as lifestyle, habits, genetic predisposition, and concomitant disease states.

Because the majority of drugs associated with clinically relevant weight gain are used in the management of psychiatric disorders, most data regarding the incidence of drug-induced weight gain have been generated from this patient population. Weight loss is a common symptom of many untreated psychiatric disorders, including depression and schizophrenia. Therefore, successful

Table 53-1 Agents Implicated in Drug-Induced Weight Gain[7-275]

Drug	Incidence[a]	Level of Evidence[b]
ANTICONVULSANTS		
Carbamazepine[7-10]	4.7–5.2%[c] (16 wk)[7]	A
Gabapentin[11-14]	2.6% (26 wk)[11]	A
Pregabalin[15-22]	9% (14 wk)[15]; 11.4% (12 wk)[20]	A
Valproic acid[8,22-31]	38%[d] (32 wk)[26]	A
ANTIDEPRESSANTS		
Amitriptyline[32-39]	5.9%[39,e]	A
Bupropion[40]	NK	C
Clomipramine[41,42]	28%[41,e]; 34.8% (2.5 yr)[42]	A
Citalopram[38,42,43]	14.3% (2.5 yr)[42]	A
Desipramine[36,37,44]	NK	A
Doxepin[45,46]	NK	A
Duloxetine[47-51]	8.4–10.8% (34 wk)[48]	A
Escitalopram[47,49,52-55]	10.5–12% (32 wk)[47,53]	A
Fluoxetine[38,42,43,49,56]	6.8% (26–32 wk)[56]; 8.7% (2.5 yr)[42]	A
Fluvoxamine[42,43]	10.7% (2.5 yr)[42]	A
Imipramine[33,57-59]	8.3% (16 wk)[59]; 19.7% (long-term)[59]	A
Maprotiline[60-62]	NK	A
Mirtazapine[32,63-70]	7.5%[32,e]; 49% (8 wk)[32,f]	A
Nortriptyline[33,35,71-73]	NK	A
Paroxetine[38,42,43,48,49,56]	25.5% (26 to 32 wk)[56]; 13.8% (34 wk)[48]; 14.3% (2.5 yr)[42]	A
Phenelzine[74,75]	NK	B
Sertraline[38,42,49,56]	4.2% (26–32 wk)[56]; 4.5% (2.5 yr)[42]	A
Venlafaxine[38,49,67]	NK	B
Vilazodone[76,77]	1% (8 wk)[76]	A
Vortioxitine[78]	NK	B
ANTIPSYCHOTICS (ATYPICAL)		
Aripiprazole[79-102]	5.2–8.1% (4–6 wk)[79]; 5.2–26.3% (4–10 wk)[79,f]	A
Asenapine[103-109]	4.9–5.8% (short-term)[103]; 14.7% (1 yr)[103]	A
Brexpiprazole[110-114]	2–11% (6 wk)[110]; 20–30% (long-term)[11]	A
Cariprazine[115-116]	8–17% (6 wk)[115]	A
Clozapine[117-141]	35% (long-term)[117]	A
Iloperidone[108,142,143]	12–18% (4–6 wk)[142]	A
Lurasidone[144-148]	7% (short-term)[144]	A
Olanzapine[88,91,92,96,98,100,102,108,148,149-170]	22.2% (8 wk)[149]; 64% (long-term)[149]; 40.6% (4 wk)[149,f]; 89% (long-term)[149,f]	A
Paliperidone[102,108,143,171-177]	6–18% (6 wk)[171]; 33% (long-term)[171]	A
Quetiapine[80,102,108,159,178-195]	16% (18 mo)[159]; 8–23% (6–12 wk)[178]; 18.3% (26 wk)[178,f]	A
Risperidone[102,108,155,156,159,163,164,184,186,190,196-209]	14% (18 mo)[159]; 8.7–20.9% (3–8 wk)[196]; 32.6% (3–8 wk)[196,f]	A
Ziprasidone[80,159,210]	7% (18 mo)[16]; 10% (4–6 wk)[210]	A

Table 53-1 Agents Implicated in Drug-Induced Weight Gain[7-275] (continued)

Drug	Incidence[a]	Level of Evidence[b]
ANTIPSYCHOTICS (CONVENTIONAL)		
Chlorpromazine[133,211-216]	24.3% (6 wk)[216]	A
Fluphenazine[213,217-219]	NK	A
Haloperidol[162-164,175,202,213,214,218,220,221]	10–22% (4–6 wk)[220-221]; 39–87.5% (1–2 yr)[162,164]	A
Lithium[34,161,222-225]	9.8% (1 yr)[161]	A
Perphenazine[159,211,213,214,226-228]	12% (18 mo)[159]	A
Thioridazine[213,214,229-231]	NK	A
Thiothixene[213,214,232]	NK	A
Trifluoperazine[213,232-233]	NK	A
ANTIRETROVIRAL THERAPY		
Combined antiretroviral therapy[234-240]	NK	B
CHEMOTHERAPY		
Adjuvant chemotherapy for early-stage breast cancer[241-252]	NK	B
HORMONES		
Glucocorticoids[253-258]	NK	A
Insulin[258-265]	NK	A
Medroxyprogesterone[266-275]	NK	A

NK = not known.
[a]Weight gain of >7% of baseline weight as reported in prospective, randomized clinical trials with length of therapy listed in parenthesis.
[b]Definitions for Levels of Evidence: Level A—evidence from one or more randomized, controlled clinical trials; Level B—evidence from nonrandomized clinical trials, prospective observational studies, cohort studies, retrospective studies, case-control studies, meta-analyses and/or postmarketing surveillance studies; and Level C—evidence from one or more published case reports or case series.
[c]Incidence of weight gain >7.5% of baseline weight over 16 weeks of therapy.
[d]Incidence of weight gain ≥10% of baseline weight over 32 weeks of therapy.
[e]Time period of treatment not specified.
[f]Children and adolescents.

treatment of these disorders with appropriate drug therapy may be associated with weight gain that returns the patient's body weight to baseline. Unfortunately, baseline body weight measurements prior to the development of psychiatric illness are typically not available, making it difficult to assess true drug-induced weight gain.

Differences in study design and methods also complicate the assessment of drug-induced weight gain. Most studies that have reported data regarding drug-induced weight gain were not specifically designed to assess this outcome. The majority of available information has been generated from adverse event data collected during prospective clinical trials or from retrospective observational studies. These studies include differing criteria for patient inclusion and exclusion, inconsistent definitions of significant weight gain (e.g., >5%, >7%, >10%), variable periods of follow-up, and different methods of reporting weight gain (e.g., kilograms, body mass index) and the extent of weight gain (e.g., mean, median, range, proportion of patients gaining significant weight). Because of these limitations, it is often difficult to compare the incidence and extent of weight gain caused by different medications.

For the purpose of clinical trials, the U.S. Food and Drug Administration defines clinically relevant weight gain as an increase ≥7% of baseline weight. This corresponds to an approximate weight gain of 5 kg in a 70 kg individual. Unfortunately, statistics regarding weight gain are not collected in all clinical trials and therefore data are not available for all drugs. In some cases, clinical trials are not long enough to adequately evaluate a drug's potential to cause weight gain. When available, the incidence of weight gain ≥7% of baseline as reported during prospective, randomized clinical trials is presented in Table 53-1.[7-275]

MECHANISMS

The proposed mechanisms for drug-induced weight gain are specific to each particular class of medication, and for many drugs, the exact cause of weight gain is unknown. **Table 53-2** summarizes the mechanisms of drug-induced weight gain proposed for various drug classes.[20,265,266,277-288]

CLINICAL PRESENTATION AND DIFFERENTIAL DIAGNOSIS

The clinical presentation and extent of weight gain caused by drugs may vary depending on the drug class. The extent of weight gain associated with specific drugs and drug classes is presented in **Table 53-3**. Endocrine and psychiatric disorders as well as environmental and behavioral factors should be assessed in the process of differentiating drug-induced weight gain from weight gain due to

Table 53-2 Mechanisms of Drug-Induced Weight Gain[20,265-267,278-288]

Drug	Proposed Mechanism
Adjuvant chemotherapy for early-stage breast	NK
Anticonvulsants[20,277,278]	Enhancement of GABA: ↑ appetite and ↓ basal metabolic rate Decreased blood glucose concentrations: ↑ appetite Hyperinsulinemia and hyperleptinemia: ↑ appetite Individual genetic receptor polymorphisms
Antidepressants[279-281]	Blockade of noradrenergic (α_2) receptors: ↑ appetite Blockade of serotonin (5-HT_{2C}) receptors: ↑ appetite Blockade of histamine (H_1) receptors: ↑ sedation and ↓ physical activity Individual genetic receptor polymorphisms
Antipsychotics[279-283]	Blockade of serotonin (5-HT_{2C}) receptors: ↑ appetite Blockade of dopamine (D_2) receptors: ↑ appetite Blockade of histamine (H_1) receptors: ↑ sedation and ↓ physical activity Blockade of noradrenergic (α_1) receptors: ↑ appetite Blockade of muscarinic (M_1) receptors: ↑ appetite Individual genetic receptor polymorphisms
Antiretroviral therapy[285]	Improved health status: ↑ appetite Increases in visceral adipose tissue and trunk fat Impaired glucose homeostasis and dyslipidemia
Insulin[265,286]	Promotes glucose uptake into cells: ↑ glycemic control and ↑ energy storage
Lithium[284]	Blockade of cAMP in renal tubules: ↑ thirst (↑ consumption of high-calorie drinks) Blockade of dopamine (D_2) receptors: ↑ appetite Inhibition of thyroid hormone synthesis: ↓ basal metabolic rate Enhancement of GABA: ↑ appetite and ↓ basal metabolic rate
Lithium[284]	Blockade of cAMP in renal tubules: ↑ thirst (↑ consumption of high-calorie drinks) Blockade of dopamine (D_2) receptors: ↑ appetite Inhibition of thyroid hormone synthesis: ↓ basal metabolic rate Enhancement of GABA: ↑ appetite and ↓ basal metabolic rate
Steroid hormones[266,287,288]	Hypercortisolemia and hyperinsulinemia: ↑ appetite and ↑ energy storage

5-HT = 5-hydroxytryptamine, cAMP = cyclic adenosine monophosphate, GABA = gamma-aminobutyric acid, NK = not known.

Table 53-3 Extent of Weight Gain Reported with Selected Drugs and Drug Classes

Drug	Extent of Weight Gain Reported in the Literature[a]
ANTICONVULSANTS	
Carbamazepine	7–15 kg over 2 mo[8] >7.5% over 4 mo[11]
Gabapentin	6–15% over 6 mo[13] 5 to >10% over 12 mo[15]
Pregabalin	4 kg over 6 mo[19] 5.2 kg over 24 mo[16]
Valproic acid	5.8 kg over 32 wk[26]; 8–49 kg over 7.1 yr[25]
ANTIDEPRESSANTS	
Amitriptyline	0.9–13.6 kg over 8 wk[36]
Bupropion	10 kg over 1 mo[40]
Citalopram	6.9 kg over 12 mo[43]
Clomipramine	4.9 kg over 2.5 yr[42]
Desipramine	0.9–9.5 kg over 8 wk[36]
Doxepin	2.7 kg over 9–13 wk[45,46]
Duloxetine	0.61 kg over 8 mo[47]
Escitalopram	1.83 kg over 8 mo[47]
Fluoxetine	5.2–7.7 kg over 8–12 mo[43,56]
Fluvoxamine	6.3 kg over 12 mo[43]
Imipramine	2.3 kg/mo of therapy[57]
Maprotiline	4.2 kg over 4 wk[62]
Mirtazapine	2.4–16 kg over 1–5 mo[63-65]
Nortriptyline	1.82 kg over 6 mo[73]
Paroxetine	8.2–14.1 kg over 8–12 mo[43,56]
Phenelzine	>6.8 kg over 4–16 wk[74]
Sertraline	8.6 kg over 8 mo[56]
Vilazodone	1.7 kg over 52 wk[77]
Vortioxitine	0.6 kg over 52 wk[78]
ATYPICAL ANTIPSYCHOTICS	
Aripiprazole	1.7–4.3 kg over 2–3 mo[80,95]
Asenapine	2.63 kg over 7.6 mo[106]
Brexpiprazole	1.5–1.9 kg over 6 wk[114]
Clozapine	4.45 kg over 10 wk[290] 7.5–10.9 kg over 6 mo to 1 yr[120,125,128,130,133,134]
Iloperidone	2.5 kg over 6 wk[143]
Olanzapine	4.15 kg over 10 wk[290] 4.1–12 kg over 6 mo to 1 yr[150,152,153,157,159,160,162-164]
Paliperidone	2.17 kg over 6 mo[175]
Quetiapine	3.4 kg over 1 yr[181]
Risperidone	2.1 kg over 10 wk[290] 2.3–8.9 kg over 1 yr[164,199-202]
Ziprasidone	1.2 kg over 3 mo[290]
CONVENTIONAL ANTIPSYCHOTICS	
Chlorpromazine	2.58 kg over 10 wk[290] 6.5 kg over 1 yr[133]
Haloperidol	0.48 kg over 10 wk[290] 4.2–9.7 kg over 1–2 yr[162,164,202]
Lithium	1.4–11.5 kg over 1–6 yr[161,222-224]
Thioridazine	3.19 kg over 10 wk[290]
ADJUVANT CHEMOTHERAPY	
Adjuvant chemotherapy for early-stage breast cancer	2.3–12.3 kg 1–2 yr after treatment[246,247]
HORMONES	
Depot medroxyprogesterone	4.3–9.4 kg over 1–5 yr[266-275]
Insulin	2.6–8 kg over 2 mo to 1 yr[259,261,262,265]
Prednisone	2.6–13 kg over 1 yr[253-255]

[a]Reported as mean weight gain unless otherwise noted.

other causes. **Table 53-4** lists conditions to consider in the differential diagnosis of drug-induced weight gain.

ANTICONVULSANTS

Anticonvulsant agents, including carbamazepine, gabapentin, pregabalin, and valproic acid are commonly associated with weight gain in children and adults.[7-31] Anticonvulsant-induced weight gain is generally characterized by an increased appetite and increased calorie consumption.[20] A case series of four patients with epilepsy who were receiving carbamazepine therapy describes weight gain ranging from 7 to 15 kg after 2 months of therapy.[7] A double-blind, randomized study designed to assess efficacy of carbamazepine add-on therapy in patients receiving phenytoin for partial seizures reported weight gain of >7.5% of baseline weight

Table 53-4 Conditions to Consider in the Differential Diagnosis of Drug-Induced Weight Gain[4]

Endocrine disorders

- Cushing syndrome
- Growth hormone deficiency
- Hypothyroidism
- Insulinoma
- Leptin deficiency

Environmental and behavioral factors

- Overconsumption of calories
- Sedentary lifestyle
- Smoking cessation

Psychiatric disorders

- Binge eating disorder
- Depression
- Schizophrenia

in 4.7% of patients after 16 weeks.[9] A retrospective chart review of 63 patients receiving carbamazepine for bipolar I disorder reported a mean (SD) body weight gain of 3.41 (±8.81) kg after 10 years of therapy.[10]

Gabapentin has been reported to cause dose-dependent increases in weight.[11-14] In a randomized, dose-controlled trial of 275 patients (doses ranging from 600 to 2,400 mg/day), 16 patients (6%) experienced weight gain as an adverse event; 7 (2.6% of the total sample) of these patients experienced a weight gain >7% of baseline weight after 26 weeks of therapy.[11] In a review of 44 patients treated with high-dose gabapentin (mean dose 3,520 mg/day) for intractable seizures, 34% gained 5–10% of baseline weight and 23% gained >10% of baseline weight over a period of at least 12 months.[13] One patient who was receiving 6,000 mg of gabapentin per day discontinued treatment after gaining 27 kg during 1 year of treatment.

Pregabalin has also been reported to cause dose-dependent weight gain.[15-22] During clinical trials assessing the efficacy of pregabalin for treatment of partial seizures, weight gain was reported in 9–20% of patients.[15,16] In a retrospective analysis of 101 patients with epilepsy who were treated with pregabalin add-on therapy for at least 1 year, 26 (25.7%) experienced weight gain greater than 10% of baseline weight.[16] In a 6-month, randomized, controlled trial specifically designed to assess weight gain associated with pregabalin therapy for epilepsy, 41% (25 of 61) of patients experienced a weight gain >5 kg.[17]

Valproic acid and valproate are well recognized as causes of weight gain, with numerous reports in the literature describing significant weight gain in adults and children.[8,22-31] In their review of 16 clinical trials, Jallon and Picard[20] noted that the incidence of weight gain with valproic acid varied from 4% to 71%. The magnitude of weight gain reported in the literature has ranged from 2 to 49 kg during long-term valproate therapy.[22-31] In a prospective, randomized clinical trial specifically designed to assess weight changes associated with valproate as compared with lamotrigine, the average weight gain in patients randomly assigned to the valproate group was 5.8 kg over 32 weeks of treatment, with 38% of patients experiencing a ≥10% increase in weight from baseline.[26]

ANTIDEPRESSANTS

Weight gain induced by tricyclic antidepressant (TCA) medications has been reported to be dose-dependent, treatment-duration-dependent, and typically associated with increased appetite and cravings for sweets and other carbohydrates.[34,37,289] A review of studies evaluating weight gain associated with amitriptyline, nortriptyline, and imipramine reported the average weight increase to be 0.57–1.37 kg per month of therapy.[34] In comparison to other TCAs, amitriptyline has been associated with the largest degree of weight gain.[34-39]

The tetracyclic antidepressants maprotiline and mirtazapine have also been reported to cause significant weight gain in psychiatric patients.[61-70] Mirtazapine increases appetite and has been associated with weight increases ranging from 2.4 kg over 4 weeks of treatment to 16 kg over 5 months of therapy.[62-64] During short-term clinical trials, 7.5% of adult patients and 49% of children receiving mirtazapine experienced a weight gain ≥7% of baseline weight.[32]

Serotonin reuptake inhibitors and mixed serotonergic and noradrenergic antidepressants have been reported to induce small amounts of weight loss during short-term clinical trials.[49] However, the weight loss observed during the early weeks of therapy may be followed by weight gain with long-term treatment.[42,43,47-49,56] Based on available literature, paroxetine appears to be the most likely to induce significant weight gain, followed by sertraline and citalopram.[42,43,49]

Although bupropion is generally viewed as the antidepressant of choice for patients who are overweight or obese because of its propensity to cause weight loss, a recent case report described a woman with major depressive disorder who gained 11 kg over the first month of therapy.[40] This case report may be an anomaly due to the extremely low body weight of the patient at baseline (i.e., 35 kg) and the volume of literature reporting weight loss with bupropion.

Finally, the monoamine oxidase inhibitor (MAOI) phenelzine has been reported to cause clinically significant weight gain, but other drugs within the MAOI class of antidepressants have not been associated with this effect.[74,75]

ANTIPSYCHOTICS

The drug class with the strongest association with significant weight gain is the antipsychotics. A landmark meta-analysis evaluated data regarding weight gain associated with antipsychotics from over 80 clinical trials.[290] Clozapine was associated with the greatest extent of weight gain, with an average gain of 4.45 kg over 10 weeks of treatment in patients receiving standard doses. Olanzapine, risperidone, and ziprasidone were associated with average weight gains of 4.15 kg, 2.10 kg, and 0.04 kg, respectively. Significant mean weight increases of 0.48 kg, 2.58 kg, and 3.19 kg were reported in association with the conventional antipsychotics haloperidol, chlorpromazine, and thioridazine, respectively. In this analysis, placebo treatment was associated with an average weight loss of 0.74 kg over 10 weeks. The investigators used a 10-week treatment period for comparisons because weight measurement data were available at this time point for most patients. Bak et al.[102] conducted a meta-analysis to evaluate longer treatment durations. Longer duration of treatment was associated with greater weight gain for all agents, except ziprasidone and aripiprazole, which appear to have the least should be amount of weight effects.

Average weight gains ranging from 7.5 to 10.9 kg over 6 months to 1 year of therapy have been reported in patients receiving clozapine.[120,125,128,129,133,134] In one study, 21% of outpatients with schizophrenia experienced a weight gain of ≥20% of baseline weight, and 58% of outpatients experienced weight gains of ≥10% of baseline weight during 1 year of clozapine therapy.[125] Additional case reports have documented marked weight gains ranging from 30 to 50 kg associated with clozapine therapy.[119,132,135] In patients receiving olanzapine, average weight gains of 4.1–12 kg have been reported following 6 months to 1 year of treatment.[149,150,152,153,157,159,160,162-164] Of patients receiving long-term therapy with olanzapine during clinical trials (median treatment period, 238 days), 56% experienced a weight gain of ≥7% of baseline weight.[149]

Although conflicting data exist, antipsychotic-induced weight gain does not appear to be dose-related.[291] Weight gain induced by clozapine and olanzapine is associated with increased appetite, carbohydrate craving, and binge eating in some patients.[121,132,292] Based on available information regarding atypical antipsychotic agents, it appears that clozapine and olanzapine are associated with the greatest degree of weight gain.[102,108] Weight gain with olanzapine and clozapine can progress over 6 months to 1 year of therapy before reaching a plateau, with most weight gain occurring during the first 12 weeks.[122,123,153] However, some reports have suggested that clozapine-induced weight gain may persist for up to 3–4 years.[122,131] As compared with other atypical antipsychotics, ziprasidone, aripiprazole, and lurasidone appear to be associated with the smallest degree of weight gain.[102,143,145]

LITHIUM

Weight gain is a common adverse effect of lithium therapy, occurring in up to 65% of patients during long-term treatment.[222-225,284] The average weight gain induced by lithium has been reported to range from 4.5 to 11.5 kg over 1 to 6 years.[222-224] Weight increases of up to 28 kg have been described in the literature.[222] However, an expert panel from The Endocrine Society conducted a meta-analysis of 54 different drugs that did not confirm an association between weight gain and lithium.[258] Women and patients with elevated baseline BMI may be more likely to gain weight with lithium therapy than other patients. Weight gain induced by lithium occurs primarily within the first 2 years of therapy before stabilizing and is characterized by an increase in appetite and thirst, resulting in overconsumption of high-calorie beverages.[222,223,293]

ANTIRETROVIRAL THERAPY

Historically, weight gain associated with antiretroviral therapy has been viewed as highly beneficial and associated with improved health status. In recent years, however, significant advances in the management of human immunodeficiency viral infection have resulted in the availability of highly effective therapies shown to reduce morbidity and mortality.[234] Initiation of combined antiretroviral therapy (cART) has been associated with increases in body weight as well as the risk of cardiovascular disease and diabetes.[234-240] Although the exact cause of weight gain in this patient population has not been confirmed, initiation of cART appears to be associated. Weight gain with cART is associated with increased visceral adipose tissue resulting in impaired glucose homeostasis, dyslipidemia, and an increased risk of cardiovascular disease.[285] In a retrospective review of 681 patients, 20% of patients who initiated cART advanced from a normal or overweight status, to an overweight or obese status following 24 months of therapy.[234] Weight gain in patients who have initiated cART appears to be greatest in the first year of treatment, in women, in those with lower baseline CD4 concentrations, and in those who are receiving protease inhibitors as a component of cART.[236]

CHEMOTHERAPY IN EARLY-STAGE BREAST CANCER

Observational studies conducted in women with early-stage breast cancer have reported significant weight increases in the majority of patients receiving adjuvant chemotherapy.[241-252] Weight gain associated with adjuvant chemotherapy in this patient population has been reported to range from 2.5 to 6.2 kg during the treatment phase, and from 2.3 to 12.3 kg for 1–2 years after treatment.[246,247] Specific drugs reported to be associated with weight gain in this patient population include tamoxifen, prednisone, cyclophosphamide, methotrexate, and fluorouracil.[243,244] In contrast, some studies have reported no significant increases in weight in women who have received adjuvant chemotherapy regimens consisting of cyclophosphamide alone or in combination with paclitaxel.[294] The exact cause of weight gain in patients with early-stage breast cancer is poorly understood but may be related to the underlying disease state, increased calorie consumption, and decreased physical activity.[295,296]

HORMONES

Weight gain is well documented as a consequence of therapy with exogenously administered hormones, including glucocorticoids, insulin, and sex-steroid analogs. In fact, some steroid hormones are specifically used to promote weight gain in certain patient populations.[297-300] Daily oral prednisone therapy has been associated with dose-dependent increases in weight ranging from 2.6 to 13 kg over 1 year of treatment.[253,254] Glucocorticoid-induced weight gain is characterized by central adiposity, which is associated with increased health risks as compared with peripheral obesity.[4,287,288]

Insulin therapy is associated with an increase in body weight in patients diagnosed with both type 1 and type 2 diabetes.[259-265] Weight gain is more common in patients receiving intensive insulin therapy than in those receiving conventional therapy.[259-261,264] Weight gain has been reported to range from 2.6 to 8 kg over 2 months to 1 year of insulin therapy.[259,261,262,265] Although sulfonylurea and thiazolidinedione drugs have been reported to cause increases in weight, particularly when used in combination with insulin, the weight gain associated with these agents alone does not typically exceed 5 kg.[286,301,302]

Conflicting literature exists regarding the significance of weight gain associated with oral contraceptives.[303] Depot medroxyprogesterone has been reported to induce weight gain ranging from 4.3 to 9.4 kg over treatment periods varying in length from 1 to 5 years.[266-275] Adolescents and women with elevated baseline BMI appear to be at increased risk for weight gain associated with hormonal contraceptives.[270,271]

RISK FACTORS

The incidence and extent of drug-induced weight gain differ significantly between patients and across drug classes. Potential risk factors for drug-induced weight gain are listed in **Table 53-5**.

Table 53-5 Risk Factors for Drug-Induced Weight Gain[20,49,222,254,256,268,280,282,284,285,287,291,305-309]

Anticonvulsants[20]

- Dose-dependent (valproic acid, gabapentin)
- Female sex (valproic acid)

Antidepressants[49,279,304]

- Dose-dependent
- Genetic polymorphisms
- Increased treatment duration
- Low baseline BMI
- Weight increases during first week of therapy

Antipsychotic[221,279,281,283,290,305-307]

- Children and adolescents
- Genetic polymorphisms
- Increased treatment duration (clozapine)
- Low baseline BMI
- Positive treatment response[a]
- Treatment with clozapine or olanzapine

Adjuvant chemotherapy for early-stage breast cancer[308]

- Multiagent chemotherapy regimens of long duration
- Premenopausal status

Glucocorticoids[254,255]

- Dose-dependent
- Increased treatment duration

Insulin[286]

- Intensive insulin therapy

Lithium[279,284]

- Elevated baseline BMI
- Female sex

Medroxyprogesterone (depot)[267]

- Adolescents with elevated baseline BMI

BMI = body mass index.
[a]Indicates inconsistent reports in the literature.

MORBIDITY AND MORTALITY

Obesity is a chronic disease that contributes significantly to overall morbidity and mortality.[4,5,309] Epidemiologic data suggest that morbidity and mortality begin to increase with a BMI ≥25.[310] Increased morbidity has also been reported with modest weight increases, even when weight remains within the healthy weight range (BMI, 18–24).[1-4] Obesity is directly linked to the development of hypertension, hyperlipidemia, and type 2 diabetes and is considered an independent risk factor for the development of coronary heart disease.[4] Importantly, obesity may be the second most common factor contributing to preventable death in the United States, second only to cigarette smoking.[311] Obesity and overweight play significant roles in the development of gallbladder disease, degenerative joint disease, sleep apnea, and certain types of cancers. In addition to these health risks, overweight and obesity are associated with a significant psychological burden, potentially leading to depression and other psychological conditions. Therefore, drug-induced weight gain, particularly to the extent that it contributes to overweight or obesity, may be associated with an increased risk of morbidity and mortality.

PREVENTION

Prevention of drug-induced weight gain is achieved primarily through the implementation of counseling strategies that instruct patients and caregivers about behavioral modification, a proper weight-maintenance diet, and routine exercise prior to initiation of the potentially causative agent.[312-315] Studies specifically evaluating the clinical effectiveness of behavioral and dietary interventions to minimize or prevent antipsychotic-induced weight gain have reported small differences in weight changes between patients receiving behavioral dietary interventions and those receiving standard care.[316-318] These interventions appear most effective when they include a combination of cognitive behavioral therapy, reduced caloric consumption, and increased physical activity; when they are implemented at the time of initiation of antipsychotic therapy; and when patients are able to adhere to the therapy for long-term.[316-318] Small studies have also evaluated the efficacy of drug treatment for the prevention of antipsychotic-induced weight gain.[319-327] In general, these studies have reported only modest results. No significant differences in degree of weight gain were reported in association with the concomitant use of drugs such as fluoxetine, nizatidine, and famotidine in patients receiving olanzapine therapy.[319-322] However, evidence suggests that the addition of metformin, topiramate, or zonisamide may reduce weight gain or promote weight loss in patients receiving psychiatric medications.[323-325] Additional studies are needed to define the role of pharmacotherapy for the prevention of drug-induced weight gain. At present, behavioral and dietary interventions are the mainstay for prevention.

For antipsychotic medications, a joint consensus statement issued by the American Diabetes Association, the American Psychiatric Association, the American Association of Clinical Endocrinologists, and the North American Association for the Study of Obesity, provides specific recommendations for patient monitoring with regard to weight.[312] The panel recommends collection of baseline personal and family history regarding obesity and measurement of height, weight, and waist circumference to determine whether the patient is currently overweight or obese or at risk to become overweight or obese in the future. Selection of an antipsychotic agent with less likelihood to cause significant weight gain may be preferable for at-risk patients. The patient, family members, and caregivers should also be informed of the potential for significant weight gain and the subsequent increased risk of diabetes and dyslipidemia. Body weight should then be reassessed at 4, 8, and 12 weeks after the initiation of therapy and quarterly thereafter. The panel recommends switching the antipsychotic agent to another medication with less propensity to cause weight gain if the patient gains >5% of baseline weight during any time in therapy. Approaches to help prevent drug-induced weight gain are reviewed in **Table 53-6**.[293,312-315]

Table 53-6 Approaches to Help Prevent Drug-Induced Weight Gain[293,312-315]

- Consider patients' baseline height, weight, waist circumference, and risk factors for weight gain when selecting drug therapy
- Educate the patient, family, and caregivers regarding diet, physical activity, and behavior modification
- If patient gains >5% of baseline weight, switch to another agent that is less likely to cause weight gain
- Monitor weight regularly and frequently
- Refer patients to weight-management programs or nutritional counseling

MANAGEMENT

The first step in managing clinically relevant drug-induced weight gain is to consider discontinuation of the causative drug and substituting another agent within the same drug class that is associated with less weight gain. Unfortunately, this option may not always be practical or possible. Potential alternatives to consider for agents implicated as the cause of clinically relevant drug-induced weight gain are listed in **Table 53-7**.[326]

If discontinuing the offending drug is not feasible, behavioral modification in combination with a low-calorie diet and increased physical activity has proven effective for some obese patients taking antipsychotic agents.[316,317] A 1-year study of standard nutrition, exercise, and behavioral interventions in patients with schizophrenia who had gained weight while receiving antipsychotic agents reported an average weight loss of 3 kg, while a comparison group of similar schizophrenic patients receiving usual care experienced an average weight increase of 3.2 kg.[327] Current guidelines recommend a low-calorie diet that reduces daily caloric intake by 500–750 kcal and in combination with increased physical activity and behavioral modification.[6] A realistic treatment goal for the above recommendations is a 5–10% reduction in body weight over 6 months of therapy, which correlates to a loss of approximately 1–2 lb per week.[6]

Antiobesity drug therapy is generally recommended as an adjunct to behavioral modification,

Table 53-7 Potential Alternatives for Agents Implicated in Drug-Induced Weight Gain[326]

Anticonvulsants

- Lamotrigine
- Levetiracetam
- Phenytoin
- Topiramate
- Zonisamide

Antidepressants

- Bupropion[a]

Antipsychotics

- Aripiprazole
- Lurasidone
- Ziprasidone

Glucocorticoids

- Disease-modifying antirheumatic drugs (DMARDs)
- Nonsteroidal anti-inflammatory drugs (NSAIDs)

Medications for type 2 diabetes

- Amylin analogs[b]
- Glucagon-like peptide-1 (GLP-1) receptor agonists
- Metformin
- Sodium-glucose cotransporter 2 (SGLT-2) inhibitors

Medroxyprogesterone depot

- Oral contraceptives[c]

[a]Although most data support weight loss, one case has reported significant weight gain.[40]
[b]Used in combination with insulin.
[c]Conflicting data exist suggesting decreased efficacy in patients with BMI >27 kg/m^2.

a low-calorie diet, and increased physical activity when the combination of these three interventions has failed to produce sufficient weight loss in patients with BMI measurements ≥30 or those with BMI ≥27 who have at least one comorbid condition.[6] Few data exist regarding the efficacy of pharmacotherapy for the treatment of drug-induced weight gain. However, case reports and small studies have reported some success associated with use of amantadine, metformin, orlistat, topiramate, and zonisamide in psychiatric patients with drug-induced weight gain.[319,324,325] Studies have also reported that the adjunctive aripiprazole may decrease weight in patients experiencing significant weight gain associated with stable doses of clozapine or olanzapine.[328-330] Although it appears that some patients may benefit from pharmacotherapy when the combination of behavioral modification, low-calorie diet, and increased physical activity has failed to produce sufficient weight loss, further studies are needed to better define the role of pharmacotherapy in the management of drug-induced weight gain.

INFORMATION FOR PATIENTS

Patients who are to receive medications that may cause clinically relevant weight gain should be informed of the potential for this drug-induced disease prior to initiation of therapy. Moreover, patients should be encouraged to begin a weight-maintenance diet plan and exercise routine prior to the initiation of therapy to help minimize potential weight gain. Appropriate education is a critical component in successful weight management. Therefore, patients should be provided with behavior modification information and education related to appropriate dietary choices and lifestyle modification. In addition, patients should be instructed to monitor their weight to detect any changes during drug therapy.

REFERENCES

1. Willett WC, Manson JE, Stampfer MJ et al. Weight, weight changes, and coronary heart disease in women: risk within the "normal" weight range. *JAMA.* 1995; 273:461-5.
2. Rimm EB, Stampfer MJ, Giovannucci E et al. Body size and fat distribution as predictors of coronary heart disease among middle-aged and older US men. *Am J Epidemiol.* 1995; 141:1117-27.
3. Colditz GA, Willett WC, Rotnitzky A et al. Weight gain as a risk factor for clinical diabetes mellitus in women. *Ann Intern Med.* 1995; 122:481-6.
4. National Heart, Lung, and Blood Institute. Clinical guidelines on the identification, evaluation, and treatment of overweight and obesity in adults—The evidence report. *Obes Res* 1998; 6(suppl 2): S51-209.
5. National Heart, Lung, and Blood Institute. Managing overweight and obesity in adults: systemic evidence review from the Obesity Expert Panel, 2013. https://www.nhlbi.nih.gov/health-topics/managing-overweight-obesity-in-adults (accessed 2018 Apr 4).
6. Jensen MD, Ryan DH, Apovian CM et al. 2013 AHA/ACC/TOS guideline for the management of overweight and obesity in adults: a report of the American College of Cardiology/American Heart Association Task Force on Practice Guidelines and The Obesity Society. *Circulation.* 2014; 129(suppl 2):S102-38.
7. Lampl Y, Eshel Y, Rapaport A et al. Weight gain, increased appetite, and excessive food intake induced by carbamazepine. *Clin Neuropharmacol.* 1991; 14:251-5.
8. Corman CL, Leung NM, Guberman AH. Weight gain in epileptic patients during treatment with valproic acid: a retrospective study. *Can J Neurol Sci.* 1997: 24:240-4.

9. Hogan RE, Bertrand ME, Deaton RL et al. Total percentage body weight changes during add-on therapy with tiagabine, carbamazepine, and phenytoin. *Epilepsy Res.* 2000; 41:23-8.
10. Chen CH, Lin SK. Carbamazepine treatment of bipolar disorder: a retrospective evaluation of naturalistic long-term outcomes. *BMC Psychiatry.* 2012; 12:47.
11. Beydoun A, Fisher J, Labar DR et al. Gabapentin monotherapy: a 26-week, double-blind, dose-controlled, multicenter study of conversion from polytherapy in outpatients with refractory complex partial or secondarily generalized seizures. *Neurology.* 1997; 49:746-52.
12. Baulac M, Calvacanti D, Semah F et al. Gabapentin add-on therapy with adaptable dosages in 610 patients with partial epilepsy: an open, observation study. *Seizure.* 1998; 7:55-62.
13. DeToledo JC, Toledo C, De Cerce J et al. Changes in body weight with chronic, high dose gabapentin therapy. *Ther Drug Monit.* 1997; 19:394-6.
14. Jensen MP, Irving G, Rauck R et al. Long-term safety of gastroretentive gabapentin in postherpetic neuralgia patients. *Clin J Pain.* 2013; 29:770-4.
15. Lyrica package insert. New York, NY: Parke-Davis Division of Pfizer Inc; 2016.
16. Beydoun AM, Uthman BM, Kugler AR et al. Safety and efficacy of two pregabalin regimens for add-on treatment of partial epilepsy. *Neurology.* 2005; 64:475-80.
17. Carreno M, Maestro I, Molins A et al. Pregabalin as add-on therapy for refractory partial seizures in every day clinical practice. *Seizure.* 2007; 16:709-12.
18. Hoppe C, Rademacher M, Hoffmann JM. Bodyweight gain under pregabalin therapy in epilepsy: mitigation by counseling patients? *Seizure.* 2008; 17:327-32.
19. Siddall PJ, Cousins MJ, Otte A et al. Pregabalin in central neuropathic pain associated with spinal cord injury: a placebo-controlled trial. *Neurology.* 2007; 67:1792-800.
20. Jallon P, Picard F. Body weight gain and anticonvulsants: a comparative review. *Drug Saf.* 2001; 24:969-78.
21. Tzellos TG, Toulis KA, Goulis DG et al. Gabapentin and pregabalin in the treatment of fibromyalgia: a systematic review and a meta-analysis. *J Clin Pharm Ther.* 2010; 35:639-56.
22. Chen B, Choi H, Hirsch LJ et al. Cosmetic side effects of antiepileptic drugs in adults with epilepsy. *Epilepsy Behav.* 2015; 42:129-37.
23. Dinesen J, Lennart G, Andersen T et al. Weight gain during treatment with valproate. *Acta Neurol Scand.* 1984; 70:65-9.
24. Mattson, RH, Cramer JA, Collins JF et al. A comparison of valproate with carbamazepine for the treatment of complex partial seizures and secondarily generalized tonic-clonic seizures in adults. *N Engl J Med.* 1992; 327:765-71.
25. Isojarvi JIT, Laatikainen TH, Knip M et al. Obesity and endocrine disorders in women taking valproate for epilepsy. *Ann Neurol.* 1996; 39:579-84.
26. Biton V, Mirza W, Montouris G et al. Weight change associated with valproate and lamotrigine monotherapy in patients with epilepsy. *Neurology.* 2001; 56:172-7.
27. Privitera MD, Brodie MH, Mattson RH et al. Topiramate, carbamazepine, and valproate monotherapy: double-blind comparison in newly diagnosed epilepsy. *Acta Neurol Scand.* 2003; 107:165-75.
28. Pickrell WO, Lacey AS, Thomas RH et al. Weight change associated with antiepileptic drugs. *J Neurol Neurosurg Psychiatry.* 2013; 84:796-9.
29. Petty SJ, Kantor S, Lawrence KM et al. Weight and fat distribution in patients taking valproate: a valproate-discordant gender-matched twin and sibling pair study. *Epilepsia.* 2014; 55:1551-7.
30. Kanemura H, Sano F, Maeda Y et al. Valproate sodium enhances body weight gain in patients with childhood epilepsy: a pathogenic mechanisms and open-label clinical trial of behavior therapy. *Seizure.* 2012; 21:496-500.
31. Tokgoz H, Aydin K, Oran B et al. Plasma leptin, neuropeptide Y, ghrelin, and adiponectin levels and carotid artery intima media thickness in epileptic children treated with valproate. *Childs Nerv Syst.* 2012; 28:1049-53.
32. Remeron package insert. West Orange, NJ: Organon USA Inc; 2015.
33. Berken GH, Weinstein DO, Stern WC. Weight gain: a side effect of tricyclic antidepressants. *J Affect Disord.* 1984; 7:133-8.
34. Garland E, Remich RA, Zis A. Weight gain with antidepressants and lithium. *J Clin Psychopharmacol.* 1988; 8:323-30.
35. Fernstrom M, Kupfer DJ. Antidepressant-induced weight gain: a comparison study of four medications. *Psychiatry Res.* 1988; 26:265-71.
36. Szarek BL, Brandt DM. A comparison of weight changes with fluoxetine, desipramine, and amitriptyline: a retrospective study of psychiatric inpatients *J Nerv Ment Dis.* 1993; 181:702-4.
37. Serretti A, Mandelli L. Antidepressants and body weight: a comprehensive review and meta-analysis. *J Clin Psychiatry.* 2010; 71:1259-72.
38. Blumenthal SR, Castro VM, Clements CC et al. An electronic health records study of long-term weight gain following antidepressant use. *JAMA Psychiatry.* 2014; 71:889-96.
39. Dodick DW, Freitag F, Banks J et al. Topiramate versus amitriptyline in migraine prevention: a 26-week, multicenter, randomized, double-blind, double-dummy, parallel-group noninferiority trial in adult migraineurs. *Clin Ther.* 2009; 31:542-59.
40. Hou YC, Lai CH. Bupropion-related weight gain in a fresh depression patient. *J Neuropsychiatry Clin Neurosci.* 2014; 26:E52-3.
41. Anafranil package insert. Hazelwood, MO: Mallinckrodt Inc; 2014.
42. Maina G, Albert U, Salvi V et al. Weight gain during long-term treatment of obsessive-compulsive disorder: a prospective comparison between serotonin reuptake inhibitors. *J Clin Psychiatry.* 2004; 65:1365-71.
43. Dannon PN, Iancu I, Lowengrub K et al. A naturalistic long-term comparison study of selective serotonin reuptake inhibitors in the treatment of panic disorder. *Clin Neuropharmacol.* 2007; 30:326-34.
44. Garland E, Remich RA. Desipramine and weight gain. *J Clin Psychiatry.* 1987; 48:498-9.
45. Feighner J, Hendrickson G, Miller L et al. Double-blind comparison of doxepin versus bupropion in outpatients with a major depressive disorder. *J Clin Psychopharmacol.* 1986; 6:27-32.
46. Ferguson JM, Mendels J, Manowitz NR. Dothiepin versus doxepin in major depression: results of a multicenter, placebo-controlled trial: Prothiaden Collaborative Study Group. *J Clin Psychiatry.* 1994; 55:258-63.
47. Pigott TA, Prakash A, Arnold LM et al. Duloxetine versus escitalopram and placebo: an 8-month double-blind trial in patients with major depressive disorder. *Curr Med Res Opin.* 2007; 23:1303-18.
48. Nelson JC, Pritchett YL, Martynov O et al. The safety and tolerability of duloxetine compared with paroxetine and placebo: a pooled analysis of 4 clinical trials. *Prim Care Companion J Clin Psychiatry.* 2006; 8:212-9.
49. Uguz F, Sahingoz M, Gungor B et al. Weight gain and associated factors in patients using newer antidepressants. *Gen Hosp Psychiatry.* 2015; 37:46-8.
50. Dunner DL, Wilson M, Fava M et al. Long-term tolerability and effectiveness of duloxetine in the treatment of major depressive disorder. *Depress Anxiety.* 2008; 25:E1-8.
51. Gaynor P, McCarberg B, Zheng W et al. Weight change with long-term duloxetine use in chronic painful conditions: an analysis of 16 clinical studies. *Int J Clin Pract.* 2011; 65:341-9.
52. Holzer L, Paiva G, Halfon O. Quetiapine-induced weight gain and escitalopram. *Am J Psychiatry.* 2005; 162:192-3.
53. Wade AG, Crawford GM, Yellowlees A et al. Efficacy safety and tolerability of escitalopram in doses up to 50 mg in major depressive disorder (MDD): an open-label, pilot study. *BMC Psychiatry.* 2011; 16:11:42.

54. Uher R, Farmer A, Henigsberg N et al. Adverse reactions to antidepressants. *Br J Psychiatry*. 2009; 195:202-10.
55. Jeong JH, Bahk WM, Woo YS et al. Efficacy and safety of generic escitalopram (Lexacure(®)) in patients with major depressive disorder: a 6-week multicenter, randomized, rater-blinded, escitalopram-comparative, non-inferiority study. *Neuropsychiatr Dis Treat*. 2015; 11:2557-64.
56. Fava M, Judge R, Hoog SL et al. Fluoxetine versus sertraline and paroxetine in major depressive disorder: changes in weight with long-term treatment. *J Clin Psychiatry*. 2000; 61:863-7.
57. Fernstrom M, Krowinski R, Kupker D. Chronic imipramine treatment and weight gain. *Psychiatry Res*. 1986; 17:269-73.
58. Mavissakalian M, Perel J, Guo S. Specific side effects of long-term imipramine management of panic disorder. *J Clin Psychopharmacol*. 2002; 22:155-61.
59. Sussman N, Ginsberg DL, Bikoff J. Effects of nefazodone on body weight: a pooled analysis of selective serotonin reuptake inhibitor- and imipramine-controlled trials. *J Clin Psychiatry*. 2001; 62:256-60.
60. Nakra BP, Grossberg GT. Carbohydrate craving and weight gain with maprotiline. *Psychosomatics*. 1986; 27:376-81.
61. Vaz-Serra A, Fiqueira ML, Firmino H et al. Multicenter double-blind study of moclobemide and maprotiline. *Clin Neuropharmacol*. 1994; 17:S38-49.
62. Pinar M, Gulsun M, Tasci I et al. Maprotiline-induced weight gain in depressive disorder: changes in circulating ghrelin and adiponectin levels and insulin sensitivity. *Prog Neuropsychopharmacol Biol Psychiatry*. 2008; 32:135-9.
63. Kraus T, Haack M, Schuld A et al. Body weight, the tumor necrosis factor system, and leptin production during treatment with mirtazapine or venlafaxine. *Pharmacopsychiatry*. 2002; 35:220-5.
64. Abraham G. Massive weight gain and hostility force mirtazapine stoppage. *Can J Psychiatry*. 2002; 47:582.
65. Fisfalen ME, Hsiung RC. Glucose dysregulation and mirtazapine-induced weight gain. *Am J Psychiatry*. 2003; 160:797.
66. Yeephu S, Suthisisang C, Suttiruksa S et al. Efficacy and safety of mirtazapine in fibromyalgia syndrome patients: a randomized placebo-controlled pilot study. *Ann Pharmacother*. 2013; 47:921-32.
67. Bet PM, Hugtenburg JG, Penninx, B et al. Side effects of antidepressants during long-term use in a naturalistic setting. *Eur Neuropsychopharmacol*. 2013; 23:1443-51.
68. Chiu HW, Li TC. Rapid weight gain during mirtazapine treatment. *J Neuropsychiatry Clin Neurosci*. 2011; 23:E7.
69. Watanabe N, Omori IM, Nakagawa A et al. Safety reporting and adverse-event profile of mirtazapine described in randomized controlled trials in comparison with other classes of antidepressants in the acute-phase treatment of adults with depression: systematic review and meta-analysis. *CNS Drugs*. 2010; 24:35-53.
70. Danileviciute V, Sveikata A, Adomaitiene V et al. Efficacy, tolerability, and preference of mirtazapine orally disintegrating tablets in depressed patients: a 17-week naturalistic study in Lithuania. *Medicina*. 2009; 45:778-84.
71. Paradis C, Stack J, George C et al. Nortriptyline and weight change in depressed patients over 60. *J Clin Psychopharmacol*. 1992; 12:246-50.
72. Uher R, Farmer A, Henigsberg N et al. Adverse reactions to antidepressants. *Br J Psychiatry*. 2009; 196:202-10.
73. Uher R, Mors O, Hauser J et al. Changes in body weight during pharmacological treatment of depression. *Int J Neuropsychopharmacol*. 2011; 14:367-75.
74. Rabkin J, Quitkin F, Harrison W et al. Adverse reactions to monoamine oxidase inhibitors: part I. A comparative study. *J Clin Psychopharmacol*. 1984; 4:270-8.
75. Rabkin JG, Quitkin FM, McGrath P et al. Adverse reactions to monoamine oxidase inhibitors: part II. Treatment correlates and clinical management. *J Clin Psychopharmacol*. 1985; 5:2-9.
76. Croft HA, Pomara N, Gommoll C et al. Efficacy and safety of vilazodone in major depressive disorder: a randomized, double-blind, placebo-controlled trial. *J Clin Psychiatry*. 2014; 75:1291-8.
77. Robinson DS, Kajdasz DK, Gallipoli S et al. A 1-year open-label study assessing the safety and tolerability of vilazodone in patients with major depressive disorder. *J Clin Psychopharmacol*. 2011; 31:643-6.
78. Alam MY, Jacobsen PL, Chen Y et al. Safety, tolerability, and efficacy of vortioxetine (Lu AA21004) in major depressive disorder: results of an open-label, flexible-dose, 52-week extension study. *Int Clin Psychopharmacol*. 2013; 29:33-44.
79. Abilify package insert. Tokyo, Japan: Otsuka American Pharmaceutical Inc; 2016.
80. Perez-Iglesias R, Ortiz-Garcia O, Amado JA et al. Comparison of metabolic effects of aripiprazole, quetiapine and ziprasidone after 12 weeks of treatment in first treated episode of psychosis. *Schizophr Res*. 2014; 159:90-4.
81. Mankoski R, Stockton g, Manos G et al. Aripiprazole treatment of irritability associated with autistic disorder and the relationship between prior antipsychotic exposure, adverse events, and weight change. *J Child Adolesc Psychopharmacol*. 2013; 23:572-6.
82. Fleischhacker WW, Sanchez R, Johnson B et al. Long-term safety and tolerability of aripiprazole once-monthly in maintenance treatment of patients with schizophrenia. *Int Clin Psychopharmacol*. 2013; 28:171-6.
83. Almandil NB, Liu Y, Murray ML et al. Weight gain and other metabolic adverse effects associated with atypical antipsychotic treatment of children and adolescents: a systematic review and meta-analysis. *Paediatr Drugs*. 2013; 15:139-50.
84. Zhang Y, Dai G. Efficacy and metabolic influence of paliperidone ER, aripiprazole, and ziprasidone to patients with first-episode schizophrenia through 52 weeks follow-up in China. *Hum Psychopharmacol*. 2012; 27:605-14.
85. Wenzel C, Kleimann A, Bokemeyer S et al. Aripiprazole for the treatment of Tourette syndrome: a case series of 100 patients. *J Clin Psychopharmacol*. 2012; 32:548-50.
86. Jeong HG, Lee MS, Ko YH et al. Combination treatment with aripiprazole and valproic acid for acute mania: an 8-week, single-blind, randomized controlled trial. *Clin Neuropharmacol*. 2012; 35:97-102.
87. Jindal KC, Singh GP, Munjal V. Aripiprazole versus olanzapine in the treatment of schizophrenia: a clinical study from India. *Int J Psychiatry Clin Pract*. 2013; 17:21-9.
88. Woo YS, Bahk WM, Chung MY et al. Aripiprazole plus divalproex for recently manic or mixed patients with bipolar I disorder: a 6-month randomized, placebo-controlled, double-blind maintenance trial. *Hum Psychopharmacol*. 2011; 26543-53.
89. de Arce Cordon R, Eding E, Marques-Teixeira J et al. Descriptive analyses of the aripiprazole arm in the risperidone long-acting injectable versus quetiapine relapse prevention trial (Consta TRE). *Eur Arch Psychiatry Clin Neurosci*. 2012; 262:139-49.
90. Hou Y, Lai C. Aripiprazole-related body-weight gain and nutritional counseling. *J Neuropsychiatry Clin Neurosci*. 2011; 23:E44-5.
91. Lee SY, Park MH, Patkar AA et al. A retrospective comparison of BMI changes and the potential risk factors among schizophrenic inpatients treated with aripiprazole, olanzapine, quetiapine, or risperidone. *Prog Neuropsychopharmacol Biol Psychiatry*. 2011; 35:490-6.
92. Osuntokun O, Millen B, Xu W et al. Metabolic parameters in patients treated with olanzapine or other atypical antipsychotics. *J Psychopharmacol*. 2011; 25:630-8.
93. Lyon GJ, Samar S, Jummani R et al. Aripiprazole in children and adolescents with Tourette's disorder: an open-label safety and tolerability study. *J Child Adolesc Psychopharmacol*. 2009; 19:623-33.
94. Correll CU, Manu P, Olshanskiy V et al. Cardiometabolic risk of second-generation antipsychotic medications during first-time use in children and adolescents. *JAMA*. 2009; 302:1765-73.
95. Fava M, Wisniewski SR, Thase ME. Metabolic assessment of aripiprazole as adjunctive therapy in major depressive disorder: a pooled analysis of 2 studies. *J Clin Psychopharmacol*. 2009; 29:362-7.

96. Kane JM, Osuntokun O, Kryzhanovskaya LA. A 28-week, randomized, double-blind study of olanzapine versus aripiprazole in the treatment of schizophrenia. *J Clin Psychiatry*. 2009; 70:572-81.
97. Kwon JS, Jang JH Kang DH. Long-term efficacy and safety of aripiprazole in patients with schizophrenia, schizophreniform disorder, or schizoaffective disorder: a 26-week prospective study. *Psychiatry Clin Neurosci*. 2009; 63:73-81.
98. Fleischhacker WW, McQuade RD, Marcus RN et al. A double-blind, randomized comparative study of aripiprazole and olanzapine in patients with schizophrenia. *Biol Psychiatry*. 2009; 65:510-7.
99. Kerwin R, Millet B, Herman E et al. A multicenter, randomized, naturalistic, open-label study between aripiprazole and standard of care in the management of community-treated schizophrenic patients Schizophrenia Trial of Aripiprazole: (STAR) study. *Eur Psychiatry*. 2007; 22:433-43.
100. McQuade RD, Stock E, Marcus R et al. A comparison of weight change during treatment of olanzapine or aripiprazole: results from a randomized, double-blind study. *J Clin Psychiatry*. 2004; 65:47-56.
101. Potkin SG, Saha AR, Kuhawa MH et al. Aripiprazole, an antipsychotic with a novel mechanism of action, and risperidone vs placebo in patients with schizophrenia and schizoaffective disorder. *Arch Gen Psychiatry*. 2003; 60:681-90.
102. Bak M, Fransen A, Janssen J et al. Almost all antipsychotics result in weight gain: a meta-analysis. *PloS One*. 2014; 9:e94112.
103. Saphris package insert. Whitehouse Station, NJ: Merck and Co Inc; 2013.
104. Findling RL, Landbloom RP, Mackle M et al. Safety and efficacy from an 8 week double-blind trial and a 26 week open-label extension of asenapine in adolescents with schizophrenia. *J Child Adolesc Psychopharmacol*. 2015; 25:384-96.
105. Findling RL, Landbloom RL, Szegedi A et al. Asenapine for the acute treatment to pediatric manic or mixed episode of bipolar I disorder. *J Am Acad Child Adolesc Psychiatry*. 2015; 54:1032-41.
106. Worthington MA, El-Mallakh RS. A naturalistic retrospective review of weight gain in bipolar patients treated with second-generation antipsychotics. *J Clin Psychopharmacol*. 2015; 35:192-3.
107. Kemp DE, Zhao J, Cazorla P et al. Weight change and metabolic effects of asenapine in patients with schizophrenia and bipolar disorder. *J Clin Psychiatry*. 2014; 75:238-45.
108. Leucht S, Cipriani A, Spineli L et al. Comparative efficacy and tolerability of 15 antipsychotic drugs in schizophrenia: a multiple-treatments meta-analysis. *Lancet*. 2013; 382:951-62.
109. Vita A, DePeri L, Siracusano A et al. Efficacy and tolerability of asenapine for acute mania in bipolar I disorder: meta-analyses of randomized controlled trials. *Int Clin Psychopharmacol*. 2013; 28:219-27.
110. Rexulti package insert. Tokyo, Japan: Otsuka American Pharmaceutical Inc; 2015.
111. Thase, ME, Youakim JM, Skuban A et al. Efficacy and safety of adjunctive brexpiprazole 2 mg in major depressive disorder: a phase 3, randomized, placebo-controlled study in patients with inadequate response to antidepressants. *J Clin Psychiatry*. 2015; 76:1224-31.
112. Citrome L. Brexpiprazole for schizophrenia and as adjunct for major depressive disorder: a systematic review of the efficacy and safety profile for this newly approved antipsychotic—what is the number needed to treat, number needed to harm and likelihood to be helped or harmed? *Int J Clin Pract*. 2015; 69:978-97.
113. Correll CU, Skuban A, Ouyang J et al. Efficacy and safety of brexpiprazole for the treatment of acute schizophrenia: a 6-week randomized, double-blind placebo-controlled trial. *Am J Psychiatry*. 2015; 172:870-80.
114. Kane JM, Skuban A, Ouyang J et al. A multicenter, randomized, double-blind controlled phase 3 trial of fixed-dose brexipiprazole for the treatment of adults and acute schizophrenia. *Schizophr Res*. 2015; 164:127-35.
115. Vraylar package insert. Parsippany, NJ: Actavis Pharma Inc; 2015.
116. Durgam S, Earley W, Lipschitz A et al. An 8-week randomized, double-blind, placebo-controlled evaluation of the safety and efficacy of cariprazine in patients with bipolar I depression. *Am J Psychiatry*. 2016; 173271-81.
117. Clozaril package insert. East Hanover, NJ: Novartis Pharmaceuticals Corporation; 2015.
118. Leppig M, Bosch B, Naber D et al. Clozapine in the treatment of 121 outpatients. *Psychopharmacology*. 1989; 99(suppl):S77-9.
119. Cohen S, Chiles J, MacNauthton A. Weight gain associated with clozapine. *Am J Psychiatry*. 1990; 147:503-4.
120. Lamberti S, Terrance B, Schwarzkopt F. Weight gain among schizophrenic patients treated with clozapine. *Am J Psychiatry*. 1992; 149:689-90.
121. Leadbetter R, Shutty M, Pavalonis D et al. Clozapine-induced weight gain: prevalence and clinical relevance. *Am J Psychiatry*. 1992; 149:68-72.
122. Umbricht D, Pollack S, Kane J. Clozapine and weight gain. *J Clin Psychiatry*. 1994; 55:157-60.
123. Hummer M, Kemmler G, Kurz M et al. Weight gain induced by clozapine. *Eur Neuropsychopharmacol*. 1995; 5:437-40.
124. John JP, Chengappa KN, Baker RW et al. Assessment of changes in both weight and frequency of use of medications for the treatment of gastrointestinal symptoms among clozapine-treated patients. *Ann Clin Psychiatry*. 1995; 7:119-25.
125. Bustillo JR, Buchanan RW, Irsh D et al. Differential effect of clozapine on weight: a controlled study. *Am J Psychiatry*. 1996; 153:817-9.
126. Bondolfi G, Dufour H, Patris M et al. Risperidone versus clozapine in treatment resistant chronic schizophrenia: a randomized double-blind study. *Am J Psychiatry*. 1998; 155:499-504.
127. Frankenburg FR, Zanarini MC, Kando J et al. Clozapine and body mass change. *Biol Psychiatry*. 1998; 43:520-4.
128. Briffa D, Meehan T. Weight changes during clozapine treatment. *Aust N Z J Psychiatry*. 1998; 32:718-21.
129. Bai Y, Lin C, Chen J et al. Weight gain among patients on clozapine. *Psychiatr Serv*. 1999; 50:704-5.
130. Spivak B, Musin E, Mester R et al. The effect of long-term antipsychotic treatment on the body weight of patients suffering from chronic schizophrenia: clozapine versus classical antipsychotic agents. *Int Clin Psychopharmacol*. 1999; 14:229-32.
131. Henderson DC, Cagliero E, Gray C et al. Clozapine, diabetes mellitus, weight gain, and lipid abnormalities: a five-year naturalistic study. *Am J Psychiatry*. 2000; 157:975-81.
132. Theisen FM, Cichon S, Linden A et al. Clozapine and weight gain. *Am J Psychiatry*. 2001; 158:816.
133. Lieberman JA, Phillips M, Gu H et al. Atypical and conventional antipsychotic drugs in treatment-naïve first-episode schizophrenia: a 52-week randomized trial of clozapine vs chlorpromazine. *Neuropsychopharmacology*. 2003; 28:995-1003.
134. Covell NH, Weissman EM, Essock SM. Weight gain with clozapine compared to first generation antipsychotic medications. *Schizophr Bull*. 2004; 30:229-40.
135. Wehmeir PM, Gebhardt S, Schmidtke J et al. Clozapine weight gain in a pair of monozygotic twins concordant for schizophrenia and mild mental retardation. *Psychiatry Res*. 2005; 133:273-6.
136. Rummel-Kluge C, Komossa K, Schwarz S et al. Head-to-head comparisons of metabolic side effects of second-generation antipsychotics in the treatment of schizophrenia: a systematic review and meta-analysis. *Schizophr Res*. 2010; 123:225-33.
137. Guo X, Fang M, Zhai J et al. Effectiveness of maintenance treatments with atypical and typical antipsychotics in stable schizophrenia with early stage: 1-year naturalistic study. *Psychopharmacology (Berl)*. 2011; 216:474-84.
138. Gao K, Kemp DE, Fein E et al. Number needed to treat to harm for discontinuation due to adverse events in the treatment to bipolar depression and major depressive disorder, and generalized anxiety disorder with atypical antipsychotics. *J Clin Psychiatry*. 2011; 72:1062-71.

139. Schuster JP, Raucher-Chene D, Lemogne C et al. Impact of switching or initiating antipsychotic treatment of body weight during a 6-month follow-up in a cohort of patients with schizophrenia. *J Clin Psychopharmacol.* 2012; 32:672-7.
140. Kelly AC, Sheitman BB, Hamer RM et al. A naturalistic comparison of the long-term metabolic adverse effects of clozapine versus other antipsychotics for patients with psychotic illnesses. *J Clin Psychopharmacol.* 2014; 34:441-5.
141. Schneider C, Corrigall R, Hayes D et al. Systematic review of the efficacy and tolerability of clozapine in the treatment of youth with early onset schizophrenia. *Eur Psychiatry.* 2014; 29:1-10.
142. Fanapt package insert. East Hanover, NJ: Novartis Pharmaceuticals Corporation; 2014.
143. De Hert M, Yu W, Detraux J et al. Bodyweight and metabolic adverse effects of asenapine, iloperidone, lurasidone, and paliperidone in the treatment of schizophrenia and bipolar disorder: a systematic review and exploratory meta-analysis. *CNS Drugs.* 2012; 26:733-59.
144. Latuda package insert. Takeno, Kawagoe, Saitama, Japan: Bushu Pharmaceuticals Ltd.; 2010.
145. Meyer JM, Mao Y, Pikalov A et al. Weight change during long-term treatment with lurasidone: pooled analysis of studies in patients with schizophrenia. *Int Clin Psychopharmacol.* 2015; 30:342-50.
146. Nasrallah HA, Silva R, Phillips D et al. Lurasidone for the treatment of acutely psychotic patients with schizophrenia: a 6-week, randomized, placebo-controlled study. *J Psychiatr Res.* 2013; 47:670-7.
147. Loebel A, Cucchiaro J, Sarma K et al. Efficacy and safety of lurasidone 80 mg/day and 160 mg/day in the treatment of schizophrenia: a randomized, double-blind, placebo- and active-controlled trial. *Schizophr Res.* 2013; 145:101-9.
148. Meltzer HY, Cucchiaro J Silva R et al. Lurasidone in the treatment of schizophrenia: a randomized, double-blind, placebo- and olanzapine-controlled study. *Am J Psychiatry.* 2011; 168:957-67.
149. Zyprexa package insert. Indianapolis, IN: Eli Lilly and Company; 2015.
150. Nemeroff CB. Dosing the antipsychotic medication olanzapine. *J Clin Psychiatry.* 1997; 58(suppl 10):45-9.
151. Osser DN, Najarian DM, Dufresne RL. Olanzapine increases weight and serum triglyceride levels. *J Clin Psychiatry.* 1999; 60:767-70.
152. Tran PV, Tollefson GD, Sanger TM et al. Olanzapine versus haloperidol in the treatment of schizoaffective disorder. *Br J Psychiatry.* 1999; 174:15-22.
153. Kinon BJ, Basson BR, Gilmore JA, Tollefson GD. Long-term olanzapine treatment: weight change and weight-related health factors in schizophrenia. *J Clin Psychiatry.* 2001; 62:92-100.
154. Haapasalo-Pesu KM, Saarijarvi S. Olanzapine induces remarkable weight gain in adolescent patients. *Eur Child Adolesc Psychiatry.* 2001; 10:205-8.
155. Ganguli R, Brar J, Ayrton Z. Weight gain over 4 months in schizophrenia patients: a comparison of olanzapine and risperidone. *Schizophr Research.* 2001; 49:261-7.
156. Farwell WR, Stump TE, Wang J et al. Weight gain and new onset diabetes associated with olanzapine and risperidone. *J Gen Intern Med.* 2004; 19:1200-5.
157. Haberfellner EM, Rittmannsberger H. Weight gain during long-term treatment with olanzapine: a case series. *Int Clin Psychopharmacol.* 2004; 19:251-3.
158. Hennen J, Perlis RH, Sachs G et al. Weight gain during treatment of bipolar I patients with olanzapine. *J Clin Psychiatry.* 2004; 64:1679-87.
159. Lieberman JA, Stroup TS, McEnvoy JP et al. Effectiveness of antipsychotic drugs in patients with chronic schizophrenia. *New Engl J Med.* 2005; 353:1209-33.
160. Tohen M, Chengappa KNR, Suppes T et al. Relapse prevention in bipolar I disorder: 18-month comparison of olanzapine plus mood stabilizers versus mood stabilizers alone. *Br J Psychiatry.* 2004; 184:337-45.
161. Tohen M, Greil W, Calabrese JR et al Olanzapine versus lithium in the maintenance treatment of bipolar disorder: a 12-month, randomized, double-blind controlled clinical trial. *Am J Psychiatry.* 2005; 162:1281-90.
162. Zipurski RB, Gu H, Green AI et al. Course and predictors of weight gain in people with first-episode psychosis treated with olanzapine or haloperidol. *Br J Psychiatry.* 2005; 187:537-43.
163. Saddichha S, Manjunatha N, Ameen S et al. Effect of olanzapine, risperidone, and haloperidol treatment on weight and body mass index in first-episode schizophrenia patients in India: a randomized, double-blind, controlled, prospective study. *J Clin Psychiatry.* 2007; 68:1793-8.
164. Perez-Iglesias R, Crespo-Facorro B, Martinez-Garcia O et al. Weight gain induced by haloperidol, risperidone, and olanzapine after 1 year: findings of a randomized clinical trial in a drug-naïve population. *Schizopr Res.* 2008; 99:13-22.
165. Schoemaker J, Naber D, Vrijland P et al. Long-term assessment of asenapine vs. olanzapine in patients with schizophrenia or schizoaffective disorder. *Pharmacopsychiatry.* 2010; 43:138-46.
166. Detke HC, Zhao F, Witte MM. Efficacy of olanzapine long-acting injection in patients with acute exacerbated schizophrenia: an insight from effect size comparison with historical data. *BMC Psychiatry.* 2012; 12:51.
167. Park S, Yi KK, Kim MS et al. Effects of ziprasidone and olanzapine in body composition and metabolic parameters: an open-label comparative pilot study. *Behav Brian Funct.* 2013; 9:27
168. Katagiri H, Tohen M, McDonnell DP et al. Efficacy and safety of olanzapine for treatment of patients with bipolar depression: Japanese subpopulation analysis of a randomized, double-blind, placebo-controlled study. *BMC Psychiatry.* 2013; 13:138.
169. Kimmel RJ, Levy MR. Profound hypertriglyceridemia and weight gain in the first week following initiation of olanzapine: a case report with implications for lipid monitoring guidelines. *Psychosomatics.* 2013; 54:392-4.
170. McDonnell DP, Landry J, Detke HC. Long-term safety and efficacy of olanzapine long-acting injection in patients with schizophrenia or schizoaffective disorder: a 6-year, multinational, single-arm, open label study. *Int Clin Psychopharmacol.* 2014; 29:322-31.
171. Invega package insert. Titusville, NJ: Janssen, LP; 2016.
172. Harrington CA, English C. Tolerability of paliperidone: a meta-analysis of randomized, controlled trials. *Int Clin Psychopharmacol.* 2010; 25:334-41.
173. Kim SW, yoon JS, Kim YS et al. The effect of paliperidone extended release on subjective well-being and responses in patients with schizophrenia. *Prog Neuropsychopharmacol Biol Psychiatry.* 2012; 38:228-35.
174. Sliwa JK, Fu DJ, Bossie CA et al. Body mass index and metabolic parameters in patients with schizophrenia during long-term treatment with paliperidone palmitate. *BMC Psychiatry.* 2014; 14:52.
175. McEvoy JP, Byerly M, Hamer RM et al. Effectiveness of paliperidone palmitate vs haloperidol decanoate for maintenance treatment of schizophrenia: a randomized clinical trial. *JAMA.* 2014; 311:1978-87.
176. Savitz AJ, Lane R, Nuamah I et al. Efficacy and safety of paliperidone extended release in adolescents with schizophrenia: a randomized, double-blind study. *J Am Acad Child Adolesc Psychiatry.* 2015; 54:126-37.
177. Kotler M, Dilbaz N, Rosa F et al. A flexible-dose study of paliperidone ER in patients with nonacute schizophrenia previously treated unsuccessfully with oral olanzapine. *J Psychiatr Pract.* 2016; 22:9-21.
178. Seroquel package insert. Wilmington, DE: AstraZeneca Pharmaceuticals LP; 2013.
179. Tariot PN, Salzman C, Yeung PP et al. Long-term use of quetiapine in elderly patients with psychotic disorders. *Clin Ther.* 2000; 22:1068-84.

180. McConville BJ, Arvanitis LA, Thyrum PT et al. Pharmacokinetics, tolerability, and clinical effectiveness of quetiapine fumarate: an open-label trial in adolescents with psychotic disorders. *J Clin Psychiatry*. 2000; 61:252-60.
181. Kasper S, Brecher M, Fitton L et al. Maintenance of long-term efficacy and safety of quetiapine in the open-label treatment of schizophrenia. *Int Clin Psychopharmacol*. 2004; 19:281-9.
182. Vieta E, Mullen J, Brecher M et al. Quetiapine monotherapy for mania associated with bipolar disorder: combined analysis of two international double-blind randomized, placebo-controlled studies. *Curr Med Res Opin*. 2005; 21:923-34.
183. Kopala LC, Good KP, Milliken H et al. Treatment of a first episode of psychotic illness with quetiapine: an analysis of 2 year outcomes. *Schizophr Res*. 2006; 81:29-39.
184. Potkin SG, Gharabawi GM, Greenspan AJ et al. A double-blind comparison of risperidone, quetiapine and placebo in patients with schizophrenia experiencing an acute exacerbation requiring hospitalization. *Schizophr Res*. 2006; 85:254-65.
185. McEvoy JP, Lieberman JA, Perkins DO et al. Efficacy and tolerability of olanzapine, quetiapine, and risperidone in the treatment of early psychosis: a randomized, double-blind 52-week comparison. *Am J Psychiatry*. 2007; 164:1050-60.
186. Langosch JM, Drieling T, Biedermann NC et al. Efficacy of quetiapine monotherapy in rapid-cycling bipolar disorder in comparison with sodium valproate. *J Clin Psychopharmacol*. 2008; 28:555-60.
187. Sajatovic M, Calabrese JR, Mullen J. Quetiapine for the treatment of bipolar mania in older adults. *Bipolar Disord*. 2008; 10:622-71.
188. Zheng L, Mack WJ, Dagerman KS et al. Metabolic changes associated with second-generation antipsychotic use in Alzheimer's disease patients: the CATIE-AD study. *Am J Psychiatry*. 2009; 166:583-90.
189. Patel JK, Buckley PF, Woolson S et al. Metabolic profiles of second-generation antipsychotics in early psychosis: findings from the CAFE study. *Schizophr Res*. 2009; 111:9-16.
190. Swadi HS, Craig BJ, Pirwani NZ et al. A trial of quetiapine compared with risperidone in the treatment of first onset psychosis among 15- to 18-year-old adolescents. *Int Clin Psychopharmacol*. 2010; 25:1-6.
191. Suppes R, Datto C, Minkwitz M et al. Effectiveness of the extended release formulation of quetiapine as monotherapy for the treatment of acute bipolar depression. *J Affect Disord*. 2010; 121:106-15.
192. Honer WG, MacEwan GW, Gendron A et al. A randomized, double-blind, placebo-controlled study of the safety and tolerability of high-dose quetiapine in patients with persistent symptoms of schizophrenia or schizoaffective disorder. *J Clin Psychiatry*. 2012; 73:13-20.
193. Sheehan DV, Harnett-Sheehan K, Hidalgo RB et al. Randomized, placebo-controlled trial of quetiapine XR and divalproex ER monotherapies in the treatment of the anxious bipolar patient. *J Affect Disord*. 2013; 145:83-94.
194. Chue P, Malla A, Bouchard RH et al. The long-term clinical benefit and effectiveness of switching to once-daily quetiapine extended release in patients with schizophrenia. *Curr Med Res Opin*. 2013; 29:227-39.
195. Findling RL, Rathak S, Earley WR et al. Safety, tolerability, and efficacy of quetiapine in youth with schizophrenia or bipolar I disorder: a 26-week, open-label, continuation study. *J Child Adolesc Psychopharmacol*. 2013; 23:490-501.
196. Risperdal package insert. Titusville, NJ: Janssen Pharmaceuticals Inc; 2016.
197. Penn JV, Martini J, Radka D. Weight gain associated with risperidone. *J Clin Psychopharmacol*. 1996; 16:259-60.
198. Buitelaar JK. Open-label treatment with risperidone of 26 psychiatrically-hospitalized patients and adolescents with mixed diagnoses and aggressive behavior. *J Child Adolesc Psychopharmacol*. 2000; 10:19-26.
199. Cohen S, Glazewski R, Khan S et al. Weight gain with risperidone among patients with mental retardation: effect of calorie restriction. *J Clin Psychiatry*. 2001; 62:114-6.
200. Hellings JA, Zarcone JR, Crandall K et al. Weight gain in a controlled study of risperidone in children, adolescents, and adults with mental retardation and autism. *J Child Adolesc Psychiatry*. 2001; 11:229-38.
201. Csernansky JB, Mahmoud, R, Brenner R. A comparison of risperidone and haloperidol for the prevention of relapse in patients with schizophrenia. *N Engl J Med*. 2002; 346:16-22.
202. Scholler N, Rabinowitz J, Davidson M et al Risperidone and haloperidol in first-episode psychosis: a long-term randomized trial. *Am J Psychiatry*. 2005; 162:947-53.
203. Maayan LA, Vakhrusheva J. Risperidone associated weight, leptin, and anthropometric changes in children and adolescents with psychotic disorders in early treatment. *Hum Psychopharmacol*. 2010; 25:133-8.
204. Verma S, Subramaniam M Abdin E et al. Safety and efficacy of long-acting injectable risperidone in patients with schizophrenia spectrum disorders: a 6-month open-label trial in Asian patients. *Hum Psychopharmacol*. 2010; 25:230-5.
205. Xiang YT, Wang CY, Ungvari GS et al. Weight changes and their associations with demographic and clinical characteristics in risperidone maintenance treatment for schizophrenia. *Pharmacopsychiatry*. 2011; 44:135-41.
206. Krystal JH, Rosenheck RA, Cramer JA et al. Adjunctive risperidone treatment for antidepressant-resistant symptoms of chronic military service-related PTSD: a randomized trial. *JAMA*. 2011; 306:493-502.
207. Covell NH, McEvoy HP, Schooler NR et al. Effectiveness of switching from long-acting injectable fluphenazine or haloperidol decanoate to long-acting injectable risperidone microspheres: an open-label, randomized controlled trial. *J Clin Psychiatry*. 2012; 73:669-75.
208. Song X, Fan X, Li X et al. Changes in pro-inflammatory cytokines and body weight during 6-month risperidone treatment in drug naive, first-episode schizophrenia. *Psychopharmacology (Berl)*. 2014; 231:319-25.
209. Lee NY, Kim SH, Cho SJ et al. A prospective, open-label study to evaluate symptomatic remission in schizophrenia with risperidone long-acting injectable in Korea. *Int Clin Psychopharmacol*. 2014; 29:279-87.
210. Geodon package insert. New York, NY: Roerig Division of Pfizer Inc; 2015.
211. Amdisen A. Drug produced obesity: experiences with chlorpromazine, perphenazine and clopenthixol. *Dan Med Bull*. 1964; 11:184-9.
212. Clark ML, Huber WK, Sullivan J et al. Evaluation of loxapine succinate in chronic schizophrenia. *Dis Nerv Syst*. 1972; 12:783-91.
213. Doss FW. The effect of antipsychotic drugs on body weight: a retrospective review. *J Clin Psychiatry*. 1979; 40:528-30.
214. Harris E, Eth S. Weight gain during neuroleptic treatment. *Int J Nurs Stud*. 1981; 18:171-5.
215. Kane J, Honifeld G, Singer J et al. Clozapine for the treatment resistant schizophrenic: a double-blind comparison with chlorpromazine. *Arch Gen Psych*. 1988; 45:789-96.
216. Dossenbach M, Treuer R, Kryzhanovskaya L et al. Olanzapine versus chlorpromazine in the treatment of schizophrenia: a pooled analysis of four 6-week, randomized, open-label studies in the Middle East and North Africa. *J Clin Psychopharmacol*. 2007; 27:329-37.
217. Marriott P, Pansa M, Hiep A. Depot fluphenazine maintenance treatment associated with weight changes. *Compr Psychiatry*. 1981; 22:320-5.
218. Cookson JC, Kennedy NM, Gribbon D. Weight gain and prolactin levels in patients on long-term antipsychotic medication: a double-blind comparative trial of haloperidol decanoate and fluphenazine decanoate. *Int Clin Psychopharmacol*. 1986; 1 (suppl 1):41-51.

219. Dossenbach MR, Folnegovic-Smalc V, Hotujac L et al. Double-blind randomized comparison of olanzapine versus fluphenazine in the long-term treatment of schizophrenia. *Prog Neuropsychopharmacol Biol Psychiatry*. 2004; 28:311-8.
220. Kane JM, Carson WH, Saha AR et al. Efficacy and safety of aripiprazole and haloperidol versus placebo in patients with schizophrenia and schizoaffective disorder. *J Clin Psych*. 2002; 63:763-71.
221. Saddichha S, Ameen S, Akkhtar S. Predictors of antipsychotic-induced weight gain in first-episode psychosis. *J Clin Psychopharmacol*. 2008; 28:27-31.
222. Kerry RJ, Liebling LI, Owen G. Weight changes in lithium responders. *Acta Psychiatr Scand*. 1970; 46:238-43.
223. Vendsborg P, Bech P, Rafaelsen O. Lithium treatment and weight gain. *Acta Psychiatr Scand*. 1976; 53:139-47.
224. Peslow E, Dunner D, Fieve R et al. Lithium carbonate and weight gain. *J Affect Disord*. 1980; 2:303-10.
225. McKnight RF, Adida M, Budge K et al. Lithium toxicity profile: a systematic review and meta-analysis. *Lancet*. 2012; 379:721-8.
226. Korsgaard S, Skausing O. Increase in weight after treatment with depot neuroleptics. *Acta Psychiatr Scand*. 1979; 59:139-44.
227. Hoyberg OJ, Fensbo C, Remvig J et al. Risperidone versus perphenazine in the treatment of chronic schizophrenic patients with acute exacerbations. *Acta Psychiatr Scand*. 1993; 88:395-402.
228. Strassnig M, Miewald J, Keshavan M et al. Weight gain in newly diagnosed first-episode psychosis patients and healthy comparisons: one-year analysis. *Schizophr Res*. 2007; 93:90-8.
229. Pfister AK. Weight gain from combined phenothiazine and tricyclic therapy. *JAMA*. 1978; 239:1959.
230. McCreadie RG, Todd N, Livingston M et al. A double-blind comparative study of remoxipride and thioridazine in the acute phase of schizophrenia. *Acta Psychiatr Scand*. 1998; 78:49-56.
231. Keks N, McGrath J, Lamber T. The Australian multicentre double-blind comparative study of remoxipride and thioridazine in schizophrenia. *Acta Psychiatr Scand*. 1994; 90:358-65.
232. Deneber HC, Turns D. Double blind comparison of thiothixene and trifluoperazine in acute schizophrenia. *Psychosomatics*. 1972; 13:100-4.
233. Bishop MP, Buddington RW, Robinson WG et al. A comparison of SKF-7261 and trifluoperazine (Stelazine) in the treatment of chronic schizophrenic patients. *J Neuropsychiatr*. 1963; 4:28-32.
234. Tate T, Willig AL, Willig JH et al. HIV infection and obesity: where did all the wasting go? *Antivir Ther*. 2012; 17:1281-9.
235. Erlandson KM, Kitch D, Tierney C et al. Weight and lean body mass change with antiretroviral initiation and impact on bone mineral density. *AIDS*. 2013; 24;27:2069-79.
236. Lakey W, Yang LY, Yancy W et al. Short communication: from wasting to obesity: initial antiretroviral therapy and weight gain in HIV-infected persons. *AIDS Res Hum Retroviruses*. 2013; 29:435-40.
237. Achhra AC, Mocroft A, Reiss P et al. Short-term weight gain after antiretroviral therapy initiation and subsequent risk of cardiovascular disease and diabetes: the DAD study. *HIV Med*. 2015.
238. Yuh, Tate J, Butt AA et al. Weight change after antiretroviral therapy and mortality. *Clin Infect Dis*. 2015; 60:1852-9.
239. Mave V, Erlandson KM, Gupte N et al. Inflammation and change in body weight with antiretroviral therapy initiation in a multinational cohort of HIV-infected adults. *J Infect Dis*. 2016; Mar 8. pii: jiw096.
240. Koethe JR, Jenkins CA, Lau B et al. Rising obesity prevalence and weight gain among adults starting antiretroviral therapy in the United States and Canada. *AIDS Res Hum Retroviruses*. 2016; 32:50-8.
241. Dixon J, Moritz D, Baker F. Breast cancer and weight gain: an unexpected finding. *Oncol Nurs Forum*. 1978; 5:5-7.
242. Heasman KZ, Sutherland HJ, Campbell JA et al. Weight gain during adjuvant chemotherapy for breast cancer. *Breast Cancer Res Treat*. 1985; 5:195-200.
243. Huntington MO. Weight gain in patients receiving adjuvant chemotherapy for carcinoma of the breast. *Cancer*. 1985; 56:472-4.
244. Chlebowski RT, Weiner JM, Reynolds R et al. Long-term survival following relapse after 5-FU, but not CMF adjuvant breast cancer therapy. *Breast Cancer Res Treat*. 1986; 7:23-9.
245. Goodwin PJ, Panzarella T, Boyd NF et al. Weight gain in women with localized breast cancer: a descriptive study. *Breast Cancer Res Treat*. 1988; 11:59-66.
246. Levine EG, Raczynski JM, Carpenter JT. Weight gain with breast cancer adjuvant treatment. *Cancer*. 1991; 67:1954-9.
247. McInnes JA, Knobf MK. Weight gain and quality of life in women treated with adjuvant chemotherapy for early-stage breast cancer. *Oncol Nurs Forum*. 2001; 28:675-84.
248. Costa LJ, Varella PC, del Giglio A et al. Weight changes during chemotherapy of breast cancer. *Sao Paulo Med J*. 2002; 120:113-7.
249. Makari-Judson G, Judson CH, Mertens WC. Longitudinal patterns of weight gain after breast cancer diagnosis: observations beyond the first year. *Breast J*. 2007; 13:258-65.
250. Gordon AM, Hurwitz S, Shapiro CL et al. Premature ovarian failure and body composition changes with adjuvant chemotherapy for breast cancer. *Menopause*. 2011; 18:1244-8.
251. Nissen MJ, Shapiro A, Swenson KK. Changes in weight and body composition in women receiving chemotherapy for breast cancer. *Clin Breast Cancer*. 2011; 11:52-60.
252. Basaran G, Turhal NS, Cabuk D et al. Weight gain after adjuvant chemotherapy in patients with early breast cancer in Istanbul Turkey. *Med Oncol*. 2011; 28:409-15.
253. Kyle V, Hazleman BL. Treatment of polymyalgia rheumatica and giant cell arteritis: relation between steroid dose and steroid associated side effects. *Ann Rheum Dis*. 1989; 48:662-6.
254. Prummel MF, Mourits MP, Blank L et al. Randomized double-blind trial of prednisone versus radiotherapy in Graves' ophthalmopathy. *Lancet*. 1993; 342:949-54.
255. Wung PK, Anderson T, Fontaine KR et al. Effects of glucocorticoids on weight change during the treatment of Wegener's granulomatosis. *Arthritis Rheum*. 2008; 59:746-53.
256. Rogers CC, Alloway RR, Hanaway M et al. Body weight alterations under early corticosteroid withdrawal and chronic corticosteroid therapy with modern immunosuppression. *Transplant Proc*. 2005; 37:800-1.
257. Berthon BS, MacDonald-Wicks LK, Wood LG. A systematic review of the effect of oral glucocorticoids on energy intake, appetite, and body weight in humans. *Nutr Res*. 2014; 34:179-90.
258. Domecq JP, Prutsky G, Leppin A et al. Drugs commonly associated with weight change: a systematic review and meta-analysis. *J Clin Endocrinol Metab*. 2015; 100:363-70.
259. Yki-Jarvinen H, Kauppila M, Kujansuu E et al. Comparison of insulin regimens in patients with non-insulin-depending diabetes mellitus. *N Eng J Med*. 1992; 327:1426-33.
260. The Diabetes Control and Complications Trial Research Group. Weight gain associated with intensive therapy in the diabetes control and complications trial. *Diabetes Care*. 1993; 11:567-73.
261. Carlson MG, Campbell PJ. Intensive insulin therapy and weight gain in IDDM. *Diabetes*. 1993; 42:1700-7.
262. Chow CC, Sorensen JP, Tsang LWW et al. Comparison of insulin with or without continuation of oral hypoglycaemic agents in the treatment of secondary failure in NIDDM patients. *Diabetes Care*. 1995; 18:307-14.
263. The Diabetes Control and Complications Trial Research Group. Adverse events and their association with treatment regimens in the diabetes control and complications trial. *Diabetes Care*. 1995; 18:1415-27.
264. UK Prospective Diabetes Study (UKPDS) Group. Intensive blood glucose control with sulphonylureas or insulin compared with conventional treatment and risk of complications in patients with type 2 diabetes (UKPDS 33). *Lancet*. 1998; 352:837-53.

265. Makimattila S, Nikkila K, Yki-Jarvinen H. Causes of weight gain during insulin therapy with and without metformin in patients with type II diabetes. *Diabetologia.* 1999; 42:406-12.
266. Amatayakul K, Sivasomboon B, Thanangkul O. A study of the mechanism of weight gain in medroxyprogesterone acetate users. *Contraception.* 1980; 22:605-22.
267. Risser WL, Gefter LR, Barratt MS et al. Weight change in adolescents who used hormonal contraception. *J Adolesc Health.* 1999; 24:433-6.
268. Espey E, Steinhardt J, Ogburn T et al. Depo-provera associated with weight gain in Navajo women. *Contraception.* 2000; 62:55-8.
269. Bahamondes L, Del Castillo S, Tabares G et al. Comparison of weight increase in users of depot medroxyprogesterone acetate and copper IUD up to 5 years. *Contraception.* 2001; 64:223-5.
270. Mangan SA, Larsen PG, Hudson S. Overweight teens at increased risk for weight gain while using depot medroxyprogesterone acetate. *J Pediatr Adolesc Gynecol.* 2002; 15:79-82.
271. Bonny AE, Ziegler J, Harvey R et al. Weight gain in obese and nonobese adolescent girls initiating depot medroxyprogesterone, oral contraceptive pills, or no hormonal contraceptive method. *Arch Pediatr Adolesc Med.* 2006; 160:40-5.
272. Westoff C, Jain JK, Milsom I et al. Changes in weight with depot medroxyprogesterone acetate subcutaneous injection 104 mg/0.65 mL. *Contraception.* 2007; 75:261-7.
273. Lopez LM, Edleman A, Chen M et al. Progestin-only contraceptives: effects on weight. *Cochrane Database Syst Rev.* 2013; 7:CD008815.
274. Dal'Ava N, Bahamondes L, Bahamondes MV et al. Body weight and body composition of depot medroxyprogesterone acetate users. *Contraception.* 2014; 90:182-7.
275. DepoProvera package insert. Pharmacia and Upjohn Company, Division of Pfizer Inc; New York, NY; 2016.
276. Ogden CL, Carroll MD, Kit BK et al. Prevalence of childhood and adult obesity in the United States, 2011-2012. *JAMA.* 2014; 311:806-14.
277. Hamed SA. Leptin and insulin homeostasis in epilepsy: relation to weight adverse conditions. *Epilepsy Res.* 2007; 75:1-9.
278. Chukwu J, Delanty N, Webb D et al. Weight change, genetics and antiepileptic drugs. *Expert Rev Clin Pharmacol.* 2014; 7:43-51.
279. Zimmermann U, Kraus T, Himmerich H et al. Epidemiology, implications and mechanisms underlying drug-induced weight gain in psychiatric patients. *J Psychiatr Res.* 2003; 37:193-220.
280. Virk S, Schwartz TL, Jindal N et al. Psychiatric medication induced obesity: an aetiologic review. *Obes Rev.* 2004; 5:167-70.
281. Himmerich H, Minkwitz J, Kirkby KC. Weight gain and metabolic changes during treatment with antipsychotics and antidepressants. *Endocr Metab Immune Disord Drug Targets.* 2015; 15:252-60.
282. McIntyre RS, Mancini DA, Basile VA. Mechanisms of antipsychotic-induced weight gain. *J Clin Psychiatry.* 2001; 62(suppl):23-9.
283. Ma X, Maimaitirexiati T, Zhang R et al. HTR2C polymorphisms, olanzapine-induced weight gain and antipsychotic-induced metabolic syndrome in schizophrenia patients: a meta-analysis. *Int J Psychiatry Clin Pract.* 2014; 18:229-42.
284. Baptista R, Teneud L, Contreras Q et al. Lithium and body weight gain. *Pharmacopsychiatry.* 1995; 28:35-44.
285. Standley TL, Grinspoon SK. Body composition and metabolic changes in HIV-infected patients. *J Infect Dis.* 2012; 205(suppl 3): S383-90.
286. Hermansen K, Mortensen LS. Bodyweight changes associated with antihyperglycemic agents in type 2 diabetes mellitus. *Drug Saf.* 2007; 30:1127-42.
287. Horber FF, Zurcher RM, Herren H et al. Altered body fat distribution in patients with glucocorticoid treatment and in patients on long-term dialysis. *Am J Clin Nutr.* 1986; 43:758-69.
288. Nordborg E, Schaufelberger C, Bosaeus I. The effect of glucocorticoids on fat and lean tissue masses in giant cell arteritis. *Scand J Rheumatol.* 1998; 27:106-11.
289. Yergani V, Rohl R, Aleem A et al. Carbohydrate craving and increased appetite associated with antidepressant therapy. *Can J Psychiatry.* 1988; 33:606-10.
290. Allison DB, Mentore JL, Moonseong H et al. Antipsychotic-induced weight gain: a comprehensive research synthesis. *Am J Psychiatry.* 1999; 156:1686-96.
291. Gentile S. Long-term treatment with atypical antipsychotics and the risk of weight gain: a literature analysis. *Drug Saf.* 2006; 29:303-19.
292. Theisen FM, Linden A, Konig IR et al. Spectrum of binge eating symptomatology in patients treated with clozapine and olanzapine. *J Neural Transm.* 2003; 110:111-21.
293. Livingstone C, Rampes H. Lithium: a review of its metabolic adverse effects. *J Psychopharmacol.* 2006; 20:347-55.
294. Freedman RJ, Aziz N, Albanes D et al. Weight and body composition changes during and after adjuvant chemotherapy in women with breast cancer. *J Clin Endocrinol Metab.* 2004; 89:2248-53.
295. Denmark-Wahnefried W, Hars V, Conaway MR et al. Reduced rates of metabolism and decreased physical activity in breast cancer patients receiving adjuvant chemotherapy. *Am J Clin Nutr.* 1997; 65:1495-501.
296. Harvie MN, Campbell IT, Baildam A, Howell A. Energy balance in early breast cancer patients receiving adjuvant chemotherapy. *Breast Cancer Res Treat.* 2004; 83:201-10.
297. Demling RH, DeSanti L. Oxandrolone, an anabolic steroid, significantly increases the rate of weight gain in the recovery phase after major burns. *J Trauma.* 1997; 43:47-51.
298. Karcic E, Philpot C, Morley JE. Treating malnutrition with megestrol acetate: literature review and review of our experience. *Nutr Health Aging.* 2002; 6:191-200.
299. Mwamburi DM, Gerrior J, Wilson IB et al. Combination megestrol acetate, oxandrolone, and dietary advice restores weight in human immunodeficiency virus. *Nutr Clin Pract.* 2004; 19:395-402.
300. Cuerda C, Zugasti A, Breton I et al. Treatment with nandrolone decanoate and megestrol acetate in HIV-infected men. *Nutr Clin Pract.* 2005; 20:93-7.
301. Actos package insert. Deerfield, IL: Takeda Pharmaceuticals America Inc; 2013.
302. Avandia package insert. Research Triangle Park, NC: GlaxoSmithKline; 2014.
303. Pelkman C. Hormones and weight change. *J Reprod Med.* 2002; 47(suppl):791-4.
304. Himmerich H, Schuld A, Haack M et al. Early prediction of changes in weight during six weeks of treatment with antidepressants. *J Clin Psych Res.* 2004; 38:485-9.
305. Reynolds GP, Hill MK, Kirk SL et al. The 5-HT_{2C} receptor and antipsychotic-induced weight gain-mechanisms and genetics. *J Psychopharmacol.* 2006; 20(suppl):15-8.
306. Yu H, Wang L, Lv L et al. Genome-wide association study suggested the PTPRD polymorphisms were associated with weight gain effects of atypical antipsychotic medications. *Schizophr Bull.* 2015; pii:sbv179.
307. Czerwensky F, Leucht S, Steimer W. Association of the common MC4R rs17782313 polymorphism with antipsychotic-related weight gain. *J Clin Psychopharmacol.* 2013; 33:74-9.
308. Demark-Wahnefried W, Rimer B, Winer EP. Weight gain in women diagnosed with breast cancer. *J Am Diet Assoc.* 1997; 97:519-29.
309. Field AE, Coakley EH, Must A et al. Impact of overweight on the risk of developing common chronic diseases during a 10-year period. *Arch Intern Med.* 2001; 161:1581-6.
310. The global BMI Mortality Collaboration. Body-mass index and all-cause mortality: individual-participant-data meta-analysis of 239 prospective studies in four continents. *Lancet.* 2016.

311. Danaei G, Ding EL, Mozaffarian D et al. The preventable causes of death in the United States: comparative risk assessment of dietary lifestyle, and metabolic risk factors. *PLoS Med.* 2009; 6:e1000058.
312. American Diabetes Association, American Psychiatric Association, American Association of Clinical Endocrinologists, and North American Association for the Study of Obesity. Consensus development conference on antipsychotic drugs and obesity and diabetes. *Obes Res.* 2004; 12:362-6.
313. Ananth J, Venkatesh R, Burgoyne K et al. Atypical antipsychotic induced weight gain: pathophysiology and management. *Ann Clin Psychiatry.* 2004; 16:75-85.
314. Wirshing DA. Schizophrenia and obesity: impact of antipsychotic medications. *J Clin Psychiatry.* 2004; 65(suppl 18):13-26.
315. Henderson DC. Weight gain with atypical antipsychotics: evidence and insights. *J Clin Psychiatry.* 2007; 65(suppl 12):18-26.
316. Werneke U, Taylor D, Sanders TA et al. Behavioral interventions for antipsychotic-induced appetite changes. *Curr Psychiatry Rep.* 2013; 15:347.
317. Bonfioli E, Berti L, Gross C et al. Health promotion lifestyle interventions for weight management in psychosis: a systematic review and meta-analysis of randomized controlled trials. *BMC Psychiatry.* 2012; 12:78.
318. Gabriele JM, Dubbert PM, Reeves RR. Efficacy of behavioural interventions in managing atypical antipsychotic weight gain. *Obes Rev.* 2009; 10:442-55.
319. Das C, Mendez G, Jagasis S et al. Second generation antipsychotic use in schizophrenia and associated weight gain: a critical review and meta-analysis of behavioral and pharmacologic treatments. *Ann Clin Psychiatry.* 2012; 24:225-39.
320. Poyurovsky M, Pashinian A, Maayan et al. Olanzapine-induced weight gain in patients with first-episode schizophrenia: a double-blind, placebo-controlled study of fluoxetine addition. *Am J Psychiatry.* 2002; 159:1058-60.
321. Cavazzoni P, Tanaka Y, Roychowdhury SM et al. Nizatidine for prevention of weight gain with olanzapine: a double-blind placebo-controlled trial. *Eur Neuropsychopharmacol.* 2003; 13:81-5.
322. Poyurovsky M, Tal V, Maayan R et al. The effect of famotidine addition on olanzapine-induced weight gain in first-episode schizophrenia patients: a double-blind placebo-controlled pilot study. *Eur Neuropsychopharmacol.* 2004; 14:332-6.
323. Newall H, Myles N, Ward PB et al. Efficacy of metformin for prevention of weight gain in psychiatric populations: a review. *Int Clin Psychopharmacol.* 2012; 27:69-75.
324. Mahmood S, Booker I, Huang J et al. Effect of topiramate on weight gain in patients receiving atypical antipsychotic agents. *J Clin Psychopharmacol.* 2013; 33:90-4.
325. Ghanizadeh A, Nikseresht MS, Sahraian A. The effect of zonisamide on antipsychotic-associated weight gain in patients with schizophrenia: a randomized, double-blind, placebo-controlled clinical trial. *Schizophr Res.* 2013; 147:110-5.
326. Apovian CM, Aronne LJ, Bessesen DH et al. Pharmacological management of obesity: an endocrine society clinical practice guideline. *J Clin Endocrinol Metab.* 2015; 100:342-62.
327. Menza M. Vreeland B, Minksy S et al. Managing atypical antipsychotic-associated weight gain: 12-month data on a multimodal weight control program. *J Clin Psychiatry.* 2004; 65:471-7.
328. Masopust J, Tuma I, Libiger J. Adjunctive aripiprazole decreased metabolic side effects of clozapine treatment. *Neuro Endocrinol Lett.* 2008; 29:435-7.
329. Henderson DC, Fan X, Copeland PM et al. Aripiprazole added to overweight and obese olanzapine-treated schizophrenia patients. *J Clin Psychopharmacol.* 2009; 29:165-9.
330. Englisch S, Weinbrenner A, Inta D et al. Aripiprazole for the management of olanzapine-induced weight gain. *Pharmacopsychiatry.* 2009; 42:166-7.

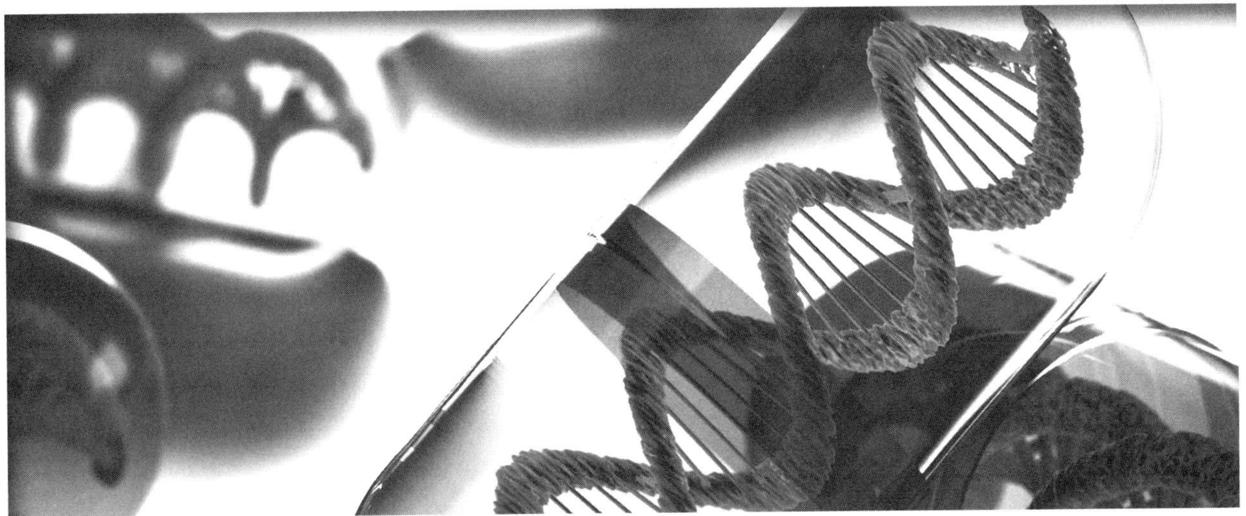

CHAPTER 54

Temperature Dysregulation

Susan M. Wilson and Ian A. Ross

Normal human body temperature ranges from 36.7°C to 37°C measured orally. Axillary temperatures and those measured rectally are 1°C lower and 1°C higher, respectively. Intraindividual body temperature varies throughout the day and over time, and slight variations may also be noted between individuals. The anterior hypothalamus maintains body temperature within a relatively narrow range by sensing core body temperature and adjusting (homeostatic) mechanisms in the autonomic nervous system. Central dopaminergic and serotonergic pathways are also involved in temperature regulation via the autonomic nervous system. A relative decrease in serum dopamine concentrations or alterations in serotonin balance may lead to autonomic impairment and dysregulation in body temperature. Drugs may act as antigens to induce an immune-mediated response, causing the release of endogenous pyrogens such as interleukin-1 and tumor necrosis factor from leukocytes, resulting in a febrile response.

Drug-induced hyperthermia may be divided into five general categories: altered thermoregulatory mechanisms, drug administration–related fever, fevers relating to the pharmacologic action of the drug, idiosyncratic reactions, and hypersensitivity reactions.[1]

A drug may alter thermoregulation by disrupting central dopamine or serotonin homeostasis, or via peripheral alteration of normal hypothalamic temperature balance, creating an imbalance of increased heat production and reduced heat dissipation.[2] Two such drug-induced dysregulation diseases—neuroleptic malignant syndrome (NMS) and serotonin syndrome—will be discussed in subsequent sections. A rare, but serious, late effect of salicylate toxicity is fever resultant of excess heat production due to an uncoupling of mitochondrial oxidative phosphorylation.[3] Additionally, drugs may affect thermoregulation via modulation of peripheral factors that help maintain normal body temperature, including cutaneous and regional blood flow, hormonal responses, shivering, and sweating.[4-6] Drugs such as anticholinergics, sympathomimetics, prostaglandins, general anesthetics, and thyroid supplements that affect these peripheral factors directly or indirectly will not be discussed in detail in this chapter.

Drug administration–related fever is caused by pyrogens or endotoxins and is often encountered in association with agents derived from microbial products. These pyrogens induce an immune-mediated response causing the release of cytokines such as interleukin-1 and tumor necrosis factor from leukocytes, leading to fever. Examples include fever during amphotericin B and bleomycin infusion. Further, an administration-related response associated with fever may occur in association with drugs given intravenously (phlebitis) or intramuscularly (sterile abscess). Pentazocine and paraldehyde are known to induce such a response when administered intramuscularly.

Fevers relating to the pharmacologic action of drugs are most commonly observed in the treatment of infections or cancer as pyrogen is released from damaged or dying cells. The classic example is the Jarisch–Herxheimer reaction that occurs during the treatment of syphilis. Patients taking clozapine may experience fever potentially due to the immunomodulating effects of increased concentrations of interleukin-6 and tumor necrosis factor.[7,8]

Malignant hyperthermia is a specific idiosyncratic reaction that results in the development of severe fever and muscle damage in susceptible individuals receiving causative drugs. Approximately 5–8% of patients treated with the antiretroviral drug abacavir experience a hypersensitivity reaction characterized by fever, rash, malaise, gastrointestinal, and respiratory symptoms that has been linked to the major histocompatibility complex allele HLA-B*5701. Reactions can be severe enough that screening prior to therapy initiation is required for safe use.[9,10]

Finally, the most common cause of drug-induced hyperthermia is a hypersensitivity reaction. The reaction is mediated through immunologic mechanisms and caused by drugs or their metabolites, most commonly antibiotics.[1]

Conditions to consider in the differential diagnosis of the drug-induced hyperthermia include primary central nervous system disorders (infection, tumors, ischemic or hemorrhagic stroke, trauma, seizures), systemic diseases (infections, cancer, metabolic conditions, endocrinopathies, autoimmune disorders), and toxins (carbon monoxide, phenols, strychnine, tetanus). Drug reaction with eosinophilia and systemic symptoms (DRESS), discussed in Chapter 6: Drug Allergy and Cutaneous Diseases, is another condition in which hyperthermia is often observed. A comparison of the signs and symptoms of the various drug-induced hyperthermic conditions is presented in **Table 54-1**.

Although antipyretics are effective in the treatment of hyperthermia due to drug fever and serum sickness-like reaction, careful temperature monitoring during their use is very important. The mechanism of fever in these cases is a hypothalamus-mediated increase in the body's core temperature. Antipyretics are not effective for the treatment of hyperthermia secondary to NMS, serotonin syndrome, or malignant hyperthermia because the hyperthermia represents an alteration in thermoregulatory balance and hypermetabolism and not a fever.

Drug-induced hypothermia is much less common than hyperthermia and is associated more commonly with illicit drugs rather than with prescription or nonprescription medications. Agents with agonist activity at the gamma-aminobutyric acid (GABA) receptor, such as gamma-hydroxybutyrate (GHB), are often associated with hypothermic effects. GABA is a primary inhibitory central neurotransmitter. GABA, dopamine, serotonin, and opioid peptides are mediators in temperature regulation; the primary effect of GABA is to decrease temperature.

HYPERTHERMIA DUE TO DRUG FEVER

A diagnosis of "drug fever" is generally established when there is a febrile response to a medication, no other cause of the fever may be elucidated, and the fever resolves upon discontinuation of the suspect agent.[1,11] Drug fever tends to be a diagnosis of exclusion following a review of a patient's drug therapy, clinical presentation characteristics, and laboratory values. An early presumptive diagnosis of drug fever and initiation of treatment may reduce unnecessary further evaluation and patient discomfort.

CAUSATIVE AGENTS

Although any drug has the potential to cause drug fever, certain medications should be considered with a higher level of suspicion. Drugs

Table 54-1 Comparison of Signs and Symptoms Associated with Drug-Induced Hyperthermia

Characteristic	Drug Fever	SSLR	NMS	SS	MH
Dose related	N	N	Y	Y	N
Usual onset from drug initiation	7–10 days	7–21 days	Days to weeks	24 hours	Minutes
Symptom resolution with drug withdrawal	Within 72 hours	4–14 days	24–72 hours	24–72 hours	Minutes to hours
Altered consciousness	N	N	Y	Y	Y
Behavior changes	N	N	Y	Y	N
Fever	Y	Y	Y	Y	Y
Hemodynamic alterations	N	N	Y	Y	Y
Hyper-reflexia	N	N	N	Y	N
Increased creatine kinase	N	N	Y	Y	Y
Increased white cell count	Y	Y	N	Y	N
Muscle rigidity	N	N	Y	N	Y
Myoclonus	N	N	N	Y	N
Myoglobinuria	N	N	Y	Y	Y
Rhabdomyolysis	N	N	Y	Y	Y
Tachycardia	N	N	Y	Y	Y
Tachypnea/hypercarbia	N	N	Y	Y	Y
Tremor	N	N	N	Y	N

MH = malignant hyperthermia, N = not usually associated with this disease, NMS = neuroleptic malignant syndrome, SS = serotonin syndrome, SSLR = serum sickness-like reaction, Y = may be observed with this disease.

that have been reported to cause drug fever are listed in **Table 54-2**.[12-133] Anticonvulsants, certain antihypertensive drugs, antiarrhythmic agents, and antibiotics are the drugs most commonly associated with drug fever. Antibiotics account for approximately one third of cases.[134] Of the antibiotics, penicillins and cephalosporins are most often implicated. Antibiotics that are rarely or have never been reported to cause drug fever include chloramphenicol, clindamycin, and aminoglycosides.[1,19]

EPIDEMIOLOGY

The true incidence of drug fever is unknown because of underreporting and misdiagnosis. It has been estimated that a drug is the cause of fever in approximately 5–15% of hospitalized patients.[135-137] The incidence is even higher in patients receiving antimicrobials other than antibiotics, such as antiviral agents, and in patients receiving other classes of medications, particularly anticonvulsant and cardiovascular drugs.[16] It has been postulated that the incidence of drug fever is higher in older patients and in female patients; however, this has not been substantiated.[16,135] It has been demonstrated that drug fever due to antibiotics is more likely to occur in younger patients.[19]

MECHANISMS

Drug fever has been hypothesized to be a type III hypersensitivity immune response reaction, based on the time course of the onset of symptoms, the clinical presentation, which may include eosinophilia, and its usual recurrence with rechallenge.[1,19,136,138,139] Drugs or their metabolites may be directly antigenic or act as haptens and combine with endogenous proteins, which become antigens. The immune response may include release of immune mediators and cause the release of pyrogens, thereby inducing fever.

Table 54-2 Agents Implicated in Drug Fever[4]

Drug	Incidence	Level of Evidence[a]
3,4-methylenedioxymethamphetamine (MDMA; ecstasy)[12]	NK	C
6-mercaptopurine[13,14]	NK	C
Acyclovir[15]	NK	C
Allopurinol[16]	NK	C
Amitriptyline[17]	NK	C
Amphetamines[18]	NK	C
Ampicillin[16,19]	NK	C
Amoxicillin–clavulanate[20]	NK	C
Asparaginase[21]	NK	C
Aspirin[1,16]	NK	C
Azathioprine[22-30]	NK	C
Benztropine[31]	NK	C
Bleomycin[32,33]	NK	C
Carbamazepine[34,35]	NK	C
Carbenicillin[36,37]	NK	C
Cefoperazone[19]	NK	C
Cefazolin[38]	NK	C
Cefotaxime[19]	NK	C
Ceftazidime[37]	NK	C
Ceftizoxime[19]	NK	C
Ceftriaxone[39]	NK	C
Cefuroxime[19]	NK	C
Cephalexin[38]	NK	C
Chlorpromazine[40]	NK	C
Chlorambucil[41]	NK	C
Cimetidine[42]	NK	C
Cisplatin[43]	NK	C
Clofibrate[44]	NK	C
Cloxacillin[45]	NK	C
Cytosine[46,47]	NK	C
Diltiazem[48]	NK	C
Daunorubicin[16]	NK	C
Dobutamine[49,50]	NK	C
Doxepin[17]	NK	C
Erythromycin[38]	NK	C
Everolimus[51]	NK	C
Fluoroquinolones[52]	NK	C
Fluoxetine[17]	NK	C
Folic acid[53]	NK	C
Furosemide[54]	NK	C
Ganciclovir[55]	NK	C
Haloperidol[56]	NK	C
Heparin[57]	NK	C
Hydralazine[16]	NK	C
Hydrochlorothiazide[38]	NK	C
Hydroxyurea[58-69]	NK	C
Ibuprofen[70]	NK	C
Imipenem–cilastatin[37,71]	NK	C
Imipramine[17]	NK	C
Isoniazid[72-76]	NK	C
Levamisole[77]	NK	C
Lysergic acid diethylamide (LSD)[78,79]	NK	C
Maprotiline[17]	NK	C
Mebendazole[80]	NK	C
Methicillin[16]	NK	C
Methotrexate[26]	NK	C
Methyldopa[16,81-87]	NK	C
Metoclopramide[88]	NK	C
Mezlocillin[36,37]	NK	C
Minocycline[89]	NK	C
Mycophenolate[90]	NK	C
Nafcillin[37]	NK	C
Naproxen[38]	NK	C
Nifedipine[91]	NK	C
Nitrofurantoin[16,92]	NK	C
Oxacillin[93]	NK	C
Penicillin[1,16,37]	NK	C
Phenobarbital[92]	NK	C
Phenytoin[1,16]	NK	C
Piperacillin[19,36,37]	NK	C
Potassium iodide[1,95,96]	NK	C
Primidone[92]	NK	C
Procainamide[16,97-99]	NK	C
Procarbazine[100]	NK	C
Propafenone[101]	NK	C
Propylthiouracil[16,102-106]	NK	C
Pyrazinamide[107]	NK	C
Quinidine[16,99,108-114]	NK	C
Quinine[110]	NK	C
Ranitidine[115]	NK	C
Rifampin[76,116]	NK	C
Sirolimus[117]	NK	C

Table 54-2 Agents Implicated in Drug Fever[4] (continued)

Drug	Incidence	Level of Evidence[a]	Drug	Incidence	Level of Evidence[a]
Stavudine[118]	NK	C	Tolmetin[126]	NK	C
Streptomycin[119]	NK	C	Trazodone[17]	NK	C
Streptozocin[120,121]	NK	C	Triameterene[127,128]	NK	C
Sulfonamides[1,16,108,122,123]	NK	C	Trifluoperazine[129]	NK	C
Teicoplanin[124]	NK	C	Trimethoprim–sulfamethoxazole[38,130]	NK	C
Tetracycline[16]	NK	C	Vancomycin[16,131]	NK	C
Theophylline[38]	NK	C	Vincristine[132]	NK	C
Thioridazine[125]	NK	C	Zoledronic acid[133]	NK	C
Ticarcillin[38]	NK	C			

NK = not known.

[a]Definitions for Levels of Evidence: Level A—evidence from one or more randomized, controlled clinical trials; Level B—evidence from nonrandomized clinical trials, prospective observational studies, cohort studies, retrospective studies, case-control studies, meta-analyses and/or postmarketing surveillance studies; and Level C—evidence from one or more published case reports or case series.

Table 54-3 Signs and Symptoms of Drug Fever

- More common
  - Fever
  - Headache
  - Leukocytosis
  - Myalgias
  - Relative sense of well-being
- Less common
  - Elevated erythrocyte sedimentation rate
  - Elevated liver function tests (aspartate aminotransferase, alanine aminotransferase) and alkaline phosphatase
  - Eosinophilia
  - Maculopapular rash
  - Relative bradycardia
  - Thrombocytopenia

CLINICAL PRESENTATION AND DIFFERENTIAL DIAGNOSIS

Signs and symptoms of drug fever are presented in **Table 54-3**. The onset of fever is generally 7–10 days from the time of initiation of therapy with the culprit drug. The time of onset may vary by drug class, with the shortest time interval observed with antineoplastic agents (mean of 6 days) and antimicrobials (mean of 7.8 days) and a much longer time interval observed with central nervous system agents (mean of 18.5 days) and cardiac drugs (mean of 44.7 days).[16] Because of this variability, assessment of the temporal relationship between drug initiation and fever onset does not generally aid in the diagnosis. Patients who have been previously sensitized have symptoms much more quickly, usually within hours of reintroduction of the offending drug.

The pattern of fever varies as well and may present as continuous, remittent, intermittent, or hectic.[1,16,17,19,135] Hectic fever is variable or fluctuating; the use of antipyretics or other cooling measures may contribute to this pattern. Chills and rigors may occasionally accompany fever, mimicking the symptoms of sepsis, thereby complicating the diagnosis. Patients may experience a low maximum temperature (T_{max}), or it may be as high as 43°C.[7] No strong association has been made between T_{max} and any patient characteristics, except an inverse relationship between T_{max} and age.[7] Higher temperatures have been observed in patients taking antineoplastic agents; however, this may have been due to the underlying disease.

Cutaneous manifestations are observed in 18–29% of patients during or following drug fever.[1,16,19] After discontinuation of the offending agent, a maculopapular rash can occur that may have an urticarial component with or without petechiae.[16,19,36,58,101,137,140]

Although heart rate typically increases with fever, with drug fever heart rate may not increase to the extent expected relative to the temperature elevation. This "relative bradycardia" in patients without another explanation (e.g., those taking β-blockers or with second- or third-degree heart block) has been used as evidence favoring the diagnosis of drug fever, particularly in patients for whom infection or sepsis is being ruled out.[135,136] Although some patients may experience headache or myalgias, another common observation in patients with drug fever is the sense of well-being relative to the degree of hyperthermia; often patients feel well and are not aware of the fever.[16]

Laboratory abnormalities that may occur with drug fever include leukocytosis, thrombocytopenia, eosinophilia, and markedly elevated erythrocyte sedimentation rate and serum aspartate aminotransferase, alanine aminotransferase, and alkaline phosphatase concentrations.[16,19,36,58,88,101,128,141]

Differential diagnosis of drug fever is difficult because of the inconsistent and nonspecific signs and symptoms described above. Patients often undergo an extensive evaluation and treatment for infection, including blood cultures, radiologic studies, antibiotics, and antipyretic therapy. Multiple studies highlight the cost of diagnostic exclusion and a late diagnosis of drug fever, citing an average of five blood cultures per patient and 2.85 radiological examinations, with an attributed length-of-stay increase of 5.5–8.7 days and an average cost of $9,022 per patient.[140,142] A reasonable effort should be made to rule out other causes (**Table 54-4**). However, depending on the severity of illness, a trial of discontinuing potential fever-inducing medications may be considered.

Table 54-4 Conditions to Consider in the Differential Diagnosis of Drug Fever

- Drug withdrawal (alcohol, benzodiazepines, levodopa)
- Endocrine disorders
- Heat stroke
- Hematologic or solid organ malignancy
- Infection
- Sepsis

RISK FACTORS

Risk factors for the development of drug fever have not been fully elucidated. Patients with a prior drug allergy and those with a history of atopic disease have not been shown to be more susceptible to drug fever.[16] A higher incidence of drug fever has been noted in patients with active HIV infection as well as those with cystic fibrosis. This increased incidence may be due in part to increased use of antibiotics and antiretrovirals in these patient populations.[143-145] Patients with glucose-6-phosphate dehydrogenase deficiency may be at higher risk for drug fever associated with methyldopa because of drug accumulation and higher serum concentrations.[87] Younger patients may be at higher risk for drug fever secondary to antibiotic administration.[19,135]

MORBIDITY AND MORTALITY

The clinical course for patients with drug fever may range from full recovery following very mild illness to significant morbidity and mortality. Drug fever may be the first sign of a hypersensitivity reaction that can prove fatal, even though a direct relationship is rare. In one evaluation of 290 cases of drug fever, 10 patients died.[16] Those who died were more likely to have higher temperatures and an underlying diagnosis of cancer.[16] Most other reviews and cases in the literature have not reported death as a common event associated with drug fever. Continuing the offending agent after a fever appears may put a patient at risk for more serious sequelae, including organ dysfunction, as the syndrome may be expected to worsen. Progression of disease and organ dysfunction is the most probable cause of death due to drug fever.

PREVENTION

The recurrence of drug fever may be prevented by avoiding the offending agent and using an alternative drug if possible. Cross-sensitivity between drugs in the same class is a theoretical concern but has not been reported after the reaction has completely resolved. Given the possibility of recurrence, choosing an agent from another class may be warranted if treatment is to continue. However, after discontinuation of the offending agent, a secondary immune reaction may be observed if the patient is taking another immune sensitizing drug.[1] The mechanism by which this occurs is not well understood but is not thought to be mediated via cross-allergenicity, as these drugs are often pharmacologically unrelated.[137] Desensitization protocols should be implemented in patients for whom no other treatment options are possible. Desensitization is usually accomplished by administering very small doses of the drug via the intravenous or oral route. The dose is gradually increased over hours or days until the full therapeutic dose may be safely administered. In addition to general desensitization guidelines, specific desensitization protocols have been published for many drugs that cause drug fever, including acyclovir, allopurinol, aspirin, imipenem–cilastatin, isoniazid, penicillin, rifampin, ticarcillin–clavulanate, trimethoprim–sulfamethoxazole, chlorambucil, and vancomycin.[146-148]

MANAGEMENT

Discontinuation of the suspected causative agent is the primary treatment, as drug-induced fever is unlikely to remit otherwise (**Table 54-5**). The fever generally resolves within 72 hours of discontinuation of the offending drug, and no other treatment may be necessary. Rarely, 4–5 days may be required for resolution of fever if drug or metabolite elimination is prolonged. For patients receiving therapy with multiple medications and for whom the fever-inducing drug is not known, it is advisable to discontinue all non-life-sustaining medications, particularly those of higher suspicion, including all antimicrobial drugs, if possible. Medications may be reintroduced cautiously, one at a time, if necessary after fever abatement. Corticosteroids may be used to help prevent or treat fever and other manifestations of drug fever if continuation or reintroduction of a particular potential culprit drug is necessary. Corticosteroids are also indicated in patients with severe systemic manifestations of drug fever, including vital organ involvement. Corticosteroids should be used judiciously, particularly in patients with concomitant infection or increased risk of infection or in those with pre-existing immunosuppression from disease or other drug therapy. Antipyretics should be avoided to facilitate monitoring of the patient's response to discontinuation of suspected sensitizing medications and should be reserved for use as a comfort measure, if necessary.

The risks and benefits of rechallenge should be weighed prior to reintroduction of the suspected agent. Although patients have been rechallenged with relatively few serious sequelae, there is a potential for the occurrence of a faster onset, more severe drug fever reaction upon rechallenge.[16]

Following discontinuation of the suspected culprit drug or drugs, patients with presumed drug fever should be monitored for resolution of signs and symptoms, most importantly fever. Resolution should occur within 72 hours (**Table 54-6**). Patients should also be monitored for signs and symptoms of infection just in case the diagnosis of drug fever was incorrect or in case concomitant infection is present.

Table 54-5 Management of Drug Fever and Serum Sickness-Like Reaction

- Discontinue suspected agent
- Discontinue all non-life-sustaining therapies
- Antihistamines may be considered for rash-associated pruritus
- Corticosteroids for treatment of severe systemic signs and symptoms

Table 54-6 Monitoring Parameters for Patients in Whom Drug Fever or Serum Sickness-Like Reaction Develops

- Blood urea nitrogen and serum creatinine concentrations
- Coagulation profile
- Heart rate
- Liver function tests (aspartate aminotransferase, alanine aminotransferase) and alkaline phosphatase
- Platelet count
- Pulse oximetry
- Respiratory rate
- Serum electrolyte concentrations
- Temperature
- White cell count with differential

INFORMATION FOR PATIENTS

General education of patients receiving a new prescription for a medication that may cause drug fever is imperative. This is particularly important for those receiving prescriptions for antibiotics, anticonvulsants, and other drugs associated with a higher incidence of drug fever. Patients should be counseled regarding the approximate time of onset and signs and symptoms to watch for and should be instructed about when to seek medical attention. Onset of fever within hours of initiating drug therapy, particularly with a drug to which the patient has been previously exposed, requires medical evaluation. A fever that is not associated with other symptoms of infection, and one that is temporally related to the initiation of drug therapy, should prompt the patient to contact a healthcare professional. Clinicians should instruct patients to be aware of a fever and the corresponding time interval expected for each drug class. Patients receiving antibiotics, central nervous system agents, or cardiac drugs should report a fever that presents within 7–10 days, 3 weeks, or 4–6 weeks, respectively, after initiation of therapy. Finally, patients with a history of safe antibiotic use or a prior experience with drug fever should be instructed to keep this information in their health records and to provide this information to prescribers and other healthcare professionals.

HYPERTHERMIA DUE TO SERUM SICKNESS-LIKE REACTION

Serum sickness occurs after the administration of heterologous antitoxin serum. When the syndrome is associated with any other antigenic source, it is known as a serum sickness-like reaction (SSLR).[149,150] Drugs are the most common cause of SSLR. Although antibiotics are commonly implicated, SSLR has been reported in association with a wide variety of medications. SSLR may be a form of drug fever, may accompany drug fever, or may be an extension of drug fever.

CAUSATIVE AGENTS

When SSLR was first described, the primary drugs implicated were those containing antigenic (foreign) material such as antitoxins, vaccines, antivenom, and murine monoclonal antibodies.[151-165] The advent of recombinant human-derived biologic agents has minimized cases of antigenic SSLR. Most recent reports of SSLR have been described in association with antibiotics, classically cefaclor. Rare cases of humanized monoclonal antibody-mediated SSLR have been reported. Drugs that have been reported to induce SSLR are listed in **Table 54-7**.[166-233]

EPIDEMIOLOGY

It is difficult to determine the incidence of SSLR, and most available information is related to antibiotic-associated SSLR. It has been estimated that SSLR occurs in approximately 0.2% of drug courses and in 0.5% of pediatric patients receiving multiple courses of antibiotics.[170] Serum sickness accounts for up to 68% of drug-induced reactions reported in association with cefaclor.[189] One review of antibiotic use found five cases of SSLR in 3,553 courses of cefaclor; five cases in 5,597 courses of amoxicillin; one case in 13,487 courses of trimethoprim–sulfamethoxazole; and one case in 2,325 courses of penicillin.[171] The relative risk of SSLR associated with antibiotic therapy was 65.1. The risk of SSLR associated with cefaclor was 14.8 relative to amoxicillin.

MECHANISMS

Like drug fever, SSLR is probably a type III hypersensitivity reaction, although there may also be a complement independent mechanism whereby the fragment crystallizable (Fc) region of an antibody reacts directly with the gamma receptors of leucocytes.[234-236] The parent drug, reactive metabolites, or a combination of the drug and endogenous proteins may form soluble immune complexes or antigens. These circulating soluble immune complexes deposit in tissues, most commonly joints, and activate an inflammatory response causing the release of mediators such as histamine, serotonin, complement, and platelet-activating factor. This leads

Table 54-7 Agents Implicated in Drug-Induced Serum Sickness-Like Reaction

Drug	Incidence	Level of Evidence[a]
6-mercaptopurine[166]	NK	C
Adalimumab[230]	NK	C
Alemtuzumab[231]	NK	C
Amoxicillin[167-172]	0.089%	B
Antithymocyte globulin (equine or murine)[155]	NK	C
Bupropion[173-177]	NK	C
Carbamazepine[178]	NK	C
Cefaclor[170,179-189]	0.141%	B
Cefazolin[190]	NK	C
Cefprozil[191]	NK	C
Ceftriaxone[192]	NK	C
Cefuroxime[192,193]	NK	C
Cephalexin[169]	NK	C
Ciprofloxacin[194,195]	NK	C
Clopidogrel[196,197]	NK	C
Fluoxetine[198-201]	NK	C
Griseofulvin[202]	NK	C
Infliximab[159,160,203]	NK	C
Insulin[232]	NK	C
Iron dextran[204]	NK	C
Itraconazole[205]	NK	C
Meropenem[206]	NK	C
Metronidazole[207]	NK	C
Minocycline[208-212]	NK	C
N-acetylcysteine[213]	NK	C
Natalizumab[214]	NK	C
Omalizumab[233]	NK	C
Penicillin[170,171,215]	0.043%	B
Propranolol[216]	NK	C
Rifampin[217]	NK	C
Rituximab[156-158,218-224]	NK	C
Streptokinase[225-228]	NK	C
Sulfonamides with trimethoprim[169,171]	0.007%	B
Ticlopidine[229]	NK	C

NK = not known.

[a]Definitions for Levels of Evidence: Level A—evidence from one or more randomized, controlled clinical trials; Level B—evidence from nonrandomized clinical trials, prospective observational studies, cohort studies, retrospective studies, case-control studies, meta-analyses and/or postmarketing surveillance studies; and Level C—evidence from one or more published case reports or case series.

to tissue injury and the clinical manifestations of serum sickness.

CLINICAL PRESENTATION AND DIFFERENTIAL DIAGNOSIS

The onset of SSLR after primary exposure to a causative drug is usually 6–21 days but may be as long as 4–6 weeks.[198,209,237] The onset following secondary exposure is much shorter, usually 1–4 days.[200,201] The reaction may occur even after discontinuation of a causative agent, and diagnosis can be considerably more difficult in this situation.[173,198] Fever, malaise, and lymphadenopathy are the cardinal symptoms of SSLR (**Table 54-8**). Patients may also experience arthralgias, particularly in the major joints, and myalgias, commonly in the hands and feet. Urticaria and morbilliform or purpuric rashes are common.[179,212,228,238] Edema may occur, usually in the hands and feet or the face and neck, and patients may experience headache or blurred vision. Laboratory abnormalities may include leukocytosis with or without a left shift, increases in aspartate aminotransferase, alanine aminotransferase, lactate dehydrogenase, alkaline phosphatase,

Table 54-8 Signs and Symptoms Associated with Drug-Induced Serum Sickness-Like Reaction

- Arthralgias
- Edema
- Fever
- Increased C-reactive protein
- Increased erythrocyte sedimentation rate
- Increased liver transaminases (aspartate aminotransferase, alanine aminotransferase), lactate dehydrogenase, and alkaline phosphatase
- Increased serum creatinine
- Leukocytosis
- Lymphadenopathy
- Malaise
- Morbilliform or purpuric rash
- Myalgias
- Urticaria

Table 54-9 Conditions to Consider in the Differential Diagnosis of Drug-Induced Serum Sickness-Like Reaction

- DRESS
- Drug withdrawal (alcohol, benzodiazepines, levodopa)
- Endocrine disorders
- Heat stroke
- Hematologic or solid organ malignancy
- Infection
- Reactive or systemic juvenile idiopathic arthritis
- Systemic lupus erythematosus

DRESS = drug reaction with eosinophilia and systemic symptoms.

serum creatinine, erythrocyte sedimentation rate, and C-reactive protein, although these are inconsistent findings. Proper diagnosis requires careful questioning of patients with the suggestive signs and symptoms. Other conditions to consider in the differential diagnosis include febrile illness, reactive or systemic juvenile idiopathic arthritis, systemic lupus erythematosus, or drug-induced hyperthermic conditions (**Table 54-9**). In general, the presence of fever, arthralgias, and lymphadenopathy, although not always present, are useful clues to the diagnosis of drug-induced SSLR.

RISK FACTORS

Risk factors for the development of SSLR in children prescribed amoxicillin or cefaclor include younger age (<5 years), longer course of antibiotic therapy, and multiple courses of antibiotics.[171] Risk factors in adults for SSLR due to drugs other than antibiotics have not been identified although some reports suggest a greater likelihood of developing SSLR with higher dosages of antitoxins or antivenoms, intermittent heterologous protein exposure (versus continuous exposure), and concomitant hypergammaglobulinemia with monoclonal antibody administration.[165,221,239]

MORBIDITY AND MORTALITY

In general, the course and outcome of drug-induced SSLR are benign. Hospitalization may be required for patients with significant arthralgic involvement due to disability and for supportive therapy.

PREVENTION

An initial event of drug-induced SSLR is unlikely to be effectively prevented. Judicious antibiotic use, particularly in children, is recommended. The use of cefaclor is associated with a higher incidence of occurrence as compared with that due to other antibiotics; however, this is not reason enough to avoid the use of this agent.

For secondary prevention of SSLR, the offending agent should not be administered again. Another drug from the same pharmacologic class may be initiated, with close monitoring and thorough patient education. There are no data demonstrating a risk of cross-reactivity, and there are cases reported in which another drug from the same class was used without sequelae.[179,240] Fluoxetine, as well as rituximab, desensitization has been implemented successfully in patients with a previous SSLR reaction.[201,241]

MANAGEMENT

Discontinuation of the causative drug is the primary treatment (Table 54-5), and typically signs and symptoms of SSLR will begin to abate within 72 hours.[198] In general, drug-induced SSLR resolves 4–14 days after the discontinuation of therapy, although it may take up to 1 month to completely resolve.[212] Medical management may include antihistamines for urticaria and pruritus and in more severe or worsening cases corticosteroids.[174] Steroids have proven very successful in rapidly reversing symptoms, including rash, joint pain, and facial swelling or edema. Corticosteroids may be administered intravenously or orally in a fixed or tapering regimen over 5–14 days.[174,176,179,187,188,194-196,198,204,205,209,217,218,225] In rare cases, in which discontinuation of the offending agent is not possible, plasmapheresis is an option.[232] Monitoring parameters in patients with SSLR include those listed in Table 54-6, in addition to resolution of rash, pruritus, and arthralgias.

INFORMATION FOR PATIENTS

Patient education is similar for drug fever and drug-induced SSLR. Patients should be aware of the potential for drug-induced SSLR, the approximate onset, signs and symptoms, and when to seek additional medical intervention. Worsening fever, lymphadenopathy, and any joint pain or rash should prompt patients to contact a healthcare professional for further instructions. Patients with a previous history of SSLR should keep this information in their health records and provide this information to prescribers and other healthcare professionals to avoid re-exposure.

HYPERTHERMIA DUE TO NEUROLEPTIC MALIGNANT SYNDROME

First described in 1960, NMS is a serious, idiosyncratic reaction to certain medications, primarily neuroleptics, that results in a relative dopamine depletion causing muscle rigidity, hyperthermia, autonomic instability, and altered mental status.[242] Although NMS is an uncommon disorder, the sequelae may be serious, particularly if the condition is unrecognized and left untreated.

CAUSATIVE AGENTS

Hundreds of cases of NMS have been reported in the literature, most secondary to neuroleptic agents, particularly haloperidol.[243-246] Other agents that inhibit dopamine have been implicated, including prochlorperazine, metoclopramide, lithium, and anticonvulsants.[246-265] Drugs that have been associated with NMS are listed in **Table 54-10.**[243-326] The older, higher-potency antipsychotic agents such as haloperidol and fluphenazine are more likely to induce NMS than the newer, atypical agents such as risperidone and olanzapine, although this may be because there is more experience with and exposure to the older drugs.

Table 54-10 Agents Implicated in Drug-Induced Neuroleptic Malignant Syndrome[197]

Drug	Incidence	Level of Evidence[a]
Amoxapine[261,266]	NK	C
Aripiprazole[267-273]	NK	C
Carbamazepine[262-264]	NK	C
Chlorpromazine[247,254,255]	NK	C
Clozapine[264,274,277-283]	NK	C
Donepezil[284]	NK	C
Droperidol[247,248,285-288]	NK	C
Fluphenazine[289,290]	NK	C
Haloperidol[243-246]	NK	C
Iloperidone[327]	NK	C
Lamotrigine[328]	NK	C
Lithium[246,253-261,271,291]	NK	C
Lorazepam[292]	NK	C
Loxapine[274,293]	NK	C
Metoclopramide[248-252]	NK	C
Molindone[246,294,295]	NK	C
Olanzapine[257,296-308]	NK	C
Paliperidone[309,329]	NK	C
Perphenazine[310-312]	NK	C
Phenelzine[244,253]	NK	C
Phenytoin[265]	NK	C
Prochlorperazine[247]	NK	C
Promethazine[266,289,313]	NK	C
Quetiapine[307,314-317]	NK	C
Risperidone[259,261,283,307,318,319]	NK	C
Thioridazine[260,294,320]	NK	C
Thiothixene[321,322]	NK	C
Trifluoperazine[294,318,322-325]	NK	C
Valproic acid[330]	NK	C
Ziprasidone[291,326]	NK	C

NK = not known.

[a]Definitions for Levels of Evidence: Level A—evidence from one or more randomized, controlled clinical trials; Level B—evidence from nonrandomized clinical trials, prospective observational studies, cohort studies, retrospective studies, case-control studies, meta-analyses and/or postmarketing surveillance studies; and Level C—evidence from one or more published case reports or case series.

EPIDEMIOLOGY

The reported incidence of NMS ranges from 0.02 to 3.23% in patients treated with neuroleptics.[336-343] The true incidence may be higher because of a lack of recognition and underreporting. Retrospective analysis reports the incidence of NMS can be as high as 12%.[344,345] The reported number of NMS cases is decreasing, perhaps because of the availability of newer, lower-potency antipsychotics.[346] NMS occurs approximately twice as commonly in men than in women and has been reported to occur more frequently in young and middle-aged adults, with an average age at occurrence of 40 years, although conflicting evidence exists.[341,343] It should be noted that the apparent higher occurrence in younger male patients may be secondary to a higher incidence of schizophrenia in this population and subsequent higher use of neuroleptics.[347] Patients with pre-existing psychomotor agitation and mental retardation are significantly more likely to develop NMS.[348,349]

MECHANISMS

NMS is a dose-related idiosyncratic reaction that is a result of a relative depletion of dopamine in the central nervous system. NMS may also involve the serotonergic and cholinergic systems. Inhibition of dopaminergic systems in the central nervous system, namely the anterior hypothalamus, and metabolic changes in peripheral skeletal muscle lead to a sustained muscle contraction, resultant heat production, and inappropriate vasoconstriction, decreasing heat dissipation and leading to hyperthermia. This occurs as a result of drug-induced antagonism of dopamine receptors or transmission blockade but has also been reported after changing antipsychotic medications or with the addition of new medications to a neuroleptic regimen that alter additional neurotransmitters such as serotonin. Typical antipsychotics have a greater specificity to antagonize D_2 dopamine receptors, whereas atypical antipsychotics are believed to be more selective toward D_3 and D_4. One proposed mechanism for the decreased incidence of NMS with atypical agents is their ability to also inhibit 5-hydroxytryptamine receptor 2A.[347] Abrupt discontinuation of anti-Parkinsonian agents such as dopamine precursors carbidopa–levodopa and dopamine agonists amantadine, ropinirole, pramipexole, or bromocriptine can produce a subtype of NMS known as Parkinsonism hyperpyrexia syndrome. In these cases, NMS resolves after reinitiation of therapy with these drugs.[255,350-355]

CLINICAL PRESENTATION AND DIFFERENTIAL DIAGNOSIS

NMS usually occurs within hours to months after the initiation of neuroleptic therapy or following a dose increase but may take up to a year or longer to manifest. In most cases, NMS develops within the first 4 weeks of therapy with the offending agent. Classic signs and symptoms of NMS (**Table 54-11**) develop progressively over 1–3 days and include hyperthermia, severe muscle rigidity (described as lead-pipe

Table 54-11 Signs and Symptoms Associated with Drug-Induced Neuroleptic Malignant Syndrome

- Autonomic dysfunction
  - Hypertension or fluctuating blood pressure
  - Hyperthermia
  - Tachycardia
  - Tachypnea
- Diaphoresis
- Electrolyte abnormalities
  - Hypocalcemia
  - Hypokalemia
  - Hypomagnesemia
- Increased serum creatine kinase
- Leukocytosis with or without a left shift
- Mental status changes
  - Coma
  - Delirium
  - Obtundation
  - Stupor
- Metabolic acidosis
- Muscle rigidity[a] (lead-pipe rigidity)
- Rhabdomyolysis and myoglobinuria

[a]This classic sign may not always be observed in patients with neuroleptic malignant syndrome caused by atypical antipsychotics.

rigidity), autonomic dysfunction (tachycardia, tachypnea, hypertension or fluctuating blood pressure, diaphoresis), and mental status changes (delirium, stupor, obtundation, coma). There tends to be a particular pattern to the onset of the signs of NMS, which may help in early diagnosis and recognition. In more than 80% of cases, mental status changes and rigidity (or serum creatine kinase [CK] elevations) can be expected to precede autonomic dysfunction and hyperthermia.[351] Other signs that may be observed include increased CK concentrations, leukocytosis with or without a left shift, and electrolyte abnormalities (hypocalcemia, hypokalemia, hypomagnesemia). Increased CK concentrations have been found in over 95% of reported cases and may be demonstrated in patients without the classic muscle rigidity.[322,336,356] Elevated CK may also be a function of repeated intramuscular injections to control agitation as well as combativeness against physical restraints. Rhabdomyolysis and resultant myoglobinuria may develop and, without intervention, may progress to renal failure and metabolic acidosis. Temperature elevation may follow other signs and symptoms, and the absence of hyperthermia should not preclude the consideration of NMS. Temperatures of over 38°C are seen in 87% of patients. Temperatures in excess of 40°C occur with a prevalence of 40%.[357] NMS is often confused with heat stroke because both may cause mental status changes and because neuroleptics are a risk factor for both conditions. In contrast to those with NMS, patients with heat stroke present with hot, dry skin, hypotension, and limb flaccidity. Temperature elevation may not be as pronounced in association with the atypical antipsychotics, particularly risperidone and paliperidone.[309,319,358,359] In addition, NMS induced by atypical antipsychotics may be associated with a longer time to onset and the absence of muscle rigidity.[307,360,361] The presence of CK elevations in these patients may be particularly useful in the diagnosis.[360] The clinical presentation in children differs slightly from adults in that children may exhibit more dystonia and less tremor.[369]

Because NMS has various manifestations, differential diagnosis must include many neurologic, psychiatric, systemic, and drug-induced disorders. Catatonia may be an early sign of NMS and may be confused with the underlying illness, leading the clinician to increase the dose of the neuroleptic, which may worsen the condition. Patients with preexisting catatonia may be at increased risk for NMS, but there is some speculation that NMS and catatonia are part of the same neurochemical syndrome or that NMS is an exacerbation of catatonia.[362-366] Catatonia is usually treated with neuroleptics, and therefore NMS may be more likely to develop because of continued treatment, rapid dose escalation, or higher usage of parenteral neuroleptics. The initial presentation may be helpful for differentiating catatonia from NMS: lethal catatonia often begins with extreme psychotic excitement, often over weeks, with more dystonic movements whereas NMS usually begins with muscle rigidity, although there are exceptions. It should be recognized that there is a relationship between the two syndromes, and in patients with catatonia or NMS with catatonic signs or symptoms, consideration should be given to alternative therapy, such as benzodiazepines or electroconvulsive therapy (ECT).

Abrupt withdrawal of certain medications has been described to produce a NMS-like syndrome. As mentioned previously, cessation of dopaminergic agents can produce the Parkinsonism hyperpyrexia syndrome. Reinstitution of therapy is usually sufficient to alleviate symptoms.[355] Another NMS-like picture occurs in patients who abruptly discontinue therapy with baclofen.[331-335] In the majority of these cases, patients were receiving baclofen intrathecally.[331-333] Patients who have used cocaine may also present with symptoms similar to NMS, including agitation, delirium, and hyperthermia, but often without rigidity. It has been theorized that cocaine enhances dopamine reuptake, such that decreasing serum cocaine levels produces a relative decrease in dopamine transmission.[355]

Serotonin syndrome, anticholinergic delirium, sympathomimetic overdose, pheochromocytoma, thyrotoxicosis, status epilepticus, and lithium toxicity are other disorders with signs and symptoms that overlap with NMS (**Table 54-12**). In one review of 28 patients who met criteria for NMS, 22 also met diagnostic criteria for serotonin syndrome.[311] Another review compared signs and symptoms of

Table 54-12 Conditions to Consider in the Differential Diagnosis of Drug-Induced Neuroleptic Malignant Syndrome

- Status epilepticus
- Anticholinergic toxicity
- Drug withdrawal (alcohol, benzodiazepines, baclofen)
- Endocrine disorders
- Heat stroke
- Hematologic or solid organ malignancy
- Infection
- Lithium toxicity
- Parkinsonism hyperpyrexia syndrome
- Pheochromocytoma
- Sepsis
- Serotonin syndrome
- Thyrotoxicosis

Table 54-13 Risk Factors for Drug-Induced Neuroleptic Malignant Syndrome

Drug-related

- Cotreatment with lithium
- Faster dose escalation
- Higher dose
- Intramuscular route
- Multiple dopamine antagonists

Patient-related

- Alzheimer disease
- Bipolar disease
- Catatonia
- Dehydration
- Exhaustion
- Family history
- Mental retardation
- Psychomotor agitation

NMS induced by olanzapine with the 10 "classical" signs and symptoms of serotonin syndrome. Three or more signs and symptoms of serotonin syndrome were identified in 11 of the 17 patients, indicating considerable overlap between these drug-induced diseases.[367,368]

Despite the creation of rating scales and scoring criteria, there are no universally accepted diagnostic criteria for NMS.[347,370,371] Although it is hypothesized that serum analysis of dopamine and serotonin metabolites can aid in differential diagnosis, other reports cite no clear relationship between NMS and serum antipsychotic levels.[372,373] NMS remains a diagnosis of exclusion. Identification of the causative agent aids in the differential diagnosis. Correct diagnosis is essential, as chlorpromazine, a common treatment option for serotonin syndrome, may worsen signs and symptoms in a patient with NMS.

RISK FACTORS

In a case-control study, higher neuroleptic dose, faster dose escalation, more intramuscular neuroleptic injections, and a greater degree of psychomotor agitation were found to be risk factors for NMS (**Table 54-13**).[374] The incidence of NMS in patients with a high degree of psychomotor agitation may be over-reported due to increased likelihood of higher neuroleptic doses, rapid titration, and frequent intramuscular injections. Other reported risk factors for the development of NMS include use of multiple medications that reduce dopamine transmission, dehydration, concomitant infection, lithium use, exhaustion, pre-existing brain disorder (bipolar disease, delirium tremens, postoperative delirium, Alzheimer disease, and mental retardation), and catatonia, although many patients treated with neuroleptics may possess some of these factors.[338-340,347-350,355,362-364,375-379] In addition, there has been one report of NMS in a patient with bilateral subdural hematoma who had been stable on a neuroleptic agent for 10 years.[262] It is clear that the use of drugs with higher potency, at higher doses, administration via the parenteral route, and history of a prior episode increase the risk for the development of NMS.[249,336,337,341,346,362,374,380,381] There have been reports of NMS cases within families, indicating a possible genetic link, although this link has not been established conclusively. Overexpression of a specific dopamine D_2 receptor gene allele is believed to be related to decreased dopamine receptor function and dopaminergic activity. Involvement of the D_2 receptor may also explain why atypical antipsychotics appear to have a lower propensity to cause NMS.[382-385]

MORBIDITY AND MORTALITY

If left untreated or mistreated because of misdiagnosis, NMS can result in very serious sequelae, including permanent disability, coma, and death.[386,387] Mortality has been reported to occur in 4–20% of patients as a consequence of NMS and results from progression of the clinical syndrome.[248,336-338,388] The resultant acute renal failure due to ischemia and rhabdomyolysis, respiratory failure, metabolic acidosis, and electrolyte imbalances may be irreversible and fatal. Venous thromboembolism (VTE) is a major risk for patients with NMS. Although the exact incidence is not known, patients are at higher risk for VTE due to a multitude of factors including immobility, hypovolemia, and increased activation of coagulation factors. Pulmonary embolism is the cause of death in 23% of patients.[389] The rate of mortality has declined over time because of prompt recognition, discontinuation of the offending agent, supportive care, and drug therapy management and is now estimated to be about 10%.[255,339,378] Patients with organic brain disease have a mortality as high as 38.5%. Multiple case reports suggest persistent neurologic functional declines following NMS in patients with underlying traumatic brain injury.[390] There is suggestion of reduced mortality with use of atypical compared to typical antipsychotics.[369,412]

PREVENTION

Because NMS is an idiosyncratic reaction, avoidance is difficult. Recommendations for prevention are listed in **Table 54-14**. The lowest possible dose of neuroleptic drugs should be used to control patient behavior. Patients who are receiving high doses of parenteral neuroleptics or who are having the dose adjusted upward should be well hydrated and monitored for signs and symptoms. Patients with a history of NMS should optimally be treated with an alternative agent, such as a newer, atypical antipsychotic, a drug with lower potency, or a lower dose of the same agent, and treatment should not be initiated or reinitiated until at least 2 weeks after signs and symptoms have resolved.[391-393]

Table 54-14 Approaches to Help Prevent Drug-Induced Neuroleptic Malignant Syndrome

- Avoid lithium cotreatment
- Ensure adequate hydration for patients undergoing active dose escalation
- Rechallenge no sooner than 2 weeks after signs and symptoms have resolved
- Titrate dose slowly
- Use atypical neuroleptics
- Use lowest dose of neuroleptic possible

Overall rates of NMS recurrence are 30–50% following reintroduction of dopamine antagonists.[355] One study reported the experience with rechallenge in 15 patients with a prior NMS episode.[391] Ten patients were successfully rechallenged initially; four of five patients who were unsuccessfully rechallenged underwent a second rechallenge, which was successful in two cases. One of the patients who had a failure was rechallenged a third time, and on that occasion therapy with the neuroleptic drug was successfully initiated and maintained. Overall, neuroleptic agents were tolerated in 13 of the 15 patients with a prior history of NMS. The time from the resolution of signs and symptoms to the rechallenge attempt correlated significantly with success. Twelve of 13 rechallenges were successful if the rechallenge was attempted more than 2 weeks after the signs and symptoms of NMS had resolved, whereas six of seven that were attempted in less than 2 weeks were unsuccessful.[391] Similar results have been reported in other cases of attempted rechallenge.[392,393] Neither the specific neuroleptic agent used nor the dose was found to be a significant factor related to successful rechallenge; however, most rechallenges were attempted with lower-potency agents or lower doses of the same drug.[391] Others have noted that the use of lower-potency agents improves the success of rechallenge as well: 47% and 83% of patients had a relapse when given a drug of equal potency, but only 15% and 10% had a relapse when a lower-potency agent was used.[340,394] Administration of an atypical neuroleptic (clozapine) was used successfully in a patient with three prior episodes of NMS associated with haloperidol, lithium, and molindone.[247] There are other reports of successful atypical antipsychotic rechallenge in 16 of 20 patients who had NMS with atypical antipsychotics.[360,395] Eleven of the patients were successfully rechallenged with the same agent without recurrence of symptoms.

In a patient with a history of NMS, adequate hydration should be maintained, the lowest possible dose of neuroleptic should be used, and the dose should be titrated upward slowly. The use of the parenteral route, particularly depot intramuscular injections, should be avoided. Avoidance of concurrent lithium use may also reduce reoccurrence.[355] Electroconvulsive therapy, as opposed to drugs, should be considered in patients requiring management of an acute psychotic episode and a recent NMS diagnosis (especially of less than 2 weeks).

MANAGEMENT

Strategies for NMS management are presented in **Table 54-15**. In some cases, NMS is a self-limiting disease with signs and symptoms resolving as soon as 7–10 days after the causative drug is discontinued. Therapy should be initiated when rigidity, mental status, and autonomic changes are apparent and the temperature is ≥38°C. However, treatment may be initiated if a presumptive diagnosis of NMS is made prior to the onset of hyperthermia in the presence of other progressing signs and symptoms. One review of published cases reported a mortality rate of 9.7% in patients who received drug therapy (dantrolene, bromocriptine, levodopa, amantadine) as compared with 21% in patients who did not receive any specific drug therapy intervention.[396] Use of dopamine agonists has also been shown to reverse symptoms faster than supportive care alone.[347]

All medications that cause dopamine-depleting or antagonistic effects should be discontinued, particularly any antipsychotic agents that have been initiated recently, or for which the dose has recently been increased. Supportive measures include fluid, electrolyte, and acid–base management. Rapid cooling measures, including cooled intravenous solutions, surface cooling, ice bath, and ice water gastric lavage should be used for management of significant temperature elevation.[347]

Bromocriptine, amantadine, other dopamine agonists, and dantrolene have been used successfully in NMS management. Bromocriptine is considered the drug of initial choice. Doses of 2.5 mg 3 times daily, titrated to a maximum of 45 mg/day, should be administered orally for 10 days, although a longer duration of treatment may be required.[266,296,342,355,394-400] Treatment with bromocriptine should be continued until signs and symptoms resolve, after which the dose should be tapered gradually over 1 week.[347] Improvement in signs and symptoms is usually observed within 24–72 hours. Potential side effects of bromocriptine include the potential to worsen psychosis and cause significant hypotension and vomiting.[354]

Amantadine is a treatment alternative for NMS. The recommended dose is 100–200 mg orally twice daily and should be continued for 10 days after signs and symptoms are controlled, after which the dose should be tapered to avoid rebound NMS.[252,401-404]

Dantrolene has been used successfully to treat NMS symptoms by relieving muscle rigidity and heat generation via inhibition of calcium release from the endoplasmic reticulum.[261,405-411] Often patients are unable to take oral medications during NMS, necessitating use of the intravenous route. Dantrolene therapy is recommended if the temperature exceeds 40°C, rhabdomyolysis is suspected,

Table 54-15 Management of Drug-Induced Neuroleptic Malignant Syndrome

- Discontinue suspected agent
- Cooling measures and other supportive care
  - Cooled intravenous fluids
  - Fluid and electrolyte replacement as needed
  - Ice water nasogastric lavage or bath
  - Surface cooling
- Bromocriptine 2.5 mg orally 3 times daily up to 45 mg daily for up to 10 days after symptoms abate; then taper over 1 week
- Amantadine 100–200 mg orally 2 times daily for up to 10 days after symptoms abate; then taper
- Dantrolene 1–2.5 mg/kg intravenously 4 times daily until symptoms abate, then 1 mg/kg intravenously every 4–6 hours until able to take orally; oral dosage 1–2 mg/kg 4 times daily for 10 days; then taper
- Benzodiazepines
  - Lorazepam 2–4 mg intravenously or orally as needed for control of symptoms
  - Diazepam 5 mg intravenously or orally as needed for control of symptoms
- Electroconvulsive therapy

cardiorespiratory or renal failure is imminent, and administration of dopamine agonists has not been successful.[339] These patients have severe NMS and are at high risk of serious morbidity or death and require the most rigorous intervention.[375,412] Dantrolene should be administered at a dose of 1–2.5 mg/kg intravenously 4 times daily until signs and symptoms have been adequately controlled or a cumulative dose of 10 mg/kg is reached. [354,413] Maintenance therapy is 1 mg/kg infused every 4–6 hours to prevent reoccurrence. When the patient is able to take oral medications, dantrolene may be administered at a dose of 1–2 mg/kg every 6 hours orally for another 10 days, and then the dose may be tapered. Intravenous dantrolene is a highly alkaline solution and can cause significant phlebitis. Dantrolene therapy is also associated with hepatotoxicity and should be avoided in patients with liver disease.[354,355] Although combination therapy of a dopamine agonist (bromocriptine or amantadine) plus dantrolene has not shown any proven advantage, it may be considered in refractory or extremely severe cases, as this approach offers treatment with drugs with different mechanisms of action.[409-411,414,415]

Although they successfully control some of the signs and symptoms of NMS, anticholinergic agents are not recommended because they inhibit heat dissipation and may worsen hyperthermia.[338,379,414,415] Hyperthermia in NMS is not prostaglandin-mediated so there is no use for antipyretics such as NSAIDs, aspirin, or acetaminophen.[347] If symptoms are severe and unable to be controlled, requiring intubation or paralysis, the use of a nondepolarizing neuromuscular blocker is preferred over a depolarizing agent. Pancuronium with concomitant diazepam administration was reported to be effective for cessation of muscle rigidity in a patient with NMS in whom treatment with anticholinergics failed but who was not treated with dantrolene.[416] Carbidopa–levodopa may also be effective because of its dopamine agonist properties.[410,411,417] Intravenous diazepam may be used to manage involuntary movements, fever, tachycardia, hypertension, muscle rigidity, tremor, and diaphoresis associated with NMS.[418,419] Benzodiazepines may be useful as adjunct therapy for suspected catatonia and for treatment of agitation.[420-422] ECT may be considered for the treatment of NMS refractory to other therapies, although there are no prospective comparative studies.[423-430] One retrospective review of NMS cases demonstrated a mortality rate of 10.3% in patients who underwent ECT, as compared with 21% in patients who received no specific intervention, a difference that did not reach statistical significance.[396] ECT should be considered the therapy of choice in patients with suspected catatonia.

Resolution of mental status changes, muscle rigidity, serum CK concentrations, acid–base abnormalities, and myoglobinuria should be closely monitored. Progression of these signs and symptoms requires more aggressive management. Monitoring parameters for patients with NMS are listed in **Table 54-16**.

With appropriate care, symptoms should resolve within 6–10 days of treatment.[354] Signs and symptoms may persist longer and may be more difficult to manage in patients who have received intramuscular (depot) antipsychotic agents, sometimes necessitating continued treatment for 2–3 weeks, although one case of NMS secondary to long-acting risperidone injection resolved in 10 days.[355,375,385] A residual catatonic state has been described in several patients for 1–6 months after resolution of hyperthermic signs and symptoms.[387] Rigidity and mental status changes persisted in these patients for unknown reasons.

Table 54-16 Monitoring Parameters for Patients with Drug-Induced Neuroleptic Malignant Syndrome or Drug-Induced Serotonin Syndrome

- Coagulation profile
- Heart rate
- Mental status
- Muscle rigidity (NMS)
- Myoclonus (SS)
- Pulse oximetry
- Respiratory rate
- Serum creatinine and blood urea nitrogen concentrations
- Serum creatine kinase concentrations (NMS)
- Serum electrolyte concentrations
- Temperature
- Urine myoglobin concentrations
- White cell count with differential

NMS = neuroleptic malignant syndrome, SS = serotonin syndrome.

INFORMATION FOR PATIENTS

Patient education may be uniquely difficult in the patient population treated with neuroleptic agents. Despite the potential obstacles, patients and caregivers should be alerted to the signs and symptoms of NMS and instructed when to seek medical attention. Patients and caregivers should be instructed to call a healthcare professional or visit a healthcare facility in the event of sudden onset of muscle rigidity, tachycardia, tachypnea, diaphoresis, or mental status changes. It is particularly important to stress to patients that medications should not be discontinued if signs and symptoms develop and to seek medical attention to ensure that a proper diagnosis is achieved.

HYPERTHERMIA DUE TO SEROTONIN SYNDROME

Serotonin syndrome is a potentially serious and occasionally fatal complication of therapy with drugs that cause an increase in serotonergic activity. Serotonergic neurons are associated with behavioral, motor, and thermoregulation.[355] Fever is one common component of the syndrome. With the significant increase in the number of patients treated with selective serotonin (5-hydroxytryptamine [5-HT]) reuptake inhibitors (SSRIs) and nonselective (serotonin-norepinephrine) reuptake inhibitors (SNRIs), it may be expected that the prevalence of this drug-induced disease will continue to increase.

CAUSATIVE AGENTS

Any drug that causes a direct or indirect increase in the effective serotonin concentration in the central nervous system has the potential to induce serotonin syndrome. Drugs that have been reported to cause serotonin syndrome are listed in **Table 54-17**.[431-531] Included are cases in which drugs were used in combination and the specific causative agent could not be conclusively determined. In addition, paroxetine and fluoxetine are inhibitors of the cytochrome P-450 2D6 enzyme and may increase serum concentrations of serotonergic metabolites when used in combination with trazadone and nefazadone; the combination should be used cautiously. Selective and nonselective SSRIs have been implicated in numerous case reports of serotonin syndrome, as have selective and nonselective monoamine oxidase inhibitors (MAOIs) alone and in combination with opioids. Linezolid has nonselective MAOI properties and has been reported to precipitate serotonin syndrome when combined with a serotonergic agent but also when used with a synthetic opioid analgesic without the presence of an SSRI.[469]

EPIDEMIOLOGY

The incidence of serotonin syndrome is not known but may be as high as 14% in cases of SSRI overdose.[532] Serotonin syndrome has also been reported following ingestion of a single therapeutic dose.[486] However, the true incidence may be relatively low, considering the widespread use of medications, alone and in combination, known to disrupt serotonin balance. One retrospective review examined the use of SSRIs and linezolid, a weak inhibitor of MAO, and found that 3% of patients had a high likelihood of having experienced serotonin syndrome without definitive diagnosis.[466] In another retrospective review of the records of 262 hospitalized patients treated with meperidine, 10% were receiving concomitant SSRIs; serotonin syndrome did not develop in any of them.[533] The sample size in this report was small, and the SSRI doses were not discussed. Although there is an increased awareness of the triggering factors for serotonin syndrome, the disease is still not commonly considered in patients presenting with suspicious signs and symptoms. SSRIs are being prescribed with increased frequency; however, there is declining use of MAOIs, resulting in an unknown net effect on the true incidence of this drug-induced disease.

MECHANISMS

Mechanisms by which drugs cause serotonin syndrome are presented in **Table 54-18**. Excessive serotonergic activity in the peripheral and central nervous system is responsible for serotonin syndrome.[534] Fever in serotonin syndrome is due to a

Table 54-17 Agents Implicated in Drug-Induced Serotonin Syndrome

Drug	Incidence	Level of Evidence[a]
3,4-methylenedioxymethamphetamine (MDMA; ecstasy)[433-441,522]	NK	C
Dexamphetamine[432]	NK	C
L-tryptophan[431]	NK	C
Levodopa[442]	NK	C
MAO INHIBITORS		
Isocarbazid[443,444]	NK	C
Linezolid[457-469,524]	NK	C
Methylene blue[525-527]	NK	C
Moclobemide (reversible MAO inhibitor)[435,450-456,522]	NK	C
Rasagiline[523]	NK	C
Selegiline[445]	NK	C
Tranylcypromine[446-449]	NK	C
SNRIs		
Duloxetine[468,478]	NK	C
Milnacipran[528]	NK	C
Venlafaxine[432,446,447,450,462,467,495,500-510]	NK	C
SSRIs		
Citalopram[432,456,457,470-472]	NK	C
Escitalopram[479]	NK	C
Fluoxetine[461,465,470,471,480-483]	NK	C
Fluvoxamine[478,484-487]	NK	C
Paroxetine[386,458,487-491]	NK	C
Sertraline[443,459,460,477,493-499]	NK	C
Trazodone[444,462,494,500]	NK	C
Nefazadone[472,483,488]	NK	C
TCAs		
Amitriptyline[504,505]	NK	C
Clomipramine[448,511]	NK	C
Imipramine[445]	NK	C
Nortriptyline[449]	NK	C
Amantadine[499,512]	NK	C
Buprenorphine[515]	NK	C
Buspirone[513,524]	NK	C
Dextromethorphan[472,489,514]	NK	C
Fentanyl[477,516]	NK	C
Hypericum perforatum (St. John's Wort)[513,520,521]	NK	C
Lithium[502,509]	NK	C
Meperidine[474,481,504,516]	NK	C
Metaxalone[529]	NK	C
Oxycodone[478]	NK	C
Sibutramine[516,517]	NK	C
Tramadol[475,482,490,518,519]	NK	C
Ziprasidone[530,531]	NK	C
Metoclopramide + venlafaxine[495]	NK	C

MAO = monoamine oxidase, NK = not known, SNRI = serotonin norepinephrine reuptake inhibitor, SSRI = selective serotonin reuptake inhibitor, TCA = tricyclic antidepressant.
[a]Definitions for Levels of Evidence: Level A—evidence from one or more randomized, controlled clinical trials; Level B—evidence from nonrandomized clinical trials, prospective observational studies, cohort studies, retrospective studies, case-control studies, meta-analyses and/or postmarketing surveillance studies; and Level C—evidence from one or more published case reports or case series.

combination of neuromuscular effects combined with altered hypothalamic homeostasis.[355] Seven 5-HT receptor subtypes have been identified, and it is believed that 5-HT_{1A} and 5-HT_{2A} are involved specifically with the adverse sequelae encountered with serotonin syndrome.[535,536] Although controversy exists regarding which of these two receptors is most responsible for the syndrome, it is likely that both of these receptor subtypes, and possibly others, are involved in the clinical manifestations of serotonin syndrome. The syndrome generally occurs after initiating therapy with, or increasing the dose of, a drug with one or more of the following actions: (1) inhibition of serotonin metabolism; (2) potentiation of serotonin activity; (3) direct activation of serotonin receptors; (4) inhibition of serotonin uptake; and (5) increase of substrate supply. Substrate supply may be increased through supplementation with over-the-counter products or consumption of foods such as wine or cheese known to have high levels of the serotonin precursor tryptophan.[537] Serotonin syndrome has been associated with single-drug therapy; however, because it is a dose-dependent phenomenon,

Table 54-18 Mechanisms of Drug-Induced Serotonin Syndrome

Drug	Mechanism
3,4-methylenedioxy-methamphetamine (MDMA; ecstasy)	Increase 5-HT synthesis or release Inhibit 5-HT reuptake
Dexamphetamine	Increase 5-HT synthesis or release Inhibit 5-HT reuptake
L-tryptophan	Increase 5-HT synthesis or release
Levodopa	Increase 5-HT synthesis or release
MAO INHIBITORS	
Isocarboxazid	Increase 5-HT synthesis or release Inhibit 5-HT metabolism
Linezolid	Increase 5-HT synthesis or release
Methylene blue	Increase 5-HT synthesis or release Inhibit 5-HT metabolism
Moclobemide (reversible MAO inhibitor)	Increase 5-HT synthesis or release Inhibit 5-HT metabolism
Rasagiline	Inhibit 5-HT metabolism
Selegiline	Increase 5-HT synthesis or release Inhibit 5-HT metabolism
Tranylcypromine	Increase 5-HT synthesis or release Inhibit 5-HT metabolism
SNRIs	
Duloxetine	Inhibit 5-HT reuptake
Milnacipran	Inhibit 5-HT reuptake
Venlafaxine	Inhibit 5-HT reuptake
SSRIs	
Citalopram	Inhibit 5-HT reuptake
Escitalopram	Inhibit 5-HT reuptake
Fluoxetine	Inhibit 5-HT reuptake
Fluvoxamine	Inhibit 5-HT reuptake
Paroxetine	Inhibit 5-HT reuptake
Sertraline	Inhibit 5-HT reuptake
Trazadone	Inhibit 5-HT reuptake
Nefazadone	Inhibit 5-HT reuptake
TCAs	
Amitriptyline	Inhibit 5-HT reuptake
Clomipramine	Inhibit 5-HT reuptake
Imipramine	Inhibit 5-HT reuptake
Nortriptyline	Inhibit 5-HT reuptake
Amantadine	Increase 5-HT synthesis or release
Buprenorphine	Mechanism unknown
Buspirone	Postsynaptic receptor stimulation
Dextromethorphan	Inhibit 5-HT reuptake
Fentanyl	Inhibit 5-HT reuptake and/or other unknown
Hypericum perforatum (St. John's Wort)	Inhibit 5-HT reuptake Inhibit 5-HT metabolism
Lithium	Postsynaptic receptor stimulation
Meperidine	Inhibit 5-HT reuptake and/or other unknown
Metaxalone	Increase 5-HT synthesis or release
Oxycodone	Inhibit 5-HT reuptake and/or other unknown
Sibutramine	Inhibit 5-HT reuptake and/or other unknown
Tramadol	Inhibit 5-HT reuptake and/or other unknown
Ziprasidone	Increase 5-HT synthesis or release Inhibit 5-HT metabolism
Metoclopramide + venlafaxine	Inhibit 5-HT reuptake

5-HT = 5-hydroxytryptamine, MAO = monoamine oxidase, SNRI = serotonin norepinephrine reuptake inhibitor, SSRI = selective serotonin reuptake inhibitor, TCA = tricyclic antidepressant.

combinations of drugs in particular are associated with the development of the syndrome. Both a combination of drugs that have a similar effect on serotonin as well as pharmacokinetic drug interactions, resulting in an increase at the serotonin receptor, can lead to excessive serotonergic effects.[472,491] There is much debate as to the potential for the antimigraine "triptan" class of drugs to trigger serotonin syndrome given their ability to act as 5-HT_{1B} and 5-HT_{1D} agonists.[538,539] Serotonin syndrome may also be precipitated by the addition of other drugs that inhibit cytochrome P450 2D6 or 3A4, such as ritonavir, leading to an increased drug concentration in an otherwise stable regimen. In one case, serotonin syndrome occurred in a patient taking a maintenance dose of sertraline after the addition of erythromycin.[493,534] Some drugs inhibit the metabolism of SSRIs while some SSRIs inhibit cytochrome P450 2D6, which metabolizes other drugs with serotonergic effects such as dextromethorphan. In general, opioid analgesics are thought to inhibit the reuptake of serotonin, thereby increasing the risk of serotonin syndrome when combined with agents that have serotonergic activity. There may be other mechanisms involved, however, as serotonin syndrome has been reported with oxycodone and buprenorphine, which do not inhibit the reuptake of serotonin.[477,515] Other neurotransmitters such as *N*-methyl-d-aspartate antagonists or GABA may play a role.[537]

CLINICAL PRESENTATION AND DIFFERENTIAL DIAGNOSIS

The onset of the signs and symptoms of serotonin syndrome may be almost immediate, with approximately 60% of cases presenting within 6 hours after the offending agent has been initiated, the dose increased, or the serum concentration increased by a drug–drug interaction. Serotonin syndrome manifests as a succession of signs and symptoms that progress rapidly over the course of hours and may be highly variable, making identification and diagnosis difficult. Serotonin syndrome is most appropriately thought of as a spectrum of diseases and has been classified into severity categories to aid in earlier or more accurate diagnosis.[535,540,541] Some of the signs and symptoms associated with milder forms of serotonin syndrome (tremor, confusion, incoordination) may be difficult to distinguish from the underlying illness.[535] The more severe symptoms of serotonin toxicity (temperature >38.5°C, myoclonus, diarrhea) are generally observed in overdose situations or when an MAOI or a serotonin-releasing agent is used in combination with an SSRI.[535,542]

Signs and symptoms of serotonin syndrome are listed in **Table 54-19** and may be divided into three categories for patient assessment: autonomic dysfunction (fever, shivering, diaphoresis, diarrhea, tachycardia, labile blood pressure); neuromuscular hyperactivity (clonus, myoclonus, hyper-reflexia, incoordination, tremor); and mental status changes (confusion, agitation, mania possibly progressing to hallucinations, obtundation, coma). Autonomic dysfunction and mental status changes appear in 40% of patients. One half of patients show evidence of neuromuscular hyperactivity.[537,543]

Table 54-19 Signs and Symptoms Associated with Serotonin Syndrome

- Autonomic dysfunction
  - Diaphoresis
  - Diarrhea
  - Hyperthermia
  - Labile blood pressure
  - Shivering
  - Tachycardia
- Electrolyte abnormalities
  - Hypocalcemia
  - Hypomagnesemia
  - Hyponatremia
- Elevated aspartate aminotransferase and alanine aminotransferase
- Elevated creatine kinase
- Leukocytosis
- Mental status changes
  - Agitation
  - Coma
  - Confusion
  - Mania
  - Obtundation
- Neuromuscular hyperactivity
  - Clonus
  - Hyper-reflexia (greater in lower extremities)
  - Incoordination
  - Myoclonus
  - Tremor
- Rhabdomyolysis and myoglobinuria

Sternbach's original criteria for diagnosis of serotonin syndrome are the presence of at least three symptoms temporally related to a suspect medication; other causes have been ruled out; and a neuroleptic agent has not been started or dose increased prior to the onset of signs and symptoms (indicating possible NMS).[535] Problems with the Sternbach criteria may exist and include the weight of mental status changes in the criteria, causing patients with abnormal mental states to be misdiagnosed and a diagnosis of serotonin syndrome to be missed in patients with mild serotonin toxicity. Others have determined that serotonin syndrome may be misdiagnosed in patients with infection using Sternbach's criteria.[466] Because of this lack of sensitivity, diagnostic decision rules have been developed based on the evaluation of 2,222 cases of serotonin overdose reported to the Hunter Area Toxicology Service.[542] These criteria are simpler and include primarily clonus, agitation, diaphoresis, tremor, hyper-reflexia, hypertonia, and hyperthermia. The Hunter criteria have a sensitivity of 84% compared to 75% with the Sternbach criteria. The most important sign in the Hunter criteria is clonus and, if spontaneously present in a patient taking a serotonergic agent, is by itself adequate to make the diagnosis. It is important to note that the diagnostics decision rules were developed from data in patients with overdoses and have not yet been validated to be sensitive and specific for patients with serotonin syndrome at therapeutic doses of serotonergic agents. Fulminant cases of serotonin syndrome may progress to seizures, rhabdomyolysis, renal failure, and death.

Other conditions to consider in the differential diagnosis of serotonin syndrome include infection, sepsis, heat stroke, drug or alcohol withdrawal, sympathomimetic overdose, thyrotoxicosis, anticholinergic fever, and NMS (**Table 54-20**). Although both NMS and serotonin syndrome may present with some common symptoms—including catatonia, tremors, rigidity, and hyperthermia—differences may aid in the diagnosis. Proper diagnosis is essential; bromocriptine is a treatment considered for NMS but should be strictly avoided in patients with serotonin syndrome because it may worsen the condition. The rigidity associated with serotonin syndrome may be less pronounced than that due to NMS and usually occurs in the lower extremities as compared with NMS (described as lead-pipe rigidity) and is not usually limited to the lower extremities. With NMS, the progression of signs and symptoms occurs over the course of days, and there may be a lower incidence of tremors, clonus, and myoclonus. There are usually no gastrointestinal symptoms; however, hyperthermia may be more common. Like NMS, no specific laboratory test exists to confirm a diagnosis of serotonin syndrome.[534] Serotonin concentrations at the synaptic cleft are responsible for toxicity and do not correlate with serum levels.[355] There is some evidence to support the use of urinary 5-HT concentrations as adjuncts to clinical decision making.[544] The most reliable method for appropriate diagnosis is an accurate medication history, including starting dates and doses of medications that increase serotonergic activity and specific information regarding dose escalation, if available.

Table 54-20 Conditions to Consider in the Differential Diagnosis of Drug-Induced Serotonin Syndrome

- Anticholinergic toxicity
- Drug withdrawal (alcohol, benzodiazepines, levodopa)
- Endocrine disorders
- Heat stroke
- Hematologic or solid organ malignancy
- Infection
- Neuroleptic malignant syndrome
- Sepsis
- Sympathomimetic overdose
- Thyrotoxicosis

RISK FACTORS

No patient-specific risk factors for the development of serotonin syndrome have been definitively identified, although increased age and female sex may be predisposing factors (**Table 54-21**). In addition, risk factors may include endogenous or acquired defects in MAO activity that lead to impairment in SSRI metabolism, such as those occurring in patients with cardiovascular diseases (including hypertension and hyperlipidemia), liver disease, pulmonary disease, and in those who smoke cigarettes. Genetic variation in the ability to metabolize

Table 54-21 Risk Factors for Drug-Induced Serotonin Syndrome

Drug-related

- Higher total daily dose
- Higher-potency agents
- Rapid dose escalation
- Use of concomitant drugs that increase serotonin activity

Patient-related

- Endogenous or acquired defects in MAO activity
- Female sex
- Older age
- Poor metabolizers of SSRIs

MAO = monoamine oxidase, SSRI = selective serotonin reuptake inhibitor.

serotonergic drugs and activities of MAO isoenzymes may predispose patients to serotonin syndrome. Approximately 7% of individuals are poor metabolizers of SSRIs.[545] This genetic predisposition may enhance a patient's sensitivity to serotonergic agents and increase the propensity for the development of serotonin syndrome.

Other potential risk factors for serotonin syndrome are drug-specific features including drug potency, total daily dose, rapid dose escalation, and use of concomitant agents that may increase serotonin activity or interact with serotonergic agents.

MORBIDITY AND MORTALITY

Most patients fully recover following discontinuation of the causative agent and implementation of supportive care; however, deaths have been reported due to serotonin syndrome.[434,435,442,445,451,457,511] Deaths are reported more often in association with intentional overdose of SSRIs alone or in combination with an MAOI. Mortality from serotonin syndrome ranges between 2–12%.[347] Death from serotonin syndrome generally occurs secondary to multiple organ dysfunction, including rhabdomyolysis leading to renal failure, disseminated intravascular coagulopathy, adult respiratory distress syndrome, and cardiovascular collapse from muscular hyperactivity and hyperthermia. With prompt intervention, however, patients usually recover without long-term sequelae.

PREVENTION

Keys to the prevention of serotonin syndrome are careful initiation and dose escalation of SSRIs, in addition to appropriate patient education regarding drug-induced diseases, drug interactions, and recognition of signs and symptoms of toxicity (**Table 54-22**). SSRI therapy should be initiated at a low dosage and titrated upward slowly, particularly in elderly patients or those with impairment of liver or renal function.

Following discontinuation of the culprit drug, a washout period of at least 5–7 days prior to initiating therapy with an MAOI or another SSRI is important; the duration should be determined based on the half-life of the active compound. A washout period of 5 weeks or longer may be necessary for SSRIs with very long half-lives or those with active metabolites such as fluoxetine, sertraline, and clomipramine. In addition, if delayed elimination is suspected in selected patients, a longer drug-free period is warranted. MAOIs inhibit the metabolism of SSRIs and, therefore, directly increase serotonin concentrations at the site of activity. MAOIs should be discontinued at least 4 weeks prior to starting therapy with an SSRI. Moclobemide, a reversible MAOI, requires a much shorter washout period because of its very short half-life; 24 hours may be sufficient. Concomitant use of agents that increase serum serotonin concentrations should be avoided.[534] Appropriate dose adjustments should be made in older patients and in those with renal or hepatic impairment, in addition to closer monitoring of these patients for signs or symptoms of toxicity.

Table 54-22 Approaches to Help Prevent Drug-Induced Serotonin Syndrome

- Adjust dose appropriately for elderly patients and those with hepatic dysfunction or chronic kidney disease
- Be aware of drug interactions and avoid if possible
- Carefully initiate and titrate serotonergic agents
- Carefully switch from one serotonergic agent to another
- Ensure adequate washout period when switching from MAOI to serotonergic agents or serotonergic agents to MAOI

MAOI = monoamine oxidase inhibitor.

MANAGEMENT

Discontinuation of the offending agent is imperative, as is supportive care, which often results in resolution of signs and symptoms within 24 hours without additional pharmacotherapeutic intervention (**Table 54-23**). Fluid therapy should be implemented in patients in whom diaphoresis has been a significant clinical symptom, in addition to those requiring cooling augmentation.

Although there are no clinical trials that have specifically evaluated the efficacy of any therapeutic intervention for serotonin syndrome, several drugs have anecdotally been reported to be successful. Cyproheptadine, a histamine[1] (H^1) antagonist with

Table 54-23 Management of Drug-Induced Serotonin Syndrome

- Discontinue suspected agent
- Supportive care
  - Cooled fluids
  - Fluid replacement for patients with severe diaphoresis or rhabdomyolysis
  - Surface cooling
- Cyproheptadine 12-mg loading dose followed by 2 mg every 2 hours until symptoms are controlled; 4–8 mg every 6 hours for up to 48 hours for maintenance
- Chlorpromazine 50–100 mg intramuscularly as a single dose, repeat dose every 6 hours if symptoms return; may be given orally if able
- Lorazepam or diazepam may be added to the above therapy in refractory cases as needed to control signs and symptoms
- Benzodiazepine, propofol, or dexmedetomidine infusions may be used for patients requiring sedation and mechanical ventilation
- Neuromuscular blocking agents may be considered for patients with sustained myoclonus or severe hyperthermia

nonselective anti–5-HT and anticholinergic properties, has been a successful treatment for serotonin syndrome. In some reports, cyproheptadine has not been found to alter the time course of serotonin syndrome but may relieve signs and symptoms.[546] Others have indicated that cyproheptadine can shorten the duration of some symptoms of serotonin syndrome, including tachycardia, tremor, neuromuscular features, and anxiety.[432] The recommended dose of cyproheptadine for the management of serotonin syndrome is a loading dose of 12 mg followed by 2 mg orally (or via nasogastric tube) every 2 hours until symptoms are controlled then 4–8 mg every 6 hours.[355] In children, 0.25 mg/kg/day has been administered. It has been suggested that these doses are lower than those required to adequately block the 5-HT_{2A} receptors and that 30 mg is a more optimal dose in an adult, potentially explaining some reported treatment failures.[547,548] However, doses of 12–32 mg are likely sufficient to bind 85–95% of serotonin receptors, and alternative treatment or diagnosis should be considered if there has been no response after 32 mg.[347,355] In most cases, the duration of therapy has been no longer than 48 hours, with many patients receiving only a single dose. Cyproheptadine should be avoided in patients in whom anticholinergic toxicity has not been ruled out. The drug may cause hypotension, and fluid therapy may be used, if necessary, for management.

Chlorpromazine has been used in the management of serotonin syndrome, although far less commonly than cyproheptadine and benzodiazepines.[547] In addition to having antimuscarinic effects, chlorpromazine inhibits dopamine, α-adrenergic, and 5-HT_2 receptors. Chlorpromazine is available as an injectable agent and, therefore, may be considered in more severe cases and in cases in which more prompt onset of the effect is desired. Chlorpromazine should not be used in patients with suspected NMS, because dopamine receptor inhibition could worsen the condition. Chlorpromazine should be considered in cases of cyproheptadine failure or in cases with a significant hyperpyrexial or behavioral manifestation. The suggested dose of chlorpromazine is 50–100 mg intramuscularly initially and then every 6 hours. The drug may be administered orally, intramuscularly, or intravenously.[449,547] Single-dose therapy has generally been effective, but the dose may be repeated if signs or symptoms return. Patients receiving chlorpromazine should be adequately hydrated, as it may cause hypotension due to α_2-adrenergic receptor antagonism.[547] Dantrolene has been used successfully in two cases but has also been theorized to increase serotonin levels and decrease metabolism. Routine use in serotonin syndrome is not recommended.[549-551]

Other therapies have been used as either adjunctive therapy or in cases of cyproheptadine failure. Benzodiazepines have been used in the treatment of serotonin syndrome and should be strongly considered in patients with anxiety or agitation. Single-dose therapy has been used, but multiple doses may be administered as needed for management of symptoms. Lorazepam and diazepam have been used alone and in combination with prochlorperazine and propranolol to control the symptoms of serotonin syndrome.[448,489,495,516,520,552] Propranolol has also been used as monotherapy and is thought to possess some 5-HT_{1a}-receptor blocking activity.[508,552,553] Caution should be used when attempting to treat both hypertension or hypotension in this patient population as the blood pressure tends to be quite labile. Preference should be given to short-acting, titratable, agents. Antipsychotics, such as haloperidol, should be avoided for treatment of agitation as they possess anticholinergic activity and may worsen heat dissipation. Propofol has been used for serotonin syndrome as well. One case describes rapid resolution of tachycardia and neuromuscular tone and normalization of reflexes with the use of propofol starting at 10 mcg/kg/min and titrated up to 30 mcg/kg/min in a patient with serotonin syndrome due to intentional dextromethorphan ingestion.[514] Signs and symptoms returned when the propofol was discontinued 2 hours after presentation but again resolved after propofol was restarted. The propofol infusion was continued for an additional 8 hours. Dexmedetomidine has also been used with success in serotonin syndrome.[554] Neuromuscular blockade may be considered for patients with severe serotonin syndrome who experience sustained myoclonus and hyperthermia >41.1°C.[355,452,489] Up to 25% of patients may require intubation, sedation, and mechanical ventilation.[347] Serotonin syndrome should be treated aggressively if symptoms are worsening and in overdose situations, as the disease may be fatal. Signs and symptoms must be monitored closely; Table 54-16 lists important monitoring parameters for patients with serotonin syndrome.

INFORMATION FOR PATIENTS

Patients should be instructed to notify healthcare professionals of all prescription and nonprescription medications and herbal products that they are taking. Healthcare providers should ensure that patients are aware of potential drug interactions, specific medications that should be avoided (such as nonprescription cough medications that contain dextromethorphan), and should instruct patients to ask a pharmacist if they have any questions regarding safe combinations of medications. Clinicians should encourage patients to follow the dosage regimen prescribed closely and accurately and not to increase any doses unless specifically instructed to by the prescriber. Patients should be aware of the signs and symptoms of serotonin syndrome and should be instructed about when to seek medical attention. Development of fever, shivering or diaphoresis, or myoclonus or any mental status changes should prompt patients or caregivers to contact a healthcare facility for further evaluation and treatment.

MALIGNANT HYPERTHERMIA

Malignant hyperthermia is a rare but serious idiosyncratic reaction observed primarily in association with the administration of inhaled anesthetics. Hyperthermia occurs quickly, is often severe, and may be associated with muscle weakness, increased muscular tone, and damage including rhabdomyolysis and metabolic acidosis. Early recognition and intervention are crucial in the management of this drug-induced disease.

CAUSATIVE AGENTS

Drugs that have been reported to cause malignant hyperthermia are listed in **Table 54-24.**[555-604] Inhalational anesthetics, with the exception of nitrous

Table 54-24 Agents Implicated in Drug-Induced Malignant Hyperthermia

Drug	Incidence	Level of Evidence[a]
ANESTHETICS, INHALED	NK	C
Desflurane[555-563]	NK	C
Enflurane[540-566]	NK	C
Halothane[567-574]	NK	C
Isoflurane[575-589]	NK	C
Methoxyflurane[590]	NK	C
Sevoflurane[572,591-598]	NK	C
DEPOLARIZING SKELETAL MUSCLE RELAXANTS	NK	C
Succinylcholine[472,555-558,563,567,599-604]	NK	C

NK = not known.

[a]Definitions for Levels of Evidence: Level A—evidence from one or more randomized, controlled clinical trials; Level B—evidence from nonrandomized clinical trials, prospective observational studies, cohort studies, retrospective studies, case-control studies, meta-analyses and/or postmarketing surveillance studies; and Level C—evidence from one or more published case reports or case series.

oxide, and depolarizing neuromuscular blocking drugs (skeletal muscle relaxants) are the drug classes most frequently implicated in the development of malignant hyperthermia. The agents most commonly reported to cause malignant hyperthermia include halothane, enflurane, isoflurane, and succinylcholine. Succinylcholine may increase the risk, worsen the severity, and shorten the onset time of malignant hyperthermia when used in combination with inhaled anesthetics.[555-558] Succinylcholine may also cause malignant hyperthermia independently.

EPIDEMIOLOGY

Malignant hyperthermia is a genetically linked, life-threatening condition that is observed in all ethnic groups and is more common in men than in women.[605,606] On average, malignant hyperthermia may be observed with the third exposure to a triggering agent, although it is possible to occur with the first use in a susceptible patient. Malignant hyperthermia is more common in children under 15 years of age, with an incidence of 1 in 8,000 to 1 in 15,000, as compared with an estimated incidence of 1 in 40,000 to 1 in 150,000 in adults.[605-607]

MECHANISMS

Heterogenic mutations in the ryanodine receptor (*RYR1*) and dihydropyridine receptor (*CACNA1S*) genes, and other mutations yet to be fully characterized, are involved in the etiology of malignant hyperthermia.[608] The RYR1 receptor is a calcium channel located in the sarcoplasmic reticulum membrane. Disruptions in this channel lead to malignant hyperthermia susceptibility. Although not all of the genetic loci involved have been identified, it is known that malignant hyperthermia occurs because of a defect in the regulation of intracellular calcium metabolism, specifically the proteins involved in excitation–contraction coupling, the dihydropyridine–ryanodine receptor complex, such that the sarcoplasmic reticulum of skeletal muscle releases calcium inappropriately in response to an inducing drug.[608-610] The increase in calcium concentration may lead to unregulated actin and myosin cross-bridging, resulting in sustained muscle contraction. This muscle rigidity results in increased oxygen consumption, hypoxia, excessive heat production and muscle damage, and the clinical presentation of malignant hyperthermia.

CLINICAL PRESENTATION AND DIFFERENTIAL DIAGNOSIS

Although highly variable, the classic presentation of malignant hyperthermia is sudden, severe hyperthermia with muscle rigidity, metabolic acidosis, and rhabdomyolysis (**Table 54-25**). The onset of symptoms is very rapid, beginning within minutes to several hours after drug initiation and up to 1 hour after discontinuation.[611] Hyperthermia may be delayed and may occur after other symptoms (rigidity and tachycardia). Temperature may acutely increase in excess of 1°C every 5 minutes up to maximum temperatures of 46°C or higher.[605,612] With the more modern use of less potent inhalational agents, this course has been described to be more insidious or attenuated, with a delayed onset and slower clinical progression.[613,614]

Early signs and symptoms of malignant hyperthermia may include masseter-muscle rigidity (particularly in children), tachycardia, and a sudden,

Table 54-25 Signs and Symptoms Associated with Drug-Induced Malignant Hyperthermia

- Muscle pain, weakness in jaw, chest, and extremities
- Muscle contraction
- Initial signs
  - Hyperthermia
  - Increase in end-tidal carbon dioxide
  - Masseter-muscle rigidity
  - Metabolic acidosis
  - Tachycardia
- Signs as syndrome progresses
  - Cardiac dysrhythmias
  - Hyperkalemia, hypercalcemia, hyperphosphatemia
  - Hypotension
  - Metabolic and respiratory acidosis
  - Pulmonary edema
  - Rhabdomyolysis and renal failure

dramatic increase in end-tidal carbon dioxide ($ETCO_2$) to >55 mm Hg. The increase in $ETCO_2$ is a sensitive indicator of the disease but may be less dramatic and more gradual in patients who do not receive succinylcholine. Muscle pain, weakness, and increased tone in the jaw, chest, and extremities may occur and are often severe and refractory to therapy with neuromuscular blocking agents. Muscle contraction and subsequent muscle damage results in the release of CK and myoglobin, which may contribute to the development of rhabdomyolysis and renal failure.

As the syndrome progresses, pulmonary edema, hypotension, heart failure, electrolyte abnormalities (hyperkalemia, hypercalcemia, hyperphosphatemia), metabolic and respiratory acidosis (pH <7.25 and partial pressure of CO_2 [$paCO_2$] >60 mm Hg), and the resultant dysrhythmias may be observed. The $paCO_2$ may exceed 100 mm Hg and pH may decline to <7 in severe cases. A presumptive diagnosis is made based on signs and symptoms temporally related to the administration of inhalational anesthetics or succinylcholine. Definitive diagnosis of malignant hyperthermia requires the European in vitro contracture test (IVCT), or the modified caffeine halothane contracture test (CHCT) used in North America. These tests require a muscle biopsy, which is exposed to halothane or caffeine to determine the contracture threshold. The patient is diagnosed as being susceptible to malignant hyperthermia based on the threshold at which the muscle is reactive.[615] This test is not necessary as a confirmation of diagnosis for patients in whom the typical signs and symptoms have developed.[616,617] Rather, optimal use of this test is as a screen for susceptible individuals (based on family history) prior to use of triggering agents. DNA testing is also an option for specific, at-risk individuals; guidelines for testing have been published.[618,619]

In addition, a clinical grading scale for malignant hyperthermia has been developed to aid in the diagnosis and for predicting susceptibility to this drug-induced disease.[620] This scale was developed by an international panel of malignant hyperthermia experts using anonymous polling and questionnaires to minimize bias and subjective influence. Clinical indicators were developed with points for each indicator as well as scoring rules. The clinical grading scale allows for objective determination of the likelihood of a malignant hyperthermia diagnosis and is an extremely valuable tool. Differential diagnosis includes hypoxia due to atelectasis, bronchial obstruction, sepsis, and pulmonary mechanical failure, although these conditions are not generally associated with the degree of temperature elevation that occurs in patients with malignant hyperthermia (**Table 54-26**).

Table 54-26 Conditions to Consider in the Differential Diagnosis of Drug-Induced Malignant Hyperthermia

- Atelectasis
- Bronchial obstruction
- Drug withdrawal (alcohol, benzodiazepines, levodopa)
- Endocrine disorders
- Heat stroke
- Hematologic or solid organ malignancy
- Infection
- Pulmonary mechanical failure
- Sepsis

RISK FACTORS

Malignant hyperthermia is an idiosyncratic reaction and therefore is difficult to predict. However, because the disorder is genetically linked, patients with a family history of malignant hyperthermia are at significantly higher risk than those without a family history (**Table 54-27**). Younger patients, males, and those with central core disease tend to be predisposed to this drug-induced disease. The type of surgical procedure may also be associated with differences in incidence of malignant hyperthermia. Eye, head, neck, and musculoskeletal surgeries are associated with the highest risk.[606]

Table 54-27 Risk Factors for Drug-Induced Malignant Hyperthermia

- Eye, head, or neck surgeries
- Family history of malignant hyperthermia
- Male sex
- Muscular dystrophies/diseases
- Young age (<15 yr)

Certain muscular diseases, including Duchenne muscular dystrophy, Becker's muscular dystrophy, Wolf–Hirschhorn syndrome, kyphoscoliosis, myotonic dystrophy, and others have been linked to a predisposition to malignant hyperthermia.[621,622]

Elevated resting serum CK concentrations have been used in the past as a means to try to identify patients at risk for malignant hyperthermia and research exploring the relationship between resting CK levels and malignant hyperthermia is ongoing.[623,624] Currently, however, use of this screening method is not routinely recommended.[625]

Table 54-28 Approaches to Help Prevent Drug- Induced Malignant Hyperthermia

- Avoid use of triggering agents, if possible, in selected patients
- Carefully screen patient and family members prior to use of anesthesia
- Use genetic testing in specifically targeted patients
- Use in vitro contracture test in appropriate patients
- Use medical alerting devices in patients with a history of malignant hyperthermia or who are at high risk
- Use nitrous oxide, bupivacaine, barbiturates, opiates and nondepolarizing skeletal muscle relaxants

MORBIDITY AND MORTALITY

In the past, mortality associated with malignant hyperthermia was high, exceeding 60%.[626,627] With early recognition and appropriate intervention, mortality has decreased substantially and currently may be as low as 7%.[628-630] Early implementation of therapy with dantrolene and shorter duration of anesthesia (<30 minutes) may be associated with enhanced survival (87%); patients who receive anesthesia for longer than 30 minutes have been found to have lower survival rates (43–61%).[631] The prognosis has been found to be worse for men than for women for unknown reasons, although an increased muscle mass in men may be contributory.[605,606]

The risk of death has also been associated with the maximum temperature, the rate of rise of temperature, and the duration of hyperthermia.[631] Hyperthermia may cause agitation, confusion, disorientation, combativeness, lethargy, seizures, coma, and death. Rhabdomyolysis and disseminated intravascular coagulation may lead to acute tubular necrosis. Volume depletion, tissue injury, and hypoxia may lead to shock, organ dysfunction, and organ failure. Cardiac dysrhythmias, such as ventricular fibrillation due to hyperkalemia, may occur, are often difficult to treat, and may result in cardiac arrest and death.[632,633]

PREVENTION

The key to the prevention of malignant hyperthermia is avoidance of the use of inhaled anesthetics and depolarizing neuromuscular blocking agents in patients with a personal history or a strong family history of the condition (**Table 54-28**) and flushing of the anesthesia machine prior to use in these individuals. Appropriate patient screening regarding family members with a history of malignant hyperthermia or death during surgery or general anesthesia should be performed. Patients at risk may be given the opportunity for an IVCT or CHCT to determine susceptibility to triggering agents. Drugs that have been used safely in susceptible patients (those with a history of malignant hyperthermia or those with a strong family history) include nitrous oxide, bupivacaine, barbiturates, opiates, propofol, and nondepolarizing muscle relaxants.[599,634,635]

It has been suggested that prophylaxis with oral dantrolene may be effective for the prevention of malignant hyperthermia in susceptible individuals, although no data from randomized, controlled trials are available.[636-639] In one study, oral dantrolene was administered at a dose of 5 mg/kg in three or four divided doses with the last dose administered 4 hours preoperatively to 10 patients who were susceptible to malignant hyperthermia.[637] None of the patients experienced malignant hyperthermia, but some experienced drowsiness and weakness due to dantrolene administration.[636] Malignant hyperthermia has also been prevented via the administration of dantrolene 100 mg 4 times daily for 3 days before surgery and 100 mg on the day of surgery.[638] Two cases of malignant hyperthermia despite oral dantrolene administration have been reported, although in these cases the administered doses were lower than recommended.[640,641] Dantrolene prophylaxis is not expected to be completely successful and may cause significant muscle weakness resulting in temporary disability, a factor that should be considered in the decision about whether to attempt prophylaxis.[639,642,643] Several cases have been reported in which patients were successfully anesthetized without prophylactic administration of dantrolene when triggering agents were not used and patients were monitored very closely.[635,644] Currently, the use of dantrolene prophylaxis in susceptible patients is not recommended because the risk of malignant hyperthermia when triggering agents are avoided is low and because of the potential adverse effects associated with dantrolene.

MANAGEMENT

Early recognition and intervention is crucial. All suspected medications must be immediately discontinued, the surgical procedure stopped as soon as feasible, and the patient removed from the anesthesia machine and hyperventilated with 100% oxygen (**Table 54-29**). Ongoing anesthesia can be provided using intravenous anesthetics, opioids and nondepolarizing muscle relaxants. Control of fever, acidosis, hypermetabolism, and hypercarbia is imperative. Administration of intravenous fluids will aid in the prevention of acute tubular necrosis and metabolic acidosis from the hypermetabolic state and in maintaining cardiac output. Hypercarbia and hypoxemia should be treated with aggressive oxygen management and hyperventilation. Rapid cooling measures such as cooling blankets, ice packs, ice water gastric lavage, and intravenous fluids should be implemented. Shivering may occur from rapid temperature decrease and should be treated with chlorpromazine, opioids, benzodiazepines, and when necessary, paralysis with mechanical ventilation for severe, refractory shivering to control oxygen utilization. In addition to fluid resuscitation and electrolyte and acid–base management, patients may require treatment with procainamide, amiodarone, or β-blockers to control tachydysrhythmias that may develop. Calcium channel blockers should not be used due to a potential for hyperkalemia in association with dantrolene administration.

Table 54-29 Management of Drug-Induced Malignant Hyperthermia

- Discontinue suspected agent
- Cooling measures and other supportive care
  - Cooled intravenous fluids
  - Ice water nasogastric or rectal lavage
  - Surface cooling
- Fluid and electrolyte replacement as needed
- Continuous ventilatory management
- Dantrolene 2.5 mg/kg intravenously as needed to control signs and symptoms (up to 10 mg/kg; doses up to 30 mg/kg may be used in severe, refractory cases)
- Nondepolarizing neuromuscular blocking drugs, benzodiazepines, chlorpromazine as needed for refractory shivering or rigidity

Dantrolene is a specific ryanodine receptor antagonist that inhibits calcium release from the endoplasmic reticulum, which dramatically alters the course of malignant hyperthermia. In one study of 11 patients with malignant hyperthermia to whom dantrolene was administered, 100% of patients survived.[645] In one retrospective medical record review, the mortality rate was 8.9% in 79 patients who received intravenous dantrolene prior to cardiac arrest, as compared to a mortality rate of 25.4% in 375 patients who did not receive dantrolene—a 16.6% absolute reduction in mortality.[631] Rapid dantrolene administration after recognition of the syndrome is critical, as a favorable outcome is related to a shorter elapsed time from symptom onset to time of drug administration. Dantrolene should be administered as an intravenous dose of 2–2.5 mg/kg initially, repeated as necessary up to 10 mg/kg until signs and symptoms begin to abate, which is expected to occur within minutes of dantrolene administration. Higher doses of up to 30 mg/kg may be administered in severe, refractory cases although reaching these higher doses without improvement suggests the diagnosis of malignant hyperthermia should be reassessed.

Two formulations of dantrolene are currently available, a 20-mg vial and a 250-mg vial. Both preparations require reconstitution with sterile water for injection; no other diluent is recommended. The 20-mg vial requires 60 mL of sterile water and shaking until a clear solution is achieved, and the 250-mg vial requires 5 mL of sterile water and will result in an orange suspension. Both are to be administered via intravenous push for emergency management of malignant hyperthermia. It should be noted that the 250-mg vial is currently more costly but may be more convenient in the critical setting of malignant hyperthermia because only one vial and 5 mL of sterile water are needed compared to 10–12 vials of the 20-mg per vial and 60 mL sterile water for each vial. The currently recommended initial doses are higher than those that were recommended previously (1 mg/kg) because of diminished circulation in patients with malignant hyperthermia and so a more aggressive approach is warranted.[569,646] The duration of treatment in the cases reported has varied considerably, from single-dose therapy to multiple days of therapy.

After the patient has stabilized, dantrolene may be administered orally at a dose of 50–300 mg per day in divided doses or 1–2 mg/kg 4 times daily for several days (at least 36 hours) to prevent recurrence.[647] Dantrolene has been used successfully and safely in pregnant patients who are susceptible to malignant hyperthermia and are undergoing caesarean section.[648-655] Dantrolene may cause dizziness, diplopia, dysarthria, a sensation of swelling of the eyes and tongue, and subjective (but not objective) weakness.[569,631,643] Patients have been successfully managed without the use of dantrolene with only supportive and cooling therapies but this approach is not recommended.[614,656,657]

Close monitoring for improvement of signs and symptoms as well as any signs of recurrence is important for a successful outcome in patients with malignant hyperthermia. Appropriate monitoring parameters are listed in **Table 54-30**. Patients who may be susceptible but are not given triggering agents can be safely monitored with the standard procedures used for nonsusceptible patients.[658]

Table 54-30 Monitoring Parameters for Patients with Drug-Induced Malignant Hyperthermia

- Blood gases
- Coagulation profile
- Continuous cardiac rhythm
- Continuous central temperature
- End-tidal carbon dioxide
- Heart rate
- Mental status
- Metabolic panel including serum carbon dioxide concentration
- Muscle rigidity
- Pulse oximetry
- Respiratory rate
- Serum creatinine and blood urea nitrogen concentrations
- Serum creatine kinase concentrations
- Serum electrolyte concentrations
- Urine myoglobin concentrations

INFORMATION FOR PATIENTS

Patients should be questioned regarding a history of malignant hyperthermia or a problem with anesthesia and should be instructed to alert all healthcare professionals of this risk. In addition, family members of patients with a prior episode should be made aware of their potential risk. Patients at risk should be given the opportunity for an IVCT to determine susceptibility to triggering agents. Various options for anesthesia, as well as the risks and benefits of those options in addition to prophylaxis with dantrolene, should be discussed with patients at risk prior to any surgery. A medical alerting device is recommended for those with a history of malignant hyperthermia or who have a significant family history and positive IVCT in the event that emergency surgery is needed. Finally, patients should be offered the opportunity to register with the Malignant Hyperthermia Association of the United States (MHAUS) by calling 1-800-MH-HYPER (1-800-644-9737) or visiting the website at www.mhaus.org. The website provides patient and healthcare professional information in addition to resources for susceptibility testing, hotline contact information, and for obtaining an Emergency Medical Identification Card.

HYPOTHERMIA

Drug-induced hypothermia occurs much less frequently than hyperthermia. Hypothermia can be defined as a core body temperature <35°C.[572] Although drug-induced hypothermia can occur with certain prescription drugs, it is most commonly associated with illicit drug use.

CAUSATIVE AGENTS

Baclofen, GHB, and gamma-butyrolactone (GBL), is converted to GHB after ingestion, are structurally related to GABA and may cause hypothermia in overdose.[660-667] GHB is best known as the "date rape" drug but is also contained within body-building supplements and marketed for recreational purposes. GBL is found in industrial and household solvents and other products, including dietary supplements marketed for sleep and for enhancing sexual and athletic performance. Although the U.S. Food and Drug Administration requested a voluntary recall of GBL-containing products in 1999, it may still be available via the Internet in products labeled as dietary supplements listed as "dihydro-2(3H)-furanone," "4-butanolide," "2(3H)-furanone, dihydro," "tetrahydro-2-furanone," and "butyrolactone gamma." Street names for both GHB and GBL are listed in **Table 54-31**. Drugs associated with hypothermia are listed in **Table 54-32**.[660-667,669-679] It has been suggested that antipsychotics can cause hypothermia but clear data to substantiate the claim are lacking.[668] Additional data continue to emerge indicating hypothermia related to antipsychotics to be a true effect, although not well understood.[669,670,674-677,679] Atypical antipsychotics account for 55% of the cases of reported drug-induced hypothermia.[668] Reports also exist of patients experiencing hypothermia following general anesthesia secondary to vasodilation, impaired shivering, and cool operating rooms.[680] Additional reports implicate intrathecal morphine and some benzodiazepines as potential culprits.[659,668,671,673,678]

EPIDEMIOLOGY

The incidence of drug-induced hypothermia is unknown. With regard to hypothermia related to antipsychotic use, a 2007 article analyzing the World Health Organization international database found 480 cases of antipsychotic-related hypothermia. Oral risperidone was the most common agent associated, with 27% of cases, and clozapine second, with 14%.[668]

Table 54-31 Street Names for Gamma-Hydroxybutyrate and Gamma-Butyrolactone

Gamma-hydroxybutyrate (GHB)

- Bedtime Scoop
- Cherry Meth
- Easy Lay
- Fantasy
- "G"
- G-juice
- GBH
- G-riffic
- Gamma Oh
- Gamma Ten
- Georgia Home Boy
- Gook
- Great Hormones at Bedtime
- Grievous Bodily Harm
- Jib
- Liquid E
- Liquid Ecstasy
- Liquid G
- Liquid X
- Organic Quaalude
- Salty Water
- Scoop
- Sleep
- Sleep-500
- Soap
- Somatomax
- Vita G

Gamma-butyrolactone (GBL)

- Blue Nitro
- Blue Nitro Vitality
- Fire Water
- GH Revitalizer
- Gamma G
- Re-energize
- Remforce
- RenewTrient
- Revivarant
- Revivarant G

MECHANISMS

Temperature balance occurs via the anterior hypothalamus, with stimulation and inhibition from a variety of neurotransmitters in a complex process. Dopamine and serotonin receptors are involved in thermoregulatory balance. Although

Table 54-32 Agents Implicated in Drug-Induced Hypothermia

Drug	Incidence	Level of Evidence[a]
Baclofen[663]	NK	C
Cannabinoids[666]	NK	C
Chlorpromazine[669,670]	NK	C
Clobazam[671]	NK	C
Clozapine[659,668,670]	NK	C
Diazepam[672,673]	NK	C
Gamma-butyrolactone (GBL)[666]	NK	C
Gamma-hydroxybutyrate (GHB)[660-662,664,667]	NK	C
Haloperidol[674,675]	NK	C
Olanzapine[676,677]	NK	C
Opioids[666,678]	NK	C
Promethazine[670]	NK	C
Risperidone[668,679]	NK	C
Thioridazine[675]	NK	C

NK = not known.

[a]Definitions for Levels of Evidence: Level A—evidence from one or more randomized, controlled clinical trials; Level B—evidence from nonrandomized clinical trials, prospective observational studies, cohort studies, retrospective studies, case-control studies, meta-analyses and/or postmarketing surveillance studies; and Level C—evidence from one or more published case reports or case series.

both D_1 and D_2 receptor subtypes are involved in temperature regulation, the more prominent effect of dopamine receptor stimulation is lowering of temperature, and the more prominent effect of dopamine receptor antagonism is that of elevating temperature. Cannabinoid and opioid-induced hypothermia is mediated via dopaminergic pathways. In addition, opioids may decrease body temperature through agonism of opiate receptors in the hypothalamus and vasodilation. A relative increase in serotonin concentrations increases temperature. GABA and baclofen inhibit the release of excitatory neurotransmitters, including serotonin and dopamine, resulting in a net effect of hypothermia.

Antipsychotic-induced hypothermia is poorly understood. Although dopaminergic and serotonergic antagonism would seemingly lead to hyperthermia as in NMS, these agents have been implicated on multiple accounts to cause hypothermia. Due to the propensity of atypical antipsychotic agents to produce more hypothermia than typical agents, it is proposed that there is some component mediated by serotonin because atypical agents have stronger 5-HT_2 antagonism.[668] Additional theories suggest that agents such as chlorpromazine, clozapine, promethazine, and risperidone lower body temperature through alpha sympatholytic impairment of skin vessel vasoconstriction thus increasing heat dissipation.[670] Impaired vasoconstriction has also been hypothesized for some benzodiazepine-mediated cases.[679] Antipsychotic agents may also indirectly create temperature disturbances by altering the behavioral response to environmental temperature changes.[659] The intricacy in the balance of factors is not fully understood, highlighted by the ability of the same antipsychotic being capable of producing both hyperthermia and hypothermia. Antipyretic agents such as acetaminophen, aspirin, and other nonsteroidal anti-inflammatory drugs decrease temperature in febrile patients in whom the thermoregulatory set point has been raised. However, these drugs have no effect on temperature in afebrile patients.

CLINICAL PRESENTATION AND DIFFERENTIAL DIAGNOSIS

Drug-induced effects other than hypothermia associated with overdose of these agents are generally more clinically significant (**Table 54-33**). In one series of cases of intentional baclofen overdose, it was reported that six of eight patients were hypothermic (temperature ≤35.5°C).[663] Other clinical signs included bradycardia, hypertension, hyporeflexia, apnea requiring intubation, and coma. Two patients experienced seizures. Hypertension and seizures were managed, and patients were treated for the possibility of co-ingestion of other drugs. Otherwise, treatment was supportive. All patients recovered without permanent sequelae within 5 days of ingestion.

Seventy cases of GHB overdose in which body temperature was reported have been reviewed.[660] The mean (±SD) initial temperature was 35.8 ± 1.1°C (range, 32–39); 48 patients had an initial

Table 54-33 Signs and Symptoms of Drug-Induced Hypothermia

- Bradycardia
- Chills
- Combativeness
- Decreased motivation
- Hyporeflexia
- Hypotension
- Hypothermia
- Nausea
- Personal neglect
- Respiratory depression
- Tremors or twitching
- Vomiting
- Weight loss

temperature of ≤36°C, and 22 had an initial temperature of ≤35°C. Alcohol or other drugs were usually co-ingested, impairing detection of specific drug-induced signs and symptoms. In addition to hypothermia, commonly reported clinical signs and symptoms of GHB and GBL ingestion include hypotension, respiratory depression, central nervous system depression, bradycardia, nausea, vomiting, combativeness, and tremors or twitching. Co-ingestion of other substances must be strongly considered in the differential diagnosis as well as hypothyroidism.

Patients with hypothermia secondary to antipsychotic use may present with nonspecific symptoms similar to those of their underlying disease, such as decreased motivation, poor personal hygiene, hostility, weight loss, and possibly chills.[659,674,676]

RISK FACTORS

There are no known risk factors for the development of drug-induced hypothermia related to illicit drugs. Based on the cases reported, the disease appears to be dose-related, and therefore individuals taking these products and drugs in larger quantities or more frequently may be at higher risk. Organic brain disease such as mental retardation and epilepsy appear to place patients treated with antipsychotic agents at higher risk for hypothermia.[681] Patients with schizophrenia have also been shown to display impaired thermoregulation at baseline without medication. Levels of the thermoregulatory peptide neurotensin are decreased in the cerebral spinal fluid of these patients but increase to normal levels with antipsychotic treatment.[682,683] It is unclear whether a diagnosis of schizophrenia would place a patient at higher risk for drug-induced hypothermia. Patients also appear to be at higher risk for hypothermia during the first few days following the initiation of a new antipsychotic regimen or dosage increase.[684]

MORBIDITY AND MORTALITY

Most patients with drug-induced hypothermia recover without permanent sequelae. However, severe symptoms have developed in some, including seizures, apnea, and coma.[660-665] In summaries of reported GBL overdose cases (41 patients) and GHB cases at a single facility (88 patients), no deaths were reported.[660,664] Most patients fully recover without significant intervention within hours of ingestion. Deaths have rarely been reported in other cases of sole GHB ingestion.[665,667] Most cases of antipsychotic-induced hypothermia resolve within 24–36 hours.[671]

PREVENTION

The key to prevention of illicit drug-induced hypothermia is avoidance of the use of these drugs. Tighter control of the contents of products available over the Internet and patient awareness are advisable. Because baclofen is often used in children and adolescents, secured storage may help reduce the occurrence of hypothermia due to overdose of this drug. There is no clear way to reduce the risk of antipsychotic-induced hypothermia. Atypical agents appear to have a higher incidence of hypothermia but have a better safety profile in general compared to typical agents.

MANAGEMENT

Drug-induced hypothermia secondary to ingestion of these drugs is generally mild and does not require specific intervention apart from cessation of the offending substance. If hypothermia is secondary to antipsychotic use and continued therapy is needed, reinitiation at a lower dose or an alternative agent is recommended.[671,674] In one rare case of persistent hypothermia following intrathecal morphine administration, temperature normalized following a single oral dose of lorazepam. Other causes of hypothermia should be evaluated and treated, if applicable. Although warming patients is usually not necessary, if hypothermia is severe or if large amounts of fluids are to be administered, blankets and warmed fluid replacement to prevent further body cooling may be used. Supportive measures should be implemented, including intubation and mechanical ventilation (in patients with severe respiratory depression or for airway protection) as well as cardiac monitoring for arrhythmias. Concomitant management of known or suspected co-ingestants is imperative; toxicology screens should be performed and blood alcohol concentrations should be determined.

INFORMATION FOR PATIENTS

Patient information should include warnings about the use of illicit drugs, particularly those that may be available through the Internet, health facilities, and other sources with the potential for hidden ingredients. Patients who are hospitalized because of illicit drug use should receive drug counseling prior to discharge and be offered information regarding treatment programs. Patients or caregivers of those receiving antipsychotic therapy should notify healthcare providers in the event of declining mental status or motivation. Patients should also maintain an accurate history of any adverse drug events in their health history and offer this information to healthcare providers.

REFERENCES

1. Cluff LE, Johnson JE. Drug fever. *Prog Allergy.* 1964; 8:149-94.
2. Lee-Chiong TL Jr, Stitt JT. Disorders of temperature regulation. *Compr Ther.* 1995; 21:697.
3. Eyer F, Zilker T. Bench to bedside review: mechanisms and management of hyperthermia due to toxicity. *Crit Care.* 2007; 11:236.
4. Knudsen JF, Thambi LR, Kapcala LP, Racoosin JA. Oligohydrosis and fever in pediatric patients treated with zonisamide. *Pediatr Neurol.* 2003; 28:184.
5. Karachristianou S, Papamichalis E, Sarantopoulos A et al. Hypohidrosis induced by topiramate in an adult patient. *Epileptic Disord.* 2013 Jun; 15:203-6.
6. Diaz M, Becker DE. Thermoregulation: physiological and clinical considerations during sedation and general anesthesia. *Anesth Prog.* 2010 Spring; 57:25-32.
7. Pollmacher T, Hinze-Selch D, Mullington J. Effects of clozapine on plasma cytokine and soluble cytokine receptor levels. *J Clin Psychopharmacol.* 1996; 16:403-9.
8. Maes M, Bosmans E, Kenis G et al. In vivo immunomodulatory effects of clozapine in schizophrenia. *Schizophr Res.* 1997; 26:221-5.
9. Hetherington S, McGuirk S, Powell G et al. Hypersensitivity reactions during therapy with the nucleoside reverse transcriptase inhibitor abacavir. *Clin Ther.* 2001; 23:1603-14.
10. Hughes CA, Foisy MM, Dewhurst N et al. Abacavir hypersensitivity reaction: an update. *Ann Pharmacother.* 2008; 42:387-96.
11. Hanson MA. Drug fever. Remember to consider it in diagnosis. *Postgrad Med.* 1991; 89:167.
12. Dar KJ, McBrien ME. MDMA-induced hyperthermia: report of a fatality and review of current therapy. *Intensive Care Med.* 1996; 22:995-6.
13. Herrmann R, Manegold C, Fritze D. Fever due to 6-mercaptopurine. *Cancer Treat Rep.* 1982; 66:1785.
14. Rehr EL, Swanson KA, Kern JA. Mercaptopurine-induced fever in a patient with Crohn's disease. *Ann Pharmacother.* 1992; 26:907-9.
15. Shea BF, Harbison MA, Sesin GP et al. Acyclovir-associated fever: a case report. *Pharmacotherapy.* 1987; 7:54-5.
16. Mackowiak PA, LeMaistre CF. Drug fever: critical appraisal of conventional concepts: an analysis of 51 episodes in two Dallas hospitals and 97 episodes reported in the English literature. *Ann Intern Med.* 1987; 106:728-33.
17. Zajecka J, Guy C, Solomon B. Antidepressant drug fever. *J Clin Psychopharmacol.* 1991; 11:73-4.
18. Ginsberg MD, Hertzman M, Schmidt-Nowara WW. Amphetamine intoxication with coagulopathy, hyperthermia, and reversible renal failure: a syndrome resembling heatstroke. *Ann Intern Med.* 1970; 73:81-5.
19. Oizumi K, Onuma K, Watanabe A et al. Clinical study of drug fever induced by parenteral administration of antibiotics. *J Exp Med.* 1989; 159:45-56.
20. Obwegeser J, Junz J, Wüst J et al. Clinical efficacy of amoxicillin/clavulanate in laparoscopically confirmed salpingitis. *J Antimicrob Chemother.* 1989; 24:165-76.
21. Smithson WA, Gronert GA, Moss KK. Dantrolene and potentially fatal hyperthermia secondary to Lasparaginase. *Cancer Treat Rep.* 1983; 67:318-9.
22. Sabeel A, Al Meshari K, Abutaleb N et al. Drug fever induced by azathioprine in a hemodialysis patient. *Nephrol Dial Transplant.* 1998; 13:1004-5.
23. Redon J, Pascual JM, Michavila J et al. Drug fever. *Ann Intern Med.* 1987; 107:264.
24. Kissel JT, Levy RJ, Mendell JR et al. Azathioprine toxicity in neuromuscular disease. *Neurology.* 1986; 36:35-9.
25. Jeurissen MEC, Boerbooms AM, Van de Putte LBA et al. Azathioprine induced fever, chills, rash, and hepatotoxicity in rheumatoid arthritis. *Ann Rheum Dis.* 1990; 49:25-7.
26. Blanco R, Martinez-Taboada VM, Gonzales-Gay MA et al. Acute febrile toxic reaction in patients with refractory rheumatoid arthritis who are receiving combined therapy with methotrexate and azathioprine. *Arthritis Rheum.* 1996; 39:1016-20.
27. Saway PA, Heck LW, Bonner JR et al. Azathioprine hypersensitivity: case report and review of the literature. *Am J Med.* 1988; 84:960-4.
28. Stetter M, Schmidi M, Krapf R. Azathioprine hypersensitivity mimicking Goodpasture's syndrome. *Am J Kidney Dis.* 1994; 23:874-7.
29. Vandepitte K, Vanreterghem Y, Michielsen P. Azathioprine hypersensitivity in a renal transplant recipient. *Transpl Int.* 1990; 3:47-8.
30. Smak Gregoor PJ, van Saase JL, Weimar W et al. Fever and rigors as sole symptoms of azathioprine hypersensitivity. *Neth J Med.* 1995; 47:288-90.

31. Goldstein MR, Kasper R. Hyperpyrexia and coma due to overdose of benztropine. *South Med J.* 1968; 61:984-9.
32. Rosenfelt F, Palmer J, Weinstein I et al. Fatal hyperpyrexial response to bleomycin following prior therapy: a case report and literature review. *Yale J Biol Med.* 1982; 55:529-31.
33. Carter JJ, McLaughlin ML, Bern MM. Bleomycin-induced fatal hyperpyrexia. *Am J Med.* 1983; 74:523-5.
34. Stewart CR, Vengrow MI, Riley TL. Double quotidian fever caused by carbamazepine. *N Engl J Med.* 1980; 302:1262.
35. Sheridan WP, King RW, Gerstman M. Fever as an adverse reaction to carbamazepine. *Aust N Z J Med.* 1982; 12:520-2.
36. Lang R, Lishner M, Ravid M. Adverse reactions to prolonged treatment with high doses of carbenicillin and ureidopenicillins. *Rev Infect Dis.* 1991; 13:68-72.
37. Pleasants RA, Walker TR, Samuelson WM. Allergic reactions to parenteral beta-lactam antibiotics in patients with cystic fibrosis. *Chest.* 1994; 106:1124-8.
38. Harris LF, Holdsambeck HK. Drug fever: surprisingly common and costly. *Ala Med.* 1986; 56:19-22.
39. Hirata-Dulas CAI, Stein DJ, Guay DRP et al. A randomized study of ciprofloxacin versus ceftriaxone in the treatment of nursing home-acquired lower respiratory tract infections. *J Am Geriatr Soc.* 1991; 39:979-85.
40. Greenblatt DJ, Greenblatt GR. Chlorpromazine and hyperpyrexia: a reminder that this drug affects the mechanisms which regulate body temperature. *Clin Pediatr.* 1973; 8:504-5.
41. Sawitsky A, Boklan BF, Benjamin Z. Drug fever produced by chlorambucil. *N Y State J Med.* 1971; 71:2434-6.
42. Corbett CL, Holdsworth CD. Fever, abdominal pain, and leukopenia during treatment with cimetidine. *Br Med J.* 1978; 1:753-4.
43. Ashford RE, McLachlan A, Nelson I et al. Pyrexia after cisplatin. *Lancet.* 1980; 2:691-2.
44. Beckner RR, Canada AT, Ockene IS. Fever due to clofibrate. *N Engl J Med.* 1979; 301:1345-6.
45. Portnoy J, Torchinsky A, Mendelson J et al. Febrile reactions after cloxacillin. *Can Med Assoc J.* 1975; 112:280.
46. Rose MS, Bateman DN. Pyrexia with cytosine arabinoside. *BMJ.* 1972; 4:115.
47. Shipp MA, Takvorian RC, Canellos GP. High-dose cytosine arabinoside: active agent in treatment of non-Hodgkin's lymphoma. *Am J Med.* 1984; 77:845-50.
48. Dominguez EA, Hamill RJ. Drug-induced fever due to diltiazem. *Arch Intern Med.* 1991; 151:1869-70.
49. Chapman SA, Stephan T, Lake KD et al. Fever induced by dobutamine infusion. *Am J Cardiol.* 1994; 74:517.
50. Robison-Strane SR, Bubik JS. Dobutamine-induced fever. *Ann Pharmacother.* 1992; 26:1523-4.
51. Dorschner L, Speich R, Ruschitzka F et al. Everolimus-induced drug fever after heart transplantation. *Transplantation.* 2004; 78:303-4.
52. Wolfson JS, Hooper DC. Overview of fluoroquinolone safety. *Am J Med.* 1991; 91(suppl 6A):S153-61.
53. Sesin GP, Kirschenbaum H. Folic acid hypersensitivity and fever: a case report. *Am J Hosp Pharm.* 1979; 36:1565-7.
54. Garty BZ. Furosemide-associated fever: drug fever or dehydration fever? *J Pediatr.* 1997; 130: 499-500.
55. Weisenthal RW, Sinclair SH, Frank I et al. Long-term outpatient treatment of CMV retinitis with ganciclovir in AIDS patients. *Br J Ophthalmol.* 1989; 73:996-1001.
56. Greenblatt DJ, Gross PL, Harris J et al. Fatal hyperthermia following haloperidol therapy of sedative-hypnotic withdrawal. *J Clin Psychiatry.* 1978; 39:673-5.
57. Forni AL, Murray HW. Drug fever induced by heparin. *Am J Med.* 1992; 92:107.
58. Van der Klooster JM, Sućec PM, Stiegelis WF et al. Fever caused by hydroxyurea: a report of three cases and review of the literature. *Neth J Med.* 1997; 51:114-8.
59. Najean Y. Unwanted side effect of hydroxyurea. *Ann Hematol.* 1996; 72:101.
60. Starmans-Kool MJF, Fickers MMF, Pannebakker MAG. An unwanted side effect of hydroxyurea in a patient with idiopathic myelofibrosis. *Ann Hematol.* 1995; 70:279-80.
61. Lossos IS, Matzner Y. Hydroxyurea-induced fever: case report and review of the literature. *Ann Pharmacother.* 1995; 29:132-3.
62. Jacobs P, Wood L, Foster J. Hydroxyurea hypersensitivity reaction. *S Afr Med J.* 1989; 75:506.
63. Blonk MC, Ossenkoppele GJ. Hydroxyurea as a cause of drug fever in chronic myeloid leukaemia. *Neth J Med.* 1988; 32:240-2.
64. Sharon R, Tatarsky I, Ben-Arieh Y. Treatment of polycythemia vera with hydroxyurea. *Cancer.* 1986; 57:718-20.
65. Bauman JL, Shulruff S, Hasegawa GR et al. Fever caused by hydroxyurea. *Arch Intern Med.* 1981; 141:260-1.
66. Folan DW. Severe reaction to hydroxyurea. *Cutis.* 1977; 20:95.
67. Moshella SL, Greenwald MA. Psoriasis with hydroxyurea: an 18-month study of 60 patients. *Arch Dermatol.* 1973; 107:363-8.
68. Braester A, Quitt M. Hydroxyurea as a cause of drug fever. *Acta Haematol.* 2000; 104:50-1.
69. Lannemyr O, Kutti J. Hydroxyurea as a cause of drug fever in essential thrombocythaemia. *Eur J Haematol.* 1999; 62:354-5.
70. Mandell B, Shen HS, Hepburn B. Fever from ibuprofen in a patient with lupus erythematosus. *Ann Intern Med.* 1976; 85:209-10.
71. Chiodini PL, Geddes AM, Smith EG et al. Imipenem/cilastatin in the treatment of serious bacterial infections. *Rev Infect Dis.* 1985; 7(suppl 3):S490-5.
72. Committee on therapy of the American Trudeau Society. The toxicity of isoniazid. *Am Rev Tuberc.* 1953; 68:302-5.
73. Davis RS, Stoler BS. Febrile reaction to INH. *N Engl J Med.* 1977; 297:337.
74. Jacobs NF Jr, Thompson SE III. Spiking fever from isoniazid simulating a septic process. *JAMA.* 1977; 238:1759-60.
75. Dasta JF, Prior JA, Kurzrok S. Isoniazid-induced fever. *Chest.* 1979; 75:196-7.
76. Holland CL, Malasky C, Ogunkoya A et al. Rapid oral desensitization to isoniazid and rifampin. *Chest.* 1990; 98:1518-9.
77. Yust I, Vaardinou N, Fiersteter E et al. Levamisole induced allergy. *Lancet.* 1977; 1:457.
78. Friedman SA, Hirsch SE. Extreme hyperthermia after LSD ingestion. *JAMA.* 1971; 217:549-50.
79. Klock JC, Boerner U, Becker CE. Coma, hyperthermia, and bleeding associated with massive LSD overdose: a report of eight cases. *Clin Toxicol.* 1975; 8:191-203.
80. Harris A. Pyrexia and mebendazole. *Br Med J.* 1979; 2:1365.
81. Tallgren LG, Servo C. Hyperpyrexia in association with administration of L-alpha methyldopa: a report of two cases. *Acta Med Scand.* 1969; 186:223-6.
82. Glontz GE, Saslaw S. Methyldopa fever. *Arch Intern Med.* 1968; 122:445-7.
83. Klein HO, Kaminsky N. Methyldopa fever: recurrence of symptoms with resumption of therapy. *NY State J Med.* 1973; 73:448-51.
84. Parker WA. Methyldopa hyperpyrexia. *JAMA.* 1974; 228:1097.
85. Chan W. Less common side effects of methyldopa. *Med J Aust.* 1977; 2:14-5.
86. Mainzer E. A reminder—fever due to methyldopa. *N Engl J Med.* 1980; 302:174.
87. Valnes K, Hillestad L, Hansen T et al. Alpha-methyldopa and drug fever: a study of the metabolism of x-methyldopa in patients and normal subjects. *Acta Med Scand.* 1978; 204:21-5.
88. Wandless I, Evans JG, Jackson M. Fever associated with metoclopramide-induced dystonia. *Lancet.* 1980; 1:1255-6.
89. Gorad DA. Late-onset drug fever associated with minocycline. *Postgrad Med J.* 1990; 66:404-5.

90. Chueh SC, Hong JC, Huang CY et al. Drug fever caused by mycophenolate mofetil in a renal transplant recipient: a case report. *Transplant Proc.* 2000; 32:1925-6.
91. Caraway RD. Febrile reaction following nifedipine therapy. *Am Heart J.* 1984; 108:611.
92. Israel HL, Diamond P. Recurrent pulmonary infiltration and pleural effusion due to nitrofurantoin sensitivity. *N Engl J Med.* 1962; 266:1024-6.
93. Vittorio CC, Muglia JJ. Anticonvulsant hypersensitivity syndrome. *Arch Intern Med.* 1995; 155:2285.
94. Caldwell JR, Cluff LE. Adverse reactions to antimicrobial agents. *JAMA.* 1974; 230:77-80.
95. Horn B, Kabins SA. Iodide fever. *Am J Med Sci.* 1972; 264:467-71.
96. Kurtz SC, Aber RC. Potassium iodide as a cause of prolonged fever. *Arch Intern Med.* 1982; 142:1543-4.
97. Dole RR. Adverse drug reaction: chills and fever due to procainamide. *J Maine Med Assoc.* 1968; 59:28.
98. Pierach CA. Drug fever due to procainamide. *Minn Med.* 1969; 52:813-6.
99. Grenadier E, Keidar S, Marmor A et al. Quinidine and procainamide induced fever in the same patient. *Practitioner.* 1979; 222:685-6.
100. Jones SE, Morre M, Blank N et al. Hypersensitivity to procarbazine (Matulane) manifested by fever and pleuropulmonary reaction. *Cancer.* 1972; 29:498-500.
101. O'Rourke DJ, Palac RT, Holzberger PT et al. Propafenone-induced drug fever in the absence of agranulocytosis. *Clin Cardiol.* 1997; 20:662-4.
102. Astwood EB. Medical treatment of hyperthyroidism. *Bull New Engl Med Cent.* 1944; 6:1.
103. Gabrilove JL, Kent MJ. Sensitivity to thiouracil. *JAMA.* 1944; 124:504-5.
104. Moore FD. Toxic manifestations of thiouracil therapy: a cooperative study. *JAMA.* 1946; 130:315-9.
105. VanWinkle W, Hardy SM, Hazel GR et al. The chemical toxicity of thiouracil: a survey of 5745 cases. *JAMA.* 1946; 130:343-7.
106. Williams RH, Clute HM. Thiouracil in the treatment of thyrotoxicosis: a report of seventy-two cases. *N Engl J Med.* 1944; 230:657-67.
107. Fang Y, Xiao H, Tang S et al. Clinical features and treatment of drug fever caused by anti-tuberculosis drugs. *Clin Respir J.* 2016 Jul; 10:449-54. http://www.ncbi.nlm.nih.gov/m/pubmed/25401489/ (accessed 2018 Mar 5).
108. Lysy J. Oren R. Drug fever with a shift to the left. *DICP.* 1990; 24:782.
109. Foley RE, Parada EA. Drug fever of quinidine: report of a case and review of the literature. *Lahey Clin Found Bull.* 1966; 15:49-52.
110. Schultz M, Zinneman HH, Hall WH. Drug fever caused by quinine and quinidine. *Minn Med.* 1973; 56:668-70.
111. Abrams J. Quinidine fever: an unusual manifestation of quinidine allergy. *Chest.* 1973; 64:120-2.
112. Savran SV, Flamm MD Jr. Fever as a toxic reaction to quinidine. *N Engl J Med.* 1975; 292:427.
113. Tiliakos N, Waites TF. Multiform quinidine toxicity. *South Med J.* 1981; 74:1267-8.
114. Bedell SE, Kang JL. Leukocytosis and left shift associated with quinine fever. *Am J Med.* 1984; 77:345-6.
115. Hiraide A, Yoshioka T, Ohshima S. IgE-mediated drug fever due to histamine H_2-receptor blockers. *Drug Saf.* 1990; 5:455-7.
116. Cook SV, Fujiwara PI, Frieden TR. Rates and risk factors for discontinuation of rifampicin. *Int J Tuberc Lung Dis.* 2000; 4:118-22.
117. Schacherer D, Zeitoun M, Buttner R et al. Sirloimus-induced drug fever and ciclosporin-induced leukoencephalopathia with seizures in one liver transplant recipient. *World J Gastroenterol.* 2007; 13:6090-3.
118. Wax JR, Mueller S. Puerperal febrile morbidity associated with the reverse transcriptase inhibitor stavudine. *J Matern Fetal Med.* 1997; 6:118-9.
119. Feldbaum JS, Silverstein H. Streptomycin drug fever during treatment of bilateral Meniere's disease. *Arch Otolaryngol.* 1984; 110:538-39.
120. Shah KA, Greenwald E, Levin J et al. Streptozocin-induced eosinophilia and fever: a case report. *Cancer Treat Rep.* 1982; 66:1449-50.
121. Garnick MB, Ernst T, Martinez F. Acute febrile reaction to streptozocin. *N Engl J Med.* 1984; 311:798.
122. Wiener I, Rubin DA, Martinex E et al. QT prolongation and paroxysmal ventricular tachycardia occurring during fever following trimethoprim-sulfamethoxazole administration. *Mt Sinai J Med.* 1981; 48:53-5.
123. Wofsy CB. Use of trimethoprim-sulfamethoxazole in the treatment of Pneumocystis carinii pneumonia in patients with acquired immunodeficiency syndrome. *Rev Infect Dis.* 1987; 9(suppl 2):S184-94.
124. Greenberg RN. Treatment of bone, joint, and vascular-access-associated gram-positive bacterial infections with teicoplanin. *Antimicrob Agents Chemother.* 1990; 34:2392-7.
125. Jacknowitz AI. Thioridazine-induced hyperpyrexia: a case report. *Am J Hosp Pharm.* 1979; 36:674-8.
126. Brown JR, Weir AB. Drug fever from tolmetin administration. *JAMA.* 1978; 239:24.
127. Safdi MA. Fever secondary to triamterene therapy. *N Engl J Med.* 1980; 303:701.
128. Nolan PJ, D'Arcy G. Triamterene drug fever and hepatitis. *Med J Aust.* 1987; 147:262.
129. Shapiro MF. Despair, trifluoperazine, exercise, and temperature of 108°F. *Am J Psychiatry.* 1967; 124:705-7.
130. Lysy J, Oren R. Drug fever with shift to the left. *DICP* 1990; 24:782.
131. Smith, PF, Taylor CT. Vancomycin-induced neutropenia associated with fever: similarities between two immune-mediated drug reactions. *Pharmacotherapy.* 1999; 19:240-4.
132. Ishii E, Hara T, Mizuno Y, Ueda K. Vincristine-induced fever in children with leukemia and lymphoma. *Cancer.* 1988; 61:660-2.
133. Rizos EC, Milionis HJ, Elisaf MS. Fever with rash following zoledronic acid administration. *Clin Exp Rheumatol.* 2006; 24:455.
134. Mackowiak PA. Drug fever; mechanisms, maxims and misconceptions. *Am J Med Sci.* 1987; 294:275.
135. Lipsky BA, Hirschmann JV. Drug fever. *JAMA.* 1981; 245:851-4.
136. Kumar KL, Reuler JB. Drug fever. *West J Med.* 1986; 144:753-7.
137. Cunha BA. Drug fever the importance of recognition. *Postgrad Med.* 1986; 80:123-9.
138. Tierney L. Drug fever. *Am J Med Sci.* 1972; 264:473-4.
139. Neilsen JL, Lund NO. Drug fever due to nomifensine treatment in patients with endogenous depression. *Int Pharmacopsychiatry.* 1981; 16:66-8.
140. Johnson DH, Cunha BA. Drug fever. *Infect Dis Clin North Am.* 1996; 10:85-91.
141. Cunha BA. Antibiotic side effects. *Med Clin North Am.* 2001; 85:149-85.
142. Classen DC, Pestotnik SL, Evans RS et al. Adverse drug events in hospitalized patients. Excess length of stay, extra costs, and attributable mortality. *JAMA.* 1997; 277:301-6.
143. Bayard PJ, Berger TG, Jacobson MA. Drug hypersensitivity reactions and human immunodeficiency virus disease. *J Acquir Immune Defic Syndr.* 1992; 5:1237.
144. Mijch AM, Hoy JF. Unexplained fever and drug reactions as clues to HIV infection. *Med J Aust.* 1993; 158:188.
145. Pleasants RA, Walker TR, Samuelson WM. Allergic reactions to parenteral beta-lactam antibiotics in patients with cystic fibrosis. *Chest.* 1994; 106:1124.
146. Gruchalla RS. Acute drug desensitization. *Clin Exp Allergy.* 1998; 28(suppl 4):63-4.
147. Weber E, Knowles SR, Berger S et al. Rapid desensitization for chlorambucil drug fever. *Haematologica.* 2007; 92:77.
148. Castells M. Rapid desensitization for hypersensitivity reactions to medications. *Immunol Allergy Clin North Am.* 2009; 29:585.

149. Von Pirquet C, Schick B. *Serum sickness*. Baltimore, MD: Williams and Wilkins; 1951.
150. Buhner D, Grant JA. Serum sickness. *Dermatol Clin.* 1985; 3:107-17.
151. Reisman RE, Livingston A. Late-onset allergic reactions, including serum sickness, after insect stings. *J Allergy Clin Immunol.* 1989; 84:331-7.
152. Warrington RJ, Martens CJ, Rubin M et al. Immunologic studies in subjects with a serum sickness-like illness after immunization with human diploid cell rabies vaccine. *J Allergy Clin Immunol.* 1987; 79:605-10.
153. Bielory L, Gascon P, Lawley TJ et al. Human serum sickness: a prospective analysis of 35 patients treated with equine anti-thymocyte globulin for bone marrow failure. *Medicine.* 1988; 67:40-57.
154. Arkachaisri T. Serum sickness and hepatitis B vaccine including review of the literature. *J Med Assoc Thai.* 2002; 85(suppl 2): S607-12.
155. Boothpur R, Hardinger KL, Skelton RN et al. Serum sickness after treatment with rabbit antithymocyte globulin in kidney transplant recipients with previous rabbit exposure. *Am J Kidney Dis.* 2010; 55:141.
156. Karmacharya P, Poudel DR, Pathak R et al. Rituximab-induced serum sickness: a systematic review. *Semin Arthritis Rheum.* 2015; 45:334-40.
157. Tanriover B, Chuang P, Fishbach B et al. Polyclonal antibody-induced serum sickness in renal transplant recipients: treatment with therapeutic plasma exchange. *Transplantation.* 2005; 80:279.
158. Hansel TT, Kropshofer H, Singer T et al. The safety and side effects of monoclonal antibodies. *Nat Rev Drug Discov.* 2010; 9:325.
159. Hamzaoglu H, Cooper J, Alsahli M et al. Safety of infliximab in Crohn's disease: a large single-center experience. *Inflamm Bowel Dis.* 2010; 16:2109.
160. Vermeire S, Van Assche G, Rutgeerts P. Serum sickness, encephalitis and other complications of anti-cytokine therapy. *Best Pract Res Clin Gastroenterol.* 2009; 23:101.
161. Bonds RS, Kelly BC. Severe serum sickness after H1N1 influenza vaccination. *Am J Med Sci.* 2013; 345:412.
162. Warrington RJ, Martens CJ, Rubin M et al. Immunologic studies in subjects with a serum sickness-like illness after immunization with human diploid cell rabies vaccine. *J Allergy Clin Immunol.* 1987; 79:605.
163. Wise RP, Iskander J, Pratt RD et al. Postlicensure safety surveillance for 7-valent pneumococcal conjugate vaccine. *JAMA.* 2004; 292:1702.
164. Milstein JB, Gross TP, Kuritsky JN. Adverse reactions reported following receipt of Haemophilus influenzae type B vaccine: an analysis after 1 year of marketing. *Pediatrics.* 1987; 80:270.
165. Black RE, Gunn RA. Hypersensitivity reactions associated with botulinal antitoxin. *Am J Med.* 1980; 69:567.
166. Andersen JM, Tiede J. Serum sickness associated with 6-mercaptopurine in a patient with Crohn's disease. *Pharmacotherapy.* 1997; 17:173-6.
167. Chopra R, Roberts J, Warrington RJ. Severe delayed-onset hypersensitivity reactions to amoxicillin in children. *Can Med Assoc J.* 1989; 140:921-3.
168. Schiano CM. Augmentin as a cause of serum-sickness-like reaction: the urticaria-arthralgia syndrome. *Immunol Allergy Pract.* 1989; 11:25-7.
169. Platt R, Dreis MW, Kennedy DL et al. Serum sickness-like reactions to amoxicillin, cefaclor, cephalexin, and trimethoprim-sulfamethoxazole. *J Infect Dis.* 1988; 158:474-7.
170. Tatum AJ, Ditto AM, Patterson R. Severe serum sickness-like reaction to oral penicillin drugs: three case reports. *Ann Allergy Asthma Immunol.* 2001; 86:330-4.
171. Heckbert SR, Stryker WS, Coltin KL et al. Serum sickness in children after antibiotic exposure: estimates of occurrence and morbidity in a health maintenance organization population. *Am J Epidemiol.* 1990; 132:336-42.
172. Lin B, Strehlow M. Images in emergency medicine: serum sickness-like reaction to amoxicillin. *Ann Emerg Med.* 2007; 50:350, 359.
173. Yolles JC, Armenta WA, Alao AO. Serum sickness induced by bupropion. *Ann Pharmacother.* 1999; 33:931-3.
174. McCollom RA, Elbe DHT, Ritchie AH. Bupropion-induced serum sickness-like reaction. *Ann Pharmacother.* 2000; 34:471-3.
175. Wooltorton E. Bupropion (Zyban, Wellbutrin SR): reports of deaths, seizures, serum sickness. *CMAJ.* 2002; 166:68.
176. Davis JS, Boyle MJ, Hannaford R et al. Bupropion and serum sickness-like reaction. *Med J Aust.* 2001; 174:479-80.
177. Tripathi A, Greenberger PA. Bupropion hydrochloride induced serum sickness-like reaction. *Ann Allergy Asthma Immunol.* 1999; 83:165-6.
178. Hosoda N, Sunaoshi W, Shirai H et al. Anticarbamazepine antibody induced by carbamazepine in a patient with severe serum sickness. *Arch Dis Child.* 1991; 66:722-3.
179. Vial T, Pont J, Pham E et al. Cefaclor-associated serum sickness-like disease: eight cases and review of the literature. *Ann Pharmacother.* 1992; 26:910-4.
180. McCue JD. Delayed detection of serum sickness caused by oral antimicrobials. *Adv Ther.* 1990; 7:22-7.
181. Leng M, Anderson PO. Serum sickness with cefaclor. *Drug Intell Clin Pharm.* 1985; 19:186-7.
182. Ackley AM, Felsher J. Adverse reaction to cefaclor. *South Med J.* 1981; 74:1550.
183. Callahan CW, Musci MN, Sanatucci TF. Cefaclor serum sickness-like reactions: report of a case and review of the literature. *J Am Osteopath Assoc.* 1985: 450-2.
184. Johnson T, Stern C, Field C. Serum sickness in a child treated with cefaclor. *J Ark Med Soc.* 1983; 80:110.
185. Lovell SJ, Reid WD. Serum sickness with cefaclor. *Can Med Assoc J.* 1982; 126:1032.
186. Murray DL, Singer DA, Singer AG et al. Cefaclor: a cluster of adverse reactions. *N Engl J Med.* 1980; 303:1003.
187. Hebert AA, Sigman ES, Levey M. Serum sickness-like reactions from cefaclor in children. *J Am Acad Dermatol.* 1991; 25:805-8.
188. Yerushalmi J, Azulunov A, Halevy S. Serum sickness-like reactions. *Cutis.* 2002; 69:395-7.
189. Boyd IW. Cefaclor-associated serum sickness. *Med J Aust.* 1998; 169:443-4.
190. Brucculeri M, Charlton M, Serur D. Serum sickness-like reaction associated with cefazolin. *BMC Clin Pharmacol.* 2006; 6:3.
191. Lowery N, Kearns GL, Young RA et al. Serum sickness-like reactions associated with cefprozil therapy. *J Pediatr.* 1994; 125:325-8.
192. Baniasadi S, Fahimi F, Mansouri D. Serum sickness-like reaction associated with cefuroxime and ceftriaxone. *Ann Pharmacother.* 2007; 41:1318-9.
193. Katta R, Anusuri V. Serum sickness-like reaction to cefuroxime: a case report and review of the literature. *J Drugs Dermatol.* 2007; 6:747-8.
194. Slama TG. Serum sickness-like illness associated with ciprofloxacin. *Antimicrob Agents Chemother.* 1990; 34:904-5.
195. Guharoy SR. Serum sickness secondary to ciprofloxacin use. *Vet Hum Toxicol.* 1994; 36:540-1.
196. Phillips EJ, Knowles SR, Shear NH. Serum sickness-like reaction associated with clopidogrel. *J Clin Pharmacol.* 2003; 56:583.
197. Garg A, Radvan J, Jopkinson N. Clopidogrel associated with acute arthritis. *Br Med J.* 2000; 320:483.
198. Shapiro LE, Knowles SR, Shear NG. Fluoxetine-induced serum sickness-like reaction. *Ann Pharmacother.* 1997; 31:927.
199. Miller L, Bowman R, Mann D et al. A case of fluoxetine-induced serum sickness. *Am J Psychiatry.* 1989; 146:1616-7.
200. Vincent A, Doubille M, Baruch P. Serum sickness induced by fluoxetine. *Am J Psychiatry.* 1991; 148:1602-3.
201. Leznoff A, Binkley KE, Joffee RT et al. Adverse cutaneous reactions associated with fluoxetine strategy for reintroduction of this drug in selected patients. *J Clin Psychopharmacol.* 1992; 12:355-7.
202. Colton RL, Amir J, Mimouni M et al. Serum sickness-like reaction associated with griseofulvin. *Ann Pharmacother.* 2004; 38:609-11.

203. Gamarra RM, McGraw SD, Drelichman VS et al. Serum sickness-like reactions in patients receiving intravenous infliximab. *J Emerg Med.* 2006; 30:41-4.
204. Bielory L. Serum sickness from iron-dextran administration. *Acta Haematol.* 1990; 83:166-8.
205. Park H, Knowles S, Shear NH. Serum sickness-like reaction to itraconazole. *Ann Pharmacother.* 1998; 32:1249.
206. Ralph ED, John M, Rieder MJ et al. Serum sickness-like reaction possibly associated with meropenem use. *Clin Infect Dis.* 2003; 36:149-51.
207. Weart CW, Hyman LC. Serum sickness associated with metronidazole. *South Med J.* 1983; 76:410-1.
208. Landau M, Eyal S, Brenner S. Minocycline-induced serum sickness-like reaction. *J Eur Acad Dermatol Venereol.* 2000; 14:65-8.
209. Levenson T, Masood D, Patterson R. Minocycline-induced serum sickness. *Allergy Asthma Proc.* 1996; 17:79-81.
210. Malakar S, Dhar S, Malakar RS. Is serum sickness an uncommon adverse effect of minocycline treatment? *Arch Dermatol.* 2001; 137:100-1.
211. Puyana J, Urena V, Quirce S et al. Serum sickness-like syndrome associated with minocycline therapy. *Allergy.* 1990; 45:313-5.
212. Knowles SR, Shapiro L, Shear NH. Serious adverse reactions induced by minocycline. *Arch Dermatol.* 1996; 132:934-9.
213. Mohammed S, Jamal AZ, Robison LR. Serum sickness-like illness associated with *N*-acetylcysteine therapy. *Ann Pharmacother.* 1994; 28:285.
214. Krumbholz M, Pellkofer H, Gold F et al. Delayed allergic reaction to evodopamy associated with early formation of neutralizing antibodies. *Arch Neurol.* 2007; 64:1331-3.
215. Erffmeyer JE. Penicillin allergy. *Clin Rev Allergy.* 1986; 4:171-88.
216. Yen MC, Pisczek JE, Mintzer DL. Serum sickness-like syndrome associated with propranolol therapy. *Postgrad Med.* 1983; 74:291-4.
217. Parra FM, Elias MJP, Cuevas M et al. Serum sickness-like illness associated with rifampicin. *Ann Allergy.* 1994; 73:123-5.
218. Herishanu Y. Rituximab-induced serum sickness. *Am J Hematol.* 2002; 70:329-34.
219. D'Arcy CA, Mannik M. Serum sickness secondary to treatment with the murine-human chimeric antibody IDEC-C2B8 (rituximab). *Arthritis Rheum.* 2001; 44:1717-8.
220. Todd DJ, Helfgott SM. Serum sickness following treatment with rituximab. *J Rheumatol.* 2007; 34:430-3.
221. Finger E, Scheinberg M. Development of serum sickness-like symptoms after rituximab infusion in two patients with severe hypergammaglobulinemia. *J Clin Rheumatol.* 2007; 13:94-5.
222. Catuogno M, Rezai S, Priori R et al. Serum sickness associated with rituximab in a patient with hepatitis C virus-related mixed cryoglobinaemia. *Rheumatology (Oxford).* 2005; 44:406.
223. Gottenberg JE, Guillevin L, Lambotte O et al. Tolerance and short term efficacy of rituximab in 43 patients with systemic autoimmune diseases. *Ann Rheum Dis.* 2005; 64:913-20.
224. Hellerstedt B, Ahmed A. Delayed-type hypersensitivity reaction or serum sickness after rituximab treatment. *Ann Oncol.* 2003; 14:1792.
225. Totty WG, Romano T, Benian GM et al. Serum sickness following streptokinase therapy. *AJR Am J Roentgenol.* 1982; 138;143-4.
226. McGrath KG, Zeffren B, Alexander J et al. Allergic reactions to streptokinase consistent with anaphylactic or antigen-antibody complex-mediated damage. *J Allergy Clin Immunol.* 1985; 76:453-7.
227. Schweitzer DH, Van der Wall EE, Bosker HA et al. Serum sickness-like illness as a complication after streptokinase therapy for acute myocardial infarction. *Cardiology.* 1991; 78:68-71.
228. Clesham GJ, Terry HJ, Jalihal S et al. Serum sickness and purpura following intravenous streptokinase. *J Royal Soc Med.* 1992; 85:638-9.
229. Dakik H, Salti I, Haidar R et al. Ticlopidine associated with acute arthritis. *Br Med J.* 2002; 324:27.
230. Russo EA, Iacucci M, Lindsay JO et al. Survey on the use of adalimumab as maintenance therapy in Crohn's disease in England and Ireland. *Eur J Gastroenterol Hepatol.* 2010; 22:334.
231. Abu-Elmagd KM, Costa G, Bond GJ et al. A decade of experience with a single dose of rabbit antithymocyte globulin or alemtuzumab pretreatment for intestinal and multivisceral transplantation. *Clin Transpl.* 2012; 155-66.
232. Bayraktar F, Akinci B, Demirkan F et al. Serum sickness-like reactions associated with type III insulin allergy responding to plasmapheresis. *Diabet Med.* 2009; 26:659.
233. Pilette C, Coppens N, Houssiau FA, Rodenstein DO. Severe serum sickness-like syndrome after omalizumab therapy for asthma. *J Allergy Clin Immunol.* 2007; 120:972.
234. Sylvestre DL, Ravetch JV. Fc receptors initiate the Arthus reaction: redefining the inflammatory cascade. *Science.* 1994; 265:1095.
235. Clynes R, Dumitru C, Ravetch JV. Uncoupling of immune complex formation and kidney damage in autoimmune glomerulonephritis. *Science.* 1998; 279:1052.
236. Ravetch JV, Clynes RA. Divergent roles for Fc receptors and complement in vivo. *Annu Rev Immunol.* 1998; 16:421.
237. Roujeau JC, Stern RS. Severe adverse cutaneous reactions to drugs. *N Engl J Med.* 1994; 331:1272-85.
238. Prussick R, Knowles S, Shear N. Cutaneous drug reactions. *Curr Probl Dermatol.* 1994; 6:83-122.
239. Borden J, Fonkalsrud E, Newcomer V. Snake bite: treatment by isolation perfusion technique. *Surgery.* 1961; 49:303.
240. Bengtsson B, Lundmark J, Walinder J. No crossover reactions to citalopram or paroxetine among patients hypersensitive to zimeldine. *Br J Psychiatry.* 1991; 158:853-5.
241. Faft ML, Petrov AA. Desensitization protocol for rituximab-induced serum sickness. *Curr Drug Saf.* 2014; 9:240.
242. Delay J, Pichot P, Lempérière T et al. Un neuroleptique majeur non phénothiazinique et non réserpinique, l'haloperidol, dans le traitement des psychoses. *Ann Med Psychol (Paris).* 1960; 118:145-52.
243. Amdurski S, Radwan M, Levi A et al. A therapeutic trial of amantadine in haloperidol-induced neuroleptic malignant syndrome. *J Clin Psychiatry.* 1987; 48:69-73.
244. Hermesh H, Huberman M, Radvan H et al. Recurrent neuroleptic malignant syndrome due to tiapride and haloperidol: the possible role of D-2 dopamine receptors. *J Nerv Ment Dis.* 1984; 172:692-5.
245. Lannas PA, Pachar JV. A fatal case of neuroleptic malignant syndrome. *Med Sci Law.* 1993; 33:68-88.
246. Stoudemire A, Clayton L. Successful use of clozapine in a patient with a history of neuroleptic malignant syndrome. *J Neuropsychiatry Clin Neurosci.* 1989; 1:303.
247. Bernstein WB, Scherokman B. Neuroleptic malignant syndrome in a patient with acquired immunodeficiency syndrome. *Acta Neurol Scand.* 1986; 73:636-7.
248. Shaw A, Matthews EE. Postoperative neuroleptic malignant syndrome. *Anaesthesia.* 1995; 50:246-7.
249. Patel P, Bristow G. Postoperative neuroleptic malignant syndrome: a case report. *Can J Anaesth.* 1987; 34:515-8.
250. Bakri YN, Khan R, Subhi J et al. Neuroleptic malignant syndrome associated with metoclopramide antiemetic therapy. *Gynecol Oncol.* 1992; 189-90.
251. Donnet A, Harle JR, Dumont JC et al. Neuroleptic malignant syndrome induced by metoclopramide. *Biomed Pharmacother.* 1991; 45:461-2.
252. Henderson A, Longdon P. Fulminant metoclopramide induced neuroleptic malignant syndrome rapidly responsive to intravenous dantrolene. *Aust N Z J Med.* 1991; 21:742-3.
253. Heyland D, Sauve M. Neuroleptic malignant syndrome without the use of neuroleptics. *CMAJ.* 1991; 145:817-9.
254. Lev R, Clark RF. Neuroleptic malignant syndrome presenting without fever: case report and review of the literature. *J Emerg Med.* 1994; 12:49-55.
255. Susman VL, Addonizio G. Reinduction of neuroleptic malignant syndrome by lithium. *J Clin Psychopharmacol.* 1987; 7:334-41.

256. Gill J, Singh H, Nugent K. Acute lithium intoxication and neuroleptic malignant syndrome. *Pharmacotherapy.* 2003; 23:811-5.

257. Berry N, Pradhan S, Sagar R et al. Neuroleptic malignant syndrome in an adolescent receiving olanzapine-lithium combination therapy. *Pharmacotherapy.* 2003; 23:255-9.

258. Ananth J, Johnson KM, Levander EM et al. Diabetic ketoacidosis, neuroleptic malignant syndrome, and myocardial infarction in a patient taking risperidone and lithium carbonate. *J Clin Psychiatry.* 2004; 65:724.

259. Sparrow P, Murnaghan D, Kearney P et al. Acute cardiac failure in neuroleptic malignant syndrome. *Eur J Heart Fail.* 2003; 5:575-8.

260. Bourgeois JA, Kahn DR. Neuroleptic malignant syndrome following administration of risperidone and lithium. *J Clin Psychopharmacol.* 2003; 23:315-7.

261. Gupta S, Racaniello AA. Neuroleptic malignant syndrome associated with amoxapine and lithium in an older adult. *Ann Clin Psychiatry.* 2000; 12:107-9.

262. Nisijima K, Kusakabe Y, Ohtuka K et al. Addition of carbamazepine to long-term treatment with neuroleptics may induce neuroleptic malignant syndrome. *Biol Psychiatry.* 1998; 4:930-1.

263. O'Griofa FM, Voris JC. Neuroleptic malignant syndrome associated with carbamazepine. *South Med J.* 1991; 84:1378-80.

264. Muller T, Becker T, Fritze J. Neuroleptic malignant syndrome after clozapine plus carbamazepine. *Lancet.* 1988; 2:1500.

265. Woolf DC. Neuroleptic malignant syndrome associated with phenytoin intoxication. *S Afr Med J.* 1988; 7:620-1.

266. Taylor NE, Schwartz HI. Neuroleptic malignant syndrome following amoxapine overdose. *J Nerv Ment Dis.* 1988; 176:249-51.

267. Chakraborty N, Johnston T. Aripiprazole and neuroleptic malignant syndrome. *Int Clin Psychopharmacol.* 2004; 19:351-3.

268. Strawn JR. Aripiprazole and the neuroleptic malignant syndrome. *Schizophr Res.* 2006; 85:298-9.

269. Brunelle J, Guigueno S, Gouin P et al. Aripiprazole and neuroleptic malignant syndrome. *J Clin Psychopharmacol.* 2007; 27:212-3.

270. Evcimen H, Alici-Evcimen Y, Basil B et al. Neuroleptic malignant syndrome induced by low dose aripiprazole in first episode psychosis. *J Psychiatr Pract.* 2007; 13:117-9.

271. Ali S, Pearlman RL, Upadhyay A et al. Neuroleptic malignant syndrome with aripiprazole and lithium: a case report. *J Clin Psychopharmacol.* 2006; 26:434-6.

272. Srephichit S, Sanchez R, Bourgeois JA. Neuroleptic malignant syndrome and aripiprazole in an antipsychotic-naïve patient. *J Clin Psychopharmacol.* 2006; 26:94-5.

273. Palakurthi HB, Parvin MM, Kaplan S. Neuroleptic malignant syndrome from aripiprazole in an agitated pediatric patient. *Clin Neuropharmacol.* 2007; 30:47-51.

274. Duggal HS. Clozapine-induced neuroleptic malignant syndrome and subdural hematoma. *J Neuropsychiatry Clin Neurosci.* 2004; 16:118-9.

275. Tenebein M. The neuroleptic malignant syndrome: occurrence in a 15-year-old boy and recovery with bromocriptine therapy. *Pediatr Neurosci.* 1985–86; 12:161-4.

276. Lew TY, Tollefson G. Chlorpromazine-induced neuroleptic malignant syndrome and its response to diazepam. *Biol Psychiatry.* 1983; 18:1441-6.

277. Tsai G, Crisostomo G, Rosenblatt ML et al. Neuroleptic malignant syndrome associated with clozapine treatment. *Ann Clin Psychiatry.* 1995; 7:91-5.

278. Miller DD, Sharafuddin MJA, Kathol RG. A case of clozapine-induced neuroleptic malignant syndrome. *J Clin Psychiatry.* 1991; 52:99-101.

279. Anderson ES, Powers PS. Neuroleptic malignant syndrome associated with clozapine use. *J Clin Psychiatry.* 1991; 52:102-4.

280. Daa Gupta K, Young A. Clozapine-induced neuroleptic malignant syndrome. *J Clin Psychiatry.* 1991; 52:105-7.

281. Thornberg SA, Ereshefsky L. Neuroleptic malignant syndrome associated with clozapine monotherapy. *Pharmacotherapy.* 1993; 13:510-4.

282. Goates MG, Escobar J. An apparent neuroleptic malignant syndrome without extrapyramidal symptoms upon initiation of clozapine therapy: report of a case and results of a clozapine rechallenge. *J Clin Psychopharmacol.* 1992; 12:139-40.

283. Najib J. Neuroleptic malignant syndrome: a case report and review of treatment. *Hosp Pharm.* 1997; 32:512-8.

284. Matsumota T, Kawanishi C, Isojima D et al. Neuroleptic malignant syndrome induced by donepezil. *Int J Neuropsychopharmacol.* 2004; 7:101-3.

285. So PC. Neuroleptic malignant syndrome induced by droperidol. *Hong Kong Med J.* 2001; 7:101-3.

286. Edgar J. Droperidol-induced neuroleptic malignant syndrome. *Hosp Med.* 1999; 60:448-9.

287. Portel L, Hilbert G, Gruson D et al. Malignant hyperthermia and neuroleptic syndrome in a patient during treatment for acute asthma. *Acta Anaesthesiol Scand.* 1999; 43:107-10.

288. Burke C, Fulda GJ, Castellano J. Neuroleptic malignant syndrome in a trauma patient. *J Trauma.* 1995; 39:796-8.

289. Meltzer HY. Rigidity, hyperpyrexia and coma following fluphenazine enanthate. *Psychopharmacologia.* 1973; 29:337-46.

290. Aruna AS, Murungi JH. Fluphenazine-induced neuroleptic malignant syndrome in a schizophrenic patient. *Ann Pharmacother.* 2005; 39:1131-5.

291. Borovicka MC, Bond LC, Gaughan KM. Ziprasidone and lithium-induced neuroleptic malignant syndrome. *Ann Pharmacother.* 2006; 40:139-42.

292. Duggal HS. Neuroleptic malignant syndrome precipitated by promethazine and lorazepam. *Aust N Z J Psychiatry.* 2001; 35:250-1.

293. Ewert AL, Loek J, Wells B et al. Neuroleptic malignant syndrome associated with loxapine. *J Clin Psychiatry.* 1983; 44:37-8.

294. Gradon JD. Neuroleptic malignant syndrome possibly caused by molindone hydrochloride. *Drug Intell Clin Pharm.* 1991; 25:1071-2.

295. Slack T, Stoudemire A. Reinstitution of neuroleptic treatment with molindone in a patient with a history of neuroleptic malignant syndrome. *Gen Hosp Psychiatry.* 1989; 11:365-7.

296. Filice GA, McDougall BC, Ercan-Fang N et al. Neuroleptic malignant syndrome associated with olanzapine. *Ann Pharmacother.* 1998; 32:1158-9.

297. Goveas JS, Hermida A. Olanzapine induced "typical" neuroleptic malignant syndrome. *J Clin Psychopharmacol.* 2003; 23:101-2.

298. Stanfield SC, Privette T. Neuroleptic malignant syndrome associated with olanzapine therapy: a case report. *J Emerg Med.* 2000; 19:355-7.

299. Burkhard PR, Vingerhoets FJ, Alberque C et al. Olanzapine-induced neuroleptic malignant syndrome. *Arch Gen Psychiatry.* 1999; 56:101-2.

300. Johnon V, Bruxner G. Neuroleptic malignant syndrome associated with olanzapine. *Aust N Z J Psychiatry.* 1998; 32:884-6.

301. Moltz DA, Coeytaux RR. Case report: possible neuroleptic malignant syndrome associated with olanzapine. *J Clin Psychopharmacol.* 1998; 18:485-6.

302. Hanel RA, Sandmann MC, Kranich M et al. Neuroleptic malignant syndrome: a case report of a recurrence related to olanzapine. *Arq Neuropsiquiatr.* 1998; 56:833-7.

303. Margolese HC, Chouinard G. Olanzapine-induced neuroleptic malignant syndrome with mental retardation. *Am J Psychiatry.* 1999; 156:1836.

304. Levenson JL. Neuroleptic malignant syndrome after the initiation of olanzapine. *J Clin Psychopharmacol.* 1999; 19:477-8.

305. Nyfort-Hansen K, Alderman CP. Possible neuroleptic malignant syndrome associated with olanzapine. *Ann Pharmacother.* 2000; 34:667.

306. Kunz M, Gomes FA, Tramontina JF et al. Late-onset neuroleptic malignant syndrome in a patient using olanzapine. *J Clin Psychopharmacol.* 2007; 27:303-4.

307. Chungh DS, Kim BN, Cho SC. Neuroleptic malignant syndrome due to three atypical antipsychotics in a child. *J Psychopharmacol.* 2005; 19:422-5.
308. Stevens DL, Lee MR, Padua Y. Olanzapine-associated neuroleptic malignant syndrome in a patient receiving concomitant rivastigmine therapy. *Pharmacotherapy.* 2008; 28:403-5.
309. Duggal HS. Possible neuroleptic malignant syndrome associated with paliperidone. *J Neuropsychiatry Clin Neurosci.* 2007; 19:477-8.
310. Zohar Y, Talmi YP, Sabo R et al. Neuroleptic malignant syndrome during perphenazine treatment in a patient with head and neck cancer: a case report. *Otolaryngol Head Neck Surg.* 1992; 106;206-8.
311. Guerrero RM, Shifrar KA. Diagnosis and treatment of neuroleptic malignant syndrome. *Clin Pharm.* 1988; 7:697-701.
312. Nielsen D, Aunsholt NA, Andersen PT. Neuroleptic malignant syndrome during perphenazine treatment. *Pharmacol Toxicol.* 1987; 60:221-2.
313. Chan-Tack KM. Neuroleptic malignant syndrome due to promethazine. *South Med J.* 1999; 92:1017-8.
314. Hatch CD, Lund BC, Perry PJ. Failed challenge with quetiapine after neuroleptic malignant syndrome with conventional antipsychotics. *Pharmacotherapy.* 2001; 21:1003-6.
315. Stanley AK, Hunter J. Possible neuroleptic malignant syndrome with quetiapine. *Br J Psychiatry.* 2000; 176:497.
316. Kobayashi A, Kawanishi C, Matsumura T et al. Quetiapine-induced neuroleptic malignant syndrome in dementia with Lewy bodies: a case report. *Prog Neuropsychopharmacol Biol Psychiatry.* 2006; 30:1170-2.
317. Matsumoto R, Kitabayashi Y, Nakatomi Y et al. Neuroleptic malignant syndrome induced by quetiapine and fluvoxamine. *Am J Psychiatry.* 2005; 162:812.
318. Sechi G, Agnetti V, Masuri R et al. Risperidone, neuroleptic malignant syndrome and probable dementia with Lewy bodies. *Prog Neuropsychopharmacol Biol Psychiatry.* 2000; 24:1043-51.
319. Norris B, Angeles V, Eisenstein R et al. Neuroleptic malignant syndrome with delayed onset of fever following risperidone administration. *Ann Pharmacother.* 2006; 40:2260-4.
320. Zammit GK, Sullivan TB. Thioridazine and neuroleptic malignant syndrome. *Biol Psychiatry.* 1987; 22:1296-7.
321. Petzinger GM, Bressman SB. A case of tetrabenazine induced neuroleptic malignant syndrome after prolonged treatment. *Mov Disord.* 1997; 12:246-8.
322. Levenson JL. Neuroleptic malignant syndrome. *Am J Psychiatry.* 1985; 142:1137-45.
323. Lappa A, Podesta M, Capelli O et al. Successful treatment of a complicated case of neuroleptic malignant syndrome. *Intensive Care Med.* 2002; 28:976-7.
324. Lee MK, Ong SB, Tan CT et al. Neuroleptic malignant syndrome in Malaysia: a university hospital experience. *Med J Malaysia.* 1992; 47:200-7.
325. Montalto M. A malignant reaction to trifluoperazine (Stelazine). *Aust Fam Physician.* 1990; 19:1589-90.
326. Ozen ME, Yumru M, Savas HA et al. Neuroleptic malignant syndrome induced by ziprasidone on the second day of treatment. *World J Biol Psychiatry.* 2007; 8:42-4.
327. Guanci N, Aggarwal R, Schleifer S. Atypical neuroleptic malignant syndrome associated with iloperidone administration. *Psychosomatics.* 2012; 53:603-5.
328. Ishioka M, Yasui-Furukori N, Hashimoto K, Sugawara N. Neuroleptic malignant syndrome induced by lamotrigine. *Clin Neuropharmacol.* 2013; 36:131-2.
329. Ozdemir A, Aksoy-Poyraz C, Kilic-Yener E. Possible paliperidone-induced neuroleptic malignant syndrome: a case report. *J Neuropsychiatry Clin Neurosci.* 2012; 24:E22-3.
330. Verma R, Junewar V, Rathaur BP. An atypical case of neuroleptic malignant syndrome precipitated by valproate. *BMJ Rep.* 2014; 2014. pii: bcr2013202578.
331. Meythaler JM, Roper JF, Brunner RC. Cyproheptadine for intrathecal baclofen withdrawal. *Arch Phys Med Rehab.* 2003; 84:638-42.
332. Reeves RK, Stolp-Smith, KA, Christopherson MW. Hyperthermia, rhabdomyolysis, and disseminated intravascular coagulation associated with baclofen pump catheter failure. *Arch Phys Med Rehab.* 1998; 79:353-6.
333. Kao LW, Amin Y, Kirk MA et al. Intrathecal baclofen withdrawal mimicking sepsis. *J Emerg Med.* 2003; 24:423-7.
334. Turner MR, Gainsborough N. Neuroleptic malignant-like syndrome after abrupt withdrawal of baclofen. *J Psychopharmacol.* 2001; 15:61-3.
335. Mandac BR, Hurvita EA, Nelson VS. Hyperthermia associated with baclofen withdrawal and increased spasticity. *Arch Phys Med Rehab.* 1993; 74:96-7.
336. Rosebush P, Stewart T. A prospective analysis of 24 episodes of NMS. *Am J Psychiatry.* 1989; 146:717-25.
337. Dickey W. The neuroleptic malignant syndrome. *Prog Neurobiol.* 1991; 36:425-36.
338. Caroff SN. The neuroleptic malignant syndrome. *J Clin Psychiatry.* 1980; 41:79-83.
339. Gratz SS, Levinson DF, Simpson GM. The treatment and management of neuroleptic malignant syndrome. *Prog Neuropsychopharmacol Biol Psychiatry.* 1992; 16:425-43.
340. Shalev A, Munitz H. The neuroleptic malignant syndrome: agent and host interaction. *Acta Psychiatr Scand.* 1986; 73:337-47.
341. Deng MZ, Chen GQ, Phillips MR. Neuroleptic malignant syndrome in 12 of 9,792 Chinese inpatients exposed to neuroleptics: a prospective study. *Am J Psychiatry.* 1990; 147:1149-55.
342. Totten VY, Hirschenstein E, Hew P. Neuroleptic malignant syndrome presenting without initial fever: a case report. *J Emerg Med.* 1994; 12:43-7.
343. Wells AJ, Sommi RW, Crismon ML. Neuroleptic rechallenge after neuroleptic malignant syndrome: case report and literature review. *Drug Intell Clin Pharm.* 1988; 22:475-80.
344. Gurrera RJ, Simpson JC, Tsuang MT. Meta-analytic evidence of systematic bias in estimates of neuroleptic malignant syndrome incidence. *Compr Psychiatry.* 2007; 48:205-11.
345. Atityanjee, Aderibigbe YA, Matthews T. Epidemiology of neuroleptic malignant syndrome. *Clin Neuropharmacol.* 1999; 22:151-8.
346. Keck PE, Pope HG, McElroy SL. Frequency and presentation of neuroleptic malignant syndrome: a prospective study. *Am J Psychiatry.* 1987; 144:1344-6.
347. Paden MS, Franjic L, Halcomb E. Hyperthermia caused by drug interactions and adverse reactions. *Emerg Med Clin.* 2013; 31:1035-44.
348. Keck PE, Pope HG, Cohen BM et al. Risk factors for neuroleptic malignant syndrome: a case-control study. *Arch Gen Psychiatry.* 1989; 6:914-8.
349. Viejo LF, Morales V, Puñal P et al. Risk factors in neuroleptic malignant syndrome: a case-control study. *Acta Psychiatr Scand.* 2003; 107:45-9.
350. Velamoor VR, Swamy GN, Parmar RS et al. Management of suspected neuroleptic malignant syndrome. *Can J Psychiatry.* 1995; 40:545-50.
351. Velamoor VR, Norman RM, Caroff SN et al. Progression of symptoms in neuroleptic malignant syndrome. *J Nerv Ment Dis.* 1994; 182:168-73.
352. Ito T, Shibata K, Watanabe A, Akabane J. Neuroleptic malignant syndrome following withdrawal of amantadine in a patient with influenza A encephalopathy. *Eur J Pediatr.* 2001; 160:401.
353. Freidman JH, Feinberg SS, Feldman RG. A Neuroleptic malignant-like syndrome due to levodopa therapy withdrawal. *JAMA.* 1985; 254:2792-5.
354. Musselman ME, Saely S. Diagnosis and treatment of drug-induced hyperthermia. *Am J Health-Syst Pharm.* 2013; 70:34-42.

355. McAllen KJ, Schwartz DR. Adverse drug reactions resulting in hyperthermia in the intensive care unit. *Crit Care Med.* 2010; 38(suppl 6):S244-52.
356. Caroff SN, Mann SC, Lazarus A et al. Neuroleptic malignant syndrome: diagnostic issues. *Psychiatr Ann.* 1991; 21:130-47.
357. Caroff SN, Mann SC. Neuroleptic malignant syndrome. *Med Clin North Am.* 1993; 77:185.
358. Caroff SN, Mann SC, Campbell C. Atypical antipsychotics and neuroleptic malignant syndrome. *Psychiatr Ann.* 2000; 5:314-21.
359. Farver DK. Neuroleptic malignant syndrome induced by atypical antipsychotics. *Expert Opin Drug Saf.* 2003; 2:21-35.
360. Ananth J, Parameswaran S, Gunatilake S et al. Neuroleptic malignant syndrome and atypical antipsychotic drugs. *J Clin Psychiatry.* 2004; 65:464-70.
361. David M, Remy C. Case report: possible neuroleptic malignant syndrome associated with olanzapine. *J Clin Psychopharmacol.* 1998; 18:485-6.
362. White DAC, Robins AH. Catatonia: harbinger of the neuroleptic malignant syndrome. *Br J Psychiatry.* 1991; 158:419-21.
363. White DAC. Catatonia and the neuroleptic malignant syndrome: a single entity? *Br J Psychiatry.* 1992; 161:558-60.
364. Woodbury MM, Woodbury MA. Neuroleptic-induced catatonia as a stage in the progression toward neuroleptic malignant syndrome. *J Am Acad Child Adolesc Psychiatry.* 1992; 31:1161-4.
365. Mann SC, Caroff SN, Bleier HR et al. Lethal catatonia. *Am J Psychiatry.* 1986; 143:1374-81.
366. Osman AA, Khurasani MH. Lethal catatonia and neuroleptic malignant syndrome: a dopamine receptor shut-down hypothesis. *Br J Psychiatry.* 1994; 165:548-50.
367. Carroll BT, Graham KT, Thalassinos AJ. A common pathogenesis of the serotonin syndrome, catatonia, and neuroleptic malignant syndrome. *J Neuropsychiatry Clin Neurosci.* 2001; 13:150.
368. Kogoj A, Velikonja I. Olanzapine induced neuroleptic malignant syndrome: a case review. *Hum Psychopharmacol.* 2003; 18:301-9.
369. Silva RR, Munoz DM, Alpert M et al. Neuroleptic malignant syndrome in children and adolescents. *J Am Acad Child Adolesc Psychiatry.* 1999; 38:187-94.
370. Sachdev PS. A rating scale for neuroleptic malignant syndrome. *Psychiatry Res.* 2005; 135:249-56.
371. Guerrera RJ, Caroff SN, Cohen A et al. An international consensus study of neuroleptic malignant syndrome diagnostic criteria using the Delphi method. *J Clin Psychiatry.* 2011; 72:1222.
372. Sokoro AH, Zivot J, Ariano RE. Neuroleptic malignant syndrome versus serotonin syndrome: the search for a diagnostic tool. *Ann Pharmacother.* 2011; 45:E50.
373. Yamashita T, Fujii Y, Misawa F. Neuroleptic malignant syndrome associated with risperidone long-acting injection: a case report. *J Clin Psychopharmacol.* 2013; 33:127-9.
374. Connelly MA, Fowler EK. Neuroleptic malignant syndrome. *J Am Board Fam Pract.* 1992; 5:327-31.
375. Caroff SN, Mann SC. Neuroleptic malignant syndrome. *Med Clin North Am.* 1993; 77:185-202.
376. Lazarus A. Neuroleptic malignant syndrome and preexisting brain damage. *J Neuropsychiatry Clin Neurosci.* 1992; 4:185-7.
377. Stockman M, Olson J, Gorbien M. Neuroleptic malignant syndrome with clozapine use in pre-senilin-1 Alzheimer's disease. *J Am Geriatr Soc.* 2001; 49:S89-90.
378. Heiman-Patterson TD. Neuroleptic malignant syndrome and malignant hyperthermia: important issues for the medical consultant. *Med Clin North Am.* 1993; 77:477-92.
379. Kornhuber J, Weller M. Neuroleptic malignant syndrome. *Curr Opin Neurol.* 1994; 7:353-57.
380. Addonizio G, Susman VL, Roth SD. Neuroleptic malignant syndrome: review and analysis of 115 cases. *Biol Psychiatry.* 1987; 22:1004-20.
381. Parikh AM, Camara EG. Neuroleptic malignant syndrome. *Am Fam Physician.* 1988; 37:296-8.
382. Hermesh H, Aizenberg D, Lapidot M et al. Risk of malignant hyperthermia among patients with neuroleptic malignant syndrome and their families. *Am J Psychiatry.* 1988; 145:1431-4.
383. Deuschal G, Oepen G, Hermle L et al. Neuroleptic malignant syndrome: observations on altered consciousness. *Pharmacopsychiatry.* 1987; 20:168-79.
384. Otani K, Horiuchi M, Kondo T et al. Is the predisposition to neuroleptic malignant syndrome genetically transmitted? *Br J Psychiatry.* 1991; 158:850-3.
385. Mihara K, Kondo T, Suzuki A et al. Relationship between functional dopamine D2 and D3 receptors gene polymorphisms and neuroleptic malignant syndrome. *Am J Med Genet B Neuropsychiatr Genet.* 2003; 117B:57-60.
386. Allsop P, Twigley AJ. The neuroleptic malignant syndrome: case report with review of the literature. *Anaesthesia.* 1987; 42:49-53.
387. Caroff SN, Mann SC, Keck PE et al. Residual catatonic state following neuroleptic malignant syndrome. *J Clin Psychopharmacol.* 2000; 20:257-9.
388. Nakamura M, Yasunaga H, Miyata H et al. Mortality of neuroleptic malignant syndrome induced by typical and atypical antipsychotic drugs: a propensity-matched analysis from the Japanese Diagnosis Procedure Combination database. *J Clin Psychiatry.* 2012; 73:427.
389. Bhanushali MJ, Tuite PJ. The evaluation and management of patients with neuroleptic malignant syndrome. *Neurol Clin.* 2004; 22:389-411.
390. Labuda A, Cullen N. Brain injury following neuroleptic malignant syndrome: case report and review of the literature. *Brain Inj.* 2006; 20:775-8.
391. Rosebush P, Stewart TD, Glenberg AJ. Twenty neuroleptic challenges after neuroleptic malignant syndrome in 15 patients. *J Clin Psychiatry.* 1989; 50:295-8.
392. Harsch HH. Neuroleptic malignant syndrome: physiological and laboratory findings in a series of nine cases. *J Clin Psychiatry.* 1987; 48:328-33.
393. Pelonero AL, Levenson JL, Silverman JJ. Neuroleptic therapy following neuroleptic malignant syndrome. *Psychosomatics.* 1988; 26:946-8.
394. Caroff SN, Mann SC. Neuroleptic malignant syndrome. *Psychopharmacol Bull.* 1998; 24:25-9.
395. Anbalagan E, Ithman M, Lauriello J. Rechallenging clozapine after neuroleptic malignant syndrome. *Psychiatr Q.* 2014; 85:345-8.
396. Davis JM, Janicak PG, Sakkas P et al. Electroconvulsive therapy in the treatment of the neuroleptic malignant syndrome. *Convuls Ther.* 1991; 7:111-20.
397. Janati A, Webb T. Successful treatment of neuroleptic malignant syndrome with bromocriptine. *South Med J.* 1986; 79:1567-70.
398. Mueller PS, Vester JW, Fermaglich J. Neuroleptic malignant syndrome: successful treatment with bromocriptine. *JAMA.* 1983; 249:386-8.
399. Dhib-Jalbut S, Hesselbrock R, Mouradian MM et al. Bromocriptine treatment of neuroleptic malignant syndrome. *Aust N Z J Med.* 1983; 13:70-3.
400. Reeves RR, Mack JE, Torres RA. Neuroleptic malignant syndrome during a change from haloperidol to risperidone. *Ann Pharmacother.* 2001; 35:698-701.
401. McCarron MM, Boettger ML, Peck JJ. A case of neuroleptic malignant syndrome successfully treated with amantadine. *J Clin Psychiatry.* 1982; 43:381-2.
402. Gangadhar BN, Desai NG, Channabasavanna SM. Amantadine in the neuroleptic malignant syndrome. *J Clin Psychiatry.* 1984; 45:526.
403. Kontaxakis VP, Vaidakis NM, Christodoulou GN et al. Neuroleptic-induced catatonia or a mild form of neuroleptic malignant syndrome? *Neuropsychobiology.* 1990; 23:38-40.
404. Woo J, Teoh R, Vallance-Owen J. Neuroleptic malignant syndrome successfully treated with amantadine. *Postgrad Med J.* 1986; 62:809-10.

405. Khan A, Jaffe JH, Nelson WH et al. Resolution of neuroleptic malignant syndrome with dantrolene sodium: case report. *J Clin Psychiatry.* 1985; 46:244-6.
406. Coons DJ, Hillman FJ, Marshall RW. Treatment of neuroleptic malignant syndrome with dantrolene sodium: a case report. *Am J Psychiatry.* 1982; 139:944-5.
407. Nisijima K, Ishiguro T. Does dantrolene influence central dopamine and serotonin metabolism in the neuroleptic malignant syndrome? A retrospective study. *Biol Psychiatry.* 1993; 33:45-8.
408. Tsutsumi Y, Yamamoto K, Matsuura S et al. The treatment of neuroleptic malignant syndrome using dantrolene sodium. *Psychiatry Clin Neurosci.* 1998; 52:433-8.
409. Schneiderhan ME, Marken PA. An atypical course of neuroleptic malignant syndrome. *J Clin Pharmacol.* 1994; 34:325-34.
410. Ebadi M, Pfeiffer RF, Murrin LC. Pathogenesis and treatment of neuroleptic malignant syndrome. *Gen Pharm.* 1990; 21:367-86.
411. Lazarus A. Therapy of neuroleptic malignant syndrome. *Psychiatric Dev.* 1986; 4:19-30.
412. Shalev A, Hermesh H, Munitz H. Mortality from neuroleptic malignant syndrome. *J Clin Psychiatry.* 1989; 50:18-25.
413. Carbone JR. The neuroleptic malignant and serotonin syndromes. *Emerg Med Clin North Am.* 2000; 18:317-25.
414. Sakkas P, Davis JM, Hua J et al. Pharmacotherapy of neuroleptic malignant syndrome. *Psychiatr Ann.* 1991; 21:157-64.
415. Sakkas P, Davis JM, Janicak PG et al. Drug treatment of the neuroleptic malignant syndrome. *Psychopharmacol Bull.* 1991; 27:381-4.
416. Sangal R, Dimitrijevic R. Neuroleptic malignant syndrome: successful treatment with pancuronium. *JAMA.* 1985; 254:2795-6.
417. Harris M, Nora L, Tanner CM. Neuroleptic malignant syndrome responsive to carbidopa/levodopa support for a dopaminergic pathogenesis. *Clin Neuropharmacol.* 1987; 10:186-9.
418. Kumar V. A case of neuroleptic malignant syndrome treated with diazepam. *Can J Psychiatry.* 1987; 32:815-6.
419. O'Brien P. Neuroleptic malignant syndrome treated with diazepam. *Can J Psychiatry.* 1988; 33:780.
420. Rosebush P, Hildebrand A, Furlong B et al. Catatonic syndrome in a general psychiatric inpatient population: frequency, clinical presentation, and response to lorazepam. *J Clin Psychiatry.* 1990; 51:357-62.
421. Ungvari GS, Leung CM, Wong MK et al. Benzodiazepines in the treatment of catatonic syndrome. *Acta Psychiatr Scand.* 1994; 89:285-8.
422. Fricchione GL, Cassem NH, Hooterman D et al. Intravenous lorazepam in neuroleptic-induced catatonia. *J Clin Psychopharmacol.* 1983; 3:338-42.
423. Scheftner WA, Shulman RB. Treatment choice in neuroleptic malignant syndrome. *Convuls Ther.* 1992; 8:267-79.
424. Lazarus A. Treatment of neuroleptic malignant syndrome with electroconvulsive therapy. *J Nerv Ment Dis.* 1986; 174:47-9.
425. Addonizio G, Susman VL. ECT as a treatment alternative for patients with symptoms of neuroleptic malignant syndrome. *J Clin Psychiatry.* 1987; 48:102-5.
426. Trollor JN, Sachdev PS. Electroconvulsive treatment of neuroleptic malignant syndrome: a review and report of cases. *Aust N Z J Psychiatry.* 1999; 33:650-9.
427. Harland CC, O'Leary MM, Winters R et al. Neuroleptic malignant syndrome: a case for electroconvulsive therapy. *Postgrad Med J.* 1990; 66:49-51.
428. Hermesh H, Aizenberg D, Weizman A. A successful electroconvulsive treatment of neuroleptic malignant syndrome. *Acta Psychiatr Scand.* 1987; 75:237-9.
429. Jessee SS, Anderson GF. ECT in the neuroleptic malignant syndrome: case report. *J Clin Psychiatry.* 1983; 44:37-8.
430. Hashim H, Zeb-un-Nisa, Alrukn SA, Al Madani AA. Drug resistant neuroleptic malignant syndrome and the role of electroconvulsive therapy. *JPMA.* 2014; 64:471-3.
431. Oates JA, Sjoerdsma A. Neurologic effects of tryptophan in a patient receiving a monoamine oxidase inhibitor. *Neurology.* 1960; 10:1076-8.
432. Prior FH, Isbister GK, Dawson AH et al. Serotonin toxicity with therapeutic doses of dexamphetamine and venlafaxine. *Med J Aust.* 2002; 176:240-1.
433. Parrott AC. Recreational ecstasy/MDMA, the serotonin syndrome, and serotonergic neurotoxicity. *Pharmacol Biochem Behav.* 2002; 71:837-44.
434. Mueller PD, Korey WS. Death by "ecstasy;" the serotonin syndrome? *Ann Emerg Med.* 1998; 32:377-80.
435. Vuori E, Henry JA, Ojanpera I et al. Death following ingestion of MDMA (ecstasy) and moclobemide. *Addiction.* 2003; 98:365-8.
436. Martin TL, Chiasson DA, Kish SJ. Does hyperthyroidism increase risk of death due to the ingestion of ecstasy? *J Forensic Sci.* 2007; 52:951-3.
437. Garcia-Algar, O, López N, Bonet M et al. 3,4methylenedioxymethamphetimine (MDMA) intoxication in an infant chronically exposed to cocaine. *Ther Drug Monit.* 2005; 27:409-11.
438. Melian AM, Burillo-Putze G, Campo CG et al. Accidental ecstasy poisoning in a toddler. *Pediatr Emerg Care.* 2004; 20:534-5.
439. Chang YJ, Lai MW, Kong MS et al. Accidental ingestion of Ecstasy in a toddler. *J Formos Med Assoc.* 2005; 104:946-7.
440. Duffy MR, Swart M. Severe Ecstasy poisoning in a toddler. *Anaesthesia.* 2006; 61:498-501.
441. Eifinger F, Roth B, Kröner L et al. Severe Ecstasy poisoning in an 8-month-old infant. *Eur J Pediatr.* 2008; 167:1067-70.
442. Avarello TP, Cottone S. Serotonin syndrome: a reported case. *Neurol Sci.* 2002; 23(suppl 2):S55-6.
443. Brannan SK, Talley BJ, Bowden CL. Sertraline and isocarboxazid cause serotonin syndrome. *J Clin Psychopharmacol.* 1995; 15:144.
444. Bodner RA, Lynch T, Lewis L et al. Serotonin syndrome. *Neurology.* 1995; 45:219-23.
445. Hinds NP, Hillier CE, Wiles CM. Possible serotonin syndrome arising from an interaction between nortriptyline and selegiline in a lady with Parkinsonism. *J Neurol.* 2000; 247:811.
446. Otte W, Birkenhager TK, van den Broek WW. Fatal interaction between tranylcypromine and imipramine. *Eur Psychiatry.* 2003; 18:264-5.
447. Hodgman MJ, Martin RG, Krenzelok EP. Serotonin syndrome due to venlafaxine and maintenance tranylcypromine therapy. *Hum Exp Toxicol.* 1997; 16:14-7.
448. Brubacher JR, Hoffman RS, Lurin MJ. Serotonin syndrome from venlafaxine-tranylcypromine interaction. *Vet Hum Toxicol.* 1996; 38:358-61.
449. Gillman PK. Serotonin syndrome treated with chlorpromazine. *J Clin Psychopharmacol.* 1997; 17:128-9.
450. Roxanas MG, Machado JF. Serotonin syndrome in combined moclobemide and venlafaxine ingestion. *Med J Aust.* 1998; 168:523-4.
451. Ferrer-Dufol A, Perez-Arados C, Murillo ED et al. Fatal serotonin syndrome caused by moclobemideclomipramine overdose. *Clin Toxicol.* 1998; 36:31-2.
452. FitzSimmons CR, Metha S. Serotonin syndrome caused by overdose with paroxetine and moclobemide. *J Accid Emerg Med.* 1999; 16:293-5.
453. Butzkueven H. A case of serotonin syndrome induced by moclobemide during an extreme heatwave. *Aust N Z J Med.* 1997; 27:603-4.
454. Fischer P. Serotonin syndrome in the elderly after antidepressive monotherapy. *J Clin Psychopharmacol.* 1995; 15:440-2.
455. Francois B, Marquet P, Desachy A et al. Serotonin syndrome due to an overdose of moclobemide and clomipramine: a potentially life threatening association. *Intensive Care Med.* 1997; 23:122-4.
456. Dams R, Benijts TH, Lambert WE et al. A fatal case of serotonin syndrome after combined moclobemidecitalopram intoxication. *J Anal Toxicol.* 2001; 25:147-51.
457. Bernard L, Stern R, Lew D et al. Serotonin syndrome after concomitant treatment with linezolid and citalopram. *Clin Infect Dis.* 2003; 36:1197.

458. Wigen CL, Goetz MB. Serotonin syndrome and linezolid. *Clin Infect Dis*. 2002; 34:1651-2.
459. Lavery S, Ravi H, McDaniel WW et al. Linezolid and serotonin syndrome. *Psychosomatics*. 2001; 42:432-4.
460. Clark DB, Andrus MR, Byrd DC. Drug interactions between linezolid and selective serotonin reuptake inhibitors: case report involving sertraline and review of the literature. *Pharmacotherapy*. 2006; 26:269-76.
461. Steinberg M, Morin K. Mild serotonin syndrome associated with concurrent linezolid and fluoxetine. *Am J Health-Syst Pharm*. 2007; 64:59-62.
462. Bergeron L, Boulé M, Perreault S. Serotonin toxicity associated with concomitant use of linezolid. *Ann Pharmacother*. 2005; 39:956-61.
463. Strouse TB, Kerrihard TN, Forscher CA et al. Serotonin syndrome precipitated by linezolid in a medically ill patient on duloxetine. *J Clin Psychopharmacol*. 2006; 26:681-3.
464. DeBellis RJ, Schaefer OP, Liquori M et al. Linezolid associated serotonin syndrome after concomitant treatment with citalopram and mirtazapine in a critically ill bone marrow transplant recipient. *J Intensive Care Med*. 2005; 20:351-3.
465. Morales N, Vermette H. Serotonin syndrome associated with linezolid treatment after discontinuation of fluoxetine. *Psychosomatics*. 2005; 46:274-5.
466. Taylor JJ, Wilson JW, Estes LL. Linezolid and serotonergic drug interactions: a retrospective survey. *Clin Infect Dis*. 2006; 43:180-7.
467. Packer S, Berman SA. Serotonin syndrome precipitated by the monoamine oxidase inhibitor linezolid. *Am J Psychiatry*. 2007; 164;346-7.
468. Jimenez-Genchi A. Immediate switching from moclobemide to duloxetine may induce serotonin syndrome. *J Clin Psychiatry*. 2006; 67:1821-2.
469. Das PK, Warkentin DI, Hewko R et al. Serotonin syndrome after concomitant treatment with linezolid and meperidine. *Clin Infect Dis*. 2008; 46:264-5.
470. Chechani V. Serotonin syndrome presenting as hypotonic coma and apnea: potentially fatal complications of selective serotonin receptor inhibitor therapy. *Crit Care Med*. 2002; 30:473-6.
471. Birmes P, Coppin D, Schmitt L et al. Serotonin syndrome: a brief review. *CMAJ*. 2003; 168:1439-42.
472. Ener RA, Meglathery SB, Van Decker WA et al. Serotonin syndrome and other serotonergic disorders. *Pain Med*. 2003; 4:63-74.
473. Tseng WP, Tsai JH, Wu MT et al. Citalopram-induced serotonin syndrome: a case report. *Kaohsiung J Med Sci*. 2005; 21:326-8.
474. Altman EM, Manos GH. Serotonin syndrome associated with citalopram and meperidine. *Psychosomatics*. 2007; 48:361-3.
475. Mahlberg R, Kunz D, Sasse J et al. Serotonin syndrome with tramadol and citalopram. *Am J Psychiatry*. 2004; 161:1129.
476. Ailawadhi S, Sung KW, Carlson LA et al. Serotonin syndrome caused by interaction between citalopram and fentanyl. *J Clin Pharm Ther*. 2007; 32:199-202.
477. Tomaselli G, Modestin J. Repetition of serotonin syndrome after reexposure to SSRI: a case report. *Pharmacopsychiatry*. 2004; 37:236-8.
478. Karunatilake H, Buckley NA. Serotonin syndrome induced by fluvoxamine and oxycodone. *Ann Pharmacother*. 2006; 40:155-7.
479. Huska MT, Catalano G, Catalano MC. Serotonin syndrome associated with the use of escitalopram. *CNS Spectr*. 2007; 12:270-4.
480. Benazzi F. Serotonin syndrome with mirtazapinefluoxetine combination. *Int J Geriatr Psychiatry*. 1998; 13:495-6.
481. Tissot TA. Probable meperidine-induced serotonin syndrome in a patient with a history of fluoxetine use. *Anesthesiology*. 2003; 98:1511-2.
482. Kesavan S, Sobala GM. Serotonin syndrome with fluoxetine plus tramadol. *J R Soc Med*. 1999; 92:474-5.
483. Smith DL, Wenegrat BG. A case report of serotonin syndrome associated with combined nefazodone and fluoxetine. *J Clin Psychiatry*. 2000; 61:146-7.
484. Mullins ME, Horowitz BZ. Serotonin syndrome after a single dose of fluvoxamine. *Ann Emerg Med*. 1999; 34:806-7.
485. Demers JC, Malone M. Serotonin syndrome induced by fluvoxamine and mirtazapine. *Ann Pharmacother*. 2001; 35:1217-20.
486. Gill M, LoVecchio F, Selden B. Serotonin syndrome in a child after a single dose of fluvoxamine. *Ann Emerg Med*. 1999; 33:457-9.
487. Satoh K, Takano S, Onogi T et al. Serotonin syndrome caused by minimum doses of SSRIs in a patient with spinal cord injury. *Fukushima J Med Sci*. 2006; 52:29-33.
488. John L, Perrault M, Tao T et al. Serotonin syndrome associated with nefazodone and paroxetine. *Ann Emerg Med*. 1997; 29:278-89.
489. Skop BP, Finkelstein JA, Mareth TR et al. The serotonin syndrome associated with paroxetine, an over-the-counter cold remedy, and vascular disease. *Am J Emerg Med*. 1994; 12:642-4.
490. Egberts AC, ter Borgh J, Brodie-Meijer CC. Serotonin syndrome attributed to tramadol addition to paroxetine therapy. *Int Clin Psychopharmacol*. 1997; 12:181-2.
491. Jaber BL, Lobon LF, Madias NE. The serotonin syndrome complicating co-prescription of paroxetine and clarithromycin. *Am J Med*. 2006; 119:E3.
492. Horowitz BZ, Mullins ME. Cyproheptadine for serotonin syndrome in an accidental pediatric sertraline ingestion. *Pediatr Emerg Care*. 1999; 15:325-7.
493. Lee DO, Lee CD. Serotonin syndrome in a child associated with erythromycin and sertraline. *Pharmacotherapy*. 1999; 19:894-6.
494. Adson DE, Erickson-Birkedahl S, Kotlyar M. An unusual presentation of sertraline and trazodone overdose. *Ann Pharmacother*. 2001; 35:1375-7.
495. Fisher AA, Davis MW. Serotonin syndrome caused by selective serotonin reuptake-inhibitors-metoclopramide interaction. *Ann Pharmacother*. 2002; 36:67-71.
496. DeVane CL. Pharmacokinetics of the newer antidepressants: clinical relevance. *Am J Med*. 1994; 97(suppl 6A):S13-23.
497. Leonard HL, March J, Rickler KC et al. Pharmacology of the selective serotonin reuptake inhibitors in children and adolescents. *J Am Acad Child Adolesc Psychiatry*. 1997; 36:725-36.
498. Pao M, Tipnis T. Serotonin syndrome after sertraline overdose in a 5-year-old girl. *Arch Pediatr Adolesc Med*. 1997; 151:1064-7.
499. Dike GL. Triphasic waves in serotonin syndrome. *J Neurol Neurosurg Psychiatry*. 1997; 62:200.
500. McCue RE, Joseph M. Venlafaxine and trazodone-induced serotonin syndrome. *Am J Psychiatry*. 2001; 158:2008-9.
501. Kolecki P. Isolated venlafaxine-induced serotonin syndrome. *J Emerg Med*. 1997; 15:491-3.
502. Mekler G, Woggon B. Serotonin syndrome caused by venlafaxine and lithium. *Pharmacopsychiatry*. 1997; 30:27273.
503. Pan JJ, Shen WW. Serotonin syndrome induced by low-dose venlafaxine. *Ann Pharmacother*. 2003; 37:209-11.
504. Dougherty JA, Young H, Shafi T. Serotonin syndrome induced by amitriptyline, meperidine, and venlafaxine. *Ann Pharmacother*. 2002; 36:1647-8.
505. Perry NK. Venlafaxine-induced serotonin syndrome with relapse following amitriptyline. *Postgrad Med J*. 2000; 76:254-6.
506. Connor H. Serotonin syndrome after single doses of co-amoxiclav during treatment with venlafaxine. *J R Soc Med*. 2003; 96:233-4.
507. Kolecki P. Venlafaxine-induced serotonin syndrome occurring after abstinence from phenelzine for more than two weeks. *J Toxicol Clin Toxicol*. 1997; 35:211-2.
508. Dimellis D. Serotonin syndrome produced by a combination of venlafaxine and mirtazapine. *World J Biol Psychiatry*. 2002; 3:167.
509. Adan-Manes J, Novalbos J, López-Rodríguez R et al. Lithium and venlafaxine interaction: a case of serotonin syndrome. *J Clin Pharm Ther*. 2007; 32:529-31.
510. Liau CH, Shen WW, Su KP. Venlafaxine-associated serotonin syndrome and manic episode in a geriatric depressive patient. *Psychiatry Clin Neurosci*. 2006; 60:121-2.

511. Rosebush PI, Margetts P, Mazurek MF. Serotonin syndrome as a result of clomipramine monotherapy. *J Clin Psychopharmacol.* 1999; 19:285-7.
512. Cheng P, Hung S, Lin L. Amantadine-induced serotonin syndrome in a patient with renal failure. *Am J Emerg Med.* 2008; 26:112.E5-6.
513. Dannawi M. Possible serotonin syndrome after combination of buspirone and St. John's Wort. *J Psychopharmacol.* 2002; 16:401.
514. Ganetsky M, Babu KM, Boyer EW. Serotonin syndrome in dextromethorphan ingestion responsive to propofol therapy. *Pediatr Emerg Care.* 2007; 23:829-31.
515. Isenberg D, Wong, SC, Curtis JA. Serotonin syndrome triggered by a single dose of suboxone. *Am J Emerg Med.* 2008; 26:840. E3-5.
516. Giese SY, Neborsky R. Serotonin syndrome: potential consequences of Meridia combined with Demerol or fentanyl. *Plast Reconstr Surg.* 2001; 107:293-4.
517. Trakas K, Shear NH. Serotonin syndrome risk with antiobesity drug. *Can J Clin Pharmacol.* 2000; 7:216.
518. Duggal HS, Fetchko J. Serotonin syndrome and atypical antipsychotics. *Am J Psychiatry.* 2002; 159:672-3.
519. Vizcaychipi MP, Walker S, Palazzo M. Serotonin syndrome triggered by tramadol. *Br J Anaesth.* 2007; 99:919.
520. Parker V, Wong AH, Boon HS et al. Adverse reactions to St. John's Wort. *Can J Psychiatry.* 2001; 46:77-9.
521. Bryant SM, Kolodchak J. Serotonin syndrome resulting from an herbal detox cocktail. *Am J Emerg Med.* 2004; 22:625-6.
522. Pilgrim JL, Gerostamoulos D, Woodford N, Drummer OH. Serotonin toxicity involving MDMA (ecstasy) and moclobemide. *Forensic Sci Int.* 2012; 215:184-8.
523. Fernandes C, Reddy P, Kessel B. Rasagiline-induced serotonin syndrome. *Movement Disorders.* 2011; 26:766-7.
524. Morrison EK, Rowe AS. Probable drug-drug interaction leading to serotonin syndrome in a patient treated with concomitant buspirone and linezolid in the setting of therapeutic hypothermia. *J Clin Pharm Ther.* 2012; 37:610-3.
525. Top WM, Gillman PK, De Langen CJ, Kooy A. Fatal methylene blue associated serotonin toxicity. *Neth J Med.* 2014; 72:179-81.
526. Shopes E, Gerard W, Baughman J. Methylene blue encephalopathy: a case report and review of published cases. *AANA Journal.* 2013; 81:215-21.
527. Ng BK, Cameron AJ. The role of methylene blue in serotonin syndrome: a systematic review. *Psychosomatics.* 2010; 51:194-200.
528. Huskey AM, Thomas CC, Waddell JA. Occurrence of milnacipran-associated morbilliform rash and serotonin toxicity. *Ann of Pharmacotherapy.* 2013; 47:E32.
529. Bosak AR, Skolnik AB. Serotonin syndrome associated with metaxalone overdose. *J Med Toxicol.* 2014; 10:402-5.
530. Palekar N, Eisman J. Serotonin syndrome with ziprasidone and sertraline. *J Neuropsychiatry Clin Neurosci.* 2013; 25:E1.
531. Lin PY, Hong CJ, Tsai SJ. Serotonin syndrome caused by ziprasidone alone. *Psychiatry Clin Neurosci.* 2010; 64:338-9.
532. Isbister GK, Bowe SJ, Dawson A et al. Relative toxicity of selective serotonin reuptake inhibitors (SSRIs) in overdose. *J Toxicol Clin Toxicol.* 2004; 42:277-85.
533. Weiner AL. Meperidine as a potential cause of serotonin syndrome in the emergency department. *Acad Emerg Med.* 1999; 6:156-8.
534. Ables AZ, Nagubilli R. Prevention, diagnosis, and management of serotonin syndrome. *Am Fam Physician.* 2010; 81:1139-42.
535. Sternbach H. The serotonin syndrome. *Am J Psychiatry.* 1991; 148:705-13.
536. Glennon RA, Darmani NA, Martin BR. Multiple populations of serotonin receptors may modulate the behavioral effects of serotonergic agents. *Life Sci.* 1991; 48:2493-8.
537. Iqbal MM, Basil MJ, Kaplan J, Iqbal T. Overview of serotonin syndrome. *Ann of Clin Psychiatry.* 2012; 24:310-8.
538. Rolan PE. Drug interactions with triptans: which are clinically significant? *CNS Drugs.* 2012; 26:949-57.
539. Gillman PK. Triptans, serotonin agonists, and serotonin syndrome: a review. *Headache.* 2010; 50:264-72.
540. Radomski JW, Dursun SM, Revely MA et al. An exploratory approach to the serotonin syndrome: an update of clinical phenomenology and revised diagnostic criteria. *Med Hypotheses.* 2000; 55:218-24.
541. Hegerl U, Bottlender R, Galliant J et al. The serotonin syndrome scale: first results on validity. *Eur Arch Psychiatry Clin Neurosci.* 1998; 248:96-103.
542. Dunkley EJC, Isbister GK, Sibbritt D et al. The Hunter Serotonin Toxicity Criteria: simple and accurate diagnostic decision rules for serotonin toxicity. *Q J Med.* 2003; 96:635-42.
543. Walsh J. Serotonin syndrome. *Anaesthesia Tutorial of the Week.* 2010; 1-5.
544. Brvar M, Stajer D, Kozelj G et al. Urinary serotonin level is associated with serotonin syndrome after moclobemide, sertraline, and citalopram overdose. *Clin Toxicol.* 2007; 45:458-60.
545. Brosen K, Hansen JG, Nielsen KK et al. Inhibition by paroxetine of desipramine metabolism in extensive but not in poor metabolizers of sparteine. *Eur J Clin Pharmacol.* 1993; 32:692-8.
546. Meltzer HY, Lee MA, Ranjan R et al. Relapse following clozapine withdrawal: effect of neuroleptic drugs and cyproheptadine. *Psychopharmacology (Berl).* 1996; 194:176-81.
547. Gillman PK. The serotonin syndrome and its treatment. *J Psychopharmacol.* 1999; 13:100-9.
548. Kapur S, Zipursky RB, Jones C et al. Cyproheptadine: a potent in vivo serotonin antagonist. *Am J Psychiatry.* 1997; 154:884.
549. Brennan D, MacManus M, Howe J et al. Neuroleptic malignant syndrome without neuroleptics. *Br J Psychiatry.* 1998; 152:578-9.
550. Kline SS, Mauro LS, Scala-Barnett DM et al. Serotonin syndrome versus neuroleptic malignant syndrome as a cause of death. *Clin Pharmacol.* 1989; 8:510-4.
551. Nisiijima K, Ishiguro T. Does dantrolene influence central dopamine and serotonin metabolism in the neuroleptic malignant syndrome? A retrospective study. *Biol Psychiatry.* 1993; 33:45-8.
552. Dursun SM, Burke JG, Nielsen F et al. SSRI-related toxic serotonin syndrome: improvement by discontinuation of treatment and propranolol. *Eur Psych.* 1997; 12:321.
553. Guze BH, Baxter LR Jr. The serotonin syndrome: case responsive to propranolol. *J Clin Psychopharmacol.* 1986; 6:119-20.
554. Rushton WF, Charlton NP. Dexmedetomidine in the treatment of serotonin syndrome. *Ann of Pharmacotherapy.* 2014; 48:1651-4.
555. Garrido S, Fraga M, Martin MJ et al. Malignant hyperthermia during desflurane-succinylcholine anaesthesia for orthopedic surgery. *Anesthesiology.* 1999; 90:1208-9.
556. Celebioglu B. A case of suspected malignant hyperthermia during desflurane administration. *Anesth Analg.* 1998; 86:916.
557. Lowes R, Mayhew JF. A suspected malignant hyperthermia episode during desflurane anesthesia. *Anesth Analg.* 1998; 86:449-50.
558. Michalek-Sauberer A, Fricker R, Gradwohl I et al. A case of suspected malignant hyperthermia during desflurane administration. *Anesth Analg.* 1997; 85:461-2.
559. Hoenemann CW, Halene-Holtgraeve TB, Booke M et al. Delayed onset of malignant hyperthermia in desflurane anesthesia. *Anesth Analg.* 2003; 96:165-7.
560. Allen GC, Brubaker CL. Human malignant hyperthermia associated with desflurane anesthesia. *Anesth Analg.* 1998; 86:1328-31.
561. Papadimos TJ, Almasri M, Padgett JC et al. A suspected case of delayed onset malignant hyperthermia with desflurane anesthesia. *Anesth Analg.* 2004; 98:548-9.
562. Lane JE, Brooks AG, Logan MS et al. An unusual case of malignant hyperthermia during desflurane anesthesia in an African-American patient. *Anesth Analg.* 2000; 91:1032-4.
563. Fu ES, Scharf JE, Mangar D et al. Malignant hyperthermia involving the administration of desflurane. *Can J Anesth.* 1996; 43:687-90.

564. Oikkonen M, Rosenberg PH, Bjorkenheim JM et al. Spinal block, after dantrolene pretreatment, for resection of a thigh muscle herniation in a young malignant hyperthermia susceptible man. *Acta Anaesthesiol Scand.* 1987; 31:309-11.

565. Ward RJ, Eisele JW, Reay DT et al. Hemolysis and hyperkalemia complicate malignant hyperpyrexia during anesthetic death. *J Forensic Sci.* 1986; 31:543-5.

566. Caropreso PR. Gittleman MA, Reilly DJ et al. Malignant hyperthermia associated with enflurane anesthesia. *Arch Surg.* 1975; 110:1491-3.

567. Kimura H, Yoshida K, Ohsawa M et al. An autopsy case of malignant hyperthermia. *Forensic Sci Int.* 1985; 27:25-30.

568. Smith CA, Carvill KA, Eckert T 3rd. Suspected malignant hyperthermia in a 13-month old: today's typical episode—report. *AANA J.* 1997; 65:247-9.

569. Blank JW, Boggs SD. Successful treatment of an episode of malignant hyperthermia using a large dose of dantrolene. *J Clin Anesth.* 1993; 5:69-72.

570. Dodd MJ, Phattiyakul P, Silpasuvan S. Suspected malignant hyperthermia in a strabismus patient: a case report. *Arch Ophthalmol.* 1981; 99:1247-50.

571. Ahmed AE, Usman M. Malignant hyperthermia: a case report. *Middle East J Anesthesiol.* 1994; 12:573-8.

572. Vorrakitpokatorn P, Limsakul A. Drug-induced hyperthermia and rhabdomyolysis during the perioperative period: report of three patients. *J Med Assoc Thai.* 2002; 85(suppl 3):S884-92.

573. Melvoll R, Stovner J, Whittaker M. Suxamethonium-induced jaw stiffness and myalgia associated with atypical cholinesterase: case report. *Can Anaesth Soc J.* 1980; 27:283-5.

574. Theilade D, Rosendal T. Malignant hyperpyrexia: a case report of successful treatment and subsequent uneventful general anaesthesia. *Anaesthesia.* 1978; 33:606-10.

575. Karger B, Teige K. Fatal malignant hyperthermia: delayed onset and atypical course. *Forensic Sci Int.* 2002; 129:187-90.

576. Ramirez JA, Cheetham ED, Laurence AS et al. Suxamthonium, masseter spasm and later malignant hyperthermia. *Anaesthesia.* 1998; 53:1111-6.

577. Liao YC, Wang JJ, Chien CC et al. Suspected malignant hyperthermia during isoflurane anesthesia: a case report. *Acta Anaesthesiol Sin.* 1998; 36:53-8.

578. Christiaens F, Gepts E, D'Haese J et al. Malignant hyperthermia suggestive hypermetabolic syndrome at emergence from anesthesia. *Acta Anaesthesiol Belg.* 1995; 46:93-7.

579. Struebing VL. Differential diagnosis of malignant hyperthermia: a case report. *AANA J.* 1995; 63:455-60.

580. Chambers FA, Casey W, Dowling F et al. Malignant hyperthermia during isoflurane anaesthesia. *Can J Anaesth.* 1994; 41:355-6.

581. Prescott RJ, Roberts SP, Williams G. Malignant hyperpyrexia: a rare cause of postoperative death. *J Clin Pathol.* 1992; 45:361-3.

582. McGuire N, Easy WR. Malignant hyperthermia during isoflurane anaesthesia. *Anaethesia.* 1990; 45:124-7.

583. Meluch AM, Sibert KS, Bloch EC. Malignant hyperthermia following isoflurane anesthesia in an American Lumbee Indian. *N C Med J.* 1989; 50:485-7.

584. Thomas DW, Dev VJ, Whitehead MJ. Malignant hyperpyrexia and evodopae: a case report. *Br J Anaesth.* 1987; 59:1196-8.

585. Johannesson G, Veel T, Rogstadius J. Malignant hyperthermia during isoflurane anaesthesia: a case report. *Acta Anaesthesiol Scand.* 1987; 31:231-2.

586. Jensen AG, Bach V, Werner MU et al. A fatal case of malignant hyperthermia following isoflurane anaesthesia. *Acta Anaesthesiol Scand.* 1986; 30:293-4.

587. Boheler J, Hamrick JC Jr, McKnight RL et al. Isoflurane and malignant hyperthermia. *Anesth Analg.* 1982; 61:712-3.

588. Joseph MM, Shah K, Biljoen JF. Malignant hyperthermia associated with isoflurane anesthesia. *Anesth Analg.* 1982; 61:711-2.

589. Pandya AB, O'Leary CE. Development of malignant hyperthermia post-cardiopulmonary bypass during surgery for mitral valve replacement. *J Cardiothorac Vasc Anesth.* 2003; 17:625-8.

590. Bergman JA. Idiopathic malignant hyperthermia. Review and report of a case. *Arch Ophthalmol.* 1975; 93:232-4.

591. Nishiyama K, Kitahara A, Natsume H et al. Malignant hyperthermia in a patient with Graves' disease during subtotal thyroidectomy. *Endocr J.* 2001; 48:227-32.

592. Snoeck MM, Gielen MJ, Tangerman A et al. Contractures in skeletal muscle of malignant hyperthermia susceptible patients after in vitro exposure to sevoflurane. *Acta Anaesthesiol Scand.* 2000; 44:334-7.

593. Maeda H, Iranami H, Hatano Y. Delayed recovery from muscle weakness due to malignant hyperthermia during sevoflurane anesthesia. *Anesthesiology.* 1997; 87:425-6.

594. Kanaya N, Nakayama M, Nakae Y et al. Hyperthermia during sevoflurane anaesthesia in arthrogryposis multiplex congenital with central nervous system dysfunction. *Paediatr Anaes.* 1996; 6:428-9.

595. Ducart A, Adnet P, Renaud B et al. Malignant hyperthermia during sevoflurane administration. *Anesth Analg.* 1995; 80:609-11.

596. Otsuka H, Kemmotsu O. Malignant hyperthermia during sevoflurane anesthesia. *Anesth Analg.* 1992; 75:867.

597. Ochiai R, Toyoda Y, Nishio I et al. Possible association of malignant hyperthermia with sevoflurane anesthesia. *Anesth Analg.* 1992; 74:616-8.

598. Otsuka H, Komura Y, Mayumi T et al. Malignant hyperthermia during sevoflurane anesthesia in a child with central core disease. *Anesthesiology.* 1991; 75:699-701.

599. Kelly D, Brull SJ. Neuroleptic malignant syndrome and mivacurium: a safe alternative to succinylcholine? *Can J Anaesth.* 1994; 41:845-9.

600. Gürgey A, Altay C, Ozgen S. Malignant hyperthermia in a patient with sickle cell anemia. *Turk J Pediatr.* 1989; 31:245-7.

601. Larsen UT, Juhl B, Hein-Sorensen O et al. Complications during anaesthesia in patients with Duchenne's muscular dystrophy (a retrospective study). *Can J Anaesth.* 1989; 36:418-22.

602. Wang JM, Stanley TH. Duchenne muscular dystrophy and malignant hyperthermia: two case reports. *Can Anaesth Soc J.* 1986; 33:492-7.

603. Kimura H, Yoshida K, Ohsawa M et al. An autopsy case of malignant hyperthermia. *Forensic Sci Int.* 1985; 27:25-30.

604. Kalow W. Succinylcholine and malignant hyperthermia. *Fed Proc.* 1972; 31:1270-5.

605. Johnson C, Edleman KJ. Malignant hyperthermia: A review. *J Perinatol.* 1992; 12:61-71.

606. Strazis KP, Fox AW. Malignant hyperthermia: a review of published cases. *Anesth Analg.* 1993; 77:297-304.

607. Sessler DI. Malignant hyperthermia. *J Pediatr.* 1986; 109:9-14.

608. MacLennan D, Duff C, Zorzato F et al. Ryanodine receptor gene is a candidate for predisposition to malignant hyperthermia. *Nature.* 1990; 343:559-61.

609. Iaizzo PA, Klein W, Lehmann-Horn F. Fura-2 detected myoplasmic calcium and its correlation with contracture force in skeletal muscle from normal and malignant hyperthermia susceptible pigs. *Pflugers Arch.* 1988; 411:648-53.

610. Mickelson JR, Gallant EM, Litterer LA et al. Abnormal sacrcoplasmic reticulum ryanodine receptor in malignant hyperthermia. *J Biol Chem.* 1988; 263:9310-5.

611. Litman RS, Flood CD, Kaplan RF et al. Postoperative malignant hyperthermia: an analysis of cases from the North American Malignant Hyperthermia Registry. *Anesthesiology.* 2008; 109:825-9.

612. Dubrow JT, Wackym PA, Abul-Rasool IH et al. Malignant hyperthermia: experience in the management of 8 children. *J Pediatr Surg.* 1989; 24:163-6.

613. Heytens L, Forget P, Scholtès JL et al. The changing face of malignant hyperthermia: less fulminant, more insidious. *Anaesth Intensive Care.* 2015; 43:1-6.

614. Larach MG, Gronert GA, Allen GC et al. Clinical presentation, treatment, and complications of malignant hyperthermia in North America from 1987 to 2006. *Anesth Analg.* 2010; 110:498-507.

615. Larach MG. Standardization of the caffeine halothane muscle contracture test. North American Malignant Hyperthermia Group. *Anesth Analg.* 1989; 69:511-5.
616. Kalow W, Britt BA, Richter A. The caffeine test of isolated human muscle in relation to malignant hyperthermia. *Can Anaesth Soc J.* 1977; 24:678-94.
617. Gronert GA. Muscle contractures and adenosine triphosphate depletion in procine malignant hyperthermia. *Anesth Analg.* 1979; 58:367-71.
618. Urwyler A, Deufel T, McCarthy T et al. Guidelines for molecular genetic detection of susceptibility to malignant hyperthermia. *Br J Anaesth.* 2001; 86:283-7.
619. Girard T, Treves S, Vronkov E et al. Molecular genetic testing for malignant hyperthermia susceptibility. *Anesthesiology.* 2004; 100:1076-80.
620. Larach MG, Localio AR, Allen GC et al. A clinical grading scale to predict malignant hyperthermia susceptibility. *Anesthesiology.* 1994; 80:771-9.
621. Brownell AK. Malignant hyperthermia: relationship to other diseases. *Br J Anaesth.* 1988; 60:303-8.
622. Ohkoshi N, Yoshizawa T, Mizusawa H et al. Malignant hyperthermia in a patient with Becker muscular dystrophy: dystrophin analysis and caffeine contracture study. *Neuromuscul Disord.* 1995; 5:53-8.
623. Britt BA, Endrenyi L, Peters PL et al. Screening of malignant hyperthermia susceptible families by creatine phosphokinase measurement and other clinical investigations. *Can Anaesth Soc J.* 1976; 23:263-84.
624. Kasi PM. Malignant hyperthermia and idiopathic HyperCKemia. *Case Rep Med.* 2011; 211:194-298.
625. Malandrini A, Orrico A, Gaudiano C et al. Muscle biopsy and in vitro contracture test in subjects with idiopathic HyperCKemia. *Anesthesiology.* 2008; 109:625-8.
626. Stovner J, Innes KR, Holen A. Ten cases of malignant hyperthermia in Norway. *Can Anaesth Soc J.* 1976; 23:518-26.
627. Jardon OM. Physiologic stress, heat stroke, malignant hyperthermia: a perspective. *Mil Med.* 1982; 147:8-14.
628. Gronert GA. Malignant hyperthermia. *Anesthesiology.* 1980; 53:395-423.
629. Tomarken JL, Britt BA. Malignant hyperthermia. *Ann Emerg Med.* 1987; 16:1253-65.
630. Duncan PG. Availability of dantrolene in Canadian hospitals. *Can Anaesth Soc J.* 1985; 32:205-9.
631. Britt BA. Dantrolene. *Can Anaesth Soc J.* 1984; 31:61-75.
632. Britt BA, Kalow W. Malignant hyperthermia: a statistical review. *Can Anaesth Soc J.* 1970; 17:293-315.
633. Felice-Johnson J, Sudds T, Bennett G. Malignant hyperthermia: current perspectives. *Am J Hosp Pharm.* 1981; 38:646-51.
634. Wackym PA, Blackwell KE. Malignant hyperthermia in the otology patient: the UCLA experience. *Am J Otol.* 1994; 15:371-5.
635. Lucy SJ. Anaesthesia for caesarean delivery of a malignant hyperthermia susceptible parturient. *Can J Anaesth.* 1994; 41:1220-6.
636. Friessen CM, Brodsky JB, Dillingham MF. Successful use of dantrolene sodium in human malignant hyperthermia syndrome: a case report. *Can Anaesth Soc J.* 1979; 26:319-21.
637. Allen GC, Cattran CB, Peterson RG et al. Plasma levels of dantrolene following oral administration in malignant hyperthermia-susceptible patients. *Anesthesiology.* 1988; 69:900-4.
638. Pandit SK, Kothary SP, Cohen PJ. Orally administered dantrolene for prophylaxis of malignant hyperthermia. *Anesthesiology.* 1979; 50:156-8.
639. Watson CB, Reierson N, Norfleet EA. Clinically significant muscle weakness induced by oral dantrolene sodium prophylaxis for malignant hyperthermia. *Anesthesiology.* 1986; 65:312-4.
640. Fitzgibbon DC. Malignant hyperthermia following preoperative oral administration of dantrolene. *Anesthesiology.* 1981; 54:73-5.
641. Ruhland D, Hinkle AJ. Malignant hyperthermia after oral and intravenous pretreatment with dantrolene in a patient susceptible to malignant hyperthermia. *Anesthesiology.* 1984; 60:159-60.
642. Gronert GA. Puzzles in malignant hyperthermia. *Anesthesiology.* 1981; 54:1-2.
643. Wedel DJ. Quinlan JG, Iaizzo PA. Clinical effects of intravenously administered dantrolene. *Mayo Clin Proc.* 1995; 70:241-6.
644. Hackl W, Mauritz W, Winkler M et al. Anaesthesia in malignant hyperthermia-susceptible patients without dantrolene prophylaxis: a report of 30 cases. *Acta Anaesthesiol Scand.* 1990; 34:534-7.
645. Kolb ME, Horne ML, Martz R. Dantrolene in human malignant hyperthermia: a multicenter study. *Anesthesiology.* 1982; 56:254-62.
646. Flewellen EH, Nelson TE, Jones WP et al. Dantrolene dose response in awake man: implications for management of malignant hyperthermia. *Anesthesiology.* 1983; 59:275-80.
647. Short JA, Cooper CM. Suspected recurrence of malignant hyperthermia after post-extubation shivering in the intensive care unit, 18 h after tonsillectomy. *Br J Anaesth.* 1999; 82:945-7.
648. Shime J, Gare D, Andrews J et al. Dantrolene in pregnancy: lack of adverse effects on the fetus and newborn infant. *Am J Obstet Gynecol.* 1988; 159:831-4.
649. Douglas MJ, McMorland GH. The anaesthetic management of the malignant hyperthermia susceptible parturient. *Can Anaesth Soc J.* 1986; 33:371-8.
650. Willatts SM. Malignant hyperthermia susceptibility: management during pregnancy and labour. *Anaesthesia.* 1979; 34:41-6.
651. Wadhwha RK. Obstetric anesthesia for a patient with malignant hyperthermia susceptibility. *Anesthesiology.* 1997; 46:63-4.
652. Khalil SN, Williams JP, Bourke DL. Management of a malignant hyperthermia susceptible patient in labor with 2-chloroprocaine epidural anesthesia. *Anesth Analg.* 1983; 62:119-21.
653. Cupryn JP, Kennedy A, Byrick RJ. Malignant hyperthermia in pregnancy. *Am J Obstet Gynecol.* 1984; 150:327-8.
654. Lips FJ, Newland M, Dutton G. Malignant hyperthermia triggered by cyclopropane during Cesarean section. *Anesthesiology.* 1982; 56:144-6.
655. Gibbs JM. Unexplained hyperpyrexia during labor. *Anaesth Intensive Care.* 1984; 12:375.
656. Koo BS, Kim YK, Kim YI et al. A suspected malignant hyperthermia managed without dantrolene sodium. *Korean J Anessthesiol.* 2014; 67(suppl):S81-2.
657. Ratzlaff EH, Jenkins, LC. Malignant hyperthermia: a case report of successful management. *Can Anaesth Soc J.* 1972; 19:549-56.
658. Barnes C, Stowell KM, Bulger T et al. Safe duration of postoperative monitoring for malignant hyperthermia patients administered non-triggering anaesthesia: an update. *Anaesth Intensive Care.* 2015; 43:98-104.
659. Kreuzer P, Landgrebe M, Wittman M et al. Hypothermia associated with antipsychotic drug use: a clinical case series and review of current literature. *J Clin Pharmacol.* 2012; 52:1090-7.
660. Chin RL, Sporer KA, Cullison B et al. Clinical course of gamma-hydroxybutyrate overdose. *Ann Emerg Med.* 1998; 31:716-22.
661. Ross TM. Gamma-hydroxybutyrate overdose: two cases illustrate the unique aspects of this dangerous recreational drug. *J Emerg Nurs.* 1995; 21:374-6.
662. Suner S, Szlatenyi C, Wang R. Pediatric gamma-hydroxybutyrate intoxication. *Acad Emerg Med.* 1997; 4:1041-5.
663. Perry HE, Wright RO, Michael SS et al. Baclofen overdose: drug experimentation in a group of adolescents. *Pediatrics.* 1998; 101:1045-8.
664. US Centers for Disease Control. Gamma-hydroxy butyrate use: New York and Texas 1995–1996. *MMWR Morb Mortal Wkly Rep.* 1997; 46:281-3.
665. US Centers for Disease Control. Adverse events associated with ingestion of gamma-butyrolactone: Minnesota, New Mexico, and Texas, 1998–1999. *MMWR Morb Mortal Wkly Rep.* 1999; 48:137-40.

666. Wenger T, Moldrich G. The role of endocannabinoids in the hypothalamic regulation of visceral function. *Prostaglandins Leukot Essent Fatty Acids.* 2002; 66:301-7.
667. James C. Another case of gamma-hydroxybutyrate (GHB) overdose. *J Emerg Nurs.* 1996; 22:97.
668. Van Marum RJ, Wegewijs MA, Loonen AJM et al. Hypothermia following antipsychotic drug use. *Eur J Clin Pharmacol.* 2007; 63:627-31.
669. Lopez-Munoz F, Alamo C, Cuenca E et al. History of the discovery and clinical introduction of chlorpromazine. *Ann Clin Psychiatry.* 2005; 17:113-35.
670. Eikenboom HC, Janssens AR, Rosekrans PC, Molendijk W. Hypothermia during use of pipamperone. *Ned Tijdschr Geneeskd.* 1997; 141:301-3.
671. DiFazio MP, Lavenstein B, Demarest S. Profound hypothermia secondary to clobazam use in epilepsy: a novel association. *Neuroscience and Medicine.* 2014; 5:15-9.
672. Irvine RE. Hypothermia due to diazepam. *BMJ.* 1966; 2:1007.
673. Hostler D, Northington WE, Callaway CW. High-dose diazepam facilitates core cooling during cold saline infusion in healthy volunteers. *Appl Physiol Nutr Metab.* 2009; 34:582-6.
674. Signorelli MS, Nalis F, Battiato M, Aguglia E. What about temperature? Haloperidol-induced hypotermia. *BMJ Case Rep* published online: 19 September 2013.
675. Hagg S, Mjorndal T, Lindqvist L. Repeated episodes of hypothermia in a subject treated with halperidol, levomepromazine, olanzapine, and thioridazine. *J Clin Psychopharmacol.* 2001; 21:113-5.
676. Kreuzer P, Landgrebe M, Hajak G et al. A case of severe hypothermia following single-dose administration of olanzapine: a case report. *J Clin Pharmacol.* 2012; 52:266-8.
677. Fukunishi I, Sato Y, Kino K, Shirai T, Kitaoka T. Hypothermia in a hemodialysis patient treated with olanzapine monotherapy. *J Clin Psychopharmacol.* 2003; 23:314.
678. Ryan KF, Price JW, Warriner CB, Choi PT. Persistent hypothermia after intrathecal morphine: case report and literature review. *Can J Anesth.* 2012; 59:384-8.
679. Bookstaver BP, Miller AD. Possible long-acting risperidone-induced hypothermia precipitating phenytoin toxicity in an elderly patient. *JCPT.* 2011; 36:426-9.
680. Kurz A, Sessler DI, Schroeder M, Kurz M. Thermoregulatory response thresholds during spinal anesthesia. *Anesth Analg.* 1993; 77:721-6.
681. Young DM. Risk factors for hypothermia in psychiatric patients. *Ann Clin Psychiatry.* 1996; 8:93-7.
682. Shiloh R, Weizman A, Epstien Y et al. Abnormal thermoregulation in drug-free male schizophrenia patients. *Eur Neuropsychopharmacol.* 2001; 11:285-8.
683. Sharma RP, Janicak PG, Bissette G, Nermeroff CB. CSF neurotensin concentrations and antipsychotic treatment in schizophrenia and schizoaffective disorder. *Am J Psychiatry.* 1997; 154:1019-21.
684. Van Marum RJ, Jansen S, Ponssen HH. Antipsychotic medication as a cause of deep hypothermia. *Ned Tijdschr Geneeskd.* 2003; 147:1201-4.

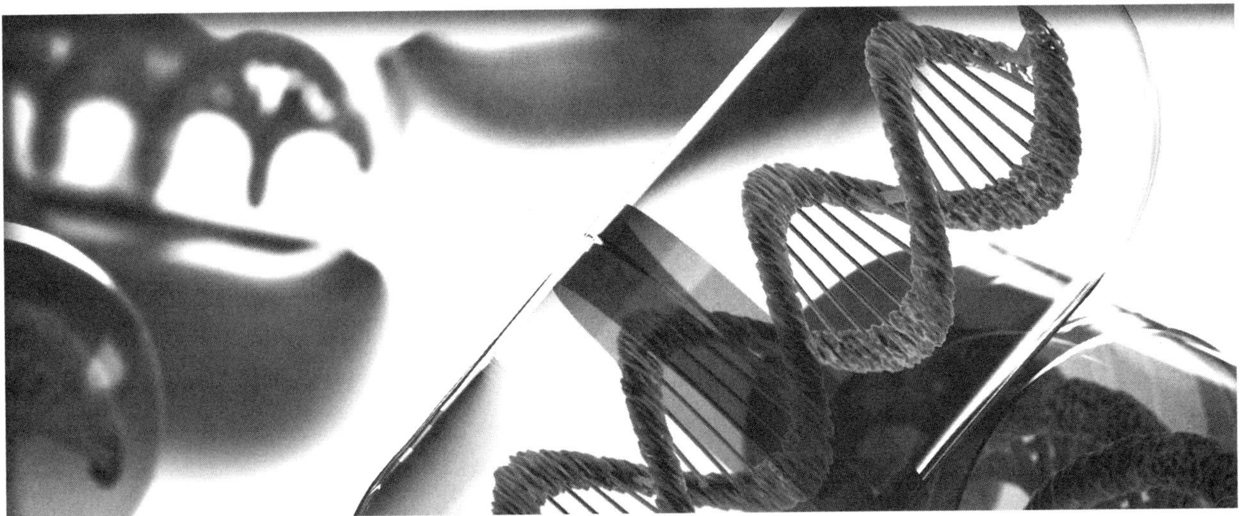

CHAPTER 55

Ototoxicity

Monica L. Miller

Ototoxicity is a broad term defining toxicity induced by certain drugs or chemicals that affect the cochlea, vestibular cells, or the acoustic nerve.[1-3] Damage to these structures can lead to a sensorineural hearing loss.[4] This type of hearing loss can be associated with aging as well as medications.[4] Symptoms associated with ototoxicity include hearing loss, tinnitus, hyperacusis, and vertigo.[5] Hearing loss can range from partial to complete and may occur in one or both ears. Tinnitus is defined as hearing a sound without a source.[6] Hyperacusis is defined as auditory acuity that may be associated with painful sensitivity or sounds that are "normal volume" that are so loud they are painful.[7] Vertigo is a symptom defined as illusionary movement where patients may feel as if they or surrounding objects are moving when in actuality, both are stationary.[6] Patients with tinnitus often report hearing buzzing, ringing, or hissing sounds. Vertigo and tinnitus, like hearing loss, range in severity.

CAUSATIVE AGENTS

Drugs that have been reported to cause ototoxicity are listed in **Table 55-1**.[1, 8-242] Common drug classes associated with auditory toxicity include aminoglycosides, diuretics, nonsteroidal anti-inflammatory drugs (NSAIDs), and platinum-based chemotherapeutic agents. Otic administration of aminoglycoside antibiotics is not generally associated with ototoxicity except in patients with a perforated tympanic membrane.[243]

The data regarding the ototoxic potential of vancomycin are mixed. In the past, early formulations had impurities that may have caused ototoxicity and could have accounted for a higher reported incidence.[244,245] Further, vancomycin and aminoglycosides have frequently been administered concomitantly to patients with serious infections.[244,245] Today, reports of vancomycin ototoxicity are rare, except when patients have other risk factors.[243] A study of patients receiving only vancomycin revealed a mild, reversible hearing loss in 3% of patients.[232]

Opioids and opiates have also been reported to cause ototoxicity, principally sensorineural hearing loss that can either be reversible or permanent.[4,174,246] Methadone is the most commonly implicated, but there are also reports of ototoxicity with codeine–acetaminophen, hydrocodone–acetaminophen, morphine, oxymorphone, and propoxyphene.[4,10,246] Ototoxicity has been associated with both acute and chronic use of these

Table 55-1 Agents Implicated in Drug-Induced Ototoxicity[1,8-242]

Drug	Incidence	Level of Evidence[a]
Abacavir[8,b]	NK	C
Acetaminophen[10,d]	NK	C
Acetazolamide[9,c]	NK	B
Alfuzosin hydrochloride[11,b]	2%	B
Amikacin[12-16,d]	0–28.5%	B
Aminocaproic acid[18,c]	NK	B
Aminophylline[19,20,b]	NK	B
Amiodarone[17,b]	NK	C
Amitriptyline[21,22,c,d]	NK	B
Amlodipine[23,b]	0.1–1%	C
Amphotericin B[24,d]	NK	B
Ampicillin[25,d]	NK	C
Aripiprazole[26,b]	1–10%	B
Aspirin[27-30,b,d]	0.3–1.7% 50–75% if dose >4 g/day	B
Atazanavir[31,b]	0.1–1%	B
Atropine[32,d]	NK	C
Azithromycin[1,33-36,d]	14–26% (in patients with HIV)	C
Aztreonam[37,d]	3%	C
Bacitracin[38,c]	NK	C
Bleomycin[39,d]	NK	B
Bromocriptine[40,b]	NK	B
Bumetanide[41,b,c]	1.1–1.7%	B
Bupivacaine[42,c]	NK	B
Bupropion[43,44,d]	NK	C
Candesartan cilexetil[45,b]	NK	A
Capreomycin[46,d]	NK	B
Captopril[47,b]	NK	B
Carbamazepine[48,c,d]	0.2%	B
Carboplatin[49-52,d]	15–82%	B
Carvediolol[53,b]	NK	B
Chloramphenicol[55,d]	NK	B
Chlorhexidine[56,d]	NK	B
Chloroquine[57,c,d]	NK	B
Chlorthalidone[58,c]	NK	B
Ciclopirox[54,d]	NK	C
Cidofovir[59,d]	NK	C
Ciprofloxacin[60,b]	NK	B
Cisplatin[61-66,d]	4–97%	B
Clarithromycin[67,68,c]	NK	C
Clindamycin[69,d]	NK	C
Clonazepam[70,b]	NK	B

Table 55-1 Agents Implicated in Drug-Induced Ototoxicity[1,8-242] (continued)

Drug	Incidence	Level of Evidence[a]
Codeine[9,d]	NK	C
Cycloserine[71,b]	NK	B
Cyclosporine[72,d]	2%	B
Cytarabine[73,b]	NK	B
Danazol[74,d]	NK	C
Dantrolene[75,b]	NK	B
Dapsone[76,c]	NK	B
Deferoxamine[77,78,c,d]	29–50%	B
Desipramine[79,c]	NK	B
Diazepam[80,b,c,d]	NK	B
Diclofenac[82,b,c]	NK	B
Didanosine[83,d]	NK	C
Diflunisal[84,c]	1–3%	B
Diltiazem[85,b]	NK	B
Donepezil[86,b]	10%	B
Doxepin[87,c]	NK	C
Doxycycline[88,b]	up to 77%	B
Efavirenz[89,90,d]	NK	C
Enalapril[91,92,d]	NK	C
Enalaprilat[92,d]	NK	C
Erlotinib[93,d]	NK	C
Erythromycin[35,94,95,b,c,d]	32%	B
Ethacrynic acid[96,b,c]	NK	B
Ethionamide[97,d]	NK	C
Etidronate[98,99,c,d]	NK	C
Etodolac[82,c]	NK	B
Famotidine[100,b,c]	NK	C
Fenofibrate[101,b]	NK	C
Fenoprofen[82,c]	NK	B
Flecainide[102,c]	3%	B
Fludarabine[103,d]	NK	C
Fluoxetine[104,b]	NK	C
Furosemide[96,105,106,b,c]	3–6.4% 50–100% if injected rapidly	B
Gentamicin[107-120,d]	0–63%	B
Glycerin[121,d]	NK	C
Hepatitis B vaccine[122,d]	NK	C
Hyaluronidase[128,b]	NK	B
Hydrochlorothiazide[c,d]	NK	B
Hydrocodone–acetaminophen[123,124,d]	NK	C
Hydroxychloroquine[125-127,d]	NK	C
Ibuprofen[82,b,c]	NK	B

Table 55-1 Agents Implicated in Drug-Induced Ototoxicity[1,8-242] (continued)

Drug	Incidence	Level of Evidence[a]
Ifosfamide[129,d]	NK	B
Imipramine[130,c]	NK	C
Indomethacin[82,b,c]	NK	B
Interferon[131,132,c,d]	39.5%	B
Irbesartan[133,b]	NK	A
Isoniazid[134,b,c]	16.6%[e]	B
Isotretinoin[135,c,d]	NK	C
Itraconazole[136,b]	NK	B
Kanamycin[137,d]	5–26.9%	B
Ketoconazole[138,c]	NK	B
Ketoprofen[82,c]	NK	C
Ketorolac[139,d]	NK	C
Lacosamide[140,b]	NK	B
Lamivudine[141,142,d]	NK	C
Lamotrigine[143,144,b]	NK	B
Leflunomide[145,c]	NK	C
Lidocaine[146,c]	NK	B
Lisinopril[147,b]	NK	B
Lithium[148,c]	NK	B
Lorazepam[81,b,c,d]	NK	B
Lovastatin[149,b]	NK	C
Mannitol[150,d]	NK	C
Mefenamic acid[151,b,c,d]	NK	C
Mefloquine[152,c,d]	NK	C
Methylergonovine[153,b,c]	NK	C
Metronidazole[154,d]	NK	C
Minocycline[155,156,b]	14–60%	B
Minoxidil[157,d]	NK	C
Mirtazapine[158,c,d]	1%	B
Misoprostol[159,b,c,d]	NK	C
Moxifloxacin[160,d]	NK	C
Muromonab-CD3[161,d]	NK	C
Nabumetone[162,b]	NK	C
Naproxen[163,d]	NK	C
Neomycin[164,d]	up to 60%	B
Nicardipine[85,165,b,c]	NK	C
Nicotine[166,b]	NK	B
Nifedipine[85,165,b,c]	NK	B
Nimodipine[85,165,c]	NK	B
Nitroprusside[167,168,d]	NK	B
Norfloxacin[169,c,d]	NK	C
Nortriptyline[80,c]	NK	C

Table 55-1 Agents Implicated in Drug-Induced Ototoxicity[1,8-242] (continued)

Drug	Incidence	Level of Evidence[a]
Omeprazole[170,c]	<1%	C
Oxaprozin[171,c,d]	<1%	B
Oxcarbazepine[172,b]	NK	B
Oxymorphone[173,d]	NK	C
Paclitaxel[174,d]	NK	C
Pamidronate[99,b,c,d]	NK	C
Pancuronium[175,d]	60%[f]	C
Paromomycin[176,d]	NK	C
Paroxetine[177,b]	NK	B
Phenobarbital[178,b]	NK	B
Phenylbutazone[82,b,c,d]	NK	B
Phenytoin[179,b]	NK	B
Piroxicam[180,181,c,d]	NK	C
Polymixin B[182,b]	NK	B
Potassium iodide[183,d,g]	NK	C
Prazosin[184,c]	1%	B
Prednisolone[185,b]	NK	B
Pregabalin[186,187,b]	NK	B
Primaquine[188,b]	NK	B
Promethazine[189,b]	NK	B
Propoxyphene[191,d,h]	NK	C
Propylthiouracil[190,d]	NK	C
Quinidine[192,c]	NK	B
Quinine[193,194,b,d]	20%	B
Ramipril[195,b]	2.2%	B
Rifampin[97,196,b]	NK	B
Rimantadine[197,c]	0.3–1%	B
Ritonavir[198,b]	2.6%	B
Ropinirole[199,b]	NK	B
Salicylates[200,c]	NK	B
Sertraline[80,c]	NK	C
Sildenafil[201,202,c,d]	<2%	C
Spectinomycin[203,b]	NK	C
Stavudine[141,142,d]	NK	C
Streptomycin[204,b,d]	4–75%	B
Sulfasalazine[205,c,d]	NK	B
Sulindac[82,c]	NK	C
Tacrolimus[206,d]	NK	C
Tadalafil[207,b]	NK	C
Temazepam[81,b]	1.2%	B
Telmisartan[23,b]	0.3–1%	B
Terazosin[208,b,c]	NK	B

Table 55-1 Agents Implicated in Drug-Induced Ototoxicity[1,8-242] (continued)

Drug	Incidence	Level of Evidence[a]
Tetracaine[209,b]	NK	B
Tetracycline[156,157,b,c]	11–14%	B
Thalidomide[210,211,b]	NK	B
Thiabendazole[212,c]	NK	B
Thiethylperazine[213,c]	NK	B
Tiagabine[215,b]	NK	B
Ticlopidine[214,c]	NK	B
Tigecycline[216,c]	NK	B
Timolol[217,b]	NK	C
Tobramycin[218,b,d]	0–43%	B
Tolmetin[82,c,d]	<3%	C
Topiramate[219,220,b]	NK	C
Torsemide[96,105,106,c]	NK	B
Tramadol[221-224,b]	NK	A, B
Tranylcypromine[225,c]	NK	B
Trazodone[226,b]	NK	C
Valproic acid[227,228,c,d]	1–7%	B
Valsartan[229,b]	<1%	B
Vancomycin[230-232,d]	NK	B
Varenicline[233,b]	NK	C
Venlafaxine[80,c,i]	NK	C
Verapamil[165,b]	NK	C
Vinblastine[234,d]	NK	C
Vincristine[235,d]	NK	B
Vindesine[236,b,c]	<0.05%	A
Vinorelbine[237,c]	NK	A
Vitamin A[238,d,h]	NK	C
Zalcitabine[239,240,d]	NK	C
Zidovudine[141,142,d]	NK	B
Zolipidem[241,b]	NK	B
Zonisamide[242,b]	NK	B

[a]Definitions for Levels of Evidence: Level A—evidence from one or more randomized, controlled clinical trials; Level B—evidence from nonrandomized clinical trials, prospective observational studies, cohort studies, retrospective studies, case-control studies, meta-analyses and/or postmarketing surveillance studies; and Level C—evidence from one or more published case reports or case series.
[b]Vertigo.
[c]Tinnitus.
[d]Ototoxicity.
[e]Of patients with end-stage kidney disease.
[f]Associated with cumulative dose and extended duration.
[g]Associated with accidental topical administration.
[h]In overdose.
[i]Associated with withdrawal symptoms.

medications. Methadone, in particular, has been associated with bilateral sensorineural hearing loss. In most cases, ototoxicity resolved after discontinuation of the drug, although one report noted persistent hearing loss 9 months later.[4,246-248] There are several case reports of heroin-induced ototoxicity leading to reversible or permanent hearing loss.[249-251]

EPIDEMIOLOGY

Drug-induced ototoxicity was first documented in the 17th century in association with quinine therapy, and salicylate ototoxicity was first reported in the 19th century.[251-253] The overall incidence of drug-induced auditory toxicity is not known, but there are known incidence rates with some individual drugs. The incidence of aminoglycoside-induced ototoxicity varies from 0% to >60% depending on the specific agent and the method of assessment.[9,114] The incidence of ototoxicity associated with chemotherapeutic agents is high, especially when dose-intense chemotherapy is administered.[46,148,149] The reported incidence of drug-induced auditory disorders associated with specific agents, where available, is included in Table 55-1.[1,8-242]

MECHANISMS

Drug-induced auditory disorders result from a number of mechanisms (**Table 55-2**[15,27,106,252,254-265]). Ototoxicity generally results from damage to the cochlea (leading to changes in hearing) or the vestibulum (leading to disorders of balance).[266,267] Architectural changes that can be caused by drugs closely resemble the damage caused by noise and aging.[4,268] The actual causes of the structural changes may be multifactorial.

Aminoglycosides can cause the formation of reactive oxygen species that overwhelm the body's natural detoxification systems (glutathione, superoxide dismutase).[257,261,262] The physical changes in the inner ear induced by aminoglycosides include a decreased number of hair cells.[13,254,255] Loss of spiral ganglion—cells that conduct nerve impulses from the cochlea to the brain—has also been observed following aminoglycoside administration.[262,263]

Diuretics can cause temporary profound hearing loss through disruption of the homeostasis of the endocochlear fluid resulting in depression of the endocochlear potential.[252,255,256] The endocochlear fluid, endocochlear potential, and endolymph all are parts of the ear that allow sound to be converted into nerve impulses.[263] Although loop diuretics used alone generally cause only temporary hearing loss, they can potentiate the toxicity of other ototoxic agents, possibly by increasing their concentrations in the endolymph fluid covering hair cells resulting in much higher hair cell exposure.[252,255,263-265]

Table 55-2 Mechanisms of Drug-Induced Ototoxicity[15,27,106 252,254-265]

Drug	Mechanism(s)
Aminoglycosides	Formation of reactive oxygen species
Aminoglycosides and chemotherapeutic agents	Decreased number of hair cells Loss of spiral ganglion
Chemotherapeutic agents	Changes in mitochondrial function Direct cell death
Chemotherapeutic agents and diuretics	Reduction in endocochlear potential
Diuretics	Disruption of endocochlear fluid homeostasis Disruption of endolymph homeostatis
Opioids, quinine, and salicylates	Decreased cochlear blood flow
Salicylates	Activation of NMDA receptors

NMDA = *N*-methyl-D-aspartate.

The primary mechanism of quinine and salicylate ototoxicity is thought to be decreased cochlear blood flow due to inhibition of prostaglandin synthesis.[252,255] This hearing loss is generally reversible and usually occurs only with high doses of the culprit agents.[256] Salicylate ototoxicity may also be caused by increasing labyrinthine pressure or vasoconstriction.[200] In addition, activation of *N*-methyl-D-aspartate (NMDA) receptors has been implicated in salicylate-induced tinnitus.[26] Similarly, it is thought that opioids reduce cochlear blood flow as a result of vasoconstriction leading to cochlear ischemia and hearing loss.[269]

Cancer chemotherapeutic agents damage the inner ear in a number ways. These drugs may cause direct cell death, disturb the homeostasis of the endolymph, or cause degeneration of hair cells.[254,255,270,271] In addition, cisplatin may impair function of the stria vascularis by reducing endocochlear potential. In the normal inner ear, the stria vascularis maintains the electrochemical gradient between the endolymph and the perilymph.[256] Cisplatin also reduces the number of spiral ganglion cells in areas of the cochlea that may otherwise appear normal.[262,270] Change in mitochondrial function has also been noted with cisplatin ototoxicity.[270]

CLINICAL PRESENTATION AND DIFFERENTIAL DIAGNOSIS

Patient symptom reporting is generally the initiating event in the diagnosis of drug-induced ear disorders. Ototoxicity can result in cochleotoxicity, which leads to changes in hearing, and/or vestibulotoxicity, resulting in disorders of balance. Hearing and balance changes may be present simultaneously. Vestibular symptoms include vertigo, nausea, oscillopsia (problematic ocular fixation), dizziness, lightheadedness, and gait disturbance.[115,272] Common symptoms and symptoms of drug-induced ototoxicity are presented in **Table 55-3**.[9,115,252]

Diagnosis of ototoxicity can be challenging due to the variability in symptom severity and inconsistent presentation among patients. The primary reason for delayed diagnosis is the propensity for hearing loss to develop initially at frequencies above those used in daily conversation.[273] Initial symptoms may include perceived fullness in the ear, tinnitus, difficulty hearing the television or radio, or difficulty talking on the telephone.[115] **Table 55-4** lists the

Table 55-3 Signs and Symptoms Associated with Drug-Induced Ototoxicity[9,115,252]

- Difficulty hearing television or conversation
- Disequilibrium
- Frank hearing loss
- Fullness in the ear
- Gait disturbance
- Lightheadedness
- Oscillopsia
- Tinnitus

Table 55-4 Conditions to Consider in the Differential Diagnosis of Drug-Induced Ototoxicity[274-276]

Hearing Loss (sensorineural)

- Acoustic neuroma
- Autoimune disease
- Barotrauma
- Cerebrovascular ischemia/stroke
- Meniere disease
- Meningioma
- Meningitis
- Multiple sclerosis
- Noise exposure
- Ototoxic medications
- Penetrating trauma
- Presbycusis
- Viral infections

Tinnitus

- Cerebrovascular ischemia/stroke
- Chronic renal failure
- Diabetes
- Fibrous dysplasia
- Hypercholesterolemia
- Hypertension
- Infection
- Medications
- Osteogensis imperfecta
- Otosclerosis
- Paget disease
- Rheumatoid arthritis
- Sarcoid
- Sickle cell anemia
- Stroke
- Systemic lupus erythematos
- Thyroid disease
- Tumors

Vertigo

- Acoustic neuroma
- Benign paroxysmal positional vertigo
- Cogan syndrome
- Herpes zoster oticus
- Labyrinthine concussion
- Medications
- Meniere disease
- Otitis media
- Perilymphatic fistula
- Recurrent vestibulopathy
- Semicircular canal dehiscensce syndrome
- Vestibular neuritis

conditions that should be considered in the differential diagnosis of drug-induced ototoxicity.[274,275]

Baseline audiometric testing for all patients receiving a drug with a potential to cause ototoxicity has been recommended. This is not always done, however, due to the large number of drugs known to cause ototoxicity, the cost of testing, and inconsistent practices or prescreening.[273,277] At a minimum, efforts should be made to do baseline audiometric testing and testing during treatment for those patients receiving medications with the highest risk of ototoxicity. In addition, audiometric monitoring of selected high-risk patient populations (e.g., children who are still developing language skills) may allow detection of ototoxicity at an early stage so that disability can be prevented.[278]

There are three main approaches currently used for monitoring: ototoxicity basic audiologic assessment, high frequency audiometry, and otoacoustic emission.[279] The latter two methods are becoming more widely used to evaluate ototoxicity because they are less resource-intense and are easier for patients even when critically ill.[279] However, none of these assessment approaches is appropriate for all patients.

Table 55-5 Risk Factors for Drug-Induced Ototoxicity[16,45-51,61,77,109,114,115,117,204,252,256,280-287]

- Age
- Bacteremia
- Concomitant or prior exposure to ototoxic drugs
- Cranial radiation
- Cumulative dose
- Decreased serum albumin concentration
- Decreased serum hemoglobin concentration, hematocrit, and red blood cell count
- Diet (magnesium and zinc deficiency, low protein)
- Duration of therapy >14 days
- Electrolyte imbalances
- Elevated serum iron concentration
- Elevated temperature
- Genetic mutation in mitochondrial RNA
- Hepatic dysfunction
- High daily dose
- Hypovolemia
- Meningitis
- Neonatal intensive care unit
- Noise exposure
- Pre-existing hearing problems
- Renal dysfunction

RNA = ribonucleic acid.

RISK FACTORS

Risk factors for drug-induced ototoxicity are listed in **Table 55-5**.[16,45-51,61,77,109,114,115,117,204,252,256,280-287] High drug doses (e.g., with NSAIDs, diuretics) and, in some cases, cumulative doses (e.g., with aminoglycoside antibiotics, oncologic agents) are occasionally predictors of ototoxicity.[38] Rapid administration of intravenous (IV) loop diuretics is a risk factor for ototoxicity.[267]

Familial groupings of individuals at increased risk for aminoglycoside ototoxicity have been reported.[205] Several point mutations (A1555G, T deletion at 961) in the mitochondrial 12S rRNA of selected families was confirmed to predispose members to both familial deafness and aminoglycoside-induced ototoxicity. At least one of the mutations facilitates binding of the aminoglycoside to the mitochondrial RNA.[283] Studies indicate that development of ototoxicity is due to changed mitochondrial protein synthesis.[204,267,283]

Factors reported to increase the risk of aminoglycoside ototoxicity include total dose administered, duration of administration >14 days, dehydration, hypotension, metabolic acidosis, hypokalemia, hypomagnesemia, renal dysfunction, hepatic dysfunction, and concomitant administration of other ototoxic agents.[27,106,107,120,158,267,288] Gentamicin and tobramycin peak concentrations >12 mg/L and trough concentrations >2 mg/L, have been reported to increase the risk of ototoxicity.[288] Similarly, peak serum amikacin concentrations >35 mg/L and trough concentrations >10 mg/L have been reported to increase the risk of ototoxicity.[288]

Vancomycin ototoxicity does not occur in animal models, and some studies indicate that it is related to concomitant use of other ototoxic medications.[244,245] However, evidence from the 1950s suggested that peak serum vancomycin concentrations >80 mg/L were associated with hearing loss.[244] There is also a case report of a neonate who received an accidental overdose of vancomycin (serum concentrations >100 mg/L for 4 days) who subsequently had no evidence of hearing loss.[285] Reversible tinnitus has been reported in patients with serum vancomycin concentrations >40 mg/L.[284,288]

Animal research and limited human studies suggest low-protein diets and lower serum albumin concentrations increase the risk for cisplatin-induced ototoxicity.[280] In a small group of patients who participated in audiometric testing prior to cisplatin therapy, those with poorer health status as indicated by lower serum albumin concentration and anemia experienced a higher rate of hearing loss than those in better health.[289] Low serum albumin concentrations may lead to higher unbound cisplatin concentrations increasing the risk of ototoxicity; however, apoptosis of cochlear cells and avid cisplatin tissue binding are more problematic than decreased levels of albumin.[290] Decreased blood flow and oxygen availability secondary to anemia may play a role in developing hearing loss due to reduced metabolism.[289]

Elevated blood concentrations of metals such as iron can potentiate the formation of the reactive oxygen species.[291,292] Iron accumulation in transfusion-dependent patients has been associated with end organ damage in some patient populations, and deferoxamine is frequently used to decrease the iron burden. Sensorineural hearing loss has been reported in 3.8–57% of these patients.[293] Some investigators attribute the hearing deficit to iron overload, while others ascribe it to deferoxamine. Chiodo and colleagues found no association between risk of ototoxicity and serum ferritin and hemoglobin concentrations.[77,79] One study found an association between higher doses of deferoxamine given less frequently compared to lower doses administered daily.[77] Iron may also play a role in ototoxicity induced by aminoglycosides by forming complexes with the drugs. These complexes serve as precursors to free radical formation.[292] The risk of ototoxicity associated with furosemide is increased with prolonged duration of therapy.[294]

MORBIDITY AND MORTALITY

The exact incidence of ototoxicity has not been quantified, but it is approximated that millions of patients are exposed to ototoxic medications annually. Hearing loss and, sometimes, tinnitus due to ototoxicity can cause permanent disability.[295] In children, hearing difficulties impact social, emotional, and cognitive development.[36] Children with hearing problems have delayed language development and reading skills. Hearing loss also causes social and emotional challenges for adults including decreased quality of life due to struggles with communicating, cognitive decline, social isolation, and development of depression.[296]

PREVENTION

Prevention of drug-induced ototoxicity requires appropriate risk assessment and close monitoring.[297] Methods of prevention are listed in **Table 55-6**.[288-308] Administration of numerous chemicals to provide

Table 55-6 Approaches to Help Prevent Drug-Induced Ototoxicity[288-308]

Currently Available

- Avoid rapid intravenous infusions
- Close monitoring
- Limiting therapy duration
- Limiting total dose
- Risk assessment

Investigational

- α-MSH
- α-tocopherol
- Amifostine
- Ethacrynic acid
- Glial derived neurotrophic factor
- Glutathione
- Intensity-modulated radiation therapy
- Iron chelators
- Melatonin
- *N*-acetylcysteine
- Neurotrophic peptide ORG 2766
- Salicylates
- Sodium thiosulfate
- Superoxide dismutase

MSH = melanocyte-stimulating hormone.

protection from ototoxicity and enhance recovery of hearing are under investigation.[277,289] Included in this group are drugs commonly used for other indications.[271,289,290,296,304,305,309-314] Acetylcysteine protects auditory neurons and hair cells from cisplatin ototoxicity in vitro.[305] Concomitant administration of the nutritional supplement α-tocopherol with gentamicin has delayed progression of hearing loss and preserved vestibular function in animals.[301] Other promising experimental agents include diethyldithiocarbamate, glutathione, and methionine.[289,296] No drugs are currently U.S. Food and Drug Administration (FDA)–approved specifically for prevention of drug-induced ototoxicity.

Judicious administration of aminoglycosides to only those patients with serious infections and limiting the duration of exposure can help prevent permanent hearing loss. Unfortunately, in the current era of more widespread antimicrobial resistance, the use of aminoglycosides in combination with other antibiotics is sometimes required in the treatment of serious infections such as *Pseudomonas aeruginosa*.

Prevention of cancer chemotherapy-induced ototoxicity is complicated. A primary concern with the use of preventive measures is the possibility that the anti-tumor activity of the antineoplastic agent could be compromised. Several strategies for retaining the cytotoxic properties of cancer chemotherapy agents while reducing the incidence of ototoxicity are in the early stages of testing. These include compartmentalization of medication, timed dosing, and localized cranial radiation.[296,297,307]

There are some data supporting the use of sodium thiosulfate to protect children and adults from ototoxicity during carboplatin treatment. Sodium thiosulfate provided protection from ototoxicity when administered in a dose of at least 16 g/m^2 4 hours after carboplatin treatment.[315]

Salicylates and ethacrynic acid—drugs that may themselves cause temporary hearing loss—have actually shown promise for protecting from drug-induced ototoxicity caused by other agents when administration is timed appropriately. Animal data revealed salicylates can chelate iron and serve as an antioxidant against gentamicin-induced hearing loss without affecting antibiotic efficacy.[299] Administration of ethacrynic acid when serum gentamicin concentrations are highest in the cochlear fluid facilitates excretion, leading to loss of fewer outer hair cells and lower compound action potential thresholds.[304]

MANAGEMENT

Treatment of reversible ototoxicity as with salicylate- or furosemide-induced tinnitus involves simply discontinuing therapy with the offending agent.[252] Generally, tinnitus resolves within several days.[29] When offending medications cannot be discontinued and/or damage is permanent, specific treatment measures are indicated. For patients who experience permanent drug-induced hearing loss, options include hearing aids and cochlear implants.[257]

Several options for the treatment of tinnitus have been explored, although evidence of the effectiveness of drugs in the treatment of this condition is largely anecdotal. Agents that are well-known causes of tinnitus have also been used in its treatment (e.g., benzodiazepines, furosemide, lidocaine, prednisone, metformin), albeit with limited success.[109,308] Anesthetics, antidepressants, anticonvulsants, anxiolytics, antihistamines, diuretics, and antispasmodics have all been studied but had little to no benefit and were associated with adverse effects.[304,308-314] There have been several antioxidants that have been shown some efficacy of alleviating ototoxicity; however, to date there are no human trials with these medications.[316-320]

The use of frequency masking devices and patient counseling on ways to live with tinnitus remain the mainstays of treatment for this disorder.[304,314] Frequency masking devices produce a sound that masks the tinnitus sound patients hear.[311] The device emits a frequency that is similar in pitch to the tinnitus sound effectively blocking out that sound.[311] These devices can be incorporated into hearing aids or used separately, and patients who utilize them report good success in masking their tinnitus.[311]

There is continuing research on treatment options for vestibular dysfunction. Antihistamines such as diphenhydramine, meclizine, and promethazine have been shown to provide some benefit for patients suffering from vestibular dysfunction.[321] Other treatment options include trimethadione and scopolamine patches.[321] Vestibular rehabilitation exercises are often required to help patients learn adaptation to residual reflexes or substitution of ocular and proprioception cues.[121]

INFORMATION FOR PATIENTS

Patients who are taking drugs known to cause auditory disorders should be instructed to consult their healthcare provider should they notice a change in hearing acuity or unusual sounds in the ears which might include ringing, buzzing, clicking, hissing, or roaring.[322] Patients should be instructed to avoid concomitant use of drugs known to cause ototoxicity for the duration of their treatment with a potentially ototoxic medication.[323,324] It would also be reasonable for healthcare providers to review medication lists to identify any other ototoxic medications and evaluate their continued need. Information about the warning signs of ototoxicity such as dizziness, ringing in the ears, worsening of tinnitus, unexplained ear pressure, and any abnormal hearing changes should be communicated to the patient when they start medications known to cause ototoxicity.[324] Patients should also be instructed to keep hydrated, avoid caffeine, and avoid loud music or noises while taking ototoxic medications.[324]

REFERENCES

1. Mick P, Westerberg BD. Sensorineural hearing loss as a probable serious adverse drug reaction associated with low-dose oral azithromycin. *J Otolaryngol.* 2007; 36:257-63.
2. Roth SM, Williams SM, Jiang L et al. Susceptibility genes for gentamicin-induced vestibular dysfunction. *J Vestib Res.* 2008; 18:59-68.
3. Knoll C, Smith RJ, Shores C, Blatt J. Hearing genes and cisplatin deafness: a pilot study. *Laryngoscope.* 2006; 116:72-4.
4. Shaw KA, Babu KM, Hack JB. Methadone, another cause of opioid-associated hearing loss: a case report. *J Emerg Med.* 2011; 41:635-9.
5. Cianfrone G, Pentangelo D, Cianfrone F et al. Pharmacological drugs inducing ototoxicity, vestibular symptoms and tinnitus: an updated guide. *Eur Rev Med Pharmacol Sci.* 2011; 15:601-36.
6. Lalwani, AK. Disorders of hearing. In: Kasper D, Fauci A, Longo D et al. (eds). *Harrison's manual of medicine.* 19th ed. New York: McGraw-Hill; 2014.
7. Tyler RS, Pienkowski M, Roncancio ER et al. A review of hyperacusis and future directions: part I. Definitions and manifestations. *Am J Audiol.* 2014; 23:402-19.
8. Thein P, Kalinec GM, Park C, Kalinec F. In vitro assessment of antiretroviral drugs demonstrates potential for ototoxicity. *Hear Res.* 2014; 310:27-35.
9. Seligmann H, Podoshin L, Ben-David J et al. Drug-induced tinnitus and other hearing disorders. *Drug Saf.* 1996; 14:198-212.
10. Blakley BW, Schilling H. Deafness associated with acetaminophen and codeine abuse. *J. Otolaryngol Head Neck Surg.* 2008; 7:507-9.
11. Lukacs B, Grange JC, Comet D, McCarthy C. Three-year prospective study of 3228 clinical BPH patients treated with alfuzosin in general practice. *Prostate Cancer Prostatic Dis.* 1998; 1:276-83.
12. Barclay ML, Kirkpatrick CMJ, Begg EJ. Once daily aminoglycoside therapy: is it less toxic than multiple daily doses and how should it be monitored? *Clin Pharmacokinet.* 1999; 36:89-98.
13. Aran JM, Erre JP, Da Costa DL et al. Acute and chronic effects of aminoglycosides on cochlear hair cells. *Ann N Y Acad Sci.* 1999; 884:60-8.
14. Nakashima T, Teranishi M, Hibi T et al. Vestibular and cochlear toxicity of aminoglycosides—a review. *Acta Otolaryngol.* 2000; 120:904-11.
15. Beubien AR, Desjardins S, Ormsby E, Bayne et al. Delay in hearing loss following drug administration: a consistent feature of amikacin ototoxicity. *Acta Otolaryngol.* 1990; 109:345-52.
16. Saxena AK, Panhotra BR, Naguib M. Sudden irreversible sensory-neural hearing loss in a patient with diabetes receiving amikacin as an antibiotic-heparin lock. *Pharmacother.* 2002; 105-8.
17. Arbusow V, Strupp M, Brandt T. Amiodarone-induced severe prolonged head-positional vertigo and vomiting. *Neurology.* 1998; 51:917.
18. Amicar, aminocaproic acid [product information]. Florence, KY: Xanodyne Pharmacal; 2001.
19. Camarata SJ, Weil MH, Hanashiro PK et al. Cardiac arrest in the critically ill: I—a study of predisposing causes in 132 patients. *Circulation.* 1971; 44:688-95.
20. Gult JE. A fatal reaction to aminophylline given intravenously. *Med J Aust.* 1964; 51:148.
21. Feder R. Tinnitus associated with amitriptyline. *J Clin Psychiatry.* 1990; 51:85-6.
22. Mendis D, Johnston M. An unusual case of prolonged tinnitus following low-dose amitriptyline. *J Psychopharmacol.* 2008; 22:574-5.
23. Faruqui AA. Evaluation of safety and efficacy of telmisartan-amlodipine combination in treating hypertension. *J Indian Med Assoc.* 2008; 106:612-4.
24. Brummett RE. Effects of antibiotics-diuretic interactions in the guinea pig model of ototoxicity. *Rev Infect Dis.* 1981; 3(suppl):S216-23.
25. Jones FE, Hanson DR. H influenza meningitis treated with ampicillin or chloramphenicol, and subsequent hearing loss. *Dev Med Child Neurol.* 1977; 19:593-7.
26. Hirose T, Uwahodo Y, Yamada S et al. Mechanism of action of aripiprazole predicts clinical efficacy and a favorable side-effect profile. *J Psychopharmacol.* 2004; 18:375-83.
27. Guitton MJ, Caston J, Ruel J et al. Salicylate induces tinnitus through activation of cochlear NMDA receptors. *J Neurosci.* 2003; 23:3944-52.
28. Cazals Y. Auditory sensori-neural alterations induced by salicylate. *Prog Neurobiol.* 2000; 62:583-631.
29. Brien J. Ototoxicity associated with salicylates. *Drug Saf.* 1993; 9:143-8.
30. Koren G. Hearing loss in a woman on aspirin: the silent pharmacokinetic parameter. *Ther Drug Monitor.* 2009; 31:1-2.
31. Bentuè-Ferre D, Arvieux C, Tribut O et al. Clinical pharmacology, efficacy and safety of atazanavir: a review. *Expert Opin Drug Metab Toxicol.* 2009; 5:1455-68.

32. Tjernstrom O, Andreasson L, Groth P et al. Effect of atropine on the eustachian tube function. *ORL J Otorhinolaryngol Relat Spec.* 1985; 47:95-100.
33. Bizjak ED, Huag III MT, Schilz RJ et al. Intravenous azithromycin-induced ototoxicity. *Pharmacother.* 1999; 19:245-8.
34. Ress BD, Gross EM. Irreversible sensorineural hearing loss as a result of azithromycin ototoxicity: a case report. *Ann Otol Rhinol Laryngol.* 2000; 109:435-7.
35. Tseng AL, Dolovich L, Salit IE. Azithromycin-related ototoxicity in patients infected with human immunodeficiency virus. *Clin Infect Dis.* 1997; 24:76-7.
36. Prinicipi N, Esposito S. Comparative tolerability of erythromycin and newer macrolide antibacterials in paediatric patients. *Drug Saf.* 1999; 20:25-41.
37. Moore RD, Lerner SA, Levine DP. Nephrotoxicity and ototoxicity of aztreonam vs aminoglycoside therapy in seriously ill nonneutropenic patients. *J Infect Dis.* 1992; 165:683-8.
38. Zintel HA, Ma RA, Nichols AC et al. The absorption, distribution, excretion and toxicity of bacitracin in man. *Am J Med Sci.* 1949; 218:439-45.
39. Marina N, Chang KW, Malogolowkin M et al. Amifostine does not protect against the ototoxicity of high-dose cisplatin combined with etoposide and bleomycin in pediatric germ-cell tumors: a Children's Oncology Group study. *Cancer.* 2005; 104:841-7.
40. Lanthier PL, Morgan MY, Ballantyne J. Bromocriptine-associated ototoxicity. *J Laryngol Otol.* 1984; 98:399-404.
41. Ward A, Heel RC. Bumetanide: a review of its pharmacodynamic and pharmacokinetic properties and therapeutic use. *Drugs.* 1984; 28:426-64.
42. Hussain SS, Heard CM, Bembridge JL. Hearing loss following spinal anaesthesia with bupivacaine. *Clin Otolaryngol Allied Sci.* 1996; 21:449-54.
43. Szuba MP, Leuchter AF. Falling backward in two elderly patients taking bupropion. *J Clin Psychiatry.* 1992; 53:157-9.
44. Settle EC. Tinnitus related to bupropion treatment. *J Clin Psychiatry.* 1991; 52:352.
45. Neldham S, Forsen B. Antihypertensive treatment in elderly patients aged 75 years or over: a 24-week study of the tolerability of candesartan cilexetil in relation to hydrochlorothiazide. *Drugs Aging.* 2001; 18:225-32.
46. Huitema AD, Spaander M, Mathot RA et al. Relationship between exposure and toxicity in high-dose chemotherapy with cyclophosphamide, thiotepa and carboplatin. *Ann Oncol.* 2002; 13:374-84.
47. El-Mehairy MM, Shaker A, Ramadan M et al. Control of essential hypertension with captopril, an angiotensin converting enzyme inhibitor. *Br J Clin Pharmacol.* 1981; 11:469-75.
48. Kobayashi T, Nisijima K, Ehara Y et al. Pitch perception shift: a rare side effect of carbamazepine. *Psychiatry Clin Neurosci.* 2001; 55:415-7.
49. Cavaletti G, Bogliun G, Zincone A et al. Neuro- and ototoxicity of high-dose carboplatin treatment in poor prognosis ovarian cancer patients. *Anticancer Res.* 1998; 18:3797-802.
50. Parsons SK, Neault MW, Lehmann LE et al. Severe ototoxicity following carboplatin-containing conditioning regimen for autologous marrow transplantation for neuroblastoma. *Bone Marrow Transplant.* 1998; 22:669-74.
51. Landier W. Hearing loss related to ototoxicity in children with cancer. *J Ped Oncol Nurs.* 1998; 15:195-206.
52. Salvinelli F, Casale M, Vincenzi B et al. Bilateral irreversible hearing loss associated with the combination of carboplatin and paclitaxel chemotherapy: a unusual side effect. *J Exp Clin Cancer Res.* 2003; 22:155-8.
53. McTavish D, Campoli-Richards D, Sorkin EM. Carvedilol: a review of its pharmacodynamic and pharmacokinetic properties and therapeutic efficacy. *Drugs.* 1993; 45:232-58.
54. Baylancicek S, Serin GM, Ciprut A et al. Ototoxic effect of topical ciclopirox as an antimycotic preparation. *Otol Neurotol.* 2008; 29:910-3.
55. Iqbal SM, Srivatsav CB. Chloramphenicol ototoxicity. *J Laryngol Otol.* 1984; 98:523-5.
56. Peridex, chlorhexidine [product information]. Phoenix, AZ: Zila Pharmaceuticals; 2000.
57. Belai N, Gebrehiwet S, Fitsum Y et al. Hydrochlorothiazide and risk of hearing disorder: a case series. *J Med Case Rep.* 2018; 12:135.
58. Norris CH. Drugs affecting the inner ear. A review of their clinical efficacy, mechanisms of action, toxicity and place in therapy. *Drugs.* 1988; 36:754-72.
59. Safrin SF. Reinforcement of guidelines to prevent nephrotoxicity with Vistide use, and reports of uveitis/iritis, hearing loss. Foster City, CA: Gilead Sciences; 1998. Letter.
60. Lode H, Borner K, Koeppe P. Pharmacodynamics of fluoroquinolones. *Clin Infect Dis.* 1998; 27:33-9.
61. Kollmannsberger C, Kuzcyk M, Mayer F et al Late toxicity following curative treatment of testicular cancer. *Semin Surg Oncol.* 1999; 17:275-81.
62. Sakamoto M, Kaga K, Tomokazu K. Extended high-frequency ototoxicity induced by the first administration of cisplatin. *Otolaryngol Head Neck Surg.* 2000; 122:828-33.
63. Huddart RA, Lau FN, Guerrero-Urbano T et al. Accelerated chemotherapy in the treatment of urothelial cancer. *Clin Oncol.* 2001; 13:279-83.
64. Gogas H, Shapiro F, Aghajanian C et al. The impact of diabetes mellitus on the toxicity of therapy for advanced ovarian cancer. *Gynecol Oncol.* 1996; 61:22-6.
65. Brandt T. Bilateral vestibulopathy revisited. *Eur J Med Res.* 1996; 1:361-8.
66. Mota LA, Melo MS, Santos MH et al. Cisplatin ototoxicity: series of case. *Rev Assoc Med Bras.* 2007; 53:370-3.
67. Roussel G, Igual J; GETIM. Clarithromycin with minocycline and clofazimine for *Mycobacterium avium intracellulare* complex lung disease in patients without the acquired immune deficiency syndrome. *Int J Tuberc Lung Dis.* 1998; 2:462-70.
68. Uzun C. Tinnitus due to clarithromycin. *J Laryngol Otol.* 2003; 117:1006-7.
69. Scissors B, Shwayder T. Topical clindamycin reproducibly causing tinnitus in a 14-year-old boy. *J Am Acad Dermatol.* 2005; 54:S243-44.
70. Jenner P, Pratt JA, Marsden CD. Mechanism of action of clonazepam in myoclonus in relation to effects on GABA and 5-HT. *Adv Neurol.* 1986; 43:629-43.
71. Seromycin, cycloserine [product information]. Indianapolis, IN: Eli Lilly and Company; 1995.
72. Sandimmune, cyclosporine [product information]. East Hanover, NJ: Novartis Pharmaceuticals Corporation; 1999.
73. Cersosimo RJ, Carter RT, Matthews SJ et al. Acute cerebellar syndrome, conjunctivitis, and hearing loss associated with low-dose cytarabine administration. *Drug Intell Clin Pharm.* 1987; 21:798-803.
74. Enyeart JJ, Price WA. Bilateral sensorineural hearing loss from danazol therapy: a case report. *J Reprod Med.* 1984; 29:351-3.
75. Pace-Balzan A, Ramsden RT. Sudden bilateral sensorineural hearing loss during treatment with dantrolene sodium (Dantrium). *J Laryngol Otol.* 1988; 102:57-8.
76. Dapsone [product information]. Princeton, NJ: Jacobus Pharmaceutical; 1997.
77. Chiodo AA, Alberti PW, Sher GD et al. Desferrioxamine ototoxicity in an adult transfusion-dependent population. *J Otolaryngol.* 1997; 26:116-22.
78. Cases A, Kelly J, Sabater F et al. Ocular and auditory toxicity in hemodialyzed patients receiving desferrioxamine. *Nephron.* 1990; 56:19-23.
79. Karimi M, Asadi-Pooya AA, Dhademi B et al. Evaluation of the incidence of sensorineural hearing loss in beta-thalassemia major patients under regular chelation therapy with desferrioxamine. *Acta Haematol.* 2002; 108:79-83.

80. Robinson SK, Viirre ES, Stein MB. Antidepressant therapy in tinnitus. *Hear Res.* 2007; 226:221-31.
81. Busto U, Sellers EM, Naranjo CA et al. Withdrawal reaction after long-term therapeutic use of benzodiazepines. *N Engl J Med.* 1986; 315:854-9.
82. Jung TT, Rhee CK, Lee CS et al. Ototoxicity of salicylate, nonsteroidal anti-inflammatory drugs and quinine. *Otolaryngol Clin North Am.* 1993; 26:791-810.
83. Vogeser M, Colebunders R, Depraetere K et al. Deafness caused by didanosine. *Eur J Clin Microbiol Infect Dis.* 1998; 17:214-5.
84. Dolobid, diflunisal [product information]. West Point, PA: Merck and Co; 1997.
85. Narvaez M, Figueras A, Capella D. Tinnitus with calcium-channel blockers. *Lancet.* 1994; 343: 1229-30.
86. McCain KR, Sawyer TS, Spiller HA. Evaluation of centrally acting cholinesterase inhibitor exposures in adults. *Ann Pharmacother.* 2007; 41:1632-7.
87. Golden RN, Evans DL, Nau CH Jr. Doxepin and tinnitus. *South Med J.* 1983; 76:1204-5.
88. Pages F, Boutin JP, Meynard JB et al. Tolerability of doxycycline monohydrate salt vs. chloroquine-proguanil in malaria chemoprophylaxis. *Trop Med Int Health.* 2002; 7:919-24.
89. Simdon J, Watters D, Bartlett S et al. Ototoxicity associated with the use of nucleoside analog reverse transcriptase inhibitors: a report of 3 possible cases and review of the literature. *Clin Infect Dis.* 2001; 32:1623-7.
90. Sustiva [product information]. Princeton, NJ: Bristol-Myers Squibb Company; 2004.
91. Inman WH, Rawson NS. Deafness with enalapril and prescription event monitoring. *Lancet.* 1987;1:872.
92. Menne J, Haller H. Fixed-dose lercanidipine/enalapril for hypertension. *Drugs Today (Barc).* 2008; 44:261-70.
93. Koutras AK, Mastronikolis NS, Evans TR J et al. Irreversible ototoxicity associated with the use of erlotinib in a patient with pancreatic cancer. *Acta Oncologica.* 2008; 47:1171-3.
94. Sacristan JA, de Cos MA, Soto J et al. Ototoxicity of erythromycin in man: electrophysiologic approach. *Am J Otol.* 1993; 14:186-8.
95. Swanson DJ, Sung RJ, Fine MJ et al. Erythromycin ototoxicity: prospective assessment with serum concentrations and audiograms in a study of patients with pneumonia. *Am J Med.* 1992; 92:61-8.
96. Ikeda K, Oshima T, Hidaka H et al. Molecular and clinical implications of loop diuretic ototoxicity. *Hear Res.* 1997; 107:1-8.
97. Newton RW. Side effects of drugs used to treat tuberculosis. *Scott Med J.* 1975; 20:47-9.
98. Yeşil S, Çömlekçi A, Güneri A. Further hearing loss during osteoporosis treatment with etidronate. *Postgrad Med J.* 1998; 74:363-4.
99. Reid IR, Mills DA, Wattie DJ. Ototoxicity associated with intravenous bisphosphonate administration. *Calcif Tissue Int.* 1995; 56:584-5.
100. Bernal Sahagun F, Barinagarrementeria AR, Barrera Rios L et al. Treatment of duodenal ulcer with famotidine. *Rev Gastroenterol Mex.* 1989; 54:13-7.
101. Asquer JC, Corda C, Le Malicot K, Jessent V. Effects of atorvastatin 10 mg and fenofibrate 200 mg on the low-density lipoprotein profile in dyslipidemic patients: a 12-week, multicenter, randomized, open-label, parallel-group study. *Curr Ther Res Clin Exp.* 2009; 70:71-93.
102. Gentzkow GD, Sullivan JY. Extracardiac adverse effects of flecainide. *Am J Cardiol.* 1984; 53:101B-105B.
103. O'Brien RK, Sparling TG. Gentamicin and fludarabine ototoxicity. *Ann Pharmacother.* 1995; 29:200-1.
104. Cunningham M, Cunningham K, Lydiard RB. Eye tics and subjective hearing impairment during fluoxetine therapy. *Am J Psychiatry.* 1990; 147:947-8.
105. Tudball CF, Cook DJ. Potentiators and bolus intravenous furosemide. *Lancet.* 2001; 358:1373.
106. Quick CA, Hoppe W. Permanent deafness associated with furosemide administration. *Ann Otol.* 1975; 84:94-101.
107. Govaerts PJ, Claes J, Van De Heyning PH et al. Aminoglycoside-induced ototoxicity. *Toxicol Lett.* 1990; 52:227-51.
108. Knoderer CA, Everett JA, Buss WF. Clinical issues surrounding once-daily aminoglycoside dosing in children. *Pharmacother.* 2003; 23:44-56.
109. Bates DE, Beaumont SJ, Baylis BW. Ototoxicity induced by gentamicin and furosemide. *Ann Pharmacother.* 2002; 36:446-51.
110. Rizzi MD, Hirose K. Aminoglycoside ototoxicity. *Curr Opin Otolaryngol Head Neck Surg.* 2007; 15:352-7.
111. Wong DL, Rutka JA. Do aminoglycoside otic preparations cause ototoxicity in the presence of tympanic membrane perforations? *Otolaryngol Head Neck Surg.* 1997; 116:404-10.
112. Mulheran M, Degg C, Burr S et al. Occurrence and risk of cochleotoxicity in cystic fibrosis patients receiving repeated high-dose aminoglycoside therapy. *Antimicrob Agents Chemother.* 2001; 45:2502-9.
113. Hinojosa R, Nelson EG, Lerner SA et al. Aminoglycoside ototoxicity: a human temporal bone study. *Laryngoscope.* 2001; 111:1797-805.
114. Minor LB. Gentamicin-induced bilateral vestibular hypofunction. *JAMA.* 1998; 279:541-4.
115. Warkentin D, Ippoliti C, Bruton J et al. Toxicity of single daily dose gentamicin in stem cell transplantation. *Bone Marrow Transplant,* 1999; 24:57-61.
116. Kirkpatrick CMJ, Duffull BS, Begg EJ. Once-daily aminoglycoside therapy: potential ototoxicity (letter). *Antimicrob Agents Chemother.* 1997; 41:879-80.
117. Smith PF. Are vestibular hair cells excited to death by aminoglycoside antibiotics? *J Vestib Res.* 2000; 10:1-5.
118. Ohler KH, Menke JA, Fuller L. Use of higher dose extended interval aminoglycosides in a neonatal intensive care unit. *Am J Perinatol.* 2000; 17:285-90.
119. Walsted A. Unpredictable hearing loss after intratympanic gentamicin treatment for vertigo: a new theory. *Acta Otolaryngol.* 2001; 121:42-4.
120. Triggs E, Charles B. Pharmacokinetics and therapeutic drug monitoring of gentamicin in the elderly. *Clin Pharmacokinet.* 1999; 37:331-41.
121. Bodo G, Rozsa L, Shea JJ. Temporary loss of hearing after salt loading in glycerol test. *Am J Otol.* 1984; 5:16-9.
122. Biacabe B, Erminy M, Bonfils P. A case report of fluctuant sensorineural hearing loss after hepatitis B vaccination. *Auris Nasus Larynx.* 1997; 24:357-60.
123. Oh AK, Ishiyama A, Baloh RW. Deafness associated with abuse of hydrocodone/acetaminophen. *Neurology.* 2000; 54:2345.
124. Ho T, Vrabec JT, Burton AW. Hydrocodone use and sensorineural hearing loss. *Pain Physician.* 2007; 10:467-72.
125. Coutinho MB, Duarte I. Hydroxychloroquine ototoxicity in a child with idiopathic pulmonary haemosiderosis. *Int J Ped Otorhinolaryngol.* 2002; 62:53-7.
126. Johansen PB, Gran JT. Ototoxicity due to hydroxychloroquine: report of two cases. *Clin Exp Rheumatol.* 1998; 16:472-2.
127. Seckin U, Ozoran K, Ikinciogullary A et al. Hydroxychloroquine ototoxicity in a patient with rheumatoid arthritis. *Rheumatol Int.* 2000; 19:203-4.
128. Vitrase hyophylized (ovine), hyaluronidase for injection [product information]. Irvine, CA: Allergan; 2004.
129. Perez EA, Sowray PC, Gardner SL et al. Phase I study of high dose cisplatin, ifosfamide and etoposide. *Cancer Chemother Pharmacol.* 1994; 34:331-4.
130. Laird LK, Lydiard RB. Imipramine-related tinnitus. *J Clin Psychiatry.* 1989; 50:146.
131. Kanda Y, Shigeno K, Matsuo H et al. Interferon-induced sudden hearing loss. *Audiology.* 1995; 24:98-102.

132. Johnson K, Sargent LA, Galizio C et al. Interferon-alpha-2b/ribavirin-induced vestibulocochlear toxicity with dysautonomia in a chronic hepatitis C patient. *Dur J Gastrenterol Hepatol.* 2008; 20:1110-4.

133. Forni V, Wuerzner G, Pruijm M, Burnier M. Long-term use and tolerability of irbesartan for control of hypertension. *Integr Blood Press Control.* 2011; 4:17-26.

134. Altiparmak MR, Pamuk ON, Pamuk GE et al. Is isoniazid ototoxic in patients undergoing hemodialysis. *Nephron.* 2002; 92:478-80.

135. Yaman M, Albayram S, Altintas A et al. A cerebellar demyelinating lesion following treatment of acne with isotretinoin. *Clin Exp Dermatol.* 2008; 33:118-21.

136. Cosata I, Castanet J, Lacour JP et al. Vertigo and hypokalemia. Two rare side effects of itraconazole. *Therapie.* 1994; 49:149.

137. Johnson AH, Hamilton CH. Kanamycin ototoxicity-possible potentiation by other drug. *South Med J.* 1970; 63:511-3.

138. Graybill JR, Drutz DJ. Ketoconazole: a major innovation for treatment of fungal disease. *Ann Intern Med.* 1980; 93:921-3.

139. Schaab KC, Dickinson ET, Setzen G. Acute sensorineural hearing loss following intravenous ketorolac administration. *J Emerg Med.* 1995; 13:509-13.

140. Beydoun A, D'Souza J, Hebert D, Doty P. Lacosamide: pharmacology, mechanisms of action and pooled efficacy and safety data in partial-onset seizures. *Expert Rev Neurother.* 2009; 9:33-42.

141. Rey D, L'Heritier A, Lang JM. Severe ototoxicity in health care worker who received postexposure prophylaxis with stavudine, lamivudine and nevirapine after occupational exposure to HIV. *Clin Infect Dis.* 2002; 34:418-9.

142. Kakuda TN. Pharmacology of nucleoside and nucleotide reverse transcriptase inhibitor-induced mitochondrial toxicity. *Clin Ther.* 2000; 22:685-708.

143. Vohora D, Saraogi P, Yazdani MA et al. Recent advances in adjunctive therapy for epilepsy: Focus on sodium channel blockers as third-generation antiepileptic drugs. *Drug Today (Barc).* 2010; 46:265-77.

144. Lofton AL, Klein-Schwartz W. Evaluation of lamotrigine toxicity reported to poison centers. *Ann Pharmacother.* 2004; 38:1811-5.

145. Van Roon EN, Jansent A, Mourad L et al. Leflunomide in active rheumatoid arthritis: a prospective study in daily practice. *Br J Clin Pharmacol.* 2004; 58:201-8.

146. Lidoderm, lidocaine patch 5% [product information]. Chadds Ford, PA: Endo Pharmaceuticals; 2005.

147. Zannad F, van den Broek SA, Bory M. Comparison of treatment with lisinopril versus enalapril for congestive heart failure. *Am J Cardiol.* 1992; 70:78C-83C.

148. Lewis DA. Lithium and internal medicine and psychiatry: an outline. *J Clin Psychiatry.* 1982; 43:8.

149. Ahmad S. Vestibular vertigo and lovastatin therapy. *South Med J.* 1996; 89:257-8.

150. Heidland A, Wigand ME. Einfluss hoher rurosemiddosen auf die gehorfunktion bei uramie. *Klin Wschr.* 1970; 48:1052.

151. Morris DL, Fletcher A. Hyperacusis after treatment with mefanamic acid. *Br Med J.* 1986; 293:823.

152. Wise M, Toovey S. Reversible hearing loss in temporal association with chemoprophylactic mefloquine use. *Travel Med Infect Dis.* 2007; 5:385-8.

153. Methergine, (methylergonovine maleate) [product information. East Hanover, NJ: Novartis Pharmaceuticals Corporation; 2004.

154. Iqbal SM, Murthy JG, Banerjee et al. Metronidazole ototoxicity: report of two cases. *J Laryngol and Otol.* 1999; 113:355-7.

155. Fanning WL, Gump DW. Distressing side-effects of minocycline hydrochloride. *Arch Intern Med.* 1976; 136:761-2.

156. Corbacella E, Lanzoni I, Ding D et al. Minocycline attenuates gentamicin induced hair cell loss in neonatal cochlear cultures. *Hear Res.* 2004; 197:11-8.

157. Toriumi dM, Konior RJ, Berktold RE. Severe hypertrichosis of the external ear canal during minoxidil therapy. *Arch Otolaryngol Head Neck Surg.* 1988; 114:918-9.

158. Remeron, mirtazapine [product information]. West Orange, NJ: Organon; 2002.

159. Cytotec, misoprostol [product information]. Shokie, IL: GD Searle and Company; 2002.

160. Daniel SJ, Duval M, Sahmkow S et al. Ototoxicity of topical moxifloxacin in a chinchilla animal model. *Laryngoscope.* 2007; 117:2201-5.

161. Hartnick CJ, Cohen AF, Smith RV. Reversible sensorineural hearing loss after renal transplant immunosuppression with OKT3 (muromonab-CD3). *Ann Otol Rhinol Laryngol.* 1997; 106:640-2.

162. Jackson RE, Mitchell FN, Brindley DA. Safety evaluation of nabumetone in United States clinical trials. *Am J Med.* 1987; 83(suppl 4B):115-20.

163. McKinnon BJ, Lassen LF. Naproxen-associated sudden sensorineural hearing loss. *Mil Med.* 1998; 163:792-3.

164. Gilbert TB, Jacobs SC, Quaddoura AA. Deafness and prolonged neuromuscular blockade following single-dose peritoneal neomycin irrigation. *Can J Anaesth.* 1998; 45:568-570.

165. Meyer JS, Hardenberg J. Clinical effectiveness of calcium entry blockers in prophylactic treatment of migraine and cluster headaches. *Headache.* 1983; 23:266-77.

166. Sonderskov J, Olsen J, Sabroe S et al. Nicotine patches in smoking cessation: a randomized trial among over-the-counter customers in Denmark. *Am J Epidemiol.* 1997; 145:309-18.

167. Ruan RS, Leong SK, Yeoh KH. Ototoxicity of sodium nitroprusside. *Hear Res.* 1997; 114:169-78.

168. Ruan RS, Leong SK, Yeoh KH. Ototoxity of sodium nitroprusside is not due to nitric oxide. *Exp Neurol.* 1999; 158:192-201.

169. Thomas RJ. Neurotoxicity of antibacterial therapy. *S Med J.* 1994; 87:869-74.

170. Prilosec, omeprazole delayed-release capsules [product information]. Wilmington, DE: AstraZeneca; 2001.

171. Lussier A, LeBel E, Tetreault L. Gastrointestinal blood loss of oxaprozin and aspirin with placebo control. *J Clin Pharmacol.* 1982; 22:173-8.

172. Vohora D, Saraogi P, Yazdani MA et al. Recent advances in adjunctive therapy for epilepsy: Focus on sodium channel blockers as third-generation antiepileptic drugs. *Drug Today (Barc).* 2010; 46:265-77.

173. Boyle KL, Rosenbaum CD. Oxymorphone insufflation associated with acute sensorineural hearing loss: case files of the University of Massachusetts Medical Toxicology Fellowship. *J Med Toxicol.* 2013; 9:179-83.

174. Tibaldi C, Pazzagli I, Berrettini S et al. A case of ototoxicity in a patient with metastatic carcinoma of the breast treated with paclitaxel and vinorelbine. *Eur J Cancer.* 1998; 34:1133-4.

175. Cheung PY, Tyebkhan JM, Peliowski A et al. Prolonged use of pancuronium bromide and sensorineural hearing loss in childhood survivors of congenital diaphragmatic hernia. *J Pediatr.* 1999; 135:233-9.

176. Kewitz H. Rare but serious risks associated with non-narcotic analgesics: clinical experience. *Med Toxicol.* 1986; 1(suppl 1):86-92.

177. Fitzgerald KT, Bronstein AC. Selective serotonin reuptake inhibitor exposure. *Top Companion Anim Med.* 2013; 28:13-7.

178. Phenobarbital [product information]. Indianapolis, IN: Eli Lilly and Company; 1994.

179. Hwang WJ, Tsai JJ. Acute phenytoin intoxication: causes, symptoms, misdiagnoses and outcomes. *Kaohsiung J Med Sci.* 2004; 20):580-5.

180. Bassoumi T, Miled I, Benzartis S. Drug-induced toxic hearing loss (piroxicam and natural sulfo-conjugated estrogens): 2 case reports. *Rev Larngol Otol Rhino (Bord).* 2001; 122:185-6.

181. Vernick DM, Kelly JH. Sudden hearing loss associated with piroxicam. *Am J Otol.* 1986; 7:97-8.

182. Coly-Mycin M injection, colistimethate sodium injection [product information]. Bristol, TN: Monarch Pharmaceuticals; 2005.

183. Boudewyns A, Claes J. Acute cochleovestibular toxicity due to topical application of potassium iodide. *Eur Arch Otorhinolaryngol.* 2001; 258:109-11.
184. Minipress oral capsules, prazosin hydrochloride oral capsules [product information]. New York: Pfizer Labs; 2009.
185. Prelone syrup oral liquid, prednisolone oral liquid [product information]. Pompano Beach, FL: Aero Pharmaceuticals; 2003.
186. Zaccara G, Gangemi P, Perucca P, Specchio L. The adverse event profile of pregabalin: a systematic review and meta-analysis of randomized controlled trials. *Epilepsia.* 2011; 52:826-36.
187. Uthman BM, Almas M, Emir B et al. Pregabalin or placebo used adjunctively with levetiracetam in refractory partial-onset epilepsy: a post hoc efficacy and safety analysis in combined clinical trials. *Curr Med Res Opin.* 2011; 27:1285-93.
188. Glappaththy GN, Omari AA, Tharyan P. Primaquine for preventing relapses in people with Plasmodium vivax malaria. *Cochrane Database Syst Rev.* 2007; 24:CD004389.
189. Phenergan tablets, suppositories, promethazine HCl tablets, suppositories [product information]. Philadelphia: Wyeth Pharmaceuticals; 2004.
190. Fong PC, Pun KK, Tai YT et al. Propylthiouracil hypersensitivity with circumstantial evidence for drug-induced reversible sensorineural deafness: a case report. *Horm Res.* 1991; 35:132-6.
191. Lupin AJ, Harley CH. Inner ear damage related to propoxyphene injection. *Can Med Assoc J.* 1976; 114:596.
192. Brummett RE. Drug-induced ototoxicity. *Drugs.* 1980; 19:412-28.
193. Roche RJ, Silamut K, Pukrittayakamee S et al. Quinine induces reversible high-tone hearing loss. *Br J Clin Pharmacol.* 1990; 29:780-2.
194. Tange RA, Dreschler WA, Claessen FA et al. Ototoxic reactions of quinine in healthy persons and patients with *Plasmodium falciparum* infection. *Auris Nasus Larynx.* 1997; 24:131-6.
195. Schreiner M, Berendes B, Verho M et al. Antihypertensive efficacy, tolerance and safety of long-term treatment with ramipril in patients with mild-to-moderate essential hypertension. *J Cardiovasc Pharmacol.* 1991; 18(suppl 2):S137-40.
196. Girling DJ. Adverse effects of antituberculosis drugs. *Drugs.* 1982; 23:56-74.
197. Flumadine, rimantadine [product information]. St Louis, MO: Forest Pharmaceuticals; 2000.
198. Norvir (ritonavir) [product information]. North Chicago, IL: Abbott Laboratories; 2003.
199. Titlic M, Tonkic A, Jukic I et al. Side effects of ropinirole in patients with idiopathic Parkinson's disease. *Bratisl Lek Listy.* 2008; 109:273-5.
200. Grosser T, Smyth E, FitzGerald G. Pharmacotherapy of inflammation, fever, pain and gout. In: Brunton LL, Hilal-Dandan R, Knollmann BC, eds. *Goodman and Gilman's: the pharmacological basis of therapeutics.* 13th ed. New York: McGraw Hill; 2017. http://accesspharmacy.mhmedical.com/content.aspx?bookid=2189§ionid=170271972 (accessed 2018 Mar 7).
201. Hamzavi J, Scchmetterer L, Formanek M. Vestibular symptoms as complication of sildenafil: a case report. *Wein Klin Worchenschr.* 2002; 114:54-5.
202. Buranakitjaroen P, Mangklabruks A, Leungwattanakij S et al. Efficacy and safety of sildenafil in Asian males with erectile dysfunction and cardiovascular risk. *J Med Assoc Thai.* 2007; 90:1100-8.
203. Casano RAMS, Johnson DF, Bykhovskaya Y et al. Inherited susceptibility to aminoglycoside ototoxicity: genetic heterogeneity and clinical implications. *Am J Otolaryngol.* 1999; 20:151-6.
204. Gardner JC, Goliath R, Viljoen D et al. Familial streptomycin ototoxicity in a South African family: a mitochondrial disorder. *J Med Genet* 1997; 34:904-6.
205. Savastano M, Marioni G, Bernini G et al. Tinnitus and bilateral sensorineural hearing loss: ankylosing spondylitis or a side effect of sulfasalazine treatment. *Acta Otolaryngol.* 2005; 125:671-3.
206. Min DI, Ku YM, Rayhill S et al. Sudden hearing loss associated with tacrolimus in a kidney-pancreas allograft recipient. *Pharmacother.* 1999; 19:891-3.
207. Maddox PT, Saunders J, Chandrasekhar SS. Sudden hearing loss from PDE-5 inhibitors: a possible cellular stress etiology. *Laryngoscope.* 2009; 119:1586-9.
208. Lepor H, Jones K, Williford W. The mechanism of adverse events associated with terazosin: an analysis of the Veterans Affairs Cooperative Study. *J Urol.* 2000; 163:1134-7.
209. Hoffman RA, Li CL. Tetracaine topical anesthesia for myringotomy. *Laryngoscope.* 2001; 111:1636-8.
210. Rajkumar SV, Gertz MA, Lacy MQ et al. Thalidomide as an initial therapy for early-stage myeloma. *Leukemia.* 2003; 17:775-9.
211. Lazzerini M, Matelossi S, Marchetti F et al. Efficacy and safety of thalidomide in children and young adults with intractable inflammatory bowel disease; long-term results. *Aliment Pharmacol Ther.* 2007; 25:419-27.
212. Mintezol, thiabendazole tablets and suspension [product information]. West Point, PA: Merck and Company; 2003.
213. Torecan, thiethylperazine [product information]. Ridgefield, CT: Boehringer Ingelheim; 1995.
214. Ticlid, ticlopidine [product information]. Nutley, NJ: Roche Laboratories; 2001.
215. Chmielewska B, Stelmasiak Z. Effectiveness of adjunctive therapy with tiagabine in mentally disabled patients with epilepsy. *Ann Univ Mariae Curie Sklodowska Med.* 2002; 57:226-36.
216. Wallace RJ, Dukart G, Brown-Elliot BA et al. Clinical experience in 52 patients with tigecycline-containing regimens for salvage treatment of *Mycobacterium abscessus* and *Mycobacterium chelonae* infections. *J Antimicrob Chemother.* 2014; 69:1945-53.
217. Munroe WP, Rindone JP, Kershner RM. Systemic side effects associated with the ophthalmic administration of timolol. *Drug Intell Clin Pharm.* 1985; 19:85-9.
218. Bragonier R, Brown NM. The pharmacokinetics and toxicity of once-daily tobramycin therapy in children with cystic fibrosis. *J Antimicrob Chemother.* 1998; 42:103-6.
219. Lofton AL, Klein-Schwartz W. Evaluation of toxicity of topiramate exposures reported to poison centers. *Hum Exp Toxicol.* 2005; 24:591-5.
220. Wisniewski M, Kukasik-Glebocka M, Anand JS. Acute topiramate overdose-clinical manifestations. *Clin Toxicol (Phila).* 2009; 47:317-20.
221. Chang JK, Yu CT, Lee MY et al. Tramadol/acetaminophen combination as add-on therapy in the treatment of patients with ankylosing spondylitis. *Clin Rheumatol.* 2013; 32:341-7.
222. Fishman RL, Kistler CJ, Ellerbusch MT et al. Efficacy and safety of 12 weeks of osteoarthritic pain therapy with once-daily tramadol. *J Opioid Manag.* 2007; 3:273-80.
223. Pascual ML, Fleming RR, Gana TJ, Vorsanger GJ. Open-label study of safety and effectiveness of long-term therapy with extended-release tramadol in the management of chronic nonmalignant pain. *Curr Med Res Opin.* 2007; 23:2531-42.
224. Monigin F, Yakusevich V, Kope A et al. Efficacy and safety assessment of a novel once-daily tablet formulation of tramadol: a randomized, controlled study versus twice-daily tramadol in patients with osteoarthritis of the knee. *Clin Drug Investig.* 2004; 24:545-58.
225. Parnate, tranylcypromine [product information]. Philadelphia: Smith Kline and French Labs; 1996.
226. Desyrel, trazodone [product information]. Princeton, NJ: Apothecon; 1998.
227. Armon C, Brown E, Carwile S et al. Sensorineural hearing loss: a reversible effect of valproic acid. *Neurology.* 1990; 40:1896-8.
228. Hori A, Kataoka S, Sakai K et al. Valproic acid-induced hearing loss and tinnitus. *Intern Med.* 2003; 42:1153-4.
229. Diovan HCT, valsartan and hydrochlorothiazide [product information]. East Hanover, NJ: Novartis Pharmaceuticals Corporation; 2002.

230. Gendeh BS, Gibb AG, Aziz NS et al. Vancomycin administration in continuous ambulatory peritoneal dialysis: the risk of ototoxicity. *Otolaryngol Head Neck Surg.* 1998; 118:551-8.
231. Kilbanov OM, Filicko JE, DeSimone JA et al. Sensorineural hearing loss associated with intrathecal vancomycin. *Ann Pharmacother.* 2003; 37:61-5.
232. Elting LS, Rubenstein EB, Kurtin D et al. Mississippi mud in the 1990s: risks and outcomes of vancomycin associated toxicity in general oncology practice. *Cancer.* 1998; 83:2497-607.
233. Pirmoradi P, Roshan S, Nadeem SS. Neuropsychiatric disturbance after initiation of varenicline in a patient with a history of alcohol abuse and major depression. *Am J Health-Syst Pharm.* 2008; 65:1624-6.
234. Moss PE, Hickman S, Harrison BR. Ototoxicity associated with vinblastine. *Ann Pharmacother.* 1999; 33:423-5.
235. Lugassy G, Shapira A. Sensori-neural hearing loss associated with vincristine treatment. *Blut.* 1990; 61:320-1.
236. Obrist R, Paravicini U, Hartmann D et al. A clinical trial with special reference to neurological side effects. *Cancer Chemother Pharmacol.* 1979; 2:233-7.
237. Gatineau M, Rixe O, Chevalier TL. Tirapazamine with cisplatin and vinorelbine in patients with advanced non-small-cell lung cancer: a phase I/II study. *Clin Lung Cancer.* 2005; 6:293-8.
238. Cohen HN, Fogelman I, Boyle IT et al. Deafness due to hypervitaminosis D. *Lancet.* 1979; 1:985.
239. Martinez OP, French MAH. Acoustic neuropathy associated with zalcitabine-induced peripheral neuropathy. *AIDS.* 1993; 7:901-2. Letter.
240. Monte S, Fenwick JD, Monteiro EF. Irreversible ototoxicity associated with zalcitabine. *Int J STD AIDS.* 1997; 8:201-2.
241. Ganzoni E, Gugger M. Safety profile of zolpidem: two studies of 3805 patients by Swiss practitioners. *Praxis (Bern).* 1999; 88:1120-7.
242. Shinnar S, Pellock JM, Conry JA. Open-label, long-term safety study of zonisamide administered to children and adolescents with epilepsy. *Eur J Paediatr Neurol.* 2009; 13:3-9.
243. Simdon J, Watters D, Bartlett S et al. *Clin Infect Dis.* 2001; 33:2101-2. Reply.
244. Geraci lE. Heilman FR, Nichols DR, Wellman WE. Antibiotic therapy of bacterial endocarditis. VII. Vancomycin for acute micrococcal endocarditis: preliminary report. *Mayo Clin Proc.* 1958; 33:172-8.
245. Cantu TG, Yamanaka-Yuen NA, Leitman PS. Serum vancomycin concentrations: reappraisal of their clinical value. *Clin Infect Dis.* 1994; 18:533-43.
246. Vorasubin N, Calzada AP, Ishiyama A. Methadone-induced bilateral severe sensorineural hearing loss. *Am J Otolaryngol.* 2013; 34:735-8.
247. van Gaalen FA, Compier EA, Fogteloo AJ. Sudden hearing loss after a methadone overdose. *Eur Arch Otorhinolaryngol.* 2009; 266:773-4.
248. Christenson BJ, Marjala AR. Two cases of sudden sensorineural hearing loss after methadone overdose. *Ann Pharmacother.* 2010; 44:207-10.
249. Ishiyama A, Ishiyama G, Baloh RW, Evans CJ. Heroin-induced reversible profound deafness and vestibular dysfunction. *Addiction.* 2001; 96:1363-4.
250. Schrock A, Jakob M, Wirz S, Bootz F. Sudden sensorineural hearing loss after heroin injection. *Eur Arch Otorhinolaryngol.* 2008; 265:603-6.
251. Kortequee S, Agada FO, Coatesworth AP. Sudden sensorineural hearing loss following intracarotid injection of heroin. *Int J Clin Pract Suppl.* 2005; 147:128-9.
252. Tange RA. Ototoxicity. *Adverse Drug React Toxicol Rev.* 1998; 17:75-89.
253. Iurato S, Henderson D, Quranta A et al. Ototoxicity: basic science and clinical application: introduction. *Ann N Y Acad Sci.* 1999; 884:ix-xi.
254. Aran JM. Current perspectives on inner ear toxicity. *Otolaryngol Head Neck Surg.* 1995; 112:133-44.
255. Brown RD, Henley CM, Penny JE et al. Link between functional and morphological changes in the inner ear—functional changes produced by ototoxic agents and their interactions. *Arch Toxicol Suppl.* 1985; 8:240-50.
256. Matz GJ. Clinical perspectives on ototoxic drugs. *Ann Otol Rhinol Laryngol.* 1990; 99:39-41.
257. Anniko M. Principles in cochlear toxicity. *Arch Toxicol Suppl.* 1985; 8:221-39.
258. Wu WJ, Sha SH, Schacht J. Recent advances in understanding aminoglycoside ototoxicity and its prevention. *Audiol Neurootol.* 2002; 7:171-4.
259. Evans P, Halliwell B. Free radicals and hearing: cause, consequence and criteria. *Ann N Y Acad Sci* 1999; 884:19-40.
260. Kopke R, Allen KA, Henderson D et al. A radical demise: toxins and trauma share common pathways in hair cell death. *Ann N Y Acad Sci.* 1999; 884:171-91.
261. Wang S, Bian Q, Liu Z et al. Capability of serum to convert streptomycin to cytotoxin in patients with aminoglycoside-induced hearing loss. *Hear Res.* 1999; 137:1-7.
262. Sone M, Schachern PA, Papraella MM. Loss of spiral ganglion cells as a primary manifestation of aminoglycoside ototoxicity. *Hear Res.* 1998; 115:217-23.
263. Dallos P. Overview: cochlear neurophysiology. In: Dallos P, Popper AN, Fay RR, eds. *The cochlea.* New York: Springer; 1996:1-43.
264. Horn KL, Langley LR, Gates GA. Effect of ethacrynic acid on the stria vascularis. *Arch Otolaryngol.* 1977; 103:539-41.
265. Schulman A. The cochleovestibular system/ototoxicity/clinical issues. *Ann N Y Acad Sci.* 1999; 884:433-6.
266. Nguyen KD, Lopez I, Ishiyama G, Ishiyama A. Review of opioid-associated hearing loss and possible mechanism of opioid-mediated endothelin-1-dependent cochlear vasoconstriction. *J Otol Rhinol.* 2014; 3:1-7.
267. Huang MY, Schacht J. Drug-induced ototoxicity: pathogenesis and prevention. *Med Toxicol Adverse Drug Exp.* 1989; 4:452-67.
268. Palomar Garcia V, Palomar Asenjo V. Are some ear drops ototoxic or potentially ototoxic? *Acta Otolaryngol.* 2001; 121:565-8.
269. Serra A, Grasso DL, Cocuzza S et al. Normal and altered cytoarchitecture of the inner ear. *Ann N Y Acad Sci.* 1999; 884:69-84.
270. Hamers FP, Wijbenga J, Wolters FL et al. Cisplatin ototoxicity involves organ of corti, stria vascularis and spiral ganglion: modulation by αMSH and ORG 2766. *Audiol Neurootol.* 2003; 8:305-15.
271. Vlasits AL, Simon JA, Failble DW et al. Screen of FDA-approved drug library reveals compounds that protect hair cells from aminoglycosides and cisplatin. *Hear Res.* 2012; 294:153-65.
272. Rascol O, Hain TC, Brefel C et al. Antivertigo medications and drug-induced vertigo: a pharmacological review. *Drugs.* 1995; 50:777-91.
273. Ganesan P, Schmiedge J, Manchaiah V et al. Ototoxicity: a challenge in diagnosis and treatment. *J Audiol Otol.* 2018; 22:59-68.
274. Weber PC. Evaluation of hearing loss in adults. http://www.uptodate.com/online/content/topic.do?topicKey=prim_ent/6751&selectedTitle=1~150&source=search_result# (accessed 2018 Mar 9).
275. Dinces EA. Pathogenesis and diagnosis of tinnitus. http://www.uptodate.com/online/content/topic.do?topicKey=prim_ent/8404&selectedTitle=1~150&source=search_result (accessed 2018 Mar 9).

276. Furman JM. Pathophysiology, etiology, and differential diagnosis of vertigo. http://www.uptodate.com/online/content/topic.do?topicKey=genneuro/7125&selectedTitle=1~150&source=search_result (accessed 2018 Mar 9).
277. Campbell KCM, Durrant J. Audiologic monitoring for ototoxicity. *Otolaryngol Clin N Am.* 1993; 26:903-14.
278. Blakely BW, Gupta AK, Myers SF et al. Risk factors for ototoxicity due to cisplatin. *Arch Otolaryngol Head Neck Surg.* 1994; 120:541-6.
279. Durrant JD, Rodgers G, Myers EN et al. Hearing loss—risk factors for cisplatin ototoxicity? Observations. *Am J Otol.* 1990; 11:375-77.
280. Lautermann J, Song B, McLaren J et al. Diet is a risk factor in cisplatin ototoxicity. *Hear Res.* 1995; 88:47-53.
281. Gunther T, Rebentisch E, Vormann J et al. Enhanced ototoxicity of gentamicin and salicylate caused by magnesium deficiency and zinc deficiency. *Biol Trace Elem Res.* 1988; 16:43-50.
282. Guan MX, Fischel-Ghodsian N, Attardi G. A biochemical basis for the inherited susceptibility to aminoglycoside ototoxicity. *Hum Mol Genet.* 2000; 9:1787-93.
283. Conlon BJ, Smith DW. Supplemental iron exacerbates aminoglycoside ototoxicity in vivo. *Hear Res.* 1998; 115:1-5.
284. Tan WH, Brown N, Kelsall AW et al. Dose regimen for vancomycin not needing peak levels? *Arch Dis Child Fetal Neonatal Ed.* 2002; 87:214-6.
285. de Hoog M, van Zanten BA, Hop WC et al. Newborn hearing screening: tobramycin and vancomycin are not risk factors for hearing loss. *J Pediatr.* 2003; 142:41-6.
286. de Hoog M, Mouton JW, van den Anker JN. Vancomycin: pharmacokinetics and administration regimens in neonates. *Clin Pharmacokinet.* 2004; 43:417-40.
287. Hammett-Stabler CA, Johns T. Laboratory guidelines for monitoring of antimicrobial drugs. *Clinical Chemistry.* 1998; 44:1129-40.
288. Saunders NJ. Why monitor peak vancomycin concentrations? *Lancet.* 1994; 344:1748-50.
289. Blakely BW, Cohen JI, Doolittle ND et al. Strategies for prevention of toxicity caused by platinum-based chemotherapy: review and summary of the Annual Meeting of the Blood–Brain Barrier Disruption Program, Gleneden Beach, Oregon, March 10, 2001. *Laryngoscope.* 2002; 112:1997-2001.
290. Cooper LB, Chan DK, Roediger FC et al. AAV mediated delivery of the caspase inhibitor XIAP protects against cisplatin toxicity. *Otol Neurotol.* 2006; 27:484-90.
291. Dehne N, Lautermann J, Petrat F et al. Cisplatin ototoxicity: involvement of iron and enhanced formation of superoxide anion radicals. *Toxicol Appl Pharmacol.* 2001; 174:27-34.
292. Conlon BJ, Perry BP, Smith DW. Attenuation of neomycin ototoxicity by iron chelation. *Laryngoscope.* 1998; 108:284-7.
293. Chao Y, Wu K, Lin C et al. Audiologic and vestibular assessment in patients with β-thalassemia major receiving long-term transfusion therapy. *Pediatr Blood Cancer.* 2013; 60:1963-6.
294. Borradori C, Fawer CL, Buclin T et. al. Risk factors of sensorineural hearing loss in preterm infants. *Biol Neonate.* 1997; 71:1-10.
295. Kelly WN. Potential risks and prevention, part 2: drug-induced permanent disabilities. *Am J Health-Syst Pharm.* 2001; 58:1325-9.
296. Doolittle ND, Muldoon LL, Brummett RE et al. Delayed sodium thiosulfate as an otoprotectant against carboplatin-induced hearing loss in patients with malignant brain tumors. *Clin Cancer Res.* 2001; 7:493-500.
297. Huang E, Teh BS, Strother DR et al. Intensity-modulated radiation therapy for pediatric medulloblastoma: early report on the reduction of ototoxicity. *Int J Radiation Oncology Biol Phys.* 2002; 52:599-605.
298. Rybak LP, Husain K, Morris C et al. Effect of protective agents against cisplatin ototoxicity. *Am J Otol.* 2000; 21:513-20.
299. Sha SH, Schacht J. Salicylate attenuates gentamicin-induced ototoxicity. *Lab Invest.* 1999; 79:807.
300. Smoorenburg GF, De Groot JC, Hamers FP et al. Protection and spontaneous recovery from cisplatin-induced hearing loss. *Ann N Y Acad Sci.* 1999; 884:193-210.
301. Fetoni AR, Sergi B, Scarano E et al. Protective effects of alpha-tocopherol against gentamicin-induced oto-vestibulo toxicity: an experimental study. *Acta Otolaryngol.* 2003; 123:192-7.
302. Cronin S, Uberti JP, Ayash LJ et al. Use of amifostine as a chemoprotectant during high-dose chemotherapy in autologous peripheral blood stem cell transplantation. *Bone Marrow Transplant.* 2000; 26:1247-49.
303. Grandishar WJ, Stephenson P, Glover DJ et al. A phase II trial of cisplatin plus WR-2721 (amifostine) for metastatic breast carcinoma: an Eastern Cooperative Oncology Group study. *Cancer.* 2001; 92:2517-22.
304. Ding D, McFadden SL, Browne RW et al. Late dosing with ethacrynic acid can reduce gentamicin concentration in perilymph and protect cochlear hair cells. *Hear Res.* 2003; 185:90-6.
305. Feghali JG, Liu W, van de Water TR. L-N-acetyl-cysteine protection against cisplatin-induced auditory neuronal and hair cell toxicity. *Laryngoscope.* 2001; 111:1147-55.
306. Li G, Sha SH, Zotova E et al. Salicylate protects hearing and kidney function from cisplatin toxicity without compromising its oncolytic action. *Lab Invest.* 2002; 82:585-96.
307. Neuwelt EA, Brummett RE, Doolittle ND et al. First evidence of otoprotection against carboplatin-induced hearing loss with a two-compartment system in patients with central nervous system malignancy using sodium thiosulfate. *J Pharmacol Exp Therapeutics.* 1998; 286:77-84.
308. Suzuki M, Yagi M, Brown JN et al. Effect of transgenic GDNF expression on gentamicin-induced cochlear and vestibular toxicity. *Gene Ther.* 2000; 7:1046-54.
309. Sanchez-Borges M, Capriles-Hulett A. Atopy is a risk factor for non-steroidal anti-inflammatory drug sensitivity. *Ann Allergy Asthma Immunol.* 2000; 84:101-6.
310. Seidman MD, Babu S. Alternative medications and other treatments for tinnitus: facts from fiction. *Otolaryngol Clin North Am.* 2003; 36:359-81.
311. Vernon JA, Meikle MB. Masking devices and alprazolam treatment for tinnitus. *Otolaryngol Clin North Am.* 2003; 36:307-20.
312. Bauer CA, Brozoski TJ. Effect of gabapentin on the sensation and impact of tinnitus. *The Larngyscope.* 2006; 116:675-81.
313. Bauer SA, Brozoski TJ. Gabapentin. *Prog Brain Res.* 2007; 166:287-301.
314. Mazurek B, Heidemarie H, Szczepek AJ et al. Evaluation of vardenafil for the treatment of subjective tinnitus: a controlled pilot study. *J Neg Res in BioMed.* 2009; 8:1-12.
315. Freyer DR, Chen L, Krailo MD et al. Effects of sodium thiosulfate versus observation on development of cisplatin-induced hearing loss in children with cancer (ACCL0431): a multicenter, randomized, controlled, open-label, phase 3 trial. *Lancet Oncol.* 2017; 18:63-74.
316. Fang B, Xiao H. Rapamycin alleviates cisplatin-induced ototoxicity in vivo. *Biochem Biophys Res Commun.* 2014; 448:443-7.
317. Kim Sj, Ho Hur J, Park C et al. Bucillamine prevents cisplatin-induced ototoxicity through induction of glutathione and antioxidant genes. *Exp Mol Med.* 2015; 20:e142.
318. Shi L, An Y, Wang A et al. The protective effect of Salvia miltiorrhiza on gentamicin-induced ototoxicity. *Am J Otolatyngol.* 2014; 35:171-9.
319. Lee SH, Kim HS, An YS et al. Protective effect of resveratrol against cisplatin-induced ototoxicity in HEI-OC1 auditory cells. *Int J Pediatr Otorhinolaryngol.* 2015; 79:58-62.

320. Aksoy F, Dogan R, Ozturan O et al. Protective effect of trimetazidine on amikacin-induced ototoxicity in rats. *Int J Pediatr Otorhinolaryngol.* 2014; 78:663-9.

321. Soto E, Vega R. Neuropharmacology of vestibular system disorders. *Curr Neuropharmacol.* 2010; 8:26-40.

322. WebMD Symptom Checker. Hearing loss, itching or burning, ringing in ears and sensitive to noise. https://symptomchecker.webmd.com/multiple-symptoms?symptoms=hearing-loss%7Citching-or-burning%7Cringing-in-ears%7Csensitive-to-noise&symptomids=116%7C129%7C193%7C199&locations=4%7C4%7C4%7C4 (accessed 2018 Mar 9).

323. Ryan W, Sachin D. Drug-induced ototoxicity. *Clin Exp Pharmacol.* 2014; 4:e132.

324. American Academy of Audiology. https://www.audiology.org/publications-resources/document-library/audiologic-guidelines-diagnosis-management-tinnitus-patients (accessed 2018 Mar 9).

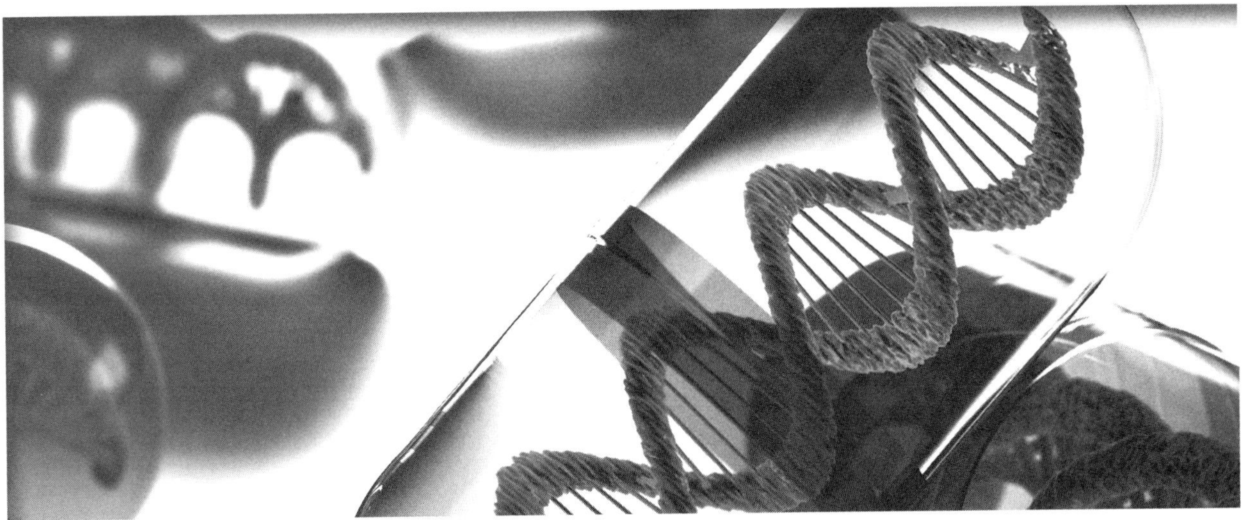

CHAPTER 56

Oral Manifestations of Systemically Administered Drugs

Ashley H. Meredith

Many commonly prescribed drugs have associated dental and oral manifestations that are often nonspecific and can vary in significance. Undesirable effects can mimic other disease processes, as is often the case with erythema multiforme, or may be very characteristic of a particular agent, such as gingival hyperplasia secondary to the anticonvulsant phenytoin. Several systemic drugs and medication classes have been implicated in causing clinically significant oral manifestations. The drug-induced diseases covered in this chapter include color changes of the oral mucosa and teeth, taste disorders, gingival hyperplasia, oral erythema multiforme, oral lichenoid drug reactions, and osteonecrosis of the jaw.

COLOR CHANGES OF THE ORAL MUCOSA AND TEETH

Color changes within the oral cavity may be classified as extrinsic (i.e., superficial discoloration) or intrinsic (i.e., within the mucosa or tooth structure).[1] Extrinsic discoloration rarely leads to clinically significant disease.

CAUSATIVE AGENTS

Any surface within the oral cavity is subject to discoloration due to medications. The most commonly impacted areas include the teeth and palate. Substances reported to cause color changes of the teeth include coffee, tobacco, tetracycline, minocycline, and fluoride.[2] Color changes of the oral mucosa have been associated with oral contraceptives, minocycline, chloroquine, phenytoin, and amiodarone.[3-9] In patients with HIV disease, diffuse or macular pigmentation has been reported within the oral mucosa with clofazimine, zidovudine, or ketoconazole treatment.[18] Drugs reported to cause color changes of the oral mucosa and teeth are listed in **Table 56-1**.[3-36]

Table 56-1 Agents Implicated in Drug-Induced Color Changes of the Oral Mucosa and Teeth[3-36]

Drug	Incidence	Level of Evidence[a]
5-fluorouracil[10-12]	<1%	B
Amiodarone[9-11,13]	<1%	B
Bismuth[10,14]	NK	B
Bleomycin[10-13]	8–40%	B
Busulfan[10,12-14]	<1%	B
Carotene[10-12]	NK	C
Chlorhexidine[11,12,14]	56%	B
Chloroquine[7,10,13-15]	<1%	B
Chlorpromazine[10,13,17]	<1%	C
Clofazimine[10-14,18]	75–100%	C
Copper[14]	NK	C
Cyclophosphamide[10-14,19-21]	NK	B
Docetaxel[19-21]	NK	B
Doxorubicin[10,12-14,19-21]	NK	B
Enalapril[14]	<1%	C
Fosinopril[14]	NK	C
Gold[10,22]	NK	B
Heroin[11-14]	NK	C
Hydroxychloroquine[10,13,16,23]	<1%	B
Hydroxyurea[13]	<1%	C
Imatinib[24,25]	NK	B
Iron[14]	NK	C
Ketoconazole[11-13]	NK	B
Lansoprazole[25]	<1%	C
Lead[10,14]	NK	C
Lisinopril[14]	NK	C
Manganese[14]	NK	C
Methyldopa[14]	<1%	C
Minocycline[5,6,10-12,14,27-32]	10–20%	A
Nicotine[11,12]	NK	B
Oral contraceptives[3,4,10-14]	NK	B
Pentamidine[14]	NK	C
Perindopril[14]	NK	C
Phenytoin[8,14]	NK	B
Premarin[11,12,33]	<1%	C
Propafenone[14]	NK	C
Quinacrine[10,13,14]	4–37%	B
Quinapril[14]	NK	C
Ramipril[14]	NK	C
Silver[14]	NK	C
Tacrolimus[13,34]	NK	C
Terbinafine[14]	NK	C
Tetracycline[10-13,27,29]	3–4%	A
Thallium[14]	NK	C

Table 56-1 Agents Implicated in Drug-Induced Color Changes of the Oral Mucosa and Teeth[3-36] (continued)

Drug	Incidence	Level of Evidence[a]
Tin[14]	NK	C
Trandolapril[14]	NK	C
Zidovudine[11-14,18,35,36]	NK	B
Zopiclone[14]	NK	C

NK = not known.
[a]Definitions for Levels of Evidence: Level A—evidence from one or more randomized, controlled clinical trials; Level B—evidence from nonrandomized clinical trials, prospective observational studies, cohort studies, retrospective studies, case-control studies, meta-analyses and/or postmarketing surveillance studies; and Level C—evidence from one or more published case reports or case series.

EPIDEMIOLOGY

The overall incidence of drug-induced color changes of the oral mucosa and teeth is unknown. The incidence of minocycline-induced hyperpigmentation increases with higher doses and longer durations of exposure. It has been reported to occur in 10% of patients after 1 year and increases to 20% after 4 years of treatment with minocycline 100–200 mg per day.[31]

MECHANISMS

Color changes of the teeth can be caused by physical contact with a substance that causes external staining (e.g., coffee or tobacco) or may be due to changes that occur during tooth formation, as is the case with the tetracyclines.[2] **Table 56-2** describes mechanisms of drug-induced color changes of the oral mucosa and teeth.[25,37,38] The proposed mechanism by which antimalarial agents induce color changes involves deposition of melanin or iron within the mucosal tissues.[1] Minocycline- and tetracycline-related color changes of the teeth are a result of a direct chelation with calcium and incorporation into hydroxyapatite as a stable organophosphate complex during tooth formation.[1,39] Additional mechanisms for drug-induced color changes of the oral mucosa and teeth include deposition of pigmented metabolic drug products within the mucosal tissues, increased melanin production and deposition, and deposition of exogenous materials.[7,16,37,40]

Table 56-2 Mechanisms of Drug-Induced Color Changes of the Oral Mucosa and Teeth[25,37,38]

Drug	Mechanism(s)
Amiodarone	• Increased lipofuscin production[37]
Antimalarials	• Increased melanin production[37]
Clofazamine	• Chelated medication metabolite(s)[37]
Heavy metals (i.e., arsenic, bismuth, lead, mercury, silver, gold)	• Peripheral metal accumulation in the oral mucosa[38]
Hormones	• Increased melanin production[37]
Imatinib	• Chelated medication metabolite[25]
Tetracyclines	• Increased melanin production[37] • Formation of iron complex[37] • Stained bone[37]

CLINICAL PRESENTATION AND DIFFERENTIAL DIAGNOSIS

The signs and symptoms of drug-induced color changes of the oral mucosa and teeth are somewhat variable (**Table 56-3**).[10] Pigmentation can range from light brown to black, with brown lesions typically related to superficial pigmentation and black/gray lesions related to deeper pigment location.[13,40] More intense colors are found in patients who smoke.[41] Any area within the oral mucosa may be impacted, with the buccal and gingival mucosa and

Table 56-3 Signs and Symptoms of Drug-Induced Oral Manifestations of Systemic Drugs

Signs	Symptoms
COLOR CHANGES OF THE ORAL MUCOSA AND TEETH	
Diffuse hyperpigmented lesion(s) of various colors (i.e., blue-gray, brown, red) Histologic exam[10]: • Increased melanin in all epidermal layers • Pigment granules within dermis	Generally asymptomatic
DRUG-INDUCED TASTE DISORDERS	
No objective signs present	Absence of normal taste sensations (i.e., excessively sweet, bitter, salty or metallic tastes)
DRUG-INDUCED GINGIVAL HYPERPLASIA[154]	
Localized or generalized gingival enlargement Firm nodular enlargement Lobulated gingival appearance Noninflamed, firm, and fibrous gingiva Edematous, erythematous, and bleeding gingiva	Bleeding Pain Impaired oral hygiene[125] Difficulty chewing[125] Speech interference[125]
DRUG-INDUCED ORAL ERYTHEMA MULTIFORME[172,189,190]	
Diffuse macules that blister and form ulcers Intraoral lesions Swollen, cracked, bleeding, and crusted lips Targetoid lesion (central necrotic area)	Fever Pain
DRUG-INDUCED ORAL LICHENOID REACTIONS[230]	
Oral ulcerations with Wickham's striae[2,74] Swollen, red, and ulcerated lesions[229] White reticular striae or plaques[229]	Pain Roughness on lining of the mouth Sensitivity to hot or spicy foods Slow onset of ulcers
DRUG-INDUCED OSTEONECROSIS OF THE JAW[241]	
Cutaneous fistula Exposed bone Mobile teeth Mucosal fistula	Delayed tissue healing[266,267] Pain

hard palate most commonly affected.[31,40] Areas of hyperpigmentation may be diffuse or multifocal.[37] Patients presenting with tetracycline-related tooth discoloration typically have a brownish color on the front teeth and a yellow color on the back teeth. This difference is due to daily light exposure, which is more intense in the front portion of the mouth as opposed to the back.

When a patient presents with complaints of color changes within the oral cavity, multiple diagnoses must be considered in addition to drug-induced disease. **Table 56-4** lists conditions to consider in the differential diagnosis of drug-induced color changes of the oral mucosa and teeth.[7,13] The differential diagnosis should include conditions such as Addison disease, vitamin B_{12} deficiency, and melanoma. Addison disease and vitamin B_{12} deficiency can be ruled out with blood tests.[7] If the index of suspicion for melanoma is high, this diagnosis can be investigated via incisional biopsy of the hyperpigmented area. Pigmentation of the oral cavity may be due to exogenous causes such as tattoo pigment, pencil lead, or amalgam, a common product used in dental restorations. Amalgam use as part of dental

Table 56-4 Conditions to Consider in the Differential Diagnosis of Drug-Induced Oral Manifestations of Systemic Drugs

Drug-induced color changes of the oral mucosa and teeth

- Acquired melanocytic nevi[13]
- Embedded foreign material (i.e., tattoo pigment, amalgam dental restoration material, pencil lead)[13]
- Endogenous sources (i.e., hemoglobin, bilirubin)[13]
- Physiological conditions (i.e., Addison disease, Peutz–Jeghers syndrome, Laugier–Hunziker syndrome)[13]
- Postinflammatory pigmentation[13]
- Primary and metastatic melanoma[13]
- Tobacco use[13]
- Vitamin B_{12} deficiency[7]

Drug-induced taste disorders[43]

- Gingivitis
- Lead or copper poisoning
- Recent dental procedures
- Thrush
- Upper respiratory tract infection
- Zinc deficiency

Drug-induced gingival hyperplasia[156]

- Gingivitis
- Hormonal conditions (i.e., pregnancy, hypothyroidism)
- Leukemia (i.e., acute monocytic, lymphocytic, myelocytic)
- Nutritional conditions (i.e., vitamin C deficiency)

Drug-induced oral erythema multiforme[187]

- Bullous pemphigoid
- Cutaneous small-vessel vasculitis
- Fixed drug eruptions
- Paraneoplastic pemphigus
- Polymorphous light eruption
- Stevens–Johnson syndrome
- Sweet syndrome
- Rowell syndrome
- Urticaria

Drug-induced oral lichenoid reactions[201,222,231]

- Candidiasis
- Chronic ulcerative stomatitis
- Desquamative gingivitis
- Graft versus host disease following allogenic bone marrow or stem cell transplant
- Lupus erythematosis
- Lichenoid dysplasia
- Mucous membrane pemphigoid
- Oral hairy leukoplakia
- Oral lichen planus
- Pemphigus vulgaris
- Poor oral hygiene
- Proliferative verrucous leukoplakia
- Squamous cell carcinoma

Drug-induced osteonecrosis of the jaw[249]

- Fungal infection
- Osteoradionecrosis

restoration can result in the generation of corrosive products, such as silver sulfide, resulting in grayish-black discoloration. Pigmented lesions often require a biopsy to establish a definitive diagnosis.[13]

RISK FACTORS

Few specific risk factors for drug-induced color changes of the oral mucosa and teeth exist (**Table 56-5**). Trauma, hormonal changes, medication, and radiation can cause increased melanin production and lead to an increased incidence of oral pigmentation.[42] The administration of medications known to induce color changes should be limited if patients are known to have increased melanin production. Given the mechanism by which the tetracyclines cause color changes of the teeth, age and developmental stage should be considered as risk factors for this adverse effect.

MORBIDITY AND MORTALITY

No cases of morbidity or mortality associated with drug-induced color changes of the mucosa or teeth have been reported. The clinical consequences are mostly cosmetic, but the impact that the cosmetic changes may have on a patient's quality of life must be considered.

PREVENTION

The most effective prevention strategy for drug-induced color changes of the oral mucosa and teeth is limiting patients' exposure (dose and duration) to

Table 56-5 Risk Factors for Drug-Induced Oral Manifestations of Systemic Drugs

Color changes of the oral mucosa and teeth

- Age of the patient
- Chronic inflammation
- Duration of medication exposure
- Early stages of tooth development (tetracycline-induced)
- Hormonal changes
- Increased melanin production
- Trauma
- Trimester of pregnancy

Drug-induced taste disorders

- Concomitant chemotherapy[89]
- Female sex[61]
- Lower body-mass index[71]
- Older age[84,90-92]
- Radiation
- Vitamin D deficiency[93]
- Zinc deficiency[89]

Drug-induced gingival hyperplasia[126]

- Duration of treatment
- Male sex
- Plaque-induced inflammation
- Poor oral hygiene
- Young age

Drug-induced oral erythema multiforme

- Human leukocyte antigen (HLA) types: HLA-DQ3, HLA-B15(B62), HLA-B35, HLA-A33, HLA-DR53, HLA-DQB1*0301[179]
- Male sex[195]
- Younger age[195]

Drug-induced oral lichenoid reactions

- Female sex[233]
- Medication contains a thiol chemical group[208,228]

Drug-induced osteonecrosis of the jaw

- Cancer that has metastasized to the bone[266]
- Combination treatment with bisphosphonate and bevacizumab or sunitinib[251]
- Dental extractions[266]
- Intravenous bisphosphonate administration[249]
- Length of exposure to bisphosphonates (>6 months)[240,257]
- Multiple myeloma[266]
- Overall poor oral health[266]
- Surgical bone manipulation[266]
- Presence of oral infections[266]
- Trauma from dentures[266]

drugs known to carry this risk. Drugs of the tetracycline class should be avoided (to the extent medically possible) in women during the last half of pregnancy and in all children up to the age of 8 years.

MANAGEMENT

Drug-induced color changes of the oral mucosa are benign, and no treatment is required once diagnosed. The pigmentation should resolve within a few months of medication discontinuation.[37] Tetracycline-induced pigmentation is irreversible, but the intensity may decrease over the years following discontinuation.[31]

INFORMATION FOR PATIENTS

When patients present with medication-induced color changes of the oral mucosa and teeth, healthcare providers should reassure the patient that it is a completely benign condition and is not commonly associated with long-term effects (unless due to tetracyclines).

TASTE DISORDERS

Three primary taste disorders exist: hypogeusia, ageusia, and dysgeusia. Hypogeusia is a decreased sensitivity to tastes, and ageusia is a total loss of taste perception. Dysgeusia is the distortion or misinterpretation of a taste while eating (i.e., tasting sour instead of sweet) or taste confusion.[43] Patients with dysgeusia may have an exaggerated sense of sweet, bitter, salty, or metallic tastes.[44,45]

CAUSATIVE AGENTS

Many drugs have been associated with disorders of taste including clarithromycin, terbinafine, furosemide, boceprevir, and telaprevir (**Table 56-6**).[14,43,46-72]

EPIDEMIOLOGY

Hypogeusia, ageusia, and dysgeusia are often grouped together and labeled simply as "taste changes" or "taste disorders." Medication-induced taste changes have been reported to account for 0.4% of reported

Table 56-6 Agents Implicated in Drug-Induced Taste Disorders[14,43,46-72]

Drug	Incidence	Level of Evidence[a]
5-fluorouracil[14,43,47-49,52]	NK	B
Acetazolamide[14,43,47-49]	NK	B
Allopurinol[14,43,47-49]	NK	B
Alprazolam[53]	NK	C
Amlodipine[53]	<0.1%	C
Amoxicillin–clavulanic acid[46]	NK	B
Amphetamines[43,47-49]	NK	B
Amphotericin B[14,43,47-49]	NK	B
Aspirin[14,47-49]	NK	B
Atorvastatin[14,47]	NK	C
Azathioprine[14,54]	NK	C
Azithromycin[46]	<1%	B
Beceprovir[50]	18–43%	C
β-lactam antibiotics[43,47-49]	NK	B
Botulinim toxin A[47-49]	NK	C
Bupivacaine[47-49]	NK	C
Captopril[14,43,47-49,55]	2–4%	B
Carbamazepine[43,47-49]	NK	B
Carboplatin[43,52]	1%	C
Ceftriaxone[47-49]	<1%	C
Chlorhexidine[43,56]	NK	C
Cisplatin[14,43,47-49,52]	NK	B
Clarithromycin[14,46-49]	0.4–18.9%	B
Crizotinib[57-59]	26%	A
Cyclophosphamide[52]	NK	C
Diltiazem[14,43]	< %	C
Dipyridamole[14,43,47-49]	NK	B
Disulfiram[47-49]	NK	C
Docetaxel[60]	NK	C
Doxorubicin[52]	NK	C
EDTA[14,43]	NK	C
Enalapril[14,43]	0.5–2.9%	C
Eprosartan[47-49]	NK	C
Ergocalciferol[47-49]	NK	C
Eszopiclone[61,62]	26–62%	A
Ethambutol[14,43,47-49]	NK	B
Ethionamide[14,43]	NK	C
Ferrous sulfate[47-49]	1.1%	C
Fluoxetine[47-49]	NK	C
Flurazepam[43,47-49]	NK	C
Furosemide[47-49]	NK	C
Interferon α[43]	1%	C
Isosorbide dinitrate[14,43]	NK	C

Table 56-6 Agents Implicated in Drug-Induced Taste Disorders[14,43,46-72] (continued)

Drug	Incidence	Level of Evidence[a]
Isotretinoin[43,63]	NK	C
Lamotrigine[47-49]	NK	C
Levamisole[43]	7%	C
Levodopa[14,43,47-49]	>3%	B
Levofloxacin[46]	8–10%	B
Lisinopril[14,43,47,55]	NK	B
Lithium[14,43,47-49,64]	NK	B
Losartan[14,43,47,65]	NK	B
Metformin[47-49]	NK	C
Methocarbamol[47-49]	NK	C
Methyldopa[47-49]	NK	C
Metolazone[47-49]	NK	C
Metronidazole[14,43,47-49,66]	2–9%	B
Moxifloxacin[46]	0.1≤1%	B
Nifedipine[14,43,47-49,67]	NK	B
Nitroglycerin[14,43]	NK	C
Olanzapine[53]	NK	C
Paclitaxel[60]	NK	C
Penicillamine[14,43,47-49]	12%	B
Pentamidine[14,43,47-49,68]	NK	B
Pergolide[14,43]	1.6%	C
Pravastatin[47]	NK	C
Procainamide[47-49]	3–4%	C
Procaine penicillin G[14,43,47-49]	NK	B
Propafenone[14,43,47-49]	>5%	B
Propylthiouracil[14,43]	NK	C
Protease inhibitors[46,69]	NK	B
Ramipril[14]	NK	C
Risperidone[47-49,70]	NK	A
Selegiline[14,43]	1≥3%	C
Simvastatin[47]	NK	C
Sulfasalazine[14,43,47-49]	NK	B
Sulfisoxazole[47-49]	NK	C
Sulindac[47-49]	NK	C
Sumatriptan[47-49]	13.5–24.5%	C
Sunitinib[46]	21–47%	B
Telaprevir[51]	27%	B
Terbinafine[14,43,46-49,71]	2.8–9%	B
Tetracycline[14,43,47-49,72]	NK	B
Vitamin D[47-49]	NK	C
Zopiclone[14,47-49]	15–30%	B

EDTA = ethylenediaminetetraacetic acid, NK = not known.

[a]Definitions for Levels of Evidence: Level A—evidence from one or more randomized, controlled clinical trials; Level B—evidence from nonrandomized clinical trials, prospective observational studies, cohort studies, retrospective studies, case-control studies, meta-analyses and/or postmarketing surveillance studies; and Level C—evidence from one or more published case reports or case series.

adverse drug events, and this adverse event occurs more often in elderly patients, with a reported incidence of up to 33%.[46,47] Medications are thought to be the cause for up to 25% of all reported taste disturbances.[73] Cardiovascular agents carry a risk of causing taste disorders of approximately 2%.[74] Taste disorders have been reported in approximately 56% of cancer patients receiving chemotherapy alone, 66% of patients receiving radiation alone, and 76% in patients receiving both chemotherapy and radiation.[75,76]

MECHANISMS

Multiple mechanisms exist that may explain how medications cause taste disturbances (**Table 56-7**).[43] Taste disorders may be secondary to hyposalivation as a result of damage to the salivary glands, change in chemical composition of the saliva, or via other mechanisms such as drug-receptor inhibition, alteration of neurotransmitter function, neuron action potential disruption, or dysfunctional sensory modulation in the brain.[46,55,77,78] Chemotherapy may cause taste disturbances due to higher rates of cell turnover and taste bud cell death.[76,79]

Table 56-7 Mechanisms of Drug-Induced Taste Disorders

Drug	Mechanism(s)[43]
Acetazolamide Tetracycline	• Dysfunction of taste bud or neuron
Allopurinol Dipyridamole Lithium	• Alteration of secondary messenger systems that leads to misinterpretation of tastes
Amphetamines	• Decreased taste threshold
Captopril Enalapril Lisinopril	• Excess bradykinin accumulation • Zinc deficiency
β-lactam antibiotics EDTA Penicillamine Propylthiouracil	• Zinc chelation
5-fluorouracil	• Mucosal toxicity
Diltiazem Nifedipine	• Decreased calcium-mediated neurotransmission

EDTA = ethylenediaminetetraacetic acid.

Taste disturbances related to radiation are a result of damage to the nerves responsible for processing taste function, anatomic changes, and a direct decrease in taste bud density due to cytotoxic and antiproliferative effects.[76,79-83]

CLINICAL PRESENTATION AND DIFFERENTIAL DIAGNOSIS

Taste disorders often present with patients complaining of strange tastes, changes to the taste of food, or lack of taste (Table 56-3). Symptoms may begin suddenly or have a gradual onset. When related to radiation therapy, taste disorders peak 3–4 weeks after the start of treatment.[84]

Differential diagnoses for taste disorders include upper respiratory tract infections, dental causes, or structural changes (Table 56-4).[43,85,86] Tests to rule out nondrug causes may include computed tomography and magnetic resonance imaging to look for structural changes that may be contributing to the taste disorder and to assess neurologic or intracranial causes.[87] Simple taste testing based on exposure to substances known to produce certain tastes, such as salty or sweet, can be completed to confirm the diagnosis of dysgeusia and other taste disorders.[88]

RISK FACTORS

Many nonspecific risk factors exist that may predispose patients to taste disorders (Table 56-5).[61,71,84,90-93] Some data suggest women may be more sensitive to taste disturbances related to medications.[61] Lower body mass index is thought to increase the risk from lipophilic drugs, such as terbinafine.[71] Older age is associated with an increased risk due to a decreased quality of taste buds and higher number of daily medications to treat chronic medical conditions.[90-92] Zinc and vitamin D deficiencies have been linked to taste disturbances, particularly when patients are receiving chemotherapy.[89,93] Higher doses of radiation may be associated with more severe symptoms.[84]

MORBIDITY AND MORTALITY

Overall, taste disturbances can lead to decreased appetite, poor food choices, and decreased intake contributing to malnutrition, worsening of medical conditions impacted by dietary choices, and impaired immune function.[49] Taste disturbances do not directly cause morbidity and mortality; however, it has been estimated that up to 20% of deaths in cancer patients may be attributed to malnourishment resulting from decreased enjoyment of food.[94] Studies in cancer patients yield conflicting results concerning the impact taste disturbances have on quality of life. Some studies have found that approximately 50% of patients list taste disturbances in their top three treatment-related complaints, although other studies refute those reports.[84]

PREVENTION

Limiting drug exposure (dose and duration of treatment) is the most effective means for preventing all of the oral manifestations of systemically administered drugs. Unfortunately, no specific methods for the prevention of taste disturbances have been identified.

MANAGEMENT

Taste disturbances are best treated with removal of the offending agent.[14] Resolution of symptoms may take months due to accumulated metabolites. Small trials have reported improvement in symptoms with the use of alpha lipoic acid (200 mg given orally 3 times daily) or zinc supplementation (50 mg given orally 3 times daily), particularly if zinc deficiency is identified.[95-97] For chemotherapy patients with a documented decreased 25-hydroxyvitamin D level, daily supplementation with 2,000 units of vitamin D_3 (cholecalciferol) orally was found to be successful in reducing treatment-related taste disorders.[93] Clonazapem has been found to be effective for some types of dysgeusia due to its action on gamma-aminobutyric acid receptors.[98]

If taste disturbances persist following removal of the offending agent, masking techniques such as the use of breath mints or sugarless chewing gum may be utilized. These approaches may have limited efficacy, however, due to loss of flavor from the underlying taste disturbance. Lozenges containing the local anesthetic dyclonine (e.g., Sucrets) may provide temporary relief.[44] A case report found improvement in dysgeusia when patients held an ice cube in the mouth before meals.[99] Patients may also see improvement with the use of plastic utensils, eating food cold, and, in severe cases, use of an oral suspension composed of lidocaine, aluminum-magnesium hydroxide, and diphenhydramine.[60]

INFORMATION FOR PATIENTS

Patients with drug-induced disturbances of taste should understand that the disorder could cause them to either eat too much and gain weight or eat too little and lose weight. Flavor enhancement can increase food enjoyment, even in the presence of taste disturbances; however, if salt or sugar is used, it may have an impact on chronic conditions such as hypertension or diabetes. Techniques such as marinating meats before cooking, using low-calorie sweeteners for sweetness, and using lemon juice for sourness can sometimes improve taste and help increase caloric intake. It is important for patients to make a conscious effort to maintain proper nutrition, utilizing supplements and dietary guidelines.[100-103]

GINGIVAL HYPERPLASIA

Gingival hyperplasia often begins as a painless enlargement that is usually generalized throughout the mouth. There is an accumulation of extracellular components within the gingival connective tissue associated with various degrees of chronic inflammation.

CAUSATIVE AGENTS

There is a definitive link between medications and gingival hyperplasia. Multiple medications have been reported to cause gingival hyperplasia, including cyclosporine, sodium valproate, nifedipine,

Table 56-8 Agents Implicated in Drug-Induced Gingival Hyperplasia[14,104-144]

Drug	Incidence	Level of Evidence[a]
Amlodipine[14,121-125]	2–10%	B
Carbamazepine[126]	NK	C
Co-trimoxazole[14]	NK	C
Cyclosporine[14,104-109,127-131]	4–16%	A
Diltiazem[14,117-119,125]	21–76%	A
Diphenoxylate[14]	NK	C
Erythromycin[14,132]	NK	C
Ethosuximide[14,125]	NK	C
Felodipine[14,125]	<0.5%	C
Interferon α[14,133]	NK	C
Ketoconazole[14]	NK	C
Lamotrigine[14,134]	NK	C
Lithium[14,135-138]	NK	B
Mephenytoin[13,125]	NK	C
Methsuximide[125]	NK	C
Nicardipine[125]	NK	C
Nifedipine[14,111-117,121,122,125,129]	0.5–40%	A
Nimodipine[125]	NK	C
Nisoldipine[125]	<1%	C
Oral contraceptives[14]	NK	C
Phenobarbital[14,139]	NK	C
Phensuximide[125]	NK	C
Phenytoin[14,120,125,134]	10–80%	B
Primidone[14]	NK	C
Sertraline[14]	NK	C
Sodium valproate[14,110,125,140]	NK	B
Tacrolimus[127,141]	NK	C
Topiramate[14]	NK	C
Tranexamic acid[142]	NK	C
Verapamil[14,125,143]	19%	B
Vigabatrin[14,144]	<1%	C

NK - not known.
[a]Definitions for Levels of Evidence: Level A—evidence from one or more randomized, controlled clinical trials; Level B—evidence from nonrandomized clinical trials, prospective observational studies, cohort studies, retrospective studies, case-control studies, meta-analyses and/or postmarketing surveillance studies; and Level C—evidence from one or more published case reports or case series.

diltiazem, verapamil, amlodipine, large doses of progesterone, and, most classically, phenytoin (**Table 56-8**).[14,104-144]

EPIDEMIOLOGY

The incidence of medication-induced gingival hyperplasia varies with medication class and specific agents within those classes. The incidence of gingival hyperplasia associated with calcium-channel blockers ranges from 3% to 6%, with some reports suggesting an incidence as high as 80%.[124,145] Up to 50% of patients treated with phenytoin will experience this gingival hyperplasia after the first 3 months of treatment.[146-148] Cyclosporine-induced gingival hyperplasia can affect 25–50% of adults and 70–97% of children.[149]

Table 56-9 Mechanisms of Drug-Induced Gingival Hyperplasia

Drug	Mechanism(s)[125]
Anticonvulsants	• Down regulation of epidermal growth factor receptor metabolism • Increased production and secretion of collagenase • Increased production of platelet-derived growth factor • Increased rate of cell growth • Interference of folic acid absorption and metabolism
Cyclosporine	• Altered gingival fibroblast metabolism • Immunogenetic predisposition (presence of HLA-DR2) • Increase in protein synthesis and cell proliferation • Increased activation of growth factors • Increased platelet-derived growth factor messenger RNA
Calcium-channel blockers	• Increased cell proliferation rate • Increased collagen synthesis • Interferences of calcium transport and calcium-dependent processes (i.e., collagenolytic effects of inflammatory cells, synthesis of collagenase)

RNA = ribonucleic acid.

MECHANISMS

The primary mechanism of drug-induced gingival hyperplasia is thought to relate to inflammation. (**Table 56-9**).[125] Inflammation may develop due to direct toxic effects of the drug in gingival fluid[150] or may be plaque-induced.[151,152] Decreased cellular folic acid uptake leads to decreased activity of collagenase and upregulation of keratinocyte growth factor, resulting in gingival overgrowth.[150,153] Once overgrown tissue develops, bacteria persist in pockets unable to be reached with a toothbrush or dental floss, which further perpetuates the cycle of inflammation.[154]

CLINICAL PRESENTATION AND DIFFERENTIAL DIAGNOSIS

Gingival hyperplasia is characterized by increased gingival mass and volume that can be localized or generalized (Table 56-3).[125,154,155] Initial presentation may be a firm nodular enlargement which progresses to an enlarged, lobulated appearance. Gingival hyperplasia related to the use of calcium-channel blockers usually begins about 2–3 months after treatment initiation.[155] Cyclosporine-induced gingival hyperplasia is more likely to cause bleeding from the gums as compared to gingival hyperplasia caused by phenytoin.[149]

Differential diagnosis for drug-induced gingival hyperplasia includes systemic conditions such as certain types of leukemia, hereditary gingival fibromatosis, sarcoidosis, Crohn disease, Wegener granulomatosis, amyloidosis, pregnancy, hypothyroidism, or vitamin C deficiency (Table 56-4).[156] In patients with leukemia, other features of the gingival hyperplasia include oral ulcers, spontaneous bleeding, and candidiasis. When gingival hyperplasia is due to vitamin C deficiency, the gums often have a bluish-red color, with a smooth, shiny surface that bleeds easily.[157] In addition to decreased serum ascorbic acid levels (<2 mcg/mL), patients may have elevated levels of high-sensitivity C-reactive protein.[158] Additional conditions to rule out include gingival cysts and pregnancy-induced hyperplasia.[157] A biopsy with histologic exam may be necessary in some instances to establish the proper diagnoses.

RISK FACTORS

Underlying gingival inflammation due to poor oral hygiene and dental plaques may increase risk of drug-induced gingival hyperplasia (Table 56-5).[126,139,159] Men are more likely to develop gingival hyperplasia than women.[160] Exposure to a combination of medications such as cyclosporine and calcium-channel blockers may increase risk.[128,129] A prior history of developing gingival hyperplasia, weight gain, acne, hirsutism, or alopecia with the use of an anti-epileptic medication is associated with an increased risk of experiencing the same or additional side effects with repeat medication exposure or use of a different medication (37% chance with prior history versus 3% chance with no prior history).[134]

Genetic mutations are thought to play a role in the development of gingival hyperplasia. Mutations in the cytochrome P450 2C9 (CYP2C9), an enzyme encoded by the *CYP2C9* gene, have been associated with an increased risk of phenytoin-induced gingival hyperplasia (specifically, variant genotypes CYP2C9FNx012 and FNx013).[161] Polymorphisms of certain genes that modify the inflammatory response (e.g., MDR1 G2677T/A) have been associated with an increased likelihood of developing gingival hyperplasia due to calcium-channel blockers.[162]

MORBIDITY AND MORTALITY

The aesthetic effects of gingival hyperplasia are often all that are considered, but the presence of this drug-induced disease can lead to difficulty with speaking and chewing, worsened oral hygiene, and even malnutrition.[139,150,159] Although the medications do not typically affect the underlying bone, accumulation of bacteria within the pockets created by the gingival hyperplasia may lead to periodontitis and bone and tooth loss.[154] Children in particular may develop abnormal swallowing and have difficulty with speech and chewing.[163]

PREVENTION

Limiting the length and amount of drug exposure is the most effective method for prevention of all oral manifestations of systemically administered drugs (**Table 56-10**).[164,165]

Limited data suggest that the addition of folic acid to patients receiving phenytoin therapy may prevent the development of gingival hyperplasia.[164,165] Because dental plaque plays such a large role in the development of gingival inflammation, patients receiving medications known to have a high incidence of gingival hyperplasia should be encouraged to follow a strict oral hygiene regimen, including plaque removal.[126]

Table 56-10 Approaches to Help Prevent Drug-Induced Gingival Hyperplasia

Drug	Approach
All	• Limit exposure (dose and duration) to drugs known to cause gingival hyperplasia • Prevent plaque-induced inflammation by good oral hygiene and preventative dental care
Phenytoin	• Folic acid supplementation[164,165]

MANAGEMENT

Primary treatment includes discontinuing the offending agent and performing good oral care. Surgery is usually unnecessary, but if required, gingivectomy or periodontal flap procedures would be the preferred options.[150,166] Nonsurgical dental procedures, such as scaling and root planing of dental plaques and calculi, may help reduce the inflammatory component of gingival hyperplasia.[154] For patients in whom discontinuing the offending agent is not a feasible option, there have been reports of improvement in gingival hyperplasia symptoms with the use of azithromycin 250 mg orally for 3–5 days.[167-171]

INFORMATION FOR PATIENTS

Healthcare providers should be knowledgeable about medications known to induce gingival hyperplasia. When patients are prescribed an agent with the potential to cause this drug-induced disease, they should be educated regarding the importance of good oral care to help minimize risk.

ORAL ERYTHEMA MULTIFORME

Drug-induced erythema multiforme (EM) is an adverse reaction to systemic drugs that manifests as skin lesions. Erythema multiforme can be categorized as minor, major, or oral based on the severity and number of sites involved. EM minor is typically a localized eruption of the skin with minimal or no mucosal involvement, while EM major is more severe, potentially life-threatening, and often includes extensive mucosal involvement. With oral EM, patients have typical oral and lip lesions without lesions elsewhere on the skin.

CAUSATIVE AGENTS

The most common triggers of EM include the sulfa drugs and anticonvulsants; however, multiple other medications such as allopurinol, carbamazepine, and clindamycin, have also been implicated.[14,172-175] **Table 56-11** lists drugs associated with oral EM.[14,22,172-185]

EPIDEMIOLOGY

Although the prevalence of EM is estimated to be <1% (estimated incidence of 0.8–6 cases per million individuals per year), it is thought to account for about 6% of all autoimmune disease of the oral mucosa.[175,186] Approximately 90% of the cases of EM (all types) are triggered by an underlying herpes simplex virus (HSV) infection. Mucosal lesions may occur in 25–60% of patients with EM. Drug-induced EM accounts for <10% of all cases and usually presents as an isolated episode, rather than a recurrent or persistent condition.[187]

Table 56-11 Agents Implicated in Drug-Induced Oral Erythema Multiforme[14,22,172-185]

Drug	Incidence	Level of Evidence[a]
Abacavir[176]	NK	C
Acetaminophen[175,177]	NK	C
Acetylsalicylic acid[14]	NK	C
Adalimumab[178]	NK	C
Allopurinol[14,172,175,179]	<3%	B
Amlodipine[14]	1–3.8%	C
Amoxicillin–clavulanic acid[175]	NK	C
Arsenic[14,175]	NK	C
Atazanavir[176]	NK	C
Atropine[14]	NK	C
Barbiturates[179,180]	NK	C
Barium contrast[175]	NK	C
Busulfan[14,172,175]	NK	C
Carbamazepine[14,173,174,175,179]	NK	B
Cefuroxime[175]	Rare	C
Cephalosporins[175,179]	NK	C
Chloramphenicol[14]	NK	C
Chlorpropamide[14,175,179]	NK	C
Ciprofloxacin[175]	1%	C
Clindamycin[14,175,179]	NK	C
Co-trimoxazole[14,174]	NK	C
Codeine[14,175,179]	NK	C
Cyclophosphamide[175]	NK	C
Darunavir[176]	NK	C
Delavirdine[176]	NK	C
Diclofenac[14,174,175]	NK	C
Didanosine[176]	NK	C
Digoxin[14,175]	NK	C

Table 56-11 Agents Implicated in Drug-Induced Oral Erythema Multiforme[14,22,172-185] (continued)

Drug	Incidence	Level of Evidence[a]
Diltiazem[14]	<0.1%	C
Dimenhydrinate[181]	NK	C
DTaP vaccine[180]	NK	C
Efavirenz[176]	0.1%	C
Ethambutol[14,175,179]	NK	C
Etravirine[176]	<0.5%	C
Fluconazole[14]	NK	C
Fluorouracil[14]	NK	C
Fosamprenavir[176]	NK	C
Furosemide[14,175,182]	NK	B
Gold[14,22,175,179]	NK	B
Griseofulvin[14]	NK	C
Hepatitis B vaccine[14,180]	NK	C
Hydralazine[175]	NK	C
Ibuprofen[174,175]	<1%	C
Indapamide[14]	NK	C
Infliximab[178,183]	Rare	C
Iodides[175]	NK	C
Ketoprofen[175]	NK	C
Lamotrigine[172]	<0.1%	C
Levofloxacin[179]	NK	C
Meclofenamic acid[14]	<0.1%	C
Methotrexate[175]	NK	C
Metoprolol[175]	Rare	C
Minoxidil[14,175]	NK	C
MMR vaccine[14,180]	NK	C
Naproxen[175]	NK	C
Nevirapine[176]	NK	C
Nifedipine[14]	NK	C
Omeprazole[14]	NK	C
Oral contraceptives[175,180]	NK	C
Penicillins[14,172,175,179,180]	NK	B
Phenylbutazone[14,175,179]	NK	C
Phenytoin[14,172,174,175,179,180]	NK	B
Piroxicam[14,175,179]	NK	C
Progesterone[14,172,175]	NK	C
Protease inhibitors[172,175,179]	NK	C
Quinine[14]	NK	C
Raltegravir[176]	NK	C
Retinol[14,184]	NK	C
Rifampin[14,175,179,180]	NK	C
Salicylates[174,175]	NK	C

Table 56-11 Agents Implicated in Drug-Induced Oral Erythema Multiforme[14,22,172-185] (continued)

Drug	Incidence	Level of Evidence[a]
Saquinavir mesylate[176]	NK	C
Sorafenib[185]	0.1≤1%	C
Streptomycin[14]	NK	C
Sulfadiazine[175]	NK	C
Sulfasalazine[14,175]	NK	C
Sulindac[14]	<1%	C
Sulphonamides[172,174,175,180]	NK	C
TB skin test[175,180]	NK	C
Tetracycline[14,175,179]	NK	C
Theophylline[14]	NK	C
Thiabendazole[175]	NK	C
Tipranavir[176]	NK	C
Tolbutamide[14,175,178]	NK	C
Trimethoprim–sulfamethoxazole[175,178]	NK	C
Valdecoxib[175]	NK	C
Valproic acid[175]	NK	C
Vancomycin[14,175,180]	NK	C
Verapamil[14,175]	NK	C
Zidovudine[14,176]	NK	C

NK = not known.

[a]Definitions for Levels of Evidence: Level A—evidence from one or more randomized, controlled clinical trials; Level B—evidence from nonrandomized clinical trials, prospective observational studies, cohort studies, retrospective studies, case-control studies, meta-analyses and/or postmarketing surveillance studies; and Level C—evidence from one or more published case reports or case series.

MECHANISMS

The exact mechanisms responsible for drug-induced oral EM are unknown (**Table 56-12**).[172,187] Erythema multiforme is a Type 4 hypersensitivity reaction that involves T-lymphocyte-induced apoptosis in epithelial keratinocytes, which leads to cell necrosis.[172] A component of the mechanism is a cell-mediated immune reaction against an antigen.[187] It has been found that the epidermal destruction with drug-induced EM is due to the cytokine tumor necrosis factor alpha, perforin, and granzyme B.[187,188]

Table 56-12 Mechanisms of Drug-Induced Oral Erythema Multiforme

- Cell-mediated immune reaction against an antigen[187]
- Epidermal destruction due to the action of tumor necrosis factor alpha, perforin, and granzyme B[187]
- Hypersensitivity reaction[172]
- T-lymphocyte induced apoptosis[172]

CLINICAL PRESENTATION AND DIFFERENTIAL DIAGNOSIS

Clinical presentation can vary from patient to patient, with lesions changing and evolving throughout the course of an eruption (Table 56-3).[172,189,190] Fever may or may not be present prior to the onset of lesions, but oral EM often presents acutely, with no prodrome and no widespread cutaneous involvement.[180] The earliest lesions usually resemble insect bites or urticaria, which may then enlarge and transform into the characteristic targetoid lesion.[187,191] These lesions include a central area of necrosis surrounded by a red inflammatory area and a lighter erythematous periphery.[189,190] Oral lesions may also present as erythema with some edema and progress to superficial erosions.[189] The initial occurrence of oral EM is typically limited to oral mucosal ulcerations and lip lesions, without any skin lesions or systemic symptoms. Subsequent episodes may involve more extensive body areas.[174,180,192] In oral EM, the skin and mucosal surface of the lips are the most commonly affected areas of the oral cavity.[175] Lips may become swollen, cracked, bloody, and crusted.[172]

Conditions to consider in the differential diagnosis of oral EM include urticaria, Stevens–Johnson syndrome, fixed drug eruptions, Sweet syndrome, Rowell syndrome, herpes infection, and autoimmune lesions (i.e., pemphigus vulgaris, bullous pemphigoid) (Table 56-4).[187] The diagnosis of EM is generally made based on patients' clinical presentation. There is typically little need for culture or other laboratory testing.[193]

RISK FACTORS

HSV 1 and 2 are very common triggers of EM (reported in up to 90% of EM cases). Mycoplasma pneumonia infection may also trigger an EM eruption.[194] There is, however, no evidence to suggest infection with these agents increases the risk of drug-induced oral EM. Adults in their 20s are most at risk for EM, with a slightly higher risk in men than in women.[195] There appears to be a genetic component to erythema multiforme, with a link to specific human leukocyte antigen (HLA) types HLA-DQ3, HLA-B15 (B62), HLA-B35, HLA-A33, HLA-DR53, and HLA-DQB1*0301 (Table 56-5).[179,195]

MORBIDITY AND MORTALITY

Mortality from oral EM has not been reported. Although initial reactions may be limited to the oral cavity, repeat outbreaks may cause more widespread lesions. Systemic EM can progress to Stevens–Johnson syndrome, an extensive blistering disease of two or more mucous membranes that causes the top layer of affected skin to be shed. Stevens–Johnson syndrome can be life-threatening. Pain caused by mucosal erosions in patients with EM can lead to poor oral intake of food and fluids. Esophagitis with esophageal strictures and upper airway erosions that lead to pneumonia are rare complications.[187,190]

PREVENTION

Limiting the length and amount of drug exposure is the most effective method for prevention of all oral manifestations of systemically administered drugs. No other specific preventive measures for drug-induced oral EM have been identified.

MANAGEMENT

In general, no specific treatment is needed for drug-induced oral EM, as lesions typically resolve in 2–4 weeks following removal of the offending agent. Severe cases may be associated with poor oral intake, requiring hospital admission for pain management and fluid and electrolyte replacement. Erythrocyte sedimentation rate, white blood cell count, and liver enzymes may be elevated in severe cases.[189,190] Oral anesthetic solutions (e.g., viscous lidocaine) and antiseptic rinses (e.g., chlorhexidine) can be used for temporary relief of healing oral lesions. Severe mucosal EM may require an oral corticosteroid burst (e.g., prednisone 40–60 mg/day tapered over 2–4 weeks).[187] Occasionally, systemic and/or topical antibiotics may be required to prevent secondary infection.

INFORMATION FOR PATIENTS

Patients with underlying HSV infections are at an increased risk of developing drug-induced oral EM. Patients receiving drugs known to be associated with oral EM should be instructed to notify their healthcare provider immediately if and when oral lesions begin to develop.

ORAL LICHENOID DRUG REACTIONS

Lichen planus (LP) is a chronic mucocutaneous inflammatory disorder of unknown etiology for which there currently is no cure. Oral lichenoid reactions (OLRs) are a variant of LP that can be due to drug exposure, local contact hypersensitivity, altered self-antigens, or superantigens. Oral lichenoid lesions can present with a wide range of features.

CAUSATIVE AGENTS

Drugs that may be associated with OLRs include nonsteroidal anti-inflammatory drugs, angiotensin converting enzyme inhibitors, allopurinol, methyldopa, β-blockers, glipizide, ketoconazole, sulfasalazine, and lithium, among others (**Table 56-13**).[14,72,196-221]

EPIDEMIOLOGY

The incidence of OLRs is not clear. They may occur as a result of systemic drug exposure or local allergic contact.[201] OLRs may be clinically indistinguishable from oral LP, leading to difficulty with accurate diagnosis.

MECHANISMS

OLRs represent a hypersensitivity disorder to circulating antigens or local irritants.[225] There is a component of T-cell mediation via an autoimmune process in which $CD8^+$ T cells trigger apoptosis of oral epithelial basal cells. Medication-related OLRs are thought to be due, at least in part, to the active thiol group found in the chemical structure of certain medications.[208,228] Another potential factor

Table 56-13 Agents Implicated in Drug-Induced Oral Lichenoid Reactions

Drug	Incidence	Level of Evidence[a]
Abatacept[202]	NK	C
Adalimumab[203,204]	NK	C
Allopurinol[14,72,198,200,205,206]	NK	B
Aminosalicylate sodium[201]	NK	C
Amlodipine[72]	NK	C
Amphotericin B[201,207]	NK	C
Aspirin[201,207]	NK	C
Atenolol[196,200,201]	NK	C
Atorvastatin[72]	NK	C
BCG vaccine[14]	NK	C
Bismuth[72,201,207]	NK	C
Captopril[14,72,205,206,208]	NK	B
Carbamazepine[14,72,201,206,207,209]	NK	B
Certolizumab[203,210,211]	NK	B
Chloroquine[14,72,201,205-207]	NK	B
Chlorpropamide[14,72,201,205,206]	NK	B
Cholera vaccine[14]	NK	C
Cimetidine[207]	NK	C
Cinnarizine[14,206,212]	NK	C
Clofibrate[14]	NK	C
Clonazepam[207]	NK	C
Colchicine[14]	NK	C
Dactinomycin[201,207]	NK	C
Dapsone[14,72,205]	NK	C
Diazepam[207]	NK	C
Diflunisal[201,206]	NK	C
Enalapril[72,196,200,201,206]	NK	B
Erythromycin[72]	NK	C

Table 56-13 Agents Implicated in Drug-Induced Oral Lichenoid Reactions (continued)

Drug	Incidence	Level of Evidence[a]
Etanercept[202]	NK	C
Ethionamide[14]	NK	C
Fenclofenac[72,206,207]	NK	C
Furosemide[72]	NK	C
Gabapentin[72]	NK	C
Glipizide[201]	NK	C
Gold salts[14,72,201,205,206]	20%	B
Griseofulvin[14]	NK	C
Hepatitis B vaccine[14,213]	NK	C
Hydrochlorothiazide[196,197,199,201,206,214]	NK	B
Hydroxychloroquine[14,72,201,207]	NK	C
Ibuprofen[201,207]	NK	C
Imatinib[201,215-217]	NK	C
Indomethacin[201,206]	NK	C
Infliximab[203,210,211]	NK	C
Insulin[201,207]	NK	C
Interferon α[14,72,133,218]	NK	C
Isoniazid[201,207]	NK	C
Ketoconazole[14,72,201,206,207]	NK	C
Labetalol[14,72,205,206]	<1%	C
Lisinopril[14,214]	NK	C
Lithium[14,201,206,207]	NK	C
Lorazepam[14,207]	NK	C
Mercury[14,72]	NK	C
Metformin[14]	<1%	C
Methyldopa[14,72,196,199-201,205,206]	NK	B
Metoprolol[196,200,201]	NK	C
Metronidazole[14]	NK	C
Naproxen[14,201,206,207]	<1%	C
Obinutuzumab[219]	NK	C
Omeprazole[207]	NK	C
Oral contraceptives[14]	NK	C
Oxcarbazepine[201,207]	NK	C
Penicillamine[14,72,201,205,206]	NK	C
Penicillins[14]	NK	C
Phenindione[14]	NK	C
Phenobarbital[220]	NK	C
Phenylbutazone[14]	<1%	C
Phenytoin[14,201,20]	NK	C
Piroxicam[14]	NK	C
Prazosin[14]	<1%	C
Procainamide[14,206]	NK	C
Propranolol[14,72,205,206]	NK	C

Table 56-13 Agents Implicated in Drug-Induced Oral Lichenoid Reactions (continued)

Drug	Incidence	Level of Evidence[a]
Propylthiouracil[14]	NK	C
Quinacrine[72,206]	20%	C
Quinidine[14,72,201,206,207]	<1%	C
Quinine[14,201,206,207]	NK	C
Ranitidine[207]	NK	C
Rifampin[14,201,207]	NK	C
Rituximab[221]	<1%	C
Sertraline[72]	NK	C
Sildenafil[72]	<1%	C
Spironolactone[72,206]	NK	C
Streptomycin[14,72,201,207]	NK	C
Sulfasalazine[201,206]	NK	C
Sulfonamides[14]	NK	C
Sulindac[201]	NK	C
Temazepam[207]	NK	C
Tetracyclines[14,72,201,205-207]	NK	B
Thalidomide[222]	<1%	C
Thyroxine[207]	NK	C
Tolbutamide[14,72,201,205]	NK	C
Tricyclic antidepressants[201,207]	NK	C
Triprolidine[14,72]	NK	C
Valproate sodium[201]	NK	C
Zidovudine[201,207]	NK	C

BCG = Bacillus Calmette–Guérin, NK = not known.
[a]Definitions for Levels of Evidence: Level A—evidence from one or more randomized, controlled clinical trials; Level B—evidence from nonrandomized clinical trials, prospective observational studies, cohort studies, retrospective studies, case-control studies, meta-analyses and/or postmarketing surveillance studies; and Level C—evidence from one or more published case reports or case series.

for the development of OLRs is related to polymorphisms of cytochrome P450 enzymes (CYP), specifically involving CYP-2D6, which leads to decreased metabolism of some medications (**Table 56-14**).[224-227]

Table 56-14 Mechanisms of Drug-Induced Oral Lichenoid Reactions

- Cytochrome P450 (CYP)-2D6 polymorphisms leading to decreased metabolism of medications[226,227]
- Cytokine upregulation and lymphocyte recruitment[224]
- Hypersensitivity reaction to antigens or local irritants[223,225]
- Mast cell degranulation[224]
- T-cell mediated destruction of epithelial basal cells[224]

CLINICAL PRESENTATION AND DIFFERENTIAL DIAGNOSIS

OLRs are commonly associated with ulcerations along the buccal mucosa and lateral borders of the tongue that contain characteristic white striations known as Wickham striae (Table 56-3).[2,74,229,230] Pain usually accompanies the development of the ulcerations, although they may present as asymptomatic white reticular striae and plaques or painful swollen, red, eroded, or ulcerated lesions.[229] The onset may be slow and patients may initially report a roughness on the lining of the mouth and sensitivity to hot or spicy foods as their first symptoms.[230]

The principal condition to consider in the differential diagnosis of an OLR is oral LP (Table 56-4).[201,222,231] Other conditions to rule out would include malignancy, graft versus host disease, lupus erythematosus, and chronic ulcerative stomatitis.[222] It has been suggested that a diagnosis based on a history of recent exposure to an inducing medication combined with consistent physical findings is appropriate, although well-established ulcerations may persist long after the culprit medication is discontinued.[200,232] Biopsy of lesions caused by OLRs should contain immunoglobulin M and occasionally immunoglobulin A, immunoglobulin G, complement component 3, and colloid bodies containing fibrin.[206] Histopathological features of the biopsy specimen may include hyperkeratosis, basal cell degeneration, and band-like inflammatory cell infiltration.[229]

RISK FACTORS

Few known risk factors have been linked to the development of OLRs (Table 56-5).[208,228,233] OLRs are more common in women, with a highest risk between the ages of 30 and 70 years.[233] There may be a higher incidence of this reaction when medications contain a thiol group as part of their chemical structure.[208,228]

MORBIDITY AND MORTALITY

Mortality is unlikely with OLRs. The presence of OLRs have been associated with moderate-to-high levels of self-reported anxiety.[234]

PREVENTION

Limiting drug exposure (dose and duration) is the most effective method for prevention of all oral manifestations of systemically administered drugs, including OLRs.

MANAGEMENT

The most effective management strategy is removal of the causative agent. If this cannot be accomplished, the use of topical corticosteroids is recommended to help control symptoms. Corticosteroids are believed to act through their anti-inflammatory and immune-modulating properties. Beneficial results with medium- to super-potency topical agents such as clobetasol propionate 0.05% and betamethasone propionate 0.05% have been reported.[201] Topical aloe vera has also been studied and may provide some pain relief.[235,236] Mucosal protectants such as milk of magnesia may provide temporary relief. Immunosuppressive agents may be necessary in severe cases.[230] Topical tacrolimus has been studied and found to be an effective option for reducing signs and symptoms of OLRs as an alternative to topical steroids, particularly if patients are at risk for oral candidiasis.[237] Topical acitretin may be used as well.[237,238] Good oral hygiene should be encouraged to avoid infections.[239]

INFORMATION FOR PATIENTS

Reactions typically occur within the first 3 months of medication exposure but may be delayed up to a year.[201] Patients receiving drugs known to be associated with OLRs should be instructed to report any signs or symptoms of oral ulceration to their healthcare provider.

OSTEONECROSIS OF THE JAW

Cases of osteonecrosis of the jaw have become more common over the last decade due primarily to the widespread use of bisphosphonates.

CAUSATIVE AGENTS

Drug-induced osteonecrosis of the jaw has been commonly associated with the use of bisphosphonates, denosumab, bevacizumab, and sunitinib. These and other agents implicated in drug-induced osteonecrosis of the jaw are listed in **Table 56-15.**[240-254]

EPIDEMIOLOGY

The risk of osteonecrosis varies by causative agent. It has been reported in 5–12% of patients receiving bisphosphonates for treatment of metastatic

Table 56-15 Agents Implicated in Drug-Induced Osteonecrosis of the Jaw

Drug	Incidence	Level of Evidence[a]
Alendronate[241,249]	0.017–0.03%	C
Bevacizumab[243-245,250,251]	NK	B
Denosumab[242,251]	1.8%	C
Etidronate[249]	NK	C
Ibandronate[249]	NK	C
Pamidronate[241,249,252,253]	Up to 18%	B
Risedronate[249]	NK	C
Sunitinib[243,246-251,254]	<1%	B
Tiludronate[249]	NK	C
Zoledronic acid[241,249,252]	1.6–2.8%	B

NK = not known.

[a]Definitions for Levels of Evidence: Level A—evidence from one or more randomized, controlled clinical trials; Level B—evidence from nonrandomized clinical trials, prospective observational studies, cohort studies, retrospective studies, case-control studies, meta-analyses and/or postmarketing surveillance studies; and Level C—evidence from one or more published case reports or case series.

malignancies.[255,256] The incidence in patients receiving zoledronic acid has been reported to be about 10%, with cumulative hazard ranging from 1% in the first year to 21% by 3 years. The overall risk with pamidronate appears to be lower, with a cumulative hazard ranging from 0% in the first year of treatment to 4% in the third year of treatment.[256,257] The reported incidence of bevacizumab- and sunitinib-induced osteonecrosis (<0.001%) is significantly less than that reported for bisphosphonates.[258]

MECHANISMS

The mandible and maxilla have a greater blood supply (leading to relatively high concentrations of the drugs associated with osteonecrosis) and faster turnover than other bones. Multiple mechanisms are thought to possibly play a role in bisphosphonate-induced osteonecrosis of the jaw, including osteoclast inhibition leading to loss of maintenance of the capillary network within the bone and to insufficient bone deposition and remodeling, downregulation of matrix metalloproteinases, and increased osteoclast apoptosis and prevention of osteoclast development from bone marrow precursors and monocytes.[259-262] A spontaneous mucosal breakdown, injury, or invasive jaw surgery can cause bone exposure and failure of healing in necrotic bone.[241]

Osteonecrosis caused by denosumab, bevacizumab, and sunitinib is related to a drug-induced decrease in bone turnover and inhibition of host defense mechanisms. Denosumab is known to act on receptor activator of nuclear factor kappa-B ligand (RANKL) to inhibit the formation and activity of osteoclasts.[263-265] Bevacizumab targets vascular endothelial growth factor (VEGF) and prevents blood vessel growth, and sunitinib interferes with VEGF receptors leading to inhibition of neoangiogenesis.[250,254] Possible mechanisms for drug-induced osteonecrosis of the jaw are listed in **Table 56-16.**[259-265]

Table 56-16 Mechanisms of Drug-Induced Osteonecrosis of the Jaw

Drug	Mechanism(s)
Bisphosphonates	• Down-regulation of matrix metalloproteinases[260] • Increased osteoclastic apoptosis • Osteoclast inhibition leading to insufficient bone deposition and remodeling[259] • Prevention of osteoclast development[261,262]
Bevacizumab	• Prevention of blood vessel growth via VEGF[250]
Denosumab	• Inhibition of formation and activity of osteoclasts via RANKL[263-265]
Sunitinib	• Inhibition of neoangiogenesis via VEGF[254]

RANKL = receptor activator of nuclear factor kappa-B ligand, VEGF = vascular endothelial growth factor.

CLINICAL PRESENTATION AND DIFFERENTIAL DIAGNOSIS

Clinical presentation of drug-induced osteonecrosis of the jaw may include asymptomatic exposed bone discovered on oral exam, exposed bone with associated pain, mobile teeth, cutaneous fistula, mucosal fistula, or bone exposed through the skin (Table 56-3).[241,266,267] Absent or delayed tissue healing after dental extractions may be one of the first signs.[266,267] Early stages of drug-induced osteonecrosis cannot be detected via x-ray.[266] Oral lesions may form with as little as 4 months of exposure to bisphosphonates, but the average time to onset is 9–14 months following medication initiation.[241,268,269] The time course for onset of osteonecrosis due to the nonbisphosphonates has not been fully elucidated. Osteonecrosis can affect both the maxilla and the mandible, with the mandible affected more often.[240] Once osteonecrosis has developed, colonization or infection with *Actinomyces* may occur. Actinomycosis is a chronic, polymicrobial infection that leads to frequent abscess formulation and multiple fistulae.[270,271]

Conditions to consider in the differential diagnoses of drug-induced osteonecrosis include fungal infection secondary to immunocompromised status in patients receiving chemotherapy and osteoradionecrosis (Table 56-4).[249]

RISK FACTORS

The greatest risk factors for the development of drug-induced osteonecrosis of the jaw include a duration of exposure to causative agents >6 months and the formulation of the bisphosphonate selected (Table 56-5).[240,249,251,257,266] Intravenous bisphosphonate administration has been associated with a greater risk than oral preparations.[249] One meta-analysis found that of 383 reports of bisphosphonate-associated osteonecrosis, 94% of the patients were receiving an intravenous bisphosphonate (primarily as treatment for various forms of cancer) while only 15 patients were receiving an oral bisphosphonate for the treatment of osteoporosis.[269] Combination treatment with a bisphosphonate and bevacizumab or sunitinib has been shown to increase the risk of osteonecrosis development while decreasing the latency period.[251] Additional risk factors include the presence of multiple myeloma, cancer that has metastasized to the bone, dental extractions, surgical bone manipulation, trauma from dentures, presence of oral infections, and overall poor oral health.[266]

MORBIDITY AND MORTALITY

Mortality attributed directly to drug-induced osteonecrosis has not been reported. However, drug-induced osteonecrosis often progresses despite treatment, leading to additional complications associated with cancer treatment and nutrition.[266]

Symptoms may range from nonexistent to severe, with severe cases causing pain, sequestration of bone, and sinus tracts that drain to the skin surface.[240,272] Necrotic exposed bone typically remains structurally strong enough to support normal daily jaw function, but may become secondarily infected, leading to pain, cellulitis, and fistula formation.[241] Paresthesia may develop if the area of osteonecrosis impacts the trigeminal nerve.[268]

PREVENTION

Limiting drug exposure (duration and dose) is the most effective method for prevention of all oral manifestations of systemically administered drugs. **Table 56-17** suggests additional steps that can be considered.[241,249] Whenever possible, dental work

Table 56-17 Approaches to Help Prevent Drug-Induced Osteonecrosis of the Jaw

Drug	Prevention
Bisphosphonates	• Avoid bisphosphonate initiation within 1 month of invasive dental procedures (i.e., tooth removal, periodontal surgery, root canal)[241] • Avoid tooth removal whenever possible[241] • Completion of dental care prior to treatment initiation[249] • Dental surveillance every 4 months while receiving bisphosphonate treatment[241]

should be completed prior to initiating therapy with drugs known to cause osteonecrosis. The goal is to control existing oral disease (to help eliminate factors that could cause mucosal irritation) and to obviate the need for invasive dental procedures in the near future.[241,249] Bisphosphonate therapy should not be initiated within 1 month of invasive dental procedures (e.g., tooth removal, periodontal surgery, root canal therapy) to allow for bone recovery and healing. Dental surveillance every 4 months for patients receiving bisphosphonate therapy is recommended. In patients receiving bisphosphonate treatment, tooth removal should be avoided, and, if unavoidable, amputation of the crown and root canal treatment is a better option than full tooth extraction. If a tooth is demonstrating mild-to-moderate mobility, it should be splinted rather than removed. If the mobility is severe or an abscess is present, it is likely that osteonecrosis is already present and removal of the tooth and treatment with antibiotics is the best option.[241]

Screening to identify patients at risk for developing osteonecrosis is recommended. Assessment should include inquiries regarding current or past history of bisphosphonate use, changes in the mouth including odor, swelling, or discharge, and/or the presence of jaw pain or toothache.[268]

MANAGEMENT

Treatment of bisphosphonate-induced osteonecrosis of the jaw should be directed at eliminating or controlling pain and preventing progression of the exposed bone. Patients with exposed bone should be treated with long-term systemic antibiotics (e.g., penicillin, clindamycin) and an oral antimicrobial rinse (e.g., chlorhexidine gluconate) and should be closely followed. Antibiotics may need to be continued for more than a year and metronidazole may be necessary for patients who do not respond adequately to an initial course of antibiotics.[241,249] Extensive debridement may lead to larger areas of exposed, painful, and infected bone and should be avoided. Complete healing may not occur, but painful symptoms can be alleviated. If osteonecrosis of the jaw leads to the development of a cellulitis requiring intravenous antibiotics, treatment should include ampicillin–clavulanate, ciprofloxacin, or erythromycin, along with metronidazole.[241] There is no clear evidence demonstrating that discontinuation of bisphosphonate therapy leads to improved short-term healing because exposure persists due to the extended half-life of the medications. Bisphosphonate therapy should be discontinued in patients who develop osteonecrosis of the jaw except when a cancer-related indication for continued therapy exists.[241,266]

No specific treatment recommendations are available for osteonecrosis caused by nonbisphosphonate medications. Precautions should be taken when performing dental surgery or periodontal treatment in patients receiving bevacizumab, sunitinib, and denosumab.[251]

In contrast to radiation-induced osteoradionecrosis, hyperbaric oxygen therapy is not an effective treatment option for drug-induced osteonecrosis of the jaw.[268] Attempts to revascularize the bone may appear promising (with favorable initial response and healing), but long-term success is unlikely due to the extended period of time the drug remains concentrated within the bone.[273]

INFORMATION FOR PATIENTS

The risk of drug-induced osteonecrosis of the jaw is highest in patients receiving intravenous bisphosphonates for cancer treatment. The risk of developing this complication as a result of orally administered drugs used to treat osteoporosis is small. Patients receiving drugs known to be associated with osteonecrosis of the jaw should be encouraged to talk to their healthcare provider if they notice any changes such as ulceration, loose teeth, or exposed bone. Patients should be advised not to discontinue treatment with bisphosphonates without first talking to their healthcare provider.

REFERENCES

1. Abdollahi M, Rahimi R, Radfar M. Current opinion on drug-induced oral reactions: a comprehensive review. *J Contemp Dent Pract.* 2008; 9:1-15.
2. Felder RS, Millar SB, Henry RH. Oral manifestations of drug therapy. *Special Care in Dentistry.* 1988; 8:119-24.
3. Hay KD, Reade PC. Spectrum of oral disease induced by drugs and other bioactive agents. *Drugs.* 1983; 26:268-77.
4. Hertz RS, Beckstead PC, Brown WJ. Epithelial melanosis of the gingiva possibly resulting from the use of oral contraceptives. *J Am Dent Assoc.* 1980; 100:713-4.
5. Salman RA, Salman DG, Glickman RS et al. Minocycline-inducted pigmentation of the oral cavity. *J Oral Med.* 1985; 40:154-7.
6. Beehner ME, Houston GD, Young JD. Oral pigmentation secondary to minocycline therapy. *J Oral Maxillofac Surg.* 1986; 44:582-4.
7. de Melo Filho MR, Dias da Silva CA, da Rocha Dourado M et al. Palate hyperpigmentation caused by prolonged use of the antimalarial chloroquine. *Head and Neck Pathol.* 2012; 6:48-50.
8. McAllan LH, Adkins KF. Drug-induced palatal pigmentation. *Aust Dent J.* 1986; 31:1-4.
9. Bucknall CA, Keeton BR, Curry PV et al. Intravenous and oral amiodarone for children with arrhythmias. *Br Heart J.* 1986; 56:278-84.
10. Granstein RD, Sober AJ. Drug- and heavy metal-induced hyperpigmentation. *J Am Acad Dermatol.* 1981; 5:1-18.
11. Lenane P, Powell FC. Oral pigmentation. *J Eur Acad Dermatol Venerol.* 2000; 14:448-65.
12. Kauzman A, Pavone M, Blanas N, Bradley G. Pigmented lesions of the oral cavity: review, differential diagnosis, and case presentation. *J Can Dent Assoc.* 2004; 70:682-3.
13. Muller S. Melanin-associated pigmented lesions of the oral mucosa: presentation, differential diagnosis, and treatment. *Dermatologic Therapy.* 2010; 23:220-9.
14. Scully C, Bagan JV. Adverse drug reactions in the orofacial region. *Crit Rev Oral Biol Med.* 2004; 15:221-39.
15. Giansanti JS, Tillery DE, Olansky S. Oral mucosal pigmentation resulting from antimalarial therapy. *Oral Surg Oral Med Oral Pathol.* 1971; 31:66-9.
16. Kleinegger CL, Hammond HL, Finkelstein MW. Oral mucosal hyperpigmentation secondary to antimalarial drug therapy. *Oral Surg Oral Med Oral Pathol Oral Radiol Endod.* 2000; 90:189-94.
17. Vogel RI, Deasy MJ. Extrinsic discoloration of the oral mucosa. *J Oral Med.* 1977; 32:14-6.
18. Schiodt M. Less common oral lesions associated with HIV infection: prevalence and classification. *Oral Dis.* 1997; 3:S208-13.
19. Alfreijat M. Tongue hyperpigmentation associated with chemotherapy. *J Community Hosp Intern Med Perspect.* 2013; 3:3-4.
20. Blaya M, Saba N. Images in clinical medicine. Chemotherapy induced hyperpigmentation of the tongue. *N Engl J Med.* 2011; 365:e20.
21. Casamiquela KM, Cohen PR. Chemotherapy-associated tongue hyperpigmentation and blue lunula. *J Drugs Dermatol.* 2013; 12:223-6.
22. Laeijendecker R, van Joost T. Oral manifestations of gold allergy. *J Am Acad Dermatol.* 1994; 30:205-9.
23. Veraldi S, Schianchi-Veraldi R, Scarabelli G. Pigmentation of the gums following hydroxychloroquine therapy. *Cutis.* 1992; 49:281-2.
24. Arora B, Kumar L, Sharma A et al. Pigmentary changes in chronic myeloid leukemia patients treated with imatinib mesylate. *Ann Oncol.* 2004; 15:358-9.
25. Li CC, Malik SM, Blaeser BF et al. Mucosal pigmentation caused by imatinib: report of three cases. *Head Neck Pathol.* 2012; 6:290-5.
26. Greco S, Mazzaglia G, Caputi AP, Pagliaro L. Glossitis, stomatitis, and black tongue with lansoprazole plus clarithromycin and other antibiotics. *Ann Pharmacother.* 1997; 31:1548.
27. Chiappinelli JA, Walton RE. Tooth discoloration resulting from long-term tetracycline therapy. *Quintessence Int.* 1992; 23:539-41.
28. Treister NS, Magalnick D, Woo SB. Oral mucosal pigmentation secondary to minocycline therapy: report of two cases and a review of the literature. *Oral Surg Oral Med Oral Pathol Oral Radiol Endod.* 2004; 97:718-25.
29. Westbury LW, Najera A. Minocycline-induced intraoral pharmacogenic pigmentation: case reports and review of the literature. *J Periodontol.* 1997; 68:84-91.
30. Chu P, Van SL, Yen TS, Berger TG. Minocycline hyperpigmentation localized to the lips: an unusual fixed drug reaction? *J Am Acad Dermatol.* 1994; 30:802-3.
31. Eisen D. Minocycline-induced oral pigmentation. *Lancet.* 1997; 349:400.
32. Meyerson MA, Cohen PR, Hymes SR. Lingual hyperpigmentation associated with minocycline therapy. *Oral Surg Oral Med Oral Pathol Oral Radiol Endod.* 1995; 79:180-4.
33. Perusse R, Morency R. Oral pigmentation induced by Premarin. *Cutis.* 1991; 48:61-4.
34. Fricain JC, Sibaud V, Campana F et al. Mucosal pigmentation after oral lichen planus treatment with topical tacrolimus. *Dermatology.* 2005; 210:229-32.
35. Ficarra G, Shillitoe EJ, Adler-Storthz K et al. Oral melanotic macules in patients infected with human immunodeficiency virus. *Oral Surg Oral Med Oral Pathol.* 1990; 70:748-55.
36. Tadini G, D'Orso M, Cusini M, Alessi E. Oral mucosa pigmentation: a new side effect of azidothymidine therapy in patients with acquired immunodeficiency syndrome. *Arch Dermatol.* 1991; 127:267-8.
37. Lerman MA, Karimbux N, Guze KA, Woo SB. Pigmentation of the hard palate. *Oral Surg Oral Med Oral Pathol Oral Radiol Endod.* 2009; 107:8-12.
38. Meleti M, Vescovi P, Mooi WJ, van der Waal I. Pigmented lesions of the oral mucosa and perioral tissues: a flow-chart for the diagnosis and some recommendations for the management. *Oral Surg Oral Med Oral Pathol Oral Radiol Endod.* 2008; 105:606-16.
39. Tredwin CJ, Scully C, Bagan-Sebastian JV. Drug-induced disorders of teeth. *J Dent Res.* 2005; 84:596-602.
40. Gaeta GM, Satriano RA, Baroni A. Oral pigmented lesions. *Clin Dermatol.* 2002; 20:286-8.
41. Eisen D. Disorders of pigmentation in the oral cavity. *Clin Dermatol.* 2000; 18:579-87.
42. Amir E, Gorsky M, Buchner A et al. Physiologic pigmentation of the oral mucosa in Israeli children. *Oral Surg Oral Med Oral Pathol Oral Radiol Endod.* 1991; 71:396-8.
43. Ackerman BH, Kasbekar N. Disturbances of taste and smell induced by drugs. *Pharmacotherapy.* 1997; 17:482-96.
44. Mott AE, Grushka M, Sessle BJ. Diagnosis and management of taste disorders and burning mouth syndrome. *Dent Clin North Am.* 1993; 37:33-71.
45. Seiden AM, Duncan HJ, Smith DV. Office management of taste and smell disorders. *Otolaryngol Clin North Am.* 1992; 25:817-35.
46. Tuccori M, Lapi F, Testi A et al. Drug-induced taste and smell alterations: a case/non-case evaluation of an Italian database and spontaneous adverse drug reaction reporting. *Drug Saf.* 2011; 34:849-59.
47. Doty RL, Shah M, Bromley SM. Drug-induced taste disorders. *Drug Saf.* 2008; 31:199-215.
48. Guidice M. Taste disturbance linked to drug use. Drug-induced disease. *Can Pharm J.* 2006; 139:70-3.
49. Briggs ER. Taste disturbances related to medication use. *Consult Pharm.* 2009; 24:538-43.
50. Poordad F, Mccone J, Bacon BR et al. Boceprevir for untreated chronic HCV genotype 1 infection. *N Engl J Med.* 2011; 364:1195-206.
51. Kumada H, Toyota J, Okanoue T et al. Telaprevir with peginterferon and ribavirin for treatment-naïve patients chronically infected with HCV of genotype 1 in Japan. *J Hepatol.* 2012; 56:78-84.

52. Wickham RS, Rehwaldt M, Kefer C et al. Taste changes experienced by patients receiving chemotherapy. *Oncol Nurs Forum.* 1999; 26:697-706.
53. Seymour R, Rudralingham M. Oral and dental adverse drug reactions. *Periodontology.* 2000; 2008; 46:9-26.
54. Ellul P, Vella V, Vassallo M. Reversible dysgeuisia attributed to azathioprine. *Am J Gastroenterol.* 2007; 102:689.
55. Henkin RI. Drug-induced taste and smell disorders. Incidence, mechanisms and management related primarily to treatment of sensory receptor dysfunction. *Drug Saf.* 1994; 11:318-77.
56. Schaupp H, Wohnaut H. Disturbances of taste from oral disinfectants. *HNO.* 1978; 26:335-41.
57. Awad MM, Shaw AT. ALK inhibitors in non-small cell lung cancer: crizotinib and beyond. *Clin Adv Hematol Oncol.* 2014; 12:429-39.
58. Koizumi T, Fukushima T, Tatai T et al. Successful treatment of crizotinib-induced dysgeusia by switching to alectinib in ALK-positive non-small cell lung cancer. *Lung Cancer.* 2015; 88:112-3.
59. Shaw AT1, Kim DW, Nakagawa K et al. Crizotinib versus chemotherapy in advanced ALK-positive lung cancer. *N Engl J Med.* 2013; 368:2385-94.
60. Speck RM, DeMichele A, Farra JT et al. Taste alteration in breast cancer patients treated with taxane chemotherapy: experience, effect and coping strategies. *Support Care Cancer.* 2013; 21:549-55.
61. Doty RL, Treem J, Tourbier I, Mirza N. A double-blind study of the influences of eszopiclone on dysgeusia and taste function. *Pharmacol Biochem Behav.* 2009; 94:312-8.
62. Krystal AD, Walsh JK, Laska E et al. Sustained efficacy of eszopiclone over 6 months of nightly treatment: results of a randomized, double-blind, placebo-controlled study in adults with chronic insomnia. *Sleep.* 2003; 26:793-9.
63. Halpern SM, Tood PM, Kirby JD. Loss of taste associated with isotretinoin. *Br J Dermatol.* 1996; 134:378.
64. Terao T, Watanabe S, Hoaki N, Hoaki T. Strange taste and mild lithium intoxication. *BMJ Case Reports.* 2011.
65. Heeringa M, Van PE. Reversible dysgeusia attributed to losartan. *Ann Intern Med.* 1998; 129:72. Letter.
66. Ohnishi K, Sakamoto N, Kobayashi K et al. Subjective adverse reactions to metronidazole in patients with amebiasis. *Parasitol Int.* 2014; 63:698-700.
67. Levenson JL, Kennedy K. Dysosmia, dysgeusia and nifedipine. *Ann Intern Med.* 1985; 102:135-6.
68. Glover J, Dibble S, Miaskowski C, Geibert R. Changes in taste associated with intravenous administration of pentamidine. *J Assoc Nurses AIDS Care.* 1995; 6:43-8.
69. Porter SR, Scully C. HIV topic update: protease inhibitor therapy and oral health care. *Oral Dis.* 1998; 4:159-63.
70. Tyssen A, Remmerie B, Eng C et al. Rapidly disintegrating risperidone in subjects with schizophrenia or schizoaffective disorder: a summary of ten phase I clinical trials assessing taste, tablet disintegration time, bioequivalence, and tolerability. *Clin Ther.* 2007; 29:290-304.
71. Stricker BH, Van Riemsdijk MM, Sturkenboom MC, Ottervanger JP. Taste loss to terbinafine: a case-control study of potential risk factors. *Br J Clin Pharmacol.* 1996; 42:313-8.
72. Abdollahi M, Radfar M. A review of drug-induced oral reactions. *J Contemp Dent Pract.* 2003; 4:10-31.
73. Tomita H, Yoshikawa T. Drug-related taste disturbances. *Acta Otolaryngol Suppl.* 2002; 116-121.
74. Habbab KM, Mole DR, Porter SR. Potential oral manifestations of cardiovascular drugs. *Oral Dis.* 2010; 16:769-73.
75. Epstein JB, Barasch A. Taste disorders in cancer patients: pathogenesis, and approach to assessment and management. *Oral Oncol.* 2010; 46:77-81.
76. Hovan AJ, Williams PM, Stevenson-Moore P et al. A systematic review of dysgeusia induced by cancer therapies. *Support Care Cancer.* 2010; 18:1081-7.
77. Boerr CC, Correa ME, Miranda EC, de Souza CA. Taste disorders and oral evaluation in patients undergoing allogeneic hematopoietic SCT. *Bone Marrow Transplant.* 2010; 45:705-11.
78. Epstein JB, Phillips N, Parry J et al. Quality of life, taste, olfactory and oral function following high-dose chemotherapy and allogeneic hematopoietic cell transplantation. *Bone Marrow Transplant.* 2002; 30:785-92.
79. Want H, Zhou M, Brand J, Huange L. Inflammation and taste disorders: mechanisms in taste buds. *Ann NY Acad Sci.* 2009; 1179:596-603.
80. Mossman KL. Gustatory tissue injury in man: radiation dose response relationships and mechanisms of taste loss. *Br J Cancer Suppl.* 1986; 7:9-11.
81. Conger AD. Loss and recovery of taste acuity in patients irradiated to the oral cavity. *Radiat Res.* 1973; 53:338-47.
82. Miller IJ, Reed FE. Variations in human taste bud density and taste intensity perception. *Physiol Behav.* 1990; 47:12:13-9.
83. Zuniga JR, Davis SH, Englehardt R et al. Taste performance on the anterior human tongue varies with fungiform taste bud density. *Chem Senses.* 1993; 18:449-60.
84. Irune E, Dwivedi RC, Nutting CM, Harrington KJ. Treatment-related dysgeusia in head and neck cancer patients. *Cancer Treatment Reviews.* 2014; 40:1106-17.
85. Souder E, Yoder L. Olfaction: the neglected sense. *J Neurosci Nurs.* 1992; 124:55-62.
86. Nan S, Ching V, Grushka M. Taste disorders: a review. *J Can Dent Assoc.* 2013; 79:d86.
87. Bromley SM. Smell and taste disorders: a primary care approach. *Am Fam Physician.* 2000; 61:427-36, 438.
88. Hummel T, Rissom K, Reden J et al. Effects of olfactory training in patients with olfactory loss. *Laryngoscope.* 2009; 119:496-9.
89. McClain CJ, McClain ML, Boosalis MG, Henning B. Zinc and the stress response. *Scand J Work Environ Health.* 1993; 19(suppl 1):132-3.
90. Hoffman HJ, Ishii EK, Macturk RH. Age-related changes in the prevalence of smell/taste problems among the United States adult population. Results of the 1994 disability supplement to the National Health Interview Survey (NHIS). *Ann NY Acad Sci.* 1998; 855:716-22.
91. Shiffman SS. Taste and smell losses in normal aging and disease. *JAMA.* 1997; 278:1357-62.
92. Mistretta CM. Aging effects on anatomy and neurophysiology of taste and smell. *Gerodontology.* 1984; 3:131-6.
93. Fink M. Vitamin D deficiency is a cofactor of chemotherapy-induced mucocutaneous toxicity and dysgeusia. *J Clin Oncol.* 2011; 29:e81-2.
94. Hong JH, Omur-Ozbek P, Stanek BT et al. Taste and odor abnormalities in cancer patients. *J Support Oncol.* 2009; 7:58-65.
95. Femiano F, Scully C, Gombos F. Idiopathic dysgeusia; an open trial of alpha lipoic acid (ALA) therapy. *Int J Oral Maxillofac Surg.* 2002; 31:625-8.
96. Heckmann SM, Hujoel P, Habiger S et al. Zinc gluconate in the treatment of dysgeusia—a randomized clinical trial. *J Dent Res.* 2005; 84:35-8.
97. Takaoka T, Sarukura N, Ueda C et al. Effects of zinc supplementation on serum zinc concentration and ratio of apo/holo-activities of angiotensin converting enzyme in patients with taste impairment. *Auris Nasus Larynx.* 2010; 37:190-4.
98. Grushka M, Epstein J, Mott A. An open-label, dose escalation pilot study of the effect of clonazepam in burning mouth syndrome. *Oral Surg Oral Med Oral Pathol Radiol Endod.* 1998; 86:557-61.
99. Fujiyama R, Ishitobi S, Honda K et al. Ice cube stimulation helps to improve dysgeusia. *Odontology.* 2010; 98:82-4.
100. Patient handout. Information from your family doctor. Are you having trouble with smelling and tasting? *Am Fam Physician.* 2000; 61:438.
101. Ravasco P. Aspects of taste and compliance in patients with cancer. *Eur J Oncol Nurs.* 2005; 9(suppl 2):S84-91.

102. Shiffman SS, Warsick ZS. Flavor enhancement of foods for the elderly can reverse anorexia. *Neurobiol Aging.* 1988; 9:24-6.
103. Shiffman SS, Warsick ZS. Effect of flavor enhancement of foods for the elderly nutritional status: food intake, biochemical indices, and anthropometric measures. *Physiol Behav.* 1993; 53:395-402.
104. Tyldesley WR, Rotter E. Gingival hyperplasia induced by cyclosporine A. *Br Dent J.* 1984; 157:305-9.
105. Rostock MH, Fry HR, Turner JE. Severe gingival overgrowth associated with cyclosporine therapy. *J Periodontol.* 1986; 57:294-9.
106. Daley TD, Wysocki GP. Cyclosporine therapy, its significance to the periodontist. *J Periodontol* 1984; 55:708-12.
107. Bennet JA, Christian JM. Cyclosporine-induced gingival hyperplasia: case report and literature review. *J Am Dent Assoc.* 1985; 111:272-3.
108. Wysocki GP, Gretzinger HA, Laupacis A et al. Fibrous hyperplasia of the gingiva: a side effect of cyclosporine A therapy. *Oral Surg Oral Med Oral Pathol.* 1983; 55:274-8.
109. Rateitschak-Pluss EM, Hefti A, Lortscher R, Thiel G. Initial observation that cyclosporine-A induces gingival enlargement in man. *J Clin Periodontol.* 1983; 10:237-46.
110. Syrjanen SM, Syrjanen KJ. Hyperplastic gingivitis in a child receiving sodium valproate treatment. *Proc Finn Dent Soc.* 1979; 75:95.
111. Lederman D, Lumerman H, Reuben S, Freedman PD. Gingival hyperplasia associated with nifedipine therapy. Report of a case. *Oral Surg Oral Med Oral Pathol.* 1984; 57:620-2.
112. Lucas RM, Howell LP, Wall BA. Nifedipine-induced gingival hyperplasia, a histochemical and ultrastructural study. *J Periodontol.* 1985; 56:211-5.
113. Van der Wall EE, Tuinzing DB, Hes J. Gingival hyperplasia induced by nifedipine, an arterial vasodilating drug. *Oral Surg Oral Med Oral Path.* 1985; 60:38-40.
114. Fletcher P. Nifedipine (Procardia) and gingival hyperplasia; a new diagnostic concern for practitioners. *Bull Ninth Dist Dent Soc.* 1986; 70:52-4.
115. Bencini PL, Crosti C, Sala F et al. Gingival hyperplasia by nifedipine. Report of a case. *Acta Derm Venereol.* 1985; 65:362-5.
116. Ramon Y, Behar S, Kishon Y, Engelberg IS. Gingival hyperplasia caused by nifedipine—a preliminary report. *Int J Cardiol.* 1984; 5:195-206.
117. Fattore L, Stablein M, Bredfelt G et al. Gingival hyperplasia: side effect of nifedipine and diltiazem. *Spec Care Dent.* 1991; 11:107-9.
118. Giustiniani S, Robustelli dell Cuna F, Marieni M. Hyperplastic gingivitis during diltiazem therapy. *Int J Cardiol.* 1987; 15:247-9.
119. Bowman J, Levy B, Grubb R. Gingival overgrowth inducted by diltiazem. *Oral Surg Oral Med Oral Pathol.* 1988; 65:183-5.
120. Seymour RA. Selected side effects. 7. Phenytoin and gingival overgrowth. *Prescribers J.* 1992; 170:376-9.
121. Pradhan S, Mishra P. Gingival enlargement in antihypertensive medication. *JNMA J Nepal Med Assoc.* 2009; 48:149-52.
122. Westbrook P, Bednarczyk EM, Carlson M et al. Regression of nifedipine-induced gingival hyperplasia following switch to a same class calcium channel blocker, isradipine. *J Periodontol.* 1997; 68:645-50.
123. Ellis JS, Seymour RA, Thomason JM et al. Gingival sequestration of amlodipine and amlodipine-induced gingival overgrowth. *Lancet.* 1993; 341:1102-3.
124. Bhatia V, Mittal A, Parida AK et al. Amlodipine induced gingival hyperplasia: a rare entity. *Int J Cardiol.* 2007; 122:e23-4.
125. Hallmon WW, Rossmann JA. The role of drugs in the pathogenesis of gingival overgrowth. *Periodontol 2000.* 1999; 21:176-96.
126. Nakib N, Ashrafi SS. Drug-induced gingival overgrowth. *Dis Mon.* 2011; 57:225-30.
127. Lee L, Miller PA, Maxymiw WG et al. Intraoral pyogenic granuloma after allogeneic bone marrow transplant. Report of three cases. *Oral Surg Oral Med Oral Pathol.* 1994; 78:607-10.
128. Cebeci I, Kantarci A, Firatli E et al. The effect of verapamil on the prevalence and severity of cyclosporine-induced gingival overgrowth in renal allograft recipients. *J Periodontol.* 1996; 67:1201-5.
129. Jackson C, Babich S. Gingival hyperplasia: interaction between cyclosporine A and nifedipine? A case report. *NY State Dent J.* 1997; 63:46-8.
130. Qunibi WY, Akhtar M, Ginn E, Smith P. Kaposi's sarcoma in cyclosporine-induced gingival hyperplasia. *Am J Kidney Dis.* 1988; 11:349-52.
131. Seymour RA, Jacobs DJ. Cyclosporine and the gingival tissues. *J Clin Periodontol.* 1992; 19:1-11.
132. Valsecchi R, Cainelli T. Gingival hyperplasia induced by erythromycin. *Acta Derm Venereol.* 1992; 72:157.
133. Cotler SJ, Wartell CF, Larson AM et al. Pretreatment symptoms and dosing regimen predict side-effects of interferon therapy for hepatitis C. *J Viral Hepat.* 2000; 7:211-7.
134. Chen B, Choi H, Hirsch LJ et al. Cosmetic side effects of antiepileptic drugs in adults with epilepsy. *Epilepsy Behav.* 2015; 42:129-37.
135. Chacko RC, Marsh BJ, Marmion J et al. Lithium side effects in elderly bipolar outpatients. *Hillside J Clin Psychiatry.* 1987; 9:79-88.
136. Christodoulou GN, Siafakas A, Rinieris PM. Side-effects of lithium. *Acta Psychiatr Belg.* 1977; 77:260-6.
137. Friedlander AH, Birch NJ. Dental conditions in patients with bipolar disorder on long-term lithium maintenance therapy. *Spec Care Dentist.* 1990; 10:148-51.
138. Tohen M, Chengappa KN, Suppes T et al. Efficacy of olanzapine in combination with valproate or lithium in the treatment of mania in patients partially nonresponsive to valproate or lithium monotherapy. *Arch Gen Psychiatry.* 2002; 59:62-9.
139. Gregoriou AP, Schneider PE, Shaw PR. Phenobarbital-induced gingival overgrowth? Report of two cases and complications in management. *ASDC J Dent Child.* 1995; 63:408-13.
140. Behari M, Gingival hyperplasia due to sodium valproate. *J Neurol Neurosurg Psychiatry.* 1991; 45:279-80.
141. Al-Mohaya M, Treister N, Al-Khadra O et al. Calcineurin inhibitor-associated oral inflammatory polyps after transplantation. *J Oral Pathol Med.* 2007; 36:570-4.
142. Diamond JP, Chandna A, Williams C et al. Tranexamic acid-associated ligneous conjunctivitis with gingival and peritoneal lesions. *Br J Opthalmol.* 1991; 75:753-4.
143. Pernu HE, Oikarinen K, Hietanen J, Knuuttila M. Verapamil-induced gingival overgrowth: a clinical, histologic, and biochemical approach. *J Oral Pathol Med.* 1989; 18:422-5.
144. Katz J, Givol N, Chausha G et al. Vigabatrin-induced gingival overgrowth. *J Clin Periodontol.* 1997; 24:180-2.
145. Kataoka M, Kido J, Shinohara Y, Nagata T. Drug-induced gingival overgrowth—a review. *Biol Pharm Bull.* 2005; 28:1817-21.
146. Angelopoulos AP, Goaz PW. Incidence of diphenylhydantoin gingival hyperplasia. *Oral Surg Oral Med Oral Pathol.* 1972; 34:898-906.
147. Seymour RA. Drug-induced gingival overgrowth. *Adverse Drug React Toxicol Rev.* 1993; 12:215-32.
148. Prasad VN, Chawla HS, Goyal A et al. Incidence of phenytoin induced gingival overgrowth in epileptic children: a six month evaluation. *J Indian Soc Pedod Prev Dent.* 2002; 20:73-80.
149. Seymore R, Heasman P. Drugs and the periodontium. *J Clin Periodontol.* 1988: 15;1-16.
150. Aldemir NM, Begenik H, Emre H et al. Amlodipine-induced gingival hyperplasia in chronic renal failure: a case report. *African Health Sciences.* 2012; 4:576-8.
151. Seymour RA, Thomason JM, Ellis JS. The pathogenesis of drug-induced gingival hyperplasia. *J Clin Periodontol.* 1996; 23:165-75.
152. Brown RS, Beaver WT, Bottomley WK. On the mechanism of drug-induced gingival hyperplasia. *J Oral Pathol Med.* 1991; 20:201-9.

153. Arya R, Gulati S, Kabra M et al. Folic acid supplementation prevents phenytoin-induced gingival overgrowth in children. *Neurology*. 2011; 76:1338-43.
154. Livada R, Shiloah J. Calcium channel blocker-induced gingival enlargement. *J Hum Hypertension*. 2014; 28:10-14.
155. Meraw SJ, Sheridan PJ. Medically induced gingival hyperplasia. *Mayo Clin Proc*. 1998; 73:1196-9.
156. Fisekciogly E. Idiopathic gingival hyperplasia: clinical features and differential diagnosis. *J Can Dent Assoc*. 2011; 77:b148.
157. Agrawal AA. Gingival enlargements: differential diagnosis and review of literature. *World J Clin Cases*. 2015; 3:779-88.
158. Kubota Y, Moriyama Y, Yamagishi K et al. Serum vitamin C concentration and hs-CRP level in middle-aged Japanese men and women. *Atherosclerosis*. 2010; 208:496-500.
159. Matharu MS, Van Vilet JA, Ferrari MD, Goadsby PJ. Verapamil induced gingival enlargement in cluster headache. *J Neural Neurosurg Psychiatry*. 2005; 76:124-7.
160. Tavassoli S, Yamalik N, Caglayan F et al. The clinical effects of nifedipine on periodontal status. *J Periodontal*. 1998; 69:108-12.
161. Charles NS, Chavan R, Moon N et al. Drug-induced gingival overgrowth: the genetic dimension. *N Am J Med Sci*. 2014; 6:478-80.
162. Meisel P, Giebal J, Kunert-Keil C et al. MDR1 gene polymorphisms and risk of gingival hyperplasia induced by calcium antagonists. *Clin Pharmacol Ther*. 2006; 79:62-71.
163. Shetty AK, Shah HJ, Patil MA, Jhota KN. Idiopathic gingival enlargement and its management. *J Indian Soc Periodontol*. 2010; 14:263-5.
164. Singh Nayyar A, Khan M, Vijayalakshmi KR, Subhas GT et al. A study on gingival enlargement and folic acid levels in phenytoin-treated epileptic patients: testing hypotheses. *Surg Neurol Int*. 2013; 4:133.
165. Sener U, Zorlu Y, Karaguzel O et al. Effects of common antiepileptic drug monotherapy on serum levels of homocysteine, vitamin B12, folic acid and vitamin B6. *Seizure*. 2006; 15:79-85.
166. Camargo PM, Melnick PR, Pirih FQ et al. Treatment of drug-induced gingival enlargement: aesthetic and functional considerations. *Periodontol 2000*. 2001; 27:131-8.
167. Fourtounas C, Vlachojannis JG. Gingival hyperplasia and calcium channel blockers. *J Clin Hypertension*. 2009; 11:111.
168. Wahlstrom E, Zamora JU, Teichman S. Improvement in cyclosporine-associated gingival hyperplasia with azithromycin therapy. *N Engl J Med*. 1995; 332:753-4.
169. Gomez E, Sanchez-Nunez M, Sanchez JE et al. Treatment of cyclosporine-induced gingival hyperplasia with azithromycin. *Nephrol Dial Transplant*. 1997; 12:2694-7.
170. Nash MM, Zaltzman JS. Efficacy of azithromycin in the treatment of cyclosporine-induced gingival hyperplasia in renal transplant recipients. *Transplantation*. 1998; 65:1611-5.
171. Tokgoz B, Sari HI, Yildiz O et al. Effects of azithromycin on cyclosporine-induced gingival hyperplasia in renal transplant patients. *Transplant Proc*. 2004; 36:2699.
172. Scully C, Bagan J. Oral mucosal diseases: erythema multiforme. *Br J Oral Maxillofac Surg*. 2008; 46:90-5.
173. Roberts DL, Marks R. Skin reactions to carbamazepine. *Arch Dermatol*. 1981; 117:273-5.
174. Joseph TI, Vargheese G, George D, Sathvan P. Drug induced oral erythema multiforme: a rare and less recognized variant of erythema multiforme. *J Oral Maxillofac Pathol*. 2012; 16:145-8.
175. Sanchis JM, Bagan JV, Gavalda C et al. Erythema multiforme: diagnosis, clinical manifestations and treatment in a retrospective study of 22 patients. *J Oral Pathol Med*. 2010; 39:747-52.
176. Diz Dios P, Scully C. Antiretroviral therapy: effects on orofacial health and health care. *Oral Dis*. 2014; 20:136-45.
177. Wetter DA, Davis MDP. Recurrent erythema multiforme: clinical characteristics, etiologic associations, and treatment in a series of 48 patients at Mayo Clinic, 2000 to 2007. *J Am Acad Dermatol*. 2010; 62:45-53.
178. Ahdout J, Haley JC, Chiu MW. Erythema multiforme during anti-tumor necrosis factor treatment for plaque psoriasis. *J Am Acad Dermatol*. 2010; 62:874-9.
179. Isik SR, Karakaya G, Erkin G, Kalyoncu AF. Multidrug-induced erythema multiforme. *J Investig Allergol Clin Immunol*. 2007; 17:196-8.
180. Jawetz RE, Elkin A, Michael L et al. Erythema multiforme limited to the oral mucosa in a teenager on oral contraceptive therapy. *J Pediatr Adolesc Gynecol*. 2007; 20:309-13.
181. Tan DSY, Sklar GE. Erythema multiforme secondary to dimenhydrinate in a patient with previous similar reactions to pamabrom. *Ann Pharmacother*. 2014; 48:425-8.
182. Atkinson JC, Shiroky JB, Macynski A, Fox PC. Effects of furosemide on the oral cavity. *Gerodontology*. 1989; 8:23-6.
183. Edwards D, Boritz E, Cowen EW, Brown RS. Erythema multiforme major following treatment with infliximab. *Oral Surg Oral Med Oral Pathol Oral Radiol*. 2013; 115:e36-40.
184. Goodman GE, Alberts DS, Earnst DL, Meyskens FL. Phase I trial of retinol in cancer patients. *J Clin Oncol*. 1983; 1:394-9.
185. MacGregor JL, Silvers DN, Grossman ME, Sherman WH. Sorafenib-induced erythema multiforme. *J Am Acad Dermatol*. 2007; 56:527-8.
186. Arisawa EA, Almeida JD, Carvalho YR, Cabral LA. Clinic pathological analysis of oral mucous autoimmune disease: a 27-year study. *Med Oral Patol Oral Cir Bucal*. 2008; 13:e94-7.
187. Sokumbi O, Wetter DA. Clinical features, diagnosis, and treatment of erythema multiforme: a review for the practicing dermatologist. *Int J Dermatol*. 2012; 51:889-902.
188. Aurelian L, Ono F, Burnett J. Herpes simplex virus (HSV)-associated erythema multiforme (HAEM): a viral disease with an autoimmune component. *Dermatol Online J*. 2003; 9:1.
189. Huff JC, Weston WL, Tonnesen MG. Erythema multiforme: a critical review of characteristics, diagnostic criteria, and causes. *J Am Acad Dermatol*. 1983; 8:763-75.
190. Huff JC. Erythema multiforme. *Dermatol Clin*. 1985; 3:141-52.
191. Bastuji-Garin S, Rzany B, Stern RS et al. Clinical classification of cases of toxic epidermal necrolysis, Stevens-Johnson syndrome, and erythema multiforme. *Arch Dermatol*. 1993; 129:92-6.
192. Ayangco L, Rogers RS. Oral manifestations of erythema multiforme. *Dermatol Clin*. 2003; 21:195-205.
193. Ladizinski B, Lee KC. Oral ulcers and targetoid lesions on the palms. *JAMA*. 2014; 311:1152-3.
194. Schifter M, Yeoh S-C, Coleman H, Georgiou A. Oral mucosal diseases: the inflammatory dermatoses. *Aust Dent J*. 2010; 55 (suppl 1):23-38.
195. Al-Johani KA, Fedel S, Porter SR. Erythema multiforme and related disorders. *Oral Surg Oral Med Oral Pathol Oral Radiol Endod*. 2007; 103:642-54.
196. Korstanje MJ. Drug-induced mouth disorders. *Clin Exp Dermatol*. 1995; 20:10-8.
197. Sugerman PB, Savage NW, Zhou X et al. Oral lichen planus. *Clin Dermatol*. 2000; 18:533-9.
198. Chau NY, Reade PC, Rich AM, Hay KD. Allopurinol-amplified lichenoid reactions of the oral mucosa. *Oral Surg Oral Med Oral Pathol*. 1984; 58:397-400.
199. Brooks SL. Lichenoid reaction of oral mucosa and skin to methyldopa. *J Oral Med*. 1982; 37:42-4.
200. McCartan BE, McCreary CE. Oral lichenoid drug eruptions. *Oral Dis*. 1997; 3:58-63.
201. Schlosser BJ. Lichen planus and lichenoid reactions of the oral mucosa. *Dermatol Ther*. 2010; 23:251-67.
202. Asarch A, Gottlieb AB, Lee J et al. Lichen planus-like eruptions: an emerging side effect of tumor necrosis factor-alpha antagonists. *J Am Acad Dermatol*. 2009; 61:104-11.
203. Andrade P, Lopes S, Albuquerque A et al. Oral lichen planus in IBD patients: a paradoxical adverse effect of anti-TNF-α therapy. *Dig Dis Sci*. 2015; 60:2746-9.

204. De Simone C, Caldarola G, D'Agostino M et al. Lichenoid reaction induced by adalimumab. *JEADV*. 2008; 22:626-7.
205. Scully C, Beyli M, Ferreiro MC et al. Update on oral lichen planus: etiopathogenesis and management. *Crit Rev Oral Biol Med*. 1998; 9:86-122.
206. Thompson DF, Skaehill PA. Drug-induced lichen planus. *Pharmacotherapy*. 1994; 14:561-71.
207. Woo V, Bonks J, Borukhova L, Zegarelli D. Oral lichenoid drug eruption: a report of a pediatric case and review of the literature. *Pediatr Dermatol*. 2009; 26:458-64.
208. Reinhardt LA, Wilkin JK, Kirkendall WM. Lichenoid eruption produced by captopril. *Cutis*. 1983; 31:98-9.
209. Artico G, Bruno IS, Seo J et al. Lichenoid reaction to carbamazepine in the oral mucosa: case report. *An Bras Dermatol*. 2011; 86:S152-5.
210. Moccioaro F, Orlando A, Renna S et al. Oral lichen planus after certolizumab pegol treatment in a patient with Crohn's disease. *J Crohns Colitis*. 2011; 5:173-4.
211. Moss AC, Treister NS, Marsee DK, Cheifetz AS. Clinical challenges and images in GI. Oral lichenoid reaction in a patient with Crohn's disease receiving infliximab. *Gastroenterology*. 2007; 132:488.
212. Gordon CR, Gonen A, Nachum Z et al. The effects of dimenhydrinate, cinnarizine and transdermal scopolamine on performance. *J Psychopharmacol*. 2001; 15:167-72.
213. Maillefert JF, Farge P, Gazet-Maillefert MP, Tavernier C. Mental nerve neuropathy as a result of hepatitis B vaccination. *Oral Surg Oral Med Oral Pathol Oral Radiol Endod*. 1997; 83:663-4.
214. Baricevic M, Mravak Sipetic M, Situm M et al. Oral bullous eruption after taking Lisinopril—case report and literature review. *Cent Eur J Med*. 2013; 125:408-11.
215. Lim DS, Muir J. Oral lichenoid reaction to imatinib (STI 572, Gleevec). *Dermatology*. 2002; 205:169-71.
216. Pascual JC, Matarredona J, Miralles J et al. Oral and cutaneous lichenoid reaction secondary to imatinib: report of two cases. *Int J Dermatol*. 2006; 45:1471-3.
217. Brazzelli V, Muzio F, Mann G et al. Photo induced dermatitis and oral lichenoid reaction in a chronic myeloid leukemia patient treated with imatinib mesylate. *Photodermatol Photoimmunol Photomed*. 2012; 28:2-5.
218. Read SJ, Crawford DH, Pender MP. Trigeminal sensory neuropathy induced by interferon-alpha therapy. *Aust NZ J Med*. 1995; 25:54.
219. Bakkour W, Coulson IH. GA101 (a novel anti-CD20 monoclonal antibody)-induced lichenoid eruption. *Dermatol Ther (Heidelb)*. 2012; 2:3.
220. Chaabane A, Fadhel NB, Chadli Z et al. Phenobarbital-induced DRESS: a lichenoid picture. *Iran J Allergy Asthma Immunol*. 2014; 13:453-5.
221. Kuten-Shorrer M, Hochberg EP, Woo SB. Lichenoid mucosal reaction to rituximab. *The Oncologist*. 2014; 19:e12-3.
222. Wright J. Diagnosis and management of oral lichenoid reactions. *CDA Journal*. 2007; 35:412-6.
223. McCartan BE, Healy CM. The reported prevalence of oral lichen planus: a review and critique. *J Oral Pathol Med*. 2008; 37:447-53.
224. Lavanya N, Jayanthi P, Rao UK, Ranganathan K. Oral lichen planus: an update on pathogenesis and treatment. *J Oral Maxillofac Pathol*. 2011; 15:127-32.
225. Spolarich AE. Risk management strategies for reducing oral adverse drug events. *J Evid Base Dent Pract*. 2014; 14S:87-94.
226. Kragelund C, Hansen C, Reibel J et al. Polymorphic drug metabolizing CYP-enzymes—a pathogenic factor in oral lichen planus? *J Oral Pathol Med*. 2009; 38:63-71.
227. Kragelund C, Hansen C, Reibel J et al. Can the genotype or phenotype of two polymorphic drug metabolizing cytochrome P450-enzymes identify oral lichenoid drug eruptions? *J Oral Pathol Med*. 2010; 39:497-505.
228. Breathnack SM. Mechanisms of drug eruptions: Part I. *Australas J Dermatol*. 1995; 36:121-7.
229. Kaomongkolgit R. Oral lichenoid drug reaction associated with antihypertensive and hypoglycemic drugs. *J Drugs Dermatol*. 2010; 9:73-5.
230. Ismail SB, Kumar SKS, Zain RB. Oral lichen planus and lichenoid reactions: etiopathogenesis, diagnosis, management and malignant transformation. *J Oral Sci*. 2007; 49:89-106.
231. Muller S. Oral manifestations of dermatologic disease: a focus on lichenoid lesions. *Head and Neck Pathol*. 2011; 5:36-40.
232. Yuan A, Woo SB. Adverse drug events in the oral cavity. *Oral Surg Oral Med Oral Pathol Oral Radiol*. 2015; 119:35-47.
233. Bascones-Martinez A, Garcia-Garcia V, Meurman JK, Requena-Caballero L. Immune-mediated diseases: what can be found in the oral cavity? *Int J Dermatol*. 2015; 54:258-70.
234. Barbosa NC, Silveira EJD, de A. Lima EN et al. Factors associated with clinical characteristics and symptoms in a case series of oral lichen planus. *Int J Dermatol*. 2015; 54:e1-6.
235. Thongprasom K, Carrozzo M, Furness S, Lodi G. Interventions for treating oral lichen planus. *Cochrane Database Syst Rev*. 2011; 7:CD001168.
236. Keenan AV, Ferraiolo D. Insufficient evidence for effectiveness of any treatment for oral lichen planus. *Evid Based Dent*. 2011; 12:85-6.
237. Lozada-Nur FI, Sroussi HY. Tacrolimus powder in Orabase 0.1% for the treatment of oral lichen planus and oral lichenoid lesions: an open clinical trial. *Oral Surg Oral Med Oral Pathol Oral Radiol Endod*. 2006; 102:744-9.
238. Dalmau J, Peramiquel L, Puig L et al. Imatinib-associated lichenoid eruption: acitretin treatment allows maintained antineoplastic effect. *Br J Dermatol*. 2006; 154:1213-6.
239. Zelickson BD, Rogers RS III. Drug reactions involving the mouth. *Clin Dermatol*. 1986; 4:98-109.
240. Ruggiero SL, Mehrotra B. Bisphosphonate-related osteonecrosis of the jaw: diagnosis, prevention, and management. *Annu Rev Med*. 2009; 60:85-9.
241. Marx RE, Sawatari Y, Fortin M, Broumand V. Bisphosphonate-induced exposed bone (osteonecrosis/osteoporosis) of the jaws: risk factors, recognition, prevention and treatment. *J Oral Maxillofac Surg*. 2005; 63:1567-75.
242. Rachner TD, Platzbecker U, Felsenberg D, Hofbauer LC. Osteonecrosis of the jaw after osteoporosis therapy with denosumab following long-term bisphosphonate therapy. *Mayo Clin Proc*. 2013; 88:418-9.
243. Estilo CL, Fornier M, Farooki A et al. Osteonecrosis of the jaw related to bevacizumab. *J Clin Oncol*. 2008; 26:4037-8.
244. Guarneri V, Miles D, Robert N et al. Bevacizumab and osteonecrosis of the jaw: incidence and association with bisphosphonate therapy in three large prospective trials in advanced breast cancer. *Breast Cancer Res Treat*. 2010; 122:181-8.
245. Katsenos S, Christophylakis C, Psathakis K. Osteonecrosis of the jaw in a patient with advanced non-small-cell lung cancer receiving bevacizumab. *Arch Bronconeumol*. 2012; 48:218-9.
246. Hoefert S, Eufinger H. Sunitinib may raise the risk of bisphosphonate-related osteonecrosis of the jaw: presentation of three cases. *Oral Surg Oral Med Oral Pathol Oral Radiol Endod*. 2010; 110:463-9.
247. Koch FP, Walter C, Hansen T et al. Osteonecrosis of the jaw related to sunitinib. *Oral Maxillofac Surg*. 2011; 15:63-6.
248. Fleissig Y, Regev E, Lehman H. Sunitinib related osteonecrosis of jaw: a case report. *Oral Surg Oral Med Oral Pathol Oral Radiol*. 2012; 113:e1-3.
249. Markiewicz MR, Margarone JR III, Campbell JH, Aguirre A. Bisphosphonate-associated osteonecrosis of the jaws. A review of current knowledge. *J Am Dent Assoc*. 2005; 136:1669-74.
250. Greuter S, Schmid F, Ruhstaller T, Thuerlimann B. Bevacizumab-associated osteonecrosis of the jaw. *Ann Oncol*. 2008; 19:2091-2.

251. Troeltzsch M, Woodlock T, Kriegelstein S et al. Physiology and pharmacology of nonbisphosphonate drugs implicated in osteonecrosis of the jaw. *J Can Dent Assoc.* 2012; 78:c85.
252. Marx RE. Pamidronate (Aredia) and zoledronate (Zometa) induced avascular necrosis of the jaws: a growing epidemic. *J Oral Maxillofac Surg.* 2003; 61:1115-7.
253. Zarychanski R, Elphee E, Walton P, Johnston J. Osteonecrosis of the jaw associated with pamidronate therapy. *Am J Hematol.* 2006; 81:73-5.
254. Brunello A, Saia G, Bedognia A, Scaglione D, Basso U. Worsening of osteonecrosis of the jaw during treatment with sunitinib in a patient with metastatic renal cell carcinoma. *Bone.* 2009; 44:173-5.
255. Reid IR, Cornish J. Epidemiology and pathogenesis of osteonecrosis of the jaw. *Nat Rev Rheumatol.* 2012; 8:90-6.
256. Durie BGM, Katz M, McCoy J, Crowley J. Osteonecrosis of the jaw and bisphosphonates. *N Engl J Med.* 2005: 353;99. Letter.
257. Bamias A, Kastritis E, Bamia C et al. Osteonecrosis of the jaw in cancer after treatment with bisphosphonates: incidence and risk factors. *J Clin Oncol.* 2005; 23:8580-7.
258. [No authors listed]. Bevacizumab, sunitinib: osteonecrosis of the jaw. *Prescrire Int.* 2011; 20:155.
259. Odvina CV, Zerwekh JE, Rao DS et al. Severely suppressed bone turnover: a potential complication of alendronate therapy. *J Clin Endocrinol Metab.* 2005; 90:1294-301.
260. Teronen O, Laitinen M, Salo T et al. Inhibition of matrix metalloproteinases by bisphosphonates may in part explain their effects in the treatment of multiple myeloma. *Blood.* 2000; 96:4006-7.
261. Hughes DE, Wright KR, Uy HL et al. Bisphosphonates promote apoptosis in murine osteoclasts in vitro and in vivo. *J Bone Miner Res.* 1995; 10:1478-87.
262. Hughes DE, MacDonald BR, Russel RG, Gowen M. Inhibition of osteoclast-like cell formation by bisphosphonates in long-term cultures of human bone marrow. *J Clin Invest.* 1989; 83:1930-5.
263. Pazianas M. Osteonecrosis of the jaw and the role of macrophages. *J Natl Cancer Inst.* 2011; 103:232-40.
264. Sopeck AT, Lipton A, Body JJ et al. Denosumab compared with zoledronic acid for the treatment of bone metastases in patients with advanced breast cancer: a randomized, double-blind study. *J Clin Oncol.* 2010; 28:5132-9.
265. Compston J. Pathophysiology of atypical femoral fractures and osteonecrosis of the jaw. *Osteoporos Int.* 2011; 22:2951-61.
266. Migliorati CA, Schubert MM, Peterson DE, Seneda LM. Bisphosphonate-associated osteonecrosis of mandibular and maxillary bone: an emerging oral complication of supportive cancer therapy. *Cancer.* 2005; 104:83-93.
267. Bagan JV, Murillo J, Jimenez Y et al. Avascular jaw osteonecrosis in association with cancer chemotherapy: series of 10 cases. *J Oral Pathol Med.* 2005; 34:120-3.
268. Melo MD, Obeid G. Osteonecrosis of the jaws in patients with a history of receiving bisphosphonate therapy: strategies for prevention and early recognition. *J Am Dent Assoc.* 2005; 136:1675-81.
269. Woo SB, Hellstein JW, Kalmar JR. Systematic review: bisphosphonates and osteonecrosis of the jaws. *Ann Intern Med.* 2006; 144:753-61.
270. Hansen T, Kunkel M, Springer E et al. Actinomycosis of the jaws—histopathological study of 45 patients shows significant involvement in bisphosphonate-associated osteonecrosis and infected osteoradionecrosis. *Virchows Arch.* 2007; 451:1009-17.
271. Smith MH, Harms PW, Newton DWet al. Mandiubular Actinomyces osteomyelitis complicating florid cemento-osseous dysplasia: case report. *BMC Oral Health.* 2011; 11:21.
272. Hellstein JW, Marek CL. Bisphosphonate osteochemonecrois (bisphossy jaw): is this phossy jaw of the 21st century? *J Oral Maxillofac Surg.* 2005; 63:682-9.
273. Russell RG, Rogers MJ, Frith JC et al. The pharmacology of bisphosphonates and new insights into their mechanism of action. *J Bone Miner Res.* 1999; 14(suppl 2):53-65.

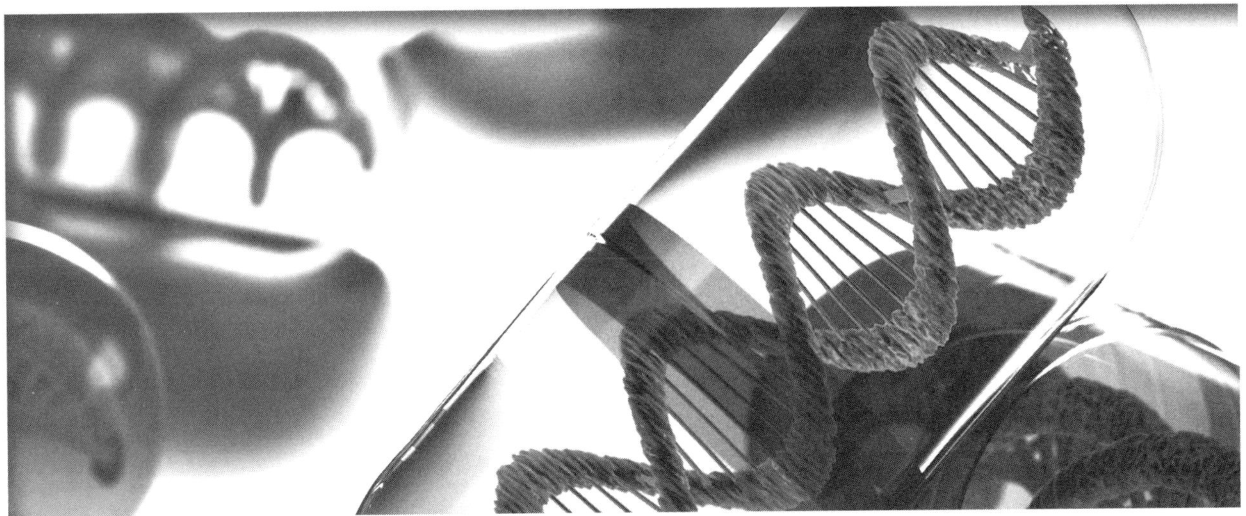

CHAPTER 57

Neoplastic Diseases

Sandra Cuellar and Christina Mactal Haaf

Malignancy is an unfortunate known consequence of some medications. These malignancies can be aggressive and often lead to significant morbidity and mortality.[1,2] The agents most often implicated include those that alter the immune response (e.g., immunosuppressants), those that affect cellular proliferation (e.g., hormones, chemotherapeutic agents), and those that cause mutations (e.g., alkylating agents).

Drug-induced malignancies are difficult to study because they may not emerge until long after treatment with the culprit agent is completed. In addition, drug-induced malignancies may not occur frequently enough to permit definitive assignment of causality to particular agents. Many medications are given in combination, which can add to the difficulty in making a determination of causation, as can a number of patient-specific factors, including age and the presence of concomitant disease states.

Research in oncology has led to the unprecedented development of novel treatment and management strategies that incorporate tumor biology and cytogenetics. The field of oncology is dynamic and changes in management algorithms occur frequently. Therefore, referring to National Comprehensive Cancer Network (NCCN) for current national treatment guidelines is recommended for healthcare providers who treat patients diagnosed with cancer.

LEUKEMIA

Therapy-related leukemia can arise from either lymphocytes or myeloid cells. The occurrence of acute lymphoblastic leukemia (ALL) after chemotherapy is rare; reports indicate these represent 1.2–2.5% of adult ALL cases.[3] The most common form of secondary leukemia is myeloid leukemia, which represents 8–10% of all acute myeloid leukemias (AML).[3] The World Health Organization updated the classification of myeloid neoplasms and acute leukemia in 2016.[4] In general, therapy-related myeloid neoplasms (t-MN) represent a heterogeneous and poorly defined group of patients with multiple and varied poor prognostic features. Patients with t-MN have poorer survival compared to those with de novo AML, myelodysplastic syndrome (MDS), or myelodysplastic syndrome/myeloproliferative neoplasm (MDS/MPN). MDS/MPN are forms of bone marrow failure that often evolve to AML.[5]

CAUSATIVE AGENTS

Table 57-1 lists the agents implicated in therapy-related leukemia; the most notorious include the alkylating agents and topoisomerase inhibitors. Several other culprits exist for t-MN. Those include azathioprine, lenalidomide (immunomodulatory agent), olaparib (poly ADP-ribose polymerase inhibitor), granulocyte colony-stimulating factor (G-CSF), and tumor necrosis factor (TNF) alpha inhibitors. TNF alpha inhibitors (infliximab, etanercept, adalimumab, certolizumab pegol, golimumab) have primarily been implicated in the development of lymphomas; however, case reports of AML have been observed in postmarketing settings.[6]

The alkylating agents associated with t-MDS/t-AML include cyclophosphamide, ifosfamide, mechlorethamine, melphalan, busulfan, nitrosoureas, chlorambucil, dacarbazine, and platinum compounds such as cisplatin.[7,8] Mechlorethamine and melphalan are associated with a higher rate of t-AML than other alkylators. Previous Hodgkin lymphoma chemotherapy regimens that included mechlorethamine resulted in high rates of t-AML, whereas more modern doxorubicin-based regimens

Table 57-1 Agents Implicated in Drug-Induced Neoplastic Diseases

Drug	Incidence	Level of Evidence[a]
LEUKEMIA[b]		
Azathioprine	NK	C
Cisplatin	NK	C
Cyclophosphamide/doxorubicin[147]	0.24–0.48%	B
Etoposide[12]	0.6%	B
Filgrastim (G-CSF)[25]	Up to 0.7%	B
Lenalidomide[30]	Up to 5.3%	B
MOPP[9]	2.9%	B
Olaparib[23]	1%	B
TNF alpha inhibitors	NK	C
LYMPHOMA[c]		
Antithymocyte globulin[148]	3%[d]	A
Azathioprine[148]	2.7%[e]	B
Cyclosporine[148]	2.4%[f]	B
Muromonab CD3 (OKT3)[149,150]	Up to 1.8%	B
Tacrolimus[148]	0.1%	B
TNF alpha inhibitors[151]	0.7%	A
SKIN CANCER[c]		
Antithymocyte globulin[149,150]	0.2%	B
Azathioprine[152]	11.2%[g]	B
BRAF inhibitors (dabrafenib, vemurafenib)[153]	15–30%	A
Cyclosporine[154]	1.2%[h]	B
Oral contraceptives[155,156]	6%	C
Muromonab CD3 (OKT3)[157]	1%	B
Selenium[68]	17%	A
Tacrolimus[158]	1.27%[i]	B
TNF alpha inhibitors[159]	Up to 30%	B
Voriconazole[160]	20%	B

Table 57-1 Agents Implicated in Drug-Induced Neoplastic Diseases (continued)

Drug	Incidence	Level of Evidence[a]
BREAST CANCER		
Estrogen[88]	0.86%[j]	B
Estrogen + progestin[88,90]	0.41%[k] 1.53%[j]	A B
ENDOMETRIAL CANCER		
Estrogen[120]	Up to 40%[l]	B
Tamoxifen[161]	1.62%	A
BLADDER CANCER		
Cyclophosphamide[136]	Up to 10%[m]	B
Pioglitazone[133]	0.23%	B

BRAF = B-rapidly accelerated fibrosarcoma, G-CSF = granulocyte colony-stimulating factor, MOPP = mechlorethamine, vincristine, prednisone, and procarbazine, NK = not known, TNF = tumor necrosis factor.

[a]Definitions for Levels of Evidence: Level A—evidence from one or more randomized, controlled clinical trials; Level B—evidence from nonrandomized clinical trials, prospective observational studies, cohort studies, retrospective studies, case-control studies, meta-analyses and/or post-marketing surveillance studies; and Level C—evidence from one or more published case reports or case series.

[b]Incidence figures reported are often combined acute myelogenous leukemia/myelodysplastic syndrome.

[c]With the exception of BRAF inhibitors used for the treatment of skin cancer, the incidence figures for lymphoma and skin cancer are variable depending on organ transplanted, cumulative dose of immunosuppressants, concomitant immunosuppressants, and time since transplant. Intensity and duration of immunosuppression seem to be more closely correlated with risk than is use of any individual agent. Figures represented are for medication given in combination with other drugs on the list, as it is rare for these medications to be given alone. Refer to footnotes for details and text for further explanation.

[d]As induction prior to renal transplant, after 20 years of follow-up. Maintenance immunosuppressants included cyclosporine, prednisone, and azathioprine. Patients receiving same regimen without antithymocyte globulin induction had a 3% incidence after same duration of follow-up.

[e]Renal transplant recipients, at average follow-up of 86.5 months, combined with prednisolone.

[f]Renal transplant recipients, "normal dose" (trough concentrations 150–250 ng/mL) after mean follow-up of 5.5 yr of use alone (5%), with azathioprine (77%) or with prednisolone (18%). Lower incidence in comparator group (lymphoma, 0.86%; skin cancer, 14.7%) randomly assigned to "low-dose" cyclosporine (trough concentrations 75–125 ng/mL).

[g]Renal transplant recipients, at 2 yr, with mycophenolate mofetil and no induction.

[h]Renal transplant recipients, 17% also received azathioprine (follow-up variable; maximum, 10 yr).

[i]Renal transplant recipients, at 3 yr. Meta-analysis, all regimens included azathioprine or mycophenolate with or without steroids.

[j]After ≥10 yr of use.

[k]After average of 5.6 yr of use.

[l]Following only 1 year of unopposed estrogen use.

[m]Following median dose of 113 g, after 15 yr of follow-up.

consisting of doxorubicin (Adriamycin), bleomycin, vinblastine, and dacarbazine (often referred to as ABVD) are not associated with increased risk.[7] Bhatia et al.[9] found the cumulative probability of leukemia 15 years after diagnosis of Hodgkin lymphoma to be 2.9% in patients who received mechlorethamine, vincristine, procarbazine, and prednisone (MOPP) as compared to 0.9% among patients who received ABVD for Hodgkin lymphoma. Therefore, the MOPP regimen is obsolete and ABVD is the standard of care for patients diagnosed with Hodgkin lymphoma. The topoisomerase inhibitors associated with t-AML include the epipodophyllotoxins (e.g., etoposide, teniposide) and the intercalating agents, mitoxantrone and doxorubicin. Mitoxantrone- and doxorubicin-associated t-AML have been reported in the literature; however, the incidence is not well defined.[10] The administration schedule of epipodophyllotoxins may be as important as, or even more important than, the cumulative dose. This theory of schedule-dependent elevated risk is plausible because epipodophyllotoxins are cell cycle-specific agents and differences in antitumor effect have been noted for different schedules. For example, administration of etoposide daily for 5 days is more active than 24-hour continuous infusion of the same total dose. Results from a study conducted by Pui et al.[11] suggested that patients who received weekly or twice weekly administration for prolonged periods were approximately 12 times more likely to develop AML versus other less frequent schedules. A Cancer Therapy Evaluation Program review also supported the theory that cumulative dose may not be as important as schedule. In their study, the likelihood of t-AML after treatment with epipodophyllotoxins was not dose-dependent. The 6-year cumulative incidence of t-AML in groups that received low (1.5 g/m^2), moderate (1.5–2.99 g/m^2), and higher (≥3 g/m^2) cumulative doses of etoposide was 3.3%, 0.7%, and 2.2%, respectively.[12] The risk of t-AML from regimens that include epipodophyllotoxins (such as etoposide) at doses of 5 g/m^2 or less administered daily for 2–5 days does not appear to increase. Therefore, most etoposide containing chemotherapy regimens include daily administration for 3–5 days.[10,12]

EPIDEMIOLOGY

According to the American Cancer Society, about 60,000 new cases of leukemia (all types) will be diagnosed in 2018. The exact incidence of therapy-related MDS/AML is unknown. Reports suggest that therapy-related MDS/AML account for 5–20% of all AML cases, which are the result of exposure to chemotherapy and/or radiation for treatment of a primary malignancy.[7,13,29] The incidence of MDS is not well defined in the literature. Therapy-induced ALL occurs less frequently than t-AML (incidence of approximately 1.2% versus 2.5%).[3]

t-AML is reported following the treatment of a variety of malignancies, including Hodgkin and non-Hodgkin lymphoma (NHL), ALL, breast cancer, ovarian cancer, and multiple myeloma. The incidence of t-AML after treatment of these diseases varies greatly, with the highest risk reported in patients who have been treated for Hodgkin lymphoma. In these patients, the incidence of AML may be 10- to 80-fold greater than that in the general population. The cumulative risk for MDS/AML in Hodgkin lymphoma is reported to be 0.3–10.2%, with a lower incidence associated with the doxorubicin-based regimen (ABVD) and a higher incidence related to use of a mechlorethamine-containing regimen such as MOPP. The cumulative incidence of MDS and/or AML among patients with breast cancer treated with the topoisomerase II-targeting drug, doxorubicin, and the deoxyribonucleic acid (DNA) alkylating agent, cyclophosphamide, has been reported to be 0.27%.[14] In a more recent study, the cumulative frequency was 0.24% at 5 years and 0.48% at 10 years. Patients included in the latter study were treated with four cycles of doxorubicin plus cyclophosphamide. Overall, the risk in breast cancer patients is small, and benefits outweigh risk. Testicular cancer represents another solid tumor in which there is an increased risk of t-AML after chemotherapy use at a cumulative dose of 650 mg of cisplatin (approximate relative risk of 3.2, 95% CI 1–8.4). The increased risk appears to be related to the cumulative dose of cisplatin rather than etoposide, with larger doses of cisplatin (≥1,000 mg) associated with approximately a sixfold increased risk. As with patients with other cancer types, patients with testicular cancer may receive therapies such as radiotherapy known to increase the risk of developing leukemia.[15]

Other chemotherapy agents such as azathioprine have also been linked to leukemogenesis. Azathioprine is classified as an antimetabolite. Unlike alkylating agents, antimetabolites do not damage DNA. Reports have largely involved patients with prolonged use of azathioprine to treat autoimmune conditions. The reported cumulative doses of azathioprine have varied from 19 to 400 g and the duration of use varied from 2 to 12 years. It is unclear whether the association between azathioprine and t-MN is dose/duration related. Published reports suggest that patients who develop t-MN may have other risk factors (e.g., use of other immunosuppressants and/or concomitant autoimmune diseases) that may contribute to the development of t-MN.[16]

The incidence of other therapy-related neoplasms such as AML and MDS has been reported with the use of lenalidomide in multiple myeloma patients.[17] Although other immunomodulatory agents, such as thalidomide and pomalidomide, are used to treat multiple myeloma, secondary neoplasms have been primarily reported with lenalidomide use in the maintenance treatment setting. In patients with multiple myeloma, maintenance therapy is proposed to control the proliferation of residual malignant cells after transplantation.[17-19] There are postmarketing case reports of t-MN with thalidomide and pomalidomide, and these agents are not used in the maintenance setting.[20,21] In clinical trials, patients treated with lenalidomide for multiple myeloma had increased risk of development of AML and MDS. One of the landmark trials that investigated lenalidomide maintenance therapy was among the first to report secondary malignancies. The pivotal phase III study was conducted in newly diagnosed multiple myeloma patients who received autologous stem cell transplants followed by consolidation treatment with lenalidomide (25 mg per day, on days 1–21 of each 28-day cycle for two cycles), followed by maintenance therapy with lenalidomide (10 mg per day for first 3 months, increased to 15 mg if tolerated). Treatment with lenalidomide continued until the patient progressed or unacceptable toxic effects occurred. The incidence of hematologic cancers (AML, MDS, Hodgkin lymphoma, and non-Hodgkin lymphoma) was 4% compared to 2% in the placebo arm. Of the patients who had secondary malignancies, several had received induction therapy with dexamethasone, cyclophosphamide, etoposide, and cisplatin or had undergone two transplantations and received lenalidomide maintenance therapy for at least 2 years.[17] The frequency of hematologic cancers was reported to be 5.3% in the newly diagnosed multiple myeloma patients who received lenalidomide in combination with oral melphalan. The frequency was approximately 5.2% following high-dose intravenous melphalan and autologous stem cell transplant. The reported frequency of AML/MDS was lowest (0.4%) when lenalidomide was combined with dexamethasone alone.[22] In the aforementioned studies, all patients had previous DNA damaging chemotherapy that might contribute to AML/MDS rates. This makes it difficult to ascertain which therapy is responsible for secondary malignancy.

Olaparib is a novel agent approved in the United States in 2014 for treatment of BRCA positive advanced ovarian cancer. MDS/AML was reported in 1% (22 of 2,618) of patients treated with olaparib across clinical trials. The duration of olaparib therapy varied from <6 months to >2 years.[23] All patients had previous DNA damaging chemotherapy, which may contribute to AML/MDS rates.

Knowledge of TNF alpha inhibitor–induced myeloid neoplasms, such as leukemia, is limited to information gleaned from case reports.[6]

MECHANISMS

In general, t-MN is thought to result from mutations induced by chemotherapy or by selection of a clone that has an increased risk of a mutation due to a certain phenotype (**Table 57-2**).[24] With respect to specific chromosome deletions, at least one and possibly two alleles of a tumor-suppressor gene may need to be deleted or inactivated. However, balanced translocations (e.g., involving the *MLL* gene at 11q23) can produce activation of fusion oncogenes that transform hematopoietic progenitor cells. The latter type of genetic transformation is thought to require a relatively smaller number of genetic events before becoming leukemogenic, perhaps explaining why t-AML associated with the use of topoisomerase inhibitors occurs earlier than with alkylating agents.[24]

Topoisomerase inhibitors block either the topoisomerase I or II enzyme, resulting in a permanent DNA strand break. Although the chromosomal breakage is important to the antineoplastic activity of these agents, it is also thought that these breakages result in chromosomal translocations that lead to secondary leukemia. In locations critical to transcription, such as the *MLL* gene, a change in the genomic function due to a translocation is likely important in the genesis of secondary AML. The rearrangements in the *MLL* gene occur within undifferentiated cells and can therefore result in lymphoid (e.g., in conjunction with chromosome 4) and myeloid (e.g., in conjunction with chromosome 9) leukemia.[7] The induction of t-AML with colony-stimulating factor use is thought to be related to the potential to promote proliferation of cells previously damaged by chemotherapy.[24] Patients diagnosed with congenital neutropenia experience lifelong low neutrophil counts and require long-term treatment with G-CSF. Long-term effects have been investigated in this population of patients. Although the data are unclear, a higher leukemic transformation rate (approximately 21%) has been reported

Table 57-2 Selected Mechanisms of Drug-Induced Neoplastic Diseases

Drug	Mechanism
LEUKEMIA	
Carmustine Chlorambucil Cyclophosphamide Mechlorethamine Melphalan	Cause DNA strand breaks resulting in chromosomal translocations/damage and alteration of key genes
Doxorubicin Epirubicin Etoposide Mitoxantrone Teniposide	Induce translocations producing activation of oncogenes that transform hematopoietic cells
Filgrastim (G-CSF) Sargramostim (GM-CSF)	Induce proliferation of hematopoietic cells previously damaged by chemotherapy
LYMPHOMA	
Cyclosporine	Increases TGF-β and VEGF
Antithymocyte globulin Azathioprine Cyclosporine Muromonab CD3 (OKT3) Tacrolimus	Suppression of immune surveillance, allowing proliferation of oncogenic viruses and inhibiting clearance of abnormal cells
SKIN CANCER	
Cyclosporine	Increases TGF-β and VEGF
Antithymocyte globulin Azathioprine Cyclosporine Muromonab CD3 (OKT3) Tacrolimus	Suppression of immunosurveillance, allowing proliferation of oncogenic viruses and inhibiting clearance of abnormal cells
BREAST CANCER	
Estrogen	Covalent binding to DNA may cause mutations; metabolites act as tumor promoters; causes tumor cell proliferation via estrogen receptors
Progestin	Causes tumor cell proliferation via progesterone receptors
ENDOMETRIAL CANCER	
Estrogen	Induces proliferation of endometrium, which can transform to cancer
Tamoxifen	Induces proliferation of endometrium, which can transform to cancer; increases activation of pro-oncoenic genes; induces high mitotic rate in endometrial polyps
BLADDER CANCER	
Cyclophosphamide	Metabolites form DNA adducts, leading to mutation and carcinomatosis
Pioglitazone	Agonism of PPARs on urothelial cells in bladder

PPAR = peroxisome proliferator-activated receptor, TGF-β = transforming growth factor beta, VEGF = vascular endothelial growth factor.

in patients with severe congenital neutropenia. It is important to note that leukemic transformation has been reported in this patient population prior to G-CSF therapy. The precise role of G-CSF therapy in leukemic transformation remains unknown.[25]

The mechanism by which lenalidomide may increase risk of AML and MDS has not been fully elucidated. Unlike cytotoxic chemotherapy, lenalidomide shows no mutagenic potential in extensive genotoxicity studies performed during its development. Other complex issues in this patient population that may contribute to secondary neoplasms include treatment factors (previous alkylating agents, stem cell transplant, radiotherapy), myeloma-related factors, and host-related factors.[18,22,26]

Poly ADP ribose polymerase inhibitors are a relatively newer drug class in oncology. These agents have been investigated for use in several solid tumors, especially breast cancer and ovarian cancer. t-MN have been reported with olaparib use; however, the mechanism has not been fully elucidated. Previous therapy with alkylating agents may also contribute to secondary neoplasms in the ovarian cancer population.[23]

The mechanism by which G-CSF can cause leukemic transformation is not fully elucidated. The use of G-CSF is not limited to the oncology population, but also occurs with patients who have severe congenital neutropenia (SCN). These patients experience neutropenia for life and require long-term treatment with G-CSF. The SCN international registry reported a 10-year follow-up of SCN patients (n = 526) treated with G-CSF. They found that 21% of patients with SCN developed leukemia while being treated with G-CSF.[25]

Understanding the mechanism by which TNF-alpha inhibitors induce myeloid neoplasms is challenging for several reasons. Patients treated with TNF-alpha inhibitors likely have disease-related risk factors that predispose them for higher risk of cancer (such has previous therapies) as well as diseases that are associated with chronic inflammation that leads to chronic cellular proliferation. As a result, these patients are at higher risk for malignant processes. Diseases with chronic inflammation have been associated with a higher risk of development of both hematologic and solid tumor malignancies. Examples of diseases associated with chronic inflammation include rheumatoid arthritis, Crohn disease, and psoriasis.[6,27]

CLINICAL PRESENTATION AND DIFFERENTIAL DIAGNOSIS

Signs and symptoms of t-MN are listed in **Table 57-3**. The diagnostic workup is identical for either de novo or t-AML and includes a complete blood cell count (CBC) with differential followed by a bone marrow biopsy or aspiration. t-AML typically occurs earlier than other types of secondary cancers, with time to presentation dependent on the causative agent used. There is usually a longer latency (3–8 years) between exposure to alkylating agents and the occurrence of t-AML compared to topoisomerase inhibitor-induced malignancy (typically presenting in 2–3 years). Patients who develop alkylator-related AML often present with MDS, although this rarely occurs in patients with AML-associated topoisomerase inhibitor use. Cytogenetic abnormalities are present in approximately 80% of patients with t-AML/t-MDS. The most commonly identified chromosomal abnormalities differ between drug classes. The most common abnormalities after treatment with alkylating agents are found in either chromosome 5, chromosome 7, or both, each of which undergoes complete or partial deletion. Balanced translocations involving the *MLL* gene on the 11q23 locus are the most common abnormalities with the use of topoisomerase inhibitors.[24]

Conditions that should be considered in the differential diagnosis of drug-induced myeloid neoplasms are listed in **Table 57-4**.

Table 57-3 Signs and Symptoms Associated with Drug-Induced Neoplastic Diseases

Leukemia

- Anemia
- Bone pain
- Bruising/bleeding
- Dyspnea on exertion
- Fatigue
- Fever/chills
- Leukopenia/leukocytosis
- Lymphadenopathy
- Thrombocytopenia
- Weight loss

Lymphoma

- Abdominal pain
- Anemia
- Chest pain
- Fatigue
- Fever
- Hepatosplenomegaly
- Lymphadenopathy
- Neutropenia
- Night sweats
- Thrombocytopenia

Skin cancer

- Abnormal sensation in skin
- Abnormal skin lesion (asymmetric, irregular border, abnormal color and/or texture, size >6 mm)
- Skin lesion that rapidly changes
- Skin ulceration, crusting

Breast cancer

- Abnormality in breast tissue (e.g., lump, erythema, induration)
- Breast pain/tenderness
- Nipple pain/tenderness
- Nipple retraction/discharge
- Upper extremity edema

Endometrial cancer

- Dysuria
- Pelvic pain
- Vaginal bleeding

Bladder cancer

- Dysuria
- Flank pain
- Hematuria
- Increased urinary frequency

Table 57-4 Conditions to Consider in the Differential Diagnosis of Drug-Induced Neoplastic Diseases

Leukemia

- Aplastic anemia
- Infection

Lymphoma

- Infection

Skin cancer

- Nonmalignant dermatologic disorder (e.g., psoriasis, eczema, actinic keratoses, seborrheic keratoses)

Breast cancer

- Nonmalignant breast cyst/calcification
- Nonmalignant dermatologic disorder
- Other malignancy (e.g., soft tissue tumors)

Endometrial cancer

- Endometriosis
- Pelvic inflammatory disease
- Uterine fibroids

Bladder cancer

- Hemorrhagic cystitis
- Urinary tract infection

RISK FACTORS

Risk factors for t-MN are listed in **Table 57-5**. Although the main risk factors for t-MN are exposure to certain types of anticancer drugs or radiation therapy, data also reveal a greater risk among patients with a prior cancer in general. This suggests an inherent increased susceptibility in this patient population, and several genetic factors thought possibly to confer increased risk are now being studied. Because t-AML develops in only a small proportion of patients exposed to alkylating agents or topoisomerase inhibitors, there are likely host factors that are critical to the development of this drug-induced disease. Polymorphisms in drug-metabolizing enzymes may be involved in susceptibility to t-AML. For example, the CYP3A4 wild-type genotype may result in increased production of reactive intermediate metabolites of epipodophyllotoxins that can damage DNA. Additionally, an increased rate of t-AML has been found among carriers of homozygous mutations in the *NQO1* gene.[7]

Table 57-5 Risk Factors for Drug-Induced Neoplastic Diseases

Leukemia

- History of malignancy
- Host factors resulting in individual susceptibility: polymorphisms in drug metabolizing enzymes

Lymphoma

- Advanced age
- Intense immunosuppression
- Long duration of immunosuppression
- Pretransplantation Epstein–Barr virus seronegativity
- Use of induction agents

Skin cancer

- Advanced age
- Exposure of skin to ultraviolet light
- Intense immunosuppression
- Light-colored skin
- Long duration of immunosuppression
- Prior skin cancer

Breast cancer

- Advanced age
- Body-mass index <25[a]
- Use of HRT, greater cumulative exposure to HRT, long duration of HRT

Endometrial cancer

- Conjugated estrogen use
- Greater cumulative exposure to estrogen and/or tamoxifen
- Long duration of estrogen use
- Obesity
- Pelvic radiation
- Pre-existing abnormal endometrial pathology

Bladder cancer

- Advanced age
- Extended duration of treatment with cyclophosphamide
- High cumulative doses of cyclophosphamide
- Smoking
- Extended duration of treatment with pioglitazone

HRT = hormone replacement therapy.
[a]Body-mass index is the weight in kilograms divided by the square of the height in meters.

MORBIDITY AND MORTALITY

The course of t-MN is progressive and the disease is typically resistant to the chemotherapeutic approaches used in the treatment of de novo leukemia. In general, t-MN is a fatal disease owing to marked and persistent cytopenias. Persistence of the underlying cancer can complicate treatment of the t-MN. Prior anticancer treatment can complicate the delivery of dose-intensive chemotherapy targeted at the t-MN by possibly causing significant organ and/or hematopoietic compromise. In addition, the high rate of cytogenetic abnormalities found in patients with t-MN often results in the abrupt development of drug resistance.[24]

PREVENTION

The primary preventive approach for t-MN involves avoiding the use of agents known to be linked to t-MN (Table 57-1) if possible. In the management of Hodgkin lymphoma, the preferred regimen, ABVD, contains agents with lower risks of t-MN development. This strategy has led to a much lower incidence of t-AML among patients treated for Hodgkin lymphoma. A similar approach has also been instituted in pediatric patients being treated for ALL, for whom epipodophyllotoxins have been removed from most first-line chemotherapy protocols. Sometimes drugs in the same class can deliver equivalent efficacy with lower leukemogenic risk. Examples include using cyclophosphamide (lower risk) instead of busulfan and substituting doxorubicin (lower risk) for mitoxantrone.

As previously noted, drug scheduling (e.g., with the epipodophyllotoxins) and cumulative dosing (e.g., with epirubicin and cisplatin) appear to be important factors to consider when designing chemotherapy regimens to mitigate the risk of drug-induced leukemia. Whether or not more judicious use of colony-stimulating factors (CSF) such as G-CSF should be considered is still debated. Although not negligible, the contribution of CSF to the absolute risk of drug-induced leukemia appears to be smaller than that of many chemotherapy agents.[24]

MANAGEMENT

There is little information available regarding optimal treatment of patients with t-MN. It is likely that a complete remission (CR) will be achieved in less than half of all cases, as compared with a CR rate of 65–80% in de novo AML patients 60 years of age or younger and 40–60% in patients older than 60 years of age. For patients who are candidates, the most likely curative approach is hematopoietic stem cell transplantation (HSCT). Small studies have reported 20–30% survival with HSCT. Patients over 40 years of age have a higher rate of transplant-related mortality.[28] Favorable, intermediate, and unfavorable karyotypes have been identified for cytogenetic abnormalities. Patients with secondary AML have a greater predominance of unfavorable types than patients with de novo AML (approximately 80% versus 20%). Mean survival among patients with secondary AML and the favorable type was approximately 27 months, but those with unfavorable features had a mean survival of only 6 months. With respect to specific cytogenetics, patients with secondary AML and abnormalities of chromosomes 5 and 7 appear to fare the worst.[24]

Treatment for patients with t-AML and a normal karyotype should follow standard AML management protocols with consideration of HSCT. Treatment consists of induction chemotherapy followed by consolidation therapy. For patients with unfavorable cytogenetics, either investigational chemotherapy approaches or HSCT (or both) should be considered.[24,29] The NCCN provides the most up-to-date guidelines for health professionals on the management of myeloid leukemia cancers.

INFORMATION FOR PATIENTS

All patients receiving chemotherapy agents/regimens with a known potential for t-MN should be apprised of the risk and possible consequences at the outset. Patients diagnosed with t-MN should receive candid information regarding the likely outcome in relation to their risk group. Any treatment options should be carefully and thoroughly explained. Although it is important for patients to fully understand the seriousness of the disease so they can plan accordingly, it is also important for them to know that supportive measures are available and will be used to their fullest extent.

LYMPHOMA

There are two settings in which medication use has been associated with an increased risk of developing lymphomas: in transplant recipients and in patients treated for autoimmune disorders. The reported incidence of this drug-induced malignancy in immunosuppressed organ transplant recipients varies widely among the different registries and centers but may be as high as 50% after 6 years of follow-up. Lymphoproliferative disorders such as NHL and, less often, Hodgkin lymphoma occur in up to 20% of organ-transplant recipients.[2] Cases of these secondary malignancies have also been reported following lenalidomide maintenance use after stem cell transplantation in multiple myeloma patients.[30] The use of TNF-alpha blockers (adalimumab, certolizumab pegol, etanercept, golimumab, and infliximab) also poses an increased risk of lymphoma development, and this led to mandated boxed warnings in package inserts for these medications in 2009. Additionally, the U.S. Food and Drug Administration (FDA) released a safety announcement in 2011 describing cases of hepatosplenic T-cell lymphoma (HSTCL) occurring primarily in adolescents and young adults treated for Crohn disease and ulcerative colitis with tumor TNF-alpha blockers, azathioprine, or mercaptopurine.[31] This lethal T-cell lymphoproliferative disorder is rare and has been reported to have a clear association with immunosuppression with either an immunomodulator or combined immunosuppression with a TNF-alpha inhibitor and an immunomodulator.[32]

CAUSATIVE AGENTS

Immunosuppressive agents have been implicated in the development of lymphoma (Table 57-1).[22] Agents used in high doses for induction to facilitate transplant and as treatment for acute rejection are associated with a higher incidence of lymphoma in the first year after transplantation.[33,34] These agents include antithymocyte globulin and muromonab CD3 (OKT3), which was removed from the U.S. market in 2010. Maintenance immunosuppressants, including the calcineurin inhibitors, cyclosporine and tacrolimus, and the antimetabolite, azathioprine, are also associated with an increased risk of drug-induced malignancy. Although there are no reports of lymphoma with sirolimus or temsirolimus, a manufacturer of everolimus has a boxed warning alerting prescribers to the possible development of both skin cancer and lymphoma when the drug is used in the solid organ transplant setting.[35]

EPIDEMIOLOGY

In the first year after surgery, kidney transplant recipients have a 20 times increased risk of lymphoma and heart transplant recipients a 120 times increased risk, as compared with the general population.[34] The difference between the two groups is thought to be related to the more aggressive immunosuppression used in heart transplantation. Risk persists over time, with lymphoma developing in 1.6% of kidney transplant recipients over 10 years and 5.6% of heart–lung recipients over 5 years.[33] OKT3 or antithymocyte globulin induction increases the risk of lymphoma primarily during the first year after transplantation.[33,34] The majority of immunosuppressant-induced lymphomas are of B-cell origin, and 28% of patients have central nervous system involvement.[36] Patients <10 or >60 years of age have the highest risk for lymphoma.[33]

Post-transplant lymphoproliferative disorders (PTLD) are potentially fatal lymphoid and/or plasmacytic proliferations that develop in solid organ or allogeneic hematopoietic cell transplant patients due to immunosuppression. B cells that multiply in the absence of normal T-cell immune function in the stem cell transplant population are thought to be infected with the Epstein–Barr virus (EBV). Thus, PTLD generally refers to an EBV-induced B-cell proliferation that develops after a solid organ transplant or allogeneic HSCT. The incidence of EBV-PTLD after allogeneic HSCT ranges between 0.5% and 17%.[37]

Of the cancer cases related to the use of TNF-alpha inhibitors that were reported to the FDA from 1998 to 2008, half were Hodgkin and non-Hodgkin lymphomas, with 10 cases of HSTCL.[38] A meta-analysis in rheumatoid arthritis patients treated with TNF-alpha inhibitors found no increased risk of lymphoma when compared to nonexposed patients.[39]

MECHANISMS

There are multiple mechanisms by which immunosuppressants are thought to cause malignancy (Table 57-2). Calcineurin inhibitors such as cyclosporine can promote malignant growth by increasing the amount of tumor growth factor (TGF) and vascular endothelial growth factor (VEGF).[40] Immunosurveillance is suppressed in patients receiving immunosuppressants. Oncogenic viruses are not as readily cleared as in nonimmunosuppressed individuals. These factors together provide an optimal environment for malignant transformation of cells by viruses and subsequent proliferation of those cells. Specifically, cases of lymphoma in the post-solid organ and allogeneic stem cell transplantation settings have been associated with proliferation of the EBV within B lymphocytes.[2,37]

T lymphocytes and natural killer cells endogenously produce the cytokine TNF-alpha as part of a cell-mediated immune response during infections and cause tumor cell lysis. TNF-alpha was recognized in 1975 for its ability to lyse tumors in laboratory models, raising the concern that inhibition of this cytokine may lead to cancer development.[41] Conflicting clinical data exist regarding the role of TNF-alpha inhibition in the development of malignancy.[42]

CLINICAL PRESENTATION AND DIFFERENTIAL DIAGNOSIS

Symptoms of lymphoma can include fatigue, weight loss, lymphadenopathy, and night sweats (Table 57-3). Diagnosis is made by node, tissue, or bone marrow biopsy; CBC with differential; and imaging studies (Table 57-4). NHL after immunosuppressive therapy is associated with increased extranodal involvement as compared to lymphomas in the general population.[36] In some patient subsets, extranodal disease occurs within or near the transplanted organ. Examples include disease of the liver in liver transplant recipients and disease of the lungs in heart, lung, or heart–lung transplant recipients.[34,35]

RISK FACTORS

Risk factors for drug-induced lymphoma are described in Table 57-5. The incidence of lymphoproliferative disorders increases proportionately with increasing dose and duration of immunosuppressant medications. Therefore, transplant procedures in which patients require the highest doses of immunosuppressants and the most aggressive antirejection strategies, such as heart and lung, are associated with the highest incidence of lymphoma.[34] This intensity–risk relationship was demonstrated by a prospective randomized trial of low-dose versus standard-dose cyclosporine therapy in kidney transplant recipients. A higher frequency of malignancy was found in the higher-dose group.[43] A study of heart transplant recipients revealed that cumulative doses of OKT3 (a medication no longer available in the United States) >75 mg imparted a 35.7% risk of lymphoma as compared with 6.2% in patients who received ≤75 mg.[44]

Advancing age and pretransplantation EBV seronegativity are additional risk factors.[45] Young children are more likely than adults to be EBV-seronegative prior to transplantation and are at risk for initial EBV exposure during or after transplantation. This puts them at high risk for post-transplantation lymphoma.[46]

MORBIDITY AND MORTALITY

Malignancy-related mortality after organ transplantation ranges from 10% to 47%. NHL after organ transplantation is more aggressive than in the general population, most likely because of the necessity to maintain immunosuppression and an advanced stage at presentation. First-year lymphoma-related mortality in kidney and heart transplant recipients was reported at 40% and 50%, respectively.[33]

PREVENTION

Approaches to preventing drug-induced lymphoma are described in **Table 57-6**. Because drug-induced lymphoma is associated with the use of intense

Table 57-6 Approaches to Help Prevent Drug-Induced Neoplastic Diseases

Leukemia

- Avoid use of mechlorethamine in the treatment of Hodgkin lymphoma
- Avoid weekly scheduling of etoposide/teniposide and avoid use when other agents are equally effective
- Consider using cyclophosphamide instead of busulfan in chemotherapeutic regimens
- Consider using doxorubicin instead of mitoxantrone in chemotherapeutic regimens
- Limit cumulative dose of cisplatin in the treatment of testicular cancer
- Limit cumulative dose of epirubicin in the treatment of breast cancer

Lymphoma

- Consider using basiliximab for induction instead of antithymocyte globulin
- Consider using everolimus or sirolimus instead of cyclosporine or tacrolimus for maintenance immunosuppression
- Limit cumulative dose of cyclosporine or tacrolimus
- Monitor EBV levels for possible reactivation
- Use antiviral prophylaxis for 3 months after organ transplantation

Skin cancer

- Avoid ultraviolet light
- Consider using everolimus or sirolimus instead of cyclosporine or tacrolimus for maintenance immunosuppression
- Consider using mycophenolate mofetil instead of azathioprine for maintenance immunosuppression

Breast cancer

- Avoid use of HRT

Endometrial cancer

- Avoid use of tamoxifen
- Consider use of aromatase inhibitors instead of tamoxifen for the treatment of breast cancer
- Do not use tamoxifen for longer than 5 yr
- Use progestin concomitantly for at least 10 days /month with estrogen when used for HRT

Bladder cancer

- Limit cumulative dose cyclophosphamide to <20 g
- Use mesna as uroprotectant with cyclophosphamide[a]
- Avoid pioglitazone use for ≥24 months

HRT = hormone replacement therapy.
[a]Unproven in humans.

immunosuppression, transplant recipients should be maintained on the lowest possible doses of immunosuppressant drugs for the shortest possible time to reduce overall risk. There is some evidence that sirolimus, a mammalian target-of-rapamycin (mTOR) inhibitor, has antiangiogenic effects and is associated with fewer post-transplantation malignancies than cyclosporine or tacrolimus (0.6% versus 1.81% at a mean follow-up of 2.3 years). Induction with an interleukin-2 antibody such as basiliximab has not been definitively associated with an increased risk of lymphoma and may be an option to improve outcomes.[47] Antiviral prophylaxis with acyclovir for 3 months after transplantation has been shown in one study to be associated with a reduced incidence of post-transplantation lymphoma in heart transplant recipients, suggesting the potential utility of antiviral agents as a preventive strategy.[48] Acyclovir use in this setting is questionable due to the absence of activity against EBV associated with PTLD.[49]

MANAGEMENT

Dose reduction or discontinuation of immunosuppression is the primary method used to manage post-transplantation lymphoma; however, the risk of organ rejection must be carefully considered.[46] Surgical excision of localized lesions has been used with favorable results.[50] The anti-CD20 monoclonal antibody rituximab is an option for the treatment of B-cell lymphomas. Two studies in which patients with drug-induced lymphoma received rituximab 375 mg/m^2 once weekly for 4 weeks reported CR rates of 53–88%.[51,52]

Chemotherapy may be an option for patients who do not respond to reduction of immunosuppression. A primary treatment regimen for lymphoma consisting of cyclophosphamide, doxorubicin, vincristine (Oncovin), and prednisone (often referred to as CHOP) has been successfully used in the post-transplantation lymphoma population.[53] Many centers use anthracycline-based regimens, adjusting chemotherapy doses as necessary to address patient comorbidities.[54,55]

INFORMATION FOR PATIENTS

Patients should be educated regarding the possible adverse effects associated with drugs that will be used after transplantation, including the risk of lymphoma with immunosuppressants. Patients in whom post-transplantation lymphoma develops should receive candid counseling regarding the prognosis, available treatments, and the risks and benefits associated with each of the treatment options.

SKIN CANCER

Basal cell carcinoma (BCC) is the most commonly diagnosed skin cancer (approximately 80% of new cases), while 16% are squamous cell carcinoma (SCC), 2% melanoma, and <1% are Merkel cell carcinoma, Kaposi sarcoma, cutaneous lymphoma, skin adnexal tumors, or various sarcomas. Basal cell carcinoma and SCC are not reported to cancer registries because these cancers rarely metastasize and almost all cases can be cured, making incidence estimates more difficult.[13] Skin cancer is the most common malignancy in patients receiving immunosuppressive medications to prevent rejection of transplanted organs, with SCC the most common cutaneous malignancy in this population.[56]

CAUSATIVE AGENTS

Several medications are associated with the development of skin cancer, including TNF-alpha blockers, B-rapidly accelerated fibrosarcoma (BRAF) inhibitors, mitogen-activated protein kinases (MEKs), and extracellular signal–regulated kinases. (Table 57-1). Additionally, recent reviews found that the short-term use of several commonly prescribed medications that cause photosensitivity may enhance the risk of skin cancers such as BCC, SCC, and cutaneous lymphoma.[57,58]

It is thought that the level of immunosuppression itself, and not any one particular drug, is responsible for the increased risk of skin cancer in the transplant setting.[2,59,60] Patients who are recipients of transplanted organs or allogeneic stem cells receive the highest doses of immunosuppressant medications and are at the highest risk for drug-induced skin cancer.[61,62] It appears that it is the concomitant use of multiple therapies including immunosuppressants, myeloablative chemotherapy, and radiation that is responsible for SCC and BCC in allogeneic HSCT recipients.[62]

Currently available BRAF inhibitors, dabrafenib and vemurafenib, as well as MEK inhibitors, cobimetinib and trametinib, have revolutionized treatment and survival of metastatic melanoma in patients with the BRAF mutation but are associated with up to a 33% incidence of SCC, 6% incidence of BCC, and 2.4% incidence of new primary melanoma.[63-67]

Selenium supplementation among patients with a prior history of nonmelanoma skin cancer (NMSC) has been implicated as a potential cause of SCC in a double-blind trial. SCC has also been reported in case reports of oral contraceptives users.[68]

EPIDEMIOLOGY

Skin cancer occurs in organ transplant recipients at a rate of 12–90 times the frequency observed in the general population.[2] Patients with nonrenal transplants are 3 times more likely to develop skin cancer than those with renal transplants.[59] This is likely due to a strong relationship between skin cancer risk and intensity of immunosuppression, because kidney transplant recipients typically require less immunosuppression. In addition, transplant recipients are more likely than patients in the general population to present with multiple lesions. Older patients tend to present with skin cancer sooner after transplantation than younger patients. However, the incidence of skin cancer in all transplant patients increases linearly with time after transplantation.[59]

MECHANISMS

As with immunosuppression-induced lymphomas, reduced immunosurveillance plays a role in post-transplantation skin cancers (Table 57-2). Apoptosis of cells damaged by ultraviolet light may not occur as efficiently in immunosuppressed individuals as in the general population. The damaged cells remain and proliferate as skin cancer. Unchecked proliferation of human papillomavirus (HPV) has also been implicated, and studies have reported that skin lesions in organ transplant recipients are positive for HPV DNA in up to 100% of cases.[2,69,70] Although HPV vaccination has been recommended for solid organ transplant recipients who meet the FDA indication, poor immunogenicity has been reported in the post-transplant patient setting.[71,72] HPV has not been detected in skin lesions of patients treated with BRAF inhibitors. It is not known whether patients receiving anti-TNF-alpha therapy have an altered response to HPV vaccination.[73]

Although TNF-alpha may be a part of cell-mediated immune response, ultimately causing tumor cell lysis, clinical data regarding the role of TNF-alpha inhibition in the development of malignancy are conflicting. Meta-analyses support an increased risk of NMSC with the use of these medications although two large cohort studies revealed no statistical difference in the development of overall increased risk of NMSC between TNF-alpha inhibitor users and nonusers.[39,42,74]

CLINICAL PRESENTATION AND DIFFERENTIAL DIAGNOSIS

Multiple other skin disorders can resemble drug-induced skin cancer (Table 57-4). Patients can present with multiple lesions that can be rapidly recurring (Table 57-3). Although lesions can occur anywhere on the body, they most frequently are found in areas exposed to sunlight.[63] Approximately 70% of skin cancers in both men and women occur on the head, neck, and upper extremities.[61,62]

Although in the general population BCC is more common than SCC, the opposite is true in immunosuppressed patients. In 1,293 kidney transplant recipients in whom skin cancer developed, 71% had SCC, 52% had BCC, and 3% had melanoma (some patients had more than one type of skin cancer).[39]

An SCC:BCC ratio of 2.2:1 was found in a group of 48 heart transplant patients in whom skin cancer developed.[60] The reported median time to first appearance of cutaneous squamous cell carcinomas and keratoacanthomas in melanoma patients treated with BRAF inhibitors was approximately 8 weeks.[66,67]

The incidence of skin cancer increases linearly with time, with an incidence of 2.2%, 7.2%, and 8.9% at 5, 10, and 14 years, respectively, reported in kidney transplant recipients.[61] As noted previously, the incidence of skin cancer is higher in heart transplant recipients, with reported rates of 12%, 27%, and 44% at 5, 10, and 14 years, respectively.[60]

RISK FACTORS

As in the general population, persons with lighter skin are at a greater risk for drug-induced skin malignancies than those with darker skin. Exposure to ultraviolet light and advanced age are additional risks (Table 57-5)[41,60,61] As with post-transplantation lymphomas, there is a correlation between intensity and duration of immunosuppression and the development of skin cancer.[34,41,59] In a retrospective study of 262 patients, those who received cyclosporine in addition to azathioprine and prednisolone had NMSC at a rate of 48 cases per 1,000 patient-years, as compared with 27 cases per 1,000 patient-years in the azathioprine-plus-prednisolone-only group.[75] Patients who have had a prior skin cancer are at greater risk than those who have not.[41,76]

Ras protein mutation is a possible risk factor for developing SCC in patients treated with BRAF inhibitors, as this mutation was present in approximately 60% of cases in patients treated with vemurafenib.[46] Other possible risk factors associated with cutaneous SCC observed in vemurafenib clinical studies are age ≥65 years, history of prior malignancy, and chronic sun exposure.

Establishing the risk of the development of skin malignancies in patients receiving TNF-alpha inhibitors is challenging because most of these medications have been studied in patients with rheumatoid arthritis or ulcerative colitis, populations that are at increased risk for developing site-specific cancers. In addition, TNF-alpha inhibitor studies in these groups often allowed concomitant medications (e.g., cyclophosphamide or methotrexate), which augment malignancy risk.[1,43,74] There are fewer studies with certolizumab pegol and golimumab. Therefore, it is unknown if these newer TNF-alpha inhibitors pose the same risks of cancer development as adalimumab, etanercept, and infliximab.[77]

MORBIDITY AND MORTALITY

Mortality due to post-transplantation skin cancer has been reported to be 5%, which is higher than the 1–2% reported for the general population. Although the majority of lethal skin cancers in the general population are melanomas, SCC is the primary skin cancer responsible for death in the transplant population.[59] Skin cancers in transplant recipients are also typically more aggressive than those found in the general population: 6% of patients in the Cincinnati Transplant Tumor Registry had metastases, nearly three-fourths of which were from SCC.[59] A multicenter study of 68 patients with metastatic skin cancer (primarily SCC) reported a relapse rate of 29% after treatment and a 3-year survival rate of 54%.[78]

Patients' risk of mortality does not appear to be affected by treatment with BRAF inhibitors or TNF-alpha inhibitors. Progression-free survival among 134 patients with metastatic melanoma was not statistically different among patients who had developed a SCC and those who had not after 4 months of BRAF inhibitor therapy.[70] The overall survival in a study of rheumatoid arthritis patients treated with either adalimumab, etanercept, or infliximab (with or without concomitant disease-modifying antirheumatic drugs) and subsequently diagnosed with a solid tumor was not statistically different than survival in TNF-alpha treatment-naïve patients.[79]

PREVENTION

Methods to help prevent drug-induced skin cancer are presented in Table 57-6. Although there are no chemoprevention studies in subjects who have received TNF-alpha inhibitors or BRAF inhibitors, it would be prudent to suggest the same recommendation for skin cancer prevention that apply to the general population (i.e., sun avoidance and routine monitoring for unusual or new skin lesions).

Because of the strong relationship between intensity of immunosuppression and risk of skin cancer, maintaining patients on the lowest possible doses of immunosuppressants or using alternative agents may decrease the incidence in recipients of solid organ transplants. Azathioprine, when used as part of the immunosuppressive regimen in renal transplant patients, was linked to an increased risk of developing aggressive SCC.[80] Mycophenolate mofetil rather than azathioprine use in the immunosuppressive regimen may reduce the risk of skin cancer in some solid organ transplant recipients.[48,81] Additionally, the development of NMSC in the transplanted population has been associated with azathioprine use compared to those who did not receive this medication.[82] There has been some evidence that the mTOR inhibitors, sirolimus and everolimus, are associated with fewer cases of NMSC than cyclosporine or tacrolimus; however, long-term data are lacking.[76,83] Further studies are required to assess the impact of immunosuppressive therapy modifications on malignancies of the skin in solid organ transplant recipients.

MANAGEMENT

General treatment options for skin cancer include surgical excision of the lesion, immunotherapy, targeted therapy, chemotherapy, or radiation.[84] Surgery or radiation may not be plausible, however, in patients with multiple lesions or metastases. In these cases of transplanted patients, reduction of immunosuppression is an option, although the benefits of this approach are not as clear as they are in patients with drug-induced lymphoma. The risks of organ rejection must be carefully considered.[85] In 2006, guidelines for immunosuppressant dose reduction were released by a task force of the International Transplant Skin Cancer Collaborative and Skin Care for Organ Transplant Patients Europe.[86] The degree of dose reduction of immunosuppressants recommended for multiple clinical scenarios is outlined in these guidelines.

New primary SCC in melanoma patients treated with BRAF inhibitors can be treated with standard ablative or excisional surgical methods without interruption of the BRAF dosing regimen; for patients with multiple lesions, curettage, electrodesiccation, or cryosurgery has been suggested.[85]

Systemic therapy is typically reserved for cases in which surgical excision with or without radiation is either unsuccessful or deemed not beneficial.

INFORMATION FOR PATIENTS

Patients receiving immunosuppressive therapy for prevention of transplant rejection should be warned of the increased risk of skin cancer. They should be instructed to protect their skin from sun damage by use of sunscreen year-round and should also use protective clothing such as long-sleeved garments and hats. It is important to note that use of sunscreen does not negate the risk of skin cancer, so even with its use patients should still make every attempt to minimize their exposure to sunlight. Patients should never use tanning beds. Patients should inspect their own skin regularly for changes and also should be checked regularly by a dermatologist.[84]

Patients who are to receive BRAF inhibitors should be screened for skin cancer prior to initiation of therapy, every 2 months during treatment, and again following completion of therapy.[66,67]

BREAST CANCER

The American Cancer Society estimates that breast cancer kills nearly 41,000 women in the United States annually with nearly 253,000 new cases of this malignancy diagnosed.[13] This makes breast cancer the most common malignancy among women. Breast cancer can be drug-induced.[13]

CAUSATIVE AGENTS

Agents implicated in the development of breast cancer are listed in Table 57-1. The association between drug use and breast cancer development has been reported in patients receiving combination estrogen and progestin hormone-replacement therapy (HRT), estrogen-only HRT (ET), or oral contraceptives (OC). Menopausal state and exogenous hormone use may influence the risk of breast cancer development depending on the type of product used.

EPIDEMIOLOGY

Numerous studies have shown an association between a longer duration of HRT use and breast cancer development.[87] The Million Women Study, an observational study of 1,084,110 women, revealed a 43% increased risk of breast cancer among the 550,172 who received HRT versus those who did not.[88] The Women's Health Initiative (WHI), a randomized, controlled trial involving 16,608 women, found those receiving combination HRT had a 26% higher risk of invasive breast cancer than patients in the control group.[89] Further analysis of these cases revealed a higher rate of invasive tubular (8%) and lobular (22%) breast cancers found in women using HRT compared with nonusers. The rate of breast cancer development in women receiving HRT exceeded that of control patients after approximately 3–4 years of use.[90] Other studies have demonstrated similar patterns.[91,92] Breast cancer risk declines after HRT use is discontinued.

The association between OC use and breast cancer is less clear. A large meta-analysis of mostly case-control studies that included 53,297 women with breast cancer and 100,239 women without breast cancer demonstrated a relative risk for breast cancer of 1.24 in current users of OC.[93] The risk did not approach that of women who had never used OC until 10 or more years after use was discontinued. The median year of first use in these pooled studies was 1968, with the majority of breast cancers subsequently diagnosed in the 1980s. The majority of women included in these studies used OC when estrogen doses were much higher than in those currently marketed, making extrapolation of these results to modern OC difficult. In 1996, the reported increase in relative risk accounted for few additional cancer diagnoses as compared with women who had never used OC: 0.5, 1.5, and 4.7 additional cases per 10,000 women who used OC between the ages of 16–19, 20–24, and 25–29 years, respectively.[94] A 2002 case-control study that included 4,575 women with breast cancer and 4,682 without showed no increased risk with current or former OC use.[93] A more recent meta-analysis of over 850,000 women demonstrated an insignificant association between OC use and breast cancer among women who are BRCA1 or BRCA2 mutation carriers compared to the general population.[95]

There are multiple theories as to how hormones can cause breast cancer (Table 57-2). Estrogen metabolites may covalently bind to DNA and cause mutations.[96] In vitro, quinone metabolites of equine estrogens (present in the most common oral formulations of HRT) act as carcinogens and tumor promoters.[97] Estrogens, progestins, and their metabolites can act on estrogen and progesterone receptors (ER/PR) on breast cancer cells, stimulating proliferation.[98,99] This mechanism is supported by the observation that hormone use has been significantly associated with the development of ER/PR positive breast cancers in multiple studies.[90,100]

CLINICAL PRESENTATION AND DIFFERENTIAL DIAGNOSIS

Breast cancer most often presents as a painless lump within the breast tissue (Table 57-3). Any suspicious lump, whether painful or not, should be assessed by physical examination and imaged using mammography or other techniques, such as ultrasound. Breast cancer is confirmed by biopsy of affected tissue and nodes. Other conditions to consider in the differential diagnosis include benign breast disease or calcification and other malignancies. Although statistically significant increases in the risk of breast cancer are not typically found during the first 3–4 years of combination HRT, women have been diagnosed as early as during the first year.[90,94,100]

RISK FACTORS

Multiple risk factors associated with this hormone-induced malignancy are listed in Table 57-5. Although it appears that use of any HRT can lead to breast cancer, multiple studies have demonstrated an increased risk of all types of breast cancer in women receiving combination HRT as compared with estrogen-only HRT.[88,101-103]

A shorter time (<5 years) between menopause and HRT initiation is associated with a significant increase in the rate of breast cancer.[13] Incidence also increases linearly with greater cumulative exposure to HRT and with age.[91,103]

Although increased breast cancer risk ratios have been associated with obese, postmenopausal women who never took estrogen–progestin therapy, some studies have shown an inverse correlation between body-mass index (BMI; calculated as the weight in kilograms divided by the square of the height in meters) and risk, such that women taking HRT with a BMI <25 have a higher relative risk than those with BMI >25.[104,105]

Studies of risk in women with a family history of breast cancer or carriers of the BRCA1 mutation and the use of OC report conflicting results.[95]

MORBIDITY AND MORTALITY

The 5-year survival rate of American women with breast cancer ranges from close to 100% for those with stages 0 and I disease to 22% for those with metastatic disease.[106] Women receiving HRT in the WHI study were found to have tumors that were larger, more likely to be node-positive, and diagnosed at a more advanced stage than controls.[90] Data from a large prospective cohort of 374,465 women found that those who used combination HRT for at least 5 years had a relative risk of invasive tumor of 1.51 as compared with women who had never used HRT.[103] Consistent with these findings, a 2013 overview of the results from the two Women's Health Initiative hormone therapy trials with extended postintervention follow-up revealed not only an increased breast cancer incidence in women using HRT but also diagnoses at higher cancer stages.[107] Despite this reported increased risk of occurrence, other studies have shown a better prognosis for patients who have a history of HRT use, with higher overall and disease-free survival rates.[108,109] Schuetz et al.[110] reported 5-year survival rates of 92.8% and 82.2% in HRT users and nonusers, respectively; in addition, metastases were more likely to occur in non-HRT patients. Most recently, researchers have found that postmenopausal women in the WHI who used HRT for a median of 5.6 years did not have an increased risk of cancer mortality during a cumulative follow-up of 18 years.[111]

PREVENTION

Avoidance of HRT may prevent drug-induced breast cancer, and available evidence suggests that the benefits of HRT should be carefully weighed against the increased breast cancer risk.[112] Patients at highest risk for breast cancer, especially those with a personal history of breast cancer and those with a strong family history, could use ET to relieve moderate-to-severe menopausal symptoms. Patients who take ET should also be informed of the increased risk of endometrial cancer.[112] In the Million Women Study cohort, women who discontinued use of HRT for at least 1 year had a breast cancer risk comparable to that of women who had never used HRT.[88]

American Cancer Society recommendations for lowering breast cancer risk for all women includes maintaining a consistent healthy weight, incorporating 150 minutes of moderate or 75 minutes of vigorous activity each week, and limiting or avoiding alcohol use. Breastfeeding for several months following delivery may also lower breast cancer risk.[113]

MANAGEMENT

Estrogen and progestin products should be discontinued in any patient diagnosed with breast cancer. Appropriate treatment of any malignancy depends on multiple factors at diagnosis, including stage, patient age, and the presence of comorbidities. Surgical excision with radiation therapy is an option for localized disease. Estrogen antagonists, such as tamoxifen, and aromatase inhibitors may be used depending on the hormone receptor status of the cancer. Chemotherapy, usually taxane- and/or anthracycline-based regimens with or without trastuzumab, are indicated for many patients. Radiation therapy is also commonly used in many cases.[114]

INFORMATION FOR PATIENTS

Patients who are receiving or are considering taking estrogens or combined estrogen and progestin products should be educated regarding the risks and benefits of these medications, including the increased risk of breast cancer with HRT. An increased risk of breast cancer has been observed with many HRT regimens, and it can be concluded that none is without risk.[88,90] It is best, therefore, to avoid HRT preparations altogether whenever possible.

ENDOMETRIAL CANCER

Endometrial cancer, also referred to as uterine carcinoma, is the most common malignancy of the female genital tract in the United States. More than 61,000 women are diagnosed with endometrial cancer annually and nearly 11,000 of those die from the disease.[13]

CAUSATIVE AGENTS

Hormonal therapy with estrogen and tamoxifen, an antiestrogen, has been implicated in the development of endometrial cancer (Table 57-1).

EPIDEMIOLOGY

Approximately 75% of women with endometrial cancer are postmenopausal with the median age of diagnosis of 62 years. A diagnosis of endometrial cancer before the age of 40 years is uncommon, accounting for about 5% of endometrial cancer cases.[115] Women who have used estrogen-only HRT are reported to have a relative risk of 2.7 for endometrial cancer as opposed to those never exposed, with 22.6 and 8 carcinomas per 10,000 person-years, respectively.[116] There is a linear association between duration of estrogen use and increased risk of endometrial cancer, with relative risk rising by 0.58 for each year of use. In addition, an elevated risk of endometrial cancer remains even 10 years after discontinuation of estrogen-only HRT.

Patients who receive tamoxifen for breast cancer are also at risk for endometrial cancer. Studies have found a relative risk approximately 2–3 times higher than the risk in an age-matched population. The rate of endometrial cancer occurrence among patients taking tamoxifen 20 mg/day was 1.6 per 1,000 patient-years, compared to 0.2 per 1,000 patient-years among those taking placebo. Even though endometrial cancer risk is higher in tamoxifen users, the benefits of breast cancer survival outweigh the small risk of endometrial cancer. A study extending tamoxifen use to 10 years reported similar outcomes in terms of improved breast cancer survival versus a small risk of endometrial cancer development.[117]

MECHANISMS

Estrogen causes hyperplasia of the endometrium, which, if unchecked, can develop into cancer (Table 57-2). Progestins inhibit this growth, likely explaining why combination estrogen and progestin HRT imparts a lower risk of endometrial cancer than estrogen-alone HRT.

Tamoxifen has antiestrogen effects in the breast, yet also has agonist activity on the endometrium via ERs. The agonist effect in the endometrium can result in benign endometrial proliferation, hyperplasia, polyp formation, invasive carcinoma, or uterine sarcoma.[118] Another proposed mechanism by which tamoxifen is carcinogenic relates to its ability to cause DNA damage. Tamoxifen is metabolized to several estrogenic metabolites and reactive intermediates. These reactive intermediates may form protein or DNA adducts to cause DNA damage. Therefore, tamoxifen may also cause malignancy by genotoxicity.[118]

CLINICAL PRESENTATION AND DIFFERENTIAL DIAGNOSIS

Endometrial cancer can present as abnormal vaginal bleeding, dysuria, or pelvic pain (Table 57-3). Conditions to consider in the differential diagnosis include uterine fibroids, endometriosis, and pelvic inflammatory disease (Table 57-4). When endometrial cancer is suspected, a pelvic examination is typically the first diagnostic procedure performed. A Papanicolaou test might also be performed. The uterus can be imaged using transvaginal ultrasound, and the physician may perform a biopsy of the endometrial tissue.[119] In one case-control study, 40% of patients in whom endometrial cancer developed were diagnosed within 5 years of starting tamoxifen, 42% within 5–9 years of starting, and 18% after 10 or more years of treatment initiation.[120]

RISK FACTORS

Risk factors for drug-induced endometrial cancer are listed in Table 57-5. Longer duration of estrogen use is associated with increasing risk, with a relative risk of 1.4 after 1 year of use and 9.5 after 10 years of use as compared with those never treated with estrogen. Conjugated estrogens are associated with a higher risk of endometrial cancer than are synthetic estrogens, with relative risks of 2.5 and 1.3, respectively.[120]

Postmenopausal women with pre-existing abnormal endometrial pathologies may be more likely to have endometrial cancer after tamoxifen therapy than patients without these pathologies. The American College of Obstetricians and Gynecologists (ACOG) review of tamoxifen-induced endometrial cancer cases concluded that etiology may be both dose- and duration-dependent.[121] There are reports that patients who use tamoxifen at a higher dose (40 mg/day) are more likely to develop more aggressive tumors. There are two sets of data regarding duration of tamoxifen use in breast cancer patients: data for patients with 5 years of tamoxifen use and data for 10 years of tamoxifen use in postmenopausal women. Five years of adjuvant tamoxifen use produces an absolute 15-year endometrial cancer risk of about 2–3% and use for 10 years produces an additional risk by year 15 of about 2%.[117,122,123]

MORBIDITY AND MORTALITY

In general, the overall survival rates for endometrial cancer are favorable if diagnosed during an early stage (0–II). Overall 5-year survival decreases significantly in women diagnosed with stage III or IV disease. According to the American Cancer Society, the 5-year survival rates for stage III range from 47% to 58% and stage IV from 15% to17%.[124]

A review of three large case-control studies of tamoxifen-induced endometrial cancer (after 5 years of adjuvant therapy) revealed less favorable morphological subtypes of endometrial cancer than found in other populations and thus a relatively poor prognosis.[125] The 3-year survival in tamoxifen-induced endometrial cancer patients is 75% versus 94% in the general population. A large case-control study of endometrial cancer following tamoxifen use for breast cancer found that stage III and IV endometrial cancers occurred more frequently in long-term tamoxifen users than nonusers. The study also found that long-term users experienced significantly higher risk of developing malignant mixed mesodermal or sarcomas of the endometrium than those not taking tamoxifen (15.4% versus 2.9%; $P < 0.2$).[126]

PREVENTION

Multiple studies have demonstrated that women taking progestin with estrogen for at least 10 days per month do not have an elevated risk of endometrial cancer (Table 57-6).[120,127-129] Progestins counteract the proliferative effects of estrogen on endometrial tissue. However, combined estrogen–progestin HRT increases the risk of breast cancer, as previously described. Therefore, the risks and benefits of estrogen-only versus combination HRT must be carefully considered before either is used.

Avoiding the use of tamoxifen is the best method to prevent drug-induced endometrial cancer. Substitution of raloxifene can be considered in patients for whom tamoxifen is utilized as chemoprevention. Raloxifene is a selective ER modulator similar to tamoxifen; however, it does not exert the same degree of agonist effects on the uterus as tamoxifen. The Study of Tamoxifen and Raloxifene trial demonstrated raloxifene as a drug of choice for reducing the risk of breast cancer among postmenopausal women because of a better adverse event profile compared to tamoxifen.[130] Tamoxifen has been shown to be highly effective in treatment of ER+ breast cancer. The benefits and risks of its use must be weighed carefully on a case-by-case basis. Some studies suggest that the aromatase inhibitors may have efficacy in the treatment of ER+ breast cancer comparable to that of tamoxifen but without the risk of secondary endometrial cancer. Following discontinuation of tamoxifen, patients continue to have an increased risk of endometrial cancer for at least 5 years.[122]

MANAGEMENT

Endometrial cancer is primarily treated surgically with hysterectomy and bilateral salpingo-oophorectomy. Pelvic radiation or vaginal brachytherapy are adjuvant treatment options, depending on the stage of the disease. For more advanced stages of endometrial cancer, chemotherapy may be used. The NCCN provides the most up-to-date guidelines on the management of endometrial cancer.[114]

INFORMATION FOR PATIENTS

In 2014 the ACOG provided specific recommendations regarding the use of tamoxifen and the development of endometrial cancer. The guidance was in response to new data demonstrating benefit with tamoxifen use extended to 10 years in breast cancer. Recommendations include informing women about the risks of endometrial changes such as proliferation, endometrial hyperplasia, endometrial malignancy, and uterine sarcoma. Women should be advised to promptly report any abnormal vaginal bleeding, bloody vaginal discharge, or spotting. In addition, postmenopausal women taking tamoxifen should be closely monitored for symptoms of endometrial cancer or hyperplasia. Premenopausal women treated with tamoxifen have no increased risk of endometrial cancer and, therefore, require no additional monitoring beyond routine gynecologic care.[117]

Women taking estrogens should also be informed of their increased risk of endometrial cancer. If a decision is made to use one of the drugs known to increase the risk of endometrial cancer, patients should be advised to seek immediate medical attention if they experience symptoms of endometrial carcinoma. Patients should also understand the importance of undergoing an annual gynecologic examination.

BLADDER CANCER

According to the American Cancer Society, nearly 82,000 people in the United States are diagnosed with bladder cancer annually and approximately 17,000 of these will succumb to the disease. The median age of diagnosis is 65 years, and the disease is rarely diagnosed in individuals younger than 40 years of age. Currently, no established methods exist for screening or prevention.[131,132]

CAUSATIVE AGENTS

Cyclophosphamide has long been known to cause cancer of the bladder when used to treat malignant or nonmalignant conditions (Table 57-1). Another agent with links to bladder cancer is pioglitazone (an oral antidiabetic agent in the thiazolidinedione class). Although a link between pioglitazone and bladder cancer was not identified when the drug was approved in 1999, accumulating postmarketing evidence has led to an update in the package insert to reflect this cancer risk.[132,133]

EPIDEMIOLOGY

Risk for bladder cancer after cyclophosphamide use varies with cumulative drug dose.[134] NHL patients receiving 20–49 g of cyclophosphamide have a sixfold increased risk of bladder cancer; those receiving 50 g or more have a 14.5-fold increased risk as compared with controls.[135] In the noncancer setting, the absolute risk of bladder cancer in a cohort of patients treated with cyclophosphamide for granulomatosis with polyangiitis, formerly known as Wegener granulomatosis, was found to be 10% at 16 years after diagnosis.[136]

Postmarketing observational studies have suggested a link between long-term use (>24 months) of pioglitazone and the development of bladder cancer. One retrospective cohort from the French health insurance database demonstrated increased risk of bladder cancer (overall HR 1.22, 95% CI 1.05–1.43; exposure >24 months 1.34, 95% CI 1.04–1.79), which led to the suspension of pioglitazone use France in June 2011.[137,138] In 2003, the manufacturer and the FDA agreed to a 10-year observational study to evaluate the risk of bladder cancer with pioglitazone in diabetic patients. The 5-year interim analysis found that patients who received pioglitazone for longer than 24 months had a small but statistically significant elevated risk of bladder cancer (HR 1.4, 95% CI 1.0–2.0), a finding that has been confirmed in most, but not all, other studies. One study found patients who received pioglitazone for <24 months did not experience an increased risk and these authors concluded there was no statistically significant association between pioglitazone and bladder cancer.[139] However, in a study of 145,806 newly diagnosed diabetic patients treated with antidiabetic drugs and followed for 14 years, pioglitazone was associated with a 63% increased risk of bladder cancer. Rosiglitazone was not associated with increased risk, suggesting bladder cancer is drug-specific and not a class effect.[140] Pioglitazone is still available in the United States, and the package insert includes a warning regarding bladder cancer risk.[133,141]

MECHANISMS

Two metabolites of cyclophosphamide, acrolein and phosphoramide mustard, are thought to cause bladder cancer (Table 57-2). Both metabolites form DNA adducts, which can lead to mutation and subsequent carcinomatosis. Acrolein has been shown to cause urinary bladder papilloma formation in both animals and humans.[134] In one series, many samples of human bladder tumor tissue were found to contain mutations of tumor-suppressor gene *p53* that were consistent with known phosphoramide mustard–induced changes.[142]

The mechanism by which pioglitazone may induce bladder tumors has not been fully elucidated. One potential mechanism has been described from animal studies and involves the agonist nature of pioglitazone on the peroxisome proliferator-activated receptors (PPARs) found on urothelial cells. In theory, this direct agonist activity may be the cause of bladder carcinogenesis.[143,144]

CLINICAL PRESENTATION AND DIFFERENTIAL DIAGNOSIS

Symptoms of bladder cancer are very nonspecific and include hematuria and dysuria (Table 57-3). In patients with more advanced bladder cancer, upper obstruction or pain may also occur.[132]

RISK FACTORS

Higher cumulative doses of cyclophosphamide (both oral and intravenous), especially doses >20 g, place a patient at increased risk for bladder cancer (Table 57-5). In addition to dose-dependent risk, some literature suggests that antecedent hemorrhagic cystitis may be associated with a future increased risk of bladder cancer.[134] Cigarette smoking and aromatic amine exposure (from the manufacture of certain plastics, dyes, or pesticides) are additional risk factors for cancer of the bladder.[145] Pioglitazone use over 24 months has also been linked with increased risk of bladder cancer.[139,141]

MORBIDITY AND MORTALITY

Specific mortality rates from cyclophosphamide-induced bladder cancer have not been reported. In general, the 5-year survival rate for those diagnosed with local disease is good compared with those diagnosed with advanced disease. The 5-year survival rate for local disease is 70% versus 8% for advanced disease.[131]

PREVENTION

Methods to prevent cyclophosphamide-induced bladder cancer are presented in Table 57-6. Mesna, a drug commonly given in combination with high-dose cyclophosphamide to prevent hemorrhagic cystitis, has been associated with a reduction in the incidence of cyclophosphamide-induced bladder tumors in rats, although this effect has not been proven in humans.[146] There are no published data regarding the effect of mesna on the rate of secondary bladder cancer in patients so the use of mesna for this indication has not been established.[134]

Avoiding the use of cyclophosphamide may be the best preventive strategy when alternative therapies are available. When the drug must be given, using a cumulative dose of <20 g is desirable because this amount may not be associated with an increased relative risk of bladder cancer.[134,136] Patients who require prolonged treatment and cumulative doses of >20 g of cyclophosphamide could theoretically benefit from the concurrent administration of mesna, although, as noted, conclusive evidence is lacking.

Some literature suggests the risk of bladder cancer may increase with pioglitazone therapy lasting longer than 24 months. Therefore, prevention strategies would include avoiding the use of this medication or avoiding its use for >24 months.[133] Over the past decade several new agents have been approved for the management of type 2 diabetes mellitus. Therefore, pioglitazone avoidance is a reasonable option for healthcare professionals concerned with pioglitazone-associated bladder cancer.

MANAGEMENT

Transurethral tumor resection can be used for patients with localized bladder cancer. When the musculature of the bladder is involved, radical cystectomy is a common treatment. Patients may receive intravesical therapy with Bacillus Calmette-Guerin or intravesical chemotherapy in the adjuvant setting. Depending on the depth of invasion, neoadjuvant chemotherapy can be considered. Concomitant radiotherapy may also be used in select patients. The NCCN provides the most up-to-date guidelines for health professionals on the management of bladder cancer.[132]

INFORMATION FOR PATIENTS

Patients who receive cyclophosphamide or pioglitazone should be warned about the increased risk of bladder cancer. They should be advised to immediately report abnormal urinary symptoms, including hematuria and dysuria. Although there are no specific recommendations for bladder cancer screening, it may be reasonable to screen patients receiving long-term cyclophosphamide therapy using urinalysis and urine cytology.

REFERENCES

1. Gutierrez-Dalmau A, Campistol JM. Immunosuppressive therapy and malignancy in organ transplant recipients: a systematic review. *Drugs*. 2007; 67:1167-98.
2. Sheil AG, Disney AP, Mathew TH, Amiss N. De novo malignancy emerges as a major cause of morbidity and late failure in renal transplantation. *Transplant Proc*. 1993; 25:1383-4.
3. Giri S, Chi M, Johnson B et al. Secondary acute lymphoblastic leukemia is an independent predictor of poor prognosis. *Leuk Res*. 2015; 39:1342-6.
4. Arber DA, Orazi A, Hasserjian R et al. The 2016 revision to the world health organization classification of myeloid neoplasms and acute leukemia. *Blood*. 2016; 127:2391-405.
5. National Comprehensive Cancer Network. Myleodysplastic syndrome (Version 1.2018). https://www.nccn.org/professionals/physician_gls/pdf/mds.pdf (accessed 2018 Feb 9).
6. Chen Y, Sun J, Yang Y et al. Malignancy risk of anti-tumor necrosis factor alpha blockers: an overview of systematic reviews and meta-analyses. *Clin Rheumatol*. 2016; 35:1-18.
7. Leone G, Mele L, Pulsoni A et al. The incidence of secondary leukemias. *Haematologica*. 1999; 84:937-45.
8. Schneider DT, Hilgenfeld E, Schwabe D et al. Acute myelogenous leukemia after treatment for malignant germ cell tumors in children. *J Clin Oncol*. 1999; 17:3226-33.
9. Bhatia S, Robison LL, Oberlin O et al. Breast cancer and other second neoplasms after childhood Hodgkin's disease. *N Engl J Med*. 1996; 334:745-51.
10. Hijiya N, Ness KK, Ribeiro RC, Hudson MM. Acute leukemia as a secondary malignancy in children and adolescents: current findings and issues. *Cancer*. 2009; 115:23-35.
11. Pui CH, Ribeiro RC, Hancock ML et al. Acute myeloid leukemia in children treated with epipodophyllotoxins for acute lymphoblastic leukemia. *N Engl J Med*. 1991; 325:1682-7.
12. Smith MA, Rubinstein L, Anderson JR et al. Secondary leukemia or myelodysplastic syndrome after treatment with epipodophyllotoxins. *J Clin Oncol*. 1999; 17:569-77.
13. American Cancer Society. *Global cancer facts and figures*. 3rd ed. https://www.cancer.org/content/dam/cancer-org/research/cancer-facts-and-statistics/global-cancer-facts-and-figures/global-cancer-facts-and-figures-3rd-edition.pdf (accessed 2018 Feb 9).
14. Smith RE, Bryant J, DeCillis A, Anderson S. National Surgical Adjuvant Breast and Bowel Project Experience. Acute myeloid leukemia and myelodysplastic syndrome after doxorubicin-cyclophosphamide adjuvant therapy for operable breast cancer: the national surgical adjuvant breast and bowel project experience. *J Clin Oncol*. 2003; 21:1195-204.

15. Travis LB, Andersson M, Gospodarowicz M et al. Treatment-associated leukemia following testicular cancer. *J Natl Cancer Inst.* 2000; 92:1165-71.
16. Kwong YL. Azathioprine: association with therapy-related myelodysplastic syndrome and acute myeloid leukemia. *J Rheumatol.* 2010; 37:485-90.
17. Attal M, Lauwers-Cances V, Marit G et al. Lenalidomide maintenance after stem-cell transplantation for multiple myeloma. *N Engl J Med.* 2012; 366:1782-91.
18. Palumbo A, Hajek R, Delforge M et al. Continuous lenalidomide treatment for newly diagnosed multiple myeloma. *N Engl J Med.* 2012; 366:1759-69.
19. McCarthy PL, Owzar K, Hofmeister CC et al. Lenalidomide after stem-cell transplantation for multiple myeloma. *N Engl J Med.* 2012; 366:1770-81.
20. Pomalidomide package insert. Summit, NJ: Celgene Corp; 2016.
21. Thalomid package insert. Summit, NJ: Celgene; 1998.
22. Dimopoulos MA, Richardson PG, Brandenburg N et al. A review of second primary malignancy in patients with relapsed or refractory multiple myeloma treated with lenalidomide. *Blood.* 2012; 119:2764-7.
23. Lynparza package insert. Wilmington, DE: AstraZeneca Pharmaceutical LP; 2014.
24. Larson RA. Etiology and management of therapy-related myeloid leukemia. *Hematology Am Soc Hematol Educ Program.* 2007: 453-9.
25. Mehta HM, Malandra M, Corey SJ. G-CSF and GM-CSF in neutropenia. *J Immunol.* 2015; 195:1341-9.
26. Yang J, Terebelo HR, Zonder JA. Secondary primary malignancies in multiple myeloma: an old NEMESIS revisited. *Adv Hematol.* 2012; 2012:801495.
27. Raval G, Mehta P. TNF-alpha inhibitors: are they carcinogenic? *Drug Healthc Patient Saf.* 2010; 2:241-7.
28. Döhner H, Weisdorf DJ, Bloomfield CD. Acute myeloid leukemia. *N Engl J Med.* 2015 Sep 17; 373:1136-52.
29. National Comprehensive Cancer Network. Acute myeloid leukemia. Version 1, 2018. http://www.nccn.org/professionals/physician_gls/pdf/aml.pdf (accessed 2018 Feb 9).
30. Revlimid package insert. Summit, NJ: Celgene Corp; 2005.
31. US Food and Drug Administration. FDA drug safety communication: safety review update on reports of hepatosplenic T-cell lymphoma in adolescents and young adults receiving tumor necrosis factor (TNF) blockers, azathioprine and/or mercaptopurine. http://wayback.archive-it.org/7993/20161022203927/http://www.fda.gov/Drugs/DrugSafety/ucm250913.htm (accessed 2018 Feb 13).
32. Parakkal D, Sifuentes H, Semer R, Ehrenpreis ED. Hepatosplenic T-cell lymphoma in patients receiving TNF-alpha inhibitor therapy: expanding the groups at risk. *Eur J Gastroenterol Hepatol.* 2011; 23:1150-6.
33. Opelz G, Dohler B. Lymphomas after solid organ transplantation: a collaborative transplant study report. *Am J Transplant.* 2004; 4:222-30.
34. Opelz G, Schwarz V, Henderson R et al. Non-Hodgkin's lymphoma after kidney or heart transplantation: frequency of occurrence during the first posttransplant year. *Transpl Int.* 1994; 7 (suppl 1):S353-6.
35. Zortress package insert. East Hanover, NJ: Novartis Pharmaceuticals Corp; 2015.
36. Penn I. Cancers complicating organ transplantation. *N Engl J Med.* 1990; 323:1767-9.
37. Rasche L, Kapp M, Einsele H, Mielke S. EBV-induced post transplant lymphoproliferative disorders: a persisting challenge in allogeneic hematopoetic SCT. *Bone Marrow Transplant.* 2014; 49:163-7.
38. US Food and Drug Administration. Information for healthcare professionals: tumor necrosis factor (TNF) blockers (marketed as Remicade, Enbrel, Humira, Cimzia, and Simponi). http://wayback.archive-it.org/7993/20161022204118/http://www.fda.gov/Drugs/DrugSafety/PostmarketDrugSafetyInformationforPatientsandProviders/DrugSafetyInformationforHeathcareProfessionals/ucm174474.htm (accessed 2018 Feb 13).
39. Mariette X, Matucci-Cerinic M, Pavelka K et al. Malignancies associated with tumour necrosis factor inhibitors in registries and prospective observational studies: a systematic review and meta-analysis. *Ann Rheum Dis.* 2011; 70:1895-904.
40. Hojo M, Morimoto T, Maluccio M et al. Cyclosporine induces cancer progression by a cell-autonomous mechanism. *Nature.* 1999; 397:530-4.
41. Carswell EA, Old LJ, Kassel RL et al. An endotoxin-induced serum factor that causes necrosis of tumors. *Proc Natl Acad Sci USA.* 1975; 72:3666-70.
42. Cohen RB, Dittrich KA. Anti-TNF therapy and malignancy—a critical review. *Can J Gastroenterol.* 2001; 15:376-84.
43. Dantal J, Hourmant M, Cantarovich D et al. Effect of long-term immunosuppression in kidney-graft recipients on cancer incidence: randomised comparison of two cyclosporin regimens. *Lancet.* 1998; 351:623-8.
44. Swinnen LJ, Costanzo-Nordin MR, Fisher SG et al. Increased incidence of lymphoproliferative disorder after immunosuppression with the monoclonal antibody OKT3 in cardiac-transplant recipients. *N Engl J Med.* 1990; 323:1723-8.
45. Penn I. Malignancies induced by drug therapy: a review. *IARC Sci Publ.* 1986; 78:13-27.
46. Everly MJ, Bloom RD, Tsai DE, Trofe J. Posttransplant lymphoproliferative disorder. *Ann Pharmacother.* 2007; 41:1850-8.
47. Koyawala N, Silber JH, Rosenbaum PR et al. Comparing outcomes between antibody induction therapies in kidney transplantation. *J Am Soc Nephrol.* 2017; 28:2188-200.
48. Crespo-Leiro MG, Alonso-Pulpon L, Vazquez de Prada JA et al. Malignancy after heart transplantation: incidence, prognosis and risk factors. *Am J Transplant.* 2008; 8:1031-9.
49. Weikert BC, Blumberg EA. Viral infection after renal transplantation: surveillance and management. *Clin J Am Soc Nephrol.* 2008; 3(suppl 2):S76-86.
50. Dror Y, Greenberg M, Taylor G et al. Lymphoproliferative disorders after organ transplantation in children. *Transplantation.* 1999; 67:990-8.
51. Ganne V, Siddiqi N, Kamaplath B et al. Humanized anti-CD20 monoclonal antibody (rituximab) treatment for post-transplant lymphoproliferative disorder. *Clin Transplant.* 2003; 17:417-22.
52. Oertel SH, Verschuuren E, Reinke P et al. Effect of anti-CD 20 antibody rituximab in patients with post-transplant lymphoproliferative disorder (PTLD). *Am J Transplant.* 2005; 5:2901-6.
53. Garrett TJ, Chadburn A, Barr ML et al. Posttransplantation lymphoproliferative disorders treated with cyclophosphamide-doxorubicin-vincristine-prednisone chemotherapy. *Cancer.* 1993; 72:2782-5.
54. Fohrer C, Caillard S, Koumarianou A et al. Long-term survival in post-transplant lymphoproliferative disorders with a dose-adjusted ACVBP regimen. *Br J Haematol.* 2006; 134:602-12.
55. Suryanarayan K, Natkunam Y, Berry G et al. Modified cyclophosphamide, hydroxydaunorubicin, vincristine, and prednisone therapy for posttransplantation lymphoproliferative disease in pediatric patients undergoing solid organ transplantation. *J Pediatr Hematol Oncol.* 2001; 23:452-5.
56. Chockalingam R, Downing C, Tyring SK. Cutaneous squamous cell carcinomas in organ transplant recipients. *J Clin Med.* 2015; 4:1229-39.
57. Kaae J, Boyd HA, Hansen AV et al. Photosensitizing medication use and risk of skin cancer. *Cancer Epidemiol Biomarkers Prev.* 2010; 19:2942-9.
58. Robinson SN, Zens MS, Perry AE et al. Photosensitizing agents and the risk of non-melanoma skin cancer: a population-based case-control study. *J Invest Dermatol.* 2013; 133:1950-5.
59. Penn I. Post-transplant malignancy: the role of immunosuppression. *Drug Saf.* 2000; 23:101-13.

60. Fortina AB, Piaserico S, Caforio AL et al. Immunosuppressive level and other risk factors for basal cell carcinoma and squamous cell carcinoma in heart transplant recipients. *Arch Dermatol.* 2004; 140:1079-85.
61. Moloney FJ, Comber H, O'Lorcain P et al. A population-based study of skin cancer incidence and prevalence in renal transplant recipients. *Br J Dermatol.* 2006; 154:498-504.
62. Leisenring W, Friedman DL, Flowers ME et al. Nonmelanoma skin and mucosal cancers after hematopoietic cell transplantation. *J Clin Oncol.* 2006; 24:1119-26.
63. Su F, Viros A, Milagre C et al. RAS mutations in cutaneous squamous-cell carcinomas in patients treated with BRAF inhibitors. *N Engl J Med.* 2012; 366:207-15.
64. Cotellic package insert. San Francisco, CA: Genentech Pharmaceuticals Corp; 2016.
65. Mekinist package insert. East Hanover, NJ: Novartis Pharmaceuticals Corp; 2017.
66. Tafinlar package insert. East Hanover, NJ: Novartis Pharmaceuticals Corp; 2017.
67. Zelboraf package insert. San Francisco, CA: Genentech Pharmaceuticals Corp; 2017.
68. Duffield-Lillico AJ, Slate EH, Reid ME et al. Selenium supplementation and secondary prevention of nonmelanoma skin cancer in a randomized trial. *J Natl Cancer Inst.* 2003; 95:1477-81.
69. Pfister H. Chapter 8: Human papillomavirus and skin cancer. *J Natl Cancer Inst Monogr.* 2003; 31:52-6.
70. Anforth R, Menzies A, Byth K et al. Factors influencing the development of cutaneous squamous cell carcinoma in patients on BRAF inhibitor therapy. *J Am Acad Dermatol.* 2015; 72:809-15.e1.
71. Danziger-Isakov L, Kumar D, AST Infectious diseases community of practice. Vaccination in solid organ transplantation. *Am J Transplant.* 2013; 13(suppl 4):311-17.
72. Falchook GS, Rady P, Konopinski JC et al. Merkel cell polyomavirus and human papilloma virus in proliferative skin lesions arising in patients treated with BRAF inhibitors. *Arch Dermatol Res.* 2016; 308:357-65.
73. Nordgaard-Lassen I, Dahlerup JF, Belard E et al. Guidelines for screening, prophylaxis and critical information prior to initiating anti-TNF-alpha treatment. *Dan Med J.* 2012; 59:C4480.
74. Askling J, Fahrbach K, Nordstrom B et al. Cancer risk with tumor necrosis factor alpha (TNF) inhibitors: meta-analysis of randomized controlled trials of adalimumab, etanercept, and infliximab using patient level data. *Pharmacoepidemiol Drug Saf.* 2011; 20:119-30.
75. Glover MT, Deeks JJ, Raftery MJ et al. Immunosuppression and risk of non-melanoma skin cancer in renal transplant recipients. *Lancet.* 1997; 349:398.
76. Kauffman HM, Cherikh WS, Cheng Y et al. Maintenance immunosuppression with target-of-rapamycin inhibitors is associated with a reduced incidence of de novo malignancies. *Transplantation.* 2005; 80:883-9.
77. Singh JA, Hossain A, Tanjong Ghogomu E et al. Biologics or tofacitinib for rheumatoid arthritis in incomplete responders to methotrexate or other traditional disease-modifying anti-rheumatic drugs: A SYStematic review and network meta-analysis. *Cochrane Database Syst Rev.* 2016; 5:CD012183.
78. Martinez JC, Otley CC, Stasko T et al. Defining the clinical course of metastatic skin cancer in organ transplant recipients: a multicenter collaborative study. *Arch Dermatol.* 2003; 139:301-6.
79. Mercer LK, Lunt M, Low AL et al. Risk of solid cancer in patients exposed to anti-tumour necrosis factor therapy: results from the British Society for Rheumatology biologics register for rheumatoid arthritis. *Ann Rheum Dis.* 2015; 74:1087-93.
80. Ducroux E, Martin C, Bouwes Bavinck JN et al. Risk of aggressive skin cancers after kidney retransplantation in patients with previous posttransplant cutaneous squamous cell carcinomas: a retrospective study of 53 cases. *Transplantation.* 2017; 101:e133-41.
81. O'Neill JO, Edwards LB, Taylor DO. Mycophenolate mofetil and risk of developing malignancy after orthotopic heart transplantation: analysis of the transplant registry of the International Society for Heart and Lung Transplantation. *J Heart Lung Transplant.* 2006; 25:1186-91.
82. Perez HC, Benavides X, Perez JS et al. Basic aspects of the pathogenesis and prevention of non-melanoma skin cancer in solid organ transplant recipients: a review. *Int J Dermatol.* 2017; 56:370-8.
83. Mathew T, Kreis H, Friend P. Two-year incidence of malignancy in sirolimus-treated renal transplant recipients: results from five multicenter studies. *Clin Transplant.* 2004; 18:446-9.
84. American Cancer Society. Treating melanoma skin cancer. https://www.cancer.org/cancer/melanoma-skin-cancer/treating.html (accessed 2018 Feb 13).
85. Tang N, Ratner D. Managing cutaneous side effects from targeted molecular inhibitors for melanoma and nonmelanoma skin cancer. *Dermatol Surg.* 2016; 42(suppl 1):S40-8.
86. Otley CC, Berg D, Ulrich C et al. Reduction of immunosuppression for transplant-associated skin cancer: expert consensus survey. *Br J Dermatol.* 2006; 154:395-400.
87. Collaborative Group on Hormonal Factors in Breast Cancer. Breast cancer and hormone replacement therapy: collaborative reanalysis of data from 51 epidemiological studies of 52,705 women with breast cancer and 108,411 women without breast cancer. *Lancet.* 1997; 350:1047-59.
88. Beral V, Million Women Study Collaborators. Breast cancer and hormone-replacement therapy in the Mllion Women Study. *Lancet.* 2003; 362:419-27.
89. Rossouw JE, Anderson GL, Prentice RL et al. Risks and benefits of estrogen plus progestin in healthy postmenopausal women: principal results from the Women's Health Initiative randomized controlled trial. *JAMA.* 2002; 288:321-33.
90. Chlebowski RT, Hendrix SL, Langer RD et al. Influence of estrogen plus progestin on breast cancer and mammography in healthy postmenopausal women: the Women's Health Initiative randomized trial. *JAMA.* 2003; 289:3243-53.
91. Newcomer LM, Newcomb PA, Potter JD et al. Postmenopausal hormone therapy and risk of breast cancer by histologic type (United States). *Cancer Causes Control.* 2003; 14:225-33.
92. Rosenberg LU, Magnusson C, Lindstrom E et al. Menopausal hormone therapy and other breast cancer risk factors in relation to the risk of different histological subtypes of breast cancer: a case-control study. *Breast Cancer Res.* 2006; 8:R11.
93. Marchbanks PA, McDonald JA, Wilson HG et al. Oral contraceptives and the risk of breast cancer. *N Engl J Med.* 2002; 346:2025-32.
94. Collaborative Group on Hormonal Factors in Breast Cancer. Breast cancer and hormonal contraceptives: collaborative reanalysis of individual data on 53 297 women with breast cancer and 100 239 women without breast cancer from 54 epidemiological studies. *Lancet.* 1996; 347:1713-27.
95. Moorman PG, Havrilesky LJ, Gierisch JM et al. Oral contraceptives and risk of ovarian cancer and breast cancer among high-risk women: a systematic review and meta-analysis. *J Clin Oncol.* 2013; 31:4188-98.
96. Yager JD. Endogenous estrogens as carcinogens through metabolic activation. *J Natl Cancer Inst Monogr.* 2000; 27:67-73.
97. Pisha E, Lui X, Constantinou AI, Bolton JL. Evidence that a metabolite of equine estrogens, 4-hydroxyequilenin, induces cellular transformation in vitro. *Chem Res Toxicol.* 2001; 14:82-90.
98. Yager JD, Davidson NE. Estrogen carcinogenesis in breast cancer. *N Engl J Med.* 2006; 354:270-82.
99. Bolton JL, Thatcher GR. Potential mechanisms of estrogen quinone carcinogenesis. *Chem Res Toxicol.* 2008; 21:93-101.
100. Chen WY, Manson JE, Hankinson SE et al. Unopposed estrogen therapy and the risk of invasive breast cancer. *Arch Intern Med.* 2006; 166:1027-32.

101. Schairer C, Lubin J, Troisi R et al. Menopausal estrogen and estrogen-progestin replacement therapy and breast cancer risk. *JAMA*. 2000; 283:485-91.
102. Ross RK, Paganini-Hill A, Wan PC, Pike MC. Effect of hormone replacement therapy on breast cancer risk: estrogen versus estrogen plus progestin. *J Natl Cancer Inst*. 2000; 92:328-32.
103. Kerlikowske K, Miglioretti DL, Ballard-Barbash R et al. Prognostic characteristics of breast cancer among postmenopausal hormone users in a screened population. *J Clin Oncol*. 2003; 21:4314-21.
104. Munsell MF, Sprague BL, Berry DA et al. Body mass index and breast cancer risk according to postmenopausal estrogen-progestin use and hormone receptor status. *Epidemiol Rev*. 2014; 36:114-36.
105. Lahmann PH, Hoffmann K, Allen N et al. Body size and breast cancer risk: findings from the European Prospective Investigation Into Cancer and Nutrition (EPIC). *Int J Cancer*. 2004; 111:762-71.
106. American Cancer Society. Breast Cancer Survival Rates. https://www.cancer.org/cancer/breast-cancer/understanding-a-breast-cancer-diagnosis/breast-cancer-survival-rates.html (accessed 2018 Feb 13).
107. Manson JE, Chlebowski RT, Stefanick ML et al. Menopausal hormone therapy and health outcomes during the intervention and extended poststopping phases of the Women's Health Initiative randomized trials. *JAMA*. 2013; 310:1353-68.
108. Christante D, Pommier S, Garreau J et al. Improved breast cancer survival among hormone replacement therapy users is durable after 5 years of additional follow-up. *Am J Surg*. 2008; 196:505-11.
109. Cheek J, Lacy J, Toth-Fejel S et al. The impact of hormone replacement therapy on the detection and stage of breast cancer. *Arch Surg*. 2002; 137:1015-9; discussion 1019-21.
110. Schuetz F, Diel IJ, Pueschel M et al. Reduced incidence of distant metastases and lower mortality in 1072 patients with breast cancer with a history of hormone replacement therapy. *Am J Obstet Gynecol*. 2007; 196:342.e1-342.e9.
111. Manson JE, Aragaki AK, Rossouw JE et al. Menopausal hormone therapy and long-term all-cause and cause-specific mortality: the Women's Health Initiative randomized trials. *JAMA*. 2017; 318:927-38.
112. American Cancer Society. Menopausal hormone therapy and cancer risk. https://www.cancer.org/cancer/cancer-causes/medical-treatments/menopausal-hormone-replacement-therapy-and-cancer-risk.html (accessed 2018 Feb 13).
113. American Cancer Society. Breast cancer risk and prevention. https://www.cancer.org/cancer/breast-cancer/risk-and-prevention/can-i-lower-my-risk.html (accessed 2018 Feb 13).
114. National Comprehensive Cancer Network. Breast cancer (Version 4.2018 – February 7, 2018). http://www.nccn.org/professionals/physician_gls/pdf/breast.pdf (accessed 2018 Feb 13).
115. National Comprehensive Cancer Network. Uterine cancer (Version 1.2018). http://www.nccn.org/professionals/physician_gls/pdf/uterine.pdf (accessed 2018 Feb 6).
116. Lacey JV Jr, Brinton LA, Lubin JH et al. Endometrial carcinoma risks among menopausal estrogen plus progestin and unopposed estrogen users in a cohort of postmenopausal women. *Cancer Epidemiol Biomarkers Prev*. 2005; 14:1724-31.
117. Committee Opinion No. 601. Tamoxifen and uterine cancer. *Obstet Gynecol*. 2014; 123:1394-7.
118. Hu R, Hilakivi-Clarke L, Clarke R. Molecular mechanisms of tamoxifen-associated endometrial cancer (review). *Oncol Lett*. 2015; 9:1495-501.
119. Visser NCM, Reijnen C, Massuger LFAG et al. Accuracy of endometrial sampling in endometrial carcinoma: a systematic review and meta-analysis. *Obstet Gynecol*. 2017; 130:803-13.
120. Grady D, Gebretsadik T, Kerlikowske K et al. Hormone replacement therapy and endometrial cancer risk: a meta-analysis. *Obstet Gynecol*. 1995; 85:304-13.
121. Berliere M, Charles A, Galant C, Donnez J. Uterine side effects of tamoxifen: a need for systematic pretreatment screening. *Obstet Gynecol*. 1998; 91:40-4.
122. Swerdlow AJ, Jones ME, British Tamoxifen Second Cancer Study Group. Tamoxifen treatment for breast cancer and risk of endometrial cancer: a case-control study. *J Natl Cancer Inst*. 2005; 97:375-84.
123. Davies C, Pan H, Godwin J et al. Long-term effects of continuing adjuvant tamoxifen to 10 years versus stopping at 5 years after diagnosis of oestrogen receptor-positive breast cancer: ATLAS, a randomised trial. *Lancet*. 2013; 381:805-16.
124. American Cancer Society. Endometrial cancer survival rates, by stage. https://www.cancer.org/cancer/endometrial-cancer/detection-diagnosis-staging/survival-rates.html (accessed 2018 Feb 9).
125. Jones ME, van Leeuwen FE, Hoogendoorn WE et al. Endometrial cancer survival after breast cancer in relation to tamoxifen treatment: pooled results from three countries. *Breast Cancer Res*. 2012; 14:R91.
126. Bland AE, Calingaert B, Secord AA et al. Relationship between tamoxifen use and high risk endometrial cancer histologic types. *Gynecol Oncol*. 2009; 112:150-4.
127. Lacey JV Jr, Leitzmann MF, Chang SC et al. Endometrial cancer and menopausal hormone therapy in the National Institutes of Health-AARP diet and health study cohort. *Cancer*. 2007; 109:1303-11.
128. Doherty JA, Cushing-Haugen KL, Saltzman BS et al. Long-term use of postmenopausal estrogen and progestin hormone therapies and the risk of endometrial cancer. *Am J Obstet Gynecol*. 2007; 197:139.e1-139.e7.
129. Pike MC, Peters RK, Cozen W et al. Estrogen-progestin replacement therapy and endometrial cancer. *J Natl Cancer Inst*. 1997; 89:1110-6.
130. Vogel VG. The NSABP study of tamoxifen and raloxifene (STAR) trial. *Expert Rev Anticancer Ther*. 2009; 9:51-60.
131. American Cancer Society. Cancer facts and figures. https://www.cancer.org/content/dam/cancer-org/research/cancer-facts-and-statistics/annual-cancer-facts-and-figures/2018/cancer-facts-and-figures-2018.pdf (accessed 2018 Feb 9).
132. National Comprehensive Cancer Network. Bladder cancer (Version 2.2018). http://www.nccn.org/professionals/physician_gls/pdf/bladder.pdf (accessed 2018 Feb 9).
133. Actos package insert. Deerfield, IL: Takeda Pharmaceuticals; 2017.
134. Monach PA, Arnold LM, Merkel PA. Incidence and prevention of bladder toxicity from cyclophosphamide in the treatment of rheumatic diseases: a data-driven review. *Arthritis Rheum*. 2010; 62:9-21.
135. Travis LB, Curtis RE, Glimelius B et al. Bladder and kidney cancer following cyclophosphamide therapy for non-Hodgkin's lymphoma. *J Natl Cancer Inst*. 1995; 87:524-30.
136. Knight A, Askling J, Granath F et al. Urinary bladder cancer in Wegener's granulomatosis: risks and relation to cyclophosphamide. *Ann Rheum Dis*. 2004; 63:1307-11.
137. Azoulay L, Yin H, Filion KB et al. The use of pioglitazone and the risk of bladder cancer in people with type 2 diabetes: nested case-control study. *BMJ*. 2012; 344:e3645.
138. US Food and Drug Administration. FDA drug safety communication: ongoing safety review of actos (pioglitazone) and potential increased risk of bladder cancer after two years exposure. http://www.fda.gov/drugs/DrugSafety/ucm226214.htm (accessed 2018 Jul 27).
139. Lewis JD, Ferrara A, Peng T et al. Risk of bladder cancer among diabetic patients treated with pioglitazone: interim report of a longitudinal cohort study. *Diabetes Care*. 2011; 34:916-22.
140. Tuccori M, Filion KB, Yin H et al. Pioglitazone use and risk of bladder cancer: population based cohort study. *BMJ*. 2016; 352:i1541.
141. Lewis JD, Habel LA, Quesenberry CP et al. Pioglitazone use and risk of bladder cancer and other common cancers in persons with diabetes. *JAMA*. 2015; 314:265-77.

142. Talar-Williams C, Hijazi YM, Walther MM et al. Cyclophosphamide-induced cystitis and bladder cancer in patients with Wegener granulomatosis. *Ann Intern Med.* 1996; 124:477-84.
143. Yoshimura R, Matsuyama M, Segawa Y et al. Expression of peroxisome proliferator-activated receptors (PPARs) in human urinary bladder carcinoma and growth inhibition by its agonists. *Int J Cancer.* 2003; 104:597-602.
144. Guan YF, Zhang YH, Breyer RM et al. Expression of peroxisome proliferator-activated receptor gamma (PPARgamma) in human transitional bladder cancer and its role in inducing cell death. *Neoplasia.* 1999; 1:330-9.
145. Pelucchi C, Bosetti C, Negri E et al. Mechanisms of disease: the epidemiology of bladder cancer. *Nat Clin Pract Urol.* 2006; 3:327-40.
146. Habs MR, Schmahl D. Prevention of urinary bladder tumors in cyclophosphamide-treated rats by additional medication with the uroprotectors sodium 2-mercaptoethane sulfonate (mesna) and disodium 2,2'-dithio-bis-ethane sulfonate (dimesna). *Cancer.* 1983; 51:606-9.
147. Wolff AC, Blackford AL, Visvanathan K et al. Risk of marrow neoplasms after adjuvant breast cancer therapy: the National Comprehensive Cancer Network experience. *J Clin Oncol.* 2015; 33:340-8.
148. Na R, Laaksonen MA, Grulich AE et al. Iatrogenic immunosuppression and risk of non-Hodgkin lymphoma in solid organ transplantation: a population-based cohort study in Australia. *Br J Haematol.* 2016; 174:550-62.
149. Hall EC, Engels EA, Pfeiffer RM, Segev DL. Association of antibody induction immunosuppression with cancer after kidney transplantation. *Transplantation.* 2015; 99:1051-7.
150. Crespo-Leiro MG, Alonso-Pulpon L, Arizon JM et al. Influence of induction therapy, immunosuppressive regimen and anti-viral prophylaxis on development of lymphomas after heart transplantation: data from the Spanish post-heart transplant tumour registry. *J Heart Lung Transplant.* 2007; 26:1105-9.
151. Maxwell LJ, Zochling J, Boonen A et al. TNF-alpha inhibitors for ankylosing spondylitis. *Cochrane Database Syst Rev.* 2015; (4):CD005468.
152. Coghill AE, Johnson LG, Berg D et al. Immunosuppressive medications and squamous cell skin carcinoma: nested case-control study within the Skin Cancer after Organ Transplant (SCOT) cohort. *Am J Transplant.* 2016; 16:565-73.
153. Su F, Viros A, Milagre C et al. RAS mutations in cutaneous squamous-cell carcinomas in patients treated with BRAF inhibitors. *N Engl J Med.* 2012; 366:207-15.
154. Frei U, Bode U, Repp H et al. Malignancies under cyclosporine after kidney transplantation: analysis of a 10-year period. *Transplant Proc.* 1993; 25(1 Pt 2):1394-6.
155. Asgari MM, Efird JT, Warton EM, Friedman GD. Potential risk factors for cutaneous squamous cell carcinoma include oral contraceptives: results of a nested case-control study. *Int J Environ Res Public Health.* 2010; 7:427-42.
156. Applebaum KM, Nelson HH, Zens MS et al. Oral contraceptives: a risk factor for squamous cell carcinoma? *J Invest Dermatol.* 2009; 129:2760-5.
157. Marcen R, Galeano C, Fernandez-Rodriguez A et al. Effects of the new immunosuppressive agents on the occurrence of malignancies after renal transplantation. *Transplant Proc.* 2010; 42:3055-7.
158. Cowlrick I, Delventhal H, Kaipainen K et al. Three-year follow-up of malignancies in tacrolimus-treated renal recipients—an analysis of European multicentre studies. *Clin Transplant.* 2008; 22:372-7.
159. Raaschou P, Simard JF, Asker Hagelberg C et al. Rheumatoid arthritis, anti-tumour necrosis factor treatment, and risk of squamous cell and basal cell skin cancer: cohort study based on nationwide prospectively recorded data from Sweden. *BMJ.* 2016; 352:i262.
160. Feist A, Lee R, Osborne S et al. Increased incidence of cutaneous squamous cell carcinoma in lung transplant recipients taking long-term voriconazole. *J Heart Lung Transplant.* 2012; 31:1177-81.
161. Nolvadex package insert. Wilmington, DE: AstraZeneca Pharmaceutical LP; 2004.

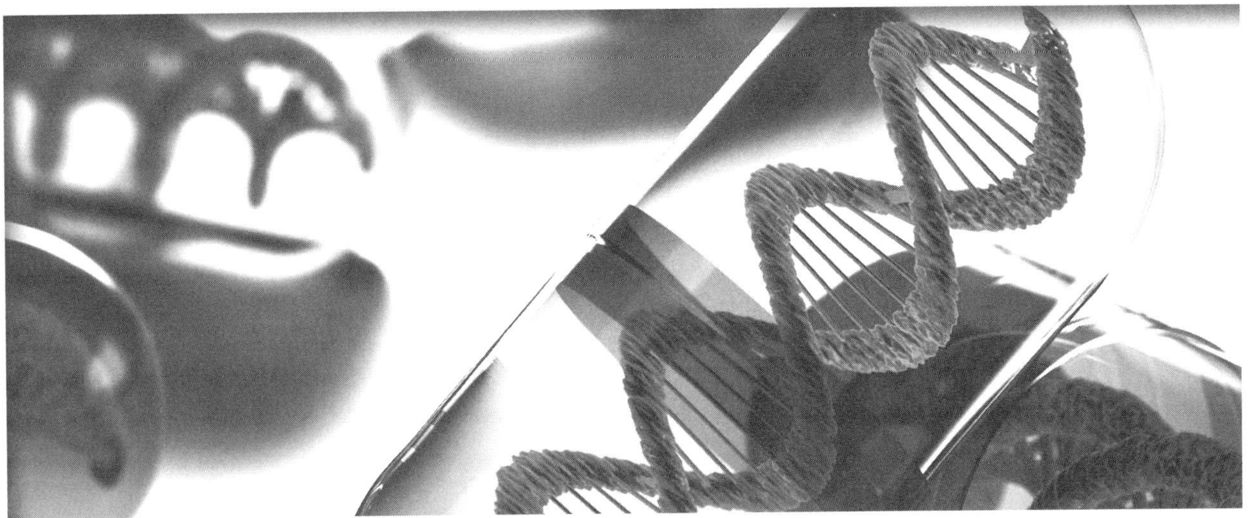

CHAPTER 58

Teratogenicity

Kylie N. Barnes

Teratogenic exposure is defined as exposure to an exogenous agent that can modify normal embryonic or fetal functional or structural development.[1] An exposure to a substance may increase risk; however, some exposures may have no impact at all. When evaluating the risk of drug-induced teratogenicity, it is important to consider exposure level, which includes the dose of the drug and the extent to which a patient may be concomitantly exposed to other substances associated with the same developmental risks. For example, a pregnant woman who is a cigarette smoker (known to be associated with low birth weight) exposed to a drug known to increase the risk for low birth weight is at greater risk of having a low birth weight infant born as a result of the exposure to two teratogens.[2] Although teratogenic exposure is often associated principally with an increased risk of major congenital anomalies (defects incompatible with life or requiring major corrective surgery), they are also associated with an increased risk for adverse pregnancy outcomes, including spontaneous abortion, stillbirth, minor structural anomalies (e.g., ear tags, extra digits, bent or curved fingers known as clinodactyly), preterm birth, intrauterine growth restrictions (IUGRs), and behavioral or cognitive deficits.

Some prescription and over-the-counter medications can be teratogenic. Additionally, recreational drugs, alcohol, nicotine, some chemicals, maternal infections and conditions during pregnancy, chromosomal disorders, and heredity may also have a negative impact on fetal development.[2-7] Due to ethical concerns, clinical studies specifically evaluating drug-induced teratogenicity in humans are lacking, and information regarding patients' direct exposure to medications during pregnancy can be limited.

For many medications, information regarding effects on pregnancy and the developing fetus are based on experimental animal studies and human data are unavailable. Animal data can be useful in indicating potential adverse effects; however, interpretation of this information requires an understanding of the differences in pharmacokinetics of the drug in the animal model and in humans, and that information is not always available. Although case reports of adverse effects of medications administered during pregnancy are available in the medical literature and/or through U.S. Food and Drug Administration (FDA) surveillance documents, these reports often lack critical information regarding concomitant exposure to other potential teratogens and potential environmental exposures. As a result, causality assessment is often very difficult. In 1965, a list of criteria for causation was published that focuses on the strength of association, consistency of the association, specificity, temporal relationship, coherence, biologic gradient, biologic plausibility, experimentation and analogy assessing other cause-effect relationships. This list for causation is often used as a baseline for practitioners to help assess teratogenic causality.[8] All criteria do not have to be met to consider an association as causal; however, the more criteria met, the greater the odds of causal relationship. In all cases, it is also important to take into consideration maternal physiological changes and their impact on drug metabolism, the fetal developmental stage at the time of proposed drug exposure, and the impact confounding variables may have on the fetus.

Retrospective and prospective data are also available from pregnancy registries that collect information regarding exposure to specific drugs or groups of drugs. Typically these registries monitor for major birth defects and can be good sources of early information regarding a new drug. Although sample size in these registries is often insufficient to prove an association between a suspect drug and a teratogenic effect, trends may be identified.

Case-controlled studies that retrospectively evaluate a specific outcome or a particular birth defect are available for some medications, and these often allow for collection of information about potential confounding variables (e.g., age; socioeconomic status; use of alcohol, tobacco, and/or illicit drugs). A major limitation in case-controlled studies is recall bias wherein women who have a negative pregnancy outcome are more likely to recall details of their pregnancy and exposures than those who had a normal outcome. It is also difficult to evaluate an agent for increased risk retrospectively, when the full pattern of the anomaly is not well understood.

Because specific, unambiguous data regarding a medication's potential for teratogenicity are not always available, evaluating the risk versus benefit of using a given drug to treat a specific condition in a given patient can constitute a significant challenge for clinicians.

HISTORY AND REVIEW OF TERATOGENICITY

Prior to the 1940s, it was generally believed the placenta provided a protective barrier for the developing embryo and fetus. Naively, clinicians believed that mothers could be exposed to agents and they would not impact normal gestational development. An Australian ophthalmologist, Norman Gregg, first raised the idea that exposure to an agent during pregnancy could cause harm to the developing fetus after he noticed an increasing number of children diagnosed with congenital cataracts shortly after a rubella epidemic. His findings led to further investigations that identified additional developmental abnormalities associated with fetal rubella infection, including congenital heart defects, hearing deficits, poor growth, and thrombocytopenia.[9]

During the early 1960s, an Australian obstetrician and a German geneticist together observed that first trimester maternal use of thalidomide, a sedative-hypnotic agent, was associated with the appearance of a characteristic pattern of limb reduction anomalies and other defects.[10,11] Thalidomide had undergone testing in rodents during product development and had not shown any effect on limbs. Early studies were not well conducted, however, and later work revealed intravenous administration of thalidomide in rats produced skeletal abnormalities involving the ribs, vertebra, hips, and tail.[12] Additional studies in rabbits showed an increased sensitivity to thalidomide embryo toxicity as compared to rats, a difference that was determined to be due to pharmacokinetic variation between the species.[12] As a result of slow detection of risk, many babies were born with severe deformities of the arms and legs, as well as other life-altering malformations. This finding led to the realization that therapeutic agents could induce malformations and cause harm. New concerns regarding other drugs and potential for harm began surfacing.

Today, many obstetricians and other healthcare providers instruct patients to avoid exposure to all medications during pregnancy due to concerns for potential harm to the developing fetus. Despite this advice, drug use during pregnancy is fairly common. Studies have shown that approximately 70% of women use at least one prescription medication during their pregnancy and over 90% use at least one prescription or an over-the-counter medication.[13] In many cases, these medications are essential for the health of the mother or fetus; however, in other cases, the exposure could be avoided.

Roughly 50% of women of reproductive age rely on the Internet for their health information, and they are more likely to share prescription medications with and/or borrow prescription medications from others. These factors increase concern regarding medication exposure during pregnancy—especially exposure that may occur before the pregnancy is known.[14]

In this chapter, we focus on mechanisms of placental drug transfer and the drugs known to cause major fetal structural or functional abnormalities. Birth defects that are due to other causes (e.g., hereditary, chromosomal deficits, maternal illness, or chronic conditions) will be noted when known to have a significant impact on fetal development.

MECHANISMS OF PLACENTAL TRANSFER

Classification of mammalian placentas is based on the number of layers between maternal and fetal blood; the layers include the hemochorial (rat, rabbit, guinea pig), endotheliochorial (cat, dog), and epitheliochorial (sheep, pig, horse).[15] Human placentas are of the hemochorial type in which fetal tissue is in direct contact with maternal blood.[15] The different structural types of the various mammalian placentas affects their function, including the transfer and metabolism of drugs. Variation makes it difficult to utilize data from animal studies to predict how a human fetus might respond to maternal drug exposure. This variability also helps explain why data may show no fetal impact of drug exposure during pregnancy in one species but significant impact in others.

The human placenta begins forming during early pregnancy at the point of implantation, just shortly after conception, and immediately helps with general nutrient exchange between the mother and fetus. By the end of the first trimester, the placental circulation has fully developed, and the placenta separates the blood supplies from the mother and the fetus.[16] The placenta receives its own blood supply and perfusion by both the mother and fetal circulations. The main purpose of the placenta is to provide nourishment and oxygen to the fetus. Many nutrients, including glucose, amino acids, and vitamins are delivered through the placenta from the mother to the fetus through specific transport mechanisms. The placenta also helps facilitate the removal of metabolic waste products from fetal blood, delivering the waste to the maternal circulation for removal. The placenta undergoes significant change throughout pregnancy. As pregnancy progresses, the placenta thins and increases in surface area to keep up with the nutritional and energy demands of the growing fetus. At 28 weeks gestation, the average placental exchange area is 3.4 m^2 and increases to an impressive 12.6 m^2 by term. The diffusion distance is also impacted throughout the pregnancy, starting at 50–100 micrometers around 8 weeks, decreasing to 4–5 micrometers at pregnancy term.[16]

Almost all drugs the mother takes during pregnancy will enter into fetal circulation via passive diffusion through the placenta, although the extent varies. Additionally, there are active transporters on both the fetal and maternal side of the placenta that actively pump some drugs across the placenta.[17] The extent of placental transfer depends on the molecular weight of the drug, the extent of drug binding to the plasma protein, and the overall lipophilicity of the drug. Most drugs with a molecular weight <600 Da cross the placenta, while drugs >1,000 Da cross very poorly (e.g., heparin, insulin).[16] Of note, larger drugs (e.g., monoclonal antibodies) pass through the placenta through active transport in a linear fashion, with minimal transport occurring during the first trimester and maximum transport occurring during the third trimester.[18] Drugs whose molecular weights fall between 500 and 1,000 Da typically have incomplete transfer across the placenta, and the amount of drug transfer can vary.[16]

Nonionized drugs have a tendency to cross the placenta more readily than ionized drugs. Fetal blood often has a lower pH than maternal blood.

Hydrogen ions bind to the nonionized form of the drug leading to ion trapping and resulting in higher drug concentrations in the fetal blood. This becomes particularly important with the local anesthetics, which are mostly weak bases. Fetal acidosis produces higher fetal drug concentrations because of binding of hydrogen ions to nonionized forms of the drug, leading to trapping of the local anesthetic in fetal circulation.

In general, highly lipophilic drugs have increased placental transfer. However, extreme lipophilicity may actually impede transfer as highly lipophilic substances may accumulate in the placenta. In these cases, the drug is absorbed by placental tissue, where it is stored, and it is not readily released into fetal circulation.

FACTORS AFFECTING TERATOGENICITY

Factors to consider when evaluating patients and drugs for teratogenicity risk include maternal physiologic changes that can impact drug levels throughout pregnancy, fetal susceptibility to the drug based on the developmental stage at the time of exposure, and the anticipated exposure level (the dose of the drug and the extent to which the patient may be concomitantly exposed to other substances associated with the same developmental risks).

Throughout pregnancy, a woman's body undergoes many changes, including physiological changes that can impact drug metabolism and clearance. These changes can also influence medication dosing, requiring in some cases larger doses than typically seen in the nonpregnant population.

The impact of drug exposure on a developing fetus is highly dependent on the timing of exposure. The term *gestational timing* is often used to describe the timeframe within which an exposure must occur to have an impact on fetal development. For example, the critical window for an agent to interfere with the closure of the neural tube during fetal embryology is between days 21 and 28 after conception.[19] For a drug to induce an increased risk of neural tube defects, the mother must take it prior to the second month of pregnancy. If the mother does not start taking the drug until later in pregnancy, the critical window has passed, and development of a neural tube defect would not be due to exposure to the drug. Drugs can have a different impact on development throughout different stages of pregnancy as well. For example, when warfarin is taken by a mother during the first 6–9 weeks of pregnancy, there is an increased pattern of nasal hypoplasia and skeletal abnormalities.[1] However, when warfarin is taken later in pregnancy, an increased risk in central nervous system (CNS) abnormalities is observed. The increased risk of nasal hypoplasia and skeletal abnormalities is likely due to vitamin K deficiency, whereas the CNS abnormalities are due directly to complications from fetal bleeding when warfarin is used during the second and third trimesters.[20] Interestingly, exposure during the first 2–4 weeks after conception poses little risk for harm. Early embryonic cells are able to replace themselves if there is damage due to exposure to a causative agent. If the magnitude of cell loss or damage is too great, however, spontaneous abortion can result.[21]

Congenital anomalies are defined as abnormalities that are present at birth, although they may be diagnosed in utero, at the time of birth, or months or years after the child is born. In the United States, birth defects occur in 1 of every 33 babies each year (3%), affecting an estimated 120,000 babies annually. Birth defects are also the leading cause of infant deaths, accounting for 20% of all infant deaths.[22] Typically, the anomalies are structural in nature; however, they may not always be inherently visible, as in mental retardation. Often birth defects are present at the time of conception and are due to genetic or chromosomal abnormalities as, for example, with Down syndrome. However they can also develop as a result of exposures or disruptions during the embryonic period or early fetal period, as with spina bifida, or result from exposures throughout gestation due to maternal pre-existing conditions (e.g., diabetes, hypertension, and psychological disorders), environmental exposures, and drug exposures. Defects can vary from a minor to a major anomaly.

CONDITIONS ASSOCIATED WITH TERATOGENICITY

LEARNING DISABILITIES

Learning disabilities are conditions characterized by an inconsistency between potential and actual levels of intellectual ability. They can involve disabilities or impairments in physical, learning, language, or behavior areas and include issues with concentration, attention, language development, or visual and aural information processing. For children with learning disabilities, struggles can include the ability to use or understand spoken or written language, complete math problems, coordinate movements, or focus their attention on specific tasks. They typically begin during the developmental period and usually persist throughout life.[23]

CAUSATIVE AGENTS

Learning disabilities can either be congenital or acquired; however, no single cause has been identified. Prenatal exposure to anticonvulsant drugs, specifically valproic acid monotherapy, has been associated with reduced cognitive ability, autistic spectrum disorders including childhood autism, Asperger syndrome, atypical autism, and additional educational needs in exposed children.[24-26] A recent prospective observational study evaluated 224 children exposed to anticonvulsant drugs during the prenatal period for 6 years of follow-up and found children exposed to valproic acid did poorly on measures of verbal and memory abilities and had lower IQs at age 6 when compared to children exposed to other anticonvulsant agents.[26] Phenytoin exposure has been associated with mental deficiency and an average IQ score 10 points lower in children when compared to children not exposed to phenytoin.[27,28] Additionally, some studies have suggested risk for developmental delay after prenatal exposure to carbamazepine; however, other studies have not confirmed this finding.[26,29,30]

EPIDEMIOLOGY

Recent data estimate 8–10% of American children under 18 years of age have some type of learning disability.[31] The incidence of drug-induced learning disabilities is unknown.

MECHANISMS

The cause(s) of learning disabilities is not known. Possible causes include heredity, teratogenicity, problems during pregnancy and birth (e.g., lack of oxygen, premature labor), or incidents after birth (e.g., head injury, nutritional deprivation). One theory suggests that learning disabilities occur as a result of small disturbances in brain development in areas dealing with language.[32] The effects of antiepileptic drugs on cognition and neurological development are not well known; however, animal studies have shown that in utero exposure can induce both anatomical and behavioral anomalies. The exact mechanism for the behavioral anomalies is not known, although evidence suggests the mechanism is multifactorial and results from folate deficiency, ischemia, neuronal suppression, detrimental effects of reactive intermediates, and antiepileptic drug-induced neuronal apoptosis leading to dysfunction in remaining neurons.[33] It is important to note that learning disabilities are not caused by economic disadvantage, environmental factors, or cultural differences.

CLINICAL PRESENTATION AND DIFFERENTIAL DIAGNOSIS

Learning disabilities include a spectrum of disorders that affect the way the brain is able to process information and can vary greatly in severity. Children with learning disabilities usually have average or above average intelligence but struggle with some aspects of learning. Identifying letters of the alphabet may be an easy task for the child, but putting the letters together to read may become confusing and difficult. Children with learning disabilities may present as frustrated, angry, or depressed and may have poor self-image due to struggles accomplishing tasks they see their peers mastering with little difficulty.

Learning disabilities are usually discovered during the first years of elementary school as the child is beginning to learn to read and write. To obtain a diagnosis, a specialist must formally evaluate the child at 5–7 years of age, and then the tests are repeated as the child gets older. If problems are noticed or suspected at younger ages, testing is usually delayed because learning styles and speed varies greatly during the early years of childhood development, and results are often inconclusive.

RISK FACTORS

Maternal social history is important, as smoking, alcohol, and cocaine exposure in utero have been linked to developmental delays in children. Additionally, other factors in an infant's environment including poor nutrition and exposure to toxins such as lead in water or paint can increase risk for development of a learning disability.[34]

MORBIDITY AND MORTALITY

Learning disabilities can be an isolated learning problem with little impact on a child's life or can occur as several overlapping learning disabilities that have lasting implications and are lifelong conditions. The extent of impact a learning disability can have depends on the learning disability itself, when it is detected, and the resources available for help. Children born with a learning disability may require a variety of treatments throughout life to manage that disability. The most common treatment for learning disabilities is special education. Once a learning disability is suspected, trained educators will perform diagnostic testing and evaluations to assess the child's academic and intellectual performance and potential. The exact approach for treatment will vary per child, but is centered on teaching learning skills by building on abilities and strengths, while compensating for disabilities and weaknesses. Depending on the child's limitations, other health professionals such as speech and language therapists may be added to the care team. If the child struggles with attention and/or concentration, behavioral therapy and pharmacotherapy may be added.[35]

LOW BIRTH WEIGHT

Low birth weight is defined as an infant born weighing <2,500 grams, or 5.5 pounds, and can occur because an infant is born too small, too early, or a combination of both. An infant's weight at birth often correlates closely with their gestational age and is a good predictor of both short- and long-term outcomes.[36] When an infant is born smaller than the usual size for a baby born at the same number of weeks gestation, the term *small for gestational age* is used. Small for gestational age babies have birth weights below the 10th percentile when compared to babies of the same gestational age.[37] Additionally, small for gestational age babies may be born premature, at term, or post-term and may be equally small all over, or be of normal length, but lower in body weight and mass. When compared to infants born at a normal weight, low birth weight infants carry a higher risk for many health problems, are at higher risk of developing infections, and may potentially suffer from delayed motor and social development or learning disabilities.

CAUSATIVE AGENTS

Maternal exposure to phenytoin, corticosteroids, and warfarin have been linked to lower birth weights in infants.[38-40] Calcium-channel blockers, angiotensin-converting enzyme inhibitors, and beta-adrenergic receptor blockers have been associated with IUGR leading to infant lower birth weight; however, it is difficult to determine whether the increased risk is due to the medication exposure or the underlying disease state.[41-48]

EPIDEMIOLOGY

In 2014, the overall incidence of low birth weight in infants in the United States was 8% (318,847 out of 3,988,076 registered live births, or roughly 1 in 12).[49] The overall incidence of drug-induced low birth weight or small for gestational age births is unknown, but it is likely very low. An estimated 70% of low birth weight babies are born prematurely, or prior to 37 weeks gestation.[49] One-fourth to one-third of infants born with a low birth weight are found to have sustained IUGR.[50] IUGR affects

3–9% of pregnancies and is the leading cause of perinatal mortality and morbidity.[51]

Maternal corticosteroid use has been associated in some studies with lowering birth weight, but recent literature indicates impact may be minimal after one or two short courses of therapy.[38,52] A randomized trial evaluating the impact of a single rescue antenatal steroid course compared to placebo in 113 cases showed no difference in birth weight.[53] In a study evaluating single versus repeat courses of antenatal corticosteroid courses in pregnant patients, repeat dosing was associated with decreased birth weight below the 10th percentile when compared to a single course ($p = 0.048$), causing the data and safety monitoring committee to stop the trial early.[39]

Calcium-channel blockers and beta-adrenergic blockers have both been associated with intrauterine IUGR and low birth weight. It can be difficult to determine true causality because chronic hypertension has also been linked to IUGR, low birth weight, and premature birth.[40] Calcium-channel blockers, specifically nifedipine, have been associated with changes in infant birth weight. However, in a study of 145 pregnant women receiving nifedipine or placebo, there was no significant difference between the two groups in the percentage of infants weighing less than the 10th percentile (OR 0.8, 95% CI 0.4–1.4) or in the mean birth weight.[41] Similarly, beta-blockers, in particular atenolol, have been linked to fetal growth restriction when taken in early pregnancy.[42] A retrospective study of 78 pregnancies exposed to atenolol showed atenolol use associated with fetal growth restrictions, specifically when used in early pregnancy and continued through delivery.[43] Another randomized trial evaluated atenolol 100 mg daily compared to placebo when given prior to 24 weeks gestation in normotensive women with high cardiac output to help prevent development of pre-eclampsia. The results were similar, with infants exposed to atenolol weighing 440 g less than infants in the placebo group ($p = 0.02$).[44] The smallest infants were born to mothers treated with atenolol who also experienced the largest reductions in cardiac output. An additional retrospective study evaluating 158 pregnancies in women with cardiovascular disease found a significant difference in the incidence of fetal growth restrictions between beta-blockers and placebo ($p < 0.05$). The beta-blocker group included propranolol, metoprolol, atenolol, and bisoprolol, and the incidence of fetal growth restriction varied depending on the agent used (35%, 17%, 33%, and 0%, respectively).[45]

Conversely, a recent meta-analysis (7 studies of 802 women) evaluating use of antihypertensive medications, including beta-blockers, calcium-channel blockers, and others, for chronic hypertension in pregnancy showed no difference in birth weight (weighted mean difference 60 g, 95% CI 200–80 g).[47] A common theme raised by many authors is that fetal growth changes are likely impacted by many factors other than just maternal blood pressure. Before initiating therapy for hypertension, it is important to consider the mother's starting blood pressure, timing of gestation relative to the start of drug therapy, and the treatment goal.[54]

MECHANISMS

The two most common reasons for low birth weight are premature birth and IUGR.[55] Understandably, babies born prior to full term are at greater risk for lower birth weight. Growth-restricted babies, on the other hand, may have a lower birth weight for a number of reasons. Some growth-restricted babies may be small simply because their parents are small. Others may have a lower birth weight because something stopped or slowed their growth during development. The cause of IUGR is not always known, but risk factors have been identified. Maternal hypertension, for example, can cause the small blood vessels in the placenta to tighten, allowing less blood and nutrients to cross to the baby. This can potentially cause delayed or restricted growth for the developing fetus.[56]

CLINICAL PRESENTATION AND DIFFERENTIAL DIAGNOSIS

As defined above, low birth weight infants are those born weighing <2,500 grams, or 5.5 pounds. Infants born small for gestational age have birth weights below the 10th percentile when compared to other babies of the same gestational age. A careful exposure history is necessary to determine whether or not drugs were the likely or possible cause of low birth weight. Other causes may be ruled in or out based on the timing of delivery, the mother's health status, and/or other conditions present at birth.

RISK FACTORS

Risks factors for drug-induced low birth weight include exposure to known causative agents during pregnancy; however, the exact cause of low birth weight, or fetal growth restriction, is not always known. Chromosomal disorders, such as trisomy 21, have also been linked to an increased risk of low birth weight. Additionally, several maternal conditions have also been linked to an increased risk, including hyperthyroidism and hypertension, maternal infections during pregnancy, including cytomegalovirus, rubella, chickenpox, and toxoplasmosis, lack of weight gain for the mother during pregnancy, a previous preterm birth, maternal age <15 or >35, and social and economic factors (low income, low educational status, stress, domestic violence or abuse, and unmarried status).[49,57,58]

Maternal cigarette smoking has also been associated with a decrease in infant birth weight of approximately 135–300 g.[59,60] Interestingly, when smoking cessation can occur prior to the third trimester, the effect on decreased birth weight is reduced.[61] A reduction in birth weight is also associated with maternal alcohol consumption, even in amounts as little as 2 drinks per day.[62] Use of cocaine has been associated with a restriction in growth leading to lower birth weights and to a reduction in head circumference.[63]

MORBIDITY AND MORTALITY

Birth weight is an indicator of fetal growth, and low birth weight predicts short-term survival in newborns more reliably than any other characteristic. Small body size at birth is also an important predictor of long-term health. The incidence of morbidity, hospitalizations, or death associated with drug-induced low birth weight in infants is more difficult to determine.[64] Research has shown an estimated 1.1 million babies die annually from complications of preterm birth.[65] Additionally, low birth weight increases the infant's risk of developing diabetes and cardiovascular diseases later in life.[66,67] Many cohort studies have demonstrated an inverse relationship between birth weight and adult morbidity and mortality from cardiovascular diseases.[66] However, available data do not consider environmental factors, social factors, or genetic factors that may contribute to fetal development.

OROFACIAL CLEFTS

Cleft lip and cleft palate are birth defects that occur when a baby's lip or mouth does not form properly during fetal development. Together, these anomalies are commonly referred to as orofacial clefts. The lip forms between weeks 4 and 7 of pregnancy, as tissue and cells from each side of the head grow together to form the face. A cleft lip occurs when the tissue that forms the lip does not completely join together before birth. As a result, the lip remains open and appears split (**Figure 58-1**). The opening can be a small slit along the lip line or can be a large opening that extends up into the nose. The palate forms between weeks 6 and 9 of pregnancy, as tissues form together to make the roof of the mouth. A cleft palate

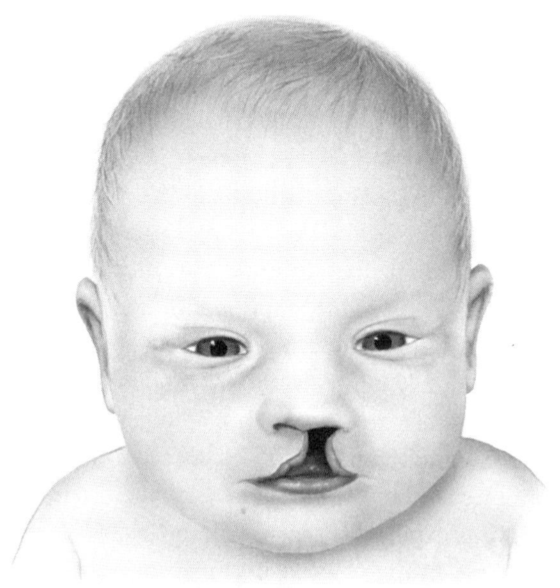

FIGURE 58-1 Cleft Lip

Source: Centers for Disease Control and Prevention, National Center on Birth Defects and Developmental Disabilities. http://www.cdc.gov/ncbddd/birthdefects/cleftlip.html.

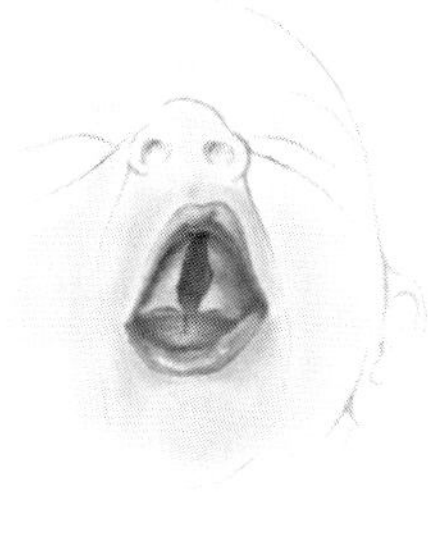
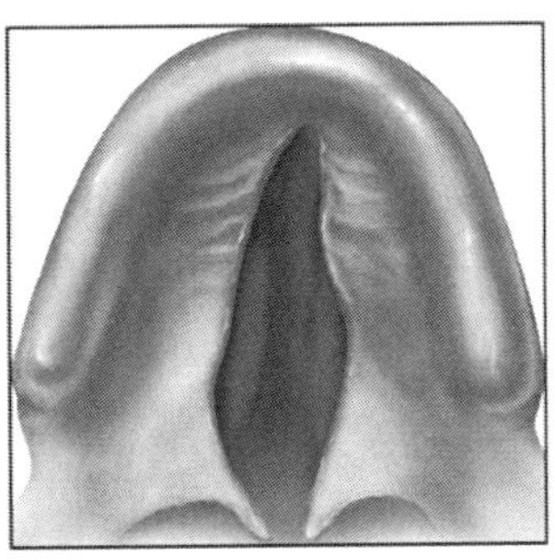

FIGURE 58-2 Cleft Palate

Source: Centers for Disease Control and Prevention, National Center on Birth Defects and Developmental Disabilities. http://www.cdc.gov/ncbddd/birthdefects/cleftlip.html.

occurs when there is a disruption in the joining of the tissues, resulting in an opening of the palate. The extent of the opening can vary, with the front and back of the palate remaining open, or only a small part of the palate remaining open (**Figure 58-2**).

CAUSATIVE AGENTS

Several medications have been linked to orofacial cleft development when used in early pregnancy. Prenatal exposure to drugs, including phenytoin, primidone, carbamazepine, oxcarbazepine, phenobarbital, ethosuximide, valproic acid, topiramate, lamotrigine, mycophenolate, isotretinoin, corticosteroids (topically and systemically), benzodiazepines, and beta-2 agonists, have been associated with an increased risk of orofacial cleft.[68-74]

EPIDEMIOLOGY

It is estimated that about 2,650 babies are born with a cleft palate and 4,440 babies are born with a cleft lip with or without a cleft palate every year in the United States (a total of about 1 in 600 babies).[75] The overall incidence of drug-induced orofacial clefts is unknown. The incidence of orofacial clefts associated with use of specific agents during pregnancy, where known, is discussed in further detail below.

A large meta-analysis designed to compare safety during pregnancy evaluated 96 studies involving 58,461 patients exposed to antiepileptic medications during pregnancy, including ethosuximide, primidone, topiramate, phenobarbital, phenytoin, carbamazepine, oxcarbazepine, gabapentin, and levetiracetam used as monotherapy and in combination therapy. The following monotherapies were associated with significantly more cases of cleft lip and/or cleft palate when compared to control: ethosuximide (OR 22.22, 95% CI 4.56–87.64), primidone (OR 7.68, 95% CI 1.41–29.27), topiramate (OR 6.12, 95% CI 1.89–19.05), phenobarbital (OR 5.75, 95% CI 2.41–14.08), phenytoin (OR 3.11, 95% CI 1.31–7.72), and valproic acid (OR 3.26, 95% CI 1.38–5.58). Additionally, the following combination therapies were associated with significantly more cases of cleft lip and/or cleft palate when compared to control: phenobarbital, phenytoin and primidone (OR 11.5, 95% CI 1.70–63.48), phenytoin and primodone (OR 16.75, 95% CI 3.02–77.19), carbamazepine and phenobarbital (OR 18.51, 95% CI 3.34–94.21), and carbamazepine and valproic acid (OR 19.12, 95% CI 3.74–88.68).[72]

A large study evaluated 4,459 cases of valproic acid exposure during pregnancy and identified 50 cases of orofacial cleft. Thirteen cases occurred in 1,282 valproic acid monotherapy-exposed pregnancies. Nine of those patients experienced isolated cleft palate, and four developed cleft lip and cleft palate, representing an 11.3-fold and 3.5-fold increase risk for isolated cleft palate and cleft lip and palate, respectively.[76]

Maternal lamotrigine use has also been associated with an increase in cleft palate development, with rates ranging between 2% and 5.6%.[77] A review of 684 women taking lamotrigine as monotherapy during pregnancy found that 16 of the infants had a major malformation. Of those, five had oral clefts (7.3 per 1,000) with three cases of isolated cleft palate, one case of isolated cleft lip, and one case of cleft lip and palate. This represents a 10.4-fold increase (95% CI 4.3–24.9) in isolated left palate development when compared to 206,224 unexposed infants surveyed at birth.[78] However, most studies have demonstrated much lower risks. One study conducted in the United Kingdom reported only one infant (0.1%) with cleft palate identified among 1,151 mothers exposed to lamotrigine.[79] In another study, only one infant was born with oral cleft among 1,558 lamotrigine-exposed mothers.[80]

Mycophenolate is an immunosuppressant used in transplant patients to prevent rejection and in autoimmune conditions to help reduce inflammation. Maternal use of mycophenolate during pregnancy has been linked to several malformations, including craniofacial malformations with orofacial clefts. Craniofacial malformations were reported in 12 of 14 infants exposed to mycophenolate during development.[73, 81-91] Seven of the infants had an orofacial cleft with four cases of cleft lip and palate, two cases of cleft palate, and one case of bilateral oblique facial cleft.

Isotretinoin was approved for use in the United States in 1982. Shortly after approval, several publications appeared warning of the human teratogenic potential associated with isotretinoin use during pregnancy or in women who may become pregnant. From September 1982 through July 1984, the FDA and Centers for Disease Control and Prevention (CDC) received reports of 154 isotretinoin-exposed pregnancies. In total, 95 were electively aborted, 12 aborted spontaneously, 21 had major malformations, and 26 infants were born without major defects. Of the 21 infants with major malformations, 3 were stillborn and 9 expired shortly after birth.[92-97] Malformations observed in the 21 infants included CNS defects, craniofacial defects, cardiovascular defects, brachial-arch mesenchymal-tissue defects, thymal defects, spina bifida, nystagmus, hepatic abnormalities, hydroureter, decreased muscle tone, large scrotal sac, and limb reduction.[98-102]

Data from the National Birth Defects Prevention Study (NBDPS) that investigated deliveries from 1997 to 2002 demonstrated an increased risk of cleft lip with or without cleft palate (OR 1.7, 95% CI 1.1–2.6) but not cleft palate only (OR 0.5, 95% CI 0.2–1.3) from maternal corticosteroid use.[103] Data collected between 2003 and 2009 showed an association between corticosteroids and cleft lip and palate (OR 1.0, 95% CI 0.7–1.4).[104]

Results of studies searching for a link between maternal benzodiazepine use and infant orofacial cleft development have been mixed. A positive association has mostly been found in retrospective case-control analyses, which raises concerns of recall bias. A meta-analysis evaluating all studies from 1966 to 1998 found no association between benzodiazepine exposure during pregnancy and cleft development (OR 1.19, 95% CI 0.34–4.15).[74] An additional review of 1,979 infants whose mothers reported taking benzodiazepines during pregnancy did not show an increased risk in orofacial clefts.[105] However, a more recent meta-analysis of over 1 million pregnancies found a twofold increased risk of oral cleft development in infants of mothers exposed to benzodiazepines during pregnancy.[106]

Bronchodilators are often needed to treat patients with asthma during pregnancy. A few studies have looked for an association between bronchodilator use during pregnancy and development of orofacial clefts. One study utilized the NBDPS to compare 2,711 infants born with orofacial clefts to 6,482 infants born without defects. Information regarding maternal medication use from 3 months before pregnancy to delivery was evaluated and reviewed. Albuterol was the most commonly used bronchodilator in this population and was used by 88.7% of the mothers who were exposed to bronchodilators. An association between bronchodilator use and cleft lip development was observed (adjusted OR 1.77, 95% CI 1.08–2.88). A trend toward an increased cleft palate development risk was also observed, but statistical significance was not achieved (adjusted OR 1.53, 95% CI 0.99–2.37). Maternal albuterol use was associated with cleft lip development (adjusted OR 1.79, 95% CI 1.07–2.99) and cleft palate development (adjusted OR 1.65, 95% CI 1.06–2.58). The authors were careful to note that it is unclear from their study if the increased risk of orofacial clefts is due to maternal exposure to bronchodilators, an increased severity of asthma, a combination of these factors, or chance.[107]

MECHANISMS

The mechanism of orofacial cleft development is not well understood, but it occurs when there is failure of the fusion of nasal processes and/or palatal shelves.[108] The exact etiology of cleft palate and lip development remains unknown; however, there are several risk factors associated with an increased prevalence. It is hypothesized that anything that disrupts cell proliferation, migration, adhesion, differentiation, or apoptosis involved in the growth and fusion on the face and palate before the end of week 6 of gestation can lead to development of a cleft lip and or cleft palate. Similar to most congenital malformations, genetics and chromosome disorders play a role in the increased risk of developing clefts. The teratogenic mechanism of isotretinoin is thought to result from an adverse effect on the initial differentiation and migration of cephalic neural crest cells.[109,110]

CLINICAL PRESENTATION AND DIFFERENTIAL DIAGNOSIS

Orofacial clefts, specifically cleft lip with or without cleft palate, are typically diagnosed during pregnancy through routine ultrasound. Some may be diagnosed after the baby is born, and this is often the case with cleft palates. Certain types of cleft palate (e.g., submucous cleft palates and bifid uvula) may not be diagnosed until later in life due to difficulty with detection. Children with clefts often suffer from abnormal nasal speech and speech difficulties, which can lead to further evaluation and discovery of the malformation. Differential diagnosis includes facial teratoma, frontonasal dysplasia, premaxillary agenesis, and amniotic band syndrome.[111]

RISK FACTORS

Exposure to known causative agents during pregnancy increases the risk of orofacial clefts. In addition, an association has been identified between maternal well-being throughout the pregnancy and the development of fetal orofacial clefts. There is an association between maternal weight and cleft development with an increased risk of malformation in both over- and underweight patients.[112,113] Febrile infections during early pregnancy have also been associated with development of clefts in the fetus.[114] Interestingly, acetaminophen use during the first trimester of pregnancy appears to reduce the risk of cleft development and appeared to decrease the risk of development in women who reported concomitant febrile infections in early pregnancy.[115] Pregestational diabetes has also been linked to oral cleft development.[116] The key to prevention is achieving well-controlled blood glucose levels prior to and during early pregnancy.

Vitamin and mineral deficiencies, specifically vitamin B_6 and zinc deficiencies, have also been associated with an increased risk of orofacial clefts.[117,118] Smoking and alcohol exposure during pregnancy have been tied to increased risk of orofacial clefts, as have maternal amphetamine, cocaine, and ecstasy use.[119,120]

MORBIDITY AND MORTALITY

Children born with facial clefts have a significantly increased mortality risk compared to the baseline population.[121] One cohort study of 432,238 live births found a mortality rate of 36 per 1,000 cleft births.[121] More than 90% had anomalies in other organ systems in addition to the orofacial cleft, and those anomalies likely impacted the reported mortality rate. Treatments for children born with orofacial clefts will vary depending on the severity of the cleft. It is generally recommended that children have surgery to repair a cleft lip within the first 12 months of life and surgery to repair cleft palate within the first 18 months.[122] Often children will need additional surgeries as they get older and their facial structures continue to grow and develop. Depending on the cleft type, the child may face problems feeding and/or speaking clearly, may experience an increased risk for ear infections, and may have dental and hearing issues.

CONGENITAL HEART DEFECTS

Congenital heart defects represent the most common type of birth defect, and there are several different types of congenital cardiac malformations that may be present at birth. These vary in presentation and can affect both the structure and the function of the heart.

CAUSATIVE AGENTS

Maternal exposure to valproic acid, thalidomide, isotretinoin, lithium, risperidone, and selective serotonin reuptake inhibitors (SSRIs) during pregnancy has been associated with a possible increased risk for heart defects in the neonate.[123-126] A relatively low prevalence of congenital heart defects and the relatively small number of expectant mothers exposed to these drugs makes it difficult to obtain large enough samples to prove true associations.

EPIDEMIOLOGY

Congenital heart defects occur in 50–150 births per every 10,000.[127] The overall incidence of drug-induced congenital heart defects is unknown. The incidence of cardiac malformations associated with use of specific agents during pregnancy, where known, is discussed in further detail below.

Maternal valproic acid use during pregnancy has been linked to cardiac defects in the developing fetus, specifically anomalies of great vessels, patent ductus arteriosus, valvular aortic stenosis, ventricular septal defect, atrial septal defect, and Tetralogy of Fallot.[128-134] One large cohort study evaluated 1,565 expectant mothers exposed to valproic acid and compared findings to controls not exposed to any antiepileptic therapy. Investigators found an increased risk for atrial septal defects (adjusted OR 2.5, 95% CI 1.4–4.4); however, there was no increased risk for other cardiac defects.[135]

Thalidomide exposure during pregnancy has frequently been linked to cardiovascular abnormalities, including ventricular septal defects, atrial septal defects, Tetralogy of Fallot, cor triloculare, pericardial effusion, hypertrophy of atrium and ventricle, coarctation of the aorta, and systolic murmurs.[125,136-139] Cardiac defects occurring after thalidomide exposure have also been identified as a major cause of early death. Thalidomide-associated early death occurs in 30% of infants at birth and occurs in up to 6% of the survivors.[140] Overall, exposure to thalidomide during pregnancy has been associated with an estimated 20–50% increased risk of congenital malformation development.[140]

Exposure to isotretinoin during pregnancy has been linked to several cardiovascular malformations, including transposition of the great vessels, Tetralogy of Fallot, double-outlet right ventricle, truncus arteriosus communis, ventricular septal defects, and atrial septal defects.[126] It is difficult to determine the true incidence of isotretinoin-induced malformation because many pregnancies that occur in exposed patients are aborted either electively or spontaneously.

In a cohort study of 1,360,101 pregnant women, risperidone was associated with a small increased risk in cardiac malformations (RR 1.26, 95% CI 0.88–1.81) when risk was evaluated independently of potential confounders. Specifics of the malformation were not specified, however.[123] The authors expressed concern for potential selection bias, as the cohort only analyzed live births, potentially missing any malformation documented in early pregnancy that resulted in spontaneous abortions, stillbirths, or planned terminations.

Some literature suggests an association between lithium and an increased risk of Ebstein anomaly, which results in a downward displacement of the tricuspid valve within the right ventricle. In one study of 225 case reports of infants exposed to lithium during pregnancy, a total of 18 infants were found to have a cardiovascular birth defect. Six of these were Ebstein anomaly (1:20,000 births or 0.5% of all cardiac heart defects).[141] Another cohort study evaluated 59 infants exposed to lithium throughout pregnancy and found that 4 were born with a congenital heart defect but none had Ebstein anomaly.[142] Two additional studies evaluated 233 infants born with Ebstein anomaly and found that none of the mothers had been exposed to lithium during their pregnancies.[143,144] The Motherisk Program conducted a prospective, controlled study of 148 women treated with lithium during the first trimester of pregnancy and found that the incidence of infants born with major malformations to women exposed to lithium was no higher than those in the control group.[145] Although early data suggested an association between lithium exposure and Ebstein anomaly, more recent work suggests the risk for Ebstein anomaly with lithium is much lower than originally estimated.

Prior to 2005, SSRIs were considered relatively safe for use during pregnancy. In general, their use had not been found to carry an increased risk of major malformations over the baseline of 1–3%

found in the general population. Since then, several studies found SSRIs associated with an increased risk for cardiovascular malformations—in particular, ventricular septal defects.[146,147] The first studies suggested paroxetine might be associated with an increased risk for septal defects.[146,147] A population-based prevalence study was done and evaluated 2,062 women with SSRI prescriptions during early pregnancy compared to 213,712 women with no SSRI prescriptions. A total of 362 infants were diagnosed with a cardiac malformation and 9 of these were infants whose mothers took SSRIs during pregnancy. SSRI use was associated with an increased risk of cardiac malformations (OR 1.7, 95% CI 1.1–2.5). Sertraline was associated with a threefold increased risk (OR 3, 95% CI 1.4–6.4). SSRI use was associated with an increased risk of septal defects (OR 1.4, 95% CI 0.8–2.3), as was sertraline (OR 3.3, 95% CI 1.5–7.5) after adjusting for maternal smoking status, maternal age, birth order, and birth age.[148] Two additional studies also found an elevated risk of septal defects associated with sertraline use.[149,150]

Some studies have reported a slight risk of cardiac malformation when paroxetine or fluoxetine has been used during the first trimester of pregnancy, but a number of other studies report no increased risk.[124] One study observed a relationship between the dose of paroxetine used during pregnancy and the risk of cardiac malformation, although that finding was not replicated in a subsequent study.[151,152] A meta-analysis conducted in 2010 reported an increased prevalence of cardiac malformations (OR 1.46, 95% CI 1.17–1.82) after paroxetine use in the first trimester of pregnancy.[153] NBDPS completed an analysis that found paroxetine and fluoxetine use during pregnancy was associated with a high risk of several subtypes of congenital heart anomalies. Paroxetine was associated with atrial septal defects (OR 1.9, 95% CI 1.1–3.0) and right ventricular outflow tract obstruction defects (RVOTO) (OR 2.4, 95% CI 1.4–3.9). Fluoxetine was associated with RVOTO (OR 2.0, 95% CI 1.4–3.1) and ventricular septal defects (OR 1.4, 95% CI 1.0–1.9).[154] Studies have not found the same risks for cardiac malformation with sertraline exposure.[154]

Interestingly, studies have found infants born to women exposed to SSRIs undergo approximately twice as many echocardiograms in the first year of life when compared to infants not exposed to SSRI therapy. This likely leads to an increased chance for diagnosis of a cardiac malformation.[155] An estimated 85–90% of ventricular septal defects close spontaneously during infancy.[156] The likelihood of finding a ventricular septal defect, whether the child was exposed to SSRIs during development or not, would be expected to decrease when the assessment is done later in childhood. This creates an additional opportunity for bias in research results.

MECHANISMS

The exact cause of most cardiac malformations is unknown, but most are due to sporadic genetic causes such as focal mutations and DNA segment deletions or additions.[157] Down syndrome has been linked to congenital heart disease in roughly 45% of cases, although researchers have not been able to isolate a single gene on chromosome 21 that is responsible for heart defects.[158] Family history also seems to play a large role and can often help identify heritable defects.

CLINICAL PRESENTATION AND DIFFERENTIAL DIAGNOSIS

Infants with congenital heart defects will present differently depending on the defect's type and severity. Some signs and symptoms may include tachypnea, cyanosis, fatigue, and poor blood circulation; however, many heart defects cause few or no signs or symptoms.[159] Babies who have congenital heart defects may have cyanosis and tire easily during feeding times, which may lead to slower weight gain. Older children with congenital heart defects may tire more easily or get short of breath during physical activity when compared to other children.

Severe congenital heart defects are generally detectable and diagnosed during pregnancy via fetal echocardiography around weeks 18–22 gestation, or very soon after birth. Depending on the defect's severity, cardiac catheterization or surgery may be required to repair damage. When the defect is less severe, it is often not diagnosed until the child is older. Minor defects that have no signs or symptoms are often diagnosed based on results from a physical exam or tests completed for other complaints.

RISK FACTORS

Several maternal factors have been linked to the development of fetal congenital heart defects, including pre-existing uncontrolled diabetes, obesity, rubella, and influenza.[160] Additionally, maternal smoking and the use of cocaine and marijuana have also been linked to cardiovascular defects. Children who acquire HIV infections from their mothers during pregnancy are at increased risk for cardiovascular defects, but children born to mothers infected with HIV and treated are not at increased risk.[160]

MORBIDITY AND MORTALITY

The incidence of morbidity or mortality associated with drug-induced congenital cardiac malformations is unknown. In general, depending on the degree of malformation, surgical repair may be necessary within the first few days after delivery. Additional surgeries may be required throughout development as the heart continues to grow. In severe cases, heart transplant may be necessary. Not all infants with congenital heart defects will require treatment. Some may only require observation and periodic reevaluation of cardiac function.

LIMB DEFICIENCY DEFECTS

Limb deficiency defects vary greatly and can be characterized by total or partial absence of a limb or smaller defects such as a missing finger or toe. They can occur as a single malformation or in conjunction with other anomalies. Limb development is complex and starts as a small limb bud on the 26th day after fertilization with the upper limb developing about 24 hours before the lower.[161]

CAUSATIVE AGENTS

Prenatal exposure to several medications has been linked to an increased risk of limb malformation. Although thalidomide is perhaps best known for this teratogenic effect, misoprostol, valproic acid, aminopterin, methotrexate, phenytoin, and isotretinoin have all been associated with limb reduction.[162-166]

EPIDEMIOLOGY

Limb deficiency defects are rare, occurring in only 3–8 infants per 10,000 live births, and it is estimated at least 30% are associated with congenital malformations.[167-172] The most common type of limb defect is caused by vascular disruption and occurs in an estimated 2.2 infants per 10,000 births.[169] The overall incidence of drug-induced limb deficiencies is unknown.

Thalidomide exposure during pregnancy has been linked to limb reduction defects which are described as bilateral and usually grossly symmetrical. Exposure has been associated with approximately 20% incidence of polydactyly, syndactyly, and limb reduction defects.[173]

Maternal use of misoprostol has been correlated with terminal vascular disruption limb anomalies in the developing fetus.[174] The most common limb defects following misoprostol exposure include terminal transverse defects in the arms and legs, including terminal limb amputation with constriction rings, fusion of fingers with constriction rings, clubfoot, and arthrogryposis.[175-177]

In 2000, a study estimated the risk of valproic acid-induced limb deficiencies that utilized data from the Spanish Collaborative Study of Congenital Malformations. A total of 22,294 malformed infants were compared to 21,937 control infants. A total of 57 infants with malformations had been exposed to valproic acid compared to 10 infant controls with no history of valproic acid exposure (OR 5.62, 95% CI 2.78–11.71, p <0.0000001). Congenital limb defects occurred in 21 of the 57 infants exposed to valproic acid (36.8%) and included overlapping digits, clubfoot, clinodactyly, arachnodactyly, hip dislocation, pre- and postaxial polydactyly, and limb deficiencies. Based on the prevalence of limb deficiencies of 6.88 per 10,000 live births in their population, the authors estimated the risk of limb deficiencies after valproic acid exposure during the first trimester to be about 0.42%.[178]

Aminopterin, an antineoplastic drug with immunosuppressive properties often used in chemotherapy regimens, was used unsuccessfully in the 1950s and 1960s as an abortifacient agent. It has been associated with clubfoot, short forearm development, and syndactyly, although the incidence is difficult to estimate because the data are limited.[179,180]

Maternal methotrexate exposure has been associated with an increased risk for total transverse limb deficiencies, with clubfoot, short limbs, hypodactyly, and syndactyly being most commonly reported.[181-183] A disproportionality analysis found total transverse limb deficiencies in 22 cases, 6.41%, compared to only 0.85% in the general population, supporting a possible association with methotrexate exposure and limb deficiencies.[184]

Phenytoin exposure during pregnancy has well-documented teratogenic effects on skeletal tissues leading to limb defects, including hypoplasia of distal phalanges, shortness of metacarpals, cone-shaped epiphyses, limited movements at interphalangeal joints, and tapering fingers with nail hypoplasia.[185-187] It is estimated that one-third of children exposed to phenytoin in utero will suffer from fetal growth restrictions leading to small head, will develop minor dysmorphic craniofacial features, and/or will have limb defects.[174]

Isotretinoin has also been linked to limb deficiency defects, specifically limb reduction. A case report in 1985 first reported limb reduction deformities secondary to isotretinoin exposure in a male infant born with reductions in all four limbs. There was some evidence suggesting the defects were secondary to amniotic bands.[188,189] There have been additional subsequent reports describing cases of infants born with limb reductions following exposure to isotretinoin in utero.[190]

MECHANISMS

The exact cause of limb defects is unknown, although it is thought to be due to disruptive events, including amniotic bands or vascular disruptions that can lead to in utero amputation or hypoperfusion of the developing limb.[191] Cases of limb defects caused by exposure to misoprostol during pregnancy are thought to be related to the induction of uterine contractions that deform the embryo. This results in vascular disruption, hemorrhage in various tissues that leads to hypoperfusion within the entire embryo, resulting in cellular death.[174,192]

CLINICAL PRESENTATION AND DIFFERENTIAL DIAGNOSIS

Limb deficiency defects can present in a variety of ways, including complete absence of the limb, failure of a portion of the limb to separate (most commonly seen in fingers or toes), duplication (most commonly seen in fingers or toes), overgrowth where the limb is much larger than normal, undergrowth where the limb is much smaller than normal, or congenital constriction band syndrome, which causes immobilization, constrictions of the limbs, amputations, and other deformities. Most limb deficiencies are diagnosed on visual inspection at birth and are immediately recognized and identified.

RISK FACTORS

The majority of limb defects are caused by genetic or chromosomal disorders; however, there are other known associated risks as well. Pregestational maternal diabetes and maternal obesity have been identified as possible risk factors for disorders of limb development, although the data regarding the effects of obesity are inconsistent.[112,193-197] Additionally, certain sets of limb deformities have been linked to other birth defects such as those involving the heart, omphalocele, and gastroschisis.[198]

MORBIDITY AND MORTALITY

The incidence of morbidity or death associated with drug-induced limb deficiencies is unknown. Infants born with limb reduction defects will face many obstacles and difficulties throughout development, and the extent of impact will depend on the limb(s) affected and the size of the reduction. Problems include difficulties performing motor skills, need for assistance with daily activities and self-care, limitations in movement, and potential for emotional and social issues due to physical appearance. The use of prosthetics and orthotics may be beneficial for patients with limitations due to limb reduction. In some cases, surgery and rehabilitation with physical and or occupational therapy may be needed. Although children born with limb reductions may face many obstacles and encounter difficulties throughout life, with proper treatment and care they are able to live healthy and productive lives and most manage well in everyday life.[199]

GASTROSCHISIS

Gastroschisis is a defect that occurs in developing fetuses that results in extrusion of the intestines out of the abdominal wall and into the amniotic space. Typically, the intestines protrude to the right of the umbilicus and the anomaly can be detected in utero via ultrasound. The size of hole can vary, and sometimes organs, such as the stomach and liver, can also protrude outside of the baby's body (**Figure 58-3**).

CAUSATIVE AGENTS

Prenatal exposure to several medications has been associated with an increased risk of gastroschisis. Evidence, although weak, suggests that women taking anti-inflammatory doses of aspirin or taking acetaminophen in combination with other medications may be at increased risk.[200] Literature has also linked prenatal pseudoephedrine use to gastroschisis, although, again, evidence is weak and reports are inconsistent.[201,202]

EPIDEMIOLOGY

In the United States, gastroschisis occurs in 1–2 of every 10,000 births, and the incidence has increased over the last three decades.[203] The overall incidence of drug-induced gastroschisis is unknown and difficult to estimate based on available literature.

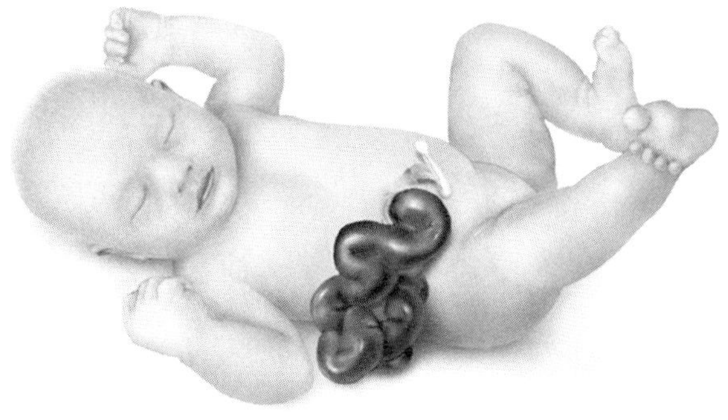

FIGURE 58-3 Gastroschisis

Source: Centers for Disease Control and Prevention, National Center on Birth Defects and Developmental Disabilities. http://www.cdc.gov/ncbddd/birthdefects/gastroschisis.html.

A retrospective study evaluating 206 cases of gastroschisis looked at the relationship between maternal use of cough, cold, and analgesic medications and development of gastroschisis. Risk of gastroschisis development was elevated in patients exposed to aspirin (OR 2.7, 95% CI 1.2–5.9). Risk was slightly elevated in infants whose mothers took acetaminophen during pregnancy (OR 1.5, 95% CI 1.1–2.2) but was significantly elevated in those exposed to acetaminophen in combination with pseudoephedrine (OR 4.2, 95% CI 1.9–9.2).[200]

Three case-control studies examined pseudoephedrine monotherapy exposure in children born with gastroschisis. In all three studies, exposure to pseudoephedrine was associated with an increased odds ratio. In one study, the risk of gastroschisis was increased 4.2-fold in women taking pseudoephedrine in combination with paracetamol (95% CI 1.9–9.2).[204] However, two other studies reported data from over 400 pregnant women who took pseudoephedrine during the first trimester, and neither study found an increase in the incidence of birth defects.[205,206]

MECHANISMS

The exact cause of gastroschisis is unknown, although it is thought to be due to a vascular disruption causing a weakness in the body wall, possibly to the right umbilical vein or the right vitelline artery.[207,208] Other proposed mechanisms include defective growth, cellular death, or impaired cellular fusion that leads to extrusion of the intestines through the defective area and into the amniotic fluid.[209] Furthermore, genetic or chromosomal changes that occur in utero cannot be ruled out as a potential cause.

CLINICAL PRESENTATION AND DIFFERENTIAL DIAGNOSIS

Gastroschisis is typically diagnosed during routine anatomy ultrasound conducted around 20 weeks gestation.[210] The ultrasonography can be performed to detect signs of intestinal injury, decreased peristalsis, and/or bowel distension. In rare scenarios, gastroschisis may not be diagnosed until after delivery. An omphalocele, another abdominal wall defect, is an umbilical cord hernia with a wall defect <4 cm. Maternal elevations of serum alpha-fetoprotein are associated with abdominal wall defects, and levels are generally higher in cases of gastroschisis compared to omphalocele. This difference can aid in initial diagnosis.[211] The differential diagnosis of gastroschisis includes normal physiological gut herniation, ruptured omphalocele, umbilical cord cysts, or loops of normal umbilical cord.[212]

RISK FACTORS

The most consistently observed link to gastroschisis is a mother's age of <20 years, although the reason for this is unclear.[213-215] The impact of maternal prepregnancy body mass index on the development of gastroschisis has been evaluated. One study noted an increased risk in underweight mothers when compared to normal weight mothers.[216] In addition, two other studies found a lower risk in mothers who were overweight or obese when compared to normal weight women, advancing the theory that maternal prepregnancy weight has an impact on fetal development.[112,113] Maternal cigarette smoking has also been linked to an increased risk of both gastroschisis and small-bowel atresia, with risk increasing with the number of cigarettes smoked. A study of 205 gastroschisis cases and 127 small-bowel atresia cases found maternal cigarette smoking to have an increased odds ratio of 2.1 (95% CI 1.0–4.4) for gastroschisis and 2.8 (95% CI 1.1–6.9) for small-bowel atresia.[217] Other risk factors for gastroschisis include maternal alcohol consumption and exposure to illicit drugs, specifically marijuana, cocaine, and methamphetamine.[214,217-220]

MORBIDITY AND MORTALITY

The incidence of morbidity or mortality associated with drug-induced gastroschisis is unknown. In general, the survival rate for those with gastroschisis is remarkably high, exceeding 90% after surgical closure; however, babies tend to suffer varying degrees of morbidity depending on the severity of bowel injury.[221] Infants with gastroschisis may struggle with feeding, digesting food, and absorbing nutrients after eating. The extent of dysfunction usually depends on the magnitude of intestinal inflammation and ischemic injury caused by amniotic fluid exposure and compression from the abdominal wall. The inflamed intestine often has prolonged transit time and decreased absorption of carbohydrates, fats, and proteins. As the inflammation subsides, transit time and absorption return to normal over 4–6 weeks, although total parenteral nutrition is often required during healing. Some may require additional surgeries throughout childhood and in severe cases, may endure intestinal failure.

NEURAL TUBE DEFECTS

Neural tube defects are a collection of anomalies of the CNS that develop within the first 28 days after conception. They occur due to incomplete closure of the neural tube during embryogenesis, causing exposure to neural elements.[222] The most common neural tube defects are spina bifida, meningomyelocele, anencephaly, and encephalocele.

Spina bifida can occur at any point along the spine. The spinal area around the opening does not form properly, leaving the spinal cord exposed (**Figure 58-4**). Often, this leads to damage to the spinal column and surrounding nerves. The severity is determined by the size and location of the opening in the spine and whether nerve damage is involved.

With anencephaly the upper portion of the neural tube does not close completely and the forebrain and cerebrum do not form. Additionally, the remaining portions of the brain are often not covered by bone or skin and are exposed at birth (**Figure 58-5**).

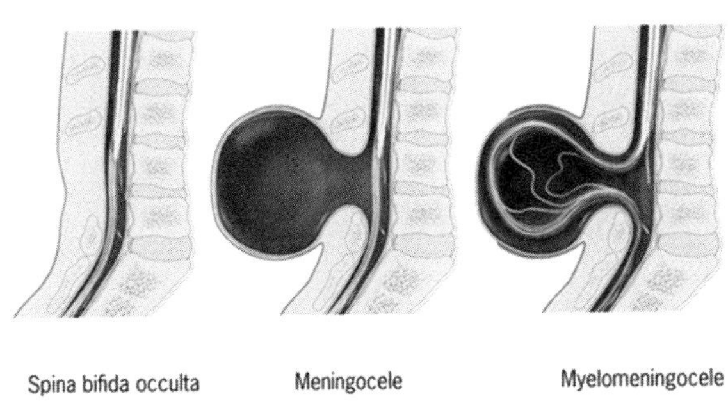

FIGURE 58-4 Spina Bifida

Source: Centers for Disease Control and Prevention, National Center on Birth Defects and Developmental Disabilities. http://www.cdc.gov/ncbddd/spinabifida/facts.html.

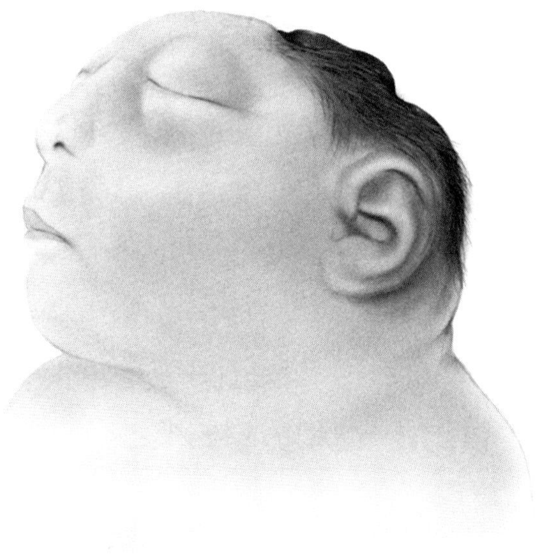

FIGURE 58-5 Anencephaly

Source: Centers for Disease Control and Prevention, National Center on Birth Defects and Developmental Disabilities. http://www.cdc.gov/ncbddd/birthdefects/anencephaly.html.

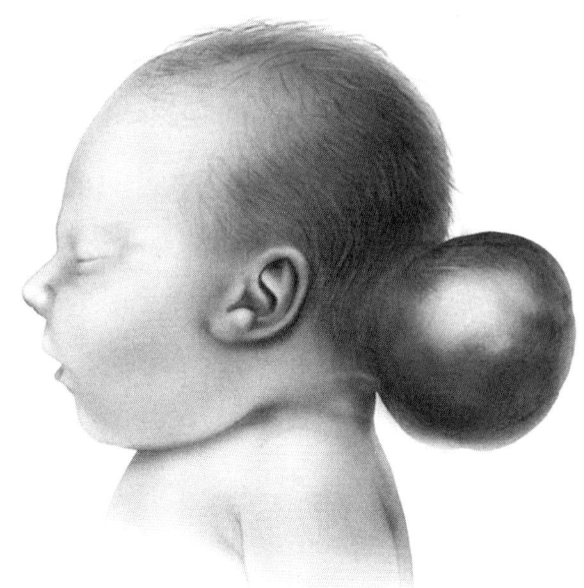

FIGURE 58-6 Encephalocele

Source: Centers for Disease Control and Prevention, National Center on Birth Defects and Developmental Disabilities. http://www.cdc.gov/ncbddd/birthdefects/encephalocele.html.

Encephalocele is a rare neural tube defect associated with a sac-like protrusion at either the upper part of the skull, the area between the forehead and nose, or the back of the skull. The brain protrudes through these openings in the skull (**Figure 58-6**). The condition is typically diagnosed at birth, but occasionally a small encephalocele can protrude into the nose and forehead region and can go undetected.

CAUSATIVE AGENTS

Several antiepileptic medications, in particular valproic acid and carbamazepine, interfere with the body's ability to utilize folate and folic acid and are associated with a higher risk for neural tube defects.[222]

EPIDEMIOLOGY

Annually, more than 300,000 babies are born worldwide with neural tube defects, making this one of the most commonly encountered birth defects. The highest incidence reported is in Northern China (3.7 cases per 1,000 live births).[223] In the United States, the incidence is much lower with a frequency of about 2 per 1,000 live births. The most recent U.S. data estimate the incidence of spina bifida at 1 case per 2,858 live births annually, anencephaly at 1 case per 4,859 live births annually, and encephalocele at 1 case per 12,235 live births annually.[224] The frequency of neural tube defects is decreasing due to the prophylactic prenatal administration of folate, implementation of universal maternal serum alpha-fetoprotein screening, and highly reliable ultrasound diagnosis.[225] The estimated risk of neural tube defects in infants with prenatal exposure to valproic acid is 5–9%, with higher doses associated with higher risks.[226,227]

MECHANISMS

The exact cause of neural tube defects is not known with many factors likely playing a role, including chromosomal disorders, genetic syndromes, nutrition, and/or exposure to environmental teratogens. Phenytoin and carbamazepine induce cytochrome P450 enzymes and are associated with a reduction in serum and red blood cell folate concentrations of up to 90%.[228] Although data are conflicting, it is thought that valproic acid may interfere with folate metabolism by inhibiting glutamate formyl transferase, an enzyme mediating the production of folinic acid.[229] Research has found that folic acid supplementation before and during pregnancy can greatly reduce the risk of neural tube defect development.

CLINICAL PRESENTATION AND DIFFERENTIAL DIAGNOSIS

Neural tube defects are generally diagnosed prior to birth through laboratory tests or imaging. Prenatal ultrasound is routinely used during pregnancy and can detect almost all types of neural tube defects.[230] Ultrasound will typically reveal a defect in the dorsal aspect of the spine which usually has an overlying cystic mass. The differential diagnosis includes sacrococcygeal teratoma, lumbosacral lipoma, sirenomelia, limb-body stalk anomaly, and amniotic band syndrome.[231]

Infants born with a known or suspected neural tube defect will undergo a variety of tests and procedures to help understand the severity of the defect and to assess for the presence of complications. Evaluation typically will include x-rays, magnetic resonance imaging, computed tomography scans, and measurement of head circumference. In addition, the infant's vigor, motor and sensory functioning, and urinary stream will be monitored and evaluated.[232]

Babies born with spina bifida often develop hydrocephalus (i.e., extra fluid in and around the brain). This can lead to swelling in the ventricles of the brain and cause the head to swell. It can be diagnosed during a routine prenatal ultrasound, but it is often not discovered until infancy or early childhood. The most common symptoms of hydrocephalus is a large head that is growing rapidly, a bulging anterior fontanelle, irritability, seizures, and delays in development. Close monitoring is required in an effort to prevent brain injury, and often a shunt is needed to allow drainage of the fluid and relieve pressure on the brain.

RISK FACTORS

Maternal uncontrolled pregestational diabetes and obesity have been linked to increased risk for development of neural tube defects.[233] Some studies have also suggested that defects are more common among infants of mothers who were exposed to high temperatures that may occur during a febrile illness or using a hot tub or sauna during the first 4–6 weeks of pregnancy.[234] Women who are pregnant or may become pregnant should avoid using hot tubs or saunas. Folate deficiency is the most clearly established risk factor for development of a neural tube defect. Folic acid supplementation is critical for the prevention of neural tube defects and should be an important part of preconception and prenatal care for all women of childbearing age. Due to increased risk associated with folate deficiency, the CDC recommends 0.4 mg/day of folic acid from diet or supplements for all women capable of becoming pregnant to reduce the risk for neural tube defects. Women with a history of pregnancy with a neural tube defect should take 4 mg of folic acid beginning 1 month prior to conception and throughout the first trimester of pregnancy.[235]

MORBIDITY AND MORTALITY

The morbidity and mortality arising from neural tube defects depends on the type of defect present. Anencephaly is incompatible with life.[236] The life of infants born with anencephaly is usually limited to a few hours and rarely can last more than 2 days. The brain stem in these patients consists of poorly differentiated neural tissue that is not able to sustain life.

The prognosis for neonates diagnosed with encephalocele is dependent on whether there is herniation of brain tissue into the meningeal sac. If brain tissue herniation is present, there is a high mortality rate.[237]

The prognosis of neonates with spina bifida depends on the size and location of the lesion. Generally, the lower the location of the lesion on the back and the smaller the size, the better the infant's outcome will be. Mortality is reported to be at least 15% in the first year of life, usually due to decline in respiratory function secondary to hindbrain herniation.[237] Additionally, patients often have lower limb paresis, bladder denervation, renal failure, and progressive obstructive hydrocephaly.

MICROCEPHALY

Microcephaly is a CNS defect wherein the baby's head is much smaller than would normally be expected. It is defined as a head circumference 2–3 standard deviations below the mean for the gestational age on standardized charts.[238] This is typically due to a failure of the baby's head to grow properly or growth stopping after birth (**Figure 58-7**).

CAUSATIVE AGENTS

Use of antiepileptic drugs, including carbamazepine, lamotrigine, phenytoin, valproic acid, and topiramate, as well as mycophenolate and methotrexate, has been associated with an increased risk of microcephaly.[184,239-241]

EPIDEMIOLOGY

Microcephaly is estimated to occur in 2–12 babies of every 10,000 live births in the United States. It can be an isolated malformation or occur in conjunction with other major and minor birth defects.[242]

Although the exact incidence of drug-induced microcephaly is unknown, some data regarding specific drug exposure and incidence are available. One study evaluated 329 pregnant women with epilepsy who were treated with monotherapy using carbamazepine, lamotrigine, phenytoin, or valproic acid. Authors observed microcephaly rates of 12–13% in newborns of mothers exposed to any of the anticonvulsants: however, the rates decreased to 3% when the children reached 24 months of age and 2% at 36 months of age.[239] Carbamazepine had the highest incidence of microcephaly (24%) in neonates and 12-month-old infants (15 out of 63 exposed) and valproic acid was the next highest at 18% (7 out of 40 exposed). However, total rates of microcephaly at 24 months and 36 months for children exposed to all study drugs were similar to population rates for microcephaly. Similar results of higher microcephaly rates with carbamazepine and valproic acid monotherapy have been reported in previous studies, although these studies did not follow patients past 18 months of age to determine if the impact was long-term or resolved.[243,244] The clinical

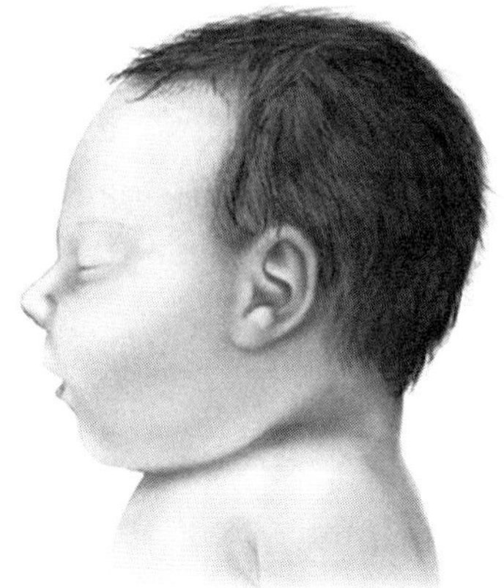

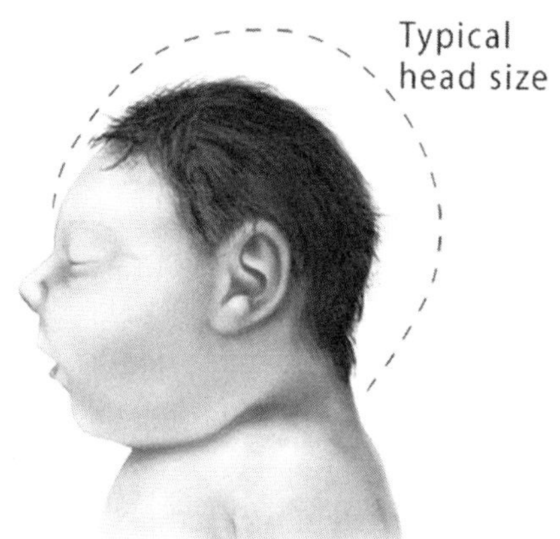

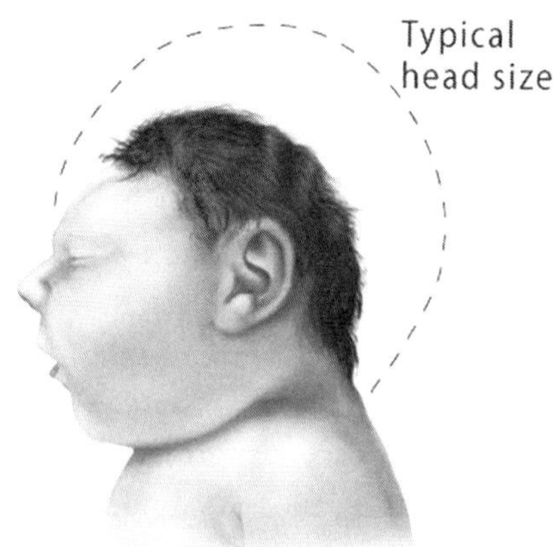

FIGURE 58-7 Microcephaly

Source: Centers for Disease Control and Prevention, National Center on Birth Defects and Developmental Disabilities. http://www.cdc.gov/ncbddd/birthdefects/microcephaly.html.

implications of early microcephaly are unclear, and it appears the effect is not permanent or regulates with time. An additional study evaluating the impact of antiepileptic drug exposure on newborn head circumference reported a significant reduction of mean body-weight adjusted head circumference after exposure to carbamazepine and valproic acid monotherapy (standard deviation 0.15, $p < 0.0001$, and standard deviation 0.10, $p = 0.04$, respectively). No effect on body-weight adjusted head circumference was seen for phenytoin, clonazepam, lamotrigine, or gabapentin. Additionally, the study reported a significant increase in the occurrence of microcephaly for any antiepileptic drug polytherapy (OR 2.85, 95% CI 1.74–4.78), suggesting risk is greatest in patients exposed to multiple antiepileptic drugs during pregnancy.[243]

A cohort study compared 2,600 children exposed to antiepileptic drugs during pregnancy to 771,412 unexposed children born to women without epilepsy. The study found infants exposed to topiramate had a considerable risk of microcephaly (11.4%) compared to 2.4% in those who weren't exposed (OR 4.8, 95% CI 2.5–9.3).[240]

Mycophenolate was linked to risk for microcephaly in one case. Microcephaly was mild, and the child had various other malformations.[241]

Maternal methotrexate exposure during pregnancy has also been linked to microcephaly. Three published cases describe infants with microcephaly (in addition to various other malformations) following maternal exposure to methotrexate for either abortion or during treatment for breast cancer.[245,246] Hyoun et al.[184] completed a disproportionality analysis and found microcephaly occurred with an incidence of 0.87% after methotrexate exposure—an incidence not disproportionate to that found in the general population.

MECHANISMS

The cause of microcephaly is not fully understood; however, it is known that this defect is multifactorial and is the common end point of a group of heterogeneous conditions that interfere with the growth of the brain. It occurs as a result of abnormal cell division and proliferation.[247]

CLINICAL PRESENTATION AND DIFFERENTIAL DIAGNOSIS

The key diagnostic feature of microcephaly is an infant with a head circumference >3 standard deviations below the mean. The head may appear smaller than normal on visual inspection and biometric parameters other than head circumference may also be small (e.g., biparietal diameter, cerebellar diameter). A reduced frontal lobe distance, sloping forehead, or a large subarachnoid space may also be present.[248] The differential diagnosis includes anencephaly, hydrocephaly, and brain atrophy.[249]

RISK FACTORS

Although the direct cause of microcephaly is unknown, certain maternal infections such as rubella, toxoplasmosis, cytomegalovirus, and Zika virus are associated with the development of fetal microcephaly.[250] The defect is also linked to genetic changes, although the genetic sequencing is currently unknown. Neonates whose mothers were malnourished during pregnancy are at increased risk. Maternal alcohol consumption and exposure to cocaine during pregnancy have also been linked to an increased risk of microcephaly.[251,252]

MORBIDITY AND MORTALITY

The overall impact of microcephaly varies depending on the severity. Some children only suffer from mild disabilities while others, especially those who are growing and developing normally, will have normal intelligence levels and continue to meet major milestones. There is no treatment that will return the size of the child's head to normal size or shape. Treatment is focused on preventing and minimizing complications and may include speech, physical, and occupational therapy as well as medications to control seizures and hyperactivity if and when present.

FETAL ALCOHOL SPECTRUM DISORDERS

Fetal alcohol spectrum disorders (FASD) is a group of conditions caused by alcohol consumption during pregnancy. Those conditions include fetal alcohol syndrome (FAS), alcohol-related neurodevelopmental disorder, and alcohol-related birth defects. The effects of alcohol exposure can include both physical and mental defects and can cause problems with development, behavior, and learning. Often, children with FASD have a mix of problems rather than one single issue. The conditions can affect each person differently and can vary in severity. The most severe of the alcohol-related disabilities is FAS, and individuals diagnosed are found to have growth problems (e.g., low pre- and postbirth weight and size), facial dysmorphia (e.g., small head, small eyes, underdevelopment of the upper lip, indistinct groove between the lip and nose, and/or flattened cheekbones), and CNS abnormalities (e.g., delayed brain development, intellectual impairment).[253]

CAUSATIVE AGENTS

Prenatal exposure to alcohol is associated with development of FASD.

EPIDEMIOLOGY

An accurate estimate of the prevalence of FASDs is lacking; however, the CDC has completed studies that have documented 0.2–1.5 infants with FAS for every 1,000 live births in certain areas of the United States.[254] Authors who combined community studies and expert estimates have stated the incidence might be as high as 2–5 for every 100 schoolchildren.[255,256] One report found that alcohol was used by 1 of every 10 pregnant women and 1 in 33 pregnant women described binge drinking within the last 30 days. Among those women who reported drinking during pregnancy, the highest use was in unmarried college graduates 35–44 years of age.[257]

MECHANISMS

The exact mechanism of harm secondary to alcohol exposure during pregnancy is not fully understood. Alcohol easily passes across the placenta to the developing fetus, and alcohol metabolism is much slower in the fetus compared to adults. As a result, the alcohol remains in the baby's blood much longer than in the mother's blood, which leads to possible irreversible harm to the baby's development. One recent study evaluated the effects of prenatal alcohol exposure on cognitive development in childhood and found that children with prenatal alcohol exposure have poorer axon packing density and/or myelination. The authors suggested this impairment in white matter is the likely cause of changes in information processing speed and eyeblink conditioning that commonly occur in children with FAS.[258]

CLINICAL PRESENTATION AND DIFFERENTIAL DIAGNOSIS

Diagnosis of FASD can be difficult because it mostly relies on infant or child clinical presentation and maternal reporting of alcohol use. Additionally, other disorders (e.g., attention deficit hyperactivity disorder) present with symptoms similar to those of FASD, which likely has led to underdiagnosis. Practitioners most often look for abnormal facial features, lower than average height, weight, or both, CNS problems, and history of prenatal alcohol exposure to help rule in or rule out FASD (**Table 58-1**).

RISK FACTORS

It is important to note that no amount of alcohol has been determined to be safe during pregnancy, and data support the "Not a Single Drop" approach for pregnant women. It is uncertain whether moderate drinking throughout pregnancy imparts more

Table 58-1 Potential Symptoms of Fetal Alcohol Spectrum Disorders[269]

- Abnormal facial features (e.g., smooth ridge between the nose and upper lip)
- Difficulty in school, especially with mathematics
- Attention deficit or hyperactivity disorders
- Poor memory
- Poor reasoning and judgment skills
- Intellectual disability or low IQ
- Learning disabilities
- Speech and language delays
- Vision or hearing problems
- Low body weight
- Shorter-than-average height
- Microcephaly
- Issues with coordination
- Problems with the heart, kidney, or bones
- Sleep and sucking problems as a baby

IQ = intelligence quotient.

or less risk than binge drinking. Some data suggest that the dose of alcohol consumed does matter and has an impact on development of FASD; however, more information is needed to confirm that finding.[259] The timing of alcohol exposure during pregnancy is important. Although consumption at any time during pregnancy is not safe, alcohol is the most harmful when consumed during the first 3 months of pregnancy.[260]

MORBIDITY AND MORTALITY

The incidence of morbidity or mortality associated with FASD and FAS is unknown. Without early diagnosis, individuals with prenatal alcohol exposure are at a high risk for a number of secondary disabilities, including mental illness, homelessness, substance abuse, and unemployment. An estimated 60% of people with FASD end up being charged, arrested, convicted, or otherwise in trouble with the law, and up to 50% end up in detention, jail, prison, or a psychiatric or drug and alcohol inpatient setting at some point in their lives.[261] Additionally, it is well documented that patients with FASD or FAS-related conditions, such as mental disorders, attention deficit hyperactivity disorder, and learning disabilities, have higher mortality rates and shorter life expectancy.[262-265]

One study found the life expectancy for people with FAS was 34 years (95% CI 31–37 years).[266] The leading causes of death included suicide (15%), accidents (14%), poisoning by illegal drugs or alcohol (7%), diseases of the nervous system and respiratory system (8% each), diseases of the digestive system (7%), congenital malformations (7%), mental and behavioral disorders (4%), and disease of the circulatory system (4%).[266]

Treatment of FASD and FAS is typically focused on symptom management and may include medications, behavior and education therapy, and parental education/support.

MISCELLANEOUS MALFORMATIONS

This chapter highlights many of the major congenital anomalies; however, there are many other malformations that are associated with teratogens and can occur during fetal development. **Table 58-2** lists additional teratogens.

PREVENTION OF TERATOGENICITY

Primary prevention is a key component of avoiding congenital anomalies associated with teratogens. Teratogencity could be avoided in women who are able to completely refrain from taking medications during pregnancy, particularly during the first trimester of pregnancy. However, this is not always possible. Women with chronic diseases (e.g., diabetes, hypertension) often require pharmacotherapy prior to and throughout pregnancy to maintain their health.

Avoiding alcohol, illicit drugs, and tobacco, maintaining adequate nutrition (which should include taking a daily multivitamin that contains at least 0.4 mg of folic acid), and maintaining a healthy body weight are all essential to the primary prevention of birth defects.

It is important for women with chronic diseases to work with their healthcare providers to control their conditions prior to conception. This is particularly important for patients with diabetes, hypertension, and thyroid disorders. Medications with known risks for development of congenital anomalies should typically be discontinued prior to conception. When this is not possible (e.g., patients receiving anticonvulsant therapy for epilepsy), a careful risk versus benefit analysis should be done to determine the best approach for each individual patient. Ultimately, each patient's care plan must be individualized to determine what is best for both maternal and fetal well-being.

Secondary prevention measures are utilized to assist with early detection, treatment, and management of an existing disorder. Goals are focused on reducing, and in some cases, preventing morbidity. Early prenatal care including ultrasound screening and fetal surveillance during the first and/or second trimester is important when there is a concern for a congenital anomaly. Transferring care of the mother to a maternal fetal care center or high-risk obstetrics clinic designed for optimal fetal and neonatal care can be invaluable and should be considered

Table 58-2 Drugs with Known Teratogenic Effects[a]

Drug	Teratogenic Effects
ACE inhibitors	Fetal growth restriction, fetal hypotension, fetal renal defects leading to anuria, anuria-associated oligohydramnios, renal tubular dysplasia, craniofacial deformation, microcephaly, encephalocele, pericardial effusion, IUGR, prematurity, small bladder, and echogenic bowel associated with exposure in 2nd and 3rd trimester[270-274]
Cocaine	Miscarriage, prematurity, fetal growth restriction; developmental issues of the urinary and genital tract, heart, limbs, and face; severe neurobehavioral and neurophysiologic problems that may persist for months; placental abruption; and potential increased risk for sudden infant death syndrome during the first few months after birth[275-287]
Finasteride	Prostate and external genital developmental disruption in animal studies[288]
Flutamide	Inhibition of Wolffian duct and prostate development; feminization of external genitalia in males in animal studies[289]
Lithium	Ebstein's anomaly and other cardiovascular abnormalities including atrial flutter, bradycardia, and cardiomegaly[290-295]
Methimazole	Choanal and esophageal atresia and aplasia cutitis, associated with 1st trimester use[296]
Methotrexate	Exposure during first 6–8 weeks postconception: associated with IUGR; hypoplastic supraorbital ridges; small, low-set ears; micrognathia; limb deformities; and mental retardation Exposure during 2nd and 3rd trimesters: associated with fetal toxicity and increased mortality[297-303]
NSAIDs	Exposure during time of conception has been associated with blocking blastocyst implantation in animals Exposure after 30 weeks gestation associated with an increased risk of premature closure of the fetal ductus arteriosus, persistent pulmonary hypertension in the newborn, and oligohydramnios[304-308]
Progestins/testosterones	Exposure prior to 10th–11th week of gestation associated with masculinization of female genitalia, clitoral hypertrophy, fused or partial fused labia, possible absent vagina[309]
Retinoids/vitamin A >18,000 units per day	Translocation of the forebrain and posteriorization of the hindbrain, disruption in CNS development, microtia, low-set ears, small mouth, facial dysmorphism[126,310-315]
Tetracyclines	Discoloration of teeth and bones in children when used after 16 weeks of gestation, maternal liver toxicity[316-323]
Tobacco	IUGR, placenta previa, abruption placentae, decreased maternal thyroid function, premature rupture of membranes, low birth weight, perinatal mortality, ectopic pregnancy Children born to mothers who smoke during pregnancy at increased risk for asthma, infantile colic, and childhood obesity[324-330]
Warfarin	Exposure during the 1st trimester (critical period being weeks 6–9 gestation) often results in fetal warfarin syndrome, which consists of nasal hypoplasia, neonatal respiratory distress, low birth weight, eye defects including blindness, optic atrophy, and microphthalmia, hypoplasia of the extremities, developmental retardation, seizures, scoliosis, deafness, congenital heart disease, and death[331-334]

[a]Many of the major drug-induced congenital anomalies are discussed in the text. This table lists additional known teratogenic effects.

where available. Delivery plans and postbirth plans including treatment and management for the infant should be discussed.

MANAGEMENT OF TERATOGENICITY

Due to the unpredictable nature and unknown etiologies of birth defects, it will likely be a long time before these can be avoided completely. Whenever possible, a comprehensive team should manage neonates and infants with congenital anomalies, and support should extend beyond the pediatric age. There is growing concern regarding the quality of life available to those with congenital anomalies, especially when the birth defect is visible to others. Visible birth defects can cause stereotyping, bullying, lack of self-esteem, and psychosocial issues, especially among school-aged children where physical appearance and "fitting in" are extremely important. Although some individuals are able to adjust to their differences, others face many of these issues well into adulthood.

A team of supportive healthcare providers needs to be established and available throughout the individual's life. At the time a structural defect is identified during pregnancy, the team will likely include obstetricians, neonatologists, geneticists, pediatricians, pharmacists, and pediatric surgeons to deal with the maternal and fetal complexities. Nonstructural defects will require a team of healthcare providers as well. The team should provide education to the prospective parents regarding fetal outcomes; possible interventions; appropriate setting, time, and route of delivery; and expected postnatal outcomes.[267] Some information may not be known until delivery, but support and care for the patient and family should be a primary concern. More than 50% of parents feel that counseling from a religious person should be available especially when critical decisions regarding possible termination of pregnancy are required.[268] Psychological care for the patient and caregivers should also be considered to help individuals adjust to life with their disability. This is especially important in patients with a visible defect. Open communications between team members and the family involved are key to continued success in promoting improved quality of life and managing the impact of the anomaly.

INFORMATION FOR PATIENTS

Providing information to patients regarding risks associated with medication use during pregnancy requires preparation and strong communication skills. Patients and their family members often have a lot of questions regarding the associated risks of drug exposure and rely heavily on information they find on the Internet, television, or from acquaintances.

Healthcare providers need to be prepared to answer questions regarding the drug the patient is taking, how the drug can impact pregnancy and the developing fetus, and the impact of not treating or controlling the underlying condition the drug was prescribed to treat. Additionally, information regarding confounding risk factors (e.g., maternal cigarette smoking, alcohol use, and illicit drug use) should be provided and discussed.

Patients need to understand there is a balance between risks and benefits when determining whether to take certain drugs during pregnancy. For example, phenytoin is known to increase the risk of orofacial cleft formation in infants whose mothers take the drug throughout pregnancy. However, untreated seizure disorders during pregnancy are linked to decreased fetal oxygen delivery and can increase the risks for stillbirths, miscarriages, and serious developmental delays. In this scenario, the benefits of phenytoin therapy likely outweigh the risks of orofacial cleft development. These risks and benefits must be communicated clearly to patients so they are able to make informed decisions and take an active role in their health and pregnancy management. The following databases and references include information regarding teratology:

- Reprotox.org
- Clinical Teratology Web (TERIS) is available at depts.washington.edu/terisdb/terisweb/index.html.
- Briggs GG, Freeman RK, Towers CV, Forinash AB. *Drugs in Pregnancy and Lactation: A Reference Guide to Fetal and Neonatal Risk.* 11th ed. Philadelphia, PA: Wolters Kluwer Health, 2015.
- The Organization of Teratology Information Specialists (OTIS) is available at http://mothertobaby.org/benefits-otis/.

Clinicians and patients should be encouraged to participate in pregnancy registries that are open for enrollment to increase the pool of information available.

REFERENCES

1. Obican S, Scialli AR. Teratogenic exposures. *Am J Med Genet C Semin Med Genet.* 2011; 157:150-69.
2. Zhou S, Rosenthal DG, Sherman S et al. Physical, behavioral, and cognitive effects of prenatal tobacco and postnatal secondhand smoke exposure. *Curr Probl Pediatr Adolesc Health Care.* 2014; 44:219-41.
3. Wickstrom R. Effects of nicotine during pregnancy: human and experimental evidence. *Curr Neuropharmacol.* 2007; 5:213-22.

4. Wendell AD. Overview and epidemiology of substance abuse in pregnancy. *Clin Obstet Gynecol.* 2013; 56:91-6.
5. Schempf AH, Strobino DM. Illicit drug use and adverse birth outcomes: is it drugs or context? *J Urban Health.* 2008; 85:858-73.
6. Shiono PH, Klebanoff MA, Nugent RP et al. The impact of cocaine and marijuana use on low birth weight and preterm birth: a multicenter study. *Am J Obstet Gynecol.* 1995; 172(1 Pt 1):19-27.
7. Ganapathy V, Prasad PD, Ganapathy ME et al. Drugs of abuse and placental transport. *Adv Drug Deliv Rev.* 1999; 1:99-110.
8. Hill AB. The environment and disease: association or causation? *Proc R Soc Med.* 1965; 58:295-300.
9. Forrest JM, Turnbull FM, Sholler GF et al. Gregg's congenital rubella patients 60 years later. *Med J Aust.* 2002 Dec 2–16; 177:664-7.
10. McBride WG. Teratogenic action of thalidomide. *Lancet.* 1978 Jun 24; 1:1362.
11. Lenz W. A short history of thalidomide embryopathy. *Teratology.* 1988 Sep; 38:203-15.
12. Schumacher H, Blake DA, Gillette JR. Disposition of thalidomide in rabbits and rats. *J Pharmacol Exp Ther.* 1968; 160:201-11.
13. Mitchell AA, Gilboa SM, Werler MM et al. Medication use during pregnancy, with particular focus on prescription drugs: 1976-2008. *Am J Obstet Gynecol.* 2011; 205:51.e1-51.e8
14. Petersen EE, Rasmussen SA, Daniel KL et al. Prescription medication borrowing and sharing among women of reproductive age. *J Womens Health (Larchmt).* 2008; 17:1073-80.
15. van der Aa EM, Peereboom-Stegeman JHJC, Noordhoek J et al. Mechanisms of drug transfer across the placenta. *Pharm World Sci.* 1998; 20:139-48.
16. Syme MR, Paxton JW, Keelan JA. Drug transfer and metabolism by the human placenta. *Clin Pharmacokinet.* 2004; 43:487-514.
17. Ganapathy V, Prasad PD, Ganapathy ME et al. Placental transporters relevant to drug distribution across the maternal-fetal interface. *J Pharmacol Exp Ther.* 2000; 294:413-20.
18. Kane SV, Acquah LA. Placental transport of immunoglobulins: a clinical review for gastroenterologists who prescribe therapeutic monoclonal antibodies to women during contraception and pregnancy. *Am J Gastroenterol.* 2009; 104:228-33.
19. Auger N, Fraser WD, Arbour L et al. Elevated ambient temperatures and risk of neural tube defects. *Occup Environ Med.* 2017; 74:315-20.
20. Schaefer C, Hannemann D, Meister R et al. Vitamin K antagonists and pregnancy outcome. A multi-centre prospective study. *Thromb Haemost.* 2006; 95:949-57.
21. Wilson JG, Fraser FC. *Handbook of teratology.* Vol. 1–4. New York and London: Plenum Press; 1997:476-91.
22. Centers for Disease Control and Prevention. Update on overall prevalence of major birth defects—Atlanta, Georgia. 1978–2005. *MMWR Morb Mortal Wkly Rep.* 2008; 56:1-5.
23. Holm V. Developmental disabilities: delivery of medical care for children and adults. *JAMA.* 1989; 262:2935-6.
24. Williams G, King J, Cunningham M et al. Fetal valproate syndrome and autism: additional evidence of an association. *Dev Med Child Neurol.* 2001; 43:202-6.
25. Christensen J, Gronborg TK, Sorensen MJ et al. Prenatal valproate exposure and risk of autism spectrum disorders and childhood autism. *JAMA.* 2013; 309:1696-703.
26. Meador KJ, Baker GA, Browning N et al. Fetal antiepileptic drug exposure and cognitive outcomes at age 6 years (NEAD study): a prospective observational study. *Lancet Neurol.* 2013; 12:244-52.
27. Hanson JW. Teratogen update: fetal hydantoin effects. *Teratology.* 1986; 33:349-53.
28. Scolnik D, Nulman I, Rovert J et al. Neurodevelopment of children exposed in utero to phenytoin and carbamazepine monotherapy. *JAMA.* 1994; 271:767-70.
29. Adab N, Kini U, Vinten J et al. The longer term outcome of children born to mothers with epilepsy. *J Neurol Neurosurg Psychiatry.* 2004; 75:1575-83.
30. Adab N, Jacoby A, Smith D et al. Additional educational needs in children born to mothers with epilepsy. *J Neurol Neurosurg Psychiatry.* 2001; 70:15-21.
31. National Institute of Neurological Disorders and Stroke. Learning disabilities. https://www.ninds.nih.gov/Disorders/All-Disorders/Learning-Disabilities-Information-Page (accessed 2017 Dec 12).
32. American Speech-Language-Hearing Association. Language-based learning disabilities: Causes and number. http://www.asha.org/public/speech/disorders/LBLD.htm (accessed 2017 Dec 11).
33. Meador K, Baker GA, Browning N et al. Foetal antiepileptic drug exposure and verbal versus non-verbal abilities at three years of age. *Brain.* 2011; 34:396-404.
34. National Center for Learning Disabilities. The navigator: a comprehensive resource guide about learning disabilities for the pediatric professional community and parents. http://ldnavigator.ncld.org/#/ld-defined/etiology-of-ld (accessed 2017 Dec 11).
35. Learning Disabilities Association of America. Support and resources for professionals. https://ldaamerica.org/professionals/ (accessed 2017 Dec 11).
36. Martin JA, Hamilton BE, Osterman MJK et al. Births: final data for 2013. *Natl Vital Stat Rep.* 2015; 64:1-65.
37. Resnik R, Creasy RK. Intrauterine growth restriction. In: *Creasy and Resnik's maternal fetal medicine.* 7th ed. Philadelphia, PA: Elsevier Saunders; 2014:743-55.
38. Bloom SL, Sheffield JS, McIntire DD et al. Antenatal dexamethasone and decreased birth weight. *Obstet Gynecol.* 2001; 97:485-90.
39. Wapner RJ, Sorokin Y, Mele L et al. Long-term outcomes after repeat doses of antenatal corticosteroids. *N Engl J Med.* 2007; 357:1190-8.
40. Report on the National High Blood Pressure Education Program Working on High Blood Pressure in Pregnancy. *Am J Obstet Gynecol.* 2000; 183:S1-22.
41. Parazzini F, Benedetto C, Bortolus R et al. Nifedipine versus expectant management in mild to moderate hypertension in pregnancy. *BJOG.* 1998; 105:718-22.
42. Magee LA, Omstein MP, von Dsadelszen P. Fortnightly review: management of hypertension in pregnancy. *BMJ.* 1999; 318:1332-6.
43. Lydakis C, Lip GY, Beevers M et al. Atenolol and fetal growth in pregnancies complicated by hypertension. *Am J Hypertens.* 1999; 12:541-7.
44. Easterling TR, Brateng D, Schmucker B et al. Prevention of preeclampsia: a randomized trial of atenolol in hyperdynamic patients before onset of hypertension. *Obstet Gynecol.* 1999; 93:725-33.
45. Tanaka K, Tanaka H, Kamiya C et al. Beta-blockers and fetal growth restriction in pregnant women with cardiovascular disease. *Circ J.* 2016; 80:2221-6.
46. Pryde PG, Sedman AB, Nugent CE, Barr M Jr. Angiotensin-converting enzyme inhibitor fetopathy. *J Am Soc Nephrol.* 1993; 3:1575-82.
47. Webster LM, Conti-Ramsden F, Seed PT et al. Impact of antihypertensive treatment on maternal and perinatal outcomes in pregnancy complicated by chronic hypertension: a systemic review and meta-analysis. *J Am Heart Assoc.* 2017; 6. pii: e005526.
48. Hamilton BE, Martin JA, Osterman MJK et al. Births: Final data for 2014. *Natl Vital Stat Rep.* 2015; 64:1-64.
49. March of Dimes. Low birthweight. www.marchofdimes.org/complications/low-birthweight.aspx (accessed 2017 Dec 11).
50. Kramer MS. Determinants of low birth weight: methodological assessment and meta-analysis. *Bull World Health Organ.* 1987; 65:663-737.
51. Miller SL, Huppi PS, Mallard C. The consequences of fetal growth restriction on brain structure and neurodevelopmental outcome. *J Physiol.* 2016; 594:807-23.
52. Magann EF, Haram K, Ounpraseuth S et al. Use of antenatal corticosteroids in special circumstances: a comprehensive review. *Acta Obstet Gynecol Scand.* 2017; 96:385-409.

53. McEvoy C, Schilling D, Peters D et al. Respiratory compliance in preterm infants after a single rescue course of antenatal steroids: a randomized controlled trial. *Am J Obstet Gynecol.* 2010; 202:544.e1-9.
54. Churchill D, Bayliss H, Beevers G. Fetal growth restriction. *Lancet.* 2000; 355:1366-7.
55. Goldenberg RL, Culhane JF, Iams JD et al. Epidemiology and causes of preterm birth. *Lancet.* 2008; 371:75-84.
56. Trudinger BJ, Giles WB, Cook CM et al. Fetal umbilical artery flow velocity waveforms and placental resistance: clinical significance. *Br J Obstet Gynaecol.* 1985; 92:23-30.
57. Aoyama K, Endo T, Saito T et al. Maternal and placental risk factors for light-for-gestational-age births. *J Obstet Gynaecol Res.* 2016; 42:831-6.
58. Centers for Disease Control and Prevention. Low birth weight and the environment. Reproductive and birth outcomes. ephtracking.cdc.gov/showRbLBWGrowthRetardationEnv.action (accessed 2017 Dec 12).
59. Wen SW, Goldenberg RL, Cutter GR et al. Smoking, maternal age, fetal growth, and gestational age at delivery. *Am J Obstet Gynecol.* 1990; 162:53-8.
60. Cliver SP, Goldenberg RL, Cutter GR et al. The effect of cigarette smoking on neonatal anthropometric measurements. *Obstet Gynecol.* 1995; 85:625-30.
61. Kallen K. Maternal smoking during pregnancy and infant head circumference at birth. *Early Hum Dev.* 2000; 58:197-204.
62. Little BB, Snell LM. Brain growth among fetuses exposed to cocaine in utero: asymmetrical growth retardation. *Obstet Gynecol.* 1991; 77:361-4.
63. Heinonen S, Taipale P, Saarikoski S. Weights of placenta from small-for-gestational age infants revisited. *Placenta.* 2001; 22:399-404.
64. Wilcox AJ. On the importance—and the unimportance—of birthweight. *Int J Epidemiol.* 2001; 30:1233-41.
65. March of Dimes, The Partnership for Maternal, Newborn and Child Health, Save the Children, WHO. Born too soon: the global action report on preterm birth. Geneva: World Health Organization; 2012. http://whqlibdoc.who.int/publications/2012/9789241503433_eng.pdf (accessed 2017 Dec 12).
66. Risnes KR, Vatten LJ, Baker JL et al. Birthweight and mortality in adulthood: a systematic review and metaanalysis. *Int J Epidemiol.* 2011; 40:647-61.
67. Larroque B, Bertrais S, Czernichow P, Leger J. School difficulties in 20-year-olds who were born small for gestational age at term in a regional cohort study. *Pediatrics.* 2001; 108:111-15.
68. Dansky LV, Finnell RH. Parental epilepsy, anticonvulsant drugs and reproductive outcome: epidemiologic and experimental findings spanning three decades; 2: human studies. *Reprod Toxicol.* 1991; 5:301-35.
69. Nguyen HT, Sharma V, McIntyre RS. Teratogenesis associated with antibipolar agents. *Adv Ther.* 2009; 26:281-94.
70. Xiao WL, Liu XY, Liu YS et al. The relationship between maternal corticosteroid use and orofacial clefts—a meta-analysis. *Reprod Toxicol.* 2017; 69:99-105.
71. Dolk H, Wang H, Loane M et al. Lamotrigine use in pregnancy and risk of orofacial cleft and other congenital anomalies. *Neurology.* 2016; 86:1716-25.
72. Veroniki AA, Cogo E, Rios P et al. Comparative safety of antiepileptic drugs during pregnancy: a systematic review and network meta-analysis of congenital malformations and prenatal outcomes. *BMC Med.* 2017; 15:95.
73. Anderka MT, Lin AE, Abuelo DN et al. Reviewing the evidence for mycophenolate mofetil as a new teratogen: case report and review of the literature. *Am J Med Genet A.* 2009; 149A:1241-8.
74. Dolovich LR, Addis A, Vaillancourt JM et al. Benzodiazepine use in pregnancy and major malformations or oral cleft: meta-analysis of cohort and case-control studies. *BMJ.* 1998; 26:839-43.
75. Parker SE, Mai CT, Canfield MA et al. for the National Birth Defects Prevention Network. Updated national birth prevalence estimates for selected birth defects in the United States, 2004-2006. Birth Defects Research (Part A): *Clin and Mol Teratol.* 2010; 88:1008-16.
76. Jackson A, Bromley R, Morrow J et al. In utero exposure to valproate increases the risk of isolated cleft palate. *Arch Dis Child Fetal Neonatal Ed.* 2016; 101:F207-11.
77. Holmes LB, Hernandez-Diaz S. Newer anticonvulsants: lamotrigine, topiramate and gabapentin. *Birth Defects Res A Clin Mol Teratol.* 2012; 94:599-606.
78. Holmes LB, Baldwin EJ, Smith CR et al. Increased frequency of isolated cleft palate in infants exposed to lamotrigine during pregnancy. *Neurology.* 2008; 70(22 Pt 2):2152-8.
79. Hunt SJ, Craig JJ, Morrow JL. Increased frequency of isolated cleft palate in infants exposed to lamotrigine during pregnancy. *Neurology.* 2009; 72:1108.
80. Cunnington M, Tennis P, International Lamotrigine Pregnancy Registry Scientific Advisory Committee. Lamotrigine and the risk of malformations in pregnancy. *Neurology.* 2005; 64:955-60.
81. Pergola PE, Kancharla A, Riley DJ. Kidney transplantation during the first trimester of pregnancy: immunosuppression with mycophenolate mofetil, tacrolimus and prednisone. *Transplantation.* 2001; 71:994-7.
82. LeRay C, Coulomb A, Elefant E et al. Mycophenolate mofetil in pregnancy after renal transplantation: a case of major fetal malformations. *Obstet Gynecol.* 2004; 103:1091-4.
83. Kallen B, Westgren M, Aberg A et al. Pregnancy outcome after maternal organ transplantation in Sweden. *Br J Obstet Gynaecol.* 2005; 112:904-9.
84. Sifontis NM, Coscia LA, Constantinescu S et al. Pregnancy outcomes in solid organ transplant with exposure to mycophenolate mofetil or sirolimus. *Transplantation.* 2006; 82:1698-1702.
85. Perez-Ayes A, Ledo A, Boso V et al. In utero exposure to mycophenolate mofetil: a characteristic phenotype? *Am J Med Genet Part A.* 2007; 146A:1-7.
86. Sebaaly ZE, Charpentier B, Snanoudj R. Fetal malformations associated with mycophenolate mofetil for lupus nephritis. *Nephrol Dial Transplant.* 2007; 22:2722-32.
87. Tjeertes IFA, Bastiaans DET, van Ganzewinkel CJLM et al. Neonatal anemia and hydrops fetalis after maternal mycophenolate mofetil use. *J Perinatol.* 2007; 27:62-4.
88. Ang GS, Simpson SA, Reddy AR. Mycophenolate mofetil embryopathy may be dose and timing dependent. *Am J Med Genet Part A.* 2008; 146A:1963-6.
89. Schoner K, Steinhard J, Figiel J et al. Severe facial clefts in acrofacial dystosis: a consequence of prenatal exposure to mycophenolate mofetil? *Obstet Gynecol.* 2008; 111:483-6.
90. Velinov M, Zellers N. The fetal mycophenolate mofetil syndrome. *Clin Dysmorphol.* 2008; 17:77-8.
91. Vila JHA, da Silva JP, Guilhen CJ et al. Even low dose of mycophenolate mofetil in a mother recipient of heart transplant can seriously damage the fetus. *Transplantation.* 2008; 86:369-70.
92. Perry MD, McEvoy GK. Isotretinoin: new therapy for severe acne. *Clin Pharm.* 1983; 2:12-9.
93. Henderson IWD, Rice WB. Accutane. *Can Med Assoc J.* 1983; 129:682.
94. Shalita AR, Cunningham WJ, Leyden JJ et al. Isotretinoin treatment of acne and related disorders: an update. *J Am Acad Dermatol.* 1983; 9:629-38.
95. Conner CS. Isotretinoin: a reappraisal. *Drug Intell Clin Pharm.* 1984; 18:308-9.
96. Ward A, Brogden RN, Heel RC et al. Isotretinoin. A review of its pharmacological properties and therapeutic efficacy in acne and other skin disorders. *Drugs.* 1984; 28:6-37.
97. Lammer EJ, Chen DT, Hoar RM et al. Retinoic acid embryopathy. *N Engl J Med.* 1985; 313:837-41.

98. Stern RS, Rosa F, Baum C. Isotretinoin and pregnancy. *J Am Acad Dermatol.* 1984; 10:851-4.
99. Marwick C. More cautionary labeling appears on isotretinoin. *JAMA*. 1984; 251:3208-9.
100. Zarowny DP. Accutane Roche: risk of teratogenic effects. *CMAJ.* 1984; 131:273.
101. Robertson R, MacLeod PM. Accutane-induced teratogensis. *CMAJ.* 1985; 133:1147-8.
102. Willhite CC, Hill RM, Irving DW. Isotretinoin-induced craniofacial malformations in humans and hamsters. *J Craniofac Genet Dev Biol.* 1986; 2(suppl):193-209.
103. Carmichael SL, Shaw GM, Ma C et al. Maternal corticosteroid use and orofacial clefts. *Am J Obstet Gynecol.* 2007; 197:585.e1-7; discussion 683-4, e1-7.
104. Skuladottir H, Wilcox AJ, Ma C et al. Corticosteroid use and risk of orofacial clefts. *Birth Defects Res A Clin Mol Teratol.* 2014; 100:499-506.
105. Wikner BN, Stiller CO, Bergman U et al. Use of benzodiazepines and benzodiazepine receptor agonists during pregnancy: neonatal outcome and congenital malformations. *Pharmacoepidemiol Drug Saf.* 2007; 16:1203-10.
106. Enato E, Moretti M, Koren G. The fetal safety of benzodiazepines: an updated meta-analysis. *J Obstet Gynaecol Can.* 2011; 33:46-8.
107. Munsie JW, Lin S, Browne ML et al. Maternal bronchodilator use and the risk of orofacial clefts. *Hum Reprod.* 2011; 26:3147-54.
108. Palmieri A, Avantaggiato A, Brunelli G et al. Drugs and nonsyndromic orofacial cleft: an update. *Braz J Oral Sci.* 2008; 7:1470-5.
109. Lammer EJ, Chen DT, Hoar RM et al. Retinoic acid embryopathy. *N Engl J Med.* 1985; 313:837-41.
110. Webster WS, Johnston MC, Lammer EJ et al. Isotretinoin embryopathy and the cranial neural crest: an in vivo and in vitro study. *J Craniofac Genet Dev Biol.* 1986; 6:211-22.
111. Dulay AT. Imaging of the face and neck: cleft lip and palate. In: Creasy and Resnik's *Maternal fetal medicine.* 7th ed. Philadelphia, PA: Elsevier Saunders; 2014:264-7.
112. Waller DK, Shaw GM, Rasmussen SA et al. Prepregnancy obesity as a risk factor for structural birth defects. *Arch Pediatr Adolesc Med.* 2007; 161:745-50.
113. Stothard KJ, Tennant PW, Bell R et al. Maternal overweight and obesity and the risk of congenital anomalies: a systemic review and meta-analysis. *JAMA*. 2009; 301:636-50.
114. Metneki J, Puho E, Czeizel AE. Maternal disease and isolated orofacial clefts in Hungary. *Birth Defects Res A Clin Mol Teratol.* 2005; 73:617-23.
115. Feldkamp ML, Meyer RE, Krikov S et al. Acetaminophen use in pregnancy and risk of birth defects: finding from the National Birth Defects Prevention Study. *Obstet Gynecol.* 2010; 115:109-15.
116. Spilson SV, Kim HJ, Chung KC. Association between maternal diabetes mellitus and newborn oral cleft. *Ann Plast Surg.* 2001; 47:477-81.
117. Munger RG, Sauberlich HE, Corcoran C et al. Maternal vitamin B-6 and folate status and risk of oral cleft birth defects in the Philippines. *Birth Defects Res A Clin Mol Teratol.* 2004; 70:464-71.
118. Tamura T, Munger RG, Corcoran C et al. Plasma zinc concentrations of mothers and the risk of nonsyndromic oral clefts in their children: a case-control study in the Philippines. *Birth Defects Res A Clin Mol Teratol.* 2005; 73:612-6.
119. Mossey PA, Shaw WC, Munger RG et al. Global oral health inequalities: challenges in the prevention and management of orofacial clefts and potential solutions. *Adv Dent Res.* 2011; 23:247-58.
120. Little J, Cardy A, Arslan MT et al. United Kingdom-based case-control study. Smoking and orofacial clefts: a United Kingdom-based case-control study. *Cleft Palate Craniofac J.* 2004; 41:381-6.
121. Kang SL, Narayanan CS, Kelsall W. Mortality among infants born with orofacial clefts in a single cleft network. *Cleft Palate Craniofac J.* 2012; 49:508-11.
122. American Cleft Palate-Craniofacial Association. *Parameters for evaluation and treatment of patients with cleft lip/palate or other craniofacial anomalies.* Rev ed. Chapel Hill, NC; Nov 2009: 1-34. http://www.cleftline.org/wp-content/uploads/2012/03/Parameters.pdf (accessed 2017 Dec 11).
123. Huybrechts KF, Hernandez-Diaz S, Patorno E et al. Antipsychotic use in pregnancy and the risk for congenital malformations. *JAMA Psychiatry*. 2016; 73:938-46.
124. Daud AN, Bergman JE, Kerstjens-Frederikse WS et al. The risk of congenital heart anomalies following prenatal exposure to serotonin reuptake inhibitors—is pharmacogenetics the key? *Int J Mol Sci.* 2016; 17. pii:E1333.
125. Lenz W. Thalidomide and congenital abnormalities. *Lancet*. 1962; 1:45.
126. Anonymous. Birth defects caused by isotretinoin—New Jersey. *MMWR Morb Mortal Wkly Rep.* 1988; 18:543-52.
127. Oyen N, Poulsen G, Boyd HA et al. National time trends in congenital heart defects, Denmark, 1977-2005. *Am Heart J.* 2009; 157:467-73.
128. Nau H, Rating D, Koch S et al. Valproic acid and its metabolites: placental transfer, neonatal pharmacokinetics, transfer via mother's milk and clinical status in neonates and epileptic mothers. *J Pharmacol Exp Ther.* 1981; 219:768-77.
129. Thomas D, Buchanan N. Teratogenic effects of anticonvulsants. *J Pediatr.* 1981; 99:163.
130. Clay SA, McVie R, Chen H. Possible teratogenic effect of valproic acid. *J Pediatr.* 1981; 99:828.
131. Bailey CJ, Pool RW, Poskitt EME et al. Valproic acid and fetal abnormality. *Br Med J.* 1983; 286:190.
132. Jager-Roman E, Deichi A, Jakob S et al. Fetal growth, major malformations, and minor anomalies in infants born to women receiving valproic acid. *J Pediatr.* 1986; 108:997-1004.
133. Legius E, Jaeken J, Eggermont E. Sodium valproate, pregnancy, and infantile fatal liver failure. *Lancet.* 1987; 2:1518-9.
134. DiLiberti JH, Farndon PA, Dennis NR et al. The fetal valproate syndrome. *Am J Med Genet.* 1984; 19:473-81.
135. Jentink J, Loane MA, Dolk H et al. Valproic acid monotherapy in pregnancy and major congenital malformations. *N Engl J Med.* 2010; 362:2185-93.
136. Pfeiffer RA, Kosenow W. Thalidomide and congenital abnormalities. *Lancet.* 1962; 1:45-6.
137. Speirs AL. Thalidomide and congenital abnormalities. *Lancet.* 1962; 1:303-5.
138. Owen R, Smith A. Cor triloculare and thalidomide. *Lancet.* 1962; 2:836.
139. Stromland K, Miller MT. Thalidomide embryopathy: revisited 27 years later. *Acta Ophthalmol.* 1993; 71:238-45.
140. Newman CGH. The thalidomide syndrome: risks of exposure and spectrum of malformations. *Clin Perinatol.* 1986; 13:555-73.
141. Schou M. What happened later to the lithium babies? A follow-up study of children born without malformations. *Acta Psychiatr Scand.* 1976; 54:193-7.
142. Kallen B, Tandberg A. Lithium and pregnancy. A cohort study on manic-depressive women. *Acta Psychiatr Scand.* 1983; 68:134-9.
143. Kallen B. Comments on teratogen update: lithium. *Teratology.* 1988; 38:597.
144. Cohen LS, Friedman JM, Jefferson JW et al. A reevaluation of risk of in utero exposure to lithium. *JAMA.* 1994; 271:146-50.
145. Jacobson SJ, Ceolin L, Kaur P et al. Prospective multicenter study of pregnancy outcome after lithium exposure during first trimester. *Lancet.* 1992; 339:530-3.
146. Cole JA, Ephross SA, Cosmatos IS et al. Paroxetine in the first trimester and the prevalence of congenital malformations. *Pharmacoepidemiol Drug Saf.* 2007; 16:1075-85.
147. Kallen B, Otterbald Olausson P. Antidepressant drugs during pregnancy and infant congenital heart defect. *Reprod Toxicol.* 2006; 21:221-2.
148. Kornum JB, Nielsen RB, Pedersen L et al. Use of selective serotonin reuptake inhibitors during early pregnancy and risk of congenital malformations: updated analysis. *Clin Epidemiol.* 2010; 2:29-36.

149. Pedersen LH, Henriksen TB, Vestergaard M et al. Selective serotonin reuptake inhibitors in pregnancy and congenital malformations: population based cohort study. *BMJ*. 2009; 339:b3569.
150. Louik C, Lin AE, Werler MM et al. First-trimester use of selective serotonin-reuptake inhibitors and the risk of birth defects. *N Engl J Med*. 2007; 356:2675-83.
151. Berard A, Ramos E, Rey E et al. First trimester exposure to paroxetine and risk of cardiac malformations in infants: the importance of dosage. *Birth Defects Res B Dev Reprod Toxicol*. 2007; 80:18-27.
152. Jimeneaz-Solem E, Andersen JT, Petersen M et al. Exposure to selective serotonin reuptake inhibitors and the risk of congenital malformations: a nationwide cohort study. *BMJ Open*. 2012; 2. pii: e001148.
153. Wurst KE, Poole C, Ephross SA et al. First trimester paroxetine use and the prevalence of congenital, specifically cardiac, defects: a meta-analysis of epidemiological studies. *Birth Defects Res A Clin Mol Teratol*. 2010; 88:159-70.
154. Reefhuis J, Devine O, Friedman JM et al. Specific SSRIs and birth defects: Bayesian analysis to interpret new data in the context of previous reports. *BMJ*. 2015; 351:h3190.
155. Bar-Oz B, Einarson T, Einarson A et al. Paroxetine and congenital malformations: meta-analysis and consideration of potential confounding factors. *Clin Ther*. 2007; 29:918-26.
156. Du ZD, Roguin N, Barak M et al. High prevalence of muscular ventricular septal defect in preterm neonates. *Am J Cardiol*. 1996; 78:1183-5.
157. Matok I, Pupco A, Koren G. Drug exposure in pregnancy and heart disease. *J Cardiovasc Pharmacol*. 2011; 58:20-4.
158. Vis JC, Duffels MGJ, Winter MM et al. Down syndrome: a cardiovascular perspective. *J Intellect Disabil Res*. 2009; 53:419-25.
159. Rao PS. Diagnosis and management of cyanotic congenital heart disease: part I. *Indian J Pediatr*. 2009; 76:57-70.
160. Jenkins KJ, Correa A, Feinstein JA et al. Noninherited risk factors and congenital cardiovascular defects: current knowledge: a scientific statement from the American Heart Association Council on Cardiovascular Disease in the Young: endorsed by the American Academy of Pediatrics. *Circulation*. 2007; 115:2995-3014.
161. Flatt AE. *The care of congenital hand anomalies*. St. Louis, MO: VB Mosby Company; 1977.
162. da Silva Dal Pizzol T, Knop FP, Mengue SS. Prenatal exposure to misoprostol and congenital anomalies: systematic review and meta-analysis. *Reprod Toxicol*. 2006; 22:666-71.
163. TERIS, The Teratogen Information System. Shepard Summary. http://depts.washington.edu/terisdb/terisweb/index.html (accessed 2017 Jan 14).
164. Alessandri JL, Isidor B, David A et al. Tibial developmental field defect in valproic acid embryopathy: report on three cases. *Am J Med Genet A*. 2010; 152A:2805-9.
165. Honein MA, Paulozzi LJ, Erikson JD. Continued occurrence of Accutane-exposed pregnancies. *Teratology*. 2001; 64:142-7.
166. Evermann D. Hands and feet. In: Stevenson Re, Hall JG, eds. *Human malformations and related anomalies*. New York: Oxford University Press; 2006:935-96.
167. Stevenson RE, Hall JG. *Human malformations and related anomalies*. New York: Oxford University Press; 2006:835-933.
168. Froster-Iskenius UG, Baird PA. Limb reduction defects in over one million consecutive live births. *Teratology*. 1989; 39:127-35.
169. Gold NB, Westgate MN, Holmes LB. Anatomic and etiological classification of congenital limb deficiencies. *Am J Med Genet A*. 2011; 155A:1225-35.
170. McGuirk CK, Westgate MN, Holmes LB. Limb deficiencies in newborn infants. *Pediatrics*. 2001; 108:E64.
171. Kallen B, Rahmani TM, Winberg J. Infants with congenital limb reduction registered in the Swedish Register of Congenital Malformations. *Teratology*. 1984; 29:73-85.
172. Rosana A, Botto LD, Botting B et al. Infant mortality and congenital anomalies from 1950 to 1994: an international perspective. *J Epidemiol Community Health*. 2000; 54:660-6.
173. McBride WB. Thalidomide and congenital abnormalities. *Lancet*. 1961; 2:1358.
174. Alexander PG, Clark KL, Tuan RS. Prenatal exposure to environmental factors and congenital limb defects. *Birth Defects Res C Embryo Today*. 2016; 108:243-73.
175. Genest DR, Di Salvo D, Rosenblatt MJ et al. Terminal transverse limb defects with tethering and omphalocele in a 17 week fetus following first trimester misoprostol exposure. *Clin Dysmorphol*. 1999; 8:53-8.
176. Coelho KE, Sarmento MF, Veiga CM et al. Misoprostol embryotoxicity: clinical evaluation of fifteen patients with arthrogryposis. *Am J Med Genet* .2000; 95:297-301.
177. Holmes LB. Teratogen-induced limb defects. *Am J Med Genet*. 2002; 112:297-303.
178. Rodriguez-Pinilla E, Arroyo I, Fondevilla J et al. Prenatal exposure to valproic acid during pregnancy and limb deficiencies: a case-control study. *Am J Med Genet*. 2000; 90:376-81.
179. Shaw EB, Rees EL. Fetal damage due to aminopterin ingestion: follow-up at 17 ½ years of age. *Am J Dis Child*. 1980; 134:1172-3.
180. Shaw EB. Fetal damage due to maternal aminopterin ingestion: follow-up at age 9 years. *Am J Dis Child*. 1972; 124:93-4.
181. Adam MP, Manning MA, Beck AE et al. Methotrexate/misoprostol embryopathy: report of four cases resulting from failed medical abortion. *Am J Med Genet A*. 2003; 123:72-8.
182. Buckley LM, Bullaboy CA, Leichtman L et al. *Arthritis Rheum*. 1997; 40:971-3.
183. Kozma C, Ramasethu J. Methotrexate and misoprostol teratogenicity: further expansion of the clinical manifestations. *Am J Med Genet*. 2011; 155:1723-8.
184. Hyoun SC, Obican SG, Scialli AR. Teratogen update: methotrexate. *Birth Defects Res A Clin Mol Teratol*. 2012; 94:187-207.
185. Loughnan PM, Gold H, Vance JC. Phenytoin teratogenicity in man. *Lancet*. 1973; 1:70-2.
186. Adams J, Vorhees CV, Middaugh LD. Developmental neurotoxicity of anticonvulsants: human and animal evidence on phenytoin. *Neurotoxicol Teratol*. 1990; 12:203-14.
187. Holmes LB, Harvey EA, Coull BA et al. The teratogenicity of anticonvulsant drugs. *N Engl J Med*. 2001; 344:1132-8.
188. McBride WG. Isotretinoin and reduction deformities. *Lancet*. 1985; 2:503.
189. Lammer EJ, Flannery DB, Barr M. Does isotretinoin cause limb reduction defects? *Lancet*. 1985; 2:328.
190. Rizzo R, Lammer EJ, Parono E et al. Limb reduction defects in humans associated with prenatal isotretinoin exposure. *Teratology*. 1991; 44:599-604.
191. Tayel SM, Fawzia MM, Al Naqeeb NA et al. A morpho-etiological description of congenital limb anomalies. *Ann Saudi Med*. 2005; 25:219-27.
192. Fonseca W, Misago C, Kanji N. Misoprostol plus mifepristone. *Lancet*. 1991; 338:1594.
193. Aberg A, Westbom L, Kallen B. Congenital malformations among infants whose mothers had gestational diabetes or preexisting diabetes. *Early Hum Dev*. 2001; 61:85-95.
194. Correa A, Gilboa SM, Besser LM et al. Diabetes mellitus and birth defects. *Am J Obstet Gynecol*. 2008; 199:237-9.
195. Moore LL, Singer MR, Bradlee ML et al. A prospective study of the risk of congenital defects associated with maternal obesity and diabetes mellitus. *Epidemiology*. 2000; 11:689-94.
196. Shaw GM, Todoroff K, Schaffer DM et al. Maternal height and prepregnancy body mass as risk factors for selected congenital anomalies. *Paediatr Perinat Epidemiol*. 2000; 14:234-39.
197. Watkins ML, Rasmussen SA, Honein MA et al. Maternal obesity and risk for birth defects. *Pediatrics*. 2003; 111(5 Part 2):1152-8.
198. Rosano A, Botto LD, Olney RS et al. Limb defects associated with major congenital anomalies: clinical and epidemiological study from the International Clearinghouse for Birth Defects Monitoring Systems. *Am J Med Genet*. 2000; 93:110-6.

199. Johansen H, Dammann B, Oinaes Andersen L et al. Children with congenital limb deficiency in Norway: issues related to school life and health-related quality of life. A cross-sectional study. *Disabil Rehabil.* 2016; 38:1803-10.
200. Werler MM, Sheehan JE, Mitchell AA. Maternal medication use and risks of gastroschisis and small intestinal atresia. *Am J Epidemiol.* 2002; 155:26-31.
201. Werler MM, Mitchell AA, Shapiro S. Demographic, reproductive, medical, and environmental factors in relation to gastroschisis. *Teratology.* 1992; 45:353-60.
202. Torfs CP, Katz EA, Bateson TF et al. Maternal medications and environmental exposures as risk factors for gastroschisis. *Teratology.* 1996; 54:84-92.
203. Seattle Children's Hospital Research Foundation. Digestive and gastrointestinal conditions: gastroschisis. http://www.seattlechildrens.org/medical-conditions/digestive-gastrointestinal-conditions/gastroschisis/ (accessed 2017 Dec 11).
204. Anonymous. Gastroschisis and pseudoephedrine during pregnancy. *Prescrire Int.* 2004; 13:141-3.
205. Aselton P, Jick H, Milunsky A et al. First-trimester drug use and congenital disorders. *Obstet Gynecol.* 1985; 65:451-5.
206. Jick H, Holmes LB, Hunter JR et al. First-trimester drug use and congenital disorders. *JAMA.* 1981; 246:343-6.
207. deVries PA. The pathogenesis of gastroschisis and omphalocele. *J Pediatr Surg.* 1980; 153:245-51.
208. Hoyme HE, Higginbottom MC, Jones KL. The vascular pathogenesis of gastroschisis: intrauterine interruption of the omphalomesenteric artery. *J Pediatr.* 1981; 98:228-31.
209. Vermeij-Keers C, Hartwig NG, van der Werff JF. Embryonic development of the ventral body wall and its congenital malformations. *Semin Pediatr Surg.* 1996; 5:82-9.
210. Finnish Medical Society Duodecim. Ultrasound scanning during pregnancy. *EBM Guidelines.* 2008; Feb 15.
211. Midrio P, Stefanutti G, Mussap M et al. Aminoexchange for fetuses with gastroschisis: is it effective? *J Pediatr Surg.* 2007; 42:777-82.
212. Wolf RB. Abdominal imaging: 24D gastroschisis. In: *Creasy and Resnik's maternal fetal medicine.* 7th ed. Philadelphia, PA: Elsevier Saunders; 2014:334-6.
213. Reefhuis J, Hoein MA. Maternal age and non-chromosomal birth defects, Atlanta—1968-2000: teenager or thirty-something, who is at risk? *Birth Defects Res A Clin Mol Teratol.* 2004; 70:572-9.
214. Torfs CP, Velie EM, Oechsli FW et al. A population-based study of gastroschisis: demographic, pregnancy, and lifestyle risk factors. *Teratology.* 1994; 50:44-53.
215. Rittler M, Castilla EE, Chambers C et al. Risk for gastroschisis in primigravidity, length of sexual cohabitation, and change in paternity. *Birth Defects Res A Clin Mol Teratol.* 2007; 79:483-7.
216. Lam PK, Torfs CP, Brand RJ. A low pregnancy body mass index is a risk factor for an offspring with gastroschisis. *Epidemiology.* 1999; 10:717-21.
217. Werler MM, Sheehan JE, Mitchell AA. Association of vasoconstrictive exposures with risks of gastroschisis and small intestinal atresia. *Epidemiology.* 2003; 14:349-54.
218. Haddow JE, Palomaki GE, Holman MS. Young maternal age and smoking during pregnancy as risk factors for gastroschisis. *Teratology.* 1993; 47:225-28.
219. Martinez-Frias ML, Rodriguez-Pinilla E, Prieto L. Prenatal exposure to salicylates and gastroschisis: a case-control study. *Teratology.* 1997; 56:241-3.
220. Draper ES, Rankin J, Tonks AM et al. Recreational drug use: a major risk factor for gastroschisis? *Am J Epidemiol.* 2008; 167:485-91.
221. Boyd PA, Tonks AM, Rankin J et al. Monitoring the prenatal detection of structural fetal congenital anomalies in England and Wales: register-based study. *J Med Screen.* 2011; 18:2-7.
222. Botto LD, Moore CA, Khoury MJ et al. Neural-tube defects. *N Engl J Med.* 1999; 341:1509-19.
223. Marks JD, Khoshnood B. Epidemiology of common neurosurgical diseases in the neonate. *Neurosurg Clin N Am.* 1998; 9:63-72.
224. Parker SE, Mai CT, Canfield MA et al. Updated National Birth Prevalence estimates for selected birth defects in the United States, 2004-2006. *Birth Defects Res A Clin Mol Teratol.* 2010; 88:1008-16.
225. Manning FA. Imaging in the diagnosis of fetal anomalies. In: *Creasy and Resnik's maternal fetal medicine.* 6th ed. Philadelphia, PA: Elsevier Saunders; 2009:275-303.
226. Omtzigt J, Los FJ, Hagenaarz AM et al. Prenatal diagnosis of spina bifida aperta after first-trimester valproate exposure. *Prenat Diagn.* 1992; 12:893-7.
227. Jager-Roman E. Fetal growth, major malformations, and minor anomalies in infants born to women receiving valproic acid. *J Pediatr.* 1986; 108:997-1004.
228. Ogawa Y, Kaneko S, Otani K et al. Serum folic acid levels in epileptic mothers and their relationship to congenital malformations. *Epilepsy Res.* 1991; 8:75-8.
229. Wegner C, Nau H. Alteration of embryonic folate metabolism by valproic acid during organogenesis: implications for mechanism of teratogenesis. *Neurology.* 1992; 42(4 suppl 5):17-24.
230. Centers for Disease Control and Prevention. Spina bifida: facts. http://www.cdc.gov/ncbddd/spinabifida/facts.html (accessed 2017 Dec 11).
231. Wolf RB. Skeletal imaging: 26C neural tube defect. In: *Creasy and Resnik's maternal fetal medicine.* 7th ed. Philadelphia, PA: Elsevier Saunders; 2014:367-9.
232. Sandler A. *Living with spina bifida: a guide for families and professional.* Chapel Hill, NC: University of North Carolina Press; 2004.
233. Chescheir N, American College of Obstetricians and Gynecologists (ACOG) Committee on Practice Bulletins-Obstetric. ACOG practice bulletin: Neural tube defects, Number 44. *Int J Gynaecol Obstet.* 2003; 83:123-33.
234. Moretti M, Bar-Oz B, Fried S et al. Maternal hyperthermia and the risk for neural tube defects in offspring: systematic review and meta-analysis. *Epidemiology.* 2005; 16:216-9.
235. Centers for Disease Control and Prevention. Folic acid: occurrence and prevention. http://www.cdc.gov/ncbddd/folicacid/recommendations.html (accessed 2017 Dec 11).
236. Walters J, Ashwal S, Masek T. Anecephaly: where do we now stand? *Semin Neurol.* 1997; 17:249-55.
237. Kiymaz N, Yilmaz N, Demir I et al. Prognostic factors in patients with occipital encephalocele. *Pediatr Neurosurg.* 2010; 46:6-11.
238. Abuelo D. Microcephaly syndromes. *Semin Pediatr Neurol.* 2007; 14:118-27.
239. Pennell PB, Klein AM, Browning N et al. Differential effects of antiepileptic drugs on neonatal outcomes. *Epilepsy Behav.* 2012; 24:449-56.
240. Veiby G, Daltveit AK, Engelsen BA et al. Fetal growth restriction and birth defects with newer and older antiepileptic drugs during pregnancy. *J Neurol.* 2014; 261:579-88.
241. Anderka MT, Lin AE, Abuelo DN et al. Reviewing the evidence for mycophenolate mofetil as a new teratogen: case report and review of the literature. *Am J Med Genet A.* 2009; 149A:1241-8.
242. National Birth Defects Prevention Network. Major birth defects data from population-based birth defects surveillance programs in the United States, 2006-2010. *Birth Defects Res A Clin Mol Teratol.* 2013; 97:S1-172.
243. Almgren M, Kallen B, Lavebratt C. Population-based study of antiepileptic drug exposure in utero—influence on head circumference in newborns. *Seizure.* 2009; 18:672-5.
244. Hiilesmaa VK, Teramo K, Granstrom ML et al. Fetal head growth retardation associated with maternal antiepileptic drugs. *Lancet.* 1981; 318:165-7.
245. Bawle EV, Conard JV, Weiss L. Adult and two children with fetal methotrexate syndrome. *Teratology.* 1998; 57:51-5.
246. Zand DJ, Blance C, Coleman B et al. In utero methotrexate exposure resulting in long bone aplasia. *Am J Hum Genet.* 2003; 73:591.

247. Pang T, Atefy R, Sheen V. Malformations of cortical development. *Neurologist.* 2008; 14:181-91.
248. Pilu G, Falco P, Milano V et al. Prenatal diagnosis of microcephaly assisted by vaginal sonography and power Doppler. *Ultrasound Obstet Gynecol.* 1998; 11:357-60.
249. Monteagudo A, Timor-Tritsch IE. Central nervous system imaging: 20M microcephaly. In: *Creasy and Resnik's maternal fetal medicine.* 7th ed. Philadelphia, PA: Elsevier Saunders; 2014. Supplemental chapter available online through www.expertconsult.com.
250. Cordiero MT, Pena LJ, Brito CA et al. Positive IgM for Zika virus in the cerebrospinal fluid of 30 neonates with microcephaly in Brazil. *Lancet.* 2016; 387:1811-2.
251. Feldman HS, Jones KL, Lindsay S et al. Prenatal alcohol exposure patterns and alcohol-related birth defects and growth deficiencies: a prospective study. *Alcohol Clin Exp Res.* 2012; 36:670-6.
252. Kesrouani A, Fallet C, Vuillard E et al. Pathologic and laboratory correlation in microcephaly associated with prenatal cocaine exposure. *Early Hum Dev.* 2001; 63:79-81.
253. Centers for Disease Control and Prevention. Fetal alcohol syndrome: guidelines for referral and diagnosis. http://www.cdc.gov/ncbddd/fasd/documents/FAS_guidelines_accessible.pdf (accessed 2017 Dec 12).
254. Centers for Disease Control and Prevention. Fetal alcohol syndrome—Alaska, Arizona, Colorado, and New York, 1995-1997. *MMWR Morb Mortal Wkly Rep.* 2002; 51:433-5.
255. May PA, Baete A, Russo J et al. Prevalence and characteristics of fetal alcohol spectrum disorders. *Pediatrics.* 2014; 134:855-66.
256. May PA, Gossage JP, Kalberg WO et al. Prevalence and epidemiologic characteristics of FASD from various research methods with an emphasis on recent in-school studies. *Dev Disabil Res Rev.* 2009; 15:176-92.
257. Tan CH, Clark HD, Cheal NE et al. Alcohol use and binge drinking among women of childbearing age—United States, 2011-2013. *MMWR Morb Mortal Wkly Rep.* 2015; 64:1042-6.
258. Fan J, Jacobson SW, Taylor PA et al. White matter deficits mediate effects of prenatal alcohol exposure on cognitive development in childhood. *Hum Brain Mapp.* 2016; 37:2943-58.
259. Gemma S, Vichi S, Testai E. Metabolic and genetic factors contributing to alcohol induced effects and fetal alcohol syndrome. *Neurosci Biobehav Rev.* 2007; 31:221-9.
260. Carlo WA. Fetal alcohol syndrome. In: Kliegman RM, Stanton BF, St. Geme JW III et al., eds. *Nelson textbook of pediatrics.* 19th ed. Philadelphia, PA: Saunders Elsevier; 2011: chap 100.2.
261. Streissguth AP, Bookstein FL, Barr HM et al. Risk factors for adverse life outcomes in fetal alcohol syndrome and fetal alcohol effects. *J Dev and Behav Pediatr.* 2004; 25:228-38.
262. Nordentoft M, Wahlbeck K, Hallgren J et al. Excess mortality, causes of death and life expectancy in 270,770 patients with recent onset of mental disorders in Denmark, Finland, and Sweden. *PLoS One.* 2013; 8:e55176.
263. Wahlbeck K, Westman J, Nordentoft M et al. Outcomes of Nordic mental health systems: life expectancy of patients with mental disorders. *Br J Psychiatry.* 2011; 199:453-8.
264. Dalsgaard S, Ostergaard SD, Leckman JF et al. Mortality in children, adolescents, and adults with attention deficit hyperactivity disorder: a nationwide cohort study. *Lancet.* 2015; 385:2190-6.
265. Patja K, Iivanainen M, Vesala H et al. Life expectancy of people with intellectual disability: a 35-year follow-up study. *J Intellect Disabil Res.* 2000; 44(Pt 5):591-9.
266. Thanh NX, Jonsson E. Life expectancy of people with fetal alcohol syndrome. *J Popul Ther Clin Pharmacol.* 2016; 23:e53-9.
267. Lakhoo K. Fetal counselling for surgical congenital malformations. *Early Hum Dev.* 2012; 88:9-13.
268. Patel P, Farley J, Impey L et al. Evaluation of a fetomaternal-surgical clinic for prenatal counselling of surgical anomalies. *Pediatr Surg Int.* 2008; 24:391-4.
269. Centers for Disease Control and Prevention. Fetal alcohol spectrum disorders: facts about FASDs. https://www.cdc.gov/ncbddd/fasd/facts.html. (accessed 2017 Dec 11).
270. Pryde PG, Nugent CE, Sedman AB et al. ACE inhibitor fetopathy (abstract). *Am J Obstet Gynecol.* 1992; 166:348.
271. Cooper WO, Hernandez-Diaz S, Arbogast PG et al. Major congenital malformations after first-trimester exposure to ACE-inhibitors. *N Engl J Med.* 2006; 354:2443-51.
272. Barr M Jr. Teratogen update: angiotensin-converting enzyme inhibitors. *Teratology.* 1994; 50:399-409.
273. Shotan A, Widerhorn J, Hurst A et al. Risks of angiotensin-converting enzyme inhibition during pregnancy: experimental and clinical evidence, potential mechanisms, and recommendations for use. *Am J Med.* 1994; 96:451-6.
274. Robillard JE, Nakamura KT, Matherne GP et al. Renal hemodynamics and functional adjustments to postnatal life. *Semin Perinatol.* 1988; 12:143-50.
275. Frank DA, Zuckerman BS, Amaro H et al. Cocaine use during pregnancy: prevalence and correlates. *Pediatrics.* 1988; 82:888-95.
276. Neerhof MG, MacGregor SN, Retzky SS et al. Cocaine abuse during pregnancy: peripartum prevalence and perinatal outcome. *Am J Obstet Gynecol.* 1989; 161:633-8.
277. Chasnoff IJ, Burns KA, Burns WJ. Cocaine use in pregnancy: perinatal morbidity and mortality. *Neurotoxicol Teratol.* 1987; 9:291-3.
278. Chasnoff IJ, Chisum GM, Kaplan WE. Maternal cocaine use and genitourinary tract malformations. *Teratology.* 1988; 37:201-4.
279. Ryan L, Ehrlich S, Finnegan L. Cocaine abuse in pregnancy: effects on the fetus and newborn. *Neurotoxicol Teratol.* 1987; 9:295-9.
280. Little BB, Snell LM, Klein VR et al. Cocaine abuse during pregnancy: maternal and fetal implications. *Obstet Gynecol.* 1989; 73:157-60.
281. MacGregor SN, Keith LG, Chasnoff IJ et al. Cocaine use during pregnancy: adverse perinatal outcome. *Am J Obset Gynecol.* 1987; 157:686-90.
282. Chasnoff IJ, Griffith DR, MacGregor S et al. Temporal patterns of cocaine use in pregnancy: perinatal outcome. *JAMA.* 1989; 261:1741-4.
283. Chasnoff IJ, Burns WJ, Schnoll SH et al. Cocaine use in pregnancy. *N Engl J Med.* 1985; 313:666-9.
284. LeBlanc PE, Parekh AJ, Naso B et al. Effects of intrauterine exposure to alkaloidal cocaine ("crack"). *Am J Dis Child.* 1987; 141:937-8.
285. Dixon SD, Coen RW, Crutchfield S. Visual dysfunction in cocaine-exposed infants (Abstract). *Pediatr Res.* 1987; 21:359A.
286. Hume RF Jr, O'Donnell KJ, Staner CL et al. In utero cocaine exposure: observations of fetal behavioral state may predict neonatal outcome. *Am J Obstet Gynecol.* 1989; 161:685-90.
287. Chasnoff IJ, Hunt CE, Kletter R et al. Prenatal cocaine exposure is associated with respiratory pattern abnormalities. *Am J Dis Child.* 1989; 143:583-7.
288. Finasteride package insert. Whitehouse Station, NJ: Merck and Co, Inc; 2011. https://www.merck.com/product/usa/pi_circulars/p/proscar/proscar_pi.pdf (accessed 2017 Dec 11).
289. Eulexin (flutamide) product information. Kenilworth, NJ: Schering Laboratories; 2011.
290. Weinstein MR, Goldfield MD. Cardiovascular malformations with lithium use during pregnancy. *Am J Psychiatry.* 1975; 132:529-31.
291. Weinstein MR. Recent advances in clinical psychopharmacology. I. Lithium carbonate. *Hosp Form.* 1977; 12:759-62.
292. Rane A, Tomson G, Bjarke B. Effects of maternal lithium therapy in a newborn infant. *J Pediatr.* 1978; 93:296-7.
293. Arnon RG, Marin-Garcia J, Peeden JN. Tricuspid valve regurgitation and lithium carbonate toxicity in a newborn infant. *Am J Dis Child.* 1981; 135:941-3.
294. Piton M, Barthe ML, Laloum D et al. Acute lithium intoxication. Report of two cases: mother and her newborn. *Therapie.* 1973; 28:1123-44.

295. Wilson N, Forfar JC, Godman MJ. Atrial flutter in the newborn resulting from maternal lithium ingestion. *Arch Dis Child.* 1983; 58:538-9.
296. Azizi F, Amouzegar A. Management of hyperthyroidism during pregnancy and lactation. *Eur J Endocrinol.* 2011; 164:871-6.
297. Del Campo M, Kosaki K, Bennett FC et al. Developmental delay in fetal aminopterin/methotrexate syndrome. *Teratology.* 1999; 60:10-2.
298. Milunsky A, Graef JW, Gaynor MF. Methotrexate-induced congenital malformations. *J Pediatr.* 1968; 72:790-5.
299. Powell HR, Ekert H. Methotrexate-induced congenital malformations. *Med J Aust.* 1971; 2:1076-7.
300. Warkany J. Teratogenicity of folic acid antagonists. *Cancer Bull.* 1981; 33:76-7.
301. Kozlowski RD, Steinbrunner JV, MacKenzie AH et al. Outcome of first-trimester exposure to low-dose methotrexate in eight patients with rheumatic disease. *Am J Med.* 1990; 88:589-92.
302. Buckley LM, Bullaboy CA, Leichtman L et al. Multiple congenital anomalies associated with weekly low-dose methotrexate treatment of mother. *Arthritis Rheum.* 1997: 40:971-3.
303. Bawle EV, Conard JV, Weiss L. Adult and two children with fetal methotrexate syndrome. *Teratology.* 1998; 57:51-5.
304. Levin DL. Effects of inhibition of prostaglandin synthesis on fetal development, oxygenation, and the fetal circulation. *Semin Perinatol.* 1980; 4:35-44.
305. Van Marter LJ, Leviton A, Allred EN et al. Persistent pulmonary hypertension of the newborn and smoking and aspirin and nonsteroidal anti-inflammatory drug consumption during pregnancy. *Pediatrics.* 1996; 97:658-63.
306. Alano MA, Ngougmna E, Ostrea EM Jr et al. Analysis of nonsteroidal anti-inflammatory drugs in meconium and its relations to persistent pulmonary hypertension of the newborn. *Pediatrics.* 2001; 107:519-23.
307. Fuchs F. Prevention of prematurity. *Am J Obstet Gynecol.* 1976; 126:809-20.
308. Dawood MY. Nonsteroidal anti-inflammatory drugs and reproduction. *Am J Obstet Gynecol.* 1993; 169:1255-65.
309. Reilly WA. Hormone therapy during pregnancy: effects on the fetus and newborn. *Q Rev Pediatr.* 1958; 13:198-202.
310. Zile MH. Vitamin A and embryonic development: an overview. *J Nutr.* 1998; 128:455S-8S.
311. Shirazi M, Abbariki E, Pirjani R et al. Congenital microtia in a neonate due to maternal isotretinoin exposure 1 month before pregnancy: case report. *J Obstet Gynaecol Res.* 2015; 41:975-8.
312. Lammer EJ, Chen DT, Hoar RM et al. Retinoic acid embryopathy. *N Engl J Med.* 1985; 313:837-41.
313. Fernhoff PM, Lammer EJ. Craniofacial features of isotretinoin embrypathy. *J Pediatr.* 1984; 105:595-7.
314. Anonymous. Isotretinoin—a newly recognized human teratogen. *MMWR Morb Mortal Wkly Rep.* 1984; 33:171-3.
315. Anonymous. Update on birth defects with isotretinoin. *FDA Drug Bull.* 1984; 14:15-6.
316. Cohlan SQ, Bevelander G, Bross S. Effect of tetracycline on bone growth in the premature infant. In: Finland M, Savage G, eds. *Antimicrobial agents and chemotherapy.* Ann Arbor, MI: Braun-Bramfield; 1961:340-7.
317. Harcourt JK, Johnson NW, Storey E. In vivo incorporation of tetracycline in the teeth of man. *Arch Oral Biol.* 1962; 7:431-7.
318. Rendle-Short TJ. Tetracycline in teeth and bone. *Lancet.* 1962; 1:1188.
319. Douglas AC. The deposition of tetracycline in human nails and teeth: a complication of long term treatment. *Br J Dis Chest.* 1963; 57:44-7.
320. Kutscher AH, Zegarelli EV, Tovell HM et al. Discoloration of teeth induced by tetracycline. *JAMA.* 1963; 184:586-7.
321. Kline AH, Blattner RJ, Lunin M. Transplacental effect of tetracyclines on teeth. *JAMA.* 1964; 188:178-80.
322. Schultz JC, Adamson JS Jr, Workman WW et al. Fatal liver disease after intravenous administration of tetracycline in high dosage. *N Engl J Med.* 1963; 269:999-1004.
323. Wenk RE, Gebhardt FC, Behagavan BS et al. Tetracycline associated fatty liver of pregnancy, including possible pregnancy risk after chronic dermatologic use of tetracycline. *J Reprod Med.* 1981; 26:135-41.
324. US Department of Health and Human Services. The health consequences of smoking: a report of the Surgeon General. Washington, DC: HHS; 2004.
325. McDonald SD, Walker MC, Ohlsson A et al. The effect of tobacco exposure on maternal and fetal thyroid function. *Eur J Obstet Gynecol Reprod Biol.* 2008; 140:38-42.
326. Castles A, Adams EK, Melvin CL et al. Effects of smoking during pregnancy. Five meta-analyses. *Am J Prev Med.* 1999; 16:208-15.
327. Spinillo A, Nicola S, Piazzi G et al. Epidemiological correlates of preterm premature rupture of membranes. *Int J Gynaecol Obstet.* 1994; 47:7-15.
328. Li YF, Langholz B, Salam MT et al. Maternal and grandmaternal smoking patterns are associated with early childhood asthma. *Chest.* 2005; 127:1232-41.
329. Sondergaard C, Henriksen TB, Obel C et al. Smoking during pregnancy and infantile colic. *Pediatrics.* 2001; 108:342-6.
330. von Kries R, Toschke AM, Koletzko B et al. Maternal smoking during pregnancy and childhood obesity. *Am J Epidemiol.* 2002; 156:954-61.
331. DiSaia PJ. Pregnancy and delivery of a patient with a Starr-Edwards mitral valve prosthesis. *Obstet Gynecol.* 1966; 28:469-71.
332. Hall JG, Pauli RM, Wilson KM. Maternal and fetal sequelae of anticoagulation during pregnancy. *Am J Med.* 1980; 68:122-40.
333. Baillie M, Allen ED. Elkington AR. The congenital warfarin syndrome: a case report. *Br J Ophthalmol.* 1980; 64:633-5.
334. Harrod MJE, Sherrod PS. Warfarin embryopathy in siblings. *Obstet Gynecol.* 1981; 57:673-6.

INDEX

Figures and tables are indicated by "f" and "t" following page numbers.

AAD. *See* Antibiotic-associated diarrhea
AAN (American Academy of Neurology), 264–265
Abacavir
acidosis and, 1003t
allergic and hypersensitivity reactions to, 75t, 88, 112
anxiety and, 400t, 403
cutaneous diseases and, 111t, 113t
genetic variability and, 16t
genetic variations affecting, 36t
glucose/insulin dysregulation and, 690
human leukocyte antigen and, 37, 38
malignant hyperthermia and, 1186
myocardial ischemia/acute coronary syndromes and, 472t
nausea/vomiting and, 909t
neutropenia/agranulocytosis and, 1089t
oral erythema multiforme and, 1266t
osteoporosis/osteomalacia and, 1127
ototoxicity and, 1234t
pharmacogenomic tests for, 35
Abatacept, 1270t
Abciximab, 238t, 239, 1029t, 1050t, 1052t, 1053
Abiraterone, 698t, 836t
Absolute neutrophil count (ANC), 1087, 1092, 1094, 1096
ABVD regimen, 1285, 1286, 1291
Acebutolol
alopecia and, 168t
hypotension and, 632t, 638t
photosensitivity and, 144t
sinus bradycardia/atrioventricular block and, 577t
systemic lupus erythematosus and, 124t, 128t, 132
ACE inhibitors. *See* Angiotensin-converting enzyme inhibitors
Acenocoumarol, 1029t
Acetaminophen
acidosis and, 1002t
asthma/bronchospasm and, 452t, 453, 455t, 461
chronic kidney disease and, 968–970, 973, 976
cutaneous diseases and, 101, 102–103t
drug interactions with, 39
hemolytic anemia and, 1105t
hepatic/cholestatic diseases and, 846t, 853, 856, 864–866
hypothermia and, 1216
myocardial ischemia/acute coronary syndromes and, 489
neutropenia/agranulocytosis and, 1089t
oral erythema multiforme and, 1266t
ototoxicity and, 1233, 1234–1235t
pancreatitis and, 878t, 881
peripheral neuropathy and, 288
smoking and, 32
teratogenicity of, 1321, 1326
thrombocytopenia and, 1050t, 1052t
vaginal bleeding disorders and, 797
Acetate, 1013–1014t
Acetazolamide
acidosis and, 1003t
aplastic anemia and, 1100t
delirium and, 326t
hirsutism and, 194, 195t, 199t
neutropenia/agranulocytosis and, 1089t
ototoxicity and, 1234t
peripheral neuropathy and, 281t
photosensitivity and, 144t
tardive dyskinesia and, 265
taste disorders and, 1259t, 1261t
visual disturbances and, 296t
Acetohydroxamic acid, 1066t, 1070t
Acetylcholine
cognitive disorders and, 359, 360
delirium and, 329
myocardial ischemia/acute coronary syndromes and, 473t
myopathy and, 1153
psychosis and, 418
sexual dysfunction and, 766
in sleep cycles, 349
Acetylcholinesterase inhibitors, 335
Acetylcysteine, 440, 1243
Acetyl-L-carnitine, 286, 287t, 288
Acetylsalicylic acid. *See* Aspirin
Acid–base disorders. *See* Acidosis; Alkalosis
Acidosis, 1001–1011
anion gap metabolic, 1002t, 1004t, 1007t
causative agents of, 1001, 1002–1003t
clinical presentation of, 1005–1007, 1006t
differential diagnosis of, 1006, 1007t
epidemiology of, 1001
ketoacidosis, 1002t, 1004t
lactic, 1002t, 1004, 1004t, 1007–1008, 1010–1011
management of, 1008–1011, 1009f, 1010t, 1011f
mechanisms of, 1001, 1004–1005, 1004t
morbidity and mortality for, 1007
patient education on, 1011
prevention of, 1007–1008, 1008t
renal tubular, 1003–1004t, 1004, 1006, 1010, 1011f
respiratory, 1001, 1003–1004t, 1005–1007, 1007–1008t, 1010–1011
risk factors for, 1007, 1008t
Acitretin, 166, 173t, 791, 1273
Acne, 102t, 105, 107t, 108, 114, 114t, 384
ACOG (American College of Obstetricians and Gynecologists), 626, 1302, 1303
Aconite, 573t
Aconite alkaloids, 524–525t, 525
ACTH. *See* Adrenocorticotropic hormone
Actinomycin, 847t, 907t
Activated charcoal, 245, 580, 587–588, 701t, 1039
Acute akathisia. *See* Akathisia
Acute coronary syndromes. *See* Myocardial ischemia/acute coronary syndromes
Acute dystonia. *See* Dystonia
Acute hypertension, 232, 240
Acute interstitial nephritis (AIN), 955–957
causative agents of, 943t, 956
clinical presentation of, 946t, 956
differential diagnosis of, 956
epidemiology of, 956
management of, 957
mechanisms of, 945t, 956
morbidity and mortality for, 956
overview, 955
patient education on, 957
prevention of, 956–957
risk factors for, 956
Acute kidney injury (AKI), 941–960
acute interstitial nephritis, 955–957
acute tubular necrosis, 949–955
community-acquired, 941–942, 944
defined, 941
glomerulonephritis, 958–960
hemodynamic-mediated, 942–949
hospital-acquired, 941–942
nephrolithiasis, 957–958
Acute lymphoblastic leukemia (ALL), 1283, 1286, 1291
Acute myeloid leukemia (AML), 1283–1287, 1289–1292
Acute tubular necrosis (ATN), 949–955
causative agents of, 943t, 949–950
clinical presentation of, 946t, 951
differential diagnosis of, 951
epidemiology of, 950
management of, 955
mechanisms of, 950–951
morbidity and mortality for, 952
patient education on, 955
prevention of, 952–955
risk factors for, 951–952
Acyclovir, 168t, 196t, 944–945t, 957, 967, 1188t, 1191, 1295
Adalimumab
alopecia and, 173t
depression and, 383
hepatic/cholestatic diseases and, 852t
interstitial lung disease/pulmonary fibrosis and, 433t
oral erythema multiforme and, 1266t
oral lichenoid reactions and, 1270t
serum sickness-like reactions and, 1193t
sexual dysfunction and, 761t
skin cancer and, 1297
systemic lupus erythematosus and, 126t
thyroid diseases and, 698–699t, 701t, 710
valvular/pericardial heart disease and, 660t, 662
visual disturbances and, 296t
Addison disease, 734–735
Adefovir, 966, 966t, 970t, 1003t, 1050t
Adenosine
acute kidney injury and, 951, 953
atrial fibrillation/atrial flutter and, 581, 582–583t, 583–586, 585t
atrial tachycardia and, 591
AV node re-entrant tachycardia and, 594
hypotension and, 644
monomorphic ventricular tachycardia and, 524–525t, 525–526
myocardial ischemia/acute coronary syndromes and, 472t, 477t, 479
sinus bradycardia/atrioventricular block and, 570t, 573t, 577–579
structural similarities with hydralazine, 127

INDEX

ADHD (attention deficit/hyperactivity disorder) agents, 219*t*, 221–222, 401
Adjuvant chemotherapy, 1167–1169*t*, 1172, 1173*t*
Adolescents. *See* Pediatric patients
Ado-trastuzumab, 169*t*, 836*t*
Adrenal diseases. *See* Hypothalamic, pituitary, and adrenal diseases
Adrenergic β-receptor blockers. *See* β-adrenergic receptor blockers (β-blockers)
Adrenocorticotropic hormone (ACTH)
  Cushing syndrome and, 731*t*, 732
  cutaneous diseases and, 108
  hirsutism and, 194, 195*t*, 199*t*
  hypersensitivity reactions to, 77*t*
  pancreatitis and, 882
  primary adrenal insufficiency and, 735
  secondary adrenal insufficiency and, 735, 741
  stimulation test for, 738
  synthesis of, 729
Adverse drug reactions (ADRs). *See also* Drug-induced diseases
  allergies. *See* Drug allergies
  categorization of, 23, 59–60
  causality/correlation in, 23
  differential diagnosis of, 51, 63–65
  documentation of, 65–66
  drug–drug interactions, 38–40, 39*t*
  food–drug interactions, 40–41
  gender differences in, 31–32
  hospital admissions due to, 28
  hypersensitivity. *See* Drug hypersensitivity reactions (DHRs)
  manifestations of, 19
  in medication histories, 60, 62
  mortality associated with, 29
  Naranjo Scale for, 64, 65, 65*t*
  in new drug approval process, 48
  9 points of consideration for, 63–64
  postmarketing surveillance for. *See* Postmarketing surveillance
  prevalence of, 4
  probability ratings for, 64, 64–65*t*, 65
  quantitative impact of, 23
  reporting systems for, 24, 49–56, 66–67
  risk-benefit balance of, 20
  teratogens and. *See* Teratogenicity
  WHO-UMC system for, 64, 64*t*, 65
Adverse Event Reporting System (AERS), 4, 6, 24, 31, 381, 882
Adverse events, defined, 66. *See also* Adverse drug reactions (ADRs)
AEDs. *See* Antiepileptic drugs
AERD (aspirin-exacerbated respiratory disease), 453, 455, 457–463
AERS. *See* Adverse Event Reporting System
Afatinib, 169*t*
Aflatoxin, 849*t*
Ageusia, 1258
Aging populations. *See* Elderly populations
Agranulocytosis. *See* Neutropenia and agranulocytosis
AHA. *See* American Heart Association
AHS (anticonvulsant hypersensitivity syndrome), 87, 95, 109
AIA. *See* Aspirin-induced asthma
AIDS. *See* HIV/AIDS
AIN. *See* Acute interstitial nephritis
Ajmaline, 547*t*, 548, 847*t*
Akathisia (acute and tardive), 254–259
  causative agents of, 254, 255*t*, 405
  clinical presentation of, 256–258, 257*t*
  differential diagnosis of, 257, 257*t*
  epidemiology of, 254–255
  management of, 258–259, 259*t*
  mechanisms of, 255–256, 256*t*
  morbidity and mortality for, 258
  overview, 253–254
  patient education on, 259
  prevention of, 258, 258*t*
  risk factors for, 258, 258*t*
AKI. *See* Acute kidney injury
Alanine aminotransferase (ALT), 859, 862, 868, 1058
Albiglutide, 879*t*
Albumin, 364, 784, 787, 868–871, 1242
Albuterol
  acidosis and, 1002*t*
  anxiety and, 404
  atrial fibrillation/atrial flutter and, 582*t*, 584
  atrial tachycardia and, 588–589*t*, 589
  AV node re-entrant tachycardia and, 592–594, 592–594*t*
  myocardial ischemia/acute coronary syndromes and, 473*t*
  psychosis and, 416*t*, 418*t*
  teratogenicity of, 1320
  visual disturbances and, 296*t*
Alcohol use
  anxiety and, 409
  atrial fibrillation/atrial flutter and, 581, 582–583*t*, 584–586, 585–586*t*
  Brugada syndrome and, 547, 547*t*, 549
  cognitive disorders and, 362
  delirium and, 326*t*, 330, 337
  diarrhea and, 825, 827
  duration of detection in urine, 420*t*
  gout/hyperuricemia and, 1139, 1146
  heart failure and, 516
  hepatic/cholestatic diseases and, 864
  hyperprolactinemia and, 744*t*
  hypertrichosis and, 197*t*
  hypotension and, 643, 648
  intracerebral hemorrhage and, 238–240, 238*t*, 240*t*, 244*t*
  macrocytic anemia and, 1107, 1108
  in medication histories, 60
  nausea/vomiting and, 915
  osteoporosis/osteomalacia and, 1125, 1126, 1128, 1130
  pancreatitis and, 887, 890, 892
  peripheral neuropathy and, 281*t*, 285
  psychosis and, 417*t*, 423
  as risk factor for drug-induced diseases, 33
  sexual dysfunction and, 771, 772, 798
  sleep disorders and, 349–350*t*
  stroke and, 230–231*t*, 232, 233, 235*t*
  teratogenicity and, 1311, 1316, 1318, 1321, 1327, 1331–1333
  withdrawal treatment protocols, 424*t*
Aldesleukin, 698*t*, 907*t*, 1065*t*, 1067, 1069*t*
Aldosterone
  acidosis and, 1003*t*
  alcohol use and, 232
  alkalosis and, 1012–1013
  function of, 729
  hypertension and, 620
  hypoaldosteronism/hyperaldosteronism, 751
  hypotension and, 637
  primary adrenal insufficiency and, 734
Alectinib, 144*t*
Alemtuzumab, 7*t*, 169*t*, 172*t*, 698–699*t*, 701*t*, 710, 715, 983*t*, 1193*t*
Alendronate
  atrial fibrillation/atrial flutter and, 581, 582*t*, 584
  hepatic/cholestatic diseases and, 848*t*
  osteonecrosis of jaw and, 1274*t*
  osteoporosis/osteomalacia and, 1129*t*, 1130
  upper gastrointestinal ulceration and, 812–814, 816, 818
  visual disturbances and, 296*t*
Alfalfa, 144*t*
Alfentanil, 906*t*
Alfuzosin, 296*t*, 472*t*, 632*t*, 639*t*, 1050*t*, 1234*t*
Aliskiren, 633*t*, 638*t*, 942
Alitretinoin, 144*t*
Alkaline phosphatase (ALP), 859, 862
Alkalosis, 1012–1018
  causative agents of, 1012, 1013*t*
  clinical presentation of, 1014–1015, 1015*t*
  differential diagnosis of, 1015, 1016*t*
  epidemiology of, 1012
  management of, 1016–1017, 1018*f*, 1018*t*
  mechanisms of, 1012–1014, 1014*t*
  morbidity and mortality for, 1015–1016
  patient education on, 1017
  respiratory, 1012–1017, 1013–1016*t*
  risk factors for, 1015, 1017*t*
Alkylating agents
  chemotherapy-induced anemia and, 1101*t*, 1109, 1109*t*
  infertility and, 783*t*, 786*t*, 800
  leukemia and, 1284, 1289, 1290
  neutropenia/agranulocytosis and, 1087, 1091
  sexual dysfunction and, 767, 770
  vaginal bleeding disorders and, 782*t*, 785*t*
ALL (acute lymphoblastic leukemia), 1283, 1286, 1291
Allergic-mediated blood disorders, 75*t*, 80, 83–84, 83*t*
Allergic reactions. *See* Drug allergies
Allodynia, 1141
Allopurinol
  acute kidney injury and, 943–944*t*, 957
  allergic and hypersensitivity reactions to, 74–75*t*, 85, 88, 109–110
  alopecia and, 171*t*
  cutaneous diseases and, 101, 102–103*t*, 111, 111*t*, 113*t*
  drug fever and, 1188*t*, 1191
  genetic variations affecting, 36*t*
  gout/hyperuricemia and, 1136–1137, 1136*t*, 1144, 1145
  hepatic/cholestatic diseases and, 852*t*
  myocardial ischemia/acute coronary syndromes and, 473*t*
  neutropenia/agranulocytosis and, 1089*t*
  oral erythema multiforme and, 1266, 1266*t*
  oral lichenoid reactions and, 1270, 1270*t*
  peripheral neuropathy and, 281*t*
  systemic lupus erythematosus and, 126*t*
  taste disorders and, 1259*t*, 1261*t*
  visual disturbances and, 296*t*, 316
Allopurinol hypersensitivity syndrome, 109–110
Allyl compounds, 849*t*
Aloe vera, 698*t*, 850*t*, 1273
Alogliptin, 506, 509, 879*t*, 884
Alopecia, 165–193. *See also* Alopecia areata
  androgenetic, 165, 176, 180, 181–182*t*, 183–186, 184*t*
  causative agents of, 166–177, 167–174*t*
  clinical presentation of, 165, 176*f*, 180–183, 181–182*t*
  differential diagnosis of, 183, 184*t*

epidemiology of, 177–178
management of, 186–192, 187–189t
mechanisms of, 178–180, 179–180t
morbidity and mortality for, 185
patient education on, 192–193
prevention of, 185–186, 185t
psoriatic, 179t, 180
risk factors for, 183–184, 184t
scarring, 174, 177, 179t, 184t
traction, 183, 184t
trichotillomania and, 183, 184t
Alopecia areata
clinical presentation of, 180, 181–182t, 183
defined, 166
differential diagnosis of, 184t
management of, 187–188t, 191, 192
mechanisms of, 178, 179t, 180
Alosetron, 7t, 39t, 836t
ALP (alkaline phosphatase), 859, 862
Alpha lipoic acid, 1262
α1-proteinase inhibitor, 7t
α-adrenergic agonists, 633t, 645t, 646, 747, 759t
α-adrenergic antagonists, 748t, 759–761t, 764–765t, 766
α-glucosidase inhibitors, 515, 822–823t
α-melanocyte-stimulating hormone, 1242t
$α_1$-antagonists, 502t
$α_1$-receptor inhibitors, 488
α-receptor agonists, 452t, 620t, 621, 625t, 626, 627
5-α reductase inhibitors, 188t, 190, 193, 206t, 207, 382, 758–760t, 763–764t
α-tocopherol, 868, 1242t, 1243
$α_2$-adrenergic receptor agonists, 647
$α_2$-adrenergic receptor antagonists, 647
$α_2$-agonists, 348t, 350t
$α_2$-reductase inhibitors, 205
Alprazolam, 144t, 327t, 329t, 368, 380, 407, 1259t
Alprenolol, 1050t
Alprostadil, 761t, 765t
ALT (alanine aminotransferase), 859, 862, 868, 1058
Alteplase, 662, 663t, 664, 1029t
Altretamine, 169t, 907t
Aluminum-containing antacids, 835, 1151
Aluminum hydroxide, 701t, 1013–1014t
Aluminum-magnesium hydroxide, 1262
Alverine, 850t
Alvimopan, 7t, 840, 840t, 841
Alzheimer disease agents, 633t
Amanitin, 849t
Amantadine
akathisia and, 259
delirium and, 327t, 329t
depression and, 390
drug interactions with, 40
dystonia and, 270
heart failure and, 502t, 509
hepatic/cholestatic diseases and, 851t
neuroleptic malignant syndrome and, 1196, 1200, 1200t
parkinsonism and, 273
photosensitivity and, 144t
psychosis and, 416t, 418t
serotonin syndrome and, 1203–1204t
SIADH and, 983t
sleep disorders and, 348t
tardive dyskinesia and, 264
torsades de pointes and, 533t, 539t
visual disturbances and, 296t
weight gain and, 1175
Ambrisentan, 7t
Amenorrhea and oligomenorrhea, 793–795
causative agents of, 782t, 793
clinical presentation of, 787t, 793
differential diagnosis of, 788t, 793–794
epidemiology of, 793
management of, 790t, 794
mechanisms of, 785t, 793
morbidity and mortality for, 794
patient education on, 794–795
prevention of, 789t, 794
risk factors for, 788t, 794
American Academy of Neurology (AAN), 264–265
American Cancer Society, 929, 1286, 1298, 1300, 1302, 1303
American College of Obstetricians and Gynecologists (ACOG), 626, 1302, 1303
American Diabetes Association, 506, 513, 689, 1174
American Heart Association (AHA)
blood pressure classification guidelines from, 618–619, 619t
on cocaine-induced chest pain, 488
on glitazone use, 506, 513
on musculoskeletal pain, 489
on NSAID use, 476
on phosphodiesterase-5 inhibitors and nitrate therapy, 484
on risk factors for acute coronary syndrome, 479
on stepped-care approach, 231
on stroke risk factors, 234
on thiazolidinedione use, 476
American Psychiatric Association, 264, 336, 1174
Amifostine
acute kidney injury and, 954–955
heart failure and, 515
hypotension and, 635t, 640t, 641–642, 645t
nausea/vomiting and, 907t
ototoxicity and, 1242t
peripheral neuropathy and, 287t
Amikacin, 1234t, 1241
Amiloride, 633t, 638t, 993, 993t, 1003t
ε-aminocaproic acid, 221
Aminocaproic acid
heart failure and, 502t, 509
myopathy and, 1150t, 1152, 1152t, 1156
ototoxicity and, 1234t
thromboembolic diseases and, 1064t, 1067, 1068t
Aminoglutethimide
alopecia and, 173t, 179t
hepatic/cholestatic diseases and, 847t
neutropenia/agranulocytosis and, 1089t
SIADH and, 983t
systemic lupus erythematosus and, 126t
thrombocytopenia and, 1050t
Aminoglycosides
acidosis and, 1003t
acute kidney injury and, 943t, 945t, 949–953, 955
alkalosis and, 1013–1014t
chronic kidney disease and, 965
delirium and, 328t
diarrhea and, 823t
drug fever and, 1187
drug interactions with, 38
ototoxicity and, 1233, 1239, 1239t, 1241–1243
Aminolevulinic acid, 144t
Aminopenicillins, 87, 90, 101, 103t
Aminophylline, 218t, 953, 1234t
Aminopterin, 1324–1325
Aminosalicylate sodium, 1270t
Aminosalicylic acids, 943t, 1050t
Amiodarone
alopecia and, 167t
asthma/bronchospasm and, 452t
atrial fibrillation/atrial flutter and, 582–583t, 583–587, 585t, 587t
atrial tachycardia and, 590, 591
bleeding disorders and, 1031
Brugada syndrome and, 549
cognitive disorders and, 358t
color changes of oral mucosa and teeth and, 1253, 1254–1255t
delirium and, 326t
depression and, 385
diabetes insipidus and, 991t
drug interactions with, 38
heart failure and, 507, 511, 513
hepatic/cholestatic diseases and, 847t, 861t, 864
hypotension and, 634t, 640t, 645t
interstitial lung disease/pulmonary fibrosis and, 432t, 435t, 436–441
iodine content of, 706t
malignant hyperthermia and, 1213
monomorphic ventricular tachycardia and, 523, 524–525t, 530
myopathy and, 1150t, 1151, 1155
ototoxicity and, 1234t
pancreatitis and, 878t, 885
peripheral neuropathy and, 280t
photosensitivity and, 144t, 152, 154, 155
sexual dysfunction and, 759t
SIADH and, 981, 983t
sinus bradycardia/atrioventricular block and, 570t, 572, 573t, 577
systemic lupus erythematosus and, 124t
thrombocytopenia and, 1050t, 1052t
thyroid diseases and, 698–699t, 701t, 704–705, 708, 710, 713–716
torsades de pointes and, 532t, 540t, 541
visual disturbances and, 295, 296t, 313, 315–317
Amisulpride, 533t, 539t, 570t, 577t
Amitriptyline
akathisia and, 259
alopecia and, 172t
Brugada syndrome and, 547t
cognitive disorders and, 365
delirium and, 326t, 329t
drug fever and, 1188t
heart failure and, 504t, 510t
hyperprolactinemia and, 743t
hypotension and, 634t, 639t
ototoxicity and, 1234t
peripheral neuropathy and, 288
photosensitivity and, 144t
serotonin syndrome and, 1203–1204t
SIADH and, 982t
sinus bradycardia/atrioventricular block and, 573t, 578t
torsades de pointes and, 533t, 540t
weight gain and, 1166t, 1169t, 1170
AML (acute myeloid leukemia), 1283–1287, 1289–1292
Amlodipine
asthma/bronchospasm and, 463
gingival hyperplasia and, 1263, 1263t
glucose/insulin dysregulation and, 688
heart failure and, 505, 510, 515
hypotension and, 632t, 639t
oral erythema multiforme and, 1266t
oral lichenoid reactions and, 1270t
ototoxicity and, 1234t
photosensitivity and, 144t
taste disorders and, 1259t

INDEX

Amoxapine
- akathisia and, 255–256*t*, 258*t*
- alopecia and, 172*t*
- depression and, 392
- dystonia and, 269*t*
- hyperprolactinemia and, 743*t*
- neuroleptic malignant syndrome and, 1195*t*
- neutropenia/agranulocytosis and, 1089*t*
- parkinsonism and, 271*t*, 273*t*
- seizures and, 221
- SIADH and, 982*t*
- tardive dyskinesia and, 260*t*, 264*t*

Amoxicillin
- cutaneous diseases and, 111*t*
- hepatic/cholestatic diseases and, 846*t*
- myocardial ischemia/acute coronary syndromes and, 472*t*
- serum sickness-like reactions and, 1192, 1193*t*, 1194
- systemic lupus erythematosus and, 130
- torsades de pointes and, 542
- upper gastrointestinal ulceration and, 809

Amoxicillin–clavulanate, 37, 846*t*, 861*t*, 1188*t*
Amoxicillin–clavulanic acid, 1259*t*, 1266*t*
Amphetamine aspartate, 167*t*
Amphetamine derivatives, 748*t*
Amphetamines
- alkalosis and, 1013–1014*t*
- alopecia and, 167*t*, 179*t*
- anxiety and, 400*t*, 401, 405*t*, 409
- drug fever and, 1188*t*
- duration of detection in urine, 420*t*
- growth hormone deficiency and, 748
- hepatic/cholestatic diseases and, 851*t*
- hypertension and, 618*t*, 620*t*
- intracerebral hemorrhage and, 238*t*, 240*t*
- myocardial ischemia/acute coronary syndromes and, 473*t*, 477*t*
- psychosis and, 415, 416*t*, 418*t*
- as risk factor for drug-induced diseases, 33
- seizures and, 219
- sexual dysfunction and, 783*t*, 786*t*
- stroke and, 230–231*t*, 232
- taste disorders and, 1259*t*, 1261*t*
- teratogenicity of, 1321
- thyroid diseases and, 701*t*
- visual disturbances and, 296*t*

Amphotericin, 472*t*, 846*t*
Amphotericin B
- acidosis and, 1003*t*
- acute kidney injury and, 943*t*, 945*t*, 949–953, 955
- allergic reactions to, 72*t*
- chronic kidney disease and, 965
- diabetes insipidus and, 991, 991*t*
- drug fever and, 1186
- heart failure and, 502*t*, 509
- oral lichenoid reactions and, 1270*t*
- ototoxicity and, 1234*t*
- taste disorders and, 1259*t*
- thrombocytopenia and, 1050*t*

Amphotericin B colloidal complex, 950, 953
Amphotericin B deoxycholate, 23, 943*t*
Amphotericin B lipid-based formulations, 23, 943*t*, 949–950, 953
Amphotericin B liposomal, 950, 953, 991, 991*t*
Ampicillin
- acute kidney injury and, 943*t*, 959
- allergic reactions to, 87
- cutaneous diseases and, 111*t*
- drug fever and, 1188*t*
- heart failure and, 503*t*, 509
- hepatic/cholestatic diseases and, 846*t*
- ototoxicity and, 1234*t*
- pancreatitis and, 878*t*, 882
- thrombocytopenia and, 1050*t*
- upper gastrointestinal ulceration and, 809

Ampicillin–clavulanate, 1276
Amprenavir, 92
Amsacrine, 169*t*, 847*t*
Amygdalin, 1002*t*
Amylin analogs, 1175*t*
Amyl nitrate, 634*t*, 640*t*
ANA (antinuclear antibody test), 130–135
Anabolic steroids
- alopecia and, 167*t*, 176, 179*t*, 180
- anxiety and, 400*t*, 402
- cutaneous diseases and, 108
- hirsutism and, 198, 199*t*
- hypertrichosis and, 198
- myocardial ischemia/acute coronary syndromes and, 473*t*
- osteoporosis/osteomalacia and, 1129*t*
- psychosis and, 415, 416*t*, 418*t*
- sexual dysfunction and, 758*t*, 762–763*t*, 765*t*

Anagen effluvium, 176, 178–183, 179*t*, 181–182*t*, 184*t*
Anagrelide, 144*t*, 432*t*, 502*t*, 510*t*, 1026*t*, 1029*t*
Analgesic nephropathy, 965, 966*t*, 968–970, 970*t*, 972–976, 974*t*
Analgesics
- acute kidney injury and, 958
- for caffeine withdrawal, 411
- chronic kidney disease and, 965, 966*t*, 968–970, 970*t*, 972–976, 974*t*
- hepatic/cholestatic diseases and, 846*t*
- myocardial ischemia/acute coronary syndromes and, 472*t*, 486, 487*t*, 489
- opioid. *See* Opioid analgesics
- ovarian hyperstimulation and, 789, 790*t*
- peripheral neuropathy and, 288
- seizures and, 218*t*, 220
- thrombocytopenia and, 1049
- visual disturbances and, 313

Analogies, in epidemiology, 23
Anaphylaxis
- causative agents, 72–73*t*, 95–96
- clinical presentation of, 82–83, 83*t*
- differential diagnosis of, 84*t*
- epidemiology of, 76–77
- hospital admissions due to, 25
- as immediate reaction, 80
- management of, 98–100, 99*t*
- mechanisms of, 81
- risk factors for, 86

Anastrozole, 126*t*, 169*t*, 1064*t*, 1068*t*, 1123*t*
ANC (absolute neutrophil count), 1087, 1092, 1094, 1096
Andexanet alfa, 245
Androgen antagonists, 798
Androgen-deprivation therapy, 358*t*
Androgenetic alopecia, 165, 176, 180, 181–182*t*, 183–186, 184*t*
Androgenic agents, 1065*t*, 1068–1069*t*
Androgenic steroids, 102*t*
Androgens
- alopecia and, 167*t*, 176, 179*t*, 183, 190
- anxiety and, 403
- hepatic/cholestatic diseases and, 848*t*
- hirsutism and, 193–194, 198, 199*t*
- primary adrenal insufficiency and, 734
- secondary adrenal insufficiency and, 735
- sexual dysfunction and, 763
- thyroid diseases and, 701*t*

Anemia, 1099–1111
- aplastic, 1100–1104
- chemotherapy-induced, 1109–1111
- defined, 1099
- hemolytic, 83–84, 86, 1104–1107
- macrocytic, 1107–1109
- microcytic, 1102*t*
- normocytic, 1102*t*
- overview, 1099–1100

Anencephaly, 1327–1329, 1328*f*
Anesthetics
- acidosis and, 1003*t*
- alopecia and, 179*t*
- cognitive disorders and, 359*t*
- general, 850*t*
- hepatic/cholestatic diseases and, 864
- hypotension and, 634*t*
- hypothermia and, 1215
- inhaled. *See* Inhaled anesthetics
- intravenous, 907*t*
- local, 530, 1262, 1314
- malignant hyperthermia and, 1209–1210, 1209*t*, 1212–1214
- myocardial ischemia/acute coronary syndromes and, 472*t*
- nausea/vomiting and, 906–907*t*, 911*t*, 913–914, 921, 923
- ototoxicity and, 1243
- seizures and, 218*t*, 220, 226
- spinal, 911*t*, 914
- taste disorders and, 1262
- topical, 818

Angina pectoris, 471, 474–475, 480–485, 481*t*, 487*t*, 488–489
Angioedema, 32, 72–73*t*, 77–83, 83–84*t*, 87, 96–98, 99*t*
Angiotensin-converting enzyme (ACE) inhibitors
- acidosis and, 1003*t*
- acute kidney injury and, 942, 943*t*, 944–949, 945*t*, 952, 953
- alopecia and, 167*t*, 179*t*
- anxiety and, 403
- asthma/bronchospasm and, 451, 452*t*, 455*t*, 457–458*t*, 457–464, 461*t*
- chronic kidney disease and, 975–976
- comorbidity and, 34
- cutaneous diseases and, 103*t*, 109
- delirium and, 327*t*
- depression and, 378
- drug-induced hospitalizations from, 26, 26*t*
- drug interactions with, 40
- genetic variability and, 15, 16, 16*t*
- glucose/insulin dysregulation and, 682*t*, 685*t*
- gout/hyperuricemia and, 1138
- heart failure and, 512, 515, 516
- hepatic/cholestatic diseases and, 847*t*
- hypersensitivity reactions to, 32, 77, 77*t*, 81–83, 87, 96–97
- hypertension and, 625
- hypotension and, 632*t*, 642–644, 645*t*
- myocardial ischemia/acute coronary syndromes and, 472*t*, 486, 489
- oral lichenoid reactions and, 1270
- ovarian hyperstimulation and, 789
- pancreatitis and, 878*t*, 880, 886*t*, 887, 891
- psychosis and, 416*t*, 422
- sexual dysfunction and, 772
- SIADH and, 981, 983*t*
- systemic lupus erythematosus and, 132
- teratogenicity of, 1316, 1334*t*

Angiotensin-receptor blockers (ARBs)
- acidosis and, 1003*t*
- acute kidney injury and, 942, 943*t*, 944–949, 945*t*, 953
- asthma/bronchospasm and, 454, 463
- drug interactions with, 40
- gout/hyperuricemia and, 1138
- heart failure and, 516
- hepatic/cholestatic diseases and, 847*t*
- hypersensitivity reactions to, 77*t*, 96–97
- hypertension and, 625
- hypotension and, 632*t*
- pancreatitis and, 878*t*, 880
- sexual dysfunction and, 772

Angiotensin-receptor neprilysin inhibitors, 633*t*

Angiotensin II, 620, 647, 945

Angiotensin II receptor antagonists. *See* Angiotensin-receptor blockers (ARBs)

Anidulafungin, 296*t*

Aniline derivatives, 849*t*

Anion gap metabolic acidosis, 1002*t*, 1004*t*, 1007*t*

Anions, 1002*t*, 1004, 1004*t*, 1013*t*

Anorectic agents, 659, 662–663

Antacids
- alkalosis and, 1013
- constipation and, 835
- heart failure and, 503*t*, 510*t*
- myopathy and, 1151, 1153, 1156
- pancreatitis and, 881
- upper gastrointestinal ulceration and, 818

Anthracyclines
- alopecia and, 185
- breast cancer and, 1300
- heart failure and, 501, 502*t*, 507, 508, 511, 514, 514*t*, 515
- infertility and, 783*t*, 786*t*
- lymphoma and, 1295
- nausea/vomiting and, 925, 926
- neutropenia/agranulocytosis and, 1087, 1091

Anthralin cream, 187*t*, 191

Antiadrenergic agents, 378, 515

Antiandrogens, 190–194, 205–207, 432*t*, 759*t*, 1064*t*, 1068*t*, 1071

Antianginal agents, 634*t*

Antianxiety agents, 175, 761*t*

Antiarrhythmics
- alopecia and, 167*t*, 179*t*
- atrial fibrillation/atrial flutter and, 583, 587
- cognitive disorders and, 358*t*, 359
- delirium and, 326*t*
- drug fever and, 1187
- food interactions with, 41
- heart failure and, 501, 502*t*, 504, 504*t*, 507, 511, 513, 514*t*
- hypotension and, 634*t*
- monomorphic ventricular tachycardia and, 523, 525, 528–529
- neutropenia/agranulocytosis and, 1087
- seizures and, 218*t*
- systemic lupus erythematosus and, 133
- thyroid diseases and, 716
- torsades de pointes and, 538

Antiasthmatics, 326*t*

Antibacterial agents, 125*t*, 150, 951–952, 1095

Antibiotic-associated diarrhea (AAD), 821, 822–823*t*, 823, 825, 827, 830

Antibiotics. *See also specific antibiotics*
- acute kidney injury and, 952, 956
- anxiety and, 403
- aplastic anemia and, 1100, 1103
- β-lactam. *See* β-lactam antibiotics
- carbapenems. *See* Carbapenems
- cephalosporin. *See* Cephalosporins
- cognitive disorders and, 358*t*
- constipation and, 836*t*
- delirium and, 333
- depression and, 377, 384
- diarrhea and. *See* Antibiotic-associated diarrhea (AAD)
- drug fever and, 1187, 1190, 1192
- drug-induced hospitalizations from, 26*t*
- fluoroquinolone. *See* Fluoroquinolones
- food interactions with, 41
- hepatic/cholestatic diseases and, 870–871
- hypersensitivity reactions and, 1186
- infertility and, 800
- macrolides, 220, 328*t*, 541–542, 822*t*, 823
- neutropenia/agranulocytosis and, 1087, 1094, 1095
- oral erythema multiforme and, 1269
- osteonecrosis of jaw and, 1276
- penicillins. *See* Penicillins
- psychosis and, 422
- quinolones, 101, 220
- seizures and, 218*t*
- serum sickness-like reactions and, 1192, 1194
- sulfonamide, 92–95, 93*f*
- thrombocytopenia and, 1052
- vulvovaginal candidiasis and, 782*t*, 785*t*, 790–792

Antibody formation, 709–710

Anticancer agents. *See* Antineoplastic agents

Anticholinergics
- cognitive disorders and, 358–359*t*, 359–361, 364, 366–368
- constipation and, 835, 836–837*t*
- delirium and, 325, 328*t*, 329, 331–333, 335
- nausea/vomiting and, 927, 927*t*
- neuroleptic malignant syndrome and, 1201
- psychosis and, 415, 416*t*, 418*t*, 421, 422, 424*t*
- seizures and, 219, 220
- sexual dysfunction and, 764–765*t*, 766
- sleep disorders and, 353
- visual disturbances and, 295, 296*t*, 315, 329

Anticoagulants
- alopecia and, 166, 167*t*, 179*t*, 183–184
- bleeding disorders and, 1025–1026, 1026*t*, 1028, 1029*t*, 1032–1033, 1038–1039
- cutaneous diseases and, 105
- dosing and pharmacokinetic properties of, 1035–1036, 1035*t*
- hepatic/cholestatic diseases and, 868
- intracerebral hemorrhage and, 237–238, 240, 242*t*, 243–246, 244*t*
- ovarian hyperstimulation and, 789, 790*t*
- reversal algorithms, 1036, 1038*f*
- stroke and, 236–237
- thrombocytopenia and, 1057–1059
- thromboembolic diseases and, 1063, 1064*t*, 1067, 1068*t*, 1071, 1075–1078
- upper gastrointestinal ulceration and, 814
- valvular/pericardial heart disease and, 662
- visual disturbances and, 313

Anticonvulsant hypersensitivity syndrome (AHS), 87, 95, 109

Anticonvulsants. *See also* Seizures
- alopecia and, 168*t*, 179*t*
- anxiety and, 402, 404, 411
- aplastic anemia and, 1100
- aromatic, 95, 109, 111*t*, 113*t*
- cognitive disorders and, 358–359*t*, 361, 365, 367
- constipation and, 835
- delirium and, 325, 326*t*
- depression and, 376*t*
- drug fever and, 1187, 1192
- drug-induced hospitalizations from, 26*t*
- gingival hyperplasia and, 1264*t*
- hepatic/cholestatic diseases and, 861*t*
- hydantoin, 133
- hypersensitivity reactions to, 87, 95, 109
- hypertrichosis and, 196*t*
- neuroleptic malignant syndrome and, 1195
- oral erythema multiforme and, 1266
- ototoxicity and, 1243
- psychosis and, 418*t*
- sexual dysfunction and, 764*t*, 772
- SIADH and, 981
- sleep disorders and, 348*t*
- suicidality and, 375, 387
- systemic lupus erythematosus and, 124*t*, 130, 133
- teratogenicity of, 1315
- thrombocytopenia and, 1049
- weight gain and, 1166*t*, 1168–1169*t*, 1169–1170, 1173*t*, 1175*t*

Antidepressants
- alopecia and, 175
- anxiety and, 405, 410
- constipation and, 835, 836–837*t*
- cyclic, 219
- delirium and, 325, 326–327*t*
- diarrhea and, 821, 822*t*
- drug-induced depression and, 376*t*
- drug interactions with, 33
- food interactions with, 41
- glucose/insulin dysregulation and, 680*t*, 684*t*
- hyperprolactinemia and, 742, 743–744*t*
- hypotension and, 634*t*
- intracerebral hemorrhage and, 239
- MAOIs. *See* Monoamine oxidase inhibitors
- myocardial ischemia/acute coronary syndromes and, 472*t*
- ototoxicity and, 1243
- seizures and, 218*t*, 219–221
- sexual dysfunction and, 758–765*t*, 761, 772, 783*t*, 786*t*, 797, 798, 800
- SIADH and, 981, 985, 988
- sleep disorders and, 352, 353
- SNRIs. *See* Serotonin–norepinephrine reuptake inhibitors
- SSRIs. *See* Selective serotonin reuptake inhibitors
- suicidality and, 375, 380, 387, 389–391
- TCAs. *See* Tricyclic antidepressants
- tetracyclic, 218*t*, 759–760*t*, 1170
- thyroid diseases and, 713
- visual disturbances and, 313
- weight gain and, 1166*t*, 1168–1169*t*, 1170–1171, 1173*t*, 1175*t*

Antidiabetic therapies, 26*t*, 634*t*, 884, 1175*t*, 1304

Antidiuretic hormone. *See* Syndrome of inappropriate antidiuretic hormone secretion (SIADH); Vasopressin

Antidotes, for drug-induced psychosis, 424, 424*t*

Antiemetics
- akathisia and, 254, 255, 255*t*
- cognitive disorders and, 359
- delirium and, 325
- dystonia and, 266*t*, 269
- hyperprolactinemia and, 742, 743–744*t*, 745
- hypotension and, 634*t*
- nausea/vomiting and, 910, 919–930
- neutropenia/agranulocytosis and, 1096
- ovarian hyperstimulation and, 789, 790*t*
- parkinsonism and, 271*t*, 273
- tardive dyskinesia and, 260*t*, 261–263

INDEX

Antiepileptic drugs (AEDs)
- akathisia and, 255*t*
- alopecia and, 175, 178
- cognitive disorders and, 367
- cutaneous diseases and, 111
- depression and, 378–379, 386, 389
- dystonia and, 270
- hepatic/cholestatic diseases and, 864
- hypotension and, 634*t*
- infertility and, 783*t*, 786*t*, 800, 802
- osteoporosis/osteomalacia and, 1121*t*, 1122, 1123*t*, 1126*t*, 1127
- pancreatitis and, 883
- parkinsonism and, 271*t*
- peripheral neuropathy and, 289
- psychosis and, 422
- seizures and, 217, 218*t*, 221, 224–226
- sexual dysfunction and, 783*t*, 786*t*
- SIADH and, 983*t*
- side effects of, 254
- systemic lupus erythematosus and, 133
- tardive dyskinesia and, 262
- teratogenicity of, 1315, 1319, 1328, 1330–1331
- vaginal bleeding disorders and, 782*t*, 785*t*, 793
- visual disturbances and, 312

Antiestrogens, 176, 381, 781, 783, 1300, 1301

Antifibrinolytic drugs, 221, 1039

Antifungal agents
- acute kidney injury and, 949, 955
- alopecia and, 168*t*, 177, 179*t*
- cognitive disorders and, 358*t*
- delirium and, 333
- imidazole, 103*t*
- neutropenia/agranulocytosis and, 1095
- systemic lupus erythematosus and, 125*t*
- vulvovaginal candidiasis and, 792

Antigen-presenting cells (APCs), 78, 79, 87, 105

Antihistamines
- for allergic reactions, 100
- asthma/bronchospasm and, 461
- cognitive disorders and, 359
- constipation and, 835, 837*t*
- cutaneous diseases and, 113
- delirium and, 325
- heart failure and, 515
- hypotension and, 634*t*
- nausea/vomiting and, 927, 927*t*
- ototoxicity and, 1243–1244
- ovarian hyperstimulation and, 789, 790*t*
- photosensitivity and, 143, 155
- seizures and, 219
- serum sickness-like reactions and, 1194
- sexual dysfunction and, 759*t*, 764*t*
- visual disturbances and, 295

Antihyperglycemics, 501, 505–506, 511, 513, 821, 822*t*

Antihyperlipidemics, 313

Antihypertensives
- acute kidney injury and, 942
- constipation and, 836*t*
- delirium and, 327*t*
- depression and, 378, 385, 391
- drug fever and, 1187
- food interactions with, 41
- gout/hyperuricemia and, 1138
- hyperprolactinemia and, 742, 743*t*
- hypertension and, 618*t*, 621, 625
- hypertrichosis and, 196*t*
- hypotension and, 632–633*t*, 637, 644, 647, 648
- sexual dysfunction and, 761, 766, 772, 783*t*, 786*t*, 797–800
- stroke and, 236
- systemic lupus erythematosus and, 135
- teratogenicity of, 1317
- vaginal bleeding disorders and, 782*t*, 785*t*

Anti-infectives
- anxiety and, 399, 403
- cutaneous diseases and, 101
- depression and, 375, 376*t*, 377
- myocardial ischemia/acute coronary syndromes and, 472*t*
- nausea/vomiting and, 909*t*
- peripheral neuropathy and, 280*t*
- visual disturbances and, 313

Anti-inflammatory agents. *See also* Nonsteroidal anti-inflammatory drugs (NSAIDS)
- alopecia and, 191
- aplastic anemia and, 1100
- gout/hyperuricemia and, 1141, 1145
- hemolytic anemia and, 1104
- hepatic/cholestatic diseases and, 846*t*
- interstitial lung disease/pulmonary fibrosis and, 433
- pancreatitis and, 887
- systemic lupus erythematosus and, 135

Antimalarial agents
- anxiety and, 403
- color changes of oral mucosa and teeth and, 1255, 1255*t*
- cutaneous diseases and, 109
- depression and, 377
- myopathy and, 1151
- seizures and, 218*t*, 226
- systemic lupus erythematosus and, 135
- visual disturbances and, 295, 313, 318–319

Antimetabolites
- chemotherapy-induced anemia and, 1109
- infertility and, 800
- leukemia and, 1286
- lymphoma and, 1293
- macrocytic anemia and, 1107
- neutropenia/agranulocytosis and, 1087, 1091

Antimicrobial agents
- acute kidney injury and, 949
- cutaneous diseases and, 100–101
- delirium and, 328*t*
- diarrhea and, 828
- drug fever and, 1187, 1189, 1191
- hepatic/cholestatic diseases and, 846–847*t*
- hypotension and, 634–635*t*
- interstitial lung disease/pulmonary fibrosis and, 433
- ototoxicity and, 1243
- pancreatitis and, 885
- thrombocytopenia and, 1049
- upper gastrointestinal ulceration and, 811

Antimicrotubular agents, 1101*t*, 1109*t*

Antimigraine agents, 376*t*, 380, 472*t*, 477*t*, 1204

Antimitotic drugs, 1091

Antimonials, 846*t*, 878*t*

Antimuscarinic agents
- akathisia and, 258, 259
- dystonia and, 265–266, 268–270
- parkinsonism and, 273
- tardive dyskinesia and, 261, 262, 265

Antineoplastic agents. *See also* Chemotherapy agents
- alopecia and, 177
- atrial fibrillation/atrial flutter and, 581
- cognitive disorders and, 358–359*t*
- constipation and, 835, 836*t*
- diarrhea and, 821, 822–823*t*, 823, 825
- drug fever and, 1189
- drug-induced hospitalizations from, 26*t*
- heart failure and, 514
- infertility and, 800
- myocardial ischemia/acute coronary syndromes and, 472*t*
- neutropenia/agranulocytosis and, 1087, 1091
- osteoporosis/osteomalacia and, 1121*t*, 1123*t*
- ototoxicity and, 1243
- peripheral neuropathy and, 279, 280*t*, 288
- seizures and, 218*t*, 221, 223, 226
- sexual dysfunction and, 762*t*, 765*t*, 767, 770–771, 774
- thromboembolic diseases and, 1065*t*, 1069*t*, 1071
- vaginal bleeding disorders and, 793
- visual disturbances and, 313

Antinuclear antibody test (ANA), 130–135

Antiobesity drug therapy, 1174–1175

Antioxidants, 437, 856, 866, 953, 1158, 1243

Antiparkinson agents
- cognitive disorders and, 358*t*, 359, 362
- delirium and, 325
- heart failure and, 510*t*
- hypotension and, 635*t*
- neuroleptic malignant syndrome and, 1196
- parkinsonism and, 273
- sexual dysfunction and, 759*t*, 764*t*
- sleep disorders and, 348*t*, 350*t*

Antiplatelet drugs
- aplastic anemia and, 1100*t*
- bleeding disorders and, 1025, 1026*t*, 1029, 1029*t*, 1033, 1039
- intracerebral hemorrhage and, 239–245
- myocardial ischemia/acute coronary syndromes and, 480, 486, 487*t*
- neutropenia/agranulocytosis and, 1087

Antipsychotics
- alopecia and, 179*t*
- anxiety and, 400*t*, 405, 410
- atypical. *See* Atypical antipsychotics
- butyrophenone, 266
- cognitive disorders and, 358–359*t*, 359, 369
- constipation and, 835, 836*t*
- conventional, 742, 743*t*, 745–746, 1167*t*, 1169*t*, 1171
- delirium and, 325, 326*t*, 335–338, 340
- dystonia and, 265, 268
- hyperprolactinemia and, 742, 743–744*t*, 745–747
- hypertrichosis and, 197*t*, 199
- hypotension and, 635*t*, 642, 645*t*
- hypothermia and, 1215–1218
- myocardial ischemia/acute coronary syndromes and, 472*t*
- neuroleptic malignant syndrome and, 1195, 1196, 1200, 1201
- neutropenia/agranulocytosis and, 1088
- phenothiazine. *See* Phenothiazines
- psychosis and, 418, 423, 424
- seizures and, 218*t*, 221, 225
- serotonin syndrome and, 1209
- sexual dysfunction and, 757, 758–760*t*, 761, 763–764*t*, 772, 783*t*, 786*t*, 797–800
- SIADH and, 982–983*t*, 985
- sleep disorders and, 353
- suicidality and, 375, 380
- tardive dyskinesia and, 260, 262, 264, 265
- thromboembolic diseases and, 1066*t*, 1067, 1070*t*
- torsades de pointes and, 540–542
- typical. *See* Typical antipsychotics
- visual disturbances and, 295
- weight gain and, 1166–1169*t*, 1170–1174, 1173*t*, 1175*t*

Antipyretics
chronic kidney disease and, 966t, 968, 970t, 972t, 974t
drug fever and, 1186, 1190, 1191
hypothermia and, 1216
serum sickness-like reactions and, 1186
Antipyrine, 701t
Antiretroviral therapy. *See also* Highly active antiretroviral therapy (HAART)
alopecia and, 183
cognitive disorders and, 358t, 362
combined, 1172
diarrhea and, 823t
drug fever and, 1190
hyperprolactinemia and, 744t
myopathy and, 1151, 1154, 1159
osteoporosis/osteomalacia and, 1121t, 1123t
peripheral neuropathy and, 279, 283, 285, 288, 289
sexual dysfunction and, 797, 798
thyroid diseases and, 701, 704
weight gain and, 1167–1168t, 1172
Antirheumatic agents, 174, 178, 1049, 1087, 1175t
Antiserotonergic agents, 256, 259
Antispasmodics, 359, 1243
Antithrombotic therapy, 235, 245–246, 476, 1028, 1057
Antithymocyte globulin (OKT3), 1193t, 1284t, 1288t, 1292–1294
Antithyroid agents. *See* Thyroid medications
Antitoxins, 1192, 1194
Antituberculosis agents, 288, 377, 710, 1138
Antitussives, 464
Antivascular endothelin growth factor agents, 620t
Antivenoms, 1192, 1194
Antivirals
alopecia and, 168t, 179t
chronic kidney disease and, 966–967
delirium and, 333
depression and, 376t, 377–378
drug fever and, 1187
hypertrichosis and, 196t
lymphoma and, 1295
in sulfa drug class, 92
Anxiety, 399–411
causative agents of, 399–404, 400–401t
clinical presentation of, 406–408, 406t, 408t
differential diagnosis of, 407, 407t
epidemiology of, 404, 404t
management of, 410–411
mechanisms of, 404–406, 405t
morbidity and mortality for, 409–410
patient education on, 411
prevention of, 410, 410t
risk factors for, 408–409, 408t
Anxiolytics, 486, 631, 1243
APCs (antigen-presenting cells), 78, 79, 87, 105
Apixaban
alopecia and, 167t
bleeding disorders and, 1029t
intracerebral hemorrhage and, 237, 238t, 245
thromboembolic diseases and, 1076, 1077t
valvular/pericardial heart disease and, 661t, 662
Aplastic anemia, 1100–1104
causative agents of, 1100, 1100t
clinical presentation of, 1101–1102, 1102t
differential diagnosis of, 1102, 1102t
epidemiology of, 1100
management of, 1103–1104
mechanisms of, 1100–1101, 1101t
morbidity and mortality for, 1102–1103
patient education on, 1104
prevention of, 1103, 1103t
risk factors for, 1102, 1103t
Apomorphine, 418t
Aprepitant, 926, 922, 923, 924t
Aprindine, 847t
Aprotinin, 8, 72t, 1064t, 1067, 1068t
ARBs. *See* Angiotensin-receptor blockers
Arbutamine, 472t
Argatroban, 472t, 1029t, 1058
Aripazine, 245
Aripiprazole
acidosis and, 1002t
alopecia and, 172t
anxiety and, 400t, 405
constipation and, 836t
delirium and, 338
depression and, 376t
hypertrichosis and, 197t
hypotension and, 635t, 639t
neuroleptic malignant syndrome and, 1195t
ototoxicity and, 1234t
photosensitivity and, 144t
sexual dysfunction and, 765t, 772
SIADH and, 982t
tardive dyskinesia and, 265
thyroid diseases and, 710
torsades de pointes and, 533t, 540t
visual disturbances and, 296t
weight gain and, 1166t, 1169t, 1170, 1175, 1175t
Aripiprazole lauroxil, 635t
Aristolochic acid (Chinese herbs), 965, 966t, 969–976, 970t, 972t, 974t
Armodafinil, 400t, 409
Aromatase inhibitors
alopecia and, 176
breast cancer and, 1300
depression and, 376t, 381–382
endometrial cancer and, 1303
osteoporosis/osteomalacia and, 1121t, 1123t
thromboembolic diseases and, 1064t, 1068t
Aromatic amines, 132
Aromatic anticonvulsants, 95, 109, 111t, 113t
Arrhythmias. *See* Supraventricular arrhythmias; Ventricular arrhythmias
Arsenic, 171t, 177, 1255t, 1266t
Arsenicals, 849t
Arsenic trioxide, 524t, 532t, 539t, 907t
Ascorbic acid, 810t, 811, 1105t
Asenapine, 1166t, 1169t
Asparaginase. *See also* L-asparaginase
drug fever and, 1188t
hepatic/cholestatic diseases and, 847t
pancreatitis and, 878t, 886t
thromboembolic diseases and, 1065t, 1069t, 1075t
Aspartame, 72t
Aspartate aminotransferase (AST), 862, 865, 868, 1058
Aspirin. *See also* Aspirin-induced asthma (AIA)
adverse events associated with, 20
allergic and hypersensitivity reactions to, 72t, 77t, 81, 97–98
bleeding disorders and, 1025–1027, 1026t, 1029, 1029t, 1030, 1033, 1039
cardioprotective effects of, 50
chronic kidney disease and, 968
comorbidity and, 34
drug fever and, 1188t, 1191
glucose/insulin dysregulation and, 688
gout/hyperuricemia and, 1136t, 1137
heart failure and, 510t
hepatic/cholestatic diseases and, 846t
hypothermia and, 1216
intracerebral hemorrhage and, 238t, 240t, 242t, 243, 244
monomorphic ventricular tachycardia and, 524t
myocardial ischemia/acute coronary syndromes and, 472t, 479, 480, 486, 487t, 488, 489
neutropenia/agranulocytosis and, 1089t
oral erythema multiforme and, 1266t
oral lichenoid reactions and, 1270t
ototoxicity and, 1234t
pancreatitis and, 881, 886t, 887–888
sinus bradycardia/atrioventricular block and, 578
stroke and, 236
for systemic lupus erythematosus, 135
taste disorders and, 1259t
teratogenicity of, 1326
thrombocytopenia and, 1053, 1056
thromboembolic diseases and, 1075
thyroid diseases and, 701t
upper gastrointestinal ulceration and, 809–818, 810–811t, 816t
vaginal bleeding disorders and, 796
visual disturbances and, 297t
Aspirin desensitization, 461–462
Aspirin-exacerbated respiratory disease (AERD), 453, 455, 457–463
Aspirin-induced asthma (AIA)
causative agents of, 451, 452t
clinical presentation of, 457–459
as drug allergy or hypersensitivity reaction, 82, 87, 98
epidemiology of, 453
management of, 462
mechanisms of, 455, 455t, 456, 456f
morbidity and mortality for, 460
prevention of, 461, 461t
risk factors for, 458t, 459–460
Aspirin tetrad, 455
AST (aspartate aminotransferase), 862, 865, 868, 1058
Astemizole, 541
Asthma and bronchospasm, 451–464. *See also* Aspirin-induced asthma (AIA)
causative agents of, 72–73t, 451, 452–453t
clinical presentation of, 457–459, 457t
differential diagnosis of, 457, 458t
epidemiology of, 451, 453–454
management of, 218t, 462–463
mechanisms of, 455–457, 455t, 456f
morbidity and mortality for, 460–461
patient education on, 463–464
prevention of, 461–462, 461t
risk factors for, 458t, 459–460
Atazanavir, 168t, 533t, 539t, 1234t, 1266t
Atenolol
alopecia and, 168t
delirium and, 327t
hyperprolactinemia and, 743t
hypotension and, 632t, 638t, 646t
oral lichenoid reactions and, 1270t
sinus bradycardia/atrioventricular block and, 577t, 579
systemic lupus erythematosus and, 124t
teratogenicity of, 1317
ATN. *See* Acute tubular necrosis
Atomoxetine, 219t, 221, 400t, 401, 646t, 647, 761t, 984t
Atorvastatin
alopecia and, 171t
constipation and, 836t

INDEX

Atorvastatin (continued)
intracerebral hemorrhage and, 239
myopathy and, 1157
oral lichenoid reactions and, 1270*t*
pancreatitis and, 878*t*, 886*t*
peripheral neuropathy and, 280*t*
sleep disorders and, 348*t*
systemic lupus erythematosus and, 124*t*
taste disorders and, 1259*t*
visual disturbances and, 297*t*
Atovaquone-proguanil, 144*t*
Atracurium, 72*t*, 636*t*, 638*t*, 644
Atrial fibrillation/atrial flutter, 581–588
causative agents for, 581, 582–583*t*
clinical presentation of, 584–585, 584*t*
differential diagnosis of, 585, 585*t*
epidemiology of, 581, 583
management of, 586–588, 587*t*
mechanisms of, 583–584, 583*t*
morbidity and mortality for, 586
patient education on, 588
prevention of, 586, 586*t*
risk factors for, 585–586, 585*t*
Atrial tachycardia, 588–592
causative agents of, 588, 588*t*
clinical presentation of, 589, 589*t*
differential diagnosis of, 589, 589*t*
epidemiology of, 588
management of, 590–591, 591*t*
mechanisms of, 589, 589*t*
morbidity and mortality for, 590
patient education on, 591–592
prevention of, 590, 590*t*
risk factors for, 589–590, 589*t*
Atrioventricular (AV) block. *See* Sinus bradycardia/atrioventricular block
Atrioventricular node re-entrant tachycardia (AVNRT), 592–595
causative agents of, 592, 592*t*
clinical presentation of, 593, 593*t*
differential diagnosis of, 593, 593*t*
epidemiology of, 592
management of, 594, 595*t*
mechanisms of, 592–593
morbidity and mortality for, 594
patient education on, 594–595
prevention of, 594, 594*t*
risk factors for, 593–594, 593*t*
Atropine, 317, 328–329*t*, 472*t*, 530, 580, 1234*t*, 1256*t*
Attention deficit/hyperactivity disorder (ADHD) agents, 219*t*, 221–222, 401
Atypical antipsychotics
acidosis and, 1002*t*
akathisia and, 254–256, 255–256*t*, 258, 258*t*, 259
alopecia and, 175
delirium and, 336, 340
development of, 254
dystonia and, 266*t*, 269, 269*t*, 270
glucose/insulin dysregulation and, 679, 680*t*, 683, 684*t*, 690
hypothermia and, 1215–1217
neuroleptic malignant syndrome and, 1195–1199
neutropenia/agranulocytosis and, 1088
parkinsonism and, 270–273, 271*t*, 273*t*
sexual dysfunction and, 758–760*t*, 761*t*, 764*t*
stroke and, 233
tardive dyskinesia and, 260*t*, 261, 263–265, 264*t*
torsades de pointes and, 541, 542
weight gain and, 1166*t*, 1169*t*, 1170
Auranofin, 1089*t*
Aurothiopropanosulfonate, 432*t*
Autism, 21, 29, 1315
Autoantibodies, 1052–1053, 1106
AV (atrioventricular) block. *See* Sinus bradycardia/atrioventricular block
Avelumab, 7*t*
AVNRT. *See* Atrioventricular node re-entrant tachycardia
Axelopran, 840–841
Axicabtagene, 7*t*
Axitinib, 169*t*, 698–699*t*, 709, 836*t*, 883
Azacitidine, 432*t*, 660*t*, 907*t*
Azaribine, 473*t*
Azathioprine
allergic reactions to, 72*t*
alopecia and, 172*t*
cutaneous diseases and, 102*t*, 108
drug fever and, 1188*t*
genetic variations affecting, 36*t*
gout/hyperuricemia and, 1145
hepatic/cholestatic diseases and, 852*t*, 866
hyperprolactinemia and, 744*t*
interstitial lung disease/pulmonary fibrosis and, 440
leukemia and, 1284, 1284*t*, 1286
lymphoma and, 1284*t*, 1288*t*, 1292, 1293
macrocytic anemia and, 1108*t*
pancreatitis and, 878*t*, 879, 880, 886*t*, 891, 891*t*
pharmacogenomic tests for, 35
photosensitivity and, 144*t*
skin cancer and, 1284*t*, 1288*t*, 1297, 1298
taste disorders and, 1259*t*
upper gastrointestinal ulceration and, 815
Azilsartan, 632*t*
Azimilide, 538
Azithromycin
cutaneous diseases and, 103*t*
delirium and, 328*t*
gingival hyperplasia and, 1265
myocardial ischemia/acute coronary syndromes and, 472*t*, 474
ototoxicity and, 1234*t*
SIADH and, 984*t*
taste disorders and, 1259*t*
torsades de pointes and, 532*t*, 542
Azole antifungals, 792, 846*t*
Azole antiparasitics, 846*t*
Aztreonam, 90, 92, 1234*t*

Bacillus Calmette-Guerin (BCG) vaccine, 197*t*, 1270*t*
Bacitracin, 1234*t*
Baclofen
anxiety and, 400*t*
asthma/bronchospasm and, 463
hypothermia and, 1215–1217, 1216*t*
neuroleptic malignant syndrome and, 1197
peripheral neuropathy and, 288
seizures and, 217
sexual dysfunction and, 759–760*t*, 783*t*, 786*t*
sinus bradycardia/atrioventricular block and, 570*t*, 577*t*
tardive dyskinesia and, 265
Balsalazide, 660*t*, 662
Barbiturates
acidosis and, 1003*t*
anxiety and, 400*t*, 402
cognitive disorders and, 359*t*, 360, 362
cutaneous diseases and, 102*t*
depression and, 379
duration of detection in urine, 420*t*
hepatic/cholestatic diseases and, 851*t*
hypotension and, 643
malignant hyperthermia and, 1212, 1212*t*
oral erythema multiforme and, 1266*t*
seizures and, 226
visual disturbances and, 297*t*, 313
Barium contrast, 1266*t*
Basal cell carcinoma (BCC), 1295–1297
Basiliximab, 72*t*, 1065*t*, 1069*t*, 1295
BCG (Bacillus Calmette-Guerin) vaccine, 197*t*, 1270*t*
BCNU. *See* Carmustine
BCNU/CCNU, 847*t*
Beclomethasone, 473*t*, 739
Beclomethasone dipropionate, 731*t*, 736*t*, 738
Beers Criteria, 31, 368
Belatacept, 172*t*, 836*t*
Benazepril, 144*t*, 167*t*, 632*t*, 638*t*, 878*t*
Bendamustine, 907*t*
Benoxaprofen, 197*t*
Benzalkonium chloride, 452*t*, 454, 455*t*
Benzocaine, 144*t*, 472*t*
Benzodiazepines
acidosis and, 1003*t*, 1011*t*
akathisia and, 259
anxiety and, 400*t*, 402, 404, 405*t*, 407, 410, 411
cognitive disorders and, 358–359*t*, 360–362, 364, 366–369
delirium and, 325, 327*t*, 333, 336, 337
depression and, 378, 380
duration of detection in urine, 420*t*
dystonia and, 270
hepatic/cholestatic diseases and, 851*t*, 871
hypothermia and, 1215, 1216
malignant hyperthermia and, 1213, 1213*t*
myocardial ischemia/acute coronary syndromes and, 487*t*, 488, 489
nausea/vomiting and, 927, 927*t*
neuroleptic malignant syndrome and, 1197, 1200*t*, 1201
psychosis and, 417*t*, 423, 424, 424*t*
secondary adrenal insufficiency and, 737
seizures and, 95, 217, 218*t*, 224–226
serotonin syndrome and, 1208, 1208*t*
sexual dysfunction and, 758–759*t*
sleep disorders and, 352–353
teratogenicity of, 1319, 1320
visual disturbances and, 313, 315
withdrawal from, 421, 424*t*
Benzonatate, 297*t*
Benzphetamine, 167*t*
Benztropine, 328–329*t*, 348*t*, 1188*t*
Bepridil, 432*t*
Bergamot oil, 144*t*
Beryllium, 849*t*
β-adrenergic agonists, 747, 748*t*
β_2-adrenergic agonists, 635*t*, 1002*t*, 1319
β-adrenergic receptor blockers (β-blockers)
akathisia and, 258, 259
alopecia and, 168*t*, 178, 179*t*
anxiety and, 400*t*, 404, 410
asthma/bronchospasm and, 451, 452*t*, 453–457, 455*t*, 458*t*, 459–464, 461*t*
atrial fibrillation/atrial flutter and, 586
atrial tachycardia and, 591
comorbidity and, 34
cutaneous diseases and, 103*t*, 106, 109
delirium and, 327*t*
depression and, 376*t*, 378, 391
drug interactions with, 40
dystonia and, 270

glucose/insulin dysregulation and, 680t, 682t, 684–685t
heart failure and, 501, 502t, 504t, 509, 510, 512, 516
hepatic/cholestatic diseases and, 847t
hypertension and, 620t, 621, 625–627, 625t
hypertrichosis and, 196t
hypotension and, 632t, 643, 645t, 647
malignant hyperthermia and, 1213
myocardial ischemia/acute coronary syndromes and, 472t, 477t, 480, 485, 486, 487t, 488, 489
oral lichenoid reactions and, 1270
psychosis and, 422
sexual dysfunction and, 758–759t, 761, 763–764t, 767, 772
sinus bradycardia/atrioventricular block and, 569, 570t, 572, 573–574t, 576–577, 579, 580
sleep disorders and, 348t, 350t, 351
smoking and, 33
teratogenicity of, 1316, 1317
thyroid diseases and, 716, 717
visual disturbances and, 313
β-carotene, 850t
Betahistine, 452t
Betaine glucuronate, 868
β-lactam antibiotics
acute kidney injury and, 943t, 956
allergic reactions to, 74t, 84, 87, 89–90, 89t
diarrhea and, 821
drug interactions with, 38
neutropenia/agranulocytosis and, 1088, 1089t, 1091t, 1094
taste disorders and, 1259t, 1261t
upper gastrointestinal ulceration and, 809
Betamethasone, 195–196t, 473t, 474, 731t, 736t, 739t, 741
Betamethasone propionate, 1273
Betaxolol, 168t, 462, 577t, 632t, 638t
Betel nut, 221
Bevacizumab
alopecia and, 169t
constipation and, 836t
heart failure and, 502t, 508, 512
hypertension and, 618t
osteonecrosis of jaw and, 1273–1276, 1274t
systemic lupus erythematosus and, 126t
thromboembolic diseases and, 1065t, 1069t
thyroid diseases and, 698t, 715
visual disturbances and, 297t
Bexarotene, 144t, 191, 698t, 701t, 710, 714
Bezafibrate, 878t
Bicalutamide, 144t, 432t, 836t, 1123t
Bicarbonate
acidosis and, 1001, 1004–1006, 1009, 1010
alkalosis and, 1012–1017
upper gastrointestinal ulceration and, 812, 817
Biguanides, 822–823t, 1002t
Bile acid sequestrants, 836t, 869
Bimatoprost, 197, 197t
Biologic agents
alopecia and, 176, 178
anaphylaxis and, 95–96
heart failure and, 501, 502t, 507–508, 511–512, 514, 514t
hypotension and, 635t
interstitial lung disease/pulmonary fibrosis and, 433
serum sickness-like reactions and, 1192
Biologic gradient, 22
Biostatistical analysis, 21
Bipolar disorder, 378–380
Birth control. *See* Contraceptives
Birth defects. *See* Teratogenicity
Bisacodyl, 840t
Bishop's weed, 144t, 297t
Bismuth, 171t, 177, 1254–1255t, 1270t
Bismuth subsalicylate, 827t, 829
Bisoprolol, 512, 632t, 638t, 1317
Bisphosphonates
atrial fibrillation/atrial flutter and, 581, 583, 584
constipation and, 836t
osteonecrosis of jaw and, 1273–1276, 1274–1275t
osteoporosis/osteomalacia and, 1129, 1129t, 1130
upper gastrointestinal ulceration and, 809–812, 810–811t, 814, 816, 816t, 818–819
visual disturbances and, 312, 318
Bisulfites, 455
Bitter melon, 682t, 685t
Bitter orange, 144t, 297t, 400t, 404, 409
Bivalirudin, 239, 487t, 1029t, 1032, 1033, 1058
Black box warnings, 38, 230, 261, 475, 841, 922
Black cohosh, 850t
Black mustard, 297t
Bladder cancer, 1303–1305
causative agents of, 1285t, 1303
clinical presentation of, 1290t, 1304
differential diagnosis of, 1290t, 1304
epidemiology of, 1303–1304
management of, 1305
mechanisms of, 1288t, 1304
morbidity and mortality for, 1304
patient education on, 1305
prevention of, 1294t, 1304–1305
risk factors for, 1291t, 1304
Bleeding diathesis, 240
Bleeding disorders, 1025–1039
causative agents of, 1025–1026, 1026t
clinical presentation of, 1030–1031, 1030t
definitions of, 1027, 1027t
differential diagnosis of, 1030, 1031t
epidemiology of, 1026–1028
management of, 1036–1037t, 1036–1039, 1038f
mechanisms of, 1028–1030, 1028f, 1029t
morbidity and mortality for, 1032–1034
patient education on, 1039
prevention of, 1034–1035t, 1034–1036
risk factors for, 1031–1032, 1031–1032t
Bleomycin
alopecia and, 169t, 176
color changes of oral mucosa and teeth and, 1254t
drug fever and, 1186, 1188t
hepatic/cholestatic diseases and, 847t
infertility and, 783t, 786t
interstitial lung disease/pulmonary fibrosis and, 431, 432t, 434, 435t, 437–440
leukemia and, 1285
myocardial ischemia/acute coronary syndromes and, 472t
ototoxicity and, 1234t
thromboembolic diseases and, 1065t, 1069t
Blood disorders, allergic-mediated, 75t, 80, 83–84, 83t
Blood modifiers, 472t
Blood pressure classification guidelines, 618–619, 619t, 621
Blue cohosh, 502t, 510t
Boceprevir, 173t, 179t, 1258, 1259t
Bone marrow aplasia, 1109
Bone remodeling, 1120, 1122, 1126
Bortezomib
alopecia and, 169t
hepatic/cholestatic diseases and, 847t
interstitial lung disease/pulmonary fibrosis and, 437
pancreatitis and, 878t, 883
peripheral neuropathy and, 280t, 282t, 285, 286, 288
SIADH and, 983t
Bosentan, 7t, 636t, 640t, 852t
Boston Collaborative Drug Surveillance Program, 94, 104, 219
Bosutinib, 907t, 1087
Botulinum toxin, 265, 270, 297t, 1066t, 1070t, 1259t
Bradykinin, 82, 96, 457, 460, 887
BRAF (B-rapidly accelerated fibrosarcoma) inhibitors, 1284t, 1295–1298
B-rapidly accelerated fibrosarcoma (BRAF) inhibitors, 1284t, 1295–1298
BRCA gene mutation, 1299, 1300
Breakthrough bleeding, 793, 794
Breast cancer, 1298–1301
causative agents of, 1285t, 1298–1299
clinical presentation of, 1290t, 1299
differential diagnosis of, 1290t, 1299
epidemiology of, 1299
management of, 1300
mechanisms of, 1288t
morbidity and mortality for, 1300
patient education on, 1301
prevention of, 1294t, 1300
risk factors for, 1291t, 1299–1300
Brentuximab, 169t, 878t, 883–884, 886t
Bretylium, 634t
Brexpiprazole, 400t, 405, 635t, 1166t, 1169t
Brinzolamide, 1003t
Brodalumab, 7t
Bromelin, 452t
Bromfenac, 846t
Bromides, 108
Bromine, 701t
Bromocriptine
alopecia and, 171t, 175
anxiety and, 408
delirium and, 327t, 329t
heart failure and, 502t, 509
hyperprolactinemia and, 746
hypotension and, 635t, 640t
interstitial lung disease/pulmonary fibrosis and, 432t
myocardial ischemia/acute coronary syndromes and, 473t
nausea/vomiting and, 911t
neuroleptic malignant syndrome and, 1196, 1200, 1200t
ototoxicity and, 1234t
psychosis and, 418t
serotonin syndrome and, 1206
sexual dysfunction and, 783t, 786t
sleep disorders and, 348t
thromboembolic diseases and, 1066t, 1070t
thyroid diseases and, 701t
valvular/pericardial heart disease and, 659, 660t, 663
visual disturbances and, 297t
Brompheniramine, 1089t
Bronchodilators, 404, 454, 460–461, 1320
Bronchospasm. *See* Asthma and bronchospasm
Brown v. American Home Products Corporation Diet Drugs (2000), 9, 9t
Brugada syndrome, 546–549
causative agents of, 546, 547t
clinical presentation of, 547–548, 547t
differential diagnosis of, 548

INDEX

Brugada syndrome, (continued)
epidemiology of, 546
management of, 549
mechanisms of, 546–547
morbidity and mortality for, 548
patient education on, 549
prevention of, 549
risk factors for, 548, 548t
Budesonide, 171t, 196t, 731t, 732, 736t, 738, 739, 879
Buflomedil, 502t
Buformin, 1002t
Bulk-forming laxatives, 840, 840t
Bumetanide, 633t, 638t, 878t, 1234t
Bupivacaine
Brugada syndrome and, 547t
hypotension and, 634t
malignant hyperthermia and, 1212, 1212t
monomorphic ventricular tachycardia and, 524–525t, 530
ototoxicity and, 1234t
sinus bradycardia/atrioventricular block and, 570t, 573t
taste disorders and, 1259t
visual disturbances and, 297t
Buprenorphine, 7t, 533t, 539t, 906t, 1203–1204t, 1205
Bupropion
allergic reactions to, 74t, 84
alopecia and, 172t
anxiety and, 400t, 405t, 409
constipation and, 836t
delirium and, 327t
depression and, 391, 392
hypertension and, 618t
monomorphic ventricular tachycardia and, 524t
myocardial ischemia/acute coronary syndromes and, 472t
nausea/vomiting and, 909t
ototoxicity and, 1234t
psychosis and, 416t, 418t, 422
seizures and, 218t, 219–221, 222t
serum sickness-like reactions and, 1193t
sexual dysfunction and, 765t, 772
SIADH and, 982t, 990
sleep disorders and, 349, 349–350t, 353
systemic lupus erythematosus and, 126t, 132
weight gain and, 1166t, 1169t, 1170, 1175t
Burning bush, 297t
Buspirone, 172t, 175, 761t, 1203–1204t
Busulfan
alopecia and, 169t, 177
color changes of oral mucosa and teeth and, 1254t
hepatic/cholestatic diseases and, 848t
interstitial lung disease/pulmonary fibrosis and, 431, 432t
leukemia and, 1284, 1291
nausea/vomiting and, 907t
oral erythema multiforme and, 1266t
osteoporosis/osteomalacia and, 1123t
seizures and, 218t
sexual dysfunction and, 759t
valvular/pericardial heart disease and, 660–661t, 662
visual disturbances and, 297t, 316
Butane, 473t
4-butanolide, 1213
Butorphanol, 906t
Butyrolactone gamma, 1213
Butyrophenones, 266, 541, 743t, 927t, 929
CA-AKI (community-acquired acute kidney injury), 941–942, 944
Cabazitaxel, 169t
Cabergoline
alopecia and, 171t
heart failure and, 502–503t, 510t
hyperprolactinemia and, 746
valvular/pericardial heart disease and, 659–664, 660t, 663t, 668–669t, 668–670
Cabozantinib, 7t, 169t, 635t, 698–699t
Cade oil, 850t
Caffeine
anxiety and, 400t, 401, 404, 405t, 407–409, 411
atrial fibrillation/atrial flutter and, 582t
atrial tachycardia and, 588–589t, 589
AV node re-entrant tachycardia and, 592t
chronic kidney disease and, 973
diarrhea and, 825, 827
in food–drug interactions, 40
hypertension and, 618t, 620t
hypotension and, 644
infertility and, 783t, 786t, 800–802
intracerebral hemorrhage and, 240, 242
malignant hyperthermia and, 1211
monomorphic ventricular tachycardia and, 527f
myocardial ischemia/acute coronary syndromes and, 473t
osteoporosis/osteomalacia and, 1128, 1130
psychosis and, 416t, 425
seizures and, 225, 231t
sleep disorders and, 349t
upper gastrointestinal ulceration and, 810
Calcineurin inhibitors, 620t, 624–625, 967–969, 972–975, 1292–1293
Calcipotriene, 144t
Calcitonin, 823t, 1129t, 1130
Calcium
acute kidney injury and, 951
osteoporosis/osteomalacia and, 1122, 1128, 1129, 1130
pancreatitis and, 878t, 888
sinus bradycardia/atrioventricular block and, 580
Calcium carbonate, 701t, 881, 1013–1014t
Calcium-channel blockers
acute kidney injury and, 953
alopecia and, 168t, 179t
asthma/bronchospasm and, 463
atrial fibrillation/atrial flutter and, 586
constipation and, 835
delirium and, 327t
depression and, 378
gingival hyperplasia and, 1263–1265, 1264t
glucose/insulin dysregulation and, 680t, 684t
gout/hyperuricemia and, 1138
heart failure and, 501, 502t, 504, 504t, 505, 509–511, 515
hepatic/cholestatic diseases and, 847t
hypertension and, 625
hypotension and, 632–633t
myocardial ischemia/acute coronary syndromes and, 472t, 478, 485, 488–489
sexual dysfunction and, 759t, 772
sinus bradycardia/atrioventricular block and, 574, 580
systemic lupus erythematosus and, 124t, 132
teratogenicity of, 1316, 1317
thyroid diseases and, 716
torsades de pointes and, 544
visual disturbances and, 297t, 313
Calcium gluconate, 1066t, 1070t
Calcium iodide, 706t
Calcium polycarbophil, 840t
Calcium salts, 287, 287t
Calcium supplements, 835
Camellia senesis, 850t
Camphor, 850t
Camptothecins, 1101t, 1109t
Canagliflozin, 144t, 1002t, 1121t, 1123t
Cancer, 1283–1305. *See also* Antineoplastic agents; Chemotherapy agents
bladder cancer, 1303–1305
breast cancer, 1298–1301
in cost-of-illness model, 28
delirium and, 333
endometrial cancer, 1301–1303
leukemia, 1283–1292
lymphoma, 1292–1295
overview, 1283
risk factors for, 32
skin cancer, 1295–1298
Cancer treatment-induced diarrhea (CTID), 821, 827–828, 827t
Candesartan, 632t, 638t
Candesartan cilexetil, 1234t
Cangrelor, 1029, 1029t
Cannabinoids, 33, 287t, 415, 473t, 912, 929, 1216, 1216t
Cannabis. *See* Marijuana
Canthaxanthin, 297t
Capecitabine, 126t, 280t, 472t, 570t, 577t, 848t, 881, 1109t
Capreomycin, 1234t
Capsaicin, 289, 473t
Captopril
acute kidney injury and, 942
allergic and hypersensitivity reactions to, 76
alopecia and, 167t
aplastic anemia and, 1100t
cutaneous diseases and, 103t
delirium and, 327t
hemolytic anemia and, 1105t
hypotension and, 632t, 638t
myocardial ischemia/acute coronary syndromes and, 472t
neutropenia/agranulocytosis and, 1089t, 1093
oral lichenoid reactions and, 1270t
ototoxicity and, 1234t
pancreatitis and, 878t, 880, 886t, 887
photosensitivity and, 144t
systemic lupus erythematosus and, 124t
taste disorders and, 1259t, 1261t
thrombocytopenia and, 1050t
Carbamazepine
akathisia and, 255–256t, 258t
allergic reactions to, 75t, 88, 95, 112
alopecia and, 168t, 175, 178
aplastic anemia and, 1100t
asthma/bronchospasm and, 452t
AV node re-entrant tachycardia and, 592t
cognitive disorders and, 360, 365, 367, 369
cutaneous diseases and, 101, 102–103t, 111–112, 111t, 113t
depression and, 378
drug fever and, 1188t
genetic variability and, 16t
genetic variations affecting, 36t
gingival hyperplasia and, 1263t
heart failure and, 502t, 510t
hemolytic anemia and, 1105t
hepatic/cholestatic diseases and, 851t, 861t
hirsutism and, 195t, 199t
human leukocyte antigen and, 38

neuroleptic malignant syndrome and, 1195*t*
neutropenia/agranulocytosis and, 1089*t*
oral erythema multiforme and, 1266, 1266*t*
oral lichenoid reactions and, 1270*t*
osteoporosis/osteomalacia and, 1122, 1123*t*, 1127
ototoxicity and, 1234*t*
pancreatitis and, 878*t*, 883
peripheral neuropathy and, 286–287, 287*t*, 289
pharmacogenomic tests for, 35
photosensitivity and, 144*t*
psychosis and, 416*t*
seizures and, 218*t*, 224
serum sickness-like reactions and, 1193*t*
sexual dysfunction and, 758*t*, 762–763*t*
SIADH and, 981, 983*t*, 985, 988–990, 988*t*
sinus bradycardia/atrioventricular block and, 570*t*, 573*t*, 578*t*
skin reactions related to, 32
sleep disorders and, 348*t*
systemic lupus erythematosus and, 124*t*
tardive dyskinesia and, 254
taste disorders and, 1259*t*
teratogenicity of, 1315, 1319, 1328, 1330, 1331
thrombocytopenia and, 1050*t*
thyroid diseases and, 699*t*, 701*t*, 715
vaginal bleeding disorders and, 793
visual disturbances and, 297–298*t*, 312, 315
weight gain and, 1166*t*, 1169–1170, 1169*t*
Carbapenems
allergic reactions to, 90, 92
diarrhea and, 822*t*
hepatic/cholestatic diseases and, 846*t*
seizures and, 218*t*, 220, 222, 222*t*, 224–226
Carbenicillin, 1188*t*
Carbidopa-levodopa, 273, 348*t*, 631, 635*t*, 640*t*, 702*t*, 1196, 1201
Carbimazole, 173*t*, 175, 178, 703*t*, 848*t*, 885, 1089*t*
Carbonic anhydrase inhibitors, 92, 1003*t*, 1088
Carbon monoxide diffusing capacity (DL_{CO}), 435–436, 438–440
Carbon tetrachloride, 849*t*, 866
Carboplatin
acute kidney injury and, 943*t*, 950
allergic reactions to, 72*t*
alopecia and, 169*t*, 177
cognitive disorders and, 358*t*
genetic variability and, 16*t*
hepatic/cholestatic diseases and, 848*t*
myocardial ischemia/acute coronary syndromes and, 472*t*
nausea/vomiting and, 907*t*, 916*t*, 925
ototoxicity and, 1234*t*, 1243
peripheral neuropathy and, 280*t*
SIADH and, 983*t*
taste disorders and, 1259*t*
thromboembolic diseases and, 1065*t*, 1069*t*
Carboprost, 452*t*
Carboxymethylcellulose, 72*t*
Carcinogenic effects, 60
Cardiac Arrhythmia Suppression Trial (CAST), 528
Cardiovascular agents
anxiety and, 399
atrial fibrillation/atrial flutter and, 581
depression and, 375, 376*t*, 378
drug fever and, 1187, 1189, 1192
drug-induced hospitalizations from, 26, 26*t*
hepatic/cholestatic diseases and, 847*t*
interstitial lung disease/pulmonary fibrosis and, 433
myocardial ischemia/acute coronary syndromes and, 472*t*
neutropenia/agranulocytosis and, 1088
parkinsonism and, 271*t*
peripheral neuropathy and, 280–281*t*
systemic lupus erythematosus and, 124–125*t*
taste disorders and, 1261
Carfilzomib, 7*t*
Carglumic acid, 7*t*
Cariprazine, 400*t*, 405, 1166*t*
Carisoprodol, 400*t*, 402, 404, 405*t*, 407
Carmustine
chronic kidney disease and, 966*t*, 970*t*
hepatic/cholestatic diseases and, 848*t*
hypotension and, 635*t*, 640*t*
interstitial lung disease/pulmonary fibrosis and, 432*t*, 434, 436, 437, 439, 440
leukemia and, 1288*t*
myocardial ischemia/acute coronary syndromes and, 472*t*
nausea/vomiting and, 907*t*, 916*t*
visual disturbances and, 298*t*
Carnitine, 515
Carnitine palmitoyltransferase II, 1157
Carotene, 1254*t*
Carp capsules, 850*t*
cART (combined antiretroviral therapy), 1172
Carteolol, 572, 577*t*
Carvedilol
alopecia and, 168*t*
heart failure and, 512, 515
hypotension and, 632*t*, 638*t*
myocardial ischemia/acute coronary syndromes and, 488
ototoxicity and, 1234*t*
photosensitivity and, 144*t*
sinus bradycardia/atrioventricular block and, 578*t*
sleep disorders and, 348*t*
Cascara sagrada, 850*t*
Caspofungin, 846*t*
CAST (Cardiac Arrhythmia Suppression Trial), 528
Catatonia, 267, 1197, 1198, 1201, 1206
Catecholamines
acidosis and, 1002*t*
adrenal glands in secretion of, 729
alkalosis and, 1013*t*
heart failure and, 511, 512
hypotension and, 643, 647
intracerebral hemorrhage and, 240
stroke and, 232
Cathinones, 415
Causality, determination of, 22–23
Causative agents
of acidosis, 1001, 1002–1003*t*
of acute interstitial nephritis, 943*t*, 956
of acute tubular necrosis, 943*t*, 949–950
of akathisia, 254, 255*t*, 405
of alkalosis, 1012, 1013*t*
of alopecia, 166–177, 167–174*t*
of amenorrhea and oligomenorrhea, 782*t*, 793
of anxiety, 399–404, 400–401*t*
of aplastic anemia, 1100, 1100*t*
of asthma and bronchospasm, 72–73*t*, 451, 452–453*t*
of atrial fibrillation/atrial flutter, 581, 582–583*t*
of atrial tachycardia, 588, 588*t*
of AV node re-entrant tachycardia, 592, 592*t*
of bladder cancer, 1285*t*, 1303
of bleeding disorders, 1025–1026, 1026*t*
of Brugada syndrome, 546, 547*t*
of cancer breast, 1285*t*, 1298–1299
of chemotherapy-induced anemia, 1109, 1109*t*
of chronic kidney disease, 965–967, 966*t*
of cognitive disorders, 357, 358*t*
of color changes of oral mucosa and teeth, 1253, 1254–1255*t*
of congenital heart defects, 1321–1322
of constipation, 835, 836*t*
of Cushing syndrome, 730, 731*t*
of cutaneous diseases, 100–104, 102–104*t*
of delirium, 325, 326–328*t*
of depression, 375–377, 376–377*t*
of diabetes insipidus, 991, 991*t*
of diarrhea, 821–822, 822*t*
of drug allergies, 71–76, 72–75*t*
of drug fever, 1186–1187, 1188–1189*t*
of dysmenorrhea, 782*t*, 796
of dystonia, 265, 266*t*
of endometrial cancer, 1285*t*, 1301
of female sexual dysfunction, 783*t*, 797–798
of fetal alcohol spectrum disorders, 1332
of gastroschisis, 1326
of gingival hyperplasia, 1253, 1262–1263, 1263*t*
of glomerulonephritis, 943*t*, 958
of glucose and insulin dysregulation, 679–681, 680–683*t*
of gout and hyperuricemia, 1135, 1136*t*
of growth hormone deficiency, 747, 748*t*
of heart failure, 501–505, 502–504*t*
of hemodynamic-mediated AKI, 942, 943–944*t*
of hemolytic anemia, 86, 1104, 1105–1106*t*, 1109
of hepatic and cholestatic diseases, 845, 846–853*t*
of hirsutism, 194, 195*t*
of hyperprolactinemia, 742, 743–744*t*
of hypersensitivity reactions, 76, 77*t*, 1186
of hypertension, 617, 618*t*
of hypertrichosis, 193–197, 196–197*t*
of hypotension, 631, 632–636*t*
of hypothermia, 1186, 1215, 1216*t*
of infertility, 762*t*, 783*t*, 800
of interstitial lung disease/pulmonary fibrosis, 431, 432–433*t*
of intracerebral hemorrhage, 232, 237–239, 238*t*
of learning disabilities, 1315
of leukemia, 1284–1286, 1284*t*
of limb deficiency defects, 1324
of low birth weight, 1316
of lymphoma, 1284*t*, 1292–1293
of macrocytic anemia, 1107, 1108*t*
of male sexual dysfunction, 757–761, 758–762*t*
of malignant hyperthermia, 1186, 1209–1210, 1209*t*
of menorrhagia and menometrorrhagia, 782*t*, 795
of microcephaly, 1330
of monomorphic ventricular tachycardia, 523, 524*t*
of myocardial ischemia/acute coronary syndromes, 471–474, 472–473*t*
of myopathy, 1150–1151, 1150*t*
of nausea and vomiting, 905–910, 906–909*t*
of nephrolithiasis, 944*t*, 957
of neural tube defects, 1328
of neuroleptic malignant syndrome, 1195, 1195*t*
of neutropenia and agranulocytosis, 1087–1088, 1089–1090*t*
of oral erythema multiforme, 1266, 1266–1268*t*
of oral lichenoid reactions, 1270, 1270–1272*t*
of orofacial clefts, 1319, 1335
of osteonecrosis of jaw, 1273, 1274*t*
of osteoporosis and osteomalacia, 1120, 1121*t*
of ototoxicity, 1233–1239, 1234–1238*t*
of ovarian hyperstimulation, 781, 782*t*
of pancreatitis, 877–879, 878–879*t*
of parkinsonism, 270, 271*t*

INDEX

Causative agents (continued)
of peripheral neuropathy, 279, 280–281t, 1155
of photosensitivity, 143, 144–148t
of psychosis, 415, 416–417t
of secondary adrenal insufficiency, 735, 736t
of seizures, 217, 218–219t
of serotonin syndrome, 1202, 1203t
of serum sickness-like reactions, 74t, 95, 1192, 1193t
of SIADH, 981, 982–984t
of sinus bradycardia/atrioventricular block, 569–572, 570–571t, 573t
of skin cancer, 1284t, 1295–1296
of sleep disorders, 347, 348–349t
of stroke, 229–231, 230t
of systemic lupus erythematosus, 123, 124–127t, 662
of tardive dyskinesia, 259, 260t
of taste disorders, 1258, 1259–1260t
of thrombocytopenia, 1049–1050, 1050–1051t
of thromboembolic diseases, 1063, 1064–1066t
of thyroid diseases, 697–701, 698–700t, 704
of torsades de pointes, 530–531, 532–534t
of upper gastrointestinal ulceration, 809–810, 810t
of valvular and pericardial heart disease, 659–662, 660–661t
of visual disturbances, 295–313, 296–312t
of vulvovaginal candidiasis, 782t, 790–791
of weight gain, 1165, 1166–1167t
CCLE (chronic cutaneous lupus erythematosus), 132
CCNU. *See* Lomustine
CDC. *See* Centers for Disease Control and Prevention
CDI. *See Clostridium difficile* infection
Cediranib, 699t
Cefaclor, 74t, 84, 92, 1192, 1193t, 1194
Cefazolin, 144t, 328t, 1101t, 1105t, 1188t, 1193t
Cefepime, 125t
Cefoperazone, 1188t
Cefotaxime, 92, 1101t, 1105t, 1188t
Cefotetan, 1101t, 1105t
Cefoxitin, 1101t, 1105t
Cefprozil, 1193t
Ceftazidime, 92, 144t, 1105t, 1188t
Ceftizoxime, 1101t, 1105t, 1188t
Ceftriaxone
alopecia and, 72t
drug fever and, 1188t
hemolytic anemia and, 1101t, 1105t
hepatic/cholestatic diseases and, 846t
serum sickness-like reactions and, 1193t
taste disorders and, 1259t
Cefuroxime
drug fever and, 1188t
hemolytic anemia and, 1101t, 1105t
oral erythema multiforme and, 1266t
serum sickness-like reactions and, 1193t
systemic lupus erythematosus and, 125t
Celandine, 850t
Celecoxib
allergic reactions to, 74t
asthma/bronchospasm and, 453, 461
cardiovascular disease associated with, 53
cutaneous diseases and, 102–103t
delirium and, 327t
heart failure and, 503t, 509, 510t
hepatic/cholestatic diseases and, 846t
hypertension and, 618t
myocardial ischemia/acute coronary syndromes and, 472t, 475
photosensitivity and, 144t
psychosis and, 416t
sexual dysfunction and, 759t
stroke and, 230
in sulfa drug class, 92
upper gastrointestinal ulceration and, 812, 817
vaginal bleeding disorders and, 790t
visual disturbances and, 298t
Celery, 298t
Centers for Disease Control and Prevention (CDC)
collaboration needs and, 14
on fetal alcohol syndrome, 1332
folic acid recommendations from, 1329
on isotretinoin-exposed pregnancies, 1320
on opioid overdose deaths, 6
on oral contraceptive risk–benefit ratio, 485
postmarketing surveillance by, 53–54, 56
Centers for Education and Research on Therapeutics (CERTs), 55
Centrally acting sympatholytics, 764t
Central nervous system (CNS) agents
alopecia and, 167t
anxiety and, 399, 401–402
cognitive disorders and, 369
depression and, 376t, 378–381
drug fever and, 1189, 1192
systemic lupus erythematosus and, 125t
Cephalexin, 328t, 1188t, 1193t
Cephalosporins
allergic reactions to, 72t, 74–75t, 87, 90, 92
cutaneous diseases and, 101, 103t
delirium and, 328t
diarrhea and, 822t
drug fever and, 1187
graded challenge procedure for, 88
hemolytic anemia and, 1104, 1105t
hepatic/cholestatic diseases and, 870
neutropenia/agranulocytosis and, 1088, 1089t
oral erythema multiforme and, 1266t
seizures and, 218t, 220
structural similarities and differences in, 93f
thrombocytopenia and, 1052t
Cephalothin, 92, 328t, 1101t, 1105t
Ceritinib, 7t, 907t
Cerivastatin, 13
Certolizumab, 126t, 173t, 1270t, 1297
CERTs (Centers for Education and Research on Therapeutics), 55
Cervical dystonia, 267, 267f
Cetirizine
allergic reactions to, 72t
alopecia and, 174t, 179t
hepatic/cholestatic diseases and, 852t
myocardial ischemia/acute coronary syndromes and, 473t
photosensitivity and, 144t
visual disturbances and, 298t
Cetuximab, 72t, 96, 102t, 169t, 196t, 432t
Chamomile, 298t, 353
Chaparral leaf, 850t
Chaso, 850t
Chaulmoogra, 298t
CHD (coronary heart disease), 514, 622, 623
Chelating agents, 196t
Chemicals, environmental, 845, 849–850t
Chemoprotectant agents, 635t
Chemoreceptor trigger zone (CTZ), 912–914, 913f
Chemotherapy agents. *See also* Chemotherapy-induced anemia (CIA); Chemotherapy-induced nausea and vomiting (CINV)
acute kidney injury and, 955
alopecia and, 169–171t, 176–178, 179t, 182, 183, 185–187
anxiety and, 399, 403
aplastic anemia and, 1100, 1101, 1101t
bladder cancer and, 1305
breast cancer and, 1300
depression and, 375, 377t, 382, 384, 388
drug-induced hospitalizations from, 26
endometrial cancer and, 1303
hepatic/cholestatic diseases and, 847–848t
hypertrichosis and, 196t
hypotension and, 635–636t
infertility and, 800–802
interstitial lung disease/pulmonary fibrosis and, 431, 433, 437
leukemia and, 1283–1287, 1291, 1292
lymphoma and, 1295
macrocytic anemia and, 1108
neutropenia/agranulocytosis and, 1087, 1091–1094, 1091t, 1095t, 1096
ototoxicity and, 1233, 1239–1240, 1239t, 1243
pancreatitis and, 881–882
peripheral neuropathy and, 279, 283, 285–289
SIADH and, 981, 983t
skin cancer and, 1296, 1298
systemic lupus erythematosus and, 132
taste disorders and, 1261, 1262
thrombocytopenia and, 1050, 1056, 1057t, 1059
thromboembolic diseases and, 1074
vaginal bleeding disorders and, 793–795
valvular/pericardial heart disease and, 662, 664, 668, 668t, 670
weight gain and, 1167–1169t, 1172, 1173t
Chemotherapy-induced anemia (CIA), 1109–1111
causative agents of, 1109, 1109t
clinical presentation of, 1102t, 1110
differential diagnosis of, 1110
epidemiology of, 1109
management of, 1111
mechanisms of, 1101t, 1110
morbidity and mortality for, 1110
patient education on, 1111
prevention of, 1110–1111
risk factors for, 1103t, 1110
Chemotherapy-induced nausea and vomiting (CINV)
causative agents of, 907–909t, 910
clinical presentation of, 916, 916t
epidemiology of, 910
management of, 928–929, 929t
mechanisms of, 911t, 914
morbidity and mortality for, 919–920
patient education on, 930–931
prevention of, 921t, 924–927, 925t
risk factors for, 33, 918–919, 918t
Chemotherapy-induced peripheral neuropathy (CIPN), 283, 285–289
Chest pain. *See* Angina pectoris
Children. *See* Pediatric patients
Chinese herbs. *See* Aristolochic acid
Chloral hydrate, 533t, 539t
Chlorambucil
anxiety and, 403
drug fever and, 1188t, 1191
hepatic/cholestatic diseases and, 848t
interstitial lung disease/pulmonary fibrosis and, 432t
leukemia and, 1284, 1288t
peripheral neuropathy and, 280t
seizures and, 218t
SIADH and, 983t
vaginal bleeding disorders and, 782t, 785t

Chloramphenicol
aplastic anemia and, 1100*t*
delirium and, 328*t*
drug fever and, 1187
hepatic/cholestatic diseases and, 846*t*, 861*t*
neutropenia/agranulocytosis and, 1089*t*
oral erythema multiforme and, 1266*t*
ototoxicity and, 1234*t*
peripheral neuropathy and, 280*t*
thrombocytopenia and, 1052*t*
visual disturbances and, 298*t*
Chlordiazepoxide, 144*t*, 424*t*, 1089*t*
Chlordiazepoxide–clidinium bromide, 1050*t*
Chlorella, 144*t*, 298*t*
Chlorhexidine, 72*t*, 1234*t*, 1254*t*, 1259*t*
Chloride channel agonists, 840
Chlormethiazole, 851*t*
Chlormezanone, 101
Chloroform, 849*t*
Chloroquine
color changes of oral mucosa and teeth and, 1253, 1254*t*
cutaneous diseases and, 103*t*
hepatic/cholestatic diseases and, 846*t*
myopathy and, 1150*t*, 1152*t*, 1153
neutropenia/agranulocytosis and, 1089*t*
oral lichenoid reactions and, 1270*t*
ototoxicity and, 1234*t*
peripheral neuropathy and, 280*t*
photosensitivity and, 144*t*
psychosis and, 416*t*, 418*t*
sinus bradycardia/atrioventricular block and, 573*t*
torsades de pointes and, 532*t*
visual disturbances and, 295, 298*t*, 312, 313, 318–319
Chlorothiazide
allergic reactions to, 94
hypotension and, 633*t*, 638*t*
pancreatitis and, 878*t*, 883
photosensitivity and, 144*t*
thrombocytopenia and, 1050*t*
Chlorpheniramine, 220, 298*t*, 852*t*, 1089*t*
Chlorpromazine
color changes of oral mucosa and teeth and, 1254*t*
delirium and, 337
drug fever and, 1188*t*
glucose/insulin dysregulation and, 680*t*
hepatic/cholestatic diseases and, 851*t*, 861*t*, 869
hypotension and, 635*t*, 639*t*
hypothermia and, 1216, 1216*t*
malignant hyperthermia and, 1213, 1213*t*
monomorphic ventricular tachycardia and, 524–525*t*
neuroleptic malignant syndrome and, 1195*t*, 1198
photosensitivity and, 144*t*, 150
seizures and, 221
serotonin syndrome and, 1208, 1208*t*
SIADH and, 982*t*, 985
systemic lupus erythematosus and, 124*t*, 127, 128*t*, 130
tardive dyskinesia and, 260
thrombocytopenia and, 1050*t*
thromboembolic diseases and, 1066*t*, 1070*t*
torsades de pointes and, 532*t*, 540*t*
visual disturbances and, 298–299*t*
weight gain and, 1167*t*, 1169*t*, 1171
Chlorpropamide
neutropenia/agranulocytosis and, 1089*t*, 1091
oral erythema multiforme and, 1266*t*
oral lichenoid reactions and, 1270*t*
photosensitivity and, 144*t*
SIADH and, 983*t*
thrombocytopenia and, 1050*t*
thyroid diseases and, 703*t*
Chlorprothixene, 125*t*
Chlorthalidone
glucose/insulin dysregulation and, 688
gout/hyperuricemia and, 1138
hypotension and, 633*t*, 638*t*
ototoxicity and, 1234*t*
pancreatitis and, 878*t*, 883
photosensitivity and, 144*t*, 150
sexual dysfunction and, 762
systemic lupus erythematosus and, 124*t*
Cholecalciferol (vitamin D_3), 890, 1122, 1126, 1262
Cholera vaccine, 1270*t*
Cholestatic injury, 855*t*, 857–858, 859*t*, 861*t*, 862. *See also* Hepatic and cholestatic diseases
Cholesterol-lowering agents, 171*t*, 179*t*
Cholestyramine
acidosis and, 1002*t*
alopecia and, 171*t*
diarrhea and, 823*t*, 827*t*, 829
hepatic/cholestatic diseases and, 869
thyroid diseases and, 701*t*
Chondroitin/chondroitin sulfate, 12, 822, 835
Chromium, 701*t*, 849*t*
Chronic allograft nephropathy, 969, 973–975
Chronic cutaneous lupus erythematosus (CCLE), 132
Chronic kidney disease (CKD), 965–976
causative agents of, 965–967, 966*t*
clinical presentation of, 970–972, 971*t*
comorbidity and, 33–34
differential diagnosis of, 971, 971*t*
epidemiology of, 967–969
management of, 975–976, 976*t*
mechanisms of, 969–970, 970*t*
morbidity and mortality for, 973–974
patient education on, 976
prevention of, 974–975, 974*t*
risk factors for, 972–973, 972*t*
Chronic thromboembolic pulmonary hypertension (CTEPH), 1074
Chrysanthemum, 144*t*
Churg-Strauss syndrome, 85
Chymopapain, 72*t*
CIA. *See* Chemotherapy-induced anemia
Ciclopirox, 1234*t*
Cidofovir, 966*t*, 970*t*, 991*t*, 1003*t*, 1234*t*
Cigarettes. *See* Smoking
Cilostazol, 1026*t*, 1029, 1029*t*
Cimetidine
allergic reactions to, 75*t*
alopecia and, 171*t*
delirium and, 328*t*
drug fever and, 1188*t*
hemolytic anemia and, 1105*t*
hyperprolactinemia and, 743*t*
myocardial ischemia/acute coronary syndromes and, 473*t*
neutropenia/agranulocytosis and, 1089*t*, 1091, 1091*t*
oral lichenoid reactions and, 1270*t*
pancreatitis and, 878*t*, 880
sexual dysfunction and, 758*t*, 762–763*t*, 765*t*, 783*t*, 786*t*
sinus bradycardia/atrioventricular block and, 570*t*, 573*t*, 577*t*
systemic lupus erythematosus and, 126*t*
thrombocytopenia and, 1050*t*
thyroid diseases and, 701*t*
visual disturbances and, 299*t*
Cinchona alkaloids, 1049
Cinnarizine, 271*t*, 273*t*, 1270*t*
Cinoxacin, 472*t*
CINV. *See* Chemotherapy-induced nausea and vomiting
CIOMS (Council for International Organizations of Medical Sciences), 51, 52
CIPN (chemotherapy-induced peripheral neuropathy), 283, 285–289
Ciprofloxacin
acute kidney injury and, 943*t*
allergic and hypersensitivity reactions to, 74*t*, 76, 77*t*, 81, 84, 87
cutaneous diseases and, 103*t*
delirium and, 328*t*
hemolytic anemia and, 1105*t*
oral erythema multiforme and, 1266*t*
osteonecrosis of jaw and, 1276
ototoxicity and, 1234*t*
pancreatitis and, 882
peripheral neuropathy and, 280*t*
photosensitivity and, 144*t*
psychosis and, 416*t*
serum sickness-like reactions and, 1193*t*
SIADH and, 984*t*
systemic lupus erythematosus and, 125*t*
torsades de pointes and, 532*t*, 539*t*
upper gastrointestinal ulceration and, 810–811*t*
visual disturbances and, 299*t*
Cisapride
asthma/bronchospasm and, 452*t*
diarrhea and, 823*t*
myocardial ischemia/acute coronary syndromes and, 473*t*, 474
regulatory actions involving, 13
restrictive drug distribution system for, 7*t*
torsades de pointes and, 532*t*, 539–540*t*, 541
Cisplatin
acidosis and, 1003*t*
acute kidney injury and, 943*t*, 945*t*, 950–952, 954–955
alkalosis and, 1013–1014*t*
allergic reactions to, 72*t*
alopecia and, 169*t*, 176
chronic kidney disease and, 966*t*, 970*t*
drug fever and, 1188*t*
genetic variability and, 16*t*
hepatic/cholestatic diseases and, 848*t*
hyperprolactinemia and, 744*t*
interstitial lung disease/pulmonary fibrosis and, 439
leukemia and, 1284, 1284*t*, 1286, 1287
myocardial ischemia/acute coronary syndromes and, 472*t*
nausea/vomiting and, 907*t*, 910, 914, 916, 916*t*, 920, 925, 926
ototoxicity and, 1234*t*, 1240, 1242, 1243
pancreatitis and, 878*t*, 881
peripheral neuropathy and, 279, 280*t*, 282, 285
seizures and, 222*t*
sexual dysfunction and, 762*t*
SIADH and, 981, 983*t*
sinus bradycardia/atrioventricular block and, 570*t*, 577*t*
stroke and, 230–231*t*, 233
taste disorders and, 1259*t*
thromboembolic diseases and, 1065*t*, 1069*t*
transport mechanisms for, 37

Citalopram
alopecia and, 172*t*
depression and, 391
hyperprolactinemia and, 743*t*
hypertrichosis and, 197*t*
monomorphic ventricular tachycardia and, 524*t*
serotonin syndrome and, 1203–1204*t*
sexual dysfunction and, 772
SIADH and, 982*t*, 990
sinus bradycardia/atrioventricular block and, 570*t*, 573*t*, 576, 577*t*
sleep disorders and, 348*t*
torsades de pointes and, 532*t*, 539–540*t*
weight gain and, 1166*t*, 1169*t*, 1171
Citrate, 1013–1014*t*
CKD. *See* Chronic kidney disease
Cladribine, 1106
Clarithromycin
delirium and, 328*t*
drug interactions with, 39*t*
genetic variability and, 16*t*
myocardial ischemia/acute coronary syndromes and, 472*t*
ototoxicity and, 1234*t*
SIADH and, 988
taste disorders and, 1258, 1259*t*
torsades de pointes and, 532*t*, 539–540*t*, 542
Clavulanic acid, 73*t*. *See also* Amoxicillin–clavulanic acid
Cleft lip/cleft palate, 1318–1319*f*, 1318–1321
Clindamycin
allergic reactions to, 75*t*
diarrhea and, 821, 822*t*
drug fever and, 1187
hepatic/cholestatic diseases and, 846*t*
neutropenia/agranulocytosis and, 1089*t*
oral erythema multiforme and, 1266, 1266*t*
ototoxicity and, 1234*t*
upper gastrointestinal ulceration and, 809, 810–811*t*
Clinical Pharmacogenetics Implementation Consortium (CPIC) guidelines, 35
Clinical presentation of disease
acidosis, 1005–1007, 1006*t*
acute interstitial nephritis, 946*t*, 956
acute tubular necrosis, 946*t*, 951
akathisia, 256–258, 257*t*
alkalosis, 1014–1015, 1015*t*
alopecia, 165, 176*f*, 180–183, 181–182*t*
amenorrhea and oligomenorrhea, 787*t*, 793
anxiety, 406–408, 406*t*, 408*t*
aplastic anemia, 1101–1102, 1102*t*
asthma and bronchospasm, 457–459, 457*t*
atrial fibrillation/atrial flutter, 584–585, 584*t*
atrial tachycardia, 589, 589*t*
AV node re-entrant tachycardia, 593, 593*t*
bladder cancer, 1290*t*, 1304
bleeding disorders, 1030–1031, 1030*t*
breast cancer, 1290*t*, 1299
Brugada syndrome, 547–548, 547*t*
chemotherapy-induced anemia, 1102*t*, 1110
chronic kidney disease, 970–972, 971*t*
cognitive disorders, 361–363, 361*t*, 363*t*
color changes of oral mucosa and teeth, 1255–1257, 1256*t*
congenital heart defects, 1323–1324
constipation, 837–838, 838*t*
Cushing syndrome, 386, 732–733, 732*t*, 749
cutaneous diseases, 106–110, 107–108*t*
delirium, 330–331, 330–331*t*, 420
depression, 386–387, 387*t*
diabetes insipidus, 992, 992*t*
diarrhea, 823–825, 824*t*
drug allergies, 82–85, 83–84*t*
drug fever, 1187*t*, 1189–1190, 1189*t*
dysmenorrhea, 787*t*, 797
dystonia, 257*t*, 266–268, 267*f*
endometrial cancer, 1290*t*, 1301–1302
female sexual dysfunction, 787*t*, 798–799
fetal alcohol spectrum disorders, 1332, 1332*t*
gastroschisis, 1326–1327, 1326*f*
gingival hyperplasia, 1256*t*, 1264
glomerulonephritis, 946*t*, 958–959
glucose and insulin dysregulation, 683, 686, 686*t*
gout and hyperuricemia, 1140–1141, 1140*t*
growth hormone deficiency, 748–749, 749*t*
heart failure, 512–513, 513*t*
hemodynamic-mediated AKI, 945–946, 946*t*
hemolytic anemia, 83–84, 1102*t*, 1106
hepatic and cholestatic, 858–862, 859–861*t*
hirsutism, 193–194, 199–201, 200–201*t*
hyperprolactinemia, 742, 744–745, 745*t*
hypertension, 621–622, 621*t*
hyperthermia, 1186, 1187*t*
hypertrichosis, 194, 198*f*, 200*t*, 201–202
hypotension, 637, 641, 641*t*
hypothermia, 1216–1217, 1217*t*
infertility, 768*t*, 769, 770, 787*t*, 801
interstitial lung disease/pulmonary fibrosis, 434–436, 435–436*t*
intracerebral hemorrhage, 233, 240–241, 241*t*
learning disabilities, 1315–1316
leukemia, 1289, 1290*t*
limb deficiency defects, 1325
low birth weight, 1317–1318
lymphoma, 1290*t*, 1293–1294
macrocytic anemia, 1102*t*, 1108
male sexual dysfunction, 767–771, 768*t*
malignant hyperthermia, 1187*t*, 1210–1211, 1210*t*
menorrhagia and menometrorrhagia, 787*t*, 795
microcephaly, 1330*f*, 1331
monomorphic ventricular tachycardia, 526–527*t*, 526–528, 527*f*
myocardial ischemia/acute coronary syndromes, 480–482, 481*t*, 483*t*
myopathy, 1153–1155, 1154*t*
nausea and vomiting, 912*t*, 915–916, 916*t*
nephrolithiasis, 946*t*, 957
neural tube defects, 1327–1328*f*, 1329
neuroleptic malignant syndrome, 1187*t*, 1196–1198, 1196*t*, 1206
neutropenia and agranulocytosis, 1092–1093, 1092*t*
oral erythema multiforme, 1253, 1256*t*, 1268–1269
oral lichenoid reactions, 1256*t*, 1272–1273
orofacial clefts, 1318–1319*f*, 1321
osteonecrosis of jaw, 1256*t*, 1275
osteoporosis and osteomalacia, 1124–1125, 1124*t*
ototoxicity, 1240–1241, 1240*t*
ovarian hyperstimulation, 784, 787*t*
pancreatitis, 888–890, 889*t*
parkinsonism, 257*t*, 262, 272
peripheral neuropathy, 282–285, 283*t*
photosensitivity, 151–152*t*, 151–153, 152*f*
psychosis, 419–420*t*, 419–421
secondary adrenal insufficiency, 737–738, 738*t*
seizures, 222–223, 223*t*
serotonin syndrome, 1187*t*, 1197–1198, 1205–1206, 1205*t*
serum sickness-like reactions, 83*t*, 1187*t*, 1193–1194, 1193*t*
SIADH, 986–988, 986*t*
sinus bradycardia/atrioventricular block, 574–576, 575*t*
skin cancer, 1290*t*, 1296–1297
sleep disorders, 349–350, 350*t*
stroke, 233–234, 233–234*t*
systemic lupus erythematosus, 129–133, 129*t*, 131–132*t*
tardive dyskinesia, 257*t*, 262
taste disorders, 1256*t*, 1261
thrombocytopenia, 83–84, 1054–1056, 1054*t*
thromboembolic diseases, 1071–1073, 1071*t*
thyroid diseases, 711–713, 711*t*
torsades de pointes, 536–537, 536–537*t*
upper gastrointestinal ulceration, 812–814, 813*t*
valvular and pericardial heart disease, 664–668, 665*t*, 666–667*f*
visual disturbances, 315–317, 316*t*
vulvovaginal candidiasis, 787*t*, 791
weight gain, 1168–1173, 1169*t*
Clinicians, 10–11, 50–51
Clioquinol, 144*t*, 706*t*
Clobazam, 125*t*, 1216*t*
Clobetasol/clobetasol propionate, 731*t*, 733, 736*t*, 739, 1273
Clofarabine, 908*t*
Clofazimine, 7*t*, 144*t*, 1253, 1254–1255*t*
Clofibrate
alopecia and, 171*t*
drug fever and, 1188*t*
hepatic/cholestatic diseases and, 861*t*
myopathy and, 1150*t*, 1152*t*
oral lichenoid reactions and, 1270*t*
peripheral neuropathy and, 280*t*
sexual dysfunction and, 763*t*
thyroid diseases and, 701*t*
Clomiphene, 299*t*, 400*t*, 403, 701*t*, 882
Clomiphene citrate, 782*t*, 784, 785*t*
Clomipramine
alopecia and, 172*t*
delirium and, 326*t*, 329*t*
depression and, 392
heart failure and, 504*t*, 510*t*
hyperprolactinemia and, 743*t*
hypotension and, 634*t*, 639*t*
neutropenia/agranulocytosis and, 1089*t*
photosensitivity and, 145*t*
serotonin syndrome and, 1203–1204*t*, 1207
SIADH and, 982*t*
thromboembolic diseases and, 1066*t*, 1070*t*
thyroid diseases and, 701*t*
weight gain and, 1166*t*, 1169*t*
Clonazepam
alopecia and, 173*t*
anxiety and, 407, 410
cognitive disorders and, 360
delirium and, 327*t*, 329*t*
oral lichenoid reactions and, 1270*t*
ototoxicity and, 1234*t*
tardive dyskinesia and, 264
taste disorders and, 1262
teratogenicity of, 1331
Clonidine
akathisia and, 259
alopecia and, 174*t*
constipation and, 836*t*
delirium and, 327*t*
depression and, 376*t*, 378, 385, 385*t*
dystonia and, 270
hypotension and, 633*t*, 639*t*, 646*t*, 647

myocardial ischemia/acute coronary syndromes and, 472t
SIADH and, 984t
sinus bradycardia/atrioventricular block and, 570t, 573–574t, 576, 577–578t
sleep disorders and, 348t
systemic lupus erythematosus and, 124t
visual disturbances and, 299t

Clopidogrel
allergic reactions to, 72t
aplastic anemia and, 1100t
bleeding disorders and, 1029, 1029t, 1031, 1031t
comorbidity and, 34
genetic variations affecting, 36t
hepatic/cholestatic diseases and, 852t
intracerebral hemorrhage and, 238t, 244
myocardial ischemia/acute coronary syndromes and, 472t, 480, 486, 489
photosensitivity and, 145t
serum sickness-like reactions and, 1193t
stroke and, 236
thrombocytopenia and, 1054
upper gastrointestinal ulceration and, 810–811t, 812, 815

Clorazepate, 327t, 329t
Clostridium difficile infection (CDI), 817, 821–823, 825–830, 827t
Clotrimazole, 790t, 792
Clotting derangements, 232–233
Cloxacillin, 809, 1188t
Cloxacillin/nafcillin, 846t

Clozapine
acidosis and, 1002t
akathisia and, 255
AV node re-entrant tachycardia and, 592t
cannabinoids and, 33
constipation and, 836t
delirium and, 326t, 329t
development of, 253–254
diabetes insipidus and, 991, 991t
drug fever and, 1186
extrapyramidal symptoms and, 254
glucose/insulin dysregulation and, 683
heart failure and, 502t, 509
hepatic/cholestatic diseases and, 851t
hypotension and, 635t, 639t
hypothermia and, 1215, 1216, 1216t
myocardial ischemia/acute coronary syndromes and, 472t
neuroleptic malignant syndrome and, 1195t
neutropenia/agranulocytosis and, 1088, 1089t, 1091, 1091t, 1093–1095, 1095t
pancreatitis and, 878t, 883, 887
parkinsonism and, 270–272
photosensitivity and, 145t
psychosis and, 424
restrictive drug distribution system for, 7t
seizures and, 218t, 221, 222t, 225
sexual dysfunction and, 765t
SIADH and, 982t, 990
sinus bradycardia/atrioventricular block and, 570t, 578t
smoking and, 32
systemic lupus erythematosus and, 125t
tardive dyskinesia and, 265
thromboembolic diseases and, 1066t, 1070t
torsades de pointes and, 533t, 540t
valvular/pericardial heart disease and, 660t, 662
weight gain and, 1166t, 1169t, 1171, 1175

CNS agents. *See* Central nervous system agents
Coagulation factor VIIA, 472t
Coal tar, 145t
Coasting phenomenon, 283, 286
Cobalamin (vitamin B_{12}), 284, 1107, 1108, 1256
Cobimetinib, 145t, 1296

Cocaine
anxiety and, 400t, 401
asthma/bronchospasm and, 452t
Brugada syndrome and, 547t
duration of detection in urine, 420t
hepatic/cholestatic diseases and, 851t, 864
hyperprolactinemia and, 744t
hypertension and, 618t, 620t
interstitial lung disease/pulmonary fibrosis and, 433
intracerebral hemorrhage and, 238t, 239, 240, 240t
monomorphic ventricular tachycardia and, 524t
neuroleptic malignant syndrome and, 1197
psychosis and, 416t
as risk factor for drug-induced diseases, 33
sexual dysfunction and, 758–759t, 761t
sinus bradycardia/atrioventricular block and, 570t, 572, 573t, 578t
sleep disorders and, 349t
stroke and, 230–231t, 231, 232
teratogenicity of, 1316, 1318, 1321, 1324, 1327, 1331, 1334t
thromboembolic diseases and, 1066t, 1070t
torsades de pointes and, 532t, 540t

Cocaine-induced myocardial ischemia/acute coronary syndrome, 474–475, 478–489, 483t, 487t

Codeine
constipation and, 836t
genetic variations affecting, 36t
hypotension and, 636t, 638t
nausea/vomiting and, 906t
oral erythema multiforme and, 1266t
ototoxicity and, 1233, 1235t
pancreatitis and, 878t, 886t

Coenzyme Q10, 515, 1158
Cognitive disorders, 357–369. *See also* Delirium; Dementia
causative agents of, 357, 358t
clinical presentation of, 361–363, 361t, 363t
differential diagnosis of, 363, 363t
epidemiology of, 357–359
management of, 368–369, 368t
mechanisms of, 359–361, 359t
morbidity and mortality for, 366
patient education on, 369
prevention of, 366–368, 366t
risk factors for, 364–366, 364t

Coherence, in epidemiology, 22

Colchicine
alopecia and, 171t
diabetes insipidus and, 991t
diarrhea and, 823t
gout/hyperuricemia and, 1141, 1144, 1145
hepatic/cholestatic diseases and, 852t, 868
interstitial lung disease/pulmonary fibrosis and, 440
myopathy and, 1150t, 1152t, 1153, 1156
neutropenia/agranulocytosis and, 1089t
oral lichenoid reactions and, 1270t
peripheral neuropathy and, 281t
thyroid diseases and, 701t
valvular/pericardial heart disease and, 670

Colesevelam, 836t
Colestipol, 701t, 836t, 869
Colistin, 452t, 943t, 950
Collagenase clostridium histolyticum, 7t
Colony-stimulating factor (CSF), 74t, 171t, 179t, 1287, 1291. *See also* Granulocyte colony-stimulating factor (G-CSF)

Color changes of oral mucosa and teeth, 1253–1258
causative agents of, 1253, 1254–1255t
clinical presentation of, 1255–1257, 1256t
differential diagnosis of, 1256–1257, 1257t
epidemiology of, 1255
management of, 1258
mechanisms of, 1255, 1255t
morbidity and mortality for, 1257
patient education on, 1258
prevention of, 1257–1258
risk factors for, 1257, 1258t

Colpachi, 850t
Combined antiretroviral therapy (cART), 1172
Comfrey, 850t
Community-acquired acute kidney injury (CA-AKI), 941–942, 944
Comorbid diseases, 33–34
Complete heart block, 569
Compound epitope formation, 1052
Congenital anomalies, defined, 1314. *See also* Teratogenicity
Congenital heart defects, 1321–1324
Conivaptan, 989–990, 989t
Conjugated estrogens, 702t, 790t, 1302
Consistency, in epidemiology, 22
Consolidated Standards of Reporting Trials (CONSORT), 15

Constipation, 835–841. *See also* Opioid-induced constipation (OIC)
causative agents of, 835, 836t
clinical presentation of, 837–838, 838t
differential diagnosis of, 837, 838t
epidemiology of, 835–837
management of, 839–841, 840t
mechanisms of, 837, 837t
morbidity and mortality for, 839
patient education on, 839, 840
prevention of, 839, 839t
risk factors for, 838–839, 838t

Contraceptives
intrauterine devices, 171t, 179t, 782t, 785t, 795, 796
oral. *See* Oral contraceptives
patches, 229
smoking and, 33

Contrast media, 219t, 965, 1066t, 1067, 1070t, 1075t. *See also* Radiocontrast media
Contrayerva, 299t
Conventional antipsychotics, 742, 743t, 745–746, 1167t, 1169t, 1171

Conventional neuroleptics
akathisia and, 254, 255, 255–256t, 258, 258t
development of, 253
dystonia and, 265–266, 266t, 268, 269, 269t
parkinsonism and, 270–273, 271t, 273t
tardive dyskinesia and, 260–263, 260t, 264t, 265

Copper, 177, 1254t
Coronary artery disease, 471, 473–475, 478–486, 489, 501
Coronary artery vasodilators, 479
Coronary heart disease (CHD), 514, 622, 623
Coronary steal, 479
Corticosteroid myopathy, 1150t, 1151, 1152t, 1153, 1155–1159

Corticosteroids
acute kidney injury and, 957, 959
allergic and hypersensitivity reactions to, 75t, 77t

INDEX

Corticosteroids (continued)
- alopecia and, 171*t*, 179*t*, 188*t*, 191
- anxiety and, 404
- asthma/bronchospasm and, 460, 461
- atrial fibrillation/atrial flutter and, 581, 586
- chronic kidney disease and, 967, 976
- cognitive disorders and, 360, 361
- Cushing syndrome and, 733, 734
- cutaneous diseases and, 101, 102*t*, 108, 113
- delirium and, 325, 326*t*
- depression and, 376*t*, 382, 386–388, 388*t*, 390, 391
- drug fever and, 1191
- drug-induced hospitalizations from, 26*t*
- food interactions with, 41
- glucose/insulin dysregulation and, 683, 688, 690
- growth hormone deficiency and, 750
- heart failure and, 502*t*
- hepatic/cholestatic diseases and, 848*t*, 866, 868
- hirsutism and, 199*t*
- hypertension and, 618*t*, 620*t*
- hypertrichosis and, 196*t*
- for immune complex diseases, 100
- inhaled, 733, 738–741, 1127
- interstitial lung disease/pulmonary fibrosis and, 439–442
- myocardial ischemia/acute coronary syndromes and, 473*t*
- myopathy and, 1150*t*, 1151, 1152*t*, 1153, 1155–1159
- nausea/vomiting and, 925, 927*t*, 929
- oral erythema multiforme and, 1269
- oral lichenoid reactions and, 1273
- osteoporosis/osteomalacia and, 1127
- pancreatitis and, 878*t*, 882, 885, 888, 891*t*
- photosensitivity and, 155
- psychosis and, 415, 416*t*, 420, 421
- secondary adrenal insufficiency and, 735, 738–741
- serum sickness-like reactions and, 1194
- sexual dysfunction and, 762*t*
- sleep disorders and, 349–350*t*
- for systemic lupus erythematosus, 135
- teratogenicity of, 1316, 1317, 1319, 1320
- thrombocytopenia and, 1059
- thyroid diseases and, 716
- topical, 734
- upper gastrointestinal ulceration and, 809–812, 810–811*t*, 814–817, 816*t*
- valvular/pericardial heart disease and, 670
- visual disturbances and, 299*t*, 313, 315–318
- vulvovaginal candidiasis and, 782*t*, 785*t*, 791

Corticotropin, 195*t*, 199*t*, 731*t*

Corticotropin-releasing hormone (CRH), 729, 734–735, 737–739, 741

Cortisol
- anxiety and, 409
- Cushing syndrome and, 729, 732
- hypertrichosis and, 198–199
- primary adrenal insufficiency and, 734
- secondary adrenal insufficiency and, 735, 737–741
- stroke and, 232

Cortisone, 195–196*t*, 385*t*, 739*t*

Cosmetic treatments
- for alopecia, 189*t*, 192
- for hirsutism and hypertrichosis, 204–205, 204–205*t*, 207–208

Cost burden of drug-induced diseases, 26–29, 27*t*

Cost-of-illness model, 27–28

Co-trimoxazole, 472*t*, 846*t*, 864, 1263*t*, 1266*t*

Cough and cold preparations, 238*t*, 517

Council for International Organizations of Medical Sciences (CIOMS), 51, 52

COX-1 inhibitors. *See* Cyclooxygenase-1 selective inhibitors

COX-2 inhibitors. *See* Cyclooxygenase-2 selective inhibitors

CPIC (Clinical Pharmacogenetics Implementation Consortium) guidelines, 35

Cremophor (polyethoxyethylated castor oil)-containing products, 77*t*, 81

CRH (corticotropin-releasing hormone), 729, 734–735, 737–739, 741

Crizotinib, 145*t*, 299*t*, 908*t*, 1259*t*

Cromolyn, 452*t*, 463

Cromolyn sodium, 515, 660*t*, 662

CSF. *See* Colony-stimulating factor

CTEPH (chronic thromboembolic pulmonary hypertension), 1074

CTID (cancer treatment-induced diarrhea), 821, 827–828, 827*t*

CTZ (chemoreceptor trigger zone), 912–914, 913*f*

Curcumin, 440

Cushing syndrome, 730–734
- causative agents of, 730, 731*t*
- clinical presentation of, 386, 732–733, 732*t*, 749
- differential diagnosis of, 732–733, 733*t*
- epidemiology of, 730
- management of, 734
- mechanisms of, 730–732, 731*t*
- morbidity and mortality for, 733
- overview, 730
- patient education on, 734
- prevention of, 733–734, 734*t*
- risk factors for, 733, 733*t*

Cutaneous diseases, 100–114
- causative agents of, 100–104, 102–104*t*
- clinical presentation of, 106–110, 107–108*t*
- differential diagnosis of, 106, 108*t*
- epidemiology of, 104–105
- management of, 113–114, 114*t*
- mechanisms of, 105–106
- morbidity and mortality for, 112
- patient education on, 114
- prevention of, 112, 113*t*
- risk factors for, 110–112, 111*t*
- systemic lupus erythematosus and, 130
- terminology related to, 100, 101*t*

Cyanoacrylate, 1064*t*, 1068*t*

Cycad nut, 849*t*

Cyclic antidepressants, 219

Cyclizine, 852*t*

Cyclobenzaprine, 145*t*, 416*t*, 418*t*, 984*t*

Cyclofenil, 848*t*

Cyclooxygenase (COX)-1 selective inhibitors, 233, 453, 455, 463, 812, 815, 945

Cyclooxygenase (COX)-2 selective inhibitors
- acute kidney injury and, 942, 944–945*t*, 945–949
- asthma/bronchospasm and, 453, 461, 463
- bleeding disorders and, 1030
- cognitive disorders and, 361
- delirium and, 327*t*
- heart failure and, 501, 503*t*, 509, 512, 516
- hypertension and, 620*t*
- myocardial ischemia/acute coronary syndromes and, 472*t*, 473, 475, 477*t*, 479, 480, 489
- stroke and, 230, 231, 233
- upper gastrointestinal ulceration and, 810*t*, 811, 812, 815, 817
- vaginal bleeding disorders and, 797
- visual disturbances and, 318

Cyclophosphamide
- alopecia and, 169*t*, 176, 177
- asthma/bronchospasm and, 452*t*
- bladder cancer and, 1285*t*, 1288*t*, 1303–1305
- cognitive disorders and, 358*t*
- color changes of oral mucosa and teeth and, 1254*t*
- depression and, 384
- diabetes insipidus and, 991*t*
- heart failure and, 502*t*, 508, 510*t*
- hepatic/cholestatic diseases and, 848*t*
- interstitial lung disease/pulmonary fibrosis and, 431, 432*t*, 439, 440
- leukemia and, 1284, 1284*t*, 1286, 1287, 1288*t*, 1291
- lymphoma and, 1295
- myocardial ischemia/acute coronary syndromes and, 472*t*
- nausea/vomiting and, 908*t*, 916*t*, 925, 926
- oral erythema multiforme and, 1266*t*
- osteoporosis/osteomalacia and, 1123*t*
- sexual dysfunction and, 759*t*
- SIADH and, 981, 983*t*, 989
- systemic lupus erythematosus and, 126*t*
- taste disorders and, 1259*t*
- valvular/pericardial heart disease and, 660–661*t*, 662, 668
- visual disturbances and, 299*t*
- weight gain and, 1172

Cycloserine, 376*t*, 377, 400*t*, 416*t*, 418*t*, 1235*t*

Cyclosporine
- acidosis and, 1003*t*
- acute kidney injury and, 943*t*, 952
- alopecia and, 172*t*, 174, 191
- aplastic anemia and, 1104
- chronic kidney disease and, 965, 966*t*, 967–969, 970*t*, 971–976, 972*t*, 974*t*
- cutaneous diseases and, 102*t*, 114
- gingival hyperplasia and, 1262–1264, 1263–1264*t*
- glucose/insulin dysregulation and, 680*t*, 684*t*, 688
- gout/hyperuricemia and, 1136*t*, 1137, 1140, 1145
- hepatic/cholestatic diseases and, 848*t*
- hirsutism and, 194, 198
- hyperprolactinemia and, 744*t*
- hypertension and, 618*t*, 620, 620*t*, 624, 625, 625*t*
- hypertrichosis and, 194, 196*t*, 198, 199, 202
- lymphoma and, 1284*t*, 1288*t*, 1292–1295
- myopathy and, 1150*t*
- osteoporosis/osteomalacia and, 1121*t*, 1123*t*, 1127
- ototoxicity and, 1235*t*
- pancreatitis and, 891*t*
- peripheral neuropathy and, 281*t*
- seizures and, 219*t*, 222*t*
- skin cancer and, 1284*t*, 1288*t*, 1297, 1298
- thrombocytopenia and, 1054, 1056
- thromboembolic diseases and, 1065*t*, 1069*t*
- thyroid diseases and, 699*t*
- upper gastrointestinal ulceration and, 815
- visual disturbances and, 299*t*

CYP2D6, 918–919, 1272

Cypress spurge, 299*t*

Cyproheptadine
- depression and, 390
- hepatic/cholestatic diseases and, 852*t*
- photosensitivity and, 145*t*
- serotonin syndrome and, 1207–1208, 1208*t*
- thyroid diseases and, 703*t*

Cyproterone, 188*t*, 190–191, 206, 206*t*, 1064*t*, 1068*t*

Cyproterone acetate, 744*t*, 848*t*

Cysteamine, 7*t*

Cysteinyl leukotrienes (CysLTs), 455, 462

Cystic fibrosis, 87

Cytarabine
anxiety and, 403
heart failure and, 503*t*, 509
hepatic/cholestatic diseases and, 848*t*
nausea/vomiting and, 908*t*, 916*t*
ototoxicity and, 1235*t*
pancreatitis and, 878*t*, 881
peripheral neuropathy and, 280*t*
sinus bradycardia/atrioventricular block and, 570*t*
valvular/pericardial heart disease and, 660–661*t*, 662, 668
visual disturbances and, 300*t*, 313
Cytokines
in allergic reactions, 79, 81, 87
in alopecia areata, 166
anxiety and, 409, 410
in atrial fibrillation/atrial flutter, 584
in bone remodeling, 1120
chronic kidney disease and, 969
depression and, 386
in hepatic and cholestatic diseases, 857
lymphoma and, 1293
in nausea and vomiting, 922
in thermoregulation, 1186
thrombocytopenia and, 1053
Cytosine, 1188*t*
Cytotoxic agents
alopecia and, 177, 178, 182
diarrhea and, 823, 825
gout/hyperuricemia and, 1136*t*, 1137–1138, 1144*t*
infertility and, 800–802
interstitial lung disease/pulmonary fibrosis and, 431
myocardial ischemia/acute coronary syndromes and, 474
neutropenia/agranulocytosis and, 1087, 1091, 1091*t*, 1092, 1094, 1095*t*
vaginal bleeding disorders and, 793, 794

Dabigatran
alopecia and, 167*t*
bleeding disorders and, 1029*t*, 1035, 1038–1039
drug interactions with, 39
intracerebral hemorrhage and, 238*t*, 245
stroke and, 237
systemic lupus erythematosus and, 126*t*
upper gastrointestinal ulceration and, 810–811*t*, 810–812, 814
valvular/pericardial heart disease and, 661*t*, 662
VTE dosing recommendations, 1077*t*
Dabrafenib, 169*t*, 1284*t*, 1296
Dacarbazine
hepatic/cholestatic diseases and, 848*t*
hypotension and, 636*t*, 640*t*
leukemia and, 1284, 1285
nausea/vomiting and, 908*t*, 916*t*
photosensitivity and, 145*t*
thromboembolic diseases and, 1065*t*, 1069*t*
Daclizumab, 967
Dactinomycin, 169*t*, 916*t*, 1270*t*
Dalbavancin, 836*t*
Dalfampridine, 7*t*
Dalteparin, 167*t*, 1034, 1055
Danaparoid, 1058, 1059
Danazol
alopecia and, 167*t*, 180
anxiety and, 403
cutaneous diseases and, 102*t*, 108
hepatic/cholestatic diseases and, 849*t*
hirsutism and, 194, 195*t*
ototoxicity and, 1235*t*
systemic lupus erythematosus and, 126*t*
thrombocytopenia and, 1050*t*
thromboembolic diseases and, 1065*t*, 1068*t*
thyroid diseases and, 701*t*
vaginal bleeding disorders and, 782*t*, 785*t*
Dantrolene
dystonia and, 270
hepatic/cholestatic diseases and, 851*t*
malignant hyperthermia and, 1212–1214, 1213*t*
neuroleptic malignant syndrome and, 1200–1201, 1200*t*
ototoxicity and, 1235*t*
photosensitivity and, 145*t*
serotonin syndrome and, 1208
valvular/pericardial heart disease and, 660*t*, 662, 664
Dapagliflozin, 634*t*, 1002*t*
Dapsone
allergic reactions to, 75*t*, 87
cutaneous diseases and, 103*t*
genetic variations affecting, 36*t*
heart failure and, 503*t*, 509
hemolytic anemia and, 1105*t*
hepatic/cholestatic diseases and, 846*t*, 861*t*
nausea/vomiting and, 930
neutropenia/agranulocytosis and, 1089*t*
oral lichenoid reactions and, 1270*t*
ototoxicity and, 1235*t*
peripheral neuropathy and, 280*t*
pharmacogenomic tests for, 35
photosensitivity and, 145*t*
psychosis and, 416*t*
visual disturbances and, 300*t*
Daptomycin, 953
Darbepoetin, 472*t*, 625*t*, 1064*t*, 1068*t*, 1075*t*, 1111*t*
Darbepoetin-α, 618*t*, 621, 626, 1111
DARRTS (Document Archiving, Reporting, and Regulatory Tracking System) system, 13
Darunavir, 92, 1266*t*
Dasatinib, 169*t*, 699*t*, 1087
Datura, 300*t*
Daunorubicin
alopecia and, 169*t*, 176
drug fever and, 1188*t*
heart failure and, 514
hepatic/cholestatic diseases and, 848*t*
nausea/vomiting and, 908*t*, 916*t*
valvular/pericardial heart disease and, 661*t*
DDIs (drug–drug interactions), 38–40, 39*t*, 153–154
Deafness. *See* Hearing loss
Decision-tree model, 28, 28*t*
Decitabine, 836*t*
Decongestants, 401
Deep vein thrombosis (DVT)
clinical presentation of, 1071–1073, 1071*t*
differential diagnosis of, 1072, 1072*t*
management of, 1076
morbidity and mortality for, 1074
overview, 1063
patient education on, 1077–1078
pretest probability of, 1072*t*
risk factors for, 1074
Deferasirox, 7*t*
Deferiprone, 7*t*
Deferoxamine, 73*t*, 300*t*, 1050*t*, 1235*t*, 1242
Defibrotide, 635*t*, 1026*t*, 1029*t*
Dehydroepiandrosterone (DHEA), 167*t*, 184, 195*t*, 199, 201
Delavirdine, 1266*t*
Delirium, 325–340
causative agents of, 325, 326–328*t*
clinical presentation of, 330–331, 330–331*t*, 420
defined, 357
differential diagnosis of, 331, 331–332*t*
epidemiology of, 325, 328–329, 357–358
management of, 335–340, 336*t*, 369
mechanisms of, 329–330, 329*t*, 360
morbidity and mortality for, 333–334, 366
patient education on, 340
prevention of, 334–335, 334*t*
risk factors for, 331–333, 332*t*
Demeclocycline, 8–9, 145*t*, 989*t*, 990, 991*t*
Dementia
clinical presentation of, 362, 363
differential diagnosis of, 331, 332*t*
management of, 340
mechanisms of, 329, 360
risk factors for, 332–334
Demographic factors related to drug-induced diseases, 31–32
Denileukin, 1065*t*, 1069*t*
Denominator, in incidence of drug-induced disease, 25
Denosumab, 126*t*, 1129*t*, 1130, 1273–1274, 1274*t*, 1276
Deoxyribonucleic acid (DNA)
acute kidney injury and, 951
bladder cancer and, 1304
breast cancer and, 1299
chemotherapy agents and, 1286, 1287, 1290
endometrial cancer and, 1301
hepatic/cholestatic diseases and, 856
macrocytic anemia and, 1107
myopathy and, 1152–1153
neoplastic injury and, 858
neutropenia/agranulocytosis and, 1091
peripheral neuropathy and, 282
in photosensitivity, 150
systemic lupus erythematosus and, 127, 130, 132
Depolarizing muscle relaxants, 1209*t*, 1210, 1212
Depot medroxyprogesterone. *See* Medroxyprogesterone depot
Depression, 375–392
causative agents of, 375–377, 376–377*t*
clinical presentation of, 386–387, 387*t*
differential diagnosis of, 387, 387*t*
epidemiology of, 377–385
management of, 390–392, 391*t*
mechanisms of, 385–386, 385*t*
morbidity and mortality for, 389
patient education on, 392
prevention of, 390, 390*t*
risk factors for, 387–389, 388*t*
Dermatologic agents, 375
Dermatomyositis, 1150, 1152*t*, 1153, 1155
Desensitization extracts, 452*t*
Desensitization procedures, 64–65, 88–90, 92, 95–96, 98, 1191
Desflurane, 850*t*, 906*t*, 1209*t*
Desglymidodrine, 646
Desipramine
alopecia and, 173*t*
Brugada syndrome and, 547*t*
delirium and, 326*t*, 329*t*
hypotension and, 634*t*, 639*t*
monomorphic ventricular tachycardia and, 524–525*t*
neutropenia/agranulocytosis and, 1089*t*
ototoxicity and, 1235*t*
photosensitivity and, 145*t*

INDEX

Desipramine (continued)
 SIADH and, 982t
 weight gain and, 1166t, 1169t
Desmopressin
 bleeding disorders and, 1039
 diabetes insipidus and, 992
 hepatic/cholestatic diseases and, 870
 hypotension and, 646t
 myocardial ischemia/acute coronary syndromes and, 473t
 thromboembolic diseases and, 1064t, 1067, 1068t
Desogestrel, 1075
Desoximetasone, 145t
Desvenlafaxine, 145t, 348t, 618t, 620t, 982t
Deutetrabenazine, 7t, 264
Dexamethasone
 alopecia and, 171t
 cognitive disorders and, 360
 Cushing syndrome and, 732
 hirsutism and, 195t
 hypertrichosis and, 196t
 leukemia and, 1287
 nausea/vomiting and, 922–927, 924t, 927–929t, 929
 pharmacologic characteristics of, 739t
 secondary adrenal insufficiency and, 736t, 741
 sinus bradycardia/atrioventricular block and, 570t
 thromboembolic diseases and, 1065t, 1069t
 thyroid diseases and, 702t
 topical, 731t
Dexamphetamine, 1203–1204t
Dexfenfluramine
 chronic kidney disease and, 973
 myocardial ischemia/acute coronary syndromes and, 473t
 valvular/pericardial heart disease and, 659, 660t, 663–664, 663t, 668–670, 668t
Dexfenfluramine-phentermine, 9
Dexlansoprazole, 966t
Dexmedetomidine, 570t, 577t, 1208t, 1209
Dexmethylphenidate, 167t, 400t, 401
Dexrazoxane, 515
Dextroamphetamine
 alopecia and, 167t
 anxiety and, 401
 growth hormone deficiency and, 748t
 myocardial ischemia/acute coronary syndromes and, 473t
 visual disturbances and, 300t
Dextromethorphan, 416t, 418t, 425, 1203–1204t, 1204t
Dextrose, 580, 870
DHEA. *See* Dehydroepiandrosterone
DHRs. *See* Drug hypersensitivity reactions
Diabetes insipidus, 991–993
 causative agents of, 991, 991t
 clinical presentation of, 992, 992t
 differential diagnosis of, 992, 992t
 epidemiology of, 991
 management of, 993, 993t
 mechanisms of, 991
 morbidity and mortality for, 993
 overview, 981
 patient education on, 993
 prevention of, 993, 993t
 risk factors for, 992–993, 993t
Diabetes mellitus, 679, 681, 683, 687–688, 690, 952
Diabetic neuropathy, 288–289
Diagnostic and Statistical Manual of Mental Disorders, 5th Edition (*DSM-5*), 256, 330, 357, 375, 399, 420
Diamorphine, 906t
Diarrhea, 821–830
 antibiotic-associated, 821, 822–823t, 823, 825, 827, 830
 cancer treatment-induced, 821, 827–828, 827t
 causative agents of, 821–822, 822t
 clinical presentation of, 823–825, 824t
 criteria for grading severity of, 828, 828t
 differential diagnosis of, 825, 826t
 epidemiology of, 822–823
 management of, 827–829, 827t
 mechanisms of, 823, 823t
 morbidity and mortality for, 826
 patient education on, 830
 prevention of, 826–827, 826t
 risk factors for, 825, 826t
Diatrizoate and iodipamide meglumine, 706t
Diatrizoate meglumine, 706t, 1050t
Diatrizoate meglumine/sodium, 706t
Diatrizoate sodium, 706t
Diazepam
 allergic reactions to, 75t
 anxiety and, 407
 cognitive disorders and, 360, 368, 369
 delirium and, 329t, 337
 drug interactions with, 39t
 hypothermia and, 1216t
 neuroleptic malignant syndrome and, 1200t, 1201
 oral lichenoid reactions and, 1270t
 ototoxicity and, 1235t
 seizures and, 226
 serotonin syndrome and, 1208, 1208t
 sinus bradycardia/atrioventricular block and, 570t, 578t
 smoking and, 32
 thrombocytopenia and, 1050t
 thyroid diseases and, 701t
 visual disturbances and, 300t
Diazoxide
 alopecia and, 174t, 179t
 glucose/insulin dysregulation and, 679, 680t, 684t
 hypertrichosis and, 194, 195, 197t, 198, 199, 202
 hypotension and, 633t, 640t
 myocardial ischemia/acute coronary syndromes and, 472t
 thrombocytopenia and, 1050t
 visual disturbances and, 300t
Dibucaine, 145t
Dichloroethylene, 849t
Dichlorphenamide, 145t
Diclofenac
 acute kidney injury and, 944
 allergic reactions to, 73t
 alopecia and, 172t
 aplastic anemia and, 1100t
 bleeding disorders and, 1033
 delirium and, 327t
 heart failure and, 510t
 hemolytic anemia and, 1105t
 hepatic/cholestatic diseases and, 846t
 human leukocyte antigen and, 37
 myocardial ischemia/acute coronary syndromes and, 472t, 475
 oral erythema multiforme and, 1266t
 ototoxicity and, 1235t
 pancreatitis and, 881
 photosensitivity and, 145t
 SIADH and, 984t
 systemic lupus erythematosus and, 126t
 thrombocytopenia and, 1050t
 upper gastrointestinal ulceration and, 813
 visual disturbances and, 300t
A Dictionary of Epidemiology (Last), 20
Didanosine
 acidosis and, 1002–1003t
 alopecia and, 168t
 diabetes insipidus and, 991t
 myocardial ischemia/acute coronary syndromes and, 472t
 oral erythema multiforme and, 1266t
 osteoporosis/osteomalacia and, 1123t
 ototoxicity and, 1235t
 pancreatitis and, 878t, 880, 886t, 890–892, 891t
 peripheral neuropathy and, 280t
Dienestrol, 790t
Dietary goitrogens, 701t, 713
Dietary supplements, 238t, 969, 970, 972–976
Diethyldithiocarbamate, 1243
Diethylpropion, 167t
Diethylstilbestrol, 1064t, 1068t
Differential diagnosis
 of acidosis, 1006, 1007t
 of acute interstitial nephritis, 956
 of acute tubular necrosis, 951
 of adverse drug reactions, 51, 63–65
 of akathisia, 257, 257t
 of alkalosis, 1015, 1016t
 of alopecia, 183, 184t
 of amenorrhea and oligomenorrhea, 788t, 793–794
 of anxiety, 407, 407t
 of aplastic anemia, 1102, 1102t
 of asthma and bronchospasm, 457, 458t
 of atrial fibrillation/atrial flutter, 585, 585t
 of atrial tachycardia, 589, 589t
 of AV node re-entrant tachycardia, 593, 593t
 of bladder cancer, 1290t, 1304
 of bleeding disorders, 1030, 1031t
 of breast cancer, 1290t, 1299
 of Brugada syndrome, 548
 of chemotherapy-induced anemia, 1110
 of chronic kidney disease, 971, 971t
 of cognitive disorders, 363, 363t
 of color changes of oral mucosa and teeth, 1256–1257, 1257t
 of congenital heart defects, 1323–1324
 of constipation, 837, 838t
 of Cushing syndrome, 732–733, 733t
 of cutaneous diseases, 106, 108t
 of delirium, 331, 331–332t
 of depression, 387, 387t
 of diabetes insipidus, 992, 992t
 of diarrhea, 825, 826t
 of drug allergies and hypersensitivity reactions, 82, 84t
 of drug fever, 1190, 1190t
 of dysmenorrhea, 788t, 797
 of dystonia, 257t, 267, 268
 of endometrial cancer, 1290t, 1301–1302
 of female sexual dysfunction, 788t, 799
 of fetal alcohol spectrum disorders, 1332
 of gastroschisis, 1326–1327
 of gingival hyperplasia, 1257t, 1264
 of glomerulonephritis, 958–959
 of glucose and insulin dysregulation, 686, 687t
 of gout and hyperuricemia, 1141, 1141t
 of growth hormone deficiency, 749, 749t
 of heart failure, 512, 513t
 of hemodynamic-mediated AKI, 946, 946t
 of hemolytic anemia, 1106
 of hepatic and cholestatic diseases, 860, 861t
 of hirsutism, 201, 201t
 of hyperprolactinemia, 744–745, 745t

of hypertension, 201t, 622, 622t
of hypertrichosis, 201, 201t
of hypotension, 641, 642t
of hypothermia, 1217
of infertility, 770t, 788t, 801
of interstitial lung disease/pulmonary fibrosis, 436, 436t
of intracerebral hemorrhage, 241, 241t
of learning disabilities, 1315–1316
of leukemia, 1289, 1290t
of limb deficiency defects, 1325
of low birth weight, 1317–1318
of lymphoma, 1290t, 1293–1294
of macrocytic anemia, 1102t, 1108
of male sexual dysfunction, 769, 770t
of malignant hyperthermia, 1211, 1211t
of menorrhagia and menometrorrhagia, 788t, 795
of microcephaly, 1331
of monomorphic ventricular tachycardia, 527, 527t
of myocardial ischemia/acute coronary syndromes, 482, 483t
of myopathy, 1154, 1154t
of nausea and vomiting, 915, 916t
of nephrolithiasis, 946t, 957
of neural tube defects, 1329
of neuroleptic malignant syndrome, 1197–1198, 1198t
of neutropenia and agranulocytosis, 1092, 1092t
of oral erythema multiforme, 1257t, 1269
of oral lichenoid reactions (OLR), 1257t, 1273
of orofacial clefts, 1321
of osteonecrosis of jaw, 1257t, 1275
of osteoporosis and osteomalacia, 1124, 1124t
of ototoxicity, 1240t, 1241
of ovarian hyperstimulation, 784, 788t
of pancreatitis, 889, 889t
of parkinsonism, 257t, 272
of peripheral neuropathy, 284–285, 284t
of photosensitivity, 151, 151t
of psychosis, 419, 419t
of secondary adrenal insufficiency, 737, 738t
of seizures, 223, 223t
of serotonin syndrome, 1206, 1206t
of serum sickness-like reactions, 84t, 1194, 1194t
of SIADH, 987, 987t
of sinus bradycardia/atrioventricular block, 575, 576t
of skin cancer, 1290t, 1296
of sleep disorders, 349, 351t
of stroke, 233, 234t
of systemic lupus erythematosus, 132, 132t
of tardive dyskinesia, 257t, 262
of taste disorders, 1257t, 1261
of thrombocytopenia, 1055, 1055t
of thromboembolic diseases, 1072, 1072t
of thyroid diseases, 711, 712, 712t
of torsades de pointes, 536–537, 537t
of upper gastrointestinal ulceration, 813–814, 813t
of valvular and pericardial heart disease, 665–668, 667t
of visual disturbances, 316, 316t
of vulvovaginal candidiasis, 788t, 791
of weight gain, 1169, 1170t
Diflunisal, 145t, 510t, 1235t, 1270t
Digitalis, 22, 26, 300t, 376t, 385, 385t
Digitalis glycoside toxicity, 589, 589t
Digitoxin, 590
DigniCap, 186, 189t
Digoxin
atrial fibrillation/atrial flutter and, 586
atrial tachycardia and, 588–590t, 588–591
cognitive disorders and, 358t, 365
comorbidity and, 34
delirium and, 326t
depression and, 378, 385
drug-induced hospitalizations from, 26t
drug interactions with, 38
genetic variability and, 16t
heart failure and, 516
monomorphic ventricular tachycardia and, 523, 524–525t, 526, 529, 530
nausea/vomiting and, 910, 911t, 930
neutropenia/agranulocytosis and, 1088, 1089t
oral erythema multiforme and, 1266t
psychosis and, 416t
sexual dysfunction and, 758–759t, 763–764t, 783t, 786t
sinus bradycardia/atrioventricular block and, 570t, 572, 573t, 577–579, 577t, 579t
thrombocytopenia and, 1050t
transport mechanisms for, 37
Digoxin immune antibody fragments, 502t, 509, 591
Dihydro-2(3H)-furanone, 1215
Dihydrocodeine, 472t, 906t
Dihydroergotamine, 472t, 646t, 647, 1066t, 1070t
Dihydrotestosterone, 183, 538, 763
Diltiazem
atrial fibrillation/atrial flutter and, 582t, 586, 587t
atrial tachycardia and, 591
drug fever and, 1188t
gingival hyperplasia and, 1263, 1263t
heart failure and, 502t, 505, 509, 510t, 515
hypertrichosis and, 196t
hypotension and, 633t, 639t
myocardial ischemia/acute coronary syndromes and, 472t, 489
oral erythema multiforme and, 1267t
ototoxicity and, 1235t
photosensitivity and, 145t
sinus bradycardia/atrioventricular block and, 570t, 572, 573t, 577, 578t, 580
systemic lupus erythematosus and, 124t
taste disorders and, 1259t, 1261t
Dimenhydrinate, 924t, 1267t
Dimethylacetamide, 849t
1,3 dimethylamylamine, 582t
Dimethylformamide, 849t
Dimethyl sulfoxide, 300t
Dinutuximab, 636t, 984t
Dioxane, 849t
Dipeptidyl peptidase 4 (DPP-4) inhibitors
glucose/insulin dysregulation and, 682t, 685t
heart failure and, 503t, 506, 511, 513, 514t
pancreatitis and, 879t, 884
Diphenhydramine
delirium and, 328t
hypotension and, 634t, 640t
nausea/vomiting and, 927t
ototoxicity and, 1243–1244
photosensitivity and, 145t
psychosis and, 416t, 425
seizures and, 219, 220
taste disorders and, 1262
torsades de pointes and, 533t
Diphenoxylate, 1263t
Diphenylcyclopropenone, 191
Diphtheria antitoxin (equine), 7t
Diphtheria-pertussis-tetanus (DTaP) vaccine, 197t, 1267t
Dipyridamole
asthma/bronchospasm and, 452t
bleeding disorders and, 1026t, 1029, 1029t
intracerebral hemorrhage and, 244
monomorphic ventricular tachycardia and, 524t, 526
myocardial ischemia/acute coronary syndromes and, 472t, 477t, 479
neutropenia/agranulocytosis and, 1088, 1089t
sinus bradycardia/atrioventricular block and, 570t, 573t, 577
stroke and, 236
taste disorders and, 1259t, 1261t
Dipyrone, 102t
Direct-acting arterial vasodilators, 645t
Disease-modifying antirheumatic drugs (DMARDs), 174, 178, 1175t
Disopyramide
glucose/insulin dysregulation and, 682t, 685t
heart failure and, 502t, 507, 510t, 511, 515
hepatic/cholestatic diseases and, 847t
monomorphic ventricular tachycardia and, 524–525t, 529
myocardial ischemia/acute coronary syndromes and, 472t
peripheral neuropathy and, 280t
sexual dysfunction and, 759t
sinus bradycardia/atrioventricular block and, 570t, 573t, 577t
systemic lupus erythematosus and, 124t
torsades de pointes and, 532t, 539t
Distal renal tubular acidosis, 1003–1004t, 1004, 1006, 1010, 1011f
Disulfiram
drug interactions with, 39t
hepatic/cholestatic diseases and, 851t
nausea/vomiting and, 915
peripheral neuropathy and, 281t
psychosis and, 416t, 418t
taste disorders and, 1259t
Diuretics
acute kidney injury and, 944t, 947–949, 952–954, 959
alkalosis and, 1012, 1015, 1017
asthma/bronchospasm and, 463
constipation and, 835, 836–837t
drug-induced hospitalizations from, 26, 26t
gout/hyperuricemia and, 1136t, 1138, 1144t
heart failure and, 508, 511, 512, 517
hepatic/cholestatic diseases and, 868, 870, 872
hypotension and, 633t, 642–644
loop. *See* Loop diuretics
myocardial ischemia/acute coronary syndromes and, 472t
myopathy and, 1150t, 1151, 1152t, 1153
nonpotassium-sparing, 34
osmotic, 636t
ototoxicity and, 1233, 1239, 1239t, 1241, 1243
ovarian hyperstimulation and, 789, 790t
photosensitivity and, 143, 150, 150t, 154
potassium-sparing, 625, 949, 1003t, 1138
sexual dysfunction and, 757, 759–760t, 761, 764t, 766
thiazide. *See* Thiazide diuretics
valvular/pericardial heart disease and, 670
DMARDs (disease-modifying antirheumatic drugs), 174, 178, 1175t
DNA. *See* Deoxyribonucleic acid
DOAC regimen, 1076

INDEX

Dobutamine
atrial fibrillation/atrial flutter and, 582–583t, 584, 585t, 586
AV node re-entrant tachycardia and, 592, 592–593t, 593
drug fever and, 1188t
hypotension and, 635t, 639t
monomorphic ventricular tachycardia and, 523, 524–525t, 529, 530
myocardial ischemia/acute coronary syndromes and, 472t
Docetaxel
allergic reactions to, 74t
alopecia and, 169t
atrial fibrillation/atrial flutter and, 582t
color changes of oral mucosa and teeth and, 1254t
interstitial lung disease/pulmonary fibrosis and, 433t, 435t
nausea/vomiting and, 908t
pancreatitis and, 881
peripheral neuropathy and, 280t
SIADH and, 983t
systemic lupus erythematosus and, 126t
taste disorders and, 1259t
thromboembolic diseases and, 1065t, 1069t
visual disturbances and, 300t, 316
Document Archiving, Reporting, and Regulatory Tracking System (DARRTS) system, 13
Documentation of drug-induced diseases, 65–66
Docusate sodium, 840t
Dofetilide
atrial fibrillation/atrial flutter and, 587, 587t
heart failure and, 507, 511, 513
restrictive drug distribution system for, 7t
torsades de pointes and, 532t, 538, 539t
Dolasetron, 473t, 533t, 918, 922, 924t, 928–929t
Domperidone, 473t, 474, 532t, 539–540t, 743t, 745
Donepezil
hypotension and, 633t, 640t
neuroleptic malignant syndrome and, 1195t
ototoxicity and, 1235t
sinus bradycardia/atrioventricular block and, 570t, 573t
systemic lupus erythematosus and, 125t
torsades de pointes and, 532t, 540t
Dopamine
acute kidney injury and, 953
alopecia and, 171t
atrial fibrillation/atrial flutter and, 582t
delirium and, 329, 332, 333
hyperprolactinemia and, 742, 745
as inhibitory factor for prolactin, 742
nausea/vomiting and, 914
neuroleptic malignant syndrome and, 1195–1198
psychosis and, 418, 419, 422
serotonin syndrome and, 1208
SIADH and, 984t
sinus bradycardia/atrioventricular block and, 580
in sleep cycles, 349
stroke and, 232
tardive dyskinesia and, 261
in thermoregulation, 1185, 1186, 1215–1216
thyroid diseases and, 701t
Dopamine agonists
alopecia and, 171t, 175, 178, 179t, 184, 186
anxiety and, 400t, 405, 405t, 408
hyperprolactinemia and, 746, 747
hypotension and, 633t, 645t
neuroleptic malignant syndrome and, 1196, 1200, 1201
parkinsonism and, 273
psychosis and, 416t, 417, 422
valvular/pericardial heart disease and, 659, 669
Dopamine antagonists
anxiety and, 400t, 405, 405t, 408, 410
hyperprolactinemia and, 745, 746
nausea/vomiting and, 927, 927t, 929
neuroleptic malignant syndrome and, 1199
psychosis and, 418, 422
Dopamine D_2 receptors, 261, 271–272, 338, 798, 912, 1196, 1198
Dopamine-receptor-blocking agents (DRBAs)
akathisia and, 255–256
dystonia and, 265–267, 269, 270
parkinsonism and, 270–273
tardive dyskinesia and, 259, 261–263
Dopaminergic agents, 327t, 415, 422, 701t, 1197
Dopexamine, 472t
Dovitinib, 570t
Down syndrome, 577, 1314, 1323
Doxapram, 1013–1014, 1013–1014t
Doxazosin, 300t, 416t, 509, 632t, 639t, 762
Doxepin
alopecia and, 173t
delirium and, 326t, 329t
drug fever and, 1188t
hypotension and, 634t, 639t
myocardial ischemia/acute coronary syndromes and, 472t
ototoxicity and, 1235t
photosensitivity and, 145t
SIADH and, 982t, 990
sleep disorders and, 353
torsades de pointes and, 533t, 540t
weight gain and, 1166t, 1169t
Doxifluridine, 169t
Doxorubicin
alopecia and, 169t, 176
atrial fibrillation/atrial flutter and, 582t
color changes of oral mucosa and teeth and, 1254t
constipation and, 836t
depression and, 384
heart failure and, 502t, 507, 510t, 511, 514, 515
hepatic/cholestatic diseases and, 848t
leukemia and, 1284–1286, 1284t, 1288t, 1291
lymphoma and, 1295
nausea/vomiting and, 908t, 916t
systemic lupus erythematosus and, 126t
taste disorders and, 1259t
vaginal bleeding disorders and, 782t, 785t
valvular/pericardial heart disease and, 661t
visual disturbances and, 300t
Doxycycline
allergic reactions to, 95
ototoxicity and, 1235t
pancreatitis and, 879t, 882
photosensitivity and, 145t, 153
SIADH and, 990
systemic lupus erythematosus and, 125t
upper gastrointestinal ulceration and, 809, 813
Doxylamine, 220
D-penicillamine
asthma/bronchospasm and, 452t
chronic kidney disease and, 966t, 970t
myopathy and, 1150, 1150t, 1151, 1152t, 1153
systemic lupus erythematosus and, 126t, 130
DPP-4 inhibitors. *See* Dipeptidyl peptidase 4 inhibitors
DRBAs. *See* Dopamine-receptor-blocking agents
DRESS (drug rash with eosinophilia and systemic symptoms), 87, 102–103t, 105, 107–108t, 109–110, 114t, 1186
Dronabinol, 400t, 416t, 418t, 929, 929t
Dronedarone
heart failure and, 502t, 507, 511
photosensitivity and, 145t
sinus bradycardia/atrioventricular block and, 570t, 577t
torsades de pointes and, 532t, 539t
Droperidol
akathisia and, 255, 255–256t, 258t
delirium and, 338
hypotension and, 634t
nausea/vomiting and, 922, 923, 924t, 927–928t, 928
neuroleptic malignant syndrome and, 1195t
torsades de pointes and, 532t
Drospirenone, 191, 206t, 1075
Drotrecogin alfa, 3
Droxidopa, 7t, 646–647, 646t
Drug allergies, 71–100
categorization of, 60
causative agents, 71–76, 72–75t
clinical presentation of, 82–85, 83–84t
comparison with hypersensitivity reactions, 71, 72t
defined, 71
differential diagnosis of, 82, 84t
epidemiology of, 76–78
Gell and Coombs classification of, 79–81, 80t
immediate vs. nonimmediate, 80–82
management of, 98–100, 99t
mechanisms of, 78–81
morbidity and mortality for, 88
patient education on, 88, 100
prevention of, 88–90, 92, 94–96
risk factors for, 85–87, 85t
Drug–drug interactions (DDIs), 38–40, 39t, 153–154
Drug fever, 1186–1192
causative agents of, 1186–1187, 1188–1189t
clinical presentation of, 1187t, 1189–1190, 1189t
differential diagnosis of, 1190, 1190t
epidemiology of, 1187
management of, 1191, 1191t
mechanisms of, 1187
morbidity and mortality for, 1190
patient education on, 1192
prevention of, 1190–1191
risk factors for, 1190
Drug hypersensitivity reactions (DHRs)
causative agents, 76, 77t, 1186
comparison with drug allergies, 71, 72t
defined, 71
differential diagnosis of, 84t
epidemiology of, 76–78
human leukocyte antigen and, 37, 38
immediate vs. nonimmediate, 81
management of, 99t
mechanisms of, 81–82
patient education on, 88, 100
prevention of, 96–98, 97t
risk factors for, 85t, 87–88
Drug-induced diseases. *See also specific diseases*
adverse reactions and. *See* Adverse drug reactions (ADRs)
comorbidity and, 33–34
cost burden of, 26–29, 27t
defined, 24
demographic factors related to, 31–32
differential diagnosis of. *See* Differential diagnosis
documentation of, 65–66
education on. *See* Patient education

epidemiology of, 21–23, 25. *See also* Epidemiology
evaluation of patients for, 60–67, 61–62*t*, 64–65*t*
gender variations in, 32, 34–38, 36*t*
levels of evidence for, 63
lifestyle factors related to, 32–33
management of. *See* Management of disease
mechanisms of. *See* Mechanisms of disease
medication errors and. *See* Medication errors
morbidity and mortality in. *See* Morbidity and mortality
nonadherence to medications and, 28, 41
postmarketing surveillance for. *See* Postmarketing surveillance
prevention of. *See* Prevention strategies
public health impact of, 21, 24–26, 29
quantitative impact of, 23
reporting systems for, 24, 66–67
risk factors for. *See* Risk factors
signs and symptoms of. *See* Clinical presentation of disease
sources of, 19–20
Drug pseudoallergies, 71
Drug-related hospitalizations, 25–29, 26*t*, 38
Drugs. *See also specific names and classes of drugs*
adverse reactions to. *See* Adverse drug reactions (ADRs)
allergies to. *See* Drug allergies
approval process for, 11–12, 48
discontinuation of, 472*t*, 480, 625*t*
duration of detection in urine, 420, 420*t*
errors related to. *See* Medication errors
fast track approval of, 59
as haptens, 1052
hypersensitivity reactions. *See* Drug hypersensitivity reactions (DHRs)
illicit. *See* Illicit drug use
metabolism pathways for, 35, 37
orphan, 48
safety of. *See* Safety of drugs
surveillance of. *See* Postmarketing surveillance
teratogenic. *See* Teratogenicity
tolerance to, 88–89
toxicity of. *See* Toxicity
transport mechanisms for, 37, 1313
withdrawal from, 415, 417*t*, 420–422, 424, 424*t*
Drug target receptors, 37
Drug tolerance, 88–89
DSM-5. *See Diagnostic and Statistical Manual of Mental Disorders,* 5th Edition
DTaP (diphtheria-pertussis-tetanus) vaccine, 197*t*, 1267*t*
D-tubocurare, 636*t*, 638*t*
D-tubocurarine, 452*t*
Dulaglutide, 879*t*
Duloxetine
constipation and, 836*t*
hepatic/cholestatic diseases and, 851*t*
hyperprolactinemia and, 743*t*
peripheral neuropathy and, 288
serotonin syndrome and, 1203–1204*t*
sexual dysfunction and, 772
SIADH and, 981, 982*t*, 990
sleep disorders and, 348*t*
smoking and, 32
visual disturbances and, 300*t*
weight gain and, 1166*t*, 1169*t*
Dutasteride, 188*t*, 190, 206*t*, 207, 503*t*
Duty to warn, 10–11
DVT. *See* Deep vein thrombosis
Dyclonine, 1262
Dysgeusia, 1258, 1261, 1262
Dysmenorrhea, 796–797
causative agents of, 782*t*, 796
clinical presentation of, 787*t*, 797
differential diagnosis of, 788*t*, 797
epidemiology of, 796
management of, 790*t*, 797
mechanisms of, 786*t*, 796
morbidity and mortality for, 797
patient education on, 797
prevention of, 789*t*, 797
risk factors for, 788*t*, 797
Dystonia (acute and tardive), 265–270
causative agents of, 265, 266*t*
cervical, 267, 267*f*
clinical presentation of, 257*t*, 266–268, 267*f*
differential diagnosis of, 257*t*, 267, 268
epidemiology of, 265–266
management of, 270, 270*t*
mechanisms of, 266
morbidity and mortality for, 269
overview, 253–254
patient education on, 270
prevention of, 269, 269*t*
risk factors for, 268, 268*t*

Echinacea, 835
Echinacea purpurea, 300*t*
Echocardiograms, transthoracic, 665, 666–667*f*
Echothiophate iodide, 706*t*
Economic costs of drug-induced diseases, 26–29, 27*t*
Ecstasy
drug fever and, 1188*t*
hepatic/cholestatic diseases and, 864
myocardial ischemia/acute coronary syndromes and, 473*t*
serotonin syndrome and, 1203–1204*t*
SIADH and, 981, 984*t*, 985–987, 989
stroke and, 230*t*
teratogenicity of, 1321
thromboembolic diseases and, 1066*t*, 1070*t*
valvular/pericardial heart disease and, 660*t*, 663*t*, 664
ECT. *See* Electroconvulsive therapy
Eculizumab, 7*t*
Edatrexate, 169*t*
Edoxaban, 238*t*, 245, 1029*t*, 1076, 1077*t*
EDTA. *See* Ethylenediaminetetraacetic acid
Education of patients. *See* Patient education
EEGs (electroencephalograms), 220, 222, 223
Efalizumab, 1050*t*
Efaproxiral, 169*t*
Efavirenz
anxiety and, 400*t*, 403, 404
depression and, 376*t*, 377–378, 385*t*, 386, 388, 388*t*, 390, 391
diabetes insipidus and, 991*t*
drug interactions with, 39*t*
oral erythema multiforme and, 1267*t*
ototoxicity and, 1235*t*
photosensitivity and, 145*t*
psychosis and, 416*t*
torsades de pointes and, 533*t*
Eflornithine, 207
EGFRs. *See* Epidermal growth factor receptor inhibitors
Ejaculation disorders
causative agents of, 760*t*
clinical presentation of, 768*t*, 769, 770
defined, 757
differential diagnosis of, 770*t*
management of, 773*t*
mechanisms of, 764–765*t*, 766–767
Elderly populations
bone loss in, 1122
cognitive disorders in, 364, 367–368
constipation among, 836–837, 839
delirium in, 333, 334
diarrhea in, 823
hypertension in, 623
hypotension in, 641
prevalence of drug-induced diseases in, 31
systemic lupus erythematosus in, 133
tardive dyskinesia in, 260, 263
taste disorders in, 1261
Electroconvulsive therapy (ECT), 265, 391, 1197, 1200, 1200*t*, 1201
Electroencephalograms (EEGs), 220, 222, 223
Electrolysis, 205, 207, 208
Electrolyte disturbances, 34, 1153
Elevated blood pressure, 617, 619*t*, 621–625. *See also* Hypertension
Eli Lilly Company v. United States Department of Justice (2009), 9*t*, 10
Eltrombopag, 171*t*, 1059
Embolic mechanisms of stroke, 231–232
Emesis. *See* Nausea and vomiting
Emetogenic agents, 910, 914, 915, 920–921, 925, 926
Emollient laxatives, 840, 840*t*
Empagliflozin, 515, 1002*t*
Emtricitabine, 991*t*
Enalapril
acute kidney injury and, 948
alopecia and, 167*t*
color changes of oral mucosa and teeth and, 1254*t*
delirium and, 327*t*
hypotension and, 632*t*, 638*t*
myocardial ischemia/acute coronary syndromes and, 472*t*, 477*t*, 478
oral lichenoid reactions and, 1270*t*
ototoxicity and, 1235*t*
pancreatitis and, 878*t*, 880, 886*t*, 887
peripheral neuropathy and, 281*t*
photosensitivity and, 145*t*
SIADH and, 983*t*
systemic lupus erythematosus and, 124*t*
taste disorders and, 1259*t*, 1261*t*
Enalaprilat, 478, 1235*t*
Encainide, 472*t*, 502*t*, 507, 510*t*, 528
Encephalocele, 1327–1329, 1328*f*
Endocrine agents, 848–849*t*
Endogenous Cushing syndrome, 730, 733
Endometrial cancer, 1301–1303
causative agents of, 1285*t*, 1301
clinical presentation of, 1290*t*, 1301–1302
differential diagnosis of, 1290*t*, 1301–1302
epidemiology of, 1301
management of, 1303
mechanisms of, 1288*t*, 1301
morbidity and mortality for, 1302
patient education on, 1303
prevention of, 1294*t*, 1302–1303
risk factors for, 1291*t*, 1302
Endothelin, 951
Endothelin-1, 232, 478
Endothelin modifiers, 636*t*
Endothelin receptor antagonists, 440
Endotoxins, 1185
End stage renal disease (ESRD), 965, 967, 968, 972, 974, 975
Enflurane, 472*t*, 850*t*, 906*t*, 1209*t*, 1210
Enoxacin, 145*t*

INDEX

Enoxaparin, 77*t*, 167*t*, 239, 487*t*, 1034, 1055
Enoximone, 582*t*, 592*t*
Entacapone, 348*t*, 635*t*, 640*t*
Entecavir, 966–967, 966*t*, 970*t*
Enteral nutrition, 1003*t*
Environmental chemicals, 845, 849–850*t*
Environmental goitrogens, 701*t*
Ephedra
  intracerebral hemorrhage and, 238*t*, 240, 240*t*, 243
  myocardial ischemia/acute coronary syndromes and, 473*t*
  seizures and, 219*t*, 221, 225
Ephedra alkaloids, 618*t*
Ephedrine
  anxiety and, 400*t*, 404, 409
  intracerebral hemorrhage and, 240
  monomorphic ventricular tachycardia and, 524*t*, 527*f*
  myocardial ischemia/acute coronary syndromes and, 473*t*
  nausea/vomiting and, 924*t*
  psychosis and, 416*t*, 418*t*
  stroke and, 232
Epidemiology
  of acidosis, 1001
  of acute interstitial nephritis, 956
  of acute tubular necrosis, 950
  of akathisia, 254–255
  of alkalosis, 1012
  of alopecia, 177–178
  of amenorrhea and oligomenorrhea, 793
  of anxiety, 404, 404*t*
  of aplastic anemia, 1100
  of asthma and bronchospasm, 451, 453–454
  of atrial fibrillation/atrial flutter, 581, 583
  of atrial tachycardia, 588
  of AV node re-entrant tachycardia, 592
  of bladder cancer, 1303–1304
  of bleeding disorders, 1026–1028
  of breast cancer, 1299
  of Brugada syndrome, 546
  of chemotherapy-induced anemia, 1109
  of chronic kidney disease, 967–969
  of cognitive disorders, 357–359
  of color changes of oral mucosa and teeth, 1255
  of congenital heart defects, 1322–1323
  of constipation, 835–837
  of Cushing syndrome, 730
  of cutaneous diseases, 104–105
  defined, 20
  of delirium, 325, 328–329, 357–358
  of depression, 377–385
  of diabetes insipidus, 991
  of diarrhea, 822–823
  of drug allergies and hypersensitivity reactions, 76–78
  of drug fever, 1187
  of drug-induced diseases, 21–23, 25
  of dysmenorrhea, 796
  of dystonia, 265–266
  of endometrial cancer, 1301
  of female sexual dysfunction, 798
  of fetal alcohol spectrum disorders, 1332
  of gastroschisis, 1326
  of gingival hyperplasia, 1263
  of glomerulonephritis, 958
  of glucose and insulin dysregulation, 681, 683
  of gout and hyperuricemia, 1135
  of growth hormone deficiency, 747
  of heart failure, 505–509
  of hemodynamic-mediated AKI, 942, 944
  of hemolytic anemia, 1104
  of hepatic and cholestatic diseases, 845, 853
  of hirsutism, 197–198
  of hyperprolactinemia, 742
  of hypertension, 617–619
  of hypertrichosis, 197–198
  of hypotension, 631, 637
  of hypothermia, 1215
  of infertility, 800
  of interstitial lung disease/pulmonary fibrosis, 433–434
  of intracerebral hemorrhage, 239–240
  of learning disabilities, 1315
  of leukemia, 1286–1287
  levels of evidence in, 20–21, 21*t*
  of limb deficiency defects, 1324–1325
  of low birth weight, 1316–1317
  of lymphoma, 1293
  of macrocytic anemia, 1107
  of male sexual dysfunction, 761–762
  of malignant hyperthermia, 1210
  of menorrhagia and menometrorrhagia, 795
  of microcephaly, 1330–1331
  of monomorphic ventricular tachycardia, 523
  in morbidity and mortality explanations, 21, 22, 25, 26
  of myocardial ischemia/acute coronary syndromes, 474–476
  of myopathy, 1151
  of nausea and vomiting, 910
  of nephrolithiasis, 957
  of neural tube defects, 1328
  of neuroleptic malignant syndrome, 1196
  of neutropenia and agranulocytosis, 1088, 1091
  of oral erythema multiforme, 1266
  of oral lichenoid reactions, 1270
  of orofacial clefts, 1319–1320
  of osteonecrosis of jaw, 1273–1274
  of osteoporosis and osteomalacia, 1120
  of ototoxicity, 1239
  of ovarian hyperstimulation, 781, 783
  overview, 20
  of pancreatitis, 879–885
  of parkinsonism, 270–271
  of peripheral neuropathy, 279
  pharmacoepidemiology, 20, 54
  of photosensitivity, 143, 148
  postmarketing surveillance as tool in, 53, 54
  of psychosis, 417
  of secondary adrenal insufficiency, 735
  of seizures, 217, 219–222
  of serotonin syndrome, 1202
  of serum sickness-like reactions, 1192
  of SIADH, 985
  of sinus bradycardia/atrioventricular block, 572
  of skin cancer, 1296
  of sleep disorders, 347
  of stroke, 231
  of systemic lupus erythematosus, 123, 127
  of tardive dyskinesia, 260–261
  of taste disorders, 1258, 1261
  of thrombocytopenia, 1050, 1052
  of thromboembolic diseases, 1063, 1066
  of thyroid diseases, 704
  of torsades de pointes, 534–535
  of upper gastrointestinal ulceration, 810–811
  of valvular and pericardial heart disease, 662–663
  of visual disturbances, 313
  of vulvovaginal candidiasis, 791
  of weight gain, 1165, 1167–1168
Epidermal growth factor receptor inhibitors (EGFRs), 102*t*, 105–106, 108, 432*t*, 433, 435*t*
Epilepsy. *See* Seizures
Epinephrine, 98, 99, 454, 473*t*, 580, 1002*t*
Epipodophyllotoxins, 1285–1286, 1291
Epirubicin
  alopecia and, 169*t*
  heart failure and, 502*t*, 510*t*
  leukemia and, 1288*t*
  myocardial ischemia/acute coronary syndromes and, 472*t*
  nausea/vomiting and, 908*t*
  photosensitivity and, 145*t*
Epitope, 1052, 1053
Eplerenone, 1003*t*
Epoetin alpha, 646*t*, 647, 1111
Epoprostenol, 636*t*, 640*t*, 645*t*, 700*t*
Eprosartan, 632*t*, 638*t*, 1259*t*
EPS. *See* Extrapyramidal symptoms
Epsilon aminocaproic acid, 1156
Eptifibatide, 1029*t*, 1050*t*, 1052*t*, 1053, 1064*t*, 1068*t*
Erectile dysfunction
  causative agents of, 757, 759–760*t*
  clinical presentation of, 768, 768*t*, 769
  defined, 757
  differential diagnosis of, 770*t*
  epidemiology of, 761–762
  management of, 773*t*
  mechanisms of, 763–764*t*, 766
Ergocalciferol, 1259*t*
Ergonovine, 472*t*, 620*t*
Ergot alkaloids
  hypertension and, 618*t*, 620*t*
  hypotension and, 547
  myocardial ischemia/acute coronary syndromes and, 474, 477*t*, 478, 485
  valvular/pericardial heart disease and, 659, 661–663
Ergotamine
  hypotension and, 647
  myocardial ischemia/acute coronary syndromes and, 472*t*
  thromboembolic diseases and, 1066*t*, 1070*t*
  valvular/pericardial heart disease and, 659–664, 660–661*t*, 663*t*, 668, 668–669*t*
Ergotamine tartrate, 646*t*
Eribulin, 169*t*, 908*t*
Erlotinib
  alopecia and, 169*t*, 177, 179*t*
  chemotherapy-induced anemia and, 1109*t*
  cutaneous diseases and, 102*t*
  hypertrichosis and, 196*t*
  interstitial lung disease/pulmonary fibrosis and, 432*t*, 438
  ototoxicity and, 1235*t*
  thyroid diseases and, 699*t*
  visual disturbances and, 300*t*
Errors. *See* Medication errors
ERT (estrogen-replacement therapy), 621
Ertapenem, 92, 328*t*
Erythematous rash, 107–108*t*
Erythromycin
  acute kidney injury and, 943*t*
  adverse effects of, 11
  comorbidity and, 34
  cutaneous diseases and, 102*t*
  diarrhea and, 823, 823*t*
  drug fever and, 1188*t*
  gingival hyperplasia and, 1263*t*
  hemolytic anemia and, 1105*t*
  hepatic/cholestatic diseases and, 846*t*

myocardial ischemia/acute coronary syndromes and, 474
nausea/vomiting and, 909*t*, 911*t*, 915, 920, 930
neutropenia/agranulocytosis and, 1089*t*
oral lichenoid reactions and, 1270*t*
osteonecrosis of jaw and, 1276
ototoxicity and, 1235*t*
pancreatitis and, 879*t*, 886*t*
serotonin syndrome and, 1204
sexual dysfunction and, 762*t*, 765*t*
torsades de pointes and, 532*t*, 536, 538, 540*t*, 541–542
upper gastrointestinal ulceration and, 810–811*t*

Erythromycin estolate, 861*t*

Erythropoiesis-stimulating agents (ESAs), 620*t*, 626, 822*t*, 1110, 1111, 1111*t*

Erythropoietin
chemotherapy-induced anemia and, 1110
dosing of, 1111*t*
hypertension and, 625*t*
hypertrichosis and, 194, 195, 196*t*, 198
myocardial ischemia/acute coronary syndromes and, 472*t*
peripheral neuropathy and, 287*t*
thromboembolic diseases and, 1064*t*, 1068*t*, 1075*t*

Erythropoietin-α, 618*t*, 621, 626

ESAs. *See* Erythropoiesis-stimulating agents

Escitalopram
alopecia and, 173*t*
serotonin syndrome and, 1203–1204*t*
sexual dysfunction and, 762*t*, 772
SIADH and, 982*t*
sinus bradycardia/atrioventricular block and, 570*t*, 577*t*
sleep disorders and, 348*t*
thromboembolic diseases and, 1066*t*, 1070*t*
thyroid diseases and, 699*t*, 710
torsades de pointes and, 532*t*, 539*t*
weight gain and, 1166*t*, 1169*t*

Esmolol, 587*t*, 632*t*, 638*t*

Esomeprazole, 126*t*, 965, 966*t*, 984*t*

ESRD. *See* End stage renal disease

Estazolam, 352

Esterified estrogens, 178

Estradiol, 538, 784, 787, 790*t*, 793, 800

Estramustine, 169*t*, 1065*t*, 1069*t*, 1075*t*

Estrogen-replacement therapy (ERT), 621

Estrogens
alopecia and, 176, 178, 180, 191
anxiety and, 400*t*, 402, 405*t*, 406
asthma/bronchospasm and, 452*t*
breast cancer and, 1285*t*, 1288*t*, 1298–1301
conjugated, 702*t*, 790*t*, 1302
depression and, 382, 385–386, 388
endometrial cancer and, 1285*t*, 1288*t*, 1301, 1302
esterified, 178
growth hormone deficiency and, 750, 751
hepatic/cholestatic diseases and, 849*t*
hyperprolactinemia and, 742, 743–744*t*
hypertension and, 618*t*, 620–621, 620*t*, 624–626
myocardial ischemia/acute coronary syndromes and, 473*t*, 475, 477*t*, 482
nausea/vomiting and, 911*t*
pancreatitis and, 878*t*, 882–883, 885, 886*t*
photosensitivity and, 145*t*
sexual dysfunction and, 758–759*t*, 762–765*t*, 790*t*, 799–800
stroke and, 229
systemic lupus erythematosus and, 126*t*
thromboembolic diseases and, 1064*t*, 1068*t*, 1071, 1074–1075, 1077
thyroid diseases and, 702*t*
torsades de pointes and, 538
vaginal bleeding disorders and, 782*t*, 785–786*t*, 794, 796

Estropipate cream, 790*t*

Eszopiclone, 352, 1259*t*

Etanercept
allergic reactions to, 74*t*
alopecia and, 173*t*
cutaneous diseases and, 103*t*, 109, 113
depression and, 383
heart failure and, 503*t*, 509, 510*t*
hepatic/cholestatic diseases and, 852*t*
interstitial lung disease/pulmonary fibrosis and, 433*t*
neutropenia/agranulocytosis and, 1089*t*
oral lichenoid reactions and, 1271*t*
skin cancer and, 1297
systemic lupus erythematosus and, 126*t*, 128*t*

Ethacrynate, 638*t*

Ethacrynic acid, 633*t*, 879*t*, 1235*t*, 1242*t*, 1243

Ethambutol
gout/hyperuricemia and, 1136*t*, 1138–1139
oral erythema multiforme and, 1267*t*
peripheral neuropathy and, 280*t*, 288
taste disorders and, 1259*t*
thrombocytopenia and, 1050*t*
visual disturbances and, 300*t*, 315

Ethanol
asthma/bronchospasm and, 452*t*
glucose/insulin dysregulation and, 681, 682*t*, 685*t*
gout/hyperuricemia and, 1136*t*, 1139, 1144*t*
hepatic/cholestatic diseases and, 852*t*
metabolism of, 33
myocardial ischemia/acute coronary syndromes and, 473*t*
nausea/vomiting and, 915
seizures and, 217, 219
sexual dysfunction and, 758–759*t*, 761–765*t*
visual disturbances and, 301*t*

Ethinyl estradiol, 191, 206*t*, 229, 702*t*, 1067, 1075

Ethinyl estradiol–levonorgestrel, 909*t*

Ethinyl estradiol–norethindrone, 909*t*

Ethiodized oil, 706*t*

Ethionamide
alopecia and, 174*t*, 179*t*
depression and, 376*t*, 377
hepatic/cholestatic diseases and, 846*t*
oral lichenoid reactions and, 1271*t*
ototoxicity and, 1235*t*
photosensitivity and, 145*t*
taste disorders and, 1259*t*
thyroid diseases and, 699*t*, 702*t*, 710

Ethionine, 849*t*

Ethosuximide, 124*t*, 254, 1089*t*, 1263*t*, 1319

Ethyl bromide/chloride, 849*t*

Ethylenediaminetetraacetic acid (EDTA), 452*t*, 454, 1055, 1259*t*, 1261*t*

Ethynodiol, 191

Ethynodiol diacetate, 206*t*

Etidronate, 301*t*, 452*t*, 1235*t*, 1274*t*

Etodolac
alopecia and, 172*t*
aplastic anemia and, 1100*t*
heart failure and, 510*t*
hemolytic anemia and, 1105*t*
hepatic/cholestatic diseases and, 846*t*
ototoxicity and, 1235*t*
upper gastrointestinal ulceration and, 817
visual disturbances and, 301*t*

Etomidate, 573*t*, 735, 736–737*t*, 737, 907*t*

Etoposide
allergic reactions to, 73*t*
alopecia and, 169*t*
hepatic/cholestatic diseases and, 848*t*
hypotension and, 636*t*, 640*t*, 645*t*
infertility and, 783*t*, 786*t*
leukemia and, 1284*t*, 1285–1287, 1288*t*
myocardial ischemia/acute coronary syndromes and, 472*t*
nausea/vomiting and, 908*t*
peripheral neuropathy and, 280*t*
SIADH and, 983*t*
thromboembolic diseases and, 1065*t*
vaginal bleeding disorders and, 782*t*, 785*t*

Etravirine, 1267*t*

Etretinate, 166, 173*t*, 852*t*, 1050*t*, 1150*t*, 1152*t*

Eucalyptus, 219*t*, 221

Evaluation of patients, 60–67, 61–62*t*, 64–65*t*

Everolimus, 169*t*, 196*t*, 432*t*, 438, 700*t*, 1188*t*, 1293, 1298

Excessive hair growth. *See* Hirsutism; Hypertrichosis

Excipients, 73*t*

Exemestane, 169*t*

Exenatide
alopecia and, 174*t*, 179*t*
nausea/vomiting and, 909*t*, 915
pancreatitis and, 879*t*, 884

Experiments, in epidemiology, 22

Extrapyramidal symptoms (EPS), 253–254, 262, 269, 271–272, 338–340

Eye disturbances. *See* Visual disturbances

Ezetimibe, 1150*t*, 1152*t*

Ezogabine, 168*t*

Factor VIII inhibitor/prothrombin complex concentrates, 472*t*

Fainting. *See* Syncope

Famotidine
delirium and, 328*t*
hemolytic anemia and, 1105*t*
hyperprolactinemia and, 743*t*
neutropenia/agranulocytosis and, 1089*t*
ototoxicity and, 1235*t*
sinus bradycardia/atrioventricular block and, 573*t*, 577*t*
thrombocytopenia and, 1050*t*
torsades de pointes and, 533*t*, 539*t*
weight gain and, 1174

FAS (fetal alcohol syndrome), 1331–1333

FASD (fetal alcohol spectrum disorders), 1331–1333, 1332*t*

Fast track drug approval, 59

Fat emulsion, 761*t*, 765*t*

FDA. *See* Food and Drug Administration, U.S.

FDAAA (Food and Drug Administration Amendments Act of 2007), 5, 55, 67

FD&C (Food, Drug, and Cosmetic) Act of 1938, 5, 47, 48

FDASIA (Food and Drug Administration Safety and Innovation Act of 2012), 5, 7, 12

FDEs (fixed drug eruptions), 102*t*, 105–108, 107–108*t*, 114*t*

Febuxostat, 171*t*, 1136–1137, 1136*t*, 1144

Federal Food and Drugs Act of 1906, 5

Felbamate
acute kidney injury and, 958
alopecia and, 168*t*
aplastic anemia and, 1100*t*
hepatic/cholestatic diseases and, 851*t*
seizures and, 218*t*, 224
SIADH and, 983*t*

INDEX

Felbamate (continued)
sleep disorders and, 348*t*
tardive dyskinesia and, 254
Feldman v. Lederle Laboratories (1984), 8, 9*t*
Felodipine, 1263*t*
gingival hyperplasia and, 1263*t*
heart failure and, 505, 510, 515
hypotension and, 633*t*, 639*t*
myocardial ischemia/acute coronary syndromes and, 472*t*
photosensitivity and, 145*t*
Females. *See* Gender differences; Gynecologic diseases
Female sexual dysfunction, 797–800
causative agents of, 783*t*, 797–798
clinical presentation of, 787*t*, 798–799
differential diagnosis of, 788*t*, 799
epidemiology of, 798
management of, 790*t*, 799–800
mechanisms of, 786*t*, 798
morbidity and mortality for, 799
patient education on, 800
prevention of, 789*t*, 799
risk factors for, 788*t*, 799
Fenclofenac, 1271*t*
Fenfluramine, 659, 660*t*, 663–664, 663*t*, 668–670, 668*t*, 852*t*
Fenfluramine–phentermine, 9
Fenofibrate, 145*t*, 849*t*, 879, 1050*t*, 1136–1137, 1152*t*, 1156, 1235*t*
Fenoldopam, 472*t*, 633*t*, 640*t*, 645*t*, 953–954
Fenoprofen, 510*t*, 956, 1235*t*
Fentanyl
alopecia and, 172*t*
constipation and, 836*t*
delirium and, 326*t*
hypotension and, 636*t*, 638*t*
nausea/vomiting and, 906*t*
restrictive drug distribution system for, 7*t*
secondary adrenal insufficiency and, 736–737*t*
serotonin syndrome and, 1203–1204*t*
SIADH and, 984*t*
Fenugreek, 682*t*, 685*t*
Ferriman–Gallwey scoring system for hirsutism, 200, 200*f*
Ferrous gluconate, 909*t*
Ferrous salts, 852*t*
Ferrous sulfate, 463, 702*t*, 809–810, 810–811*t*, 909*t*, 1259*t*
Fetal alcohol spectrum disorders (FASD), 1331–1333, 1332*t*
Fetal alcohol syndrome (FAS), 1331–1333
Fever. *See* Drug fever; Hyperthermia
FFP (fresh frozen plasma), 245, 1037*t*
Fibrates, 1150*t*, 1152, 1156
Fibrinogen inhibitors, 1053, 1057
Fibrinolytics, 661*t*, 662, 664, 668–669*t*, 669
Fidaxomicin, 829
Filgrastim, 171*t*, 1094, 1284*t*, 1288*t*
Finasteride
alopecia and, 188*t*, 190–191
depression and, 376*t*, 382
hirsutism and, 206*t*, 207
myopathy and, 1150*t*
teratogenicity of, 1334*t*
Fingolimod, 172*t*, 301*t*, 570*t*, 572–574, 573–574*t*, 582*t*
First-degree AV block, 569, 575, 578, 579
Fish oil, 680*t*, 684*t*
5 Rights of Medication Administration, 42
Fixed drug eruptions (FDEs), 102*t*, 105–108, 107–108*t*, 114*t*
Flecainide
atrial fibrillation/atrial flutter and, 582*t*, 584, 587, 587*t*
Brugada syndrome and, 546, 547*t*, 548
heart failure and, 502*t*, 507, 510*t*, 511, 515
monomorphic ventricular tachycardia and, 524–525*t*, 528–530
neutropenia/agranulocytosis and, 1091, 1091*t*
ototoxicity and, 1235*t*
sinus bradycardia/atrioventricular block and, 570*t*, 573*t*, 577–578*t*
torsades de pointes and, 532*t*, 539–540*t*
Flibanserin, 7*t*
Floxuridine, 472*t*, 848*t*
Flucloxacillin, 37, 846*t*
Fluconazole, 1267*t*
alopecia and, 168*t*, 177
bleeding disorders and, 1031
cutaneous diseases and, 102–103*t*
drug interactions with, 39*t*
myocardial ischemia/acute coronary syndromes and, 472*t*, 474
oral erythema multiforme and, 1267*t*
thrombocytopenia and, 1050*t*
torsades de pointes and, 532*t*, 539*t*
vulvovaginal candidiasis and, 790*t*, 792
Flucytosine, 145*t*, 846*t*, 1089*t*
Fludarabine, 570*t*, 577*t*, 636*t*, 640*t*, 1106, 1235*t*
Fludrocortisone, 195–196*t*, 645–648, 646*t*, 1013–1014*t*
Fluindione, 1029*t*
Flumazenil, 400*t*, 424*t*
Flunarizine, 271*t*, 273*t*
Flunitrazepam, 736–737*t*
Fluorine, 702*t*
Fluoroquinolones
allergic reactions to, 73–74*t*
anxiety and, 400*t*, 403
delirium and, 328*t*
depression and, 376*t*, 377
diarrhea and, 821, 822*t*
drug fever and, 1188*t*
glucose/insulin dysregulation and, 682*t*, 685*t*
hemolytic anemia and, 1104, 1105*t*
hepatic/cholestatic diseases and, 846*t*, 870
neutropenia/agranulocytosis and, 1095
photosensitivity and, 143, 150
psychosis and, 418*t*
seizures and, 218*t*, 222*t*, 224, 225
Fluorouracil
alopecia and, 169*t*, 176, 176*f*
color changes of oral mucosa and teeth and, 1254*t*
diarrhea and, 825, 826
heart failure and, 503*t*, 510*t*
hepatic/cholestatic diseases and, 848*t*
infertility and, 783*t*, 786*t*
myocardial ischemia/acute coronary syndromes and, 472*t*
oral erythema multiforme and, 1267*t*
peripheral neuropathy and, 280*t*
photosensitivity and, 145*t*
seizures and, 218*t*
systemic lupus erythematosus and, 126*t*
taste disorders and, 1259*t*, 1261*t*
thromboembolic diseases and, 1065*t*, 1069*t*
thyroid diseases and, 702*t*
valvular/pericardial heart disease and, 661*t*
visual disturbances and, 301*t*, 316
weight gain and, 1172
Fluoxetine
allergic reactions to, 74*t*
alopecia and, 173*t*
atrial fibrillation/atrial flutter and, 582*t*
AV node re-entrant tachycardia and, 592*t*, 594
constipation and, 836*t*
delirium and, 326*t*, 329*t*
drug fever and, 1188*t*
drug interactions with, 39*t*
hyperprolactinemia and, 743*t*
hypotension and, 646*t*, 647
myocardial ischemia/acute coronary syndromes and, 472*t*
nausea/vomiting and, 909*t*, 920
ototoxicity and, 1235*t*
photosensitivity and, 145*t*
seizures and, 220, 222*t*
serotonin syndrome and, 1202, 1203–1204*t*, 1207
serum sickness-like reactions and, 1193*t*, 1194
sexual dysfunction and, 772
SIADH and, 982*t*
sinus bradycardia/atrioventricular block and, 577–578*t*
sleep disorders and, 348*t*, 353
taste disorders and, 1259*t*
teratogenicity of, 1323
torsades de pointes and, 533*t*, 539–540*t*
visual disturbances and, 301*t*
weight gain and, 1166*t*, 1169*t*, 1174
Fluoxymesterone, 167*t*, 195*t*
Flupenthixol, 265
Fluperlapine, 265
Fluphenazine
delirium and, 326*t*
hepatic/cholestatic diseases and, 851*t*
neuroleptic malignant syndrome and, 1195, 1195*t*
photosensitivity and, 145*t*
SIADH and, 982*t*
weight gain and, 1167*t*
Flurazepam, 1259*t*
Flurbiprofen, 510*t*, 646*t*, 647
Flutamide
alopecia and, 188*t*, 190, 191
hepatic/cholestatic diseases and, 848*t*
hirsutism and, 206, 206*t*
interstitial lung disease/pulmonary fibrosis and, 432*t*
myocardial ischemia/acute coronary syndromes and, 472*t*
photosensitivity and, 145*t*
systemic lupus erythematosus and, 126*t*
teratogenicity of, 1334*t*
thromboembolic diseases and, 1064*t*, 1068*t*
Fluticasone, 74*t*, 439, 732, 733, 739
Fluticasone furoate, 731*t*
Fluticasone propionate, 731*t*, 736*t*, 738
Fluvastatin, 124*t*, 145*t*, 878*t*, 886*t*
Fluvoxamine
alopecia and, 173*t*
drug interactions with, 39*t*
hyperprolactinemia and, 743*t*
myocardial ischemia/acute coronary syndromes and, 472*t*
seizures and, 220
serotonin syndrome and, 1203–1204*t*
sexual dysfunction and, 772
SIADH and, 982*t*
sleep disorders and, 348*t*
visual disturbances and, 301*t*
weight gain and, 1166*t*, 1169*t*
Focal atrial tachycardia. *See* Atrial tachycardia

Folate, 1107, 1108, 1328, 1329
FOLFIRI regimen, 433
FOLFOX regimen, 433
Folic acid
  drug fever and, 1188*t*
  gingival hyperplasia and, 1264, 1265
  hepatic/cholestatic diseases and, 866
  macrocytic anemia and, 1107–1109
  teratogenicity of, 1328, 1329
Follicle-stimulating hormone (FSH), 767, 770, 783, 793, 800, 1065*t*, 1069*t*
Follitropin-alfa, 1065*t*, 1069*t*
Fondaparinux, 487*t*, 1026*t*, 1029*t*, 1039, 1055, 1076
Food, Drug, and Cosmetic (FD&C) Act of 1938, 5, 47, 48
Food allergies, 824–825
Food and Drug Administration, U.S. (FDA)
  Adverse Event Reporting System of, 4, 6, 24, 31, 381, 882
  on anorexiant drug–related cardiac valvulopathy, 663, 664
  on aristolochic acid, 969, 975
  on bipolar disorder, 378
  on bisphosphonates, 581, 583
  on cabergoline labeling, 662
  Center for Drug Evaluation and Research, 13
  clinically relevant weight gain as defined by, 1167
  on COX-2 inhibitors, 230, 231, 942
  on dietary supplements, 969, 975, 976
  DigniCap approval by, 186
  electrolysis approval by, 205
  on erythrocyte stimulating agents, 1111
  on estrogen labeling, 475
  fast track approval by, 59
  on GBL-containing products, 1215
  on hepatosplenic T-cell lymphoma, 1292
  on HIT treatments, 1058
  insomnia treatments approved by, 353
  interpretation of reports to, 474
  interstitial lung disease/pulmonary fibrosis therapies approved by, 431, 440
  on isotretinoin and depression, 384, 387
  medication error prevention efforts by, 42
  medication guidelines required by, 392
  MedWatch program from, 6, 15, 50, 66–67
  on metoclopramide product labeling, 261
  on montelukast-induced anxiety, 404
  on NSAIDs and stoke risk, 230, 231
  orthostatic hypotension treatments approved by, 646–647
  on pancreatitis, 884, 885
  on pergolide labeling, 661
  phenylpropanolamine banned by, 242
  postmarketing surveillance by. *See* Postmarketing surveillance
  promethazine warnings from, 922
  on quinine, 1052
  regulatory functions of, 19
  risk-benefit balance used by, 20
  on rosiglitazone, 476
  safety activities and regulations, 4–8, 4*f*, 14–15
  Science Board report from, 14, 15
  Sentinel Network of, 55, 57, 67
  SIADH treatments approved by, 989–990
  on SSRI-induced hyponatremia, 988
  on teratogenicity, 32, 1311–1312, 1320
  terfenadine-related TdP reported to, 539
  on testosterone use, 476
  on thyroid diseases in infants, 709
  varenicline advisory issued by, 402
  withdrawal of products from market, 3
Food and Drug Administration Amendments Act of 2007 (FDAAA), 5, 55, 67
Food and Drug Administration Safety and Innovation Act of 2012 (FDASIA), 5, 7, 12
Food–drug interactions, 40–41
Formoterol, 473*t*, 879
Fosamprenavir, 92, 1267*t*
Fosaprepitant, 926
Foscarnet
  acidosis and, 1003*t*
  acute kidney injury and, 944*t*, 952, 957
  allergic reactions to, 87
  diabetes insipidus and, 991*t*, 993
  heart failure and, 503*t*, 509
  SIADH and, 984*t*
  thromboembolic diseases and, 1065*t*, 1069*t*
Fosinopril, 145*t*, 632*t*, 638*t*, 1254*t*
Fosphenytoin, 88, 112, 634*t*, 640*t*, 645*t*, 991*t*
Free fatty acids, 702*t*
Fresh frozen plasma (FFP), 245, 1037*t*
FSH. *See* Follicle-stimulating hormone
2(3H)-furanone, 1215
Furosemide
  acute kidney injury and, 944*t*, 954, 957
  aplastic anemia and, 1100*t*
  AV node re-entrant tachycardia and, 592–594, 592–594*t*
  constipation and, 836*t*, 837
  drug fever and, 1188*t*
  graded challenge procedure for, 88
  hepatic/cholestatic diseases and, 870
  hypotension and, 633*t*, 638*t*
  neutropenia/agranulocytosis and, 1089*t*
  oral erythema multiforme and, 1267*t*
  oral lichenoid reactions and, 1271*t*
  osteoporosis/osteomalacia and, 1121*t*, 1123*t*
  ototoxicity and, 1235*t*, 1242, 1243
  pancreatitis and, 878*t*, 883, 886*t*, 891
  photosensitivity and, 145*t*, 150
  SIADH and, 989, 989*t*
  taste disorders and, 1258, 1259*t*
  thyroid diseases and, 702*t*
  visual disturbances and, 301*t*
Fusidic acid, 847*t*
Fusion proteins, 95
The Future of Drug Safety (IOM), 53

GABA. *See* Gamma-aminobutyric acid
Gabapentin
  alopecia and, 168*t*
  anxiety and, 400*t*, 402, 404, 407
  cognitive disorders and, 367
  depression and, 379
  hepatic/cholestatic diseases and, 852*t*
  nausea/vomiting and, 923–924
  oral lichenoid reactions and, 1271*t*
  peripheral neuropathy and, 289
  for seizure disorders, 95
  sexual dysfunction and, 759*t*
  tardive dyskinesia and, 254
  teratogenicity of, 1319, 1331
  visual disturbances and, 301*t*
  weight gain and, 1166*t*, 1169, 1169*t*, 1170, 1173*t*
Galantamine, 633*t*, 640*t*
Gallamine, 452*t*
Gamma-aminobutyric acid (GABA)
  cognitive disorders and, 360
  delirium and, 329
  depression and, 386
  dystonia and, 266
  hyperthermia and, 1186
  hypothermia and, 1215, 1216
  seizures and, 222, 226
  serotonin syndrome and, 1205
  tardive dyskinesia and, 261
Gamma-butyrolactone (GBL), 1215, 1215–1216*t*, 1217
Gamma-hydroxybutyrate (GHB), 1186, 1215–1216*t*, 1215–1217
Gamma-hydroxybutyric acid, 570*t*, 731*t*
Ganciclovir, 145*t*, 416*t*, 984*t*, 1089*t*, 1188*t*
GAO (Government Accountability Office), 12–13
Garcinia cambogia, 850*t*
Garlic, 850*t*
Gastric motility agents, 255*t*, 260*t*, 261, 266*t*, 271*t*
Gastrointestinal (GI) drugs, 26*t*, 742, 850*t*
Gastrointestinal ulceration. *See* Upper gastrointestinal ulceration
Gastroschisis, 1326–1327, 1326*f*
Gatifloxacin, 328*t*, 532*t*, 539*t*
GBL (gamma-butyrolactone), 1215, 1215–1216*t*, 1217
G-CSF. *See* Granulocyte colony-stimulating factor
Gefitinib
  alopecia and, 169*t*, 177, 179*t*
  cutaneous diseases and, 102*t*
  interstitial lung disease/pulmonary fibrosis and, 432*t*, 434, 437, 438
  restrictive drug distribution system for, 7*t*
Gell and Coombs classification of allergic reactions, 79–81, 80*t*
Gemcitabine
  alopecia and, 169*t*
  hepatic/cholestatic diseases and, 848*t*
  interstitial lung disease/pulmonary fibrosis and, 432*t*, 435*t*
  myocardial ischemia/acute coronary syndromes and, 472*t*
  systemic lupus erythematosus and, 126*t*
  thromboembolic diseases and, 1065*t*, 1069*t*
  visual disturbances and, 301*t*
Gemfibrozil
  hepatic/cholestatic diseases and, 849*t*, 868
  myopathy and, 1152*t*, 1156
  sexual dysfunction and, 759*t*, 763*t*
  systemic lupus erythematosus and, 124*t*
Gemifloxacin, 145*t*
Gender differences
  in alopecia, 178, 180, 181*t*, 183, 184
  in asthma and bronchospasm, 459–460
  in constipation, 836
  cutaneous diseases and, 111
  in drug allergies and hypersensitivity reactions, 86, 87
  gingival hyperplasia and, 1264
  in gout and hyperuricemia, 1143
  intracerebral hemorrhage and, 242–243
  in malignant hyperthermia, 1210
  in nausea and vomiting, 917
  in neuroleptic malignant syndrome, 1196
  oral erythema multiforme and, 1269
  oral lichenoid reactions and, 1273
  in prevalence of drug-induced diseases, 31–32
  systemic lupus erythematosus and, 132, 133
  taste disorders and, 1261
  in thyroid diseases, 704, 713
  torsades de pointes and, 538
General anesthetics, 850*t*
Genetic biomarkers, 16

INDEX

Genetic factors
  anemia and, 1099–1100
  anxiety and, 408–409
  in bleeding disorders, 1031
  in cognitive disorders, 365
  cutaneous diseases and, 111–112
  in drug allergies and hypersensitivity reactions, 86–87
  in drug-induced diseases, 15–16, 16*t*, 32, 34–38, 36*t*
  gingival hyperplasia and, 1265
  in hypotension, 643
  in interstitial lung disease/pulmonary fibrosis and, 437
  leukemia and, 1290
  myopathy and, 1156–1157
  in peripheral neuropathy, 285
  serotonin syndrome and, 1206–1207
  systemic lupus erythematosus and, 129
  torsades de pointes and, 540–541
Gentamicin
  acute kidney injury and, 952–953, 955
  allergic reactions to, 73*t*
  alopecia and, 174*t*, 179*t*
  neutropenia/agranulocytosis and, 1089*t*
  ototoxicity and, 1235*t*, 1241, 1243
  visual disturbances and, 301*t*, 319
Geriatric populations. *See* Elderly populations
Germander, 850*t*
Gestational timing, 1314
Gestodene, 1075
GH. *See* Growth hormone
GHB (gamma-hydroxybutyrate), 1186, 1215–1216*t*, 1215–1217
GHIH (growth hormone-inhibiting hormone), 747
GHRH (growth hormone-releasing hormone), 747, 748
GI (gastrointestinal) drugs, 26*t*, 742, 850*t*
Ginger, 924, 927
Gingival hyperplasia, 1262–1265
  causative agents of, 1253, 1262–1263, 1263*t*
  clinical presentation of, 1256*t*, 1264
  differential diagnosis of, 1257*t*, 1264
  epidemiology of, 1263
  management of, 1265
  mechanisms of, 1264, 1264*t*
  morbidity and mortality for, 1265
  patient education on, 1265
  prevention of, 1265, 1265*t*
  risk factors for, 1258*t*, 1264–1265
Ginkgo biloba, 219*t*, 221, 264, 301*t*, 524*t*, 822
Ginseng, 219*t*, 682*t*, 685*t*, 782*t*, 785*t*, 795
Glatiramer acetate, 383
Glial-derived neurotrophic factor, 1242*t*
Glimepiride, 146*t*, 983*t*
Glipizide, 35, 146*t*, 983*t*, 1270, 1271*t*
Glitazones, 503*t*, 505–506, 511, 513, 514*t*
Glomerulonephritis, 943*t*, 946*t*, 958–960
Glucagon, 98, 580, 870
Glucagon-like peptide 1 (GLP-1) receptor agonists
  diarrhea and, 822*t*
  glucose/insulin dysregulation and, 682*t*, 685*t*
  nausea/vomiting and, 911*t*, 915
  pancreatitis and, 879*t*, 884
  weight gain and, 1175*t*
Glucocorticoid excess. *See* Cushing syndrome
Glucocorticoids
  anxiety and, 400*t*, 402, 408
  cognitive disorders and, 358–359*t*, 360
  Cushing syndrome and, 730, 731*t*, 732–734
  delirium and, 329
  glucose/insulin dysregulation and, 679, 680*t*, 684*t*
  growth hormone deficiency and, 747, 748*t*
  hemolytic anemia and, 1107
  hirsutism and, 194, 206*t*, 207
  inhaled, 731*t*, 733–735, 736*t*, 738, 741, 1127
  injectable, 731*t*, 736*t*
  myopathy and, 1156
  nasal, 731*t*, 733–735, 736*t*, 738, 741
  nausea/vomiting and, 922
  oral, 731*t*, 736*t*, 739–741
  osteoporosis/osteomalacia and, 1120–1122, 1121*t*, 1123*t*, 1125–1127, 1126*t*, 1130
  pancreatitis and, 882
  pharmacologic characteristics of, 739*t*
  production of, 729
  secondary adrenal insufficiency and, 735–736, 737*t*, 738–741
  systemic, 1121*t*, 1123*t*, 1126*t*, 1127
  thyroid diseases and, 702*t*
  topical, 731*t*, 733–735, 736*t*, 739, 741
  weight gain and, 1167*t*, 1172, 1173*t*, 1175*t*
Glucosamine-chondroitin, 452*t*
Glucosamine/glucosamine sulfate, 822, 835
Glucose and insulin dysregulation, 679–690. *See also* Diabetes insipidus; Diabetes mellitus; Hyperglycemia; Hypoglycemia
  causative agents of, 679–681, 680–683*t*
  clinical presentation of, 683, 686, 686*t*
  differential diagnosis of, 686, 687*t*
  epidemiology of, 681, 683
  management of, 689–690, 690*t*
  mechanisms of, 683, 684–685*t*
  morbidity and mortality for, 688–689
  patient education on, 690
  prevention of, 689, 689*t*
  risk factors for, 687–688, 687–688*t*
Glucose Race Age Sex Pressure Stroke Severity (GRASPS) clinical risk score, 241–242
Glucose-6-phosphate dehydrogenase (G6PD) deficiency, 15, 1099–1100, 1106, 1190
Glue sniffing, 473*t*
Glue thistle, 850–851*t*
Glutamate, 261, 329, 332–333, 360, 386, 418, 1329
Glutamine, 287*t*
Glutathione
  anemia and, 1100
  chronic kidney disease and, 970
  heart failure and, 515
  hepatic/cholestatic diseases and, 856, 864, 866
  neutropenia/agranulocytosis and, 1091
  ototoxicity and, 1242*t*, 1243
Glyburide, 146*t*, 505, 983*t*, 1050*t*
Glycerin, 840*t*, 1235*t*
Glycoprotein IIb/IIIa receptor antagonists
  bleeding disorders and, 1026*t*, 1027–1029, 1029*t*, 1033, 1039
  intracerebral hemorrhage and, 238*t*, 239, 240*t*, 242*t*, 243
  myocardial ischemia/acute coronary syndromes and, 486, 487*t*
  thrombocytopenia and, 1052, 1057
Glycopyrrolate, 930
Glycyrrhizic acid, 1013–1014*t*
GM-CSF (granulocyte macrophage colony-stimulating factor), 1064*t*, 1068*t*, 1094–1096
GnRH agonists. *See* Gonadotropin-releasing hormone agonists
GnRH (gonadotropin-releasing hormone) antagonists, 758–759*t*, 763–764*t*
Goa powder, 301*t*
Goiter, 697, 704, 705, 708, 711, 713, 714
Goitrogens, 701*t*, 713
Gold
  acute kidney injury and, 943*t*, 959
  alopecia and, 172*t*, 177
  color changes of oral mucosa and teeth and, 1254–1255*t*
  hepatic/cholestatic diseases and, 853*t*
  oral erythema multiforme and, 1267*t*
  visual disturbances and, 301*t*
Gold salts
  aplastic anemia and, 1100*t*
  chronic kidney disease and, 966*t*, 970*t*
  hepatic/cholestatic diseases and, 861*t*
  oral lichenoid reactions and, 1271*t*
  peripheral neuropathy and, 281*t*
  systemic lupus erythematosus and, 126*t*
  thrombocytopenia and, 1050*t*, 1052*t*
Gold sodium thiomalate, 472*t*
Gold therapy, 174, 959, 1052–1053
Golimumab, 173*t*, 1297
Gonadotropin-releasing hormone (GnRH) agonists
  alopecia and, 171*t*, 176, 179*t*
  anxiety and, 400*t*, 403, 405*t*, 406
  depression and, 376*t*, 381, 385, 387, 390, 391
  glucose/insulin dysregulation and, 680*t*, 684*t*
  growth hormone deficiency and, 747–748, 748*t*
  hirsutism and, 206*t*, 207
  hyperprolactinemia and, 743–744*t*
  infertility and, 790*t*, 801
  osteoporosis/osteomalacia and, 1121*t*, 1123*t*
  ovarian hyperstimulation and, 781, 782*t*, 783, 785*t*, 789, 790*t*
  sexual dysfunction and, 758–759*t*, 762–765*t*
  vaginal bleeding disorders and, 794, 796
Gonadotropin-releasing hormone (GnRH) antagonists, 758–759*t*, 763–764*t*
Gonadotropins, 781, 782*t*, 783, 784, 785*t*
Gordolobo tea, 850*t*
Goserelin, 171*t*, 403, 782*t*, 785*t*, 796, 1064*t*, 1068*t*
Gotu kola, 146*t*
Gout and hyperuricemia, 1135–1146
  causative agents of, 1135, 1136*t*
  classification of, 1141, 1142–1143*t*
  clinical presentation of, 1140–1141, 1140*t*
  differential diagnosis of, 1141, 1141*t*
  epidemiology of, 1135
  management of, 171*t*, 179*t*, 1144–1145, 1145*f*
  mechanisms of, 1135–1140, 1136*t*
  morbidity and mortality for, 1143
  patient education on, 1046
  prevention of, 1143–1144, 1144*t*
  risk factors for, 1143, 1143*t*
Government Accountability Office (GAO), 12–13
Graded challenge procedures, 88–90, 92, 95, 98
Granisetron
  constipation and, 836*t*
  nausea/vomiting and, 918, 919, 922, 924*t*, 926, 928, 928–929*t*
  sexual dysfunction and, 783*t*, 786*t*
  sinus bradycardia/atrioventricular block and, 570*t*
Granulocyte colony-stimulating factor (G-CSF)
  cutaneous diseases and, 101, 102–103*t*
  leukemia and, 1284, 1287, 1289, 1291
  neutropenia/agranulocytosis and, 1094–1096
  thromboembolic diseases and, 1064*t*, 1068*t*
Granulocyte macrophage colony-stimulating factor (GM-CSF), 1064*t*, 1068*t*, 1094–1096
Granulocytopenia, 83–84
Grapefruit juice, 40–41
GRASPS (Glucose Race Age Sex Pressure Stroke Severity) clinical risk score, 241–242

Gregg, Norman, 1312
Grepafloxacin, 541
Griseofulvin
 cutaneous diseases and, 102*t*
 hepatic/cholestatic diseases and, 847*t*
 neutropenia/agranulocytosis and, 1089*t*
 oral erythema multiforme and, 1267*t*
 oral lichenoid reactions and, 1271*t*
 photosensitivity and, 146*t*
 serum sickness-like reactions and, 1193*t*
 systemic lupus erythematosus and, 125*t*, 130
Growth hormone (GH). *See also* Growth hormone deficiency
 cutaneous diseases and, 103*t*
 glucose/insulin dysregulation and, 684*t*
 synthesis of, 729, 747
 thyroid diseases and, 702*t*
Growth hormone deficiency, 747–751
 causative agents of, 747, 748*t*
 clinical presentation of, 748–749, 749*t*
 differential diagnosis of, 749, 749*t*
 epidemiology of, 747
 management of, 750, 750*t*
 mechanisms of, 747–748, 748*t*
 morbidity and mortality for, 749
 patient education on, 750–751
 prevention of, 750, 750*t*
 risk factors for, 745*t*, 749
Growth hormone-inhibiting hormone (GHIH), 747
Growth hormone-releasing hormone (GHRH), 747, 748
Guanabenz, 573*t*, 577*t*, 633*t*, 639*t*
Guanethidine, 302*t*, 376*t*, 378, 385, 385*t*, 759*t*, 765*t*
Guanfacine, 416*t*, 633*t*, 639*t*, 836*t*
Guanoxan, 124*t*
Guarana, 400*t*, 404, 405*t*, 409
Gynecologic diseases, 781–802
 infertility, 800–802
 ovarian hyperstimulation, 781–790
 sexual dysfunction, 797–800
 vaginal bleeding disorders, 793–797
 vulvovaginal candidiasis, 790–792

HA-AKI (hospital-acquired acute kidney injury), 941–942
HAART (highly active antiretroviral therapy), 701, 704, 710, 920
Hair growth, excessive. *See* Hirsutism; Hypertrichosis
Hair growth cycle, 165, 166*f*, 178
Hair loss. *See* Alopecia
Halo effect, 22
Halofantrine, 532*t*
Haloperidol
 alopecia and, 173*t*
 anxiety and, 405
 cannabinoids and, 33
 cognitive disorders and, 369
 delirium and, 326*t*, 337–340
 drug fever and, 1188*t*
 drug interactions with, 40
 dystonia and, 266
 hepatic/cholestatic diseases and, 852*t*
 hyperprolactinemia and, 742
 hypotension and, 635*t*, 639*t*
 hypothermia and, 1216*t*
 nausea/vomiting and, 924*t*, 927*t*, 929*t*
 neuroleptic malignant syndrome and, 1195, 1195*t*, 1199
 photosensitivity and, 146*t*, 154
 seizures and, 218*t*
 serotonin syndrome and, 1209
 sexual dysfunction and, 758–760*t*, 764*t*, 798
 SIADH and, 982*t*, 990
 stroke and, 230*t*
 tardive dyskinesia and, 261, 265
 thrombocytopenia and, 1051*t*
 thyroid diseases and, 702*t*
 torsades de pointes and, 532*t*, 536, 537*f*, 538, 540*t*, 542
 weight gain and, 1167*t*, 1169*t*, 1171
Halothane
 hepatic/cholestatic diseases and, 850*t*
 hypotension and, 634*t*
 malignant hyperthermia and, 1209*t*, 1210, 1211
 nausea/vomiting and, 906*t*
 sinus bradycardia/atrioventricular block and, 570*t*, 578*t*
Hansen disease, 6
Haptens
 acute kidney injury and, 956, 958
 in allergic and hypersensitivity reactions, 76, 78–79, 81
 aplastic anemia and, 1101
 in drug fever, 1187
 drugs as, 1052
 hemolytic anemia and, 1104
 neutropenia/agranulocytosis and, 1091
 photosensitivity and, 149
 systemic lupus erythematosus and, 127
Haronga, 302*t*
Health Alert Network, 53
Health care costs of drug-induced diseases, 26–29, 27*t*
Health economic assessments, 27, 27*t*
Health Insurance Portability and Accountability Act of 1996 (HIPAA), 66–67
Hearing loss, 1233, 1239–1243, 1240*t*
Heart disease. *See* Coronary heart disease (CHD); Valvular and pericardial heart disease
Heart failure, 501–517
 causative agents of, 501–505, 502–504*t*
 clinical presentation of, 512–513, 513*t*
 comorbidity with drug-induced diseases, 34
 differential diagnosis of, 512, 513*t*
 epidemiology of, 505–509
 management of, 516
 mechanisms of, 509–512, 510*t*
 morbidity and mortality for, 514–515
 patient education on, 516–517
 prevention of, 515–516, 515*t*
 risk factors for, 513–514, 514*t*
Heavy metals/toxins, 171*t*, 179*t*, 1255*t*
Hematopoietic agents, 1064*t*, 1068*t*
Hematopoietic stem cell transplantation (HSCT), 1104, 1292
Hemodynamic-mediated AKI, 942–949
 causative agents of, 942, 943–944*t*
 clinical presentation of, 945–946, 946*t*
 differential diagnosis of, 946, 946*t*
 epidemiology of, 942, 944
 management of, 948–949
 mechanisms of, 944–945, 945*t*
 morbidity and mortality for, 947–948
 patient education on, 949
 prevention of, 948, 948*t*
 risk factors for, 946–947, 947*t*
Hemolytic anemia, 1104–1107
 causative agents of, 86, 1104, 1105–1106*t*, 1109
 clinical presentation of, 83–84, 1102*t*, 1106
 differential diagnosis of, 1106
 epidemiology of, 1104
 management of, 1107
 mechanisms of, 1101*t*, 1104, 1106
 morbidity and mortality for, 1106
 patient education on, 1107
 prevention of, 1106–1107
 risk factors for, 1103*t*, 1106
Hemorrhagic stroke. *See* Intracerebral hemorrhage (ICH)
Hemostatic agents, 1037*t*, 1039, 1064*t*, 1067, 1068*t*
Henbane, 302*t*
Heparin/heparinoids. *See also* Heparin-induced thrombocytopenia (HIT); Low-molecular-weight heparin (LMWH); Unfractionated heparin
 acidosis and, 1003*t*
 allergic reactions to, 75*t*
 alopecia and, 166, 167*t*, 177, 178, 183
 contaminated, 4
 drug fever and, 1188*t*
 as inflammatory mediator, 81
 interstitial lung disease/pulmonary fibrosis and, 440
 intracerebral hemorrhage and, 238*t*, 239, 240, 240*t*, 242*t*, 243, 245
 myocardial ischemia/acute coronary syndromes and, 472*t*, 480, 486, 487*t*
 osteoporosis/osteomalacia and, 1121*t*, 1124*t*, 1126*t*
 ovarian hyperstimulation and, 789
 sexual dysfunction and, 761*t*, 765*t*
 stroke and, 235
 thromboembolic diseases and, 1064*t*, 1067, 1068*t*, 1075*t*
 thyroid diseases and, 702*t*
 visual disturbances and, 302*t*
Heparin-induced thrombocytopenia (HIT)
 causative agents of, 1050, 1051*t*, 1067
 clinical presentation of, 1054*t*, 1055
 management of, 1057–1059, 1076
 mechanisms of, 1052*t*, 1053
 morbidity and mortality for, 1056
 prevention of, 1056–1057, 1057*t*
 risk factors for, 1056, 1056*t*
Hepatic and cholestatic diseases, 845–873
 causative agents of, 845, 846–853*t*
 clinical presentation of, 858–862, 859–861*t*
 comorbidity with drug-induced diseases, 34
 differential diagnosis of, 860, 861*t*
 epidemiology of, 845, 853
 management of, 865–872, 867*t*
 mechanisms of, 854–855*t*, 855–858
 morbidity and mortality for, 865
 patient education on, 872–873
 prevention of, 865, 865*t*
 risk factors for, 862–865, 863*t*
 systemic lupus erythematosus and, 130
Hepatitis B vaccine, 126*t*, 1235*t*, 1267*t*, 1271*t*
Hepatocellular injury, 854*t*, 856–857, 862
Hepatosplenic T-cell lymphoma (HSTCL), 1292, 1293
Hepatotoxicity, 33–34, 39, 845, 853, 855–857, 865–868
HER (human epidermal growth factor receptor), 177
Herbal preparations. *See also specific substances*
 alkalosis and, 1017
 anxiety and, 399, 402
 constipation and, 835
 delirium and, 330
 diarrhea and, 822, 825, 827
 heart failure and, 517

INDEX

Herbal preparations (continued)
hepatic/cholestatic diseases and, 845, 850–851*t*
interstitial lung disease/pulmonary fibrosis and, 433
intracerebral hemorrhage and, 238*t*, 243, 246
psychosis and, 415, 420, 423
seizures and, 219*t*, 221
sexual dysfunction and, 774
thrombocytopenia and, 1049
visual disturbances and, 313
Herb paris, 302*t*
Herd immunity, 29
Heroin
acute kidney injury and, 959
asthma/bronchospasm and, 452*t*
color changes of oral mucosa and teeth and, 1254*t*
interstitial lung disease/pulmonary fibrosis and, 433
intracerebral hemorrhage and, 238*t*, 240
myocardial ischemia/acute coronary syndromes and, 473*t*
ototoxicity and, 1239
stroke and, 230–231*t*, 232
thyroid diseases and, 702*t*
Hetastarch, 75*t*
Hexachloroethane, 849*t*
Hexachlorophene, 146*t*
HIE (hyperinsulinemia-euglycemia) therapy, 580
High blood pressure. *See* Hypertension
Highly active antiretroviral therapy (HAART), 701, 704, 710, 920
Hill, Austin Bradford, 22
HIPAA (Health Insurance Portability and Accountability Act of 1996), 66–67
Hippocrates, 20
Hirsutism, 193–208
causative agents of, 194, 195*t*
clinical presentation of, 193–194, 199–201, 200–201*t*
differential diagnosis of, 201, 201*t*
epidemiology of, 197–198
Ferriman–Gallwey scoring system for, 200, 200*f*
management of, 203–207, 204–206*t*
mechanisms of, 198, 199*t*
morbidity and mortality for, 203
patient education on, 207–208
prevention of, 203, 203*t*
risk factors for, 202, 202*t*
Hirudin, 239
Histamine H_1-receptor antagonists, 98, 353, 644, 869, 1207–1208
Histamine H_2-receptor antagonists
acute kidney injury and, 943*t*
allergic reactions and, 75*t*, 98
alopecia and, 171*t*, 179*t*
cognitive disorders and, 358–359*t*, 366
delirium and, 325, 328*t*
depression and, 385
hemolytic anemia and, 1104, 1105*t*
hepatic/cholestatic diseases and, 850*t*, 864
hyperprolactinemia and, 743–744*t*
pancreatitis and, 880, 887
psychosis and, 416*t*
sexual dysfunction and, 759*t*
thrombocytopenia and, 1054
Histamines, 81, 511, 644, 1192
HIT. *See* Heparin-induced thrombocytopenia
HIV/AIDS. *See also* Antiretroviral therapy
anxiety and, 404
appetite stimulants in, 33
cognitive disorders and, 362
color changes of oral mucosa and teeth and, 1253
congenital heart defects and, 1324
cutaneous diseases and, 110, 111
delirium and, 333
depression and, 378
drug fever and, 1190
hypersensitivity reactions and, 86, 87
hypertrichosis and, 199
insulin resistance and, 690
levels of evidence for, 21
macrocytic anemia and, 1107
myopathy and, 1154, 1156, 1159
nausea/vomiting and, 920, 929–930
pancreatitis and, 879–880, 882, 890, 891
parkinsonism and, 272
peripheral neuropathy and, 279, 282, 285, 288, 289
photosensitivity and, 153
thrombocytopenia and, 1049
thyroid diseases and, 701, 704, 710
HLA. *See* Human leukocyte antigen
HMG-CoA reductase inhibitors
acute kidney injury and, 954
constipation and, 836*t*
glucose/insulin dysregulation and, 680*t*, 684*t*, 689
interstitial lung disease/pulmonary fibrosis and, 432*t*, 435*t*
psychosis and, 418*t*
sexual dysfunction and, 758*t*, 763*t*
systemic lupus erythematosus and, 124*t*, 132
HMG-CoA (hydroxy-3-methyl-glutaryl coenzyme A) reductase inhibitors, 385, 880
Hodgkin lymphoma, 1284–1286, 1291–1293
Hogweed, 302*t*
Holiday heart syndrome, 581
Hormone-replacement therapy (HRT)
alopecia and, 176, 178, 184
breast cancer and, 1298–1301
endometrial cancer and, 1301, 1302
hirsutism and, 194
hypertension and, 621
myocardial ischemia/acute coronary syndromes and, 474, 475, 482
sleep disorders and, 351
stroke and, 229, 230*t*, 235*t*
thromboembolic diseases and, 1064*t*, 1068*t*, 1074, 1075*t*
vulvovaginal candidiasis and, 782*t*, 785*t*, 791
Hormones
adrenocorticotropic. *See* Adrenocorticotropic hormone (ACTH)
alopecia and, 175–176
α-melanocyte-stimulating hormone, 1242*t*
antidiuretic. *See* Vasopressin
anxiety and, 399, 402–403, 406
color changes of oral mucosa and teeth and, 1255*t*
corticotropin-releasing, 729, 734–735, 737–739, 741
depression and, 375, 376*t*, 381–382
follicle-stimulating. *See* Follicle-stimulating hormone (FSH)
GH-inhibiting, 747
GH-releasing, 747, 748
GnRH agonists. *See* Gonadotropin-releasing hormone agonists
GnRH antagonists, 758–759*t*, 763–764*t*
growth. *See* Growth hormone; Growth hormone deficiency
hyperprolactinemia and, 743*t*
luteinizing, 729, 766, 767, 783, 793, 800
myocardial ischemia/acute coronary syndromes and, 473*t*
sex. *See* Sex hormones
steroid. *See* Steroids
thromboembolic diseases and, 1067, 1077
thyroid, 401*t*, 403, 411, 473*t*, 703*t*, 1126*t*
thyroid releasing, 697, 698*f*
thyroid stimulating, 697, 698*f*, 700–701, 704, 707–715
vaginal bleeding disorders and, 795
weight gain and, 1167*t*, 1169*t*, 1172–1173
Horse chestnut, 302*t*
Hospital-acquired acute kidney injury (HA-AKI), 941–942
Hospital admissions, drug-related, 25–29, 26*t*, 38
HPA axis. *See* Hypothalamic–pituitary–adrenal axis
HPV (human papillomavirus) vaccine, 1296
HRT. *See* Hormone-replacement therapy
HSCT (hematopoietic stem cell transplantation), 1104, 1292
HSTCL (hepatosplenic T-cell lymphoma), 1292, 1293
5-HT_3 antagonists, 836*t*
Human epidermal growth factor receptor (HER), 177
Human leukocyte antigen (HLA)
aplastic anemia and, 1104
cutaneous diseases and, 111–112
in drug allergies and hypersensitivity reactions, 32, 35, 37–38, 86, 88
malignant hyperthermia and, 1186
oral erythema multiforme and, 1269
pancreatitis and, 881
systemic lupus erythematosus and, 129, 134
Human papillomavirus (HPV) vaccine, 1296
Human relaxin, 782*t*, 785*t*, 795
Huperzine A, 302*t*
Hyaluronic acid, 302*t*
Hyaluronidase, 1235*t*
Hydantoin, 133, 197*t*
Hydralazine
acute kidney injury and, 943*t*
allergic reactions to, 74*t*, 85, 86
cutaneous diseases and, 103*t*
drug fever and, 1188*t*
drug interactions with, 40
genetic variations affecting, 36*t*
heart failure and, 503*t*, 509
hepatic/cholestatic diseases and, 847*t*
hypotension and, 633*t*, 640*t*, 644
myocardial ischemia/acute coronary syndromes and, 472*t*, 477*t*
neutropenia/agranulocytosis and, 1089*t*
oral erythema multiforme and, 1267*t*
peripheral neuropathy and, 281*t*, 285
sexual dysfunction and, 761*t*, 765*t*
systemic lupus erythematosus and, 124*t*, 127–130, 128*t*, 131*t*, 133–134
valvular/pericardial heart disease and, 661*t*, 662
Hydrazines, 126*t*, 132
Hydriodic acid syrup, 706*t*
Hydrocephaly, 1329, 1331
Hydrochlorothiazide
allergic reactions to, 94
desensitization to, 95
diabetes insipidus and, 991*t*, 993, 993*t*
drug fever and, 1188*t*
gout/hyperuricemia and, 1138
hypotension and, 633*t*, 638*t*
neutropenia/agranulocytosis and, 1089*t*
oral lichenoid reactions and, 1271*t*
ototoxicity and, 1235*t*
pancreatitis and, 878*t*, 879, 880, 883, 886*t*, 891
photosensitivity and, 146*t*, 150

systemic lupus erythematosus and, 124*t*, 132
thrombocytopenia and, 1051*t*
visual disturbances and, 302*t*
Hydrocodone, 836*t*, 906*t*, 921, 1233, 1235*t*
Hydrocortisone
alopecia and, 171*t*
for cutaneous diseases, 113
hepatic/cholestatic diseases and, 868
hirsutism and, 195*t*
hypertrichosis and, 196*t*
pharmacologic characteristics of, 739*t*
photosensitivity and, 146*t*
secondary adrenal insufficiency and, 740, 741
Hydrocortisone butyrate, 731*t*, 736*t*
Hydrocortisone sodium succinate, 452*t*
Hydromorphone, 218*t*, 636*t*, 638*t*, 736–737*t*, 836*t*, 906*t*
Hydroxocobalamin, 146*t*
3-hydroxy-3-methyl-glutaryl coenzyme A (HMG-CoA) reductase inhibitors, 385, 880
Hydroxychloroquine
color changes of oral mucosa and teeth and, 1254*t*
cutaneous diseases and, 103*t*
hepatic/cholestatic diseases and, 847*t*
myopathy and, 1150*t*, 1152*t*, 1153
neutropenia/agranulocytosis and, 1089*t*
oral lichenoid reactions and, 1271*t*
ototoxicity and, 1235*t*
seizures and, 218*t*, 225
sinus bradycardia/atrioventricular block and, 573*t*
torsades de pointes and, 533*t*
visual disturbances and, 295, 302*t*, 312, 313, 318–319
5-hydroxytryptamine (5HT). *See also* Serotonin
depression and, 378
hypotension and, 647
hypothermia and, 1216
nausea/vomiting and, 912, 914, 918–920, 922–929, 927*t*
neuroleptic malignant syndrome and, 1196
psychosis and, 418
secondary adrenal insufficiency and, 737
serotonin syndrome and, 1203, 1204, 1208
SIADH and, 986
stroke and, 232
vaginal bleeding disorders and, 795
valvular/pericardial heart disease and, 659, 663, 664, 669
5-hydroxytryptophan, 256, 302*t*, 478, 986
Hydroxyurea
color changes of oral mucosa and teeth and, 1254*t*
drug fever and, 1188*t*
hepatic/cholestatic diseases and, 848*t*
interstitial lung disease/pulmonary fibrosis and, 432*t*
macrocytic anemia and, 1107
myocardial ischemia/acute coronary syndromes and, 472*t*
pancreatitis and, 890
photosensitivity and, 146*t*
systemic lupus erythematosus and, 126*t*
Hydroxyzine, 533*t*, 761*t*
Hyoscine patches, 302*t*
Hyperacusis, 1233
Hyperaldosteronism, 751
Hyperglycemia
causative agents of, 679–681, 680–681*t*
clinical presentation of, 683, 686, 686*t*
differential diagnosis of, 686, 687*t*
epidemiology of, 681, 683
management of, 690, 690*t*, 870
mechanisms of, 683, 684*t*
morbidity and mortality for, 688–689
patient education on, 690
risk factors for, 687, 687*t*
Hyperinsulinemia-euglycemia (HIE) therapy, 580
Hyperkalemia, 946, 948, 949, 956, 959
Hyperprolactinemia, 742–747
causative agents of, 742, 743–744*t*
clinical presentation of, 742, 744–745, 745*t*
differential diagnosis of, 744–745, 745*t*
epidemiology of, 742
management of, 746, 747*t*
mechanisms of, 742, 744*t*
morbidity and mortality for, 746
patient education on, 746–747
prevention of, 746, 746*t*
risk factors for, 745–746, 745*t*
Hypersensitivity reactions. *See* Drug hypersensitivity reactions (DHRs)
Hypersensitivity syndromes, 75*t*, 84*t*, 99*t*, 109
Hypersensitivity vasculitis, 74*t*, 83–84*t*, 84–85
Hypertension, 617–627
acute, 232, 240
causative agents of, 617, 618*t*
chronic thromboembolic pulmonary, 1074
clinical presentation of, 621–622, 621*t*
differential diagnosis of, 201*t*, 622, 622*t*
epidemiology, 617–619
management of, 624–626, 625*t*, 942
mechanisms of, 619–621, 620*t*
morbidity and mortality for, 623
patient education on, 626–627
prevention of, 623–624, 624*t*
primary, 617, 622–624, 622*t*, 626
rebound, 621, 625*t*, 626, 627
risk factors for, 622–623, 622*t*
secondary, 617, 622, 622*t*, 624, 626
Hyperthermia, 1185–1212
categorization of, 1185
clinical presentation of, 1186, 1187*t*
from drug fever, 1186–1192
malignant, 1209–1214
from neuroleptic malignant syndrome, 1195–1202
from serotonin syndrome, 1202–1209
from serum sickness-like reactions, 1192–1195
Hyperthyroidism
causative agents of, 697, 699–700*t*, 700–701
clinical presentation of, 711–713, 711*t*
differential diagnosis of, 711, 712*t*
epidemiology of, 704
management of, 715*t*, 716–717
mechanisms of, 705, 707
morbidity and mortality for, 714
patient education on, 717
prevention of, 714–715
risk factors for, 713–714
Hypertrichosis, 193–208
causative agents of, 193–197, 196–197*t*
clinical presentation of, 194, 198*f*, 200*t*, 201–202
differential diagnosis of, 201, 201*t*
epidemiology of, 197–198
management of, 204–205*t*, 207
mechanisms of, 198–199, 199*t*
morbidity and mortality for, 203
patient education on, 207–208
prevention of, 203, 203*t*
risk factors for, 202, 203*t*
Hyperuricemia. *See* Gout and hyperuricemia
Hypnotics. *See* Sedative-hypnotics
Hypoaldosteronism, 751
Hypogeusia, 1258
Hypoglycemia
causative agents of, 679, 681, 682–683*t*
clinical presentation of, 686, 686*t*
differential diagnosis of, 686, 687*t*
epidemiology of, 681, 683
management of, 690, 690*t*
mechanisms of, 683, 685*t*
morbidity and mortality for, 688–689
patient education on, 690
risk factors for, 687–688, 688*t*
Hypoglycemic agents, 26*t*, 92, 761, 983*t*
Hypotension, 631–648
causative agents of, 631, 632–636*t*
clinical presentation of, 637, 641, 641*t*
differential diagnosis of, 641, 642*t*
epidemiology of, 631, 637
management of, 644–648, 645–646*t*
mechanisms of, 637, 638–640*t*
morbidity and mortality for, 643
orthostatic, 233, 631, 637, 641–648, 646*t*
patient education on, 648
prevention of, 643–644, 643*t*
risk factors for, 641–643, 642*t*
Hypothalamic, pituitary, and adrenal diseases, 729–751
Cushing syndrome, 730–734
growth hormone deficiency, 747–751
hyperprolactinemia, 742–747
hypoaldosteronism/hyperaldosteronism, 751
overview, 729
primary adrenal insufficiency, 734–735
secondary adrenal insufficiency, 734–741
Hypothalamic-pituitary-adrenal (HPA) axis
activation of, 738
anxiety and, 409
depression and, 382, 385, 386
diagnostic testing of, 732, 734
hyperprolactinemia and, 742
structure and function of, 729, 730*f*
suppression of, 734–736, 740, 741
Hypothermia, 1214–1218
causative agents of, 1186, 1215, 1216*t*
clinical presentation of, 1216–1217, 1217*t*
differential diagnosis of, 1217
epidemiology of, 1215
management of, 1217–1218
mechanisms of, 1215–1216
morbidity and mortality for, 1217
overview, 1214–1215
patient education on, 1218
prevention of, 1217
risk factors for, 1217
Hypothermia therapy, 186, 189*t*
Hypothyroidism
causative agents of, 697–701, 698–699*t*, 704
clinical presentation of, 711–712, 711*t*
differential diagnosis of, 711, 712*t*
epidemiology of, 704
management of, 715–716, 715*t*
mechanisms of, 34, 708–709
morbidity and mortality for, 714
patient education on, 717
prevention of, 714–715
risk factors for, 713–714
Hypouricemics, 313
Hypovolemia, 944–946

Ibandronate, 302*t*, 1129*t*, 1130, 1274*t*
Ibogaine, 532*t*
Ibritumomab, 7*t*

INDEX

Ibuprofen
acidosis and, 1002*t*
acute kidney injury and, 944, 947
allergic reactions to, 73*t*
alopecia and, 172*t*
aplastic anemia and, 1100*t*
asthma/bronchospasm and, 463
bleeding disorders and, 1033
constipation and, 836*t*
cutaneous diseases and, 102*t*
delirium and, 327*t*
drug fever and, 1188*t*
glucose/insulin dysregulation and, 688
gout/hyperuricemia and, 1145
heart failure and, 510*t*
hemolytic anemia and, 1105*t*
hepatic/cholestatic diseases and, 846*t*
myocardial ischemia/acute coronary syndromes and, 472*t*, 475
oral erythema multiforme and, 1267*t*
oral lichenoid reactions and, 1271*t*
ototoxicity and, 1235*t*
photosensitivity and, 146*t*, 150
SIADH and, 984*t*
systemic lupus erythematosus and, 126*t*
thrombocytopenia and, 1051*t*
upper gastrointestinal ulceration and, 811
visual disturbances and, 302*t*
Ibutilide
atrial fibrillation/atrial flutter and, 587, 587*t*
heart failure and, 507, 511, 513
hypotension and, 634*t*
monomorphic ventricular tachycardia and, 524–525*t*
sinus bradycardia/atrioventricular block and, 570*t*
torsades de pointes and, 532*t*, 535, 536, 538, 543–544
ICH. *See* Intracerebral hemorrhage
ICON (International Consensus) on Drug Allergy, 71, 80
ICS (inhaled corticosteroids), 733, 738–741, 1127
Idarubicin, 169*t*, 570*t*, 577*t*, 908*t*
Idarucizumab, 245, 1037*t*, 1038–1039
Idiosyncratic reactions, 60
Idoxuridine, 706*t*
Ifosfamide
acidosis and, 1003*t*
acute kidney injury and, 943*t*
alopecia and, 169*t*
anxiety and, 400*t*, 403
chronic kidney disease and, 966*t*, 970*t*
diabetes insipidus and, 991*t*
heart failure and, 503*t*, 509
leukemia and, 1284
nausea/vomiting and, 908*t*, 916*t*
osteoporosis/osteomalacia and, 1123*t*
ototoxicity and, 1236*t*
pancreatitis and, 879*t*, 881
peripheral neuropathy and, 280*t*
psychosis and, 416*t*
SIADH and, 983*t*
Illicit drug use. *See also specific drugs*
anxiety and, 399, 401
delirium and, 330
diarrhea and, 825
hepatic/cholestatic diseases and, 845, 851*t*, 864
hyperthermia and, 1186
hypothermia and, 1217, 1218
interstitial lung disease/pulmonary fibrosis and, 433
intracerebral hemorrhage and, 239
in medication histories, 60
myocardial ischemia/acute coronary syndromes and, 473*t*, 479, 480, 484, 485, 489
psychosis and, 415, 418, 420, 423
as risk factor for drug-induced diseases, 33
seizures and, 217
sexual dysfunction and, 774
stroke and, 231, 232, 235*t*
Illicium henryi, 221
Iloperidone, 255, 1166*t*, 1169*t*, 1195*t*
Iloprost, 7*t*, 473*t*, 636*t*, 640*t*, 1051*t*
Imatinib
alopecia and, 169*t*
aplastic anemia and, 1100*t*
bone marrow aplasia and, 1109
chemotherapy-induced anemia and, 1109*t*
color changes of oral mucosa and teeth and, 1254*t*, 1255*t*
cutaneous diseases and, 103*t*
growth hormone deficiency and, 747
heart failure and, 503*t*, 510*t*
interstitial lung disease/pulmonary fibrosis and, 433*t*, 440
nausea/vomiting and, 908*t*
neutropenia/agranulocytosis and, 1087
oral lichenoid reactions and, 1271*t*
photosensitivity and, 146*t*
SIADH and, 984*t*
thromboembolic diseases and, 1065*t*, 1069*t*
thyroid diseases and, 699–700*t*, 702*t*, 709
visual disturbances and, 303*t*
Imidazole antifungal agents, 103*t*
Imipenem, 92, 220
Imipenem-cilastatin, 909*t*, 1188*t*, 1191
Imipramine
alopecia and, 173*t*
anxiety and, 406
cognitive disorders and, 369
constipation and, 836*t*
delirium and, 326*t*, 329*t*
drug fever and, 1188*t*
heart failure and, 504*t*, 507, 510*t*
hypotension and, 634*t*, 639*t*
monomorphic ventricular tachycardia and, 524–525*t*
neutropenia/agranulocytosis and, 1089*t*
ototoxicity and, 1236*t*
photosensitivity and, 146*t*
seizures and, 220
serotonin syndrome and, 1203–1204*t*
sexual dysfunction and, 772
SIADH and, 982*t*, 990
sinus bradycardia/atrioventricular block and, 573*t*, 578*t*
torsades de pointes and, 533*t*, 540*t*
weight gain and, 1166*t*, 1169*t*, 1170
Imiquimod, 174*t*, 180*t*
Immediate drug reactions, 80–82
Immune checkpoint inhibitors, 822*t*, 825
Immune complex diseases, 81, 84, 100, 110
Immune modulators, 313, 473*t*
Immunizations. *See* Vaccines
Immunoglobulins, 230*t*, 1065*t*, 1069*t*
Immunologic agents
constipation and, 836*t*
depression and, 375, 377*t*, 382–384, 386–388, 391
thromboembolic diseases and, 1065–1066*t*, 1069–1070*t*
Immunosuppressants
alopecia and, 172*t*, 174, 179*t*, 191
aplastic anemia and, 1104
chronic kidney disease and, 967, 975
comorbidity and, 34
depression and, 382
diarrhea and, 823*t*
glucose/insulin dysregulation and, 688
hypertension and, 624
hypertrichosis and, 196*t*
lymphoma and, 1292–1295
oral lichenoid reactions and, 1273
osteoporosis/osteomalacia and, 1127
pancreatitis and, 880, 885, 890, 891*t*
seizures and, 219*t*
skin cancer and, 1295–1298
systemic lupus erythematosus and, 132, 135
thrombocytopenia and, 1050
Impila, 850*t*
Incretin-based therapies, 884–885, 888
Indapamide, 146*t*, 533*t*, 633*t*, 638*t*, 1267*t*
Indinavir
acute kidney injury and, 944–945*t*, 957, 958
alopecia and, 168*t*
chronic kidney disease and, 967
osteoporosis/osteomalacia and, 1123*t*
sexual dysfunction and, 783*t*, 786*t*
Indomethacin
alopecia and, 172*t*
anxiety and, 403–404
aplastic anemia and, 1100*t*
asthma/bronchospasm and, 463
cutaneous diseases and, 106
delirium and, 327*t*
diabetes insipidus and, 993, 993*t*
heart failure and, 510*t*
hemolytic anemia and, 1105*t*
hepatic/cholestatic diseases and, 846*t*
hypotension and, 646*t*, 647
oral lichenoid reactions and, 1271*t*
ototoxicity and, 1236*t*
peripheral neuropathy and, 281*t*
psychosis and, 416*t*
upper gastrointestinal ulceration and, 813
visual disturbances and, 303*t*
Infants. *See* Pediatric patients
Infertility, 800–802
causative agents of, 762*t*, 783*t*, 800
clinical presentation of, 768*t*, 769, 770, 787*t*, 801
differential diagnosis of, 770*t*, 788*t*, 801
epidemiology of, 800
management of, 774*t*, 790*t*, 801–802
mechanisms of, 765*t*, 767, 786*t*, 800
morbidity and mortality for, 801
patient education on, 774, 802
prevention of, 789*t*, 801
risk factors for, 788*t*, 801
Infliximab
allergic and hypersensitivity reactions to, 73–74*t*, 77*t*, 96
alopecia and, 173*t*
cutaneous diseases and, 102–103*t*, 109, 113
depression and, 383, 386
heart failure and, 502*t*, 508, 509, 512
hepatic/cholestatic diseases and, 852*t*
interstitial lung disease/pulmonary fibrosis and, 433*t*
myopathy and, 1153
neutropenia/agranulocytosis and, 1089*t*
oral erythema multiforme and, 1267*t*
oral lichenoid reactions and, 1271*t*
peripheral neuropathy and, 281*t*
serum sickness-like reactions and, 1193*t*
sinus bradycardia/atrioventricular block and, 573*t*

skin cancer and, 1297
systemic lupus erythematosus and, 126*t*, 128*t*
thromboembolic diseases and, 1065*t*, 1069*t*
thyroid diseases and, 699–700*t*, 702*t*
valvular/pericardial heart disease and, 662
Inhaled anesthetics
hepatic/cholestatic diseases and, 864
malignant hyperthermia and, 1209–1210, 1209*t*, 1212
nausea/vomiting and, 906–907*t*, 911*t*, 913, 915–916, 921, 923
Inhaled corticosteroids (ICS), 733, 738–741, 1127
Inhaled glucocorticoids, 731*t*, 733–735, 736*t*, 738, 741, 1127
Injectable glucocorticoids, 731*t*, 736*t*
Innocent bystander hypothesis, 1052
INR (international normalized ratio), 237
Insomnia, 347, 349–353
Institute for Safe Medication Practices, 24, 884
Institute of Medicine. *See* National Academy of Medicine
Insulin. *See also* Glucose and insulin dysregulation
allergic reactions to, 73*t*, 75*t*
comorbidity and, 34
hyperglycemia and, 870
hypoglycemia and, 681, 682*t*, 685*t*
oral lichenoid reactions and, 1271*t*
serum sickness-like reactions and, 1193*t*
tolerance test for, 737–738
weight gain and, 1167–1169*t*, 1172, 1173*t*
Intercalating agents, 1285
Interferon
alopecia and, 172*t*, 175, 178, 179*t*, 183
glucose/insulin dysregulation and, 680*t*, 684*t*
hepatic/cholestatic diseases and, 853*t*, 857
hypertrichosis and, 196–197*t*, 199
interstitial lung disease/pulmonary fibrosis and, 432*t*
myopathy and, 1150*t*
neutropenia/agranulocytosis and, 1093
ototoxicity and, 1236*t*
visual disturbances and, 303*t*
Interferon-2b, 74*t*
Interferon-α
alopecia and, 172*t*, 175, 178
asthma/bronchospasm and, 452*t*
cognitive disorders and, 358–359*t*
cutaneous diseases and, 103*t*
depression and, 377*t*, 382–383, 385*t*, 386–391, 388*t*
diarrhea and, 822*t*
gingival hyperplasia and, 1263*t*
heart failure and, 503*t*, 510*t*
hemolytic anemia and, 1105*t*
hypertrichosis and, 196–197*t*
myocardial ischemia/acute coronary syndromes and, 473*t*
oral lichenoid reactions and, 1271*t*
pancreatitis and, 878*t*, 884, 886*t*
peripheral neuropathy and, 281*t*
seizures and, 218*t*, 222*t*
systemic lupus erythematosus and, 126*t*, 132
taste disorders and, 1259*t*
thrombocytopenia and, 1051*t*
thromboembolic diseases and, 1065*t*, 1069*t*
thyroid diseases and, 699–700*t*, 702*t*, 704–705, 708–709, 713–714, 716–717
valvular/pericardial heart disease and, 662
Interferon-β
allergic reactions to, 96
depression and, 377*t*, 382, 383, 386
systemic lupus erythematosus and, 126*t*, 132
thromboembolic diseases and, 1065*t*, 1070*t*
thyroid diseases and, 699–700*t*, 709, 714
Interferon-γ
alopecia and, 178
cutaneous diseases and, 103*t*
thromboembolic diseases and, 1065*t*, 1069*t*
thyroid diseases and, 702*t*
Interleukin-1, 702*t*, 857, 1185, 1186
Interleukin-2
asthma/bronchospasm and, 452*t*
atrial fibrillation/atrial flutter and, 582*t*
depression and, 377*t*, 382, 384, 386
hepatic/cholestatic diseases and, 848*t*
hypotension and, 635*t*, 640*t*, 645*t*
lymphoma and, 1295
myocardial ischemia/acute coronary syndromes and, 473*t*
systemic lupus erythematosus and, 126*t*
thyroid diseases and, 702*t*, 716
visual disturbances and, 303*t*
Interleukin-3, 1065*t*, 1070*t*
Interleukin-6, 386, 439, 702*t*, 1186
Intermenstrual bleeding, 793
International Conferences on Harmonization, 52
International Consensus (ICON) on Drug Allergy, 71, 80
International normalized ratio (INR), 237
Interstitial lung disease/pulmonary fibrosis, 431–442
causative agents of, 431, 432–433*t*
clinical presentation of, 434–436, 435–436*t*
differential diagnosis of, 436, 436*t*
epidemiology of, 433–434
management of, 439–441, 441*f*
mechanisms of, 434, 435*t*
morbidity and mortality for, 438
patient education on, 441–442
prevention of, 438–439, 439*t*
risk factors for, 437–438, 437*t*
Intra-arterial thrombolytic agents, 238*t*
Intracerebral hemorrhage (ICH), 237–246
causative agents of, 232, 237–239, 238*t*
clinical presentation of, 233, 240–241, 241*t*
differential diagnosis of, 241, 241*t*
epidemiology of, 239–240
management of, 244–246
mechanisms of, 232, 240, 240*t*
morbidity and mortality for, 244
patient education on, 246
prevention of, 244, 244*t*
risk factors for, 241–244, 242*t*
Intranasal oxymetazoline, 230*t*
Intranasal phenoxazoline, 230*t*
Intrauterine contraceptive devices (IUDs), 171*t*, 179*t*, 782*t*, 785*t*, 795, 796
Intravenous immunoglobulin G (IVIG), 76, 113–114, 473*t*, 829
Iocetamic acid, 706*t*
Iodamide meglumine, 706*t*
Iodides, 102*t*, 108, 704, 706*t*, 708, 1267*t*
Iodinated compounds, 699–700*t*, 702*t*
Iodinated glycerol, 705, 706*t*
Iodinated radiocontrast dyes, 219*t*, 452*t*, 700*t*, 703*t*, 709, 716–717
Iodine, 175, 705, 706*t*, 708, 711, 713, 714
Iodine-containing vitamins, 706*t*
Iodipamide meglumine, 706*t*
Iodixanol, 706*t*
Iodized organic oils, 706*t*
Iodized salt, 706*t*
Iodoform gauze, 706*t*
Iodoquinol, 706*t*
Iohexol, 706*t*, 1066*t*, 1070*t*
Iomeprol, 1066*t*, 1070*t*
Iopamidol, 706*t*, 1066*t*, 1070*t*
Iopromide, 706*t*
Iothalamate, 1066*t*, 1070*t*
Iothalamate meglumine, 706*t*
Iothalamate sodium, 706*t*
Ioversol, 473*t*, 706*t*
Ioxaglate, 1066*t*, 1070*t*
Ioxaglate meglumine/sodium, 706*t*
Ipecac, 1150*t*, 1152*t*
Ipecac syrup, 929
Ipilimumab, 170*t*, 699–700*t*, 825
Ipratropium/ipratropium bromide, 463, 582*t*, 592, 592*t*
Irbesartan, 632*t*, 638*t*, 878*t*, 1236*t*
Irinotecan
alopecia and, 170*t*
diarrhea and, 823, 825, 826
genetic variations affecting, 36*t*
hepatic/cholestatic diseases and, 848*t*
metabolic pathway for, 35, 37
nausea/vomiting and, 908*t*, 916*t*
sinus bradycardia/atrioventricular block and, 570*t*
thromboembolic diseases and, 1065*t*, 1069*t*
Iron chelators, 1103, 1242*t*
Iron dextran, 1193*t*
Iron overdose, 1002*t*
Iron preparations, 73*t*, 836*t*, 920, 1254*t*
Iron supplements, 909*t*
Isavuconazonium, 168*t*
Ischemia. *See* Myocardial ischemia/acute coronary syndromes
Ischemic stroke. *See* Stroke
Isocarboxazid, 40, 982*t*, 1203–1204*t*
Isoflurane, 472*t*, 634*t*, 850*t*, 906*t*, 1209*t*, 1210
Isometheptene mucate, 230*t*
Isoniazid
acidosis and, 1002*t*
allergic reactions to, 73*t*
alopecia and, 174*t*, 180*t*
cutaneous diseases and, 108
drug fever and, 1188*t*, 1191
drug interactions with, 39, 39*t*
genetic variations affecting, 36*t*
gout/hyperuricemia and, 1138
hemolytic anemia and, 1105*t*
hepatic/cholestatic diseases and, 847*t*, 864
neutropenia/agranulocytosis and, 1090*t*
oral lichenoid reactions and, 1271*t*
ototoxicity and, 1236*t*
pancreatitis and, 878*t*, 882, 886*t*
peripheral neuropathy and, 280*t*, 282, 282*t*, 285, 286, 288
psychosis and, 416*t*
seizures and, 219, 220, 222*t*
systemic lupus erythematosus and, 124*t*, 127, 128*t*, 129, 133
thrombocytopenia and, 1051*t*
valvular/pericardial heart disease and, 661*t*, 662
visual disturbances and, 303*t*
Isopropamide iodide, 706*t*
Isoproterenol, 454, 473*t*, 544–545, 747, 748*t*
Isosorbide dinitrate, 40, 472*t*, 505, 634*t*, 640*t*, 1259*t*
Isosorbide mononitrate, 634*t*, 640*t*
Isotonic glucose solutions, 1151
Isotretinoin
allergic reactions to, 74*t*
alopecia and, 166, 173*t*

INDEX

Isotretinoin (continued)
- asthma/bronchospasm and, 452*t*
- depression and, 377*t*, 384, 385, 385*t*, 387, 388
- ototoxicity and, 1236*t*
- photosensitivity and, 146*t*
- restrictive drug distribution system for, 7*t*
- sexual dysfunction and, 758*t*
- taste disorders and, 1260*t*
- teratogenicity of, 1319–1322, 1324, 1325
- thyroid diseases and, 702*t*
- visual disturbances and, 303*t*

Isradipine, 472*t*, 570*t*, 577*t*, 633*t*, 639*t*

Itraconazole
- allergic reactions to, 74*t*
- Cushing syndrome and, 733
- heart failure and, 503*t*, 510*t*
- ototoxicity and, 1236*t*
- pancreatitis and, 879*t*
- photosensitivity and, 146*t*
- serum sickness-like reactions and, 1193*t*
- torsades de pointes and, 533*t*, 539, 539*t*

Intrauterine growth restrictions (IUGRs), 1316–1317

IUDs. *See* Intrauterine contraceptive devices

Ivabradine
- atrial fibrillation/atrial flutter and, 582*t*, 584
- heart failure and, 510
- hypertension and, 618*t*
- sinus bradycardia/atrioventricular block and, 570*t*, 572, 574, 574*t*, 577*t*
- torsades de pointes and, 533*t*, 539*t*

IVIG (intravenous immunoglobulin G), 76, 113–114, 473*t*, 829

Ivy gourd, 682*t*, 685*t*

Ixabepilone, 170*t*, 472*t*

Jaw. *See* Osteonecrosis of jaw

Jones v. Irvin and K-Mart (1986), 9*t*, 11

Ju bu huan, 850*t*

The Jungle (Sinclair), 5

Kanamycin, 1236*t*

Karela. *See* Bitter melon

Kava, 303*t*, 353, 851*t*

Kefauver–Harris Amendments of 1962, 5

Kelp, 699*t*, 705, 706*t*, 708

Ketamine
- myocardial ischemia/acute coronary syndromes and, 472*t*
- nausea/vomiting and, 907*t*, 914
- peripheral neuropathy and, 288
- psychosis and, 416*t*, 418, 418*t*
- sexual dysfunction and, 783*t*, 786*t*
- sinus bradycardia/atrioventricular block and, 570*t*, 578*t*

Ketoacidosis, 1002*t*, 1004*t*

Ketoconazole
- color changes of oral mucosa and teeth and, 1253, 1254*t*
- drug interactions with, 39
- gingival hyperplasia and, 1263*t*
- myocardial ischemia/acute coronary syndromes and, 472*t*
- oral lichenoid reactions and, 1270, 1271*t*
- ototoxicity and, 1236*t*
- photosensitivity and, 146*t*
- secondary adrenal insufficiency and, 735–737, 736–737*t*
- sexual dysfunction and, 758*t*, 762–763*t*, 765*t*
- thyroid diseases and, 702*t*
- torsades de pointes and, 533*t*, 539

Ketoprofen
- allergic reactions to, 73*t*
- alopecia and, 172*t*
- asthma/bronchospasm and, 463
- delirium and, 327*t*
- heart failure and, 510*t*
- oral erythema multiforme and, 1267*t*
- photosensitivity and, 146*t*, 150

Ketorolac, 172*t*, 303*t*, 815, 846*t*, 958, 1236*t*

Kidney disease. *See* Acute kidney injury (AKI); Chronic kidney disease (CKD)

Labetalol
- hyperprolactinemia and, 743*t*
- hypotension and, 632*t*, 638*t*
- myocardial ischemia/acute coronary syndromes and, 488
- myopathy and, 1150*t*
- oral lichenoid reactions and, 1271*t*
- sleep disorders and, 348*t*
- stroke and, 236
- systemic lupus erythematosus and, 124*t*

Lacidipine, 472*t*

Lacosamide, 416*t*, 524*t*, 1236*t*

Lactic acidosis, 1002*t*, 1004, 1004*t*, 1007–1008, 1010–1011

Lactulose, 822, 823, 840*t*, 871

Lamivudine, 168*t*, 280*t*, 879*t*, 1002*t*, 1123*t*, 1236*t*

Lamotrigine
- allergic reactions to, 75*t*, 95
- alopecia and, 168*t*
- cutaneous diseases and, 101, 102–104*t*, 111, 111*t*, 113*t*
- delirium and, 326*t*
- depression and, 378, 379
- gingival hyperplasia and, 1263*t*
- hepatic/cholestatic diseases and, 852*t*
- monomorphic ventricular tachycardia and, 524*t*
- neuroleptic malignant syndrome and, 1195*t*
- oral erythema multiforme and, 1267*t*
- osteoporosis/osteomalacia and, 1127
- ototoxicity and, 1236*t*
- peripheral neuropathy and, 289
- SIADH and, 983*t*
- sleep disorders and, 348*t*
- systemic lupus erythematosus and, 124*t*
- taste disorders and, 1260*t*
- teratogenicity of, 1319, 1330, 1331
- visual disturbances and, 303*t*, 312, 313
- weight gain and, 1175*t*

LAMPS (large automated multipurpose population-based systems), 55–56

Lansoprazole, 126*t*, 533*t*, 966*t*, 1254*t*

Lantana camara, 851*t*

Lapatinib, 170*t*, 177, 179*t*, 187, 472*t*, 508, 1109*t*

Large automated multipurpose population-based systems (LAMPS), 55–56

Laser therapy, 189*t*, 192, 205, 207, 208

L-asparaginase
- allergic reactions to, 72*t*
- glucose/insulin dysregulation and, 680*t*, 684*t*
- myocardial ischemia/acute coronary syndromes and, 472*t*
- pancreatitis and, 881, 887, 892
- thyroid diseases and, 702*t*

Last, John, 20

Latanoprost, 197, 197*t*

Laxatives
- abuse of, 840
- acidosis and, 1002*t*
- alkalosis and, 1013–1014*t*, 1017
- bulk-forming, 840, 840*t*
- emollient, 840, 840*t*
- lubricant, 840*t*
- myopathy and, 1150*t*, 1152*t*
- osmotic, 840, 840*t*
- saline, 840, 840*t*
- stimulant, 839, 840, 840*t*, 920, 930

L-carnitine, 682*t*, 685*t*, 868, 1009

Lead, 171*t*, 177, 1254–1255*t*, 1316

Learning disabilities, 1315–1316

Leflunomide
- acidosis and, 1003*t*
- alopecia and, 172*t*, 174
- hepatic/cholestatic diseases and, 846*t*
- macrocytic anemia and, 1108*t*
- ototoxicity and, 1236*t*
- peripheral neuropathy and, 281*t*
- photosensitivity and, 146*t*
- regulatory actions involving, 13

Legal environment for drug safety, 8–11, 9*t*

Lemon oil, 146*t*

Lenalidomide
- alopecia and, 170*t*
- interstitial lung disease/pulmonary fibrosis and, 432*t*, 435*t*
- leukemia and, 1284, 1284*t*, 1286–1287, 1289
- lymphoma and, 1292
- restrictive drug distribution system for, 7*t*
- thromboembolic diseases and, 1065*t*, 1069*t*, 1075*t*
- thyroid diseases and, 699–700*t*, 702*t*, 715

Lenvatinib, 7*t*, 170*t*, 908*t*

Lepirudin, 73*t*, 1058

Leprosy, 6

Letrozole, 170*t*, 176, 1064*t*, 1068*t*, 1123*t*

Leucovorin, 825, 826

Leukemia, 1283–1292
- acute lymphoblastic, 1283, 1286, 1291
- acute myeloid, 1283–1287, 1289–1292
- causative agents of, 1284–1286, 1284*t*
- clinical presentation of, 1289, 1290*t*
- differential diagnosis of, 1289, 1290*t*
- epidemiology of, 1286–1287
- management of, 1291–1292
- mechanisms of, 1287–1289, 1288*t*
- morbidity and mortality for, 1291
- overview, 1283
- patient education on, 1292
- prevention of, 1291, 1294*t*
- risk factors for, 1290, 1291*t*

Leukocytoclastic vasculitis, 85

Leukotriene antagonists, 74*t*, 463

Leuprolide
- anxiety and, 403
- depression and, 385*t*, 390
- myocardial ischemia/acute coronary syndromes and, 473*t*
- myopathy and, 1150*t*
- thromboembolic diseases and, 1064*t*, 1068*t*
- vaginal bleeding disorders and, 796

Leuprolide acetate, 126*t*, 699–700*t*

Leuprorelin, 73*t*, 700*t*

Levamisole, 983*t*, 1051*t*, 1188*t*, 1260*t*

Levels of evidence, 20–21, 21*t*, 63

Levetiracetam
- alopecia and, 168*t*
- depression and, 376*t*, 379, 388
- dystonia and, 270
- osteoporosis/osteomalacia and, 1127
- psychosis and, 416*t*

sexual dysfunction and, 758*t*, 772
SIADH and, 983*t*, 988
tardive dyskinesia and, 265
teratogenicity of, 1319
weight gain and, 1175*t*
Levodopa. *See also* Carbidopa–levodopa
alopecia and, 171*t*, 175
anxiety and, 400*t*, 405
delirium and, 327*t*, 329*t*
dystonia and, 270
gout/hyperuricemia and, 1136*t*, 1139
nausea/vomiting and, 911*t*
neutropenia/agranulocytosis and, 1090*t*
psychosis and, 418*t*
serotonin syndrome and, 1203–1204*t*
systemic lupus erythematosus and, 126*t*
taste disorders and, 1260*t*
Levofloxacin
cutaneous diseases and, 104*t*
delirium and, 328*t*
drug interactions with, 40
hemolytic anemia and, 1105*t*
hypersensitivity reactions to, 77*t*
hypotension and, 635*t*, 640*t*, 645*t*
oral erythema multiforme and, 1267*t*
peripheral neuropathy and, 280*t*
photosensitivity and, 146*t*
taste disorders and, 1260*t*
torsades de pointes and, 532*t*, 538, 539*t*
Levomepromazine, 532*t*, 539*t*
Levomethadyl, 541
Levomilnacipran, 982*t*
Levonorgestrel, 782*t*, 785*t*, 795, 909*t*, 1067
Levosimendan, 472*t*, 524*t*, 582*t*
Levothyroxine
alopecia and, 173*t*
hepatic/cholestatic diseases and, 849*t*
iodine content of, 707*t*
osteoporosis/osteomalacia and, 1121*t*, 1123*t*
psychosis and, 416*t*
thyroid diseases and, 703*t*, 709, 710, 715, 716
LH. *See* Luteinizing hormone
Libido disorders
causative agents of, 757, 758*t*, 798
clinical presentation of, 767–768, 768*t*, 769
defined, 757
differential diagnosis of, 770*t*
management of, 773*t*
mechanisms of, 763, 763*t*, 766
Licorice, 304*t*, 503*t*, 510*t*, 517, 618*t*, 620*t*, 1151
Lidocaine
allergic reactions to, 75*t*
anxiety and, 400*t*
cognitive disorders and, 358*t*, 365
comorbidity and, 34
delirium and, 326*t*
heart failure and, 502*t*, 510*t*
monomorphic ventricular tachycardia and, 530
ototoxicity and, 1236*t*
peripheral neuropathy and, 289
psychosis and, 416*t*
seizures and, 218*t*
sinus bradycardia/atrioventricular block and, 571*t*, 578*t*
taste disorders and, 1262
Lifestyle factors related to drug-induced diseases, 32–33
Lily of the valley, 304*t*
Limb deficiency defects, 1324–1326
Lime oil, 146*t*
Linagliptin, 879*t*
Linezolid
acidosis and, 1002*t*
aplastic anemia and, 1100*t*
delirium and, 328*t*
peripheral neuropathy and, 280*t*, 282*t*
serotonin syndrome and, 1202, 1203–1204*t*
thrombocytopenia and, 1051–1052*t*, 1056, 1056*t*
visual disturbances and, 304*t*
Linghzi, 851*t*
Linifanib, 699*t*
Liothyronine, 173*t*, 369, 707*t*
Liotrix, 707*t*
Lipokinetix, 851*t*
5-lipoxygenase inhibitors, 462
Liraglutide, 879*t*, 884, 909*t*, 915
Lisdexamfetamine, 167*t*
Lisinopril
alopecia and, 167*t*
color changes of oral mucosa and teeth and, 1254*t*
glucose/insulin dysregulation and, 688
hypotension and, 632*t*, 638*t*
myocardial ischemia/acute coronary syndromes and, 472*t*
oral lichenoid reactions and, 1271*t*
ototoxicity and, 1236*t*
pancreatitis and, 878*t*, 879, 880, 886*t*
photosensitivity and, 146*t*
SIADH and, 983*t*
systemic lupus erythematosus and, 125*t*
taste disorders and, 1260–1261*t*
Lithium
acidosis and, 1003*t*
acute kidney injury and, 943*t*, 945*t*, 959
akathisia and, 255–256*t*, 258*t*
alopecia and, 173*t*, 175, 178, 183
Brugada syndrome and, 547*t*
chronic kidney disease and, 965, 966*t*, 968–970, 970*t*, 972–976, 972*t*, 974*t*
cognitive disorders and, 358*t*, 365, 367–369
cutaneous diseases and, 102–103*t*, 108, 109
delirium and, 327*t*
depression and, 391
diabetes insipidus and, 991–993, 991*t*
gingival hyperplasia and, 1263*t*
monomorphic ventricular tachycardia and, 524*t*
myocardial ischemia/acute coronary syndromes and, 473*t*
nausea/vomiting and, 909*t*
neuroleptic malignant syndrome and, 1195, 1195*t*, 1199, 1200
oral lichenoid reactions and, 1270, 1271*t*
ototoxicity and, 1236*t*
peripheral neuropathy and, 281*t*
serotonin syndrome and, 1203–1204*t*
sexual dysfunction and, 758–759*t*, 761*t*
side effects of, 254
systemic lupus erythematosus and, 125*t*, 133
tardive dyskinesia and, 262
taste disorders and, 1260–1261*t*
teratogenicity of, 1321–1322, 1334*t*
thromboembolic diseases and, 1066*t*, 1070*t*
thyroid diseases and, 699–700*t*, 702*t*, 704, 707–709, 713–714, 717
visual disturbances and, 304*t*
weight gain and, 1167–1169*t*, 1171–1172, 1173*t*
Liver diseases. *See* Hepatic and cholestatic diseases
LLLT (low-level laser therapy), 189*t*, 192
LMWH. *See* Low-molecular-weight heparin
Lobaplatin, 170*t*
Local anesthetics, 530, 1262, 1314
Lomefloxacin, 146*t*, 280*t*
Lomitapide, 7*t*, 849*t*
Lomustine, 384, 432*t*, 908*t*, 916*t*, 966*t*, 970*t*
Loop diuretics
acute kidney injury and, 943–944*t*, 947, 953, 954
alkalosis and, 1013–1014*t*
gout/hyperuricemia and, 1138
graded challenge procedure for, 95
heart failure and, 505, 511
hepatic/cholestatic diseases and, 847*t*
ototoxicity and, 1239, 1241
pancreatitis and, 883
sexual dysfunction and, 759*t*, 764*t*
SIADH and, 989*t*
in sulfa drug class, 92
Loperamide, 39, 533*t*, 827*t*, 828
Lopinavir, 984*t*, 1051*t*
Loratadine, 146*t*, 539*t*, 853*t*, 1013–1014*t*
Lorazepam
anxiety and, 407, 410
cognitive disorders and, 369
delirium and, 327*t*, 329*t*, 337
hypothermia and, 1218
nausea/vomiting and, 929, 929*t*
neuroleptic malignant syndrome and, 1195*t*, 1200*t*
oral lichenoid reactions and, 1271*t*
ototoxicity and, 1236*t*
seizures and, 226
serotonin syndrome and, 1208, 1208*t*
SIADH and, 984*t*
visual disturbances and, 304*t*
Lorcainide, 502*t*, 507, 510*t*
Lorcaserin, 664
Losartan
acute kidney injury and, 942
asthma/bronchospasm and, 452*t*, 454
gout/hyperuricemia and, 1138
hypotension and, 632*t*, 638*t*
pancreatitis and, 878*t*
photosensitivity and, 146*t*
taste disorders and, 1260*t*
Lovage, 304*t*
Lovastatin
alopecia and, 171*t*
ototoxicity and, 1236*t*
pancreatitis and, 878*t*, 886*t*
photosensitivity and, 146*t*
sleep disorders and, 348*t*
systemic lupus erythematosus and, 124*t*
visual disturbances and, 304*t*
Low birth weight, 1311, 1316–1318
Low blood pressure. *See* Hypotension
Low-level laser therapy (LLLT), 189*t*, 192
Low-molecular-weight heparin (LMWH)
alopecia and, 166, 178
bleeding disorders and, 1026*t*, 1028, 1029*t*, 1032, 1036
intracerebral hemorrhage and, 238*t*, 239, 240*t*, 242*t*, 245
myocardial ischemia/acute coronary syndromes and, 486
osteoporosis/osteomalacia and, 1121*t*, 1124*t*
ovarian hyperstimulation and, 789
thrombocytopenia and, 1052*t*, 1055–1058, 1056–1057*t*
thromboembolic diseases and, 1064*t*, 1067, 1075, 1076
Loxapine, 326*t*, 547*t*, 582*t*, 635*t*, 639*t*, 852*t*, 1195*t*
LSD (lysergic acid diethylamide), 415, 418, 473*t*, 1188*t*
L-tryptophan, 1203–1204*t*

Lubiprostone, 840, 840*t*
Lubricant laxatives, 840*t*
Lugol's solution, 706*t*
Lupus. *See* Systemic lupus erythematosus (SLE)
Lupus diathesis, 129, 133
Lupus-like reactions, 84, 86
Lurasidone, 254, 376*t*, 635*t*, 639*t*, 1166*t*, 1171, 1175*t*
Luteinizing hormone (LH), 729, 766, 767, 783, 793, 800
Lymphoma, 1292–1295
  causative agents of, 1284*t*, 1292–1293
  clinical presentation of, 1290*t*, 1293–1294
  differential diagnosis of, 1290*t*, 1293–1294
  epidemiology of, 1293
  hepatosplenic T-cell, 1292, 1293
  Hodgkin, 1284–1286, 1291–1293
  management of, 1295
  mechanisms of, 1288*t*, 1293
  morbidity and mortality for, 1294
  non-Hodgkin, 1286, 1292–1294, 1303
  patient education on, 1295
  post-transplant lymphoproliferative disorders, 1293, 1295
  prevention of, 1294–1295, 1294*t*
  risk factors for, 1291*t*, 1294
Lysergic acid diethylamide (LSD), 415, 418, 473*t*, 1188*t*
Lysine-aspirin, 459

Macitentan, 7*t*
Macrocytic anemia, 1107–1109
  causative agents of, 1107, 1108*t*
  clinical presentation of, 1102*t*, 1108
  differential diagnosis of, 1102*t*, 1108
  epidemiology of, 1107
  management of, 1108–1109
  mechanisms of, 1101*t*, 1107–1108
  morbidity and mortality for, 1108
  patient education on, 1109
  prevention of, 1108
  risk factors for, 1103*t*, 1108
Macrolides, 220, 328*t*, 541–542, 822*t*, 823, 1088
Magnesium
  acute kidney injury and, 955
  diarrhea and, 822, 823
  hypotension and, 636*t*, 640*t*
  myopathy and, 1151, 1153, 1156
  torsades de pointes and, 543–544
Magnesium hydroxide, 1013–1014*t*
Magnesium salts, 287, 287*t*, 840*t*
Ma huang, 219*t*, 225, 243, 415, 425, 851*t*
Major depressive disorder (MDD), 375, 379, 380, 386–390
Male pattern baldness. *See* Androgenetic alopecia
Males. *See* Gender differences
Male sexual dysfunction, 757–775
  causative agents of, 757–761, 758–762*t*
  clinical presentation of, 767–771, 768*t*
  differential diagnosis of, 769, 770*t*
  epidemiology of, 761–762
  management of, 772–774, 773–774*t*
  mechanisms of, 763–765*t*, 763–767
  morbidity and mortality for, 771
  patient education on, 774–775
  prevention of, 771–772, 772*t*
  risk factors for, 771, 771*t*
Malignant hyperthermia, 1209–1214
  causative agents of, 1186, 1209–1210, 1209*t*
  clinical presentation of, 1187*t*, 1210–1211, 1210*t*
  differential diagnosis of, 1211, 1211*t*
  epidemiology of, 1210
  management of, 1213–1214, 1213–1214*t*
  mechanisms of, 1210
  morbidity and mortality for, 1212
  patient education on, 1214
  prevention of, 1212–1213, 1212*t*
  risk factors for, 1211–1212, 1211*t*
Malotilate, 868
Mammalian target-of-rapamycin (mTOR) inhibitors, 432*t*, 680*t*, 684*t*, 1295, 1298
Management of disease
  acidosis, 1008–1011, 1009*f*, 1010*t*, 1011*f*
  acute interstitial nephritis, 957
  acute tubular necrosis, 955
  akathisia, 258–259, 259*t*
  alkalosis, 1016–1017, 1018*f*, 1018*t*
  alopecia, 186–192, 187–189*t*
  amenorrhea and oligomenorrhea, 790*t*, 794
  anxiety, 410–411
  aplastic anemia, 1103–1104
  asthma and bronchospasm, 218*t*, 462–463
  atrial fibrillation/atrial flutter, 586–588, 587*t*
  atrial tachycardia, 590–591, 591*t*
  AV node re-entrant tachycardia, 594, 595*t*
  bladder cancer, 1305
  bleeding disorders, 1036–1037*t*, 1036–1039, 1038*f*
  breast cancer, 1300
  Brugada syndrome, 549
  chemotherapy-induced anemia, 1111
  chronic kidney disease, 975–976, 976*t*
  cognitive disorders, 368–369, 368*t*
  color changes of oral mucosa and teeth, 1258
  constipation, 839–841, 840*t*
  Cushing syndrome, 734
  cutaneous diseases, 113–114, 114*t*
  delirium, 335–340, 336*t*, 369
  depression, 390–392, 391*t*
  diabetes insipidus, 993, 993*t*
  diarrhea, 827–829, 827*t*
  drug allergies, 98–100, 99*t*
  drug fever, 1191, 1191*t*
  dysmenorrhea, 790*t*, 797
  dystonia, 270, 270*t*
  endometrial cancer, 1303
  female sexual dysfunction, 790*t*, 799–800
  gingival hyperplasia, 1265
  glomerulonephritis, 959
  glucose and insulin dysregulation, 689–690, 690*t*
  gout and hyperuricemia, 171*t*, 179*t*, 1144–1145, 1145*f*
  growth hormone deficiency, 750, 750*t*
  heart failure, 516
  hemodynamic-mediated AKI, 948–949
  hemolytic anemia, 1107
  hepatic and cholestatic, 865–872, 867*t*
  hirsutism, 203–207, 204–206*t*
  hyperprolactinemia, 746, 747*t*
  hypertension, 624–626, 625*t*, 942
  hypertrichosis, 204–205*t*, 207
  hypotension, 644–648, 645–646*t*
  hypothermia, 1217–1218
  infertility, 774*t*, 801–802
  interstitial lung disease/pulmonary fibrosis, 439–441, 441*f*
  intracerebral hemorrhage, 244–246
  leukemia, 1291–1292
  lymphoma, 1295
  macrocytic anemia, 1108–1109
  male sexual dysfunction, 772–774, 773–774*t*
  malignant hyperthermia, 1213–1214, 1213–1214*t*
  menorrhagia and menometrorrhagia, 790*t*, 796
  monomorphic ventricular tachycardia, 530, 531*f*
  myocardial ischemia/acute coronary syndromes, 485–489, 487*t*
  myopathy, 1158–1159
  nausea and vomiting, 927–929*t*, 927–930
  nephrolithiasis, 958
  neuroleptic malignant syndrome, 1200–1201, 1200–1201*t*
  neutropenia and agranulocytosis, 1095–1096
  oral erythema multiforme, 1269
  oral lichenoid reactions, 1273
  osteonecrosis of jaw, 1276
  osteoporosis and osteomalacia, 1129–1130, 1129*t*
  ototoxicity, 1243–1244
  ovarian hyperstimulation, 787–790, 790*t*
  pancreatitis, 892
  parkinsonism, 273, 273*t*
  peripheral neuropathy, 287–289
  photosensitivity, 155, 155*t*
  psychosis, 423–424, 424*t*
  secondary adrenal insufficiency, 740–741, 740*t*
  seizures, 225–226
  serotonin syndrome, 1201*t*, 1207–1209, 1208*t*
  serum sickness-like reactions, 1191*t*, 1194
  SIADH, 989–990, 989*t*
  sinus bradycardia/atrioventricular block, 579–580, 579*t*
  skin cancer, 1298
  sleep disorders, 352–353
  stroke, 235–237
  systemic lupus erythematosus, 135, 135*t*
  tardive dyskinesia, 264–265, 265*t*
  taste disorders, 1262
  teratogenicity, 1334–1335
  thrombocytopenia, 1057–1059
  thromboembolic diseases, 237, 1076–1077
  thyroid diseases, 715–717, 715*t*
  torsades de pointes, 544–545, 545*f*
  upper gastrointestinal ulceration, 818
  valvular and pericardial heart disease, 669–670, 670*t*
  visual disturbances, 318–319
  vulvovaginal candidiasis, 790*t*, 792
  weight gain, 1174–1175, 1175*t*
Mandrake, 304*t*
Manganese, 1254*t*
Mannitol
  acute kidney injury and, 953, 954
  heart failure and, 503*t*, 509
  hepatic/cholestatic diseases and, 871
  hypotension and, 636*t*, 638*t*
  ototoxicity and, 1236*t*
Manufacturers, role in postmarketing surveillance, 50–52
MAOIs. *See* Monoamine oxidase inhibitors
Maprotiline
  depression and, 392
  drug fever and, 1188*t*
  myocardial ischemia/acute coronary syndromes and, 472*t*
  photosensitivity and, 146*t*
  seizures and, 220, 222*t*
  weight gain and, 1166*t*, 1169*t*, 1170
Margosa oil, 851*t*
Marijuana
  duration of detection in urine, 420*t*
  myocardial ischemia/acute coronary syndromes and, 473*t*
  nausea/vomiting and, 929
  as risk factor for drug-induced diseases, 33
  sexual dysfunction and, 759*t*, 761*t*
  stroke and, 230*t*

teratogenicity of, 1324, 1326
visual disturbances and, 304t
Masterwort, 304t
Maternity status. *See* Pregnancy
MDD (major depressive disorder), 375, 379, 380, 386–390
MDMA (methylenedioxymethamphetamine). *See* Ecstasy
MDR-TB (multidrug resistant tuberculosis), 288
MDS (myelodysplastic syndrome), 1283, 1286–1287, 1289
Measles, 29
Measles, mumps, and rubella (MMR) vaccine, 21, 1267t
Measles vaccine, 197t
Mebendazole, 1090t, 1188t
Mechanisms of disease
acidosis, 1001, 1004–1005, 1004t
acute interstitial nephritis, 945t, 956
acute tubular necrosis, 950–951
akathisia, 255–256, 256t
alkalosis, 1012–1014, 1014t
alopecia, 178–180, 179–180t
amenorrhea and oligomenorrhea, 785t, 793
anxiety, 404–406, 405t
aplastic anemia, 1100–1101, 1101t
asthma and bronchospasm, 455–457, 455t, 456f
atrial fibrillation/atrial flutter, 583–584, 583t
atrial tachycardia, 589, 589t
AV node re-entrant tachycardia, 592–593
bladder cancer, 1288t, 1304
bleeding disorders, 1028–1030, 1028f, 1029t
breast cancer, 1288t
Brugada syndrome, 546–547
chemotherapy-induced anemia, 1101t, 1110
chronic kidney disease, 969–970, 970t
cognitive disorders, 359–361, 359t
color changes of oral mucosa and teeth, 1255, 1255t
congenital heart defects, 1323
constipation, 837, 837t
Cushing syndrome, 730–732, 731t
cutaneous diseases, 105–106
delirium, 329–330, 329t, 360
depression, 385–386, 385t
diabetes insipidus, 991
diarrhea, 823, 823t
drug allergies and hypersensitivity reactions, 78–82, 80t
drug fever, 1187
dysmenorrhea, 786t, 796
dystonia, 266
endometrial cancer, 1288t, 1301
female sexual dysfunction, 786t, 798
fetal alcohol spectrum disorders, 1332
gastroschisis, 1326
gingival hyperplasia, 1264, 1264t
glomerulonephritis, 958
glucose and insulin dysregulation, 683, 684–685t
gout and hyperuricemia, 1135–1140, 1136t
growth hormone deficiency, 747–748, 748t
heart failure, 509–512, 510t
hemodynamic-mediated AKI, 944–945, 945t
hemolytic anemia, 1101t, 1104, 1106
hepatic and cholestatic, 854–855t, 855–858
hirsutism, 198, 199t
hyperprolactinemia, 742, 744t
hypertension, 619–621, 620t
hypertrichosis, 198–199, 199t
hypotension, 637, 638–640t
hypothermia, 1215–1216
infertility, 765t, 767, 786t, 800
interstitial lung disease/pulmonary fibrosis, 434, 435t
intracerebral hemorrhage, 232, 240, 240t
learning disabilities, 1315
leukemia, 1287–1289, 1288t
limb deficiency defects, 1325
low birth weight, 1317
lymphoma, 1288t, 1293
macrocytic anemia, 1101t, 1107–1108
male sexual dysfunction, 763–765t, 763–767
malignant hyperthermia, 1210
menorrhagia and menometrorrhagia, 785t, 795
microcephaly, 1331
monomorphic ventricular tachycardia, 525–526, 525t
myocardial ischemia/acute coronary syndromes, 476–480, 477t
myopathy, 1151–1153, 1152t
nausea and vomiting, 910–915, 911t, 913f
nephrolithiasis, 957
neural tube defects, 1328–1329
neuroleptic malignant syndrome, 1196
neutropenia and agranulocytosis, 1091, 1091t
oral erythema multiforme, 1268, 1268t
oral lichenoid reactions, 1270, 1272, 1272t
orofacial clefts, 1320–1321
osteonecrosis of jaw, 1274, 1274t
osteoporosis and osteomalacia, 1120, 1122, 1123–1124t
ototoxicity, 1239–1240, 1239t
ovarian hyperstimulation, 783–784, 785t
pancreatitis, 885–888, 886t
parkinsonism, 271–272, 271t
peripheral neuropathy, 281–282, 282t
photosensitivity, 149–151, 149f, 150t
psychosis, 417–419, 418t
secondary adrenal insufficiency, 735–737, 737t
seizures, 222, 222t
serotonin syndrome, 1202–1205, 1204t
serum sickness-like reactions, 80, 81, 1192–1193
SIADH, 985–986
sinus bradycardia/atrioventricular block, 572, 574, 574t
skin cancer, 1288t, 1296
sleep disorders, 347, 349, 350t
stroke, 231–233, 231t
systemic lupus erythematosus, 127–129, 128t
tardive dyskinesia, 261
taste disorders, 1261, 1261t
thrombocytopenia, 1052–1054, 1052t
thromboembolic diseases, 1067–1071, 1068–1071t
thyroid diseases, 697, 698f, 701–703t, 704–710, 706–707t
torsades de pointes, 535–536
upper gastrointestinal ulceration, 811–812, 811t
valvular and pericardial heart disease, 663–664, 663t
visual disturbances, 313–315, 314–315t
vulvovaginal candidiasis, 785t, 791
weight gain, 1168, 1168t
Mechlorethamine, 304t, 908t, 916t, 1284–1286, 1288t
Meclizine, 1243–1244
Meclofenamic acid, 1267t
Medication errors
cost of, 27, 29
decision-tree model in assessment of, 28, 28t
defined, 41
monitoring systems for, 56
prevalence of, 42
reporting systems for, 24
risk factors for, 42
sources of, 19, 26, 41–42
Medication histories, 60–62, 61–62t
Medication nonadherence, 28, 41
Medications. *See* Drugs; *specific names and types of medications*
Mediterranean glue thistle, 851t
MEDMARX system, 56
Medroxyprogesterone, 176, 782t, 785t, 1013, 1167t
Medroxyprogesterone acetate (MPA), 731t, 732, 736, 736t, 741
Medroxyprogesterone depot, 1121t, 1123t, 1169t, 1172–1173, 1173t, 1175t
MedWatch program, 6, 15, 50, 66–67
Mefenamic acid, 73t, 510t, 1236t
Mefloquine
anxiety and, 400t, 403
depression and, 376t, 377
myocardial ischemia/acute coronary syndromes and, 472t
ototoxicity and, 1236t
peripheral neuropathy and, 280t
psychosis and, 416t
Megestrol, 503t, 510t, 1065t, 1069t
Megestrol acetate
glucose/insulin dysregulation and, 680t, 684t
myocardial ischemia/acute coronary syndromes and, 473t, 474
secondary adrenal insufficiency and, 731t, 732, 736, 736t, 741
Meglumine antimoniate, 878t
MEK (mitogen-activated protein kinase) inhibitors, 1295, 1296
Melanoma, 1295–1298
Melatonin, 265, 335, 337, 349, 353, 1242t
Meloxicam, 172t, 453, 461, 510t, 1051t
Melphalan, 432t, 983t, 1284, 1287, 1288t
Memantine, 571t, 577t, 984t
Men. *See* Gender differences; Male sexual dysfunction
Meningomyelocele, 1327, 1327f
Menorrhagia and menometrorrhagia, 795–796
causative agents of, 782t, 795
clinical presentation of, 787t, 795
differential diagnosis of, 788t, 795
epidemiology of, 795
management of, 790t, 796
mechanisms of, 785t, 795
morbidity and mortality for, 796
patient education on, 796
prevention of, 789t, 796
risk factors for, 788t, 796
Menthol, 452t
Meperidine
acute kidney injury and, 958
asthma/bronchospasm and, 452t
cognitive disorders and, 366
delirium and, 326t
nausea/vomiting and, 906t
psychosis and, 416t
seizures and, 218t, 222, 222t, 224
serotonin syndrome and, 1202, 1203–1204t
Mephenytoin, 124t, 1263t
Mepivacaine, 472t, 571t
Mepolizumab, 462
Meprobamate, 404, 1090t
Mequinol-tretinoin, 146t
6-mercaptopurine, 878t, 880, 886t, 891t, 1188t, 1193t
Mercaptopurine, 16, 35, 36t, 848t, 1003t, 1145, 1292

INDEX

Mercury, 171*t*, 177, 1255*t*, 1271*t*
Meropenem, 74*t*, 92, 220, 1193*t*
Mesalamine
  aplastic anemia and, 1100*t*
  cutaneous diseases and, 104*t*
  diabetes insipidus and, 991, 991*t*
  hepatic/cholestatic diseases and, 850*t*
  macrocytic anemia and, 1108*t*
  myocardial ischemia/acute coronary syndromes and, 472*t*
  pancreatitis and, 881, 891*t*
  systemic lupus erythematosus and, 126*t*
  valvular/pericardial heart disease and, 661*t*, 662, 664
Mesna, 1304–1305
Mesoridazine, 541
Metabolic acidosis. *See* Acidosis
Metabolic alkalosis. *See* Alkalosis
Metabolic myopathy. *See* Necrotizing myopathy
Metabolism of drugs, 35, 37
Metaproterenol, 582*t*
Metaxalone, 1203–1204*t*
Metergoline, 703*t*
Metformin
  acidosis and, 1002*t*, 1007, 1010
  heart failure and, 505, 506, 515
  hemolytic anemia and, 1105*t*
  hepatic/cholestatic diseases and, 849*t*
  macrocytic anemia and, 1107, 1108, 1108*t*
  nausea/vomiting and, 909*t*
  oral lichenoid reactions and, 1271*t*
  taste disorders and, 1260*t*
  thyroid diseases and, 702*t*
  visual disturbances and, 304*t*
  weight gain and, 1174, 1175, 1175*t*
Methadone
  constipation and, 836*t*
  hyperprolactinemia and, 743*t*
  myocardial ischemia/acute coronary syndromes and, 472*t*
  nausea/vomiting and, 906*t*
  ototoxicity and, 1233, 1239
  sexual dysfunction and, 763*t*, 783*t*, 786*t*
  SIADH and, 984*t*
  sinus bradycardia/atrioventricular block and, 571*t*, 578*t*
  smoking and, 32
  thyroid diseases and, 702*t*
  torsades de pointes and, 532*t*, 540*t*, 542, 544
  vaginal bleeding disorders and, 782*t*, 785*t*, 795
  as withdrawal treatment, 424*t*
Methamphetamine
  alopecia and, 167*t*
  anxiety and, 401
  monomorphic ventricular tachycardia and, 524*t*
  myocardial ischemia/acute coronary syndromes and, 473*t*, 486
  psychosis and, 417
  teratogenicity and, 1327
  visual disturbances and, 304*t*
Methanol, 304*t*
Methazolamide, 146*t*, 783*t*, 786*t*
Methicillin, 956, 1188*t*
Methimazole
  allergic reactions to, 74–75*t*
  alopecia and, 173*t*, 175
  aplastic anemia and, 1100*t*
  asthma/bronchospasm and, 452*t*
  hepatic/cholestatic diseases and, 849*t*
  neutropenia/agranulocytosis and, 1088, 1091, 1093–1094
  pancreatitis and, 885
  systemic lupus erythematosus and, 124*t*
  teratogenicity of, 1334*t*
  thyroid diseases and, 703*t*, 715–717
Methionine, 868, 1243
Methocarbamol, 1260*t*
Methohexital, 907*t*
Methotrexate
  allergic reactions to, 74*t*
  alopecia and, 170*t*, 172*t*, 174, 176, 186, 191
  asthma/bronchospasm and, 452*t*
  depression and, 384
  drug fever and, 1188*t*
  hepatic/cholestatic diseases and, 853*t*, 856, 864, 866, 868
  infertility and, 783*t*, 786*t*
  interstitial lung disease/pulmonary fibrosis and, 432*t*, 435*t*, 437, 438
  macrocytic anemia and, 1107, 1109
  myocardial ischemia/acute coronary syndromes and, 472*t*
  nausea/vomiting and, 908*t*, 916*t*
  oral erythema multiforme and, 1267*t*
  osteoporosis/osteomalacia and, 1121*t*, 1123*t*
  photosensitivity and, 146*t*, 154
  seizures and, 218*t*, 222*t*
  teratogenicity of, 1324, 1325, 1330, 1331, 1334*t*
  valvular/pericardial heart disease and, 661*t*
  visual disturbances and, 304*t*
  weight gain and, 1172
Methoxsalen, 146*t*, 150
Methoxyflurane, 861*t*, 1209*t*
Methsuximide, 1263*t*
Methyclothiazide, 146*t*
Methyl bromide/chloride/dichloride, 849*t*
Methylcellulose, 840*t*
Methyldopa
  allergic reactions to, 75*t*
  asthma/bronchospasm and, 452*t*
  color changes of oral mucosa and teeth and, 1254*t*
  delirium and, 327*t*
  depression and, 376*t*, 378, 385, 385*t*
  drug fever and, 1188*t*, 1190
  hemolytic anemia and, 1101*t*, 1105*t*, 1106
  hepatic/cholestatic diseases and, 847*t*, 861*t*
  hyperprolactinemia and, 742, 743–744*t*
  hypotension and, 633*t*, 639*t*
  neutropenia/agranulocytosis and, 1090*t*
  oral lichenoid reactions and, 1270, 1271*t*
  pancreatitis and, 878*t*, 882, 886*t*
  parkinsonism and, 271*t*, 273*t*
  photosensitivity and, 146*t*
  sexual dysfunction and, 759*t*
  SIADH and, 984*t*
  sleep disorders and, 348*t*
  systemic lupus erythematosus and, 124*t*, 127, 128*t*, 130
  tardive dyskinesia and, 265
  taste disorders and, 1260*t*
  thrombocytopenia and, 1051*t*
  vaginal bleeding disorders and, 782*t*, 785*t*
  valvular/pericardial heart disease and, 661*t*, 662
Methylene blue, 146*t*, 1105*t*, 1203–1204*t*
Methylenedioxymethamphetamine (MDMA). *See* Ecstasy
Methylergometrine, 472*t*
Methylergonovine, 472*t*, 1236*t*
Methylnaltrexone, 840, 840*t*, 841, 928
Methylphenidate
  alopecia and, 167*t*
  anxiety and, 400*t*, 401, 405*t*
  depression and, 391
  growth hormone deficiency and, 748, 748*t*
  hepatic/cholestatic diseases and, 852*t*
  myocardial ischemia/acute coronary syndromes and, 473*t*
  psychosis and, 416*t*, 418*t*
  seizures and, 219*t*, 221
  sexual dysfunction and, 761*t*
  sleep disorders and, 349*t*
  stroke and, 230–231*t*, 232
Methylprednisolone
  acute kidney injury and, 957
  alopecia and, 171*t*
  asthma/bronchospasm and, 452*t*
  atrial fibrillation/atrial flutter and, 582*t*, 586, 586*t*
  AV node re-entrant tachycardia and, 592*t*
  hirsutism and, 195*t*
  hypertrichosis and, 196*t*
  hypotension and, 644
  for immune complex diseases, 100
  nausea/vomiting and, 924*t*
  pancreatitis and, 888
  pharmacologic characteristics of, 739*t*
  sinus bradycardia/atrioventricular block and, 571*t*
  thrombocytopenia and, 1059
  thromboembolic diseases and, 1066*t*, 1070*t*
Methyltestosterone, 102*t*, 167*t*, 176, 178, 195*t*
Methylthiouracil, 124*t*
Methysergide
  hypertension and, 620*t*
  interstitial lung disease/pulmonary fibrosis and, 432*t*
  myocardial ischemia/acute coronary syndromes and, 472*t*
  systemic lupus erythematosus and, 126*t*
  thyroid diseases and, 703*t*
  valvular/pericardial heart disease and, 659, 660–661*t*, 662–664, 668, 668*t*
Metoclopramide
  akathisia and, 255, 255–256*t*, 258*t*
  anxiety and, 400*t*
  depression and, 385
  diarrhea and, 823, 823*t*
  drug fever and, 1188*t*
  dystonia and, 266*t*, 269, 269*t*
  hirsutism and, 195*t*, 199*t*
  hyperprolactinemia and, 742, 743*t*, 745
  myocardial ischemia/acute coronary syndromes and, 473*t*, 474
  nausea/vomiting and, 910, 919, 923, 927–929, 927–929*t*
  neuroleptic malignant syndrome and, 1195, 1195*t*
  neutropenia/agranulocytosis and, 1090*t*
  parkinsonism and, 271*t*, 273, 273*t*
  serotonin syndrome and, 1203–1204*t*
  sexual dysfunction and, 758*t*, 763*t*
  tardive dyskinesia and, 260*t*, 261–263, 264*t*
  thyroid diseases and, 702*t*
  torsades de pointes and, 533*t*, 539–540*t*
Metolazone, 92, 633*t*, 638*t*, 1066*t*, 1070*t*, 1260*t*
Metoprolol
  alopecia and, 168*t*
  atrial fibrillation/atrial flutter and, 587*t*
  atrial tachycardia and, 591
  comorbidity and, 34
  delirium and, 327*t*
  heart failure and, 512
  hypotension and, 632*t*, 638*t*, 646*t*
  oral erythema multiforme and, 1267*t*
  oral lichenoid reactions and, 1271*t*
  psychosis and, 417*t*

sinus bradycardia/atrioventricular block and, 578t, 579
systemic lupus erythematosus and, 125t
teratogenicity of, 1317
Metrizamide, 707t
Metronidazole
acidosis and, 1002t
bleeding disorders and, 1031
cutaneous diseases and, 102t
diarrhea and, 828–829
hepatic/cholestatic diseases and, 871
myocardial ischemia/acute coronary syndromes and, 472t
nausea/vomiting and, 909t, 911t, 915
oral lichenoid reactions and, 1271t
osteonecrosis of jaw and, 1276
ototoxicity and, 1236t
pancreatitis and, 878t, 880, 885, 886t, 891t
peripheral neuropathy and, 280t
serum sickness-like reactions and, 1193t
taste disorders and, 1260t
torsades de pointes and, 533t, 539t
visual disturbances and, 305t
Metyrapone, 180, 195t
Mevalonic acid, 866
Mexiletine, 218t, 502t, 507, 510t, 634t
Mezlocillin, 1188t
Mianserin, 259, 392
Miconazole, 790t, 792
Microcephaly, 1330–1331, 1330f
Microcytic anemia, 1102t
Midazolam, 34, 39, 77t, 226, 305t, 927t
Midodrine, 646, 646t, 647, 872
Mifepristone, 7t, 702t
Milk of magnesia, 1273
Milk thistle, 868
Milnacipran, 1203–1204t
Milrinone
atrial fibrillation/atrial flutter and, 582t
hypotension and, 636t, 640t, 644, 645t
monomorphic ventricular tachycardia and, 524t
myocardial ischemia/acute coronary syndromes and, 472t
sinus bradycardia/atrioventricular block and, 571t, 577t
Mineralocorticoids, 645, 1012, 1015, 1017
Mineral oil, 193, 840t
Minerals, 702t
Minocycline
allergic reactions to, 74–75t, 84, 85, 95
color changes of oral mucosa and teeth and, 1253, 1254t, 1255
cutaneous diseases and, 103t
drug fever and, 1188t
hemolytic anemia and, 1104
hepatic/cholestatic diseases and, 861t
ototoxicity and, 1236t
pancreatitis and, 879t, 882
photosensitivity and, 146t
serum sickness-like reactions and, 1193t
systemic lupus erythematosus and, 124t, 127–130, 128t, 133
thyroid diseases and, 700t, 710
Minoxidil
adverse effects of, 193
alopecia and, 186, 187, 187t, 190, 191
heart failure and, 503t, 510t
hirsutism and, 194, 198
hypertrichosis and, 194–195, 196–197t, 198, 202, 203
hypotension and, 633t, 640t
myocardial ischemia/acute coronary syndromes and, 472t, 477t
ototoxicity and, 1236t
Rogaine development and, 50
systemic lupus erythematosus and, 125t
thrombocytopenia and, 1051t
valvular/pericardial heart disease and, 661t, 662, 668–669t, 669
Mipomersen, 7t, 849t
Mirtazapine
akathisia and, 254, 259
delirium and, 327t
ototoxicity and, 1236t
pancreatitis and, 891
photosensitivity and, 146t
secondary adrenal insufficiency and, 736–737t, 737
sexual dysfunction and, 772
SIADH and, 982t, 990
weight gain and, 1166t, 1169t, 1170
Misoprostol, 817, 822–823t, 1236t, 1324
Mistletoe, 851t
Mitochondrial myopathy, 1150, 1152–1154, 1152t, 1159
Mitogen-activated protein kinase (MEK) inhibitors, 1295, 1296
Mitomycin, 170t, 848t
Mitomycin C, 146t, 432t, 1054
Mitotane, 702t, 735, 736–737t, 737, 741
Mitoxantrone
alopecia and, 170t
atrial fibrillation/atrial flutter and, 582t
heart failure and, 503t, 510t
leukemia and, 1285, 1288t, 1291
nausea/vomiting and, 908t
Mivacurium, 73t, 452t, 636t, 638t, 644
Mixed amphetamine salts, 401
MMR (measles, mumps, and rubella) vaccine, 21, 1267t
Mobitz type I/type II second-degree AV block, 575
Moclobemide, 743t, 1203–1204t, 1207
Modafinil, 104t, 400t, 409, 417t
Moexipril, 146t, 632t, 638t
Molindone, 743t, 852t, 1195t, 1199
Mometasone, 731t, 732, 736t, 739
Monoamine oxidase inhibitors (MAOIs)
cognitive disorders and, 360
delirium and, 327t
food interactions with, 40
hepatic/cholestatic diseases and, 852t
hypertension and, 618t, 620t
psychosis and, 417–418t
serotonin syndrome and, 1202, 1203–1204t, 1205–1207
sexual dysfunction and, 759–760t
sleep disorders and, 348t, 350t
weight gain and, 1171
Monoclonal antibodies, 95, 439, 822t, 1129t, 1192, 1194
Monomorphic ventricular tachycardia, 523–530
causative agents of, 523, 524t
clinical presentation of, 526–527t, 526–528, 527f
differential diagnosis of, 527, 527t
epidemiology of, 523
management of, 530, 531f
mechanisms of, 525–526, 525t
morbidity and mortality for, 529
patient education on, 530
prevention of, 529–530, 529t
risk factors for, 528–529, 528t
Montelukast, 385, 400t, 404, 462, 853t
MOPP regimen, 1284t, 1285, 1286
Morbidity and mortality
for acidosis, 1007
for acute interstitial nephritis, 956
for acute tubular necrosis, 952
adverse reactions and, 29
for akathisia, 258
for alkalosis, 1015–1016
for alopecia, 185
for amenorrhea and oligomenorrhea, 794
for anxiety, 409–410
for aplastic anemia, 1102–1103
for asthma and bronchospasm, 460–461
for atrial fibrillation/atrial flutter, 586
for atrial tachycardia, 590
for atrioventricular node re-entrant tachycardia, 594
for bladder cancer, 1304
for bleeding disorders, 1032–1034
for breast cancer, 1300
for Brugada syndrome, 548
for chemotherapy-induced anemia, 1110
for chronic kidney disease, 973–974
for cognitive disorders, 366
for color changes of oral mucosa and teeth, 1257
for congenital heart defects, 1324
for constipation, 839
costs for drug-related diseases, 27–28
for Cushing syndrome, 733
for cutaneous diseases, 112
for delirium, 333–334, 366
for depression, 389
for diabetes insipidus, 993
for diarrhea, 826
for drug allergies, 88
for drug fever, 1190
for dysmenorrhea, 797
for dystonia, 269
for endometrial cancer, 1302
epidemiology in explanations of, 21, 22, 25, 26
for female sexual dysfunction, 799
for fetal alcohol spectrum disorders, 1333
for gastroschisis, 1327
for gingival hyperplasia, 1265
for glomerulonephritis, 959
for glucose and insulin dysregulation, 688–689
for gout and hyperuricemia, 1143
for growth hormone deficiency, 749
for heart failure, 514–515
for hemodynamic-mediated AKI, 947–948
for hemolytic anemia, 1106
for hepatic and cholestatic diseases, 865
for hirsutism, 203
for hyperprolactinemia, 746
for hypertension, 623
for hypertrichosis, 203
for hypotension, 643
for hypothermia, 1217
for infertility, 801
for interstitial lung disease/pulmonary fibrosis, 438
for intracerebral hemorrhage, 244
for learning disabilities, 1316
for leukemia, 1291
for limb deficiency defects, 1325–1326
for low birth weight, 1318
for lymphoma, 1294
for macrocytic anemia, 1108
for male sexual dysfunction, 771
for malignant hyperthermia, 1212
for menorrhagia and menometrorrhagia, 796

INDEX

Morbidity and mortality (continued)
- for microcephaly, 1331
- for monomorphic ventricular tachycardia, 529
- for myocardial ischemia/acute coronary syndromes, 482–484
- for myopathy, 1157
- for nausea and vomiting, 919–920
- for neural tube defects, 1329
- for neuroleptic malignant syndrome, 1199
- for neutropenia and agranulocytosis, 1094
- for oral erythema multiforme, 1269
- for oral lichenoid reactions, 1273
- for orofacial clefts, 1321
- for osteonecrosis of jaw, 1275
- for osteoporosis and osteomalacia, 1126–1127
- for ototoxicity, 1242
- for ovarian hyperstimulation, 784
- for pancreatitis, 890–891, 891*t*
- for parkinsonism, 273
- for peripheral neuropathy, 285–286
- for photosensitivity, 154
- for psychosis, 422
- for secondary adrenal insufficiency, 740
- for seizures, 224–225
- for serotonin syndrome, 1207
- for serum sickness-like reactions, 1194
- for SIADH, 989
- for sinus bradycardia/atrioventricular block, 578
- for skin cancer, 1297
- for sleep disorders, 351–352
- for stroke, 234
- for systemic lupus erythematosus, 134
- for tardive dyskinesia, 263
- for taste disorders, 1262
- for thrombocytopenia, 1056
- for thromboembolic diseases, 1074
- for thyroid diseases, 714
- for torsades de pointes, 541–542
- for upper gastrointestinal ulceration, 816
- for valvular and pericardial heart disease, 669
- for visual disturbances, 317
- for vulvovaginal candidiasis, 791–792
- for weight gain, 1173

Morbidity and Mortality Weekly Report (CDC), 53

Moricizine, 502*t*, 507, 510*t*, 528

Morphine
- acute kidney injury and, 958
- atrial fibrillation/atrial flutter and, 582*t*
- comorbidity and, 34
- constipation and, 836*t*
- delirium and, 326*t*, 335
- hyperprolactinemia and, 743*t*
- hypotension and, 636*t*, 638*t*
- hypothermia and, 1215, 1218
- myocardial ischemia/acute coronary syndromes and, 472*t*, 487*t*, 489
- nausea/vomiting and, 906*t*, 928
- ototoxicity and, 1233
- seizures and, 218*t*
- SIADH and, 984*t*
- thyroid diseases and, 703*t*

Mortality. *See* Morbidity and mortality

Morus alba L, 221

Motesanib, 699*t*, 708

Mountain laurel, 305*t*

Movement disorders, 253–273
- akathisia (acute and tardive), 254–259
- dystonia (acute and tardive), 265–270
- overview, 253–254
- parkinsonism, 270–273
- tardive dyskinesia, 259–265

Moxifloxacin, 104*t*, 146*t*, 532*t*, 984*t*, 1051*t*, 1236*t*, 1260*t*

MPA. *See* Medroxyprogesterone acetate

mTOR inhibitors. *See* Mammalian target-of-rapamycin inhibitors

Mulberry, 221

Multidrug resistant tuberculosis (MDR-TB), 288

Multifocal atrial tachycardia, 588, 590, 591, 591*t*

Multiple sclerosis agents, 172*t*, 179*t*

Mumps, 29

Muromonab, 77*t*, 1066*t*, 1070*t*

Muromonab-CD3, 635*t*, 1236*t*, 1284*t*, 1288*t*, 1292

Muscarine subtype 1 (M1) receptors, 912

Muscle relaxants, 270, 1209*t*, 1210, 1212, 1212*t*, 1213

Mushroom poisoning, 851*t*, 864

Myalgia, 1149, 1151, 1155, 1159

Mycophenolate
- alopecia and, 172*t*, 174
- chronic kidney disease and, 967, 974
- depression and, 382
- drug fever and, 1188*t*
- sinus bradycardia/atrioventricular block and, 571*t*, 577*t*
- skin cancer and, 1298
- teratogenicity of, 1319, 1320, 1330, 1331
- upper gastrointestinal ulceration and, 815

Mycophenolate mofetil, 432*t*, 1127

Mycophenolic acid, 822*t*

Mydriatics, 315

Myelodysplastic syndrome (MDS), 1283, 1286–1287, 1289

Myelosuppressive therapy, 1110

Myocardial ischemia/acute coronary syndromes, 471–489
- causative agents of, 471–474, 472–473*t*
- clinical presentation of, 480–482, 481*t*, 483*t*
- cocaine-induced, 474–475, 478, 481–489, 483*t*, 487*t*
- differential diagnosis of, 482, 483*t*
- epidemiology of, 474–476
- management of, 485–489, 487*t*
- mechanisms of, 476–480, 477*t*
- morbidity and mortality for, 482–484
- patient education on, 489
- prevention of, 484–485, 484*t*
- risk factors for, 482, 483*t*

Myocilin, 317

Myopathy, 1149–1160
- causative agents of, 1150–1151, 1150*t*
- clinical presentation of, 1153–1155, 1154*t*
- corticosteroid, 1150*t*, 1151, 1152*t*, 1153, 1155–1159
- defined, 1149
- differential diagnosis of, 1154, 1154*t*
- epidemiology of, 1151
- management of, 1158–1159
- mechanisms of, 1151–1153, 1152*t*
- mitochondrial, 1150, 1152–1154, 1152*t*, 1159
- morbidity and mortality for, 1157
- necrotizing myopathy, 1150, 1152–1155, 1152*t*, 1158
- painless, 1150–1153, 1152*t*, 1155
- patient education on, 1160
- prevention of, 1157–1158, 1158*t*
- risk factors for, 1155–1157, 1156*t*

Myositis, 1149, 1151, 1157

Nabilone, 929*t*

Nab-paclitaxel, 908*t*

Nabumetone
- acute kidney injury and, 944
- alopecia and, 172*t*
- heart failure and, 510*t*
- ototoxicity and, 1236*t*
- photosensitivity and, 146*t*, 150
- upper gastrointestinal ulceration and, 817

N-acetylcysteine (NAC)
- acute kidney injury and, 954
- asthma/bronchospasm and, 452*t*, 455, 455*t*
- heart failure and, 515
- hepatic/cholestatic diseases and, 866
- hypersensitivity reactions to, 77*t*
- ototoxicity and, 1242*t*
- serum sickness-like reactions and, 1193*t*

N-acetyl-*p*-benzoquinone imine (NAPQI), 33, 39, 856, 864, 970

N-acetylprocainamide, 134

Nadolol, 168*t*, 461, 577*t*, 632*t*, 638*t*

Nadroparin, 167*t*

Nafarelin, 700*t*

Nafcillin, 125*t*, 1188*t*

Nalbuphine, 906*t*

Nalidixic acid, 147*t*, 305*t*, 1002*t*, 1051*t*

Nalmefene, 840, 840*t*

Naloxegol, 840, 840*t*

Naloxone
- for constipation, 840–841, 840*t*
- hepatic/cholestatic diseases and, 869
- nausea/vomiting and, 927*t*
- psychosis and, 424*t*
- restrictive drug distribution system for, 7*t*
- seizures and, 218*t*

Naltrexone, 174*t*, 180*t*, 349*t*

Nandrolone, 102*t*, 167*t*, 176, 195*t*, 402, 1065*t*, 1069*t*

NANSAIDs (nonaspirin nonsteroidal anti-inflammatory drugs), 239, 816

Naphazoline, 1051*t*

NAPQI. *See* *N*-acetyl-*p*-benzoquinone imine

Naproxen
- alopecia and, 172*t*
- bleeding disorders and, 1033
- comorbidity and, 34
- drug fever and, 1188*t*
- gout/hyperuricemia and, 1145
- heart failure and, 510*t*
- hepatic/cholestatic diseases and, 846*t*
- myocardial ischemia/acute coronary syndromes and, 475, 479
- oral erythema multiforme and, 1267*t*
- oral lichenoid reactions and, 1271*t*
- ototoxicity and, 1236*t*
- pancreatitis and, 881
- photosensitivity and, 147*t*, 150
- sexual dysfunction and, 760*t*, 783*t*, 786*t*
- stroke and, 230
- systemic lupus erythematosus and, 126*t*
- thrombocytopenia and, 1051*t*
- visual disturbances and, 305*t*

Naranjo Scale, 64, 65, 65*t*

Naratriptan, 380

Narcotics
- acidosis and, 1003*t*, 1005, 1007
- acute kidney injury and, 958
- delirium and, 325
- hypotension and, 643
- myocardial ischemia/acute coronary syndromes and, 489
- seizures and, 225
- sexual dysfunction and, 798
- visual disturbances and, 305*t*

Nasal decongestants, 401
Nasal glucocorticoids, 731t, 733–735, 736t, 738, 741
Natalizumab, 7t, 96, 1193t
National Academy of Medicine, 12, 19, 51, 53, 55
National Birth Defects Prevention Study (NBDPS), 1320, 1323
National Cancer Institute, 825, 826
National Comprehensive Cancer Network (NCCN), 1111, 1283, 1292, 1303, 1305
National Coordinating Council for Medication Error Reporting and Prevention, 42
National Institute for Health and Care Excellence (NICE), 333, 336
National Institute of Mental Health, 262
National Institutes of Health (NIH), 14, 230, 236, 241
Natriuretic peptides, 636t
Nausea and vomiting, 905–931
  afferent pathways of, 912, 913f
  causative agents of, 905–910, 906–909t
  chemotherapy-induced. *See* Chemotherapy-induced nausea and vomiting (CINV)
  clinical presentation of, 912t, 915–916, 916t
  differential diagnosis of, 915, 916t
  epidemiology of, 910
  management of, 927–929t, 927–930
  mechanisms of, 910–915, 911t, 913f
  morbidity and mortality for, 919–920
  opioid-induced. *See* Opioid-induced nausea and vomiting
  patient education on, 930–931
  postoperative. *See* Postoperative nausea and vomiting (PONV)
  prevention of, 920–927, 921t, 924–925t
  risk factors for, 917–918t, 917–919
NBDPS (National Birth Defects Prevention Study), 1320, 1323
NCCN. *See* National Comprehensive Cancer Network
NCS (nerve-conduction studies), 284
NDAs (New Drug Applications), 48, 51
Nebivolol, 578t, 632t, 638t
Necrotizing myopathy, 1150, 1152–1155, 1152t, 1158
Nefazodone, 772, 852t, 1202, 1203–1204t
Nefopam, 218t, 472t
Nelfinavir, 533t, 539–540t, 1123t
Neomycin, 871, 1236t
Neoplastic injury, 855t, 858, 859t, 861t, 862. *See also* Cancer
Neostigmine, 452t, 571t, 574t
NEPA (netupitant-palonosetron), 926
Nephrolithiasis, 957–958
  causative agents of, 944t, 957
  clinical presentation of, 946t, 957
  differential diagnosis of, 946t, 957
  epidemiology of, 957
  management of, 958
  mechanisms of, 957
  patient education on, 958
  prevention of, 958
  risk factors for, 958
Nephrotoxicity, 37
Neprilysin inhibitors, 516, 633t
Nerve-conduction studies (NCS), 284
Nerve growth factor (NGF)-1, 288
Nesiritide, 636t, 640t, 644, 645t
Netupitant-palonosetron (NEPA), 926
Neural tube defects, 1327–1329
  causative agents of, 1328
  clinical presentation of, 1327–1328f, 1329
  differential diagnosis of, 1329
  epidemiology of, 1328
  mechanisms of, 1328–1329
  morbidity and mortality for, 1329
  risk factors for, 1329
Neurocardiogenic syncope, 637, 641
Neurocognitive disorders. *See* Cognitive disorders
Neurokinin A, 82, 457
Neurokinin (NK-1) receptors, 912, 914, 923–927, 929
Neuroleptic malignant syndrome (NMS), 1195–1202
  causative agents of, 1195, 1195t
  clinical presentation of, 1187t, 1196–1198, 1196t, 1206
  differential diagnosis of, 1197–1198, 1198t
  epidemiology of, 1196
  management of, 1200–1201, 1200–1201t
  mechanisms of, 1196
  morbidity and mortality for, 1199
  patient education on, 1202
  prevention of, 1199–1200, 1199t
  risk factors for, 1198, 1198t
Neuroleptics, 360, 1195–1202, 1205. *See also* Conventional neuroleptics
Neuromuscular blocking agents
  hypotension and, 636t
  malignant hyperthermia and, 1211, 1212, 1213t
  myopathy and, 1156
  nausea/vomiting and, 907t, 911t, 914, 921
Neuromyopathy, 1150, 1151, 1152t, 1153, 1155
Neuropathy. *See* Peripheral neuropathy
Neuropsychiatric agents, 851–852t
Neutropenia and agranulocytosis, 1087–1096
  causative agents of, 1087–1088, 1089–1090t
  clinical presentation of, 1092–1093, 1092t
  differential diagnosis of, 1092, 1092t
  epidemiology of, 1088, 1091
  management of, 1095–1096
  mechanisms of, 1091, 1091t
  morbidity and mortality for, 1094
  patient education on, 1096
  prevention of, 1094–1095, 1095t
  risk factors for, 1093–1094, 1093t
Nevirapine
  allergic reactions to, 75t
  cutaneous diseases and, 101, 104t, 111t, 113t
  hyperprolactinemia and, 744t
  oral erythema multiforme and, 1267t
New Drug Applications (NDAs), 48, 51
New molecular entities (NMEs), 8
NGF (nerve growth factor)-1, 288
NHL (non-Hodgkin lymphoma), 1286, 1292–1294, 1303
Niacin
  acidosis and, 1002t
  glucose/insulin dysregulation and, 679, 680t, 684t
  hepatic/cholestatic diseases and, 849t, 864
  myopathy and, 1156
  visual disturbances and, 305t
Nicardipine
  gingival hyperplasia and, 1263t
  hypotension and, 633t, 639t, 644
  myocardial ischemia/acute coronary syndromes and, 478
  ototoxicity and, 1236t
  sinus bradycardia/atrioventricular block and, 571t, 573t, 577t
  stroke and, 236
NICE (National Institute for Health and Care Excellence), 333, 336
Nicotinamide hydroiodide, 707t
Nicotine. *See* Smoking
Nicotine patch, 984t
Nicotinic acid, 680t, 684t, 703t, 1136t, 1139, 1144t, 1152
Nifedipine
  alopecia and, 168t
  asthma/bronchospasm and, 463
  delirium and, 327t
  drug fever and, 1188t
  gingival hyperplasia and, 1262, 1263t
  heart failure and, 502t, 505, 509–510, 510t, 515
  hypertrichosis and, 196t
  hypotension and, 633t, 639t
  myocardial ischemia/acute coronary syndromes and, 472t, 477t, 478
  neutropenia/agranulocytosis and, 1090t
  oral erythema multiforme and, 1267t
  ototoxicity and, 1236t
  photosensitivity and, 147t
  systemic lupus erythematosus and, 124t
  tardive dyskinesia and, 265
  taste disorders and, 1260–1261t
  teratogenicity of, 1317
Niferidil, 524t
NIH (National Institutes of Health), 14, 230, 236, 241
Nilotinib, 170t, 699–700t, 883, 1087, 1109t
Nilutamide, 432t
Nimesulide, 846t
Nimodipine, 633t, 639t, 1236t, 1263t
9 points of consideration for adverse events, 63–64
Nintedanib, 440
Nisoldipine, 472t, 633t, 639t, 1263t
Nitazoxanide, 829
Nitrates, 478, 484–486, 488, 510, 574, 642–643, 645t
Nitrendipine, 953
Nitric oxide, 261, 766, 857, 866, 868
Nitroaliphatic compounds, 849t
Nitroaromatic compounds, 849t
Nitrofurantoin
  alopecia and, 174t, 180t
  drug fever and, 1188t
  hemolytic anemia and, 1105t
  hepatic/cholestatic diseases and, 847t, 861t
  interstitial lung disease/pulmonary fibrosis and, 432t, 435t
  macrocytic anemia and, 1108t
  myocardial ischemia/acute coronary syndromes and, 472t
  neutropenia/agranulocytosis and, 1090t
  peripheral neuropathy and, 280t
  sexual dysfunction and, 762t, 765t
  systemic lupus erythematosus and, 125t
Nitroglycerin
  hypotension and, 633t, 634t, 640t
  myocardial ischemia/acute coronary syndromes and, 472t, 481, 484, 487t, 488, 489
  sinus bradycardia/atrioventricular block and, 571t, 574t
  taste disorders and, 1260t
  thrombocytopenia and, 1051t
Nitroprusside
  acidosis and, 1002t
  hypotension and, 633t, 640t, 644
  myocardial ischemia/acute coronary syndromes and, 472t, 477t, 488
  ototoxicity and, 1236t
Nitrosoureas, 432t, 966t, 970t, 1284

INDEX

Nitrous oxide
  malignant hyperthermia and, 1212, 1212*t*
  nausea/vomiting and, 907*t*, 911*t*, 914, 917, 921, 923
  peripheral neuropathy and, 281*t*
  psychosis and, 417–418*t*
  seizures and, 225
Nivolumab, 825
Nizatidine, 328*t*, 1105*t*, 1174
NK-1 (neurokinin) receptors, 912, 914, 923–927, 929
NMEs (new molecular entities), 8
N-methyl-D-aspartate (NMDA), 261, 418, 1205, 1239
NMS. *See* Neuroleptic malignant syndrome
NMSC (nonmelanoma skin cancer), 1296–1298
NNRTIs (non-nucleoside reverse transcriptase inhibitors), 358*t*, 377–378, 690, 847*t*
Nonacetylated salicylates, 489, 812
Nonadherence to medications, 28, 41
Nonaspirin nonsteroidal anti-inflammatory drugs (NANSAIDs), 239, 816
Nondepolarizing muscle relaxants, 1209*t*, 1210, 1212, 1212–1213*t*, 1213
Non-Hodgkin lymphoma (NHL), 1286, 1292–1294, 1303
Noni juice, 851*t*
Nonimmediate drug reactions, 80, 81
Nonmelanoma skin cancer (NMSC), 1296–1298
Non-nucleoside reverse transcriptase inhibitors (NNRTIs), 358*t*, 377–378, 690, 847*t*
Nonpotassium-sparing diuretics, 34
Nonrapid eye movement (NREM) sleep, 347
Nonselective NSAIDs
  acute kidney injury and, 945, 947
  heart failure and, 509
  myocardial ischemia/acute coronary syndromes and, 472*t*, 475, 479, 489
  stroke and, 231
  upper gastrointestinal ulceration and, 810*t*
Nonselective opioid receptor antagonists, 840*t*
Nonsteroidal anti-inflammatory drugs (NSAIDS)
  acidosis and, 1003*t*
  acute kidney injury and, 942, 943–945*t*, 944–949, 953, 956, 958–959
  allergic and hypersensitivity reactions to, 74*t*, 77*t*, 81, 87, 97–98
  alopecia and, 172*t*, 179*t*
  anxiety and, 401*t*, 403–404
  aplastic anemia and, 1100*t*
  asthma/bronchospasm and, 451, 453, 453*t*, 455–458, 455*t*, 460, 461, 463
  bleeding disorders and, 1025, 1026, 1026*t*, 1029*t*, 1030, 1033, 1039
  chronic kidney disease and, 965, 968–970
  cognitive disorders and, 358–359*t*, 361
  constipation and, 836*t*
  cutaneous diseases and, 101, 103*t*
  delirium and, 325, 327*t*
  depression and, 385
  diarrhea and, 823*t*
  drug-induced hospitalizations from, 26*t*
  glucose/insulin dysregulation and, 688
  gout/hyperuricemia and, 1141, 1144, 1145
  heart failure and, 501, 503–504*t*, 508–509, 512, 516, 517
  hemolytic anemia and, 1105*t*
  hypertension and, 618*t*, 620*t*, 623
  hypertrichosis and, 197*t*
  hypotension and, 647
  hypothermia and, 1216
  myocardial ischemia/acute coronary syndromes and, 472*t*, 473, 475, 476, 477*t*, 485, 489
  neutropenia/agranulocytosis and, 1087, 1088, 1090*t*
  nonaspirin, 239, 816
  nonselective. *See* Nonselective NSAIDs
  oral lichenoid reactions and, 1270
  ototoxicity and, 1233
  ovarian hyperstimulation and, 789
  oxicam, 101
  pancreatitis and, 881, 887–888
  peripheral neuropathy and, 288
  photosensitivity and, 143, 150, 150*t*, 154, 155
  seizures and, 224
  sexual dysfunction and, 759*t*
  stroke and, 230, 230–231*t*, 231, 233, 235*t*
  for systemic lupus erythematosus, 135
  teratogenicity of, 1334*t*
  thrombocytopenia and, 1052, 1052*t*
  thyroid diseases and, 703*t*
  upper gastrointestinal ulceration and, 809–819, 810–811*t*, 816*t*
  vaginal bleeding disorders and, 790*t*, 797
  valvular/pericardial heart disease and, 670
  visual disturbances and, 313
  weight gain and, 1175*t*
Non-ST-segment elevation myocardial ischemia, 471
Nonsulfonylurea secretagogues, 682*t*, 685*t*
Norelgestromin/ethinyl estradiol, 229
Norepinephrine
  acidosis and, 1002*t*
  anxiety and, 406
  cocaine-induced blockade of, 478, 488
  cognitive disorders and, 360
  delirium and, 333
  depression and, 385
  heart failure and, 512
  hypertension and, 619, 621
  psychosis and, 418, 422
  sexual dysfunction and, 766, 767
  in sleep cycles, 349
Norethandrolone, 783*t*, 786*t*
Norethindrone, 176, 909*t*
Norfloxacin, 147*t*, 472*t*, 1236*t*
Norgestimate, 191, 206*t*, 229
Normal transit constipation (NTC), 837
Normocytic anemia, 1102*t*
Nortriptyline
  alopecia and, 173*t*
  Brugada syndrome and, 547*t*
  cognitive disorders and, 365
  heart failure and, 504*t*, 510*t*
  ototoxicity and, 1236*t*
  photosensitivity and, 147*t*
  serotonin syndrome and, 1203–1204*t*
  SIADH and, 982*t*
  weight gain and, 1166*t*, 1169*t*, 1170
NREM (nonrapid eye movement) sleep, 347
NSAIDS. *See* Nonsteroidal anti-inflammatory drugs
NTC (normal transit constipation), 837
Nucleoside reverse-transcriptase inhibitors (NRTIs)
  acidosis and, 1002–1003*t*, 1007, 1009–1011
  glucose/insulin dysregulation and, 680*t*, 684*t*
  hepatic/cholestatic diseases and, 847*t*
  osteoporosis/osteomalacia and, 1123*t*
  peripheral neuropathy and, 282, 282*t*
Numerator, in incidence of drug-induced disease, 25
Nutritional supplements, 415, 420, 423
Nux vomica, 221
Obesity, 1165, 1171–1175. *See also* Weight gain
Obeticholic acid, 7*t*
Obinutuzumab, 1271*t*
Ocriplasmin, 305*t*
Octreotide
  diabetes insipidus and, 991*t*
  diarrhea and, 827*t*, 828
  growth hormone deficiency and, 747
  hepatic/cholestatic diseases and, 850*t*, 871–872
  sinus bradycardia/atrioventricular block and, 571*t*
  thrombocytopenia and, 1051*t*
  thyroid diseases and, 699*t*, 703*t*
Ocular toxicities. *See* Visual disturbances
Office of the Inspector General (OIG), 13–14
Ofloxacin, 104*t*, 147*t*, 280*t*, 328*t*, 533*t*, 539*t*, 991*t*
OIC. *See* Opioid-induced constipation
Oil of cloves, 851*t*
OKT3. *See* Antithymocyte globulin
Olanzapine
  acidosis and, 1002*t*
  alopecia and, 173*t*
  cannabinoids and, 33
  constipation and, 836*t*
  delirium and, 326*t*, 329*t*, 338–340
  diabetes insipidus and, 991, 991*t*
  extrapyramidal symptoms and, 254
  glucose/insulin dysregulation and, 683, 690
  hepatic/cholestatic diseases and, 852*t*
  hyperprolactinemia and, 743*t*
  hypotension and, 635*t*, 639*t*
  hypothermia and, 1216*t*
  nausea/vomiting and, 926, 927, 929, 929*t*
  neuroleptic malignant syndrome and, 1195, 1195*t*, 1198
  neutropenia/agranulocytosis and, 1090*t*
  off-label use of, 10
  pancreatitis and, 879*t*
  parkinsonism and, 271
  photosensitivity and, 147*t*
  restrictive drug distribution system for, 7*t*
  sexual dysfunction and, 761*t*, 772
  SIADH and, 982*t*
  sinus bradycardia/atrioventricular block and, 571*t*, 578*t*
  smoking and, 32
  stroke and, 230–231*t*
  tardive dyskinesia and, 265
  taste disorders and, 1260*t*
  thromboembolic diseases and, 1066*t*, 1070*t*
  torsades de pointes and, 533*t*, 539–540*t*, 541
  weight gain and, 1169*t*, 1171, 1174, 1175
Olaparib, 7*t*, 1284, 1284*t*, 1287, 1289
Oleckna v. Daytona Discount Pharmacy (2015), 9*t*, 11
Oligomenorrhea. *See* Amenorrhea and oligomenorrhea
Olmesartan, 632*t*, 638*t*
OLR. *See* Oral lichenoid reactions
Olsalazine, 823*t*
Omacetaxine, 170*t*
Omalizumab, 73*t*, 96, 462–463, 1193*t*
Omeprazole
  chronic kidney disease and, 965, 966*t*
  cutaneous diseases and, 103*t*
  oral erythema multiforme and, 1267*t*
  oral lichenoid reactions and, 1271*t*
  ototoxicity and, 1237*t*
  pancreatitis and, 879*t*, 880
  sexual dysfunction and, 760*t*
  SIADH and, 984*t*
  systemic lupus erythematosus and, 126*t*
  thyroid diseases and, 703*t*

Omnibus Budget Reconciliation Act of 1987, 368
Onabotulinumtoxin A, 174*t*, 180*t*
Oncology. *See* Cancer
Ondansetron
  atrial fibrillation/atrial flutter and, 582*t*
  depression and, 385
  hepatic/cholestatic diseases and, 869
  hypersensitivity reactions to, 77*t*
  myocardial ischemia/acute coronary syndromes and, 473*t*
  nausea/vomiting and, 918, 919, 922, 923, 924*t*, 925–929, 927–929*t*
  torsades de pointes and, 532*t*, 539–540*t*
Ophthalmic disturbances. *See* Visual disturbances
Opioid analgesics
  cognitive disorders and, 365, 367
  delirium and, 325
  hepatic/cholestatic diseases and, 871
  nausea/vomiting and, 912, 920–921, 930
  peripheral neuropathy and, 289
  serotonin syndrome and, 1202, 1204–1205
Opioid antagonists, 927*t*, 928
Opioid-induced constipation (OIC), 6, 835, 836–837*t*, 837–841, 915, 920, 930
Opioid-induced nausea and vomiting
  causative agents of, 906*t*, 910
  clinical presentation of, 915
  epidemiology of, 910
  management of, 927–928, 927*t*
  mechanisms of, 911*t*, 912
  morbidity and mortality for, 919
  patient education on, 930
  prevention of, 920–921
  risk factors for, 917, 917*t*
Opioids
  acidosis and, 1011*t*
  akathisia and, 259
  alopecia and, 172*t*
  anxiety and, 401*t*, 402, 404, 405*t*
  cognitive disorders and, 358–359*t*, 366, 369
  constipation and. *See* Opioid-induced constipation (OIC)
  delirium and, 325, 326*t*, 335
  duration of detection in urine, 420*t*
  hyperprolactinemia and, 743–744*t*
  hypersensitivity reactions to, 77*t*, 81
  hypotension and, 636*t*, 642, 644, 645*t*
  hypothermia and, 1216, 1216*t*
  malignant hyperthermia and, 1212, 1212*t*, 1213
  myocardial ischemia/acute coronary syndromes and, 472*t*
  nausea/vomiting and. *See* Opioid-induced nausea and vomiting
  ototoxicity and, 1233, 1239, 1239*t*
  for pain. *See* Opioid analgesics
  psychosis and, 417*t*, 422, 424*t*
  risk evaluation and mitigation strategies for, 6
  secondary adrenal insufficiency and, 737
  sedation effects of, 357
  sexual dysfunction and, 758*t*, 760*t*, 763*t*
  smoking and, 33
  in thermoregulation, 1186
  thyroid diseases and, 703*t*
  vaginal bleeding disorders and, 797
  withdrawal treatment protocols, 424*t*
Opium tincture, 827*t*, 828
Oprelvekin, 1056
Oral contraceptives
  alopecia and, 171*t*, 175–176, 179*t*, 184, 186, 188*t*, 191
  breast cancer and, 1299
  color changes of oral mucosa and teeth and, 1253, 1254*t*
  cutaneous diseases and, 108
  depression and, 376*t*, 382, 386, 388, 388*t*, 391
  genetic variability and, 16*t*
  gingival hyperplasia and, 1263*t*
  glucose/insulin dysregulation and, 680*t*, 684*t*
  hepatic/cholestatic diseases and, 864
  hirsutism and, 194, 195*t*, 199*t*, 203, 205–206
  hyperaldosteronism and, 751
  hypertension and, 618*t*, 620–622, 620*t*, 624–626, 625*t*
  infertility and, 790*t*, 801
  myocardial ischemia/acute coronary syndromes and, 473–475, 473*t*, 477*t*, 480–482, 483*t*, 485
  oral erythema multiforme and, 1267*t*
  oral lichenoid reactions and, 1271*t*
  skin cancer and, 1284*t*
  smoking and, 33
  stroke and, 229–230, 230*t*, 235*t*
  systemic lupus erythematosus and, 126*t*
  tardive dyskinesia and, 262
  thromboembolic diseases and, 1064*t*, 1067, 1068*t*, 1074–1075, 1075*t*
  vaginal bleeding disorders and, 782*t*, 785*t*, 790*t*, 793, 794, 796
  visual disturbances and, 305*t*, 313
  vulvovaginal candidiasis and, 782*t*, 785*t*, 791
  weight gain and, 1172–1173, 1175*t*
Oral erythema multiforme, 1265–1269
  categorization of, 1265–1266
  causative agents of, 1266, 1266–1268*t*
  clinical presentation of, 1253, 1256*t*, 1268–1269
  differential diagnosis of, 1257*t*, 1269
  epidemiology of, 1266
  management of, 1269
  mechanisms of, 1268, 1268*t*
  morbidity and mortality for, 1269
  patient education on, 1269
  prevention of, 1269
  risk factors for, 1258*t*, 1269
Oral glucocorticoids, 731*t*, 736*t*, 739–741
Oral hypoglycemic agents, 761, 983*t*
Oral lichenoid reactions (OLR), 1269–1273
  causative agents of, 1270, 1270–1272*t*
  clinical presentation of, 1256*t*, 1272–1273
  differential diagnosis of, 1257*t*, 1273
  epidemiology of, 1270
  management of, 1273
  mechanisms of, 1270, 1272, 1272*t*
  morbidity and mortality for, 1273
  overview, 1269
  patient education on, 1273
  prevention of, 1273
  risk factors for, 1258*t*, 1273
Oral mucosa color changes. *See* Color changes of oral mucosa and teeth
Oral rehydration solution (ORS), 829
Orexin antagonists, 353
Orlistat, 822–823*t*, 823, 827, 849*t*, 879*t*, 1175
Orofacial clefts, 1318–1321
  causative agents of, 1319, 1335
  clinical presentation of, 1318–1319*f*, 1321
  differential diagnosis of, 1321
  epidemiology of, 1319–1320
  mechanisms of, 1320–1321
  morbidity and mortality for, 1321
  risk factors for, 1321
Orotic acid, 849*t*
Orphan drugs, 48
Orphenadrine, 703*t*
ORS (oral rehydration solution), 829
Orthostatic hypotension, 233, 631, 637, 641–648, 646*t*
Osmotic diuretics, 636*t*
Osmotic laxatives, 840, 840*t*
Osteomalacia. *See* Osteoporosis and osteomalacia
Osteonecrosis of jaw, 1273–1276
  causative agents of, 1273, 1274*t*
  clinical presentation of, 1256*t*, 1275
  differential diagnosis of, 1257*t*, 1275
  epidemiology of, 1273–1274
  management of, 1276
  mechanisms of, 1274, 1274*t*
  morbidity and mortality for, 1275
  patient education on, 1276
  prevention of, 1275–1276, 1275*t*
  risk factors for, 1258*t*, 1275
Osteoporosis and osteomalacia, 1119–1130
  causative agents of, 1120, 1121*t*
  clinical presentation of, 1124–1125, 1124*t*
  differential diagnosis of, 1124, 1124*t*
  epidemiology of, 1120
  management of, 1129–1130, 1129*t*
  mechanisms of, 1120, 1122, 1123–1124*t*
  morbidity and mortality for, 1126–1127
  overview, 1119–1120
  patient education on, 1130
  prevention of, 1127–1128, 1128*t*
  risk factors for, 1125–1126, 1126*t*
Ototoxicity, 1233–1244
  causative agents of, 1233–1239, 1234–1238*t*
  clinical presentation of, 1240–1241, 1240*t*
  differential diagnosis of, 1240*t*, 1241
  epidemiology of, 1239
  genetic factors and, 37
  management of, 1243–1244
  mechanisms of, 1239–1240, 1239*t*
  morbidity and mortality for, 1242
  patient education on, 1244
  prevention of, 1242–1243, 1242*t*
  risk factors for, 1241–1242, 1241*t*
Ovarian hyperstimulation, 781–790
  causative agents of, 781, 782*t*
  clinical presentation of, 784, 787*t*
  differential diagnosis of, 784, 788*t*
  epidemiology of, 781, 783
  management of, 787–790, 790*t*
  mechanisms of, 783–784, 785*t*
  morbidity and mortality for, 784
  patient education on, 790
  prevention of, 784, 787, 789*t*
  risk factors for, 784, 788*t*
Overweight, 1165, 1171–1175. *See also* Weight gain
Oxacillin, 1188*t*
Oxaliplatin
  acidosis and, 1003*t*
  allergic reactions to, 73*t*
  alopecia and, 170*t*
  chemotherapy-induced anemia and, 1109*t*
  genetic variability and, 16*t*
  hemolytic anemia and, 1109
  interstitial lung disease/pulmonary fibrosis and, 432*t*, 435*t*
  nausea/vomiting and, 908*t*
  pancreatitis and, 881
  peripheral neuropathy and, 279, 280*t*, 282*t*, 283, 285–288
  torsades de pointes and, 532*t*, 539*t*
Oxandrolone, 167*t*, 195*t*, 402
Oxaprozin, 147*t*, 172*t*, 846*t*, 1237*t*

INDEX

Oxcarbazepine
allergic reactions to, 75*t*, 95
alopecia and, 168*t*
Brugada syndrome and, 547*t*
cognitive disorders and, 360
oral lichenoid reactions and, 1271*t*
ototoxicity and, 1237*t*
peripheral neuropathy and, 286–287, 287*t*
seizures and, 218*t*, 224
SIADH and, 981, 983*t*, 985–988, 988*t*, 990
teratogenicity of, 1319
thyroid diseases and, 699*t*
Oxitropium, 463
Oxprenolol, 125*t*, 1051*t*
Oxycodone, 906*t*, 984*t*, 1203–1204*t*, 1205
Oxymetazoline, 230*t*
Oxymetholone, 167*t*, 195*t*, 402
Oxymorphone, 906*t*, 1233, 1237*t*
Oxyphenisatin, 861*t*
Oxytocin, 453*t*, 473*t*, 729, 782*t*, 786*t*, 796
Ozagrel, 463

PABA (para-aminobenzoic acid), 153, 154
Pacemakers, 572, 576–578, 580
Paclitaxel
allergic and hypersensitivity reactions to, 73*t*, 75*t*, 77*t*, 97*t*
alopecia and, 170*t*
atrial fibrillation/atrial flutter and, 582*t*
cutaneous diseases and, 102*t*
heart failure and, 503*t*, 508, 510*t*
interstitial lung disease/pulmonary fibrosis and, 433*t*, 435*t*
myocardial ischemia/acute coronary syndromes and, 472*t*
nausea/vomiting and, 908*t*
ototoxicity and, 1237*t*
pancreatitis and, 881
peripheral neuropathy and, 280*t*, 285
photosensitivity and, 147*t*
sinus bradycardia/atrioventricular block and, 571*t*, 573*t*, 577–578*t*
taste disorders and, 1260*t*
thromboembolic diseases and, 1065*t*, 1069*t*
visual disturbances and, 305*t*, 316
weight gain and, 1172
Painless myopathy, 1150–1153, 1152*t*, 1155
Pain medications. *See* Analgesics
Palbociclib, 170*t*
Paliperidone, 254, 271, 761*t*, 1166*t*, 1169*t*, 1195*t*, 1197
Palonosetron, 922, 924–927, 924*t*
Pamidronate, 305–306*t*, 1237*t*, 1274, 1274*t*
PAMORA (peripheral acting mu-opioid receptor antagonists), 840–841, 840*t*
Pancreatitis, 877–892
causative agents of, 877–879, 878–879*t*
clinical presentation of, 888–890, 889*t*
differential diagnosis of, 889, 889*t*
epidemiology of, 879–885
management of, 892
mechanisms of, 885–888, 886*t*
morbidity and mortality for, 890–891, 891*t*
patient education on, 892
prevention of, 891–892, 891*t*
risk factors for, 890, 890*t*
Pancuronium, 907*t*, 1156, 1201, 1237*t*
Pancuronium bromide, 453*t*
Panitumumab, 102*t*, 170*t*, 432*t*
Panobinostat, 7*t*

Pantoprazole
allergic reactions to, 73*t*
chronic kidney disease and, 965, 966*t*
cutaneous diseases and, 101, 104*t*
photosensitivity and, 147*t*
systemic lupus erythematosus and, 126*t*
torsades de pointes and, 533*t*, 540*t*
Papaverine, 532*t*, 761*t*, 765*t*, 771, 1002*t*, 1066*t*, 1070*t*
Para-aminobenzoic acid (PABA), 153, 154
Para-aminosalicylic acid, 125*t*, 710, 850*t*, 861*t*
Paracetamol, 1052*t*, 1326
Paraldehyde, 1186
Paraquat, 849*t*, 861*t*
Parenteral lipids, 853*t*, 868
Parenteral nutrition, 1003*t*
Parkinsonism, 270–273
causative agents of, 270, 271*t*
clinical presentation of, 257*t*, 262, 272
differential diagnosis of, 257*t*, 272
epidemiology of, 270–271
management of, 273, 273*t*
mechanisms of, 271–272, 271*t*
morbidity and mortality for, 273
overview, 253–254
patient education on, 273
prevention of, 273, 273*t*
risk factors for, 272, 272*t*
Paromomycin, 1237*t*
Paroxetine
alopecia and, 173*t*
constipation and, 836*t*
delirium and, 327*t*, 329*t*
depression and, 390
hyperprolactinemia and, 743*t*
hypotension and, 646*t*
nausea/vomiting and, 909*t*
ototoxicity and, 1237*t*
photosensitivity and, 147*t*
serotonin syndrome and, 1202, 1203–1204*t*
sexual dysfunction and, 772
SIADH and, 982*t*, 985, 988
sleep disorders and, 348*t*
teratogenicity of, 1323
thyroid diseases and, 699*t*
visual disturbances and, 306*t*
weight gain and, 1166*t*, 1169*t*, 1171
Paroxysmal atrial tachycardia, 588–591
Paroxysmal supraventricular tachycardia. *See* Atrioventricular node re-entrant tachycardia (AVNRT)
Parsnip, 306*t*
Pasireotide, 174*t*, 180*t*
Passionflower, 353
Patient education
on acidosis, 1011
on acute interstitial nephritis, 957
on acute tubular necrosis, 955
on adverse event documentation, 65–66
on akathisia, 259
on alkalosis, 1017
on alopecia, 192–193
on amenorrhea and oligomenorrhea, 794–795
on anxiety, 411
on aplastic anemia, 1104
on asthma and bronchospasm, 463–464
on atrial fibrillation/atrial flutter, 588
on atrial tachycardia, 591–592
on AV node re-entrant tachycardia, 594–595
on bladder cancer, 1305
on bleeding disorders, 1039
on breast cancer, 1301

on Brugada syndrome, 549
on chemotherapy-induced anemia, 1111
on chronic kidney disease, 976
on cognitive disorders, 369
on color changes of oral mucosa and teeth, 1258
on constipation, 839, 840
on Cushing syndrome, 734
on cutaneous diseases, 114
on delirium, 340
on depression, 392
on diabetes insipidus, 993
on diarrhea, 830
on drug allergies and hypersensitivity reactions, 88, 100
on drug fever, 1192
on dysmenorrhea, 797
on dystonia, 270
on endometrial cancer, 1303
on female sexual dysfunction, 800
on gingival hyperplasia, 1265
on glomerulonephritis, 960
on glucose and insulin dysregulation, 690
on gout and hyperuricemia, 1046
on growth hormone deficiency, 750–751
on heart failure, 516–517
on hemodynamic-mediated AKI, 949
on hemolytic anemia, 1107
on hepatic and cholestatic diseases, 872–873
on hirsutism, 207–208
on hyperprolactinemia, 746–747
on hypertension, 626–627
on hypertrichosis, 207–208
on hypotension, 648
on hypothermia, 1218
on infertility, 774, 802
on interstitial lung disease/pulmonary fibrosis, 441–442
on intracerebral hemorrhage (ICH), 246
on leukemia, 1292
on lymphoma, 1295
on macrocytic anemia, 1109
on male sexual dysfunction, 774–775
on malignant hyperthermia, 1214
on menorrhagia and menometrorrhagia, 796
on monomorphic ventricular tachycardia, 530
on myocardial ischemia/acute coronary syndromes, 489
on myopathy, 1160
on nausea and vomiting, 930–931
on nephrolithiasis, 958
on neuroleptic malignant syndrome, 1202
on neutropenia and agranulocytosis, 1096
on oral erythema multiforme, 1269
on oral lichenoid reactions, 1273
on osteonecrosis of jaw, 1276
on osteoporosis and osteomalacia, 1130
on ototoxicity, 1244
on ovarian hyperstimulation, 790
on pancreatitis, 892
on parkinsonism, 273
on peripheral neuropathy, 289
on photosensitivity, 155–156
on psychosis, 425
on secondary adrenal insufficiency, 741
on seizures, 226
on serotonin syndrome, 1209
on serum sickness-like reactions, 1195
on SIADH, 990
on sinus bradycardia/atrioventricular block, 580–581
on skin cancer, 1298

on sleep disorders, 353
on stroke, 237
on systemic lupus erythematosus, 135–136
on tardive dyskinesia, 265
on taste disorders, 1262
on teratogenicity, 1335
on thrombocytopenia, 1059
on thromboembolic diseases, 1077–1078
on thyroid diseases, 717
on torsades de pointes, 545
on upper gastrointestinal ulceration, 818–819
on valvular and pericardial heart disease, 670
on visual disturbances, 319
on vulvovaginal candidiasis, 792
on weight gain, 1175
Patients
evaluation of, 60–67, 61–62*t*, 64–65*t*
medication histories for, 60–62, 61–62*t*
physical examination of, 62–63
in postmarketing surveillance, 51
Patrinia root, 353
Pazopanib, 170*t*, 699–700*t*, 709, 908*t*
PCCs. *See* Prothrombin complex concentrates
PCP. *See* Phencyclidine
PDUFA (Prescription Drug User Fee Act of 2007), 6, 12, 14
PE. *See* Pulmonary embolism
Pediatric patients. *See also* Teratogenicity
cognitive disorders and, 362, 365
diarrhea in, 826
growth hormone deficiency in, 748–749, 749*t*
hypertrichosis in, 194, 198, 199, 202
learning disabilities in, 1315–1316
leukemia in, 1291
medication errors in, 42
in pancreatitis, 879
seizures in, 217, 219–222, 224
serum sickness-like reactions in, 1194
systemic lupus erythematosus in, 133
Pegfilgrastim, 171*t*, 1094
Peginterferon α-2a, 147*t*, 390, 822*t*
Peginterferon α-2b, 147*t*
Peginterferon β-1b, 383
PEG lavage solution, 503*t*, 510*t*
Pegylated interferon, 365, 699–700*t*, 703*t*, 707
Pembrolizumab, 825
Pemetrexed, 170*t*, 432*t*, 908*t*
Pemoline, 852*t*, 864
Penicillamine
acute kidney injury and, 943*t*, 959
allergic reactions to, 74*t*
hepatic/cholestatic diseases and, 853*t*, 861*t*
hypertrichosis and, 194, 196*t*
interstitial lung disease/pulmonary fibrosis and, 432*t*
myocardial ischemia/acute coronary syndromes and, 472*t*
neutropenia/agranulocytosis and, 1090*t*
oral lichenoid reactions and, 1271*t*
peripheral neuropathy and, 281*t*
taste disorders and, 1260–1261*t*
Penicillins
allergic and hypersensitivity reactions to, 73*t*, 75*t*, 76–77, 79, 85–90, 92, 95
cutaneous diseases and, 102*t*, 111*t*
delirium and, 328*t*
diarrhea and, 822*t*
drug fever and, 1187, 1188*t*, 1191
drug-induced hospitalizations from, 25
heart failure and, 503*t*
hemolytic anemia and, 1104
hepatic/cholestatic diseases and, 870
myocardial ischemia/acute coronary syndromes and, 472*t*
neutropenia/agranulocytosis and, 1091
oral erythema multiforme and, 1267*t*
oral lichenoid reactions and, 1271*t*
seizures and, 218*t*, 220, 222, 222*t*, 225
serum sickness-like reactions and, 1192, 1193*t*
structural similarities and differences in, 91*f*
systemic lupus erythematosus and, 125*t*
thrombocytopenia and, 1052, 1052*t*
torsades de pointes and, 542
upper gastrointestinal ulceration and, 809
Pennyroyal/pennyroyal oil, 219*t*, 221, 851*t*, 866
Pentamidine
asthma/bronchospasm and, 453*t*
color changes of oral mucosa and teeth and, 1254*t*
glucose/insulin dysregulation and, 679, 680*t*, 682*t*, 683, 684–685*t*
hepatic/cholestatic diseases and, 847*t*
hypersensitivity reactions to, 81
hypotension and, 634*t*, 640*t*, 645*t*
pancreatitis and, 878*t*, 882, 885, 886*t*, 890, 892
SIADH and, 984*t*
sinus bradycardia/atrioventricular block and, 573*t*
taste disorders and, 1260*t*
torsades de pointes and, 532*t*, 539*t*
Pentazocine, 453*t*, 571*t*, 1186
Pentobarbital, 226, 871
Pentosan, 1064*t*, 1067, 1068*t*
Pentostatin, 147*t*, 984*t*
Pentoxifylline, 853*t*, 868, 953, 1051*t*
Perchlorate, 703*t*
Percutaneous coronary intervention (PCI), 486, 488
Pergolide
alopecia and, 171*t*, 175
heart failure and, 503*t*, 510*t*
hypotension and, 635*t*, 640*t*
sleep disorders and, 348*t*
taste disorders and, 1260*t*
valvular/pericardial heart disease and, 659–661, 660*t*, 663–664, 663*t*, 668–670, 668*t*
Pericardial heart disease. *See* Valvular and pericardial heart disease
Perindopril, 472*t*, 632*t*, 638*t*, 1254*t*
Periodic Safety Update Reports, 52
Perioperative agents, 910, 912–915, 917–919, 921–924, 928, 930
Peripheral-acting arterial vasodilators, 633*t*
Peripheral acting mu-opioid receptor antagonists (PAMORA), 840–841, 840*t*
Peripheral α-blockers, 632*t*, 647
Peripheral neuropathy, 279–289
causative agents of, 279, 280–281*t*, 1155
chemotherapy-induced, 283, 285–289
clinical presentation of, 282–285, 283*t*
defined, 279
differential diagnosis of, 284–285, 284*t*
epidemiology of, 279
management of, 287–289
mechanisms of, 281–282, 282*t*
morbidity and mortality for, 285–286
patient education on, 289
prevention of, 286–287, 286–287*t*
risk factors for, 285, 285*t*
Perphenazine, 125*t*, 326*t*, 703*t*, 982*t*, 1167*t*, 1195*t*
Pertuzumab, 7*t*, 170*t*
PFTs (pulmonary function tests), 435–436, 439
P-glycoprotein (Pgp), 37, 39, 40, 969
Pharmaceutical manufacturers, 8–10, 50–52
Pharmacist duty to warn, 10–11
Pharmacodynamic drug–drug interactions, 38, 40
Pharmacoepidemiology, 20, 54
Pharmacogenomics Knowledgebase, 35
Pharmacogenomics Research Network, 35
Pharmacokinetic drug–drug interactions, 38–40
Phenacetin, 968, 970
Phenazopyridine, 1105*t*
Phencyclidine (PCP), 401, 401*t*, 415, 418, 418*t*, 851*t*
Phenelzine
delirium and, 327*t*
food interactions with, 40
myocardial ischemia/acute coronary syndromes and, 472*t*
neuroleptic malignant syndrome and, 1195*t*
peripheral neuropathy and, 281*t*
photosensitivity and, 147*t*
sexual dysfunction and, 772
SIADH and, 982*t*
sleep disorders and, 348*t*
systemic lupus erythematosus and, 125*t*
weight gain and, 1166*t*, 1169*t*, 1171
Phenformin, 1002*t*
Phenindione, 1271*t*
Phenmetrazine, 306*t*
Phenobarbital
allergic reactions to, 75*t*
alopecia and, 168*t*
cognitive disorders and, 357, 358*t*, 360, 365
cutaneous diseases and, 101, 103–104*t*, 111*t*, 113*t*
depression and, 376*t*, 379, 385*t*, 386
drug fever and, 1188*t*
gingival hyperplasia and, 1263*t*
hepatic/cholestatic diseases and, 869
macrocytic anemia and, 1109
oral lichenoid reactions and, 1271*t*
osteoporosis/osteomalacia and, 1122, 1123*t*, 1127
ototoxicity and, 1237*t*
secondary adrenal insufficiency and, 737
seizures and, 218*t*, 224, 226
sexual dysfunction and, 763*t*
tardive dyskinesia and, 254
teratogenicity of, 1319
thyroid diseases and, 703*t*
Phenolphthalein, 102*t*
Phenothiazines
delirium and, 337
dystonia and, 266
hyperprolactinemia and, 742, 743*t*
hypertrichosis and, 197*t*
hypotension and, 631
nausea/vomiting and, 927*t*, 929
neutropenia/agranulocytosis and, 1090*t*
photosensitivity and, 143, 150, 150*t*, 154
seizures and, 218*t*, 222*t*
sexual dysfunction and, 757, 758*t*, 760–765*t*
tardive dyskinesia and, 262
visual disturbances and, 316
Phenoxazoline, 230*t*
Phenprocoumon, 1029*t*
Phensuximide, 1263*t*
Phentermine, 9, 659, 660*t*, 663, 973
Phentolamine, 488, 703*t*, 747, 748*t*, 761*t*
Phenylbutazone
hepatic/cholestatic diseases and, 846*t*, 861*t*
oral erythema multiforme and, 1267*t*
oral lichenoid reactions and, 1271*t*
ototoxicity and, 1237*t*
systemic lupus erythematosus and, 126*t*
valvular/pericardial heart disease and, 661*t*, 662
visual disturbances and, 306*t*
Phenylephrine, 473*t*, 477*t*, 618*t*, 620*t*

INDEX

Phenylpropanolamine
alcohol use and, 232
atrial tachycardia and, 588*t*
AV node re-entrant tachycardia and, 592*t*
intracerebral hemorrhage and, 238*t*, 240*t*, 242–243
myocardial ischemia/acute coronary syndromes and, 473*t*
seizures and, 225
sinus bradycardia/atrioventricular block and, 573*t*
Phenytoin
acute kidney injury and, 943*t*, 959
allergic reactions to, 74–75*t*, 85, 87–88
aplastic anemia and, 1100*t*
cannabinoid interactions with, 33
cognitive disorders and, 360, 365, 367
color changes of oral mucosa and teeth and, 1253, 1254*t*
cutaneous diseases and, 101, 103–104*t*, 111*t*, 112, 113*t*
delirium and, 326*t*
depression and, 376*t*, 378, 379, 386
diabetes insipidus and, 991*t*
drug fever and, 1188*t*
drug interactions with, 38
genetic variations affecting, 36*t*
gingival hyperplasia and, 1253, 1263–1265, 1263*t*, 1265*t*
glucose/insulin dysregulation and, 680*t*, 684*t*
hepatic/cholestatic diseases and, 852*t*, 861*t*
hirsutism and, 194, 195*t*, 199*t*
hypertrichosis and, 194, 196*t*, 198, 198*f*, 199, 202
hypotension and, 634*t*, 640*t*, 645*t*
macrocytic anemia and, 1101*t*, 1107, 1108*t*, 1109
metabolic pathway for, 35
neuroleptic malignant syndrome and, 1195*t*
neutropenia/agranulocytosis and, 1090*t*
oral erythema multiforme and, 1267*t*
oral lichenoid reactions and, 1271*t*
osteoporosis/osteomalacia and, 1122, 1123*t*, 1127
ototoxicity and, 1237*t*
peripheral neuropathy and, 281*t*
secondary adrenal insufficiency and, 737
seizures and, 218*t*, 224, 226
sexual dysfunction and, 763*t*
sleep disorders and, 348*t*
systemic lupus erythematosus and, 124*t*
tardive dyskinesia and, 254
teratogenicity of, 1315–1316, 1319, 1324–1325, 1328, 1330–1331, 1335
thrombocytopenia and, 1051*t*
thyroid diseases and, 703*t*
vaginal bleeding disorders and, 793
valvular/pericardial heart disease and, 661*t*
visual disturbances and, 306*t*, 312, 315, 318
weight gain and, 1169, 1175*t*
Phosphate salts, 840*t*
Phosphodiesterase-5 inhibitors
hypotension and, 636*t*, 642
myocardial ischemia/acute coronary syndromes and, 478, 484
sexual dysfunction and, 761*t*, 765*t*, 769, 800
visual disturbances and, 312–313, 317, 318
Phosphorus, 849*t*
Photo-onycholysis, 152
Photosensitivity, 143–156
causative agents of, 143, 144–148*t*
clinical presentation of, 151–152*t*, 151–153, 152*f*
defined, 143
differential diagnosis of, 151, 151*t*
epidemiology of, 143, 148
management of, 155, 155*t*
mechanisms of, 149–151, 149*f*, 150*t*
morbidity and mortality for, 154
patient education on, 155–156
prevention of, 154–155, 154*t*
risk factors for, 153–154, 153*t*
Photosensitizing agents, 150*t*, 151, 153
Phototherapy, 191
Phototoxicity/photoallergy. *See* Photosensitivity
Physical examinations, 62–63
Physostigmine, 378, 380, 424*t*, 571*t*, 574*t*, 582*t*
Phytonadione, 73*t*
P-i concept, 79
Picotamide, 463
Pilsicainide, 547*t*, 548
Pimavanserin, 254
Pimozide, 532*t*, 540*t*, 635*t*, 639*t*, 703*t*, 982*t*
Pimpinella, 306*t*
Pindolol, 125*t*, 632*t*, 638*t*, 646*t*, 647
Pioglitazone
bladder cancer and, 1285*t*, 1288*t*, 1303–1305
heart failure and, 503*t*, 506, 510*t*
myocardial ischemia/acute coronary syndromes and, 476
osteoporosis/osteomalacia and, 1124*t*
Pipamperone, 533*t*
Piperacillin, 75*t*, 87, 90, 103*t*, 1051*t*, 1188*t*
Piperacillin–tazobactam, 328*t*, 1105*t*
Pirarubicin, 170*t*
Pirfenidone, 147*t*, 440
Piritramide, 906*t*
Piroxicam
alopecia and, 172*t*
bleeding disorders and, 1033
cutaneous diseases and, 104*t*
heart failure and, 510*t*
hepatic/cholestatic diseases and, 846*t*
oral erythema multiforme and, 1267*t*
oral lichenoid reactions and, 1271*t*
ototoxicity and, 1237*t*
pancreatitis and, 879*t*, 881
photosensitivity and, 147*t*
systemic lupus erythematosus and, 126*t*
upper gastrointestinal ulceration and, 813
Pisa syndrome, 268
Pituitary diseases. *See* Hypothalamic, pituitary, and adrenal diseases
Placental transfer mechanisms, 1313–1314
Platelet inhibitors, 1049
Platelet-rich plasma (PRP), 191
Platinum analogues, 782–783*t*, 785–786*t*, 800
Platinum-based therapies, 1101*t*, 1109*t*, 1233
Platinum compounds, 282*t*, 285, 286, 1284
Plausibility, in epidemiology, 22
Podagra, 1140
Podophyllin, 280*t*
Poisoning agents, 177
Polidocanol, 197*t*
Poly ADP ribose polymerase inhibitors, 1289
Polyarteritis nodosa, 85
Polyaspartic acid, 953
Polyethoxyethylated castor oil-containing products, 77*t*, 81
Polyethylene glycol, 840*t*, 984*t*
Polymorphisms
allergic reactions and, 86
anxiety and, 408–409
in asthma and bronchospasm, 460
cancer and, 1290
in drug response differences, 11, 34, 37–38, 365
gingival hyperplasia and, 1265
hypotension and, 643
myopathy and, 1157
oral lichenoid reactions and, 1272
racial differences in, 15–16
Polymyositis, 1150, 1152*t*, 1153, 1155, 1159
Polymyxin B, 77*t*, 1237*t*
Polysomnography (PSG), 349
Polysorbate 80, 73*t*
Pomalidomide, 7*t*, 1286–1287
Ponatinib, 1065*t*, 1069*t*, 1087
PONV. *See* Postoperative nausea and vomiting
Population-based postmarketing surveillance, 47–49, 54–56
Porfimer, 147*t*, 151, 154
Posaconazole, 533*t*, 539*t*
Postherpetic neuralgia, 288–289
Postmarketing surveillance, 47–57
clinicians in, 50–51
database for, 67
future challenges in, 56–57
importance of, 25, 47
manufacturers in, 50–52
patient role in, 51
population-based, 47–49, 54–56
proactive/sentinel, 54, 55, 57, 67
regulatory agencies in, 52–53
reporting systems for, 24, 49–56
science of, 53–56
Postoperative nausea and vomiting (PONV)
causative agents of, 910
clinical presentation of, 915–916
epidemiology of, 910
management of, 928, 928*t*
mechanisms of, 912–914
morbidity and mortality for, 919
patient education on, 930
prevention of, 921–924, 921*t*, 924*t*
risk factors for, 917–918, 917–918*t*
Post-transplant lymphoproliferative disorders (PTLD), 1293, 1295
Potassium bicarbonate–potassium citrate, 1010*t*
Potassium-channel blockers, 538
Potassium chloride, 809, 810–811*t*, 811–813, 816*t*
Potassium citrate, 1010, 1010*t*
Potassium citrate–citric acid, 1010*t*
Potassium iodide, 706–707*t*, 1188*t*, 1237*t*
Potassium perchlorate, 715, 1090*t*
Potassium-sparing diuretics, 625, 949, 1003*t*, 1138
Povidone-iodine, 73*t*, 705, 707*t*
PPIs. *See* Proton pump inhibitors
Practolol, 125*t*
Pralatrexate, 908*t*
Pramipexole
alopecia and, 175
anxiety and, 405
heart failure and, 503*t*
hyperprolactinemia and, 746
hypotension and, 635*t*, 640*t*
neuroleptic malignant syndrome and, 1196
psychosis and, 418*t*
valvular/pericardial heart disease and, 669
Pramlintide, 682*t*, 685*t*
Prasugrel, 73*t*, 1029, 1029*t*, 1033
Pravastatin, 124*t*, 171*t*, 281*t*, 878*t*, 886*t*, 1260*t*
Prazosin, 125*t*, 472*t*, 632*t*, 639*t*, 1237*t*, 1271*t*
PRCA (pure red-cell aplasia), 11
Prednisolone
acute kidney injury and, 957
Cushing syndrome and, 731*t*
heart failure and, 502*t*, 510*t*
hirsutism and, 195*t*

hypertrichosis and, 196t
ototoxicity and, 1237t
pharmacologic characteristics of, 739t
secondary adrenal insufficiency and, 741
skin cancer and, 1297
thrombocytopenia and, 1059
Prednisolone acetate, 731t, 736t
Prednisone
acute kidney injury and, 957
alopecia and, 188t, 191
cognitive disorders and, 360
delirium and, 326t, 329t
depression and, 382
hepatic/cholestatic diseases and, 866
hypertrichosis and, 196t
interstitial lung disease/pulmonary fibrosis and, 440, 441
leukemia and, 1285
lymphoma and, 1295
myopathy and, 1153, 1156, 1159
osteoporosis/osteomalacia and, 1120
pharmacologic characteristics of, 739t
photosensitivity and, 155
secondary adrenal insufficiency and, 736t, 741
sinus bradycardia/atrioventricular block and, 571t
thrombocytopenia and, 1059
thromboembolic diseases and, 1070t
thyroid diseases and, 716
weight gain and, 1169t, 1172
Pregabalin
alopecia and, 168t
anxiety and, 401t, 402, 404, 407
cognitive disorders and, 367
delirium and, 326t
depression and, 379
dystonia and, 270
heart failure and, 503t, 509
ototoxicity and, 1237t
peripheral neuropathy and, 289
sexual dysfunction and, 760t, 764t
sinus bradycardia/atrioventricular block and, 571t
visual disturbances and, 306t
weight gain and, 1166t, 1169, 1169t, 1170
Pregnancy, 32, 1313–1314. *See also* Teratogenicity
Prehypertension. *See* Elevated blood pressure
Premarin, 1254t
Premarketing data, limitations of, 47–48
Prescription Drug User Fee Act of 2007 (PDUFA), 6, 12, 14
Presyncope, 631, 637
Preventing Medication Errors (IOM), 19
Prevention strategies. *See also* Patient education
for acidosis, 1007–1008, 1008t
for acute interstitial nephritis, 956–957
for acute tubular necrosis, 952–955
for akathisia, 258, 258t
for alopecia, 185–186, 185t
for amenorrhea and oligomenorrhea, 789t, 794
for anxiety, 410, 410t
for aplastic anemia, 1103, 1103t
for asthma and bronchospasm, 461–462, 461t
for atrial fibrillation/atrial flutter, 586, 586t
for atrial tachycardia, 590, 590t
for AV node re-entrant tachycardia, 594, 594t
for bladder cancer, 1294t, 1304–1305
for bleeding disorders, 1034–1035t, 1034–1036
for breast cancer, 1294t, 1300
for Brugada syndrome, 549
for chemotherapy-induced anemia, 1110–1111
for chronic kidney disease, 974–975, 974t
for cognitive disorders, 366–368, 366t
for color changes of oral mucosa and teeth, 1257–1258
for constipation, 839, 839t
for Cushing syndrome, 733–734, 734t
for cutaneous diseases, 112, 113t
for delirium, 334–335, 334t
for depression, 390, 390t
for diabetes insipidus, 993, 993t
for diarrhea, 826–827, 826t
for drug allergies and hypersensitivity reactions, 88–90, 92, 94–98, 97t
for drug fever, 1190–1191
for dysmenorrhea, 789t, 797
for dystonia, 269, 269t
for endometrial cancer, 1294t, 1302–1303
for female sexual dysfunction, 789t, 799
for gingival hyperplasia, 1265, 1265t
for glomerulonephritis, 959
for glucose and insulin dysregulation, 689, 689t
for gout and hyperuricemia, 1143–1144, 1144t
for growth hormone deficiency, 750, 750t
for heart failure, 515–516, 515t
for hemodynamic-mediated AKI, 948, 948t
for hemolytic anemia, 1106–1107
for hepatic and cholestatic diseases, 865, 865t
for hirsutism, 203, 203t
for hyperprolactinemia, 746, 746t
for hypertension, 623–624, 624t
for hypertrichosis, 203, 203t
for hypotension, 643–644, 643t
for hypothermia, 1217
for infertility, 789t, 801
for interstitial lung disease/pulmonary fibrosis, 438–439, 439t
for intracerebral hemorrhage, 244, 244t
for leukemia, 1291, 1294t
for lymphoma, 1294–1295, 1294t
for macrocytic anemia, 1108
for male sexual dysfunction, 771–772, 772t
for malignant hyperthermia, 1212–1213, 1212t
for menorrhagia and menometrorrhagia, 789t, 796
for monomorphic ventricular tachycardia, 529–530, 529t
for myocardial ischemia/acute coronary syndromes, 484–485, 484t
for myopathy, 1157–1158, 1158t
for nausea and vomiting, 920–927, 921t, 924–925t
for nephrolithiasis, 958
for neuroleptic malignant syndrome, 1199–1200, 1199t
for neutropenia and agranulocytosis, 1094–1095, 1095t
for oral erythema multiforme, 1269
for oral lichenoid reactions, 1273
for osteonecrosis of jaw, 1275–1276, 1275t
for osteoporosis and osteomalacia, 1127–1128, 1128t
for ototoxicity, 1242–1243, 1242t
for ovarian hyperstimulation, 784, 787, 789t
for pancreatitis, 891–892, 891t
for parkinsonism, 273, 273t
for peripheral neuropathy, 286–287, 286–287t
for photosensitivity, 154–155, 154t
for psychosis, 422–423, 423t
for secondary adrenal insufficiency, 740, 740t
for seizures, 225, 225t
for serotonin syndrome, 1207, 1207t
for serum sickness-like reactions, 1194
for SIADH, 989, 989t
for sinus bradycardia/atrioventricular block, 578–579, 579t
for skin cancer, 1294t, 1297–1298
for sleep disorders, 352, 352t
for stroke, 234, 235t
for systemic lupus erythematosus, 134–135, 134t
for tardive dyskinesia, 263–264, 264t
for taste disorders, 1262
for teratogenicity, 1333–1334
for thrombocytopenia, 1056–1057, 1057t
for thromboembolic diseases, 1074–1075, 1075t
for thyroid diseases, 714–715, 715t
for torsades de pointes, 542–544, 543t
for upper gastrointestinal ulceration, 816–818, 816t
for valvular and pericardial heart disease, 669, 669t
for visual disturbances, 317–318, 318t
for vulvovaginal candidiasis, 789t, 792
for weight gain, 1173–1174, 1174t
Priapism
causative agents of, 757, 761t
clinical presentation of, 768t, 769
defined, 757
differential diagnosis of, 770t
management of, 773t
mechanisms of, 765t, 767
patient education on, 774
Primaquine, 1237t
Primary adrenal insufficiency, 734–735
Primary hypertension, 617, 622–624, 622t, 626
Primidone, 124t, 168t, 376t, 379, 1188t, 1263t, 1319
Proactive/sentinel surveillance, 54, 55, 57, 67
Probenecid, 853t, 1093, 1105t, 1136
Probiotics, 827, 829, 830
Probucol, 515
Procainamide
allergic reactions to, 75t
Brugada syndrome and, 547t, 548, 549
drug fever and, 1188t
hepatic/cholestatic diseases and, 847t
hypotension and, 634t, 640t, 645t
malignant hyperthermia and, 1213
monomorphic ventricular tachycardia and, 524–525t, 530
myopathy and, 1150t
neutropenia/agranulocytosis and, 1088, 1090–1091t, 1091
oral lichenoid reactions and, 1271t
pancreatitis and, 879t
systemic lupus erythematosus and, 124t, 127–130, 128t, 131t, 133–134
taste disorders and, 1260t
thrombocytopenia and, 1051–1052t, 1053
thromboembolic diseases and, 1066t, 1070t
torsades de pointes and, 532t, 538, 539t
valvular/pericardial heart disease and, 661t, 662
Procaine penicillin G, 1260t
Procarbazine
drug fever and, 1188t
hepatic/cholestatic diseases and, 848t
interstitial lung disease/pulmonary fibrosis and, 432t
leukemia and, 1285
nausea/vomiting and, 908t
peripheral neuropathy and, 280t
Prochlorperazine
akathisia and, 255, 255–256t, 258t
dystonia and, 266t, 269t
hepatic/cholestatic diseases and, 852t
hypotension and, 634t, 639t

INDEX

Prochlorperazine (continued)
- nausea/vomiting and, 923, 924*t*, 927–929*t*
- neuroleptic malignant syndrome and, 1195, 1195*t*
- parkinsonism and, 271*t*, 273*t*
- serotonin syndrome and, 1208
- tardive dyskinesia and, 260*t*, 261, 264*t*

Progesterone
- alkalosis and, 1013, 1013–1014*t*
- allergic reactions to, 75*t*
- alopecia and, 167*t*, 171*t*
- anxiety and, 401*t*, 402, 405*t*, 406
- depression and, 386
- gingival hyperplasia and, 1263
- hirsutism and, 195*t*
- myocardial ischemia/acute coronary syndromes and, 475
- oral erythema multiforme and, 1267*t*
- ovarian hyperstimulation and, 784, 787
- torsades de pointes and, 538, 544
- vaginal bleeding disorders and, 782*t*, 785–786*t*, 794, 796

Progestins
- alopecia and, 171*t*, 176, 180, 184, 191
- breast cancer and, 1285*t*, 1288*t*, 1298–1301
- Cushing syndrome and, 731*t*, 733
- endometrial cancer and, 1302
- hirsutism and, 194, 203, 205
- hypertension and, 621, 624, 626
- photosensitivity and, 145*t*
- secondary adrenal insufficiency and, 736, 736–737*t*
- stroke and, 229
- teratogenicity of, 1334*t*
- thromboembolic diseases and, 1067, 1075

Prohapten/hapten theory, 78–79

Prolactin, 729, 742, 798. *See also* Hyperprolactinemia

Promazine, 852*t*

Promethazine
- adverse effects related to, 10
- akathisia and, 255–256*t*, 258*t*
- hypotension and, 634*t*, 639*t*
- hypothermia and, 1216, 1216*t*
- nausea/vomiting and, 922, 924*t*, 927–929*t*
- neuroleptic malignant syndrome and, 1195*t*
- ototoxicity and, 1237*t*, 1244
- photosensitivity and, 147*t*, 150
- systemic lupus erythematosus and, 126*t*
- tardive dyskinesia and, 261

Propafenone
- asthma/bronchospasm and, 453*t*
- atrial fibrillation/atrial flutter and, 582*t*, 584, 586, 587, 587*t*
- Brugada syndrome and, 547*t*
- color changes of oral mucosa and teeth and, 1254*t*
- drug fever and, 1188*t*
- heart failure and, 502*t*, 507, 510*t*, 511, 515
- hepatic/cholestatic diseases and, 847*t*
- monomorphic ventricular tachycardia and, 524–525*t*, 528–530
- myocardial ischemia/acute coronary syndromes and, 472*t*
- neutropenia/agranulocytosis and, 1090*t*
- peripheral neuropathy and, 281*t*
- SIADH and, 984*t*
- sinus bradycardia/atrioventricular block and, 571*t*, 573*t*, 577–578*t*
- systemic lupus erythematosus and, 125*t*
- taste disorders and, 1260*t*

Propionic acid derivatives, 846*t*

Propofol
- acidosis and, 1002*t*, 1007, 1008, 1010
- asthma/bronchospasm and, 453*t*
- Brugada syndrome and, 547*t*
- cutaneous diseases and, 102*t*
- hypotension and, 634*t*, 640*t*
- malignant hyperthermia and, 1212
- myocardial ischemia/acute coronary syndromes and, 472*t*
- nausea/vomiting and, 907*t*, 921, 923
- seizures and, 218*t*, 220
- serotonin syndrome and, 1208*t*, 1209
- sinus bradycardia/atrioventricular block and, 571*t*, 573*t*, 578*t*
- torsades de pointes and, 532*t*
- visual disturbances and, 306*t*

Propolis, 306*t*

Propoxyphene, 846*t*, 906*t*, 1233, 1237*t*

Propranolol
- akathisia and, 256, 259
- alopecia and, 168*t*
- asthma/bronchospasm and, 463
- atrial fibrillation/atrial flutter and, 587*t*
- comorbidity and, 34
- cutaneous diseases and, 106
- delirium and, 328*t*
- drug interactions with, 39*t*
- heart failure and, 502*t*, 509, 510*t*
- hypotension and, 632*t*, 638*t*, 646*t*, 647
- neutropenia/agranulocytosis and, 1088, 1090*t*
- oral lichenoid reactions and, 1271*t*
- serotonin syndrome and, 1208
- serum sickness-like reactions and, 1193*t*
- sinus bradycardia/atrioventricular block and, 578*t*, 579
- sleep disorders and, 348*t*
- systemic lupus erythematosus and, 125*t*, 130
- teratogenicity of, 1317
- thyroid diseases and, 703*t*

Propylene glycol, 1002*t*, 1008, 1008*t*, 1010

Propylthiouracil
- acute kidney injury and, 943*t*
- allergic reactions to, 74–75*t*, 85
- alopecia and, 173*t*, 175
- asthma/bronchospasm and, 453*t*
- chronic kidney disease and, 966*t*, 970*t*
- drug fever and, 1188*t*
- hepatic/cholestatic diseases and, 849*t*, 861*t*
- neutropenia/agranulocytosis and, 1090*t*, 1091
- oral lichenoid reactions and, 1272*t*
- ototoxicity and, 1237*t*
- systemic lupus erythematosus and, 124*t*, 128*t*, 130
- taste disorders and, 1260–1261*t*
- thyroid diseases and, 703*t*, 715–716

Prostaglandin analogs, 194, 197, 197*t*

Prostaglandin E_2, 82, 456, 473*t*, 512, 887

Prostaglandin F_2, 473*t*

Prostaglandins
- acute kidney injury and, 945, 947
- asthma/bronchospasm and, 455–457
- chronic kidney disease and, 969, 970, 973
- hypotension and, 636*t*
- nausea/vomiting and, 912, 922
- ototoxicity and, 1239
- pancreatitis and, 887
- upper gastrointestinal ulceration and, 811–812, 815
- vaginal bleeding disorders and, 795

Prostata, 851*t*

Protamine, 73–74*t*, 76, 77*t*, 81, 1036, 1037*t*

Protamine sulfate, 245, 1064*t*, 1068*t*

Protease inhibitors
- comorbidity and, 34
- depression and, 377
- diarrhea and, 822*t*
- glucose/insulin dysregulation and, 679, 680*t*, 684*t*, 690
- hepatic/cholestatic diseases and, 847*t*
- hyperprolactinemia and, 742, 744*t*
- myocardial ischemia/acute coronary syndromes and, 472*t*, 473, 477*t*, 479
- oral erythema multiforme and, 1267*t*
- osteoporosis/osteomalacia and, 1123*t*
- sexual dysfunction and, 760*t*
- taste disorders and, 1260*t*
- thyroid diseases and, 710

Proteinuria, 34

Prothionamide, 710

Prothrombin complex concentrates (PCCs), 230*t*, 245, 1037*t*, 1064*t*, 1068*t*

Proton pump inhibitors (PPIs)
- acute kidney injury and, 943*t*
- bleeding disorders and, 1036
- chronic kidney disease and, 965–966, 966*t*
- hepatic/cholestatic diseases and, 850*t*
- myocardial ischemia/acute coronary syndromes and, 489
- myopathy and, 1150*t*, 1151, 1152*t*
- osteoporosis/osteomalacia and, 1121*t*, 1123*t*
- pancreatitis and, 880
- sexual dysfunction and, 758*t*
- systemic lupus erythematosus and, 126*t*
- upper gastrointestinal ulceration and, 817, 818

Protriptyline, 147*t*, 173*t*, 326*t*, 329*t*, 504*t*, 510*t*, 982*t*

Proximal renal tubular acidosis, 1003–1004*t*, 1004, 1006, 1010, 1011*f*

PRP (platelet-rich plasma), 191

Prucalopride, 840*t*

Pseudoallergies, 71

Pseudoephedrine
- anxiety and, 401*t*, 404, 409
- cutaneous diseases and, 102*t*
- hypertension and, 618*t*, 620*t*
- intracerebral hemorrhage and, 238*t*, 240*t*
- myocardial ischemia/acute coronary syndromes and, 473*t*
- psychosis and, 417–418*t*, 425
- stroke and, 232
- teratogenicity of, 1326

PSG (polysomnography), 349

Psilocybin, 415, 418, 864

Psoralens, 150, 150*t*, 154, 191, 194, 197*t*, 202

Psoriasis, 103*t*, 106, 107*t*, 109, 113, 114, 114*t*

Psoriatic alopecia, 179*t*, 180

Psychosis, 415–425
- causative agents of, 415, 416–417*t*
- clinical presentation of, 419–420*t*, 419–421
- defined, 415
- differential diagnosis of, 419, 419*t*
- epidemiology of, 417
- management of, 423–424, 424*t*
- mechanisms of, 417–419, 418*t*
- morbidity and mortality of, 422
- patient education on, 425
- prevention of, 422–423, 423*t*
- risk factors for, 421–422, 421*t*
- withdrawal and, 415, 417*t*, 420–422, 424, 424*t*

Psychostimulants, 254, 385

Psychotropic medications
- akathisia and, 255*t*
- alopecia and, 172–173*t*, 175, 185
- Brugada syndrome and, 549

delirium and, 336
drug-induced hospitalizations from, 26t
dystonia and, 266t
nausea/vomiting and, 909t
parkinsonism and, 271t
psychosis and, 422
tardive dyskinesia and, 260t
thromboembolic diseases and, 1066t, 1070t
Psyllium, 75t, 306t, 453t, 840t
PTLD (post-transplant lymphoproliferative disorders), 1293, 1295
$P2Y_{12}$ inhibitors, 487t, 1026t, 1029, 1029t, 1033
Public health, impact of drug-induced diseases on, 21, 24–26, 29
Pulmonary embolism (PE)
clinical presentation of, 1071–1073, 1071t
differential diagnosis of, 1072, 1072t
management of, 1076
morbidity and mortality for, 1074
overview, 1063
patient education on, 1077–1078
pretest probability of, 1072, 1072t
Pulmonary fibrosis. *See* Interstitial lung disease/ pulmonary fibrosis
Pulmonary function tests (PFTs), 435–436, 439
Pulmonary toxicity, 431, 434, 436–442
Pure red-cell aplasia (PRCA), 11
Pyrazinamide, 147t, 847t, 1136t, 1138–1140, 1188t
Pyrazolones, 968
Pyrethrin, 453t
Pyrethrum, 306t
Pyridostigmine, 571t, 573–574t, 646t, 647
Pyridoxine (Vitamin B_6)
depression and, 386
peripheral neuropathy and, 281t, 282, 286
photosensitivity and, 147t, 154
tardive dyskinesia and, 265
teratogenicity of, 1321
Pyrimethamine, 147t, 1090t
Pyrogens, 1185–1187

QT interval prolongation, 530–531, 534–544
Quantitative impact of drug-induced diseases, 23
Quetiapine
acidosis and, 1002t
alkalosis and, 1013–1014t, 1014
alopecia and, 173t
constipation and, 836t
delirium and, 326t, 329t, 338, 339
depression and, 376t
hyperprolactinemia and, 743t
hypotension and, 635t, 639t
neuroleptic malignant syndrome and, 1195t
psychosis and, 424
sexual dysfunction and, 761t, 765t, 772
SIADH and, 982t
tardive dyskinesia and, 265
thromboembolic diseases and, 1066t, 1070t
thyroid diseases and, 699t
torsades de pointes and, 534t, 539–540t
visual disturbances and, 306t
weight gain and, 1166t, 1169t
Quiescence, 1122
Quinacrine, 1090t, 1254t, 1272t
Quinapril, 167t, 632t, 638t, 878t, 1254t
Quinethazone, 147t
Quinidine
allergic reactions to, 75t
atrial tachycardia and, 590
delirium and, 326t
drug fever and, 1188t
drug interactions with, 39
genetic variability and, 16t
glucose/insulin dysregulation and, 682t, 685t
hemolytic anemia and, 1101t, 1105t
hepatic/cholestatic diseases and, 847t
hypotension and, 634t
monomorphic ventricular tachycardia and, 529
neutropenia/agranulocytosis and, 1090–1091t, 1091
oral lichenoid reactions and, 1272t
ototoxicity and, 1237t
photosensitivity and, 147t
psychosis and, 417t
sinus bradycardia/atrioventricular block and, 577, 578t
systemic lupus erythematosus and, 124t, 127, 128t, 130
thrombocytopenia and, 1051–1052t, 1052
torsades de pointes and, 532t, 538, 539–540t
upper gastrointestinal ulceration and, 809, 810t, 811, 813
Quinine
allergic reactions to, 75t
cutaneous diseases and, 102t
drug fever and, 1188t
glucose/insulin dysregulation and, 682t, 685t
hemolytic anemia and, 1101t, 1105t, 1106
neutropenia/agranulocytosis and, 1090–1091t
oral erythema multiforme and, 1267t
ototoxicity and, 1237t, 1239, 1239t
photosensitivity and, 147t
thrombocytopenia and, 1051–1052t, 1052, 1054, 1056
torsades de pointes and, 534t, 539–540t
Quinolones, 101, 220, 316
Quinupristin-dalfopristin, 984t

Rabbit syndrome, 262, 265
Rabeprazole, 966t
Racial differences
in constipation, 837
cutaneous diseases and, 111–112
in drug allergies and hypersensitivity reactions, 87
intracerebral hemorrhage and, 241
in nausea and vomiting, 917
in polymorphisms, 15–16
in prevalence of drug-induced diseases, 32, 38
systemic lupus erythematosus and, 133
Radiocontrast media
acute kidney injury and, 943t, 945t, 950–955
allergic and hypersensitivity reactions to, 76–77, 77t, 81, 87, 97t, 98
asthma/bronchospasm and, 451
iodinated, 219t, 452t, 700t, 703t, 709, 716–717
thyroid diseases and, 705, 709, 716–717
Raloxifene
depression and, 386
endometrial cancer and, 1302
osteoporosis/osteomalacia and, 1129t, 1130
thromboembolic diseases and, 1064t, 1068t, 1074, 1075t
thyroid diseases and, 703t
Raltegravir, 103t, 401t, 403, 1127, 1267t
Ramelteon, 335, 337, 353
Ramipril
acute kidney injury and, 942
alopecia and, 167t
color changes of oral mucosa and teeth and, 1254t
hypotension and, 632t, 638t
ototoxicity and, 1237t
pancreatitis and, 878t, 879
photosensitivity and, 147t
SIADH and, 983t
taste disorders and, 1260t
Ranibizumab, 1003t, 1065t, 1069t
Ranitidine
cognitive disorders and, 366
delirium and, 328t
drug fever and, 1188t
hemolytic anemia and, 1105t
neutropenia/agranulocytosis and, 1090t
oral lichenoid reactions and, 1272t
photosensitivity and, 147t
sinus bradycardia/atrioventricular block and, 571t, 577t
systemic lupus erythematosus and, 127t
thrombocytopenia and, 1051t
visual disturbances and, 307t
Ranolazine, 534t, 539t
Rapamycin, 1127
Rapid eye movement (REM) sleep, 347, 349
Rasagiline, 635t, 640t, 1203–1204t
Rasburicase, 36t, 1105t, 1138
Rashes, 100, 104–106, 107–108t
RDDS (restrictive drug distribution system), 5–7, 7t
Rebound hypertension, 621, 625t, 626, 627
Recombinant activated factor VIIa (rFVIIa), 230t, 245, 870, 1037t, 1039, 1064t, 1068t, 1075t
Recombinant human growth hormone, 680t, 684t
Recombinant proteins, 95
Recombinant tissue plasminogen activator (rt-PA), 235–237, 238t, 241, 244
Red man syndrome, 76, 97t
Regorafenib, 170t, 699t
Regulatory agencies, role in postmarketing surveillance, 52–53
Regulatory environment for drug safety, 4–8, 4*f*
Rehydration management, 829
Remifentanil, 571t, 573t, 906t
REMS. *See* Risk evaluation and mitigation strategies
REM (rapid eye movement) sleep, 347, 349
Renal disease. *See* Acute kidney injury (AKI); Chronic kidney disease (CKD); End stage renal disease (ESRD)
Renal tubular acidosis (RTA), 1003–1004t, 1004, 1006, 1010, 1011*f*
Renin, 232, 512
Renin inhibitors, 633t, 1003t
Repaglinide, 849t
Reporting systems for adverse events, 24, 49–56, 66–67
Reserpine
delirium and, 327t
depression and, 376t, 378, 385, 385t
hyperprolactinemia and, 742, 743–744t
hypotension and, 633t, 639t
parkinsonism and, 271t, 273t
sexual dysfunction and, 760t
systemic lupus erythematosus and, 125t
tardive dyskinesia and, 265
visual disturbances and, 307t
Respiratory acidosis, 1001, 1003–1004t, 1005–1007, 1007–1008t, 1010–1011
Respiratory alkalosis, 1012–1017, 1013–1016t
Restrictive drug distribution system (RDDS), 5–7, 7t
Reteplase, 663t, 1029t
Retinoic acid. *See* Tretinoin
Retinoic acid derivatives, 377t, 384–385
Retinoids
alopecia and, 166, 173t, 174, 179t, 186, 191
hypertrichosis and, 197t
teratogenicity of, 1334t
vulvovaginal candidiasis and, 791

INDEX

Retinol. *See* Vitamin A
Reversal agents, 1037*t*
Rhabdomyolysis
  clinical presentation of, 1154
  defined, 1149
  dystonia and, 267
  epidemiology of, 1151
  malignant hyperthermia and, 1209–1212
  management of, 1158, 1159
  morbidity and mortality for, 1157
  neuroleptic malignant syndrome and, 1197, 1200
  serotonin syndrome and, 1206, 1207
  statins and, 880, 888, 1151
Ribavirin
  cognitive disorders and, 365
  depression and, 390
  hemolytic anemia and, 1106*t*
  hepatic/cholestatic diseases and, 847*t*
  pancreatitis and, 879*t*, 884, 890
  thyroid diseases and, 707
Riboflavin, 1009
Rickets, 1120
Rifabutin, 125*t*, 984*t*
Rifampin
  acute kidney injury and, 943*t*, 956, 959
  allergic reactions to, 87
  cutaneous diseases and, 102*t*
  diabetes insipidus and, 991, 991*t*
  diarrhea and, 829
  drug fever and, 1188*t*, 1191
  drug interactions with, 38
  glucose/insulin dysregulation and, 680*t*, 684*t*
  hemolytic anemia and, 1106*t*
  hepatic/cholestatic diseases and, 847*t*, 869
  myopathy and, 1150*t*
  oral erythema multiforme and, 1267*t*
  oral lichenoid reactions and, 1272*t*
  ototoxicity and, 1237*t*
  secondary adrenal insufficiency and, 736–737*t*, 737
  serum sickness-like reactions and, 1193*t*
  thrombocytopenia and, 1051*t*
  thyroid diseases and, 699*t*, 703*t*
Rifaximin, 829, 871
Rilpivirine, 991*t*
Riluzole, 848*t*, 852*t*, 991*t*
Rimantadine, 1237*t*
Riociguat, 7*t*, 636*t*
Risedronate, 307*t*, 818, 1129*t*, 1130, 1274*t*
Risk evaluation and mitigation strategies (REMS), 5, 6, 12–14, 647, 1111
Risk factors
  for acidosis, 1007, 1008*t*
  for acute interstitial nephritis, 956
  for acute tubular necrosis, 951–952
  for akathisia, 258, 258*t*
  for alkalosis, 1015, 1017*t*
  for alopecia, 183–184, 184*t*
  for amenorrhea and oligomenorrhea, 788*t*, 794
  for anxiety, 408–409, 408*t*
  for aplastic anemia, 1102, 1103*t*
  for asthma and bronchospasm, 458*t*, 459–460
  for atrial fibrillation/atrial flutter, 585–586, 585*t*
  for atrial tachycardia, 589–590, 589*t*
  for AV node re-entrant tachycardia, 593–594, 593*t*
  for bladder cancer, 1291*t*, 1304
  for bleeding disorders, 1031–1032, 1031–1032*t*
  for breast cancer, 1291*t*, 1299–1300
  for Brugada syndrome, 548, 548*t*
  for chemotherapy-induced anemia, 1103*t*, 1110
  for chronic kidney disease, 972–973, 972*t*
  for cognitive disorders, 364–366, 364*t*
  for color changes of oral mucosa and teeth, 1257, 1258*t*
  for congenital heart defects, 1324
  for constipation, 838–839, 838*t*
  for Cushing syndrome, 733, 733*t*
  for cutaneous diseases, 110–112, 111*t*
  for delirium, 331–333, 332*t*
  for depression, 387–389, 388*t*
  for diabetes insipidus, 992–993, 993*t*
  for diarrhea, 825, 826*t*
  for drug allergies and hypersensitivity reactions, 85–88, 85*t*
  for drug fever, 1190
  for dysmenorrhea, 788*t*, 797
  for dystonia, 268, 268*t*
  for endometrial cancer, 1291*t*, 1302
  for female sexual dysfunction, 788*t*, 799
  for fetal alcohol spectrum disorders, 1332–1333
  for gastroschisis, 1327
  for gingival hyperplasia, 1258*t*, 1264–1265
  for glomerulonephritis, 959
  for glucose and insulin dysregulation, 687–688, 687–688*t*
  for gout and hyperuricemia, 1143, 1143*t*
  for growth hormone deficiency, 745*t*, 749
  for heart failure, 513–514, 514*t*
  for hemodynamic-mediated AKI, 946–947, 947*t*
  for hemolytic anemia, 1103*t*, 1106
  for hepatic and cholestatic diseases, 862–865, 863*t*
  for hirsutism, 202, 202*t*
  for hyperprolactinemia, 745–746, 745*t*
  for hypertension, 622–623, 622*t*
  for hypertrichosis, 202, 203*t*
  for hypotension, 641–643, 642*t*
  for hypothermia, 1217
  for infertility, 788*t*, 801
  for interstitial lung disease/pulmonary fibrosis, 437–438, 437*t*
  for intracerebral hemorrhage, 241–244, 242*t*
  for learning disabilities, 1316
  for leukemia, 1290, 1291*t*
  for limb deficiency defects, 1325
  for low birth weight, 1318
  for lymphoma, 1291*t*, 1294
  for macrocytic anemia, 1103*t*, 1108
  for male sexual dysfunction, 771, 771*t*
  for malignant hyperthermia, 1211–1212, 1211*t*
  for menorrhagia and menometrorrhagia, 788*t*, 796
  for microcephaly, 1331
  for monomorphic ventricular tachycardia, 528–529, 528*t*
  for myocardial ischemia/acute coronary syndromes, 482, 483*t*
  for myopathy, 1155–1157, 1156*t*
  for nausea and vomiting, 917–918*t*, 917–919
  for nephrolithiasis, 958
  for neural tube defects, 1329
  for neuroleptic malignant syndrome, 1198, 1198*t*
  for neutropenia and agranulocytosis, 1093–1094, 1093*t*
  for oral erythema multiforme, 1258*t*, 1269
  for oral lichenoid reactions, 1258*t*, 1273
  for orofacial clefts, 1321
  for osteonecrosis of jaw, 1258*t*, 1275
  for osteoporosis and osteomalacia, 1125–1126, 1126*t*
  for ototoxicity, 1241–1242, 1241*t*
  for ovarian hyperstimulation, 784, 788*t*
  for pancreatitis, 890, 890*t*
  for parkinsonism, 272, 272*t*
  patient evaluation of, 63
  for peripheral neuropathy, 285, 285*t*
  for photosensitivity, 153–154, 153*t*
  for psychosis, 421–422, 421*t*
  for secondary adrenal insufficiency, 738–740, 739*t*
  for seizures, 223–224, 224*t*
  for serotonin syndrome, 1206–1207, 1206*t*
  for serum sickness-like reactions, 1194
  for SIADH, 988–989, 988*t*
  for sinus bradycardia/atrioventricular block, 576–578, 576–578*t*
  for skin cancer, 1291*t*, 1297
  for sleep disorders, 350–351, 351*t*
  for stroke, 234, 234*t*
  for systemic lupus erythematosus, 133–134, 133*t*
  for tardive dyskinesia, 263, 263*t*
  for taste disorders, 1258*t*, 1261
  for thrombocytopenia, 1056, 1056*t*
  for thromboembolic diseases, 1073–1074, 1073*t*
  for thyroid diseases, 713–714, 713*t*
  for torsades de pointes, 40, 537–541, 537*t*, 539–540*t*
  for upper gastrointestinal ulceration, 814–816, 815*t*
  for valvular and pericardial heart disease, 668–669, 668*t*
  for visual disturbances, 317, 317*t*
  for vulvovaginal candidiasis, 788*t*, 791
  for weight gain, 1173, 1173*t*
Risperidone
  acidosis and, 1002*t*
  akathisia and, 255
  allergic reactions to, 73*t*
  alopecia and, 173*t*
  anxiety and, 405
  delirium and, 326*t*, 338–340
  extrapyramidal symptoms and, 254
  hepatic/cholestatic diseases and, 852*t*
  hyperprolactinemia and, 742, 743*t*, 745
  hypotension and, 635*t*, 639*t*
  hypothermia and, 1215, 1216, 1216*t*
  neuroleptic malignant syndrome and, 1195, 1195*t*, 1197, 1201
  parkinsonism and, 270–272
  photosensitivity and, 147*t*
  sexual dysfunction and, 765*t*, 772, 798
  SIADH and, 982*t*, 990
  sinus bradycardia/atrioventricular block and, 571*t*, 577–578*t*
  taste disorders and, 1260*t*
  teratogenicity of, 1321–1322
  thromboembolic diseases and, 1066*t*, 1070*t*
  torsades de pointes and, 533*t*, 539–540*t*
  visual disturbances and, 307*t*
  weight gain and, 1166*t*, 1169*t*, 1171
Ritodrine, 680*t*, 684*t*, 853*t*
Ritonavir
  Cushing syndrome and, 733
  nausea/vomiting and, 909*t*
  osteoporosis/osteomalacia and, 1123*t*, 1127
  ototoxicity and, 1237*t*
  photosensitivity and, 147*t*
  serotonin syndrome and, 1204
  SIADH and, 984*t*
  thrombocytopenia and, 1051*t*
  thyroid diseases and, 703*t*

INDEX

Rituximab
allergic and hypersensitivity reactions to, 73–74*t*, 77*t*, 96
hemolytic anemia and, 1107
interstitial lung disease/pulmonary fibrosis and, 432*t*, 438
lymphoma and, 1295
myocardial ischemia/acute coronary syndromes and, 473*t*
myopathy and, 1153
neutropenia/agranulocytosis and, 1090*t*
oral lichenoid reactions and, 1272*t*
serum sickness-like reactions and, 1193*t*, 1194
thromboembolic diseases and, 1065*t*, 1069*t*
Rivaroxaban
alopecia and, 167*t*
bleeding disorders and, 1029*t*
intracerebral hemorrhage and, 237, 238*t*, 245
thromboembolic diseases and, 1076, 1077*t*
upper gastrointestinal ulceration and, 811
valvular/pericardial heart disease and, 661*t*, 662
Rocuronium, 73*t*, 907*t*
Rofecoxib
acute kidney injury and, 942
allergic reactions to, 74*t*
cardiovascular disease associated with, 53
cognitive disorders and, 361
heart failure and, 503*t*, 509, 510*t*
myocardial ischemia/acute coronary syndromes and, 472*t*, 475
stroke and, 230, 231
withdrawal from market, 3
Rogaine, 50
Rolapitant, 926
Romiplostim, 1059
Ropinirole
alopecia and, 171*t*, 175
heart failure and, 503*t*
hyperprolactinemia and, 746
hypotension and, 635*t*, 640*t*
neuroleptic malignant syndrome and, 1196
ototoxicity and, 1237*t*
psychosis and, 418*t*
SIADH and, 984*t*
valvular/pericardial heart disease and, 669
Ropivacaine, 524–525*t*
Rosiglitazone
bladder cancer and, 1304
heart failure and, 503*t*, 505–506, 510*t*
myocardial ischemia/acute coronary syndromes and, 473, 473*t*, 476, 477*t*, 480
osteoporosis/osteomalacia and, 1124*t*
SIADH and, 983*t*
visual disturbances and, 307*t*
Rosuvastatin, 281*t*, 689
Rotigotine, 405, 418*t*
Roxithromycin, 472*t*, 474, 532*t*, 539*t*
RTA. *See* Renal tubular acidosis
rt-PA (recombinant tissue plasminogen activator), 235–237, 238*t*, 241, 244
Rue, 307*t*
Rufinamide, 379
Rule of Too, 48
Ruxolitinib, 7*t*

Sacubitril, 77*t*, 96, 633*t*
Safety of drugs, 3–16
challenges and opportunities related to, 15–16
data collection on, 15
in legal environment, 8–11, 9*t*
overview, 3–4
Periodic Safety Update Reports, 52
postmarketing surveillance for. *See* Postmarketing surveillance
public assumptions regarding, 19
recommendations for improvement, 12–15
regulatory environment for, 4–8, 4*f*
Sage, 219*t*, 221
SAI. *See* Secondary adrenal insufficiency
St. John's wort, 147*t*, 173*t*, 307*t*, 353, 703*t*, 1203–1204*t*
Sairei-to, 851*t*
Salbutamol, 454, 473*t*, 1002*t*
Salicylamides, 703*t*
Salicylates
acidosis and, 1002*t*
alkalosis and, 1013–1014*t*, 1017
aplastic anemia and, 1100*t*
chronic kidney disease and, 970
glucose/insulin dysregulation and, 681, 682*t*, 685*t*
hemolytic anemia and, 1105*t*
hypersensitivity reactions to, 97–98
nonacetylated, 489, 812
oral erythema multiforme and, 1267*t*
ototoxicity and, 1237*t*, 1239, 1239*t*, 1242*t*, 1243
pancreatitis and, 881
thyroid diseases and, 703*t*
toxicity and, 1185
Salicylic acid, 327*t*
Saline laxatives, 840, 840*t*
Salmeterol, 473*t*
Salsalate, 461, 812
Saquinavir, 147*t*, 168*t*, 1123*t*, 1268*t*
Sargramostim, 1094, 1288*t*
Sassafras, 851*t*
Saw palmetto, 822, 835, 851*t*
Saxagliptin, 503*t*, 506, 509, 879*t*, 884
Scalp cooling, 186, 189*t*
Scarring alopecia, 174, 177, 179*t*, 184*t*
SCARS (severe cutaneous adverse reactions), 101, 104–105, 111, 112
SCC (squamous cell carcinoma), 1295–1298
Schizophrenia. *See* Psychosis
SCLE (subacute cutaneous lupus erythematosus), 132
Scopolamine, 328–329*t*, 922, 924*t*, 927*t*, 929*t*, 1244
Scopolia, 307*t*
Secondary adrenal insufficiency (SAI), 734–741
causative agents of, 735, 736*t*
clinical presentation of, 737–738, 738*t*
differential diagnosis of, 737, 738*t*
epidemiology of, 735
management of, 740–741, 740*t*
mechanisms of, 735–737, 737*t*
morbidity and mortality for, 740
overview, 734–735
patient education on, 741
prevention of, 740, 740*t*
risk factors for, 738–740, 739*t*
Secondary hypertension, 617, 622, 622*t*, 624, 626
Second-degree AV block, 569, 572, 575, 578
Sedative-hypnotics, 325, 335, 351, 352, 758*t*, 763–764*t*
Sedatives, 271*t*, 797, 1005
Seizures, 217–226. *See also* Anticonvulsants
causative agents of, 217, 218–219*t*
clinical presentation of, 222–223, 223*t*
differential diagnosis of, 223, 223*t*
epidemiology of, 217, 219–222
management of, 225–226
mechanisms of, 222, 222*t*
morbidity and mortality for, 224–225
patient education on, 226
prevention of, 225, 225*t*
risk factors for, 223–224, 224*t*
Selective estrogen-receptor modulators (SERMs), 1064*t*, 1068*t*, 1071, 1129*t*
Selective serotonin reuptake inhibitors (SSRIs)
akathisia and, 254–256, 255–256*t*, 258*t*
alopecia and, 175
anxiety and, 401, 401*t*, 405*t*, 406
bleeding disorders and, 1025–1026, 1026*t*, 1029*t*, 1030, 1034
cognitive disorders and, 358–359*t*, 360, 368
delirium and, 326–327*t*
depression and, 376*t*, 390–392
diarrhea and, 822*t*
drug interactions with, 33
dystonia and, 267
hepatic/cholestatic diseases and, 852*t*
intracerebral hemorrhage and, 238*t*, 239, 240*t*, 242*t*
myocardial ischemia/acute coronary syndromes and, 472*t*
nausea/vomiting and, 911*t*
osteoporosis/osteomalacia and, 1121*t*, 1123*t*
parkinsonism and, 270
seizures and, 220
serotonin syndrome and, 1202, 1203–1204*t*, 1204–1207
sexual dysfunction and, 758–762*t*, 765*t*, 767, 799
SIADH and, 982*t*, 985, 987–990, 988*t*
sleep disorders and, 348*t*, 350*t*
stroke and, 230–231*t*, 232, 235*t*
suicides associated with, 53
tardive dyskinesia and, 262
teratogenicity of, 1321–1323
upper gastrointestinal ulceration and, 809, 810–811*t*, 811, 812, 816*t*
vaginal bleeding disorders and, 782*t*, 785*t*, 790*t*, 795, 796
weight gain and, 1170–1171
Selegiline
hypotension and, 635*t*, 640*t*
photosensitivity and, 147*t*
serotonin syndrome and, 1203–1204*t*
sleep disorders and, 348*t*
tardive dyskinesia and, 265
taste disorders and, 1260*t*
Selenium, 515, 714, 850*t*, 1284*t*, 1296
Seniors. *See* Elderly populations
Senna, 851*t*
Senna fruit, 840*t*
Sentinel surveillance, 54, 55, 57, 67
Serious adverse events, defined, 66. *See also* Adverse drug reactions (ADRs)
SERMs (selective estrogen-receptor modulators), 1064*t*, 1068*t*, 1071, 1129*t*
Serotonin. *See also* 5-hydroxytryptamine
anxiety and, 406, 409, 410
delirium and, 329
depression and, 385–386
dystonia and, 266
hyperprolactinemia and, 742
nausea/vomiting and, 913–915
psychosis and, 418, 419
serum sickness-like reactions and, 1192
in sleep cycles, 349
stroke and, 232
in thermoregulation, 1185, 1186, 1215–1216
vaginal bleeding disorders and, 795
valvular/pericardial heart disease and, 663, 664

INDEX

Serotonin antagonists, 703*t*
Serotonin–norepinephrine reuptake inhibitors (SNRIs)
akathisia and, 254
anxiety and, 401, 401*t*, 405*t*, 406
depression and, 376*t*
diarrhea and, 822*t*
serotonin syndrome and, 1203–1204*t*
sexual dysfunction and, 759–760*t*
SIADH and, 981
sleep disorders and, 348*t*, 350*t*
stroke and, 230–231*t*, 232, 235*t*
weight gain and, 1170–1171
Serotonin syndrome, 1202–1209
causative agents of, 1202, 1203*t*
clinical presentation of, 1187*t*, 1197–1198, 1205–1206, 1205*t*
differential diagnosis of, 1206, 1206*t*
epidemiology of, 1202
management of, 1201*t*, 1207–1209, 1208*t*
mechanisms of, 1202–1205, 1204*t*
morbidity and mortality for, 1207
patient education on, 1209
prevention of, 1207, 1207*t*
risk factors for, 1206–1207, 1206*t*
Sertindole, 265
Sertraline
alopecia and, 173*t*
cutaneous diseases and, 101, 104*t*
delirium and, 327*t*, 329*t*
depression and, 390, 391
gingival hyperplasia and, 1263*t*
hyperprolactinemia and, 743*t*
myocardial ischemia/acute coronary syndromes and, 472*t*
oral lichenoid reactions and, 1272*t*
ototoxicity and, 1237*t*
photosensitivity and, 147*t*
serotonin syndrome and, 1203–1204*t*, 1207
sexual dysfunction and, 772
SIADH and, 982*t*, 985
sleep disorders and, 348*t*
systemic lupus erythematosus and, 125*t*
teratogenicity of, 1323
thyroid diseases and, 699*t*, 703*t*, 710
visual disturbances and, 307*t*
weight gain and, 1166*t*, 1169*t*, 1171
Serum-sickness-like disease (SSLD), 84, 99*t*
Serum sickness-like reactions (SSLRs), 1192–1195
causative agents of, 74*t*, 95, 1192, 1193*t*
clinical presentation of, 83*t*, 1187*t*, 1193–1194, 1193*t*
differential diagnosis of, 84*t*, 1194, 1194*t*
epidemiology of, 1192
management of, 1191*t*, 1194
mechanisms of, 80, 81, 1192–1193
morbidity and mortality for, 1194
patient education on, 1195
prevention of, 1194
risk factors for, 1194
Sevelamer, 703*t*, 1002*t*, 1004*t*
Severe cutaneous adverse reactions (SCARS), 101, 104–105, 111, 112
Sevoflurane
hepatic/cholestatic diseases and, 850*t*
malignant hyperthermia and, 1209*t*
myocardial ischemia/acute coronary syndromes and, 472*t*
nausea/vomiting and, 907*t*
seizures and, 218*t*, 220, 225
sinus bradycardia/atrioventricular block and, 571*t*, 577, 578*t*
torsades de pointes and, 532*t*, 540*t*
Sex hormones, 381, 538, 741, 1122, 1172
Sex steroids, 381, 729, 746, 849*t*, 1172
Sexual dysfunction. *See* Female sexual dysfunction; Male sexual dysfunction
SGLT2 inhibitors. *See* Sodium-glucose cotransporter-2 inhibitors
Shankhapushpi, 219*t*, 221
Shark cartilage, 851*t*
Shen-min, 851*t*
Shiitake mushroom, 147*t*
Sho-saiko-to, 851*t*
SIADH. *See* Syndrome of inappropriate antidiuretic hormone secretion
Sibutramine
hepatic/cholestatic diseases and, 849*t*
hypertension and, 618*t*, 620*t*
myocardial ischemia/acute coronary syndromes and, 473*t*
psychosis and, 417–418*t*
serotonin syndrome and, 1203–1204*t*
thyroid diseases and, 700*t*
Side effects. *See* Adverse drug reactions (ADRs)
Signs and symptoms. *See* Clinical presentation of disease
Sildenafil
atrial fibrillation/atrial flutter and, 582*t*
development of, 50
hypotension and, 636*t*, 640*t*, 642
myocardial ischemia/acute coronary syndromes and, 473*t*, 478, 485
oral lichenoid reactions and, 1272*t*
ototoxicity and, 1237*t*
sexual dysfunction and, 790*t*, 798, 800
thromboembolic diseases and, 1066*t*, 1071*t*
visual disturbances and, 307*t*, 312–313
Silver, 1254–1255*t*
Silver sulfadiazine, 113
Silymarin, 868
Simeprevir, 147*t*
Simvastatin
drug interactions with, 39*t*
food interactions with, 41
intracerebral hemorrhage and, 239
myopathy and, 1151, 1157, 1158
pancreatitis and, 878*t*, 886*t*
peripheral neuropathy and, 281*t*
photosensitivity and, 147*t*
rhabdomyolysis and, 1151
systemic lupus erythematosus and, 124*t*
taste disorders and, 1260*t*
thrombocytopenia and, 1051*t*, 1054
transport mechanisms for, 37
Sinus bradycardia/atrioventricular block, 569–581
causative agents of, 569–572, 570–571*t*, 573*t*
clinical presentation of, 574–576, 575*t*
differential diagnosis of, 575, 576*t*
epidemiology of, 572
management of, 579–580, 579*t*
mechanisms of, 572, 574, 574*t*
morbidity and mortality for, 578
patient education on, 580–581
prevention of, 578–579, 579*t*
risk factors for, 576–578, 576–578*t*
Sinus pauses, 569, 572, 575, 577, 578
Sirolimus
drug fever and, 1188*t*
hepatic/cholestatic diseases and, 853*t*
interstitial lung disease/pulmonary fibrosis and, 432*t*
lymphoma and, 1293, 1295
pancreatitis and, 891*t*
skin cancer and, 1298
thrombocytopenia and, 1054, 1056
thromboembolic diseases and, 1066*t*, 1070*t*
Sitagliptin, 506, 879*t*, 884
SJS. *See* Stevens–Johnson syndrome
SJS-TEN overlap, 110
Skin cancer, 1295–1298
causative agents of, 1284*t*, 1295–1296
clinical presentation of, 1290*t*, 1296–1297
differential diagnosis of, 1290*t*, 1296
epidemiology of, 1296
management of, 1298
mechanisms of, 1288*t*, 1296
morbidity and mortality for, 1297
patient education on, 1298
prevention of, 1294*t*, 1297–1298
risk factors for, 1291*t*, 1297
Skin necrosis, 104*t*, 105, 107–108*t*
Skull cap, 851*t*
SLCO1B1, 15, 37
SLE. *See* Systemic lupus erythematosus
Sleep apnea, 351
Sleep cycles, 347, 349
Sleep disorders, 347–353
causative agents of, 347, 348–349*t*
clinical presentation of, 349–350, 350*t*
differential diagnosis of, 349, 351*t*
epidemiology of, 347
management of, 352–353
mechanisms of, 347, 349, 350*t*
morbidity and mortality for, 351–352
patient education on, 353
prevention of, 352, 352*t*
risk factors for, 350–351, 351*t*
Slow transit constipation (STC), 837
Small for gestational age infants, 1316, 1317
Smallpox vaccine, 197*t*, 473*t*
Smoking
acute kidney injury and, 947
alkalosis and, 1013*t*
anxiety and, 400*t*, 404, 409, 411
asthma/bronchospasm and, 459
bladder cancer and, 1304
cognitive disorders and, 364
color changes of oral mucosa and teeth and, 1253, 1254*t*, 1255
depression and cessation of, 381
hepatic/cholestatic diseases and, 864
interstitial lung disease/pulmonary fibrosis and, 437, 442
intracerebral hemorrhage and, 238*t*, 240, 240*t*, 244*t*
in medication histories, 60
myocardial ischemia/acute coronary syndromes and, 473, 473*t*, 479, 481, 482, 489
osteoporosis/osteomalacia and, 1126, 1128, 1130
ototoxicity and, 1236*t*
as risk factor for drug-induced diseases, 32–33
sexual dysfunction and, 771, 772
stroke and, 230–231*t*, 232–233, 235
teratogenicity and, 1311, 1316, 1318, 1321, 1324, 1327, 1334*t*
Snow, John, 20
SNRIs. *See* Serotonin–norepinephrine reuptake inhibitors
Sodium benzoate, 73*t*, 453*t*, 454

Sodium bicarbonate, 954, 1009, 1010, 1010*t*, 1013, 1013–1014*t*, 1017
Sodium-channel blockers
  atrial fibrillation/atrial flutter and, 587
  Brugada syndrome and, 546, 548
  monomorphic ventricular tachycardia and, 523, 525–526, 528–529
  peripheral neuropathy and, 286
  sinus bradycardia/atrioventricular block and, 574
Sodium chloride, 872, 953, 954, 1002*t*, 1017
Sodium citrate–citric acid, 1010*t*
Sodium-containing antacids, 503*t*, 510*t*
Sodium-glucose cotransporter-2 (SGLT2) inhibitors, 24, 682*t*, 685*t*, 1002*t*, 1175*t*
Sodium iodide, 706–707*t*
Sodium oxybate, 7*t*, 376*t*, 380
Sodium polystyrene, 812, 814
Sodium polystyrene sulfonate, 703*t*, 949, 1013–1014*t*
Sodium salicylate, 453*t*
Sodium stibogluconate, 878*t*
Sodium thiosulfate, 1002*t*, 1242*t*, 1243
Sodium valproate. *See* Valproate sodium
Solifenacin, 307*t*, 533*t*, 539*t*, 836*t*
Soluble guanylate cyclase stimulators, 636*t*
Somatostatin, 77*t*, 747
Somatostatin analogs, 680*t*, 682*t*, 684–685*t*, 747, 748*t*
Somatropin, 702*t*, 750
Sonidegib, 170*t*
Sorafenib
  alopecia and, 170*t*
  chemotherapy-induced anemia and, 1109*t*
  hypertension and, 618*t*
  hypertrichosis and, 196*t*
  interstitial lung disease/pulmonary fibrosis and, 433*t*, 438
  myocardial ischemia/acute coronary syndromes and, 472*t*
  nausea/vomiting and, 908*t*
  oral erythema multiforme and, 1268*t*
  pancreatitis and, 878*t*, 883
  thromboembolic diseases and, 1065*t*, 1069*t*
  thyroid diseases and, 699–700*t*, 707, 709
Sorbitol, 812, 814, 822, 826, 827, 1002*t*
Sotalol
  atrial fibrillation/atrial flutter and, 586
  hypotension and, 634*t*
  monomorphic ventricular tachycardia and, 524–525*t*, 530
  photosensitivity and, 147*t*
  sinus bradycardia/atrioventricular block and, 571*t*, 572, 573*t*, 577*t*
  torsades de pointes and, 532*t*, 538, 539*t*, 545
Sparfloxacin, 147*t*, 533*t*, 539*t*
Specificity, in epidemiology, 22
Spectinomycin, 1237*t*
Sphingosine 1-phosphate (S1P) receptors, 574
Spina bifida, 1314, 1320, 1327–1329, 1327*f*
Spinal anesthesia, 911*t*, 914
Spironolactone
  acidosis and, 1003*t*
  alopecia and, 188*t*, 190–191
  contraindications for, 193
  heart failure and, 516
  hepatic/cholestatic diseases and, 847*t*, 870
  hirsutism and, 206, 206*t*, 207
  hyperaldosteronism and, 751
  neutropenia/agranulocytosis and, 1090*t*
  oral lichenoid reactions and, 1272*t*
  photosensitivity and, 147*t*
  sexual dysfunction and, 758*t*, 760*t*, 762–763*t*, 765*t*
  systemic lupus erythematosus and, 125*t*
  teratogenicity of, 191
  thyroid diseases and, 703*t*
  vaginal bleeding disorders and, 782*t*, 785*t*
  visual disturbances and, 307*t*
Spontaneous adverse reactions reporting system (SRS), 49–51, 53, 55, 56
Squamous cell carcinoma (SCC), 1295–1298
SSLD (serum-sickness-like disease), 84, 99*t*
SSLRs. *See* Serum sickness-like reactions
SSRIs. *See* Selective serotonin reuptake inhibitors
Stanozolol, 167*t*, 195*t*, 402, 1013–1014*t*
Star anise, 219*t*, 221
Star fruit, 219*t*, 221
Statins
  acute kidney injury and, 954
  anxiety and, 401*t*, 403
  depression and, 385
  genetic variations affecting, 36*t*
  glucose/insulin dysregulation and, 689
  hepatic/cholestatic diseases and, 849*t*
  intracerebral hemorrhage and, 238*t*, 239, 240*t*, 242*t*
  myocardial ischemia/acute coronary syndromes and, 486, 489
  myopathy and, 1150*t*, 1151, 1152, 1152*t*, 1156–1159
  pancreatitis and, 878*t*, 880, 886*t*, 888
  peripheral neuropathy and, 279, 282*t*
  sleep disorders and, 348*t*, 350*t*
Status dystonicus, 268, 269
Stavudine, 280*t*, 704, 879*t*, 890, 1002*t*, 1189*t*, 1237*t*
STC (slow transit constipation), 837
Steatosis, 854*t*, 857, 859*t*, 862, 868
STEPS (System for Thalidomide Education and Prescribing Safety) program, 6
Steroids
  anabolic. *See* Anabolic steroids
  androgenic, 102*t*
  anxiety and, 402–403, 405*t*
  pancreatitis and, 882, 888
  psychosis and, 422
  secondary adrenal insufficiency and, 741
  sex, 381, 729, 746, 849*t*, 1172
  thrombocytopenia and, 1059
  topical, 187*t*
  weight gain and, 1168*t*, 1172
Stevens–Johnson syndrome (SJS)
  causative agents of, 49, 94, 95, 103–104*t*
  clinical presentation of, 84, 106, 107–108*t*, 109, 110
  epidemiology of, 104, 105
  genetic factors related to, 32
  management of, 113, 114*t*
  morbidity and mortality for, 112
  risk factors for, 111
Stimulant laxatives, 839, 840, 840*t*, 920, 930
Stimulants
  alopecia and, 167*t*
  anxiety and, 401, 404, 405*t*, 408, 409
  psychosis and, 417, 421, 422
  seizures and, 219, 219*t*, 221–222, 225
  sleep disorders and, 349–350*t*
Strength of association, in epidemiology, 22
Streptokinase, 73–74*t*, 307*t*, 662, 663*t*, 1064*t*, 1068*t*, 1193*t*
Streptomycin
  diabetes insipidus and, 991*t*
  drug fever and, 1189*t*
  gout/hyperuricemia and, 1138
  hemolytic anemia and, 1104
  hypertrichosis and, 197*t*
  neutropenia/agranulocytosis and, 1090*t*
  oral erythema multiforme and, 1268*t*
  oral lichenoid reactions and, 1272*t*
  ototoxicity and, 1237*t*
  systemic lupus erythematosus and, 125*t*, 130
Streptozocin
  acidosis and, 1003*t*
  chronic kidney disease and, 966*t*, 970*t*
  drug fever and, 1189*t*
  hepatic/cholestatic diseases and, 848*t*
  nausea/vomiting and, 909*t*, 916*t*
Stress testing agents, 472*t*
Stroke, 229–237. *See also* Intracerebral hemorrhage (ICH)
  causative agents of, 229–231, 230*t*
  clinical presentation of, 233–234, 233–234*t*
  in cost-of-illness model, 27–28
  differential diagnosis of, 233, 234*t*
  epidemiology of, 231
  management of, 235–237
  mechanisms of, 231–233, 231*t*
  morbidity and mortality for, 234
  patient education on, 237
  prevention of, 234, 235*t*
  risk factors for, 234, 234*t*
Strophanthus, 307*t*
Strychnine, 221
ST-segment elevation myocardial ischemia, 471, 486, 488
Subacute cutaneous lupus erythematosus (SCLE), 132
Sublingual nitrates/nitroglycerin, 481, 484–486
Substance P, 82, 457, 914
Substituted benzamide, 927*t*
Succinylcholine, 81, 571*t*, 636*t*, 638*t*, 1209*t*, 1210, 1211
Sucralfate, 703*t*, 818
Sufentanil, 906*t*
Suicide and suicidality, 53, 258, 375, 377–384, 387, 389–392, 423
Sulfacetamide, 1106*t*
Sulfadiazine, 113, 123, 127*t*, 147*t*, 945*t*, 1268*t*
Sulfa drugs, 92, 94–95, 1266
Sulfamethoxazole. *See also* Trimethoprim-sulfamethoxazole (TMP-SMX)
  acidosis and, 1003*t*
  allergic reactions to, 86, 87, 94
  cutaneous diseases and, 102*t*
  glucose/insulin dysregulation and, 682*t*, 685*t*
  hemolytic anemia and, 1106*t*
  pancreatitis and, 878*t*, 886*t*
  as prohapten, 78
Sulfanilamide, 5
Sulfapyridine, 881
Sulfasalazine
  alopecia and, 172*t*, 174, 191
  aplastic anemia and, 1100*t*
  hepatic/cholestatic diseases and, 850*t*, 866
  interstitial lung disease/pulmonary fibrosis and, 432*t*
  macrocytic anemia and, 1108*t*
  neutropenia/agranulocytosis and, 1088, 1090*t*, 1094
  oral lichenoid reactions and, 1270, 1272*t*
  ototoxicity and, 1237*t*
  pancreatitis and, 881, 887
  peripheral neuropathy and, 281*t*
  sexual dysfunction and, 762*t*, 765*t*

INDEX

Sulfasalazine (continued)
systemic lupus erythematosus and, 125*t*, 133
taste disorders and, 1260*t*
thrombocytopenia and, 1051*t*
upper gastrointestinal ulceration and, 810*t*
valvular/pericardial heart disease and, 661*t*, 662, 664
Sulfisoxazole, 94, 148*t*, 1051*t*, 1100*t*, 1108*t*, 1260*t*
Sulfites, 74*t*, 451, 453*t*, 454, 455*t*, 459
Sulfonamide antibiotics, 92–95, 93*f*
Sulfonamides
acute kidney injury and, 944*t*
allergic reactions to, 74*t*, 84, 86–87
anti-infective, 101
aplastic anemia and, 1100*t*
cutaneous diseases and, 101, 103*t*, 111*t*, 113
drug fever and, 1189*t*
hemolytic anemia and, 1106
hepatic/cholestatic diseases and, 847*t*, 861*t*
macrocytic anemia and, 1107, 1108*t*
neutropenia/agranulocytosis and, 1088, 1091, 1091*t*
oral erythema multiforme and, 1268*t*
oral lichenoid reactions and, 1272*t*
pancreatitis and, 878*t*, 882, 886*t*, 892
photosensitivity and, 143, 150, 154
in sulfa drug class, 92
systemic lupus erythematosus and, 125*t*, 128*t*, 133
thrombocytopenia and, 1052, 1052*t*
thyroid diseases and, 703*t*
visual disturbances and, 307*t*, 316
Sulfonylureas
cutaneous diseases and, 101
glucose/insulin dysregulation and, 681, 683, 683*t*, 685*t*, 688
heart failure and, 506
hepatic/cholestatic diseases and, 849*t*
hypoglycemic agents, 92
SIADH and, 981, 985
thyroid diseases and, 703*t*
weight gain and, 1172
Sulindac
alopecia and, 172*t*
aplastic anemia and, 1100*t*
asthma/bronchospasm and, 463
delirium and, 327*t*
heart failure and, 510*t*
hemolytic anemia and, 1105*t*
hepatic/cholestatic diseases and, 846*t*
oral erythema multiforme and, 1268*t*
oral lichenoid reactions and, 1272*t*
ototoxicity and, 1237*t*
pancreatitis and, 878*t*, 880, 881, 886*t*
photosensitivity and, 148*t*
taste disorders and, 1260*t*
thrombocytopenia and, 1051*t*
Sulpiride, 265, 533*t*
Sumatriptan, 73*t*, 92, 230–231*t*, 232, 380, 472*t*, 1260*t*
Sunitinib
alopecia and, 170*t*
chemotherapy-induced anemia and, 1109*t*
heart failure and, 504*t*, 510*t*
hypertension and, 618*t*
interstitial lung disease/pulmonary fibrosis and, 433*t*
nausea/vomiting and, 908*t*
osteonecrosis of jaw and, 1273–1276, 1274*t*
pancreatitis and, 883
taste disorders and, 1260*t*
thyroid diseases and, 699–700*t*, 703*t*, 707–709, 715
Superoxide dismutase, 1242*t*
Supplements. *See* Dietary supplements
Supraventricular arrhythmias, 569–595
atrial fibrillation/atrial flutter, 581–588
atrial tachycardia, 588–592
AV node re-entrant tachycardia, 592–595
sinus bradycardia/atrioventricular block, 569–581
Suramin, 280*t*
Surveillance. *See* Postmarketing surveillance
Suvorexant, 353
Suxamethonium, 73*t*
Sympatholytics, 764*t*, 772
Sympathomimetics
heart failure and, 517
intracerebral hemorrhage and, 239, 243, 246
myocardial ischemia/acute coronary syndromes and, 473*t*, 477*t*
seizures and, 219
tardive dyskinesia and, 262
Symptoms. *See* Clinical presentation of disease
Syncope, 631, 637, 641, 642*t*, 647
Syndrome of inappropriate antidiuretic hormone secretion (SIADH), 981–990
causative agents of, 981, 982–984*t*
clinical presentation of, 986–988, 986*t*
differential diagnosis of, 987, 987*t*
epidemiology of, 985
management of, 989–990, 989*t*
mechanisms of, 985–986
morbidity and mortality for, 989
overview, 981
patient education on, 990
prevention of, 989, 989*t*
risk factors for, 988–989, 988*t*
Synephrine. *See* Bitter orange
System for Thalidomide Education and Prescribing Safety (STEPS) program, 6
Systemic glucocorticoids, 1121*t*, 1123*t*, 1126*t*, 1127
Systemic lupus erythematosus (SLE), 123–136
causative agents of, 123, 124–127*t*, 662
clinical presentation of, 129–133, 129*t*, 131–132*t*
cutaneous diseases and, 111
differential diagnosis of, 132, 132*t*
epidemiology of, 123, 127
idiopathic, 130–132, 131*t*
management of, 135, 135*t*
mechanisms of, 127–129, 128*t*
morbidity and mortality for, 134
patient education on, 135–136
prevention of, 134–135, 134*t*
risk factors for, 133–134, 133*t*
valvular/pericardial heart disease and, 662, 664, 665, 670

Tachycardia. *See* Atrial tachycardia; Atrioventricular node re-entrant tachycardia (AVNRT); Monomorphic ventricular tachycardia
Tacrine, 852*t*
Tacrolimus
acidosis and, 1003*t*
alopecia and, 170*t*, 172*t*, 174
chronic kidney disease and, 965, 966*t*, 967–969, 970*t*, 971–976, 972*t*
color changes of oral mucosa and teeth and, 1254*t*
cutaneous diseases and, 102*t*
gingival hyperplasia and, 1263*t*
glucose/insulin dysregulation and, 681*t*, 684*t*, 690
gout/hyperuricemia and, 1136*t*, 1140
hepatic/cholestatic diseases and, 853*t*
hypertension and, 618*t*, 620*t*, 624, 625
hypertrichosis and, 196*t*
lymphoma and, 1284*t*, 1288*t*, 1293, 1295
oral lichenoid reactions and, 1273
osteoporosis/osteomalacia and, 1127
ototoxicity and, 1237*t*
pancreatitis and, 891*t*
peripheral neuropathy and, 281*t*
photosensitivity and, 148*t*
psychosis and, 415, 417*t*
sinus bradycardia/atrioventricular block and, 571*t*, 577–578*t*
skin cancer and, 1284*t*, 1288*t*, 1298
thrombocytopenia and, 1054, 1056
thromboembolic diseases and, 1066*t*, 1070*t*
torsades de pointes and, 533*t*, 539–540*t*
visual disturbances and, 308*t*
Tadalafil, 308*t*, 312–313, 636*t*, 640*t*, 1237*t*
Taliglucerase alfa, 7*t*
Tamoxifen
alopecia and, 170*t*, 176
asthma/bronchospasm and, 453*t*
breast cancer and, 1300
cannabinoids and, 33
depression and, 376*t*, 381, 382, 385*t*, 386
endometrial cancer and, 1285*t*, 1288*t*, 1301–1303
hepatic/cholestatic diseases and, 848*t*
myocardial ischemia/acute coronary syndromes and, 473*t*
neutropenia/agranulocytosis and, 1090*t*
ovarian hyperstimulation and, 782*t*, 785*t*, 789
pancreatitis and, 883, 886*t*, 888
stroke and, 230–231*t*, 232
systemic lupus erythematosus and, 127*t*
thrombocytopenia and, 1051*t*
thromboembolic diseases and, 1064*t*, 1068*t*, 1074, 1075*t*
thyroid diseases and, 703*t*
vaginal bleeding disorders and, 782*t*, 785*t*
visual disturbances and, 308*t*
vulvovaginal candidiasis and, 782*t*, 785*t*
weight gain and, 1172
Tamsulosin, 308*t*, 632*t*, 639*t*
Tannic acid, 850*t*
Tapentadol, 906*t*
Tardive akathisia. *See* Akathisia
Tardive dyskinesia (TDk), 259–265
causative agents of, 259, 260*t*
clinical presentation of, 257*t*, 262
differential diagnosis of, 257*t*, 262
epidemiology of, 260–261
management of, 264–265, 265*t*
mechanisms of, 261
morbidity and mortality for, 263
overview, 253–254
patient education on, 265
prevention of, 263–264, 264*t*
risk factors for, 263, 263*t*
Tardive dystonia. *See* Dystonia
Tartrazine, 453*t*
Tasimelteon, 7*t*
Taste disorders, 1258–1262
causative agents of, 1258, 1259–1260*t*
clinical presentation of, 1256*t*, 1261
differential diagnosis of, 1257*t*, 1261
epidemiology of, 1258, 1261
management of, 1262
mechanisms of, 1261, 1261*t*
morbidity and mortality for, 1262
patient education on, 1262
prevention of, 1262
risk factors for, 1258*t*, 1261
Taxanes, 127*t*, 282*t*, 288, 433*t*, 1087, 1109, 1300

Tazarotene, 148t
TCAs. *See* Tricyclic antidepressants
TDk. *See* Tardive dyskinesia
TdP. *See* Torsades de pointes
Teduglutide, 7t
Teeth. *See* Color changes of oral mucosa and teeth
Tegaserod, 7t, 473t, 840t
Teicoplanin, 103t, 1189t
Telaprevir, 1258, 1260t
Telithromycin, 847t
Telmisartan, 632t, 638t, 1237t
Telogen effluvium, 166, 175–184, 179–182t, 184t
Temazepam, 352, 1237t, 1272t
Temozolomide, 170t, 848t, 909t, 991t, 1100t
Temperature dysregulation, 1185–1218. *See also* Hyperthermia; Hypothermia
Temporality, in epidemiology, 22
Temsirolimus, 170t, 432t, 438, 836t, 1293
TEN. *See* Toxic epidermal necrolysis
Tenecteplase, 663t, 1029t
Teniposide, 73t, 170t, 848t, 1288t
Tenofovir, 966–967, 966t, 970t, 991t, 1003t, 1123t, 1127, 1150t
Tenosynovitis, 1140
Tenoxicam, 510t
Teratogenicity, 1311–1335
  causality assessment for, 22, 23, 1312
  congenital heart defects and, 1321–1324
  contraceptive use with teratogens, 191, 193, 205, 207
  defined, 1311
  factors affecting, 1314
  FDA evaluation of, 32
  fetal alcohol spectrum disorders and, 1331–1333, 1332t
  gastroschisis and, 1326–1327, 1326f
  history of, 1312–1313
  limb deficiency defects and, 1324–1326
  low birth weight and, 1311, 1316–1318
  management of, 1334–1335
  microcephaly and, 1330–1331, 1330f
  neural tube defects and, 1314, 1327–1328f, 1327–1329
  orofacial clefts and, 1318–1319f, 1318–1321, 1335
  patient education on, 1335
  placental transfer mechanisms and, 1313–1314
  prevention of, 1333–1334
  teratogenicity of, 1315–1316
  in Type D reactions, 60
Terazosin, 308t, 632t, 639t, 1237t
Terbinafine
  color changes of oral mucosa and teeth and, 1254t
  cutaneous diseases and, 103t
  hepatic/cholestatic diseases and, 847t
  myopathy and, 1150t
  photosensitivity and, 148t
  systemic lupus erythematosus and, 125t, 132
  taste disorders and, 1258, 1260t, 1261
  thrombocytopenia and, 1051t
Terbutaline
  atrial tachycardia and, 588–589t, 589
  glucose/insulin dysregulation and, 681t, 684t
  hepatic/cholestatic diseases and, 853t
  monomorphic ventricular tachycardia and, 524–525t, 529
  myocardial ischemia/acute coronary syndromes and, 473t
Terconazole, 790t, 792
Terfenadine, 473t, 538, 539, 540t, 541, 853t
Teriflunomide, 172t
Teriparatide, 1129t, 1130, 1136t, 1140, 1150t
Terlipressin, 533t, 872
Testolactone, 167t, 195t
Testosterone
  alopecia and, 167t, 176, 184
  anxiety and, 402–403
  cutaneous diseases and, 102t
  growth hormone deficiency and, 751
  hirsutism and, 194, 195t, 198, 201
  hypertension and, 618t, 620t
  myocardial ischemia/acute coronary syndromes and, 473t, 476
  sexual dysfunction and, 763, 766, 767, 769, 798
  teratogenicity of, 1334t
  torsades de pointes and, 538
  visual disturbances and, 308t
Testosterone undecanoate, 762t, 765t
Tetrabenazine
  depression and, 376t, 380, 385, 385t
  dystonia and, 270
  parkinsonism and, 271t, 273t
  restrictive drug distribution system for, 7t
  tardive dyskinesia and, 264
Tetracaine, 571t, 1238t
Tetrachloroethylene, 850t
Tetracyclic antidepressants, 218t, 759–760t, 1170
Tetracyclines
  acidosis and, 1002t, 1003t
  allergic reactions to, 95
  color changes of oral mucosa and teeth and, 8, 1253, 1254–1255t, 1255–1258
  cutaneous diseases and, 101, 102–103t
  diarrhea and, 823t
  drug fever and, 1189t
  hepatic/cholestatic diseases and, 847t, 861t
  myopathy and, 1150t
  oral erythema multiforme and, 1268t
  oral lichenoid reactions and, 1272t
  ototoxicity and, 1238t
  pancreatitis and, 878t, 882, 885, 886t
  photosensitivity and, 143, 148t, 150, 150t, 154
  systemic lupus erythematosus and, 125t
  taste disorders and, 1260–1261t
  teratogenicity of, 1334t
  upper gastrointestinal ulceration and, 809, 810–811t, 811, 816t
  visual disturbances and, 308t
Tetrahydro-2-furanone, 1215
Tetrahydrocannabinol, 33, 744t
Tetramethrin, 453t
Teucrium polium, 851t
TGF (tumor growth factor), 1293
Thalidomide
  constipation and, 836t
  glucose/insulin dysregulation and, 681t, 684t
  hepatic/cholestatic diseases and, 848t
  infertility and, 783t, 786t
  interstitial lung disease/pulmonary fibrosis and, 439, 440
  leukemia and, 1286–1287
  oral lichenoid reactions and, 1272t
  ototoxicity and, 1238t
  peripheral neuropathy and, 280t, 282t, 284
  restrictive drug distribution system for, 6, 7t
  sinus bradycardia/atrioventricular block and, 571t
  teratogenicity of, 22, 23, 1312, 1321–1322, 1324
  thromboembolic diseases and, 1065t, 1067, 1069t, 1075t
  thyroid diseases and, 699t, 702t
  vaginal bleeding disorders and, 782t, 785t
  withdrawal from market, 5
Thallium, 171t, 177, 1254t
Theophylline
  acidosis and, 1002t
  acute kidney injury and, 953
  alkalosis and, 1013–1014t, 1017
  anxiety and, 401t, 404, 405t
  asthma/bronchospasm and, 463
  atrial fibrillation/atrial flutter and, 582–583t, 584, 587–588
  atrial tachycardia and, 588, 588–590t, 590, 591
  AV node re-entrant tachycardia and, 592–594t, 594
  cognitive disorders and, 365
  delirium and, 326t
  diarrhea and, 823t
  drug fever and, 1189t
  drug-induced hospitalizations from, 26
  drug interactions with, 39t
  food interactions with, 40
  monomorphic ventricular tachycardia and, 524–525t, 529, 530
  myocardial ischemia/acute coronary syndromes and, 473t
  nausea/vomiting and, 909t
  oral erythema multiforme and, 1268t
  seizures and, 218t, 219, 222, 222t, 224, 226
  SIADH and, 984t
  sleep disorders and, 349t
Thiabendazole, 847t, 1238t, 1268t
Thiacetazone, 1138
Thiamazole, 124t, 1088
Thiamine (vitamin B_1), 265, 285, 362, 1009
Thiazide diuretics
  acute kidney injury and, 943t
  alkalosis and, 1013–1014t
  cutaneous diseases and, 101
  depression and, 378
  glucose/insulin dysregulation and, 680t, 684t
  gout/hyperuricemia and, 1138
  hepatic/cholestatic diseases and, 847t
  pancreatitis and, 878t, 886–887
  sexual dysfunction and, 759–760t, 761, 764t, 772
  SIADH and, 984t, 987
  in sulfa drug class, 92
Thiazolidinediones, 476, 849t, 1121t, 1124t, 1172
Thienopyridines, 811, 815
Thiethylperazine, 1238t
Thioamides, 703t, 716, 885, 888
Thioguanine, 848t, 880
Thiopental, 73t, 871, 907t
Thiopropazate, 265
Thioridazine
  delirium and, 326t, 329t
  drug fever and, 1189t
  hepatic/cholestatic diseases and, 852t
  hypotension and, 635t, 639t
  hypothermia and, 1216t
  monomorphic ventricular tachycardia and, 524t
  neuroleptic malignant syndrome and, 1195t
  photosensitivity and, 148t
  sexual dysfunction and, 798
  SIADH and, 983t
  sinus bradycardia/atrioventricular block and, 573t
  thromboembolic diseases and, 1066t, 1070t
  thyroid diseases and, 703t
  torsades de pointes and, 533t, 540t
  visual disturbances and, 308t
  weight gain and, 1167t, 1169t, 1171
Thiotepa, 170t, 177, 358t, 848t, 983t

Thiothixene
delirium and, 338
hypotension and, 635*t*, 639*t*
neuroleptic malignant syndrome and, 1195*t*
seizures and, 221
SIADH and, 983*t*
thrombocytopenia and, 1051*t*
weight gain and, 1167*t*
Thioxanthenes, 743*t*
Third-degree AV block, 569, 572, 575, 578
Thrombin inhibitors, 239, 487*t*, 1026*t*, 1029*t*, 1034, 1057–1058, 1076
Thrombocytopenia, 1049–1059
causative agents of, 1049–1050, 1050–1051*t*
clinical presentation of, 83–84, 1054–1056, 1054*t*
differential diagnosis of, 1055, 1055*t*
epidemiology of, 1050, 1052
management of, 1057–1059
mechanisms of, 1052–1054, 1052*t*
morbidity and mortality for, 1056
patient education for, 1059
prevention of, 1056–1057, 1057*t*
risk factors for, 1056, 1056*t*
Thromboembolic diseases, 1063–1078
causative agents of, 1063, 1064–1066*t*
clinical presentation of, 1071–1073, 1071*t*
differential diagnosis of, 1072, 1072*t*
epidemiology of, 1063, 1066
management of, 237, 1076–1077
mechanisms of, 1067–1071, 1068–1071*t*
morbidity and mortality for, 1074
patient education on, 1077–1078
prevention of, 1074–1075, 1075*t*
risk factors for, 1073–1074, 1073*t*
Thrombolytic agents
bleeding disorders and, 1025, 1026*t*, 1029*t*, 1030, 1033–1034, 1039
hepatic/cholestatic diseases and, 868
intracerebral hemorrhage and, 238*t*, 240*t*, 243, 244*t*, 245
myocardial ischemia/acute coronary syndromes and, 486, 487*t*, 488
Thrombotic thrombocytopenia purpura–hemolytic uremic syndrome (TTP-HUS), 1054, 1056
Thyroid diseases, 697–717. *See also* Hyperthyroidism; Hypothyroidism
causative agents of, 697–701, 698–700*t*, 704
clinical presentation of, 711–713, 711*t*
comorbidity with drug-induced diseases, 34
differential diagnosis of, 711, 712, 712*t*
epidemiology of, 704
management of, 715–717, 715*t*
mechanisms of, 697, 698*f*, 701–703*t*, 704–710, 706–707*t*
morbidity and mortality for, 714
patient education on, 717
prevention of, 714–715, 715*t*
risk factors for, 713–714, 713*t*
Thyroid hormones, 401*t*, 403, 411, 473*t*, 703*t*, 1126*t*
Thyroid medications
alopecia and, 173*t*, 175, 179*t*, 186
desiccated, 707*t*
neutropenia/agranulocytosis and, 1087, 1088, 1091*t*
systemic lupus erythematosus and, 124*t*
Thyroid-releasing hormone (TRH), 697, 698*f*
Thyroid-stimulating hormone (TSH), 697, 698*f*, 700–701, 704, 707–715
Thyroxine, 403, 1272*t*
Tiagabine
alopecia and, 168*t*
delirium and, 326*t*
depression and, 376*t*, 379, 385*t*
dystonia and, 270
ototoxicity and, 1238*t*
psychosis and, 417*t*
visual disturbances and, 308*t*
Tiaprofenic acid, 510*t*
Ticagrelor, 73*t*, 573*t*, 582*t*, 1029, 1029*t*, 1033
Ticarcillin, 1189*t*
Ticarcillin–clavulanate, 1191
Ticlopidine
aplastic anemia and, 1100*t*
bleeding disorders and, 1029, 1029*t*
hepatic/cholestatic diseases and, 853*t*
neutropenia/agranulocytosis and, 1090*t*, 1091, 1091*t*
ototoxicity and, 1238*t*
serum sickness-like reactions and, 1193*t*
systemic lupus erythematosus and, 125*t*
thrombocytopenia and, 1054
Tigecycline, 148*t*, 829, 878*t*, 882, 909*t*, 920, 1238*t*
Tiludronate, 308*t*, 1274*t*
Timolol, 125*t*, 168*t*, 348*t*, 454, 569, 578*t*, 1238*t*
Tin, 1255*t*
Tincture of opium, 827*t*, 828
Tinnitus, 1233, 1239, 1240, 1240*t*, 1242–1244
Tioconazole, 790*t*
Tiopronin, 853*t*
Tiotropium, 127*t*, 308*t*, 582*t*
Tipiracil, 170*t*
Tipranavir, 1268*t*
Tirofiban, 1029*t*, 1051–1052*t*, 1053
Tivantinib, 571*t*
Tivozanib, 699*t*
Tizanidine, 571*t*, 578*t*
TMP-SMX. *See* Trimethoprim–sulfamethoxazole
TNF. *See* Tumor necrosis factor
Tobacco. *See* Smoking
Tobramycin, 73*t*, 328*t*, 453*t*, 1238*t*, 1241
Tocainide
delirium and, 326*t*
heart failure and, 502*t*, 507, 510*t*
hypotension and, 634*t*
neutropenia/agranulocytosis and, 1090*t*
systemic lupus erythematosus and, 127*t*
To Err Is Human (IOM), 19, 51
Tolazamide, 148*t*
Tolbutamide, 94, 148*t*, 703*t*, 983*t*, 1268*t*, 1272*t*
Tolcapone, 635*t*, 640*t*, 852*t*, 864
Tolmetin
drug fever and, 1189*t*
hemolytic anemia and, 1105*t*
hepatic/cholestatic diseases and, 846*t*
ototoxicity and, 1238*t*
thrombocytopenia and, 1051*t*
Tolterodine, 328–329*t*, 365, 984*t*
Tolu balsam, 308*t*
Toluene, 473*t*
Tolvaptan, 872, 989*t*, 990
Topical corticosteroids, 734
Topical glucocorticoids, 731*t*, 733–735, 736*t*, 739, 741
Topiramate
acidosis and, 1003*t*
acute kidney injury and, 944*t*, 957
alopecia and, 168*t*, 175
anxiety and, 401*t*, 402, 404, 405*t*
cognitive disorders and, 358*t*, 365, 367
depression and, 376*t*, 379, 385*t*, 388–389, 388*t*
gingival hyperplasia and, 1263*t*
hepatic/cholestatic diseases and, 852*t*
osteoporosis/osteomalacia and, 1127
ototoxicity and, 1238*t*
peripheral neuropathy and, 289
seizures and, 218*t*, 224
sexual dysfunction and, 760*t*, 764*t*, 772
teratogenicity of, 1319, 1330, 1331
thromboembolic diseases and, 1066*t*, 1071*t*
visual disturbances and, 309*t*, 312
weight gain and, 1174, 1175, 1175*t*
Topoisomerase inhibitors
chemotherapy-induced anemia and, 1109
diarrhea and, 822*t*
leukemia and, 1284, 1285, 1287, 1289, 1290
neutropenia/agranulocytosis and, 1087, 1091
Topotecan, 170*t*, 848*t*, 909*t*
Toremifene, 848*t*, 1064*t*, 1068*t*
Torsades de pointes (TdP), 530–546
causative agents of, 530–531, 532–534*t*
clinical presentation of, 536–537, 536–537*t*
differential diagnosis of, 536–537, 537*t*
epidemiology of, 534–535
gender differences in, 32
management of, 544–545, 545*f*
mechanisms of, 535–536
morbidity and mortality for, 541–542
patient education on, 545
prevention of, 542–544, 543*t*
risk factors for, 40, 537–541, 537*t*, 539–540*t*
Torsemide, 148*t*, 633*t*, 638*t*, 1238*t*
Toxic epidermal necrolysis (TEN)
causative agents of, 95, 101, 103–104*t*
clinical presentation of, 107–108*t*, 109, 110
epidemiology of, 104, 105
genetic factors related to, 32
management of, 113, 114*t*
morbidity and mortality for, 112
risk factors for, 111
Toxicity
digitalis glycoside, 589, 589*t*
hepatotoxicity, 33–34, 39, 845, 853, 855–857, 865–868
nephrotoxicity, 37
ototoxicity. *See* Ototoxicity
phototoxicity. *See* Photosensitivity
pulmonary, 431, 434, 436–442
Traction alopecia, 183, 184*t*
Tramadol
cutaneous diseases and, 101, 104*t*
myocardial ischemia/acute coronary syndromes and, 489
nausea/vomiting and, 906*t*
ototoxicity and, 1238*t*
peripheral neuropathy and, 289
seizures and, 218*t*, 219, 220, 222*t*
serotonin syndrome and, 1203–1204*t*
Trametinib, 170*t*, 1296
Trandolapril, 148*t*, 632*t*, 638*t*, 1255*t*
Tranexamic acid
bleeding disorders and, 1039
cutaneous diseases and, 102*t*
gingival hyperplasia and, 1263*t*
myocardial ischemia/acute coronary syndromes and, 472*t*
seizures and, 221
thromboembolic diseases and, 1064*t*, 1067, 1068*t*
visual disturbances and, 309*t*
Transport mechanisms for drugs, 37, 1313
Transthoracic echocardiograms, 665, 666–667*f*
Tranylcypromine
alopecia and, 173*t*
delirium and, 327*t*
drug interactions with, 40

ototoxicity and, 1238*t*
serotonin syndrome and, 1203–1204*t*
SIADH and, 982*t*
sleep disorders and, 348*t*
Trastuzumab
alopecia and, 170*t*, 177, 179*t*
breast cancer and, 1300
heart failure and, 502*t*, 507–508, 511–512
visual disturbances and, 309*t*
Travoprost, 197, 197*t*
Trazodone
alopecia and, 173*t*
cognitive disorders and, 369
drug fever and, 1189*t*
hepatic/cholestatic diseases and, 852*t*
hypertrichosis and, 197*t*
hypotension and, 634*t*, 639*t*
monomorphic ventricular tachycardia and, 524–525*t*
myocardial ischemia/acute coronary syndromes and, 472*t*
ototoxicity and, 1238*t*
photosensitivity and, 148*t*
seizures and, 220
serotonin syndrome and, 1202, 1203–1204*t*
sexual dysfunction and, 765*t*
SIADH and, 982*t*
sleep disorders and, 353
torsades de pointes and, 534*t*, 540*t*
Treatment. *See* Management of disease
Treprostinil, 7*t*, 636*t*, 640*t*
Tretinoin, 148*t*, 173*t*, 191, 197*t*, 661*t*, 1066*t*, 1071*t*
TRH (thyroid-releasing hormone), 697, 698*f*
Triamcinolone, 73*t*, 171*t*, 195–196*t*, 739, 739*t*, 741
Triamcinolone acetonide, 188*t*, 731*t*, 736*t*, 738
Triamterene
acidosis and, 1003*t*
diabetes insipidus and, 991*t*
drug fever and, 1189*t*
photosensitivity and, 148*t*
systemic lupus erythematosus and, 125*t*
Triazolam, 327*t*, 329*t*, 352
Triazolopyridine, 761*t*
Trichloroethylene, 850*t*
Trichotillomania, 183, 184*t*
Tricyclic antidepressants (TCAs)
akathisia and, 254, 255, 255–256*t*, 258*t*
alopecia and, 175
anxiety and, 401, 405*t*, 406
cognitive disorders and, 359, 359*t*, 360, 362
delirium and, 325, 326*t*
depression and, 376*t*, 391, 392
drug interactions with, 33
heart failure and, 504*t*
hepatic/cholestatic diseases and, 852*t*
human leukocyte antigen and, 37
hypotension and, 631, 642, 645*t*
myocardial ischemia/acute coronary syndromes and, 472*t*
oral lichenoid reactions and, 1272*t*
peripheral neuropathy and, 289
seizures and, 218*t*, 220, 222*t*, 226
serotonin syndrome and, 1203–1204*t*
sexual dysfunction and, 758–760*t*, 765*t*
SIADH and, 982*t*
visual disturbances and, 295, 309*t*
weight gain and, 1170
Trifluoperazine, 221, 547*t*, 635*t*, 639*t*, 983*t*, 1167*t*, 1189*t*, 1195*t*
Trifluridine, 170*t*
Trihexyphenidyl, 348*t*, 984*t*
Trimethadione, 124*t*, 309*t*, 1244
Trimethobenzamide, 853*t*
Trimethoprim
acidosis and, 1003*t*
drug interactions with, 40
macrocytic anemia and, 1107
nausea/vomiting and, 930
photosensitivity and, 148*t*
SIADH and, 984*t*
Trimethoprim-sulfamethoxazole (TMP-SMX)
allergic reactions to, 75*t*
bleeding disorders and, 1031
cutaneous diseases and, 101, 104*t*
delirium and, 328*t*
drug fever and, 1189*t*, 1191
drug-induced hospitalizations from, 26
genetic variability and, 16*t*
macrocytic anemia and, 1108, 1108*t*
nausea/vomiting and, 909*t*, 915, 929–930
neutropenia/agranulocytosis and, 1088, 1090*t*
oral erythema multiforme and, 1268*t*
pancreatitis and, 882
photosensitivity and, 147*t*
psychosis and, 417*t*
serum sickness-like reactions and, 1192, 1193*t*
systemic lupus erythematosus and, 125*t*
thrombocytopenia and, 1050, 1051*t*
visual disturbances and, 307*t*
Trimipramine, 148*t*, 173*t*, 982*t*
Tripelennamine, 850*t*
Triprolidine, 1272*t*
Triptans
depression and, 376*t*, 378, 380
myocardial ischemia/acute coronary syndromes and, 474, 477*t*, 478
serotonin syndrome and, 1204
stroke and, 232
Troglitazone, 3, 10
Tropisetron, 919, 924*t*, 928*t*
Trovafloxacin, 280*t*
Troxidone, 124*t*
Tryptase, 82
Tryptophan, 154, 386, 1203
TSH. *See* Thyroid-stimulating hormone
TTP-HUS (thrombotic thrombocytopenia purpura–hemolytic uremic syndrome), 1054, 1056
Tuberculosis, 288
Tumor growth factor (TGF), 1293
Tumor necrosis factor (TNF)
in allergic reactions, 81
alopecia and, 166
cutaneous diseases and, 105, 109
in hepatic and cholestatic diseases, 857
in thermoregulation, 1185, 1186
Tumor necrosis factor alpha (TNFα), 703*t*
Tumor necrosis factor alpha (TNFα) inhibitors
depression and, 377*t*, 382, 383, 386
heart failure and, 512
hepatic/cholestatic diseases and, 852*t*
interstitial lung disease/pulmonary fibrosis and, 433, 433*t*
leukemia and, 1284, 1284*t*, 1287, 1289
lymphoma and, 1284*t*, 1292, 1293
skin cancer and, 1284*t*, 1295–1297
Tumor necrosis factor-blocking agents, 173*t*, 176, 178, 179*t*
Type A reactions, 59, 60
Type B reactions, 59–60
Type C reactions, 60
Type D reactions, 60
Typical antipsychotics
alopecia and, 175
delirium and, 336
neuroleptic malignant syndrome and, 1196, 1199
tardive dyskinesia and, 264
torsades de pointes and, 541, 542
Tyramine, 40
Tyropanoate sodium, 707*t*
Tyrosine kinase inhibitors
alopecia and, 177
chemotherapy-induced anemia and, 1101*t*
diarrhea and, 822*t*
glucose/insulin dysregulation and, 681*t*, 683–685*t*
growth hormone deficiency and, 747, 748*t*
hepatic/cholestatic diseases and, 848*t*
interstitial lung disease/pulmonary fibrosis and, 433*t*
neutropenia/agranulocytosis and, 1087
pancreatitis and, 883, 886*t*, 888
thyroid diseases and, 704, 705, 707–709

Unfractionated heparin
bleeding disorders and, 1026*t*, 1027, 1029*t*, 1032, 1036
myocardial ischemia/acute coronary syndromes and, 486
osteoporosis/osteomalacia and, 1121*t*, 1124*t*
thrombocytopenia and, 1056–1057, 1057*t*
thromboembolic diseases and, 1076
Unstable angina, 471
Upper gastrointestinal (GI) ulceration, 809–819
causative agents of, 809–810, 810*t*
clinical presentation of, 812–814, 813*t*
differential diagnosis of, 813–814, 813*t*
epidemiology of, 810–811
management of, 818
mechanisms of, 811–812, 811*t*
morbidity and mortality for, 816
patient education on, 818–819
prevention of, 816–818, 816*t*
risk factors for, 814–816, 815*t*
Uranium, 850*t*
Urethane, 850*t*
Uricosuric agents, 1136–1137, 1136*t*, 1145
Urine, detection of drugs in, 420, 420*t*
Urokinase, 77*t*, 440, 1064*t*, 1068*t*
Ursodiol, 836*t*, 868
Urticaria, 72–73*t*, 80–83, 83–84*t*, 87, 98, 99*t*, 106
Usnic acid, 851*t*
Ustekinumab, 383
Uterine carcinoma. *See* Endometrial cancer

Vaccine Adverse Event Reporting System (VAERS), 50, 66
Vaccines. *See also specific vaccines*
adverse event reporting for, 50, 66
allergic and hypersensitivity reactions to, 74–75*t*, 77*t*
autism concerns related to, 21, 29
hypertrichosis and, 195, 197*t*
serum sickness-like reactions and, 1192
Vaginal bleeding disorders, 793–797
amenorrhea and oligomenorrhea, 793–795
dysmenorrhea, 796–797
menorrhagia and menometrorrhagia, 795–796
Valacyclovir, 148*t*, 168*t*
Valbenazine, 264
Valdecoxib, 13, 104*t*, 230, 361, 472*t*, 475, 1268*t*
Valerian, 309*t*, 353, 401*t*, 402
Valerian root, 851*t*
Valganciclovir, 1090*t*

INDEX

Valproate
cognitive disorders and, 360, 362, 365, 369
parkinsonism and, 254, 270, 271*t*, 273*t*
systemic lupus erythematosus and, 124*t*
thrombocytopenia and, 1051*t*
thyroid diseases and, 699*t*
weight gain and, 1170
Valproate sodium, 103*t*, 378, 713, 761*t*, 1262, 1263*t*, 1272*t*
Valproic acid
acidosis and, 1003*t*
acute kidney injury and, 943*t*
allergic reactions to, 75*t*
alopecia and, 168*t*, 175, 178, 186
anxiety and, 411
cognitive disorders and, 358*t*, 365, 367
cutaneous diseases and, 101, 104*t*, 111
delirium and, 326*t*
depression and, 379
hepatic/cholestatic diseases and, 852*t*, 861*t*, 866, 868
hirsutism and, 194, 195*t*, 198, 199*t*
neuroleptic malignant syndrome and, 1195*t*
neutropenia/agranulocytosis and, 1090*t*
oral erythema multiforme and, 1268*t*
osteoporosis/osteomalacia and, 1123*t*
ototoxicity and, 1238*t*
pancreatitis and, 878*t*, 883, 886*t*, 887
peripheral neuropathy and, 289
photosensitivity and, 148*t*
for seizure disorders, 95
SIADH and, 983*t*
systemic lupus erythematosus and, 130
teratogenicity of, 1315, 1319, 1321–1322, 1324, 1328–1331
thrombocytopenia and, 1052*t*, 1056, 1056*t*
upper gastrointestinal ulceration and, 809, 810*t*
vaginal bleeding disorders and, 793
visual disturbances and, 309*t*
weight gain and, 1166*t*, 1169, 1169*t*, 1170, 1173*t*
Valsartan, 148*t*, 632–633*t*, 638*t*, 1238*t*
Valvular and pericardial heart disease, 659–670
causative agents of, 659–662, 660–661*t*
clinical presentation of, 664–668, 665*t*, 666–667*f*
differential diagnosis of, 665–668, 667*t*
epidemiology of, 662–663
management of, 669–670, 670*t*
mechanisms of, 663–664, 663*t*
morbidity and mortality for, 669
patient education on, 670
prevention of, 669, 669*t*
risk factors for, 668–669, 668*t*
Vancomycin
allergic and hypersensitivity reactions to, 73–75*t*, 76, 77*t*, 81, 97*t*
cutaneous diseases and, 103*t*
diarrhea and, 828–829
drug fever and, 1189*t*, 1191
hypotension and, 635*t*, 638*t*, 644, 645*t*
neutropenia/agranulocytosis and, 1090*t*, 1095
oral erythema multiforme and, 1268*t*
ototoxicity and, 1233, 1238*t*, 1241–1242
thrombocytopenia and, 1051–1052*t*
Vandetanib, 7*t*, 148*t*, 170*t*, 432*t*, 533*t*, 539*t*, 709
Vardenafil, 309*t*, 312–313, 582*t*, 636*t*, 640*t*
Varenicline
anxiety and, 401*t*, 402, 409
depression and, 376*t*, 381, 385*t*, 386, 387, 391
myocardial ischemia/acute coronary syndromes and, 473*t*
ototoxicity and, 1238*t*
Vascular endothelial growth factor (VEGF), 512, 888, 1274, 1293
Vascular injury, 855*t*, 858, 859*t*, 861*t*, 862
Vasculitis, 74*t*, 83–84*t*, 84–85, 99*t*, 232
Vasoconstriction/vasospasm, 232, 404, 478, 486–488, 1216
Vasodilators, 457, 477*t*, 478–479, 633*t*, 643–644, 645*t*, 670
Vasopressin
alcohol use and, 232
alopecia and, 174*t*, 180*t*
hepatic/cholestatic diseases and, 872
myocardial ischemia/acute coronary syndromes and, 473*t*
synthesis of, 729
vaginal bleeding disorders and, 782*t*, 786*t*, 796
Vasopressin-receptor antagonists, 989–990, 989*t*
Vasovagal syncope, 637, 647
Vatalanib, 699*t*
VEGF (vascular endothelial growth factor), 512, 888, 1274, 1293
Vemurafenib, 7*t*, 148*t*, 170*t*, 883, 886*t*, 1109*t*, 1284*t*, 1296–1297
Venencapsan, 851*t*
Venlafaxine
alopecia and, 173*t*
asthma/bronchospasm and, 453*t*
constipation and, 836*t*
delirium and, 327*t*
depression and, 391
heart failure and, 504*t*, 509
hepatic/cholestatic diseases and, 852*t*
hyperprolactinemia and, 743*t*
hypertension and, 618*t*, 620*t*
monomorphic ventricular tachycardia and, 524–525*t*
myocardial ischemia/acute coronary syndromes and, 472*t*
ototoxicity and, 1238*t*
peripheral neuropathy and, 287, 289
photosensitivity and, 148*t*
seizures and, 219
serotonin syndrome and, 1203–1204*t*
sexual dysfunction and, 772
SIADH and, 981, 982*t*, 985, 987, 988, 990
sleep disorders and, 348*t*, 349
visual disturbances and, 309*t*
weight gain and, 1166*t*
Venous thromboembolism (VTE)
clinical presentation of, 1071–1072
epidemiology of, 1063, 1067
management of, 1076–1077, 1077*t*
mechanisms of, 1067, 1071
morbidity and mortality for, 1074
overview, 1063
patient education on, 1077–1078
prevention of, 1074–1075
risk factors for, 1073–1074
Ventricular arrhythmias, 523–549
Brugada syndrome, 546–549
monomorphic ventricular tachycardia, 523–530
torsades de pointes, 530–546
Verapamil
alopecia and, 168*t*
asthma/bronchospasm and, 453*t*
atrial fibrillation/atrial flutter and, 583*t*, 586, 587*t*
atrial tachycardia and, 590, 591
AV node re-entrant tachycardia and, 594
constipation and, 836*t*
delirium and, 327*t*
drug interactions with, 38
gingival hyperplasia and, 1263, 1263*t*
heart failure and, 502*t*, 504*t*, 505, 509, 510*t*, 515
hyperprolactinemia and, 742, 743–744*t*
hypertrichosis and, 196*t*
hypotension and, 633*t*, 639*t*
myocardial ischemia/acute coronary syndromes and, 472*t*, 488–489
oral erythema multiforme and, 1268*t*
ototoxicity and, 1238*t*
sinus bradycardia/atrioventricular block and, 571*t*, 572, 573*t*, 577, 578*t*, 580
systemic lupus erythematosus and, 124*t*
Vernakalant, 634*t*
Verteporfin, 148*t*, 151, 154
Vertigo, 1233, 1240, 1240*t*
Viagra. *See* Sildenafil
Vigabatrin, 7*t*, 309*t*, 360, 376*t*, 379, 417*t*, 1263*t*
Vilazodone, 772, 982*t*, 1166*t*, 1169*t*
Vildagliptin, 879*t*
Vinblastine
alopecia and, 170*t*
anxiety and, 401*t*, 403
hypotension and, 636*t*, 640*t*
leukemia and, 1285
myocardial ischemia/acute coronary syndromes and, 472*t*
ototoxicity and, 1238*t*
pancreatitis and, 879*t*
photosensitivity and, 148*t*
SIADH and, 983*t*, 988, 988*t*
Vinca alkaloids
depression and, 386
hepatic/cholestatic diseases and, 848*t*
infertility and, 783*t*, 786*t*, 800
neutropenia/agranulocytosis and, 1087
pancreatitis and, 881
peripheral neuropathy and, 282, 282*t*
SIADH and, 981, 987
visual disturbances and, 309*t*
Vincristine
alopecia and, 170*t*, 176
depression and, 377*t*, 384, 385*t*
drug fever and, 1189*t*
hypotension and, 636*t*, 640*t*
leukemia and, 1285
lymphoma and, 1295
myocardial ischemia/acute coronary syndromes and, 472*t*
myopathy and, 1150*t*, 1151, 1155
ototoxicity and, 1238*t*
pancreatitis and, 879*t*
peripheral neuropathy and, 280*t*, 285
SIADH and, 983*t*, 988, 988*t*
Vindesine, 171*t*, 1238*t*
Vinorelbine, 171*t*, 472*t*, 983*t*, 990, 1238*t*
Vinyl chloride, 850*t*
Vismodegib, 171*t*
Visual disturbances, 295–319
causative agents of, 295–313, 296–312*t*
clinical presentation of, 315–317, 316*t*
differential diagnosis of, 316, 316*t*
epidemiology of, 313
management of, 318–319
mechanisms of, 313–315, 314–315*t*
morbidity and mortality for, 317
patient education on, 319
prevention of, 317–318, 318*t*
risk factors for, 317, 317*t*

Vitamin A (retinol)
alopecia and, 166, 174, 174*t*, 177, 184
heart failure and, 515
hepatic/cholestatic diseases and, 853*t*, 870
myopathy and, 1152
oral erythema multiforme and, 1267*t*
osteoporosis/osteomalacia and, 1121*t*, 1124*t*, 1126*t*, 1128, 1129
ototoxicity and, 1238*t*
teratogenicity of, 1334*t*
Vitamin B_1 (thiamine), 265, 285, 362, 1009
Vitamin B_6. *See* Pyridoxine
Vitamin B_{12} (cobalamin), 284, 1107, 1108, 1256
Vitamin C, 515, 792, 1264
Vitamin D, 1120, 1122, 1126, 1130, 1260*t*, 1261, 1262
Vitamin D_3 (cholecalciferol), 890, 1122, 1126, 1262
Vitamin E
alopecia and, 184
heart failure and, 515
hepatic/cholestatic diseases and, 868
myopathy and, 1152
peripheral neuropathy and, 287*t*
tardive dyskinesia and, 265
vaginal bleeding disorders and, 796
Vitamin K
characteristics of, 1037*t*
deficiencies in, 1314
hepatic/cholestatic diseases and, 869
intracerebral hemorrhage and, 245
thromboembolic diseases and, 1067
Vitamin K antagonists
bleeding disorders and, 1026, 1026*t*, 1028, 1029*t*, 1036, 1038–1039
intracerebral hemorrhage and, 237
valvular/pericardial heart disease and, 661*t*, 662, 664, 668*t*, 669
Voglibose, 849*t*
Vomiting. *See* Nausea and vomiting
Vorapaxar, 1026*t*, 1029, 1029*t*
Voriconazole
alopecia and, 168*t*, 177
cutaneous diseases and, 104*t*
diabetes insipidus and, 991*t*
drug interactions with, 39*t*
photosensitivity and, 148*t*
skin cancer and, 1284*t*
torsades de pointes and, 534*t*, 539–540*t*
visual disturbances and, 310*t*
Vorinostat, 533*t*, 539*t*
Vortioxetine, 982*t*, 1166*t*, 1169*t*
VTE. *See* Venous thromboembolism
Vulvovaginal candidiasis, 790–792
causative agents of, 782*t*, 790–791
clinical presentation of, 787*t*, 791
differential diagnosis of, 788*t*, 791
epidemiology of, 791
management of, 790*t*, 792
mechanisms of, 785*t*, 791
morbidity and mortality for, 791–792
patient education on, 792
prevention of, 789*t*, 792
risk factors for, 788*t*, 791

Wafer ash, 310*t*
Warfarin
alopecia and, 166, 167*t*, 178
bleeding disorders and, 1029*t*, 1031, 1031*t*, 1032, 1034, 1036, 1038–1039
cannabinoid interactions with, 33
comorbidity and, 34
cutaneous diseases and, 104*t*, 105, 111*t*, 113*t*
drug interactions with, 39*t*
genetic variations affecting, 36*t*
hepatic/cholestatic diseases and, 853*t*, 868
intracerebral hemorrhage and, 237, 238*t*, 240*t*, 243, 244*t*, 245, 246
metabolic pathway for, 35
sexual dysfunction and, 761*t*, 765*t*
stroke and, 237
target receptors for, 37
teratogenicity of, 1314, 1316, 1334*t*
thrombocytopenia and, 1058
thromboembolic diseases and, 1064*t*, 1067, 1068*t*, 1075, 1075*t*, 1076–1077
upper gastrointestinal ulceration and, 814
valvular/pericardial heart disease and, 662, 664
visual disturbances and, 310*t*
Warfarin-induced skin necrosis (WISN), 107–108*t*, 109–111, 114*t*
Warner Lambert v. Kent (2008), 9*t*, 10
Weight gain, 1165–1175
causative agents of, 1165, 1166–1167*t*
clinical presentation of, 1168–1173, 1169*t*
differential diagnosis of, 1169, 1170*t*
epidemiology of, 1165, 1167–1168
management of, 1174–1175, 1175*t*
mechanisms of, 1168, 1168*t*
morbidity and mortality for, 1173
patient education on, 1175
prevention of, 1173–1174, 1174*t*
risk factors for, 1173, 1173*t*
Wells criteria, 1072, 1072*t*
Wild lettuce, 353
WISN (warfarin-induced skin necrosis), 107–108*t*, 109–111, 114*t*
Withdrawal, 415, 417*t*, 420–422, 424, 424*t*
Wolff–Chaikoff effect, 705, 708
Women. *See* Gender differences; Gynecologic diseases
Women's Health Initiative (WHI), 229, 1299, 1300
World Health Organization (WHO)
on adherence interventions, 41
adverse drug reaction database of, 991
anemia as defined by, 1099
fracture risk assessment model from, 1125, 1126
on hypothermia, 1215
iodine supplement programs from, 714
leukemia classifications by, 1283
neuropathy grading scale from, 283
on osteoporosis, 1120
pancreatitis case reports received by, 880
Uppsala Monitoring Center system, 64, 64*t*, 65
Wormseed, 310*t*
Wyeth v. Levine (2009), 9*t*, 10

Xanthine oxidase inhibitors, 1136, 1137, 1145
Xenobiotics, 845, 859, 860*t*
Xylitol, 1002*t*

Yellow jasmine, 310*t*
Yi-gan san, 265
Yohimbine, 401*t*, 404, 409, 453*t*, 646*t*, 647

Zafirlukast, 127*t*, 853*t*
Zalcitabine, 168*t*, 279, 280*t*, 879*t*, 1238*t*
Zaleplon, 148*t*, 352
Zanamivir, 453*t*
Zidovudine
acidosis and, 1002*t*
allergic reactions to, 73*t*
alopecia and, 168*t*
color changes of oral mucosa and teeth and, 1253, 1255*t*
comorbidity and, 34
heart failure and, 504*t*, 509
hepatic/cholestatic diseases and, 864
hypertrichosis and, 196*t*, 199
macrocytic anemia and, 1101*t*, 1107, 1108*t*
myopathy and, 1150–1156, 1150*t*, 1152*t*, 1158, 1159
nausea/vomiting and, 909*t*
neutropenia/agranulocytosis and, 1090*t*
oral erythema multiforme and, 1268*t*
oral lichenoid reactions and, 1272*t*
osteoporosis/osteomalacia and, 1123*t*
ototoxicity and, 1238*t*
Zileuton, 462, 463
Zinc, 1261, 1262, 1321
Ziprasidone
alopecia and, 173*t*
anxiety and, 401*t*, 405, 405*t*, 406
delirium and, 326*t*, 338, 340
extrapyramidal symptoms and, 254
glucose/insulin dysregulation and, 690
hyperprolactinemia and, 743*t*
hypotension and, 635*t*, 639*t*
neuroleptic malignant syndrome and, 1195*t*
serotonin syndrome and, 1203–1204*t*
tardive dyskinesia and, 265
torsades de pointes and, 534*t*, 540*t*
weight gain and, 1166*t*, 1169*t*, 1170, 1175*t*
Zoledronic acid
atrial fibrillation/atrial flutter and, 581, 583*t*, 584
constipation and, 836*t*
drug fever and, 1189*t*
osteonecrosis of jaw and, 1274, 1274*t*
osteoporosis/osteomalacia and, 1129*t*, 1130
visual disturbances and, 310*t*
Zolmitriptan, 380, 472*t*
Zolpidem, 148*t*, 352, 367, 417–418*t*, 1238*t*
Zonisamide
acidosis and, 1003*t*
acute kidney injury and, 944*t*, 957
depression and, 379
dystonia and, 270
ototoxicity and, 1238*t*
psychosis and, 417*t*
in sulfa drug class, 92
systemic lupus erythematosus and, 124*t*
visual disturbances and, 310*t*
weight gain and, 1174, 1175, 1175*t*
Zopiclone, 1255*t*, 1260*t*